Channel Publishing
2014 Enhanced Generic ICD-10-CM
Enhanced, Coder-Helpful Features

ENHANCED FEATURES		BENEFITS FOR CODERS
✓	**Highlighted Term Differentiation** *Exclusive Feature*	✓ Selected terms within code categories and code titles have been underscored to help coders more easily and accurately identify the correct code in the Tabular List.
✓	**Further use of dashes (-)** *Exclusive Feature*	✓ All code categories and codes requiring additional digits in the Tabular List have a dash (-) at the end of last digit that helps coders be aware that additional characters are required for a complete code.
✓	**Further use of placeholder "x"** *Exclusive Feature*	✓ All codes requiring one or more "x" placeholder characters to make a complete code have been placed in advance to help coders clearly identify when these "x" placeholders are required.
✓	***Excludes ❷*** *Exclusive Feature*	✓ All Excludes2 listings have a unique graphic "❷" to more clearly identify those unique excludes notations where a coder may code both conditions, if present.
✓	***Excludes 1 and Excludes ❷ key***	✓ The short descriptions of Excludes 1 and Excludes ❷ are listed on the bottom of each page throughout the Tabular List to help coders learn the difference between the two without referring back to the introduction.
✓	**Tabular List Guide Line** *Exclusive Feature*	✓ A vertical line has been placed that aligns all 3-digit codes and 3-digit code categories to help coders follow code ranges from page to page.
✓	**Highlighted 7th digit subclassifications**	✓ Gray screen bars over the 7th digit subclassifications in the Tabular List help coders easily identify those code categories requiring a variable 7th digit.
✓	**Tab-Edge printing**	✓ Chapter-by-chapter, and section-by-section stair-stepped, tab-edge printing helps coders locate the correct section quickly.

Compare Our Features, Prices & Value to Any Other ICD-10-CM!!

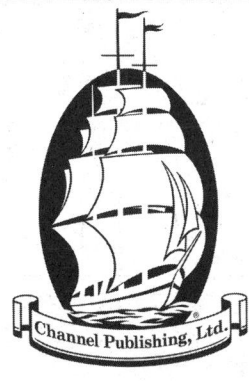

Channel Publishing, Ltd.
Reno, Nevada
1-800-248-2882
www.channelpublishing.com

Publishing Quality

ICD Code Books

Since 1986

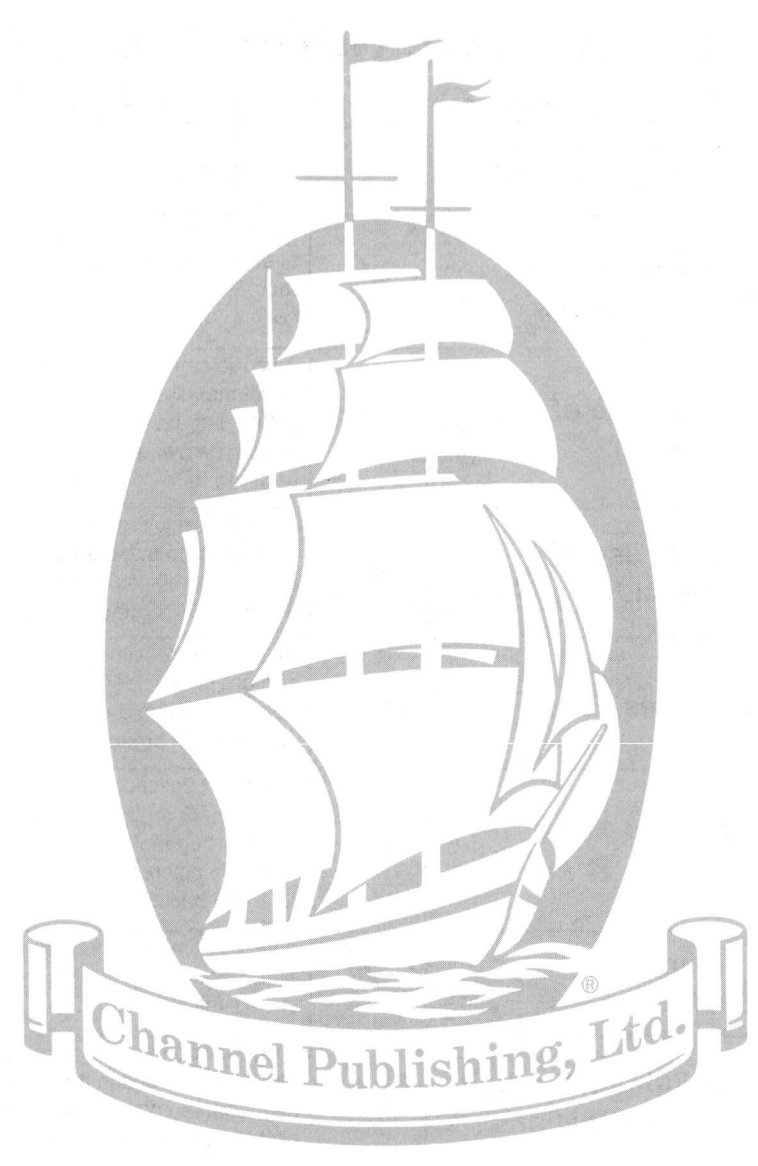

2014 ENHANCED
GENERIC
ICD-10-CM

CRAIG D. PUCKETT

2014.CM-1.V1

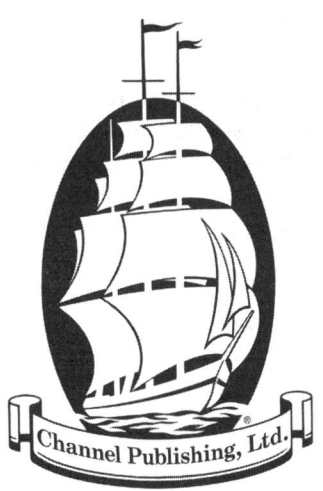

Channel Publishing, Ltd.

Complete Official ICD-10-CM Text, 2014 RELEASE
as standardized by
U.S. DEPARTMENT OF HEALTH AND HUMAN SERVICES
CENTERS FOR DISEASE CONTROL AND PREVENTION
NATIONAL CENTER FOR HEALTH STATISTICS

DISCLAIMER

Every effort has been made to ensure the accuracy and reliability of the information contained in this publication. However, complete accuracy cannot be guaranteed. The editor and publisher will not be held responsible or liable for any errors.

Corrections Identification and Reporting

In an effort to provide our customers with the best code books possible, Channel Publishing has added a "Channel Errata Page" for each of its ICD-10-CM code books on its web site: www.channelpublishing.com. These Channel Errata Pages will be updated promptly whenever an error is identified. Check the appropriate web page periodically for any changes to your Channel Publishing ICD-10-CM.

In addition, if at any time you identify a potential error, please copy the page and fax/mail/e-mail it to: Channel Publishing, Ltd., Attn: ICD-10-CM Book Production Department, 4750 Longley Lane, Suite 110, Reno, NV 89502. FAX (775) 825-5633. E-mail: info@channelpublishing.com

ICD-10-CM, Version 2014.CM-1.V1 – Published August 2013

Channel Publishing Version Key:

2014   Identifies the NCHS Release Title Year

CM-1   Identifies any changes to the 2014 CM code set and/or Official Coding Guidelines for the NCHS Version Title Year. These changes may include: Official Addenda or Errata as designated and posted by NCHS.

V1   Identifies the publication sequence of any content changes to Channel Publishing's 2014 Enhanced Generic ICD-10-CM. These content changes may include: Official Addenda or Errata as designated and posted by NCHS, and/or changes/improvements to Channel Publishing's proprietary enhanced features.

This edition contains the Complete, Official ICD-10-CM Text, 2014 Version as standardized by the U.S. Department of Health and Human Services, Centers for Disease Control and Prevention, National Center for Health Statistics.

Published by CHANNEL PUBLISHING, Ltd., Reno, Nevada

Produced by Craig Puckett, Editor; Jo Ann Jones, RHIA, CCS, Editorial Assistant; Charisse Puckett, Editorial Assistant; Amanda Rollings, Editorial Assistant

Printed in the United States of America

Additional sets may be ordered from Channel Publishing, Ltd., 4750 Longley Lane, Suite 110, Reno, Nevada 89502, 1-800-248-2882, www.channelpublishing.com

ISBN: 978-1-933053-49-3

Channel Publishing, Ltd.

Publishers of

"THE EDUCATIONAL ANNOTATION OF ICD-9-CM"
"ENHANCED GENERIC ICD-10-CM & ICD-10-PCS"

August 2013

Dear ICD-10 Colleague:

First, I would like to personally thank each and every Channel Publishing customer who has purchased and enjoyed our ICD-9-CM coding products and services over these past 27 years.

Thank you for purchasing Channel Publishing's *2014.CM-1.V1 Enhanced Generic ICD-10-CM* code book. You'll find a similar look and feel as our Generic ICD-9-CM code books. I trust you will enjoy the design, layout, and some new, coder-helpful features that we have created for you. I would also like to thank everyone who shared their ICD-10 comments and suggestions over the years from our "Preparing for ICD-10" seminars ten years ago, to those of you who called or wrote in, and those who stopped by our booth at AHIMA. We listened and made note of those comments and suggestions to bring you what we believe is an excellent ICD-10-CM code book, and at an incredibly low price.

In addition to this *2014.CM-1.V1 Enhanced Generic ICD-10-CM* code book, I'd like to talk to you about all our ICD-10 products and services. I've been coding since the mid 1970s and have experienced the transition from ICD-8 (and H-ICDA-8) to ICD-9-CM and the implementation of DRGs, so I know what it's like for coders to make these difficult transitions. And, unfortunately, the transition to ICD-10 is going to be many times more challenging and expensive.

That's why I'm so pleased to offer the high-quality ICD-10 products and services we've developed at very affordable prices. As I said when I taught Channel's "Preparing for ICD-10" coding seminars back in 2000, "you're going to have a whole sea of printed and multimedia ICD-10 products and services to choose from, and you're going to have to choose which products are going to be best suited for you." I strongly believe that the ICD-10 products and services we've developed will make this transition easier for you, both from a learning point of view and a budget point of view. And we've organized all these products and training materials into 4 logical steps to guide you through your ICD-10 training.

On the following pages you will find information and pricing on:
- Learning ICD-10-CM & ICD-10-PCS "Seminar-In-A-Box" training programs (Step 1)
  - Professional Version (teaching others)
  - Individual Version (teaching yourself)
- *Mastering ICD-10-CM & ICD-10-PCS* exercise books (Step 2)
- *Mastering the ICD-10-CM & ICD-10-PCS Guidelines* exercise books (Step 3)
- "The Last Word on ICD-10" media presentation (Step 4)
- *2014 Enhanced Generic ICD-10-CM* code books
- *2014 Enhanced Generic ICD-10-PCS* code books
- *The Educational Annotation of ICD-10-CM* and *ICD-10-PCS* code books

Once again, thank you for your purchase and I look forward to providing quality ICD-10 products and services to help you and your organization through this difficult transition from ICD-9-CM to ICD-10.

Sincerely,

Craig D. Puckett

Craig D. Puckett,
Founder, President, and Publisher

4750 Longley Lane, Suite 110 • Reno, NV 89502-5977 • (775) 825-0880 • Customer Service 1-800-248-2882 • FAX (775) 825-5633
WEB SITE: www.channelpublishing.com • E-MAIL: info@channelpublishing.com

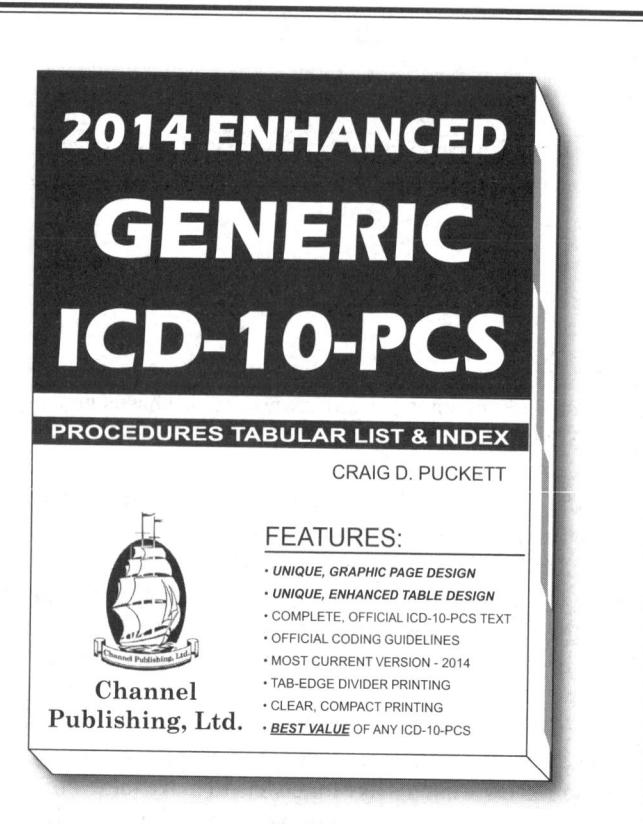
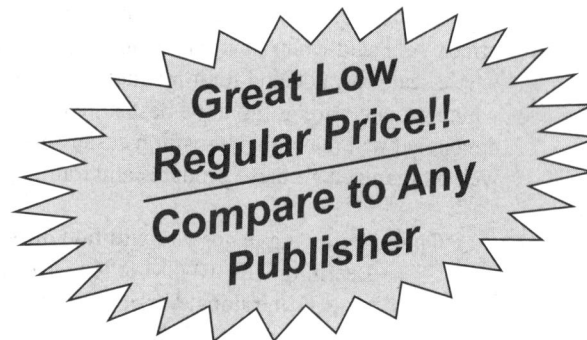

1ST - 0 Medical and Surgical		
2ND - F Hepatobiliary System and Pancreas		
3RD - B EXCISION		

EXAMPLE:	Liver biopsy
EXCISION:	Cutting out or off, without replacement, a portion of a body part.
EXPLANATION:	Qualifier "X Diagnostic" indicates biopsy ...

Body Part – 4TH	Approach – 5TH	Device – 6TH	Qualifier – 7TH
0 Liver 1 Liver, Right Lobe 2 Liver, Left Lobe 4 Gallbladder G Pancreas	0 Open 3 Percutaneous 4 Percutaneous endoscopic	Z No device	X Diagnostic Z No qualifier
5 Hepatic Duct, Right 6 Hepatic Duct, Left 8 Cystic Duct 9 Common Bile Duct C Ampulla of Vater D Pancreatic D... F Pancrea...	0 Open 3 Percutaneous 4 Percutaneous endoscopic 7 Via natural or artificial opening 8 Via natural or artificial opening endoscopic	Z No device	...nostic ...ualifier

Identifies Easy-To-Understand Example

Identifies & Defines Root Operation

Abbreviated Explanation to Help Understanding

Unique, Innovative, Enhanced, Page and Table Designs

Channel Feature Identification of section and table in the tab-edge printing

MED/SURG

0 F B

1ST - 0 Medical and Surgical		
2ND - F Hepatobiliary System and Pancreas		
3RD - C EXTIRPATION		

EXAMPLE:	Choledocholithotomy
EXTIRPATION:	Taking or cutting out solid matter from a body part.
EXPLANATION:	Abnormal byproduct or foreign body ...

Body Part – 4TH	Approach – 5TH	Device – 6TH	Qualifier – 7TH
0 Liver 1 Liver, Right Lobe 2 Liver, Left Lobe 4 Gallbladder G Pancreas	0 Open 3 Percutaneous 4 Percutaneous endoscopic	Z No device	Z No qualifier
5 Hepatic Duct, Right 6 Hepatic Duct, Left 8 Cystic Duct 9 Common Bile Duct C Ampulla of Vater D Pancreatic Duct F Pancreatic Duct, Accessory	0 Open 3 Percutaneous 4 Percutaneous endoscopic 7 Via natural or artificial opening 8 Via natural or artificial opening endoscopic	Z No device	Z No qualifier

Clearly Identifies All 7 Characters Needed To Build A Valid PCS Code

Clear, Compact, Easy To Read Type and Layout

Channel Publishing's ICD-10 Training

Channel Publishing is pleased to bring you ICD-10 training in 4 logical steps that are designed to not only teach you how to use the new code books, but to build your confidence through step-by-step practice in all areas of the new books.

STEP 1 — LEARNING THE NEW CODE BOOKS

Channel's innovative *"Seminar-In-A-Box"* programs
- **Two programs:**
  - Learning *ICD-10-CM*
  - Learning *ICD-10-PCS*
- **Two versions:**
  - **Professional Version** (Teaching others)
    - PowerPoint slide presentation
    - Instructor's manual
    - Package discounts
    - Seminar prep DVD set
    - Seminar workbook
    - ICD-10 code book
  - **Individual Version** (Teaching yourself)
    - Seminar DVD set
    - Seminar workbook
    - ICD-10 code book

STEP 2 — MASTERING THE NEW CODE BOOKS
- Coding practice exercise books (with answer key) designed to give coders confidence
- Practice quizzes and tests available for mail-in grading with CEUs
- Separate exercise books for ICD-10-CM & ICD-10-PCS

STEP 3 — MASTERING THE NEW CODING GUIDELINES
- Coding practice exercise books (with answer key) designed to give coders confidence
- Practice quizzes and tests available for mail-in grading with CEUs
- Separate exercise books for ICD-10-CM & ICD-10-PCS

STEP 4 — IMPLEMENTATION UPDATE
- A video presentation with booklet designed to bring coders completely up-to-date with any new and relevant ICD-10 information and changes, including:
  - Any new or revised code book and Coding Guideline changes
  - Current information on MS-DRGs, MCE edits, and AHA Coding Clinic™ info
  - Scheduled release - August 2014

Quality, INNOVATIVE products and services at VERY AFFORDABLE prices!!!

Channel Publishing Presents
Our Most *INNOVATIVE* ICD-10 Product
Seminar-In-A-Box (Step 1)

Channel Publishing's *"Seminar-In-A-Box"* programs (Step 1) are designed for a wide variety of facilities, consultants, and coders who need quality, affordable ICD-10 training in a flexible format using Channel's proven seminar materials and code books. The *"Seminar-In-A-Box"* programs include:

- **Two programs:**
  - Learning ICD-10-CM
  - Learning ICD-10-PCS
- **Two versions:**
  - **Professional Version includes:**
    - PowerPoint Slide Presentation
      - Includes complete set of Channel's PowerPoint seminar slides
        - Option to add slides of your own design
        - Additional instructional slides, examples, or exercises
        - Slides to identify your organization and program structure
    - Instructor's Manual — A complete Instructor's Manual in an easy-to-read and use binder that provides a detailed explanation on each teaching point
    - Package discounts — Discounts for purchasing packages of code books and seminar workbooks for re-sale or use by your attendees
    - Seminar prep DVD — A DVD of a seminar by AHIMA - Approved ICD-10-CM/PCS Trainers Craig Puckett and Jo Ann Jones that is designed for instructor preparation and review
    - Seminar Workbook — The Seminar Workbook includes a printed version of the slides and exercises to be completed by attendees and reviewed by the instructor
    - Enhanced Generic ICD-10 (CM) (PCS) code book
  - **Individual Version includes:**
    - Seminar DVD — A DVD of a seminar by AHIMA - Approved ICD-10-CM/PCS Trainers Craig Puckett and Jo Ann Jones that is designed to be viewed as if attending a live seminar (allows individuals to learn at their own pace and view the DVD, or certain segments, as often as needed)
    - Seminar Workbook — The Seminar Workbook includes a printed version of the slides and exercises to be completed and answers reviewed on the DVD
    - Enhanced Generic ICD-10 (CM) (PCS) code book

Affordable, Innovative ICD-10 Training!!!

Channel Publishing Presents
Seminar-In-A-Box Program (Step 1)

Channel Publishing's *Learning ICD-10-CM* & *Learning ICD-10-PCS Seminar-In-A-Box* programs *(Step 1)* are designed to train coders in a wide variety of settings:

Professional Version (Teaching others):
- Facilities (hospitals, clinics, insurance companies, health care industry businesses, etc.) that plan to train their own coders in-house and at their own pace and timing and/or to offer training to physicians or other groups associated with their facility
- Groups (coding roundtables, associations, etc.) who plan to train their members within the usual time frame of the group meetings
- Consultants who need an affordable set of ICD-10 training materials to train at their client facilities or who plan to offer local seminars in their areas

Individual Version (Teaching yourself):
- Individuals who would like an affordable ICD-10 training product alternative where they can teach themselves at their own pace, and review the material as often as needed

Here's what you'll learn with these Seminar-In-A-Box programs:
- All the different sections and sub-sections of each code book, including:
  - Introduction, index, tabular, and appendices
  - Conventions, formats, structures, abbreviations, and keys
  - Unique sub-sections of each code book (neoplasm table, root operations, and body part tables, etc.)
  - Coding Guidelines
- Similarities and differences to ICD-9-CM
- New features added in ICD-10-CM (laterality, two types of Excludes)
- Completely new structure for procedures (table structure, rows and columns, multiaxial)
- Exercises (with answers) to re-inforce new concept/book sections

Who should purchase a Seminar-In-A-Box program:
- Coders and managers
- Consultants
- HIM directors
- Students
- Health care related positions

Compare Our Cost Per CEU With Other Training

CEU information:
- 8 CEUs each for each program (AHIMA guidelines)
- Other organization members must contact their respective organization

Advantages of using Learning ICD-10 Seminar-In-A-Box programs:
- Flexibility to train at your own pace and on your schedule
- Quality from a known ICD-9/ICD-10 publisher
- No license fee
- Affordable
- Delay-proof

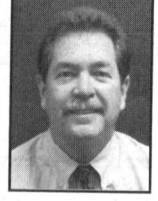

Craig Puckett, President Channel Publishing, Ltd.

AHIMA - Approved ICD-10-CM/PCS Trainer

Craig has been coding since the mid 1970s and has experienced the transition from ICD-8 to ICD-9-CM and the implementation of DRGs, so he knows what it's like for coders to make these challenging transitions. That is why he has designed and developed Channel's innovative suite of ICD-10 products and services to help coders make this difficult transition from ICD-9-CM to ICD-10.

Craig's experience in the health information field includes contract coding, consulting, and authoring of *The Educational Annotation of ICD-9-CM*, the first code book to include medical definitions, illustrations, and anatomy and physiology reviews. He is an experienced instructor who has created video workshops for ICD-9-CM and ICD-10, and seminars for both ICD-10-CM and ICD-10-PCS, including the very popular *Preparing for ICD-10* seminars held over 10 years ago.

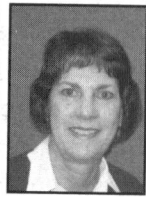

Jo Ann Jones, RHIA, CCS Manager, Coding Services

AHIMA - Approved ICD-10-CM/PCS Trainer

Jo Ann has more than 25 years experience in Health Information Management that includes coding in both rehabilitation and inpatient settings, supervisory level management, transcription, ambulatory HIM, and discharge planning. She has also contributed multiple articles to *Clinotes*.

Active in both the state and national associations, Jo Ann currently serves as Co-Chair for NvHIMA's ICD-10 Task Force, President of Northern NvHIMA, and Coding Roundtable Coordinator. Jo Ann served as President of NvHIMA from 2007-2008. As manager of Channel Coding Services, Jo Ann brings a unique insight to the challenges that coders are facing with learning and implementing ICD-10.

Affordable, Innovative ICD-10 Training!!!

Learning ICD-10-CM Seminar-In-A-Box Program

Learning ICD-10-PCS Seminar-In-A-Box Program

ICD-10-CM Seminar Outline

- Overview of seminar materials and instruction (including practice exercises)
- Implementation and "freezing" update
- Understanding the ICD-10-CM code book
  - ICD-9-CM, similarities and differences
  - Introduction, conventions, structure, format
  - Alphabetic index
  - Neoplasm and Drugs & Chemical tables
  - Coding Guidelines
  - Clinical Modifications (restructuring axes, OB ...)
  - New features (laterality, Excludes 1 & 2 ...)

- Chapter-by-chapter explanation, including unique sections/codes, and exercises
  - Chapter 1 – Infectious and parasitic diseases
  - Chapter 2 – Neoplasms
  - Chapter 3 – Blood and blood-forming organs and immune mechanism
  - Chapter 4 – Endocrine, nutritional and metabolic
  - Chapter 5 – Mental, behavioral and neurodevelopmental disorders
  - Chapter 6 – Nervous system
  - Chapter 7 – Eye and adnexa
  - Chapter 8 – Ear and mastoid process
  - Chapter 9 – Circulatory system
  - Chapter 10 – Respiratory system
  - Chapter 11 – Digestive system
  - Chapter 12 – Skin and subcutaneous tissue
  - Chapter 13 – Musculoskeletal system and connective tissues
  - Chapter 14 – Genitourinary system
  - Chapter 15 – Pregnancy, childbirth and puerperium
  - Chapter 16 – Perinatal period
  - Chapter 17 – Congenital malformations and chromosomal abnormalities
  - Chapter 18 – Symptoms, signs and abnormal clinical and laboratory findings
  - Chapter 19 – Injury and poisoning
  - Chapter 20 – External causes of morbidity
  - Chapter 21 – Factors influencing health status and contact with health services

- Developing an ongoing self-training plan to keep you on schedule and best prepared for implementation

- Tips and opportunities for keeping your new ICD-10-CM knowledge sharp and up-to-date

ICD-10-PCS Seminar Outline

- Overview of seminar materials and instruction (including practice exercises)
- Implementation and "freezing" update
- Understanding the ICD-10-PCS code book
  - Similarities and differences to ICD-9-CM
  - Introduction, conventions
  - Tabular List Tables format & structure
  - Coding Guidelines
  - Alphabetic index
  - Appendices

- Medical & Surgical Section – Root Operation explanation of similar procedure groups and exercises
  - Root Operations That Take Out Some or All of a Body Part
  - Root Operations That Take Out Solids/Fluids/Gases From a Body Part
  - Root Operations That Put In/Put Back or Move Some/All of a Body Part
  - Root Operations Involving Cutting or Separation Only
  - Root Operations That Alter the Diameter/Route of a Tubular Body Part
  - Root Operations That Always Involve a Device
  - Root Operations Involving Examination Only
  - Root Operations That Define Other Repairs
  - Root Operations That Define Other Objectives

- Medical & Surgical Section – Explanation of the 31 Body Systems sections, including the unique root operations found in each and differences

- Medical/Surgical Related Sections – Explanation of the med/surg related sections (obstetrics, placement, administration, etc.) and exercises

- Ancillary Sections – Explanation of the non-med/surg related sections (imaging, radiation therapy, mental health, etc.) and exercises

- Developing an ongoing self-training plan to keep you on schedule and best prepared for implementation

- Tips and opportunities for keeping your new ICD-10-PCS knowledge sharp and up-to-date

Affordable, Quality ICD-10 Training!!!

Channel Publishing Presents
AFFORDABLE ICD-10 Products to Complete Your Training

STEP 2
MASTERING THE NEW CODE BOOKS

Channel Publishing has developed these training exercise books to further your knowledge and understanding of the new code books. The exercises are designed to give you experience with, and confidence in, every chapter and section of the code book. The quizzes and tests will allow you an opportunity to test your knowledge, prove your competence, and receive additional CEU credits.

Mastering ICD-10-CM Exercise Book
- Thousands of practice exercises
- Answer key for all practice exercises
- Quizzes at the end of each section (Quizzes can be mailed in for grading and CEU credit certificate – additional fee applies)
- A Final Test (Final Test can be mailed in for grading and CEU credit certificate – additional fee applies)

Mastering ICD-10-PCS Exercise Book
- Thousands of practice exercises
- Answer key for all practice exercises
- Quizzes at the end of each section (Quizzes can be mailed in for grading and CEU credit certificate – additional fee applies)
- A Final Test (Final Test can be mailed in for grading and CEU credit certificate – additional fee applies)

STEP 3
MASTERING THE CODING GUIDELINES

Channel Publishing has developed these training exercise books to further your knowledge and understanding of the new coding guidelines. The exercises are designed to give you experience with, and confidence in, every section of the guidelines. The quizzes and tests will allow you an opportunity to test your knowledge, prove your competence, and receive additional CEU credits.

Mastering ICD-10-CM Guidelines Exercise Book
- Hundreds of case scenario exercises
- Answer key for all practice exercises
- Coding Guidelines included in the Introduction
- Quizzes at the end of each section (Quizzes can be mailed in for grading and CEU credit certificate – additional fee applies)
- A Final Test (Final Test can be mailed in for grading and CEU credit certificate – additional fee applies)

Mastering ICD-10-PCS Guidelines Exercise Book
- Hundreds of case scenarios exercises
- Answer key for all practice exercises
- Coding Guidelines included in the Introduction
- Quizzes at the end of each section (Quizzes can be mailed in for grading and CEU credit certificate – additional fee applies)
- A Final Test (Final Test can be mailed in for grading and CEU credit certificate – additional fee applies)

STEP 4
IMPLEMENTATION UPDATE

Channel Publishing understands that there will be a few things that will change before implementation. We are planning in advance to produce a last-minute update of anything new or revised to ICD-10 and present it to you just before implementation. This product will include a video presentation and a printed booklet.

The Last Word on ICD-10
- This presentation will include:
  - Any new codes, revisions, or errata that CMS or NCHS make official
  - Current information on MS-DRGs and MCE edits
  - Current information on the AHA Coding Clinic™ for ICD-10
  - Tips and information on implementation issues
  - A Channel logo "ICD-10 Lapel Pin" or a coffee mug with "I'm Ready for ICD-10!" (your choice)

Affordable, Innovative ICD-10 Training!!!

2013 ICD-10 TRAINING FALL SALE ORDER FORM   Sale Prices Expire 11/30/13

1. CUSTOMER INFORMATION (Ship books to address below)

☐ Organization or ☐ Individual   ATTN: Name/Title/Dept.   Customer ID #   Order Date

Shipping Address (Street address required for FedEx delivery)   E-Mail Address

City   State   Zip   Telephone   Fax

2. ORDER INFORMATION

Quantity	Product — See Web Site for Complete Product Descriptions	Regular Price	ICD-10 Training Sale Price	Total(s)
	ICD-10 CODE BOOK PRODUCTS		Sale Prices Expire 11/30/13	
	2014 Enhanced Generic ICD-10-CM – *Same Low Price!!*	$69^{95} ea.	—	
	2014 Enhanced Generic ICD-10-PCS – *Same Low Price!!*	$59^{95} ea.	—	
	ICD-10 CODING TRAINING – SEMINAR-IN-A-BOX PROGRAMS			
	(Professional Version – Includes: Power Point Slides, Instructor's Manual, DVD set, Workbook & Code Book) (Individual Version – Includes: DVD set, Workbook & Code Book - CM-12 CEUs, PCS-20 CEUs)			
	Professional Version – Learning ICD-10-CM (Step 1) – *Save Now!!*	$~~599~~^{95} ea.	$499^{95} ea.	
	Additional Learning ICD-10-CM Workbook & Book Packages	$65^{95} ea.	—	
	Professional Version – Learning ICD-10-PCS (Step 1) – *Save Now!!*	$~~699~~^{95} ea.	$499^{95} ea.	
	Additional Learning ICD-10-PCS Workbook & Book Packages	$55^{95} ea.	—	
	Individual Version – Learning ICD-10-CM (Step 1) (12 CEUs) – *Save Now!!*	$~~299~~^{95} ea.	$229^{95} ea.	
	Individual Version – Learning ICD-10-PCS (Step 1) (20 CEUs) – *Save Now!!*	$~~399~~^{95} ea.	$229^{95} ea.	
	ICD-10 CODING TRAINING – ADDITIONAL LEARNING PRODUCTS			
	Mastering ICD-10-CM Exercise Book (Step 2)	$59^{95} ea.	—	
	Mastering ICD-10-PCS Exercise Book (Step 2) *Available Fall 2013*	$59^{95} ea.	—	
	Mastering the ICD-10-CM Guidelines Exercise Book (Step 3) *Available Fall 2013*	$59^{95} ea.	—	
	Mastering the ICD-10-PCS Guidelines Exercise Book (Step 3) *Available Fall 2013*	$59^{95} ea.	—	
	The Last Word on ICD-10 (Step 4) *Available Aug 2014*	$69^{95} ea.	—	
	ICD-9-CM CODE BOOK PRODUCTS AND ACCESSORIES			
	Oct. 1, 2011 SoftCover Hospital Version The Educational Annotation of ICD-9-CM (Inc. Oct. 12 & 13)	$109^{00} ea.	—	
	Oct. 1, 2011 SoftCover Update Replacement Text (Includes Oct. 12 & 13 update information)	$69^{00} ea.	—	
	Tab Set (SoftCover only)	$16^{95} ea.	—	
	2012 Generic Hospital Version ICD-9-CM (Includes Oct. 2012 & Oct. 2013 update information)	$79^{95} ea.	—	
	2012 Generic Physician Version ICD-9-CM (Includes Oct. 2012 & Oct. 2013 update information)	$69^{95} ea.	—	
	2014 CPT™ Standard Edition	$94^{95} ea.	—	
	2014 CPT™ Professional Edition	$119^{95} ea.	—	
	Clinotes, 5th Edition Special Clearance Price	$~~77~~^{95} ea.	$19^{95} ea.	
	Expanded ICD-9-CM Table of Drugs & Chemicals, 6th Edition Special Clearance Price	$~~39~~^{95} ea.	$9^{95} ea.	
	Acrylic Bookstand ☐ One-piece ☐ Two-piece	$34^{00} ea.	—	

• OUTSIDE CONTINENTAL U.S.: Call for rates and shipping options.
Payment in U.S. Dollars.

• EXPRESS SHIPPING: Call for delivery options and rates.

ICD-10 Training Sale Prices Expire 11/30/13

Continental U.S. Shipping & Handling

Less than $50 . . . . . $7
$50-$99 . . . . $12
$100-$199 . . . . . . $19
$200-$299 . . . . . . $29
$300+ $39

Product Subtotal	
Shipping & Handling	
Nevada Res. Only Add Sales Tax	
Total Order Amount	

3. PAYMENT METHOD

☐ **Check Enclosed**

☐ **Invoice/P.O.** – Written P.O. must accompany order.

☐ **Credit Card: MC, VISA, DISC, AMEX**
(Accounts are charged on date order received)

☐☐☐☐ ☐☐☐☐ ☐☐☐☐ ☐☐☐☐

___/___
Exp. Date   Authorized Cardholder Signature

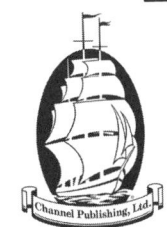

MAKE CHECKS PAYABLE AND MAIL TO:

Channel Publishing, Ltd.
4750 Longley Lane, Suite 110
Reno, NV 89502-5977
1-800-248-2882
(775) 825-0880
Fax (775) 825-5633
E-Mail: info@channelpublishing.com
Web Site: www.channelpublishing.com

THANK YOU FOR YOUR ORDER   FS99083

TABLE OF CONTENTS

Disease Index

Disease Tabular

Chapter

ICD-10-CM PREFACE (2013 Version)

Introduction

This 2014 update of the International Classification of Diseases and Related Health Problems, 10th revision, Clinical Modification (ICD-10-CM) is being published by the United States Government in recognition of its responsibility to promulgate this classification throughout the United States for morbidity coding. The International Statistical Classification of Diseases and Related Health Problems, 10th Revision (ICD-10), published by the World Health Organization (WHO), is the foundation of ICD-10-CM. ICD-10 continues to be the classification used in cause-of-death coding in the United States. The ICD-10-CM is comparable with the ICD-10. The WHO Collaborating Center for the Family of International Classifications in North America, housed at the Centers for Disease Control and Prevention's National Center for Health Statistics (NCHS), has responsibility for the implementation of ICD and other WHO-FIC classifications and serves as a liaison with the WHO, fulfilling international obligations for comparable classifications and the national health data needs of the United States.

Historical background

The historical background of ICD and ICD-10 can be found in the Introduction to the International Classification of Diseases and Related Health Problems (ICD-10), 2008, World Health Organization, Geneva, Switzerland.

Clinical modification

ICD-10-CM is the United States' clinical modification of the World Health Organization's ICD-10. The term clinical is used to emphasize the modification's intent: to serve as a useful tool in the area of classification of morbidity data for indexing of medical records, medical care review, and ambulatory and other medical care programs, as well as for basic health statistics. To describe the clinical picture of the patient the codes must be more precise than those needed only for statistical groupings and trend analysis.

Characteristics of ICD-10-CM

ICD-10-CM far exceeds its predecessors in the number of concepts and codes provided. The disease classification has been expanded to include health-related conditions and to provide greater specificity at the sixth digit level and with a seventh digit extension. The sixth and seventh characters are not optional; they are intended for use in recording the information documented in the clinical record.

ICD-10-CM extensions, interpretations, modifications, addenda, or errata other than those approved by the Centers for Disease Control and Prevention are not to be considered official and should not be utilized. Continuous maintenance of the ICD-10-CM is the responsibility of the aforementioned agencies. However, because the ICD-10-CM represents the best in contemporary thinking of clinicians, nosologists, epidemiologists, and statisticians from both public and private sectors, when future modifications are considered, advice will be sought from all stakeholders.

All official authorized addenda through October 1, 2013, have been included in this revision. The complete official authorized addenda to ICD-10-CM, including the "ICD-10-CM Official Guidelines for Coding and Reporting", can be accessed at the following website:
   http://www.cdc.gov/nchs/icd/icd10cm.htm#10update

A description of the ICD-10-CM updating and maintenance process can be found at the following website:
   http://www.cdc.gov/nchs/icd/icd9cm_maintenance.htm

INTRODUCTION TO ICD-10-CM (2014 Version)

The National Center for Health Statistics (NCHS), the Federal agency responsible for use of the International Statistical Classification of Diseases and Related Health Problems, 10th revision (ICD-10) in the United States, has developed a clinical modification of the classification for morbidity purposes. The ICD-10 is used to code and classify mortality data from death certificates, having replaced ICD-9 for this purpose as of January 1, 1999. ICD-10-CM is planned as the replacement for ICD-9-CM, volumes 1 and 2.

The ICD-10 is copyrighted by the World Health Organization (WHO), which owns and publishes the classification. WHO has authorized the development of an adaptation of ICD-10 for use in the United States for U.S. government purposes. As agreed, all modifications to the ICD-10 must conform to WHO conventions for the ICD. ICD-10-CM was developed following a thorough evaluation by a Technical Advisory Panel and extensive additional consultation with physician groups, clinical coders, and others to assure clinical accuracy and utility.

The entire draft of the Tabular List of ICD-10-CM, and the preliminary crosswalk between ICD-9-CM and ICD-10-CM were made available on the NCHS website for public comment. The public comment period ran from December 1997 through February 1998. The American Hospital Association and the American Health Information Management Association conducted a field test for ICD-10-CM in the summer of 2003, with a subsequent report. All comments and suggestions from the open comment period and the field test were reviewed, and additional modifications to ICD-10-CM were made based on these comments and suggestions. Additionally, new concepts have been added to ICD-10-CM based on the established update process for ICD-9-CM (the ICD-9-CM Coordination and Maintenance Committee) and the World Health Organization's ICD-10 (the Update and Revision Committee). This represents ICD-9-CM modifications from 2003-2009 and ICD-10 modifications from 2002-2008.

The clinical modification represents a significant improvement over ICD-9-CM and ICD-10. Specific improvements include: the addition of information relevant to ambulatory and managed care encounters; expanded injury codes; the creation of combination diagnosis/symptom codes to reduce the number of codes needed to fully describe a condition; the addition of sixth and seventh characters; incorporation of common 4th and 5th digit subclassifications; laterality; and greater specificity in code assignment. The new structure will allow further expansion than was possible with ICD-9-CM.

On January 16, 2009 HHS published a Final Rule adopting ICD-10-CM (and ICD-10-PCS) to replace ICD-9-CM in HIPAA transactions, effective implementation date of October 1, 2013 (now delayed one year to October 1, 2014). Until that time the codes in ICD-10-CM are not valid for any purpose or use.

ICD-10-CM Conventions (2014 Version)

The conventions for the ICD-10-CM are the general rules for use of the classification independent of the guidelines. These conventions are incorporated within the **Alphabetic Index** and **Tabular List** of the ICD-10-CM as instructional notes. The conventions and instructions of the classification take precedence over guidelines.

Organization of ICD-10-CM

The ICD-10-CM is divided into the Alphabetic Index, an alphabetical list of terms and their corresponding code, and the Tabular List, a chronological list of codes divided into chapters based on body system or condition.

Alphabetic Index

The Alphabetic Index consists of the following parts:
- Index of Diseases and Injury
- Table of Neoplasms
- Table of Drugs and Chemicals
- Index of External Causes of Injury

Tabular List

The Tabular List consists of the following chapters:
- Chapter 1 – Certain infectious and parasitic diseases (A00-B99)
- Chapter 2 – Neoplasms (C00-D49)
- Chapter 3 – Diseases of the blood and blood-forming organs and certain disorders involving the immune mechanism (D50-D89)
- Chapter 4 – Endocrine, nutritional and metabolic diseases (E00-E89)
- Chapter 5 – Mental, behavioral and neurodevelopmental disorders (F01-F99)
- Chapter 6 – Diseases of the nervous system (G00-G99)
- Chapter 7 – Diseases of the eye and adnexa (H00-H59)
- Chapter 8 – Diseases of the ear and mastoid process (H60-H95)
- Chapter 9 – Diseases of the circulatory system (I00-I99)
- Chapter 10 – Diseases of the respiratory system (J00-J99)
- Chapter 11 – Diseases of the digestive system (K00-K95)
- Chapter 12 – Diseases of the skin and subcutaneous tissue (L00-L99)
- Chapter 13 – Diseases of the musculoskeletal system and connective tissue M00-M99)
- Chapter 14 – Diseases of the genitourinary system (N00-N99)
- Chapter 15 – Pregnancy, childbirth and the puerperium (O00-O99)
- Chapter 16 – Certain conditions originating in the perinatal period (P00-P96)
- Chapter 17 – Congenital malformations, deformations and chromosomal abnormalities (Q00-Q99)
- Chapter 18 – Symptoms, signs and abnormal clinical and laboratory findings, not elsewhere classified (R00-R99)
- Chapter 19 – Injury, poisoning and certain other consequences of external causes (S00-T88)
- Chapter 20 – External causes of morbidity (V00-Y99)
- Chapter 21 – Factors influencing health status and contact with health services (Z00-Z99)

Appendices

There are no appendices.

How to Use ICD-10-CM, General Coding Guidelines, and Chapter-Specific Coding Guidelines

See the 2014 ICD-10-CM Official Guidelines for Coding and Reporting following this Introduction.

Characteristics of ICD-10-CM

Format and Structure:

The ICD-10-CM Tabular List contains categories, subcategories and codes. Characters for categories, subcategories and codes may be either a letter or a number. All categories are 3 characters. A three-character category that has no further subdivision is equivalent to a code. Subcategories are either 4 or 5 characters. Codes may be 3, 4, 5, 6 or 7 characters. That is, each level of subdivision after a category is a subcategory. The final level of subdivision is a code. Codes that have applicable 7th characters are still referred to as codes, not subcategories. A code that has an applicable 7th character is considered invalid without the 7th character.

The ICD-10-CM uses an indented format for ease in reference.

Use of codes for reporting purposes

For reporting purposes only codes are permissible, not categories or subcategories, and any applicable 7th character is required.

Placeholder character

The ICD-10-CM utilizes a placeholder character "x". The "x" is used as a placeholder at certain codes to allow for future expansion. An example of this is at the poisoning, adverse effect and underdosing codes, categories T36-T50.

Where a placeholder "x" exists, the "x" must be used in order for the code to be considered a valid code.

7th Characters

Certain ICD-10-CM categories have applicable 7th characters. The applicable 7th character is required for all codes within the category, or as the notes in the Tabular List instruct. The 7th character must always be the 7th character in the data field. If a code that requires a 7th character is not 6 characters, a placeholder "x" must be used to fill in the empty characters.

Abbreviations

Alphabetic Index abbreviations

NEC "Not elsewhere classifiable"
This abbreviation in the Alphabetic Index represents "other specified." When a specific code is not available for a condition, the Alphabetic Index directs the coder to the "other specified" code in the Tabular List.

NOS "Not otherwise specified"
This abbreviation is the equivalent of unspecified.

Tabular List abbreviations

NEC "Not elsewhere classifiable"
This abbreviation in the Tabular List represents "other specified." When a specific code is not available for a condition the Tabular List includes an NEC entry under a code to identify the code as the "other specified" code.

NOS "Not otherwise specified"
This abbreviation is the equivalent of unspecified.

Punctuation

[ ] Brackets are used in the Tabular List to enclose synonyms, alternative wording or explanatory phrases. Brackets are used in the Alphabetic Index to identify manifestation codes.

( ) Parentheses are used in both the Alphabetic Index and Tabular List to enclose supplementary words that may be present or absent in the statement of a disease or procedure without affecting the code number to which it is assigned. The terms within the parentheses are referred to as nonessential modifiers.

: Colons are used in the Tabular List after an incomplete term which needs one or more of the modifiers following the colon to make it assignable to a given category.

Use of "and"

When the term "and" is used in a narrative statement it represents and/or.

Other and Unspecified codes

"Other" codes

Codes titled "other" or "other specified" are for use when the information in the medical record provides detail for which a specific code does not exist. Alphabetic Index entries with NEC in the line designate "other" codes in the Tabular List. These Alphabetic Index entries represent specific disease entities for which no specific code exists so the term is included within an "other" code.

"Unspecified" codes

Codes titled "unspecified" are for use when the information in the medical record is insufficient to assign a more specific code. For those categories for which an unspecified code is not provided, the "other specified" code may represent both other and unspecified.

Includes Notes

This note appears immediately under a three character code title to further define, or give examples of, the content of the category.

Inclusion terms

List of terms is included under some codes. These terms are the conditions for which that code is to be used. The terms may be synonyms of the code title, or, in the case of "other specified" codes, the terms are a list of the various conditions assigned to that code. The inclusion terms are not necessarily exhaustive. Additional terms found only in the Alphabetic Index may also be assigned to a code.

Excludes Notes

The ICD-10-CM has two types of excludes notes. Each type of note has a different definition for use but they are all similar in that they indicate that codes excluded from each other are independent of each other.

Excludes 1

A type 1 Excludes note is a pure excludes. It means "NOT CODED HERE!" An Excludes1 note indicates that the code excluded should never be used at the same time as the code above the Excludes1 note. An Excludes1 is used when two conditions cannot occur together, such as a congenital form versus an acquired form of the same condition.

Excludes 2

A type 2 excludes note represents "Not included here". An excludes2 note indicates that the condition excluded is not part of the condition it is excluded from but a patient may have both conditions at the same time. When an Excludes2 note appears under a code it is acceptable to use both the code and the excluded code together.

Etiology/manifestation convention ("code first", "use additional code" and "in diseases classified elsewhere" notes)

Certain conditions have both an underlying etiology and multiple body system manifestations due to the underlying etiology. For such conditions, the ICD-10-CM has a coding convention that requires the underlying condition be sequenced first followed by the manifestation. Wherever such a combination exists, there is a "use additional code" note at the etiology code, and a "code first" note at the manifestation code. These instructional notes indicate the proper sequencing order of the codes, etiology followed by manifestation.

In most cases the manifestation codes will have in the code title, "in diseases classified elsewhere." Codes with this title are a component of the etiology/ manifestation convention. The code title indicates that it is a manifestation code. "In diseases classified elsewhere" codes are never permitted to be used as first-listed or principal diagnosis codes. They must be used in conjunction with an underlying condition code and they must be listed following the underlying condition. See category F02, Dementia in other diseases classified elsewhere, for an example of this convention.

There are manifestation codes that do not have "in diseases classified elsewhere" in the title. For such codes a "use additional code" note will still be present and the rules for sequencing apply.

In addition to the notes in the Tabular List, these conditions also have a specific Alphabetic Index entry structure. In the Alphabetic Index both conditions are listed together with the etiology code first followed by the manifestation codes in brackets. The code in brackets is always to be sequenced second.

An example of the etiology/manifestation convention is dementia in Parkinson's disease. In the Alphabetic Index, code G20 is listed first, followed by code F02.80 or F02.81 in brackets. Code G20 represents the underlying etiology, Parkinson's disease, and must be sequenced first, whereas codes F02.80 and F02.81 represent the manifestation of dementia in diseases classified elsewhere, with or without behavioral disturbance.

"Code first" and "Use additional code" notes are also used as sequencing rules in the classification for certain codes that are not part of an etiology/ manifestation combination.

"And"

The word "and" should be interpreted to mean either "and" or "or" when it appears in a title.

"With"

The word "with" should be interpreted to mean "associated with" or "due to" when it appears in a code title, the Alphabetic Index, or an instructional note in the Tabular List.

The word "with" in the Alphabetic Index is sequenced immediately following the main term, not in alphabetical order.

"See" and "See Also"

The "see" instruction following a main term in the Alphabetic Index indicates that another term should be referenced. It is necessary to go to the main term referenced with the "see" note to locate the correct code.

A "see also" instruction following a main term in the Alphabetic Index instructs that there is another main term that may also be referenced that may provide additional Alphabetic Index entries that may be useful. It is not necessary to follow the "see also" note when the original main term provides the necessary code.

"Code also note"

A "code also" note instructs that two codes may be required to fully describe a condition, but this note does not provide sequencing direction.

Default codes

A code listed next to a main term in the ICD-10-CM Alphabetic Index is referred to as a default code. The default code represents that condition that is most commonly associated with the main term, or is the unspecified code for the condition. If a condition is documented in a medical record (for example, appendicitis) without any additional information, such as acute or chronic, the default code should be assigned.

Syndromes

Follow the Alphabetic Index guidance when coding syndromes. In the absence of Alphabetic Index guidance, assign codes for the documented manifestations of the syndrome.

Typeface

Bold: Bold typeface is used for all codes and code titles in the Tabular List and for main terms in the Alphabetic Index.

Italics: Italicized typeface is used for all exclusion notes in the Tabular list and for "*see*" and "*see also*" instructions in the Alphabetic Index.

<u>**Underscore:**</u>   See Channel Publishing Additional *Enhanced* Features.

Channel Publishing Additional *Enhanced* Features

Highlighted Term <u>Differentiation</u>

Selected terms within code categories and code titles have been underscored to help coders more easily and accurately identify the correct code in the Tabular List.

Further use of dashes (-)

All code categories and codes requiring additional digits in the Tabular List have a dash (-) at the end of the last digit that helps coders be aware that additional characters are required for a complete code.

Further use of placeholder "x"

All codes requiring the coder to use the placeholder "x" to make a complete code have been placed in advance to clearly identify the need to use these placeholders.

Excludes ❷:

All Excludes2 listings have a graphic "❷" to help coders more clearly identify those unqiue excludes notations where a coder may code both conditions, if present.

Excludes 1 and Excludes ❷ key

The short descriptions of Excludes 1 and Excludes ❷ are listed on the bottom of each page throughout the Tabular List to help coders learn the difference between the two without referring back to the introduction.

Highlighted 7th digit subclassifications

Gray screen bars over the 7th digit subclassifications in the Tabular List help coders easily identify those code categories requiring a variable 7th digit.

Tabular List guide line

A vertical guide line has been placed that aligns with all 3-digit codes and 3-digit code categories instead of the traditional column dividing line.

Tab-Edge printing

Chapter-by-chapter, and section-by-section stair-stepped, tab-edge printing helps coders locate the correct section quickly.

2014 OFFICIAL CODING GUIDELINES

IMPORTANT NOTE REGARDING THESE PRINTED GUIDELINES

These guidelines are effective for the 2014 Version of ICD-10-CM (guidelines posted 7/11/2013). A newer version may become available after this book has been printed. Coders should periodically check the National Center for Health Statistics (NCHS) web site for the most current version.

NCHS Web Site: www.cdc.gov/nchs/icd/icd10cm.htm

Channel Publishing, Ltd.

2014 ICD-10-CM Official Guidelines for Coding and Reporting
Narrative changes appear in bold text
Items <u>underlined</u> have been moved within the guidelines
since the 2013 version
Italics are used to indicate revisions to heading changes

The Centers for Medicare and Medicaid Services (CMS) and the National Center for Health Statistics (NCHS), two departments within the U.S. Federal Government's Department of Health and Human Services (DHHS) provide the following guidelines for coding and reporting using the International Classification of Diseases, 10th Revision, Clinical Modification (ICD-10-CM). These guidelines should be used as a companion document to the official version of the ICD-10-CM as published on the NCHS website. The ICD-10-CM is a morbidity classification published by the United States for classifying diagnoses and reason for visits in all health care settings. The ICD-10-CM is based on the ICD-10, the statistical classification of disease published by the World Health Organization (WHO).

These guidelines have been approved by the four organizations that make up the Cooperating Parties for the ICD-10-CM: the American Hospital Association (AHA), the American Health Information Management Association (AHIMA), CMS, and NCHS.

These guidelines are a set of rules that have been developed to accompany and complement the official conventions and instructions provided within the ICD-10-CM itself. The instructions and conventions of the classification take precedence over guidelines. These guidelines are based on the coding and sequencing instructions in the Tabular List and Alphabetic Index of ICD-10-CM, but provide additional instruction. Adherence to these guidelines when assigning ICD-10-CM diagnosis codes is required under the Health Insurance Portability and Accountability Act (HIPAA). The diagnosis codes (Tabular List and Alphabetic Index) have been adopted under HIPAA for all healthcare settings. A joint effort between the healthcare provider and the coder is essential to achieve complete and accurate documentation, code assignment, and reporting of diagnoses and procedures. These guidelines have been developed to assist both the healthcare provider and the coder in identifying those diagnoses and procedures that are to be reported. The importance of consistent, complete documentation in the medical record cannot be overemphasized. Without such documentation accurate coding cannot be achieved. The entire record should be reviewed to determine the specific reason for the encounter and the conditions treated.

The term encounter is used for all settings, including hospital admissions. In the context of these guidelines, the term provider is used throughout the guidelines to mean physician or any qualified health care practitioner who is legally accountable for establishing the patient's diagnosis. Only this set of guidelines, approved by the Cooperating Parties, is official.

The guidelines are organized into sections. Section I includes the structure and conventions of the classification and general guidelines that apply to the entire classification, and chapter-specific guidelines that correspond to the chapters as they are arranged in the classification. Section II includes guidelines for selection of principal diagnosis for non-outpatient settings. Section III includes guidelines for reporting additional diagnoses in non-outpatient settings. Section IV is for outpatient coding and reporting. It is necessary to review all sections of the guidelines to fully understand all of the rules and instructions needed to code properly.

TABLE OF CONTENTS

TABLE OF CONTENTS

SECTION I – CONVENTIONS
Section I. A. 1.

Section I. Conventions, general coding guidelines and chapter specific guidelines

The conventions, general guidelines and chapter-specific guidelines are applicable to all health care settings unless otherwise indicated. The conventions and instructions of the classification take precedence over guidelines.

A. Conventions for the ICD-10-CM

The conventions for the ICD-10-CM are the general rules for use of the classification independent of the guidelines. These conventions are incorporated within the Alphabetic Index and Tabular List of the ICD-10-CM as instructional notes.

1. The Alphabetic Index and Tabular List

The ICD-10-CM is divided into the Alphabetic Index, an alphabetical list of terms and their corresponding code, and the Tabular List, a structured list of codes divided into chapters based on body system or condition. The Alphabetic Index consists of the following parts: the Index of Diseases and Injury, the Index of External Causes of Injury, the Table of Neoplasms and the Table of Drugs and Chemicals.

See Section I.C2. General guidelines
See Section I.C.19. Adverse effects, poisoning, underdosing and toxic effects

2. Format and Structure

The ICD-10-CM Tabular List contains categories, subcategories and codes. Characters for categories, subcategories and codes may be either a letter or a number. All categories are 3 characters. A three-character category that has no further subdivision is equivalent to a code. Subcategories are either 4 or 5 characters. Codes may be 3, 4, 5, 6 or 7 characters. That is, each level of subdivision after a category is a subcategory. The final level of subdivision is a code. Codes that have applicable 7th characters are still referred to as codes, not subcategories. A code that has an applicable 7th character is considered invalid without the 7th character.

The ICD-10-CM uses an indented format for ease in reference.

3. Use of codes for reporting purposes

For reporting purposes only codes are permissible, not categories or subcategories, and any applicable 7th character is required.

4. Placeholder character

The ICD-10-CM utilizes a placeholder character "X". The "X" is used as a placeholder at certain codes to allow for future expansion. An example of this is at the poisoning, adverse effect and underdosing codes, categories T36-T50.

Where a placeholder exists, the X must be used in order for the code to be considered a valid code.

5. 7th Characters

Certain ICD-10-CM categories have applicable 7th characters. The applicable 7th character is required for all codes within the category, or as the notes in the Tabular List instruct. The 7th character must always be the 7th character in the data field. If a code that requires a 7th character is not 6 characters, a placeholder X must be used to fill in the empty characters.

GUIDELINES

SECTION I – CONVENTIONS
Section I. A. 6.

6. **Abbreviations**

  a. **Alphabetic Index abbreviations**

   NEC "Not elsewhere classifiable"
   This abbreviation in the Alphabetic Index represents "other specified". When a specific code is not available for a condition, the Alphabetic Index directs the coder to the "other specified" code in the Tabular List.

   NOS "Not otherwise specified"
   This abbreviation is the equivalent of unspecified.

  b. **Tabular List abbreviations**

   NEC "Not elsewhere classifiable"
   This abbreviation in the Tabular List represents "other specified". When a specific code is not available for a condition the Tabular List includes an NEC entry under a code to identify the code as the "other specified" code.

   NOS "Not otherwise specified"
   This abbreviation is the equivalent of unspecified.

7. **Punctuation**

   [ ] Brackets are used in the Tabular List to enclose synonyms, alternative wording or explanatory phrases. Brackets are used in the Alphabetic Index to identify manifestation codes.

   ( ) Parentheses are used in both the Alphabetic Index and Tabular List to enclose supplementary words that may be present or absent in the statement of a disease or procedure without affecting the code number to which it is assigned. The terms within the parentheses are referred to as nonessential modifiers. **The nonessential modifiers in the Alphabetic Index to Diseases apply to subterms following a main term except when a nonessential modifier and a subentry are mutually exclusive, the subentry takes precedence. For example, in the ICD-10-CM Alphabetic Index under the main term Enteritis, "acute" is a nonessential modifier and "chronic" is a subentry. In this case, the nonessential modifier "acute" does not apply to the subentry "chronic".**

   : Colons are used in the Tabular List after an incomplete term which needs one or more of the modifiers following the colon to make it assignable to a given category.

8. **Use of "and"**

   See Section I.A.14. Use of the term "And"

9. **Other and Unspecified codes**

  a. **"Other" codes**

   Codes titled "other" or "other specified" are for use when the information in the medical record provides detail for which a specific code does not exist. Alphabetic Index entries with NEC in the line designate "other" codes in the Tabular List. These Alphabetic Index entries represent specific disease entities for which no specific code exists so the term is included within an "other" code.

  b. **"Unspecified" codes**

   Codes titled "unspecified" are for use when the information in the medical record is insufficient to assign a more specific code. For those categories for which an unspecified code is not provided, the "other specified" code may represent both other and unspecified.

   See Section I.B.18 Use of Sign/Symptom/Unspecified Codes

10. **Includes Notes**

   This note appears immediately under a three character code title to further define, or give examples of, the content of the category.

SECTION I – CONVENTIONS
Section I. A. 11.

11. **Inclusion terms**

   List of terms is included under some codes. These terms are the conditions for which that code is to be used. The terms may be synonyms of the code title, or, in the case of "other specified" codes, the terms are a list of the various conditions assigned to that code. The inclusion terms are not necessarily exhaustive. Additional terms found only in the Alphabetic Index may also be assigned to a code.

12. **Excludes Notes**

   The ICD-10-CM has two types of excludes notes. Each type of note has a different definition for use but they are all similar in that they indicate that codes excluded from each other are independent of each other.

  a. **Excludes 1**

   A type 1 Excludes note is a pure excludes note. It means "NOT CODED HERE!" An Excludes1 note indicates that the code excluded should never be used at the same time as the code above the Excludes1 note. An Excludes1 is used when two conditions cannot occur together, such as a congenital form versus an acquired form of the same condition.

  b. **Excludes 2**

   A type 2 Excludes note represents "Not included here". An Excludes2 note indicates that the condition excluded is not part of the condition represented by the code, but a patient may have both conditions at the same time. When an Excludes2 note appears under a code, it is acceptable to use both the code and the excluded code together, when appropriate.

13. **Etiology/manifestation convention ("code first", "use additional code" and "in diseases classified elsewhere" notes)**

   Certain conditions have both an underlying etiology and multiple body system manifestations due to the underlying etiology. For such conditions, the ICD-10-CM has a coding convention that requires the underlying condition be sequenced first followed by the manifestation. Wherever such a combination exists, there is a "use additional code" note at the etiology code, and a "code first" note at the manifestation code. These instructional notes indicate the proper sequencing order of the codes, etiology followed by manifestation.

   In most cases the manifestation codes will have in the code title, "in diseases classified elsewhere." Codes with this title are a component of the etiology/ manifestation convention. The code title indicates that it is a manifestation code. "In diseases classified elsewhere" codes are never permitted to be used as first-listed or principal diagnosis codes. They must be used in conjunction with an underlying condition code and they must be listed following the underlying condition. See category F02, Dementia in other diseases classified elsewhere, for an example of this convention.

   There are manifestation codes that do not have "in diseases classified elsewhere" in the title. For such codes, there is a "use additional code" note at the etiology code and a "code first" note at the manifestation code and the rules for sequencing apply.

   In addition to the notes in the Tabular List, these conditions also have a specific Alphabetic Index entry structure. In the Alphabetic Index both conditions are listed together with the etiology code first followed by the manifestation codes in brackets. The code in brackets is always to be sequenced second.

   An example of the etiology/manifestation convention is dementia in Parkinson's disease. In the Alphabetic Index, code G20 is listed first, followed by code F02.80 or F02.81 in brackets. Code G20 represents the underlying etiology, Parkinson's disease, and must be sequenced first, whereas codes F02.80 and F02.81 represent the manifestation of dementia in diseases classified elsewhere, with or without behavioral disturbance.

   "Code first" and "Use additional code" notes are also used as sequencing rules in the classification for certain codes that are not part of an etiology/ manifestation combination.
   See Section I.B.7. Multiple coding for a single condition.

SECTION I – CONVENTIONS
Section I. A. 14.

14. "And"
The word "and" should be interpreted to mean either "and" or "or" when it appears in a title.

For example, cases of "tuberculosis of bones", "tuberculosis of joints" and "tuberculosis of bones and joints" are classified to subcategory A18.0, Tuberculosis of bones and joints.

15. "With"
The word "with" should be interpreted to mean "associated with" or "due to" when it appears in a code title, the Alphabetic Index, or an instructional note in the Tabular List.

The word "with" in the Alphabetic Index is sequenced immediately following the main term, not in alphabetical order.

16. "See" and "See Also"
The "see" instruction following a main term in the Alphabetic Index indicates that another term should be referenced. It is necessary to go to the main term referenced with the "see" note to locate the correct code.

A "see also" instruction following a main term in the Alphabetic Index instructs that there is another main term that may also be referenced that may provide additional Alphabetic Index entries that may be useful. It is not necessary to follow the "see also" note when the original main term provides the necessary code.

17. "Code also note"
A "code also" note instructs that two codes may be required to fully describe a condition, but this note does not provide sequencing direction.

18. Default codes
A code listed next to a main term in the ICD-10-CM Alphabetic Index is referred to as a default code. The default code represents that condition that is most commonly associated with the main term, or is the unspecified code for the condition. If a condition is documented in a medical record (for example, appendicitis) without any additional information, such as acute or chronic, the default code should be assigned.

SECTION I – GENERAL CODING GUIDELINES
Section I. B. 1.

B. General Coding Guidelines

1. Locating a code in the ICD-10-CM
To select a code in the classification that corresponds to a diagnosis or reason for visit documented in a medical record, first locate the term in the Alphabetic Index, and then verify the code in the Tabular List. Read and be guided by instructional notations that appear in both the Alphabetic Index and the Tabular List.

It is essential to use both the Alphabetic Index and Tabular List when locating and assigning a code. The Alphabetic Index does not always provide the full code. Selection of the full code, including laterality and any applicable 7th character can only be done in the Tabular List. A dash (-) at the end of an Alphabetic Index entry indicates that additional characters are required. Even if a dash is not included at the Alphabetic Index entry, it is necessary to refer to the Tabular List to verify that no 7th character is required.

2. Level of Detail in Coding
Diagnosis codes are to be used and reported at their highest number of characters available.

ICD-10-CM diagnosis codes are composed of codes with 3, 4, 5, 6 or 7 characters. Codes with three characters are included in ICD-10-CM as the heading of a category of codes that may be further subdivided by the use of fourth and/or fifth characters and/or sixth characters, which provide greater detail.

A three-character code is to be used only if it is not further subdivided. A code is invalid if it has not been coded to the full number of characters required for that code, including the 7th character, if applicable.

3. Code or codes from A00.0 through T88.9, Z00-Z99.8
The appropriate code or codes from A00.0 through T88.9, Z00-Z99.8 must be used to identify diagnoses, symptoms, conditions, problems, complaints or other reason(s) for the encounter/visit.

4. Signs and symptoms
Codes that describe symptoms and signs, as opposed to diagnoses, are acceptable for reporting purposes when a related definitive diagnosis has not been established (confirmed) by the provider. Chapter 18 of ICD-10-CM, Symptoms, Signs, and Abnormal Clinical and Laboratory Findings, Not Elsewhere Classified (codes R00.0 - R99) contains many, but not all codes for symptoms.

See Section I.B.18 Use of Sign/Symptom/Unspecified Codes

5. Conditions that are an integral part of a disease process
Signs and symptoms that are associated routinely with a disease process should not be assigned as additional codes, unless otherwise instructed by the classification.

6. Conditions that are not an integral part of a disease process
Additional signs and symptoms that may not be associated routinely with a disease process should be coded when present.

GUIDELINES

SECTION I – GENERAL CODING GUIDELINES
Section I. B. 7.

7. **Multiple coding for a single condition**

In addition to the etiology/manifestation convention that requires two codes to fully describe a single condition that affects multiple body systems, there are other single conditions that also require more than one code. "Use additional code" notes are found in the Tabular List at codes that are not part of an etiology/manifestation pair where a secondary code is useful to fully describe a condition. The sequencing rule is the same as the etiology/manifestation pair, "use additional code" indicates that a secondary code should be added.

For example, for bacterial infections that are not included in chapter 1, a secondary code from category B95, Streptococcus, Staphylococcus, and Enterococcus, as the cause of diseases classified elsewhere, or B96, Other bacterial agents as the cause of diseases classified elsewhere, may be required to identify the bacterial organism causing the infection. A "use additional code" note will normally be found at the infectious disease code, indicating a need for the organism code to be added as a secondary code.

"Code first" notes are also under certain codes that are not specifically manifestation codes but may be due to an underlying cause. When there is a "code first" note and an underlying condition is present, the underlying condition should be sequenced first.

"Code, if applicable, any causal condition first", notes indicate that this code may be assigned as a principal diagnosis when the causal condition is unknown or not applicable. If a causal condition is known, then the code for that condition should be sequenced as the principal or first-listed diagnosis.

Multiple codes may be needed for sequela, complication codes and obstetric codes to more fully describe a condition. See the specific guidelines for these conditions for further instruction.

8. **Acute and Chronic Conditions**

If the same condition is described as both acute (subacute) and chronic, and separate subentries exist in the Alphabetic Index at the same indentation level, code both and sequence the acute (subacute) code first.

9. **Combination Code**

A combination code is a single code used to classify:
> Two diagnoses, or
> A diagnosis with an associated secondary process (manifestation)
> A diagnosis with an associated complication

Combination codes are identified by referring to subterm entries in the Alphabetic Index and by reading the inclusion and exclusion notes in the Tabular List.

Assign only the combination code when that code fully identifies the diagnostic conditions involved or when the Alphabetic Index so directs. Multiple coding should not be used when the classification provides a combination code that clearly identifies all of the elements documented in the diagnosis. When the combination code lacks necessary specificity in describing the manifestation or complication, an additional code should be used as a secondary code.

10. **Sequela (Late Effects)**

A sequela is the residual effect (condition produced) after the acute phase of an illness or injury has terminated. There is no time limit on when a sequela code can be used. The residual may be apparent early, such as in cerebral infarction, or it may occur months or years later, such as that due to a previous injury. Coding of sequela generally requires two codes sequenced in the following order: The condition or nature of the sequela is sequenced first. The sequela code is sequenced second.

SECTION I – GENERAL CODING GUIDELINES
Section I. B. 11.

An exception to the above guidelines are those instances where the code for sequela is followed by a manifestation code identified in the Tabular List and title, or the sequela code has been expanded (at the fourth, fifth or sixth character levels) to include the manifestation(s). The code for the acute phase of an illness or injury that led to the sequela is never used with a code for the late effect.

See Section I.C.9. Sequelae of cerebrovascular disease
See Section I.C.15. Sequelae of complication of pregnancy, childbirth and the puerperium
See Section I.C.19. Application of 7th characters for Chapter 19

11. **Impending or Threatened Condition**

Code any condition described at the time of discharge as "impending" or "threatened" as follows:
> If it did occur, code as confirmed diagnosis.
> If it did not occur, reference the Alphabetic Index to determine if the condition has a subentry term for "impending" or "threatened" and also reference main term entries for "Impending" and for "Threatened."
> If the subterms are listed, assign the given code.
> If the subterms are not listed, code the existing underlying condition(s) and not the condition described as impending or threatened.

12. **Reporting Same Diagnosis Code More than Once**

Each unique ICD-10-CM diagnosis code may be reported only once for an encounter. This applies to bilateral conditions when there are no distinct codes identifying laterality or two different conditions classified to the same ICD-10-CM diagnosis code.

13. **Laterality**

Some ICD-10-CM codes indicate laterality, specifying whether the condition occurs on the left, right or is bilateral. If no bilateral code is provided and the condition is bilateral, assign separate codes for both the left and right side. If the side is not identified in the medical record, assign the code for the unspecified side.

14. **Documentation for BMI, Non-pressure ulcers and Pressure Ulcer Stages**

For the Body Mass Index (BMI), depth of non-pressure chronic ulcers and pressure ulcer stage codes, code assignment may be based on medical record documentation from clinicians who are not the patient's provider (i.e., physician or other qualified healthcare practitioner legally accountable for establishing the patient's diagnosis), since this information is typically documented by other clinicians involved in the care of the patient (e.g., a dietitian often documents the BMI and nurses often documents the pressure ulcer stages). However, the associated diagnosis (such as overweight, obesity, or pressure ulcer) must be documented by the patient's provider. If there is conflicting medical record documentation, either from the same clinician or different clinicians, the patient's attending provider should be queried for clarification.

The BMI codes should only be reported as secondary diagnoses. As with all other secondary diagnosis codes, the BMI codes should only be assigned when they meet the definition of a reportable additional diagnosis (see Section III, Reporting Additional Diagnoses).

15. **Syndromes**

Follow the Alphabetic Index guidance when coding syndromes. In the absence of Alphabetic Index guidance, assign codes for the documented manifestations of the syndrome. Additional codes for manifestations that are not an integral part of the disease process may also be assigned when the condition does not have a unique code.

CHAPTER 1 – INFECTIOUS DISEASES
Section I. B. 16.

16. Documentation of Complications of Care
Code assignment is based on the provider's documentaion of the relationship between the condition and the care or procedure. The guideline extends to any complications of care, regardless of the chapter the code is located in. It is important to note that not all conditions that occur during or following medical care or surgery are classified as complications. There must be a cause-and-effect relationship between the care provided and the condition, and an indication in the documentation that it is a complication. Query the provider for clarification, if the complication is not clearly documented.

17. Borderline diagnosis
If the provider documents a "borderline" diagnosis at the time of discharge, the diagnosis is coded as confirmed, unless the classification provides a specific entry (e.g., borderline diabetes). If a borderline condition has a specific index entry in ICD-10-CM, it should be coded as such. Since borderline conditions are not uncertain diagnoses, no distinction is made between the care setting (inpatient versus outpatient). Whenever the documentation is unclear regarding a borderline condition, coders are encouraged to query for clarification.

18. Use of Sign/Symptom/Unspecified Codes
Sign/symptom and "unspecified" codes have acceptable, even necessary, uses. While specific diagnosis codes should be reported when they are supported by the available medical record documentation and clinical knowledge of the patient's health condition, there are instances when signs/symptoms or unspecified codes are the best choices for accurately reflecting the healthcare encounter. Each healthcare encounter should be coded to the level of certainty known for that encounter.

If a definitive diagnosis has not been established by the end of the encounter, it is appropriate to report codes for sign(s) and/or symptoms(s) in lieu of a definitive diagnosis. When sufficient clinical information isn't known or available about a particular health condition to assign a more specific code, it is acceptable to report the appropriate "unspecified" code (e.g., a diagnosis of pneumonia has been determined, but not the specific type). Unspecified codes should be reported when they are the codes that most accurately reflects what is known about the patient's condition at the time of that particular encounter. It would be inappropriate to select a specific code that is not supported by the medical record documentation or conduct medically unnecessary diagnostic testing in order to determine a more specific code.

C. Chapter-Specific Coding Guidelines
In addition to general coding guidelines, there are guidelines for specific diagnoses and/or conditions in the classification. Unless otherwise indicated, these guidelines apply to all health care settings. Please refer to Section II for guidelines on the selection of principal diagnosis.

1. Chapter 1: Certain Infectious and Parasitic Diseases (A00-B99)

a. Human Immunodeficiency Virus (HIV) Infections

1) Code only confirmed cases
Code only confirmed cases of HIV infection/illness. This is an exception to the hospital inpatient guideline Section II, H.

In this context, "confirmation" does not require documentation of positive serology or culture for HIV; the provider's diagnostic statement that the patient is HIV positive, or has an HIV-related illness is sufficient.

2) Selection and sequencing of HIV codes

(a) Patient admitted for HIV-related condition
If a patient is admitted for an HIV-related condition, the principal diagnosis should be B20, Human immunodeficiency virus [HIV] disease followed by additional diagnosis codes for all reported HIV-related conditions.

CHAPTER 1 – INFECTIOUS DISEASES
Section I. C. 1. a. 2) (b)

(b) Patient with HIV disease admitted for unrelated condition
If a patient with HIV disease is admitted for an unrelated condition (such as a traumatic injury), the code for the unrelated condition (e.g., the nature of injury code) should be the principal diagnosis. Other diagnoses would be B20 followed by additional diagnosis codes for all reported HIV-related conditions.

(c) Whether the patient is newly diagnosed
Whether the patient is newly diagnosed or has had previous admissions/encounters for HIV conditions is irrelevant to the sequencing decision.

(d) Asymptomatic human immunodeficiency virus
Z21, Asymptomatic human immunodeficiency virus [HIV] infection status, is to be applied when the patient without any documentation of symptoms is listed as being "HIV positive," "known HIV," "HIV test positive," or similar terminology. Do not use this code if the term "AIDS" is used or if the patient is treated for any HIV-related illness or is described as having any condition(s) resulting from his/her HIV positive status; use B20 in these cases.

(e) Patients with inconclusive HIV serology
Patients with inconclusive HIV serology, but no definitive diagnosis or manifestations of the illness, may be assigned code R75, Inconclusive laboratory evidence of human immunodeficiency virus [HIV].

(f) Previously diagnosed HIV-related illness
Patients with any known prior diagnosis of an HIV-related illness should be coded to B20. Once a patient has developed an HIV-related illness, the patient should always be assigned code B20 on every subsequent admission/encounter. Patients previously diagnosed with any HIV illness (B20) should never be assigned to R75 or Z21, Asymptomatic human immunodeficiency virus [HIV] infection status.

(g) HIV Infection in Pregnancy, Childbirth and the Puerperium
During pregnancy, childbirth or the puerperium, a patient admitted (or presenting for a health care encounter) because of an HIV-related illness should receive a principal diagnosis code of O98.7-, Human immunodeficiency [HIV] disease complicating pregnancy, childbirth and the puerperium, followed by B20 and the code(s) for the HIV-related illness(es). Codes from Chapter 15 always take sequencing priority.

Patients with asymptomatic HIV infection status admitted (or presenting for a health care encounter) during pregnancy, childbirth, or the puerperium should receive codes of O98.7- and Z21.

(h) Encounters for testing for HIV
If a patient is being seen to determine his/her HIV status, use code Z11.4, Encounter for screening for human immunodeficiency virus [HIV]. Use additional codes for any associated high risk behavior.

If a patient with signs or symptoms is being seen for HIV testing, code the signs and symptoms. An additional counseling code Z71.7, Human immunodeficiency virus [HIV] counseling, may be used if counseling is provided during the encounter for the test.

When a patient returns to be informed of his/her HIV test results and the test result is negative, use code Z71.7, Human immunodeficiency virus [HIV] counseling.

If the results are positive, see previous guidelines and assign codes as appropriate.

b. Infectious agents as the cause of diseases classified to other chapters

Certain infections are classified in chapters other than Chapter 1 and no organism is identified as part of the infection code. In these instances, it is necessary to use an additional code from Chapter 1 to identify the organism. A code from category B95, Streptococcus, Staphylococcus, and Enterococcus as the cause of diseases classified to other chapters, B96, Other bacterial agents as the cause of diseases classified to other chapters, or B97, Viral agents as the cause of diseases classified to other chapters, is to be used as an additional code to identify the organism. An instructional note will be found at the infection code advising that an additional organism code is required.

c. Infections resistant to antibiotics

Many bacterial infections are resistant to current antibiotics. It is necessary to identify all infections documented as antibiotic resistant. Assign a code from category Z16, Resistance to antimicrobial drugs, following the infection code only if the infection code does not identify drug resistance.

d. Sepsis, Severe Sepsis, and Septic Shock

1) Coding of Sepsis and Severe Sepsis

(a) Sepsis

For a diagnosis of sepsis, assign the appropriate code for the underlying systemic infection. If the type of infection or causal organism is not further specified, assign code A41.9, Sepsis, unspecified organism.

A code from subcategory R65.2, Severe sepsis, should not be assigned unless severe sepsis or an associated acute organ dysfunction is documented.

(i) Negative or inconclusive blood cultures and sepsis

Negative or inconclusive blood cultures do not preclude a diagnosis of sepsis in patients with clinical evidence of the condition, however, the provider should be queried.

(ii) Urosepsis

The term urosepsis is a nonspecific term. It is not to be considered synonymous with sepsis. It has no default code in the Alphabetic Index. Should a provider use this term, he/she must be queried for clarification.

(iii) Sepsis with organ dysfunction

If a patient has sepsis and associated acute organ dysfunction or multiple organ dysfunction (MOD), follow the instructions for coding severe sepsis.

(iv) Acute organ dysfunction that is not clearly associated with the sepsis

If a patient has sepsis and an acute organ dysfunction, but the medical record documentation indicates that the acute organ dysfunction is related to a medical condition other than the sepsis, do not assign a code from subcategory R65.2, Severe sepsis. An acute organ dysfunction must be associated with the sepsis in order to assign the severe sepsis code. If the documentation is not clear as to whether an acute organ dysfunction is related to the sepsis or another medical condition, query the provider.

(b) Severe sepsis

The coding of severe sepsis requires a minimum of 2 codes: first a code for the underlying systemic infection, followed by a code from subcategory R65.2, Severe sepsis. If the causal organism is not documented, assign code A41.9, Sepsis, unspecified organism, for the infection. Additional code(s) for the associated acute organ dysfunction are also required.

Due to the complex nature of severe sepsis, some cases may require querying the provider prior to assignment of the codes.

2) Septic shock

(a) Septic shock

Septic shock generally refers to circulatory failure associated with severe sepsis, and therefore, it represents a type of acute organ dysfunction.

For cases of septic shock, the code for the systemic infection should be sequenced first, followed by code R65.21, Severe sepsis with septic shock or code T81.12, Postprocedural septic shock. Any additional codes for the other acute organ dysfunctions should also be assigned. As noted in the sequencing instructions in the Tabular List, the code for septic shock cannot be assigned as a principal diagnosis.

3) Sequencing of severe sepsis

If severe sepsis is present on admission, and meets the definition of principal diagnosis, the underlying systemic infection should be assigned as principal diagnosis followed by the appropriate code from subcategory R65.2 as required by the sequencing rules in the Tabular List. A code from subcategory R65.2 can never be assigned as a principal diagnosis.

When severe sepsis develops during an encounter (it was not present on admission) the underlying systemic infection and the appropriate code from subcategory R65.2 should be assigned as secondary diagnoses.

Severe sepsis may be present on admission but the diagnosis may not be confirmed until sometime after admission. If the documentation is not clear whether severe sepsis was present on admission, the provider should be queried.

4) Sepsis and severe sepsis with a localized infection

If the reason for admission is both sepsis or severe sepsis and a localized infection, such as pneumonia or cellulitis, a code(s) for the underlying systemic infection should be assigned first and the code for the localized infection should be assigned as a secondary diagnosis. If the patient has severe sepsis, a code from subcategory R65.2 should also be assigned as a secondary diagnosis. If the patient is admitted with a localized infection, such as pneumonia, and sepsis/severe sepsis doesn't develop until after admission, the localized infection should be assigned first, followed by the appropriate sepsis/severe sepsis codes.

5) Sepsis due to a postprocedural infection

(a) Documentation of causal relationship
As with all postprocedural complications, code assignment is based on the provider's documentation of the relationship between the infection and the procedure.

(b) Septis due to a postprocedural infection
For such cases, the postprocedural infection code, such as, T80.2, Infections following infusion, transfusion, and therapeutic injection, T81.4, Infection following a procedure, T88.0, Infection following immunization, or O86.0, Infection of obstetric surgical wound, should be coded first, followed by the code for the specific infection. If the patient has severe sepsis the appropriate code from subcategory R65.2 should also be assigned with the additional code(s) for any acute organ dysfunction.

(c) Postprocedural infection and postprocedural septic shock
In cases where a postprocedural infection has occurred and has resulted in severe sepsis and postprocedural septic shock, the code for the precipitating complication such as code T81.4, Infection following a procedure, or O86.0, Infection of obstetrical surgical wound should be coded first followed by code R65.21, Severe sepsis with septic shock and a code for the systemic infection.

6) Sepsis and severe sepsis associated with a noninfectious process (condition)
In some cases a noninfectious process (condition), such as trauma, may lead to an infection which can result in sepsis or severe sepsis. If sepsis or severe sepsis is documented as associated with a noninfectious condition, such as a burn or serious injury, and this condition meets the definition for principal diagnosis, the code for the noninfectious condition should be sequenced first, followed by the code for the resulting infection. If severe sepsis, is present a code from subcategory R65.2 should also be assigned with any associated organ dysfunction(s) codes. It is not necessary to assign a code from subcategory R65.1, Systemic inflammatory response syndrome (SIRS) of non-infectious origin, for these cases.

If the infection meets the definition of principal diagnosis it should be sequenced before the non-infectious condition. When both the associated non-infectious condition and the infection meet the definition of principal diagnosis either may be assigned as principal diagnosis.

Only one code from category R65, Symptoms and signs specifically associated with systemic inflammation and infection, should be assigned. Therefore, when a non-infectious condition leads to an infection resulting in severe sepsis, assign the appropriate code from subcategory R65.2, Severe sepsis. Do not additionally assign a code from subcategory R65.1, Systemic inflammatory response syndrome (SIRS) of non-infectious origin.

See Section I.C.18. SIRS due to non-infectious process

7) Sepsis and septic shock complicating abortion, pregnancy, childbirth, and the puerperium
See Section I.C.15. Sepsis and septic shock complicating abortion, pregnancy, childbirth and the puerperium

8) Newborn sepsis
See Section I.C.16.f. Bacterial sepsis of Newborn

e. Methicillin Resistant *Staphylococcus aureus* (MRSA) Conditions

1) Selection and sequencing of MRSA codes

(a) Combination codes for MRSA infection
When a patient is diagnosed with an infection that is due to methicillin resistant *Staphylococcus aureus* (MRSA), and that infection that has a combination code that includes the causal organism (e.g., sepsis, pneumonia) assign the appropriate combination code for the condition (e.g., code A41.02, Sepsis due to methicillin resistant Staphylococcus aureus or code J15.212, Pneumonia due to methicillin resistant Staphylococcus aureus). Do not assign code B95.62, Methicillin resistant Staphylococcus aureus infection as the cause of the diseases classified elsewhere, as an additional code because the combination code includes the type of infection and the MRSA organism. Do not assign a code from subcategory Z16.11, Resistance to penicillins, as an additional diagnosis.

See Section C.1. for instructions on coding and sequencing of sepsis and severe sepsis

(b) Other codes for MRSA infection
When there is documentation of a current infection (e.g., wound infection, stitch abscess, urinary tract infection) due to MRSA, and that infection does not have a combination code that includes the causal organism, assign the appropriate code to identify the condition along with code B95.62, Methicillin resistant Staphylococcus aureus infection as the cause of diseases classified elsewhere for the MRSA infection. Do not assign a code from subcategory Z16.11, Resistance to penicillins.

(c) Methicillin susceptible Staphylococcus aureus (MSSA) and MRSA colonization
The condition or state of being colonized or carrying MSSA or MRSA is called colonization or carriage, while an individual person is described as being colonized or being a carrier. Colonization means that MSSA and MSRA is present on or in the body without necessarily causing illness. A positive MRSA colonization test might be documented by the provider as "MRSA screen positive" or "MRSA nasal swab positive".

Assign code Z22.322, Carrier or suspected carrier of methicillin resistant Staphylococcus aureus, for patients documented as having MRSA colonization. Assign code Z22.321, Carrier or suspected carrier of methicillin susceptible Staphylococcus aureus, for patient documented as having MSSA colonization. Colonization is not necessarily indicative of a disease process or as the cause of a specific condition the patient may have unless documented as such by the provider.

(d) MRSA colonization and infection
If a patient is documented as having both MRSA colonization and infection during a hospital admission, code Z22.322, Carrier or suspected carrier of methicillin resistant Staphylococcus aureus, and a code for the MRSA infection may both be assigned.

GUIDELINES

2. Chapter 2: Neoplasms (C00-D49)

<u>General guidelines</u>

Chapter 2 of the ICD-10-CM contains the codes for most benign and all malignant neoplasms. Certain benign neoplasms, such as prostatic adenomas, may be found in the specific body system chapters. To properly code a neoplasm it is necessary to determine from the record if the neoplasm is benign, in-situ, malignant, or of uncertain histologic behavior. If malignant, any secondary (metastatic) sites should also be determined.

Primary malignant neoplasms overlapping site boundaries

A primary malignant neoplasm that overlaps two or more contiguous (next to each other) sites should be classified to the subcategory/code .8 ('overlapping lesion'), unless the combination is specifically indexed elsewhere. For multiple neoplasms of the same site that are not contiguous such as tumors in different quadrants of the same breast, codes for each site should be assigned.

Malignant neoplasm of ectopic tissue

Malignant neoplasms of ectopic tissue are to be coded to the site of origin mentioned, e.g., ectopic pancreatic malignant neoplasms involving the stomach are coded to pancreas, unspecified (C25.9).

The neoplasm table in the Alphabetic Index should be referenced first. However, if the histological term is documented, that term should be referenced first, rather than going immediately to the Neoplasm Table, in order to determine which column in the Neoplasm Table is appropriate. For example, if the documentation indicates "adenoma," refer to the term in the Alphabetic Index to review the entries under this term and the instructional note to "see also neoplasm, by site, benign." The table provides the proper code based on the type of neoplasm and the site. It is important to select the proper column in the table that corresponds to the type of neoplasm. The Tabular List should then be referenced to verify that the correct code has been selected from the table and that a more specific site code does not exist.

See Section I.C.21. Factors influencing health status and contact with health services, Status, for information regarding Z15.0, codes for genetic susceptibility to cancer.

a. Treatment directed at the malignancy
If the treatment is directed at the malignancy, designate the malignancy as the principal diagnosis.

The only exception to this guideline is if a patient admission/encounter is solely for the administration of chemotherapy, immunotherapy or radiation therapy, assign the appropriate Z51.– code as the first-listed or principal diagnosis, and the diagnosis or problem for which the service is being performed as a secondary diagnosis.

b. Treatment of secondary site
When a patient is admitted because of a primary neoplasm with metastasis and treatment is directed toward the secondary site only, the secondary neoplasm is designated as the principal diagnosis even though the primary malignancy is still present.

c. Coding and sequencing of complications
Coding and sequencing of complications associated with the malignancies or with the therapy thereof are subject to the following guidelines:

1) Anemia associated with malignancy
When admission/encounter is for management of an anemia associated with the malignancy, and the treatment is only for anemia, the appropriate code for the malignancy is sequenced as the principal or first-listed diagnosis followed by the appropriate code for the anemia (such as code D63.0, Anemia in neoplastic disease).

2) Anemia associated with chemotherapy, immunotherapy and radiation therapy
When the admission/encounter is for management of an anemia associated with an adverse effect of the administration of chemotherapy or immunotherapy and the only treatment is for the anemia, the anemia code is sequenced first followed by the appropriate codes for the neoplasm and the adverse effect (T45.1X5, Adverse effect of antineoplastic and immunosuppressive drugs).

When the admission/encounter is for management of an anemia associated with an adverse effect of radiotherapy, the anemia code should be sequenced first, followed by the appropriate neoplasm code and code Y84.2, Radiological procedure and radiotherapy as the cause of abnormal reaction of the patient, or of later complication, without mention of misadventure at the time of the procedure.

3) Management of dehydration due to the malignancy
When the admission/encounter is for management of dehydration due to the malignancy and only the dehydration is being treated (intravenous rehydration), the dehydration is sequenced first, followed by the code(s) for the malignancy.

4) Treatment of a complication resulting from a surgical procedure
When the admission/encounter is for treatment of a complication resulting from a surgical procedure, designate the complication as the principal or first-listed diagnosis if treatment is directed at resolving the complication.

d. Primary malignancy previously excised
When a primary malignancy has been previously excised or eradicated from its site and there is no further treatment directed to that site and there is no evidence of any existing primary malignancy, a code from category Z85, Personal history of malignant neoplasm, should be used to indicate the former site of the malignancy. Any mention of extension, invasion, or metastasis to another site is coded as a secondary malignant neoplasm to that site. The secondary site may be the principal or irst-listed with the Z85 code used as a secondary code.

e. Admissions/Encounters involving chemotherapy, immunotherapy and radiation therapy

1) Episode of care involves surgical removal of neoplasm
When an episode of care involves the surgical removal of a neoplasm, primary or secondary site, followed by adjunct chemotherapy or radiation treatment during the same episode of care, the code for the neoplasm should be assigned as principal or first-listed diagnosis.

2) Patient admission/encounter solely for administration of chemotherapy, immunotherapy and radiation therapy
If a patient admission/encounter is solely for the administration of chemotherapy, immunotherapy or radiation therapy assign code Z51.0, Encounter for antineoplastic radiation therapy, or Z51.11, Encounter for antineoplastic chemotherapy, or Z51.12, Encounter for antineoplastic immunotherapy as the first-listed or principal diagnosis. If a patient receives more than one of these therapies during the same admission more than one of these codes may be assigned, in any sequence.

The malignancy for which the therapy is being administered should be assigned as a secondary diagnosis.

3) Patient admitted for radiation therapy, chemotherapy or immunotherapy and develops complications
When a patient is admitted for the purpose of radiotherapy, immunotherapy or chemotherapy and develops complications such as uncontrolled nausea and vomiting or dehydration, the principal or first-listed diagnosis is Z51.0, Encounter for antineoplastic radiation therapy, or Z51.11, Encounter for antineoplastic chemotherapy, or Z51.12, Encounter for antineoplastic immunotherapy followed by any codes for the complications.

f. **Admission/encounter to determine extent of malignancy**
When the reason for admission/encounter is to determine the extent of the malignancy, or for a procedure such as paracentesis or thoracentesis, the primary malignancy or appropriate metastatic site is designated as the principal or first-listed diagnosis, even though chemotherapy or radiotherapy is administered.

g. **Symptoms, signs, and abnormal findings listed in Chapter 18 associated with neoplasms**
Symptoms, signs, and ill-defined conditions listed in Chapter 18 characteristic of, or associated with, an existing primary or secondary site malignancy cannot be used to replace the malignancy as principal or first-listed diagnosis, regardless of the number of admissions or encounters for treatment and care of the neoplasm.

See section I.C.21. Factors influencing health status and contact with health services, Encounter for prophylactic organ removal.

h. **Admission/encounter for pain control/management**
See Section I.C.6. for information on coding admission/encounter for pain control/management.

i. **Malignancy in two or more noncontiguous sites**
A patient may have more than one malignant tumor in the same organ. These tumors may represent different primaries or metastatic disease, depending on the site. Should the documentation be unclear, the provider should be queried as to the status of each tumor so that the correct codes can be assigned.

j. **Disseminated malignant neoplasm, unspecified**
Code C80.0, Disseminated malignant neoplasm, unspecified, is for use only in those cases where the patient has advanced metastatic disease and no known primary or secondary sites are specified. It should not be used in place of assigning codes for the primary site and all known secondary sites.

k. **Malignant neoplasm without specification of site**
Code C80.1, Malignant (primary) neoplasm, unspecified, equates to Cancer, unspecified. This code should only be used when no determination can be made as to the primary site of a malignancy. This code should rarely be used in the inpatient setting.

l. **Sequencing of neoplasm codes**

   1) **Encounter for treatment of primary malignancy**
   If the reason for the encounter is for treatment of a primary malignancy, assign the malignancy as the principal/first-listed diagnosis. The primary site is to be sequenced first, followed by any metastatic sites.

   2) **Encounter for treatment of secondary malignancy**
   When an encounter is for a primary malignancy with metastasis and treatment is directed toward the metastatic (secondary) site(s) only, the metastatic site(s) is designated as the principal/first-listed diagnosis. The primary malignancy is coded as an additional code.

   3) **Malignant neoplasm in a pregnant patient**
   When a pregnant woman has a malignant neoplasm, a code from subcategory O9A.1-, Malignant neoplasm complicating pregnancy, childbirth, and the puerperium, should be sequenced first, followed by the appropriate code from Chapter 2 to indicate the type of neoplasm.

   4) **Encounter for complication associated with a neoplasm**
   When an encounter is for management of a complication associated with a neoplasm, such as dehydration, and the treatment is only for the complication, the complication is coded first, followed by the appropriate code(s) for the neoplasm.

   The exception to this guideline is anemia. When the admission/encounter is for management of an anemia associated with the

malignancy, and the treatment is only for anemia, the appropriate code for the malignancy is sequenced as the principal or first-listed diagnosis followed by code D63.0, Anemia in neoplastic disease.

   5) **Complication from surgical procedure for treatment of a neoplasm**
   When an encounter is for treatment of a complication resulting from a surgical procedure performed for the treatment of the neoplasm, designate the complication as the principal/first-listed diagnosis. See guideline regarding the coding of a current malignancy versus personal history to determine if the code for the neoplasm should also be assigned.

   6) **Pathologic fracture due to a neoplasm**
   When an encounter is for a pathological fracture due to a neoplasm, and the focus of treatment is the fracture, a code from subcategory M84.5, Pathological fracture in neoplastic disease, should be sequenced first, followed by the code for the neoplasm.

   If the focus of treatment is the neoplasm with an associated pathological fracture, the neoplasm code should be sequenced first, followed by a code from M84.5 for the pathological fracture.

m. **Current malignancy versus personal history of malignancy**
When a primary malignancy has been excised but further treatment, such as an additional surgery for the malignancy, radiation therapy or chemotherapy is directed to that site, the primary malignancy code should be used until treatment is completed.

When a primary malignancy has been previously excised or eradicated from its site, there is no further treatment (of the malignancy) directed to that site, and there is no evidence of any existing primary malignancy, a code from category Z85, Personal history of malignant neoplasm, should be used to indicate the former site of the malignancy.

See Section I.C.21. Factors influencing health status and contact with health services, History (of)

n. **Leukemia, Multiple Myeloma, and Malignant Plasma Cell Neoplasms in remission versus personal history**
The categories for leukemia, and category C90, Multiple myeloma and malignant plasma cell neoplasms, have codes indicating whether or not the leukemia has achieved remission. There are also codes Z85.6, Personal history of leukemia, and Z85.79, Personal history of other malignant neoplasms of lymphoid, hematopoietic and related tissues. If the documentation is unclear, as to whether the leukemia has achieved remission, the provider should be queried.

See Section I.C.21. Factors influencing health status and contact with health services, History (of)

o. **Aftercare following surgery for neoplasm**
See Section I.C.21. Factors influencing health status and contact with health services, Aftercare

p. **Follow-up care for completed treatment of a malignancy**
See Section I.C.21. Factors influencing health status and contact with health services, Follow-up

q. **Prophylactic organ removal for prevention of malignancy**
See Section I.C.21. Factors influencing health status and contact with health services, Prophylactic organ removal

r. **Malignant neoplasm associated with transplanted organ**
A malignant neoplasm of a transplanted organ should be coded as a transplant complication. Assign first the appropriate code from category T86.-, Complications of transplanted organs and tissue, followed by code C80.2, Malignant neoplasm associated with transplanted organ. Use an additional code for the specific malignancy.

CHAPTER 3 – BLOOD & IMMUNE DISORDERS
Section I. C. 3.

3. **Chapter 3: Disease of the blood and blood-forming organs and certain disorders involving the immune mechanism (D50-D89)**
    Reserved for future guideline expansion

CHAPTER 4 – ENDOCRINE & METABOLIC
Section I. C. 4.

4. **Chapter 4: Endocrine, Nutritional, and Metabolic Diseases (E00-E89)**

    a. **Diabetes mellitus**
        The diabetes mellitus codes are combination codes that include the type of diabetes mellitus, the body system affected, and the complications affecting that body system. As many codes within a particular category as are necessary to describe all of the complications of the disease may be used. They should be sequenced based on the reason for a particular encounter. Assign as many codes from categories E08 – E13 as needed to identify all of the associated conditions that the patient has.

    1) **Type of diabetes**
        The age of a patient is not the sole determining factor, though most type 1 diabetics develop the condition before reaching puberty. For this reason type 1 diabetes mellitus is also referred to as juvenile diabetes.

    2) **Type of diabetes mellitus not documented**
        If the type of diabetes mellitus is not documented in the medical record the default is E11.-, Type 2 diabetes mellitus.

    3) **Diabetes mellitus and the use of insulin**
        If the documentation in a medical record does not indicate the type of diabetes but does indicate that the patient uses insulin, code E11, Type 2 diabetes mellitus, should be assigned. Code Z79.4, Long-term (current) use of insulin, should also be assigned to indicate that the patient uses insulin. Code Z79.4 should not be assigned if insulin is given temporarily to bring a type 2 patient's blood sugar under control during an encounter.

    4) **Diabetes mellitus in pregnancy and gestational diabetes**
        See Section I.C.15. Diabetes mellitus in pregnancy.
        See Section I.C.15. Gestational (pregnancy induced) diabetes

    5) **Complications due to insulin pump malfunction**

        (a) **Underdose of insulin due to insulin pump failure**
             An underdose of insulin due to an insulin pump failure should be assigned to a code from subcategory T85.6, Mechanical complication of other specified internal and external prosthetic devices, implants and grafts, that specifies the type of pump malfunction, as the principal or first-listed code, followed by code T38.3x6-, Underdosing of insulin and oral hypoglycemic [antidiabetic] drugs. Additional codes for the type of diabetes mellitus and any associated complications due to the underdosing should also be assigned.

        (b) **Overdose of insulin due to insulin pump failure**
             The principal or first-listed code for an encounter due to an insulin pump malfunction resulting in an overdose of insulin, should also be T85.6-, Mechanical complication of other specified internal and external prosthetic devices, implants and grafts, followed by code T38.3x1-, Poisoning by insulin and oral hypoglycemic [antidiabetic] drugs, accidental (unintentional).

CHAPTER 4 – ENDOCRINE & METABOLIC
Section I. C. 4. a. 6)

6) **Secondary diabetes mellitus**

Codes under categories E08, Diabetes mellitus due to underlying condition, and E09, Drug or chemical induced diabetes mellitus, and E13, Other specified diabetes mellitus, identify complications/manifestations associated with secondary diabetes mellitus. Secondary diabetes is always caused by another condition or event (e.g., cystic fibrosis, malignant neoplasm of pancreas, pancreatectomy, adverse effect of drug, or poisoning).

(a) **Secondary diabetes mellitus and the use of insulin**

For patients who routinely use insulin, code Z79.4, Long-term (current) use of insulin, should also be assigned. Code Z79.4 should not be assigned if insulin is given temporarily to bring a patient's blood sugar under control during an encounter.

(b) **Assigning and sequencing secondary diabetes codes and its causes**

The sequencing of the secondary diabetes codes in relationship to codes for the cause of the diabetes is based on the Tabular List instructions for categories E08, E09 and E13.

(i) **Secondary diabetes mellitus due to pancreatectomy**

For postpancreatectomy diabetes mellitus (lack of insulin due to the surgical removal of all or part of the pancreas), assign code E89.1, Postprocedural hypoinsulinemia. Assign a code from category E13 and a code from subcategory Z90.41-, Acquired absence of pancreas, as additional codes.

(ii) **Secondary diabetes due to drugs**

Secondary diabetes may be caused by an adverse effect of correctly administered medications, poisoning or sequela of poisoning.

See section I.C.19.e for coding of adverse effects and poisoning, and section I.C.20 for external cause code reporting.

CHAPTER 5 – MENTAL & BEHAVIORAL
Section I. C. 5.

5. **Chapter 5: Mental and behavioral disorders (F01 – F99)**

a. **Pain disorders related to psychological factors**

Assign code F45.41, for pain that is exclusively related to psychological disorders. As indicated by the Excludes1 note under category G89, a code from category G89 should not be assigned with code F45.41.

Code F45.42, Pain disorders with related psychological factors, should be used should be used with a code from category G89, Pain, not elsewhere classified, if there is documentation of a psychological component for a patient with acute or chronic pain.

See Section I.C.6. Pain

b. **Mental and behavioral disorders due to psychoactive substance use**

1) **In Remission**

Selection of codes for "in remission" for categories F10-F19, Mental and behavioral disorders due to psychoactive substance use (categories F10-F19 with -.21) requires the provider's clinical judgment. The appropriate codes for "in remission" are assigned only on the basis of provider documentation (as defined in the Official Guidelines for Coding and Reporting).

2) **Psychoactive Substance Use, Abuse And Dependence**

When the provider documentation refers to use, abuse and dependence of the same substance (e.g. alcohol, opioid, cannabis, etc.), only one code should be assigned to identify the pattern of use based on the following hierarchy:
- If both use and abuse are documented, assign only the code for abuse
- If both abuse and dependence are documented, assign only the code for dependence
- If use, abuse and dependence are all documented, assign only the code for dependence
- If both use and dependence are documented, assign only the code for dependence

3) **Psychoactive Substance Use**

As with all other diagnoses, the codes for psychoactive substance use (F10.9-, F11.9-, F12.9-, F13.9-, F14.9-, F15.9-, F16.9-) should only be assigned based on provider documentation and when they meet the definition of a reportable diagnosis (see Section III, Reporting Additional Diagnoses). The codes are to be used only when the psychoactive substance use is associated with a mental or behavioral disorder, and such a relationship is documented by the provider.

CHAPTER 6 – NERVOUS SYSTEM
Section I. C. 6.

6. Chapter 6: Diseases of Nervous System and Sense Organs (G00-G99)

a. Dominant/nondominant side

Codes from category G81, Hemiplegia and hemiparesis, and subcategories, G83.1, Monoplegia of lower limb, G83.2, Monoplegia of upper limb, and G83.3, Monoplegia, unspecified, identify whether the dominant or nondominant side is affected. Should the affected side be documented, but not specified as dominant or nondominant, and the classification system does not indicate a default, code selection is as follows:

- For ambidextrous patients, the default should be dominant.
- If the left side is affected, the default is non-dominant.
- If the right side is affected, the default is dominant.

b. Pain - Category G89

1) General coding information

Codes in category G89, Pain, not elsewhere classified, may be used in conjunction with codes from other categories and chapters to provide more detail about acute or chronic pain and neoplasm-related pain, unless otherwise indicated below.

If the pain is not specified as acute or chronic, post-thoracotomy, postprocedural, or neoplasm-related, do not assign codes from category G89.

A code from category G89 should not be assigned if the underlying (definitive) diagnosis is known, unless the reason for the encounter is pain control/management and not management of the underlying condition.

When an admission or encounter is for a procedure aimed at treating the underlying condition (e.g., spinal fusion, kyphoplasty), a code for the underlying condition (e.g., vertebral fracture, spinal stenosis) should be assigned as the principal diagnosis. No code from category G89 should be assigned.

(a) Category G89 Codes as Principal or First-Listed Diagnosis

Category G89 codes are acceptable as principal diagnosis or the first-listed code:

- When pain control or pain management is the reason for the admission/encounter (e.g., a patient with displaced intervertebral disc, nerve impingement and severe back pain presents for injection of steroid into the spinal canal). The underlying cause of the pain should be reported as an additional diagnosis, if known.

- When a patient is admitted for the insertion of a neurostimulator for pain control, assign the appropriate pain code as the principal or first-listed diagnosis. When an admission or encounter is for a procedure aimed at treating the underlying condition and a neurostimulator is inserted for pain control during the same admission/encounter, a code for the underlying condition should be assigned as the principal diagnosis and the appropriate pain code should be assigned as a secondary diagnosis.

CHAPTER 6 – NERVOUS SYSTEM
Section I. C. 6. b. 1) (b)

(b) Use of Category G89 Codes in Conjunction with Site Specific Pain Codes

(i) Assigning Category G89 and Site-Specific Pain Codes

Codes from category G89 may be used in conjunction with codes that identify the site of pain (including codes from chapter 18) if the category G89 code provides additional information. For example, if the code describes the site of the pain, but does not fully describe whether the pain is acute or chronic, then both codes should be assigned.

(ii) Sequencing of Category G89 Codes with Site-Specific Pain Codes

The sequencing of category G89 codes with site-specific pain codes (including chapter 18 codes), is dependent on the circumstances of the encounter/admission as follows:

- If the encounter is for pain control or pain management, assign the code from category G89 followed by the code identifying the specific site of pain (e.g., encounter for pain management for acute neck pain from trauma is assigned code G89.11, Acute pain due to trauma, followed by code M54.2, Cervicalgia, to identify the site of pain).

- If the encounter is for any other reason except pain control or pain management, and a related definitive diagnosis has not been established (confirmed) by the provider, assign the code for the specific site of pain first, followed by the appropriate code from category G89.

2) Pain due to devices, implants and grafts

See Section I.C.19. Pain due to medical devices

3) Postoperative Pain

The provider's documentation should be used to guide the coding of postoperative pain, as well as *Section III. Reporting Additional Diagnoses and Section IV. Diagnostic Coding and Reporting in the Outpatient Setting.*

The default for post-thoracotomy and other postoperative pain not specified as acute or chronic is the code for the acute form.

Routine or expected postoperative pain immediately after surgery should not be coded.

(a) Postoperative pain not associated with specific postoperative complication

Postoperative pain not associated with a specific postoperative complication is assigned to the appropriate postoperative pain code in category G89.

(b) Postoperative pain associated with specific postoperative complication

Postoperative pain associated with a specific postoperative complication (such as painful wire sutures) is assigned to the appropriate code(s) found in Chapter 19, Injury, poisoning, and certain other consequences of external causes. If appropriate, use additional code(s) from category G89 to identify acute or chronic pain (G89.18 or G89.28).

4) Chronic pain

Chronic pain is classified to subcategory G89.2. There is no time frame defining when pain becomes chronic pain. The provider's documentation should be used to guide use of these codes.

5) Neoplasm Related Pain

Code G89.3 is assigned to pain documented as being related, associated or due to cancer, primary or secondary malignancy, or tumor. This code is assigned regardless of whether the pain is acute or chronic.

This code may be assigned as the principal or first-listed code when the stated reason for the admission/encounter is documented as pain control/pain management. The underlying neoplasm should be reported as an additional diagnosis.

When the reason for the admission/encounter is management of the neoplasm and the pain associated with the neoplasm is also documented, code G89.3 may be assigned as an additional diagnosis. It is not necessary to assign an additional code for the site of the pain.

See Section I.C.2 for instructions on the sequencing of neoplasms for all other stated reasons for the admission/encounter (except for pain control/pain management).

6) Chronic pain syndrome

Central pain syndrome (G89.0) and chronic pain syndrome (G89.4) are different than the term "chronic pain," and therefore codes should only be used when the provider has specifically documented this condition.

See Section I.C.5. Pain disorders related to psychological factors

7. Chapter 7: Diseases of Eye and Adnexa (H00-H59)

a. Glaucoma

1) Assigning Glaucoma Codes

Assign as many codes from category H40, Glaucoma, as needed to identify the type of glaucoma, the affected eye, and the glaucoma stage.

2) Bilateral glaucoma with same type and stage

When a patient has bilateral glaucoma and both eyes are documented as being the same type and stage, and there is a code for bilateral glaucoma, report only the code for the type of glaucoma, bilateral, with the seventh character for the stage.

When a patient has bilateral glaucoma and both eyes are documented as being the same type and stage, and the classification does not provide a code for bilateral glaucoma (i.e. subcategories H40.10, H40.11 and H40.20) report only one code for the type of glaucoma with the appropriate seventh character for the stage.

3) Bilateral glaucoma stage with different types or stages

When a patient has bilateral glaucoma and each eye is documented as having a different type or stage, and the classification distinguishes laterality, assign the appropriate code for each eye rather than the code for bilateral glaucoma.

When a patient has bilateral glaucoma and each eye is documented as having a different type, and the classification does not distinguish laterality (i.e. subcategories H40.10, H40.11 and H40.20), assign one code for each type of glaucoma with the appropriate seventh character for the stage.

When a patient has bilateral glaucoma and each eye is documented as having the same type, but different stage, and the classification does not distinguish laterality (i.e. subcategories H40.10, H40.11 and H40.20), assign a code for the type of glaucoma for each eye with the seventh character for the specific glaucoma stage documented for each eye.

4) Patient admitted with glaucoma and stage evolves during the admission

If a patient is admitted with glaucoma and the stage progresses during the admission, assign the code for highest stage documented.

5) Indeterminate stage glaucoma

Assignment of the seventh character "4" for "indeterminate stage" should be based on the clinical documentation. The seventh character "4" is used for glaucomas whose stage cannot be clinically determined. This seventh character should not be confused with the seventh character "0", unspecified, which should be assigned when there is no documentation regarding the stage of the glaucoma.

GUIDELINES

CHAPTER 8 – EAR AND MASTIOD PROCESS
Section I. C. 8.

8. **Chapter 8: Diseases of Ear and Mastoid Process (H60-H95)**
   Reserved for future guideline expansion

CHAPTER 9 – CIRCULATORY SYSTEM
Section I. C. 9.

9. **Chapter 9: Diseases of Circulatory System (I00-I99)**

   a. **Hypertension**

   1) **Hypertension with Heart Disease**
      Heart conditions classified to I50.- or I51.4-I51.9, are assigned to, a code from category I11, Hypertensive heart disease, when a causal relationship is stated (due to hypertension) or implied (hypertensive). Use an additional code from category I50, Heart failure, to identify the type of heart failure in those patients with heart failure.

      The same heart conditions (I50.-, I51.4-I51.9) with hypertension, but without a stated causal relationship, are coded separately. Sequence according to the circumstances of the admission/encounter.

   2) **Hypertensive Chronic Kidney Disease**
      Assign codes from category I12, Hypertensive chronic kidney disease, when both hypertension and a condition classifiable to category N18, Chronic kidney disease (CKD), are present. Unlike hypertension with heart disease, ICD-10-CM presumes a cause-and-effect relationship and classifies chronic kidney disease with hypertension as hypertensive chronic kidney disease.

      The appropriate code from category N18 should be used as a secondary code with a code from category I12 to identify the stage of chronic kidney disease.

      See Section I.C.14. Chronic kidney disease.

      If a patient has hypertensive chronic kidney disease and acute renal failure, an additional code for the acute renal failure is required.

   3) **Hypertensive Heart and Chronic Kidney Disease**
      Assign codes from combination category I13, Hypertensive heart and chronic kidney disease, when both hypertensive kidney disease and hypertensive heart disease are stated in the diagnosis. Assume a relationship between the hypertension and the chronic kidney disease, whether or not the condition is so designated. If heart failure is present, assign an additional code from category I50 to identify the type of heart failure.

      The appropriate code from category N18, Chronic kidney disease, should be used as a secondary code with a code from category I13 to identify the stage of chronic kidney disease.

      See Section I.C.14. Chronic kidney disease.

      The codes in category I13, Hypertensive heart and chronic kidney disease, are combination codes that include hypertension, heart disease and chronic kidney disease. The Includes note at I13 specifies that the conditions included at I11 and I12 are included together in I13. If a patient has hypertension, heart disease and chronic kidney disease then a code from I13 should be used, not individual codes for hypertension, heart disease and chronic kidney disease, or codes from I11 or I12.

      For patients with both acute renal failure and chronic kidney disease an additional code for acute renal failure is required.

   4) **Hypertensive Cerebrovascular Disease**
      For hypertensive cerebrovascular disease, first assign the appropriate code from categories I60-I69, followed by the appropriate hypertension code.

   5) **Hypertensive Retinopathy**
      Subcategory H35.0, Background retinopathy and retinal vascular changes, should be used with a code from category I10-I15, Hypertensive disease to include the systemic hypertension. The sequencing is based on the reason for the encounter.

6) Hypertension, Secondary

Secondary hypertension is due to an underlying condition. Two codes are required: one to identify the underlying etiology and one from category I15 to identify the hypertension. Sequencing of codes is determined by the reason for admission/encounter.

7) Hypertension, Transient

Assign code R03.0, Elevated blood pressure reading without diagnosis of hypertension, unless patient has an established diagnosis of hypertension. Assign code O13.-, Gestational [pregnancy-induced] hypertension without significant proteinuria, or O14.-, Pre-eclampsia, for transient hypertension of pregnancy.

8) Hypertension, Controlled

This diagnostic statement usually refers to an existing state of hypertension under control by therapy. Assign the appropriate code from categories I10-I15, Hypertensive diseases.

9) Hypertension, Uncontrolled

Uncontrolled hypertension may refer to untreated hypertension or hypertension not responding to current therapeutic regimen. In either case, assign the appropriate code from categories I10-I15, Hypertensive diseases.

b. Atherosclerotic Coronary Artery Disease and Angina

ICD-10-CM has combination codes for atherosclerotic heart disease with angina pectoris. The subcategories for these codes are I25.11, Atherosclerotic heart disease of native coronary artery with angina pectoris and I25.7, Atherosclerosis of coronary artery bypass graft(s) and coronary artery of transplanted heart with angina pectoris.

When using one of these combination codes it is not necessary to use an additional code for angina pectoris. A causal relationship can be assumed in a patient with both atherosclerosis and angina pectoris, unless the documentation indicates the angina is due to something other than the atherosclerosis.

If a patient with coronary artery disease is admitted due to an acute myocardial infarction (AMI), the AMI should be sequenced before the coronary artery disease.

See Section I.C.9. Acute myocardial infarction (AMI)

c. Intraoperative and Postprocedural Cerebrovascular Accident

Medical record documentation should clearly specify the cause-and-effect relationship between the medical intervention and the cerebrovascular accident in order to assign a code for intraoperative or postprocedural cerebrovascular accident.

Proper code assignment depends on whether it was an infarction or hemorrhage and whether it occurred intraoperatively or postoperatively. If it was a cerebral hemorrhage, code assignment depends on the type of procedure performed.

d. Sequelae of Cerebrovascular Disease

1) Category I69, Sequelae of Cerebrovascular disease

Category I69 is used to indicate conditions classifiable to categories I60-I67 as the causes of sequela (neurologic deficits), themselves classified elsewhere. These "late effects" include neurologic deficits that persist after initial onset of conditions classifiable to categories I60-I67. The neurologic deficits caused by cerebrovascular disease may be present from the onset or may arise at any time after the onset of the condition classifiable to categories I60-I67.

Codes from category I69, Sequelae of cerebrovascular disease, that specify hemiplegia, hemiparesis and monoplegia identify whether the dominant or nondominant side is affected. Should the affected side be documented, but not specified as dominant or nondominant, and the classification system does not indicate a default, code selection is as follows:

- For ambidextrous patients, the default should be dominant.
- If the left side is affected, the default is nondominant.
- If the right side is affected, the default is dominant.

2) Codes from category I69 with codes from I60-I67

Codes from category I69 may be assigned on a health care record with codes from I60-I67, if the patient has a current cerebrovascular disease and deficits from an old cerebrovascular disease.

3) Codes from category I69 and Personal history of transient ischemic attack (TIA) and cerebral infarction (Z86.73)

Codes from category I69 should not be assigned if the patient does not have neurologic deficits.

See Section I.C.21.c.4. History (of) for use of personal history codes

e. Acute myocardial infarction (AMI)

1) ST elevation myocardial infarction (STEMI) and non ST elevation myocardial infarction (NSTEMI)

The ICD-10-CM codes for acute myocardial infarction (AMI) identify the site, such as anterolateral wall or true posterior wall. Subcategories I21.0-I21.2 and code I21.3 are used for ST elevation myocardial infarction (STEMI). Code I21.4, Non-ST elevation (NSTEMI) myocardial infarction, is used for non ST elevation myocardial infarction (NSTEMI) and nontransmural MIs.

If NSTEMI evolves to STEMI, assign the STEMI code. If STEMI converts to NSTEMI due to thrombolytic therapy, it is still coded as STEMI.

For encounters occurring while the myocardial infarction is equal to, or less than, four weeks old, including transfers to another acute setting or a postacute setting, and the patient requires continued care for the myocardial infarction, codes from category I21 may continue to be reported. For encounters after the 4 week time frame and the patient is still receiving care related to the myocardial infarction, the appropriate aftercare code should be assigned, rather than a code from category I21. For old or healed myocardial infarctions not requiring further care, code I25.2, Old myocardial infarction, may be assigned.

2) Acute myocardial infarction, unspecified

Code I21.3, ST elevation (STEMI) myocardial infarction of unspecified site, is the default for the unspecified acute myocardial infarction. If only STEMI or transmural MI without the site is documented, assign code I21.3.

3) AMI documented as nontransmural or subendocardial but site provided

If an AMI is documented as nontransmural or subendocardial, but the site is provided, it is still coded as a subendocardial AMI.

See Section I.C.21.3 for information on coding status post administration of tPA in a different facility within the last 24 hours.

4) Subsequent acute myocardial infarction

A code from category I22, Subsequent ST elevation (STEMI) and non ST elevation (NSTEMI) myocardial infarction, is to be used when a patient who has suffered an AMI has a new AMI within the 4 week time frame of the initial AMI. A code from category I22 must be used in conjunction with a code from category I21. The sequencing of the I22 and I21 codes depends on the circumstances of the encounter.

OFFICIAL CODING GUIDELINES – 2014 ICD-10-CM   [2014.CM-1.V1

CHAPTER 10 – RESPIRATORY SYSTEM
Section I. C. 10.

CHAPTER 10 – RESPIRATORY SYSTEM
Section I. C. 10. d.

GUIDELINES

10. Chapter 10: Diseases of the Respiratory System (J00-J99)

a. **Chronic Obstructive Pulmonary Disease [COPD] and Asthma**

1) **Acute exacerbation of chronic obstructive bronchitis and asthma**
The codes in categories J44 and J45 distinguish between uncomplicated cases and those in acute exacerbation. An acute exacerbation is a worsening or a decompensation of a chronic condition. An acute exacerbation is not equivalent to an infection superimposed on a chronic condition, though an exacerbation may be triggered by an infection.

b. **Acute Respiratory Failure**

1) **Acute respiratory failure as principal diagnosis**
A code from subcategory J96.0, Acute respiratory failure, or subcategory J96.2, Acute and chronic respiratory failure, may be assigned as a principal diagnosis when it is the condition established after study to be chiefly responsible for occasioning the admission to the hospital, and the selection is supported by the Alphabetic Index and Tabular List. However, chapter-specific coding guidelines (such as obstetrics, poisoning, HIV, newborn) that provide sequencing direction take precedence.

2) **Acute respiratory failure as secondary diagnosis**
Respiratory failure may be listed as a secondary diagnosis if it occurs after admission, or if it is present on admission, but does not meet the definition of principal diagnosis.

3) **Sequencing of acute respiratory failure and another acute condition**
When a patient is admitted with respiratory failure and another acute condition, (e.g., myocardial infarction, cerebrovascular accident, aspiration pneumonia), the principal diagnosis will not be the same in every situation. This applies whether the other acute condition is a respiratory or nonrespiratory condition. Selection of the principal diagnosis will be dependent on the circumstances of admission. If both the respiratory failure and the other acute condition are equally responsible for occasioning the admission to the hospital, and there are no chapter-specific sequencing rules, the guideline regarding two or more diagnoses that equally meet the definition for principal diagnosis *(Section II, C.)* may be applied in these situations.

If the documentation is not clear as to whether acute respiratory failure and another condition are equally responsible for occasioning the admission, query the provider for clarification.

c. **Influenza due to certain identified influenza viruses**
Code only confirmed cases of influenza due to certain identified influenza viruses (category J09), and due to other identified influenza virus (category J10). This is an exception to the hospital inpatient guideline Section II, H. (Uncertain Diagnosis).

In this context, "confirmation" does not require documentation of positive laboratory testing specific for avian or other novel influenza A or other identified influenza virus. However, coding should be based on the provider's diagnostic statement that the patient has avian influenza, or other novel influenza A, for category J09, or has another particular identified strain of influenza, such as H1N1 or H3N2, but not identified as novel or variant, for category J10.

If the provider records "suspected" or "possible" or "probable" avian influenza, or novel influenza, or other identified influenza, then the appropriate influenza code from category J11, Influenza due to unidentified influenza virus, should be assigned. A code from category J09, Influenza due to certain identified influenza viruses, should not be assigned nor should a code from category J10, Influenza due to other identified influenza virus.

d. **Ventilator associated Pneumonia**

1) **Documentation of Ventilator associated Pneumonia**
As with all procedural or postprocedural complications, code assignment is based on the provider's documentation of the relationship between the condition and the procedure.

Code J95.851, Ventilator associated pneumonia, should be assigned only when the provider has documented ventilator associated pneumonia (VAP). An additional code to identify the organism (e.g., Pseudomonas aeruginosa, code B96.5) should also be assigned. Do not assign an additional code from categories J12-J18 to identify the type of pneumonia.

Code J95.851 should not be assigned for cases where the patient has pneumonia and is on a mechanical ventilator and the provider has not specifically stated that the pneumonia is ventilator-associated pneumonia. If the documentation is unclear as to whether the patient has a pneumonia that is a complication attributable to the mechanical ventilator, query the provider.

2) **Ventilator associated Pneumonia Develops after Admission**
A patient may be admitted with one type of pneumonia (e.g., code J13, Pneumonia due to Streptococcus pneumonia) and subsequently develop VAP. In this instance, the principal diagnosis would be the appropriate code from categories J12-J18 for the pneumonia diagnosed at the time of admission. Code J95.851, Ventilator associated pneumonia, would be assigned as an additional diagnosis when the provider has also documented the presence of ventilator associated pneumonia.

CHAPTER 11 – DIGESTIVE SYSTEM
Section I. C. 11.

11. **Chapter 11: Diseases of the Digestive System (K00-K94)**
    Reserved for future guideline expansion

CHAPTER 12 – SKIN & SUBCUTANEOUS TISSUE
Section I. C. 12.

12. **Chapter 12: Diseases of the Skin and Subcutaneous Tissue (L00-L99)**

   a. **Pressure ulcer stage codes**

      1) **Pressure ulcer stages**
         Codes from category L89, Pressure ulcer, are combination codes that
         identify the site of the pressure ulcer as well as the stage of the ulcer.

         The ICD-10-CM classifies pressure ulcer stages based on severity,
         which is designated by stages 1-4, unspecified stage and unstageable.

         Assign as many codes from category L89 as needed to identify all the
         pressure ulcers the patient has, if applicable.

      2) **Unstageable pressure ulcers**
         Assignment of the code for unstageable pressure ulcer (L89.--0)
         should be based on the clinical documentation. These codes are used
         for pressure ulcers whose stage cannot be clinically determined (e.g.,
         the ulcer is covered by eschar or has been treated with a skin or muscle
         graft) and pressure ulcers that are documented as deep tissue injury but
         not documented as due to trauma. This code should not be confused
         with the codes for unspecified stage (L89.--9). When there is no
         documentation regarding the stage of the pressure ulcer, assign the
         appropriate code for unspecified stage (L89.--9).

      3) **Documented pressure ulcer stage**
         Assignment of the pressure ulcer stage code should be guided by
         clinical documentation of the stage or documentation of the terms
         found in the Alphabetic Index. For clinical terms describing the
         stage that are not found in the Alphabetic Index, and there is no
         documentation of the stage, the provider should be queried.

      4) **Patients admitted with pressure ulcers documented as healed**
         No code is assigned if the documentation states that the pressure ulcer
         is completely healed.

      5) **Patients admitted with pressure ulcers documented as healing**
         Pressure ulcers described as healing should be assigned the appropriate
         pressure ulcer stage code based on the documentation in the medical
         record. If the documentation does not provide information about the
         stage of the healing pressure ulcer, assign the appropriate code for
         unspecified stage.

         If the documentation is unclear as to whether the patient has a current
         (new) pressure ulcer or if the patient is being treated for a healing
         pressure ulcer, query the provider.

      6) **Patient admitted with pressure ulcer evolving into another stage
         during the admission**
         If a patient is admitted with a pressure ulcer at one stage and it
         progresses to a higher stage, assign the code for the highest stage
         reported for that site.

CHAPTER 13 – MUSCULOSKELETAL SYSTEM
Section I. C. 13.

13. **Chapter 13: Diseases of the Musculoskeletal System and Connective Tissue (M00-M99)**

  a. **Site and laterality**

   Most of the codes within Chapter 13 have site and laterality designations. The site represents the bone, joint or the muscle involved. For some conditions where more than one bone, joint or muscle is usually involved, such as osteoarthritis, there is a "multiple sites" code available. For categories where no multiple site code is provided and more than one bone, joint or muscle is involved, multiple codes should be used to indicate the different sites involved.

   1) **Bone versus joint**

    For certain conditions, the bone may be affected at the upper or lower end, (c.g., avascular necrosis of bone, M87, Osteoporosis, M80, M81). Though the portion of the bone affected may be at the joint, the site designation will be the bone, not the joint.

  b. **Acute traumatic versus chronic or recurrent musculoskeletal conditions**

   Many musculoskeletal conditions are a result of previous injury or trauma to a site, or are recurrent conditions. Bone, joint or muscle conditions that are the result of a healed injury are usually found in chapter 13. Recurrent bone, joint or muscle conditions are also usually found in chapter 13. Any current, acute injury should be coded to the appropriate injury code from chapter 19. Chronic or recurrent conditions should generally be coded with a code from chapter 13. If it is difficult to determine from the documentation in the record which code is best to describe a condition, query the provider.

  c. **Coding of Pathologic Fractures**

   7th character A is for use as long as the patient is receiving active treatment for the fracture. Examples of active treatment are: surgical treatment, emergency department encounter, evaluation and treatment by a new physician. 7th character, D is to be used for encounters after the patient has completed active treatment. The other 7th characters, listed under each subcategory in the Tabular List, are to be used for subsequent encounters for treatment of problems associated with the healing, such as malunions, nonunions, and sequelae.

   Care for complications of surgical treatment for fracture repairs during the healing or recovery phase should be coded with the appropriate complication codes.

   See Section I.C.19. Coding of traumatic fractures.

  d. **Osteoporosis**

   Osteoporosis is a systemic condition, meaning that all bones of the musculoskeletal system are affected. Therefore, site is not a component of the codes under category M81, Osteoporosis without current pathological fracture. The site codes under category M80, Osteoporosis with current pathological fracture, identify the site of the fracture, not the osteoporosis.

   1) **Osteoporosis without pathological fracture**

    Category M81, Osteoporosis without current pathological fracture, is for use for patients with osteoporosis who do not currently have a pathologic fracture due to the osteoporosis, even if they have had a fracture in the past. For patients with a history of osteoporosis fractures, status code Z87.310, Personal history of (healed) osteoporosis fracture, should follow the code from M81.

   2) **Osteoporosis with current pathological fracture**

    Category M80, Osteoporosis with current pathological fracture, is for patients who have a current pathologic fracture at the time of an encounter. The codes under M80 identify the site of the fracture. A code from category M80, not a traumatic fracture code, should be used for any patient with known osteoporosis who suffers a fracture, even if the patient had a minor fall or trauma, if that fall or trauma would not usually break a normal, healthy bone.

CHAPTER 14 – GENITOURINARY SYSTEM
Section I. C. 14.

14. **Chapter 14: Diseases of Genitourinary System (N00-N99)**

  a. **Chronic kidney disease**

   1) **Stages of chronic kidney disease (CKD)**

    The ICD-10-CM classifies CKD based on severity. The severity of CKD is designated by stages 1-5. Stage 2, code N18.2, equates to mild CKD; stage 3, code N18.3, equates to moderate CKD; and stage 4, code N18.4, equates to severe CKD. Code N18.6, End stage renal disease (ESRD), is assigned when the provider has documented end-stage-renal disease (ESRD).

    If both a stage of CKD and ESRD are documented, assign code N18.6 only.

   2) **Chronic kidney disease and kidney transplant status**

    Patients who have undergone kidney transplant may still have some form of chronic kidney disease (CKD) because the kidney transplant may not fully restore kidney function. Therefore, the presence of CKD alone does not constitute a transplant complication. Assign the appropriate N18 code for the patient's stage of CKD and code Z94.0, Kidney transplant status. If a transplant complication such as failure or rejection or other transplant complication is documented, see section I.C.19.g for information on coding complications of a kidney transplant. If the documentation is unclear as to whether the patient has a complication of the transplant, query the provider.

   3) **Chronic kidney disease with other conditions**

    Patients with CKD may also suffer from other serious conditions, most commonly diabetes mellitus and hypertension. The sequencing of the CKD code in relationship to codes for other contributing conditions is based on the conventions in the Tabular List.

    See I.C.9. Hypertensive chronic kidney disease.
    See I.C.19. Chronic kidney disease and kidney transplant complications.

15. Chapter 15: Pregnancy, Childbirth, and the Puerperium (O00-O9A)

a. **General Rules for Obstetric Cases**

1) **Codes from chapter 15 and sequencing priority**
Obstetric cases require codes from chapter 15, codes in the range O00-O9A, Pregnancy, Childbirth, and the Puerperium. Chapter 15 codes have sequencing priority over codes from other chapters. Additional codes from other chapters may be used in conjunction with chapter 15 codes to further specify conditions. Should the provider document that the pregnancy is incidental to the encounter, then code Z33.1, Pregnant state, incidental, should be used in place of any chapter 15 codes. It is the provider's responsibility to state that the condition being treated is not affecting the pregnancy.

2) **Chapter 15 codes used only on the maternal record**
Chapter 15 codes are to be used only on the maternal record, never on the record of the newborn.

3) **Final character for trimester**
The majority of codes in Chapter 15 have a final character indicating the trimester of pregnancy. The timeframes for the trimesters are indicated at the beginning of the chapter. If trimester is not a component of a code it is because the condition always occurs in a specific trimester, or the concept of trimester of pregnancy is not applicable. Certain codes have characters for only certain trimesters because the condition does not occur in all trimesters, but it may occur in more than just one.

Assignment of the final character for trimester should be based on the provider's documentation of the trimester (or number of weeks) for the current admission/encounter. This applies to the assignment of trimester for pre-existing conditions as well as those that develop during or are due to the pregnancy. The provider's documentation of the number of weeks may be used to assign the appropriate code identifying the trimester.

Whenever delivery occurs during the current admission, and there is an "in childbirth" option for the obstetric complication being coded, the "in childbirth" code should be assigned.

4) **Selection of trimester for inpatient admissions that encompass more than one trimesters**
In instances when a patient is admitted to a hospital for complications of pregnancy during one trimester and remains in the hospital into a subsequent trimester, the trimester character for the antepartum complication code should be assigned on the basis of the trimester when the complication developed, not the trimester of the discharge. If the condition developed prior to the current admission/encounter or represents a pre-existing condition, the trimester character for the trimester at the time of the admission/encounter should be assigned.

5) **Unspecified trimester**
Each category that includes codes for trimester has a code for "unspecified trimester." The "unspecified trimester" code should rarely be used, such as when the documentation in the record is insufficient to determine the trimester and it is not possible to obtain clarification.

6) **7th character for Fetus Identification**
Where applicable, a 7th character is to be assigned for certain categories (O31, O32, O33.3 - O33.6, O35, O36, O40, O41, O60.1, O60.2, O64, and O69) to identify the fetus for which the complication code applies.

Assign 7th character "0":
• For single gestations
• When the documentation in the record is insufficient to determine the fetus affected and it is not possible to obtain clarification.
• When it is not possible to clinically determine which fetus is affected.

b. **Selection of OB Principal or First-listed Diagnosis**

1) **Routine outpatient prenatal visits**
For routine outpatient prenatal visits when no complications are present, a code from category Z34, Encounter for supervision of normal pregnancy, should be used as the first-listed diagnosis. These codes should not be used in conjunction with chapter 15 codes.

2) **Prenatal outpatient visits for high-risk patients**
For routine prenatal outpatient visits for patients with high-risk pregnancies, a code from category O09, Supervision of high-risk pregnancy, should be used as the first-listed diagnosis. Secondary chapter 15 codes may be used in conjunction with these codes if appropriate.

3) **Episodes when no delivery occurs**
In episodes when no delivery occurs, the principal diagnosis should correspond to the principal complication of the pregnancy which necessitated the encounter. Should more than one complication exist, all of which are treated or monitored, any of the complications codes may be sequenced first.

4) **When a delivery occurs**
When a delivery occurs, the principal diagnosis should correspond to the main circumstances or complication of the delivery. In cases of cesarean delivery, the selection of the principal diagnosis should be the condition established after study that was responsible for the patient's admission. If the patient was admitted with a condition that resulted in the performance of a cesarean procedure, that condition should be selected as the principal diagnosis. If the reason for the admission/encounter was unrelated to the condition resulting in the cesarean delivery, the condition related to the reason for the admission/encounter should be selected as the principal diagnosis.

5) **Outcome of delivery**
A code from category Z37, Outcome of delivery, should be included on every maternal record when a delivery has occurred. These codes are not to be used on subsequent records or on the newborn record.

c. **Pre-existing conditions versus conditions due to the pregnancy**
Certain categories in Chapter 15 distinguish between conditions of the mother that existed prior to pregnancy (pre-existing) and those that are a direct result of pregnancy. When assigning codes from Chapter 15, it is important to assess if a condition was pre-existing prior to pregnancy or developed during or due to the pregnancy in order to assign the correct code.

Categories that do not distinguish between pre-existing and pregnancy-related conditions may be used for either. It is acceptable to use codes specifically for the puerperium with codes complicating pregnancy and childbirth if a condition arises postpartum during the delivery encounter.

d. **Pre-existing hypertension in pregnancy**
Category O10, Pre-existing hypertension complicating pregnancy, childbirth and the puerperium, includes codes for hypertensive heart and hypertensive chronic kidney disease. When assigning one of the O10 codes that includes hypertensive heart disease or hypertensive chronic kidney disease, it is necessary to add a secondary code from the appropriate hypertension category to specify the type of heart failure or chronic kidney disease.

See Section I.C.9. Hypertension.

e. **Fetal Conditions Affecting the Management of the Mother**

1) **Codes from categories O35 and O36**
Codes from categories O35, Maternal care for known or suspected fetal abnormality and damage, and O36, Maternal care for other fetal problems, are assigned only when the fetal condition is actually responsible for modifying the management of the mother, i.e., by requiring diagnostic studies, additional observation, special care, or termination of pregnancy. The fact that the fetal condition exists does not justify assigning a code from this series to the mother's record.

2) **In utero surgery**
In cases when surgery is performed on the fetus, a diagnosis code from category O35, Maternal care for known or suspected fetal abnormality and damage, should be assigned identifying the fetal condition. Assign the appropriate procedure code for the procedure performed.

No code from Chapter 16, the perinatal codes, should be used on the mother's record to identify fetal conditions. Surgery performed in utero on a fetus is still to be coded as an obstetric encounter.

f. **HIV Infection in Pregnancy, Childbirth and the Puerperium**
During pregnancy, childbirth or the puerperium, a patient admitted because of an HIV-related illness should receive a principal diagnosis from subcategory O98.7-, Human immunodeficiency [HIV] disease complicating pregnancy, childbirth and the puerperium, followed by the code(s) for the HIV-related illness(es).

Patients with asymptomatic HIV infection status admitted during pregnancy, childbirth, or the puerperium should receive codes of O98.7- and Z21, Asymptomatic human immunodeficiency virus [HIV] infection status.

g. **Diabetes mellitus in pregnancy**
Diabetes mellitus is a significant complicating factor in pregnancy. Pregnant women who are diabetic should be assigned a code from category O24, Diabetes mellitus in pregnancy, childbirth, and the puerperium, first, followed by the appropriate diabetes code(s) (E08-E13) from Chapter 4.

h. **Long term use of insulin**
Code Z79.4, Long-term (current) use of insulin, should also be assigned if the diabetes mellitus is being treated with insulin.

i. **Gestational (pregnancy induced) diabetes**
Gestational (pregnancy induced) diabetes can occur during the second and third trimester of pregnancy in women who were not diabetic prior to pregnancy. Gestational diabetes can cause complications in the pregnancy similar to those of pre-existing diabetes mellitus. It also puts the woman at greater risk of developing diabetes after the pregnancy. Codes for gestational diabetes are in subcategory O24.4, Gestational diabetes mellitus. No other code from category O24, Diabetes mellitus in pregnancy, childbirth, and the puerperium, should be used with a code from O24.4.

The codes under subcategory O24.4 include diet controlled and insulin controlled. If a patient with gestational diabetes is treated with both diet and insulin, only the code for insulin-controlled is required. Code Z79.4, Long-term (current) use of insulin, should not be assigned with codes from subcategory O24.4.

An abnormal glucose tolerance in pregnancy is assigned a code from subcategory O99.81, Abnormal glucose complicating pregnancy, childbirth, and the puerperium.

j. **Sepsis and septic shock complicating abortion, pregnancy, childbirth and the puerperium**
When assigning a chapter 15 code for sepsis complicating abortion, pregnancy, childbirth, and the puerperium, a code for the specific type of infection should be assigned as an additional diagnosis. If severe sepsis is present, a code from subcategory R65.2, Severe sepsis, and code(s) for associated organ dysfunction(s) should also be assigned as additional diagnoses.

k. **Puerperal sepsis**
Code O85, Puerperal sepsis, should be assigned with a secondary code to identify the causal organism (e.g., for a bacterial infection, assign a code from category B95-B96, Bacterial infections in conditions classified elsewhere). A code from category A40, Streptococcal sepsis, or A41, Other sepsis, should not be used for puerperal sepsis. If applicable, use additional codes to identify severe sepsis (R65.2-) and any associated acute organ dysfunction.

l. **Alcohol and tobacco use during pregnancy, childbirth and the puerperium**

1) **Alcohol use during pregnancy, childbirth and the puerperium**
Codes under subcategory O99.31, Alcohol use complicating pregnancy, childbirth, and the puerperium, should be assigned for any pregnancy case when a mother uses alcohol during the pregnancy or postpartum. A secondary code from category F10, Alcohol related disorders, should also be assigned to identify manifestations of the alcohol use.

2) **Tobacco use during pregnancy, childbirth and the puerperium**
Codes under subcategory O99.33, Smoking (tobacco) complicating pregnancy, childbirth, and the puerperium, should be assigned for any pregnancy case when a mother uses any type of tobacco product during the pregnancy or postpartum. A secondary code from category F17, Nicotine dependence, Tobacco use, should also be assigned to identify the type of nicotine dependence.

m. **Poisoning, toxic effects, adverse effects and underdosing in a pregnant patient**
A code from subcategory O9A.2, Injury, poisoning and certain other consequences of external causes complicating pregnancy, childbirth, and the puerperium, should be sequenced first, followed by the appropriate injury, poisoning, toxic effect, adverse effect or underdosing code, and then the additional code(s) that specifies the condition caused by the poisoning, toxic effect, adverse effect or underdosing.

See Section I.C.19. Adverse effects, poisoning, underdosing and toxic effects.

CHAPTER 15 – PREGNANCY
Section I. C. 15. n.

n. Normal Delivery, Code O80

1) Encounter for full term uncomplicated delivery
Code O80 should be assigned when a woman is admitted for a full-term normal delivery and delivers a single, healthy infant without any complications antepartum, during the delivery, or postpartum during the delivery episode. Code O80 is always a principal diagnosis. It is not to be used if any other code from chapter 15 is needed to describe a current complication of the antenatal, delivery, or perinatal period. Additional codes from other chapters may be used with code O80 if they are not related to or are in any way complicating the pregnancy.

2) Uncomplicated delivery with resolved antepartum complication
Code O80 may be used if the patient had a complication at some point during the pregnancy, but the complication is not present at the time of the admission for delivery.

3) Outcome of delivery for O80
Z37.0, Single live birth, is the only outcome of delivery code appropriate for use with O80.

o. The Peripartum and Postpartum Periods

1) Peripartum and Postpartum periods
The postpartum period begins immediately after delivery and continues for six weeks following delivery. The peripartum period is defined as the last month of pregnancy to five months postpartum.

2) Peripartum and postpartum complication
A postpartum complication is any complication occurring within the six-week period.

3) Pregnancy-related complications after 6 week period
Chapter 15 codes may also be used to describe pregnancy-related complications after the peripartum or postpartum period if the provider documents that a condition is pregnancy related.

4) Admission for routine postpartum care following delivery outside hospital
When the mother delivers outside the hospital prior to admission and is admitted for routine postpartum care and no complications are noted, code Z39.0, Encounter for care and examination of mother immediately after delivery, should be assigned as the principal diagnosis.

5) Pregnancy associated cardiomyopathy
Pregnancy associated cardiomyopathy, code O90.3, is unique in that it may be diagnosed in the third trimester of pregnancy but may continue to progress months after delivery. For this reason, it is referred to as peripartum cardiomyopathy. Code O90.3 is only for use when the cardiomyopathy develops as a result of pregnancy in a woman who did not have pre-existing heart disease.

p. Code O94, Sequelae of complication of pregnancy, childbirth, and the puerperium

1) Code O94
Code O94, Sequelae of complication of pregnancy, childbirth, and the puerperium, is for use in those cases when an initial complication of a pregnancy develops a sequelae requiring care or treatment at a future date.

2) After the initial postpartum period
This code may be used at any time after the initial postpartum period.

3) Sequencing of Code O94
This code, like all sequela codes, is to be sequenced following the code describing the sequelae of the complication.

CHAPTER 15 – PREGNANCY
Section I. C. 15. q.

q. Termination of Pregnancy and Spontaneous abortions

1) Abortion with Liveborn Fetus
When an attempted termination of pregnancy results in a liveborn fetus, assign code Z33.2, Encounter for elective termination of pregnancy and a code from category Z37, Outcome of Delivery.

2) Retained Products of Conception following an abortion
Subsequent encounters for retained products of conception following a spontaneous abortion or elective termination of pregnancy are assigned the appropriate code from category O03, Spontaneous abortion, or codes O07.4, Failed attempted termination of pregnancy without complication and Z33.2, Encounter for elective termination of pregnancy. This advice is appropriate even when the patient was discharged previously with a discharge diagnosis of complete abortion.

3) Complications leading to abortion
Codes from Chapter 15 may be used as additional codes to identify any documented complications of the pregnancy in conjunction with codes in categories in O07 and O08.

r. Abuse in a pregnant patient
For suspected or confirmed cases of abuse of a pregnant patient, a code(s) from subcategories O9A.3, Physical abuse complicating pregnancy, childbirth, and the puerperium, O9A.4, Sexual abuse complicating pregnancy, childbirth, and the puerperium, and O9A.5, Psychological abuse complicating pregnancy, childbirth, and the puerperium, should be sequenced first, followed by the appropriate codes (if applicable) to identify any associated current injury due to physical abuse, sexual abuse, and the perpetrator of abuse.

See Section I.C.19.f. Adult and child abuse, neglect and other maltreatment.

16. **Chapter 16: Certain Conditions Originating in the Perinatal Period (P00-P96)**

For coding and reporting purposes the perinatal period is defined as before birth through the 28th day following birth. The following guidelines are provided for reporting purposes

a. **General Perinatal Rules**

1) **Use of Chapter 16 Codes**

Codes in this chapter are <u>never</u> for use on the maternal record.

Codes from Chapter 15, the obstetric chapter, are never permitted on the newborn record. Chapter 16 codes may be used throughout the life of the patient if the condition is still present.

2) **Principal Diagnosis for Birth Record**

When coding the birth episode in a newborn record, assign a code from category Z38, Liveborn infants according to place of birth and type of delivery, as the principal diagnosis. A code from category Z38 is assigned only once, to a newborn at the time of birth. If a newborn is transferred to another institution, a code from category Z38 should not be used at the receiving hospital.

A code from category Z38 is used only on the newborn record, not on the mother's record.

3) **Use of Codes from other Chapters with Codes from Chapter 16**

Codes from other chapters may be used with codes from chapter 16 if the codes from the other chapters provide more specific detail. Codes for signs and symptoms may be assigned when a definitive diagnosis has not been established. If the reason for the encounter is a perinatal condition, the code from chapter 16 should be sequenced first.

4) **Use of Chapter 16 Codes after the Perinatal Period**

Should a condition originate in the perinatal period, and continue throughout the life of the patient, the perinatal code should continue to be used regardless of the patient's age.

5) **Birth process or community acquired conditions**

If a newborn has a condition that may be either due to the birth process or community acquired and the documentation does not indicate which it is, the default is due to the birth process and the code from Chapter 16 should be used. If the condition is community-acquired, a code from Chapter 16 should not be assigned.

6) **Code all clinically significant conditions**

All clinically significant conditions noted on routine newborn examination should be coded. A condition is clinically significant if it requires:

- clinical evaluation; or
- therapeutic treatment; or
- diagnostic procedures; or
- extended length of hospital stay; or
- increased nursing care and/or monitoring; or
- has implications for future health care needs

Note: The perinatal guidelines listed above are the same as the general coding guidelines for "additional diagnoses", except for the final point regarding implications for future health care needs. Codes should be assigned for conditions that have been specified by the provider as having implications for future health care needs.

b. **Observation and Evaluation of Newborns for Suspected Conditions not Found**
Reserved for future expansion

c. **Coding Additional Perinatal Diagnoses**

1) **Assigning codes for conditions that require treatment**

Assign codes for conditions that require treatment or further investigation, prolong the length of stay, or require resource utilization.

2) **Codes for conditions specified as having implications for future health care needs**

Assign codes for conditions that have been specified by the provider as having implications for future health care needs.

Note: This guideline should not be used for adult patients.

d. **Prematurity and Fetal Growth Retardation**

Providers utilize different criteria in determining prematurity. A code for prematurity should not be assigned unless it is documented. Assignment of codes in categories P05, Disorders of newborn related to slow fetal growth and fetal malnutrition, and P07, Disorders of newborn related to short gestation and low birth weight, not elsewhere classified, should be based on the recorded birth weight and estimated gestational age. Codes from category P05 should not be assigned with codes from category P07.

When both birth weight and gestational age are available, two codes from category P07 should be assigned, with the code for birth weight sequenced before the code for gestational age.

e. **Low birth weight and immaturity status**

Codes from category P07, Disorders of newborn related to short gestation and low birth weight, not elsewhere classified, are for use for a child or adult who was premature or had a low birth weight as a newborn and this is affecting the patient's current health status.

See Section I.C.21. Factors influencing health status and contact with health services, Status.

f. **Bacterial Sepsis of Newborn**

Category P36, Bacterial sepsis of newborn, includes congenital sepsis. If a perinate is documented as having sepsis without documentation of congenital or community acquired, the default is congenital and a code from category P36 should be assigned. If the P36 code includes the causal organism, an additional code from category B95, Streptococcus, Staphylococcus, and Enterococcus as the cause of diseases classified elsewhere, or B96, Other bacterial agents as the cause of diseases classified elsewhere, should not be assigned. If the P36 code does not include the causal organism, assign an additional code from category B96. If applicable, use additional codes to identify severe sepsis (R65.2-) and any associated acute organ dysfunction.

g. **Stillbirth**

Code P95, Stillbirth, is only for use in institutions that maintain separate records for stillbirths. No other code should be used with P95. Code P95 should not be used on the mother's record.

CHAPTER 17 – CONGENITAL MALFORMATIONS
Section I. C. 17.

17. **Chapter 17: Congenital malformations, deformations, and chromosomal abnormalities (Q00-Q99)**

Assign an appropriate code(s) from categories Q00-Q99, Congenital malformations, deformations, and chromosomal abnormalities when a malformation/deformation or chromosomal abnormality is documented. A malformation/deformation/or chromosomal abnormality may be the principal/first-listed diagnosis on a record or a secondary diagnosis.

When a malformation/deformation/or chromosomal abnormality does not have a unique code assignment, assign additional code(s) for any manifestations that may be present.

When the code assignment specifically identifies the malformation/deformation/or chromosomal abnormality, manifestations that are an inherent component of the anomaly should not be coded separately. Additional codes should be assigned for manifestations that are not an inherent component.

Codes from Chapter 17 may be used throughout the life of the patient. If a congenital malformation or deformity has been corrected, a personal history code should be used to identify the history of the malformation or deformity. Although present at birth, malformation/deformation/or chromosomal abnormality may not be identified until later in life. Whenever the condition is diagnosed by the physician, it is appropriate to assign a code from codes Q00-Q99.

For the birth admission, the appropriate code from category Z38, Liveborn infants, according to place of birth and type of delivery, should be sequenced as the principal diagnosis, followed by any congenital anomaly codes, Q00-Q99.

CHAPTER 18 – SYMPTOMS & SIGNS
Section I. C. 18.

18. **Chapter 18: Symptoms, signs, and abnormal clinical and laboratory findings, not elsewhere classified (R00-R99)**

Chapter 18 includes symptoms, signs, abnormal results of clinical or other investigative procedures, and ill-defined conditions regarding which no diagnosis classifiable elsewhere is recorded. Signs and symptoms that point to a specific diagnosis have been assigned to a category in other chapters of the classification.

a. **Use of symptom codes**
Codes that describe symptoms and signs are acceptable for reporting purposes when a related definitive diagnosis has not been established (confirmed) by the provider.

b. **Use of a symptom code with a definitive diagnosis code**
Codes for signs and symptoms may be reported in addition to a related definitive diagnosis when the sign or symptom is not routinely associated with that diagnosis, such as the various signs and symptoms associated with complex syndromes. The definitive diagnosis code should be sequenced before the symptom code.

Signs or symptoms that are associated routinely with a disease process should not be assigned as additional codes, unless otherwise instructed by the classification.

c. **Combination codes that include symptoms**
ICD-10-CM contains a number of combination codes that identify both the definitive diagnosis and common symptoms of that diagnosis. When using one of these combination codes, an additional code should not be assigned for the symptom.

d. **Repeated falls**
Code R29.6, Repeated falls, is for use for encounters when a patient has recently fallen and the reason for the fall is being investigated.

Code Z91.81, History of falling, is for use when a patient has fallen in the past and is at risk for future falls. When appropriate, both codes R29.6 and Z91.81 may be assigned together.

e. **Coma scale**
The coma scale codes (R40.2-) can be used in conjunction with traumatic brain injury codes, acute cerebrovascular disease or sequelae of cerebrovascular disease codes. These codes are primarily for use by trauma registries, but they may be used in any setting where this information is collected. The coma scale codes should be sequenced after the diagnosis code(s).

These codes, one from each subcategory, are needed to complete the scale. The 7th character indicates when the scale was recorded. The 7th character should match for all three codes.

At a minimum, report the initial score documented on presentation at your facility. This may be a score from the emergency medicine technician (EMT) or in the emergency department. If desired, a facility may choose to capture multiple coma scale scores.

Assign code R40.24, Glascow coma scale, total score, when only the total score is documented in the medical record and not the individual score(s).

f. **Functional quadriplegia**
Functional quadriplegia (code R53.2) is the lack of ability to use one's limbs or to ambulate due to extreme debility. It is not associated with neurologic deficit or injury, and code R53.2 should not be used for cases of neurologic quadriplegia. It should only be assigned if functional quadriplegia is specifically documented in the medical record.

g. SIRS due to Non-Infectious Process

The systemic inflammatory response syndrome (SIRS) can develop as a result of certain non-infectious disease processes, such as trauma, malignant neoplasm, or pancreatitis. When SIRS is documented with a noninfectious condition, and no subsequent infection is documented, the code for the underlying condition, such as an injury, should be assigned, followed by code R65.10, Systemic inflammatory response syndrome (SIRS) of non-infectious origin without acute organ dysfunction, or code R65.11, Systemic inflammatory response syndrome (SIRS) of non-infectious origin with acute organ dysfunction. If an associated acute organ dysfunction is documented, the appropriate code(s) for the specific type of organ dysfunction(s) should be assigned in addition to code R65.11. If acute organ dysfunction is documented, but it cannot be determined if the acute organ dysfunction is associated with SIRS or due to another condition (e.g., directly due to the trauma), the provider should be queried.

h. Death NOS

Code R99, Ill-defined and unknown cause of mortality, is only for use in the very limited circumstance when a patient who has already died is brought into an emergency department or other healthcare facility and is pronounced dead upon arrival. It does not represent the discharge disposition of death.

19. Chapter 19: Injury, poisoning, and certain other consequences of external causes (S00-T88)

a. Application of 7th Characters in Chapter 19

Most categories in chapter 19 have a 7th character requirement for each applicable code. Most categories in this chapter have three 7th character values (with the exception of fractures): A, initial encounter, D, subsequent encounter and S, sequela. Categories for traumatic fractures have additional 7th character values.

7th character "A" initial encounter is used while the patient is receiving active treatment for the condition. Examples of active treatment are: surgical treatment, emergency department encounter, and evaluation and treatment by a new physician.

7th character "D" subsequent encounter is used for encounters after the patient has received active treatment of the condition and is receiving routine care for the condition during the healing or recovery phase. Examples of subsequent care are: cast change or removal, removal of external or internal fixation device, medication adjustment, other aftercare and follow up visits following treatment of the injury or condition.

The aftercare Z codes should not be used for aftercare for conditions such as injuries or poisonings, where 7th characters are provided to identify subsequent care. For example, for aftercare of an injury, assign the acute injury code with the 7th character "D" (subsequent encounter).

7th character "S", sequela, is for use for complications or conditions that arise as a direct result of an condition, such as scar formation after a burn. The scars are sequelae of the burn. When using 7th character "S", it is necessary to use both the injury code that precipitated the sequela and the code for the sequela itself. The "S" is added only to the injury code, not the sequela code. The 7th character "S" identifies the injury responsible for the sequela. The specific type of sequela (e.g. scar) is sequenced first, followed by the injury code.

b. Coding of Injuries

When coding injuries, assign separate codes for each injury unless a combination code is provided, in which case the combination code is assigned. Code T07, Unspecified multiple injuries should not be assigned in the inpatient setting unless information for a more specific code is not available. Traumatic injury codes (S00-T14.9) are not to be used for normal, healing surgical wounds or to identify complications of surgical wounds.

The code for the most serious injury, as determined by the provider and the focus of treatment, is sequenced first.

1) Superficial injuries

Superficial injuries such as abrasions or contusions are not coded when associated with more severe injuries of the same site.

2) Primary injury with damage to nerves/blood vessels

When a primary injury results in minor damage to peripheral nerves or blood vessels, the primary injury is sequenced first with additional code(s) for injuries to nerves and spinal cord (such as category S04), and/or injury to blood vessels (such as category S15). When the primary injury is to the blood vessels or nerves, that injury should be sequenced first.

CHAPTER 19 – INJURY & POISONING
Section I. C. 19. c.

c. **Coding of Traumatic Fractures**

The principles of multiple coding of injuries should be followed in coding fractures. Fractures of specified sites are coded individually by site in accordance with both the provisions within categories S02, S12, S22, S32, S42, S49, S52, S59, S62, S72, S79, S82, S89, S92 and the level of detail furnished by medical record content.

A fracture not indicated as open or closed should be coded to closed. A fracture not indicated whether displaced or not displaced should be coded to displaced.

More specific guidelines are as follows:

1) **Initial vs. Subsequent Encounter for Fractures**

Traumatic fractures are coded using the appropriate 7th character for initial encounter (A, B, C) while the patient is receiving active treatment for the fracture. Examples of active treatment are: surgical treatment, emergency department encounter, and evaluation and treatment by a new physician. The appropriate 7th character for initial encounter should also be assigned for a patient who delayed seeking treatment for the fracture or nonunion.

Fractures are coded using the appropriate 7th character for subsequent care for encounters after the patient has completed active treatment of the fracture and is receiving routine care for the fracture during the healing or recovery phase. Examples of fracture aftercare are: cast change or removal, removal of external or internal fixation device, medication adjustment, and follow-up visits following fracture treatment.

Care for complications of surgical treatment for fracture repairs during the healing or recovery phase should be coded with the appropriate complication codes.

Care of complications of fractures, such as malunion and nonunion, should be reported with the appropriate 7th character for subsequent care with nonunion (K, M, N,) or subsequent care with malunion (P, Q, R).

A code from category M80, not a traumatic fracture code, should be used for any patient with known osteoporosis who suffers a fracture, even if the patient had a minor fall or trauma, if that fall or trauma would not usually break a normal, healthy bone.

See Section I.C.13. Osteoporosis.

The aftercare Z codes should not be used for aftercare for traumatic fractures. For aftercare of a traumatic fracture, assign the acute fracture code with the appropriate 7th character.

2) **Multiple fractures sequencing**

Multiple fractures are sequenced in accordance with the severity of the fracture.

CHAPTER 19 – INJURY & POISONING
Section I. C. 19. d.

d. **Coding of Burns and Corrosions**

The ICD-10-CM makes a distinction between burns and corrosions. The burn codes are for thermal burns, except sunburns, that come from a heat source, such as a fire or hot appliance. The burn codes are also for burns resulting from electricity and radiation. Corrosions are burns due to chemicals. The guidelines are the same for burns and corrosions.

Current burns (T20-T25) are classified by depth, extent and by agent (X code). Burns are classified by depth as first degree (erythema), second degree (blistering), and third degree (full-thickness involvement). Burns of the eye and internal organs (T26-T28) are classified by site, but not by degree.

1) **Sequencing of burn and related condition codes**

Sequence first the code that reflects the highest degree of burn when more than one burn is present.

a. When the reason for the admission or encounter is for treatment of external multiple burns, sequence first the code that reflects the burn of the highest degree.

b. When a patient has both internal and external burns, the circumstances of admission govern the selection of the principal diagnosis or first-listed diagnosis.

c. When a patient is admitted for burn injuries and other related conditions such as smoke inhalation and/or respiratory failure, the circumstances of admission govern the selection of the principal or first-listed diagnosis.

2) **Burns of the same local site**

Classify burns of the same local site (three-character category level, T20-T28) but of different degrees to the subcategory identifying the highest degree recorded in the diagnosis.

3) **Non-healing burns**

Non-healing burns are coded as acute burns.

Necrosis of burned skin should be coded as a non-healed burn.

4) **Infected Burn**

For any documented infected burn site, use an additional code for the infection.

5) **Assign separate codes for each burn site**

When coding burns, assign separate codes for each burn site. Category T30, Burn and corrosion, body region unspecified is extremely vague and should rarely be used.

6) **Burns and Corrosions Classified According to Extent of Body Surface Involved**

Assign codes from category T31, Burns classified according to extent of body surface involved, or T32, Corrosions classified according to extent of body surface involved, when the site of the burn is not specified or when there is a need for additional data. It is advisable to use category T31 as additional coding when needed to provide data for evaluating burn mortality, such as that needed by burn units. It is also advisable to use category T31 as an additional code for reporting purposes when there is mention of a third-degree burn involving 20 percent or more of the body surface.

Categories T31 and T32 are based on the classic "rule of nines" in estimating body surface involved: head and neck are assigned nine percent, each arm nine percent, each leg 18 percent, the anterior trunk 18 percent, posterior trunk 18 percent, and genitalia one percent. Providers may change these percentage assignments where necessary to accommodate infants and children who have proportionately larger heads than adults, and patients who have large buttocks, thighs, or abdomen that involve burns.

GUIDELINES

7) **Encounters for treatment of sequela of burns**
Encounters for the treatment of the late effects of burns or corrosions (i.e., scars or joint contractures) should be coded with a burn or corrosion code with the 7th character "S" for sequela.

8) **Sequelae with a late effect code and current burn**
When appropriate, both a code for a current burn or corrosion with 7th character "A" or "D" and a burn or corrosion code with 7th character "S" may be assigned on the same record (when both a current burn and sequelae of an old burn exist). Burns and corrosions do not heal at the same rate and a current healing wound may still exist with sequela of a healed burn or corrosion.

9) **Use of an external cause code with burns and corrosions**
An external cause code should be used with burns and corrosions to identify the source and intent of the burn, as well as the place where it occurred.

e. **Adverse Effects, Poisoning, Underdosing and Toxic Effects**
Codes in categories T36-T65 are combination codes that include the substance that was taken as well as the intent. No additional external cause code is required for poisonings, toxic effects, adverse effects and underdosing codes.

1) **Do not code directly from the Table of Drugs**
Do not code directly from the Table of Drugs and Chemicals. Always refer back to the Tabular List.

2) **Use as many codes as necessary to describe**
Use as many codes as necessary to describe completely all drugs, medicinal or biological substances.

3) **If the same code would describe the causative agent**
If the same code would describe the causative agent for more than one adverse reaction, poisoning, toxic effect or underdosing, assign the code only once.

4) **If two or more drugs, medicinal or biological substances**
If two or more drugs, medicinal or biological substances are reported, code each individually unless a combination code is listed in the Table of Drugs and Chemicals.

5) **The occurrence of drug toxicity is classified in ICD-10-CM as follows:**

(a) **Adverse Effect**
When coding an adverse effect of a drug that has been correctly prescribed and properly administered, assign the appropriate code for the nature of the adverse effect followed by the appropriate code for the adverse effect of the drug (T36-T50). The code for the drug should have a 5th or 6th character "5" (for example T36.0X5-). Examples of the nature of an adverse effect are tachycardia, delirium, gastrointestinal hemorrhaging, vomiting, hypokalemia, hepatitis, renal failure, or respiratory failure.

(b) **Poisoning**
When coding a poisoning or reaction to the improper use of a medication (e.g., overdose, wrong substance given or taken in error, wrong route of administration), first assign the appropriate code from categories T36-T50. The poisoning codes have an associated intent as their 5th or 6th character accidental, intentional self-harm, assault and undetermined. Use additional code(s) for all manifestations of poisonings.

If there is also a diagnosis of abuse or dependence of the substance, the abuse or dependence is assigned as an additional code.

Examples of poisoning include:

(i) Error was made in drug prescription
Errors made in drug prescription or in the administration of the drug by provider, nurse, patient, or other person.

(ii) Overdose of a drug intentionally taken
If an overdose of a drug was intentionally taken or administered and resulted in drug toxicity, it would be coded as a poisoning.

(iii) Nonprescribed drug taken with correctly prescribed and properly administered drug
If a nonprescribed drug or medicinal agent was taken in combination with a correctly prescribed and properly administered drug, any drug toxicity or other reaction resulting from the interaction of the two drugs would be classified as a poisoning.

(iv) Interaction of drug(s) and alcohol
When a reaction results from the interaction of a drug(s) and alcohol, this would be classified as poisoning.

See Section I.C.4. if poisoning is the result of insulin pump malfunctions.

(c) **Underdosing**
Underdosing refers to taking less of a medication than is prescribed by a provider or a manufacturer's instruction. For underdosing, assign the code from categories T36-T50 (fifth or sixth character "6").

Codes for underdosing should never be assigned as principal or first-listed codes. If a patient has a relapse or exacerbation of the medical condition for which the drug is prescribed because of the reduction in dose, then the medical condition itself should be coded.

Noncompliance (Z91.12-, Z91.13-) or complication of care (Y63.61, Y63.6-Y63.9) codes are to be used with an underdosing code to indicate intent, if known.

(d) **Toxic Effects**
When a harmful substance is ingested or comes in contact with a person, this is classified as a toxic effect. The toxic effect codes are in categories T51-T65.

Toxic effect codes have an associated intent: accidental, intentional self-harm, assault and undetermined.

[2014.CM-1.V1]   **OFFICIAL CODING GUIDELINES – 2014 ICD-10-CM**

CHAPTER 19 – INJURY & POISONING	CHAPTER 19 – INJURY & POISONING
Section I. C. 19. f.	Section I. C. 19. g. 3)

GUIDELINES

f. Adult and child abuse, neglect and other maltreatment
Sequence first the appropriate code from categories T74.- (Adult and child abuse, neglect and other maltreatment, confirmed) or T76.- (Adult and child abuse, neglect and other maltreatment, suspected) for abuse, neglect and other maltreatment, followed by any accompanying mental health or injury code(s).

If the documentation in the medical record states abuse or neglect it is coded as confirmed (T74.-). It is coded as suspected if it is documented as suspected (T76.-).

For cases of confirmed abuse or neglect an external cause code from the assault section (X92-Y08) should be added to identify the cause of any physical injuries. A perpetrator code (Y07) should be added when the perpetrator of the abuse is known. For suspected cases of abuse or neglect, do not report external cause or perpetrator code.

If a suspected case of abuse, neglect or mistreatment is ruled out during an encounter code Z04.71, Encounter for examination and observation following alleged physical adult abuse, ruled out, or code Z04.72, Encounter for examination and observation following alleged physical child abuse, ruled out, should be used, not a code from T76.

If a suspected case of alleged rape or sexual abuse is ruled out during an encounter code Z04.41, Encounter for examination and observation following alleged physical adult abuse, ruled out, or code Z04.42, Encounter for examination and observation following alleged rape or sexual abuse, ruled out, should be used, not a code from T76.

See Section I.C.15. Abuse in a pregnant patient.

g. Complications of care

1) General guidelines for complications of care

(a) Documentation of complications of care

See section I.B.16. for information on documentation of complications of care.

2) Pain due to medical devices
Pain associated with devices, implants or grafts left in a surgical site (for example painful hip prosthesis) is assigned to the appropriate code(s) found in Chapter 19, Injury, poisoning, and certain other consequences of external causes. Specific codes for pain due to medical devices are found in the T code section of the ICD-10-CM. Use additional code(s) from category G89 to identify acute or chronic pain due to presence of the device, implant or graft (G89.18 or G89.28).

3) Transplant complications

(a) Transplant complications other than kidney
Codes under category T86, Complications of transplanted organs and tissues, are for use for both complications and rejection of transplanted organs. A transplant complication code is only assigned if the complication affects the function of the transplanted organ. Two codes are required to fully describe a transplant complication: the appropriate code from category T86 and a secondary code that identifies the complication.

Pre-existing conditions or conditions that develop after the transplant are not coded as complications unless they affect the function of the transplanted organs.

See I.C.21. for transplant organ removal status
See I.C.2. for malignant neoplasm associated with transplanted organ.

(b) Kidney transplant complications
Patients who have undergone kidney transplant may still have some form of chronic kidney disease (CKD) because the kidney transplant may not fully restore kidney function. Code T86.1- should be assigned for documented complications of a kidney transplant, such as transplant failure or rejection or other transplant complication. Code T86.1- should not be assigned for post kidney transplant patients who have chronic kidney (CKD) unless a transplant complication such as transplant failure or rejection is documented. If the documentation is unclear as to whether the patient has a complication of the transplant, query the provider.

Conditions that affect the function of the transplanted kidney, other than CKD, should be assigned a code from subcategory T86.1, Complications of transplanted organ, kidney, and a secondary code that identifies the complication.

For patients with CKD following a kidney transplant, but who do not have a complication such as failure or rejection, *see section I.C.14. Chronic kidney disease and kidney transplant status.*

4) Complication codes that include the external cause
As with certain other T codes, some of the complications of care codes have the external cause included in the code. The code includes the nature of the complication as well as the type of procedure that caused the complication. No external cause code indicating the type of procedure is necessary for these codes.

5) Complications of care codes within the body system chapters
Intraoperative and postprocedural complication codes are found within the body system chapters with codes specific to the organs and structures of that body system. These codes should be sequenced first, followed by a code(s) for the specific complication, if applicable.

20. Chapter 20: External Causes of Morbidity (V00-Y99)
The external causes of morbidity codes should never be sequenced as the first-listed or principal diagnosis.

External cause codes are intended to provide data for injury research and evaluation of injury prevention strategies. These codes capture how the injury or health condition happened (cause), the intent (unintentional or accidental; or intentional, such as suicide or assault), the place where the event occurred the activity of the patient at the time of the event, and the person's status (e.g., civilian, military).

There is no national requirement for mandatory ICD-10-CM external cause code reporting. Unless a provider is subject to a state-based external cause code reporting mandate or these codes are required by a particular payer, reporting of ICD-10-CM codes in Chapter 20, External Causes of Morbidity, is not required. In the absence of a mandatory reporting requirement, providers are encouraged to voluntarily report external cause codes, as they provide valuable data for injury research and evaluation of injury prevention strategies.

a. General External Cause Coding Guidelines

1) Used with any code in the range of A00.0-T88.9, Z00-Z99
An external cause code may be used with any code in the range of A00.0-T88.9, Z00-Z99, classification that is a health condition due to an external cause. Though they are most applicable to injuries, they are also valid for use with such things as infections or diseases due to an external source, and other health conditions, such as a heart attack that occurs during strenuous physical activity.

2) External cause code used for length of treatment
Assign the external cause code, with the appropriate 7th character (initial encounter, subsequent encounter or sequela) for each encounter for which the injury or condition is being treated.

3) Use the full range of external cause codes
Use the full range of external cause codes to completely describe the cause, the intent, the place of occurrence, and if applicable, the activity of the patient at the time of the event, and the patient's status, for all injuries, and other health conditions due to an external cause.

4) Assign as many external cause codes as necessary
Assign as many external cause codes as necessary to fully explain each cause. If only one external code can be recorded, assign the code most related to the principal diagnosis.

5) The selection of the appropriate external cause code
The selection of the appropriate external cause code is guided by the Alphabetic Index of External Causes and by Inclusion and Exclusion notes in the Tabular List.

6) External cause code can never be a principal diagnosis
An external cause code can never be a principal (first-listed) diagnosis.

7) Combination external cause codes
Certain of the external cause codes are combination codes that identify sequential events that result in an injury, such as a fall which results in striking against an object. The injury may be due to either event or both. The combination external cause code used should correspond to the sequence of events regardless of which caused the most serious injury.

8) No external cause code needed in certain circumstances
No external cause code from Chapter 20 is needed if the external cause and intent are included in a code from another chapter (e.g. T36.0x1- Poisoning by penicillins, accidental (unintentional)).

b. Place of Occurrence Guideline
Codes from category Y92, Place of occurrence of the external cause, are secondary codes for use after other external cause codes to identify the location of the patient at the time of injury or other condition.

A place of occurrence code is used only once, at the initial encounter for treatment. No 7th characters are used for Y92. Only one code from Y92 should be recorded on a medical record.

Do not use place of occurrence code Y92.9 if the place is not stated or is not applicable.

c. Activity Code
Assign a code from category Y93, Activity code, to describe the activity of the patient at the time the injury or other health condition occurred.

An activity code is used only once, at the initial encounter for treatment. Only one code from Y93 should be recorded on a medical record.

The activity codes are not applicable to poisonings, adverse effects, misadventures or sequela.

Do not assign Y93.9, Unspecified activity, if the activity is not stated.

A code from category Y93 is appropriate for use with external cause and intent codes if identifying the activity provides additional information about the event.

d. Place of Occurrence, Activity, and Status Codes Used with other External Cause Code
When applicable, place of occurrence, activity, and external cause status codes are sequenced after the main external cause code(s). Regardless of the number of external cause codes assigned, there should be only one place of occurrence code, one activity code, and one external cause status code assigned to an encounter.

e. If the Reporting Format Limits the Number of External Cause Codes
If the reporting format limits the number of external cause codes that can be used in reporting clinical data, report the code for the cause/intent most related to the principal diagnosis. If the format permits capture of additional external cause codes, the cause/intent, including medical misadventures, of the additional events should be reported rather than the codes for place, activity, or external status.

f. Multiple External Cause Coding Guidelines
More than one external cause code is required to fully describe the external cause of an illness or injury. The assignment of external cause codes should be sequenced in the following priority:

If two or more events cause separate injuries, an external cause code should be assigned for each cause. The first-listed external cause code will be selected in the following order:

External codes for child and adult abuse take priority over all other external cause codes.

See Section I.C.19. Child and Adult abuse guidelines.

External cause codes for terrorism events take priority over all other external cause codes except child and adult abuse.

External cause codes for cataclysmic events take priority over all other external cause codes except child and adult abuse and terrorism.

External cause codes for transport accidents take priority over all other external cause codes except cataclysmic events, child and adult abuse and terrorism.

CHAPTER 20 – EXTERNAL CAUSES
Section I. C. 20. g.

Activity and external cause status codes are assigned following all causal (intent) external cause codes.

The first-listed external cause code should correspond to the cause of the most serious diagnosis due to an assault, accident, or self-harm, following the order of hierarchy listed above.

g. Child and Adult Abuse Guideline

Adult and child abuse, neglect and maltreatment are classified as assault. Any of the assault codes may be used to indicate the external cause of any injury resulting from the confirmed abuse.

For confirmed cases of abuse, neglect and maltreatment, when the perpetrator is known, a code from Y07, Perpetrator of maltreatment and neglect, should accompany any other assault codes.

See Section I.C.19. Adult and child abuse, neglect and other maltreatment

h. Unknown or Undetermined Intent Guideline

If the intent (accident, self-harm, assault) of the cause of an injury or other condition is unknown or unspecified, code the intent as accidental intent. All transport accident categories assume accidental intent.

1) Use of undetermined intent

External cause codes for events of undetermined intent are only for use if the documentation in the record specifies that the intent cannot be determined.

i. Sequelae (Late Effects) of External Cause Guidelines

1) Sequelae external cause codes

Sequela are reported using the external cause code with the 7th character "S" for sequela. These codes should be used with any report of a late effect or sequela resulting from a previous injury.

2) Sequela external cause code with a related current injury

A sequela external cause code should never be used with a related current nature of injury code.

3) Use of sequela external cause codes for subsequent visits

Use a late effect external cause code for subsequent visits when a late effect of the initial injury is being treated. Do not use a late effect external cause code for subsequent visits for follow-up care (e.g., to assess healing, to receive rehabilitative therapy) of the injury when no late effect of the injury has been documented.

CHAPTER 20 – EXTERNAL CAUSES
Section I. C. 20. j.

j. Terrorism Guidelines

1) Cause of injury identified by the Federal Government (FBI) as terrorism

When the cause of an injury is identified by the Federal Government (FBI) as terrorism, the first-listed external cause code should be a code from category Y38, Terrorism. The definition of terrorism employed by the FBI is found at the inclusion note at the beginning of category Y38. Use additional code for place of occurrence (Y92.-). More than one Y38 code may be assigned if the injury is the result of more than one mechanism of terrorism.

2) Cause of an injury is suspected to be the result of terrorism

When the cause of an injury is suspected to be the result of terrorism a code from category Y38 should not be assigned. Suspected cases should be classified as assault.

3) Code Y38.9, Terrorism, secondary effects

Assign code Y38.9, Terrorism, secondary effects, for conditions occurring subsequent to the terrorist event. This code should not be assigned for conditions that are due to the initial terrorist act.

It is acceptable to assign code Y38.9 with another code from Y38 if there is an injury due to the initial terrorist event and an injury that is a subsequent result of the terrorist event.

k. External cause status

A code from category Y99, External cause status, should be assigned whenever any other external cause code is assigned for an encounter, including an Activity code, except for the events noted below. Assign a code from category Y99, External cause status, to indicate the work status of the person at the time the event occurred. The status code indicates whether the event occurred during military activity, whether a non-military person was at work, whether an individual including a student or volunteer was involved in a non-work activity at the time of the causal event.

A code from Y99, External cause status, should be assigned, when applicable, with other external cause codes, such as transport accidents and falls. The external cause status codes are not applicable to poisonings, adverse effects, misadventures or late effects.

Do not assign a code from category Y99 if no other external cause codes (cause, activity) are applicable for the encounter.

An external cause status code is used only once, at the initial encounter for treatment. Only one code from Y99 should be recorded on a medical record.

Do not assign code Y99.9, Unspecified external cause status, if the status is not stated.

GUIDELINES

21. Chapter 21: Factors influencing health status and contact with health services (Z00-Z99)

Note: The chapter specific guidelines provide additional information about the use of Z codes for specified encounters.

a. Use of Z codes in any healthcare setting

Z codes are for use in any healthcare setting. Z codes may be used as either a first-listed (principal diagnosis code in the inpatient setting) or secondary code, depending on the circumstances of the encounter. Certain Z codes may only be used as first-listed or principal diagnosis.

b. Z Codes indicate a reason for an encounter

Z codes are not procedure codes. A corresponding procedure code must accompany a Z code to describe any procedure performed.

c. Categories of Z Codes

1) Contact/Exposure

Category Z20 indicates contact with, and suspected exposure to, communicable diseases. These codes are for patients who do not show any sign or symptom of a disease but are suspected to have been exposed to it by close personal contact with an infected individual or are in an area where a disease is epidemic.

Category Z77, indicates contact with and suspected exposures hazardous to health.

Contact/exposure codes may be used as a first-listed code to explain an encounter for testing, or, more commonly, as a secondary code to identify a potential risk.

2) Inoculations and vaccinations

Code Z23 is for encounters for inoculations and vaccinations. It indicates that a patient is being seen to receive a prophylactic inoculation against a disease. Procedure codes are required to identify the actual administration of the injection and the type(s) of immunizations given. Code Z23 may be used as a secondary code if the inoculation is given as a routine part of preventive health care, such as a well-baby visit.

3) Status

Status codes indicate that a patient is either a carrier of a disease or has the sequelae or residual of a past disease or condition. This includes such things as the presence of prosthetic or mechanical devices resulting from past treatment. A status code is informative, because the status may affect the course of treatment and its outcome. A status code is distinct from a history code. The history code indicates that the patient no longer has the condition.

A status code should not be used with a diagnosis code from one of the body system chapters, if the diagnosis code includes the information provided by the status code. For example, code Z94.1, Heart transplant status, should not be used with a code from subcategory T86.2, Complications of heart transplant. The status code does not provide additional information. The complication code indicates that the patient is a heart transplant patient.

For encounters for weaning from a mechanical ventilator, assign a code from subcategory J96.1, Chronic respiratory failure, followed by code Z99.11, Dependence on respirator [ventilator] status.

The status Z codes/categories are:

Z14   Genetic carrier
       Genetic carrier status indicates that a person carries a gene, associated with a particular disease, which may be passed to offspring who may develop that disease. The person does not have the disease and is not at risk of developing the disease.

Z15   Genetic susceptibility to disease
       Genetic susceptibility indicates that a person has a gene that increases the risk of that person developing the disease.

       Codes from category Z15 should not be used as principal or first-listed codes. If the patient has the condition to which he/she is susceptible, and that condition is the reason for the encounter, the code for the current condition should be sequenced first. If the patient is being seen for follow-up after completed treatment for this condition, and the condition no longer exists, a follow-up code should be sequenced first, followed by the appropriate personal history and genetic susceptibility codes. If the purpose of the encounter is genetic counseling associated with procreative management, code Z31.5, Encounter for genetic counseling, should be assigned as the first-listed code, followed by a code from category Z15. Additional codes should be assigned for any applicable family or personal history.

Z16   Resistance to antimicrobial drugs
       This code indicates that a patient has a condition that is resistant to antimicrobial drug treatment. Sequence the infection code first.

Z17   Estrogen receptor status

Z18   Retained foreign body fragments

Z21   Asymptomatic HIV infection status
       This code indicates that a patient has tested positive for HIV but has manifested no signs or symptoms of the disease.

Z22   Carrier of infectious disease
       Carrier status indicates that a person harbors the specific organisms of a disease without manifest symptoms and is capable of transmitting the infection.

Z28.3 Underimmunization status

Z33.1 Pregnant state, incidental
       This code is a secondary code only for use when the pregnancy is in no way complicating the reason for visit. Otherwise, a code from the obstetric chapter is required.

Z66   Do not resuscitate
       This code may be used when it is documented by the provider that a patient is on do not resuscitate status at any time during the stay.

Z67   Blood type

Z68   Body mass index (BMI)

Z74.01 Bed confinement status

Z76.82 Awaiting organ transplant status

Z78   Other specified health status
       Code Z78.1, Physical restraint status, may be used when it is documented by the provider that a patient has been put in restraints during the current encounter. Please note that this code should not be reported when it is documented by the provider that a patient is temporarily restrained during a procedure.

© 2013 Channel Publishing Ltd

Z79   Long-term (current) drug therapy
Codes from this category indicate a patient's continuous use of a prescribed drug (including such things as aspirin therapy) for the long-term treatment of a condition or for prophylactic use. It is not for use for patients who have addictions to drugs. This subcategory is not for use of medications for detoxification or maintenance programs to prevent withdrawal symptoms in patients with drug dependence (e.g., methadone maintenance for opiate dependence). Assign the appropriate code for the drug dependence instead.

Assign a code from Z79 if the patient is receiving a medication for an extended period as a prophylactic measure (such as for the prevention of deep vein thrombosis) or as treatment of a chronic condition (such as arthritis) or a disease requiring a lengthy course of treatment (such as cancer). Do not assign a code from category Z79 for medication being administered for a brief period of time to treat an acute illness or injury (such as a course of antibiotics to treat acute bronchitis).

Z88   Allergy status to drugs, medicaments and biological substances
Except: Z88.9, Allergy status to unspecified drugs, medicaments and biological substances status

Z89   Acquired absence of limb

Z90   Acquired absence of organs, not elsewhere classified

Z91.0- Allergy status, other than to drugs and biological substances

Z92.82 Status post administration of tPA (rtPA) in a different facility within the last 24 hours prior to admission to a current facility
Assign code Z92.82, Status post administration of tPA (rtPA) in a different facility within the last 24 hours prior to admission to current facility, as a secondary diagnosis when a patient is received by transfer into a facility and documentation indicates they were administered tissue plasminogen activator (tPA) within the last 24 hours prior to admission to the current facility.

This guideline applies even if the patient is still receiving the tPA at the time they are received into the current facility.

The appropriate code for the condition for which the tPA was administered (such as cerebrovascular disease or myocardial infarction) should be assigned first.
Code Z92.82 is only applicable to the receiving facility record and not to the transferring facility record.

Z93   Artificial opening status

Z94   Transplanted organ and tissue status

Z95   Presence of cardiac and vascular implants and grafts

Z96   Presence of other functional implants

Z97   Presence of other devices

Z98   Other postprocedural states
Assign code Z98.85, Transplanted organ removal status, to indicate that a transplanted organ has been previously removed. This code should not be assigned for the encounter in which the transplanted organ is removed. The complication necessitating removal of the transplant organ should be assigned for that encounter.

See section I.C19. for information on the coding of organ transplant complications.

Z99   Dependence on enabling machines and devices, not elsewhere classified
Note: Categories Z89-Z90 and Z93-Z99 are for use only if there are no complications or malfunctions of the organ or tissue replaced, the amputation site or the equipment on which the patient is dependent.

4) History (of)
There are two types of history Z codes, personal and family. Personal history codes explain a patient's past medical condition that no longer exists and is not receiving any treatment, but that has the potential for recurrence, and therefore may require continued monitoring.

Family history codes are for use when a patient has a family member(s) who has had a particular disease that causes the patient to be at higher risk of also contracting the disease.

Personal history codes may be used in conjunction with follow-up codes and family history codes may be used in conjunction with screening codes to explain the need for a test or procedure. History codes are also acceptable on any medical record regardless of the reason for visit. A history of an illness, even if no longer present, is important information that may alter the type of treatment ordered.

The history Z code categories are:
Z80   Family history of primary malignant neoplasm
Z81   Family history of mental and behavioral disorders
Z82   Family history of certain disabilities and chronic diseases (leading to disablement)
Z83   Family history of other specific disorders
Z84   Family history of other conditions
Z85   Personal history of malignant neoplasm
Z86   Personal history of certain other diseases
Z87   Personal history of other diseases and conditions
Z91.4- Personal history of psychological trauma, not elsewhere classified
Z91.5   Personal history of self-harm
Z91.8- Other specified personal risk factors, not elsewhere classified
Exception:
Z91.83, Wandering in diseases classified elsewhere
Z92   Personal history of medical treatment
Except: Z92.0, Personal history of contraception
Except: Z92.82, Status post administration of tPA (rtPA) in a different facility within the last 24 hours prior to admission to a current facility

5) Screening
Screening is the testing for disease or disease precursors in seemingly well individuals so that early detection and treatment can be provided for those who test positive for the disease (e.g., screening mammogram).

The testing of a person to rule out or confirm a suspected diagnosis because the patient has some sign or symptom is a diagnostic examination, not a screening. In these cases, the sign or symptom is used to explain the reason for the test.

A screening code may be a first-listed code if the reason for the visit is specifically the screening exam. It may also be used as an additional code if the screening is done during an office visit for other health problems. A screening code is not necessary if the screening is inherent to a routine examination, such as a pap smear done during a routine pelvic examination.

Should a condition be discovered during the screening then the code for the condition may be assigned as an additional diagnosis.

The Z code indicates that a screening exam is planned. A procedure code is required to confirm that the screening was performed.

The screening Z codes/categories:
Z11   Encounter for screening for infectious and parasitic diseases
Z12   Encounter for screening for malignant neoplasms
Z13   Encounter for screening for other diseases and disorders
Except: Z13.9, Encounter for screening, unspecified
Z36   Encounter for antenatal screening for mother

GUIDELINES

6) Observation

There are two observation Z code categories. They are for use in very limited circumstances when a person is being observed for a suspected condition that is ruled out. The observation codes are not for use if an injury or illness or any signs or symptoms related to the suspected condition are present. In such cases the diagnosis/symptom code is used with the corresponding external cause code.

The observation codes are to be used as principal diagnosis only. Additional codes may be used in addition to the observation code but only if they are unrelated to the suspected condition being observed.

Codes from subcategory Z03.7, Encounter for suspected maternal and fetal conditions ruled out, may either be used as a first-listed or as an additional code assignment depending on the case. They are for use in very limited circumstances on a maternal record when an encounter is for a suspected maternal or fetal condition that is ruled out during that encounter (for example, a maternal or fetal condition may be suspected due to an abnormal test result). These codes should not be used when the condition is confirmed. In those cases, the confirmed condition should be coded. In addition, these codes are not for use if an illness or any signs or symptoms related to the suspected condition or problem are present. In such cases the diagnosis/symptom code is used.

Additional codes may be used in addition to the code from subcategory Z03.7, but only if they are unrelated to the suspected condition being evaluated.

Codes from subcategory Z03.7 may not be used for encounters for antenatal screening of mother. *See Section I.C.21. Screening.*

For encounters for suspected fetal condition that are inconclusive following testing and evaluation, assign the appropriate code from category O35, O36, O40 or O41.

The observation Z code categories:

Z03   Encounter for medical observation for suspected diseases and conditions ruled out
Z04   Encounter for examination and observation for other reasons
      Except: Z04.9, Encounter for examination and observation for unspecified reason

7) Aftercare

Aftercare visit codes cover situations when the initial treatment of a disease has been performed and the patient requires continued care during the healing or recovery phase, or for the long-term consequences of the disease. The aftercare Z code should not be used if treatment is directed at a current, acute disease. The diagnosis code is to be used in these cases. Exceptions to this rule are codes Z51.0, Encounter for antineoplastic radiation therapy, and codes from subcategory Z51.1, Encounter for antineoplastic chemotherapy and immunotherapy. These codes are to be first-listed, followed by the diagnosis code when a patient's encounter is solely to receive radiation therapy, chemotherapy, or immunotherapy for the treatment of a neoplasm. If the reason for the encounter is more than one type of antineoplastic therapy, code Z51.0 and a code from subcategory Z51.1 may be assigned together, in which case one of these codes would be reported as a secondary diagnosis.

The aftercare Z codes should also not be used for aftercare for injuries. For aftercare of an injury, assign the acute injury code with the appropriate 7th character (for subsequent encounter).

The aftercare codes are generally first-listed to explain the specific reason for the encounter. An aftercare code may be used as an additional code when some type of aftercare is provided in addition to the reason for admission and no diagnosis code is applicable. An example of this would be the closure of a colostomy during an encounter for treatment of another condition.

Aftercare codes should be used in conjunction with other aftercare codes or diagnosis codes to provide better detail on the specifics of an aftercare encounter visit, unless otherwise directed by the classification. Should a patient receive multiple types of antineoplastic therapy during the same encounter, code Z51.0, Encounter for antineoplastic radiation therapy, and codes from subcategory Z51.1, Encounter for antineoplastic chemotherapy and immunotherapy, may be used together on a record. The sequencing of multiple aftercare codes depends on the circumstances of the encounter.

Certain aftercare Z code categories need a secondary diagnosis code to describe the resolving condition or sequelae. For others, the condition is included in the code title.

Additional Z code aftercare category terms include fitting and adjustment, and attention to artificial openings.

Status Z codes may be used with aftercare Z codes to indicate the nature of the aftercare. For example code Z95.1, Presence of aortocoronary bypass graft, may be used with code Z48.812, Encounter for surgical aftercare following surgery on the circulatory system, to indicate the surgery for which the aftercare is being performed. A status code should not be used when the aftercare code indicates the type of status, such as using Z43.0, Encounter for attention to tracheostomy, with Z93.0, Tracheostomy status.

The aftercare Z category/codes:

Z42   Encounter for plastic and reconstructive surgery following medical procedure or healed injury
Z43   Encounter for attention to artificial openings
Z44   Encounter for fitting and adjustment of external prosthetic device
Z45   Encounter for adjustment and management of implanted device
Z46   Encounter for fitting and adjustment of other devices
Z47   Orthopedic aftercare
Z48   Encounter for other postprocedural aftercare
Z49   Encounter for care involving renal dialysis
Z51   Encounter for other aftercare

8) Follow-up

The follow-up codes are used to explain continuing surveillance following completed treatment of a disease, condition, or injury. They imply that the condition has been fully treated and no longer exists. They should not be confused with aftercare codes, or injury codes with a 7th character for subsequent encounter, that explain ongoing care of a healing condition or its sequelae. Follow-up codes may be used in conjunction with history codes to provide the full picture of the healed condition and its treatment. The follow-up code is sequenced first, followed by the history code.

A follow-up code may be used to explain multiple visits. Should a condition be found to have recurred on the follow-up visit, then the diagnosis code for the condition should be assigned in place of the follow-up code.

The follow-up Z code categories:

Z08   Encounter for follow-up examination after completed treatment for malignant neoplasm
Z09   Encounter for follow-up examination after completed treatment for conditions other than malignant neoplasm
Z39   Encounter for maternal postpartum care and examination

9) Donor

Codes in category Z52, Donors of organs and tissues, are used for living individuals who are donating blood or other body tissue. These codes are only for individuals donating for others, not for self-donations. They are not used to identify cadaveric donations.

CHAPTER 21 – FACTORS INFLUENCING HEALTH
Section I. C. 21. c. 10)

10) Counseling

Counseling Z codes are used when a patient or family member receives assistance in the aftermath of an illness or injury, or when support is required in coping with family or social problems. They are not used in conjunction with a diagnosis code when the counseling component of care is considered integral to standard treatment.

The counseling Z codes/categories:

Z30.0-	Encounter for general counseling and advice on contraception
Z31.5	Encounter for genetic counseling
Z31.6-	Encounter for general counseling and advice on procreation
Z32.2	Encounter for childbirth instruction
Z32.3	Encounter for childcare instruction
Z69	Encounter for mental health services for victim and perpetrator of abuse
Z70	Counseling related to sexual attitude, behavior and orientation
Z71	Persons encountering health services for other counseling and medical advice, not elsewhere classified
Z76.81	Expectant mother prebirth pediatrician visit

11) Encounters for Obstetrical and Reproductive Services

See Section I.C.15. Pregnancy, Childbirth, and the Puerperium, for further instruction on the use of these codes.

Z codes for pregnancy are for use in those circumstances when none of the problems or complications included in the codes from the Obstetrics chapter exist (a routine prenatal visit or postpartum care). Codes in category Z34, Encounter for supervision of normal pregnancy, are always first-listed and are not to be used with any other code from the OB chapter.

Codes in category Z3A, Weeks of gestation, may be assigned to provide additional information about the pregnancy. **The date of the admission should be used to determine weeks of gestation for inpatient admissions that encompass more than one gestational week.**

The outcome of delivery, category Z37, should be included on all maternal delivery records. It is always a secondary code. Codes in category Z37 should not be used on the newborn record.

Z codes for family planning (contraceptive) or procreative management and counseling should be included on an obstetric record either during the pregnancy or the postpartum stage, if applicable.

Z codes/categories for obstetrical and reproductive services:

Z30	Encounter for contraceptive management
Z31	Encounter for procreative management
Z32.2	Encounter for childbirth instruction
Z32.3	Encounter for childcare instruction
Z33	Pregnant state
Z34	Encounter for supervision of normal pregnancy
Z36	Encounter for antenatal screening of mother
Z3A	Weeks of gestation
Z37	Outcome of delivery
Z39	Encounter for maternal postpartum care and examination
Z76.81	Expectant mother prebirth pediatrician visit

12) Newborns and Infants

See Section I.C.16. Newborn (Perinatal) Guidelines, for further instruction on the use of these codes.

Newborn Z codes/categories:

Z76.1	Encounter for health supervision and care of foundling
Z00.1-	Encounter for routine child health examination
Z38	Liveborn infants according to place of birth and type of delivery

CHAPTER 21 – FACTORS INFLUENCING HEALTH
Section I. C. 21. c. 13)

13) Routine and administrative examinations

The Z codes allow for the description of encounters for routine examinations, such as, a general check-up, or, examinations for administrative purposes, such as, a pre-employment physical. The codes are not to be used if the examination is for diagnosis of a suspected condition or for treatment purposes. In such cases the diagnosis code is used. During a routine exam, should a diagnosis or condition be discovered, it should be coded as an additional code. Pre-existing and chronic conditions and history codes may also be included as additional codes as long as the examination is for administrative purposes and not focused on any particular condition.

Some of the codes for routine health examinations distinguish between "with" and "without" abnormal findings. Code assignment depends on the information that is known at the time the encounter is being coded. For example, if no abnormal findings were found during the examination, but the encounter is being coded before test results are back, it is acceptable to assign the code for "without abnormal findings." When assigning a code for "with abnormal findings," additional code(s) should be assigned to identify the specific abnormal finding(s).

Pre-operative examination and pre-procedural laboratory examination Z codes are for use only in those situations when a patient is being cleared for a procedure or surgery and no treatment is given.

The Z codes/categories for routine and administrative examinations:

Z00	Encounter for general examination without complaint, suspected or reported diagnosis
Z01	Encounter for other special examination without complaint, suspected or reported diagnosis
Z02	Encounter for administrative examination Except: Z02.9, Encounter for administrative examinations, unspecified
Z32.0-	Encounter for pregnancy test

14) Miscellaneous Z codes

The miscellaneous Z codes capture a number of other health care encounters that do not fall into one of the other categories. Certain of these codes identify the reason for the encounter; others are for use as additional codes that provide useful information on circumstances that may affect a patient's care and treatment.

Prophylactic Organ Removal

For encounters specifically for prophylactic removal of an organ (such as prophylactic removal of breasts due to a genetic susceptibility to cancer or a family history of cancer), the principal or first-listed code should be a code from category Z40, Encounter for prophylactic surgery, followed by the appropriate codes to identify the associated risk factor (such as genetic susceptibility or family history).

If the patient has a malignancy of one site and is having prophylactic removal at another site to prevent either a new primary malignancy or metastatic disease, a code for the malignancy should also be assigned in addition to a code from subcategory Z40.0, Encounter for prophylactic surgery for risk factors related to malignant neoplasms. A Z40.0 code should not be assigned if the patient is having organ removal for treatment of a malignancy, such as the removal of the testes for the treatment of prostate cancer.

Miscellaneous Z codes/categories:

Z28	Immunization not carried out Except: Z28.3, Underimmunization status
Z40	Encounter for prophylactic surgery
Z41	Encounter for procedures for purposes other than remedying health state Except: Z41.9, Encounter for procedure for purposes other than remedying health state, unspecified
Z53	Persons encountering health services for specific procedures and treatment, not carried out

Z55   Problems related to education and literacy
Z56   Problems related to employment and unemployment
Z57   Occupational exposure to risk factors
Z58   Problems related to physical environment
Z59   Problems related to housing and economic circumstances
Z60   Problems related to social environment
Z62   Problems related to upbringing
Z63   Other problems related to primary support group, including family circumstances
Z64   Problems related to certain psychosocial circumstances
Z65   Problems related to other psychosocial circumstances
Z72   Problems related to lifestyle
Z73   Problems related to life management difficulty
Z74   Problems related to care provider dependency
     Except: Z74.01, Bed confinement status
Z75   Problems related to medical facilities and other health care
Z76.0   Encounter for issue of repeat prescription
Z76.3   Healthy person accompanying sick person
Z76.4   Other boarder to healthcare facility
Z76.5   Malingerer [conscious simulation]
Z91.1-   Patient's noncompliance with medical treatment and regimen
Z91.83   Wandering in diseases classified elsewhere
Z91.89   Other specified personal risk factors, not elsewhere classified

15) Nonspecific Z codes

Certain Z codes are so non-specific, or potentially redundant with other codes in the classification, that there can be little justification for their use in the inpatient setting. Their use in the outpatient setting should be limited to those instances when there is no further documentation to permit more precise coding. Otherwise, any sign or symptom or any other reason for visit that is captured in another code should be used.

Nonspecific Z codes/categories:
Z02.9   Encounter for administrative examinations, unspecified
Z04.9   Encounter for examination and observation for unspecified reason
Z13.9   Encounter for screening, unspecified
Z41.9   Encounter for procedure for purposes other than remedying health state, unspecified
Z52.9   Donor of unspecified organ or tissue
Z86.59   Personal history of other mental and behavioral disorders
Z88.9   Allergy status to unspecified drugs, medicaments and biological substances status
Z92.0   Personal history of contraception

16) Z Codes That May Only be Principal/First-Listed Diagnosis

The following Z codes/categories may only be reported as the principal/first-listed diagnosis, except when there are multiple encounters on the same day and the medical records for the encounters are combined:

Z00   Encounter for general examination without complaint, suspected or reported diagnosis
Z01   Encounter for other special examination without complaint, suspected or reported diagnosis
Z02   Encounter for administrative examination
Z03   Encounter for medical observation for suspected diseases and conditions ruled out
Z04   Encounter for examination and observation for other reasons
Z31.81   Encounter for male factor infertility in female patient
Z31.82   Encounter for Rh incompatibility status
Z31.83   Encounter for assisted reproductive fertility procedure cycle
Z31.84   Encounter for fertility preservation procedure
Z34   Encounter for supervision of normal pregnancy
Z39   Encounter for maternal postpartum care and examination
Z38   Liveborn infants according to place of birth and type of delivery
Z42   Encounter for plastic and reconstructive surgery following medical procedure or healed injury
Z51.0   Encounter for antineoplastic radiation therapy
Z51.1-   Encounter for antineoplastic chemotherapy and immunotherapy
Z52   Donors of organs and tissues
     Except: Z52.9, Donor of unspecified organ or tissue
Z76.1   Encounter for health supervision and care of foundling
Z76.2   Encounter for health supervision and care of other healthy infant and child
Z99.12   Encounter for respirator [ventilator] dependence during power failure

SECTION II – PRINCIPAL DIAGNOSIS
Section II. A.

Section II. Selection of Principal Diagnosis

The circumstances of inpatient admission always govern the selection of principal diagnosis. The principal diagnosis is defined in the Uniform Hospital Discharge Data Set (UHDDS) as "that condition established after study to be chiefly responsible for occasioning the admission of the patient to the hospital for care."

The UHDDS definitions are used by hospitals to report inpatient data elements in a standardized manner. These data elements and their definitions can be found in the July 31, 1985, Federal Register (Vol. 50, No, 147), pp. 31038-40.

Since that time the application of the UHDDS definitions has been expanded to include all non-outpatient settings (acute care, short term, long term care and psychiatric hospitals; home health agencies; rehab facilities; nursing homes, etc).

In determining principal diagnosis the coding conventions in the ICD-10-CM, the Tabular List and Alphabetic Index take precedence over these official coding guidelines. *(See Section I.A., Conventions for the ICD-10-CM)*

The importance of consistent, complete documentation in the medical record cannot be overemphasized. Without such documentation the application of all coding guidelines is a difficult, if not impossible, task.

A. Codes for symptoms, signs, and ill-defined conditions
    Codes for symptoms, signs, and ill-defined conditions from Chapter 18 are not to be used as principal diagnosis when a related definitive diagnosis has been established.

B. Two or more interrelated conditions, each potentially meeting the definition for principal diagnosis.
    When there are two or more interrelated conditions (such as diseases in the same ICD-10-CM chapter or manifestations characteristically associated with a certain disease) potentially meeting the definition of principal diagnosis, either condition may be sequenced first, unless the circumstances of the admission, the therapy provided, the Tabular List, or the Alphabetic Index indicate otherwise.

C. Two or more diagnoses that equally meet the definition for principal diagnosis
    In the unusual instance when two or more diagnoses equally meet the criteria for principal diagnosis as determined by the circumstances of admission, diagnostic workup and/or therapy provided, and the Alphabetic Index, Tabular List, or another coding guidelines does not provide sequencing direction, any one of the diagnoses may be sequenced first.

D. Two or more comparative or contrasting conditions.
    In those rare instances when two or more contrasting or comparative diagnoses are documented as "either/or" (or similar terminology), they are coded as if the diagnoses were confirmed and the diagnoses are sequenced according to the circumstances of the admission. If no further determination can be made as to which diagnosis should be principal, either diagnosis may be sequenced first.

E. A symptom(s) followed by contrasting/comparative diagnoses
    When a symptom(s) is followed by contrasting/comparative diagnoses, the symptom code is sequenced first. **However, if the symptom code is integral to the conditions listed, no code for the symptom is reported.** All the contrasting/comparative diagnoses should be coded as additional diagnoses.

F. Original treatment plan not carried out
    Sequence as the principal diagnosis the condition, which after study occasioned the admission to the hospital, even though treatment may not have been carried out due to unforeseen circumstances.

SECTION II – PRINCIPAL DIAGNOSIS
Section II. G.

G. Complications of surgery and other medical care
    When the admission is for treatment of a complication resulting from surgery or other medical care, the complication code is sequenced as the principal diagnosis. If the complication is classified to the T80-T88 series and the code lacks the necessary specificity in describing the complication, an additional code for the specific complication should be assigned.

H. Uncertain Diagnosis
    If the diagnosis documented at the time of discharge is qualified as "probable", "suspected", "likely", "questionable", "possible", or "still to be ruled out", or other similar terms indicating uncertainty, code the condition as if it existed or was established. The bases for these guidelines are the diagnostic workup, arrangements for further workup or observation, and initial therapeutic approach that correspond most closely with the established diagnosis.

    Note: This guideline is applicable only to inpatient admissions to short-term, acute, long-term care and psychiatric hospitals.

I. Admission from Observation Unit

    1. Admission Following Medical Observation
        When a patient is admitted to an observation unit for a medical condition, which either worsens or does not improve, and is subsequently admitted as an inpatient of the same hospital for this same medical condition, the principal diagnosis would be the medical condition which led to the hospital admission.

    2. Admission Following Post-Operative Observation
        When a patient is admitted to an observation unit to monitor a condition (or complication) that develops following outpatient surgery, and then is subsequently admitted as an inpatient of the same hospital, hospitals should apply the Uniform Hospital Discharge Data Set (UHDDS) definition of principal diagnosis as "that condition established after study to be chiefly responsible for occasioning the admission of the patient to the hospital for care."

J. Admission from Outpatient Surgery
    When a patient receives surgery in the hospital's outpatient surgery department and is subsequently admitted for continuing inpatient care at the same hospital, the following guidelines should be followed in selecting the principal diagnosis for the inpatient admission:
        • If the reason for the inpatient admission is a complication, assign the complication as the principal diagnosis.
        • If no complication, or other condition, is documented as the reason for the inpatient admission, assign the reason for the outpatient surgery as the principal diagnosis.
        • If the reason for the inpatient admission is another condition unrelated to the surgery, assign the unrelated condition as the principal diagnosis.

K. Admission/Encounters for Rehabilitation
    When the purpose for the admission/encounter is rehabilitation, sequence first the code for the condition for which the service is being performed. For example, for an admission/encounter for rehabilitation right-sided dominant hemiplegia following a cerebrovascular infarction, report code I69.351, Hemiplegia and hemiparesis following cerebral infarction affecting right dominant side, as the first-listed or principal diagnosis.

    If the condition for which the rehabilitation service is no longer present, report the appropriate aftercare code as the first-listed or principal diagnosis. For example, if a patient with severe degenerative osteoarthritis of the hip, underwent hip replacement and the current encounter/admission is for rehabilitation, report code Z47.1, Aftercare following joint replacement surgery, as the principal diagnosis.

    See Section I.C.21.c.7, Factors influencing health status and contact with health services, Aftercare

SECTION III – ADDITIONAL DIAGNOSES
Section III. A.

Section III. Reporting Additional Diagnoses

GENERAL RULES FOR OTHER (ADDITIONAL) DIAGNOSES

For reporting purposes the definition for "other diagnoses" is interpreted as additional conditions that affect patient care in terms of requiring:

- clinical evaluation; or
- therapeutic treatment; or
- diagnostic procedures; or
- extended length of hospital stay; or
- increased nursing care and/or monitoring.

The UHDDS item #11-b defines Other Diagnoses as "all conditions that coexist at the time of admission, that develop subsequently, or that affect the treatment received and/or the length of stay. Diagnoses that relate to an earlier episode which have no bearing on the current hospital stay are to be excluded." UHDDS definitions apply to inpatients in acute care, short-term, long term care and psychiatric hospital setting. The UHDDS definitions are used by acute care short-term hospitals to report inpatient data elements in a standardized manner. These data elements and their definitions can be found in the July 31, 1985, Federal Register (Vol. 50, No, 147), pp. 31038-40.

Since that time the application of the UHDDS definitions has been expanded to include all non-outpatient settings (acute care, short term, long term care and psychiatric hospitals; home health agencies; rehab facilities; nursing homes, etc).

The following guidelines are to be applied in designating "other diagnoses" when neither the Alphabetic Index nor the Tabular List in ICD-10-CM provide direction. The listing of the diagnoses in the patient record is the responsibility of the attending provider.

A. Previous conditions

If the provider has included a diagnosis in the final diagnostic statement, such as the discharge summary or the face sheet, it should ordinarily be coded. Some providers include in the diagnostic statement resolved conditions or diagnoses and status-post procedures from previous admission that have no bearing on the current stay. Such conditions are not to be reported and are coded only if required by hospital policy.

However, history codes (categories Z80-Z87) may be used as secondary codes if the historical condition or family history has an impact on current care or influences treatment.

B. Abnormal findings

Abnormal findings (laboratory, x-ray, pathologic, and other diagnostic results) are not coded and reported unless the provider indicates their clinical significance. If the findings are outside the normal range and the attending provider has ordered other tests to evaluate the condition or prescribed treatment, it is appropriate to ask the provider whether the abnormal finding should be added.

Please note: This differs from the coding practices in the outpatient setting for coding encounters for diagnostic tests that have been interpreted by a provider.

C. Uncertain Diagnosis

If the diagnosis documented at the time of discharge is qualified as "probable", "suspected", "likely", "questionable", "possible", or "still to be ruled out" or other similar terms indicating uncertainty, code the condition as if it existed or was established. The bases for these guidelines are the diagnostic workup, arrangements for further workup or observation, and initial therapeutic approach that correspond most closely with the established diagnosis.

Note: This guideline is applicable only to inpatient admissions to short-term, acute, long-term care and psychiatric hospitals.

SECTION IV – OUTPATIENT GUIDELINES
Section IV. A.

Section IV. Diagnostic Coding and Reporting Guidelines for Outpatient Services

These coding guidelines for outpatient diagnoses have been approved for use by hospitals/ providers in coding and reporting hospital-based outpatient services and provider-based office visits.

Information about the use of certain abbreviations, punctuation, symbols, and other conventions used in the ICD-10-CM Tabular List (code numbers and titles), can be found in Section IA of these guidelines, under "Conventions Used in the Tabular List." **Section I.B. contains general guidelines that apply to the entire classification. Section I.C. contains chapter-specific guidelines that correspond to the chapters as they are arranged in the classification.** Information about the correct sequence to use in finding a code is also described in Section I.

The terms encounter and visit are often used interchangeably in describing outpatient service contacts and, therefore, appear together in these guidelines without distinguishing one from the other.

Though the conventions and general guidelines apply to all settings, coding guidelines for outpatient and provider reporting of diagnoses will vary in a number of instances from those for inpatient diagnoses, recognizing that:

The Uniform Hospital Discharge Data Set (UHDDS) definition of principal diagnosis applies only to inpatients in acute, short-term, long-term care and psychiatric hospitals.

Coding guidelines for inconclusive diagnoses (probable, suspected, rule out, etc.) were developed for inpatient reporting and do not apply to outpatients.

A. Selection of first-listed condition

In the outpatient setting, the term first-listed diagnosis is used in lieu of principal diagnosis.

In determining the first-listed diagnosis the coding conventions of ICD-10-CM, as well as the general and disease specific guidelines take precedence over the outpatient guidelines.

Diagnoses often are not established at the time of the initial encounter/visit. It may take two or more visits before the diagnosis is confirmed.

The most critical rule involves beginning the search for the correct code assignment through the Alphabetic Index. Never begin searching initially in the Tabular List as this will lead to coding errors.

1. Outpatient Surgery

When a patient presents for outpatient surgery (same day surgery), code the reason for the surgery as the first-listed diagnosis (reason for the encounter), even if the surgery is not performed due to a contraindication.

2. Observation Stay

When a patient is admitted for observation for a medical condition, assign a code for the medical condition as the first-listed diagnosis.

When a patient presents for outpatient surgery and develops complications requiring admission to observation, code the reason for the surgery as the first reported diagnosis (reason for the encounter), followed by codes for the complications as secondary diagnoses.

B. Codes from A00.0 through T88.9, Z00-Z99

The appropriate code(s) from A00.0 through T88.9, Z00-Z99 must be used to identify diagnoses, symptoms, conditions, problems, complaints, or other reason(s) for the encounter/visit.

SECTION IV – OUTPATIENT GUIDELINES
Section IV. C.

C. Accurate reporting of ICD-10-CM diagnosis codes

For accurate reporting of ICD-10-CM diagnosis codes, the documentation should describe the patient's condition, using terminology which includes specific diagnoses as well as symptoms, problems, or reasons for the encounter. There are ICD-10-CM codes to describe all of these.

D. Codes that describe symptoms and signs

Codes that describe symptoms and signs, as opposed to diagnoses, are acceptable for reporting purposes when a diagnosis has not been established (confirmed) by the provider. Chapter 18 of ICD-10-CM, Symptoms, Signs, and Abnormal Clinical and Laboratory Findings Not Elsewhere Classified (codes R00-R99) contain many, but not all codes for symptoms.

E. Encounters for circumstances other than a disease or injury

ICD-10-CM provides codes to deal with encounters for circumstances other than a disease or injury. The Factors Influencing Health Status and Contact with Health Services codes (Z00-Z99) are provided to deal with occasions when circumstances other than a disease or injury are recorded as diagnosis or problems.

See Section I.C.21. Factors influencing health status and contact with health services.

F. Level of Detail in Coding

1. **ICD-10-CM codes with 3, 4, 5, 6 or 7 characters**

   ICD-10-CM is composed of codes with 3, 4, 5, 6 or 7 characters. Codes with three characters are included in ICD-10-CM as the heading of a category of codes that may be further subdivided by the use of fourth, fifth, sixth or seventh characters to provide greater specificity.

2. **Use of full number of *characters* required for a code**

   A three-character code is to be used only if it is not further subdivided. A code is invalid if it has not been coded to the full number of characters required for that code, including the 7th character, if applicable.

G. ICD-10-CM code for the diagnosis, condition, problem, or other reason for encounter/visit

List first the ICD-10-CM code for the diagnosis, condition, problem, or other reason for encounter/visit shown in the medical record to be chiefly responsible for the services provided. List additional codes that describe any coexisting conditions. In some cases the first-listed diagnosis may be a symptom when a diagnosis has not been established (confirmed) by the physician.

H. Uncertain diagnosis

Do not code diagnoses documented as "probable", "suspected," "questionable," "rule out," or "working diagnosis" or other similar terms indicating uncertainty. Rather, code the condition(s) to the highest degree of certainty for that encounter/visit, such as symptoms, signs, abnormal test results, or other reason for the visit.

Please note: This differs from the coding practices used by short-term, acute care, long-term care and psychiatric hospitals.

I. Chronic diseases

Chronic diseases treated on an ongoing basis may be coded and reported as many times as the patient receives treatment and care for the condition(s)

J. Code all documented conditions that coexist

Code all documented conditions that coexist at the time of the encounter/visit, and require or affect patient care treatment or management. Do not code conditions that were previously treated and no longer exist. However, history codes (categories Z80-Z87) may be used as secondary codes if the historical condition or family history has an impact on current care or influences treatment.

SECTION IV – OUTPATIENT GUIDELINES
Section IV. K.

K. Patients receiving diagnostic services only

For patients receiving diagnostic services only during an encounter/visit, sequence first the diagnosis, condition, problem, or other reason for encounter/visit shown in the medical record to be chiefly responsible for the outpatient services provided during the encounter/visit. Codes for other diagnoses (e.g., chronic conditions) may be sequenced as additional diagnoses.

For encounters for routine laboratory/radiology testing in the absence of any signs, symptoms, or associated diagnosis, assign Z01.89, Encounter for other specified special examinations. If routine testing is performed during the same encounter as a test to evaluate a sign, symptom, or diagnosis, it is appropriate to assign both the Z code and the code describing the reason for the non-routine test.

For outpatient encounters for diagnostic tests that have been interpreted by a physician, and the final report is available at the time of coding, code any confirmed or definitive diagnosis(es) documented in the interpretation. Do not code related signs and symptoms as additional diagnoses.

Please note: This differs from the coding practice in the hospital inpatient setting regarding abnormal findings on test results.

L. Patients receiving therapeutic services only

For patients receiving therapeutic services only during an encounter/visit, sequence first the diagnosis, condition, problem, or other reason for encounter/visit shown in the medical record to be chiefly responsible for the outpatient services provided during the encounter/visit. Codes for other diagnoses (e.g., chronic conditions) may be sequenced as additional diagnoses.

The only exception to this rule is that when the primary reason for the admission/encounter is chemotherapy or radiation therapy, the appropriate Z code for the service is listed first, and the diagnosis or problem for which the service is being performed listed second.

M. Patients receiving preoperative evaluations only

For patients receiving preoperative evaluations only, sequence first a code from subcategory Z01.81, Encounter for pre-procedural examinations, to describe the pre-op consultations. Assign a code for the condition to describe the reason for the surgery as an additional diagnosis. Code also any findings related to the pre-op evaluation.

N. Ambulatory surgery

For ambulatory surgery, code the diagnosis for which the surgery was performed. If the postoperative diagnosis is known to be different from the preoperative diagnosis at the time the diagnosis is confirmed, select the postoperative diagnosis for coding, since it is the most definitive.

O. Routine outpatient prenatal visits

See Section I.C.15. Routine outpatient prenatal visits.

P. Encounters for general medical examinations with abnormal findings

The subcategories for encounters for general medical examinations, Z00.0-, provide codes for with and without abnormal findings. Should a general medical examination result in an abnormal finding, the code for general medical examination with abnormal finding should be assigned as the **first-listed** diagnosis. A secondary code for the abnormal finding should also be coded.

Q. Encounters for routine health screenings

See Section I.C.21. Factors influencing health status and contact with health services, Screening

Appendix I
Present on Admission Reporting Guidelines

Introduction

These guidelines are to be used as a supplement to the *ICD-10-CM Official Guidelines for Coding and Reporting* to facilitate the assignment of the Present on Admission (POA) indicator for each diagnosis and external cause of injury code reported on claim forms (UB-04 and 837 Institutional).

These guidelines are not intended to replace any guidelines in the main body of the *ICD-10-CM Official Guidelines for Coding and Reporting*. The POA guidelines are not intended to provide guidance on when a condition should be coded, but rather, how to apply the POA indicator to the final set of diagnosis codes that have been assigned in accordance with Sections I, II, and III of the official coding guidelines. Subsequent to the assignment of the ICD-10-CM codes, the POA indicator should then be assigned to those conditions that have been coded.

As stated in the Introduction to the ICD-10-CM Official Guidelines for Coding and Reporting, a joint effort between the healthcare provider and the coder is essential to achieve complete and accurate documentation, code assignment, and reporting of diagnoses and procedures. The importance of consistent, complete documentation in the medical record cannot be overemphasized. Medical record documentation from any provider involved in the care and treatment of the patient may be used to support the determination of whether a condition was present on admission or not. In the context of the official coding guidelines, the term "provider" means a physician or any qualified healthcare practitioner who is legally accountable for establishing the patient's diagnosis.

These guidelines are not a substitute for the provider's clinical judgment as to the determination of whether a condition was/was not present on admission. The provider should be queried regarding issues related to the linking of signs/symptoms, timing of test results, and the timing of findings.

General Reporting Requirements

All claims involving inpatient admissions to general acute care hospitals or other facilities that are subject to a law or regulation mandating collection of present on admission information.

Present on admission is defined as present at the time the order for inpatient admission occurs – conditions that develop during an outpatient encounter, including emergency department, observation, or outpatient surgery, are considered as present on admission.

POA indicator is assigned to principal and secondary diagnoses (as defined in Section II of the Official Guidelines for Coding and Reporting) and the external cause of injury codes.

Issues related to inconsistent, missing, conflicting or unclear documentation must still be resolved by the provider.

If a condition would not be coded and reported based on UHDDS definitions and current official coding guidelines, then the POA indicator would not be reported.

Reporting Options
Y - Yes
N - No
U - Unknown
W – Clinically undetermined
Unreported/Not used (or "1" for Medicare usage) – (Exempt from POA reporting)

Reporting Definitions
Y = present at the time of inpatient admission
N = not present at the time of inpatient admission
U = documentation is insufficient to determine if condition is present on admission
W = provider is unable to clinically determine whether condition was present on admission or not

Timeframe for POA Identification and Documentation

There is no required timeframe as to when a provider (per the definition of "provider" used in these guidelines) must identify or document a condition to be present on admission. In some clinical situations, it may not be possible for a provider to make a definitive diagnosis (or a condition may not be recognized or reported by the patient) for a period of time after admission. In some cases it may be several days before the provider arrives at a definitive diagnosis. This does not mean that the condition was not present on admission. Determination of whether the condition was present on admission or not will be based on the applicable POA guideline as identified in this document, or on the provider's best clinical judgment.

If at the time of code assignment the documentation is unclear as to whether a condition was present on admission or not, it is appropriate to query the provider for clarification.

Assigning the POA Indicator

Condition is on the "Exempt from Reporting" list
Leave the "present on admission" field blank if the condition is on the list of ICD-10-CM codes for which this field is not applicable. This is the only circumstance in which the field may be left blank.

POA Explicitly Documented
Assign Y for any condition the provider explicitly documents as being present on admission.

Assign N for any condition the provider explicitly documents as not present at the time of admission.

Conditions diagnosed prior to inpatient admission
Assign "Y" for conditions that were diagnosed prior to admission (example: hypertension, diabetes mellitus, asthma)

Conditions diagnosed during the admission but clearly present before admission
Assign "Y" for conditions diagnosed during the admission that were clearly present but not diagnosed until after admission occurred.

Diagnoses subsequently confirmed after admission are considered present on admission if at the time of admission they are documented as suspected, possible, rule out, differential diagnosis, or constitute an underlying cause of a symptom that is present at the time of admission.

Condition develops during outpatient encounter prior to inpatient admission
Assign Y for any condition that develops during an outpatient encounter prior to a written order for inpatient admission.

Documentation does not indicate whether condition was present on admission
Assign "U" when the medical record documentation is unclear as to whether the condition was present on admission. "U" should not be routinely assigned and used only in very limited circumstances. Coders are encouraged to query the providers when the documentation is unclear.

Documentation states that it cannot be determined whether the condition was or was not present on admission
Assign "W" when the medical record documentation indicates that it cannot be clinically determined whether or not the condition was present on admission.

APPENDIX I – POA GUIDELINES
Appendix I.

Chronic condition with acute exacerbation during the admission

If a single code identifies both the chronic condition and the acute exacerbation, see POA guidelines pertaining to combination codes.

If a single code only identifies the chronic condition and not the acute exacerbation (e.g., acute exacerbation of chronic leukemia), assign "Y."

Conditions documented as possible, probable, suspected, or rule out at the time of discharge

If the final diagnosis contains a possible, probable, suspected, or rule out diagnosis, and this diagnosis was based on signs, symptoms or clinical findings suspected at the time of inpatient admission, assign "Y."

If the final diagnosis contains a possible, probable, suspected, or rule out diagnosis, and this diagnosis was based on signs, symptoms or clinical findings that were not present on admission, assign "N".

Conditions documented as impending or threatened at the time of discharge

If the final diagnosis contains an impending or threatened diagnosis, and this diagnosis is based on symptoms or clinical findings that were present on admission, assign "Y".

If the final diagnosis contains an impending or threatened diagnosis, and this diagnosis is based on symptoms or clinical findings that were not present on admission, assign "N".

Acute and Chronic Conditions

Assign "Y" for acute conditions that are present at time of admission and N for acute conditions that are not present at time of admission.

Assign "Y" for chronic conditions, even though the condition may not be diagnosed until after admission.

If a single code identifies both an acute and chronic condition, see the POA guidelines for combination codes.

Combination Codes

Assign "N" if any part of the combination code was not present on admission (e.g., COPD with acute exacerbation and the exacerbation was not present on admission; gastric ulcer that does not start bleeding until after admission; asthma patient develops status asthmaticus after admission)

Assign "Y" if all parts of the combination code were present on admission (e.g., patient with acute prostatitis admitted with hematuria)

If the final diagnosis includes comparative or contrasting diagnoses, and both were present, or suspected, at the time of admission, assign "Y".

For infection codes that include the causal organism, assign "Y" if the infection (or signs of the infection) was present on admission, even though the culture results may not be known until after admission (e.g., patient is admitted with pneumonia and the provider documents pseudomonas as the causal organism a few days later).

APPENDIX I – POA GUIDELINES
Appendix I.

Same Diagnosis Code for Two or More Conditions

When the same ICD-10-CM diagnosis code applies to two or more conditions during the same encounter (e.g. two separate conditions classified to the same ICD-10-CM diagnosis code):

Assign "Y" if all conditions represented by the single ICD-10-CM code were present on admission (e.g. bilateral unspecified age-related cataracts).

Assign "N" if any of the conditions represented by the single ICD-10-CM code was not present on admission (e.g. traumatic secondary and recurrent hemorrhage and seroma is assigned to a single code T79.2, but only one of the conditions was present on admission).

Obstetrical conditions

Whether or not the patient delivers during the current hospitalization does not affect assignment of the POA indicator. The determining factor for POA assignment is whether the pregnancy complication or obstetrical condition described by the code was present at the time of admission or not.

If the pregnancy complication or obstetrical condition was present on admission (e.g., patient admitted in preterm labor), assign "Y".

If the pregnancy complication or obstetrical condition was not present on admission (e.g., 2nd degree laceration during delivery, postpartum hemorrhage that occurred during current hospitalization, fetal distress develops after admission), assign "N".

If the obstetrical code includes more than one diagnosis and any of the diagnoses identified by the code were not present on admission assign "N" (e.g., Category O11, Pre-existing hypertension with pre-eclampsia).

Perinatal conditions

Newborns are not considered to be admitted until after birth. Therefore, any condition present at birth or that developed in utero is considered present at admission and should be assigned "Y". This includes conditions that occur during delivery (e.g., injury during delivery, meconium aspiration, exposure to streptococcus B in the vaginal canal).

Congenital conditions and anomalies

Assign "Y" for congenital conditions and anomalies except for categories Q00-Q99, Congenital anomalies, which are on the exempt list. Congenital conditions are always considered present on admission.

External cause of injury codes

Assign "Y" for any external cause code representing an external cause of morbidity that occurred prior to inpatient admission (e.g., patient fell out of bed at home, patient fell out of bed in emergency room prior to admission).

Assign "N" for any external cause code representing an external cause of morbidity that occurred during inpatient hospitalization (e.g., patient fell out of hospital bed during hospital stay, patient experienced an adverse reaction to a medication administered after inpatient admission).

APPENDIX I – POA GUIDELINES
Appendix I.

**Categories and Codes
Exempt from
Diagnosis Present on Admission Requirement**

Note: "Diagnosis present on admission" for these code categories are exempt because they represent circumstances regarding the healthcare encounter or factors influencing health status that do not represent a current disease or injury or are always present on admission.

B90-B94	Sequelae of infectious and parasitic diseases
E64	Sequelae of malnutrition and other nutritional deficiencies
I25.2	Old myocardial infarction
I69	Sequelae of cerebrovascular disease
O09	Supervision of high risk pregnancy
O66.5	Attempted application of vacuum extractor and forceps
O80	Encounter for full-term uncomplicated delivery
O94	Sequelae of complication of pregnancy, childbirth, and the puerperium
P00	Newborn (suspected to be) affected by maternal conditions that may be unrelated to present pregnancy
Q00-Q99	Congenital malformations, deformations and chromosomal abnormalities
S00-T88.9	Injury, poisoning and certain other consequences of external causes with 7th character representing subsequent encounter or sequela
V00-V09	Pedestrian injured in transport accident
	Except V00.81- Accident with wheelchair (powered)
	Except V00.83- Accident with motorized mobility scooter
V10-V19	Pedal cycle rider injured in transport accident
V20-V29	Motorcycle cycle rider injured in transport accident
V30-V39	Occupant of three-wheeled motor vehicle injured in transport accident
V40-V49	Car occupant injured in transport accident
V50-V59	Occupant of pick-up truck or van injured in transport accident
V60-V69	Occupant of heavy transport vehicle injured in transport accident
V70-V79	Bus occupant injured in transport accident
V80-V89	Other land transport accidents
V90-V94	Water transport accidents
V95-V97	Air and space transport accidents
V98-V99	Other and unspecified transport accidents
W09	Fall on and from playground equipment
W14	Fall from tree
W15	Fall from cliff
W17.0	Fall into well
W17.1	Fall into storm drain or manhole
W18.01	Striking against sports equipment with subsequent fall
W21	Striking against or struck by sports equipment
W30	Contact with agricultural machinery
W31	Contact with other and unspecified machinery
W32-W34	Accidental handgun discharge and malfunction
W35-W40	Exposure to inanimate mechanical forces
W52	Crushed, pushed or stepped on by crowd or human stampede
W56	Contact with nonvenomous marine animal
W58	Contact with crocodile or alligator
W61	Contact with birds (domestic) (wild)
W62	Contact with nonvenomous amphibians
W89	Exposure to man-made visible and ultraviolet light

X02	Exposure to controlled fire in building or structure
X03	Exposure to controlled fire, not in building or structure
X04	Exposure to ignition of highly flammable material
X52	Prolonged stay in weightless environment
X71	Intentional self-harm by drowning and submersion
	Except X71.0- Intentional self-harm by drowning and submersion while in bath tub
X72	Intentional self-harm by handgun discharge
X73	Intentional self-harm by rifle, shotgun and larger firearm discharge
X74	Intentional self-harm by other and unspecified firearm and gun discharge
X75	Intentional self-harm by explosive material
X76	Intentional self-harm by smoke, fire and flames
X77	Intentional self-harm by steam, hot vapors and hot objects
X81	Intentional self-harm by jumping or lying in front of moving object
X82	Intentional self-harm by crashing of motor vehicle
X83	Intentional self-harm by other specified means
Y03	**Assault by crashing of motor vehicle**
Y07	**Perpetrator of assault, maltreatment and neglect**
Y08.8	**Assault by strike by sports equipment**
Y21	Drowning and submersion, undetermined intent
Y22	Handgun discharge, undetermined intent
Y23	Rifle, shotgun and larger firearm discharge, undetermined intent
Y24	Other and unspecified firearm discharge, undetermined intent
Y30	Falling, jumping or pushed from a high place, undetermined intent
Y32	**Assault by crashing of motor vehicle, undetermined intent**
Y36	Operations of war
Y37	Military operations
Y92	Place of occurrence of the external cause
Y93	Activity code
Y99	External cause status
Z00	Encounter for general examination without complaint, suspected or reported diagnosis
Z01	Encounter for other special examination without complaint, suspected or reported diagnosis
Z02	Encounter for administrative examination
Z03	Encounter for medical observation for suspected diseases and conditions ruled out
Z08	Encounter for follow-up examination following completed treatment for malignant neoplasm
Z09	Encounter for follow-up examination after completed treatment for conditions other than malignant neoplasm
Z11	Encounter for screening for infectious and parasitic diseases
Z11.8	Encounter for screening for other infectious and parasitic diseases
Z12	Encounter for screening for malignant neoplasms
Z13	Encounter for screening for other diseases and disorders
Z13.4	Encounter for screening for certain developmental disorders in childhood
Z13.5	Encounter for screening for eye and ear disorders
Z13.6	Encounter for screening for cardiovascular disorders
Z13.83	Encounter for screening for respiratory disorder NEC
Z13.89	Encounter for screening for other disorder (Inclusion term - Encounter for screening for genitourinary disorders)
Z13.89	Encounter for screening for other disorder
Z14	Genetic carrier
Z15	Genetic susceptibility to disease
Z17	Estrogen receptor status
Z18	Retained foreign body fragments
Z22	Carrier of infectious disease
Z23	Encounter for immunization
Z28	Immunization not carried out and underimmunization status
Z28.3	Underimmunization status
Z30	Encounter for contraceptive management
Z31	Encounter for procreative management

APPENDIX I – POA GUIDELINES
Appendix I.

Z34	Encounter for supervision of normal pregnancy
Z36	Encounter for antenatal screening of mother
Z37	Outcome of delivery
Z38	Liveborn infants according to place of birth and type of delivery
Z39	Encounter for maternal postpartum care and examination
Z41	Encounter for procedures for purposes other than remedying health state
Z42	Encounter for plastic and reconstructive surgery following medical procedure or healed injury
Z43	Encounter for attention to artificial openings
Z44	Encounter for fitting and adjustment of external prosthetic device
Z45	Encounter for adjustment and management of implanted device
Z46	Encounter for fitting and adjustment of other devices
Z47.8	Encounter for other orthopedic aftercare
Z49	Encounter for care involving renal dialysis
Z51	Encounter for other aftercare
Z51.5	Encounter for palliative care
Z51.8	Encounter for other specified aftercare
Z52	Donors of organs and tissues
Z59	Problems related to housing and economic circumstances
Z63	Other problems related to primary support group, including family circumstances
Z65	Problems related to other psychosocial circumstances
Z65.8	Other specified problems related to psychosocial circumstances
Z67.1-Z67.9	Blood type
Z68	Body mass index (BMI)
Z72	Problems related to lifestyle
Z74.01	Bed confinement status
Z76	Persons encountering health services in other circumstances
Z77.110 -Z77.128	Environmental pollution and hazards in the physical environment
Z78	Other specified health status
Z79	Long term (current) drug therapy
Z80	Family history of primary malignant neoplasm
Z81	Family history of mental and behavioral disorders
Z82	Family history of certain disabilities and chronic diseases (leading to disablement)
Z83	Family history of other specific disorders
Z84	Family history of other conditions
Z85	Personal history of primary malignant neoplasm
Z86	Personal history of certain other diseases
Z87	Personal history of other diseases and conditions
Z87.828	Personal history of other (healed) physical injury and trauma
Z87.891	Personal history of nicotine dependence
Z88	Allergy status to drugs, medicaments and biological substances
Z89	Acquired absence of limb
Z90.710	Acquired absence of both cervix and uterus
Z91.0	Allergy status, other than to drugs and biological substances
Z91.4	Personal history of psychological trauma, not elsewhere classified
Z91.5	Personal history of self-harm
Z91.8	Other specified risk factors, not elsewhere classified
Z92	Personal history of medical treatment
Z93	Artificial opening status
Z94	Transplanted organ and tissue status
Z95	Presence of cardiac and vascular implants and grafts
Z97	Presence of other devices
Z98	Other postprocedural states
Z99	Dependence on enabling machines and devices, not elsewhere classified

GUIDELINES

A

Aarskog's syndrome Q87.1
Abandonment — *see* Maltreatment
Abasia (-astasia) (hysterical) F44.4
Abderhalden-Kaufmann-Lignac syndrome (cystinosis) E72.04
Abdomen, abdominal — *see also* condition
　acute R10.0
　angina K55.1
　muscle deficiency syndrome Q79.4
Abdominalgia — *see* Pain, abdominal
Abduction contracture, hip or other joint — *see* Contraction, joint
Aberrant (congenital) — *see also* Malposition, congenital
　adrenal gland Q89.1
　artery (peripheral) Q27.8
　　basilar NEC Q28.1
　　cerebral Q28.3
　　coronary Q24.5
　　digestive system Q27.8
　　eye Q15.8
　　lower limb Q27.8
　　precerebral Q28.1
　　pulmonary Q25.79
　　renal Q27.2
　　retina Q14.1
　　specified site NEC Q27.8
　　subclavian Q27.8
　　upper limb Q27.8
　　vertebral Q28.1
　breast Q83.8
　endocrine gland NEC Q89.2
　hepatic duct Q44.5
　pancreas Q45.3
　parathyroid gland Q89.2
　pituitary gland Q89.2
　sebaceous glands, mucous membrane, mouth, congenital Q38.6
　spleen Q89.09
　subclavian artery Q27.8
　thymus (gland) Q89.2
　thyroid gland Q89.2
　vein (peripheral) NEC Q27.8
　　cerebral Q28.3
　　digestive system Q27.8
　　lower limb Q27.8
　　precerebral Q28.1
　　specified site NEC Q27.8
　　upper limb Q27.8
Aberration
　distantial — *see* Disturbance, visual
　mental F99
Abetalipoproteinemia E78.6
Abiotrophy R68.89
Ablatio, ablation
　retinae — *see* Detachment, retina
Ablepharia, ablepharon Q10.3
Abnormal, abnormality, abnormalities — *see also* Anomaly
　acid-base balance (mixed) E87.4
　albumin R77.0
　alphafetoprotein R77.2
　alveolar ridge K08.9
　anatomical relationship Q89.9
　apertures, congenital, diaphragm Q79.1
　auditory perception H93.29-
　　diplacusis — *see* Diplacusis
　　hyperacusis — *see* Hyperacusis
　　recruitment — *see* Recruitment, auditory
　　threshold shift — *see* Shift, auditory threshold
　autosomes Q99.9
　　fragile site Q95.5
　basal metabolic rate R94.8
　biosynthesis, testicular androgen E29.1
　bleeding time R79.1
　blood level (of)
　　cobalt R79.0
　　copper R79.0
　　iron R79.0
　　lithium R78.89
　　magnesium R79.0
　　mineral NEC R79.0
　　zinc R79.0
　blood pressure
　　elevated R03.0
　　low reading (nonspecific) R03.1
　blood sugar R73.09
　blood-gas level R79.81
　bowel sounds R19.15
　　absent R19.11
　　hyperactive R19.12
　brain scan R94.02
　breathing R06.9

Abnormal, abnormality, abnormalities (*see also* Anomaly) — *continued*
　caloric test R94.138
　cerebrospinal fluid R83.9
　　cytology R83.6
　　drug level R83.2
　　enzyme level R83.0
　　hormones R83.1
　　immunology R83.4
　　microbiology R83.5
　　nonmedicinal level R83.3
　　specified type NEC R83.8
　chemistry, blood R79.9
　　C-reactive protein R79.82
　　drugs — *see* Findings, abnormal, in blood
　　gas level R79.81
　　minerals R79.0
　　pancytopenia D61.818
　　PTT R79.1
　　specified NEC R79.89
　　toxins — *see* Findings, abnormal, in blood
　chest sounds (friction) (rales) R09.89
　chromosome, chromosomal Q99.9
　　with more than three X chromosomes, female Q97.1
　　analysis result R89.8
　　　bronchial washings R84.8
　　　cerebrospinal fluid R83.8
　　　cervix uteri NEC R87.89
　　　nasal secretions R84.8
　　　nipple discharge R89.8
　　　peritoneal fluid R85.89
　　　pleural fluid R84.8
　　　prostatic secretions R86.8
　　　saliva R85.89
　　　seminal fluid R86.8
　　　sputum R84.8
　　　synovial fluid R89.8
　　　throat scrapings R84.8
　　　vagina R87.89
　　　vulva R87.89
　　　wound secretions R89.8
　　dicentric replacement Q93.2
　　ring replacement Q93.2
　　sex Q99.8
　　　female phenotype Q97.9
　　　　specified NEC Q97.8
　　　male phenotype Q98.9
　　　　specified NEC Q98.8
　　　structural male Q98.6
　　specified NEC Q99.8
　clinical findings NEC R68.89
　coagulation D68.9
　　newborn, transient P61.6
　　profile R79.1
　　time R79.1
　communication — *see* Fistula
　conjunctiva, vascular H11.41-
　coronary artery Q24.5
　cortisol-binding globulin E27.8
　course, eustachian tube Q17.8
　creatinine clearance R94.4
　cytology
　　anus R85.619
　　　atypical squamous cells cannot exclude high grade squamous intraepithelial lesion (ASC-H) R85.611
　　　atypical squamous cells of undetermined significance (ASC-US) R85.610
　　　cytologic evidence of malignancy R85.614
　　　high grade squamous intraepithelial lesion (HGSIL) R85.613
　　　human papillomavirus (HPV) DNA test
　　　　high risk positive R85.81
　　　　low risk postive R85.82
　　　inadequate smear R85.615
　　　low grade squamous intraepithelial lesion (LGSIL) R85.612
　　　satisfactory anal smear but lacking transformation zone R85.616
　　　specified NEC R85.618
　　　unsatisfactory smear R85.615
　　female genital organs — *see* Abnormal, Papanicolaou (smear)
　dark adaptation curve H53.61
　dentofacial NEC — *see* Anomaly, dentofacial
　development, developmental Q89.9
　　central nervous system Q07.9

Abnormal, abnormality, abnormalities (*see also* Anomaly) — *continued*
　diagnostic imaging
　　abdomen, abdominal region NEC R93.5
　　biliary tract R93.2
　　breast R92.8
　　central nervous system NEC R90.89
　　cerebrovascular NEC R90.89
　　coronary circulation R93.1
　　digestive tract NEC R93.3
　　gastrointestinal (tract) R93.3
　　genitourinary organs R93.8
　　head R93.0
　　heart R93.1
　　intrathoracic organ NEC R93.8
　　limbs R93.6
　　liver R93.2
　　lung (field) R91.8
　　musculoskeletal system NEC R93.7
　　retroperitoneum R93.5
　　site specified NEC R93.8
　　skin and subcutaneous tissue R93.8
　　skull R93.0
　　urinary organs R93.4
　direction, teeth, fully erupted M26.30
　ear ossicles, acquired NEC H74.39-
　　ankylosis — *see* Ankylosis, ear ossicles
　　discontinuity — *see* Discontinuity, ossicles, ear
　　partial loss — *see* Loss, ossicles, ear (partial)
　Ebstein Q22.5
　echocardiogram R93.1
　echoencephalogram R90.81
　echogram — *see* Abnormal, diagnostic imaging
　electro-oculogram [EOG] R94.110
　electrocardiogram [ECG] [EKG] R94.31
　electroencephalogram [EEG] R94.01
　electrolyte — *see* Imbalance, electrolyte
　electromyogram [EMG] R94.131
　electrophysiological intracardiac studies R94.39
　electroretinogram [ERG] R94.111
　erythrocytes
　　congenital, with perinatal jaundice D58.9
　feces (color) (contents) (mucus) R19.5
　finding — *see* Findings, abnormal, without diagnosis
　fluid
　　amniotic — *see* Abnormal, specimen, specified
　　cerebrospinal — *see* Abnormal, cerebrospinal fluid
　　peritoneal — *see* Abnormal, specimen, digestive organs
　　pleural — *see* Abnormal, specimen, respiratory organs
　　synovial — *see* Abnormal, specimen, specified
　　thorax (bronchial washings) (pleural fluid) — *see* Abnormal, specimen, respiratory organs
　　vaginal — *see* Abnormal, specimen, female genital organs
　form
　　teeth K00.2
　　uterus — *see* Anomaly, uterus
　function studies
　　auditory R94.120
　　bladder R94.8
　　brain R94.09
　　cardiovascular R94.30
　　ear R94.128
　　endocrine NEC R94.7
　　eye NEC R94.118
　　kidney R94.4
　　liver R94.5
　　nervous system
　　　central NEC R94.09
　　　peripheral NEC R94.138
　　pancreas R94.8
　　placenta R94.8
　　pulmonary R94.2
　　special senses NEC R94.128
　　spleen R94.8
　　thyroid R94.6
　　vestibular R94.121
　gait — *see* Gait
　　hysterical F44.4
　gastrin secretion E16.4
　globulin R77.1
　　cortisol-binding E27.8
　　thyroid-binding E07.89
　glomerular, minor (*see also* N00-N07 with fourth character .0) N05.0
　glucagon secretion E16.3
　glucose tolerance (test) (non-fasting) R73.09

Abnormal, abnormality, abnormalities (*see also* Anomaly) — *continued*
　gravitational (G) forces or states (effect of) T75.81
　hair (color) (shaft) L67.9
　　specified NEC L67.8
　hard tissue formation in pulp (dental) K04.3
　head movement R25.0
　heart
　　rate R00.9
　　　specified NEC R00.8
　　shadow R93.1
　　sounds NEC R01.2
　hemoglobin (disease) (*see also* Disease, hemoglobin) D58.2
　　trait — *see* Trait, hemoglobin, abnormal
　histology NEC R89.7
　immunological findings R89.4
　　in serum R76.9
　　　specified NEC R76.8
　increase in appetite R63.2
　involuntary movement — *see* Abnormal, movement, involuntary
　jaw closure M26.51
　karyotype R89.8
　kidney function test R94.4
　knee jerk R29.2
　leukocyte (cell) (differential) NEC D72.9
　liver
　loss of
　　height R29.890
　　weight R63.4
　mammogram NEC R92.8
　　calcification (calculus) R92.1
　　microcalcification R92.0
　Mantoux test R76.11
　movement (disorder) — *see also* Disorder, movement
　　head R25.0
　　involuntary R25.9
　　　fasciculation R25.3
　　　of head R25.0
　　　spasm R25.2
　　　specified type NEC R25.8
　　　tremor R25.1
　myoglobin (Aberdeen) (Annapolis) R89.7
　neonatal screening P09
　oculomotor study R94.113
　palmar creases Q82.8
　Papanicolaou (smear)
　　anus R85.619
　　　atypical squamous cells cannot exclude high grade squamous intraepithelial lesion (ASC-H) R85.611
　　　atypical squamous cells of undetermined significance (ASC-US) R85.610
　　　cytologic evidence of malignancy R85.614
　　　high grade squamous intraepithelial lesion (HGSIL) R85.613
　　　human papillomavirus (HPV) DNA test
　　　　high risk positive R85.81
　　　　low risk postive R85.82
　　　inadequate smear R85.615
　　　low grade squamous intraepithelial lesion (LGSIL) R85.612
　　　satisfactory anal smear but lacking transformation zone R85.616
　　　specified NEC R85.618
　　　unsatisfactory smear R85.615
　　bronchial washings R84.6
　　cerebrospinal fluid R83.6
　　cervix R87.619
　　　atypical squamous cells cannot exclude high grade squamous intraepithelial lesion (ASC-H) R87.611
　　　atypical squamous cells of undetermined significance (ASC-US) R87.610
　　　cytologic evidence of malignancy R87.614
　　　high grade squamous intraepithelial lesion (HGSIL) R87.613
　　　inadequate smear R87.615
　　　low grade squamous intraepithelial lesion (LGSIL) R87.612
　　　non-atypical endometrial cells R87.619
　　　satisfactory cervical smear but lacking transformation zone R87.616
　　　specified NEC R87.618
　　　thin preparaton R87.619
　　　unsatisfactory smear R87.615
　　nasal secretions R84.6
　　nipple discharge R89.6

DISEASE INDEX

Abnormal, abnormality, abnormalities (see also Anomaly) — continued
Papanicolaou (smear) — continued
  peritoneal fluid R85.69
  pleural fluid R84.6
  prostatic secretions R86.6
  saliva R85.69
  seminal fluid R86.6
  sites NEC R89.6
  sputum R84.6
  synovial fluid R89.6
  throat scrapings R84.6
  vagina R87.629
    atypical squamous cells cannot exclude high grade squamous intraepithelial lesion (ASC-H) R87.621
    atypical squamous cells of undetermined significance (ASC-US) R87.620
    cytologic evidence of malignancy R87.624
    high grade squamous intraepithelial lesion (HGSIL) R87.623
    inadequate smear R87.625
    low grade squamous intraepithelial lesion (LGSIL) R87.622
    specified NEC R87.628
    thin preparation R87.629
    unsatisfactory smear R87.625
  vulva R87.69
  wound secretions R89.6
partial thromboplastin time (PTT) R79.1
pelvis (bony) — see Deformity, pelvis
percussion, chest (tympany) R09.89
periods (grossly) — see Menstruation
phonocardiogram R94.39
plantar reflex R29.2
plasma
  protein R77.9
    specified NEC R77.8
  viscosity R70.1
pleural (folds) Q34.0
posture R29.3
product of conception O02.9
  specified type NEC O02.89
prothrombin time (PT) R79.1
pulmonary
  artery, congenital Q25.79
  function, newborn P28.89
  test results R94.2
pulsations in neck R00.2
pupillary H21.56-
  function (reaction) (reflex) — see Anomaly, pupil, function
radiological examination — see Abnormal, diagnostic imaging
red blood cell(s) (morphology) (volume) R71.8
reflex — see Reflex
renal function test R94.4
response to nerve stimulation R94.130
retinal correspondence H53.31
retinal function study R94.111
rhythm, heart — see also Arrhythmia
saliva — see Abnormal, specimen, digestive organs
scan
  kidney R94.4
  liver R93.2
  thyroid R94.6
secretion
  gastrin E16.4
  glucagon E16.3
semen, seminal fluid — see Abnormal, specimen, male genital organs
serum level (of)
  acid phosphatase R74.8
  alkaline phosphatase R74.8
  amylase R74.8
  enzymes R74.9
    specified NEC R74.8
  lipase R74.8
  triacylglycerol lipase R74.8
shape
  gravid uterus — see Anomaly, uterus
sinus venosus Q21.1
size, tooth, teeth K00.2
spacing, tooth, teeth, fully erupted M26.30
specimen
  digestive organs (peritoneal fluid) (saliva) R85.9
    cytology R85.69
    drug level R85.2
    enzyme level R85.0
    histology R85.7
    hormones R85.1

Abnormal, abnormality, abnormalities (see also Anomaly) — continued
specimen — continued
  digestive organs (peritoneal fluid) (saliva) R85.9 — continued
    immunology R85.4
    microbiology R85.5
    nonmedicinal level R85.3
    specified type NEC R85.89
  female genital organs (secretions) (smears) R87.9
    cytology R87.69
    cervix R87.619
      human papillomavirus (HPV) DNA test
        high risk positive R87.810
        low risk positive R87.820
      inadequate (unsatisfactory) smear R87.615
      non-atypical endometrial cells R87.618
      specified NEC R87.618
    vagina R87.629
      human papillomavirus (HPV) DNA test
        high risk positive R87.811
        low risk positive R87.821
      inadequate (unsatisfactory) smear R87.625
    vulva R87.69
    drug level R87.2
    enzyme level R87.0
    histological R87.7
    hormones R87.1
    immunology R87.4
    microbiology R87.5
    nonmedicinal level R87.3
    specified type NEC R87.89
  male genital organs (prostatic secretions) (semen) R86.9
    cytology R86.6
    drug level R86.2
    enzyme level R86.0
    histological R86.7
    hormones R86.1
    immunology R86.4
    microbiology R86.5
    nonmedicinal level R86.3
    specified type NEC R86.8
  nipple discharge — see Abnormal, specimen, specified
  respiratory organs (bronchial washings) (nasal secretions) (pleural fluid) (sputum) R84.9
    cytology R84.6
    drug level R84.2
    enzyme level R84.0
    histology R84.7
    hormones R84.1
    immunology R84.4
    microbiology R84.5
    nonmedicinal level R84.3
    specified type NEC R84.8
  specified organ, system and tissue NOS R89.9
    cytology R89.6
    drug level R89.2
    enzyme level R89.0
    histology R89.7
    hormones R89.1
    immunology R89.4
    microbiology R89.5
    nonmedicinal level R89.3
    specified type NEC R89.8
  synovial fluid — see Abnormal, specimen, specified
  thorax (bronchial washings) (pleural fluids) — see Abnormal, specimen, respiratory organs
  vagina (secretion) (smear) R87.629
  vulva (secretion) (smear) R87.69
  wound secretion — see Abnormal, specimen, specified
spermatozoa — see Abnormal, specimen, male genital organs
sputum (amount) (color) (odor) R09.3
stool (color) (contents) (mucus) R19.5
  bloody K92.1
  guaiac positive R19.5
synchondrosis Q78.8
thermography (see also Abnormal, diagnostic imaging) R93.8
thyroid-binding globulin E07.89
tooth, teeth (form) (size) K00.2
toxicology (findings) R78.9
transport protein E88.09
tumor marker NEC R97.8
ultrasound results — see Abnormal, diagnostic imaging

Abnormal, abnormality, abnormalities (see also Anomaly) — continued
umbilical cord complicating delivery O69.9
urination NEC R39.19
urine (constituents) R82.90
  bile R82.2
  cytological examination R82.8
  drugs R82.5
  fat R82.0
  glucose R81
  heavy metals R82.6
  hemoglobin R82.3
  histological examination R82.8
  ketones R82.4
  microbiological examination (culture) R82.7
  myoglobin R82.1
  positive culture R82.7
  protein — see Proteinuria
  specified substance NEC R82.99
    chromoabnormality NEC R82.91
  substances nonmedical R82.6
uterine hemorrhage — see Hemorrhage, uterus
vectorcardiogram R94.39
visually evoked potential (VEP) R94.112
white blood cells D72.9
  specified NEC D72.89
X-ray examination — see Abnormal, diagnostic imaging
Abnormity (any organ or part) — see Anomaly
Abocclusion M26.29
  hemolytic disease (newborn) P55.1
  incompatibility reaction ABO — see Complication(s), transfusion, incompatibility reaction, ABO
Abolition, language R48.8
Aborter, habitual or recurrent — see Loss (of), pregnancy, recurrent
Abortion (complete) (spontaneous) O03.9
with
  retained products of conception — see Abortion, incomplete
attempted (elective) (failed) O07.4
  complicated by O07.30
    afibrinogenemia O07.1
    cardiac arrest O07.36
    chemical damage of pelvic organ(s) O07.34
    circulatory collapse O07.31
    cystitis O07.38
    defibrination syndrome O07.1
    electrolyte imbalance O07.33
    embolism (air) (amniotic fluid) (blood clot) (fat) (pulmonary) (septic) (soap) O07.2
    endometritis O07.0
    genital tract and pelvic infection O07.0
    hemolysis O07.1
    hemorrhage (delayed) (excessive) O07.1
    infection
      genital tract or pelvic O07.0
      urinary tract tract O07.38
    intravascular coagulation O07.1
    laceration of pelvic organ(s) O07.34
    metabolic disorder O07.33
    oliguria O07.32
    oophoritis O07.0
    parametritis O07.0
    pelvic peritonitis O07.0
    perforation of pelvic organ(s) O07.34
    renal failure or shutdown O07.32
    salpingitis or salpingo-oophoritis O07.0
    sepsis O07.37
    shock O07.31
    specified condition NEC O07.39
    tubular necrosis (renal) O07.32
    uremia O07.32
    urinary tract infection O07.38
    venous complication NEC O07.35
      embolism (air) (amniotic fluid) (blood clot) (fat) (pulmonary) (septic) (soap) O07.2
complicated (by) (following) O03.80
  afibrinogenemia O03.6
  cardiac arrest O03.86
  chemical damage of pelvic organ(s) O03.84
  circulatory collapse O03.81
  cystitis O03.88
  defibrination syndrome O03.6
  electrolyte imbalance O03.83

Abortion (complete) (spontaneous) O03.9 — continued
complicated (by) (following) O03.80 — continued
  embolism (air) (amniotic fluid) (blood clot) (fat) (pulmonary) (septic) (soap) O03.7
  endometritis O03.5
  genital tract and pelvic infection O03.5
  hemolysis O03.6
  hemorrhage (delayed) (excessive) O03.6
  infection
    genital tract or pelvic O03.5
    urinary tract O03.88
  intravascular coagulation O03.6
  laceration of pelvic organ(s) O03.84
  metabolic disorder O03.83
  oliguria O03.82
  oophoritis O03.5
  parametritis O03.5
  pelvic peritonitis O03.5
  perforation of pelvic organ(s) O03.84
  renal failure or shutdown O03.82
  salpingitis or salpingo-oophoritis O03.5
  sepsis O03.87
  shock O03.81
  specified condition NEC O03.89
  tubular necrosis (renal) O03.82
  uremia O03.82
  urinary tract infection O03.88
  venous complication NEC O03.85
    embolism (air) (amniotic fluid) (blood clot) (fat) (pulmonary) (septic) (soap) O03.7
failed — see Abortion, attempted
habitual or recurrent N96
  with current abortion — see categories O03-O06
  care in current pregnancy O26.2-
  without current pregnancy N96
incomplete (spontaneous) O03.4
  complicated (by) (following) O03.30
    afibrinogenemia O03.1
    cardiac arrest O03.36
    chemical damage of pelvic organ(s) O03.34
    circulatory collapse O03.31
    cystitis O03.38
    defibrination syndrome O03.1
    electrolyte imbalance O03.33
    embolism (air) (amniotic fluid) (blood clot) (fat) (pulmonary) (septic) (soap) O03.2
    endometritis O03.0
    genital tract and pelvic infection O03.0
    hemolysis O03.1
    hemorrhage (delayed) (excessive) O03.1
    infection
      genital tract or pelvic O03.0
      urinary tract O03.38
    intravascular coagulation O03.1
    laceration of pelvic organ(s) O03.34
    metabolic disorder O03.33
    oliguria O03.32
    oophoritis O03.0
    parametritis O03.0
    pelvic peritonitis O03.0
    perforation of pelvic organ(s) O03.34
    renal failure or shutdown O03.32
    salpingitis or salpingo-oophoritis O03.0
    sepsis O03.37
    shock O03.31
    specified condition NEC O03.39
    tubular necrosis (renal) O03.32
    uremia O03.32
    urinary infection O03.38
    venous complication NEC O03.35
      embolism (air) (amniotic fluid) (blood clot) (fat) (pulmonary) (septic) (soap) O03.2
induced (encounter for) Z33.2
  complicated by O04.80
    afibrinogenemia O04.6
    cardiac arrest O04.86
    chemical damage of pelvic organ(s) O04.84
    circulatory collapse O04.81
    cystitis O04.88
    defibrination syndrome O04.6
    electrolyte imbalance O04.83
    embolism (air) (amniotic fluid) (blood clot) (fat) (pulmonary) (septic) (soap) O04.7
    endometritis O04.5
    genital tract and pelvic infection O04.5
    hemolysis O04.6

Abortion (complete) (spontaneous) O03.9 — *continued*
  induced (encounter for) Z33.2 — *continued*
    complicated by O04.80 — *continued*
      hemorrhage (delayed) (excessive) O04.6
      infection
        genital tract or pelvic O04.5
        urinary tract O04.88
      intravascular coagulation O04.6
      laceration of pelvic organ(s) O04.84
      metabolic disorder O04.83
      oliguria O04.82
      oophoritis O04.5
      parametritis O04.5
      pelvic peritonitis O04.5
      perforation of pelvic organ(s) O04.84
      renal failure or shutdown O04.82
      salpingitis or salpingo-oophoritis O04.5
      sepsis O04.87
      shock O04.81
      specified condition NEC O04.89
      tubular necrosis (renal) O04.82
      uremia O04.82
      urinary tract infection O04.88
      venous complication NEC O04.85
        embolism (air) (amniotic fluid) (blood clot) (fat) (pulmonary) (septic) (soap) O04.7
  missed O02.1
  spontaneous — *see* Abortion (complete) (spontaneous)
  threatened O20.0
  threatened (spontaneous) O20.0
  tubal O00.1
Abortus fever A23.1
Aboulomania F60.7
Abrami's disease D59.8
Abramov-Fiedler myocarditis (acute isolated myocarditis) I40.1
Abrasion T14.8
  abdomen, abdominal (wall) S30.811
  alveolar process S00.512
  ankle S90.51-
  antecubital space — *see* Abrasion, elbow
  anus S30.817
  arm (upper) S40.81-
  auditory canal — *see* Abrasion, ear
  auricle — *see* Abrasion, ear
  axilla — *see* Abrasion, arm
  back, lower S30.810
  breast S20.11-
  brow S00.81
  buttock S30.810
  calf — *see* Abrasion, leg
  canthus — *see* Abrasion, eyelid
  cheek S00.81
    internal S00.512
  chest wall — *see* Abrasion, thorax
  chin S00.81
  clitoris S30.814
  cornea S05.0-
  costal region — *see* Abrasion, thorax
  dental K03.1
  digit(s)
    foot — *see* Abrasion, toe
    hand — *see* Abrasion, finger
  ear S00.41-
  elbow S50.31-
  epididymis S30.813
  epigastric region S30.811
  epiglottis S10.11
  esophagus (thoracic) S27.818
    cervical S10.11
  eyebrow — *see* Abrasion, eyelid
  eyelid S00.21-
  face S00.81
  finger(s) S60.41-
    index S60.41-
    little S60.41-
    middle S60.41-
    ring S60.41-
  flank S30.811
  foot (except toe(s) alone) S90.81-
    toe — *see* Abrasion, toe
  forearm S50.81-
    elbow only — *see* Abrasion, elbow
  forehead S00.81
  genital organs, external
    female S30.816
    male S30.815
  groin S30.811
  gum S00.512
  hand S60.51-

Abrasion — *continued*
  head S00.91
    ear — *see* Abrasion, ear
    eyelid — *see* Abrasion, eyelid
    lip S00.511
    nose S00.31
    oral cavity S00.512
    scalp S00.01
    specified site NEC S00.81
  heel — *see* Abrasion, foot
  hip S70.21-
  inguinal region S30.811
  interscapular region S20.419
  jaw S00.81
  knee S80.21-
  labium (majus) (minus) S30.814
  larynx S10.11
  leg (lower) S80.81-
    knee — *see* Abrasion, knee
    upper — *see* Abrasion, thigh
  lip S00.511
  lower back S30.810
  lumbar region S30.810
  malar region S00.81
  mammary — *see* Abrasion, breast
  mastoid region S00.81
  mouth S00.512
  nail
    finger — *see* Abrasion, finger
    toe — *see* Abrasion, toe
  nape S10.81
  nasal S00.31
  neck S10.91
    specified site NEC S10.81
    throat S10.11
  nose S00.31
  occipital region S00.01
  oral cavity S00.512
  orbital region — *see* Abrasion, eyelid
  palate S00.512
  palm — *see* Abrasion, hand
  parietal region S00.01
  pelvis S30.810
  penis S30.812
  perineum
    female S30.814
    male S30.810
  periocular area — *see* Abrasion, eyelid
  phalanges
    finger — *see* Abrasion, finger
    toe — *see* Abrasion, toe
  pharynx S10.11
  pinna — *see* Abrasion, ear
  popliteal space — *see* Abrasion, knee
  prepuce S30.812
  pubic region S30.810
  pudendum
    female S30.816
    male S30.815
  sacral region S30.810
  scalp S00.01
  scapular region — *see* Abrasion, shoulder
  scrotum S30.813
  shin — *see* Abrasion, leg
  shoulder S40.21-
  skin NEC T14.8
  sternal region S20.319
  submaxillary region S00.81
  submental region S00.81
  subungual
    finger(s) — *see* Abrasion, finger
    toe(s) — *see* Abrasion, toe
  supraclavicular fossa S10.81
  supraorbital S00.81
  temple S00.81
  temporal region S00.81
  testis S30.813
  thigh S70.31-
  thorax, thoracic (wall) S20.91
    back S20.41-
    front S20.31-
  throat S10.11
  thumb S60.31-
  toe(s) (lesser) S90.416
    great S90.41-
  tongue S00.512
  tooth, teeth (dentifrice) (habitual) (hard tissues) (occupational) (ritual) (traditional) K03.1
  trachea S10.11
  tunica vaginalis S30.813
  tympanum, tympanic membrane — *see* Abrasion, ear
  uvula S00.512
  vagina S30.814
  vocal cords S10.11
  vulva S30.814
  wrist S60.81-
Abrism — *see* Poisoning, food, noxious, plant

Abruptio placentae O45.9-
  with
    afibrinogenemia O45.01-
    coagulation defect O45.00-
      specified NEC O45.09-
    disseminated intravascular coagulation O45.02-
    hypofibrinogenemia O45.01-
    specified NEC O45.8-
Abruption, placenta — *see* Abruptio placentae
Abscess (connective tissue) (embolic) (fistulous) (infective) (metastatic) (multiple) (pernicious) (pyogenic) (septic) L02.91
  with
    diverticular disease (intestine) K57.80
      with bleeding K57.81
      large intestine K57.20
        with
          bleeding K57.21
          small intestine K57.40
            with bleeding K57.41
      small intestine K57.00
        with
          bleeding K57.01
          large intestine K57.40
            with bleeding K57.41
    lymphangitis — *code by* site under Abscess
  abdomen, abdominal
    cavity K65.1
    wall L02.211
  abdominopelvic K65.1
  accessory sinus — *see* Sinusitis
  adrenal (capsule) (gland) E27.8
  alveolar K04.7
    with sinus K04.6
  amebic A06.4
    brain (and liver or lung abscess) A06.6
    genitourinary tract A06.82
    liver (without mention of brain or lung abscess) A06.4
    lung (and liver) (without mention of brain abscess) A06.5
    specified site NEC A06.89
    spleen A06.89
  anerobic A48.0
  ankle — *see* Abscess, lower limb
  anorectal K61.2
  antecubital space — *see* Abscess, upper limb
  antrum (chronic) (Highmore) — *see* Sinusitis, maxillary
  anus K61.0
  apical (tooth) K04.7
    with sinus (alveolar) K04.6
  appendix K35.3
  areola (acute) (chronic) (nonpuerperal) N61
    puerperal, postpartum or gestational — *see* Infection, nipple
  arm (any part) — *see* Abscess, upper limb
  artery (wall) I77.89
  atheromatous I77.2
  auricle, ear — *see* Abscess, ear, external
  axilla (region) L02.41-
    lymph gland or node L04.2
  back (any part, except buttock) L02.212
  Bartholin's gland N75.1
    with
      abortion — *see* Abortion, by type
        complicated by, sepsis
      ectopic or molar pregnancy O08.0
    following ectopic or molar pregnancy O08.0
  Bezold's — *see* Mastoiditis, acute
  bilharziasis B65.1
  bladder (wall) — *see* Cystitis, specified type NEC
  bone (subperiosteal) — *see also* Osteomyelitis, specified type NEC
    accessory sinus (chronic) — *see* Sinusitis
    chronic or old — *see* Osteomyelitis, chronic
    jaw (lower) (upper) M27.2
    mastoid — *see* Mastoiditis, acute, subperiosteal
    petrous — *see* Petrositis
    spinal (tuberculous) A18.01
      nontuberculous — *see* Osteomyelitis, vertebra
  bowel K63.0

Abscess (connective tissue) (embolic) (fistulous) (infective) (metastatic) (multiple) (pernicious) (pyogenic) (septic) L02.91 — *continued*
  brain (any part) (cystic) (otogenic) G06.0
    amebic (with abscess of any other site) A06.6
    gonococcal A54.82
    pheomycotic (chromomycotic) B43.1
    tuberculous A17.81
  breast (acute) (chronic) (nonpuerperal) N61
    newborn P39.0
    puerperal, postpartum, gestational — *see* Mastitis, obstetric, purulent
  broad ligament N73.2
    acute N73.0
    chronic N73.1
  Brodie's (localized) (chronic) M86.8x-
  bronchi J98.09
  buccal cavity K12.2
  bulbourethral gland N34.0
  bursa M71.00
    ankle M71.07-
    elbow M71.02-
    foot M71.07-
    hand M71.04-
    hip M71.05-
    knee M71.06-
    multiple sites M71.09
    pharyngeal J39.1
    shoulder M71.01-
    specified site NEC M71.08
    wrist M71.03-
  buttock L02.31
  canthus — *see* Blepharoconjunctivitis
  cartilage — *see* Disorder, cartilage, specified type NEC
  cecum K35.3
  cerebellum, cerebellar G06.0
    sequelae G09
  cerebral (embolic) G06.0
    sequelae G09
  cervical (meaning neck) L02.11
    lymph gland or node L04.0
  cervix (stump) (uteri) — *see* Cervicitis
  cheek (external) L02.01
    inner K12.2
  chest J86.9
    with fistula J86.0
    wall L02.213
  chin L02.01
  choroid — *see* Inflammation, chorioretinal
  circumtonsillar J36
  cold (lung) (tuberculous) — *see also* Tuberculosis, abscess, lung
    articular — *see* Tuberculosis, joint
  colon (wall) K63.0
  colostomy K94.02
  conjunctiva — *see* Conjunctivitis, acute
  cornea H16.31-
  corpus
    cavernosum N48.21
    luteum — *see* Oophoritis
  Cowper's gland N34.0
  cranium G06.0
  cul-de-sac (Douglas') (posterior) — *see* Peritonitis, pelvic, female
  cutaneous — *see* Abscess, by site
  dental K04.7
    with sinus (alveolar) K04.6
  dentoalveolar K04.7
    with sinus K04.6
  diaphragm, diaphragmatic K65.1
  Douglas' cul-de-sac or pouch — *see* Peritonitis, pelvic, female
  Dubois A50.59
  ear (middle) — *see also* Otitis, media, suppurative
    acute — *see* Otitis, media, suppurative, acute
    external H60.0-
  entamebic — *see* Abscess, amebic
  enterostomy K94.02
  epididymis N45.4
  epidural G06.2
    brain G06.0
    spinal cord G06.1
  epiglottis J38.7
  epiploon, epiploic K65.1
  erysipelatous — *see* Erysipelas
  esophagus K20.8
  ethmoid (bone) (chronic) (sinus) J32.2
  external auditory canal — *see* Abscess, ear, external
  extradural G06.2
    brain G06.0
      sequelae G09
    spinal cord G06.1

Abscess (connective tissue) (embolic) (fistulous) (infective) (metastatic) (multiple) (pernicious) (pyogenic) (septic) L02.91 — *continued*
- extraperitoneal K68.19
- eye — *see* Endophthalmitis, purulent
- eyelid H00.03-
- face (any part, except ear, eye and nose) L02.01
- fallopian tube — *see* Salpingitis
- fascia M72.8
- fauces J39.1
- fecal K63.0
- femoral (region) — *see* Abscess, lower limb
- filaria, filarial — *see* Infestation, filarial
- finger (any) — *see* Abscess, hand
  - nail — *see* Cellulitis, finger
- foot L02.61-
- forehead L02.01
- frontal sinus (chronic) J32.1
- gallbladder K81.0
- genital organ or tract
  - female (external) N76.4
  - male N49.9
    - multiple sites N49.8
    - specified NEC N49.8
- gestational mammary O91.11-
- gestational subareolar O91.11-
- gingival K05.21
- gland, glandular (lymph) (acute) — *see* Lymphadenitis, acute
- gluteal (region) L02.31
- gonorrheal — *see* Gonococcus
- groin L02.214
- gum K05.21
- hand L02.51-
- head NEC L02.811
  - face (any part, except ear, eye and nose) L02.01
- heart — *see* Carditis
- heel — *see* Abscess, foot
- helminthic — *see* Infestation, helminth
- hepatic (cholangitic) (hematogenic) (lymphogenic) (pylephlebitic) K75.0
  - amebic A06.4
- hip (region) — *see* Abscess, lower limb
- ileocecal K35.3
- ileostomy (bud) K94.12
- iliac (region) L02.214
  - fossa K35.3
- infraclavicular (fossa) — *see* Abscess, upper limb
- inguinal (region) L02.214
  - lymph gland or node L04.1
- intestine, intestinal NEC K63.0
  - rectal K61.1
- intra-abdominal (*see also* Abscess, peritoneum) K65.1
  - postoperative T81.4
  - retroperitoneal K68.11
- intracranial G06.0
- intramammary — *see* Abscess, breast
- intraorbital — *see* Abscess, orbit
- intraperitoneal K65.1
- intrasphincteric (anus) K61.4
- intraspinal G06.1
- intratonsillar J36
- ischiorectal (fossa) K61.3
- jaw (bone) (lower) (upper) M27.2
- joint — *see* Arthritis, pyogenic or pyemic
  - spine (tuberculous) A18.01
    - nontuberculous — *see* Spondylopathy, infective
- kidney N15.1
  - with calculus N20.0
    - with hydronephrosis N13.6
  - puerperal (postpartum) O86.21
- knee — *see also* Abscess, lower limb
  - joint M00.9
- labium (majus) (minus) N76.4
- lacrimal
  - caruncle — *see* Inflammation, lacrimal, passages, acute
  - gland — *see* Dacryoadenitis
  - passages (duct) (sac) — *see* Inflammation, lacrimal, passages, acute
- lacunar N34.0
- larynx J38.7
- lateral (alveolar) K04.7
  - with sinus K04.6
- leg (any part) — *see* Abscess, lower limb
- lens H27.8
- lingual K14.0
  - tonsil J36
- lip K13.0
- Littre's gland N34.0

Abscess (connective tissue) (embolic) (fistulous) (infective) (metastatic) (multiple) (pernicious) (pyogenic) (septic) L02.91 — *continued*
- liver (cholangitic) (hematogenic) (lymphogenic) (pylephlebitic) (pyogenic) K75.0
  - amebic (due to Entamoeba histolytica) (dysenteric) (tropical) A06.4
    - with
      - brain abscess (and liver or lung abscess) A06.6
      - lung abscess A06.5
- loin (region) L02.211
- lower limb L02.41-
  - lumbar (tuberculous) A18.01
  - nontuberculous L02.212
- lung (miliary) (putrid) J85.2
  - with pneumonia J85.1
    - due to specified organism (see Pneumonia, in (due to))
  - amebic (with liver abscess) A06.5
    - with
      - brain abscess A06.6
      - pneumonia A06.5
- lymph, lymphatic, gland or node (acute) — *see also* Lymphadenitis, acute
  - mesentery I88.0
- malar M27.2
- mammary gland — *see* Abscess, breast
- marginal, anus K61.0
- mastoid — *see* Mastoiditis, acute
- maxilla, maxillary M27.2
  - molar (tooth) K04.7
    - with sinus K04.6
  - premolar K04.7
  - sinus (chronic) J32.0
- mediastinum J85.3
- meibomian gland — *see* Hordeolum
- meninges G06.2
- mesentery, mesenteric K65.1
- mesosalpinx — *see* Salpingitis
- mons pubis L02.215
- mouth (floor) K12.2
- muscle — *see* Myositis, infective
- myocardium I40.0
- nabothian (follicle) — *see* Cervicitis
- nasal J32.9
- nasopharyngeal J39.1
- navel L02.216
  - newborn P38.9
    - with mild hemorrhage P38.1
    - without hemorrhage P38.9
- neck (region) L02.11
  - lymph gland or node L04.0
- nephritic — *see* Abscess, kidney
- nipple N61
  - associated with
    - lactation — *see* Pregnancy, complicated by,
    - pregnancy — *see* Pregnancy, complicated by
- nose (external) (fossa) (septum) J34.0
  - sinus (chronic) — *see* Sinusitis
- omentum K65.1
- operative wound T81.4
- orbit, orbital — *see* Cellulitis, orbit
- otogenic G06.0
- ovary, ovarian (corpus luteum) — *see* Oophoritis
- oviduct — *see* Oophoritis
- palate (soft) K12.2
  - hard M27.2
- palmar (space) — *see* Abscess, hand
- pancreas (duct) — *see* Pancreatitis, acute
- parafrenal N48.21
- parametric, parametrium N73.2
  - acute N73.0
  - chronic N73.1
- paranephric N15.1
- parapancreatic — *see* Pancreatitis, acute
- parapharyngeal J39.0
- pararectal K61.1
- parasinus — *see* Sinusitis
- parauterine (*see also* Disease, pelvis, inflammatory) N73.2
- paravaginal — *see* Vaginitis
- parietal region (scalp) L02.811
- parodontal K05.21
- parotid (duct) (gland) K11.3
  - region K12.2
- pectoral (region) L02.213
- pelvis, pelvic
  - female — *see* Disease, pelvis, inflammatory
  - male, peritoneal K65.1

Abscess (connective tissue) (embolic) (fistulous) (infective) (metastatic) (multiple) (pernicious) (pyogenic) (septic) L02.91 — *continued*
- penis N48.21
  - gonococcal (accessory gland) (periurethral) A54.1
- perianal K61.0
- periapical K04.7
  - with sinus (alveolar) K04.6
- periappendicular K35.3
- pericardial I30.1
- pericecal K35.3
- pericemental K05.21
- pericholecystic — *see* Cholecystitis, acute
- pericoronal K05.21
- peridental K05.21
- perimetric (*see also* Disease, pelvis, inflammatory) N73.2
- perinephric, perinephritic — *see* Abscess, kidney
- perineum, perineal (superficial) L02.215
  - urethra N34.0
- periodontal (parietal) K05.21
  - apical K04.7
- periosteum, periosteal — *see also* Osteomyelitis, specified type NEC
  - with osteomyelitis — *see also* Osteomyelitis, specified type NEC
    - acute — *see* Osteomyelitis, acute
    - chronic — *see* Osteomyelitis, chronic
- peripharyngeal J39.0
- peripleuritic J86.9
  - with fistula J86.0
- periprostatic N41.2
- perirectal K61.1
- perirenal (tissue) — *see* Abscess, kidney
- perisinuous (nose) — *see* Sinusitis
- peritoneum, peritoneal (perforated) (ruptured) K65.1
  - with appendicitis K35.3
  - pelvic
    - female — *see* Peritonitis, pelvic, female
    - male K65.1
  - postoperative T81.4
  - puerperal, postpartum, childbirth O85
  - tuberculous A18.31
- peritonsillar J36
- perityphlic K35.3
- periureteral N28.89
- periurethral N34.0
  - gonococcal (accessory gland) (periurethral) A54.1
- periuterine (*see also* Disease, pelvis, inflammatory) N73.2
- perivesical — *see* Cystitis, specified type NEC
- petrous bone — *see* Petrositis
- phagedenic NOS L02.91
  - chancroid A57
- pharynx, pharyngeal (lateral) J39.1
- pilonidal L05.01
- pituitary (gland) E23.6
- pleura J86.9
  - with fistula J86.0
- popliteal — *see* Abscess, lower limb
- postcecal K35.3
- postlaryngeal J38.7
- postnasal J34.0
- postoperative (any site) T81.4
  - retroperitoneal K68.11
- postpharyngeal J39.0
- posttonsillar J36
- post-typhoid A01.09
- pouch of Douglas — *see* Peritonitis, pelvic, female
- premammary — *see* Abscess, breast
- prepatellar — *see* Abscess, lower limb
- prostate N41.2
  - gonococcal (acute) (chronic) A54.22
- psoas muscle K68.12
- puerperal — *code by* site under Puerperal, abscess
- pulmonary — *see* Abscess, lung
- pulp, pulpal (dental) K04.0
- rectovaginal septum K63.0
- rectovesical — *see* Cystitis, specified type NEC
- rectum K61.1
- renal — *see* Abscess, kidney
- retina — *see* Inflammation, chorioretinal
- retrobulbar — *see* Abscess, orbit
- retrocecal K65.1
- retrolaryngeal J38.7
- retromammary — *see* Abscess, breast
- retroperitoneal NEC K68.19
  - postprocedural K68.11

Abscess (connective tissue) (embolic) (fistulous) (infective) (metastatic) (multiple) (pernicious) (pyogenic) (septic) L02.91 — *continued*
- retropharyngeal J39.0
- retrouterine — *see* Peritonitis, pelvic, female
- retrovesical — *see* Cystitis, specified type NEC
- root, tooth K04.7
  - with sinus (alveolar) K04.6
- round ligament (*see also* Disease, pelvis, inflammatory) N73.2
- rupture (spontaneous) NOS L02.91
- sacrum (tuberculous) A18.01
  - nontuberculous M46.28
- salivary (duct) (gland) K11.3
- scalp (any part) L02.811
- scapular — *see* Osteomyelitis, specified type NEC
- sclera — *see* Scleritis
- scrofulous (tuberculous) A18.2
- scrotum N49.2
- seminal vesicle N49.0
- septal, dental K04.7
  - with sinus (alveolar) K04.6
- serous — *see* Periostitis
- shoulder (region) — *see* Abscess, upper limb
- sigmoid K63.0
- sinus (accessory) (chronic) (nasal) — *see also* Sinusitis
  - intracranial venous (any) G06.0
- Skene's duct or gland N34.0
- skin — *see* Abscess, by site
- specified site NEC L02.818
- spermatic cord N49.1
- sphenoidal (sinus) (chronic) J32.3
- spinal cord (any part) (staphylococcal) G06.1
  - tuberculous A17.81
- spine (column) (tuberculous) A18.01
  - epidural G06.1
  - nontuberculous — *see* Osteomyelitis, vertebra
- spleen D73.3
  - amebic A06.89
- stitch T81.4
- subarachnoid G06.2
  - brain G06.0
  - spinal cord G06.1
- subareolar — *see* Abscess, breast
- subcecal K35.3
- subcutaneous — *see also* Abscess, by site
  - pheomycotic (chromomycotic) B43.2
- subdiaphragmatic K65.1
- subdural G06.2
  - brain G06.0
    - sequelae G09
  - spinal cord G06.1
- subgaleal L02.811
- subhepatic K65.1
- sublingual K12.2
  - gland K11.3
- submammary — *see* Abscess, breast
- submandibular (region) (space) (triangle) K12.2
  - gland K11.3
- submaxillary (region) L02.01
  - gland K11.3
- submental L02.01
  - gland K11.3
- subperiosteal — *see* Osteomyelitis, specified type NEC
- subphrenic K65.1
  - postoperative T81.4
- suburethral N34.0
- sudoriparous L75.8
- supraclavicular (fossa) — *see* Abscess, upper limb
- suprapelvic, acute N73.0
- suprarenal (capsule) (gland) E27.8
- sweat gland L74.8
- tear duct — *see* Inflammation, lacrimal, passages, acute
- temple L02.01
- temporal region L02.01
- temporosphenoidal G06.0
- tendon (sheath) M65.00
  - ankle M65.07-
  - foot M65.07-
  - forearm M65.03-
  - hand M65.04-
  - lower leg M65.06-
  - pelvic region M65.05-
  - shoulder region M65.01-
  - specified site NEC M65.08
  - thigh M65.05-
  - upper arm M65.02-

Abscess (connective tissue) (embolic) (fistulous) (infective) (metastatic) (multiple) (pernicious) (pyogenic) (septic) L02.91 — *continued*
testis N45.4
thigh — *see* Abscess, lower limb
thorax J86.9
  with fistula J86.0
throat J39.1
thumb — *see also* Abscess, hand
  nail — *see* Cellulitis, finger
thymus (gland) E32.1
thyroid (gland) E06.0
toe (any) — *see also* Abscess, foot
  nail — *see* Cellulitis, toe
tongue (staphylococcal) K14.0
tonsil(s) (lingual) J36
tonsillopharyngeal J36
tooth, teeth (root) K04.7
  with sinus (alveolar) K04.6
  supporting structures NEC K05.21
trachea J39.8
trunk L02.219
  abdominal wall L02.211
  back L02.212
  chest wall L02.213
  groin L02.214
  perineum L02.215
  umbilicus L02.216
tubal — *see* Salpingitis
tuberculous — *see* Tuberculosis, abscess
tubo-ovarian — *see* Salpingo-oophoritis
tunica vaginalis N49.1
umbilicus L02.216
upper
  limb L02.41-
  respiratory J39.8
urethral (gland) N34.0
urinary N34.0
uterus, uterine (wall) — *see also* Endometritis
  ligament (*see also* Disease, pelvis, inflammatory) N73.2
  neck — *see* Cervicitis
uvula K12.2
vagina (wall) — *see* Vaginitis
vaginorectal — *see* Vaginitis
vas deferens N49.1
vermiform appendix K35.3
vertebra (column) (tuberculous) A18.01
  nontuberculous — *see* Osteomyelitis, vertebra
vesical — *see* Cystitis, specified type NEC
vesico-uterine pouch — *see* Peritonitis, pelvic, female
vitreous (humor) — *see* Endophthalmitis, purulent
vocal cord J38.3
von Bezold's — *see* Mastoiditis, acute
vulva N76.4
vulvovaginal gland N75.1
web space — *see* Abscess, hand
wound T81.4
wrist — *see* Abscess, upper limb
Absence (of) (organ or part) (complete or partial)
adrenal (gland) (congenital) Q89.1
  acquired E89.6
albumin in blood E88.09
alimentary tract (congenital) Q45.8
  upper Q40.8
alveolar process (acquired) — *see* Anomaly, alveolar
ankle (acquired) Z89.44-
anus (congenital) Q42.3
  with fistula Q42.2
aorta (congenital) Q25.4
appendix, congenital Q42.8
arm (acquired) Z89.20-
  above elbow Z89.22-
    congenital (with hand present) — *see* Agenesis, arm, with hand present and hand — *see* Agenesis, forearm, and hand
  below elbow Z89.21-
    congenital (with hand present) — *see* Agenesis, arm, with hand present and hand — *see* Agenesis, forearm, and hand
  congenital — *see* Defect, reduction, upper limb
  shoulder (following explantation of shoulder joint prosthesis) (joint) (with or without presence of antibiotic-impregnated cement spacer) Z89.23-
    congenital (with hand present) — *see* Agenesis, arm, with hand present

Absence (of) (organ or part) (complete or partial) — *continued*
artery (congenital) (peripheral) Q27.8
  brain Q28.3
  coronary Q24.5
  pulmonary Q25.79
  specified NEC Q27.8
  umbilical Q27.0
atrial septum (congenital) Q21.1
auditory canal (congenital) (external) Q16.1
auricle (ear), congenital Q16.0
bile, biliary duct, congenital Q44.5
bladder (acquired) Z90.6
  congenital Q64.5
bowel sounds R19.11
brain Q00.0
  part of Q04.3
breast(s) (and nipple(s)) (acquired) Z90.1-
  congenital Q83.8
broad ligament Q50.6
bronchus (congenital) Q32.4
canaliculus lacrimalis, congenital Q10.4
cerebellum (vermis) Q04.3
cervix (acquired) (with uterus) Z90.710
  with remaining uterus Z90.712
  congenital Q51.5
chin, congenital Q18.8
cilia (congenital) Q10.3
  acquired — *see* Madarosis
clitoris (congenital) Q52.6
coccyx, congenital Q76.49
cold sense R20.8
congenital
  lumen — *see* Atresia
  organ or site NEC — *see* Agenesis
  septum — *see* Imperfect, closure
corpus callosum Q04.0
cricoid cartilage, congenital Q31.8
diaphragm (with hernia), congenital Q79.1
digestive organ(s) or tract, congenital Q45.8
  acquired NEC Z90.49
  upper Q40.8
ductus arteriosus Q28.8
duodenum (acquired) Z90.49
  congenital Q41.0
ear, congenital Q16.9
  acquired H93.8-
  auricle Q16.0
  external Q16.0
  inner Q16.5
  lobe, lobule Q17.8
  middle, except ossicles Q16.4
    ossicles Q16.3
  ossicles Q16.3
ejaculatory duct (congenital) Q55.4
endocrine gland (congenital) NEC Q89.2
  acquired E89.89
epididymis (congenital) Q55.4
  acquired Z90.79
epiglottis, congenital Q31.8
esophagus (congenital) Q39.8
  acquired (partial) Z90.49
eustachian tube (congenital) Q16.2
extremity (acquired) Z89.9
  congenital Q73.0
  knee (following explantation of knee joint prosthesis) (joint) (with or without presence of antibiotic-impregnated cement spacer) Z89.52-
  lower (above knee) Z89.619
    below knee Z89.51-
  upper — *see* Absence, arm
eye (acquired) Z90.01
  congenital Q11.1
  muscle (congenital) Q10.3
eyeball (acquired) Z90.01
eyelid (fold) (congenital) Q10.3
  acquired Z90.01
face, specified part NEC Q18.8
fallopian tube(s) (acquired) Z90.79
  congenital Q50.6
family member (causing problem in home) NEC (*see also* Disruption, family) Z63.32
femur, congenital — *see* Defect, reduction, lower limb, longitudinal, femur
fibrinogen (congenital) D68.2
  acquired D65
finger(s) (acquired) Z89.02-
  congenital — *see* Agenesis, hand
foot (acquired) Z89.43-
  congenital — *see* Agenesis, foot
forearm (acquired) — *see* Absence, arm, below elbow
gallbladder (acquired) Z90.49
  congenital Q44.0

Absence (of) (organ or part) (complete or partial) — *continued*
gamma globulin in blood D80.1
  hereditary D80.0
genital organs
  acquired (female) (male) Z90.79
  female, congenital Q52.8
    external Q52.71
    internal NEC Q52.8
  male, congenital Q55.8
genitourinary organs, congenital NEC
  female Q52.8
  male Q55.8
globe (acquired) Z90.01
  congenital Q11.1
glottis, congenital Q31.8
hand and wrist (acquired) Z89.11-
  congenital — *see* Agenesis, hand
head, part (acquired) NEC Z90.09
heat sense R20.8
hip (following explantation of hip joint prosthesis) (joint) (with or without presence of antibiotic-impregnated cement spacer) Z89.62-
hymen (congenital) Q52.4
ileum (acquired) Z90.49
  congenital Q41.2
immunoglobulin, isolated NEC D80.3
  IgA D80.2
  IgG D80.3
  IgM D80.4
incus (acquired) — *see* Loss, ossicles, ear
  congenital Q16.3
inner ear, congenital Q16.5
intestine (acquired) (small) Z90.49
  congenital Q41.9
    specified NEC Q41.8
  large Z90.49
    congenital Q42.9
      specified NEC Q42.8
iris, congenital Q13.1
jejunum (acquired) Z90.49
  congenital Q41.1
joint
  acquired
    hip (following explantation of hip joint prosthesis) (with or without presence of antibiotic-impregnated cement spacer) Z89.62-
    knee (following explantation of knee joint prosthesis) (with or without presence of antibiotic-impregnated cement spacer) Z89.52-
    shoulder (following explantation of shoulder joint prosthesis) (with or without presence of antibiotic-impregnated cement spacer) Z89.23-
  congenital NEC Q74.8
kidney(s) (acquired) Z90.5
  congenital Q60.2
    bilateral Q60.1
    unilateral Q60.0
knee (following explantation of knee joint prosthesis) (joint) (with or without presence of antibiotic-impregnated cement spacer) Z89.52-
labyrinth, membranous Q16.5
larynx (congenital) Q31.8
  acquired Z90.02
leg (acquired) (above knee) Z89.61-
  below knee (acquired) Z89.51-
  congenital — *see* Defect, reduction, lower limb
lens (acquired) — *see also* Aphakia
  congenital Q12.3
  post cataract extraction Z98.4-
limb (acquired) — *see* Absence, extremity
lip Q38.6
liver (congenital) Q44.7
lung (fissure) (lobe) (bilateral) (unilateral) (congenital) Q33.3
  acquired (any part) Z90.2
menstruation — *see* Amenorrhea
muscle (congenital) (pectoral) Q79.8
  ocular Q10.3
neck, part Q18.8
neutrophil — *see* Agranulocytosis
nipple(s) (with breast(s)) (acquired) Z90.1-
  congenital Q83.2
nose (congenital) Q30.1
  acquired Z90.09
organ
  of Corti, congenital Q16.5
  or site, congenital NEC Q89.8
    acquired NEC Z90.89
osseous meatus (ear) Q16.4

Absence (of) (organ or part) (complete or partial) — *continued*
ovary (acquired)
  bilateral Z90.722
  congenital
    bilateral Q50.02
    unilateral Q50.01
  unilateral Z90.721
oviduct (acquired)
  bilateral Z90.722
  congenital Q50.6
  unilateral Z90.721
pancreas (congenital) Q45.0
  acquired Z90.410
    complete Z90.410
    partial Z90.411
    total Z90.410
parathyroid gland (acquired) E89.2
  congenital Q89.2
patella, congenital Q74.1
penis (congenital) Q55.5
  acquired Z90.79
pericardium (congenital) Q24.8
pituitary gland (congenital) Q89.2
  acquired E89.3
prostate (acquired) Z90.79
  congenital Q55.4
pulmonary valve Q22.0
punctum lacrimale (congenital) Q10.4
radius, congenital — *see* Defect, reduction, upper limb, longitudinal, radius
rectum (congenital) Q42.1
  with fistula Q42.0
  acquired Z90.49
respiratory organ NOS Q34.9
rib (acquired) Z90.89
  congenital Q76.6
sacrum, congenital Q76.49
salivary gland(s), congenital Q38.4
scrotum, congenital Q55.29
seminal vesicles (congenital) Q55.4
  acquired Z90.79
septum
  atrial (congenital) Q21.1
  between aorta and pulmonary artery Q21.4
  ventricular (congenital) Q20.4
sex chromosome
  female phenotype Q97.8
  male phenotype Q98.8
skull bone (congenital) Q75.8
  with
    anencephaly Q00.0
    encephalocele — *see* Encephalocele
    hydrocephalus Q03.9
      with spina bifida — *see* Spina bifida, by site, with hydrocephalus
    microcephaly Q02
spermatic cord, congenital Q55.4
spine, congenital Q76.49
spleen (congenital) Q89.01
  acquired Z90.81
sternum, congenital Q76.7
stomach (acquired) (partial) Z90.3
  congenital Q40.2
superior vena cava, congenital Q26.8
teeth, tooth (congenital) K00.0
  acquired (complete) K08.109
    class I K08.101
    class II K08.102
    class III K08.103
    class IV K08.104
    due to
      caries K08.139
        class I K08.131
        class II K08.132
        class III K08.133
        class IV K08.134
      periodontal disease K08.129
        class I K08.121
        class II K08.122
        class III K08.123
        class IV K08.124
      specified NEC K08.199
        class I K08.191
        class II K08.192
        class III K08.193
        class IV K08.194
      trauma K08.119
        class I K08.111
        class II K08.112
        class III K08.113
        class IV K08.114
    partial K08.409
      class I K08.401
      class II K08.402
      class III K08.403
      class IV K08.404

DISEASE INDEX

Absence (of) (organ or part) (complete or partial) — *continued*
  teeth, tooth (congenital) K00.0 — *continued*
    acquired (complete) K08.109 — *continued*
      partial K08.409 — *continued*
        due to
          caries K08.439
            class I K08.431
            class II K08.432
            class III K08.433
            class IV K08.434
          periodontal disease K08.429
            class I K08.421
            class II K08.422
            class III K08.423
            class IV K08.424
          specified NEC K08.499
            class I K08.491
            class II K08.492
            class III K08.493
            class IV K08.494
          trauma K08.419
            class I K08.411
            class II K08.412
            class III K08.413
            class IV K08.414
  tendon (congenital) Q79.8
  testis (congenital) Q55.0
    acquired Z90.79
  thumb (acquired) Z89.01-
    congenital — *see* Agenesis, hand
  thymus gland Q89.2
  thyroid (gland) (acquired) E89.0
    cartilage, congenital Q31.8
    congenital E03.1
  toe(s) (acquired) Z89.42-
    with foot — *see* Absence, foot and ankle
    congenital — *see* Agenesis, foot
    great Z89.41-
  tongue, congenital Q38.3
  trachea (cartilage), congenital Q32.1
  transverse aortic arch, congenital Q25.4
  tricuspid valve Q22.4
  umbilical artery, congenital Q27.0
  upper arm and forearm with hand present, congenital — *see* Agenesis, arm, with hand present
  ureter (congenital) Q62.4
    acquired Z90.6
  urethra, congenital Q64.5
  uterus (acquired) Z90.710
    with cervix Z90.710
    with remaining cervical stump Z90.711
    congenital Q51.0
  uvula, congenital Q38.5
  vagina, congenital Q52.0
  vas deferens (congenital) Q55.4
    acquired Z90.79
  vein (peripheral) congenital NEC Q27.8
    cerebral Q28.3
    digestive system Q27.8
    great Q26.8
    lower limb Q27.8
    portal Q26.5
    precerebral Q28.1
    specified site NEC Q27.8
    upper limb Q27.8
  vena cava (inferior) (superior), congenital Q26.8
  ventricular septum Q20.4
  vertebra, congenital Q76.49
  vulva, congenital Q52.71
  wrist (acquired) Z89.12-
Absorbent system disease I87.8
Absorption
  carbohydrate, disturbance K90.4
  chemical — *see* Table of Drugs and Chemcials
    through placenta (newborn) P04.9
      environmental substance P04.6
      nutritional substance P04.5
      obstetric anesthetic or analgesic drug P04.0
  drug NEC — *see* Table of Drugs and Chemicals
    addictive
      through placenta (newborn) P04.49
        cocaine P04.41
    medicinal
      through placenta (newborn) P04.1
    through placenta (newborn) P04.1
      obstetric anesthetic or analgesic drug P04.0
  fat, disturbance K90.4
    pancreatic K90.3
  noxious substance — *see* Table of Drugs and Chemicals
  protein, disturbance K90.4

Absorption — *continued*
  starch, disturbance K90.4
  toxic substance — *see* Table of Drugs and Chemicals
  uremic — *see* Uremia
Abstinence symptoms, syndrome
  alcohol F10.239
    with delirium F10.231
  cocaine F14.23
  neonatal P96.1
  nicotine — *see* Dependence, drug, nicotine, with, withdrawal
  opioid F11.93
    with dependence F11.23
  psychoactive NEC F19.939
    with
      delirium F19.931
      dependence F19.239
        with
          delirium F19.231
            perceptual disturbance F19.232
          uncomplicated F19.230
        perceptual disturbance F19.932
      uncomplicated F19.930
  sedative F13.939
    with
      delirium F13.931
      dependence F13.239
        with
          delirium F13.231
            perceptual disturbance F13.232
          uncomplicated F13.230
        perceptual disturbance F13.932
      uncomplicated F13.930
  stimulant NEC F15.93
    with dependence F15.23
Abulia R68.89
Abulomania F60.7
Abuse
  adult — *see* Maltreatment, adult
    as reason for
      couple seeking advice (including offender) Z63.0
  alcohol (non-dependent) F10.10
    with
      anxiety disorder F10.180
      intoxication F10.129
        with delirium F10.121
        uncomplicated F10.120
      mood disorder F10.14
      other specified disorder F10.188
      psychosis F10.159
        delusions F10.150
        hallucinations F10.151
      sexual dysfunction F10.181
      sleep disorder F10.182
      unspecified disorder F10.19
    counseling and surveillance Z71.41
  amphetamine (or related substance) — *see* Abuse, drug, stimulant NEC
  analgesics (non-prescribed) (over the counter) F55.8
  antacids F55.0
  antidepressants — *see* Abuse, drug, psychoactive NEC
  anxiolytic — *see* Abuse, drug, sedative
  barbiturates — *see* Abuse, drug, sedative
  caffeine — *see* Abuse, drug, stimulant NEC
  cannabis, cannabinoids — *see* Abuse, drug, cannabis
  child — *see* Maltreatment, child
  cocaine — *see* Abuse, drug, cocaine
  drug NEC (non-dependent) F19.10
    with sleep disorder F19.182
    amphetamine type — *see* Abuse, drug, stimulant NEC
    analgesics (non-prescribed) (over the counter) F55.8
    antacids F55.0
    antidepressants — *see* Abuse, drug, psychoactive NEC
    anxiolytics — *see* Abuse, drug, sedative
    barbiturates — *see* Abuse, drug, sedative
    caffeine — *see* Abuse, drug, stimulant NEC
    cannabis F12.10
      with
        anxiety disorder F12.180
        intoxication F12.129
          with
            delirium F12.121
            perceptual disturbance F12.122
          uncomplicated F12.120
        other specified disorder F12.188
        psychosis F12.159
          delusions F12.150
          hallucinations F12.151
        unspecified disorder F12.19

Abuse — *continued*
  drug NEC (non-dependent) F19.10 — *continued*
    cocaine F14.10
      with
        anxiety disorder F14.180
        intoxication F14.129
          with
            delirium F14.121
            perceptual disturbance F14.122
          uncomplicated F14.120
        mood disorder F14.14
        other specified disorder F14.188
        psychosis F14.159
          delusions F14.150
          hallucinations F14.151
        sexual dysfunction F14.181
        sleep disorder F14.182
        unspecified disorder F14.19
    counseling and surveillance Z71.51
    hallucinogen F16.10
      with
        anxiety disorder F16.180
        flashbacks F16.183
        intoxication F16.129
          with
            delirium F16.121
            perceptual disturbance F16.122
          uncomplicated F16.120
        mood disorder F16.14
        other specified disorder F16.188
        perception disorder, persisting F16.183
        psychosis F16.159
          delusions F16.150
          hallucinations F16.151
        unspecified disorder F16.19
    hashish — *see* Abuse, drug, cannabis
    herbal or folk remedies F55.1
    hormones F55.3
    hypnotics — *see* Abuse, drug, sedative
    inhalant F18.10
      with
        anxiety disorder F18.180
        dementia, persisting F18.17
        intoxication F18.129
          with delirium F18.121
          uncomplicated F18.120
        mood disorder F18.14
        other specified disorder F18.188
        psychosis F18.159
          delusions F18.150
          hallucinations F18.151
        unspecified disorder F18.19
    laxatives F55.2
    LSD — *see* Abuse, drug, hallucinogen
    marihuana — *see* Abuse, drug, cannabis
    morphine type (opioids) — *see* Abuse, drug, opioid
    opioid F11.10
      with
        intoxication F11.129
          with
            delirium F11.121
            perceptual disturbance F11.122
          uncomplicated F11.120
        mood disorder F11.14
        other specified disorder F11.188
        psychosis F11.159
          delusions F11.150
          hallucinations F11.151
        sexual dysfunction F11.181
        sleep disorder F11.182
        unspecified disorder F11.19
    PCP (phencyclidine) (or related substance) — *see* Abuse, drug, hallucinogen
    psychoactive NEC F19.10
      with
        amnestic disorder F19.16
        anxiety disorder F19.180
        dementia F19.17
        intoxication F19.129
          with
            delirium F19.121
            perceptual disturbance F19.122
          uncomplicated F19.120
        mood disorder F19.14
        other specified disorder F19.188
        psychosis F19.159
          delusions F19.150
          hallucinations F19.151
        sexual dysfunction F19.181
        sleep disorder F19.182
        unspecified disorder F19.19

Abuse — *continued*
  drug NEC (non-dependent) F19.10 — *continued*
    sedative, hypnotic or anxiolytic F13.10
      with
        anxiety disorder F13.180
        intoxication F13.129
          with delirium F13.121
          uncomplicated F13.120
        mood disorder F13.14
        other specified disorder F13.188
        psychosis F13.159
          delusions F13.150
          hallucinations F13.151
        sexual dysfunction F13.181
        sleep disorder F13.182
        unspecified disorder F13.19
    solvent — *see* Abuse, drug, inhalant
    steroids F55.3
    stimulant NEC F15.10
      with
        anxiety disorder F15.180
        intoxication F15.129
          with
            delirium F15.121
            perceptual disturbance F15.122
          uncomplicated F15.120
        mood disorder F15.14
        other specified disorder F15.188
        psychosis F15.159
          delusions F15.150
          hallucinations F15.151
        sexual dysfunction F15.181
        sleep disorder F15.182
        unspecified disorder F15.19
    tranquilizers — *see* Abuse, drug, sedative
    vitamins F55.4
  hallucinogens — *see* Abuse, drug, hallucinogen
  hashish — *see* Abuse, drug, cannabis
  herbal or folk remedies F55.1
  hormones F55.3
  hypnotic — *see* Abuse, drug, sedative
  inhalant — *see* Abuse, drug, inhalant
  laxatives F55.2
  LSD — *see* Abuse, drug, hallucinogen
  marihuana — *see* Abuse, drug, cannabis
  morphine type (opioids) — *see* Abuse, drug, opioid
  non-psychoactive substance NEC F55.8
    antacids F55.0
    folk remedies F55.1
    herbal remedies F55.1
    hormones F55.3
    laxatives F55.2
    steroids F55.3
    vitamins F55.4
  opioids — *see* Abuse, drug, opioid
  PCP (phencyclidine) (or related substance) — *see* Abuse, drug, hallucinogen
  physical (adult) (child) — *see* Maltreatment
  psychoactive substance — *see* Abuse, drug, psychoactive NEC
  psychological (adult) (child) — *see* Maltreatment
  sedative — *see* Abuse, drug, sedative
  sexual — *see* Maltreatment
  solvent — *see* Abuse, drug, inhalant
  steroids F55.3
  vitamins F55.4
Acalculia R48.8
  developmental F81.2
Acanthamebiasis (with) B60.10
  conjunctiva B60.12
  keratoconjunctivitis B60.13
  meningoencephalitis B60.11
  other specified B60.19
Acanthocephaliasis B83.8
Acanthocheilonemiasis B74.4
Acanthocytosis E78.6
Acantholysis L11.9
Acanthosis (acquired) (nigricans) L83
  benign Q82.8
  congenital Q82.8
  seborrheic L82.1
    inflamed L82.0
  tongue K14.3
Acapnia E87.3
Acarbia E87.2
Acardia, acardius Q89.8
Acardiacus amorphus Q89.8
Acardiotrophia I51.4
Acariasis B88.0
  scabies B86
Acarodermatitis (urticarioides) B88.0
Acarophobia F40.218
Acatalasemia, acatalasia E80.3
Acathisia (drug induced) G25.71

Accelerated atrioventricular conduction I45.6

Accentuation of personality traits (type A) Z73.1

Accessory (congenital)
adrenal gland Q89.1
anus Q43.4
appendix Q43.4
atrioventricular conduction I45.6
auditory ossicles Q16.3
auricle (ear) Q17.0
biliary duct or passage Q44.5
bladder Q64.79
blood vessels NEC Q27.9
coronary Q24.5
bone NEC Q79.8
breast tissue, axilla Q83.1
carpal bones Q74.0
cecum Q43.4
chromosome(s) NEC (nonsex) Q92.9
with complex rearrangements NEC Q92.5
seen only at prometaphase Q92.8
13 — see Trisomy, 13
18 — see Trisomy, 18
21 — see Trisomy, 21
partial Q92.9
sex
female phenotype Q97.8
coronary artery Q24.5
cusp(s), heart valve NEC Q24.8
pulmonary Q22.3
cystic duct Q44.5
digit(s) Q69.9
ear (auricle) (lobe) Q17.0
endocrine gland NEC Q89.2
eye muscle Q10.3
eyelid Q10.3
face bone(s) Q75.8
fallopian tube (fimbria) (ostium) Q50.6
finger(s) Q69.0
foreskin N47.8
frontonasal process Q75.8
gallbladder Q44.1
genital organ(s)
female Q52.8
external Q52.79
internal NEC Q52.8
male Q55.8
genitourinary organs NEC Q89.8
female Q52.8
male Q55.8
hallux Q69.2
heart Q24.8
valve NEC Q24.8
pulmonary Q22.3
hepatic ducts Q44.5
hymen Q52.4
intestine (large) (small) Q43.4
kidney Q63.0
lacrimal canal Q10.6
leaflet, heart valve NEC Q24.8
ligament, broad Q50.6
liver Q44.7
duct Q44.5
lobule (ear) Q17.0
lung (lobe) Q33.1
muscle Q79.8
navicular of carpus Q74.0
nervous system, part NEC Q07.8
nipple Q83.3
nose Q30.8
organ or site not listed — see Anomaly, by site
ovary Q50.31
oviduct Q50.6
pancreas Q45.3
parathyroid gland Q89.2
parotid gland (and duct) Q38.4
pituitary gland Q89.2
preauricular appendage Q17.0
prepuce N47.8
renal arteries (multiple) Q27.2
rib Q76.6
cervical Q76.5
roots (teeth) K00.2
salivary gland Q38.4
sesamoid bones Q74.8
foot Q74.2
hand Q74.0
skin tags Q82.8
spleen Q89.09
sternum Q76.7
submaxillary gland Q38.4
tarsal bones Q74.2
teeth, tooth K00.1
tendon Q79.8
thumb Q69.1
thymus gland Q89.2
thyroid gland Q89.2

Accessory (congenital) — continued
toes Q69.2
tongue Q38.3
tooth, teeth K00.1
tragus Q17.0
ureter Q62.5
urethra Q64.79
urinary organ or tract NEC Q64.8
uterus Q51.2
vagina Q52.10
valve, heart NEC Q24.8
pulmonary Q22.3
vertebra Q76.49
vocal cords Q31.8
vulva Q52.79

Accident
birth — see Birth, injury
cardiac — see Infarct, myocardium
cerebral I63.9
cerebrovascular (embolic) (ischemic) (thrombotic) I63.9
aborted I63.9
hemorrhagic — see Hemorrhage, intracranial, intracerebral
old (without sequelae) Z86.73
with sequelae (of) — see Sequelae, infarction, cerebral
coronary — see Infarct, myocardium
craniovascular I63.9
vascular, brain I63.9

Accidental — see condition

Accommodation (disorder) — see also condition
hysterical paralysis of F44.89
insufficiency of H52.4
paresis — see Paresis, of accommodation
spasm — see Spasm, of accommodation

Accouchement — see Delivery

Accreta placenta O43.21-

Accretio cordis (nonrheumatic) I31.0

Accretions, tooth, teeth K03.6

Acculturation difficulty Z60.3

Accumulation secretion, prostate N42.89

Acephalia, acephalism, acephalus, acephaly Q00.0

Acephalobrachia monster Q89.8

Acephalochirus monster Q89.8

Acephalogaster Q89.8

Acephalostomus monster Q89.8

Acephalothorax Q89.8

Acerophobia F40.298

Acetonemia R79.89
in Type 1 diabetes E10.10
with coma E10.11

Acetonuria R82.4

Achalasia (cardia) (esophagus) K22.0
congenital Q39.5
pylorus Q40.0
sphincteral NEC K59.8

Ache(s) — see Pain

Acheilia Q38.6

Achilloburitis — see Tendinitis, Achilles

Achillodynia — see Tendinitis, Achilles

Achlorhydria, achlorhydric (neurogenic) K31.83
anemia D50.8
diarrhea K31.83
psychogenic F45.8
secondary to vagotomy K91.1

Achluophobia F40.228

Acholia K82.8

Acholuric jaundice (familial) (splenomegalic) — see also Spherocytosis
acquired D59.8

Achondrogenesis Q77.0

Achondroplasia (osteosclerosis congenita) Q77.4

Achroma, cutis L80

Achromat(ism), achromatopsia (acquired) (congenital) H53.51

Achromia, congenital — see Albinism

Achromia parasitica B36.0

Achylia gastrica K31.89
psychogenic F45.8

Acid
burn — see Corrosion
deficiency
amide nicotinic E52
ascorbic E54
folic E53.8
nicotinic E52
pantothenic E53.8
intoxication E87.2
peptic disease K30
phosphatase deficiency E83.39
stomach K30
psychogenic F45.8

Acidemia E87.2
argininosuccinic E72.22
isovaleric E71.110
metabolic (newborn) P19.9
first noted before onset of labor P19.0
first noted during labor P19.1
noted at birth P19.2
methylmalonic E71.120
pipecolic E72.3
propionic E71.121

Acidity, gastric (high) K30
psychogenic F45.8

Acidocytopenia — see Agranulocytosis

Acidocytosis D72.1

Acidopenia — see Agranulocytosis

Acidosis (lactic) (respiratory) E87.2
in Type 1 diabetes E10.10
with coma E10.11
kidney, tubular N25.89
lactic E87.2
metabolic NEC E87.2
with respiratory acidosis E87.4
late, of newborn P74.0
mixed metabolic and respiratory, newborn P84
newborn P84
renal (hyperchloremic) (tubular) N25.89
respiratory E87.2
complicated by
metabolic
acidosis E87.4
alkalosis E87.4

Aciduria
argininosuccinic E72.22
glutaric (type I) E72.3
type II E71.313
type III E71.5-
orotic (congenital) (hereditary) (pyrimidine deficiency) E79.8
anemia D53.0

Acladiosis (skin) B36.0

Aclasis, diaphyseal Q78.6

Acleistocardia Q21.1

Aclusion — see Anomaly, dentofacial, malocclusion

Acne L70.9
artificialis L70.8
atrophica L70.2
cachecticorum (Hebra) L70.8
conglobata L70.1
cystic L70.0
decalvans L66.2
excoriée des jeunes filles L70.5
frontalis L70.2
indurata L70.0
infantile L70.4
keloid L73.0
lupoid L70.2
necrotic, necrotica (miliaris) L70.2
neonatal L70.4
nodular L70.0
occupational L70.8
picker's L70.5
pustular L70.0
rodens L70.2
rosacea L71.9
specified NEC L70.8
tropica L70.3
varioliformis L70.2
vulgaris L70.0

Acnitis (primary) A18.4

Acosta's disease T70.29

Acoustic — see condition

Acousticophobia F40.298

Acquired — see also condition
immunodeficiency syndrome (AIDS) B20

Acrania Q00.0

Acroangiodermatitis I78.9

Acroasphyxia, chronic I73.89

Acrobystitis N47.7

Acrocephalopolysyndactyly Q87.0

Acrocephalosyndactyly Q87.0

Acrocephaly Q75.0

Acrochondrohyperplasia — see Syndrome, Marfan's

Acrocyanosis I73.8
newborn P28.2
meaning transient blue hands and feet — omit code

Acrodermatitis L30.8
atrophicans (chronica) L90.4
continua (Hallopeau) L40.2
enteropathica (hereditary) E83.2
Hallopeau's L40.2
infantile papular L44.4
perstans L40.2
pustulosa continua L40.2
recalcitrant pustular L40.2

Acrodynia — see Poisoning, mercury

Acromegaly, acromegalia E22.0

Acromelalgia I73.81

Acromicria, acromikria Q79.8

Acronyx L60.0

Acropachy, thyroid — see Thyrotoxicosis

Acroparesthesia (simple) (vasomotor) I73.89

Acropathy, thyroid — see Thyrotoxicosis

Acrophobia F40.241

Acroposthitis N47.7

Acroscleriasis, acroscleroderma, acrosclerosis — see Sclerosis, systemic

Acrosphacelus I96

Acrospiroma, eccrine — see Neoplasm, skin, benign

Acrostealgia — see Osteochondropathy

Acrotrophodynia — see Immersion

ACTH ectopic syndrome E24.3

Actinic — see condition

Actinobacillosis, actinobacillus A28.8
mallei A24.0
muris A25.1

Actinomyces israelii (infection) — see Actinomycosis

Actinomycetoma (foot) B47.1

Actinomycosis, actinomycotic A42.9
with pneumonia A42.0
abdominal A42.1
cervicofacial A42.2
cutaneous A42.89
gastrointestinal A42.1
pulmonary A42.0
sepsis A42.7
specified site NEC A42.89

Actinoneuritis G62.82

Action, heart
disorder I49.9
irregular I49.9
psychogenic F45.8

Activated protein C resistance D68.51

Active — see condition

Acute — see also condition
abdomen R10.0
gallbladder — see Cholecystitis, acute

Acyanotic heart disease (congenital) Q24.9

Acystia Q64.5

Adair-Dighton syndrome (brittle bones and blue sclera, deafness) Q78.0

Adamantinoblastoma — see Ameloblastoma

Adamantinoma — see also Cyst, calcifying odontogenic
long bones C40.90
lower limb C40.2-
upper limb C40.0-
malignant C41.1
jaw (bone) (lower) C41.1
upper C41.0
tibial C40.2-

Adamantoblastoma — see Ameloblastoma

Adams-Stokes(-Morgagni) disease or syndrome I45.9

Adaption reaction — see Disorder, adjustment

Addiction (see also Dependence) F19.20
alcohol, alcoholic (ethyl) (methyl) (wood) (without remission) F10.20
with remission F10.21
drug — see Dependence, drug
ethyl alcohol (without remission) F10.20
with remission F10.21
heroin — see Dependence, drug, opioid
methyl alcohol (without remission) F10.20
with remission F10.21
methylated spirit (without remission) F10.20
with remission F10.21
morphine(-like substances) — see Dependence, drug, opioid
nicotine — see Dependence, drug, nicotine
opium and opioids — see Dependence, drug, opioid
tobacco — see Dependence, drug, nicotine

Addison-Biermer anemia (pernicious) D51.0

Addisonian crisis E27.2

Addison's
anemia (pernicious) D51.0
disease (bronze) or syndrome E27.1
tuberculous A18.7
keloid L94.0

Addison-Schilder complex E71.528

Additional — see also Accessory
chromosome(s) Q99.8
21 — see Trisomy, 21
sex — see Abnormal, chromosome, sex

Adduction contracture, hip or other joint — see Contraction, joint

Adenitis — see also Lymphadenitis
acute, unspecified site L04.9
axillary I88.9
acute L04.2
chronic or subacute I88.1

D I S E A S E   I N D E X

Adenitis (see also Lymphadenitis) — continued
  Bartholin's gland N75.8
  bulbourethral gland — see Urethritis
  cervical I88.9
    acute L04.0
    chronic or subacute I88.1
  chancroid (Hemophilus ducreyi) A57
  chronic, unspecified site I88.1
  Cowper's gland — see Urethritis
  due to Pasteurella multocida (p. septica)
    A28.0
  epidemic, acute B27.09
  gangrenous L04.9
  gonorrheal NEC A54.89
  groin I88.9
    acute L04.1
    chronic or subacute I88.1
  infectious (acute) (epidemic) B27.09
  inguinal I88.9
    acute L04.1
    chronic or subacute I88.1
  lymph gland or node, except mesenteric
    I88.9
    acute — see Lymphadenitis, acute
    chronic or subacute I88.1
  mesenteric (acute) (chronic) (nonspecific)
    (subacute) I88.0
  parotid gland (suppurative) — see
    Sialoadenitis
  salivary gland (any) (suppurative) — see
    Sialoadenitis
  scrofulous (tuberculous) A18.2
  Skene's duct or gland — see Urethritis
  strumous, tuberculous A18.2
  subacute, unspecified site I88.1
  sublingual gland (suppurative) — see
    Sialoadenitis
  submandibular gland (suppurative) — see
    Sialoadenitis
  submaxillary gland (suppurative) — see
    Sialoadenitis
  tuberculous — see Tuberculosis, lymph
    gland
  urethral gland — see Urethritis
  Wharton's duct (suppurative) — see
    Sialoadenitis
Adenoacanthoma — see Neoplasm,
  malignant, by site
Adenoameloblastoma — see Cyst, calcifying
  odontogenic
Adenocarcinoid (tumor) — see Neoplasm,
  malignant, by site
Adenocarcinoma — see also Neoplasm,
  malignant, by site
  acidophil
    specified site — see Neoplasm,
      malignant, by site
    unspecified site C75.1
  adrenal cortical C74.0
  alveolar — see Neoplasm, lung, malignant
  apocrine
    breast — see Neoplasm, breast,
      malignant
    in situ
      breast D05.8-
      specified site NEC — see Neoplasm,
        skin, in situ
      unspecified site D04.9
    specified site NEC — see Neoplasm,
      skin, malignant
    unspecified site C44.99
  basal cell
    specified site — see Neoplasm, skin,
      malignant
    unspecified site C08.9
  basophil
    specified site — see Neoplasm,
      malignant, by site
    unspecified site C75.1
  bile duct type C22.1
    liver C22.1
    specified site NEC — see Neoplasm,
      malignant, by site
    unspecified site C22.1
  bronchiolar — see Neoplasm, lung,
    malignant
  bronchioloalveolar — see Neoplasm, lung,
    malignant
  ceruminous C44.29-
  cervix, in situ (see also Carcinoma, cervix
    uteri, in situ) D06.9
  chromophobe
    specified site — see Neoplasm,
      malignant, by site
    unspecified site C75.1
  diffuse type
    specified site — see Neoplasm,
      malignant, by site
    unspecified site C16.9

Adenocarcinoma (see also Neoplasm,
  malignant, by site) — continued
  duct
    infiltrating
      with Paget's disease — see Neoplasm,
        breast, malignant
      specified site — see Neoplasm,
        malignant, by site
      unspecified site (female) C50.91-
        male C50.92-
      specified site — see Neoplasm,
        malignant, by site
      unspecified site
        female C56.9
        male C61
    eosinophil
      specified site — see Neoplasm,
        malignant, by site
      unspecified site C75.1
    follicular
      with papillary C73
      moderately differentiated C73
      specified site — see Neoplasm,
        malignant, by site
      trabecular C73
      unspecified site C73
      well differentiated C73
    Hurthle cell C73
    in
      adenomatous
        polyposis coli C18.9
    infiltrating duct
      with Paget's disease — see Neoplasm,
        breast, malignant
      specified site — see Neoplasm, by site,
        malignant
      unspecified site (female) C50.91-
        male C50.92-
    inflammatory
      specified site — see Neoplasm, by site,
        malignant
      unspecified site (female) C50.91-
        male C50.92-
    intestinal type
      specified site — see Neoplasm, by site,
        malignant
      unspecified site C16.9
    intracystic papillary
    intraductal
      breast D05.1-
      noninfiltrating
        breast D05.1-
        papillary
          with invasion
            specified site — see Neoplasm,
              by site, malignant
            unspecified site (female)
              C50.91-
              male C50.92-
          breast D05.1-
          specified site NEC — see
            Neoplasm, in situ, by site
          unspecified site D05.1-
        specified site NEC — see Neoplasm,
          in situ, by site
        unspecified site D05.1-
      papillary
        with invasion
          specified site — see Neoplasm,
            malignant, by site
          unspecified site (female) C50.91-
            male C50.92-
        breast D05.1-
        specified site — see Neoplasm, in
          situ, by site
        unspecified site D05.1-
      specified site NEC — see Neoplasm, in
        situ, by site
      unspecified site D05.1-
    islet cell
      with exocrine, mixed
        specified site — see Neoplasm,
          malignant, by site
        unspecified site C25.9
      pancreas C25.4
      specified site NEC — see Neoplasm,
        malignant, by site
      unspecified site C25.4
    lobular
      in situ
        breast D05.0-
        specified site NEC — see Neoplasm,
          in situ, by site
        unspecified site D05.0-
      specified site — see Neoplasm,
        malignant, by site
      unspecified site (female) C50.91-
        male C50.92-

Adenocarcinoma (see also Neoplasm,
  malignant, by site) — continued
  mucoid — see also Neoplasm, malignant,
    by site
    cell
      specified site — see Neoplasm,
        malignant, by site
      unspecified site C75.1
    nonencapsulated sclerosing C73
    papillary
      with follicular C73
      follicular variant C73
      intraductal (noninfiltrating)
        with invasion
          specified site — see Neoplasm,
            malignant, by site
          unspecified site (female) C50.91-
            male C50.92-
        breast D05.1-
        specified site NEC — see Neoplasm,
          in situ, by site
        unspecified site D05.1-
      serous
        specified site — see Neoplasm,
          malignant, by site
        unspecified site C56.9
    papillocystic
      specified site — see Neoplasm,
        malignant, by site
      unspecified site C56.9
    pseudomucinous
      specified site — see Neoplasm,
        malignant, by site
      unspecified site C56.9
    renal cell C64-
    sebaceous — see Neoplasm, skin,
      malignant
    serous — see also Neoplasm, malignant, by
      site
      papillary
        specified site — see Neoplasm,
          malignant, by site
        unspecified site C56.9
    sweat gland — see Neoplasm, skin,
      malignant
    water-clear cell C75.0
Adenocarcinoma-in-situ — see also
  Neoplasm, in situ, by site
  breast D05.9-
Adenofibroma
  clear cell — see Neoplasm, benign, by site
  endometrioid D27.9
    borderline malignancy D39.10
    malignant C56-
  mucinous
    specified site — see Neoplasm, benign,
      by site
    unspecified site D27.9
  papillary
    specified site — see Neoplasm, benign,
      by site
    unspecified site D27.9
  prostate — see Enlargement, enlarged,
    prostate
  serous
    specified site — see Neoplasm, benign,
      by site
    unspecified site D27.9
  specified site — see Neoplasm, benign, by
    site
  unspecified site D27.9
Adenofibrosis
  breast — see Fibroadenosis, breast
  endometrioid N80.0
Adenoiditis (chronic) J35.02
  with tonsillitis J35.03
  acute J03.90
    recurrent J03.91
    specified organism NEC J03.80
      recurrent J03.81
    staphylococcal J03.80
      recurrent J03.81
    streptococcal J03.00
      recurrent J03.01
Adenoids — see condition
Adenolipoma — see Neoplasm, benign, by
  site
Adenolipomatosis, Launois-Bensaude
  E88.89
Adenolymphoma
  specified site — see Neoplasm, benign, by
    site
  unspecified site D11.9
Adenoma — see also Neoplasm, benign, by
  site
  acidophil
    specified site — see Neoplasm, benign,
      by site
    unspecified site D35.2

Adenoma (see also Neoplasm, benign, by
  site) — continued
  acidophil-basophil, mixed
    specified site — see Neoplasm, benign,
      by site
    unspecified site D35.2
  adrenal (cortical) D35.00
    clear cell D35.00
    compact cell D35.00
    glomerulosa cell D35.00
    heavily pigmented variant D35.00
    mixed cell D35.00
  alpha-cell
    pancreas D13.7
    specified site NEC — see Neoplasm,
      benign, by site
    unspecified site D13.7
  alveolar D14.30
  apocrine
    breast D24-
    specified site NEC — see Neoplasm,
      skin, benign, by site
    unspecified site D23.9
  basal cell D11.9
  basophil
    specified site — see Neoplasm, benign,
      by site
    unspecified site D35.2
  basophil-acidophil, mixed
    specified site — see Neoplasm, benign,
      by site
    unspecified site D35.2
  beta-cell
    pancreas D13.7
    specified site NEC — see Neoplasm,
      benign, by site
    unspecified site D13.7
  bile duct D13.4
    common D13.5
    extrahepatic D13.5
    intrahepatic D13.4
    specified site NEC — see Neoplasm,
      benign, by site
    unspecified site D13.4
  black D35.00
  bronchial D38.1
    cylindroid type — see Neoplasm, lung,
      malignant
  ceruminous D23.2-
  chief cell D35.1
  chromophobe
    specified site — see Neoplasm, benign,
      by site
    unspecified site D35.2
  colloid
    specified site — see Neoplasm, benign,
      by site
    unspecified site D34
  duct
  eccrine, papillary — see Neoplasm, skin,
    benign
  endocrine, multiple
    single specified site — see Neoplasm,
      uncertain behavior, by site
    two or more specified sites D44-
    unspecified site D44.9
  endometrioid — see also Neoplasm, benign
    borderline malignancy — see Neoplasm,
      uncertain behavior, by site
  eosinophil
    specified site — see Neoplasm, benign,
      by site
    unspecified site D35.2
  fetal
    specified site — see Neoplasm, benign,
      by site
    unspecified site D34
  follicular
    specified site — see Neoplasm, benign,
      by site
    unspecified site D34
  hepatocellular D13.4
  Hurthle cell D34
  islet cell
    pancreas D13.7
    specified site NEC — see Neoplasm,
      benign, by site
    unspecified site D13.7
  liver cell D13.4
  macrofollicular
    specified site — see Neoplasm, benign,
      by site
    unspecified site D34
  malignant, malignum — see Neoplasm,
    malignant, by site
  microcystic
    pancreas D13.7
    specified site NEC — see Neoplasm,
      benign, by site
    unspecified site D13.7

DISEASE INDEX

Adenoma *(see also* Neoplasm, benign, by site*) — continued*
microfollicular
specified site — *see* Neoplasm, benign, by site
unspecified site D34
mucoid cell
specified site — *see* Neoplasm, benign, by site
unspecified site D35.2
multiple endocrine
single specified site — *see* Neoplasm, uncertain behavior, by site
two or more specified sites D44-
unspecified site D44.9
nipple D24-
papillary — *see also* Neoplasm, benign, by site
eccrine — *see* Neoplasm, skin, benign, by site
Pick's tubular
specified site — *see* Neoplasm, benign, by site
unspecified site
female D27.9
male D29.20
pleomorphic
carcinoma in — *see* Neoplasm, salivary gland, malignant
specified site — *see* Neoplasm, malignant, by site
unspecified site C08.9
polypoid — *see also* Neoplasm, benign
adenocarcinoma in — *see* Neoplasm, malignant, by site
adenocarcinoma in situ — *see* Neoplasm, in situ, by site
prostate — *see* Neoplasm, benign, prostate
rete cell D29.20
sebaceous — *see* Neoplasm, skin, benign
Sertoli cell
specified site — *see* Neoplasm, benign, by site
unspecified site
female D27.9
male D29.20
skin appendage — *see* Neoplasm, skin, benign
sudoriferous gland — *see* Neoplasm, skin, benign
sweat gland — *see* Neoplasm, skin, benign
testicular
specified site — *see* Neoplasm, benign, by site
unspecified site
female D27.9
male D29.20
tubular — *see also* Neoplasm, benign, by site
adenocarcinoma in — *see* Neoplasm, malignant, by site
adenocarcinoma in situ — *see* Neoplasm, in situ, by site
Pick's
specified site — *see* Neoplasm, benign, by site
unspecified site
female D27.9
male D29.20
tubulovillous — *see also* Neoplasm, benign, by site
adenocarcinoma in — *see* Neoplasm, malignant, by site
adenocarcinoma in situ — *see* Neoplasm, in situ, by site
villous — *see* Neoplasm, uncertain behavior, by site
adenocarcinoma in — *see* Neoplasm, malignant, by site
adenocarcinoma in situ — *see* Neoplasm, in situ, by site
water-clear cell D35.1
Adenomatosis
endocrine (multiple) E31.20
single specified site — *see* Neoplasm, uncertain behavior, by site
erosive of nipple D24-
pluriendocrine — *see* Adenomatosis, endocrine
pulmonary D38.1
malignant — *see* Neoplasm, lung, malignant
specified site — *see* Neoplasm, benign, by site
unspecified site D12.6

Adenomatous
goiter (nontoxic) E04.9
with hyperthyroidism — *see* Hyperthyroidism, with, goiter, nodular
toxic — *see* Hyperthyroidism, with, goiter, nodular
Adenomyoma — *see also* Neoplasm, benign, by site
prostate — *see* Enlarged, prostate
Adenomyometritis N80.0
Adenomyosis N80.0
Adenopathy (lymph gland) R59.9
generalized R59.1
inguinal R59.0
localized R59.0
mediastinal R59.0
mesentery R59.0
syphilitic (secondary) A51.49
tracheobronchial R59.0
tuberculous A15.4
primary (progressive) A15.7
tuberculous — *see also* Tuberculosis, lymph gland
tracheobronchial A15.4
primary (progressive) A15.7
Adenosalpingitis — *see* Salpingitis
Adenosarcoma — *see* Neoplasm, malignant, by site
Adenosclerosis I88.8
Adenosis (sclerosing) breast — *see* Fibroadenosis, breast
Adenovirus, as cause of disease classified elsewhere B97.0
Adentia (complete) (partial) — *see* Absence, teeth
Adherent — *see also* Adhesions
labia (minora) N90.89
pericardium (nonrheumatic) I31.0
rheumatic I09.2
placenta (with hemorrhage) O72.0
without hemorrhage O73.0
prepuce, newborn N47.0
scar (skin) L90.5
tendon in scar L90.5
Adhesions, adhesive (postinfective) K66.0
with intestinal obstruction K56.5
abdominal (wall) — *see* Adhesions, peritoneum
appendix K38.8
bile duct (common) (hepatic) K83.8
bladder (sphincter) N32.89
bowel — *see* Adhesions, peritoneum
cardiac I31.0
rheumatic I09.2
cecum — *see* Adhesions, peritoneum
cervicovaginal N88.1
congenital Q52.8
postpartal O90.89
old N88.1
cervix N88.1
ciliary body NEC — *see* Adhesions, iris
clitoris N90.89
colon — *see* Adhesions, peritoneum
common duct K83.8
congenital — *see also* Anomaly, by site
fingers — *see* Syndactylism, complex, fingers
omental, anomalous Q43.3
peritoneal Q43.3
tongue (to gum or roof of mouth) Q38.3
conjunctiva (acquired) H11.21-
congenital Q15.8
cystic duct K82.8
diaphragm — *see* Adhesions, peritoneum
due to foreign body — *see* Foreign body
duodenum — *see* Adhesions, peritoneum
ear
middle H74.1-
epididymis N50.8
epidural — *see* Adhesions, meninges
epiglottis J38.7
eyelid H02.59
female pelvis N73.6
gallbladder K82.8
globe H44.89
heart I31.0
rheumatic I09.2
ileocecal (coil) — *see* Adhesions, peritoneum
ileum — *see* Adhesions, peritoneum
intestine — *see also* Adhesions, peritoneum
with obstruction K56.5
intra-abdominal — *see* Adhesions, peritoneum
iris H21.50-
anterior H21.51-
goniosynechiae H21.52-
posterior H21.54-
to corneal graft T85.89

Adhesions, adhesive (postinfective) K66.0 — *continued*
joint — *see* Ankylosis
knee M23.8x
temporomandibular M26.61
labium (majus) (minus), congenital Q52.5
liver — *see* Adhesions, peritoneum
lung J98.4
mediastinum J98.5
meninges (cerebral) (spinal) G96.12
congenital Q07.8
tuberculous (cerebral) (spinal) A17.0
mesenteric — *see* Adhesions, peritoneum
nasal (septum) (to turbinates) J34.89
ocular muscle — *see* Strabismus, mechanical
omentum — *see* Adhesions, peritoneum
ovary N73.6
congenital (to cecum, kidney or omentum) Q50.39
paraovarian N73.6
pelvic (peritoneal)
female N73.6
postprocedural N99.4
male — *see* Adhesions, peritoneum
postpartal (old) N73.6
tuberculous A18.17
penis to scrotum (congenital) Q55.8
periappendiceal — *see also* Adhesions, peritoneum
pericardium (nonrheumatic) I31.0
focal I31.8
rheumatic I09.2
tuberculous A18.84
pericholecystic K82.8
perigastric — *see* Adhesions, peritoneum
periovarian N73.6
periprostatic N42.89
perirectal — *see* Adhesions, peritoneum
perirenal N28.89
peritoneum, peritoneal (postinfective) (postprocedural) K66.0
with obstruction (intestinal) K56.5
congenital Q43.3
pelvic, female N73.6
postprocedural N99.4
postpartal, pelvic N73.6
to uterus N73.6
peritubal N73.6
periureteral N28.89
periuterine N73.6
perivesical N32.89
perivesicular (seminal vesicle) N50.8
pleura, pleuritic J94.8
tuberculous NEC A15.6
pleuropericardial J94.8
postoperative (gastrointestinal tract) K66.0
with obstruction K91.3
due to foreign body accidentally left in wound — *see* Foreign body, accidentally left during a procedure
pelvic peritoneal N99.4
urethra — *see* Stricture, urethra, postprocedural
vagina N99.2
postpartal, old (vulva or perineum) N90.89
preputial, prepuce N47.5
pulmonary J98.4
pylorus — *see* Adhesions, peritoneum
sciatic nerve — *see* Lesion, nerve, sciatic
seminal vesicle N50.8
shoulder (joint) — *see* Capsulitis, adhesive
sigmoid flexure — *see* Adhesions, peritoneum
spermatic cord (acquired) N50.8
congenital Q55.4
spinal canal G96.12
stomach — *see* Adhesions, peritoneum
subscapular — *see* Capsulitis, adhesive
temporomandibular M26.61
tendinitis — *see also* Tenosynovitis, specified type NEC
shoulder — *see* Capsulitis, adhesive
testis N44.8
tongue, congenital (to gum or roof of mouth) Q38.3
acquired K14.8
trachea J39.8
tubo-ovarian N73.6
tunica vaginalis N44.8
uterus N73.6
internal N85.6
to abdominal wall N73.6
vagina (chronic) N89.5
postoperative N99.2
vitreomacular H43.82-
vitreous H43.89
vulva N90.89
Adiaspiromycosis B48.8

Adie(-Holmes) pupil or syndrome — *see* Anomaly, pupil, function, tonic pupil
Adiponecrosis neonatorum P83.8
Adiposis — *see also* Obesity
cerebralis E23.6
dolorosa E88.2
Adiposity — *see also* Obesity
heart — *see* Degeneration, myocardial
localized E65
Adiposogenital dystrophy E23.6
Adjustment
disorder — *see* Disorder, adjustment
implanted device — *see* Encounter (for), adjustment (of)
prosthesis, external — *see* Fitting
reaction — *see* Disorder, adjustment
Administration of tPA (rtPA) in a different facility within the last 24 hours prior to admission to current facility Z92.82
Admission (for) — *see also* Encounter (for)
adjustment (of)
artificial
arm Z44.00-
complete Z44.01-
partial Z44.02-
eye Z44.2
leg Z44.10-
complete Z44.11-
partial Z44.12-
brain neuropacemaker Z46.2
implanted Z45.42
breast
implant Z45.81
prosthesis (external) Z44.3
colostomy belt Z46.89
contact lenses Z46.0
cystostomy device Z46.6
dental prosthesis Z46.3
device NEC
abdominal Z46.89
implanted Z45.89
cardiac Z45.09
defibrillator (with synchronous cardiace pacemaker) Z45.02
pacemaker Z45.018
pulse generator Z45.010
hearing device Z45.328
bone conduction Z45.320
cochlear Z45.321
infusion pump Z45.1
nervous system Z45.49
CSF drainage Z45.41
hearing device — *see* Admission, adjustment, device, implanted, hearing device
neuropacemaker Z45.42
visual substitution Z45.31
specified NEC Z45.89
vascular access Z45.2
visual substitution Z45.31
nervous system Z46.2
implanted — *see* Admission, adjustment, device, implanted, nervous system
orthodontic Z46.4
prosthetic Z44.9
arm — *see* Admission, adjustment, artificial, arm
breast Z44.3
dental Z46.3
eye Z44.2
leg — *see* Admission, adjustment, artificial, leg
specified type NEC Z44.8
substitution
auditory Z46.2
implanted — *see* Admission, adjustment, device, implanted, hearing device
nervous system Z46.2
implanted — *see* Admission, adjustment, device, implanted, nervous system
visual Z46.2
implanted Z45.31
urinary Z46.6
hearing aid Z46.1
implanted — *see* Admission, adjustment, device, implanted, hearing device
ileostomy device Z46.89
intestinal appliance or device NEC Z46.89
neuropacemaker (brain) (peripheral nerve) (spinal cord) Z46.2
implanted Z45.42
orthodontic device Z46.4
orthopedic (brace) (cast) (device) (shoes) Z46.89

D I S E A S E   I N D E X

Admission (for) *(see also* Encounter (for)) — continued
  adjustment (of) — *continued*
    pacemaker
      cardiac Z45.018
        pulse generator Z45.010
      nervous system Z46.2
        implanted Z45.42
    portacath (port-a-cath) Z45.2
    prosthesis Z44.9
      arm — *see* Admission, adjustment, artificial, arm
      breast Z44.3
      dental Z46.3
      eye Z44.2
      leg — *see* Admission, adjustment, artificial, leg
      specified NEC Z44.8
    spectacles Z46.0
  aftercare *(see also* Aftercare) Z51.89
    postpartum
      immediately after delivery Z39.0
      routine follow-up Z39.2
    radiation therapy (antineoplastic) Z51.0
  attention to artificial opening (of) Z43.9
    artificial vagina Z43.7
    colostomy Z43.3
    cystostomy Z43.5
    enterostomy Z43.4
    gastrostomy Z43.1
    ileostomy Z43.2
    jejunostomy Z43.4
    nephrostomy Z43.6
    specified site NEC Z43.8
      intestinal tract Z43.4
      urinary tract Z43.6
    tracheostomy Z43.0
    ureterostomy Z43.6
    urethrostomy Z43.6
  breast augmentation or reduction Z41.1
  breast reconstruction following mastectomy Z42.1
  change of
    dressing (nonsurgical) Z48.00
    neuropacemaker device (brain) (peripheral nerve) (spinal cord) Z46.2
      implanted Z45.42
    surgical dressing Z48.01
  circumcision, ritual or routine (in absence of diagnosis) Z41.2
  clinical research investigation (control) (normal comparison) (participant) Z00.6
  contraceptive management Z30.9
  cosmetic surgery NEC Z41.1
  counseling — *see also* Counseling
    dietary Z71.3
    HIV Z71.7
    human immunodeficiency virus Z71.7
    nonattending third party Z71.0
    procreative management NEC Z31.69
  delivery, full-term, uncomplicated O80
    cesarean, without indication O82
  dietary surveillance and counseling Z71.3
  ear piercing Z41.3
  examination at health care facility (adult) *(see also* Examination) Z00.00
    with abnormal findings Z00.01
    clinical research investigation (control) (normal comparison) (participant) Z00.6
    dental Z01.20
      with abnormal findings Z01.21
    donor (potential) Z00.5
    ear Z01.10
      with abnormal findings NEC Z01.118
    eye Z01.00
      with abnormal findings Z01.01
    general, specified reason NEC Z00.8
    hearing Z01.10
      with abnormal findings NEC Z01.118
    postpartum checkup Z39.2
    psychiatric (general) Z00.8
      requested by authority Z04.6
    vision Z01.00
      with abnormal findings Z01.01
  fitting (of)
    artificial
      arm — *see* Admission, adjustment, artificial, arm
      eye Z44.2
      leg — *see* Admission, adjustment, artificial, leg
    brain neuropacemaker Z46.2
      implanted Z45.42
    breast prosthesis (external) Z44.3
    colostomy belt Z46.89
    contact lenses Z46.0
    cystostomy device Z46.6
    dental prosthesis Z46.3

Admission (for) *(see also* Encounter (for)) — continued
  fitting (of) — *continued*
    dentures Z46.3
    device NEC
      abdominal Z46.89
      nervous system Z46.2
        implanted — *see* Admission, adjustment, device, implanted, nervous system
    orthodontic Z46.4
    prosthetic Z44.9
      breast Z44.3
      dental Z46.3
      eye Z44.2
    substitution
      auditory Z46.2
        implanted — *see* Admission, adjustment, device, implanted, hearing device
      nervous system Z46.2
        implanted — *see* Admission, adjustment, device, implanted, nervous system
      visual Z46.2
        implanted Z45.31
    hearing aid Z46.1
    ileostomy device Z46.89
    intestinal appliance or device NEC Z46.89
    neuropacemaker (brain) (peripheral nerve) (spinal cord) Z46.2
      implanted Z45.42
    orthodontic device Z46.4
    orthopedic device (brace) (cast) (shoes) Z46.89
    prosthesis Z44.9
      arm — *see* Admission, adjustment, artificial, arm
      breast Z44.3
      dental Z46.3
      eye Z44.2
      leg — *see* Admission, adjustment, artificial, leg
      specified type NEC Z44.8
    spectacles Z46.0
  follow-up examination Z09
  intrauterine device management Z30.431
    initial prescription Z30.014
  mental health evaluation Z00.8
    requested by authority Z04.6
  observation — *see* Observation
  Papanicolaou smear, cervix Z12.4
    for suspected malignant neoplasm Z12.4
  plastic and reconstructive surgery following medical procedure or healed injury NEC Z42.8
  plastic surgery, cosmetic NEC Z41.1
  postpartum observation
    immediately after delivery Z39.0
    routine follow-up Z39.2
  poststerilization (for restoration) Z31.0
    aftercare Z31.42
  procreative management Z31.9
  prophylactic (measure)
    organ removal Z40.00
      breast Z40.01
      ovary Z40.02
      specified organ NEC Z40.09
      testes Z40.09
    vaccination Z23
  psychiatric examination (general) Z00.8
    requested by authority Z04.6
  radiation therapy (antineoplastic) Z51.0
  reconstructive surgery following medical procedure or healed injury NEC Z42.8
  removal of
    cystostomy catheter Z43.5
    drains Z48.03
    dressing (nonsurgical) Z48.00
    intrauterine contraceptive device Z30.432
    neuropacemaker (brain) (peripheral nerve) (spinal cord) Z46.2
      implanted Z45.42
    staples Z48.02
    surgical dressing Z48.01
    sutures Z48.02
    ureteral stent Z46.6
  respirator [ventilator] use during power failure Z99.12
  restoration of organ continuity (poststerilization) Z31.0
    aftercare Z31.42
  sensitivity test — *see also* Test, skin
    allergy NEC Z01.82
    Mantoux Z11.1

Admission (for) *(see also* Encounter (for)) — continued
  tuboplasty following previous sterilization Z31.0
    aftercare Z31.42
  vasoplasty following previous sterilization Z31.0
    aftercare Z31.42
  vision examination Z01.00
    with abnormal findings Z01.01
  waiting period for admission to other facility Z75.1
Adnexitis (suppurative) — *see* Salpingo-oophoritis
Adolescent X-linked adrenoleukodystrophy E71.521
Adrenal (gland) — *see* condition
Adrenalism, tuberculous A18.7
Adrenalitis, adrenitis E27.8
  autoimmune E27.1
  meningococcal, hemorrhagic A39.1
Adrenarche, premature E27.0
Adrenocortical syndrome — *see* Cushing's, syndrome
Adrenogenital syndrome E25.9
  acquired E25.8
  congenital E25.0
  salt loss E25.0
Adrenogenitalism, congenital E25.0
Adrenoleukodystrophy E71.529
  neonatal E71.511
  X-linked E71.529
    Addison only phenotype E71.528
    Addison-Schilder E71.528
    adolescent E71.521
    adrenomyeloneuropathy E71.522
    childhood cerebral E71.520
    other specified E71.528
Adrenomyeloneuropathy E71.522
Adventitious bursa — *see* Bursopathy, specified type NEC
Adverse effect — *see* Table of Drugs and Chemicals, categories T36-T50, with 6th character 5
Advice — *see* Counseling
Adynamia (episodica) (hereditary) (periodic) G72.3
Aeration lung imperfect, newborn — *see* Atelectasis
Aero-otitis media T70.0
Aerobullosis T70.3
Aerocele — *see* Embolism, air
Aerodermectasia
  subcutaneous (traumatic) T79.7
Aerodontalgia T70.29
Aeroembolism T70.3
Aerogenes capsulatus infection A48.0
Aerophagy, aerophagia (psychogenic) F45.8
Aerophobia F40.228
Aerosinusitis T70.1
Aerotitis T70.0
Affection — *see* Disease
Afibrinogenemia *(see also* Defect, coagulation) D68.8
  acquired D65
  congenital D68.2
  following ectopic or molar pregnancy O08.1
  in abortion — *see* Abortion, by type, complicated by, afibrinogenemia
  puerperal O72.3
African
  sleeping sickness B56.9
  tick fever A68.1
  trypanosomiasis B56.9
    gambian B56.0
    rhodesian B56.1
Aftercare *(see also* Care) Z51.89
  following surgery (for) (on)
    amputation Z47.81
    attention to
      drains Z48.03
      dressings (nonsurgical) Z48.00
        surgical Z48.01
      sutures Z48.02
    circulatory system Z48.812
    delayed (planned) wound closure Z48.1
    digestive system Z48.815
    explantation of joint prosthesis (staged procedure)
      hip Z47.32
      knee Z47.33
      shoulder Z47.31
    genitourinary system Z48.816
    joint replacement Z47.1
    neoplasm Z48.3
    nervous system Z48.811
    oral cavity Z48.814

Aftercare *(see also* Care) Z51.89 — continued
  following surgery (for) (on) — *continued*
    organ transplant
      bone marrow Z48.290
      heart Z48.21
      heart-lung Z48.280
      kidney Z48.22
      liver Z48.23
      lung Z48.24
      multiple organs NEC Z48.288
      specified NEC Z48.298
    orthopedic NEC Z47.89
    planned wound closure Z48.1
    removal of internal fixation device Z47.2
    respiratory system Z48.813
    scoliosis Z47.82
    sense organs Z48.810
    skin and subcutaneous tissue Z48.817
    specified body system
      circulatory Z48.812
      digestive Z48.815
      genitourinary Z48.816
      nervous Z48.811
      oral cavity Z48.814
      respiratory Z48.813
      sense organs Z48.810
      skin and subcutaneous tissue Z48.817
      teeth Z48.814
    specified NEC Z48.89
    spinal Z48.89
    teeth Z48.814
  fracture — *code to* fracture with seventh character D
  involving
    removal of
      drains Z48.03
      dressings (nonsurgical) Z48.00
      staples Z48.02
      surgical dressings Z48.01
      sutures Z48.02
  neuropacemaker (brain) (peripheral nerve) (spinal cord) Z46.2
    implanted Z45.42
  orthopedic NEC Z47.89
  postprocedural — *see* Aftercare, following surgery
After-cataract — *see* Cataract, secondary
Agalactia (primary) O92.3
  elective, secondary or therapeutic O92.5
Agammaglobulinemia (acquired) (secondary) (nonfamilial) D80.1
  with
    immunoglobulin-bearing B-lymphocytes D80.1
    lymphopenia D81.9
  autosomal recessive (Swiss type) D80.0
  Bruton's X-linked D80.0
  common variable (CVAgamma) D80.1
  congenital sex-linked D80.0
  hereditary D80.0
  lymphopenic D81.9
  Swiss type (autosomal recessive) D80.0
  X-linked (with growth hormone deficiency)(Bruton) D80.0
Aganglionosis (bowel) (colon) Q43.1
Age (old) — *see* Senility
Agenesis
  adrenal (gland) Q89.1
  alimentary tract (complete) (partial) NEC Q45.8
    upper Q40.8
  anus, anal (canal) Q42.3
    with fistula Q42.2
  aorta Q25.4
  appendix Q42.8
  arm (complete) Q71.0-
    with hand present Q71.1-
  artery (peripheral) Q27.9
    brain Q28.3
    coronary Q24.5
    pulmonary Q25.79
    specified NEC Q27.8
    umbilical Q27.0
  auditory (canal) (external) Q16.1
  auricle (ear) Q16.0
  bile duct or passage Q44.5
  bladder Q64.5
  bone Q79.9
  brain Q00.0
    part of Q04.3
  breast (with nipple present) Q83.8
    with absent nipple Q83.0
  bronchus Q32.4
  canaliculus lacrimalis Q10.4
  carpus — *see* Agenesis, hand
  cartilage Q79.9
  cecum Q42.8
  cerebellum Q04.3

Agenesis — *continued*
  cervix Q51.5
  chin Q18.8
  cilia Q10.3
  circulatory system, part NOS Q28.9
  clavicle Q74.0
  clitoris Q52.6
  coccyx Q76.49
  colon Q42.9
    specified NEC Q42.8
  corpus callosum Q04.0
  cricoid cartilage Q31.8
  diaphragm (with hernia) Q79.1
  digestive organ(s) or tract (complete)
      (partial) NEC Q45.8
    upper Q40.8
  ductus arteriosus Q28.8
  duodenum Q41.0
  ear Q16.9
    auricle Q16.0
    lobe Q17.8
  ejaculatory duct Q55.4
  endocrine (gland) NEC Q89.2
  epiglottis Q31.8
  esophagus Q39.8
  eustachian tube Q16.2
  eye Q11.1
    adnexa Q15.8
  eyelid (fold) Q10.3
  face
    bones NEC Q75.8
    specified part NEC Q18.8
  fallopian tube Q50.6
  femur — *see* Defect, reduction, lower limb,
      longitudinal, femur
  fibula — *see* Defect, reduction, lower limb,
      longitudinal, fibula
  finger (complete) (partial) — *see* Agenesis,
      hand
  foot (and toes) (complete) (partial) Q72.3-
  forearm (with hand present) — *see*
      Agenesis, arm, with hand present
      and hand Q71.2-
  gallbladder Q44.0
  gastric Q40.2
  genitalia, genital (organ(s))
    female Q52.8
      external Q52.71
      internal NEC Q52.8
    male Q55.8
  glottis Q31.8
  hair Q84.0
  hand (and fingers) (complete) (partial)
      Q71.3-
  heart Q24.8
    valve NEC Q24.8
      pulmonary Q22.0
  hepatic Q44.7
  humerus — *see* Defect, reduction, upper
      limb
  hymen Q52.4
  ileum Q41.2
  incus Q16.3
  intestine (small) Q41.9
    large Q42.9
      specified NEC Q42.8
  iris (dilator fibers) Q13.1
  jaw M26.09
  jejunum Q41.1
  kidney(s) (partial) Q60.2
    bilateral Q60.1
    unilateral Q60.0
  labium (majus) (minus) Q52.71
  labyrinth, membranous Q16.5
  lacrimal apparatus Q10.4
  larynx Q31.8
  leg (complete) Q72.0-
    with foot present Q72.1-
    lower leg (with foot present) — *see*
        Agenesis, leg, with foot present
        and foot Q72.2-
  lens Q12.3
  limb (complete) Q73.0
    lower — *see* Agenesis, leg
    upper — *see* Agenesis, arm
  lip Q38.0
  liver Q44.7
  lung (fissure) (lobe) (bilateral) (unilateral)
      Q33.3
  mandible, maxilla M26.09
  metacarpus — *see* Agenesis, hand
  metatarsus — *see* Agenesis, foot
  muscle Q79.8
    eyelid Q10.3
    ocular Q15.8
  musculoskeletal system NEC Q79.8
  nail(s) Q84.3
  neck, part Q18.8
  nerve Q07.8
  nervous system, part NEC Q07.8

Agenesis — *continued*
  nipple Q83.2
  nose Q30.1
  nuclear Q07.8
  organ
    of Corti Q16.5
    or site not listed — *see* Anomaly, by site
  osseous meatus (ear) Q16.1
  ovary
    bilateral Q50.02
    unilateral Q50.01
  oviduct Q50.6
  pancreas Q45.0
  parathyroid (gland) Q89.2
  parotid gland(s) Q38.4
  patella Q74.1
  pelvic girdle (complete) (partial) Q74.2
  penis Q55.5
  pericardium Q24.8
  pituitary (gland) Q89.2
  prostate Q55.4
  punctum lacrimale Q10.4
  radioulnar — *see* Defect, reduction, upper
      limb
  radius — *see* Defect, reduction, upper limb,
      longitudinal, radius
  rectum Q42.1
    with fistula Q42.0
  renal Q60.2
    bilateral Q60.1
    unilateral Q60.0
  respiratory organ NEC Q34.8
  rib Q76.6
  roof of orbit Q75.8
  round ligament Q52.8
  sacrum Q76.49
  salivary gland Q38.4
  scapula Q74.0
  scrotum Q55.29
  seminal vesicles Q55.4
  septum
    atrial Q21.1
    between aorta and pulmonary artery
        Q21.4
    ventricular Q20.4
  shoulder girdle (complete) (partial) Q74.0
  skull (bone) Q75.8
    with
      anencephaly Q00.0
      encephalocele — *see* Encephalocele
      hydrocephalus Q03.9
        with spina bifida — *see* Spina
            bifida, by site, with
            hydrocephalus
      microcephaly Q02
  spermatic cord Q55.4
  spinal cord Q06.0
  spine Q76.49
  spleen Q89.01
  sternum Q76.7
  stomach Q40.2
  submaxillary gland(s) (congenital) Q38.4
  tarsus — *see* Agenesis, foot
  tendon Q79.8
  testicle Q55.0
  thymus (gland) Q89.2
  thyroid (gland) E03.1
    cartilage Q31.8
  tibia — *see* Defect, reduction, lower limb,
      longitudinal, tibia
  tibiofibular — *see* Defect, reduction, lower
      limb, specified type NEC
  toe (and foot) (complete) (partial) — *see*
      Agenesis, foot
  tongue Q38.3
  trachea (cartilage) Q32.1
  ulna — *see* Defect, reduction, upper limb,
      longitudinal, ulna
  upper limb — *see* Agenesis, arm
  ureter Q62.4
  urethra Q64.5
  urinary tract NEC Q64.8
  uterus Q51.0
  uvula Q38.5
  vagina Q52.0
  vas deferens Q55.4
  vein(s) (peripheral) Q27.9
    brain Q28.3
    great NEC Q26.8
    portal Q26.5
    vena cava (inferior) (superior) Q26.8
  vermis of cerebellum Q04.3
  vertebra Q76.49
  vulva Q52.71
Ageusia R43.2
Agitated — *see* condition
Agitation R45.1
Aglossia (congenital) Q38.3
Aglossia-adactylia syndrome Q87.0

Aglycogenosis E74.00
Agnosia (body image) (other senses) (tactile)
    R48.1
  developmental F88
  verbal R48.1
    auditory R48.1
      developmental F80.2
    developmental F80.2
    visual (object) R48.3
Agoraphobia F40.00
  with panic disorder F40.01
  without panic disorder F40.02
Agrammatism R48.8
Agranulocytopenia — *see* Agranulocytosis
Agranulocytosis (chronic) (cyclical)
    (genetic) (infantile) (periodic)
    (pernicious) (*see also* Neutropenia)
    D70.9
  congenital D70.0
  cytoreductive cancer chemotherapy sequela
      D70.1
  drug-induced D70.2
    due to cytoreductive cancer
        chemotherapy D70.1
  due to infection D70.3
  secondary D70.4
    drug-induced D70.2
      due to cytoreductive cancer
          chemotherapy D70.1
Agraphia (absolute) R48.8
  with alexia R48.0
  developmental F81.81
Ague (dumb) — *see* Malaria
Agyria Q04.3
Ahumada-del Castillo syndrome E23.0
Aichmophobia F40.298
AIDS (related complex) B20
Ailment heart — *see* Disease, heart
Ailurophobia F40.218
Ainhum (disease) L94.6
AIPHI (acute idiopathic pulmonary
    hemorrhage in infants (over 28 days
    old)) R04.81
Air
  anterior mediastinum J98.2
  compressed, disease T70.3
  conditioner lung or pneumonitis J67.7
  embolism (artery) (cerebral) (any site)
      T79.0
    with ectopic or molar pregnancy O08.2
    due to implanted device NEC — *see*
        Complications, by site and type,
        specified NEC
    following
      abortion — *see* Abortion by type,
          complicated by, embolism
      ectopic or molar pregnancy O08.2
    infusion, therapeutic injection or
        transfusion T80.0
    in pregnancy, childbirth or puerperium
        — *see* Embolism, obstetric
    traumatic T79.0
  hunger, psychogenic F45.8
  rarefied, effects of — *see* Effect, adverse,
      high altitude
  sickness T75.3
Airplane sickness T75.3
Akathisia (drug-induced) (treatment-
    induced) G25.71
  neuroleptic induced (acute) G25.71
Akinesia R29.898
Akinetic mutism R41.89
Akureyri's disease G93.3
Alactasia, congenital E73.0
Alagille's syndrome Q44.7
Alastrim B03
Albers-Schönberg syndrome Q78.2
Albert's syndrome — *see* Tendinitis,
    Achilles
Albinism, albino E70.30
  with hematologic abnormality E70.339
    Chédiak-Higashi syndrome E70.330
    Hermansky-Pudlak syndrome E70.331
    other specified E70.338
  I E70.320
  II E70.321
  ocular E70.319
    autosomal recessive E70.311
    other specified E70.318
    X-linked E70.310
  oculocutaneous E70.329
    other specified E70.328
    tyrosinase (ty) negative E70.320
    tyrosinase (ty) positive E70.321
  other specified E70.39
Albinismus E70.30
Albright(-McCune)(-Sternberg) syndrome
    Q78.1
Albuminous — *see* condition

Albuminuria, albuminuric (acute) (chronic)
    (subacute) (*see also* Proteinuria) R80.9
  complicating pregnancy — *see* Proteinuria,
      gestational
  with
    gestational hypertension — *see* Pre-
        eclampsia
    pre-existing hypertension — *see*
        Hypertension, complicating
        pregnancy, pre-existing, with,
        pre-eclampsia
  gestational — *see* Proteinuria, gestational
      with
      gestational hypertension — *see* Pre-
          eclampsia
      pre-existing hypertension — *see*
          Hypertension, complicating
          pregnancy, pre-existing, with,
          pre-eclampsia
  orthostatic R80.2
  postural R80.2
  pre-eclamptic — *see* Pre-eclampsia
  scarlatinal A38.8
Albuminurophobia F40.298
Alcaptonuria E70.29
Alcohol, alcoholic, alcohol-induced
  addiction (without remission) F10.20
    with remission F10.21
  amnestic disorder, persisting F10.96
    with dependence F10.26
  brain syndrome, chronic F10.97
    with dependence F10.27
  cardiopathy I42.6
  counseling and surveillance Z71.41
    family member Z71.42
  delirium (acute) (tremens) (withdrawal)
      F10.231
    with intoxication F10.921
      in
        abuse F10.121
        dependence F10.221
  dementia F10.97
    with dependence F10.27
  deterioration F10.97
    with dependence F10.27
  hallucinosis (acute) F10.951
    in
      abuse F10.151
      dependence F10.251
  insanity F10.959
  intoxication (acute) (without dependence)
      F10.129
    with
      delirium F10.121
      dependence F10.229
        with delirium F10.221
        uncomplicated F10.220
      uncomplicated F10.120
  jealousy F10.988
  Korsakoff's, Korsakov's, Korsakow's
      F10.26
  liver K70.9
    acute — *see* Disease, liver, alcoholic,
        hepatitis
  mania (acute) (chronic) F10.959
  paranoia, paranoid (type) psychosis
      F10.950
  pellagra E52
  poisoning, accidental (acute) NEC — *see*
      Table of Drugs and Chemicals,
      alcohol, poisoning
  psychosis — *see* Psychosis, alcoholic
  withdrawal (without convulsions) F10.239
    with delirium F10.231
Alcoholism (chronic) (without remission)
    F10.20
  with
    psychosis — *see* Psychosis, alcoholic
    remission F10.21
  Korsakov's F10.96
    with dependence F10.26
Alder (-Reilly) anomaly or syndrome
    (leukocyte granulation) D72.0
Aldosteronism E26.9
  familial (type I) E26.02
  glucocorticoid-remediable E26.02
  primary (due to (bilateral) adrenal
      hyperplasia) E26.09
  primary NEC E26.09
  secondary E26.1
  specified NEC E26.89
Aldosteronoma D44.10
Aldrich(-Wiskott) syndrome (eczema-
    thrombocytopenia) D82.0
Alektorophobia F40.218
Aleppo boil B55.1
Aleukemic — *see* condition

DISEASE INDEX

Aleukia
congenital D70.0
hemorrhagica D61.9
congenital D61.09
splenica D73.1
Alexia R48.0
developmental F81.0
secondary to organic lesion R48.0
Algoneurodystrophy M89.00
ankle M89.07-
foot M89.07-
forearm M89.03-
hand M89.04-
lower leg M89.06-
multiple sites M89.0-
shoulder M89.01-
specified site NEC M89.08
thigh M89.05-
upper arm M89.02-
Algophobia F40.298
Alienation, mental — see Psychosis
Alkalemia E87.3
Alkalosis E87.3
metabolic E87.3
with respiratory acidosis E87.4
respiratory E87.3
Alkaptonuria E70.29
Allen-Masters syndrome N83.8
Allergy, allergic (reaction) (to) T78.40
air-borne substance NEC (rhinitis) J30.89
alveolitis (extrinsic) J67.9
due to
Aspergillus clavatus J67.4
Cryptostroma corticale J67.6
organisms (fungal, thermophilic actinomycete) growing in ventilation (air conditioning) systems J67.7
specified type NEC J67.8
anaphylactic reaction or shock T78.2
angioneurotic edema T78.3
animal (dander) (epidermal) (hair) (rhinitis) J30.81
bee sting (anaphylactic shock) — see Toxicity, venom, arthropod, bee
biological — see Allergy, drug
colitis K52.2
dander (animal) (rhinitis) J30.81
dandruff (rhinitis) J30.81
dental restorative material (existing) K08.55
dermatitis — see Dermatitis, contact, allergic
diathesis — see History, allergy
drug, medicament & biological (any) (external) (internal) T78.40
correct substance properly administered — see Table of Drugs and Chemicals, by drug, adverse effect
wrong substance given or taken NEC (by accident) — see Table of Drugs and Chemicals, by drug, poisoning
due to pollen J30.1
dust (house) (stock) (rhinitis) J30.89
with asthma — see Asthma, allergic extrinsic
eczema — see Dermatitis, contact, allergic
epidermal (animal) (rhinitis) J30.81
feathers (rhinitis) J30.89
food (any) (ingested) NEC T78.1
anaphylactic shock — see Shock, anaphylactic, due to food
dermatitis — see Dermatitis, due to, food
dietary counseling and surveillance Z71.3
in contact with skin L23.6
rhinitis J30.5
status (without reaction) Z91.018
eggs Z91.012
milk products Z91.011
peanuts Z91.010
seafood Z91.013
specified NEC Z91.018
gastrointestinal K52.2
grain J30.1
grass (hay fever) (pollen) J30.1
asthma — see Asthma, allergic extrinsic
hair (animal) (rhinitis) J30.81
history (of) — see History, allergy
horse serum — see Allergy, serum
inhalant (rhinitis) J30.89
pollen J30.1
kapok (rhinitis) J30.89
medicine — see Allergy, drug
milk protein K52.2
nasal, seasonal due to pollen J30.1
pneumonia J82
pollen (any) (hay fever) J30.1
asthma — see Asthma, allergic extrinsic
primrose J30.1

Allergy, allergic (reaction) (to) T78.40 — continued
primula J30.1
purpura D69.0
ragweed (hay fever) (pollen) J30.1
asthma — see Asthma, allergic extrinsic
rose (pollen) J30.1
seasonal NEC J30.2
Senecio jacobae (pollen) J30.1
serum (see also Reaction, serum) T80.69
anaphylactic shock T80.59
shock (anaphylactic) T78.2
due to
adverse effect of correct medicinal substance properly administered T88.6
administration of blood and blood products T80.51
immunization T80.52
serum NEC T80.59
vaccination T80.52
specific NEC T78.49
tree (any) (hay fever) (pollen) J30.1
asthma — see Asthma, allergic extrinsic
upper respiratory J30.9
urticaria L50.0
vaccine — see Allergy, serum
wheat — see Allergy, food
Allescheriasis B48.2
Alligator skin disease Q80.9
Allocheiria, allochiria R20.8
Almeida's disease — see Paracoccidioidomycosis
Alopecia (hereditaria) (seborrheica) L65.9
androgenic L64.9
drug-induced L64.0
specified NEC L64.8
areata L63.9
ophiasis L63.2
specified NEC L63.8
totalis L63.0
universalis L63.1
cicatricial L66.9
specified NEC L66.8
circumscripta L63.2
congenital, congenitalis Q84.0
due to cytotoxic drugs NEC L65.8
mucinosa L65.2
postinfective NEC L65.8
postpartum L65.0
premature L64.8
specific (syphilitic) A51.32
specified NEC L65.8
syphilitic (secondary) A51.32
totalis (capitis) L63.0
universalis (entire body) L63.1
X-ray L58.1
Alpers' disease G31.81
Alpine sickness T70.29
Alport syndrome Q87.81
ALTE (apparent life threatening event) in newborn and infant R68.13
Alteration (of), Altered
awareness, transient R40.4
mental status R41.82
pattern of family relationships affecting child Z62.898
sensation
following
cerebrovascular disease I69.998
cerebral infarction I69.398
intracerebral hemorrhage I69.198
nontraumatic intracranial hemorrhage NEC I69.298
specified disease NEC I69.898
subarachnoid hemorrhage I69.098
Alternating — see condition
Altitude, high (effects) — see Effect, adverse, high altitude
Aluminosis (of lung) J63.0
Alveolitis
allergic (extrinsic) — see Pneumonitis, hypersensitivity
due to
Aspergillus clavatus J67.4
Cryptostroma corticale J67.6
fibrosing (cryptogenic) (idiopathic) J84.112
jaw M27.3
sicca dolorosa M27.3
Alveolus, alveolar — see condition
Alymphocytosis D72.810
thymic (with immunodeficiency) D82.1
Alymphoplasia, thymic D82.1
Alzheimer's disease or sclerosis — see Disease, Alzheimer's
Amastia (with nipple present) Q83.8
with absent nipple Q83.0
Amathophobia F40.228

Amaurosis (acquired) (congenital) — see also Blindness
fugax G45.3
hysterical F44.6
Leber's congenital H35.50
uremic — see Uremia
Amaurotic idiocy (infantile) (juvenile) (late) E75.4
Amaxophobia F40.248
Ambiguous genitalia Q56.4
Amblyopia (congenital) (ex anopsia) (partial) (suppression) H53.00-
anisometropic — see Amblyopia, refractive
deprivation H53.01-
hysterical F44.6
nocturnal — see also Blindness, night
vitamin A deficiency E50.5
refractive H53.02-
strabismic H53.03-
tobacco H53.8
toxic NEC H53.8
uremic — see Uremia
Ameba, amebic (histolytica) — see also Amebiasis
abscess (liver) A06.4
Amebiasis A06.9
with abscess — see Abscess, amebic
acute A06.0
chronic (intestine) A06.1
with abscess — see Abscess, amebic
cutaneous A06.7
cutis A06.7
cystitis A06.81
genitourinary tract NEC A06.82
hepatic — see Abscess, liver, amebic
intestine A06.0
nondysenteric colitis A06.2
skin A06.7
specified site NEC A06.89
Ameboma (of intestine) A06.3
Amelia Q73.0
lower limb — see Agenesis, leg
upper limb — see Agenesis, arm
Ameloblastoma — see also Cyst, calcifying odontogenic
long bones C40.9-
lower limb C40.2-
upper limb C40.0-
malignant C41.1
jaw (bone) (lower) C41.1
upper C41.0
tibial C40.2-
Amelogenesis imperfecta K00.5
nonhereditaria (segmentalis) K00.4
Amenorrhea N91.2
hyperhormonal E28.8
primary N91.0
secondary N91.1
Amentia — see Disability, intellectual
Meynert's (nonalcoholic) F04
American
leishmaniasis B55.2
mountain tick fever A93.2
Ametropia — see Disorder, refraction
Amianthosis J61
Amimia R48.8
Amino-acid disorder E72.9
anemia D53.0
Aminoacidopathy E72.9
Aminoaciduria E72.9
Amnesia R41.3
anterograde R41.1
auditory R48.8
dissociative F44.0
hysterical F44.0
postictal in epilepsy — see Epilepsy
psychogenic F44.0
retrograde R41.2
transient global G45.4
Amnes(t)ic syndrome (post-traumatic) F04
induced by
alcohol F10.96
with dependence F10.26
psychoactive NEC F19.96
with
abuse F19.16
dependence F19.26
sedative F13.96
with dependence F13.26
Amnion, amniotic — see condition
Amnionitis — see Pregnancy, complicated by
Amok F68.8
Amoral traits F60.89
Ampulla
lower esophagus K22.8
phrenic K22.8

Amputation — see also Absence, by site, acquired
neuroma (postoperative) (traumatic) — see Complications, amputation stump, neuroma
stump (surgical)
abnormal, painful, or with complication (late) — see Complications, amputation stump
healed or old NOS Z89.9
traumatic (complete) (partial)
arm (upper) (complete) S48.91-
at
elbow S58.01-
partial S58.02-
shoulder joint (complete) S48.01-
partial S48.02-
between
elbow and wrist (complete) S58.11-
partial S58.12-
shoulder and elbow (complete) S48.11-
partial S48.12-
partial S48.92-
breast (complete) S28.21-
partial S28.22-
clitoris (complete) S38.211
partial S38.212
ear (complete) S08.11-
partial S08.12-
finger (complete) (metacarpophalangeal) S68.11-
index S68.11-
little S68.11-
middle S68.11-
partial S68.12-
index S68.12-
little S68.12-
middle S68.12-
ring S68.12-
ring S68.11-
thumb — see Amputation, traumatic, thumb
transphalangeal (complete) S68.61-
index S68.61-
little S68.61-
middle S68.61-
partial S68.62-
index S68.62-
little S68.62-
middle S68.62-
ring S68.62-
ring S68.61-
foot (complete) S98.91-
at ankle level S98.01-
partial S98.02-
midfoot S98.31-
partial S98.32-
partial S98.92-
forearm (complete) S58.91-
at elbow level (complete) S58.01-
partial S58.02-
between elbow and wrist (complete) S58.11-
partial S58.12-
partial S58.92-
genital organ(s) (external)
female (complete) S38.211
partial S38.212
male
penis (complete) S38.221
partial S38.222
scrotum (complete) S38.231
partial S38.232
testes (complete) S38.231
partial S38.232
hand (complete) (wrist level) S68.41-
finger(s) alone — see Amputation, traumatic, finger
partial S68.42-
thumb alone — see Amputation, traumatic, thumb
transmetacarpal (complete) S68.71-
partial S68.72-
head
ear — see Amputation, traumatic, ear
nose (partial) S08.812
complete S08.811
part S08.89
scalp S08.0
hip (and thigh) (complete) S78.91-
at hip joint (complete) S78.01-
partial S78.02-
between hip and knee (complete) S78.11-
partial S78.12-
partial S78.92-
labium (majus) (minus) (complete) S38.21-
partial S38.21-

Amputation (see also Absence, by site, acquired) — continued
  traumatic (complete) (partial) — continued
    leg (lower) S88.91-
      at knee level S88.01-
        partial S88.02-
      between knee and ankle S88.11-
        partial S88.12-
      partial S88.92-
    nose (partial) S08.812
      complete S08.811
    penis (complete) S38.221
      partial S38.222
    scrotum (complete) S38.231
      partial S38.232
    shoulder — see Amputation, traumatic, arm
      at shoulder joint — see Amputation, traumatic, arm, at shoulder joint
    testes (complete) S38.231
      partial S38.232
    thigh — see Amputation, traumatic, hip
    thorax, part of S28.1
      breast — see Amputation, traumatic, breast
    thumb (complete)
      (metacarpophalangeal) S68.01-
      partial S68.02-
      transphalangeal (complete) S68.51-
        partial S68.52-
    toe (lesser) S98.13-
      great S98.11-
        partial S98.12-
      more than one S98.21-
        partial S98.22-
      partial S98.14-
    vulva (complete) S38.211
      partial S38.212
Amputee (bilateral) (old) Z89.9
Amsterdam dwarfism Q87.1
Amusia R48.8
  developmental F80.89
Amyelencephalus, amyelencephaly Q00.0
Amyelia Q06.0
Amygdalitis — see Tonsillitis
Amygdalolith J35.8
Amyloid heart (disease) E85.4 [I43]
Amyloidosis (generalized) (primary) E85.9
  with lung involvement E85.4 [J99]
  familial E85.2
  genetic E85.2
  heart E85.4 [I43]
  hemodialysis-associated E85.3
  liver E85.4 [K77]
  localized E85.4
  neuropathic heredofamilial E85.1
  non-neuropathic heredofamilial E85.0
  organ limited E85.4
  Portuguese E85.1
  pulmonary E85.4 [J99]
  secondary systemic E85.3
  skin (lichen) (macular) E85.4 [L99]
  specified NEC E85.8
  subglottic E85.4 [J99]
Amylopectinosis (brancher enzyme deficiency) E74.03
Amylophagia — see Pica
Amyoplasia congenita Q79.8
Amyotonia M62.89
  congenita G70.2
Amyotrophia, amyotrophy, amyotrophic G71.8
  congenita Q79.8
  diabetic — see Diabetes, amyotrophy
  lateral sclerosis G12.21
  neuralgic G54.5
  spinal progressive G12.21
Anacidity, gastric K31.83
  psychogenic F45.8
Anaerosis of newborn P28.89
Analbuminemia E88.09
Analgesia — see Anesthesia
Analphalipoproteinemia E78.6
Anaphylactic
  purpura D69.0
  shock or reaction — see Shock, anaphylactic
Anaphylactoid shock or reaction — see Shock, anaphylactic
Anaphylactoid syndrome of pregnancy O88.01-
Anaphylaxis — see Shock, anaphylactic
Anaplasia cervix (see also Dysplasia, cervix) N87.9
Anaplasmosis, human A77.49
Anarthria R47.1

Anasarca R60.1
  cardiac — see Failure, heart, congestive
  lung J18.2
  newborn P83.2
  nutritional E43
  pulmonary J18.2
  renal N04.9
Anastomosis
  aneurysmal — see Aneurysm
  arteriovenous ruptured brain I60.8
  intestinal K63.89
    complicated NEC K91.89
      involving urinary tract N99.89
  retinal and choroidal vessels (congenital) Q14.8
Anatomical narrow angle H40.03-
Ancylostoma, ancylostomiasis (braziliense) (caninum) (ceylanicum) (duodenale) B76.0
  Necator americanus B76.1
Andersen's disease (glycogen storage) E74.09
Anderson-Fabry disease E75.21
Andes disease T70.29
Andrews' disease (bacterid) L08.89
Androblastoma
  benign
    specified site — see Neoplasm, benign, by site
    unspecified site
      female D27.9
      male D29.20
  malignant
    specified site — see Neoplasm, malignant, by site
    unspecified site
      female C56.9
      male C62.90
  specified site — see Neoplasm, uncertain behavior, by site
  tubular
    with lipid storage
      specified site — see Neoplasm, benign, by site
      unspecified site
        female D27.9
        male D29.20
    specified site — see Neoplasm, benign, by site
    unspecified site
      female D27.9
      male D29.20
  unspecified site
    female D39.10
    male D40.10
Androgen insensitivity syndrome (see also Syndrome, androgen insensitivity) E34.50
Androgen resistance syndrome (see also Syndrome, androgen insensitivity) E34.50
Android pelvis Q74.2
  with disproportion (fetopelvic) O33.3
    causing obstructed labor O65.3
Androphobia F40.290
Anectasis, pulmonary (newborn) — see Atelectasis
Anemia (essential) (general) (hemoglobin deficiency) (infantile) (primary) (profound) D64.9
  with (due to) (in)
    disorder of
      anaerobic glycolysis D55.2
      pentose phosphate pathway D55.1
    koilonychia D50.9
  achlorhydric D50.8
  achrestic D53.1
  Addison(-Biermer) (pernicious) D51.0
  agranulocytic — see Agranulocytosis
  amino-acid-deficiency D53.0
  aplastic D61.9
    congenital D61.09
    drug-induced D61.1
    due to
      drugs D61.1
      external agents NEC D61.2
      infection D61.2
      radiation D61.2
    idiopathic D61.3
    red cell (pure) D60.9
      chronic D60.0
      congenital D61.01
      specified type NEC D60.8
      transient D60.1
    specified type NEC D61.89
    toxic D61.2
  aregenerative
    congenital D61.09
  asiderotic D50.9
  atypical (primary) D64.9

Anemia (essential) (general) (hemoglobin deficiency) (infantile) (primary) (profound) D64.9 — continued
  Baghdad spring D55.0
  Balantidium coli A07.0
  Biermer's (pernicious) D51.0
  blood loss (chronic) D50.0
    acute D62
  bothriocephalus B70.0 [D63.8]
  brickmaker's B76.9 [D63.8]
  cerebral I67.89
  childhood D58.9
  chlorotic D50.8
  chronic
    blood loss D50.0
    hemolytic D58.9
      idiopathic D59.9
    simple D53.9
  chronica congenita aregenerativa D61.09
  combined system disease NEC D51.0 [G32.0]
    due to dietary vitamin B12 deficiency D51.3 [G32.0]
  complicating pregnancy, childbirth or puerperium — see Pregnancy, complicated by (management affected by), anemia
  congenital P61.4
    aplastic D61.09
    due to isoimmunization NOS P55.9
    dyserythropoietic, dyshematopoietic D64.4
    following fetal blood loss P61.3
    Heinz body D58.2
    hereditary hemolytic NOS D58.9
    pernicious D51.0
    spherocytic D58.0
  Cooley's (erythroblastic) D56.1
  cytogenic D51.0
  deficiency D53.9
    2, 3 diphosphoglycurate mutase D55.2
    2, 3 PG D55.2
    6 phosphogluconate dehydrogenase D55.1
    6-PGD D55.1
    amino-acid D53.0
    combined B12 and folate D53.1
    enzyme D55.9
      drug-induced (hemolytic) D59.2
      glucose-6-phosphate dehydrogenase (G6PD) D55.0
      glycolytic D55.2
      nucleotide metabolism D55.3
      related to hexose monophosphate (HMP) shunt pathway NEC D55.1
      specified type NEC D55.8
    erythrocytic glutathione D55.1
    folate D52.9
      dietary D52.0
      drug-induced D52.1
    folic acid D52.9
      dietary D52.0
      drug-induced D52.1
    G SH D55.1
    G6PD D55.0
    GGS-R D55.1
    glucose-6-phosphate dehydrogenase D55.0
    glutathione reductase D55.1
    glyceraldehyde phosphate dehydrogenase D55.2
    hexokinase D55.2
    iron D50.9
      secondary to blood loss (chronic) D50.0
    nutritional D53.9
      with
        poor iron absorption D50.8
        specified deficiency NEC D53.8
    phosphofructo-aldolase D55.2
    phosphoglycerate kinase D55.2
    PK D55.2
    protein D53.0
    pyruvate kinase D55.2
    transcobalamin II D51.2
    triose-phosphate isomerase D55.2
    vitamin B12 NOS D51.9
      dietary D51.3
      due to
        intrinsic factor deficiency D51.0
        selective vitamin B12 malabsorption with proteinuria D51.1
      pernicious D51.0
      specified type NEC D51.8
  Diamond-Blackfan (congenital hypoplastic) D61.01
  dibothriocephalus B70.0 [D63.8]
  dimorphic D53.1

Anemia (essential) (general) (hemoglobin deficiency) (infantile) (primary) (profound) D64.9 — continued
  diphasic D53.1
  Diphyllobothrium (Dibothriocephalus) B70.0 [D63.8]
  due to (in) (with)
    antineoplastic chemotherapy D64.81
    blood loss (chronic) D50.0
      acute D62
    chemotherapy, antineoplastic D64.81
    chronic disease classified elsewhere NEC D63.8
    chronic kidney disease D63.1
    deficiency
      amino-acid D53.0
      copper D53.8
      folate (folic acid) D52.9
        dietary D52.0
        drug-induced D52.1
      molybdenum D53.8
      protein D53.0
      zinc D53.8
    dietary vitamin B12 deficiency D51.3
    disorder of
      glutathione metabolism D55.1
      nucleotide metabolism D55.3
    drug — see Anemia, by type — see also Table of Drugs and Chemicals
    end stage renal disease D63.1
    enzyme disorder D55.9
    fetal blood loss P61.3
    fish tapeworm (D.latum) infestation B70.0 [D63.8]
    hemorrhage (chronic) D50.0
      acute D62
    impaired absorption D50.9
    loss of blood (chronic) D50.0
      acute D62
    myxedema E03.9 [D63.8]
    Necator americanus B76.1 [D63.8]
    prematurity P61.2
    selective vitamin B12 malabsorption with proteinuria D51.1
    transcobalamin II deficiency D51.2
  Dyke-Young type (secondary) (symptomatic) D59.1
  dyserythropoietic (congenital) D64.4
  dyshematopoietic (congenital) D64.4
  Egyptian B76.9 [D63.8]
  elliptocytosis — see Elliptocytosis
  enzyme-deficiency, drug-induced D59.2
  epidemic (see also Ancylostomiasis) B76.9 [D63.8]
  erythroblastic
    familial D56.1
    newborn (see also Disease, hemolytic) P55.9
    of childhood D56.1
  erythrocytic glutathione deficiency D55.1
  erythropoietin-resistant anemia (EPO resistant anemia) D63.1
  Faber's (achlorhydric anemia) D50.9
  factitious (self-induced blood letting) D50.0
  familial erythroblastic D56.1
  Fanconi's (congenital pancytopenia) D61.09
  favism D55.0
  fish tapeworm (D. latum) infestation B70.0 [D63.8]
  folate (folic acid) deficiency D52.9
  glucose-6-phosphate dehydrogenase (G6PD) deficiency D55.0
  glutathione-reductase deficiency D55.1
  goat's milk D52.0
  granulocytic — see Agranulocytosis
  Heinz body, congenital D58.2
  hemolytic D58.9
    acquired D59.9
      with hemoglobinuria NEC D59.6
      autoimmune NEC D59.1
      infectious D59.4
      specified type NEC D59.8
      toxic D59.4
    acute D59.9
      due to enzyme deficiency specified type NEC D55.8
      Lederer's D59.1
    autoimmune D59.1
      drug-induced D59.0
    chronic D58.9
      idiopathic D59.9
    cold type (secondary) (symptomatic) D59.1
    congenital (spherocytic) — see Spherocytosis

DISEASE INDEX

Aneurysm (anastomotic) (artery) (cirsoid) (diffuse) (false) (fusiform) (multiple) (saccular) I72.9 — *continued*
  interauricular septum — *see* Aneurysm, heart
  interventricular septum — *see* Aneurysm, heart
  intrathoracic (nonsyphilitic) I71.2
    ruptured I71.1
    syphilitic A52.01
  lower limb I72.4
  lung (pulmonary artery) I28.1
  mediastinal (nonsyphilitic) I72.8
    syphilitic A52.09
  miliary (congenital) I67.1
    ruptured — *see* Hemorrhage, intracerebral, subarachnoid, intracranial
  mitral (heart) (valve) I34.8
  mural — *see* Aneurysm, heart
  mycotic I72.9
    endocardial (any valve) I33.0
    ruptured, brain — *see* Hemorrhage, intracerebral, subarachnoid
  myocardium — *see* Aneurysm, heart
  neck I72.0
  pancreaticoduodenal I72.8
  patent ductus arteriosus Q25.0
  peripheral NEC I72.8
    congenital Q27.8
      digestive system Q27.8
      lower limb Q27.8
      specified site NEC Q27.8
      upper limb Q27.8
  popliteal (artery) (ruptured) I72.4
  precerebral, congenital (nonruptured) Q28.1
  pulmonary I28.1
    arteriovenous Q25.72
      acquired I28.0
    syphilitic A52.09
    valve (heart) — *see* Endocarditis, pulmonary
  racemose (peripheral) I72.9
    congenital — *see* Aneurysm, congenital
  radial I72.1
  Rasmussen NEC A15.0
  renal (artery) I72.2
  retina — *see also* Disorder, retina, microaneurysms
    congenital Q14.1
    diabetic — *see* Diabetes, microaneurysms, retinal
  sinus of Valsalva Q25.4
  specified NEC I72.8
  spinal (cord) I72.8
    syphilitic (hemorrhage) A52.09
  splenic I72.8
  subclavian (artery) (ruptured) I72.8
    syphilitic A52.09
  superior mesenteric I72.8
  syphilitic (aorta) A52.01
    central nervous system A52.05
    congenital (late) A50.54 [I79.0]
    spine, spinal A52.09
  thoracoabdominal (aorta) I71.6
    ruptured I71.5
    syphilitic A52.01
  thorax, thoracic (aorta) (arch) (nonsyphilitic) I71.2
    ruptured I71.1
    syphilitic A52.01
  traumatic (complication) (early), specified site — *see* Injury, blood vessel
  tricuspid (heart) (valve) I07.8
  ulnar I72.1
  upper limb (ruptured) I72.1
  valve, valvular — *see* Endocarditis
  venous (*see also* Varix) I86.8
    congenital Q27.8
      digestive system Q27.8
      lower limb Q27.8
      specified site NEC Q27.8
      upper limb Q27.8
  ventricle — *see* Aneurysm, heart
  visceral NEC I72.8
Angelman syndrome Q93.5
Anger R45.4
Angiectasis, angiectopia I99.8
Angiitis I77.6
  allergic granulomatous M30.1
  hypersensitivity M31.0
  necrotizing M31.9
    specified NEC M31.8
  nervous system, granulomatous I67.7

Angina (attack) (cardiac) (chest) (heart) (pectoris) (syndrome) (vasomotor) I20.9
  with
    atherosclerotic heart disease — *see* Arteriosclerosis, coronary (artery)
    documented spasm I20.1
  abdominal K55.1
  accelerated — *see* Angina, unstable
  agranulocytic — *see* Agranulocytosis
  angiospastic — *see* Angina, with, documented spasm
  aphthous B08.5
  crescendo — *see* Angina, unstable
  croupous J05.0
  cruris I73.9
  de novo effort — *see* Angina, unstable
  diphtheritic, membranous A36.0
  equivalent I20.8
  exudative, chronic J37.0
  following acute myocardial infarction I23.7
  gangrenous diphtheritic A36.0
  intestinal K55.1
  Ludovici K12.2
  Ludwig's K12.2
  malignant diphtheritic A36.0
  membranous J05.0
    diphtheritic A36.0
    Vincent's A69.1
  mesenteric K55.1
  monocytic — *see* Mononucleosis, infectious
  of effort — *see* Angina, specified NEC
  phlegmonous J36
    diphtheritic A36.0
  post-infarctional I23.7
  pre-infarctional — *see* Angina, unstable
  Prinzmetal — *see* Angina, with, documented spasm
  progressive — *see* Angina, unstable
  pseudomembranous A69.1
  pultaceous, diphtheritic A36.0
  spasm-induced — *see* Angina, with, documented spasm
  specified NEC I20.8
  stable I20.9
  stenocardia — *see* Angina, specified NEC
  stridulous, diphtheritic A36.2
  tonsil J36
  trachealis J05.0
  unstable I20.0
  variant — *see* Angina, with, documented spasm
  Vincent's A69.1
  worsening effort — *see* Angina, unstable
Angioblastoma — *see* Neoplasm, connective tissue, uncertain behavior
Angiocholecystitis — *see* Cholecystitis, acute
Angiocholitis (*see also* Cholecystitis, acute) K83.0
Angiodysgenesis spinalis G95.19
Angiodysplasia (cecum) (colon) K55.20
  with bleeding K55.21
    duodenum (and stomach) K31.819
      with bleeding K31.811
    stomach (and duodenum) K31.819
      with bleeding K31.811
Angioedema (allergic) (any site) (with urticaria) T78.3
  hereditary D84.1
Angioendothelioma — *see* Neoplasm, uncertain behavior, by site
  benign D18.00
    intra-abdominal D18.03
    intracranial D18.02
    skin D18.01
    specified site NEC D18.09
  bone — *see* Neoplasm, bone, malignant
  Ewing's — *see* Neoplasm, bone, malignant
Angioendotheliomatosis C85.8-
Angiofibroma — *see also* Neoplasm, benign, by site
  juvenile
    specified site — *see* Neoplasm, benign, by site
    unspecified site D10.6
Angiohemophilia (A) (B) D68.0
Angioid streaks (choroid) (macula) (retina) H35.33
Angiokeratoma — *see* Neoplasm, skin, benign
  corporis diffusum E75.21
Angioleiomyoma — *see* Neoplasm, connective tissue, benign
Angiolipoma — *see also* Lipoma
  infiltrating — *see* Lipoma
Angioma — *see also* Hemangioma, by site
  capillary I78.1
  hemorrhagicum hereditaria I78.0
  intra-abdominal D18.03
  intracranial D18.02

Angioma — *see also* Hemangioma, by site — *continued*
  malignant — *see* Neoplasm, connective tissue, malignant
  plexiform D18.00
    intra-abdominal D18.03
    intracranial D18.02
    skin D18.01
    specified site NEC D18.09
  senile I78.1
  serpiginosum L81.7
  skin D18.01
  specified site NEC D18.09
  spider I78.1
  stellate I78.1
  venous Q28.3
Angiomatosis Q82.8
  bacillary A79.89
  encephalotrigeminal Q85.8
  hemorrhagic familial I78.0
  hereditary familial I78.0
  liver K76.4
Angiomyolipoma — *see* Lipoma
Angiomyoliposarcoma — *see* Neoplasm, connective tissue, malignant
Angiomyoma — *see* Neoplasm, connective tissue, benign
Angiomyosarcoma — *see* Neoplasm, connective tissue, malignant
Angiomyxoma — *see* Neoplasm, connective tissue, uncertain behavior
Angioneurosis F45.8
Angioneurotic edema (allergic) (any site) (with urticaria) T78.3
  hereditary D84.1
Angiopathia, angiopathy I99.9
  cerebral I67.9
    amyloid E85.4 [I68.0]
  diabetic (peripheral) — *see* Diabetes, angiopathy
  peripheral I73.9
    diabetic — *see* Diabetes, angiopathy
    specified type NEC I73.89
  retinae syphilitica A52.05
  retinalis (juvenilis)
    diabetic — *see* Diabetes, retinopathy
    proliferative — *see* Retinopathy, proliferative
Angiosarcoma — *see also* Neoplasm, connective tissue, malignant
  liver C22.3
Angiosclerosis — *see* Arteriosclerosis
Angiospasm (peripheral) (traumatic) (vessel) I73.9
  brachial plexus G54.0
  cerebral G45.9
  cervical plexus G54.2
  nerve
    arm — *see* Mononeuropathy, upper limb
    axillary G54.0
      median — *see* Lesion, nerve, median
      ulnar — *see* Lesion, nerve, ulnar
    axillary G54.0
    leg — *see* Mononeuropathy, lower limb
    median — *see* Lesion, nerve, median
    plantar — *see* Lesion, nerve, plantar
    ulnar — *see* Lesion, nerve, ulnar
Angiospastic disease or edema I73.9
Angiostrongyliasis
  due to
    Parastrongylus
      cantonensis B83.2
      costaricensis B81.3
    intestinal B81.3
Anguillulosis — *see* Strongyloidiasis
Angulation
  cecum — *see* Obstruction, intestine
  coccyx (acquired) (*see also* subcategory) M43.8
    congenital NEC Q76.49
  femur (acquired) — *see also* Deformity, limb, specified type NEC, thigh
    congenital Q74.2
  intestine (large) (small) — *see* Obstruction, intestine
  sacrum (acquired) (*see also* subcategory) M43.8
    congenital NEC Q76.49
  sigmoid (flexure) — *see* Obstruction, intestine
  spine — *see* Dorsopathy, deforming, specified NEC
  tibia (acquired) — *see also* Deformity, limb, specified type NEC, lower leg
    congenital Q74.2
  ureter N13.5
    with infection N13.6
  wrist (acquired) — *see also* Deformity, limb, specified type NEC, forearm
    congenital Q74.0

Angulus infectiosus (lips) K13.0
Anhedonia R45.84
Anhidrosis L74.4
Anhydration, anhydremia E86.0
  with
    hypernatremia E87.0
    hyponatremia E87.1
Anhydremia E86.0
  with
    hypernatremia E87.0
    hyponatremia E87.1
Anidrosis L74.4
Aniridia (congenital) Q13.1
Anisakiasis (infection) (infestation) B81.0
Anisakis larvae infestation B81.0
Aniseikonia H52.32
Anisocoria (pupil) H57.02
  congenital Q13.2
Anisocytosis R71.8
Anisometropia (congenital) H52.31
Ankle — *see* condition
Ankyloblepharon (eyelid) (acquired) — *see also* Blepharophimosis
  filiforme (adnatum) (congenital) Q10.3
  total Q10.3
Ankyloglossia Q38.1
Ankylosis (fibrous) (osseous) (joint) M24.60
  ankle M24.67-
  arthrodesis status Z98.1
  cricoarytenoid (cartilage) (joint) (larynx) J38.7
  dental K03.5
  ear ossicles H74.31-
  elbow M24.62-
  foot M24.67-
  hand M24.64-
  hip M24.65-
  incostapedial joint (infectional) — *see* Ankylosis, ear ossicles
  jaw (temporomandibular) M26.61
  knee M24.66-
  lumbosacral (joint) M43.27
  postoperative (status) Z98.1
  produced by surgical fusion, status Z98.1
  sacro-iliac (joint) M43.28
  shoulder M24.61-
  spine (joint) — *see also* Fusion, spine
    spondylitic — *see* Spondylitis, ankylosing
  surgical Z98.1
  temporomandibular M26.61
  tooth, teeth (hard tissues) K03.5
  wrist M24.63-
Ankylostoma — *see* Ancylostoma
Ankylostomiasis — *see* Ancylostomiasis
Ankylurethria — *see* Stricture, urethra
Annular — *see also* condition
  detachment, cervix N88.8
  organ or site, congenital NEC — *see* Distortion
  pancreas (congenital) Q45.1
Anodontia (complete) (partial) (vera) K00.0
  acquired K08.10
Anomaly, anomalous (congenital) (unspecified type) Q89.9
  abdominal wall NEC Q79.59
  acoustic nerve Q07.8
  adrenal (gland) Q89.1
  Alder (-Reilly) (leukocyte granulation) D72.0
  alimentary tract Q45.9
    upper Q40.9
  alveolar M26.70
    hyperplasia M26.79
      mandibular M26.72
      maxillary M26.71
    hypoplasia M26.79
      mandibular M26.74
      maxillary M26.73
    ridge (process) M26.79
    specified NEC M26.79
  ankle (joint) Q74.2
  anus Q43.9
  aorta (arch) NEC Q25.4
    coarctation (preductal) (postductal) Q25.1
  aortic cusp or valve Q23.9
  appendix Q43.8
  apple peel syndrome Q41.1
  aqueduct of Sylvius Q03.0
    with spina bifida — *see* Spina bifida, with hydrocephalus
  arm Q74.0
  arteriovenous NEC
    coronary Q24.5
    gastrointestinal Q27.33
      acquired — *see* Angiodysplasia

DISEASE INDEX

Anomaly, anomalous (congenital)
(unspecified type) Q89.9 — *continued*
artery (peripheral) Q27.9
basilar NEC Q28.1
cerebral Q28.3
coronary Q24.5
digestive system Q27.8
eye Q15.8
great Q25.9
specified NEC Q25.8
lower limb Q27.8
peripheral Q27.9
specified NEC Q27.8
pulmonary NEC Q25.79
renal Q27.2
retina Q14.1
specified site NEC Q27.8
subclavian Q27.8
umbilical Q27.0
upper limb Q27.8
vertebral NEC Q28.1
aryteno-epiglottic folds Q31.8
atrial
bands or folds Q20.8
septa Q21.1
atrioventricular
excitation I45.6
septum Q21.0
auditory canal Q17.8
auricle
ear Q17.8
causing impairment of hearing Q16.9
heart Q20.8
Axenfeld's Q15.0
back Q89.9
band
atrial Q20.8
heart Q24.8
ventricular Q24.8
Bartholin's duct Q38.4
biliary duct or passage Q44.5
bladder Q64.70
absence Q64.5
diverticulum Q64.6
exstrophy Q64.10
cloacal Q64.12
extroversion Q64.19
specified type NEC Q64.19
supravesical fissure Q64.11
neck obstruction Q64.31
specified type NEC Q64.79
bone Q79.9
arm Q74.0
face Q75.9
leg Q74.2
pelvic girdle Q74.2
shoulder girdle Q74.0
skull Q75.9
with
anencephaly Q00.0
encephalocele — *see*
Encephalocele
hydrocephalus Q03.9
with spina bifida — *see* Spina
bifida, by site, with
hydrocephalus
microcephaly Q02
brain (multiple) Q04.9
vessel Q28.3
breast Q83.9
broad ligament Q50.6
bronchus Q32.4
bulbus cordis Q21.9
bursa Q79.9
canal of Nuck Q52.4
canthus Q10.3
capillary Q27.9
cardiac Q24.9
chambers Q20.9
specified NEC Q20.8
septal closure Q21.9
specified NEC Q21.8
valve NEC Q24.8
pulmonary Q22.3
cardiovascular system Q28.8
carpus Q74.0
caruncle, lacrimal Q10.6
cascade stomach Q40.2
cauda equina Q06.3
cecum Q43.9
cerebral Q04.9
vessels Q28.3
cervix Q51.9
Chédiak-Higashi(-Steinbrinck) (congenital
gigantism of peroxidase granules)
E70.330
cheek Q18.9
chest wall Q67.8
bones Q76.9
chin Q18.9

Anomaly, anomalous (congenital)
(unspecified type) Q89.9 — *continued*
chordae tendineae Q24.8
choroid Q14.3
plexus Q07.8
chromosomes, chromosomal Q99.9
D(1) — *see* condition, chromosome 13
E(3) — *see* condition, chromosome 18
G — *see* condition, chromosome 21
sex
female phenotype Q97.8
gonadal dysgenesis (pure) Q99.1
Klinefelter's Q98.4
male phenotype Q98.9
Turner's Q96.9
specified NEC Q99.8
cilia Q10.3
circulatory system Q28.9
clavicle Q74.0
clitoris Q52.6
coccyx Q76.49
colon Q43.9
common duct Q44.5
communication
coronary artery Q24.5
left ventricle with right atrium Q21.0
concha (ear) Q17.3
connection
portal vein Q26.5
pulmonary venous Q26.4
partial Q26.3
total Q26.2
renal artery with kidney Q27.2
cornea (shape) Q13.4
coronary artery or vein Q24.5
cranium — *see* Anomaly, skull
cricoid cartilage Q31.8
cystic duct Q44.5
dental
alveolar — *see* Anomaly, alveolar
arch relationship M26.20
specified NEC M26.29
dentofacial M26.9
alveolar — *see* Anomaly, alveolar
dental arch relationship M26.20
specified NEC M26.29
functional M26.50
specified NEC M26.59
jaw size M26.00
macrogenia M26.05
mandibular
hyperplasia M26.03
hypoplasia M26.04
maxillary
hyperplasia M26.01
hypoplasia M26.02
microgenia M26.06
specified type NEC M26.09
jaw-cranial base relationship M26.10
asymmetry M26.12
maxillary M26.11
specified type NEC M26.19
malocclusion M26.4
dental arch relationship NEC M26.29
jaw size — *see* Anomaly, dentofacial,
jaw size
jaw-cranial base relationship — *see*
Anomaly, dentofacial, jaw-cranial
base relationship
specified type NEC M26.89
temporomandibular joint M26.60
adhesions M26.61
ankylosis M26.61
arthralgia M26.62
articular disc M26.63
specified type NEC M26.69
tooth position, fully erupted M26.30
specified NEC M26.39
dermatoglyphic Q82.8
diaphragm (apertures) NEC Q79.1
digestive organ(s) or tract Q45.9
lower Q43.9
upper Q40.9
distance, interarch (excessive) (inadequate)
M26.25
distribution, coronary artery Q24.5
ductus
arteriosus Q25.0
botalli Q25.0
duodenum Q43.9
dura (brain) Q04.9
spinal cord Q06.9
ear (external) Q17.9
causing impairment of hearing Q16.9
inner Q16.5
middle (causing impairment of hearing)
Q16.4
ossicles Q16.3
Ebstein's (heart) (tricuspid valve) Q22.5
ectodermal Q82.9

Anomaly, anomalous (congenital)
(unspecified type) Q89.9 — *continued*
Eisenmenger's (ventricular septal defect)
Q21.8
ejaculatory duct Q55.4
elbow Q74.0
endocrine gland NEC Q89.2
epididymis Q55.4
epiglottis Q31.8
esophagus Q39.9
eustachian tube Q17.8
eye Q15.9
anterior segment Q13.9
specified NEC Q13.89
posterior segment Q14.9
specified NEC Q14.8
ptosis (eyelid) Q10.0
specified NEC Q15.8
eyebrow Q18.8
eyelid Q10.3
ptosis Q10.0
face Q18.9
bone(s) Q75.9
fallopian tube Q50.6
fascia Q79.9
femur NEC Q74.2
fibula NEC Q74.2
finger Q74.0
fixation, intestine Q43.3
flexion (joint) NOS Q74.9
hip or thigh Q65.89
foot NEC Q74.2
varus (congenital) Q66.3
foramen
Botalli Q21.1
ovale Q21.1
forearm Q74.0
forehead Q75.8
form, teeth K00.2
fovea centralis Q14.1
frontal bone — *see* Anomaly, skull
gallbladder (position) (shape) (size) Q44.1
Gartner's duct Q52.4
gastrointestinal tract Q45.9
genitalia, genital organ(s) or system
female Q52.9
external Q52.70
internal NOS Q52.9
male Q55.9
hydrocele P83.5
specified NEC Q55.8
genitourinary NEC
female Q52.9
male Q55.9
Gerbode Q21.0
glottis Q31.8
granulation or granulocyte, genetic
(constitutional) (leukocyte) D72.0
gum Q38.6
gyri Q07.9
hair Q84.2
hand Q74.0
hard tissue formation in pulp K04.3
head — *see* Anomaly, skull
heart Q24.9
auricle Q20.8
bands or folds Q24.8
fibroelastosis cordis I42.4
obstructive NEC Q22.6
patent ductus arteriosus (Botalli) Q25.0
septum Q21.9
auricular Q21.1
interatrial Q21.1
interventricular Q21.0
with pulmonary stenosis or atresia,
dextraposition of aorta and
hypertrophy of right ventricle
Q21.3
specified NEC Q21.8
ventricular Q21.0
with pulmonary stenosis or atresia,
dextraposition of aorta and
hypertrophy of right ventricle
Q21.3
tetralogy of Fallot Q21.3
valve NEC Q24.8
aortic
bicuspid valve Q23.1
insufficiency Q23.1
stenosis Q23.0
subaortic Q24.4
mitral
insufficiency Q23.3
stenosis Q23.2
pulmonary Q22.3
atresia Q22.0
insufficiency Q22.2

Anomaly, anomalous (congenital)
(unspecified type) Q89.9 — *continued*
heart Q24.9 — *continued*
valve NEC Q24.8 — *continued*
pulmonary Q22.3 — *continued*
stenosis Q22.1
infundibular Q24.3
subvalvular Q24.3
tricuspid
atresia Q22.4
stenosis Q22.4
ventricle Q20.8
heel NEC Q74.2
Hegglin's D72.0
hemianencephaly Q00.0
hemicephaly Q00.0
hemicrania Q00.0
hepatic duct Q44.5
hip NEC Q74.2
hourglass stomach Q40.2
humerus Q74.0
hydatid of Morgagni
female Q50.5
male (epididymal) Q55.4
testicular Q55.29
hymen Q52.4
hypersegmentation of neutrophils,
hereditary D72.0
hypophyseal Q89.2
ileocecal (coil) (valve) Q43.9
ileum Q43.9
ilium NEC Q74.2
integument Q84.9
specified NEC Q84.8
interarch distance (excessive) (inadequate)
M26.25
intervertebral cartilage or disc Q76.49
intestine (large) (small) Q43.9
with anomalous adhesions, fixation or
malrotation Q43.3
iris Q13.2
ischium NEC Q74.2
jaw — *see* Anomaly, dentofacial
alveolar — *see* Anomaly, alveolar
jaw-cranial base relationship — *see*
Anomaly, dentofacial, jaw-cranial
base relationship
jejunum Q43.8
joint Q74.9
specified NEC Q74.8
Jordan's D72.0
kidney(s) (calyx) (pelvis) Q63.9
artery Q27.2
specified NEC Q63.8
Klippel-Feil (brevicollis) Q76.1
knee Q74.1
labium (majus) (minus) Q52.70
labyrinth, membranous Q16.5
lacrimal apparatus or duct Q10.6
larynx, laryngeal (muscle) Q31.9
web(bed) Q31.0
lens Q12.9
leukocytes, genetic D72.0
granulation (constitutional) D72.0
lid (fold) Q10.3
ligament Q79.9
broad Q50.6
round Q52.8
limb Q74.9
lower NEC Q74.2
reduction deformity — *see* Defect,
reduction, lower limb
upper Q74.0
lip Q38.0
liver Q44.7
duct Q44.5
lower limb NEC Q74.2
lumbosacral (joint) (region) Q76.49
kyphosis — *see* Kyphosis, congenital
lordosis — *see* Lordosis, congenital
lung (fissure) (lobe) Q33.9
mandible — *see* Anomaly, dentofacial
maxilla — *see* Anomaly, dentofacial
May (-Hegglin) D72.0
meatus urinarius NEC Q64.79
meningeal bands or folds Q07.9
constriction of Q07.8
spinal Q06.9
meninges Q07.9
cerebral Q04.8
spinal Q06.9
meningocele Q05.9
mesentery Q45.9
metacarpus Q74.0
metatarsus NEC Q74.2
middle ear Q16.4
ossicles Q16.3

Anomaly, anomalous (congenital)
(unspecified type) Q89.9 — *continued*
mitral (leaflets) (valve) Q23.9
insufficiency Q23.3
specified NEC Q23.8
stenosis Q23.2
mouth Q38.6
multiple NEC Q89.7
muscle Q79.9
eyelid Q10.3
musculoskeletal system, except limbs Q79.9
myocardium Q24.8
Müllerian — *see also* Anomaly, by site
uterus NEC Q51.818
nail Q84.6
narrowness, eyelid Q10.3
nasal sinus (wall) Q30.8
neck (any part) Q18.9
nerve Q07.9
acoustic Q07.8
optic Q07.8
nervous system (central) Q07.9
nipple Q83.9
nose, nasal (bones) (cartilage) (septum) (sinus) Q30.9
specified NEC Q30.8
ocular muscle Q15.8
omphalomesenteric duct Q43.0
opening, pulmonary veins Q26.4
optic
disc Q14.2
nerve Q07.8
opticociliary vessels Q13.2
orbit (eye) Q10.7
organ Q89.9
of Corti Q16.5
origin
artery
innominate Q25.8
pulmonary Q25.79
renal Q27.2
subclavian Q25.8
osseous meatus (ear) Q16.1
ovary Q50.39
oviduct Q50.6
palate (hard) (soft) NEC Q38.5
pancreas or pancreatic duct Q45.3
papillary muscles Q24.8
parathyroid gland Q89.2
paraurethral ducts Q64.79
parotid (gland) Q38.4
patella Q74.1
Pelger-Huët (hereditary hyposegmentation) D72.0
pelvic girdle NEC Q74.2
pelvis (bony) NEC Q74.2
rachitic E64.3
penis (glans) Q55.69
pericardium Q24.8
peripheral vascular system Q27.9
Peter's Q13.4
pharynx Q38.8
pigmentation L81.9
congenital Q82.8
pituitary (gland) Q89.2
pleural (folds) Q34.0
portal vein Q26.5
connection Q26.5
position, tooth, teeth, fully erupted M26.30
specified NEC M26.39
precerebral vessel Q28.1
prepuce Q55.69
prostate Q55.4
pulmonary Q33.9
artery NEC Q25.79
valve Q22.3
atresia Q22.0
insufficiency Q22.2
specified type NEC Q22.3
stenosis Q22.1
infundibular Q24.3
subvalvular Q24.3
venous connection Q26.4
partial Q26.3
total Q26.2
pupil Q13.2
function H57.00
anisocoria H57.02
Argyll Robertson pupil H57.01
miosis H57.03
mydriasis H57.04
specified type NEC H57.09
tonic pupil H57.05-
pylorus Q40.3
radius Q74.0
rectum Q43.9

Anomaly, anomalous (congenital)
(unspecified type) Q89.9 — *continued*
reduction (extremity) (limb)
femur (longitudinal) — *see* Defect, reduction, lower limb, longitudinal, femur
fibula (longitudinal) — *see* Defect, reduction, lower limb, longitudinal, fibula
lower limb — *see* Defect, reduction, lower limb
radius (longitudinal) — *see* Defect, reduction, upper limb, longitudinal, radius
tibia (longitudinal) — *see* Defect, reduction, lower limb, longitudinal, tibia
ulna (longitudinal) — *see* Defect, reduction, upper limb, longitudinal, ulna
upper limb — *see* Defect, reduction, upper limb
refraction — *see* Disorder, refraction
renal Q63.9
artery Q27.2
pelvis Q63.9
specified NEC Q63.8
respiratory system Q34.9
specified NEC Q34.8
retina Q14.1
rib Q76.6
cervical Q76.5
Rieger's Q13.81
rotation — *see* Malrotation
hip or thigh Q65.89
round ligament Q52.8
sacroiliac (joint) NEC Q74.2
sacrum NEC Q76.49
kyphosis — *see* Kyphosis, congenital
lordosis — *see* Lordosis, congenital
saddle nose, syphilitic A50.57
salivary duct or gland Q38.4
scapula Q74.0
scrotum — *see* Malformation, testis and scrotum
sebaceous gland Q82.9
seminal vesicles Q55.4
sense organs NEC Q07.8
sex chromosomes NEC — *see also* Anomaly, chromosomes
female phenotype Q97.8
male phenotype Q98.9
shoulder (girdle) (joint) Q74.0
sigmoid (flexure) Q43.9
simian crease Q82.8
sinus of Valsalva Q25.4
skeleton generalized Q78.9
skin (appendage) Q82.9
skull Q75.9
with
anencephaly Q00.0
encephalocele — *see* Encephalocele
hydrocephalus Q03.9
with spina bifida — *see* Spina bifida, by site, with hydrocephalus
microcephaly Q02
specified organ or site NEC Q89.8
spermatic cord Q55.4
spine, spinal NEC Q76.49
column NEC Q76.49
kyphosis — *see* Kyphosis, congenital
lordosis — *see* Lordosis, congenital
cord Q06.9
nerve root Q07.8
spleen Q89.09
agenesis Q89.01
stenonian duct Q38.4
sternum NEC Q76.7
stomach Q40.3
submaxillary gland Q38.4
tarsus NEC Q74.2
tendon Q79.9
testis — *see* Malformation, testis and scrotum
thigh NEC Q74.2
thorax (wall) Q67.8
bony Q76.9
throat Q38.8
thumb Q74.0
thymus gland Q89.2
thyroid (gland) Q89.2
cartilage Q31.8
tibia NEC Q74.2
saber A50.56
toe Q74.2
tongue Q38.3

Anomaly, anomalous (congenital)
(unspecified type) Q89.9 — *continued*
tooth, teeth K00.9
eruption K00.6
position, fully erupted M26.30
spacing, fully erupted M26.30
trachea (cartilage) Q32.1
tragus Q17.9
tricuspid (leaflet) (valve) Q22.9
atresia or stenosis Q22.4
Ebstein's Q22.5
Uhl's (hypoplasia of myocardium, right ventricle) Q24.8
ulna Q74.0
umbilical artery Q27.0
union
cricoid cartilage and thyroid cartilage Q31.8
thyroid cartilage and hyoid bone Q31.8
trachea with larynx Q31.8
upper limb NEC Q74.0
urachus Q64.4
ureter Q62.8
obstructive NEC Q62.39
cecoureterocele Q62.32
orthotopic ureterocele Q62.31
urethra Q64.70
absence Q64.5
double Q64.74
fistula to rectum Q64.73
obstructive Q64.39
stricture Q64.32
prolapse Q64.71
specified type NEC Q64.79
urinary tract Q64.9
uterus Q51.9
with only one functioning horn Q51.4
uvula Q38.5
vagina Q52.4
valleculae Q31.8
valve (heart) NEC Q24.8
coronary sinus Q24.5
inferior vena cava Q24.8
pulmonary Q22.3
sinus coronario Q24.5
venae cavae inferioris Q24.8
vas deferens Q55.4
vascular Q27.9
brain Q28.3
ring Q25.4
vein(s) (peripheral) Q27.9
brain Q28.3
cerebral Q28.3
coronary Q24.5
developmental Q28.3
great Q26.9
specified NEC Q26.8
vena cava (inferior) (superior) Q26.9
venous — *see* Anomaly, vein(s)
venous return Q26.8
ventricular
bands or folds Q24.8
septa Q21.0
vertebra Q76.49
kyphosis — *see* Kyphosis, congenital
lordosis — *see* Lordosis, congenital
vesicourethral orifice Q64.79
vessel(s) Q27.9
optic papilla Q14.2
precerebral Q28.1
vitelline duct Q43.0
vitreous body or humor Q14.0
vulva Q52.70
wrist (joint) Q74.0
Anomia R48.8
Anonychia (congenital) Q84.3
acquired L60.8
Anophthalmos, anophthalmus (congenital) (globe) Q11.1
acquired Z90.01
Anopia, anopsia H53.46-
quadrant H53.46-
Anorchia, anorchism, anorchidism Q55.0
Anorexia R63.0
hysterical F44.89
nervosa F50.00
atypical F50.9
binge-eating type F50.2
with purging F50.02
restricting type F50.01
Anorgasmy, psychogenic (female) F52.31
male F52.32
Anosmia R43.0
hysterical F44.6
postinfectional J39.8
Anosognosia R41.89
Anosteoplasia Q78.9
Anovulatory cycle N97.0
Anoxemia R09.02
newborn P84

Anoxia (pathological) R09.02
altitude T70.29
cerebral G93.1
complicating
anesthesia (general) (local) or other sedation T88.59
in labor and delivery O74.3
in pregnancy O29.21-
postpartum, puerperal O89.2
delivery (cesarean) (instrumental) O75.4
during a procedure G97.81
newborn P84
resulting from a procedure G97.82
due to
drowning T75.1
high altitude T70.29
heart — *see* Insufficiency, coronary
intrauterine P84
myocardial — *see* Insufficiency, coronary
newborn P84
spinal cord G95.11
systemic (by suffocation) (low content in atmosphere) — *see* Asphyxia, traumatic
Anteflexion — *see* Anteversion
Antenatal
care (normal pregnancy) Z34.90
screening (encounter for) of mother Z36
Antepartum — *see* condition
Anterior — *see* condition
Antero-occlusion M26.220
Anteversion
cervix — *see* Anteversion, uterus
femur (neck), congenital Q65.89
uterus, uterine (cervix) (postinfectional) (postpartal, old) N85.4
congenital Q51.818
in pregnancy or childbirth — *see* Pregnancy, complicated by
Anthophobia F40.228
Anthracosilicosis J60
Anthracosis (lung) (occupational) J60
lingua K14.3
Anthrax A22.9
with pneumonia A22.1
cerebral A22.8
colitis A22.2
cutaneous A22.0
gastrointestinal A22.2
inhalation A22.1
intestinal A22.2
meningitis A22.8
pulmonary A22.1
respiratory A22.1
sepsis A22.7
specified manifestation NEC A22.8
Anthropoid pelvis Q74.2
with disproportion (fetopelvic) O33.0
Anthropophobia F40.10
generalized F40.11
Antibodies, maternal (blood group) — *see* Isoimmunization, affecting management of pregnancy
anti-D — *see* Isoimmunization, affecting management of pregnancy, Rh
newborn P55.0
Antibody
anticardiolipin R76.0
with
hemorrhagic disorder D68.312
hypercoagulable state D68.61
antiphosphatidylglycerol R76.0
with
hemorrhagic disorder D68.312
hypercoagulable state D68.61
antiphosphatidylinositol R76.0
with
hemorrhagic disorder D68.312
hypercoagulable state D68.61
antiphosphatidylserine R76.0
with
hemorrhagic disorder D68.312
hypercoagulable state D68.61
antiphospholipid R76.0
with
hemorrhagic disorder D68.312
hypercoagulable state D68.61
Anticardiolipin syndrome D68.61
Anticoagulant, circulating (intrinsic) (*see also* Disorder, hemorrhagic) D68.318
drug-induced (extrinsic) (*see also* Disorder, hemorrhagic) D68.32
Antidiuretic hormone syndrome E22.2
Antimonial cholera — *see* Poisoning, antimony
Antiphospholipid
antibody
with hemorrhagic disorder D68.312
syndrome D68.61

Antisocial personality F60.2
Antithrombinemia — see Circulating anticoagulants
Antithromboplastinemia D68.318
Antithromboplastinogenemia D68.318
Antitoxin complication or reaction — see Complications, vaccination
Antlophobia F40.228
Antritis J32.0
　maxilla J32.0
　　acute J01.00
　　　recurrent J01.01
　stomach K29.60
　　with bleeding K29.61
Antrum, antral — see condition
Anuria R34
　calculous (impacted) (recurrent) (see also Calculus, urinary) N20.9
　following
　　abortion — see Abortion, by type, complicated by, renal failure
　　ectopic or molar pregnancy O08.4
　newborn P96.0
　postprocedural N99.0
　postrenal N13.8
　traumatic (following crushing) T79.5
Anus, anal — see condition
Anusitis K62.89
Anxiety F41.9
　depression F41.8
　episodic paroxysmal F41.0
　generalized F41.1
　hysteria F41.8
　neurosis F41.1
　panic type F41.0
　reaction F41.1
　separation, abnormal (of childhood) F93.0
　specified NEC F41.8
　state F41.1
Aorta, aortic — see condition
Aortectasia — see Ectasia, aorta
　with aneurysm — see Aneurysm, aorta
Aortitis (nonsyphilitic) (calcific) I77.6
　arteriosclerotic I70.0
　Doehle-Heller A52.02
　luetic A52.02
　rheumatic — see Endocarditis, acute, rheumatic
　specific (syphilitic) A52.02
　syphilitic A52.02
　　congenital A50.54 [I79.1]
Apathetic thyroid storm — see Thyrotoxicosis
Apathy R45.3
Apeirophobia F40.228
Apepsia K30
　psychogenic F45.8
Aperistalsis, esophagus K22.0
Apertognathia M26.29
Apert's syndrome Q87.0
Aphagia R13.0
　psychogenic F50.9
Aphakia (acquired) (postoperative) H27.0-
　congenital Q12.3
Aphasia (amnestic) (global) (nominal) (semantic) (syntactic) R47.01
　acquired, with epilepsy (Landau-Kleffner syndrome) — see Epilepsy, specified NEC
　auditory (developmental) F80.2
　developmental (receptive type) F80.2
　　expressive type F80.1
　　Wernicke's F80.2
　following
　　cerebrovascular disease I69.920
　　　cerebral infarction I69.320
　　　intracerebral hemorrhage I69.120
　　　nontraumatic intracranial hemorrhage NEC I69.220
　　　specified disease NEC I69.820
　　　subarachnoid hemorrhage I69.020
　primary progressive G31.01 [F02.80]
　　with behavioral disturbance G31.01 [F02.81]
　progressive isolated G31.01 [F02.80]
　　with behavioral disturbance G31.01 [F02.81]
　sensory F80.2
　syphilis, tertiary A52.19
　Wernicke's (developmental) F80.2
Aphonia (organic) R49.1
　hysterical F44.4
　psychogenic F44.4
Aphthae, aphthous — see also condition
　Bednar's K12.0
　cachectic K14.0
　epizootic B08.8
　fever B08.8
　oral (recurrent) K12.0
　stomatitis (major) (minor) K12.0

Aphthae, aphthous (see also condition) — continued
　thrush B37.0
　ulcer (oral) (recurrent) K12.0
　　genital organ(s) NEC
　　　female N76.6
　　　male N50.8
　　larynx J38.7
Apical — see condition
Apiphobia F40.218
Aplasia — see also Agenesis
　abdominal muscle syndrome Q79.4
　alveolar process (acquired) — see Anomaly, alveolar
　　congenital Q38.6
　aorta (congenital) Q25.4
　axialis extracorticalis (congenita) E75.29
　bone marrow (myeloid) D61.9
　　congenital D61.01
　brain Q00.0
　　part of Q04.3
　bronchus Q32.4
　cementum K00.4
　cerebellum Q04.3
　cervix (congenital) Q51.5
　congenital pure red cell D61.01
　corpus callosum Q04.0
　cutis congenita Q84.8
　erythrocyte congenital D61.01
　extracortical axial E75.29
　eye Q11.1
　fovea centralis (congenital) Q14.1
　gallbladder, congenital Q44.0
　iris Q13.1
　labyrinth, membranous Q16.5
　limb (congenital) Q73.8
　　lower — see Defect, reduction, lower limb
　　upper — see Agenesis, arm
　lung, congenital (bilateral) (unilateral) Q33.3
　pancreas Q45.0
　parathyroid-thymic D82.1
　Pelizaeus-Merzbacher E75.29
　penis Q55.5
　prostate Q55.4
　red cell (with thymoma) D60.9
　　acquired D60.9
　　　due to drugs D60.9
　　adult D60.9
　　chronic D60.0
　　congenital D61.01
　　constitutional D61.01
　　due to drugs D60.9
　　hereditary D61.01
　　of infants D61.01
　　primary D61.01
　　pure D61.01
　　　due to drugs D60.9
　　specified type NEC D60.8
　　transient D60.1
　round ligament Q52.8
　skin Q84.8
　spermatic cord Q55.4
　spleen Q89.01
　testicle Q55.0
　thymic, with immunodeficiency D82.1
　thyroid (congenital) (with myxedema) E03.1
　uterus Q51.0
　ventral horn cell Q06.1
Apnea, apneic (of) (spells) R06.81
　newborn NEC P28.4
　　obstructive P28.4
　　sleep (central) (obstructive) (primary) P28.3
　prematurity P28.4
　sleep G47.30
　　central (primary) G47.31
　　　in conditions classified elsewhere G47.37
　　obstructive (adult) (pediatric) G47.33
　　primary central G47.31
　　specified NEC G47.39
Apneumatosis, newborn P28.0
Apocrine metaplasia (breast) — see Dysplasia, mammary, specified type NEC
Apophysitis (bone) — see also Osteochondropathy
　calcaneus M92.8
　juvenile M92.9
Apoplectiform convulsions (cerebral ischemia) I67.82
Apoplexia, apoplexy, apoplectic
　adrenal A39.1
　heart (auricle) (ventricle) — see Infarct, myocardium
　heat T67.0

Apoplexia, apoplexy, apoplectic — continued
　hemorrhagic (stroke) — see Hemorrhage, intracranial
　meninges, hemorrhagic — see Hemorrhage, intracranial, subarachnoid
　uremic N18.9 [I68.8]
Appearance
　bizarre R46.1
　specified NEC R46.89
　very low level of personal hygiene R46.0
Appendage
　epididymal (organ of Morgagni) Q55.4
　intestine (epiploic) Q43.8
　preauricular Q17.0
　testicular (organ of Morgagni) Q55.29
Appendicitis (pneumococcal) (retrocecal) K37
　with
　　perforation or rupture K35.2
　　peritoneal abscess K35.3
　　peritonitis K35.2
　　　generalized (with perforation or rupture) K35.2
　　　localized (with perforation or rupture) K35.3
　acute (catarrhal) (fulminating) (gangrenous) (obstructive) (retrocecal) (suppurative) K35.80
　　with
　　　peritoneal abscess K35.3
　　　peritonitis K35.2
　　　　generalized (with perforation or rupture) K35.2
　　　　localized (with perforation or rupture) K35.3
　　specified NEC K35.89
　amebic A06.89
　chronic (recurrent) K36
　exacerbation — see Appendicitis, acute
　gangrenous — see Appendicitis, acute
　healed (obliterative) K36
　interval K36
　neurogenic K36
　obstructive K36
　recurrent K36
　relapsing K36
　subacute (adhesive) K36
　subsiding K36
　suppurative — see Appendicitis, acute
　tuberculous A18.32
Appendicopathia oxyurica B80
Appendix, appendicular — see also condition
　epididymis Q55.4
　Morgagni
　　female Q50.5
　　male (epididymal) Q55.4
　　testicular Q55.29
　testis Q55.29
Appetite
　depraved — see Pica
　excessive R63.2
　lack or loss (see also Anorexia) R63.0
　　nonorganic origin F50.8
　　psychogenic F50.8
　perverted (hysterical) — see Pica
Apple peel syndrome Q41.1
Apprehension state F41.1
Apprehensiveness, abnormal F41.9
Approximal wear K03.0
Apraxia (classic) (ideational) (ideokinetic) (ideomotor) (motor) (verbal) R48.2
　following
　　cerebrovascular disease I69.990
　　　cerebral infarction I69.390
　　　intracerebral hemorrhage I69.190
　　　nontraumatic intracranial hemorrhage NEC I69.290
　　　specified disease NEC I69.890
　　　subarachnoid hemorrhage I69.090
　oculomotor, congenital H51.8
Aptyalism K11.7
Apudoma — see Neoplasm, uncertain behavior, by site
Aqueous misdirection H40.83-
Arabicum elephantiasis — see Infestation, filarial
Arachnitis — see Meningitis
Arachnodactyly — see Syndrome, Marfan's
Arachnoiditis (acute) (adhesive) (basal) (brain) (cerebrospinal) — see Meningitis
Arachnophobia F40.210
Arboencephalitis, Australian A83.4
Arborization block (heart) I45.5
ARC (AIDS-related complex) B20
Arches — see condition
Arcuate uterus Q51.810
Arcuatus uterus Q51.810

Arcus (cornea) senilis — see Degeneration, cornea, senile
Arc-welder's lung J63.4
Areflexia R29.2
Areola — see condition
Argentaffinoma — see also Neoplasm, uncertain behavior, by site
　malignant — see Neoplasm, malignant, by site
　syndrome E34.0
Argininemia E72.21
Arginosuccinic aciduria E72.22
Argyll Robertson phenomenon, pupil or syndrome (syphilitic) A52.19
　atypical H57.09
　nonsyphilitic H57.09
Argyria, argyriasis
　conjunctival H11.13-
　from drug or medicament — see Table of Drugs and Chemicals, by substance
Argyrosis, conjunctival H11.13-
Arhinencephaly Q04.1
Ariboflavinosis E53.0
Arm — see condition
Arnold-Chiari disease, obstruction or syndrome (type II) Q07.00
　with
　　hydrocephalus Q07.02
　　　with spina bifida Q07.03
　　spina bifida Q07.01
　　　with hydrocephalus Q07.03
　type III — see Encephalocele
　type IV Q04.8
Aromatic amino-acid metabolism disorder E70.9
　specified NEC E70.8
Arousals, confusional G47.51
Arrest, arrested
　cardiac I46.9
　　complicating
　　　abortion — see Abortion, by type, complicated by, cardiac arrest
　　　anesthesia (general) (local) or other sedation — see Table of Drugs and Chemicals, by drug,
　　　　in labor and delivery O74.2
　　　　in pregnancy O29.11-
　　　　postpartum, puerperal O89.1
　　　　delivery (cesarean) (instrumental) O75.4
　　due to
　　　cardiac condition I46.2
　　　specified condition NEC I46.8
　　intraoperative I97.71-
　　newborn P29.81
　　postprocedural I97.12-
　　　obstetric procedure O75.4
　cardiorespiratory — see Arrest, cardiac
　circulatory — see Arrest, cardiac
　deep transverse O64.0
　development or growth
　　bone — see Disorder, bone, development or growth
　　child R62.50
　　tracheal rings Q32.1
　epiphyseal
　　complete
　　　femur M89.15-
　　　humerus M89.12-
　　　tibia M89.16-
　　　ulna M89.13-
　　forearm M89.13-
　　　specified NEC M89.13-
　　　ulna — see Arrest, epiphyseal, by type, ulna
　　lower leg M89.16-
　　　specified NEC M89.168
　　　tibia — see Arrest, epiphyseal, by type, tibia
　　partial
　　　femur M89.15-
　　　humerus M89.12-
　　　tibia M89.16-
　　　ulna M89.13-
　　specified NEC M89.18
　granulopoiesis — see Agranulocytosis
　growth plate — see Arrest, epiphyseal
　heart — see Arrest, cardiac
　legal, anxiety concerning Z65.3
　physeal — see Arrest, epiphyseal
　respiratory R09.2
　　newborn P28.81
　sinus I45.5
　spermatogenesis (complete) — see Azoospermia
　　incomplete — see Oligospermia
　transverse (deep) O64.0

DISEASE INDEX

Arrhenoblastoma
  benign
    specified site — *see* Neoplasm, benign, by site
    unspecified site
      female D27.9
      male D29.20
  malignant
    specified site — *see* Neoplasm, malignant, by site
    unspecified site
      female C56.9
      male C62.90
  specified site — *see* Neoplasm, uncertain behavior, by site
  unspecified site
    female D39.10
    male D40.10
Arrhythmia (auricle) (cardiac) (juvenile) (nodal) (reflex) (sinus) (supraventricular) (transitory) (ventricle) I49.9
  block I45.9
  extrasystolic I49.49
  newborn
    bradycardia P29.12
    occurring before birth P03.819
      before onset of labor P03.810
      during labor P03.811
    tachycardia P29.11
  psychogenic F45.8
  specified NEC I49.8
  vagal R55
  ventricular re-entry I47.0
Arrillaga-Ayerza syndrome (pulmonary sclerosis with pulmonary hypertension) I27.0
Arsenical pigmentation L81.8
  from drug or medicament — *see* Table of Drugs and Chemicals
Arsenism — *see* Poisoning, arsenic
Arterial — *see* condition
Arteriofibrosis — *see* Arteriosclerosis
Arteriolar sclerosis — *see* Arteriosclerosis
Arteriolith — *see* Arteriosclerosis
Arteriolitis I77.6
  necrotizing, kidney I77.5
  renal — *see* Hypertension, kidney
Arteriolosclerosis — *see* Arteriosclerosis
Arterionephrosclerosis — *see* Hypertension, kidney
Arteriopathy I77.9
Arteriosclerosis, arteriosclerotic (diffuse) (obliterans) (of) (senile) (with calcification) I70.90
  aorta I70.0
  arteries of extremities — *see* Arteriosclerosis, extremities
  brain I67.2
  bypass graft
    coronary — *see* Arteriosclerosis, coronary, bypass graft
    extremities — *see* Arteriosclerosis, extremities, bypass graft
  cardiac — *see* Disease, heart, ischemic, atherosclerotic
  cardiopathy — *see* Disease, heart, ischemic, atherosclerotic
  cardiorenal — *see* Hypertension, cardiorenal
  cardiovascular — *see* Disease, heart, ischemic, atherosclerotic
  carotid (*see also* Occlusion, artery, carotid) I65.2-
  central nervous system I67.2
  cerebral I67.2
  cerebrovascular I67.2
  coronary (artery) I25.10
    bypass graft I25.810
      with
        angina pectoris I25.709
          with documented spasm I25.701
          specified type NEC I25.708
          unstable I25.700
        ischemic chest pain I25.709
      autologous artery I25.810
        with
          angina pectoris I25.729
            with documented spasm I25.721
            specified type I25.728
            unstable I25.720
          ischemic chest pain I25.729

Arteriosclerosis, arteriosclerotic (diffuse) (obliterans) (of) (senile) (with calcification) I70.90 — *continued*
  coronary (artery) I25.10 — *continued*
    bypass graft I25.810 — *continued*
      autologous vein I25.810
        with
          angina pectoris I25.719
            with documented spasm I25.711
            specified type I25.718
            unstable I25.710
          ischemic chest pain I25.719
      nonautologous biological I25.810
        with
          angina pectoris I25.739
            with documented spasm I25.731
            specified type I25.738
            unstable I25.730
          ischemic chest pain I25.739
      specified type NEC I25.810
        with
          angina pectoris I25.799
            with documented spasm I25.791
            specified type I25.798
            unstable I25.790
          ischemic chest pain I25.799
    due to
      calcified coronary lesion (severely) I25.84
      lipid rich plaque I25.83
    native vessel
      with
        angina pectoris I25.119
          with documented spasm I25.111
          specified type NEC I25.118
          unstable I25.110
        ischemic chest pain I25.119
    transplanted heart I25.811
      bypass graft I25.812
        with
          angina pectoris I25.769
            with documented spasm I25.761
            specified type I25.768
            unstable I25.760
          ischemic chest pain I25.769
        native coronary artery I25.811
          with
            angina pectoris I25.759
              with documented spasm I25.751
              specified type I25.758
              unstable I25.750
            ischemic chest pain I25.759
  extremities (native arteries) I70.209
    bypass graft I70.309
      autologous vein graft I70.409
        leg I70.409
          with
            gangrene (and intermittent claudication, rest pain and ulcer) I70.469
            intermittent claudication I70.419
            rest pain (and intermittent claudication) I70.429
          bilateral I70.403
            with
              gangrene (and intermittent claudication, rest pain and ulcer) I70.463
              intermittent claudication I70.413
              rest pain (and intermittent claudication) I70.423
              specified type NEC I70.493
          left I70.402
            with
              gangrene (and intermittent claudication, rest pain and ulcer) I70.462
              intermittent claudication I70.412
              rest pain (and intermittent claudication) I70.422
              ulceration (and intermittent claudication and rest pain) I70.449
              ankle I70.443
              calf I70.442
              foot site NEC I70.445
              heel I70.444
              lower leg NEC I70.448
              midfoot I70.444
              thigh I70.441
              specified type NEC I70.492

Arteriosclerosis, arteriosclerotic (diffuse) (obliterans) (of) (senile) (with calcification) I70.90 — *continued*
  extremities (native arteries) I70.209 — *continued*
    bypass graft I70.309 — *continued*
      autologous vein graft I70.409 — *continued*
        leg I70.309 — *continued*
          right I70.401
            with
              gangrene (and intermittent claudication, rest pain and ulcer) I70.461
              intermittent claudication I70.411
              rest pain (and intermittent claudication) I70.421
              ulceration (and intermittent claudication and rest pain) I70.439
              ankle I70.433
              calf I70.432
              foot site NEC I70.435
              heel I70.434
              lower leg NEC I70.438
              midfoot I70.434
              thigh I70.431
            specified type NEC I70.491
          specified type NEC I70.499
        specified NEC I70.408
          with
            gangrene (and intermittent claudication, rest pain and ulcer) I70.468
            intermittent claudication I70.418
            rest pain (and intermittent claudication) I70.428
            ulceration (and intermittent claudication and rest pain) I70.45
          specified type NEC I70.498
      leg I70.309
        with
          gangrene (and intermittent claudication, rest pain and ulcer) I70.369
          intermittent claudication I70.319
          rest pain (and intermittent claudication) I70.329
        bilateral I70.303
          with
            gangrene (and intermittent claudication, rest pain and ulcer) I70.363
            intermittent claudication I70.313
            rest pain (and intermittent claudication) I70.323
            specified type NEC I70.393
        left I70.302
          with
            gangrene (and intermittent claudication, rest pain and ulcer) I70.362
            intermittent claudication I70.312
            rest pain (and intermittent claudication) I70.322
            ulceration (and intermittent claudication and rest pain) I70.349
            ankle I70.343
            calf I70.342
            foot site NEC I70.345
            heel I70.344
            lower leg NEC I70.348
            midfoot I70.344
            thigh I70.341
          specified type NEC I70.392
        right I70.301
          with
            gangrene (and intermittent claudication, rest pain and ulcer) I70.361
            intermittent claudication I70.311
            rest pain (and intermittent claudication) I70.321
            ulceration (and intermittent claudication and rest pain) I70.339
            ankle I70.333
            calf I70.332
            foot site NEC I70.335
            heel I70.334
            lower leg NEC I70.338
            midfoot I70.334
            thigh I70.331

Arteriosclerosis, arteriosclerotic (diffuse) (obliterans) (of) (senile) (with calcification) I70.90 — *continued*
  extremities (native arteries) I70.209 — *continued*
    bypass graft I70.309 — *continued*
      leg I70.309 — *continued*
        right I70.301 — *continued*
          specified type NEC I70.391
        specified type NEC I70.399
    nonautologous biological graft I70.509
      leg I70.509
        with
          gangrene (and intermittent claudication, rest pain and ulcer) I70.569
          intermittent claudication I70.519
          rest pain (and intermittent claudication) I70.529
        bilateral I70.503
          with
            gangrene (and intermittent claudication, rest pain and ulcer) I70.563
            intermittent claudication I70.513
            rest pain (and intermittent claudication) I70.523
            specified type NEC I70.593
        left I70.502
          with
            gangrene (and intermittent claudication, rest pain and ulcer) I70.562
            intermittent claudication I70.512
            rest pain (and intermittent claudication) I70.522
            ulceration (and intermittent claudication and rest pain) I70.549
            ankle I70.543
            calf I70.542
            foot site NEC I70.545
            heel I70.544
            lower leg NEC I70.548
            midfoot I70.544
            thigh I70.541
          specified type NEC I70.592
        right I70.501
          with
            gangrene (and intermittent claudication, rest pain and ulcer) I70.561
            intermittent claudication I70.511
            rest pain (and intermittent claudication) I70.521
            ulceration (and intermittent claudication and rest pain) I70.539
            ankle I70.533
            calf I70.532
            foot site NEC I70.535
            heel I70.534
            lower leg NEC I70.538
            midfoot I70.534
            thigh I70.531
          specified type NEC I70.591
        specified type NEC I70.599
    specified NEC I70.508
      with
        gangrene (and intermittent claudication, rest pain and ulcer) I70.568
        intermittent claudication I70.518
        rest pain (and intermittent claudication) I70.528
        ulceration (and intermittent claudication and rest pain) I70.55
      specified type NEC I70.598

DISEASE INDEX

Arteriosclerosis, arteriosclerotic (diffuse) (obliterans) (of) (senile) (with calcification) I70.90 — *continued*
  extremities (native arteries) I70.209 — *continued*
    bypass graft I70.309 — *continued*
      nonbiological graft I70.609
        leg I70.609
          with
            gangrene (and intermittent claudication, rest pain and ulcer) I70.669
            intermittent claudication I70.619
            rest pain (and intermittent claudication) I70.629
          bilateral I70.603
            with
              gangrene (and intermittent claudication, rest pain and ulcer) I70.663
              intermittent claudication I70.613
              rest pain (and intermittent claudication) I70.623
            specified type NEC I70.693
          left I70.602
            with
              gangrene (and intermittent claudication, rest pain and ulcer) I70.662
              intermittent claudication I70.612
              rest pain (and intermittent claudication) I70.622
              ulceration (and intermittent claudication and rest pain) I70.649
                ankle I70.643
                calf I70.642
                foot site NEC I70.645
                heel I70.644
                lower leg NEC I70.648
                midfoot I70.644
                thigh I70.641
            specified type NEC I70.692
          right I70.601
            with
              gangrene (and intermittent claudication, rest pain and ulcer) I70.661
              intermittent claudication I70.611
              rest pain (and intermittent claudication) I70.621
              ulceration (and intermittent claudication and rest pain) I70.639
                ankle I70.633
                calf I70.632
                foot site NEC I70.635
                heel I70.634
                lower leg NEC I70.638
                midfoot I70.634
                thigh I70.631
            specified type NEC I70.691
        specified type NEC I70.699
      specified NEC I70.608
        with
          gangrene (and intermittent claudication, rest pain and ulcer) I70.668
          intermittent claudication I70.618
          rest pain (and intermittent claudication) I70.628
          ulceration (and intermittent claudication and rest pain) I70.65
          specified type NEC I70.698
      specified graft NEC I70.709
        leg I70.709
          with
            gangrene (and intermittent claudication, rest pain and ulcer) I70.769
            intermittent claudication I70.719
            rest pain (and intermittent claudication) I70.729
          bilateral I70.703
            with
              gangrene (and intermittent claudication, rest pain and ulcer) I70.763
              intermittent claudication I70.713
              rest pain (and intermittent claudication) I70.723
            specified type NEC I70.793

Arteriosclerosis, arteriosclerotic (diffuse) (obliterans) (of) (senile) (with calcification) I70.90 — *continued*
  extremities (native arteries) I70.209 — *continued*
    bypass graft I70.309 — *continued*
      specified graft NEC I70.709 — *continued*
        leg I70.709 — *continued*
          left I70.702
            with
              gangrene (and intermittent claudication, rest pain and ulcer) I70.762
              intermittent claudication I70.712
              rest pain (and intermittent claudication) I70.722
              ulceration (and intermittent claudication and rest pain) I70.749
                ankle I70.743
                calf I70.742
                foot site NEC I70.745
                heel I70.744
                lower leg NEC I70.748
                midfoot I70.744
                thigh I70.741
            specified type NEC I70.792
          right I70.701
            with
              gangrene (and intermittent claudication, rest pain and ulcer) I70.761
              intermittent claudication I70.711
              rest pain (and intermittent claudication) I70.721
              ulceration (and intermittent claudication and rest pain) I70.739
                ankle I70.733
                calf I70.732
                foot site NEC I70.735
                heel I70.734
                lower leg NEC I70.738
                midfoot I70.734
                thigh I70.731
            specified type NEC I70.791
        specified type NEC I70.799
      specified NEC I70.708
        with
          gangrene (and intermittent claudication, rest pain and ulcer) I70.768
          intermittent claudication I70.718
          rest pain (and intermittent claudication) I70.728
          ulceration (and intermittent claudication and rest pain) I70.75
          specified type NEC I70.798
    specified NEC I70.308
      with
        gangrene (and intermittent claudication, rest pain and ulcer) I70.368
        intermittent claudication I70.318
        rest pain (and intermittent claudication) I70.328
        ulceration (and intermittent claudication and rest pain) I70.35
        specified type NEC I70.398
    leg I70.209
      with
        gangrene (and intermittent claudication, rest pain and ulcer) I70.269
        intermittent claudication I70.219
        rest pain (and intermittent claudication) I70.229
      bilateral I70.203
        with
          gangrene (and intermittent claudication, rest pain and ulcer) I70.263
          intermittent claudication I70.213
          rest pain (and intermittent claudication) I70.223
          specified type NEC I70.293
      left I70.202
        with
          gangrene (and intermittent claudication, rest pain and ulcer) I70.262
          intermittent claudication I70.212
          rest pain (and intermittent claudication) I70.222

Arteriosclerosis, arteriosclerotic (diffuse) (obliterans) (of) (senile) (with calcification) I70.90 — *continued*
  extremities (native arteries) I70.209 — *continued*
    leg I70.209 — *continued*
      left I70.202 — *continued*
        with — *continued*
          ulceration (and intermittent claudication and rest pain) I70.249
            ankle I70.243
            calf I70.242
            foot site NEC I70.245
            heel I70.244
            lower leg NEC I70.248
            midfoot I70.244
            thigh I70.241
        specified type NEC I70.292
      right I70.201
        with
          gangrene (and intermittent claudication, rest pain and ulcer) I70.261
          intermittent claudication I70.211
          rest pain (and intermittent claudication) I70.221
          ulceration (and intermittent claudication and rest pain) I70.239
            ankle I70.233
            calf I70.232
            foot site NEC I70.235
            heel I70.234
            lower leg NEC I70.238
            midfoot I70.234
            thigh I70.231
        specified type NEC I70.291
      specified type NEC I70.299
    specified site NEC I70.208
      with
        gangrene (and intermittent claudication, rest pain and ulcer) I70.268
        intermittent claudication I70.218
        rest pain (and intermittent claudication) I70.228
        ulceration (and intermittent claudication and rest pain) I70.25
        specified type NEC I70.298
  generalized I70.91
  heart (disease) — *see* Arteriosclerosis, coronary (artery),
  kidney — *see* Hypertension, kidney
  medial — *see* Arteriosclerosis, extremities
  mesenteric (artery) K55.1
  myocarditis I51.4
  Mönckeberg's — *see* Arteriosclerosis, extremities
  peripheral (of extremities) — *see* Arteriosclerosis, extremities
  pulmonary (idiopathic) I27.0
  renal (arterioles) — *see also* Hypertension, kidney
    artery I70.1
  retina (vascular) I70.8 [H35.0-]
  specified artery NEC I70.8
  spinal (cord) G95.19
  vertebral (artery) I67.2
Arteriospasm I73.9
Arteriovenous — *see* condition
Arteritis I77.6
  allergic M31.0
  aorta (nonsyphilitic) I77.6
    syphilitic A52.02
  aortic arch M31.4
  brachiocephalic M31.4
  brain I67.7
    syphilitic A52.04
  cerebral I67.7
    in
      diseases classified elsewhere I68.2
      systemic lupus erythematosus M32.19
    listerial A32.89
    syphilitic A52.04
    tuberculous A18.89
  coronary (artery) I25.89
    rheumatic I01.8
      chronic I09.89
    syphilitic A52.06
  cranial (left) (right), giant cell M31.6
  deformans — *see* Arteriosclerosis
  giant cell NEC M31.6
    with polymyalgia rheumatica M31.5
  necrosing or necrotizing M31.9
    specified NEC M31.8
  nodosa M30.0
  obliterans — *see* Arteriosclerosis

Arteritis I77.6 — *continued*
  pulmonary I28.8
  rheumatic — *see* Fever, rheumatic
  senile — *see* Arteriosclerosis
  suppurative I77.2
  syphilitic (general) A52.09
    brain A52.04
    coronary A52.06
    spinal A52.09
  temporal, giant cell M31.6
  young female aortic arch syndrome M31.4
Artery, arterial — *see also* condition
  abscess I77.89
  single umbilical Q27.0
Arthralgia (allergic) — *see also* Pain, joint
  in caisson disease T70.3
  temporomandibular M26.62
Arthritis, arthritic (acute) (chronic) (nonpyogenic) (subacute) M19.90
  allergic — *see* Arthritis, specified form NEC
  ankylosing (crippling) (spine) — *see also* Spondylitis, ankylosing
    sites other than spine — *see* Arthritis, specified form NEC
  atrophic — *see* Osteoarthritis
    spine — *see* Spondylitis, ankylosing
  back — *see* Spondylopathy, inflammatory
  blennorrhagic (gonococcal) A54.42
  Charcot's — *see* Arthropathy, neuropathic
    diabetic — *see* Diabetes, arthropathy, neuropathic
    syringomyelic G95.0
  chylous (filarial) (see also category M01) B74.9
  climacteric (any site) NEC — *see* Arthritis, specified form NEC
  crystal(-induced) — *see* Arthritis, in, crystals
  deformans — *see* Osteoarthritis
  degenerative — *see* Osteoarthritis
  due to or associated with
    acromegaly E22.0
    brucellosis — *see* Brucellosis
    caisson disease T70.3
    diabetes — *see* Diabetes, arthropathy
    dracontiasis (see also category M01) B72
    enteritis NEC
      regional — *see* Enteritis, regional
    erysipelas (see also category M01) A46
    erythema
      epidemic A25.1
      nodosum L52
    filariasis NOS B74.9
    glanders A24.0
    helminthiasis (see also category M01) B83.9
    hemophilia D66 [M36.2]
    Henoch-(Schönlein) purpura D69.0 [M36.4]
    human parvovirus (see also category M01) B97.6
    infectious disease NEC — *see* category M01
    leprosy (see also category M01) (see also Leprosy) A30.9
    Lyme disease A69.23
    mycobacteria (see also category M01) A31.8
    parasitic disease NEC (see also category M01) B89
    paratyphoid fever (see also category M01) (see also Fever, paratyphoid) A01.4
    rat bite fever (see also category M01) A25.1
    regional enteritis — *see* Enteritis, regional
    respiratory disorder NOS J98.9
    serum sickness (see also Reaction, serum) T80.69
    syringomyelia G95.0
    typhoid fever A01.04
  epidemic erythema A25.1
  febrile — *see* Fever, rheumatic
  gonococcal A54.42
  gouty (acute) — *see* Gout, idiopathic
  in (due to)
    acromegaly (see also subcategory M14.8-) E22.0
    amyloidosis (see also subcategory M14.8-) E85.4
    bacterial disease (see also subcategory M01) A49.9
    Behçet's syndrome M35.2
    caisson disease (see also subcategory M14.8-) T70.3
    coliform bacilli (Escherichia coli) — *see* Arthritis, in, pyogenic organism NEC

Arthritis, arthritic (acute) (chronic) (nonpyogenic) (subacute) M19.90 — *continued*
in (due to) — *continued*
  crystals M11.9
    dicalcium phosphate — *see* Arthritis, in, crystals, specified type NEC
    hydroxyapatite M11.0-
    pyrophosphate — *see* Arthritis, in, crystals, specified type NEC
    specified type NEC M11.80
      ankle M11.87-
      elbow M11.82-
      foot joint M11.87-
      hand joint M11.84-
      hip M11.85-
      knee M11.86-
      multiple sites M11.8-
      shoulder M11.81-
      vertebrae M11.88
      wrist M11.83-
  dermatoarthritis, lipoid E78.81
  dracontiasis (dracunculiasis) (*see also* category M01) B72
  endocrine disorder NEC (*see also* subcategory M14.8-) E34.9
  enteritis, infectious NEC (*see also* category M01) A09
    specified organism NEC (*see also* category M01) A08.8
  erythema
    multiforme (*see also* subcategory M14.8-) L51.9
    nodosum (*see also* subcategory M14.8-) L52
  gout — *see* Gout, idiopathic
  helminthiasis NEC (*see also* category M01) B83.9
  hemochromatosis (*see also* subcategory M14.8-) E83.118
  hemoglobinopathy NEC D58.2 [M36.3]
  hemophilia NEC D66 [M36.2]
  Hemophilus influenzae M00.8- [B96.3]
  Henoch(-Schönlein) purpura D69.0 [M36.4]
  hyperparathyroidism NEC (*see also* subcategory M14.8-) E21.3
  hypersensitivity reaction NEC T78.49 [M36.4]
  hypogammaglobulinemia (*see also* subcategory M14.8-) D80.1
  hypothyroidism NEC (*see also* subcategory M14.8-) E03.9
  infection — *see* Arthritis, pyogenic or pyemic
    spine — *see* Spondylopathy, infective
  infectious disease NEC — *see* category M01
  leprosy (*see also* category M01) A30.9
  leukemia NEC C95.9-[M36.1]
  lipoid dermatoarthritis E78.81
  Lyme disease A69.23
  Mediterranean fever, familial (*see also* subcategory M14.8-) E85.0
  Meningococcus A39.83
  metabolic disorder NEC (*see also* subcategory M14.8-) E88.9
  multiple myelomatosis C90.0-[M36.1]
  mumps B26.85
  mycosis NEC (*see also* category M01) B49
  myelomatosis (multiple) C90.0-[M36.1]
  neurological disorder NEC G98.0
  ochronosis (*see also* subcategory M14.8-) E70.29
  O'nyong-nyong (*see also* category M01) A92.1
  parasitic disease NEC (*see also* category M01) B89
  paratyphoid fever (*see also* category M01) A01.4
  Pseudomonas — *see* Arthritis, pyogenic, bacterial NEC
  psoriasis L40.50
  pyogenic organism NEC — *see* Arthritis, pyogenic, bacterial NEC
  Reiter's disease — *see* Reiter's disease
  respiratory disorder NEC (*see also* subcategory M14.8-) J98.9
  reticulosis, malignant (*see also* subcategory M14.8-) C86.0
  rubella B06.82
  Salmonella (arizonae) (cholerae-suis) (enteritidis) (typhimurium) A02.23
  sarcoidosis D86.86
  specified bacteria NEC — *see* Arthritis, pyogenic, bacterial NEC
  sporotrichosis B42.82
  syringomyelia G95.0
  thalassemia NEC D56.9 [M36.3]

Arthritis, arthritic (acute) (chronic) (nonpyogenic) (subacute) M19.90 — *continued*
in (due to) — *continued*
  tuberculosis — *see* Tuberculosis, arthritis
  typhoid fever A01.04
  urethritis, Reiter's — *see* Reiter's disease
  viral disease NEC (*see also* category M01) B34.9
infectious or infective — *see also* Arthritis, pyogenic or pyemic
  spine — *see* Spondylopathy, infective
juvenile M08.90
  with systemic onset — *see* Still's disease
  ankle M08.97-
  elbow M08.92-
  foot joint M08.97-
  hand joint M08.94-
  hip M08.95-
  knee M08.96-
  multiple site M08.99
  pauciarticular M08.40
    ankle M08.47-
    elbow M08.42-
    foot joint M08.47-
    hand joint M08.44-
    hip M08.45-
    knee M08.46-
    shoulder M08.41-
    vertebrae M08.48
    wrist M08.43-
  psoriatic L40.54
  rheumatoid — *see* Arthritis, rheumatoid, juvenile
  shoulder M08.91-
  specified type NEC M08.80
    ankle M08.87-
    elbow M08.82-
    foot joint M08.87-
    hand joint M08.84-
    hip M08.85-
    knee M08.86-
    multiple site M08.89
    shoulder M08.81-
    specified joint NEC M08.88
    vertebrae M08.88
    wrist M08.83-
  wrist M08.93-
meaning osteoarthritis — *see* Osteoarthritis
meningococcal A39.83
menopausal (any site) NEC — *see* Arthritis, specified form NEC
mutilans (psoriatic) L40.52
mycotic NEC (*see also* category M01) B49
neuropathic (Charcot) — *see* Arthropathy, neuropathic
  diabetic — *see* Diabetes, arthropathy, neuropathic
  nonsyphilitic NEC G98.0
  syringomyelic G95.0
ochronotic (*see also* subcategory M14.8-) E70.29
palindromic (any site) — *see* Rheumatism, palindromic
pneumococcal M00.10
  ankle M00.17-
  elbow M00.12-
  foot joint — *see* Arthritis, pneumococcal, ankle
  hand joint M00.14-
  hip M00.15-
  knee M00.16-
  multiple site M00.19
  shoulder M00.11-
  vertebra M00.18
  wrist M00.13-
postdysenteric — *see* Arthropathy, postdysenteric
postmeningococcal A39.84
postrheumatic, chronic — *see* Arthropathy, postrheumatic, chronic
primary progressive — *see also* Arthritis, specified form NEC
  spine — *see* Spondylitis, ankylosing
psoriatic L40.50
purulent (any site except spine) — *see* Arthritis, pyogenic or pyemic
  spine — *see* Spondylopathy, infective
pyogenic or pyemic (any site except spine) M00.9
  bacterial NEC M00.80
    ankle M00.87-
    elbow M00.82-
    foot joint — *see* Arthritis, pyogenic, bacterial NEC, ankle
    hand joint M00.84-
    hip M00.85-
    knee M00.86-

Arthritis, arthritic (acute) (chronic) (nonpyogenic) (subacute) M19.90 — *continued*
pyogenic or pyemic (any site except spine) M00.9 — *continued*
  bacterial NEC M00.80 — *continued*
    multiple site M00.89
    shoulder M00.81-
    vertebra M00.88
    wrist M00.83-
  pneumococcal — *see* Arthritis, pneumococcal
  spine — *see* Spondylopathy, infective
  staphylococcal — *see* Arthritis, staphylococcal
  streptococcal — *see* Arthritis, streptococcal NEC
  pneumococcal — *see* Arthritis, pneumococcal
reactive — *see* Reiter's disease
rheumatic — *see also* Arthritis, rheumatoid
  acute or subacute — *see* Fever, rheumatic
rheumatoid M06.9
  with
    carditis — *see* Rheumatoid, carditis
    endocarditis — *see* Rheumatoid, carditis
    heart involvement NEC — *see* Rheumatoid, carditis
    lung involvement — *see* Rheumatoid, lung
    myocarditis — *see* Rheumatoid, carditis
    myopathy — *see* Rheumatoid, myopathy
    pericarditis — *see* Rheumatoid, carditis
    polyneuropathy — *see* Rheumatoid, polyneuropathy
    rheumatoid factor — *see* Arthritis, rheumatoid, seropositive
    splenoadenomegaly and leukopenia — *see* Felty's syndrome
    vasculitis — *see* Rheumatoid, vasculitis
    visceral involvement NEC — *see* Rheumatoid, arthritis, with involvement of organs NEC
  juvenile (with or without rheumatoid factor) M08.00
    ankle M08.07-
    elbow M08.02-
    foot joint M08.07-
    hand joint M08.04-
    hip M08.05-
    knee M08.06-
    multiple site M08.09
    shoulder M08.01-
    vertebra M08.08
    wrist M08.03-
  seronegative M06.00
    ankle M06.07-
    elbow M06.02-
    foot joint M06.07-
    hand joint M06.04-
    hip M06.05-
    knee M06.06-
    multiple site M06.09
    shoulder M06.01-
    vertebra M06.08
    wrist M06.03-
  seropositive M05.9
    specified NEC M05.80
      ankle M05.87-
      elbow M05.82-
      foot joint M05.87-
      hand joint M05.84-
      hip M05.85-
      knee M05.86-
      multiple sites M05.89
      shoulder M05.81-
      vertebra — *see* Spondylitis, ankylosing
      wrist M05.83-
    without organ involvement M05.70
      ankle M05.77-
      elbow M05.72-
      foot joint M05.77-
      hand joint M05.74-
      hip M05.75-
      knee M05.76-
      multiple sites M05.79
      shoulder M05.71-
      vertebra — *see* Spondylitis, ankylosing
      wrist M05.73-

Arthritis, arthritic (acute) (chronic) (nonpyogenic) (subacute) M19.90 — *continued*
rheumatoid M06.9 — *continued*
  specified type NEC M06.80
    ankle M06.87-
    elbow M06.82-
    foot joint M06.87-
    hand joint M06.84-
    hip M06.85-
    knee M06.86-
    multiple site M06.89
    shoulder M06.81-
    vertebra M06.88
    wrist M06.83-
  spine — *see* Spondylitis, ankylosing
rubella B06.82
scorbutic (*see also* subcategory M14.8-) E54
senile or senescent — *see* Osteoarthritis
septic (any site except spine) — *see* Arthritis, pyogenic or pyemic
  spine — *see* Spondylopathy, infective
serum (nontherapeutic) (therapeutic) — *see* Arthropathy, postimmunization
specified form NEC M13.80
  ankle M13.87-
  elbow M13.82-
  foot joint M13.87-
  hand joint M13.84-
  hip M13.85-
  knee M13.86-
  multiple site M13.89
  shoulder M13.81-
  specified joint NEC M13.88
  wrist M13.83-
  spine — *see also* Spondylopathy, inflammatory
  infectious or infective NEC — *see* Spondylopathy, infective
  Marie-Strümpell — *see* Spondylitis, ankylosing
  pyogenic — *see* Spondylopathy, infective
  rheumatoid — *see* Spondylitis, ankylosing
  traumatic (old) — *see* Spondylopathy, traumatic
tuberculous A18.01
staphylococcal M00.00
  ankle M00.07-
  elbow M00.02-
  foot joint — *see* Arthritis, staphylococcal, ankle
  hand joint M00.04-
  hip M00.05-
  knee M00.06-
  multiple site M00.09
  shoulder M00.01-
  vertebra M00.08
  wrist M00.03-
streptococcal NEC M00.20
  ankle M00.27-
  elbow M00.22-
  foot joint — *see* Arthritis, streptococcal, ankle
  hand joint M00.24-
  hip M00.25-
  knee M00.26-
  multiple site M00.29
  shoulder M00.21-
  vertebra M00.28
  wrist M00.23-
suppurative — *see* Arthritis, pyogenic or pyemic
syphilitic (late) A52.16
  congenital A50.55 [M12.80]
syphilitica deformans (Charcot) A52.16
temporomandibular M26.69
toxic of menopause (any site) — *see* Arthritis, specified form NEC
transient — *see* Arthropathy, specified form NEC
traumatic (chronic) — *see* Arthropathy, traumatic
tuberculous A18.02
  spine A18.01
uratic — *see* Gout, idiopathic
urethritica (Reiter's) — *see* Reiter's disease
vertebral — *see* Spondylopathy, inflammatory
villous (any site) — *see* Arthropathy, specified form NEC
Arthrocele — *see* Effusion, joint
Arthrodesis status Z98.1
Arthrodynia — *see also* Pain, joint
Arthrodysplasia Q74.9
Arthrofibrosis, joint — *see* Ankylosis
Arthrogryposis (congenital) Q68.8
  multiplex congenita Q74.3

DISEASE INDEX

Arthrokatadysis M24.7
Arthropathy (see also Arthritis) M12.9
  Charcot's — see Arthropathy, neuropathic
    diabetic — see Diabetes, arthropathy,
      neuropathic
    syringomyelic G95.0
  cricoarytenoid J38.7
  crystal(-induced) — see Arthritis, in,
    crystals
  diabetic NEC — see Diabetes, arthropathy
  distal interphalangeal, psoriatic L40.51
  enteropathic M07.60
    ankle M07.67-
    elbow M07.62-
    foot joint M07.67-
    hand joint M07.64-
    hip M07.65-
    knee M07.66-
    multiple site M07.69
    shoulder M07.61-
    vertebra M07.68
    wrist M07.63-
  following intestinal bypass M02.00
    ankle M02.07-
    elbow M02.02-
    foot joint M02.07-
    hand joint M02.04-
    hip M02.05-
    knee M02.06-
    multiple site M02.09
    shoulder M02.01-
    vertebra M02.08
    wrist M02.03-
  gouty — see also Gout, idiopathic
    in (due to)
      Lesch-Nyhan syndrome E79.1
        [M14.-]
      sickle-cell disorders D57- [M14.8-]
  hemophilic NEC D66 [M36.2]
    in (due to)
      hyperparathyroidism NEC E21.3
        [M14.-]
      metabolic disease NOS E88.9 [M14.-]
  in (due to)
    acromegaly E22.0 [M14.-]
    amyloidosis E85.4 [M14.-]
    blood disorder NOS D75.9 [M36.3]
    diabetes — see Diabetes, arthropathy
    endocrine disease NOS E34.9 [M14.-]
    erythema
      multiforme L51.9 [M14.-]
      nodosum L52 [M14.-]
    hemochromatosis E83.118 [M14.-]
    hemoglobinopathy NEC D58.2 [M36.3]
    hemophilia NEC D66 [M36.2]
    Henoch-Schönlein purpura D69.0
      [M36.4]
    hyperthyroidism E05.90 [M14.-]
    hypothyroidism E03.9 [M14.-]
    infective endocarditis I33.0 [M12.80]
    leukemia NEC C95.9-[M36.1]
    malignant histiocytosis C96.A [M36.1]
    metabolic disease NOS E88.9 [M14.-]
    multiple myeloma C90.0-[M36.1]
    neoplastic disease NOS (see also
      Neoplasm) D49.9 [M36.1]
    nutritional deficiency (see also
      subcategory M14.8-) E63.9
    psoriasis NOS L40.50
    sarcoidosis D86.86
    syphilis (late) A52.77
      congenital A50.55 [M12.80]
    thyrotoxicosis (see also subcategory
      M14.8-) E05.90
    ulcerative colitis K51.90 [M07.60]
    viral hepatitis (postinfectious) NEC
      B19.9 [M12.80]
    Whipple's disease (see also subcategory
      M14.8-) K90.81
  Jaccoud — see Arthropathy, postrheumatic,
    chronic
  juvenile — see Arthritis, juvenile
    psoriatic L40.54
  mutilans (psoriatic) L40.52
  neuropathic (Charcot) M14.60
    ankle M14.67-
    diabetic — see Diabetes, arthropathy,
      neuropathic
    elbow M14.62-
    foot joint M14.67-
    hand joint M14.64-
    hip M14.65-
    knee M14.66-
    multiple site M14.69
    nonsyphilitic NEC G98.0
    shoulder M14.61-
    syringomyelic G95.0
    vertebra M14.68
    wrist M14.63-

Arthropathy (see also Arthritis) M12.9 —
  continued
  osteopulmonary — see Osteoarthropathy,
    hypertrophic, specified NEC
  postdysenteric M02.10
    ankle M02.17-
    elbow M02.12-
    foot joint M02.17-
    hand joint M02.14-
    hip M02.15-
    knee M02.16-
    multiple site M02.19
    shoulder M02.11-
    vertebra M02.18
    wrist M02.13-
  postimmunization M02.20
    ankle M02.27-
    elbow M02.22-
    foot joint M02.27-
    hand joint M02.24-
    hip M02.25-
    knee M02.26-
    multiple site M02.29
    shoulder M02.21-
    vertebra M02.28
    wrist M02.23-
  postinfectious NEC B99 [M12.80]
    in (due to)
      enteritis due to Yersinia enterocolitica
        A04.6 [M12.80]
      syphilis A52.77
      viral hepatitis NEC B19.9 [M12.80]
  postrheumatic, chronic (Jaccoud) M12.00
    ankle M12.07-
    elbow M12.02-
    foot joint M12.07-
    hand joint M12.04-
    hip M12.05-
    knee M12.06-
    multiple site M12.09
    shoulder M12.01-
    specified joint NEC M12.08
    vertebrae M12.08
    wrist M12.03-
  psoriatic NEC L40.59
    interphalangeal, distal L40.51
  reactive M02.9
    in (due to)
      infective endocarditis I33.0 [M02.9]
    specified type NEC M02.80
      ankle M02.87-
      elbow M02.82-
      foot joint M02.87-
      hand joint M02.84-
      hip M02.85-
      knee M02.86-
      multiple site M02.89
      shoulder M02.81-
      vertebra M02.88
      wrist M02.83-
  specified form NEC M12.80
    ankle M12.87-
    elbow M12.82-
    foot joint M12.87-
    hand joint M12.84-
    hip M12.85-
    knee M12.86-
    multiple site M12.89
    shoulder M12.81-
    specified joint NEC M12.88
    vertebrae M12.88
    wrist M12.83-
  syringomyelic G95.0
  tabes dorsalis A52.16
  tabetic A52.16
  transient — see Arthropathy, specified form
    NEC
  traumatic M12.50
    ankle M12.57-
    elbow M12.52-
    foot joint M12.57-
    hand joint M12.54-
    hip M12.55-
    knee M12.56-
    multiple site M12.59
    shoulder M12.51-
    specified joint NEC M12.58
    vertebrae M12.58
    wrist M12.53-
Arthropyosis — see Arthritis, pyogenic or
  pyemic
Arthrosis (deformans) (degenerative)
  (localized) (see also Osteoarthritis)
  M19.90
  spine — see Spondylosis
Arthus' phenomenon or reaction T78.41
  due to
    drug — see Table of drugs and
      chemicals, by drug
Articular — see condition

Articulation, reverse (teeth) M26.24
Artificial
  insemination complication — see
    Complications, artificial, fertilization
  opening status (functioning) (without
    complication) Z93.9
    anus (colostomy) Z93.3
    colostomy Z93.3
    cystostomy Z93.50
      appendico-vesicostomy Z93.52
      cutaneous Z93.51
      specified NEC Z93.59
    enterostomy Z93.4
    gastrostomy Z93.1
    ileostomy Z93.2
    intestinal tract NEC Z93.4
    jejunostomy Z93.4
    nephrostomy Z93.6
    specified site NEC Z93.8
    tracheostomy Z93.0
    ureterostomy Z93.6
    urethrostomy Z93.6
    urinary tract NEC Z93.6
    vagina Z93.8
    vagina status Z93.8
Arytenoid — see condition
Asbestosis (occupational) J61
Ascariasis B77.9
  with
    complications NEC B77.89
    intestinal complications B77.0
    pneumonia, pneumonitis B77.81
Ascaridosis, ascaridiasis — see Ascariasis
Ascaris (infection) (infestation)
  (lumbricoides) — see Ascariasis
Ascending — see condition
ASC-H (atypical squamous cells cannot
  exclude high grade squamous
  intraepithelial lesion on cytologic smear)
  anus R85.611
  cervix R87.611
  vagina R87.621
Aschoff's bodies — see Myocarditis,
  rheumatic
Ascites (abdominal) R18.8
  cardiac I50.9
  chylous (nonfilarial) I89.8
    filarial — see Infestation, filarial
  due to
    cirrhosis, alcoholic K70.31
    hepatitis
      alcoholic K70.11
      chronic active K71.51
    S. japonicum B65.2
  heart I50.9
  malignant R18.0
  pseudochylous R18.8
  syphilitic A52.74
  tuberculous A18.31
ASC-US (atypical squamous cells of
  undetermined significance on cytologic
  smear)
  anus R85.610
  cervix R87.610
  vagina R87.620
Aseptic — see condition
Asherman's syndrome N85.6
Asialia K11.7
Asiatic cholera — see Cholera
Asimultagnosia (simultanagnosia) R48.3
Askin's tumor — see Neoplasm, connective
  tissue, malignant
Asocial personality F60.2
Asomatognosia R41.4
Aspartylglucosaminuria E77.1
Asperger's disease or syndrome F84.5
Aspergilloma — see Aspergillosis
Aspergillosis (with pneumonia) B44.9
  bronchopulmonary, allergic B44.81
  disseminated B44.7
  generalized B44.7
  pulmonary NEC B44.1
    allergic B44.81
    invasive B44.0
  specified NEC B44.89
  tonsillar B44.2
Aspergillus (flavus) (fumigatus) (infection)
  (terreus) — see Aspergillosis
Aspermatogenesis — see Azoospermia
Aspermia (testis) — see Azoospermia
Asphyxia, asphyxiation (by) R09.01
  antenatal P84
  birth P84
  bunny bag — see Asphyxia, due to,
    mechanical threat to breathing,
    trapped in bed clothes
  crushing S28.0
  drowning T75.1
  gas, fumes, or vapor — see Table of Drugs
    and Chemicals

Asphyxia, asphyxiation (by) R09.01 —
  continued
  inhalation — see Inhalation
  intrauterine P84
  local I73.00
    with gangrene I73.01
  mucus — see also Foreign body,
    respiratory tract, causing asphyxia
  newborn P84
  pathological R09.01
  postnatal P84
    mechanical — see Asphyxia, due to,
      mechanical threat to breathing
  prenatal P84
  reticularis R23.1
  strangulation — see Asphyxia, due to,
    mechanical threat to breathing
  submersion T75.1
  traumatic T71.9
    due to
      crushed chest S28.0
      foreign body (in) — see Foreign body,
        respiratory tract, causing
        asphyxia
      low oxygen content of ambient air
        T71.20
        due to
          being trapped in
            low oxygen environment
              T71.29
            in car trunk T71.221
              circumstances
                undetermined
                  T71.224
              done with intent to harm
                by
                  another person
                    T71.223
                  self T71.222
            in refrigerator T71.231
              circumstances
                undetermined
                  T71.234
              done with intent to harm
                by
                  another person
                    T71.233
                  self T71.232
            cave-in T71.21
      mechanical threat to breathing
        (accidental) T71.191
        circumstances undetermined
          T71.194
        done with intent to harm by
          another person T71.193
          self T71.192
        hanging T71.161
        circumstances undetermined
          T71.164
        done with intent to harm by
          another person T71.163
          self T71.162
        plastic bag T71.121
        circumstances undetermined
          T71.124
        done with intent to harm by
          another person T71.123
          self T71.122
      smothering
        in furniture T71.151
          circumstances undetermined
            T71.154
          done with intent to harm by
            another person T71.153
            self T71.152
        under
          another person's body
            T71.141
          circumstances
            undetermined T71.144
          done with intent to harm
            T71.143
        pillow T71.111
          circumstances
            undetermined T71.114
          done with intent to harm by
            another person T71.113
            self T71.112
        trapped in bed clothes T71.131
        circumstances undetermined
          T71.134
        done with intent to harm by
          another person T71.133
          self T71.132
  vomiting, vomitus — see Foreign body,
    respiratory tract, causing asphyxia

Aspiration
amniotic (clear) fluid (newborn) P24.10
  with
    pneumonia (pneumonitis) P24.11
    respiratory symptoms P24.11
blood
  newborn (without respiratory symptoms) P24.20
    with
      pneumonia (pneumonitis) P24.21
      respiratory symptoms P24.21
    specified age NEC — *see* Foreign body, respiratory tract
bronchitis J69.0
food or foreign body (with asphyxiation) — *see* Asphyxia, food
liquor (amnii) (newborn) P24.10
  with
    pneumonia (pneumonitis) P24.11
    respiratory symptoms P24.11
meconium (newborn) (without respiratory symptoms) P24.00
  with
    pneumonitis (pneumonitis) P24.01
    respiratory symptoms P24.01
milk (newborn) (without respiratory symptoms) P24.30
  with
    pneumonia (pneumonia) P24.31
    respiratory symptoms P24.31
  specified age NEC — *see* Foreign body, respiratory tract
mucus — *see also* Foreign body, by site, causing asphyxia
  newborn P24.10
    with
      pneumonia (pneumonitis) P24.11
      respiratory symptoms P24.11
neonatal P24.9
  specific NEC (without respiratory symptoms) P24.80
    with
      pneumonia (pneumonitis) P24.81
      respiratory symptoms P24.81
  newborn P24.9
    specific NEC (without respiratory symptoms) P24.80
      with
        pneumonia (pneumonitis) P24.81
        respiratory symptoms P24.81
pneumonia J69.0
pneumonitis J69.0
syndrome of newborn — *see* Aspiration, by substance, with pneumonia
vernix caseosa (newborn) P24.80
  with
    pneumonia (pneumonitis) P24.81
    respiratory symptoms P24.81
vomitus — *see also* Foreign body, respiratory tract
  newborn (without respiratory symptoms) P24.30
    with
      pneumonia (pneumonitis) P24.31
      respiratory symptoms P24.31
Asplenia (congenital) Q89.01
postsurgical Z90.81
Assam fever B55.0
Assault, sexual — *see* Maltreatment
Assmann's focus NEC A15.0
Astasia(-abasia) (hysterical) F44.4
Asteatosis cutis L85.3
Astereognosia, astereognosis R48.1
Asterixis R27.8
in liver disease K71.3
Asteroid hyalitis — *see* Deposit, crystalline
Asthenia, asthenic R53.1
cardiac (*see also* Failure, heart) I50.9
  psychogenic F45.8
cardiovascular (*see also* Failure, heart) I50.9
  psychogenic F45.8
heart (*see also* Failure, heart) I50.9
  psychogenic F45.8
hysterical F44.4
myocardial (*see also* Failure, heart) I50.9
  psychogenic F45.8
nervous F48.8
neurocirculatory F45.8
neurotic F48.8
psychogenic F48.8
psychoneurotic F48.8
psychophysiologic F48.8
reaction (psychophysiologic) F48.8
senile R54
Asthenopia — *see also* Discomfort, visual
hysterical F44.6
psychogenic F44.6
Asthenospermia — *see* Abnormal, specimen, male genital organs

Asthma, asthmatic (bronchial) (catarrh) (spasmodic) J45.909
with
  chronic obstructive bronchitis J44.9
    with
      acute lower respiratory infection J44.0
      exacerbation (acute) J44.1
  chronic obstructive pulmonary disease J44.9
    with
      acute lower respiratory infection J44.0
      exacerbation (acute) J44.1
  exacerbation (acute) J45.901
  hay fever — *see* Asthma, allergic extrinsic
  rhinitis, allergic — *see* Asthma, allergic extrinsic
  status asthmaticus J45.902
allergic extrinsic J45.909
  with
    exacerbation (acute) J45.901
    status asthmaticus J45.902
atopic — *see* Asthma, allergic extrinsic
cardiac — *see* Failure, ventricular, left
cardiobronchial I50.1
childhood J45.909
  with
    exacerbation (acute) J45.901
    status asthmaticus J45.902
chronic obstructive J44.9
  with
    acute lower respiratory infection J44.0
    exacerbation (acute) J44.1
collier's J60
cough variant J45.991
detergent J69.8
due to
  detergent J69.8
  inhalation of fumes J68.3
eosinophilic J82
extrinsic, allergic — *see* Asthma, allergic extrinsic
grinder's J62.8
hay — *see* Asthma, allergic extrinsic
heart I50.1
idiosyncratic — *see* Asthma, nonallergic
intermittent (mild) J45.20
  with
    exacerbation (acute) J45.21
    status asthmaticus J45.22
intrinsic, nonallergic — *see* Asthma, nonallergic
Kopp's E32.8
late-onset J45.909
  with
    exacerbation (acute) J45.901
    status asthmaticus J45.902
mild intermittent J45.20
  with
    exacerbation (acute) J45.21
    status asthmaticus J45.22
mild persistent J45.30
  with
    exacerbation (acute) J45.31
    status asthmaticus J45.32
Millar's (laryngismus stridulus) J38.5
miner's J60
mixed J45.909
  with
    exacerbation (acute) J45.901
    status asthmaticus J45.902
moderate persistent J45.40
  with
    exacerbation (acute) J45.41
    status asthmaticus J45.42
nervous — *see* Asthma, nonallergic
nonallergic (intrinsic) J45.909
  with
    exacerbation (acute) J45.901
    status asthmaticus J45.902
persistent
  mild J45.30
    with
      exacerbation (acute) J45.31
      status asthmaticus J45.32
  moderate J45.40
    with
      exacerbation (acute) J45.41
      status asthmaticus J45.42
  severe J45.50
    with
      exacerbation (acute) J45.51
      status asthmaticus J45.52
platinum J45.998
pneumoconiotic NEC J64
potter's J62.8
predominantly allergic J45.909
psychogenic F54

Asthma, asthmatic (bronchial) (catarrh) (spasmodic) J45.909 — *continued*
pulmonary eosinophilic J82
red cedar J67.8
Rostan's I50.1
sandblaster's J62.8
sequoiosis J67.8
severe persistent J45.50
  with
    exacerbation (acute) J45.51
    status asthmaticus J45.52
specified NEC J45.998
stonemason's J62.8
thymic E32.8
tuberculous — *see* Tuberculosis, pulmonary
Wichmann's (laryngismus stridulus) J38.5
wood J67.8
Astigmatism (compound) (congenital) H52.20-
irregular H52.21-
regular H52.22-
Astraphobia F40.220
Astroblastoma
specified site — *see* Neoplasm, malignant, by site
unspecified site C71.9
Astrocytoma (cystic)
anaplastic
  specified site — *see* Neoplasm, malignant, by site
  unspecified site C71.9
fibrillary
  specified site — *see* Neoplasm, malignant, by site
  unspecified site C71.9
fibrous
  specified site — *see* Neoplasm, malignant, by site
  unspecified site C71.9
gemistocytic
  specified site — *see* Neoplasm, malignant, by site
  unspecified site C71.9
juvenile
  specified site — *see* Neoplasm, malignant, by site
  unspecified site C71.9
pilocytic
  specified site — *see* Neoplasm, malignant, by site
  unspecified site C71.9
piloid
  specified site — *see* Neoplasm, malignant, by site
  unspecified site C71.9
protoplasmic
  specified site — *see* Neoplasm, malignant, by site
  unspecified site C71.9
specified site NEC — *see* Neoplasm, malignant, by site
subependymal D43.2
  giant cell
    specified site — *see* Neoplasm, uncertain behavior, by site
    unspecified site D43.2
  specified site — *see* Neoplasm, uncertain behavior, by site
  unspecified site D43.2
unspecified site C71.9
Astroglioma
specified site — *see* Neoplasm, malignant, by site
unspecified site C71.9
Asymbolia R48.8
Asymmetry — *see also* Distortion
between native and reconstructed breast N65.1
face Q67.0
jaw (lower) — *see* Anomaly, dentofacial, jaw-cranial base relationship, asymmetry
Asynergia, asynergy R27.8
ventricular I51.89
Asystole (heart) — *see* Arrest, cardiac
At risk
for falling Z91.81
Ataxia, ataxy, ataxic R27.0
acute R27.8
brain (hereditary) G11.9
cerebellar (hereditary) G11.9
  with defective DNA repair G11.3
  alcoholic G31.2
  early-onset G11.1
  in
    alcoholism G31.2
    myxedema E03.9 [G13.2]
    neoplastic disease (*see also* Neoplasm) D49.9 [G13.1]

Ataxia, ataxy, ataxic R27.0 — *continued*
cerebellar (hereditary) G11.9 — *continued*
  in — *continued*
    specified disease NEC G32.81
  late-onset (Marie's) G11.2
cerebral (hereditary) G11.9
congenital nonprogressive G11.0
family, familial — *see* Ataxia, hereditary
following
  cerebrovascular disease I69.993
    cerebral infarction I69.393
    intracerebral hemorrhage I69.193
    nontraumatic intracranial hemorrhage NEC I69.293
    specified disease NEC I69.893
    subarachnoid hemorrhage I69.093
Friedreich's (heredofamilial) (cerebellar) (spinal) G11.1
gait R26.0
  hysterical F44.4
general R27.8
gluten M35.9 [G32.81]
  with celiac disease K90.0 [G32.81]
hereditary G11.9
  with neuropathy G60.2
  cerebellar — *see* Ataxia, cerebellar
  spastic G11.4
  specified NEC G11.8
  spinal (Friedreich's) G11.1
heredofamilial — *see* Ataxia, hereditary
Hunt's G11.1
hysterical F44.4
locomotor (progressive) (syphilitic) (partial) (spastic) A52.11
  diabetic — *see* Diabetes, ataxia
Marie's (cerebellar) (heredofamilial) (late-onset) G11.2
nonorganic origin F44.4
nonprogressive, congenital G11.0
psychogenic F44.4
Roussy-Lévy G60.0
Sanger-Brown's (hereditary) G11.2
spastic hereditary G11.4
spinal
  hereditary (Friedreich's) G11.1
  progressive (syphilitic) A52.11
spinocerebellar, X-linked recessive G11.1
telangiectasia (Louis-Bar) G11.3
Ataxia-telangiectasia (Louis-Bar) G11.3
Atelectasis (massive) (partial) (pressure) (pulmonary) J98.11
newborn P28.10
  due to resorption P28.11
  partial P28.19
  primary P28.0
  secondary P28.19
primary (newborn) P28.0
tuberculous — *see* Tuberculosis, pulmonary
Atelocardia Q24.9
Atelomyelia Q06.1
Atheroembolism
of
  extremities
    lower I75.02-
    upper I75.01-
  kidney I75.81
  specified NEC I75.89
Atheroma, atheromatous (*see also* Arteriosclerosis) I70.90
aorta, aortic I70.0
  valve (*see also* Endocarditis, aortic) I35.8
aorto-iliac I70.0
artery — *see* Arteriosclerosis
basilar (artery) I67.2
carotid (artery) (common) (internal) I67.2
cerebral (arteries) I67.2
coronary (artery) I25.10
  with angina pectoris — *see* Arteriosclerosis, coronary (artery),
  degeneration — *see* Arteriosclerosis
heart, cardiac — *see* Disease, heart, ischemic, atherosclerotic
mitral (valve) I34.8
myocardium, myocardial — *see* Disease, heart, ischemic, atherosclerotic
pulmonary valve (heart) (*see also* Endocarditis, pulmonary) I37.8
tricuspid (heart) (valve) I36.8
valve, valvular — *see* Endocarditis
vertebral (artery) I67.2

Atheromatosis — see Arteriosclerosis
Atherosclerosis — see also Arteriosclerosis
  coronary
    artery I25.10
      with angina pectoris — see
        Arteriosclerosis, coronary
        (artery)
      due to
        calcified coronary lesion (severely)
          I25.84
        lipid rich plaque I25.83
    transplanted heart I25.811
    bypass graft I25.812
      with angina pectoris — see
        Arteriosclerosis, coronary
        (artery)
      native coronary artery I25.811
        with angina pectoris — see
          Arteriosclerosis, coronary
          (artery)
Athetosis (acquired) R25.8
  bilateral (congenital) G80.3
  congenital (bilateral) (double) G80.3
  double (congenital) G80.3
  unilateral R25.8
Athlete's
  foot B35.3
  heart I51.7
Athrepsia E41
Athyrea (acquired) — see also
    Hypothyroidism
  congenital E03.1
Atonia, atony, atonic
  bladder (sphincter) (neurogenic) N31.2
  capillary I78.8
  cecum K59.8
    psychogenic F45.8
  colon — see Atony, intestine
  congenital P94.2
  esophagus K22.8
  intestine K59.8
    psychogenic F45.8
  stomach K31.89
    neurotic or psychogenic F45.8
  uterus (during labor) O62.2
    with hemorrhage (postpartum) O72.1
    postpartum (with hemorrhage) O72.1
      without hemorrhage O75.89
Atopy — see History, allergy
Atransferrinemia, congenital E88.09
Atresia, atretic
  alimentary organ or tract NEC Q45.8
    upper Q40.8
  ani, anus, anal (canal) Q42.3
    with fistula Q42.2
  aorta (arch) (ring) Q25.2
  aortic (orifice) (valve) Q23.0
    arch Q25.2
    congenital with hypoplasia of ascending
      aorta and defective development of
      left ventricle (with mitral stenosis)
      Q23.4
    in hypoplastic left heart syndrome Q23.4
  aqueduct of Sylvius Q03.0
    with spina bifida — see Spina bifida,
      with hydrocephalus
  artery NEC Q27.8
    cerebral Q28.3
    coronary Q24.5
    digestive system Q27.8
    eye Q15.8
    lower limb Q27.8
    pulmonary Q25.5
    specified site NEC Q27.8
    umbilical Q27.0
    upper limb Q27.8
  auditory canal (external) Q16.1
  bile duct (common) (congenital) (hepatic)
    Q44.2
    acquired — see Obstruction, bile duct
  bladder (neck) Q64.39
    obstruction Q64.31
  bronchus Q32.4
  cecum Q42.8
  cervix (acquired) N88.2
    congenital Q51.828
    in pregnancy or childbirth — see
      Anomaly, cervix, in pregnancy or
      childbirth
      causing obstructed labor O65.5
  choana Q30.0
  colon Q42.9
    specified NEC Q42.8
  common duct Q44.2
  cricoid cartilage Q31.8
  cystic duct Q44.2
    acquired K82.8
      with obstruction K82.0
  digestive organs NEC Q45.8
  duodenum Q41.0

Atresia, atretic — continued
  ear canal Q16.1
  ejaculatory duct Q55.4
  epiglottis Q31.8
  esophagus Q39.0
    with tracheoesophageal fistula Q39.1
  eustachian tube Q17.8
  fallopian tube (congenital) Q50.6
    acquired N97.1
  follicular cyst N83.0
  foramen of
    Luschka Q03.1
      with spina bifida — see Spina
        bifida, with hydrocephalus
    Magendie Q03.1
      with spina bifida — see Spina
        bifida, with hydrocephalus
  gallbladder Q44.1
  genital organ
    external
      female Q52.79
      male Q55.8
    internal
      female Q52.8
      malc Q55.8
  glottis Q31.8
  gullet Q39.0
    with tracheoesophageal fistula Q39.1
  heart valve NEC Q24.8
    pulmonary Q22.0
    tricuspid Q22.4
  hymen Q52.3
    acquired (postinfective) N89.6
  ileum Q41.2
  intestine (small) Q41.9
    large Q42.9
      specified NEC Q42.8
  iris, filtration angle Q15.0
  jejunum Q41.1
  lacrimal apparatus Q10.4
  larynx Q31.8
  meatus urinarius Q64.33
  mitral valve Q23.2
    in hypoplastic left heart syndrome Q23.4
  nares (anterior) (posterior) Q30.0
  nasopharynx Q34.8
  nose, nostril Q30.0
    acquired J34.89
  organ or site NEC Q89.8
  osseous meatus (ear) Q16.1
  oviduct (congenital) Q50.6
    acquired N97.1
  parotid duct Q38.4
    acquired K11.8
  pulmonary (artery) Q25.5
    valve Q22.0
  pulmonic Q22.0
  pupil Q13.2
  rectum Q42.1
    with fistula Q42.0
  salivary duct Q38.4
    acquired K11.8
  sublingual duct Q38.4
    acquired K11.8
  submandibular duct Q38.4
    acquired K11.8
  submaxillary duct Q38.4
    acquired K11.8
  thyroid cartilage Q31.8
  trachea Q32.1
  tricuspid valve Q22.4
  ureter Q62.10
    pelvic junction Q62.11
    vesical orifice Q62.12
  ureteropelvic junction Q62.11
  ureterovesical orifice Q62.12
  urethra (valvular) Q64.39
    stricture Q64.32
  urinary tract NEC Q64.8
  uterus Q51.818
    acquired N85.8
  vagina (congenital) Q52.4
    acquired (postinfectional) (senile) N89.5
  vas deferens Q55.3
  vascular NEC Q27.8
    cerebral Q28.3
    digestive system Q27.8
    lower limb Q27.8
    specified site NEC Q27.8
    upper limb Q27.8

Atresia, atretic — continued
  vein NEC Q27.8
    digestive system Q27.8
    great Q26.8
    lower limb Q27.8
    portal Q26.5
    pulmonary Q26.3
    specified site NEC Q27.8
    upper limb Q27.8
  vena cava (inferior) (superior) Q26.8
  vesicourethral orifice Q64.31
  vulva Q52.79
    acquired N90.5
Atrichia, atrichosis — see Alopecia
At risk
  for falling Z91.81
Atrophia — see also Atrophy
  cutis senilis L90.8
    due to radiation L57.8
  gyrata of choroid and retina H31.23
  senilis R54
    dermatological L90.8
      due to radiation (nonionizing) (solar)
        L57.8
  unguium L60.3
    congenita Q84.6
Atrophie blanche (en plaque) (de Milian)
    L95.0
Atrophoderma, atrophodermia (of) L90.9
  diffusum (idiopathic) L90.4
  maculatum L90.8
    et striatum L90.8
      due to syphilis A52.79
    syphilitic A51.39
  neuriticum L90.8
  Pasini and Pierini L90.3
  pigmentosum Q82.1
  reticulatum symmetricum faciei L66.4
  senile L90.8
    due to radiation (nonionizing) (solar)
      L57.8
  vermiculata (cheeks) L66.4
Atrophy, atrophic (of)
  adrenal (capsule) (gland) E27.49
    primary (autoimmune) E27.1
  alveolar process or ridge (edentulous)
    K08.20
  anal sphincter (disuse) N81.84
  appendix K38.8
  arteriosclerotic — see Arteriosclerosis
  bile duct (common) (hepatic) K83.8
  bladder N32.89
    neurogenic N31.8
  blanche (en plaque) (of Milian) L95.0
  bone (senile) NEC — see also Disorder,
    bone, specified type NEC
    due to
      tabes dorsalis (neurogenic) A52.11
  brain (cortex) (progressive) G31.9
    frontotemporal circumscribed G31.01
      [F02.80]
      with behavioral disturbance G31.01
        [F02.81]
    senile NEC G31.1
  breast N64.2
    obstetric — see Disorder, breast,
      specified type NEC
  buccal cavity K13.79
  cardiac — see Degeneration, myocardial
  cartilage (infectional) (joint) — see
    Disorder, cartilage, specified NEC
  cerebellar — see Atrophy, brain
  cerebral — see Atrophy, brain
  cervix (mucosa) (senile) (uteri) N88.8
    menopausal N95.8
  Charcot-Marie-Tooth G60.0
  choroid (central) (macular) (myopic)
    (retina) H31.10-
    diffuse secondary H31.12-
    gyrate H31.23
    senile H31.11-
  ciliary body — see Atrophy, iris
  conjunctiva (senile) H11.89
  corpus cavernosum N48.89
  cortical — see Atrophy, brain
  cystic duct K82.8
  Déjérine-Thomas G23.8
  disuse NEC — see Atrophy, muscle
  Duchenne-Aran G12.21
  ear H93.8-
  edentulous alveolar ridge K08.20
  endometrium (senile) N85.8
    cervix N88.8
  enteric K63.89
  epididymis N50.8
  eyeball — see Disorder, globe, degenerated
    condition, atrophy
  eyelid (senile) — see Disorder, eyelid,
    degenerative

Atrophy, atrophic (of) — continued
  facial (skin) L90.9
  fallopian tube (senile) N83.32
    with ovary N83.33
  fascioscapulohumeral (Landouzy-Déjérine)
    G71.0
  fatty, thymus (gland) E32.8
  gallbladder K82.8
  gastric K29.40
    with bleeding K29.41
  gastrointestinal K63.89
  glandular I89.8
  globe H44.52-
  gum K06.0
  hair L67.8
  heart (brown) — see Degeneration,
    myocardial
  hemifacial Q67.4
    Romberg G51.8
  infantile E41
    paralysis, acute — see Poliomyelitis,
      paralytic
  intestine K63.89
  iris (essential) (progressive) H21.26-
    specified NEC H21.29
  kidney (senile) (terminal) (see also
    Sclerosis, renal) N26.1
    congenital or infantile Q60.5
      bilateral Q60.4
      unilateral Q60.3
    hydronephrotic — see Hydronephrosis
  lacrimal gland (primary) H04.14-
    secondary H04.15-
  Landouzy-Déjérine G71.0
  laryngitis, infective J37.0
  larynx J38.7
  Leber's optic (hereditary) H47.22
  lip K13.0
  liver (yellow) K72.90
    with coma K72.91
    acute, subacute K72.00
      with coma K72.01
    chronic K72.10
      with coma K72.11
  lung (senile) J98.4
  macular (dermatological) L90.8
    syphilitic, skin A51.39
      striated A52.79
  mandible (edentulous) K08.20
    minimal K08.21
    moderate K08.22
    severe K08.23
  maxilla (edentulous) K08.20
    minimal K08.24
    moderate K08.25
    severe K08.26
  muscle, muscular (diffuse) (general)
    (idiopathic) (primary) M62.50
    ankle M62.57-
    Duchenne-Aran G12.21
    foot M62.57-
    forearm M62.53-
    hand M62.54-
    infantile spinal G12.0
    lower leg M62.56-
    multiple sites M62.59
    myelopathic — see Atrophy, muscle,
      spinal
    myotonic G71.11
    neuritic G58.9
    neuropathic (peroneal) (progressive)
      G60.0
    pelvic (disuse) N81.84
    peroneal G60.0
    progressive (bulbar) G12.21
      adult G12.1
      infantile (spinal) G12.0
      spinal G12.9
        adult G12.1
        infantile G12.0
    pseudohypertrophic G71.0
    shoulder region M62.51-
    specified site NEC M62.58
    spinal G12.9
      adult form G12.1
      Aran-Duchenne G12.21
      childhood form, type II G12.1
      distal G12.1
      hereditary NEC G12.1
      infantile, type I (Werdnig-Hoffmann)
        G12.0
      juvenile form, type III (Kugelberg-
        Welander) G12.1
      progressive G12.21
      scapuloperoneal form G12.1
      specified NEC G12.8
    syphilitic A52.78
    thigh M62.55-
    upper arm M62.52-

DISEASE INDEX

Atrophy, atrophic (of) — *continued*
  myocardium — *see* Degeneration, myocardial
  myometrium (senile) N85.8
    cervix N88.8
  myopathic NEC — *see* Atrophy, muscle
  myotonia G71.11
  nail L60.3
  nasopharynx J31.1
  nerve — *see also* Disorder, nerve
    abducens — *see* Strabismus, paralytic, sixth nerve
    accessory G52.8
    acoustic or auditory — *see* subcategory H93.3
    cranial G52.9
      eighth (auditory) — *see* subcategory H93.3
      eleventh (accessory) G52.8
      fifth (trigeminal) G50.8
      first (olfactory) G52.0
      fourth (trochlear) — *see* Strabismus, paralytic, fourth nerve
      second (optic) H47.20
      sixth (abducens) — *see* Strabismus, paralytic, sixth nerve
      tenth (pneumogastric) (vagus) G52.2
      third (oculomotor) — *see* Strabismus, paralytic, third nerve
      twelfth (hypoglossal) G52.3
    hypoglossal G52.3
    oculomotor — *see* Strabismus, paralytic, third nerve
    olfactory G52.0
    optic (papillomacular bundle)
      syphilitic (late) A52.15
        congenital A50.44
    pneumogastric G52.2
    trigeminal G50.8
    trochlear — *see* Strabismus, paralytic, fourth nerve
    vagus (pneumogastric) G52.2
  neurogenic, bone, tabetic A52.11
  nutritional E41
  old age R54
  olivopontocerebellar G23.8
  optic (nerve) H47.20
    glaucomatous H47.23-
    hereditary H47.22
    primary H47.21-
    specified type NEC H47.29-
    syphilitic (late) A52.15
      congenital A50.44
  orbit H05.31-
  ovary (senile) N83.31
    with fallopian tube N83.33
  oviduct (senile) — *see* Atrophy, fallopian tube
  palsy, diffuse (progressive) G12.22
  pancreas (duct) (senile) K86.8
  parotid gland K11.0
  pelvic muscle N81.84
  penis N48.89
  pharynx J39.2
  plurilglandular E31.8
    autoimmune E31.0
  polyarthritis M15.9
  prostate N42.89
  pseudohypertrophic (muscle) G71.0
  renal (*see also* Sclerosis, renal) N26.1
  retina, retinal (postinfectional) H35.89
  rhinitis J31.0
  salivary gland K11.0
  scar L90.5
  sclerosis, lobar (of brain) G31.09 [F02.80]
    with behavioral disturbance G31.09 [F02.81]
  scrotum N50.8
  seminal vesicle N50.8
  senile R54
    due to radiation (nonionizing) (solar) L57.8
  skin (patches) (spots) L90.9
    degenerative (senile) L90.8
    due to radiation (nonionizing) (solar) L57.8
    senile L90.8
  spermatic cord N50.8
  spinal (acute) (cord) G95.89
    muscular — *see* Atrophy, muscle, spinal
    paralysis G12.20
      acute — *see* Poliomyelitis, paralytic
      meaning progressive muscular atrophy G12.21

Atrophy, atrophic (of) — *continued*
  spine (column) — *see* Spondylopathy, specified NEC
  spleen (senile) D73.0
  stomach K29.40
    with bleeding K29.41
  striate (skin) L90.6
    syphilitic A52.79
  subcutaneous L90.9
  sublingual gland K11.0
  submandibular gland K11.0
  submaxillary gland K11.0
  Sudeck's — *see* Algoneurodystrophy
  suprarenal (capsule) (gland) E27.49
    primary E27.1
  systemic affecting central nervous system in
    myxedema E03.9 [G13.2]
    neoplastic disease (*see also* Neoplasm) D49.9 [G13.1]
    specified disease NEC G13.8
  tarso-orbital fascia, congenital Q10.3
  testis N50.0
  thenar, partial — *see* Syndrome, carpal tunnel
  thymus (fatty) E32.8
  thyroid (gland) (acquired) E03.4
    with cretinism E03.1
    congenital (with myxedema) E03.1
  tongue (senile) K14.8
    papillae K14.4
  trachea J39.8
  tunica vaginalis N50.8
  turbinate J34.89
  tympanic membrane (nonflaccid) H73.82-
    flaccid H73.81-
  upper respiratory tract J39.8
  uterus, uterine (senile) N85.8
    cervix N88.8
    due to radiation (intended effect) N85.8
      adverse effect or misadventure N99.89
  vagina (senile) N95.2
  vas deferens N50.8
  vascular I99.8
  vertebra (senile) — *see* Spondylopathy, specified NEC
  vulva (senile) N90.5
  Werdnig-Hoffmann G12.0
  yellow — *see* Failure, hepatic

Attack, attacks
  with alteration of consciousness (with automatisms) — *see* Epilepsy, localization-related, symptomatic, with complex partialseizures
  Adams-Stokes I45.9
  akinetic — *see* Epilepsy, generalized, specified NEC
  angina — *see* Angina
  atonic — *see* Epilepsy, generalized, specified NEC
  benign shuddering G25.83
  cataleptic — *see* Catalepsy
  coronary — *see* Infarct, myocardium
  cyanotic, newborn P28.2
  drop NEC R55
  epileptic — *see* Epilepsy
  heart — *see* infarct, myocardium
  hysterical F44.9
  jacksonian — *see* Epilepsy, localization-related, symptomatic, with simple partial seizures
  myocardium, myocardial — *see* Infarct, myocardium
  myoclonic — *see* Epilepsy, generalized, specified NEC
  panic F41.0
  psychomotor — *see* Epilepsy, localization-related, symptomatic, with complex partial seizures
  salaam — *see* Epilepsy, spasms
  schizophreniform, brief F23
  shuddering, benign G25.83
  Stokes-Adams I45.9
  syncope R55
  transient ischemic (TIA) G45.9
    specified NEC G45.8
  unconsciousness R55
    hysterical F44.89
  vasomotor R55
  vasovagal (paroxysmal) (idiopathic) R55
  without alteration of consciousness — *see* Epilepsy, localization-related, symptomatic, with simple partial seizures

Attention (to)
  artificial
    opening (of) Z43.9
      digestive tract NEC Z43.4
        colon Z43.3
        ilium Z43.2
        stomach Z43.1
      specified NEC Z43.8
      trachea Z43.0
      urinary tract NEC Z43.6
        cystostomy Z43.5
        nephrostomy Z43.6
        ureterostomy Z43.6
        urethrostomy Z43.6
      vagina Z43.7
  colostomy Z43.3
  cystostomy Z43.5
  deficit disorder or syndrome F98.8
    with hyperactivity — *see* Disorder, attention-deficit hyperactivity
  gastrostomy Z43.1
  ileostomy Z43.2
  jejunostomy Z43.4
  nephrostomy Z43.6
  surgical dressings Z48.01
  sutures Z48.02
  tracheostomy Z43.0
  ureterostomy Z43.6
  urethrostomy Z43.6
Attrition
  gum K06.0
  tooth, teeth (excessive) (hard tissues) K03.0
Atypical, atypism — *see also* condition
  cells (on cytolgcial smear) (endocervical) (endometrial) (glandular)
    cervix R87.619
    vagina R87.629
  cervical N87.9
  endometrium N85.9
    hyperplasia N85.00
  parenting situation Z62.9
Auditory — *see* condition
Aujeszky's disease B33.8
Aurantiasis, cutis E67.1
Auricle, auricular — *see also* condition
  cervical Q18.2
Auriculotemporal syndrome G50.8
Austin Flint murmur (aortic insufficiency) I35.1
Australian
  Q fever A78
  X disease A83.4
Autism, autistic (childhood) (infantile) F84.0
  atypical F84.9
Autodigestion R68.89
Autoerythrocyte sensitization (syndrome) D69.2
Autographism L50.3
Autoimmune
  disease (systemic) M35.9
  inhibitors to clotting factors D68.311
  lymphoproliferative syndrome [ALPS] D89.82
  thyroiditis E06.3
Autointoxication R68.89
Automatism G93.89
  with temporal sclerosis G93.81
  epileptic — *see* Epilepsy, localization-related, symptomatic, with complex partial seizures
  paroxysmal, idiopathic — *see* Epilepsy, localization-related, symptomatic, with complex partial seizures
Autonomic, autonomous
  bladder (neurogenic) N31.2
  hysteria seizure F44.5
Autosensitivity, erythrocyte D69.2
Autosensitization, cutaneous L30.2
Autosome — *see* condition by chromosome involved
Autotopagnosia R48.1
Autotoxemia R68.89
Autumn — *see* condition
Avellis' syndrome G46.8
Aversion
  oral R63.3
    newborn P92-
    nonorganic origin F98.2
  sexual F52.1
Aviator's
  disease or sickness — *see* Effect, adverse, high altitude
  ear T70.0

Avitaminosis (multiple) (*see also* Deficiency, vitamin) E56.9
  B E53.9
    with
      beriberi E51.11
      pellagra E52
  B12 E53.8
  B2 E53.0
  B6 E53.1
  D E55.9
    with rickets E55.0
  G E53.0
  K E56.1
  nicotinic acid E52
AVNRT (atrioventricular nodal re-entrant tachycardia) I47.1
AVRT (atrioventricular nodal re-entrant tachycardia) I47.1
Avulsion (traumatic)
  blood vessel — *see* Injury, blood vessel
  bone — *see* Fracture, by site
  cartilage — *see also* Dislocation, by site
    symphyseal (inner), complicating delivery O71.6
  external site other than limb — *see* Wound, open, by site
  eye S05.7-
  head (intracranial)
    external site NEC S08.89
    scalp S08.0
  internal organ or site — *see* Injury, by site
  joint — *see also* Dislocation, by site
    capsule — *see* Sprain, by site
  kidney S37.06-
  ligament — *see* Sprain, by site
  limb — *see also* Amputation, traumatic, by site
    skin and subcutaneous tissue — *see* Wound, open, by site
  muscle — *see* Injury, muscle
  nerve (root) — *see* Injury, nerve
  scalp S08.0
  skin and subcutaneous tissue — *see* Wound, open, by site
  spleen S36.032
  symphyseal cartilage (inner), complicating delivery O71.6
  tendon — *see* Injury, muscle
  tooth S03.2
Awareness of heart beat R00.2
Axenfeld's
  anomaly or syndrome Q15.0
  degeneration (calcareous) Q13.4
Axilla, axillary — *see also* condition
  breast Q83.1
Axonotmesis — *see* Injury, nerve
Ayerza's disease or syndrome (pulmonary artery sclerosis with pulmonary hypertension) I27.0
Azoospermia (organic) N46.01
  due to
    drug therapy N46.021
    efferent duct obstruction N46.023
    infection N46.022
    radiation N46.024
    specified cause NEC N46.029
    systemic disease N46.025
Azotemia R79.89
  meaning uremia N19
Aztec ear Q17.3
Azygos
  continuation inferior vena cava Q26.8
  lobe (lung) Q33.1

B

Baastrup's disease — see Kissing spine
Babesiosis B60.0
Babington's disease (familial hemorrhagic telangiectasia) I78.0
Babinski's syndrome A52.79
Baby
 crying constantly R68.11
 floppy (syndrome) P94.2
Bacillary — see condition
Bacilluria N39.0
Bacillus — see also Infection, bacillus
 abortus infection A23.1
 anthracis infection A22.9
 coli infection (see also Escherichia coli) B96.20
 Flexner's A03.1
 mallei infection A24.0
 Shiga's A03.0
 suipestifer infection — see Infection, salmonella
Back — see condition
Backache (postural) M54.9
 sacroiliac M53.3
 specified NEC M54.89
Backflow — see Reflux
Backward reading (dyslexia) F81.0
Bacteremia R78.81
 with sepsis — see Sepsis
Bactericholia — see Cholecystitis, acute
Bacterid, bacteride (pustular) L40.3
Bacterium, bacteria, bacterial
 agent NEC, as cause of disease classified elsewhere B96.89
 in blood — see Bacteremia
 in urine — see Bacteriuria
Bacteriuria, bacteruria N39.0
 asymptomatic N39.0
Bacteroides
 fragilis, as cause of disease classified elsewhere B96.6
Bad
 heart — see Disease, heart
 trip
  due to drug abuse — see Abuse, drug, hallucinogen
  due to drug dependence — see Dependence, drug, hallucinogen
Baelz's disease (cheilitis glandularis apostematosa) K13.0
Baerensprung's disease (eczema marginatum) B35.6
Bagasse disease or pneumonitis J67.1
Bagassosis J67.1
Baker's cyst — see Cyst, Baker's
Bakwin-Krida syndrome (craniometaphyseal dysplasia) Q78.5
Balancing side interference M26.56
Balanitis (circinata) (erosiva) (gangrenosa) (phagedenic) (vulgaris) N48.1
 amebic A06.82
 candidal B37.42
 due to Haemophilus ducreyi A57
 gonococcal (acute) (chronic) A54.09
 xerotica obliterans N48.0
Balanoposthitis N47.6
 gonococcal (acute) (chronic) A54.09
 ulcerative (specific) A63.8
Balanorrhagia — see Balanitis
Balantidiasis, balantidiosis A07.0
Bald tongue K14.4
Baldness — see also Alopecia
 male-pattern — see Alopecia, androgenic
Balkan grippe A78
Balloon disease — see Effect, adverse, high altitude
Balo's disease (concentric sclerosis) G37.5
Bamberger-Marie disease — see Osteoarthropathy, hypertrophic, specified type NEC
Bancroft's filariasis B74.0
Band(s)
 adhesive — see Adhesions, peritoneum
 anomalous or congenital — see also Anomaly, by site
  heart (atrial) (ventricular) Q24.8
  intestine Q43.3
  omentum Q43.3
 cervix N88.1
 constricting, congenital Q79.8
 gallbladder (congenital) Q44.1
 intestinal (adhesive) — see Adhesions, peritoneum
 obstructive
  intestine K56.5
  peritoneum K56.5

Band(s) — continued
 periappendiceal, congenital Q43.3
 peritoneal (adhesive) — see Adhesions, peritoneum
 uterus N73.6
  internal N85.6
 vagina N89.5
Bandemia D72.825
Bandl's ring (contraction), complicating delivery O62.4
Bang's disease (brucella abortus) A23.1
Bangkok hemorrhagic fever A91
Bankruptcy, anxiety concerning Z59.8
Bannister's disease T78.3
 hereditary D84.1
Banti's disease or syndrome (with cirrhosis) (with portal hypertension) K76.6
Bar, median, prostate — see Enlargement, enlarged, prostate
Barcoo disease or rot — see Ulcer, skin
Barlow's disease E54
Barodontalgia T70.29
Baron Münchausen syndrome — see Disorder, factitious
Barosinusitis T70.1
Barotitis T70.0
Barotrauma T70.29
 odontalgia T70.29
 otitic T70.0
 sinus T70.1
Barraquer(-Simons) disease or syndrome (progressive lipodystrophy) E88.1
Barrel chest M95.4
Barrett's
 disease — see Barrett's, esophagus
 esophagus K22.70
  with dysplasia K22.719
   high grade K22.711
   low grade K22.710
  without dysplasia K22.70
 syndrome — see Barrett's, esophagus
 ulcer K22.10
  with bleeding K22.11
  without bleeding K22.10
Barré-Guillain disease or syndrome G61.0
Barré-Liéou syndrome (posterior cervical sympathetic) M53.0
Bársony (-Polgár) (-Teschendorf) syndrome (corkscrew esophagus) K22.4
Barth syndrome E78.71
Bartholinitis (suppurating) N75.8
 gonococcal (acute) (chronic) (with abscess) A54.1
Barton's fracture S52.56-
Bartonellosis A44.9
 cutaneous A44.1
 mucocutaneous A44.1
 specified NEC A44.8
 systemic A44.0
Bartter's syndrome E26.81
Basal — see condition
Basan's (hidrotic) ectodermal dysplasia Q82.4
Baseball finger — see Dislocation, finger
Basedow's disease (exophthalmic goiter) — see Hyperthyroidism, with, goiter
Basic — see condition
Basilar — see condition
Bason's (hidrotic) ectodermal dysplasia Q82.4
Basopenia — see Agranulocytosis
Basophilia D72.824
Basophilism (cortico-adrenal) (Cushing's) (pituitary) E24.0
Bassen-Kornzweig disease or syndrome E78.6
Bat ear Q17.5
Bateman's
 disease B08.1
 purpura (senile) D69.2
Bathing cramp T75.1
Bathophobia F40.248
Batten(-Mayou) disease E75.4
 retina E75.4 [H36]
Batten-Steinert syndrome G71.11
Battered — see Maltreatment
Battey Mycobacterium infection A31.0
Battle exhaustion F43.0
Battledore placenta O43.19-
Baumgarten-Cruveilhier cirrhosis, disease or syndrome K74.69
Bauxite fibrosis (of lung) J63.1
Bayle's disease (general paresis) A52.17
Bazin's disease (primary) (tuberculous) A18.4
Beach ear — see Swimmer's, ear
Beaded hair (congenital) Q84.1

Béal conjunctivitis or syndrome B30.2
Beard's disease (neurasthenia) F48.8
Beat(s)
 atrial, premature I49.1
 ectopic I49.49
 elbow — see Bursitis, elbow
 escaped, heart I49.49
 hand — see Bursitis, hand
 knee — see Bursitis, knee
 premature I49.40
  atrial I49.1
  auricular I49.1
  supraventricular I49.1
Beau's
 disease or syndrome — see Degeneration, myocardial
 lines (transverse furrows on fingernails) L60.4
Bechterew's syndrome — see Spondylitis, ankylosing
Becker's
 cardiomyopathy I42.8
 disease
  idiopathic mural endomyocardial disease I42.3
  myotonia congenita, recessive form G71.12
 dystrophy G71.0
 pigmented hairy nevus D22.5
Beck's syndrome (anterior spinal artery occlusion) I65.8
Beckwith-Wiedemann syndrome Q87.3
Bed confinement status Z74.01
Bed sore — see Ulcer, pressure, by site
Bedbug bite(s) — see Bite(s), by site, superficial, insect
Bedclothes, asphyxiation or suffocation by — see Asphyxia, traumatic, due to, mechanical, trapped
Bednar's
 aphthae K12.0
 tumor — see Neoplasm, malignant, by site
Bedridden Z74.01
Bedsore — see Ulcer, pressure, by site
Bedwetting — see Enuresis
Bee sting (with allergic or anaphylactic shock) — see Toxicity, venom, arthropod, bee
Beer drinker's heart (disease) I42.6
Begbie's disease (exophthalmic goiter) — see Hyperthyroidism, with, goiter
Behavior
 antisocial
  adult Z72.811
  child or adolescent Z72.810
 disorder, disturbance — see Disorder, conduct
 disruptive — see Disorder, conduct
 drug seeking Z72.89
 inexplicable R46.2
 marked evasiveness R46.5
 obsessive-compulsive R46.81
 overactivity R46.3
 poor responsiveness R46.4
 self-damaging (life-style) Z72.89
 sleep-incompatible Z72.821
 slowness R46.4
 specified NEC R46.89
 strange (and inexplicable) R46.2
 suspiciousness R46.5
 type A pattern Z73.1
 undue concern or preoccupation with stressful events R46.6
 verbosity and circumstantial detail obscuring reason for contact R46.7
Behçet's disease or syndrome M35.2
Behr's disease — see Degeneration, macula
Beigel's disease or morbus (white piedra) B36.2
Bejel A65
Bekhterev's syndrome — see Spondylitis, ankylosing
Belching — see Eructation
Bell's
 mania F30.8
 palsy, paralysis G51.0
  infant or newborn P11.3
 spasm G51.3
Bence Jones albuminuria or proteinuria NEC R80.3
Bends T70.3
Benedikt's paralysis or syndrome G46.3
Benign — see also condition
 prostatic hyperplasia — see Hyperplasia, prostate
Bennett's fracture (displaced) S62.21-

Benson's disease — see Deposit, crystalline
Bent
 back (hysterical) F44.4
 nose M95.0
  congenital Q67.4
Bereavement (uncomplicated) Z63.4
Berger's disease — see Nephropathy, IgA
Bergeron's disease (hysterical chorea) F44.4
Beriberi (dry) E51.11
 heart (disease) E51.12
 polyneuropathy E51.11
 wet E51.12
  involving circulatory system E51.11
Berlin's disease or edema (traumatic) S05.8x-
Berlock (berloque) dermatitis L56.2
Bernard-Horner syndrome G90.2
Bernard-Soulier disease or thrombopathia D69.1
Bernhardt(-Roth) disease — see Mononeuropathy, lower limb, meralgia paresthetica
Bernheim's syndrome — see Failure, heart, congestive
Bertielliasis B71.8
Berylliosis (lung) J63.2
Besnier-Boeck(-Schaumann) disease — see Sarcoidosis
Besnier's
 lupus pernio D86.3
 prurigo L20.0
Best's disease H35.50
Bestiality F65.89
Betalipoproteinemia, broad or floating E78.2
Beta-mercaptolactate-cysteine disulfiduria E72.09
Betting and gambling Z72.6
 pathological (compulsive) F63.0
Bezoar T18.9
 intestine T18.3
 stomach T18.2
Bezold's abscess — see Mastoiditis, acute
Bianchi's syndrome R48.8
Bicornate or bicornis uterus Q51.3
 in pregnancy or childbirth O34.59-
  causing obstructed labor O65.5
Bicuspid aortic valve Q23.1
Biedl-Bardet syndrome Q87.89
Bielschowsky(-Jansky) disease E75.4
Biermer's (pernicious) anemia or disease D51.0
Biett's disease L93.0
Bifid (congenital)
 apex, heart Q24.8
 clitoris Q52.6
 kidney Q63.8
 nose Q30.2
 patella Q74.1
 scrotum Q55.29
 toe NEC Q74.2
 tongue Q38.3
 ureter Q62.8
 uterus Q51.3
 uvula Q35.7
Biforis uterus (suprasimplex) Q51.3
Bifurcation (congenital)
 gallbladder Q44.1
 kidney pelvis Q63.8
 renal pelvis Q63.8
 rib Q76.6
 tongue, congenital Q38.3
 trachea Q32.1
 ureter Q62.8
 urethra Q64.74
 vertebra Q76.49
Big spleen syndrome D73.1
Bigeminal pulse R00.8
Bilateral — see condition
Bile
 duct — see condition
 pigments in urine R82.2
Bilharziasis — see also Schistosomiasis
 chyluria B65.0
 cutaneous B65.3
 galacturia B65.0
 hematochyluria B65.0
 intestinal B65.1
 lipemia B65.9
 lipuria B65.0
 oriental B65.2
 piarhemia B65.9
 pulmonary NOS B65.9 [J99]
  pneumonia B65.9 [J17]
 tropical hematuria B65.0
 vesical B65.0
Biliary — see condition

Bilirubin metabolism disorder E80.7
　specified NEC E80.6
Bilirubinemia, familial nonhemolytic E80.4
Bilirubinuria R82.2
Biliuria R82.2
Bilocular stomach K31.2
Binswanger's disease I67.3
Biparta, bipartite
　carpal scaphoid Q74.0
　patella Q74.1
　vagina Q52.10
Bird
　face Q75.8
　fancier's disease or lung J67.2
Birth
　complications in mother — *see* Delivery, complicated
　compression during NOS P15.9
　defect — *see* Anomaly
　immature (less than 37 completed weeks) — *see* Preterm, newborn
　　extremely (less than 28 completed weeks) — *see* Immaturity, extreme
　inattention, at or after — *see* Maltreatment, child, neglect
　injury NOS P15.9
　　basal ganglia P11.1
　　brachial plexus NEC P14.3
　　brain (compression) (pressure) P11.2
　　central nervous system NOS P11.9
　　cerebellum P11.1
　　cerebral hemorrhage P10.1
　　external genitalia P15.5
　　eye P15.3
　　face P15.4
　　fracture
　　　bone P13.9
　　　　specified NEC P13.8
　　　clavicle P13.4
　　　femur P13.2
　　　humerus P13.3
　　　long bone, except femur P13.3
　　　radius and ulna P13.3
　　　skull P13.0
　　　spine P11.5
　　　tibia and fibula P13.3
　　intracranial P11.2
　　　laceration or hemorrhage P10.9
　　　　specified NEC P10.8
　　intraventricular hemorrhage P10.2
　　laceration
　　　brain P10.1
　　　by scalpel P15.8
　　　peripheral nerve P14.9
　　liver P15.0
　　meninges
　　　brain P11.1
　　　spinal cord P11.5
　　nerve
　　　brachial plexus P14.3
　　　cranial NEC (except facial) P11.4
　　　facial P11.3
　　　peripheral P14.9
　　　phrenic (paralysis) P14.2
　　paralysis
　　　facial nerve P11.3
　　　spinal P11.5
　　penis P15.5
　　rupture
　　　spinal cord P11.5
　　scalp P12.9
　　scalpel wound P15.8
　　scrotum P15.5
　　skull NEC P13.1
　　　fracture P13.0
　　specified type NEC P15.8
　　spinal cord P11.5
　　spine P11.5
　　spleen P15.1
　　sternomastoid (hematoma) P15.2
　　subarachnoid hemorrhage P10.3
　　subcutaneous fat necrosis P15.6
　　subdural hemorrhage P10.0
　　tentorial tear P10.4
　　testes P15.5
　　vulva P15.5
　lack of care, at or after — *see* Maltreatment, child, neglect
　neglect, at or after — *see* Maltreatment, child, neglect
　palsy or paralysis, newborn, NOS (birth injury) P14.9
　premature (infant) — *see* Preterm, newborn
　shock, newborn P96.89
　trauma — *see* Birth, injury

Birth — *continued*
　weight
　　4000 grams to 4499 grams P08.1
　　4500 grams or more P08.0
　　low (2499 grams or less) — *see* Low, birthweight
　　extremely (999 grams or less) — *see* Low, birthweight, extreme
Birthmark Q82.5
Birt-Hogg-Dube syndrome Q87.89
Bisalbuminemia E88.09
Biskra's button B55.1
Bite(s) (animal) (human)
　abdomen, abdominal
　　wall S31.159
　　　with penetration into peritoneal cavity S31.659
　　　epigastric region S31.152
　　　　with penetration into peritoneal cavity S31.652
　　　left
　　　　lower quadrant S31.154
　　　　　with penetration into peritoneal cavity S31.654
　　　　upper quadrant S31.151
　　　　　with penetration into peritoneal cavity S31.651
　　　periumbilic region S31.155
　　　　with penetration into peritoneal cavity S31.655
　　　right
　　　　lower quadrant S31.153
　　　　　with penetration into peritoneal cavity S31.653
　　　　upper quadrant S31.150
　　　　　with penetration into peritoneal cavity S31.650
　　　superficial NEC S30.871
　　　　insect S30.861
　alveolar (process) — *see* Bite, oral cavity
　amphibian (venomous) — *see* Venom, bite, amphibian
　animal — *see also* Bite, by site
　　venomous — *see* Venom
　ankle S91.05-
　　superficial NEC S90.57-
　　　insect S90.56-
　antecubital space — *see* Bite, elbow
　anus S31.835
　　superficial NEC S30.877
　　　insect S30.867
　arm (upper) S41.15-
　　lower — *see* Bite, forearm
　　superficial NEC S40.87-
　　　insect S40.86-
　arthropod NEC — *see* Venom, bite, arthropod
　auditory canal (external) (meatus) — *see* Bite, ear
　auricle, ear — *see* Bite, ear
　axilla — *see* Bite, arm
　back — *see also* Bite, thorax, back
　　lower S31.050
　　　with penetration into retroperitoneal space S31.051
　　　superficial NEC S30.870
　　　　insect S30.860
　bedbug — *see* Bite(s), by site, superficial, insect
　breast S21.05-
　　superficial NEC S20.17-
　　　insect S20.16-
　brow — *see* Bite, head, specified site NEC
　buttock S31.805
　　left S31.825
　　right S31.815
　　superficial NEC S30.870
　　　insect S30.860
　calf — *see* Bite, leg
　canaliculus lacrimalis — *see* Bite, eyelid
　canthus, eye — *see* Bite, eyelid
　centipede — *see* Toxicity, venom, arthropod, centipede
　cheek (external) S01.45-
　　internal — *see* Bite, oral cavity
　　superficial NEC S00.87
　　　insect S00.86
　chest wall — *see* Bite, thorax
　chigger B88.0
　chin — *see* Bite, head, specified site NEC
　clitoris — *see* Bite, vulva
　costal region — *see* Bite, thorax
　digit(s)
　　hand — *see* Bite, finger
　　toe — *see* Bite, toe
　ear (canal) (external) S01.35-
　　superficial NEC S00.47-
　　　insect S00.46-

Bite(s) (animal) (human) — *continued*
　elbow S51.05-
　　superficial NEC S50.37-
　　　insect S50.36-
　epididymis — *see* Bite, testis
　epigastric region — *see* Bite, abdomen
　epiglottis — *see* Bite, neck, specified site NEC
　esophagus, cervical S11.25
　　superficial NEC S10.17
　　　insect S10.16
　eyebrow — *see* Bite, eyelid
　eyelid S01.15-
　　superficial NEC S00.27-
　　　insect S00.26-
　face NEC — *see* Bite, head, specified site NEC
　finger(s) S61.259
　　with
　　　damage to nail S61.359
　　index S61.258
　　　with
　　　　damage to nail S61.358
　　　left S61.251
　　　　with
　　　　　damage to nail S61.351
　　　right S61.250
　　　　with
　　　　　damage to nail S61.350
　　　superficial NEC S60.478
　　　　insect S60.46-
　　little S61.25-
　　　with
　　　　damage to nail S61.35-
　　　superficial NEC S60.47-
　　　　insect S60.46-
　　middle S61.25-
　　　with
　　　　damage to nail S61.35-
　　　superficial NEC S60.47-
　　　　insect S60.46-
　　ring S61.25-
　　　with
　　　　damage to nail S61.35-
　　　superficial NEC S60.47-
　　　　insect S60.46-
　　superficial NEC S60.479
　　　insect S60.469
　　thumb — *see* Bite, thumb
　flank — *see* Bite, abdomen, wall
　flea — *see* Bite, by site, superficial, insect
　foot (except toe(s) alone) S91.35-
　　superficial NEC S90.87-
　　　insect S90.86-
　　toe — *see* Bite, toe
　forearm S51.85-
　　elbow only — *see* Bite, elbow
　　superficial NEC S50.87-
　　　insect S50.86-
　forehead — *see* Bite, head, specified site NEC
　genital organs, external
　　female S31.552
　　　superficial NEC S30.876
　　　　insect S30.866
　　　vagina and vulva — *see* Bite, vulva
　　male S31.551
　　　penis — *see* Bite, penis
　　　scrotum — *see* Bite, scrotum
　　　superficial NEC S30.875
　　　　insect S30.865
　　　testes — *see* Bite, testis
　groin — *see* Bite, abdomen, wall
　gum — *see* Bite, oral cavity
　hand S61.45-
　　finger — *see* Bite, finger
　　superficial NEC S60.57-
　　　insect S60.56-
　　thumb — *see* Bite, thumb
　head S01.95
　　cheek — *see* Bite, cheek
　　ear — *see* Bite, ear
　　eyelid — *see* Bite, eyelid
　　lip — *see* Bite, lip
　　nose — *see* Bite, nose
　　oral cavity — *see* Bite, oral cavity
　　scalp — *see* Bite, scalp
　　specified site NEC S01.85
　　　superficial NEC S00.87
　　　　insect S00.86
　　superficial NEC S00.97
　　　insect S00.96
　　temporomandibular area — *see* Bite, cheek
　heel — *see* Bite, foot
　hip S71.05-
　　superficial NEC S70.27-
　　　insect S70.26-

Bite(s) (animal) (human) — *continued*
　hymen S31.45
　hypochondrium — *see* Bite, abdomen, wall
　hypogastric region — *see* Bite, abdomen, wall
　inguinal region — *see* Bite, abdomen, wall
　insect — *see* Bite, by site, superficial, insect
　instep — *see* Bite, foot
　interscapular region — *see* Bite, thorax, back
　jaw — *see* Bite, head, specified site NEC
　knee S81.05-
　　superficial NEC S80.27-
　　　insect S80.26-
　labium (majus) (minus) — *see* Bite, vulva
　lacrimal duct — *see* Bite, eyelid
　larynx S11.015
　　superficial NEC S10.17
　　　insect S10.16
　leg (lower) S81.85-
　　ankle — *see* Bite, ankle
　　foot — *see* Bite, foot
　　knee — *see* Bite, knee
　　superficial NEC S80.87-
　　　insect S80.86-
　　toe — *see* Bite, toe
　　upper — *see* Bite, thigh
　lip S01.551
　　superficial NEC S00.571
　　　insect S00.561
　lizard (venomous) — *see* Venom, bite, reptile
　loin — *see* Bite, abdomen, wall
　lower back — *see* Bite, back, lower
　lumbar region — *see* Bite, back, lower
　malar region — *see* Bite, head, specified site NEC
　mammary — *see* Bite, breast
　marine animals (venomous) — *see* Toxicity, venom, marine animal
　mastoid region — *see* Bite, head, specified site NEC
　mouth — *see* Bite, oral cavity
　nail
　　finger — *see* Bite, finger
　　toe — *see* Bite, toe
　nape — *see* Bite, neck, specified site NEC
　nasal (septum) (sinus) — *see* Bite, nose
　nasopharynx — *see* Bite, head, specified site NEC
　neck S11.95
　　involving
　　　cervical esophagus — *see* Bite, esophagus, cervical
　　　larynx — *see* Bite, larynx
　　　pharynx — *see* Bite, pharynx
　　　thyroid gland S11.15
　　　trachea — *see* Bite, trachea
　　specified site NEC S11.85
　　　superficial NEC S10.87
　　　　insect S10.86
　　superficial NEC S10.97
　　　insect S10.96
　　throat S11.85
　　　superficial NEC S10.17
　　　　insect S10.16
　nose (septum) (sinus) S01.25
　　superficial NEC S00.37
　　　insect S00.36
　occipital region — *see* Bite, scalp
　oral cavity S01.552
　　superficial NEC S00.572
　　　insect S00.562
　orbital region — *see* Bite, eyelid
　palate — *see* Bite, oral cavity
　palm — *see* Bite, hand
　parietal region — *see* Bite, scalp
　pelvis S31.050
　　with penetration into retroperitoneal space S31.051
　　superficial NEC S30.870
　　　insect S30.860
　penis S31.25
　　superficial NEC S30.872
　　　insect S30.862
　perineum
　　female — *see* Bite, vulva
　　male — *see* Bite, pelvis
　periocular area (with or without lacrimal passages) — *see* Bite, eyelid
　phalanges
　　finger — *see* Bite, finger
　　toe — *see* Bite, toe
　pharynx S11.25
　　superficial NEC S10.17
　　　insect S10.16
　pinna — *see* Bite, ear

Bite(s) (animal) (human) — *continued*
  poisonous — *see* Venom
  popliteal space — *see* Bite, knee
  prepuce — *see* Bite, penis
  pubic region — *see* Bite, abdomen, wall
  rectovaginal septum — *see* Bite, vulva
  red bug B88.0
  reptile NEC — *see also* Venom, bite, reptile
    nonvenomous — *see* Bite, by site
    snake — *see* Venom, bite, snake
  sacral region — *see* Bite, back, lower
  sacroiliac region — *see* Bite, back, lower
  salivary gland — *see* Bite, oral cavity
  scalp S01.05
    superficial NEC S00.07
      insect S00.06
  scapular region — *see* Bite, shoulder
  scrotum S31.35
    superficial NEC S30.873
      insect S30.863
  sea-snake (venomous) — *see* Toxicity, venom, snake, sea snake
  shin — *see* Bite, leg
  shoulder S41.05-
    superficial NEC S40.27-
      insect S40.26-
  snake — *see also* Venom, bite, snake
    nonvenomous — *see* Bite, by site
  spermatic cord — *see* Bite, testis
  spider (venomous) — *see* Toxicity, venom, spider
    nonvenomous — *see* Bite, by site, superficial, insect
  sternal region — *see* Bite, thorax, front
  submaxillary region — *see* Bite, head, specified site NEC
  submental region — *see* Bite, head, specified site NEC
  subungual
    finger(s) — *see* Bite, finger
    toe — *see* Bite, toe
  superficial — *see* Bite, by site, superficial, insect
  supraclavicular fossa S11.85
  supraorbital — *see* Bite, head, specified site NEC
  temple, temporal region — *see* Bite, head, specified site NEC
  temporomandibular area — *see* Bite, cheek
  testis S31.35
    superficial NEC S30.873
      insect S30.863
  thigh S71.15-
    superficial NEC S70.37-
      insect S70.36-
  thorax, thoracic (wall) S21.95
    back S21.25-
      with penetration into thoracic cavity S21.45-
    breast — *see* Bite, breast
    front S21.15-
      with penetration into thoracic cavity S21.35-
    superficial NEC S20.97
      back S20.47-
      front S20.37-
      insect S20.96
        back S20.46-
        front S20.36-
  throat — *see* Bite, neck, throat
  thumb S61.05-
    with
      damage to nail S61.15-
    superficial NEC S60.37-
      insect S60.36-
  thyroid S11.15
    superficial NEC S10.87
      insect S10.86
  toe(s) S91.15-
    with
      damage to nail S91.25-
    great S91.15-
      with
        damage to nail S91.25-
    lesser S91.15-
      with
        damage to nail S91.25-
    superficial NEC S90.47-
      great S90.47-
      insect S90.46-
        great S90.46-
  tongue S01.552
  trachea S11.025
    superficial NEC S10.17
      insect S10.16

Bite(s) (animal) (human) — *continued*
  tunica vaginalis — *see* Bite, testis
  tympanum, tympanic membrane — *see* Bite, ear
  umbilical region S31.155
  uvula — *see* Bite, oral cavity
  vagina — *see* Bite, vulva
  venomous — *see* Venom
  vocal cords S11.035
    superficial NEC S10.17
      insect S10.16
  vulva S31.45
    superficial NEC S30.874
      insect S30.864
  wrist S61.55-
    superficial NEC S60.87-
      insect S60.86-
Biting, cheek or lip K13.1
Biventricular failure (heart) I50.9
Björck (-Thorson) syndrome (malignant carcinoid) E34.0
Black
  death A20.9
  eye S00.1-
  hairy tongue K14.3
  heel (foot) S90.3-
  lung (disease) J60
  palm (hand) S60.22-
Blackfan-Diamond anemia or syndrome (congenital hypoplastic anemia) D61.01
Blackhead L70.0
Blackout R55
Bladder — *see* condition
Blast (air) (hydraulic) (immersion) (underwater)
  blindness S05.8x-
  injury
    abdomen or thorax — *see* Injury, by site
    ear (acoustic nerve trauma) — *see* Injury, nerve, acoustic, specified type NEC
    syndrome NEC T70.8
Blastoma — *see* Neoplasm, malignant, by site
  pulmonary — *see* Neoplasm, lung, malignant
Blastomycosis, blastomycotic B40.9
  Brazilian — *see* Paracoccidioidomycosis
  cutaneous B40.3
  disseminated B40.7
  European — *see* Cryptococcosis
  generalized B40.7
  keloidal B48.0
  North American B40.9
  primary pulmonary B40.0
  pulmonary B40.2
    acute B40.0
    chronic B40.1
  skin B40.3
  South American — *see* Paracoccidioidomycosis
  specified NEC B40.89
Blebitis, postprocedural H59.40
  stage 1 H59.41
  stage 2 H59.42
  stage 3 H59.43
Bleb(s) R23.8
  emphysematous (lung) (solitary) J43.9
  endophthalmitis H59.43
  filtering (vitreous), after glaucoma surgery Z98.83
  inflamed (infected), postprocedural H59.40
    stage 1 H59.41
    stage 2 H59.42
    stage 3 H59.43
  lung (ruptured) J43.9
    congenital — *see* Atelectasis
    newborn P25.8
  subpleural (emphysematous) J43.9
Bleeder (familial) (hereditary) — *see* Hemophilia
Bleeding — *see also* Hemorrhage
  anal K62.5
  anovulatory N97.0
  atonic, following delivery O72.1
  capillary I78.8
    puerperal O72.2
  contact (postcoital) N93.0
  due to uterine subinvolution N85.3
  ear — *see* Otorrhagia
  excessive, associated with menopausal onset N92.4
  familial — *see* Defect, coagulation
  following intercourse N93.0
  gastrointestinal K92.2
  hemorrhoids — *see* Hemorrhoids

Bleeding (*see also* Hemorrhage) — *continued*
  intermenstrual (regular) N92.3
    irregular N92.1
  intraoperative — *see* Complication, intraoperative, hemorrhage
  irregular N92.6
  menopausal N92.4
  newborn, intraventricular — *see* Newborn, affected by, hemorrhage, intraventricular
  nipple N64.59
  nose R04.0
  ovulation N92.3
  postclimacteric N95.0
  postcoital N93.0
  postmenopausal N95.0
  postoperative — *see* Complication, postprocedural, hemorrhage
  preclimacteric N92.4
  puberty (excessive, with onset of menstrual periods) N92.2
  rectum, rectal K62.5
    newborn P54.2
  tendencies — *see* Defect, coagulation
  throat R04.1
  tooth socket (post-extraction) K91.840
  umbilical stump P51.9
  uterus, uterine NEC N93.9
    climacteric N92.4
    dysfunctional of functional N93.8
    menopausal N92.4
    preclimacteric or premenopausal N92.4
    unrelated to menstrual cycle N93.9
  vagina, vaginal (abnormal) N93.9
    dysfunctional or functional N93.8
    newborn P54.6
  vicarious N94.89
Blennorrhagia, blennorrhagic — *see* Gonorrhea
Blennorrhea (acute) (chronic) — *see also* Gonorrhea
  inclusion (neonatal) (newborn) P39.1
  lower genitourinary tract (gonococcal) A54.00
  neonatorum (gonococcal ophthalmia) A54.31
Blepharelosis — *see* Entropion
Blepharitis (angularis) (ciliaris) (eyelid) (marginal) (nonulcerative) H01.009
  herpes zoster B02.39
  left H01.006
    lower H01.005
    upper H01.004
  right H01.003
    lower H01.002
    upper H01.001
  squamous H01.029
    left H01.026
      lower H01.025
      upper H01.024
    right H01.023
      lower H01.022
      upper H01.021
  ulcerative H01.019
    left H01.016
      lower H01.015
      upper H01.014
    right H01.013
      lower H01.012
      upper H01.011
Blepharochalasis H02.30
  congenital Q10.0
  left H02.36
    lower H02.35
    upper H02.34
  right H02.33
    lower H02.32
    upper H02.31
Blepharoclonus H02.59
Blepharoconjunctivitis H10.50-
  angular H10.52-
  contact H10.53-
  ligneous H10.51-
Blepharophimosis (eyelid) H02.529
  congenital Q10.3
  left H02.526
    lower H02.525
    upper H02.524
  right H02.523
    lower H02.522
    upper H02.521
Blepharoptosis H02.40-
  congenital Q10.0
  mechanical H02.41-
  myogenic H02.42-
  neurogenic H02.43-
  paralytic H02.43-

Blepharopyorrhea, gonococcal A54.39
Blepharospasm G24.5
  drug induced G24.01
Blighted ovum O02.0
Blind — *see also* Blindness
  bronchus (congenital) Q32.4
  loop syndrome K90.2
    congenital Q43.8
  sac, fallopian tube (congenital) Q50.6
  spot, enlarged — *see* Defect, visual field, localized, scotoma, blind spot area
  tract or tube, congenital NEC — *see* Atresia, by site
Blindness (acquired) (congenital) (both eyes) H54.0
  blast S05.8x-
  color — *see* Deficiency, color vision
  concussion S05.8x-
  cortical H47.619
    left brain H47.612
    right brain H47.611
  day H53.11
  due to injury (current episode) S05.9-
    sequelae — *code to* injury with seventh character S
  eclipse (total) — *see* Retinopathy, solar
  emotional (hysterical) F44.6
  face H53.16
  hysterical F44.6
  legal (both eyes) (USA definition) H54.8
  mind R48.8
  night H53.60
    abnormal dark adaptation curve H53.61
    acquired H53.62
    congenital H53.63
    specified type NEC H53.69
    vitamin A deficiency E50.5
  one eye (other eye normal) H54.40
    left (normal vision on right) H54.42
      low vision on right H54.12
    low vision, other eye H54.10
    right (normal vision on left) H54.41
      low vision on left H54.11
  psychic R48.8
  river B73.01
  snow — *see* Photokeratitis
  sun, solar — *see* Retinopathy, solar
  transient — *see* Disturbance, vision, subjective, loss, transient
  traumatic (current episode) S05.9-
  word (developmental) F81.0
    acquired R48.0
    secondary to organic lesion R48.0
Blister (nonthermal)
  abdominal wall S30.821
  alveolar process S00.522
  ankle S90.52-
  antecubital space — *see* Blister, elbow
  anus S30.827
  arm (upper) S40.82-
  auditory canal — *see* Blister, ear
  auricle — *see* Blister, ear
  axilla — *see* Blister, arm
  back, lower S30.820
  beetle dermatitis L24.89
  breast S20.12-
  brow S00.82
  calf — *see* Blister, leg
  canthus — *see* Blister, eyelid
  cheek S00.82
    internal S00.522
  chest wall — *see* Blister, thorax
  chin S00.82
  costal region — *see* Blister, thorax
  digit(s)
    foot — *see* Blister, toe
    hand — *see* Blister, finger
  due to burn — *see* Burn, by site, second degree
  ear S00.42-
  elbow S50.32-
  epiglottis S10.12
  esophagus, cervical S10.12
  eyebrow — *see* Blister, eyelid
  eyelid S00.22-
  face S00.82
  fever B00.1
  finger(s) S60.429
    index S60.42-
    little S60.42-
    middle S60.42-
    ring S60.42-
  foot (except toe(s) alone) S90.82-
    toe — *see* Blister, toe

Blister (nonthermal) — *continued*
  forearm S50.82-
    elbow only — *see* Blister, elbow
  forehead S00.82
  fracture — *omit code*
  genital organ
    female S30.826
    male S30.825
  gum S00.522
  hand S60.52-
  head S00.92
    ear — *see* Blister, ear
    eyelid — *see* Blister, eyelid
    lip S00.521
    nose S00.32
    oral cavity S00.522
    scalp S00.02
    specified site NEC S00.82
  heel — *see* Blister, foot
  hip S70.22-
  interscapular region S20.429
  jaw S00.82
  knee S80.22-
  larynx S10.12
  leg (lower) S80.82-
    knee — *see* Blister, knee
    upper — *see* Blister, thigh
  lip S00.521
  malar region S00.82
  mammary — *see* Blister, breast
  mastoid region S00.82
  mouth S00.522
  multiple, skin, nontraumatic R23.8
  nail
    finger — *see* Blister, finger
    toe — *see* Blister, toe
  nasal S00.32
  neck S10.92
    specified site NEC S10.82
    throat S10.12
  nose S00.32
  occipital region S00.02
  oral cavity S00.522
  orbital region — *see* Blister, eyelid
  palate S00.522
  palm — *see* Blister, hand
  parietal region S00.02
  pelvis S30.820
  penis S30.822
  periocular area — *see* Blister, eyelid
  phalanges
    finger — *see* Blister, finger
    toe — *see* Blister, toe
  pharynx S10.12
  pinna — *see* Blister, ear
  popliteal space — *see* Blister, knee
  scalp S00.02
  scapular region — *see* Blister, shoulder
  scrotum S30.823
  shin — *see* Blister, leg
  shoulder S40.22-
  sternal region S20.329
  submaxillary region S00.82
  submental region S00.82
  subungual
    finger(s) — *see* Blister, finger
    toe(s) — *see* Blister, toe
  supraclavicular fossa S10.82
  supraorbital S00.82
  temple S00.82
  temporal region S00.82
  testis S30.823
  thermal — *see* Burn, second degree, by site
  thigh S70.32-
  thorax, thoracic (wall) S20.92
    back S20.42-
    front S20.32-
  throat S10.12
  thumb S60.32-
  toe(s) S90.42-
    great S90.42-
  tongue S00.522
  trachea S10.12
  tympanum, tympanic membrane — *see* Blister, ear
  upper arm — *see* Blister, arm (upper)
  uvula S00.522
  vagina S30.824
  vocal cords S10.12
  vulva S30.824
  wrist S60.52-
Bloating R14.0
Bloch-Sulzberger disease or syndrome Q82.3

Block, blocked
  alveolocapillary J84.10
  arborization (heart) I45.5
  arrhythmic I45.9
  atrioventricular (incomplete) (partial) I44.30
    with atrioventricular dissociation I44.2
    complete I44.2
      congenital Q24.6
    congenital Q24.6
    first degree I44.0
    second degree (types I and II) I44.1
    specified NEC I44.39
    third degree I44.2
    types I and II I44.1
  auriculoventricular — *see* Block, atrioventricular
  bifascicular (cardiac) I45.2
  bundle-branch (complete) (false) (incomplete) I45.4
    bilateral I45.2
    left I44.7
      with right bundle branch block I45.2
      hemiblock I44.60
        anterior I44.4
        posterior I44.5
      incomplete I44.7
        with right bundle branch block I45.2
    right I45.10
      with
        left bundle branch block I45.2
        left fascicular block I45.2
      specified NEC I45.19
    Wilson's type I45.19
  cardiac I45.9
  conduction I45.9
    complete I44.2
  fascicular (left) I44.60
    anterior I44.4
    posterior I44.5
    right I45.0
    specified NEC I44.69
  foramen Magendie (acquired) G91.1
    congenital Q03.1
      with spina bifida — *see* Spina bifida, by site, with hydrocephalus
  heart I45.9
    bundle branch I45.4
      bilateral I45.2
    complete (atrioventricular) I44.2
    congenital Q24.6
    first degree (atrioventricular) I44.0
    second degree (atrioventricular) I44.1
    specified type NEC I44.5
    third degree (atrioventricular) I44.2
  hepatic vein I82.0
  intraventricular (nonspecific) I45.4
    bundle branch
      bilateral I45.2
  kidney N28.9
    postcystoscopic or postprocedural N99.0
  Mobitz (types I and II) I44.1
  myocardial — *see* Block, heart
  nodal I45.5
  organ or site, congenital NEC — *see* Atresia, by site
  portal (vein) I81
  second degree (types I and II) I44.1
  sinoatrial I45.5
  sinoauricular I45.5
  third degree I44.2
  trifascicular I45.3
  tubal N97.1
  vein NOS I82.90
  Wenckebach (types I and II) I44.1
Blockage — *see* Obstruction
Blocq's disease F44.4
Blood
  constituents, abnormal R78.9
  disease D75.9
  donor — *see* Donor, blood
  dyscrasia D75.9
    with
      abortion — *see* Abortion, by type, complicated by, hemorrhage
      ectopic pregnancy O08.1
      molar pregnancy O08.1
    following ectopic or molar pregnancy O08.1
    newborn P61.9
    puerperal, postpartum O72.3
  flukes NEC — *see* Schistosomiasis
  in
    feces K92.1
      occult R19.5
    urine — *see* Hematuria

Blood — *continued*
  mole O02.0
  occult in feces R19.5
  pressure
    decreased, due to shock following injury T79.4
    examination only Z01.30
    fluctuating I99.8
    high — *see* Hypertension
      borderline R03.0
      incidental reading, without diagnosis of hypertension R03.0
    low — *see also* Hypotension
      incidental reading, without diagnosis of hypotension R03.1
  spitting — *see* Hemoptysis
  staining cornea — *see* Pigmentation, cornea, stromal
  transfusion
    reaction or complication — *see* Complications, transfusion
  type
    A (Rh positive) Z67.10
      Rh negative Z67.11
    AB (Rh positive) Z67.30
      Rh negative Z67.31
    B (Rh positive) Z67.20
      Rh negative Z67.21
    O (Rh positive) Z67.40
      Rh negative Z67.41
    Rh (positive) Z67.90
      negative Z67.91
  vessel rupture — *see* Hemorrhage
  vomiting — *see* Hematemesis
Blood-forming organs, disease D75.9
Bloodgood's disease — *see* Mastopathy, cystic
Bloom(-Machacek)(-Torre) syndrome Q82.8
Blount's disease or osteochondrosis — *see* Osteochondrosis, juvenile, tibia
Blue
  baby Q24.9
  diaper syndrome E72.09
  dome cyst (breast) — *see* Cyst, breast
  dot cataract Q12.0
  nevus D22.9
  sclera Q13.5
    with fragility of bone and deafness Q78.0
  toe syndrome I75.02-
Blueness — *see* Cyanosis
Blues, postpartal O90.6
  baby O90.6
Blurring, visual H53.8
Blushing (abnormal) (excessive) R23.2
BMI — *see* Body, mass index
Boarder, hospital NEC Z76.4
  accompanying sick person Z76.3
  healthy infant or child Z76.2
  foundling Z76.1
Bockhart's impetigo L01.02
Bodechtel-Guttman disease (subacute sclerosing panencephalitis) A81.1
Boder-Sedgwick syndrome (ataxia-telangiectasia) G11.3
Body, bodies
  Aschoff's — *see* Myocarditis, rheumatic
  asteroid, vitreous — *see* Deposit, crystalline
  cytoid (retina) — *see* Occlusion, artery, retina
  drusen (degenerative) (macula) (retinal) — *see also* Degeneration, macula, drusen
    optic disc — *see* Drusen, optic disc
  foreign — *see* Foreign body
  loose
    joint, except knee — *see* Loose, body, joint
      knee M23.4-
    sheath, tendon — *see* Disorder, tendon, specified type NEC
  mass index (BMI)
    adult
      19 or less Z68.1
      20.0-20.9 Z68.20
      21.0-21.9 Z68.21
      22.0-22.9 Z68.22
      23.0-23.9 Z68.23
      24.0-24.9 Z68.24
      25.0-25.9 Z68.25
      26.0-26.9 Z68.26
      27.0-27.9 Z68.27
      28.0-28.9 Z68.28
      29.0-29.9 Z68.29
      30.0-30.9 Z68.30
      31.0-31.9 Z68.31
      32.0-32.9 Z68.32

Body, bodies — *continued*
  mass index (BMI) — *continued*
    adult — *continued*
      33.0-33.9 Z68.33
      34.0-34.9 Z68.34
      35.0-35.9 Z68.35
      36.0-36.9 Z68.36
      37.0-37.9 Z68.37
      38.0-38.9 Z68.38
      39.0-39.9 Z68.39
      40.0-44.9 Z68.41
      45.0-49.9 Z68.42
      50.0-59.9 Z68.43
      60.0-69.9 Z68.44
      70 and over Z68.45
    pediatric
      5th percentile to less than 85th percentile for age Z68.52
      85th percentile to less than 95th percentile for age Z68.53
      greater than or equal to ninety-fifth percentile for age Z68.54
      less than fifth percentile for age Z68.51
  Mooser's A75.2
  rice — *see also* Loose, body, joint
    knee M23.4-
  rocking F98.4
Boeck's
  disease or sarcoid — *see* Sarcoidosis
  lupoid (miliary) D86.3
Boerhaave's syndrome (spontaneous esophageal rupture) K22.3
Boggy
  cervix N88.8
  uterus N85.8
Boil — *see also* Furuncle, by site
  Aleppo B55.1
  Baghdad B55.1
  Delhi B55.1
  lacrimal
    gland — *see* Dacryoadenitis
    passages (duct) (sac) — *see* Inflammation, lacrimal, passages, acute
  Natal B55.1
  orbit, orbital — *see* Abscess, orbit
  tropical B55.1
Bold hives — *see* Urticaria
Bombé, iris — *see* Membrane, pupillary
Bone — *see* condition
Bonnevie-Ullrich syndrome Q87.1
Bonnier's syndrome — *see* subcategory H81.8
Bonvale dam fever T73.3
Bony block of joint — *see* Ankylosis
BOOP (bronchiolitis obliterans organized pneumonia) J84.89
Borderline
  diabetes mellitus R73.09
  hypertension R03.0
  osteopenia M85.8-
  pelvis, with obstruction during labor O65.1
  personality F60.3
Borna disease A83.9
Bornholm disease B33.0
Boston exanthem A88.0
Botalli, ductus (patent) (persistent) Q25.0
Bothriocephalus latus infestation B70.0
Botulism (foodborne intoxication) A05.1
  infant A48.51
  non-foodborne A48.52
  wound A48.52
Bouba — *see* Yaws
Bouchard's nodes (with arthropathy) M15.2
Bouffée délirante F23
Bouillaud's disease or syndrome (rheumatic heart disease) I01.9
Bourneville's disease Q85.1
Boutonniere deformity (finger) — *see* Deformity, finger, boutonniere
Bouveret(-Hoffmann) syndrome (paroxysmal tachycardia) I47.9
Bovine heart — *see* Hypertrophy, cardiac
Bowel — *see* condition
Bowen's
  dermatosis (precancerous) — *see* Neoplasm, skin, in situ
  disease — *see* Neoplasm, skin, in situ
  epithelioma — *see* Neoplasm, skin, in situ
  type
    epidermoid carcinoma-in-situ — *see* Neoplasm, skin, in situ
    intraepidermal squamous cell carcinoma — *see* Neoplasm, skin, in situ

Bowing
femur — *see also* Deformity, limb, specified type NEC, thigh
  congenital Q68.3
fibula — *see also* Deformity, limb, specified type NEC, lower leg
  congenital Q68.4
forearm — *see* Deformity, limb, specified type NEC, forearm
leg(s), long bones, congenital Q68.5
radius — *see* Deformity, limb, specified type NEC, forearm
tibia — *see also* Deformity, limb, specified type NEC, lower leg
Bowleg(s) (acquired) M21.16-
  congenital Q68.5
  rachitic E64.3
Boyd's dysentery A03.2
Brachial — *see* condition
Brachycardia R00.1
Brachycephaly Q75.0
Bradley's disease A08.19
Bradyarrhythmia, cardiac I49.8
Bradycardia (sinoatrial) (sinus) (vagal) R00.1
  neonatal P29.12
  reflex G90.09
  tachycardia syndrome I49.5
Bradykinesia R25.8
Bradypnea R06.89
Bradytachycardia I49.5
Brailsford's disease or osteochondrosis — *see* Osteochondrosis, juvenile, radius
Brain — *see also* condition
  death G93.82
  syndrome — *see* Syndrome, brain
Branched-chain amino-acid disorder E71.2
Branchial — *see* condition
  cartilage, congenital Q18.2
Branchiogenic remnant (in neck) Q18.0
Brandt's syndrome (acrodermatitis enteropathica) E83.2
Brash (water) R12
Bravais-jacksonian epilepsy — *see* Epilepsy, localization-related, symptomatic, with simple partial seizures
Braxton Hicks contractions — *see* False, labor
Brazilian leishmaniasis B55.2
BRBPR K62.5
Break, retina (without detachment) H33.30-
  with retinal detachment — *see* Detachment, retina
  horseshoe tear H33.31-
  multiple H33.33-
  round hole H33.32-
Breakdown
device, graft or implant (*see also* Complications, by site and type, mechanical) T85.618
  arterial graft NEC — *see* Complication, cardiovascular device, mechanical, vascular
  breast (implant) T85.41
  catheter NEC T85.618
    cystostomy T83.010
    dialysis (renal) T82.41
      intraperitoneal T85.611
    infusion NEC T82.514
      spinal (epidural) (subdural) T85.610
    urinary (indwelling) T83.018
  electronic (electrode) (pulse generator) (stimulator)
    bone T84.310
    cardiac T82.119
      electrode T82.110
      pulse generator T82.111
      specified type NEC T82.118
    nervous system — *see* Complication, prosthetic device, mechanical, electronic nervous system stimulator
    urinary — *see* Complication, genitourinary, device, urinary, mechanical
  fixation, internal (orthopedic) NEC — *see* Complication, fixation device, mechanical
  gastrointestinal — *see* Complications, prosthetic device, mechanical, gastrointestinal device
  genital NEC T83.418
    intrauterine contraceptive device T83.31
    penile prosthesis T83.410

Breakdown — *continued*
device, graft or implant (*see also* Complications, by site and type, mechanical) T85.618 — *continued*
  heart NEC — *see* Complication, cardiovascular device, mechanical
  joint prosthesis — *see* Complications..., joint prosthesis,internal, mechanical, by site
  ocular NEC — *see* Complications, prosthetic device, mechanical, ocular device
  orthopedic NEC — *see* Complication, orthopedic, device, mechanical
  specified NEC T85.618
  sutures, permanent T85.612
    used in bone repair — *see* Complications, fixation device, internal (orthopedic), mechanical
  urinary NEC — *see also* Complication, genitourinary, device, urinary, mechanical
    graft T83.21
  vascular NEC — *see* Complication, cardiovascular device, mechanical
  ventricular intracranial shunt T85.01
nervous F48.8
perineum O90.1
respirator J95.850
  specified NEC J95.859
ventilator J95.850
  specified NEC J95.859
Breast — *see also* condition
buds E30.1
  in newborn P96.89
dense R92.2
nodule N63
Breath
foul R19.6
holder, child R06.89
holding spell R06.89
shortness R06.02
Breathing
labored — *see* Hyperventilation
mouth R06.5
  causing malocclusion M26.5
periodic R06.3
high altitude G47.32
Breathlessness R06.81
Breda's disease — *see* Yaws
Breech presentation (mother) O32.1
causing obstructed labor O64.1
footling O32.8
  causing obstructed labor O64.8
incomplete O32.8
  causing obstructed labor O64.8
Breisky's disease N90.4
Brennemann's syndrome I88.0
Brenner
tumor (benign) D27.9
  borderline malignancy D39.1-
  malignant C56
  proliferating D39.1-
Bretonneau's disease or angina A36.0
Breus' mole O02.0
Brevicollis Q76.49
Brickmakers' anemia B76.9 [D63.8]
Bridge, myocardial Q24.5
Bright red blood per rectum (BRBPR) K62.5
Bright's disease — *see also* Nephritis
arteriosclerotic — *see* Hypertension, kidney
Brill-Symmers' disease C82.90
Brill(-Zinsser) disease (recrudescent typhus) A75.1
  flea-borne A75.2
  louse-borne A75.1
Brion-Kayser disease — *see* Fever, parathyroid
Briquet's disorder or syndrome F45.0
Brissaud's
infantilism or dwarfism E23.0
motor-verbal tic F95.2
Brittle
bones disease Q78.0
nails L60.3
  congenital Q84.6
Broad — *see also* condition
beta disease E78.2
ligament laceration syndrome N83.8
Broad- or floating-betalipoproteinemia E78.2
Brock's syndrome (atelectasis due to enlarged lymph nodes) J98.19
Brocq-Duhring disease (dermatitis herpetiformis) L13.0
Brodie's abscess or disease M86.8x-

Broken
arches — *see also* Deformity, limb, flat foot
arm (meaning upper limb) — *see* Fracture, arm
back — *see* Fracture, vertebra
bone — *see* Fracture
implant or internal device — *see* Complications, by site and type, mechanical
leg (meaning lower limb) — *see* Fracture, leg
nose S02.2
tooth, teeth — *see* Fracture, tooth
Bromhidrosis, bromidrosis L75.0
Bromidism, bromism G92
chronic (dependence) F13.20
due to
  correct substance properly administered — *see* Table of Drugs and Chemicals, by drug, adverse effect
  overdose or wrong substance given or taken — *see* Table of Drugs and Chemicals, by drug, poisoning
Bromidrosiphobia F40.298
Bronchi, bronchial — *see* condition
Bronchiectasis (cylindrical) (diffuse) (fusiform) (localized) (saccular) J47.9
with
  acute
    bronchitis J47.0
    lower respiratory infection J47.0
  exacerbation (acute) J47.1
congenital Q33.4
tuberculous NEC — *see* Tuberculosis, pulmonary
Bronchiolectasis — *see* Bronchiectasis
Bronchiolitis (acute) (infective) (subacute) J21.9
with
  bronchospasm or obstruction J21.9
  influenza, flu or grippe — *see* Influenza, with, respiratory manifestations NEC
chemical (chronic) J68.4
  acute J68.0
chronic (fibrosing) (obliterative) J44.9
due to
  external agent — *see* Bronchitis, acute, due to
  human metapneumovirus J21.1
  respiratory syncytial virus J21.0
  specified organism NEC J21.8
fibrosa obliterans J44.9
influenzal — *see* Influenza, with, respiratory manifestations NEC
obliterans J42
  with organizing pneumonia (BOOP) J84.89
obliterative (chronic) (subacute) J44.9
  due to chemicals, gases, fumes or vapors (inhalation) J68.4
  due to fumes or vapors J68.4
respiratory, interstitial lung disease J84.115
Bronchitis (diffuse) (fibrinous) (hypostatic) (infective) (membranous) J40
with
  influenza, flu or grippe — *see* Influenza, with, respiratory manifestations NEC
  obstruction (airway) (lung) J44.9
  tracheitis (15 years of age and above) J40
    acute or subacute J20.9
    chronic J42
    under 15 years of age J20.9
acute or subacute (with bronchospasm or obstruction) J20.9
  with
    bronchiectasis J47.0
    chronic obstructive pulmonary disease J44.0
    chemical (due to gases, fumes or vapors) J68.0
  due to
    fumes or vapors J68.0
    Haemophilus influenzae J20.1
    Mycoplasma pneumoniae J20.0
    radiation J70.0
    specified organism NEC J20.8
    Streptococcus J20.2
    virus
      coxsackie J20.3
      echovirus J20.7
      parainfluenzae J20.4
      respiratory syncytial J20.5
      rhinovirus J20.6
  viral NEC J20.8

Bronchitis (diffuse) (fibrinous) (hypostatic) (infective) (membranous) J40 — *continued*
allergic (acute) J45.909
  with
    exacerbation (acute) J45.901
    status asthmaticus J45.902
arachidic T17.528
aspiration (due to fumes or vapors) J68.0
asthmatic J45.9
  chronic J44.9
    with
      acute lower respiratory infection J44.0
      exacerbation (acute) J44.1
capillary — *see* Pneumonia, broncho
caseous (tuberculous) A15.5
Castellani's A69.8
catarrhal (15 years of age and above) J40
  acute — *see* Bronchitis, acute
  chronic J41.0
  under 15 years of age J20.9
chemical (acute) (subacute) J68.0
  chronic J68.4
  due to fumes or vapors J68.0
    chronic J68.4
chronic J42
  with
    airways obstruction J44.9
    tracheitis (chronic) J42
  asthmatic (obstructive) J44.9
  catarrhal J41.0
  chemical (due to fumes or vapors) J68.4
  due to
    chemicals, gases, fumes or vapors (inhalation) J68.4
    radiation J70.1
    tobacco smoking J41.0
  emphysematous J44.9
  mucopurulent J41.1
  non-obstructive J41.0
  obliterans J44.9
  obstructive J44.9
  purulent J41.1
  simple J41.0
croupous — *see* Bronchitis, acute
due to gases, fumes or vapors (chemical) J68.0
emphysematous (obstructive) J44.9
exudative — *see* Bronchitis, acute
fetid J41.1
grippal — *see* Influenza, with, respiratory manifestations NEC
in those under 15 years age — *see* Bronchitis, acute
  chronic — *see* Bronchitis, chronic
influenzal — *see* Influenza, with, respiratory manifestations NEC
mixed simple and mucopurulent J41.8
moulder's J62.8
mucopurulent (chronic) (recurrent) J41.1
  acute or subacute J20.9
  simple (mixed) J41.8
obliterans (chronic) J44.9
obstructive (chronic) (diffuse) J44.9
pituitous J41.1
pneumococcal, acute or subacute J20.2
pseudomembranous, acute or subacute — *see* Bronchitis, acute
purulent (chronic) (recurrent) J41.1
  acute or subacute — *see* Bronchitis, acute
putrid J41.1
senile (chronic) J42
simple and mucopurulent (mixed) J41.8
smokers' J41.0
spirochetal NEC A69.8
subacute — *see* Bronchitis, acute
suppurative (chronic) J41.1
  acute or subacute — *see* Bronchitis, acute
tuberculous A15.5
under 15 years of age — *see* Bronchitis, acute
  chronic — *see* Bronchitis, chronic
viral NEC, acute or subacute (*see also* Bronchitis, acute) J20.8
Bronchoalveolitis J18.0
Bronchoaspergillosis B44.1
Bronchocele meaning goiter E04.0
Broncholithiasis J98.09
  tuberculous NEC A15.5
Bronchomalacia J98.09
  congenital Q32.2
Bronchomycosis NOS B49 [J99]
  candidal B37.1
Bronchopleuropneumonia — *see* Pneumonia, broncho
Bronchopneumonia — *see* Pneumonia, broncho

DISEASE INDEX

Bronchopneumonitis — *see* Pneumonia, broncho
Bronchopulmonary — *see* condition
Bronchopulmonitis — *see* Pneumonia, broncho
Bronchorrhagia (*see* Hemoptysis)
Bronchorrhea J98.09
  acute J20.9
  chronic (infective) (purulent) J42
Bronchospasm (acute) J98.01
  with
    bronchiolitis, acute J21.9
    bronchitis, acute (conditions in J20) — *see* Bronchitis, acute
  due to external agent — *see* condition, respiratory, acute, due to
  exercise induced J45.990
Bronchospirochetosis A69.8
  Castellani A69.8
Bronchostenosis J98.09
Bronchus — *see* condition
Brontophobia F40.220
Bronze baby syndrome P83.8
Brooke's tumor — *see* Neoplasm, skin, benign
Brown enamel of teeth (hereditary) K00.5
Brown-Séquard disease, paralysis or syndrome G83.81
Brown's sheath syndrome H50.61-
Bruce sepsis A23.0
Brucellosis (infection) A23.9
  abortus A23.1
  canis A23.3
  dermatitis A23.9
  melitensis A23.0
  mixed A23.8
  sepsis A23.9
    melitensis A23.0
    specified NEC A23.8
  suis A23.2
Bruck-de Lange disease Q87.1
Bruck's disease — *see* Deformity, limb
Brugsch's syndrome Q82.8
Bruise (skin surface intact) — *see also* Contusion
  with
    open wound — *see* Wound, open
  internal organ — *see* Injury, by site
  newborn P54.5
  scalp, due to birth injury, newborn P12.3
  umbilical cord O69.5
Bruit (arterial) R09.89
  cardiac R01.1
Brush burn — *see* Abrasion, by site
Bruton's X-linked agammaglobulinemia D80.0
Bruxism
  psychogenic F45.8
  sleep related G47.63
Bubbly lung syndrome P27.0
Bubo I88.8
  blennorrhagic (gonococcal) A54.89
  chancroidal A57
  climatic A55
  due to Haemophilus ducreyi A57
  gonococcal A54.89
  indolent (nonspecific) I88.8
  inguinal (nonspecific) I88.8
    chancroidal A57
    climatic A55
    due to H. ducreyi A57
    infective I88.8
  scrofulous (tuberculous) A18.2
  soft chancre A57
  suppurating — *see* Lymphadenitis, acute
  syphilitic (primary) A51.0
    congenital A50.07
  tropical A55
  virulent (chancroidal) A57
Bubonic plague A20.0
Bubonocele — *see* Hernia, inguinal
Buccal — *see* condition
Buchanan's disease or osteochondrosis M91.0
Buchem's syndrome (hyperostosis corticalis) M85.2
Bucket-handle fracture or tear (semilunar cartilage) — *see* Tear, meniscus
Budd-Chiari syndrome (hepatic vein thrombosis) I82.0
Budgerigar fancier's disease or lung J67.2
Buds
  breast E30.1
  in newborn P96.89
Buerger's disease (thromboangiitis obliterans) I73.1
Bulbar — *see* condition
Bulbus cordis (left ventricle) (persistent) Q21.8

Bulimia (nervosa) F50.2
  atypical F50.9
  normal weight F50.9
Bulky
  stools R19.5
  uterus N85.2
Bulla(e) R23.8
  lung (emphysematous) (solitary) J43.9
  newborn P25.8
Bullet wound — *see also* Wound, open
  fracture — *code as* Fracture, by site
  internal organ — *see* Injury, by site
Bundle
  branch block (complete) (false) (incomplete) — *see* Block, bundle-branch
  of His — *see* condition
Bunion — *see* Deformity, toe, hallux valgus
Buphthalmia, buphthalmos (congenital) Q15.0
Burdwan fever B55.0
Bürger-Grütz disease or syndrome E78.3
Buried
  penis (congenital) Q55.64
    acquired N48.83
  roots K08.3
Burke's syndrome K86.8
Burkitt
  cell leukemia C91.0-
  lymphoma (malignant) C83.7-
    small noncleaved, diffuse C83.7-
    spleen C83.77
    undifferentiated C83.7-
  tumor C83.7-
  type
    acute lymphoblastic leukemia C91.0-
    undifferentiated C83.7-
Burn (electricity) (flame) (hot gas, liquid or hot object) (radiation) (steam) (thermal) T30.0
  abdomen, abdominal (muscle) (wall) T21.02
    first degree T21.12
    second degree T21.22
    third degree T21.32
  above elbow T22.039
    first degree T22.139
    left T22.032
      first degree T22.132
      second degree T22.232
      third degree T22.332
    right T22.031
      first degree T22.131
      second degree T22.231
      third degree T22.331
    second degree T22.239
    third degree T22.339
  acid (caustic) (external) (internal) — *see* Corrosion, by site
  alimentary tract NEC T28.2
    esophagus T28.1
    mouth T28.0
    pharynx T28.0
  alkaline (caustic) (external) (internal) — *see* Corrosion, by site
  ankle T25.019
    first degree T25.119
    left T25.012
      first degree T25.112
      second degree T25.212
      third degree T25.312
    multiple with foot — *see* Burn, lower, limb, multiple, ankle and foot
    right T25.011
      first degree T25.111
      second degree T25.211
      third degree T25.311
    second degree T25.219
    third degree T25.319
  anus — *see* Burn, buttock
  arm (lower) (upper) — *see* Burn, upper, limb
  axilla T22.049
    first degree T22.149
    left T22.042
      first degree T22.142
      second degree T22.242
      third degree T22.342
    right T22.041
      first degree T22.141
      second degree T22.241
      third degree T22.341
    second degree T22.249
    third degree T22.349
  back (lower) T21.04
    first degree T21.14
    second degree T21.24
    third degree T21.34

Burn (electricity) (flame) (hot gas, liquid or hot object) (radiation) (steam) (thermal) T30.0 — *continued*
  back (lower) T21.04 — *continued*
    upper T21.03
      first degree T21.13
      second degree T21.23
      third degree T21.33
  blisters — *code as* Burn, second degree, by site
  breast(s) — *see* Burn, chest wall
  buttock(s) T21.05
    first degree T21.15
    second degree T21.25
    third degree T21.35
  calf T24.039
    first degree T24.139
    left T24.032
      first degree T24.132
      second degree T24.232
      third degree T24.332
    right T24.031
      first degree T24.131
      second degree T24.231
      third degree T24.331
    second degree T24.239
    third degree T24.339
  canthus (eye) — *see* Burn, eyelid
  caustic acid or alkaline — *see* Corrosion, by site
  cervix T28.3
  cheek T20.06
    first degree T20.16
    second degree T20.26
    third degree T20.36
  chemical (acids) (alkalines) (caustics) (external) (internal) — *see* Corrosion, by site
  chest wall T21.01
    first degree T21.11
    second degree T21.21
    third degree T21.31
  chin T20.03
    first degree T20.13
    second degree T20.23
    third degree T20.33
  colon T28.2
  conjunctiva (and cornea) — *see* Burn, cornea
  cornea (and conjunctiva) T26.1-
    chemical — *see* Corrosion, cornea
  corrosion (external) (internal) — *see* Corrosion, by site
  deep necrosis of underlying tissue — *code as* Burn, third degree, by site
  dorsum of hand T23.069
    first degree T23.169
    left T23.062
      first degree T23.162
      second degree T23.262
      third degree T23.362
    right T23.061
      first degree T23.161
      second degree T23.261
      third degree T23.361
    second degree T23.269
    third degree T23.369
  due to ingested chemical agent — *see* Corrosion, by site
  ear (auricle) (external) (canal) T20.01
    first degree T20.11
    second degree T20.21
    third degree T20.31
  elbow T22.029
    first degree T22.129
    left T22.022
      first degree T22.122
      second degree T22.222
      third degree T22.322
    right T22.021
      first degree T22.121
      second degree T22.221
      third degree T22.321
    second degree T22.229
    third degree T22.329
  epidermal loss — *code as* Burn, second degree, by site
  erythema, erythematous — *code as* Burn, first degree, by site
  esophagus T28.1
  extent (percentage of body surface)
    10-19 percent T31.10
      with 0-9 percent third degree burns T31.10
      with 10-19 percent third degree burns T31.11

Burn (electricity) (flame) (hot gas, liquid or hot object) (radiation) (steam) (thermal) T30.0 — *continued*
  extent (percentage of body surface) — *continued*
    20-29 percent T31.20
      with 0-9 percent third degree burns T31.20
      with 10-19 percent third degree burns T31.21
      with 20-29 percent third degree burns T31.22
    30-39 percent T31.30
      with 0-9 percent third degree burns T31.30
      with 10-19 percent third degree burns T31.31
      with 20-29 percent third degree burns T31.32
      with 30-39 percent third degree burns T31.33
    40-49 percent T31.40
      with 0-9 percent third degree burns T31.40
      with 10-19 percent third degree burns T31.41
      with 20-29 percent third degree burns T31.42
      with 30-39 percent third degree burns T31.43
      with 40-49 percent third degree burns T31.44
    50-59 percent T31.50
      with 0-9 percent third degree burns T31.50
      with 10-19 percent third degree burns T31.51
      with 20-29 percent third degree burns T31.52
      with 30-39 percent third degree burns T31.53
      with 40-49 percent third degree burns T31.54
      with 50-59 percent third degree burns T31.55
    60-69 percent T31.60
      with 0-9 percent third degree burns T31.60
      with 10-19 percent third degree burns T31.61
      with 20-29 percent third degree burns T31.62
      with 30-39 percent third degree burns T31.63
      with 40-49 percent third degree burns T31.64
      with 50-59 percent third degree burns T31.65
      with 60-69 percent third degree burns T31.66
    70-79 percent T31.70
      with 0-9 percent third degree burns T31.70
      with 10-19 percent third degree burns T31.71
      with 20-29 percent third degree burns T31.72
      with 30-39 percent third degree burns T31.73
      with 40-49 percent third degree burns T31.74
      with 50-59 percent third degree burns T31.75
      with 60-69 percent third degree burns T31.76
      with 70-79 percent third degree burns T31.77
    80-89 percent T31.80
      with 0-9 percent third degree burns T31.80
      with 10-19 percent third degree burns T31.81
      with 20-29 percent third degree burns T31.82
      with 30-39 percent third degree burns T31.83
      with 40-49 percent third degree burns T31.84
      with 50-59 percent third degree burns T31.85
      with 60-69 percent third degree burns T31.86
      with 70-79 percent third degree burns T31.87
      with 80-89 percent third degree burns T31.88

Burn (electricity) (flame) (hot gas, liquid or hot object) (radiation) (steam) (thermal) T30.0 — continued
  extent (percentage of body surface) — continued
    90 percent or more T31.90
      with 0-9 percent third degree burns T31.90
      with 10-19 percent third degree burns T31.91
      with 20-29 percent third degree burns T31.92
      with 30-39 percent third degree burns T31.93
      with 40-49 percent third degree burns T31.94
      with 50-59 percent third degree burns T31.95
      with 60-69 percent third degree burns T31.96
      with 70-79 percent third degree burns T31.97
      with 80-89 percent third degree burns T31.98
      with 90 percent or more third degree burns T31.99
    less than 10 percent T31.0
  extremity — see Burn, limb
  eye(s) and adnexa T26.4-
    with resulting rupture and destruction of eyeball T26.2-
    conjunctival sac — see Burn, cornea
    cornea — see Burn, cornea
    lid — see Burn, eyelid
    periocular area — see Burn, eyelid
    specified site NEC T26.3-
  eyeball — see Burn, eye
  eyelid(s) T26.0-
    chemical — see Corrosion, eyelid
  face — see Burn, head
  finger T23.029
    first degree T23.129
    left T23.022
      first degree T23.122
      second degree T23.222
      third degree T23.322
    multiple sites (without thumb) T23.039
      with thumb T23.049
        first degree T23.149
        left T23.042
          first degree T23.142
          second degree T23.242
          third degree T23.342
        right T23.041
          first degree T23.141
          second degree T23.241
          third degree T23.341
        second degree T23.249
        third degree T23.349
      first degree T23.139
      left T23.032
        first degree T23.132
        second degree T23.232
        third degree T23.332
      right T23.031
        first degree T23.131
        second degree T23.231
        third degree T23.331
      second degree T23.239
      third degree T23.339
    right T23.021
      first degree T23.121
      second degree T23.221
      third degree T23.321
    second degree T23.229
    third degree T23.329
  flank — see Burn, abdominal wall
  foot T25.029
    first degree T25.129
    left T25.022
      first degree T25.122
      second degree T25.222
      third degree T25.322
    multiple with ankle — see Burn, lower, limb, multiple, ankle and foot
    right T25.021
      first degree T25.121
      second degree T25.221
      third degree T25.321
    second degree T25.229
    third degree T25.329
  forearm T22.019
    first degree T22.119
    left T22.012
      first degree T22.112
      second degree T22.212
      third degree T22.312

Burn (electricity) (flame) (hot gas, liquid or hot object) (radiation) (steam) (thermal) T30.0 — continued
  forearm T22.019 — continued
    right T22.011
      first degree T22.111
      second degree T22.211
      third degree T22.311
    second degree T22.219
    third degree T22.319
  forehead T20.06
    first degree T20.16
    second degree T20.26
    third degree T20.36
  fourth degree — code as Burn, third degree, by site
  friction — see Burn, by site
  from swallowing caustic or corrosive substance NEC — see Corrosion, by site
  full thickness skin loss — code as Burn, third degree, by site
  gastrointestinal tract NEC T28.2
    from swallowing caustic or corrosive substance T28.7
  genital organs
    external
      female T21.07
        first degree T21.17
        second degree T21.27
        third degree T21.37
      male T21.06
        first degree T21.16
        second degree T21.26
        third degree T21.36
    internal T28.3
      from caustic or corrosive substance T28.8
  groin — see Burn, abdominal wall
  hand(s) T23.009
    back — see Burn, dorsum of hand
    finger — see Burn, finger
    first degree T23.109
    left T23.002
      first degree T23.102
      second degree T23.202
      third degree T23.302
    multiple sites with wrist T23.099
      first degree T23.199
      left T23.092
        first degree T23.192
        second degree T23.292
        third degree T23.392
      right T23.091
        first degree T23.191
        second degree T23.291
        third degree T23.391
      second degree T23.299
      third degree T23.399
    palm — see Burn, palm
    right T23.001
      first degree T23.101
      second degree T23.201
      third degree T23.301
    second degree T23.209
    third degree T23.309
    thumb — see Burn, thumb
  head (and face) (and neck) T20.00
    cheek — see Burn, cheek
    chin — see Burn, chin
    ear — see Burn, ear
    eye(s) only — see Burn, eye
    first degree T20.10
    forehead — see Burn, forehead
    lip — see Burn, lip
    multiple sites T20.09
      first degree T20.19
      second degree T20.29
      third degree T20.39
    neck — see Burn, neck
    nose — see Burn, nose
    scalp — see Burn, scalp
    second degree T20.20
    third degree T20.30
  hip(s) — see Burn, lower, limb
  inhalation — see Burn, respiratory tract
    caustic or corrosive substance (fumes) — see Corrosion, respiratory tract
  internal organ(s) T28.40
    alimentary tract T28.2
      esophagus T28.1
    eardrum T28.41
    esophagus T28.1
      from caustic or corrosive substance (swallowing) NEC — see Corrosion, by site
    genitourinary T28.3
    mouth T28.0

Burn (electricity) (flame) (hot gas, liquid or hot object) (radiation) (steam) (thermal) T30.0 — continued
  internal organ(s) T28.40 — continued
    pharynx T28.0
    respiratory tract — see Burn, respiratory tract
    specified organ NEC T28.49
  interscapular region — see Burn, back, upper
  intestine (large) (small) T28.2
  knee T24.029
    first degree T24.129
    left T24.022
      first degree T24.122
      second degree T24.222
      third degree T24.322
    right T24.021
      first degree T24.121
      second degree T24.221
      third degree T24.321
    second degree T24.229
    third degree T24.329
  labium (majus) (minus) — see Burn, genital organs, external, female
  lacrimal apparatus, duct, gland or sac — see Burn, eye, specified site NEC
  larynx T27.0
    with lung T27.1
  leg(s) (lower) (upper) — see Burn, lower, limb
  lightning — see Burn, by site
  limb(s)
    lower (except ankle or foot alone) — see Burn, lower, limb
    upper — see Burn, upper limb
  lip(s) T20.02
    first degree T20.12
    second degree T20.22
    third degree T20.32
  lower
    back — see Burn, back
    limb T24.009
      ankle — see Burn, ankle
      calf — see Burn, calf
      first degree T24.109
      foot — see Burn, foot
      hip — see Burn, thigh
      knee — see Burn, knee
      left T24.002
        first degree T24.102
        second degree T24.202
        third degree T24.302
      multiple sites, except ankle and foot T24.099
        ankle and foot T25.099
          first degree T25.199
          left T25.092
            first degree T25.192
            second degree T25.292
            third degree T25.392
          right T25.091
            first degree T25.191
            second degree T25.291
            third degree T25.391
          second degree T25.299
          third degree T25.399
        first degree T24.199
        left T24.092
          first degree T24.192
          second degree T24.292
          third degree T24.392
        right T24.091
          first degree T24.191
          second degree T24.291
          third degree T24.391
        second degree T24.299
        third degree T24.399
      right T24.001
        first degree T24.101
        second degree T24.201
        third degree T24.301
      second degree T24.209
      thigh — see Burn, thigh
      third degree T24.309
      toe — see Burn, toe
  lung (with larynx and trachea) T27.1
  mouth T28.0
  neck T20.07
    first degree T20.17
    second degree T20.27
    third degree T20.37
  nose (septum) T20.04
    first degree T20.14
    second degree T20.24
    third degree T20.34
  ocular adnexa — see Burn, eye
  orbit region — see Burn, eyelid
  palm T23.059
    first degree T23.159

Burn (electricity) (flame) (hot gas, liquid or hot object) (radiation) (steam) (thermal) T30.0 — continued
  palm T23.059 — continued
    left T23.052
      first degree T23.152
      second degree T23.252
      third degree T23.352
    right T23.051
      first degree T23.151
      second degree T23.251
      third degree T23.351
    second degree T23.259
    third degree T23.359
  partial thickness — code as Burn, unspecified degree, by site
  pelvis — see Burn, trunk
  penis — see Burn, genital organs, external, male
  perineum
    female — see Burn, genital organs, external, female
    male — see Burn, genital organs, external, male
  periocular area — see Burn, eyelid
  pharynx T28.0
  rectum T28.2
  respiratory tract T27.3
    larynx — see Burn, larynx
    specified part NEC T27.2
    trachea — see Burn, trachea
  sac, lacrimal — see Burn, eye, specified site NEC
  scalp T20.05
    first degree T20.15
    second degree T20.25
    third degree T20.35
  scapular region T22.069
    first degree T22.169
    left T22.062
      first degree T22.162
      second degree T22.262
      third degree T22.362
    right T22.061
      first degree T22.161
      second degree T22.261
      third degree T22.361
    second degree T22.269
    third degree T22.369
  sclera — see Burn, eye, specified site NEC
  scrotum — see Burn, genital organs, external, male
  shoulder T22.059
    first degree T22.159
    left T22.052
      first degree T22.152
      second degree T22.252
      third degree T22.352
    right T22.051
      first degree T22.151
      second degree T22.251
      third degree T22.351
    second degree T22.259
    third degree T22.359
  stomach T28.2
  temple — see Burn, head
  testis — see Burn, genital organs, external, male
  thigh T24.019
    first degree T24.119
    left T24.012
      first degree T24.112
      second degree T24.212
      third degree T24.312
    right T24.011
      first degree T24.111
      second degree T24.211
      third degree T24.311
    second degree T24.219
    third degree T24.319
  thorax (external) — see Burn, trunk
  throat (meaning pharynx) T28.0
  thumb(s) T23.019
    first degree T23.119
    left T23.012
      first degree T23.112
      second degree T23.212
      third degree T23.312
    multiple sites with fingers T23.049
      first degree T23.149
      left T23.042
        first degree T23.142
        second degree T23.242
        third degree T23.342
      right T23.041
        first degree T23.141
        second degree T23.241
        third degree T23.341
      second degree T23.249
      third degree T23.349

DISEASE INDEX

Burn (electricity) (flame) (hot gas, liquid or hot object) (radiation) (steam) (thermal) T30.0 — continued
- thumb(s) T23.019 — continued
  - right T23.011
    - first degree T23.111
    - second degree T23.211
    - third degree T23.311
  - second degree T23.219
  - third degree T23.319
- toe T25.039
  - first degree T25.139
  - left T25.032
    - first degree T25.132
    - second degree T25.232
    - third degree T25.332
  - right T25.031
    - first degree T25.131
    - second degree T25.231
    - third degree T25.331
  - second degree T25.239
  - third degree T25.339
- tongue T28.0
- tonsil(s) T28.0
- trachea T27.0
  - with lung T27.1
- trunk T21.00
  - abdominal wall — see Burn, abdominal wall
  - anus — see Burn, buttock
  - axilla — see Burn, upper limb
  - back — see Burn, back
  - breast — see Burn, chest wall
  - buttock — see Burn, buttock
  - chest wall — see Burn, chest wall
  - first degree T21.10
  - flank — see Burn, abdominal wall
  - genital
    - female — see Burn, genital organs, external, female
    - male — see Burn, genital organs, external, male
  - groin — see Burn, abdominal wall
  - interscapular region — see Burn, back, upper
  - labia — see Burn, genital organs, external, female
  - lower back — see Burn, back
  - penis — see Burn, genital organs, external, male
  - perineum
    - female — see Burn, genital organs, external, female
    - male — see Burn, genital organs, external, male
  - scapula region — see Burn, scapular region
  - scrotum — see Burn, genital organs, external, male
  - second degree T21.20
  - specified site NEC T21.09
    - first degree T21.19
    - second degree T21.29
    - third degree T21.39
  - testes — see Burn, genital organs, external, male
  - third degree T21.30
  - upper back — see Burn, back, upper
  - vulva — see Burn, genital organs, external, female
- unspecified site with extent of body surface involved specified
  - 10-19 per cent (0-9 percent third degree) T31.10
    - with 10-19 percent third degree T31.11
  - 20-29 per cent (0-9 percent third degree) T31.20
    - with
      - 10-19 percent third degree T31.21
      - 20-29 percent third degree T31.22
  - 30-39 per cent (0-9 percent third degree) T31.30
    - with
      - 10-19 percent third degree T31.31
      - 20-29 percent third degree T31.32
      - 30-39 percent third degree T31.33
  - 40-49 per cent (0-9 percent third degree) T31.40
    - with
      - 10-19 percent third degree T31.41
      - 20-29 percent third degree T31.42
      - 30-39 percent third degree T31.43
      - 40-49 percent third degree T31.44

Burn (electricity) (flame) (hot gas, liquid or hot object) (radiation) (steam) (thermal) T30.0 — continued
- unspecified site with extent of body surface involved specified — continued
  - 50-59 per cent (0-9 percent third degree) T31.50
    - with
      - 10-19 percent third degree T31.51
      - 20-29 percent third degree T31.52
      - 30-39 percent third degree T31.53
      - 40-49 percent third degree T31.54
      - 50-59 percent third degree T31.55
  - 60-69 per cent (0-9 percent third degree) T31.60
    - with
      - 10-19 percent third degree T31.61
      - 20-29 percent third degree T31.62
      - 30-39 percent third degree T31.63
      - 40-49 percent third degree T31.64
      - 50-59 percent third degree T31.65
      - 60-69 percent third degree T31.66
  - 70-79 per cent (0-9 percent third degree) T31.70
    - with
      - 10-19 percent third degree T31.71
      - 20-29 percent third degree T31.72
      - 30-39 percent third degree T31.73
      - 40-49 percent third degree T31.74
      - 50-59 percent third degree T31.75
      - 60-69 percent third degree T31.76
      - 70-79 percent third degree T31.77
  - 80-89 per cent (0-9 percent third degree) T31.80
    - with
      - 10-19 percent third degree T31.81
      - 20-29 percent third degree T31.82
      - 30-39 percent third degree T31.83
      - 40-49 percent third degree T31.84
      - 50-59 percent third degree T31.85
      - 60-69 percent third degree T31.86
      - 70-79 percent third degree T31.87
      - 80-89 percent third degree T31.88
  - 90 per cent or more (0-9 percent third degree) T31.90
    - with
      - 10-19 percent third degree T31.91
      - 20-29 percent third degree T31.92
      - 30-39 percent third degree T31.93
      - 40-49 percent third degree T31.94
      - 50-59 percent third degree T31.95
      - 60-69 percent third degree T31.96
      - 70-79 percent third degree T31.97
      - 80-89 percent third degree T31.98
      - 90-99 percent third degree T31.99
  - less than 10 per cent T31.0
- upper limb T22.00
  - above elbow — see Burn, above elbow
  - axilla — see Burn, axilla
  - elbow — see Burn, elbow
  - first degree T22.10
  - forearm — see Burn, forearm
  - hand — see Burn, hand
  - interscapular region — see Burn, back, upper
  - multiple sites T22.099
    - first degree T22.199
    - left T22.092
      - first degree T22.192
      - second degree T22.292
      - third degree T22.392
    - right T22.091
      - first degree T22.191
      - second degree T22.291
      - third degree T22.391
    - second degree T22.299
    - third degree T22.399
  - scapular region — see Burn, scapular region
  - second degree T22.20
  - shoulder — see Burn, shoulder
  - third degree T22.30
  - wrist — see Burn, wrist
- uterus T28.3
- vagina T28.3
- vulva — see Burn, genital organs, external, female
- wrist T23.079
  - first degree T23.179
  - left T23.072
    - first degree T23.172
    - second degree T23.272
    - third degree T23.372
  - multiple sites with hand T23.099
    - first degree T23.199
    - left T23.092
      - first degree T23.192
      - second degree T23.292
      - third degree T23.392

Burn (electricity) (flame) (hot gas, liquid or hot object) (radiation) (steam) (thermal) T30.0 — continued
- wrist T23.079 — continued
  - multiple sites with hand T23.099 — continued
    - right T23.091
      - first degree T23.191
      - second degree T23.291
      - third degree T23.391
    - second degree T23.299
    - third degree T23.399
  - right T23.071
    - first degree T23.171
    - second degree T23.271
    - third degree T23.371
  - second degree T23.279
  - third degree T23.379

Burnett's syndrome E83.52
Burn-out (state) Z73.0
Burning
- feet syndrome E53.9
- sensation R20.8
- tongue K14.6

Burns' disease or osteochondrosis — see Osteochondrosis, juvenile, ulna
Bursa — see condition
Bursitis M71.9
- Achilles — see Tendinitis, Achilles
- adhesive — see Bursitis, specified NEC
- ankle — see Enthesopathy, lower limb, ankle, specified type NEC
- calcaneal — see Enthesopathy, foot, specified type NEC
- collateral ligament, tibial — see Bursitis, tibial collateral
- due to use, overuse, pressure — see also Disorder, soft tissue, due to use, specified type NEC
  - specified NEC — see Disorder, soft tissue, due to use, specified NEC
- Duplay's M75.0
- elbow NEC M70.3-
  - olecranon M70.2-
- finger — see Disorder, soft tissue, due to use, specified type NEC, hand
- foot — see Enthesopathy, foot, specified type NEC
- gonococcal A54.49
- gouty — see Gout, idiopathic
- hand M70.1-
- hip NEC M70.7-
  - trochanteric M70.6-
- infective NEC M71.10
  - abscess — see Abscess, bursa
  - ankle M71.17-
  - elbow M71.12-
  - foot M71.17-
  - hand M71.14-
  - hip M71.15-
  - knee M71.16-
  - multiple sites M71.19
  - shoulder M71.11-
  - specified site NEC M71.18
  - wrist M71.13-
- ischial — see Bursitis, hip
- knee NEC M70.5-
  - prepatellar M70.4-
- occupational NEC — see also Disorder, soft tissue, due to, use
- olecranon — see Bursitis, elbow, olecranon
- pharyngeal J39.1
- popliteal — see Bursitis, knee
- prepatellar M70.4-
- radiohumeral M77.8
- rheumatoid M06.20
  - ankle M06.27-
  - elbow M06.22-
  - foot joint M06.27-
  - hand joint M06.24-
  - hip M06.25-
  - knee M06.26-
  - multiple site M06.29
  - shoulder M06.21-
  - vertebra M06.28
  - wrist M06.23-
- scapulohumeral — see Bursitis, shoulder
- semimembranous muscle (knee) — see Bursitis, knee
- shoulder M75.5-
  - adhesive — see Capsulitis, adhesive
- specified NEC M71.50
  - ankle M71.57-
  - due to use, overuse or pressure — see Disorder, soft tissue, due to, use
  - elbow M71.52-
  - foot M71.57-
  - hand M71.54-

Bursitis M71.9 — continued
- specified NEC M71.50 — continued
  - hip M71.55-
  - knee M71.56-
  - shoulder — see Bursitis, shoulder
  - specified site NEC M71.58
  - tibial collateral M76.4-
  - wrist M71.53-
- subacromial — see Bursitis, shoulder
- subcoracoid — see Bursitis, shoulder
- subdeltoid — see Bursitis, shoulder
- syphilitic A52.78
- Thornwaldt, Tornwaldt J39.2
- tibial collateral — see Bursitis, tibial collateral
- toe — see Enthesopathy, foot, specified type NEC
- trochanteric (area) — see Bursitis, hip, trochanteric
- wrist — see Bursitis, hand

Bursopathy M71.9
- specified type NEC M71.80
  - ankle M71.87-
  - elbow M71.82-
  - foot M71.87-
  - hand M71.84-
  - hip M71.85-
  - knee M71.86-
  - multiple sites M71.89
  - shoulder M71.81-
  - specified site NEC M71.88
  - wrist M71.83-

Burst stitches or sutures (complication of surgery) T81.31
- external operation wound T81.31
- internal operation wound T81.32

Buruli ulcer A31.1
Bury's disease L95.1
Buschke's
- disease B45.3
- scleredema — see Sclerosis, systemic

Busse-Buschke disease B45.3
Buttock — see condition
Button
- Biskra B55.1
- Delhi B55.1
- oriental B55.1

Buttonhole deformity (finger) — see Deformity, finger, boutonniere
Bwamba fever A92.8
Byssinosis J66.0
Bywaters' syndrome T79.5

C

D I S E A S E   I N D E X

Cachexia R64
- cancerous R64
- cardiac — *see* Disease, heart
- dehydration E86.0
  - with
    - hypernatremia E87.0
    - hyponatremia E87.1
- due to malnutrition R64
- exophthalmic — *see* Hyperthyroidism
- heart — *see* Disease, heart
- hypophyseal E23.0
- hypopituitary E23.0
- lead — *see* Poisoning, lead
- malignant R64
- marsh — *see* Malaria
- nervous F48.8
- old age R54
- paludal — *see* Malaria
- pituitary E23.0
- renal N28.9
- saturnine — *see* Poisoning, lead
- senile R54
- Simmonds' E23.0
- splenica D73.0
- strumipriva E03.4
- tuberculous NEC — *see* Tuberculosis

Café, au lait spots L81.3
Caffey's syndrome Q78.8
Caisson disease T70.3
Cake kidney Q63.1
Caked breast (puerperal, postpartum) O92.79
Calabar swelling B74.3
Calcaneal spur — *see* Spur, bone, calcaneal
Calcaneo-apophysitis M92.8
Calcareous — *see* condition
Calcicosis J62.8
Calciferol (vitamin D) deficiency E55.9
- with rickets E55.0

Calcification
- adrenal (capsule) (gland) E27.49
  - tuberculous E35 [B90.8]
- aorta I70.0
- artery (annular) — *see* Arteriosclerosis
- auricle (ear) — *see* Disorder, pinna, specified type NEC
- basal ganglia G23.8
- bladder N32.89
  - due to Schistosoma hematobium B65.0
- brain (cortex) — *see* Calcification, cerebral
- bronchus J98.09
- bursa M71.40
  - ankle M71.47-
  - elbow M71.42-
  - foot M71.47-
  - hand M71.44-
  - hip M71.45-
  - knee M71.46-
  - multiple sites M71.49
  - shoulder M75.3-
  - specified site NEC M71.48
  - wrist M71.43-
- cardiac — *see* Degeneration, myocardial
- cerebral (cortex) G93.89
  - artery I67.2
- cervix (uteri) N88.8
- choroid plexus G93.89
- conjunctiva — *see* Concretion, conjunctiva
- corpora cavernosa (penis) N48.89
- cortex (brain) — *see* Calcification, cerebral
- dental pulp (nodular) K04.2
- dentinal papilla K00.4
- fallopian tube N83.8
- falx cerebri G96.19
- gallbladder K82.8
- general E83.59
- heart — *see* Degeneration, myocardial
  - valve — *see* Endocarditis
- idiopathic infantile arterial (IIAC) Q28.8
- intervertebral cartilage or disc (postinfective) — *see* Disorder, disc, specified NEC
- intracranial — *see* Calcification, cerebral
- joint — *see* Disorder, joint, specified type NEC
- kidney N28.89
  - tuberculous N29 [B90.1]
- larynx (senile) J38.7
- lens — *see* Cataract, specified NEC
- lung (active) (postinfectional) J98.4
  - tuberculous B90.9

Calcification — *continued*
- lymph gland or node (postinfectional) I89.8
  - tuberculous (*see also* Tuberculosis, lymph gland) B90.8
- mammographic R92.1
- massive (paraplegic) — *see* Myositis, ossificans, in, quadriplegia
- medial — *see* Arteriosclerosis, extremities
- meninges (cerebral) (spinal) G96.19
- metastatic E83.59
- muscle M61.9
  - due to burns — *see* Myositis, ossificans, in, burns
  - paralytic — *see* Myositis, ossificans, in, quadriplegia
  - specified type NEC M61.40
    - ankle M61.47-
    - foot M61.47-
    - forearm M61.43-
    - hand M61.44-
    - lower leg M61.46-
    - multiple sites M61.49
    - pelvic region M61.45-
    - shoulder region M61.41-
    - specified site NEC M61.48
    - thigh M61.45-
    - upper arm M61.42-
- myocardium, myocardial — *see* Degeneration, myocardial
- Mönckeberg's — *see* Arteriosclerosis, extremities
- ovary N83.8
- pancreas K86.8
- penis N48.89
- periarticular — *see* Disorder, joint, specified type NEC
- pericardium (*see also* Pericarditis) I31.1
- pineal gland E34.8
- pleura J94.8
  - postinfectional J94.8
  - tuberculous NEC B90.9
- pulpal (dental) (nodular) K04.2
- sclera H15.89
- spleen D73.89
- subcutaneous L94.2
- suprarenal (capsule) (gland) E27.49
- tendon (sheath) — *see also* Tenosynovitis, specified type NEC
  - with bursitis, synovitis or tenosynovitis — *see* Tendinitis, calcific
- trachea J39.8
- ureter N28.89
- vitreous — *see* Deposit, crystalline

Calcified — *see* Calcification
Calcinosis (interstitial) (tumoral) (universalis) E83.59
- with Raynaud's phenomenon, esophageal dysfunction, sclerodactyly, telangiectasia (CREST syndrome) M34.1
- circumscripta (skin) L94.2
- cutis L94.2

Calciphylaxis (*see also* Calcification, by site) E83.59
Calcium
- deposits — *see* Calcification, by site
- metabolism disorder E83.50
- salts or soaps in vitreous — *see* Deposit, crystalline

Calciuria R82.99
Calculi — *see* Calculus
Calculosis, intrahepatic — *see* Calculus, bile duct
Calculus, calculi, calculous
- ampulla of Vater — *see* Calculus, bile duct
- anuria (impacted) (recurrent) (*see also* Calculus, urinary) N20.9
- appendix K38.1
- bile duct (common) (hepatic) K80.50
  - with
    - calculus of gallbladder — *see* Calculus, gallbladder and bile duct
    - cholangitis K80.30
      - with
        - cholecystitis — *see* Calculus, bile duct, with cholecystitis
        - obstruction K80.31
      - acute K80.32
        - with
          - chronic cholangitis K80.36
            - with obstruction K80.37
          - obstruction K80.33
      - chronic K80.34
        - with
          - acute cholangitis K80.36
            - with obstruction K80.37
          - obstruction K80.35

Calculus, calculi, calculous — *continued*
- bile duct (common) (hepatic) K80.50 — *continued*
  - with — *continued*
    - cholecystitis (with cholangitis) K80.40
      - with obstruction K80.41
      - acute K80.42
        - with
          - chronic cholecystitis K80.46
            - with obstruction K80.47
          - obstruction K80.43
      - chronic K80.44
        - with
          - acute cholecystitis K80.46
            - with obstruction K80.47
          - obstruction K80.45
    - obstruction K80.51
  - biliary — *see also* Calculus, gallbladder
    - specified NEC K80.80
      - with obstruction K80.81
  - bilirubin, multiple — *see* Calculus, gallbladder
  - bladder (encysted) (impacted) (urinary) (diverticulum) N21.0
  - bronchus J98.09
  - calyx (kidney) (renal) — *see* Calculus, kidney
  - cholesterol (pure) (solitary) — *see* Calculus, gallbladder
  - common duct (bile) — *see* Calculus, bile duct
  - conjunctiva — *see* Concretion, conjunctiva
  - cystic N21.0
    - duct — *see* Calculus, gallbladder
  - dental (subgingival) (supragingival) K03.6
  - diverticulum
    - bladder N21.0
    - kidney N20.0
  - epididymis N50.8
  - gallbladder K80.20
    - with
      - bile duct calculus — *see* Calculus, gallbladder and bile duct
      - cholecystitis K80.10
        - with obstruction K80.11
        - acute K80.00
          - with
            - chronic cholecystitis K80.12
              - with obstruction K80.13
            - obstruction K80.01
        - chronic K80.10
          - with
            - acute cholecystitis K80.12
              - with obstruction K80.13
            - obstruction K80.11
      - specified NEC K80.18
        - with obstruction K80.19
    - obstruction K80.21
  - gallbladder and bile duct K80.70
    - with
      - cholecystitis K80.60
        - with obstruction K80.61
        - acute K80.62
          - with
            - chronic cholecystitis K80.66
              - with obstruction K80.67
            - obstruction K80.63
        - chronic K80.64
          - with
            - acute cholecystitis K80.66
              - with obstruction K80.67
            - obstruction K80.65
      - obstruction K80.71
  - hepatic (duct) — *see* Calculus, bile duct
  - hepatobiliary K80.80
    - with obstruction K80.81
  - ileal conduit N21.8
  - intestinal (impaction) (obstruction) K56.49
  - kidney (impacted) (multiple) (pelvis) (recurrent) (staghorn) N20.0
    - with calculus, ureter N20.2
    - congenital Q63.8
  - lacrimal passages — *see* Dacryolith
  - liver (impacted) — *see* Calculus, bile duct
  - lung J98.4
  - mammographic R92.1
  - nephritic (impacted) (recurrent) — *see* Calculus, kidney
  - nose J34.89
  - pancreas (duct) K86.8
  - parotid duct or gland K11.5
  - pelvis, encysted — *see* Calculus, kidney
  - prostate N42.0
  - pulmonary J98.4
  - pyelitis (impacted) (recurrent) N20.0
    - with hydronephrosis N13.2
  - pyelonephritis (impacted) (recurrent) — *see* category N20
    - with hydronephrosis N13.2

Calculus, calculi, calculous — *continued*
- renal (impacted) (recurrent) — *see* Calculus, kidney
- salivary (duct) (gland) K11.5
- seminal vesicle N50.8
- staghorn — *see* Calculus, kidney
- Stensen's duct K11.5
- stomach K31.89
- sublingual duct or gland K11.5
  - congenital Q38.4
- submandibular duct, gland or region K11.5
- submaxillary duct, gland or region K11.5
- suburethral N21.8
- tonsil J35.8
- tooth, teeth (subgingival) (supragingival) K03.6
- tunica vaginalis N50.8
- ureter (impacted) (recurrent) N20.1
  - with calculus, kidney N20.2
    - with hydronephrosis N13.2
      - with infection N13.6
- urethra (impacted) N21.1
- urinary (duct) (impacted) (passage) (tract) N20.9
  - with hydronephrosis N13.2
    - with infection N13.6
  - in (due to)
    - lower N21.9
      - specified NEC N21.8
  - vagina N89.8
  - vesical (impacted) N21.0
  - Wharton's duct K11.5
  - xanthine E79.8 [N22]

Calicectasis N28.89
Caliectasis N28.89
California
- disease B38.9
- encephalitis A83.5

Caligo cornea — *see* Opacity, cornea, central
Callositas, callosity (infected) L84
Callus (infected) L84
- bone — *see* Osteophyte
  - excessive, following fracture — *code as* Sequelae of fracture

Calorie deficiency or malnutrition (*see also* Malnutrition) E46
Calvities — *see* Alopecia, androgenic
Calvé-Perthes disease — *see* Legg-Calvé-Perthes disease
Calvé's disease — *see* Osteochondrosis, juvenile, spine
Cameroon fever — *see* Malaria
Camptocormia (hysterical) F44.4
Camurati-Engelmann syndrome Q78.3
Canal — *see also* condition
- atrioventricular common Q21.2

Canaliculitis (lacrimal) (acute) (subacute) H04.33-
- Actinomyces A42.89
- chronic H04.42-

Canavan's disease E75.29
Canceled procedure (surgical) Z53.9
- because of
  - contraindication Z53.09
    - smoking Z53.01
  - left against medical advice (AMA) Z53.21
  - patient's decision Z53.20
    - for reasons of belief or group pressure Z53.1
    - specified reason NEC Z53.29
  - specified reason NEC Z53.8

Cancer — *see also* Neoplasm, by site, malignant
- bile duct type liver C22.1
- blood — *see* Leukemia
- breast (*see also* Neoplasm, breast, malignant) C50.91-
- hepatocellular C22.0
- lung (*see also* Neoplasm, lung, malignant) C34.90-
- ovarian (*see also* Neoplasm ovary, malignant) C56.9-
- unspecified site (primary) C80.1

Cancer (o)phobia F45.29
Cancerous — *see* Neoplasm, malignant, by site
Cancrum oris A69.0
Candidiasis, candidal B37.9
- balanitis B37.42
- bronchitis B37.1
- cheilitis B37.83
- congenital P37.5
- cystitis B37.41
- disseminated B37.7
- endocarditis B37.6
- enteritis B37.82

Candidiasis, candidal B37.9 — *continued*
  esophagitis B37.81
  intertrigo B37.2
  lung B37.1
  meningitis B37.5
  mouth B37.0
  nails B37.2
  neonatal P37.5
  onychia B37.2
  oral B37.0
  osteomyelitis B37.89
  otitis externa B37.84
  paronychia B37.2
  perionyxis B37.2
  pneumonia B37.1
  proctitis B37.82
  pulmonary B37.1
  pyelonephritis B37.49
  sepsis B37.7
  skin B37.2
  specified site NEC B37.89
  stomatitis B37.0
  systemic B37.7
  urethritis B37.41
  urogenital site NEC B37.49
  vagina B37.3
  vulva B37.3
  vulvovaginitis B37.3
Candidid L30.2
Candidosis — *see* Candidiasis
Candiru infection or infestation B88.8
Canities (premature) L67.1
  congenital Q84.2
Canker (mouth) (sore) K12.0
  rash A38.9
Cannabinosis J66.2
Canton fever A75.9
Cantrell's syndrome Q87.89
Capillariasis (intestinal) B81.1
  hepatic B83.8
Capillary — *see* condition
Caplan's syndrome — *see* Rheumatoid, lung
Capsule — *see* condition
Capsulitis (joint) — *see also* Enthesopathy
  adhesive (shoulder) M75.0-
  hepatic K65.8
  labyrinthine — *see* Otosclerosis, specified NEC
  thyroid E06.9
Caput
  crepitus Q75.8
  medusae I86.8
  succedaneum P12.81
Car sickness T75.3
Carapata (disease) A68.0
Carate — *see* Pinta
Carbon lung J60
Carbuncle L02.93
  abdominal wall L02.231
  anus K61.0
  auditory canal, external — *see* Abscess, ear, external
  auricle ear — *see* Abscess, ear, external
  axilla L02.43-
  back (any part) L02.232
  breast N61
  buttock L02.33
  cheek (external) L02.03
  chest wall L02.233
  chin L02.03
  corpus cavernosum N48.21
  ear (any part) (external) (middle) — *see* Abscess, ear, external
  external auditory canal — *see* Abscess, ear, external
  eyelid — *see* Abscess, eyelid
  face NEC L02.03
  femoral (region) — *see* Carbuncle, lower limb
  finger — *see* Carbuncle, hand
  flank L02.231
  foot L02.63-
  forehead L02.03
  genital — *see* Abscess, genital
  gluteal (region) L02.33
  groin L02.234
  hand L02.53-
  head NEC L02.831
  heel — *see* Carbuncle, foot
  hip — *see* Carbuncle, lower limb
  kidney — *see* Abscess, kidney
  knee — *see* Carbuncle, lower limb
  labium (majus) (minus) N76.4
  lacrimal
    gland — *see* Dacryoadenitis
    passages (duct) (sac) — *see* Inflammation, lacrimal, passages, acute

Carbuncle L02.93 — *continued*
  leg — *see* Carbuncle, lower limb
  lower limb L02.43-
  malignant A22.0
  navel L02.236
  neck L02.13
  nose (external) (septum) J34.0
  orbit, orbital — *see* Abscess, orbit
  palmar (space) — *see* Carbuncle, hand
  partes posteriores L02.33
  pectoral region L02.233
  penis N48.21
  perineum L02.235
  pinna — *see* Abscess, ear, external
  popliteal — *see* Carbuncle, lower limb
  scalp L02.831
  seminal vesicle N49.0
  shoulder — *see* Carbuncle, upper limb
  specified site NEC L02.838
  temple (region) L02.03
  thumb — *see* Carbuncle, hand
  toe — *see* Carbuncle, foot
  trunk L02.239
    abdominal wall L02.231
    back L02.232
    chest wall L02.233
    groin L02.234
    perineum L02.235
    umbilicus L02.236
  umbilicus L02.236
  upper limb L02.43-
  urethra N34.0
  vulva N76.4
Carbunculus — *see* Carbuncle
Carcinoid (tumor) — *see* Tumor, carcinoid
Carcinoidosis E34.0
Carcinoma (malignant) — *see also* Neoplasm, by site, malignant
  acidophil
    specified site — *see* Neoplasm, malignant, by site
    unspecified site C75.1
  acidophil-basophil, mixed
    specified site — *see* Neoplasm, malignant, by site
    unspecified site C75.1
  adnexal (skin) — *see* Neoplasm, skin, malignant
  adrenal cortical C74.0-
  alveolar — *see* Neoplasm, lung, malignant
    cell — *see* Neoplasm, lung, malignant
  ameloblastic C41.1
    upper jaw (bone) C41.0
  apocrine
    breast — *see* Neoplasm, breast, malignant
    specified site NEC — *see* Neoplasm, skin, malignant
    unspecified site C44.99
  basal cell (pigmented) (*see also* Neoplasm, skin, malignant) C44.91
    fibro-epithelial — *see* Neoplasm, skin, malignant
    morphea — *see* Neoplasm, skin, malignant
    multicentric — *see* Neoplasm, skin, malignant
  basal-squamous cell, mixed — *see* Neoplasm, skin, malignant
  basaloid
  basophil
    specified site — *see* Neoplasm, malignant, by site
    unspecified site C75.1
  basophil-acidophil, mixed
    specified site — *see* Neoplasm, malignant, by site
    unspecified site C75.1
  basosquamous — *see* Neoplasm, skin, malignant
  bile duct
    with hepatocellular, mixed C22.0
    liver C22.1
    specified site NEC — *see* Neoplasm, malignant, by site
    unspecified site C22.1
  branchial or branchiogenic C10.4
  bronchial or bronchogenic — *see* Neoplasm, lung, malignant
  bronchiolar — *see* Neoplasm, lung, malignant
  bronchioloalveolar — *see* Neoplasm, lung, malignant
  C cell
    specified site — *see* Neoplasm, malignant, by site
    unspecified site C73

Carcinoma (malignant) (*see also* Neoplasm, by site, malignant) — *continued*
  ceruminous C44.29-
  cervix uteri
    in situ D06.9
      endocervix D06.0
      exocervix D06.1
      specified site NEC D06.7
  chorionic
    specified site — *see* Neoplasm, malignant, by site
    unspecified site
      female C58
      male C62.90
  chromophobe
    specified site — *see* Neoplasm, malignant, by site
    unspecified site C75.1
  cloacogenic
    specified site — *see* Neoplasm, malignant, by site
    unspecified site C21.2
  diffuse type
    specified site — *see* Neoplasm, malignant, by site
    unspecified site C16.9
  duct (cell)
    with Paget's disease — *see* Neoplasm, breast, malignant
    infiltrating
      with lobular carcinoma (in situ)
        specified site — *see* Neoplasm, malignant, by site
        unspecified site (female) C50.91- male C50.92-
      specified site — *see* Neoplasm, malignant, by site
      unspecified site (female) C50.91- male C50.92-
  ductal
    with lobular
      specified site — *see* Neoplasm, malignant, by site
      unspecified site (female) C50.91- male C50.92-
  ductular, infiltrating
    specified site — *see* Neoplasm, malignant, by site
    unspecified site (female) C50.91- male C50.92-
  embryonal
    liver C22.7
  endometrioid
    specified site — *see* Neoplasm, malignant, by site
    unspecified site
      female C56.9
      male C61
  eosinophil
    specified site — *see* Neoplasm, malignant, by site
    unspecified site C75.1
  epidermoid — *see also* Neoplasm, skin, malignant
    in situ, Bowen's type — *see* Neoplasm, skin, in situ
  fibroepithelial, basal cell — *see* Neoplasm, skin, malignant
  follicular
    with papillary (mixed) C73
    moderately differentiated C73
    pure follicle C73
    specified site — *see* Neoplasm, malignant, by site
    trabecular C73
    unspecified site C73
    well differentiated C73
  generalized, with unspecified primary site C80.0
  glycogen-rich — *see* Neoplasm, breast, malignant
  granulosa cell C56-
  hepatic cell C22.0
  hepatocellular C22.0
    with bile duct, mixed C22.0
    fibrolamellar C22.0
  hepatocholangiolitic C22.0
  Hurthle cell C73
  in
    adenomatous
      polyposis coli C18.9
    pleomorphic adenoma — *see* Neoplasm, salivary glands, malignant
    situ — *see* Carcinoma-in-situ

Carcinoma (malignant) (*see also* Neoplasm, by site, malignant) — *continued*
  infiltrating
    duct
      with lobular
        specified site — *see* Neoplasm, malignant, by site
        unspecified site (female) C50.91- male C50.92-
      with Paget's disease — *see* Neoplasm, breast, malignant
      specified site — *see* Neoplasm, malignant
      unspecified site (female) C50.91- male C50.92-
    ductular
      specified site — *see* Neoplasm, malignant
      unspecified site (female) C50.91- male C50.92-
    lobular
      specified site — *see* Neoplasm, malignant
      unspecified site (female) C50.91- male C50.92-
  inflammatory
    specified site — *see* Neoplasm, malignant
    unspecified site (female) C50.91- male C50.92-
  intestinal type
    specified site — *see* Neoplasm, malignant, by site
    unspecified site C16.9
  intracystic
    noninfiltrating — *see* Neoplasm, in situ, by site
  intraductal (noninfiltrating)
    with Paget's disease — *see* Neoplasm, breast, malignant
    breast D05.1-
    papillary
      with invasion
        specified site — *see* Neoplasm, malignant, by site
        unspecified site (female) C50.91- male C50.92-
      breast D05.1-
      specified site NEC — *see* Neoplasm, in situ, by site
      unspecified site (female) D05.1-
    specified site NEC — *see* Neoplasm, in situ, by site
    unspecified site (female) D05.1-
  intraepidermal — *see* Neoplasm, in situ
    squamous cell, Bowen's type — *see* Neoplasm, skin, in situ
  intraepithelial — *see* Neoplasm, in situ, by site
    squamous cell — *see* Neoplasm, in situ, by site
  intraosseous C41.1
    upper jaw (bone) C41.0
  islet cell
    with exocrine, mixed
      specified site — *see* Neoplasm, malignant, by site
      unspecified site C25.9
    pancreas C25.4
    specified site NEC — *see* Neoplasm, malignant, by site
    unspecified site C25.4
  juvenile, breast — *see* Neoplasm, breast, malignant
  large cell
    small cell
      specified site — *see* Neoplasm, malignant, by site
      unspecified site C34.90
  Leydig cell (testis)
    specified site — *see* Neoplasm, malignant, by site
    unspecified site
      female C56.9
      male C62.90
  lipid-rich (female) C50.91- male C50.92-
  liver cell C22.0
  liver NEC C22.7
  lobular (infiltrating)
    with intraductal
      specified site — *see* Neoplasm, malignant, by site
      unspecified site (female) C50.91- male C50.92-
    noninfiltrating
      breast D05.0-
      specified site NEC — *see* Neoplasm, in situ, by site
      unspecified site D05.0-

Carcinoma (malignant) (*see also* Neoplasm, by site, malignant) — *continued*
　lobular (infiltrating) — *continued*
　　specified site — *see* Neoplasm, malignant, by site
　　unspecified site (female) C50.91-
　　　male C50.92-
　medullary
　　with
　　　amyloid stroma
　　　　specified site — *see* Neoplasm, malignant, by site
　　　　unspecified site C73
　　　lymphoid stroma
　　　　specified site — *see* Neoplasm, malignant, by site
　　　　unspecified site (female) C50.91-
　　　　　male C50.92-
　Merkel cell C4A.9
　　anal margin C4A.51
　　anal skin C4A.51
　　canthus C4A.1-
　　ear and external auricular canal C4A.2-
　　external auricular canal C4A.2-
　　eyelid, including canthus C4A.1-
　　face C4A.30
　　　specified NEC C4A.39
　　hip C4A.7-
　　lip C4A.0
　　lower limb, including hip C4A.7-
　　neck C4A.4
　　nodal presentation C7B.1
　　nose C4A.31
　　overlapping sites C4A.8
　　perianal skin C4A.51
　　scalp C4A.4
　　secondary C7B.1
　　shoulder C4A.6-
　　skin of breast C4A.52
　　trunk NEC C4A.59
　　upper limb, including shoulder C4A.6-
　　visceral metastatic C7B.1
　metastatic — *see* Neoplasm, secondary, by site
　metatypical — *see* Neoplasm, skin, malignant
　morphea, basal cell — *see* Neoplasm, skin, malignant
　mucoid
　　cell
　　　specified site — *see* Neoplasm, malignant, by site
　　　unspecified site C75.1
　neuroendocrine — *see also* Tumor, neuroendocrine
　　high grade, any site C7A.1
　　poorly differentiated, any site C7A.1
　nonencapsulated sclerosing C73
　noninfiltrating
　　intracystic — *see* Neoplasm, in situ, by site
　　intraductal
　　　breast D05.1-
　　　papillary
　　　　breast D05.1-
　　　　specified site NEC — *see* Neoplasm, in situ, by site
　　　　unspecified site D05.1-
　　　specified site — *see* Neoplasm, in situ, by site
　　　unspecified site D05.1-
　　lobular
　　　breast D05.0-
　　　specified site NEC — *see* Neoplasm, in situ, by site
　　　unspecified site (female) D05.0-
　oat cell
　　specified site — *see* Neoplasm, malignant, by site
　　unspecified site C34.90
　odontogenic C41.1
　　upper jaw (bone) C41.0
　papillary
　　with follicular (mixed) C73
　　follicular variant C73
　　intraductal (noninfiltrating)
　　　with invasion
　　　　specified site — *see* Neoplasm, malignant, by site
　　　　unspecified site (female) C50.91-
　　　　　male C50.92-
　　　breast D05.1-
　　　specified site NEC — *see* Neoplasm, in situ, by site
　　　unspecified site D05.1-

Carcinoma (malignant) (*see also* Neoplasm, by site, malignant) — *continued*
　papillary — *continued*
　　serous
　　　specified site — *see* Neoplasm, malignant, by site
　　　surface
　　　　specified site — *see* Neoplasm, malignant, by site
　　　　unspecified site C56.9
　　　unspecified site C56.9
　　papillocystic
　　　specified site — *see* Neoplasm, malignant, by site
　　　unspecified site C56.9
　parafollicular cell
　　specified site — *see* Neoplasm, malignant, by site
　　unspecified site C73
　pilomatrix — *see* Neoplasm, skin, malignant
　pseudomucinous
　　specified site — *see* Neoplasm, malignant, by site
　　unspecified site C56.9
　renal cell C64-
　Schmincke — *see* Neoplasm, nasopharynx, malignant
　Schneiderian
　　specified site — *see* Neoplasm, malignant, by site
　　unspecified site C30.0
　sebaceous — *see* Neoplasm, skin, malignant
　secondary — *see also* Neoplasm, secondary, by site
　　Merkel cell C7B.1
　secretory, breast — *see* Neoplasm, breast, malignant
　serous
　　papillary
　　　specified site — *see* Neoplasm, malignant, by site
　　　unspecified site C56.9
　　surface, papillary
　　　specified site — *see* Neoplasm, malignant, by site
　　　unspecified site C56.9
　Sertoli cell
　　specified site — *see* Neoplasm, malignant, by site
　　unspecified site C62.90
　　　female C56.9
　　　male C62.90
　skin appendage — *see* Neoplasm, skin, malignant
　small cell
　　fusiform cell
　　　specified site — *see* Neoplasm, malignant, by site
　　　unspecified site C34.90
　　intermediate cell
　　　specified site — *see* Neoplasm, malignant, by site
　　　unspecified site C34.90
　　large cell
　　　specified site — *see* Neoplasm, malignant, by site
　　　unspecified site C34.90
　solid
　　with amyloid stroma
　　　specified site — *see* Neoplasm, malignant, by site
　　　unspecified site C73
　　microinvasive
　　　specified site — *see* Neoplasm, malignant, by site
　　　unspecified site C53.9
　sweat gland — *see* Neoplasm, skin, malignant
　theca cell C56-
　thymic C37
　unspecified site (primary) C80.1
　water-clear cell C75.0

Carcinoma-in-situ — *see also* Neoplasm, in situ, by site
　breast NOS D05.9-
　　specified type NEC D05.8-
　epidermoid — *see also* Neoplasm, in situ, by site
　　with questionable stromal invasion
　　　cervix D06.9
　　specified site NEC — *see* Neoplasm, in situ, by site
　　unspecified site D06.9
　Bowen's type — *see* Neoplasm, skin, in situ

Carcinoma-in-situ (*see also* Neoplasm, in situ, by site) — *continued*
　intraductal
　　breast D05.1-
　　specified site NEC — *see* Neoplasm, in situ, by site
　　unspecified site D05.1-
　lobular
　　with
　　　infiltrating duct
　　　　breast (female) C50.91-
　　　　　male C50.92-
　　　　specified site NEC — *see* Neoplasm, malignant
　　　　unspecified site (female) C50.91-
　　　　　male C50.92-
　　　intraductal
　　　　breast D05.8-
　　　　specified site NEC — *see* Neoplasm, in situ, by site
　　　　unspecified site (female) D05.8-
　　breast D05.0-
　　specified site NEC — *see* Neoplasm, in situ, by site
　　unspecified site D05.0-
　squamous cell — *see also* Neoplasm, in situ, by site
　　with questionable stromal invasion
　　　cervix D06.9
　　specified site NEC — *see* Neoplasm, in situ, by site
　　unspecified site D06.9
Carcinomaphobia F45.29
Carcinomatosis C80.0
　peritonei C78.6
　unspecified site (primary) (secondary) C80.0
Carcinosarcoma — *see* Neoplasm, malignant, by site
　embryonal — *see* Neoplasm, malignant, by site
Cardia, cardial — *see* condition
Cardiac — *see also* condition
　death, sudden — *see* Arrest, cardiac
　pacemaker
　　in situ Z95.0
　　management or adjustment Z45.018
　tamponade I31.4
Cardialgia — *see* Pain, precordial
Cardiectasis — *see* Hypertrophy, cardiac
Cardiochalasia K21.9
Cardiomalacia I51.5
Cardiomegalia glycogenica diffusa E74.02 [I43]
Cardiomegaly — *see also* Hypertrophy, cardiac
　congenital Q24.8
　glycogen E74.02 [I43]
　idiopathic I51.7
Cardiomyoliposis I51.5
Cardiomyopathy (familial) (idiopathic) I42.9
　alcoholic I42.6
　amyloid E85.4 [I43]
　arteriosclerotic — *see* Disease, heart, ischemic, atherosclerotic
　beriberi E51.12
　cobalt-beer I42.6
　congenital I42.4
　congestive I42.0
　constrictive NOS I42.5
　dilated I42.0
　due to
　　alcohol I42.6
　　beriberi E51.12
　　cardiac glycogenosis E74.02 [I43]
　　drugs I42.7
　　external agents NEC I42.7
　　Friedreich's ataxia G11.1
　　myotonia atrophica G71.11 [I43]
　　progressive muscular dystrophy G71.0
　glycogen storage E74.02 [I43]
　hypertensive — *see* Hypertension, heart
　hypertrophic (nonobstructive) I42.2
　　obstructive I42.1
　　　congenital Q24.8
　in
　　Chagas' disease (chronic) B57.2
　　　acute B57.0
　　sarcoidosis D86.85
　ischemic I25.5
　metabolic E88.9 [I43]
　　thyrotoxic E05.90 [I43]
　　　with thyroid storm E05.91 [I43]
　newborn I42.8
　　congenital I42.4

Cardiomyopathy (familial) (idiopathic) I42.9 — *continued*
　nutritional E63.9 [I43]
　　beriberi E51.12
　obscure of Africa I42.8
　peripartum O90.3
　postpartum O90.3
　restrictive NEC I42.5
　rheumatic I09.0
　secondary I42.9
　stress induced I51.81
　takotsubo I51.81
　thyrotoxic E05.90 [I43]
　　with thyroid storm E05.91 [I43]
　toxic NEC I42.7
　tuberculous A18.84
　viral B33.24
Cardionephritis — *see* Hypertension, cardiorenal
Cardionephropathy — *see* Hypertension, cardiorenal
Cardionephrosis — *see* Hypertension, cardiorenal
Cardiopathia nigra I27.0
Cardiopathy (*see also* Disease, heart) I51.9
　idiopathic I42.9
　mucopolysaccharidosis E76.3 [I52]
Cardiopericarditis — *see* Pericarditis
Cardiophobia F45.29
Cardiorenal — *see* condition
Cardiorrhexis — *see* Infarct, myocardium
Cardiosclerosis — *see* Disease, heart, ischemic, atherosclerotic
Cardiosis — *see* Disease, heart
Cardiospasm (esophagus) (reflex) (stomach) K22.0
　congenital Q39.5
　with megaesophagus Q39.5
Cardiostenosis — *see* Disease, heart
Cardiosymphysis I31.0
Cardiovascular — *see* condition
Carditis (acute) (bacterial) (chronic) (subacute) I51.89
　meningococcal A39.50
　rheumatic — *see* Disease, heart, rheumatic
　rheumatoid — *see* Rheumatoid, carditis
　viral B33.20
Care (of) (for) (following)
　child (routine) Z76.2
　family member (handicapped) (sick)
　　creating problem for family Z63.6
　　provided away from home for holiday relief Z75.5
　　unavailable, due to
　　　absence (person rendering care) (sufferer) Z74.2
　　　inability (any reason) of person rendering care Z74.2
　foundling Z76.1
　holiday relief Z75.5
　improper — *see* Maltreatment
　lack of (at or after birth) (infant) — *see* Maltreatment, child, neglect
　lactating mother Z39.1
　palliative Z51.5
　postpartum
　　immediately after delivery Z39.0
　　routine follow-up Z39.2
　respite Z75.5
　unavailable, due to
　　absence of person rendering care Z74.2
　　inability (any reason) of person rendering care Z74.2
　well-baby Z76.2
Caries
　bone NEC A18.03
　dental K02.9
　　arrested (coronal) (root) K02.3
　　chewing surface
　　　limited to enamel K02.51
　　　penetrating into dentin K02.52
　　　penetrating into pulp K02.53
　　coronal surface
　　　chewing surface
　　　　limited to enamel K02.51
　　　　penetrating into dentin K02.52
　　　　penetrating into pulp K02.53
　　　pit and fissure surface
　　　　limited to enamel K02.51
　　　　penetrating into dentin K02.52
　　　　penetrating into pulp K02.53
　　　smooth surface
　　　　limited to enamel K02.61
　　　　penetrating into dentin K02.62
　　　　penetrating into pulp K02.63
　　pit and fissure surface
　　　limited to enamel K02.51
　　　penetrating into dentin K02.52
　　　penetrating into pulp K02.53

Caries — *continued*
  dental K02.9 — *continued*
    root K02.7
    smooth surface
      limited to enamel K02.61
      penetrating into dentin K02.62
      penetrating into pulp K02.63
  external meatus — *see* Disorder, ear, external, specified type NEC
  hip (tuberculous) A18.02
  initial (tooth)
    chewing surface K02.51
    pit and fissure surface K02.51
    smooth surface K02.61
  knee (tuberculous) A18.02
  labyrinth — *see* subcategory H83.8
  limb NEC (tuberculous) A18.03
  mastoid process (chronic) — *see* Mastoiditis, chronic
    tuberculous A18.03
  middle ear — *see* subcategory H74.8
  nose (tuberculous) A18.03
  orbit (tuberculous) A18.03
  ossicles, ear — *see* Abnormal, ear ossicles
  petrous bone — *see* Petrositis
  root (dental) (tooth) K02.7
  sacrum (tuberculous) A18.01
  spine, spinal (column) (tuberculous) A18.01
  syphilitic A52.77
    congenital (early) A50.02 [M90.80]
  tooth, teeth — *see* Caries, dental
  tuberculous A18.03
  vertebra (column) (tuberculous) A18.01
Carious teeth — *see* Caries, dental
Carneous mole O02.0
Carnitine insufficiency E71.40
Carotid body or sinus syndrome G90.01
Carotidynia G90.01
Carotinemia (dietary) E67.1
Carotinosis (cutis) (skin) E67.1
Carpal tunnel syndrome — *see* Syndrome, carpal tunnel
Carpenter's syndrome Q87.0
Carpopedal spasm — *see* Tetany
Carr-Barr-Plunkett syndrome Q97.1
Carrier (suspected) of
  amebiasis Z22.1
  bacterial disease NEC Z22.39
    diphtheria Z22.2
    intestinal infectious NEC Z22.1
      typhoid Z22.0
    meningococcal Z22.31
    sexually transmitted Z22.4
    specified NEC Z22.39
    staphylococcal (Methicillin susceptible) Z22.321
      Methicillin resistant Z22.322
    streptococcal Z22.338
      group B Z22.330
    typhoid Z22.0
  cholera Z22.1
  diphtheria Z22.2
  gastrointestinal pathogens NEC Z22.1
  genetic Z14.8
    cystic fibrosis Z14.1
    hemophilia A (asymptomatic) Z14.01
      symptomatic Z14.02
  gonorrhea Z22.4
  HAA (hepatitis Australian-antigen) Z22.59
  HB(c)(s)-AG Z22.51
  hepatitis (viral) Z22.50
    Australia-antigen (HAA) Z22.59
    B surface antigen (HBsAg) Z22.51
      with acute delta-(super)infection B17.0
    C Z22.52
    specified NEC Z22.59
  human T-cell lymphotropic virus type-1 (HTLV-1) infection Z22.6
  infectious organism Z22.9
    specified NEC Z22.8
  meningococci Z22.31
  Salmonella typhosa Z22.0
  serum hepatitis — *see* Carrier, hepatitis
  staphylococci (Methicillin susceptible) Z22.321
    Methicillin resistant Z22.322
  streptococci Z22.338
    group B Z22.330
  syphilis Z22.4
  typhoid Z22.0
  venereal disease NEC Z22.4
Carrion's disease A44.0
Carter's relapsing fever (Asiatic) A68.1
Cartilage — *see* condition
Caruncle (inflamed)
  conjunctiva (acute) — *see* Conjunctivitis, acute
  labium (majus) (minus) N90.89

Caruncle (inflamed) — *continued*
  lacrimal — *see* Inflammation, lacrimal, passages
  myrtiform N89.8
  urethral (benign) N36.2
Cascade stomach K31.2
Caseation lymphatic gland (tuberculous) A18.2
Cassidy (-Scholte) syndrome (malignant carcinoid) E34.0
Castellani's disease A69.8
Castration, traumatic, male S38.231
Casts in urine R82.99
Cat
  cry syndrome Q93.4
  ear Q17.3
  eye syndrome Q92.8
Catabolism, senile R54
Catalepsy (hysterical) F44.2
  schizophrenic F20.2
Cataplexy (idiopathic) — *see* Narcolepsy
Cataract (cortical) (immature) (incipient) H26.9
  with
    neovascularization — *see* Cataract, complicated
  age-related — *see* Cataract, senile
  anterior
    and posterior axial embryonal Q12.0
    pyramidal Q12.0
  associated with
    galactosemia E74.21 [H28]
    myotonic disorders G71.19 [H28]
  blue Q12.0
  central Q12.0
  cerulean Q12.0
  complicated H26.20
    with
      neovascularization H26.21-
      ocular disorder H26.22-
      glaucomatous flecks H26.23-
  congenital Q12.0
  coraliform Q12.0
  coronary Q12.0
  crystalline Q12.0
  diabetic — *see* Diabetes, cataract
  drug-induced H26.3-
  due to
    ocular disorder — *see* Cataract, complicated
    radiation H26.8
  electric H26.8
  extraction status Z98.4-
  glass-blower's H26.8
  heat ray H26.8
  heterochromic — *see* Cataract, complicated
  hypermature — *see* Cataract, senile, morgagnian type
  in (due to)
    chronic iridocyclitis — *see* Cataract, complicated
    diabetes — *see* Diabetes, cataract
    endocrine disease E34.9 [H28]
    eye disease — *see* Cataract, complicated
    hypoparathyroidism E20.9 [H28]
    malnutrition-dehydration E46 [H28]
    metabolic disease E88.9 [H28]
    myotonic disorders G71.19 [H28]
    nutritional disease E63.9 [H28]
  infantile — *see* Cataract, presenile
  irradiational — *see* Cataract, specified NEC
  juvenile — *see* Cataract, presenile
  malnutrition-dehydration E46 [H28]
  morgagnian — *see* Cataract, senile, morgagnian type
  myotonic G71.19 [H28]
  myxedema E03.9 [H28]
  nuclear
    embryonal Q12.0
    sclerosis — *see* Cataract, senile, nuclear
  presenile H26.00-
    combined forms H26.06-
    cortical H26.01-
      lamellar — *see* Cataract, presenile, cortical
    nuclear H26.03-
    specified NEC H26.09
    subcapsular polar (anterior) H26.04-
      posterior H26.05-
    zonular — *see* Cataract, presenile, cortical
  secondary H26.40
    Soemmering's ring H26.41-
    specified NEC H26.49-
    to eye disease — *see* Cataract, complicated
  senile H25.9
    brunescens — *see* Cataract, senile, nuclear

Cataract (cortical) (immature) (incipient) H26.9 — *continued*
  senile H25.9 — *continued*
    combined forms H25.81-
    coronary — *see* Cataract, senile, incipient
    cortical H25.01-
    hypermature — *see* Cataract, senile, morgagnian type
    incipient (mature) (total) H25.09-
      cortical — *see* Cataract, senile, cortical
      subcapsular — *see* Cataract, senile, subcapsular
    morgagnian type (hypermature) H25.2-
    nuclear (sclerosis) H25.1-
    polar subcapsular (anterior) (posterior) — *see* Cataract, senile, incipient
    punctate — *see* Cataract, senile, incipient
    specified NEC H25.89
    subcapsular polar (anterior) H25.03-
      posterior H25.04-
  snowflake — *see* Diabetes, cataract
  specified NEC H26.8
  toxic — *see* Cataract, drug-induced
  traumatic H26.10-
    localized H26.11-
    partially resolved H26.12-
    total H26.13-
  zonular (perinuclear) Q12.0
Cataracta — *see also* Cataract
  brunescens — *see* Cataract, senile, nuclear
  centralis pulverulenta Q12.0
  cerulea Q12.0
  complicata — *see* Cataract, complicated
  congenita Q12.0
  coralliformis Q12.0
  coronaria Q12.0
  diabetic — *see* Diabetes, cataract
  membranacea
    accreta — *see* Cataract, secondary
    congenita Q12.0
  nigra — *see* Cataract, senile, nuclear
  sunflower — *see* Cataract, complicated
Catarrh, catarrhal (acute) (febrile) (infectious) (inflammation) (*see also* condition) J00
  bronchial — *see* Bronchitis
  chest — *see* Bronchitis
  chronic J31.0
  due to congenital syphilis A50.03
  enteric — *see* Enteritis
  eustachian H68.009
  fauces — *see* Pharyngitis
  gastrointestinal — *see* Enteritis
  gingivitis K05.00
    nonplaque induced K05.01
    plaque induced K05.00
  hay — *see* Fever, hay
  intestinal — *see* Enteritis
  larynx, chronic J37.0
  liver B15.9
    with hepatic coma B15.0
  lung — *see* Bronchitis
  middle ear, chronic — *see* Otitis, media, nonsuppurative, chronic, serous
  mouth K12.1
  nasal (chronic) — *see* Rhinitis
  nasobronchial J31.1
  nasopharyngeal (chronic) J31.1
    acute J00
  pulmonary — *see* Bronchitis
  spring (eye) (vernal) — *see* Conjunctivitis, acute, atopic
  summer (hay) — *see* Fever, hay
  throat J31.2
  tubotympanal — *see also* Otitis, media, nonsuppurative
    chronic — *see* Otitis, media, nonsuppurative, chronic, serous
Catatonia (schizophrenic) F20.2
Catatonic
  disorder due to known physiologic condition F06.1
  schizophrenia F20.2
  stupor R40.1
Cat-scratch — *see also* Abrasion
  disease or fever A28.1
Cauda equina — *see* condition
Cauliflower ear M95.1-
Causalgia (upper limb) G56.4-
  lower limb G57.7-
Cause
  external, general effects T75.89
Caustic burn — *see* Corrosion, by site
Cavare's disease (familial periodic paralysis) G72.3

Cave-in, injury
  crushing (severe) — *see* Crush
  suffocation — *see* Asphyxia, traumatic, due to low oxygen, due to cave-in
Cavernitis (penis) N48.29
Cavernositis N48.29
Cavernous — *see* condition
Cavitation of lung — *see also* Tuberculosis, pulmonary
  nontuberculous J98.4
Cavities, dental — *see* Caries, dental
Cavity
  lung — *see* Cavitation of lung
  optic papilla Q14.2
  pulmonary — *see* Cavitation of lung
Cavovarus foot, congenital Q66.1
Cavus foot (congenital) Q66.7
  acquired — *see* Deformity, limb, foot, specified NEC
Cazenave's disease L10.2
Cecitis K52.9
  with perforation, peritonitis, or rupture K65.8
Cecum — *see* condition
Celiac
  artery compression syndrome I77.4
  disease K90.0
  infantilism K90.0
Cell(s), cellular — *see also* condition
  in urine R82.99
Cellulitis (diffuse) (phlegmonous) (septic) (suppurative) L03.90
  abdominal wall L03.311
  anaerobic A48.0
  ankle — *see* Cellulitis, lower limb
  anus K61.0
  arm — *see* Cellulitis, upper limb
  auricle (ear) — *see* Cellulitis, ear
  axilla L03.11-
  back (any part) L03.312
  broad ligament
    acute N73.0
  buttock L03.317
  cervical (meaning neck) L03.221
  cervix (uteri) — *see* Cervicitis
  cheek (external) L03.211
    internal K12.2
  chest wall L03.313
  chronic L03.90
  clostridial A48.0
  corpus cavernosum N48.22
  digit
    finger — *see* Cellulitis, finger
    toe — *see* Cellulitis, toe
  Douglas' cul-de-sac or pouch
    acute N73.0
  drainage site (following operation) T81.4
  ear (external) H60.1-
  eosinophilic (granulomatous) L98.3
  erysipelatous — *see* Erysipelas
  external auditory canal — *see* Cellulitis, ear
  eyelid — *see* Abscess, eyelid
  face NEC L03.211
  finger (intrathecal) (periosteal) (subcutaneous) (subcuticular) L03.01-
  foot — *see* Cellulitis, lower limb
  gangrenous — *see* Gangrene
  genital organ NEC
    female (external) N76.4
    male N49.9
      multiple sites N49.8
      specified NEC N49.8
  gluteal (region) L03.317
  gonococcal A54.89
  groin L03.314
  hand — *see* Cellulitis, upper limb
  head NEC L03.811
    face (any part, except ear, eye and nose) L03.211
  heel — *see* Cellulitis, lower limb
  hip — *see* Cellulitis, lower limb
  jaw (region) L03.211
  knee — *see* Cellulitis, lower limb
  labium (majus) (minus) — *see* Vulvitis
  lacrimal passages — *see* Inflammation, lacrimal, passages
  larynx J38.7
  leg — *see* Cellulitis, lower limb
  lip K13.0
  lower limb L03.11-
    toe — *see* Cellulitis, toe
  mouth (floor) K12.2
  multiple sites, so stated L03.90
  nasopharynx J39.1
  navel L03.316
    newborn P38.9
      with mild hemorrhage P38.1
      without hemorrhage P38.9
  neck (region) L03.221
  nose (septum) (external) J34.0

Cellulitis (diffuse) (phlegmonous) (septic) (suppurative) L03.90 — *continued*
orbit, orbital H05.01-
palate (soft) K12.2
pectoral (region) L03.313
pelvis, pelvic (chronic)
female (*see also* Disease, pelvis, inflammatory) N73.2
acute N73.0
following ectopic or molar pregnancy O08.0
male K65.0
penis N48.22
perineal, perineum L03.315
perirectal K61.1
peritonsillar J36
periurethral N34.0
periuterine (*see also* Disease, pelvis, inflammatory) N73.2
acute N73.0
pharynx J39.1
rectum K61.1
retroperitoneal K68.9
round ligament
acute N73.0
scalp (any part) L03.811
scrotum N49.2
seminal vesicle N49.0
shoulder — *see* Cellulitis, upper limb
specified site NEC L03.818
submandibular (region) (space) (triangle) K12.2
gland K11.3
submaxillary (region) K12.2
gland K11.3
thigh — *see* Cellulitis, lower limb
thumb (intrathecal) (periosteal) (subcutaneous) (subcuticular) — *see* Cellulitis, finger
toe (intrathecal) (periosteal) (subcutaneous) (subcuticular) L03.03-
tonsil J36
trunk L03.319
abdominal wall L03.311
back (any part) L03.312
buttock L03.317
chest wall L03.313
groin L03.314
perineal, perineum L03.315
umbilicus L03.316
tuberculous (primary) A18.4
umbilicus L03.316
upper limb L03.11-
axilla — *see* Cellulitis, axilla
finger — *see* Cellulitis, finger
thumb — *see* Cellulitis, finger
vaccinal T88.0
vocal cord J38.3
vulva — *see* Vulvitis
wrist — *see* Cellulitis, upper limb
Cementoblastoma, benign — *see* Cyst, calcifying odontogenic
Cementoma — *see* Cyst, calcifying odontogenic
Cementoperiostitis — *see* Periodontitis
Cementosis K03.4
Central auditory processing disorder H93.25
Central pain syndrome G89.0
Cephalematocele, cephal (o)hematocele
newborn P52.8
birth injury P10.8
traumatic — *see* Hematoma, brain
Cephalematoma, cephalhematoma (calcified)
newborn (birth injury) P12.0
traumatic — *see* Hematoma, brain
Cephalgia, cephalalgia — *see also* Headache
histamine G44.009
intractable G44.001
not intractable G44.009
trigeminal autonomic (TAC) NEC G44.099
intractable G44.091
not intractable G44.099
Cephalic — *see* condition
Cephalitis — *see* Encephalitis
Cephalocele — *see* Encephalocele
Cephalomenia N94.89
Cephalopelvic — *see* condition
Cerclage (with cervical incompetence) in pregnancy — *see* Incompetence, cervix, in pregnancy
Cerebellitis — *see* Encephalitis
Cerebellum, cerebellar — *see* condition
Cerebral — *see* condition
Cerebritis — *see* Encephalitis

Cerebro-hepato-renal syndrome Q87.89
Cerebromalacia — *see* Softening, brain
sequelae of cerebrovascular disease I69.398
Cerebroside lipidosis E75.22
Cerebrospasticity (congenital) G80.1
Cerebrospinal — *see* condition
Cerebrum — *see* condition
Ceroid-lipofuscinosis, neuronal E75.4
Cerumen (accumulation) (impacted) H61.2-
Cervical — *see also* condition
auricle Q18.2
dysplasia in pregnancy — *see* Abnormal, cervix, in pregnancy or childbirth
erosion in pregnancy — *see* Abnormal, cervix, in pregnancy or childbirth
fibrosis in pregnancy — *see* Abnormal, cervix, in pregnancy or childbirth
fusion syndrome Q76.1
rib Q76.5
shortening (complicating pregnancy) O26.87-
Cervicalgia M54.2
Cervicitis (acute) (chronic) (nonvenereal) (senile (atrophic)) (subacute) (with ulceration) N72
with
abortion — *see* Abortion, by type
complicated by genital tract and pelvic infection
ectopic pregnancy O08.0
molar pregnancy O08.0
chlamydial A56.09
gonococcal A54.03
herpesviral A60.03
puerperal (postpartum) O86.11
syphilitic A52.76
trichomonal A59.09
tuberculous A18.16
Cervicocolpitis (emphysematosa) (*see also* Cervicitis) N72
Cervix — *see* condition
Cesarean delivery, previous, affecting management of pregnancy O34.21
Céstan(-Chenais) paralysis or syndrome G46.3
Céstan-Raymond syndrome I65.8
Cestode infestation B71.9
specified type NEC B71.8
Cestodiasis B71.9
Chabert's disease A22.9
Chacaleh E53.8
Chafing L30.4
Chagas' (-Mazza) disease (chronic) B57.2
with
cardiovascular involvement NEC B57.2
digestive system involvement B57.30
megacolon B57.32
megaesophagus B57.31
other specified B57.39
megacolon B57.32
megaesophagus B57.31
myocarditis B57.2
nervous system involvement B57.40
meningitis B57.41
meningoencephalitis B57.42
other specified B57.49
specified organ involvement NEC B57.5
acute (with) B57.1
cardiovascular NEC B57.0
myocarditis B57.0
Chagres fever B50.9
Chairridden Z74.09
Chalasia (cardiac sphincter) K21.9
Chalazion H00.19
left H00.16
lower H00.15
upper H00.14
right H00.13
lower H00.12
upper H00.11
Chalcosis — *see also* Disorder, globe, degenerative, chalcosis
cornea — *see* Deposit, cornea
crystalline lens — *see* Cataract, complicated
retina H35.89
Chalicosis (pulmonum) J62.8
Chancre (any genital site) (hard) (hunterian) (mixed) (primary) (seronegative) (seropositive) (syphilitic) A51.0
congenital A50.07
conjunctiva NEC A51.2
Ducrey's A57
extragenital A51.2
eyelid A51.2
lip A51.2

Chancre (any genital site) (hard) (hunterian) (mixed) (primary) (seronegative) (seropositive) (syphilitic) A51.0 — *continued*
nipple A51.2
Nisbet's A57
of
carate A67.0
pinta A67.0
yaws A66.0
palate, soft A51.2
phagedenic A57
simple A57
soft A57
bubo A57
palate A51.2
urethra A51.0
yaws A66.0
Chancroid (anus) (genital) (penis) (perineum) (rectum) (urethra) (vulva) A57
Chandler's disease (osteochondritis dissecans, hip) — *see* Osteochondritis, dissecans, hip
Change(s) (in) (of) — *see also* Removal
arteriosclerotic — *see* Arteriosclerosis
bone — *see also* Disorder, bone
diabetic — *see* Diabetes, bone change
bowel habit R19.4
cardiorenal (vascular) — *see* Hypertension, cardiorenal
cardiovascular — *see* Disease, cardiovascular
circulatory I99.9
cognitive (mild) (organic) R41.89
color, tooth, teeth
during formation K00.8
posteruptive K03.7
contraceptive device Z30.433
corneal membrane H18.30
Bowman's membrane fold or rupture H18.31-
Descemet's membrane
fold H18.32-
rupture H18.33-
coronary — *see* Disease, heart, ischemic
degenerative, spine or vertebra — *see* Spondylosis
dental pulp, regressive K04.2
dressing (nonsurgical) Z48.00
surgical Z48.01
heart — *see* Disease, heart
hip joint — *see* Derangement, joint, hip
hyperplastic larynx J38.7
hypertrophic
nasal sinus J34.89
turbinate, nasal J34.3
upper respiratory tract J39.8
indwelling catheter Z46.6
inflammatory — *see also* Inflammation
sacroiliac M46.1
job, anxiety concerning Z56.1
joint — *see* Derangement, joint
life — *see* Menopause
mental status R41.82
minimal (glomerular) (*see also* N00-N07 with fourth character .0) N05.0
myocardium, myocardial — *see* Degeneration, myocardial
of life — *see* Menopause
pacemaker Z45.018
pulse generator Z45.010
personality (enduring) F68.8
due to (secondary to)
general medical condition F07.0
secondary (nonspecific) F60.89
regressive, dental pulp K04.2
renal — *see* Disease, renal
retina H35.9
myopic H44.2-
sacroiliac joint M53.3
senile (*see also* condition) R54
sensory R20.8
skin R23.9
acute, due to ultraviolet radiation L56.9
specified NEC L56.8
chronic, due to nonionizing radiation L57.9
specified NEC L57.8
cyanosis R23.0
flushing R23.2
pallor R23.1
petechiae R23.3
specified change NEC R23.8
swelling — *see* Mass, localized
texture R23.4

Change(s) (in) (of) (*see also* Removal) — *continued*
trophic
arm — *see* Mononeuropathy, upper limb
leg — *see* Mononeuropathy, lower limb
vascular I99.9
vasomotor I73.9
voice R49.9
psychogenic F44.4
specified NEC R49.8
Changing sleep-work schedule, affecting sleep G47.26
Changuinola fever A93.1
Chapping skin T69.8
Charcôt-Marie-Tooth disease, paralysis or syndrome G60.0
Charcôt's
arthropathy — *see* Arthropathy, neuropathic
cirrhosis K74.3
disease (tabetic arthropathy) A52.16
joint (disease) (tabetic) A52.16
diabetic — *see* Diabetes, with, arthropathy
syringomyelic G95.0
syndrome (intermittent claudication) I73.9
CHARGE association Q89.8
Charley-horse (quadriceps) M62.831
traumatic (quadriceps) S76.11-
Charlouis' disease — *see* Yaws
Cheadle's disease E54
Checking (of)
cardiac pacemaker (battery) (electrode(s)) Z45.018
pulse generator Z45.010
intrauterine contraceptive device Z30.431
Check-up — *see* Examination
Chédiak-Higashi(-Steinbrinck) syndrome (congenital gigantism of peroxidase granules) E70.330
Cheek — *see* condition
Cheese itch B88.0
Cheese-washer's lung J67.8
Cheese-worker's lung J67.8
Cheilitis (acute) (angular) (catarrhal) (chronic) (exfoliative) (gangrenous) (glandular) (infectional) (suppurative) (ulcerative) (vesicular) K13.0
actinic (due to sun) L56.8
other than from sun L59.8
candidal B37.83
Cheilodynia K13.0
Cheiloschisis — *see* Cleft, lip
Cheilosis (angular) K13.0
with pellagra E52
due to
vitamin B2 (riboflavin) deficiency E53.0
Cheiromegaly M79.89
Cheiropompholyx L30.1
Cheloid — *see* Keloid
Chemical burn — *see* Corrosion, by site
Chemodectoma — *see* Paraganglioma, nonchromaffin
Chemosis, conjunctiva — *see* Edema, conjunctiva
Chemotherapy (session) (for)
cancer Z51.11
neoplasm Z51.11
Cherubism M27.8
Chest — *see* condition
Cheyne-Stokes breathing (respiration) R06.3
Chiari's
disease or syndrome (hepatic vein thrombosis) I82.0
malformation
type I G93.5
type II — *see* Spina bifida
net Q24.8
Chicago disease B40.9
Chickenpox — *see* Varicella
Chiclero ulcer or sore B55.1
Chigger (infestation) B88.0
Chignon (disease) B36.8
newborn (from vacuum extraction) (birth injury) P12.1
Chilaiditi's syndrome (subphrenic displacement, colon) Q43.3
Chilblain(s) (lupus) T69.1
Child
custody dispute Z65.3
Childbirth — *see* Delivery
Childhood
cerebral X-linked adrenoleukodystrophy E71.520
period of rapid growth Z00.2

DISEASE INDEX

Chill(s) R68.83
  with fever R50.9
  congestive in malarial regions B54
  without fever R68.83
Chilomastigiasis A07.8
Chimera 46,XX/46,XY Q99.0
Chin — *see* condition
Chinese dysentery A03.9
Chionophobia F40.228
Chitral fever A93.1
Chlamydia, chlamydial A74.9
  cervicitis A56.09
  conjunctivitis A74.0
  cystitis A56.01
  endometritis A56.11
  epididymitis A56.19
  female
    pelvic inflammatory disease A56.11
    pelviperitonitis A56.11
  orchitis A56.19
  peritonitis A74.81
  pharyngitis A56.4
  proctitis A56.3
  psittaci (infection) A70
  salpingitis A56.11
  sexually-transmitted infection NEC A56.8
  specified NEC A74.89
  urethritis A56.01
  vulvovaginitis A56.02
Chlamydiosis — *see* Chlamydia
Chloasma (skin) (idiopathic) (symptomatic)
  L81.1
  eyelid H02.719
    hyperthyroid E05.90 [H02.719]
      with thyroid storm E05.91 [H02.719]
    left H02.716
      lower H02.715
      upper H02.714
    right H02.713
      lower H02.712
      upper H02.711
Chloroma C92.3-
Chlorosis D50.9
  Egyptian B76.9 [D63.8]
  miner's B76.9 [D63.8]
Chlorotic anemia D50.8
Chocolate cyst (ovary) N80.1
Choked
  disc or disk — *see* Papilledema
  on food, phlegm, or vomitus NOS — *see*
    Foreign body, by site
  while vomiting NOS — *see* Foreign body,
    by site
Chokes (resulting from bends) T70.3
Choking sensation R09.89
Cholangiectasis K83.8
Cholangiocarcinoma
  with hepatocellular carcinoma, combined
    C22.0
  liver C22.1
  specified site NEC — *see* Neoplasm,
    malignant, by site
  unspecified site C22.1
Cholangiohepatitis K83.8
  due to fluke infestation B66.1
Cholangiohepatoma C22.0
Cholangiolitis (acute) (chronic)
  (extrahepatic) (gangrenous)
  (intrahepatic) K83.0
  paratyphoidal — *see* Fever, paratyphoid
  typhoidal A01.09
Cholangioma D13.4
  malignant — *see* Cholangiocarcinoma
Cholangitis (ascending) (primary) (recurrent)
  (sclerosing) (secondary) (stenosing)
  (suppurative) K83.0
  with calculus, bile duct — *see* Calculus,
    bile duct, with cholangitis
  chronic nonsuppurative destructive K74.3
Cholecystectasia K82.8
Cholecystitis K81.9
  with
    calculus, stones in
      bile duct (common) (hepatic) — *see*
        Calculus, bile duct, with
        cholecystitis
      cystic duct — *see* Calculus,
        gallbladder, with cholecystitis
      gallbladder — *see* Calculus,
        gallbladder, with cholecystitis
      choledocholithiasis — *see* Calculus, bile
        duct, with cholecystitis
      cholelithiasis — *see* Calculus,
        gallbladder, with cholecystitis

Cholecystitis K81.9 — *continued*
  acute (emphysematous) (gangrenous)
    (suppurative) K81.0
    with
      calculus, stones in
        cystic duct — *see* Calculus,
          gallbladder, with cholecystitis,
          acute
        gallbladder — *see* Calculus,
          gallbladder, with cholecystitis,
          acute
        choledocholithiasis — *see* Calculus,
          bile duct, with cholecystitis,
          acute
        cholelithiasis — *see* Calculus,
          gallbladder, with cholecystitis,
          acute
      chronic cholecystitis K81.2
        with gallbladder calculus K80.12
          with obstruction K80.13
    chronic K81.1
      with acute cholecystitis K81.2
        with gallbladder calculus K80.12
          with obstruction K80.13
    emphysematous (acute) — *see*
      Cholecystitis, acute
    gangrenous — *see* Cholecystitis, acute
    paratyphoidal, current A01.4
    suppurative — *see* Cholecystitis, acute
    typhoidal A01.09
Cholecystolithiasis — *see* Calculus,
  gallbladder
Choledochitis (suppurative) K83.0
Choledocholith — *see* Calculus, bile duct
Choledocholithiasis (common duct) (hepatic
  duct) — *see* Calculus, bile duct
  cystic — *see* Calculus, gallbladder
  typhoidal A01.09
Cholelithiasis (cystic duct) (gallbladder)
  (impacted) (multiple) — *see* Calculus,
  gallbladder
  bile duct (common) (hepatic) — *see*
    Calculus, bile duct
  hepatic duct — *see* Calculus, bile duct
  specified NEC K80.80
    with obstruction K80.81
Cholemia — *see also* Jaundice
  familial (simple) (congenital) E80.4
  Gilbert's E80.4
Choleperitoneum, choleperitonitis K65.3
Cholera (Asiatic) (epidemic) (malignant)
  A00.9
  antimonial — *see* Poisoning, antimony
  classical A00.0
  due to Vibrio cholerae 01 A00.9
    biovar cholerae A00.0
    biovar el tor A00.1
    el tor A00.1
  el tor A00.1
Cholerine — *see* Cholera
Cholestasis NEC K83.1
  with hepatocyte injury K71.0
  due to total parenteral nutrition (TPN)
    K76.89
  pure K71.0
Cholesteatoma (ear) (middle) (with reaction)
  H71.9-
  attic H71.0-
  external ear (canal) H60.4-
  mastoid H71.2-
  postmastoidectomy cavity (recurrent) —
    see Complications,
    postmastoidectomy, recurrent
    cholesteatoma
  recurrent (postmastoidectomy) — *see*
    Complications, postmastoidectomy,
    recurrent cholesteatoma
  tympanum H71.1-
Cholesteatosis, diffuse H71.3-
Cholesteremia E78.0
Cholesterin in vitreous — *see* Deposit,
  crystalline
Cholesterol
  deposit
    retina H35.89
    vitreous — *see* Deposit, crystalline
  elevated (high) E78.0
    with elevated (high) triglycerides E78.2
    screening for Z13.220
  imbibition of gallbladder K82.4
Cholesterolemia (essential) (familial)
  (hereditary) (pure) E78.0
Cholesterolosis, cholesterosis (gallbladder)
  K82.4
  cerebrotendinous E75.5
Cholocolic fistula K82.3
Choluria R82.2

Chondritis M94.8x9
  aurical H61.03-
  costal (Tietze's) M94.0
  external ear H61.03-
  patella, posttraumatic — *see*
    Chondromalacia, patella
  pinna H61.03-
  purulent M94.8x-
  tuberculous NEC A18.02
    intervertebral A18.01
Chondroblastoma — *see also* Neoplasm,
  bone, benign
  malignant — *see* Neoplasm, bone,
    malignant
Chondrocalcinosis M11.20
  ankle M11.27-
  elbow M11.22-
  familial M11.10
    ankle M11.17-
    elbow M11.12-
    foot joint M11.17-
    hand joint M11.14-
    hip M11.15-
    knee M11.16-
    multiple site M11.19
    shoulder M11.11-
    vertebrae M11.18
    wrist M11.13-
  foot joint M11.27-
  hand joint M11.24-
  hip M11.25-
  knee M11.26-
  multiple site M11.29
  shoulder M11.21-
  specified type NEC M11.20
    ankle M11.27-
    elbow M11.22-
    foot joint M11.27-
    hand joint M11.24-
    hip M11.25-
    knee M11.26-
    multiple site M11.29
    shoulder M11.21-
    vertebrae M11.28
    wrist M11.23-
  vertebrae M11.28
  wrist M11.23-
Chondrodermatitis nodularis helicis or
  anthelicis — *see* Perichondritis, ear
Chondrodysplasia Q78.9
  with hemangioma Q78.4
  calcificans congenita Q77.3
  fetalis Q77.4
  metaphyseal (Jansen's) (McKusick's)
    (Schmid's) Q78.5
  punctata Q77.3
Chondrodystrophy, chondrodystrophia
  (familial) (fetalis) (hypoplastic) Q78.9
  calcificans congenita Q77.3
  myotonic (congenital) G71.13
  punctata Q77.3
Chondroectodermal dysplasia Q77.6
Chondrogenesis imperfecta Q77.4
Chondrolysis M94.35-
Chondroma — *see also* Neoplasm, cartilage,
  benign
  juxtacortical — *see* Neoplasm, bone,
    benign
  periosteal — *see* Neoplasm, bone, benign
Chondromalacia (systemic) M94.20
  acromioclavicular joint M94.21-
  ankle M94.27-
  elbow M94.22-
  foot joint M94.27-
  glenohumeral joint M94.21-
  hand joint M94.24-
  hip M94.25-
  knee M94.26-
    patella M22.4-
  multiple sites M94.29
  patella M22.4-
  rib M94.28
  sacroiliac joint M94.259
  shoulder M94.21-
  sternoclavicular joint M94.21-
  vertebral joint M94.28
  wrist M94.23-
Chondromatosis — *see also* Neoplasm,
  cartilage, uncertain behavior
  internal Q78.4
Chondromyxosarcoma — *see* Neoplasm,
  cartilage, malignant
Chondro-osteodysplasia (Morquio-
  Brailsford type) E76.219
Chondro-osteodystrophy E76.29
Chondro-osteoma — *see* Neoplasm, bone,
  benign
Chondropathia tuberosa M94.0

Chondrosarcoma — *see* Neoplasm,
  cartilage, malignant
  juxtacortical — *see* Neoplasm, bone,
    malignant
  mesenchymal — *see* Neoplasm, connective
    tissue, malignant
  myxoid — *see* Neoplasm, cartilage,
    malignant
Chordee (nonvenereal) N48.89
  congenital Q54.4
  gonococcal A54.09
Chorditis (fibrinous) (nodosa) (tuberosa)
  J38.2
Chordoma — *see* Neoplasm, vertebral
  (column), malignant
Chorea (chronic) (gravis) (posthemiplegic)
  (senile) (spasmodic) G25.5
  with
    heart involvement I02.0
      active or acute (conditions in I01-)
        I02.0
      rheumatic I02.9
        with valvular disorder I02.0
    rheumatic heart disease (chronic)
      (inactive) (quiescent) — *code to*
      rheumatic heart condition involved
  drug-induced G25.4
  habit F95.8
  hereditary G10
  Huntington's G10
  hysterical F44.4
  minor I02.9
    with heart involvement I02.0
  progressive G25.5
    hereditary G10
  rheumatic (chronic) I02.9
    with heart involvement I02.0
  Sydenham's I02.9
    with heart involvement — *see* Chorea,
      with rheumatic heart disease
  nonrheumatic G25.5
Choreoathetosis (paroxysmal) G25.5
Chorioadenoma (destruens) D39.2
Chorioamnionitis O41.12-
Chorioangioma D26.7
Choriocarcinoma — *see* Neoplasm,
  malignant, by site
  combined with
    embryonal carcinoma — *see* Neoplasm,
      malignant, by site
    other germ cell elements — *see*
      Neoplasm, malignant, by site
    teratoma — *see* Neoplasm, malignant,
      by site
  specified site — *see* Neoplasm, malignant,
    by site
  unspecified site
    female C58
    male C62.90
Chorioencephalitis (acute) (lymphocytic)
  (serous) A87.2
Chorioepithelioma — *see* Choriocarcinoma
Choriomeningitis (acute) (lymphocytic)
  (serous) A87.2
Chorionepithelioma — *see* Choriocarcinoma
Chorioretinitis — *see also* Inflammation,
  chorioretinal
  disseminated — *see also* Inflammation,
    chorioretinal, disseminated
    in neurosyphilis A52.19
  Egyptian B76.9 [D63.8]
  focal — *see also* Inflammation,
    chorioretinal, focal
  histoplasmic B39.9 [H32]
  in (due to)
    histoplasmosis B39.9 [H32]
    syphilis (secondary) A51.43
      late A52.71
    toxoplasmosis (acquired) B58.01
      congenital (active) P37.1 [H32]
    tuberculosis A18.53
  juxtapapillary, juxtapapillaris — *see*
    Inflammation, chorioretinal, focal,
    juxtapapillary
  leprous A30.9 [H32]
  miner's B76.9 [D63.8]
  progressive myopia (degeneration) H44.2-
  syphilitic (secondary) A51.43
    congenital (early) A50.01 [H32]
      late A50.32
    late A52.71
  tuberculous A18.53
Chorioretinopathy, central serous H35.71-
Choroid — *see* condition
Choroideremia H31.21
Choroiditis — *see* Chorioretinitis
Choroidopathy — *see* Disorder, choroid
Choroidoretinitis — *see* Chorioretinitis

D I S E A S E   I N D E X

Choroidoretinopathy, central serous — *see* Chorioretinopathy, central serous
Christian-Weber disease M35.6
Christmas disease D67
Chromaffinoma — *see also* Neoplasm, benign, by site
  malignant — *see* Neoplasm, malignant, by site
Chromatopsia — *see* Deficiency, color vision
Chromhidrosis, chromidrosis L75.1
Chromoblastomycosis — *see* Chromomycosis
Chromoconversion R82.91
Chromomycosis B43.9
  brain abscess B43.1
  cerebral B43.1
  cutaneous B43.0
  skin B43.0
  specified NEC B43.8
  subcutaneous abscess or cyst B43.2
Chromophytosis B36.0
Chromosome — *see* condition by chromosome involved
  D(1) — *see* condition, chromosome 13
  E(3) — *see* condition, chromosome 18
  G — *see* condition, chromosome 21
Chromotrichomycosis B36.8
Chronic — *see* condition
  fracture — *see* Fracture, pathological
Churg-Strauss syndrome M30.1
Chyle cyst, mesentery I89.8
Chylocele (nonfilarial) I89.8
  filarial (*see also* Infestation, filarial) B74.9 [N51]
  tunica vaginalis N50.8
    filarial (*see also* Infestation, filarial) B74.9 [N51]
Chylomicronemia (fasting) (with hyperprebetalipoproteinemia) E78.3
Chylopericardium I31.3
  acute I30.9
Chylothorax (nonfilarial) I89.8
  filarial (*see also* Infestation, filarial) B74.9 [J91.8]
Chylous — *see* condition
Chyluria (nonfilarial) R82.0
  due to
    bilharziasis B65.0
    Brugia (malayi) B74.1
      timori B74.2
    schistosomiasis (bilharziasis) B65.0
    Wuchereria (bancrofti) B74.0
  filarial — *see* Infestation, filarial
Cicatricial (deformity) — *see* Cicatrix
Cicatrix (adherent) (contracted) (painful) (vicious) (*see also* Scar) L90.5
  adenoid (and tonsil) J35.8
  alveolar process M26.79
  anus K62.89
  auricle — *see* Disorder, pinna, specified type NEC
  bile duct (common) (hepatic) K83.8
  bladder N32.89
  bone — *see* Disorder, bone, specified type NEC
  brain G93.89
  cervix (postoperative) (postpartal) N88.1
  common duct K83.8
  cornea H17.9
    tuberculous A18.59
  duodenum (bulb), obstructive K31.5
  esophagus K22.2
  eyelid — *see* Disorder, eyelid function
  hypopharynx J39.2
  lacrimal passages — *see* Obstruction, lacrimal
  larynx J38.7
  lung J98.4
  middle ear — *see* subcategory H74.8
  mouth K13.79
  muscle M62.89
    with contracture — *see* Contraction, muscle NEC
  nasopharynx J39.2
  palate (soft) K13.79
  penis N48.89
  pharynx J39.2
  prostate N42.89
  rectum K62.89
  retina — *see* Scar, chorioretinal
  semilunar cartilage — *see* Derangement, meniscus
  seminal vesicle N50.8
  skin L90.5
    infected L08.89
    postinfective L90.5
    tuberculous B90.8

Cicatrix (adherent) (contracted) (painful) (vicious) (*see also* Scar) L90.5 — *continued*
  specified site NEC L90.5
  throat J39.2
  tongue K14.8
  tonsil (and adenoid) J35.8
  trachea J39.8
  tuberculous NEC B90.9
  urethra N36.8
  uterus N85.8
  vagina N89.8
    postoperative N99.2
  vocal cord J38.3
  wrist, constricting (annular) L90.5
CIDP (chronic inflammatory demyelinating polyneuropathy) G61.81
CIN — *see* Neoplasia, intraepithelial, cervix
Cinchonism — *see* Deafness, ototoxic
  correct substance properly administered — *see* Table of Drugs and Chemicals, by drug, adverse effect
  overdose or wrong substance given or taken — *see* Table of Drugs and Chemicals, by drug, poisoning
Circle of Willis — *see* condition
Circular — *see* condition
Circulating anticoagulants (see also Disorder, hemorrhagic) D68.318
  due to drugs (*see also* Disorder, hemorrhagic) D68.32
  following childbirth O72.3
Circulation
  collateral, any site I99.8
  defective (lower extremity) I99.8
    congenital Q28.9
  embryonic Q28.9
  failure (peripheral) R57.9
    newborn P29.89
  fetal, persistent P29.3
  heart, incomplete P29.9
Circulatory system — *see* condition
Circulus senilis (cornea) — *see* Degeneration, cornea, senile
Circumcision (in absence of medical indication) (ritual) (routine) Z41.2
Circumscribed — *see* condition
Circumvallate placenta O43.11-
Cirrhosis, cirrhotic (hepatic) (liver) K74.60
  alcoholic K70.30
    with ascites K70.31
  atrophic — *see* Cirrhosis, liver
  Baumgarten-Cruveilhier K74.69
  biliary (cholangiolitic) (cholangitic) (hypertrophic) (obstructive) (pericholangiolitic) K74.5
    due to
      Clonorchiasis B66.1
      flukes B66.3
    primary K74.3
    secondary K74.4
  cardiac (of liver) K76.1
  Charcot's K74.3
  cholangiolitic, cholangitic, cholostatic (primary) K74.3
  congestive K76.1
  Cruveilhier-Baumgarten K74.69
  cryptogenic (liver) K74.69
  due to
    hepatolenticular degeneration E83.01
    Wilson's disease E83.01
    xanthomatosis E78.2
  fatty K76.0
    alcoholic K70.0
  Hanot's (hypertrophic) K74.3
  hepatic — *see* Cirrhosis, liver
  hypertrophic K74.3
  Indian childhood K74.69
  kidney — *see* Sclerosis, renal
  Laennec's K70.30
    with ascites K70.31
    alcoholic K70.30
      with ascites K70.31
    nonalcoholic K74.69
  liver K74.60
    alcoholic K70.30
      with ascites K70.31
    fatty K76.0
    congenital P78.81
    syphilitic A52.74
  lung (chronic) J84.10
  macronodular K74.69
    alcoholic K70.30
      with ascites K70.31
  micronodular K74.69
    alcoholic K70.30
      with ascites K70.31
  mixed type K74.69
  monolobular K74.3

Cirrhosis, cirrhotic (hepatic) (liver) K74.60 — *continued*
  nephritis — *see* Sclerosis, renal
  nutritional K74.69
    alcoholic K70.30
      with ascites K70.31
  obstructive — *see* Cirrhosis, biliary
  ovarian N83.8
  pancreas (duct) K86.8
  pigmentary E83.110
  portal K74.69
    alcoholic K70.30
      with ascites K70.31
  postnecrotic K74.69
    alcoholic K70.30
      with ascites K70.31
  pulmonary J84.10
  renal — *see* Sclerosis, renal
  spleen D73.2
  stasis K76.1
  Todd's K74.3
  unilobar K74.3
  xanthomatous (biliary) K74.5
    due to xanthomatosis (familial) (metabolic) (primary) E78.2
Cistern, subarachnoid R93.0
Citrullinemia E72.23
Citrullinuria E72.23
Civatte's disease or poikiloderma L57.3
Clam digger's itch B65.3
Clammy skin R23.1
Clap — *see* Gonorrhea
Clarke-Hadfield syndrome (pancreatic infantilism) K86.8
Clark's paralysis G80.9
Clastothrix L67.8
Claude Bernard-Horner syndrome G90.2
  traumatic — *see* Injury, nerve, cervical sympathetic
Claude's disease or syndrome G46.3
Claudicatio venosa intermittens I87.8
Claudication, intermittent I73.9
  cerebral (artery) G45.9
  spinal cord (arteriosclerotic) G95.19
    syphilitic A52.09
  venous (axillary) I87.8
Claustrophobia F40.240
Clavus (infected) L84
Clawfoot (congenital) Q66.89
  acquired — *see* Deformity, limb, clawfoot
Clawhand (acquired) — *see also* Deformity, limb, clawhand
  congenital Q68.1
Clawtoe (congenital) Q66.89
  acquired — *see* Deformity, toe, specified NEC
Clay eating — *see* Pica
Cleansing of artificial opening — *see* Attention to, artificial, opening
Cleft (congenital) — *see also* Imperfect, closure
  alveolar process M26.79
  branchial (cyst) (persistent) Q18.2
  cricoid cartilage, posterior Q31.8
  lip (unilateral) Q36.9
    with cleft palate Q37.9
      hard Q37.1
        with soft Q37.5
      soft Q37.3
        with hard Q37.5
    bilateral Q36.0
      with cleft palate Q37.8
        hard Q37.0
          with soft Q37.4
        soft Q37.2
          with hard Q37.4
    median Q36.1
  nose Q30.2
  palate Q35.9
    with cleft lip (unilateral) Q37.9
      bilateral Q37.8
    hard Q35.1
      with
        cleft lip (unilateral) Q37.1
          bilateral Q37.0
        soft Q35.5
          with cleft lip (unilateral) Q37.5
            bilateral Q37.4
    medial Q35.5
    soft Q35.3
      with
        cleft lip (unilateral) Q37.3
          bilateral Q37.2
        hard Q35.5
          with cleft lip (unilateral) Q37.5
            bilateral Q37.4
  penis Q55.69
  scrotum Q55.29
  thyroid cartilage Q31.8
  uvula Q35.7

Cleidocranial dysostosis Q74.0
Cleptomania F63.2
Clicking hip (newborn) R29.4
Climacteric (female) — *see also* Menopause
  arthritis (any site) NEC — *see* Arthritis, specified form NEC
  depression (single episode) F32.8
  male (symptoms) (syndrome) NEC N50.8
  paranoid state F22
  polyarthritis NEC — *see* Arthritis, specified form NEC
  symptoms (female) N95.1
Clinical research investigation (clinical trial) (control subject) (normal comparison) (participant) Z00.6
Clitoris — *see* condition
Cloaca (persistent) Q43.7
Clonorchiasis, clonorchis infection (liver) B66.1
Clonus R25.8
Closed bite M26.29
Clostridium (C.) perfringens, as cause of disease classified elsewhere B96.7
Closure
  congenital, nose Q30.0
  cranial sutures, premature Q75.0
  defective or imperfect NEC — *see* Imperfect, closure
  fistula, delayed — *see* Fistula
  foramen ovale, imperfect Q21.1
  hymen N89.6
  interauricular septum, defective Q21.1
  interventricular septum, defective Q21.0
  lacrimal duct — *see also* Stenosis, lacrimal, duct
    congenital Q10.5
  nose (congenital) Q30.0
    acquired M95.0
  of artificial opening — *see* Attention to, artificial, opening
  primary angle, without glaucoma damage H40.06-
  vagina N89.5
  valve — *see* Endocarditis
  vulva N90.5
Clot (blood) — *see also* Embolism
  artery (obstruction) (occlusion) — *see* Embolism
  bladder N32.89
  brain (intradural or extradural) — *see* Occlusion, artery, cerebral
  circulation I74.9
  heart — *see also* Infarct, myocardium
    not resulting in infarction I24.0
  vein — *see* Thrombosis
Clouded state R40.1
  epileptic — *see* Epilepsy, specified NEC
  paroxysmal — *see* Epilepsy, specified NEC
Cloudy antrum, antra J32.0
Clouston's (hidrotic) ectodermal dysplasia Q82.4
Clubbed nail pachydermoperiostosis M89.40 [L62]
Clubbing of finger(s) (nails) R68.3
Clubfinger R68.3
  congenital Q68.1
Clubfoot (congenital) Q66.89
  acquired — *see* Deformity, limb, clubfoot
  equinovarus Q66.0
  paralytic — *see* Deformity, limb, clubfoot
Clubhand (congenital) (radial) Q71.4-
  acquired — *see* Deformity, limb, clubhand
Clubnail R68.3
  congenital Q84.6
Clump, kidney Q63.1
Clumsiness, clumsy child syndrome F82
Cluttering F80.81
Clutton's joints A50.51 [M12.80]
Coagulation, intravascular (diffuse) (disseminated) — *see also* Defibrination syndrome
  complicating abortion — *see* Abortion, by type, complicated by, intravascular coagulation
  following ectopic or molar pregnancy O08.1
Coagulopathy — *see also* Defect, coagulation
  consumption D65
  intravascular D65
  newborn P60
Coalition
  calcaneo-scaphoid Q66.89
  tarsal Q66.89
Coalminer's
  elbow — *see* Bursitis, elbow, olecranon
  lung or pneumoconiosis J60
Coalworker's lung or pneumoconiosis J60

Coarctation
aorta (preductal) (postductal) Q25.1
pulmonary artery Q25.71
Coated tongue K14.3
Coats' disease (exudative retinopathy) — see Retinopathy, exudative
Cocainism — see Dependence, drug, cocaine
Coccidioidomycosis B38.9
cutaneous B38.3
disseminated B38.7
generalized B38.7
meninges B38.4
prostate B38.81
pulmonary B38.2
acute B38.0
chronic B38.1
skin B38.3
specified NEC B38.89
Coccidioidosis — see Coccidioidomycosis
Coccidiosis (intestinal) A07.3
Coccydynia, coccygodynia M53.3
Coccyx — see condition
Cochin-China diarrhea K90.1
Cockayne's syndrome Q87.1
Cock's peculiar tumor L72.3
Cocked up toe — see Deformity, toe, specified NEC
Codman's tumor — see Neoplasm, bone, benign
Coenurosis B71.8
Coffee-worker's lung J67.8
Cogan's syndrome H16.32-
oculomotor apraxia H51.8
Coitus, painful (female) N94.1
male N53.12
psychogenic F52.6
Cold J00
with influenza, flu, or grippe — see Influenza, with, respiratory manifestations NEC
agglutinin disease or hemoglobinuria (chronic) D59.1
bronchial — see Bronchitis
chest — see Bronchitis
common (head) J00
effects of T69.9
specified effect NEC T69.8
excessive, effects of T69.9
specified effect NEC T69.8
exhaustion from T69.8
exposure to T69.9
specified effect NEC T69.8
head J00
injury syndrome (newborn) P80.0
on lung — see Bronchitis
rose J30.1
sensitivity, auto-immune D59.1
virus J00
Coldsore B00.1
Colibacillosis A49.8
as the cause of other disease (see also Escherichia coli) B96.20
generalized A41.50
Colic (bilious) (infantile) (intestinal) (recurrent) (spasmodic) R10.83
abdomen R10.83
psychogenic F45.8
appendix, appendicular K38.8
bile duct — see Calculus, bile duct
biliary — see Calculus, bile duct
common duct — see Calculus, bile duct
cystic duct — see Calculus, gallbladder
Devonshire NEC — see Poisoning, lead
gallbladder — see Calculus, gallbladder
gallstone — see Calculus, gallbladder
gallbladder or cystic duct — see Calculus, gallbladder
hepatic (duct) — see Calculus, bile duct
hysterical F45.8
kidney N23
lead NEC — see Poisoning, lead
mucous K58.9
with diarrhea K58.0
psychogenic F54
nephritic N23
painter's NEC — see Poisoning, lead
pancreas K86.8
psychogenic F45.8
renal N23
saturnine NEC — see Poisoning, lead
ureter N23
urethral N36.8
due to calculus N21.1
uterus NEC N94.89
menstrual — see Dysmenorrhea
worm NOS B83.9
Colicystitis — see Cystitis

Colitis (acute) (catarrhal) (chronic) (noninfective) (hemorrhagic) (see also Enteritis) K52.9
allergic K52.2
amebic (acute) (see also Amebiasis) A06.0
nondysenteric A06.2
anthrax A22.2
bacillary — see Infection, Shigella
balantidial A07.0
Clostridium difficile A04.7
coccidial A07.3
collagenous K52.89
cystica superficialis K52.89
dietary counseling and surveillance (for) Z71.3
dietetic K52.2
drug-induced K52.1
due to radiation K52.0
eosinophilic K52.82
food hypersensitivity K52.2
giardial A07.1
granulomatous — see Enteritis, regional, large intestine
infectious — see Enteritis, infectious
ischemic K55.9
acute (fulminant) (subacute) K55.0
chronic K55.1
due to mesenteric artery insufficiency K55.1
fulminant (acute) K55.0
left sided K51.50
with
abscess K51.514
complication K51.519
specified NEC K51.518
fistula K51.513
obstruction K51.512
rectal bleeding K51.511
lymphocytic K52.89
membranous
psychogenic F54
microscopic (collagenous) (lymphocytic) K52.89
mucous — see Syndrome, irritable, bowel
psychogenic F54
noninfective K52.9
specified NEC K52.89
polyposa — see Polyp, colon, inflammatory
protozoal A07.9
pseudomembranous A04.7
pseudomucinous — see Syndrome, irritable, bowel
regional — see Enteritis, regional, large intestine
segmental — see Enteritis, regional, large intestine
septic — see Enteritis, infectious
spastic K58.9
with diarrhea K58.0
psychogenic F54
staphylococcal A04.8
foodborne A05.0
subacute ischemic K55.0
thromboulcerative K55.0
toxic NEC K52.1
due to Clostridium difficile A04.7
transmural — see Enteritis, regional, large intestine
trichomonal A07.8
tuberculous (ulcerative) A18.32
ulcerative (chronic) K51.90
with
complication K51.919
abscess K51.914
fistula K51.913
obstruction K51.912
rectal bleeding K51.911
specified complication NEC K51.918
enterocolitis — see Enterocolitis, ulcerative
ileocolitis — see Ileocolitis, ulcerative
mucosal proctocolitis — see Proctocolitis, mucosal
proctitis — see Proctitis, ulcerative
pseudopolyposis — see Polyp, colon, inflammatory
psychogenic F54
rectosigmoiditis — see Rectosigmoiditis, ulcerative
specified type NEC K51.80
with
complication K51.819
abscess K51.814
fistula K51.813
obstruction K51.812
rectal bleeding K51.811
specified complication NEC K51.818

Collagenosis, collagen disease (nonvascular) (vascular) M35.9
cardiovascular I42.8
reactive perforating L87.1
specified NEC M35.8
Collapse R55
adrenal E27.2
cardiorespiratory R57.0
cardiovascular R57.0
newborn P29.89
circulatory (peripheral) R57.9
during or after labor and delivery O75.1
following ectopic or molar pregnancy O08.3
newborn P29.89
during or
after labor and delivery O75.1
resulting from a procedure, not elsewhere classified T81.10
external ear canal — see Stenosis, external ear canal
general R55
heart — see Disease, heart
heat T67.1
hysterical F44.89
labyrinth, membranous (congenital) Q16.5
lung (massive) (see also Atelectasis) J98.19
pressure due to anesthesia (general) (local) or other sedation T88.2
during labor and delivery O74.1
in pregnancy O29.02-
postpartum, puerperal O89.09
myocardial — see Disease, heart
nervous F48.8
neurocirculatory F45.8
nose M95.0
postoperative T81.10
pulmonary (see also Atelectasis) J98.19
newborn — see Atelectasis
trachea J39.8
tracheobronchial J98.09
valvular — see Endocarditis
vascular (peripheral) R57.9
during or after labor and delivery O75.1
following ectopic or molar pregnancy O08.3
newborn P29.89
vertebra M48.50-
cervical region M48.52-
cervicothoracic region M48.53-
in (due to)
metastasis — see Collapse, vertebra, in, specified disease NEC
osteoporosis (see also Osteoporosis) M80.88
cervical region M80.88
cervicothoracic region M80.88
lumbar region M80.88
lumbosacral region M80.88
multiple sites M80.88
occipito-atlanto-axial region M80.88
sacrococcygeal region M80.88
thoracic region M80.88
thoracolumbar region M80.88
specified disease NEC M48.50-
cervical region M48.52-
cervicothoracic region M48.53-
lumbar region M48.56-
lumbosacral region M48.57-
occipito-atlanto-axial region M48.51-
sacrococcygeal region M48.58-
thoracic region M48.54-
thoracolumbar region M48.55-
lumbar region M48.56-
lumbosacral region M48.57-
occipito-atlanto-axial region M48.51-
sacrococcygeal region M48.58-
thoracic region M48.54-
thoracolumbar region M48.55-
Collateral — see also condition
circulation (venous) I87.8
dilation, veins I87.8
Colles' fracture S52.53-
Collet(-Sicard) syndrome G52.7
Collier's asthma or lung J60
Collodion baby Q80.2
Colloid nodule (of thyroid) (cystic) E04.1
Coloboma (iris) Q13.0
eyelid Q10.3
fundus Q14.8
lens Q12.2
optic disc (congenital) Q14.2
acquired H47.31-
Coloenteritis — see Enteritis
Colon — see condition

Colonization
MRSA (Methicillin resistant Staphylococcus aureus) Z22.322
MSSA (Methicillin susceptible Staphylococcus aureus) Z22.321
status — see Carrier (suspected) of
Coloptosis K63.4
Color blindness — see Deficiency, color vision
Colostomy
attention to Z43.3
fitting or adjustment Z46.89
malfunctioning K94.03
status Z93.3
Colpitis (acute) — see Vaginitis
Colpocele N81.5
Colpocystitis — see Vaginitis
Colpospasm N94.2
Column, spinal, vertebral — see condition
Coma R40.20
with
motor response (none) R40.231
abnormal R40.233
extension R40.232
flexion withdrawal R40.234
localizes pain R40.235
obeys commands R40.236
opening of eyes (never) R40.211
in response to
pain R40.212
sound R40.213
spontaneous R40.214
verbal response (none) R40.221
confused conversation R40.224
inappropriate words R40.223
incomprehensible words R40.222
oriented R40.225
eclamptic — see Eclampsia
epileptic — see Epilepsy
Glasgow, scale score — see Glasgow coma scale
hepatic — see Failure, hepatic, by type, with coma
hyperglycemic (diabetic) — see Diabetes, coma
hyperosmolar (diabetic) — see Diabetes, coma
hypoglycemic (diabetic) — see Diabetes, coma, hypoglycemic
nondiabetic E15
in diabetes — see Diabetes, coma
insulin-induced — see Coma, hypoglycemic
myxedematous E03.5
newborn P91.5
persistent vegetative state R40.3
specified NEC, without documented Glasgow coma scale score, or with partial Glasgow coma scale score reported R40.244
Comatose — see Coma
Combat fatigue F43.0
Combined — see condition
Comedo, comedones (giant) L70.0
Comedocarcinoma — see also Neoplasm, breast, malignant
noninfiltrating
breast D05.8-
specified site — see Neoplasm, in situ, by site
unspecified site D05.8-
Comedomastitis — see Ectasia, mammary duct
Comminuted fracture — code as Fracture, closed
Common
arterial trunk Q20.0
atrioventricular canal Q21.2
atrium Q21.1
cold (head) J00
truncus (arteriosus) Q20.0
variable immunodeficiency — see Immunodeficiency, common variable
ventricle Q20.4
Commotio, commotion (current)
brain — see Injury, intracranial, concussion
cerebri — see Injury, intracranial, concussion
retinae S05.8x-
spinal cord — see Injury, spinal cord, by region
spinalis — see Injury, spinal cord, by region

D I S E A S E   I N D E X

Communication
between
  base of aorta and pulmonary artery Q21.4
  left ventricle and right atrium Q20.5
  pericardial sac and pleural sac Q34.8
  pulmonary artery and pulmonary vein, congenital Q25.72
  congenital between uterus and digestive or urinary tract Q51.7
Compartment syndrome (deep) (posterior) (traumatic) T79.A0
abdomen T79.A3
lower extremity (hip, buttock, thigh, leg, foot, toes) T79.A2
nontraumatic
  abdomen M79.A3
  lower extremity (hip, buttock, thigh, leg, foot, toes) M79.A2-
  specified site NEC M79.A9
  upper extremity (shoulder, arm, forearm, wrist, hand, fingers) M79.A1-
specified site NEC T79.A9
upper extremity (shoulder, arm, forearm, wrist, hand, fingers) T79.A1
Compensation
failure — see Disease, heart
neurosis, psychoneurosis — see Disorder, factitious
Complaint — see also Disease
bowel, functional K59.9
  psychogenic F45.8
intestine, functional K59.9
  psychogenic F45.8
kidney — see Disease, renal
miners' J60
Complete — see condition
Complex
Addison-Schilder E71.528
cardiorenal — see Hypertension, cardiorenal
Costen's M26.69
disseminated mycobacterium avium-intracellulare (DMAC) A31.2
Eisenmenger's (ventricular septal defect) I27.89
hypersexual F52.8
jumped process, spine — see Dislocation, vertebra
primary, tuberculous A15.7
Schilder-Addison E71.528
subluxation (vertebral) M99.19
  abdomen M99.19
  acromioclavicular M99.17
  cervical region M99.11
  cervicothoracic M99.11
  costochondral M99.18
  costovertebral M99.18
  head region M99.10
  hip M99.15
  lower extremity M99.16
  lumbar region M99.13
  lumbosacral M99.13
  occipitocervical M99.10
  pelvic region M99.15
  pubic M99.15
  rib cage M99.18
  sacral region M99.14
  sacrococcygeal M99.14
  sacroiliac M99.14
  specified NEC M99.19
  sternochondral M99.18
  sternoclavicular M99.17
  thoracic region M99.12
  thoracolumbar M99.12
  upper extremity M99.17
Taussig-Bing (transposition, aorta and overriding pulmonary artery) Q20.1
Complication(s) (from) (of)
accidental puncture or laceration during a procedure (of) — see Complications, intraoperative (intraprocedural), puncture or laceration
amputation stump (surgical) (late) NEC T87.9
  dehiscence T87.81
  infection or inflammation T87.40
    lower limb T87.4-
    upper limb T87.4-
  necrosis T87.50
    lower limb T87.5-
    upper limb T87.5-
  neuroma T87.30
    lower limb T87.3-
    upper limb T87.3-
  specified type NEC T87.89

Complication(s) (from) (of) — continued
anastomosis (and bypass) — see also Complications, prosthetic device or implant
  intestinal (internal) NEC K91.89
    involving urinary tract N99.89
  urinary tract (involving intestinal tract) N99.89
  vascular — see Complications, cardiovascular device or implant
anesthesia, anesthetic (see also Anesthesia, complication) T88.59
brain, postpartum, puerperal O89.2
cardiac
  in
    labor and delivery O74.2
    pregnancy O29.19-
  postpartum, puerperal O89.1
central nervous system
  in
    labor and delivery O74.3
    pregnancy O29.29-
  postpartum, puerperal O89.2
difficult or failed intubation T88.4
  in pregnancy O29.6-
failed sedation (conscious) (moderate) during procedure T88.52
hyperthermia, malignant T88.3
hypothermia T88.51
intubation failure T88.4
malignant hyperthermia T88.3
pulmonary
  in
    labor and delivery O74.1
    pregnancy NEC O29.09-
  postpartum, puerperal O89.09
shock T88.2
spinal and epidural
  in
    labor and delivery NEC O74.6
      headache O74.5
    pregnancy NEC O29.5x-
  postpartum, puerperal NEC O89.5
    headache O89.4
anti-reflux device — see Complications, esophageal anti-reflux device
aortic (bifurcation) graft — see Complications, graft, vascular
aortocoronary (bypass) graft — see Complications, coronary artery (bypass) graft
aortofemoral (bypass) graft — see Complications, extremity artery (bypass) graft
arteriovenous
  fistula, surgically created T82.9
    embolism T82.818
    fibrosis T82.828
    hemorrhage T82.838
    infection or inflammation T82.7
    mechanical
      breakdown T82.510
      displacement T82.520
      leakage T82.530
      malposition T82.520
      obstruction T82.590
      perforation T82.590
      protrusion T82.590
    pain T82.848
    specified type NEC T82.898
    stenosis T82.858
    thrombosis T82.868
  shunt, surgically created T82.9
    embolism T82.818
    fibrosis T82.828
    hemorrhage T82.838
    infection or inflammation T82.7
    mechanical
      breakdown T82.511
      displacement T82.521
      leakage T82.531
      malposition T82.521
      obstruction T82.591
      perforation T82.591
      protrusion T82.591
    pain T82.848
    specified type NEC T82.898
    stenosis T82.858
    thrombosis T82.868
arthroplasty — see Complications, joint prosthesis
artificial
  fertilization or insemination N98.9
    attempted introduction (of)
      embryo in embryo transfer N98.3
      ovum following in vitro fertilization N98.2
    hyperstimulation of ovaries N98.1
    infection N98.0
    specified NEC N98.8

Complication(s) (from) (of) — continued
artificial — continued
  heart T82.9
    embolism T82.817
    fibrosis T82.827
    hemorrhage T82.837
    infection or inflammation T82.7
    mechanical
      breakdown T82.512
      displacement T82.522
      leakage T82.532
      malposition T82.522
      obstruction T82.592
      perforation T82.592
      protrusion T82.592
    pain T82.847
    specified type NEC T82.897
    stenosis T82.857
    thrombosis T82.867
  opening
    cecostomy — see Complications, colostomy
    colostomy — see Complications, colostomy
    cystostomy — see Complications, cystostomy
    enterostomy — see Complications, enterostomy
    gastrostomy — see Complications, gastrostomy
    ileostomy — see Complications, enterostomy
    jejunostomy — see Complications, enterostomy
    nephrostomy — see Complications, stoma, urinary tract
    tracheostomy — see Complications, tracheostomy
    ureterostomy — see Complications, stoma, urinary tract
    urethrostomy — see Complications, stoma, urinary tract
balloon implant or device
  gastrointestinal T85.9
    embolism T85.81
    fibrosis T85.82
    hemorrhage T85.83
    infection and inflammation T85.79
    pain T85.84
    specified type NEC T85.89
    stenosis T85.85
    thrombosis T85.86
  vascular (counterpulsation) T82.9
    embolism T82.818
    fibrosis T82.828
    hemorrhage T82.838
    infection or inflammation T82.7
    mechanical
      breakdown T82.513
      displacement T82.523
      leakage T82.533
      malposition T82.523
      obstruction T82.593
      perforation T82.593
      protrusion T82.593
    pain T82.848
    specified type NEC T82.898
    stenosis T82.858
    thrombosis T82.868
bariatric procedure
  gastric band procedure K95.09
    infection K95.01
  specified procedure NEC K95.89
    infection K95.81
bile duct implant (prosthetic) T85.9
  embolism T85.81
  fibrosis T85.82
  hemorrhage T85.83
  infection and inflammation T85.79
  mechanical
    breakdown T85.510
    displacement T85.520
    malfunction T85.510
    malposition T85.520
    obstruction T85.590
    perforation T85.590
    protrusion T85.590
    specified NEC T85.590
  pain T85.84
  specified type NEC T85.89
  stenosis T85.85
  thrombosis T85.86
bladder device (auxiliary) — see Complications, genitourinary, device or implant, urinary system
bleeding (postoperative) — see Complication, postoperative, hemorrhage
  intraoperative — see Complication, intraoperative, hemorrhage

Complication(s) (from) (of) — continued
blood vessel graft — see Complications, graft, vascular
bone
  device NEC T84.9
    embolism T84.81
    fibrosis T84.82
    hemorrhage T84.83
    infection or inflammation T84.7
    mechanical
      breakdown T84.318
      displacement T84.328
      malposition T84.328
      obstruction T84.398
      perforation T84.398
      protrusion T84.398
    pain T84.84
    specified type NEC T84.89
    stenosis T84.85
    thrombosis T84.86
  graft — see Complications, graft, bone
  growth stimulator (electrode) — see Complications, electronic stimulator device, bone
  marrow transplant — see Complications, transplant, bone, marrow
brain neurostimulator (electrode) — see Complications, electronic stimulator device, brain
breast implant (prosthetic) T85.9
  capsular contracture T85.44
  embolism T85.81
  fibrosis T85.82
  hemorrhage T85.83
  infection and inflammation T85.79
  mechanical
    breakdown T85.41
    displacement T85.42
    leakage T85.43
    malposition T85.42
    obstruction T85.49
    perforation T85.49
    protrusion T85.49
    specified NEC T85.49
  pain T85.84
  specified type NEC T85.89
  stenosis T85.85
  thrombosis T85.86
bypass — see also Complications, prosthetic device or implant
  aortocoronary — see Complications, coronary artery (bypass) graft
  arterial — see also Complications, graft, vascular
  extremity — see Complications, extremity artery (bypass) graft
cardiac — see also Disease, heart
  device, implant or graft T82.9
    embolism T82.817
    fibrosis T82.827
    hemorrhage T82.837
    infection or inflammation T82.7
      valve prosthesis T82.6
    mechanical
      breakdown T82.519
        specified device NEC T82.518
      displacement T82.529
        specified device NEC T82.528
      leakage T82.539
        specified device NEC T82.538
      malposition T82.529
        specified device NEC T82.528
      obstruction T82.599
        specified device NEC T82.598
      perforation T82.599
        specified device NEC T82.598
      protrusion T82.599
        specified device NEC T82.598
    pain T82.847
    specified type NEC T82.897
    stenosis T82.857
    thrombosis T82.867
cardiovascular device, graft or implant T82.9
  aortic graft — see Complications, graft, vascular
  arteriovenous
    fistula, artificial — see Complication, arteriovenous, fistula, surgically created
    shunt — see Complication, arteriovenous, shunt, surgically created
  artificial heart — see Complication, artificial, heart
  balloon (counterpulsation) device — see Complication, balloon implant, vascular

Complication(s) (from) (of) — *continued*
cardiovascular device, graft or implant
  T82.9 — *continued*
  carotid artery graft — *see*
    Complications, graft, vascular
  coronary bypass graft — *see*
    Complication, coronary artery
    (bypass) graft
  dialysis catheter (vascular) — *see*
    Complication, catheter, dialysis
  electronic T82.9
    electrode T82.9
      embolism T82.817
      fibrosis T82.827
      hemorrhage T82.837
      infection T82.7
      mechanical
        breakdown T82.110
        displacement T82.120
        leakage T82.190
        obstruction T82.190
        perforation T82.190
        protrusion T82.190
        specified type NEC T82.190
      pain T82.847
      specified NEC T82.897
      stenosis T82.857
      thrombosis T82.867
    embolism T82.817
    fibrosis T82.827
    hemorrhage T82.837
    infection T82.7
    mechanical
      breakdown T82.119
      displacement T82.129
      leakage T82.199
      obstruction T82.199
      perforation T82.199
      protrusion T82.199
      specified type NEC T82.199
    pain T82.847
    pulse generator T82.9
      embolism T82.817
      fibrosis T82.827
      hemorrhage T82.837
      infection T82.7
      mechanical
        breakdown T82.111
        displacement T82.121
        leakage T82.191
        obstruction T82.191
        perforation T82.191
        protrusion T82.191
        specified type NEC T82.191
      pain T82.847
      specified NEC T82.897
      stenosis T82.857
      thrombosis T82.867
    specified condition NEC T82.897
    specified device NEC T82.9
      embolism T82.817
      fibrosis T82.827
      hemorrhage T82.837
      infection T82.7
      mechanical
        breakdown T82.118
        displacement T82.128
        leakage T82.198
        obstruction T82.198
        perforation T82.198
        protrusion T82.198
        specified type NEC T82.198
      pain T82.847
      specified NEC T82.897
      stenosis T82.857
      thrombosis T82.867
    stenosis T82.857
    thrombosis T82.867
  extremity artery graft — *see*
    Complication, extremity artery
    (bypass) graft
  femoral artery graft — *see* Complication,
    extremity artery (bypass) graft
  heart
    transplant — *see* Complication,
      transplant, heart
    valve — *see* Complication, prosthetic
      device, heart valve
      graft — *see* Complication, heart,
        valve, graft
  heart-lung transplant — *see*
    Complication, transplant, heart,
    with lung
  infection or inflammation T82.7
  umbrella device — *see* Complication,
    umbrella device, vascular
  vascular graft (or anastomosis) — *see*
    Complication, graft, vascular
  carotid artery (bypass) graft — *see*
    Complications, graft, vascular

Complication(s) (from) (of) — *continued*
catheter (device) NEC — *see also*
  Complications, prosthetic device or
  implant
  cystostomy T83.9
    embolism T83.81
    fibrosis T83.82
    hemorrhage T83.83
    infection and inflammation T83.59
    mechanical
      breakdown T83.010
      displacement T83.020
      leakage T83.030
      malposition T83.020
      obstruction T83.090
      perforation T83.090
      protrusion T83.090
      specified NEC T83.090
    pain T83.84
    specified type NEC T83.89
    stenosis T83.85
    thrombosis T83.86
  dialysis (vascular) T82.9
    embolism T82.818
    fibrosis T82.828
    hemorrhage T82.838
    infection and inflammation T82.7
    intraperitoneal — *see* Complications,
      catheter, intraperitoneal
    mechanical
      breakdown T82.41
      displacement T82.42
      leakage T82.43
      malposition T82.42
      obstruction T82.49
      perforation T82.49
      protrusion T82.49
    pain T82.848
    specified type NEC T82.898
    stenosis T82.858
    thrombosis T82.868
  epidural infusion T85.9
    embolism T85.81
    fibrosis T85.82
    hemorrhage T85.83
    infection and inflammation T85.79
    mechanical
      breakdown T85.610
      displacement T85.620
      leakage T85.630
      malfunction T85.610
      malposition T85.620
      obstruction T85.690
      perforation T85.690
      protrusion T85.690
      specified NEC T85.690
    pain T85.84
    specified type NEC T85.89
    stenosis T85.85
    thrombosis T85.86
  intraperitoneal dialysis T85.9
    embolism T85.81
    fibrosis T85.82
    hemorrhage T85.83
    infection and inflammation T85.71
    mechanical
      breakdown T85.611
      displacement T85.621
      leakage T85.631
      malfunction T85.611
      malposition T85.621
      obstruction T85.691
      perforation T85.691
      protrusion T85.691
      specified NEC T85.691
    pain T85.84
    specified type NEC T85.89
    stenosis T85.85
    thrombosis T85.86
  intravenous infusion T82.9
    embolism T82.818
    fibrosis T82.828
    hemorrhage T82.838
    infection or inflammation T82.7
    mechanical
      breakdown T82.514
      displacement T82.524
      leakage T82.534
      malposition T82.524
      obstruction T82.594
      perforation T82.594
      protrusion T82.594
    pain T82.848
    specified type NEC T82.898
    stenosis T82.858
    thrombosis T82.868

Complication(s) (from) (of) — *continued*
catheter (device) NEC *(see also*
  Complications, prosthetic device or
  implant) — *continued*
  subdural infusion T85.9
    embolism T85.81
    fibrosis T85.82
    hemorrhage T85.83
    infection and inflammation T85.79
    mechanical
      breakdown T85.610
      displacement T85.620
      leakage T85.630
      malfunction T85.610
      malposition T85.620
      obstruction T85.690
      perforation T85.690
      protrusion T85.690
      specified NEC T85.690
    pain T85.84
    specified type NEC T85.89
    stenosis T85.85
    thrombosis T85.86
  urethral, indwelling T83.9
    displacement T83.028
    embolism T83.81
    fibrosis T83.82
    hemorrhage T83.83
    infection and inflammation T83.51
    leakage T83.038
    malposition T83.028
    mechanical
      breakdown T83.018
    obstruction (mechanical) T83.098
    pain T83.84
    perforation T83.098
    protrusion T83.098
    specified type NEC T83.098
    stenosis T83.85
    thrombosis T83.86
  urinary (indwelling) — *see*
    Complications, catheter, urethral,
    indwelling
cecostomy (stoma) — *see* Complications,
  colostomy
cesarean delivery wound NEC O90.89
  disruption O90.0
  hematoma O90.2
  infection (following delivery) O86.0
chemotherapy (antineoplastic) NEC T88.7
chin implant (prosthetic) — *see*
  Complication, prosthetic device or
  implant, specified NEC
circulatory system I99.8
  intraoperative I97.88
  postprocedural I97.89
    following cardiac surgery I97.19-
      postcardiotomy syndrome I97.0
    hypertension I97.3
    lymphedema after mastectomy I97.2
    postcardiotomy syndrome I97.0
    specified NEC I97.89
colostomy (stoma) K94.00
  hemorrhage K94.01
  infection K94.02
  malfunction K94.03
  mechanical K94.03
  specified complication NEC K94.09
contraceptive device, intrauterine — *see*
  Complications, intrauterine,
  contraceptive device
cord (umbilical) — *see* Complications,
  umbilical cord
corneal graft — *see* Complications, graft,
  cornea
coronary artery (bypass) graft T82.9
  atherosclerosis — *see* Arteriosclerosis,
    coronary (artery)
  embolism T82.818
  fibrosis T82.828
  hemorrhage T82.838
  infection and inflammation T82.7
  mechanical
    breakdown T82.211
    displacement T82.212
    leakage T82.213
    malposition T82.212
    obstruction T82.218
    perforation T82.218
    protrusion T82.218
    specified NEC T82.218
  pain T82.848
  specified type NEC T82.897
  stenosis T82.858
  thrombosis T82.868
counterpulsation device (balloon), intra-
  aortic — *see* Complications, balloon
  implant, vascular

Complication(s) (from) (of) — *continued*
cystostomy (stoma) N99.518
  catheter — *see* Complications, catheter,
    cystostomy
  hemorrhage N99.510
  infection N99.511
  malfunction N99.512
  specified type NEC N99.518
delivery (*see also* Complications, obstetric)
  O75.9
  procedure (instrumental) (manual)
    (surgical) O75.4
  specified NEC O75.89
dialysis (peritoneal) (renal) — *see also*
  Complications, infusion
  catheter (vascular) — *see* Complication,
    catheter, dialysis
  peritoneal, intraperitoneal — *see*
    Complications, catheter,
    intraperitoneal
dorsal column (spinal) neurostimulator —
  see Complications, electronic
  stimulator device, spinal cord
drug NEC T88.7
ear procedure — *see also* Disorder, ear
  intraoperative H95.88
    hematoma — *see* Complications,
      intraoperative, hemorrhage
      (hematoma) (of), ear
    hemorrhage — *see* Complications,
      intraoperative, hemorrhage
      (hematoma) (of), ear
    laceration — *see* Complications,
      intraoperative, puncture or
      laceration, ear
    specified NEC H95.88
  postoperative H95.89
    external ear canal stenosis H95.81-
    hematoma — *see* Complications,
      postprocedural, hemorrhage
      (hematoma) (of), ear
    hemorrhage — *see* Complications,
      postprocedural, hemorrhage
      (hematoma) (of), ear
    postmastoidectomy — *see*
      Complications,
      postmastoidectomy
    specified NEC H95.89
ectopic pregnancy O08.9
  damage to pelvic organs O08.6
  embolism O08.2
  genital infection O08.0
  hemorrhage (delayed) (excessive) O08.1
  metabolic disorder O08.5
  renal failure O08.4
  shock O08.3
  specified type NEC O08.0
  venous complication NEC O08.7
electronic stimulator device
  bladder (urinary) — *see* Complications,
    electronic stimulator device,
    urinary
  bone T84.9
    breakdown T84.310
    displacement T84.320
    embolism T84.81
    fibrosis T84.82
    hemorrhage T84.83
    infection or inflammation T84.7
    malfunction T84.310
    malposition T84.320
    mechanical NEC T84.390
    obstruction T84.390
    pain T84.84
    perforation T84.390
    protrusion T84.390
    specified type NEC T84.89
    stenosis T84.85
    thrombosis T84.86
  brain T85.9
    embolism T85.81
    fibrosis T85.82
    hemorrhage T85.83
    infection and inflammation T85.79
    mechanical
      breakdown T85.110
      displacement T85.120
      leakage T85.190
      malposition T85.120
      obstruction T85.190
      perforation T85.190
      protrusion T85.190
      specified NEC T85.190
    pain T85.84
    specified type NEC T85.89
    stenosis T85.85
    thrombosis T85.86

D I S E A S E I N D E X

Complication(s) (from) (of) — continued
electronic stimulator device — continued
  cardiac (defibrillator) (pacemaker) —
    see Complications, cardiovascular
    device or implant, electronic
  muscle T84.9
    breakdown T84.418
    displacement T84.428
    embolism T84.81
    fibrosis T84.82
    hemorrhage T84.83
    infection or inflammation T84.7
    mechanical NEC T84.498
    pain T84.84
    specified type NEC T84.89
    stenosis T84.85
    thrombosis T84.86
  nervous system T85.9
    brain — see Complications, electronic
      stimulator device, brain
    embolism T85.81
    fibrosis T85.82
    hemorrhage T85.83
    infection and inflammation T85.79
    mechanical
      breakdown T85.118
      displacement T85.128
      leakage T85.199
      malposition T85.128
      obstruction T85.199
      perforation T85.199
      protrusion T85.199
      specified NEC T85.199
    pain T85.84
    peripheral nerve — see
      Complications, electronic
      stimulator device, peripheral
      nerve
    specified type NEC T85.89
    spinal cord — see Complications,
      electronic stimulator device,
      spinal cord
    stenosis T85.85
    thrombosis T85.86
  peripheral nerve T85.9
    embolism T85.81
    fibrosis T85.82
    hemorrhage T85.83
    infection and inflammation T85.79
    mechanical
      breakdown T85.111
      displacement T85.121
      leakage T85.191
      malposition T85.121
      obstruction T85.191
      perforation T85.191
      protrusion T85.191
      specified NEC T85.191
    pain T85.84
    specified type NEC T85.89
    stenosis T85.85
    thrombosis T85.86
  spinal cord T85.9
    embolism T85.81
    fibrosis T85.82
    hemorrhage T85.83
    infection and inflammation T85.79
    mechanical
      breakdown T85.112
      displacement T85.122
      leakage T85.192
      malposition T85.122
      obstruction T85.192
      perforation T85.192
      protrusion T85.192
      specified NEC T85.192
    pain T85.84
    specified type NEC T85.89
    stenosis T85.85
    thrombosis T85.86
  urinary T83.9
    embolism T83.81
    fibrosis T83.82
    hemorrhage T83.83
    infection and inflammation T83.59
    mechanical
      breakdown T83.110
      displacement T83.120
      malposition T83.120
      perforation T83.190
      protrusion T83.190
      specified NEC T83.190
    pain T83.84
    specified type NEC T83.89
    stenosis T83.85
    thrombosis T83.86

Complication(s) (from) (of) — continued
electroshock therapy T88.9
  specified NEC T88.8
endocrine E34.9
  postprocedural
    adrenal hypofunction E89.6
    hypoinsulinemia E89.1
    hypoparathyroidism E89.2
    hypopituitarism E89.3
    hypothyroidism E89.0
    ovarian failure E89.40
      asymptomatic E89.40
      symptomatic E89.41
    specified NEC E89.89
    testicular hypofunction E89.5
endodontic treatment NEC M27.59
enterostomy (stoma) K94.10
  hemorrhage K94.11
  infection K94.12
  malfunction K94.13
  mechanical K94.13
  specified complication NEC K94.19
episiotomy, disruption O90.1
esophageal anti-reflux device T85.9
  embolism T85.81
  fibrosis T85.82
  hemorrhage T85.83
  infection and inflammation T85.79
  mechanical
    breakdown T85.511
    displacement T85.521
    malfunction T85.511
    malposition T85.521
    obstruction T85.591
    perforation T85.591
    protrusion T85.591
    specified NEC T85.591
  pain T85.84
  specified type NEC T85.89
  stenosis T85.85
  thrombosis T85.86
esophagostomy K94.30
  hemorrhage K94.31
  infection K94.32
  malfunction K94.33
  mechanical K94.33
  specified complication NEC K94.39
extracorporeal circulation T80.90
extremity artery (bypass) graft T82.9
  arteriosclerosis — see Arteriosclerosis,
    extremities, bypass graft
  embolism T82.818
  fibrosis T82.828
  hemorrhage T82.838
  infection and inflammation T82.7
  mechanical
    breakdown T82.318
      femoral artery T82.312
    displacement T82.328
      femoral artery T82.322
    leakage T82.338
      femoral artery T82.332
    malposition T82.328
      femoral artery T82.322
    obstruction T82.398
      femoral artery T82.392
    perforation T82.398
      femoral artery T82.392
    protrusion T82.398
      femoral artery T82.392
  pain T82.848
  specified type NEC T82.898
  stenosis T82.858
  thrombosis T82.868
eye H57.9
  corneal graft — see Complications,
    graft, cornea
  implant (prosthetic) T85.9
    embolism T85.81
    fibrosis T85.82
    hemorrhage T85.83
    infection and inflammation T85.79
    mechanical
      breakdown T85.318
      displacement T85.328
      leakage T85.398
      malposition T85.328
      obstruction T85.398
      perforation T85.398
      protrusion T85.398
      specified NEC T85.398
    pain T85.84
    specified type NEC T85.89
    stenosis T85.85
    thrombosis T85.86
  intraocular lens — see Complications,
    intraocular lens
  orbital prosthesis — see Complications,
    orbital prosthesis

Complication(s) (from) (of) — continued
female genital N94.9
  device, implant or graft NEC — see
    Complications, genitourinary,
    device or implant, genital tract
femoral artery (bypass) graft — see
  Complication, extremity artery
  (bypass) graft
fixation device, internal (orthopedic) T84.9
  infection and inflammation T84.60
    arm T84.61-
      humerus T84.61-
      radius T84.61-
      ulna T84.61-
    leg T84.629
      femur T84.62-
      fibula T84.62-
      tibia T84.62-
    specified site NEC T84.69
    spine T84.63
  mechanical
    breakdown
      limb T84.119
        carpal T84.210
        femur T84.11-
        fibula T84.11-
        humerus T84.11-
        metacarpal T84.210
        metatarsal T84.213
        phalanx
          foot T84.213
          hand T84.210
        radius T84.11-
        tarsal T84.213
        tibia T84.11-
        ulna T84.11-
      specified bone NEC T84.218
      spine T84.216
    displacement
      limb T84.129
        carpal T84.220
        femur T84.12-
        fibula T84.12-
        humerus T84.12-
        metacarpal T84.220
        metatarsal T84.223
        phalanx
          foot T84.223
          hand T84.220
        radius T84.12-
        tarsal T84.223
        tibia T84.12-
        ulna T84.12-
      specified bone NEC T84.228
      spine T84.226
    malposition — see Complications,
      fixation device, internal,
      mechanical, displacement
    obstruction — see Complications,
      fixation device, internal,
      mechanical, specified type NEC
    perforation — see Complications,
      fixation device, internal,
      mechanical, specified type NEC
    protrusion — see Complications,
      fixation device, internal,
      mechanical, specified type NEC
    specified type NEC
      limb T84.199
        carpal T84.290
        femur T84.19-
        fibula T84.19-
        humerus T84.19-
        metacarpal T84.290
        metatarsal T84.293
        phalanx
          foot T84.293
          hand T84.290
        radius T84.19-
        tarsal T84.293
        tibia T84.19-
        ulna T84.19-
      specified bone NEC T84.298
      vertebra T84.296
  specified type NEC T84.89
    embolism T84.81
    fibrosis T84.82
    hemorrhage T84.83
    pain T84.84
    specified complication NEC T84.89
    stenosis T84.85
    thrombosis T84.86

Complication(s) (from) (of) — continued
following
  acute myocardial infarction NEC I23.8
    aneurysm (false) (of cardiac wall) (of
      heart wall) (ruptured) I23.3
    angina I23.7
    atrial
      septal defect I23.1
      thrombosis I23.6
    cardiac wall rupture I23.3
    chordae tendinae rupture I23.4
    defect
      septal
        atrial (heart) I23.1
        ventricular (heart) I23.2
    hemopericardium I23.0
    papillary muscle rupture I23.5
    rupture
      cardiac wall I23.3
        with hemopericardium I23.0
      chordae tendineae I23.4
      papillary muscle I23.5
    specified NEC I23.8
    thrombosis
      atrium I23.6
      auricular appendage I23.6
      ventricle (heart) I23.6
    ventricular
      septal defect I23.2
      thrombosis I23.6
  ectopic or molar pregnancy O08.9
    cardiac arrest O08.81
    sepsis O08.82
    specified type NEC O08.89
    urinary tract infection O08.83
  termination of pregnancy — see
    Abortion
gastrointestinal K92.9
  bile duct prosthesis — see
    Complications, bile duct implant
  esophageal anti-reflux device — see
    Complications, esophageal anti-
    reflux device
  postoperative
    colostomy — see Complications,
      colostomy
    dumping syndrome K91.1
    enterostomy — see Complications,
      enterostomy
    gastrostomy — see Complications,
      gastrostomy
    malabsorption NEC K91.2
    obstruction K91.3
    postcholecystectomy syndrome K91.5
    specified NEC K91.89
    vomiting after GI surgery K91.0
  prosthetic device or implant
    bile duct prosthesis — see
      Complications, bile duct implant
    esophageal anti-reflux device — see
      Complications, esophageal anti-
      reflux device
    specified type NEC
      embolism T85.81
      fibrosis T85.82
      hemorrhage T85.83
      mechanical
        breakdown T85.518
        displacement T85.528
        malfunction T85.518
        malposition T85.528
        obstruction T85.598
        perforation T85.598
        protrusion T85.598
        specified NEC T85.598
      pain T85.84
      specified complication NEC
        T85.89
      stenosis T85.85
      thrombosis T85.86
gastrostomy (stoma) K94.20
  hemorrhage K94.21
  infection K94.22
  malfunction K94.23
  mechanical K94.23
  specified complication NEC K94.29
genitourinary
  device or implant T83.9
    genital tract T83.9
      infection or inflammation T83.6
      intrauterine contraceptive device —
        see Complications,
        intrauterine, contraceptive
        device
      mechanical — see Complications,
        by device, mechanical
      mesh — see Complications, mesh
      penile prosthesis — see
        Complications, prosthetic
        device, penile

Complication(s) (from) (of) — continued
genitourinary — continued
  device or implant T83.9 — continued
   genital tract T83.9 — continued
    specified type NEC T83.89
     embolism T83.81
     fibrosis T83.82
     hemorrhage T83.83
     pain T83.84
     specified complication NEC
      T83.89
     stenosis T83.85
     thrombosis T83.86
    vaginal mesh — see Complications,
     mesh
  urinary system T83.9
   cystostomy catheter — see
    Complication, catheter,
    cystostomy
   electronic stimulator — see
    Complications, electronic
    stimulator device, urinary
   indwelling urethral catheter — see
    Complications, catheter,
    urethral, indwelling
   infection or inflammation T83.59
    indwelling urinary catheter
     T83.51
   kidney transplant — see
    Complication, transplant,
    kidney
   organ graft — see Complication,
    graft, urinary organ
   specified type NEC T83.89
    embolism T83.81
    fibrosis T83.82
    hemorrhage T83.83
    mechanical T83.198
     breakdown T83.118
     displacement T83.128
     malfunction T83.118
     malposition T83.128
     obstruction T83.198
     perforation T83.198
     protrusion T83.198
     specified NEC T83.198
    pain T83.84
    specified complication NEC
     T83.89
    stenosis T83.85
    thrombosis T83.86
   sphincter implant — see
    Complications, implant,
    urinary sphincter
postprocedural
  pelvic peritoneal adhesions N99.4
  renal failure N99.0
  specified NEC N99.89
  stoma — see Complications, stoma,
   urinary tract
  urethral stricture — see Stricture,
   urethra, postprocedural
  vaginal
   adhesions N99.2
   vault prolapse N99.3
graft (bypass) (patch) — see also
  Complications, prosthetic device or
  implant
  aorta — see Complications, graft,
   vascular
  arterial — see Complication, graft,
   vascular
  bone T86.839
   failure T86.831
   infection T86.832
   mechanical T84.318
    breakdown T84.318
    displacement T84.328
    protrusion T84.398
    specified type NEC T84.398
   rejection T86.830
   specified type NEC T86.838
  carotid artery — see Complications,
   graft, vascular
  cornea T86.849
   failure T86.841
   infection T86.842
   mechanical T85.398
    breakdown T85.318
    displacement T85.328
    protrusion T85.398
    specified type NEC T85.398
   rejection T86.840
   retroprosthetic membrane T85.398
   specified type NEC T86.848
  femoral artery (bypass) — see
   Complication, extremity artery
   (bypass) graft

Complication(s) (from) (of) — continued
graft (bypass) (patch) (see also
  Complications, prosthetic device or
  implant) — continued
  genital organ or tract — see
   Complications, genitourinary,
   device or implant, genital tract
  muscle T84.9
   breakdown T84.410
   displacement T84.420
   embolism T84.81
   fibrosis T84.82
   hemorrhage T84.83
   infection and inflammation T84.7
   mechanical NEC T84.490
   pain T84.84
   specified type NEC T84.89
   stenosis T84.85
   thrombosis T84.86
  nerve — see Complication, prosthetic
   device or implant, specified NEC
  skin — see Complications, prosthetic
   device or implant, skin graft
  tendon T84.9
   breakdown T84.410
   displacement T84.420
   embolism T84.81
   fibrosis T84.82
   hemorrhage T84.83
   infection and inflammation T84.7
   mechanical NEC T84.490
   pain T84.84
   specified type NEC T84.89
   stenosis T84.85
   thrombosis T84.86
  urinary organ T83.9
   embolism T83.81
   fibrosis T83.82
   hemorrhage T83.83
   infection and inflammation T83.59
    indwelling urinary catheter T83.51
   mechanical
    breakdown T83.21
    displacement T83.22
    leakage T83.23
    malposition T83.22
    obstruction T83.29
    perforation T83.29
    protrusion T83.29
    specified NEC T83.29
   pain T83.84
   specified type NEC T83.89
   stenosis T83.85
   thrombosis T83.86
  vascular T82.9
   embolism T82.818
   femoral artery — see Complication,
    extremity artery (bypass) graft
   fibrosis T82.828
   hemorrhage T82.838
   mechanical
    breakdown T82.319
     aorta (bifurcation) T82.310
     carotid artery T82.311
     specified vessel NEC T82.318
    displacement T82.329
     aorta (bifurcation) T82.320
     carotid artery T82.321
     specified vessel NEC T82.328
    leakage T82.339
     aorta (bifurcation) T82.330
     carotid artery T82.331
     specified vessel NEC T82.338
    malposition T82.329
     aorta (bifurcation) T82.320
     carotid artery T82.321
     specified vessel NEC T82.328
    obstruction T82.399
     aorta (bifurcation) T82.390
     carotid artery T82.391
     specified vessel NEC T82.398
    perforation T82.399
     aorta (bifurcation) T82.390
     carotid artery T82.391
     specified vessel NEC T82.398
    protrusion T82.399
     aorta (bifurcation) T82.390
     carotid artery T82.391
     specified vessel NEC T82.398
    pain T82.848
    specified complication NEC T82.898
    stenosis T82.858
    thrombosis T82.868
heart I51.9
  assist device
   infection and inflammation T82.7
   following acute myocardial infarction —
    see Complications, following, acute
    myocardial infarction

Complication(s) (from) (of) — continued
heart I51.9 — continued
  postoperative — see Complications,
   circulatory system
  transplant — see Complication,
   transplant, heart
   and lung(s) — see Complications,
    transplant, heart, with lung
  valve
   graft (biological) T82.9
    embolism T82.817
    fibrosis T82.827
    hemorrhage T82.837
    infection and inflammation T82.7
    mechanical T82.228
     breakdown T82.221
     displacement T82.222
     leakage T82.223
     malposition T82.222
     obstruction T82.228
     perforation T82.228
     protrusion T82.228
    pain T82.847
    specified type NEC T82.897
    stenosis T82.857
    thrombosis T82.867
   prosthesis T82.9
    embolism T82.817
    fibrosis T82.827
    hemorrhage T82.837
    infection or inflammation T82.6
    mechanical T82.09
     breakdown T82.01
     displacement T82.02
     leakage T82.03
     malposition T82.02
     obstruction T82.09
     perforation T82.09
     protrusion T82.09
    pain T82.847
    specified type NEC T82.897
     mechanical T82.09
    stenosis T82.857
    thrombosis T82.867
hematoma
  intraoperative — see Complication,
   intraoperative, hemorrhage
  postprocedural — see Complication,
   postprocedural, hemorrhage
hemodialysis — see Complications,
  dialysis
hemorrhage
  intraoperative — see Complication,
   intraoperative, hemorrhage
  postprocedural — see Complication,
   postprocedural, hemorrhage
ileostomy (stoma) — see Complications,
  enterostomy
immunization (procedure) — see
  Complications, vaccination
implant — see also Complications, by site
  and type
  urinary sphincter T83.9
   embolism T83.81
   fibrosis T83.82
   hemorrhage T83.83
   infection and inflammation T83.59
   mechanical
    breakdown T83.111
    displacement T83.121
    leakage T83.191
    malposition T83.121
    obstruction T83.191
    perforation T83.191
    protrusion T83.191
    specified NEC T83.191
   pain T83.84
   specified type NEC T83.89
   stenosis T83.85
   thrombosis T83.86
infusion (procedure) T80.90
  air embolism T80.0
  blood — see Complications, transfusion
  catheter — see Complications, catheter
  infection T80.29
  pump — see Complications,
   cardiovascular, device or implant
  sepsis T80.29
  serum reaction (see also Reaction,
   serum) T80.69
   anaphylactic shock (see also Shock,
    anaphylactic) T80.59
  specified type NEC T80.89
inhalation therapy NEC T81.81

Complication(s) (from) (of) — continued
injection (procedure) T80.90
  drug reaction — see Reaction, drug
  infection T80.29
  sepsis T80.29
  serum (prophylactic) (therapeutic) — see
   Complications, vaccination
  specified type NEC T80.89
  vaccine (any) — see Complications,
   vaccination
inoculation (any) — see Complications,
  vaccination
insulin pump
  infection and inflammation T85.72
  mechanical
   breakdown T85.614
   displacement T85.624
   leakage T85.633
   malposition T85.624
   obstruction T85.694
   perforation T85.694
   protrusion T85.694
   specified NEC T85.694
intestinal pouch NEC K91.858
intraocular lens (prosthetic) T85.9
  embolism T85.81
  fibrosis T85.82
  hemorrhage T85.83
  infection and inflammation T85.79
  mechanical
   breakdown T85.21
   displacement T85.22
   malposition T85.22
   obstruction T85.29
   perforation T85.29
   protrusion T85.29
   specified NEC T85.29
  pain T85.84
  specified type NEC T85.89
  stenosis T85.85
  thrombosis T85.86
intraoperative (intraprocedural)
  cardiac arrest
   during cardiac surgery I97.710
   during other surgery I97.711
  cardiac functional disturbance NEC
   during cardiac surgery I97.790
   during other surgery I97.791
  hemorrhage (hematoma) (of)
   circulatory system organ or structure
    during cardiac bypass I97.411
    during cardiac catheterization
     I97.410
    during other circulatory system
     procedure I97.418
    during other procedure I97.42
   digestive system organ
    during procedure on digestive
     system K91.61
    during procedure on other organ
     K91.62
   ear
    during procedure on ear and
     mastoid process H95.21
    during procedure on other organ
     H95.22
   endocrine system organ or structure
    during procedure on endocrine
     system organ or structure
     E36.01
    during procedure on other organ
     E36.02
   eye and adnexa
    during ophthalmic procedure
     H59.11-
    during other procedure H59.12-
   genitourinary organ or structure
    during procedure on genitourinary
     organ or structure N99.61
    during procedure on other organ
     N99.62
   mastoid process
    during procedure on ear and
     mastoid process H95.21
    during procedure on other organ
     H95.22
   musculoskeletal structure
    during musculoskeletal surgery
     M96.810
    during non-orthopedic surgery
     M96.811
    during orthopedic surgery M96.810
   nervous system
    during a nervous system procedure
     G97.31
    during other procedure G97.32

DISEASE INDEX

DISEASE INDEX

Complication(s) (from) (of) — *continued*
intraoperative (intraprocedural) — *continued*
  hemorrhage (hematoma) (of) — *continued*
    respiratory system
      during other procedure J95.62
      during procedure on respiratory system organ or structure J95.61
    skin and subcutaneous tissue
      during a dermatologic procedure L76.01
      during a procedure on other organ L76.02
    spleen
      during a procedure on other organ D78.02
      during a procedure on the spleen D78.01
  puncture or laceration (accidental) (unintentional) (of)
    brain
      during a nervous system procedure G97.48
      during other procedure G97.49
    circulatory system organ or structure
      during circulatory system procedure I97.51
      during other procedure I97.52
    digestive system
      during procedure on digestive system K91.71
      during procedure on other organ K91.72
    ear
      during procedure on ear and mastoid process H95.31
      during procedure on other organ H95.32
    endocrine system organ or structure
      during procedure on endocrine system organ or structure E36.11
      during procedure on other organ E36.12
    eye and adnexa
      during ophthalmic procedure H59.21-
      during other procedure H59.22-
    genitourinary organ or structure
      during procedure on genitourinary organ or structure N99.71
      during procedure on other organ N99.72
    mastoid process
      during procedure on ear and mastoid process H95.31
      during procedure on other organ H95.32
    musculoskeletal structure
      during musculoskeletal surgery M96.820
      during non-orthopedic surgery M96.821
      during orthopedic surgery M96.820
    nervous system
      during a nervous system procedure G97.48
      during other procedure G97.49
    respiratory system
      during other procedure J95.72
      during procedure on respiratory system organ or structure J95.71
    skin and subcutaneous tissue
      during a dermatologic procedure L76.11
      during a procedure on other organ L76.12
    spleen
      during a procedure on other organ D78.12
      during a procedure on the spleen D78.11
  specified NEC
    circulatory system I97.88
    digestive system K91.81
    ear H95.88
    endocrine system E36.8
    eye and adnexa H59.88
    genitourinary system N99.81
    mastoid process H95.88
    musculoskeletal structure M96.89
    nervous system G97.81
    respiratory system J95.88
    skin and subcutaneous tissue L76.81
    spleen D78.81

Complication(s) (from) (of) — *continued*
intraperitoneal catheter (dialysis) (infusion) — *see* Complications, catheter, intraperitoneal
intrauterine
  contraceptive device
    embolism T83.81
    fibrosis T83.82
    hemorrhage T83.83
    infection and inflammation T83.6
    mechanical
      breakdown T83.31
      displacement T83.32
      malposition T83.32
      obstruction T83.39
      perforation T83.39
      protrusion T83.39
      specified NEC T83.39
    pain T83.84
    specified type NEC T83.89
    stenosis T83.85
    thrombosis T83.86
  procedure (fetal), to newborn P96.5
jejunostomy (stoma) — *see* Complications, enterostomy
joint prosthesis, internal T84.9
  breakage (fracture) T84.01-
  dislocation T84.02-
  fracture T84.01-
  infection or inflammation T84.50
    hip T84.5-
    knee T84.5-
    specified joint NEC T84.59
  instability T84.02-
  malposition — *see* Complications, joint prosthesis, mechanical, displacement
  mechanical
    breakage, broken T84.01-
    dislocation T84.02-
    fracture T84.01-
    instability T84.02-
    leakage — *see* Complications, joint prosthesis, mechanical, specified NEC
    loosening T84.039
      hip T84.03-
      knee T84.03-
      specified joint NEC T84.038
    obstruction — *see* Complications, joint prosthesis, mechanical, specified NEC
    perforation — *see* Complications, joint prosthesis, mechanical, specified NEC
    periprosthetic
      fracture T84.049
        hip T84.04-
        knee T84.04-
        other specified joint T84.048
      osteolysis T84.059
        hip T84.05-
        knee T84.05-
        other specified joint T84.058
    protrusion — *see* Complications, joint prosthesis, mechanical, specified NEC
    specified complication NEC T84.099
      hip T84.09-
      knee T84.09-
      other specified joint T84.098
    subluxation T84.02-
      wear of articular bearing surface T84.069
      hip T84.06-
      knee T84.06-
      other specified joint T84.068
  specified joint NEC T84.89
    embolism T84.81
    fibrosis T84.82
    hemorrhage T84.83
    pain T84.84
    specified complication NEC T84.89
    stenosis T84.85
    thrombosis T84.86
  subluxation T84.02-
kidney transplant — *see* Complications, transplant, kidney
labor O75.9
  specified NEC O75.89
liver transplant (immune or nonimmune) — *see* Complications, transplant, liver
lumbar puncture G97.1
  cerebrospinal fluid leak G97.0
  headache or reaction G97.1
lung transplant — *see* Complications, transplant, lung
  and heart — *see* Complications, transplant, lung, with heart

Complication(s) (from) (of) — *continued*
male genital N50.9
  device, implant or graft — *see* Complications, genitourinary, device or implant, genital tract
  postprocedural or postoperative — *see* Complications, genitourinary, postprocedural
  specified NEC N99.89
mastoid (process) procedure
  intraoperative H95.88
    hematoma — *see* Complications, intraoperative, hemorrhage (hematoma) (of), mastoid process
    hemorrhage — *see* Complications, intraoperative, hemorrhage (hematoma) (of), mastoid process
    laceration — *see* Complications,intraoperative, puncture or laceration, mastoid process
    specified NEC H95.88
  postmastoidectomy — *see* Complications, postmastoidectomy
  postoperative H95.89
    external ear canal stenosis H95.81-
    hematoma — *see* Complications, postprocedural, hemorrhage (hematoma) (of), mastoid process
    hemorrhage — *see* Complications, postprocedural, hemorrhage (hematoma) (of), mastoid process
    postmastoidectomy — *see* Complications, postmastoidectomy
    specified NEC H95.89
mastoidectomy cavity — *see* Complications, postmastoidectomy
mechanical — *see* Complications, by site and type, mechanical
medical procedures (*see also* Complication(s), intraoperative) T88.9
metabolic E88.9
  postoperative E89.89
    specified NEC E89.89
molar pregnancy NOS O08.9
  damage to pelvic organs O08.6
  embolism O08.2
  genital infection O08.0
  hemorrhage (delayed) (excessive) O08.1
  metabolic disorder O08.5
  renal failure O08.4
  shock O08.3
  specified type NEC O08.0
  venous complication NEC O08.7
musculoskeletal system — *see also* Complication, intraoperative (intraprocedural), by site
  device, implant or graft NEC — *see* Complications, orthopedic, device or implant
  internal fixation (nail) (plate) (rod) — *see* Complications, fixation device, internal
  joint prosthesis — *see* Complications, joint prosthesis
  post radiation M96.89
    kyphosis M96.3
    scoliosis M96.5
    specified complication NEC M96.89
  postoperative (postprocedural) M96.89
    with osteoporosis — *see* Osteoporosis
    fracture following insertion of device — *see* Fracture, following insertion of orthopedic implant, joint prosthesis or boneplate
    joint instability after prosthesis removal M96.89
    lordosis M96.4
    postlaminectomy syndrome NEC M96.1
      kyphosis M96.3
    pseudarthrosis M96.0
    specified complication NEC M96.89
nephrostomy (stoma) — *see* Complications, stoma, urinary tract, external NEC

Complication(s) (from) (of) — *continued*
nervous system G98.8
  central G96.9
  device, implant or graft — *see also* Complication, prosthetic device or implant, specified NEC
    electronic stimulator (electrode(s)) — *see* Complications, electronic stimulator device
    ventricular shunt — *see* Complications, ventricular shunt
  electronic stimulator (electrode(s)) — *see* Complications, electronic stimulator device
  postprocedural G97.82
    intracranial hypotension G97.2
    specified NEC G97.82
    spinal fluid leak G97.0
  newborn, due to intrauterine (fetal) procedure P96.5
nonabsorbable (permanent) sutures — *see* Complication, sutures, permanent
obstetric O75.9
  procedure (instrumental) (manual) (surgical) specified NEC O75.4
  specified NEC O75.89
  surgical wound NEC O90.89
    hematoma O90.2
    infection O86.0
ocular lens implant — *see* Complications, intraocular lens
ophthalmologic
  postprocedural bleb — *see* Blebitis
orbital prosthesis T85.9
  embolism T85.81
  fibrosis T85.82
  hemorrhage T85.83
  infection and inflammation T85.79
  mechanical
    breakdown T85.31-
    displacement T85.32-
    malposition T85.32-
    obstruction T85.39-
    perforation T85.39-
    protrusion T85.39-
    specified NEC T85.39-
  pain T85.84
  specified type NEC T85.89
  stenosis T85.85
  thrombosis T85.86
organ or tissue transplant (partial) (total) — *see* Complications, transplant
orthopedic — *see also* Disorder, soft tissue
  device or implant T84.9
    bone
      device or implant — *see* Complication, bone, device NEC
      graft — *see* Complication, graft, bone
    breakdown T84.418
    displacement T84.428
    electronic bone stimulator — *see* Complications, electronic stimulator device, bone
    embolism T84.81
    fibrosis T84.82
    fixation device — *see* Complication, fixation device, internal
    hemorrhage T84.83
    infection or inflammation T84.7
    joint prosthesis — *see* Complication, joint prosthesis, internal
    malfunction T84.418
    malposition T84.428
    mechanical NEC T84.498
    muscle graft — *see* Complications, graft, muscle
    obstruction T84.498
    pain T84.84
    perforation T84.498
    protrusion T84.498
    specified complication NEC T84.89
    stenosis T84.85
    tendon graft — *see* Complications, graft, tendon
    thrombosis T84.86
  fracture (following insertion of device) — *see* Fracture, following insertion of orthopedic implant, joint prosthesis or boneplate
  postprocedural M96.89
    fracture — *see* Fracture, following insertion of orthopedic implant, joint prosthesis or bone plate
    postlaminectomy syndrome NEC M96.1
      kyphosis M96.3
      lordosis M96.4

Complication(s) (from) (of) — *continued*
orthopedic — *see also* Disorder, soft tissue — *continued*
  postprocedural M96.89 — *continued*
  postradiation
    kyphosis M96.2
    scoliosis M96.5
  pseudarthrosis post-fusion M96.0
  specified type NEC M96.89
pacemaker (cardiac) — *see* Complications, cardiovascular device or implant, electronic
pancreas transplant — *see* Complications, transplant, pancreas
penile prosthesis (implant) — *see* Complications, prosthetic device, penile
perfusion NEC T80.90
perineal repair (obstetrical) NEC O90.89
  disruption O90.1
  hematoma O90.2
  infection (following delivery) O86.0
phototherapy T88.9
  specified NEC T88.8
postmastoidectomy NEC H95.19-
  cyst, mucosal H95.13-
  granulation H95.12-
  inflammation, chronic H95.11-
  recurrent cholesteatoma H95.0-
postoperative — *see* Complications, postprocedural
  circulatory — *see* Complications, circulatory system
  ear — *see* Complications, ear
  endocrine — *see* Complications, endocrine
  eye — *see* Complications, eye
  lumbar puncture G97.1
    cerebrospinal fluid leak G97.0
  nervous system (central) (peripheral) — *see* Complications, nervous system
  respiratory system — *see* Complications, respiratory system
postprocedural — *see also* Complications, surgical procedure
  cardiac arrest
    following cardiac surgery I97.120
    following other surgery I97.121
  cardiac functional disturbance NEC
    following cardiac surgery I97.190
    following other surgery I97.191
  cardiac insufficiency
    following cardiac surgery I97.110
    following other surgery I97.111
  chorioretinal scars following retinal surgery H59.81-
  following cataract surgery
    cataract (lens) fragments H59.02-
    cystoid macular edema H59.03-
    specified NEC H59.09-
    vitreous (touch) syndrome H59.01-
  heart failure
    following cardiac surgery I97.130
    following other surgery I97.131
  hemorrhage (hematoma) (of)
    circulatory system organ or structure
      following a cardiac bypass I97.611
      following a cardiac catheterization I97.610
      following other circulatory system procedure I97.618
      following other procedure I97.62
    digestive system
      following procedure on digestive system K91.840
      following procedure on other organ K91.841
    ear
      following other procedure H95.42
      following procedure on ear and mastoid process H95.41
    endocrine system
      following endocrine system procedure E89.810
      following other procedure E89.811
    eye and adnexa
      following ophthalmic procedure H59.31-
      following other procedure H59.32-
    genitourinary organ or structure
      following procedure on genitourinary organ or structure N99.820
      following procedure on other organ N99.821
    mastoid process
      following other procedure H95.42
      following procedure on ear and mastoid process H95.41

Complication(s) (from) (of) — *continued*
postprocedural (*see also* Complications, surgical procedure) — *continued*
  hemorrhage (hematoma) (of) — *continued*
    musculoskeletal structure
      following musculoskeletal surgery M96.830
      following non-orthopedic surgery M96.831
      following orthopedic surgery M96.830
    nervous system
      following a nervous system procedure G97.51
      following other procedure G97.52
    respiratory system
      following other procedure J95.831
      following procedure on respiratory system organ or structure J95.830
    skin and subcutaneous tissue
      following a dermatologic procedure L76.21
      following a procedure on other organ L76.22
    spleen
      following procedure on other organ D78.22
      following procedure on the spleen D78.21
  specified NEC
    circulatory system I97.89
    digestive K91.89
    ear H95.89
    endocrine E89.89
    eye and adnexa H59.89
    genitourinary N99.89
    mastoid process H95.89
    metabolic E89.89
    musculoskeletal structure M96.89
    nervous system G97.82
    respiratory system J95.89
    skin and subcutaneous tissue L76.82
    spleen D78.89
pregnancy NEC — *see* Pregnancy, complicated by
prosthetic device or implant T85.9
  bile duct — *see* Complications, bile duct implant
  breast — *see* Complications, breast implant
  cardiac and vascular NEC — *see* Complications, cardiovascular device or implant
  corneal transplant — *see* Complications, graft, cornea
  electronic nervous system stimulator — *see* Complications, electronic stimulator device
  epidural infusion catheter — *see* Complications, catheter, epidural
  esophageal anti-reflux device — *see* Complications, esophageal anti-reflux device
  genital organ or tract — *see* Complications, genitourinary, device or implant, genital tract
  heart valve — *see* Complications, heart, valve, prosthesis
  infection or inflammation T85.79
    intestine transplant T86.892
    liver transplant T86.43
    lung transplant T86.812
    pancreas transplant T86.892
    skin graft T86.822
  intraocular lens — *see* Complications, intraocular lens
  intraperitoneal (dialysis) catheter — *see* Complications, catheter, intraperitoneal
  joint — *see* Complications, joint prosthesis, internal
  mechanical NEC T85.698
    dialysis catheter (vascular) — *see also* Complication, catheter, dialysis, mechanical
    peritoneal — *see* Complication, catheter, intraperitoneal, mechanical
    gastrointestinal device T85.598
    ocular device T85.398
    subdural (infusion) catheter T85.690
    suture, permanent T85.692
      that for bone repair — *see* Complications, fixation device, internal (orthopedic), mechanical

Complication(s) (from) (of) — *continued*
prosthetic device or implant T85.9 — *continued*
  mechanical NEC T85.698 — *continued*
    ventricular shunt
      breakdown T85.01
      displacement T85.02
      leakage T85.03
      malposition T85.02
      obstruction T85.09
      perforation T85.09
      protrusion T85.09
      specified NEC T85.09
    mesh
      erosion (to surrounding organ or tissue) T83.718
        vaginal (into pelvic floor muscles) T83.711
      exposure (to surrounding organ or tissue) T83.728
        vaginal (into vagina) (through vaginal wall) T83.721
    orbital — *see* Complications, orbital prosthesis
    penile T83.9
      embolism T83.81
      fibrosis T83.82
      hemorrhage T83.83
      infection and inflammation T83.6
      mechanical
        breakdown T83.410
        displacement T83.420
        leakage T83.490
        malposition T83.420
        obstruction T83.490
        perforation T83.490
        protrusion T83.490
        specified NEC T83.490
      pain T83.84
      specified type NEC T83.89
      stenosis T83.85
      thrombosis T83.86
    prosthetic materials NEC
      erosion (to surrounding organ or tissue) T83.718
        vaginal (into pelvic floor muscles) T83.711
      exposure (to surrounding organ or tissue) T83.728
        vaginal (into vagina) (through vaginal wall) T83.721
    skin graft T86.829
      artificial skin or decellularized allodermis
        embolism T85.81
        fibrosis T85.82
        hemorrhage T85.83
        infection and inflammation T85.79
        mechanical
          breakdown T85.613
          displacement T85.623
          malfunction T85.613
          malposition T85.623
          obstruction T85.693
          perforation T85.693
          protrusion T85.693
          specified NEC T85.693
        pain T85.84
        specified type NEC T85.89
        stenosis T85.85
        thrombosis T85.86
      failure T86.821
      infection T86.822
      rejection T86.820
      specified NEC T86.828
    specified NEC T85.9
      embolism T85.81
      fibrosis T85.82
      hemorrhage T85.83
      infection and inflammation T85.79
      mechanical
        breakdown T85.618
        displacement T85.628
        leakage T85.638
        malfunction T85.618
        malposition T85.628
        obstruction T85.698
        perforation T85.698
        protrusion T85.698
        specified NEC T85.698
      pain T85.84
      specified type NEC T85.89
      stenosis T85.85
      thrombosis T85.86
    subdural infusion catheter — *see* Complications, catheter, subdural
    sutures — *see* Complications, sutures
    urinary organ or tract NEC — *see* Complications, genitourinary, device or implant, urinary system

Complication(s) (from) (of) — *continued*
prosthetic device or implant T85.9 — *continued*
  vascular — *see* Complications, cardiovascular device or implant
  ventricular shunt — *see* Complications, ventricular shunt (device)
puerperium — *see* Puerperal
puncture, spinal G97.1
  cerebrospinal fluid leak G97.0
  headache or reaction G97.1
pyelogram N99.89
radiation
  kyphosis M96.2
  scoliosis M96.5
reattached
  extremity (infection) (rejection)
    lower T87.1x-
    upper T87.0x-
  specified body part NEC T87.2
reconstructed breast
  asymmetry between native and reconstructed breast N65.1
  deformity N65.0
  disproportion between native and reconstructed breast N65.1
  excess tissue N65.0
  misshappen N65.0
reimplant NEC — *see also* Complications, prosthetic device or implant
  limb (infection) (rejection) — *see* Complications, reattached, extremity
  organ (partial) (total) — *see* Complications, transplant
  prosthetic device NEC — *see* Complications, prosthetic device
renal N28.9
  allograft — *see* Complications, transplant, kidney
  dialysis — *see* Complications, dialysis
respirator
  mechanical J95.850
  specified NEC J95.859
respiratory system J98.9
  device, implant or graft — *see* Complication, prosthetic device or implant, specified NEC
  lung transplant — *see* Complications, prosthetic device or implant, lung transplant
  postoperative J95.89
    air leak J95.812
    Mendelson's syndrome (chemical pneumonitis) J95.4
    pneumothorax J95.811
    pulmonary insufficiency (acute) (after nonthoracic surgery) J95.2
      chronic J95.3
      following thoracic surgery J95.1
    respiratory failure (acute) J95.821
      acute and chronic J95.822
    specified NEC J95.89
    subglottic stenosis J95.5
    tracheostomy complication — *see* Complications, tracheostomy
  therapy T81.89
sedation during labor and delivery O74.9
  cardiac O74.2
  central nervous system O74.3
  pulmonary NEC O74.1
shunt — *see also* Complications, prosthetic device or implant
  arteriovenous — *see* Complications, arteriovenous, shunt
  ventricular (communicating) — *see* Complications, ventricular shunt
skin
  graft T86.829
    failure T86.821
    infection T86.822
    rejection T86.820
    specified type NEC T86.828
spinal
  anesthesia — *see* Complications, anesthesia, spinal
  catheter (epidural) (subdural) — *see* Complications, catheter
  puncture or tap G97.1
    cerebrospinal fluid leak G97.0
    headache or reaction G97.1

DISEASE INDEX

Complication(s) (from) (of) — *continued*
stent
  bile duct — *see* Complications, bile duct prosthesis
  urinary T83.9
    embolism T83.81
    fibrosis T83.82
    hemorrhage T83.83
    infection and inflammation T83.59
    mechanical
      breakdown T83.112
      displacement T83.122
      leakage T83.192
      malposition T83.122
      obstruction T83.192
      perforation T83.192
      protrusion T83.192
      specified NEC T83.192
    pain T83.84
    specified type NEC T83.89
    stenosis T83.85
    thrombosis T83.86
stoma
  digestive tract
    colostomy — *see* Complications, colostomy
    enterostomy — *see* Complications, enterostomy
    esophagostomy — *see* Complications, esophagostomy
    gastrostomy — *see* Complications, gastrostomy
  urinary tract N99.538
    cystostomy — *see* Complications, cystostomy
    external NOS N99.528
      hemorrhage N99.520
      infection N99.521
      malfunction N99.522
      specified type NEC N99.528
    hemorrhage N99.530
    infection N99.531
    malfunction N99.532
    specified type NEC N99.538
stomach banding — *see* Complication(s), bariatric procedure
stomach stapling — *see* Complication(s), bariatric procedure
surgical material, nonabsorbable — *see* Complication, suture, permanent
surgical procedure (on) T81.9
  amputation stump (late) — *see* Complications, amputation stump
  cardiac — *see* Complications, circulatory system
  cholesteatoma, recurrent — *see* Complications, postmastoidectomy, recurrent cholesteatoma
  circulatory (early) — *see* Complications, circulatory system
  digestive system — *see* Complications, gastrointestinal
  dumping syndrome (postgastrectomy) K91.1
  ear — *see* Complications, ear
  elephantiasis or lymphedema I97.89
    postmastectomy I97.2
  emphysema (surgical) T81.82
  endocrine — *see* Complications, endocrine
  eye — *see* Complications, eye
  fistula (persistent postoperative) T81.83
  foreign body inadvertently left in wound (sponge) (suture) (swab) — *see* Foreign body, accidentally left during aprocedure
  gastrointestinal — *see* Complications, gastrointestinal
  genitourinary NEC N99.89
  hematoma
    intraoperative — *see* Complication, intraoperative, hemorrhage
    postprocedural — *see* Complication, postprocedural, hemorrhage
  hemorrhage
    intraoperative — *see* Complication, intraoperative, hemorrhage
    postprocedural — *see* Complication, postprocedural, hemorrhage
  hepatic failure K91.82
  hyperglycemia (postpancreatectomy) E89.1
  hypoinsulinemia (postpancreatectomy) E89.1
  hypoparathyroidism (postparathyroidectomy) E89.2
  hypopituitarism (posthypophysectomy) E89.3
  hypothyroidism (post-thyroidectomy) E89.0

Complication(s) (from) (of) — *continued*
surgical procedure (on) T81.9 — *continued*
  intestinal obstruction K91.3
  intracranial hypotension following ventricular shunting (ventriculostomy) G97.2
  lymphedema I97.89
    postmastectomy I97.2
  malabsorption (postsurgical) NEC K91.2
    osteoporosis — *see* Osteoporosis, postsurgical malabsorption
  mastoidectomy cavity NEC — *see* Complications, postmastoidectomy
  metabolic E89.89
    specified NEC E89.89
  musculoskeletal — *see* Complications, musculoskeletal system
  nervous system (central) (peripheral) — *see* Complications, nervous system
  ovarian failure E89.40
    asymptomatic E89.40
    symptomatic E89.41
  peripheral vascular — *see* Complications, surgical procedure, vascular
  postcardiotomy syndrome I97.0
  postcholecystectomy syndrome K91.5
  postcommissurotomy syndrome I97.0
  postgastrectomy dumping syndrome K91.1
  postlaminectomy syndrome NEC M96.1
    kyphosis M96.3
  postmastectomy lymphedema syndrome I97.2
  postmastoidectomy cholesteatoma — *see* Complications, postmastoidectomy, recurrent cholesteatoma
  postvagotomy syndrome K91.1
  postvalvulotomy syndrome I97.0
  pulmonary insufficiency (acute) J95.2
    chronic J95.3
    following thoracic surgery J95.1
  reattached body part — *see* Complications, reattached
  respiratory — *see* Complications, respiratory system
  shock (hypovolemic) T81.19
  spleen (postoperative) D78.89
    intraoperative D78.81
  stitch abscess T81.4
  subglottic stenosis (postsurgical) J95.5
  testicular hypofunction E89.5
  transplant — *see* Complications, organ or tissue transplant
  urinary NEC N99.89
  vaginal vault prolapse (posthysterectomy) N99.3
  vascular (peripheral)
    artery T81.719
      mesenteric T81.710
      renal T81.711
      specified NEC T81.718
    vein T81.72
  wound infection T81.4
suture, permanent (wire) NEC T85.9
  with repair of bone — *see* Complications, fixation device, internal
  embolism T85.81
  fibrosis T85.82
  hemorrhage T85.83
  infection and inflammation T85.79
  mechanical
    breakdown T85.612
    displacement T85.622
    malfunction T85.612
    malposition T85.622
    obstruction T85.692
    perforation T85.692
    protrusion T85.692
    specified NEC T85.692
  pain T85.84
  specified type NEC T85.89
  stenosis T85.85
  thrombosis T85.86
tracheostomy J95.00
  granuloma J95.09
  hemorrhage J95.01
  infection J95.02
  malfunction J95.03
  mechanical J95.03
  obstruction J95.03
  specified type NEC J95.09
  tracheo-esophageal fistula J95.04
transfusion (blood) (lymphocytes) (plasma) T80.92
  air emblism T80.0
  circulatory overload E87.71
  febrile nonhemolytic transfusion reaction R50.84

Complication(s) (from) (of) — *continued*
transfusion (blood) (lymphocytes) (plasma) T80.92 — *continued*
  hemochromatosis E83.111
  hemolysis T80.89
  hemolytic reaction (antigen unspecified) T80.919
  incompatibility reaction (antigen unspecified) T80.919
    ABO T80.30
      delayed serologic (DSTR) T80.39
      hemolytic transfusion reaction (HTR) (unspecified time after transfusion) T80.319
        acute (AHTR) (less than 24 hours after transfusion) T80.310
        delayed (DHTR) (24 hours or more after transfusion) T80.311
      specified NEC T80.39
    acute (antigen unspecified) T80.910
    delayed (antigen unspecified) T80.911
    delayed serologic (DSTR) T80.89
    Non-ABO (minor antigens (Duffy) (Kell) (Kidd) (Lewis) (M) (N) (P) (S)) T80.A0
      delayed serologic (DSTR) T80.A9
      hemolytic transfusion reaction (HTR) (unspecified time after transfusion) T80.A19
        acute (AHTR) (less than 24 hours after transfusion) T80.A10
        delayed (DHTR) (24 hours or more after transfusion) T80.A11
      specified NEC T80.A9
    Rh (antigens (C) (c) (D) (E) (e)) (factor) T80.40
      delayed serologic (DSTR) T80.49
      hemolytic transfusion reaction (HTR) (unspecified time after transfusion) T80.419
        acute (AHTR) (less than 24 hours after transfusion) T80.410
        delayed (DHTR) (24 hours or more after transfusion) T80.411
      specified NEC T80.49
  infection T80.29
    acute T80.22
  reaction NEC T80.89
  sepsis T80.29
  shock T80.89
transplant T86.90
  bone T86.839
    failure T86.831
    infection T86.832
    rejection T86.830
    specified type NEC T86.838
  bone marrow T86.00
    failure T86.02
    infection T86.03
    rejection T86.01
    specified type NEC T86.09
  cornea T86.849
    failure T86.841
    infection T86.842
    rejection T86.840
    specified type NEC T86.848
  failure T86.92
  heart T86.20
    with lung T86.30
    cardiac allograft vasculopathy T86.290
      failure T86.32
      infection T86.33
      rejection T86.31
      specified type NEC T86.39
    failure T86.22
    infection T86.23
    rejection T86.21
    specified type NEC T86.298
  infection T86.93
  intestine T86.859
    failure T86.851
    infection T86.852
    rejection T86.850
    specified type NEC T86.858
  kidney T86.10
    failure T86.12
    infection T86.13
    rejection T86.11
    specified type NEC T86.19
  liver T86.40
    failure T86.42
    infection T86.43
    rejection T86.41
    specified type NEC T86.49

Complication(s) (from) (of) — *continued*
transplant T86.90 — *continued*
  lung T86.819
    with heart T86.30
      failure T86.32
      infection T86.33
      rejection T86.31
      specified type NEC T86.39
    failure T86.811
    infection T86.812
    rejection T86.810
    specified type NEC T86.818
  malignant neoplasm C80.2
  pancreas T86.899
    failure T86.891
    infection T86.892
    rejection T86.890
    specified type NEC T86.898
  peripheral blood stem cells T86.5
  post-transplant lymphoproliferative disorder (PTLD) D47.Z1
  rejection T86.91
  skin T86.829
    failure T86.821
    infection T86.822
    rejection T86.820
    specified type NEC T86.828
  specified
    tissue T86.899
      failure T86.891
      infection T86.892
      rejection T86.890
      specified type NEC T86.898
    type NEC T86.99
  stem cell (from peripheral blood) (from umbilical cord) T86.5
  umbilical cord stem cells T86.5
trauma (early) T79.9
  specified NEC T79.8
ultrasound therapy NEC T88.9
umbilical cord NEC
  complicating delivery O69.9
    specified NEC O69.89
umbrella device, vascular T82.9
  embolism T82.818
  fibrosis T82.828
  hemorrhage T82.838
  infection or inflammation T82.7
  mechanical
    breakdown T82.515
    displacement T82.525
    leakage T82.535
    malposition T82.525
    obstruction T82.595
    perforation T82.595
    protrusion T82.595
  pain T82.848
  specified type NEC T82.898
  stenosis T82.858
  thrombosis T82.868
urethral catheter — *see* Complications, catheter, urethral, indwelling
vaccination T88.1
  anaphylaxis NEC T80.52
  arthropathy — *see* Arthropathy, postimmunization
  cellulitis T88.0
  encephalitis or encephalomyelitis G04.02
  infection (general) (local) NEC T88.0
  meningitis G03.8
  myelitis G04.89
  protein sickness T80.62
  rash T88.1
  reaction (allergic) T88.1
    serum T80.62
  sepsis T88.0
  serum intoxication, sickness, rash, or other serum reaction NEC T80.62
    anaphylactic shock T80.52
  shock (allergic) (anaphylactic) T80.52
  vaccinia (generalized) (localized) T88.1
vas deferens device or implant — *see* Complications, genitourinary, device or implant, genital tract
vascular I99.9
  device or implant T82.9
    embolism T82.818
    fibrosis T82.828
    hemorrhage T82.838
    infection or inflammation T82.7
    mechanical
      breakdown T82.519
        specified device NEC T82.518
      displacement T82.529
        specified device NEC T82.528
      leakage T82.539
        specified device NEC T82.538
      malposition T82.529
        specified device NEC T82.528

Complication(s) (from) (of) — *continued*
  vascular I99.9 — *continued*
    device or implant T82.9 — *continued*
      mechanical — *continued*
        obstruction T82.599
          specified device NEC T82.598
        perforation T82.599
          specified device NEC T82.598
        protrusion T82.599
          specified device NEC T82.598
      pain T82.848
      specified type NEC T82.898
      stenosis T82.858
      thrombosis T82.868
    dialysis catheter — *see* Complication, catheter, dialysis
    following infusion, therapeutic injection or transfusion T80.1
  graft T82.9
    embolism T82.818
    fibrosis T82.828
    hemorrhage T82.838
    mechanical
      breakdown T82.319
        aorta (bifurcation) T82.310
        carotid artery T82.311
        specified vessel NEC T82.318
      displacement T82.329
        aorta (bifurcation) T82.320
        carotid artery T82.321
        specified vessel NEC T82.328
      leakage T82.339
        aorta (bifurcation) T82.330
        carotid artery T82.331
        specified vessel NEC T82.338
      malposition T82.329
        aorta (bifurcation) T82.320
        carotid artery T82.321
        specified vessel NEC T82.328
      obstruction T82.399
        aorta (bifurcation) T82.390
        carotid artery T82.391
        specified vessel NEC T82.398
      perforation T82.399
        aorta (bifurcation) T82.390
        carotid artery T82.391
        specified vessel NEC T82.398
      protrusion T82.399
        aorta (bifurcation) T82.390
        carotid artery T82.391
        specified vessel NEC T82.398
    pain T82.848
    specified complication NEC T82.898
    stenosis T82.858
    thrombosis T82.868
  postoperative — *see* Complications, postoperative, circulatory
  vena cava device (filter) (sieve) (umbrella) — *see* Complications, umbrella device, vascular
  ventilation therapy NEC T81.81
  ventilator
    mechanical J95.850
    specified NEC J95.859
  ventricular (communicating) shunt (device) T85.9
    embolism T85.81
    fibrosis T85.82
    hemorrhage T85.83
    infection and inflammation T85.79
    mechanical
      breakdown T85.01
      displacement T85.02
      leakage T85.03
      malposition T85.02
      obstruction T85.09
      perforation T85.09
      protrusion T85.09
      specified NEC T85.09
    pain T85.84
    specified type NEC T85.89
    stenosis T85.85
    thrombosis T85.86
  wire suture, permanent (implanted) — *see* Complications, suture, permanent
Compressed air disease T70.3
Compression
  with injury — *code by* nature of injury
  artery I77.1
    celiac, syndrome I77.4
  brachial plexus G54.0
  brain (stem) G93.5
    due to
      contusion (diffuse) — *see* Injury, intracranial, diffuse
        focal — *see* Injury, intracranial, focal
      injury NEC — *see* Injury, intracranial, diffuse

Compression — *continued*
  brain (stem) G93.5 — *continued*
    traumatic — *see* Injury, intracranial, diffuse
  bronchus J98.09
  cauda equina G83.4
  celiac (artery) (axis) I77.4
  cerebral — *see* Compression, brain
  cervical plexus G54.2
  cord
    spinal — *see* Compression, spinal
    umbilical — *see* Compression, umbilical cord
  cranial nerve G52.9
    eighth — *see* subcategory H93.3
    eleventh G52.8
    fifth G50.8
    first G52.0
    fourth — *see* Strabismus, paralytic, fourth nerve
    ninth G52.1
    second — *see* Disorder, nerve, optic
    seventh G52.8
    sixth — *see* Strabismus, paralytic, third nerve
    tenth G52.2
    third — *see* Strabismus, paralytic, third nerve
    twelfth G52.3
  diver's squeeze S70.3
  during birth (newborn) P15.9
  esophagus K22.2
  eustachian tube — *see* Obstruction, eustachian tube, cartilaginous
  facies Q67.1
  fracture — *see* Fracture
  heart — *see* Disease, heart
  intestine — *see* Obstruction, intestine
  laryngeal nerve, recurrent G52.2
    with paralysis of vocal cords and larynx J38.00
      bilateral J38.02
      unilateral J38.01
  lumbosacral plexus G54.1
  lung J98.4
  lymphatic vessel I89.0
  medulla — *see* Compression, brain
  nerve (*see also* Disorder, nerve) G58.9
    arm NEC — *see* Mononeuropathy, upper limb
    axillary G54.0
    cranial — *see* Compression, cranial nerve
    leg NEC — *see* Mononeuropathy, lower limb
    median (in carpal tunnel) — *see* Syndrome, carpal tunnel
    optic — *see* Disorder, nerve, optic
    plantar — *see* Lesion, nerve, plantar
    posterior tibial (in tarsal tunnel) — *see* Syndrome, tarsal tunnel
    root or plexus NOS (in) G54.9
      intervertebral disc disorder NEC — *see* Disorder, disc, with, radiculopathy
      with myelopathy — *see* Disorder, disc, with, myelopathy
      neoplastic disease (*see also* Neoplasm) D49.9 [G55]
      spondylosis — *see* Spondylosis, with radiculopathy
    sciatic (acute) — *see* Lesion, nerve, sciatic
    sympathetic G90.8
    traumatic — *see* Injury, nerve
    ulnar — *see* Lesion, nerve, ulnar
    upper extremity NEC — *see* Mononeuropathy, upper limb
  spinal (cord) G95.20
    by displacement of intervertebral disc NEC — *see* Disorder, disc, with, myelopathy
    nerve root NOS G54.9
      due to displacement of intervertebral disc NEC — *see* Disorder, disc, with, radiculopathy
      with myelopathy — *see* Disorder, disc, with, myelopathy
    specified NEC G95.29
    spondylogenic (cervical) (lumbar, lumbosacral) (thoracic) — *see* Spondylosis, with myelopathy NEC
    anterior — *see* Syndrome, anterior, spinal artery, compression
    traumatic — *see* Injury, spinal cord, by region
  subcostal nerve (syndrome) — *see* Mononeuropathy, upper limb, specified NEC

Compression — *continued*
  sympathetic nerve NEC G90.8
  syndrome T79.5
  trachea J39.8
  ulnar nerve (by scar tissue) — *see* Lesion, nerve, ulnar
  umbilical cord
    complicating delivery O69.2
      cord around neck O69.1
      prolapse O69.0
      specified NEC O69.2
  ureter N13.5
  vein I87.1
  vena cava (inferior) (superior) I87.1
Compulsion, compulsive
  gambling F63.0
  neurosis F42
  personality F60.5
  states F42
  swearing F42
    in Gilles de la Tourette's syndrome F95.2
  tics and spasms F95.9
Concato's disease (pericardial polyserositis) A19.9
  nontubercular I31.1
  pleural — *see* Pleurisy, with effusion
Concavity chest wall M95.4
Concealed penis Q55.69
Concern (normal) about sick person in family Z63.6
Concrescence (teeth) K00.2
Concretio cordis I31.1
  rheumatic I09.2
Concretion — *see also* Calculus
  appendicular K38.1
  canaliculus — *see* Dacryolith
  clitoris N90.89
  conjunctiva H11.12-
  eyelid — *see* Disorder, eyelid, specified type NEC
  lacrimal passages — *see* Dacryolith
  prepuce (male) N47.8
  salivary gland (any) K11.5
  seminal vesicle N50.8
  tonsil J35.8
Concussion (brain) (cerebral) (current) S06.0x-
  blast (air) (hydraulic) (immersion) (underwater)
    abdomen or thorax — *see* Injury, blast, by site
    ear with acoustic nerve injury — *see* Injury, nerve, acoustic, specified type NEC
  cauda equina S34.3
  conus medullaris S34.02
  ocular S05.8x-
  spinal (cord)
    cervical S14.0
    lumbar S34.01
    sacral S34.02
    thoracic S24.0
  syndrome F07.81
Condition — *see* Disease
Conditions arising in the perinatal period — *see* Newborn, affected by
Conduct disorder — *see* Disorder, conduct
Condyloma A63.0
  acuminatum A63.0
  gonorrheal A54.09
  latum A51.31
  syphilitic A51.31
    congenital A50.07
  venereal, syphilitic A51.31
Conflagration — *see also* Burn
  asphyxia (by inhalation of gases, fumes or vapors) (*see also* Table of Drugs and Chemicals) T59.9-
Conflict (with) — *see also* Discord
  family Z73.9
  marital Z63.0
    involving divorce or estrangement Z63.5
  parent-child Z62.820
    parent-adopted child Z62.821
    parent-biological child Z62.820
    parent-foster child Z62.822
  social role NEC Z73.5
Confluent — *see* condition
Confusion, confused R41.0
  epileptic F05
  mental state (psychogenic) F44.89
  psychogenic F44.89
  reactive (from emotional stress, psychological trauma) F44.89
Confusional arousals G47.51
Congelation T69.9
Congenital — *see also* condition
  aortic septum Q25.4
  intrinsic factor deficiency D51.0
  malformation — *see* Anomaly

Congestion, congestive
  bladder N32.89
  bowel K63.89
  brain G93.89
  breast N64.59
  bronchial J98.09
  catarrhal J31.0
  chest R09.89
  chill, malarial — *see* Malaria
  circulatory NEC I99.8
  duodenum K31.89
  eye — *see* Hyperemia, conjunctiva
  facial, due to birth injury P15.4
  general R68.89
  glottis J37.0
  heart — *see* Failure, heart, congestive
  hepatic K76.1
  hypostatic (lung) — *see* Edema, lung
  intestine K63.89
  kidney N28.89
  labyrinth — *see* subcategory H83.8
  larynx J37.0
  liver K76.1
  lung R09.89
    active or acute — *see* Pneumonia
    malaria, malarial — *see* Malaria
  nasal R09.81
  nose R09.81
  orbit, orbital — *see also* Exophthalmos
    inflammatory (chronic) — *see* Inflammation, orbit
  ovary N83.8
  pancreas K86.8
  pelvic, female N94.89
  pleural J94.8
  prostate (active) N42.1
  pulmonary — *see* Congestion, lung
  renal N28.89
  retina H35.81
  seminal vesicle N50.1
  spinal cord G95.19
  spleen (chronic) D73.2
  stomach K31.89
  trachea — *see* Tracheitis
  urethra N36.8
  uterus N85.8
    with subinvolution N85.3
  venous (passive) I87.8
  viscera R68.89
Congestive — *see* Congestion
Conical
  cervix (hypertrophic elongation) N88.4
  cornea — *see* Keratoconus
  teeth K00.2
Conjoined twins Q89.4
Conjugal maladjustment Z63.0
  involving divorce or estrangement Z63.5
Conjunctiva — *see* condition
Conjunctivitis (staphylococcal) (streptococcal) NOS H10.9
  Acanthamoeba B60.12
  acute H10.3-
    atopic H10.1-
    chemical (*see also* Corrosion, cornea) H10.21-
    mucopurulent H10.02-
      follicular H10.01-
    pseudomembranous H10.22-
    serous except viral H10.23-
      viral — *see* Conjunctivitis, viral
    toxic H10.21-
  adenoviral (acute) (follicular) B30.1
  allergic (acute) — *see* Conjunctivitis, acute, atopic
    chronic H10.45
      vernal H10.44
  anaphylactic — *see* Conjunctivitis, acute, atopic
  Apollo B30.3
  atopic (acute) — *see* Conjunctivitis, acute, atopic
  blennorrhagic (gonococcal) (neonatorum) A54.31
  Béal's B30.2
  chemical (acute) (*see also* Corrosion, cornea) H10.21-
  chlamydial A74.0
    due to trachoma A71.1
    neonatal P39.1
  chronic (nodosa) (petrificans) (phlyctenular) H10.40-
    allergic H10.45
      vernal H10.44
    follicular H10.43-
      giant papillary H10.41-
      simple H10.42-
      vernal H10.44
  coxsackievirus 24 B30.3
  diphtheritic A36.86

DISEASE INDEX

Conjunctivitis (staphylococcal) (streptococcal) NOS H10.9 — *continued*
- due to
  - dust — *see* Conjunctivitis, acute, atopic
  - filariasis B74.9
  - mucocutaneous leishmaniasis B55.2
- enterovirus type 70 (hemorrhagic) B30.3
- epidemic (viral) B30.9
  - hemorrhagic B30.3
- gonococcal (neonatorum) A54.31
- granular (trachomatous) A71.1
  - sequelae (late effect) B94.0
- hemorrhagic (acute) (epidemic) B30.3
- herpes zoster B02.31
- in (due to)
  - Acanthamoeba B60.12
  - adenovirus (acute) (follicular) B30.1
  - Chlamydia A74.0
  - coxsackievirus 24 B30.3
  - diphtheria A36.86
  - enterovirus type 70 (hemorrhagic) B30.3
  - filariasis B74.9
  - gonococci A54.31
  - herpes (simplex) virus B00.53
    - zoster B02.31
  - infectious disease NEC B99
  - meningococci A39.89
  - mucocutaneous leishmaniasis B55.2
  - rosacea L71.9
  - syphilis (late) A52.71
  - zoster B02.31
- inclusion A74.0
- infantile P39.1
  - gonococcal A54.31
- Koch-Weeks' — *see* Conjunctivitis, acute, mucopurulent
- light — *see* Conjunctivitis, acute, atopic
- ligneous — *see* Blepharoconjunctivitis, ligneous
- meningococcal A39.89
- mucopurulent — *see* Conjunctivitis, acute, mucopurulent
- neonatal P39.1
  - gonococcal A54.31
- Newcastle B30.8
- of Béal B30.2
- parasitic
  - filariasis B74.9
  - mucocutaneous leishmaniasis B55.2
- Parinaud's H10.89
- petrificans H10.89
- rosacea L71.9
- specified NEC H10.89
- swimming-pool B30.1
- trachomatous A71.1
  - acute A71.0
  - sequelae (late effect) B94.0
- traumatic NEC H10.89
- tuberculous A18.59
- tularemic A21.1
- tularensis A21.1
- viral B30.9
  - due to
    - adenovirus B30.1
    - enterovirus B30.3
    - specified NEC B30.8
Conjunctivochalasis H11.82-
Connective tissue — *see* condition
Conn's syndrome E26.01
Conradi(-Hunermann) disease Q77.3
Consanguinity Z84.3
- counseling Z71.89
Conscious simulation (of illness) Z76.5
Consecutive — *see* condition
Consolidation lung (base) — *see* Pneumonia, lobar
Constipation (atonic) (neurogenic) (simple) (spastic) K59.00
- drug-induced — *see* Table of Drugs and Chemicals
- outlet dysfunction K59.02
- psychogenic F45.8
- slow transit K59.01
- specified NEC K59.09
Constitutional — *see also* condition
- substandard F60.7
Constitutionally substandard F60.7
Constriction — *see also* Stricture
- auditory canal — *see* Stenosis, external ear canal
- bronchial J98.09
- duodenum K31.5
- esophagus K22.2
- external
  - abdomen, abdominal (wall) S30.841
  - alveolar process S00.542
  - ankle S90.54-
  - antecubital space — *see* Constriction, external, forearm
  - arm (upper) S40.84-

Constriction (*see also* Stricture) — *continued*
- external — *continued*
  - auricle — *see* Constriction, external, ear
  - axilla — *see* Constriction, external, arm
  - back, lower S30.840
  - breast S20.14-
  - brow S00.84
  - buttock S30.840
  - calf — *see* Constriction, external, leg
  - canthus — *see* Constriction, external, eyelid
  - cheek S00.84
    - internal S00.542
  - chest wall — *see* Constriction, external, thorax
  - chin S00.84
  - clitoris S30.844
  - costal region — *see* Constriction, external, thorax
  - digit(s)
    - foot — *see* Constriction, external, toe
    - hand — *see* Constriction, external, finger
  - ear S00.44-
  - elbow S50.34-
  - epididymis S30.843
  - epigastric region S30.841
  - esophagus, cervical S10.14
  - eyebrow — *see* Constriction, external, eyelid
  - eyelid S00.24-
  - face S00.84
  - finger(s) S60.44-
    - index S60.44-
    - little S60.44-
    - middle S60.44-
    - ring S60.44-
  - flank S30.841
  - foot (except toe(s) alone) S90.84-
    - toe — *see* Constriction, external, toe
  - forearm S50.84-
    - elbow only — *see* Constriction, external, elbow
  - forehead S00.84
  - genital organs, external
    - female S30.846
    - male S30.845
  - groin S30.841
  - gum S00.542
  - hand S60.54-
  - head S00.94
    - ear — *see* Constriction, external, ear
    - eyelid — *see* Constriction, external, eyelid
    - lip S00.541
    - nose S00.34
    - oral cavity S00.542
    - scalp S00.04
    - specified site NEC S00.84
  - heel — *see* Constriction, external, foot
  - hip S70.24-
  - inguinal region S30.841
  - interscapular region S20.449
  - jaw S00.84
  - knee S80.24-
  - labium (majus) (minus) S30.844
  - larynx S10.14
  - leg (lower) S80.84-
    - knee — *see* Constriction, external, knee
    - upper — *see* Constriction, external, thigh
  - lip S00.541
  - lower back S30.840
  - lumbar region S30.840
  - malar region S00.84
  - mammary — *see* Constriction, external, breast
  - mastoid region S00.84
  - mouth S00.542
  - nail
    - finger — *see* Constriction, external, finger
    - toe — *see* Constriction, external, toe
  - nasal S00.34
  - neck S10.94
    - specified site NEC S10.84
    - throat S10.14
  - nose S00.34
  - occipital region S00.04
  - oral cavity S00.542
  - orbital region — *see* Constriction, external, eyelid
  - palate S00.542
  - palm — *see* Constriction, external, hand
  - parietal region S00.04
  - pelvis S30.840
  - penis S30.842

Constriction (*see also* Stricture) — *continued*
- external — *continued*
  - perineum
    - female S30.844
    - male S30.840
  - periocular area — *see* Constriction, external, eyelid
  - phalanges
    - finger — *see* Constriction, external, finger
    - toe — *see* Constriction, external, toe
  - pharynx S10.14
  - pinna — *see* Constriction, external, ear
  - popliteal space — *see* Constriction, external, knee
  - prepuce S30.842
  - pubic region S30.840
  - pudendum
    - female S30.846
    - male S30.845
  - sacral region S30.840
  - scalp S00.04
  - scapular region — *see* Constriction, external, shoulder
  - scrotum S30.843
  - shin — *see* Constriction, external, leg
  - shoulder S40.24-
  - sternal region S20.349
  - submaxillary region S00.84
  - submental region S00.84
  - subungual
    - finger(s) — *see* Constriction, external, finger
    - toe(s) — *see* Constriction, external, toe
  - supraclavicular fossa S10.84
  - supraorbital S00.84
  - temple S00.84
  - temporal region S00.84
  - testis S30.843
  - thigh S70.34-
  - thorax, thoracic (wall) S20.94
    - back S20.44-
    - front S20.34-
  - throat S10.14
  - thumb S60.34-
  - toe(s) (lesser) S90.44-
    - great S90.44-
  - tongue S00.542
  - trachea S10.14
  - tunica vaginalis S30.843
  - uvula S00.542
  - vagina S30.844
  - vulva S30.844
  - wrist S60.84-
- gallbladder — *see* Obstruction, gallbladder
- intestine — *see* Obstruction, intestine
- larynx J38.6
  - congenital Q31.8
    - specified NEC Q31.8
    - subglottic Q31.1
- organ or site, congenital NEC — *see* Atresia, by site
- prepuce (acquired) (congenital) N47.1
- pylorus (adult hypertrophic) K31.1
  - congenital or infantile Q40.0
  - newborn Q40.0
- ring dystocia (uterus) O62.4
- spastic — *see also* Spasm
  - ureter N13.5
- ureter N13.5
  - with infection N13.6
- urethra — *see* Stricture, urethra
- visual field (peripheral) (functional) — *see* Defect, visual field
Constrictive — *see* condition
Consultation
- medical — *see* Counseling, medical
- religious Z71.81
- specified reason NEC Z71.89
- spiritual Z71.81
- without complaint or sickness Z71.9
  - feared complaint unfounded Z71.1
  - specified reason NEC Z71.89
Consumption — *see* Tuberculosis
Contact (with) — *see also* Exposure (to)
- acariasis Z20.7
- AIDS virus Z20.6
- air pollution Z77.110
- algae and algae toxins Z77.121
- algae bloom Z77.121
- anthrax Z20.810
- aromatic (hazardous) compounds NEC Z77.028
- aromatic amines Z77.020
- aromatic dyes NOS Z77.028
- arsenic Z77.010
- asbestos Z77.090
- bacterial disease NEC Z20.818
- benzene Z77.021

Contact (with) (*see also* Exposure (to)) — *continued*
- blue-green algae bloom Z77.121
- body fluids (potentially hazardous) Z77.21
- brown tide Z77.121
- chemicals (chiefly nonmedicinal) (hazardous) NEC Z77.098
- cholera Z20.09
- chromium compounds Z77.018
- communicable disease Z20.9
  - bacterial NEC Z20.818
  - specified NEC Z20.89
  - viral NEC Z20.828
- cyanobacteria bloom Z77.121
- dyes Z77.098
- Escherichia coli (E. coli) Z20.01
- fiberglass — *see* Table of Drugs and Chemicals, fiberglass
- German measles Z20.4
- gonorrhea Z20.2
- hazardous metals NEC Z77.018
- hazardous substances NEC Z77.29
- hazards in the physical environment NEC Z77.128
- hazards to health NEC Z77.9
- HIV Z20.6
- HTLV-III/LAV Z20.6
- human immunodeficiency virus (HIV) Z20.6
- infection Z20.9
  - specified NEC Z20.89
- infestation (parasitic) NEC Z20.7
- intestinal infectious disease NEC Z20.09
  - Escherichia coli (E. coli) Z20.01
- lead Z77.011
- meningococcus Z20.811
- mold (toxic) Z77.120
- nickel dust Z77.018
- noise Z77.122
- parasitic disease Z20.7
- pediculosis Z20.7
- pfiesteria piscicida Z77.121
- poliomyelitis Z20.89
- pollution
  - air Z77.110
  - environmental NEC Z77.118
  - soil Z77.112
  - water Z77.111
- polycyclic aromatic hydrocarbons Z77.028
- rabies Z20.3
- radiation, naturally occurring NEC Z77.123
- radon Z77.123
- red tide (Florida) Z77.121
- rubella Z20.4
- sexually-transmitted disease Z20.2
- smallpox (laboratory) Z20.89
- syphilis Z20.2
- tuberculosis Z20.1
- uranium Z77.012
- varicella Z20.820
- venereal disease Z20.2
- viral disease NEC Z20.828
- viral hepatitis Z20.5
- water pollution Z77.111
Contamination, food — *see* Intoxication, foodborne
Contraception, contraceptive
- advice Z30.09
- counseling Z30.09
- device (intrauterine) (in situ) Z97.5
  - causing menorrhagia T83.83
  - checking Z30.431
  - complications — *see* Complications, intrauterine, contraceptive device
  - in place Z97.5
  - initial prescription Z30.014
  - reinsertion Z30.433
  - removal Z30.432
  - replacement Z30.433
- emergency (postcoital) Z30.012
- initial prescription Z30.019
  - injectable Z30.013
  - intrauterine device Z30.014
  - pills Z30.011
  - postcoital (emergency) Z30.012
  - specified type NEC Z30.018
  - subdermal implantable Z30.019
- maintenance Z30.40
  - examination Z30.8
  - injectable Z30.42
  - intrauterine device Z30.431
  - pills Z30.41
  - specified type NEC Z30.49
  - subdermal implantable Z30.49
- management Z30.9
  - specified NEC Z30.8
- postcoital (emergency) Z30.012
- prescription Z30.019
  - repeat Z30.40

© 2013 Channel Publishing Ltd

Contraception, contraceptive — *continued*
　sterilization Z30.2
　surveillance (drug) — *see* Contraception, maintenance
Contraction(s), contracture, contracted
　Achilles tendon — *see also* Short, tendon, Achilles
　　congenital Q66.89
　amputation stump (surgical) (flexion) (late) (next proximal joint) T87.89
　anus K59.8
　bile duct (common) (hepatic) K83.8
　bladder N32.89
　　neck or sphincter N32.0
　bowel, cecum, colon or intestine, any part — *see* Obstruction, intestine
　Braxton Hicks — *see* False, labor
　breast implant, capsular T85.44
　bronchial J98.09
　burn (old) — *see* Cicatrix
　cervix — *see* Stricture, cervix
　cicatricial — *see* Cicatrix
　conjunctiva, trachomatous, active A71.1
　　sequelae (late effect) B94.0
　Dupuytren's M72.0
　eyelid — *see* Disorder, eyelid function
　fascia (lata) (postural) M72.8
　　Dupuytren's M72.0
　　palmar M72.0
　　plantar M72.2
　finger NEC — *see also* Deformity, finger
　　congenital Q68.1
　　joint — *see* Contraction, joint, hand
　flaccid — *see* Contraction, paralytic
　gallbladder K82.0
　heart valve — *see* Endocarditis
　hip — *see* Contraction, joint, hip
　hourglass
　　bladder N32.89
　　　congenital Q64.79
　　gallbladder K82.0
　　　congenital Q44.1
　　stomach K31.89
　　　congenital Q40.2
　　　psychogenic F45.8
　　uterus (complicating delivery) O62.4
　hysterical F44.4
　internal os — *see* Stricture, cervix
　joint (abduction) (acquired) (adduction) (flexion) (rotation) M24.50
　　ankle M24.57-
　　congenital NEC Q68.8
　　　hip Q65.89
　　elbow M24.52-
　　foot joint M24.57-
　　hand joint M24.54-
　　hip M24.55-
　　　congenital Q65.89
　　hysterical F44.4
　　knee M24.56-
　　shoulder M24.51-
　　wrist M24.53-
　kidney (granular) (secondary) N26.9
　　congenital Q63.8
　　hydronephritic — *see* Hydronephrosis Page N26.2
　　pyelonephritic — *see* Pyelitis, chronic
　　tuberculous A18.11
　ligament — *see also* Disorder, ligament
　　congenital Q79.8
　muscle (postinfective) (postural) NEC M62.40
　　with contracture of joint — *see* Contraction, joint
　　ankle M62.47-
　　congenital Q79.8
　　　sternocleidomastoid Q68.0
　　extraocular — *see* Strabismus
　　eye (extrinsic) — *see* Strabismus
　　foot M62.47-
　　forearm M62.43-
　　hand M62.44-
　　hysterical F44.4
　　ischemic (Volkmann's) T79.6
　　lower leg M62.46-
　　multiple sites M62.49
　　pelvic region M62.45-
　　posttraumatic — *see* Strabismus, paralytic
　　psychogenic F45.8
　　　conversion reaction F44.4
　　shoulder region M62.41-
　　specified site NEC M62.48
　　thigh M62.45-
　　upper arm M62.42-
　neck — *see* Torticollis
　ocular muscle — *see* Strabismus
　organ or site, congenital NEC — *see* Atresia, by site
　outlet (pelvis) — *see* Contraction, pelvis

Contraction(s), contracture, contracted — *continued*
　palmar fascia M72.0
　paralytic
　　joint — *see* Contraction, joint
　　muscle — *see also* Contraction, muscle NEC
　　ocular — *see* Strabismus, paralytic
　pelvis (acquired) (general) M95.5
　　with disproportion (fetopelvic) O33.1
　　　causing obstructed labor O65.1
　　　inlet O33.2
　　　mid-cavity O33.3
　　　outlet O33.3
　plantar fascia M72.2
　premature
　　atrium I49.1
　　auriculoventricular I49.49
　　heart I49.49
　　junctional I49.2
　　supraventricular I49.1
　　ventricular I49.3
　prostate N42.89
　pylorus NEC — *see also* Pylorospasm
　　psychogenic F45.8
　rectum, rectal (sphincter) K59.8
　ring (Bandl's) (complicating delivery) O62.4
　scar — *see* Cicatrix
　spine — *see* Dorsopathy, deforming
　sternocleidomastoid (muscle), congenital Q68.0
　stomach K31.89
　　hourglass K31.89
　　　congenital Q40.2
　　　psychogenic F45.8
　　psychogenic F45.8
　tendon (sheath) M62.40
　　with contracture of joint — *see* Contraction, joint
　　　Achilles — *see* Short, tendon, Achilles
　　ankle M62.47-
　　　Achilles — *see* Short, tendon, Achilles
　　foot M62.47-
　　forearm M62.43-
　　hand M62.44-
　　lower leg M62.46-
　　multiple sites M62.49
　　neck M62.48
　　pelvic region M62.45-
　　shoulder region M62.41-
　　specified site NEC M62.48
　　thigh M62.45-
　　thorax M62.48
　　trunk M62.48
　　upper arm M62.42-
　toe — *see* Deformity, toe, specified NEC
　ureterovesical orifice (postinfectional) N13.5
　　with infection N13.6
　urethra — *see also* Stricture, urethra
　　orifice N32.0
　uterus N85.8
　　abnormal NEC O62.9
　　clonic (complicating delivery) O62.4
　　dyscoordinate (complicating delivery) O62.4
　　hourglass (complicating delivery) O62.4
　　hypertonic O62.4
　　hypotonic NEC O62.2
　　inadequate
　　　primary O62.0
　　　secondary O62.1
　　incoordinate (complicating delivery) O62.4
　　poor O62.2
　　tetanic (complicating delivery) O62.4
　vagina (outlet) N89.5
　vesical N32.89
　　neck or urethral orifice N32.0
　visual field — *see* Defect, visual field, generalized
　Volkmann's (ischemic) T79.6
Contusion (skin surface intact) T14.8
　abdomen, abdominal (muscle) (wall) S30.1
　adnexa, eye NEC S05.8x-
　adrenal gland S37.812
　alveolar process S00.532
　ankle S90.0-
　antecubital space — *see* Contusion, forearm
　anus S30.3
　arm (upper) S40.02-
　　lower (with elbow) — *see* Contusion, forearm
　auditory canal — *see* Contusion, ear
　auricle — *see* Contusion, ear
　axilla — *see* Contusion, arm, upper
　back — *see also* Contusion, thorax, back
　　lower S30.0

Contusion (skin surface intact) T14.8 — *continued*
　bile duct S36.13
　bladder S37.22
　bone NEC T14.8
　brain (diffuse) — *see* Injury, intracranial, diffuse
　　focal — *see* Injury, intracranial, focal
　brainstem S06.38-
　breast S20.0-
　broad ligament S37.892
　brow S00.83
　buttock S30.0
　canthus, eye S00.1-
　cauda equina S34.3
　cerebellar, traumatic S06.37-
　cerebral S06.33-
　　left side S06.32-
　　right side S06.31-
　cheek S00.83
　　internal S00.532
　chest (wall) — *see* Contusion, thorax
　chin S00.83
　clitoris S30.23
　colon — *see* Injury, intestine, large, contusion
　common bile duct S36.13
　conjunctiva S05.1-
　　with foreign body (in conjunctival sac) — *see* Foreign body, conjunctival sac
　conus medullaris (spine) S34.139
　cornea — *see* Contusion, eyeball
　　with foreign body — *see* Foreign body, cornea
　corpus cavernosum S30.21
　cortex (brain) (cerebral) — *see* Injury, intracranial, diffuse
　　focal — *see* Injury, intracranial, focal
　costal region — *see* Contusion, thorax
　cystic duct S36.13
　diaphragm S27.802
　duodenum S36.420
　ear S00.43-
　elbow S50.0-
　　with forearm — *see* Contusion, forearm
　epididymis S30.22
　epigastric region S30.1
　epiglottis S10.0
　esophagus (thoracic) S27.812
　　cervical S10.0
　eyeball S05.1-
　eyebrow S00.1-
　eyelid (and periocular area) S00.1-
　face NEC S00.83
　fallopian tube S37.529
　　bilateral S37.522
　　unilateral S37.521
　femoral triangle S30.1
　finger(s) S60.00
　　with damage to nail (matrix) S60.10
　　index S60.02-
　　　with damage to nail S60.12-
　　little S60.05-
　　　with damage to nail S60.15-
　　middle S60.03-
　　　with damage to nail S60.13-
　　ring S60.04-
　　　with damage to nail S60.14-
　　thumb — *see* Contusion, thumb
　flank S30.1
　foot (except toe(s) alone) S90.3-
　　toe — *see* Contusion, toe
　forearm S50.1-
　　elbow only — *see* Contusion, elbow
　forehead S00.83
　gallbladder S36.122
　genital organs, external
　　female S30.202
　　male S30.201
　globe (eye) — *see* Contusion, eyeball
　groin S30.1
　gum S00.532
　hand S60.22-
　　finger(s) — *see* Contusion, finger
　　wrist — *see* Contusion, wrist
　head S00.93
　　ear — *see* Contusion, ear
　　eyelid — *see* Contusion, eyelid
　　lip S00.531
　　nose S00.33
　　oral cavity S00.532
　　scalp S00.03
　　specified part NEC S00.83
　heel — *see* Contusion, foot
　hepatic duct S36.13
　hip S70.0-
　ileum S36.428
　iliac region S30.1
　inguinal region S30.1

Contusion (skin surface intact) T14.8 — *continued*
　interscapular region S20.229
　intra-abdominal organ S36.92
　　colon — *see* Injury, intestine, large, contusion
　　liver S36.112
　　pancreas — *see* Contusion, pancreas
　　rectum S36.62
　　small intestine — *see* Injury, intestine, small, contusion
　　specified organ NEC S36.892
　　spleen — *see* Contusion, spleen
　　stomach S36.32
　iris (eye) — *see* Contusion, eyeball
　jaw S00.83
　jejunum S36.428
　kidney S37.01-
　　major (greater than 2 cm) S37.02-
　　minor (less than 2 cm) S37.01-
　knee S80.0-
　labium (majus) (minus) S30.23
　lacrimal apparatus, gland or sac S05.8x-
　larynx S10.0
　leg (lower) S80.1-
　　knee — *see* Contusion, knee
　lens — *see* Contusion, eyeball
　lip S00.531
　liver S36.112
　lower back S30.0
　lumbar region S30.0
　lung S27.329
　　bilateral S27.322
　　unilateral S27.321
　malar region S00.83
　mastoid region S00.83
　membrane, brain — *see* Injury, intracranial, diffuse
　　focal — *see* Injury, intracranial, focal
　mesentery S36.892
　mesosalpinx S37.892
　mouth S00.532
　muscle — *see* Contusion, by site
　nail
　　finger — *see* Contusion, finger, with damage to nail
　　toe — *see* Contusion, toe, with damage to nail
　nasal S00.33
　neck S10.93
　　specified site NEC S10.83
　　throat S10.0
　nerve — *see* Injury, nerve
　newborn P54.5
　nose S00.33
　occipital
　　lobe (brain) — *see* Injury, intracranial, diffuse
　　　focal — *see* Injury, intracranial, focal
　　region (scalp) S00.03
　orbit (region) (tissues) S05.1-
　ovary S37.429
　　bilateral S37.422
　　unilateral S37.421
　palate S00.532
　pancreas S36.229
　　body S36.221
　　head S36.220
　　tail S36.222
　parietal
　　lobe (brain) — *see* Injury, intracranial, diffuse
　　　focal — *see* Injury, intracranial, focal
　　region (scalp) S00.03
　pelvic organ S37.92
　　adrenal gland S37.812
　　bladder S37.22
　　fallopian tube — *see* Contusion, fallopian tube
　　kidney — *see* Contusion, kidney
　　ovary — *see* Contusion, ovary
　　prostate S37.822
　　specified organ NEC S37.892
　　ureter S37.12
　　urethra S37.32
　　uterus S37.62
　pelvis S30.0
　penis S30.21
　perineum
　　female S30.23
　　male S30.0
　periocular area S00.1-
　peritoneum S36.81
　periurethral tissue — *see* Contusion, urethra
　pharynx S10.0

Contusion (skin surface intact) T14.8 — *continued*
  pinna — *see* Contusion, ear
  popliteal space — *see* Contusion, knee
  prepuce S30.21
  prostate S37.822
  pubic region S30.1
  pudendum
    female S30.202
    male S30.201
  quadriceps femoris — *see* Contusion, thigh
  rectum S36.62
  retroperitoneum S36.892
  round ligament S37.892
  sacral region S30.0
  scalp S00.03
    due to birth injury P12.3
  scapular region — *see* Contusion, shoulder
  sclera — *see* Contusion, eyeball
  scrotum S30.22
  seminal vesicle S37.892
  shoulder S40.01-
  skin NEC T14.8
  small intestine — *see* Injury, intestine, small, contusion
  spermatic cord S30.22
  spinal cord — *see* Injury, spinal cord, by region
    cauda equina S34.3
    conus medullaris S34.139
  spleen S36.029
    major S36.021
    minor S36.020
  sternal region S20.219
  stomach S36.32
  subconjunctival S05.1-
  subcutaneous NEC T14.8
  submaxillary region S00.83
  submental region S00.83
  subperiosteal NEC T14.8
  subungual
    finger — *see* Contusion, finger, with damage to nail
    toe — *see* Contusion, toe, with damage to nail
  supraclavicular fossa S10.83
  supraorbital S00.83
  suprarenal gland S37.812
  temple (region) S00.83
  temporal
    lobe (brain) — *see* Injury, intracranial, diffuse
    focal — *see* Injury, intracranial, focal
    region S00.83
  testis S30.22
  thigh S70.1-
  thorax (wall) S20.20
    back S20.22-
    front S20.21-
  throat S10.0
  thumb S60.01-
    with damage to nail S60.11-
  toe(s) (lesser) S90.12-
    with damage to nail S90.22-
    great S90.11-
      with damage to nail S90.21-
      specified type NEC S90.221
  tongue S00.532
  trachea (cervical) S10.0
    thoracic S27.52
  tunica vaginalis S30.22
  tympanum, tympanic membrane — *see* Contusion, ear
  ureter S37.12
  urethra S37.32
  urinary organ NEC S37.892
  uterus S37.62
  uvula S00.532
  vagina S30.23
  vas deferens S37.892
  vesical S37.22
  vocal cord(s) S10.0
  vulva S30.23
  wrist S60.21-
Conus (congenital) (any type) Q14.8
  cornea — *see* Keratoconus
  medullaris syndrome G95.81
Conversion hysteria, neurosis or reaction F44.9
Converter, tuberculosis (test reaction) R76.11
Conviction (legal), anxiety concerning Z65.0
  with imprisonment Z65.1

Convulsions (idiopathic) (*see also* Seizure(s)) R56.9
  apoplectiform (cerebral ischemia) I67.82
  benign neonatal (familial) — *see* Epilepsy, generalized, idiopathic
  dissociative F44.5
  epileptic — *see* Epilepsy
  epileptiform, epileptoid — *see* Seizure, epileptiform
  ether (anesthetic) — *see* Table of Drugs and Chemicals, by drug
  febrile R56.00
    with status epilepticus G40.901
    complex R56.01
      with status epilepticus G40.901
    simple R56.00
  hysterical F44.5
  infantile P90
    epilepsy — *see* Epilepsy
  jacksonian — *see* Epilepsy, localization-related, symptomatic, with simple partial seizures
  myoclonic G25.3
  neonatal, benign (familial) — *see* Epilepsy, generalized, idiopathic
  newborn P90
  obstetrical (nephritic) (uremic) — *see* Eclampsia
  paretic A52.17
  post traumatic R56.1
  psychomotor — *see* Epilepsy, localization-related, symptomatic, with complex partial seizures
  recurrent R56.9
  reflex R25.8
  scarlatinal A38.8
  tetanus, tetanic — *see* Tetanus
  thymic E32.8
Convulsive — *see also* Convulsions
Cooley's anemia D56.1
Coolie itch B76.9
Cooper's
  disease — *see* Mastopathy, cystic
  hernia — *see* Hernia, abdomen, specified site NEC
Copra itch B88.0
Coprophagy F50.8
Coprophobia F40.298
Coproporphyria, hereditary E80.29
Cor
  biloculare Q20.8
  bovis, bovinum — *see* Hypertrophy, cardiac
  pulmonale (chronic) I27.81
    acute I26.09
  triatriatum, triatriatum Q24.2
  triloculare Q20.8
    biatrium Q20.4
    biventriculare Q21.1
Corbus' disease (gangrenous balanitis) N48.1
Cord — *see also* condition
  around neck (tightly) (with compression) complicating delivery O69.1
  bladder G95.89
    tabetic A52.19
Cordis ectopia Q24.8
Corditis (spermatic) N49.1
Corectopia Q13.2
Cori's disease (glycogen storage) E74.03
Corkhandler's disease or lung J67.3
Corkscrew esophagus K22.4
Corkworker's disease or lung J67.3
Corn (infected) L84
Cornea — *see also* condition
  donor Z52.5
  plana Q13.4
Cornelia de Lange syndrome Q87.1
Cornu cutaneum L85.8
Cornual gestation or pregnancy O00.8
Coronary (artery) — *see* condition
Coronavirus, as cause of disease classified elsewhere B97.29
  SARS-associated B97.21
Corpora — *see also* condition
  amylacea, prostate N42.89
  cavernosa — *see* condition
Corpulence — *see* Obesity
Corpus — *see* condition
Corrected transposition Q20.5

Corrosion (injury) (acid) (caustic) (chemical) (lime) (external) (internal) T30.4
  abdomen, abdominal (muscle) (wall) T21.42
    first degree T21.52
    second degree T21.62
    third degree T21.72
  above elbow T22.439
    first degree T22.539
    left T22.432
      first degree T22.532
      second degree T22.632
      third degree T22.732
    right T22.431
      first degree T22.531
      second degree T22.631
      third degree T22.731
    second degree T22.639
    third degree T22.739
  alimentary tract NEC T28.7
  ankle T25.419
    first degree T25.519
    left T25.412
      first degree T25.512
      second degree T25.612
      third degree T25.712
    multiple with foot — *see* Corrosion, lower, limb, multiple, ankle and foot
    right T25.411
      first degree T25.511
      second degree T25.611
      third degree T25.711
    second degree T25.619
    third degree T25.719
  anus — *see* Corrosion, buttock
  arm(s) (meaning upper limb(s)) — *see* Corrosion, upper limb
  axilla T22.449
    first degree T22.549
    left T22.442
      first degree T22.542
      second degree T22.642
      third degree T22.742
    right T22.441
      first degree T22.541
      second degree T22.641
      third degree T22.741
    second degree T22.649
    third degree T22.749
  back (lower) T21.44
    first degree T21.54
    second degree T21.64
    third degree T21.74
    upper T21.43
      first degree T21.53
      second degree T21.63
      third degree T21.73
  blisters — *code as* Corrosion, second degree, by site
  breast(s) — *see* Corrosion, chest wall
  buttock(s) T21.45
    first degree T21.55
    second degree T21.65
    third degree T21.75
  calf T24.439
    first degree T24.539
    left T24.432
      first degree T24.532
      second degree T24.632
      third degree T24.732
    right T24.431
      first degree T24.531
      second degree T24.631
      third degree T24.731
    second degree T24.639
    third degree T24.739
  canthus (eye) — *see* Corrosion, eyelid
  cervix T28.8
  cheek T20.46
    first degree T20.56
    second degree T20.66
    third degree T20.76
  chest wall T21.41
    first degree T21.51
    second degree T21.61
    third degree T21.71
  chin T20.43
    first degree T20.53
    second degree T20.63
    third degree T20.73
  colon T28.7
  conjunctiva (and cornea) — *see* Corrosion, cornea
  cornea (and conjunctiva) T26.6-
  deep necrosis of underlying tissue — *code as* Corrosion, third degree, by site

Corrosion (injury) (acid) (caustic) (chemical) (lime) (external) (internal) T30.4 — *continued*
  dorsum of hand T23.469
    first degree T23.569
    left T23.462
      first degree T23.562
      second degree T23.662
      third degree T23.762
    right T23.461
      first degree T23.561
      second degree T23.661
      third degree T23.761
    second degree T23.669
    third degree T23.769
  ear (auricle) (external) (canal) T20.41
    drum T28.91
    first degree T20.51
    second degree T20.61
    third degree T20.71
  elbow T22.429
    first degree T22.529
    left T22.422
      first degree T22.522
      second degree T22.622
      third degree T22.722
    right T22.421
      first degree T22.521
      second degree T22.621
      third degree T22.721
    second degree T22.629
    third degree T22.729
  entire body — *see* Corrosion, multiple body regions
  epidermal loss — *code as* Corrosion, second degree, by site
  epiglottis T27.4
  erythema, erythematous — *code as* Corrosion, first degree, by site
  esophagus T28.6
  extent (percentage of body surface)
    10-19 per cent (0-9 percent third degree) T32.10
      with 10-19 percent third degree T32.11
    20-29 per cent (0-9 percent third degree) T32.20
      with
        10-19 percent third degree T32.21
        20-29 percent third degree T32.22
    30-39 per cent (0-9 percent third degree) T32.30
      with
        10-19 percent third degree T32.31
        20-29 percent third degree T32.32
        30-39 percent third degree T32.33
    40-49 per cent (0-9 percent third degree) T32.40
      with
        10-19 percent third degree T32.41
        20-29 percent third degree T32.42
        30-39 percent third degree T32.43
        40-49 percent third degree T32.44
    50-59 per cent (0-9 percent third degree) T32.50
      with
        10-19 percent third degree T32.51
        20-29 percent third degree T32.52
        30-39 percent third degree T32.53
        40-49 percent third degree T32.54
        50-59 percent third degree T32.55
    60-69 per cent (0-9 percent third degree) T32.60
      with
        10-19 percent third degree T32.61
        20-29 percent third degree T32.62
        30-39 percent third degree T32.63
        40-49 percent third degree T32.64
        50-59 percent third degree T32.65
        60-69 percent third degree T32.66
    70-79 per cent (0-9 percent third degree) T32.70
      with
        10-19 percent third degree T32.71
        20-29 percent third degree T32.72
        30-39 percent third degree T32.73
        40-49 percent third degree T32.74
        50-59 percent third degree T32.75
        60-69 percent third degree T32.76
        70-79 percent third degree T32.77
    80-89 per cent (0-9 percent third degree) T32.80
      with
        10-19 percent third degree T32.81
        20-29 percent third degree T32.82
        30-39 percent third degree T32.83

Corrosion (injury) (acid) (caustic) (chemical) (lime) (external) (internal) T30.4 — *continued*
extent (percentage of body surface) — *continued*
  80-89 per cent (0-9 percent third degree) T32.80 — *continued*
    with — *continued*
      40-49 percent third degree T32.84
      50-59 percent third degree T32.85
      60-69 percent third degree T32.86
      70-79 percent third degree T32.87
      80-89 percent third degree T32.88
  90 per cent or more (0-9 percent third degree) T32.90
    with
      10-19 percent third degree T32.91
      20-29 percent third degree T32.92
      30-39 percent third degree T32.93
      40-49 percent third degree T32.94
      50-59 percent third degree T32.95
      60-69 percent third degree T32.96
      70-79 percent third degree T32.97
      80-89 percent third degree T32.98
      90-99 percent third degree T32.99
  less than 10 per cent T32.0
extremity — *see* Corrosion, limb
eye(s) and adnexa T26.9-
  with resulting rupture and destruction of eyeball T26.7-
  conjunctival sac — *see* Corrosion, cornea
  cornea — *see* Corrosion, cornea
  lid — *see* Corrosion, eyelid
  periocular area — *see* Corrosion eyelid
  specified site NEC T26.8-
eyeball — *see* Corrosion, eye
eyelid(s) T26.5-
face — *see* Corrosion, head
finger T23.429
  first degree T23.529
  left T23.422
    first degree T23.522
    second degree T23.622
    third degree T23.722
  multiple sites (without thumb) T23.439
    with thumb T23.449
      first degree T23.549
      left T23.442
        first degree T23.542
        second degree T23.642
        third degree T23.742
      right T23.441
        first degree T23.541
        second degree T23.641
        third degree T23.741
      second degree T23.649
      third degree T23.749
    first degree T23.539
    left T23.432
      first degree T23.532
      second degree T23.632
      third degree T23.732
    right T23.431
      first degree T23.531
      second degree T23.631
      third degree T23.731
    second degree T23.639
    third degree T23.739
  right T23.421
    first degree T23.521
    second degree T23.621
    third degree T23.721
  second degree T23.629
  third degree T23.729
flank — *see* Corrosion, abdomen
foot T25.429
  first degree T25.529
  left T25.422
    first degree T25.522
    second degree T25.622
    third degree T25.722
  multiple with ankle — *see* Corrosion, lower, limb, multiple, ankle and foot
  right T25.421
    first degree T25.521
    second degree T25.621
    third degree T25.721
  second degree T25.629
  third degree T25.729
forearm T22.419
  first degree T22.519
  left T22.412
    first degree T22.512
    second degree T22.612
    third degree T22.712
  right T22.411
    first degree T22.511
    second degree T22.611
    third degree T22.711

Corrosion (injury) (acid) (caustic) (chemical) (lime) (external) (internal) T30.4 — *continued*
forearm T22.419 — *continued*
  second degree T22.619
  third degree T22.719
forehead T20.46
  first degree T20.56
  second degree T20.66
  third degree T20.76
fourth degree — *code as* Corrosion, third degree, by site
full thickness skin loss — *code as* Corrosion, third degree, by site
gastrointestinal tract NEC T28.7
genital organs
  external
    female T21.47
      first degree T21.57
      second degree T21.67
      third degree T21.77
    male T21.46
      first degree T21.56
      second degree T21.66
      third degree T21.76
  internal T28.8
groin — *see* Corrosion, abdominal wall
hand(s) T23.409
  back — *see* Corrosion, dorsum of hand
  finger — *see* Corrosion, finger
  first degree T23.509
  left T23.402
    first degree T23.502
    second degree T23.602
    third degree T23.702
  multiple sites with wrist T23.499
    first degree T23.599
    left T23.492
      first degree T23.592
      second degree T23.692
      third degree T23.792
    right T23.491
      first degree T23.591
      second degree T23.691
      third degree T23.791
    second degree T23.699
    third degree T23.799
  palm — *see* Corrosion, palm
  right T23.401
    first degree T23.501
    second degree T23.601
    third degree T23.701
  second degree T23.609
  third degree T23.709
  thumb — *see* Corrosion, thumb
head (and face) (and neck) T20.40
  cheek — *see* Corrosion, cheek
  chin — *see* Corrosion, chin
  ear — *see* Corrosion, ear
  eye(s) only — *see* Corrosion, eye
  first degree T20.50
  forehead — *see* Corrosion, forehead
  lip — *see* Corrosion, lip
  multiple sites T20.49
    first degree T20.59
    second degree T20.69
    third degree T20.79
  neck — *see* Corrosion, neck
  nose — *see* Corrosion, nose
  scalp — *see* Corrosion, scalp
  second degree T20.60
  third degree T20.70
hip(s) — *see* Corrosion, lower, limb
inhalation — *see* Corrosion, respiratory tract
internal organ(s) *(see also* Corrosion, by site)* T28.90
  alimentary tract T28.7
    esophagus T28.6
  esophagus T28.6
  genitourinary T28.8
  mouth T28.5
  pharynx T28.5
  specified organ NEC T28.99
interscapular region — *see* Corrosion, back, upper
intestine (large) (small) T28.7
knee T24.429
  first degree T24.529
  left T24.422
    first degree T24.522
    second degree T24.622
    third degree T24.722

Corrosion (injury) (acid) (caustic) (chemical) (lime) (external) (internal) T30.4 — *continued*
knee T24.429 — *continued*
  right T24.421
    first degree T24.521
    second degree T24.621
    third degree T24.721
  second degree T24.629
  third degree T24.729
labium (majus) (minus) — *see* Corrosion, genital organs, external, female
lacrimal apparatus, duct, gland or sac — *see* Corrosion, eye, specified site NEC
larynx T27.4
  with lung T27.5
leg(s) (meaning lower limb(s)) — *see* Corrosion, lower limb
limb(s)
  lower — *see* Corrosion, lower, limb
  upper — *see* Corrosion, upper limb
lip(s) T20.42
  first degree T20.52
  second degree T20.62
  third degree T20.72
lower
  back — *see* Corrosion, back
  limb T24.409
    ankle — *see* Corrosion, ankle
    calf — *see* Corrosion, calf
    first degree T24.509
    foot — *see* Corrosion, foot
    hip — *see* Corrosion, thigh
    knee — *see* Corrosion, knee
    left T24.402
      first degree T24.502
      second degree T24.602
      third degree T24.702
    multiple sites, except ankle and foot T24.499
      ankle and foot T25.499
        first degree T25.599
        left T25.492
          first degree T25.592
          second degree T25.692
          third degree T25.792
        right T25.491
          first degree T25.591
          second degree T25.691
          third degree T25.791
        second degree T25.699
        third degree T25.799
      first degree T24.599
      left T24.492
        first degree T24.592
        second degree T24.692
        third degree T24.792
      right T24.491
        first degree T24.591
        second degree T24.691
        third degree T24.791
      second degree T24.699
      third degree T24.799
    right T24.401
      first degree T24.501
      second degree T24.601
      third degree T24.701
    second degree T24.609
    thigh — *see* Corrosion, thigh
    third degree T24.709
lung (with larynx and trachea) T27.5
mouth T28.5
neck T20.47
  first degree T20.57
  second degree T20.67
  third degree T20.77
nose (septum) T20.44
  first degree T20.54
  second degree T20.64
  third degree T20.74
ocular adnexa — *see* Corrosion, eye
orbit region — *see* Corrosion, eyelid
palm T23.459
  first degree T23.559
  left T23.452
    first degree T23.552
    second degree T23.652
    third degree T23.752
  right T23.451
    first degree T23.551
    second degree T23.651
    third degree T23.751
  second degree T23.659
  third degree T23.759
partial thickness — *code as* Corrosion, unspecified degree, by site

Corrosion (injury) (acid) (caustic) (chemical) (lime) (external) (internal) T30.4 — *continued*
pelvis — *see* Corrosion, trunk
penis — *see* Corrosion, genital organs, external, male
perineum
  female — *see* Corrosion, genital organs, external, female
  male — *see* Corrosion, genital organs, external, male
periocular area — *see* Corrosion, eyelid
pharynx T28.5
rectum T28.7
respiratory tract T27.7
  larynx — *see* Corrosion, larynx
  specified part NEC T27.6
  trachea — *see* Corrosion, larynx
sac, lacrimal — *see* Corrosion, eye, specified site NEC
scalp T20.45
  first degree T20.55
  second degree T20.65
  third degree T20.75
scapular region T22.469
  first degree T22.569
  left T22.462
    first degree T22.562
    second degree T22.662
    third degree T22.762
  right T22.461
    first degree T22.561
    second degree T22.661
    third degree T22.761
  second degree T22.669
  third degree T22.769
sclera — *see* Corrosion, eye, specified site NEC
scrotum — *see* Corrosion, genital organs, external, male
shoulder T22.459
  first degree T22.559
  left T22.452
    first degree T22.552
    second degree T22.652
    third degree T22.752
  right T22.451
    first degree T22.551
    second degree T22.651
    third degree T22.751
  second degree T22.659
  third degree T22.759
stomach T28.7
temple — *see* Corrosion, head
testis — *see* Corrosion, genital organs, external, male
thigh T24.419
  first degree T24.519
  left T24.412
    first degree T24.512
    second degree T24.612
    third degree T24.712
  right T24.411
    first degree T24.511
    second degree T24.611
    third degree T24.711
  second degree T24.619
  third degree T24.719
thorax (external) — *see* Corrosion, trunk
throat (meaning pharynx) T28.5
thumb(s) T23.429
  first degree T23.519
  left T23.412
    first degree T23.512
    second degree T23.612
    third degree T23.712
  multiple sites with fingers T23.449
    first degree T23.549
    left T23.442
      first degree T23.542
      second degree T23.642
      third degree T23.742
    right T23.441
      first degree T23.541
      second degree T23.641
      third degree T23.741
    second degree T23.649
    third degree T23.749
  right T23.411
    first degree T23.511
    second degree T23.611
    third degree T23.711
  second degree T23.619
  third degree T23.719

DISEASE INDEX

Corrosion (injury) (acid) (caustic) (chemical) (lime) (external) (internal) T30.4 — *continued*
toe T25.439
  first degree T25.539
  left T25.432
    first degree T25.532
    second degree T25.632
    third degree T25.732
  right T25.431
    first degree T25.531
    second degree T25.631
    third degree T25.731
  second degree T25.639
  third degree T25.739
tongue T28.5
tonsil(s) T28.5
total body — *see* Corrosion, multiple body regions
trachea T27.4
  with lung T27.5
trunk T21.40
  abdominal wall — *see* Corrosion, abdominal wall
  anus — *see* Corrosion, buttock
  axilla — *see* Corrosion, upper limb
  back — *see* Corrosion, back
  breast — *see* Corrosion, chest wall
  buttock — *see* Corrosion, buttock
  chest wall — *see* Corrosion, chest wall
  first degree T21.50
  flank — *see* Corrosion, abdominal wall
  genital
    female — *see* Corrosion, genital organs, external, female
    male — *see* Corrosion, genital organs, external, male
  groin — *see* Corrosion, abdominal wall
  interscapular region — *see* Corrosion, back, upper
  labia — *see* Corrosion, genital organs, external, female
  lower back — *see* Corrosion, back
  penis — *see* Corrosion, genital organs, external, male
  perineum
    female — *see* Corrosion, genital organs, external, female
    male — *see* Corrosion, genital organs, external, male
  scapular region — *see* Corrosion, upper limb
  scrotum — *see* Corrosion, genital organs, external, male
  second degree T21.60
  shoulder — *see* Corrosion, upper limb
  specified site NEC T21.49
    first degree T21.59
    second degree T21.69
    third degree T21.79
  testes — *see* Corrosion, genital organs, external, male
  third degree T21.70
  upper back — *see* Corrosion, back, upper
  vagina T28.8
  vulva — *see* Corrosion, genital organs, external, female
unspecified site with extent of body surface involved specified
  10-19 per cent (0-9 percent third degree) T32.10
    with 10-19 percent third degree T32.11
  20-29 per cent (0-9 percent third degree) T32.20
    with
      10-19 percent third degree T32.21
      20-29 percent third degree T32.22
  30-39 per cent (0-9 percent third degree) T32.30
    with
      10-19 percent third degree T32.31
      20-29 percent third degree T32.32
      30-39 percent third degree T32.33
  40-49 per cent (0-9 percent third degree) T32.40
    with
      10-19 percent third degree T32.41
      20-29 percent third degree T32.42
      30-39 percent third degree T32.43
      40-49 percent third degree T32.44
  50-59 per cent (0-9 percent third degree) T32.50
    with
      10-19 percent third degree T32.51
      20-29 percent third degree T32.52
      30-39 percent third degree T32.53
      40-49 percent third degree T32.54
      50-59 percent third degree T32.55

Corrosion (injury) (acid) (caustic) (chemical) (lime) (external) (internal) T30.4 — *continued*
unspecified site with extent of body surface involved specified — *continued*
  60-69 per cent (0-9 percent third degree) T32.60
    with
      10-19 percent third degree T32.61
      20-29 percent third degree T32.62
      30-39 percent third degree T32.63
      40-49 percent third degree T32.64
      50-59 percent third degree T32.65
      60-69 percent third degree T32.66
  70-79 per cent (0-9 percent third degree) T32.70
    with
      10-19 percent third degree T32.71
      20-29 percent third degree T32.72
      30-39 percent third degree T32.73
      40-49 percent third degree T32.74
      50-59 percent third degree T32.75
      60-69 percent third degree T32.76
      70-79 percent third degree T32.77
  80-89 per cent (0-9 percent third degree) T32.80
    with
      10-19 percent third degree T32.81
      20-29 percent third degree T32.82
      30-39 percent third degree T32.83
      40-49 percent third degree T32.84
      50-59 percent third degree T32.85
      60-69 percent third degree T32.86
      70-79 percent third degree T32.87
      80-89 percent third degree T32.88
  90 per cent or more (0-9 percent third degree) T32.90
    with
      10-19 percent third degree T32.91
      20-29 percent third degree T32.92
      30-39 percent third degree T32.93
      40-49 percent third degree T32.94
      50-59 percent third degree T32.95
      60-69 percent third degree T32.96
      70-79 percent third degree T32.97
      80-89 percent third degree T32.98
      90-99 percent third degree T32.99
  less than 10 per cent T32.0
upper limb (axilla) (scapular region) T22.40
  above elbow — *see* Corrosion, above elbow
  axilla — *see* Corrosion, axilla
  elbow — *see* Corrosion, elbow
  first degree T22.50
  forearm — *see* Corrosion, forearm
  hand — *see* Corrosion, hand
  interscapular region — *see* Corrosion, back, upper
  multiple sites T22.499
    first degree T22.599
    left T22.492
      first degree T22.592
      second degree T22.692
      third degree T22.792
    right T22.491
      first degree T22.591
      second degree T22.691
      third degree T22.791
    second degree T22.699
    third degree T22.799
  scapular region — *see* Corrosion, scapular region
  second degree T22.60
  shoulder — *see* Corrosion, shoulder
  third degree T22.70
  wrist — *see* Corrosion, hand
uterus T28.8
vagina T28.8
vulva — *see* Corrosion, genital organs, external, female
wrist T23.479
  first degree T23.579
  left T23.472
    first degree T23.572
    second degree T23.672
    third degree T23.772
  multiple sites with hand T23.499
    first degree T23.599
    left T23.492
      first degree T23.592
      second degree T23.692
      third degree T23.792
    right T23.491
      first degree T23.591
      second degree T23.691
      third degree T23.791
    second degree T23.699
    third degree T23.799

Corrosion (injury) (acid) (caustic) (chemical) (lime) (external) (internal) T30.4 — *continued*
wrist T23.479 — *continued*
  right T23.471
    first degree T23.571
    second degree T23.671
    third degree T23.771
  second degree T23.679
  third degree T23.779
Corrosive burn — *see* Corrosion
Corsican fever — *see* Malaria
Cortical — *see* condition
Cortico-adrenal — *see* condition
Coryza (acute) J00
  with grippe or influenza — *see* Influenza, with, respiratory manifestations NEC
  syphilitic
    congenital (chronic) A50.05
Costen's syndrome or complex M26.69
Costiveness — *see* Constipation
Costochondritis M94.0
Cot death R99
Cotard's syndrome F22
Cotia virus B08.8
Cotton wool spots (retinal) H35.81
Cotungo's disease — *see* Sciatica
Cough (affected) (chronic) (epidemic) (nervous) R05
  with hemorrhage — *see* Hemoptysis
  bronchial R05
    with grippe or influenza — *see* Influenza, with, respiratory manifestations NEC
  functional F45.8
  hysterical F45.8
  laryngeal, spasmodic R05
  psychogenic F45.8
  smokers' J41.0
  tea taster's B49
Counseling (for) Z71.9
  abuse NEC
    perpetrator Z69.82
    victim Z69.81
  alcohol abuser Z71.41
    family Z71.42
  child abuse
    nonparental
      perpetrator Z69.021
      victim Z69.020
    parental
      perpetrator Z69.011
      victim Z69.010
  consanguinity Z71.89
  contraceptive Z30.09
  dietary Z71.3
  drug abuser Z71.51
    family member Z71.52
  family Z71.89
  fertility preservation (prior to cancer therapy) (prior to removal of gonads) Z31.62
  for non-attending third party Z71.0
    related to sexual behavior or orientation Z70.2
  genetic NEC Z31.5
  health (advice) (education) (instruction) — *see* Counseling, medical
  human immunodeficiency virus (HIV) Z71.7
  impotence Z70.1
  insulin pump use Z46.81
  medical (for) Z71.9
    boarding school resident Z59.3
    consanguinity Z71.89
    feared complaint and no disease found Z71.1
    human immunodeficiency virus (HIV) Z71.7
    institutional resident Z59.3
    on behalf of another Z71.0
      related to sexual behavior or orientation Z70.2
    person living alone Z60.2
    specified reason NEC Z71.89
  natural family planning
    procreative Z31.61
    to avoid pregnancy Z30.02
  perpetrator (of)
    abuse NEC Z69.82
    child abuse
      non-parental Z69.021
      parental Z69.011
    rape NEC Z69.82
    spousal abuse Z69.12

Counseling (for) Z71.9 — *continued*
  procreative NEC Z31.69
    fertility preservation (prior to cancer therapy) (prior to removal of gonads) Z31.62
    using natural family planning Z31.61
  promiscuity Z70.1
  rape victim Z69.81
  religious Z71.81
  sex, sexual (related to) Z70.9
    attitude(s) Z70.0
    behavior or orientation Z70.1
    combined concerns Z70.3
    non-responsiveness Z70.1
    on behalf of third party Z70.2
    specified reason NEC Z70.8
  specified reason NEC Z71.89
  spiritual Z71.81
  spousal abuse (perpetrator) Z69.12
    victim Z69.11
  substance abuse Z71.89
    alcohol Z71.41
    drug Z71.51
    tobacco Z71.6
  tobacco use Z71.6
  use (of)
    insulin pump Z46.81
  victim (of)
    abuse Z69.81
    child abuse
      by parent Z69.010
      non-parental Z69.020
    rape NEC Z69.81
Coupled rhythm R00.8
Couvelaire syndrome or uterus (complicating delivery) O45.8x-
Cowper's gland — *see* condition
Cowperitis — *see* Urethritis
Cowpox B08.010
  due to vaccination T88.1
Coxa
  magna M91.4-
  plana M91.2-
  valga (acquired) — *see also* Deformity, limb, specified type NEC, thigh
    congenital Q65.81
    sequelae (late effect) of rickets E64.3
  vara (acquired) — *see also* Deformity, limb, specified type NEC, thigh
    congenital Q65.82
    sequelae (late effect) of rickets E64.3
Coxalgia, coxalgic (nontuberculous) — *see also* Pain, joint, hip
  tuberculous A18.02
Coxitis — *see* Monoarthritis, hip
Coxsackie (virus) (infection) B34.1
  as cause of disease classified elsewhere B97.11
  carditis B33.20
  central nervous system NEC A88.8
  endocarditis B33.21
  enteritis A08.39
  meningitis (aseptic) A87.0
  myocarditis B33.22
  pericarditis B33.23
  pharyngitis B08.5
  pleurodynia B33.0
  specific disease NEC B33.8
Crabs, meaning pubic lice B85.3
Crack baby P04.41
Cracked nipple N64.0
  associated with
    lactation O92.13
    pregnancy O92.11-
    puerperium O92.12
Cracked tooth K03.81
Cradle cap L21.0
Craft neurosis F48.8
Cramp(s) R25.2
  abdominal — *see* Pain, abdominal
  bathing T75.1
  colic R10.83
    psychogenic F45.8
  due to immersion T75.1
  fireman T67.2
  heat T67.2
  immersion T75.1
  intestinal — *see* Pain, abdominal
    psychogenic F45.8
  leg, sleep related G47.62
  limb (lower) (upper) NEC R25.2
    sleep related G47.62
  linotypist's F48.8
  organic G25.89
  muscle (limb) (general) R25.2
    due to immersion T75.1
    psychogenic F45.8

Cramp(s) R25.2 — *continued*
occupational (hand) F48.8
  organic G25.89
salt-depletion E87.1
sleep related, leg G47.62
stoker's T67.2
swimmer's T75.1
telegrapher's F48.8
  organic G25.89
typist's F48.8
  organic G25.89
uterus N94.89
  menstrual — *see* Dysmenorrhea
writer's F48.8
  organic G25.89
Cranial — *see* condition
Craniocleidodysostosis Q74.0
Craniofenestria (skull) Q75.8
Craniolacunia (skull) Q75.8
Craniopagus Q89.4
Craniopathy, metabolic M85.2
Craniopharyngeal — *see* condition
Craniopharyngioma D44.4
Craniorachischisis (totalis) Q00.1
Craniaschisis Q75.8
Craniostenosis Q75.0
Craniosynostosis Q75.0
Craniotabes (cause unknown) M83.8
neonatal P96.3
rachitic E64.3
syphilitic A50.56
Cranium — *see* condition
Craw-craw — *see* Onchocerciasis
Creaking joint — *see* Derangement, joint,
  specified type NEC
Creeping
eruption B76.9
palsy or paralysis G12.22
Crenated tongue K14.8
Creotoxism A05.9
Crepitus
caput Q75.8
joint — *see* Derangement, joint, specified
  type NEC
Crescent or conus choroid, congenital
  Q14.3
CREST syndrome M34.1
Cretin, cretinism (congenital) (endemic)
  (nongoitrous) (sporadic) E00.9
pelvis
  with disproportion (fetopelvic) O33.0
    causing obstructed labor O65.0
type
  hypothyroid E00.1
  mixed E00.2
  myxedematous E00.1
  neurological E00.0
Creutzfeldt-Jakob disease or syndrome
  (with dementia) A81.00
familial A81.09
iatrogenic A81.09
specified NEC A81.09
sporadic A81.09
variant (vCJD) A81.01
Cri-du-chat syndrome Q93.4
Crib death R99
Cribriform hymen Q52.3
Crigler-Najjar disease or syndrome E80.5
Crime, victim of Z65.4
Crimean hemorrhagic fever A98.0
Criminalism F60.2
Crisis
abdomen R10.0
acute reaction F43.0
addisonian E27.2
adrenal (cortical) E27.2
celiac K90.0
Dietl's N13.8
emotional — *see also* Disorder, adjustment
  acute reaction to stress F43.0
  specific to childhood and adolescence
    F93.8
glaucomatocyclitic — *see* Glaucoma,
  secondary, inflammation
heart — *see* Failure, heart
nitritoid I95.2
  correct substance properly administered
    — *see* Table of Drugs and
    Chemicals, by drug, adverse effect
  overdose or wrong substance given or
    taken — *see* Table of Drugs and
    Chemicals, by drug, poisoning
oculogyric H51.8
  psychogenic F45.8
Pel's (tabetic) A52.11

Crisis — *continued*
psychosexual identity F64.2
renal N28.0
sickle-cell D57.00
  with
    acute chest syndrome D57.01
    splenic sequestration D57.02
state (acute reaction) F43.0
tabetic A52.11
thyroid — *see* Thyrotoxicosis with thyroid
  storm
thyrotoxic — *see* Thyrotoxicosis with
  thyroid storm
Crocq's disease (acrocyanosis) I73.89
Crohn's disease — *see* Enteritis, regional
Crooked septum, nasal J34.2
Cross syndrome E70.328
Crossbite (anterior) (posterior) M26.24
Cross-eye — *see* Strabismus, convergent
  concomitant
Croup, croupous (catarrhal) (infectious)
  (inflammatory) (nondiphtheritic) J05.0
bronchial J20.9
diphtheritic A36.2
false J38.5
spasmodic J38.5
  diphtheritic A36.2
stridulous J38.5
  diphtheritic A36.2
Crouzon's disease Q75.1
Crowding, tooth, teeth, fully erupted
  M26.31
CRST syndrome M34.1
Cruchet's disease A85.8
Cruelty in children — *see also* Disorder,
  conduct
Crural ulcer — *see* Ulcer, lower limb
Crush, crushed, crushing T14.8
abdomen S38.1
ankle S97.0-
arm (upper) (and shoulder) S47-
  axilla — *see* Crush, arm
back, lower S38.1
buttock S38.1
cheek S07.0
chest S28.0
cranium S07.1
ear S07.0
elbow S57.0-
extremity
  lower
    ankle — *see* Crush, ankle
    below knee — *see* Crush, leg
    foot — *see* Crush, foot
    hip — *see* Crush, hip
    knee — *see* Crush, knee
    thigh — *see* Crush, thigh
    toe — *see* Crush, toe
  upper
    below elbow S67.9-
    elbow — *see* Crush, elbow
    finger — *see* Crush, finger
    forearm — *see* Crush, forearm
    hand — *see* Crush, hand
    thumb — *see* Crush, thumb
    upper arm — *see* Crush, arm
    wrist — *see* Crush, wrist
face S07.0
finger(s) S67.1-
  with hand (and wrist) — *see* Crush,
    hand, specified site NEC
  index S67.19-
  little S67.19-
  middle S67.19-
  ring S67.19-
  thumb — *see* Crush, thumb
foot S97.8-
  toe — *see* Crush, toe
forearm S57.8-
genitalia, external
  female S38.002
    vagina S38.03
    vulva S38.03
  male S38.001
    penis S38.01
    scrotum S38.02
    testis S38.02
hand (except fingers alone) S67.2-
  with wrist S67.4-
head S07.9
  specified NEC S07.8
heel — *see* Crush, foot
hip S77.0-
  with thigh S77.2-
internal organ (abdomen, chest, or pelvis)
  NEC T14.8
knee S87.0-

Crush, crushed, crushing — *continued*
labium (majus) (minus) S38.03
larynx S17.0
leg (lower) S87.8-
  knee — *see* Crush, knee
lip S07.0
lower
  back S38.1
  leg — *see* Crush, leg
neck S17.9
nerve — *see* Injury, nerve
nose S07.0
pelvis S38.1
penis S38.01
scalp S07.8
scapular region — *see* Crush, arm
scrotum S38.02
severe, unspecified site T14.8
shoulder (and upper arm) — *see* Crush,
  arm
skull S07.1
syndrome (complication of trauma) T79.5
testis S38.02
thigh S77.1-
  with hip S77.2-
throat S17.8
thumb S67.0-
  with hand (and wrist) — *see* Crush,
    hand, specified site NEC
toe(s) S97.10-
  great S97.11-
  lesser S97.12-
trachea S17.0
vagina S38.03
vulva S38.03
wrist S67.3-
  with hand S67.4-
Crusta lactea L21.0
Crusts R23.4
Crutch paralysis — *see* Injury, brachial
  plexus
Cruveilhier's atrophy or disease G12.8
Cruveilhier-Baumgarten cirrhosis, disease
  or syndrome K74.69
Crying (constant) (continuous) (excessive)
child, adolescent, or adult R45.83
infant (baby) (newborn) R68.11
Cryofibrinogenemia D89.2
Cryoglobulinemia (essential) (idiopathic)
  (mixed) (primary) (purpura) (secondary)
  (vasculitis) D89.1
with lung involvement D89.1 [J99]
Cryptitis (anal) (rectal) K62.89
Cryptococcosis, cryptococcus (infection)
  (neoformans) B45.9
bone B45.3
cerebral B45.1
cutaneous B45.2
disseminated B45.7
generalized B45.7
meningitis B45.1
meningocerebralis B45.1
osseous B45.3
pulmonary B45.0
skin B45.2
specified NEC B45.8
Cryptopapillitis (anus) K62.89
Cryptophthalmos Q11.2
syndrome Q87.0
Cryptorchid, cryptorchism,
  cryptorchidism Q53.9
bilateral Q53.20
  abdominal Q53.21
  perineal Q53.22
unilateral Q53.10
  abdominal Q53.11
  perineal Q53.12
Cryptosporidiosis A07.2
hepatobiliary B88.8
respiratory B88.8
Cryptostromosis J67.6
Crystalluria R82.99
Cubitus
congenital Q68.8
valgus (acquired) M21.0-
  congenital Q68.8
  sequelae (late effect) of rickets E64.3
varus (acquired) M21.1-
  congenital Q68.8
  sequelae (late effect) of rickets E64.3
Cultural deprivation or shock Z60.3
Curling esophagus K22.4
Curling's ulcer — *see* Ulcer, peptic, acute
Curschmann (-Batten) (-Steinert) disease
  or syndrome G71.11

Curse, Ondine's — *see* Apnea, sleep
Curvature
organ or site, congenital NEC — *see*
  Distortion
penis (lateral) Q55.61
Pott's (spinal) A18.01
radius, idiopathic, progressive (congenital)
  Q74.0
spine (acquired) (angular) (idiopathic)
  (incorrect) (postural) — *see*
  Dorsopathy, deforming
  congenital Q67.5
  due to or associated with
    Charcot-Marie-Tooth disease (*see*
      also subcategory M49.8) G60.0
    osteitis
      deformans M88.88
      fibrosa cystica (*see also*
        subcategory M49.8) E21.0
    tuberculosis (Pott's curvature) A18.01
  sequelae (late effect) of rickets E64.3
  tuberculous A18.01
Cushing's
syndrome or disease E24.9
  drug-induced E24.2
  iatrogenic E24.2
  pituitary-dependent E24.0
  specified NEC E24.8
ulcer — *see* Ulcer, peptic, acute
Cushingoid due to steroid therapy E24.2
correct substance properly administered —
  see Table of Drugs and Chemicals, by
  drug, adverse effect
overdose or wrong substance given or
  taken — *see* Table of Drugs and
  Chemicals, by drug, poisoning
Cusp, Carabelli — omit code
Cut (external) — *see also* Laceration
muscle — *see* Injury, muscle
Cutaneous — *see also* condition
hemorrhage R23.3
larva migrans B76.9
Cutis — *see also* condition
hyperelastica Q82.8
  acquired L57.4
laxa (hyperelastica) — *see* Dermatolysis
marmorata R23.8
osteosis L94.2
pendula — *see* Dermatolysis
rhomboidalis nuchae L57.2
verticis gyrata Q82.8
  acquired L91.8
Cyanosis R23.0
due to
  patent foramen botalli Q21.1
    persistent foramen ovale Q21.1
enterogenous D74.8
paroxysmal digital — *see* Raynaud's
  disease
  with gangrene I73.01
retina, retinal H35.89
Cyanotic heart disease I24.9
congenital Q24.9
Cycle
anovulatory N97.0
menstrual, irregular N92.6
Cyclencephaly Q04.9
Cyclical vomiting (*see also* Vomiting,
  cyclical) G43.A0
psychogenic F50.8
Cyclitis (*see also* Iridocyclitis) H20.9
chronic — *see* Iridocyclitis, chronic
Fuchs' heterochromic H20.81-
granulomatous — *see* Iridocyclitis, chronic
lens-induced — *see* Iridocyclitis, lens-
  induced
posterior H30.2-
Cycloid personality F34.0
Cyclophoria H50.54
Cyclopia, cyclops Q87.0
Cyclopism Q87.0
Cyclosporiasis A07.4
Cyclothymia F34.0
Cyclothymic personality F34.0
Cyclotropia H50.41-
Cylindroma — *see also* Neoplasm,
  malignant, by site
eccrine dermal — *see* Neoplasm, skin,
  benign
skin — *see* Neoplasm, skin, benign
Cylindruria R82.99
Cynanche
diphtheritic A36.2
tonsillaris J36
Cynophobia F40.218
Cynorexia R63.2
Cyphosis — *see* Kyphosis
Cyprus fever — *see* Brucellosis

DISEASE INDEX

Cyst (colloid) (mucous) (simple) (retention)
- adenoid (infected) J35.8
- adrenal gland E27.8
  - congenital Q89.1
- air, lung J98.4
- allantoic Q64.4
- alveolar process (jaw bone) M27.40
- amnion, amniotic O41.8x-
- anterior
  - chamber (eye) — see Cyst, iris
  - nasopalatine K09.1
- antrum J34.1
- anus K62.89
- apical (tooth) (periodontal) K04.8
- appendix K38.8
- arachnoid, brain (acquired) G93.0
  - congenital Q04.6
- arytenoid J38.7
- Baker's M71.2-
  - ruptured M66.0
  - tuberculous A18.02
- Bartholin's gland N75.0
- bile duct (common) (hepatic) K83.5
- bladder (multiple) (trigone) N32.89
- blue dome (breast) — see Cyst, breast
- bone (local) NEC M85.60
  - aneurysmal M85.50
    - ankle M85.57-
    - foot M85.57-
    - forearm M85.53-
    - hand M85.54-
    - jaw M27.49
    - lower leg M85.56-
    - multiple site M85.59
    - neck M85.58
    - rib M85.58
    - shoulder M85.51-
    - skull M85.58
    - specified site NEC M85.58
    - thigh M85.55-
    - toe M85.57-
    - upper arm M85.52-
    - vertebra M85.58
  - solitary M85.40
    - ankle M85.47-
    - fibula M85.46-
    - foot M85.47-
    - hand M85.44-
    - humerus M85.42-
    - jaw M27.49
    - neck M85.48
    - pelvis M85.45-
    - radius M85.43-
    - rib M85.48
    - shoulder M85.41-
    - skull M85.48
    - specified site NEC M85.48
    - tibia M85.46-
    - toe M85.47-
    - ulna M85.43-
    - vertebra M85.48
  - specified type NEC M85.60
    - ankle M85.67-
    - foot M85.67-
    - forearm M85.63-
    - hand M85.64-
    - jaw M27.40
      - developmental (nonodontogenic) K09.1
        - odontogenic K09.0
      - latent M27.0
    - lower leg M85.66-
    - multiple site M85.69
    - neck M85.68
    - rib M85.68
    - shoulder M85.61-
    - skull M85.68
    - specified site NEC M85.68
    - thigh M85.65-
    - toe M85.67-
    - upper arm M85.62-
    - vertebra M85.68
- brain (acquired) G93.0
  - congenital Q04.6
  - hydatid B67.99 [G94]
  - third ventricle (colloid), congenital Q04.6
- branchial (cleft) Q18.0
- branchiogenic Q18.0
- breast (benign) (blue dome) (pedunculated) (solitary) N60.0-
  - involution — see Dysplasia, mammary, specified type NEC
  - sebaceous — see Dysplasia, mammary, specified type NEC

Cyst (colloid) (mucous) (simple) (retention) — continued
- broad ligament (benign) N83.8
- bronchogenic (mediastinal) (sequestration) J98.4
  - congenital Q33.0
- buccal K09.8
- bulbourethral gland N36.8
- bursa, bursal NEC M71.30
  - with rupture — see Rupture, synovium
  - ankle M71.37-
  - elbow M71.32-
  - foot M71.37-
  - hand M71.34-
  - hip M71.35-
  - multiple sites M71.39
  - pharyngeal J39.2
  - popliteal space — see Cyst, Baker's
  - shoulder M71.31-
  - specified site NEC M71.38
  - wrist M71.33-
- calcifying odontogenic D16.5
  - upper jaw (bone) (maxilla) D16.4
- canal of Nuck (female) N94.89
  - congenital Q52.4
- canthus — see Cyst, conjunctiva
- carcinomatous — see Neoplasm, malignant, by site
- cauda equina G95.89
- cavum septi pellucidi — see Cyst, brain
- celomic (pericardium) Q24.8
- cerebellopontine (angle) — see Cyst, brain
- cerebellum — see Cyst, brain
- cerebral — see Cyst, brain
- cervical lateral Q18.1
- cervix NEC N88.8
  - embryonic Q51.6
  - nabothian N88.8
- chiasmal optic NEC — see Disorder, optic, chiasm
- chocolate (ovary) N80.1
- choledochus, congenital Q44.4
- chorion O41.8x-
- choroid plexus G93.0
- ciliary body — see Cyst, iris
- clitoris N90.7
- colon K63.89
- common (bile) duct K83.5
- congenital NEC Q89.8
  - adrenal gland Q89.1
  - epiglottis Q31.8
  - esophagus Q39.8
  - fallopian tube Q50.4
  - kidney Q61.00
    - more than one (multiple) Q61.02
      - specified as polycystic Q61.3
        - adult type Q61.2
        - infantile type NEC Q61.19
          - collecting duct dilation Q61.11
    - solitary Q61.01
  - larynx Q31.8
  - liver Q44.6
  - lung Q33.0
  - mediastinum Q34.1
  - ovary Q50.1
  - oviduct Q50.4
  - periurethral (tissue) Q64.79
  - prepuce Q55.69
  - salivary gland (any) Q38.4
  - sublingual Q38.6
  - submaxillary gland Q38.6
  - thymus (gland) Q89.2
  - tongue Q38.3
  - ureterovesical orifice Q62.8
  - vulva Q52.79
- conjunctiva H11.44-
- cornea H18.89-
- corpora quadrigemina G93.0
- corpus
  - albicans N83.29
  - luteum (hemorrhagic) (ruptured) N83.1
- Cowper's gland (benign) (infected) N36.8
- cranial meninges G93.0
- craniobuccal pouch E23.6
- craniopharyngeal pouch E23.6
- cystic duct K82.8
- Cysticercus — see Cysticercosis
- Dandy-Walker Q03.1
  - with spina bifida — see Spina bifida
- dental (root) K04.8
  - developmental K09.0
  - eruption K09.0
  - primordial K09.0
- dentigerous (mandible) (maxilla) K09.0

Cyst (colloid) (mucous) (simple) (retention) — continued
- dermoid — see Neoplasm, benign, by site
  - with malignant transformation C56-
  - implantation
    - external area or site (skin) NEC L72.0
    - iris — see Cyst, iris, implantation
    - vagina N89.8
    - vulva N90.7
  - mouth K09.8
  - oral soft tissue K09.8
  - sacrococcygeal — see Cyst, pilonidal
- developmental K09.1
  - odontogenic K09.0
  - oral region (nonodontogenic) K09.1
  - ovary, ovarian Q50.1
- dura (cerebral) G93.0
  - spinal G96.19
- ear (external) Q18.1
- echinococcal — see Echinococcus
- embryonic
  - cervix uteri Q51.6
  - fallopian tube Q50.4
  - vagina Q51.6
- endometrium, endometrial (uterus) N85.8
  - ectopic — see Endometriosis
- enterogenous Q43.8
- epidermal, epidermoid (inclusion) (see also Cyst, skin) L72.0
  - mouth K09.8
  - oral soft tissue K09.8
- epididymis N50.3
- epiglottis J38.7
- epiphysis cerebri E34.8
- epithelial (inclusion) L72.0
- epoophoron Q50.5
- eruption K09.0
- esophagus K22.8
- ethmoid sinus J34.1
- external female genital organs NEC N90.7
- eye NEC H57.8
  - congenital Q15.8
- eyelid (sebaceous) H02.829
  - infected — see Hordeolum
  - left H02.826
    - lower H02.825
    - upper H02.824
  - right H02.823
    - lower H02.822
    - upper H02.821
- fallopian tube N83.8
  - congenital Q50.4
- fimbrial (twisted) Q50.4
- fissural (oral region) K09.1
  - nabothian N88.8
- follicle (graafian) (hemorrhagic) N83.0
  - nabothian N88.8
- follicular (atretic) (hemorrhagic) (ovarian) N83.0
  - dentigerous K09.0
  - odontogenic K09.0
  - skin L72.9
    - specified NEC L72.8
- frontal sinus J34.1
- gallbladder K82.8
- ganglion — see Ganglion
- Gartner's duct Q52.4
- gingiva K09.0
- gland of Moll — see Cyst, eyelid
- globulomaxillary K09.1
- graafian follicle (hemorrhagic) N83.0
- granulosal lutein (hemorrhagic) N83.1
- hemangiomatous D18.00
  - intra-abdominal D18.03
  - intracranial D18.02
  - skin D18.01
  - specified site NEC D18.09
- hydatid (see also Echinococcus) B67.90
  - brain B67.99 [G94]
  - liver (see also Cyst, liver, hydatid) B67.8
  - lung NEC B67.99 [J99]
  - Morgagni
    - female Q50.5
    - male (epididymal) Q55.4
      - testicular Q55.29
  - specified site NEC B67.99
- hymen N89.8
  - embryonic Q52.4
- hypopharynx J39.2
- hypophysis, hypophyseal (duct) (recurrent) E23.6
  - cerebri E23.6
- implantation (dermoid)
  - external area or site (skin) NEC L72.0
  - iris — see Cyst, iris, implantation
  - vagina N89.8
  - vulva N90.7

Cyst (colloid) (mucous) (simple) (retention) — continued
- incisive canal K09.1
- inclusion (epidermal) (epithelial) (epidermoid) (squamous) L72.0
  - not of skin — code under Cyst, by site
- intestine (large) (small) K63.89
- intracranial — see Cyst, brain
- intraligamentous — see also Disorder, ligament
  - knee — see Derangement, knee
- intrasellar E23.6
- iris H21.309
  - exudative H21.31-
  - idiopathic H21.30-
  - implantation H21.32-
  - parasitic H21.33-
  - pars plana (primary) H21.34-
    - exudative H21.35-
- jaw (bone) M27.40
  - aneurysmal M27.49
  - developmental (odontogenic) K09.0
  - fissural K09.1
  - hemorrhagic M27.49
  - traumatic M27.49
- joint NEC — see Disorder, joint, specified type NEC
- kidney (acquired) N28.1
  - calyceal — see Hydronephrosis
  - congenital Q61.00
    - more than one (multiple) Q61.02
      - specified as polycystic Q61.3
        - adult type (autosomal dominant) Q61.2
        - infantile type (autosomal recessive) NEC Q61.19
          - collecting duct dilation Q61.11
  - pyelogenic — see Hydronephrosis
  - simple N28.1
  - solitary (single) Q61.01
    - acquired N28.1
- labium (majus) (minus) N90.7
  - sebaceous N90.7
- lacrimal — see also Disorder, lacrimal system, specified NEC
  - gland H04.13-
  - passages or sac — see Disorder, lacrimal system, specified NEC
- larynx J38.7
- lateral periodontal K09.0
- lens H27.8
  - congenital Q12.8
- lip (gland) K13.0
- liver (idiopathic) (simple) K76.89
  - congenital Q44.6
  - hydatid B67.8
    - granulosus B67.0
    - multilocularis B67.5
- lung J98.4
  - congenital Q33.0
  - giant bullous J43.9
- lutein N83.1
- lymphangiomatous D18.1
- lymphoepithelial, oral soft tissue K09.8
- macula — see Degeneration, macula, hole
- malignant — see Neoplasm, malignant, by site
- mammary gland — see Cyst, breast
- mandible M27.40
  - dentigerous K09.0
  - radicular K04.8
- maxilla M27.40
  - dentigerous K09.0
  - radicular K04.8
- medial, face and neck Q18.8
- median
  - anterior maxillary K09.1
  - palatal K09.1
- mediastinum, congenital Q34.1
- meibomian (gland) — see Chalazion
  - infected — see Hordeolum
- membrane, brain G93.0
- meninges (cerebral) G93.0
  - spinal G96.19
- meniscus, knee — see Derangement, knee, meniscus, cystic
- mesentery, mesenteric K66.8
  - chyle I89.8
- mesonephric duct
  - female Q50.5
  - male Q55.4
- milk N64.89
- Morgagni (hydatid)
  - female Q50.5
  - male (epididymal) Q55.4
    - testicular Q55.29
- mouth K09.8

DISEASE INDEX

Cyst (colloid) (mucous) (simple) (retention) — *continued*
- Müllerian duct Q50.4
  - appendix testis Q55.29
  - cervix Q51.6
  - fallopian tube Q50.4
  - female Q50.4
  - male Q55.29
  - prostatic utricle Q55.4
  - vagina (embryonal) Q52.4
- multilocular (ovary) D39.10
  - benign — *see* Neoplasm, benign, by site
- myometrium N85.8
- nabothian (follicle) (ruptured) N88.8
- nasoalveolar K09.1
- nasolabial K09.1
- nasopalatine (anterior) (duct) K09.1
- nasopharynx J39.2
- neoplastic — *see* Neoplasm, uncertain behavior, by site
  - benign — *see* Neoplasm, benign, by site
- nervous system NEC G96.8
- neuroenteric (congenital) Q06.8
- nipple — *see* Cyst, breast
- nose (turbinates) J34.1
  - sinus J34.1
- odontogenic, developmental K09.0
- omentum (lesser) K66.8
  - congenital Q45.8
- ora serrata — *see* Cyst, retina, ora serrata
- oral
  - region K09.9
    - developmental (nonodontogenic) K09.1
    - specified NEC K09.8
  - soft tissue K09.9
    - specified NEC K09.8
- orbit H05.81-
- ovary, ovarian (twisted) N83.20
  - adherent N83.20
  - chocolate N80.1
  - corpus
    - albicans N83.29
    - luteum (hemorrhagic) N83.1
  - dermoid D27.9
  - developmental Q50.1
  - due to failure of involution NEC N83.20
  - endometrial N80.1
  - follicular (graafian) (hemorrhagic) N83.0
  - hemorrhagic N83.20
  - in pregnancy or childbirth O34.8-
    - with obstructed labor O65.5
  - multilocular D39.10
  - pseudomucinous D27.9
  - retention N83.29
  - serous N83.20
  - specified NEC N83.29
  - theca lutein (hemorrhagic) N83.1
  - tuberculous A18.18
- oviduct N83.8
- palate (median) (fissural) K09.1
- palatine papilla (jaw) K09.1
- pancreas, pancreatic (hemorrhagic) (true) K86.2
  - congenital Q45.2
  - false K86.3
- paralabral
  - hip M24.85-
  - shoulder S43.43-
- paramesonephric duct Q50.4
  - female Q50.4
  - male Q55.29
- paranephric N28.1
- paraphysis, cerebri, congenital Q04.6
- parasitic B89
- parathyroid (gland) E21.4
- paratubal N83.8
- paraurethral duct N36.8
- paroophoron Q50.5
- parotid gland K11.6
- parovarian Q50.5
- pelvis, female N94.89
  - in pregnancy or childbirth O34.8-
    - causing obstructed labor O65.5
- penis (sebaceous) N48.89
- periapical K04.8
- pericardial, congenital Q24.8
  - acquired (secondary) I31.8
- pericoronal K09.0
- periodontal K04.8
  - lateral K09.0
- peripelvic (lymphatic) N28.1
- peritoneum K66.8
  - chylous I89.8
- periventricular, acquired, newborn P91.1

Cyst (colloid) (mucous) (simple) (retention) — *continued*
- pharynx (wall) J39.2
- pilar L72.11
- pilonidal (infected) (rectum) L05.91
  - with abscess L05.01
  - malignant C44.59-
- pituitary (duct) (gland) E23.6
- placenta O43.19-
- pleura J94.8
- popliteal — *see* Cyst, Baker's
- porencephalic Q04.6
  - acquired G93.0
- postanal (infected) — *see* Cyst, pilonidal
- postmastectomy cavity (mucosal) — *see* Complications, postmastoidectomy, cyst
- preauricular Q18.1
- prepuce N47.4
  - congenital Q55.69
- primordial (jaw) K09.0
- prostate N42.83
- pseudomucinous (ovary) D27.9
- pupillary, miotic H21.27-
- radicular (residual) K04.8
- radiculodental K04.8
- ranular K11.8
- Rathke's pouch E23.6
- rectum (epithelium) (mucous) K62.89
- renal — *see* Cyst, kidney
- residual (radicular) K04.8
- retention (ovary) N83.29
  - salivary gland K11.6
- retina H33.19-
  - ora serrata H33.11-
  - parasitic H33.12-
- retroperitoneal K68.9
- sacrococcygeal (dermoid) — *see* Cyst, pilonidal
- salivary gland or duct (mucous extravasation or retention) K11.6
- Sampson's N80.1
- sclera H15.89
- scrotum L72.9
  - sebaceous L72.3
- sebaceous (duct) (gland) L72.3
  - breast — *see* Dysplasia, mammary, specified type NEC
  - eyelid — *see* Cyst, eyelid
  - genital organ NEC
    - female N94.89
    - male N50.8
  - scrotum L72.3
- semilunar cartilage (knee) (multiple) — *see* Derangement, knee, meniscus, cystic
- seminal vesicle N50.8
- serous (ovary) N83.20
- sinus (accessory) (nasal) J34.1
- Skene's gland N36.8
- skin L72.9
  - breast — *see* Dysplasia, mammary, specified type NEC
  - epidermal, epidermoid L72.0
  - epithelial L72.0
  - eyelid — *see* Cyst, eyelid
  - genital organ NEC
    - female N90.7
    - male N50.8
  - inclusion L72.0
  - scrotum L72.9
  - sebaceous L72.3
  - sweat gland or duct L74.8
- solitary
  - bone — *see* Cyst, bone, solitary
  - jaw M27.40
  - kidney N28.1
- spermatic cord N50.8
- sphenoid sinus J34.1
- spinal meninges G96.19
- spleen NEC D73.4
  - congenital Q89.09
  - hydatid (*see also* Echinococcus) B67.99 [D77]
- Stafne's M27.0
- subarachnoid intrasellar R93.0
- subcutaneous, pheomycotic (chromomycotic) B43.2
- subdural (cerebral) G93.0
  - spinal cord G96.19
- sublingual gland K11.6
- submandibular gland K11.6
- submaxillary gland K11.6
- suburethral N36.8
- suprarenal gland E27.8
- suprasellar — *see* Cyst, brain
- sweat gland or duct L74.8
- synovial — *see also* Cyst, bursa
  - ruptured — *see* Rupture, synovium
- tarsal — *see* Chalazion

Cyst (colloid) (mucous) (simple) (retention) — *continued*
- tendon (sheath) — *see* Disorder, tendon, specified type NEC
- testis N44.2
  - tunica albuginea N44.1
- theca lutein (ovary) N83.1
- Thornwaldt's J39.2
- thymus (gland) E32.8
- thyroglossal duct (infected) (persistent) Q89.2
- thyroid (gland) E04.1
- thyrolingual duct (infected) (persistent) Q89.2
- tongue K14.8
- tonsil J35.8
- tooth — *see* Cyst, dental
- Tornwaldt's J39.2
- trichilemmal (proliferating) L72.12
- trichodermal L72.12
- tubal (fallopian) N83.8
  - inflammatory — *see* Salpingitis, chronic
- tubo-ovarian N83.8
  - inflammatory N70.13
- tunica
  - albuginea testis N44.1
  - vaginalis N50.8
- turbinate (nose) J34.1
- Tyson's gland N48.89
- urachus, congenital Q64.4
- ureter N28.89
- ureterovesical orifice N28.89
- urethra, urethral (gland) N36.8
- uterine ligament N83.8
- uterus (body) (corpus) (recurrent) N85.8
  - embryonic Q51.818
    - cervix Q51.6
- vagina, vaginal (implantation) (inclusion) (squamous cell) (wall) N89.8
  - embryonic Q52.4
- vallecula, vallecular (epiglottis) J38.7
- vesical (orifice) N32.89
- vitreous body H43.89
- vulva (implantation) (inclusion) N90.7
  - congenital Q52.79
  - sebaceous gland N90.7
- vulvovaginal gland N90.7
- wolffian
  - female Q50.5
  - male Q55.4

Cystadenocarcinoma — *see* Neoplasm, malignant, by site
- bile duct C22.1
- endometrioid — *see* Neoplasm, malignant, by site
  - specified site — *see* Neoplasm, malignant, by site
  - unspecified site
    - female C56.9
    - male C61
- mucinous
  - papillary
    - specified site — *see* Neoplasm, malignant, by site
    - unspecified site C56.9
  - specified site — *see* Neoplasm, malignant, by site
  - unspecified site C56.9
- papillary
  - mucinous
    - specified site — *see* Neoplasm, malignant, by site
    - unspecified site C56.9
  - pseudomucinous
    - specified site — *see* Neoplasm, malignant, by site
    - unspecified site C56.9
  - serous
    - specified site — *see* Neoplasm, malignant, by site
    - unspecified site C56.9
  - specified site — *see* Neoplasm, malignant, by site
  - unspecified site C56.9
- pseudomucinous
  - papillary
    - specified site — *see* Neoplasm, malignant, by site
    - unspecified site C56.9
  - specified site — *see* Neoplasm, malignant, by site
  - unspecified site C56.9
- serous
  - papillary
    - specified site — *see* Neoplasm, malignant, by site
    - unspecified site C56.9
  - specified site — *see* Neoplasm, malignant, by site
  - unspecified site C56.9

Cystadenofibroma
- clear cell — *see* Neoplasm, benign, by site
- endometrioid D27.9
  - borderline malignancy D39.1-
  - malignant C56-
- mucinous
  - specified site — *see* Neoplasm, benign, by site
  - unspecified site D27.9
- serous
  - specified site — *see* Neoplasm, benign, by site
  - unspecified site D27.9
- specified site — *see* Neoplasm, benign, by site
- unspecified site D27.9

Cystadenoma — *see also* Neoplasm, benign, by site
- bile duct D13.4
- endometrioid — *see* Neoplasm, benign, by site
  - borderline malignancy — *see* Neoplasm, uncertain behavior, by site
- malignant — *see* Neoplasm, malignant, by site
- mucinous
  - borderline malignancy
    - ovary C56-
    - specified site NEC — *see* Neoplasm, uncertain behavior, by site
    - unspecified site C56.9
  - papillary
    - borderline malignancy
      - ovary C56-
      - specified site NEC — *see* Neoplasm, uncertain behavior, by site
      - unspecified site C56.9
    - specified site — *see* Neoplasm, benign, by site
    - unspecified site D27.9
  - specified site — *see* Neoplasm, benign, by site
  - unspecified site D27.9
- papillary
  - borderline malignancy
    - ovary C56-
    - specified site NEC — *see* Neoplasm, uncertain behavior, by site
    - unspecified site C56.9
  - lymphomatosum
    - specified site — *see* Neoplasm, benign, by site
    - unspecified site D11.9
  - mucinous
    - borderline malignancy
      - ovary C56-
      - specified site NEC — *see* Neoplasm, uncertain behavior, by site
      - unspecified site C56.9
    - specified site — *see* Neoplasm, benign, by site
    - unspecified site D27.9
  - pseudomucinous
    - borderline malignancy
      - ovary C56-
      - specified site NEC — *see* Neoplasm, uncertain behavior, by site
      - unspecified site C56.9
    - specified site — *see* Neoplasm, benign, by site
    - unspecified site D27.9
  - serous
    - borderline malignancy
      - ovary C56-
      - specified site NEC — *see* Neoplasm, uncertain behavior, by site
      - unspecified site C56.9
    - specified site — *see* Neoplasm, benign, by site
    - unspecified site D27.9
  - specified site — *see* Neoplasm, benign, by site
  - unspecified site D27.9

D I S E A S E   I N D E X

Cystadenoma — *see also* Neoplasm, benign, by site — *continued*
  pseudomucinous
    borderline malignancy
      ovary C56-
      specified site NEC — *see* Neoplasm, uncertain behavior, by site
      unspecified site C56.9
    papillary
      borderline malignancy
        ovary C56-
        specified site NEC — *see* Neoplasm, uncertain behavior, by site
        unspecified site C56.9
      specified site — *see* Neoplasm, benign, by site
      unspecified site D27.9
    specified site — *see* Neoplasm, benign, by site
    unspecified site D27.9
  serous
    borderline malignancy
      ovary C56-
      specified site NEC — *see* Neoplasm, uncertain behavior, by site
      unspecified site C56.9
    papillary
      borderline malignancy
        ovary C56-
        specified site NEC — *see* Neoplasm, uncertain behavior, by site
        unspecified site C56.9
      specified site — *see* Neoplasm, benign, by site
      unspecified site D27.9
    specified site — *see* Neoplasm, benign, by site
    unspecified site D27.9
Cystathionine synthase deficiency E72.11
Cystathioninemia E72.19
Cystathioninuria E72.19
Cystic — *see also* condition
  breast (chronic) — *see* Mastopathy, cystic
  corpora lutea (hemorrhagic) N83.1
  duct — *see* condition
  eyeball (congenital) Q11.0
  fibrosis — *see* Fibrosis, cystic
  kidney (congenital) Q61.9
    adult type Q61.2
    infantile type NEC Q61.19
      collecting duct dilatation Q61.11
    medullary Q61.5
  liver, congenital Q44.6
  lung disease J98.4
    congenital Q33.0
  mastitis, chronic — *see* Mastopathy, cystic
  medullary, kidney Q61.5
  meniscus — *see* Derangement, knee, meniscus, cystic
  ovary N83.20
Cysticercosis, cysticerciasis B69.9
  with
    epileptiform fits B69.0
    myositis B69.81
  brain B69.0
  central nervous system B69.0
  cerebral B69.0
  ocular B69.1
  specified NEC B69.89
Cysticercus cellulose infestation — *see* Cysticercosis
Cystinosis (malignant) E72.04
Cystinuria E72.01
Cystitis (exudative) (hemorrhagic) (septic) (suppurative) N30.90
  with
    fibrosis — *see* Cystitis, chronic, interstitial
    hematuria N30.91
    leukoplakia — *see* Cystitis, chronic, interstitial
    malakoplakia — *see* Cystitis, chronic, interstitial
    metaplasia — *see* Cystitis, chronic, interstitial
    prostatitis N41.3
  acute N30.00
    with hematuria N30.01
    of trigone N30.30
      with hematuria N30.31
  allergic — *see* Cystitis, specified type NEC
  amebic A06.81
  bilharzial B65.9 [N33]
  blennorrhagic (gonococcal) A54.01

Cystitis (exudative) (hemorrhagic) (septic) (suppurative) N30.90 — *continued*
  bullous — *see* Cystitis, specified type NEC
  calculous N21.0
  chlamydial A56.01
  chronic N30.20
    with hematuria N30.21
    interstitial N30.10
      with hematuria N30.11
    of trigone N30.30
      with hematuria N30.31
    specified NEC N30.20
      with hematuria N30.21
  cystic(a) — *see* Cystitis, specified type NEC
  diphtheritic A36.85
  echinococcal
    granulosus B67.39
    multilocularis B67.69
  emphysematous — *see* Cystitis, specified type NEC
  encysted — *see* Cystitis, specified type NEC
  eosinophilic — *see* Cystitis, specified type NEC
  follicular — *see* Cystitis, of trigone
  gangrenous — *see* Cystitis, specified type NEC
  glandularis — *see* Cystitis, specified type NEC
  gonococcal A54.01
  incrusted — *see* Cystitis, specified type NEC
  interstitial (chronic) — *see* Cystitis, chronic, interstitial
  irradiation N30.40
    with hematuria N30.41
  irritation — *see* Cystitis, specified type NEC
  malignant — *see* Cystitis, specified type NEC
  of trigone N30.30
    with hematuria N30.31
  panmural — *see* Cystitis, chronic, interstitial
  polyposa — *see* Cystitis, specified type NEC
  prostatic N41.3
  puerperal (postpartum) O86.22
  radiation — *see* Cystitis, irradiation
  specified type NEC N30.80
    with hematuria N30.81
  subacute — *see* Cystitis, chronic
  submucous — *see* Cystitis, chronic, interstitial
  syphilitic (late) A52.76
  trichomonal A59.03
  tuberculous A18.12
  ulcerative — *see* Cystitis, chronic, interstitial
Cystocele(-urethrocele)
  female N81.10
    with prolapse of uterus — *see* Prolapse, uterus
    lateral N81.12
    midline N81.11
    paravaginal N81.12
  in pregnancy or childbirth O34.8-
    causing obstructed labor O65.5
  male N32.89
Cystolithiasis N21.0
Cystoma — *see also* Neoplasm, benign, by site
  endometrial, ovary N80.1
  mucinous
    specified site — *see* Neoplasm, benign, by site
    unspecified site D27.9
  serous
    specified site — *see* Neoplasm, benign, by site
    unspecified site D27.9
  simple (ovary) N83.29
Cystoplegia N31.2
Cystoptosis N32.89
Cystopyelitis — *see* Pyelonephritis
Cystorrhagia N32.89
Cystosarcoma phyllodes D48.6-
  benign D24-
  malignant — *see* Neoplasm, breast, malignant
Cystostomy
  attention to Z43.5
  complication — *see* Complications, cystostomy
  status Z93.50
    appendico-vesicostomy Z93.52
    cutaneous Z93.51
    specified NEC Z93.59

Cystourethritis — *see* Urethritis
Cystourethrocele — *see also* Cystocele
  female N81.10
    with uterine prolapse — *see* Prolapse, uterus
    lateral N81.12
    midline N81.11
    paravaginal N81.12
  male N32.89
Cytomegalic inclusion disease
  congenital P35.1
Cytomegalovirus infection B25.9
Cytomycosis (reticuloendothelial) B39.4
Cytopenia D75.9
  refractory
    with multilineage dysplasia D46.A
      and ring sideroblasts (RCMD RS) D46.B
Czerny's disease (periodic hydrarthrosis of the knee) — *see* Effusion, joint, knee

D

Da Costa's syndrome F45.8
Daae (-Finsen) disease (epidemic pleurodynia) B33.0
Dabney's grip B33.0
Dacryoadenitis, dacryadenitis H04.00-
　acute H04.01-
　chronic H04.02-
Dacryocystitis H04.30-
　acute H04.32-
　chronic H04.41-
　neonatal P39.1
　phlegmonous H04.31-
　syphilitic A52.71
　　congenital (early) A50.01
　trachomatous, active A71.1
　　sequelae (late effect) B94.0
Dacryocystoblenorrhea — see Inflammation, lacrimal, passages, chronic
Dacryocystocele — see Disorder, lacrimal system, changes
Dacryolith, dacryolithiasis H04.51-
Dacryoma — see Disorder, lacrimal system, changes
Dacryopericystitis — see Dacryocystitis
Dacryops H04.11-
Dacryostenosis — see also Stenosis, lacrimal
　congenital Q10.5
Dactylitis
　bone — see Osteomyelitis
　sickle-cell D57.00
　　Hb C D57.219
　　Hb SS D57.00
　　specified NEC D57.819
　skin L08.9
　syphilitic A52.77
　tuberculous A18.03
Dactylolysis spontanea (ainhum) L94.6
Dactylosymphysis Q70.9
　fingers — see Syndactylism, complex, fingers
　toes — see Syndactylism, complex, toes
Damage
　arteriosclerotic — see Arteriosclerosis
　brain (nontraumatic) G93.9
　　anoxic, hypoxic P11.2
　　　resulting from a procedure G97.82
　　child NEC G80.9
　　due to birth injury P11.2
　cardiorenal (vascular) — see Hypertension, cardiorenal
　cerebral NEC — see Damage, brain
　coccyx, complicating delivery O71.6
　coronary — see Disease, heart, ischemic
　eye, birth injury P15.3
　liver (nontraumatic) K76.9
　　alcoholic K70.9
　　due to drugs — see Disease, liver, toxic
　　toxic — see Disease, liver, toxic
　medication T88.7
　pelvic
　　joint or ligament, during delivery O71.6
　　organ NEC
　　　during delivery O71.5
　　　following ectopic or molar pregnancy O08.6
　renal — see Disease, renal
　subendocardium, subendocardial — see Degeneration, myocardial
　vascular I99.9
Dana-Putnam syndrome (subacute combined sclerosis with pernicious anemia) — see Degeneration, combined
Danbolt (-Cross) syndrome (acrodermatitis enteropathica) E83.2
Dandruff L21.0
Dandy-Walker syndrome Q03.1
　with spina bifida — see Spina bifida
Danlos' syndrome Q79.6
Darier-Roussy sarcoid D86.3
Darier(-White) disease (congenital) Q82.8
　meaning erythema annulare centrifugum L53.1
Darling's disease or histoplasmosis B39.4
Darwin's tubercle Q17.8
Dawson's (inclusion body) encephalitis A81.1
De Beurmann(-Gougerot) disease B42.1
De la Tourette's syndrome F95.2
De Lange's syndrome Q87.1
De Morgan's spots (senile angiomas) I78.1

De Quervain's
　disease (tendon sheath) M65.4
　syndrome E34.51
　thyroiditis (subacute granulomatous thyroiditis) E06.1
De Toni-Fanconi(-Debré) syndrome E72.09
　with cystinosis E72.04
Dead
　fetus, retained (mother) O36.4
　　early pregnancy O02.1
　labyrinth — see subcategory H83.2
　ovum, retained O02.0
Deaf nonspeaking NEC H91.3
Deafmutism (acquired) (congenital) NEC H91.3
　hysterical F44.6
　syphilitic, congenital (see also subcategory H94.8) A50.09
Deafness (acquired) (complete) (hereditary) (partial) H91.9-
　with blue sclera and fragility of bone Q78.0
　auditory fatigue — see Deafness, specified type NEC
　aviation T70.0
　　nerve injury — see Injury, nerve, acoustic, specified type NEC
　boilermaker's — see subcategory H83.3
　central — see Deafness, sensorineural
　conductive H90.2
　　and sensorineural, mixed H90.8
　　　bilateral H90.6
　　bilateral H90.0
　　unilateral H90.1-
　congenital H90.5
　　with blue sclera and fragility of bone Q78.0
　due to toxic agents — see Deafness, ototoxic
　emotional (hysterical) F44.6
　functional (hysterical) F44.6
　high frequency H91.9-
　hysterical F44.6
　low frequency H91.9-
　mental R48.8
　mixed conductive and sensorineural H90.8
　　bilateral H90.6
　　unilateral H90.7-
　nerve — see Deafness, sensorineural
　neural — see Deafness, sensorineural
　noise-induced (see also subcategory) H83.3
　　nerve injury — see Injury, nerve, acoustic, specified type NEC
　nonspeaking H91.3
　ototoxic — see subcategory H91.0
　perceptive — see Deafness, sensorineural
　psychogenic (hysterical) F44.6
　sensorineural H90.5
　　and conductive, mixed H90.8
　　　bilateral H90.6
　　bilateral H90.3
　　unilateral H90.4-
　sensory — see Deafness, sensorineural
　specified type NEC — see subcategory H91.8
　sudden (idiopathic) H91.2-
　syphilitic A52.15
　transient ischemic H93.01-
　traumatic — see Injury, nerve, acoustic, specified type NEC
　word (developmental) H93.25
Death (cause unknown) (of) (unexplained) (unspecified cause) R99
　brain G93.82
　cardiac (sudden) (with successful resuscitation) — code to underlying disease
　　family history of Z82.41
　　personal history of Z86.74
　family member (assumed) Z63.4
Debility (chronic) (general) (nervous) R53.81
　congenital or neonatal NOS P96.9
　nervous R53.81
　old age R54
　senile R54
Débove's disease (splenomegaly) R16.1
Decalcification
　bone — see Osteoporosis
　teeth K03.89
Decapsulation, kidney N28.89
Decay
　dental — see Caries, dental
　senile R54
　tooth, teeth — see Caries, dental
Deciduitis (acute)
　following ectopic or molar pregnancy O08.0
Decline (general) — see Debility
　cognitive, age-associated R41.81

Decompensation
　cardiac (acute) (chronic) — see Disease, heart
　cardiovascular — see Disease, cardiovascular
　heart — see Disease, heart
　hepatic — see Failure, hepatic
　myocardial (acute) (chronic) — see Disease, heart
　respiratory J98.8
Decompression sickness T70.3
Decrease(d)
　absolute neutrophile count — see Neutropenia
　blood
　　platelets — see Thrombocytopenia
　　pressure R03.1
　　　due to shock following injury T79.4
　　　operation T81.19
　estrogen E28.39
　　postablative E89.40
　　　asymptomatic E89.40
　　　symptomatic E89.41
　fragility of erythrocytes D58.8
　function
　　lipase (pancreatic) K90.3
　　ovary in hypopituitarism E23.0
　　parenchyma of pancreas K86.8
　　pituitary (gland) (anterior) (lobe) E23.0
　　　posterior (lobe) E23.0
　functional activity R68.89
　glucose R73.09
　hematocrit R71.0
　hemoglobin R71.0
　leukocytes D72.819
　　specified NEC D72.818
　libido R68.82
　lymphocytes D72.810
　platelets D69.6
　respiration, due to shock following injury T79.4
　sexual desire R68.82
　tear secretion NEC — see Syndrome, dry eye
　tolerance
　　fat K90.4
　　glucose R73.09
　　pancreatic K90.3
　　salt and water E87.8
　vision NEC H54.7
　white blood cell count D72.819
　　specified NEC D72.818
Decubitus (ulcer) — see Ulcer, pressure, by site
　cervix N86
Deepening acetabulum — see Derangement, joint, specified type NEC, hip
Defect, defective Q89.9
　3-beta-hydroxysteroid dehydrogenase E25.0
　11-hydroxylase E25.0
　21-hydroxylase E25.0
　abdominal wall, congenital Q79.59
　antibody immunodeficiency D80.9
　aorticopulmonary septum Q21.4
　atrial septal (ostium secundum type) Q21.1
　　following acute myocardial infarction (current complication) I23.1
　　ostium primum type Q21.2
　atrioventricular
　　canal Q21.2
　　septum Q21.2
　auricular septal Q21.1
　bilirubin excretion NEC E80.6
　biosynthesis, androgen (testicular) E29.1
　bulbar septum Q21.0
　catalase E80.3
　cell membrane receptor complex (CR3) D71
　circulation I99.9
　　congenital Q28.9
　　newborn Q28.9
　coagulation (factor) (see also Deficiency, factor) D68.9
　　with
　　　ectopic pregnancy O08.1
　　　molar pregnancy O08.1
　　acquired D68.4
　　antepartum with hemorrhage — see Hemorrhage, antepartum, with coagulation defect
　　due to
　　　liver disease D68.4
　　　vitamin K deficiency D68.4
　　hereditary NEC D68.2
　　intrapartum I67.0
　　newborn, transient P61.6
　　postpartum O72.3
　　specified type NEC D68.8

　complement system D84.1
　conduction (heart) I45.9
　　bone — see Deafness, conductive
　congenital, organ or site not listed — see Anomaly, by site
　coronary sinus Q21.1
　cushion, endocardial Q21.2
　degradation, glycoprotein E77.1
　dental bridge, crown, fillings — see Defect, dental restoration
　dental restoration K08.50
　　specified NEC K08.59
　dentin (hereditary) K00.5
　Descemet's membrane, congenital Q13.89
　developmental — see also Anomaly
　　cauda equina Q06.3
　diaphragm
　　with elevation, eventration or hernia — see Hernia, diaphragm
　　congenital Q79.1
　　　with hernia Q79.0
　　　gross (with hernia) Q79.0
　ectodermal, congenital Q82.9
　Eisenmenger's Q21.8
　enzyme
　　catalase E80.3
　　peroxidase E80.3
　esophagus, congenital Q39.9
　extensor retinaculum M62.89
　fibrin polymerization D68.2
　filling
　　bladder R93.4
　　kidney R93.4
　　stomach R93.3
　　ureter R93.4
　Gerbode Q21.0
　glycoprotein degradation E77.1
　Hageman (factor) D68.2
　hearing — see Deafness
　high grade F70
　interatrial septal Q21.1
　interauricular septal Q21.1
　interventricular septal Q21.0
　　with dextroposition of aorta, pulmonary stenosis and hypertrophy of right ventricle Q21.3
　　in tetralogy of Fallot Q21.3
　learning (specific) — see Disorder, learning
　lymphocyte function antigen-1 (LFA-1) D84.0
　lysosomal enzyme, post-translational modification E77.0
　major osseous M89.70
　　ankle M89.77-
　　carpus M89.74-
　　clavicle M89.71-
　　femur M89.75-
　　fibula M89.76-
　　fingers M89.74-
　　foot M89.77-
　　forearm M89.73-
　　hand M89.74-
　　humerus M89.72-
　　lower leg M89.76-
　　metacarpus M89.74-
　　metatarsus M89.77-
　　multiple sites M89.79
　　pelvic region M89.75-
　　pelvis M89.75-
　　radius M89.73-
　　scapula M89.71-
　　shoulder region M89.71-
　　specified NEC M89.78
　　tarsus M89.77-
　　thigh M89.75-
　　tibia M89.76-
　　toes M89.77-
　　ulna M89.73-
　mental — see Disability, intellectual
　modification, lysosomal enzymes, post-translational E77.0
　obstructive, congenital
　　renal pelvis Q62.39
　　ureter Q62.39
　　　atresia — see Atresia, ureter
　　　cecoureterocele Q62.32
　　　megaureter Q62.2
　　　orthotopic ureterocele Q62.31
　osseous, major M89.70
　　ankle M89.77-
　　carpus M89.74-
　　clavicle M89.71-
　　femur M89.75-
　　fibula M89.76-
　　fingers M89.74-
　　foot M89.77-

D I S E A S E   I N D E X

Defect, defective Q89.9 — *continued*
  osseous, major M89.70 — *continued*
    forearm M89.73-
    hand M89.74-
    humerus M89.72-
    lower leg M89.76-
    metacarpus M89.74-
    metatarsus M89.77-
    multiple sites M89.9
    pelvic region M89.75-
    pelvis M89.75-
    radius M89.73-
    scapula M89.71-
    shoulder region M89.71-
    specified NEC M89.78
    tarsus M89.77-
    thigh M89.75-
    tibia M89.76-
    toes M89.77-
    ulna M89.73-
  osteochondral NEC (*see also* Deformity)
    M95.8
  ostium
    primum Q21.2
    secundum Q21.1
  peroxidase E80.3
  placental blood supply — *see* Insufficiency,
    placental
  platelets, qualitative D69.1
    constitutional D68.0
  postural NEC, spine — *see* Dorsopathy,
    deforming
  reduction
    limb Q73.8
      lower Q72.9-
        absence — *see* Agenesis, leg
          foot — *see* Agenesis, foot
        longitudinal
          femur Q72.4-
          fibula Q72.6-
          tibia Q72.5-
          specified type NEC Q72.89-
        split foot Q72.7-
        specified type NEC Q73.8
      upper Q71.9-
        absence — *see* Agenesis, arm
          forearm — *see* Agenesis, forearm
          hand — *see* Agenesis, hand
        lobster-claw hand Q71.6-
        longitudinal
          radius Q71.4-
          ulna Q71.5-
        specified type NEC Q71.89-
  renal pelvis Q63.8
    obstructive Q62.39
  respiratory system, congenital Q34.9
  restoration, dental K08.50
    specified NEC K08.59
  retinal nerve bundle fibers H35.89
  septal (heart) NOS Q21.9
    acquired (atrial) (auricular) (ventricular)
      (old) I51.0
    atrial Q21.1
      concurrent with acute myocardial
        infarction — *see* Infarct,
        myocardium
      following acute myocardial infarction
        (current complication) I23.1
    ventricular (*see also* Defect, ventricular
      septal) Q21.0
  sinus venosus Q21.1
  speech R47.9
    developmental F80.9
    specified NEC R47.89
  Taussig-Bing (aortic transposition and
    overriding pulmonary artery) Q20.1
  teeth, wedge K03.1
  vascular (local) I99.9
    congenital Q27.9
  ventricular septal Q21.0
    concurrent with acute myocardial
      infarction — *see* Infarct,
      myocardium
    following acute myocardial infarction
      (current complication) I23.2
    in tetralogy of Fallot Q21.3
  vision NEC H54.7
  visual field H53.40
    bilateral
      heteronymous H53.47
      homonymous H53.46-
    generalized contraction H53.48-
    localized
      arcuate H53.43-
      scotoma (central area) H53.41-
        blind spot area H53.42-
      sector H53.43-
      specified type NEC H53.45-

Defect, defective Q89.9 — *continued*
  voice R49.9
    specified NEC R49.8
  wedge, tooth, teeth (abrasion) K03.1
Deferentitis N49.1
  gonorrheal (acute) (chronic) A54.23
Defibrination (syndrome) D65
  antepartum — *see* Hemorrhage,
    antepartum, with coagulation defect,
    disseminated intravascular
    coagulation
  following ectopic or molar pregnancy
    O08.1
  intrapartum O67.0
  newborn P60
  postpartum O72.3
Deficiency, deficient
  3-beta hydroxysteroid dehydrogenase
    E25.0
  5-alpha reductase (with male
    pseudohermaphroditism) E29.1
  11-hydroxylase E25.0
  21-hydroxylase E25.0
  abdominal muscle syndrome Q79.4
  AC globulin (congenital) (hereditary)
    D68.2
    acquired D68.4
  accelerator globulin (Ac G) (blood) D68.2
  acid phosphatase E83.39
  activating factor (blood) D68.2
  adenosine deaminase (ADA) D81.3
  aldolase (hereditary) E74.19
  alpha-1-antitrypsin E88.01
  amino-acids E72.9
  anemia — *see* Anemia
  aneurin E51.9
  anti-hemophilic
    factor (A) D66
      B D67
      C D68.1
    globulin (AHG) NEC D66
  antibody with
    hyperimmunoglobulinemia D80.6
    near-normal immunoglobins D80.6
  antidiuretic hormone E23.2
  antithrombin (antithrombin III) D68.59
  ascorbic acid E54
  attention (disorder) (syndrome) F98.8
    with hyperactivity — *see* Disorder,
      attention-deficit hyperactivity
  autoprothrombin
    C D68.2
    I D68.2
    II D67
  beta-glucuronidase E76.29
  biotin E53.8
  biotin-dependent carboxylase D81.819
  biotinidase D81.810
  brancher enzyme (amylopectinosis) E74.03
  C1 esterase inhibitor (C1-INH) D84.1
  calciferol E55.9
    with
      adult osteomalacia M83.8
      rickets — *see* Rickets
  calcium (dietary) E58
  calorie, severe E43
    with marasmus E41
    and kwashiorkor E42
  cardiac — *see* Insufficiency, myocardial
  carnitine E71.40
    due to
      hemodialysis E71.43
      inborn errors of metabolism E71.42
      Valproic acid therapy E71.43
    iatrogenic E71.43
    muscle palmitytransferase E71.314
    primary E71.41
    secondary E71.448
  carotene E50.9
  central nervous system G96.8
  ceruloplasmin (Wilson) E83.01
  choline E53.8
  Christmas factor D67
  chromium E61.4
  clotting (blood) (*see also* Deficiency,
    coagulation factor) D68.9
  clotting factor NEC (hereditary) (*see also*
    Deficiency, factor) D68.2
  coagulation NOS D68.9
    with
      ectopic pregnancy O08.1
      molar pregnancy O08.1
    acquired (any) D68.4
    antepartum hemorrhage — *see*
      Hemorrhage, antepartum, with
      coagulation defect
    clotting factor NEC (*see also*
      Deficiency, factor) D68.2

Deficiency, deficient — *continued*
  coagulation NOS D68.9 — *continued*
    due to
      hyperprothrombinemia D68.4
      liver disease D68.4
      vitamin K deficiency D68.4
    newborn, transient P61.6
    postpartum O72.3
    specified NEC D68.8
  cognitive F09
  color vision H53.50
    achromatopsia H53.51
    acquired H53.52
    deuteranomaly H53.53
    protanomaly H53.54
    specified type NEC H53.59
    tritanomaly H53.55
  combined glucocorticoid and
    mineralocorticoid E27.49
  contact factor D68.2
  copper (nutritional) E61.0
  corticoadrenal E27.40
    primary E27.1
  craniofacial axis Q75.0
  cyanocobalamin E53.8
  debrancher enzyme (limit dextrinosis)
    E74.03
  dehydrogenase
    long chain/very long chain acyl CoA
      E71.310
    medium chain acyl CoA E71.311
    short chain acyl CoA E71.312
  diet E63.9
  dihydropyrimidine dehydrogenase (DPD)
    E88.89
  disaccharidase E73.9
  edema — *see* Malnutrition, severe
  endocrine E34.9
  energy-supply — *see* Malnutrition
  enzymes, circulating NEC E88.09
  ergosterol E55.9
    with
      adult osteomalacia M83.8
      rickets — *see* Rickets
  essential fatty acid (EFA) E63.0
  factor — *see also* Deficiency, coagulation
    I (congenital) (hereditary) D68.2
    II (congenital) (hereditary) D68.2
    V (congenital) (hereditary) D68.2
    VII (congenital) (hereditary) D68.2
    VIII (congenital) (functional)
      (hereditary) (with functional
      defect) D66
      with vascular defect D68.0
    IX (congenital) (functional) (hereditary)
      (with functional defect) D67
    X (congenital) (hereditary) D68.2
    XI (congenital) (hereditary) D68.1
    XII (congenital) (hereditary) D68.2
    XIII (congenital) (hereditary) D68.2
    Hageman D68.2
    multiple (congenital) D68.8
      acquired D68.4
  femoral, proximal focal (congenital) — *see*
    Defect, reduction, lower limb,
    longitudinal, femur
  fibrin-stabilizing factor (congenital)
    (hereditary) D68.2
    acquired D68.4
  fibrinase D68.2
  fibrinogen (congenital) (hereditary) D68.2
    acquired D65
  folate E53.8
  folic acid E53.8
  foreskin N47.3
  fructokinase E74.11
  fructose 1,6-diphosphatase E74.19
  fructose-1-phosphate aldolase E74.19
  galactokinase E74.29
  galactose-1-phosphate uridyl transferase
    E74.29
  gammaglobulin in blood D80.1
    hereditary D80.0
  glass factor D68.2
  glucocorticoid E27.49
    mineralocorticoid E27.49
  glucose-6-phosphatase E74.01
  glucose-6-phosphate dehydrogenase
    anemia D55.0
  glucuronyl transferase E80.5
  glycogen synthetase E74.09
  gonadotropin (isolated) E23.0
  growth hormone (idiopathic) (isolated)
    E23.0
  Hageman factor D68.2
  hemoglobin D64.9
  hepatophosphorylase E74.09
  homogentisate 1,2-dioxygenase E70.29

Deficiency, deficient — *continued*
  hormone
    anterior pituitary (partial) NEC E23.0
      growth E23.0
    growth (isolated) E23.0
    pituitary E23.0
    testicular E29.1
  hypoxanthine-(guanine)-
    phosphoribosyltransferase (HG-PRT)
    (total H-PRT) E79.1
  immunity D84.9
    cell-mediated D84.8
      with thrombocytopenia and eczema
        D82.0
    combined D81.9
    humoral D80.9
    IgA (secretory) D80.2
    IgG D80.3
    IgM D80.4
  immuno — *see* Immunodeficiency
  immunoglobulin, selective
    A (IgA) D80.2
    G (IgG) (subclasses) D80.3
    M (IgM) D80.4
  inositol (B complex) E53.8
  intrinsic
    factor (congenital) D51.0
    sphincter N36.42
      with urethral hypermobility N36.43
  iodine E61.8
    congenital syndrome — *see* Syndrome,
      iodine-deficiency, congenital
  iron E61.1
    anemia D50.9
  kalium E87.6
  kappa-light chain D80.8
  labile factor (congenital) (hereditary)
    D68.2
    acquired D68.4
  lacrimal fluid (acquired) — *see also*
    Syndrome, dry eye
    congenital Q10.6
  lactase
    congenital E73.0
    secondary E73.1
  Laki-Lorand factor D68.2
  lecithin cholesterol acyltransferase E78.6
  lipocaic K86.8
  lipoprotein (familial) (high density) E78.6
  liver phosphorylase E74.09
  lysosomal alpha-1, 4 glucosidase E74.02
  magnesium E61.2
  major histocompatibility complex
    class I D81.6
    class II D81.7
  manganese E61.3
  menadione (vitamin K) E56.1
    newborn P53
  mental (familial) (hereditary) — *see*
    Disability, intellectual
  methylenetetrahydrofolate reductase
    (MTHFR) E72.12
  mineral NEC E61.8
  mineralocorticoid E27.49
    with glucocorticoid E27.49
  molybdenum (nutritional) E61.5
  moral F60.2
  multiple nutrient elements E61.7
  muscle
    carnitine (palmityltransferase) E71.314
    phosphofructokinase E74.09
  myoadenylate deaminase E79.2
  myocardial — *see* Insufficiency,
    myocardial
  myophosphorylase E74.04
  NADH diaphorase or reductase
    (congenital) D74.0
  NADH-methemoglobin reductase
    (congenital) D74.0
  natrium E87.1
  niacin (amide) (-tryptophan) E52
  nicotinamide E52
  nicotinic acid E52
  number of teeth — *see* Anodontia
  nutrient element E61.9
    multiple E61.7
    specified NEC E61.8
  nutrition, nutritional E63.9
    sequelae — *see* Sequelae, nutritional
      deficiency
    specified NEC E63.8
  ornithine transcarbamylase E72.4
  ovarian E28.39
  oxygen — *see* Anoxia
  pantothenic acid E53.8
  parathyroid (gland) E20.9
  perineum (female) N81.89
  phenylalanine hydroxylase E70.1
  phosphoenolpyruvate carboxykinase E74.4

Deficiency, deficient — *continued*
phosphofructokinase E74.19
phosphomannomutase E74.8
phosphomannose isomerase E74.8
phosphomannosyl mutase E74.8
phosphorylase kinase, liver E74.09
pituitary hormone (isolated) E23.0
plasma thromboplastin
   antecedent (PTA) D68.1
   component (PTC) D67
platelet NEC D69.1
   constitutional D68.0
polyglandular E31.8
   autoimmune E31.0
potassium (K) E87.6
prepuce N47.3
proaccelerin (congenital) (hereditary)
   D68.2
   acquired D68.4
proconvertin factor (congenital)
   (hereditary) D68.2
   acquired D68.4
protein (*see also* Malnutrition) E46
   anemia D53.0
   C D68.59
   S D68.59
prothrombin (congenital) (hereditary)
   D68.2
   acquired D68.4
Prower factor D68.2
pseudocholinesterase E88.09
PTA (plasma thromboplastin antecedent)
   D68.1
PTC (plasma thromboplastin component)
   D67
purine nucleoside phosphorylase (PNP)
   D81.5
pyracin (alpha) (beta) E53.1
pyridoxal E53.1
pyridoxamine E53.1
pyridoxine (derivatives) E53.1
pyruvate
   carboxylase E74.4
   dehydrogenase E74.4
riboflavin (vitamin B2) E53.0
salt E87.1
secretion
   ovary E28.39
   salivary gland (any) K11.7
   urine R34
selenium (dietary) E59
serum antitrypsin, familial E88.01
short stature homeobox gene (SHOX)
   with
      dyschondrosteosis Q78.8
      short stature (idiopathic) E34.3
      Turner's syndrome Q96.9
sodium (Na) E87.1
SPCA (factor VII) D68.2
sphincter, intrinsic N36.42
   with urethral hypermobility N36.43
stable factor (congenital) (hereditary)
   D68.2
   acquired D68.4
Stuart-Prower (factor X) D68.2
sucrase E74.39
sulfatase E75.29
sulfite oxidase E72.19
thiamin, thiaminic (chloride) E51.9
   beriberi (dry) E51.11
      wet E51.12
thrombokinase D68.2
   newborn P53
thyroid (gland) — *see* Hypothyroidism
tocopherol E56.0
tooth bud K00.0
transcobalamine II (anemia) D51.2
vanadium E61.6
vascular I99.9
vasopressin E23.2
viosterol — *see* Deficiency, calciferol
vitamin (multiple) NOS E56.9
   A E50.9
      with
         Bitot's spot (corneal) E50.1
         follicular keratosis E50.8
         keratomalacia E50.4
         manifestations NEC E50.8
         night blindness E50.5
         scar of cornea, xerophthalmic
           E50.6
         xeroderma E50.8
         xerophthalmia E50.7
         xerosis
           conjunctival E50.0
              and Bitot's spot E50.1
           cornea E50.2
              and ulceration E50.3
      sequelae E64.1

Deficiency, deficient — *continued*
vitamin (multiple) NOS E56.9 —
   continued
   B (complex) NOS E53.9
      with
         beriberi (dry) E51.11
           wet E51.11
         pellagra E52
   B1 NOS E51.9
      beriberi (dry) E51.11
         with circulatory system
           manifestations E51.11
         wet E51.12
   B12 E53.8
   B2 (riboflavin) E53.0
   B6 E53.1
   C E54
      sequelae E64.2
   D E55.9
      with
         adult osteomalacia M83.8
         rickets — *see* Rickets
      25-hydroxylase E83.32
   E E56.0
   folic acid E53.8
   G E53.0
   group B E53.9
      specified NEC E53.8
   H (biotin) E53.8
   K E56.1
      of newborn P53
   nicotinic E52
   P E56.8
   PP (pellagra-preventing) E52
   specified NEC E56.8
   thiamin E51.9
      beriberi — *see* Beriberi
zinc, dietary E60
Deficit — *see also* Deficiency
attention and concentration R41.840
   disorder — *see* Attention, deficit
cognitive communication R41.841
cognitive NEC R41.89
   following
      cerebral infarction I69.31
      cerebrovascular disease I69.91
         specified disease NEC I69.81
      intracerebral hemorrhage I69.11
      nontraumatic intracranial hemorrhage
         NEC I69.21
      subarachnoid hemorrhage I69.01
concentration R41.840
executive function R41.844
frontal lobe R41.844
neurologic NEC R29.818
   ischemic
      reversible (RIND) I63.9
      prolonged (PRIND) I63.9
oxygen R09.02
prolonged reversible ischemic neurologic
   (PRIND) I63.9
psychomotor R41.843
visuospatial R41.842
Deflection
radius — *see* Deformity, limb, specified
   type NEC, forearm
septum (acquired) (nasal) (nose) J34.2
spine — *see* Curvature, spine
turbinate (nose) J34.2
Defluvium
capillorum — *see* Alopecia
ciliorum — *see* Madarosis
unguium L60.8
Deformity Q89.9
abdomen, congenital Q89.9
abdominal wall
   acquired M95.8
   congenital Q79.59
acquired (unspecified site) M95.9
adrenal gland Q89.1
alimentary tract, congenital Q45.9
   upper Q40.9
ankle (joint) (acquired) — *see also*
   Deformity, limb, lower leg
   abduction — *see* Contraction, joint,
      ankle
   congenital Q68.8
   contraction — *see* Contraction, joint,
      ankle
   specified type NEC — *see* Deformity,
      limb, foot, specified NEC
anus (acquired) K62.89
   congenital Q43.9
aorta (arch) (congenital) Q25.4
   acquired I77.89
aortic
   arch, acquired I77.89
   cusp or valve (congenital) Q23.8
      acquired (*see also* Endocarditis,
         aortic) I35.8

Deformity Q89.9 — *continued*
arm (acquired) (upper) — *see also*
   Deformity, limb, upper arm
   congenital Q68.8
   forearm — *see* Deformity, limb, forearm
artery (congenital) (peripheral) NOS Q27.9
   acquired I77.89
   coronary (acquired) I25.9
      congenital Q24.5
   umbilical Q27.0
atrial septal Q21.1
auditory canal (external) (congenital)
   — *see also* Malformation, ear, external
   acquired — *see* Disorder, ear, external,
      specified type NEC
auricle
   ear (congenital) — *see also*
      Malformation, ear, external
      acquired — *see* Disorder, pinna,
         deformity
back — *see* Dorsopathy, deforming
bile duct (common) (congenital) (hepatic)
   Q44.5
   acquired K83.8
biliary duct or passage (congenital) Q44.5
   acquired K83.8
bladder (neck) (trigone) (sphincter)
   (acquired) N32.89
   congenital Q64.79
bone (acquired) NOS M95.9
   congenital Q79.9
   turbinate M95.0
brain (congenital) Q04.9
   acquired G93.89
   reduction Q04.3
breast (acquired) N64.89
   congenital Q83.9
   reconstructed N65.0
bronchus (congenital) Q32.4
   acquired NEC J98.09
bursa, congenital Q79.9
canaliculi (lacrimalis) (acquired) — *see*
   also Disorder, lacrimal system,
      changes
   congenital Q10.6
canthus, acquired — *see* Disorder, eyelid,
   specified type NEC
capillary (acquired) I78.8
cardiovascular system, congenital Q28.9
caruncle, lacrimal (acquired) — *see also*
   Disorder, lacrimal system, changes
   congenital Q10.6
cascade, stomach K31.2
cecum (congenital) Q43.9
   acquired K63.89
cerebral, acquired G93.89
   congenital Q04.9
cervix (uterus) (acquired) NEC N88.8
   congenital Q51.9
cheek (acquired) M95.2
   congenital Q18.9
chest (acquired) (wall) M95.4
   congenital Q67.8
   sequelae (late effect) of rickets E64.3
chin (acquired) M95.2
   congenital Q18.9
choroid (congenital) Q14.3
   acquired H31.8
   plexus Q07.8
      acquired G96.19
cicatricial — *see* Cicatrix
cilia, acquired — *see* Disorder, eyelid,
   specified type NEC
clavicle (acquired) M95.8
   congenital Q68.8
clitoris (congenital) Q52.6
   acquired N90.89
clubfoot — *see* Clubfoot
coccyx (acquired) — *see* subcategory
   M43.8
colon (congenital) Q43.9
   acquired K63.89
concha (ear), congenital — *see also*
   Malformation, ear, external
   acquired — *see* Disorder, pinna,
      deformity
cornea (acquired) H18.70
   congenital Q13.4
   descemetocele — *see* Descemetocele
   ectasia — *see* Ectasia, cornea
   specified NEC H18.79-
   staphyloma — *see* Staphyloma, cornea
coronary artery (acquired) I25.9
   congenital Q24.5
cranium (acquired) — *see* Deformity, skull
cricoid cartilage (congenital) Q31.8
   acquired J38.7

Deformity Q89.9 — *continued*
cystic duct (congenital) Q44.5
   acquired K82.8
Dandy-Walker Q03.1
   with spina bifida — *see* Spina bifida
diaphragm (congenital) Q79.1
   acquired J98.6
digestive organ NOS Q45.9
ductus arteriosus Q25.0
duodenal bulb K31.89
duodenum (congenital) Q43.9
   acquired K31.89
dura — *see* Deformity, meninges
ear (acquired) — *see also* Disorder, pinna,
   deformity
   congenital (external) Q17.9
      internal Q16.5
      middle Q16.4
         ossicles Q16.3
      ossicles Q16.3
ectodermal (congenital) NEC Q84.9
ejaculatory duct (congenital) Q55.4
   acquired N50.8
elbow (joint) (acquired) — *see also*
   Deformity, limb, upper arm
   congenital Q68.8
   contraction — *see* Contraction, joint,
      elbow
endocrine gland NEC Q89.2
epididymis (congenital) Q55.4
   acquired N50.8
epiglottis (congenital) Q31.8
   acquired J38.7
esophagus (congenital) Q39.9
   acquired K22.8
eustachian tube (congenital) NEC Q17.8
eye, congenital Q15.9
eyebrow (congenital) Q18.8
eyelid (acquired) — *see also* Disorder,
   eyelid, specified type NEC
   congenital Q10.3
face (acquired) M95.2
   congenital Q18.9
fallopian tube, acquired N83.8
femur (acquired) — *see* Deformity, limb,
   specified type NEC, thigh
fetal
   with fetopelvic disproportion O33.7
   causing obstructed labor O66.3
finger (acquired) M20.00-
   boutonniere M20.02-
   congenital Q68.1
   flexion contracture — *see* Contraction,
      joint, hand
   mallet finger M20.01-
   specified NEC M20.09-
   swan-neck M20.03-
flexion (joint) (acquired) (*see also*
   Deformity, limb, flexion) M21.20
   congenital NOS Q74.9
      hip Q65.89
foot (acquired) — *see also* Deformity,
   limb, lower leg
   cavovarus (congenital) Q66.1
   congenital NOS Q66.9
      specified type NEC Q66.89
   specified type NEC — *see* Deformity,
      limb, foot, specified NEC
   valgus (congenital) Q66.6
      acquired — *see* Deformity, valgus,
         ankle
   varus (congenital) NEC Q66.3
      acquired — *see* Deformity, varus,
         ankle
forearm (acquired) — *see also* Deformity,
   limb, forearm
   congenital Q68.8
forehead (acquired) M95.2
   congenital Q75.8
frontal bone (acquired) M95.2
   congenital Q75.8
gallbladder (congenital) Q44.1
   acquired K82.8
gastrointestinal tract (congenital) NOS
   Q45.9
   acquired K63.89
genitalia, genital organ(s) or system NEC
   female (congenital) Q52.9
      acquired N94.89
      external Q52.70
   male (congenital) Q55.9
      acquired N50.8
globe (eye) (congenital) Q15.8
   acquired H44.89
gum, acquired NEC K06.8
hand (acquired) — *see* Deformity, limb,
   hand
   congenital Q68.1
head (acquired) M95.2
   congenital Q75.8

D I S E A S E I N D E X

Deformity Q89.9 — *continued*
  heart (congenital) Q24.9
    septum Q21.9
      auricular Q21.1
      ventricular Q21.0
    valve (congenital) NEC Q24.8
      acquired — *see* Endocarditis
  heel (acquired) — *see* Deformity, foot
  hepatic duct (congenital) Q44.5
    acquired K83.8
  hip (joint) (acquired) — *see also*
    Deformity, limb, thigh
    congenital Q65.9
    due to (previous) juvenile
      osteochondrosis — *see* Coxa, plana
    flexion — *see* Contraction, joint, hip
  hourglass — *see* Contraction, hourglass
  humerus (acquired) M21.82-
    congenital Q74.0
  hypophyseal (congenital) Q89.2
  ileocecal (coil) (valve) (acquired) K63.89
  ileum (congenital) Q43.9
    acquired K63.89
  ilium (acquired) M95.5
    congenital Q74.2
  integument (congenital) Q84.9
  intervertebral cartilage or disc (acquired)
    — *see* Disorder, disc, specified NEC
  intestine (large) (small) (congenital) NOS
    Q43.9
    acquired K63.89
  intrinsic minus or plus (hand) — *see*
    Deformity, limb, specified type NEC,
    forearm
  iris (acquired) H21.89
    congenital Q13.2
  ischium (acquired) M95.5
    congenital Q74.2
  jaw (acquired) (congenital) M26.9
  joint (acquired) NEC M21.90
    congenital Q68.8
    elbow M21.92-
    hand M21.94-
    hip M21.95-
    knee M21.96-
    shoulder M21.92-
    wrist M21.93-
  kidney(s) (calyx) (pelvis) (congenital)
    Q63.9
    acquired N28.89
    artery (congenital) Q27.2
      acquired I77.89
  Klippel-Feil (brevicollis) Q76.1
  knee (acquired) NEC — *see also*
    Deformity, limb, lower leg
    congenital Q68.2
  labium (majus) (minus) (congenital)
    Q52.79
    acquired N90.89
  lacrimal passages or duct (congenital) NEC
    Q10.6
    acquired — *see* Disorder, lacrimal
      system, changes
  larynx (muscle) (congenital) Q31.8
    acquired J38.7
    web (glottic) Q31.0
  leg (upper) (acquired) NEC — *see also*
    Deformity, limb, thigh
    congenital Q68.8
    lower leg — *see* Deformity, limb, lower
      leg
  lens (acquired) H27.8
    congenital Q12.9
  lid (fold) (acquired) — *see also* Disorder,
    eyelid, specified type NEC
    congenital Q10.3
  ligament (acquired) — *see* Disorder,
    ligament
    congenital Q79.9
  limb (acquired) M21.90
    clawfoot M21.53-
    clawhand M21.51-
    clubfoot M21.54-
    clubhand M21.52-
    congenital, except reduction deformity
      Q74.9
    flat foot M21.4-
    flexion M21.20
      ankle M21.27-
      elbow M21.22-
      finger M21.24-
      hip M21.25-
      knee M21.26-
      shoulder M21.21-
      toe M21.27-
      wrist M21.23-

Deformity Q89.9 — *continued*
  limb (acquired) M21.90 — *continued*
    foot
      claw — *see* Deformity, limb, clawfoot
      club — *see* Deformity, limb, clubfoot
      drop M21.37-
      flat — *see* Deformity, limb, flat foot
      specified NEC M21.6x-
    forearm M21.93-
    hand M21.94-
    lower leg M21.96-
    specified type NEC M21.80
      forearm M21.83-
      lower leg M21.86-
      thigh M21.85-
      upper arm M21.82-
    thigh M21.95-
    unequal length M21.70
      short site is
        femur M21.75-
        fibula M21.76-
        humerus M21.72-
        radius M21.73-
        tibia M21.76-
        ulna M21.73-
    upper arm M21.92-
    valgus — *see* Deformity, valgus
    varus — *see* Deformity, varus
    wrist drop M21.33-
  lip (acquired) NEC K13.0
    congenital Q38.0
  liver (congenital) Q44.7
    acquired K76.89
  lumbosacral (congenital) (joint) (region)
    Q76.49
    acquired — *see* subcategory M43.8
    kyphosis — *see* Kyphosis, congenital
    lordosis — *see* Lordosis, congenital
  lung (congenital) Q33.9
    acquired J98.4
  lymphatic system, congenital Q89.9
  Madelung's (radius) Q74.0
  mandible (acquired) (congenital) M26.9
  maxilla (acquired) (congenital) M26.9
  meninges or membrane (congenital) Q07.9
    cerebral Q04.8
      acquired G96.19
    spinal cord (congenital) G96.19
      acquired G96.19
  metacarpus (acquired) — *see* Deformity,
    limb, forearm
    congenital Q74.0
  metatarsus (acquired) — *see* Deformity,
    foot
    congenital Q66.9
  middle ear (congenital) Q16.4
    ossicles Q16.3
  mitral (leaflets) (valve) I05.8
    parachute Q23.2
    stenosis, congenital Q23.2
  mouth (acquired) K13.79
    congenital Q38.6
  multiple, congenital NEC Q89.7
  muscle (acquired) M62.89
    congenital Q79.9
      sternocleidomastoid Q68.0
  musculoskeletal system (acquired) M95.9
    congenital Q79.9
    specified NEC M95.8
  nail (acquired) L60.8
    congenital Q84.6
  nasal — *see* Deformity, nose
  neck (acquired) M95.3
    congenital Q18.9
      sternocleidomastoid Q68.0
  nervous system (congenital) Q07.9
  nipple (congenital) Q83.9
    acquired N64.89
  nose (acquired) (cartilage) M95.0
    bone (turbinate) M95.0
    congenital Q30.9
      bent or squashed Q67.4
    saddle M95.0
      syphilitic A50.57
    septum (acquired) J34.2
      congenital Q30.8
    sinus (wall) (congenital) Q30.8
      acquired M95.0
    syphilitic (congenital) A50.57
      late A52.73
  ocular muscle (congenital) Q10.3
    acquired — *see* Strabismus, mechanical
  opticociliary vessels (congenital) Q13.2

Deformity Q89.9 — *continued*
  orbit (eye) (acquired) H05.30
    atrophy — *see* Atrophy, orbit
    congenital Q10.7
    due to
      bone disease NEC H05.32-
      trauma or surgery H05.33-
    enlargement — *see* Enlargement, orbit
    exostosis — *see* Exostosis, orbit
  organ of Corti (congenital) Q16.5
  ovary (congenital) Q50.39
    acquired N83.8
  oviduct, acquired N83.8
  palate (congenital) Q38.5
    acquired M27.8
    cleft (congenital) — *see* Cleft, palate
  pancreas (congenital) Q45.3
    acquired K86.8
  parathyroid (gland) Q89.2
  parotid (gland) (congenital) Q38.4
    acquired K11.8
  patella (acquired) — *see* Disorder, patella,
    specified NEC
  pelvis, pelvic (acquired) (bony) M95.5
    with disproportion (fetopelvic) O33.0
      causing obstructed labor O65.0
    congenital Q74.2
    rachitic sequelae (late effect) E64.3
  penis (glans) (congenital) Q55.69
    acquired N48.89
  pericardium (congenital) Q24.8
    acquired — *see* Pericarditis
  pharynx (congenital) Q38.8
    acquired J39.2
  pinna, acquired — *see also* Disorder, pinna,
    deformity
    congenital Q17.9
  pituitary (congenital) Q89.2
  posture — *see* Dorsopathy, deforming
  prepuce (congenital) Q55.69
    acquired N47.8
  prostate (congenital) Q55.4
    acquired N42.89
  pupil (congenital) Q13.2
    acquired — *see* Abnormality, pupillary
  pylorus (congenital) Q40.3
    acquired K31.89
  rachitic (acquired), old or healed E64.3
  radius (acquired) — *see also* Deformity,
    limb, forearm
    congenital Q68.8
  rectum (congenital) Q43.9
    acquired K62.89
  reduction (extremity) (limb), congenital
    (*see also* condition and site) Q73.8
    brain Q04.3
    lower — *see* Defect, reduction, lower
      limb
    upper — *see* Defect, reduction, upper
      limb
  renal — *see* Deformity, kidney
  respiratory system (congenital) Q34.9
  rib (acquired) M95.4
    congenital Q76.6
      cervical Q76.5
  rotation (joint) (acquired) — *see* Deformity,
    limb, specified site NEC
    congenital Q74.9
    hip — *see* Deformity, limb, specified
      type NEC, thigh
      congenital Q65.89
  sacroiliac joint (congenital) Q74.2
    acquired — *see* subcategory M43.8
  sacrum (acquired) — *see* subcategory
    M43.8
  saddle
    back — *see* Lordosis
    nose M95.0
      syphilitic A50.57
  salivary gland or duct (congenital) Q38.4
    acquired K11.8
  scapula (acquired) M95.8
    congenital Q68.8
  scrotum (congenital) — *see also*
    Malformation, testis and scrotum
    acquired N50.8
  seminal vesicles (congenital) Q55.4
    acquired N50.8
  septum, nasal (acquired) J34.2
  shoulder (joint) (acquired) — *see*
    Deformity, limb, upper arm
    congenital Q74.0
    contraction — *see* Contraction, joint,
      shoulder
  sigmoid (flexure) (congenital) Q43.9
    acquired K63.89
  skin (congenital) Q82.9

Deformity Q89.9 — *continued*
  skull (acquired) M95.2
    congenital Q75.8
    with
      anencephaly Q00.0
      encephalocele — *see*
        Encephalocele
      hydrocephalus Q03.9
        with spina bifida — *See* Spina
          bifida, by site, with
          hydrocephalus
      microcephaly Q02
  soft parts, organs or tissues (of pelvis)
    in pregnancy or childbirth NEC O34.8-
      causing obstructed labor O65.5
  spermatic cord (congenital) Q55.4
    acquired N50.8
    torsion — *see* Torsion, spermatic cord
  spinal — *see* Dorsopathy, deforming
    column (acquired) — *see* Dorsopathy,
      deforming
      congenital Q67.5
    cord (congenital) Q06.9
      acquired G95.89
    nerve root (congenital) Q07.9
  spine (congenital) — *see also* Dorsopathy,
    deforming
    congenital Q67.5
    rachitic E64.3
    specified NEC — *see* Dorsopathy,
      deforming, specified NEC
  spleen
    acquired D73.89
    congenital Q89.09
  Sprengel's (congenital) Q74.0
  sternocleidomastoid (muscle), congenital
    Q68.0
  sternum (acquired) M95.4
    congenital NEC Q76.7
  stomach (congenital) Q40.3
    acquired K31.89
  submandibular gland (congenital) Q38.4
  submaxillary gland (congenital) Q38.4
    acquired K11.8
  talipes — *see* Talipes
  testis (congenital) — *see also*
    Malformation, testis and scrotum
    acquired N44.8
    torsion — *see* Torsion, testis
  thigh (acquired) — *see also* Deformity,
    limb, thigh
    congenital NEC Q68.8
  thorax (acquired) (wall) M95.4
    congenital Q67.8
    sequelae of rickets E64.3
  thumb (acquired) — *see also* Deformity,
    finger
    congenital NEC Q68.1
  thymus (tissue) (congenital) Q89.2
  thyroid (gland) (congenital) Q89.2
    cartilage Q31.8
      acquired J38.7
  tibia (acquired) — *see also* Deformity,
    limb, specified type NEC, lower leg
    congenital NEC Q68.8
    saber (syphilitic) A50.56
  toe (acquired) M20.6-
    congenital Q66.9
    hallux rigidus M20.2-
    hallux valgus M20.1-
    hallux varus M20.3-
    hammer toe M20.4-
    specified NEC M20.5x-
  tongue (congenital) Q38.3
    acquired K14.8
  tooth, teeth K00.2
  trachea (rings) (congenital) Q32.1
    acquired J39.8
  transverse aortic arch (congenital) Q25.4
  tricuspid (leaflets) (valve) I07.8
    atresia or stenosis Q22.4
    Ebstein's Q22.5
  trunk (acquired) M95.8
    congenital Q89.9
  ulna (acquired) — *see also* Deformity,
    limb, forearm
    congenital NEC Q68.8
  urachus, congenital Q64.4
  ureter (opening) (congenital) Q62.8
    acquired N28.89
  urethra (congenital) Q64.79
    acquired N36.8
  urinary tract (congenital) Q64.9
    urachus Q64.4
  uterus (congenital) Q51.9
    acquired N85.8
  uvula (congenital) Q38.5
  vagina (acquired) N89.8
    congenital Q52.4

Deformity Q89.9 — *continued*
   valgus NEC M21.00
      ankle M21.07-
      elbow M21.02-
      hip M21.05-
      knee M21.06-
   valve, valvular (congenital) (heart) Q24.8
      acquired — *see* Endocarditis
   varus NEC M21.10
      ankle M21.17-
      elbow M21.12-
      hip M21.15-
      knee M21.16-
      tibia — *see* Osteochondrosis, juvenile, tibia
   vas deferens (congenital) Q55.4
      acquired N50.8
   vein (congenital) Q27.9
      great Q26.9
   vertebra — *see* Dorsopathy, deforming
   vertical talus (congenital) Q66.80
      left foot Q66.82
      right foot Q66.81
   vesicourethral orifice (acquired) N32.89
      congenital NEC Q64.79
   vessels of optic papilla (congenital) Q14.2
   visual field (contraction) — *see* Defect, visual field
   vitreous body, acquired H43.89
   vulva (congenital) Q52.79
      acquired N90.89
   wrist (joint) (acquired) — *see also* Deformity, limb, forearm
      congenital Q68.8
      contraction — *see* Contraction, joint, wrist

Degeneration, degenerative
   adrenal (capsule) (fatty) (gland) (hyaline) (infectional) E27.8
   amyloid (*see also* Amyloidosis) E85.9
   anterior cornua, spinal cord G12.29
   anterior labral S43.49-
   aorta, aortic I70.0
      fatty I77.89
   aortic valve (heart) — *see* Endocarditis, aortic
   arteriovascular — *see* Arteriosclerosis
   artery, arterial (atheromatous) (calcareous) — *see also* Arteriosclerosis
      cerebral, amyloid E85.4 [I68.0]
      medial — *see* Arteriosclerosis, extremities
   articular cartilage NEC — *see* Derangement, joint, articular cartilage, by site
   atheromatous — *see* Arteriosclerosis
   basal nuclei or ganglia G23.9
      specified NEC G23.8
   bone NEC — *see* Disorder, bone, specified type NEC
   brachial plexus G54.0
   brain (cortical) (progressive) G31.9
      alcoholic G31.2
      arteriosclerotic I67.2
      childhood G31.9
         specified NEC G31.89
      cystic G31.89
         congenital Q04.6
      in
         alcoholism G31.2
         beriberi E51.2
         cerebrovascular disease I67.9
         congenital hydrocephalus Q03.9
            with spina bifida — *see also* Spina bifida
         Fabry-Anderson disease E75.21
         Gaucher's disease E75.22
         Hunter's syndrome E76.1
         lipidosis
            cerebral E75.4
            generalized E75.6
         mucopolysaccharidosis — *see* Mucopolysaccharidosis
         myxedema E03.9 [G32.89]
         neoplastic disease (*see also* Neoplasm) D49.6 [G32.89]
         Niemann-Pick disease E75.249 [G32.89]
         sphingolipidosis E75.3 [G32.89]
         vitamin B12 deficiency E53.8 [G32.89]
      senile NEC G31.1
   breast N64.89
   Bruch's membrane — *see* Degeneration, choroid
   capillaries (fatty) I78.8
      amyloid E85.8 [I79.8]
   cardiac — *see also* Degeneration, myocardial
      valve, valvular — *see* Endocarditis

Degeneration, degenerative — *continued*
   cardiorenal — *see* Hypertension, cardiorenal
   cardiovascular — *see also* Disease, cardiovascular
      renal — *see* Hypertension, cardiorenal
   cerebellar NOS G31.9
      alcoholic G31.2
      primary (hereditary) (sporadic) G11.9
   cerebral — *see* Degeneration, brain
   cerebrovascular I67.9
      due to hypertension I67.4
   cervical plexus G54.2
   cervix N88.8
      due to radiation (intended effect) N88.8
         adverse effect or misadventure N99.89
   chamber angle H21.21-
   changes, spine or vertebra — *see* Spondylosis
   chorioretinal — *see also* Degeneration, choroid
      hereditary H31.20
   choroid (colloid) (drusen) H31.10-
      atrophy — *see* Atrophy, choroidal
      hereditary — *see* Dystrophy, choroidal, hereditary
   ciliary body H21.22-
   cochlear — *see* subcategory H83.8
   combined (spinal cord) (subacute) E53.8 [G32.0]
      with anemia (pernicious) D51.0 [G32.0]
         due to dietary vitamin B12 deficiency D51.3 [G32.0]
      in (due to)
         vitamin B12 deficiency E53.8 [G32.0]
         anemia D51.9 [G32.0]
   conjunctiva H11.10
      concretions — *see* Concretion, conjunctiva
      deposits — *see* Deposit, conjunctiva
      pigmentations — *see* Pigmentation, conjunctiva
      pinguecula — *see* Pinguecula
      xerosis — *see* Xerosis, conjunctiva
   cornea H18.40
      calcerous H18.43
         band keratopathy H18.42-
      familial, hereditary — *see* Dystrophy, cornea
      hyaline (of old scars) H18.49
      keratomalacia — *see* Keratomalacia
      nodular H18.45-
      peripheral H18.46-
      senile H18.41-
      specified type NEC H18.49
   cortical (cerebellar) (parenchymatous) G31.89
      alcoholic G31.2
      diffuse, due to arteriopathy I67.2
   corticobasal G31.85
   cutis L98.8
      amyloid E85.4 [L99]
   dental pulp K04.2
   disc disease — *see* Degeneration, intervertebral disc NEC
   dorsolateral (spinal cord) — *see* Degeneration, combined
   extrapyramidal G25.9
   eye, macular — *see also* Degeneration, macula
      congenital or hereditary — *see* Dystrophy, retina
   facet joints — *see* Spondylosis
   fatty
      liver NEC K76.0
         alcoholic K70.0
   grey matter (brain) (Alpers') G31.81
   heart — *see also* Degeneration, myocardial
      amyloid E85.4 [I43]
      atheromatous — *see* Disease, heart, ischemic, atherosclerotic
      ischemic — *see* Disease, heart, ischemic
   hepatolenticular (Wilson's) E83.01
   hepatorenal K76.7
   hyaline (diffuse) (generalized)
      localized — *see* Degeneration, by site
   infrapatellar fat pad M79.4
   intervertebral disc NOS
      with
         myelopathy — *see* Disorder, disc, with, myelopathy
         radiculitis or radiculopathy — *see* Disorder, disc, with, radiculopathy

Degeneration, degenerative — *continued*
   intervertebral disc NOS — *continued*
      cervical, cervicothoracic — *see* Disorder, disc, cervical, degeneration
         with
            myelopathy — *see* Disorder, disc, cervical, with myelopathy
            neuritis, radiculitis or radiculopathy — *see* Disorder, disc, cervical, with neuritis
      lumbar region M51.36
         with
            myelopathy M51.06
            neuritis, radiculitis, radiculopathy or sciatica M51.16
      lumbosacral region M51.37
         with
            neuritis, radiculitis, radiculopathy or sciatica M51.17
      sacrococcygeal region M53.3
      thoracic region M51.34
         with
            myelopathy M51.04
            neuritis, radiculitis, radiculopathy M51.14
      thoracolumbar region M51.35
         with
            myelopathy M51.05
            neuritis, radiculitis, radiculopathy M51.15
   intestine, amyloid E85.4
   iris (pigmentary) H21.23-
   ischemic — *see* Ischemia
   joint disease — *see* Osteoarthritis
   kidney N28.89
      amyloid E85.4 [N29]
      cystic, congenital Q61.9
      fatty N28.89
      polycystic Q61.3
         adult type (autosomal dominant) Q61.2
         infantile type (autosomal recessive) NEC Q61.19
            collecting duct dilatation Q61.11
   Kuhnt-Junius (*see also* Degeneration, macula) H35.32
   lens — *see* Cataract
   lenticular (familial) (progressive) (Wilson's) (with cirrhosis of liver) E83.01
   liver (diffuse) NEC K76.89
      amyloid E85.4 [K77]
      cystic K76.89
         congenital Q44.6
      fatty NEC K76.0
         alcoholic K70.0
      hypertrophic K76.89
      parenchymatous, acute or subacute K72.00
         with coma K72.01
      pigmentary K76.89
      toxic (acute) K71.9
   lung J98.4
   lymph gland I89.8
      hyaline I89.8
   macula, macular (acquired) (age-related) (senile) H35.30
      angioid streaks H35.33
      atrophic age-related H35.31
      congenital or hereditary — *see* Dystrophy, retina
      cystoid H35.35-
      drusen H35.36-
      exudative H35.32
      hole H35.34-
      nonexudative H35.31
      puckering H35.37-
      toxic H35.38-
   membranous labyrinth, congenital (causing impairment of hearing) Q16.5
   meniscus — *see* Derangement, meniscus
   mitral — *see* Insufficiency, mitral
   Mönckeberg's — *see* Arteriosclerosis, extremities
   motor centers, senile G31.1
   multi-system G90.3
   mural — *see* Degeneration, myocardial
   muscle (fatty) (fibrous) (hyaline) (progressive) M62.89
      heart — *see* Degeneration, myocardial
   myelin, central nervous system G37.9
   myocardial, myocardium (fatty) (hyaline) (senile) I51.5
      with rheumatic fever (conditions in I00) I09.0
         active, acute or subacute I01.2
            with chorea I02.0
         inactive or quiescent (with chorea) I09.0

Degeneration, degenerative — *continued*
   myocardial, myocardium (fatty) (hyaline) (senile) I51.5 — *continued*
      hypertensive — *see* Hypertension, heart
      rheumatic — *see* Degeneration, myocardial, with rheumatic fever
      syphilitic A52.06
   nasal sinus (mucosa) J32.9
      frontal J32.1
      maxillary J32.0
   nerve — *see* Disorder, nerve
   nervous system G31.9
      alcoholic G31.2
      amyloid E85.4 [G99.8]
      autonomic G90.9
      fatty G31.89
      specified NEC G31.89
   nipple N64.89
   olivopontocerebellar (hereditary) (familial) G23.8
   osseous labyrinth — *see* subcategory H83.8
   ovary N83.8
      cystic N83.20
      microcystic N83.20
   pallidal pigmentary (progressive) G23.0
   pancreas K86.8
      tuberculous A18.83
   penis N48.89
   pigmentary (diffuse) (general)
      localized — *see* Degeneration, by site
      pallidal (progressive) G23.0
   pineal gland E34.8
   pituitary (gland) E23.6
   popliteal fat pad M79.4
   posterolateral (spinal cord) — *see* Degeneration, combined
   pulmonary valve (heart) I37.8
   pulp (tooth) K04.2
   pupillary margin H21.24-
   renal — *see* Degeneration, kidney
   retina H35.9
      hereditary (cerebroretinal) (congenital) (juvenile) (macula) (peripheral) (pigmentary) — *see* Dystrophy, retina
      Kuhnt-Junius (*see also* Degeneration, macula) H35.32
      macula (cystic) (exudative) (hole) (nonexudative) (pseudohole) (senile) (toxic) — *see* Degeneration, macula
      peripheral H35.40
         lattice H35.41-
         microcystoid H35.42-
         paving stone H35.43-
         secondary
            pigmentary H35.45-
            vitreoretinal H35.46-
         senile reticular H35.44-
      pigmentary (primary) — *see also* Dystrophy, retina
         secondary — *see* Degeneration, retina, peripheral, secondary
      posterior pole — *see* Degeneration, macula
   saccule, congenital (causing impairment of hearing) Q16.5
   senile R54
      brain G31.1
      cardiac, heart or myocardium — *see* Degeneration, myocardial
      motor centers G31.1
      vascular — *see* Arteriosclerosis
   sinus (cystic) — *see also* Sinusitis
      polypoid J33.1
   skin L98.8
      amyloid E85.4 [L99]
      colloid L98.8
   spinal (cord) G31.89
      amyloid E85.4 [G32.89]
      combined (subacute) — *see* Degeneration, combined
      dorsolateral — *see* Degeneration, combined
      familial NEC G31.89
      fatty G31.89
      funicular — *see* Degeneration, combined
      posterolateral — *see* Degeneration, combined
      subacute combined — *see* Degeneration, combined
      tuberculous A17.81
   spleen D73.0
      amyloid E85.4 [D77]
   stomach K31.89
   striatonigral G23.2
   suprarenal (capsule) (gland) E27.8
   synovial membrane (pulpy) — *see* Disorder, synovium, specified type NEC

D I S E A S E   I N D E X

Degeneration, degenerative — *continued*
  tapetoretinal — *see* Dystrophy, retina
  thymus (gland) E32.8
    fatty E32.8
  thyroid (gland) E07.89
  tricuspid (heart) (valve) I07.9
  tuberculous NEC — *see* Tuberculosis
  turbinate J34.89
  uterus (cystic) N85.8
  vascular (senile) — *see* Arteriosclerosis
    hypertensive — *see* Hypertension
  vitreoretinal, secondary — *see*
      Degeneration, retina, peripheral,
      secondary, vitreoretinal
  vitreous (body) H43.81-
  Wallerian — *see* Disorder, nerve
  Wilson's hepatolenticular E83.01
Deglutition
  paralysis R13.0
    hysterical F44.4
  pneumonia J69.0
Degos' disease I77.89
Dehiscence (of)
  amputation stump T87.81
  cesarean wound O90.0
  closure of
    cornea T81.31
    craniotomy T81.32
    fascia (muscular) (superficial) T81.32
    internal organ or tissue T81.32
    laceration (external) (internal) T81.33
    ligament T81.32
    mucosa T81.31
    muscle or muscle flap T81.32
    ribs or rib cage T81.32
    skin and subcutaneous tissue (full-
      thickness) (superficial) T81.31
    skull T81.32
    sternum (sternotomy) T81.32
    tendon T81.32
    traumatic laceration (external) (internal)
      T81.33
  episiotomy O90.1
  operation wound NEC T81.31
    external operation wound (superficial)
      T81.31
    internal operation wound (deep) T81.32
  perineal wound (postpartum) O90.1
  traumatic injury wound repair T81.33
  wound T81.30
    traumatic repair T81.33
Dehydration E86.0
  hypertonic E87.0
  hypotonic E87.1
  newborn P74.1
Déjérine-Roussy syndrome G89.0
Déjérine-Sottas disease or neuropathy
  (hypertrophic) G60.0
Déjérine-Thomas atrophy G23.8
Delay, delayed
  any plane in pelvis
    complicating delivery O66.9
  birth or delivery NOS O63.9
  closure, ductus arteriosus (Botalli) P29.3
  coagulation — *see* Defect, coagulation
  conduction (cardiac) (ventricular) I45.9
  delivery, second twin, triplet, etc O63.2
  development R62.50
    global F88
    intellectual (specific) F81.9
    language F80.9
      due to hearing loss F80.4
    learning F81.9
    pervasive F84.9
    physiological R62.50
      specified stage NEC R62.0
    reading F81.0
    sexual E30.0
    speech F80.9
      due to hearing loss F80.4
    spelling F81.81
  gastric emptying K30
  menarche E30.0
  menstruation (cause unknown) N91.0
  milestone R62.0
  passage of meconium (newborn) P76.0
  primary respiration P28.9
  puberty (constitutional) E30.0
  separation of umbilical cord P96.82
  sexual maturation, female E30.0
  sleep phase syndrome G47.21
  union, fracture — *see* Fracture, by site
  vaccination Z28.9
Deletion(s)
  autosome Q93.9
    identified by fluorescence in situ
      hybridization (FISH) Q93.89
    identified by in situ hybridization (ISH)
      Q93.89

Deletion(s) — *continued*
  chromosome
    with complex rearrangements NEC
      Q93.7
    part of NEC Q93.5
    seen only at prometaphase Q93.89
    short arm
      22q11.2 Q93.81
      4 Q93.3
      5p Q93.4
    specified NEC Q93.89
  long arm chromosome 18 or 21 Q93.89
    with complex rearrangements NEC
      Q93.7
  microdeletions NEC Q93.88
Delhi boil or button B55.1
Delinquency (juvenile) (neurotic) F91.8
  group Z72.810
Delinquent immunization status Z28.3
Delirium, delirious (acute or subacute) (not
  alcohol- or drug-induced) (with
  dementia) R41.0
  alcoholic (acute) (tremens) (withdrawal)
    F10.921
    with intoxication F10.921
      in
        abuse F10.121
        dependence F10.221
  due to (secondary to)
    alcohol
      intoxication F10.921
        in
          abuse F10.121
          dependence F10.221
      withdrawal F10.231
    amphetamine intoxication F15.921
      in
        abuse F15.121
        dependence F15.221
    anxiolytic
      intoxication F13.921
        in
          abuse F13.121
          dependence F13.221
      withdrawal F13.231
    cannabis intoxication (acute) F12.921
      in
        abuse F12.121
        dependence F12.221
    cocaine intoxication (acute) F14.921
      in
        abuse F14.121
        dependence F14.221
    general medical condition F05
    hallucinogen intoxication F16.921
      in
        abuse F16.121
        dependence F16.221
    hypnotic
      intoxication F13.921
        in
          abuse F13.121
          dependence F13.221
      withdrawal F13.231
    inhalant intoxication (acute) F18.921
      in
        abuse F18.121
        dependence F18.221
    multiple etiologies F05
    opioid intoxication (acute) F11.921
      in
        abuse F11.121
        dependence F11.221
    phencyclidine intoxication (acute)
      F16.921
      in
        abuse F16.121
        dependence F16.221
    psychoactive substance NEC
      intoxication (acute) F19.921
      in
        abuse F19.121
        dependence F19.221
    sedative
      intoxication F13.921
        in
          abuse F13.121
          dependence F13.221
      withdrawal F13.231
    unknown etiology F05
  exhaustion F43.0
  hysterical F44.89
  postprocedural (postoperative) F05
  puerperal F05
  thyroid — *see* Thyrotoxicosis with thyroid
    storm
  traumatic — *see* Injury, intracranial
  tremens (alcohol-induced) F10.231
    sedative-induced F13.231

Delivery (childbirth) (labor)
  arrested active phase O62.1
  cesarean (for)
    abnormal
      pelvis (bony) (deformity) (major)
        NEC with disproportion
        (fetopelvic) O33.0
        with obstructed labor O65.0
      presentation or position O32.9
    abruptio placentae (*see also* Abruptio
      placentae) O45.9-
    acromion presentation O32.2
    atony, uterus O62.2
    breech presentation O32.1
      incomplete O32.8
    brow presentation O32.3
    cephalopelvic disproportion O33.9
    cerclage O34.3-
    chin presentation O32.3
    cicatrix of cervix O34.4-
    contracted pelvis (general)
      inlet O33.2
      outlet O33.3
    cord presentation or prolapse O69.0
    cystocele O34.8-
    deformity (acquired) (congenital)
      pelvic organs or tissues NEC O34.8-
      pelvis (bony) NEC O33.0
    disproportion NOS O33.9
    eclampsia — *see* Eclampsia
    face presentation O32.3
    failed
      forceps O66.5
      induction of labor O61.9
        instrumental O61.1
        mechanical O61.1
        medical O61.0
        specified NEC O61.8
        surgical O61.1
      trial of labor NOS O66.40
        following previous cesarean
          delivery O66.41
      vacuum extraction O66.5
      ventouse O66.5
    fetal-maternal hemorrhage O43.01-
    hemorrhage (intrapartum) O67.9
      with coagulation defect O67.0
      specified cause NEC O67.8
    high head at term O32.4
    hydrocephalic fetus O33.6
    incarceration of uterus O34.51-
    incoordinate uterine action O62.4
    increased size, fetus O33.5
    inertia, uterus O62.2
      primary O62.0
      secondary O62.1
    lateroversion, uterus O34.59-
    mal lie O32.9
    malposition
      fetus O32.9
      pelvic organs or tissues NEC O34.8-
      uterus NEC O34.59-
    malpresentation NOS O32.9
    oblique presentation O32.2
    occurring after 37 completed weeks of
      gestation but before 39 completed
      weeks of gestation due to
      (spontaneous) onset of labor
      O75.82
    oversize fetus O33.5
    pelvic tumor NEC O34.8-
    placenta previa O44.1-
      without hemorrhage O44.0-
    placental insufficiency O36.51-
    planned, occurring after 37 completed
      weeks of gestation but before 39
      completed weeks of gestation due
      to (spontaneous) onset of labor
      O75.82
    polyp, cervix O34.4-
      causing obstructed labor O65.5
    poor dilatation, cervix O62.0
    pre-eclampsia O14.9-
      mild O14.0-
      moderate O14.0-
      severe
        with hemolysis, elevated liver
          enzymes and low platelet
          count (HELLP) O14.2-
    previous
      cesarean delivery O34.21
      surgery (to)
        cervix O34.4-
        gynecological NEC O34.8-
        rectum O34.7-
        uterus O34.29
        vagina O34.6-

Delivery (childbirth) (labor) — *continued*
  cesarean (for) — *continued*
    prolapse
      arm or hand O32.2
      uterus O34.52-
    prolonged labor NOS O63.9
    rectocele O34.8-
    retroversion
      uterus O34.53-
    rigid
      cervix O34.4-
      pelvic floor O34.8-
      perineum O34.7-
      vagina O34.6-
      vulva O34.7-
    sacculation, pregnant uterus O34.59-
    scar(s)
      cervix O34.4-
      cesarean delivery O34.21
      uterus O34.29
    Shirodkar suture in situ O34.3-
    shoulder presentation O32.2
    stenosis or stricture, cervix O34.4-
    streptococcus B carrier state O99.824
    transverse presentation or lie O32.2
    tumor, pelvic organs or tissues NEC
      O34.8-
      cervix O34.4-
    umbilical cord presentation or prolapse
      O69.0
    without indication O82
  completely normal case O80
  complicated O75.9
    by
      abnormal, abnormality (of)
        forces of labor O62.9
          specified type NEC O62.8
        glucose O99.814
        uterine contractions NOS O62.9
      abruptio placentae (*see also* Abruptio
        placentae) O45.9-
      abuse
        physical O9A.32
        psychological O9A.52
        sexual O9A.42
      adherent placenta O72.0
        without hemorrhage O73.0
      alcohol use O99.314
      anemia (pre-existing) O99.02
      anesthetic death O74.8
      annular detachment of cervix O71.3
      atony, uterus O62.2
      attempted vacuum extraction and
        forceps O66.5
      Bandl's ring O62.4
      bariatric surgery status O99.844
      biliary tract disorder O26.62
      bleeding — *see* Delivery, complicated
        by, hemorrhage
      blood disorder NEC O99.12
      cervical dystocia (hypotonic) O62.2
        primary O62.0
        secondary O62.1
      circulatory system disorder O99.42
      compression of cord (umbilical) NEC
        O69.2
      condition NEC O99.89
      contraction, contracted ring O62.4
      cord (umbilical)
        around neck
          with compression O69.1
          without compression O69.81
        bruising O69.5
        complication O69.9
          specified NEC O69.89
        compression NEC O69.2
        entanglement O69.2
          without compression O69.82
        hematoma O69.5
        presentation O69.0
        prolapse O69.0
        short O69.3
        thrombosis (vessels) O69.5
        vascular lesion O69.5
      Couvelaire uterus O45.8x-
      damage to (injury) NEC
        perineum O71.82
        periurethral tissue O71.82
        vulva O71.82
      delay following rupture of membranes
        (spontaneous) — *see* Pregnancy,
        complicated by, premature
        rupture of membranes
      depressed fetal heart tones O76

Delivery (childbirth) (labor) — *continued*
complicated O75.9 — *continued*
by — *continued*
diabetes O24.92
gestational O24.429
diet controlled O24.420
insulin controlled O24.424
pre-existing O24.32
specified NEC O24.82
type 1 O24.02
type 2 O24.12
diastasis recti (abdominis) O71.89
dilatation
bladder O66.8
cervix incomplete, poor or slow O62.0
disease NEC O99.89
disruptio uteri — *see* Delivery, complicated by, rupture, uterus
drug use O99.324
dysfunction, uterus NOS O62.9
hypertonic O62.4
hypotonic O62.2
primary O62.0
secondary O62.1
incoordinate O62.4
eclampsia O15.1
embolism (pulmonary) — *see* Embolism, obstetric
endocrine, nutritional or metabolic disease NEC O99.284
failed
attempted vaginal birth after previous cesarean delivery O66.41
induction of labor O61.9
instrumental O61.1
mechanical O61.1
medical O61.0
specified NEC O61.8
surgical O61.1
trial of labor O66.40
female genital mutilation O65.5
fetal
abnormal acid-base balance O68
acidemia O68
acidosis O68
alkalosis O68
death, early O02.1
deformity O66.3
heart rate or rhythm (abnormal) (non-reassuring) O76
hypoxia O77.8
stress O77.9
due to drug administration O77.1
electrocardiographic evidence of O77.8
specified NEC O77.8
ultrasound evidence of O77.8
fever during labor O75.2
gastric banding status O99.844
gastric bypass status O99.844
gastrointestinal disease NEC O99.62
gestational diabetes O24.429
diet controlled O24.420
insulin (and diet) controlled O24.424
gonorrhea O98.22
hematoma O71.7
ischial spine O71.7
pelvic O71.7
vagina O71.7
vulva or perineum O71.7
hemorrhage (uterine) O67.9
associated with
afibrinogenemia O67.0
coagulation defect O67.0
hyperfibrinolysis O67.0
hypofibrinogenemia O67.0
due to
low-lying placenta O44.1-
placenta previa O44.1-
premature separation of placenta (normally implanted) (*see also* Abruptio placentae) O45.9-
retained placenta O72.0
uterine leiomyoma O67.8
placenta NEC O67.8
postpartum NEC (atonic) (immediate) O72.1
with retained or trapped placenta O72.0
delayed O72.2
secondary O72.2
third stage O72.0
hourglass contraction, uterus O62.4

Delivery (childbirth) (labor) — *continued*
complicated O75.9 — *continued*
by — *continued*
hypertension, hypertensive (pre-existing) — *see* Hypertension, complicated by, childbirth (labor)
hypotension O26.5-
incomplete dilatation (cervix) O62.0
incoordinate uterus contractions O62.4
inertia, uterus O62.2
during latent phase of labor O62.0
primary O62.0
secondary O62.1
infection (maternal) O98.92
carrier state NEC O99.834
gonorrhea O98.22
human immunodeficiency virus (HIV) O98.72
sexually transmitted NEC O98.32
specified NEC O98.82
syphilis O98.12
tuberculosis O98.02
viral hepatitis O98.42
viral NEC O98.52
injury (to mother) (*see also* Delivery, complicated, by, damage to) O71.9
nonobstetric O9A.22
caused by abuse — *see* Delivery, complicated by, abuse
intrauterine fetal death, early O02.1
inversion, uterus O71.2
laceration (perineal) O70.9
anus (sphincter) O70.4
with third degree laceration O70.2
with mucosa O70.3
without third degree laceration O70.4
bladder (urinary) O71.5
bowel O71.5
cervix (uteri) O71.3
fourchette O70.0
hymen O70.0
labia O70.0
pelvic
floor O70.1
organ NEC O71.5
perineum, perineal O70.9
first degree O70.0
fourth degree O70.3
muscles O70.1
second degree O70.1
skin O70.0
slight O70.0
third degree O70.2
peritoneum (pelvic) O71.5
rectovaginal (septum) (without perineal laceration) O71.4
with perineum O70.2
with anal or rectal mucosa O70.3
specified NEC O71.89
sphincter ani — *see* Delivery, complicated, by, laceration, anus (sphincter)
urethra O71.5
uterus O71.81
before labor O71.81
vagina, vaginal (deep) (high) (without perineal laceration) O71.4
with perineum O70.0
muscles, with perineum O70.1
vulva O70.0
liver disorder O26.62
malignancy O9A.12
malnutrition O25.2
malposition, malpresentation
without obstruction (*see also* Delivery, complicated by, obstruction) O32.9
breech O32.1
compound O32.6
face (brow) (chin) O32.3
footling O32.8
high head O32.4
oblique O32.2
specified NEC O32.8
transverse O32.2
unstable lie O32.0
placenta (with hemorrhage) O44.1-
without hemorrhage O44.0-
uterus or cervix O65.5
meconium in amniotic fluid O77.0
mental disorder NEC O99.344
metrorrhexis — *see* Delivery, complicated by, rupture, uterus

Delivery (childbirth) (labor) — *continued*
complicated O75.9 — *continued*
by — *continued*
nervous system disorder O99.354
obesity (pre-existing) O99.214
obesity surgery status O99.844
obstetric trauma O71.9
specified NEC O71.89
obstructed labor
due to
breech (complete) (frank) presentation O64.1
incomplete O64.8
brow presenation O64.3
buttock presentation O64.1
chin presentation O64.2
compound presentation O64.5
contracted pelvis O65.1
deep transverse arrest O64.0
deformed pelvis O65.0
dystocia (fetal) O66.9
due to
conjoined twins O66.3
fetal
abnormality NEC O66.3
ascites O66.3
hydrops O66.3
meningomyelocele O66.3
sacral teratoma O66.3
tumor O66.3
hydrocephalic fetus O66.3
shoulder O66.0
face presentation O64.2
fetopelvic disproportion O65.4
footling presentation O64.8
impacted shoulders O66.0
incomplete rotation of fetal head O64.0
large fetus O66.2
locked twins O66.1
malposition O64.9
specified NEC O64.8
malpresentation O64.9
specified NEC O64.8
multiple fetuses NEC O66.6
pelvic
abnormality (maternal) O65.9
organ O65.5
specified NEC O65.8
contraction
inlet O65.2
mid-cavity O65.3
outlet O65.3
persistent (position)
occipitoiliac O64.0
occipitoposterior O64.0
occipitosacral O64.0
occipitotransverse O64.0
prolapsed arm O64.4
shoulder presentation O64.4
specified NEC O66.8
pathological retraction ring, uterus O62.4
penetration, pregnant uterus by instrument O71.1
perforation — *see* Delivery, complicated by, laceration
placenta, placental
ablatio (*see also* Abruptio placentae) O45.9-
abnormality O43.9-
specified NEC O43.89-
abruptio (*see also* Abruptio placentae) O45.9-
accreta O43.21-
adherent (with hemorrhage) O72.0
without hemorrhage O73.0
detachment (premature) (*see also* Abruptio placentae) O45.9-
disorder O43.9-
specified NEC O43.89-
hemorrhage NEC O67.8
increta O43.22-
low (implantation) O44.1-
without hemorrhage O44.0-
malformation O43.10-
malposition O44.1-
without hemorrhage O44.0-
percreta O43.23-
previa (central) (lateral) (low) (marginal) (partial) (total) O44.1-
without hemorrhage O44.0-
retained (with hemorrhage) O72.0
without hemorrhage O73.0
separation (premature) O45.9-
specified NEC O45.8x-
vicious insertion O44.1-
precipitate labor O62.3

Delivery (childbirth) (labor) — *continued*
complicated O75.9 — *continued*
by — *continued*
premature rupture, membranes (*see also* Pregnancy, complicated by, premature rupture of membranes) O42.90
prolapse
arm or hand O32.2
cord (umbilical) O69.0
foot or leg O32.8
uterus O34.52-
prolonged labor O63.9
first stage O63.0
second stage O63.1
protozoal disease (maternal) O98.62
respiratory disease NEC O99.52
retained membranes or portions of placenta O72.2
without hemorrhage O73.1
retarded birth O63.9
retention of secundines (with hemorrhage) O72.0
without hemorrhage O73.0
partial O72.2
without hemorrhage O73.1
rupture
bladder (urinary) O71.5
cervix O71.3
pelvic organ NEC O71.5
urethra O71.5
uterus (during or after labor) O71.1
before labor O71.0-
separation, pubic bone (symphysis pubis) O71.6
shock O75.1
shoulder presentation O64.4
skin disorder NEC O99.72
spasm, cervix O62.4
stenosis or stricture, cervix O65.5
streptococcus B carrier state O99.824
subluxation of symphysis (pubis) O26.72
syphilis (maternal) O98.12
tear — *see* Delivery, complicated by, laceration
tetanic uterus O62.4
trauma (obstetrical) (*see also* Delivery, complicated, by, damage to) O71.9
non-obstetric O9A.22
periurethral O71.82
specified NEC O71.89
tuberculosis (maternal) O98.02
tumor, pelvic organs or tissues NEC O65.5
umbilical cord around neck
with compression O69.1
without compression O69.81
uterine inertia O62.2
during latent phase of labor O62.0
primary O62.0
secondary O62.1
vasa previa O69.4
velamentous insertion of cord O43.12-
specified complication NEC O75.89
delayed NOS O63.9
following rupture of membranes artificial O75.5
second twin, triplet, etc. O63.2
forceps, low following failed vacuum extraction O66.5
missed (at or near term) O36.4
normal O80
obstructed — *see* Delivery, complicated by, obstruction
precipitate O62.3
preterm (*see also* Pregnancy, complicated by, preterm labor) O60.10
spontaneous O80
term pregnancy NOS O80
uncomplicated O80
vaginal, following previous cesarean delivery O34.21
Delusions (paranoid) — *see* Disorder, delusional
Dementia (degenerative (primary)) (old age) (persisting) F03.90
with
aggressive behavior F03.91
behavioral disturbance F03.91
combative behavior F03.91
Lewy bodies G31.83 [F02.80]
with behavioral disturbance G31.83 [F02.81]
Parkinsonism G31.83 [F02.80]
with behavioral disturbance G31.83 [F02.81]

DISEASE INDEX

Dementia (degenerative (primary)) (old age) (persisting) F03 — *continued*
with — *continued*
  Parkinson's disease G20 [F02.80]
    with behavioral disturbance G20 [F02.81]
  violent behavior F03.91
alcoholic F10.97
  with dependence F10.27
Alzheimer's type — *see* Disease, Alzheimer's
arteriosclerotic — *see* Dementia, vascular
atypical, Alzheimer's type — *see* Disease, Alzheimer's, specified NEC
congenital — *see* Disability, intellectual
frontal (lobe) G31.09 [F02.80]
  with behavioral disturbance G31.09 [F02.81]
frontotemporal G31.09 [F02.80]
  with behavioral disturbance G31.09 [F02.81]
  specified NEC G31.09 [F02.80]
    with behavioral disturbance G31.09 [F02.81]
in (due to)
  with behavioral disturbance G31.83 [F02.81]
  alcohol F10.97
    with dependence F10.27
  Alzheimer's disease — *see* Disease, Alzheimer's
  arteriosclerotic brain disease — *see* Dementia, vascular
  cerebral lipidoses E75-[F02.80]
    with behavioral disturbance E75-[F02.81]
  Creutzfeldt-Jakob disease (*see also* Creutzfeldt-Jakob disease or syndrome (with dementia)) A81.00
  epilepsy G40-[F02.80]
    with behavioral disturbance G40-[F02.81]
  hepatolenticular degeneration E83.01 [F02.80]
    with behavioral disturbance E83.01 [F02.81]
  human immunodeficiency virus (HIV) disease B20 [F02.80]
    with behavioral disturbance B20 [F02.81]
  Huntington's disease or chorea G10
  hypercalcemia E83.52 [F02.80]
    with behavioral disturbance E83.52 [F02.81]
  hypothyroidism, acquired E03.9 [F02.80]
    with behavioral disturbance E03.9 [F02.81]
    due to iodine deficiency E01.8 [F02.80]
      with behavioral disturbance E01.8 [F02.81]
  inhalants F18.97
    with dependence F18.27
  multiple
    etiologies F03
    sclerosis G35 [F02.80]
      with behavioral disturbance G35 [F02.81]
  neurosyphilis A52.17 [F02.80]
    with behavioral disturbance A52.17 [F02.81]
    juvenile A50.49 [F02.80]
      with behavioral disturbance A50.49 [F02.81]
  niacin deficiency E52 [F02.80]
    with behavioral disturbance E52 [F02.81]
  paralysis agitans G20 [F02.80]
    with behavioral disturbance G20 [F02.81]
  Parkinson's disease G20 [F02.80]
  pellagra E52 [F02.80]
    with behavioral disturbance E52 [F02.81]
  Pick's G31.01 [F02.80]
    with behavioral disturbance G31.01 [F02.81]
  polyarteritis nodosa M30.0 [F02.80]
    with behavioral disturbance M30.0 [F02.81]
  psychoactive drug F19.97
    with dependence F19.27
    inhalants F18.97
      with dependence F18.27
    sedatives, hypnotics or anxiolytics F13.97
      with dependence F13.27

Dementia (degenerative (primary)) (old age) (persisting) F03 — *continued*
in (due to) — *continued*
  sedatives, hypnotics or anxiolytics F13.97
    with dependence F13.27
  systemic lupus erythematosus M32-[F02.80]
    with behavioral disturbance M32-[F02.81]
  trypanosomiasis
    African B56.9 [F02.80]
      with behavioral disturbance B56.9 [F02.81]
  unknown etiology F03
  vitamin B12 deficiency E53.8 [F02.80]
    with behavioral disturbance E53.8 [F02.81]
  volatile solvents F18.97
    with dependence F18.27
infantile, infantilis F84.3
Lewy body G31.83 [F02.80]
  with behavioral disturbance G31.83 [F02.81]
multi-infarct — *see* Dementia, vascular
paralytica, paralytic (syphilitic) A52.17 [F02.80]
  with behavioral disturbance A52.17 [F02.81]
  juvenilis A50.45
paretic A52.17
praecox — *see* Schizophrenia
presenile F03
  Alzheimer's type — *see* Disease, Alzheimer's, early onset
  primary degenerative F03
progressive, syphilitic A52.17
senile F03
  with acute confusional state F05
  Alzheimer's type — *see* Disease, Alzheimer's, late onset
  depressed or paranoid type F03
vascular (acute onset) (mixed) (multi-infarct) (subcortical) F01.50
  with behavioral disturbance F01.51
Demineralization, bone — *see* Osteoporosis
Demodex folliculorum (infestation) B88.0
Demophobia F40.248
Demoralization R45.3
Demyelination, demyelinization
central nervous system G37.9
  specified NEC G37.8
corpus callosum (central) G37.1
disseminated, acute G36.9
  specified NEC G36.8
global G35
in optic neuritis G36.0
Dengue (classical) (fever) A90
hemorrhagic A91
sandfly A93.1
Dennie-Marfan syphilitic syndrome A50.45
Dens evaginatus, in dente or invaginatus K00.2
Dense breasts R92.2
Density
increased, bone (disseminated) (generalized) (spotted) — *see* Disorder, bone, density and structure, specified type NEC
lung (nodular) J98.4
Dental — *see also* condition
examination Z01.20
  with abnormal findings Z01.21
restoration
  aesthetically inadequate or displeasing K08.56
  defective K08.50
    specified NEC K08.59
  failure of marginal integrity K08.51
  failure of periodontal anatomical integrity K08.54
Dentia praecox K00.6
Denticles (pulp) K04.2
Dentigerous cyst K09.0
Dentin
irregular (in pulp) K04.3
opalescent K00.5
secondary (in pulp) K04.3
sensitive K03.89
Dentinogenesis imperfecta K00.5
Dentinoma — *see* Cyst, calcifying odontogenic
Dentition (syndrome) K00.7
delayed K00.6
difficult K00.7
precocious K00.6
premature K00.6
retarded K00.6

Dependence (on) (syndrome) F19.20
with remission F19.21
alcohol (ethyl) (methyl) (without remission) F10.20
  with
    amnestic disorder, persisting F10.26
    anxiety disorder F10.280
    dementia, persisting F10.27
    intoxication F10.229
      with delirium F10.221
      uncomplicated F10.220
    mood disorder F10.24
    psychotic disorder F10.259
      with
        delusions F10.250
        hallucinations F10.251
    remission F10.21
    sexual dysfunction F10.281
    sleep disorder F10.282
    specified disorder NEC F10.288
    withdrawal F10.239
      with
        delirium F10.231
        perceptual disturbance F10.232
      uncomplicated F10.230
  counseling and surveillance Z71.41
amobarbital — *see* Dependence, drug, sedative
amphetamine(s) (type) — *see* Dependence, drug, stimulant NEC
amytal (sodium) — *see* Dependence, drug, sedative
analgesic NEC F55.8
anesthetic (agent) (gas) (general) (local) NEC — *see* Dependence, drug, psychoactive NEC
anxiolytic NEC — *see* Dependence, drug, sedative
barbital(s) — *see* Dependence, drug, sedative
barbiturate(s) (compounds) (drugs classifiable to T42) — *see* Dependence, drug, sedative
benzedrine — *see* Dependence, drug, stimulant NEC
bhang — *see* Dependence, drug, cannabis
bromide(s) NEC — *see* Dependence, drug, sedative
caffeine — *see* Dependence, drug, stimulant NEC
cannabis (sativa) (indica) (resin) (derivatives) (type) — *see* Dependence, drug, cannabis
chloral (betaine) (hydrate) — *see* Dependence, drug, sedative
chlordiazepoxide — *see* Dependence, drug, sedative
coca (leaf) (derivatives) — *see* Dependence, drug, cocaine
cocaine — *see* Dependence, drug, cocaine
codeine — *see* Dependence, drug, opioid
combinations of drugs F19.20
dagga — *see* Dependence, drug, cannabis
demerol — *see* Dependence, drug, opioid
dexamphetamine — *see* Dependence, drug, stimulant NEC
dexedrine — *see* Dependence, drug, stimulant NEC
dextro-nor-pseudo-ephedrine — *see* Dependence, drug, stimulant NEC
dextromethorphan — *see* Dependence, drug, opioid
dextromoramide — *see* Dependence, drug, opioid
dextrorphan — *see* Dependence, drug, opioid
diazepam — *see* Dependence, drug, sedative
dilaudid — *see* Dependence, drug, opioid
D-lysergic acid diethylamide — *see* Dependence, drug, hallucinogen
drug NEC F19.20
  with sleep disorder F19.282
  cannabis F12.20
    with
      anxiety disorder F12.280
      intoxication F12.229
        with
          delirium F12.221
          perceptual disturbance F12.222
        uncomplicated F12.220
      other specified disorder F12.288
      psychosis F12.259
        delusions F12.250
        hallucinations F12.251
      unspecified disorder F12.29
    in remission F12.21

Dependence (on) (syndrome) F19.20 — *continued*
drug NEC F19.20 — *continued*
  cocaine F14.20
    with
      anxiety disorder F14.280
      intoxication F14.229
        with
          delirium F14.221
          perceptual disturbance F14.222
        uncomplicated F14.220
      mood disorder F14.24
      other specified disorder F14.288
      psychosis F14.259
        delusions F14.250
        hallucinations F14.251
      sexual dysfunction F14.281
      sleep disorder F14.282
      unspecified disorder F14.29
      withdrawal F14.23
    in remission F14.21
    withdrawal symptoms in newborn P96.1
  counseling and surveillance Z71.51
  hallucinogen F16.20
    with
      anxiety disorder F16.280
      flashbacks F16.283
      intoxication F16.229
        with delirium F16.221
        uncomplicated F16.220
      mood disorder F16.24
      other specified disorder F16.288
      perception disorder, persisting F16.283
      psychosis F16.259
        delusions F16.250
        hallucinations F16.251
      unspecified disorder F16.29
    in remission F16.21
  in remission F19.21
  inhalant F18.20
    with
      anxiety disorder F18.280
      dementia, persisting F18.27
      intoxication F18.229
        with delirium F18.221
        uncomplicated F18.220
      mood disorder F18.24
      other specified disorder F18.288
      psychosis F18.259
        delusions F18.250
        hallucinations F18.251
      unspecified disorder F18.29
    in remission F18.21
  nicotine F17.200
    with disorder F17.209
      remission F17.201
      specified disorder NEC F17.208
      withdrawal F17.203
    chewing tobacco F17.220
      with disorder F17.229
      remission F17.221
      specified disorder NEC F17.228
      withdrawal F17.223
    cigarettes F17.210
      with disorder F17.219
      remission F17.211
      specified disorder NEC F17.218
      withdrawal F17.213
    specified product NEC F17.290
      with disorder F17.299
      remission F17.291
      specified disorder NEC F17.298
      withdrawal F17.293
  opioid F11.20
    with
      intoxication F11.229
        with
          delirium F11.221
          perceptual disturbance F11.222
        uncomplicated F11.220
      mood disorder F11.24
      other specified disorder F11.288
      psychosis F11.259
        delusions F11.250
        hallucinations F11.251
      sexual dysfunction F11.281
      sleep disorder F11.282
      unspecified disorder F11.29
      withdrawal F11.23
    in remission F11.21

Dependence (on) (syndrome) F19.20 — *continued*
drug NEC F19.20
  psychoactive NEC F19.20
    with
      amnestic disorder F19.26
      anxiety disorder F19.280
      dementia F19.27
      intoxication F19.229
        with
          delirium F19.221
          perceptual disturbance F19.222
        uncomplicated F19.220
      mood disorder F19.24
      other specified disorder F19.288
      psychosis F19.259
        delusions F19.250
        hallucinations F19.251
      sexual dysfunction F19.281
      sleep disorder F19.282
      unspecified disorder F19.29
      withdrawal F19.239
        with
          delirium F19.231
          perceptual disturbance F19.232
        uncomplicated F19.230
  sedative, hypnotic or anxiolytic F13.20
    with
      amnestic disorder F13.26
      anxiety disorder F13.280
      dementia, persisting F13.27
      intoxication F13.229
        with delirium F13.221
        uncomplicated F13.220
      mood disorder F13.24
      other specified disorder F13.288
      psychosis F13.259
        delusions F13.250
        hallucinations F13.251
      sexual dysfunction F13.281
      sleep disorder F13.282
      unspecified disorder F13.29
      withdrawal F13.239
        with
          delirium F13.231
          perceptual disturbance F13.232
        uncomplicated F13.230
    in remission F13.21
  stimulant NEC F15.20
    with
      anxiety disorder F15.280
      intoxication F15.229
        with
          delirium F15.221
          perceptual disturbance F15.222
        uncomplicated F15.220
      mood disorder F15.24
      other specified disorder F15.288
      psychosis F15.259
        delusions F15.250
        hallucinations F15.251
      sexual dysfunction F15.281
      sleep disorder F15.282
      unspecified disorder F15.29
      withdrawal F15.23
    in remission F15.21
  ethyl
    alcohol (without remission) F10.20
      with remission F10.21
    bromide — *see* Dependence, drug, sedative
  carbamate F19.20
  chloride F19.20
  morphine — *see* Dependence, drug, opioid
  ganja — *see* Dependence, drug, cannabis
  glue (airplane) (sniffing) — *see* Dependence, drug, inhalant
  glutethimide — *see* Dependence, drug, sedative
  hallucinogenics — *see* Dependence, drug, hallucinogen
  hashish — *see* Dependence, drug, cannabis
  hemp — *see* Dependence, drug, cannabis
  heroin (salt) (any) — *see* Dependence, drug, opioid
  hypnotic NEC — *see* Dependence, drug, sedative
  Indian hemp — *see* Dependence, drug, cannabis
  inhalants — *see* Dependence, drug, inhalant
  khat — *see* Dependence, drug, stimulant NEC
  laudanum — *see* Dependence, drug, opioid

Dependence (on) (syndrome) F19.20 — *continued*
LSD(-25) (derivatives) — *see* Dependence, drug, hallucinogen
luminal — *see* Dependence, drug, sedative
lysergic acid — *see* Dependence, drug, hallucinogen
maconha — *see* Dependence, drug, cannabis
marihuana — *see* Dependence, drug, cannabis
meprobamate — *see* Dependence, drug, sedative
mescaline — *see* Dependence, drug, hallucinogen
methadone — *see* Dependence, drug, opioid
methamphetamine(s) — *see* Dependence, drug, stimulant NEC
methaqualone — *see* Dependence, drug, sedative
methyl
  alcohol (without remission) F10.20
    with remission F10.21
  bromide — *see* Dependence, drug, sedative
  morphine — *see* Dependence, drug, opioid
  phenidate — *see* Dependence, drug, stimulant NEC
  sulfonal — *see* Dependence, drug, sedative
morphine (sulfate) (sulfite) (type) — *see* Dependence, drug, opioid
narcotic (drug) NEC — *see* Dependence, drug, opioid
nembutal — *see* Dependence, drug, sedative
neraval — *see* Dependence, drug, sedative
neravan — *see* Dependence, drug, sedative
neurobarb — *see* Dependence, drug, sedative
nicotine — *see* Dependence, drug, nicotine
nitrous oxide F19.20
nonbarbiturate sedatives and tranquilizers with similar effect — *see* Dependence, drug, sedative
on
  artificial heart (fully implantable) (mechanical) Z95.812
  aspirator Z99.0
  care provider (because of) Z74.9
    impaired mobility Z74.09
    need for
      assistance with personal care Z74.1
      continuous supervision Z74.3
    no other household member able to render care Z74.2
    specified reason NEC Z74.8
  machine Z99.89
    enabling NEC Z99.89
    specified type NEC Z99.89
  renal dialysis (hemodialysis) (peritoneal) Z99.2
  respirator Z99.11
  ventilator Z99.11
  wheelchair Z99.3
opiate — *see* Dependence, drug, opioid
opioids — *see* Dependence, drug, opioid
opium (alkaloids) (derivatives) (tincture) — *see* Dependence, drug, opioid
oxygen (long-term) (supplemental) Z99.81
paraldehyde — *see* Dependence, drug, sedative
paregoric — *see* Dependence, drug, opioid
PCP (phencyclidine) (see also Abuse, drug, hallucinogen) F16.20
pentobarbital — *see* Dependence, drug, sedative
pentobarbitone (sodium) — *see* Dependence, drug, sedative
pentothal — *see* Dependence, drug, sedative
peyote — *see* Dependence, drug, hallucinogen
phencyclidine (PCP) (and related substances) (see also Abuse, drug, hallucinogen) F16.20
phenmetrazine — *see* Dependence, drug, stimulant NEC
phenobarbital — *see* Dependence, drug, sedative
polysubstance F19.20
psilocibin, psilocin, psilocyn, psilocyline — *see* Dependence, drug, hallucinogen
psychostimulant NEC — *see* Dependence, drug, stimulant NEC
secobarbital — *see* Dependence, drug, sedative
seconal — *see* Dependence, drug, sedative

Dependence (on) (syndrome) F19.20 — *continued*
sedative NEC — *see* Dependence, drug, sedative
specified drug NEC — *see* Dependence, drug
stimulant NEC — *see* Dependence, drug, stimulant NEC
substance NEC — *see* Dependence, drug
supplemental oxygen Z99.81
tobacco — *see* Dependence, drug, nicotine
  counseling and surveillance Z71.6
tranquilizer NEC — *see* Dependence, drug, sedative
vitamin B6 E53.1
volatile solvents — *see* Dependence, drug, inhalant
Dependency
care-provider Z74.9
passive F60.7
reactions (persistent) F60.7
Depersonalization (in neurotic state) (neurotic) (syndrome) F48.1
Depletion
extracellular fluid E86.9
plasma E86.1
potassium E87.6
  nephropathy N25.89
salt or sodium E87.1
  causing heat exhaustion or prostration T67.4
  nephropathy N28.9
volume NOS E86.9
Deployment (current) (military) status Z56.82
in theater or in support of military war, peacekeeping and humanitarian operations Z56.82
personal history of Z91.82
  military war, peacekeeping and humanitarian deployment (current or past conflict) Z91.82
returned from Z91.82
Depolarization, premature I49.40
atrial I49.1
junctional I49.2
specified NEC I49.49
ventricular I49.3
Deposit
bone in Boeck's sarcoid D86.89
calcareous, calcium — *see* Calcification
cholesterol
  retina H35.89
  vitreous (body) (humor) — *see* Deposit, crystalline
conjunctiva H11.11-
cornea H18.00-
  argentous H18.02-
  due to metabolic disorder H18.03-
  Kayser-Fleischer ring H18.04-
  pigmentation — *see* Pigmentation, cornea
crystalline, vitreous (body) (humor) H43.2-
hemosiderin in old scars of cornea — *see* Pigmentation, cornea, stromal
metallic in lens — *see* Cataract, specified NEC
skin R23.8
tooth, teeth (betel) (black) (green) (materia alba) (orange) (tobacco) K03.6
urate, kidney — *see* Calculus, kidney
Depraved appetite — *see* Pica
Depressed
HDL cholesterol E78.6
Depression (acute) (mental) F32.9
agitated (single episode) F32.2
anaclitic — *see* Disorder, adjustment
anxiety F41.8
  persistent F34.1
arches — *see also* Deformity, limb, flat foot
atypical (single episode) F32.8
basal metabolic rate R94.8
bone marrow D75.89
central nervous system R09.2
cerebral R29.818
  newborn P91.4
cerebrovascular I67.9
chest wall M95.4
climacteric (single episode) F32.8
endogenous (without psychotic symptoms) F33.2
  with psychotic symptoms F33.3
functional activity R68.89
hysterical F44.89
involutional (single episode) F32.8
major F32.9
  with psychotic symptoms F32.3
  recurrent — *see* Disorder, depressive, recurrent

Depression (acute) (mental) F32.9 — *continued*
manic-depressive — *see* Disorder, depressive, recurrent
masked (single episode) F32.8
medullary G93.89
menopausal (single episode) F32.8
metatarsus — *see* Depression, arches
monopolar F33.9
nervous F34.1
neurotic F34.1
nose M95.0
postnatal F53
postpartum F53
post-psychotic of schizophrenia F32.8
post-schizophrenic F32.8
psychogenic (reactive) (single episode) F32.9
psychoneurotic F34.1
psychotic (single episode) F32.3
  recurrent F33.3
reactive (psychogenic) (single episode) F32.9
  psychotic (single episode) F32.3
recurrent — *see* Disorder, depressive, recurrent
respiratory center G93.89
seasonal — *see* Disorder, depressive, recurrent
senile F03
severe, single episode F32.2
situational F43.21
skull Q67.4
specified NEC (single episode) F32.8
sternum M95.4
visual field — *see* Defect, visual field
vital (recurrent) (without psychotic symptoms) F33.2
  with psychotic symptoms F33.3
  single episode F32.2
Deprivation
cultural Z60.3
effects NOS T73.9
  specified NEC T73.8
emotional NEC Z65.8
  affecting infant or child — *see* Maltreatment, child, psychological
food T73.0
protein — *see* Malnutrition
sleep Z72.820
social Z60.4
  affecting infant or child — *see* Maltreatment, child, psychological
specified NEC T73.8
vitamins — *see* Deficiency, vitamin
water T73.1
Derangement
ankle (internal) — *see* Derangement, joint, ankle
cartilage (articular) NEC — *see* Derangement, joint, articular cartilage, by site
  recurrent — *see* Dislocation, recurrent
cruciate ligament, anterior, current injury — *see* Sprain, knee, cruciate, anterior
elbow (internal) — *see* Derangement, joint, elbow
hip (joint) (internal) (old) — *see* Derangement, joint, hip
joint (internal) M24.9
  ankylosis — *see* Ankylosis
  articular cartilage M24.10
    ankle M24.17-
    elbow M24.12-
    foot M24.17-
    hand M24.14-
    hip M24.15-
    knee NEC M23.9-
    loose body — *see* Loose, body
    shoulder M24.11-
    wrist M24.13-
  contracture — *see* Contraction, joint
  current injury — *see also* Dislocation
    knee, meniscus or cartilage — *see* Tear, meniscus
  dislocation
    pathological — *see* Dislocation, pathological
    recurrent — *see* Dislocation, recurrent
  knee — *see* Derangement, knee
  ligament — *see* Disorder, ligament
  loose body — *see* Loose, body
  recurrent — *see* Dislocation, recurrent
  specified type NEC M24.80
    ankle M24.87-
    elbow M24.82-
    foot joint M24.87-
    hand joint M24.84-
    hip M24.85-
    shoulder M24.81-

Derangement — *continued*
joint (internal) M24.9 — *continued*
specified type NEC M24.80 — *continued*
wrist M24.83-
temporomandibular M26.69
knee (recurrent) M23.9-
ligament disruption, spontaneous M23.60-
anterior cruciate M23.61-
capsular M23.67-
instability, chronic M23.5-
lateral collateral M23.64-
medial collateral M23.63-
posterior cruciate M23.62-
loose body M23.4-
meniscus M23.30-
cystic M23.00-
lateral M23.002
anterior horn M23.04-
posterior horn M23.05-
specified NEC M23.06-
medial M23.005
anterior horn M23.01-
posterior horn M23.02-
specified NEC M23.03-
degenerate — *see* Derangement, knee, meniscus, specified NEC
detached — *see* Derangement, knee, meniscus, specified NEC
due to old tear or injury M23.20-
lateral M23.20-
anterior horn M23.24-
posterior horn M23.25-
specified NEC M23.26-
medial M23.20-
anterior horn M23.21-
posterior horn M23.22-
specified NEC M23.23-
retained — *see* Derangement, knee, meniscus, specified NEC
specified NEC M23.30-
lateral M23.30-
anterior horn M23.34-
posterior horn M23.35-
specified NEC M23.36-
medial M23.30-
anterior horn M23.31-
posterior horn M23.32-
specified NEC M23.33-
old M23.8x-
specified NEC — *see subcategory* M23.8
low back NEC — *see* Dorsopathy, specified NEC
meniscus — *see* Derangement, knee, meniscus
mental — *see* Psychosis
patella, specified NEC — *see* Disorder, patella, derangement NEC
semilunar cartilage (knee) — *see* Derangement, knee, meniscus, specified NEC
shoulder (internal) — *see* Derangement, joint, shoulder
Dercum's disease E88.2
Derealization (neurotic) F48.1
Dermal — *see* condition
Dermaphytid — *see* Dermatophytosis
Dermatitis (eczematous) L30.9
ab igne L59.0
acarine B88.0
actinic (due to sun) L57.8
other than from sun L59.8
allergic — *see* Dermatitis, contact, allergic
ambustionis, due to burn or scald — *see* Burn
amebic A06.7
ammonia L22
arsenical (ingested) L27.8
artefacta L98.1
psychogenic F54
atopic L20.9
psychogenic F54
specified NEC L20.89
autoimmune progesterone L30.8
berlock, berloque L56.2
blastomycotic B40.3
blister beetle L24.89
bullous, bullosa L13.9
mucosynechial, atrophic L12.1
seasonal L30.8
specified NEC L13.8
calorica L59.0
due to burn or scald — *see* Burn
caterpillar L24.89
cercarial B65.3
combustionis L59.0
due to burn or scald — *see* Burn
congelationis T69.1

Dermatitis (eczematous) L30.9 — *continued*
contact (occupational) L25.9
allergic L23.9
due to
adhesives L23.1
cement L23.5
chemical products NEC L23.5
chromium L23.0
cosmetics L23.2
dander (cat) (dog) L23.81
drugs in contact with skin L23.3
dyes L23.4
food in contact with skin L23.6
hair (cat) (dog) L23.81
insecticide L23.5
metals L23.0
nickel L23.0
plants, non-food L23.7
plastic L23.5
rubber L23.5
specified agent NEC L23.89
due to
cement L25.3
chemical products NEC L25.3
cosmetics L25.0
dander (cat) (dog) L23.81
drugs in contact with skin L25.1
dyes L25.2
food in contact with skin L25.4
hair (cat) (dog) L23.81
plants, non-food L25.5
specified agent NEC L25.8
irritant L24.9
due to
cement L25.3
chemical products NEC L24.5
cosmetics L24.3
detergents L24.0
drugs in contact with skin L24.4
food in contact with skin L24.6
oils and greases L24.1
plants, non-food L24.7
solvents L24.2
specified agent NEC L24.89
contusiformis L52
diabetic — *see* E08-E13 with .620
diaper L22
diphtheritica A36.3
dry skin L85.3
due to
acetone (contact) (irritant) L24.2
acids (contact) (irritant) L24.5
adhesive(s) (allergic) (contact) (plaster) L23.1
irritant L24.5
alcohol (irritant) (skin contact) (substances in category T51) L24.2
taken internally L27.8
alkalis (contact) (irritant) L24.5
arsenic (ingested) L27.8
carbon disulfide (contact) (irritant) L24.2
caustics (contact) (irritant) L24.5
cement (contact) L25.3
cereal (ingested) L27.2
chemical(s) NEC L25.3
taken internally L27.8
chlorocompounds L24.2
chromium (contact) (irritant) L24.81
coffee (ingested) L27.2
cold weather L30.8
cosmetics (contact) L25.0
allergic L23.2
irritant L24.3
cyclohexanes L24.2
dander (cat) (dog) L23.81
Demodex species B88.0
Dermanyssus gallinae B88.0
detergents (contact) (irritant) L24.0
dichromate L24.81
drugs and medicaments (generalized) (internal use) L27.0
external — *see* Dermatitis, due to, drugs, in contact with skin
in contact with skin L25.1
allergic L23.3
irritant L24.4
localized skin eruption L27.1
specified substance — *see* Table of Drugs and Chemicals
dyes (contact) L25.2
allergic L23.4
irritant L24.89
epidermophytosis — *see* Dermatophytosis
esters L24.2
external irritant NEC L24.9
fish (ingested) L27.2
flour (ingested) L27.2
food (ingested) L27.2
in contact with skin L25.4

Dermatitis (eczematous) L30.9 — *continued*
due to — *continued*
fruit (ingested) L27.2
furs (allergic) (contact) L23.81
glues — *see* Dermatitis, due to, adhesives
glycols L24.2
greases NEC (contact) (irritant) L24.1
hair (cat) (dog) L23.81
hot
objects and materials — *see* Burn
weather or places L59.0
hydrocarbons L24.2
infrared rays L59.8
ingestion, ingested substance L27.9
chemical NEC L27.8
drugs and medicaments — *see* Dermatitis, due to, drugs
food L27.2
specified NEC L27.8
insecticide in contact with skin L24.5
internal agent L27.9
drugs and medicaments (generalized) — *see* Dermatitis, due to, drugs
food L27.2
irradiation — *see* Dermatitis, due to, radioactive substance
ketones L24.2
lacquer tree (allergic) (contact) L23.7
light (sun) NEC L57.8
acute L56.8
other L59.8
Liponyssoides sanguineus B88.0
low temperature L30.8
meat (ingested) L27.2
metals, metal salts (contact) (irritant) L24.81
milk (ingested) L27.2
nickel (contact) (irritant) L24.81
nylon (contact) (irritant) L24.5
oils NEC (contact) (irritant) L24.1
paint solvent (contact) (irritant) L24.2
petroleum products (contact) (irritant) (substances in T52.0) L24.2
plants NEC (contact) L25.5
allergic L23.7
irritant L24.7
plasters (adhesive) (any) (allergic) (contact) L23.1
irritant L24.5
plastic (contact) L25.3
preservatives (contact) — *see* Dermatitis, due to, chemical, in contact with skin
primrose (allergic) (contact) L23.7
primula (allergic) (contact) L23.7
radiation L59.8
nonionizing (chronic exposure) L57.8
sun NEC L57.8
acute L56.8
radioactive substance L58.9
acute L58.0
chronic L58.1
radium L58.9
acute L58.0
chronic L58.1
ragweed (allergic) (contact) L23.7
Rhus (allergic) (contact) (diversiloba) (radicans) (toxicodendron) (venenata) (verniciflua) L23.7
rubber (contact) L24.5
Senecio jacobaea (allergic) (contact) L23.7
solvents (contact) (irritant) (substances in category T52) L24.2
specified agent NEC (contact) L25.8
allergic L23.89
irritant L24.89
sunshine NEC L57.8
acute L56.8
tetrachlorethylene (contact) (irritant) L24.2
toluene (contact) (irritant) L24.2
turpentine (contact) L24.2
ultraviolet rays (sun NEC) (chronic exposure) L57.8
acute L56.8
vaccine or vaccination L27.0
specified substance — *see* Table of Drugs and Chemicals
varicose veins — *see* Varix, leg, with, inflammation
X-rays L58.9
acute L58.0
chronic L58.1
dyshydrotic L30.1
dysmenorrheica N94.6
escharotica — *see* Burn
exfoliative, exfoliativa (generalized) L26
neonatorum L00

Dermatitis (eczematous) L30.9 — *continued*
eyelid — *see also* Dermatosis, eyelid
allergic H01.119
left H01.116
lower H01.115
upper H01.114
right H01.113
lower H01.112
upper H01.111
contact — *see* Dermatitis, eyelid, allergic
due to
Demodex species B88.0
herpes (zoster) B02.39
simplex B00.59
eczematous H01.139
left H01.136
lower H01.135
upper H01.134
right H01.133
lower H01.132
upper H01.131
facta, factitia, factitial L98.1
psychogenic F54
flexural NEC L20.82
friction L30.4
fungus B36.9
specified type NEC B36.8
gangrenosa, gangrenous infantum L08.0
harvest mite B88.0
heat L59.0
herpesviral, vesicular (ear) (lip) B00.1
herpetiformis (bullous) (erythematous) (pustular) (vesicular) L13.0
juvenile L12.2
senile L12.0
hiemalis L30.8
hypostatic, hypostatica — *see* Varix, leg, with, inflammation
infectious eczematoid L30.3
infective L30.3
irritant — *see* Dermatitis, contact, irritant
Jacquet's (diaper dermatitis) L22
Leptus B88.0
lichenified NEC L28.0
medicamentosa (generalized) (internal use) — *see* Dermatitis, due to drugs
mite B88.0
multiformis L13.0
juvenile L12.2
napkin L22
neurotica L13.0
nummular L30.0
papillaris capillitii L73.0
pellagrous E52
perioral L71.0
photocontact L56.2
polymorpha dolorosa L13.0
pruriginosa L13.0
pruritic NEC L30.8
psychogenic F54
purulent L08.0
pustular
contagious B08.02
subcorneal L13.1
pyococcal L08.0
pyogenica L08.0
repens L40.2
Ritter's (exfoliativa) L00
Schamberg's L81.7
schistosome B65.3
seasonal bullous L30.8
seborrheic L21.9
infantile L21.1
specified NEC L21.8
sensitization NOS L23.9
septic L08.0
solare L57.8
specified NEC L30.8
stasis I87.2
with varicose ulcer — *see* Varix, leg, with ulcer, with inflammation
due to postthrombotic syndrome — *see* Syndrome, postthrombotic
suppurative L08.0
traumatic NEC L30.4
trophoneurotica L13.0
ultraviolet (sun) (chronic exposure) L57.8
acute L56.8
varicose — *see* Varix, leg, with, inflammation
vegetans L10.1
verrucosa B43.0
vesicular, herpesviral B00.1
Dermatoarthritis, lipoid E78.81

Dermatochalasis, eyelid H02.839
  left H02.836
    lower H02.835
    upper H02.834
  right H02.833
    lower H02.832
    upper H02.831
Dermatofibroma (lenticulare) — *see* Neoplasm, skin, benign
  protuberans — *see* Neoplasm, skin, uncertain behavior
Dermatofibrosarcoma (pigmented) (protuberans) — *see* Neoplasm, skin, malignant
Dermatographia L50.3
Dermatolysis (exfoliativa) (congenital) Q82.8
  acquired L57.4
  eyelids — *see* Blepharochalasis
  palpebrarum — *see* Blepharochalasis
  senile L57.4
Dermatomegaly NEC Q82.8
Dermatomucosomyositis M33.10
  with
    myopathy M33.12
    respiratory involvement M33.11
    specified organ involvement NEC M33.19
Dermatomycosis B36.9
  furfuracea B36.0
  specified type NEC B36.8
Dermatomyositis (acute) (chronic) — *see also* Dermatopolymyositis
  in (due to) neoplastic disease (*see also* Neoplasm) D49.9 [M36.0]
Dermatoneuritis of children — *see* Poisoning, mercury
Dermatophilosis A48.8
Dermatophytid L30.2
Dermatophytide — *see* Dermatophytosis
Dermatophytosis (epidermophyton) (infection) (Microsporum) (tinea) (Trichophyton) B35.9
  beard B35.0
  body B35.4
  capitis B35.0
  corporis B35.4
  deep-seated B35.8
  disseminated B35.8
  foot B35.3
  granulomatous B35.8
  groin B35.6
  hand B35.2
  nail B35.1
  perianal (area) B35.6
  scalp B35.0
  specified NEC B35.8
Dermatopolymyositis M33.90
  with
    myopathy M33.92
    respiratory involvement M33.91
    specified organ involvement NEC M33.99
  in neoplastic disease (*see also* Neoplasm) D49.9 [M36.0]
  juvenile M33.00
    with
      myopathy M33.02
      respiratory involvement M33.01
      specified organ involvement NEC M33.09
    specified NEC M33.10
      myopathy M33.12
      respiratory involvement M33.11
      specified organ involvement NEC M33.19
Dermatopolyneuritis — *see* Poisoning, mercury
Dermatorrhexis Q79.6
  acquired L57.4
Dermatosclerosis — *see also* Scleroderma
  localized L94.0
Dermatosis L98.9
  Andrews' L08.89
  Bowen's — *see* Neoplasm, skin, in situ
  bullous L13.9
    specified NEC L13.8
  exfoliativa L26
  eyelid (noninfectious)
    dermatitis — *see* Dermatitis, eyelid
    discoid lupus erythematosus — *see* Lupus, erythematosus, eyelid
    xeroderma — *see* Xeroderma, acquired, eyelid
  factitial L98.1
  febrile neutrophilic L98.2

Dermatosis L98.9 — *continued*
  gonococcal A54.89
  herpetiformis L13.0
    juvenile L12.2
  linear IgA L13.8
  menstrual NEC L98.8
  neutrophilic, febrile L98.2
  occupational — *see* Dermatitis, contact
  papulosa nigra L82.1
  pigmentary L81.9
    progressive L81.7
    Schamberg's L81.7
  psychogenic F54
  purpuric, pigmented L81.7
  pustular, subcorneal L13.1
  transient acantholytic L11.1
Dermographia, dermographism L50.3
Dermoid (cyst) — *see also* Neoplasm, benign, by site
  with malignant transformation C56-
  due to radiation (nonionizing) L57.8
Dermopathy
  infiltrative with thyrotoxicosis — *see* Thyrotoxicosis
  nephrogenic fibrosing L90.8
Descemet's membrane — *see* condition
Descemetocele H18.73-
Descending — *see* condition
Descensus uteri — *see* Prolapse, uterus
Desert
  rheumatism B38.0
  sore — *see* Ulcer, skin
Desertion (newborn) — *see* Maltreatment
Desmoid (extra-abdominal) (tumor) — *see* Neoplasm, connective tissue, uncertain behavior
  abdominal D48.1
Despondency F32.9
Desquamation, skin R23.4
Destruction, destructive — *see also* Damage
  articular facet — *see also* Derangement, joint, specified type NEC
    knee M23.8x-
    vertebra — *see* Spondylosis
  bone — *see also* Disorder, bone, specified type NEC
    syphilitic A52.77
  joint — *see also* Derangement, joint, specified type NEC
    sacroiliac M53.3
  rectal sphincter K62.89
  septum (nasal) J34.89
  tuberculous NEC — *see* Tuberculosis
  tympanum, tympanic membrane (nontraumatic) — *see* Disorder, tympanic membrane, specified NEC
  vertebral disc — *see* Degeneration, intervertebral disc
Destructiveness — *see also* Disorder, conduct
  adjustment reaction — *see* Disorder, adjustment
Desultory labor O62.2
Detachment
  cartilage — *see* Sprain
  cervix, annular N88.8
    complicating delivery O71.3
  choroid (old) (postinfectional) (simple) (spontaneous) H31.40-
    hemorrhagic H31.41-
    serous H31.42-
  ligament — *see* Sprain
  meniscus (knee) — *see also* Derangement, knee, meniscus, specified NEC
    current injury — *see* Tear, meniscus
    due to old tear or injury — *see* Derangement, knee, meniscus, due to old tear
  retina (without retinal break) (serous) H33.2-
    with retinal:
      break H33.00-
        giant H33.03-
        multiple H33.02-
        single H33.01-
      dialysis H33.04-
    pigment epithelium — *see* Degeneration, retina, separation of layers, pigment epithelium detachment
    rhegmatogenous — *see* Detachment, retina, with retinal, break
    specified NEC H33.8
    total H33.05-
    traction H33.4-
  vitreous (body) H43.81
Detergent asthma J69.8

Deterioration
  epileptic F06.8
  general physical R53.81
  heart, cardiac — *see* Degeneration, myocardial
  mental — *see* Psychosis
  myocardial, myocardium — *see* Degeneration, myocardial
  senile (simple) R54
Deuteranomaly (anomalous trichromat) H53.53
Deuteranopia (complete) (incomplete) H53.53
Development
  abnormal, bone Q79.9
  arrested R62.50
    bone — *see* Arrest, development or growth, bone
    child R62.50
    due to malnutrition E45
  defective, congenital — *see also* Anomaly, by site
    cauda equina Q06.3
    left ventricle Q24.8
      in hypoplastic left heart syndrome Q23.4
    valve Q24.8
      pulmonary Q22.3
  delayed (*see also* Delay, development) R62.50
    arithmetical skills F81.2
    language (skills) (expressive) F80.1
    learning skill F81.9
    mixed skills F88
    motor coordination F82
    reading F81.0
    specified learning skill NEC F81.89
    speech F80.9
    spelling F81.81
    written expression F81.81
  imperfect, congenital — *see also* Anomaly, by site
    heart Q24.9
    lungs Q33.6
  incomplete
    bronchial tree Q32.4
    organ or site not listed — *see* Hypoplasia, by site
    respiratory system Q34.9
  sexual, precocious NEC E30.1
  tardy, mental (*see also* Disability, intellectual) F79
Developmental — *see* condition
  testing, child — *see* Examination, child
Devergie's disease (pityriasis rubra pilaris) L44.0
Deviation (in)
  conjugate palsy (eye) (spastic) H51.0
  esophagus (acquired) K22.8
  eye, skew H51.8
  midline (jaw) (teeth) (dental arch) M26.29
    specified site NEC — *see* Malposition
  nasal septum J34.2
    congenital Q67.4
  opening and closing of the mandible M26.53
  organ or site, congenital NEC — *see* Malposition, congenital
  septum (nasal) (acquired) J34.2
    congenital Q67.4
  sexual F65.9
    bestiality F65.89
    erotomania F52.8
    exhibitionism F65.2
    fetishism, fetishistic F65.0
      transvestism F65.1
    frotteurism F65.81
    masochism F65.51
    multiple F65.89
    necrophilia F65.89
    nymphomania F52.8
    pederosis F65.4
    pedophilia F65.4
    sadism, sadomasochism F65.52
    satyriasis F52.8
    specified type NEC F65.89
    transvestism F64.1
    voyeurism F65.3
  teeth, midline M26.29
  trachea J39.8
  ureter, congenital Q62.61
Devic's disease G36.0
Device
  cerebral ventricle (communicating) in situ Z98.2
  contraceptive — *see* Contraceptive, device
  drainage, cerebrospinal fluid, in situ Z98.2
Devil's
  grip B33.0
  pinches (purpura simplex) D69.2

Devitalized tooth K04.99
Devonshire colic — *see* Poisoning, lead
Dextraposition, aorta Q20.3
  in tetralogy of Fallot Q21.3
Dextrinosis, limit (debrancher enzyme deficiency) E74.03
Dextrocardia (true) Q24.0
  with
    complete transposition of viscera Q89.3
    situs inversus Q89.3
Dextrotransposition, aorta Q20.3
d-glycericacidemia E72.59
Dhat syndrome F48.8
Dhobi itch B35.6
Diabetes, diabetic (mellitus) (sugar) E11.9
  with
    amyotrophy E11.44
    arthropathy NEC E11.618
    autonomic (poly)neuropathy E11.43
    cataract E11.36
    Charcôt's joints E11.610
    chronic kidney disease E11.22
    circulatory complication NEC E11.59
    complication E11.8
      specified NEC E11.69
    dermatitis E11.620
    foot ulcer E11.621
    gangrene E11.52
    gastroparesis E11.43
    glomerulonephrosis, intracapillary E11.21
    glomerulosclerosis, intercapillary E11.21
    hyperglycemia E11.65
    hyperosmolarity E11.00
      with coma E11.01
    hypoglycemia E11.649
      with coma E11.641
    kidney complications NEC E11.29
    Kimmelstiel-Wilson disease E11.21
    loss of protective sensation (LOPS) — *see* Diabetes, by type, with neuropathy
    mononeuropathy E11.41
    myasthenia E11.44
    necrobiosis lipoidica E11.620
    nephropathy E11.21
    neuralgia E11.42
    neurologic complication NEC E11.49
    neuropathic arthropathy E11.610
    neuropathy E11.42
    ophthalmic complication NEC E11.39
    oral complication NEC E11.638
    periodontal disease E11.630
    peripheral angiopathy E11.51
      with gangrene E11.52
    polyneuropathy E11.42
    renal complication NEC E11.29
    renal tubular degeneration E11.29
    retinopathy E11.319
      with macular edema E11.311
      nonproliferative E11.329
        with macular edema E11.321
        mild E11.329
          with macular edema E11.321
        moderate E11.339
          with macular edema E11.331
        severe E11.349
          with macular edema E11.341
      proliferative E11.359
        with macular edema E11.351
    skin complication NEC E11.628
    skin ulcer NEC E11.622
  bronzed E83.110
  complicating pregnancy — *see* Pregnancy, complicated by, diabetes
  dietary counseling and surveillance Z71.3
  due to drug or chemical E09.9
    with
      amyotrophy E09.44
      arthropathy NEC E09.618
      autonomic (poly)neuropathy E09.43
      cataract E09.36
      Charcôt's joints E09.610
      chronic kidney disease E09.22
      circulatory complication NEC E09.59
      complication E09.8
        specified NEC E09.69
      dermatitis E09.620
      foot ulcer E09.621
      gangrene E09.52
      gastroparesis E09.43
      glomerulonephrosis, intracapillary E09.21
      glomerulosclerosis, intercapillary E09.21

D I S E A S E I N D E X

Diabetes, diabetic (mellitus) (sugar) E11.9 — continued
  due to drug or chemical E09.9 — continued
    with — continued
      hyperglycemia E09.65
      hyperosmolarity E09.00
        with coma E09.01
      hypoglycemia E09.649
        with coma E09.641
      ketoacidosis E09.10
        with coma E09.11
      kidney complications NEC E09.29
      Kimmelstiel-Wilson disease E09.21
      mononeuropathy E09.41
      myasthenia E09.44
      necrobiosis lipoidica E09.620
      nephropathy E09.21
      neuralgia E09.42
      neurologic complication NEC E09.49
      neuropathic arthropathy E09.610
      neuropathy E09.40
      ophthalmic complication NEC E09.39
      oral complication NEC E09.638
      periodontal disease E09.630
      peripheral angiopathy E09.51
        with gangrene E09.52
      polyneuropathy E09.42
      renal complication NEC E09.29
      renal tubular degeneration E09.29
      retinopathy E09.319
        with macular edema E09.311
        nonproliferative E09.329
          with macular edema E09.321
          mild E09.329
            with macular edema E09.321
          moderate E09.339
            with macular edema E09.331
          severe E09.349
            with macular edema E09.341
        proliferative E09.359
          with macular edema E09.351
      skin complication NEC E09.628
      skin ulcer NEC E09.622
  due to underlying condition E08.9
    with
      amyotrophy E08.44
      arthropathy NEC E08.618
      autonomic (poly)neuropathy E08.43
      cataract E08.36
      Charcôt's joints E08.610
      chronic kidney disease E08.22
      circulatory complication NEC E08.59
      complication E08.8
        specified NEC E08.69
      dermatitis E08.620
      foot ulcer E08.621
      gangrene E08.52
      gastroparesis E08.43
      glomerulonephrosis, intracapillary E08.21
      glomerulosclerosis, intercapillary E08.21
      hyperglycemia E08.65
      hyperosmolarity E08.00
        with coma E08.01
      hypoglycemia E08.649
        with coma E08.641
      ketoacidosis E08.10
        with coma E08.11
      kidney complications NEC E08.29
      Kimmelstiel-WIlson disease E08.21
      mononeuropathy E08.41
      myasthenia E08.44
      necrobiosis lipoidica E08.620
      nephropathy E08.21
      neuralgia E08.42
      neurologic complication NEC E08.49
      neuropathic arthropathy E08.610
      neuropathy E08.40
      ophthalmic complication NEC E08.39
      oral complication NEC E08.638
      periodontal disease E08.630
      peripheral angiopathy E08.51
        with gangrene E08.52
      polyneuropathy E08.42
      renal complication NEC E08.29
      renal tubular degeneration E08.29
      retinopathy E08.319
        with macular edema E08.311
        nonproliferative E08.329
          with macular edema E08.321
          mild E08.329
            with macular edema E08.321
          moderate E08.339
            with macular edema E08.331
          severe E08.349
            with macular edema E08.341
        proliferative E08.359
          with macular edema E08.351

Diabetes, diabetic (mellitus) (sugar) E11.9 — continued
  due to underlying condition E08.9 — continued
    with — continued
      skin complication NEC E08.628
      skin ulcer NEC E08.622
  gestational (in pregnancy) O24.419
    affecting newborn P70.0
    diet controlled O24.410
    in childbirth O24.429
      diet controlled O24.420
      insulin (and diet) controlled O24.424
    insulin (and diet) controlled O24.414
    puerperal O24.439
      diet controlled O24.430
      insulin (and diet) controlled O24.434
  hepatogenous E13.9
  inadequately controlled — code to Diabetes, by type, with hyperglycemia
  insipidus E23.2
    nephrogenic N25.1
    pituitary E23.2
    vasopressin resistant N25.1
  insulin dependent — code to type of diabetes
  juvenile-onset — see Diabetes, type 1
  ketosis-prone — see Diabetes, type 1
  latent R73.09
  neonatal (transient) P70.2
  non-insulin dependent — code to type of diabetes
  out of control — code to Diabetes, by type, with hyperglycemia
  phosphate E83.39
  poorly controlled — code to Diabetes, by type, with hyperglycemia
  postpancreatectomy — see Diabetes, specified type NEC
  postprocedural — see Diabetes, specified type NEC
  secondary diabetes mellitus NEC — see Diabetes, specified type NEC
  specified type NEC E13.9
    with
      amyotrophy E13.44
      arthropathy NEC E13.618
      autonomic (poly)neuropathy E13.43
      cataract E13.36
      Charcôt's joints E13.610
      chronic kidney disease E13.22
      circulatory complication NEC E13.59
      complication E13.8
        specified NEC E13.69
      dermatitis E13.620
      foot ulcer E13.621
      gangrene E13.52
      gastroparesis E13.43
      glomerulonephrosis, intracapillary E13.21
      glomerulosclerosis, intercapillary E13.21
      hyperglycemia E13.65
      hyperosmolarity E13.00
        with coma E13.01
      hypoglycemia E13.649
        with coma E13.641
      ketoacidosis E13.10
        with coma E13.11
      kidney complications NEC E13.29
      Kimmelstiel-Wilson disease E13.21
      mononeuropathy E13.41
      myasthenia E13.44
      necrobiosis lipoidica E13.620
      nephropathy E13.21
      neuralgia E13.42
      neurologic complication NEC E13.49
      neuropathic arthropathy E13.610
      neuropathy E13.40
      ophthalmic complication NEC E13.39
      oral complication NEC E13.638
      periodontal disease E13.630
      peripheral angiopathy E13.51
        with gangrene E13.52
      polyneuropathy E13.42
      renal complication NEC E13.29
      renal tubular degeneration E13.29
      retinopathy E13.319
        with macular edema E13.311
        nonproliferative E13.329
          with macular edema E13.321
          mild E13.329
            with macular edema E13.321
          moderate E13.339
            with macular edema E13.331
          severe E13.349
            with macular edema E13.341
        proliferative E13.359
          with macular edema E13.351
      skin complication NEC E13.628

Diabetes, diabetic (mellitus) (sugar) E11.9 — continued
  specified type NEC E13.9 — continued
    with — continued
      skin ulcer NEC E13.622
  steroid-induced — see Diabetes, due to, drug or chemical
  type 1 E10.9
    with
      amyotrophy E10.44
      arthropathy NEC E10.618
      autonomic (poly)neuropathy E10.43
      cataract E10.36
      Charcôt's joints E10.610
      chronic kidney disease E10.22
      circulatory complication NEC E10.59
      complication E10.8
        specified NEC E10.69
      dermatitis E10.620
      foot ulcer E10.621
      gangrene E10.52
      gastroparesis E10.43
      glomerulonephrosis, intracapillary E10.21
      glomerulosclerosis, intercapillary E10.21
      hyperglycemia E10.65
      hypoglycemia E10.649
        with coma E10.641
      ketoacidosis E10.10
        with coma E10.11
      kidney complications NEC E10.29
      Kimmelstiel-Wilson disease E10.21
      mononeuropathy E10.41
      myasthenia E10.44
      necrobiosis lipoidica E10.620
      nephropathy E10.21
      neuralgia E10.42
      neurologic complication NEC E10.49
      neuropathic arthropathy E10.610
      neuropathy E10.40
      ophthalmic complication NEC E10.39
      oral complication NEC E10.638
      periodontal disease E10.630
      peripheral angiopathy E10.51
        with gangrene E10.52
      polyneuropathy E10.42
      renal complication NEC E10.29
      renal tubular degeneration E10.29
      retinopathy E10.319
        with macular edema E10.311
        nonproliferative E10.329
          with macular edema E10.321
          mild E10.329
            with macular edema E10.321
          moderate E10.339
            with macular edema E10.331
          severe E10.349
            with macular edema E10.341
        proliferative E10.359
          with macular edema E10.351
      skin complication NEC E10.628
      skin ulcer NEC E10.622
  type 2 E11.9
    with
      amyotrophy E11.44
      arthropathy NEC E11.618
      autonomic (poly)neuropathy E11.43
      cataract E11.36
      Charcôt's joints E11.610
      chronic kidney disease E11.22
      circulatory complication NEC E11.59
      complication E11.8
        specified NEC E11.69
      dermatitis E11.620
      foot ulcer E11.621
      gangrene E11.52
      gastroparesis E11.43
      glomerulonephrosis, intracapillary E11.21
      glomerulosclerosis, intercapillary E11.21
      hyperglycemia E11.65
      hyperosmolarity E11.00
        with coma E11.01
      hypoglycemia E11.649
        with coma E11.641
      kidney complications NEC E11.29
      Kimmelstiel-Wilson disease E11.21
      mononeuropathy E11.41
      myasthenia E11.44
      necrobiosis lipoidica E11.620
      nephropathy E11.21
      neuralgia E11.42
      neurologic complication NEC E11.49
      neuropathic arthropathy E11.610
      neuropathy E11.40
      ophthalmic complication NEC E11.39
      oral complication NEC E11.638

Diabetes, diabetic (mellitus) (sugar) E11.9 — continued
  type 2 E11.9 — continued
    with — continued
      periodontal disease E11.630
      peripheral angiopathy E11.51
        with gangrene E11.52
      polyneuropathy E11.42
      renal complication NEC E11.29
      renal tubular degeneration E11.29
      retinopathy E11.319
        with macular edema E11.311
        nonproliferative E11.329
          with macular edema E11.321
          mild E11.329
            with macular edema E11.321
          moderate E11.339
            with macular edema E11.331
          severe E11.349
            with macular edema E11.341
        proliferative E11.359
          with macular edema E11.351
      skin complication NEC E11.628
      skin ulcer NEC E11.622
Diacyclothrombopathia D69.1
Diagnosis deferred R69
Dialysis (intermittent) (treatment)
  noncompliance (with) Z91.15
  renal (hemodialysis) (peritoneal), status Z99.2
  retina, retinal — see Detachment, retina, with retinal, dialysis
Diamond-Blackfan anemia (congenital hypoplastic) D61.01
Diamond-Gardener syndrome (autoerythrocyte sensitization) D69.2
Diaper rash L22
Diaphoresis (excessive) R61
Diaphragm — see condition
Diaphragmalgia R07.1
Diaphragmatitis, diaphragmitis J98.6
Diaphysial aclasis Q78.6
Diaphysitis — see Osteomyelitis, specified type NEC
Diarrhea, diarrheal (disease) (infantile) (inflammatory) R19.7
  achlorhydric K31.83
  allergic K52.2
  amebic (see also Amebiasis) A06.0
    with abscess — see Abscess, amebic
    acute A06.0
    chronic A06.1
    nondysenteric A06.2
  bacillary — see Dysentery, bacillary
  balantidial A07.0
  cachectic NEC K52.89
  Chilomastix A07.8
  choleriformis A00.1
  chronic (noninfectious) K52.9
  coccidial A07.3
  Cochin-China K90.1
    strongyloidiasis B78.0
  Dientamoeba A07.8
  dietetic K52.2
  drug-induced K52.1
  due to
    bacteria A04.9
      specified NEC A04.8
    Campylobacter A04.5
    Capillaria philippinensis B81.1
    Clostridium difficile A04.7
    Clostridium perfringens (C) (F) A04.8
    Cryptosporidium A07.2
    drugs K52.1
    Escherichia coli A04.4
      enteroaggregative A04.4
      enterohemorrhagic A04.3
      enteroinvasive A04.2
      enteropathogenic A04.0
      enterotoxigenic A04.1
      specified NEC A04.4
    food hypersensitivity K52.2
    Necator americanus B76.1
    S. japonicum B65.2
    specified organism NEC A08.8
      bacterial A04.8
      viral A08.39
    Staphylococcus A04.8
    Trichuris trichiuria B79
    virus — see Enteritis, viral
    Yersinia enterocolitica A04.6
  dysenteric A09
  endemic A09
  epidemic A09
  flagellate A07.9
  Flexner's (ulcerative) A03.1
  functional K59.1
    following gastrointestinal surgery K91.89
    psychogenic F45.8

Diarrhea, diarrheal (disease) (infantile) (inflammatory) R19.7 — *continued*
  Giardia lamblia A07.1
  giardial A07.1
  hill K90.1
  infectious A09
  malarial — *see* Malaria
  mite B88.0
  mycotic NEC B49
  neonatal (noninfectious) P78.3
  nervous F45.8
  neurogenic K59.1
  noninfectious K52.9
  postgastrectomy K91.1
  postvagotomy K91.1
  protozoal A07.9
    specified NEC A07.8
  psychogenic F45.8
  specified
    bacterium NEC A04.8
    virus NEC A08.39
  strongyloidiasis B78.0
  toxic K52.1
  trichomonal A07.8
  tropical K90.1
  tuberculous A18.32
  viral — *see* Enteritis, viral
Diastasis
  cranial bones M84.88
    congenital NEC Q75.8
  joint (traumatic) — *see* Dislocation
  muscle M62.00
    ankle M62.07-
    congenital Q79.8
    foot M62.07-
    forearm M62.03-
    hand M62.04-
    lower leg M62.06-
    pelvic region M62.05-
    shoulder region M62.01-
    specified site NEC M62.08
    thigh M62.05-
    upper arm M62.02-
  recti (abdomen)
    complicating delivery O71.89
    congenital Q79.59
Diastema, tooth, teeth, fully erupted M26.32
Diastematomyelia Q06.2
Diataxia, cerebral G80.4
Diathesis
  allergic — *see* History, allergy
  bleeding (familial) D69.9
  cystine (familial) E72.00
  gouty — *see* Gout
  hemorrhagic (familial) D69.9
    newborn NEC P53
  spasmophilic R29.0
Diaz's disease or osteochondrosis (juvenile) (talus) — *see* Osteochondrosis, juvenile, tarsus
Dibothriocephalus, dibothriocephaliasis (latus) (infection) (infestation) B70.0
  larval B70.1
Dicephalus, dicephaly Q89.4
Dichotomy, teeth K00.2
Dichromat, dichromatopsia (congenital) — *see* Deficiency, color vision
Dichuchwa A65
Dicroceliasis B66.2
Didelphia, didelphys — *see* Double uterus
Didymytis N45.1
  with orchitis N45.3
Dietary
  inadequacy or deficiency E63.9
  surveillance and counseling Z71.3
Dietl's crisis N13.8
Dieulafoy lesion (hemorrhagic)
  duodenum K31.82
  esophagus K22.8
  intestine (colon) K63.81
  stomach K31.82
Difficult, difficulty (in)
  acculturation Z60.3
  feeding R63.3
    newborn P92.9
      breast P92.5
      specified NEC P92.8
    nonorganic (infant or child) F98.29
  intubation, in anesthesia T88.4
  mechanical, gastroduodenal stoma K91.89
    causing obstruction K91.3
  reading (developmental) F81.0
    secondary to emotional disorders F93.9
  spelling (specific) F81.81
    with reading disorder F81.89
    due to inadequate teaching Z55.8

Difficult, difficulty (in) — *continued*
  swallowing — *see* Dysphagia
  walking R26.2
  work
    conditions NEC Z56.5
    schedule Z56.3
Diffuse — *see* condition
Di George's syndrome (thymic hypoplasia) D82.1
Di Guglielmo's disease C94.0-
Digestive — *see* condition
Dihydropyrimidine dehydrogenase disease (DPD) E88.89
Diktyoma — *see* Neoplasm, malignant, by site
Dilaceration, tooth K00.4
Dilatation
  anus K59.8
    venule — *see* Hemorrhoids
  aorta (focal) (general) — *see* Ectasia, aorta
    with aneuysm — *see* Aneurysm, aorta
  artery — *see* Aneurysm
  bladder (sphincter) N32.89
    congenital Q64.79
  blood vessel I99.8
  bronchial J47.9
    with
      exacerbation (acute) J47.1
      lower respiratory infection J47.0
  calyx (due to obstruction) — *see* Hydronephrosis
  capillaries I78.8
  cardiac (acute) (chronic) — *see also* Hypertrophy, cardiac
    congenital Q24.8
    valve NEC Q24.8
      pulmonary Q22.3
    valve — *see* Endocarditis
  cavum septi pellucidi Q06.8
  cervix (uteri) — *see also* Incompetency, cervix
    incomplete, poor, slow complicating delivery O62.0
  colon K59.3
    congenital Q43.1
    psychogenic F45.8
  common duct (acquired) K83.8
    congenital Q44.5
  cystic duct (acquired) K82.8
    congenital Q44.5
  duct, mammary — *see* Ectasia, mammary duct
  duodenum K59.8
  esophagus K22.8
    congenital Q39.5
    due to achalasia K22.0
  eustachian tube, congenital Q17.8
  gallbladder K82.8
  gastric — *see* Dilatation, stomach
  heart (acute) (chronic) — *see also* Hypertrophy, cardiac
    congenital Q24.8
    valve — *see* Endocarditis
  ileum K59.8
    psychogenic F45.8
  jejunum K59.8
    psychogenic F45.8
  kidney (calyx) (collecting structures) (cystic) (parenchyma) (pelvis) (idiopathic) N28.89
  lacrimal passages or duct — *see* Disorder, lacrimal system, changes
  lymphatic vessel I89.0
  mammary duct — *see* Ectasia, mammary duct
  Meckel's diverticulum (congenital) Q43.0
    malignant — *see* Table of Neoplasms, small intestine, malignant
  myocardium (acute) (chronic) — *see* Hypertrophy, cardiac
  organ or site, congenital NEC — *see* Distortion
  pancreatic duct K86.8
  pericardium — *see* Pericarditis
  pharynx J39.2
  prostate N42.89
  pulmonary
    artery (idiopathic) I28.8
    valve, congenital Q22.3
  pupil H57.04
  rectum K59.3
  saccule, congenital Q16.5
  salivary gland (duct) K11.8
  sphincter ani K62.89
  stomach K31.89
    acute K31.0
    psychogenic F45.8
  submaxillary duct K11.8
  trachea, congenital Q32.1

Dilatation — *continued*
  ureter (idiopathic) N28.82
    congenital Q62.2
    due to obstruction N13.4
  urethra (acquired) N36.8
  vasomotor I73.9
  vein I86.8
  ventricular, ventricle (acute) (chronic) — *see also* Hypertrophy, cardiac
    cerebral, congenital Q04.8
    venule NEC I86.8
  vesical orifice N32.89
Dilated, dilation — *see* Dilatation
Diminished, diminution
  hearing (acuity) — *see* Deafness
  sense or sensation (cold) (heat) (tactile) (vibratory) R20.8
  vision NEC H54.7
  vital capacity R94.2
Diminuta taenia B71.0
Dimitri-Sturge-Weber disease Q85.8
Dimple
  parasacral, pilonidal or postanal — *see* Cyst, pilonidal
Dioctophyme renalis (infection) (infestation) B83.8
Dipetalonemiasis B74.4
Diphallus Q55.69
Diphtheria, diphtheritic (gangrenous) (hemorrhagic) A36.9
  carrier (suspected) Z22.2
  cutaneous A36.3
  faucial A36.0
  infection of wound A36.3
  laryngeal A36.2
  myocarditis A36.81
  nasal, anterior A36.89
  nasopharyngeal A36.1
  neurological complication A36.89
  pharyngeal A36.0
  specified site NEC A36.89
  tonsillar A36.0
Diphyllobothriasis (intestine) B70.0
  larval B70.1
Diplacusis H93.22-
Diplegia (upper limbs) G83.0
  congenital (cerebral) G80.8
  facial G51.0
  lower limbs G82.20
  spastic G80.1
Diplococcus, diplococcal — *see* condition
Diplopia H53.2
Dipsomania F10.20
  with
    psychosis — *see* Psychosis, alcoholic
  remission F10.21
Dipylidiasis B71.1
Direction, teeth, abnormal, fully erupted M26.30
Dirofilariasis B74.8
Dirt-eating child F98.3
Disability, disabilities
  heart — *see* Disease, heart
  intellectual F79
    with
      autistic features F84.9
    mild (I.Q. 50-69) F70
    moderate (I.Q. 35-49) F71
    profound (I.Q. under 20) F73
    severe (I.Q. 20-34) F72
    specified level NEC F78
  knowledge acquisition F81.9
  learning F81.9
  limiting activities Z73.6
  spelling, specific F81.81
Disappearance of family member Z63.4
Disarticulation — *see* Amputation
  meaning traumatic amputation — *see* Amputation, traumatic
Discharge (from)
  abnormal finding in — *see* Abnormal, specimen
  breast (female) (male) N64.52
  diencephalic autonomic idiopathic — *see* Epilepsy, specified NEC
  ear — *see also* Otorrhea
    blood — *see* Otorrhagia
  excessive urine R35.8
  nipple N64.52
  penile R36.9
  postnasal R09.82
  prison, anxiety concerning Z65.2
  urethral R36.9
    hematospermia R36.1
    without blood R36.0
  vaginal N89.8
Discitis, diskitis M46.40
  cervical region M46.42
  cervicothoracic region M46.43
  lumbar region M46.46

Discitis, diskitis M46.40 — *continued*
  lumbosacral region M46.47
  multiple sites M46.49
  occipito-atlanto-axial region M46.41
  pyogenic — *see* Infection, intervertebral disc, pyogenic
  sacrococcygeal region M46.48
  thoracic region M46.44
  thoracolumbar region M46.45
Discoid
  meniscus (congenital) Q68.6
  semilunar cartilage (congenital) — *see* Derangement, knee, meniscus, specified NEC
Discoloration
  nails L60.8
  teeth (posteruptive) K03.7
    during formation K00.8
Discomfort
  chest R07.89
  visual H53.14-
Discontinuity, ossicles, ear H74.2-
Discord (with)
  boss Z56.4
  classmates Z55.4
  counselor Z64.4
  employer Z56.4
  family Z63.8
  fellow employees Z56.4
  in-laws Z63.1
  landlord Z59.2
  lodgers Z59.2
  neighbors Z59.2
  probation officer Z64.4
  social worker Z64.4
  teachers Z55.4
  workmates Z56.4
Discordant connection
  atrioventricular (congenital) Q20.5
  ventriculoarterial Q20.3
Discrepancy
  centric occlusion maximum intercuspation M26.55
  leg length (acquired) — *see* Deformity, limb, unequal length
    congenital — *see* Defect, reduction, lower limb
  uterine size date O26.84-
Discrimination
  ethnic Z60.5
  political Z60.5
  racial Z60.5
  religious Z60.5
  sex Z60.5
Disease, diseased — *see also* Syndrome
  absorbent system I87.8
  acid-peptic K30
  Acosta's T70.29
  Adams-Stokes (-Morgagni) (syncope with heart block) I45.9
  Addison's anemia (pernicious) D51.0
  adenoids (and tonsils) J35.9
  adrenal (capsule) (cortex) (gland) (medullary) E27.9
    hyperfunction E27.0
    specified NEC E27.8
  ainhum L94.6
  airway
    obstructive, chronic J44.9
      due to
        cotton dust J66.0
        specific organic dusts NEC J66.8
    reactive — *see* Asthma
  akamushi (scrub typhus) A75.3
  Albers-Schönberg (marble bones) Q78.2
  Albert's — *see* Tendinitis, Achilles
  alimentary canal K63.9
  alligator-skin Q80.9
    acquired L85.0
  alpha heavy chain C88.3
  alpine T70.29
  altitude T70.20
  alveolar ridge
    edentulous K06.9
      specified NEC K06.8
  alveoli, teeth K08.9
  Alzheimer's G30.9 [F02.80]
    with behavioral disturbance G30.9 [F02.81]
    early onset G30.0 [F02.80]
      with behavioral disturbance G30.0 [F02.81]
    late onset G30.1 [F02.80]
      with behavioral disturbance G30.1 [F02.81]
    specified NEC G30.8 [F02.80]
      with behavioral disturbance G30.8 [F02.81]
  amyloid — *see* Amyloidosis
  Andersen's (glycogenosis IV) E74.09

DISEASE INDEX

Disease, diseased (*see also* Syndrome) — *continued*

Andes T70.29
Andrews' (bacterid) L08.89
angiospastic I73.9
  cerebral G45.9
  vein I87.8
anterior
  chamber H21.9
  horn cell G12.29
antiglomerular basement membrane (anti-GBM) antibody M31.0
  tubulo-interstitial nephritis N12
antral — *see* Sinusitis, maxillary
anus K62.9
  specified NEC K62.89
aorta (nonsyphilitic) I77.9
  syphilitic NEC A52.02
aortic (heart) (valve) I35.9
  rheumatic I06.9
Apollo B30.3
aponeuroses — *see* Enthesopathy
appendix K38.9
  specified NEC K38.8
aqueous (chamber) H21.9
Arnold-Chiari — *see* Arnold-Chiari disease
arterial I77.9
  occlusive — *see* Occlusion, by site
    due to stricture or stenosis I77.1
arteriocardiorenal — *see* Hypertension, cardiorenal
arteriolar (generalized) (obliterative) I77.9
arteriorenal — *see* Hypertension, kidney
arteriosclerotic — *see also* Arteriosclerosis
  cardiovascular — *see* Disease, heart, ischemic, atherosclerotic
  coronary (artery) — *see* Disease, heart, ischemic, atherosclerotic
  heart — *see* Disease, heart, ischemic, atherosclerotic
artery I77.9
  cerebral I67.9
  coronary I25.10
    with angina pectoris — *see* Arteriosclerosis, coronary (artery),
arthropod-borne NOS (viral) A94
  specified type NEC A93.8
atticoantral, chronic H66.20
  left H66.22
    with right H66.23
  right H66.21
    with left H66.23
auditory canal — *see* Disorder, ear, external
auricle, ear NEC — *see* Disorder, pinna
Australian X A83.4
autoimmune (systemic) NOS M35.9
  hemolytic (cold type) (warm type) D59.1
    drug-induced D59.0
  thyroid E06.3
aviator's — *see* Effect, adverse, high altitude
Ayala's Q78.5
Ayerza's (pulmonary artery sclerosis with pulmonary hypertension) I27.0
Babington's (familial hemorrhagic telangiectasia) I78.0
bacterial A49.9
  specified NEC A48.8
  zoonotic A28.9
    specified type NEC A28.8
Baelz's (cheilitis glandularis apostematosa) K13.0
bagasse J67.1
balloon — *see* Effect, adverse, high altitude
Bang's (brucella abortus) A23.1
Bannister's T78.3
barometer makers' — *see* Poisoning, mercury
Barraquer (-Simons') (progressive lipodystrophy) E88.1
Barrett's — *see* Barrett's, esophagus
Bartholin's gland N75.9
basal ganglia G25.9
  degenerative G23.9
    specified NEC G23.8
  specified NEC G25.89
Basedow's (exophthalmic goiter) — *see* Hyperthyroidism, with, goiter (diffuse)
Bateman's B08.1
Batten-Steinert G71.11
Battey A31.0
Beard's (neurasthenia) F48.8
Becker
  idiopathic mural endomyocardial I42.3
  myotonia congenita G71.12

Disease, diseased (*see also* Syndrome) — *continued*

Begbie's (exophthalmic goiter) — *see* Hyperthyroidism, with, goiter (diffuse)
behavioral, organic F07.9
Beigel's (white piedra) B36.2
Benson's — *see* Deposit, crystalline
Bernard-Soulier (thrombopathy) D69.1
Bernhardt (-Roth) — *see* Mononeuropathy, lower limb, meralgia paresthetica
Biermer's (pernicious anemia) D51.0
bile duct (common) (hepatic) K83.9
  with calculus, stones — *see* Calculus, bile duct
  specified NEC K83.8
biliary (tract) K83.9
  specified NEC K83.8
Billroth's — *see* Spina bifida
bird fancier's J67.2
black lung J60
bladder N32.9
  in (due to)
    schistosomiasis (bilharziasis) B65.0 [N33]
  specified NEC N32.89
bleeder's D66
blood D75.9
  forming organs D75.9
  vessel I99.9
Bloodgood's — *see* Mastopathy, cystic
Bodechtel-Guttmann (subacute sclerosing panencephalitis) A81.1
bone — *see also* Disorder, bone
  aluminum M83.4
  fibrocystic NEC
    jaw M27.49
bone-marrow D75.9
Borna A83.9
Bornholm (epidemic pleurodynia) B33.0
Bouchard's (myopathic dilatation of the stomach) K31.0
Bouillaud's (rheumatic heart disease) I01.9
Bourneville (-Brissaud) (tuberous sclerosis) Q85.1
Bouveret (-Hoffmann) (paroxysmal tachycardia) I47.9
bowel K63.9
  functional K59.9
    psychogenic F45.8
brain G93.9
  arterial, artery I67.9
  arteriosclerotic I67.2
  congenital Q04.9
  degenerative — *see* Degeneration, brain
  inflammatory — *see* Encephalitis
  organic G93.9
    arteriosclerotic I67.2
  parasitic NEC B71.9 [G94]
  senile NEC G31.1
  specified NEC G93.89
breast (*see also* Disorder, breast) N64.9
  cystic (chronic) — *see* Mastopathy, cystic
  fibrocystic — *see* Mastopathy, cystic
  Paget's
    female, unspecified side C50.91-
    male, unspecified side C50.92-
  specified NEC N64.89
Breda's — *see* Yaws
Bretonneau's (diphtheritic malignant angina) A36.0
Bright's — *see* Nephritis
  arteriosclerotic — *see* Hypertension, kidney
Brill's (recrudescent typhus) A75.1
Brill-Zinsser (recrudescent typhus) A75.1
Brion-Kayser — *see* Fever, paratyphoid
broad
  beta E78.2
  ligament (noninflammatory) N83.9
    inflammatory — *see* Disease, pelvis, inflammatory
    specified NEC N83.8
Brocq's
  meaning
    dermatitis herpetiformis L13.0
    prurigo L28.2
Brocq-Duhring (dermatitis herpetiformis) L13.0
bronchopulmonary J98.4
bronchus NEC J98.09
bronze Addison's E27.1
  tuberculous A18.7
budgerigar fancier's J67.2
Buerger's (thromboangiitis obliterans) I73.1
bullous L13.9
  chronic of childhood L12.2
  specified NEC L13.8

Disease, diseased (*see also* Syndrome) — *continued*

Bürger-Grütz (essential familial hyperlipemia) E78.3
bursa — *see* Bursopathy
caisson T70.3
California — *see* Coccidioidomycosis
capillaries I78.9
  specified NEC I78.8
Carapata A68.0
cardiac — *see* Disease, heart
cardiopulmonary, chronic I27.9
cardiorenal (hepatic) (hypertensive) (vascular) — *see* Hypertension, cardiorenal
cardiovascular (atherosclerotic) I25.10
  with angina pectoris — *see* Arteriosclerosis, coronary (artery),
  congenital Q28.9
  hypertensive — *see* Hypertension, heart
  newborn P29.9
    specified NEC P29.89
  renal (hypertensive) — *see* Hypertension, cardiorenal
  syphilitic (asymptomatic) A52.00
cartilage — *see* Disorder, cartilage
Castellani's A69.8
cat-scratch A28.1
Cavare's (familial periodic paralysis) G72.3
cecum K63.9
celiac (adult) (infantile) K90.0
cellular tissue L98.9
central core G71.2
cerebellar, cerebellum — *see* Disease, brain
cerebral — *see also* Disease, brain
  degenerative — *see* Degeneration, brain
cerebrospinal G96.9
cerebrovascular I67.9
  acute I67.89
    embolic I63.4-
    thrombotic I63.3-
  arteriosclerotic I67.2
  specified NEC I67.89
cervix (uteri) (noninflammatory) N88.9
  inflammatory — *see* Cervicitis
  specified NEC N88.8
Chabert's A22.9
Chandler's (osteochondritis dissecans, hip) — *see* Osteochondritis, dissecans, hip
Charlouis — *see* Yaws
Chédiak-Steinbrinck (-Higashi) (congenital gigantism of peroxidase granules) E70.330
chest J98.9
Chiari's (hepatic vein thrombosis) I82.0
Chicago B40.9
Chignon B36.8
chigo, chigoe B88.1
childhood granulomatous D71
Chinese liver fluke B66.1
chlamydial A74.9
  specified NEC A74.89
cholecystic K82.9
choroid H31.9
  specified NEC H31.8
Christmas D67
chronic bullous of childhood L12.2
chylomicron retention E78.3
ciliary body H21.9
  specified NEC H21.89
circulatory (system) NEC I99.8
  newborn P29.9
  syphilitic A52.00
    congenital A50.54
coagulation factor deficiency (congenital) — *see* Defect, coagulation
coccidioidal — *see* Coccidioidomycosis
cold
  agglutinin or hemoglobinuria D59.1
    paroxysmal D59.6
  hemagglutinin (chronic) D59.1
collagen NOS (nonvascular) (vascular) M35.9
  specified NEC M35.8
colon K63.9
  functional K59.9
    congenital Q43.2
  ischemic K55.0
combined system — *see* Degeneration, combined
compressed air T70.3
Concato's (pericardial polyserositis) A19.9
  nontubercular I31.1
  pleural — *see* Pleurisy, with effusion
conjunctiva H11.9
  chlamydial A74.0
  specified NEC H11.89
  viral B30.9
    specified NEC B30.8

Disease, diseased (*see also* Syndrome) — *continued*

connective tissue, systemic (diffuse) M35.9
  in (due to)
    hypogammaglobulinemia D80.1 [M36.8]
    ochronosis E70.29 [M36.8]
  specified NEC M35.8
Conor and Bruch's (boutonneuse fever) A77.1
Cooper's — *see* Mastopathy, cystic
Cori's (glycogenosis III) E74.03
corkhandler's or corkworker's J67.3
cornea H18.9
  specified NEC H18.89-
coronary (artery) — *see* Disease, heart, ischemic, atherosclerotic
  congenital Q24.5
  ostial, syphilitic (aortic) (mitral) (pulmonary) A52.03
corpus cavernosum N48.9
  specified NEC N48.89
Cotugno's — *see* Sciatica
coxsackie (virus) NEC B34.1
cranial nerve NOS G52.9
Creutzfeldt-Jakob — *see* Creutzfeldt-Jakob disease or syndrome
Crocq's (acrocyanosis) I73.89
Crohn's — *see* Enteritis, regional
Curschmann G71.11
cystic
  breast (chronic) — *see* Mastopathy, cystic
  kidney, congenital Q61.9
  liver, congenital Q44.6
  lung J98.4
    congenital Q33.0
cytomegalic inclusion (generalized) B25.9
  with pneumonia B25.0
  congenital P35.1
cytomegaloviral B25.9
  specified NEC B25.8
Czerny's (periodic hydrarthrosis of the knee) — *see* Effusion, joint, knee
Daae (-Finsen) (epidemic pleurodynia) B33.0
Darling's — *see* Histoplasmosis capsulati
de Quervain's (tendon sheath) M65.4
  thyroid (subacute granulomatous thyroiditis) E06.1
Débove's (splenomegaly) R16.1
deer fly — *see* Tularemia
Degos' I77.89
demyelinating, demyelinizating (nervous system) G37.9
  multiple sclerosis G35
  specified NEC G37.8
dense deposit (*see also* N00-N07 with fourth character .6) N05.6
deposition, hydroxyapatite — *see* Disease, hydroxyapatite deposition
Devergie's (pityriasis rubra pilaris) L44.0
Devic's G36.0
diaphorase deficiency D74.0
diaphragm J98.6
diarrheal, infectious NEC A09
digestive system K92.9
  specified NEC K92.89
disc, degenerative — *see* Degeneration, intervertebral disc
discogenic — *see also* Displacement, intervertebral disc NEC
  with myelopathy — *see* Disorder, disc, with, myelopathy
diverticular — *see* Diverticula
Dubois (thymus) A50.59 [E35]
Duchenne's
  muscular dystrophy G71.0
  pseudohypertrophy, muscles G71.0
Duchenne-Griesinger G71.0
ductless glands E34.9
Duhring's (dermatitis herpetiformis) L13.0
duodenum K31.9
  specified NEC K31.89
Dupré's (meningism) R29.1
Dupuytren's (muscle contracture) M72.0
Durand-Nicholas-Favre (climatic bubo) A55
Duroziez's (congenital mitral stenosis) Q23.2
ear — *see* Disorder, ear
Eberth's — *see* Fever, typhoid
Ebola (virus) A98.4
Ebstein's heart Q22.5
Echinococcus — *see* Echinococcus
echovirus NEC B34.1

Disease, diseased (see also Syndrome) — continued

Eddowes' (brittle bones and blue sclera) Q78.0
edentulous (alveolar) ridge K06.9
  specified NEC K06.8
Edsall's T67.2
Eichstedt's (pityriasis versicolor) B36.0
Ellis-van Creveld (chondroectodermal dysplasia) Q77.6
end stage renal (ESRD) N18.6
  due to hypertension I12.0
endocrine glands or system NEC E34.9
endomyocardial (eosinophilic) I42.3
English (rickets) E55.0
enteroviral, enterovirus NEC B34.1
  central nervous system NEC A88.8
epidemic B99.9
  specified NEC B99.8
epididymis N50.9
Erb (-Landouzy) G71.0
Erdheim-Chester (ECD) E88.89
esophagus K22.9
  functional K22.4
    psychogenic F45.8
  specified NEC K22.8
Eulenburg's (congenital paramyotonia) G71.19
eustachian tube — see Disorder, eustachian tube
external
  auditory canal — see Disorder, ear, external
  ear — see Disorder, ear, external
extrapyramidal G25.9
  specified NEC G25.89
eye H57.9
  anterior chamber H21.9
  inflammatory NEC H57.8
  muscle (external) — see Strabismus
  specified NEC H57.8
  syphilitic — see Oculopathy, syphilitic
eyeball H44.9
  specified NEC H44.89
eyelid — see Disorder, eyelid
  specified NEC — see Disorder, eyelid, specified type NEC
eyeworm of Africa B74.3
facial nerve (seventh) G51.9
  newborn (birth injury) P11.3
Fahr (of brain) G23.8
Fahr Volhard (of kidney) I12-
fallopian tube (noninflammatory) N83.9
  inflammatory — see Salpingo-oophoritis
  specified NEC N83.8
familial periodic paralysis G72.3
Fanconi's (congenital pancytopenia) D61.09
fascia NEC — see also Disorder, muscle
  inflammatory — see Myositis
  specified NEC M62.89
Fauchard's (periodontitis) — see Periodontitis
Favre-Durand-Nicolas (climatic bubo) A55
Fede's K14.0
Feer's — see Poisoning, mercury
female pelvic inflammatory (see also Disease, pelvis, inflammatory) N73.9
  syphilitic (secondary) A51.42
  tuberculous A18.17
Fernels' (aortic aneurysm) I71.9
fibrocaseous of lung — see Tuberculosis, pulmonary
fibrocystic — see Fibrocystic disease
Fiedler's (leptospiral jaundice) A27.0
fifth B08.3
file-cutter's — see Poisoning, lead
fish-skin Q80.9
  acquired L85.0
Flajani (-Basedow) (exophthalmic goiter) — see Hyperthyroidism, with, goiter (diffuse)
flax-dresser's J66.1
fluke — see Infestation, fluke
foot-and-mouth B08.8
foot process N04.9
Forbes' (glycogenosis III) E74.03
Fordyce's (ectopic sebaceous glands) (mouth) Q38.6
Fordyce-Fox (apocrine miliaria) L75.2
Forestier's (rhizomelic pseudopolyarthritis) M35.3
  meaning ankylosing hyperostosis — see Hyperostosis, ankylosing
Fothergill's
  neuralgia — see Neuralgia, trigeminal
  scarlatina anginosa A38.9

Disease, diseased (see also Syndrome) — continued

Fournier (gangrene) N49.3
  female N76.89
fourth B08.8
Fox (-Fordyce) (apocrine miliaria) L75.2
Francis' — see Tularemia
Franklin C88.2
Frei's (climatic bubo) A55
Friedreich's
  combined systemic or ataxia G11.1
  myoclonia G25.3
frontal sinus — see Sinusitis, frontal
fungus NEC B49
Gaisböck's (polycythemia hypertonica) D75.1
gallbladder K82.9
  calculus — see Calculus, gallbladder
  cholecystitis — see Cholecystitis
  cholesterolosis K82.4
  fistula — see Fistula, gallbladder
  hydrops K82.1
  obstruction — see Obstruction, gallbladder
  perforation K82.2
  specified NEC K82.8
gamma heavy chain C88.2
Gamna's (siderotic splenomegaly) D73.2
Gamstorp's (adynamia episodica hereditaria) G72.3
Gandy-Nanta (siderotic splenomegaly) D73.2
ganister J62.8
gastric — see Disease, stomach
gastroesophageal reflux (GERD) K21.9
  with esophagitis K21.0
gastrointestinal (tract) K92.9
  amyloid E85.4
  functional K59.9
    psychogenic F45.8
  specified NEC K92.89
Gee (-Herter) (-Heubner) (-Thaysen) (nontropical sprue) K90.0
genital organs
  female N94.9
  male N50.9
Gerhardt's (erythromelalgia) I73.81
Gibert's (pityriasis rosea) L42
Gierke's (glycogenosis I) E74.01
Gilles de la Tourette's (motor-verbal tic) F95.2
gingiva K06.9
  specified NEC K06.8
gland (lymph) I89.9
Glanzmann's (hereditary hemorrhagic thrombasthenia) D69.1
glass-blower's (cataract) — see Cataract, specified NEC
  salivary gland hypertrophy K11.1
Glisson's — see Rickets
globe H44.9
  specified NEC H44.89
glomerular — see also Glomerulonephritis
  with edema — see Nephrosis
  acute — see Nephritis, acute
  chronic — see Nephritis, chronic
  minimal change N05.0
  rapidly progressive N01.9
glycogen storage E74.00
  Andersen's E74.09
  Cori's E74.03
  Forbes' E74.03
  generalized E74.00
  glucose-6-phosphatase deficiency E74.01
  heart E74.02 [I43]
  hepatorenal E74.09
  Hers' E74.09
  liver and kidney E74.09
  McArdle's E74.04
  muscle phosphofructokinase E74.09
  myocardium E74.02 [I43]
  Pompe's E74.02
  Tauri's E74.09
  type 0 E74.09
  type I E74.01
  type II E74.02
  type III E74.03
  type IV E74.09
  type V E74.04
  type VI-XI E74.09
  Von Gierke's E74.01
Goldstein's (familial hemorrhagic telangiectasia) I78.0
gonococcal NOS A54.9
graft-versus-host (GVH) D89.813
  acute D89.810
  acute on chronic D89.812
  chronic D89.811

Disease, diseased (see also Syndrome) — continued

grainhandler's J67.8
granulomatous (childhood) (chronic) D71
Graves' (exophthalmic goiter) — see Hyperthyroidism, with, goiter (diffuse)
Griesinger's — see Ancylostomiasis
Grisel's M43.6
Gruby's (tinea tonsurans) B35.0
Guillain-Barré G61.0
Guinon's (motor-verbal tic) F95.2
gum K06.9
gynecological N94.9
H (Hartnup's) E72.02
Haff — see Poisoning, mercury
Hageman (congenital factor XII deficiency) D68.2
hair (color) (shaft) L67.9
  follicles L73.9
    specified NEC L73.8
Hamman's (spontaneous mediastinal emphysema) J98.2
hand, foot and mouth B08.4
Hansen's — see Leprosy
Hantavirus, with pulmonary manifestations B33.4
  with renal manifestations A98.5
Harada's H30.81-
Hart's (pellagra-cerebellar ataxia-renal aminoaciduria) E72.02
Hartnup (pellagra-cerebellar ataxia-renal aminoaciduria) E72.02
Hashimoto's (struma lymphomatosa) E06.3
Hb — see Disease, hemoglobin
heart (organic) I51.9
  with
    pulmonary edema (acute) (see also Failure, ventricular, left) I50.1
    rheumatic fever (conditions in I00)
      active I01.9
        with chorea I02.0
        specified NEC I01.8
      inactive or quiescent (with chorea) I09.9
        specified NEC I09.89
  amyloid E85.4 [I43]
  aortic (valve) I35.9
  arteriosclerotic or sclerotic (senile) — see Disease, heart, ischemic, atherosclerotic
  artery, arterial — see Disease, heart, ischemic, atherosclerotic
  beer drinkers' I42.6
  beriberi (wet) E51.12
  black I27.0
  congenital Q24.9
    cyanotic Q24.9
    specified NEC Q24.8
  coronary — see Disease, heart, ischemic
  cryptogenic I51.9
  fibroid — see Myocarditis
  functional I51.89
    psychogenic F45.8
  glycogen storage E74.02 [I43]
  gonococcal A54.83
  hypertensive — see Hypertension, heart
  hyperthyroid (see also Hyperthyroidism) E05.90 [I43]
    with thyroid storm E05.91 [I43]
  ischemic (chronic or with a stated duration of over 4 weeks) I25.9
    atherosclerotic (of) I25.10
      with angina pectoris — see Arteriosclerosis, coronary (artery)
      coronary artery bypass graft — see Arteriosclerosis, coronary (artery),
    cardiomyopathy I25.5
    diagnosed on ECG or other special investigation, but currently presenting no symptoms I25.6
    silent I25.6
    specified form NEC I25.89
  kyphoscoliotic I27.1
  meningococcal A39.50
    endocarditis A39.51
    myocarditis A39.52
    pericarditis A39.53
  mitral I05.9
    specified NEC I05.8
  muscular — see Degeneration, myocardial
  psychogenic (functional) F45.8
  pulmonary (chronic) I27.9
    in schistosomiasis B65.9 [I52]
    specified NEC I27.89

Disease, diseased (see also Syndrome) — continued

heart (organic) I51.9 — continued
  rheumatic (chronic) (inactive) (old) (quiescent) (with chorea) I09.9
    active or acute I01.9
      with chorea (acute) (rheumatic) (Sydenham's) I02.0
    specified NEC I09.89
  senile — see Myocarditis
  syphilitic A52.06
    aortic A52.03
    aneurysm A52.01
    congenital A50.54 [I52]
  thyrotoxic (see also Thyrotoxicosis) E05.90 [I43]
    with thyroid storm E05.91 [I43]
  valve, valvular (obstructive) (regurgitant) — see also Endocarditis
    congenital NEC Q24.8
    pulmonary Q22.3
  vascular — see Disease, cardiovascular
heavy chain NEC C88.2
  alpha C88.3
  gamma C88.2
  mu C88.2
Hebra's
  pityriasis
    maculata et circinata L42
    rubra pilaris L44.0
  prurigo L28.2
hematopoietic organs D75.9
hemoglobin or Hb
  abnormal (mixed) NEC D58.2
    with thalassemia D56.9
  AS genotype D57.3
  Bart's D56.0
  C (Hb-C) D58.2
    with other abnormal hemoglobin NEC D58.2
    elliptocytosis D58.1
    Hb-S D57.2-
    sickle-cell D57.2-
    thalassemia D56.8
    Constant Spring D58.2
  D (Hb-D) D58.2
  E (Hb-E) D58.2
  E-beta thalassemia D56.5
  elliptocytosis D58.1
  H (Hb-H) (thalassemia) D56.0
    with other abnormal hemoglobin NEC D56.9
    Constant Spring D58.2
  I thalassemia D56.9
  M D74.0
  S or SS D57.1
  SC D57.2-
  SD D57.8-
  SE D57.8-
  spherocytosis D58.0
  unstable, hemolytic D58.2
hemolytic (newborn) P55.9
  autoimmune (cold type) (warm type) D59.1
  drug-induced D59.0
  due to
    incompatibility
      ABO (blood group) P55.1
      blood (group) (Duffy) (K(ell)) (Kidd) (Lewis) (M) (S) NEC P55.8
      Rh (blood group) (factor) P55.0
      Rh negative mother P55.0
    specified type NEC P55.8
  unstable hemoglobin D58.2
hemorrhagic D69.9
  newborn P53
Henoch (-Schönlein) (purpura nervosa) D69.0
hepatic — see Disease, liver
hepatobiliary K83.9
  toxic K71.9
hepatolenticular E83.01
heredodegenerative NEC
  spinal cord G95.89
herpesviral, disseminated B00.7
Hers' (glycogenosis VI) E74.09
Herter (-Gee) (-Heubner) (nontropical sprue) K90.0
Heubner-Herter (nontropical sprue) K90.0
high fetal gene or hemoglobin thalassemia D56.9
Hildenbrand's — see Typhus
hip (joint) M25.9
  congenital Q65.89
  suppurative M00.9
  tuberculous A18.02
His (-Werner) (trench fever) A79.0

Disease, diseased (see also Syndrome) — continued

Hodgson's I71.2
  ruptured I71.1
Holla — see Spherocytosis
hookworm B76.9
  specified NEC B76.8
host-versus-graft D89.813
  acute D89.810
  acute on chronic D89.812
  chronic D89.811
human immunodeficiency virus (HIV) B20
Huntington's G10
Hutchinson's (cheiropompholyx) — see Hutchinson's disease
hyaline (diffuse) (generalized)
  membrane (lung) (newborn) P22.0
  adult J80
hydatid — see Echinococcus
hydroxyapatite deposition M11.00
  ankle M11.07-
  elbow M11.02-
  foot joint M11.07-
  hand joint M11.04-
  hip M11.05-
  knee M11.06-
  multiple site M11.09
  shoulder M11.01-
  vertebra M11.08
  wrist M11.03-
hyperkinetic — see Hyperkinesia
hypertensive — see Hypertension
hypophysis E23.7
I-cell E77.0
Iceland G93.3
immune D89.9
immunoproliferative (malignant) C88.9
  small intestinal C88.3
  specified NEC C88.8
inclusion B25.9
  salivary gland B25.9
infectious, infective B99.9
  congenital P37.9
    specified NEC P37.8
    viral P35.9
      specified type NEC P35.8
  specified NEC B99.8
inflammatory
  penis N48.29
    abscess N48.21
    cellulitis N48.22
  prepuce N47.7
    balanoposthitis N47.6
  tubo-ovarian — see Salpingo-oophoritis
intervertebral disc — see also Disorder, disc
  with myelopathy — see Disorder, disc, with, myelopathy
  cervical, cervicothoracic — see Disorder, disc, cervical
    with
      myelopathy — see Disorder, disc, cervical, with myelopathy
      neuritis, radiculitis or radiculopathy — see Disorder, disc, cervical, with neuritis
    specified NEC — see Disorder, disc, cervical, specified type NEC
  lumbar (with)
    myelopathy M51.06
    neuritis, radiculitis, radiculopathy or sciatica M51.16
    specified NEC M51.86
  lumbosacral (with)
    neuritis, radiculitis, radiculopathy or sciatica M51.17
    specified NEC M51.87
  specified NEC — see Disorder, disc, specified NEC
  thoracic (with)
    myelopathy M51.04
    neuritis, radiculitis or radiculopathy M51.14
    specified NEC M51.84
  thoracolumbar (with)
    myelopathy M51.05
    neuritis, radiculitis or radiculopathy M51.15
    specified NEC M51.85
intestine K63.9
  functional K59.9
    psychogenic F45.8
    specified NEC K59.8
  organic K63.9
  protozoal A07.9
  specified NEC K63.89
iris H21.9
  specified NEC H21.89

Disease, diseased (see also Syndrome) — continued

iron metabolism or storage E83.10
island (scrub typhus) A75.3
itai-itai — see Poisoning, cadmium
Jakob-Creutzfeldt — see Creutzfeldt-Jakob disease or syndrome
jaw M27.9
  fibrocystic M27.49
  specified NEC M27.8
jigger B88.1
joint — see also Disorder, joint
  Charcot's — see Arthropathy, neuropathic (Charcot)
  degenerative — see Osteoarthritis
    multiple M15.9
    spine — see Spondylosis
  hypertrophic — see Osteoarthritis
  sacroiliac M53.3
  specified NEC — see Disorder, joint, specified type NEC
  spine NEC — see Dorsopathy
  suppurative — see Arthritis, pyogenic or pyemic
Jourdain's (acute gingivitis) K05.00
  nonplaque induced K05.01
  plaque induced K05.00
Kaschin-Beck (endemic polyarthritis) M12.10
  ankle M12.12-
  elbow M12.12-
  foot joint M12.17-
  hand joint M12.14-
  hip M12.15-
  knee M12.16-
  multiple site M12.19
  shoulder M12.11-
  vertebra M12.18
  wrist M12.13-
Katayama B65.2
Kedani (scrub typhus) A75.3
Keshan E59
kidney (functional) (pelvis) N28.9
  chronic N18.9
    hypertensive — see Hypertension, kidney
    stage 1 N18.1
    stage 2 (mild) N18.2
    stage 3 (moderate) N18.3
    stage 4 (severe) N18.4
    stage 5 N18.5
  complicating pregnancy — see Pregnancy, complicated by, renal disease
  cystic (congenital) Q61.9
  diabetic — see E08-E13 with .22
  fibrocystic (congenital) Q61.8
  hypertensive — see Hypertension, kidney
  in (due to)
    schistosomiasis (bilharziasis) B65.9 [N29]
  multicystic Q61.4
  polycystic Q61.3
    adult type Q61.2
    childhood type NEC Q61.19
      collecting duct dilatation Q61.11
Kimmelstiel (-Wilson) (intercapillary polycystic (congenital) glomerulosclerosis) — see E08-E13 with .21
Kimura D21.9
  specified site — see Neoplasm, connective tissue, benign
Kinnier Wilson's (hepatolenticular degeneration) E83.01
kissing — see Mononucleosis, infectious
Klebs' (see also Glomerulonephritis) N05.-
Klippel-Feil (brevicollis) Q76.1
Köhler-Pellegrini-Stieda (calcification, knee joint) — see Bursitis, tibial collateral
Kok Q89.8
König's (osteochondritis dissecans) — see Osteochondritis, dissecans
Korsakoff's (nonalcoholic) F04
  alcoholic F10.96
    with dependence F10.26
Kostmann's (infantile genetic agranulocytosis) D70.0
kuru A81.81
Kyasanur Forest A98.2
labyrinth, ear — see Disorder, ear, inner
lacrimal system — see Disorder, lacrimal system
Lafora's — see Epilepsy, generalized, idiopathic
Lancereaux-Mathieu (leptospiral jaundice) A27.0
Landry's G61.0

Disease, diseased (see also Syndrome) — continued

Larrey-Weil (leptospiral jaundice) A27.0
larynx J38.7
legionnaires' A48.1
  nonpneumonic A48.2
Lenegre's I44.2
lens H27.9
  specified NEC H27.8
Lev's (acquired complete heart block) I44.2
Lewy body (dementia) G31.83 [F02.80]
  with behavioral disturbance G31.83 [F02.81]
Lichtheim's (subacute combined sclerosis with pernicious anemia) D51.0
Lightwood's (renal tubular acidosis) N25.89
Lignac's (cystinosis) E72.04
lip K13.0
lipid-storage E75.6
  specified NEC E75.5
Lipschütz's N76.6
liver (chronic) (organic) K76.9
  alcoholic (chronic) K70.9
    acute — see Disease, liver, alcoholic, hepatitis
    cirrhosis K70.30
      with ascites K70.31
    failure K70.40
      with coma K70.41
    fatty liver K70.0
    fibrosis K70.2
    hepatitis K70.10
      with ascites K70.11
    sclerosis K70.2
  cystic, congenital Q44.6
  drug-induced (idiosyncratic) (toxic) (predictable) (unpredictable) — see Disease, liver, toxic
  end stage K72.90
    due to hepatitis — see Hepatitis
  fatty, nonalcoholic (NAFLD) K76.0
    alcoholic K70.0
  fibrocystic (congenital) Q44.6
  fluke
    Chinese B66.1
    oriental B66.1
    sheep B66.3
  glycogen storage E74.09 [K77]
  in (due to)
    schistosomiasis (bilharziasis) B65.9 [K77]
  inflammatory K75.9
    alcoholic K70.1
    specified NEC K75.89
  polycystic (congenital) Q44.6
  toxic K71.9
    with
      cholestasis K71.0
      cirrhosis (liver) K71.7
      fibrosis (liver) K71.7
      focal nodular hyperplasia K71.8
      hepatic granuloma K71.8
      hepatic necrosis K71.10
        with coma K71.11
      hepatitis NEC K71.6
        acute K71.2
        chronic
          active K71.50
            with ascites K71.51
          lobular K71.4
          persistent K71.3
      lupoid K71.50
        with ascites K71.51
      peliosis hepatis K71.8
      veno-occlusive disease (VOD) of liver K71.8
  veno-occlusive K76.5
Lobo's (keloid blastomycosis) B48.0
Lobstein's (brittle bones and blue sclera) Q78.0
Ludwig's (submaxillary cellulitis) K12.2
lumbosacral region M53.87
lung J98.4
  black J60
  congenital Q33.9
  cystic J98.4
    congenital Q33.0
  fibroid (chronic) — see Fibrosis, lung
  fluke B66.4
    oriental B66.4
  in
    amyloidosis E85.4 [J99]
    sarcoidosis D86.0
    Sjögren's syndrome M35.02
    systemic
      lupus erythematosus M32.13
      sclerosis M34.81

Disease, diseased (see also Syndrome) — continued

lung J98.4 — continued
  interstitial J84.9
    of childhood, specified NEC J84.848
    respiratory bronchiolitis J84.115
    specified NEC J84.89
  obstructive (chronic) J44.9
    with
      acute
        bronchitis J44.0
        exacerbation NEC J44.1
        lower respiratory infection J44.0
    alveolitis, allergic J67.9
    asthma J44.9
    bronchiectasis J47.9
      with
        exacerbation (acute) J47.1
        lower respiratory infection J47.0
    bronchitis J44.9
      with
        exacerbation (acute) J44.1
        lower respiratory infection J44.0
    emphysema J44.9
    hypersensitivity pneumonitis J67.9
    decompensated J44.1
      with
        exacerbation (acute) J44.1
  polycystic J98.4
    congenital Q33.0
  rheumatoid (diffuse) (interstitial) — see Rheumatoid, lung
Lutembacher's (atrial septal defect with mitral stenosis) Q21.1
Lyme A69.20
lymphatic (gland) (system) (channel) (vessel) I89.9
lymphoproliferative D47.9
  specified NEC D47.Z9
  T-gamma D47.Z9
  X-linked D82.3
Magitot's M27.2
malarial — see Malaria
malignant — see also Neoplasm, malignant, by site
Manson's B65.1
maple bark J67.6
maple-syrup-urine E71.0
Marburg (virus) A98.3
Marion's (bladder neck obstruction) N32.0
Marsh's (exophthalmic goiter) — see Hyperthyroidism, with, goiter (diffuse)
mastoid (process) — see Disorder, ear, middle
Mathieu's (leptospiral jaundice) A27.0
Maxcy's A75.2
McArdle (-Schmid-Pearson) (glycogenosis V) E74.04
mediastinum J98.5
medullary center (idiopathic) (respiratory) G93.89
Meige's (chronic hereditary edema) Q82.0
meningococcal — see Infection, meningococcal
mental F99
  organic F09
mesenchymal M35.9
mesenteric embolic K55.0
metabolic, metabolism E88.9
  bilirubin E80.7
metal-polisher's J62.8
metastatic (see also Neoplasm, secondary, by site) C79.9
microvascular — code to condition
microvillus
  atrophy Q43.8
  inclusion (MVD) Q43.8
middle ear — see Disorder, ear, middle
Mikulicz' (dryness of mouth, absent or decreased lacrimation) K11.8
Milroy's (chronic hereditary edema) Q82.0
Minamata — see Poisoning, mercury
minicore G71.2
Minor's G95.19
Minot's (hemorrhagic disease, newborn) P53
Minot-von Willebrand-Jürgens (angiohemophilia) D68.0
Mitchell's (erythromelalgia) I73.81
mitral (valve) I05.9
  nonrheumatic I34.9
mixed connective tissue M35.1
moldy hay J67.0
Monge's T70.29
Morgagni's (syndrome) (hyperostosis frontalis interna) M85.2

Disease, diseased (see also Syndrome) —
continued
Morgagni-Adams-Stokes (syncope with heart block) I45.9
Morton's (with metatarsalgia) — see Lesion, nerve, plantar
Morvan's G60.8
motor neuron (bulbar) (familial) (mixed type) (spinal) G12.20
amyotrophic lateral sclerosis G12.21
progressive bulbar palsy G12.22
specified NEC G12.29
moyamoya I67.5
mu heavy chain disease C88.2
multicore G71.2
muscle — see also Disorder, muscle
inflammatory — see Myositis
ocular (external) — see Strabismus
musculoskeletal system, soft tissue — see also Disorder, soft tissue
specified NEC — see Disorder, soft tissue, specified type NEC
mushroom workers' J67.5
mycotic B49
myelodysplastic, not classified C94.6
myeloproliferative, not classified C94.6
chronic D47.1
myocardium, myocardial (see also Degeneration, myocardial) I51.5
primary (idiopathic) I42.9
myoneural G70.9
Naegeli's D69.1
nails L60.9
specified NEC L60.8
Nairobi (sheep virus) A93.8
nasal J34.9
nemaline body G71.2
nerve — see Disorder, nerve
nervous system G98.8
autonomic G90.9
central G96.9
specified NEC G96.8
congenital Q07.9
parasympathetic G90.9
specified NEC G98.8
sympathetic G90.9
vegetative G90.9
neuromuscular system G70.9
Newcastle B30.8
Nicolas (-Durand)-Favre (climatic bubo) A55
nipple N64.9
Paget's C50.01-
female C50.01-
male C50.02-
Nishimoto (-Takeuchi) I67.5
nonarthropod-borne NOS (viral) B34.9
enterovirus NEC B34.1
nonautoimmune hemolytic D59.4
drug-induced D59.2
Nonne-Milroy-Meige (chronic hereditary edema) Q82.0
nose J34.9
nucleus pulposus — see Disorder, disc
nutritional E63.9
oast-house-urine E72.19
ocular
herpesviral B00.50
zoster B02.30
obliterative vascular I77.1
Ohara's — see Tularemia
Opitz's (congestive splenomegaly) D73.2
Oppenheim-Urbach (necrobiosis lipoidica diabeticorum) — see E08-E13 with .620
optic nerve NEC — see Disorder, nerve, optic
orbit — see Disorder, orbit
Oriental liver fluke B66.1
Oriental lung fluke B66.4
Ormond's N13.5
Oropouche virus A93.0
Osler-Rendu (familial hemorrhagic telangiectasia) I78.0
osteofibrocystic E21.0
Otto's M24.7
outer ear — see Disorder, ear, external
ovary (noninflammatory) N83.9
cystic N83.20
inflammatory — see Salpingo-oophoritis
polycystic E28.2
specified NEC N83.8
Owren's (congenital) — see Defect, coagulation
pancreas K86.9
cystic K86.2
fibrocystic E84.9
specified NEC K86.8
panvalvular I08.9
specified NEC I08.8

Disease, diseased (see also Syndrome) —
continued
parametrium (noninflammatory) N83.9
parasitic B89
cerebral NEC B71.9 [G94]
intestinal NOS B82.9
mouth B37.0
skin NOS B88.9
specified type — see Infestation
tongue B37.0
parathyroid (gland) E21.5
specified NEC E21.4
Parkinson's G20
parodontal K05.6
Parrot's (syphilitic osteochondritis) A50.02
Parry's (exophthalmic goiter) — see Hyperthyroidism, with, goiter (diffuse)
Parson's (exophthalmic goiter) — see Hyperthyroidism, with, goiter (diffuse)
Paxton's (white piedra) B36.2
pearl-worker's — see Osteomyelitis, specified type NEC
Pellegrini-Stieda (calcification, knee joint) — see Bursitis, tibial collateral
pelvis, pelvic
female NOS N94.9
specified NEC N94.89
gonococcal (acute) (chronic) A54.24
inflammatory (female) N73.9
acute N73.0
chronic N73.1
specified NEC N73.8
syphilitic (secondary) A51.42
late A52.76
tuberculous A18.17
organ, female N94.9
peritoneum, female NEC N94.89
penis N48.9
inflammatory N48.29
abscess N48.21
cellulitis N48.22
specified NEC N48.89
periapical tissues NOS K04.90
periodontal K05.6
specified NEC K05.5
periosteum — see Disorder, bone, specified type NEC
peripheral
arterial I73.9
autonomic nervous system G90.9
nerves — see Polyneuropathy
vascular NOS I73.9
peritoneum K66.9
pelvic, female NEC N94.89
specified NEC K66.8
Petit's — see Hernia, abdomen, specified site NEC
pharynx J39.2
specified NEC J39.2
Phocas' — see Mastopathy, cystic
photochromogenic (acid-fast bacilli) (pulmonary) A31.0
nonpulmonary A31.9
Pick's G31.01 [F02.80]
with behavioral disturbance G31.01 [F02.81]
pigeon fancier's J67.2
pineal gland E34.8
pink — see Poisoning, mercury
Pinkus' (lichen nitidus) L44.1
pinworm B80
Piry virus A93.8
pituitary (gland) E23.7
pituitary-snuff-taker's J67.8
pleura (cavity) J94.9
specified NEC J94.8
pneumatic drill (hammer) T75.21
Pollitzer's (hidradenitis suppurativa) L73.2
polycystic
kidney or renal Q61.3
adult type Q61.2
childhood type NEC Q61.19
collecting duct dilatation Q61.11
liver or hepatic Q44.6
lung or pulmonary J98.4
congenital Q33.0
ovary, ovaries E28.2
spleen Q89.09
polyethylene T84.05-
Pompe's (glycogenosis II) E74.02
Posadas-Wernicke B38.9
Potain's (pulmonary edema) — see Edema, lung

Disease, diseased (see also Syndrome) —
continued
prepuce N47.8
inflammatory N47.7
balanoposthitis N47.6
Pringle's (tuberous sclerosis) Q85.1
prion, central nervous system A81.9
specified NEC A81.89
prostate N42.9
specified NEC N42.89
protozoal B64
acanthamebiasis — see Acanthamebiasis
African trypanosomiasis — see African trypanosomiasis
babesiosis B60.0
Chagas disease — see Chagas disease
intestine, intestinal A07.9
leishmaniasis — see Leishmaniasis
malaria — see Malaria
naegleriasis B60.2
pneumocystosis B59
specified organism NEC B60.8
toxoplasmosis — see Toxoplasmosis
pseudo-Hurler's E77.0
psychiatric F99
psychotic — see Psychosis
Puente's (simple glandular cheilitis) K13.0
puerperal (see also Puerperal) O90.89
pulmonary — see also Disease, lung
artery I28.9
chronic obstructive J44.9
with
acute bronchitis J44.0
exacerbation (acute) J44.1
lower respiratory infection (acute) J44.0
decompensated J44.1
with
exacerbation (acute) J44.1
heart I27.9
specified NEC I27.89
hypertensive (vascular) I27.0
valve I37.9
rheumatic I09.89
pulp (dental) K04.90
pulseless M31.4
Putnam's (subacute combined sclerosis with pernicious anemia) D51.0
Pyle (-Cohn) (craniometaphyseal dysplasia) Q78.5
ragpicker's or ragsorter's A22.1
Raynaud's — see Raynaud's disease
reactive airway — see Asthma
Reclus' (cystic) — see Mastopathy, cystic
rectum K62.9
specified NEC K62.89
Refsum's (heredopathia atactica polyneuritiformis) G60.1
renal (functional) (pelvis) (see also Disease, kidney) N28.9
with
edema — see Nephrosis
glomerular lesion — see Glomerulonephritis
with edema — see Nephrosis
interstitial nephritis N12
acute N28.9
chronic (see also Disease, kidney, chronic) N18.9
cystic, congenital Q61.9
diabetic — see E08-E13 with .22
end-stage (failure) N18.6
due to hypertension I12.0
fibrocystic (congenital) Q61.8
hypertensive — see Hypertension, kidney
lupus M32.14
phosphate-losing (tubular) N25.0
polycystic (congenital) Q61.3
adult type Q61.2
childhood type NEC Q61.19
collecting duct dilatation Q61.11
rapidly progressive N01.9
subacute N01.9
Rendu-Osler-Weber (familial hemorrhagic telangiectasia) I78.0
renovascular (arteriosclerotic) — see Hypertension, kidney
respiratory (tract) J98.9
acute or subacute NOS J06.9
due to
chemicals, gases, fumes or vapors (inhalation) J68.3
external agent J70.9
specified NEC J70.8
radiation J70.0
smoke inhalation J70.5
noninfectious J39.8

Disease, diseased (see also Syndrome) —
continued
respiratory (tract) J98.9 — continued
chronic NOS J98.9
due to
chemicals, gases, fumes or vapors J68.4
external agent J70.9
specified NEC J70.8
radiation J70.1
newborn P27.9
specified NEC P27.8
due to
chemicals, gases, fumes or vapors J68.9
acute or subacute NEC J68.3
chronic J68.4
external agent J70.9
specified NEC J70.8
newborn P28.9
specified type NEC P28.89
upper J39.9
acute or subacute J06.9
noninfectious NEC J39.8
specified NEC J39.8
streptococcal J06.9
retina, retinal H35.9
Batten's or Batten-Mayou E75.4 [H36]
specified NEC H35.89
rheumatoid — see Arthritis, rheumatoid
rickettsial NOS A79.9
specified type NEC A79.89
Riga (-Fede) (cachectic aphthae) K14.0
Riggs' (compound periodontitis) — see Periodontitis
Ritter's L00
Rivalta's (cervicofacial actinomycosis) A42.2
Robles' (onchocerciasis) B73.01
Roger's (congenital interventricular septal defect) Q21.0
Rosenthal's (factor XI deficiency) D68.1
Ross River B33.1
Rossbach's (hyperchlorhydria) K30
Rotes Quérol — see Hyperostosis, ankylosing
Roth (-Bernhardt) — see Mononeuropathy, lower limb, meralgia paresthetica
Runeberg's (progressive pernicious anemia) D51.0
sacroiliac NEC M53.3
salivary gland or duct K11.9
inclusion B25.9
specified NEC K11.8
virus B25.9
sandworm B76.9
Schimmelbusch's — see Mastopathy, cystic
Schmorl's — see Schmorl's disease or nodes
Schönlein (-Henoch) (purpura rheumatica) D69.0
Schottmüller's — see Fever, paratyphoid
Schultz's (agranulocytosis) — see Agranulocytosis
Schwalbe-Ziehen-Oppenheim G24.1
Schwartz-Jampel G71.13
sclera H15.9
specified NEC H15.89
scrofulous (tuberculous) A18.2
scrotum N50.9
sebaceous glands L73.9
semilunar cartilage, cystic — see also Derangement, knee, meniscus, cystic
seminal vesicle N50.9
serum NEC (see also Reaction, serum) T80.69
sexually transmitted A64
anogenital
herpesviral infection — see Herpes, anogenital
warts A63.0
chancroid A57
chlamydial infection — see Chlamydia
gonorrhea — see Gonorrhea
granuloma inguinale A58
specified organism NEC A63.8
syphilis — see Syphilis
trichomoniasis — see Trichomoniasis
Sézary C84.1-
shimamushi (scrub typhus) A75.3
shipyard B30.0
sickle-cell D57.1
with crisis (vasoocclusive pain) D57.00
with
acute chest syndrome D57.01
splenic sequestration D57.02
elliptocytosis D57.8-

Disease, diseased (see also Syndrome) — continued
  sickle-cell D57.1 — continued
    Hb-C D57.20
      with crisis (vasoocclusive pain) D57.219
        with
          acute chest syndrome D57.211
          splenic sequestration D57.212
      without crisis D57.20
    Hb-SD D57.80
      with crisis D57.819
        with
          acute chest syndrome D57.811
          splenic sequestration D57.812
    Hb-SE D57.80
      with crisis D57.819
        with
          acute chest syndrome D57.811
          splenic sequestration D57.812
    specified NEC D57.80
      with crisis D57.819
        with
          acute chest syndrome D57.811
          splenic sequestration D57.812
    spherocytosis D57.80
      with crisis D57.819
        with
          acute chest syndrome D57.811
          splenic sequestration D57.812
    thalassemia D57.40
      with crisis (vasoocclusive pain) D57.419
        with
          acute chest syndrome D57.411
          splenic sequestration D57.412
      without crisis D57.40
  silo-filler's J68.8
    bronchitis J68.0
    pneumonitis J68.0
    pulmonary edema J68.1
  simian B B00.4
  Simons' (progressive lipodystrophy) E88.1
  sin nombre virus B33.4
  sinus — see Sinusitis
  Sirkari's B55.0
  sixth B08.20
    due to human herpesvirus 6 B08.21
    due to human herpesvirus 7 B08.22
  skin L98.9
    due to metabolic disorder NEC E88.9 [L99]
    specified NEC L98.8
  slim (HIV) B20
  small vessel I73.9
  Sneddon-Wilkinson (subcorneal pustular dermatosis) L13.1
  South African creeping B88.0
  spinal (cord) G95.9
    congenital Q06.9
    specified NEC G95.89
  spine — see also Spondylopathy
    joint — see Dorsopathy
    tuberculous A18.01
  spinocerebellar (hereditary) G11.9
    specified NEC G11.8
  spleen D73.9
    amyloid E85.4 [D77]
    organic D73.9
    polycystic Q89.09
    postinfectional D73.89
  sponge-diver's — see Toxicity, venom, marine animal, sea anemone
  Startle Q89.8
  Steinert's G71.11
  Sticker's (erythema infectiosum) B08.3
  Stieda's (calcification, knee joint) — see Bursitis, tibial collateral
  Stokes' (exophthalmic goiter) — see Hyperthyroidism, with, goiter (diffuse)
  Stokes-Adams (syncope with heart block) I45.9
  stomach K31.9
    functional, psychogenic F45.8
    specified NEC K31.89
  stonemason's J62.8
  storage
    glycogen — see Disease, glycogen storage
    mucopolysaccharide — see Mucopolysaccharidosis
  striatopallidal system NEC G25.89
  Stuart's (congenital factor X deficiency) D68.2
  Stuart-Prower (congenital factor X deficiency) D68.2
  subcutaneous tissue — see Disease, skin
  supporting structures of teeth K08.9
    specified NEC K08.8

Disease, diseased (see also Syndrome) — continued
  suprarenal (capsule) (gland) E27.9
    hyperfunction E27.0
    specified NEC E27.8
  sweat glands L74.9
    specified NEC L74.8
  Sweeley-Klionsky E75.21
  Swift (-Feer) — see Poisoning, mercury
  swimming-pool granuloma A31.1
  Sylvest's (epidemic pleurodynia) B33.0
  sympathetic nervous system G90.9
  synovium — see Disorder, synovium
  syphilitic — see Syphilis
  systemic tissue mast cell C96.2
  tanapox (virus) B08.71
  Tangier E78.6
  Tarral-Besnier (pityriasis rubra pilaris) L44.0
  Tauri's E74.09
  tear duct — see Disorder, lacrimal system
  tendon, tendinous — see also Disorder, tendon
    nodular — see Trigger finger
  terminal vessel I73.9
  testis N50.9
  thalassemia Hb-S — see Disease, sickle-cell, thalassemia
  Thaysen-Gee (nontropical sprue) K90.0
  Thomsen G71.12
  throat J39.2
    septic J02.0
  thromboembolic — see Embolism
  thymus (gland) E32.9
    specified NEC E32.8
  thyroid (gland) E07.9
    heart (see also Hyperthyroidism) E05.90 [I43]
      with thyroid storm E05.91 [I43]
    specified NEC E07.89
  Tietze's M94.0
  tongue K14.9
    specified NEC K14.8
  tonsils, tonsillar (and adenoids) J35.9
  tooth, teeth K08.9
    hard tissues K03.9
      specified NEC K03.89
    pulp NEC K04.99
    specified NEC K08.8
  Tourette's F95.2
  trachea NEC J39.8
  tricuspid I07.9
    nonrheumatic I36.9
  triglyceride-storage E75.5
  trophoblastic — see Mole, hydatidiform
  tsutsugamushi A75.3
  tube (fallopian) (noninflammatory) N83.9
    inflammatory — see Salpingitis
    specified NEC N83.8
  tuberculous NEC — see Tuberculosis
  tubo-ovarian (noninflammatory) N83.9
    inflammatory — see Salpingo-oophoritis
    specified NEC N83.8
  tubotympanic, chronic — see Otitis, media, suppurative, chronic, tubotympanic
  tubulo-interstitial N15.9
    specified NEC N15.8
  tympanum — see Disorder, tympanic membrane
  Uhl's Q24.8
  Underwood's (sclerema neonatorum) P83.0
  Unverricht (-Lundborg) — see Epilepsy, generalized, idiopathic
  Urbach-Oppenheim (necrobiosis lipoidica diabeticorum) — see E08-E13 with .620
  ureter N28.9
    in (due to)
      schistosomiasis (bilharziasis) B65.0 [N29]
  urethra N36.9
    specified NEC N36.8
  urinary (tract) N39.9
    bladder N32.9
      specified NEC N32.89
    specified NEC N39.8
  uterus (noninflammatory) N85.9
    infective — see Endometritis
    inflammatory — see Endometritis
    specified NEC N85.8
  uveal tract (anterior) H21.9
    posterior H31.9
  vagabond's B85.1
  vagina, vaginal (noninflammatory) N89.9
    inflammatory NEC N76.89
    specified NEC N89.8
  valve, valvular I38
    multiple I08.9
      specified NEC I08.8

Disease, diseased (see also Syndrome) — continued
  van Creveld-von Gierke (glycogenosis I) E74.01
  vas deferens N50.9
  vascular I99.9
    arteriosclerotic — see Arteriosclerosis
    ciliary body NEC — see Disorder, iris, vascular
    hypertensive — see Hypertension
    iris NEC — see Disorder, iris, vascular
    obliterative I77.1
      peripheral I73.9
    occlusive I99.8
    peripheral (occlusive) I73.9
      in diabetes mellitus — see E08-E13 with .51
  vasomotor I73.9
  vasospastic I73.9
  vein I87.9
  venereal (see also Disease, sexually transmitted) A64
    chlamydial NEC A56.8
      anus A56.3
      genitourinary NOS A56.2
      pharynx A56.4
      rectum A56.3
    fifth A55
    sixth A55
    specified nature or type NEC A63.8
  vertebra, vertebral — see also Spondylopathy
    disc — see Disorder, disc
  vibration — see Vibration, adverse effects
  viral, virus (see also Disease, by type of virus) B34.9
    arbovirus NOS A94
    arthropod-borne NOS A94
    congenital P35.9
      specified NEC P35.8
    Hanta (with renal manifestations) (Dobrava) (Puumala) (Seoul) A98.5
      with pulmonary manifestations (Andes) (Bayou) (Bermejo) (Black Creek Canal) (Choclo) (Juquitiba) (Laguna negra) (Lechiguanas) (New York) (Oran) (Sin nombre) B33.4
    Hantaan (Korean hemorrhagic fever) A98.5
    human immunodeficiency (HIV) B20
    Kunjin A83.4
    nonarthropod-borne NOS B34.9
    Powassan A84.8
    Rocio (encephalitis) A83.6
    Sin nombre (Hantavirus) (cardio)-pulmonary syndrome) B33.4
    Tahyna B33.8
    vesicular stomatitis A93.8
  vitreous H43.9
    specified NEC H43.89
  vocal cord J38.3
  Volkmann's, acquired T79.6
  von Eulenburg's (congenital paramyotonia) G71.19
  von Gierke's (glycogenosis I) E74.01
  von Graefe's — see Strabismus, paralytic, ophthalmoplegia, progressive
  von Willebrand (-Jürgens) (angiohemophilia) D68.0
  Vrolik's (osteogenesis imperfecta) Q78.0
  vulva (noninflammatory) N90.9
    inflammatory NEC N76.89
    specified NEC N90.89
  Wallgren's (obstruction of splenic vein with collateral circulation) I87.8
  Wassilieff's (leptospiral jaundice) A27.0
  wasting NEC R64
    due to malnutrition E41
  Waterhouse-Friderichsen A39.1
  Wegner's (syphilitic osteochondritis) A50.02
  Weil's (leptospiral jaundice of lung) A27.0
  Weir Mitchell's (erythromelalgia) I73.81
  Werdnig-Hoffmann G12.0
  Wermer's E31.21
  Werner-His (trench fever) A79.0
  Werner-Schultz (neutropenic splenomegaly) D73.81
  Wernicke-Posadas B38.9
  whipworm B79
  white blood cells D72.9
    specified NEC D72.89
  white matter R90.82
  white-spot, meaning lichen sclerosus et atrophicus L90.0
    penis N48.0
    vulva N90.4
  Wilkie's K55.1

Disease, diseased (see also Syndrome) — continued
  Wilkinson-Sneddon (subcorneal pustular dermatosis) L13.1
  Willis' — see Diabetes
  Wilson's (hepatolenticular degeneration) E83.01
  woolsorter's A22.1
  yaba monkey tumor B08.72
  yaba pox (virus) B08.72
  zoonotic, bacterial A28.9
    specified type NEC A28.8
Disfigurement (due to scar) L90.5
Disgerminoma — see Dysgerminoma
DISH (diffuse idiopathic skeletal hyperostosis) — see Hyperostosis, ankylosing
Disinsertion, retina — see Detachment, retina
Dislocatable hip, congenital Q65.6
Dislocation (articular)
  with fracture — see Fracture
  acromioclavicular (joint) S43.10-
    with displacement
      100%-200% S43.12-
      more than 200% S43.13-
    inferior S43.14-
    posterior S43.15-
  ankle S93.0-
  astragalus — see Dislocation, ankle
  atlantoaxial S13.121
  atlantooccipital S13.111
  atloidooccipital S13.111
  breast bone S23.29
  capsule, joint — code by site under Dislocation
  carpal (bone) — see Dislocation, wrist
  carpometacarpal (joint) NEC S63.05-
    thumb S63.04-
  cartilage (joint) — code by site under Dislocation
  cervical spine (vertebra) — see Dislocation, vertebra, cervical
  chronic — see Dislocation, recurrent
  clavicle — see Dislocation, acromioclavicular joint
  coccyx S33.2
  congenital NEC Q68.8
  coracoid — see Dislocation, shoulder
  costal cartilage S23.29
  costochondral S23.29
  cricoarytenoid articulation S13.29
  cricothyroid articulation S13.29
  dorsal vertebra — see Dislocation, vertebra, thoracic
  ear ossicle — see Discontinuity, ossicles, ear
  elbow S53.10-
    congenital Q68.8
    pathological — see Dislocation, pathological NEC, elbow
    radial head alone — see Dislocation, radial head
    recurrent — see Dislocation, recurrent, elbow
    traumatic S53.10-
      anterior S53.11-
      lateral S53.14-
      medial S53.13-
      posterior S53.12-
      specified type NEC S53.19-
  eye, nontraumatic — see Luxation, globe
  eyeball, nontraumatic — see Luxation, globe
  femur
    distal end — see Dislocation, knee
    proximal end — see Dislocation, hip
  fibula
    distal end — see Dislocation, ankle
    proximal end — see Dislocation, knee
  finger S63.25-
    index S63.25-
    interphalangeal S63.27-
      distal S63.29-
        index S63.29-
        little S63.29-
        middle S63.29-
        ring S63.29-
      index S63.27-
      little S63.27-
      middle S63.27-
      proximal S63.28-
        index S63.28-
        little S63.28-
        middle S63.28-
        ring S63.28-
      ring S63.27-
    little S63.25-

Dislocation (articular) — *continued*
finger S63.25- — *continued*
  metacarpophalangeal S63.26-
    index S63.26-
    little S63.26-
    middle S63.26-
    ring S63.26-
  middle S63.25-
  recurrent — *see* Dislocation, recurrent, finger
  ring S63.25-
  thumb — *see* Dislocation, thumb
foot S93.30-
  recurrent — *see* Dislocation, recurrent, foot
  specified site NEC S93.33-
  tarsal joint S93.31-
  tarsometatarsal joint S93.32-
  toe — *see* Dislocation, toe
fracture — *see* Fracture
glenohumeral (joint) — *see* Dislocation, shoulder
glenoid — *see* Dislocation, shoulder
habitual — *see* Dislocation, recurrent
hip S73.00-
  anterior S73.03-
    obturator S73.02-
  central S73.04-
  congenital (total) Q65.2
    bilateral Q65.1
    partial Q65.5
      bilateral Q65.4
      unilateral Q65.3-
    unilateral Q65.0-
  developmental M24.85-
  pathological — *see* Dislocation, pathological NEC, hip
  posterior S73.01-
  recurrent — *see* Dislocation, recurrent, hip
humerus, proximal end — *see* Dislocation, shoulder
incomplete — *see* Subluxation, by site
incus — *see* Discontinuity, ossicles, ear
infracoracoid — *see* Dislocation, shoulder
innominate (pubic junction) (sacral junction) S33.39
  acetabulum — *see* Dislocation, hip
interphalangeal (joint(s))
  finger S63.279
    distal S63.29-
      index S63.29-
      little S63.29-
      middle S63.29-
      ring S63.29-
    index S63.27-
    little S63.27-
    middle S63.27-
    proximal S63.28-
      index S63.28-
      little S63.28-
      middle S63.28-
      ring S63.28-
    ring S63.27-
  foot or toe — *see* Dislocation, toe
  thumb S63.12-
    distal joint S63.14-
    proximal joint S63.13-
jaw (cartilage) (meniscus) S03.0
joint prosthesis — *see* Complications, joint prosthesis, mechanical, displacement, by site
knee S83.106
  cap — *see* Dislocation, patella
  congenital Q68.2
  old M23.8x-
  patella — *see* Dislocation, patella
  pathological — *see* Dislocation, pathological NEC, knee
  proximal tibia
    anteriorly S83.11-
    laterally S83.14-
    medially S83.13-
    posteriorly S83.12-
  recurrent — *see also* Derangement, knee, specified NEC
  specified type NEC S83.19-
lacrimal gland H04.16-
lens (complete) H27.10
  anterior H27.12-
  congenital Q12.1
  ocular implant — *see* Complications, intraocular lens
  partial H27.11-
  posterior H27.13-
  traumatic S05.8x-
ligament — *code by* site under Dislocation
lumbar (vertebra) — *see* Dislocation, vertebra, lumbar

Dislocation (articular) — *continued*
lumbosacral (vertebra) — *see also* Dislocation, vertebra, lumbar
  congenital Q76.49
mandible S03.0
meniscus (knee) — *see* Tear, meniscus
  other sites — *code by* site under Dislocation
metacarpal (bone)
  distal end — *see* Dislocation, finger
  proximal end S63.06-
metacarpophalangeal (joint)
  finger S63.26-
    index S63.26-
    little S63.26-
    middle S63.26-
    ring S63.26-
    thumb S63.11-
metatarsal (bone) — *see* Dislocation, foot
metatarsophalangeal (joint(s)) — *see* Dislocation, toe
midcarpal (joint) S63.03-
midtarsal (joint) — *see* Dislocation, foot
neck S13.20
  specified site NEC S13.29
  vertebra — *see* Dislocation, vertebra, cervical
nose (septal cartilage) S03.1
occipitoatloid S13.111
old — *see* Derangement, joint, specified type NEC
ossicles, ear — *see* Discontinuity, ossicles, ear
partial — *see* Subluxation, by site
patella S83.006
  congenital Q74.1
  lateral S83.01-
  recurrent (nontraumatic) M22.0-
    incomplete M22.1-
  specified type NEC S83.09-
pathological NEC M24.30
  ankle M24.37-
  elbow M24.32-
  foot joint M24.37-
  hand joint M24.34-
  hip M24.35-
  knee M24.36-
  lumbosacral joint — *see* subcategory M53.2
  pelvic region — *see* Dislocation, pathological, hip
  sacroiliac — *see* subcategory M53.2
  shoulder M24.31-
  wrist M24.33-
pelvis NEC S33.30
  specified NEC S33.39
phalanx
  finger or hand — *see* Dislocation, finger
  foot or toe — *see* Dislocation, toe
prosthesis, internal — *see* Complications, prosthetic device, by site, mechanical
radial head S53.006
  anterior S53.01-
  posterior S53.02-
  specified type NEC S53.09-
radiocarpal (joint) S63.02-
radiohumeral (joint) — *see* Dislocation, radial head
radioulnar (joint)
  distal S63.01-
  proximal — *see* Dislocation, elbow
radius
  distal end — *see* Dislocation, wrist
  proximal end — *see* Dislocation, radial head
recurrent M24.40
  ankle M24.47-
  elbow M24.42-
  finger M24.44-
  foot joint M24.47-
  hand joint M24.44-
  hip M24.45-
  knee M24.46-
    patella — *see* Dislocation, patella, recurrent
  patella — *see* Dislocation, patella, recurrent
  sacroiliac — *see* subcategory M53.2
  shoulder M24.41-
  toe M24.47-
  vertebra (*see also* subcategory) M43.5
    atlantoaxial M43.4
      with myelopathy M43.3
  wrist M24.43-
rib (cartilage) S23.29
sacrococcygeal S33.2
sacroiliac (joint) (ligament) S33.2
  congenital Q74.2
  recurrent — *see* subcategory M53.2

Dislocation (articular) — *continued*
sacrum S33.2
scaphoid (bone) (hand) (wrist) — *see* Dislocation, wrist
  foot — *see* Dislocation, foot
scapula — *see* Dislocation, shoulder, girdle, scapula
semilunar cartilage, knee — *see* Tear, meniscus
septal cartilage (nose) S03.1
septum (nasal) (old) J34.2
sesamoid bone — *code by* site under Dislocation
shoulder (blade) (ligament) (joint) (traumatic) S43.006
  acromioclavicular — *see* Dislocation, acromioclavicular
  chronic — *see* Dislocation, recurrent, shoulder
  congenital Q68.8
  girdle S43.30-
    scapula S43.31-
    specified site NEC S43.39-
  humerus S43.00-
    anterior S43.01-
    inferior S43.03-
    posterior S43.02-
  pathological — *see* Dislocation, pathological NEC, shoulder
  recurrent — *see* Dislocation, recurrent, shoulder
  specified type NEC S43.08-
spine
  cervical — *see* Dislocation, vertebra, cervical
  congenital Q76.49
  due to birth trauma P11.5
  lumbar — *see* Dislocation, vertebra, lumbar
  thoracic — *see* Dislocation, vertebra, thoracic
spontaneous — *see* Dislocation, pathological
sternoclavicular (joint) S43.206
  anterior S43.21-
  posterior S43.22-
sternum S23.29
subglenoid — *see* Dislocation, shoulder
symphysis pubis S33.4
talus — *see* Dislocation, ankle
tarsal (bone(s)) (joint(s)) — *see* Dislocation, foot
tarsometatarsal (joint(s)) — *see* Dislocation, foot
temporomandibular (joint) S03.0
thigh, proximal end — *see* Dislocation, hip
thorax S23.20
  specified site NEC S23.29
  vertebra — *see* Dislocation, vertebra thumb S23.20
thumb S63.10-
  interphalangeal joint — *see* Dislocation, interphalangeal (joint), thumb
  metacarpophalangeal joint — *see* Dislocation, metacarpophalangeal (joint), thumb
thyroid cartilage S13.29
tibia
  distal end — *see* Dislocation, ankle
  proximal end — *see* Dislocation, knee
tibiofibular (joint)
  distal — *see* Dislocation, ankle
  superior — *see* Dislocation, knee
toe(s) S93.106
  great S93.10-
    interphalangeal joint S93.11-
    metatarsophalangeal joint S93.12-
  interphalangeal joint S93.119
  lesser S93.106
    interphalangeal joint S93.11-
    metatarsophalangeal joint S93.12-
  metatarsophalangeal joint S93.12-
tooth S03.2
trachea S23.29
ulna
  distal end S63.07-
  proximal end — *see* Dislocation, elbow
ulnohumeral (joint) — *see* Dislocation, elbow
vertebra (articular process) (body) (traumatic)
  cervical S13.101
    atlantoaxial joint S13.121
    atlantooccipital joint S13.111
    atloidooccipital joint S13.111

Dislocation (articular) — *continued*
vertebra (articular process) (body) (traumatic) — *continued*
  cervical S13.101 — *continued*
    joint between
      C0 and C1 S13.111
      C1 and C2 S13.121
      C2 and C3 S13.131
      C3 and C4 S13.141
      C4 and C5 S13.151
      C5 and C6 S13.161
      C6 and C7 S13.171
      C7 and T1 S13.181
    occipitoatloid joint S13.111
  congenital Q76.49
  lumbar S33.101
    joint between
      L1 and L2 S33.111
      L2 and L3 S33.121
      L3 and L4 S33.131
      L4 and L5 S33.141
  nontraumatic — *see* Displacement, intervertebral disc
  partial — *see* Subluxation, by site
  recurrent NEC — *see* subcategory M43.5
  thoracic S23.101
    joint between
      T1 and T2 S23.111
      T10 and T11 S23.161
      T11 and T12 S23.163
      T12 and L1 S23.171
      T2 and T3 S23.121
      T3 and T4 S23.123
      T4 and T5 S23.131
      T5 and T6 S23.133
      T6 and T7 S23.141
      T7 and T8 S23.143
      T8 and T9 S23.151
      T9 and T10 S23.153
wrist (carpal bone) S63.006
  carpometacarpal joint — *see* Dislocation, carpometacarpal (joint)
  distal radioulnar joint — *see* Dislocation, radioulnar (joint), distal
  metacarpal bone, proximal — *see* Dislocation, metacarpal (bone), proximal end
  midcarpal — *see* Dislocation, midcarpal (joint)
  radiocarpal joint — *see* Dislocation, radiocarpal (joint)
  recurrent — *see* Dislocation, recurrent, wrist
  specified site NEC S63.09-
  ulna — *see* Dislocation, ulna, distal end
xiphoid cartilage S23.29
Disorder (of) — *see also* Disease
acantholytic L11.9
  specified NEC L11.8
acute
  psychotic — *see* Psychosis, acute
  stress F43.0
adjustment (grief) F43.20
  with
    anxiety F43.22
      with depressed mood F43.23
    conduct disturbance F43.24
      with emotional disturbance F43.25
    depressed mood F43.21
      with anxiety F43.23
    other specified symptom F43.29
adrenal (capsule) (gland) (medullary) E27.9
  specified NEC E27.8
adrenogenital E25.9
  drug-induced E25.8
  iatrogenic E25.8
  idiopathic E25.8
adult personality (and behavior) F69
  specified NEC F68.8
affective (mood) — *see* Disorder, mood
aggressive, unsocialized F91.1
alcohol-related F10.99
  with
    amnestic disorder, persisting F10.96
    anxiety disorder F10.980
    dementia, persisting F10.97
    intoxication F10.929
      with delirium F10.921
        uncomplicated F10.920
    mood disorder F10.94
    other specified F10.988
    psychotic disorder F10.959
      with
        delusions F10.950
        hallucinations F10.951
    sexual dysfunction F10.981
    sleep disorder F10.982

Disorder (of) *(see also* Disease*)* — *continued*
- allergic — *see* Allergy
- alveolar NEC J84.09
- amino-acid
  - cystathioninuria E72.19
  - cystinosis E72.04
  - cystinuria E72.01
  - glycinuria E72.09
  - homocystinuria E72.11
  - metabolism — *see* Disturbance, metabolism, amino-acid
  - specified NEC E72.8
  - neonatal, transitory P74.8
  - renal transport NEC E72.09
  - transport NEC E72.09
- amnesic, amnestic
  - alcohol-induced F10.96
    - with dependence F10.26
  - due to (secondary to) general medical condition F04
  - psychoactive NEC-induced F19.96
    - with
      - abuse F19.16
      - dependence F19.26
  - sedative, hypnotic or anxiolytic-induced F13.96
    - with dependence F13.26
- anaerobic glycolysis with anemia D55.2
- anxiety F41.9
  - due to (secondary to)
    - alcohol F10.980
    - amphetamine F15.980
      - in
        - abuse F15.180
        - dependence F15.280
    - anxiolytic F13.980
      - in
        - abuse F13.180
        - dependence F13.280
    - caffeine F15.980
      - in
        - abuse F15.180
        - dependence F15.280
    - cannabis F12.980
      - in
        - abuse F12.180
        - dependence F12.280
    - cocaine F14.980
      - in
        - abuse F14.180
        - dependence F14.180
    - general medical condition F06.4
    - hallucinogen F16.980
      - in
        - abuse F16.180
        - dependence F16.280
    - hypnotic F13.980
      - in
        - abuse F13.180
        - dependence F13.280
    - inhalant F18.980
      - in
        - abuse F18.180
        - dependence F18.280
    - phencyclidine F16.980
      - in
        - abuse F16.180
        - dependence F16.280
    - psychoactive substance NEC F19.980
      - in
        - abuse F19.180
        - dependence F19.280
    - sedative F13.980
      - in
        - abuse F13.180
        - dependence F13.280
    - volatile solvents F18.980
      - in
        - abuse F18.180
        - dependence F18.280
  - generalized F41.1
  - mixed
    - with depression (mild) F41.8
    - specified NEC F41.3
  - organic F06.4
  - phobic F40.9
    - of childhood F40.8
  - specified NEC F41.8
- aortic valve — *see* Endocarditis, aortic
- aromatic amino-acid metabolism E70.9
  - specified NEC E70.8
- arteriole NEC I77.89
- artery NEC I77.89
- articulation — *see* Disorder, joint
- attachment (childhood)
  - disinhibited F94.2
  - reactive F94.1

Disorder (of) *(see also* Disease*)* — *continued*
- attention-deficit hyperactivity (adolescent) (adult) (child) F90.9
  - combined type F90.2
  - hyperactive type F90.1
  - inattentive type F90.0
  - specified type NEC F90.8
- attention-deficit without hyperactivity (adolescent) (adult) (child) F90.0
- auditory processing (central) H93.25
- autistic F84.0
- autonomic nervous system G90.9
  - specified NEC G90.8
- avoidant, child or adolescent F40.10
- balance
  - acid-base E87.8
    - mixed E87.4
  - electrolyte E87.8
  - fluid NEC E87.8
- behavioral (disruptive) — *see* Disorder, conduct
- beta-amino-acid metabolism E72.8
- bile acid and cholesterol metabolism E78.70
  - Barth syndrome E78.71
  - other specified E78.79
  - Smith-Lemli-Opitz syndrome E78.72
- bilirubin excretion E80.6
- binocular
  - movement H51.9
    - convergence
      - excess H51.12
      - insufficiency H51.11
    - internuclear ophthalmoplegia — *see* Ophthalmoplegia, internuclear
    - palsy of conjugate gaze H51.0
    - specified type NEC H51.8
  - vision NEC — *see* Disorder, vision, binocular
- bipolar (I) F31.9
  - current episode
    - depressed F31.9
      - with psychotic features F31.5
      - without psychotic features F31.30
        - mild F31.31
        - moderate F31.32
        - severe (without psychotic features) F31.4
          - with psychotic features F31.5
    - hypomanic F31.0
    - manic F31.9
      - with psychotic features F31.2
      - without psychotic features F31.10
        - mild F31.11
        - moderate F31.12
        - severe (without psychotic features) F31.13
          - with psychotic features F31.2
    - mixed F31.60
      - mild F31.61
      - moderate F31.62
      - severe (without psychotic features) F31.63
        - with psychotic features F31.64
      - severe depression (without psychotic features) F31.4
        - with psychotic features F31.5
  - II F31.81
  - in remission (currently) F31.70
    - in full remission
      - most recent episode
        - depressed F31.76
        - hypomanic F31.72
        - manic F31.74
        - mixed F31.78
    - in partial remission
      - most recent episode
        - depressed F31.75
        - hypomanic F31.71
        - manic F31.73
        - mixed F31.77
  - organic F06.30
  - single manic episode F30.9
    - mild F30.11
    - moderate F30.12
    - severe (without psychotic symptoms) F30.13
      - with psychotic symptoms F30.2
  - specified NEC F31.89
- bladder N32.9
  - functional NEC N31.9
  - in schistosomiasis B65.0 [N33]
  - specified NEC N32.89
- bleeding D68.9
- blood D75.9
  - in congenital early syphilis A50.09 [D77]
- body dysmorphic F45.22

Disorder (of) *(see also* Disease*)* — *continued*
- bone M89.9
  - continuity M84.9
    - specified type NEC M84.80
      - ankle M84.87-
      - fibula M84.86-
      - foot M84.87-
      - hand M84.84-
      - humerus M84.82-
      - neck M84.88
      - pelvis M84.859
      - radius M84.83-
      - rib M84.88
      - shoulder M84.81-
      - skull M84.88
      - thigh M84.85-
      - tibia M84.86-
      - ulna M84.83-
      - vertebra M84.88
  - density and structure M85.9
    - cyst — *see also* Cyst, bone, specified type NEC
      - aneurysmal — *see* Cyst, bone, aneurysmal
      - solitary — *see* Cyst, bone, solitary
    - diffuse idiopathic skeletal hyperostosis — *see* Hyperostosis, ankylosing
    - fibrous dysplasia (monostotic) — *see* Dysplasia, fibrous, bone
    - fluorosis — *see* Fluorosis, skeletal
    - hyperostosis of skull M85.2
    - osteitis condensans — *see* Osteitis, condensans
    - specified type NEC M85.8-
      - ankle M85.87-
      - foot M85.87-
      - forearm M85.83-
      - hand M85.84-
      - lower leg M85.86-
      - multiple sites M85.89
      - neck M85.88
      - rib M85.88
      - shoulder M85.81-
      - skull M85.88
      - thigh M85.85-
      - upper arm M85.82-
      - vertebra M85.88
  - development and growth NEC M89.20
    - carpus M89.24-
    - clavicle M89.21-
    - femur M89.25-
    - fibula M89.26-
    - finger M89.24-
    - humerus M89.22-
    - ilium M89.259
    - ischium M89.259
    - metacarpus M89.24-
    - metatarsus M89.27-
    - multiple sites M89.29
    - neck M89.28
    - radius M89.23-
    - rib M89.28
    - scapula M89.21-
    - skull M89.28
    - tarsus M89.27-
    - tibia M89.26-
    - toe M89.27-
    - ulna M89.23-
    - vertebra M89.28
  - specified type NEC M89.8x-
- brachial plexus G54.0
- branched-chain amino-acid metabolism E71.2
  - specified NEC E71.19
- breast N64.9
  - agalactia — *see* Agalactia
  - associated with
    - lactation O92.70
      - specified NEC O92.79
    - pregnancy O92.20
      - specified NEC O92.29
    - puerperium O92.20
      - specified NEC O92.29
  - cracked nipple — *see* Cracked nipple
  - galactorrhea — *see* Galactorrhea
  - hypogalactia O92.4
  - lactation disorder NEC O92.79
  - mastitis — *see* Mastitis
  - nipple infection — *see* Infection, nipple
  - retracted nipple — *see* Retraction, nipple
  - specified type NEC N64.89
- Briquet's F45.0
- bullous, in diseases classified elsewhere L14
- cannabis use
  - due to drug abuse — *see* Abuse, drug, cannabis
  - due to drug dependence — *see* Dependence, drug, cannabis

Disorder (of) *(see also* Disease*)* — *continued*
- carbohydrate
  - absorption, intestinal NEC E74.39
  - metabolism (congenital) E74.9
    - specified NEC E74.8
- cardiac, functional I51.89
- carnitine metabolism E71.40
- cartilage M94.9
  - articular NEC — *see* Derangement, joint, articular cartilage
  - chondrocalcinosis — *see* Chondrocalcinosis
  - specified type NEC M94.8x-
    - articular — *see* Derangement, joint, articular cartilage
    - multiple sites M94.8x0
- catatonic
  - due to (secondary to) known physiological condition F06.1
  - organic F06.1
- central auditory processing H93.25
- cervical
  - region NEC M53.82
  - root (nerve) NEC G54.2
- character NOS F60.9
- childhood disintegrative NEC F84.3
- cholesterol and bile acid metabolism E78.70
  - Barth syndrome E78.71
  - other specified E78.79
  - Smith-Lemli-Opitz syndrome E78.72
- choroid H31.9
  - atrophy — *see* Atrophy, choroid
  - degeneration — *see* Degeneration, choroid
  - detachment — *see* Detachment, choroid
  - dystrophy — *see* Dystrophy, choroid
  - hemorrhage — *see* Hemorrhage, choroid
  - rupture — *see* Rupture, choroid
  - scar — *see* Scar, chorioretinal
  - solar retinopathy — *see* Retinopathy, solar
  - specified type NEC H31.8
- ciliary body — *see* Disorder, iris
  - degeneration — *see* Degeneration, ciliary body
- coagulation (factor) *(see also* Defect, coagulation) D68.9
  - newborn, transient P61.6
- coccyx NEC M53.3
- cognitive F09
  - due to (secondary to) general medical condition F09
  - persisting R41.89
    - due to
      - alcohol F10.97
        - with dependence F10.27
      - anxiolytics F13.97
        - with dependence F13.27
      - hypnotics F13.97
        - with dependence F13.27
      - sedatives F13.97
        - with dependence F13.27
      - specified substance NEC F19.97
        - with
          - abuse F19.17
          - dependence F19.27
- communication F80.9
- conduct (childhood) F91.9
  - adjustment reaction — *see* Disorder, adjustment
  - adolescent onset type F91.2
  - childhood onset type F91.1
  - compulsive F63.9
  - confined to family context F91.0
  - depressive F91.8
  - group type F91.2
  - hyperkinetic — *see* Disorder, attention-deficit hyperactivity
  - oppositional defiance F91.3
  - socialized F91.2
  - solitary aggressive type F91.1
  - specified NEC F91.8
  - unsocialized (aggressive) F91.1
- conduction, heart I45.9
- congenital glycosylation (CDG) E74.8
- conjunctiva H11.9
  - infection — *see* Conjunctivitis
- connective tissue, localized L94.9
  - specified NEC L94.8
- conversion — *see* Disorder, dissociative
- convulsive (secondary) — *see* Convulsions

DISEASE INDEX

Disorder (of) (see also Disease) — continued
cornea H18.9
  deformity — see Deformity, cornea
  degeneration — see Degeneration, cornea
  deposits — see Deposit, cornea
  due to contact lens H18.82-
    specified as edema — see Edema, cornea
  edema — see Edema, cornea
  keratitis — see Keratitis
  keratoconjunctivitis — see Keratoconjunctivitis
  membrane change — see Change, corneal membrane
  neovascularization — see Neovascularization, cornea
  scar — see Opacity, cornea
  specified type NEC H18.89-
  ulcer — see Ulcer, cornea
corpus cavernosum N48.9
cranial nerve — see Disorder, nerve, cranial
cyclothymic F34.0
defiant oppositional F91.3
delusional (persistent) (systematized) F22
  induced F24
depersonalization F48.1
depressive F32.9
  major F32.9
    with psychotic symptoms F32.3
    in remission (full) F32.5
      partial F32.4
    recurrent F33.9
    single episode F32.9
      mild F32.0
      moderate F32.1
      severe (without psychotic symptoms) F32.2
        with psychotic symptoms F32.3
  organic F06.31
  recurrent F33.9
    current episode
      mild F33.0
      moderate F33.1
      severe (without psychotic symptoms) F33.2
        with psychotic symptoms F33.3
    in remission F33.40
      full F33.42
      partial F33.41
    specified NEC F33.8
  single episode — see Episode, depressive
developmental F89
  arithmetical skills F81.2
  coordination (motor) F82
  expressive writing F81.81
  language F80.9
    expressive F80.1
    mixed receptive and expressive F80.2
    receptive type F80.2
    specified NEC F80.89
  learning F81.9
    arithmetical F81.2
    reading F81.0
  mixed F88
  motor coordination or function F82
  pervasive F84.9
    specified NEC F84.8
  phonological F80.0
  reading F81.0
  scholastic skills — see also Disorder, learning
    mixed F81.89
  specified NEC F88
  speech F80.9
    articulation F80.0
    specified NEC F80.89
  written expression F81.81
diaphragm J98.6
digestive (system) K92.9
  newborn P78.9
    specified NEC P78.89
  postprocedural — see Complication, gastrointestinal
  psychogenic F45.8
disc (intervertebral) M51.9
  with
    myelopathy
      cervical region M50.00
      cervicothoracic region M50.03
      high cervical region M50.01
      lumbar region M51.06
      mid-cervical region M50.02
      sacrococcygeal region M53.3
      thoracic region M51.04
      thoracolumbar region M51.05

Disorder (of) (see also Disease) — continued
disc (intervertebral) M51.9 — continued
  with — continued
    radiculopathy
      cervical region M50.10
      cervicothoracic region M50.13
      high cervical region M50.11
      lumbar region M51.16
      lumbosacral region M51.17
      mid-cervical region M50.12
      sacrococcygeal region M53.3
      thoracic region M51.14
      thoracolumbar region M51.15
  cervical M50.90
    with
      myelopathy M50.00
        C2-C3 M50.01
        C3-C4 M50.01
        C4-C5 M50.02
        C5-C6 M50.02
        C6-C7 M50.02
        C7-T1 M50.03
        cervicothoracic region M50.03
        high cervical region M50.01
        mid-cervical region M50.02
      neuritis, radiculitis or radiculopathy M50.10
        C2-C3 M50.11
        C3-C4 M50.11
        C4-C5 M50.12
        C5-C6 M50.12
        C6-C7 M50.12
        C7-T1 M50.13
        cervicothoracic region M50.13
        high cervical region M50.11
        mid-cervical region M50.12
    C2-C3 M50.91
    C3-C4 M50.91
    C4-C5 M50.92
    C5-C6 M50.92
    C6-C7 M50.92
    C7-T1 M50.93
    cervicothoracic region M50.93
    degeneration M50.30
      C2-C3 M50.31
      C3-C4 M50.31
      C4-C5 M50.32
      C5-C6 M50.32
      C6-C7 M50.32
      C7-T1 M50.33
      cervicothoracic region M50.33
      high cervical region M50.31
      mid-cervical region M50.32
    displacement M50.20
      C2-C3 M50.21
      C3-C4 M50.21
      C4-C5 M50.22
      C5-C6 M50.22
      C6-C7 M50.22
      C7-T1 M50.23
      cervicothoracic region M50.23
      high cervical region M50.21
      mid-cervical region M50.22
    high cervical region M50.91
    mid-cervical region M50.92
    specified type NEC M50.80
      C2-C3 M50.81
      C3-C4 M50.81
      C4-C5 M50.82
      C5-C6 M50.82
      C6-C7 M50.82
      C7-T1 M50.83
      cervicothoracic region M50.83
      high cervical region M50.81
      mid-cervical region M50.82
  specified NEC
    lumbar region M51.86
    lumbosacral region M51.87
    sacrococcygeal region M53.3
    thoracic region M51.84
    thoracolumbar region M51.85
disinhibited attachment (childhood) F94.2
disintegrative, childhood NEC F84.3
disruptive behavior F98.9
dissocial personality F60.2
dissociative F44.9
  affecting
    motor function F44.4
      and sensation F44.7
    sensation F44.6
      and motor function F44.7
  brief reactive F43.0
  due to (secondary to) general medical condition F06.8
  mixed F44.7
  organic F06.8
  other specified NEC F44.89
double heterozygous sickling — see Disease, sickle-cell
dream anxiety F51.5

Disorder (of) (see also Disease) — continued
drug induced hemorrhagic D68.32
drug related F19.99
  abuse — see Abuse, drug
  dependence — see Dependence, drug
dysmorphic body F45.1
dysthymic F34.1
ear H93.9-
  bleeding — see Otorrhagia
  deafness — see Deafness
  degenerative H93.09-
  discharge — see Otorrhea
  external H61.9-
    auditory canal stenosis — see Stenosis, external ear canal
    exostosis — see Exostosis, external ear canal
    impacted cerumen — see Impaction, cerumen
    otitis — see Otitis, externa
    perichondritis — see Perichondritis, ear
    pinna — see Disorder, pinna
    specified type NEC H61.89-
      in diseases classified elsewhere H62.8x-
  inner H83.9-
    vestibular dysfunction — see Disorder, vestibular function
  middle H74.9-
    adhesive H74.1-
    ossicle — see Abnormal, ear ossicles
    polyp — see Polyp, ear (middle)
    specified NEC, in diseases classified elsewhere H75.8-
  postprocedural — see Complications, ear, procedure
  specified NEC, in diseases classified elsewhere H94.8-
eating (adult) (psychogenic) F50.9
  anorexia — see Anorexia
  bulimia F50.2
  child F98.29
    pica F98.3
    rumination disorder F98.21
  pica F50.8
    childhood F98.3
electrolyte (balance) NEC E87.8
  with
    abortion — see Abortion by type
    complicated by specified condition NEC
    ectopic pregnancy O08.5
    molar pregnancy O08.5
    acidosis (metabolic) (respiratory) E87.2
    alkalosis (metabolic) (respiratory) E87.3
elimination, transepidermal L87.9
  specified NEC L87.8
emotional (persistent) F34.9
  of childhood F93.9
    specified NEC F93.8
endocrine E34.9
  postprocedural E89.89
  specified NEC E89.89
erectile (male) (organic) (see also Dysfunction, sexual, male, erectile) N52.9
  nonorganic F52.21
  erythematous — see Erythema
esophagus K22.9
  functional K22.4
  psychogenic F45.8
eustachian tube H69.9-
  infection — see Salpingitis, eustachian
  obstruction — see Obstruction, eustachian tube
  patulous — see Patulous, eustachian tube
  specified NEC H69.8-
extrapyramidal G25.9
  in diseases classified elsewhere — see category G26
  specified type NEC G25.89
eye H57.9
  postprocedural — see Complication, postprocedural, eye
eyelid H02.9
  cyst — see Cyst, eyelid
  degenerative H02.70
    chloasma — see Chloasma, eyelid
    madarosis — see Madarosis
    specified type NEC H02.79
    vitiligo — see Vitiligo, eyelid
    xanthelasma — see Xanthelasma
  dermatochalasis — see Dermatochalasis
  edema — see Edema, eyelid
  elephantiasis — see Elephantiasis, eyelid
  foreign body, retained — see Foreign body, retained, eyelid

Disorder (of) (see also Disease) — continued
eyelid H02.9 — continued
  function H02.59
    abnormal innervation syndrome — see Syndrome, abnormal innervation
    blepharochalasis — see Blepharochalasis
    blepharoclonus — see Blepharoclonus
    blepharophimosis — see Blepharophimosis
    blepharoptosis — see Blepharoptosis
    lagophthalmos — see Lagophthalmos
    lid retraction — see Retraction, lid
  hypertrichosis — see Hypertrichosis, eyelid
  specified type NEC H02.89
  vascular H02.879
    left H02.876
      lower H02.875
      upper H02.874
    right H02.873
      lower H02.872
      upper H02.871
factitious F68.10
  with predominantly
    physical symptoms F68.12
      with psychological symptoms F68.13
    psychological symptoms F68.11
      with physical symptoms F68.13
factor, coagulation — see Defect, coagulation
fatty acid
  metabolism E71.30
    specified NEC E71.39
  oxidation
    LCAD E71.310
    MCAD E71.311
    SCAD E71.312
    specified deficiency NEC E71.318
feeding (infant or child) (see also Disorder, eating) R63.3
feigned (with obvious motivation) Z76.5
  without obvious motivation — see Disorder, factitious
female
  hypoactive sexual desire F52.0
  orgasmic F52.31
  sexual arousal F52.22
fibroblastic M72.9
  specified NEC M72.8
fluency
  adult onset F98.5
  childhood onset F80.81
  following
    cerebral infarction I69.323
    cerebrovascular disease I69.923
      specified disease NEC I69.823
    intracerebral hemorrhage I69.123
    nontraumatic intracranial hemorrhage NEC I69.223
    subarachnoid hemorrhage I69.023
  in conditions classified elsewhere R47.82
fluid balance E87.8
follicular (skin) L73.9
  specified NEC L73.8
fructose metabolism E74.10
  essential fructosuria E74.11
  fructokinase deficiency E74.11
  fructose-1, 6-diphosphatase deficiency E74.19
  hereditary fructose intolerance E74.12
  other specified E74.19
functional polymorphonuclear neutrophils D71
gallbladder, biliary tract and pancreas in diseases classified elsewhere K87
gamma-glutamyl cycle E72.8
gastric (functional) K31.9
  motility K30
  psychogenic F45.8
  secretion K30
gastrointestinal (functional) NOS K92.9
  newborn P78.9
  psychogenic F45.8
gender-identity or -role F64.9
  childhood F64.2
  effect on relationship F66
  of adolescence or adulthood (nontranssexual) F64.1
  specified NEC F64.8
  uncertainty F66
genitourinary system
  female N94.9
  male N50.9
  psychogenic F45.8

Disorder (of) (see also Disease) — continued
globe H44.9
  degenerated condition H44.50
    absolute glaucoma H44.51-
    atrophy H44.52-
    leucocoria H44.53-
  degenerative H44.30
    chalcosis H44.31-
    myopia H44.2-
    siderosis H44.32-
    specified type NEC H44.39-
  endophthalmitis — see Endophthalmitis
  foreign body, retained — see Foreign
    body, intraocular, old, retained
  hemophthalmos — see Hemophthalmos
  hypotony H44.40
    due to
      ocular fistula H44.42-
        specified disorder NEC H44.43-
      flat anterior chamber H44.41-
      primary H44.44-
  luxation — see Luxation, globe
  specified type NEC H44.89
glomerular (in) N05.9
  amyloidosis E85.4 [N08]
  cryoglobulinemia D89.1 [N08]
  disseminated intravascular coagulation
    D65 [N08]
  Fabry's disease E75.21 [N08]
  familial lecithin cholesterol
    acyltransferase deficiency E78.6
    [N08]
  Goodpasture's syndrome M31.0
  hemolytic-uremic syndrome D59.3
  Henoch (-Schönlein) purpura D69.0
    [N08]
  malariae malaria B52.0
  microscopic polyangiitis M31.7 [N08]
  multiple myeloma C90.0-[N08]
  mumps B26.83
  schistosomiasis B65.9 [N08]
  sepsis NEC A41.- [N08]
    streptococcal A40.- [N08]
  sickle-cell disorders D57-[N08]
  strongyloidiasis B78.9 [N08]
  subacute bacterial endocarditis I33.0
    [N08]
  syphilis A52.75
  systemic lupus erythematosus M32.14
  thrombotic thrombocytopenic purpura
    M31.1 [N08]
  Waldenström macroglobulinemia C88.0
    [N08]
  Wegener's granulomatosis M31.31
gluconeogenesis E74.4
glucosaminoglycan metabolism — see
  Disorder, metabolism,
  glucosaminoglycan
glycine metabolism E72.50
  d-glycericacidemia E72.59
  hyperhydroxyprolinemia E72.59
  hyperoxaluria E72.53
  hyperprolinemia E72.59
  non-ketotic hyperglycinemia E72.51
  oxalosis E72.53
  oxaluria E72.53
  sarcosinemia E72.59
  trimethylaminuria E72.52
glycoprotein metabolism E77.9
  specified NEC E77.8
habit (and impulse) F63.9
  involving sexual behavior NEC F65.9
  specified NEC F63.89
heart action I49.9
hematological D75.9
  newborn (transient) P61.9
    specified NEC P61.8
hematopoietic organs D75.9
hemorrhagic NEC D69.9
  drug-induced D68.32
  due to
    extrinsic circulating anticoagulants
      D68.32
    increase in
      anti-IIa D68.32
      anti-Xa D68.32
    intrinsic
      circulating anticoagulants D68.318
      increase in
        antithrombin D68.318
        anti-VIIIa D68.318
        anti-IXa D68.318
        anti-XIa D68.318
  following childbirth O72.3
hemostasis — see Defect, coagulation
histidine metabolism E70.40
  histidinemia E70.41
  other specified E70.49
hyperkinetic — see Disorder, attention-
  deficit hyperactivity

Disorder (of) (see also Disease) — continued
hyperleucine-isoleucinemia E71.19
hypervalinemia E71.19
hypoactive sexual desire F52.0
hypochondriacal F45.20
  body dysmorphic F45.22
  neurosis F45.21
  other specified F45.29
identity
  dissociative F44.81
  of childhood F93.8
immune mechanism (immunity) D89.9
  specified type NEC D89.89
impaired renal tubular function N25.9
  specified NEC N25.89
impulse (control) F63.9
inflammatory
  pelvic, in diseases classified elsewhere
    — see category N74
  penis N48.29
    abscess N48.21
    cellulitis N48.22
  integument, newborn P83.9
    specified NEC P83.8
intermittent explosive F63.81
internal secretion pancreas — see
  Increased, secretion, pancreas,
  endocrine
intestine, intestinal
  carbohydrate absorption NEC E74.39
    postoperative K91.2
  functional NEC K59.9
    postoperative K91.89
  psychogenic F45.8
  vascular K55.9
    chronic K55.1
    specified NEC K55.8
intraoperative (intraprocedural) — see
  Complications, intraoperative
involuntary emotional expression (IEED)
  F48.2
iris H21.9
  adhesions — see Adhesions, iris
  atrophy — see Atrophy, iris
  chamber angle recession — see
    Recession, chamber angle
  cyst — see Cyst, iris
  degeneration — see Degeneration, iris
  in diseases classified elsewhere H22
  iridodialysis — see Iridodialysis
  iridoschisis — see Iridoschisis
  miotic pupillary cyst — see Cyst,
    pupillary
  pupillary
    abnormality — see Abnormality,
      pupillary
    membrane — see Membrane,
      pupillary
  specified type NEC H21.89
  vascular NEC H21.1x-
iron metabolism E83.10
  specified NEC E83.19
isovaleric acidemia E71.110
jaw, developmental M27.0
  temporomandibular — see Anomaly,
    dentofacial, temporomandibular
    joint
joint M25.9
  derangement — see Derangement, joint
  effusion — see Effusion, joint
  fistula — see Fistula, joint
  hemarthrosis — see Hemarthrosis
  instability — see Instability, joint
  osteophyte — see Osteophyte
  pain — see Pain, joint
  psychogenic F45.8
  specified type NEC M25.80
    ankle M25.87-
    elbow M25.82-
    foot joint M25.87-
    hand joint M25.84-
    hip M25.85-
    knee M25.86-
    shoulder M25.81-
    wrist M25.83-
  stiffness — see Stiffness, joint
ketone metabolism E71.32
kidney N28.9
  functional (tubular) N25.9
  in
    schistosomiasis B65.9 [N29]
  tubular function N25.9
    specified NEC N25.89
lacrimal system H04.9
  changes H04.69
    fistula — see Fistula, lacrimal

Disorder (of) (see also Disease) — continued
lacrimal system H04.9 — continued
  gland H04.19
    atrophy — see Atrophy, lacrimal
      gland
    cyst — see Cyst, lacrimal, gland
    dacryops — see Dacryops
    dislocation — see Dislocation,
      lacrimal gland
    dry eye syndrome — see Syndrome,
      dry eye
    infection — see Dacryoadenitis
    granuloma — see Granuloma, lacrimal
    inflammation — see Inflammation,
      lacrimal
    obstruction — see Obstruction, lacrimal
    specified NEC H04.89
lactation NEC O92.79
language (developmental) F80.9
  expressive F80.1
  mixed receptive and expressive F80.2
  receptive F80.2
late luteal phase dysphoric N94.89
learning (specific) F81.9
  acalculia R48.8
  alexia R48.0
  mathematics F81.2
  reading F81.0
  specified NEC F81.89
  spelling F81.81
  written expression F81.81
lens H27.9
  aphakia — see Aphakia
  cataract — see Cataract
  dislocation — see Dislocation, lens
  specified type NEC H27.8
ligament M24.20
  ankle M24.27-
  attachment, spine — see Enthesopathy,
    spinal
  elbow M24.22-
  foot joint M24.27-
  hand joint M24.24-
  hip M24.25-
  knee — see Derangement, knee,
    specified NEC
  shoulder M24.21-
  vertebra M24.28
  wrist M24.23-
ligamentous attachments — see also
  Enthesopathy
  spine — see Enthesopathy, spinal
lipid
  metabolism, congenital E78.9
  storage E75.6
    specified NEC E75.5
lipoprotein
  deficiency (familial) E78.6
  metabolism E78.9
    specified NEC E78.89
liver K76.9
  malarial B54 [K77]
low back — see also Dorsopathy, specified
  NEC
lumbosacral
  plexus G54.1
  root (nerve) NEC G54.4
lung, interstitial, drug-induced J70.4
  acute J70.2
  chronic J70.3
lymphoproliferative, post-transplant
  (PTLD) D47.Z1
lysine and hydroxylysine metabolism
  E72.3
male
  erectile (organic) (see also Dysfunction,
    sexual, male, erectile) N52.9
    nonorganic F52.21
  hypoactive sexual desire F52.0
  orgasmic F52.32
manic F30.9
  organic F06.33
mastoid — see also Disorder, ear, middle
  postprocedural — see Complications,
    ear, procedure
meniscus — see Derangement, knee,
  meniscus
menopausal N95.9
  specified NEC N95.8
menstrual N92.6
  psychogenic F45.8
  specified NEC N92.5
mental (or behavioral) (nonpsychotic) F99
  due to (secondary to)
    amphetamine
      due to drug abuse — see Abuse,
        drug, stimulant
      due to drug dependence — see
        Dependence, drug, stimulant

Disorder (of) (see also Disease) — continued
mental (or behavioral) (nonpsychotic) F99
  — continued
  due to (secondary to) — continued
    brain disease, damage and
      dysfunction F09
    caffeine use
      due to drug abuse — see Abuse,
        drug, stimulant
      due to drug dependence — see
        Dependence, drug, stimulant
    cannabis use
      due to drug abuse — see Abuse,
        drug, cannabis
      due to drug dependence — see
        Dependence, drug, cannabis
    general medical condition F09
    sedative or hypnotic use
      due to drug abuse — see Abuse,
        drug, sedative
      due to drug dependence — see
        Dependence, drug, sedative
    tobacco (nicotine) use — see
      Dependence, drug, nicotine
  following drug abuse or brain damage F07.9
  frontal lobe syndrome F07.0
  personality change F07.0
  postconcussional syndrome F07.81
  specified NEC F07.89
  infancy, childhood or adolescence F98.9
  neurotic — see Neurosis
  organic or symptomatic F09
  presenile, psychotic F03
  problem NEC
  psychoneurotic — see Neurosis
  psychotic — see Psychosis
  puerperal F53
  senile, psychotic NEC F03
metabolic, amino acid, transitory, newborn
  P74.8
metabolism NOS E88.9
  amino-acid E72.9
    aromatic E70.9
      albinism — see Albinism
      histidine E70.40
        histidinemia E70.41
        other specified E70.49
      hyperphenylalaninemia E70.1
        classical phenylketonuria E70.0
      other specified E70.8
      tryptophan E70.5
      tyrosine E70.20
        hypertyrosinemia E70.21
        other specified E70.29
    branched chain E71.2
      3-methylglutaconic aciduria
        E71.111
      hyperleucine-isoleucinemia E71.19
      hypervalinemia E71.19
      isovaleric acidemia E71.110
      maple syrup urine disease E71.0
      methylmalonic acidemia E71.120
      organic aciduria NEC E71.118
      other specified E71.19
      proprionate NEC E71.128
      propionic acidemia E71.121
    glycine E72.50
      d-glycericacidemia E72.59
      hyperhydroxyprolinemia E72.59
      hyperoxaluria E72.53
      hyperprolinemia E72.59
      non-ketotic hyperglycinemia
        E72.51
      other specified E72.59
      sarcosinemia E72.59
      trimethylaminuria E72.52
    hydroxylysine E72.3
    lysine E72.3
    ornithine E72.4
    other specified E72.8
      beta-amino acid E72.8
      gamma-glutamyl cycle E72.8
      straight-chain E72.8
      sulfur-bearing E72.10
        homocystinuria E72.11
        methylenetetrahydrofolate
          reductase deficiency E72.12
      other specified E72.19
  bile acid and cholesterol metabolism
    E78.70
  bilirubin E80.7
    specified NEC E80.6
  calcium E83.50
    hypercalcemia E83.52
    hypocalcemia E83.51
    other specified E83.59
  carbohydrate E74.9
    specified NEC E74.8
  cholesterol and bile acid metabolism
    E78.70

Disorder (of) *(see also* Disease*)* — *continued*
metabolism NOS E88.9 — *continued*
  congenital E88.9
  copper E83.00
    specified type NEC E83.09
    Wilson's disease E83.01
  cystinuria E72.01
  fructose E74.10
  galactose E74.20
  glucosaminoglycan E76.9
    mucopolysaccharidosis — *see*
      Mucopolysaccharidosis
    specified NEC E76.8
  glutamine E72.8
  glycine E72.50
  glycogen storage (hepatorenal) E74.09
  glycoprotein E77.9
    specified NEC E77.8
  glycosaminoglycan E76.9
    specified NEC E76.8
  in labor and delivery O75.89
  iron E83.10
  isoleucine E71.19
  leucine E71.19
  lipoid E78.9
  lipoprotein E78.9
    specified NEC E78.89
  magnesium E83.40
    hypermagnesemia E83.41
    hypomagnesemia E83.42
    other specified E83.49
  mineral E83.9
    specified NEC E83.89
  mitochondrial E88.40
    MELAS syndrome E88.41
    MERRF syndrome (myoclonic
      epilepsy associated with
      ragged-red fibers) E88.42
    other specified E88.49
  ornithine E72.4
  phosphatases E83.30
  phosphorus E83.30
    acid phosphatase deficiency E83.39
    hypophosphatasia E83.39
    hypophosphatemia E83.39
      familial E83.31
    other specified E83.39
    pseudovitamin D deficiency E83.32
  plasma protein NEC E88.09
  porphyrin — *see* Porphyria
  postprocedural E89.89
    specified NEC E89.89
  purine E79.9
    specified NEC E79.8
  pyrimidine E79.9
    specified NEC E79.8
  pyruvate E74.4
  serine E72.8
  sodium E87.8
  specified NEC E88.89
  threonine E72.8
  valine E71.19
  zinc E83.2
methylmalonic acidemia E71.120
micturition NEC R39.19
  feeling of incomplete emptying R39.14
  hesitancy R39.11
  poor stream R39.12
  psychogenic F45.8
  split stream R39.13
  straining R39.16
  urgency R39.15
mitochondrial metabolism E88.40
mitral (valve) — *see* Endocarditis, mitral
mixed
  anxiety and depressive F41.8
  of scholastic skills (developmental)
    F81.89
  receptive expressive language F80.2
mood F39
  bipolar — *see* Disorder, bipolar
  depressive — *see* Disorder, depressive
  due to (secondary to)
    alcohol F10.94
    amphetamine F15.94
      in
        abuse F15.14
        dependence F15.24
    anxiolytic F13.94
      in
        abuse F13.14
        dependence F13.24
    cocaine F14.94
      in
        abuse F14.14
        dependence F14.24
    general medical condition F06.30

Disorder (of) *(see also* Disease*)* — *continued*
mood F39 — *continued*
  due to (secondary to) — *continued*
    hallucinogen F16.94
      in
        abuse F16.14
        dependence F16.24
    hypnotic F13.94
      in
        abuse F13.14
        dependence F13.24
    inhalant F18.94
      in
        abuse F18.14
        dependence F18.24
    opioid F11.94
      in
        abuse F11.14
        dependence F11.24
    phencyclidine (PCP) F16.94
      in
        abuse F16.14
        dependence F16.24
    physiological condition F06.30
      with
        depressive features F06.31
        major depressive-like episode
          F06.32
        manic features F06.33
        mixed features F06.34
    psychoactive substance NEC F19.94
      in
        abuse F19.14
        dependence F19.24
    sedative F13.94
      in
        abuse F13.14
        dependence F13.24
    volatile solvents F18.94
      in
        abuse F18.14
        dependence F18.24
  manic episode F30.9
    with psychotic symptoms F30.2
    in remission (full) F30.4
      partial F30.3
    specified type NEC F30.8
    without psychotic symptoms F30.10
      mild F30.11
      moderate F30.12
      severe F30.13
  organic F06.30
    right hemisphere F07.89
  persistent F34.9
    cyclothymia F34.0
    dysthymia F34.1
    specified type NEC F34.8
  recurrent F39
  right hemisphere organic F07.89
movement G25.9
  drug-induced G25.70
    akathisia G25.71
    specified NEC G25.79
  hysterical F44.4
  in diseases classified elsewhere — *see*
    category G26
  periodic limb G47.61
    sleep related G47.61
  sleep related NEC G47.69
  specified NEC G25.89
  stereotyped F98.4
  treatment-induced G25.9
multiple personality F44.81
muscle M62.9
  attachment, spine — *see* Enthesopathy,
    spinal
  in trichinellosis — *see* Trichinellosis,
    with muscle disorder
  psychogenic F45.8
  specified type NEC M62.89
  tone, newborn P94.9
    specified NEC P94.8
muscular
  attachments — *see also* Enthesopathy
    spine — *see* Enthesopathy, spinal
  urethra N36.44
musculoskeletal system, soft tissue — *see*
  Disorder, soft tissue
  postprocedural M96.89
  psychogenic F45.8
myoneural G70.9
  due to lead G70.1
  specified NEC G70.89
  toxic G70.1
myotonic NEC G71.19
nail, in diseases classified elsewhere L62
neck region NEC — *see* Dorsopathy,
  specified NEC

Disorder (of) *(see also* Disease*)* — *continued*
nerve G58.9
  abducent NEC — *see* Strabismus,
    paralytic, sixth nerve
  accessory G52.8
  acoustic — *see* subcategory H93.3
  auditory — *see* subcategory H93.3
  auriculotemporal G50.8
  axillary G54.0
  cerebral — *see* Disorder, nerve, cranial
  cranial G52.9
    eighth — *see* subcategory H93.3
    eleventh G52.8
    fifth G50.9
    first G52.0
    fourth NEC — *see* Strabismus,
      paralytic, fourth nerve
    multiple G52.7
    ninth G52.1
    second NEC — *see* Disorder, nerve,
      optic
    seventh NEC G51.8
    sixth NEC — *see* Strabismus,
      paralytic, sixth nerve
    specified NEC G52.8
    tenth G52.2
    third NEC — *see* Strabismus,
      paralytic, third nerve
    twelfth G52.3
  entrapment — *see* Neuropathy,
    entrapment
  facial G51.9
    specified NEC G51.8
  femoral — *see* Lesion, nerve, femoral
  glossopharyngeal NEC G52.1
  hypoglossal G52.3
  intercostal G58.0
  lateral
    cutaneous of thigh — *see*
      Mononeuropathy, lower limb,
      meralgia paresthetica
    popliteal — *see* Lesion, nerve,
      popliteal
  lower limb — *see* Mononeuropathy,
    lower limb
  medial popliteal — *see* Lesion, nerve,
    popliteal, medial
  median NEC — *see* Lesion, nerve,
    median
  multiple G58.7
  oculomotor NEC — *see* Strabismus,
    paralytic, third nerve
  olfactory G52.0
  optic NEC H47.09-
    hemorrhage into sheath — *see*
      Hemorrhage, optic nerve
    ischemic H47.01-
  peroneal — *see* Lesion, nerve, popliteal
  phrenic G58.8
  plantar — *see* Lesion, nerve, plantar
  pneumogastric G52.2
  posterior tibial — *see* Syndrome, tarsal
    tunnel
  radial — *see* Lesion, nerve, radial
  recurrent laryngeal G52.2
  root G54.9
    cervical G54.2
    lumbosacral G54.1
    specified NEC G54.8
    thoracic G54.3
  sciatic NEC — *see* Lesion, nerve, sciatic
  specified NEC G58.8
    lower limb — *see* Mononeuropathy,
      lower limb, specified NEC
    upper limb — *see* Mononeuropathy,
      upper limb, specified NEC
  sympathetic G90.9
  tibial — *see* Lesion, nerve, popliteal,
    medial
  trigeminal G50.9
    specified NEC G50.8
  trochlear NEC — *see* Strabismus,
    paralytic, fourth nerve
  ulnar — *see* Lesion, nerve, ulnar
  upper limb — *see* Mononeuropathy,
    upper limb
  vagus G52.2
nervous system G98.8
  autonomic (peripheral) G90.9
    specified NEC G90.8
  central G96.9
    specified NEC G96.8
  parasympathetic G90.9
  specified NEC G98.8
  sympathetic G90.9
  vegetative G90.9
neurohypophysis NEC E23.3
neurological NEC R29.818

Disorder (of) *(see also* Disease*)* — *continued*
neuromuscular G70.9
  hereditary NEC G71.9
  specified NEC G70.89
  toxic G70.1
neurotic F48.9
  specified NEC F48.8
neutrophil, polymorphonuclear D71
nicotine use — *see* Dependence, drug,
  nicotine
nightmare F51.5
nose J34.9
  specified NEC J34.89
obsessive-compulsive F42
odontogenesis NOS K00.9
opioid use
  with
    opiod-induced psychotic disorder
      F11.959
      with
        delusions F11.950
        hallucinations F11.951
  due to drug abuse — *see* Abuse, drug,
    opioid
  due to drug dependence — *see*
    Dependence, drug, opioid
oppositional defiant F91.3
optic
  chiasm H47.49
    due to
      inflammatory disorder H47.41
      neoplasm H47.42
      vascular disorder H47.43
  disc H47.39-
    coloboma — *see* Coloboma, optic disc
    drusen — *see* Drusen, optic disc
    pseudopapilledema — *see*
      Pseudopapilledema
  radiations — *see* Disorder, visual,
    pathway
  tracts — *see* Disorder, visual, pathway
orbit H05.9
  cyst — *see* Cyst, orbit
  deformity — *see* Deformity, orbit
  edema — *see* Edema, orbit
  enophthalmos — *see* Enophthalmos
  exophthalmos — *see* Exophthalmos
  hemorrhage — *see* Hemorrhage, orbit
  inflammation — *see* Inflammation, orbit
  myopathy — *see* Myopathy, extraocular
    muscles
  retained foreign body — *see* Foreign
    body, orbit, old
  specified type NEC H05.89
organic
  anxiety F06.4
  catatonic F06.1
  delusional F06.2
  dissociative F06.8
  emotionally labile (asthenic) F06.8
  mood (affective) F06.30
  schizophrenia-like F06.2
orgasmic (female) F52.31
  male F52.32
ornithine metabolism E72.4
overanxious F41.1
  of childhood F93.8
pain
  with related psychological factors
    F45.42
  exclusively related to psychological
    factors F45.41
pancreatic internal secretion E16.9
  specified NEC E16.8
panic F41.0
  with agoraphobia F40.01
papulosquamous L44.9
  in diseases classified elsewhere L45
  specified NEC L44.8
paranoid F22
  induced F24
  shared F24
parathyroid (gland) E21.5
  specified NEC E21.4
parietoalveolar NEC J84.09
paroxysmal, mixed R56.9
patella M22.9-
  chondromalacia — *see* Chondromalacia,
    patella
  derangement NEC M22.3x-
  recurrent
    dislocation — *see* Dislocation, patella,
      recurrent
    subluxation — *see* Dislocation,
      patella, recurrent, incomplete
  specified NEC M22.8x-
  patellofemoral M22.2x-
pentose phosphate pathway with anemia
  D55.1

DISEASE INDEX

Disorder (of) *(see also* Disease) — *continued*
perception, due to hallucinogens F16.983
  in
    abuse F16.183
    dependence F16.283
peripheral nervous system NEC G64
peroxisomal E71.50
  biogenesis
    neonatal adrenoleukodystrophy E71.511
    specified disorder NEC E71.518
    Zellweger syndrome E71.510
  rhizomelic chondrodysplasia punctata E71.540
  specified form NEC E71.548
    group 1 E71.518
    group 2 E71.53
    group 3 E71.542
  X-linked adrenoleukodystrophy E71.529
    adolescent E71.521
    adrenomyeloneuropathy E71.522
    childhood E71.520
    specified form NEC E71.528
  Zellweger-like syndrome E71.541
persistent
  (somatoform) pain F45.41
  affective (mood) F34.9
personality *(see also* Personality) F60.9
  affective F34.0
  aggressive F60.3
  amoral F60.2
  anankastic F60.5
  antisocial F60.2
  anxious F60.6
  asocial F60.2
  asthenic F60.7
  avoidant F60.6
  borderline F60.3
  change (secondary) due to general medical condition F07.0
  compulsive F60.5
  cyclothymic F34.0
  dependent (passive) F60.7
  depressive F34.1
  dissocial F60.2
  emotional instability F60.3
  expansive paranoid F60.0
  explosive F60.3
  following organic brain damage F07.9
  histrionic F60.4
  hyperthymic F34.0
  hypothymic F34.1
  hysterical F60.4
  immature F60.89
  inadequate F60.7
  labile F60.3
  mixed (nonspecific) F60.89
  moral deficiency F60.2
  narcissistic F60.81
  negativistic F60.89
  obsessional F60.5
  obsessive(-compulsive) F60.5
  organic F07.9
  overconscientious F60.5
  paranoid F60.0
  passive(-dependent) F60.7
  passive-aggressive F60.89
  pathological NEC F60.9
  pseudosocial F60.2
  psychopathic F60.2
  schizoid F60.1
  schizotypal F21
  self-defeating F60.7
  specified NEC F60.89
  type A F60.5
  unstable (emotional) F60.3
pervasive, developmental F84.9
phobic anxiety, childhood F40.8
phosphate-losing tubular N25.0
pigmentation L81.9
  choroid, congenital Q14.3
  diminished melanin formation L81.6
  iron L81.8
  specified NEC L81.8
pinna (noninfective) H61.10-
  deformity, acquired H61.11-
  hematoma H61.12-
  perichondritis — *see* Perichondritis, ear
  specified type NEC H61.19-
pituitary gland E23.7
  iatrogenic (postprocedural) E89.3
  specified NEC E23.6
platelets D69.1

Disorder (of) *(see also* Disease) — *continued*
plexus G54.9
  specified NEC G54.8
polymorphonuclear neutrophils D71
porphyrin metabolism — *see* Porphyria
post-transplant lymphoproliferative D47.Z1
post-traumatic stress (PTSD) F43.10
  acute F43.11
  chronic F43.12
postconcussional F07.81
posthallucinogen perception F16.983
  in
    abuse F16.183
    dependence F16.283
postmenopausal N95.9
  specified NEC N95.8
postprocedural (postoperative) — *see* Complications, postprocedural
premenstrual dysphoric (PMDD) N94.3
prepuce N47.8
propionic acidemia E71.121
prostate N42.9
  specified NEC N42.89
psychogenic NOS *(see also* condition) F45.9
  anxiety F41.8
  appetite F50.9
  asthenic F48.8
  cardiovascular (system) F45.8
  compulsive F42
  cutaneous F54
  depressive F32.9
  digestive (system) F45.8
  dysmenorrheic F45.8
  dyspneic F45.8
  endocrine (system) F54
  eye NEC F45.8
  feeding — *see* Disorder, eating
  functional NEC F45.8
  gastric F45.8
  gastrointestinal (system) F45.8
  genitourinary (system) F45.8
  heart (function) (rhythm) F45.8
  hyperventilatory F45.8
  hypochondriacal — *see* Disorder, hypochondriacal
  intestinal F45.8
  joint F45.8
  learning F81.9
  limb F45.8
  lymphatic (system) F45.8
  menstrual F45.8
  micturition F45.8
  monoplegic NEC F44.4
  motor F44.4
  muscle F45.8
  musculoskeletal F45.8
  neurocirculatory F45.8
  obsessive F42
  occupational F48.8
  organ or part of body NEC F45.8
  paralytic NEC F44.4
  phobic F40.9
  physical NEC F45.8
  rectal F45.8
  respiratory (system) F45.8
  rheumatic F45.8
  sexual (function) F52.9
  skin (allergic) (eczematous) F54
  sleep F51.9
  specified part of body NEC F45.8
  stomach F45.8
psychological F99
  associated with
    disease classified elsewhere F54
    sexual
      development F66
      relationship F66
      uncertainty about gender identity F66
psychomotor NEC F44.4
  hysterical F44.4
psychoneurotic — *see also* Neurosis
  mixed NEC F48.8
psychophysiologic — *see* Disorder, somatoform
psychosexual F65.9
  development F66
  identity of childhood F64.2
psychosomatic NOS — *see* Disorder, somatoform
  multiple F45.0
  undifferentiated F45.1
psychotic — *see* Psychosis
  transient (acute) F23
puberty E30.9
  specified NEC E30.8

Disorder (of) *(see also* Disease) — *continued*
pulmonary (valve) — *see* Endocarditis, pulmonary
purine metabolism E79.9
pyrimidine metabolism E79.9
pyruvate metabolism E74.4
reactive attachment (childhood) F94.1
reading R48.0
  developmental (specific) F81.0
receptive language F80.2
receptor, hormonal, peripheral *(see also* Syndrome, androgen insensitivity) E34.50
recurrent brief depressive F33.8
reflex R29.2
refraction H52.7
  aniseikonia H52.32
  anisometropia H52.31
  astigmatism — *see* Astigmatism
  hypermetropia — *see* Hypermetropia
  myopia — *see* Myopia
  presbyopia H52.4
  specified NEC H52.6
relationship F68.8
  due to sexual orientation F66
REM sleep behavior G47.52
renal function, impaired (tubular) N25.9
resonance R49.9
  specified NEC R49.8
respiratory function, impaired — *see also* Failure, respiration
  postprocedural — *see* Complication, postoperative, respiratory system
  psychogenic F45.8
retina H35.9
  angioid streaks H35.33
  changes in vascular appearance H35.01-
  degeneration — *see* Degeneration, retina
  dystrophy (hereditary) — *see* Dystrophy, retina
  edema H35.81
  hemorrhage — *see* Hemorrhage, retina
  ischemia H35.82
  macular degeneration — *see* Degeneration, macula
  microaneurysms H35.04-
  microvascular abnormality NEC H35.09
  neovascularization — *see* Neovascularization, retina
  retinopathy — *see* Retinopathy
  separation of layers H35.70
    central serous chorioretinopathy H35.71-
    pigment epithelium detachment (serous) H35.72-
    hemorrhagic H35.73-
  specified type NEC H35.89
  telangiectasis — *see* Telangiectasis, retina
  vasculitis — *see* Vasculitis, retina
retroperitoneal K68.9
right hemisphere organic affective F07.89
rumination (infant or child) F98.21
sacrum, sacrococcygeal NEC M53.3
schizoaffective F25.9
  bipolar type F25.0
  depressive type F25.1
  manic type F25.0
  mixed type F25.0
  specified NEC F25.8
schizoid of childhood F84.5
schizophreniform F20.81
  brief F23
schizotypal (personality) F21
secretion, thyrocalcitonin E07.0
seizure *(see also* Epilepsy) G40.909
  intractable G40.919
    with status epilepticus G40.911
semantic pragmatic F80.89
  with autism F84.0
sense of smell R43.1
  psychogenic F45.8
separation anxiety, of childhood F93.0
sexual
  arousal, female F52.22
  aversion F52.1
  function, psychogenic F52.9
  maturation F66
  nonorganic F52.9
  preference *(see also* Deviation, sexual) F65.9
    fetishistic transvestism F65.1
  relationship F66
shyness, of childhood and adolescence F40.10
sibling rivalry F93.8

Disorder (of) *(see also* Disease) — *continued*
sickle-cell (sickling) (homozygous) — *see* Disease, sickle-cell
  heterozygous D57.3
  specified type NEC D57.8-
  trait D57.3
sinus (nasal) J34.9
  specified NEC J34.89
skin L98.9
  atrophic L90.9
    specified NEC L90.8
  granulomatous L92.9
    specified NEC L92.8
  hypertrophic L91.9
    specified NEC L91.8
  infiltrative NEC L98.6
  newborn P83.9
    specified NEC P83.8
  psychogenic (allergic) (eczematous) F54
sleep G47.9
  breathing-related — *see* Apnea, sleep
  circadian rhythm G47.20
    advance sleep phase type G47.22
    delayed sleep phase type G47.21
    due to
      alcohol
        abuse F10.182
        dependence F10.282
        use F10.982
      amphetamines
        abuse F15.182
        dependence F15.282
        use F15.982
      caffeine
        abuse F15.182
        dependence F15.282
        use F15.982
      cocaine
        abuse F14.182
        dependence F14.282
        use F14.982
      drug NEC
        abuse F19.182
        dependence F19.282
        use F19.982
      opioid
        abuse F11.182
        dependence F11.282
        use F11.982
      psychoactive substance NEC
        abuse F19.182
        dependence F19.282
        use F19.982
      sedative, hypnotic, or anxiolytic
        abuse F13.182
        dependence F13.282
        use F13.982
      stimulant NEC
        abuse F15.182
        dependence F15.282
        use F15.982
    free running type G47.24
    in conditions classified elsewhere G47.27
    irregular sleep wake type G47.23
    jet lag type G47.25
    shift work type G47.26
    specified NEC G47.29
  due to
    alcohol
      abuse F10.182
      dependence F10.282
      use F10.982
    amphetamine
      abuse F15.182
      dependence F15.282
      use F15.982
    anxiolytic
      abuse F13.182
      dependence F13.282
      use F13.982
    caffeine
      abuse F15.182
      dependence F15.282
      use F15.982
    cocaine
      abuse F14.182
      dependence F14.282
      use F14.982
    drug NEC
      abuse F19.182
      dependence F19.282
      use F19.982
    hypnotic
      abuse F13.182
      dependence F13.282
      use F13.982

Disorder (of) (see also Disease) — continued
sleep G47.9 — continued
  due to — continued
    opioid
      abuse F11.182
      dependence F11.282
      use F11.982
    psychoactive substance NEC
      abuse F19.182
      dependence F19.282
      use F19.982
    sedative
      abuse F13.182
      dependence F13.282
      use F13.982
    stimulant NEC
      abuse F15.182
      dependence F15.282
      use F15.982
  emotional F51.9
  excessive somnolence — see Hypersomnia
  hypersomnia type — see Hypersomnia
  initiating or maintaining — see Insomnia
  nightmares F51.5
  nonorganic F51.9
    specified NEC F51.8
  parasomnia type G47.50
  specified NEC G47.8
  terrors F51.4
  walking F51.3
sleep-wake pattern or schedule — see Disorder, sleep, circadian rhythm
social
  anxiety of childhood F40.10
  functioning in childhood F94.9
  specified NEC F94.8
soft tissue M79.9
  ankle M79.9
  due to use, overuse and pressure M70.90
    ankle M70.97-
    bursitis — see Bursitis
    foot M70.97-
    forearm M70.93-
    hand M70.94-
    lower leg M70.96-
    multiple sites M70.99
    pelvic region M70.95-
    shoulder region M70.91-
    specified site NEC M70.98
    specified type NEC M70.80
      ankle M70.87-
      foot M70.87-
      forearm M70.83-
      hand M70.84-
      lower leg M70.86-
      multiple sites M70.89
      pelvic region M70.85-
      shoulder region M70.81-
      specified site NEC M70.88
      thigh M70.85-
      upper arm M70.82-
    thigh M70.95-
    upper arm M70.92-
  foot M79.9
  forearm M79.9
  hand M79.9
  lower leg M79.9
  multiple sites M79.9
  occupational — see Disorder, soft tissue, due to use, overuse and pressure
  pelvic region M79.9
  shoulder region M79.9
  specified type NEC M79.89
  thigh M79.9
  upper arm M79.9
somatization F45.0
somatoform F45.9
  pain (persistent) F45.41
  somatization (multiple) (long-lasting) F45.0
  specified NEC F45.8
  undifferentiated F45.1
somnolence, excessive — see Hypersomnia
specific
  arithmetical F81.2
  developmental, of motor F82
  reading F81.0
  speech and language F80.9
  spelling F81.81
  written expression F81.81
speech R47.9
  articulation (functional) (specific) F80.0
  developmental F80.9
  specified NEC R47.89
  spelling (specific) F81.81

Disorder (of) (see also Disease) — continued
spine — see also Dorsopathy
  ligamentous or muscular attachments, peripheral — see Enthesopathy, spinal
  specified NEC — see Dorsopathy, specified NEC
stereotyped, habit or movement F98.4
stomach (functional) — see Disorder, gastric
stress F43.9
  post-traumatic F43.10
    acute F43.11
    chronic F43.12
sulfur-bearing amino-acid metabolism E72.10
sweat gland (eccrine) L74.9
  apocrine L75.9
    specified NEC L75.8
  specified NEC L74.8
synovium M67.90
  acromioclavicular M67.91-
  ankle M67.97-
  elbow M67.92-
  foot M67.97-
  forearm M67.93-
  hand M67.94-
  hip M67.95-
  knee M67.96-
  multiple sites M67.99
  rupture — see Rupture, synovium
  shoulder M67.91-
  specified type NEC M67.80
    acromioclavicular M67.81-
    ankle M67.87-
    elbow M67.82-
    foot M67.87-
    hand M67.84-
    hip M67.85-
    knee M67.86-
    multiple sites M67.89
    wrist M67.83-
  synovitis — see Synovitis
  upper arm M67.92-
  wrist M67.93-
temperature regulation, newborn P81.9
  specified NEC P81.8
temporomandibular joint — see Anomaly, dentofacial, temporomandibular joint
tendon M67.90
  acromioclavicular M67.91-
  ankle M67.97-
  contracture — see Contracture, tendon
  elbow M67.92-
  foot M67.97-
  forearm M67.93-
  hand M67.94-
  hip M67.95-
  knee M67.96-
  multiple sites M67.99
  rupture — see Rupture, tendon
  shoulder M67.91-
  specified type NEC M67.80
    acromioclavicular M67.81-
    ankle M67.87-
    elbow M67.82-
    foot M67.87-
    hand M67.84-
    hip M67.85-
    knee M67.86-
    multiple sites M67.89
    trunk M67.88
    wrist M67.83-
  synovitis — see Synovitis
  tendinitis — see Tendinitis
  tenosynovitis — see Tenosynovitis
  trunk M67.98
  upper arm M67.92-
  wrist M67.93-
thoracic root (nerve) NEC G54.3
thyrocalcitonin hypersecretion E07.0
thyroid (gland) E07.9
  function NEC, neonatal, transitory P72.2
  iodine-deficiency related E01.8
  specified NEC E07.89
tic — see Tic
tooth K08.9
  development K00.9
    specified NEC K00.8
  eruption K00.6
Tourette's F95.2
trance and possession F44.89
tricuspid (valve) — see Endocarditis, tricuspid
tryptophan metabolism E70.5
tubular, phosphate-losing N25.0

Disorder (of) (see also Disease) — continued
tubulo-interstitial (in)
  brucellosis A23.9 [N16]
  cystinosis E72.04
  diphtheria A36.84
  glycogen storage disease E74.00 [N16]
  leukemia NEC C95.9-[N16]
  lymphoma NEC C85.9-[N16]
  mixed cryoglobulinemia D89.1 [N16]
  multiple myeloma C90.0-[N16]
  Salmonella infection A02.25
  sarcoidosis D86.84
  sepsis A41.9 [N16]
    streptococcal A40.9 [N16]
  systemic lupus erythematosus M32.15
  toxoplasmosis B58.83
  transplant rejection T86.91 [N16]
  Wilson's disease E83.01 [N16]
tubulo-renal function, impaired N25.9
  specified NEC N25.89
tympanic membrane H73.9-
  atrophy — see Atrophy, tympanic membrane
  infection — see Myringitis
  perforation — see Perforation, tympanum
  specified NEC H73.89-
unsocialized aggressive F91.1
urea cycle metabolism E72.20
  argininemia E72.21
  arginosuccinic aciduria E72.22
  citrullinemia E72.23
  ornithine transcarbamylase deficiency E72.4
  other specified E72.29
ureter (in) N28.9
  schistosomiasis B65.0 [N29]
  tuberculosis A18.11
urethra N36.9
  specified NEC N36.8
urinary system N39.9
  specified NEC N39.8
valve, heart
  aortic — see Endocarditis, aortic
  mitral — see Endocarditis, mitral
  pulmonary — see Endocarditis, pulmonary
  rheumatic
    aortic — see Endocarditis, aortic, rheumatic
    mitral — see Endocarditis, mitral
    pulmonary — see Endocarditis, pulmonary, rheumatic
    tricuspid — see Endocarditis, tricuspid
  tricuspid — see Endocarditis, tricuspid
vestibular function H81.9-
  specified NEC — see subcategory H81.8-
  in diseases classified elsewhere H82-
  vertigo — see Vertigo
vision, binocular H53.30
  abnormal retinal correspondence H53.31
  diplopia H53.2
  fusion with defective stereopsis H53.32
  simultaneous perception H53.33
  suppression H53.34
visual
  cortex
    blindness H47.619
      left brain H47.612
      right brain H47.611
    due to
      inflammatory disorder H47.629
        left brain H47.622
        right brain H47.621
      neoplasm H47.639
        left brain H47.632
        right brain H47.631
      vascular disorder H47.649
        left brain H47.642
        right brain H47.641
  pathway H47.9
    due to
      inflammatory disorder H47.51-
      neoplasm H47.52-
      vascular disorder H47.53-
  optic chiasm — see Disorder, optic, chiasm
vitreous body H43.9
  crystalline deposits — see Deposit, crystalline
  degeneration — see Degeneration, vitreous
  hemorrhage — see Hemorrhage, vitreous
  opacities — see Opacity, vitreous
  prolapse — see Prolapse, vitreous
  specified type NEC H43.89
voice R49.9
  specified type NEC R49.8

Disorder (of) (see also Disease) — continued
volatile solvent use
  due to drug abuse — see Abuse, drug, inhalant
  due to drug dependence — see Dependence, drug, inhalant
white blood cells D72.9
  specified NEC D72.89
withdrawing, child or adolescent F40.10
Disorientation R41.0
Displacement, displaced
acquired traumatic of bone, cartilage, joint, tendon NEC — see Dislocation
adrenal gland (congenital) Q89.1
appendix, retrocecal (congenital) Q43.8
auricle (congenital) Q17.4
bladder (acquired) N32.89
  congenital Q64.19
brachial plexus (congenital) Q07.8
brain stem, caudal (congenital) Q04.8
canaliculus (lacrimalis), congenital Q10.6
cardia through esophageal hiatus (congenital) Q40.1
cerebellum, caudal (congenital) Q04.8
cervix — see Malposition, uterus
colon (congenital) Q43.3
device, implant or graft (see also Complications, by site and type, mechanical) T85.628
  arterial graft NEC — see Complication, cardiovascular device, mechanical, vascular
  breast (implant) T85.42
  catheter NEC T85.628
    dialysis (renal) T82.42
    intraperitoneal T85.621
    infusion NEC T82.524
      spinal (epidural) (subdural) T85.620
    urinary (indwelling) T83.028
      cystostomy T83.020
  electronic (electrode) (pulse generator) (stimulator) — see Complication, electronic stimulator
  fixation, internal (orthopedic) NEC — see Complication, fixation device, mechanical
  gastrointestinal — see Complications, prosthetic device, mechanical, gastrointestinal device
  genital NEC T83.428
    intrauterine contraceptive device T83.32
    penile prosthesis T83.420
  heart NEC — see Complication, cardiovascular device, mechanical
  joint prosthesis — see Complications, joint prosthesis, mechanical
  ocular — see Complications, prosthetic device, mechanical, ocular device
  orthopedic NEC — see Complication, orthopedic, device or graft, mechanical
  specified NEC T85.628
  urinary NEC — see also Complication, genitourinary, device, urinary, mechanical
    graft T83.22
  vascular NEC — see Complication, cardiovascular device, mechanical
  ventricular intracranial shunt T85.02
electronic stimulator
  bone T84.320
  cardiac — see Complications, cardiac device, electronic
  nervous system — see Complication, prosthetic device, mechanical, electronic nervous system stimulator
  urinary — see Complications, electronic stimulator, urinary
esophageal mucosa into cardia of stomach, congenital Q39.8
esophagus (acquired) K22.8
  congenital Q39.8
eyeball (acquired) (lateral) (old) — see Displacement, globe
  congenital Q15.8
  current — see Avulsion, eye
fallopian tube (acquired) N83.4
  congenital Q50.6
  opening (congenital) Q50.6
gallbladder (congenital) Q44.1
gastric mucosa (congenital) Q40.2
globe (acquired) (old) (lateral) H05.21-
  current — see Avulsion, eye
heart (congenital) Q24.8
  acquired I51.89
hymen (upward) (congenital) Q52.4

DISEASE INDEX

Displacement, displaced — continued
intervertebral disc NEC
  with myelopathy — see Disorder, disc, with, myelopathy
  cervical, cervicothoracic (with) M50.20
    myelopathy — see Disorder, disc, cervical, with myelopathy
    neuritis, radiculitis or radiculopathy — see Disorder, disc, cervical, with neuritis
  due to trauma — see Dislocation, vertebra
  lumbar region M51.26
    with
      myelopathy M51.06
      neuritis, radiculitis, radiculopathy or sciatica M51.16
  lumbosacral region M51.27
    with
      neuritis, radiculitis, radiculopathy or sciatica M51.17
  sacrococcygeal region M53.3
  thoracic region M51.24
    with
      myelopathy M51.04
      neuritis, radiculitis, radiculopathy M51.14
  thoracolumbar region M51.25
    with
      myelopathy M51.05
      neuritis, radiculitis, radiculopathy M51.15
intrauterine device T83.32
kidney (acquired) N28.83
  congenital Q63.2
lachrymal, lacrimal apparatus or duct (congenital) Q10.6
lens, congenital Q12.1
macula (congenital) Q14.1
Meckel's diverticulum Q43.0
  malignant — see Table of Neoplasms, small intestine, malignant
nail (congenital) Q84.6
  acquired L60.8
opening of Wharton's duct in mouth Q38.4
organ or site, congenital NEC — see Malposition, congenital
ovary (acquired) N83.4
  congenital Q50.39
  free in peritoneal cavity (congenital) Q50.39
  into hernial sac N83.4
oviduct (acquired) N83.4
  congenital Q50.6
parathyroid (gland) E21.4
parotid gland (congenital) Q38.4
punctum lacrimale (congenital) Q10.6
sacro-iliac (joint) (congenital) Q74.2
  current injury S33.2
  old — see subcategory M53.2
salivary gland (any) (congenital) Q38.4
spleen (congenital) Q89.09
stomach, congenital Q40.2
sublingual duct Q38.4
tongue (downward) (congenital) Q38.3
tooth, teeth, fully erupted M26.30
  horizontal M26.33
  vertical M26.34
trachea (congenital) Q32.1
ureter or ureteric opening or orifice (congenital) Q62.62
uterine opening of oviducts or fallopian tubes Q50.6
uterus, uterine — see Malposition, uterus
ventricular septum Q21.0
  with rudimentary ventricle Q20.4

Disproportion
between native and reconstructed breast N65.1
fiber-type G71.2

Disruptio uteri — see Rupture, uterus

Disruption (of)
ciliary body NEC H21.89
closure of
  cornea T81.31
  craniotomy T81.32
  fascia (muscular) (superficial) T81.32
  internal organ or tissue T81.32
  laceration (external) (internal) T81.33
  ligament T81.32
  mucosa T81.31
  muscle or muscle flap T81.32
  ribs or rib cage T81.32
  skin and subcutaneous tissue (full-thickness) (superficial) T81.31
  skull T81.32
  sternum (sternotomy) T81.32
  tendon T81.32
  traumatic laceration (external) (internal) T81.33

Disruption (of) — continued
family Z63.8
  due to
    absence of family member due to military deployment Z63.31
    absence of family member NEC Z63.32
    alcoholism and drug addiction in family Z63.72
    bereavement Z63.4
    death (assumed) or disappearance of family member Z63.4
    divorce or separation Z63.5
    drug addiction in family Z63.72
    return of family member from military deployment (current or past conflict) Z63.71
    stressful life events NEC Z63.79
iris NEC H21.89
ligament(s) — see also Sprain
  knee
    current injury — see Dislocation, knee
    old (chronic) — see Derangement, knee, ligament, instability, chronic
    spontaneous NEC — see Derangement, knee, disruption ligament
ossicular chain — see Discontinuity, ossicles, ear
pelvic ring (stable) S32.810
  unstable S32.811
traumatic injury wound repair T81.33
wound T81.30
  episiotomy O90.1
  operation T81.31
    cesarean O90.0
    external operation wound (superficial) T81.31
    internal operation wound (deep) T81.32
  perineal (obstetric) O90.1
  traumatic injury repair T81.33

Dissatisfaction with
employment Z56.9
school environment Z55.4

Dissecting — see condition

Dissection
aorta I71.00
  abdominal I71.02
  thoracic I71.01
  thoracoabdominal I71.03
artery
  carotid I77.71
  cerebral (nonruptured) I67.0
    ruptured — see Hemorrhage, intracranial, subarachnoid
  coronary I25.42
  iliac I77.72
  renal I77.73
  specified NEC I77.79
  vertebral I77.74
traumatic — see Wound, open, by site
vascular I99.8
wound — see Wound, open

Disseminated — see condition

Dissociation
auriculoventricular or atrioventricular (AV) (any degree) (isorhythmic) I45.89
  with heart block I44.2
interference I45.89

Dissociative reaction, state F44.9

Dissolution, vertebra — see Osteoporosis

Distension, distention
abdomen R14.0
bladder N32.89
cecum K63.89
colon K63.89
gallbladder K82.8
intestine K63.89
kidney N28.89
liver K76.89
seminal vesicle N50.8
stomach K31.89
  acute K31.0
  psychogenic F45.8
ureter — see Dilatation, ureter
uterus N85.8

Disto-occlusion (Division I) (Division II) M26.212

Distoma hepaticum infestation B66.3

Distomiasis B66.9
bile passages B66.3
hemic B65.9
hepatic B66.3
  due to Clonorchis sinensis B66.1
intestinal B66.5
liver B66.3
  due to Clonorchis sinensis B66.1
lung B66.4
pulmonary B66.4

Distomolar (fourth molar) K00.1

Distortion(s) (congenital)
adrenal (gland) Q89.1
arm NEC Q68.8
bile duct or passage Q44.5
bladder Q64.79
brain Q04.9
cervix (uteri) Q51.9
chest (wall) Q67.8
  bones Q76.8
clavicle Q74.0
clitoris Q52.6
coccyx Q76.49
common duct Q44.5
coronary Q24.5
cystic duct Q44.5
ear (auricle) (external) Q17.3
  inner Q16.5
  middle Q16.4
    ossicles Q16.3
endocrine NEC Q89.2
eustachian tube Q17.8
eye (adnexa) Q15.8
face bone(s) NEC Q75.8
fallopian tube Q50.6
femur NEC Q68.8
fibula NEC Q68.8
finger(s) Q68.1
foot Q66.9
genitalia, genital organ(s)
  female Q52.8
    external Q52.79
    internal NEC Q52.8
gyri Q04.8
hand bone(s) Q68.1
heart (auricle) (ventricle) Q24.8
  valve (cusp) Q24.8
hepatic duct Q44.5
humerus NEC Q68.8
hymen Q52.4
intrafamilial communications Z63.8
jaw NEC M26.89
labium (majus) (minus) Q52.79
leg NEC Q68.8
lens Q12.8
liver Q44.7
lumbar spine Q76.49
  with disproportion O33.8
    causing obstructed labor O65.0
lumbosacral (joint) (region) Q76.49
  kyphosis — see Kyphosis, congenital
  lordosis — see Lordosis, congenital
nerve Q07.8
nose Q30.8
organ
  of Corti Q16.5
  or site not listed — see Anomaly, by site
ossicles, ear Q16.3
oviduct Q50.6
pancreas Q45.3
parathyroid (gland) Q89.2
pituitary (gland) Q89.2
radius NEC Q68.8
sacroiliac joint Q74.2
sacrum Q76.49
scapula Q74.0
shoulder girdle Q74.0
skull bone(s) NEC Q75.8
  with
    anencephalus Q00.0
    encephalocele — see Encephalocele
    hydrocephalus Q03.9
      with spina bifida — see Spina bifida, with hydrocephalus
    microcephaly Q02
spinal cord Q06.8
spine Q76.49
  kyphosis — see Kyphosis, congenital
  lordosis — see Lordosis, congenital
spleen Q89.09
sternum NEC Q76.7
thorax (wall) Q67.8
  bony Q76.8
thymus (gland) Q89.2
thyroid (gland) Q89.2
tibia NEC Q68.8
toe(s) Q66.9
tongue Q38.3
trachea (cartilage) Q32.1
ulna NEC Q68.8

Distortion(s) (congenital) — continued
ureter Q62.8
urethra Q64.79
  causing obstruction Q64.39
uterus Q51.9
vagina Q52.4
vertebra Q76.49
  kyphosis — see Kyphosis, congenital
  lordosis — see Lordosis, congenital
visual — see also Disturbance, vision
  shape and size H53.15
vulva Q52.79
wrist (bones) (joint) Q68.8

Distress
abdomen — see Pain, abdominal
acute respiratory (adult) (child) J80
epigastric R10.13
fetal P84
  complicating pregnancy — see Stress, fetal
gastrointestinal (functional) K30
  psychogenic F45.8
intestinal (functional) NOS K59.9
  psychogenic F45.8
maternal, during labor and delivery O75.0
respiratory R06.00
  adult J80
  child J80
  newborn P22.9
    specified NEC P22.8
  orthopnea R06.01
  psychogenic F45.8
  shortness of breath R06.02
  specified type NEC R06.09

Distribution vessel, atypical Q27.9
coronary artery Q24.5
precerebral Q28.1

Distichiasis L68.8

Disturbance(s) — see also Disease
absorption K90.9
  calcium E58
  carbohydrate K90.4
  fat K90.4
    pancreatic K90.3
  protein K90.4
  starch K90.4
  vitamin — see Deficiency, vitamin
acid-base equilibrium E87.8
  mixed E87.4
activity and attention (with hyperkinesis) — see Disorder, attention-deficit hyperactivity
amino acid transport E72.00
assimilation, food K90.9
auditory nerve, except deafness — see subcategory H93.3
behavior — see Disorder, conduct
blood clotting (mechanism) (see also Defect, coagulation) D68.9
cerebral
  nerve — see Disorder, nerve, cranial
  status, newborn P91.9
    specified NEC P91.8
circulatory I99.9
conduct (see also Disorder, conduct) F91.9
  adjustment reaction — see Disorder, adjustment
  compulsive F63.9
  disruptive F91.9
  hyperkinetic — see Disorder, attention-deficit hyperactivity
  socialized F91.2
  specified NEC F91.8
  unsocialized F91.1
coordination R27.8
cranial nerve — see Disorder, nerve, cranial
deep sensibility — see Disturbance, sensation
digestive K30
  psychogenic F45.8
electrolyte — see also Imbalance, electrolyte
  newborn, transitory P74.4
    hyperammonemia P74.6
    potassium balance P74.3
    sodium balance P74.2
    specified type NEC P74.4
emotions specific to childhood and adolescence F93.9
  with
    anxiety and fearfulness NEC F93.8
    elective mutism F94.0
    oppositional disorder F91.3
    sensitivity (withdrawal) F40.10
    shyness F40.10
    social withdrawal F40.10
  involving relationship problems F93.8
  mixed F93.8
  specified NEC F93.8

Disturbance(s) *(see also* Disease) — *continued*
endocrine (gland) E34.9
  neonatal, transitory P72.9
    specified NEC P72.8
equilibrium R42
fructose metabolism E74.10
gait — *see* Gait
  hysterical F44.4
  psychogenic F44.4
gastrointestinal (functional) K30
  psychogenic F45.8
habit, child F98.9
hearing, except deafness and tinnitus — *see* Abnormal, auditory perception
heart, functional (conditions in I44-I50)
  due to presence of (cardiac) prosthesis I97.19-
  postoperative I97.89
    cardiac surgery I97.19-
hormones E34.9
innervation uterus (parasympathetic) (sympathetic) N85.8
keratinization NEC
  gingiva K05.10
    nonplaque induced K05.11
    plaque induced K05.10
  lip K13.0
  oral (mucosa) (soft tissue) K13.29
  tongue K13.29
learning (specific) — *see* Disorder, learning
memory — *see* Amnesia
  mild, following organic brain damage F06.8
mental F99
  associated with diseases classified elsewhere F54
metabolism E88.9
  with
    abortion — *see* Abortion, by type with other specified complication
    ectopic pregnancy O08.5
    molar pregnancy O08.5
  amino-acid E72.9
    aromatic E70.9
    branched-chain E71.2
    straight-chain E72.8
    sulfur-bearing E72.10
  ammonia E72.20
  arginine E72.21
  arginosuccinic acid E72.22
  carbohydrate E74.9
  cholesterol E78.9
  citrulline E72.23
  cystathionine E72.19
  general E88.9
  glutamine E72.8
  histidine E70.40
  homocystine E72.19
  hydroxylysine E72.3
  in labor or delivery O75.89
  iron E83.10
  lipoid E78.9
  lysine E72.3
  methionine E72.19
  neonatal, transitory P74.9
    calcium and magnesium P71.9
      specified type NEC P71.8
    carbohydrate metabolism P70.9
      specified type NEC P70.8
    specified NEC P74.8
  ornithine E72.4
  phosphate E83.39
  sodium NEC E87.8
  threonine E72.8
  tryptophan E70.5
  tyrosine E70.20
  urea cycle E72.20
motor R29.2
nervous, functional R45.0
neuromuscular mechanism (eye), due to syphilis A52.15
nutritional E63.9
  nail L60.3
ocular motion H51.9
  psychogenic F45.8
oculogyric H51.8
  psychogenic F45.8
oculomotor H51.9
  psychogenic F45.8
olfactory nerve R43.1
optic nerve NEC — *see* Disorder, nerve, optic
oral epithelium, including tongue NEC K13.29

Disturbance(s) *(see also* Disease) — *continued*
perceptual due to
  alcohol withdrawal F10.232
  amphetamine intoxication F15.922
    in
      abuse F15.122
      dependence F15.222
  anxiolytic withdrawal F13.232
  cannabis intoxication (acute) F12.922
    in
      abuse F12.122
      dependence F12.222
  cocaine intoxication (acute) F14.922
    in
      abuse F14.122
      dependence F14.222
  hypnotic withdrawal F13.232
  opioid intoxication (acute) F11.922
    in
      abuse F11.122
      dependence F11.222
  phencyclidine intoxication (acute) F19.922
    in
      abuse F19.122
      dependence F19.222
  sedative withdrawal F13.232
personality (pattern) (trait) *(see also* Disorder, personality) F60.9
following organic brain damage F07.9
polyglandular E31.9
  specified NEC E31.8
potassium balance, newborn P74.3
psychogenic F45.9
psychomotor F44.4
psychophysical visual H53.16
pupillary — *see* Anomaly, pupil, function
reflex R29.2
rhythm, heart I49.9
salivary secretion K11.7
sensation (cold) (heat) (localization) (tactile discrimination) (texture) (vibratory) NEC R20.9
  hysterical F44.6
  skin R20.9
    anesthesia R20.0
    hyperesthesia R20.3
    hypoesthesia R20.1
    paresthesia R20.2
    specified type NEC R20.8
  smell R43.9
    and taste (mixed) R43.8
    anosmia R43.0
    parosmia R43.1
    specified NEC R43.8
  taste R43.9
    and smell (mixed) R43.8
    parageusia R43.2
    specified NEC R43.8
sensory — *see* Disturbance, sensation
situational (transient) — *see also* Disorder, adjustment
  acute F43.0
sleep G47.9
  nonorganic origin F51.9
smell — *see* Disturbance, sensation, smell
sociopathic F60.2
sodium balance, newborn P74.2
speech R47.9
  developmental F80.9
  specified NEC R47.89
stomach (functional) K31.9
sympathetic (nerve) G90.9
taste — *see* Disturbance, sensation, taste
temperature
  regulation, newborn P81.9
    specified NEC P81.8
  sense R20.8
    hysterical F44.6
tooth
  eruption K00.6
  formation K00.4
  structure, hereditary NEC K00.5
touch — *see* Disturbance, sensation
vascular I99.9
  arteriosclerotic — *see* Arteriosclerosis
vasomotor I73.9
vasospastic I73.9
vision, visual H53.9
  following
    cerebral infarction I69.398
    cerebrovascular disease I69.998
    intracerebral hemorrhage I69.198
    nontraumatic intracranial hemorrhage NEC I69.298
    specified disease NEC I69.898
    specified NEC I69.898
    subarachnoid hemorrhage I69.098

Disturbance(s) *(see also* Disease) — *continued*
vision, visual H53.9 — *continued*
  psychophysical H53.16
  specified NEC H53.8
  subjective H53.10
    day blindness H53.11
    discomfort H53.14-
    distortions of shape and size H53.15
    loss
      sudden H53.13-
      transient H53.12-
    specified type NEC H53.19
voice R49.9
  psychogenic F44.4
  specified NEC R49.8
Diuresis R35.8
Diver's palsy, paralysis or squeeze T70.3
Diverticulitis (acute) K57.92
  bladder — *see* Cystitis
  ileum — *see* Diverticulitis, intestine, small
  intestine K57.92
    with
      abscess, perforation or peritonitis K57.80
        with bleeding K57.81
      bleeding K57.93
    congenital Q43.8
    large K57.32
      with
        abscess, perforation or peritonitis K57.20
          with bleeding K57.21
        bleeding K57.33
      small intestine K57.52
        with
          abscess, perforation or peritonitis K57.40
            with bleeding K57.41
          bleeding K57.53
    small K57.12
      with
        abscess, perforation or peritonitis K57.00
          with bleeding K57.01
        bleeding K57.13
      large intestine K57.52
        with
          abscess, perforation or peritonitis K57.40
            with bleeding K57.41
          bleeding K57.53
Diverticulosis K57.90
  with bleeding K57.91
  large intestine K57.30
    with
      bleeding K57.31
      small intestine K57.50
        with bleeding K57.51
  small intestine K57.10
    with
      bleeding K57.11
      large intestine K57.50
        with bleeding K57.51
Diverticulum, diverticula (multiple) K57.90
  appendix (noninflammatory) K38.2
  bladder (sphincter) N32.3
    congenital Q64.6
  bronchus (congenital) Q32.4
    acquired J98.09
  calyx, calyceal (kidney) N28.89
  cardia (stomach) K31.4
  cecum — *see* Diverticulosis, intestine, large
    congenital Q43.8
  colon — *see* Diverticulosis, intestine, large
    congenital Q43.8
  duodenum — *see* Diverticulosis, intestine, small
    congenital Q43.8
  epiphrenic (esophagus) K22.5
  esophagus (congenital) Q39.6
    acquired (epiphrenic) (pulsion) (traction) K22.5
  eustachian tube — *see* Disorder, eustachian tube, specified NEC
  fallopian tube N83.8
  gastric K31.4
  heart (congenital) Q24.8
  ileum — *see* Diverticulosis, intestine, small
  jejunum — *see* Diverticulosis, intestine, small
  kidney (pelvis) (calyces) N28.89
    with calculus — *see* Calculus, kidney
  Meckel's (displaced) (hypertrophic) Q43.0
    malignant — *see* Table of Neoplasms, small intestine, malignant
  midthoracic K22.5
  organ or site, congenital NEC — *see* Distortion

Diverticulum, diverticula (multiple) K57.90 — *continued*
  pericardium (congenital) (cyst) Q24.8
    acquired I31.8
  pharyngoesophageal (congenital) Q39.6
    acquired K22.5
  pharynx (congenital) Q38.7
  rectosigmoid — *see* Diverticulosis, intestine, large
    congenital Q43.8
  rectum — *see* Diverticulosis, intestine, large
  Rokitansky's K22.5
  seminal vesicle N50.8
  sigmoid — *see* Diverticulosis, intestine, large
    congenital Q43.8
  stomach (acquired) K31.4
    congenital Q40.2
  trachea (acquired) J39.8
  ureter (acquired) N28.89
    congenital Q62.8
  ureterovesical orifice N28.89
  urethra (acquired) N36.1
    congenital Q64.79
  ventricle, left (congenital) Q24.8
  vesical N32.3
    congenital Q64.6
  Zenker's (esophagus) K22.5
Division
  cervix uteri (acquired) N88.8
  glans penis Q55.69
  labia minora (congenital) Q52.79
  ligament (partial or complete) (current) — *see also* Sprain
    with open wound — *see* Wound, open
  muscle (partial or complete) (current) — *see also* Injury, muscle
    with open wound — *see* Wound, open
  nerve (traumatic) — *see* Injury, nerve
  spinal cord — *see* Injury, spinal cord, by region
  vein I87.8
Divorce, causing family disruption Z63.5
Dix-Hallpike neurolabyrinthitis — *see* Neuronitis, vestibular
Dizziness R42
  hysterical F44.89
  psychogenic F45.8
DMAC (disseminated mycobacterium aviumintracellulare complex) A31.2
DNR (do not resuscitate) Z66
Doan-Wiseman syndrome (primary splenic neutropenia) — *see* Agranulocytosis
Doehle-Heller aortitis A52.02
Dog bite — *see* Bite
Dohle body panmyelopathic syndrome D72.0
Dolichocephaly Q67.2
Dolichocolon Q43.8
Dolichostenomelia — *see* Syndrome, Marfan's
Donohue's syndrome E34.8
Donor (organ or tissue) Z52.9
  blood (whole) Z52.000
    autologous Z52.010
    specified component (lymphocytes) (platelets) NEC Z52.008
      autologous Z52.018
      specified donor NEC Z52.098
    specified donor NEC Z52.090
    stem cells Z52.001
      autologous Z52.011
      specified donor NEC Z52.091
  bone Z52.20
    autologous Z52.21
    marrow Z52.3
    specified type NEC Z52.29
  cornea Z52.5
  egg (Oocyte) Z52.819
    age 35 and over Z52.812
      anonymous recipient Z52.812
      designated recipient Z52.813
    under age 35 Z52.810
      anonymous recipient Z52.810
      designated recipient Z52.811
  kidney Z52.4
  liver Z52.6
  lung Z52.89
  lymphocyte — *see* Donor, blood, specified components NEC
  Oocyte — *see* Donor, egg
  platelets Z52.008
  potential, examination of Z00.5
  semen Z52.89
  skin Z52.10
    autologous Z52.11
    specified type NEC Z52.19
  specified organ or tissue NEC Z52.89
  sperm Z52.89

DISEASE INDEX

Donovanosis A58
Dorsalgia M54.9
  psychogenic F45.41
  specified NEC M54.89
Dorsopathy M53.9
  deforming M43.9
    specified NEC — see subcategory
      M43.8
  specified NEC M53.80
    cervical region M53.82
    cervicothoracic region M53.83
    lumbar region M53.86
    lumbosacral region M53.87
    occipito-atlanto-axial region M53.81
    sacrococcygeal region M53.88
    thoracic region M53.84
    thoracolumbar region M53.85
Double
  albumin E88.09
  aortic arch Q25.4
  auditory canal Q17.8
  auricle (heart) Q20.8
  bladder Q64.79
  cervix Q51.820
    with doubling of uterus (and vagina)
      Q51.10
      with obstruction Q51.11
  inlet ventricle Q20.4
  kidney with double pelvis (renal) Q63.0
  meatus urinarius Q64.75
  monster Q89.4
  outlet
    left ventricle Q20.2
    right ventricle Q20.1
  pelvis (renal) with double ureter Q62.5
  tongue Q38.3
  ureter (one or both sides) Q62.5
    with double pelvis (renal) Q62.5
  urethra Q64.74
  urinary meatus Q64.75
  uterus Q51.2
    with
      doubling of cervix (and vagina)
        Q51.10
        with obstruction Q51.11
    in pregnancy or childbirth O34.59-
      causing obstructed labor O65.5
  vagina Q52.10
    with doubling of uterus (and cervix)
      Q51.10
      with obstruction Q51.11
  vision H53.2
  vulva Q52.79
Douglas' pouch, cul-de-sac — see condition
Down syndrome Q90.9
  meiotic nondisjunction Q90.0
  mitotic nondisjunction Q90.1
  mosaicism Q90.1
  translocation Q90.2
DPD (dihydropyrimidine dehydrogenase
  deficiency) E88.89
Dracontiasis B72
Dracunculiasis, dracunculosis B72
Dream state, hysterical F44.89
Drepanocytic anemia — see Disease, sickle-
  cell
Dresbach's syndrome (elliptocytosis) D58.1
Dreschlera (hawaiiensis) (infection) B43.8
Dressler's syndrome I24.1
Drift, ulnar — see Deformity, limb, specified
  type NEC, forearm
Drinking (alcohol)
  excessive, to excess NEC (without
    dependence) F10.10
  habitual (continual) (without remission)
    F10.20
    with remission F10.21
Drip, postnasal (chronic) R09.82
  due to
    allergic rhinitis — see Rhinitis, allergic
    common cold J00
    gastroesophageal reflux — see Reflux,
      gastroesophageal
    nasopharyngitis — see Nasopharyngitis
    other know condition — code to
      condition
    sinusitis — see Sinusitis
Droop
  facial R29.810
    cerebrovascular disease I69.992
      cerebral infarction I69.392
      intracerebral hemorrhage I69.192
      nontraumatic intracranial hemorrhage
        NEC I69.292
      specified disease NEC I69.892
      subarachnoid hemorrhage I69.092

Drop (in)
  attack NEC R55
  finger — see Deformity, finger
  foot — see Deformity, limb, foot, drop
  hematocrit (precipitous) R71.0
  hemoglobin R71.0
  toe — see Deformity, toe, specified NEC
  wrist — see Deformity, limb, wrist drop
Dropped heart beats I45.9
Dropsy, dropsical — see also Hydrops
  abdomen R18.8
  brain — see Hydrocephalus
  cardiac, heart — see Failure, heart,
    congestive
  gangrenous — see Gangrene
  heart — see Failure, heart, congestive
  kidney — see Nephrosis
  lung — see Edema, lung
  newborn due to isoimmunization P56.0
  pericardium — see Pericarditis
Drowned, drowning (near) T75.1
Drowsiness R40.0
Drug
  abuse counseling and surveillance Z71.51
  addiction — see Dependence
  dependence — see Dependence
  habit — see Dependence
  harmful use — see Abuse, drug
  induced fever R50.2
  overdose — see Table of Drugs and
    Chemicals, by drug, poisoning
  poisoning — see Table of Drugs and
    Chemicals, by drug, poisoning
  resistant organism infection (see also
    Resistant, organism, to, drug) Z16.30
  therapy
    long term (current) (prophylactic) — see
      Therapy, drug long-term (current)
      (prophylactic)
    short term — omit code
  wrong substance given or taken in error —
    see Table of Drugs and Chemicals, by
    drug, poisoning
Drunkenness (without dependence) F10.129
  acute in alcoholism F10.229
  chronic (without remission) F10.20
    with remission F10.21
  pathological (without dependence) F10.129
    with dependence F10.229
  sleep F51.9
Drusen
  macula (degenerative) (retina) — see
    Degeneration, macula, drusen
  optic disc H47.32-
Dry, dryness — see also condition
  larynx J38.7
  mouth R68.2
    due to dehydration E86.0
  nose J34.89
  socket (teeth) M27.3
  throat J39.2
DSAP L56.5
Duane's syndrome H50.81-
Dubin-Johnson disease or syndrome E80.6
Dubois' disease (thymus gland) A50.59
  [E35]
Dubowitz' syndrome Q87.1
Duchenne-Aran muscular atrophy G12.21
Duchenne-Griesinger disease G71.0
Duchenne's
  disease or syndrome
    motor neuron disease G12.22
    muscular dystrophy G71.0
  locomotor ataxia (syphilitic) A52.11
  paralysis
    birth injury P14.0
    due to or associated with
      motor neuron disease G12.22
      muscular dystrophy G71.0
Ducrey's chancre A57
Duct, ductus — see condition
Duhring's disease (dermatitis herpetiformis)
  L13.0
Dullness, cardiac (decreased) (increased)
  R01.2
Dumb ague — see Malaria
Dumbness — see Aphasia
Dumdum fever B55.0
Dumping syndrome (postgastrectomy)
  K91.1
Duodenitis (nonspecific) (peptic) K29.80
  with bleeding K29.81
Duodenocholangitis — see Cholangitis
Duodenum, duodenal — see condition
Duplay's bursitis or periarthritis — see
  Tendinitis, calcific, shoulder

Duplication, duplex — see also Accessory
  alimentary tract Q45.8
  anus Q43.4
  appendix (and cecum) Q43.4
  biliary duct (any) Q44.5
  bladder Q64.79
  cecum (and appendix) Q43.4
  cervix Q51.820
  chromosome NEC
    with complex rearrangements NEC
      Q92.5
    seen only at prometaphase Q92.8
  cystic duct Q44.5
  digestive organs Q45.8
  esophagus Q39.8
  frontonasal process Q75.8
  intestine (large) (small) Q43.4
  kidney Q63.0
  liver Q44.7
  pancreas Q45.3
  penis Q55.69
  respiratory organs NEC Q34.8
  salivary duct Q38.4
  spinal cord (incomplete) Q06.2
  stomach Q40.2
Dupré's disease (meningism) R29.1
Dupuytren's contraction or disease M72.0
Durand-Nicolas-Favre disease A55
Durotomy (inadvertent) (incidental) G97.41
Duroziez's disease (congenital mitral
  stenosis) Q23.2
Dutton's relapsing fever (West African)
  A68.1
Dwarfism E34.3
  achondroplastic Q77.4
  congenital E34.3
  constitutional E34.3
  hypochondroplastic Q77.4
  hypophyseal E23.0
  infantile E34.3
  Laron-type E34.3
  Lorain(-Levi) type E23.0
  metatropic Q77.8
  nephrotic-glycosuric (with
    hypophosphatemic rickets) E72.09
  nutritional E45
  pancreatic K86.8
  pituitary E23.0
  renal N25.0
  thanatophoric Q77.1
Dyke-Young anemia (secondary)
  (symptomatic) D59.1
Dysacusis — see Abnormal, auditory
  perception
Dysadrenocortism E27.9
  hyperfunction E27.0
Dysarthria R47.1
  following
    cerebral infarction I69.322
    cerebrovascular disease I69.922
      specified disease NEC I69.822
    intracerebral hemorrhage I69.122
    nontraumatic intracranial hemorrhage
      NEC I69.222
    subarachnoid hemorrhage I69.022
Dysautonomia (familial) G90.1
Dysbarism T70.3
Dysbasia R26.2
  angiosclerotica intermittens I73.9
  hysterical F44.4
  lordotica (progressiva) G24.1
  nonorganic origin F44.4
  psychogenic F44.4
Dysbetalipoproteinemia (familial) E78.2
Dyscalculia R48.8
  developmental F81.2
Dyschezia K59.00
Dyschondroplasia (with hemangiomata)
  Q78.4
Dyschromia (skin) L81.9
Dyscollagenosis M35.9
Dyscranio-pygo-phalangy Q87.0
Dyscrasia
  blood (with) D75.9
    antepartum hemorrhage — see
      Hemorrhage, antepartum, with
      coagulation defect
    intrapartum hemorrhage O67.0
    newborn P61.9
      specified type NEC P61.8
    puerperal, postpartum O72.3
  polyglandular, pluriglandular E31.9
Dysendocrinism E34.9

Dysentery, dysenteric (catarrhal) (diarrhea)
  (epidemic) (hemorrhagic) (infectious)
  (sporadic) (tropical) A09
  abscess, liver A06.4
  amebic (see also Amebiasis) A06.0
    with abscess — see Abscess, amebic
    acute A06.0
    chronic A06.1
  arthritis (see also category M01) A09
    bacillary (see also category M01) A03.9
  bacillary A03.9
    arthritis (see also category M01) A03.9
    Boyd A03.2
    Flexner A03.1
    Schmitz(-Stutzer) A03.0
    Shiga(-Kruse) A03.0
    Shigella A03.9
      boydii A03.2
      dysenteriae A03.0
      flexneri A03.1
      group A A03.0
      group B A03.1
      group C A03.2
      group D A03.3
      sonnei A03.3
      specified type NEC A03.8
    Sonne A03.3
    specified type NEC A03.8
  balantidial A07.0
  Balantidium coli A07.0
  Boyd's A03.2
  candidal B37.82
  Chilomastix A07.8
  Chinese A03.9
  coccidial A07.3
  Dientamoeba (fragilis) A07.8
  Embadomonas A07.8
  Entamoeba, entamebic — see Dysentery,
    amebic
  Flexner's A03.1
  Flexner-Boyd A03.2
  Giardia lamblia A07.1
  Hiss-Russell A03.1
  Lamblia A07.1
  leishmanial B55.0
  malarial — see Malaria
  metazoal B82.0
  monilial B37.82
  protozoal A07.9
  Salmonella A02.0
  schistosomal B65.1
  Schmitz(-Stutzer) A03.0
  Shiga(-Kruse) A03.0
  Shigella NOS — see Dysentery, bacillary
  Sonne A03.3
  strongyloidiasis B78.0
  trichomonal A07.8
  viral (see also Enteritis, viral) A08.4
Dysequilibrium R42
Dysesthesia R20.8
  hysterical F44.6
Dysfibrinogenemia (congenital) D68.2
Dysfunction
  adrenal E27.9
    hyperfunction E27.0
  autonomic
    due to alcohol G31.2
    somatoform F45.8
  bladder N31.9
    neurogenic NOS — see Dysfunction,
      bladder, neuromuscular
    neuromuscular NOS N31.9
      atonic (motor) (sensory) N31.2
      autonomous N31.2
      flaccid N31.2
      nonreflex N31.2
      reflex N31.1
      specified NEC N31.8
      uninhibited N31.0
  bleeding, uterus N93.8
  cerebral G93.89
  colon K59.9
    psychogenic F45.8
  colostomy K94.03
  cystic duct K82.8
  cystostomy (stoma) — see Complications,
    cystostomy
  ejaculatory N53.19
    anejaculatory orgasm N53.13
    painful N53.12
    premature F52.4
    retarded N53.11
  endocrine NOS E34.9
  endometrium N85.8
  enterostomy K94.13
  gallbladder K82.8
  gastrostomy (stoma) K94.23
  gland, glandular NOS E34.9
  heart I51.89
  hemoglobin D75.89

Dysfunction — *continued*
hepatic K76.89
hypophysis E23.7
hypothalamic NEC E23.3
ileostomy (stoma) K94.13
jejunostomy (stoma) K94.13
kidney — *see* Disease, renal
labyrinthine — *see* subcategory H83.2
left ventricular, following sudden
   emotional stress I51.81
liver K76.89
male — *see* Dysfunction, sexual, male
orgasmic (female) F52.31
  male F52.32
ovary E28.9
  specified NEC E28.8
papillary muscle I51.89
parathyroid E21.4
physiological NEC R68.89
  psychogenic F59
pineal gland E34.8
pituitary (gland) E23.3
platelets D69.1
polyglandular E31.9
  specified NEC E31.8
psychophysiologic F59
psychosexual F52.9
  with
    dyspareunia F52.6
    premature ejaculation F52.4
    vaginismus F52.5
pylorus K31.9
rectum K59.9
  psychogenic F45.8
reflex (sympathetic) — *see* Syndrome,
  pain, complex regional I
segmental — *see* Dysfunction, somatic
senile R54
sexual (due to) R37
  alcohol F10.981
  amphetamine F15.981
    in
      abuse F15.181
      dependence F15.281
  anxiolytic F13.981
    in
      abuse F13.181
      dependence F13.281
  cocaine F14.981
    in
      abuse F14.181
      dependence F14.281
  excessive sexual drive F52.8
  failure of genital response (male) F52.21
    female F52.22
  female N94.9
    aversion F52.1
    dyspareunia N94.1
      psychogenic F52.6
    frigidity F52.22
    nymphomania F52.8
    orgasmic F52.31
    psychogenic F52.9
      aversion F52.1
      dyspareunia F52.6
      frigidity F52.22
      nymphomania F52.8
      orgasmic F52.31
      vaginismus F52.5
    vaginismus N94.2
      psychogenic F52.5
  hypnotic F13.981
    in
      abuse F13.181
      dependence F13.281
  inhibited orgasm (female) F52.31
    male F52.32
  lack
    of sexual enjoyment F52.1
    or loss of sexual desire F52.0
  male N53.9
    anejaculatory orgasm N53.13
    ejaculatory N53.19
      painful N53.12
      premature F52.4
      retarded N53.11
    erectile N52.9
      drug induced N52.2
      due to
        disease classified elsewhere
          N52.1
        drug N52.2
      postoperative (postprocedural)
        N52.39
      following
        prostatectomy N52.34
          radical N52.31
        radical cystectomy N52.32
        urethral surgery N52.33

Dysfunction — *continued*
sexual (due to) R37 — *continued*
  male N53.9 — *continued*
    erectile N52.9 — *continued*
      psychogenic F52.21
      specified cause NEC N52.8
      vasculogenic
        arterial insufficiency N52.01
          with corporo-venous occlusive
            N52.03
        corporo-venous occlusive
          N52.02
          with arterial insufficiency
            N52.03
    impotence — *see* Dysfunction, sexual,
      male, erectile
    psychogenic F52.9
      aversion F52.1
      erectile F52.21
      orgasmic F52.32
      premature ejaculation F52.4
      satyriasis F52.8
      specified type NEC F52.8
    specified type NEC N53.8
  nonorganic F52.9
    specified NEC F52.8
  opioid F11.981
    in
      abuse F11.181
      dependence F11.281
  orgasmic dysfunction (female) F52.31
    male F52.32
  premature ejaculation F52.4
  psychoactive substances NEC F19.981
    in
      abuse F19.181
      dependence F19.281
  psychogenic F52.9
  sedative F13.981
    in
      abuse F13.181
      dependence F13.281
  sexual aversion F52.1
  vaginismus (nonorganic) (psychogenic)
    F52.5
sinoatrial node I49.5
somatic M99.09
  abdomen M99.09
  acromioclavicular M99.07
  cervical region M99.01
  cervicothoracic M99.01
  costochondral M99.08
  costovertebral M99.08
  head region M99.00
  hip M99.05
  lower extremity M99.06
  lumbar region M99.03
  lumbosacral M99.03
  occipitocervical M99.00
  pelvic region M99.05
  pubic M99.05
  rib cage M99.08
  sacral region M99.04
  sacrococcygeal M99.04
  sacroiliac M99.04
  specified NEC M99.09
  sternochondral M99.08
  sternoclavicular M99.07
  thoracic region M99.02
  thoracolumbar M99.02
  upper extremity M99.07
somatoform autonomic F45.8
stomach K31.89
  psychogenic F45.8
suprarenal E27.9
  hyperfunction E27.0
symbolic R48.9
  specified type NEC R48.8
temporomandibular (joint) M26.69
  joint-pain syndrome M26.62
testicular (endocrine) E29.9
  specified NEC E29.8
thymus E32.9
thyroid E07.9
ureterostomy (stoma) — *see*
  Complications, stoma, urinary tract
urethrostomy (stoma) — *see*
  Complications, stoma, urinary tract
uterus, complicating delivery O62.9
  hypertonic O62.4
  hypotonic O62.2
    primary O62.0
    secondary O62.1
ventricular I51.9
  with congestive heart failure I50.9
  left, reversible, following sudden
    emotional stress I51.81

Dysgenesis
gonadal (due to chromosomal anomaly)
  Q96.9
  pure Q99.1
renal Q60.5
  bilateral Q60.4
  unilateral Q60.3
reticular D72.0
tidal platelet D69.3
Dysgerminoma
specified site — *see* Neoplasm, malignant,
  by site
unspecified site
  female C56.9
  male C62.90
Dysgeusia R43.2
Dysgraphia R27.8
Dyshidrosis, dysidrosis L30.1
Dyskaryotic cervical smear R87.619
Dyskeratosis L85.8
cervix — *see* Dysplasia, cervix
congenital Q82.8
uterus NEC N85.8
Dyskinesia G24.9
biliary (cystic duct or gallbladder) K82.8
drug induced
  orofacial G24.01
esophagus K22.4
hysterical F44.4
intestinal K59.8
nonorganic origin F44.4
orofacial (idiopathic) G24.4
  drug induced G24.01
psychogenic F44.4
subacute, drug induced G24.01
tardive G24.01
  neuroleptic induced G24.01
trachea J39.8
tracheobronchial J98.09
Dyslalia (developmental) F80.0
Dyslexia R48.0
developmental F81.0
Dyslipidemia E78.5
depressed HDL cholesterol E78.6
elevated fasting triglycerides E78.1
Dysmaturity — *see also* Light for dates
pulmonary (newborn) (Wilson-Mikity)
  P27.0
Dysmenorrhea (essential) (exfoliative)
  N94.6
congestive (syndrome) N94.6
primary N94.4
psychogenic F45.8
secondary N94.5
Dysmetabolic syndrome X E88.81
Dysmetria R27.8
Dysmorphism (due to)
alcohol Q86.0
exogenous cause NEC Q86.8
hydantoin Q86.1
warfarin Q86.2
Dysmorphophobia (nondelusional) F45.22
delusional F22
Dysnomia R47.01
Dysorexia R63.0
psychogenic F50.8
Dysostosis
cleidocranial, cleidocranialis Q74.0
craniofacial Q75.1
Fairbank's (idiopathic familial generalized
  osteophytosis) Q78.9
mandibulofacial (incomplete) Q75.4
multiplex E76.01
oculomandibular Q75.5
Dyspareunia (female) N94.1
male N53.12
nonorganic F52.6
psychogenic F52.6
secondary N94.1
Dyspepsia R10.13
atonic K30
functional (allergic) (congenital)
  (gastrointestinal) (occupational)
  (reflex) K30
intestinal K59.8
nervous F45.8
neurotic F45.8
psychogenic F45.8

Dysphagia R13.10
cervical R13.19
following
  cerebral infarction I69.391
  cerebrovascular disease I69.991
  intracerebral hemorrhage I69.191
  nontraumatic intracranial hemorrhage
    NEC I69.291
  specified disease NEC I69.891
  specified NEC I69.891
  subarachnoid hemorrhage I69.091
functional (hysterical) F45.8
hysterical F45.8
nervous (hysterical) F45.8
neurogenic R13.19
oral phase R13.11
oropharyngeal phase R13.12
pharyneal phase R13.13
pharyngoesophageal phase R13.14
psychogenic F45.8
sideropenic D50.1
spastica K22.4
specified NEC R13.19
Dysphagocytosis, congenital D71
Dysphasia R47.02
developmental
  expressive type F80.1
  receptive type F80.2
following
  cerebrovascular disease I69.921
    cerebral infarction I69.321
    intracerebral hemorrhage I69.121
    nontraumatic intracranial hemorrhage
      NEC I69.221
    specified disease NEC I69.821
    subarachnoid hemorrhage I69.021
Dysphonia R49.0
functional F44.4
hysterical F44.4
psychogenic F44.4
spastica J38.3
Dysphoria, postpartal O90.6
Dyspituitarism E23.3
Dysplasia — *see also* Anomaly
acetabular, congenital Q65.89
alveolar capillary, with vein misalignment
  J84.843
anus (histologically confirmed) (mild)
  (moderate) K62.82
  severe D01.3
arrhythmogenic right ventricular I42.8
arterial, fibromuscular I77.3
asphyxiating thoracic (congenital) Q77.2
brain Q07.9
bronchopulmonary, perinatal P27.1
cervix (uteri) N87.9
  mild N87.0
  moderate N87.1
  severe D06.9
chondroectodermal Q77.6
colon D12.6
craniometaphyseal Q78.5
dentinal K00.5
diaphyseal, progressive Q78.3
dystrophic Q77.5
ectodermal (anhidrotic) (congenital)
  (hereditary) Q82.4
  hydrotic Q82.8
epithelial, uterine cervix — *see* Dysplasia,
  cervix
eye (congenital) Q11.2
fibrous
  bone NEC (monostotic) M85.00
    ankle M85.07-
    foot M85.07-
    forearm M85.03-
    hand M85.04-
    lower leg M85.06-
    multiple site M85.09
    neck M85.08
    rib M85.08
    shoulder M85.01-
    skull M85.08
    specified site NEC M85.08
    thigh M85.05-
    toe M85.07-
    upper arm M85.02-
    vertebra M85.08
  diaphyseal, progressive Q78.3
  jaw M27.8
  polyostotic Q78.1
florid osseous — *see also* Cyst, calcifying
  odontogenic
high grade, focal D12.6
hip, congenital Q65.89
joint, congenital Q74.8
kidney Q61.4
  multicystic Q61.4
leg Q74.2

Dysplasia *(see also* Anomaly*)* — *continued*
lung, congenital (not associated with short gestation) Q33.6
mammary (gland) (benign) N60.9-
  cyst (solitary) — *see* Cyst, breast
  cystic — *see* Mastopathy, cystic
  duct ectasia — *see* Ectasia, mammary duct
  fibroadenosis — *see* Fibroadenosis, breast
  fibrosclerosis — *see* Fibrosclerosis, breast
  specified type NEC N60.8-
metaphyseal (Jansen's) (McKusick's) (Schmid's) Q78.5
muscle Q79.8
oculodentodigital Q87.0
periapical (cemental) (cemento-osseous) — *see* Cyst, calcifying odontogenic
periosteum — *see* Disorder, bone, specified type NEC
polyostotic fibrous Q78.1
prostate *(see also* Neoplasia, intraepithelial, prostate) N42.3
  severe D07.5
renal Q61.4
  multicystic Q61.4
retinal, congenital Q14.1
right ventricular, arrhythmogenic I42.8
septo-optic Q04.4
skin L98.8
spinal cord Q06.1
spondyloepiphyseal Q77.7
thymic, with immunodeficiency D82.1
vagina N89.3
  mild N89.0
  moderate N89.1
  severe NEC D07.2
vulva N90.3
  mild N90.0
  moderate N90.1
  severe NEC D07.1
Dyspnea (nocturnal) (paroxysmal) R06.00
asthmatic (bronchial) J45.909
  with
    bronchitis J45.909
      with
        exacerbation (acute) J45.901
        status asthmaticus J45.902
      chronic J44.9
      exacerbation (acute) J45.901
      status asthmaticus J45.902
cardiac — *see* Failure, ventricular, left
cardiac — *see* Failure, ventricular, left
functional F45.8
hyperventilation R06.4
hysterical F45.8
newborn P28.89
orthopnea R06.01
psychogenic F45.8
shortness of breath R06.02
specified type NEC R06.09
Dyspraxia R27.8
developmental (syndrome) F82
Dysproteinemia E88.09
Dysreflexia, autonomic G90.4
Dysrhythmia
cardiac I49.9
  newborn
    bradycardia P29.12
      occurring before birth P03.819
        before onset of labor P03.810
        during labor P03.811
      tachycardia P29.11
    postoperative I97.89
cerebral or cortical — *see* Epilepsy
Dyssomnia — *see* Disorder, sleep
Dyssynergia
biliary K83.8
bladder sphincter N36.44
cerebellaris myoclonica (Hunt's ataxia) G11.1
Dysthymia F34.1
Dysthyroidism E07.9
Dystocia O66.9
affecting newborn P03.1
cervical (hypotonic) O62.2
  affecting newborn P03.6
  primary O62.0
  secondary O62.1
contraction ring O62.4
fetal O66.9
  abnormality NEC O66.3
  conjoined twins O66.3
  oversize O66.2
maternal O66.9
positional O64.9
shoulder (girdle) O66.0
  causing obstructed labor O66.0
uterine NEC O62.4

Dystonia G24.9
deformans progressiva G24.1
drug induced NEC G24.09
  acute G24.02
  specified NEC G24.09
familial G24.1
idiopathic G24.1
  familial G24.1
  nonfamilial G24.2
  orofacial G24.4
lenticularis G24.8
musculorum deformans G24.1
neuroleptic induced (acute) G24.02
orofacial (idiopathic) G24.4
oromandibular G24.4
  due to drug G24.01
specified NEC G24.8
torsion (familial) (idiopathic) G24.1
  acquired G24.8
  genetic G24.1
  symptomatic (nonfamilial) G24.2
Dystonic movements R25.8
Dystrophy, dystrophia
adiposogenital E23.6
Becker's type G71.0
cervical sympathetic G90.2
choroid (hereditary) H31.20
  central areolar H31.22
  choroideremia H31.21
  gyrate atrophy H31.23
  specified type NEC H31.29
cornea (hereditary) H18.50
  endothelial H18.51
  epithelial H18.52
  granular H18.53
  lattice H18.54
  macular H18.55
  specified type NEC H18.59
Duchenne's type G71.0
due to malnutrition E45
Erb's G71.0
Fuchs' H18.51
Gower's muscular G71.0
hair L67.8
infantile neuraxonal G31.89
Landouzy-Déjérine G71.0
Leyden-Möbius G71.0
muscular G71.0
  benign (Becker type) G71.0
  congenital (hereditary) (progressive) (with specific morphological abnormalities of the muscle fiber) G71.0
    myotonic G71.11
  distal G71.0
  Duchenne type G71.0
  Emery-Dreifuss G71.0
  Erb type G71.0
  facioscapulohumeral G71.0
  Gower's G71.0
  hereditary (progressive) G71.0
  Landouzy-Déjérine type G71.0
  limb-girdle G71.0
  myotonic G71.11
  progressive (hereditary) G71.0
    Charcot-Marie(-Tooth) type G60.0
  pseudohypertrophic (infantile) G71.0
  severe (Duchenne type) G71.0
myocardium, myocardial — *see* Degeneration, myocardial
myotonic, myotonica G71.11
nail L60.3
  congenital Q84.6
nutritional E45
ocular G71.0
oculocerebrorenal E72.03
oculopharyngeal G71.0
ovarian N83.8
polyglandular E31.8
reflex (neuromuscular) (sympathetic) — *see* Syndrome, pain, complex regional I
retinal (hereditary) H35.50
  in
    lipid storage disorders E75.6 [H36]
    systemic lipidoses E75.6 [H36]
  involving
    pigment epithelium H35.54
    sensory area H35.53
  pigmentary H35.52
  vitreoretinal H35.51
Salzmann's nodular — *see* Degeneration, cornea, nodular
scapuloperoneal G71.0
skin NEC L98.8
sympathetic (reflex) — *see* Syndrome, pain, complex regional I
  cervical G90.2
tapetoretinal H35.54

Dystrophy, dystrophia — *continued*
thoracic, asphyxiating Q77.2
unguium L60.3
  congenital Q84.6
vitreoretinal H35.51
vulva N90.4
yellow (liver) — *see* Failure, hepatic
Dysuria R30.0
psychogenic F45.8

© 2013 Channel Publishing Ltd

E

Eales' disease H35.06-
Ear — see also condition
  piercing Z41.3
  tropical B36.8
  wax (impacted) H61.20
    left H61.22
      with right H61.23
    right H61.21
      with left H61.23
Earache — see subcategory H92.0
Early satiety R68.81
Eaton-Lambert syndrome — see Syndrome, Lambert-Eaton
Eberth's disease (typhoid fever) A01.00
Ebola virus disease A98.4
Ebstein's anomaly or syndrome (heart) Q22.5
Eccentro-osteochondrodysplasia E76.29
Ecchondroma — see Neoplasm, bone, benign
Ecchondrosis D48.0
Ecchymosis R58
  conjunctiva — see Hemorrhage, conjunctiva
  eye (traumatic) — see Contusion, eyeball
  eyelid (traumatic) — see Contusion, eyelid
  newborn P54.5
  spontaneous R23.3
  traumatic — see Contusion
Echinococciasis — see Echinococcus
Echinococcosis — see Echinococcus
Echinococcus (infection) B67.90
  granulosus B67.4
    bone B67.2
    liver B67.0
    lung B67.1
    multiple sites B67.32
    specified site NEC B67.39
    thyroid B67.31 [E35]
  liver NOS B67.8
    granulosus B67.0
    multilocularis B67.5
  lung NEC B67.99
    granulosus B67.1
    multilocularis B67.69
  multilocularis B67.7
    liver B67.5
    multiple sites B67.61
    specified site NEC B67.69
  specified site NEC B67.99
    granulosus B67.39
    multilocularis B67.69
  thyroid NEC B67.99
    granulosus B67.31 [E35]
    multilocularis B67.69 [E35]
Echinorhynchiasis B83.8
Echinostomiasis B66.8
Echolalia R48.8
Echovirus, as cause of disease classified elsewhere B97.12
Eclampsia, eclamptic (coma) (convulsions) (delirium) (with hypertension) NEC O15.9
  during labor and delivery O15.1
  postpartum O15.2
  pregnancy O15.0-
  puerperal O15.2
Economic circumstances affecting care Z59.9
Economo's disease A85.8
Ectasia, ectasis
  annuloaortic I35.8
  aorta I77.819
    with aneurysm — see Aneurysm, aorta
    abdominal I77.811
    thoracic I77.810
    thoracoabdominal I77.812
  breast — see Ectasia, mammary duct
  capillary I78.8
  cornea H18.71-
  gastric antral vascular (GAVE) K31.819
    with hemorrhage K31.811
    without hemorrhage K31.819
  mammary duct N60.4-
  salivary gland (duct) K11.8
  sclera — see Sclerectasia
Ecthyma L08.0
  contagiosum B08.02
  gangrenosum L08.0
  infectiosum B08.02

Ectocardia Q24.8
Ectodermal dysplasia (anhidrotic) Q82.4
Ectodermosis erosiva pluriorificialis L51.1
Ectopic, ectopia (congenital)
  abdominal viscera Q45.8
    due to defect in anterior abdominal wall Q79.59
  ACTH syndrome E24.3
  adrenal gland Q89.1
  anus Q43.5
  atrial beats I49.1
  beats I49.49
    atrial I49.1
    ventricular I49.3
  bladder Q64.10
  bone and cartilage in lung Q33.5
  brain Q04.8
  breast tissue Q83.8
  cardiac Q24.8
  cerebral Q04.8
  cordis Q24.8
  endometrium — see Endometriosis
  gastric mucosa Q40.2
  gestation — see Pregnancy, by site
  heart Q24.8
  hormone secretion NEC E34.2
  kidney (crossed) (pelvis) Q63.2
  lens, lentis Q12.1
  mole — see Pregnancy, by site
  organ or site NEC — see Malposition, congenital
  pancreas Q45.3
  pregnancy — see Pregnancy, ectopic
  pupil — see Abnormality, pupillary
  renal Q63.2
  sebaceous glands of mouth Q38.6
  spleen Q89.09
  testis Q53.00
    bilateral Q53.02
    unilateral Q53.01
  thyroid Q89.2
  tissue in lung Q33.5
  ureter Q62.63
  ventricular beats I49.3
  vesicae Q64.10
Ectromelia Q73.8
  lower limb — see Defect, reduction, limb, lower, specified type NEC
  upper limb — see Defect, reduction, limb, upper, specified type NEC
Ectropion H02.109
  cervix N86
    with cervicitis N72
    congenital Q10.1
  eyelid (paralytic) H02.109
    cicatricial H02.119
      left H02.116
        lower H02.115
        upper H02.114
      right H02.113
        lower H02.112
        upper H02.111
    congenital Q10.1
    left H02.106
      lower H02.105
      upper H02.104
    mechanical H02.129
      left H02.126
        lower H02.125
        upper H02.124
      right H02.123
        lower H02.122
        upper H02.121
    right H02.103
      lower H02.102
      upper H02.101
    senile H02.139
      left H02.136
        lower H02.135
        upper H02.134
      right H02.133
        lower H02.132
        upper H02.131
    spastic H02.149
      left H02.146
        lower H02.145
        upper H02.144
      right H02.143
        lower H02.142
        upper H02.141
  iris H21.89
  lip (acquired) K13.0
    congenital Q38.0
  urethra N36.8
  uvea H21.89

Eczema (acute) (chronic) (erythematous) (fissum) (rubrum) (squamous) (see also Dermatitis) L30.9
  contact — see Dermatitis, contact
  dyshidrotic L30.1
  external ear — see Otitis, externa, acute, eczematoid
  flexural L20.82
  herpeticum B00.0
  hypertrophicum L28.0
  hypostatic — see Varix, leg, with, inflammation
  impetiginous L01.1
  infantile (due to any substance) L20.83
    intertriginous L21.1
    seborrheic L21.1
  intertriginous NEC L30.4
    infantile L21.1
  intrinsic (allergic) L20.84
  lichenified NEC L28.0
  marginatum (hebrae) B35.6
  pustular L30.3
  stasis — see Varix, leg, with, inflammation
  vaccination, vaccinatum T88.1
  varicose — see Varix, leg, with, inflammation
Eczematid L30.2
Eddowes(-Spurway) syndrome Q78.0
Edema, edematous (infectious) (pitting) (toxic) R60.9
  with nephritis — see Nephrosis
  allergic T78.3
  amputation stump (surgical) (sequelae (late effect)) T87.89
  angioneurotic (allergic) (any site) (with urticaria) T78.3
    hereditary D84.1
  angiospastic I73.9
  Berlin's (traumatic) S05.8x-
  brain (cytotoxic) (vasogenic) G93.6
    due to birth injury P11.0
    newborn (anoxia or hypoxia) P52.4
      birth injury P11.0
    traumatic — see Injury, intracranial, cerebral edema
  cardiac — see Failure, heart, congestive
  cardiovascular — see Failure, heart, congestive
  cerebral — see Edema, brain
  cerebrospinal — see Edema, brain
  cervix (uteri) (acute) N88.8
    puerperal, postpartum O90.89
  chronic hereditary Q82.0
  circumscribed, acute T78.3
    hereditary D84.1
  conjunctiva H11.42-
  cornea H18.2-
    idiopathic H18.22-
    secondary H18.23-
      due to contact lens H18.21-
  due to
    lymphatic obstruction I89.0
    salt retention E87.0
  epiglottis — see Edema, glottis
  essential, acute T78.3
    hereditary D84.1
  extremities, lower — see Edema, legs
  eyelid NEC H02.849
    left H02.846
      lower H02.845
      upper H02.844
    right H02.843
      lower H02.842
      upper H02.841
  familial, hereditary Q82.0
  famine — see Malnutrition, severe
  generalized R60.1
  glottis, glottic, glottidis (obstructive) (passive) J38.4
    allergic T78.3
      hereditary D84.1
  heart — see Failure, heart, congestive
  heat T67.7
  hereditary Q82.0
  inanition — see Malnutrition, severe
  intracranial G93.6
  iris H21.89
  joint — see Effusion, joint
  larynx — see Edema, glottis
  legs R60.0
    due to venous obstruction I87.1
    hereditary Q82.0
  localized R60.0
    due to venous obstruction I87.1
  lower limbs — see Edema, legs

Edema, edematous (infectious) (pitting) (toxic) R60.9 — continued
  lung J81.1
    with heart condition or failure — see Failure, ventricular, left
    acute J81.0
      chemical (acute) J68.1
        chronic J68.1
    chronic J81.1
      due to
        chemicals, gases, fumes or vapors (inhalation) J68.1
        external agent J70.9
          specified NEC J70.8
        radiation J70.1
    due to
      chemicals, fumes or vapors (inhalation) J68.1
      external agent J70.9
        specified NEC J70.8
      high altitude T70.29
      near drowning T75.1
      radiation J70.0
    meaning failure, left ventricle I50.1
  lymphatic I89.0
    due to mastectomy I97.2
  macula H35.81
    cystoid, following cataract surgery — see Complications, postprocedural, following cataract surgery
    diabetic — see Diabetes, by type, with, retinopathy, with macular edema
  malignant — see Gangrene, gas
  Milroy's Q82.0
  nasopharynx J39.2
  newborn P83.30
    hydrops fetalis — see Hydrops, fetalis
    specified NEC P83.39
  nutritional — see also Malnutrition, severe
    with dyspigmentation, skin and hair E40
  optic disc or nerve — see Papilledema
  orbit H05.22-
  pancreas K86.8
  papilla, optic — see Papilledema
  penis N48.89
  periodic T78.3
    hereditary D84.1
  pharynx J39.2
  pulmonary — see Edema, lung
  Quincke's T78.3
    hereditary D84.1
  renal — see Nephrosis
  retina H35.81
    diabetic — see Diabetes, by type, with, retinopathy, with macular edema
  salt E87.0
  scrotum N50.8
  seminal vesicle N50.8
  spermatic cord N50.8
  spinal (cord) (vascular) (nontraumatic) G95.19
  starvation — see Malnutrition, severe
  stasis — see Hypertension, venous, (chronic)
  subglottic — see Edema, glottis
  supraglottic — see Edema, glottis
  testis N44.8
  tunica vaginalis N50.8
  vas deferens N50.8
  vulva (acute) N90.89
Edentulism — see Absence, teeth, acquired
Edsall's disease T67.2
Educational handicap Z55.9
  specified NEC Z55.8
Edward's syndrome — see Trisomy, 18
Effect(s) (of) (from) — see Effect, adverse NEC
Effect, adverse
  abnormal gravitational (G) forces or states T75.81
  abuse — see Maltreatment
  air pressure T70.9
    specified NEC T70.8
  altitude (high) — see Effect, adverse, high altitude
  anesthesia (see also Anesthesia) T88.59
    in labor and delivery O74.9
    in pregnancy NEC O29.3-
    local, toxic
      in labor and delivery O74.4
      postpartum, puerperal O89.3
    postpartum, puerperal O89.9
    specified NEC T88.59
      in labor and delivery O74.8
      postpartum, puerperal O89.8

DISEASE INDEX

Effect, adverse — *continued*
  anesthesia (*see also* Anesthesia) T88.59 — *continued*
    spinal and epidural T88.59
      headache T88.59
        in labor and delivery O74.5
        postpartum, puerperal O89.4
      specified NEC
        in labor and delivery O74.6
        postpartum, puerperal O89.5
  antitoxin — *see* Complications, vaccination
  atmospheric pressure T70.9
    due to explosion T70.8
    high T70.3
    low — *see* Effect, adverse, high altitude
    specified effect NEC T70.8
  biological, correct substance properly administered — *see* Effect, adverse, drug
  blood (derivatives) (serum) (transfusion) — *see* Complications, transfusion
  chemical substance — *see* Table of Drugs and Chemicals
  cold (temperature) (weather) T69.9
    chilblains T69.1
    frostbite — *see* Frostbite
    specified effect NEC T69.8
  drugs and medicaments T88.7
    specified drug — *see* Table of Drugs and Chemicals, by drug, adverse effect
    specified effect — *code to* condition
  electric current, electricity (shock) T75.4
    burn — *see* Burn
  exertion (excessive) T73.3
  exposure — *see* Exposure
  external cause NEC T75.89
  foodstuffs T78.1
    allergic reaction — *see* Allergy, food
    causing anaphylaxis — *see* Shock, anaphylactic, due to, food
    noxious — *see* Poisoning, food, noxious
  gases, fumes, or vapors T59.9-
    specified agent — *see* Table of Drugs and Chemicals
  glue (airplane) sniffing
    due to drug abuse — *see* Abuse, drug, inhalant
    due to drug dependence — *see* Dependence, drug, inhalant
  heat — *see* Heat
  high altitude NEC T70.29
    anoxia T70.29
    on
      ears T70.0
      sinuses T70.1
    polycythemia D75.1
  high pressure fluids T70.4
  hot weather — *see* Heat
  hunger T73.0
  immersion, foot — *see* Immersion
  immunization — *see* Complications, vaccination
  immunological agents — *see* Complications, vaccination
  infrared (radiation) (rays) NOS T66
    dermatitis or eczema L59.8
  infusion — *see* Complications, infusion
  lack of care of infants — *see* Maltreatment, child
  lightning — *see* Lightning
  medical care T88.9
    specified NEC T88.8
  medicinal substance, correct, properly administered — *see* Effect, adverse, drug
  motion T75.3
  noise, on inner ear — *see* subcategory H83.3
  overheated places — *see* Heat
  psychosocial, of work environment Z56.5
  radiation (diagnostic) (infrared) (natural source) (therapeutic) (ultraviolet) (X-ray) NOS T66
    dermatitis or eczema — *see* Dermatitis, due to, radiation
    fibrosis of lung J70.1
    pneumonitis J70.0
    pulmonary manifestations
      acute J70.0
      chronic J70.1
    skin L59.9
  radioactive substance NOS

Effect, adverse — *continued*
  reduced temperature T69.9
    immersion foot or hand — *see* Immersion
    specified effect NEC T69.8
  serum NEC (*see also* Reaction, serum) T80.69
  specified NEC T78.8
    external cause NEC T75.89
  strangulation — *see* Asphyxia, traumatic
  submersion T75.1
  thirst T73.1
  toxic — *see* Toxicity
  transfusion — *see* Complications, transfusion
  ultraviolet (radiation) (rays) NOS T66
    burn — *see* Burn
    dermatitis or eczema — *see* Dermatitis, due to, ultraviolet rays
      acute L56.8
  vaccine (any) — *see* Complications, vaccination
  vibration — *see* Vibration, adverse effects
  water pressure NEC T70.9
    specified NEC T70.8
  weightlessness T75.82
  whole blood — *see* Complications, transfusion
  work environment Z56.5
Effects, late — *see* Sequelae
Effluvium
  anagen L65.1
  telogen L65.0
Effort syndrome (psychogenic) F45.8
Effusion
  amniotic fluid — *see* Pregnancy, complicated by, prematue rupture of membranes
  brain (serous) G93.6
  bronchial — *see* Bronchitis
  cerebral G93.6
  cerebrospinal — *see also* Meningitis
    vessel G93.6
  chest — *see* Effusion, pleura
  chylous, chyliform (pleura) J94.0
  intracranial G93.6
  joint M25.40
    ankle M25.47-
    elbow M25.42-
    foot joint M25.47-
    hand joint M25.44-
    hip M25.45-
    knee M25.46-
    shoulder M25.41-
    specified joint NEC M25.48
    wrist M25.43-
  malignant pleural J91.0
  meninges — *see* Meningitis
  pericardium, pericardial (noninflammatory) I31.3
    acute — *see* Pericarditis, acute
  peritoneal (chronic) R18.8
  pleura, pleurisy, pleuritic, pleuropericardial J90
    chylous, chyliform J94.0
    due to systemic lupus erythematosis M32.13
    influenzal — *see* Influenza, with, respiratory manifestations NEC
    malignant J91.0
    newborn P28.89
    tuberculous NEC A15.6
      primary (progressive) A15.7
  spinal — *see* Meningitis
  thorax, thoracic — *see* Effusion, pleura
Egg shell nails L60.3
  congenital Q84.6
Egyptian splenomegaly B65.1
Ehlers-Danlos syndrome Q79.6
Ehrlichiosis A77.40
  due to
    E. chafeensis A77.41
    E. sennetsu A79.81
    specified organism NEC A77.49
Eichstedt's disease B36.0
Eisenmenger's
  complex or syndrome I27.89
  defect Q21.8
Ejaculation
  painful N53.12
  premature F52.4
  retarded N53.11
  retrograde N53.14
  semen, painful N53.12
    psychogenic F52.6

Ekbom's syndrome (restless legs) G25.81
Ekman's syndrome (brittle bones and blue sclera) Q78.0
Elastic skin Q82.8
  acquired L57.4
Elastofibroma — *see* Neoplasm, connective tissue, benign
Elastoma (juvenile) Q82.8
  Miescher's L87.2
Elastomyofibrosis I42.4
Elastosis
  actinic, solar L57.8
  atrophicans (senile) L57.4
  perforans serpiginosa L87.2
  senilis L57.4
Elbow — *see* condition
Electric current, electricity, effects (concussion) (fatal) (nonfatal) (shock) T75.4
  burn — *see* Burn
Electric feet syndrome E53.8
Electrocution T75.4
  from electroshock gun (taser) T75.4
Electrolyte imbalance E87.8
  with
    abortion — *see* Abortion, by type, complicated by, electrolyte imbalance
    ectopic pregnancy O08.5
    molar pregnancy O08.5
Elephantiasis (nonfilarial) I89.0
  arabicum — *see* Infestation, filarial
  bancrofti B74.0
  congenital (any site) (hereditary) Q82.0
  due to
    Brugia (malayi) B74.1
      timori B74.2
    mastectomy I97.2
    Wuchereria (bancrofti) B74.0
  eyelid H02.859
    left H02.856
      lower H02.855
      upper H02.854
    right H02.853
      lower H02.852
      upper H02.851
  filarial, filariensis — *see* Infestation, filarial
  glandular I89.0
  graecorum A30.9
  lymphangiectatic I89.0
  lymphatic vessel I89.0
    due to mastectomy I97.2
  scrotum (nonfilarial) I89.0
  streptococcal I89.0
  surgical I97.89
    postmastectomy I97.2
  telangiectodes I89.0
  vulva (nonfilarial) N90.89
Elevated, elevation
  antibody titer R76.0
  basal metabolic rate R94.8
  blood pressure — *see also* Hypertension
    reading (incidental) (isolated) (nonspecific), no diagnosis of hypertension R03.0
  blood sugar R73.9
  body temperature (of unknown origin) R50.9
  cancer antigen 125 [CA 125] R97.1
  carcinoembryonic antigen [CEA] R97.0
  cholesterol E78.0
    with high triglycerides E78.2
  conjugate, eye H51.0
  C-reactive protein (CRP) R79.82
  diaphragm, congenital Q79.1
  erythrocyte sedimentation rate R70.0
  fasting glucose R73.01
  fasting triglycerides E78.1
  finding on laboratory examination — *see* Findings, abnormal, inconclusive, without diagnosis, by type of exam
  GFR (glomerular filtration rate) — *see* Findings, abnormal, inconclusive, without diagnosis, by type of exam
  glucose tolerance (oral) R73.02
  immunoglobulin level R76.8
  indoleacetic acid R82.5
  lactic acid dehydrogenase (LDH) level R74.0
  leukocytes D72.829
  lipoprotein a level E78.8

Elevated, elevation — *continued*
  liver function
    study R94.5
    test R79.89
      alkaline phosphatase R74.8
      aminotransferase R74.0
      bilirubin R17
      hepatic enzyme R74.8
      lactate dehydrogenase R74.0
  lymphocytes D72.820
  prostate specific antigen [PSA] R97.2
  Rh titer — *see* Complication(s), transfusion, incompatibility reaction, Rh (factor)
  scapula, congenital Q74.0
  sedimentation rate R70.0
  SGOT R74.0
  SGPT R74.0
  transaminase level R74.0
  triglycerides E78.1
    with high cholesterol E78.2
  tumor associated antigens [TAA] NEC R97.8
  tumor specific antigens [TSA] NEC R97.8
  urine level of
    17-ketosteroids R82.5
    catecholamine R82.5
    indoleacetic acid R82.5
    steroids R82.5
    vanillylmandelic acid (VMA) R82.5
  venous pressure I87.8
  white blood cell count D72.829
    specified NEC D72.828
Elliptocytosis (congenital) (hereditary) D58.1
  Hb C (disease) D58.1
  hemoglobin disease D58.1
  sickle-cell (disease) D57.8-
    trait D57.3
Ellison-Zollinger syndrome E16.4
Ellis-van Creveld syndrome (chondroectodermal dysplasia) Q77.6
Elongated, elongation (congenital) — *see also* Distortion
  bone Q79.9
  cervix (uteri) Q51.828
    acquired N88.4
    hypertrophic N88.4
  colon Q43.8
  common bile duct Q44.5
  cystic duct Q44.5
  frenulum, penis Q55.69
  labia minora (acquired) N90.6
  ligamentum patellae Q74.1
  petiolus (epiglottidis) Q31.8
  tooth, teeth K00.2
  uvula Q38.6
Eltor cholera A00.1
Emaciation (due to malnutrition) E41
Embadomoniasis A07.8
Embedded tooth, teeth K01.0
  root only K08.3
Embolic — *see* condition
Embolism (multiple) (paradoxical) I74.9
  air (any site) (traumatic) T79.0
    following
      abortion — *see* Abortion by type complicated by embolism
      ectopic pregnancy O08.2
      infusion, therapeutic injection or transfusion T80.0
      molar pregnancy O08.2
      procedure NEC
        artery T81.719
          mesenteric T81.710
          renal T81.711
          specified NEC T81.718
        vein T81.72
    in pregnancy, childbirth or puerperium — *see* Embolism, obstetric
  amniotic fluid (pulmonary) — *see also* Embolism, obstetric
    following
      abortion — *see* Abortion by type complicated by embolism
      ectopic pregnancy O08.2
      molar pregnancy O08.2
  aorta, aortic I74.10
    abdominal I74.09
      saddle I74.01
    bifurcation I74.09
    saddle I74.01
    thoracic I74.11

Embolism (multiple) (paradoxical) I74.9 — *continued*
artery I74.9
  auditory, internal I65.8
  basilar — *see* Occlusion, artery, basilar
  carotid (common) (internal) — *see*
    Occlusion, artery, carotid
  cerebellar (anterior inferior) (posterior
    inferior) (superior) I66.3
  cerebral — *see* Occlusion, artery,
    cerebral
  choroidal (anterior) I66.8
  communicating posterior I66.8
  coronary — *see also* Infarct,
    myocardium
    not resulting in infarction I24.0
  extremity I74.4
    lower I74.3
    upper I74.2
  hypophyseal I66.8
  iliac I74.5
  limb I74.4
    lower I74.3
    upper I74.2
  mesenteric (with gangrene) K55.0
  ophthalmic — *see* Occlusion, artery,
    retina
  peripheral I74.4
  pontine I66.8
  precerebral — *see* Occlusion, artery,
    precerebral
  pulmonary — *see* Embolism, pulmonary
  renal N28.0
  retinal — *see* Occlusion, artery, retina
  septic I76
  specified NEC I74.8
  vertebral — *see* Occlusion, artery,
    vertebral
basilar (artery) I65.1
blood clot
  following
    abortion — *see* Abortion by type
      complicated by embolism
    ectopic or molar pregnancy O08.2
  in pregnancy, childbirth or puerperium
    — *see* Embolism, obstetric
brain — *see also* Occlusion, artery, cerebral
  following
    abortion — *see* Abortion by type
      complicated by embolism
    ectopic or molar pregnancy O08.2
    puerperal, postpartum, childbirth — *see*
      Embolism, obstetric
capillary I78.8
cardiac — *see also* Infarct, myocardium
  not resulting in infarction I24.0
carotid (artery) (common) (internal) — *see*
  Occlusion, artery, carotid
cavernous sinus (venous) — *see* Embolism,
  intracranial venous sinus
cerebral — *see* Occlusion, artery, cerebral
cholesterol — *see* Atheroembolism
coronary (artery or vein) (systemic) — *see*
  Occlusion, coronary
due to device, implant or graft — *see also*
  Complications, by site and type,
  specified NEC
  arterial graft NEC T82.818
  breast (implant) T85.81
  catheter NEC T85.81
    dialysis (renal) T82.818
      intraperitoneal T85.81
    infusion NEC T82.818
      spinal (epidural) (subdural) T85.81
    urinary (indwelling) T83.81
  electronic (electrode) (pulse generator)
    (stimulator)
    bone T84.81
    cardiac T82.817
    nervous system (brain) (peripheral
      nerve) (spinal) T85.81
    urinary T83.81
  fixation, internal (orthopedic) NEC
    T84.81
  gastrointestinal (bile duct) (esophagus)
    T85.81
  genital NEC T83.81
  heart (graft) (valve) T82.817
  joint prosthesis T84.81
  ocular (corneal graft) (orbital implant)
    T85.81
  orthopedic (bone graft) NEC T86.838
  specified NEC T85.81
  urinary (graft) NEC T83.81
  vascular NEC T82.818
  ventricular intracranial shunt T85.81

Embolism (multiple) (paradoxical) I74.9 — *continued*
extremities
  lower — *see* Embolism, vein, lower
    extremity
    arterial I74.3
  upper I74.2
eye H34.9
fat (cerebral) (pulmonary) (systemic) T79.1
  complicating delivery — *see* Embolism,
    obstetric
  following
    abortion — *see* Abortion by type
      complicated by embolism
    ectopic or molar pregnancy O08.2
  following
    abortion — *see* Abortion by type
      complicated by embolism
    ectopic or molar pregnancy O08.2
    infusion, therapeutic injection or
      transfusion
      air T80.0
heart (fatty) — *see also* Infarct,
  myocardium
  not resulting in infarction I24.0
hepatic (vein) I82.0
in pregnancy, childbirth or puerperium —
  see Embolism, obstetric
intestine (artery) (vein) (with gangrene)
  K55.0
intracranial — *see also* Occlusion, artery,
  cerebral
  venous sinus (any) G08
    nonpyogenic I67.6
intraspinal venous sinuses or veins G08
  nonpyogenic G95.19
kidney (artery) N28.0
lateral sinus (venous) — *see* Embolism,
  intracranial, venous sinus
leg — *see* Embolism, vein, lower extremity
  arterial I74.3
longitudinal sinus (venous) — *see*
  Embolism, intracranial, venous sinus
lung (massive) — *see* Embolism,
  pulmonary
meninges I66.8
mesenteric (artery) (vein) (with gangrene)
  K55.0
obstetric (in) (pulmonary)
  childbirth O88.82
    air O88.02
    amniotic fluid O88.12
    blood clot O88.22
    fat O88.82
    pyemic O88.32
    septic O88.32
    specified type NEC O88.82
  pregnancy O88.81-
    air O88.01-
    amniotic fluid O88.11-
    blood clot O88.21-
    fat O88.81-
    pyemic O88.31-
    septic O88.31-
    specified type NEC O88.81-
  puerperal O88.83
    air O88.03
    amniotic fluid O88.13
    blood clot O88.23
    fat O88.83
    pyemic O88.33
    septic O88.33
    specified type NEC O88.83
ophthalmic — *see* Occlusion, artery, retina
penis N48.81
peripheral artery NOS I74.4
pituitary E23.6
popliteal (artery) I74.3
portal (vein) I81
postoperative, postrpocedural
  artery T81.719
    mesenteric T81.710
    renal T81.711
    specified NEC T81.718
  vein T81.72
precerebral artery — *see* Occlusion, artery,
  precerebral
puerperal — *see* Embolism, obstetric
pulmonary (acute) (artery) (vein) I26.99
  with acute cor pulmonale I26.09
  chronic I27.82
  following
    abortion — *see* Abortion by type
      complicated by embolism
    ectopic or molar pregnancy O08.2
  healed or old Z86.711

Embolism (multiple) (paradoxical) I74.9 — *continued*
pulmonary (acute) (artery) (vein) I26.99 — *continued*
  in pregnancy, childbirth or puerperium
    — *see* Embolism, obstetric
  personal history of Z86.711
  saddle I26.92
    with acute cor pulmonale I26.02
  septic I26.90
    with acute cor pulmonale I26.01
pyemic (multiple) I76
  following
    abortion — *see* Abortion by type
      complicated by embolism
    ectopic or molar pregnancy O08.2
  Hemophilus influenzae A41.3
  pneumococcal A40.3
    with pneumonia J13
  puerperal, postpartum, childbirth (any
    organism) — *see* Embolism,
    obstetric
  specified organism NEC A41.89
  staphylococcal A41.2
  streptococcal A40.9
renal (artery) N28.0
  vein I82.3
retina, retinal — *see* Occlusion, artery,
  retina
saddle
  abdominal aorta I74.01
  pulmonary artery I26.92
    with acute cor pulmonale I26.02
septic (arterial) I76
  complicating abortion — *see* Abortion,
    by type, complicated by, embolism
sinus — *see* Embolism, intracranial, venous
  sinus
soap complicating abortion — *see*
  Abortion, by type, complicated by,
  embolism
spinal cord G95.19
  pyogenic origin G06.1
spleen, splenic (artery) I74.8
upper extremity I74.2
vein (acute) I82.90
  antecubital I82.61-
    chronic I82.71-
  axillary I82.A1-
    chronic I82.A2-
  basilic I82.61-
    chronic I82.71-
  brachial I82.62-
    chronic I82.72-
  brachiocephalic (innominate) I82.290
    chronic I82.291
  cephalic I82.61-
    chronic I82.71-
  chronic I82.91
  deep (DVT) I82.40-
    calf I82.4Z-
      chronic I82.5Z-
    lower leg I82.4Z-
      chronic I82.5Z-
    thigh I82.4Y-
      chronic I82.5Y-
    upper leg I82.4Y-
      chronic I82.5Y-
  femoral I82.41-
    chronic I82.51-
  iliac (iliofemoral) I82.42-
    chronic I82.52-
  innominate I82.290
    chronic I82.291
  internal jugular I82.C1-
    chronic I82.C2-
  lower extremity
    deep I82.40-
      chronic I82.50-
      specified NEC I82.49-
        chronic NEC I82.59-
    distal
      deep I82.4Z-
    proximal
      deep I82.4Y-
        chronic I82.5Y-
    superficial I82.81-
  popliteal I82.43-
    chronic I82.53-
  radial I82.62-
    chronic I82.72-
  renal I82.3
  saphenous (greater) (lesser) I82.81-
  specified NEC I82.890
    chronic NEC I82.891
  subclavian I82.B1-
    chronic I82.B2-
  thoracic NEC I82.290
    chronic I82.291

Embolism (multiple) (paradoxical) I74.9 — *continued*
vein (acute) I82.90 — *continued*
  tibial I82.44-
    chronic I82.54-
  ulnar I82.62-
    chronic I82.72-
  upper extremity I82.60-
    chronic I82.70-
    deep I82.62-
      chronic I82.72-
    superficial I82.61-
      chronic I82.71-
  vena cava
    inferior (acute) I82.220
      chronic I82.221
    superior (acute) I82.210
      chronic I82.211
  venous sinus G08
  vessels of brain — *see* Occlusion, artery,
    cerebral
Embolus — *see* Embolism
Embryoma — *see also* Neoplasm, uncertain
  behavior, by site
  benign — *see* Neoplasm, benign, by site
    kidney C64-
    liver C22.0
  malignant — *see also* Neoplasm,
    malignant, by site
    kidney C64-
    liver C22.0
    testis C62.9-
      descended (scrotal) C62.1-
      undescended C62.0-
  testis C62.9-
    descended (scrotal) C62.1-
    undescended C62.0-
Embryonic
  circulation Q28.9
  heart Q28.9
  vas deferens Q55.4
Embryopathia NOS Q89.9
Embryotoxon Q13.4
Emesis — *see* Vomiting
Emotional lability R45.86
Emotionality, pathological F60.3
Emotogenic disease — *see* Disorder,
  psychogenic
Emphysema (atrophic) (bullous) (chronic)
  (interlobular) (lung) (obstructive)
  (pulmonary) (senile) (vesicular) J43.9
  cellular tissue (traumatic) T79.7
    surgical T81.82
  centrilobular J43.2
  compensatory J98.3
  congenital (interstitial) P25.0
  conjunctiva H11.89
  connective tissue (traumatic) T79.7
    surgical T81.82
  due to chemicals, gases, fumes or vapors
    J68.4
  eyelid(s) — *see* Disorder, eyelid, specified
    type NEC
    surgical T81.82
    traumatic T79.7
  interstitial J98.2
    congenital P25.0
    perinatal period P25.0
  laminated tissue T79.7
    surgical T81.82
  mediastinal J98.2
    newborn P25.2
  orbit, orbital — *see* Disorder, orbit,
    specified type NEC
  panacinar J43.1
  panlobular J43.1
  specified NEC J43.8
  subcutaneous (traumatic) T79.7
    nontraumatic J98.2
    postprocedural T81.82
    surgical T81.82
  surgical T81.82
  thymus (gland) (congenital) E32.8
  traumatic (subcutaneous) T79.7
  unilateral J43.0
Empty nest syndrome Z60.0
Empyema (acute) (chest) (double) (pleura)
  (supradiaphragmatic) (thorax) J86.9
  with fistula J86.0
  accessory sinus (chronic) — *see* Sinusitis
  antrum (chronic) — *see* Sinusitis, maxillary
  brain (any part) — *see* Abscess, brain
  ethmoidal (chronic) (sinus) — *see*
    Sinusitis, ethmoidal
  extradural — *see* Abscess, extradural
  frontal (chronic) (sinus) — *see* Sinusitis,
    frontal
  gallbladder K81.0

D I S E A S E   I N D E X

Empyema (acute) (chest) (double) (pleura) (supradiaphragmatic) (thorax) J86.9 — *continued*
  mastoid (process) (acute) — *see* Mastoiditis, acute
  maxilla, maxillary M27.2
    sinus — *see* Sinusitis, maxillary
  nasal sinus (chronic) — *see* Sinusitis
  sinus (accessory) (chronic) (nasal) — *see* Sinusitis
  sphenoidal (sinus) (chronic) — *see* Sinusitis, sphenoidal
  subarachnoid — *see* Abscess, extradural
  subdural — *see* Abscess, subdural
  tuberculous A15.6
  ureter — *see* Ureteritis
  ventricular — *see* Abscess, brain
En coup de sabre lesion L94.1
Enamel pearls K00.2
Enameloma K00.2
Enanthema, viral B09
Encephalitis (chronic) (hemorrhagic) (idiopathic) (nonepidemic) (spurious) (subacute) G04.90
  acute (*see also* Encephalitis, viral) A86
    disseminated G04.00
      infectious G04.01
      noninfectious G04.81
      postimmunization (postvaccination) G04.02
      postinfectious G04.01
    inclusion body A85.8
    necrotizing hemorrhagic G04.30
      postimmunization G04.32
      postinfectious G04.31
      specified NEC G04.39
  arboviral, arbovirus NEC A85.2
  arthropod-borne NEC (viral) A85.2
  Australian A83.4
  California (virus) A83.5
  Central European (tick-borne) A84.1
  Czechoslovakian A84.1
  Dawson's (inclusion body) A81.1
  diffuse sclerosing A81.1
  disseminated, acute G04.00
  due to
    cat scratch disease A28.1
    human immunodeficiency virus (HIV) disease B20 [G05.3]
    malaria — *see* Malaria
    rickettsiosis — *see* Rickettsiosis
    smallpox inoculation G04.02
    typhus — *see* Typhus
  Eastern equine A83.2
  endemic (viral) A86
  epidemic NEC (viral) A86
  equine (acute) (infectious) (viral) A83.9
    Eastern A83.2
    Venezuelan A92.2
    Western A83.1
  Far Eastern (tick-borne) A84.0
  following vaccination or other immunization procedure G04.02
  herpes zoster B02.0
  herpesviral B00.4
    due to herpesvirus 6 B10.01
    due to herpesvirus 7 B10.09
    specified NEC B10.09
  Ilheus (virus) A83.8
  in (due to)
    actinomycosis A42.82
    adenovirus A85.1
    African trypanosomiasis B56.9 [G05.3]
    Chagas' disease (chronic) B57.42
    cytomegalovirus B25.8
    enterovirus A85.0
    herpes (simplex) virus B00.4
      due to herpesvirus 6 B10.01
      due to herpesvirus 7 B10.09
      specified NEC B10.09
    infectious disease NEC B99 [G05.3]
    influenza — *see* Influenza, with, encephalopathy
    listeriosis A32.12
    measles B05.0
    mumps B26.2
    naegleriasis B60.2
    parasitic disease NEC B89 [G05.3]
    poliovirus A80.9 [G05.3]
    rubella B06.01
    syphilis
      congenital A50.42
      late A52.14
    systemic lupus erythematosus M32.19
    toxoplasmosis (acquired) B58.2
      congenital P37.1
    tuberculosis A17.82
    zoster B02.0

Encephalitis (chronic) (hemorrhagic) (idiopathic) (nonepidemic) (spurious) (subacute) G04.90 — *continued*
  inclusion body A81.1
  infectious (acute) (virus) NEC A86
  Japanese (B type) A83.0
  La Crosse A83.5
  lead — *see* Poisoning, lead
  lethargica (acute) (infectious) A85.8
  louping ill A84.8
  lupus erythematosus, systemic M32.19
  lymphatica A87.2
  Mengo A85.8
  meningococcal A39.81
  Murray Valley A83.4
  otitic NEC H66.40 [G05.3]
  parasitic NOS B71.9
  periaxial G37.0
  periaxialis (concentrica) (diffuse) G37.5
  postchickenpox B01.11
  postexanthematous NEC B09
  postimmunization G04.02
  postinfectious NEC G04.01
  postmeasles B05.0
  postvaccinal G04.02
  postvaricella B01.11
  postviral NEC A86
  Powassan A84.8
  Rasmussen G04.81
  Rio Bravo A85.8
  Russian
    autumnal A83.0
    spring-summer (taiga) A84.0
  saturnine — *see* Poisoning, lead
  specified NEC G04.81
  St. Louis A83.3
  subacute sclerosing A81.1
  summer A83.0
  suppurative G04.81
  tick-borne A84.9
  Torula, torular (cryptococcal) B45.1
  toxic NEC G92
  trichinosis B75 [G05.3]
  type
    B A83.0
    C A83.3
  van Bogaert's A81.1
  Venezuelan equine A92.2
  Vienna A85.8
  viral, virus A86
    arthropod-borne NEC A85.2
    mosquito-borne A83.9
      Australian X disease A83.4
      California virus A83.5
      Eastern equine A83.2
      Japanese (B type) A83.0
      Murray Valley A83.4
      specified NEC A83.8
      St. Louis A83.3
      type B A83.0
      type C A83.3
      Western equine A83.1
    tick-borne A84.9
      biundulant A84.1
      central European A84.1
      Czechoslovakian A84.1
      diphasic meningoencephalitis A84.1
      Far Eastern A84.0
      Russian spring-summer (taiga) A84.0
      specified NEC A84.8
    specified type NEC A85.8
  Western equine A83.1
Encephalocele Q01.9
  frontal Q01.0
  nasofrontal Q01.1
  occipital Q01.2
  specified NEC Q01.8
Encephalocystocele — *see* Encephalocele
Encephaloduroarteriomyosynangiosis (EDAMS) I67.5
Encephalomalacia (brain) (cerebellar) (cerebral) — *see* Softening, brain
Encephalomeningitis — *see* Meningoencephalitis
Encephalomeningocele — *see* Encephalocele
Encephalomeningomyelitis — *see* Meningoencephalitis
Encephalomyelitis (*see also* Encephalitis) G04.90
  acute disseminated G04.00
    infectious G04.01
    noninfectious G04.81
    postimmunization G04.02
    postinfectious G04.01

Encephalomyelitis (*see also* Encephalitis) G04.90 — *continued*
  acute necrotizing hemorrhagic G04.30
    postimmunization G04.32
    postinfectious G04.31
    specified NEC G04.39
  benign myalgic G93.3
  equine A83.9
    Eastern A83.2
    Venezuelan A92.2
    Western A83.1
  in diseases classified elsewhere G05.3
  myalgic, benign G93.3
  postchickenpox B01.11
  postinfectious NEC G04.01
  postmeasles B05.0
  postvaccinal G04.02
  postvaricella B01.11
  rubella B06.01
  specified NEC G04.81
  Venezuelan equine A92.2
Encephalomyelocele — *see* Encephalocele
Encephalomyelomeningitis — *see* Meningoencephalitis
Encephalomyelopathy G96.9
Encephalomyeloradiculitis (acute) G61.0
Encephalomyeloradiculoneuritis (acute) (Guillain-Barré) G61.0
Encephalomyeloradiculopathy G96.9
Encephalopathia hyperbilirubinemica, newborn P57.9
  due to isoimmunization (conditions in P55) P57.0
Encephalopathy (acute) G93.40
  acute necrotizing hemorrhagic G04.30
    postimmunization G04.32
    postinfectious G04.31
    specified NEC G04.39
  alcoholic G31.2
  anoxic — *see* Damage, brain, anoxic
  arteriosclerotic I67.2
  centrolobar progressive (Schilder) G37.0
  congenital Q07.9
  degenerative, in specified disease NEC G32.89
  demyelinating callosal G37.1
  due to
    drugs (*see also* Table of drugs and chemicals) G92
    hepatic — *see* Failure, hepatic
  hyperbilirubinemic, newborn P57.9
    due to isoimmunization (conditions in P55) P57.0
  hypertensive I67.4
  hypoglycemic E16.2
  hypoxic — *see* Damage, brain, anoxic
  hypoxic ischemic P91.60
    mild P91.61
    moderate P91.62
    severe P91.63
  in (due to) (with)
    birth injury P11.1
    hyperinsulinism E16.1 [G94]
    influenza — *see* Influenza, with, encephalopathy
    lack of vitamin (*see also* Deficiency, vitamin) E56.9 [G32.89]
    neoplastic disease (*see also* Neoplasm) D49.9 [G13.1]
    serum (*see also* Reaction, serum) T80.69
    syphilis A52.17
    trauma (postconcussional) F07.81
      current injury — *see* Injury, intracranial
    vaccination G04.02
  lead — *see* Poisoning, lead
  metabolic G93.41
    drug-induced G92
    toxic G92
  myoclonic, early, symptomatic — *see* Epilepsy, generalized, specified NEC
  necrotizing, subacute (Leigh) G31.82
  pellagrous E52 [G32.89]
  portosystemic — *see* Failure, hepatic
  postcontusional F07.81
    current injury — *see* Injury, intracranial, diffuse
  posthypoglycemic (coma) E16.1 [G94]
  postradiation G93.89
  saturnine — *see* Poisoning, lead
  septic G93.41
  specified NEC G93.49
  spongiform, subacute (viral) A81.09
  toxic NEC
    metabolic G92
  traumatic (postconcussional) F07.81
    current injury — *see* Injury, intracranial
  vitamin B deficiency NEC E53.9 [G32.89]
    vitamin B1 E51.2
  Wernicke's E51.2

Encephalorrhagia — *see* Hemorrhage, intracranial, intracerebral
Encephalosis, posttraumatic F07.81
Enchondroma — *see also* Neoplasm, bone, benign
Enchondromatosis (cartilaginous) (multiple) Q78.4
Encopresis R15.9
  functional F98.1
  nonorganic origin F98.1
  psychogenic F98.1
Encounter (with health service) (for) Z76.89
  adjustment and management (of)
    breast implant Z45.81
    implanted device NEC Z45.89
    myringotomy device (stent) (tube) Z45.82
  administrative purpose only Z02.9
    examination for
      adoption Z02.82
      armed forces Z02.3
      disability determination Z02.71
      driving license Z02.4
      employment Z02.1
      insurance Z02.6
      medical certificate NEC Z02.79
      paternity testing Z02.81
      residential institution admission Z02.2
      school admission Z02.0
      sports Z02.5
    specified reason NEC Z02.89
  aftercare — *see* Aftercare
  antenatal screening Z36
  assisted reproductive fertility procedure cycle Z31.83
  blood typing Z01.83
    Rh typing Z01.83
  breast augmentation or reduction Z41.1
  breast implant exchange (different material) (different size) Z45.81
  breast reconstruction following mastectomy Z42.1
  check-up — *see* Examination
  chemotherapy for neoplasm Z51.11
  colonoscopy, screening Z12.11
  counseling — *see* Counseling
  delivery, full-term, uncomplicated O80
    cesarean, without indication O82
  ear piercing Z41.3
  examination — *see* Examination
  expectant parent(s) (adoptive) pre-birth pediatrician visit Z76.81
  fertility preservation procedure (prior to cancer therapy) (prior to removal of gonads) Z31.84
  fitting (of) — *see* Fitting (and adjustment) (of)
  genetic
    counseling Z31.5
    testing — *see* Test, genetic
  hearing conservation and treatment Z01.12
  immunotherapy for neoplasm Z51.12
  in vitro fertilization cycle Z31.83
  instruction (in)
    child care (postpartal) (prenatal) Z32.3
    childbirth Z32.2
    natural family planning
      procreative Z31.61
      to avoid pregnancy Z30.02
  insulin pump titration Z46.81
  joint prosthesis insertion following prior explantation of joint prosthesis (staged procedure)
    hip Z47.32
    knee Z47.33
    shoulder Z47.31
  laboratory (as part of a general medical examination) Z00.00
    with abnormal findings Z00.01
  mental health services (for)
    abuse NEC
      perpetrator Z69.82
      victim Z69.81
    child abuse
      nonparental
        perpetrator Z69.021
        victim Z69.020
      parental
        perpetrator Z69.011
        victim Z69.010
    spousal or partner abuse
      perpetrator Z69.12
      victim Z69.11
  observation (for) (ruled out)
    exposure to (suspected)
      anthrax Z03.810
      biological agent NEC Z03.818
  pediatrician visit, by expectant parent(s) (adoptive) Z76.81

DISEASE INDEX

Encounter (with health service) (for) Z76.89
— *continued*
  plastic and reconstructive surgery
    following medical procedure or
    healed injury NEC Z42.8
  pregnancy
    supervision of — *see* Pregnancy,
      supervision of
    test Z32.00
      result negative Z32.02
      result positive Z32.01
  radiation therapy (antineoplastic) Z51.0
  radiological (as part of a general medical
    examination) Z00.00
    with abnormal findings Z00.01
  reconstructive surgery following medical
    procedure or healed injury NEC
    Z42.8
  removal (of) — *see also* Removal
    artificial
      arm Z44.00-
        complete Z44.01-
        partial Z44.02-
      eye Z44.2-
      leg Z44.10-
        complete Z44.11-
        partial Z44.12-
    breast implant Z45.81
      tissue expander (without synchronous
        insertion of permanent implant)
        Z45.81
    device Z46.9
      specified NEC Z46.89
    external
      fixation device — *code to* fracture
        with seventh character D
      prosthesis, prosthetic device Z44.9
        breast Z44.3-
        specified NEC Z44.8
    implanted device NEC Z45.89
    insulin pump Z46.81
    internal fixation device Z47.2
    myringotomy device (stent) (tube)
      Z45.82
    nervous system device NEC Z46.2
      brain neuropacemaker Z46.2
      visual substitution device Z46.2
        implanted Z45.31
    non-vascular catheter Z46.82
    orthodontic device Z46.4
    stent
      ureteral Z46.6
    urinary device Z46.6
  repeat cervical smear to confirm findings
    of recent normal smear following
    initial abnormal smear Z01.42
  respirator [ventilator] use during power
    failure Z99.12
  Rh typing Z01.83
  screening — *see* Screening
  specified NEC Z76.89
  sterilization Z30.2
  suspected condition, ruled out
    amniotic cavity and membrane Z03.71
    cervical shortening Z03.75
    fetal anomaly Z03.73
    fetal growth Z03.74
    maternal and fetal conditions NEC
      Z03.79
    oligohydramnios Z03.71
    placental problem Z03.72
    polyhydramnios Z03.71
  suspected exposure (to), ruled out
    anthrax Z03.810
    biological agents NEC Z03.818
  termination of pregnancy, elective Z33.2
  testing — *see* Test
  therapeutic drug level monitoring Z51.81
  titration, insulin pump Z46.81
  to determine fetal viability of pregnancy
    O36.80
  training
    insulin pump Z46.81
  X-ray of chest (as part of a general medical
    examination) Z00.00
    with abnormal findings Z00.01
Encystment — *see* Cyst
Endarteritis (bacterial, subacute) (infective)
  I77.6
  brain I67.7
  cerebral or cerebrospinal I67.7
  deformans — *see* Arteriosclerosis
  embolic — *see* Embolism
  obliterans — *see also* Arteriosclerosis
    pulmonary I28.8
  pulmonary I28.8
  retina — *see* Vasculitis, retina
  senile — *see* Arteriosclerosis

Endarteritis (bacterial, subacute) (infective)
  I77.6 — *continued*
  syphilitic A52.09
    brain or cerebral A52.04
    congenital A50.54 [I79.8]
  tuberculous A18.89
Endemic — *see* condition
Endocarditis (chronic) (marantic)
  (nonbacterial) (thrombotic) (valvular)
  I38
  with rheumatic fever (conditions in I00)
    active — *see* Endocarditis, acute,
      rheumatic
    inactive or quiescent (with chorea) I09.1
  acute or subacute I33.9
    infective I33.0
    rheumatic (aortic) (mitral) (pulmonary)
      (tricuspid) I01.1
      with chorea (acute) (rheumatic)
        (Sydenham's) I02.0
  aortic (heart) (nonrheumatic) (valve) I35.8
    with
      mitral disease I08.0
        with tricuspid (valve) disease I08.3
        active or acute I01.1
          with chorea (acute) (rheumatic)
            (Sydenham's) I02.0
      rheumatic fever (conditions in I00)
        active — *see* Endocarditis, acute,
          rheumatic
        inactive or quiescent (with chorea)
          I06.9
      tricuspid (valve) disease I08.2
        with mitral disease I08.3
    acute or subacute I33.9
    arteriosclerotic I35.8
    rheumatic I06.9
      with mitral disease I08.0
        with tricuspid (valve) disease I08.3
        active or acute I01.1
          with chorea (acute) (rheumatic)
            (Sydenham's) I02.0
      active or acute I01.1
        with chorea (acute) (rheumatic)
          (Sydenham's) I02.0
      specified NEC I06.8
    specified cause NEC I35.8
    syphilitic A52.03
  arteriosclerotic I38
  atypical verrucous (Libman-Sacks) M32.11
  bacterial (acute) (any valve) (subacute)
    I33.0
  candidal B37.6
  congenital Q24.8
  constrictive I33.0
  Coxiella burnetii A78 [I39]
  Coxsackie B33.21
  due to
    prosthetic cardiac valve T82.6
    Q fever A78 [I39]
    Serratia marcescens I33.0
    typhoid (fever) A01.02
  gonococcal A54.83
  infectious or infective (acute) (any valve)
    (subacute) I33.0
  lenta (acute) (any valve) (subacute) I33.0
  Libman-Sacks M32.11
  listerial A32.82
  Löffler's I42.3
  malignant (acute) (any valve) (subacute)
    I33.0
  meningococcal A39.51
  mitral (chronic) (double) (fibroid) (heart)
    (inactive) (valve) (with chorea) I05.9
    with
      aortic (valve) disease I08.0
        with tricuspid (valve) disease I08.3
        active or acute I01.1
          with chorea (acute) (rheumatic)
            (Sydenham's) I02.0
      rheumatic fever (conditions in I00)
        active — *see* Endocarditis, acute,
          rheumatic
        inactive or quiescent (with chorea)
          I05.9
      tricuspid (valve) disease I08.1
        with aortic (valve) disease I08.3
    active or acute I01.1
      with chorea (acute) (rheumatic)
        (Sydenham's) I02.0
    bacterial I33.0
    arteriosclerotic I34.8
    nonrheumatic I34.8
      acute or subacute I33.9
    specified NEC I05.8
  monilial B37.6
  multiple valves I08.9
    specified disorders I08.8
  mycotic (acute) (any valve) (subacute)
    I33.0

Endocarditis (chronic) (marantic)
  (nonbacterial thrombotic) (valvular) I38
  — *continued*
  pneumococcal (acute) (any valve)
    (subacute) I33.0
  pulmonary (chronic) (heart) (valve) I37.8
    with rheumatic fever (conditions in I00)
      active — *see* Endocarditis, acute,
        rheumatic
      inactive or quiescent (with chorea)
        I09.89
        with aortic, mitral or tricuspid
          disease I08.8
    acute or subacute I33.9
      rheumatic I01.1
        with chorea (acute) (rheumatic)
          (Sydenham's) I02.0
    arteriosclerotic I37.8
    congenital Q22.2
    rheumatic (chronic) (inactive) (with
      chorea) I09.89
      active or acute I01.1
        with chorea (acute) (rheumatic)
          (Sydenham's) I02.0
    syphilitic A52.03
  purulent (acute) (any valve) (subacute)
    I33.0
  Q fever A78 [I39]
  rheumatic (chronic) (inactive) (with
    chorea) I09.1
    active or acute (aortic) (mitral)
      (pulmonary) (tricuspid) I01.1
      with chorea (acute) (rheumatic)
        (Sydenham's) I02.0
  rheumatoid — *see* Rheumatoid, carditis
  septic (acute) (any valve) (subacute) I33.0
  streptococcal (acute) (any valve)
    (subacute) I33.0
  subacute — *see* Endocarditis, acute
  suppurative (acute) (any valve) (subacute)
    I33.0
  syphilitic A52.03
  toxic I33.9
  tricuspid (chronic) (heart) (inactive)
    (rheumatic) (valve) (with chorea)
    I07.9
    with
      aortic (valve) disease I08.2
      mitral (valve) disease I08.3
      mitral (valve) disease I08.1
        aortic (valve) disease I08.3
      rheumatic fever (conditions in I00)
        active — *see* Endocarditis, acute,
          rheumatic
        inactive or quiescent (with chorea)
          I07.8
    active or acute I01.1
      with chorea (acute) (rheumatic)
        (Sydenham's) I02.0
    arteriosclerotic I36.8
    nonrheumatic I36.8
      acute or subacute I33.9
    specified cause, except rheumatic I36.8
  tuberculous — *see* Tuberculosis,
    endocarditis
  typhoid A01.02
  ulcerative (acute) (any valve) (subacute)
    I33.0
  vegetative (acute) (any valve) (subacute)
    I33.0
  verrucous (atypical) (nonbacterial)
    (nonrheumatic) M32.11
Endocardium, endocardial — *see also*
  condition
  cushion defect Q21.2
Endocervicitis — *see also* Cervicitis
  due to intrauterine (contraceptive) device
    T83.6
  hyperplastic N72
Endocrine — *see* condition
Endocrinopathy, pluriglandular E31.9
Endodontic
  overfill M27.52
  underfill M27.53
Endodontitis K04.0
Endomastoiditis — *see* Mastoiditis
Endometrioma N80.9
Endometriosis N80.9
  appendix N80.5
  bladder N80.8
  bowel N80.5
  broad ligament N80.3
  cervix N80.0
  colon N80.5
  cul-de-sac (Douglas') N80.3
  exocervix N80.0
  fallopian tube N80.2

Endometriosis N80.9 — *continued*
  female genital organ NEC N80.8
  gallbladder N80.8
  in scar of skin N80.6
  internal N80.0
  intestine N80.5
  lung N80.8
  myometrium N80.0
  ovary N80.1
  parametrium N80.3
  pelvic peritoneum N80.3
  peritoneal (pelvic) N80.3
  rectovaginal septum N80.4
  rectum N80.5
  round ligament N80.3
  skin (scar) N80.6
  specified site NEC N80.8
  stromal D39.0
  umbilicus N80.8
  uterus (internal) N80.0
  vagina N80.4
  vulva N80.8
Endometritis (decidual) (nonspecific)
  (purulent) (senile) (atrophic)
  (suppurative) N71.9
  with ectopic pregnancy O08.0
  acute N71.0
  blenorrhagic (gonococcal) (acute) (chronic)
    A54.24
  cervix, cervical (with erosion or ectropion)
    — *see also* Cervicitis
    hyperplastic N72
  chlamydial A56.11
  chronic N71.1
  following
    abortion — *see* Abortion by type
      complicated by genital infection
    ectopic or molar pregnancy O08.0
  gonococcal, gonorrheal (acute) (chronic)
    A54.24
  hyperplastic (see also Hyperplasia,
    endometrial) N85.00-
    cervix N72
  puerperal, postpartum, childbirth O86.12
  subacute N71.0
  tuberculous A18.17
Endometrium — *see* condition
Endomyocardiopathy, South African I42.3
Endomyocarditis — *see* Endocarditis
Endomyofibrosis I42.3
Endomyometritis — *see* Endometritis
Endopericarditis — *see* Endocarditis
Endoperineuritis — *see* Disorder, nerve
Endophlebitis — *see* Phlebitis
Endophthalmia — *see* Endophthalmitis,
  purulent
Endophthalmitis (acute) (infective)
  (metastatic) (subacute) H44.009
  bleb associated H59.4 — *see also* Bleb,
    inflamed (infected), postprocedural
  gonorrheal A54.39
  in (due to)
    cysticercosis B69.1
    onchocerciasis B73.01
    toxocariasis B83.0
  panuveitis — *see* Panuveitis
  parasitic H44.12-
  purulent H44.00-
    panophthalmitis — *see* Panophthalmitis
    vitreous abscess H44.02-
  specified NEC H44.19
  sympathetic — *see* Uveitis, sympathetic
Endosalpingioma D28.2
Endosalpingiosis N94.89
Endosteitis — *see* Osteomyelitis
Endothelioma, bone — *see* Neoplasm, bone,
  malignant
Endotheliosis (hemorrhagic infectional)
  D69.8
Endotoxemia — *code to* condition
Endotrachelitis — *see* Cervicitis
Engelmann(-Camurati) syndrome Q78.3
English disease — *see* Rickets
Engman's disease L30.3
Engorgement
  breast N64.59
    newborn P83.4
    puerperal, postpartum O92.79
  lung (passive) — *see* Edema, lung
  pulmonary (passive) — *see* Edema, lung
  stomach K31.89
  venous, retina — *see* Occlusion, retina,
    vein, engorgement

D
I
S
E
A
S
E

I
N
D
E
X

Entomophobia F40.218
Entomophthoromycosis B46.8
Entrance, air into vein — see Embolism, air
Entrapment, nerve — see Neuropathy, entrapment
Entropion (eyelid) (paralytic) H02.009
  cicatricial H02.019
    left H02.016
      lower H02.015
      upper H02.014
    right H02.013
      lower H02.012
      upper H02.011
  congenital Q10.2
  left H02.006
    lower H02.005
    upper H02.004
  mechanical H02.029
    left H02.026
      lower H02.025
      upper H02.024
    right H02.023
      lower H02.022
      upper H02.021
  right H02.003
    lower H02.002
    upper H02.001
  senile H02.039
    left H02.036
      lower H02.035
      upper H02.034
    right H02.033
      lower H02.032
      upper H02.031
  spastic H02.049
    left H02.046
      lower H02.045
      upper H02.044
    right H02.043
      lower H02.042
      upper H02.041
Enucleated eye (traumatic, current) S05.7-
Enuresis R32
  functional F98.0
  habit disturbance F98.0
  nocturnal N39.44
    psychogenic F98.0
  nonorganic origin F98.0
  psychogenic F98.0
Eosinopenia — see Agranulocytosis
Eosinophilia (allergic) (hereditary) (idiopathic) (secondary) D72.1
  with
    angiolymphoid hyperplasia (ALHE) D18.01
  infiltrative J82
  Löffler's J82
  peritoneal — see Peritonitis, eosinophilic
  pulmonary NEC J82
  tropical (pulmonary) J82
Eosinophilia-myalgia syndrome M35.8
Ependymitis (acute) (cerebral) (chronic) (granular) — see Encephalomyelitis
Ependymoblastoma
  specified site — see Neoplasm, malignant, by site
  unspecified site C71.9
Ependymoma (epithelial) (malignant)
  anaplastic
    specified site — see Neoplasm, malignant, by site
    unspecified site C71.9
  benign
    specified site — see Neoplasm, benign, by site
    unspecified site D33.2
  myxopapillary D43.2
    specified site — see Neoplasm, uncertain behavior, by site
    unspecified site D43.2
  papillary D43.2
    specified site — see Neoplasm, uncertain behavior, by site
    unspecified site D43.2
  specified site — see Neoplasm, malignant, by site
  unspecified site C71.9
Ependymopathy G93.89
Ephelis, ephelides L81.2
Epiblepharon (congenital) Q10.3
Epicanthus, epicanthic fold (eyelid) (congenital) Q10.3
Epicondylitis (elbow)
  lateral M77.1-
  medial M77.0-
Epicystitis — see Cystitis
Epidemic — see condition
Epidermidalization, cervix — see Dysplasia, cervix

Epidermis, epidermal — see condition
Epidermodysplasia verruciformis B07.8
Epidermolysis
  bullosa (congenital) Q81.9
    acquired L12.30
      drug-induced L12.31
      specified cause NEC L12.35
    dystrophica Q81.2
    letalis Q81.1
    simplex Q81.0
    specified NEC Q81.8
  necroticans combustiformis L51.2
    due to drug — see Table of Drugs and Chemicals, by drug
Epidermophytid — see Dermatophytosis
Epidermophytosis (infected) — see Dermatophytosis
Epididymis — see condition
Epididymitis (acute) (nonvenereal) (recurrent) (residual) N45.1
  with orchitis N45.3
  blennorrhagic (gonococcal) A54.23
  caseous (tuberculous) A18.15
  chlamydial A56.19
  filarial (see also Infestation, filarial) B74.9 [N51]
  gonococcal A54.23
  syphilitic A52.76
  tuberculous A18.15
Epididymo-orchitis (see also Epididymitis) N45.3
Epidural — see condition
Epigastrium, epigastric — see condition
Epigastrocele — see Hernia, ventral
Epiglottis — see condition
Epiglottitis, epiglottiditis (acute) J05.10
  with obstruction J05.11
  chronic J37.0
Epignathus Q89.4
Epilepsia partialis continua (see also Kozhevnikof's epilepsy) G40.1-
Epilepsy, epileptic, epilepsia (attack) (cerebral) (convulsion) (fit) (seizure) G40.909

Note: The following terms are to be considered equivalent to intractable: pharmacoresistant (pharmacologically resistant), treatment resistant, refractory (medically) and poorly controlled

  with
    complex partial seizures — see Epilepsy, localization-related, symptomatic, with complex partial seizures
    grand mal seizures on awakening — see Epilepsy, generalized, specified NEC
    myoclonic absences — see Epilepsy, generalized, specified NEC
    myoclonic-astatic seizures — see Epilepsy, generalized, specified NEC
    simple partial seizures — see Epilepsy, localization-related, symptomatic, with simple partial seizures
  akinetic — see Epilepsy, generalized, specified NEC
  benign childhood with centrotemporal EEG spikes — see Epilepsy, localization-related, idiopathic
  benign myoclonic in infancy G40.80-
  Bravais-jacksonian — see Epilepsy, localization-related, symptomatic, with simple partial seizures
  childhood
    with occipital EEG paroxysms — see Epilepsy, localization-related, idiopathic
    absence G40.A09
      intractable G40.A19
        with status epilepticus G40.A11
        without status epilepticus G40.A19
      not intractable G40.A09
        with status epilepticus G40.A01
        without status epilepticus G40.A09
  climacteric — see Epilepsy, specified NEC
  cysticercosis B69.0
  deterioration (mental) F06.8
  due to syphilis A52.19
  focal — see Epilepsy, localization-related, symptomatic, with simple partial seizures
  generalized
    idiopathic G40.309
      intractable G40.319
        with status epilepticus G40.311
        without status epilepticus G40.319
      not intractable G40.309
        with status epilepticus G40.301
        without status epilepticus G40.309

Epilepsy, epileptic, epilepsia (attack) (cerebral) (convulsion) (fit) (seizure) G40.909 — continued
  generalized — continued
    specified NEC G40.409
      intractable G40.419
        with status epilepticus G40.411
        without status epilepticus G40.419
      not intractable G40.409
        with status epilepticus G40.401
        without status epilepticus G40.409
  impulsive petit mal — see Epilepsy, juvenile myoclonic
  intractable G40.919
    with status epilepticus G40.911
    without status epilepticus G40.919
  juvenile absence G40.A09
    intractable G40.A19
      with status epilepticus G40.A11
      without status epilepticus G40.A19
    not intractable G40.A09
      with status epilepticus G40.A01
      without status epilepticus G40.A09
  juvenile myoclonic G40.B09
    intractable G40.B19
      with status epilepticus G40.B11
      without status epilepticus G40.B19
    not intractable G40.B09
      with status epilepticus G40.B01
      without status epilepticus G40.B09
  localization-related (focal) (partial)
    idiopathic G40.009
      with seizures of localized onset G40.009
        intractable G40.019
          with status epilepticus G40.011
          without status epilepticus G40.019
        not intractable G40.009
          with status epilepticus G40.001
          without status epilepticus G40.009
    symptomatic
      with complex partial seizures G40.209
        intractable G40.219
          with status epilepticus G40.211
          without status epilepticus G40.219
        not intractable G40.209
          with status epilepticus G40.201
          without status epilepticus G40.209
      with simple partial seizures G40.109
        intractable G40.119
          with status epilepticus G40.111
          without status epilepticus G40.119
        not intractable G40.109
          with status epilepticus G40.101
          without status epilepticus G40.109
  myoclonus, myoclonic (progressive) — see Epilepsy, generalized, specified NEC
  not intractable G40.909
    with status epilepticus G40.901
    without status epilepticus G40.909
  on awakening — see Epilepsy, generalized, specified NEC
  parasitic NOS B71.9 [G94]
  partialis continua (see also Kozhevnikof's epilepsy) G40.1-
  peripheral — see Epilepsy, specified NEC
  procursiva — see Epilepsy, localization-related, symptomatic, with simple partial seizures
  progressive (familial) myoclonic — see Epilepsy, generalized, idiopathic
  reflex — see Epilepsy, specified NEC
  related to
    alcohol G40.509
      not intractable G40.509
        with status epilepticus G40.501
        without status epilepticus G40.509
    drugs G40.509
      not intractable G40.509
        with status epilepticus G40.501
        without status epilepticus G40.509
    external causes G40.509
      not intractable G40.509
        with status epilepticus G40.501
        without status epilepticus G40.509
    hormonal changes G40.509
      not intractable G40.509
        with status epilepticus G40.501
        without status epilepticus G40.509
    sleep deprivation G40.509
      not intractable G40.509
        with status epilepticus G40.501
        without status epliepticus G40.509

Epilepsy, epileptic, epilepsia (attack) (cerebral) (convulsion) (fit) (seizure) G40.909 — continued
  related to — continued
    stress G40.509
      not intractable G40.509
        with status epilepticus G40.501
        without status epliepticus G40.509
  somatomotor — see Epilepsy, localization-related, symptomatic, with simple partial seizures
  somatosensory — see Epilepsy, localization-related, symptomatic, with simple partial seizures
  spasms G40.822
    intractable G40.824
      with status epilepticus G40.823
      without status epilepticus G40.824
    not intractable G40.822
      with status epilepticus G40.821
      without status epilepticus G40.822
  specified NEC G40.802
    intractable G40.804
      with status epilepticus G40.803
      without status epilepticus G40.804
    not intractable G40.802
      with status epilepticus G40.801
      without status epilepticus G40.802
  syndromes
    generalized
      idiopathic G40.309
        intractable G40.319
          with status epilepticus G40.311
          without status epilepticus G40.319
        not intractable G40.309
          with status epilepticus G40.301
          without status epilepticus G40.309
      specified NEC G40.409
        intractable G40.419
          with status epilepticus G40.411
          without status epilepticus G40.419
        not intractable G40.409
          with status epilepticus G40.401
          without status epilepticus G40.409
    localization-related (focal) (partial)
      idiopathic G40.009
        with seizures of localized onset G40.009
          intractable G40.019
            with status epilepticus G40.011
            without status epilepticus G40.019
          not intractable G40.009
            with status epilepticus G40.001
            without status epilepticus G40.009
    symptomatic
      with complex partial seizures G40.209
        intractable G40.219
          with status epilepticus G40.211
          without status epilepticus G40.219
        not intractable G40.209
          with status epilepticus G40.201
          without status epilepticus G40.209
      with simple partial seizures G40.109
        intractable G40.119
          with status epilepticus G40.111
          without status epilepticus G40.119
        not intractable G40.109
          with status epilepticus G40.101
          without status epilepticus G40.109
    specified NEC G40.802
      intractable G40.804
        with status epilepticus G40.803
        without status epilepticus G40.804
      not intractable G40.802
        with status epilepticus G40.801
        without status epilepticus G40.802
  tonic(-clonic) — see Epilepsy, generalized, specified NEC
  twilight F05
  uncinate (gyrus) — see Epilepsy, localization-related, symptomatic, with complex partial seizures

D I S E A S E   I N D E X

Epilepsy, epileptic, epilepsia (attack) (cerebral) (convulsion) (fit) (seizure) G40.909 — *continued*
  Unverricht (-Lundborg) (familial myoclonic) — *see* Epilepsy, generalized, idiopathic
  visceral — *see* Epilepsy, specified NEC
  visual — *see* Epilepsy, specified NEC
Epiloia Q85.1
Epimenorrhea N92.0
Epipharyngitis — *see* Nasopharyngitis
Epiphora H04.20-
  due to
    excess lacrimation H04.21-
    insufficient drainage H04.22-
Epiphyseal arrest — *see* Arrest, epiphyseal
Epiphyseolysis, epiphysiolysis — *see* Osteochondropathy
Epiphysitis — *see also* Osteochondropathy
  juvenile M92.9
  syphilitic (congenital) A50.02
Epiplocele — *see* Hernia, abdomen
Epiploitis — *see* Peritonitis
Epiplosarcomphalocele — *see* Hernia, umbilicus
Episcleritis (suppurative) H15.10-
  in (due to)
    syphilis A52.71
    tuberculosis A18.51
  nodular H15.12-
  periodica fugax H15.11-
    angioneurotic — *see* Edema, angioneurotic
  syphilitic (late) A52.71
  tuberculous A18.51
Episode
  affective, mixed F39
  depersonalization (in neurotic state) F48.1
  depressive F32.9
    major F32.9
      mild F32.0
      moderate F32.1
      severe (without psychotic symptoms) F32.2
        with psychotic symptoms F32.3
    recurrent F33.9
    brief F33.8
    specified NEC F32.8
  hypomanic F30.8
  manic F30.9
    with
      psychotic symptoms F30.2
      remission (full) F30.4
        partial F30.3
    other specified F30.8
    recurrent F31.89
    without psychotic symptoms F30.10
      mild F30.11
      moderate F30.12
      severe (without psychotic symptoms) F30.13
        with psychotic symptoms F30.2
  psychotic F23
    organic F06.8
  schizophrenic (acute) NEC, brief F23
Epispadias (female) (male) Q64.0
Episplenitis D73.89
Epistaxis (multiple) R04.0
  hereditary I78.0
  vicarious menstruation N94.89
Epithelioma (malignant) — *see also* Neoplasm, malignant, by site
  adenoides cysticum — *see* Neoplasm, skin, benign
  basal cell — *see* Neoplasm, skin, malignant
  benign — *see* Neoplasm, benign, by site
  Bowen's — *see* Neoplasm, skin, in situ
  calcifying, of Malherbe — *see* Neoplasm, skin, benign
  external ear — *see* Neoplasm, skin, malignant
  intraepidermal, Jadassohn — *see* Neoplasm, skin, benign
  squamous cell — *see* Neoplasm, malignant, by site
Epitheliomatosis pigmented Q82.1
Epitheliopathy, multifocal placoid pigment H30.14-
Epithelium, epithelial — *see* condition
Epituberculosis (with atelectasis) (allergic) A15.7
Eponychia Q84.6
Epstein's
  nephrosis or syndrome — *see* Nephrosis
  pearl K09.8
Epulis (gingiva) (fibrous) (giant cell) K06.8
Equinia A24.0
Equinovarus (congenital) (talipes) Q66.0
  acquired — *see* Deformity, limb, clubfoot

Equivalent
  convulsive (abdominal) — *see* Epilepsy, specified NEC
  epileptic (psychic) — *see* Epilepsy, localization-related, symptomatic, with complex partial seizures
Erb(-Duchenne) paralysis (birth injury) (newborn) P14.0
Erb-Goldflam disease or syndrome G70.00
  with exacerbation (acute) G70.01
  in crisis G70.01
Erb's
  disease G71.0
  palsy, paralysis (brachial) (birth) (newborn) P14.0
  spinal (spastic) syphilitic A52.17
  pseudohypertrophic muscular dystrophy G71.0
Erdheim's syndrome (acromegalic macrospondylitis) E22.0
Erection, painful (persistent) — *see* Priapism
Ergosterol deficiency (vitamin D) E55.9
  with
    adult osteomalacia M83.8
    rickets — *see* Rickets
Ergotism — *see also* Poisoning, food, noxious, plant
  from ergot used as drug (migraine therapy) — *see* Table of Drugs and Chemicals
Erosio interdigitalis blastomycetica B37.2
Erosion
  artery I77.2
    without rupture I77.89
  bone — *see* Disorder, bone, density and structure, specified NEC
  bronchus J98.09
  cartilage (joint) — *see* Disorder, cartilage, specified type NEC
  cervix (uteri) (acquired) (chronic) (congenital) N86
    with cervicitis N72
  cornea (nontraumatic) — *see* Ulcer, cornea
    recurrent H18.83-
    traumatic — *see* Abrasion, cornea
  dental (idiopathic) (occupational) (due to diet, drugs or vomiting) K03.2
  duodenum, postpyloric — *see* Ulcer, duodenum
  esophagus K22.10
    with bleeding K22.11
  gastric — *see* Ulcer, stomach
  gastrojejunal — *see* Ulcer, gastrojejunal
  implanted mesh — *see* Complications, mesh
  intestine K63.3
  lymphatic vessel I89.8
  pylorus, pyloric (ulcer) — *see* Ulcer, stomach
  spine, aneurysmal A52.09
  stomach — *see* Ulcer, stomach
  teeth (idiopathic) (occupational) (due to diet, drugs or vomiting) K03.2
  urethra N36.8
  uterus N85.8
Erotomania F52.8
Error
  metabolism, inborn — *see* Disorder, metabolism
  refractive — *see* Disorder, refraction
Eructation R14.2
  nervous or psychogenic F45.8
Eruption
  creeping B76.9
  drug (generalized) (taken internally) L27.0
    fixed L27.1
    in contact with skin — *see* Dermatitis, due to drugs
    localized L27.1
  Hutchinson, summer L56.4
  Kaposi's varicelliform B00.0
  napkin L22
  polymorphous light (sun) L56.4
  recalcitrant pustular L13.8
  ringed R23.8
  skin (nonspecific) R21
    creeping (meaning hookworm) B76.9
    due to inoculation/vaccination (generalized) (*see also* Dermatitis, due to, vaccine) L27.0
      localized L27.1
    erysipeloid A26.0
    feigned L98.1
    Kaposi's varicelliform B00.0
    lichenoid L28.0
    meaning dermatitis — *see* Dermatitis
    toxic NEC L53.0
  tooth, teeth, abnormal (incomplete) (late) (premature) (sequence) K00.6
  vesicular R23.8

Erysipelas (gangrenous) (infantile) (newborn) (phlegmonous) (suppurative) A46
  external ear A46 [H62.40]
  puerperal, postpartum O86.89
Erysipeloid A26.9
  cutaneous (Rosenbach's) A26.0
  disseminated A26.8
  sepsis A26.7
  specified NEC A26.8
Erythema, erythematous (infectional) (inflammation) L53.9
  ab igne L59.0
  annulare (centrifugum) (rheumaticum) L53.1
  arthriticum epidemicum A25.1
  brucellum — *see* Brucellosis
  chronic figurate NEC L53.3
  chronicum migrans (Borrelia burgdorferi) A69.20
  diaper L22
  due to
    chemical NEC L53.0
      in contact with skin L24.5
    drug (internal use) — *see* Dermatitis, due to, drugs
  elevatum diutinum L95.1
  endemic E52
  epidemic, arthritic A25.1
  figuratum perstans L53.3
  gluteal L22
  heat — *code by* site under Burn, first degree
  ichthyosiforme congenitum bullous Q80.3
  in diseases classified elsewhere L54
  induratum (nontuberculous) L52
    tuberculous A18.4
  infectiosum B08.3
  intertrigo L30.4
  iris L51.9
  marginatum L53.2
    in (due to) acute rheumatic fever I00
  medicamentosum — *see* Dermatitis, due to, drugs
  migrans A26.0
    chronicum A69.20
    tongue K14.1
  multiforme (major) (minor) L51.9
    bullous, bullosum L51.1
    conjunctiva L51.1
    nonbullous L51.0
    pemphigoides L12.0
    specified NEC L51.8
  napkin L22
  neonatorum P83.8
    toxic P83.1
  nodosum L52
    tuberculous A18.4
  palmar L53.8
  pernio T69.1
  rash, newborn P83.8
  scarlatiniform (recurrent) (exfoliative) L53.8
  solare L55.0
  specified NEC L53.8
  toxic, toxicum NEC L53.0
    newborn P83.1
  tuberculous (primary) A18.4
Erythematous, erythematosus — *see* condition
Erythermalgia (primary) I73.81
Erythralgia I73.81
Erythrasma L08.1
Erythredema (polyneuropathy) — *see* Poisoning, mercury
Erythremia (acute) C94.0-
  chronic D45
  secondary D75.1
Erythroblastopenia (*see also* Aplasia, red cell) D60.9
  congenital D61.01
Erythroblastophthisis D61.09
Erythroblastosis (fetalis) (newborn) P55.9
  due to
    ABO (antibodies) (incompatibility) (isoimmunization) P55.1
    Rh (antibodies) (incompatibility) (isoimmunization) P55.0
Erythrocyanosis (crurum) I73.89
Erythrocythemia — *see* Erythremia
Erythrocytosis (megalosplenic) (secondary) D75.1
  familial D75.0
  oval, hereditary — *see* Elliptocytosis
  secondary D75.1
  stress D75.1

Erythroderma (secondary) (*see also* Erythema) L53.9
  bullous ichthyosiform, congenital Q80.3
  desquamativum L21.1
  ichthyosiform, congenital (bullous) Q80.3
  neonatorum P83.8
  psoriaticum L40.8
Erythrodysesthesia, palmar plantar (PPE) L27.1
Erythrogenesis imperfecta D61.09
Erythroleukemia C94.0-
Erythromelalgia I73.81
Erythrophagocytosis D75.89
Erythrophobia F40.298
Erythroplakia, oral epithelium, and tongue K13.29
Erythroplasia (Queyrat) D07.4
  specified site — *see* Neoplasm, skin, in situ
  unspecified site D07.4
Escherichia coli (E. coli), as cause of disease classified elsewhere B96.20
  non-O157 Shiga toxin-producing (with known O group) B96.22
  non-Shiga toxin-producing B96.29
  O157 with confirmation of Shiga toxin when H antigen is unknown, or is not H7 B96.21
  O157:H- (nonmotile) with confirmation of Shiga toxin B96.21
  O157:H7 with or without confirmation of Shiga toxin-production B96.21
  Shiga toxin-producing (with unspecified O group) (STEC) B96.23
  O157 B96.21
  O157:H7 with or without confirmation of Shiga toxin-production B96.21
  specified NEC B96.22
  specified NEC B96.29
Esophagismus K22.4
Esophagitis (acute) (alkaline) (chemical) (chronic) (infectional) (necrotic) (peptic) (postoperative) K20.9
  candidal B37.81
  due to gastrointestinal reflux disease K21.0
  eosinophilic K20.0
  reflux K21.0
  specified NEC K20.8
  tuberculous A18.83
  ulcerative K22.10
    with bleeding K22.11
Esophagocele K22.5
Esophagomalacia K22.8
Esophagospasm K22.4
Esophagostenosis K22.2
Esophagostomiasis B81.8
Esophagotracheal — *see* condition
Esophagus — *see* condition
Esophoria H50.51
  convergence, excess H51.12
  divergence, insufficiency H51.8
Esotropia — *see* Strabismus, convergent concomitant
Espundia B55.2
Essential — *see* condition
Esthesioneuroblastoma C30.0
Esthesioneurocytoma C30.0
Esthesioneuroepithelioma C30.0
Esthiomene A55
Estivo-autumnal malaria (fever) B50.9
Estrangement (marital) Z63.5
  parent-child NEC Z62.890
Estriasis — *see* Myiasis
Ethanolism — *see* Alcoholism
Etherism — *see* Dependence, drug, inhalant
Ethmoid, ethmoidal — *see* condition
Ethmoiditis (chronic) (nonpurulent) (purulent) — *see also* Sinusitis, ethmoidal
  influenzal — *see* Influenza, with, respiratory manifestations NEC
  Woakes' J33.1
Ethylism — *see* Alcoholism
Eulenburg's disease (congenital paramyotonia) G71.19
Eumycetoma B47.0
Eunuchoidism E29.1
  hypogonadotropic E23.0
European blastomycosis — *see* Cryptococcosis
Eustachian — *see* condition
Evaluation (for) (of)
  development state
    adolescent Z00.3
    period of
      delayed growth in childhood Z00.70
        with abnormal findings Z00.71
      rapid growth in childhood Z00.2
    puberty Z00.3

Evaluation (for) (of) — *continued*
growth and developmental state (period of rapid growth) Z00.2
delayed growth Z00.70
with abnormal findings Z00.71
mental health (status) Z00.8
requested by authority Z04.6
period of
delayed growth in childhood Z00.70
with abnormal findings Z00.71
rapid growth in childhood Z00.2
suspected condition — *see* Observation
Evans syndrome D69.41
Event, apparent life threatening in newborn and infant (ALTE) R68.13
Eventration — *see also* Hernia, ventral
colon into chest — *see* Hernia, diaphragm
diaphragm (congenital) Q79.1
Eversion
bladder N32.89
cervix (uteri) N86
with cervicitis N72
foot NEC — *see also* Deformity, valgus, ankle
congenital Q66.6
punctum lacrimale (postinfectional) (senile) H04.52-
ureter (meatus) N28.89
urethra (meatus) N36.8
uterus N81.4
Evidence
cytologic
of malignancy on anal smear R85.614
of malignancy on cervical smear R87.614
of malignancy on vaginal smear R87.624
Evisceration
birth injury P15.8
traumatic NEC
eye — *see* Enucleated eye
Evulsion — *see* Avulsion
Ewing's sarcoma or tumor — *see* Neoplasm, bone, malignant
Examination (for) (following) (general) (of) (routine) Z00.00
with abnormal findings Z00.01
abuse, physical (alleged), ruled out
adult Z04.71
child Z04.72
adolescent (development state) Z00.3
alleged rape or sexual assault (victim), ruled out
adult Z04.41
child Z04.42
allergy Z01.82
annual (adult) (periodic) (physical) Z00.00
with abnormal findings Z00.01
gynecological Z01.419
with abnormal findings Z01.411
antibody response Z01.84
blood — *see* Examination, laboratory
blood pressure Z01.30
with abnormal findings Z01.31
cancer staging — *see* Neoplasm, malignant, by site
cervical Papanicolaou smear Z12.4
as part of routine gynecological examination Z01.419
with abnormal findings Z01.411
child (over 28 days old) Z00.129
with abnormal findings Z00.121
under 28 days old — *see* Newborn, examination
clinical research control or normal comparison (control) (participant) Z00.6
contraceptive (drug) maintenance (routine) Z30.8
device (intrauterine) Z30.431
dental Z01.20
with abnormal findings Z01.21
developmental — *see* Examination, child
donor (potential) Z00.5
ear Z01.10
with abnormal findings NEC Z01.118
eye Z01.00
with abnormal findings Z01.01
follow-up (routine) (following) Z09
chemotherapy NEC Z09
malignant neoplasm Z08
fracture Z09
malignant neoplasm Z08
postpartum Z39.2
psychotherapy Z09
radiotherapy NEC Z09
malignant neoplasm Z08
surgery NEC Z09
malignant neoplasm Z08

Examination (for) (following) (general) (of) (routine) Z00.00 — *continued*
following
accident NEC Z04.3
transport Z04.1
work Z04.2
assault, alleged, ruled out
adult Z04.71
child Z04.72
motor vehicle accident Z04.1
treatment (for) Z09
combined NEC Z09
fracture Z09
malignant neoplasm Z08
malignant neoplasm Z08
mental disorder Z09
specified condition NEC Z09
gynecological Z01.419
with abnormal findings Z01.411
for contraceptive maintenance Z30.8
health — *see* Examination, medical
hearing Z01.10
with abnormal findings NEC Z01.118
following failed hearing screening Z01.110
immunity status testing Z01.84
laboratory (as part of a general medical examination) Z00.00
with abnormal findings Z00.01
preprocedural Z01.812
lactating mother Z39.1
medical (adult) (for) (of) Z00.00
with abnormal findings Z00.01
administrative purpose only Z02.9
specified NEC Z02.89
admission to
armed forces Z02.3
old age home Z02.2
prison Z02.89
residential institution Z02.2
school Z02.0
following illness or medical treatment Z02.0
summer camp Z02.89
adoption Z02.82
blood alcohol or drug level Z02.83
camp (summer) Z02.89
clinical research, normal subject (control) (participant) Z00.6
control subject in clinical research (normal comparison) (participant) Z00.6
donor (potential) Z00.5
driving license Z02.4
general (adult) Z00.00
with abnormal findings Z00.01
immigration Z02.89
insurance purposes Z02.6
marriage Z02.89
medicolegal reasons NEC Z04.8
naturalization Z02.89
participation in sport Z02.5
paternity testing Z02.81
population survey Z00.8
pre-employment Z02.1
pre-operative — *see* Examination, pre-procedural
pre-procedural
cardiovascular Z01.810
respiratory Z01.811
specified NEC Z01.818
preschool children
for admission to school Z02.0
prisoners
for entrance into prison Z02.89
recruitment for armed forces Z02.3
specified NEC Z00.8
sport competition Z02.5
medicolegal reason NEC Z04.8
newborn — *see* Newborn, examination
pelvic (annual) (periodic) Z01.419
with abnormal findings Z01.411
period of rapid growth in childhood Z00.2
periodic (adult) (annual) (routine) Z00.00
with abnormal findings Z00.01
physical (adult) — *see also* Examination, medical Z00.00
sports Z02.5
postpartum
immediately after delivery Z39.0
routine follow-up Z39.2
pre-chemotherapy (antineoplastic) Z01.818
prenatal (normal pregnancy) (*see also* Pregnancy, normal) Z34.9-
pre-procedural (pre-operative)
cardiovascular Z01.810
laboratory Z01.812
respiratory Z01.811
specified NEC Z01.818

Examination (for) (following) (general) (of) (routine) Z00.00 — *continued*
prior to chemotherapy (antineoplastic) Z01.818
psychiatric NEC Z00.8
follow-up not needing further care Z09
requested by authority Z04.6
radiological (as part of a general medical examination) Z00.00
with abnormal findings Z00.01
repeat cervical smear to confirm findings of recent normal smear following initial abnormal smear Z01.42
skin (hypersensitivity) Z01.82
special (*see also* Examination, by type) Z01.89
specified type NEC Z01.89
specified type or reason NEC Z04.8
teeth Z01.20
with abnormal findings Z01.21
urine — *see* Examination, laboratory
vision Z01.00
with abnormal findings Z01.01
Exanthem, exanthema — *see also* Rash
with enteroviral vesicular stomatitis B08.4
Boston A88.0
epidemic with meningitis A88.0 [G02]
subitum B08.20
due to human herpesvirus 6 B08.21
due to human herpesvirus 7 B08.22
viral, virus B09
specified type NEC B08.8
Excess, excessive, excessively
alcohol level in blood R78.0
androgen (ovarian) E28.1
attrition, tooth, teeth K03.0
carotene, carotin (dietary) E67.1
cold, effects of T69.9
specified effect NEC T69.8
convergence H51.12
crying
in child, adolescent, or adult R45.83
in infant R68.11
development, breast N62
divergence H51.8
drinking (alcohol) NEC (without dependence) F10.10
habitual (continual) (without remission) F10.20
eating R63.2
estrogen E28.0
fat — *see also* Obesity
in heart — *see* Degeneration, myocardial
localized E65
foreskin N47.8
gas R14.0
glucagon E16.3
heat — *see* Heat
intermaxillary vertical dimension of fully erupted teeth M26.37
interocclusal distance of fully erupted teeth M26.37
kalium E87.5
large
colon K59.3
congenital Q43.8
infant P08.0
organ or site, congenital NEC — *see* Anomaly, by site
long
organ or site, congenital NEC — *see* Anomaly, by site
menstruation (with regular cycle) N92.0
with irregular cycle N92.1
napping G72.821
natrium E87.0
number of teeth K00.1
nutrient (dietary) NEC R63.2
potassium (K) E87.5
salivation K11.7
secretion — *see also* Hypersecretion
milk O92.6
sputum R09.3
sweat R61
sexual drive F52.8
short
organ or site, congenital NEC — *see* Anomaly, by site
umbilical cord in labor or delivery O69.3
skin, eyelid (acquired) — *see* Blepharochalasis
congenital Q10.3
sodium (Na) E87.0
spacing of fully erupted teeth M26.32
sputum R09.3
sweating R61
thirst R63.1
due to deprivation of water T73.1
tuberosity of jaw M26.07

Excess, excessive, excessively — *continued*
vitamin
A (dietary) E67.0
administered as drug (prolonged intake) — *see* Table of Drugs and Chemicals, vitamins, adverse effect
overdose or wrong substance given or taken — *see* Table of Drugs and Chemicals, vitamins, poisoning
D (dietary) E67.3
administered as drug (prolonged intake) — *see* Table of Drugs and Chemicals, vitamins, adverse effect
overdose or wrong substance given or taken — *see* Table of Drugs and Chemicals, vitamins, poisoning
weight
gain R63.5
loss R63.4
Excitability, abnormal, under minor stress (personality disorder) F60.3
Excitation
anomalous atrioventricular I45.6
psychogenic F30.8
reactive (from emotional stress, psychological trauma) F30.8
Excitement
hypomanic F30.8
manic F30.9
mental, reactive (from emotional stress, psychological trauma) F30.8
state, reactive (from emotional stress, psychological trauma) F30.8
Excoriation (traumatic) — *see also* Abrasion
neurotic L98.1
Exfoliation
due to erythematous conditions according to extent of body surface involved L49.0
10-19 percent of body surface L49.1
20-29 percent of body surface L49.2
30-39 percent of body surface L49.3
40-49 percent of body surface L49.4
50-59 percent of body surface L49.5
60-69 percent of body surface L49.6
70-79 percent of body surface L49.7
80-89 percent of body surface L49.8
90-99 percent of body surface L49.9
less than 10 percent of body surface L49.0
teeth, due to systemic causes K08.0
Exfoliative — *see* condition
Exhaustion, exhaustive (physical NEC) R53.83
battle F43.0
cardiac — *see* Failure, heart
delirium F43.0
due to
cold T69.8
excessive exertion T73.3
exposure T73.2
neurasthenia F48.8
heart — *see* Failure, heart
heat (*see also* Heat, exhaustion) T67.5
due to
salt depletion T67.4
water depletion T67.3
maternal, complicating delivery O75.81
mental F48.8
myocardium, myocardial — *see* Failure, heart
nervous F48.8
old age R54
psychogenic F48.8
psychosis F43.0
senile R54
vital NEC Z73.0
Exhibitionism F65.2
Exocervicitis — *see* Cervicitis
Exomphalos Q79.2
meaning hernia — *see* Hernia, umbilicus
Exophoria H50.52
convergence, insufficiency H51.11
divergence, excess H51.8
Exophthalmos H05.2-
congenital Q15.8
constant NEC H05.24-
displacement, globe — *see* Displacement, globe
due to thyrotoxicosis (hyperthyroidism) — *see* Hyperthyroidism, with, goiter (diffuse)
dysthyroid — *see* Hyperthyroidism, with, goiter (diffuse)
goiter — *see* Hyperthyroidism, with, goiter (diffuse)
intermittent NEC H05.25-

Exophthalmos H05.2- — *continued*
 malignant — *see* Hyperthyroidism, with, goiter (diffuse)
 orbital
  edema — *see* Edema, orbit
  hemorrhage — *see* Hemorrhage, orbit
 pulsating NEC H05.26-
 thyrotoxic, thyrotropic — *see* Hyperthyroidism, with, goiter (diffuse)
Exostosis — *see also* Disorder, bone
 cartilaginous — *see* Neoplasm, bone, benign
 congenital (multiple) Q78.6
 external ear canal H61.81-
 gonococcal A54.49
 jaw (bone) M27.8
 multiple, congenital Q78.6
 orbit H05.35-
 osteocartilaginous — *see* Neoplasm, bone, benign
 syphilitic A52.77
Exotropia — *see* Strabismus, divergent concomitant
Explanation of
 investigation finding Z71.2
 medication Z71.89
Exposure (to) (*see also* Contact, with) T75.89
 acariasis Z20.7
 AIDS virus Z20.6
 air pollution Z77.110
 algae and algae toxins Z77.121
 algae bloom Z77.121
 anthrax Z20.810
 aromatic (hazardous) compounds NEC Z77.028
 aromatic amines Z77.020
 aromatic dyes NOS Z77.028
 arsenic Z77.010
 asbestos Z77.090
 bacterial disease NEC Z20.818
 benzene Z77.021
 blue-green algae bloom Z77.121
 body fluids (potentially hazardous) Z77.21
 brown tide Z77.121
 chemicals (chiefly nonmedicinal) (hazardous) NEC Z77.098
 cholera Z20.09
 chromium compounds Z77.018
 cold, effects of T69.9
  specified effect NEC T69.8
 communicable disease Z20.9
  bacterial NEC Z20.818
  specified NEC Z20.89
  viral NEC Z20.828
 cyanobacteria bloom Z77.121
 disaster Z65.5
 discrimination Z60.5
 dyes Z77.098
 effects of T73.9
 environmental tobacco smoke (acute) (chronic) Z77.22
 Escherichia coli (E. coli) Z20.01
 exhaustion due to T73.2
 fiberglass — *see* Table of Drugs and Chemicals, fiberglass
 German measles Z20.4
 gonorrhea Z20.2
 hazardous metals NEC Z77.018
 hazardous substances NEC Z77.29
 hazards in the physical environment NEC Z77.128
 hazards to health NEC Z77.9
 human immunodeficiency virus (HIV) Z20.6
 human T-lymphotropic virus type-1 (HTLV-1) Z20.89
 implanted
  mesh — *see* Complications, mesh
  prosthetic materials NEC — *see* Complications, prosthetic materials NEC
 infestation (parasitic) NEC Z20.7
 intestinal infectious disease NEC Z20.09
  Escherichia coli (E. coli) Z20.01
 lead Z77.011
 meningococcus Z20.811
 mold (toxic) Z77.120
 nickel dust Z77.018
 noise Z77.122

Exposure (to) (*see also* Contact, with) T75.89 — *continued*
 occupational
  air contaminants NEC Z57.39
  dust Z57.2
  environmental tobacco smoke Z57.31
  extreme temperature Z57.6
  noise Z57.0
  radiation Z57.1
  risk factors Z57.9
   specified NEC Z57.8
  toxic agents (gases) (liquids) (solids) (vapors) in agriculture Z57.4
  toxic agents (gases) (liquids) (solids) (vapors) in industry NEC Z57.5
  vibration Z57.7
 parasitic disease NEC Z20.7
 pediculosis Z20.7
 persecution Z60.5
 pfiesteria piscicida Z77.121
 poliomyelitis Z20.89
 pollution
  air Z77.110
  environmental NEC Z77.118
  soil Z77.112
  water Z77.111
 polycyclic aromatic hydrocarbons Z77.028
 prenatal (drugs) (toxic chemicals) — *see* Newborn, affected by (suspected to be), noxious substances transmitted viaplacenta or breast milk
 rabies Z20.3
 radiation, naturally occurring NEC Z77.123
 radon Z77.123
 red tide (Florida) Z77.121
 rubella Z20.4
 second hand tobacco smoke (acute) (chronic) Z77.22
  in the perinatal period P96.81
 sexually-transmitted disease Z20.2
 smallpox (laboratory) Z20.89
 syphilis Z20.2
 terrorism Z65.4
 torture Z65.4
 tuberculosis Z20.1
 uranium Z77.012
 varicella Z20.820
 venereal disease Z20.2
 viral disease NEC Z20.828
 war Z65.5
 water pollution Z77.111
Exsanguination — *see* Hemorrhage
Exstrophy
 abdominal contents Q45.8
 bladder Q64.10
  cloacal Q64.12
  specified type NEC Q64.19
  supravesical fissure Q64.11
Extensive — *see* condition
Extra — *see also* Accessory
 marker chromosomes (normal individual) Q92.61
  in abnormal individual Q92.62
 rib Q76.6
  cervical Q76.5
Extrasystoles (supraventricular) I49.49
 atrial I49.1
 auricular I49.1
 junctional I49.2
 ventricular I49.3
Extrauterine gestation or pregnancy — *see* Pregnancy, by site
Extravasation
 blood R58
 chyle into mesentery I89.8
 pelvicalyceal N13.8
 pyelosinus N13.8
 urine (from ureter) R39.0
 vesicant agent
  antineoplastic chemotherapy T80.810
  other agent NEC T80.818
Extremity — *see* condition, limb
Extrophy — *see* Exstrophy
Extroversion
 bladder Q64.19
 uterus N81.4
  complicating delivery O71.2
  postpartal (old) N81.4
Extruded tooth (teeth) M26.34
Extrusion
 breast implant (prosthetic) T85.42
 eye implant (globe) (ball) T85.328
 intervertebral disc — *see* Displacement, intervertebral disc
 ocular lens implant (prosthetic) — *see* Complications, intraocular lens
 vitreous — *see* Prolapse, vitreous

Exudate
 pleural — *see* Effusion, pleura
 retina H35.89
Exudative — *see* condition
Eye, eyeball, eyelid — *see* condition
Eyestrain — *see* Disturbance, vision, subjective
Eyeworm disease of Africa B74.3

F

Faber's syndrome (achlorhydric anemia)
   D50.9
Fabry(-Anderson) disease E75.21
Faciocephalalgia, autonomic (see also
   Neuropathy, peripheral, autonomic)
   G90.09
Factor(s)
   psychic, associated with diseases classified
      elsewhere F54
   psychological
      affecting physical conditions F54
      or behavioral
         affecting general medical condition
            F54
         associated with disorders or diseases
            classified elsewhere F54
Fahr disease (of brain) G23.8
Fahr Volhard disease (of kidney) I12-
Failure, failed
   abortion — see Abortion, attempted
   aortic (valve) I35.8
      rheumatic I06.8
   attempted abortion — see Abortion,
      attempted
   biventricular I50.9
   bone marrow — see Anemia, aplastic
   cardiac — see Failure, heart
   cardiorenal (chronic) I50.9
      hypertensive I13.2
   cardiorespiratory (see also Failure, heart)
      R09.2
   cardiovascular (chronic) — see Failure,
      heart
   cerebrovascular I67.9
   cervical dilatation in labor O62.0
   circulation, circulatory (peripheral) R57.9
      newborn P29.89
   compensation — see Disease, heart
   compliance with medical treatment or
      regimen — see Noncompliance
   congestive — see Failure, heart, congestive
   dental implant (endosseous) M27.69
      due to
         failure of dental prosthesis M27.63
         lack of attached gingiva M27.62
         occlusal trauma (poor prosthetic
            design) M27.62
         parafunctional habits M27.62
         periodontal infection (peri-
            implantitis) M27.62
         poor oral hygiene M27.62
      osseointegration M27.61
         due to
            complications of systemic disease
               M27.61
            poor bone quality M27.61
         iatrogenic M27.61
         post-osseointegration
            biological M27.62
            due to complications of systemic
               disease M27.62
            iatrogenic M27.62
            mechanical M27.63
         pre-integration M27.61
         pre-osseointegration M27.61
      specified NEC M27.69
   descent of head (at term) of pregnancy
      (mother) O32.4
   endosseous dental implant — see Failure,
      dental implant
   engagement of head (term of pregnancy)
      (mother) O32.4
   erection (penile) (see also Dysfunction,
      sexual, male, erectile) N52.9
      nonorgqanic F52.21
   examination(s), anxiety concerning Z55.2
   expansion terminal respiratory units
      (newborn) (primary) P28.0
   forceps NOS (with subsequent cesarean
      delivery) O66.5
   gain weight (child over 28 days old)
      R62.51
      adult R62.7
      newborn P92.6
   genital response (male) F52.21
      female F52.22

Failure, failed — continued
   heart (acute) (senile) (sudden) I50.9
      with
         acute pulmonary edema — see
            Failure, ventricular, left
         decompensation — see Failure, heart,
            congestive
         dilatation — see Disease, heart
      arteriosclerotic I70.90
      biventricular I50.9
      combined left-right sided I50.9
      compensated I50.9
      complicating
         anesthesia (general) (local) or other
            sedation
            in labor and delivery O74.2
            in pregnancy O29.12-
            postpartum, puerperal O89.1
         delivery (cesarean) (instrumental)
            O75.4
      congestive (compensated)
         (decompensated) I50.9
         with rheumatic fever (conditions in
            I00)
            active I01.8
            inactive or quiescent (with chorea)
               I09.81
         newborn P29.0
         rheumatic (chronic) (inactive) (with
            chorea) I09.81
            active or acute I01.8
               with chorea I02.0
      decompensated I50.9
      degenerative — see Degeneration,
         myocardial
      diastolic (congestive) I50.30
         acute (congestive) I50.31
            and (on) chronic (congestive)
               I50.33
         chronic (congestive) I50.32
            and (on) acute (congestive) I50.33
         combined with systolic (congestive)
            I50.40
            acute (congestive) I50.41
               and (on) chronic (congestive)
                  I50.43
            chronic (congestive) I50.42
               and (on) acute (congestive)
                  I50.43
      due to presence of cardiac prosthesis
         I97.13-
      following cardiac surgery I97.13-
      high output NOS I50.9
      hypertensive — see Hypertension, heart
      left (ventricular) — see Failure,
         ventricular, left
      low output (syndrome) NOS I50.9
      newborn P29.0
      organic — see Disease, heart
      peripartum O90.3
      postprocedural I97.13-
      rheumatic (chronic) (inactive) I09.9
      right (ventricular) (secondary to left
         heart failure) — see Failure, heart,
         congestive
      systolic (congestive) I50.20
         acute (congestive) I50.21
            and (on) chronic (congestive)
               I50.23
         chronic (congestive) I50.22
            and (on) acute (congestive) I50.23
         combined with diastolic (congestive)
            I50.40
            acute (congestive) I50.41
               and (on) chronic (congestive)
                  I50.43
            chronic (congestive) I50.42
               and (on) acute (congestive)
                  I50.43
      thyrotoxic (see also Thyrotoxicosis)
         E05.90 [I43]
         with thyroid storm E05.91 [I43]
      valvular — see Endocarditis
   hepatic K72.90
      with coma K72.91
      acute or subacute K72.00
         with coma K72.01
         due to drugs K71.10
            with coma K71.11
         alcoholic (acute) (chronic) (subacute)
            K70.40
            with coma K70.41
      chronic K72.10
         with coma K72.11
         due to drugs (acute) (subacute)
            (chronic) K71.10
            with coma K71.11

Failure, failed — continued
   hepatic K72.90 — continued
      due to drugs (acute) (subacute) (chronic)
         K71.10
         with coma K71.11
      postprocedural K91.82
   hepatorenal K76.7
   induction (of labor) O61.9
      abortion — see Abortion, attempted
      by
         oxytocic drugs O61.0
         prostaglandins O61.0
      instrumental O61.1
      mechanical O61.1
      medical O61.0
      specified NEC O61.8
      surgical O61.1
   intubation during anesthesia T88.4
      in pregnancy O29.6-
      labor and delivery O74.7
      postpartum, puerperal O89.6
   involution, thymus (gland) E32.0
   kidney (see also Disease, kidney, chronic)
      N19
      acute (see also Failure, renal, acute)
         N17.9-
      diabetic — see E08-E13 with .22
   lactation (complete) O92.3
      partial O92.4
   Leydig's cell, adult E29.1
   liver — see Failure, hepatic
   menstruation at puberty N91.0
   mitral I05.8
   myocardial, myocardium (see also Failure,
      heart) I50.9
      chronic (see also Failure, heart,
         congestive) I50.9
      congestive (see also Failure, heart,
         congestive) I50.9
   orgasm (female) (psychogenic) F52.31
      male F52.32
   ovarian (primary) E28.39
      iatrogenic E89.40
         asymptomatic E89.40
         symptomatic E89.41
      postprocedural (postablative)
         (postirradiation) (postsurgical)
         E89.40
         asymptomatic E89.40
         symptomatic E89.41
   ovulation causing infertility N97.0
   polyglandular, autoimmune E31.0
   prosthetic joint implant — see
      Complications, joint prosthesis,
      mechanical, breakdown, by site
   renal N19
      with
         tubular necrosis (acute) N17.0
      acute N17.9
         with
            cortical necrosis N17.1
            medullary necrosis N17.2
            tubular necrosis N17.0
         specified NEC N17.8
      chronic N18.9
         hypertensive — see Hypertension,
            kidney
      congenital P96.0
      end stage (chronic) N18.6
         due to hypertension I12.0
      following
         abortion — see Abortion by type
            complicated by specified
            condition NEC
         crushing T79.5
         ectopic or molar pregnancy O08.4
         labor and delivery (acute) O90.4
      hypertensive — see Hypertension,
         kidney
      postprocedural N99.0
   respiration, respiratory J96.90
      with
         hypercapnia J96.92
         hypoxia J96.91
      acute J96.00
         with
            hypercapnia J96.02
            hypoxia J96.01
      acute and (on) chronic J96.20
         with
            hypercapnia J96.22
            hypoxia J96.21
      center G93.89
      chronic J96.10
         with
            hypercapnia J96.12
            hypoxia J96.11
      newborn P28.5
      postprocedural (acute) J95.821
         acute and chronic J95.822

Failure, failed — continued
   rotation
      cecum Q43.3
      colon Q43.3
      intestine Q43.3
      kidney Q63.2
   sedation (conscious) (moderate) during
      procedure T88.52
      history of Z92.83
   segmentation — see also Fusion
      fingers — see Syndactylism, complex,
         fingers
      vertebra Q76.49
         with scoliosis Q76.3
   seminiferous tubule, adult E29.1
   senile (general) R54
   sexual arousal (male) F52.21
      female F52.22
   testicular endocrine function E29.1
   to thrive (child over 28 days old) R62.51
      adult R62.7
      newborn P92.6
   transplant T86.92
      bone T86.831
         marrow T86.02
      cornea T86.841
      heart T86.22
         with lung(s) T86.32
      intestine T86.851
      kidney T86.12
      liver T86.42
      lung(s) T86.811
         with heart T86.32
      pancreas T86.891
      skin (allograft) (autograft) T86.821
      specified organ or tissue NEC T86.891
      stem cell (peripheral blood) (umbilical
         cord) T86.5
   trial of labor (with subsequent cesarean
      delivery) O66.40
      following previous cesarean delivery
         O66.41
   tubal ligation N99.89
   urinary — see Disease, kidney, chronic
   vacuum extraction NOS (with subsequent
      cesarean delivery) O66.5
   vasectomy N99.89
   ventouse NOS (with subsequent cesarean
      delivery) O66.5
   ventricular (see also Failure, heart) I50.9
      left I50.1
         with rheumatic fever (conditions in
            I00)
            active I01.8
               with chorea I02.0
            inactive or quiescent (with chorea)
               I09.81
         rheumatic (chronic) (inactive) (with
            chorea) I09.81
            active or acute I01.8
               with chorea I02.0
      right (see also Failure, heart, congestive)
         I50.9
   vital centers, newborn P91.8
Fainting (fit) R55
Fallen arches — see Deformity, limb, flat
   foot
Falling, falls (repeated) R29.6
   any organ or part — see Prolapse
Fallopian
   insufflation Z31.41
   tube — see condition
Fallot's
   pentalogy Q21.8
   tetrad or tetralogy Q21.3
   triad or trilogy Q22.3
False — see also condition
   croup J38.5
   joint — see Nonunion, fracture
   labor (pains) O47.9
      at or after 37 completed weeks of
         gestation O47.1
      before 37 completed weeks of gestation
         O47.0-
   passage, urethra (prostatic) N36.5
   pregnancy F45.8
Family, familial — see also condition
   disruption Z63.8
      involving divorce or separation Z63.5
   Li-Fraumeni (syndrome) Z15.01
   planning advice Z30.09
   problem Z63.9
      specified NEC Z63.8
   retinoblastoma C69.2-
Famine (effects of) T73.0
   edema — see Malnutrition, severe

D
I
S
E
A
S
E

I
N
D
E
X

D I S E A S E   I N D E X

Fanconi (-de Toni) (-Debré) syndrome E72.09
   with cystinosis E72.04
Fanconi's anemia (congenital pancytopenia) D61.09
Farber's disease or syndrome E75.29
Farcy A24.0
Farmer's
   lung J67.0
   skin L57.8
Farsightedness — see Hypermetropia
Fascia — see condition
Fasciculation R25.3
Fasciitis M72.9
   diffuse (eosinophilic) M35.4
   infective M72.8
      necrotizing M72.6
   necrotizing M72.6
   nodular M72.4
   perirenal (with ureteral obstruction) N13.5
      with infection N13.6
   plantar M72.2
   specified NEC M72.8
   traumatic (old) M72.8
      current — code by site under Sprain
Fascioliasis B66.3
Fasciolopsis, fasciolopsiasis (intestinal) B66.5
Fascioscapulohumeral myopathy G71.0
Fast pulse R00.0
Fat
   embolism — see Embolism, fat
   excessive — see also Obesity
      in heart — see Degeneration, myocardial
   in stool R19.5
   localized (pad) E65
      heart — see Degeneration, myocardial
      knee M79.4
      retropatellar M79.4
   necrosis
      breast N64.1
      mesentery K65.4
      omentum K65.4
   pad E65
      knee M79.4
Fatigue R53.83
   auditory deafness — see Deafness
   chronic R53.82
   combat F43.0
   general R53.83
      psychogenic F48.8
   heat (transient) T67.6
   muscle M62.89
   myocardium — see Failure, heart
   neoplasm-related R53.0
   nervous, neurosis F48.8
   operational F48.8
   psychogenic (general) F48.8
   senile R54
   voice R49.8
Fatness — see Obesity
Fatty — see also condition
   apron E65
   degeneration — see Degeneration, fatty
   heart (enlarged) — see Degeneration, myocardial
   liver NEC K76.0
      alcoholic K70.0
      nonalcoholic K76.0
   necrosis — see Degeneration, fatty
Fauces — see condition
Fauchard's disease (periodontitis) — see Periodontitis
Faucitis J02.9
Favism (anemia) D55.0
Favus — see Dermatophytosis
Fazio-Londe disease or syndrome G12.1
Fear complex or reaction F40.9
Fear of — see Phobia
Feared complaint unfounded Z71.1
Febris, febrile — see also Fever
   flava (see also Fever, yellow) A95.9
   melitensis A23.0
   pestis — see Plague
   recurrens — see Fever, relapsing
   rubra A38.9
Fecal
   incontinence R15.9
   smearing R15.1
   soiling R15.1
   urgency R15.2
Fecalith (impaction) K56.41
   appendix K38.1
   congenital P76.8
Fede's disease K14.0

Feeble rapid pulse due to shock following injury T79.4
Feeble-minded F70
Feeding
   difficulties R63.3
   problem R63.3
      newborn P92.9
         specified NEC P92.8
      nonorganic (adult) — see Disorder, eating
Feeling (of)
   foreign body in throat R09.89
Feer's disease — see Poisoning, mercury
Feet — see condition
Feigned illness Z76.5
Feil-Klippel syndrome (brevicollis) Q76.1
Feinmesser's (hidrotic) ectodermal dysplasia Q82.4
Felinophobia F40.218
Felon — see also Cellulitis, digit
   with lymphangitis — see Lymphangitis, acute, digit
Felty's syndrome M05.00
   ankle M05.07-
   elbow M05.02-
   foot joint M05.07-
   hand joint M05.04-
   hip M05.05-
   knee M05.06-
   multiple site M05.09
   shoulder M05.01-
   vertebra — see Spondylitis, ankylosing
   wrist M05.03-
Female genital mutilation status (FGM) N90.810
   specified NEC N90.818
   type I (clitorectomy status) N90.811
   type II (clitorectomy with excision of labia minora status) N90.812
   type III (infibulation status) N90.813
   type IV N90.818
Female genital cutting status — see Female genital mutilation status (FGM)
Femur, femoral — see condition
Fenestration, fenestrated — see also Imperfect, closure
   aortico-pulmonary Q21.4
   cusps, heart valve NEC Q24.8
      pulmonary Q22.3
   pulmonic cusps Q22.3
Fernell's disease (aortic aneurysm) I71.9
Fertile eunuch syndrome E23.0
Fetid
   breath R19.6
   sweat L75.0
Fetishism F65.0
   transvestic F65.1
Fetus, fetal — see also condition
   alcohol syndrome (dysmorphic) Q86.0
   compressus O31.0-
   hydantoin syndrome Q86.1
   lung tissue P28.0
   papyraceous O31.0-
Fever (inanition) (of unknown origin) (persistent) (with chills) (with rigor) R50.9
   abortus A23.1
   Aden (dengue) A90
   African tick-borne A68.1
   American
      mountain (tick) A93.2
      spotted A77.0
   aphthous B08.8
   arbovirus, arboviral A94
      hemorrhagic A94
      specified NEC A93.8
   Argentinian hemorrhagic A96.0
   Assam B55.0
   Australian Q A78
   Bangkok hemorrhagic A91
   Barmah forest A92.8
   Bartonella A44.0
   bilious, hemoglobinuric B50.8
   blackwater B50.8
   blister B00.1
   Bolivian hemorrhagic A96.1
   Bonvale dam T73.3
   boutonneuse A77.1
   brain — see Encephalitis
   Brazilian purpuric A48.4
   breakbone A90
   Bullis A77.0
   Bunyamwera A92.8
   Burdwan B55.0
   Bwamba A92.8
   Cameroon — see Malaria

Fever (inanition) (of unknown origin) (persistent) (with chills) (with rigor) R50.9 — continued
   Canton A75.9
   catarrhal (acute) J00
      chronic J31.0
   cat-scratch A28.1
   Central Asian hemorrhagic A98.0
   cerebral — see Encephalitis
   cerebrospinal meningococcal A39.0
   Chagres B50.9
   Chandipura A92.8
   Changuinola A93.1
   Charcot's (biliary) (hepatic) (intermittent) — see Calculus, bile duct
   Chikungunya (viral) (hemorrhagic) A92.0
   Chitral A93.1
   Colombo — see Fever, paratyphoid
   Colorado tick (virus) A93.2
   congestive (remittent) — see Malaria
   Congo virus A98.0
   continued malarial B50.9
   Corsican — see Malaria
   Crimean-Congo hemorrhagic A98.0
   Cyprus — see Brucellosis
   dandy A90
   deer fly — see Tularemia
   dengue (virus) A90
      hemorrhagic A91
      sandfly A93.1
   desert B38.0
   drug induced R50.2
   due to
      conditions classified elsewhere R50.81
      heat T67.0
   enteric A01.00
   enteroviral exanthematous (Boston exanthem) A88.0
   ephemeral (of unknown origin) R50.9
   epidemic hemorrhagic A98.5
   erysipelatous — see Erysipelas
   estivo-autumnal (malarial) B50.9
   famine A75.0
   five day A79.0
   following delivery O86.4
   Fort Bragg A27.89
   gastroenteric A01.00
   gastromalarial — see Malaria
   Gibraltar — see Brucellosis
   glandular — see Mononucleosis, infectious
   Guama (viral) A92.8
   Haverhill A25.1
   hay (allergic) J30.1
      with asthma (bronchial) J45.909
         with
            exacerbation (acute) J45.901
            status asthmaticus J45.902
         due to
            allergen other than pollen J30.89
            pollen, any plant or tree J30.1
   heat (effects) T67.0
   hematuric, bilious B50.8
   hemoglobinuric (malarial) (bilious) B50.8
   hemorrhagic (arthropod-borne) NOS A94
      with renal syndrome A98.5
      arenaviral A96.9
         specified NEC A96.8
      Argentinian A96.0
      Bangkok A91
      Bolivian A96.1
      Central Asian A98.0
      Chikungunya A92.0
      Crimean-Congo A98.0
      dengue (virus) A91
      epidemic A98.5
      Junin (virus) A96.0
      Korean A98.5
      Kyasanur forest A98.2
      Machupo (viral) A96.1
      mite-borne A93.8
      mosquito-borne A92.8
      Omsk A98.1
      Philippine A91
      Russian A98.5
      Singapore A91
      Southeast Asia A91
      Thailand A91
      tick-borne NEC A93.8
      viral A99
         specified NEC A98.8
   hepatic — see Cholecystitis
   herpetic — see Herpes
   icterohemorrhagic A27.0
   Indiana A93.8
   infective B99.9
      specified NEC B99.8

Fever (inanition) (of unknown origin) (persistent) (with chills) (with rigor) R50.9 — continued
   intermittent (bilious) — see also Malaria of unknown origin R50.9
      pernicious B50.9
   iodide R50.2
   Japanese river A75.3
   jungle — see also Malaria
      yellow A95.0
   Junin (virus) hemorrhagic A96.0
   Katayama B65.2
   kedani A75.3
   Kenya (tick) A77.1
   Kew Garden A79.1
   Korean hemorrhagic A98.5
   Lassa A96.2
   Lone Star A77.0
   Machupo (virus) hemorrhagic A96.1
   malaria, malarial — see Malaria
   Malta A23.9
   Marseilles A77.1
   marsh — see Malaria
   Mayaro (viral) A92.8
   Mediterranean (see also Brucellosis) A23.9
      familial E85.0
      tick A77.1
   meningeal — see Meningitis
   Meuse A79.0
   Mexican A75.2
   mianeh A68.1
   miasmatic — see Malaria
   mosquito-borne (viral) A92.9
      hemorrhagic A92.8
   mountain — see also Brucellosis
      meaning Rocky Mountain spotted fever A77.0
      tick (American) (Colorado) (viral) A93.2
   Mucambo (viral) A92.8
   mud A27.9
   Neapolitan — see Brucellosis
   neutropenic D70.9
   newborn P81.9
      environmental P81.0
   Nine-Mile A78
   non-exanthematous tick A93.2
   North Asian tick-borne A77.2
   O'nyong-nyong (viral) A92.1
   Omsk hemorrhagic A98.1
   Oropouche (viral) A93.0
   Oroya A44.0
   paludal — see Malaria
   Panama (malarial) B50.9
   Pappataci A93.1
   paratyphoid A01.4
      A A01.1
      B A01.2
      C A01.3
   parrot A70
   periodic (Mediterranean) E85.0
   persistent (of unknown origin) R50.9
   petechial A39.0
   pharyngoconjunctival B30.2
   Philippine hemorrhagic A91
   phlebotomus A93.1
   Piry (virus) A93.8
   Pixuna (viral) A92.8
   Plasmodium ovale B53.0
   polioviral (nonparalytic) A80.4
   Pontiac A48.2
   postimmunization R50.83
   postoperative R50.82
      due to infection T81.4
   posttransfusion R50.84
   postvaccination R50.83
   presenting with conditions classified elsewhere R50.81
   pretibial A27.89
   puerperal O86.4
   Q A78
   quadrilateral A78
   quartan (malaria) B52.9
   Queensland (coastal) (tick) A77.3
   quintan A79.0
   rabbit — see Tularemia
   rat-bite A25.9
      due to
         Spirillum A25.0
         Streptobacillus moniliformis A25.1
   recurrent — see Fever, relapsing
   relapsing (Borrelia) A68.9
      Carter's (Asiatic) A68.1
      Dutton's (West African) A68.1
      Koch's A68.9
      louse-borne A68.0
      Novy's
         louse-borne A68.0
         tick-borne A68.1
      Obermeyer's (European) A68.0
      tick-borne A68.1

DISEASE INDEX

Fever (inanition) (of unknown origin) (persistent) (with chills) (with rigor) R50.9 — *continued*
  remittent (bilious) (congestive) (gastric) — *see* Malaria
  rheumatic (active) (acute) (chronic) (subacute) I00
    with central nervous system involvement I02.9
    active with heart involvement — *see* category I01
    inactive or quiescent with
      cardiac hypertrophy I09.89
      carditis I09.9
      endocarditis I09.1
        aortic (valve) I06.9
          with mitral (valve) disease I08.0
        mitral (valve) I05.9
          with aortic (valve) disease I08.0
        pulmonary (valve) I09.89
        tricuspid (valve) I07.8
      heart disease NEC I09.89
      heart failure (congestive) (conditions in I50.9) I09.81
      left ventricular failure (conditions in I50.1) I09.81
      myocarditis, myocardial degeneration (conditions in I51.4) I09.0
      pancarditis I09.9
      pericarditis I09.2
  Rift Valley (viral) A92.4
  Rocky Mountain spotted A77.0
  rose J30.1
  Ross River B33.1
  Russian hemorrhagic A98.5
  San Joaquin (Valley) B38.0
  sandfly A93.1
  Sao Paulo A77.0
  scarlet A38.9
  seven day (leptospirosis) (autumnal) (Japanese) A27.89
  dengue A90
  shin-bone A79.0
  Singapore hemorrhagic A91
  solar A90
  Songo A98.5
  sore B00.1
  South African tick-bite A68.1
  Southeast Asia hemorrhagic A91
  spinal — *see* Meningitis
  spirillary A25.0
  splenic — *see* Anthrax
  spotted A77.9
    American A77.0
    Brazilian A77.0
    cerebrospinal meningitis A39.0
    Colombian A77.0
    due to Rickettsia
      australis A77.3
      conorii A77.1
      rickettsii A77.0
      sibirica A77.2
      specified type NEC A77.8
    Ehrlichiosis A77.40
      due to
        E. chafeensis A77.41
        specified organism NEC A77.49
    Rocky Mountain A77.0
  steroid R50.2
  streptobacillary A25.1
  subtertian B50.9
  Sumatran mite A75.3
  sun A90
  swamp A27.9
  swine A02.8
  sylvatic, yellow A95.0
  Tahyna B33.8
  tertian — *see* Malaria, tertian
  Thailand hemorrhagic A91
  thermic T67.0
  three-day A93.1
  tick
    American mountain A93.2
    Colorado A93.2
    Kemerovo A93.8
    Mediterranean A77.1
    mountain A93.2
    nonexanthematous A93.2
    Quaranfil A93.8
  tick-bite NEC A93.8
  tick-borne (hemorrhagic) NEC A93.8
  trench A79.0
  tsutsugamushi A75.3
  typhogastric A01.00

Fever (inanition) (of unknown origin) (persistent) (with chills) (with rigor) R50.9 — *continued*
  typhoid (abortive) (hemorrhagic) (intermittent) (malignant) A01.00
    complicated by
      arthritis A01.04
      heart involvement A01.02
      meningitis A01.01
      osteomyelitis A01.05
      pneumonia A01.03
      specified NEC A01.09
  typhomalarial — *see* Malaria
  typhus — *see* Typhus (fever)
  undulant — *see* Brucellosis
  unknown origin R50.9
  uveoparotid D86.89
  valley B38.0
  Venezuelan equine A92.2
  vesicular stomatitis A93.8
  viral hemorrhagic — *see* Fever, hemorrhagic, by type of virus
  Volhynian A79.0
  Wesselsbron (viral) A92.8
  West
    African B50.8
    Nile (viral) A92.30
      with
        complications NEC A92.39
        cranial nerve disorders A92.32
        encephalitis A92.31
        encephalomyelitis A92.31
        neurologic manifestation NEC A92.32
        optic neuritis A92.32
        polyradiculitis A92.32
  Whitmore's — *see* Melioidosis
  Wolhynian A79.0
  worm B83.9
  yellow A95.9
    jungle A95.0
    sylvatic A95.0
    urban A95.1
  Zika (viral) A92.8
Fibrillation
  atrial or auricular (established) I48.91
    chronic I48.2
    paroxysmal I48.0
    permanent I48.2
    persistent I48.1
  cardiac I49.8
  heart I49.8
  muscular M62.89
  ventricular I49.01
Fibrin
  ball or bodies, pleural (sac) J94.1
  chamber, anterior (eye) (gelatinous exudate) — *see* Iridocyclitis, acute
Fibrinogenolysis — *see* Fibrinolysis
Fibrinogenopenia D68.8
  acquired D65
  congenital D68.2
Fibrinolysis (hemorrhagic) (acquired) D65
  antepartum hemorrhage — *see* Hemorrhage, antepartum, with coagulation defect
  following
    abortion — *see* Abortion by type complicated by hemorrhage
    ectopic or molar pregnancy O08.1
  intrapartum O67.0
  newborn, transient P60
  postpartum O72.3
Fibrinopenia (hereditary) D68.2
  acquired D68.4
Fibrinopurulent — *see* condition
Fibrinous — *see* condition
Fibroadenoma
  cellular intracanalicular D24-
  giant D24-
  intracanalicular
    cellular D24-
    giant D24-
    specified site — *see* Neoplasm, benign, by site
    unspecified site D24-
  juvenile D24-
  pericanalicular
    specified site — *see* Neoplasm, benign, by site
    unspecified site D24-
  phyllodes D24-
  prostate D29.1
  specified site NEC — *see* Neoplasm, benign, by site
  unspecified site D24-
Fibroadenosis, breast (chronic) (cystic) (diffuse) (periodic) (segmental) N60.2-

Fibroangioma — *see also* Neoplasm, benign, by site
  juvenile
    specified site — *see* Neoplasm, benign, by site
    unspecified site D10.6
Fibrochondrosarcoma — *see* Neoplasm, cartilage, malignant
Fibrocystic
  disease — *see also* Fibrosis, cystic
    breast — *see* Mastopathy, cystic
    jaw M27.49
    kidney (congenital) Q61.8
    liver Q44.6
    pancreas E84.9
  kidney (congenital) Q61.8
Fibrodysplasia ossificans progressiva — *see* Myositis, ossificans, progressiva
Fibroelastosis (cordis) (endocardial) (endomyocardial) I42.4
Fibroid (tumor) — *see also* Neoplasm, connective tissue, benign
  disease, lung (chronic) — *see* Fibrosis, lung
  heart (disease) — *see* Myocarditis
  in pregnancy or childbirth O34.1-
    causing obstructed labor O65.5
  induration, lung (chronic) — *see* Fibrosis, lung
  lung — *see* Fibrosis, lung
  pneumonia (chronic) — *see* Fibrosis, lung
  uterus D25.9
Fibrolipoma — *see* Lipoma
Fibroliposarcoma — *see* Neoplasm, connective tissue, malignant
Fibroma — *see also* Neoplasm, connective tissue, benign
  ameloblastic — *see* Cyst, calcifying odontogenic
  bone (nonossifying) — *see* Disorder, bone, specified type NEC
    ossifying — *see* Neoplasm, bone, benign
  cementifying — *see* Neoplasm, bone, benign
  chondromyxoid — *see* Neoplasm, bone, benign
  desmoplastic — *see* Neoplasm, connective tissue, uncertain behavior
  durum — *see* Neoplasm, connective tissue, benign
  fascial — *see* Neoplasm, connective tissue, benign
  invasive — *see* Neoplasm, connective tissue, uncertain behavior
  molle — *see* Lipoma
  myxoid — *see* Neoplasm, connective tissue, benign
  nasopharynx, nasopharyngeal (juvenile) D10.6
  nonosteogenic (nonossifying) — *see* Dysplasia, fibrous
  odontogenic (central) — *see* Cyst, calcifying odontogenic
  ossifying — *see* Neoplasm, bone, benign
  periosteal — *see* Neoplasm, bone, benign
  soft — *see* Lipoma
Fibromatosis M72.9
  abdominal — *see* Neoplasm, connective tissue, uncertain behavior
  aggressive — *see* Neoplasm, connective tissue, uncertain behavior
  congenital generalized — *see* Neoplasm, connective tissue, uncertain behavior
  Dupuytren's M72.0
  gingival K06.1
  palmar (fascial) M72.0
  plantar (fascial) M72.2
  pseudosarcomatous (proliferative) (Myositis) (subcutaneous) M72.4
  retroperitoneal D48.3
  specified NEC M72.8
Fibromyalgia M79.7
Fibromyoma — *see also* Neoplasm, connective tissue, benign
  uterus (corpus) — *see also* Leiomyoma, uterus
    in pregnancy or childbirth — *see* Fibroid, in pregnancy or childbirth causing obstructed labor O65.5
Fibromyositis M79.7
Fibromyxolipoma D17.9
Fibromyxoma — *see* Neoplasm, connective tissue, benign
Fibromyxosarcoma — *see* Neoplasm, connective tissue, malignant
Fibro-odontoma, ameloblastic — *see* Cyst, calcifying odontogenic

Fibro-osteoma — *see* Neoplasm, bone, benign
Fibroplasia, retrolental H35.17-
Fibropurulent — *see* condition
Fibrosarcoma — *see also* Neoplasm, connective tissue, malignant
  ameloblastic C41.1
    upper jaw (bone) C41.0
  congenital — *see* Neoplasm, connective tissue, malignant
  fascial — *see* Neoplasm, connective tissue, malignant
  infantile — *see* Neoplasm, connective tissue, malignant
  odontogenic C41.1
    upper jaw (bone) C41.0
  periosteal — *see* Neoplasm, bone, malignant
Fibrosclerosis
  breast N60.3-
  multifocal M35.5
  penis (corpora cavernosa) N48.6
Fibrosis, fibrotic
  adrenal (gland) E27.8
  amnion O41.8x-
  anal papillae K62.89
  arteriocapillary — *see* Arteriosclerosis
  bladder N32.89
    interstitial — *see* Cystitis, chronic, interstitial
    localized submucosal — *see* Cystitis, chronic, interstitial
    panmural — *see* Cystitis, chronic, interstitial
  breast — *see* Fibrosclerosis, breast
  capillary (*see also* Arteriosclerosis) I70.90
    lung (chronic) — *see* Fibrosis, lung
  cardiac — *see* Myocarditis
  cervix N88.8
  chorion O41.8x-
  corpus cavernosum (sclerosing) N48.6
  cystic (of pancreas) E84.9
    with
      distal intestinal obstruction syndrome E84.19
      fecal impaction E84.19
      intestinal manifestations NEC E84.19
      pulmonary manifestations E84.0
      specified manifestations NEC E84.8
    due to device, implant or graft (*see also* Complications, by site and type, specified NEC) T85.82
      arterial graft NEC T82.828
      breast (implant) T85.82
      catheter NEC T85.82
        dialysis (renal) T82.828
          intraperitoneal T85.82
        infusion NEC T82.828
          spinal (epidural) (subdural) T85.82
        urinary (indwelling) T83.82
      electronic (electrode) (pulse generator) (stimulator)
        bone T84.82
        cardiac T82.827
        nervous system (brain) (peripheral nerve) (spinal) T85.82
        urinary T83.82
      fixation, internal (orthopedic) NEC T84.82
      gastrointestinal (bile duct) (esophagus) T85.82
      genital NEC T83.82
      heart NEC T82.827
      joint prosthesis T84.82
      ocular (corneal graft) (orbital implant) NEC T85.82
      orthopedic NEC T84.82
      specified NEC T85.82
      urinary NEC T83.82
      vascular NEC T82.828
      ventricular intracranial shunt T85.82
  ejaculatory duct N50.8
  endocardium — *see* Endocarditis
  endomyocardial (tropical) I42.3
  epididymis N50.8
  eye muscle — *see* Strabismus, mechanical
  heart — *see* Myocarditis
  hepatic — *see* Fibrosis, liver
  hepatolienal (portal hypertension) K76.6
  hepatosplenic (portal hypertension) K76.6
  infrapatellar fat pad M79.4
  intrascrotal N50.8
  kidney N26.9
  liver K74.0
    with sclerosis K74.2
    alcoholic K70.2

Fistula (cutaneous) L98.8 — *continued*
breast N61
  puerperal, postpartum or gestational, due
    to mastitis (purulent) — *see*
      Mastitis, obstetric, purulent
bronchial J86.0
bronchocutaneous, bronchomediastinal,
  bronchopleural,
  bronchopleuromediastinal (infective)
  J86.0
  tuberculous NEC A15.5
bronchoesophageal J86.0
  congenital Q39.2
    with atresia of esophagus Q39.1
bronchovisceral J86.0
buccal cavity (infective) K12.2
cecosigmoidal K63.2
cecum K63.2
cerebrospinal (fluid) G96.0
cervical, lateral Q18.1
cervicoaural Q18.1
cervicosigmoidal N82.4
cervicovesical N82.1
cervix N82.8
chest (wall) J86.0
cholecystenteric — *see* Fistula, gallbladder
cholecystocolic — *see* Fistula, gallbladder
cholecystocolonic — *see* Fistula,
  gallbladder
cholecystoduodenal — *see* Fistula,
  gallbladder
cholecystogastric — *see* Fistula,
  gallbladder
cholecystointestinal — *see* Fistula,
  gallbladder
choledochoduodenal — *see* Fistula, bile
  duct
cholocolic K82.3
coccyx — *see* Sinus, pilonidal
colon K63.2
colostomy K94.09
common duct — *see* Fistula, bile duct
congenital, site not listed — *see* Anomaly,
  by site
coronary, arteriovenous I25.41
  congenital Q24.5
costal region J86.0
cul-de-sac, Douglas' N82.8
cystic duct — *see also* Fistula, gallbladder
  congenital Q44.5
dental K04.6
diaphragm J86.0
duodenum K31.6
ear (external) (canal) — *see* Disorder, ear,
  external, specified type NEC
enterocolic K63.2
enterocutaneous K63.2
enterouterine N82.4
  congenital Q51.7
enterovaginal N82.4
  congenital Q52.2
  large intestine N82.3
  small intestine N82.2
enterovesical N32.1
epididymis N50.8
  tuberculous A18.15
esophagobronchial J86.0
  congenital Q39.2
    with atresia of esophagus Q39.1
esophagocutaneous K22.8
esophagopleural-cutaneous J86.0
esophagotracheal J86.0
  congenital Q39.2
    with atresia of esophagus Q39.1
esophagus K22.8
  congenital Q39.2
    with atresia of esophagus Q39.1
ethmoid — *see* Sinusitis, ethmoidal
eyeball (cornea) (sclera) — *see* Disorder,
  globe, hypotony
eyelid H01.8
fallopian tube, external N82.5
fecal K63.2
  congenital Q43.6
from periapical abscess K04.6
frontal sinus — *see* Sinusitis, frontal
gallbladder K82.3
  with calculus, cholelithiasis, stones —
    see Calculus, gallbladder
gastric K31.6
gastrocolic K31.6
  congenital Q40.2
  tuberculous A18.32
gastroenterocolic K31.6
gastroesophageal K31.6
gastrojejunal K31.6
gastrojejunocolic K31.6

Fistula (cutaneous) L98.8 — *continued*
genital tract (female) N82.9
  specified NEC N82.8
  to intestine NEC N82.4
  to skin N82.5
hepatic artery-portal vein, congenital Q26.6
hepatopleural J86.0
hepatopulmonary J86.0
ileorectal or ileosigmoidal K63.2
ileovaginal N82.2
ileovesical N32.1
ileum K63.2
in ano K60.3
  tuberculous A18.32
inner ear (labyrinth) — *see* subcategory
  H83.1
intestine NEC K63.2
intestinocolonic (abdominal) K63.2
intestinoureteral N28.89
intestinouterine N82.4
intestinovaginal N82.4
large intestine N82.3
  small intestine N82.2
intestinovesical N32.1
ischiorectal (fossa) K61.3
jejunum K63.2
joint M25.10
  ankle M25.17-
  elbow M25.12-
  foot joint M25.17-
  hand joint M25.14-
  hip M25.15-
  knee M25.16-
  shoulder M25.11-
  specified joint NEC M25.18
  tuberculous — *see* Tuberculosis, joint
  vertebrae M25.18
  wrist M25.13-
kidney N28.89
labium (majus) (minus) N82.8
labyrinth — *see* subcategory H83.1
lacrimal (gland) (sac) H04.61-
lacrimonasal duct — *see* Fistula, lacrimal
laryngotracheal, congenital Q34.8
larynx J38.7
lip K13.0
  congenital Q38.0
lumbar, tuberculous A18.01
lung J86.0
lymphatic I89.8
mammary (gland) N61
mastoid (process) (region) — *see*
  Mastoiditis, chronic
maxillary J32.0
medial, face and neck Q18.8
mediastinal J86.0
mediastinobronchial J86.0
mediastinocutaneous J86.0
middle ear — *see* subcategory H74.8
mouth K12.2
nasal J34.89
  sinus — *see* Sinusitis
nasopharynx J39.2
nipple N64.0
nose J34.89
oral (cutaneous) K12.2
  maxillary J32.0
  nasal (with cleft palate) — *see* Cleft,
    palate
orbit, orbital — *see* Disorder, orbit,
  specified type NEC
oroantral J32.0
oviduct, external N82.5
palate (hard) M27.8
pancreatic K86.8
pancreaticoduodenal K86.8
parotid (gland) K11.4
  region K12.2
penis N48.89
perianal K60.3
pericardium (pleura) (sac) — *see*
  Pericarditis
pericecal K63.2
perineorectal K60.4
perineosigmoidal K63.2
perineum, perineal (with urethral
  involvement) NEC N36.0
  tuberculous A18.13
  ureter N28.89
perirectal K60.4
  tuberculous A18.32
peritoneum K65.9
pharyngoesophageal J39.2
pharynx J39.2
  branchial cleft (congenital) Q18.0
pilonidal (infected) (rectum) — *see* Sinus,
  pilonidal
pleura, pleural, pleurocutaneous,
  pleuroperitoneal J86.0
  tuberculous NEC A15.6

Fistula (cutaneous) L98.8 — *continued*
pleuropericardial I31.8
portal vein-hepatic artery, congenital Q26.6
postauricular H70.81-
postoperative, persistent T81.83
  specified site — *see* Fistula, by site
preauricular (congenital) Q18.1
prostate N42.89
pulmonary J86.0
  arteriovenous I28.0
    congenital Q25.72
  tuberculous — *see* Tuberculosis,
    pulmonary
pulmonoperitoneal J86.0
rectolabial N82.4
rectosigmoid (intercommunicating) K63.2
rectoureteral N28.89
rectourethral N36.0
  congenital Q64.73
rectouterine N82.4
  congenital Q51.7
rectovaginal N82.3
  congenital Q52.2
  tuberculous A18.18
rectovesical N32.1
  congenital Q64.79
rectovesicovaginal N82.3
rectovulval N82.4
  congenital Q52.79
rectum (to skin) K60.4
  congenital Q43.6
    with absence, atresia and stenosis
      Q42.0
  tuberculous A18.32
renal N28.89
retroauricular — *see* Fistula, postauricular
salivary duct or gland (any) K11.4
  congenital Q38.4
scrotum (urinary) N50.8
  tuberculous A18.15
semicircular canals — *see* subcategory
  H83.1
sigmoid K63.2
  to bladder N32.1
sinus — *see* Sinusitis
skin L98.8
  to genital tract (female) N82.5
splenocolic D73.89
stercoral K63.2
stomach K31.6
sublingual gland K11.4
submandibular gland K11.4
submaxillary (gland) K11.4
  region K12.2
thoracic J86.0
  duct I89.8
thoracoabdominal J86.0
thoracogastric J86.0
thoracointestinal J86.0
thorax J86.0
thyroglossal duct Q89.2
thyroid E07.89
trachea, congenital (external) (internal)
  Q32.1
tracheoesophageal J86.0
  congenital Q39.2
    with atresia of esophagus Q39.1
  following tracheostomy J95.04
traumatic arteriovenous — *see* Injury,
  blood vessel, by site
tuberculous — *code by* site under
  Tuberculosis
typhoid A01.09
umbilicourinary Q64.8
urachus, congenital Q64.4
ureter (persistent) N28.89
ureteroabdominal N28.89
ureterorectal N28.89
ureterosigmoido-abdominal N28.89
ureterovaginal N82.1
ureterovesical N32.2
urethra N36.0
  congenital Q64.79
  tuberculous A18.13
urethroperineal N36.0
urethroperineovesical N32.2
urethrorectal N36.0
  congenital Q64.73
urethroscrotal N50.8
urethrovaginal N82.1
urethrovesical N32.2
urinary (tract) (persistent) (recurrent)
  N36.0
uteroabdominal N82.5
  congenital Q51.7
uteroenteric, uterointestinal N82.4
  congenital Q51.7

Fistula (cutaneous) L98.8 — *continued*
uterorectal N82.4
  congenital Q51.7
uteroureteric N82.1
uterourethral Q51.7
uterovaginal N82.8
uterovesical N82.1
  congenital Q51.7
uterus N82.8
vagina (postpartal) (wall) N82.8
vaginocutaneous (postpartal) N82.5
vaginointestinal NEC N82.4
  large intestine N82.3
  small intestine N82.2
vaginoperineal N82.5
vasocutaneous, congenital Q55.7
vesical NEC N32.2
vesicoabdominal N32.2
vesicocervicovaginal N82.1
vesicocolic N32.1
vesicocutaneous N32.2
vesicoenteric N32.1
vesicointestinal N32.1
vesicometrorectal N82.4
vesicoperineal N32.2
vesicorectal N32.1
  congenital Q64.79
vesicosigmoidal N32.1
vesicosigmoidovaginal N82.3
vesicoureteral N32.2
vesicoureterovaginal N82.1
vesicourethral N32.2
vesicourethrorectal N32.1
vesicouterine N82.1
  congenital Q51.7
vesicovaginal N82.0
vulvorectal N82.4
  congenital Q52.79
Fit R56.9
epileptic — *see* Epilepsy
fainting R55
hysterical F44.5
newborn P90
Fitting (and adjustment) (of)
artificial
  arm — *see* Admission, adjustment,
    artificial, arm
  breast Z44.3
  eye Z44.2
  leg — *see* Admission, adjustment,
    artificial, leg
automatic implantable cardiac defibrillator
  (with synchronous cardiac
  pacemaker) Z45.02
brain neuropacemaker Z46.2
  implanted Z45.42
cardiac defibrillator — *see* Fitting (and
  adjustment) (of), automatic
  implantable cardiac defibrillator
catheter, non-vascular Z46.82
colostomy belt Z46.89
contact lenses Z46.0
cystostomy device Z46.6
defibrillator, cardiac — *see* Fitting (and
  adjustment) (of), automatic
  implantable cardiac defibrillator
dentures Z46.3
device NOS Z46.9
  abdominal Z46.89
  gastrointestinal NEC Z46.59
  implanted NEC Z45.89
  nervous system Z46.2
    implanted — *see* Admission,
      adjustment, device, implanted,
      nervous system
  orthodontic Z46.4
  orthoptic Z46.0
  orthotic Z46.89
  prosthetic (external) Z44.9
    breast Z44.3
    dental Z46.3
    eye Z44.2
    specified NEC Z44.8
  specified NEC Z46.89
substitution
  auditory Z46.2
    implanted — *see* Admission,
      adjustment, device, implanted,
      hearing device
  nervous system Z46.2
    implanted — *see* Admission,
      adjustment, device, implanted,
      nervous system
  visual Z46.2
    implanted Z45.31
urinary Z46.6

Fitting (and adjustment) (of) — *continued*
  gastric lap band Z46.51
  gastrointestinal appliance NEC Z46.59
  glasses (reading) Z46.0
  hearing aid Z46.1
  ileostomy device Z46.89
  insulin pump Z46.81
  intestinal appliance NEC Z46.89
  myringotomy device (stent) (tube) Z45.82
  neuropacemaker Z46.2
    implanted Z45.42
  non-vascular catheter Z46.82
  orthodontic device Z46.4
  orthopedic device (brace) (cast) (corset) (shoes) Z46.89
  pacemaker (cardiac) Z45.018
    nervous system (brain) (peripheral nerve) (spinal cord) Z46.2
      implanted Z45.42
    pulse generator Z45.010
  portacath (port-a-cath) Z45.2
  prosthesis (external) Z44.9
    arm — *see* Admission, adjustment, artificial, arm
    breast Z44.3
    dental Z46.3
    eye Z44.2
    leg — *see* Admission, adjustment, artificial, leg
    specified NEC Z44.8
  spectacles Z46.0
  wheelchair Z46.89
Fitz's syndrome (acute hemorrhagic pancreatitis) K85.8
Fitzhugh-Curtis syndrome
  due to
    Chlamydia trachomatis A74.81
    Neisseria gonorrhorea (gonococcal peritonitis) A54.85
Fixation
  joint — *see* Ankylosis
  larynx J38.7
  stapes — *see* Ankylosis, ear ossicles
    deafness — *see* Deafness, conductive
  uterus (acquired) — *see* Malposition, uterus
  vocal cord J38.3
Flabby ridge K06.8
Flaccid — *see also* condition
  palate, congenital Q38.5
Flail
  chest S22.5
    newborn (birth injury) P13.8
  joint (paralytic) M25.20
    ankle M25.27-
    elbow M25.22-
    foot joint M25.27-
    hand joint M25.24-
    hip M25.25-
    knee M25.26-
    shoulder M25.21-
    specified joint NEC M25.28
    wrist M25.23-
Flajani's disease — *see* Hyperthyroidism, with, goiter (diffuse)
Flap, liver K71.3
Flashbacks (residual to hallucinogen use) F16.283
Flat
  chamber (eye) — *see* Disorder, globe, hypotony, flat anterior chamber
  chest, congenital Q67.8
  foot (acquired) (fixed type) (painful) (postural) — *see also* Deformity, limb, flat foot
    congenital (rigid) (spastic) (everted)) Q66.5-
    rachitic sequelae (late effect) E64.3
  organ or site, congenital NEC — *see* Anomaly, by site
  pelvis M95.5
    with disproportion (fetopelvic) O33.0
      causing obstructed labor O65.0
    congenital Q74.2
Flatau-Schilder disease G37.0
Flatback syndrome M40.30
  lumbar region M40.36
  lumbosacral region M40.37
  thoracolumbar region M40.35
Flattening
  head, femur M89.8x5
  hip — *see* Coxa, plana
  lip (congenital) Q18.8
  nose (congenital) Q67.4
    acquired M95.0

Flatulence R14.3
  psychogenic F45.8
Flatus R14.3
  vaginalis N89.8
Flax-dresser's disease J66.1
Flea bite — *see* Injury, bite, by site, superficial, insect
Flecks, glaucomatous (subcapsular) — *see* Cataract, complicated
Fleischer(-Kayser) ring (cornea) H18.04-
Fleshy mole O02.0
Flexibilitas cerea — *see* Catalepsy
Flexion
  amputation stump (surgical) T87.89
  cervix — *see* Malposition, uterus
  contracture, joint — *see* Contraction, joint
  deformity, joint (*see also* Deformity, limb, flexion) M21.20
    hip, congenital Q65.89
  uterus — *see also* Malposition, uterus
    lateral — *see* Lateroversion, uterus
Flexner's dysentery A03.1
Flexner-Boyd dysentery A03.2
Flexure — *see* Flexion
Flint murmur (aortic insufficiency) I35.1
Floater, vitreous — *see* Opacity, vitreous
Floating
  cartilage (joint) — *see also* Loose, body, joint
    knee — *see* Derangement, knee, loose body
  gallbladder, congenital Q44.1
  kidney N28.89
    congenital Q63.8
  spleen D73.89
Flooding N92.0
Floor — *see* condition
Floppy
  baby syndrome (nonspecific) P94.2
  iris syndrome (intraoperative) (IFIS) H21.81
  nonrheumatic mitral valve syndrome I34.1
Flu — *see also* Influenza
  avian (*see also* Influenza, due to, identified novel influenza A virus) J09.X2
  bird (*see also* Influenza, due to, identified novel influenza A virus) J09.X2
  intestinal NEC A08.4
  swine (viruses that normally cause infections in pigs) (*see also* Influenza, due to, identified novel influenza A virus) J09.X2
Fluctuating blood pressure I99.8
Fluid
  abdomen R18.8
  chest J94.8
  heart — *see* Failure, heart, congestive
  joint — *see* Effusion, joint
  loss (acute) E86.9
    with
      hypernatremia E87.0
      hyponatremia E87.1
  lung — *see* Edema, lung
  overload E87.70
    specified NEC E87.79
  peritoneal cavity R18.8
  pleural cavity J94.8
  retention R60.9
Flukes NEC — *see also* Infestation, fluke
  blood NEC — *see* Schistosomiasis
  liver B66.3
Fluor (vaginalis) N89.8
  trichomonal or due to Trichomonas (vaginalis) A59.00
Fluorosis
  dental K00.3
  skeletal M85.10
    ankle M85.17-
    foot M85.17-
    forearm M85.13-
    hand M85.14-
    lower leg M85.16-
    multiple site M85.19
    neck M85.18
    rib M85.18
    shoulder M85.11-
    skull M85.18
    specified site NEC M85.18
    thigh M85.15-
    toe M85.17-
    upper arm M85.12-
    vertebra M85.18
Flush syndrome E34.0
Flushing R23.2
  menopausal N95.1

Flutter
  atrial or auricular I48.92
    atypical I48.4
    type I I48.3
    type II I48.4
    typical I48.3
  heart I49.8
    atrial or auricular I48.92
      atypical I48.4
      type I I48.3
      type II I48.4
      typical I48.3
    ventricular I49.02
  ventricular I49.02
FNHTR (febrile nonhemolytic transfusion reaction) R50.84
Fochier's abscess — *code by* site under Abscess
Focus, Assmann's — *see* Tuberculosis, pulmonary
Fogo selvagem L10.3
Foix-Alajouanine syndrome G95.19
Fold, folds (anomalous) — *see also* Anomaly, by site
  Descemet's membrane — *see* Change, corneal membrane, Descemet's, fold
  epicanthic Q10.3
  heart Q24.8
Folie à deux F24
Follicle
  cervix (nabothian) (ruptured) N88.8
  graafian, ruptured, with hemorrhage N83.0
  nabothian N88.8
Follicular — *see* condition
Folliculitis (superficial) L73.9
  abscedens et suffodiens L66.3
  cyst N83.0
  decalvans L66.2
  deep — *see* Furuncle, by site
  gonococcal (acute) (chronic) A54.01
  keloid, keloidalis L73.0
  pustular L01.02
  ulerythematosa reticulata L66.4
Folliculome lipidique
  specified site — *see* Neoplasm, benign, by site
  unspecified site
    female D27.9
    male D29.20
Følling's disease E70.0
Follow-up — *see* Examination, follow-up
Fong's syndrome (hereditary osteo-onychodysplasia) Q78.5
Food
  allergy L27.2
  asphyxia (from aspiration or inhalation) — *see* Foreign body, by site
  choked on — *see* Foreign body, by site
  deprivation T73.0
    specified kind of food NEC E63.8
  intoxication — *see* Poisoning, food
  lack of T73.0
  poisoning — *see* Poisoning, food
  rejection NEC — *see* Disorder, eating
  strangulation or suffocation — *see* Foreign body, by site
  toxemia — *see* Poisoning, food
Foot — *see* condition
Foramen ovale (nonclosure) (patent) (persistent) Q21.1
Forbes' glycogen storage disease E74.03
Fordyce's disease (mouth) Q38.6
Fordyce-Fox disease L75.2
Forearm — *see* condition
Foreign body
  with
    laceration — *see* Laceration, by site, with foreign body
    puncture wound — *see* Puncture, by site, with foreign body
  accidentally left following a procedure T81.509
  aspiration T81.506
    resulting in
      adhesions T81.516
      obstruction T81.526
      perforation T81.536
      specified complication NEC T81.596
  cardiac catheterization T81.505
    resulting in
      acute reaction T81.60
        aseptic peritonitis T81.61
        specified NEC T81.69
      adhesions T81.515
      obstruction T81.525
      perforation T81.535
      specified complication NEC T81.595

Foreign body — *continued*
  accidentally left following a procedure T81.509 — *continued*
    causing
      acute reaction T81.60
        aseptic peritonitis T81.61
        specified complication NEC T81.69
      adhesions T81.519
      aseptic peritonitis T81.61
      obstruction T81.529
      perforation T81.539
      specified complication NEC T81.599
    endoscopy T81.504
      resulting in
        adhesions T81.514
        obstruction T81.524
        perforation T81.534
        specified complication NEC T81.594
    immunization T81.503
      resulting in
        adhesions T81.513
        obstruction T81.523
        perforation T81.533
        specified complication NEC T81.593
    infusion T81.501
      resulting in
        adhesions T81.511
        obstruction T81.521
        perforation T81.531
        specified complication NEC T81.591
    injection T81.503
      resulting in
        adhesions T81.513
        obstruction T81.523
        perforation T81.533
        specified complication NEC T81.593
    kidney dialysis T81.502
      resulting in
        adhesions T81.512
        obstruction T81.522
        perforation T81.532
        specified complication NEC T81.592
    packing removal T81.507
      resulting in
        acute reaction T81.60
          aseptic peritonitis T81.61
          specified NEC T81.69
        adhesions T81.517
        obstruction T81.527
        perforation T81.537
        specified complication NEC T81.597
    puncture T81.506
      resulting in
        adhesions T81.516
        obstruction T81.526
        perforation T81.536
        specified complication NEC T81.596
    specified procedure NEC T81.508
      resulting in
        acute reaction T81.60
          aseptic peritonitis T81.61
          specified NEC T81.69
        adhesions T81.518
        obstruction T81.528
        perforation T81.538
        specified complication NEC T81.598
    surgical operation T81.500
      resulting in
        acute reaction T81.60
          aseptic peritonitis T81.61
          specified NEC T81.69
        adhesions T81.510
        obstruction T81.520
        perforation T81.530
        specified complication NEC T81.590
    transfusion T81.501
      resulting in
        adhesions T81.511
        obstruction T81.521
        perforation T81.531
        specified complication NEC T81.591
  alimentary tract T18.9
  anus T18.5
  colon T18.4
  esophagus — *see* Foreign body, esophagus
  mouth T18.0
  multiple sites T18.8
  rectosigmoid (junction) T18.5

Foreign body — *continued*
  alimentary tract T18.9 — *continued*
    rectum T18.5
    small intestine T18.3
    specified site NEC T18.8
    stomach T18.2
  anterior chamber (eye) S05.5-
  auditory canal — *see* Foreign body,
    entering through orifice, ear
  bronchus T17.508
    causing
      asphyxiation T17.500
        food (bone) (seed) T17.520
        gastric contents (vomitus) T17.510
        specified type NEC T17.590
      injury NEC T17.508
        food (bone) (seed) T17.528
        gastric contents (vomitus) T17.518
        specified type NEC T17.598
  canthus — *see* Foreign body, conjunctival
    sac
  ciliary body (eye) S05.5-
  conjunctival sac T15.1-
  cornea T15.0-
  entering through orifice
    accessory sinus T17.0
    alimentary canal T18.9
      multiple parts T18.8
      specified part NEC T18.8
    alveolar process T18.0
    antrum (Highmore's) T17.0
    anus T18.5
    appendix T18.4
    auditory canal — *see* Foreign body,
      entering through orifice, ear
    auricle — *see* Foreign body, entering
      through orifice, ear
    bladder T19.1
    bronchioles — *see* Foreign body,
      respiratory tract, specified site NEC
    bronchus (main) — *see* Foreign body,
      bronchus
    buccal cavity T18.0
    canthus (inner) — *see* Foreign body,
      conjunctival sac
    cecum T18.4
    cervix (canal) (uteri) T19.3
    colon T18.4
    conjunctival sac — *see* Foreign body,
      conjunctival sac
    cornea — *see* Foreign body, cornea
    digestive organ or tract NOS T18.9
      multiple parts T18.8
      specified part NEC T18.8
    duodenum T18.3
    ear (external) T16-
    esophagus — *see* Foreign body,
      esophagus
    eye (external) NOS T15.9-
      conjunctival sac — *see* Foreign body,
        conjunctival sac
      cornea — *see* Foreign body, cornea
      specified part NEC T15.8-
    eyeball — *see also* Foreign body,
      entering through orifice, eye,
      specified part NEC
      with penetrating wound — *see*
        Puncture, eyeball
    eyelid — *see also* Foreign body,
      conjunctival sac
      with
        laceration — *see* Laceration, eyelid,
          with foreign body
        puncture — *see* Puncture, eyelid,
          with foreign body
        superficial injury — *see* Foreign
          body, superficial, eyelid
    gastrointestinal tract T18.9
      multiple parts T18.8
      specified part NEC T18.8
    genitourinary tract T19.9
      multiple parts T19.8
      specified part NEC T19.8
    globe — *see* Foreign body, entering
      through orifice, eyeball
    gum T18.0
    Highmore's antrum T17.0
    hypopharynx — *see* Foreign body,
      pharynx
    ileum T18.3
    intestine (small) T18.3
      large T18.4
    lacrimal apparatus (punctum) — *see*
      Foreign body, entering through
      orifice, eye, specified part NEC
    large intestine T18.4
    larynx — *see* Foreign body, larynx
    lung — *see* Foreign body, respiratory
      tract, specified site NEC
    maxillary sinus T17.0

Foreign body — *continued*
  entering through orifice — *continued*
    mouth T18.0
    nasal sinus T17.0
    nasopharynx — *see* Foreign body,
      pharynx
    nose (passage) T17.1
    nostril T17.1
    oral cavity T18.0
    palate T18.0
    penis T19.4
    pharynx — *see* Foreign body, pharynx
    piriform sinus — *see* Foreign body,
      pharynx
    rectosigmoid (junction) T18.5
    rectum T18.5
    respiratory tract — *see* Foreign body,
      respiratory tract
    sinus (accessory) (frontal) (maxillary)
      (nasal) T17.0
      piriform — *see* Foreign body, pharynx
    small intestine T18.3
    stomach T18.2
    suffocation by — *see* Foreign body, by
      site
    tear ducts or glands — *see* Foreign body,
      entering through orifice, eye,
      specified part NEC
    throat — *see* Foreign body, pharynx
    tongue T18.0
    tonsil, tonsillar (fossa) — *see* Foreign
      body, pharynx
    trachea — *see* Foreign body, trachea
    ureter T19.8
    urethra T19.0
    uterus (any part) T19.3
    vagina T19.2
    vulva T19.2
  esophagus T18.108
    causing
      injury NEC T18.108
        food (bone) (seed) T18.128
        gastric contents (vomitus) T18.118
        specified type NEC T18.198
      tracheal compression T18.100
        food (bone) (seed) T18.120
        gastric contents (vomitus) T18.110
        specified type NEC T18.190
  felling of, in throat R09.89
  fragment — *see* Retained, foreign body
    fragments (type of)
  genitourinary tract T19.9
    bladder T19.1
    multiple parts T19.8
    penis T19.4
    specified site NEC T19.8
    urethra T19.0
    uterus T19.3
      IUD Z97.5
    vagina T19.2
      contraceptive device Z97.5
    vulva T19.2
  granuloma (old) (soft tissue) — *see also*
    Granuloma, foreign body
    skin L92.3
  in
    laceration — *see* Laceration, by site,
      with foreign body
    puncture wound — *see* Puncture, by site,
      with foreign body
    soft tissue (residual) M79.5
  inadvertently left in operation wound —
    see Foreign body, accidentally left
    during a procedure
  ingestion, ingested NOS T18.9
  inhalation or inspiration — *see* Foreign
    body, by site
  internal organ, not entering through a
    natural orifice — *code as* specific
    injury with foreign body
  intraocular S05.5-
    old, retained (nonmagnetic) H44.70-
      anterior chamber H44.71-
      ciliary body H44.72-
      iris H44.72-
      lens H44.73-
      magnetic H44.60-
        anterior chamber H44.61-
        ciliary body H44.62-
        iris H44.62-
        lens H44.63-
        posterior wall H44.64-
        specified site NEC H44.69-
        vitreous body H44.65-
      posterior wall H44.74-
      specified site NEC H44.79-
      vitreous body H44.75-
    iris — *see* Foreign body, intraocular

Foreign body — *continued*
  lacrimal punctum — *see* Foreign body,
    entering through orifice, eye,
    specified part NEC
  larynx T17.308
    causing
      asphyxiation T17.300
        food (bone) (seed) T17.320
        gastric contents (vomitus) T17.310
        specified type NEC T17.390
      injury NEC T17.308
        food (bone) (seed) T17.328
        gastric contents (vomitus) T17.318
        specified type NEC T17.398
  lens — *see* Foreign body, intraocular
  ocular muscle S05.4-
    old, retained — *see* Foreign body, orbit,
      old
  old or residual
    soft tissue (residual) M79.5
  operation wound, left accidentally — *see*
    Foreign body, accidentally left during
    a procedure
  orbit S05.4-
    old, retained H05.5-
  pharynx T17.208
    causing
      asphyxiation T17.200
        food (bone) (seed) T17.220
        gastric contents (vomitus) T17.210
        specified type NEC T17.290
      injury NEC T17.208
        food (bone) (seed) T17.228
        gastric contents (vomitus) T17.218
        specified type NEC T17.298
  respiratory tract T17.908
    bronchioles — *see* Foreign body,
      respiratory tract, specified site NEC
    bronchus — *see* Foreign body, bronchus
    causing
      asphyxiation T17.900
        food (bone) (seed) T17.920
        gastric contents (vomitus) T17.910
        specified type NEC T17.990
      injury NEC T17.908
        food (bone) (seed) T17.928
        gastric contents (vomitus) T17.918
        specified type NEC T17.998
    larynx — *see* Foreign body, larynx
    lung — *see* Foreign body, respiratory
      tract, specified site NEC
    multiple parts — *see* Foreign body,
      respiratory tract, specified site NEC
    nasal sinus T17.0
    nasopharynx — *see* Foreign body,
      pharynx
    nose T17.1
    nostril T17.1
    pharynx — *see* Foreign body, pharynx
    specified site NEC T17.808
      causing
        asphyxiation T17.800
          food (bone) (seed) T17.820
          gastric contents (vomitus)
            T17.810
          specified type NEC T17.890
        injury NEC T17.808
          food (bone) (seed) T17.828
          gastric contents (vomitus)
            T17.818
          specified type NEC T17.898
    throat — *see* Foreign body, pharynx
    trachea — *see* Foreign body, trachea
  retained (old) (nonmagnetic) (in)
    anterior chamber (eye) — *see* Foreign
      body, intraocular, old, retained,
      anterior chamber
      magnetic — *see* Foreign body,
        intraocular, old, retained,
        magnetic, anterior chamber
    ciliary body — *see* Foreign body,
      intraocular, old, retained, ciliary
      body
      magnetic — *see* Foreign body,
        intraocular, old, retained,
        magnetic, ciliary body
    eyelid H02.819
      left H02.816
        lower H02.815
        upper H02.814
      right H02.813
        lower H02.812
        upper H02.811
    fragments — *see* Retained, foreign body
      fragments (type of)

Foreign body — *continued*
  retained (old) (nonmagnetic) (in) —
    continued
    globe — *see* Foreign body, intraocular,
      old, retained
      magnetic — *see* Foreign body,
        intraocular, old, retained,
        magnetic
    intraocular — *see* Foreign body,
      intraocular, old, retained
      magnetic — *see* Foreign body,
        intraocular, old, retained,
        magnetic
    iris — *see* Foreign body, intraocular, old,
      retained, iris
      magnetic — *see* Foreign body,
        intraocular, old, retained,
        magnetic, iris
    lens — *see* Foreign body, intraocular, old,
      retained, lens
      magnetic — *see* Foreign body,
        intraocular, old, retained,
        magnetic, lens
    muscle — *see* Foreign body, retained,
      soft tissue
    orbit — *see* Foreign body, orbit, old
    posterior wall of globe — *see* Foreign
      body, intraocular, old, retained,
      posterior wall
      magnetic — *see* Foreign body,
        intraocular, old, retained,
        magnetic, posterior wall
    retrobulbar — *see* Foreign body, orbit,
      old, retrobulbar
    soft tissue M79.5
    vitreous — *see* Foreign body,
      intraocular, old, retained, vitreous
      body
      magnetic — *see* Foreign body,
        intraocular, old, retained,
        magnetic, vitreous body
  retina S05.5-
  superficial, without open wound
    abdomen, abdominal (wall) S30.851
    alveolar process S00.552
    ankle S90.55-
    antecubital space — *see* Foreign body,
      superficial, forearm
    anus S30.857
    arm (upper) S40.85-
    auditory canal — *see* Foreign body,
      superficial, ear
    auricle — *see* Foreign body, superficial,
      ear
    axilla — *see* Foreign body, superficial,
      arm
    back, lower S30.850
    breast S20.15-
    brow S00.85
    buttock S30.850
    calf — *see* Foreign body, superficial, leg
    canthus — *see* Foreign body, superficial,
      eyelid
    cheek S00.85
      internal S00.552
    chest wall — *see* Foreign body,
      superficial, thorax
    chin S00.85
    clitoris S30.854
    costal region — *see* Foreign body,
      superficial, thorax
    digit(s)
      foot — *see* Foreign body, superficial,
        toe
      hand — *see* Foreign body, superficial,
        finger
    ear S00.45-
    elbow S50.35-
    epididymis S30.853
    epigastric region S30.851
    epiglottis S10.15
    esophagus, cervical S10.15
    eyebrow — *see* Foreign body,
      superficial, eyelid
    eyelid S00.25-
    face S00.85
    finger(s) S60.459
      index S60.45-
      little S60.45-
      middle S60.45-
      ring S60.45-
    flank S30.851
    foot (except toe(s) alone) S90.85-
      toe — *see* Foreign body, superficial,
        toe
    forearm S50.85-
      elbow only — *see* Foreign body,
        superficial, elbow

Foreign body — *continued*
  superficial, without open wound — *continued*
    forehead S00.85
    genital organs, external
      female S30.856
      male S30.855
    groin S30.851
    gum S00.552
    hand S60.55-
    head S00.95
      ear — *see* Foreign body, superficial, ear
      eyelid — *see* Foreign body, superficial, eyelid
      lip S00.551
      nose S00.35
      oral cavity S00.552
      scalp S00.05
      specified site NEC S00.85
    heel — *see* Foreign body, superficial, foot
    hip S70.25-
    inguinal region S30.851
    interscapular region S20.459
    jaw S00.85
    knee S80.25-
    labium (majus) (minus) S30.854
    larynx S10.15
    leg (lower) S80.85-
      knee — *see* Foreign body, superficial, knee
      upper — *see* Foreign body, superficial, thigh
    lip S00.551
    lower back S30.850
    lumbar region S30.850
    malar region S00.85
    mammary — *see* Foreign body, superficial, breast
    mastoid region S00.85
    mouth S00.552
    nail
      finger — *see* Foreign body, superficial, finger
      toe — *see* Foreign body, superficial, toe
    nape S10.85
    nasal S00.35
    neck S10.95
      specified site NEC S10.85
      throat S10.15
    nose S00.35
    occipital region S00.05
    oral cavity S00.552
    orbital region — *see* Foreign body, superficial, eyelid
    palate S00.552
    palm — *see* Foreign body, superficial, hand
    parietal region S00.05
    pelvis S30.850
    penis S30.852
    perineum
      female S30.854
      male S30.850
    periocular area — *see* Foreign body, superficial, eyelid
    phalanges
      finger — *see* Foreign body, superficial, finger
      toe — *see* Foreign body, superficial, toe
    pharynx S10.15
    pinna — *see* Foreign body, superficial, ear
    popliteal space — *see* Foreign body, superficial, knee
    prepuce S30.852
    pubic region S30.850
    pudendum
      female S30.856
      male S30.855
    sacral region S30.850
    scalp S00.05
    scapular region — *see* Foreign body, superficial, shoulder
    scrotum S30.853
    shin — *see* Foreign body, superficial, leg
    shoulder S40.25-
    sternal region S20.359
    submaxillary region S00.85
    submental region S00.85
    subungual
      finger(s) — *see* Foreign body, superficial, finger
      toe(s) — *see* Foreign body, superficial, toe

Foreign body — *continued*
  superficial, without open wound — *continued*
    supraclavicular fossa S10.85
    supraorbital S00.85
    temple S00.85
    temporal region S00.85
    testis S30.853
    thigh S70.35-
    thorax, thoracic (wall) S20.95
      back S20.45-
      front S20.35-
    throat S10.15
    thumb S60.35-
    toe(s) (lesser) S90.456
      great S90.45-
    tongue S00.552
    trachea S10.15
    tunica vaginalis S30.853
    tympanum, tympanic membrane — *see* Foreign body, superficial, ear
    uvula S00.552
    vagina S30.854
    vocal cords S10.15
    vulva S30.854
    wrist S60.85-
  swallowed T18.9
  trachea T17.408
    causing
      asphyxiation T17.400
        food (bone) (seed) T17.420
        gastric contents (vomitus) T17.410
        specified type NEC T17.490
      injury NEC T17.408
        food (bone) (seed) T17.428
        gastric contents (vomitus) T17.418
        specified type NEC T17.498
  type of fragment — *see* Retained, foreign body fragments (type of)
  vitreous (humor) S05.5-
Forestier's disease (rhizomelic pseudopolyarthritis) M35.3
  meaning ankylosing hyperostosis — *see* Hyperostosis, ankylosing
Formation
  hyalin in cornea — *see* Degeneration, cornea
  sequestrum in bone (due to infection) — *see* Osteomyelitis, chronic
  valve
    colon, congenital Q43.8
    ureter (congenital) Q62.39
Formication R20.2
Fort Bragg fever A27.89
Fossa — *see also* condition
  pyriform — *see* condition
Foster-Kennedy syndrome H47.14-
Fothergill's
  disease (trigeminal neuralgia) — *see also* Neuralgia, trigeminal
  scarlatina anginosa A38.9
Foul breath R19.6
Foundling Z76.1
Fournier disease or gangrene N49.3
  female N76.89
Fourth
  cranial nerve — *see* condition
  molar K00.1
Foville's (peduncular) disease or syndrome G46.3
Fox-(Fordyce) disease (apocrine miliaria) L75.2
Fracture, burst — *see* Fracture, traumatic, by site
Fracture, chronic — *see* Fracture, pathological
Fracture, insufficiency — *see* Fracture, pathologic, by site
Fracture, pathological (pathologic) — *see also* **Fracture, traumatic** M84.40
  ankle M84.47-
  carpus M84.44-
  clavicle M84.41-
  dental implant M27.63
  dental restorative material K08.539
    with loss of material K08.531
    without loss of material K08.530
  due to
    neoplastic disease NEC (*see also* Neoplasm) M84.50
      ankle M84.57-
      carpus M84.54-
      clavicle M84.51-
      femur M84.55-
      fibula M84.56-
      finger M84.54-

Fracture, pathological (pathologic) — *see also* **Fracture, traumatic** M84.40 — *continued*
  due to — *continued*
    neoplastic disease NEC (*see also* Neoplasm) M84.50 — *continued*
      hip M84.559
      humerus M84.52-
      ilium M84.550
      ischium M84.550
      metacarpus M84.54-
      metatarsus M84.57-
      neck M84.58
      pelvis M84.550
      radius M84.53-
      rib M84.58
      scapula M84.51-
      skull M84.58
      specified site NEC M84.58
      tarsus M84.57-
      tibia M84.56-
      toe M84.57-
      ulna M84.53-
      vertebra M84.58
    osteoporosis M80.80
      disuse — *see* Osteoporosis, specified type NEC, with pathological fracture
      drug-induced — *see* Osteoporosis, drug induced, with pathological fracture
      idiopathic — *see* Osteoporosis, specified type NEC, with pathological fracture
      postmenopausal — *see* Osteoporosis, postmenopausal, with pathological fracture
      postoophorectomy — *see* Osteoporosis, postoophorectomy, with pathological fracture
      postsurgical malabsorption — *see* Osteoporosis, specified type NEC, with pathological fracture
      specified cause NEC — *see* Osteoporosis, specified type NEC, with pathological fracture
    specified disease NEC M84.60
      ankle M84.67-
      carpus M84.64-
      clavicle M84.61-
      femur M84.65-
      fibula M84.66-
      finger M84.64-
      hip M84.65-
      humerus M84.62-
      ilium M84.650
      ischium M84.650
      metacarpus M84.64-
      metatarsus M84.67-
      neck M84.68
      radius M84.63-
      rib M84.68
      scapula M84.61-
      skull M84.68
      tarsus M84.67-
      tibia M84.66-
      toe M84.67-
      ulna M84.63-
      vertebra M84.68
  femur M84.45-
  fibula M84.46-
  finger M84.44-
  hip M84.459
  humerus M84.42-
  ilium M84.454
  ischium M84.454
  joint prosthesis — *see* Complications, joint prosthesis, mechanical, breakdown, by site
  periprosthetic — *see* Complications, joint prosthesis, mechanical, periprosthetic, fracture, by site
  metacarpus M84.44-
  metatarsus M84.47-
  neck M84.48
  pelvis M84.454
  radius M84.43-
  restorative material (dental) K08.539
    with loss of material K08.531
    without loss of material K08.530
  rib M84.48
  scapula M84.41-
  skull M84.48
  tarsus M84.47-
  tibia M84.46-
  toe M84.47-
  ulna M84.43-
  vertebra M84.48

Fracture, traumatic (abduction) (adduction) (separation) (*see also* **Fracture, pathological**) T14.8
  acetabulum S32.40-
    column
      anterior (displaced) (iliopubic) S32.43-
        nondisplaced S32.436
      posterior (displaced) (ilioischial) S32.443
        nondisplaced S32.44-
    dome (displaced) S32.48-
      nondisplaced S32.48
    specified NEC S32.49-
    transverse (displaced) S32.45-
      with associated posterior wall fracture (displaced) S32.46-
        nondisplaced S32.46-
      nondisplaced S32.45-
    wall
      anterior (displaced) S32.41-
        nondisplaced S32.41-
      medial (displaced) S32.47-
        nondisplaced S32.47-
      posterior (displaced) S32.42-
        with associated transverse fracture (displaced) S32.46-
          nondisplaced S32.46-
        nondisplaced S32.42-
  acromion — *see* Fracture, scapula, acromial process
  ankle S82.899
    bimalleolar (displaced) S82.84-
      nondisplaced S82.84-
    lateral malleolus only (displaced) S82.6-
      nondisplaced S82.6-
    medial malleolus (displaced) S82.5-
      associated with Maisonneuve's fracture — *see* Fracture, Maisonneuve's
      nondisplaced S82.5-
    talus — *see* Fracture, tarsal, talus
    trimalleolar (displaced) S82.85-
      nondisplaced S82.85-
  arm (upper) — *see also* Fracture, humerus, shaft
    humerus — *see* Fracture, humerus
    radius — *see* Fracture, radius
    ulna — *see* Fracture, ulna
  astragalus — *see* Fracture, tarsal, talus
  atlas — *see* Fracture, neck, cervical vertebra, first
  axis — *see* Fracture, neck, cervical vertebra, second
  back — *see* Fracture, vertebra
  Barton's — *see* Barton's fracture
  base of skull — *see* Fracture, skull, base
  basicervical (basal) (femoral) S72.0
  Bennett's — *see* Bennett's fracture
  bimalleolar — *see* Fracture, ankle, bimalleolar
  blow-out S02.3
  bone NEC T14.8
    birth injury P13.9
    following insertion of orthopedic implant, joint prosthesis or bone plate — *see* Fracture, following insertion of orthopedic implant, joint prosthesis or bone plate
    in (due to) neoplastic disease NEC — *see* Fracture, pathological, due to, neoplastic disease
    pathological (cause unknown) — *see* Fracture, pathological
  breast bone — *see* Fracture, sternum
  bucket handle (semilunar cartilage) — *see* Tear, meniscus
  burst — *see* Fracture, traumatic, by site
  calcaneus — *see* Fracture, tarsal, calcaneus
  carpal bone(s) S62.10-
    capitate (displaced) S62.13-
      nondisplaced S62.13-
    cuneiform — *see* Fracture, carpal bone, triquetrum
    hamate (body) (displaced) S62.143
      hook process (displaced) S62.15-
        nondisplaced S62.15-
      nondisplaced S62.14-
    larger multangular — *see* Fracture, carpal bones, trapezium
    lunate (displaced) S62.12-
      nondisplaced S62.12-
    navicular S62.00-
      distal pole (displaced) S62.01-
        nondisplaced S62.01-
      middle third (displaced) S62.02-
        nondisplaced S62.02-
      proximal third (displaced) S62.03-
        nondisplaced S62.03-

Fracture, traumatic (abduction) (adduction) (separation) (*see also* **Fracture, pathological**) T14.8 — *continued*
carpal bone(s) S62.10- — *continued*
  navicular S62.00- — *continued*
    volar tuberosity — *see* Fracture, carpal bones, navicular, distal pole
  os magnum — *see* Fracture, carpal bones, capitate
  pisiform (displaced) S62.16-
    nondisplaced S62.16-
  semilunar — *see* Fracture, carpal bones, lunate
  smaller multangular — *see* Fracture, carpal bones, trapezoid
  trapezium (displaced) S62.17-
    nondisplaced S62.17-
  trapezoid (displaced) S62.18-
    nondisplaced S62.18-
  triquetrum (displaced) S62.11-
    nondisplaced S62.11-
  unciform — *see* Fracture, carpal bones, hamate
cervical — *see* Fracture, vertebra, cervical
clavicle S42.00-
  acromial end (displaced) S42.03-
    nondisplaced S42.03-
  birth injury P13.4
  lateral end — *see* Fracture, clavicle, acromial end
  shaft (displaced) S42.02-
    nondisplaced S42.02-
  sternal end (anterior) (displaced) S42.01-
    nondisplaced S42.01-
    posterior S42.01-
coccyx S32.2
collapsed — *see* Collapse, vertebra
collar bone — *see* Fracture, clavicle
Colles' — *see* Colles' fracture
compression, not due to trauma — *see* Collapse, vertebra
coronoid process — *see* Fracture, ulna, upper end, coronoid process
corpus cavernosum penis S39.840
costochondral cartilage S23.41
costochondral, costosternal junction — *see* Fracture, rib
cranium — *see* Fracture, skull
cricoid cartilage S12.8
cuboid (ankle) — *see* Fracture, tarsal, cuboid
cuneiform
  foot — *see* Fracture, tarsal, cuneiform
  wrist — *see* Fracture, carpal, triquetrum
delayed union — *see* Delay, union, fracture
dental restorative material K08.539
  with loss of material K08.531
  without loss of material K08.530
due to
  birth injury — *see* Birth, injury, fracture
  osteoporosis — *see* Osteoporosis, with fracture
Dupuytren's — *see* Fracture, ankle, lateral malleolus
elbow S42.40-
ethmoid (bone) (sinus) — *see* Fracture, skull, base
face bone S02.92
fatigue — *see also* Fracture, stress
  vertebra M48.40
    cervical region M48.42
    cervicothoracic region M48.43
    lumbar region M48.46
    lumbosacral region M48.47
    occipito-atlanto-axial region M48.41
    sacrococcygeal region M48.48
    thoracic region M48.44
    thoracolumbar region M48.45
femur, femoral S72.9-
  basicervical (basal) S72.0
  birth injury P13.2
  capital epiphyseal S79.01-
  condyles, epicondyles — *see* Fracture, femur, lower end
  distal end — *see* Fracture, femur, lower end
  epiphysis
    head — *see* Fracture, femur, upper end, epiphysis
    lower — *see* Fracture, femur, lower end, epiphysis
    upper — *see* Fracture, femur, upper end, epiphysis
  following insertion of implant, prosthesis or plate M96.66-

Fracture, traumatic (abduction) (adduction) (separation) (*see also* **Fracture, pathological**) T14.8 — *continued*
femur, femoral S72.9- — *continued*
  head — *see* Fracture, femur, upper end, head
  intertrochanteric — *see* Fracture, femur, trochanteric
  intratrochanteric — *see* Fracture, femur, trochanteric
  lower end S72.40-
    condyle (displaced) S72.41-
      lateral (displaced) S72.42-
        nondisplaced S72.42-
      medial (displaced) S72.43-
        nondisplaced S72.43-
      nondisplaced S72.41-
    epiphysis (displaced) S72.44-
      nondisplaced S72.44-
    physeal S79.10-
      Salter-Harris
        Type I S79.11-
        Type II S79.12-
        Type III S79.13-
        Type IV S79.14-
      specified NEC S79.19-
    specified NEC S72.49-
    supracondylar (displaced) S72.45-
      with intracondylar extension (displaced) S72.46-
        nondisplaced S72.46-
      nondisplaced S72.45-
    torus S72.47-
  neck — *see* Fracture, femur, upper end, neck
  pertrochanteric — *see* Fracture, femur, trochanteric
  shaft (lower third) (middle third) (upper third) S72.30-
    comminuted (displaced) S72.35-
      nondisplaced S72.35-
    oblique (displaced) S72.33-
      nondisplaced S72.33-
    segmental (displaced) S72.36-
      nondisplaced S72.36-
    specified NEC S72.39-
    spiral (displaced) S72.34-
      nondisplaced S72.34-
    transverse (displaced) S72.32-
      nondisplaced S72.32-
  specified site NEC — *see* subcategory S72.8
  subcapital (displaced) S72.01-
  subtrochanteric (region) (section) (displaced) S72.2-
    nondisplaced S72.2-
  transcervical — *see* Fracture, femur, upper end, neck
  transtrochanteric — *see* Fracture, femur, trochanteric
  trochanteric S72.10-
    apophyseal (displaced) S72.13-
      nondisplaced S72.13-
    greater trochanter (displaced) S72.11-
      nondisplaced S72.11-
    intertrochanteric (displaced) S72.14-
      nondisplaced S72.14-
    lesser trochanter (displaced) S72.12-
      nondisplaced S72.12-
  upper end S72.00-
    apophyseal (displaced) S72.13-
      nondisplaced S72.13-
    cervicotrochanteric — *see* Fracture, femur, upper end, neck, base
    epiphysis (displaced) S72.02-
      nondisplaced S72.02-
    head S72.05-
      articular (displaced) S72.06-
        nondisplaced S72.06-
      specified NEC S72.09-
    intertrochanteric (displaced) S72.14-
      nondisplaced S72.14-
    intracapsular S72.01-
    midcervical (displaced) S72.03-
      nondisplaced S72.03-
    neck S72.00-
      base (displaced) S72.04-
        nondisplaced S72.04-
      specified NEC S72.09-
    pertrochanteric — *see* Fracture, femur, upper end, trochanteric
    physeal S79.00-
      Salter-Harris type I S79.01-
      specified NEC S79.09-
    subcapital (displaced) S72.01-

Fracture, traumatic (abduction) (adduction) (separation) (*see also* **Fracture, pathological**) T14.8 — *continued*
femur, femoral S72.9- — *continued*
  upper end S72.00- — *continued*
    subtrochanteric (displaced) S72.2-
      nondisplaced S72.2-
    transcervical — *see* Fracture, femur, upper end, midcervical
    trochanteric S72.10-
      greater (displaced) S72.11-
        nondisplaced S72.11-
      lesser (displaced) S72.12-
        nondisplaced S72.12-
fibula (shaft) (styloid) S82.40-
  comminuted (displaced) S82.45-
    nondisplaced S82.45-
  following insertion of implant, prosthesis or plate M96.67-
  involving ankle or malleolus — *see* Fracture, fibula, lateral malleolus
  lateral malleolus (displaced) S82.6-
    nondisplaced S82.6-
  lower end
    physeal S89.30-
      Salter-Harris
        Type I S89.31-
        Type II S89.32-
      specified NEC S89.39-
    specified NEC S82.83-
    torus S82.82-
  oblique (displaced) S82.43-
    nondisplaced S82.43-
  segmental (displaced) S82.46-
    nondisplaced S82.46-
  specified NEC S82.49-
  spiral (displaced) S82.44-
    nondisplaced S82.44-
  transverse (displaced) S82.42-
    nondisplaced S82.42-
  upper end
    physeal S89.20-
      Salter-Harris
        Type I S89.21-
        Type II S89.22-
      specified NEC S89.29-
    specified NEC S82.83-
    torus S82.81-
finger (except thumb) S62.60-
  distal phalanx (displaced) S62.63-
    nondisplaced S62.66-
  index S62.60-
    distal phalanx (displaced) S62.63-
      nondisplaced S62.66-
    medial phalanx (displaced) S62.62-
      nondisplaced S62.65-
    proximal phalanx (displaced) S62.61-
      nondisplaced S62.64-
  little S62.60-
    distal phalanx (displaced) S62.63-
      nondisplaced S62.66-
    medial phalanx (displaced) S62.62-
      nondisplaced S62.65-
    proximal phalanx (displaced) S62.61-
      nondisplaced S62.64-
  medial phalanx (displaced) S62.62-
    nondisplaced S62.65-
  middle S62.60-
    distal phalanx (displaced) S62.63-
      nondisplaced S62.66-
    medial phalanx (displaced) S62.62-
      nondisplaced S62.65-
    proximal phalanx (displaced) S62.61-
      nondisplaced S62.64-
  proximal phalanx (displaced) S62.61-
    nondisplaced S62.64-
  ring S62.60-
    distal phalanx (displaced) S62.63-
      nondisplaced S62.66-
    medial phalanx (displaced) S62.62-
      nondisplaced S62.65-
    proximal phalanx (displaced) S62.61-
      nondisplaced S62.64-
  thumb — *see* Fracture, thumb
following insertion (intraoperative) (postoperative) of orthopedic implant, joint prosthesis or bone plate M96.69
  femur M96.66-
  fibula M96.67-
  humerus M96.62-
  pelvis M96.65
  radius M96.63-
  specified bone NEC M96.69
  tibia M96.67-
  ulna M96.63-

Fracture, traumatic (abduction) (adduction) (separation) (*see also* **Fracture, pathological**) T14.8 — *continued*
foot S92.90-
  astragalus — *see* Fracture, tarsal, talus
  calcaneus — *see* Fracture, tarsal, calcaneus
  cuboid — *see* Fracture, tarsal, cuboid
  cuneiform — *see* Fracture, tarsal, cuneiform
  metatarsal — *see* Fracture, metatarsal
  navicular — *see* Fracture, tarsal, navicular
  talus — *see* Fracture, tarsal, talus
  tarsal — *see* Fracture, tarsal
  toe — *see* Fracture, toe
forearm S52.9-
  radius — *see* Fracture, radius
  ulna — *see* Fracture, ulna
fossa (anterior) (middle) (posterior) S02.19
frontal (bone) (skull) S02.0
  sinus S02.19
glenoid (cavity) (scapula) — *see* Fracture, scapula, glenoid cavity
greenstick — *see* Fracture, by site
hallux — *see* Fracture, toe, great
hand S62.9-
  carpal — *see* Fracture, carpal bone
  finger (except thumb) — *see* Fracture, finger
  metacarpal — *see* Fracture, metacarpal
  navicular (scaphoid) (hand) — *see* Fracture, carpal bone, navicular
  thumb — *see* Fracture, thumb
healed or old
  with complications — *code by* Nature of the complication
heel bone — *see* Fracture, tarsal, calcaneus
Hill-Sachs S42.29-
hip — *see* Fracture, femur, neck
humerus S42.30-
  anatomical neck — *see* Fracture, humerus, upper end
  articular process — *see* Fracture, humerus, lower end
  capitellum — *see* Fracture, humerus, lower end, condyle, lateral
  distal end — *see* Fracture, humerus, lower end
  epiphysis
    lower — *see* Fracture, humerus, lower end, physeal
    upper — *see* Fracture, humerus, upper end, physeal
  external condyle — *see* Fracture, humerus, lower end, condyle, lateral
  following insertion of implant, prosthesis or plate M96.62-
  great tuberosity — *see* Fracture, humerus, upper end, greater tuberosity
  intercondylar — *see* Fracture, humerus, lower end
  internal epicondyle — *see* Fracture, humerus, lower end, epicondyle, medial
  lesser tuberosity — *see* Fracture, humerus, upper end, lesser tuberosity
  lower end S42.40-
    condyle
      lateral (displaced) S42.45-
        nondisplaced S42.45-
      medial (displaced) S42.46-
        nondisplaced S42.46-
    epicondyle
      lateral (displaced) S42.43-
        nondisplaced S42.43-
      medial (displaced) S42.44-
        incarcerated S42.44-
        nondisplaced S42.44-
    physeal S49.10-
      Salter-Harris
        Type I S49.11-
        Type II S49.12-
        Type III S49.13-
        Type IV S49.14-
      specified NEC S49.19-
    specified NEC (displaced) S42.49-
      nondisplaced S42.49-
    supracondylar (simple) (displaced) S42.41-
      comminuted (displaced) S42.42-
        nondisplaced S42.42-
      nondisplaced S42.41-
    torus S42.48-
    transcondylar (displaced) S42.47-
      nondisplaced S42.47-

DISEASE INDEX

Fracture, traumatic (abduction) (adduction) (separation) (*see also* **Fracture, pathological**) T14.8 — *continued*
humerus S42.30- — *continued*
proximal end — *see* Fracture, humerus, upper end
shaft S42.30-
comminuted (displaced) S42.35-
nondisplaced S42.35-
greenstick S42.31-
oblique (displaced) S42.33-
nondisplaced S42.33-
segmental (displaced) S42.36-
nondisplaced S42.36-
specified NEC S42.39-
spiral (displaced) S42.34-
nondisplaced S42.34-
transverse (displaced) S42.32-
nondisplaced S42.32-
supracondylar — *see* Fracture, humerus, lower end
surgical neck — *see* Fracture, humerus, upper end, surgical neck
trochlea — *see* Fracture, humerus, lower end, condyle, medial
tuberosity — *see* Fracture, humerus, upper end
upper end S42.20-
anatomical neck — *see* Fracture, humerus, upper end, specified NEC
articular head — *see* Fracture, humerus, upper end, specified NEC
epiphysis — *see* Fracture, humerus, upper end, physeal
greater tuberosity (displaced) S42.25-
nondisplaced S42.25-
lesser tuberosity (displaced) S42.26-
nondisplaced S42.26-
physeal S49.00-
Salter-Harris
Type I S49.01-
Type II S49.02-
Type III S49.03-
Type IV S49.04-
specified NEC S49.09-
specified NEC (displaced) S42.29-
nondisplaced S42.29-
surgical neck (displaced) S42.21-
four-part S42.24-
nondisplaced S42.21-
three-part S42.23-
two-part (displaced) S42.22-
nondisplaced S42.22-
torus S42.27-
transepiphyseal — *see* Fracture, humerus, upper end, physeal
hyoid bone S12.8
ilium S32.30-
with disruption of pelvic ring — *see* Disruption, pelvic ring
avulsion (displaced) S32.31-
nondisplaced S32.31-
specified NEC S32.39-
impaction, impacted — *code as* Fracture, by site
innominate bone — *see* Fracture, ilium
instep — *see* Fracture, foot
ischium S32.60-
with disruption of pelvic ring — *see* Disruption, pelvic ring
avulsion (displaced) S32.61-
nondisplaced S32.61-
specified NEC S32.69-
jaw (bone) (lower) — *see* Fracture, mandible
upper — *see* Fracture, maxilla
joint prosthesis — *see* Complications, joint prosthesis, mechanical, breakdown, by site
periprosthetic — *see* Complications, joint prosthesis, mechanical, periprosthesis, fracture, by site
knee cap — *see* Fracture, patella
larynx S12.8
late effects — *see* Sequelae, fracture
leg (lower) S82.9-
ankle — *see* Fracture, ankle
femur — *see* Fracture, femur
fibula — *see* Fracture, fibula
malleolus — *see* Fracture, ankle
patella — *see* Fracture, patella
specified site NEC S82.89-
tibia — *see* Fracture, tibia
lumbar spine — *see* Fracture, vertebra, lumbar
lumbosacral spine S32.9

Fracture, traumatic (abduction) (adduction) (separation) (*see also* **Fracture, pathological**) T14.8 — *continued*
Maisonneuve's (displaced) S82.86-
nondisplaced S82.86-
malar bone (*see also* Fracture, maxilla) S02.400
malleolus — *see* Fracture, ankle
malunion — *see* Fracture, by site
mandible (lower jaw (bone)) S02.609
alveolus S02.67
angle (of jaw) S02.65
body, unspecified S02.600
condylar process S02.61
coronoid process S02.63
ramus, unspecified S02.64
specified site NEC S02.69
subcondylar process S02.62
symphysis S02.66
manubrium (sterni) S22.21
dissociation from sternum S22.23
march — *see* Fracture, traumatic, stress, by site
maxilla, maxillary (bone) (sinus) (superior) (upper jaw) S02.401
alveolus S02.42
inferior — *see* Fracture, mandible
LeFort I S02.411
LeFort II S02.412
LeFort III S02.413
metacarpal S62.309
base (displaced) S62.319
nondisplaced S62.349
fifth S62.30-
base (displaced) S62.31-
nondisplaced S62.34-
neck (displaced) S62.33-
nondisplaced S62.36-
shaft (displaced) S62.32-
nondisplaced S62.35-
specified NEC S62.398
first S62.20-
base NEC (displaced) S62.23-
nondisplaced S62.23-
Bennett's — *see* Bennett's fracture
neck (displaced) S62.25-
nondisplaced S62.25-
shaft (displaced) S62.24-
nondisplaced S62.24-
specified NEC S62.29-
fourth S62.30-
base (displaced) S62.31-
nondisplaced S62.34-
neck (displaced) S62.33-
nondisplaced S62.36-
shaft (displaced) S62.32-
nondisplaced S62.35-
specified NEC S62.39-
neck (displaced) S62.33-
nondisplaced S62.36-
Rolando's — *see* Rolando's fracture
second S62.30-
base (displaced) S62.31-
nondisplaced S62.34-
neck (displaced) S62.33-
nondisplaced S62.36-
shaft (displaced) S62.32-
nondisplaced S62.35-
specified NEC S62.39-
shaft (displaced) S62.32-
nondisplaced S62.35-
specified NEC S62.399
third S62.30-
base (displaced) S62.31-
nondisplaced S62.34-
neck (displaced) S62.33-
nondisplaced S62.36-
shaft (displaced) S62.32-
nondisplaced S62.35-
specified NEC S62.39-
metastatic — *see* Fracture, pathological, due to, neoplastic disease — *see also* Neoplasm
metatarsal bone S92.30-
fifth (displaced) S92.35-
nondisplaced S92.35-
first (displaced) S92.31-
nondisplaced S92.31-
fourth (displaced) S92.34-
nondisplaced S92.34-
second (displaced) S92.32-
nondisplaced S92.32-
third (displaced) S92.33-
nondisplaced S92.33-
Monteggia's — *see* Monteggia's fracture
multiple
hand (and wrist) NEC — *see* Fracture, by site
ribs — *see* Fracture, rib, multiple

Fracture, traumatic (abduction) (adduction) (separation) (*see also* **Fracture, pathological**) T14.8 — *continued*
nasal (bone(s)) S02.2
navicular (scaphoid) (foot) — *see also* Fracture, tarsal, navicular
hand — *see* Fracture, carpal, navicular
neck S12.9
cervical vertebra S12.9
fifth (displaced) S12.400
nondisplaced S12.401
specified type NEC (displaced) S12.490
nondisplaced S12.491
first (displaced) S12.000
burst (stable) S12.01
unstable S12.02
lateral mass (displaced) S12.040
nondisplaced S12.041
nondisplaced S12.001
posterior arch (displaced) S12.030
nondisplaced S12.031
specified type NEC (displaced) S12.090
nondisplaced S12.091
fourth (displaced) S12.300
nondisplaced S12.301
specified type NEC (displaced) S12.390
nondisplaced S12.391
second (displaced) S12.100
dens (anterior) (displaced) (type II) S12.110
nondisplaced S12.112
posterior S12.111
specified type NEC (displaced) S12.120
nondisplaced S12.121
nondisplaced S12.101
specified type NEC (displaced) S12.190
nondisplaced S12.191
seventh (displaced) S12.600
nondisplaced S12.601
specified type NEC (displaced) S12.690
displaced S12.691
sixth (displaced) S12.500
nondisplaced S12.501
specified type NEC (displaced) S12.590
displaced S12.591
third (displaced) S12.200
nondisplaced S12.201
specified type NEC (displaced) S12.290
displaced S12.291
hyoid bone S12.8
larynx S12.8
specified site NEC S12.8
thyroid cartilage S12.8
trachea S12.8
neoplastic NEC — *see* Fracture, pathological, due to, neoplastic disease
neural arch — *see* Fracture, vertebra
newborn — *see* Birth, injury, fracture
nontraumatic — *see* Fracture, pathological
nonunion — *see* Nonunion, fracture
nose, nasal (bone) (septum) S02.2
occiput — *see* Fracture, skull, base, occiput
odontoid process — *see* Fracture, neck, cervical vertebra, second
olecranon (process) (ulna) — *see* Fracture, ulna, upper end, olecranon process
orbit, orbital (bone) (region) S02.8
floor (blow-out) S02.3
roof S02.19
os
calcis — *see* Fracture, tarsal, calcaneus
magnum — *see* Fracture, carpal, capitate
pubis — *see* Fracture, pubis
palate S02.8
parietal bone (skull) S02.0
patella S82.00-
comminuted (displaced) S82.04-
nondisplaced S82.04-
longitudinal (displaced) S82.02-
nondisplaced S82.02-
osteochondral (displaced) S82.01-
nondisplaced S82.01-
specified NEC S82.09-
transverse (displaced) S82.03-
nondisplaced S82.03-
pedicle (of vertebral arch) — *see* Fracture, vertebra

Fracture, traumatic (abduction) (adduction) (separation) (*see also* **Fracture, pathological**) T14.8 — *continued*
pelvis, pelvic (bone) S32.9
acetabulum — *see* Fracture, acetabulum
circle — *see* Disruption, pelvic ring
following insertion of implant, prosthesis or plate M96.65
ilium — *see* Fracture, ilium
ischium — *see* Fracture, ischium
multiple
with disruption of pelvic ring (circle) — *see* Disruption, pelvic ring
without disruption of pelvic ring (circle) S32.82
pubis — *see* Fracture, pubis
sacrum — *see* Fracture, sacrum
specified site NEC S32.89
phalanx
foot — *see* Fracture, toe
hand — *see* Fracture, finger
pisiform — *see* Fracture, carpal, pisiform
pond — *see* Fracture, skull
prosthetic device, internal — *see* Complications, prosthetic device, by site, mechanical
pubis S32.50-
with disruption of pelvic ring — *see* Disruption, pelvic ring
specified site NEC S32.59-
superior rim S32.51-
radius S52.9-
distal end — *see* Fracture, radius, lower end
following insertion of implant, prosthesis or plate M96.63-
head — *see* Fracture, radius, upper end, head
lower end S52.50-
Barton's — *see* Barton's fracture
Colles' — *see* Colles' fracture
extraarticular NEC S52.55-
intraarticular NEC S52.57-
physeal S59.20-
Salter-Harris
Type I S59.21-
Type II S59.22-
Type III S59.23-
Type IV S59.24-
specified NEC S59.29-
Smith's — *see* Smith's fracture
specified NEC S52.59-
styloid process (displaced) S52.51-
nondisplaced S52.51-
torus S52.52-
neck — *see* Fracture, radius, upper end
proximal end — *see* Fracture, radius, upper end
shaft S52.30-
bent bone S52.38-
comminuted (displaced) S52.35-
nondisplaced S52.35-
Galeazzi's — *see* Galeazzi's fracture
greenstick S52.31-
oblique (displaced) S52.33-
nondisplaced S52.33-
segmental (displaced) S52.36-
nondisplaced S52.36-
specified NEC S52.39-
spiral (displaced) S52.34-
nondisplaced S52.34-
transverse (displaced) S52.32-
nondisplaced S52.32-
upper end S52.10-
head (displaced) S52.12-
nondisplaced S52.12-
neck (displaced) S52.13-
nondisplaced S52.13-
physeal S59.10-
Salter-Harris
Type I S59.11-
Type II S59.12-
Type III S59.13-
Type IV S59.14-
specified NEC S59.19-
specified NEC S52.18-
torus S52.11-
ramus
inferior or superior, pubis — *see* Fracture, pubis
mandible — *see* Fracture, mandible
restorative material (dental) K08.539
with loss of material K08.531
without loss of material K08.530
rib S22.3-
with flail chest — *see* Flail, chest
multiple S22.4-
with flail chest — *see* Flail, chest
root, tooth — *see* Fracture, tooth

Fracture, traumatic (abduction) (adduction) (separation) (*see also* **Fracture, pathological**) T14.8 — *continued*
sacrum S32.10
 specified NEC S32.19
 Type
  1 S32.14
  2 S32.15
  3 S32.16
  4 S32.17
 Zone
  I S32.119
   displaced (minimally) S32.111
    severely S32.112
   nondisplaced S32.110
  II S32.129
   displaced (minimally) S32.121
    severely S32.122
   nondisplaced S32.120
  III S32.139
   displaced (minimally) S32.131
    severely S32.132
   nondisplaced S32.130
scaphoid (hand) — *see also* Fracture, carpal, navicular
 foot — *see* Fracture, tarsal, navicular
scapula S42.10-
 acromial process (displaced) S42.12-
  nondisplaced S42.12-
 body (displaced) S42.11-
  nondisplaced S42.11-
 coracoid process (displaced) S42.13-
  nondisplaced S42.13-
 glenoid cavity (displaced) S42.14-
  nondisplaced S42.14-
 neck (displaced) S42.15-
  nondisplaced S42.15-
 specified NEC S42.19-
semilunar bone, wrist — *see* Fracture, carpal, lunate
sequelae — *see* Sequelae, fracture
sesamoid bone
 hand — *see* Fracture, carpal
 other — *code by* site under Fracture
shepherd's — *see* Fracture, tarsal, talus
shoulder (girdle) S42.9-
 blade — *see* Fracture, scapula
sinus (ethmoid) (frontal) S02.19
skull S02.91
 base S02.10
  occiput S02.119
   condyle S02.113
    type I S02.110
    type II S02.111
    type III S02.112
   specified NEC S02.118
  specified NEC S02.19
 birth injury P13.0
 frontal bone S02.0
 parietal bone S02.0
 specified site NEC S02.8
 temporal bone S02.19
 vault S02.0
Smith's — *see* Smith's fracture
sphenoid (bone) (sinus) S02.19
spine — *see* Fracture, vertebra
spinous process — *see* Fracture, vertebra
spontaneous (cause unknown) — *see* Fracture, pathological
stave (of thumb) — *see* Fracture, metacarpal, first
sternum S22.20
 with flail chest — *see* Flail, chest
 body S22.22
 manubrium S22.21
 xiphoid (process) S22.24
stress M84.30
 ankle M84.37-
 carpus M84.34-
 clavicle M84.31-
 femoral neck M84.359
 femur M84.35-
 fibula M84.36-
 finger M84.34-
 hip M84.359
 humerus M84.32-
 ilium M84.350
 ischium M84.350
 metacarpus M84.34-
 metatarsus M84.37-
 neck — *see* Fracture, fatigue, vertebra
 pelvis M84.350
 radius M84.33-
 rib M84.38
 scapula M84.31-
 skull M84.38
 tarsus M84.37-
 tibia M84.36-
 toe M84.37-
 ulna M84.33-

Fracture, traumatic (abduction) (adduction) (separation) (*see also* **Fracture, pathological**) T14.8 — *continued*
stress M84.30 — *continued*
 vertebra — *see* Fracture, fatigue, vertebra
supracondylar, elbow — *see* Fracture, humerus, lower end, supracondylar
symphysis pubis — *see* Fracture, pubis
talus (ankle bone) — *see* Fracture, tarsal, talus
tarsal bone(s) S92.20-
 astragalus — *see* Fracture, tarsal, talus
 calcaneus S92.00-
  anterior process (displaced) S92.02-
   nondisplaced S92.02-
  body (displaced) S92.01-
   nondisplaced S92.01-
  extraarticular NEC (displaced) S92.05-
   nondisplaced S92.05-
  intraarticular (displaced) S92.06-
   nondisplaced S92.06-
  tuberosity (displaced) S92.04-
   avulsion (displaced) S92.03-
    nondisplaced S92.03-
   nondisplaced S92.04-
 cuboid (displaced) S92.21-
  nondisplaced S92.21-
 cuneiform
  intermediate (displaced) S92.23-
   nondisplaced S92.23-
  lateral (displaced) S92.22-
   nondisplaced S92.22-
  medial (displaced) S92.24-
   nondisplaced S92.24-
 navicular (displaced) S92.25-
  nondisplaced S92.25-
 scaphoid — *see* Fracture, tarsal, navicular
 talus S92.10-
  avulsion (displaced) S92.15-
   nondisplaced S92.15-
  body (displaced) S92.12-
   nondisplaced S92.12-
  dome (displaced) S92.14-
   nondisplaced S92.14-
  head (displaced) S92.12-
   nondisplaced S92.12-
  lateral process (displaced) S92.14-
   nondisplaced S92.14-
  neck (displaced) S92.11-
   nondisplaced S92.11-
  posterior process (displaced) S92.13-
   nondisplaced S92.13-
  specified NEC S92.19-
 temporal bone (styloid) S02.19
thorax (bony) S22.9
 with flail chest — *see* Flail, chest
 rib S22.3-
  multiple S22.4-
   with flail chest — *see* Flail, chest
 sternum S22.20
  body S22.22
  manubrium S22.21
  xiphoid process S22.24
 vertebra (displaced) S22.009
  burst (stable) S22.001
   unstable S22.002
  eighth S22.069
   burst (stable) S22.061
    unstable S22.062
   specified type NEC S22.068
   wedge compression S22.060
  eleventh S22.089
   burst (stable) S22.081
    unstable S22.082
   specified type NEC S22.088
   wedge compression S22.080
  fifth S22.059
   burst (stable) S22.051
    unstable S22.052
   specified type NEC S22.058
   wedge compression S22.050
  first S22.019
   burst (stable) S22.011
    unstable S22.012
   specified type NEC S22.018
   wedge compression S22.010
  fourth S22.049
   burst (stable) S22.041
    unstable S22.042
   specified type NEC S22.048
   wedge compression S22.040

Fracture, traumatic (abduction) (adduction) (separation) (*see also* **Fracture, pathological**) T14.8 — *continued*
thorax (bony) S22.9 — *continued*
 vertebra (displaced) S22.009 — *continued*
  ninth S22.079
   burst (stable) S22.071
    unstable S22.072
   specified type NEC S22.078
   wedge compression S22.070
  nondisplaced S22.001
  second S22.029
   burst (stable) S22.021
    unstable S22.022
   specified type NEC S22.028
   wedge compression S22.020
  seventh S22.069
   burst (stable) S22.061
    unstable S22.062
   specified type NEC S22.068
   wedge compression S22.060
  sixth S22.059
   burst (stable) S22.051
    unstable S22.052
   specified type NEC S22.058
   wedge compression S22.050
  specified type NEC S22.008
  tenth S22.079
   burst (stable) S22.071
    unstable S22.072
   specified type NEC S22.078
   wedge compression S22.070
  third S22.039
   burst (stable) S22.031
    unstable S22.032
   specified type NEC S22.038
   wedge compression S22.030
  twelfth S22.089
   burst (stable) S22.081
    unstable S22.082
   specified type NEC S22.088
   wedge compression S22.080
  wedge compression S22.000
thumb S62.50-
 distal phalanx (displaced) S62.52-
  nondisplaced S62.52-
 proximal phalanx (displaced) S62.51-
  nondisplaced S62.51-
thyroid cartilage S12.8
tibia (shaft) S82.20-
 comminuted (displaced) S82.25-
  nondisplaced S82.25-
 condyles — *see* Fracture, tibia, upper end
 distal end — *see* Fracture, tibia, lower end
 epiphysis
  lower — *see* Fracture, tibia, lower end
  upper — *see* Fracture, tibia, upper end
 following insertion of implant, prosthesis or plate M96.67-
 head (involving knee joint) — *see* Fracture, tibia, upper end
 intercondyloid eminence — *see* Fracture, tibia, upper end
 involving ankle or malleolus — *see* Fracture, ankle, medial malleolus
 lower end S82.30-
  physeal S89.10-
   Salter-Harris
    Type I S89.11-
    Type II S89.12-
    Type III S89.13-
    Type IV S89.14-
   specified NEC S89.19-
  pilon (displaced) S82.87-
   nondisplaced S82.87-
  specified NEC S82.39-
  torus S82.31-
 malleolus — *see* Fracture, ankle, medial malleolus
 oblique (displaced) S82.23-
  nondisplaced S82.23-
 pilon — *see* Fracture, tibia, lower end, pilon
 proximal end — *see* Fracture, tibia, upper end
 segmental (displaced) S82.26-
  nondisplaced S82.26-
 specified NEC S82.29-
 spine — *see* Fracture, upper end, spine
 spiral (displaced) S82.24-
  nondisplaced S82.24-
 transverse (displaced) S82.22-
  nondisplaced S82.22-

Fracture, traumatic (abduction) (adduction) (separation) (*see also* **Fracture, pathological**) T14.8 — *continued*
tibia (shaft) S82.20- — *continued*
 tuberosity — *see* Fracture, tibia, upper end, tuberosity
 upper end S82.10-
  bicondylar (displaced) S82.14-
   nondisplaced S82.14-
  lateral condyle (displaced) S82.12-
   nondisplaced S82.12-
  medial condyle (displaced) S82.13-
   nondisplaced S82.13-
  physeal S89.00-
   Salter-Harris
    Type I S89.01-
    Type II S89.02-
    Type III S89.03-
    Type IV S89.04-
   specified NEC S89.09-
  plateau — *see* Fracture, tibia, upper end, bicondylar
  specified NEC S82.19-
  spine (displaced) S82.11-
   nondisplaced S82.11-
  torus S82.16-
  tuberosity (displaced) S82.15-
   nondisplaced S82.15-
toe S92.91-
 great (displaced) S92.40-
  distal phalanx (displaced) S92.42-
   nondisplaced S92.42-
  nondisplaced S92.40-
  proximal phalanx (displaced) S92.41-
   nondisplaced S92.41-
  specified NEC S92.49-
 lesser (displaced) S92.50-
  distal phalanx (displaced) S92.53-
   nondisplaced S92.53-
  medial phalanx (displaced) S92.52-
   nondisplaced S92.52-
  nondisplaced S92.50-
  proximal phalanx (displaced) S92.51-
   nondisplaced S92.51-
  specified NEC S92.59-
tooth (root) S02.5
trachea (cartilage) S12.8
transverse process — *see* Fracture, vertebra
trapezium or trapezoid bone — *see* Fracture, carpal
trimalleolar — *see* Fracture, ankle, trimalleolar
triquetrum (cuneiform of carpus) — *see* Fracture, carpal, triquetrum
trochanter — *see* Fracture, femur, trochanteric
tuberosity (external) — *code by* site under Fracture
ulna (shaft) S52.20-
 bent bone S52.28-
 coronoid process — *see* Fracture, ulna, upper end, coronoid process
 distal end — *see* Fracture, ulna, lower end
 following insertion of implant, prosthesis or plate M96.63-
 head S52.00-
 lower end S52.60-
  physeal S59.00-
   Salter-Harris
    Type I S59.01-
    Type II S59.02-
    Type III S59.03-
    Type IV S59.04-
   specified NEC S59.09-
  specified NEC S52.69-
  styloid process (displaced) S52.61-
   nondisplaced S52.61-
  torus S52.62-
 proximal end — *see* Fracture, ulna, upper end
 shaft S52.20-
  comminuted (displaced) S52.25-
   nondisplaced S52.25-
  greenstick S52.21-
  Monteggia's — *see* Monteggia's fracture
  oblique (displaced) S52.23-
   nondisplaced S52.23-
  segmental (displaced) S52.26-
   nondisplaced S52.26-
  specified NEC S52.29-
  spiral (displaced) S52.24-
   nondisplaced S52.24-
  transverse (displaced) S52.22-
   nondisplaced S52.22-

Fracture, traumatic (abduction) (adduction) (separation) (*see also* **Fracture, pathological**) T14.8 — *continued*
ulna (shaft) S52.20- — *continued*
  upper end S52.00-
    coronoid process (displaced) S52.04-
    nondisplaced S52.04-
    olecranon process (displaced) S52.02-
      with intraarticular extension S52.03-
      nondisplaced S52.02-
        with intraarticular extension S52.03-
    specified NEC S52.09-
    torus S52.01-
unciform — *see* Fracture, carpal, hamate
vault of skull S02.0
vertebra, vertebral (arch) (body) (column) (neural arch) (pedicle) (spinous process) (transverse process)
  atlas — *see* Fracture, neck, cervical vertebra, first
  axis — *see* Fracture, neck, cervical vertebra, second
  cervical (teardrop) S12.9
    axis — *see* Fracture, neck, cervical vertebra, second
    first (atlas) — *see* Fracture, neck, cervical vertebra, first
    second (axis) — *see* Fracture, neck, cervical vertebra, second
  chronic M84.48
  coccyx S32.2
  dorsal — *see* Fracture, thorax, vertebra
  lumbar S32.009
    burst (stable) S32.001
      unstable S32.002
    fifth S32.059
      burst (stable) S32.051
        unstable S32.052
      specified type NEC S32.058
      wedge compression S32.050
    first S32.019
      burst (stable) S32.011
        unstable S32.012
      specified type NEC S32.018
      wedge compression S32.010
    fourth S32.049
      burst (stable) S32.041
        unstable S32.042
      specified type NEC S32.048
      wedge compression S32.040
    second S32.029
      burst (stable) S32.021
        unstable S32.022
      specified type NEC S32.028
      wedge compression S32.020
    specified type NEC S32.008
    third S32.039
      burst (stable) S32.031
        unstable S32.032
      specified type NEC S32.038
      wedge compression S32.030
    wedge compression S32.000
  metastatic — *see* Collapse, vertebra, in, specified disease NEC — *see also* Neoplasm
  newborn (birth injury) P11.5
  sacrum S32.10
    specified NEC S32.19
    Type
      1 S32.14
      2 S32.15
      3 S32.16
      4 S32.17
    Zone
      I S32.119
        displaced (minimally) S32.111
          severely S32.112
        nondisplaced S32.110
      II S32.129
        displaced (minimally) S32.121
          severely S32.122
        nondisplaced S32.120
      III S32.139
        displaced (minimally) S32.131
          severely S32.132
        nondisplaced S32.130
  thoracic — *see* Fracture, thorax, vertebra

Fracture, traumatic (abduction) (adduction) (separation) (*see also* **Fracture, pathological**) T14.8 — *continued*
vertex S02.0
vomer (bone) S02.2
wrist S62.10-
  carpal — *see* Fracture, carpal bone
  navicular (scaphoid) (hand) — *see* Fracture, carpal, navicular
xiphisternum, xiphoid (process) S22.24
zygoma S02.402
Fragile, fragility
autosomal site Q95.5
bone, congenital (with blue sclera) Q78.0
capillary (hereditary) D69.8
hair L67.8
nails L60.3
non-sex chromosome site Q95.5
X chromosome Q99.2
Fragilitas
crinium L67.8
ossium (with blue sclerae) (hereditary) Q78.0
unguium L60.3
  congenital Q84.6
Fragments, cataract (lens), following cataract surgery H59.02-
retained foreign body — *see* Retained, foreign body fragments (type of)
Frailty (frail) R54
mental R41.81
Frambesia, frambesial (tropica) — *see also* Yaws
initial lesion or ulcer A66.0
primary A66.0
Frambeside
gummatous A66.4
of early yaws A66.2
Frambesioma A66.1
Franceschetti-Klein(-Wildervanck) disease or syndrome Q75.4
Francis' disease — *see* Tularemia
Frank's essential thrombocytopenia D69.3
Franklin disease C88.2
Fraser's syndrome Q87.0
Freckle(s) L81.2
malignant melanoma in — *see* Melanoma
melanotic (Hutchinson's) — *see* Melanoma, in situ
retinal D49.81
Frederickson's hyperlipoproteinemia, type
I and V E78.3
IIA E78.0
IIB and III E78.2
IV E78.1
Freeman Sheldon syndrome Q87.0
Freezing (*see also* Effect, adverse, cold) T69.9
Frei's disease A55
Freiberg's disease (infraction of metatarsal head or osteochondrosis) — *see* Osteochondrosis, juvenile, metatarsus
Fremitus, friction, cardiac R01.2
Frenum, frenulum
external os Q51.828
tongue (shortening) (congenital) Q38.1
Frequency micturition (nocturnal) R35.0
psychogenic F45.8
Frey's syndrome
auriculotemporal G50.8
hyperhidrosis L74.52
Friction
burn — *see* Burn, by site
fremitus, cardiac R01.2
precordial R01.2
sounds, chest R09.89
Friderichsen-Waterhouse syndrome or disease A39.1
Friedländer's B (bacillus) NEC (*see also* condition) A49.8
Friedreich's
ataxia G11.1
combined systemic disease G11.1
facial hemihypertrophy Q67.4
sclerosis (cerebellum) (spinal cord) G11.1
Frigidity F52.22
Fröhlich's syndrome E23.6
Frontal — *see also* condition
lobe syndrome F07.0

Frostbite (superficial) T33.90
with
  partial thickness skin loss — *see* Frostbite (superficial), by site
  tissue necrosis T34.90
abdominal wall T33.3
  with tissue necrosis T34.3
ankle T33.81-
  with tissue necrosis T34.81-
arm T33.4-
  with tissue necrosis T34.4-
  finger(s) — *see* Frostbite, finger
  hand — *see* Frostbite, hand
  wrist — *see* Frostbite, wrist
ear T33.01-
  with tissue necrosis T34.01-
face T33.09
  with tissue necrosis T34.09
finger T33.53-
  with tissue necrosis T34.53-
foot T33.82-
  with tissue necrosis T34.82-
hand T33.52-
  with tissue necrosis T34.52-
head T33.09
  with tissue necrosis T34.09
  ear — *see* Frostbite, ear
  nose — *see* Frostbite, nose
hip (and thigh) T33.6-
  with tissue necrosis T34.6-
knee T33.7-
  with tissue necrosis T34.7-
leg T33.9-
  with tissue necrosis T34.9-
  ankle — *see* Frostbite, ankle
  foot — *see* Frostbite, foot
  knee — *see* Frostbite, knee
  lower T33.7-
    with tissue necrosis T34.7-
  thigh — *see* Frostbite, hip
  toe — *see* Frostbite, toe
limb
  lower T33.99
    with tissue necrosis T34.99
  upper — *see* Frostbite, arm
neck T33.1
  with tissue necrosis T34.1
nose T33.02
  with tissue necrosis T34.02
pelvis T33.3
  with tissue necrosis T34.3
specified site NEC T33.99
  with tissue necrosis T34.99
thigh — *see* Frostbite, hip
thorax T33.2
  with tissue necrosis T34.2
toes T33.83-
  with tissue necrosis T34.83-
trunk T33.99
  with tissue necrosis T34.99
wrist T33.51-
  with tissue necrosis T34.51-
Frotteurism F65.81
Frozen (*see also* Effect, adverse, cold) T69.9
pelvis (female) N94.89
  male K66.8
shoulder — *see* Capsulitis, adhesive
Fructokinase deficiency E74.11
Fructose 1,6 diphosphatase deficiency E74.19
Fructosemia (benign) (essential) E74.12
Fructosuria (benign) (essential) E74.11
Fuchs'
black spot (myopic) H44.2-
dystrophy (corneal endothelium) H18.51
heterochromic cyclitis — *see* Cyclitis, Fuchs' heterochromic
Fucosidosis E77.1
Fugue R68.89
dissociative F44.1
hysterical (dissociative) F44.1
postictal in epilepsy — *see* Epilepsy
reaction to exceptional stress (transient) F43.0
Fulminant, fulminating — *see* condition
Functional — *see also* condition
bleeding (uterus) N93.8
Functioning, intellectual, borderline R41.83
Fundus — *see* condition
Fungemia NOS B49
Fungus, fungous
cerebral G93.89
disease NOS B49
infection — *see* Infection, fungus
Funiculitis (acute) (chronic) (endemic) N49.1
gonococcal (acute) (chronic) A54.23
tuberculous A18.15

Funnel
breast (acquired) M95.4
  congenital Q67.6
  sequelae (late effect) of rickets E64.3
chest (acquired) M95.4
  congenital Q67.6
  sequelae (late effect) of rickets E64.3
pelvis (acquired) M95.5
  with disproportion (fetopelvic) O33.3
    causing obstructed labor O65.3
  congenital Q74.2
FUO (fever of unknown origin) R50.9
Furfur L21.0
microsporon B36.0
Furrier's lung J67.8
Furrowed K14.5
nail(s) (transverse) L60.4
  congenital Q84.6
tongue K14.5
  congenital Q38.3
Furuncle L02.92
abdominal wall L02.221
ankle — *see* Furuncle, lower limb
antecubital space — *see* Furuncle, upper limb
anus K61.0
arm — *see* Furuncle, upper limb
auditory canal, external — *see* Abscess, ear, external
auricle (ear) — *see* Abscess, ear, external
axilla (region) L02.42-
back (any part) L02.222
breast N61
buttock L02.32
cheek (external) L02.02
chest wall L02.223
chin L02.02
corpus cavernosum N48.21
ear, external — *see* Abscess, ear, external
external auditory canal — *see* Abscess, ear, external
eyelid — *see* Abscess, eyelid
face L02.02
femoral (region) — *see* Furuncle, lower limb
finger — *see* Furuncle, hand
flank L02.221
foot L02.62-
forehead L02.02
gluteal (region) L02.32
groin L02.224
hand L02.52-
head L02.821
  face L02.02
hip — *see* Furuncle, lower limb
kidney — *see* Abscess, kidney
knee — *see* Furuncle, lower limb
labium (majus) (minus) N76.4
lacrimal
  gland — *see* Dacryoadenitis
  passages (duct) (sac) — *see* Inflammation, lacrimal, passages, acute
leg (any part) — *see* Furuncle, lower limb
lower limb L02.42-
malignant A22.0
mouth K12.2
navel L02.226
neck L02.12
nose J34.0
orbit, orbital — *see* Abscess, orbit
palmar (space) — *see* Furuncle, hand
partes posteriores L02.32
pectoral region L02.223
penis N48.21
perineum L02.225
pinna — *see* Abscess, ear, external
popliteal — *see* Furuncle, lower limb
prepatellar — *see* Furuncle, lower limb
scalp L02.821
seminal vesicle N49.0
shoulder — *see* Furuncle, upper limb
specified site NEC L02.828
submandibular K12.2
temple (region) L02.02
thumb — *see* Furuncle, hand
toe — *see* Furuncle, foot
trunk L02.229
  abdominal wall L02.221
  back L02.222
  chest wall L02.223
  groin L02.224
  perineum L02.225
  umbilicus L02.226
umbilicus L02.226
upper limb L02.42-
vulva N76.4

Furunculosis — see Furuncle
Fused — see Fusion, fused
Fusion, fused (congenital)
  astragaloscaphoid Q74.2
  atria Q21.1
  auditory canal Q16.1
  auricles, heart Q21.1
  binocular with defective stereopsis H53.32
  bone Q79.8
  cervical spine M43.22
  choanal Q30.0
  commissure, mitral valve Q23.2
  cusps, heart valve NEC Q24.8
    mitral Q23.2
    pulmonary Q22.1
    tricuspid Q22.4
  ear ossicles Q16.3
  fingers Q70.0-
  hymen Q52.3
  joint (acquired) — see also Ankylosis
    congenital Q74.8
  kidneys (incomplete) Q63.1
  labium (majus) (minus) Q52.5
  larynx and trachea Q34.8
  limb, congenital Q74.8
    lower Q74.2
    upper Q74.0
  lobes, lung Q33.8
  lumbosacral (acquired) M43.27
    arthrodesis status Z98.1
    congenital Q76.49
    postprocedural status Z98.1
  nares, nose, nasal, nostril(s) Q30.0
  organ or site not listed — see Anomaly, by
    site
  ossicles Q79.9
    auditory Q16.3
  pulmonic cusps Q22.1
  ribs Q76.6
  sacroiliac (joint) (acquired) M43.28
    arthrodesis status Z98.1
    congenital Q74.2
    postprocedural status Z98.1
  spine (acquired) NEC M43.20
    arthrodesis status Z98.1
    cervical region M43.22
    cervicothoracic region M43.23
    congenital Q76.49
    lumbar M43.26
    lumbosacral region M43.27
    occipito-atlanto-axial region M43.21
    postoperative status Z98.1
    sacrococcygeal region M43.28
    thoracic region M43.24
    thoracolumbar region M43.25
  sublingual duct with submaxillary duct at
    opening in mouth Q38.4
  testes Q55.1
  toes Q70.2-
  tooth, teeth K00.2
  trachea and esophagus Q39.8
  twins Q89.4
  vagina Q52.4
  ventricles, heart Q21.0
  vertebra (arch) — see Fusion, spine
  vulva Q52.5
Fusospirillosis (mouth) (tongue) (tonsil)
  A69.1
Fussy baby R68.12

G

Gain in weight (abnormal) (excessive) — see
  also Weight, gain
Gaisböck's disease (polycythemia
  hypertonica) D75.1
Gait abnormality R26.9
  ataxic R26.0
  falling R29.6
  hysterical (ataxic) (staggering) F44.4
  paralytic R26.1
  spastic R26.1
  specified type NEC R26.89
  staggering R26.0
  unsteadiness R26.81
  walking difficulty NEC R26.2
Galactocele (breast) N64.89
  puerperal, postpartum O92.79
Galactokinase deficiency E74.29
Galactophoritis N61
  gestational, puerperal, postpartum O91.2-
Galactorrhea O92.6
  not associated with childbirth N64.3
Galactosemia (classic) (congenital) E74.21
Galactosuria E74.29
Galacturia R82.0
  schistosomiasis (bilharziasis) B65.0
Galeazzi's fracture S52.37-
Galen's vein — see condition
Galeophobia F40.218
Gall duct — see condition
Gallbladder — see also condition
  acute K81.0
Gallop rhythm R00.8
Gallstone (colic) (cystic duct) (gallbladder)
  (impacted) (multiple) — see also
  Calculus, gallbladder
  with
    cholecystitis — see Calculus,
      gallbladder, with cholecystitis
    bile duct (common) (hepatic) — see
      Calculus, bile duct
    causing intestinal obstruction K56.3
    specified NEC K80.80
      with obstruction K80.81
Gambling Z72.6
  pathological (compulsive) F63.0
Gammopathy (of undetermined significance
  [MGUS]) D47.2
  associated with lymphoplasmacytic
    dyscrasia D47.2
  monoclonal D47.2
  polyclonal D89.0
Gamna's disease (siderotic splenomegaly)
  D73.1
Gamophobia F40.298
Gampsodactylia (congenital) Q66.7
Gamstorp's disease (adynamia episodica
  hereditaria) G72.3
Gandy-Nanta disease (siderotic
  splenomegaly) D73.1
Gang
  membership offenses Z72.810
Gangliocytoma D36.10
Ganglioglioma — see Neoplasm, uncertain
  behavior, by site
Ganglion (compound) (diffuse) (joint)
  (tendon (sheath)) M67.40
  ankle M67.47-
  foot M67.47-
  forearm M67.43-
  hand M67.44-
  lower leg M67.46-
  multiple sites M67.49
  of yaws (early) (late) A66.6
  pelvic region M67.45-
  periosteal — see Periostitis
  shoulder region M67.41-
  specified site NEC M67.48
  thigh region M67.45-
  tuberculous A18.09
  upper arm M67.42-
  wrist M67.43-
Ganglioneuroblastoma — see Neoplasm,
  nerve, malignant
Ganglioneuroma D36.10
  malignant — see Neoplasm, nerve,
    malignant
Ganglioneuromatosis D36.10
Ganglionitis
  fifth nerve — see Neuralgia, trigeminal
  gasserian (postherpetic) (postzoster)
    B02.21
  geniculate G51.1
    newborn (birth injury) P11.3
    postherpetic, postzoster B02.21
  herpes zoster B02.21

Ganglionitis — continued
  postherpetic geniculate B02.21
Gangliosidosis E75.10
  GM1 E75.19
  GM2 E75.00
    other specified E75.09
    Sandhoff disease E75.01
    Tay-Sachs disease E75.02
  GM3 E75.19
  mucolipidosis IV E75.11
Gangosa A66.5
Gangrene, gangrenous (connective tissue)
  (dropsical) (dry) (moist) (skin) (ulcer)
  (see also Necrosis) I96
  with diabetes (mellitus) — see Diabetes,
    gangrene
  abdomen (wall) I96
  alveolar M27.3
  appendix K35.80
    with
      perforation or rupture K35.2
      peritoneal abscess K35.3
      peritonitis NEC K35.3
        generalized (with perforation or
          rupture) K35.2
        localized (with perforation or
          rupture) K35.3
  arteriosclerotic (general) (senile) — see
    Arteriosclerosis, extremities, with,
    gangrene
  auricle I96
  Bacillus welchii A48.0
  bladder (infectious) — see Cystitis,
    specified type NEC
  bowel, cecum, or colon — see Gangrene,
    intestine
  Clostridium perfringens or welchii A48.0
  cornea H18.89-
  corpora cavernosa N48.29
    noninfective N48.89
  cutaneous, spreading I96
  decubital — see Ulcer, pressure, by site
  diabetic (any site) — see Diabetes,
    gangrene
  emphysematous — see Gangrene, gas
  epidemic — see Poisoning, food, noxious,
    plant
  epididymis (infectional) N45.1
  erysipelas — see Erysipelas
  extremity (lower) (upper) I96
  Fournier N49.3
    female N76.89
  fusospirochetal A69.0
  gallbladder — see Cholecystitis, acute
  gas (bacillus) A48.0
    following
      abortion — see Abortion by type
        complicated by infection
      ectopic or molar pregnancy O08.0
  glossitis K14.0
  hernia — see Hernia, by site, with gangrene
  intestine, intestinal (hemorrhagic)
    (massive) K55.0
    with
      mesenteric embolism K55.0
      obstruction — see Obstruction,
        intestine
  laryngitis J04.0
  limb (lower) (upper) I96
  lung J85.0
    spirochetal A69.8
  lymphangitis I89.1
  Meleney's (synergistic) — see Ulcer, skin
  mesentery K55.0
    with
      embolism K55.0
      intestinal obstruction — see
        Obstruction, intestine
  mouth A69.0
  ovary — see Oophoritis
  pancreas K85.9
  penis N48.29
    noninfective N48.89
  perineum I96
  pharynx — see also Pharyngitis
    Vincent's A69.1
  presenile I73.1
  progressive synergistic — see Ulcer, skin
  pulmonary J85.0
  pulpal (dental) K04.1
  quinsy J36
  Raynaud's (symmetric gangrene) I73.01
  retropharyngeal J39.2
  scrotum N49.3
    noninfective N50.8
  senile (atherosclerotic) — see
    Arteriosclerosis, extremities, with,
    gangrene

Gangrene, gangrenous (connective tissue)
  (dropsical) (dry) (moist) (skin) (ulcer)
  (see also Necrosis) I96 — continued
  spermatic cord N49.1
    noninfective N50.8
  spine I96
  spirochetal NEC A69.8
  spreading cutaneous I96
  stomatitis A69.0
  symmetrical I73.01
  testis (infectional) N45.2
    noninfective N44.8
  throat — see also Pharyngitis
    diphtheritic A36.0
    Vincent's A69.1
  thyroid (gland) E07.89
  tooth (pulp) K04.1
  tuberculous NEC — see Tuberculosis
  tunica vaginalis N49.1
    noninfective N50.8
  umbilicus I96
  uterus — see Endometritis
  uvulitis K12.2
  vas deferens N49.1
    noninfective N50.8
  vulva N76.89
Ganister disease J62.8
Ganser's syndrome (hysterical) F44.89
Gardner-Diamond syndrome
  (autoerythrocyte sensitization) D69.2
Gargoylism E76.01
**Garré's disease, osteitis (sclerosing),
  osteomyelitis** — see Osteomyelitis,
  specified type NEC
Garrod's pad, knuckle M72.1
Gartner's duct
  cyst Q52.4
  persistent Q50.6
Gas R14.3
  asphyxiation, inhalation, poisoning,
    suffocation NEC — see Table of
    Drugs and Chemicals
  excessive R14.0
  gangrene A48.0
    following
      abortion — see Abortion by type
        complicated by infection
      ectopic or molar pregnancy O08.0
  on stomach R14.0
  pains R14.1
Gastralgia — see also Pain, abdominal
Gastrectasis K31.0
  psychogenic F45.8
Gastric — see condition
Gastrinoma
  malignant
    pancreas C25.4
    specified site NEC — see Neoplasm,
      malignant, by site
    unspecified site C25.4
  specified site — see Neoplasm, uncertain
    behavior
  unspecified site D37.9
Gastritis (simple) K29.70
  with bleeding K29.71
  acute (erosive) K29.00
    with bleeding K29.01
  alcoholic K29.20
    with bleeding K29.21
  allergic K29.60
    with bleeding K29.61
  atrophic (chronic) K29.40
    with bleeding K29.41
  chronic (antral) (fundal) K29.50
    with bleeding K29.51
    atrophic K29.40
      with bleeding K29.41
    superficial K29.30
      with bleeding K29.31
  dietary counseling and surveillance Z71.3
  due to diet deficiency E63.9
  eosinophilic K52.81
  giant hypertrophic K29.60
    with bleeding K29.61
  granulomatous K29.60
    with bleeding K29.61
  hypertrophic (mucosa) K29.60
    with bleeding K29.61
  nervous F54
  spastic K29.60
    with bleeding K29.61
  specified NEC K29.60
    with bleeding K29.61
  superficial chronic K29.30
    with bleeding K29.31
  tuberculous A18.83
  viral NEC A08.4

DISEASE INDEX

Gastrocarcinoma — see Neoplasm, malignant, stomach
Gastrocolic — see condition
Gastrodisciasis, gastrodiscoidiasis B66.8
Gastroduodenitis K29.90
  with bleeding K29.91
  virus, viral A08.4
    specified type NEC A08.39
Gastrodynia — see Pain, abdominal
Gastroenteritis (acute) (chronic) (noninfectious) (see also Enteritis) K52.9
  allergic K52.2
  dietetic K52.2
  drug-induced K52.1
  due to
    Cryptosporidium A07.2
    drugs K52.1
    food poisoning — see Intoxication, foodborne
    radiation K52.0
  eosinophilic K52.81
  epidemic (infectious) A09
  food hypersensitivity K52.2
  infectious — see Enteritis, infectious
  influenzal — see Influenza, with gastroenteritis
  noninfectious K52.9
    specified NEC K52.89
  rotaviral A08.0
  Salmonella A02.0
  toxic K52.1
  viral NEC A08.4
    acute infectious A08.39
      type Norwalk A08.11
    infantile (acute) A08.39
    Norwalk agent A08.11
    rotaviral A08.0
    severe of infants A08.39
    specified type NEC A08.39
Gastroenteropathy (see also Gastroenteritis) K52.9
  acute, due to Norovirus A08.11
  acute, due to Norwalk agent A08.11
  infectious A09
Gastroenteroptosis K63.4
Gastroesophageal laceration-hemorrhage syndrome K22.6
Gastrointestinal — see condition
Gastrojejunal — see condition
Gastrojejunitis (see also Enteritis) K52.9
Gastrojejunocolic — see condition
Gastroliths K31.89
Gastromalacia K31.89
Gastroparalysis K31.84
  diabetic — see Diabetes, gastroparalysis
Gastroparesis K31.84
  diabetic — see Diabetes, by type, with gastroparesis
Gastropathy K31.9
  congestive portal K31.89
  erythematous K29.70
  exudative K90.89
  portal hypertensive K31.89
Gastroptosis K31.89
Gastrorrhagia K92.2
  psychogenic F45.8
Gastroschisis (congenital) Q79.3
Gastrospasm (neurogenic) (reflex) K31.89
  neurotic F45.8
  psychogenic F45.8
Gastrostaxis — see Gastritis, with bleeding
Gastrostenosis K31.89
Gastrostomy
  attention to Z43.1
  status Z93.1
Gastrosuccorrhea (continuous) (intermittent) K31.89
  neurotic F45.8
  psychogenic F45.8
Gatophobia F40.218
Gaucher's disease or splenomegaly (adult) (infantile) E75.22
Gee(-Herter)(-Thaysen) disease (nontropical sprue) K90.0
Gélineau's syndrome G47.419
  with cataplexy G47.411
Gemination, tooth, teeth K00.2
Gemistocytoma
  specified site — see Neoplasm, malignant, by site
  unspecified site C71.9
General, generalized — see condition
Genetic
  carrier (status)
    cystic fibrosis Z14.1
    hemophilia A (asymptomatic) Z14.01
      symptomatic Z14.02
    specified NEC Z14.8

Genetic — continued
  susceptibility to disease NEC Z15.89
    malignant neoplasm Z15.09
      breast Z15.01
      endometrium Z15.04
      ovary Z15.02
      prostate Z15.03
      specified type NEC Z15.09
    multiple endocrine neoplasia Z15.81
Genital — see condition
Genito-anorectal syndrome A55
Genitourinary system — see condition
Genu
  congenital Q74.1
  extrorsum (acquired) — see also Deformity, varus, knee
    congenital Q74.1
    sequelae (late effect) of rickets E64.3
  introrsum (acquired) — see also Deformity, valgus, knee
    congenital Q74.1
    sequelae (late effect) of rickets E64.3
  rachitic (old) E64.3
  recurvatum (acquired) — see also Deformity, limb, specified type NEC, lower leg
    congenital Q68.2
    sequelae (late effect) of rickets E64.3
  valgum (acquired) (knock-knee) M21.06-
    congenital Q74.1
    sequelae (late effect) of rickets E64.3
  varum (acquired) (bowleg) M21.16-
    congenital Q74.1
    sequelae (late effect) of rickets E64.3
Geographic tongue K14.1
Geophagia — see Pica
Geotrichosis B48.3
  stomatitis B48.3
Gephyrophobia F40.242
Gerbode defect Q21.0
GERD (gastroesophageal reflux disease) K21.9
Gerhardt's
  disease (erythromelalgia) I73.81
  syndrome (vocal cord paralysis) J38.00
    bilateral J38.02
    unilateral J38.01
German measles — see also Rubella
  exposure to Z20.4
Germinoblastoma (diffuse) C85.9-
  follicular C82.9-
Germinoma — see Neoplasm, malignant, by site
Gerontoxon — see Degeneration, cornea, senile
Gerstmann's syndrome R48.8
  developmental F81.2
Gerstmann-Sträussler-Scheinker syndrome (GSS) A81.82
Gestation (period) — see also Pregnancy
  ectopic — see Pregnancy, by site
  multiple O30.9-
    greater than quadruplets — see Pregnancy, multiple (gestation), specified NEC
    specified NEC — see Pregnancy, multiple (gestation), specified NEC
Gestational
  mammary abscess O91.11-
  purulent mastitis O91.11-
  subareolar abscess O91.11-
Ghon tubercle, primary infection A15.7
Ghost
  teeth K00.4
  vessels (cornea) H16.41-
Ghoul hand A66.3
Gianotti-Crosti disease L44.4
Giant
  cell
    epulis K06.8
    peripheral granuloma K06.8
  esophagus, congenital Q39.5
  kidney, congenital Q63.3
  urticaria T78.3
    hereditary D84.1
Giardiasis A07.1
Gibert's disease or pityriasis L42
Giddiness R42
  hysterical F44.89
  psychogenic F45.8
Gierke's disease (glycogenosis I) E74.01
Gigantism (cerebral) (hypophyseal) (pituitary) E22.0
  constitutional E34.4
Gilbert's disease or syndrome E80.4

Gilchrist's disease B40.9
Gilford-Hutchinson disease E34.8
Gilles de la Tourette's disease or syndrome (motor-verbal tic) F95.2
Gingivitis K05.10
  acute (catarrhal) K05.00
    necrotizing A69.1
    nonplaque induced K05.01
    plaque induced K05.00
  chronic (desquamative) (hyperplastic) (simple marginal) (ulcerative) K05.10
    nonplaque induced K05.11
    plaque induced K05.10
  expulsiva — see Periodontitis
  necrotizing ulcerative (acute) A69.1
  pellagrous E52
    acute necrotizing A69.1
  Vincent's A69.1
Gingivoglossitis K14.0
Gingivopericementitis — see Periodontitis
Gingivosis — see Gingivitis, chronic
Gingivostomatitis K05.10
  herpesviral B00.2
  necrotizing ulcerative (acute) A69.1
Gland, glandular — see condition
Glanders A24.0
Glanzmann (-Naegeli) disease or thrombasthenia D69.1
Glasgow coma scale
  total score
    3-8 R40.243
    9-12 R40.242
    13-15 R40.241
Glass-blower's disease (cataract) — see Cataract, specified NEC
Glaucoma H40.9
  with
    increased episcleral venous pressure H40.81-
    pseudoexfoliation of lens — see Glaucoma, open angle, primary, capsular
  absolute H44.51-
  angle-closure (primary) H40.20-
    acute (attack) (crisis) H40.21-
    chronic H40.22-
    intermittent H40.23-
    residual stage H40.24-
  borderline H40.00-
  capsular (with pseudoexfoliation of lens) — see Glaucoma, open angle, primary, capsular
  childhood Q15.0
  closed angle — see Glaucoma, angle-closure
  congenital Q15.0
  corticosteroid-induced — see Glaucoma, secondary, drugs
  hypersecretion H40.82-
  in (due to)
    amyloidosis E85.4 [H42]
    aniridia Q13.1 [H42]
    concussion of globe — see Glaucoma, secondary, trauma
    dislocation of lens — see Glaucoma, secondary
    disorder of lens NEC — see Glaucoma, secondary
    drugs — see Glaucoma, secondary, drugs
    endocrine disease NOS E34.9 [H42]
    eye
      inflammation — see Glaucoma, secondary, inflammation
      trauma — see Glaucoma, secondary, trauma
    hypermature cataract — see Glaucoma, secondary
    iridocyclitis — see Glaucoma, secondary, inflammation
    lens disorder — see Glaucoma, secondary,
    Lowe's syndrome E72.03 [H42]
    metabolic disease NOS E88.9 [H42]
    ocular disorders NEC — see Glaucoma, secondary
    onchocerciasis B73.02
    pupillary block — see Glaucoma, secondary
    retinal vein occlusion — see Glaucoma, secondary
    Rieger's anomaly Q13.81 [H42]
    rubeosis of iris — see Glaucoma, secondary
    tumor of globe — see Glaucoma, secondary
  infantile Q15.0
  low tension — see Glaucoma, open angle, primary, low-tension
  malignant H40.83-

Glaucoma H40.9 — continued
  narrow angle — see Glaucoma, angle-closure
  newborn Q15.0
  noncongestive (chronic) — see Glaucoma, open angle
  nonobstructive — see Glaucoma, open angle
  obstructive — see also Glaucoma, angle-closure
    due to lens changes — see Glaucoma, secondary
  open angle H40.10-
    primary H40.11-
      capsular (with pseudoexfoliation of lens) H40.14-
      low-tension H40.12-
      pigmentary H40.13-
      residual stage H40.15-
  phacolytic — see Glaucoma, secondary
  pigmentary — see Glaucoma, open angle, primary, pigmentary
  postinfectious — see Glaucoma, secondary, inflammation
  secondary (to) H40.5-
    drugs H40.6-
    inflammation H40.4-
    trauma H40.3-
  simple (chronic) H40.11-
  simplex H40.11-
  specified type NEC H40.89
  suspect H40.00-
  syphilitic A52.71
  traumatic — see also Glaucoma, secondary, trauma
    newborn (birth injury) P15.3
  tuberculous A18.59
Glaucomatous flecks (subcapsular) — see Cataract, complicated
Glazed tongue K14.4
Gleet (gonococcal) A54.01
Glénard's disease K63.4
Glioblastoma (multiforme)
  with sarcomatous component
    specified site — see Neoplasm, malignant, by site
    unspecified site C71.9
  giant cell
    specified site — see Neoplasm, malignant, by site
    unspecified site C71.9
  specified site — see Neoplasm, malignant, by site
  unspecified site C71.9
Glioma (malignant)
  astrocytic
    specified site — see Neoplasm, malignant, by site
    unspecified site C71.9
  mixed
    specified site — see Neoplasm, malignant, by site
    unspecified site C71.9
  nose Q30.8
  specified site NEC — see Neoplasm, malignant, by site
  subependymal D43.2
    specified site — see Neoplasm, uncertain behavior, by site
    unspecified site D43.2
  unspecified site C71.9
Gliomatosis cerebri C71.0
Glioneuroma — see Neoplasm, uncertain behavior, by site
Gliosarcoma
  specified site — see Neoplasm, malignant, by site
  unspecified site C71.9
Gliosis (cerebral) G93.89
  spinal G95.89
Glisson's disease — see Rickets
Globinuria R82.3
Globus (hystericus) F45.8
Glomangioma D18.00
  intra-abdominal D18.03
  intracranial D18.02
  skin D18.01
  specified site NEC D18.09
Glomangiomyoma D18.00
  intra-abdominal D18.03
  intracranial D18.02
  skin D18.01
  specified site NEC D18.09
Glomangiosarcoma — see Neoplasm, connective tissue, malignant
Glomerular
  disease in syphilis A52.75
  nephritis — see Glomerulonephritis
Glomerulitis — see Glomerulonephritis

© 2013 Channel Publishing, Ltd.

Glomerulonephritis (see also Nephritis) N05.9
with
  edema — see Nephrosis
  minimal change N05.0
  minor glomerular abnormality N05.0
acute N00.9
chronic N03.9
crescentic (diffuse) NEC (see also N00-N07 with fourth character .7) N05.7
dense deposit (see also N00-N07 with fourth character .6) N05.6
diffuse
  crescentic (see also N00-N07 with fourth character .7) N05.7
  endocapillary proliferative (see also N00-N07 with fourth character .4) N05.4
  membranous (see also N00-N07 with fourth character .2) N05.2
  mesangial proliferative (see also N00-N07 with fourth character .3) N05.3
  mesangiocapillary (see also N00-N07 with fourth character .5) N05.5
  sclerosing N05.8
endocapillary proliferative (diffuse) NEC (see also N00-N07 with fourth character .4) N05.4
extracapillary NEC (see also N00-N07 with fourth character .7) N05.7
focal (and segmental) (see also N00-N07 with fourth character .1) N05.1
hypocomplementemic — see Glomerulonephritis, membranoproliferative
IgA — see Nephropathy, IgA
immune complex (circulating) NEC N05.8
in (due to)
  amyloidosis E85.4 [N08]
  bilharziasis B65.9 [N08]
  cryoglobulinemia D89.1 [N08]
  defibrination syndrome D65 [N08]
  diabetes mellitus — see Diabetes, glomerulosclerosis
  disseminated intravascular coagulation D65 [N08]
  Fabry(-Anderson) disease E75.21 [N08]
  Goodpasture's syndrome M31.0
  hemolytic-uremic syndrome D59.3
  Henoch(-Schönlein) purpura D69.0 [N08]
  lecithin cholesterol acyltransferase deficiency E78.6 [N08]
  microscopic polyangiitis M31.7 [N08]
  multiple myeloma C90.0-[N08]
  Plasmodium malariae B52.0
  schistosomiasis B65.9 [N08]
  sepsis A41.9 [N08]
    streptococcal A40-[N08]
  sickle-cell disorders D57-[N08]
  strongyloidiasis B78.9 [N08]
  subacute bacterial endocarditis I33.0 [N08]
  syphilis (late) congenital A50.59 [N08]
  systemic lupus erythematosus M32.14
  thrombotic thrombocytopenic purpura M31.1 [N08]
  typhoid fever A01.09
  Waldenström macroglobulinemia C88.0 [N08]
  Wegener's granulomatosis M31.31
latent or quiescent N03.9
lobular, lobulonodular — see Glomerulonephritis, membranoproliferative
membranoproliferative (diffuse)(type 1 or 3) (see also N00-N07 with fourth character .5) N05.5
  dense deposit (type 2) NEC (see also N00-N07 with fourth character .6) N05.6
  membranous (diffuse) NEC (see also N00-N07 with fourth character .2) N05.2
mesangial
  IgA/IgG — see Nephropathy, IgA
  proliferative (diffuse) NEC (see also N00-N07 with fourth character .3) N05.3
mesangiocapillary (diffuse) NEC (see also N00-N07 with fourth character .5) N05.5
necrotic, necrotizing NEC (see also N00-N07 with fourth character .8) N05.8
nodular — see Glomerulonephritis, membranoproliferative

Glomerulonephritis (see also Nephritis) N05.9 — continued
poststreptococcal NEC N05.9
  acute N00.9
  chronic N03.9
  rapidly progressive N01.9
proliferative NEC (see also N00-N07 with fourth character .8) N05.8
  diffuse (lupus) M32.14
rapidly progressive N01.9
sclerosing, diffuse N05.8
specified pathology NEC (see also N00-N07 with fourth character .8) N05.8
subacute N01.9
Glomerulopathy — see Glomerulonephritis
Glomerulosclerosis — see also Sclerosis, renal
intercapillary (nodular) (with diabetes) — see Diabetes, glomerulosclerosis
intracapillary — see Diabetes, glomerulosclerosis
Glossagra K14.6
Glossalgia K14.6
Glossitis (chronic superficial) (gangrenous) (Moeller's) K14.0
areata exfoliativa K14.1
atrophic K14.4
benign migratory K14.1
cortical superficial, sclerotic K14.0
Hunter's D51.0
interstitial, sclerous K14.0
median rhomboid K14.2
pellagrous E52
superficial, chronic K14.0
Glossocele K14.8
Glossodynia K14.6
exfoliativa K14.4
Glossoncus K14.8
Glossopathy K14.9
Glossophytia K14.3
Glossoplegia K14.8
Glossoptosis K14.8
Glossopyrosis K14.6
Glossotrichia K14.3
Glossy skin L90.8
Glottis — see condition
Glottitis (see also Laryngitis) J04.0
Glucagonoma
pancreas
  benign D13.7
  malignant C25.4
  uncertain behavior D37.8
specified site NEC
  benign — see Neoplasm, benign, by site
  malignant — see Neoplasm, malignant, by site
  uncertain behavior — see Neoplasm, uncertain behavior, by site
unspecified site
  benign D13.7
  malignant C25.4
  uncertain behavior D37.8
Glucoglycinuria E72.51
Glucose-galactose malabsorption E74.39
Glue
ear — see Otitis, media, nonsuppurative, chronic, mucoid
sniffing (airplane) — see Abuse, drug, inhalant
  dependence — see Dependence, drug, inhalant
Glutaric aciduria E72.3
Glycinemia E72.51
Glycinuria (renal) (with ketosis) E72.09
Glycogen
infiltration — see Disease, glycogen storage
storage disease — see Disease, glycogen storage
Glycogenosis (diffuse) (generalized) — see also Disease, glycogen storage
cardiac E74.02 [I43]
diabetic, secondary — see Diabetes, glycogenosis, secondary
pulmonary interstitial J84.842
Glycopenia E16.2
Glycosuria R81
renal E74.8
Gnathostoma spinigerum (infection) (infestation), gnathostomiasis (wandering swelling) B83.1

Goiter (plunging) (substernal) E04.9
with
  hyperthyroidism (recurrent) — see Hyperthyroidism, with, goiter
  thyrotoxicosis — see Hyperthyroidism, with, goiter
adenomatous — see Goiter, nodular
cancerous C73
congenital (nontoxic) E03.0
  diffuse E03.0
  parenchymatous E03.0
  transitory, with normal functioning P72.0
cystic E04.2
  due to iodine-deficiency E01.1
due to
  enzyme defect in synthesis of thyroid hormone E07.1
  iodine-deficiency (endemic) E01.2
dyshormonogenetic (familial) E07.1
endemic (iodine-deficiency) E01.2
  diffuse E01.0
  multinodular E01.1
exophthalmic — see Hyperthyroidism, with, goiter
iodine-deficiency (endemic) E01.2
  diffuse E01.0
  multinodular E01.1
  nodular E01.1
lingual Q89.2
lymphadenoid E06.3
malignant C73
multinodular (cystic) (nontoxic) E04.2
  toxic or with hyperthyroidism E05.20
    with thyroid storm E05.21
neonatal NEC P72.0
nodular (nontoxic) (due to) E04.9
  with
    hyperthyroidism E05.20
      with thyroid storm E05.21
    thyrotoxicosis E05.20
      with thyroid storm E05.21
  endemic E01.1
  iodine-deficiency E01.1
  sporadic E04.9
  toxic E05.20
    with thyroid storm E05.21
nontoxic E04.9
  diffuse (colloid) E04.0
  multinodular E04.2
  simple E04.0
  specified NEC E04.8
  uninodular E04.1
simple E04.0
toxic — see Hyperthyroidism, with, goiter
uninodular (nontoxic) E04.1
  toxic or with hyperthyroidism E05.10
    with thyroid storm E05.11
Goiter-deafness syndrome E07.1
Goldberg syndrome Q89.8
Goldberg-Maxwell syndrome E34.51
Goldblatt's hypertension or kidney I70.1
Goldenhar(-Gorlin) syndrome Q87.0
Goldflam-Erb disease or syndrome G70.00
with exacerbation (acute) G70.01
in crisis G70.01
Goldscheider's disease Q81.8
Goldstein's disease (familial hemorrhagic telangiectasia) I78.0
Golfer's elbow — see Epicondylitis, medial
Gonadoblastoma
specified site — see Neoplasm, uncertain behavior, by site
unspecified site
  female D39.10
  male D40.10
Gonecystitis — see Vesiculitis
Gongylonemiasis B83.8
Goniosynechiae — see Adhesions, iris, goniosynechiae
Gonococcemia A54.86
Gonococcus, gonococcal (disease) (infection) (see also condition) A54.9
anus A54.6
bursa, bursitis A54.49
conjunctiva, conjunctivitis (neonatorum) A54.31
endocardium A54.83
eye A54.30
  conjunctivitis A54.31
  iridocyclitis A54.32
  keratitis A54.33
  newborn A54.31
  other specified A54.39
fallopian tubes (acute) (chronic) A54.24

Gonococcus, gonococcal (disease) (infection) (see also condition) A54.9 — continued
genitourinary (organ) (system) (tract) (acute)
  lower A54.00
    with abscess (accessory gland) (periurethral) A54.1
  upper (see also condition) A54.29
heart A54.83
iridocyclitis A54.32
joint A54.42
lymphatic (gland) (node) A54.89
meninges, meningitis A54.81
musculoskeletal A54.40
  arthritis A54.42
  osteomyelitis A54.43
  other specified A54.49
  spondylopathy A54.41
pelviperitonitis A54.24
pelvis (acute) (chronic) A54.24
pharynx A54.5
proctitis A54.6
pyosalpinx (acute) (chronic) A54.24
rectum A54.6
skin A54.89
specified site NEC A54.89
tendon sheath A54.49
throat A54.5
urethra (acute) (chronic) A54.01
  with abscess (accessory gland) (periurethral) A54.1
vulva (acute) (chronic) A54.02
Gonocytoma
specified site — see Neoplasm, uncertain behavior, by site
unspecified site
  female D39.10
  male D40.10
Gonorrhea (acute) (chronic) A54.9
Bartholin's gland (acute) (chronic) (purulent) A54.02
  with abscess (accessory gland) (periurethral) A54.1
bladder A54.01
cervix A54.03
conjunctiva, conjunctivitis (neonatorum) A54.31
contact Z20.2
Cowper's gland (with abscess) A54.1
exposure to Z20.2
fallopian tube (acute) (chronic) A54.24
kidney (acute) (chronic) A54.21
lower genitourinary tract A54.00
  with abscess (accessory gland) (periurethral) A54.1
ovary (acute) (chronic) A54.24
pelvis (acute) (chronic) A54.24
  female pelvic inflammatory disease A54.24
penis A54.09
prostate (acute) (chronic) A54.22
seminal vesicle (acute) (chronic) A54.23
specified site not listed (see also Gonococcus) A54.89
spermatic cord (acute) (chronic) A54.23
urethra A54.01
  with abscess (accessory gland) (periurethral) A54.1
vagina A54.02
vas deferens (acute) (chronic) A54.23
vulva A54.02
Goodall's disease A08.19
Goodpasture's syndrome M31.0
Gopalan's syndrome (burning feet) E53.0
Gorlin-Chaudry-Moss syndrome Q87.0
Gottron's papules L94.4
Gougerot-Blum syndrome (pigmented purpuric lichenoid dermatitis) L81.7
Gougerot-Carteaud disease or syndrome (confluent reticulate papillomatosis) L83
Gougerot's syndrome (trisymptomatic) L81.7
Gouley's syndrome (constrictive pericarditis) I31.1
Goundou A66.6

D I S E A S E   I N D E X

Gout, chronic (*see also* **Gout, gouty**) M1A.9
  drug-induced M1A.20
    ankle M1A.27-
    elbow M1A.22-
    foot joint M1A.27-
    hand joint M1A.24-
    hip M1A.25-
    knee M1A.26-
    multiple site M1A.29-
    shoulder M1A.21-
    vertebrae M1A.28
    wrist M1A.23-
  idiopathic M1A.00
    ankle M1A.07-
    elbow M1A.02-
    foot joint M1A.07-
    hand joint M1A.04-
    hip M1A.05-
    knee M1A.06-
    multiple site M1A.09
    shoulder M1A.01-
    vertebrae M1A.08
    wrist M1A.03-
  in (due to) renal impairment M1A.30
    ankle M1A.37-
    elbow M1A.32-
    foot joint M1A.37-
    hand joint M1A.34-
    hip M1A.35-
    knee M1A.36-
    multiple site M1A.39
    shoulder M1A.31-
    vertebrae M1A.38
    wrist M1A.33-
  lead-induced M1A.10
    ankle M1A.17-
    elbow M1A.12-
    foot joint M1A.17-
    hand joint M1A.14-
    hip M1A.15-
    knee M1A.16-
    multiple site M1A.19
    shoulder M1A.11-
    vertebrae M1A.18
    wrist M1A.13-
  primary — *see* Gout, chronic, idiopathic
  saturnine — *see* Gout, chronic, lead-induced
  secondary NEC M1A.40
    ankle M1A.47-
    elbow M1A.42-
    foot joint M1A.47-
    hand joint M1A.44-
    hip M1A.45-
    knee M1A.46-
    multiple site M1A.49
    shoulder M1A.41-
    vertebrae M1A.48
    wrist M1A.43-
  syphilitic (*see also* subcategory M14.8-) A52.77
  tophi M1A.9
Gout, gouty (acute) (attack) (flare) (*see also* **Gout, chronic**) M10.9
  drug-induced M10.20
    ankle M10.27-
    elbow M10.22-
    foot joint M10.27-
    hand joint M10.24-
    hip M10.25-
    knee M10.26-
    multiple site M10.29
    shoulder M10.21-
    vertebrae M10.28
    wrist M10.23-
  idiopathic M10.00
    ankle M10.07-
    elbow M10.02-
    foot joint M10.07-
    hand joint M10.04-
    hip M10.05-
    knee M10.06-
    multiple site M10.09
    shoulder M10.01-
    vertebrae M10.08
    wrist M10.03-
  in (due to) renal impairment M10.30
    ankle M10.37-
    elbow M10.32-
    foot joint M10.37-
    hand joint M10.34-
    hip M10.35-
    knee M10.36-
    multiple site M10.39
    shoulder M10.31-
    vertebrae M10.38
    wrist M10.33-

Gout, gouty (acute) (attack) (flare) (*see also* **Gout, chronic**) M10.9 — *continued*
  lead-induced M10.10
    ankle M10.17-
    elbow M10.12-
    foot joint M10.17-
    hand joint M10.14-
    hip M10.15-
    knee M10.16-
    multiple site M10.19
    shoulder M10.11-
    vertebrae M10.18
    wrist M10.13-
  primary — *see* Gout, idiopathic
  saturnine — *see* Gout, lead-induced
  secondary NEC M10.40
    ankle M10.47-
    elbow M10.42-
    foot joint M10.47-
    hand joint M10.44-
    hip M10.45-
    knee M10.46-
    multiple site M10.49
    shoulder M10.41-
    vertebrae M10.48
    wrist M10.43-
  syphilitic (*see also* subcategory M14.8-) A52.77
  tophi — *see* Gout, chronic
Gower's
  muscular dystrophy G71.0
  syndrome (vasovagal attack) R55
Gradenigo's syndrome — *see* Otitis, media, suppurative, acute
Graefe's disease — *see* Strabismus, paralytic, ophthalmoplegia, progressive
Graft-versus-host disease D89.813
  acute D89.810
  acute on chronic D89.812
  chronic D89.811
Grain mite (itch) B88.0
Grainhandler's disease or lung J67.8
Grand mal — *see* Epilepsy, generalized, specified NEC
Grand multipara status only (not pregnant) Z64.1
  pregnant — *see* Pregnancy, complicated by, grand multiparity
Granite worker's lung J62.8
Granular — *see also* condition
  inflammation, pharynx J31.2
  kidney (contracting) — *see* Sclerosis, renal
  liver K74.69
Granulation tissue (abnormal) (excessive) L92.9
  postmastoidectomy cavity — *see* Complications, postmastoidectomy, granulation
Granulocytopenia (primary) (malignant) — *see* Agranulocytosis
Granuloma L92.9
  abdomen K66.8
    from residual foreign body L92.3
    pyogenicum L98.0
  actinic L57.5
  annulare (perforating) L92.0
  apical K04.5
  aural — *see* Otitis, externa, specified NEC
  beryllium (skin) L92.3
  bone
    eosinophilic C96.6
    from residual foreign body — *see* Osteomyelitis, specified type NEC
    lung C96.6
  brain (any site) G06.0
    schistosomiasis B65.9 [G07]
  canaliculus lacrimalis — *see* Granuloma, lacrimal
  candidal (cutaneous) B37.2
  cerebral (any site) G06.0
  coccidioidal (primary) (progressive) B38.7
    lung B38.1
    meninges B38.4
  colon K63.89
  conjunctiva H11.22-
  dental K04.5
  ear, middle — *see* Cholesteatoma
  eosinophilic C96.6
    bone C96.6
    lung C96.6
    oral mucosa K13.4
    skin L92.2
  eyelid H01.8
  facial(e) L92.2

Granuloma L92.9 — *continued*
  foreign body (in soft tissue) NEC M60.20
    ankle M60.27-
    foot M60.27-
    forearm M60.23-
    hand M60.24-
    in operation wound — *see* Foreign body, accidentally left during a procedure
    lower leg M60.26-
    pelvic region M60.25-
    shoulder region M60.21-
    skin L92.3
    specified site NEC M60.28
    subcutaneous tissue L92.3
    thigh M60.25-
    upper arm M60.22-
  gangraenescens M31.2
  genito-inguinale A58
  giant cell (central) (reparative) (jaw) M27.1
    gingiva (peripheral) K06.8
  gland (lymph) I88.8
  hepatic NEC K75.3
    in (due to)
      berylliosis J63.2 [K77]
      sarcoidosis D86.89
  Hodgkin C81.9
  ileum K63.89
  infectious B99.9
    specified NEC B99.8
  inguinale (Donovan) (venereal) A58
  intestine NEC K63.89
  intracranial (any site) G06.0
  intraspinal (any part) G06.1
  iridocyclitis — *see* Iridocyclitis, chronic
  jaw (bone) (central) M27.1
    reparative giant cell M27.1
  kidney (*see also* Infection, kidney) N15.8
  lacrimal H04.81-
  larynx J38.7
  lethal midline (faciale(e)) M31.2
  liver NEC — *see* Granuloma, hepatic
  lung (infectious) — *see also* Fibrosis, lung
    coccidioidal B38.1
    eosinophilic C96.6
  Majocchi's B35.8
  malignant (facial(e)) M31.2
  mandible (central) M27.1
  midline (lethal) M31.2
  monilial (cutaneous) B37.2
  nasal sinus — *see* Sinusitis
  operation wound T81.89
    foreign body — *see* Foreign body, accidentally left during a procedure
    stitch T81.89
    talc — *see* Foreign body, accidentally left during a procedure
  oral mucosa K13.4
  orbit, orbital H05.11-
  paracoccidioidal B41.8
  penis, venereal A58
  periapical K04.5
  peritoneum K66.8
    due to ova of helminths NOS (*see also* Helminthiasis) B83.9 [K67]
  postmastoidectomy cavity — *see* Complications, postmastoidectomy, recurrent cholesteatoma
  prostate N42.89
  pudendi (ulcerating) A58
  pulp, internal (tooth) K03.3
  pyogenic, pyogenicum (of) (skin) L98.0
    gingiva K06.8
    maxillary alveolar ridge K04.5
    oral mucosa K13.4
  rectum K62.89
  reticulohistiocytic D76.3
  rubrum nasi L74.8
  Schistosoma — *see* Schistosomiasis
  septic (skin) L98.0
  silica (skin) L92.3
  sinus (accessory) (infective) (nasal) — *see* Sinusitis
  skin L92.9
    from residual foreign body L92.3
    pyogenicum L98.0
  spine
    syphilitic (epidural) A52.19
    tuberculous A18.01
  stitch (postoperative) T81.89
  suppurative (skin) L98.0
  swimming pool A31.1
  talc — *see also* Granuloma, foreign body
    in operation wound — *see* Foreign body, accidentally left during a procedure
  telangiectaticum (skin) L98.0

Granuloma L92.9 — *continued*
  tracheostomy J95.09
  trichophyticum B35.8
  tropicum A66.4
  umbilicus L92.9
  urethra N36.8
  uveitis — *see* Iridocyclitis, chronic
  vagina A58
  venereum A58
  vocal cord J38.3
Granulomatosis L92.9
  lymphoid C83.8-
  miliary (listerial) A32.89
  necrotizing, respiratory M31.30
  progressive septic D71
  specified NEC L92.8
  Wegener's M31.30
    with renal involvement M31.31
Granulomatous tissue (abnormal) (excessive) L92.9
Granulosis rubra nasi L74.8
Graphite fibrosis (of lung) J63.3
Graphospasm F48.8
  organic G25.89
Grating scapula M89.8x1
Gravel (urinary) — *see* Calculus, urinary
Graves' disease — *see* Hyperthyroidism, with, goiter
Gravis — *see* condition
Grawitz tumor C64-
Gray syndrome (newborn) P93.0
Grayness, hair (premature) L67.1
  congenital Q84.2
Green sickness D50.8
Greenfield's disease
  meaning
    concentric sclerosis (encephalitis periaxialis concentrica) G37.5
    metachromatic leukodystrophy E75.25
Greenstick fracture — code as Fracture, by site
Grey syndrome (newborn) P93.0
Grief F43.21
  prolonged F43.29
  reaction (*see also* Disorder, adjustment) F43.20
Griesinger's disease B76.9
Grinder's lung or pneumoconiosis J62.8
Grinding, teeth
  psychogenic F45.8
  sleep related G47.63
Grip
  Dabney's B33.0
  devil's B33.0
Grippe, grippal — *see also* Influenza
  Balkan A78
  summer, of Italy A93.1
Grisel's disease M43.6
Groin — *see* condition
Grooved tongue K14.5
Ground itch B76.9
Grover's disease or syndrome L11.1
Growing pains, children R29.898
Growth (fungoid) (neoplastic) (new) — *see also* Neoplasm
  adenoid (vegetative) J35.8
  benign — *see* Neoplasm, benign, by site
  malignant — *see* Neoplasm, malignant, by site
  rapid, childhood Z00.2
  secondary — *see* Neoplasm, secondary, by site
Gruby's disease B35.0
Gubler-Millard paralysis or syndrome G46.3
Guerin-Stern syndrome Q74.3
Guidance, insufficient anterior (occlusal) M26.54
Guillain-Barré disease or syndrome G61.0
  sequelae G65.0
Guinea worms (infection) (infestation) B72
Guinon's disease (motor-verbal tic) F95.2
Gull's disease E03.4
Gum — *see* condition
Gumboil K04.7
  with sinus K04.6
Gumma (syphilitic) A52.79
  artery A52.09
    cerebral A52.04
  bone A52.77
    of yaws (late) A66.6
  brain A52.19
  cauda equina A52.19
  central nervous system A52.3
  ciliary body A52.71
  congenital A50.59

Gumma (syphilitic) A52.79 — *continued*
eyelid A52.71
heart A52.06
intracranial A52.19
iris A52.71
kidney A52.75
larynx A52.73
leptomeninges A52.19
liver A52.74
meninges A52.19
myocardium A52.06
nasopharynx A52.73
neurosyphilitic A52.3
nose A52.73
orbit A52.71
palate (soft) A52.79
penis A52.76
pericardium A52.06
pharynx A52.73
pituitary A52.79
scrofulous (tuberculous) A18.4
skin A52.79
specified site NEC A52.79
spinal cord A52.19
tongue A52.79
tonsil A52.73
trachea A52.73
tuberculous A18.4
ulcerative due to yaws A66.4
ureter A52.75
yaws A66.4
bone A66.6
Gunn's syndrome Q07.8
Gunshot wound — *see also* Wound, open
fracture — *code as* Fracture, by site
internal organs — *see* Injury, by site
Gynandrism Q56.0
Gynandroblastoma
specified site — *see* Neoplasm, uncertain behavior, by site
unspecified site
female D39.10
male D40.10
Gynecological examination (periodic) (routine) Z01.419
with abnormal findings Z01.411
Gynecomastia N62
Gynephobia F40.291
Gyrate scalp Q82.8

H

H (Hartnup's) disease E72.02
Haas' disease or osteochondrosis (juvenile) (head of humerus) — *see* Osteochondrosis, juvenile, humerus
Habit, habituation
bad sleep Z72.821
chorea F95.8
disturbance, child F98.9
drug — *see* Dependence, drug
irregular sleep Z72.821
laxative F55.2
spasm — *see* Tic
tic — *see* Tic
Haemophilus (H.) influenzae, as cause of disease classified elsewhere B96.3
Haff disease — *see* Poisoning, mercury
Hageman's factor defect, deficiency or disease D68.2
Haglund's disease or osteochondrosis (juvenile) (os tibiale externum) — *see* Osteochondrosis, juvenile, tarsus
Hailey-Hailey disease Q82.8
Hair — *see also* condition
plucking F63.3
in stereotyped movement disorder F98.4
tourniquet syndrome — *see also* Constriction, external, by site
finger S60.44-
penis S30.842
thumb S60.34-
toe S90.44-
Hairball in stomach T18.2
Hair-pulling, pathological (compulsive) F63.3
Hairy black tongue K14.3
Half vertebra Q76.49
Halitosis R19.6
Hallerman-Streiff syndrome Q87.0
Hallervorden-Spatz disease G23.0
Hallopeau's acrodermatitis or disease L40.2
Hallucination R44.3
auditory R44.0
gustatory R44.2
olfactory R44.2
specified NEC R44.2
tactile R44.2
visual R44.1
Hallucinosis (chronic) F28
alcoholic (acute) F10.951
in
abuse F10.151
dependence F10.251
drug-induced F19.951
cannabis F12.951
cocaine F14.951
hallucinogen F16.151
in
abuse F19.151
cannabis F12.151
cocaine F14.151
hallucinogen F16.151
inhalant F18.151
opioid F11.151
sedative, anxiolytic or hypnotic F13.151
stimulant NEC F15.151
dependence F19.251
cannabis F12.251
cocaine F14.251
hallucinogen F16.251
inhalant F18.251
opioid F11.251
sedative, anxiolytic or hypnotic F13.251
stimulant NEC F15.251
inhalant F18.951
opioid F11.951
sedative, anxiolytic or hypnotic F13.951
stimulant NEC F15.951
organic F06.0
Hallux
deformity (acquired) NEC M20.5x-
limitus M20.5x-
malleus (acquired) NEC M20.3-
rigidus (acquired) M20.2-
congenital Q74.2
sequelae (late effect) of rickets E64.3
valgus (acquired) M20.1-
congenital Q66.6
varus (acquired) M20.3-
congenital Q66.3
Halo, visual H53.19

Hamartoma, hamartoblastoma Q85.9
epithelial (gingival), odontogenic, central or peripheral — *see* Cyst, calcifying odontogenic
Hamartosis Q85.9
Hamman-Rich syndrome J84.114
Hammer toe (acquired) NEC — *see also* Deformity, toe, hammer toe
congenital Q66.89
sequelae (late effect) of rickets E64.3
Hand — *see* condition
Hand-foot syndrome L27.1
Handicap, handicapped
educational Z55.9
specified NEC Z55.8
Hand-Schüller-Christian disease or syndrome C96.5
Hanging (asphyxia) (strangulation) (suffocation) — *see* Asphyxia, traumatic, due to mechanical threat
Hangnail — *see also* Cellulitis, digit
with lymphangitis — *see* Lymphangitis, acute, digit
Hangover (alcohol) F10.129
Hanhart's syndrome Q87.0
Hanot's cirrhosis or disease K74.3
Hanot-Chauffard(-Troisier) syndrome E83.19
Hansen's disease — *see* Leprosy
Hantaan virus disease (Korean hemorrhagic fever) A98.5
Hantavirus disease (with renal manifestations) (Dobrava) (Puumala) (Seoul) A98.5
with pulmonary manifestations (Andes) (Bayou) (Bermejo) (Black Creek Canal) (Choclo) (Juquitiba) (Laguna negra) (Lechiguanas) (New York) (Oran) (Sin nombre) B33.4
Happy puppet syndrome Q93.5
Harada's disease or syndrome H30.81-
Hardening
artery — *see* Arteriosclerosis
brain G93.89
Harelip (complete) (incomplete) — *see* Cleft, lip
Harlequin (newborn) Q80.4
Harley's disease D59.6
Harmful use (of)
alcohol F10.10
anxiolytics — *see* Abuse, drug, sedative
cannabinoids — *see* Abuse, drug, cannabis
cocaine — *see* Abuse, drug, cocaine
drug — *see* Abuse, drug
hallucinogens — *see* Abuse, drug, hallucinogen
hypnotics — *see* Abuse, drug, sedative
opioids — *see* Abuse, drug, opioid
PCP (phencyclidine) — *see* Abuse, drug, hallucinogen
sedatives — *see* Abuse, drug, sedative
stimulants NEC — *see* Abuse, drug, stimulant
Harris' lines — *see* Arrest, epiphyseal
Hartnup's disease E72.02
Harvester's lung J67.0
Harvesting ovum for in vitro fertilization Z31.83
Hashimoto's disease or thyroiditis E06.3
Hashitoxicosis (transient) E06.3
Hassal-Henle bodies or warts (cornea) H18.49
Haut mal — *see* Epilepsy, generalized, specified NEC
Haverhill fever A25.1
Hay fever (*see also* Fever, hay) J30.1
Hayem-Widal syndrome D59.8
Haygarth's nodes M15.8
Haymaker's lung J67.0
Hb (abnormal)
Bart's disease D56.0
disease — *see* Disease, hemoglobin
trait — *see* Trait
Head — *see* condition
Headache R51
allergic NEC G44.89
associated with sexual activity G44.82
chronic daily R51
cluster G44.009
chronic G44.029
intractable G44.021
not intractable G44.029
episodic G44.019
intractable G44.011
not intractable G44.019
intractable G44.001
not intractable G44.009

Headache R51 — *continued*
cough (primary) G44.83
daily chronic R51
drug-induced NEC G44.40
intractable G44.41
not intractable G44.40
exertional (primary) G44.84
histamine G44.009
intractable G44.001
not intractable G44.009
hypnic G44.81
lumbar puncture G97.1
medication overuse G44.40
intractable G44.41
not intractable G44.40
menstrual — *see* Migraine, menstrual
migraine (type) (*see also* Migraine) G43.909
nasal septum R51
neuralgiform, short lasting unilateral, with conjunctival injection and tearing (SUNCT) G44.059
intractable G44.051
not intractable G44.059
new daily persistent (NDPH) G44.52
orgasmic G44.82
periodic syndromes in adults and children G43.C0
with refractory migraine G43.C1
intractable G43.C19
not intractable G43.C09
without refractory migraine G43.C0
post-traumatic G44.309
acute G44.319
intractable G44.311
not intractable G44.319
chronic G44.329
intractable G44.321
not intractable G44.329
intractable G44.301
not intractable G44.309
postspinal puncture G97.1
pre-menstrual — *see* Migraine, menstrual
preorgasmic G44.82
primary
cough G44.83
exertional G44.84
stabbing G44.85
thunderclap G44.53
rebound G44.40
intractable G44.41
not intractable G44.40
short lasting unilateral neuralgiform, with conjunctival injection and tearing (SUNCT) G44.059
intractable G44.051
not intractable G44.059
specified syndrome NEC G44.89
spinal and epidural anesthesia-induced T88.59
in labor and delivery O74.5
in pregnancy O29.4-
postpartum, puerperal O89.4
spinal fluid loss (from puncture) G97.1
stabbing (primary) G44.85
tension(-type) G44.209
chronic G44.229
intractable G44.221
not intractable G44.229
episodic G44.219
intractable G44.211
not intractable G44.219
intractable G44.201
not intractable G44.209
thunderclap (primary) G44.53
vascular NEC G44.1
Healthy
infant
accompanying sick mother Z76.3
receiving care Z76.2
person accompanying sick person Z76.3
Hearing examination Z01.10
with abnormal findings NEC Z01.118
following failed hearing screening Z01.110
for hearing conservation and treatment Z01.12
Heart — *see* condition
Heart beat
abnormality R00.9
specified NEC R00.8
awareness R00.2
rapid R00.0
slow R00.1
Heartburn R12
psychogenic F45.8

DISEASE INDEX

Heat (effects) T67.9
  apoplexy T67.0
  burn (see also Burn) L55.9
  collapse T67.1
  cramps T67.2
  dermatitis or eczema L59.0
  edema T67.7
  erythema — code by site under Burn, first
    degree
  excessive T67.9
    specified effect NEC T67.8
  exhaustion T67.5
    anhydrotic T67.3
    due to
      salt (and water) depletion T67.4
      water depletion T67.3
        with salt depletion T67.4
  fatigue (transient) T67.6
  fever T67.0
  hyperpyrexia T67.0
  prickly L74.0
  prostration — see Heat, exhaustion
  pyrexia T67.0
  rash L74.0
  specified effect NEC T67.8
  stroke T67.0
  sunburn — see Sunburn
  syncope T67.1
Heavy-for-dates NEC (infant) (4000g to
    4499g) P08.1
  exceptionally (4500g or more) P08.0
Hebephrenia, hebephrenic (schizophrenia)
    F20.1
Heberden's disease or nodes (with
    arthropathy) M15.1
Hebra's
  pityriasis L26
  prurigo L28.2
Heel — see condition
Heerfordt's disease D86.89
Hegglin's anomaly or syndrome D72.0
Heilmeyer-Schoner disease D45
Heine-Medin disease A80.9
Heinz body anemia, congenital, D58.2
Heliophobia F40.228
Heller's disease or syndrome F84.3
HELLP syndrome (hemolysis, elevated liver
    enzymes and low platelet count) O14.2-
Helminthiasis — see also Infestation,
    helminth
  Ancylostoma B76.0
  intestinal B82.0
    mixed types (types classifiable to more
      than one of the titles B65.0-B81.3
      and B81.8) B81.4
    specified type NEC B81.8
  mixed types (intestinal) (types classifiable
    to more than one of the titles B65.0-
    B81.3 and B81.8) B81.4
  Necator (americanus) B76.1
  specified type NEC B83.8
Heloma L84
Hemangioblastoma — see Neoplasm,
    connective tissue, uncertain behavior
  malignant — see Neoplasm, connective
    tissue, malignant
Hemangioendothelioma — see also
    Neoplasm, uncertain behavior, by site
  benign D18.00
    intra-abdominal D18.03
    intracranial D18.02
    skin D18.01
    specified site NEC D18.09
  bone (diffuse) — see Neoplasm, bone,
    malignant
  epithelioid — see also Neoplasm, uncertain
    behavior, by site
    malignant — see Neoplasm, malignant,
      by site
  malignant — see Neoplasm, connective
    tissue, malignant
Hemangiofibroma — see Neoplasm, benign,
    by site
Hemangiolipoma — see Lipoma
Hemangioma D18.00
  arteriovenous D18.00
    intra-abdominal D18.03
    intracranial D18.02
    skin D18.01
    specified site NEC D18.09
  capillary D18.00
    intra-abdominal D18.03
    intracranial D18.02
    skin D18.01
    specified site NEC D18.09
  cavernous D18.00
    intra-abdominal D18.03
    intracranial D18.02
    skin D18.01
    specified site NEC D18.09

Hemangioma D18.00 — continued
  epithelioid D18.00
    intra-abdominal D18.03
    intracranial D18.02
    skin D18.01
    specified site NEC D18.09
  histiocytoid D18.00
    intra-abdominal D18.03
    intracranial D18.02
    skin D18.01
    specified site NEC D18.09
  infantile D18.00
    intra-abdominal D18.03
    intracranial D18.02
    skin D18.01
    specified site NEC D18.09
  intra-abdominal D18.03
  intracranial D18.02
  intramuscular D18.00
    intra-abdominal D18.03
    intracranial D18.02
    skin D18.01
    specified site NEC D18.09
  juvenile D18.00
  malignant — see Neoplasm,connective
    tissue, malignant
  plexiform D18.00
    intra-abdominal D18.03
    intracranial D18.02
    skin D18.01
    specified site NEC D18.09
  racemose D18.00
    intra-abdominal D18.03
    intracranial D18.02
    skin D18.01
    specified site NEC D18.09
  sclerosing — see Neoplasm,skin, benign
  simplex D18.00
    intra-abdominal D18.03
    intracranial D18.02
    skin D18.01
    specified site NEC D18.09
  skin D18.01
  specified site NEC D18.09
  venous D18.00
    intra-abdominal D18.03
    intracranial D18.02
    skin D18.01
    specified site NEC D18.09
  verrucous keratotic D18.00
    intra-abdominal D18.03
    intracranial D18.02
    skin D18.01
    specified site NEC D18.09
Hemangiomatosis (systemic) I78.8
  involving single site — see Hemangioma
Hemangiopericytoma — see also Neoplasm,
    connective tissue, uncertain behavior
  benign — see Neoplasm, connective tissue,
    benign
  malignant — see Neoplasm, connective
    tissue, malignant
Hemangiosarcoma — see Neoplasm,
    connective tissue, malignant
Hemarthrosis (nontraumatic) M25.00
  ankle M25.07-
  elbow M25.02-
  foot joint M25.07-
  hand joint M25.04-
  hip M25.05-
  in hemophilic arthropathy — see
    Arthropathy, hemophilic
  knee M25.06-
  shoulder M25.01-
  specified joint NEC M25.08
  traumatic — see Sprain, by site
  vertebrae M25.08
  wrist M25.03-
Hematemesis K92.0
  with ulcer — code by site under Ulcer, with
    hemorrhage K27.4
  newborn, neonatal P54.0
    due to swallowed maternal blood P78.2
Hematidrosis L74.8
Hematinuria — see also Hemoglobinuria
  malarial B50.8
Hematobilia K83.8
Hematocele
  female NEC N94.89
    with ectopic pregnancy O00.9
    ovary N83.8
  male N50.1
Hematochezia (see also Melena) K92.1
Hematochyluria — see also Infestation,
    filarial
  schistosomiasis (bilharziasis) B65.0
Hematocolpos (with hematometra or
    hematosalpinx) N89.7

Hematocornea — see Pigmentation, cornea,
    stromal
Hematogenous — see condition
Hematoma (traumatic) (skin surface intact)
    — see also Contusion
  with
    injury of internal organs — see Injury,
      by site
    open wound — see Wound, open
  amputation stump (surgical) (late) T87.89
  aorta, dissecting I71.00
    abdominal I71.02
    thoracic I71.01
    thoracoabdominal I71.03
  aortic intramural — see Dissection, aorta
  arterial (complicating trauma) — see
    Injury, blood vessel, by site
  auricle — see Contusion, ear
    nontraumatic — see Disorder, pinna,
      hematoma
  birth injury NEC P15.8
  brain (traumatic)
    with
      cerebral laceration or contusion
        (diffuse) — see Injury,
        intracranial, diffuse
        focal — see Injury, intracranial,
          focal
    cerebellar, traumatic S06.37-
    intracerebral, traumatic — see Injury,
      intracranial, intracerebral
      hemorrhage
    newborn NEC P52.4
      birth injury P10.1
    nontraumatic — see Hemorrhage,
      intracranial
    subarachnoid, arachnoid, traumatic —
      see Injury, intracranial,
      subarachnoid hemorrhage
    subdural, traumatic — see Injury,
      intracranial, subdural hemorrhage
  breast (nontraumatic) N64.89
  broad ligament (nontraumatic) N83.7
    traumatic S37.892
  cerebellar, traumatic S06.37-
  cerebral — see Hematoma, brain
  cerebrum S06.36-
    left S06.35-
    right S06.34-
  cesarean delivery wound O90.2
  complicating delivery (perineal) (pelvic)
    (vagina) (vulva) O71.7
  corpus cavernosum (nontraumatic) N48.89
  epididymis (nontraumatic) N50.1
  epidural (traumatic) — see Injury,
    intracranial, epidural hemorrhage
    spinal — see Injury, spinal cord, by
      region
  episiotomy O90.2
  face, birth injury P15.4
  genital organ NEC (nontraumatic)
    female (nonobstetric) N94.89
      traumatic S30.202
    male N50.1
      traumatic S30.201
  internal organs — see Injury, by site
  intracerebral, traumatic — see Injury,
    intracranial, intracerebral hemorrhage
  intraoperative — see Complications,
    intraoperative, hemorrhage
  labia (nontraumatic) (nonobstetric) N90.89
  liver (subcapsular) (nontraumatic) K76.89
    birth injury P15.0
  mediastinum — see Injury, intrathoracic
  mesosalpinx (nontraumatic) N83.7
    traumatic S37.898
  muscle — code by site under Contusion
  nontraumatic
    muscle M79.81
    soft tissue M79.81
  obstetrical surgical wound O90.2
  orbit, orbital (nontraumatic) — see also
    Hemorrhage, orbit
    traumatic — see Contusion, orbit
  pelvis (female) (nontraumatic)
    (nonobstetric) N94.89
    obstetric O71.7
    traumatic — see Injury, by site
  penis (nontraumatic) N48.89
    birth injury P15.5
  perianal (nontraumatic) K64.5
  perineal S30.23
    complicating delivery O71.7
  perirenal — see Injury, kidney
  pinna — see Contusion, ear
    nontraumatic — see Disorder, pinna,
      hematoma

Hematoma (traumatic) (skin surface intact)
    (see also Contusion) — continued
  placenta O43.89-
  postoperative (postprocedural) — see
    Complication, postprocedural,
    hemorrhage
  retroperitoneal (nontraumatic) K66.1
    traumatic S36.892
  scrotum, superficial S30.22
    birth injury P15.5
  seminal vesicle (nontraumatic) N50.1
    traumatic S37.892
  spermatic cord (traumatic) S37.892
    nontraumatic N50.1
  spinal (cord) (meninges) — see also Injury,
    spinal cord, by region
    newborn (birth injury) P11.5
  spleen D73.5
    intraoperative — see Complications,
      intraoperative, hemorrhage, spleen
    postprocedural (postoperative) — see
      Complications, postprocedural,
      hemorrhage, spleen
  sternocleidomastoid, birth injury P15.2
  sternomastoid, birth injury P15.2
  subarachnoid (traumatic) — see Injury,
    intracranial, subarachnoid hemorrhage
    newborn (nontraumatic) P52.5
      due to birth injury P10.3
    nontraumatic — see Hemorrhage,
      intracranial, subarachnoid
  subdural (traumatic) — see Injury,
    intracranial, subdural hemorrhage
    newborn (localized) P52.8
      birth injury P10.0
    nontraumatic — see Hemorrhage,
      intracranial, subdural
  superficial, newborn P54.5
  testis (nontraumatic) N50.1
    birth injury P15.5
  tunica vaginalis (nontraumatic) N50.1
  umbilical cord, complicating delivery
    O69.5
  uterine ligament (broad) (nontraumatic)
    N83.7
    traumatic S37.892
  vagina (ruptured) (nontraumatic) N89.8
    complicating delivery O71.7
  vas deferens (nontraumatic) N50.1
    traumatic S37.892
  vitreous — see Hemorrhage, vitreous
  vulva (nontraumatic) (nonobstetric)
    N90.89
    complicating delivery O71.7
    newborn (birth injury) P15.5
Hematometra N85.7
  with hematocolpos N89.7
Hematomyelia (central) G95.19
  newborn (birth injury) P11.5
  traumatic T14.8
Hematomyelitis G04.90
Hematoperitoneum — see Hemoperitoneum
Hematophobia F40.230
Hematopneumothorax — see Hemothorax
Hematopoiesis, cyclic D70.4
Hematoporphyria — see Porphyria
Hematorachis G95.19
  newborn (birth injury) P11.5
Hematosalpinx N83.6
  with
    hematocolpos N89.7
    hematometra N85.7
      with hematocolpos N89.7
  infectional — see Salpingitis
Hematospermia R36.1
Hematothorax — see Hemothorax
Hematuria R31.9
  benign (familial) (of childhood) — see also
    Hematuria, idiopathic
  essential microscopic R31.1
  due to sulphonamide, sulfonamide — see
    Table of Drugs and Chemicals, by
    drug
  endemic (see also Schistosomiasis) B65.0
  gross R31.0
  idiopathic N02.9
    with glomerular lesion
      crescentic (diffuse)
        glomerulonephritis N02.7
      dense deposit disease N02.6
      endocapillary proliferative
        glomerulonephritis N02.4
      focal and segmental hyalinosis or
        sclerosis N02.1
      membranoproliferative (diffuse)
        N02.5
      membranous (diffuse) N02.2

Hematuria R31.9 — *continued*
  idiopathic N02.9 — *continued*
    with glomerular lesion — *continued*
      mesangial proliferative (diffuse) N02.3
      mesangiocapillary (diffuse) N02.5
      minor abnormality N02.0
      proliferative NEC N02.8
      specified pathology NEC N02.8
  intermittent — *see* Hematuria, idiopathic
  malarial B50.8
  microscopic NEC R31.2
    benign essential R31.1
  paroxysmal — *see also* Hematuria, idiopathic
    nocturnal D59.5
  persistent — *see* Hematuria, idiopathic
  recurrent — *see* Hematuria, idiopathic
  tropical (*see also* Schistosomiasis) B65.0
  tuberculous A18.13
Hemeralopia (day blindness) H53.11
  vitamin A deficiency E50.5
Hemi-akinesia R41.4
Hemianalgesia R20.0
Hemianencephaly Q00.0
Hemianesthesia R20.0
Hemianopia, hemianopsia (heteronymous) H53.47
  homonymous H53.46-
  syphilitic A52.71
Hemiathetosis R25.8
Hemiatrophy R68.89
  cerebellar G31.9
  face, facial, progressive (Romberg) G51.8
  tongue K14.8
Hemiballism(us) G25.5
Hemicardia Q24.8
Hemicephalus, hemicephaly Q00.0
Hemichorea G25.5
Hemicolitis, left — *see* Colitis, left sided
Hemicrania
  congenital malformation Q00.0
  continua G44.51
  meaning migraine (*see also* Migraine) G43.909
  paroxysmal G44.039
    chronic G44.049
      intractable G44.041
      not intractable G44.049
    episodic G44.039
      intractable G44.031
      not intractable G44.039
    intractable G44.031
    not intractable G44.039
Hemidystrophy — *see* Hemiatrophy
Hemiectromelia Q73.8
Hemihypalgesia R20.8
Hemihypesthesia R20.1
Hemi-inattention R41.4
Hemimelia Q73.8
  lower limb — *see* Defect, reduction, lower limb, specified type NEC
  upper limb — *see* Defect, reduction, upper limb, specified type NEC
Hemiparalysis — *see* Hemiplegia
Hemiparesis — *see* Hemiplegia
Hemiparesthesia R20.2
Hemiparkinsonism G20
Hemiplegia G81.9-
  alternans facialis G83.89
  ascending NEC G81.90
    spinal G95.89
  congenital (cerebral) G80.8
    spastic G80.2
  embolic (current episode) I63.4-
  flaccid G81.0-
  following
    cerebrovascular disease I69.959
      cerebral infarction I69.35-
      intracerebral hemorrhage I69.15-
      nontraumatic intracranial hemorrhage NEC I69.25-
      specified disease NEC I69.85-
      stroke NOS I69.35-
      subarachnoid hemorrhage I69.05-
  hysterical F44.4
  newborn NEC P91.8
    birth injury P11.9
  spastic G81.1-
    congenital G80.2
  thrombotic (current episode) I63.3
Hemisection, spinal cord — *see* Injury, spinal cord, by region
Hemispasm (facial) R25.2
Hemisporosis B48.8
Hemitremor R25.1

Hemivertebra Q76.49
  failure of segmentation with scoliosis Q76.3
  fusion with scoliosis Q76.3
Hemochromatosis E83.119
  with refractory anemia D46.1
  due to repeated red blood cell transfusion E83.111
  hereditary (primary) E83.110
  primary E83.110
  specified NEC E83.118
Hemoglobin — *see also* condition
  abnormal (disease) — *see* Disease, hemoglobin
  AS genotype D57.3
  Constant Spring D58.2
  E-beta thalassemia D56.5
  fetal, hereditary persistence (HPFH) D56.4
  H Constant Spring D56.0
  low NOS D64.9
  S (Hb S), heterozygous D57.3
Hemoglobinemia D59.9
  due to blood transfusion T80.89
  paroxysmal D59.6
    nocturnal D59.5
Hemoglobinopathy (mixed) D58.2
  with thalassemia D56.8
  sickle-cell D57.1
    with thalassemia D57.40
      with crisis (vasoocclusive pain) D57.419
      with
        acute chest syndrome D57.411
        splenic sequestration D57.412
      without crisis D57.40
Hemoglobinuria R82.3
  with anemia, hemolytic, acquired (chronic) NEC D59.6
  cold (agglutinin) (paroxysmal) (with Raynaud's syndrome) D59.6
  due to exertion or hemolysis NEC D59.6
  intermittent D59.6
  malarial B50.8
  march D59.6
  nocturnal (paroxysmal) D59.5
  paroxysmal (cold) D59.6
    nocturnal D59.5
Hemolymphangioma D18.1
Hemolysis
  intravascular
    with
      abortion — *see* Abortion, by type, complicated by, hemorrhage
      ectopic or molar pregnancy O08.1
      hemorrhage
        antepartum — *see* Hemorrhage, antepartum, with coagulation defect
        intrapartum (*see also* Hemorrhage, complicating, delivery) O67.0
    postpartum O72.3
  neonatal (excessive) P58.9
    specified NEC P58.8
Hemolytic — *see* condition
Hemopericardium I31.2
  following acute myocardial infarction (current complication) I23.0
  newborn P54.8
  traumatic — *see* Injury, heart, with hemopericardium
Hemoperitoneum K66.1
  infectional K65.9
  traumatic S36.899
    with open wound — *see* Wound, open, with penetration into peritoneal cavity
Hemophilia (classical) (familial) (hereditary) D66
  A D66
  acquired D68.311
  autoimmune D68.311
  B D67
  C D68.1
  calcipriva (*see also* Defect, coagulation) D68.4
  nonfamilial (*see also* Defect, coagulation) D68.4
  secondary D68.311
  vascular D68.0
Hemophthalmos H44.81-
Hemopneumothorax — *see also* Hemothorax
  traumatic S27.2
Hemoptysis R04.2
  newborn P26.9
  tuberculous — *see* Tuberculosis, pulmonary

Hemorrhage, hemorrhagic (concealed) R58
  abdomen R58
  accidental antepartum — *see* Hemorrhage, antepartum
  acute idiopathic pulmonary, in infants R04.81
  adenoid J35.8
  adrenal (capsule) (gland) E27.49
    medulla E27.8
    newborn P54.4
  after delivery — *see* Hemorrhage, postpartum
  alveolar
    lung, newborn P26.8
    process K08.8
  alveolus K08.8
  amputation stump (surgical) T87.89
  anemia (chronic) D50.0
    acute D62
  antepartum (with) O46.90
    with coagulation defect O46.00-
      afibrinogenemia O46.01-
      disseminated intravascular coagulation O46.02-
      hypofibrinogenemia O46.01-
      specified defect NEC O46.09-
    before 20 weeks gestation O20.9
    specified type NEC O20.8
    threatened abortion O20.0
    due to
      abruptio placenta (*see also* Abruptio placentae) O45.9-
      leiomyoma, uterus — *see* Hemorrhage, antepartum, specified cause NEC
      placenta previa O44.1-
    specified cause NEC — *see* subcategory O46.8x-
  anus (sphincter) K62.5
  apoplexy (stroke) — *see* Hemorrhage, intracranial, intracerebral
  arachnoid — *see* Hemorrhage, intracranial, subarachnoid
  artery R58
    brain — *see* Hemorrhage, intracranial, intracerebral
  basilar (ganglion) I61.0
  bladder N32.89
  bowel K92.2
    newborn P54.3
  brain (miliary) (nontraumatic) — *see* Hemorrhage, intracranial, intracerebral
    due to
      birth injury P10.1
      syphilis A52.05
    epidural or extradural (traumatic) — *see* Injury, intracranial, epidural hemorrhage
    newborn P52.4
      birth injury P10.1
    subarachnoid — *see* Hemorrhage, intracranial, subarachnoid
    subdural — *see* Hemorrhage, intracranial, subdural
  brainstem (nontraumatic) I61.3
    traumatic S06.38-
  breast N64.59
  bronchial tube — *see* Hemorrhage, lung
  bronchopulmonary — *see* Hemorrhage, lung
  bronchus — *see* Hemorrhage, lung
  bulbar I61.5
  capillary I78.8
    primary D69.8
  cecum K92.2
  cerebellar, cerebellum (nontraumatic) I61.4
    newborn P52.6
    traumatic S06.37-
  cerebral, cerebrum — *see also* Hemorrhage, intracranial, intracerebral
    lobe I61.1
    newborn (anoxic) P52.4
      birth injury P10.1
  cerebromeningeal I61.8
  cerebrospinal — *see* Hemorrhage, intracranial, intracerebral
  cervix (uteri) (stump) NEC N88.8
  chamber, anterior (eye) — *see* Hyphema
  childbirth — *see* Hemorrhage, complicating, delivery
  choroid H31.30-
    expulsive H31.31-
  ciliary body — *see* Hyphema
  cochlea — *see* subcategory H83.8
  colon K92.2

Hemorrhage, hemorrhagic (concealed) R58
  — *continued*
  complicating
    abortion — *see* Abortion, by type, complicated by, hemorrhage
    delivery O67.9
      associated with coagulation defect (afibrinogenemia) (DIC) (hyperfibrinolysis) O67.0
      specified cause NEC O67.8
    surgical procedure — *see* Hemorrhage, intraoperative
  conjunctiva H11.3-
    newborn P54.8
  cord, newborn (stump) P51.9
  corpus luteum (ruptured) cyst N83.1
  cortical (brain) I61.1
  cranial — *see* Hemorrhage, intracranial
  cutaneous R23.3
    due to autosensitivity, erythrocyte D69.2
    newborn P54.5
  delayed
    following ectopic or molar pregnancy O08.1
    postpartum O72.2
  diathesis (familial) D69.9
  disease D69.9
    newborn P53
    specified type NEC D69.8
  due to or associated with
    afibrinogenemia or other coagulation defect (conditions in categories D65-D69)
      antepartum — *see* Hemorrhage, antepartum, with coagulation defect
      intrapartum O67.0
  dental implant M27.61
  device, implant or graft (*see also* Complications, by site and type, specified NEC) T85.83
    arterial graft NEC T82.838
    breast T85.83
    catheter NEC T85.83
      dialysis (renal) T82.838
        intraperitoneal T85.83
      infusion NEC T82.838
        spinal (epidural) (subdural) T85.83
      urinary (indwelling) T83.83
    electronic (electrode) (pulse generator) (stimulator)
      bone T84.83
      cardiac T82.837
      nervous system (brain) (peripheral nerve) (spinal) T85.83
      urinary T83.83
    fixation, internal (orthopedic) NEC T84.83
    gastrointestinal (bile duct) (esophagus) T85.83
    genital NEC T83.83
    heart NEC T82.837
    joint prosthesis T84.83
    ocular (corneal graft) (orbital implant) NEC T85.83
    orthopedic NEC T84.83
      bone graft T86.838
    specified NEC T85.83
    urinary NEC T83.83
    vascular NEC T82.838
    ventricular intracranial shunt T85.83
  duodenum, duodenal K92.2
    ulcer — *see* Ulcer, duodenum, with hemorrhage
  dura mater — *see* Hemorrhage, intracranial, subdural
  endotracheal — *see* Hemorrhage, lung
  epicranial subaponeurotic (massive), birth injury P12.2
  epidural (traumatic) — *see also* Injury, intracranial, epidural hemorrhage
    nontraumatic I62.1
  esophagus K22.8
    varix I85.01
      secondary I85.11
  excessive, following ectopic gestation (subsequent episode) O08.1
  extradural (traumatic) — *see* Injury, intracranial, epidural hemorrhage
    birth injury P10.8
    newborn (anoxic) (nontraumatic) P52.8
    nontraumatic I62.1
  eye NEC H57.8
    fundus — *see* Hemorrhage, retina
    lid — *see* Disorder, eyelid, specified type NEC

Hemorrhage, hemorrhagic (concealed) R58
— *continued*
fallopian tube N83.6
fibrinogenolysis — *see* Fibrinolysis
fibrinolytic (acquired) — *see* Fibrinolysis
from
ear (nontraumatic) — *see* Otorrhagia
tracheostomy stoma J95.01
fundus, eye — *see* Hemorrhage, retina
funis — *see* Hemorrhage, umbilicus, cord
gastric — *see* Hemorrhage, stomach
gastroenteric K92.2
newborn P54.3
gastrointestinal (tract) K92.2
newborn P54.3
genital organ, male N50.1
genitourinary (tract) NOS R31.9
gingiva K06.8
globe (eye) — *see* Hemophthalmos
graafian follicle cyst (ruptured) N83.0
gum K06.8
heart I51.89
hypopharyngeal (throat) R04.1
intermenstrual (regular) N92.3
irregular N92.1
internal (organs) NEC R58
capsule I61.0
ear — *see* subcategory H83.8
newborn P54.8
intestine K92.2
newborn P54.3
intra-abdominal R58
intra-alveolar (lung), newborn P26.8
intracerebral (nontraumatic) — *see*
Hemorrhage, intracranial,
intracerebral
intracranial (nontraumatic) I62.9
birth injury P10.9
epidural, nontraumatic I62.1
extradural, nontraumatic I62.1
intracerebral (nontraumatic) (in) I61.9
brain stem I61.3
cerebellum I61.4
hemisphere I61.2
cortical (superficial) I61.1
subcortical (deep) I61.0
intraoperative
during a nervous system procedure
G97.31
during other procedure G97.32
intraventricular I61.5
multiple localized I61.6
newborn P52.4
birth injury P10.1
postprocedural
following a nervous system
procedure G97.51
following other procedure G97.52
specified NEC I61.8
superficial I61.1
traumatic (diffuse) — *see* Injury,
intracranial, diffuse
focal — *see* Injury, intracranial,
focal
newborn P52.9
specified NEC P52.8
subarachnoid (nontraumatic) (from)
I60.9
intracranial (cerebral) artery I60.7
anterior communicating I60.2-
basilar I60.4
carotid siphon and bifurcation
I60.0-
communicating I60.7
anterior I60.2-
posterior I60.3-
middle cerebral I60.1-
posterior communicating I60.3-
specified artery NEC I60.6
vertebral I60.5-
newborn P52.5
birth injury P10.3
specified NEC I60.8
traumatic S06.6x-
subdural (nontraumatic) I62.00
acute I62.01
birth injury P10.0
chronic I62.03
newborn (anoxic) (hypoxic) P52.8
birth injury P10.0
spinal G95.19
subacute I62.02
traumatic — *see* Injury, intracranial,
subdural hemorrhage
subgaleal P12.1
traumatic — *see* Injury, intracranial,
focal brain injury

Hemorrhage, hemorrhagic (concealed) R58
— *continued*
intramedullary NEC G95.19
intraocular — *see* Hemophthalmos
intraoperative, intraprocedural — *see*
Complication, hemorrhage
(hematoma), intraoperative
(intraprocedural), by site
intrapartum — *see* Hemorrhage,
complicating, delivery
intrapelvic
female N94.89
male K66.1
intraperitoneal K66.1
intrapontine I61.3
intraprocedural — *see* Complication,
hemorrhage (hematoma),
intraoperative (intraprocedural), by
site
intrauterine N85.7
complicating delivery (see also
Hemorrhage, complicating,
delivery) O67.9
postpartum — *see* Hemorrhage,
postpartum
intraventricular I61.5
newborn (nontraumatic) (see also
Newborn, affected by, hemorrhage)
P52.3
due to birth injury P10.2
grade
1 P52.0
2 P52.1
3 P52.21
4 P52.22
intravesical N32.89
iris (postinfectional) (postinflammatory)
(toxic) — *see* Hyphema
joint (nontraumatic) — *see* Hemarthrosis
kidney N28.89
knee (joint) (nontraumatic) — *see*
Hemarthrosis, knee
labyrinth — *see* subcategory H83.8
lenticular striate artery I61.0
ligature, vessel — *see* Hemorrhage,
postoperative
liver K76.89
lung R04.89
newborn P26.9
massive P26.1
specified NEC P26.8
tuberculous — *see* Tuberculosis,
pulmonary
massive umbilical, newborn P51.0
mediastinum — *see* Hemorrhage, lung
medulla I61.3
membrane (brain) I60.8
spinal cord — *see* Hemorrhage, spinal
cord
meninges, meningeal (brain) (middle)
I60.8
spinal cord — *see* Hemorrhage, spinal
cord
mesentery K66.1
metritis — *see* Endometritis
mouth K13.79
mucous membrane NEC R58
newborn P54.8
muscle M62.89
nail (subungual) L60.8
nasal turbinate R04.0
newborn P54.8
navel, newborn P51.9
newborn P54.9
specified NEC P54.8
nipple N64.59
nose R04.0
newborn P54.8
omentum K66.1
optic nerve (sheath) H47.02-
orbit, orbital H05.23-
ovary NEC N83.8
oviduct N83.6
pancreas K86.89
parathyroid (gland) (spontaneous) E21.4
parturition — *see* Hemorrhage,
complicating, delivery
penis N48.89
pericardium, pericarditis I31.2
peritoneum, peritoneal K66.1
peritonsillar tissue J35.8
due to infection J36
petechial R23.3
due to autosensitivity, erythrocyte D69.2
pituitary (gland) E23.6
pleura — *see* Hemorrhage, lung
polioencephalitis, superior E51.2

Hemorrhage, hemorrhagic (concealed) R58
— *continued*
polymyositis — *see* Polymyositis
pons, pontine I61.3
posterior fossa (nontraumatic) I61.8
newborn P52.6
postmenopausal N95.0
postnasal R04.0
postoperative — *see* Complications,
postprocedural, hemorrhage, by site
postpartum NEC (following delivery of
placenta) O72.1
delayed or secondary O72.2
retained placenta O72.0
third stage O72.0
pregnancy — *see* Hemorrhage, antepartum
preretinal — *see* Hemorrhage, retina
prostate N42.1
puerperal — *see* Hemorrhage, postpartum
delayed or secondary O72.2
pulmonary R04.89
newborn P26.9
massive P26.1
specified NEC P26.8
tuberculous — *see* Tuberculosis,
pulmonary
purpura (primary) D69.3
rectum (sphincter) K62.5
newborn P54.2
recurring, following initial hemorrhage at
time of injury T79.2
renal N28.89
respiratory passage or tract R04.9
specified NEC R04.89
retina, retinal (vessels) H35.6-
diabetic — *see* Diabetes, retinal,
hemorrhage
retroperitoneal R58
scalp R58
scrotum N50.1
secondary (nontraumatic) R58
following initial hemorrhage at time of
injury T79.2
seminal vesicle N50.1
skin R23.3
newborn P54.5
slipped umbilical ligature P51.8
spermatic cord N50.1
spinal (cord) G95.19
newborn (birth injury) P11.5
spleen D73.5
intraoperative — *see* Complications,
intraoperative, hemorrhage, spleen
postprocedural — *see* Complications,
postprocedural, hemorrhage, spleen
stomach K92.2
newborn P54.3
ulcer — *see* Ulcer, stomach, with
hemorrhage
subarachnoid (nontraumatic) — *see*
Hemorrhage, intracranial,
subarachnoid
subconjunctival — *see also* Hemorrhage,
conjunctiva
birth injury P15.3
subcortical (brain) I61.0
subcutaneous R23.3
subdiaphragmatic R58
subdural (acute) (nontraumatic) — *see*
Hemorrhage, intracranial, subdural
subependymal
newborn P52.0
with intraventricular extension P52.1
and intracerebral extension P52.22
subhyaloid — *see* Hemorrhage, retina
subperiosteal — *see* Disorder, bone,
specified type NEC
subretinal — *see* Hemorrhage, retina
subtentorial — *see* Hemorrhage,
intracranial, subdural
subungual L60.8
suprarenal (capsule) (gland) E27.49
newborn P54.4
tentorium (traumatic) NEC — *see*
Hemorrhage, brain
newborn (birth injury) P10.4
testis N50.1
third stage (postpartum) O72.0
thorax — *see* Hemorrhage, lung
throat R04.1
thymus (gland) E32.8
thyroid (cyst) (gland) E07.89
tongue K14.8
tonsil J35.8
trachea — *see* Hemorrhage, lung

Hemorrhage, hemorrhagic (concealed) R58
— *continued*
tracheobronchial R04.89
newborn P26.0
traumatic — *code to* specific injury
cerebellar — *see* Hemorrhage, brain
intracranial — *see* Hemorrhage, brain
recurring or secondary (following initial
hemorrhage at time of injury)
T79.2
tuberculous NEC (*see also* Tuberculosis,
pulmonary) A15.0
tunica vaginalis N50.1
ulcer — *code by* site under Ulcer, with
hemorrhage K27.4
umbilicus, umbilical
cord
after birth, newborn P51.9
complicating delivery O69.5
newborn P51.9
massive P51.0
slipped ligature P51.8
stump P51.9
urethra (idiopathic) N36.8
uterus, uterine (abnormal) N93.9
climacteric N92.4
complicating delivery — *see*
Hemorrhage, complicating,
delivery
dysfunctional or functional N93.8
intermenstrual (regular) N92.3
irregular N92.1
postmenopausal N95.0
postpartum — *see* Hemorrhage,
postpartum
preclimacteric or premenopausal N92.4
prepubertal N93.8
pubertal N92.2
vagina (abnormal) N93.9
newborn P54.6
vas deferens N50.1
vasa previa O69.4
ventricular I61.5
vesical N32.89
viscera NEC R58
newborn P54.8
vitreous (humor) (intraocular) H43.1-
vulva N90.89
Hemorrhoids (bleeding) (without mention of
degree) K64.9
1st degree (grade/stage I) (without prolapse
outside of anal canal) K64.0
2nd degree (grade/stage II) (that with
prolapse with straining but retract
spontaneously) K64.1
3rd degree (grade/stage III) (that with
prolapse with straining and require
manual replacement back inside anal
canal) K64.2
4th degree (grade/stage IV) (with prolapsed
tissue that cannot be manually
replaced) K64.3
complicating
pregnancy O22.4
puerperium O87.2
external K64.4
with
thrombosis K64.5
internal (without mention of degree) K64.8
prolapsed K64.8
skin tags
anus K64.4
residual K64.4
specified NEC K64.8
strangulated (*see also* Hemorrhoids, by
degree) K64.8
thrombosed (*see also* Hemorrhoids, by
degree) K64.5
ulcerated (*see also* Hemorrhoids, by
degree) K64.8
Hemosalpinx N83.6
with
hematocolpos N89.7
hematometra N85.7
with hematocolpos N89.7
Hemosiderosis (dietary) E83.19
pulmonary, idiopathic E83.1- [J84.03]
transfusion T80.89
Hemothorax (bacterial) (nontuberculous)
J94.2
newborn P54.8
traumatic S27.1
with pneumothorax S27.2
tuberculous NEC A15.6
Henoch(-Schönlein) disease or syndrome
(purpura) D69.0
Henpue, henpuye A66.6

Hepar lobatum (syphilitic) A52.74
Hepatalgia K76.89
Hepatitis K75.9
  acute B17.9
    with coma K72.01
    with hepatic failure — *see* Failure,
      hepatic
    alcoholic — *see* Hepatitis, alcoholic
    infectious B15.9
      with hepatic coma B15.0
    viral B17.9
  alcoholic (acute) (chronic) K70.10
    with ascites K70.11
  amebic — *see* Abscess, liver, amebic
  anicteric, (viral) — *see* Hepatitis, viral
  antigen-associated (HAA) — *see* Hepatitis,
    B
  Australia-antigen (positive) — *see*
    Hepatitis, B
  autoimmune K75.4
  B B19.10
    with hepatic coma B19.11
    acute B16.9
      with
        delta-agent (coinfection) (without
          hepatic coma) B16.1
          with hepatic coma B16.0
        hepatic coma (without delta-agent
          coinfection) B16.2
    chronic B18.1
      with delta-agent B18.0
  bacterial NEC K75.89
  C (viral) B19.20
    with hepatic coma B19.21
    acute B17.10
      with hepatic coma B17.11
    chronic B18.2
  catarrhal (acute) B15.9
    with hepatic coma B15.0
  cholangiolitic K75.89
  cholestatic K75.89
  chronic K73.9
    active NEC K73.2
    lobular NEC K73.1
    persistent NEC K73.0
    specified NEC K73.8
  cytomegaloviral B25.1
  due to ethanol (acute) (chronic) — *see*
    Hepatitis, alcoholic
  epidemic B15.9
    with hepatic coma B15.0
  fulminant NEC (viral) — *see* Hepatitis,
    viral
  granulomatous NEC K75.3
  herpesviral B00.81
  history of
    B Z86.19
    C Z86.19
  homologous serum — *see* Hepatitis, viral,
    type B
  in (due to)
    mumps B26.81
    toxoplasmosis (acquired) B58.1
      congenital (active) P37.1 [K77]
  infectious, infective (acute) (chronic)
    (subacute) B15.9
    with hepatic coma B15.0
  inoculation — *see* Hepatitis, viral, type B
  interstitial (chronic) K74.69
  lupoid NEC K75.4
  malignant NEC (with hepatic failure)
    K72.90
    with coma K72.91
  neonatal giant cell P59.29
  neonatal (idiopathic) (toxic) P59.29
  newborn P59.29
  post-transfusion — *see* Hepatitis, viral,
    type B
  postimmunization — *see* Hepatitis, viral,
    type B
  reactive, nonspecific K75.2
  serum — *see* Hepatitis, viral, type B
  specified type NEC
    with hepatic failure — *see* Failure,
      hepatic
  syphilitic (late) A52.74
    congenital (early) A50.08 [K77]
      late A50.59 [K77]
    secondary A51.45
  toxic (*see also* Disease, liver, toxic) K71.6
  tuberculous A18.83

Hepatitis K75.9 — *continued*
  viral, virus B19.9
    with hepatic coma B19.0
    acute B17.9
    chronic B18.9
      specified NEC B18.8
      type
        B B18.1
          with delta-agent B18.0
        C B18.2
    congenital P35.3
    coxsackie B33.8 [K77]
    cytomegalic inclusion B25.1
    in remission, any type — *code to*
      Hepatitis, chronic, by type
    non-A, non-B B17.8
    specified type NEC (with or without
      coma) B17.8
    type
      A B15.9
        with hepatic coma B15.0
      B B19.10
        with hepatic coma B19.11
        acute B16.9
          with
            delta-agent (coinfection)
              (without hepatic coma)
              B16.1
              with hepatic coma B16.0
            hepatic coma (without delta-
              agent coinfection) B16.2
        chronic B18.1
          with delta-agent B18.0
      C B19.20
        with hepatic coma B19.21
        acute B17.10
          with hepatic coma B17.11
        chronic B18.2
      E B17.2
      non-A, non-B B17.8
Hepatization lung (acute) — *see* Pneumonia,
  lobar
Hepatoblastoma C22.2
Hepatocarcinoma C22.0
Hepatocholangiocarcinoma C22.0
Hepatocholangioma, benign D13.4
Hepatocholangitis K75.89
Hepatolenticular degeneration E83.01
Hepatoma (malignant) C22.0
  benign D13.4
  embryonal C22.0
Hepatomegaly — *see also* Hypertrophy, liver
  with splenomegaly R16.2
  congenital Q44.7
  in mononucleosis
    gammaherpesviral B27.09
    infectious specified NEC B27.89
Hepatoptosis K76.89
Hepatorenal syndrome following labor and
  delivery O90.4
Hepatosis K76.89
Hepatosplenomegaly R16.2
  hyperlipemic (Bürger-Grütz type) E78.3
    [K77]
Hereditary — *see* condition
Heredodegeneration, macular — *see*
  Dystrophy, retina
Heredopathia atactica polyneuritiformis
  G60.1
Heredosyphilis — *see* Syphilis, congenital
Herlitz' syndrome Q81.1
Hermansky-Pudlak syndrome E70.331
Hermaphrodite, hermaphroditism (true)
  Q56.0
  46,XX with streak gonads Q99.1
  46,XX/46,XY Q99.0
  46,XY with streak gonads Q99.1
  chimera 46,XX/46,XY Q99.0
Hernia, hernial (acquired) (recurrent) K46.9
  with
    gangrene — *see* Hernia, by site, with,
      gangrene
    incarceration — *see* Hernia, by site,
      with, obstruction
    irreducible — *see* Hernia, by site, with,
      obstruction
    obstruction — *see* Hernia, by site, with,
      obstruction
    strangulation — *see* Hernia, by site,
      with, obstruction
  abdomen, abdominal K46.9
    with
      gangrene (and obstruction) K46.1
      obstruction K46.0
    femoral — *see* Hernia, femoral
    incisional — *see* Hernia, incisional
    inguinal — *see* Hernia, inguinal

Hernia, hernial (acquired) (recurrent) K46.9
  — *continued*
  abdomen, abdominal K46.9 — *continued*
    specified site NEC K45.8
      with
        gangrene (and obstruction) K45.1
        obstruction K45.0
    umbilical — *see* Hernia, umbilical
    wall — *see* Hernia, ventral
  appendix — *see* Hernia, abdomen
  bladder (mucosa) (sphincter)
    congenital (female) (male) Q79.51
    female — *see* Cystocele
    male N32.89
  brain, congenital — *see* Encephalocele
  cartilage, vertebra — *see* Displacement,
    intervertebral disc
  cerebral, congenital — *see also*
    Encephalocele
    endaural Q01.8
  ciliary body (traumatic) S05.2-
  colon — *see* Hernia, abdomen
  Cooper's — *see* Hernia, abdomen,
    specified site NEC
  crural — *see* Hernia, femoral
  diaphragm, diaphragmatic K44.9
    with
      gangrene (and obstruction) K44.1
      obstruction K44.0
    congenital Q79.0
  direct (inguinal) — *see* Hernia, inguinal
  diverticulum, intestine — *see* Hernia,
    abdomen
  double (inguinal) — *see* Hernia, inguinal,
    bilateral
  due to adhesions (with obstruction) K56.5
  epigastric (*see also* Hernia, ventral) K43.9
  esophageal hiatus — *see* Hernia, hiatal
  external — *see* Hernia, inguinal
  fallopian tube N83.4
  fascia M62.89
  femoral K41.90
    with
      gangrene (and obstruction) K41.40
        not specified as recurrent K41.40
        recurrent K41.41
      obstruction K41.30
        not specified as recurrent K41.30
        recurrent K41.31
    bilateral K41.20
      with
        gangrene (and obstruction) K41.10
          not specified as recurrent K41.10
          recurrent K41.11
        obstruction K41.00
          not specified as recurrent K41.00
          recurrent K41.01
      not specified as recurrent K41.20
      recurrent K41.21
    not specified as recurrent K41.90
    recurrent K41.91
    unilateral K41.90
      with
        gangrene (and obstruction) K41.40
          not specified as recurrent K41.40
          recurrent K41.41
        obstruction K41.30
          not specified as recurrent K41.30
          recurrent K41.31
      not specified as recurrent K41.90
      recurrent K41.91
  foramen magnum G93.5
    congenital Q01.8
  funicular (umbilical) — *see also* Hernia,
    umbilicus
    spermatic (cord) — *see* Hernia, inguinal
  gastrointestinal tract — *see* Hernia,
    abdomen
  Hesselbach's — *see* Hernia, femoral,
    specified site NEC
  hiatal (esophageal) (sliding) K44.9
    with
      gangrene (and obstruction) K44.1
      obstruction K44.0
    congenital Q40.1
  hypogastric — *see* Hernia, ventral
  incarcerated — *see also* Hernia, by site,
    with obstruction
    with gangrene — *see* Hernia, by site,
      with gangrene
  incisional K43.2
    with
      gangrene (and obstruction) K43.1
      obstruction K43.0
  indirect (inguinal) — *see* Hernia, inguinal

Hernia, hernial (acquired) (recurrent) K46.9
  — *continued*
  inguinal (direct) (external) (funicular)
    (indirect) (internal) (oblique) (scrotal)
    (sliding) K40.90
    with
      gangrene (and obstruction) K40.40
        not specified as recurrent K40.40
        recurrent K40.41
      obstruction K40.30
        not specified as recurrent K40.30
        recurrent K40.31
    bilateral K40.20
      with
        gangrene (and obstruction) K40.10
          not specified as recurrent K40.10
          recurrent K40.11
        obstruction K40.00
          not specified as recurrent K40.00
          recurrent K40.01
      not specified as recurrent K40.20
      recurrent K40.21
    not specified as recurrent K40.90
    recurrent K40.91
    unilateral K40.90
      with
        gangrene (and obstruction) K40.40
          not specified as recurrent K40.40
          recurrent K40.41
      obstruction K40.30
        not specified as recurrent K40.30
        recurrent K40.31
      not specified as recurrent K40.90
      recurrent K40.91
  internal — *see also* Hernia, abdomen
    inguinal — *see* Hernia, inguinal
  interstitial — *see* Hernia, abdomen
  intervertebral cartilage or disc — *see*
    Displacement, intervertebral disc
  intestine, intestinal — *see* Hernia, by site
  intra-abdominal — *see* Hernia, abdomen
  iris (traumatic) S05.2-
  irreducible — *see also* Hernia, by site, with
    obstruction
    with gangrene — *see* Hernia, by site,
      with gangrene
  ischiatic — *see* Hernia, abdomen, specified
    site NEC
  ischiorectal — *see* Hernia, abdomen,
    specified site NEC
  lens (traumatic) S05.2-
  linea (alba) (semilunaris) — *see* Hernia,
    ventral
  Littre's — *see* Hernia, abdomen
  lumbar — *see* Hernia, abdomen, specified
    site NEC
  lung (subcutaneous) J98.4
  mediastinum J98.5
  mesenteric (internal) — *see* Hernia,
    abdomen
  midline — *see* Hernia, ventral
  muscle (sheath) M62.89
  nucleus pulposus — *see* Displacement,
    intervertebral disc
  oblique (inguinal) — *see* Hernia, inguinal
  obstructive — *see also* Hernia, by site, with
    obstruction
    with gangrene — *see* Hernia, by site,
      with gangrene
  obturator — *see* Hernia, abdomen,
    specified site NEC
  omental — *see* Hernia, abdomen
  ovary N83.4
  oviduct N83.4
  paraesophageal — *see also* Hernia,
    diaphragm
    congenital Q40.1
  parastomal K43.5
    with
      gangrene (and obstruction) K43.4
      obstruction K43.3
  paraumbilical — *see* Hernia, umbilicus
  perineal — *see* Hernia, abdomen, specified
    site NEC
  Petit's — *see* Hernia, abdomen, specified
    site NEC
  postoperative — *see* Hernia, incisional
  pregnant uterus — *see* Abnormal, uterus in
    pregnancy or childbirth
  prevesical N32.89
  properitoneal — *see* Hernia, abdomen,
    specified site NEC
  pudendal — *see* Hernia, abdomen,
    specified site NEC
  rectovaginal N81.6
  retroperitoneal — *see* Hernia, abdomen,
    specified site NEC
  Richter's — *see* Hernia, abdomen, with
    obstruction

Hernia, hernial (acquired) (recurrent) K46.9 — *continued*
Rieux's, Riex's — *see* Hernia, abdomen, specified site NEC
sac condition (adhesion) (dropsy) (inflammation) (laceration) (suppuration) — *code by* site under Hernia
sciatic — *see* Hernia, abdomen, specified site NEC
scrotum, scrotal — *see* Hernia, inguinal
sliding (inguinal) — *see also* Hernia, inguinal
hiatus — *see* Hernia, hiatal
spigelian — *see* Hernia, ventral
spinal — *see* Spina bifida
strangulated — *see also* Hernia, by site, with obstruction
with gangrene — *see* Hernia, by site, with gangrene
subxiphoid — *see* Hernia, ventral
supra-umbilicus — *see* Hernia, ventral
tendon — *see* Disorder, tendon, specified type NEC
Treitz's (fossa) — *see* Hernia, abdomen, specified site NEC
tunica vaginalis Q55.29
umbilicus, umbilical K42.9
with
gangrene (and obstruction) K42.1
obstruction K42.0
ureter N28.89
urethra, congenital Q64.79
urinary meatus, congenital Q64.79
uterus N81.4
pregnant — *see* Abnormal, uterus in pregnancy or childbirth
vaginal (anterior) (wall) — *see* Cystocele
Velpeau's — *see* Hernia, femoral
ventral K43.9
with
gangrene (and obstruction) K43.7
obstruction K43.6
incisional K43.2
with
gangrene (and obstruction) K43.1
obstruction K43.0
recurrent — *see* Hernia, incisional
specified NEC K43.9
with
gangrene (and obstruction) K43.7
obstruction K43.6
vesical
congenital (female) (male) Q79.51
female — *see* Cystocele
male N32.89
vitreous (into wound) S05.2-
into anterior chamber — *see* Prolapse, vitreous
Herniation — *see also* Hernia
brain (stem) G93.5
cerebral G93.5
mediastinum J98.5
nucleus pulposus — *see* Displacement, intervertebral disc
Herpangina B08.5
Herpes, herpesvirus, herpetic B00.9
anogenital A60.9
perianal skin A60.1
rectum A60.1
urogenital tract A60.00
cervix A60.03
male genital organ NEC A60.02
penis A60.01
specified site NEC A60.09
vagina A60.04
vulva A60.04
blepharitis (zoster) B02.39
simplex B00.59
circinatus B35.4
bullosus L12.0
conjunctivitis (simplex) B00.53
zoster B02.31
cornea B02.33
encephalitis B00.4
due to herpesvirus 6 B10.01
due to herpesvirus 7 B10.09
specified NEC B10.09
eye (zoster) B02.30
simplex B00.50
eyelid (zoster) B02.39
simplex B00.59
facialis B00.1
febrilis B00.1
geniculate ganglionitis B02.21
genital, genitalis A60.00
female A60.09
male A60.02
gestational, gestationis O26.4-
gingivostomatitis B00.2

Herpes, herpesvirus, herpetic B00.9 — *continued*
human B00.9
1 — *see* Herpes, simplex
2 — *see* Herpes, simplex
3 — *see* Varicella
4 — *see* Mononucleosis, Epstein-Barr (virus)
5 — *see* Disease, cytomegalic inclusion (generalized)
6
encephalitis B10.01
specified NEC B10.81
7
encephalitis B10.09
specified NEC B10.82
8 B10.89
infection NEC B10.89
Kaposi's sarcoma associated B10.89
iridocyclitis (simplex) B00.51
zoster B02.32
iris (vesicular erythema multiforme) L51.9
iritis (simplex) B00.51
Kaposi's sarcoma associated B10.89
keratitis (simplex) (dendritic) (disciform) (interstitial) B00.52
zoster (interstitial) B02.33
keratoconjunctivitis (simplex) B00.52
zoster B02.33
labialis B00.1
lip B00.1
meningitis (simplex) B00.3
zoster B02.1
ophthalmicus (zoster) NEC B02.30
simplex B00.50
penis A60.01
perianal skin A60.1
pharyngitis, pharyngotonsillitis B00.2
rectum A60.1
scrotum A60.02
sepsis B00.7
simplex B00.9
complicated NEC B00.89
congenital P35.2
conjunctivitis B00.53
external ear B00.1
eyelid B00.59
hepatitis B00.81
keratitis (interstitial) B00.52
myleitis B00.82
specified complication NEC B00.89
visceral B00.89
stomatitis B00.2
tonsurans B35.0
visceral B00.89
vulva A60.04
whitlow B00.89
zoster (*see also* condition) B02.9
auricularis B02.21
complicated NEC B02.8
conjunctivitis B02.31
disseminated B02.7
encephalitis B02.0
eye(lid) B02.39
geniculate ganglionitis B02.21
keratitis (interstitial) B02.33
meningitis B02.1
myelitis B02.24
neuritis, neuralgia B02.29
ophthalmicus NEC B02.30
oticus B02.21
polyneuropathy B02.23
specified complication NEC B02.8
trigeminal neuralgia B02.22
Herpesvirus (human) — *see* Herpes
Herpetophobia F40.218
Herrick's anemia — *see* Disease, sickle-cell
Hers' disease E74.09
Herter-Gee syndrome K90.0
Herxheimer's reaction R68.89
Hesitancy
of micturition R39.11
urinary R39.11
Hesselbach's hernia — *see* Hernia, femoral, specified site NEC
Heterochromia (congenital) Q13.2
cataract — *see* Cataract, complicated
cyclitis (Fuchs') — *see* Cyclitis, Fuchs' heterochromic
hair L67.1
iritis — *see* Cyclitis, Fuchs' heterochromic
retained metallic foreign body (nonmagnetic) — *see* Foreign body, intraocular, old, retained
magnetic — *see* Foreign body, intraocular, old, retained, magnetic
uveitis — *see* Cyclitis, Fuchs' heterochromic

Heterophoria — *see* Strabismus, heterophoria
Heterophyes, heterophyiasis (small intestine) B66.8
Heterotopia, heterotopic — *see also* Malposition, congenital
cerebralis Q04.8
Heterotropia — *see* Strabismus
Heubner-Herter disease K90.0
Hexadactylism Q69.9
HGSIL (cytology finding) (high grade squamous intraepithelial lesion on cytologic smear) (Pap smear finding)
anus R85.613
cervix R87.613
biopsy (histology) finding — *code to* CIN II or CIN III
vagina R87.623
biopsy (histology) finding — *code to* VAIN II or VAIN III
Hibernoma — *see* Lipoma
Hiccup, hiccough R06.6
epidemic B33.0
psychogenic F45.8
Hidden penis (congenital) Q55.64
acquired N48.83
Hidradenitis (axillaris) (suppurative) L73.2
Hidradenoma (nodular) — *see also* Neoplasm, skin, benign
clear cell — *see* Neoplasm, skin, benign
papillary — *see* Neoplasm, skin, benign
Hidrocystoma — *see* Neoplasm, skin, benign
High
altitude effects T70.20
anoxia T70.29
on
ears T70.0
sinuses T70.1
polycythemia D75.1
arch
foot Q66.7
palate, congenital Q38.5
arterial tension — *see* Hypertension
basal metabolic rate R94.8
blood pressure — *see also* Hypertension
borderline R03.0
reading (incidental) (isolated) (nonspecific), without diagnosis of hypertension R03.0
cholesterol E78.0
with high triglycerides E78.2
diaphragm (congenital) Q79.1
expressed emotional level within family Z63.8
head at term O32.4
palate, congenital Q38.5
risk
infant NEC Z76.2
sexual behavior (heterosexual) Z72.51
bisexual Z72.53
homosexual Z72.52
temperature (of unknown origin) R50.9
thoracic rib Q76.6
triglycerides E78.1
with high cholesterol E78.2
Hildenbrand's disease A75.0
Hilum — *see* condition
Hip — *see* condition
Hippel's disease Q85.8
Hippophobia F40.218
Hippus H57.09
Hirschsprung's disease or megacolon Q43.1
Hirsutism, hirsuties L68.0
Hirudiniasis
external B88.3
internal B83.4
Hiss-Russell dysentery A03.1
His-Werner disease A79.0
Histidinemia, histidinuria E70.41
Histiocytoma — *see also* Neoplasm, skin, benign
fibrous — *see also* Neoplasm, skin, benign
atypical — *see* Neoplasm, connective tissue, uncertain behavior
malignant — *see* Neoplasm, connective tissue, malignant
Histiocytosis D76.3
acute differentiated progressive C96.0
Langerhans' cell NEC C96.6
multifocal X
multisystemic (disseminated) C96.0
unisystemic C96.5
pulmonary, adult (adult PLCH) J84.82
unifocal (X) C96.6
lipid, lipoid D76.3
essential E75.29
malignant C96.A
mononuclear phagocytes NEC D76.1
Langerhans' cells C96.6

Histiocytosis D76.3 — *continued*
non-Langerhans cell D76.3
polyostotic sclerosing D76.3
sinus, with massive lymphadenopathy D76.3
syndrome NEC D76.3
X NEC C96.6
acute (progressive) C96.0
chronic C96.6
multifocal C96.5
multisystemic C96.0
unifocal C96.6
Histoplasmosis B39.9
with pneumonia NEC B39.2
African B39.5
American — *see* Histoplasmosis, capsulati
capsulati B39.4
disseminated B39.3
generalized B39.3
pulmonary B39.2
acute B39.0
chronic B39.1
Darling's B39.4
duboisii B39.5
lung NEC B39.2
History
family (of) — *see also* History, personal (of)
alcohol abuse Z81.1
allergy NEC Z84.89
anemia Z83.2
arthritis Z82.61
asthma Z82.5
blindness Z82.1
cardiac death (sudden) Z82.41
carrier of genetic disease Z84.81
chromosomal anomaly Z82.79
chronic
disabling disease NEC Z82.8
lower respiratory disease Z82.5
colonic polyps Z83.71
congenital malformations and deformations Z82.79
polycystic kidney Z82.71
consanguinity Z84.3
deafness Z82.2
diabetes mellitus Z83.3
disability NEC Z82.8
disease or disorder (of)
allergic NEC Z84.89
behavioral NEC Z81.8
blood and blood-forming organs Z83.2
cardiovascular NEC Z82.49
chronic disabling NEC Z82.8
digestive Z83.79
ear NEC Z83.52
endocrine NEC Z83.49
eye NEC Z83.518
glaucoma Z83.511
genitourinary NEC Z84.2
glaucoma Z83.511
hematological Z83.2
immune mechanism Z83.2
infectious NEC Z83.1
ischemic heart Z82.49
kidney Z84.1
mental NEC Z81.8
metabolic Z83.49
musculoskeletal NEC Z82.69
neurological NEC Z82.0
nutritional Z83.49
parasitic NEC Z83.1
psychiatric NEC Z81.8
respiratory NEC Z83.6
skin and subcutaneous tissue NEC Z84.0
specified NEC Z84.89
drug abuse NEC Z81.3
epilepsy Z82.0
genetic disease carrier Z84.81
glaucoma Z83.511
hearing loss Z82.2
human immunodeficiency virus (HIV) infection Z83.0
Huntington's chorea Z82.0
intellectual disability Z81.0
leukemia Z80.6
malignant neoplasm (of) NOS Z80.9
bladder Z80.52
breast Z80.3
bronchus Z80.1
digestive organ Z80.0
gastrointestinal tract Z80.0
genital organ Z80.49
ovary Z80.41
prostate Z80.42
specified organ NEC Z80.49
testis Z80.43
hematopoietic NEC Z80.7

History — continued
family (of) (see also History, personal (of)) — continued
  malignant neoplasm (of) NOS Z80.9 — continued
    intrathoracic organ NEC Z80.2
    kidney Z80.51
    lung Z80.1
    lymphatic NEC Z80.7
    ovary Z80.41
    prostate Z80.42
    respiratory organ NEC Z80.2
    specified site NEC Z80.8
    testis Z80.43
    trachea Z80.1
    urinary organ or tract Z80.59
      bladder Z80.52
      kidney Z80.51
  mental
    disorder NEC Z81.8
  multiple endocrine neoplasia (MEN) syndrome Z83.41
  osteoporosis Z82.62
  polycystic kidney Z82.71
  polyps (colon) Z83.71
  psychiatric disorder Z81.8
  psychoactive substance abuse NEC Z81.3
  respiratory condition NEC Z83.6
    asthma and other lower respiratory conditions Z82.5
  self-harmful behavior Z81.8
  skin condition Z84.0
  specified condition NEC Z84.89
  stroke (cerebrovascular) Z82.3
  substance abuse NEC Z81.4
    alcohol Z81.1
    drug NEC Z81.3
    psychoactive NEC Z81.3
    tobacco Z81.2
  sudden cardiac death Z82.41
  tobacco abuse Z81.2
  violence, violent behavior Z81.8
  visual loss Z82.1
personal (of) — see also History, family (of)
  abuse
    adult Z91.419
      physical and sexual Z91.410
      psychological Z91.411
    childhood Z62.819
      physical Z62.810
      psychological Z62.811
      sexual Z62.810
  alcohol dependence F10.21
  allergy (to) Z88.9
    analgesic agent NEC Z88.6
    anesthetic Z88.4
    anti-infective agent NEC Z88.3
    antibiotic agent NEC Z88.1
    contrast media Z91.041
    drugs, medicaments and biological substances Z88.9
      specified NEC Z88.8
    food Z91.018
      additives Z91.02
      eggs Z91.012
      milk products Z91.011
      peanuts Z91.010
      seafood Z91.013
      specified food NEC Z91.018
    insect Z91.038
      bee Z91.030
    latex Z91.040
    medicinal agents Z88.9
      specified NEC Z88.8
    narcotic agent NEC Z88.5
    nonmedicinal agents Z91.048
    penicillin Z88.0
    serum Z88.7
    specified NEC Z91.09
    sulfonamides Z88.2
    vaccine Z88.7
  anaphylactic shock Z87.892
  anaphylaxis Z87.892
  behavioral disorders Z86.59
  benign carcinoid tumor Z86.012
  benign neoplasm Z86.018
    brain Z86.011
    carcinoid Z86.012
    colonic polyps Z86.010
  brain injury (traumatic) Z87.820
  breast implant removal Z98.86
  calculi, renal Z87.442
  cancer — see History, personal (of), malignant neoplasm (of)
  cardiac arrest (death), successfully resuscitated Z86.74

History — continued
personal (of) (see also History, family (of)) — continued
  cerebral infarction without residual deficit Z86.73
  cervical dysplasia Z87.410
  chemotherapy for neoplastic condition Z92.21
  childhood abuse — see History, personal (of), abuse
  cleft lip (corrected) Z87.730
  cleft palate (corrected) Z87.730
  collapsed vertebra (healed) Z87.311
    due to osteoporosis Z87.310
  combat and operational stress reaction Z86.51
  congenital malformation (corrected) Z87.798
    circulatory system (corrected) Z87.74
    digestive system (corrected) NEC Z87.738
    ear (corrected) Z87.720
    eye (corrected) Z87.721
    face and neck (corrected) Z87.790
    genitourinary system (corrected) NEC Z87.718
    heart (corrected) Z87.74
    integument (corrected) Z87.76
    limb(s) (corrected) Z87.76
    musculoskeletal system (corrected) Z87.76
    neck (corrected) Z87.790
    nervous system (corrected) NEC Z87.728
    respiratory system (corrected) Z87.75
    sense organs (corrected) NEC Z87.728
    specified NEC Z87.798
  contraception Z92.0
  deployment (military) Z91.82
  diabetic foot ulcer Z86.31
  disease or disorder (of) Z87.898
    anaphylaxis Z87.892
    blood and blood-forming organs Z86.2
    circulatory system Z86.79
      specified condition NEC Z86.79
    connective tissue NEC Z87.39
    digestive system Z87.19
      colonic polyp Z86.010
      peptic ulcer disease Z87.11
      specified condition NEC Z87.19
    ear Z86.69
    endocrine Z86.39
      diabetic foot ulcer Z86.31
      gestational diabetes Z86.32
      specified type NEC Z86.39
    eye Z86.69
    genital (track) system NEC
      female Z87.42
      male Z87.438
    hematological Z86.2
    Hodgkin Z85.71
    immune mechanism Z86.2
    infectious Z86.19
      malaria Z86.13
      methicillin resistant Staphylococcus aureus (MRSA) Z86.14
      poliomyelitis Z86.12
      specified NEC Z86.19
      tuberculosis Z86.11
    mental NEC Z86.59
    metabolic Z86.39
      diabetic foot ulcer Z86.31
      gestational diabetes Z86.32
      specified type NEC Z86.39
    musculoskeletal NEC Z87.39
    nervous system Z86.69
    nutritional Z86.39
    parasitic Z86.19
    respiratory system NEC Z87.09
    sense organs Z86.69
    skin Z87.2
    specified site or type NEC Z87.898
    subcutaneous tissue Z87.2
    trophoblastic Z87.59
    urinary system NEC Z87.448
  drug dependence — see Dependence, drug, by type, in remission
  drug therapy
    antineoplastic chemotherapy Z92.21
    estrogen Z92.23
    immunosupression Z92.25
    inhaled steroids Z92.240
    monoclonal drug Z92.22
    specified NEC Z92.29
    steroid Z92.241
    systemic steroids Z92.241

History — continued
personal (of) (see also History, family (of)) — continued
  dysplasia
    cervical Z87.410
    prostatic Z87.430
    vaginal Z87.411
    vulvar Z87.412
  embolism (venous) Z86.718
    pulmonary Z86.711
  encephalitis Z86.61
  estrogen therapy Z92.23
  extracorporeal membrane oxygenation (ECMO) Z92.81
  failed conscious sedation Z92.83
  failed moderate sedation Z92.83
  fall, falling Z91.81
  fracture (healed)
    fatigue Z87.312
    fragility Z87.310
    osteoporosis Z87.310
    pathological NEC Z87.311
    stress Z87.312
    traumatic Z87.81
  gestational diabetes Z86.32
  hepatitis
    B Z86.19
    C Z86.19
  Hodgkin disease Z85.71
  hyperthermia, malignant Z88.4
  hypospadias (corrected) Z87.710
  hysterectomy Z90.710
  immunosupression therapy Z92.25
  in situ neoplasm
    breast Z86.000
    cervix uteri Z86.001
    specified NEC Z86.008
  in utero procedure during pregnancy Z98.870
  in utero procedure while a fetus Z98.871
  infection NEC Z86.19
    central nervous system Z86.61
    methicillin resistant Staphylococcus aureus (MRSA) Z86.14
    urinary (recurrent) (tract) Z87.440
  injury NEC Z87.828
  irradiation Z92.3
  kidney stones Z87.442
  leukemia Z85.6
  lymphoma (non-Hodgkin) Z85.72
  malignant melanoma (skin) Z85.820
  malignant neoplasm (of) Z85.9
    accessory sinuses Z85.22
    anus NEC Z85.048
      carcinoid Z85.040
    bladder Z85.51
    bone Z85.830
    brain Z85.841
    breast Z85.3
    bronchus NEC Z85.118
      carcinoid Z85.110
    carcinoid — see History, personal (of), malignant neoplasm, by site, carcinioid
    cervix Z85.41
    colon NEC Z85.038
      carcinoid Z85.030
    digestive organ Z85.00
      specified NEC Z85.09
    endocrine gland NEC Z85.858
    epididymis Z85.48
    esophagus Z85.01
    eye Z85.840
    gastrointestinal tract — see History, malignant neoplasm, digestive organ
    genital organ
      female Z85.40
        specified NEC Z85.44
      male Z85.45
        specified NEC Z85.49
    hematopoietic NEC Z85.79
    intrathoracic organ Z85.20
    kidney NEC Z85.528
      carcinoid Z85.520
    large intestine NEC Z85.038
      carcinoid Z85.030
    larynx Z85.21
    liver Z85.05
    lung NEC Z85.118
      carcinoid Z85.110
    mediastinum Z85.29
    Merkel cell Z85.821
    middle ear Z85.22
    nasal cavities Z85.22
    nervous system NEC Z85.848
    oral cavity Z85.819
      specified site NEC Z85.818
    ovary Z85.43
    pancreas Z85.07

History — continued
personal (of) (see also History, family (of)) — continued
  malignant neoplasm (of) Z85.9 — continued
    pelvis Z85.53
    pharynx Z85.819
      specified site NEC Z85.818
    pleura Z85.29
    prostate Z85.46
    rectosigmoid junction NEC Z85.048
      carcinoid Z85.040
    rectum NEC Z85.048
      carcinoid Z85.040
    respiratory organ Z85.20
    sinuses, accessory Z85.22
    skin NEC Z85.828
      melanoma Z85.820
      Merkel cell Z85.821
    small intestine NEC Z85.068
      carcinoid Z85.060
    soft tissue Z85.831
    specified site NEC Z85.89
    stomach NEC Z85.028
      carcinoid Z85.020
    testis Z85.47
    thymus NEC Z85.238
      carcinoid Z85.230
    thyroid Z85.850
    tongue Z85.810
    trachea Z85.12
    ureter Z85.54
    urinary organ or tract Z85.50
      specified NEC Z85.59
    uterus Z85.42
  maltreatment Z91.89
  medical treatment NEC Z92.89
  melanoma (malignant) (skin) Z85.820
  meningitis Z86.61
  mental disorder Z86.59
  Merkel cell carcinoma (skin) Z85.821
  Methicillin resistant Staphylococcus aureus (MRSA) Z86.14
  military deployment Z91.82
  military war, peacekeeping and humanitarian deployment (current or past conflict) Z91.82
  myocardial infarction (old) I25.2
  neglect (in)
    adult Z91.412
    childhood Z62.812
  neoplasm
    benign Z86.018
      brain Z86.011
      colon polyp Z86.010
    in situ
      breast Z86.000
      cervix uteri Z86.001
      specified NEC Z86.008
    malignant — see History of, malignant neoplasm
    uncertain behavior Z86.03
  nephrotic syndrome Z87.441
  nicotine dependence Z87.891
  noncompliance with medical treatment or regimen — see Noncompliance
  nutritional deficiency Z86.39
  obstetric complications Z87.59
    childbirth Z87.59
    pre-term labor Z87.51
    pregnancy Z87.59
    puerperium Z87.59
  osteoporosis fractures Z87.31
  parasuicide (attempt) Z91.5
  physical trauma NEC Z87.828
  self-harm or suicide attempt Z91.5
  pneumonia (recurrent) Z87.01
  poisoning NEC Z91.89
    self-harm or suicide attempt Z91.5
  poor personal hygiene Z91.89
  preterm labor Z87.51
  procedure during pregnancy Z98.870
  procedure while a fetus Z98.871
  prolonged reversible ischemic neurologic deficit (PRIND) Z86.73
  prostatic dysplasia Z87.430
  psychological
    abuse
      adult Z91.411
      child Z62.811
    trauma, specified NEC Z91.49
  radiation therapy Z92.3
  removal
    implant
      breast Z98.86
  renal calculi Z87.442
  respiratory condition NEC Z87.09
  retained foreign body fully removed Z87.821
  risk factors NEC Z91.89

History — *continued*
- personal (of) *(see also* History, family (of)) — *continued*
  - self-harm Z91.5
  - self-poisoning attempt Z91.5
  - sex reassignment Z87.890
  - sleep-wake cycle problem Z72.821
  - specified NEC Z87.898
  - steroid therapy (systemic) Z92.241
    - inhaled Z92.240
  - stroke without residual deficits Z86.73
  - substance abuse NEC F10-F19 with fifth character 1
  - sudden cardiac arrest Z86.74
  - sudden cardiac death successfully resuscitated Z86.74
  - suicide attempt Z91.5
  - surgery NEC Z98.89
    - sex reassignment Z87.890
    - transplant — *see* Transplant
  - thrombophlebitis Z86.72
  - thrombosis (venous) Z86.718
    - pulmonary Z86.711
  - tobacco dependence Z87.891
  - transient ischemic attack (TIA) without residual deficits Z86.73
  - trauma (physical) NEC Z87.828
    - psychological NEC Z91.49
    - self-harm Z91.5
  - traumatic brain injury Z87.820
  - unhealthy sleep-wake cycle Z72.821
  - urinary (recurrent) (tract) infection(s) Z87.440
  - urinary calculi Z87.442
  - vaginal dysplasia Z87.411
  - venous thrombosis or embolism Z86.718
    - pulmonary Z86.711
  - vulvar dysplasia Z87.412

HIV *(see also* Human, immunodeficiency virus) B20
- laboratory evidence (nonconclusive) R75
- nonconclusive test (in infants) R75
- positive, seropositive Z21

Hives (bold) *(see also* Urticaria
Hoarseness R49.0
Hobo Z59.0
Hodgkin disease — *see* Lymphoma, Hodgkin
Hodgson's disease I71.2
- ruptured I71.1
Hoffa-Kastert disease E88.89
Hoffa's disease E88.89
Hoffmann's syndrome E03.9 [G73.7]
Hoffmann-Bouveret syndrome I47.9
Hole (round)
- macula H35.34-
- retina (without detachment) — *see* Break, retina, round hole
  - with detachment — *see* Detachment, retina, with retinal, break
Holiday relief care Z75.5
Hollenhorst's plaque — *see* Occlusion, artery, retina
Hollow foot (congenital) Q66.7
- acquired — *see* Deformity, limb, foot, specified NEC
Holoprosencephaly Q04.2
Holt-Oram syndrome Q87.2
Homelessness Z59.0
Homesickness — *see* Disorder, adjustment
Homocystinemia, homocystinuria E72.11
Homogentisate 1,2-dioxygenase deficiency E70.29
Homologous serum hepatitis (prophylactic) (therapeutic) — *see* Hepatitis, viral, type B
Honeycomb lung J98.4
- congenital Q33.0
Hooded
- clitoris Q52.6
- penis Q55.69
Hookworm (anemia) (disease) (infection) (infestation) B76.9
- specified NEC B76.8
Hordeolum (eyelid) (externum) (recurrent) H00.019
- internum H00.029
  - left H00.026
    - lower H00.025
    - upper H00.024
  - right H00.023
    - lower H00.022
    - upper H00.021
- left H00.016
  - lower H00.015
  - upper H00.014
- right H00.013
  - lower H00.012
  - upper H00.011

Horn
- cutaneous L85.8
- nail L60.2
  - congenital Q84.6
Horner(-Claude Bernard) syndrome G90.2
- traumatic — *see* Injury, nerve, cervical sympathetic
Horseshoe kidney (congenital) Q63.1
Horton's headache or neuralgia G44.099
- intractable G44.091
- not intractable G44.099
Hospital hopper syndrome — *see* Disorder, factitious
Hospitalism in children — *see* Disorder, adjustment
Hostility R45.5
- towards child Z62.3
Hot flashes
- menopausal N95.1
Hourglass (contracture) — *see also* Contraction, hourglass
- stomach K31.89
  - congenital Q40.2
  - stricture K31.2
Houschold, housing circumstance affecting care Z59.9
- specified NEC Z59.8
Housemaid's knee — *see* Bursitis, prepatellar
Hudson(-Stähli) line (cornea) — *see* Pigmentation, cornea, anterior
Human
- bite (open wound) — *see also* Bite
  - intact skin surface — *see* Bite, superficial
- herpesvirus — *see* Herpes
- immunodeficiency virus (HIV) disease (infection) B20
  - asymptomatic status Z21
  - contact Z20.6
  - counseling Z71.7
  - dementia B20 [F02.80]
    - with behavioral disturbance B20 [F02.81]
  - exposure to Z20.6
  - laboratory evidence R75
  - type-2 (HIV 2) as cause of disease classified elsewhere B97.35
- papillomavirus (HPV)
  - DNA test positive
    - high risk
      - cervix R87.810
      - vagina R87.811
    - low risk
      - cervix R87.820
      - vagina R87.821
  - screening for Z11.51
- T-cell lymphotropic virus
  - type-1 (HTLV-I) infection B33.3
    - as cause of disease classified elsewhere B97.33
    - carrier Z22.6
  - type-2 (HTLV-II) as cause of disease classified elsewhere B97.34
Humidifier lung or pneumonitis J67.7
Humiliation (experience) in childhood Z62.898
Humpback (acquired) — *see* Kyphosis
Hunchback (acquired) — *see* Kyphosis
Hunger T73.0
- air, psychogenic F45.8
Hungry bone syndrome E83.81
Hunner's ulcer — *see* Cystitis, chronic, interstitial
Hunter's
- glossitis D51.0
- syndrome E76.1
Huntington's disease or chorea G10
- with dementia G10 [F02.80]
  - with behavioral disturbance G10 [F02.81]
Hunt's
- disease or syndrome (herpetic geniculate ganglionitis) B02.21
- dyssynergia cerebellaris myoclonica G11.1
- neuralgia B02.21
Hurler(-Scheie) disease or syndrome E76.02
Hurst's disease G36.1
Hurthle cell
- adenocarcinoma C73
- adenoma D34
- carcinoma C73
- tumor D34
Hutchinson's
- disease, meaning
  - angioma serpiginosum L81.7
  - pompholyx (cheiropompholyx) L30.1
  - prurigo estivalis L56.4

Hutchinson's — *continued*
- disease, meaning — *continued*
  - summer eruption or summer prurigo L56.4
  - melanotic freckle — *see* Melanoma, in situ
  - malignant melanoma in — *see* Melanoma
  - teeth or incisors (congenital syphilis) A50.52
  - triad (congenital syphilis) A50.53
Hutchinson-Boeck disease or syndrome — *see* Sarcoidosis
Hutchinson-Gilford disease or syndrome E34.8
Hyalin plaque, sclera, senile H15.89
Hyaline membrane (disease) (lung) (pulmonary) (newborn) P22.0
Hyalinosis
- cutis (et mucosae) E78.89
- focal and segmental (glomerular) *(see also* N00-N07 with fourth character .1) N05.1
Hyalitis, hyalosis, asteroid — *see also* Deposit, crystalline
- syphilitic (late) A52.71
Hydatid
- cyst or tumor — *see* Echinococcus
- mole — *see* Hydatidiform mole
- Morgagni
  - female Q50.5
  - male (epididymal) Q55.4
  - testicular Q55.29
Hydatidiform mole (benign) (complicating pregnancy) (delivered) (undelivered) O01.9
- classical O01.0
- complete O01.0
- incomplete O01.1
- invasive D39.2
- malignant D39.2
- partial O01.1
Hydatidosis — *see* Echinococcus
Hydradenitis (axillaris) (suppurative) L73.2
Hydradenoma — *see* Hidradenoma
Hydramnios O40-
Hydrancephaly, hydranencephaly Q04.3
- with spina bifida — *see* Spina bifida, with hydrocephalus
Hydrargyrism NEC — *see* Poisoning, mercury
Hydrarthrosis — *see also* Effusion, joint
- gonococcal A54.42
- intermittent M12.40
  - ankle M12.47-
  - elbow M12.42-
  - foot joint M12.47-
  - hand joint M12.44-
  - hip M12.45-
  - knee M12.46-
  - multiple site M12.49
  - shoulder M12.41-
  - specified joint NEC M12.48
  - wrist M12.43-
- of yaws (early) (late) *(see also* subcategory M14.8-) A66.6
- syphilitic (late) A52.77
  - congenital A50.55 [M12.80]
Hydremia D64.89
Hydrencephalocele (congenital) — *see* Encephalocele
Hydrencephalomeningocele (congenital) — *see* Encephalocele
Hydroa R23.8
- aestivale L56.4
- vacciniforme L56.4
Hydroadenitis (axillaris) (suppurative) L73.2
Hydrocalycosis — *see* Hydronephrosis
Hydrocele (spermatic cord) (testis) (tunica vaginalis) N43.3
- canal of Nuck N94.89
- communicating N43.2
  - congenital P83.5
- congenital P83.5
- encysted N43.0
- female NEC N94.89
- infected N43.1
- newborn P83.5
- round ligament N94.89
- specified NEC N43.2
- spinalis — *see* Spina bifida
- vulva N90.89
Hydrocephalus (acquired) (external) (internal) (malignant) (recurrent) G91.9
- aqueduct Sylvius stricture Q03.0
- causing disproportion O33.6
  - with obstructed labor O66.3
- communicating G91.0

Hydrocephalus (acquired) (external) (internal) (malignant) (recurrent) G91.9 — *continued*
- congenital (external) (internal) Q03.9
  - with spina bifida Q05.4
    - cervical Q05.0
    - dorsal Q05.1
    - lumbar Q05.2
    - lumbosacral Q05.2
    - sacral Q05.3
    - thoracic Q05.1
    - thoracolumbar Q05.1
  - specified NEC Q03.8
- due to toxoplasmosis (congenital) P37.1
- foramen Magendie block (acquired) G91.1
- congenital *(see also* Hydrocephalus, congenital) Q03.1
- in (due to)
  - infectious disease NEC B89 [G91.4]
  - neoplastic disease NEC *(see also* Neoplasm) G91.4
  - parasitic disease B89 [G91.4]
- newborn Q03.9
  - with spina bifida — *see* Spina bifida, with hydrocephalus
- noncommunicating G91.1
- normal pressure G91.2
  - secondary G91.0
- obstructive G91.1
- otitic G93.2
- post-traumatic NEC G91.3
- secondary G91.4
  - post-traumatic G91.3
- specified NEC G91.8
- syphilitic, congenital A50.49
Hydrocolpos (congenital) N89.8
Hydrocystoma — *see* Neoplasm, skin, benign
Hydroencephalocele (congenital) — *see* Encephalocele
Hydroencephalomeningocele (congenital) — *see* Encephalocele
Hydrohematopneumothorax — *see* Hemothorax
Hydromeningitis — *see* Meningitis
Hydromeningocele (spinal) — *see also* Spina bifida
- cranial — *see* Encephalocele
Hydrometra N85.8
Hydrometrocolpos N89.8
Hydromicrocephaly Q02
Hydromphalos (since birth) Q45.8
Hydromyelia Q06.4
Hydromyelocele — *see* Spina bifida
Hydronephrosis (atrophic) (early) (functionless) (intermittent) (primary) (secondary) NEC N13.30
- with
  - infection N13.6
  - obstruction (by) (of)
    - renal calculus N13.2
      - with infection N13.6
    - ureteral calculus N13.1
      - with infection N13.6
      - calculus N13.2
        - with infection N13.6
    - ureteropelvic junction (congenital) Q62.0
      - with infection N13.6
    - ureteral stricture NEC N13.1
      - with infection N13.6
- congenital Q62.0
- specified type NEC N13.39
- tuberculous A18.11
Hydropericarditis — *see* Pericarditis
Hydropericardium — *see* Pericarditis
Hydroperitoneum R18.8
Hydrophobia — *see* Rabies
Hydrophthalmos Q15.0
Hydropneumohemothorax — *see* Hemothorax
Hydropneumopericarditis — *see* Pericarditis
Hydropneumopericardium — *see* Pericarditis
Hydropneumothorax J94.8
- traumatic — *see* Injury, intrathoracic, lung
- tuberculous NEC A15.6
Hydrops R60.9
- abdominis R18.8
- articulorum intermittens — *see* Hydrarthrosis, intermittent
- cardiac — *see* Failure, heart, congestive
- causing obstructed labor (mother) O66.3
- endolymphatic H81.0-
- fetal — *see* Pregnancy, complicated by, hydrops, fetalis

Hydrops R60.9 — *continued*
  fetalis P83.2
    due to
      ABO isoimmunization P56.0
      alpha thalassemia D56.0
      hemolytic disease P56.90
        specified NEC P56.99
      isoimmunization (ABO) (Rh) P56.0
      other specified nonhemolytic disease NEC P83.2
      Rh incompatibility P56.0
    during pregnancy — *see* Pregnancy, complicated by, hydrops, fetalis
  gallbladder K82.1
  joint — *see* Effusion, joint
  labyrinth H81.0-
  newborn (idiopathic) P83.2
    due to
      ABO isoimmunization P56.0
      alpha thalassemia D56.0
      hemolytic disease P56.90
        specified NEC P56.99
      isoimmunization (ABO) (Rh) P56.0
      Rh incompatibility P56.0
  nutritional — *see* Malnutrition, severe
  pericardium — *see* Pericarditis
  pleura — *see* Hydrothorax
  spermatic cord — *see* Hydrocele
Hydropyonephrosis N13.6
Hydrorachis Q06.4
Hydrorrhea (nasal) J34.89
  pregnancy — *see* Rupture, membranes, premature
Hydrosadenitis (axillaris) (suppurative) L73.2
Hydrosalpinx (fallopian tube) (follicularis) N70.11
Hydrothorax (double) (pleura) J94.8
  chylous (nonfilarial) I89.8
    filarial (*see also* Infestation, filarial) B74.9 [J91.8]
  traumatic — *see* Injury, intrathoracic
  tuberculous NEC (non primary) A15.6
Hydroureter (*see also* Hydronephrosis) N13.4
  with infection N13.6
  congenital Q62.39
Hydroureteronephrosis — *see* Hydronephrosis
Hydrourethra N36.8
Hydroxykynureninuria E70.8
Hydroxylysinemia E72.3
Hydroxyprolinemia E72.59
Hygiene, sleep
  abuse Z72.821
  inadequate Z72.821
  poor Z72.821
Hygroma (congenital) (cystic) D18.1
  praepatellare, prepatellar — *see* Bursitis, prepatellar
Hymen — *see* condition
Hymenolepis, hymenolepiasis (diminuta) (infection) (infestation) (nana) B71.0
Hypalgesia R20.8
Hyperacidity (gastric) K31.89
  psychogenic F45.8
Hyperactive, hyperactivity F90.9
  basal cell, uterine cervix — *see* Dysplasia, cervix
  bowel sounds R19.12
  cervix epithelial (basal) — *see* Dysplasia, cervix
  child F90.9
    attention deficit — *see* Disorder, attention-deficit hyperactivity
  detrusor muscle N32.81
  gastrointestinal K31.89
    psychogenic F45.8
  nasal mucous membrane J34.3
  stomach K31.89
  thyroid (gland) — *see* Hyperthyroidism
Hyperacusis H93.23-
Hyperadrenalism E27.5
Hyperadrenocorticism E24.9
  congenital E25.0
  iatrogenic E24.2
    correct substance properly administered — *see* Table of Drugs and Chemicals, by drug, adverse effect
    overdose or wrong substance given or taken — *see* Table of Drugs and Chemicals, by drug, poisoning
  not associated with Cushing's syndrome E27.0
  pituitary-dependent E24.0
Hyperaldosteronism E26.9
  familial (type I) E26.02
  glucocorticoid-remediable E26.02
  primary (due to (bilateral) adrenal hyperplasia) E26.09

Hyperaldosteronism E26.9 — *continued*
  primary NEC E26.09
  secondary E26.1
  specified NEC E26.89
Hyperalgesia R20.8
Hyperalimentation R63.2
  carotene, carotin E67.1
  specified NEC E67.8
  vitamin
    A E67.0
    D E67.3
Hyperaminoaciduria
  arginine E72.21
  cystine E72.01
  lysine E72.3
  ornithine E72.4
Hyperammonemia (congenital) E72.20
Hyperazotemia — *see* Uremia
Hyperbetalipoproteinemia (familial) E78.0
  with prebetalipoproteinemia E78.2
Hyperbilirubinemia
  constitutional E80.6
  familial conjugated E80.6
  neonatal (transient) — *see* Jaundice, newborn
Hypercalcemia, hypocalciuric, familial E83.52
Hypercalciuria, idiopathic E83.52
Hypercapnia R06.89
  newborn P84
Hypercarotenemia, hypercarotinemia (dietary) E67.1
Hypercementosis K03.4
Hyperchloremia E87.8
Hyperchlorhydria K31.89
  neurotic F45.8
  psychogenic F45.8
Hypercholesterinemia — *see* Hypercholesterolemia
Hypercholesterolemia (essential) (familial) (hereditary) (primary) (pure) E78.0
  with hyperglyceridemia, endogenous E78.2
  dietary counseling and surveillance Z71.3
Hyperchylia gastrica, psychogenic F45.8
Hyperchylomicronemia (familial) (primary) E78.3
  with hyperbetalipoproteinemia E78.3
Hypercoagulable (state) D68.59
  activated protein C resistance D68.51
  antithrombin (III) deficiency D68.59
  factor V Leiden mutation D68.51
  primary NEC D68.59
  protein C deficiency D68.59
  protein S deficiency D68.59
  prothrombin gene mutation D68.52
  secondary D68.69
  specified NEC D68.69
Hypercoagulation (state) D68.59
Hypercorticalism, pituitary-dependent E24.0
Hypercorticosolism — *see* Cushing's, syndrome
Hypercorticosteronism E24.2
  correct substance properly administered — *see* Table of Drugs and Chemicals, by drug, adverse effect
  overdose or wrong substance given or taken — *see* Table of Drugs and Chemicals, by drug, poisoning
Hypercortisonism E24.2
  correct substance properly administered — *see* Table of Drugs and Chemicals, by drug, adverse effect
  overdose or wrong substance given or taken — *see* Table of Drugs and Chemicals, by drug, poisoning
Hyperekplexia Q89.8
Hyperelectrolytemia E87.8
Hyperemesis R11.10
  with nausea R11.2
  gravidarum (mild) O21.0
    with
      carbohydrate depletion O21.1
      dehydration O21.1
      electrolyte imbalance O21.1
      metabolic disturbance O21.1
      severe (with metabolic disturbance) O21.1
  projectile R11.12
  psychogenic F45.8
Hyperemia (acute) (passive) R68.89
  anal mucosa K62.89
  bladder N32.89
  cerebral I67.99
  conjunctiva H11.43-
  ear internal, acute — *see* subcategory H83.0
  enteric K59.8
  eye — *see* Hyperemia, conjunctiva

Hyperemia (acute) (passive) R68.89 — *continued*
  eyelid (active) (passive) — *see* Disorder, eyelid, specified type NEC
  intestine K59.8
  iris — *see* Disorder, iris, vascular
  kidney N28.89
  labyrinth — *see* subcategory H83.0
  liver (active) K76.89
  lung (passive) — *see* Edema, lung
  pulmonary (passive) — *see* Edema, lung
  renal N28.89
  retina H35.89
  stomach K31.89
Hyperesthesia (body surface) R20.3
  larynx (reflex) J38.7
    hysterical F44.89
  pharynx (reflex) J39.2
    hysterical F44.89
Hyperestrogenism (drug-induced) (iatrogenic) E28.0
Hyperexplexia Q89.8
Hyperfibrinolysis — *see* Fibrinolysis
Hyperfructosemia E74.19
Hyperfunction
  adrenal cortex, not associated with Cushing's syndrome E27.0
    medulla E27.5
      adrenomedullary E27.5
    virilism E25.9
      congenital E25.0
  ovarian E28.8
  pancreas K86.8
  parathyroid (gland) E21.3
  pituitary (gland) (anterior) E22.9
    specified NEC E22.8
  polyglandular E31.1
  testicular E29.0
Hypergammaglobulinemia D89.2
  polyclonal D89.0
  Waldenström D89.0
Hypergastrinemia E16.4
Hyperglobulinemia R77.1
Hyperglycemia, hyperglycemic (transient) R73.9
  coma — *see* Diabetes, by type, with coma
  postpancreatectomy E89.1
Hyperglyceridemia (endogenous) (essential) (familial) (hereditary) (pure) E78.1
  mixed E78.3
Hyperglycinemia (non-ketotic) E72.51
Hypergonadism
  ovarian E28.8
  testicular (primary) (infantile) E29.0
Hyperheparinemia D68.32
Hyperhidrosis, hyperidrosis R61
  focal
    primary L74.519
      axilla L74.510
      face L74.511
      palms L74.512
      soles L74.513
    secondary L74.52
  generalized R61
  localized
    primary L74.519
      axilla L74.510
      face L74.511
      palms L74.512
      soles L74.513
    secondary L74.52
  psychogenic F45.8
  secondary R61
    focal L74.52
Hyperhistidinemia E70.41
Hyperhomocysteinemia E72.11
Hyperhydroxyprolinemia E72.59
Hyperinsulinism (functional) E16.1
  with
    coma (hypoglycemic) E15
    encephalopathy E16.1 [G94]
  ectopic E16.1
  therapeutic misadventure (from administration of insulin) — *see* subcategory T38.3
Hyperkalemia E87.5
Hyperkeratosis (*see also* Keratosis) L85.9
  cervix N88.0
  due to yaws (early) (late) (palmar or plantar) A66.3
  follicularis Q82.8
    penetrans (in cutem) L87.0
  palmoplantaris climacterica L85.1
  pinta A67.1
  senile (with pruritus) L57.0
  universalis congenita Q80.8
  vocal cord J38.3
  vulva N90.4

Hyperkinesia, hyperkinetic (disease) (reaction) (syndrome) (childhood) (adolescence) — *see also* Disorder, attention-deficit hyperactivity
  heart I51.89
Hyperleucine-isoleucinemia E71.19
Hyperlipemia, hyperlipidemia E78.5
  combined E78.2
    familial E78.4
  group
    A E78.0
    B E78.1
    C E78.2
    D E78.3
  mixed E78.2
  specified NEC E78.4
Hyperlipidosis E75.6
  hereditary NEC E75.5
Hyperlipoproteinemia E78.5
  Fredrickson's type
    I E78.3
    IIa E78.0
    IIb E78.2
    III E78.2
    IV E78.1
    V E78.3
  low-density-lipoprotein-type (LDL) E78.0
  very-low-density-lipoprotein-type (VLDL) E78.1
Hyperlucent lung, unilateral J43.0
Hyperlysinemia E72.3
Hypermagnesemia E83.41
  neonatal P71.8
Hypermenorrhea N92.0
Hypermethioninemia E72.19
Hypermetropia (congenital) H52.0-
Hypermobility, hypermotility
  cecum — *see* Syndrome, irritable bowel
  coccyx — *see* subcategory M53.2
  colon — *see* Syndrome, irritable bowel
    psychogenic F45.8
  ileum K58.9
  intestine (*see also* Syndrome, irritable bowel) K58.9
    psychogenic F45.8
  meniscus (knee) — *see* Derangement, knee, meniscus
  scapula — *see* Instability, joint, shoulder
  stomach K31.89
    psychogenic F45.8
  syndrome M35.7
  urethra N36.41
    with intrinsic sphincter deficiency N36.43
Hypernasality R49.21
Hypernatremia E87.0
Hypernephroma C64-
Hyperopia — *see* Hypermetropia
Hyperorexia nervosa F50.2
Hyperornithinemia E72.4
Hyperosmia R43.1
Hyperosmolality E87.0
Hyperostosis (monomelic) — *see also* Disorder, bone, density and structure, specified NEC
  ankylosing (spine) M48.10
    cervical region M48.12
    cervicothoracic region M48.13
    lumbar region M48.16
    lumbosacral region M48.17
    multiple sites M48.19
    occipito-atlanto-axial region M48.11
    sacrococcygeal region M48.18
    thoracic region M48.14
    thoracolumbar region M48.15
  cortical (skull) M85.2
    infantile M89.8x-
  frontal, internal of skull M85.2
  interna frontalis M85.2
  skeletal, diffuse idiopathic — *see* Hyperostosis, ankylosing
  skull M85.2
    congenital Q75.8
  vertebral, ankylosing — *see* Hyperostosis, ankylosing
Hyperovarism E28.8
Hyperoxaluria (primary) E72.53
Hyperparathyroidism E21.3
  primary E21.0
  secondary (renal) N25.81
    non-renal E21.1
  specified NEC E21.2
  tertiary E21.2
Hyperpathia R20.8
Hyperperistalsis R19.2
  psychogenic F45.8
Hyperpermeability, capillary I78.8
Hyperphagia R63.2
Hyperphenylalaninemia NEC E70.1
Hyperphoria (alternating) H50.53

D I S E A S E   I N D E X

Hyperphosphatemia E83.39
Hyperpiesis, hyperpiesia — *see* Hypertension
Hyperpigmentation — *see also* Pigmentation
  melanin NEC L81.4
  postinflammatory L81.0
Hyperpinealism E34.8
Hyperpituitarism E22.9
Hyperplasia, hyperplastic
  adenoids J35.2
  adrenal (capsule) (cortex) (gland) E27.8
    with
      sexual precocity (male) E25.9
        congenital E25.0
      virilism, adrenal E25.9
        congenital E25.0
      virilization (female) E25.9
        congenital E25.0
    congenital E25.0
    salt-losing E25.0
  adrenomedullary E27.5
  angiolymphoid, eosinophilia (ALHE) D18.01
  appendix (lymphoid) K38.0
  artery, fibromuscular I77.3
  bone — *see also* Hypertrophy, bone
    marrow D75.89
  breast — *see also* Hypertrophy, breast
    ductal (atypical) N60.9-
    C-cell, thyroid E07.0
  cementation (tooth) (teeth) K03.4
  cervical gland R59.0
  cervix (uteri) (basal cell) (endometrium)
    (polypoid) — *see also* Dysplasia,
    cervix
    congenital Q51.828
  clitoris, congenital Q52.6
  denture K06.2
  endocervicitis N72
  endometrium, endometrial (adenomatous)
    (benign) (cystic) (glandular)
    (glandular-cystic) (polypoid) N85.00
    with atypia N85.02
    cervix — *see* Dysplasia, cervix
    complex (without atypia) N85.01
    simple (without atypia) N85.01
  epithelial L85.9
    focal, oral, including tongue K13.29
    nipple N62
    skin L85.9
    tongue K13.29
    vaginal wall N89.3
  crythroid D75.89
  fibromuscular of artery (carotid) (renal)
    I77.3
  genital
    female NEC N94.89
    male N50.8
  gingiva K06.1
  glandularis cystica uteri (interstitialis) (*see
    also* Hyperplasia, endometrial)
    N85.00-
  gum K06.1
  hymen, congenital Q52.4
  irritative, edentulous (alveolar) K06.2
  jaw M26.09
    alveolar M26.79
    lower M26.03
      alveolar M26.72
    upper M26.01
      alveolar M26.71
  kidney (congenital) Q63.3
  labia N90.6
    epithelial N90.3
  liver (congenital) Q44.7
    nodular, focal K76.89
  lymph gland or node R59.9
  mandible, mandibular M26.03
    alveolar M26.72
    unilateral condylar M27.8
  maxilla, maxillary M26.01
    alveolar M26.71
  myometrium, myometrial N85.2
  neuroendocrine cell, of infancy J84.841
  nose
    lymphoid J34.89
    polypoid J33.9
  oral mucosa (irritative) K13.6
  organ or site, congenital NEC — *see*
    Anomaly, by site
  ovary N83.8
  palate, papillary (irritative) K13.6
  pancreatic islet cells E16.9
    alpha E16.8
      with excess
        gastrin E16.4
        glucagon E16.3
    beta E16.1
  parathyroid (gland) E21.0

Hyperplasia, hyperplastic — *continued*
  pharynx (lymphoid) J39.2
  prostate (adenofibromatous) (nodular)
    N40.0
    with lower urinary tract symptoms
      (LUTS) N40.1
    without lower urinary tract symtpoms
      (LUTS) N40.0
  renal artery I77.89
  reticulo-endothelial (cell) D75.89
  salivary gland (any) K11.1
  Schimmelbusch's — *see* Mastopathy, cystic
  suprarenal capsule (gland) E27.8
  thymus (gland) (persistent) E32.0
  thyroid (gland) — *see* Goiter
  tonsils (faucial) (infective) (lingual)
    (lymphoid) J35.1
    with adenoids J35.3
  unilateral condylar M27.8
  uterus, uterine N85.2
    endometrium (glandular) (*see also*
      Hyperplasia, endometrial) N85.00-
  vulva N90.6
    epithelial N90.3
Hyperpnea — *see* Hyperventilation
Hyperpotassemia E87.5
Hyperprebetalipoproteinemia (familial)
  E78.1
Hyperprolactinemia E22.1
Hyperprolinemia (type I) (type II) E72.59
Hyperproteinemia E88.09
**Hyperprothrombinemia, causing
  coagulation factor deficiency** D68.4
Hyperpyrexia R50.9
  heat (effects) T67.0
  malignant, due to anesthetic T88.3
  rheumatic — *see* Fever, rheumatic
  unknown origin R50.9
Hyper-reflexia R29.2
Hypersalivation K11.7
Hypersecretion
  ACTH (not associated with Cushing's
    syndrome) E27.0
    pituitary E24.0
  adrenaline E27.5
  adrenomedullary E27.5
  androgen (testicular) E29.0
    ovarian (drug-induced) (iatrogenic)
      E28.1
  calcitonin E07.0
  catecholamine E27.5
  corticoadrenal E24.9
  cortisol E24.9
  epinephrine E27.5
  estrogen E28.0
  gastric K31.89
    psychogenic F45.8
  gastrin E16.4
  glucagon E16.3
  hormone(s)
    ACTH (not associated with Cushing's
      syndrome) E27.0
      pituitary E24.0
    antidiuretic E22.2
    growth E22.0
    intestinal NEC E34.1
    ovarian androgen E28.1
    pituitary E22.9
    testicular E29.0
    thyroid stimulating E05.80
      with thyroid storm E05.81
  insulin — *see* Hyperinsulinism
  lacrimal glands — *see* Epiphora
  medulloadrenal E27.5
  milk O92.6
  ovarian androgens E28.1
  salivary gland (any) K11.7
  thyrocalcitonin E07.0
  upper respiratory J39.8
Hypersegmentation, leukocytic, hereditary
  D72.0
**Hypersensitive, hypersensitiveness,
  hypersensitivity** — *see also* Allergy
  carotid sinus G90.01
  colon — *see* Irritable, colon
  drug T88.7
  gastrointestinal K52.2
    psychogenic F45.8
  labyrinth — *see* subcategory H83.2
  pain R20.8
  pneumonitis — *see* Pneumonitis, allergic
  reaction T78.40
    upper respiratory tract NEC J39.3
Hypersomnia (organic) G47.10
  due to
    alcohol
      abuse F10.182
      dependence F10.282
      use F10.982

Hypersomnia (organic) G47.10 — *continued*
  due to — *continued*
    amphetamines
      abuse F15.182
      dependence F15.282
      use F15.982
    caffeine
      abuse F15.182
      dependence F15.282
      use F15.982
    cocaine
      abuse F14.182
      dependence F14.282
      use F14.982
    drug NEC
      abuse F19.182
      dependence F19.282
      use F19.982
    medical condition G47.14
    mental disorder F51.13
    opioid
      abuse F11.182
      dependence F11.282
      use F11.982
    psychoactive substance NEC
      abuse F19.182
      dependence F19.282
      use F19.982
    sedative, hypnotic, or anxiolytic
      abuse F13.182
      dependence F13.282
      use F13.982
    stimulant NEC
      abuse F15.182
      dependence F15.282
      use F15.982
  idiopathic G47.11
    with long sleep time G47.11
    without long sleep time G47.12
  menstrual related G47.13
  nonorganic origin F51.11
    specified NEC F51.19
  not due to a substance or known
    physiological condition F51.11
    specified NEC F51.19
  primary F51.11
  recurrent G47.13
  specified NEC G47.19
Hypersplenia, hypersplenism D73.1
Hyperstimulation, ovaries (associated with
  induced ovulation) N98.1
Hypersusceptibility — *see* Allergy
Hypertelorism (ocular) (orbital) Q75.2
Hypertension, hypertensive (accelerated)
  (benign) (essential) (idiopathic)
  (malignant) (systemic) I10
  with
    heart involvement (conditions in I51.4 –
      I51.9 due to hypertension) — *see*
      Hypertension, heart
    kidney involvement — *see*
      Hypertension, kidney
  benign, intracranial G93.2
  borderline R03.0
  cardiorenal (disease) I13.10
    with heart failure I13.0
      with stage 1 through stage 4 chronic
        kidney disease I13.0
      with stage 5 or end stage renal disease
        I13.2
    without heart failure I13.10
      with stage 1 through stage 4 chronic
        kidney disease I13.10
      with stage 5 or end stage renal disease
        I13.11
  cardiovascular
    disease (arteriosclerotic) (sclerotic) —
      see Hypertension, heart
    renal (disease) — *see* Hypertension,
      cardiorenal
  chronic venous — *see* Hypertension,
    venous (chronic)
  complicating
    childbirth (labor) O10.92
      with
        heart disease O10.12
          with renal disease O10.32
        renal disease O10.22
          with heart disease O10.32
      essential O10.02
      secondary O10.42

Hypertension, hypertensive (accelerated)
  (benign) (essential) (idiopathic)
  (malignant) (systemic) I10 — *continued*
  complicating — *continued*
    pregnancy O16-
      with edema (*see also* Pre-eclampsia)
        O14.9-
      gestational (pregnancy induced)
        (transient) (without proteinuria)
        O13-
        with proteinuria O14.9-
          mild pre-eclampsia O14.0-
          moderate pre-eclampsia O14.0-
          severe pre-eclampsia O14.1-
            with hemolysis, elevated liver
              enzymes and low platelet
              count (HELLP) O14.2-
      pre-existing O10.91-
        with
          heart disease O10.11-
            with renal disease O10.31-
          pre-eclampsia O11-
          renal disease O10.21-
            with heart disease O10.31-
        essential O10.01-
        secondary O10.41-
      puerperium, pre-existing O10.93
        with
          heart disease O10.13
            with renal disease O10.33
          renal disease O10.23
            with heart disease O10.33
        essential O10.03
        pregnancy-induced O13.9
        secondary O10.43
  due to
    endocrine disorders I15.2
    pheochromocytoma I15.2
    renal disorders NEC I15.1
      arterial I15.0
    renovascular disorders I15.0
    specified disease NEC I15.8
  encephalopathy I67.4
  gestational (without significant proteinuria)
    (pregnancy-induced) (transient) O13-
    with significant proteinuria — *see* Pre-
      eclampsia
  Goldblatt's I70.1
  heart (disease) (conditions in I51.4-I51.9
    due to hypertension) I11.9
    with
      heart failure (congestive) I11.0
      kidney disease (chronic) — *see*
        Hypertension, cardiorenal
  intracranial (benign) G93.2
  kidney I12.9
    with
      heart disease — *see* Hypertension,
        cardiorenal
      stage 1 through stage 4 chronic
        kidney disease I12.9
      stage 5 chronic kidney disease (CKD)
        or end stage renal disease
        (ESRD) I12.0
  lesser circulation I27.0
  newborn P29.2
    pulmonary (persistent) P29.3
  ocular H40.05-
  pancreatic duct — *code to* underlying
    condition
    with chronic pancreatitis K86.1
  portal (due to chronic liver disease)
    (idiopathic) K76.6
    gastropathy K31.89
    in (due to) schistosomiasis (bilharziasis)
      B65.9 [K77]
  postoperative I97.3
  psychogenic F45.8
  pulmonary (artery) (secondary) NEC I27.2
    with
      cor pulmonale (chronic) I27.2
        acute I26.09
      right heart ventricular strain/failure
        I27.2
        acute I26.09
    of newborn (persistent) P29.3
    primary (idiopathic) I27.0
  renal — *see* Hypertension, kidney
  renovascular I15.0
  secondary NEC I15.9
    due to
      endocrine disorders I15.2
      pheochromocytoma I15.2
      renal disorders NEC I15.1
        arterial I15.0
      renovascular disorders I15.0
    specified NEC I15.8

DISEASE INDEX

Hypertension, hypertensive (accelerated) (benign) (essential) (idiopathic) (malignant) (systemic) I10 — *continued*
  venous (chronic)
    due to
      deep vein thrombosis — *see* Syndrome, postthrombotic
    idiopathic I87.309
      with
        inflammation I87.32-
          with ulcer I87.33-
        specified complication NEC I87.39-
        ulcer I87.31-
          with inflammation I87.33-
      asymptomatic I87.30-
Hypertensive urgency — *see* Hypertension
Hyperthecosis ovary E28.8
Hyperthermia (of unknown origin) — *see also* Hyperpyrexia
  malignant, due to anesthesia T88.3
  newborn P81.9
    environmental P81.0
Hyperthyroid (recurrent) — *see* Hyperthyroidism
Hyperthyroidism (latent) (pre-adult) (recurrent) E05.90
  with
    goiter (diffuse) E05.00
      nodular (multinodular) E05.20
        with thyroid storm E05.21
        uninodular E05.10
          with thyroid storm E05.11
    storm E05.91
  due to ectopic thyroid tissue E05.30
    with thyroid storm E05.31
  neonatal, transitory P72.1
  specified NEC E05.80
    with thyroid storm E05.81
Hypertony, hypertonia, hypertonicity
  bladder N31.8
  congenital P94.1
  stomach K31.89
    psychogenic F45.8
  uterus, uterine (contractions) (complicating delivery) O62.4
Hypertrichosis L68.9
  congenital Q84.2
  eyelid H02.869
    left H02.866
      lower H02.865
      upper H02.864
    right H02.863
      lower H02.862
      upper H02.861
  lanuginosa Q84.2
    acquired L68.1
  localized L68.2
  specified NEC L68.8
Hypertriglyceridemia, essential E78.1
Hypertrophy, hypertrophic
  adenofibromatous, prostate — *see* Enlargement, enlarged, prostate
  adenoids (infective) J35.2
    with tonsils J35.3
  adrenal cortex E27.8
  alveolar process or ridge — *see* Anomaly, alveolar
  anal papillae K62.89
  artery I77.89
    congenital NEC Q27.8
      digestive system Q27.8
      lower limb Q27.8
      specified site NEC Q27.8
      upper limb Q27.8
  auricular — *see* Hypertrophy, cardiac
  Bartholin's gland N75.8
  bile duct (common) (hepatic) K83.8
  bladder (sphincter) (trigone) N32.89
  bone M89.30
    carpus M89.34-
    clavicle M89.31-
    femur M89.35-
    fibula M89.36-
    finger M89.34-
    humerus M89.32-
    ilium M89.359
    ischium M89.359
    metacarpus M89.34-
    metatarsus M89.37-
    multiple sites M89.39
    neck M89.38
    radius M89.33-
    rib M89.38
    scapula M89.31-
    skull M89.38
    tarsus M89.37-
    tibia M89.36-
    toe M89.37-

Hypertrophy, hypertrophic — *continued*
  bone M89.30 — *continued*
    ulna M89.33-
    vertebra M89.38
  brain G93.89
  breast N62
    cystic — *see* Mastopathy, cystic
    newborn P83.4
    pubertal, massive N62
    puerperal, postpartum — *see* Disorder, breast, specified type NEC
    senile (parenchymatous) N62
  cardiac (chronic) (idiopathic) I51.7
    with rheumatic fever (conditions in I00)
      active I01.8
      inactive or quiescent (with chorea) I09.89
    congenital NEC Q24.8
    fatty — *see* Degeneration, myocardial
    hypertensive — *see* Hypertension, heart
    rheumatic (with chorea) I09.89
      active or acute I01.8
        with chorea I02.0
    valve — *see* Endocarditis
  cartilage — *see* Disorder, cartilage, specified type NEC
  cecum — *see* Megacolon
  cervix (uteri) N88.8
    congenital Q51.828
    elongation N88.4
  clitoris (cirrhotic) N90.89
    congenital Q52.6
  colon — *see also* Megacolon
    congenital Q43.2
  conjunctiva, lymphoid H11.89
  corpora cavernosa N48.89
  cystic duct K82.8
  duodenum K31.89
  endometrium (glandular) (*see also* Hyperplasia, endometrial) N85.00-
    cervix N88.8
  epididymis N50.8
  esophageal hiatus (congenital) Q79.1
    with hernia — *see* Hernia, hiatal
  eyelid — *see* Disorder, eyelid, specified type NEC
  fat pad E65
    knee (infrapatellar) (popliteal) (prepatellar) (retropatellar) M79.4
  foot (congenital) Q74.2
  frenulum, frenum (tongue) K14.8
    lip K13.0
  gallbladder K82.8
  gastric mucosa K29.60
    with bleeding K29.61
  gland, glandular R59.9
    generalized R59.1
    localized R59.0
  gum (mucous membrane) K06.1
  heart (idiopathic) — *see also* Hypertrophy, cardiac
    valve (*see also* Endocarditis) I38
  hemifacial Q67.4
  hepatic — *see* Hypertrophy, liver
  hiatus (esophageal) Q79.1
  hilus gland R59.0
  hymen, congenital Q52.4
  ileum K63.89
  intestine NEC K63.89
  jejunum K63.89
  kidney (compensatory) N28.81
    congenital Q63.3
  labium (majus) (minus) N90.6
  ligament — *see* Disorder, ligament
  lingual tonsil (infective) J35.1
    with adenoids J35.3
  lip K13.0
    congenital Q18.6
  liver R16.0
    acute K76.89
    cirrhotic — *see* Cirrhosis, liver
    congenital Q44.7
    fatty — *see* Fatty, liver
  lymph, lymphatic gland R59.9
    generalized R59.1
    localized R59.0
    tuberculous — *see* Tuberculosis, lymph gland
  mammary gland — *see* Hypertrophy, breast
  Meckel's diverticulum (congenital) Q43.0
    malignant — *see* Table of Neoplasms, small intestine, malignant
  median bar — *see* Hyperplasia, prostate
  meibomian gland — *see* Chalazion
  meniscus, knee, congenital Q74.1
  metatarsal head — *see* Hypertrophy, bone, metatarsus
  metatarsus — *see* Hypertrophy, bone, metatarsus

Hypertrophy, hypertrophic — *continued*
  mucous membrane
    alveolar ridge K06.2
    gum K06.1
    nose (turbinate) J34.3
  muscle M62.89
  muscular coat, artery I77.89
  myocardium — *see also* Hypertrophy, cardiac
    idiopathic I42.2
  myometrium N85.2
  nail L60.2
    congenital Q84.5
  nasal J34.89
    alae J34.89
    bone J34.89
    cartilage J34.89
    mucous membrane (septum) J34.3
    sinus J34.89
    turbinate J34.3
  nasopharynx, lymphoid (infectional) (tissue) (wall) J35.2
  nipple N62
  organ or site, congenital NEC — *see* Anomaly, by site
  ovary N83.8
  palate (hard) M27.8
    soft K13.79
  pancreas, congenital Q45.3
  parathyroid (gland) E21.0
  parotid gland K11.1
  penis N48.89
  pharyngeal tonsil J35.2
  pharynx J39.2
    lymphoid (infectional) (tissue) (wall) J35.2
  pituitary (anterior) (fossa) (gland) E23.6
  prepuce (congenital) N47.8
    female N90.89
  prostate — *see* Enlargement, enlarged, prostate
    congenital Q55.4
  pseudomuscular G71.0
  pylorus (adult) (muscle) (sphincter) K31.1
    congenital or infantile Q40.0
  rectal, rectum (sphincter) K62.89
  rhinitis (turbinate) J31.0
  salivary gland (any) K11.1
    congenital Q38.4
  scaphoid (tarsal) — *see* Hypertrophy, bone, tarsus
  scar L91.0
  scrotum N50.8
  seminal vesicle N50.8
  sigmoid — *see* Megacolon
  skin L91.9
    specified NEC L91.8
  spermatic cord N50.8
  spleen — *see* Splenomegaly
  spondylitis — *see* Spondylosis
  stomach K31.89
  sublingual gland K11.1
  submandibular gland K11.1
  suprarenal cortex (gland) E27.8
  synovial NEC M67.20
    acromioclavicular M67.21-
    ankle M67.27-
    elbow M67.22-
    foot M67.27-
    hand M67.24-
    hip M67.25-
    knee M67.26-
    multiple sites M67.29
    specified site NEC M67.28
    wrist M67.23-
  tendon — *see* Disorder, tendon, specified type NEC
  testis N44.8
    congenital Q55.29
  thymic, thymus (gland) (congenital) E32.0
  thyroid (gland) — *see* Goiter
  toe (congenital) Q74.2
    acquired — *see also* Deformity, toe, specified NEC
  tongue K14.8
    congenital Q38.2
    papillae (foliate) K14.3
  tonsils (faucial) (infective) (lingual) (lymphoid) J35.1
    with adenoids J35.3
  tunica vaginalis N50.8
  ureter N28.89
  urethra N36.8
  uterus N85.2
    neck (with elongation) N88.4
    puerperal O90.89
  uvula K13.79
  vagina N89.8
  vas deferens N50.8
  vein I87.8

Hypertrophy, hypertrophic — *continued*
  ventricle, ventricular (heart) — *see also* Hypertrophy, cardiac
    congenital Q24.8
      in tetralogy of Fallot Q21.3
  verumontanum N36.8
  vocal cord J38.3
  vulva N90.6
    stasis (nonfilarial) N90.6
Hypertropia H50.2-
Hypertyrosinemia E70.21
Hyperuricemia (asymptomatic) E79.0
Hypervalinemia E71.19
Hyperventilation (tetany) R06.4
  hysterical F45.8
  psychogenic F45.8
  syndrome F45.8
Hypervitaminosis (dietary) NEC E67.8
  A E67.0
    administered as drug (prolonged intake) — *see* Table of Drugs and Chemicals, vitamins, adverse effect
    overdose or wrong substance given or taken — *see* Table of Drugs and Chemicals, vitamins, poisoning
  B6 E67.2
  D E67.3
    administered as drug (prolonged intake) — *see* Table of Drugs and Chemicals, vitamins, adverse effect
    overdose or wrong substance given or taken — *see* Table of Drugs and Chemicals, vitamins, poisoning
  K E67.8
    administered as drug (prolonged intake) — *see* Table of Drugs and Chemicals, vitamins, adverse effect
    overdose or wrong substance given or taken — *see* Table of Drugs and Chemicals, vitamins, poisoning
Hypervolemia E87.70
  specified NEC E87.79
Hypesthesia R20.1
  cornea — *see* Anesthesia, cornea
Hyphema H21.0-
  traumatic S05.1-
Hypo-osmolality E87.1
Hypo-ovarianism, hypo-ovarism E28.39
Hypoacidity, gastric K31.89
  psychogenic F45.8
Hypoadrenalism, hypoadrenia E27.40
  primary E27.1
  tuberculous A18.7
Hypoadrenocorticism E27.40
  pituitary E23.0
  primary E27.1
Hypoalbuminemia E88.09
Hypoaldosteronism E27.40
Hypoalphalipoproteinemia E78.6
Hypobarism T70.29
Hypobaropathy T70.29
Hypobetalipoproteinemia (familial) E78.6
Hypocalcemia E83.51
  dietary E58
  neonatal P71.1
    due to cow's milk P71.0
  phosphate-loading (newborn) P71.1
Hypochloremia E87.8
Hypochlorhydria K31.89
  neurotic F45.8
  psychogenic F45.8
Hypochondria, hypochondriac, hypochondriasis (reaction) F45.21
  sleep F51.03
Hypochondrogenesis Q77.0
Hypochondroplasia Q77.4
Hypochromasia, blood cells D50.8
Hypodontia — *see* Anodontia
Hypoeosinophilia D72.89
Hypoesthesia R20.1
Hypofibrinogenemia D68.8
  acquired D65
  congenital (hereditary) D68.2
Hypofunction
  adrenocortical E27.40
    drug-induced E27.3
    postprocedural E89.6
    primary E27.1
  adrenomedullary, postprocedural E89.6
  cerebral R29.818
  corticoadrenal NEC E27.40
  intestinal K59.8
  labyrinth — *see* subcategory H83.2
  ovary E28.39
  pituitary (gland) (anterior) E23.0
  testicular E29.1
    postprocedural (postsurgical) (postirradiation) (iatrogenic) E89.5
Hypogalactia O92.4

D I S E A S E   I N D E X

Hypogammaglobulinemia (see also Agammaglobulinemia) D80.1
  hereditary D80.0
  nonfamilial D80.1
  transient, of infancy D80.7
Hypogenitalism (congenital) — see Hypogonadism
Hypoglossia Q38.3
Hypoglycemia (spontaneous) E16.2
  coma E15
    diabetic — see Diabetes, coma
  diabetic — see Diabetes, hypoglycemia
  dietary counseling and surveillance Z71.3
  drug-induced E16.0
    with coma (nondiabetic) E15
    due to insulin E16.0
      with coma (nondiabetic) E15
      therapeutic misadventure — see subcategory T38.3
  functional, nonhyperinsulinemic E16.1
  iatrogenic E16.0
    with coma (nondiabetic) E15
  in infant of diabetic mother P70.1
    gestational diabetes P70.0
  infantile E16.1
  leucine-induced E71.19
  neonatal (transitory) P70.4
    iatrogenic P70.3
  reactive (not drug-induced) E16.1
  transitory neonatal P70.4
Hypogonadism
  female E28.39
  hypogonadotropic E23.0
  male E29.1
  ovarian (primary) E28.39
  pituitary E23.0
  testicular (primary) E29.1
Hypohidrosis, hypoidrosis L74.4
Hypoinsulinemia, postprocedural E89.1
Hypokalemia E87.6
Hypoleukocytosis — see Agranulocytosis
Hypolipoproteinemia (alpha) (beta) E78.6
Hypomagnesemia E83.42
  neonatal P71.2
Hypomania, hypomanic reaction F30.8
Hypomenorrhea — see Oligomenorrhea
Hypometabolism R63.8
Hypomotility
  gastrointestinal (tract) K31.89
    psychogenic F45.8
  intestine K59.8
    psychogenic F45.8
  stomach K31.89
    psychogenic F45.8
Hyponasality R49.22
Hyponatremia E87.1
Hypoparathyroidism E20.9
  familial E20.8
  idiopathic E20.0
  neonatal, transitory P71.4
  postprocedural E89.2
  specified NEC E20.8
Hypoperfusion (in)
  newborn P96.89
Hypopharyngitis — see Laryngopharyngitis
Hypophoria H50.53
Hypophosphatemia, hypophosphatasia (acquired) (congenital) (renal) E83.39
  familial E83.31
Hypophyseal, hypophysis — see also condition
  dwarfism E23.0
  gigantism E22.0
Hypopiesis — see Hypotension
Hypopinealism E34.8
Hypopituitarism (juvenile) E23.0
  drug-induced E23.1
  due to
    hypophysectomy E89.3
    radiotherapy E89.3
  iatrogenic NEC E23.1
  postirradiation E89.3
  postpartum E23.0
  postprocedural E89.3
Hypoplasia, hypoplastic
  adrenal (gland), congenital Q89.1
  alimentary tract, congenital Q45.8
    upper Q40.8
  anus, anal (canal) Q42.3
    with fistula Q42.2
  aorta, aortic Q25.4
    ascending, in hypoplastic left heart syndrome Q23.4
    valve Q23.1
      in hypoplastic left heart syndrome Q23.4
  areola, congenital Q83.8
  arm (congenital) — see Defect, reduction, upper limb

Hypoplasia, hypoplastic — continued
  artery (peripheral) Q27.8
    brain (congenital) Q28.3
    coronary Q24.5
    digestive system Q27.8
    lower limb Q27.8
    pulmonary Q25.79
      functional, unilateral J43.0
    retinal (congenital) Q14.1
    specified site NEC Q27.8
    umbilical Q27.0
    upper limb Q27.8
  auditory canal Q17.8
    causing impairment of hearing Q16.9
  biliary duct or passage Q44.5
  bone NOS Q79.9
    face Q75.8
    marrow D61.9
      megakaryocytic D69.49
    skull — see Hypoplasia, skull
  brain Q02
    gyri Q04.3
    part of Q04.3
  breast (areola) N64.82
  bronchus Q32.4
  cardiac Q24.8
  carpus — see Defect, reduction, upper limb, specified type NEC
  cartilage hair Q78.5
  cecum Q42.8
  cementum K00.4
  cephalic Q02
  cerebellum Q04.3
  cervix (uteri), congenital Q51.821
  clavicle (congenital) Q74.0
  coccyx Q76.49
  colon Q42.9
    specified NEC Q42.8
  corpus callosum Q04.0
  cricoid cartilage Q31.2
  digestive organ(s) or tract NEC Q45.8
    upper (congenital) Q40.8
  ear (auricle) (lobe) Q17.2
    middle Q16.4
  enamel of teeth (neonatal) (postnatal) (prenatal) K00.4
  endocrine (gland) NEC Q89.2
  endometrium N85.8
  epididymis (congenital) Q55.4
  epiglottis Q31.2
  erythroid, congenital D61.01
  esophagus (congenital) Q39.8
  eustachian tube Q17.8
  eye Q11.2
  eyelid (congenital) Q10.3
  face Q18.8
    bone(s) Q75.8
  femur (congenital) — see Defect, reduction, lower limb, specified type NEC
  fibula (congenital) — see Defect, reduction, lower limb, specified type NEC
  finger (congenital) — see Defect, reduction, upper limb, specified type NEC
  focal dermal Q82.8
  foot — see Defect, reduction, lower limb, specified type NEC
  gallbladder Q44.0
  genitalia, genital organ(s)
    female, congenital Q52.8
      external Q52.79
      internal NEC Q52.8
    in adiposogenital dystrophy E23.6
  glottis Q31.2
  hair Q84.2
  hand (congenital) — see Defect, reduction, upper limb, specified type NEC
  heart Q24.8
  humerus (congenital) — see Defect, reduction, upper limb, specified type NEC
  intestine (small) Q41.9
    large Q42.9
      specified NEC Q42.8
  jaw M26.09
    alveolar M26.79
    lower M26.04
      alveolar M26.74
    upper M26.02
      alveolar M26.73
  kidney(s) Q60.5
    bilateral Q60.4
    unilateral Q60.3
  labium (majus) (minus), congenital Q52.79
  larynx Q31.2
  left heart syndrome Q23.4
  leg (congenital) — see Defect, reduction, lower limb

Hypoplasia, hypoplastic — continued
  limb Q73.8
    lower (congenital) — see Defect, reduction, lower limb
    upper (congenital) — see Defect, reduction, upper limb
  liver Q44.7
  lung (lobe) (not associated with short gestation) Q33.6
    associated with immaturity, low birth weight, prematurity, or short gestation P28.0
  mammary (areola), congenital Q83.8
  mandible, mandibular M26.04
    alveolar M26.74
    unilateral condylar M27.8
  maxillary M26.02
    alveolar M26.73
  medullary D61.9
  megakaryocytic D69.49
  metacarpus — see Defect, reduction, upper limb, specified type NEC
  metatarsus — see Defect, reduction, lower limb, specified type NEC
  muscle Q79.8
  nail(s) Q84.6
  nose, nasal Q30.1
  optic nerve H47.03-
  osseous meatus (ear) Q17.8
  ovary, congenital Q50.39
  pancreas Q45.0
  parathyroid (gland) Q89.2
  parotid gland Q38.4
  patella Q74.1
  pelvis, pelvic girdle Q74.2
  penis (congenital) Q55.62
  peripheral vascular system Q27.8
    digestive system Q27.8
    lower limb Q27.8
    specified site NEC Q27.8
    upper limb Q27.8
  pituitary (gland) (congenital) Q89.2
  pulmonary (not associated with short gestation) Q33.6
    artery, functional J43.0
    associated with short gestation P28.0
  radioulnar — see Defect, reduction, upper limb, specified type NEC
  radius — see Defect, reduction, upper limb
  rectum Q42.1
    with fistula Q42.0
  respiratory system NEC Q34.8
  rib Q76.6
  right heart syndrome Q22.6
  sacrum Q76.49
  scapula Q74.0
  scrotum Q55.1
  shoulder girdle Q74.0
  skin Q82.8
  skull (bone) Q75.8
    with
      anencephaly Q00.0
      encephalocele — see Encephalocele
      hydrocephalus Q03.9
        with spina bifida — see Spina bifida, by site, with hydrocephalus
      microcephaly Q02
  spinal (cord) (ventral horn cell) Q06.1
  spine Q76.49
  sternum Q76.7
  tarsus — see Defect, reduction, lower limb, specified type NEC
  testis Q55.1
  thymic, with immunodeficiency D82.1
  thymus (gland) Q89.2
    with immunodeficiency D82.1
  thyroid (gland) E03.1
    cartilage Q31.2
  tibiofibular (congenital) — see Defect, reduction, lower limb, specified type NEC
  toe — see Defect, reduction, lower limb, specified type NEC
  tongue Q38.3
  Turner's K00.4
  ulna (congenital) — see Defect, reduction, upper limb
  umbilical artery Q27.0
  unilateral condylar M27.8
  ureter Q62.8
  uterus, congenital Q51.811
  vagina Q52.4
  vascular NEC peripheral Q27.8
    brain Q28.3
    digestive system Q27.8
    lower limb Q27.8
    specified site NEC Q27.8
    upper limb Q27.8

Hypoplasia, hypoplastic — continued
  vein(s) (peripheral) Q27.8
    brain Q28.3
    digestive system Q27.8
    great Q26.8
    lower limb Q27.8
    specified site NEC Q27.8
    upper limb Q27.8
  vena cava (inferior) (superior) Q26.8
  vertebra Q76.49
  vulva, congenital Q52.79
  zonule (ciliary) Q12.8
Hypopotassemia E87.6
Hypoproconvertinemia, congenital (hereditary) D68.2
Hypoproteinemia E77.8
Hypoprothrombinemia (congenital) (hereditary) (idiopathic) D68.2
  acquired D68.4
  newborn, transient P61.6
Hypoptyalism K11.7
Hypopyon (eye) (anterior chamber) — see Iridocyclitis, acute, hypopyon
Hypopyrexia R68.0
Hyporeflexia R29.2
Hyposecretion
  ACTH E23.0
  antidiuretic hormone E23.2
  ovary E28.39
  salivary gland (any) K11.7
  vasopressin E23.2
Hyposegmentation, leukocytic, hereditary D72.0
Hyposiderinemia D50.9
Hypospadias Q54.9
  balanic Q54.0
  coronal Q54.0
  glandular Q54.0
  penile Q54.1
  penoscrotal Q54.2
  perineal Q54.3
  specified NEC Q54.8
Hypospermatogenesis — see Oligospermia
Hyposplenism D73.0
Hypostasis pulmonary, passive — see Edema, lung
Hypostatic — see condition
Hyposthenuria N28.89
Hypotension (arterial) (constitutional) I95.9
  chronic I95.89
  drug-induced I95.2
  due to (of) hemodialysis I95.3
  iatrogenic I95.89
  idiopathic (permanent) I95.0
  intra-dialytic I95.3
  intracranial, following ventricular shunting (ventriculostomy) G97.2
  maternal, syndrome (following labor and delivery) O26.5-
  neurogenic, orthostatic G90.3
  orthostatic (chronic) I95.1
    due to drugs I95.2
    neurogenic G90.3
  postoperative I95.81
  postural I95.1
  specified NEC I95.89
Hypothermia (accidental) T68
  due to anesthesia, anesthetic T88.51
  low environmental temperature T68
  neonatal P80.9
    environmental (mild) NEC P80.8
    mild P80.8
    severe (chronic) (cold injury syndrome) P80.0
    specified NEC P80.8
  not associated with low environmental temperature R68.0
Hypothyroidism (acquired) E03.9
  congenital (without goiter) E03.1
    with goiter (diffuse) E03.0
  due to
    exogenous substance NEC E03.2
    iodine-deficiency, acquired E01.8
      subclinical E02
    irradiation therapy E89.0
    medicament NEC E03.2
    P-aminosalicylic acid (PAS) E03.2
    phenylbutazone E03.2
    resorcinol E03.2
    sulfonamide E03.2
    surgery E89.0
    thiourea group drugs E03.2
  iatrogenic NEC E03.2
  iodine-deficiency (acquired) E01.8
    congenital — see Syndrome, iodine-deficiency, congenital
    subclinical E02

Hypothyroidism (acquired) E03.9 — *continued*
  neonatal, transitory P72.2
  postinfectious E03.3
  postirradiation E89.0
  postprocedural E89.0
  postsurgical E89.0
  specified NEC E03.8
  subclinical, iodine-deficiency related E02
Hypotonia, hypotonicity, hypotony
  bladder N31.2
  congenital (benign) P94.2
  eye — *see* Disorder, globe, hypotony
Hypotrichosis — *see* Alopecia
Hypotropia H50.2-
Hypoventilation R06.89
  congenital central alveolar G47.35
  sleep related
    idiopathic nonobstructive alveolar G47.34
    in conditions classified elsewhere G47.36
Hypovitaminosis — *see* Deficiency, vitamin
Hypovolemia E86.1
  surgical shock T81.19
  traumatic (shock) T79.4
Hypoxemia R09.02
  newborn P84
  sleep related, in conditions classified elsewhere G47.36
Hypoxia (*see also* Anoxia) R09.02
  cerebral, during a procedure NEC G97.81
    postprocedural NEC G97.82
  intrauterine P84
  myocardial — *see* Insufficiency, coronary
  newborn P84
  sleep-related G47.34
Hypsarhythmia — *see* Epilepsy, generalized, specified NEC
Hysteralgia, pregnant uterus O26.89-
Hysteria, hysterical (conversion) (dissociative state) F44.9
  anxiety F41.8
  convulsions F44.5
  psychosis, acute F44.9
Hysteroepilepsy F44.5

I

Ichthyoparasitism due to Vandellia cirrhosa B88.8
Ichthyosis (congenital) Q80.9
  acquired L85.0
  fetalis Q80.4
  hystrix Q80.8
  lamellar Q80.2
  lingual K13.29
  palmaris and plantaris Q82.8
  simplex Q80.0
  vera Q80.8
  vulgaris Q80.0
  X-linked Q80.1
Ichthyotoxism — *see* Poisoning, fish
  bacterial — *see* Intoxication, foodborne
Icteroanemia, hemolytic (acquired) D59.9
  congenital — *see* Spherocytosis
Icterus — *see also* Jaundice
  conjunctiva R17
  gravis, newborn P55.0
  hematogenous (acquired) D59.9
  hemolytic (acquired) D59.9
    congenital — *see* Spherocytosis
  hemorrhagic (acute) (leptospiral) (spirochetal) A27.0
    newborn P53
  infectious B15.9
    with hepatic coma B15.0
    leptospiral A27.0
    spirochetal A27.0
  neonatorum — *see* Jaundice, newborn
  newborn P59.9
  spirochetal A27.0
Ictus solaris, solis T67.0
Id reaction (due to bacteria) L30.2
Ideation
  homicidal R45.850
  suicidal R45.851
Identity disorder (child) F64.9
  gender role F64.2
  psychosexual F64.2
Idioglossia F80.0
Idiopathic — *see* condition
Idiot, idiocy (congenital) F73
  amaurotic (Bielschowsky(-Jansky)) (family) (infantile (late)) (juvenile (late)) (Vogt-Spielmeyer) E75.4
  microcephalic Q02
IgE asthma J45.909
IIAC (idiopathic infantile arterial calcification) Q28.8
Ileitis (chronic) (noninfectious) (*see also* Enteritis) K52.9
  backwash — *see* Pancolitis, ulcerative (chronic)
  infectious A09
  regional (ulcerative) — *see* Enteritis, regional, small intestine
  segmental — *see* Enteritis, regional
  terminal (ulcerative) — *see* Enteritis, regional, small intestine
Ileocolitis (*see also* Enteritis) K52.9
  infectious A09
  regional — *see* Enteritis, regional
Ileostomy
  attention to Z43.2
  malfunctioning K94.13
  status Z93.2
    with complication — *see* Complications, enterostomy
Ileotyphus — *see* Typhoid
Ileum — *see* condition
Ileus (bowel) (colon) (inhibitory) (intestine) K56.7
  adynamic K56.0
  due to gallstone (in intestine) K56.3
  duodenal (chronic) K31.5
  gallstone K56.3
  mechanical NEC K56.69
  meconium P76.0
    in cystic fibrosis E84.11
    meaning meconium plug (without cystic fibrosis) P76.0
  myxedema K59.8
  neurogenic K56.0
    Hirschsprung's disease or megacolon Q43.1
  newborn
    due to meconium P76.0
      in cystic fibrosis E84.11
      meaning meconium plug (without cystic fibrosis) P76.0
    transitory P76.1
  obstructive K56.69
  paralytic K56.0

Iliac — *see* condition
Iliotibial band syndrome M76.3-
Illiteracy Z55.0
Illness (*see also* Disease) R69
  manic-depressive — *see* Disorder, bipolar
Imbalance R26.89
  autonomic G90.8
  constituents of food intake E63.1
  electrolyte E87.8
    with
      abortion — *see* Abortion, by type, complicated by, electrolyte imbalance
      molar pregnancy O08.5
    due to hyperemesis gravidarum O21.1
    following ectopic or molar pregnancy O08.5
    neonatal, transitory NEC P74.4
      potassium P74.3
      sodium P74.2
  endocrine E34.9
  eye muscle NOS H50.9
  hormone E34.9
  hysterical F44.4
  labyrinth — *see* subcategory H83.2
  posture R29.3
  protein-energy — *see* Malnutrition
  sympathetic G90.8
Imbecile, imbecility (I.Q. 35-49) F71
Imbedding, intrauterine device T83.39
Imbibition, cholesterol (gallbladder) K82.4
Imbrication, teeth, fully erupted M26.30
Imerslund(-Gräsbeck) syndrome D51.1
Immature — *see also* Immaturity
  birth (less than 37 completed weeks) — *see* Preterm, newborn
  extremely (less than 28 completed weeks) — *see* Immaturity, extreme
  personality F60.89
Immaturity (less than 37 completed weeks) — *see also* Preterm, newborn
  extreme of newborn (less than 28 completed weeks of gestation) (less than 196 completed days of gestation) (unspecified weeks of gestation) P07.20
    gestational age
      23 completed weeks (23 weeks, 0 days through 23 weeks, 6 days) P07.22
      24 completed weeks (24 weeks, 0 days through 24 weeks, 6 days) P07.23
      25 completed weeks (25 weeks, 0 days through 25 weeks, 6 days) P07.24
      26 completed weeks (26 weeks, 0 days through 26 weeks, 6 days) P07.25
      27 completed weeks (27 weeks, 0 days through 27 weeks, 6 days) P07.26
    less than 23 completed weeks P07.21
  fetus or infant light-for-dates — *see* Light-for-dates
  lung, newborn P28.0
  organ or site NEC — *see* Hypoplasia
  pulmonary, newborn P28.0
  reaction F60.89
  sexual (female) (male), after puberty E30.0
Immersion T75.1
  foot T69.02-
  hand T69.01-
Immobile, immobility
  complete, due to severe physical disability or frailty R53.2
  intestine K59.8
  syndrome (paraplegic) M62.3
Immune reconstitution (inflammatory) syndrome [IRIS] D89.3
Immunization — *see also* Vaccination
  ABO — *see* Incompatibility, ABO
    in newborn P55.1
  complication — *see* Complications, vaccination
  encounter for Z23
  not done (not carried out) Z28.9
    because (of)
      acute illness of patient Z28.01
      allergy to vaccine (or component) Z28.04
      caregiver refusal Z28.82
      chronic illness of patient Z28.02
      contraindication NEC Z28.09
      group pressure Z28.1
      guardian refusal Z28.82
      immune compromised state of patient Z28.03
      parent refusal Z28.82

Immunization — *see also* Vaccination — *continued*
  not done (not carried out) Z28.9 — *continued*
    because (of) — *continued*
      patient's belief Z28.1
      patient had disease being vaccinated against Z28.81
      patient refusal Z28.21
      religious beliefs of patient Z28.1
      specified reason NEC Z28.89
        of patient Z28.29
      unspecified patient reason Z28.20
  Rh factor
    affecting management of pregnancy NEC O36.09-
      anti-D antibody O36.01-
    from transfusion — *see* Complication(s), transfusion, incompatibility reaction, Rh (factor)
Immunocytoma C83.0-
Immunodeficiency D84.9
  with
    adenosine-deaminase deficiency D81.3
    antibody defects D80.9
      specified type NEC D80.8
    hyperimmunoglobulinemia D80.6
    increased immunoglobulin M (IgM) D80.5
    major defect D82.9
      specified type NEC D82.8
    partial albinism D82.8
    short-limbed stature D82.2
    thrombocytopenia and eczema D82.0
  antibody with
    hyperimmunoglobulinemia D80.6
    near-normal immunoglobulins D80.6
  autosomal recessive, Swiss type D80.0
  combined D81.9
    biotin-dependent carboxylase D81.819
      biotinidase D81.810
      holocarboxylase synthetase D81.818
      specified type NEC D81.818
    severe (SCID) D81.9
      with
        low or normal B-cell numbers D81.2
        low T-and B-cell numbers D81.1
        reticular dysgenesis D81.0
    specified type NEC D81.89
  common variable D83.9
    with
      abnormalities of B-cell numbers and function D83.0
      autoantibodies to B-or T-cells D83.2
      immunoregulatory T-cell disorders D83.1
    specified type NEC D83.8
  following hereditary defective response to Epstein-Barr virus (EBV) D82.3
  selective, immunoglobulin
    A (IgA) D80.2
    G (IgG) (subclasses) D80.3
    M (IgM) D80.4
  severe combined (SCID) D81.9
  specified type NEC D84.8
  X-linked, with increased IgM D80.5
Immunotherapy (encounter for)
  antineoplastic Z51.12
Impaction, impacted
  bowel, colon, rectum (*see also* Impaction, fecal) K56.49
    by gallstone K56.3
  calculus — *see* Calculus
  cerumen (ear) (external) H61.2-
  cuspid — *see* Impaction, tooth
  dental (same or adjacent tooth) K01.1
  fecal, feces K56.41
  fracture — *see* Fracture, by site
  gallbladder — *see* Calculus, gallbladder
  gallstone(s) — *see* Calculus, gallbladder
    bile duct (common) (hepatic) — *see* Calculus, bile duct
    cystic duct — *see* Calculus, gallbladder
    in intestine, with obstruction (any part) K56.3
  intestine (calculous) NEC (*see also* Impaction, fecal) K56.49
    gallstone, with ileus K56.3
  intrauterine device (IUD) T83.39
  molar — *see* Impaction, tooth
  shoulder, causing obstructed labor O66.0
  tooth, teeth K01.1
  turbinate J34.89
Impaired, impairment (function)
  auditory discrimination — *see* Abnormal, auditory perception
  cognitive, mild, so stated G31.84
  dual sensory Z73.82
  fasting glucose R73.01

DISEASE INDEX

Impaired, impairment (function) — *continued*
glucose tolerance (oral) R73.02
hearing — *see* Deafness
heart — *see* Disease, heart
kidney N28.9
  disorder resulting from N25.9
    specified NEC N25.89
liver K72.90
  with coma K72.91
mastication K08.8
mild cognitive, so stated G31.84
mobility
  ear ossicles — *see* Ankylosis, ear ossicles
  requiring care provider Z74.09
myocardium, myocardial — *see* Insufficiency, myocardial
rectal sphincter R19.8
renal (acute) (chronic) N28.9
  disorder resulting from N25.9
    specified NEC N25.89
vision NEC H54.7
  both eyes H54.3
Impediment, speech R47.9
psychogenic (childhood) F98.8
slurring R47.81
specified NEC R47.89
Impending
coronary syndrome I20.0
delirium tremens F10.239
myocardial infarction I20.0
Imperception auditory (acquired) — *see also* Deafness
congenital H93.25
Imperfect
aeration, lung (newborn) NEC — *see* Atelectasis
closure (congenital)
  alimentary tract NEC Q45.8
    lower Q43.8
    upper Q40.8
  atrioventricular ostium Q21.2
  atrium (secundum) Q21.1
  branchial cleft or sinus Q18.0
  choroid Q14.3
  cricoid cartilage Q31.8
  cusps, heart valve NEC Q24.8
    pulmonary Q22.3
  ductus
    arteriosus Q25.0
    Botalli Q25.0
  ear drum (causing impairment of hearing) Q16.4
  esophagus with communication to bronchus or trachea Q39.1
  eyelid Q10.3
  foramen
    botalli Q21.1
    ovale Q21.1
  genitalia, genital organ(s) or system
    female Q52.8
      external Q52.79
      internal NEC Q52.8
    male Q55.8
  glottis Q31.8
  interatrial ostium or septum Q21.1
  interauricular ostium or septum Q21.1
  interventricular ostium or septum Q21.0
  larynx Q31.8
  lip — *see* Cleft, lip
  nasal septum Q30.3
  nose Q30.2
  omphalomesenteric duct Q43.0
  optic nerve entry Q14.2
  organ or site not listed — *see* Anomaly, by site
  ostium
    interatrial Q21.1
    interauricular Q21.1
    interventricular Q21.0
  palate — *see* Cleft, palate
  preauricular sinus Q18.1
  retina Q14.1
  roof of orbit Q75.8
  sclera Q13.5
  septum
    aorticopulmonary Q21.4
    atrial (secundum) Q21.1
    between aorta and pulmonary artery Q21.4
    heart Q21.9
    interatrial (secundum) Q21.1
    interauricular (secundum) Q21.1
    interventricular Q21.0
      in tetralogy of Fallot Q21.3
    nasal Q30.3

Imperfect — *continued*
closure (congenital) — *continued*
  septum — *continued*
    ventricular Q21.0
      with pulmonary stenosis or atresia, dextraposition of aorta, and hypertrophy of right ventricle Q21.3
      in tetralogy of Fallot Q21.3
  skull Q75.0
    with
      anencephaly Q00.0
      encephalocele — *see* Encephalocele
      hydrocephalus Q03.9
        with spina bifida — *see* Spina bifida, by site, with hydrocephalus
      microcephaly Q02
  spine (with meningocele) — *see* Spina bifida
  trachea Q32.1
  tympanic membrane (causing impairment of hearing) Q16.4
  uterus Q51.818
  vitelline duct Q43.0
erection — *see* Dysfunction, sexual, male, erectile
fusion — *see* Imperfect, closure
inflation, lung (newborn) — *see* Atelectasis
posture R29.3
rotation, intestine Q43.3
septum, ventricular Q21.0
Imperfectly descended testis — *see* Cryptorchid
Imperforate (congenital) — *see also* Atresia
anus Q42.3
  with fistula Q42.2
cervix (uteri) Q51.828
esophagus Q39.0
  with tracheoesophageal fistula Q39.1
hymen Q52.3
jejunum Q41.1
pharynx Q38.8
rectum Q42.1
  with fistula Q42.0
urethra Q64.39
vagina Q52.4
Impervious (congenital) — *see also* Atresia
anus Q42.3
  with fistula Q42.2
bile duct Q44.2
esophagus Q39.0
  with tracheoesophageal fistula Q39.1
intestine (small) Q41.9
  large Q42.9
    specified NEC Q42.8
rectum Q42.1
  with fistula Q42.0
ureter — *see* Atresia, ureter
urethra Q64.39
Impetiginization of dermatoses L01.1
Impetigo (any organism) (any site) (circinate) (contagiosa) (simplex) (vulgaris) L01.00
Bockhart's L01.02
bullous, bullosa L01.03
external ear L01.00 [H62.40]
follicularis L01.02
furfuracea L30.5
herpetiformis L40.1
  nonobstetrical L40.1
neonatorum L01.03
nonbullous L01.01
specified type NEC L01.09
ulcerative L01.09
Impingement (on teeth)
soft tissue
  anterior M26.81
  posterior M26.82
Implant, endometrial N80.9
Implantation
anomalous — *see* Anomaly, by site
  ureter Q62.63
cyst
  external area or site (skin) NEC L72.0
  iris — *see* Cyst, iris, implantation
  vagina N89.8
  vulva N90.7
dermoid (cyst) — *see* Implantation, cyst
Impotence (sexual) N52.9
counseling Z70.1
organic origin (*see also* Dysfunction, sexual, male, erectile) N52.9
psychogenic F52.21
Impression, basilar Q75.8
Imprisonment, anxiety concerning Z65.1
Improper care (child) (newborn) — *see* Maltreatment
Improperly tied umbilical cord (causing hemorrhage) P51.8

Impulsiveness (impulsive) R45.87
Inability to swallow — *see* Aphagia
Inaccessible, inaccessibility
health care NEC Z75.3
  due to
    waiting period Z75.2
      for admission to facility elsewhere Z75.1
  other helping agencies Z75.4
Inactive — *see* condition
Inadequate, inadequacy
aesthetics of dental restoration K08.56
biologic, constitutional, functional, or social F60.7
development
  child R62.50
  genitalia
    after puberty NEC E30.0
    congenital
      female Q52.8
        external Q52.79
        internal Q52.8
      male Q55.8
  lungs Q33.6
    associated with short gestation P28.0
  organ or site not listed — *see* Anomaly, by site
diet (causing nutritional deficiency) E63.9
eating habits Z72.4
environment, household Z59.1
family support Z63.8
food (supply) NEC Z59.4
  hunger effects T73.0
functional F60.7
household care, due to
  family member
    handicapped or ill Z74.2
    on vacation Z75.5
    temporarily away from home Z74.2
  technical defects in home Z59.1
  temporary absence from home of person rendering care Z74.2
housing (heating) (space) Z59.1
income (financial) Z59.6
intrafamilial communication Z63.8
material resources Z59.9
mental — *see* Disability, intellectual
parental supervision or control of child Z62.0
personality F60.7
pulmonary
  function R06.89
    newborn P28.5
  ventilation, newborn P28.5
sample of cytologic smear
  anus R85.615
  cervix R87.615
  vagina R87.625
social F60.7
  insurance Z59.7
  skills NEC Z73.4
supervision of child by parent Z62.0
teaching affecting education Z55.8
welfare support Z59.7
Inanition R64
with edema — *see* Malnutrition, severe
due to
  deprivation of food T73.0
  malnutrition — *see* Malnutrition
fever R50.9
Inappropriate
change in quantitative human chorionic gonadotropin (hCG) in early pregnancy O02.81
diet or eating habits Z72.4
level of quantitative human chorionic gonadotropin (hCG) for gestational age in early pregnancy O02.81
secretion
  antidiuretic hormone (ADH) (excessive) E22.2
  deficiency E23.2
  pituitary (posterior) E22.2
Inattention at or after birth — *see* Neglect
Incarceration, incarcerated
enterocele K46.0
  gangrenous K46.1
epiplocele K46.0
  gangrenous K46.1
exophthalmos K42.0
  gangrenous K42.1
hernia — *see also* Hernia, by site, with obstruction
  with gangrene — *see* Hernia, by site, with gangrene
iris, in wound — *see* Injury, eye, laceration, with prolapse
lens, in wound — *see* Injury, eye, laceration, with prolapse
omphalocele K42.0

Incarceration, incarcerated — *continued*
prison, anxiety concerning Z65.1
rupture — *see* Hernia, by site
sarcoepiplocele K46.0
  gangrenous K46.1
sarcoepiplomphalocele K42.0
  with gangrene K42.1
uterus N85.8
  gravid O34.51-
    causing obstructed labor O65.5
Incised wound
external — *see* Laceration
internal organs — *see* Injury, by site
Incision, incisional
hernia K43.2
  with
    gangrene (and obstruction) K43.1
    obstruction K43.0
  surgical, complication — *see* Complications, surgical procedure
traumatic
  external — *see* Laceration
  internal organs — *see* Injury, by site
Inclusion
azurophilic leukocytic D72.0
blennorrhea (neonatal) (newborn) P39.1
gallbladder in liver (congenital) Q44.1
Incompatibility
ABO
  affecting management of pregnancy O36.11-
    anti-A sensitization O36.11-
    anti-B sensitization O36.19-
    specified NEC O36.19-
  infusion or transfusion reaction — *see* Complication(s), transfusion, incompatibility reaction, ABO
  newborn P55.1
blood (group) (Duffy) (K(ell)) (Kidd) (Lewis) (M) (S) NEC
  affecting management of pregnancy O36.11-
    anti-A sensitization O36.11-
    anti-B sensitization O36.19-
  infusion or transfusion reaction T80.89
  newborn P55.8
divorce or estrangement Z63.5
Rh (blood group) (factor) Z31.82
  affecting management of pregnancy NEC O36.09-
    anti-D antibody O36.01-
  infusion or transfusion reaction — *see* Complication(s), transfusion, incompatibility reaction, Rh (factor)
  newborn P55.0
rhesus — *see* Incompatibility, Rh
Incompetency, incompetent, incompetence
annular
  aortic (valve) — *see* Insufficiency, aortic
  mitral (valve) I34.0
  pulmonary valve (heart) I37.1
aortic (valve) — *see* Insufficiency, aortic
cardiac valve — *see* Endocarditis
cervix, cervical (os) N88.3
  in pregnancy O34.3-
chronotropic I45.89
  with
    autonomic dysfunction G90.8
    ischemic heart disease I25.89
    left ventricular dysfunction I51.89
    sinus node dysfunction I49.8
esophagogastric (junction) (sphincter) K22.0
mitral (valve) — *see* Insufficiency, mitral
pelvic fundus N81.89
pubocervical tissue N81.82
pulmonary valve (heart) I37.1
  congenital Q22.3
rectovaginal tissue N81.83
tricuspid (annular) (valve) — *see* Insufficiency, tricuspid
valvular — *see* Endocarditis
  congenital Q24.8
vein, venous (saphenous) (varicose) — *see* Varix, leg
Incomplete — *see also* condition
bladder, emptying R33.9
defecation R15.0
expansion lungs (newborn) NEC — *see* Atelectasis
rotation, intestine Q43.3
Inconclusive
diagnostic imaging due to excess body fat of patient R93.9
findings on diagnostic imaging of breast NEC R92.8
mammogram (due to dense breasts) R92.2

Incontinence R32
  anal sphincter R15.9
  feces R15.9
    nonorganic origin F98.1
  overflow N39.490
  psychogenic F45.8
  rectal R15.9
  reflex N39.498
  stress (female) (male) N39.3
    and urge N39.46
  urethral sphincter R32
  urge N39.41
    and stress (female) (male) N39.46
  urine (urinary) R32
    continuous N39.45
      due to cognitive impairment, or severe
        physical disability or immobility
        R39.81
    functional R39.81
    mixed (stress and urge) N39.46
    nocturnal N39.44
    nonorganic origin F98.0
    overflow N39.490
    post dribbling N39.43
    reflex N39.498
    specified NEC N39.498
    stress (female) (male) N39.3
      and urge N39.46
    total N39.498
    unaware N39.42
    urge N39.41
      and stress (female) (male) N39.46
Incontinentia pigmenti Q82.3
Incoordinate, incoordination
  esophageal-pharyngeal (newborn) — see
    Dysphagia
  muscular R27.8
  uterus (action) (contractions) (complicating
    delivery) O62.4
Increase, increased
  abnormal, in development R63.8
  androgens (ovarian) E28.1
  anticoagulants (antithrombin) (anti-VIIIa)
    (anti-IXa) (anti-Xa) (anti-XIa) — see
    Circulating anticoagulants
  cold sense R20.8
  estrogen E28.0
  function
    adrenal
      cortex — see Cushing's, syndrome
      medulla E27.5
    pituitary (gland) (anterior) (lobe) E22.9
      posterior E22.2
  heat sense R20.8
  intracranial pressure (benign) G93.2
  permeability, capillaries I78.8
  pressure, intracranial G93.2
  secretion
    gastrin E16.4
    glucagon E16.3
    pancreas, endocrine E16.9
      growth hormone-releasing hormone
        E16.8
      pancreatic polypeptide E16.8
      somatostatin E16.8
      vasoactive-intestinal polypeptide
        E16.8
  sphericity, lens Q12.4
  splenic activity D73.1
  venous pressure I87.8
    portal K76.6
Increta placenta O43.22-
Incrustation, cornea, foreign body
  (lead)(zinc) — see Foreign body, cornea
Incyclophoria H50.54
Incyclotropia — see Cyclotropia
Indeterminate sex Q56.4
India rubber skin Q82.8
Indigestion (acid) (bilious) (functional) K30
  catarrhal K31.89
  due to decomposed food NOS A05.9
  nervous F45.8
  psychogenic F45.8
Indirect — see condition
Induratio penis plastica N48.6
Induration, indurated
  brain G93.89
  breast (fibrous) N64.51
    puerperal, postpartum O92.29
  broad ligament N83.8
  chancre
    anus A51.1
    congenital A50.07
    extragenital NEC A51.2
  corpora cavernosa (penis) (plastic) N48.6
  liver (chronic) K76.89
  lung (black) (chronic) (fibroid) (see also
    Fibrosis, lung) J84.10
    essential brown J84.03
  penile (plastic) N48.6

Induration, indurated — continued
  phlebitic — see Phlebitis
  skin R23.4
Inebriety (without dependence) — see
  Alcohol, intoxication
Inefficiency, kidney N28.9
Inelasticity, skin R23.4
Inequality, leg (length) (acquired) — see also
  Deformity, limb, unequal length
  congenital — see Defect, reduction, lower
    limb
  lower leg — see Deformity, limb, unequal
    length
Inertia
  bladder (neurogenic) N31.2
  stomach K31.89
    psychogenic F45.8
  uterus, uterine during labor O62.2
    during latent phase of labor O62.0
    primary O62.0
    secondary O62.1
  vesical (neurogenic) N31.2
Infancy, infantile, infantilism — see also
  condition
  celiac K90.0
  genitalia, genitals (after puberty) E30.0
  Herter's (nontropical sprue) K90.0
  intestinal K90.0
  Lorain E23.0
  pancreatic K86.8
  pelvis M95.5
    with disproportion (fetopelvic) O33.1
      causing obstructed labor O65.1
  pituitary E23.0
  renal N25.0
  uterus — see Infantile, genitalia
Infant(s) — see also Infancy
  excessive crying R68.11
  irritable child R68.12
  lack of care — see Neglect
  liveborn (singleton) Z38.2
    born in hospital Z38.00
      by cesarean Z38.01
    born outside hospital Z38.1
    multiple NEC Z38.8
      born in hospital Z38.68
        by cesarean Z38.69
      born outside hospital Z38.7
    quadruplet Z38.8
      born in hospital Z38.63
        by cesarean Z38.64
      born outside hospital Z38.7
    quintuplet Z38.8
      born in hospital Z38.65
        by cesarean Z38.66
      born outside hospital Z38.7
    triplet Z38.8
      born in hospital Z38.61
        by cesarean Z38.62
      born outside hospital Z38.7
    twin Z38.5
      born in hospital Z38.30
        by cesarean Z38.31
      born outside hospital Z38.4
  of diabetic mother (syndrome of) P70.1
    gestational diabetes P70.0
Infantile — see also condition
  genitalia, genitals E30.0
  os, uterine E30.0
  penis E30.0
  testis E29.1
  uterus E30.0
Infantilism — see Infancy
Infarct, infarction
  adrenal (capsule) (gland) E27.49
  appendices epiploicae K55.0
  bowel K55.0
  brain (stem) — see Infarct, cerebral
  breast N64.89
  brewer's (kidney) N28.0
  cardiac — see Infarct, myocardium
  cerebellar — see Infarct, cerebral
  cerebral (see also Occlusion, artery
    cerebral or precerebral, with
    infarction) I63.9
    aborted I63.9
    cortical I63.9
    due to
      cerebral venous thrombosis,
        nonpyogenic I63.6
      embolism
        cerebral arteries I63.4-
        precerebral arteries I63.1-
      occlusion NEC
        cerebral arteries I63.5-
        precerebral arteries I63.2-
      stenosis NEC
        cerebral arteries I63.5-
        precerebral arteries I63.2-

Infarct, infarction — continued
  cerebral (see also Occlusion, artery
    cerebral or precerebral, with
    infarction) I63.9 — continued
    due to — continued
      thrombosis
        cerebral artery I63.3-
        precerebral artery I63.0-
    intraoperative
      during cardiac surgery I97.810
      during other surgery I97.811
    postprocedural
      following cardiac surgery I97.820
      following other surgery I97.821
    specified NEC I63.8
  colon (acute) (agnogenic) (embolic)
    (hemorrhagic) (nonocclusive)
    (nonthrombotic) (occlusive)
    (segmental) (thrombotic) (with
    gangrene) K55.0
  coronary artery — see Infarct, myocardium
  embolic — see Embolism
  fallopian tube N83.8
  gallbladder K82.8
  heart — see Infarct, myocardium
  hepatic K76.3
  hypophysis (anterior lobe) E23.6
  impending (myocardium) I20.0
  intestine (acute) (agnogenic) (embolic)
    (hemorrhagic) (nonocclusive)
    (nonthrombotic) (occlusive)
    (thrombotic) (withgangrene) K55.0
  kidney N28.0
  liver K76.3
  lung (embolic) (thrombotic) — see
    Embolism, pulmonary
  lymph node I89.8
  mesentery, mesenteric (embolic)
    (thrombotic) (with gangrene) K55.0
  muscle (ischemic) M62.20
    ankle M62.27-
    foot M62.27-
    forearm M62.23-
    hand M62.24-
    lower leg M62.26-
    pelvic region M62.25-
    shoulder region M62.21-
    specified site NEC M62.28
    thigh M62.25-
    upper arm M62.22-
  myocardium, myocardial (acute) (with
    stated duration of 4 weeks or less)
    I21.3
    diagnosed on ECG, but presenting no
      symptoms I25.2
    healed or old I25.2
    intraoperative
      during cardiac surgery I97.790
      during other surgery I97.791
    non-Q wave I21.4
    non-ST elevation (NSTEMI) I21.4
      subsequent I22.2
    nontransmural I21.4
    past (diagnosed on ECG or other
      investigation, but currently
      presenting no symptoms) I25.2
    postprocedural
      following cardiac surgery I97.190
      following other surgery I97.191
    Q wave (see also Infarct, myocardium,
      by site) I21.3
    ST elevation (STEMI) I21.3
      anterior (anteroapical) (anterolateral)
        (anteroseptal) (Q wave) (wall)
        I21.09
        subsequent I22.0
      inferior (diaphragmatic)
        (inferolateral) (inferoposterior)
        (wall) NEC I21.19
        subsequent I22.1
      inferoposterior transmural (Q wave)
        I21.11
      involving
        coronary artery of anterior wall
          NEC I21.09
        coronary artery of inferior wall
          NEC I21.19
        diagonal coronary artery I21.02
        left anterior descending coronary
          artery I21.02
        left circumflex coronary artery
          I21.21
        left main coronary artery I21.01
        oblique marginal coronary artery
          I21.21
        right coronary artery I21.11
      lateral (apical-lateral) (basal-lateral)
        (high) I21.29
        subsequent I22.8

Infarct, infarction — continued
  myocardium, myocardial (acute) (with
    stated duration of 4 weeks or less)
    I21.3 — continued
    ST elevation (STEMI) I21.3 —
      continued
      posterior (posterobasal)
        (posterolateral) (posteroseptal)
        (true) I21.29
        subsequent I22.8
      septal I21.29
        subsequent I22.8
      specified NEC I21.29
        subsequent I22.8
    subsequent (recurrent) (reinfarction)
      I22.9
      anterior (anteroapical) (anterolateral)
        (anteroseptal) (wall) I22.0
      diaphragmatic (wall) I22.1
      inferior (diaphragmatic)
        (inferolateral) (inferoposterior)
        (wall) I22.1
      lateral (apical-lateral) (basal-lateral)
        (high) I22.8
      non-ST elevation (NSTEMI) I22.2
      posterior (posterobasal)
        (posterolateral) (posteroseptal)
        (true) I22.8
      septal I22.8
      specified NEC I22.8
      ST elevation I22.9
        anterior (anteroapical)
          (anterolateral) (anteroseptal)
          (wall) I22.0
        inferior (diaphragmatic)
          (inferolateral)
          (inferoposterior) (wall) I22.1
        specified NEC I22.8
      subendocardial I22.2
      transmural I22.9
        anterior (anteroapical)
          (anterolateral) (anteroseptal)
          (wall) I22.0
        diaphragmatic (wall) I22.1
        inferior (diaphragmatic)
          (inferolateral)
          (inferoposterior) (wall) I22.1
        lateral (apical-lateral) (basal-
          lateral) (high) I22.8
        posterior (posterobasal)
          (posterolateral) (posteroseptal)
          (true) I22.8
        specified NEC I22.8
    syphilitic A52.06
    transmural I21.3
      anterior (anteroapical) (anterolateral)
        (anteroseptal) (Q wave) (wall)
        NEC I21.09
      inferior (diaphragmatic)
        (inferolateral) (inferoposterior)
        (Q wave) (wall) NEC I21.19
      inferoposterior (Q wave) I21.11
      lateral (apical-lateral) (basal-lateral)
        (high) NEC I21.29
      posterior (posterobasal)
        (posterolateral) (posteroseptal)
        (true) NEC I21.29
      septal NEC I21.29
      specified NEC I21.29
  nontransmural I21.4
  omentum K55.0
  ovary N83.8
  pancreas K86.8
  papillary muscle — see Infarct,
    myocardium
  parathyroid gland E21.4
  pituitary (gland) E23.6
  placenta O43.81-
  prostate N42.89
  pulmonary (artery) (vein) (hemorrhagic) —
    see Embolism, pulmonary
  renal (embolic) (thrombotic) N28.0
  retina, retinal (artery) — see Occlusion,
    artery, retina
  spinal (cord) (acute) (embolic)
    (nonembolic) G95.11
  spleen D73.5
    embolic or thrombotic I74.8
  subendocardial (acute) (nontransmural)
    I21.4
  suprarenal (capsule) (gland) E27.49
  testis N50.1
  thrombotic — see also Thrombosis
    artery, arterial — see Embolism
  thyroid (gland) E07.89
  ventricle (heart) — see Infarct,
    myocardium

D I S E A S E   I N D E X

Infecting — see condition
Infection, infected, infective (opportunistic)
  B99.9
  with
    drug resistant organism — see
      Resistance (to), drug — see also
      specific organism
    lymphangitis — see Lymphangitis
    organ dysfunction (acute) R65.20
      with septic shock R65.21
  abscess (skin) — code by site under
    Abscess
  Absidia — see Mucormycosis
  Acanthamoeba — see Acanthamebiasis
  Acanthocheilonema (perstans)
    (streptocerca) B74.4
  accessory sinus (chronic) — see Sinusitis
  achorion — see Dermatophytosis
  Acremonium falciforme B47.0
  acromioclavicular M00.9
  Actinobacillus (actinomycetem-comitans)
    A28.8
    mallei A24.0
    muris A25.1
  Actinomadura B47.1
  Actinomyces (israelii) (see also
    Actinomycosis) A42.9
  Actinomycetales — see Actinomycosis
  actinomycotic NOS — see Actinomycosis
  adenoid (and tonsil) J03.90
    chronic J35.02
  adenovirus NEC
    as cause of disease classified elsewhere
      B97.0
    unspecified nature or site B34.0
  aerogenes capsulatus A48.0
  aertrycke — see Infection, salmonella
  alimentary canal NOS — see Enteritis,
    infectious
  Allescheria boydii B48.2
  Alternaria B48.8
  alveolus, alveolar (process) K04.7
  Ameba, amebic (histolytica) — see
    Amebiasis
  amniotic fluid, sac or cavity O41.10-
    chorioamnionitis O41.12-
    placentitis O41.14-
  amputation stump (surgical) — see
    Complication, amputation stump,
    infection
  Ancylostoma (duodenalis) B76.0
  Anisakiasis, Anisakis larvae B81.0
  anthrax — see Anthrax
  antrum (chronic) — see Sinusitis, maxillary
  anus, anal (papillae) (sphincter) K62.89
  arbovirus (arbor virus) A94
    specified type NEC A93.8
  artificial insemination N98.0
  Ascaris lumbricoides — see Ascariasis
  Ascomycetes B47.0
  Aspergillus (flavus) (fumigatus) (terreus)
    — see Aspergillosis
  atypical
    acid-fast (bacilli) — see Mycobacterium,
      atypical
    mycobacteria — see Mycobacterium,
      atypical
    virus A81.9
      specified type NEC A81.89
  auditory meatus (external) — see Otitis,
    externa, infective
  auricle (ear) — see Otitis, externa, infective
  axillary gland (lymph) L04.2
  Bacillus A49.9
    abortus A23.1
    anthracis — see Anthrax
    Ducrey's (any location) A57
    Flexner's A03.1
    Friedländer's NEC A49.8
    gas (gangrene) A48.0
    mallei A24.0
    melitensis A23.0
    paratyphoid, paratyphosus A01.4
      A A01.1
      B A01.2
      C A01.3
    Shiga(-Kruse) A03.0
    suipestifer — see Infection, salmonella
    swimming pool A31.1
    typhosa A01.00
    welchii — see Gangrene, gas
  bacterial NOS A49.9
    as cause of disease classified elsewhere
      B96.89
      Bacteroides fragilis [B. fragilis] B96.6
      Clostridium perfringens [C.
        perfringens] B96.7
      Enterobacter sakazakii B96.89
      Enterococcus B95.2

Infection, infected, infective (opportunistic)
  B99.9 — continued
  bacterial NOS A49.9 — continued
    as cause of disease classified elsewhere
      B96.89 — continued
      Escherichia coli [E. coli] (see also
        Escherichia coli) B96.20
      Helicobacter pylori [H.pylori] B96.81
      Hemophilus influenzae [H.
        influenzae] B96.3
      Klebsiella pneumoniae [K.
        pneumoniae] B96.1
      Mycoplasma pneumoniae [M.
        pneumoniae] B96.0
      Proteus (mirabilis) (morganii) B96.4
      Pseudomonas (aeruginosa) (mallei)
        (pseudomallei) B96.5
      Staphylococcus B95.8
        aureus (methicillin susceptible)
          (MSSA) B95.61
          methicillin resistant (MRSA)
            B95.62
        specified NEC B95.7
      Streptococcus B95.5
        group A B95.0
        group B B95.1
        pneumoniae B95.3
        specified NEC B95.4
      Vibrio vulnificus B96.82
    specified NEC A48.8
  Bacterium
    paratyphosum A01.4
      A A01.1
      B A01.2
      C A01.3
    typhosum A01.00
  Bacteroides NEC A49.8
    fragilis, as cause of disease classified
      elsewhere B96.6
  Balantidium coli A07.0
  Bartholin's gland N75.8
  Basidiobolus B46.8
  bile duct (common) (hepatic) — see
    Cholangitis
  bladder — see Cystitis
  Blastomyces, blastomycotic — see also
    Blastomycosis
    brasiliensis — see
      Paracoccidioidomycosis
    dermatitidis — see Blastomycosis
    European — see Cryptococcosis
    Loboi B48.0
    North American B40.9
    South American — see
      Paracoccidioidomycosis
  bleb, postprocedure — see Blebitis
  bone — see Osteomyelitis
  Bordetella — see Whooping cough
  Borrelia bergdorfi A69.20
  brain (see also Encephalitis) G04.90
    membranes — see Meningitis
    septic G06.0
      meninges — see Meningitis, bacterial
  branchial cyst Q18.0
  breast — see Mastitis
  bronchus — see Bronchitis
  Brucella A23.9
    abortus A23.1
    canis A23.3
    melitensis A23.0
    mixed A23.8
    specified NEC A23.8
    suis A23.2
  Brugia (malayi) B74.1
    timori B74.2
  bursa — see Bursitis, infective
  buttocks (skin) L08.9
  Campylobacter, intestinal A04.5
    as cause of disease classified elsewhere
      B96.81
  Candida (albicans) (tropicalis) — see
    Candidiasis
  candiru B88.8
  Capillaria (intestinal) B81.1
    hepatica B83.8
    philippinensis B81.1
  cartilage — see Disorder, cartilage,
    specified type NEC
  cat liver fluke B66.0
  catheter-related bloodstream (CRBSI)
    T80.211
  cellulitis — code by site under Cellulitis
  central line-associated T80.219
    bloodstream (CLABSI) T80.211
    specified NEC T80.218
  Cephalosporium falciforme B47.0
  cerebrospinal — see Meningitis
  cervical gland (lymph) L04.0
  cervix — see Cervicitis
  cesarean delivery wound (puerperal) O86.0

Infection, infected, infective (opportunistic)
  B99.9 — continued
  cestodes — see Infestation, cestodes
  chest J22
  Chilomastix (intestinal) A07.8
  Chlamydia, chlamydial A74.9
    anus A56.3
    genitourinary tract A56.2
      lower A56.00
      specified NEC A56.19
    lymphogranuloma A55
    pharynx A56.4
    psittaci A70
    rectum A56.3
    sexually transmitted NEC A56.8
  cholera — see Cholera
  Cladosporium
    bantianum (brain abscess) B43.1
    carrionii B43.0
    castellanii B36.1
    trichoides (brain abscess) B43.1
    werneckii B36.1
  Clonorchis (sinensis) (liver) B66.1
  Clostridium NEC
    bifermentans A48.0
    botulinum (food poisoning) A05.1
      infant A48.51
      wound A48.52
    difficile
      as cause of disease classified
        elsewhere B96.89
      foodborne (disease) A04.7
      gas gangrene A48.0
      necrotizing enterocolitis A04.7
      sepsis A41.4
    gas-forming NEC A48.0
    histolyticum A48.0
    novyi, causing gas gangrene A48.0
    oedematiens A48.0
    perfringens
      as cause of disease classified
        elsewhere B96.7
      due to food A05.2
      foodborne (disease) A05.2
      gas gangrene A48.0
      sepsis A41.4
    septicum, causing gas gangrene A48.0
    sordellii, causing gas gangrene A48.0
    welchii
      as cause of disease classified
        elsewhere B96.7
      foodborne (disease) A05.2
      gas gangrene A48.0
      necrotizing enteritis A05.2
      sepsis A41.4
  Coccidioides (immitis) — see
    Coccidioidomycosis
  colon — see Enteritis, infectious
  colostomy K94.02
  common duct — see Cholangitis
  congenital P39.9
    Candida (albicans) P37.5
    cytomegalovirus P35.1
    hepatitis, viral P35.3
    herpes simplex P35.2
    infectious or parasitic disease P37.9
      specified NEC P37.8
    listeriosis (disseminated) P37.2
    malaria NEC P37.4
      falciparum P37.3
    Plasmodium falciparum P37.3
    poliomyelitis P35.8
    rubella P35.0
    skin P39.4
    toxoplasmosis (acute) (subacute)
      (chronic) P37.1
    tuberculosis P37.0
    urinary (tract) P39.3
    vaccinia P35.8
    virus P35.9
      specified type NEC P35.8
  Conidiobolus B46.8
  coronavirus NEC B34.2
    as cause of disease classified elsewhere
      B97.29
    severe acute respiratory syndrome
      (SARS associated) B97.21
  corpus luteum — see Salpingo-oophoritis
  Corynebacterium diphtheriae — see
    Diphtheria
  cotia virus B08.8
  Coxiella burnetii A78
  coxsackie — see Coxsackie
  Cryptococcus neoformans — see
    Cryptococcosis
  Cryptosporidium A07.2
  Cunninghamella — see Mucormycosis
  cyst — see Cyst
  cystic duct (see also Cholecystitis) K81.9
  Cysticercus cellulosae — see Cysticercosis

Infection, infected, infective (opportunistic)
  B99.9 — continued
  cytomegalovirus, cytomegaloviral B25.9
    congenital P35.1
    maternal, maternal care for (suspected)
      damage to fetus O35.3
    mononucleosis B27.10
      with
        complication NEC B27.19
        meningitis B27.12
        polyneuropathy B27.11
  delta-agent (acute), in hepatitis B carrier
    B17.0
  dental (pulpal origin) K04.7
  Deuteromycetes B47.0
  Dicrocoelium dendriticum B66.2
  Dipetalonema (perstans) (streptocerca) B74.4
  diphtherial — see Diphtheria
  Diphyllobothrium (adult) (latum)
    (pacificum) B70.0
    larval B70.1
  Diplogonoporus (grandis) B71.8
  Dipylidium caninum B67.4
  Dirofilaria B74.8
  Dracunculus medinensis B72
  Drechslera (hawaiiensis) B43.8
  Ducrey Haemophilus (any location) A57
  due to or resulting from
    artificial insemination N98.0
    central venous catheter T80.219
      bloodstream T80.211
      exit or insertion site T80.212
      localized T80.212
      port or reservoir T80.212
      specified NEC T80.218
      tunnel T80.212
    device, implant or graft (see also
      Complications, by site and type,
      infection or inflammation) T85.79
      arterial graft NEC T82.7
      breast (implant) T85.79
      catheter NEC T85.79
        dialysis (renal) T82.7
          intraperitoneal T85.71
        infusion NEC T82.7
          spinal (epidural) (subdural) T85.79
        urinary (indwelling) T83.51
      electronic (electrode) (pulse
        generator) (stimulator)
        bone T84.7
        cardiac T82.7
        nervous system (brain) (peripheral
          nerve) (spinal) T85.79
        urinary T83.59
      fixation, internal (orthopedic) NEC —
        see Complication, fixation
        device, infection
      gastrointestinal (bile duct)
        (esophagus) T85.79
      genital NEC T83.6
      heart NEC T82.7
        valve (prosthesis) T82.6
        graft T82.7
      joint prosthesis — see Complication,
        joint prosthesis, infection
      ocular (corneal graft) (orbital implant)
        NEC T85.79
      orthopedic NEC T84.7
      specified NEC T85.79
      urinary NEC T83.59
      vascular NEC T82.7
      ventricular intracranial shunt T85.79
    Hickman catheter T80.219
      bloodstream T80.211
      localized T80.212
      specified NEC T80.218
    immunization or vaccination T88.0
    infusion, injection or transfusion NEC
      T80.29
      acute T80.22
    injury NEC — code by site under
      Wound, open
    peripherally inserted central catheter
      (PICC) T80.219
      bloodstream T80.211
      localized T80.212
      specified NEC T80.218
    portacath (port-a-cath) T80.219
      bloodstream T80.211
      localized T80.212
      specified NEC T80.218
    surgery T81.4
    triple lumen catheter T80.219
      bloodstream T80.211
      localized T80.212
      specified NEC T80.218
    umbilical venous catheter T80.219
      bloodstream T80.211
      localized T80.212
      specified NEC T80.218

Infection, infected, infective (opportunistic)
B99.9 — continued
during labor NEC O75.3
ear (middle) — see also Otitis media
  external — see Otitis, externa, infective
  inner — see subcategory H83.0
Eberthella typhosa A01.00
Echinococcus — see Echinococcus
echovirus
  as cause of disease classified elsewhere B97.12
  unspecified nature or site B34.1
endocardium I33.0
endocervix — see Cervicitis
Entamoeba — see Amebiasis
enteric — see Enteritis, infectious
Enterobacter sakazakii B96.89
Enterobius vermicularis B80
enterostomy K94.12
enterovirus B34.1
  as cause of disease classified elsewhere B97.10
    coxsackievirus B97.11
    echovirus B97.12
    specified NEC B97.19
Entomophthora B46.8
Epidermophyton — see Dermatophytosis
epididymis — see Epididymitis
episiotomy (puerperal) O86.0
Erysipelothrix (insidiosa) (rhusiopathiae) — see Erysipeloid
erythema infectiosum B08.3
Escherichia (E.) coli NEC A49.8
  as cause of disease classified elsewhere (see also Escherichia coli) B96.20
    congenital P39.8
    sepsis P36.4
    generalized A41.51
    intestinal — see Enteritis, infectious, due to, Escherichia coli
ethmoidal (chronic) (sinus) — see Sinusitis, ethmoidal
eustachian tube (ear) — see Salpingitis, eustachian
external auditory canal (meatus) NEC — see Otitis, externa, infective
eye (purulent) — see Endophthalmitis, purulent
eyelid — see Inflammation, eyelid
fallopian tube — see Salpingo-oophoritis
Fasciola (gigantica) (hepatica) (indica) B66.3
Fasciolopsis (buski) B66.5
filarial — see Infestation, filarial
finger (skin) L08.9
  nail L03.01-
    fungus B35.1
fish tapeworm B70.0
  larval B70.1
flagellate, intestinal A07.9
fluke — see Infestation, fluke
focal
  teeth (pulpal origin) K04.7
  tonsils J35.01
Fonsecaea (compactum) (pedrosoi) B43.0
food — see Intoxication, foodborne
foot (skin) L08.9
  dermatophytic fungus B35.3
Francisella tularensis — see Tularemia
frontal (sinus) (chronic) — see Sinusitis, frontal
fungus NOS B49
  beard B35.0
  dermatophytic — see Dermatophytosis
  foot B35.3
  groin B35.6
  hand B35.2
  nail B35.1
  pathogenic to compromised host only B48.8
  perianal (area) B35.6
  scalp B35.0
  skin B36.9
    foot B35.3
    hand B35.2
    toenails B35.1
Fusarium B48.8
gallbladder — see Cholecystitis
gas bacillus — see Gangrene, gas
gastrointestinal — see Enteritis, infectious
generalized NEC — see Sepsis
genital organ or tract
  female — see Disease, pelvis, inflammatory
  male N49.9
    multiple sites N49.8
    specified NEC N49.8
Ghon tubercle, primary A15.7
Giardia lamblia A07.1

Infection, infected, infective (opportunistic)
B99.9 — continued
gingiva (chronic) K05.10
  acute K05.00
    nonplaque induced K05.01
    plaque induced K05.00
    nonplaque induced K05.11
    plaque induced K05.10
glanders A24.0
glenosporopsis B48.0
Gnathostoma (spinigerum) B83.1
Gongylonema B83.8
gonococcal — see Gonococcus
gram-negative bacilli NOS A49.9
guinea worm B72
gum (chronic) K05.10
  acute K05.00
    nonplaque induced K05.01
    plaque induced K05.00
    nonplaque induced K05.11
    plaque induced K05.10
Haemophilus — see Infection, Hemophilus
heart — see Carditis
Helicobacter pylori A04.8
  as cause of disease classified elsewhere B96.81
helminths B83.9
  intestinal B82.0
    mixed (types classifiable to more than one of the titles B65.0-B81.3 and B81.8) B81.4
    specified type NEC B81.8
  specified type NEC B83.8
Hemophilus
  aegyptius, systemic A48.4
  ducrey (any location) A57
  generalized A41.3
  influenzae NEC A49.2
    as cause of disease classified elsewhere B96.3
herpes (simplex) — see also Herpes
  congenital P35.2
  disseminated B00.7
  zoster B02.9
herpesvirus, herpesviral — see Herpes
Heterophyes (heterophyes) B66.8
hip (joint) NEC M00.9
  due to internal joint prosthesis
    left T84.52
    right T84.51
  skin NEC L08.9
Histoplasma — see Histoplasmosis
  American B39.4
  capsulatum B39.4
hookworm B76.9
human
  papilloma virus A63.0
  T-cell lymphotropic virus type-1 (HTLV-1) B33.3
hydrocele N43.0
Hymenolepis B71.0
hypopharynx — see Pharyngitis
inguinal (lymph) glands L04.1
  due to soft chancre A57
intervertebral disc, pyogenic M46.30
  cervical region M46.32
  cervicothoracic region M46.33
  lumbar region M46.36
  lumbosacral region M46.37
  multiple sites M46.39
  occipito-atlanto-axial region M46.31
  sacrococcygeal region M46.38
  thoracic region M46.34
  thoracolumbar region M46.35
intestine, intestinal — see Enteritis, infectious
  specified NEC A08.8
intra-amniotic affecting newborn NEC P39.2
Isospora belli or hominis A07.3
Japanese B encephalitis A83.0
jaw (bone) (lower) (upper) M27.2
joint NEC M00.9
  due to internal joint prosthesis T84.50
kidney (cortex) (hematogenous) N15.9
  with calculus N20.0
    with hydronephrosis N13.6
  following ectopic gestation O08.83
  pelvis and ureter (cystic) N28.85
  puerperal (postpartum) O86.21
  specified NEC N15.8
Klebsiella (K.) pneumoniae NEC A49.8
  as cause of disease classified elsewhere B96.1
knee (joint) NEC M00.9
  due to internal joint prosthesis
    left T84.54
    right T84.53
  skin NEC L08.9
Koch's — see Tuberculosis

Infection, infected, infective (opportunistic)
B99.9 — continued
labia (majora) (minora) (acute) — see Vulvitis
lacrimal
  gland — see Dacryoadenitis
  passages (duct) (sac) — see Inflammation, lacrimal, passages
lancet fluke B66.2
larynx NEC J38.7
leg (skin) NOS L08.9
Legionella pneumophila A48.1
  nonpneumonic A48.2
Leishmania — see also Leishmaniasis
  aethiopica B55.1
  braziliensis B55.2
  chagasi B55.0
  donovani B55.0
  infantum B55.0
  major B55.1
  mexicana B55.1
  tropica B55.1
lentivirus, as cause of disease classified elsewhere B97.31
Leptosphaeria senegalensis B47.0
Leptospira interrogans A27.9
  autumnalis A27.89
  canicola A27.89
  hebdomadis A27.89
  icterohaemorrhagiae A27.0
  pomona A27.89
  specified type NEC A27.89
leptospirochetal NEC — see Leptospirosis
Listeria monocytogenes — see also Listeriosis
  congenital P37.2
Loa loa B74.3
  with conjunctival infestation B74.3
  eyelid B74.3
Loboa loboi B48.0
local, skin (staphylococcal) (streptococcal) L08.9
  abscess — code by site under Abscess
  cellulitis — code by site under Cellulitis
  specified NEC L08.89
  ulcer — see Ulcer, skin
Loefflerella mallei A24.0
lung (see also Pneumonia) J18.9
  atypical Mycobacterium A31.0
  spirochetal A69.8
  tuberculous — see Tuberculosis, pulmonary
  virus — see Pneumonia, viral
lymph gland — see also Lymphadenitis, acute
  mesenteric I88.0
lymphoid tissue, base of tongue or posterior pharynx, NEC (chronic) J35.03
Madurella (grisea) (mycetomii) B47.0
major
  following ectopic or molar pregnancy O08.0
  puerperal, postpartum, childbirth O85
Malassezia furfur B36.0
Malleomyces
  mallei A24.0
  pseudomallei (whitmori) — see Melioidosis
mammary gland N61
Mansonella (ozzardi) (perstans) (streptocerca) B74.4
mastoid — see Mastoiditis
maxilla, maxillary M27.2
  sinus (chronic) — see Sinusitis, maxillary
mediastinum J98.5
Medina (worm) B72
meibomian cyst or gland — see Hordeolum
meninges — see Meningitis, bacterial
meningococcal (see also condition) A39.9
  adrenals A39.1
  brain A39.81
  cerebrospinal A39.0
  conjunctiva A39.89
  endocardium A39.51
  heart A39.50
    endocardium A39.51
    myocardium A39.52
    pericardium A39.53
  joint A39.83
  meninges A39.0
  meningococcemia A39.4
    acute A39.3
    chronic A39.3
  myocardium A39.52
  pericardium A39.53
  retrobulbar neuritis A39.82
  specified site NEC A39.89

Infection, infected, infective (opportunistic)
B99.9 — continued
mesenteric lymph nodes or glands NEC I88.0
Metagonimus B66.8
metatarsophalangeal M00.9
methicillin
  resistant Staphylococcus aureus (MRSA) A49.02
  susceptible Staphylococcus aureus (MSSA) A49.01
Microsporum, microsporic — see Dermatophytosis
mixed flora (bacterial) NEC A49.8
Monilia — see Candidiasis
Monosporium apiospermum B48.2
mouth, parasitic B37.0
Mucor — see Mucormycosis
muscle NEC — see Myositis, infective
mycelium NOS B49
mycetoma B47.9
  actinomycotic NEC B47.1
  mycotic NEC B47.0
Mycobacterium, mycobacterial — see Mycobacterium
Mycoplasma NEC A49.3
  pneumoniae, as cause of disease classified elsewhere B96.0
mycotic NOS B49
  pathogenic to compromised host only B48.8
  skin NOS B36.9
myocardium NEC I40.0
nail (chronic)
  with lymphangitis — see Lymphangitis, acute, digit
  finger L03.01-
    fungus B35.1
    ingrowing L60.0
  toe L03.03-
    fungus B35.1
nasal sinus (chronic) — see Sinusitis
nasopharynx — see Nasopharyngitis
navel L08.82
Necator americanus B76.1
Neisseria — see Gonococcus
Neotestudina rosatii B47.0
newborn P39.9
  intra-amniotic NEC P39.2
  skin P39.4
  specified type NEC P39.8
nipple N61
  associated with
    lactation O91.03
    pregnancy O91.01-
    puerperium O91.02
Nocardia — see Nocardiosis
obstetrical surgical wound (puerperal) O86.0
Oesophagostomum (apiostomum) B81.8
Oestrus ovis — see Myiasis
Oidium albicans B37.9
Onchocerca (volvulus) — see Onchocerciasis
oncovirus, as cause of disease classified elsewhere B97.32
operation wound T81.4
Opisthorchis (felineus) (viverrini) B66.0
orbit, orbital — see Inflammation, orbit
orthopoxvirus NEC B08.09
ovary — see Salpingo-oophoritis
Oxyuris vermicularis B80
pancreas (acute) K85.9
  abscess — see Pancreatitis, acute
  specified NEC K85.8
papillomavirus, as cause of disease classified elsewhere B97.7
papovavirus NEC B34.4
Paracoccidioides brasiliensis — see Paracoccidioidomycosis
Paragonimus (westermani) B66.4
parainfluenza virus B34.8
parameningococcus NOS A39.9
parapoxvirus B08.60
  specified NEC B08.69
parasitic B89
Parastrongylus
  cantonensis B83.2
  costaricensis B81.3
paratyphoid A01.4
  Type A A01.1
  Type B A01.2
  Type C A01.3
paraurethral ducts N34.2
parotid gland — see Sialoadenitis
parvovirus NEC B34.3
  as cause of disease classified elsewhere B97.6

D
I
S
E
A
S
E

I
N
D
E
X

D I S E A S E   I N D E X

Infection, infected, infective (opportunistic)
B99.9 — *continued*
Pasteurella NEC A28.0
  multocida A28.0
  pestis — *see* Plague
  pseudotuberculosis A28.0
  septica (cat bite) (dog bite) A28.0
  tularensis — *see* Tularemia
pelvic, female — *see* Disease, pelvis, inflammatory
Penicillium (marneffei) B48.4
penis (glans) (retention) NEC N48.29
periapical K04.5
peridental, periodontal K05.20
  generalized K05.22
  localized K05.21
perinatal period P39.9
  specified type NEC P39.8
perineal repair (puerperal) O86.0
periorbital — *see* Inflammation, orbit
perirectal K62.89
perirenal — *see* Infection, kidney
peritoneal — *see* Peritonitis
periureteral N28.89
Petriellidium boydii B48.2
pharynx — *see also* Pharyngitis
  coxsackievirus B08.5
  posterior, lymphoid (chronic) J35.03
Phialophora
  gougerotii (subcutaneous abscess or cyst) B43.2
  jeanselmei (subcutaneous abscess or cyst) B43.2
  verrucosa (skin) B43.0
Piedraia hortae B36.3
pinta A67.9
  intermediate A67.1
  late A67.2
  mixed A67.3
  primary A67.0
pinworm B80
pityrosporum furfur B36.0
pleuro-pneumonia-like organism (PPLO) NEC A49.3
  as cause of disease classified elsewhere B96.0
pneumococcus, pneumococcal NEC A49.1
  as cause of disease classified elsewhere B95.3
  generalized (purulent) A40.3
  with pneumonia J13
Pneumocystis carinii (pneumonia) B59
Pneumocystis jiroveci (pneumonia) B59
port or reservoir T80.212
postoperative T81.4
postoperative wound T81.4
postprocedural T81.4
postvaccinal T88.0
prepuce NEC N47.7
  with penile inflammation N47.6
prion — *see* Disease, prion, central nervous system
prostate (capsule) — *see* Prostatitis
Proteus (mirabilis) (morganii) (vulgaris) NEC A49.8
  as cause of disease classified elsewhere B96.4
protozoal NEC B64
  intestinal A07.9
    specified NEC A07.8
  specified NEC B60.8
Pseudoallescheria boydii B48.2
Pseudomonas NEC A49.8
  as cause of disease classified elsewhere B96.5
  mallei A24.0
  pneumonia J15.1
  pseudomallei — *see* Melioidosis
puerperal O86.4
  genitourinary tract NEC O86.89
  major or generalized O85
  minor O86.4
  specified NEC O86.89
pulmonary — *see* Infection, lung
purulent — *see* Abscess
Pyrenochaeta romeroi B47.0
Q fever A78
rectum (sphincter) K62.89
renal — *see also* Infection, kidney
  pelvis and ureter (cystic) N28.85
reovirus, as cause of disease classified elsewhere B97.5
respiratory (tract) NEC J98.8
  acute J22
  chronic J98.8
  influenzal (upper) (acute) — *see* Influenza, with, respiratory manifestations NEC

Infection, infected, infective (opportunistic)
B99.9 — *continued*
respiratory (tract) NEC J98.8 — *continued*
  lower (acute) J22
    chronic — *see* Bronchitis, chronic
  rhinovirus J00
  syncytial virus, as cause of disease classified elsewhere B97.4
  upper (acute) NOS J06.9
    chronic J39.8
    streptococcal J06.9
    viral NOS J06.9
resulting from
  presence of internal prosthesis, implant, graft — *see* Complications, by site and type, infection
retortamoniasis A07.8
retroperitoneal NEC K68.9
retrovirus B33.3
  as cause of disease classified elsewhere B97.30
  human
    immunodeficiency, type 2 (HIV 2) B97.35
    T-cell lymphotropic
      type I (HTLV-I) B97.33
      type II (HTLV-II) B97.34
  lentivirus B97.31
  oncovirus B97.32
  specified NEC B97.39
Rhinosporidium (seeberi) B48.1
rhinovirus
  as cause of disease classified elsewhere B97.89
  unspecified nature or site B34.8
Rhizopus — *see* Mucormycosis
rickettsial NOS A79.9
roundworm (large) NEC B82.0
  Ascariasis (*see also* Ascariasis) B77.9
rubella — *see* Rubella
Saccharomyces — *see* Candidiasis
salivary duct or gland (any) — *see* Sialoadenitis
Salmonella (aertrycke) (arizonae) (callinarum) (cholerae-suis) (enteritidis) (suipestifer) (typhimurium) A02.9
  with
    (gastro)enteritis A02.0
    sepsis A02.1
    specified manifestation NEC A02.8
  due to food (poisoning) A02.9
  hirschfeldii A01.3
  localized A02.20
    arthritis A02.23
    meningitis A02.21
    osteomyelitis A02.24
    pneumonia A02.22
    pyelonephritis A02.25
    specified NEC A02.29
  paratyphi A01.4
    A A01.1
    B A01.2
    C A01.3
  schottmuelleri A01.2
  typhi, typhosa — *see* Typhoid
Sarcocystis A07.8
scabies B86
Schistosoma — *see* Infestation, Schistosoma
scrotum (acute) NEC N49.2
seminal vesicle — *see* Vesiculitis
septic
  localized, skin — *see* Abscess
sheep liver fluke B66.3
Shigella A03.9
  boydii A03.2
  dysenteriae A03.0
  flexneri A03.1
  group
    A A03.0
    B A03.1
    C A03.2
    D A03.3
  Schmitz (-Stutzer) A03.0
  schmitzii A03.0
  shigae A03.0
  sonnei A03.3
  specified NEC A03.8
shoulder (joint) NEC M00.9
  due to internal joint prosthesis T84.59
  skin NEC L08.9
sinus (accessory) (chronic) (nasal) — *see also* Sinusitis
  pilonidal — *see* Sinus, pilonidal
  skin NEC L08.89
Skene's duct or gland — *see* Urethritis

Infection, infected, infective (opportunistic)
B99.9 — *continued*
skin (local) (staphylococcal) (streptococcal) L08.9
  abscess — *code by* site under Abscess
  cellulitis — *code by* site under Cellulitis
  due to fungus B36.9
    specified type NEC B36.8
  mycotic B36.9
    specified type NEC B36.8
  newborn P39.4
  ulcer — *see* Ulcer, skin
slow virus A81.9
  specified NEC A81.89
Sparganum (mansoni) (proliferum) (baxteri) B70.1
specific — *see also* Syphilis
  to perinatal period — *see* Infection, congenital
specified NEC B99.8
spermatic cord NEC N49.1
sphenoidal (sinus) — *see* Sinusitis, sphenoidal
spinal cord NOS (*see also* Myelitis) G04.91
  abscess G06.1
  meninges — *see* Meningitis
  streptococcal G04.89
Spirillum A25.0
spirochetal NOS A69.9
  lung A69.8
  specified NEC A69.8
Spirometra larvae B70.1
spleen D73.89
Sporotrichum, Sporothrix (schenckii) — *see* Sporotrichosis
staphylococcal, unspecified site
  as cause of disease classified elsewhere B95.8
  aureus (methicillin susceptible) (MSSA) B95.61
    methicillin resistant (MRSA) B95.62
  specified NEC B95.7
  aureus (methicillin susceptible) (MSSA) A49.01
    methicillin resistant (MRSA) A49.02
  food poisoning A05.0
  generalized (purulent) A41.2
  pneumonia — *see* Pneumonia, staphylococcal
Stellantchasmus falcatus B66.8
streptobacillus moniliformis A25.1
streptococcal NEC A49.1
  as cause of disease classified elsewhere B95.5
  B genitourinary complicating
    childbirth O98.82
    pregnancy O98.81-
    puerperium O98.83
  congenital
    sepsis P36.10
      group B P36.0
      specified NEC P36.19
  generalized (purulent) A40.9
Streptomyces B47.1
Strongyloides (stercoralis) — *see* Strongyloidiasis
stump (amputation) (surgical) — *see* Complication, amputation stump, infection
subcutaneous tissue, local L08.9
suipestifer — *see* Infection, salmonella
swimming pool bacillus A31.1
Taenia — *see* Infestation, Taenia
Taeniarhynchus saginatus B68.1
tapeworm — *see* Infestation, tapeworm
tendon (sheath) — *see* Tenosynovitis, infective NEC
Ternidens diminutus B81.8
testis — *see* Orchitis
threadworm B80
throat — *see* Pharyngitis
thyroglossal duct K14.8
toe (skin) L08.9
  cellulitis L03.03-
    fungus B35.1
  nail L03.03-
    fungus B35.1
tongue NEC K14.0
  parasitic B37.0
tonsil (and adenoid) (faucial) (lingual) (pharyngeal) — *see* Tonsillitis
tooth, teeth K04.7
  periapical K04.7
  peridental, periodontal K05.20
    generalized K05.22
    localized K05.21
  pulp K04.0
  socket M27.3

Infection, infected, infective (opportunistic)
B99.9 — *continued*
TORCH — *see* Infection, congenital without active infection P00.2
Torula histolytica — *see* Cryptococcosis
Toxocara (cati) (felis) B83.0
Toxoplasma gondii — *see* Toxoplasma
trachea, chronic J42
trematode NEC — *see* Infestation, fluke
trench fever A79.0
Treponema pallidum — *see* Syphilis
Trichinella (spiralis) B75
Trichomonas A59.9
  cervix A59.09
  intestine A07.8
  prostate A59.02
  specified site NEC A59.8
  urethra A59.03
  urogenitalis A59.00
  vagina A59.01
  vulva A59.01
Trichophyton, trichophytic — *see* Dermatophytosis
Trichosporon (beigelii) cutaneum B36.2
Trichostrongylus B81.2
Trichuris (trichiura) B79
Trombicula (irritans) B88.0
Trypanosoma
  brucei
    gambiense B56.0
    rhodesiense B56.1
  cruzi — *see* Chagas' disease
tubal — *see* Salpingo-oophoritis
tuberculous NEC — *see* Tuberculosis
tubo-ovarian — *see* Salpingo-oophoritis
tunica vaginalis N49.1
tunnel T80.212
tympanic membrane NEC — *see* Myringitis
typhoid (abortive) (ambulant) (bacillus) — *see* Typhoid
typhus A75.9
  flea-borne A75.2
  mite-borne A75.3
  recrudescent A75.1
  tick-borne A77.9
    African A77.1
    North Asian A77.2
umbilicus L08.82
ureter N28.86
urethra NEC — *see* Urethritis
urinary (tract) N39.0
  bladder — *see* Cystitis
  complicating
    pregnancy O23.4-
      specified type NEC O23.3-
  kidney — *see* Infection, kidney
  newborn P39.3
  puerperal (postpartum) O86.20
  tuberculous A18.13
  urethra — *see* Urethritis
uterus, uterine — *see* Endometritis
vaccination T88.0
vaccinia not from vaccination B08.011
vagina (acute) — *see* Vaginitis
varicella B01.9
varicose veins — *see* Varix
vas deferens NEC N49.1
vesical — *see* Cystitis
Vibrio
  cholerae A00.0
    El Tor A00.1
  parahaemolyticus (food poisoning) A05.3
  vulnificus
    as cause of disease classified elsewhere B96.82
    foodborne intoxication A05.5
Vincent's (gum) (mouth) (tonsil) A69.1
virus, viral NOS B34.9
  adenovirus
    as cause of disease classified elsewhere B97.0
    unspecified nature or site B34.0
  arborvirus, arbovirus arthropod-borne A94
  as cause of disease classified elsewhere B97.89
    adenovirus B97.0
    coronavirus B97.29
      SARS-associated B97.21
    coxsackievirus B97.11
    echovirus B97.12
    enterovirus B97.10
      coxsackievirus B97.11
      echovirus B97.12
      specified NEC B97.19

Infection, infected, infective (opportunistic) B99.9 — continued
  virus, viral NOS B34.9 — continued
    as cause of disease classified elsewhere B97.89 — continued
      human
        immunodeficiency, type 2 (HIV 2) B97.35
        metapneumovirus B97.81
        T-cell lymphotropic,
          type I (HTLV-I) B97.33
          type II (HTLV-II) B97.34
      papillomavirus B97.7
      parvovirus B97.6
      reovirus B97.5
      respiratory syncytial B97.4
      retrovirus B97.30
        human
          immunodeficiency, type 2 (HIV 2) B97.35
        T-cell lymphotropic,
          type I (HTLV-I) B97.33
          type II (HTLV-II) B97.34
      lentivirus B97.31
      oncovirus B97.32
      specified NEC B97.39
    specified NEC B97.89
  central nervous system A89
    atypical A81.9
      specified NEC A81.89
    enterovirus NEC A88.8
      meningitis A87.0
    slow virus A81.9
      specified NEC A81.89
    specified NEC A88.8
  chest J98.8
  cotia B08.8
  coxsackie (see also Infection, coxsackie) B34.1
    as cause of disease classified elsewhere B97.11
  ECHO
    as cause of disease classified elsewhere B97.12
    unspecified nature or site B34.1
  encephalitis, tick-borne A84.9
  enterovirus, as cause of disease classified elsewhere B97.10
    coxsackievirus B97.11
    echovirus B97.12
    specified NEC B97.19
  exanthem NOS B09
  human metapneumovirus as cause of disease classified elsewhere B97.81
  human papilloma as cause of disease classified elsewhere B97.7
  intestine — see Enteritis, viral
  respiratory syncytial
    as cause of disease classified elsewhere B97.4
    bronchopneumonia J12.1
    common cold syndrome J00
    nasopharyngitis (acute) J00
  rhinovirus
    as cause of disease classified elsewhere B97.89
    unspecified nature or site B34.8
  slow A81.9
    specified NEC A81.89
  specified type NEC B33.8
    as cause of disease classified elsewhere B97.89
    unspecified nature or site B34.8
  unspecified nature or site B34.9
  West Nile — see Virus, West Nile
  vulva (acute) — see Vulvitis
  West Nile — see Virus, West Nile
  whipworm B79
  worms B83.9
    specified type NEC B83.8
  Wuchereria (bancrofti) B74.0
    malayi B74.1
  yatapoxvirus B08.70
    specified NEC B08.79
  yeast (see also Candidiasis) B37.9
  yellow fever — see Fever, yellow
  Yersinia
    enterocolitica (intestinal) A04.6
    pestis — see Plague
    pseudotuberculosis A28.2
  Zeis' gland — see Hordeolum
  zoonotic bacterial NOS A28.9
  Zopfia senegalensis B47.0
Infective, infectious — see condition

Infertility
  female N97.9
    age-related N97.8
    associated with
      anovulation N97.0
      cervical (mucus) disease or anomaly N88.3
      congenital anomaly
        cervix N88.3
        fallopian tube N97.1
        uterus N97.2
        vagina N97.8
      dysmucorrhea N88.3
      fallopian tube disease or anomaly N97.1
      pituitary-hypothalamic origin E23.0
      specified origin NEC N97.8
      Stein-Leventhal syndrome E28.2
      uterine disease or anomaly N97.2
      vaginal disease or anomaly N97.8
    due to
      cervical anomaly N88.3
      fallopian tube anomaly N97.1
      ovarian failure E28.39
      Stein-Leventhal syndrome E28.2
      uterine anomaly N97.2
      vaginal anomaly N97.8
    nonimplantation N97.2
    origin
      cervical N88.3
      tubal (block) (occlusion) (stenosis) N97.1
      uterine N97.2
      vaginal N97.8
  male N46.9
    azoospermia N46.01
      extratesticular cause N46.029
        drug therapy N46.021
        efferent duct obstruction N46.023
        infection N46.022
        radiation N46.024
        specified cause NEC N46.029
        systemic disease N46.025
    oligospermia N46.11
      extratesticular cause N46.129
        drug therapy N46.121
        efferent duct obstruction N46.123
        infection N46.122
        radiation N46.124
        specified cause NEC N46.129
        systemic disease N46.125
    specified type NEC N46.8

Infestation B88.9
  Acanthocheilonema (perstans) (streptocerca) B74.4
  Acariasis B88.0
    demodex folliculorum B88.0
    sarcoptes scabiei B86
    trombiculae B88.0
  Agamofilaria streptocerca B74.4
  Ancylostoma, ankylostoma (braziliense) (caninum) (ceylanicum) (duodenale) B76.0
    americanum B76.1
    new world B76.1
  Anisakis larvae, anisakiasis B81.0
  arthropod NEC B88.2
  Ascaris lumbricoides — see Ascariasis
  Balantidium coli A07.0
  beef tapeworm B68.1
  Bothriocephalus (latus) B70.0
    larval B70.1
  broad tapeworm B70.0
    larval B70.1
  Brugia (malayi) B74.1
    timori B74.2
  candiru B88.8
  Capillaria
    hepatica B83.8
    philippinensis B81.1
  cat liver fluke B66.0
  cestodes B71.9
    diphyllobothrium — see Infestation, diphyllobothrium
    dipylidiasis B71.1
    hymenolepiasis B71.0
    specified type NEC B71.8
  chigger B88.0
  chigo, chigoe B88.1
  Clonorchis (sinensis) (liver) B66.1
  coccidial A07.3
  crab-lice B85.3
  Cysticercus cellulosae — see Cysticercosis
  Demodex (folliculorum) B88.0
  Dermanyssus gallinae B88.0
  Dermatobia (hominis) — see Myiasis
  Dibothriocephalus (latus) B70.0
    larval B70.1
  Dicrocoelium dendriticum B66.2

Infestation B88.9 — continued
  Diphyllobothrium (adult) (latum) (intestinal) (pacificum) B70.0
    larval B70.1
  Diplogonoporus (grandis) B71.8
  Dipylidium caninum B67.4
  Distoma hepaticum B66.3
  dog tapeworm B67.4
  Dracunculus medinensis B72
  dragon worm B72
  dwarf tapeworm B71.0
  Echinococcus — see Echinococcus
  Echinostomum ilocanum B66.8
  Entamoeba (histolytica) — see Infection, Ameba
  Enterobius vermicularis B80
  eyelid
    in (due to)
      leishmaniasis B55.1
      loiasis B74.3
      onchocerciasis B73.09
      phthriasis B85.3
    parasitic NOS B89
  eyeworm B74.3
  Fasciola (gigantica) (hepatica) (indica) B66.3
  Fasciolopsis (buski) (intestine) B66.5
  filarial B74.9
    bancroftian B74.0
    conjunctiva B74.9
    due to
      Acanthocheilonema (perstans) (streptocerca) B74.4
      Brugia (malayi) B74.1
        timori B74.2
      Dracunculus medinensis B72
      guinea worm B72
      loa loa B74.3
      Mansonella (ozzardi) (perstans) (streptocerca) B74.4
      Onchocerca volvulus B73.00
        eye B73.00
        eyelid B73.09
      Wuchereria (bancrofti) B74.0
    Malayan B74.1
    ozzardi B74.4
    specified type NEC B74.8
  fish tapeworm B70.0
    larval B70.1
  fluke B66.9
    blood NOS — see Schistosomiasis
    cat liver B66.0
    intestinal B66.5
    lancet B66.2
    liver (sheep) B66.3
      cat B66.0
      Chinese B66.1
      due to clonorchiasis B66.1
      oriental B66.1
    lung (oriental) B66.4
    sheep liver B66.3
    specified type NEC B66.8
  fly larvae — see Myiasis
  Gasterophilus (intestinalis) — see Myiasis
  Gastrodiscoides hominis B66.8
  Giardia lamblia A07.1
  Gnathostoma (spinigerum) B83.1
  Gongylonema B83.8
  guinea worm B72
  helminth B83.9
    angiostrongyliasis B83.2
      intestinal B81.3
    gnathostomiasis B83.1
    hirudiniasis, internal B83.4
    intestinal B82.0
      angiostrongyliasis B81.3
      anisakiasis B81.0
      ascariasis — see Ascariasis
      capillariasis B81.1
      cysticercosis — see Cysticercosis
      diphyllobothriasis — see Infestation, diphyllobothriasis
      dracunculiasis B72
      echinococcus — see Echinococcosis
      enterobiasis B80
      filariasis — see Infestation, filarial
      fluke — see Infestation, fluke
      hookworm — see Infestation, hookworm
      mixed (types classifiable to more than one of the titles B65.0-B81.3 and B81.8) B81.4
      onchocerciasis — see Onchocerciasis
      schistosomiasis — see Infestation, schistosoma
      specified
        cestode NEC — see Infestation, cestode
        type NEC B81.8

Infestation B88.9 — continued
  helminth B83.9 — continued
    intestinal B82.0 — continued
      strongyloidiasis — see Strongyloidiasis
      taenia — see Infestation, taenia
      trichinellosis B75
      trichostrongyliasis B81.2
      trichuriasis B79
    specified type NEC B83.8
    syngamiasis B83.3
    visceral larva migrans B83.0
  Heterophyes (heterophyes) B66.8
  hookworm B76.9
    ancylostomiasis B76.0
    necatoriasis B76.1
    specified type NEC B76.8
  Hymenolepis (diminuta) (nana) B71.0
  intestinal NEC B82.9
  leeches (aquatic) (land) — see Hirudiniasis
  Leishmania — see Leishmaniasis
  lice, louse — see Infestation, Pediculus
  Linguatula B88.8
  Liponyssoides sanguineus B88.0
  Loa loa B74.3
    conjunctival B74.3
    eyelid B74.3
  louse — see Infestation, Pediculus
  maggots — see Myiasis
  Mansonella (ozzardi) (perstans) (streptocerca) B74.4
  Medina (worm) B72
  Metagonimus (yokogawai) B66.8
  microfilaria streptocerca — see Onchocerciasis
    eye B73.00
    eyelid B73.09
  mites B88.9
    scabic B86
  Monilia (albicans) — see Candidiasis
  mouth B37.0
  Necator americanus B76.1
  nematode NEC (intestinal) B82.0
    Ancylostoma B76.0
    conjunctiva NEC B83.9
    Enterobius vermicularis B80
    Gnathostoma spinigerum B83.1
    physaloptera B80
    specified NEC B81.8
    trichostrongylus B81.2
    trichuris (trichuria) B79
  Oesophagostomum (apiostomum) B81.8
  Oestrus ovis (see also Myiasis) B87.9
  Onchocerca (volvulus) — see Onchocerciasis
  Opisthorchis (felineus) (viverrini) B66.0
  orbit, parasitic NOS B89
  Oxyuris vermicularis B80
  Paragonimus (westermani) B66.4
  parasite, parasitic B89
    eyelid B89
    intestinal NOS B82.9
    mouth B37.0
    skin B88.9
    tongue B37.0
  Parastrongylus
    cantonensis B83.2
    costaricensis B81.3
  Pediculus B85.2
    body B85.1
    capitis (humanus) (any site) B85.0
    corporis (humanus) (any site) B85.1
    head B85.0
    mixed (classifiable to more than one of the titles B85.0-B85.3) B85.4
    pubis (any site) B85.3
  Pentastoma B88.8
  Phthirus (pubis) (any site) B85.3
    with any infestation classifiable to B85.0-B85.2 B85.4
  pinworm B80
  pork tapeworm (adult) B68.0
  protozoal NEC B64
    intestinal A07.9
      specified NEC A07.8
    specified NEC B60.8
  pubic, louse B85.3
  rat tapeworm B71.0
  red bug B88.0
  roundworm (large) NEC B82.0
    Ascariasis (see also Ascariasis) B77.9
  sandflea B88.1
  Sarcoptes scabiei B86
  scabies B86
  Schistosoma B65.9
    bovis B65.8
    cercariae B65.3
    haematobium B65.0
    intercalatum B65.8
    japonicum B65.2

Infestation B88.9 — *continued*
  Schistosoma B65.9 — *continued*
    mansoni B65.1
    mattheei B65.8
    mekongi B65.8
    specified type NEC B65.8
    spindale B65.8
  screw worms — *see* Myiasis
  skin NOS B88.9
  Sparganum (mansoni) (proliferum)
    (baxteri) B70.1
    larval B70.1
  specified type NEC B88.8
  Spirometra larvae B70.1
  Stellantchasmus falcatus B66.8
  Strongyloides stercoralis — *see*
    Strongyloidiasis
  Taenia B68.9
    diminuta B71.0
    echinococcus — *see* Echinococcus
    mediocanellata B68.1
    nana B71.0
    saginata B68.1
    solium (intestinal form) B68.0
      larval form — *see* Cysticercosis
  Taeniarhynchus saginatus B68.1
  tapeworm B71.9
    beef B68.1
    broad B70.0
      larval B70.1
    dog B67.4
    dwarf B71.0
    fish B70.0
      larval B70.1
    pork B68.0
    rat B71.0
  Ternidens diminutus B81.8
  Tetranychus molestissimus B88.0
  threadworm B80
  tongue B37.0
  Toxocara (canis) (cati) (felis) B83.0
  trematode(s) NEC — *see* Infestation, fluke
  Trichinella (spiralis) B75
  Trichocephalus B79
  Trichomonas — *see* Trichomoniasis
  Trichostrongylus B81.2
  Trichuris (trichiura) B79
  Trombicula (irritans) B88.0
  Tunga penetrans B88.1
  Uncinaria americana B76.1
  Vandellia cirrhosa B88.8
  whipworm B79
  worms B83.9
    intestinal B82.0
  Wuchereria (bancrofti) B74.0
Infiltrate, infiltration
  amyloid (generalized) (localized) — *see*
    Amyloidosis
  calcareous NEC R89.7
    localized — *see* Degeneration, by site
  calcium salt R89.7
  cardiac
    fatty — *see* Degeneration, myocardial
    glycogenic E74.02 [I43]
  corneal — *see* Edema, cornea
  eyelid — *see* Inflammation, eyelid
  glycogen, glycogenic — *see* Disease,
    glycogen storage
  heart, cardiac
    fatty — *see* Degeneration, myocardial
    glycogenic E74.02 [I43]
  inflammatory in vitreous H43.89
  kidney N28.89
  leukemic — *see* Leukemia
  liver K76.89
    fatty — *see* Fatty, liver NEC
    glycogen (*see also* Disease, glycogen
      storage) E74.03 [K77]
  lung R91.8
    eosinophilic J82
  lymphatic (*see also* Leukemia, lymphatic)
    C91.9-
    gland I88.9
  muscle, fatty M62.89
  myocardium, myocardial
    fatty — *see* Degeneration, myocardial
    glycogenic E74.02 [I43]
  on chest x-ray R91.8
  pulmonary R91.8
    with eosinophilia J82
  skin (lymphocytic) L98.6
  thymus (gland) (fatty) E32.8
  urine R39.0
  vesicant agent
    antineoplastic chemotherapy T80.810
    other agent NEC T80.818
  vitreous body H43.89

Infirmity R68.89
  senile R54
Inflammation, inflamed, inflammatory
  (with exudation)
  abducent (nerve) — *see* Strabismus,
    paralytic, sixth nerve
  accessory sinus (chronic) — *see* Sinusitis
  adrenal (gland) E27.8
  alveoli, teeth M27.3
    scorbutic E54
  anal canal, anus K62.89
  antrum (chronic) — *see* Sinusitis, maxillary
  appendix — *see* Appendicitis
  arachnoid — *see* Meningitis
  areola N61
    puerperal, postpartum or gestational —
      see Infection, nipple
  areolar tissue NOS L08.9
  artery — *see* Arteritis
  auditory meatus (external) — *see* Otitis,
    externa
  Bartholin's gland N75.8
  bile duct (common) (hepatic) or passage —
    see Cholangitis
  bladder — *see* Cystitis
  bone — *see* Osteomyelitis
  brain — *see also* Encephalitis
    membrane — *see* Meningitis
  breast N61
    puerperal, postpartum, gestational — *see*
      Mastitis, obstetric
  broad ligament — *see* Disease, pelvis,
    inflammatory
  bronchi — *see* Bronchitis
  catarrhal J00
  cecum — *see* Appendicitis
  cerebral — *see also* Encephalitis
    membrane — *see* Meningitis
  cerebrospinal
    meningococcal A39.0
  cervix (uteri) — *see* Cervicitis
  chest J98.8
  chorioretinal H30.9-
    cyclitis — *see* Cyclitis
    disseminated H30.10-
      generalized H30.13-
      peripheral H30.12-
      posterior pole H30.11-
    epitheliopathy — *see* Epitheliopathy
    focal H30.00-
      juxtapapillary H30.01-
      macular H30.04-
      paramacular — *see* Inflammation,
        chorioretinal, focal, macular
      peripheral H30.03-
      posterior pole H30.02-
    specified type NEC H30.89-
  choroid — *see* Inflammation, chorioretinal
  chronic, postmastoidectomy cavity — *see*
    Complications, postmastoidectomy,
    inflammation
  colon — *see* Enteritis
  connective tissue (diffuse) NEC — *see*
    Disorder, soft tissue, specified type
    NEC
  cornea — *see* Keratitis
  corpora cavernosa N48.29
  cranial nerve — *see* Disorder, nerve,
    cranial
  Douglas' cul-de-sac or pouch (chronic)
    N73.0
  due to device, implant or graft — *see also*
    Complications, by site and type,
    infection or inflammation
    arterial graft T82.7
    breast (implant) T85.79
    catheter T85.79
      dialysis (renal) T82.7
        intraperitoneal T85.71
      infusion T82.7
        spinal (epidural) (subdural) T85.79
      urinary (indwelling) T83.51
    electronic (electrode) (pulse generator)
      (stimulator)
      bone T84.7
      cardiac T82.7
      nervous system (brain) (peripheral
        nerve) (spinal) T85.79
      urinary T83.59
    fixation, internal (orthopedic) NEC —
      see Complication, fixation device,
      infection
    gastrointestinal (bile duct) (esophagus)
      T85.79
    genital NEC T83.6
    heart NEC T82.7
      valve (prosthesis) T82.6
        graft T82.7
    joint prosthesis — *see* Complication,
      joint prosthesis, infection

Inflammation, inflamed, inflammatory
  (with exudation) — *continued*
  due to device, implant or graft — *see also*
    Complications, by site and type,
    infection or inflammation —
    continued
    ocular (corneal graft) (orbital implant)
      NEC T85.79
    orthopedic NEC T84.7
    specified NEC T85.79
    urinary NEC T83.59
    vascular NEC T82.7
    ventricular intracranial shunt T85.79
  duodenum K29.80
    with bleeding K29.81
  dura mater — *see* Meningitis
  ear (middle) — *see also* Otitis, media
    external — *see* Otitis, externa
    inner — *see* subcategory H83.0
  epididymis — *see* Epididymitis
  esophagus K20.9
  ethmoidal (sinus) (chronic) — *see*
    Sinusitis, ethmoidal
  eustachian tube (catarrhal) — *see*
    Salpingitis, eustachian
  eyelid H01.9
    abscess — *see* Abscess, eyelid
    blepharitis — *see* Blepharitis
    chalazion — *see* Chalazion
    dermatitis (noninfectious) — *see*
      Dermatosis, eyelid
    hordeolum — *see* Hordeolum
    specified NEC H01.8
  fallopian tube — *see* Salpingo-oophoritis
  fascia — *see* Myositis
  follicular, pharynx J31.2
  frontal (sinus) (chronic) — *see* Sinusitis,
    frontal
  gallbladder — *see* Cholecystitis
  gastric — *see* Gastritis
  gastrointestinal — *see* Enteritis
  genital organ (internal) (diffuse)
    female — *see* Disease, pelvis,
      inflammatory
    male N49.9
      multiple sites N49.8
      specified NEC N49.8
  gland (lymph) — *see* Lymphadenitis
  glottis — *see* Laryngitis
  granular, pharynx J31.2
  gum K05.10
    nonplaque induced K05.11
    plaque induced K05.10
  heart — *see* Carditis
  hepatic duct — *see* Cholangitis
  ileoanal (internal) pouch K91.850
  ileum — *see also* Enteritis
    regional or terminal — *see* Enteritis,
      regional
  intestinal pouch K91.850
  intestine (any part) — *see* Enteritis
  jaw (acute) (bone) (chronic) (lower)
    (suppurative) (upper) M27.2
  joint NEC — *see* Arthritis
    sacroiliac M46.1
  kidney — *see* Nephritis
  knee (joint) M13.169
    tuberculous A18.02
  labium (majus) (minus) — *see* Vulvitis
  lacrimal
    gland — *see* Dacryoadenitis
    passages (duct) (sac) — *see also*
      Dacryocystitis
      canaliculitis — *see* Canaliculitis,
        lacrimal
  larynx — *see* Laryngitis
  leg NOS L08.9
  lip K13.0
  liver (capsule) — *see also* Hepatitis
    chronic K73.9
    suppurative K75.0
  lung (acute) — *see also* Pneumonia
    chronic J98.4
  lymph gland or node — *see* Lymphadenitis
  lymphatic vessel — *see* Lymphangitis
  maxilla, maxillary M27.2
    sinus (chronic) — *see* Sinusitis,
      maxillary
  membranes of brain or spinal cord — *see*
    Meningitis
  meninges — *see* Meningitis
  mouth K12.1
  muscle — *see* Myositis
  myocardium — *see* Myocarditis
  nasal sinus (chronic) — *see* Sinusitis
  nasopharynx — *see* Nasopharyngitis
  navel L08.82
  nerve NEC — *see* Neuralgia

Inflammation, inflamed, inflammatory
  (with exudation) — *continued*
  nipple N61
    puerperal, postpartum or gestational —
      see Infection, nipple
  nose — *see* Rhinitis
  oculomotor (nerve) — *see* Strabismus,
    paralytic, third nerve
  optic nerve — *see* Neuritis, optic
  orbit (chronic) H05.10
    acute H05.00
      abscess — *see* Abscess, orbit
      cellulitis — *see* Cellulitis, orbit
      osteomyelitis — *see* Osteomyelitis,
        orbit
      periostitis — *see* Periostitis, orbital
      tenonitis — *see* Tenonitis, eye
      granuloma — *see* Granuloma, orbit
      myositis — *see* Myositis, orbital
  ovary — *see* Salpingo-oophoritis
  oviduct — *see* Salpingo-oophoritis
  pancreas (acute) — *see* Pancreatitis
  parametrium N73.0
  parotid region L08.9
  pelvis, female — *see* Disease, pelvis,
    inflammatory
  penis (corpora cavernosa) N48.29
  perianal K62.89
  pericardium — *see* Pericarditis
  perineum (female) (male) L08.9
  perirectal K62.89
  peritoneum — *see* Peritonitis
  periuterine — *see* Disease, pelvis,
    inflammatory
  perivesical — *see* Cystitis
  petrous bone (acute) (chronic) — *see*
    Petrositis
  pharynx (acute) — *see* Pharyngitis
  pia mater — *see* Meningitis
  pleura — *see* Pleurisy
  polyp, colon (*see also* Polyp, colon,
    inflammatory) K51.40
  prostate — *see also* Prostatitis
    specified type NEC N41.8
  rectosigmoid — *see* Rectosigmoiditis
  rectum (*see also* Proctitis) K62.89
  respiratory, upper (*see also* Infection,
    respiratory, upper) J06.9
    acute, due to radiation J70.0
    chronic, due to external agent — *see*
      condition, respiratory, chronic, due
      to
    due to
      chemicals, gases, fumes or vapors
        (inhalation) J68.2
      radiation J70.1
  retina — *see* Chorioretinitis
  retrocecal — *see* Appendicitis
  retroperitoneal — *see* Peritonitis
  salivary duct or gland (any) (suppurative)
    — *see* Sialoadenitis
  scorbutic, alveoli, teeth E54
  scrotum N49.2
  seminal vesicle — *see* Vesiculitis
  sigmoid — *see* Enteritis
  sinus — *see* Sinusitis
  Skene's duct or gland — *see* Urethritis
  skin L08.9
  spermatic cord N49.1
  sphenoidal (sinus) (chronic) — *see* Sinusitis,
    sphenoidal
  spinal
    cord — *see* Encephalitis
    membrane — *see* Meningitis
    nerve — *see* Disorder, nerve
  spine — *see* Spondylopathy, inflammatory
  spleen (capsule) D73.89
  stomach — *see* Gastritis
  subcutaneous tissue L08.9
  suprarenal (gland) E27.8
  synovial — *see* Tenosynovitis
  tendon (sheath) NEC — *see* Tenosynovitis
  testis — *see* Orchitis
  throat (acute) — *see* Pharyngitis
  thymus (gland) E32.8
  thyroid (gland) — *see* Thyroiditis
  tongue K14.0
  tonsil — *see* Tonsillitis
  trachea — *see* Tracheitis
  trochlear (nerve) — *see* Strabismus,
    paralytic, fourth nerve
  tubal — *see* Salpingo-oophoritis
  tuberculous NEC — *see* Tuberculosis
  tubo-ovarian — *see* Salpingo-oophoritis
  tunica vaginalis N49.1
  tympanic membrane — *see* Tympanitis
  umbilicus, umbilical L08.82
  uterine ligament — *see* Disease, pelvis,
    inflammatory
  uterus (catarrhal) — *see* Endometritis

Inflammation, inflamed, inflammatory
(with exudation) — *continued*
uveal tract (anterior) NOS — *see also*
Iridocyclitis
posterior — *see* Chorioretinitis
vagina — *see* Vaginitis
vas deferens N49.1
vein — *see also* Phlebitis
intracranial or intraspinal (septic) G08
thrombotic I80.9
leg — *see* Phlebitis, leg
lower extremity — *see* Phlebitis, leg
vocal cord J38.3
vulva — *see* Vulvitis
Wharton's duct (suppurative) — *see*
Sialoadenitis
Inflation, lung, imperfect (newborn) — *see*
Atelectasis
Influenza (bronchial) (epidemic) (respiratory
(upper)) (unidentified influenza virus)
J11.1
with
digestive manifestations J11.2
encephalopathy J11.81
enteritis J11.2
gastroenteritis J11.2
gastrointestinal manifestations J11.2
laryngitis J11.1
myocarditis J11.82
otitis media J11.83
pharyngitis J11.1
pneumonia J11.00
specified type J11.08
respiratory manifestations NEC J11.1
specified manifestation NEC J11.89
A/H5N1 (*see also* Influenza, due to,
identified novel influenza A virus)
J09.X2
avian (*see also* Influenza, due to, identified
novel influenza A virus) J09.X2
bird (*see also* Influenza, due to, identified
novel influenza A virus) J09.X2
due to
avian (*see also* Influenza, due to,
identified novel influenza A virus)
J09.X2
identified influenza virus NEC J10.1
with
digestive manifestations J10.2
encephalopathy J10.81
enteritis J10.2
gastroenteritis J10.2
gastrointestinal manifestations
J10.2
laryngitis J10.1
myocarditis J10.82
otitis media J10.83
pharyngitis J10.1
pneumonia (unspecified type)
J10.00
with same identified influenza
virus J10.01
specified type NEC J10.08
respiratory manifestations NEC
J10.1
specified manifestation NEC
J10.89
identified novel influenza A virus
J09.X2
with
digestive manifestations J09.X3
encephalopathy J09.X9
enteritis J09.X3
gastroenteritis J09.X3
gastrointestinal manifestations
J09.X3
laryngitis J09.X2
myocarditis J09.X9
otitis media J09.X9
pharyngitis J09.X2
pneumonia J09.X1
respiratory manifestations NEC
J09.X2
specified manifestation NEC
J09.X9
upper respiratory symptoms J09.X2
novel (2009) H1N1 influenza (*see also*
Influenza, due to, identified influenza
virus NEC) J10.1
novel influenza A/H1N1 (*see also*
Influenza, due to, identified influenza
virus NEC) J10.1
of other animal origin, not bird or swine
(*see also* Influenza, due to, identified
novel influenza A virus) J09.X2
swine (viruses that normally cause
infections in pigs) (*see also* Influenza,
due to, identified novel influenza A
virus) J09.X2

Influenzal — *see* Influenza
Influenza-like disease — *see* Influenza
Infraction, Freiberg's (metatarsal head) —
see Osteochondrosis, juvenile,
metatarsus
Infraeruption of tooth (teeth) M26.34
**Infusion complication, misadventure, or
reaction** — *see* Complications, infusion
Ingestion
chemical — *see* Table of Drugs and
Chemicals, by substance, poisoning
drug or medicament
correct substance properly administered
— *see* Table of Drugs and
Chemicals, by drug, adverse effect
overdose or wrong substance given or
taken — *see* Table of Drugs and
Chemicals, by drug, poisoning
foreign body — *see* Foreign body,
alimentary tract
tularemia A21.3
Ingrowing
hair (beard) L73.1
nail (finger) (toe) L60.0
Inguinal — *see also* condition
testicle Q53.9
bilateral Q53.21
unilateral Q53.11
Inhalation
anthrax A22.1
flame T27.3
food or foreign body — *see* Foreign body,
by site
gases, fumes, or vapors NEC T59.9-
specified agent — *see* Table of Drugs
and Chemicals, by substance
liquid or vomitus — *see* Asphyxia
meconium (newborn) P24.00
with
with respiratory symptoms P24.01
pneumonia (pneumonitis) P24.01
mucus — *see* Asphyxia, mucus
oil or gasoline (causing suffocation) — *see*
Foreign body, by site
smoke J70.5
due to chemicals, gases, fumes and
vapors J68.9
steam — *see* Toxicity, vapors
stomach contents or secretions — *see*
Foreign body, by site
due to anesthesia (general) (local) or
other sedation T88.59
in labor and delivery O74.0
in pregnancy O29.01-
postpartum, puerperal O89.01
Inhibition, orgasm
female F52.31
male F52.32
Inhibitor, systemic lupus erythematosus
(presence of) D68.62
Iniencephalus, iniencephaly Q00.2
Injection, traumatic jet (air) (industrial)
(water) (paint or dye) T70.4
Injury (*see also* specified injury type) T14.90
abdomen, abdominal S39.91
blood vessel — *see* Injury, blood vessel,
abdomen
cavity — *see* Injury, intra-abdominal
contusion S30.1
internal — *see* Injury, intra-abdominal
intra-abdominal organ — *see* Injury,
intra-abdominal
nerve — *see* Injury, nerve, abdomen
open — *see* Wound, open, abdomen
specified NEC S39.81
superficial — *see* Injury, superficial,
abdomen
Achilles tendon S86.00-
laceration S86.02-
specified type NEC S86.09-
strain S86.01-
acoustic, resulting in deafness — *see*
Injury, nerve, acoustic
adrenal (gland) S37.819
contusion S37.812
laceration S37.813
specified type NEC S37.818
alveolar (process) S09.93
ankle S99.91-
contusion — *see* Contusion, ankle
dislocation — *see* Dislocation, ankle
fracture — *see* Fracture, ankle
nerve — *see* Injury, nerve, ankle
open — *see* Wound, open, ankle
specified type NEC S99.81-
sprain — *see* Sprain, ankle
superficial — *see* Injury, superficial,
ankle
anterior chamber, eye — *see* Injury, eye,
specified site NEC

Injury (*see also* specified injury type) T14.90
— *continued*
anus — *see* Injury, abdomen
aorta (thoracic) S25.00
abdominal S35.00
laceration (minor) (superficial)
S35.01
major S35.02
specified type NEC S35.09
laceration (minor) (superficial) S25.01
major S25.02
specified type NEC S25.09
arm (upper) S49.9-
blood vessel — *see* Injury, blood vessel,
arm
contusion — *see* Contusion, arm, upper
fracture — *see* Fracture, humerus
lower — *see* Injury, forearm
muscle — *see* Injury, muscle, shoulder
nerve — *see* Injury, nerve, arm
open — *see* Wound, open, arm
specified type NEC S49.8-
superficial — *see* Injury, superficial, arm
artery (complicating trauma) — *see also*
Injury, blood vessel, by site
cerebral or meningeal — *see* Injury,
intracranial
auditory canal (external) (meatus) S09.91
auricle, auris, ear S09.91
axilla — *see* Injury, shoulder
back — *see* Injury, back, lower
bile duct S36.13
birth (*see also* Birth, injury) P15.9
bladder (sphincter) S37.20
at delivery O71.5
contusion S37.22
laceration S37.23
obstetrical trauma O71.5
specified type NEC S37.29
blast (air) (hydraulic) (immersion)
(underwater) NEC T14.8
acoustic nerve trauma — *see* Injury,
nerve, acoustic
bladder — *see* Injury, bladder
brain — *see* Concussion
colon — *see* Injury, intestine, large, blast
injury
ear (primary) S09.31-
secondary S09.39-
generalized T70.8
lung — *see* Injury, intrathoracic, lung,
blast injury
multiple body organs T70.8
peritoneum S36.81
rectum S36.61
retroperitoneum S36.898
small intestine S36.419
duodenum S36.410
specified site NEC S36.418
specified
intra-abdominal organ NEC S36.898
pelvic organ NEC S37.899
blood vessel NEC T14.8
abdomen S35.9-
aorta — *see* Injury, aorta, abdominal
celiac artery — *see* Injury, blood
vessel, celiac artery
iliac vessel — *see* Injury, blood
vessel, iliac
laceration S35.91
mesenteric vessel — *see* Injury,
mesenteric
portal vein — *see* Injury, blood vessel,
portal vein
renal vessel — *see* Injury, blood
vessel, renal
specified vessel NEC S35.8x-
splenic vessel — *see* Injury, blood
vessel, splenic
vena cava — *see* Injury, vena cava,
inferior
ankle — *see* Injury, blood vessel, foot
aorta (abdominal) (thoracic) — *see*
Injury, aorta
arm (upper) NEC S45.90-
forearm — *see* Injury, blood vessel,
forearm
laceration S45.91-
specified
site NEC S45.80-
laceration S45.81-
specified type NEC S45.89-
type NEC S45.99-
superficial vein S45.30-
laceration S45.31-
specified type NEC S45.39-

Injury (*see also* specified injury type) T14.90
— *continued*
blood vessel NEC T14.8 — *continued*
axillary
artery S45.00-
laceration S45.01-
specified type NEC S45.09-
vein S45.20-
laceration S45.21-
specified type NEC S45.29-
azygos vein — *see* Injury, blood vessel,
thoracic, specified site NEC
brachial
artery S45.10-
laceration S45.11-
specified type NEC S45.19-
vein S45.20-
laceration S45.219
specified type NEC S45.29-
carotid artery (common) (external)
(internal, extracranial) S15.00-
internal, intracranial S06.8-
laceration (minor) (superficial)
S15.01-
major S15.02-
specified type NEC S15.09-
celiac artery S35.219
branch S35.299
laceration (minor) (superficial)
S35.291
major S35.292
specified NEC S35.298
laceration (minor) (superficial)
S35.211
major S35.212
specified type NEC S35.218
cerebral — *see* Injury, intracranial
deep plantar — *see* Injury, blood vessel,
plantar artery
digital (hand) — *see* Injury, blood vessel,
finger
dorsal
artery (foot) S95.00-
laceration S95.01-
specified type NEC S95.09-
vein (foot) S95.20-
laceration S95.21-
specified type NEC S95.29-
due to accidental laceration during
procedure — *see* Laceration,
accidental complicating surgery
extremity — *see* Injury, blood vessel,
limb
femoral
artery (common) (superficial) S75.00-
laceration (minor) (superficial)
S75.01-
major S75.02-
specified type NEC S75.09-
vein (hip level) (thigh level) S75.10-
laceration (minor) (superficial)
S75.11-
major S75.12-
specified type NEC S75.19-
finger S65.50-
index S65.50-
laceration S65.51-
specified type NEC S65.59-
laceration S65.51-
little S65.50-
laceration S65.51-
specified type NEC S65.59-
middle S65.50-
specified type NEC S65.59-
thumb — *see* Injury, blood vessel,
thumb
foot S95.90-
dorsal
artery — *see* Injury, blood vessel,
dorsal, artery
vein — *see* Injury, blood vessel,
dorsal, vein
laceration S95.91-
plantar artery — *see* Injury, blood
vessel, plantar artery
specified
site NEC S95.80-
laceration S95.81-
specified type NEC S95.89-
specified type NEC S95.99-
forearm S55.90-
laceration S55.91-
radial artery — *see* Injury, blood
vessel, radial artery
specified
site NEC S55.80-
laceration S55.81-
specified type NEC S55.89-
type NEC S55.99-

DISEASE INDEX

Injury (*see also* specified injury type) T14.90
— *continued*
blood vessel NEC T14.8 — *continued*
  forearm S55.90- — *continued*
    ulnar artery — *see* Injury, blood
      vessel, ulnar artery
    vein S55.20-
      laceration S55.21-
      specified type NEC S55.29-
  gastric
    artery — *see* Injury, mesenteric,
      artery, branch
    vein — *see* Injury, blood vessel,
      abdomen
  gastroduodenal artery — *see* Injury,
    mesenteric, artery, branch
  greater saphenous vein (lower leg level)
    S85.30-
    hip (and thigh) level S75.20-
      laceration (minor) (superficial)
        S75.21-
      major S75.22-
      specified type NEC S75.29-
    laceration S85.31-
    specified type NEC S85.39-
  hand (level) S65.90-
    finger — *see* Injury, blood vessel,
      finger
    laceration S65.91-
    palmar arch — *see* Injury, blood
      vessel, palmar arch
    radial artery — *see* Injury, blood
      vessel, radial artery, hand
    specified
      site NEC S65.80-
        laceration S65.81-
        specified type NEC S65.89-
      type NEC S65.99-
    thumb — *see* Injury, blood vessel,
      thumb
    ulnar artery — *see* Injury, blood
      vessel, ulnar artery, hand
  head S09.0
    intracranial — *see* Injury, intracranial
    multiple S09.0
  hepatic
    artery — *see* Injury, mesenteric, artery
    vein — *see* Injury, vena cava, inferior
  hip S75.90-
    femoral artery — *see* Injury, blood
      vessel, femoral, artery
    femoral vein — *see* Injury, blood
      vessel, femoral, vein
    greater saphenous vein — *see* Injury,
      blood vessel, greater saphenous,
      hip level
    laceration S75.91-
      specified
        site NEC S75.80-
          laceration S75.81-
          specified type NEC S75.89-
        type NEC S75.99-
  hypogastric (artery) (vein) — *see* Injury,
    blood vessel, iliac
  iliac S35.5-
    artery S35.51-
    specified vessel NEC S35.5-
    uterine vessel — *see* Injury, blood
      vessel, uterine
    vein S35.51-
  innominate — *see* Injury, blood vessel,
    thoracic, innominate
  intercostal (artery) (vein) — *see* Injury,
    blood vessel, thoracic, intercostal
  jugular vein (external) S15.20-
    internal S15.30-
      laceration (minor) (superficial)
        S15.31-
      major S15.32-
      specified type NEC S15.39-
    laceration (minor) (superficial)
      S15.21-
      major S15.22-
    specified type NEC S15.29-
  leg (level) (lower) S85.90-
    greater saphenous — *see* Injury, blood
      vessel, greater saphenous
    laceration S85.91-
    lesser saphenous — *see* Injury, blood
      vessel, lesser saphenous
    peroneal artery — *see* Injury, blood
      vessel, peroneal artery
    popliteal
      artery — *see* Injury, blood vessel,
        popliteal, artery
      vein — *see* Injury, blood vessel,
        popliteal, vein

Injury (*see also* specified injury type) T14.90
— *continued*
blood vessel NEC T14.8 — *continued*
  leg (level) (lower) S85.90- — *continued*
    specified
      site NEC S85.80-
        laceration S85.81-
        specified type NEC S85.89-
      type NEC S85.99-
    thigh — *see* Injury, blood vessel, hip
    tibial artery — *see* Injury, blood
      vessel, tibial artery
  lesser saphenous vein (lower leg level)
    S85.40-
    laceration S85.41-
    specified type NEC S85.49-
  limb
    lower — *see* Injury, blood vessel, leg
    upper — *see* Injury, blood vessel, arm
  lower back — *see* Injury, blood vessel,
    abdomen
    specified NEC — *see* Injury, blood
      vessel, abdomen, specified, site
      NEC
  mammary (artery) (vein) — *see* Injury,
    blood vessel, thoracic, specified
    site NEC
  mesenteric (inferior) (superior)
    artery — *see* Injury, mesenteric, artery
    vein — *see* Injury, mesenteric, vein
  neck S15.9
    specified site NEC S15.8
  ovarian (artery) (vein) — *see*
    subcategory S35.8
  palmar arch (superficial) S65.20-
    deep S65.30-
      laceration S65.31-
      specified type NEC S65.39-
    laceration S65.21-
    specified type NEC S65.29-
  pelvis — *see* Injury, blood vessel,
    abdomen
    specified NEC — *see* Injury, blood
      vessel, abdomen, specified, site
      NEC
  peroneal artery S85.20-
    laceration S85.21-
    specified type NEC S85.29-
  plantar artery (deep) (foot) S95.10-
    laceration S95.11-
    specified type NEC S95.19-
  popliteal
    artery S85.00-
      laceration S85.01-
      specified type NEC S85.09-
    vein S85.50-
      laceration S85.51-
      specified type NEC S85.59-
  portal vein S35.319
    laceration S35.311
    specified type NEC S35.318
  precerebral — *see* Injury, blood vessel,
    neck
  pulmonary (artery) (vein) — *see* Injury,
    blood vessel, thoracic, pulmonary
  radial artery (forearm level) S55.10-
    hand and wrist (level) S65.10-
      laceration S65.11-
      specified type NEC S65.19-
    laceration S55.11-
    specified type NEC S55.19-
  renal
    artery S35.40-
      laceration S35.41-
      specified NEC S35.49-
    vein S35.40-
      laceration S35.41-
      specified NEC S35.49-
  saphenous vein (greater) (lower leg
    level) — *see* Injury, blood vessel,
    greater saphenous
    hip and thigh level — *see* Injury,
      blood vessel, greater saphenous,
      hip level
    lesser — *see* Injury, blood vessel,
      lesser saphenous
  shoulder
    specified NEC — *see* Injury, blood
      vessel, arm, specified site NEC
    superficial vein — *see* Injury, blood
      vessel, arm, superficial vein
  specified NEC T14.8
  splenic
    artery — *see* Injury, blood vessel,
      celiac artery, branch
    vein S35.329
      laceration S35.321
      specified NEC S35.328

Injury (*see also* specified injury type) T14.90
— *continued*
blood vessel NEC T14.8 — *continued*
  subclavian — *see* Injury, blood vessel,
    thoracic, innominate
  thigh — *see* Injury, blood vessel, hip
  thoracic S25.90
    aorta S25.00
      laceration (minor) (superficial)
        S25.01
      major S25.02
      specified type NEC S25.09
    azygos vein — *see* Injury, blood
      vessel, thoracic, specified, site
      NEC
    innominate
      artery S25.10-
        laceration (minor) (superficial)
          S25.11-
        major S25.12-
        specified type NEC S25.19-
      vein S25.30-
        laceration (minor) (superficial)
          S25.31-
        major S25.32-
        specified type NEC S25.39-
    intercostal S25.50-
      laceration S25.51-
      specified type NEC S25.59-
    laceration S25.91
    mammary vessel — *see* Injury, blood
      vessel, thoracic, specified, site
      NEC
    pulmonary S25.40-
      laceration (minor) (superficial)
        S25.41-
      major S25.42-
      specified type NEC S25.49-
    specified
      site NEC S25.80-
        laceration S25.81-
        specified type NEC S25.89-
      type NEC S25.99-
    subclavian — *see* Injury, blood vessel,
      thoracic, innominate
    vena cava (superior) S25.20
      laceration (minor) (superficial)
        S25.21
      major S25.22
      specified type NEC S25.29
  thumb S65.40-
    laceration S65.41-
    specified type NEC S65.49-
  tibial artery S85.10-
    anterior S85.13-
      laceration S85.14-
      specified injury NEC S85.15-
    laceration S85.11-
    posterior S85.16-
      laceration S85.17-
      specified injury NEC S85.18-
    specified injury NEC S85.12-
  ulnar artery (forearm level) S55.00-
    hand and wrist (level) S65.00-
      laceration S65.01-
      specified type NEC S65.09-
    laceration S55.01-
    specified type NEC S55.09-
  upper arm (level) — *see* Injury, blood
    vessel, arm
    superficial vein — *see* Injury, blood
      vessel, arm, superficial vein
  uterine S35.5-
    artery S35.53-
    vein S35.53-
  vena cava — *see* Injury, vena cava
  vertebral artery S15.10-
    laceration (minor) (superficial)
      S15.11-
    major S15.12-
    specified type NEC S15.19-
  wrist (level) — *see* Injury, blood vessel,
    hand
brachial plexus S14.3
  newborn P14.3
brain (traumatic) S06.9-
  diffuse (axonal) S06.2x-
  focal S06.30-
  traumatic — *see* category S06
brainstem S06.38-
breast NOS S29.9
broad ligament — *see* Injury, pelvic organ,
  specified site NEC
bronchus, bronchi — *see* Injury,
  intrathoracic, bronchus
brow S09.90
buttock S39.92
canthus, eye S05.90
cardiac plexus — *see* Injury, nerve, thorax,
  sympathetic

Injury (*see also* specified injury type) T14.90
— *continued*
cauda equina S34.3
cavernous sinus — *see* Injury, intracranial
cecum — *see* Injury, colon
celiac ganglion or plexus — *see* Injury,
  nerve, lumbosacral, sympathetic
cerebellum — *see* Injury, intracranial
cerebral — *see* Injury, intracranial
cervix (uteri) — *see* Injury, uterus
cheek (wall) S09.93
chest — *see* Injury, thorax
childbirth (newborn) — *see also* Birth,
  injury
  maternal NEC O71.9
chin S09.93
choroid (eye) — *see* Injury, eye, specified
  site NEC
clitoris S39.94
coccyx — *see also* Injury, back, lower
  complicating delivery O71.6
colon — *see* Injury, intestine, large
common bile duct — *see* Injury, liver
conjunctiva (superficial) — *see* Injury, eye,
  conjunctiva
conus medullaris — *see* Injury, spinal,
  sacral
cord
  spermatic (pelvic region) S37.898
    scrotal region S39.848
  spinal — *see* Injury, spinal cord, by
    region
cornea — *see* Injury, eye, specified site
  NEC
  abrasion — *see* Injury, eye, cornea,
    abrasion
cortex (cerebral) — *see also* Injury,
  intracranial
  visual — *see* Injury, nerve, optic
costal region NEC S29.9
costochondral NEC S29.9
cranial
  cavity — *see* Injury, intracranial
  nerve — *see* Injury, nerve, cranial
crushing — *see* Crush
cutaneous sensory nerve
cystic duct — *see* Injury, liver
deep tissue — *see* Contusion, by site
  meaning pressure ulcer — *see* Ulcer,
    pressure, unstageable, by site
delivery (newborn) P15.9
  maternal NEC O71.9
Descemet's membrane — *see* Injury,
  eyeball, penetrating
diaphragm — *see* Injury, intrathoracic,
  diaphragm
duodenum — *see* Injury, intestine, small,
  duodenum
ear (auricle) (external) (canal) S09.91
  abrasion — *see* Abrasion, ear
  bite — *see* Bite, ear
  blister — *see* Blister, ear
  bruise — *see* Contusion, ear
  contusion — *see* Contusion, ear
  external constriction — *see* Constriction,
    external, ear
  hematoma — *see* Hematoma, ear
  inner — *see* Injury, ear, middle
  laceration — *see* Laceration, ear
  middle S09.30-
    blast — *see* Injury, blast, ear
    specified NEC S09.39-
  puncture — *see* Puncture, ear
  superficial — *see* Injury, superficial, ear
eighth cranial nerve (acoustic or auditory)
  — *see* Injury, nerve, acoustic
elbow S59.90-
  contusion — *see* Contusion, elbow
  dislocation — *see* Dislocation, elbow
  fracture — *see* Fracture, ulna, upper end
  open — *see* Wound, open, elbow
  specified NEC S59.80-
  sprain — *see* Sprain, elbow
  superficial — *see* Injury, superficial,
    elbow
eleventh cranial nerve (accessory) — *see*
  Injury, nerve, accessory
epididymis S39.94
epigastric region S39.91
epiglottis NEC S19.89
esophageal plexus — *see* Injury, nerve,
  thorax, sympathetic
esophagus (thoracic part) — *see also*
  Injury, intrathoracic, esophagus
  cervical NEC S19.85
eustachian tube S09.30-

Injury (*see also* specified injury type) T14.90
— *continued*
- eye S05.9-
  - avulsion S05.7-
  - ball — *see* Injury, eyeball
  - conjunctiva S05.0-
  - cornea
    - abrasion S05.0-
    - laceration S05.3-
      - with prolapse S05.2-
  - lacrimal apparatus S05.8x-
  - orbit penetration S05.4-
  - specified site NEC S05.8x-
- eyeball S05.8x-
  - contusion S05.1-
  - penetrating S05.6-
    - with
      - foreign body S05.5-
      - prolapse or loss of intraocular tissue S05.2-
      - without prolapse or loss of intraocular tissue S05.3-
  - specified type NEC S05.8-
- eyebrow S09.93
- eyelid S09.93
  - abrasion — *see* Abrasion, eyelid
  - contusion — *see* Contusion, eyelid
  - open — *see* Wound, open, eyelid
- face S09.93
- fallopian tube S37.509
  - bilateral S37.502
    - blast injury S37.512
    - contusion S37.522
    - laceration S37.532
    - specified type NEC S37.592
  - blast injury (primary) S37.519
    - bilateral S37.512
    - secondary — *see* Injury, fallopian tube, specified type NEC
    - unilateral S37.511
  - contusion S37.529
    - bilateral S37.522
    - unilateral S37.521
  - laceration S37.539
    - bilateral S37.532
    - unilateral S37.531
  - specified type NEC S37.599
    - bilateral S37.592
    - unilateral S37.591
  - unilateral S37.501
    - blast injury S37.511
    - contusion S37.521
    - laceration S37.531
    - specified type NEC S37.591
- fascia — *see* Injury, muscle
- fifth cranial nerve (trigeminal) — *see* Injury, nerve, trigeminal
- finger (nail) S69.9-
  - blood vessel — *see* Injury, blood vessel, finger
  - contusion — *see* Contusion, finger
  - dislocation — *see* Dislocation, finger
  - fracture — *see* Fracture, finger
  - muscle — *see* Injury, muscle, finger
  - nerve — *see* Injury, nerve, digital, finger
  - open — *see* Wound, open, finger
  - specified NEC S69.8-
  - sprain — *see* Sprain, finger
  - superficial — *see* Injury, superficial, finger
- first cranial nerve (olfactory) — *see* Injury, nerve, olfactory
- flank — *see* Injury, abdomen
- foot S99.92-
  - blood vessel — *see* Injury, blood vessel, foot
  - contusion — *see* Contusion, foot
  - dislocation — *see* Dislocation, foot
  - fracture — *see* Fracture, foot
  - muscle — *see* Injury, muscle, foot
  - open — *see* Wound, open, foot
  - specified type NEC S99.82-
  - sprain — *see* Sprain, foot
  - superficial — *see* Injury, superficial, foot
  - forceps NOS P15.9
- forearm S59.91-
  - blood vessel — *see* Injury, blood vessel, forearm
  - contusion — *see* Contusion, forearm
  - fracture — *see* Fracture, forearm
  - muscle — *see* Injury, muscle, forearm
  - nerve — *see* Injury, nerve, forearm
  - open — *see* Wound, open, forearm
  - specified NEC S59.81-
  - superficial — *see* Injury, superficial, forearm

Injury (*see also* specified injury type) T14.90
— *continued*
- forehead S09.90
- fourth cranial nerve (trochlear) — *see* Injury, nerve, trochlear
- gallbladder S36.129
  - contusion S36.122
  - laceration S36.123
  - specified NEC S36.128
- ganglion
  - celiac, coeliac — *see* Injury, nerve, lumbosacral, sympathetic
  - gasserian — *see* Injury, nerve, trigeminal
  - stellate — *see* Injury, nerve, thorax, sympathetic
  - thoracic sympathetic — *see* Injury, nerve, thorax, sympathetic
- gasserian ganglion — *see* Injury, nerve, trigeminal
- gastric artery — *see* Injury, blood vessel, celiac artery, branch
- gastroduodenal artery — *see* Injury, blood vessel, celiac artery, branch
- gastrointestinal tract — *see* Injury, intra-abdominal
  - with open wound into abdominal cavity — *see* Wound, open, with penetration into peritoneal cavity
  - colon — *see* Injury, intestine, large
  - rectum — *see* Injury, intestine, large, rectum
    - with open wound into abdominal cavity S36.61
  - small intestine — *see* Injury, intestine, small
  - specified site NEC — *see* Injury, intra-abdominal, specified, site NEC
  - stomach — *see* Injury, stomach
- genital organ(s)
  - external S39.94
    - specified NEC S39.848
  - internal S37.90
    - fallopian tube — *see* Injury, fallopian tube
    - ovary — *see* Injury, ovary
    - prostate — *see* Injury, prostate
    - seminal vesicle — *see* Injury, pelvis, organ, specified site NEC
    - uterus — *see* Injury, uterus
    - vas deferens — *see* Injury, pelvis, organ, specified site NEC
  - obstetrical trauma O71.9
- gland
  - lacrimal laceration — *see* Injury, eye, specified site NEC
  - salivary S09.90
  - thyroid NEC S19.84
- globe (eye) S05.90
  - specified NEC S05.8x-
- groin — *see* Injury, abdomen
- gum S09.90
- hand S69.9-
  - blood vessel — *see* Injury, blood vessel, hand
  - contusion — *see* Contusion, hand
  - fracture — *see* Fracture, hand
  - muscle — *see* Injury, muscle, hand
  - nerve — *see* Injury, nerve, hand
  - open — *see* Wound, open, hand
  - specified NEC S69.8-
  - sprain — *see* Sprain, hand
  - superficial — *see* Injury, superficial, hand
- head S09.90
  - with loss of consciousness S06.9-
  - specified NEC S09.8
- heart S26.90
  - with hemopericardium S26.00
    - contusion S26.01
    - laceration (mild) S26.020
      - major S26.022
      - moderate S26.021
    - specified type NEC S26.09
  - contusion S26.91
  - laceration S26.92
  - specified type NEC S26.99
  - without hemopericardium S26.10
    - contusion S26.11
    - laceration S26.12
    - specified type NEC S26.19
- heel — *see* Injury, foot
- hepatic
  - artery — *see* Injury, blood vessel, celiac artery, branch
  - duct — *see* Injury, liver
  - vein — *see* Injury, vena cava, inferior

Injury (*see also* specified injury type) T14.90
— *continued*
- hip S79.91-
  - blood vessel — *see* Injury, blood vessel, hip
  - contusion — *see* Contusion, hip
  - dislocation — *see* Dislocation, hip
  - fracture — *see* Fracture, femur, neck
  - muscle — *see* Injury, muscle, hip
  - nerve — *see* Injury, nerve, hip
  - open — *see* Wound, open, hip
  - specified NEC S79.81-
  - sprain — *see* Sprain, hip
  - superficial — *see* Injury, superficial, hip
- hymen S39.94
- hypogastric
  - blood vessel — *see* Injury, blood vessel, iliac
  - plexus — *see* Injury, nerve, lumbosacral, sympathetic
- ileum — *see* Injury, intestine, small
- iliac region S39.91
- instrumental (during surgery) — *see* Laceration, accidental complicating surgery
  - birth injury — *see* Birth, injury
  - nonsurgical — *see* Injury, by site
- obstetrical O71.9
  - bladder O71.5
  - cervix O71.3
  - high vaginal O71.4
  - perineal NOS O70.9
  - urethra O71.5
  - uterus O71.5
    - with rupture or perforation O71.1
- internal T14.8
  - aorta — *see* Injury, aorta
  - bladder (sphincter) — *see* Injury, bladder
    - with
      - ectopic or molar pregnancy O08.6
      - following ectopic or molar pregnancy O08.6
      - obstetrical trauma O71.5
  - bronchus, bronchi — *see* Injury, intrathoracic, bronchus
  - cecum — *see* Injury, intestine, large
  - cervix (uteri) — *see also* Injury, uterus
    - with ectopic or molar pregnancy O08.6
    - following ectopic or molar pregnancy O08.6
    - obstetrical trauma O71.3
  - chest — *see* Injury, intrathoracic
  - gastrointestinal tract — *see* Injury, intra-abdominal
  - heart — *see* Injury, heart
  - intestine NEC — *see* Injury, intestine
  - intrauterine — *see* Injury, uterus
  - mesentery — *see* Injury, intra-abdominal, specified, site NEC
  - pelvis, pelvic (organ) S37.90
    - following ectopic or molar pregnancy (subsequent episode) O08.6
    - obstetrical trauma NEC O71.5
    - rupture or perforation O71.1
    - specified NEC S39.83
  - rectum — *see* Injury, intestine, large, rectum
  - stomach — *see* Injury, stomach
  - ureter — *see* Injury, ureter
  - urethra (sphincter) following ectopic or molar pregnancy O08.6
  - uterus — *see* Injury, uterus
- interscapular area — *see* Injury, thorax
- intestine
  - large S36.509
    - ascending (right) S36.500
      - blast injury (primary) S36.510
        - secondary S36.590
      - contusion S36.520
      - laceration S36.530
      - specified type NEC S36.590
    - blast injury (primary) S36.519
      - ascending (right) S36.510
      - descending (left) S36.512
      - rectum S36.61
      - sigmoid S36.513
      - specified site NEC S36.518
      - transverse S36.511
    - contusion S36.529
      - ascending (right) S36.520
      - descending (left) S36.522
      - rectum S36.62
      - sigmoid S36.523
      - specified site NEC S36.528
      - transverse S36.521

Injury (*see also* specified injury type) T14.90
— *continued*
- intestine — *continued*
  - large S36.509 — *continued*
    - descending (left) S36.502
      - blast injury (primary) S36.512
        - secondary S36.592
      - contusion S36.522
      - laceration S36.532
      - specified type NEC S36.592
    - laceration S36.539
      - ascending (right) S36.530
      - descending (left) S36.532
      - rectum S36.63
      - sigmoid S36.533
      - specified site NEC S36.538
      - transverse S36.531
    - rectum S36.60
      - blast injury (primary) S36.61
        - secondary S36.69
      - contusion S36.62
      - laceration S36.63
      - specified type NEC S36.69
    - sigmoid S36.503
      - blast injury (primary) S36.513
        - secondary S36.593
      - contusion S36.523
      - laceration S36.533
      - specified type NEC S36.593
    - specified
      - site NEC S36.508
        - blast injury (primary) S36.518
          - secondary S36.598
        - contusion S36.528
        - laceration S36.538
        - specified type NEC S36.598
      - type NEC S36.599
        - ascending (right) S36.590
        - descending (left) S36.592
        - rectum S36.69
        - sigmoid S36.593
        - specified site NEC S36.598
        - transverse S36.591
    - transverse S36.501
      - blast injury (primary) S36.511
        - secondary S36.591
      - contusion S36.521
      - laceration S36.531
      - specified type NEC S36.591
  - small S36.409
    - blast injury (primary) S36.419
      - duodenum S36.410
      - secondary S36.499
        - duodenum S36.490
        - specified site NEC S36.498
      - specified site NEC S36.418
    - contusion S36.429
      - duodenum S36.420
      - specified site NEC S36.428
    - duodenum S36.400
      - blast injury (primary) S36.410
        - secondary S36.490
      - contusion S36.420
      - laceration S36.430
      - specified NEC S36.490
    - laceration S36.439
      - duodenum S36.430
      - specified site NEC S36.438
    - specified
      - site NEC S36.408
      - type NEC S36.499
        - duodenum S36.490
        - specified site NEC S36.498
  - intra-abdominal S36.90
    - adrenal gland — *see* Injury, adrenal gland
    - bladder — *see* Injury, bladder
    - colon — *see* Injury, intestine, large
    - contusion S36.92
    - fallopian tube — *see* Injury, fallopian tube
    - gallbladder — *see* Injury, gallbladder
    - intestine — *see* Injury, intestine
    - kidney — *see* Injury, kidney
    - laceration S36.93
    - liver — *see* Injury, liver
    - ovary — *see* Injury, ovary
    - pancreas — *see* Injury, pancreas
    - pelvic NOS S37.90
    - peritoneum — *see* Injury, intra-abdominal, specified, site NEC
    - prostate — *see* Injury, prostate
    - rectum — *see* Injury, intestine, large, rectum
    - retroperitoneum — *see* Injury, intra-abdominal, specified, site NEC

DISEASE INDEX

D I S E A S E   I N D E X

Injury (*see also* specified injury type) T14.90
— *continued*
  intra-abdominal S36.90 — *continued*
    seminal vesicle — *see* Injury, pelvis, organ, specified site NEC
    small intestine — *see* Injury, intestine, small
    specified
      pelvic S37.90
        specified
          site NEC S37.899
            specified type NEC S37.898
          type NEC S37.99
      site NEC S36.899
        contusion S36.892
        laceration S36.893
        specified type NEC S36.898
        type NEC S36.99
    spleen — *see* Injury, spleen
    stomach — *see* Injury, stomach
    ureter — *see* Injury, ureter
    urethra — *see* Injury, urethra
    uterus — *see* Injury, uterus
    vas deferens — *see* Injury, pelvis, organ, specified site NEC
  intracranial (traumatic) S06.9-
    cerebellar hemorrhage, traumatic — *see* Injury, intracranial, focal
    cerebral edema, traumatic S06.1x-
      diffuse S06.1x-
      focal S06.1x-
    diffuse (axonal) S06.2x-
    epidural hemorrhage (traumatic) S06.4x-
    focal brain injury S06.30-
      contusion — *see* Contusion, cerebral
      laceration — *see* Laceration, cerebral
    intracerebral hemorrhage, traumatic S06.36-
      left side S06.35-
      right side S06.34-
    subarachnoid hemorrhage, traumatic S06.6x-
    subdural hemorrhage, traumatic S06.5x-
  intraocular — *see* Injury, eyeball, penetrating
  intrathoracic S27.9
    bronchus S27.409
      bilateral S27.402
      blast injury (primary) S27.419
        bilateral S27.412
        secondary — *see* Injury, intrathoracic, bronchus, specified type NEC
        unilateral S27.411
      contusion S27.429
        bilateral S27.422
        unilateral S27.421
      laceration S27.439
        bilateral S27.432
        unilateral S27.431
      specified type NEC S27.499
        bilateral S27.492
        unilateral S27.491
      unilateral S27.401
    diaphragm S27.809
      contusion S27.802
      laceration S27.803
      specified type NEC S27.808
    esophagus (thoracic) S27.819
      contusion S27.812
      laceration S27.813
      specified type NEC S27.818
    heart — *see* Injury, heart
    hemopneumothorax S27.2
    hemothorax S27.1
    lung S27.309
      aspiration J69.0
      bilateral S27.302
      blast injury (primary) S27.319
        bilateral S27.312
        secondary — *see* Injury, intrathoracic, lung, specified type NEC
        unilateral S27.311
      contusion S27.329
        bilateral S27.322
        unilateral S27.321
      laceration S27.339
        bilateral S27.332
        unilateral S27.331
      specified type NEC S27.399
        bilateral S27.392
        unilateral S27.391
      unilateral S27.301
    pleura S27.60
      laceration S27.63
      specified type NEC S27.69

Injury (*see also* specified injury type) T14.90
— *continued*
  intrathoracic S27.9 — *continued*
    pneumothorax S27.0
    specified organ NEC S27.899
      contusion S27.892
      laceration S27.893
      specified type NEC S27.898
    thoracic duct — *see* Injury, intrathoracic, specified organ NEC
    thymus gland — *see* Injury, intrathoracic, specified organ NEC
    trachea, thoracic S27.50
      blast (primary) S27.51
      contusion S27.52
      laceration S27.53
      specified type NEC S27.59
  iris — *see* Injury, eye, specified site NEC
    penetrating — *see* Injury, eyeball, penetrating
  jaw S09.93
  jejunum — *see* Injury, intestine, small
  joint NOS T14.8
    old or residual — *see* Disorder, joint, specified type NEC
  kidney S37.00-
    acute (nontraumatic) N17.9
    contusion — *see* Contusion, kidney
    laceration — *see* Laceration, kidney
    specified NEC S37.09-
  knee S89.9-
    contusion — *see* Contusion, knee
    dislocation — *see* Dislocation, knee
    meniscus (lateral) (medial) — *see* Sprain, knee, specified site NEC
      old injury or tear — *see* Derangement, knee, meniscus, due to old injury
    open — *see* Wound, open, knee
    specified NEC S89.8-
    sprain — *see* Sprain, knee
    superficial — *see* Injury, superficial, knee
  labium (majus) (minus) S39.94
  labyrinth, ear S09.30-
  lacrimal apparatus, duct, gland, or sac — *see* Injury, eye, specified site NEC
  larynx NEC S19.81
  leg (lower) S89.9-
    blood vessel — *see* Injury, blood vessel, leg
    contusion — *see* Contusion, leg
    fracture — *see* Fracture, leg
    muscle — *see* Injury, muscle, leg
    nerve — *see* Injury, nerve, leg
    open — *see* Wound, open, leg
    specified NEC S89.8-
    superficial — *see* Injury, superficial, leg
  lens, eye — *see* Injury, eye, specified site NEC
    penetrating — *see* Injury, eyeball, penetrating
  limb NEC T14.8
  lip S09.93
  liver S36.119
    contusion S36.112
    laceration S36.113
      major (stellate) S36.116
      minor S36.114
      moderate S36.115
    specified NEC S36.118
  lower back S39.92
    specified NEC S39.82
  lumbar, lumbosacral (region) S39.92
    plexus — *see* Injury, lumbosacral plexus
  lumbosacral plexus S34.4
  lung — *see also* Injury, intrathoracic, lung
    aspiration J69.0
    transfusion-related (TRALI) J95.84
  lymphatic thoracic duct — *see* Injury, intrathoracic, specified organ NEC
  malar region S09.93
  mastoid region S09.90
  maxilla S09.93
  mediastinum — *see* Injury, intrathoracic, specified organ NEC
  membrane, brain — *see* Injury, intracranial
  meningeal artery — *see* Injury, intracranial, subdural hemorrhage
  meninges (cerebral) — *see* Injury, intracranial

Injury (*see also* specified injury type) T14.90
— *continued*
  mesenteric
    artery
      branch S35.299
        laceration (minor) (superficial) S35.291
        major S35.292
        specified NEC S35.298
      inferior S35.239
        laceration (minor) (superficial) S35.231
        major S35.232
        specified NEC S35.238
      superior S35.229
        laceration (minor) (superficial) S35.221
        major S35.222
        specified NEC S35.228
    plexus (inferior) (superior) — *see* Injury, nerve, lumbosacral, sympathetic
    vein
      inferior S35.349
        laceration S35.341
        specified NEC S35.348
      superior S35.339
        laceration S35.331
        specified NEC S35.338
  mesentery — *see* Injury, intra-abdominal, specified site NEC
  mesosalpinx — *see* Injury, pelvic organ, specified site NEC
  middle ear S09.30-
  midthoracic region NOS S29.9
  mouth S09.93
  multiple NOS T07
  muscle (and fascia) (and tendon)
    abdomen S39.001
      laceration S39.021
      specified type NEC S39.091
      strain S39.011
    abductor
      thumb, forearm level — *see* Injury, muscle, thumb, abductor
    adductor
      thigh S76.20-
        laceration S76.22-
        specified type NEC S76.29-
        strain S76.21-
    ankle — *see* Injury, muscle, foot
    anterior muscle group, at leg level (lower) S86.20-
      laceration S86.22-
      specified type NEC S86.29-
      strain S86.21-
    arm (upper) — *see* Injury, muscle, shoulder
    biceps (parts NEC) S46.20-
      laceration S46.22-
      long head S46.10-
        laceration S46.12-
        specified type NEC S46.19-
        strain S46.11-
      specified type NEC S46.29-
      strain S46.21-
    extensor
      finger(s) (other than thumb) — *see* Injury, muscle, finger by site, extensor
      forearm level, specified NEC — *see* Injury, muscle, forearm, extensor
      thumb — *see* Injury, muscle, thumb, extensor
      toe (large) (ankle level) (foot level) — *see* Injury, muscle, toe, extensor
    finger
      extensor (forearm level) S56.40-
        hand level S66.309
          laceration S66.329
          specified type NEC S66.399
          strain S66.319
        laceration S56.429
        specified type NEC S56.499
        strain S56.419
      flexor (forearm level) S56.10-
        hand level S66.109
          laceration S66.129
          specified type NEC S66.199
          strain S66.119
        laceration S56.129
        specified type NEC S56.199
        strain S56.119

Injury (*see also* specified injury type) T14.90
— *continued*
  muscle (and fascia) (and tendon) — *continued*
    finger — *continued*
      index
        extensor (forearm level)
          hand level S66.308
            laceration S66.32-
            specified type NEC S66.39-
            strain S66.31-
          specified type NEC S56.492-
        flexor (forearm level)
          hand level S66.108
            laceration S66.12-
            specified type NEC S66.19-
            strain S66.11-
          specified type NEC S56.19-
          strain S56.11-
        intrinsic S66.50-
          laceration S66.52-
          specified type NEC S66.59-
          strain S66.51-
      intrinsic S66.509
        laceration S66.529
        specified type NEC S66.599
        strain S66.519
      little
        extensor (forearm level)
          hand level S66.30-
            laceration S66.32-
            specified type NEC S66.39-
            strain S66.31-
          laceration S56.42-
          specified type NEC S56.49-
          strain S56.41-
        flexor (forearm level)
          hand level S66.10-
            laceration S66.12-
            specified type NEC S66.19-
            strain S66.11-
          laceration S56.12-
          specified type NEC S56.19-
          strain S56.11-
        intrinsic S66.50-
          laceration S66.52-
          specified type NEC S66.59-
          strain S66.51-
      middle
        extensor (forearm level)
          hand level S66.30-
            laceration S66.32-
            specified type NEC S66.39-
            strain S66.31-
          laceration S56.42-
          specified type NEC S56.49-
          strain S56.41-
        flexor (forearm level)
          hand level S66.10-
            laceration S66.12-
            specified type NEC S66.19-
            strain S66.11-
          laceration S56.12-
          specified type NEC S56.19-
          strain S56.11-
        intrinsic S66.50-
          laceration S66.52-
          specified type NEC S66.59-
          strain S66.51-
      ring
        extensor (forearm level)
          hand level S66.30-
            laceration S66.32-
            specified type NEC S66.39-
            strain S66.31-
          laceration S56.42-
          specified type NEC S56.49-
          strain S56.41-
        flexor (forearm level)
          hand level S66.10-
            laceration S66.12-
            specified type NEC S66.19-
            strain S66.11-
          laceration S56.12-
          specified type NEC S56.19-
          strain S56.11-
        intrinsic S66.50-
          laceration S66.52-
          specified type NEC S66.59-
          strain S66.51-
    flexor
      finger(s) (other than thumb) — *see* Injury, muscle, finger
      forearm level, specified NEC — *see* Injury, muscle, forearm, flexor
      thumb — *see* Injury, muscle, thumb, flexor
      toe (long) (ankle level) (foot level) — *see* Injury, muscle, toe, flexor

Injury (*see also* specified injury type) T14.90
— *continued*
muscle (and fascia) (and tendon) —
continued
foot S96.90-
intrinsic S96.20-
laceration S96.22-
specified type NEC S96.29-
strain S96.21-
laceration S96.92-
long extensor, toe — *see* Injury,
muscle, toe, extensor
long flexor, toe — *see* Injury, muscle,
toe, flexor
specified
site NEC S96.80-
laceration S96.82-
specified type NEC S96.89-
strain S96.81-
type NEC S96.99-
strain S96.91-
forearm (level) S56.90-
extensor S56.50-
laceration S56.52-
specified type NEC S56.59-
strain S56.51-
flexor S56.20-
laceration S56.22-
specified type NEC S56.29-
strain S56.21-
laceration S56.92-
specified S56.99-
site NEC S56.80-
laceration S56.82-
strain S56.81-
type NEC S56.89-
strain S56.91-
hand (level) S66.90-
laceration S66.92-
specified
site NEC S66.80-
laceration S66.82-
specified type NEC S66.89-
strain S66.81-
type NEC S66.99-
strain S66.91-
head S09.10
laceration S09.12
specified type NEC S09.19
strain S09.11
hip NEC S76.00-
laceration S76.02-
specified type NEC S76.09-
strain S76.01-
intrinsic
ankle and foot level — *see* Injury,
muscle, foot, intrinsic
finger (other than thumb) — *see*
Injury, muscle, finger by site,
intrinsic
foot (level) — *see* Injury, muscle,
foot, intrinsic
thumb — *see* Injury, muscle, thumb,
intrinsic
leg (level) (lower) S86.90-
Achilles tendon — *see* Injury, Achilles
tendon
anterior muscle group — *see* Injury,
muscle, anterior muscle group
laceration S86.92-
peroneal muscle group — *see* Injury,
muscle, peroneal muscle group
posterior muscle group — *see* Injury,
muscle, posterior muscle group,
leg level
specified
site NEC S86.80-
laceration S86.82-
specified type NEC S86.89-
strain S86.81-
type NEC S86.99-
strain S86.91-
long
extensor toe, at ankle and foot level —
see Injury, muscle, toe, extensor
flexor, toe, at ankle and foot level —
see Injury, muscle, toe, flexor
head, biceps — *see* Injury, muscle,
biceps, long head
lower back S39.002
laceration S39.022
specified type NEC S39.092
strain S39.012
neck (level) S16.9
laceration S16.2
specified type NEC S16.8
strain S16.1

Injury (*see also* specified injury type) T14.90
— *continued*
muscle (and fascia) (and tendon) —
continued
pelvis S39.003
laceration S39.023
specified type NEC S39.093
strain S39.013
peroneal muscle group, at leg level
(lower) S86.30-
laceration S86.32-
specified type NEC S86.39-
strain S86.31-
posterior muscle (group)
leg level (lower) S86.10-
laceration S86.12-
specified type NEC S86.19-
strain S86.11-
thigh level S76.30-
laceration S76.32-
specified type NEC S76.39-
strain S76.31-
quadriceps (thigh) S76.10-
laceration S76.12-
specified type NEC S76.19-
strain S76.11-
shoulder S46.90-
laceration S46.92-
rotator cuff — *see* Injury, rotator cuff
specified site NEC S46.80-
laceration S46.82-
specified type NEC S46.89-
strain S46.81-
specified type NEC S46.99-
strain S46.91-
thigh NEC (level) S76.90-
adductor — *see* Injury, muscle,
adductor, thigh
laceration S76.92-
posterior muscle (group) — *see*
Injury, muscle, posterior muscle,
thigh level
quadriceps — *see* Injury, muscle,
quadriceps
specified
site NEC S76.80-
laceration S76.82-
specified type NEC S76.89-
strain S76.81-
type NEC S76.99-
strain S76.91-
thorax (level) S29.009
back wall S29.002
front wall S29.001
laceration S29.029
back wall S29.022
front wall S29.021
specified type NEC S29.099
back wall S29.092
front wall S29.091
strain S29.019
back wall S29.012
front wall S29.011
thumb
abductor (forearm level) S56.30-
laceration S56.32-
specified type NEC S56.39-
strain S56.31-
extensor (forearm level) S56.30-
hand level S66.20-
laceration S66.22-
specified type NEC S66.29-
strain S66.21-
laceration S56.32-
specified type NEC S56.39-
strain S56.31-
flexor (forearm level) S56.00-
hand level S66.00-
laceration S66.02-
specified type NEC S66.09-
strain S66.01-
laceration S56.02-
specified type NEC S56.09-
strain S56.01-
wrist level — *see* Injury, muscle,
thumb, flexor, hand level
intrinsic S66.40-
laceration S66.42-
specified type NEC S66.49-
strain S66.41-
toe — *see also* Injury, muscle, foot
extensor, long S96.10-
laceration S96.12-
specified type NEC S96.19-
strain S96.11-
flexor, long S96.00-
laceration S96.02-
specified type NEC S96.09-
strain S96.01-

Injury (*see also* specified injury type) T14.90
— *continued*
muscle (and fascia) (and tendon) —
continued
triceps S46.30-
laceration S46.32-
specified type NEC S46.39-
strain S46.31-
wrist (and hand) level — *see* Injury,
muscle, hand
musculocutaneous nerve — *see* Injury,
nerve, musculocutaneous
myocardium — *see* Injury, heart
nape — *see* Injury, neck
nasal (septum) (sinus) S09.92
nasopharynx S09.92
neck S19.9
specified NEC S19.80
specified site NEC S19.89
nerve NEC T14.8
abdomen S34.9
peripheral S34.6
specified site NEC S34.8
abducens S04.4-
contusion S04.4-
laceration S04.4-
specified type NEC S04.4-
abducent — *see* Injury, nerve, abducens
accessory S04.7-
contusion S04.7-
laceration S04.7-
specified type NEC S04.7-
acoustic S04.6-
contusion S04.6-
laceration S04.6-
specified type NEC S04.6-
ankle S94.9-
cutaneous sensory S94.3-
specified type NEC — *see* subcategory
S94.8
anterior crural, femoral — *see* Injury,
nerve, femoral
arm (upper) S44.9-
axillary — *see* Injury, nerve, axillary
cutaneous — *see* Injury, nerve,
cutaneous, arm
median — *see* Injury, nerve, median,
upper arm
musculocutaneous — *see* Injury,
nerve, musculocutaneous
radial — *see* Injury, nerve, radial,
upper arm
specified site NEC — *see* subcategory
S44.8
ulnar — *see* Injury, nerve, ulnar, arm
auditory — *see* Injury, nerve, acoustic
axillary S44.3-
brachial plexus — *see* Injury, brachial
plexus
cervical sympathetic S14.5
cranial S04.9
contusion S04.9
eighth (acoustic or auditory) — *see*
Injury, nerve, acoustic
eleventh (accessory) — *see* Injury,
nerve, accessory
fifth (trigeminal) — *see* Injury, nerve,
trigeminal
first (olfactory) — *see* Injury, nerve,
olfactory
fourth (trochlear) — *see* Injury, nerve,
trochlear
laceration S04.9
ninth (glossopharyngeal) — *see*
Injury, nerve, glossopharyngeal
second (optic) — *see* Injury, nerve,
optic
seventh (facial) — *see* Injury, nerve,
facial
sixth (abducent) — *see* Injury, nerve,
abducens
specified
nerve NEC S04.89-
contusion S04.89-
laceration S04.89-
specified type NEC S04.89-
type NEC S04.9
tenth (pneumogastric or vagus) — *see*
Injury, nerve, vagus
third (oculomotor) — *see* Injury,
nerve, oculomotor
twelfth (hypoglossal) — *see* Injury,
nerve, hypoglossal

Injury (*see also* specified injury type) T14.90
— *continued*
nerve NEC T14.8 — *continued*
cutaneous sensory
ankle (level) S94.3-
arm (upper) (level) S44.5-
foot (level) — *see* Injury, nerve,
cutaneous sensory, ankle
forearm (level) S54.3-
hip (level) S74.2-
leg (lower level) S84.2-
shoulder (level) — *see* Injury, nerve,
cutaneous sensory, arm
thigh (level) — *see* Injury, nerve,
cutaneous sensory, hip
deep peroneal — *see* Injury, nerve,
peroneal, foot
digital
finger S64.4-
index S64.49-
little S64.49-
middle S64.49-
ring S64.49-
thumb S64.3-
toe — *see* Injury, nerve, ankle,
specified site NEC
eighth cranial (acoustic or auditory) —
see Injury, nerve, acoustic
eleventh cranial (accessory) — *see*
Injury, nerve, accessory
facial S04.5-
contusion S04.5-
laceration S04.5-
newborn P11.3
specified type NEC S04.5-
femoral (hip level) (thigh level) S74.1-
fifth cranial (trigeminal) — *see* Injury,
nerve, trigeminal
finger (digital) — *see* Injury, nerve,
digital, finger
first cranial (olfactory) — *see* Injury,
nerve, olfactory
foot S94.9-
cutaneous sensory S94.3-
deep peroneal S94.2-
lateral plantar S94.0-
medial plantar S94.1-
specified site NEC — *see* subcategory
S94.8
forearm (level) S54.9-
cutaneous sensory — *see* Injury,
nerve, cutaneous sensory,
forearm
median — *see* Injury, nerve, median
radial — *see* Injury, nerve, radial
specified site NEC — *see* subcategory
S54.8
ulnar — *see* Injury, nerve, ulnar
fourth cranial (trochlear) — *see* Injury,
nerve, trochlear
glossopharyngeal S04.89-
specified type NEC S04.89-
hand S64.9-
median — *see* Injury, nerve, median,
hand
radial — *see* Injury, nerve, radial,
hand
specified NEC — *see* subcategory
S64.8
ulnar — *see* Injury, nerve, ulnar, hand
hip (level) S74.9-
cutaneous sensory — *see* Injury,
nerve, cutaneous sensory, hip
femoral — *see* Injury, nerve, femoral
sciatic — *see* Injury, nerve, sciatic
specified site NEC — *see* subcategory
S74.8
hypoglossal S04.89-
specified type NEC S04.89-
lateral plantar S94.0-
leg (lower) S84.9-
cutaneous sensory — *see* Injury,
nerve, cutaneous sensory, leg
peroneal — *see* Injury, nerve, peroneal
specified site NEC — *see* subcategory
S84.8
tibial — *see* Injury, nerve, tibial
upper — *see* Injury, nerve, thigh
lower
back — *see* Injury, nerve, abdomen,
specified site NEC
peripheral — *see* Injury, nerve,
abdomen, peripheral
limb — *see* Injury, nerve, leg
lumbar plexus — *see* Injury, nerve,
lumbosacral, sympathetic
lumbar spinal — *see* Injury, nerve,
spinal, lumbar

Injury (*see also* specified injury type) T14.90 — *continued*
  nerve NEC T14.8 — *continued*
    lumbosacral
      plexus — *see* Injury, nerve, lumbosacral, sympathetic
      sympathetic S34.5
    medial plantar S94.1-
    median (forearm level) S54.1-
      hand (level) S64.1-
      upper arm (level) S44.1-
      wrist (level) — *see* Injury, nerve, median, hand
    musculocutaneous S44.4-
    musculospiral (upper arm level) — *see* Injury, nerve, radial, upper arm
    neck S14.9
      peripheral S14.4
      specified site NEC S14.8
      sympathetic S14.5
    ninth cranial (glossopharyngeal) — *see* Injury, nerve, glossopharyngeal
    oculomotor S04.1-
      contusion S04.1-
      laceration S04.1-
      specified type NEC S04.1-
    olfactory S04.81-
      specified type NEC S04.81-
    optic S04.01-
      contusion S04.01-
      laceration S04.01-
      specified type NEC S04.01-
    pelvic girdle — *see* Injury, nerve, hip
    pelvis — *see* Injury, nerve, abdomen, specified site NEC
    peripheral — *see* Injury, nerve, abdomen, peripheral
    peripheral NEC T14.8
      abdomen — *see* Injury, nerve, abdomen, peripheral
      lower back — *see* Injury, nerve, abdomen, peripheral
      neck — *see* Injury, nerve, neck, peripheral
      pelvis — *see* Injury, nerve, abdomen, peripheral
      specified NEC T14.8
    peroneal (lower leg level) S84.1-
      foot S94.2-
    plexus
      brachial — *see* Injury, brachial plexus
      celiac, coeliac — *see* Injury, nerve, lumbosacral, sympathetic
      mesenteric, inferior — *see* Injury, nerve, lumbosacral, sympathetic
      sacral — *see* Injury, lumbosacral plexus
      spinal
        brachial — *see* Injury, brachial plexus
        lumbosacral — *see* Injury, lumbosacral plexus
    pneumogastric — *see* Injury, nerve, vagus
    radial (forearm level) S54.2-
      hand (level) S64.2-
      upper arm (level) S44.2-
      wrist (level) — *see* Injury, nerve, radial, hand
    root — *see* Injury, nerve, spinal, root
    sacral plexus — *see* Injury, lumbosacral plexus
    sacral spinal — *see* Injury, nerve, spinal, sacral
    sciatic (hip level) (thigh level) S74.0-
    second cranial (optic) — *see* Injury, nerve, optic
    seventh cranial (facial) — *see* Injury, nerve, facial
    shoulder — *see* Injury, nerve, arm
    sixth cranial (abducent) — *see* Injury, nerve, abducens
    spinal
      plexus — *see* Injury, nerve, plexus, spinal
      root
        cervical S14.2
        dorsal S24.2
        lumbar S34.21
        sacral S34.22
        thoracic — *see* Injury, nerve, spinal, root, dorsal
    splanchnic — *see* Injury, nerve, lumbosacral, sympathetic
    sympathetic NEC — *see* Injury, nerve, lumbosacral, sympathetic
      cervical — *see* Injury, nerve, cervical sympathetic

Injury (*see also* specified injury type) T14.90 — *continued*
  nerve NEC T14.8 — *continued*
    tenth cranial (pneumogastric or vagus) — *see* Injury, nerve, vagus
    thigh (level) — *see* Injury, nerve, hip
      cutaneous sensory — *see* Injury, nerve, cutaneous sensory, hip
      femoral — *see* Injury, nerve, femoral
      sciatic — *see* Injury, nerve, sciatic
      specified NEC — *see* Injury, nerve, hip
    third cranial (oculomotor) — *see* Injury, nerve, oculomotor
    thorax S24.9
      peripheral S24.3
      specified site NEC S24.8
      sympathetic S24.4
    thumb, digital — *see* Injury, nerve, digital, thumb
    tibial (lower leg level) (posterior) S84.0-
      toe — *see* Injury, nerve, ankle
    trigeminal S04.3-
      contusion S04.3-
      laceration S04.3-
      specified type NEC S04.3-
    trochlear S04.2-
      contusion S04.2-
      laceration S04.2-
      specified type NEC S04.2-
    twelfth cranial (hypoglossal) — *see* Injury, nerve, hypoglossal
    ulnar (forearm level) S54.0-
      arm (upper) (level) S44.0-
      hand (level) S64.0-
      wrist (level) — *see* Injury, nerve, ulnar, hand
    vagus S04.89-
      specified type NEC S04.89-
    wrist (level) — *see* Injury, nerve, hand
  ninth cranial nerve (glossopharyngeal) — *see* Injury, nerve, glossopharyngeal
  nose (septum) S09.92
  obstetrical O71.9
    specified NEC O71.89
  occipital (region) (scalp) S09.90
    lobe — *see* Injury, intracranial
  optic chiasm S04.02
  optic radiation S04.03-
  optic tract and pathways S04.03-
  orbit, orbital (region) — *see* Injury, eye
    penetrating (with foreign body) — *see* Injury, eye, orbit, penetrating
    specified NEC — *see* Injury, eye, specified site NEC
  ovary, ovarian S37.409
    bilateral S37.402
      contusion S37.422
      laceration S37.432
      specified type NEC S37.492
    blood vessel — *see* Injury, blood vessel, ovarian
    contusion S37.429
      bilateral S37.422
      unilateral S37.421
    laceration S37.439
      bilateral S37.432
      unilateral S37.431
    specified type NEC S37.499
      bilateral S37.492
      unilateral S37.491
    unilateral S37.401
      contusion S37.421
      laceration S37.431
      specified type NEC S37.491
  palate (hard) (soft) S09.93
  pancreas S36.209
    body S36.201
      contusion S36.221
      laceration S36.231
        major S36.261
        minor S36.241
        moderate S36.251
      specified type NEC S36.291
    contusion S36.229
    head S36.200
      contusion S36.220
      laceration S36.230
        major S36.260
        minor S36.240
        moderate S36.250
      specified type NEC S36.290
    laceration S36.239
      major S36.269
      minor S36.249
      moderate S36.259

Injury (*see also* specified injury type) T14.90 — *continued*
  pancreas S36.209 — *continued*
    specified type NEC S36.299
    tail S36.202
      contusion S36.222
      laceration S36.232
        major S36.262
        minor S36.242
        moderate S36.252
      specified type NEC S36.292
  parietal (region) (scalp) S09.90
    lobe — *see* Injury, intracranial
  patellar ligament (tendon) S76.10-
    laceration S76.12-
    specified NEC S76.19-
    strain S76.11-
  pelvis, pelvic (floor) S39.93
    complicating delivery O70.1
    joint or ligament, complicating delivery O71.6
    organ S37.90
      with ectopic or molar pregnancy O08.6
      complication of abortion — *see* Abortion
      contusion S37.92
      following ectopic or molar pregnancy O08.6
      laceration S37.93
      obstetrical trauma NEC O71.5
      specified
        site NEC S37.899
          contusion S37.892
          laceration S37.893
          specified type NEC S37.898
        type NEC S37.99
      specified NEC S39.83
  penis S39.94
  perineum S39.94
  peritoneum S36.81
    laceration S36.893
  periurethral tissue — *see* Injury, urethra
    complicating delivery O71.82
  phalanges
    foot — *see* Injury, foot
    hand — *see* Injury, hand
  pharynx NEC S19.85
  pleura — *see* Injury, intrathoracic, pleura
  plexus
    brachial — *see* Injury, brachial plexus
    cardiac — *see* Injury, nerve, thorax, sympathetic
    celiac, coeliac — *see* Injury, nerve, lumbosacral, sympathetic
    esophageal — *see* Injury, nerve, thorax, sympathetic
    hypogastric — *see* Injury, nerve, lumbosacral, sympathetic
    lumbar, lumbosacral — *see* Injury, lumbosacral plexus
    mesenteric — *see* Injury, nerve, lumbosacral, sympathetic
    pulmonary — *see* Injury, nerve, thorax, sympathetic
  postcardiac surgery (syndrome) I97.0
  prepuce S39.94
  prostate S37.829
    contusion S37.822
    laceration S37.823
    specified type NEC S37.828
  pubic region S39.94
  pudendum S39.94
  pulmonary plexus — *see* Injury, nerve, thorax, sympathetic
  rectovaginal septum NEC S39.83
  rectum — *see* Injury, intestine, large, rectum
  retina — *see* Injury, eye, specified site NEC
    penetrating — *see* Injury, eyeball, penetrating
  retroperitoneal — *see* Injury, intra-abdominal, specified site NEC
  rotator cuff (muscle(s)) (tendon(s)) S46.00-
    laceration S46.02-
    specified type NEC S46.09-
    strain S46.01-
  round ligament — *see* Injury, pelvic organ, specified site NEC
  sacral plexus — *see* Injury, lumbosacral plexus
  salivary duct or gland S09.93
  scalp S09.90
    newborn (birth injury) P12.9
      due to monitoring (electrode) (sampling incision) P12.4
      specified NEC P12.89
        caput succedaneum P12.81

Injury (*see also* specified injury type) T14.90 — *continued*
  scapular region — *see* Injury, shoulder
  sclera — *see* Injury, eye, specified site NEC
    penetrating — *see* Injury, eyeball, penetrating
  scrotum S39.94
  second cranial nerve (optic) — *see* Injury, nerve, optic
  seminal vesicle — *see* Injury, pelvic organ, specified site NEC
  seventh cranial nerve (facial) — *see* Injury, nerve, facial
  shoulder S49.9-
    blood vessel — *see* Injury, blood vessel, arm
    contusion — *see* Contusion, shoulder
    dislocation — *see* Dislocation, shoulder
    fracture — *see* Fracture, shoulder
    muscle — *see* Injury, muscle, shoulder
    nerve — *see* Injury, nerve, shoulder
    open — *see* Wound, open, shoulder
    specified type NEC S49.8-
    sprain — *see* Sprain, shoulder girdle
    superficial — *see* Injury, superficial, shoulder
  sinus
    cavernous — *see* Injury, intracranial
    nasal S09.92
  sixth cranial nerve (abducent) — *see* Injury, nerve, abducens
  skeleton, birth injury P13.9
    specified part NEC P13.8
  skin NEC T14.8
    surface intact — *see* Injury, superficial
  skull NEC S09.90
  specified NEC T14.8
  spermatic cord (pelvic region) S37.898
    scrotal region S39.848
  spinal (cord)
    cervical (neck) S14.109
      anterior cord syndrome S14.139
        C1 level S14.131
        C2 level S14.132
        C3 level S14.133
        C4 level S14.134
        C5 level S14.135
        C6 level S14.136
        C7 level S14.137
        C8 level S14.138
      Brown-Séquard syndrome S14.149
        C1 level S14.141
        C2 level S14.142
        C3 level S14.143
        C4 level S14.144
        C5 level S14.145
        C6 level S14.146
        C7 level S14.147
        C8 level S14.148
      C1 level S14.101
      C2 level S14.102
      C3 level S14.103
      C4 level S14.104
      C5 level S14.105
      C6 level S14.106
      C7 level S14.107
      C8 level S14.108
      central cord syndrome S14.129
        C1 level S14.121
        C2 level S14.122
        C3 level S14.123
        C4 level S14.124
        C5 level S14.125
        C6 level S14.126
        C7 level S14.127
        C8 level S14.128
      complete lesion S14.119
        C1 level S14.111
        C2 level S14.112
        C3 level S14.113
        C4 level S14.114
        C5 level S14.115
        C6 level S14.116
        C7 level S14.117
        C8 level S14.118
      concussion S14.0
      edema S14.0
      incomplete lesion specified NEC S14.159
        C1 level S14.151
        C2 level S14.152
        C3 level S14.153
        C4 level S14.154
        C5 level S14.155
        C6 level S14.156
        C7 level S14.157
        C8 level S14.158

Injury (*see also* specified injury type) T14.90
— *continued*
spinal (cord) — *continued*
  cervical (neck) S14.109 — *continued*
    posterior cord syndrome S14.159
      C1 level S14.151
      C2 level S14.152
      C3 level S14.153
      C4 level S14.154
      C5 level S14.155
      C6 level S14.156
      C7 level S14.157
      C8 level S14.158
  dorsal — *see* Injury, spinal, thoracic
  lumbar S34.109
    complete lesion S34.119
      L1 level S34.111
      L2 level S34.112
      L3 level S34.113
      L4 level S34.114
      L5 level S34.115
    concussion S34.01
    edema S34.01
    incomplete lesion S34.129
      L1 level S34.121
      L2 level S34.122
      L3 level S34.123
      L4 level S34.124
      L5 level S34.125
      L1 level S34.101
      L2 level S34.102
      L3 level S34.103
      L4 level S34.104
      L5 level S34.105
  nerve root NEC
    cervical — *see* Injury, nerve, spinal,
      root, cervical
    dorsal — *see* Injury, nerve, spinal,
      root, dorsal
    lumbar S34.21
    sacral S34.22
    thoracic — *see* Injury, nerve, spinal,
      root, dorsal
  plexus
    brachial — *see* Injury, brachial plexus
    lumbosacral — *see* Injury,
      lumbosacral plexus
  sacral S34.139
    complete lesion S34.131
    incomplete lesion S34.132
  thoracic S24.109
    anterior cord syndrome S24.139
      T1 level S24.131
      T11-T12 level S24.134
      T2-T6 level S24.132
      T7-T10 level S24.133
    Brown-Séquard syndrome S24.149
      T1 level S24.141
      T11-T12 level S24.144
      T2-T6 level S24.142
      T7-T10 level S24.143
    complete lesion S24.119
      T1 level S24.111
      T11-T12 level S24.114
      T2-T6 level S24.112
      T7-T10 level S24.113
    concussion S24.0
    edema S24.0
    incomplete lesion specified NEC
      S24.159
      T1 level S24.151
      T11-T12 level S24.154
      T2-T6 level S24.152
      T7-T10 level S24.153
    posterior cord syndrome S24.159
      T1 level S24.151
      T11-T12 level S24.154
      T2-T6 level S24.152
      T7-T10 level S24.153
      T1 level S24.101
      T11-T12 level S24.104
      T2-T6 level S24.102
      T7-T10 level S24.103
  splanchnic nerve — *see* Injury, nerve,
    lumbosacral, sympathetic
  spleen S36.00
    contusion S36.029
      major S36.021
      minor S36.020
    laceration S36.039
      major (massive) (stellate) S36.032
      moderate S36.031
      superficial (capsular) (minor) S36.030
    specified type NEC S36.09
  splenic artery — *see* Injury, blood vessel,
    celiac artery, branch

Injury (*see also* specified injury type) T14.90
— *continued*
stellate ganglion — *see* Injury, nerve,
  thorax, sympathetic
sternal region S29.9
stomach S36.30
  contusion S36.32
  laceration S36.33
  specified type NEC S36.39
subconjunctival — *see* Injury, eye,
  conjunctiva
subcutaneous NEC T14.8
submaxillary region S09.93
submental region S09.93
subungual
  fingers — *see* Injury, hand
  toes — *see* Injury, foot
superficial NEC T14.8
  abdomen, abdominal (wall) S30.92
    abrasion S30.811
      bite S30.871
        insect S30.861
    contusion S30.1
    external constriction S30.841
    foreign body S30.851
  abrasion — *see* Abrasion, by site
  adnexa, eye NEC — *see* Injury, eye,
    specified site NEC
  alveolar process — *see* Injury,
    superficial, oral cavity
  ankle S90.91-
    abrasion — *see* Abrasion, ankle
    bite — *see* Bite, ankle
    blister — *see* Blister, ankle
    contusion — *see* Contusion, ankle
    external constriction — *see*
      Constriction, external, ankle
    foreign body — *see* Foreign body,
      superficial, ankle
  anus S30.98
  arm (upper) S40.92-
    abrasion — *see* Abrasion, arm
    bite — *see* Bite, superficial, arm
    blister — *see* Blister, arm (upper)
    contusion — *see* Contusion, arm
    external constriction — *see*
      Constriction, external, arm
    foreign body — *see* Foreign body,
      superficial, arm
  auditory canal (external) (meatus) — *see*
    Injury, superficial, ear
  auricle — *see* Injury, superficial, ear
  axilla — *see* Injury, superficial, arm
  back — *see also* Injury, superficial,
    thorax, back
    lower S30.91
      abrasion S30.810
      contusion S30.0
      external constriction S30.840
      superficial
        bite NEC S30.870
          insect S30.860
        foreign body S30.850
  bite NEC — *see* Bite, superficial NEC,
    by site
  blister — *see* Blister, by site
  breast S20.10-
    abrasion — *see* Abrasion, breast
    bite — *see* Bite, superficial, breast
    contusion — *see* Contusion, breast
    external constriction — *see*
      Constriction, external, breast
    foreign body — *see* Foreign body,
      superficial, breast
  brow — *see* Injury, superficial, head,
    specified NEC
  buttock S30.91
  calf — *see* Injury, superficial, leg
  canthus, eye — *see* Injury, superficial,
    periocular area
  cheek (external) — *see* Injury,
    superficial, head, specified NEC
    internal — *see* Injury, superficial, oral
      cavity
  chest wall — *see* Injury, superficial,
    thorax
  chin — *see* Injury, superficial, head NEC
  clitoris S30.95
  conjunctiva — *see* Injury, eye,
    conjunctiva
    with foreign body (in conjunctival
      sac) — *see* Foreign body,
      conjunctival sac
  contusion — *see* Contusion, by site
  costal region — *see* Injury, superficial,
    thorax
  digit(s)
    hand — *see* Injury, superficial, finger

Injury (*see also* specified injury type) T14.90
— *continued*
superficial NEC T14.8 — *continued*
  ear (auricle) (canal) (external) S00.40-
    abrasion — *see* Abrasion, ear
    bite — *see* Bite, superficial, ear
    contusion — *see* Contusion, ear
    external constriction — *see*
      Constriction, external, ear
    foreign body — *see* Foreign body,
      superficial, ear
  elbow S50.90-
    abrasion — *see* Abrasion, elbow
    bite — *see* Bite, superficial, elbow
    blister — *see* Blister, elbow
    contusion — *see* Contusion, elbow
    external constriction — *see*
      Constriction, external, elbow
    foreign body — *see* Foreign body,
      superficial, elbow
  epididymis S30.94
  epigastric region S30.92
  epiglottis — *see* Injury, superficial,
    throat
  esophagus
    cervical — *see* Injury, superficial,
      throat
  external constriction — *see* Constriction,
    external, by site
  extremity NEC T14.8
  eyeball NEC — *see* Injury, eye, specified
    site NEC
  eyebrow — *see* Injury, superficial,
    periocular area
  eyelid S00.20-
    abrasion — *see* Abrasion, eyelid
    bite — *see* Bite, superficial, eyelid
    contusion — *see* Contusion, eyelid
    external constriction — *see*
      Constriction, external, eyelid
    foreign body — *see* Foreign body,
      superficial, eyelid
  face NEC — *see* Injury, superficial,
    head, specified NEC
  finger(s) S60.949
    abrasion — *see* Abrasion, finger
    bite — *see* Bite, superficial, finger
    blister — *see* Blister, finger
    contusion — *see* Contusion, finger
    external constriction — *see*
      Constriction, external, finger
    foreign body — *see* Foreign body,
      superficial, finger
    index S60.94-
    insect bite — *see* Bite, by site,
      superficial, insect
    little S60.94-
    middle S60.94-
    ring S60.94-
  flank S30.92
  foot S90.92-
    abrasion — *see* Abrasion, foot
    bite — *see* Bite, foot
    blister — *see* Blister, foot
    contusion — *see* Contusion, foot
    external constriction — *see*
      Constriction, external, foot
    foreign body — *see* Foreign body,
      superficial, foot
  forearm S50.91-
    abrasion — *see* Abrasion, forearm
    bite — *see* Bite, forearm, superficial
    blister — *see* Blister, forearm
    contusion — *see* Contusion, forearm
    elbow only — *see* Injury, superficial,
      elbow
    external constriction — *see*
      Constriction, external, forearm
    foreign body — *see* Foreign body,
      superficial, forearm
  forehead — *see* Injury, superficial, head
    NEC
  foreign body — *see* Foreign body,
    superficial
  genital organs, external
    female S30.97
    male S30.96
  globe (eye) — *see* Injury, eye, specified
    site NEC
  groin S30.92
  gum — *see* Injury, superficial, oral
    cavity
  hand S60.92-
    abrasion — *see* Abrasion, hand
    bite — *see* Bite, superficial, hand
    contusion — *see* Contusion, hand
    external constriction — *see*
      Constriction, external, hand
    foreign body — *see* Foreign body,
      superficial, hand

Injury (*see also* specified injury type) T14.90
— *continued*
superficial NEC T14.8 — *continued*
  head S00.90
    ear — *see* Injury, superficial, ear
    eyelid — *see* Injury, superficial, eyelid
    nose S00.30
    oral cavity S00.502
    scalp S00.00
    specified site NEC S00.80
  heel — *see* Injury, superficial, foot
  hip S70.91-
    abrasion — *see* Abrasion, hip
    bite — *see* Bite, superficial, hip
    blister — *see* Blister, hip
    contusion — *see* Contusion, hip
    external constriction — *see*
      Constriction, external, hip
    foreign body — *see* Foreign body,
      superficial, hip
  iliac region — *see* Injury, superficial,
    abdomen
  inguinal region — *see* Injury, superficial,
    abdomen
  insect bite — *see* Bite, by site,
    superficial, insect
  interscapular region — *see* Injury,
    superficial, thorax, back
  jaw — *see* Injury, superficial, head,
    specified NEC
  knee S80.91-
    abrasion — *see* Abrasion, knee
    bite — *see* Bite, superficial, knee
    blister — *see* Blister, knee
    contusion — *see* Contusion, knee
    external constriction — *see*
      Constriction, external, knee
    foreign body — *see* Foreign body,
      superficial, knee
  labium (majus) (minus) S30.95
  lacrimal (apparatus) (gland) (sac) — *see*
    Injury, eye, specified site NEC
  larynx — *see* Injury, superficial, throat
  leg (lower) S80.92-
    abrasion — *see* Abrasion, leg
    bite — *see* Bite, superficial, leg
    contusion — *see* Contusion, leg
    external constriction — *see*
      Constriction, external, leg
    foreign body — *see* Foreign body,
      superficial, leg
    knee — *see* Injury, superficial, knee
  limb NEC T14.8
  lip S00.501
  lower back S30.91
  lumbar region S30.91
  malar region — *see* Injury, superficial,
    head, specified NEC
  mammary — *see* Injury, superficial,
    breast
  mastoid region — *see* Injury, superficial,
    head, specified NEC
  mouth — *see* Injury, superficial, oral
    cavity
  muscle NEC T14.8
  nail NEC T14.8
    finger — *see* Injury, superficial, finger
    toe — *see* Injury, superficial, toe
  nasal (septum) — *see* Injury, superficial,
    nose
  neck S10.90
    specified site NEC S10.80
  nose (septum) S00.30
  occipital region — *see* Injury,
    superficial, scalp
  oral cavity S00.502
  orbital region — *see* Injury, superficial,
    periocular area
  palate — *see* Injury, superficial, oral
    cavity
  palm — *see* Injury, superficial, hand
  parietal region — *see* Injury, superficial,
    scalp
  pelvis S30.91
    girdle — *see* Injury, superficial, hip
  penis S30.93
  perineum
    female S30.95
    male S30.91
  periocular area S00.20-
    abrasion — *see* Abrasion, eyelid
    bite — *see* Bite, superficial, eyelid
    contusion — *see* Contusion, eyelid
    external constriction — *see*
      Constriction, external, eyelid
    foreign body — *see* Foreign body,
      superficial, eyelid

D I S E A S E   I N D E X

Injury (see also specified injury type) T14.90
— continued
superficial NEC T14.8 — continued
  phalanges
    finger — see Injury, superficial, finger
    toe — see Injury, superficial, toe
  pharynx — see Injury, superficial, throat
  pinna — see Injury, superficial, ear
  popliteal space — see Injury, superficial, knee
  prepuce S30.93
  pubic region S30.91
  pudendum
    female S30.97
    male S30.96
  sacral region S30.91
  scalp S00.00
  scapular region — see Injury, superficial, shoulder
  sclera — see Injury, eye, specified site NEC
  scrotum S30.94
  shin — see Injury, superficial, leg
  shoulder S40.91-
    abrasion — see Abrasion, shoulder
    bite — see Bite, superficial, shoulder
    blister — see Blister, shoulder
    contusion — see Contusion, shoulder
    external constriction — see Constriction, external, shoulder
    foreign body — see Foreign body, superficial, shoulder
  skin NEC T14.8
  sternal region — see Injury, superficial, thorax, front
  subconjunctival — see Injury, eye, specified site NEC
  subcutaneous NEC T14.8
  submaxillary region — see Injury, superficial, head, specified NEC
  submental region — see Injury, superficial, head, specified NEC
  subungual
    finger(s) — see Injury, superficial, finger
    toe(s) — see Injury, superficial, toe
  supraclavicular fossa — see Injury, superficial, neck
  supraorbital — see Injury, superficial, head, specified NEC
  temple — see Injury, superficial, head, specified NEC
  temporal region — see Injury, superficial, head, specified NEC
  testis S30.94
  thigh S70.92-
    abrasion — see Abrasion, thigh
    bite — see Bite, superficial, thigh
    blister — see Blister, thigh
    contusion — see Contusion, thigh
    external constriction — see Constriction, external, thigh
    foreign body — see Foreign body, superficial, thigh
  thorax, thoracic (wall) S20.90
    abrasion — see Abrasion, thorax
    back S20.40-
    bite — see Bite, thorax, superficial
    blister — see Blister, thorax
    contusion — see Contusion, thorax
    external constriction — see Constriction, external, thorax
    foreign body — see Foreign body, superficial, thorax
    front S20.30-
  throat S10.10
    abrasion S10.11
    bite S10.17
      insect S10.16
    blister S10.12
    contusion S10.0
    external constriction S10.14
    foreign body S10.15
  thumb S60.93-
    abrasion — see Abrasion, thumb
    bite — see Bite, superficial, thumb
    blister — see Blister, thumb
    contusion — see Contusion, thumb
    external constriction — see Constriction, external, thumb
    foreign body — see Foreign body, superficial, thumb
    insect bite — see Bite, by site, superficial, insect
    specified type NEC S60.39-

Injury (see also specified injury type) T14.90
— continued
superficial NEC T14.8 — continued
  toe(s) S90.93-
    abrasion — see Abrasion, toe
    bite — see Bite, toe
    blister — see Blister, toe
    contusion — see Contusion, toe
    external constriction — see Constriction, external, toe
    foreign body — see Foreign body, superficial, toe
    great S90.93-
  tongue — see Injury, superficial, oral cavity
  tooth, teeth — see Injury, superficial, oral cavity
  trachea S10.10
  tunica vaginalis S30.94
  tympanum, tympanic membrane — see Injury, superficial, ear
  uvula — see Injury, superficial, oral cavity
  vagina S30.95
  vocal cords — see Injury, superficial, throat
  vulva S30.95
  wrist S60.91-
supraclavicular region — see Injury, neck
supraorbital S09.93
suprarenal gland (multiple) — see Injury, adrenal
surgical complication (external or internal site) — see Laceration, accidental complicating surgery
temple S09.90
temporal region S09.90
tendon — see also Injury, muscle, by site
  abdomen — see Injury, muscle, abdomen
  Achilles — see Injury, Achilles tendon
  lower back — see Injury, muscle, lower back
  pelvic organs — see Injury, muscle, pelvis
tenth cranial nerve (pneumogastric or vagus) — see Injury, nerve, vagus
testis S39.94
thigh S79.92-
  blood vessel — see Injury, blood vessel, hip
  contusion — see Contusion, thigh
  fracture — see Fracture, femur
  muscle — see Injury, muscle, thigh
  nerve — see Injury, nerve, thigh
  open — see Wound, open, thigh
  specified NEC S79.82-
  superficial — see Injury, superficial, thigh
third cranial nerve (oculomotor) — see Injury, nerve, oculomotor
thorax, thoracic S29.9
  blood vessel — see Injury, blood vessel, thorax
  cavity — see Injury, intrathoracic
  dislocation — see Dislocation, thorax
  external (wall) S29.9
    contusion — see Contusion, thorax
    nerve — see Injury, nerve, thorax
    open — see Wound, open, thorax
    specified NEC S29.8
    sprain — see Sprain, thorax
    superficial — see Injury, superficial, thorax
  fracture — see Fracture, thorax
  internal — see Injury, intrathoracic
  intrathoracic organ — see Injury, intrathoracic
  sympathetic ganglion — see Injury, nerve, thorax, sympathetic
throat (see also Injury, neck) S19.9
thumb S69.9-
  blood vessel — see Injury, blood vessel, thumb
  contusion — see Contusion, thumb
  dislocation — see Dislocation, thumb
  fracture — see Fracture, thumb
  muscle — see Injury, muscle, thumb
  nerve — see Injury, nerve, digital, thumb
  open — see Wound, open, thumb
  specified NEC S69.8-
  sprain — see Sprain, thumb
  superficial — see Injury, superficial, thumb
thymus (gland) — see Injury, intrathoracic, specified organ NEC
thyroid (gland) NEC S19.84

Injury (see also specified injury type) T14.90
— continued
toe S99.92-
  contusion — see Contusion, toe
  dislocation — see Dislocation, toe
  fracture — see Fracture, toe
  muscle — see Injury, muscle, toe
  open — see Wound, open, toe
  specified type NEC S99.82-
  sprain — see Sprain, toe
  superficial — see Injury, superficial, toe
tongue S09.93
tonsil S09.93
tooth S09.93
trachea (cervical) NEC S19.82
  thoracic — see Injury, intrathoracic, trachea, thoracic
transfusion-related acute lung (TRALI) J95.84
tunica vaginalis S39.94
twelfth cranial nerve (hypoglossal) — see Injury, nerve, hypoglossal
ureter S37.10
  contusion S37.12
  laceration S37.13
  specified type NEC S37.19
urethra (sphincter) S37.30
  at delivery O71.5
  contusion S37.32
  laceration S37.33
  specified type NEC S37.39
urinary organ S37.90
  contusion S37.92
  laceration S37.93
  specified
    site NEC S37.899
      contusion S37.892
      laceration S37.893
      specified type NEC S37.898
    type NEC S37.99
uterus, uterine S37.60
  with ectopic or molar pregnancy O08.6
  blood vessel — see Injury, blood vessel, iliac
  contusion S37.62
  laceration S37.63
    cervix at delivery O71.3
  rupture associated with obstetrics — see Rupture, uterus
  specified type NEC S37.69
uvula S09.93
vagina S39.93
  abrasion S30.814
  bite S31.45
    insect S30.864
    superficial NEC S30.874
  contusion S30.23
  crush S38.03
  during delivery — see Laceration, vagina, during delivery
  external constriction S30.844
  insect bite S30.864
  laceration S31.41
    with foreign body S31.42
  open wound S31.40
  puncture S31.43
    with foreign body S31.44
  superficial S30.95
    foreign body S30.854
vas deferens — see Injury, pelvic organ, specified site NEC
vascular NEC T14.8
vein — see Injury, blood vessel
vena cava (superior) S25.20
  inferior S35.10
    laceration (minor) (superficial) S35.11
      major S35.12
    specified type NEC S35.19
  laceration (minor) (superficial) S25.21
    major S25.22
  specified type NEC S25.29
vesical (sphincter) — see Injury, bladder
visual cortex S04.04-
vitreous (humor) S05.90
  specified NEC S05.8x-
vocal cord NEC S19.83
vulva S39.94
  abrasion S30.814
  bite S31.45
    insect S30.864
    superficial NEC S30.874
  contusion S30.23
  crush S38.03
  during delivery — see Laceration, perineum, female, during delivery
  external constriction S30.844

Injury (see also specified injury type) T14.90
— continued
vulva S39.94 — continued
  insect bite S30.864
  laceration S31.41
    with foreign body S31.42
  open wound S31.40
  puncture S31.43
    with foreign body S31.44
  superficial S30.95
    foreign body S30.854
whiplash (cervical spine) S13.4
wrist S69.9-
  blood vessel — see Injury, blood vessel, hand
  contusion — see Contusion, wrist
  dislocation — see Dislocation, wrist
  fracture — see Fracture, wrist
  muscle — see Injury, muscle, hand
  nerve — see Injury, nerve, hand
  open — see Wound, open, wrist
  specified NEC S69.8-
  sprain — see Sprain, wrist
  superficial — see Injury, superficial, wrist
Inoculation — see also Vaccination
  complication or reaction — see Complications, vaccination
Insanity, insane — see also Psychosis
  adolescent — see Schizophrenia
  confusional F28
    acute or subacute F05
  delusional F22
  senile F03
Insect
  bite — see Bite, by site, superficial, insect
  venomous, poisoning NEC (by) — see Venom, arthropod
Insensitivity
  adrenocorticotropin hormone (ACTH) E27.49
  androgen E34.50
    complete E34.51
    partial E34.52
Insertion
  cord (umbilical) lateral or velamentous O43.12-
  intrauterine contraceptive device (encounter for) — see Intrauterine contraceptive device
Insolation (sunstroke) T67.0
Insomnia (organic) G47.00
  adjustment F51.02
  adjustment disorder F51.02
  behavioral, of childhood Z73.819
    combined type Z73.812
    limit setting type Z73.811
    sleep-onset association type Z73.810
  childhood Z73.819
  chronic F51.04
    somatized tension F51.04
  conditioned F51.04
  due to
    alcohol
      abuse F10.182
      dependence F10.282
      use F10.982
    amphetamines
      abuse F15.182
      dependence F15.282
      use F15.982
    anxiety disorder F51.05
    caffeine
      abuse F15.182
      dependence F15.282
      use F15.982
    cocaine
      abuse F14.182
      dependence F14.282
      use F14.982
    depression F51.05
    drug NEC
      abuse F19.182
      dependence F19.282
      use F19.982
    medical condition G47.01
    mental disorder NEC F51.05
    opioid
      abuse F11.182
      dependence F11.282
      use F11.982
    psychoactive substance NEC
      abuse F19.182
      dependence F19.282
      use F19.982

Insomnia (organic) G47.00 — *continued*
  due to — *continued*
    sedative, hypnotic, or anxiolytic
      abuse F13.182
      dependence F13.282
      use F13.982
    stimulant NEC
      abuse F15.182
      dependence F15.282
      use F15.982
  fatal familial (FFI) A81.83
  idiopathic F51.01
  learned F51.3
  nonorganic origin F51.01
  not due to a substance or known
    physiological condition F51.01
    specified NEC F51.09
  paradoxical F51.03
  primary F51.01
  psychiatric F51.05
  psychophysiologic F51.04
  related to psychopathology F51.05
  short-term F51.02
  specified NEC G47.09
  stress-related F51.02
  transient F51.02
  without objective findings F51.02
Inspiration
  food or foreign body — *see* Foreign body,
    by site
  mucus — *see* Asphyxia, mucus
Inspissated bile syndrome (newborn) P59.1
Instability
  emotional (excessive) F60.3
  joint (post-traumatic) M25.30
    ankle M25.37-
    due to old ligament injury — *see*
      Disorder, ligament
    elbow M25.32-
    flail — *see* Flail, joint
    foot M25.37-
    hand M25.34-
    hip M25.35-
    knee M25.36-
    lumbosacral — *see* subcategory M53.2
    prosthesis — *see* Complications, joint
      prosthesis, mechanical,
      displacement, by site
    sacroiliac — *see* subcategory M53.2
    secondary to
      old ligament injury — *see* Disorder,
        ligament
      removal of joint prosthesis M96.89
    shoulder (region) M25.31-
    spine — *see* subcategory M53.2
    wrist M25.33-
  knee (chronic) M23.5-
  lumbosacral — *see* subcategory M53.2
  nervous F48.8
  personality (emotional) F60.3
  spine — *see* Instability, joint, spine
  vasomotor R55
Institutional syndrome (childhood) F94.2
Institutionalization, affecting child Z62.22
  disinhibited attachment F94.2
Insufficiency, insufficient
  accommodation, old age H52.4
  adrenal (gland) E27.40
    primary E27.1
  adrenocortical E27.40
    drug-induced E27.3
    iatrogenic E27.3
    primary E27.1
  anterior (occlusal) guidance M26.54
  anus K62.89
  aortic (valve) I35.1
    with
      mitral (valve) disease I08.0
        with tricuspid (valve) disease I08.3
      stenosis I35.2
      tricuspid (valve) disease I08.2
        with mitral (valve) disease I08.3
    congenital Q23.1
    rheumatic I06.1
      with
        mitral (valve) disease I08.0
          with tricuspid (valve) disease
            I08.3
        stenosis I06.2
          with mitral (valve) disease I08.0
            with tricuspid (valve) disease
              I08.3
        tricuspid (valve) disease I08.2
          with mitral (valve) disease I08.3
    specified cause NEC I35.1
    syphilitic A52.03

Insufficiency, insufficient — *continued*
  arterial I77.1
    basilar G45.0
    carotid (hemispheric) G45.1
    cerebral I67.81
    coronary (acute or subacute) I24.8
    mesenteric K55.1
    peripheral I73.9
    precerebral (multiple) (bilateral) G45.2
    vertebral G45.0
  arteriovenous I99.8
  biliary K83.8
  cardiac — *see also* Insufficiency,
    myocardial
    due to presence of (cardiac) prosthesis
      I97.11-
    postprocedural I97.11-
  cardiorenal, hypertensive I13.2
  cardiovascular — *see* Disease,
    cardiovascular
  cerebrovascular (acute) I67.81
    with transient focal neurological signs
      and symptoms G45.8
  circulatory NEC I99.8
    newborn P29.89
  convergence H51.11
  coronary (acute or subacute) I24.8
    chronic or with a stated duration of over
      4 weeks I25.89
  corticoadrenal E27.40
    primary E27.1
  dietary E63.9
  divergence H51.8
  food T73.0
  gastroesophageal K22.8
  gonadal
    ovary E28.39
    testis E29.1
  heart — *see also* Insufficiency, myocardial
    newborn P29.0
    valve — *see* Endocarditis
  hepatic — *see* Failure, hepatic
  idiopathic autonomic G90.09
  interocclusal distance of fully erupted teeth
    (ridge) M26.36
  kidney N28.9
    acute N28.9
    chronic N18.9
  lacrimal (secretion) H04.12-
    passages — *see* Stenosis, lacrimal
  liver — *see* Failure, hepatic
  lung — *see* Insufficiency, pulmonary
  mental (congenital) — *see* Disability,
    intellectual
  mesenteric K55.1
  mitral (valve) I34.0
    with
      aortic valve disease I08.0
        with tricuspid (valve) disease I08.3
      obstruction or stenosis I05.2
        with aortic valve disease I08.0
      tricuspid (valve) disease I08.1
        with aortic (valve) disease I08.3
    congenital Q23.3
    rheumatic I05.1
      with
        aortic valve disease I08.0
          with tricuspid (valve) disease
            I08.3
        obstruction or stenosis I05.2
          with aortic valve disease I08.0
            with tricuspid (valve)
              disease I08.3
        tricuspid (valve) disease I08.1
          with aortic (valve) disease I08.3
    active or acute I01.1
      with chorea, rheumatic
        (Sydenham's) I02.0
    specified cause, except rheumatic I34.0
  muscle — *see also* Disease, muscle
    heart — *see* Insufficiency, myocardial
  ocular NEC H50.9
  myocardial, myocardium (with
    arteriosclerosis) I50.9
    with
      rheumatic fever (conditions in I00)
        I09.0
        active, acute or subacute I01.2
          with chorea I02.0
        inactive or quiescent (with chorea)
          I09.0
    congenital Q24.8
    hypertensive — *see* Hypertension, heart
    newborn P29.0
    rheumatic I09.0
      active, acute, or subacute I01.2
    syphilitic A52.06
  nourishment T73.0
  pancreatic K86.8

Insufficiency, insufficient — *continued*
  parathyroid (gland) E20.9
  peripheral vascular (arterial) I73.9
  pituitary E23.0
  placental (mother) O36.51-
  platelets D69.6
  prenatal care affecting management of
    pregnancy O09.3-
  progressive pluriglandular E31.0
  pulmonary J98.4
    acute, following surgery (nonthoracic)
      J95.2
      thoracic J95.1
    chronic, following surgery J95.3
    following
      shock J98.4
      trauma J98.4
    newborn P28.5
    valve I37.1
      with stenosis I37.2
      congenital Q22.2
      rheumatic I09.89
        with aortic, mitral or tricuspid
          (valve) disease I08.8
  pyloric K31.89
  renal (acute) N28.9
    chronic N18.9
  respiratory R06.89
    newborn P28.5
  rotation — *see* Malrotation
  sleep syndrome F51.12
  social insurance Z59.7
  suprarenal E27.40
    primary E27.1
  tarso-orbital fascia, congenital Q10.3
  testis E29.1
  thyroid (gland) (acquired) E03.9
    congenital E03.1
  tricuspid (valve) (rheumatic) I07.1
    with
      aortic (valve) disease I08.2
        with mitral (valve) disease I08.3
      mitral (valve) disease I08.1
        with aortic (valve) disease I08.3
      obstruction or stenosis I07.2
        with aortic (valve) disease I08.2
          with mitral (valve) disease I08.3
    congenital Q22.8
    nonrheumatic I36.1
      with stenosis I36.2
  urethral sphincter R32
  valve, valvular (heart) — *see* Endocarditis
    congenital Q24.8
  vascular I99.8
    intestine K55.9
      acute K55.0
    mesenteric K55.1
    peripheral I73.9
    renal — *see* Hypertension, kidney
  velopharyngeal
    acquired K13.79
    congenital Q38.8
  venous (chronic) (peripheral) I87.2
  ventricular — *see* Insufficiency, myocardial
  welfare support Z59.7
Insufflation, fallopian Z31.41
Insular — *see* condition
Insulinoma
  pancreas
    benign D13.7
    malignant C25.4
    uncertain behavior D37.8
  specified site
    benign — *see* Neoplasm, by site, benign
    malignant — *see* Neoplasm, by site,
      malignant
    uncertain behavior — *see* Neoplasm, by
      site, uncertain behavior
  unspecified site
    benign D13.7
    malignant C25.4
    uncertain behavior D37.8
Insuloma — *see* Insulinoma
Interference
  balancing side M26.56
  non-working side M26.56
Intermenstrual — *see* condition
Intermittent — *see* condition
Internal — *see* condition
Interrogation
  cardiac defibrillator (automatic)
    (implantable) Z45.02
  cardiac pacemaker Z45.018
  cardiac (event) (loop) recorder Z45.09
  infusion pump (implanted) (intrathecal)
    Z45.1
  neurostimulator Z46.2

Interruption
  bundle of His I44.30
  phase-shift, sleep cycle — *see* Disorder,
    sleep, circadian rhythm
  sleep phase-shift, or 24 hour sleep-wake
    cycle — *see* Disorder, sleep, circadian
    rhythm
Interstitial — *see* condition
Intertrigo L30.4
  labialis K13.0
Intervertebral disc — *see* condition
Intestine, intestinal — *see* condition
Intolerance
  carbohydrate K90.4
  disaccharide, hereditary E73.0
  fat NEC K90.4
    pancreatic K90.3
  food K90.4
    dietary counseling and surveillance
      Z71.3
  fructose E74.10
    hereditary E74.12
  glucose(-galactose) E74.39
  gluten K90.0
  lactose E73.9
    specified NEC E73.8
  lysine E72.3
  milk NEC K90.4
    lactose E73.9
  protein K90.4
  starch NEC K90.4
  sucrose(-isomaltose) E74.31
Intoxicated NEC (without dependence) —
  see Alcohol, intoxication
Intoxication
  acid E87.2
  alcoholic (acute) (without dependence) —
    see Alcohol, intoxication
  alimentary canal K52.1
  amphetamine (without dependence) —
    see Abuse, drug, stimulant, with
      intoxication
    with dependence — *see* Dependence,
      drug, stimulant, with intoxication
  anxiolytic (acute) (without dependence) —
    see Abuse, drug, sedative, with
      intoxication
    with dependence — *see* Dependence,
      drug, sedative, with intoxication
  caffeine (acute) (without dependence) —
    see Abuse, drug, stimulant, with
      intoxication
    with dependence — *see* Dependence,
      drug, stimulant, with intoxication
  cannabinoids (acute) (without dependence)
    — *see* Abuse, drug, cannabis, with
      intoxication
    with dependence — *see* Dependence,
      drug, cannabis, with intoxication
  chemical — *see* Table of Drugs and
    Chemicals
    via placenta or breast milk — *see*
      Absorption, chemical, through
      placenta
  cocaine (acute) (without dependence) —
    see Abuse, drug, cocaine, with
      intoxication
    with dependence — *see* Dependence,
      drug, cocaine, with intoxication
  drug
    acute (without dependence) — *see*
      Abuse, drug, by type with
      intoxication
      with dependence — *see* Dependence,
        drug, by type with intoxication
    addictive
      via placenta or breast milk — *see*
        Absorption, drug, addictive,
        through placenta
    newborn P93.8
      gray baby syndrome P93.0
    overdose or wrong substance given or
      taken — *see* Table of Drugs and
      Chemicals, by drug, poisoning
  enteric K52.1
  foodborne A05.9
    bacterial A05.9
    classical (Clostridium botulinum) A05.1
    due to
      Bacillus cereus A05.4
      bacterium A05.9
        specified NEC A05.8
      Clostridium
        botulinum A05.1
        perfringens A05.2
        welchii A05.2

Intoxication — *continued*
foodborne A05.9 — *continued*
  due to — *continued*
    Salmonella A02.9
      with
        (gastro)enteritis A02.0
        localized infection(s) A02.20
          arthritis A02.23
          meningitis A02.21
          osteomyelitis A02.24
          pneumonia A02.22
          pyelonephritis A02.25
          specified NEC A02.29
        sepsis A02.1
        specified manifestation NEC A02.8
    Staphylococcus A05.0
    Vibrio
      parahaemolyticus A05.3
      vulnificus A05.5
  enterotoxin, staphylococcal A05.0
  noxious — *see* Poisoning, food, noxious
gastrointestinal K52.1
hallucinogenic (without dependence) — *see* Abuse, drug, hallucinogen, with intoxication
  with dependence — *see* Dependence, drug, hallucinogen, with intoxication
hypnotic (acute) (without dependence) — *see* Abuse, drug, sedative, with intoxication
  with dependence — *see* Dependence, drug, sedative, with intoxication
inhalant (acute) (without dependence) — *see* Abuse, drug, inhalant, with intoxication
  with dependence — *see* Dependence, drug, inhalant, with intoxication
meaning
  inebriation — *see* category F10
  poisoning — *see* Table of Drugs and Chemicals
methyl alcohol (acute) (without dependence) — *see* Alcohol, intoxication
opioid (acute) (without dependence) — *see* Abuse, drug, opioid, with intoxication
  with dependence — *see* Dependence, drug, opioid, with intoxication
pathologic NEC (without dependence) — *see* Alcohol, intoxication
phencyclidine (without dependence) — *see* Abuse, drug, psychoactive NEC, with intoxication
  with dependence — *see* Dependence, drug, psychoactive NEC, with intoxication
potassium (K) E87.5
psychoactive substance NEC (without dependence) — *see* Abuse, drug, psychoactive NEC, with intoxication
  with dependence — *see* Dependence, drug, psychoactive NEC, with intoxication
sedative (acute) (without dependence) — *see* Abuse, drug, sedative, with intoxication
  with dependence — *see* Dependence, drug, sedative, with intoxication
serum (*see also* Reaction, serum) T80.69
uremic — *see* Uremia
volatile solvents (acute) (without dependence) — *see* Abuse, drug, inhalant, with intoxication
  with dependence — *see* Dependence, drug, inhalant, with intoxication
water E87.79
Intracranial — *see* condition
Intrahepatic gallbladder Q44.1
Intraligamentous — *see* condition
Intrathoracic — *see also* condition
  kidney Q63.2
Intrauterine contraceptive device
  checking Z30.431
  in situ Z97.5
  insertion Z30.430
    immediately following removal Z30.433
  management Z30.431
  reinsertion Z30.433
  removal Z30.432
  replacement Z30.433
  retention in pregnancy O26.3-
Intraventricular — *see* condition
Intrinsic deformity — *see* Deformity
Intubation, difficult or failed T88.4
Intumescence, lens (eye) (cataract) — *see* Cataract

Intussusception (bowel) (colon) (enteric) (ileocecal) (ileocolic) (intestine) (rectum) K56.1
  appendix K38.8
  congenital Q43.8
  ureter (with obstruction) N13.5
Invagination (bowel, colon, intestine or rectum) K56.1
Inversion
  albumin-globulin (A-G) ratio E88.09
  bladder N32.89
  cecum — *see* Intussusception
  cervix N88.8
  chromosome in normal individual Q95.1
  circadian rhythm — *see* Disorder, sleep, circadian rhythm
  nipple N64.59
    congenital Q83.8
    gestational — *see* Retraction, nipple
    puerperal, postpartum — *see* Retraction, nipple
  nyctohemeral rhythm — *see* Disorder, sleep, circadian rhythm
  optic papilla Q14.2
  organ or site, congenital NEC — *see* Anomaly, by site
  sleep rhythm — *see* Disorder, sleep, circadian rhythm
  testis (congenital) Q55.29
  uterus (chronic) (postinfectional) (postpartal, old) N85.5
    postpartum O71.2
  vagina (posthysterectomy) N99.3
  ventricular Q20.5
Investigation (*see also* Examination) Z04.9
  clinical research subject (control) (normal comparison) (participant) Z00.6
Involuntary movement, abnormal R25.9
Involution, involutional — *see also* condition
  breast, cystic — *see* Dysplasia, mammary, specified type NEC
  depression (single episode) F32.8
    recurrent episode F33.9
  melancholia (recurrent episode) (single episode) F32.8
  ovary, senile — *see* Atrophy, ovary
  thymus failure E32.8
I.Q.
  20-34 F72
  35-49 F71
  50-69 F70
  under 20 F73
IRDS (type I) P22.0
  type II P22.1
Irideremia Q13.1
Iridis rubeosis — *see* Disorder, iris, vascular
Iridochoroiditis (panuveitis) — *see* Panuveitis
Iridocyclitis H20.9
  acute H20.0-
    hypopyon H20.05-
    primary H20.01-
    recurrent H20.02-
    secondary (noninfectious) H20.04-
      infectious H20.03-
  chronic H20.1-
  due to allergy — *see* Iridocyclitis, acute, secondary
  endogenous — *see* Iridocyclitis, acute, primary
  Fuchs' — *see* Cyclitis, Fuchs' heterochromic
  gonococcal A54.32
  granulomatous — *see* Iridocyclitis, chronic
  herpes, herpetic (simplex) B00.51
    zoster B02.32
  hypopyon — *see* Iridocyclitis, acute, hypopyon
  in (due to)
    ankylosing spondylitis M45.9
    gonococcal infection A54.32
    herpes (simplex) virus B00.51
      zoster B02.32
    infectious disease NOS B99
    parasitic disease NOS B89 [H22]
    sarcoidosis D86.83
    syphilis A51.43
    tuberculosis A18.54
    zoster B02.32
  lens-induced H20.2-
  nongranulomatous — *see* Iridocyclitis, acute
  recurrent — *see* Iridocyclitis, acute, recurrent
  rheumatic — *see* Iridocyclitis, chronic
  subacute — *see* Iridocyclitis, acute
  sympathetic — *see* Uveitis, sympathetic
  syphilitic (secondary) A51.43
  tuberculous (chronic) A18.54

Iridocyclitis H20.9- — *continued*
  Vogt-Koyanagi H20.82-
Iridocyclochoroiditis (panuveitis) — *see* Panuveitis
Iridodialysis H21.53-
Iridodonesis H21.89
Iridoplegia (complete) (partial) (reflex) H57.09
Iridoschisis H21.25-
Iris — *see also* condition
  bombé — *see* Membrane, pupillary
Iritis — *see also* Iridocyclitis
  chronic — *see* Iridocyclitis, chronic
  diabetic — *see* E08-E13 with .39
  due to
    herpes simplex B00.51
    leprosy A30.9 [H22]
  gonococcal A54.32
  gouty M10.9
  granulomatous — *see* Iridocyclitis, chronic
  lens induced — *see* Iridocyclitis, lens-induced
  papulosa (syphilitic) A52.71
  rheumatic — *see* Iridocyclitis, chronic
  syphilitic (secondary) A51.43
    congenital (early) A50.01
    late A52.71
  tuberculous A18.54
Iron — *see* condition
Iron-miner's lung J63.4
Irradiated enamel (tooth, teeth) K03.89
Irradiation effects, adverse T66
Irreducible, irreducibility — *see* condition
Irregular, irregularity
  action, heart I49.9
  alveolar process K08.8
  bleeding N92.6
  breathing R06.89
  contour of cornea (acquired) — *see* Deformity, cornea
    congenital Q13.4
  contour, reconstructed breast N65.0
  dentin (in pulp) K04.3
  eye movements H55.89
    nystagmus — *see* Nystagmus
    saccadic H55.81
  labor O62.2
  menstruation (cause unknown) N92.6
  periods N92.6
  prostate N42.9
  pupil — *see* Abnormality, pupillary
  reconstructed breast N65.0
  respiratory R06.89
  septum (nasal) J34.2
  shape, organ or site, congenital NEC — *see* Distortion
  sleep-wake pattern (rhythm) G47.23
Irritable, irritability R45.4
  bladder N32.89
  bowel (syndrome) K58.9
    with diarrhea K58.0
    psychogenic F45.8
  bronchial — *see* Bronchitis
  cerebral, in newborn P91.3
  colon K58.9
    with diarrhea K58.0
    psychogenic F45.8
  duodenum K59.8
  heart (psychogenic) F45.8
  hip — *see* Derangement, joint, specified type NEC, hip
  ileum K59.8
  infant R68.12
  jejunum K59.8
  rectum K59.8
  stomach K31.89
    psychogenic F45.8
  sympathetic G90.8
  urethra N36.8
Irritation
  anus K62.89
  axillary nerve G54.0
  bladder N32.89
  brachial plexus G54.0
  bronchial — *see* Bronchitis
  cervical plexus G54.2
  cervix — *see* Cervicitis
  choroid, sympathetic — *see* Endophthalmitis
  cranial nerve — *see* Disorder, nerve, cranial
  gastric K31.89
    psychogenic F45.8
  globe, sympathetic — *see* Uveitis, sympathetic
  labyrinth — *see* subcategory H83.2
  lumbosacral plexus G54.1
  meninges (traumatic) — *see* Injury, intracranial
    nontraumatic — *see* Meningismus

Irritation — *continued*
  nerve — *see* Disorder, nerve
  nervous R45.0
  penis N48.89
  perineum NEC L29.3
  peripheral autonomic nervous system G90.8
  peritoneum — *see* Peritonitis
  pharynx J39.2
  plantar nerve — *see* Lesion, nerve, plantar
  spinal (cord) (traumatic) — *see also* Injury, spinal cord, by region
    nerve G58.9
      root NEC — *see* Radiculopathy
    nontraumatic — *see* Myelopathy
  stomach K31.89
    psychogenic F45.8
  sympathetic nerve NEC G90.8
  ulnar nerve — *see* Lesion, nerve, ulnar
  vagina N89.8
Ischemia, ischemic I99.8
  bowel (transient)
    acute K55.0
    chronic K55.1
    due to mesenteric artery insufficiency K55.1
  brain — *see* Ischemia, cerebral
  cardiac (see Disease, heart, ischemic)
  cardiomyopathy I25.5
  cerebral (chronic) (generalized) I67.82
    arteriosclerotic I67.2
    intermittent G45.9
    newborn P91.0
    recurrent focal G45.8
    transient G45.9
  colon chronic (due to mesenteric artery insufficiency) K55.1
  coronary — *see* Disease, heart, ischemic
  demand (coronary) (*see also* Angina) I24.8
  heart (chronic or with a stated duration of over 4 weeks) I25.9
    acute or with a stated duration of 4 weeks or less I24.9
    subacute I24.9
  infarction, muscle — *see* Infarct, muscle
  intestine (large) (small) (transient) K55.9
    acute K55.0
    chronic K55.1
    due to mesenteric artery insufficiency K55.1
  kidney N28.0
  mesenteric, acute K55.0
  muscle, traumatic T79.6
  myocardium, myocardial (chronic or with a stated duration of over 4 weeks) I25.9
    acute, without myocardial infarction I24.0
    silent (asymptomatic) I25.6
    transient of newborn P29.4
  renal N28.0
  retina, retinal — *see* Occlusion, artery, retina
  small bowel
    acute K55.0
    chronic K55.1
    due to mesenteric artery insufficiency K55.1
  spinal cord G95.11
  subendocardial — *see* Insufficiency, coronary
  supply (coronary) (*see also* Angina) I25.9
    due to vasospasm I20.1
Ischial spine — *see* condition
Ischialgia — *see* Sciatica
Ischiopagus Q89.4
Ischium, ischial — *see* condition
Ischuria R34
Iselin's disease or osteochondrosis — *see* Osteochondrosis, juvenile, metatarsus
Islands of
  parotid tissue in
    lymph nodes Q38.6
    neck structures Q38.6
  submaxillary glands in
    fascia Q38.6
    lymph nodes Q38.6
    neck muscles Q38.6
Islet cell tumor, pancreas D13.7

Isoimmunization NEC — *see also*
  Incompatibility
  affecting management of pregnancy (ABO)
    (with hydrops fetalis) O36.11-
    anti-A sensitization O36.11-
    anti-B sensitization O36.19-
    anti-c sensitization O36.09-
    anti-C sensitization O36.09-
    anti-e sensitization O36.09-
    anti-E sensitization O36.09-
    Rh NEC O36.09-
      anti-D antibody O36.01-
    specified NEC O36.19-
  newborn P55.9
    with
      hydrops fetalis P56.0
      kernicterus P57.0
    ABO (blood groups) P55.1
    Rhesus (Rh) factor P55.0
    specified type NEC P55.8
Isolation, isolated
  dwelling Z59.8
  family Z63.79
  social Z60.4
Isoleucinosis E71.19
Isomerism atrial appendages (with asplenia
    or polysplenia) Q20.6
Isosporiasis, isosporosis A07.3
Isovaleric acidemia E71.110
Issue of
  medical certificate Z02.79
    for disability determination Z02.71
  repeat prescription (appliance) (glasses)
    (medicinal substance, medicament,
    medicine) Z76.0
    contraception — *see* Contraception
Itch, itching — *see also* Pruritus
  baker's L23.6
  barber's B35.0
  bricklayer's L24.5
  cheese B88.0
  clam digger's B65.3
  coolie B76.9
  copra B88.0
  dew B76.9
  dhobi B35.6
  filarial — *see* Infestation, filarial
  grain B88.0
  grocer's B88.0
  ground B76.9
  harvest B88.0
  jock B35.6
  Malabar B35.5
    beard B35.0
    foot B35.3
    scalp B35.0
  meaning scabies B86
  Norwegian B86
  perianal L29.0
  poultrymen's B88.0
  sarcoptic B86
  scabies B86
  scrub B88.0
  straw B88.0
  swimmer's B65.3
  water B76.9
  winter L29.8
Ivemark's syndrome (asplenia with
    congenital heart disease) Q89.01
Ivory bones Q78.2
Ixodiasis NEC B88.8

J

Jaccoud's syndrome — *see* Arthropathy,
    postrheumatic, chronic
Jackson's
  membrane Q43.3
  paralysis or syndrome G83.89
  veil Q43.3
Jacquet's dermatitis (diaper dermatitis) L22
Jadassohn's
  blue nevus — *see* Nevus
  intraepidermal epithelioma — *see*
    Neoplasm, skin, benign
Jadassohn-Pellizari's disease or
    anetoderma L90.2
Jaffe-Lichtenstein (-Uehlinger) syndrome
    — *see* Dysplasia, fibrous, bone NEC
Jakob-Creutzfeldt disease or syndrome —
    see Creutzfeldt-Jakob disease or
    syndrome
Jaksch-Luzet disease D64.89
Jamaican
  neuropathy G92
  paraplegic tropical ataxic-spastic syndrome
    G92
Janet's disease F48.8
Janiceps Q89.4
Jansky-Bielschowsky amaurotic idiocy
    E75.4
Japanese
  B-type encephalitis A83.0
  river fever A75.3
Jaundice (yellow) R17
  acholuric (familial) (splenomegalic) — *see*
    also Spherocytosis
    acquired D59.8
  breast-milk (inhibitor) P59.3
  catarrhal (acute) B15.9
    with hepatic coma B15.0
  cholestatic (benign) R17
  due to or associated with
    delayed conjugation P59.8
      associated with (due to) preterm
        delivery P59.0
    preterm delivery P59.0
  epidemic (catarrhal) B15.9
    with hepatic coma B15.0
    leptospiral A27.0
    spirochetal A27.0
  familial nonhemolytic (congenital)
    (Gilbert) E80.4
    Crigler-Najjar E80.5
  febrile (acute) B15.9
    with hepatic coma B15.0
    leptospiral A27.0
    spirochetal A27.0
  hematogenous D59.9
  hemolytic (acquired) D59.9
    congenital — *see* Spherocytosis
  hemorrhagic (acute) (leptospiral)
    (spirochetal) A27.0
  infectious (acute) (subacute) B15.9
    with hepatic coma B15.0
    leptospiral A27.0
    spirochetal A27.0
  leptospiral (hemorrhagic) A27.0
  malignant (without coma) K72.90
    with coma K72.91
  neonatal — *see* Jaundice, newborn
  newborn P59.9
    due to or associated with
      ABO
        antibodies P55.1
        incompatibility, maternal/fetal
          P55.1
        isoimmunization P55.1
      absence or deficiency of enzyme
        system for bilirubin conjugation
        (congenital) P59.8
      bleeding P58.1
      breast milk inhibitors to conjugation
        P59.3
        associated with preterm delivery
          P59.0
      bruising P58.0
      Crigler-Najjar syndrome E80.5
      delayed conjugation P59.8
        associated with preterm delivery
          P59.0
      drugs or toxins
        given to newborn P58.42
        transmitted from mother P58.41

Jaundice (yellow) R17 — *continued*
  newborn P59.9 — *continued*
    due to or associated with — *continued*
      excessive hemolysis P58.9
        due to
          bleeding P58.1
          bruising P58.0
          drugs or toxins
            given to newborn P58.42
            transmitted from mother
              P58.41
          infection P58.2
          polycythemia P58.3
          swallowed maternal blood P58.5
        specified type NEC P58.8
      galactosemia E74.21
      Gilbert syndrome E80.4
      hemolytic disease P55.9
        ABO isoimmunization P55.1
        Rh isoimmunization P55.0
        specified NEC P55.8
      hepatocellular damage P59.20
        specified NEC P59.29
      hereditary hemolytic anemia P58.8
      hypothyroidism, congenital E03.1
      incompatibility, maternal/fetal NOS
        P55.9
      infection P58.2
      inspissated bile syndrome P59.1
      isoimmunization NOS P55.9
      mucoviscidosis E84.9
      polycythemia P58.3
      preterm delivery P59.0
      Rh
        antibodies P55.0
        incompatibility, maternal/fetal
          P55.0
        isoimmunization P55.0
      specified cause NEC P59.8
      swallowed maternal blood P58.5
    spherocytosis (congenital) D58.0
  nonhemolytic congenital familial (Gilbert)
    E80.4
  nuclear, newborn (*see also* Kernicterus of
    newborn) P57.9
  obstructive (*see also* Obstruction, bile
    duct) K83.1
  post-immunization — *see* Hepatitis, viral,
    type, B
  post-transfusion — *see* Hepatitis, viral,
    type, B
  regurgitation (*see also* Obstruction, bile
    duct) K83.1
  serum (homologous) (prophylactic)
    (therapeutic) — *see* Hepatitis, viral,
    type, B
  spirochetal (hemorrhagic) A27.0
  symptomatic R17
    newborn P59.9
Jaw — *see* condition
Jaw-winking phenomenon or syndrome
    Q07.8
Jealousy
  alcoholic F10.988
  childhood F93.8
  sibling F93.8
Jejunitis — *see* Enteritis
Jejunostomy status Z93.4
Jejunum, jejunal — *see* condition
Jensen's disease — *see* Inflammation,
    chorioretinal, focal, juxtapapillary
Jerks, myoclonic G25.3
Jervell-Lange-Nielsen syndrome I45.81
Jeune's disease Q77.2
Jigger disease B88.1
Job's syndrome (chronic granulomatous
    disease) D71
Joint — *see also* condition
  mice — *see* Loose, body, joint
    knee M23.4-
Jordan's anomaly or syndrome D72.0
Joseph-Diamond-Blackfan anemia
    (congenital hypoplastic) D61.01
Jungle yellow fever A95.0
Jüngling's disease — *see* Sarcoidosis
Juvenile — *see* condition

K

Kahler's disease C90.0-
Kakke E51.11
Kala-azar B55.0
Kallmann's syndrome E23.0
Kanner's syndrome (autism) — *see*
    Psychosis, childhood
Kaposi's
  dermatosis (xeroderma pigmentosum)
    Q82.1
  lichen ruber L44.0
    acuminatus L44.0
  sarcoma
    colon C46.4
    connective tissue C46.1
    gastrointestinal organ C46.4
    lung C46.5-
    lymph node (multiple) C46.3
    palate (hard) (soft) C46.2
    rectum C46.4
    skin (multiple sites) C46.0
    specified site NEC C46.7
    stomach C46.4
    unspecified site C46.9
  varicelliform eruption B00.0
  vaccinia T88.1
Kartagener's syndrome or triad (sinusitis,
    bronchiectasis, situs inversus) Q89.3
Karyotype
  with abnormality except iso (Xq) Q96.2
  45,X Q96.0
  46,X
    iso (Xq) Q96.1
  46,XX Q98.3
    with streak gonads Q50.32
    hermaphrodite (true) Q99.1
    male Q98.3
  46,XY
    with streak gonads Q56.1
    female Q97.3
    hermaphrodite (true) Q99.1
  47,XXX Q97.0
  47,XXY Q98.0
  47,XYY Q98.5
Kaschin-Beck disease — *see* Disease,
    Kaschin-Beck
Katayama's disease or fever B65.2
Kawasaki's syndrome M30.3
Kayser-Fleischer ring (cornea)
    (pseudosclerosis) H18.04-
Kaznelson's syndrome (congenital
    hypoplastic anemia) D61.01
Kearns-Sayre syndrome H49.81-
Kedani fever A75.3
Kelis L91.0
Kelly (-Patterson) syndrome (sideropenic
    dysphagia) D50.1
Keloid, cheloid L91.0
  acne L73.0
  Addison's L94.0
  cornea — *see* Opacity, cornea
  Hawkin's L91.0
  scar L91.0
Keloma L91.0
Kenya fever A77.1
Keratectasia — *see also* Ectasia, cornea
  congenital Q13.4
Keratinization of alveolar ridge mucosa
  excessive K13.23
  minimal K13.22
Keratinized residual ridge mucosa
  excessive K13.23
  minimal K13.22
Keratitis (nodular) (nonulcerative) (simple)
    (zonular) H16.9
  with ulceration (central) (marginal)
    (perforated) (ring) — *see* Ulcer,
    cornea
  actinic — *see* Photokeratitis
  arborescens (herpes simplex) B00.52
  areolar H16.11-
  bullosa H16.8
  deep H16.309
    specified type NEC H16.399
  dendritic(a) (herpes simplex) B00.52
  disciform(is) (herpes simplex) B00.52
    varicella B01.81
  filamentary H16.12-
  gonococcal (congenital or prenatal) A54.33
  herpes, herpetic (simplex) B00.52
    zoster B02.33

Keratitis (nodular) (nonulcerative) (simple) (zonular) H16.9 — *continued*
in (due to)
  acanthamebiasis B60.13
  adenovirus B30.0
  exanthema (*see also* Exanthem) B09
  herpes (simplex) virus B00.52
  measles B05.81
  syphilis A50.31
  tuberculosis A18.52
  zoster B02.33
interstitial (nonsyphilitic) H16.30-
  diffuse H16.32-
  herpes, herpetic (simplex) B00.52
    zoster B02.33
  sclerosing H16.33-
  specified type NEC H16.39-
  syphilitic (congenital) (late) A50.31
  tuberculous A18.52
macular H16.11-
nummular H16.11-
oyster shuckers' H16.8
parenchymatous — *see* Keratitis, interstitial
petrificans H16.8
postmeasles B05.81
punctata
  leprosa A30.9 [H16.14-]
  syphilitic (profunda) A50.31
punctate H16.14-
purulent H16.8
rosacea L71.8
sclerosing H16.33-
specified type NEC H16.8
stellate H16.11-
striate H16.11-
superficial H16.10-
  with conjunctivitis — *see* Keratoconjunctivitis
  due to light — *see* Photokeratitis
suppurative H16.8
syphilitic (congenital) (prenatal) A50.31
trachomatous A71.1
  sequelae B94.0
tuberculous A18.52
vesicular H16.8
xerotic (*see also* Keratomalacia) H16.8
  vitamin A deficiency E50.4
Kerato-uveitis — *see* Iridocyclitis
Keratoacanthoma L85.8
Keratocele — *see* Descemetocele
Keratoconjunctivitis H16.20-
Acanthamoeba B60.13
adenoviral B30.0
epidemic B30.0
exposure H16.21-
herpes, herpetic (simplex) B00.52
  zoster B02.33
in exanthema (*see also* Exanthem) B09
infectious B30.0
lagophthalmic — *see* Keratoconjunctivitis, specified type NEC
neurotrophic H16.23-
phlyctenular H16.25-
postmeasles B05.81
shipyard B30.0
sicca (Sjogren's) M35.0-
  not Sjogren's H16.22-
specified type NEC H16.29-
tuberculous (phlyctenular) A18.52
vernal H16.26-
Keratoconus H18.60-
congenital Q13.4
stable H18.61-
unstable H18.62-
Keratocyst (dental) (odontogenic) — *see* Cyst, calcifying odontogenic
Keratoderma, keratodermia (congenital) (palmaris et plantaris) (symmetrical) Q82.8
acquired L85.1
in diseases classified elsewhere L86
climactericum L85.1
gonococcal A54.89
gonorrheal A54.89
punctata L85.2
Reiter's — *see* Reiter's disease
Keratodermatocele — *see* Descemetocele
Keratoglobus H18.79
congenital Q15.8
  with glaucoma Q15.0
Keratohemia — *see* Pigmentation, cornea, stromal
Keratoiritis — *see also* Iridocyclitis
syphilitic A50.39
tuberculous A18.54
Keratoma L57.0
palmaris and plantaris hereditarium Q82.8
senile L57.0
Keratomalacia H18.44-
vitamin A deficiency E50.4

Keratomegaly Q13.4
Keratomycosis B49
nigrans, nigricans (palmaris) B36.1
Keratopathy H18.9
band H18.42-
bullous H18.1-
bullous (aphakic), following cataract surgery H59.01-
Keratoscleritis, tuberculous A18.52
Keratosis L57.0
actinic L57.0
arsenical L85.8
congenital, specified NEC Q80.8
female genital NEC N94.89
follicularis Q82.8
  acquired L11.0
  congenita Q82.8
  et parafollicularis in cutem penetrans L87.0
  spinulosa (decalvans) Q82.8
  vitamin A deficiency E50.8
gonococcal A54.89
male genital (external) N50.8
nigricans L83
obturans, external ear (canal) — *see* Cholesteatoma, external ear
palmaris et plantaris (inherited) (symmetrical) Q82.8
  acquired L85.1
penile N48.89
pharynx J39.2
pilaris, acquired L85.8
punctata (palmaris et plantaris) L85.2
scrotal N50.8
seborrheic L82.1
  inflamed L82.0
senile L57.0
solar L57.0
tonsillaris J35.8
vagina N89.4
vegetans Q82.8
vitamin A deficiency E50.8
vocal cord J38.3
Kerion (celsi) B35.0
Kernicterus of newborn (not due to isoimmunization) P57.9
due to isoimmunization (conditions in P55.0-P55.9) P57.0
specified type NEC P57.8
Kerunoparalysis T75.09
Keshan disease E59
Ketoacidosis E87.2
diabetic — *see* Diabetes, by type, with ketoacidosis
Ketonuria R82.4
Ketosis NEC E88.89
diabetic — *see* Diabetes, by type, with ketoacidosis
Kew Garden fever A79.1
Kidney — *see* condition
Kienböck's disease — *see also* Osteochondrosis, juvenile, hand, carpal lunate
adult M93.1
Kimmelstiel (-Wilson) disease — *see* Diabetes, Kimmelstiel (-Wilson) disease
Kimura disease D21.9
specified site — *see* Neoplasm, connective tissue, benign
Kink, kinking
artery I77.1
hair (acquired) L67.8
ileum or intestine — *see* Obstruction, intestine
Lane's — *see* Obstruction, intestine
organ or site, congenital NEC — *see* Anomaly, by site
ureter (pelvic junction) N13.5
  with
    hydronephrosis N13.1
     with infection N13.6
    pyelonephritis (chronic) N11.1
  congenital Q62.39
vein(s) I87.8
  caval I87.1
  peripheral I87.1
Kinnier Wilson's disease (hepatolenticular degeneration) E83.01
Kissing spine M48.20
cervical region M48.22
cervicothoracic region M48.23
lumbar region M48.26
lumbosacral region M48.27
occipito-atlanto-axial region M48.21
thoracic region M48.24
thoracolumbar region M48.25

Klatskin's tumor C24.0
Klauder's disease A26.8
Klebs' disease (*see also* Glomerulonephritis) N05-
Klebsiella (K.) pneumoniae, as cause of disease classified elsewhere B96.1
Klein(e)-Levin syndrome G47.13
Kleptomania F63.2
Klinefelter's syndrome Q98.4
karyotype 47,XXY Q98.0
male with more than two X chromosomes Q98.1
Klippel-Feil deficiency, disease, or syndrome (brevicollis) Q76.1
Klippel's disease I67.2
Klippel-Trenaunay (-Weber) syndrome Q87.2
Klumpke(-Déjerine) palsy, paralysis (birth) (newborn) P14.1
Knee — *see* condition
Knock knee (acquired) M21.06-
congenital Q74.1
Knot(s)
intestinal, syndrome (volvulus) K56.2
surfer S89.8-
umbilical cord (true) O69.2
Knotting (of)
hair L67.8
intestine K56.2
Knuckle pad (Garrod's) M72.1
Koch's
infection — *see* Tuberculosis
relapsing fever A68.9
Koch-Weeks' conjunctivitis — *see* Conjunctivitis, acute, mucopurulent
Köebner's syndrome Q81.8
Köenig's disease (osteochondritis dissecans) — *see* Osteochondritis, dissecans
Köhler's disease
patellar — *see* Osteochondrosis, juvenile, patella
tarsal navicular — *see* Osteochondrosis, juvenile, tarsus
Köhler-Pellegrini-Steida disease or syndrome (calcification, knee joint) — *see* Bursitis, tibial collateral
Koilonychia L60.3
congenital Q84.6
Kojevnikov's, epilepsy — *see* Kozhevnikof's epilepsy
Kozhevnikof's epilepsy G40.109
intractable G40.119
  with status epilepticus G40.111
  without status epilepticus G40.119
not intractable G40.109
  with status epilepticus G40.101
  without status epilepticus G40.109
Koplik's spots B05.9
Kopp's asthma E32.8
Korsakoff's (Wernicke) disease, psychosis or syndrome (alcoholic) F10.96
with dependence F10.26
drug-induced
  due to drug abuse — *see* Abuse, drug, by type, with amnestic disorder
  due to drug dependence — *see* Dependence, drug, by type, with amnestic disorder
nonalcoholic F04
Korsakov's disease, psychosis or syndrome — *see* Korsakoff's disease
Korsakow's disease, psychosis or syndrome — *see* Korsakoff's disease
Kostmann's disease or syndrome (infantile genetic agranulocytosis) — *see* Agranulocytosis
Krabbe's
disease E75.23
syndrome, congenital muscle hypoplasia Q79.8
Kraepelin-Morel disease — *see* Schizophrenia
Kraft-Weber-Dimitri disease Q85.8
Kraurosis
ani K62.89
penis N48.0
vagina N89.8
vulva N90.4
Kreotoxism A05.9
Krukenberg's
spindle — *see* Pigmentation, cornea, posterior
tumor C79.6-
Kufs' disease E75.4
Kugelberg-Welander disease G12.1
Kuhnt-Junius degeneration (*see also* Degeneration, macula) H35.32

Kümmell's disease or spondylitis — *see* Spondylopathy, traumatic
Kupffer cell sarcoma C22.3
Kuru A81.81
Kussmaul's
disease M30.0
respiration E87.2
  in diabetic acidosis — *see* Diabetes, by type, with ketoacidosis
Kwashiorkor E40
marasmic, marasmus type E42
Kyasanur Forest disease A98.2
Kyphoscoliosis, kyphoscoliotic (acquired) (*see also* Scoliosis) M41.9
congenital Q67.5
heart (disease) I27.1
sequelae of rickets E64.3
tuberculous A18.01
Kyphosis, kyphotic (acquired) M40.209
cervical region M40.202
cervicothoracic region M40.203
congenital Q76.419
  cervical region Q76.412
  cervicothoracic region Q76.413
  occipito-atlanto-axial region Q76.411
  thoracic region Q76.414
  thoracolumbar region Q76.415
Morquio-Brailsford type (spinal) (*see also* subcategory M49.8) E76.219
postlaminectomy M96.3
postradiation therapy M96.2
postural (adolescent) M40.00
  cervicothoracic region M40.03
  thoracic region M40.04
  thoracolumbar region M40.05
secondary NEC M40.10
  cervical region M40.12
  cervicothoracic region M40.13
  thoracic region M40.14
  thoracolumbar region M40.15
sequelae of rickets E64.3
specified type NEC M40.299
  cervical region M40.292
  cervicothoracic region M40.293
  thoracic region M40.294
  thoracolumbar region M40.295
syphilitic, congenital A50.56
thoracic region M40.204
thoracolumbar region M40.205
tuberculous A18.01
Kyrle disease L87.0

L

Labia, labium — *see* condition
Labile
　blood pressure R09.89
　vasomotor system I73.9
Labioglossal paralysis G12.29
Labium leporinum — *see* Cleft, lip
Labor — *see* Delivery
Labored breathing — *see* Hyperventilation
Labyrinthitis (circumscribed) (destructive)
　(diffuse) (inner ear) (latent) (purulent)
　(suppurative) (*see also*
　subcategory)H83.0
　syphilitic A52.79
Laceration
　with abortion — *see* Abortion, by type,
　　complicated by laceration of pelvic
　　organs
　abdomen, abdominal
　　wall S31.119
　　　with
　　　　foreign body S31.129
　　　　penetration into peritoneal cavity
　　　　　S31.619
　　　　　with foreign body S31.629
　　　　epigastric region S31.112
　　　　　with
　　　　　　foreign body S31.122
　　　　　　penetration into peritoneal cavity
　　　　　　　S31.612
　　　　　　　with foreign body S31.622
　　　　left
　　　　　lower quadrant S31.114
　　　　　　with
　　　　　　　foreign body S31.124
　　　　　　　penetration into peritoneal
　　　　　　　　cavity S31.614
　　　　　　　　with foreign body S31.624
　　　　　upper quadrant S31.111
　　　　　　with
　　　　　　　foreign body S31.121
　　　　　　　penetration into peritoneal
　　　　　　　　cavity S31.611
　　　　　　　　with foreign body S31.621
　　　　periumbilic region S31.115
　　　　　with
　　　　　　foreign body S31.125
　　　　　　penetration into peritoneal cavity
　　　　　　　S31.615
　　　　　　　with foreign body S31.625
　　　　right
　　　　　lower quadrant S31.113
　　　　　　with
　　　　　　　foreign body S31.123
　　　　　　　penetration into peritoneal
　　　　　　　　cavity S31.613
　　　　　　　　with foreign body S31.623
　　　　　upper quadrant S31.110
　　　　　　with
　　　　　　　foreign body S31.120
　　　　　　　penetration into peritoneal
　　　　　　　　cavity S31.610
　　　　　　　　with foreign body S31.620
　accidental, complicating surgery — *see*
　　Complications, surgical, accidental
　　puncture or laceration
　Achilles tendon S86.02-
　adrenal gland S37.813
　alveolar (process) — *see* Laceration, oral
　　cavity
　ankle S91.01-
　　with
　　　foreign body S91.02-
　antecubital space — *see* Laceration, elbow
　anus (sphincter) S31.831
　　with
　　　ectopic or molar pregnancy O08.6
　　　foreign body S31.832
　　complicating delivery — *see* Delivery,
　　　complicated, by, laceration, anus
　　　(sphincter)
　　following ectopic or molar pregnancy
　　　O08.6
　　nontraumatic, nonpuerperal — *see*
　　　Fissure, anus
　arm (upper) S41.11-
　　with foreign body S41.12-
　　lower — *see* Laceration, forearm
　auditory canal (external) (meatus) — *see*
　　Laceration, ear
　auricle, ear — *see* Laceration, ear
　axilla — *see* Laceration, arm

Laceration — *continued*
　back — *see also* Laceration, thorax, back
　　lower S31.010
　　　with
　　　　foreign body S31.020
　　　　　with penetration into
　　　　　　retroperitoneal space
　　　　　　S31.021
　　　　penetration into retroperitoneal
　　　　　space S31.011
　bile duct S36.13
　bladder S37.23
　　with ectopic or molar pregnancy O08.6
　　following ectopic or molar pregnancy
　　　O08.6
　　obstetrical trauma O71.5
　blood vessel — *see* Injury, blood vessel
　bowel — *see also* Laceration, intestine
　　with ectopic or molar pregnancy O08.6
　　complicating abortion — *see* Abortion,
　　　by type, complicated by, specified
　　　condition NEC
　　following ectopic or molar pregnancy
　　　O08.6
　　obstetrical trauma O71.5
　brain (any part) (cortex) (diffuse)
　　(membrane) — *see also* Injury,
　　intracranial, diffuse
　　during birth P10.8
　　　with hemorrhage P10.1
　　focal — *see* Injury, intracranial, focal
　　　brain injury
　brainstem S06.38-
　breast S21.01-
　　with foreign body S21.02-
　broad ligament S37.893
　　with ectopic or molar pregnancy O08.6
　　following ectopic or molar pregnancy
　　　O08.6
　　laceration syndrome N83.8
　　obstetrical trauma O71.6
　　syndrome (laceration) N83.8
　buttock S31.801
　　with foreign body S31.802
　　left S31.821
　　　with foreign body S31.822
　　right S31.811
　　　with foreign body S31.812
　calf — *see* Laceration, leg
　canaliculus lacrimalis — *see* Laceration,
　　eyelid
　canthus, eye — *see* Laceration, eyelid
　capsule, joint — *see* Sprain
　causing eversion of cervix uteri (old) N86
　central (perineal), complicating delivery
　　O70.9
　cerebellum, traumatic S06.37-
　cerebral S06.33-
　　during birth P10.8
　　　with hemorrhage P10.1
　　left side S06.32-
　　right side S06.31-
　cervix (uteri)
　　with ectopic or molar pregnancy O08.6
　　following ectopic or molar pregnancy
　　　O08.6
　　nonpuerperal, nontraumatic N88.1
　　obstetrical trauma (current) O71.3
　　old (postpartal) N88.1
　　traumatic S37.63
　cheek (external) S01.41-
　　with foreign body S01.42-
　　internal — *see* Laceration, oral cavity
　chest wall — *see* Laceration, thorax
　chin — *see* Laceration, head, specified site
　　NEC
　chordae tendinae NEC I51.1
　　concurrent with acute myocardial
　　　infarction — *see* Infarct,
　　　myocardium
　　following acute myocardial infarction
　　　(current complication) I23.4
　clitoris — *see* Laceration, vulva
　colon — *see* Laceration, intestine, large,
　　colon
　common bile duct S36.13
　cortex (cerebral) — *see* Injury, intracranial,
　　diffuse
　costal region — *see* Laceration, thorax
　cystic duct S36.13
　diaphragm S27.803
　digit(s)
　　foot — *see* Laceration, toe
　　hand — *see* Laceration, finger
　duodenum S36.430
　ear (canal) (external) S01.31-
　　with foreign body S01.32-
　　drum S09.2-

Laceration — *continued*
　elbow S51.01-
　　with
　　　foreign body S51.02-
　epididymis — *see* Laceration, testis
　epigastric region — *see* Laceration,
　　abdomen, wall, epigastric region
　esophagus K22.8
　　traumatic
　　　cervical S11.21
　　　　with foreign body S11.22
　　　thoracic S27.813
　eye(ball) S05.3-
　　with prolapse or loss of intraocular
　　　tissue S05.2-
　　penetrating S05.6-
　eyebrow — *see* Laceration, eyelid
　eyelid S01.11-
　　with foreign body S01.12-
　face NEC — *see* Laceration, head,
　　specified site NEC
　fallopian tube S37.539
　　bilateral S37.532
　　unilateral S37.531
　finger(s) S61.219
　　with
　　　damage to nail S61.319
　　　　with
　　　　　foreign body S61.329
　　　foreign body S61.229
　　index S61.218
　　　with
　　　　damage to nail S61.318
　　　　　with
　　　　　　foreign body S61.328
　　　　foreign body S61.228
　　　left S61.211
　　　　with
　　　　　damage to nail S61.311
　　　　　　with
　　　　　　　foreign body S61.321
　　　　　foreign body S61.221
　　　right S61.210
　　　　with
　　　　　damage to nail S61.310
　　　　　　with
　　　　　　　foreign body S61.320
　　　　　foreign body S61.220
　　little S61.218
　　　with
　　　　damage to nail S61.318
　　　　　with
　　　　　　foreign body S61.328
　　　　foreign body S61.228
　　　left S61.217
　　　　with
　　　　　damage to nail S61.317
　　　　　　with
　　　　　　　foreign body S61.327
　　　　　foreign body S61.227
　　　right S61.216
　　　　with
　　　　　damage to nail S61.316
　　　　　　with
　　　　　　　foreign body S61.326
　　　　　foreign body S61.226
　　middle S61.218
　　　with
　　　　damage to nail S61.318
　　　　　with
　　　　　　foreign body S61.328
　　　　foreign body S61.228
　　　left S61.213
　　　　with
　　　　　damage to nail S61.313
　　　　　　with
　　　　　　　foreign body S61.323
　　　　　foreign body S61.223
　　　right S61.212
　　　　with
　　　　　damage to nail S61.312
　　　　　　with
　　　　　　　foreign body S61.322
　　　　　foreign body S61.222
　　ring S61.218
　　　with
　　　　damage to nail S61.318
　　　　　with
　　　　　　foreign body S61.328
　　　　foreign body S61.228
　　　left S61.215
　　　　with
　　　　　damage to nail S61.315
　　　　　　with
　　　　　　　foreign body S61.325
　　　　　foreign body S61.225

Laceration — *continued*
　finger(s) S61.219 — *continued*
　　ring S61.218 — *continued*
　　　right S61.214
　　　　with
　　　　　damage to nail S61.314
　　　　　　with
　　　　　　　foreign body S61.324
　　　　　foreign body S61.224
　flank S31.119
　　with foreign body S31.129
　foot (except toe(s) alone) S91.319
　　with foreign body S91.329
　　left S91.312
　　　with foreign body S91.322
　　right S91.311
　　　with foreign body S91.321
　　toe — *see* Laceration, toe
　forearm S51.819
　　with
　　　foreign body S51.829
　　elbow only — *see* Laceration, elbow
　　left S51.812
　　　with
　　　　foreign body S51.822
　　right S51.811
　　　with
　　　　foreign body S51.821
　forehead S01.81
　　with foreign body S01.82
　fourchette O70.0
　　with ectopic or molar pregnancy O08.6
　　complicating delivery O70.0
　　following ectopic or molar pregnancy
　　　O08.6
　gallbladder S36.123
　genital organs, external
　　female S31.512
　　　with foreign body S31.522
　　　vagina — *see* Laceration, vagina
　　　vulva — *see* Laceration, vulva
　　male S31.511
　　　with foreign body S31.521
　　　penis — *see* Laceration, penis
　　　scrotum — *see* Laceration, scrotum
　　　testis — *see* Laceration, testis
　groin — *see* Laceration, abdomen, wall
　gum — *see* Laceration, oral cavity
　hand S61.419
　　with
　　　foreign body S61.429
　　finger — *see* Laceration, finger
　　left S61.412
　　　with
　　　　foreign body S61.422
　　right S61.411
　　　with
　　　　foreign body S61.421
　　thumb — *see* Laceration, thumb
　head S01.91
　　with foreign body S01.92
　　cheek — *see* Laceration, cheek
　　ear — *see* Laceration, ear
　　eyelid — *see* Laceration, eyelid
　　lip — *see* Laceration, lip
　　nose — *see* Laceration, nose
　　oral cavity — *see* Laceration, oral cavity
　　scalp S01.01
　　　with foreign body S01.02
　　specified site NEC S01.81
　　　with foreign body S01.82
　　temporomandibular area — *see*
　　　Laceration, cheek
　heart — *see* Injury, heart, laceration
　heel — *see* Laceration, foot
　hepatic duct S36.13
　hip S71.019
　　with foreign body S71.029
　　left S71.012
　　　with foreign body S71.022
　　right S71.011
　　　with foreign body S71.021
　hymen — *see* Laceration, vagina
　hypochondrium — *see* Laceration,
　　abdomen, wall
　hypogastric region — *see* Laceration,
　　abdomen, wall
　ileum S36.438
　inguinal region — *see* Laceration,
　　abdomen, wall
　instep — *see* Laceration, foot
　internal organ — *see* Injury, by site
　interscapular region — *see* Laceration,
　　thorax, back

DISEASE INDEX

Laceration — *continued*
intestine
  large
    colon S36.539
      ascending S36.530
      descending S36.532
      sigmoid S36.533
      specified site NEC S36.538
    rectum S36.63
      transverse S36.531
  small S36.439
    duodenum S36.430
    specified site NEC S36.438
intra-abdominal organ S36.93
  intestine — *see* Laceration, intestine
  liver — *see* Laceration, liver
  pancreas — *see* Laceration, pancreas
  peritoneum S36.81
  specified site NEC S36.893
  spleen — *see* Laceration, spleen
  stomach — *see* Laceration, stomach
intracranial NEC — *see also* Injury, intracranial, diffuse
  birth injury P10.9
jaw — *see* Laceration, head, specified site NEC
jejunum S36.438
joint capsule — *see* Sprain, by site
kidney S37.03-
  major (greater than 3 cm) (massive) (stellate) S37.06-
  minor (less than 1 cm) S37.04-
  moderate (1 to 3 cm) S37.05-
    multiple S37.06-
knee S81.01-
  with foreign body S81.02-
labium (majus) (minus) — *see* Laceration, vulva
lacrimal duct — *see* Laceration, eyelid
large intestine — *see* Laceration, intestine, large
larynx S11.011
  with foreign body S11.012
leg (lower) S81.819
  with foreign body S81.829
  foot — *see* Laceration, foot
  knee — *see* Laceration, knee
  left S81.812
    with foreign body S81.822
  right S81.811
    with foreign body S81.821
  upper — *see* Laceration, thigh
ligament — *see* Sprain
lip S01.511
  with foreign body S01.521
liver S36.113
  major (stellate) S36.116
  minor S36.114
  moderate S36.115
loin — *see* Laceration, abdomen, wall
lower back — *see* Laceration, back, lower
lumbar region — *see* Laceration, back, lower
lung S27.339
  bilateral S27.332
  unilateral S27.331
malar region — *see* Laceration, head, specified site NEC
mammary — *see* Laceration, breast
mastoid region — *see* Laceration, head, specified site NEC
meninges — *see* Injury, intracranial, diffuse
meniscus — *see* Tear, meniscus
mesentery S36.893
mesosalpinx S37.893
mouth — *see* Laceration, oral cavity
muscle — *see* Injury, muscle, by site, laceration
nail
  finger — *see* Laceration, finger, with damage to nail
  toe — *see* Laceration, toe, with damage to nail
nasal (septum) (sinus) — *see* Laceration, nose
nasopharynx — *see* Laceration, head, specified site NEC
neck S11.91
  with foreign body S11.92
  involving
    cervical esophagus S11.21
      with foreign body S11.22
    larynx — *see* Laceration, larynx
    pharynx — *see* Laceration, pharynx
    thyroid gland — *see* Laceration, thyroid gland
    trachea — *see* Laceration, trachea

Laceration — *continued*
neck S11.91 — *continued*
  specified site NEC S11.81
    with foreign body S11.82
nerve — *see* Injury, nerve
nose (septum) (sinus) S01.21
  with foreign body S01.22
ocular NOS S05.3-
  adnexa NOS S01.11-
oral cavity S01.512
  with foreign body S01.522
orbit (eye) — *see* Wound, open, ocular, orbit
ovary S37.439
  bilateral S37.432
  unilateral S37.431
palate — *see* Laceration, oral cavity
palm — *see* Laceration, hand
pancreas S36.239
  body S36.231
    major S36.261
    minor S36.241
    moderate S36.251
  head S36.230
    major S36.260
    minor S36.240
    moderate S36.250
  major S36.269
  minor S36.249
  moderate S36.259
  tail S36.232
    major S36.262
    minor S36.242
    moderate S36.252
pelvic S31.010
  with
    foreign body S31.020
      penetration into retroperitoneal cavity S31.021
    penetration into retroperitoneal cavity S31.011
  floor — *see also* Laceration, back, lower
    with ectopic or molar pregnancy O08.6
    complicating delivery O70.1
    following ectopic or molar pregnancy O08.6
    old (postpartal) N81.89
  organ S37.93
    with ectopic or molar pregnancy O08.6
    adrenal gland S37.813
    bladder S37.23
    fallopian tube — *see* Laceration, fallopian tube
    following ectopic or molar pregnancy O08.6
    kidney — *see* Laceration, kidney
    obstetrical trauma O71.5
    ovary — *see* Laceration, ovary
    prostate S37.823
    specified site NEC S37.893
    ureter S37.13
    urethra S37.33
    uterus S37.63
penis S31.21
  with foreign body S31.22
perineum
  female S31.41
    with
      ectopic or molar pregnancy O08.6
      foreign body S31.42
    during delivery O70.9
      first degree O70.0
      fourth degree O70.3
      second degree O70.1
      third degree O70.2
    old (postpartal) N81.89
    postpartal N81.89
    secondary (postpartal) O90.1
  male S31.119
    with foreign body S31.129
periocular area (with or without lacrimal passages) — *see* Laceration, eyelid
peritoneum S36.893
periumbilic region — *see* Laceration, abdomen, wall, periumbilic
periurethral tissue — *see* Laceration, urethra
phalanges
  finger — *see* Laceration, finger
  toe — *see* Laceration, toe
pharynx S11.21
  with foreign body S11.22
pinna — *see* Laceration, ear

Laceration — *continued*
popliteal space — *see* Laceration, knee
prepuce — *see* Laceration, penis
prostate S37.823
pubic region S31.119
  with foreign body S31.129
pudendum — *see* Laceration, genital organs, external
rectovaginal septum — *see* Laceration, vagina
rectum S36.63
retroperitoneum S36.893
round ligament S37.893
sacral region — *see* Laceration, back, lower
sacroiliac region — *see* Laceration, back, lower
salivary gland — *see* Laceration, oral cavity
scalp S01.01
  with foreign body S01.02
scapular region — *see* Laceration, shoulder
scrotum S31.31
  with foreign body S31.32
seminal vesicle S37.893
shin — *see* Laceration, leg
shoulder S41.019
  with foreign body S41.029
  left S41.012
    with foreign body S41.022
  right S41.011
    with foreign body S41.021
small intestine — *see* Laceration, intestine, small
spermatic cord — *see* Laceration, testis
spinal cord (meninges) — *see also* Injury, spinal cord, by region
  due to injury at birth P11.5
  newborn (birth injury) P11.5
spleen S36.039
  major (massive) (stellate) S36.032
  moderate S36.031
  superficial (minor) S36.030
sternal region — *see* Laceration, thorax, front
stomach S36.33
submaxillary region — *see* Laceration, head, specified site NEC
submental region — *see* Laceration, head, specified site NEC
subungual
  finger(s) — *see* Laceration, finger, with damage to nail
  toe(s) — *see* Laceration, toe, with damage to nail
suprarenal gland — *see* Laceration, adrenal gland
temple, temporal region — *see* Laceration, head, specified site NEC
temporomandibular area — *see* Laceration, cheek
tendon — *see* Injury, muscle, by site, laceration
  Achilles S86.02-
tentorium cerebelli — *see* Injury, intracranial, diffuse
testis S31.31
  with foreign body S31.32
thigh S71.11-
  with foreign body S71.12-
thorax, thoracic (wall) S21.91
  with foreign body S21.92
  back S21.22-
    with penetration into thoracic cavity S21.42-
  front S21.12-
    with penetration into thoracic cavity S21.32-
  back S21.21-
    with
      foreign body S21.22-
        with penetration into thoracic cavity S21.42-
      penetration into thoracic cavity S21.41-
  breast — *see* Laceration, breast
  front S21.11-
    with
      foreign body S21.12-
        with penetration into thoracic cavity S21.32-
      penetration into thoracic cavity S21.31-

Laceration — *continued*
thumb S61.019
  with
    damage to nail S61.119
      with
        foreign body S61.129
    foreign body S61.029
  left S61.012
    with
      damage to nail S61.112
        with
          foreign body S61.122
      foreign body S61.022
  right S61.011
    with
      damage to nail S61.111
        with
          foreign body S61.121
      foreign body S61.021
thyroid gland S11.11
  with foreign body S11.12
toe(s) S91.119
  with
    damage to nail S91.219
      with
        foreign body S91.229
    foreign body S91.129
  great S91.113
    with
      damage to nail S91.213
        with
          foreign body S91.223
      foreign body S91.123
    left S91.112
      with
        damage to nail S91.212
          with
            foreign body S91.222
        foreign body S91.122
    right S91.111
      with
        damage to nail S91.211
          with
            foreign body S91.221
        foreign body S91.121
  lesser S91.116
    with
      damage to nail S91.216
        with
          foreign body S91.226
      foreign body S91.126
    left S91.115
      with
        damage to nail S91.215
          with
            foreign body S91.225
        foreign body S91.125
    right S91.114
      with
        damage to nail S91.214
          with
            foreign body S91.224
        foreign body S91.124
tongue — *see* Laceration, oral cavity
trachea S11.021
  with foreign body S11.022
tunica vaginalis — *see* Laceration, testis
tympanum, tympanic membrane — *see* Laceration, ear, drum
umbilical region S31.115
  with foreign body S31.125
ureter S37.13
urethra S37.33
  with or following ectopic or molar pregnancy O08.6
  obstetrical trauma O71.5
urinary organ NEC S37.893
uterus S37.63
  with ectopic or molar pregnancy O08.6
  following ectopic or molar pregnancy O08.6
  nonpuerperal, nontraumatic N85.8
  obstetrical trauma NEC O71.81
  old (postpartal) N85.8
uvula — *see* Laceration, oral cavity
vagina S31.41
  with
    ectopic or molar pregnancy O08.6
    foreign body S31.42
  during delivery O71.4
    with perineal laceration — *see* Laceration, perineum, female, during delivery
  following ectopic or molar pregnancy O08.6
  nonpuerperal, nontraumatic N89.8
  old (postpartal) N89.8

Laceration — *continued*
vas deferens S37.893
vesical — *see* Laceration, bladder
vocal cords S11.031
  with foreign body S11.032
vulva S31.41
  with
    ectopic or molar pregnancy O08.6
    foreign body S31.42
  complicating delivery O70.0
  following ectopic or molar pregnancy O08.6
  nonpuerperal, nontraumatic N90.89
  old (postpartal) N90.89
wrist S61.519
  with
    foreign body S61.529
  left S61.512
    with
      foreign body S61.522
  right S61.511
    with
      foreign body S61.521
Lack of
achievement in school Z55.3
adequate
  food Z59.4
  intermaxillary vertical dimension of fully erupted teeth M26.36
  sleep Z72.820
appetite (*see also* Anorexia) R63.0
awareness R41.9
care
  in home Z74.2
  of infant (at or after birth) T76.02
    confirmed T74.02
cognitive functions R41.9
coordination R27.9
  ataxia R27.0
  specified type NEC R27.8
development (physiological) R62.50
  failure to thrive (child over 28 days old) R62.51
    adult R62.7
    newborn P92.6
  short stature R62.52
  specified type NEC R62.59
energy R53.83
financial resources Z59.6
food T73.0
growth R62.52
heating Z59.1
housing (permanent) (temporary) Z59.0
  adequate Z59.1
learning experiences in childhood Z62.898
leisure time (affecting life-style) Z73.2
material resources Z59.9
memory — *see also* Amnesia
  mild, following organic brain damage F06.8
ovulation N97.0
parental supervision or control of child Z62.0
person able to render necessary care Z74.2
physical exercise Z72.3
play experience in childhood Z62.898
posterior occlusal support M26.57
relaxation (affecting life-style) Z73.2
sexual
  desire F52.0
  enjoyment F52.1
shelter Z59.0
sleep (adequate) Z72.820
supervision of child by parent Z62.0
support, posterior occlusal M26.57
water T73.1
Lacrimal — *see* condition
Lacrimation, abnormal — *see* Epiphora
Lacrimonasal duct — *see* condition
Lactation, lactating (breast) (puerperal, postpartum)
associated
  cracked nipple O92.13
  retracted nipple O92.03
defective O92.4
disorder NEC O92.79
excessive O92.6
failed (complete) O92.3
  partial O92.4
mastitis NEC — *see* Mastitis, obstetric
mother (care and/or examination) Z39.1
nonpuerperal N64.3
Lacticemia, excessive E87.2
Lacunar skull Q75.8
Laennec's cirrhosis K74.69
alcoholic K70.30
  with ascites K70.31
Lafora's disease — *see* Epilepsy, generalized, idiopathic

Lag, lid (nervous) — *see* Retraction, lid
Lagophthalmos (eyelid) (nervous) H02.209
cicatricial H02.219
  left H02.216
    lower H02.215
    upper H02.214
  right H02.213
    lower H02.212
    upper H02.211
keratoconjunctivitis — *see* Keratoconjunctivitis
left H02.206
  lower H02.205
  upper H02.204
mechanical H02.229
  left H02.226
    lower H02.225
    upper H02.224
  right H02.223
    lower H02.222
    upper H02.221
paralytic H02.239
  left H02.236
    lower H02.235
    upper H02.234
  right H02.233
    lower H02.232
    upper H02.231
right H02.203
  lower H02.202
  upper H02.201
Laki-Lorand factor deficiency — *see* Defect, coagulation, specified type NEC
Lalling F80.0
Lambert-Eaton syndrome — *see* Syndrome, Lambert-Eaton
Lambliasis, lambliosis A07.1
Landau-Kleffner syndrome — *see* Epilepsy, specified NEC
Landouzy-Déjérine dystrophy or facioscapulohumeral atrophy G71.0
Landouzy's disease (icterohemorrhagic leptospirosis) A27.0
Landry-Guillain-Barré, syndrome or paralysis G61.0
Landry's disease or paralysis G61.0
Lane's
band Q43.3
kink — *see* Obstruction, intestine
syndrome K90.2
Langdon Down syndrome — *see* Trisomy, 21
Lapsed immunization schedule status Z28.3
Large
baby (regardless of gestational age) (4000g to 4499g) P08.1
ear, congenital Q17.1
physiological cup Q14.2
stature R68.89
Large-for-dates NEC (infant) (4000g to 4499g) P08.1
affecting management of pregnancy O36.6-
  exceptionally (4500g or more) P08.0
Larsen-Johansson disease orosteochondrosis — *see* Osteochondrosis, juvenile, patella
Larsen's syndrome (flattened facies and multiple congenital dislocations) Q74.8
Larva migrans
cutaneous B76.9
  Ancylostoma B76.0
visceral B83.0
Laryngeal — *see* condition
Laryngismus (stridulus) J38.5
congenital P28.89
diphtheritic A36.2
Laryngitis (acute) (edematous) (fibrinous) (infective) (infiltrative) (malignant) (membranous) (phlegmonous) (pneumococcal) (pseudomembranous) (septic) (subglottic) (suppurative) (ulcerative) J04.0
with
  influenza, flu, or grippe — *see* Influenza, with, laryngitis
  tracheitis (acute) — *see* Laryngotracheitis
atrophic J37.0
catarrhal J37.0
chronic J37.0
  with tracheitis (chronic) J37.1
diphtheritic A36.2
due to external agent — *see* Inflammation, respiratory, upper, due to
H. influenzae J04.0
Hemophilus influenzae J04.0

Laryngitis (acute) (edematous) (fibrinous) (infective) (infiltrative) (malignant) (membranous) (phlegmonous)(pneumococcal) (pseudomembranous) (septic) (subglottic) (suppurative) (ulcerative) J04.0 — *continued*
hypertrophic J37.0
influenzal — *see* Influenza, with, respiratory manifestations NEC
obstructive J05.0
sicca J37.0
spasmodic J05.0
  acute J04.0
streptococcal J04.0
stridulous J05.0
syphilitic (late) A52.73
  congenital A50.59 [J99]
    early A50.03 [J99]
tuberculous A15.5
Vincent's A69.1
Laryngocele (congenital) (ventricular) Q31.3
Laryngofissure J38.7
congenital Q31.8
Laryngomalacia (congenital) Q31.5
Laryngopharyngitis (acute) J06.0
chronic J37.0
due to external agent — *see* Inflammation, respiratory, upper, due to
Laryngoplegia J38.00
bilateral J38.02
unilateral J38.01
Laryngoptosis J38.7
Laryngospasm J38.5
Laryngostenosis J38.6
Laryngotracheitis (acute) (Infectional) (infective) (viral) J04.2
atrophic J37.1
catarrhal J37.1
chronic J37.1
diphtheritic A36.2
due to external agent — *see* Inflammation, respiratory, upper, due to
Hemophilus influenzae J04.2
hypertrophic J37.1
influenzal — *see* Influenza, with, respiratory manifestations NEC
pachydermic J38.7
sicca J37.1
spasmodic J38.5
  acute J05.0
streptococcal J04.2
stridulous J38.5
syphilitic (late) A52.73
  congenital A50.59 [J99]
    early A50.03 [J99]
tuberculous A15.5
Vincent's A69.1
Laryngotracheobronchitis — *see* Bronchitis
Larynx, laryngeal — *see* condition
Lassa fever A96.2
Lassitude — *see* Weakness
Late
talker R62.0
walker R62.0
Late effect(s) — *see* Sequelae
Latent — *see* condition
Laterocession — *see* Lateroversion
Lateroflexion — *see* Lateroversion
Lateroversion
cervix — *see* Lateroversion, uterus
uterus, uterine (cervix) (postinfectional) (postpartal, old) N85.4
  congenital Q51.818
  in pregnancy or childbirth O34.59-
Lathyrism — *see* Poisoning, food, noxious, plant
Launois' syndrome (pituitary gigantism) E22.0
Launois-Bensaude adenolipomatosis E88.89
Laurence-Moon(-Bardet)-Biedl syndrome Q87.89
Lax, laxity — *see also* Relaxation
ligament(ous) — *see also* Disorder, ligament
  familial M35.7
  knee — *see* Derangement, knee
skin (acquired) L57.4
  congenital Q82.8
Laxative habit F55.2
Lazy leukocyte syndrome D70.8
Lead miner's lung J63.6

Leak, leakage
air NEC J93.82
  postprocedural J95.812
amniotic fluid — *see* Rupture, membranes, premature
blood (microscopic), fetal, into maternal circulation affecting management of pregnancy — *see* Pregnancy, complicated by
cerebrospinal fluid G96.0
  from spinal (lumbar) puncture G97.0
device, implant or graft — *see also* Complications, by site and type, mechanical
  arterial graft NEC — *see* Complication, cardiovascular device, mechanical, vascular
  breast (implant) T85.43
  catheter NEC T85.638
    dialysis (renal) T82.43
      intraperitoneal T85.631
    infusion NEC T82.534
      spinal (epidural) (subdural) T85.630
    urinary, indwelling T83.038
      cystostomy T83.030
  gastrointestinal — *see* Complications, prosthetic device, mechanical, gastrointestinal device
  genital NEC T83.498
    penile prosthesis T83.490
  heart NEC — *see* Complication, cardiovascular device, mechanical
  ocular NEC — *see* Complications, prosthetic device, mechanical, ocular device
  orthopedic NEC — *see* Complication, orthopedic, device, mechanical
  persistent air J93.82
  specified NEC T85.638
  urinary NEC — *see also* Complication, genitourinary, device, urinary, mechanical
    graft T83.23
  vascular NEC — *see* Complication, cardiovascular device, mechanical
  ventricular intracranial shunt T85.03
urine — *see* Incontinence
Leaky heart — *see* Endocarditis
Learning defect (specific) F81.9
Leather bottle stomach C16.9
Leber's
congenital amaurosis H35.50
optic atrophy (hereditary) H47.22
Lederer's anemia D59.1
Leeches (external) — *see* Hirudiniasis
Leg — *see* condition
Legg(-Calvé)-Perthes disease, syndrome or osteochondrosis M91.1-
Legionellosis A48.1
nonpneumonic A48.2
Legionnaires'
disease A48.1
  nonpneumonic A48.2
  pneumonia A48.1
Leigh's disease G31.82
Leiner's disease L21.1
Leiofibromyoma — *see* Leiomyoma
Leiomyoblastoma — *see* Neoplasm, connective tissue, benign
Leiomyofibroma — *see also* Neoplasm, connective tissue, benign
uterus (cervix) (corpus) D25.9
Leiomyoma — *see also* Neoplasm, connective tissue, benign
bizarre — *see* Neoplasm, connective tissue, benign
cellular — *see* Neoplasm, connective tissue, benign
epithelioid — *see* Neoplasm, connective tissue, benign
uterus (cervix) (corpus) D25.9
  intramural D25.1
  submucous D25.0
  subserosal D25.2
vascular — *see* Neoplasm, connective tissue, benign
Leiomyoma, leiomyomatosis (intravascular) — *see* Neoplasm, connective tissue, uncertain behavior
Leiomyosarcoma — *see also* Neoplasm, connective tissue, malignant
epithelioid — *see* Neoplasm, connective tissue, malignant
myxoid — *see* Neoplasm, connective tissue, malignant

D I S E A S E I N D E X

Leishmaniasis B55.9
  American (mucocutaneous) B55.2
    cutaneous B55.2
  Asian Desert B55.1
  Brazilian B55.2
  cutaneous (any type) B55.1
  dermal — *see also* Leishmaniasis,
    cutaneous
    post-kala-azar B55.0
  eyelid B55.1
  infantile B55.0
  Mediterranean B55.0
  mucocutaneous (American) (New World)
    B55.2
  naso-oral B55.2
  nasopharyngeal B55.2
  old world B55.1
  tegumentaria diffusa B55.1
  visceral B55.0
Leishmanoid, dermal — *see also*
  Leishmaniasis, cutaneous
  post-kala-azar B55.0
Lenegre's disease I44.2
Lengthening, leg — *see* Deformity, limb,
  unequal length
Lennert's lymphoma — *see* Lymphoma,
  Lennert's
Lennox-Gastaut syndrome G40.812
  intractable G40.814
    with status epilepticus G40.813
    without status epilepticus G40.814
  not intractable G40.812
    with status epilepticus G40.811
    without status epilepticus G40.812
Lens — *see* condition
Lenticonus (anterior) (posterior) (congenital)
  Q12.8
Lenticular degeneration, progressive
  E83.01
Lentiglobus (posterior) (congenital) Q12.8
Lentigo (congenital) L81.4
  maligna — *see also* Melanoma, in situ
    melanoma — *see* Melanoma
Lentivirus, as cause of disease classified
  elsewhere B97.31
Leontiasis
  ossium M85.2
  syphilitic (late) A52.78
    congenital A50.59
Lepothrix A48.8
Lepra — *see* Leprosy
Leprechaunism E34.8
Leprosy A30-
  with muscle disorder A30.9 [M63.80]
    ankle A30.9 [M63.8-]
    foot A30.9 [M63.8-]
    forearm A30.9 [M63.8-]
    hand A30.9 [M63.8-]
    lower leg A30.9 [M63.8-]
    multiple sites A30.9 [M63.89]
    pelvic region A30.9 [M63.8-]
    shoulder region A30.9 [M63.8-]
    specified site NEC A30.9 [M63.88]
    thigh A30.9 [M63.8-]
    upper arm A30.9 [M63.8-]
  anesthetic A30.9
  BB A30.3
  BL A30.4
  borderline (infiltrated) (neuritic) A30.3
    lepromatous A30.4
    tuberculoid A30.2
  BT A30.2
  dimorphous (infiltrated) (neuritic) A30.3
  I A30.0
  indeterminate (macular) (neuritic) A30.0
  lepromatous (diffuse) (infiltrated)
    (macular) (neuritic) (nodular) A30.5
  LL A30.5
  macular (early) (neuritic) (simple) A30.9
  maculoanesthetic A30.9
  mixed A30.3
  neural A30.9
  nodular A30.5
  primary neuritic A30.3
  specified type NEC A30.8
  TT A30.1
  tuberculoid (major) (minor) A30.1
Leptocytosis, hereditary D56.9
Leptomeningitis (chronic) (circumscribed)
  (hemorrhagic) (nonsuppurative) — *see*
  Meningitis
Leptomeningopathy G96.19
Leptospiral — *see* condition
Leptospirochetal — *see* condition

Leptospirosis A27.9
  canicola A27.89
  due to Leptospira interrogans serovar
    icterohaemorrhagiae A27.0
  icterohemorrhagica A27.0
  pomona A27.89
  Weil's disease A27.0
Leptus dermatitis B88.0
Leri's pleonosteosis Q78.8
Leri-Weill syndrome Q77.8
Leriche's syndrome (aortic bifurcation
  occlusion) I74.09
Lermoyez' syndrome — *see* Vertigo,
  peripheral NEC
Lesch-Nyhan syndrome E79.1
Leser-Trélat disease L82.1
  inflamed L82.0
Lesion(s) (nontraumatic)
  abducens nerve — *see* Strabismus,
    paralytic, sixth nerve
  alveolar process K08.9
  angiocentric immunoproliferative D47.Z9
  anorectal K62.9
  aortic (valve) I35.9
  auditory nerve — *see* subcategory H93.3
  basal ganglion G25.9
  bile duct — *see* Disease, bile duct
  biomechanical M99.9
    specified type NEC M99.89
      abdomen M99.89
      acromioclavicular M99.87
      cervical region M99.81
      cervicothoracic M99.81
      costochondral M99.88
      costovertebral M99.88
      head region M99.80
      hip M99.85
      lower extremity M99.86
      lumbar region M99.83
      lumbosacral M99.83
      occipitocervical M99.80
      pelvic region M99.85
      pubic M99.85
      rib cage M99.88
      sacral region M99.84
      sacrococcygeal M99.84
      sacroiliac M99.84
      specified NEC M99.89
      sternochondral M99.88
      sternoclavicular M99.87
      thoracic region M99.82
      thoracolumbar M99.82
      upper extremity M99.87
  bladder N32.9
  bone — *see* Disorder, bone
  brachial plexus G54.0
  brain G93.9
    congenital Q04.9
    vascular I67.9
      degenerative I67.9
      hypertensive I67.4
  buccal cavity K13.79
  calcified — *see* Calcification
  canthus — *see* Disorder, eyelid
  carate — *see* Pinta, lesions
  cardia K22.9
  cardiac (*see also* Disease, heart) I51.9
    congenital Q24.9
    valvular — *see* Endocarditis
  cauda equina G83.4
  cecum K63.9
  cerebral — *see* Lesion, brain
  cerebrovascular I67.9
    degenerative I67.9
    hypertensive I67.4
  cervical (nerve) root NEC G54.2
  chiasmal — *see* Disorder, optic, chiasm
  chorda tympani G51.8
  coin, lung R91.1
  colon K63.9
  congenital — *see* Anomaly, by site
  conjunctiva H11.9
  conus medullaris — *see* Injury, conus
    medullaris
  coronary artery — *see* Ischemia, heart
  cranial nerve G52.9
    eighth — *see* Disorder, ear
    eleventh G52.9
    fifth G50.9
    first G52.0
    fourth — *see* Strabismus, paralytic,
      fourth nerve
    seventh G51.9
    sixth — *see* Strabismus, paralytic, sixth
      nerve
    tenth G52.2
    twelfth G52.3
  cystic — *see* Cyst
  degenerative — *see* Degeneration
  duodenum K31.9

Lesion(s) (nontraumatic) — *continued*
  edentulous (alveolar) ridge, associated with
    trauma, due to traumatic occlusion
    K06.2
  en coup de sabre L94.1
  eyelid — *see* Disorder, eyelid
  gasserian ganglion G50.8
  gastric K31.9
  gastroduodenal K31.9
  gastrointestinal K63.9
  gingiva, associated with trauma K06.2
  glomerular
    focal and segmental (*see also* N00-N07
      with fourth character .1) N05.1
    minimal change (*see also* N00-N07 with
      fourth character .0) N05.0
  heart (organic) — *see* Disease, heart
  hyperchromic, due to pinta (carate) A67.1
  hyperkeratotic — *see* Hyperkeratosis
  hypothalamic E23.7
  ileocecal K63.9
  ileum K63.9
  iliohypogastric nerve G57.8-
  inflammatory — *see* Inflammation
  intestine K63.9
  intracerebral — *see* Lesion, brain
  intrachiasmal (optic) — *see* Disorder, optic,
    chiasm
  intracranial, space-occupying R90.0
  joint — *see* Disorder, joint
    sacroiliac (old) M53.3
  keratotic — *see* Keratosis
  kidney — *see* Disease, renal
  laryngeal nerve (recurrent) G52.2
  lip K13.0
  liver K76.9
  lumbosacral
    plexus G54.1
    root (nerve) NEC G54.4
  lung (coin) R91.1
  maxillary sinus J32.0
  mitral I05.9
  Morel-Lavallée — *see* Hematoma, by site
  motor cortex NEC G93.89
  mouth K13.79
  nerve G58.9
    femoral G57.2-
    median G56.1-
      carpal tunnel syndrome — *see*
        Syndrome, carpal tunnel
    plantar G57.6-
    popliteal (lateral) G57.3-
      medial G57.4-
    radial G56.3-
    sciatic G57.0-
    spinal — *see* Injury, nerve, spinal
    ulnar G56.2-
  nervous system, congenital Q07.9
  nonallopathic — *see* Lesion, biomechanical
  nose (internal) J34.89
  obstructive — *see* Obstruction
  obturator nerve G57.8-
  oral mucosa K13.70
  organ or site NEC — *see* Disease, by site
  osteolytic — *see* Osteolysis
  peptic K27.9
  periodontal, due to traumatic occlusion
    K05.5
  pharynx J39.2
  pigment, pigmented (skin) L81.9
  pinta — *see* Pinta, lesions
  polypoid — *see* Polyp
  prechiasmal (optic) — *see* Disorder, optic,
    chiasm
  primary (*see also* Syphilis, primary) A51.0
    carate A67.0
    pinta A67.0
    yaws A66.0
  pulmonary J98.4
    valve I37.9
  pylorus K31.9
  rectosigmoid K63.9
  retina, retinal H35.9
  sacroiliac (joint) (old) M53.3
  salivary gland K11.9
    benign lymphoepithelial K11.8
  saphenous nerve G57.8-
  sciatic nerve G57.0-
  secondary — *see* Syphilis, secondary
  shoulder (region) M75.9-
    specified NEC M75.8-
  sigmoid K63.9
  sinus (accessory) (nasal) J34.89
  skin L98.9
    suppurative L08.0
  SLAP S43.43-
  spinal cord G95.9
    congenital Q06.9
  spleen D73.89
  stomach K31.9

Lesion(s) (nontraumatic) — *continued*
  superior glenoid labrum S43.43-
  syphilitic — *see* Syphilis
  tertiary — *see* Syphilis, tertiary
  thoracic root (nerve) NEC G54.3
  tonsillar fossa J35.9
  tooth, teeth K08.9
    white spot
      chewing surface K02.51
      pit and fissure surface K02.51
      smooth surface K02.61
  traumatic — *see* specific type of injury by
    site
  tricuspid (valve) I07.9
    nonrheumatic I36.9
  trigeminal nerve G50.9
  ulcerated or ulcerative — *see* Ulcer, skin
  uterus N85.9
  vagus nerve G52.2
  valvular — *see* Endocarditis
  vascular I99.9
    affecting central nervous system I67.9
    following trauma NEC T14.8
    umbilical cord, complicating delivery
      O69.5
  warty — *see* Verruca
  white spot (tooth)
    chewing surface K02.51
    pit and fissure surface K02.51
    smooth surface K02.61
Lethargic — *see* condition
Lethargy R53.83
Letterer-Siwe's disease C96.0
Leukemia, leukemic C95.9-
  acute basophilic C94.8-
  acute bilineal C95.0-
  acute erythroid C94.0-
  acute lymphoblastic C91.0-
  acute megakaryoblastic C94.2-
  acute megakaryocytic C94.2-
  acute mixed lineage C95.0-
  acute monoblastic
    (monoblastic/monocytic) C93.0-
  acute monocytic (monoblastic/monocytic)
    C93.0-
  acute myeloblastic (minimal
    differentiation) (with maturation)
    C92.0-
  acute myeloid
    with
      11q23-abnormality C92.6-
      dysplasia of remaining hematopoesis
        and/or myelodysplastic disease
        in its history C92.A-
      multilineage dysplasia C92.A-
      variation of MLL-gene C92.6-
    M6(a)(b) C94.0-
    M7 C94.2-
  acute myelomonocytic C92.5-
  acute promyelocytic C92.4-
  adult T-cell (HTLV-1-associated) (acute
    variant) (chronic variant)
    (lymphomatoid variant) (smouldering
    variant) C91.5-
  aggressive NK-cell C94.8-
  AML (1/ETO) (M0) (M1) (M2) (without a
    FAB classification) C92.0-
  AML M3 C92.4-
  AML M4 (Eo with inv(16) or t(16;16))
    C92.5-
  AML M5 C93.0-
  AML M5a C93.0-
  AML M5b C93.0-
  AML Me with t(15;17) and variants C92.4-
  atypical chronic myeloid, BCR/ABL-
    negative C92.2-
  biphenotypic acute C95.0-
  blast cell C95.0-
  Burkitt-type, mature B-cell C91.A-
  chronic lymphocytic, of B-cell type C91.1-
  chronic monocytic C93.1-
  chronic myelogenous (Philadelphia
    chromosome (Ph1) positive) (t(9;22))
    (q34;q11) (with crisis of blast cells)
    C92.1-
  chronic myeloid, BCR/ABL-positive
    C92.1-
    atypical, BCR/ABL-negative C92.2-
  chronic myelomonocytic C93.1-
  chronic neutrophilic D47.1
  CMML (-1) (-2) (with eosinophilia) C93.1-
  granulocytic (*see also* Category C92)
    C92.9-
  hairy cell C91.4-
  juvenile myelomonocytic C93.3-
  lymphoid C91.9-
    specified NEC C91.Z-

Leukemia, leukemic C95.9- — *continued*
  mast cell C94.3-
  mature B-cell, Burkitt-type C91.A-
  monocytic (subacute) C93.9-
    specified NEC C93.Z-
  myelogenous (*see also* Category C92)
    C92.9-
  myeloid C92.9-
    specified NEC C92.Z-
  plasma cell C90.1-
  plasmacytic C90.1-
  prolymphocytic
    of B-cell type C91.3-
    of T-cell type C91.6-
  specified NEC C94.8-
  stem cell, of unclear lineage C95.0-
  subacute lymphocytic C91.9-
  T-cell large granular lymphocytic C91.Z-
  unspecified cell type C95.9-
    acute C95.0-
    chronic C95.1-
Leukemoid reaction (*see also* Reaction, leukemoid) D72.823-
Leukoaraiosis (hypertensive) I67.81
Leukoariosis — *see* Leukoaraiosis
Leukocoria — *see* Disorder, globe, degenerated condition, leucocoria
Leukocytopenia D72.819
Leukocytosis D72.829
  eosinophilic D72.1
Leukoderma, leukodermia NEC L81.5
  syphilitic A51.39
    late A52.79
Leukodystrophy E75.29
Leukoedema, oral epithelium K13.29
Leukoencephalitis G04.81
  acute (subacute) hemorrhagic G36.1
    postimmunization or postvaccinal G04.02
  postinfectious G04.01
  subacute sclerosing A81.1
  van Bogaert's (sclerosing) A81.1
Leukoencephalopathy (*see also* Encephalopathy) G93.49
  Binswanger's I67.3
  heroin vapor G92
  metachromatic E75.25
  multifocal (progressive) A81.2
  postimmunization and postvaccinal G04.02
  progressive multifocal A81.2
  reversible, posterior G93.6
  van Bogaert's (sclerosing) A81.1
  vascular, progressive I67.3
Leukoerythroblastosis D75.9
Leukokeratosis — *see also* Leukoplakia
  mouth K13.21
  nicotina palati K13.24
  oral mucosa K13.21
  tongue K13.21
  vocal cord J38.3
Leukokraurosis vulva(e) N90.4
Leukoma (cornea) — *see also* Opacity, cornea
  adherent H17.0-
  interfering with central vision — *see* Opacity, cornea, central
Leukomalacia, cerebral, newborn P91.2
  periventricular P91.2
Leukomelanopathy, hereditary D72.0
Leukonychia (punctata) (striata) L60.8
  congenital Q84.4
Leukopathia unguium L60.8
  congenital Q84.4
Leukopenia D72.819
  basophilic D72.818
  chemotherapy (cancer) induced D70.1
  congenital D70.0
  cyclic D70.0
  drug induced NEC D70.2
    due to cytoreductive cancer chemotherapy D70.1
  eosinophilic D72.818
  familial D70.0
  infantile genetic D70.0
  malignant D70.9
  periodic D70.0
  transitory neonatal P61.5
Leukopenic — *see* condition
Leukoplakia
  anus K62.89
  bladder (postinfectional) N32.89
  buccal K13.21
  cervix (uteri) N88.0
  esophagus K22.8
  gingiva K13.21
  hairy (oral mucosa) (tongue) K13.3

Leukoplakia — *continued*
  kidney (pelvis) N28.89
  larynx J38.7
  lip K13.21
  mouth K13.21
  oral epithelium, including tongue (mucosa) K13.21
  palate K13.21
  pelvis (kidney) N28.89
  penis (infectional) N48.0
  rectum K62.89
  syphilitic (late) A52.79
  tongue K13.21
  ureter (postinfectional) N28.89
  urethra (postinfectional) N36.8
  uterus N85.8
  vagina N89.4
  vocal cord J38.3
  vulva N90.4
Leukorrhea N89.8
  due to Trichomonas (vaginalis) A59.00
  trichomonal A59.00
Leukosarcoma C85.9-
Levocardia (isolated) Q24.1
  with situs inversus Q89.3
Levotransposition Q20.5
Lev's disease or syndrome (acquired complete heart block) I44.2
Levulosuria — *see* Fructosuria
Levurid L30.2
Lewy body(ies) (dementia) (disease) G31.83
Leyden-Moebius dystrophy G71.0
Leydig cell
  carcinoma
    specified site — *see* Neoplasm, malignant, by site
    unspecified site
      female C56.9
      male C62.9-
  tumor
    benign
      specified site — *see* Neoplasm, benign, by site
      unspecified site
        female D27-
        male D29.2-
    malignant
      specified site — *see* Neoplasm, malignant, by site
      unspecified site
        female C56-
        male C62.9-
    specified site — *see* Neoplasm, uncertain behavior, by site
    unspecified site
      female D39.1-
      male D40.1-
Leydig-Sertoli cell tumor
  specified site — *see* Neoplasm, benign, by site
  unspecified site
    female D27-
    male D29.2-
LGSIL (low grade squamous intraepithelial lesion on cytologic smear of)
  anus R85.612
  cervix R87.612
  vagina R87.622
Liar, pathologic F60.2
Libido
  decreased R68.82
Libman-Sacks disease M32.11
Lice (infestation) B85.2
  body (Pediculus corporis) B85.1
  crab B85.3
  head (Pediculus capitis) B85.0
  mixed (classifiable to more than one of the titles B85.0-B85.3) B85.4
  pubic (Phthirus pubis) B85.3
Lichen L28.0
  albus L90.0
    penis N48.0
    vulva N90.4
  amyloidosis E85.4 [L99]
  atrophicus L90.0
    penis N48.0
    vulva N90.4
  congenital Q82.8
  myxedematosus L98.5
  nitidus L44.1
  pilaris Q82.8
    acquired L85.8
  planopilaris L66.1

Lichen L28.0 — *continued*
  planus (chronicus) L43.9
    annularis L43.8
    bullous L43.1
    follicular L66.1
    hypertrophic L43.0
    moniliformis L44.3
    of Wilson L43.9
    specified NEC L43.8
    subacute (active) L43.3
    tropicus L43.3
  ruber
    acuminatus L44.0
    moniliformis L44.3
    planus L43.9
  sclerosus (et atrophicus) L90.0
    penis N48.0
    vulva N90.4
  scrofulosus (primary) (tuberculous) A18.4
  simplex (chronicus) (circumscriptus) L28.0
  striatus L44.2
  urticatus L28.2
Lichenification L28.0
Lichenoides tuberculosis (primary) A18.4
Lichtheim's disease or syndrome — *see* Degeneration, combined
Lien migrans D73.89
Ligament — *see* condition
Light
  for gestational age — *see* Light for dates
  headedness R42
Light-for-dates (infant) P05.00
  with weight of
    1000-1249 grams P05.04
    1250-1499 grams P05.05
    1500-1749 grams P05.06
    1750-1999 grams P05.07
    2000-2499 grams P05.08
    499 grams or less P05.01
    500-749 grams P05.02
    750-999 grams P05.03
  affecting management of pregnancy O36.59-
  and small-for-dates — *see* Small for dates
Lightning (effects) (stroke) (struck by) T75.00
  burn — *see* Burn
  foot E53.8
  shock T75.01
  specified effect NEC T75.09
Lightwood-Albright syndrome N25.89
Lightwood's disease or syndrome (renal tubular acidosis) N25.89
Lignac(-de Toni) (-Fanconi) (-Debré) disease or syndrome E72.09
  with cystinosis E72.04
Ligneous thyroiditis E06.5
Likoff's syndrome I20.8
Limb — *see* condition
Limbic epilepsy personality syndrome F07.0
Limitation, limited
  activities due to disability Z73.6
  cardiac reserve — *see* Disease, heart
  eye muscle duction, traumatic — *see* Strabismus, mechanical
  mandibular range of motion M26.52
Lindau(-von Hippel) disease Q85.8
Line(s)
  Beau's L60.4
  Harris' — *see* Arrest, epiphyseal
  Hudson's (cornea) — *see* Pigmentation, cornea, anterior
  Stähli's (cornea) — *see* Pigmentation, cornea, anterior
Linea corneae senilis — *see* Change, cornea, senile
Lingua
  geographica K14.1
  nigra (villosa) K14.3
  plicata K14.5
  tylosis K13.29
Lingual — *see* condition
Linguatulosis B88.8
Linitis (gastric) plastica C16.9
Lip — *see* condition
Lipedema — *see* Edema
Lipemia — *see also* Hyperlipidemia
  retina, retinalis E78.3
Lipidosis E75.6
  cerebral (infantile) (juvenile) (late) E75.4
  cerebroretinal E75.4
  cerebroside E75.22
  cholesterol (cerebral) E75.5
  glycolipid E75.21
  hepatosplenomegalic E78.3
  sphingomyelin — *see* Niemann-Pick disease or syndrome
  sulfatide E75.29

Lipoadenoma — *see* Neoplasm, benign, by site
Lipoblastoma — *see* Lipoma
Lipoblastomatosis — *see* Lipoma
Lipochondrodystrophy E76.01
Lipochrome histiocytosis (familial) D71
Lipodermatosclerosis — *see* Varix, leg, with, inflammation
  ulcerated — *see* Varix, leg, with, ulcer, with inflammation by site
Lipodystrophia progressiva E88.1
Lipodystrophy (progressive) E88.1
  insulin E88.1
  intestinal K90.81
  mesenteric K65.4
Lipofibroma — *see* Lipoma
Lipofuscinosis, neuronal (with ceroidosis) E75.4
Lipogranuloma, sclerosing L92.8
Lipogranulomatosis E78.89
Lipoid — *see also* condition
  histiocytosis D76.3
    essential E75.29
  nephrosis N04.9
  proteinosis of Urbach E78.89
Lipoidemia — *see* Hyperlipidemia
Lipoidosis — *see* Lipidosis
Lipoma D17.9
  fetal D17.9
  fat cell D17.9
  infiltrating D17.9
  intramuscular D17.9
  pleomorphic D17.9
  site classification
    arms (skin) (subcutaneous) D17.2-
    connective tissue D17.30
      intra-abdominal D17.5
      intrathoracic D17.4
      peritoneum D17.79
      retroperitoneum D17.79
      specified site NEC D17.39
      spermatic cord D17.6
    face (skin) (subcutaneous) D17.0
    genitourinary organ NEC D17.72
    head (skin) (subcutaneous) D17.0
    intra-abdominal D17.5
    intrathoracic D17.4
    kidney D17.71
    legs (skin) (subcutaneous) D17.2-
    neck (skin) (subcutaneous) D17.0
    peritoneum D17.79
    retroperitoneum D17.79
    skin D17.30
      specified site NEC D17.39
    specified site NEC D17.79
    spermatic cord D17.6
    subcutaneous D17.30
      specified site NEC D17.39
    trunk (skin) (subcutaneous) D17.1
    unspecified D17.30
  spindle cell D17.9
Lipomatosis E88.2
  dolorosa (Dercum) E88.2
  fetal — *see* Lipoma
  Launois-Bensaude E88.89
Lipomyoma — *see* Lipoma
Lipomyxoma — *see* Lipoma
Lipomyxosarcoma — *see* Neoplasm, connective tissue, malignant
Lipoprotein metabolism disorder E78.9
Lipoproteinemia E78.5
  broad-beta E78.2
  floating-beta E78.2
  hyper-pre-beta E78.1
Liposarcoma — *see also* Neoplasm, connective tissue, malignant
  dedifferentiated — *see* Neoplasm, connective tissue, malignant
  differentiated type — *see* Neoplasm, connective tissue, malignant
  embryonal — *see* Neoplasm, connective tissue, malignant
  mixed type — *see* Neoplasm, connective tissue, malignant
  myxoid — *see* Neoplasm, connective tissue, malignant
  pleomorphic — *see* Neoplasm, connective tissue, malignant
  round cell — *see* Neoplasm, connective tissue, malignant
  well differentiated type — *see* Neoplasm, connective tissue, malignant
Liposynovitis prepatellaris E88.89
Lipping, cervix N86
Lipschütz disease or ulcer N76.6
Lipuria R82.0
  schistosomiasis (bilharziasis) B65.0
Lisping F80.0

Luxation — see also Dislocation
eyeball (nontraumatic) — see Luxation, globe
birth injury P15.3
globe, nontraumatic H44.82-
lacrimal gland — see Dislocation, lacrimal gland
lens (old) (partial) (spontaneous)
congenital Q12.1
syphilitic A50.39
Lycanthropy F22
Lyell's syndrome L51.2
due to drug L51.2
correct substance properly administered — see Table of Drugs and Chemicals, by drug, adverse effect
overdose or wrong substance given or taken — see Table of Drugs and Chemicals, by drug, poisoning
Lyme disease A69.20
Lymph
gland or node — see condition
scrotum — see Infestation, filarial
Lymphadenitis I88.9
with ectopic or molar pregnancy O08.0
acute L04.9
axilla L04.2
face L04.0
head L04.0
hip L04.3
limb
lower L04.3
upper L04.2
neck L04.0
shoulder L04.2
specified site NEC L04.8
trunk L04.1
anthracosis (occupational) J60
any site, except mesenteric I88.9
chronic I88.1
subacute I88.1
breast
gestational — see Mastitis, obstetric
puerperal, postpartum (nonpurulent) O91.22
chancroidal (congenital) A57
chronic I88.1
mesenteric I88.0
due to
Brugia (malayi) B74.1
timori B74.2
chlamydial lymphogranuloma A55
diphtheria (toxin) A36.89
lymphogranuloma venereum A55
Wuchereria bancrofti B74.0
following ectopic or molar pregnancy O08.0
gonorrheal A54.89
infective — see Lymphadenitis, acute
mesenteric (acute) (chronic) (nonspecific) (subacute) I88.0
due to Salmonella typhi A01.09
tuberculous A18.39
mycobacterial A31.8
purulent — see Lymphadenitis, acute
pyogenic — see Lymphadenitis, acute
regional, nonbacterial I88.8
septic — see Lymphadenitis, acute
subacute, unspecified site I88.1
suppurative — see Lymphadenitis, acute
syphilitic (early) (secondary) A51.49
late A52.79
tuberculous — see Tuberculosis, lymph gland
venereal (chlamydial) A55
Lymphadenoid goiter E06.3
Lymphadenopathy (generalized) R59.1
angioimmunoblastic, with dysproteinemia (AILD) C86.5
due to toxoplasmosis (acquired) B58.89
congenital (acute) (subacute) (chronic) P37.1
localized R59.0
syphilitic (early) (secondary) A51.49
Lymphadenosis R59.1
Lymphangiectasis I89.0
conjunctiva H11.89
postinfectional I89.0
scrotum I89.0
Lymphangiectatic elephantiasis, nonfilarial I89.0
Lymphangioendothelioma D18.1
malignant — see Neoplasm, connective tissue, malignant
Lymphangioma D18.1
capillary D18.1
cavernous D18.1
cystic D18.1
malignant — see Neoplasm, connective tissue, malignant

Lymphangiomyoma D18.1
Lymphangioleiomyomatosis J84.81
Lymphangiomyomatosis J84.81
Lymphangiosarcoma — see Neoplasm, connective tissue, malignant
Lymphangitis I89.1
with
abscess — code by site under Abscess
cellulitis — code by site under Cellulitis
ectopic or molar pregnancy O08.0
acute L03.91
abdominal wall L03.321
ankle — see Lymphangitis, acute, lower limb
arm — see Lymphangitis, acute, upper limb
auricle (ear) — see Lymphangitis, acute, ear
axilla L03.12-
back (any part) L03.322
buttock L03.327
cervical (meaning neck) L03.222
cheek (external) L03.212
chest wall L03.323
digit
finger — see Lymphangitis, acute, finger
toe — see Lymphangitis, acute, toe
ear (external) H60.1-
external auditory canal — see Lymphangitis, acute, ear
eyelid — see Abscess, eyelid
face NEC L03.212
finger (intrathecal) (periosteal) (subcutaneous) (subcuticular) L03.02-
foot — see Lymphangitis, acute, lower limb
gluteal (region) L03.327
groin L03.324
hand — see Lymphangitis, acute, upper limb
head NEC L03.891
face (any part, except ear, eye and nose) L03.212
heel — see Lymphangitis, acute, lower limb
hip — see Lymphangitis, acute, lower limb
jaw (region) L03.212
knee — see Lymphangitis, acute, lower limb
leg — see Lymphangitis, acute, lower limb
lower limb L03.12-
toe — see Lymphangitis, acute, toe
navel L03.326
neck (region) L03.222
orbit, orbital — see Cellulitis, orbit
pectoral (region) L03.323
perineal, perineum L03.325
scalp (any part) L03.891
shoulder — see Lymphangitis, acute, upper limb
specified site NEC L03.898
thigh — see Lymphangitis, acute, lower limb
thumb (intrathecal) (periosteal) (subcutaneous) (subcuticular) — see Lymphangitis, acute, finger
toe (intrathecal) (periosteal) (subcutaneous) (subcuticular) L03.04-
trunk L03.329
abdominal wall L03.321
back (any part) L03.322
buttock L03.327
chest wall L03.323
groin L03.324
perineal, perineum L03.325
umbilicus L03.326
umbilicus L03.326
upper limb L03.12-
axilla — see Lymphangitis, acute, axilla
finger — see Lymphangitis, acute, finger
thumb — see Lymphangitis, acute, finger
wrist — see Lymphangitis, acute, upper limb
breast
gestational — see Mastitis, obstetric
chancroidal A57
chronic (any site) I89.1
due to
Brugia (malayi) B74.1
timori B74.2
Wuchereria bancrofti B74.0

Lymphangitis I89.1 — continued
following ectopic or molar pregnancy O08.89
penis
acute N48.29
gonococcal (acute) (chronic) A54.09
puerperal, postpartum, childbirth O86.89
strumous, tuberculous A18.2
subacute (any site) I89.1
tuberculous — see Tuberculosis, lymph gland
Lymphatic (vessel) — see condition
Lymphatism E32.8
Lymphedema (acquired) — see also Elephantiasis
congenital Q82.0
hereditary (chronic) (idiopathic) Q82.0
postmastectomy I97.2
praecox I89.0
secondary I89.0
surgical NEC I97.89
postmastectomy (syndrome) I97.2
Lymphoblastic — see condition
Lymphoblastoma (diffuse) — see Lymphoma, lymphoblastic (diffuse)
giant follicular — see Lymphoma, lymphoblastic (diffuse)
macrofollicular — see Lymphoma, lymphoblastic (diffuse)
Lymphocele I89.8
Lymphocytic
chorioencephalitis (acute) (serous) A87.2
choriomeningitis (acute) (serous) A87.2
meningoencephalitis A87.2
Lymphocytoma, benign cutis L98.8
Lymphocytopenia D72.810
Lymphocytosis (symptomatic) D72.820
infectious (acute) B33.8
Lymphoepithelioma — see Neoplasm, malignant, by site
Lymphogranuloma (malignant) — see also Lymphoma, Hodgkin
chlamydial A55
inguinale A55
venereum (any site) (chlamydial) (with stricture of rectum) A55
Lymphogranulomatosis (malignant) — see also Lymphoma, Hodgkin
benign (Boeck's sarcoid) (Schaumann's) D86.1
Lymphohistiocytosis, hemophagocytic (familial) D76.1
Lymphoid — see condition
Lymphoma (of) (malignant) C85.90
adult T-cell (HTLV-1-associated) (acute variant) (chronic variant) (lymphomatoid variant) (smouldering variant) C91.5-
anaplastic large cell
ALK-negative C84.7-
ALK-positive C84.6-
CD30-positive C84.6-
primary cutaneous C86.6
angioimmunoblastic T-cell C86.5
BALT C88.4
B-cell C85.1-
blastic NK-cell C86.4
B-precursor C83.5-
bronchial-associated lymphoid tissue [BALT-lymphoma] C88.4
Burkitt (atypical) C83.7-
Burkitt-like C83.7-
centrocytic C83.1-
cutaneous follicle center C82.6-
cutaneous T-cell C84.A-
diffuse follicle center C82.5-
diffuse large cell C83.3-
anaplastic C83.3-
B-cell C83.3-
CD30-positive C83.3-
centroblastic C83.3-
immunoblastic C83.3-
plasmablastic C83.3-
subtype not specified C83.3-
T-cell rich C83.3-
enteropathy-type (associated) (intestinal) T-cell C86.2
extranodal marginal zone B-cell lymphoma of mucosa-associated lymphoid tissue [MALT-lymphoma] C88.4
extranodal NK/T-cell, nasal type C86.0
follicular C82.9-
grade
I C82.0-
II C82.1-
III C82.2-
IIIa C82.3-
IIIb C82.4-
specified NEC C82.8-

Lymphoma (of) (malignant) C85.90 — continued
hepatosplenic T-cell (alpha-beta) (gamma-delta) C86.1
histiocytic C85.9-
true C96.A
Hodgkin C81.9
classical C81.7-
lymphocyte depleted C81.3-
lymphocyte-rich C81.4-
mixed cellularity C81.2-
nodular sclerosis C81.1-
specified NEC C81.7-
lymphocyte depleted classical C81.3-
lymphocyte-rich classical C81.4-
mixed cellularity classical C81.2-
nodular
lymphocyte predominant C81.0-
sclerosis classical C81.1-
intravascular large B-cell C83.8-
Lennert's C84.4-
lymphoblastic (diffuse) C83.5-
lymphoblastic B-cell C83.5-
lymphoblastic T-cell C83.5-
lymphoepithelioid C84.4-
lymphoplasmacytic C83.0-
with IgM-production C88.0
MALT C88.4
mantle cell C83.1-
mature T-cell NEC C84.4-
mature T/NK-cell C84.9-
specified NEC C84.Z-
mediastinal (thymic) large B-cell C85.2-
Mediterranean C88.3
mucosa-associated lymphoid tissue [MALT-lymphoma] C88.4
NK/T cell C84.9-
nodal marginal zone C83.0-
non-follicular (diffuse) C83.9-
specified NEC C83.8-
non-Hodgkin (see also Lymphoma, by type) C85.9-
specified NEC C85.8-
non-leukemic variant of B-CLL C83.0-
peripheral T-cell, not classified C84.4-
primary cutaneous
anaplastic large cell C86.6
CD30-positive large T-cell C86.6
primary effusion B-cell C83.8-
SALT C88.4
skin-associated lymphoid tissue [SALT-lymphoma] C88.4
small cell B-cell C83.0-
splenic marginal zone C83.0-
subcutaneous panniculitis-like T-cell C86.3
T-precursor C83.5-
true histiocytic C96.A
Lymphomatosis — see Lymphoma
Lymphopathia venereum, veneris A55
Lymphopenia D72.810
Lymphoplasmacyticleukemia — see Leukemia, chronic lymphocytic, B-cell type
Lymphoproliferation, X-linked disease D82.3
Lymphoreticulosis, benign (of inoculation) A28.1
Lymphorrhea I89.8
Lymphosarcoma (diffuse) (see also Lymphoma) C85.9-
Lymphostasis I89.8
Lypemania — see Melancholia
Lysine and hydroxylysine metabolism disorder E72.3
Lyssa — see Rabies

M

Macacus ear Q17.3
Maceration, wet feet, tropical (syndrome) T69.02-
MacLeod's syndrome J43.0
Macrocephalia, macrocephaly Q75.3
Macrocheilia, macrochilia (congenital) Q18.6
Macrocolon (see also Megacolon) Q43.1
Macrocornea Q15.8
  with glaucoma Q15.0
Macrocytic — see condition
Macrocytosis D75.89
Macrodactylia, macrodactylism (fingers) (thumbs) Q74.0
  toes Q74.2
Macrodontia K00.2
Macrogenia M26.05
Macrogenitosomia (adrenal) (male) (praecox) E25.9
  congenital E25.0
Macroglobulinemia (idiopathic) (primary) C88.0
  monoclonal (essential) D47.2
  Waldenström C88.0
Macroglossia (congenital) Q38.2
  acquired K14.8
Macrognathia, macrognathism (congenital) (mandibular) (maxillary) M26.09
Macrogyria (congenital) Q04.8
Macrohydrocephalus — see Hydrocephalus
Macromastia — see Hypertrophy, breast
Macrophthalmos Q11.3
  in congenital glaucoma Q15.0
Macropsia H53.15
Macrosigmoid K59.3
  congenital Q43.2
Macrospondylitis, acromegalic E22.0
Macrostomia (congenital) Q18.4
Macrotia (external ear) (congenital) Q17.1
Macula
  cornea, corneal — see Opacity, cornea
  degeneration (atrophic) (exudative) (senile) — see also Degeneration, macula
  hereditary — see Dystrophy, retina
Maculae ceruleae B85.1
Maculopathy, toxic — see Degeneration, macula, toxic
Madarosis (eyelid) H02.729
  left H02.726
    lower H02.725
    upper H02.724
  right H02.723
    lower H02.722
    upper H02.721
Madelung's
  deformity (radius) Q74.0
  disease
    radial deformity Q74.0
    symmetrical lipomas, neck E88.89
Madness — see Psychosis
Madura
  foot B47.9
    actinomycotic B47.1
    mycotic B47.0
Maduromycosis B47.0
Maffucci's syndrome Q78.4
Magnesium metabolism disorder — see Disorder, metabolism, magnesium
Main en griffe (acquired) — see also Deformity, limb, clawhand
  congenital Q74.0
Maintenance (encounter for)
  antineoplastic chemotherapy Z51.11
  antineoplastic radiation therapy Z51.0
  methadone F11.20
Majocchi's
  disease L81.7
  granuloma B35.8
Major — see condition
Mal de los pintos — see Pinta
Mal de mer T75.3
Malabar itch (any site) B35.5
Malabsorption K90.9
  calcium K90.89
  carbohydrate K90.4
  disaccharide E73.9
  fat K90.4
  galactose E74.20
  glucose(-galactose) E74.39
  intestinal K90.9
    specified NEC K90.89
  isomaltose E74.31
  lactose E73.9

Malabsorption K90.9 — continued
  methionine E72.19
  monosaccharide E74.39
  postgastrectomy K91.2
  postsurgical K91.2
  protein K90.4
  starch K90.4
  sucrose E74.39
  syndrome K90.9
    postsurgical K91.2
Malacia, bone (adult) M83.9
  juvenile — see Rickets
Malacoplakia
  bladder N32.89
  pelvis (kidney) N28.89
  ureter N28.89
  urethra N36.8
Malacosteon, juvenile — see Rickets
Maladaptation — see Maladjustment
Maladie de Roger Q21.0
Maladjustment
  conjugal Z63.0
    involving divorce or estrangement Z63.5
  educational Z55.4
  family Z63.9
  marital Z63.0
    involving divorce or estrangement Z63.5
  occupational NEC Z56.89
  simple, adult — see Disorder, adjustment
  situational — see Disorder, adjustment
  social Z60.9
    due to
      acculturation difficulty Z60.3
      discrimination and persecution (perceived) Z60.5
      exclusion and isolation Z60.4
      life-cycle (phase of life) transition Z60.0
      rejection Z60.4
      specified reason NEC Z60.8
Malaise R53.81
Malakoplakia — see Malacoplakia
Malaria, malarial (fever) B54
  with
    blackwater fever B50.8
      hemoglobinuric (bilious) B50.8
    hemoglobinuria B50.8
  accidentally induced (therapeutically) — code by type under Malaria
  □□d B50.9
  cerebral B50.0 [G94]
  clinically diagnosed (without parasitological confirmation) B54
  congenital NEC P37.4
    falciparum P37.3
  congestion, congestive B54
  continued (fever) B50.9
  estivo-autumnal B50.9
  falciparum B50.9
    with complications NEC B50.8
      cerebral B50.0 [G94]
    severe B50.8
  hemorrhagic B54
  malariae B52.9
    with
      complications NEC B52.8
      glomerular disorder B52.0
  malignant (tertian) — see Malaria, falciparum
  mixed infections — code to first listed type in B50-B53
  ovale B53.0
  parasitologically confirmed NEC B53.8
  pernicious, acute — see Malaria, falciparum
  Plasmodium (P.)
    falciparum NEC — see Malaria, falciparum
    malariae NEC B52.9
      with Plasmodium
        falciparum (and or vivax) — see Malaria, falciparum
        vivax — see also Malaria, vivax
        and falciparum — see Malaria, falciparum
    ovale B53.0
      with Plasmodium malariae — see also Malaria, malariae
      and vivax — see also Malaria, vivax
      and falciparum — see Malaria, falciparum
    simian B53.1
      with Plasmodium malariae — see also Malaria, malariae
      and vivax — see also Malaria, vivax
      and falciparum — see Malaria, falciparum

Malaria, malarial (fever) B54 — continued
  Plasmodium (P.) — continued
    vivax NEC B51.9
      with Plasmodium falciparum — see Malaria, falciparum
    quartan — see Malaria, malariae
    quotidian — see Malaria, falciparum
    recurrent B54
    remittent B54
    specified type NEC (parasitologically confirmed) B53.8
    spleen B54
    subtertian (fever) — see Malaria, falciparum
    tertian (benign) — see also Malaria, vivax
      malignant B50.9
    tropical B50.9
    typhoid B54
    vivax B51.9
      with
        complications NEC B51.8
        ruptured spleen B51.0
Malassez's disease (cystic) N50.8
Malassimilation K90.9
Maldescent, testis Q53.9
  bilateral Q53.20
    abdominal Q53.21
    perineal Q53.22
  unilateral Q53.10
    abdominal Q53.11
    perineal Q53.12
Maldevelopment — see also Anomaly
  brain Q07.9
  colon Q43.9
  hip Q74.2
    congenital dislocation Q65.2
      bilateral Q65.1
      unilateral Q65.0-
  mastoid process Q75.8
  middle ear Q16.4
    except ossicles Q16.4
    ossicles Q16.3
  ossicles Q16.3
  spine Q76.49
  toe Q74.2
Male type pelvis Q74.2
  with disproportion (fetopelvic) O33.3
    causing obstructed labor O65.3
Malformation (congenital) — see also Anomaly
  adrenal gland Q89.1
  affecting multiple systems with skeletal changes NEC Q87.5
  alimentary tract Q45.9
    specified type NEC Q45.8
    upper Q40.9
      specified type NEC Q40.8
  aorta Q25.9
    atresia Q25.2
    coarctation (preductal) (postductal) Q25.1
    patent ductus arteriosus Q25.0
    specified type NEC Q25.4
    stenosis (supravalvular) Q25.3
  aortic valve Q23.9
    specified NEC Q23.8
  arteriovenous, aneurysmatic (congenital) Q27.30
    brain Q28.2
    cerebral Q28.2
    peripheral Q27.30
      digestive system Q27.33
      lower limb Q27.32
      other specified site Q27.39
      renal vessel Q27.34
      upper limb Q27.31
    precerebral vessels (nonruptured) Q28.0
  auricle
    ear (congenital) Q17.3
      acquired H61.119
        left H61.112
          with right H61.113
        right H61.111
          with left H61.113
  bile duct Q44.5
  bladder Q64.79
    aplasia Q64.5
    diverticulum Q64.6
    exstrophy — see Exstrophy, bladder
    neck obstruction Q64.31
  bone Q79.9
    face Q75.9
      specified type NEC Q75.8
    skull Q75.9
      specified type NEC Q75.8
  brain (multiple) Q04.9
    arteriovenous Q28.2
    specified type NEC Q04.8

Malformation (congenital) (see also Anomaly) — continued
  branchial cleft Q18.2
  breast Q83.9
    specified type NEC Q83.8
  broad ligament Q50.6
  bronchus Q32.4
  bursa Q79.9
  cardiac
    chambers Q20.9
      specified type NEC Q20.8
    septum Q21.9
      specified type NEC Q21.8
  cerebral Q04.9
    vessels Q28.3
  cervix uteri Q51.9
    specified type NEC Q51.828
  Chiari
    Type I G93.5
    Type II Q07.01
  choroid (congenital) Q14.3
    plexus Q07.8
  circulatory system Q28.9
  cochlea Q16.5
  cornea Q13.4
  coronary vessels Q24.5
  corpus callosum (congenital) Q04.0
  diaphragm Q79.1
  digestive system NEC, specified type NEC Q45.8
  dura Q07.9
    brain Q04.9
    spinal Q06.9
  ear Q17.9
    causing impairment of hearing Q16.9
    external Q17.9
      accessory auricle Q17.0
      causing impairment of hearing Q16.9
      absence of
        auditory canal Q16.1
        auricle Q16.0
      macrotia Q17.1
      microtia Q17.2
      misplacement Q17.4
      misshapen NEC Q17.3
      prominence Q17.5
      specified type NEC Q17.8
    inner Q16.5
    middle Q16.4
      absence of eustachian tube Q16.2
      ossicles (fusion) Q16.3
    ossicles Q16.3
    specified type NEC Q17.8
  epididymis Q55.4
  esophagus Q39.9
    specified type NEC Q39.8
  eye Q15.9
    lid Q10.3
    specified NEC Q15.8
  fallopian tube Q50.6
  genital organ — see Anomaly, genitalia
  great
    artery Q25.9
      aorta — see Malformation, aorta
      pulmonary artery — see Malformation, pulmonary, artery
      specified type NEC Q25.8
    vein Q26.9
      anomalous
        portal venous connection Q26.5
        pulmonary venous connection Q26.4
        partial Q26.3
        total Q26.2
      persistent left superior vena cava Q26.1
      portal vein-hepatic artery fistula Q26.6
      specified type NEC Q26.8
      vena cava stenosis, congenital Q26.0
  gum Q38.6
  hair Q84.2
  heart Q24.9
    specified type NEC Q24.8
  integument Q84.9
    specified type NEC Q84.8
  internal ear Q16.5
  intestine Q43.9
    specified type NEC Q43.8
  iris Q13.2
  joint Q74.9
    ankle Q74.2
    lumbosacral Q76.49
    sacroiliac Q74.2
    specified type NEC Q74.8

Malformation (congenital) (see also Anomaly) — continued
kidney Q63.9
  accessory Q63.0
  giant Q63.3
  horseshoe Q63.1
  hydronephrosis Q62.0
  malposition Q63.2
  specified type NEC Q63.8
lacrimal apparatus Q10.6
lingual Q38.3
lip Q38.0
liver Q44.7
lung Q33.9
meninges or membrane (congenital) Q07.9
  cerebral Q04.8
  spinal (cord) Q06.9
middle ear Q16.4
  ossicles Q16.3
mitral valve Q23.9
  specified NEC Q23.8
Mondini's (congenital) (malformation, cochlea) Q16.5
mouth (congenital) Q38.6
multiple types NEC Q89.7
musculoskeletal system Q79.9
myocardium Q24.8
nail Q84.6
nervous system (central) Q07.9
nose Q30.9
  specified type NEC Q30.8
optic disc Q14.2
orbit Q10.7
ovary Q50.39
palate Q38.5
parathyroid gland Q89.2
pelvic organs or tissues NEC
  in pregnancy or childbirth O34.8-
    causing obstructed labor O65.5
penis Q55.69
  aplasia Q55.5
  curvature (lateral) Q55.61
  hypoplasia Q55.62
pericardium Q24.8
peripheral vascular system Q27.9
  specified type NEC Q27.8
pharynx Q38.8
precerebral vessels Q28.1
prostate Q55.4
pulmonary
  arteriovenous Q25.72
  artery Q25.9
    atresia Q25.5
    specified type NEC Q25.79
    stenosis Q25.6
  valve Q22.3
renal artery Q27.2
respiratory system Q34.9
retina Q14.1
scrotum — see Malformation, testis and scrotum
seminal vesicles Q55.4
sense organs NEC Q07.9
skin Q82.9
specified NEC Q89.8
spinal
  cord Q06.9
  nerve root Q07.8
spine Q76.49
  kyphosis — see Kyphosis, congenital
  lordosis — see Lordosis, congenital
spleen Q89.09
stomach Q40.3
  specified type NEC Q40.2
teeth, tooth K00.9
tendon Q79.9
testis and scrotum Q55.20
  aplasia Q55.0
  hypoplasia Q55.1
  polyorchism Q55.21
  retractile testis Q55.22
  scrotal transposition Q55.23
  specified NEC Q55.29
thorax, bony Q76.9
throat Q38.8
thyroid gland Q89.2
tongue (congenital) Q38.3
  hypertrophy Q38.2
  tie Q38.1
trachea Q32.1
tricuspid valve Q22.9
  specified type NEC Q22.8
umbilical cord NEC (complicating delivery) O69.89
umbilicus Q89.9
ureter Q62.8
  agenesis Q62.4
  duplication Q62.5
  malposition — see Malposition, congenital, ureter

Malformation (congenital) (see also Anomaly) — continued
ureter Q62.8 — continued
  obstructive defect — see Defect, obstructive, ureter
  vesico-uretero-renal reflux Q62.7
urethra Q64.79
  aplasia Q64.5
  duplication Q64.74
  posterior valves Q64.2
  prolapse Q64.71
  stricture Q64.32
urinary system Q64.9
uterus Q51.9
  specified type NEC Q51.818
vagina Q52.4
vas deferens Q55.4
  atresia Q55.3
vascular system, peripheral Q27.9
  venous — see Anomaly, vein(s)
vulva Q52.70
Malfunction — see also Dysfunction
cardiac electronic device T82.119
  electrode T82.110
  pulse generator T82.111
  specified type NEC T82.118
catheter device NEC T85.618
  cystostomy T83.010
  dialysis (renal) (vascular) T82.41
    intraperitoneal T85.611
  infusion NEC T82.514
    spinal (epidural) (subdural) T85.610
  urinary, indwelling T83.018
colostomy K94.03
  valve K94.03
cystostomy (stoma) N99.512
  catheter T83.010
enteric stoma K94.13
enterostomy K94.13
esophagostomy K94.33
gastroenteric K31.89
gastrostomy K94.23
ileostomy K94.13
  valve K94.13
jejunostomy K94.13
pacemaker — see Malfunction, cardiac electronic device
prosthetic device, internal — see Complications, prosthetic device, by site, mechanical
tracheostomy J95.03
urinary device NEC — see Complication, genitourinary, device, urinary, mechanical
valve
  colostomy K94.03
  heart T82.09
  ileostomy K94.13
vascular graft or shunt NEC — see Complication, cardiovascular device, mechanical, vascular
ventricular (communicating shunt) T85.01
Malherbe's tumor — see Neoplasm, skin, benign
Malibu disease L98.8
Malignancy — see also Neoplasm, malignant, by site
unspecified site (primary) C80.1
Malignant — see condition
Malingerer, malingering Z76.5
Mallet finger (acquired) — see Deformity, finger, mallet finger
  congenital Q74.0
  sequelae of rickets E64.3
Malleus A24.0
Mallory's bodies R89.7
Mallory-Weiss syndrome K22.6
Malnutrition E46
degree
  first E44.1
  mild (protein) E44.1
  moderate (protein) E44.0
  second E44.0
  severe (protein-energy) E43
    intermediate form E42
    with
      kwashiorkor (and marasmus) E42
      marasmus E41
  third E43
following gastrointestinal surgery K91.2
intrauterine
  light-for-dates — see Light for dates
  small-for-dates — see Small for dates
lack of care, or neglect (child) (infant) T76.02
  confirmed T74.02
malignant E40

Malnutrition E46 — continued
protein E46
  calorie E46
    mild E44.1
    moderate E44.0
    severe E43
      intermediate form E42
      with
        kwashiorkor (and marasmus) E42
        marasmus E41
  energy E46
    mild E44.1
    moderate E44.0
    severe E43
      intermediate form E42
      with
        kwashiorkor (and marasmus) E42
        marasmus E41
severe (protein-energy) E43
  with
    kwashiorkor (and marasmus) E42
    marasmus E41
Malocclusion (teeth) M26.4
Angle's M26.219
  class I M26.211
  class II M26.212
  class III M26.213
due to
  abnormal swallowing M26.59
  mouth breathing M26.59
  tongue, lip or finger habits M26.59
temporomandibular (joint) M26.69
Malposition
cervix — see Malposition, uterus
congenital
  adrenal (gland) Q89.1
  alimentary tract Q45.8
    lower Q43.8
    upper Q40.8
  aorta Q25.4
  appendix Q43.8
  arterial trunk Q20.0
  artery (peripheral) Q27.8
    coronary Q24.5
    digestive system Q27.8
    lower limb Q27.8
    pulmonary Q25.79
    specified site NEC Q27.8
    upper limb Q27.8
  auditory canal Q17.8
    causing impairment of hearing Q16.9
  auricle (ear) Q17.4
    causing impairment of hearing Q16.9
    cervical Q18.2
  biliary duct or passage Q44.5
  bladder (mucosa) — see Exstrophy, bladder
  brachial plexus Q07.8
  brain tissue Q04.8
  breast Q83.8
  bronchus Q32.4
  cecum Q43.8
  clavicle Q74.0
  colon Q43.8
  digestive organ or tract NEC Q45.8
    lower Q43.8
    upper Q40.8
  ear (auricle) (external) Q17.4
    ossicles Q16.3
  endocrine (gland) NEC Q89.2
  epiglottis Q31.8
  eustachian tube Q17.8
  eye Q15.8
  facial features Q18.8
  fallopian tube Q50.6
  finger(s) Q68.1
    supernumerary Q69.0
  foot Q66.9
  gallbladder Q44.1
  gastrointestinal tract Q45.8
  genitalia, genital organ(s) or tract
    female Q52.8
      external Q52.79
      internal NEC Q52.8
    male Q55.8
  glottis Q31.8
  hand Q68.1
  heart Q24.8
    dextrocardia Q24.0
      with complete transposition of viscera Q89.3
  hepatic duct Q44.5
  hip (joint) Q65.89
  intestine (large) (small) Q43.8
    with anomalous adhesions, fixation or malrotation Q43.3
  joint NEC Q68.8
  kidney Q63.2

Malposition — continued
congenital — continued
  larynx Q31.8
  limb Q68.8
    lower Q68.8
    upper Q68.8
  liver Q44.7
  lung (lobe) Q33.8
  nail(s) Q84.6
  nerve Q07.8
  nervous system NEC Q07.8
  nose, nasal (septum) Q30.8
  organ or site not listed — see Anomaly, by site
  ovary Q50.39
  pancreas Q45.3
  parathyroid (gland) Q89.2
  patella Q74.1
  peripheral vascular system Q27.8
  pituitary (gland) Q89.2
  respiratory organ or system NEC Q34.8
  rib (cage) Q76.6
    supernumerary in cervical region Q76.5
  scapula Q74.0
  shoulder Q74.0
  spinal cord Q06.8
  spleen Q89.09
  sternum NEC Q76.7
  stomach Q40.2
  symphysis pubis Q74.2
  thymus (gland) Q89.2
  thyroid (gland) (tissue) Q89.2
    cartilage Q31.8
  toe(s) Q66.9
    supernumerary Q69.2
  tongue Q38.3
  trachea Q32.1
  ureter Q62.60
    deviation Q62.61
    displacement Q62.62
    ectopia Q62.63
    specified type NEC Q62.69
  uterus Q51.818
  vein(s) (peripheral) Q27.8
    great Q26.8
  vena cava (inferior) (superior) Q26.8
device, implant or graft (see also Complications, by site and type, mechanical) T85.628
  arterial graft NEC — see Complication, cardiovascular device, mechanical, vascular
  breast (implant) T85.42
  catheter NEC T85.628
    cystostomy T83.020
    dialysis (renal) T82.42
      intraperitoneal T85.621
    infusion NEC T82.524
      spinal (epidural) (subdural) T85.620
    urinary, indwelling T83.028
  electronic (electrode) (pulse generator) (stimulator)
    bone T84.320
    cardiac T82.129
    electrode T82.120
    pulse generator T82.121
    specified type NEC T82.128
    nervous system — see Complication, prosthetic device, mechanical, electronic nervous system stimulator
    urinary — see Complication, genitourinary, device, urinary, mechanical
  fixation, internal (orthopedic) NEC — see Complication, fixation device, mechanical
  gastrointestinal — see Complications, prosthetic device, mechanical, gastrointestinal device
  genital NEC T83.428
    intrauterine contraceptive device T83.32
    penile prosthesis T83.420
  heart NEC — see Complication, cardiovascular device, mechanical
  joint prosthesis — see Complication, joint prosthesis, mechanical
  ocular NEC — see Complications, prosthetic device, mechanical, ocular device
  orthopedic NEC — see Complication, orthopedic, device, mechanical
  specified NEC T85.628
  urinary NEC — see also Complication, genitourinary, device, urinary, mechanical
    graft T83.22

DISEASE INDEX

Malposition — *continued*
device, implant or graft (*see also*
Complications, by site and type,
mechanical) *continued*
vascular NEC — *see* Complication,
cardiovascular device, mechanical
ventricular intracranial shunt T85.02
fetus — *see* Pregnancy, complicated by
(management affected by),
presentation, fetal
gallbladder K82.8
gastrointestinal tract, congenital Q45.8
heart, congenital NEC Q24.8
joint prosthesis — *see* Complications, joint
prosthesis, mechanical, displacement,
by site
stomach K31.89
congenital Q40.2
tooth, teeth, fully erupted M26.30
uterus (acute) (acquired) (adherent)
(asymptomatic) (postinfectional)
(postpartal, old) N85.4
anteflexion or anteversion N85.4
congenital Q51.818
flexion N85.4
lateral — *see* Lateroversion, uterus
inversion N85.5
lateral (flexion) (version) — *see*
Lateroversion, uterus
in pregnancy or childbirth — *see*
subcategory O34.5
retroflexion or retroversion — *see*
Retroversion, uterus
Malposture R29.3
Malrotation
cecum Q43.3
colon Q43.3
intestine Q43.3
kidney Q63.2
Malta fever — *see* Brucellosis
Maltreatment
adult
abandonment
confirmed T74.01
suspected T76.01
confirmed T74.91
history of Z91.419
neglect
confirmed T74.01
suspected T76.01
physical abuse
confirmed T74.11
suspected T76.11
psychological abuse
confirmed T74.31
history of Z91.411
suspected T76.31
sexual abuse
confirmed T74.21
suspected T76.21
suspected T76.91
child
abandonment
confirmed T74.02
suspected T76.02
confirmed T74.92
history of — *see* History, personal (of),
abuse
neglect
confirmed T74.02
history of — *see* History, personal
(of), abuse
suspected T76.02
physical abuse
confirmed T74.12
history of — *see* History, personal
(of), abuse
suspected T76.12
psychological abuse
confirmed T74.32
history of — *see* History, personal
(of), abuse
suspected T76.32
sexual abuse
confirmed T74.22
history of — *see* History, personal
(of), abuse
suspected T76.22
suspected T76.92
personal history of Z91.89
Maltworker's lung J67.4
Malunion, fracture — *see* Fracture, by site
Mammillitis N61
puerperal, postpartum O91.02
Mammitis — *see* Mastitis
Mammogram (examination) Z12.39
routine Z12.31
Mammoplasia N62

Management (of)
bone conduction hearing device
(implanted) Z45.320
cardiac pacemaker NEC Z45.018
cerebrospinal fluid drainage device Z45.41
cochlear device (implanted) Z45.321
contraceptive Z30.9
specified NEC Z30.8
implanted device Z45.9
specified NEC Z45.89
infusion pump Z45.1
procreative Z31.9
male factor infertility in female Z31.81
specified NEC Z31.89
prosthesis (external) (*see also* Fitting)
Z44.9
implanted Z45.9
specified NEC Z45.89
renal dialysis catheter Z49.01
vascular access device Z45.2
Mangled — *see* specified injury by site
Mania (monopolar) — *see also* Disorder,
mood, manic episode
with psychotic symptoms F30.2
Bell's F30.8
chronic (recurrent) F31.89
hysterical F44.89
puerperal F30.8
recurrent F31.89
without psychotic symptoms F30.10
mild F30.11
moderate F30.12
severe F30.13
**Manic-depressive insanity, psychosis, or
syndrome** — *see* Disorder, bipolar
Mannosidosis E77.1
Manson's
disease B65.1
schistosomiasis B65.1
Mansonelliasis, mansonellosis B74.4
Manual — *see* condition
Maple-bark-stripper's lung (disease) J67.6
Maple-syrup-urine disease E71.0
Marable's syndrome (celiac artery
compression) I77.4
Marasmus E41
due to malnutrition E41
intestinal E41
nutritional E41
senile R54
tuberculous NEC — *see* Tuberculosis
Marble
bones Q78.2
skin R23.8
Marburg virus disease A98.3
March
fracture — *see* Fracture, traumatic, stress,
by site
hemoglobinuria D59.6
Marchesani(-Weill) syndrome Q87.0
**Marchiafava(-Bignami) syndrome or
disease** G37.1
Marchiafava-Micheli syndrome D59.5
Marcus Gunn's syndrome Q07.8
Marfan's syndrome — *see* Syndrome,
Marfan's
Marie-Bamberger disease — *see*
Osteoarthropathy, hypertrophic,
specified NEC
**Marie-Charcot-Tooth neuropathic
muscular atrophy** G60.0
Marie's
cerebellar ataxia (late-onset) G11.2
disease or syndrome (acromegaly) E22.0
**Marie-Strümpell arthritis, disease or
spondylitis** — *see* Spondylitis,
ankylosing
Marion's disease (bladder neck obstruction)
N32.0
Marital conflict Z63.0
Mark
port wine Q82.5
raspberry Q82.5
strawberry Q82.5
stretch L90.6
tattoo L81.8
Marker heterochromatin — *see* Extra,
marker chromosomes
Maroteaux-Lamy syndrome (mild) (severe)
E76.29
Marrow
arrest D61.9
poor function D75.89
Marseilles fever A77.1
Marsh fever — *see* Malaria
Marsh's disease (exophthalmic goiter)
E05.00
with storm E05.01
Marshall's (hidrotic) ectodermal dysplasia
Q82.4

**Masculinization (female) with adrenal
hyperplasia** E25.9
congenital E25.0
Masculinovoblastoma D27.
Masochism (sexual) F65.51
Mason's lung J62.8
Mass
abdominal R19.00
epigastric R19.06
generalized R19.07
left lower quadrant R19.04
left upper quadrant R19.02
periumbilic R19.05
right lower quadrant R19.03
right upper quadrant R19.01
specified site NEC R19.09
breast N63
chest R22.2
cystic — *see* Cyst
ear H93.8-
head R22.0
intra-abdominal (diffuse) (generalized) —
see Mass, abdominal
kidney N28.89
liver R16.0
localized (skin) R22.9
chest R22.2
head R22.0
limb
lower R22.4-
upper R22.3-
neck R22.1
trunk R22.2
lung R91.8
malignant — *see* Neoplasm, malignant, by
site
neck R22.1
pelvic (diffuse) (generalized) — *see* Mass,
abdominal
specified organ NEC — *see* Disease, by
site
splenic R16.1
substernal thyroid — *see* Goiter
superficial (localized) R22.9
umbilical (diffuse) (generalized) R19.09
Massive — *see* condition
Mast cell
disease, systemic tissue D47.0
leukemia C94.3-
sarcoma C96.2
tumor D47.0
malignant C96.2
Mastalgia N64.4
Masters-Allen syndrome N83.8
Mastitis (acute) (diffuse) (nonpuerperal)
(subacute) N61
chronic (cystic) — *see* Mastopathy, cystic
cystic (Schimmelbusch's type) — *see*
Mastopathy, cystic
fibrocystic — *see* Mastopathy, cystic
infective N61
newborn P39.0
interstitial, gestational or puerperal — *see*
Mastitis, obstetric
neonatal (noninfective) P83.4
infective P39.0
obstetric (interstitial) (nonpurulent)
associated with
lactation O91.23
pregnancy O91.21-
puerperium O91.22
purulent
associated with
lactation O91.13
pregnancy O91.11-
puerperium O91.12
periductal — *see* Ectasia, mammary duct
phlegmonous — *see* Mastopathy, cystic
plasma cell — *see* Ectasia, mammary duct
Mastocytoma D47.0
malignant C96.2
Mastocytosis Q82.2
aggressive systemic C96.2
indolent systemic D47.0
malignant C96.2
systemic, associated with clonal
hematopoetic non-mast-cell disease
(SM-AHNMD) D47.0
Mastodynia N64.4
Mastoid — *see* condition
Mastoidalgia — *see* subcategory H92.0
Mastoiditis (coalescent) (hemorrhagic)
(suppurative) H70.9-
acute, subacute H70.00-
complicated NEC H70.09-
subperiosteal H70.01-
chronic (necrotic) (recurrent) H70.1-

Mastoiditis (coalescent) (hemorrhagic)
(suppurative) H70.9- — *continued*
in (due to)
infectious disease NEC B99 [H75.-]
parasitic disease NEC B89 [H75.-]
tuberculosis A18.03
petrosis — *see* Petrositis
postauricular fistula — *see* Fistula,
postauricular
specified NEC H70.89-
tuberculous A18.03
Mastopathy, mastopathia N64.9
chronica cystica — *see* Mastopathy, cystic
cystic (chronic) (diffuse) N60.1-
with epithelial proliferation N60.3-
diffuse cystic — *see* Mastopathy, cystic
estrogenic, oestrogenica N64.89
ovarian origin N64.89
Mastoplasia, mastoplastia N62
Masturbation (excessive) F98.8
Maternal care (for) — *see* Pregnancy
(complicated by) (management affected
by)
Matheiu's disease (leptospiral jaundice)
A27.0
Mauclaire's disease or osteochondrosis —
see Osteochondrosis, juvenile, hand,
metacarpal
Maxcy's disease A75.2
Maxilla, maxillary — *see* condition
May(-Hegglin) anomaly or syndrome
D72.0
McArdle(-Schmid)(-Pearson) disease
(glycogen storage) E74.04
McCune-Albright syndrome Q78.1
McQuarrie's syndrome (idiopathic familial
hypoglycemia) E16.2
Meadow's syndrome Q86.1
Measles (black) (hemorrhagic) (suppressed)
B05.9
with
complications NEC B05.89
encephalitis B05.0
intestinal complications B05.4
keratitis (keratoconjunctivitis) B05.81
meningitis B05.1
otitis media B05.3
pneumonia B05.2
French — *see* Rubella
German — *see* Rubella
Liberty — *see* Rubella
Meat-wrappers' asthma J68.9
Meatitis, urethral — *see* Urethritis
Meatus, meatal — *see* condition
Meckel's diverticulitis, diverticulum
(displaced) (hypertrophic) Q43.0
malignant — *see* Table of Neoplasms,
small intestine, malignant
Meckel-Gruber syndrome Q61.9
Meconium
ileus, newborn P76.0
in cystic fibrosis E84.11
meaning meconium plug (without cystic
fibrosis) P76.0
obstruction, newborn P76.0
due to fecaliths P76.0
in mucoviscidosis E84.11
peritonitis P78.0
plug syndrome (newborn) NEC P76.0
Median — *see also* condition
arcuate ligament syndrome I77.4
bar (prostate) (vesical orifice) — *see*
Hyperplasia, prostate
rhomboid glossitis K14.2
Mediastinal shift R93.8
Mediastinitis (acute) (chronic) J98.5
syphilitic A52.73
tuberculous A15.8
Mediastinopericarditis — *see also*
Pericarditis
acute I30.9
adhesive I31.0
chronic I31.8
rheumatic I09.2
Mediastinum, mediastinal — *see* condition
Medicine poisoning — *see* Table of Drugs
and Chemicals, by drug, poisoning
Mediterranean
fever — *see* Brucellosis
familial E85.0
tick A77.1
kala-azar B55.0
leishmaniasis B55.0
tick fever A77.1
Medulla — *see* condition
Medullary cystic kidney Q61.5

Medullated fibers
optic (nerve) Q14.8
retina Q14.1
Medulloblastoma
desmoplastic C71.6
specified site — see Neoplasm, malignant, by site
unspecified site C71.6
Medulloepithelioma — see also Neoplasm, malignant, by site
teratoid — see Neoplasm, malignant, by site
Medullomyoblastoma
specified site — see Neoplasm, malignant, by site
unspecified site C71.6
Meekeren-Ehlers-Danlos syndrome Q79.6
Megacolon (acquired) (functional) (not Hirschsprung's disease) (in) K59.3
Chagas' disease B57.32
congenital, congenitum (aganglionic) Q43.1
Hirschsprung's (disease) Q43.1
toxic NEC K59.3
due to Clostridium difficile A04.7
Megaesophagus (functional) K22.0
congenital Q39.5
in (due to) Chagas' disease B57.31
Megalencephaly Q04.5
Megalerythema (epidemic) B08.3
Megaloappendix Q43.8
Megalocephalus, megalocephaly NEC Q75.3
Megalocornea Q15.8
with glaucoma Q15.0
Megalocytic anemia D53.91
Megalodactylia (fingers) (thumbs) (congenital) Q74.0
toes Q74.2
Megaloduodenum Q43.8
Megaloesophagus (functional) K22.0
congenital Q39.5
Megalogastria (acquired) K31.89
congenital Q40.2
Megalophthalmos Q11.3
Megalopsia H53.15
Megalosplenia — see Splenomegaly
Megaloureter N28.82
congenital Q62.2
Megarectum K62.89
Megasigmoid K59.3
congenital Q43.2
Megaureter N28.82
congenital Q62.2
Megavitamin-B6 syndrome E67.2
Megrim — see Migraine
Meibomian
cyst, infected — see Hordeolum
gland — see condition
sty, stye — see Hordeolum
Meibomitis — see Hordeolum
Meige's syndrome Q82.0
Meige-Milroy disease (chronic hereditary edema) Q82.0
Melalgia, nutritional E53.8
Melancholia F32.9
climacteric (single episode) F32.8
recurrent episode F33.9
hypochondriac F45.29
intermittent (single episode) F32.8
recurrent episode F33.9
involutional (single episode) F32.8
recurrent episode F33.9
menopausal (single episode) F32.8
recurrent episode F33.9
puerperal F32.8
reactive (emotional stress or trauma) F32.3
recurrent F33.9
senile F03
stuporous (single episode) F32.8
recurrent episode F33.9
Melanemia R79.89
Melanoameloblastoma — see Neoplasm, bone, benign
Melanoblastoma — see Melanoma
Melanocarcinoma — see Melanoma
Melanocytoma, eyeball D31.4-
Melanocytosis, neurocutaneous Q82.8
Melanoderma, melanodermia L81.4
Melanodontia, infantile K03.89
Melanodontoclasia K03.89
Melanoepithelioma — see Melanoma
Melanoma (malignant) C43.9
acral lentiginous, malignant — see Melanoma, skin, by site
amelanotic — see Melanoma, skin, by site
balloon cell — see Melanoma, skin, by site
benign — see Nevus
desmoplastic, malignant — see Melanoma, skin, by site

Melanoma (malignant) C43.9 — continued
epithelioid cell — see Melanoma, skin, by site
with spindle cell, mixed — see Melanoma, skin, by site
in
giant pigmented nevus — see Melanoma, skin, by site
Hutchinson's melanotic freckle — see Melanoma, skin, by site
junctional nevus — see Melanoma, skin, by site
precancerous melanosis — see Melanoma, skin, by site
in situ D03.9
abdominal wall D03.59
ala nasi D03.39
ankle D03.7-
anus, anal (margin) (skin) D03.51
arm D03.6-
auditory canal D03.2-
auricle (ear) D03.2-
auricular canal (external) D03.2-
axilla, axillary fold D03.59
back D03.59
breast D03.52
brow D03.39
buttock D03.59
canthus (eye) D03.1-
cheek (external) D03.39
chest wall D03.59
chin D03.39
choroid D03.8
conjunctiva D03.8
ear (external) D03.2-
external meatus (ear) D03.2-
eye D03.8
eyebrow D03.39
eyelid (lower) (upper) D03.1-
face D03.30
specified NEC D03.39
female genital organ (external) NEC D03.8
finger D03.6-
flank D03.59
foot D03.7-
forearm D03.6-
forehead D03.39
foreskin D03.8
gluteal region D03.59
groin D03.59
hand D03.6-
heel D03.7-
helix D03.2-
hip D03.7-
interscapular region D03.59
iris D03.8
jaw D03.39
knee D03.7-
labium (majus) (minus) D03.8
lacrimal gland D03.8
leg D03.7-
lip (lower) (upper) D03.0
lower limb NEC D03.7-
male genital organ (external) NEC D03.8
nail D03.9
finger D03.6-
toe D03.7-
neck D03.4
nose (external) D03.39
orbit D03.8
penis D03.8
perianal skin D03.51
perineum D03.51
pinna D03.2-
popliteal fossa or space D03.7-
prepuce D03.8
pudendum D03.8
retina D03.8
retrobulbar D03.8
scalp D03.4
scrotum D03.8
shoulder D03.6-
specified site NEC D03.8
submammary fold D03.52
temple D03.39
thigh D03.7-
toe D03.7-
trunk NEC D03.59
umbilicus D03.59
upper limb NEC D03.6-
vulva D03.8
juvenile — see Nevus
malignant, of soft parts except skin — see Neoplasm, connective tissue, malignant

Melanoma (malignant) C43.9 — continued
metastatic
breast C79.81
genital organ C79.82
specified site NEC C79.89
neurotropic, malignant — see Melanoma, skin, by site
nodular — see Melanoma, skin, by site
regressing, malignant — see Melanoma, skin, by site
skin C43.9
abdominal wall C43.59
ala nasi C43.31
ankle C43.7-
anus, anal (skin) C43.51
arm C43.6-
auditory canal (external) C43.2-
auricle (ear) C43.2-
auricular canal (external) C43.2-
axilla, axillary fold C43.59
back C43.59
breast (female) (male) C43.52
brow C43.39
buttock C43.59
canthus (eye) C43.1-
cheek (external) C43.39
chest wall C43.59
chin C43.39
ear (external) C43.2-
elbow C43.6-
external meatus (ear) C43.2-
eyebrow C43.39
eyelid (lower) (upper) C43.1-
face C43.30
specified NEC C43.39
female genital organ (external) NEC C51.9
finger C43.6-
flank C43.59
foot C43.7-
forearm C43.6-
forehead C43.39
foreskin C60.0
glabella C43.39
gluteal region C43.59
groin C43.59
hand C43.6-
heel C43.7-
helix C43.2-
hip C43.7-
interscapular region C43.59
jaw (external) C43.39
knee C43.7-
labium C51.9
majus C51.0
minus C51.1
leg C43.7-
lip (lower) (upper) C43.0
lower limb NEC C43.7-
male genital organ (external) NEC C63.9
nail
finger C43.6-
toe C43.7-
nasolabial groove C43.39
nates C43.59
neck C43.4
nose (external) C43.31
overlapping site C43.8
palpebra C43.1-
penis C60.9
perianal skin C43.51
perineum C43.51
pinna C43.2-
popliteal fossa or space C43.7-
prepuce C60.0
pudendum C51.9
scalp C43.4
scrotum C63.2
shoulder C43.6-
skin NEC C43.9
submammary fold C43.52
temple C43.39
thigh C43.7-
toe C43.7-
trunk NEC C43.59
umbilicus C43.59
upper limb NEC C43.6-
vulva C51.9
overlapping sites C51.8
spindle cell
with epithelioid, mixed — see Melanoma, skin, by site
type A C69.4-
type B C69.4-
superficial spreading — see Melanoma, skin, by site
Melanosarcoma — see also Melanoma
epithelioid cell — see Melanoma

Melanosis L81.4
addisonian E27.1
tuberculous A18.7
adrenal E27.1
colon K63.89
conjunctiva — see Pigmentation, conjunctiva
congenital Q13.89
cornea (presenile) (senile) — see also Pigmentation, cornea
congenital Q13.4
eye NEC H57.8
congenital Q15.8
lenticularis progressiva Q82.1
liver K76.89
precancerous — see also Melanoma, in situ
malignant melanoma in — see Melanoma
Riehl's L81.4
sclera H15.89
congenital Q13.89
suprarenal E27.1
tar L81.4
toxic L81.4
Melanuria R82.99
MELAS syndrome E88.41
Melasma L81.1
adrenal (gland) E27.1
suprarenal (gland) E27.1
Melena K92.1
with ulcer — code by site under Ulcer, with hemorrhage K27.4
due to swallowed blood P78.2
newborn, neonatal P54.1
due to swallowed maternal blood P78.2
Meleney's
gangrene (cutaneous) — see Ulcer, skin
ulcer (chronic undermining) — see Ulcer, skin
Melioidosis A24.9
acute A24.1
chronic A24.2
fulminating A24.1
pneumonia A24.1
pulmonary (chronic) A24.2
acute A24.1
subacute A24.2
sepsis A24.1
specified NEC A24.3
subacute A24.2
Melitensis, febris A23.0
Melkersson(-Rosenthal) syndrome G51.2
Mellitus, diabetes — see Diabetes
Melorheostosis (bone) — see Disorder, bone, density and structure, specified NEC
Meloschisis Q18.4
Melotia Q17.4
Membrana
capsularis lentis posterior Q13.89
epipapillaris Q14.2
Membranacea placenta O43.19-
Membranaceous uterus N85.8
Membrane(s), membranous — see also condition
cyclitic — see Membrane, pupillary
folds, congenital — see Web
Jackson's Q43.3
over face of newborn P28.9
premature rupture — see Rupture, membranes, premature
pupillary H21.4-
persistent Q13.89
retained (with hemorrhage) (complicating delivery) O72.2
without hemorrhage O73.1
secondary cataract — see Cataract, secondary
unruptured (causing asphyxia) — see Asphyxia, newborn
vitreous — see Opacity, vitreous, membranes and strands
Membranitis — see Chorioamnionitis
Memory disturbance, lack or loss — see also Amnesia
mild, following organic brain damage F06.8
Menadione deficiency E56.1
Menarche
delayed E30.0
precocious E30.1
Mendacity, pathologic F60.2
Mendelson's syndrome (due to anesthesia) J95.4
in labor and delivery O74.0
in pregnancy O29.01-
obstetric O74.0
postpartum, puerperal O89.01
Ménétrier's disease or syndrome K29.60
with bleeding K29.61

Ménière's disease, syndrome or vertigo H81.0-
Meninges, meningeal — see condition
Meningioma — see also Neoplasm, meninges, benign
  angioblastic — see Neoplasm, meninges, benign
  angiomatous — see Neoplasm, meninges, benign
  endotheliomatous — see Neoplasm, meninges, benign
  fibroblastic — see Neoplasm, meninges, benign
  fibrous — see Neoplasm, meninges, benign
  hemangioblastic — see Neoplasm, meninges, benign
  hemangiopericytic — see Neoplasm, meninges, benign
  malignant — see Neoplasm, meninges, malignant
  meningiothelial — see Neoplasm, meninges, benign
  meningotheliomatous — see Neoplasm, meninges, benign
  mixed — see Neoplasm, meninges, benign
  multiple — see Neoplasm, meninges, uncertain behavior
  papillary — see Neoplasm, meninges, uncertain behavior
  psammomatous — see Neoplasm, meninges, benign
  syncytial — see Neoplasm, meninges, benign
  transitional — see Neoplasm, meninges, benign
Meningiomatosis (diffuse) — see Neoplasm, meninges, uncertain behavior
Meningism — see Meningismus
Meningismus (infectional) (pneumococcal) R29.1
  due to serum or vaccine R29.1
  influenzal — see Influenza, with, manifestations NEC
Meningitis (basal) (basic) (brain) (cerebral) (cervical) (congestive) (diffuse) (hemorrhagic) (infantile) (membranous)(metastatic) (nonspecific) (pontine) (progressive) (simple) (spinal) (subacute) (sympathetic) (toxic) G03.9
  abacterial G03.0
  actinomycotic A42.81
  adenoviral A87.1
  arbovirus A87.8
  aseptic (acute) G03.0
  bacterial G00.9
    Escherichia coli (E. coli) G00.8
    Friedländer (bacillus) G00.8
    gram-negative G00.9
    H. influenzae G00.0
    Klebsiella G00.8
    pneumococcal G00.1
    specified organism NEC G00.8
    staphylococcal G00.3
    streptococcal (acute) G00.2
  benign recurrent (Mollaret) G03.2
  candidal B37.5
  caseous (tuberculous) A17.0
  cerebrospinal A39.0
  chronic NEC G03.1
  clear cerebrospinal fluid NEC G03.0
  coxsackievirus A87.0
  cryptococcal B45.1
  diplococcal (gram positive) A39.0
  echovirus A87.0
  enteroviral A87.0
  eosinophilic B83.2
  epidemic NEC A39.0
  Escherichia coli (E. coli) G00.8
  fibrinopurulent G00.9
    specified organism NEC G00.8
  Friedländer (bacillus) G00.8
  gonococcal A54.81
  gram-negative cocci G00.9
  gram-positive cocci G00.9
  H. influenzae G00.0
  Haemophilus (influenzae) G00.0
  in (due to)
    adenovirus A87.1
    African trypanosomiasis B56.9 [G02]
    anthrax A22.8
    bacterial disease NEC A48.8 [G01]
    Chagas' disease (chronic) B57.41
    chickenpox B01.0
    coccidioidomycosis B38.4
    Diplococcus pneumoniae G00.1
    enterovirus A87.0
    herpes (simplex) virus B00.3
      zoster B02.1
    infectious mononucleosis B27.92
    leptospirosis A27.81

Meningitis (basal) (basic) (brain) (cerebral) (cervical) (congestive) (diffuse) (hemorrhagic) (infantile) (membranous)(metastatic) (nonspecific) (pontine) (progressive) (simple) (spinal) (subacute) (sympathetic) (toxic) G03.9 — continued
  in (due to) — continued
    Listeria monocytogenes A32.11
    Lyme disease A69.21
    measles B05.1
    mumps (virus) B26.1
    neurosyphilis (late) A52.13
    parasitic disease NEC B89 [G02]
    poliovirus A80.9 [G02]
    preventive immunization, inoculation or vaccination G03.8
    rubella B06.02
    Salmonella infection A02.21
    specified cause NEC G03.8
    typhoid fever A01.01
    varicella B01.0
    viral disease NEC A87.8
    whooping cough A37.90
    zoster B02.1
  infectious G00.9
  influenzal (H. influenzae) G00.0
  Klebsiella G00.8
  leptospiral (aseptic) A27.81
  lymphocytic (acute) (benign) (serous) A87.2
  meningococcal A39.0
  Mima polymorpha G00.8
  Mollaret (benign recurrent) G03.2
  monilial B37.5
  mycotic NEC B49 [G02]
  Neisseria A39.0
  nonbacterial G03.0
  nonpyogenic NEC G03.0
  ossificans G96.19
  pneumococcal G00.1
  poliovirus A80.9 [G02]
  postmeasles B05.1
  purulent G00.9
    specified organism NEC G00.8
  pyogenic G00.9
    specified organism NEC G00.8
  Salmonella (arizonae) (Cholerae-Suis) (enteritidis) (typhimurium) A02.21
  septic G00.9
    specified organism NEC G00.8
  serosa circumscripta NEC G03.0
  serous NEC G93.2
  specified organism NEC G00.8
  sporotrichosis B42.81
  staphylococcal G00.3
  sterile G03.0
  streptococcal (acute) G00.2
  suppurative G00.9
    specified organism NEC G00.8
  syphilitic (late) (tertiary) A52.13
    acute A51.41
    congenital A50.41
    secondary A51.41
  Torula histolytica (cryptococcal) B45.1
  traumatic (complication of injury) T79.8
  tuberculous A17.0
  typhoid A01.01
  viral NEC A87.9
  Yersinia pestis A20.3
Meningocele (spinal) — see also Spina bifida
  with hydrocephalus — see Spina bifida, by site, with hydrocephalus
  acquired (traumatic) G96.19
  cerebral — see Encephalocele
Meningocerebritis — see Meningoencephalitis
Meningococcemia A39.4
  acute A39.2
  chronic A39.3
Meningococcus, meningococcal (see also condition) A39.9
  adrenalitis, hemorrhagic A39.1
  carrier (suspected) of Z22.31
  meningitis (cerebrospinal) A39.0
Meningoencephalitis (see also Encephalitis) G04.90
  acute NEC (see also Encephalitis, viral) A86
  bacterial NEC G04.2
  California A83.5
  diphasic A84.1
  eosinophilic B83.2
  epidemic A39.81
  herpesviral, herpetic B00.4
    due to herpesvirus 6 B10.01
    due to herpesvirus 7 B10.09
    specified NEC B10.09

Meningoencephalitis (see also Encephalitis) G04.90 — continued
  in (due to)
    blastomycosis NEC B40.81
    diseases classified elsewhere G05.3
    free-living amebae B60.2
    H. influenzae G00.0
    Hemophilus influenzae (H .influenzae) G04.2
    herpes B00.4
      due to herpesvirus 6 B10.01
      due to herpesvirus 7 B10.09
      specified NEC B10.09
    Lyme disease A69.22
    mercury — see subcategory T56.1
    mumps B26.2
    Naegleria (amebae) (organisms) (fowleri) B60.2
    Parastrongylus cantonensis B83.2
    toxoplasmosis (acquired) B58.2
      congenital P37.1
  infectious (acute) (viral) A86
  influenzal (H. influenzae) G04.2
  Listeria monocytogenes A32.12
  lymphocytic (serous) A87.2
  mumps B26.2
  parasitic NEC B89 [G05.3]
  pneumococcal G00.1
  primary amebic B60.2
  specific (syphilitic) A52.14
  specified organism NEC G04.81
  staphylococcal G04.2
  streptococcal G04.2
  syphilitic A52.14
  toxic NEC G92
    due to mercury — see subcategory T56.1
  tuberculous A17.82
  virus NEC A86
Meningoencephalocele — see also Encephalocele
  syphilitic A52.19
  congenital A50.49
Meningoencephalomyelitis — see also Meningoencephalitis
  acute NEC (viral) A86
    disseminated G04.00
      postimmunization or postvaccination G04.02
      postinfectious G04.01
  due to
    actinomycosis A42.82
    Torula B45.1
    Toxoplasma or toxoplasmosis (acquired) B58.2
      congenital P37.1
  postimmunization or postvaccination G04.02
Meningoencephalomyelopathy G96.9
Meningoencephalopathy G96.9
Meningomyelitis — see also Meningoencephalitis
  bacterial NEC G04.2
  blastomycotic NEC B40.81
  cryptococcal B45.1
  in diseases classified elsewhere G05.4
  meningococcal A39.81
  syphilitic A52.14
  tuberculous A17.82
Meningomyelocele — see also Spina bifida
  syphilitic A52.19
Meningomyeloneuritis — see Meningoencephalitis
Meningoradiculitis — see Meningitis
Meningovascular — see condition
Menkes' disease or syndrome E83.09
  meaning maple-syrup-urine disease E71.0
Menometrorrhagia N92.1
Menopause, menopausal (asymptomatic) (state) Z78.0
  arthritis (any site) NEC — see Arthritis, specified form NEC
  bleeding N92.4
  depression (single episode) F32.8
    agitated (single episode) F32.2
      recurrent episode F33.9
    psychotic (single episode) F32.8
      recurrent episode F33.9
    recurrent episode F33.9
    melancholia (single episode) F32.8
      recurrent episode F33.9
  paranoid state F22
  premature E28.319
    asymptomatic E28.319
      postirradiation E89.40
      postsurgical E89.40
    symptomatic E28.310
      postirradiation E89.41
      postsurgical E89.41
  psychosis NEC F28
  symptomatic N95.1

Menopause, menopausal (asymptomatic) (state) Z78.0 — continued
  toxic polyarthritis NEC — see Arthritis, specified form NEC
Menorrhagia (primary) N92.0
  climacteric N92.4
    menopausal N92.4
  menopausal N92.4
  postclimacteric N95.0
  postmenopausal N95.0
  preclimacteric or premenopausal N92.4
  pubertal (menses retained) N92.2
Menostaxis N92.0
Menses, retention N94.89
Menstrual — see Menstruation
Menstruation
  absent — see Amenorrhea
  anovulatory N97.0
  cycle, irregular N92.6
  delayed N91.0
  disorder N93.9
    psychogenic F45.8
  during pregnancy O20.8
  excessive (with regular cycle) N92.0
    with irregular cycle N92.1
    at puberty N92.2
  frequent N92.0
  infrequent — see Oligomenorrhea
  irregular N92.6
    specified NEC N92.5
  latent N92.5
  membranous N92.5
  painful (see also Dysmenorrhea) N94.6
    primary N94.4
    psychogenic F45.8
    secondary N94.5
  passage of clots N92.0
  precocious E30.1
  protracted N92.5
  rare — see Oligomenorrhea
  retained N94.89
  retrograde N92.5
  scanty — see Oligomenorrhea
  suppression N94.89
  vicarious (nasal) N94.89
Mental — see also condition
  deficiency — see Disability, intellectual
  deterioration — see Psychosis
  disorder — see Disorder, mental
  exhaustion F48.8
  insufficiency (congenital) — see Disability, intellectual
  observation without need for further medical care Z03.89
  retardation — see Disability, intellectual
  subnormality — see Disability, intellectual
  upset — see Disorder, mental
Meralgia paresthetica G57.1-
Mercurial — see condition
Mercurialism — see subcategory T56.1
MERFF syndrome (myoclonic epilepsy associated with ragged-red fiber) E88.42
Merkel cell tumor — see Carcinoma, Merkel cell
Merocele — see Hernia, femoral
Meromelia
  lower limb — see Defect, reduction, lower limb
    intercalary
      femur — see Defect, reduction, lower limb, specified type NEC
        tibiofibular (complete)
          (incomplete) — see Defect, reduction, lower limb
  upper limb — see Defect, reduction, upper limb
    intercalary, humeral, radioulnar — see Agenesis, arm, with hand present
Merzbacher-Pelizaeus disease E75.29
Mesaortitis — see Aortitis
Mesarteritis — see Arteritis
Mesencephalitis — see Encephalitis
Mesenchymoma — see also Neoplasm, connective tissue, uncertain behavior
  benign — see Neoplasm, connective tissue, benign
  malignant — see Neoplasm, connective tissue, malignant
Mesenteritis
  retractile K65.4
  sclerosing K65.4
Mesentery, mesenteric — see condition
Mesio-occlusion M26.213
Mesiodens, mesiodentes K00.1
Mesocolon — see condition
Mesonephroma (malignant) — see Neoplasm, malignant, by site
  benign — see Neoplasm, benign, by site
Mesophlebitis — see Phlebitis
Mesostromal dysgenesia Q13.89

DISEASE INDEX

Mesothelioma (malignant) C45.9
  benign
    mesentery D19.1
    mesocolon D19.1
    omentum D19.1
    peritoneum D19.1
    pleura D19.0
    specified site NEC D19.7
    unspecified site D19.9
  biphasic C45.9
    benign
      mesentery D19.1
      mesocolon D19.1
      omentum D19.1
      peritoneum D19.1
      pleura D19.0
      specified site NEC D19.7
      unspecified site D19.9
  cystic D48.4
  epithelioid C45.9
    benign
      mesentery D19.1
      mesocolon D19.1
      omentum D19.1
      peritoneum D19.1
      pleura D19.0
      specified site NEC D19.7
      unspecified site D19.9
  fibrous C45.9
    benign
      mesentery D19.1
      mesocolon D19.1
      omentum D19.1
      peritoneum D19.1
      pleura D19.0
      specified site NEC D19.7
      unspecified site D19.9
  site classification
    liver C45.7
    lung C45.7
    mediastinum C45.7
    mesentery C45.1
    mesocolon C45.1
    omentum C45.1
    pericardium C45.2
    peritoneum C45.1
    pleura C45.0
      parietal C45.0
    retroperitoneum C45.7
    specified site NEC C45.7
    unspecified C45.9
Metabolic syndrome E88.81
Metagonimiasis B66.8
Metagonimus infestation (intestine) B66.8
Metal
  pigmentation L81.8
  polisher's disease J62.8
Metamorphopsia H53.15
Metaplasia
  apocrine (breast) — see Dysplasia, mammary, specified type NEC
  cervix (squamous) — see Dysplasia, cervix
  endometrium (squamous) (uterus) N85.8
  esophagus
  kidney (pelvis) (squamous) N28.89
  myelogenous D73.1
  myeloid (agnogenic) (megakaryocytic) D73.1
  spleen D73.1
  squamous cell, bladder N32.89
Metastasis, metastatic
  abscess — see Abscess
  calcification E83.59
  cancer
    from specified site — see Neoplasm, malignant, by site
    to specified site — see Neoplasm, secondary, by site
  deposits (in) — see Neoplasm, secondary, by site
  disease (see also Neoplasm, secondary, by site) C79.9
  spread (to) — see Neoplasm, secondary, by site
Metastrongyliasis B83.8
Metatarsalgia M77.4-
  anterior G57.6-
  Morton's G57.6-
Metatarsus, metatarsal — see also condition
  valgus (abductus), congenital Q66.6
  varus (adductus) (congenital) Q66.2
Methadone use F11.20
Methemoglobinemia D74.9
  acquired (with sulfhemoglobinemia) D74.8
  congenital D74.0
  enzymatic (congenital) D74.0
  Hb M disease D74.0
  hereditary D74.0
  toxic D74.8

Methemoglobinuria — see Hemoglobinuria
Methioninemia E72.19
Methylmalonic acidemia E71.120
Metritis (catarrhal) (hemorrhagic) (septic) (suppurative) — see also Endometritis
  cervical — see Cervicitis
Metropathia hemorrhagica N93.8
Metroperitonitis — see Peritonitis, pelvic, female
Metrorrhagia N92.1
  climacteric N92.4
  menopausal N92.4
  postpartum NEC (atonic) (following delivery of placenta) O72.1
    delayed or secondary O72.2
  preclimacteric or premenopausal N92.4
  psychogenic F45.8
Metrorrhexis — see Rupture, uterus
Metrosalpingitis N70.91
Metrostaxis N93.8
Metrovaginitis — see Endometritis
Meyer-Schwickerath and Weyers syndrome Q87.0
Meynert's amentia (nonalcoholic) F04
  alcoholic F10.96
    with dependence F10.26
Mibelli's disease (porokeratosis) Q82.8
Mice, joint — see Loose, body, joint
  knee M23.4-
Micrencephalon, micrencephaly Q02
Microalbuminuria R80.9
Microaneurysm, retinal — see also Disorder, retina, microaneurysms
  diabetic — see E08-E13 with .31
Microangiopathy (peripheral) I73.9
  thrombotic M31.1
Microcalcifications, breast R92.0
Microcephalus, microcephalic, microcephaly Q02
  due to toxoplasmosis (congenital) P37.1
Microcheilia Q18.7
Microcolon (congenital) Q43.8
Microcornea (congenital) Q13.4
Microcytic — see condition
Microdeletions NEC Q93.88
Microdontia K00.2
Microdrepanocytosis D57.40
  with crisis (vasoocclusive pain) D57.419
    with
      acute chest syndrome D57.411
      splenic sequestration D57.412
Microembolism
  atherothrombotic — see Atheroembolism
  retinal — see Occlusion, artery, retina
Microencephalon Q02
Microfilaria streptocerca infestation — see Onchocerciasis
Microgastria (congenital) Q40.2
Microgenia M26.06
Microgenitalia, congenital
  female Q52.8
  male Q55.8
Microglioma — see Lymphoma, non-Hodgkin, specified NEC
Microglossia (congenital) Q38.3
Micrognathia, micrognathism (congenital) (mandibular) (maxillary) M26.09
Microgyria (congenital) Q04.3
Microinfarct of heart — see Insufficiency, coronary
Microlentia (congenital) Q12.8
Microlithiasis, alveolar, pulmonary J84.02
Micromastia N64.82
Micromyelia (congenital) Q06.8
Micropenis Q55.62
Microphakia (congenital) Q12.8
Microphthalmos, microphthalmia (congenital) Q11.2
  due to toxoplasmosis P37.1
Micropsia H53.15
Microscopic polyangiitis (polyarteritis) M31.7
Microsporidiosis B60.8
  intestinal A07.8
Microsporon furfur infestation B36.0
Microsporosis — see also Dermatophytosis
  nigra B36.1
Microstomia (congenital) Q18.5
Microtia (congenital) (external ear) Q17.2
Microtropia H50.40
Microvillus inclusion disease (MVD) (MVID) Q43.8
Micturition
  disorder NEC R39.19
    psychogenic F45.8
  frequency R35.0
    psychogenic F45.8
  hesitancy R39.11
  incomplete emptying R39.14
  nocturnal R35.1

Micturition — continued
  painful R30.9
    dysuria R30.0
    psychogenic F45.8
    tenesmus R30.12
  poor stream R39.12
  split stream R39.13
  straining R39.16
  urgency R39.15
Mid plane — see condition
Middle
  ear — see condition
  lobe (right) syndrome J98.19
Miescher's elastoma L87.2
Mietens' syndrome Q87.2
Migraine (idiopathic) G43.909
  with aura (acute-onset) (prolonged) (typical) (without headache) G43.109
    with refractory migraine G43.119
      with status migrainosus G43.111
      without status migrainosus G43.919
    intractable G43.119
      with status migrainosus G43.111
      without status migrainosus G43.119
    not intractable G43.109
      with status migrainosus G43.101
      without status migrainosus G43.109
    persistent G43.509
      with cerebral infarction G43.609
        with refractory migraine G43.619
          with status migrainosus G43.611
          without status migrainosus G43.619
        intractable G43.619
          with status migrainosus G43.611
          without status migrainosus G43.619
        not intractable G43.609
          with status migrainosus G43.601
          without status migrainosus G43.609
        without refractory migraine G43.609
          with status migrainosus G43.601
          without status migrainosus G43.609
      without cerebral infarction G43.509
        with refractory migraine G43.519
          with status migrainosus G43.511
          without status migrainosus G43.519
        intractable G43.519
          with status migrainosus G43.511
          without status migrainosus G43.519
        not intractable G43.509
          with status migrainosus G43.501
          without status migrainosus G43.509
        without refractory migraine G43.509
          with status migrainosus G43.501
          without status migrainosus G43.509
    without mention of refractory migraine G43.109
      with status migrainosus G43.101
      without status migrainosus G43.109
  with refractory migraine G43.919
    with status migrainosus G43.911
    without status migrainosus G43.919
  abdominal G43.D0
    with refractory migraine G43.D1
    intractable G43.D1
    not intractable G43.D0
    without refractory migraine G43.D0
  basilar — see Migraine, with aura
  classical — see Migraine, with aura
  common — see Migraine, without aura
  complicated G43.109
  equivalents — see Migraine, with aura
  familial — see Migraine, hemiplegic
  hemiplegic G43.409
    with refractory migraine G43.419
      with status migrainosus G43.411
      without status migrainosus G43.419
    intractable G43.419
      with status migrainosus G43.411
      without status migrainosus G43.419
    not intractable G43.409
      with status migrainosus G43.401
      without status migrainosus G43.409
    without refractory migraine G43.409
      with status migrainosus G43.401
      without status migrainosus G43.409
  intractable G43.919
    with status migrainosus G43.911
    without status migrainosus G43.919

Migraine (idiopathic) G43.909 — continued
  menstrual G43.D09
    with refractory migraine G43.839
      with status migrainosus G43.831
      without status migrainosus G43.839
    intractable G43.839
      with status migrainosus G43.831
      without status migrainosus G43.839
    not intractable G43.829
      with status migrainosus G43.821
      without status migrainosus G43.829
    without refractory migraine G43.829
      with status migrainosus G43.821
      without status migrainosus G43.829
  menstrually related — see Migraine, menstrual
  not intractable G43.909
    with status migrainosus G43.901
    without status migrainosus G43.919
  ophthalmoplegic G43.B0
    with refractory migraine G43.B1
    intractable G43.B1
    not intractable G43.B0
    without refractory migraine G43.B0
  persistent aura (with, without) cerebral infarction — see Migraine, with aura, persistent
  preceded or accompanied by transient focal neurological phenomena — see Migraine, with aura
  pre-menstrual — see Migraine, menstrual
  pure menstrual — see Migraine, menstrual
  retinal — see Migraine, with aura
  specified NEC G43.809
    intractable G43.819
      with status migrainosus G43.811
      without status migrainosus G43.819
    not intractable G43.809
      with status migrainosus G43.801
      without status migrainosus G43.809
  sporadic — see Migraine, hemiplegic
  transformed — see Migraine, without aura, chronic
  triggered seizures — see Migraine, with aura
  without aura G43.009
    with refractory migraine G43.019
      with status migrainosus G43.011
      without status migrainosus G43.019
    chronic G43.709
      with refractory migraine G43.719
        with status migrainosus G43.711
        without status migrainosus G43.719
      intractable
        with status migrainosus G43.711
        without status migrainosus G43.719
      not intractable
        with status migrainosus G43.701
        without status migrainosus G43.709
      without refractory migraine G43.709
        with status migrainosus G43.701
        without status migrainosus G43.709
    intractable
      with status migrainosus G43.011
      without status migrainosus G43.019
    not intractable
      with status migrainosus G43.001
      without status migrainosus G43.009
    without mention of refractory migraine G43.009
      with status migrainosus G43.001
      without status migrainosus G43.009
  without refractory migraine G43.909
    with status migrainosus G43.901
    without status migrainosus G43.909
Migrant, social Z59.0
Migration, anxiety concerning Z60.3
Migratory, migrating — see also condition
  person Z59.0
  testis Q55.29
Mikity-Wilson disease or syndrome P27.0
Mikulicz' disease or syndrome K11.8
Miliaria L74.3
  alba L74.1
  apocrine L75.2
  crystallina L74.1
  profunda L74.2
  rubra L74.0
  tropicalis L74.2
Miliary — see condition
Milium L72.0
  colloid L57.8

DISEASE INDEX

Milk
  crust L21.0
  excessive secretion O92.6
  poisoning — *see* Poisoning, food, noxious
  retention O92.79
  sickness — *see* Poisoning, food, noxious
  spots I31.0
Milk-alkali disease or syndrome E83.52
Milk-leg (deep vessels) (nonpuerperal) — *see*
    Embolism, vein, lower extremity
  complicating pregnancy O22.3-
  puerperal, postpartum, childbirth O87.1
Milkman's disease or syndrome M83.8
Milky urine — *see* Chyluria
Millar's asthma J38.5
**Millard-Gubler(-Foville) paralysis or
    syndrome** G46.3
Miller Fisher syndrome G61.0
Mills' disease — *see* Hemiplegia
Millstone maker's pneumoconiosis J62.8
Milroy's disease (chronic hereditary edema)
    Q82.0
Minamata disease T26.1-
Miners' asthma or lung J60
Minkowski-Chauffard syndrome — *see*
    Spherocytosis
Minor — *see* condition
Minor's disease (hematomyelia) G95.19
Minot's disease (hemorrhagic disease),
    newborn P53
**Minot-von Willebrand-Jurgens disease or
    syndrome** (angiohemophilia) D68.0
Minus (and plus) hand (intrinsic) — *see*
    Deformity, limb, specified type NEC,
    forearm
Miosis (pupil) H57.03
Mirizzi's syndrome (hepatic duct stenosis)
    K83.1
Mirror writing F81.0
Misadventure (of) (prophylactic)
    (therapeutic) (*see also* Complications)
    T88.9
  administration of insulin (by accident) —
    see subcategory T38.3
  infusion — *see* Complications, infusion
  local applications (of fomentations,
    plasters, etc.) T88.9
    burn or scald — *see* Burn
    specified NEC T88.8
  medical care (early) (late) T88.9
    adverse effect of drugs or chemicals —
      see Table of Drugs and Chemicals
    specified NEC T88.8
  surgical procedure (early) (late) — *see*
    Complications, surgical procedure
  transfusion — *see* Complications,
    transfusion
  vaccination or other immunological
    procedure — *see* Complications,
    vaccination
Miscarriage O03.9
Misdirection, aqueous H40.83-
Misperception, sleep state F51.02
Misplaced, misplacement
  ear Q17.4
  kidney (acquired) N28.89
    congenital Q63.2
  organ or site, congenital NEC — *see*
    Malposition, congenital
Missed
  abortion O02.1
  delivery O36.4
Missing — *see* Absence
Misuse of drugs F19.99
Mitchell's disease (erythromelalgia) I73.81
Mite(s) (infestation) B88.9
  diarrhea B88.0
  grain (itch) B88.0
  hair follicle (itch) B88.0
  in sputum B88.0
Mitral — *see* condition
Mittelschmerz N94.0
Mixed — *see* condition
MNGIE (mitochondrial neurogastrointestinal
    encephalopathy) syndrome E88.49
Mobile, mobility
  cecum Q43.3
  excessive — *see* Hypermobility
  gallbladder, congenital Q44.1
  kidney N28.89
  organ or site, congenital NEC — *see*
    Malposition, congenital
Mobitz heart block (atrioventricular) I44.1

Moebius, Möbius
  disease (ophthalmoplegic migraine) — *see*
    Migraine, ophthalmoplegic
  syndrome Q87.0
    congenital oculofacial paralysis (with
      other anomalies) Q87.0
    ophthalmoplegic migraine — *see*
      Migraine, ophthalmoplegic
Moeller's glossitis K14.0
Mohr's syndrome (Types I and II) Q87.0
Mola destruens D39.2
Molar pregnancy O02.0
Molarization of premolars K00.2
Molding, head (during birth) — *omit code*
Mole (pigmented) — *see also* Nevus
  blood O02.0
  Breus' O02.0
  cancerous — *see* Melanoma
  carneous O02.0
  destructive D39.2
  fleshy O02.0
  hydatid, hydatidiform (benign)
      (complicating pregnancy) (delivered)
      (undelivered) O01.9
    classical O01.0
    complete O01.0
    incomplete O01.1
    invasive D39.2
    malignant D39.2
    partial O01.1
  intrauterine O02.0
  invasive (hydatidiform) D39.2
  malignant
    meaning
      malignant hydatidiform mole D39.2
      melanoma — *see* Melanoma
  nonhydatidiform O02.0
  nonpigmented — *see* Nevus
  pregnancy NEC O02.0
  skin — *see* Nevus
  tubal O00.1
  vesicular — *see* Mole, hydatidiform
Molimen, molimina (menstrual) N94.3
Molluscum contagiosum (epitheliale) B08.1
**Mönckeberg's arteriosclerosis, disease, or
    sclerosis** — *see* Arteriosclerosis,
    extremities
Mondini's malformation (cochlea) Q16.5
Mondor's disease I80.8
Monge's disease T70.29
Monilethrix (congenital) Q84.1
Moniliasis (*see also* Candidiasis) B37.9
  neonatal P37.5
Monitoring (encounter for)
  therapeutic drug level Z51.81
Monkey malaria B53.1
Monkeypox B04
Monoarthritis M13.10
  ankle M13.17-
  elbow M13.12-
  foot joint M13.17-
  hand joint M13.14-
  hip M13.15-
  knee M13.16-
  shoulder M13.11-
  wrist M13.13-
Monoblastic — *see* condition
Monochromat(ism), monochromatopsia
    (acquired) (congenital) H53.51
Monocytic — *see* condition
Monocytopenia D72.818
Monocytosis (symptomatic) D72.821
Monomania — *see* Psychosis
Mononeuritis G58.9
  cranial nerve — *see* Disorder, nerve,
    cranial
  femoral nerve G57.2-
  lateral
    cutaneous nerve of thigh G57.1-
    popliteal nerve G57.3-
  lower limb G57.9-
    specified nerve NEC G57.8-
  medial popliteal nerve G57.4-
  median nerve G56.1-
  multiplex G58.7
  plantar nerve G57.6-
  posterior tibial nerve G57.5-
  radial nerve G56.3-
  sciatic nerve G57.0-
  specified NEC G58.8
  tibial nerve G57.4-
  ulnar nerve G56.2-
  upper limb G56.9-
    specified nerve NEC G56.8-
  vestibular — *see* subcategory H93.3

Mononeuropathy G58.9
  carpal tunnel syndrome — *see* Syndrome,
    carpal tunnel
  diabetic NEC — *see* E08-E13 with .41
  femoral nerve — *see* Lesion, nerve,
    femoral
  ilioinguinal nerve G57.8-
  in diseases classified elsewhere — *see*
    category G59
  intercostal G58.0
  lower limb G57.9-
    causalgia — *see* Causalgia, lower limb
    femoral nerve — *see* Lesion, nerve,
      femoral
    meralgia paresthetica G57.1-
    plantar nerve — *see* Lesion, nerve,
      plantar
    popliteal nerve — *see* Lesion, nerve,
      popliteal
    sciatic nerve — *see* Lesion, nerve, sciatic
    specified NEC G57.8-
    tarsal tunnel syndrome — *see* Syndrome,
      tarsal tunnel
  median nerve — *see* Lesion, nerve, median
  multiplex G58.7
  obturator nerve G57.8-
  popliteal nerve — *see* Lesion, nerve,
    popliteal
  radial nerve — *see* Lesion, nerve, radial
  saphenous nerve G57.8-
  specified NEC G58.8
  tarsal tunnel syndrome — *see* Syndrome,
    tarsal tunnel
  tuberculous A17.83
  ulnar nerve — *see* Lesion, nerve, ulnar
  upper limb G56.9-
    carpal tunnel syndrome — *see*
      Syndrome, carpal tunnel
    causalgia — *see* Causalgia
    median nerve — *see* Lesion, nerve,
      median
    radial nerve — *see* Lesion, nerve, radial
    specified site NEC G56.8-
    ulnar nerve — *see* Lesion, nerve, ulnar
Mononucleosis, infectious B27.90
  with
    complication NEC B27.99
    meningitis B27.92
    polyneuropathy B27.91
  cytomegaloviral B27.10
    with
      complication NEC B27.19
      meningitis B27.12
      polyneuropathy B27.11
  Epstein-Barr (virus) B27.00
    with
      complication NEC B27.09
      meningitis B27.02
      polyneuropathy B27.01
  gammaherpesviral B27.00
    with
      complication NEC B27.09
      meningitis B27.02
      polyneuropathy B27.01
  specified NEC B27.80
    with
      complication NEC B27.89
      meningitis B27.82
      polyneuropathy B27.81
Monoplegia G83.3-
  congenital (cerebral) G80.8
    spastic G80.1
  embolic (current episode) I63.4
  following
    cerebrovascular disease
      cerebral infarction
        lower limb I69.34-
        upper limb I69.33-
      intracerebral hemorrhage
        lower limb I69.14-
        upper limb I69.13-
      lower limb I69.94-
      nontraumatic intracranial hemorrhage
        NEC
        lower limb I69.24-
        upper limb I69.23-
      specified disease NEC
        lower limb I69.84-
        upper limb I69.83-
      stroke NOS
        lower limb I69.34-
        upper limb I69.33-
      subarachnoid hemorrhage
        lower limb I69.04-
        upper limb I69.03-
      upper limb I69.93-
  hysterical (transient) F44.4
  lower limb G83.1-
  psychogenic (conversion reaction) F44.4
  thrombotic (current episode) I63.3

Monoplegia G83.3- — *continued*
  transient R29.818
  upper limb G83.2-
Monorchism, monorchidism Q55.0
Monosomy (*see also* Deletion, chromosome)
    Q93.9
  specified NEC Q93.89
  whole chromosome
    meiotic nondisjunction Q93.0
    mitotic nondisjunction Q93.1
    mosaicism Q93.1
  X Q96.9
Monster, monstrosity (single) Q89.7
  acephalic Q00.0
  twin Q89.4
Monteggia's fracture(-dislocation) S52.27-
Moore's syndrome — *see* Epilepsy, specified
    NEC
Mooren's ulcer (cornea) — *see* Ulcer,
    cornea, Mooren's
Mooser's bodies A75.2
Mooser-Neill reaction A75.2
Morbidity not stated or unknown R69
Morbilli — *see* Measles
Morbus — *see also* Disease
  angelicus, anglorum E55.0
  Beigel B36.2
  caducus — *see* Epilepsy
  celiacus K90.0
  comitialis — *see* Epilepsy
  cordis (*see also* Disease, heart) I51.9
    valvulorum — *see* Endocarditis
  coxae senilis M16.9
    tuberculous A18.02
  hemorrhagicus neonatorum P53
  maculosus neonatorum P54.5
Morel-Kraepelin disease — *see*
    Schizophrenia
Morel-Moore syndrome M85.2
Morel(-Stewart)(-Morgagni) syndrome
    M85.2
Morgagni's
  cyst, organ, hydatid, or appendage
    female Q50.5
    male (epididymal) Q55.4
      testicular Q55.29
  syndrome M85.2
Morgagni-Stewart-Morel syndrome M85.2
Morgagni-Stokes-Adams syndrome I45.9
Morgagni-Turner(-Albright) syndrome
    Q96.9
Moria F07.0
Moron (I.Q. 50-69) F70
Morphea L94.0
Morphinism (without remission) F11.20
  with remission F11.21
Morphinomania (without remission) F11.20
  with remission F11.21
**Morquio(-Ullrich)(-Brailsford) disease or
    syndrome** — *see*
    Mucopolysaccharidosis
Mortification (dry) (moist) — *see* Gangrene
Morton's metatarsalgia (neuralgia)
    (neuroma) (syndrome) G57.6-
Morvan's disease or syndrome G60.8
Mosaicism, mosaic (autosomal)
    (chromosomal)
  45,X/46,XX Q96.3
  45,X/other cell lines NEC with abnormal
    sex chromosome Q96.4
  sex chromosome
    female Q97.8
    lines with various numbers of X
      chromosomes Q97.2
    male Q98.7
  XY Q96.3
Moschowitz' disease M31.1
Mother yaw A66.0
Motion sickness (from travel, any vehicle)
    (from roundabouts or swings) T75.3
Mottled, mottling, teeth (enamel) (endemic)
    (nonendemic) K00.3
Mounier-Kuhn syndrome Q32.4
  with bronchiectasis J47.9
    exacerbation (acute) J47.1
    lower respiratory infection J47.0
  acquired J98.09
    with bronchiectasis J47.9
      with
        exacerbation (acute) J47.1
        lower respiratory infection J47.0
Mountain
  sickness T70.29
    with polycythemia , acquired (acute)
      D75.1
  tick fever A93.2
Mouse, joint — *see* Loose, body, joint
  knee M23.4-
Mouth — *see* condition

Movable
coccyx — see subcategory M53.2
kidney N28.89
congenital Q63.8
spleen D73.89
Movements, dystonic R25.8
Moyamoya disease I67.5
MRSA (methacillin resistant Staphylococcus aureus)
infection A49.02
as the cause of diseases classified elsewhere B95.62
sepsis A41.02
MSSA (methacillin susceptible Staphylococcus aureus)
infection A49.01
as the cause of diseases classified elsewhere B95.61
sepsis A41.01
Mucha-Habermann disease L41.0
Mucinosis (cutaneous) (focal) (papular) (reticular erythematous) (skin) L98.5
oral K13.79
Mucocele
appendix K38.8
buccal cavity K13.79
gallbladder K82.1
lacrimal sac, chronic H04.43-
nasal sinus J34.1
nose J34.1
salivary gland (any) K11.6
sinus (accessory) (nasal) J34.1
turbinate (bone) (middle) (nasal) J34.1
uterus N85.8
Mucolipidosis
I E77.1
II, III E77.0
IV E75.11
Mucopolysaccharidosis E76.3
beta-glucuronidase deficiency E76.29
cardiopathy E76.3 [I52]
Hunter's syndrome E76.1
Hurler's syndrome E76.01
Hurler-Scheie syndrome E76.02
Maroteaux-Lamy syndrome E76.29
Morquio syndrome E76.219
A E76.210
B E76.211
classic E76.210
Sanfilippo syndrome E76.22
Scheie's syndrome E76.03
specified NEC E76.29
type
I
Hurler's syndrome E76.01
Hurler-Scheie syndrome E76.02
Scheie's syndrome E76.03
II E76.1
III E76.22
IV E76.219
IVA E76.210
IVB E76.211
VI E76.29
VII E76.29
Mucormycosis B46.5
cutaneous B46.3
disseminated B46.4
gastrointestinal B46.2
generalized B46.4
pulmonary B46.0
rhinocerebral B46.1
skin B46.3
subcutaneous B46.3
Mucositis (ulcerative) K12.30
due to drugs NEC K12.32
gastrointestinal K92.81
mouth (oral) (oropharyngeal) K12.30
due to antineoplastic therapy K12.31
due to drugs NEC K12.32
due to radiation K12.33
specified NEC K12.39
viral K12.39
nasal J34.81
oral cavity — see Mucositis, mouth
oral soft tissues — see Mucositis, mouth
vagina and vulva N76.81
Mucositis necroticans agranulocytica — see Agranulocytosis
Mucous — see also condition
patches (syphilitic) A51.39
congenital A50.07
Mucoviscidosis E84.9
with meconium obstruction E84.11
Mucus
asphyxia or suffocation — see Asphyxia, mucus
in stool R19.5
plug — see Asphyxia, mucus
Muguet B37.0

Mulberry molars (congenital syphilis) A50.52
Müllerian mixed tumor
specified site — see Neoplasm, malignant, by site
unspecified site C54.9
Multicystic kidney (development) Q61.4
Multiparity (grand) Z64.1
affecting management of pregnancy, labor and delivery (supervision only) O09.4-
requiring contraceptive management — see Contraception
Multipartita placenta O43.19-
Multiple, multiplex — see also condition
digits (congenital) Q69.9
endocrine neoplasia — see Neoplasia, endocrine, multiple (MEN)
personality F44.81
Mumps B26.9
arthritis B26.85
complication NEC B26.89
encephalitis B26.2
hepatitis B26.81
meningitis (aseptic) B26.1
meningoencephalitis B26.2
myocarditis B26.82
oophoritis B26.89
orchitis B26.0
pancreatitis B26.3
polyneuropathy B26.84
Mumu (see also Infestation, filarial) B74.9 [N51]
Münchhausen's syndrome — see Disorder, factitious
Münchmeyer's syndrome — see Myositis, ossificans, progressiva
Mural — see condition
Murmur (cardiac) (heart) (organic) R01.1
abdominal R19.15
aortic (valve) — see Endocarditis, aortic
benign R01.0
diastolic — see Endocarditis
Flint I35.1
functional R01.0
Graham Steell I37.1
innocent R01.0
mitral (valve) — see Insufficiency, mitral
nonorganic R01.0
presystolic, mitral — see Insufficiency, mitral
pulmonic (valve) I37.8
systolic (valvular) — see Endocarditis
tricuspid (valve) I07.9
valvular — see Endocarditis
Murri's disease (intermittent hemoglobinuria) D59.6
Muscle, muscular — see also condition
carnitine (palmityltransferase) deficiency E71.314
Musculoneuralgia — see Neuralgia
Mushroom-workers' (pickers') disease or lung J67.5
Mushrooming hip — see Derangement, joint, specified NEC, hip
Mutation(s)
factor V Leiden D68.51
prothrombin gene D68.52
surfactant, of lung J84.83
Mutism — see also Aphasia
deaf (acquired) (congenital) NEC H91.3
elective (adjustment reaction) (childhood) F94.0
hysterical F44.4
selective (childhood) F94.0
MVD (microvillus inclusion disease) Q43.8
MVID (microvillus inclusion disease) Q43.8
Myalgia M79.1
epidemic (cervical) B33.0
traumatic NEC T14.8
Myasthenia G70.9
congenital G70.2
cordis — see Failure, heart
developmental G70.2
gravis G70.00
with exacerbation (acute) G70.01
in crisis G70.01
neonatal, transient P94.0
pseudoparalytica G70.00
with exacerbation (acute) G70.01
in crisis G70.01
stomach, psychogenic F45.8
syndrome
in
diabetes mellitus — see E08-E13 with .44
neoplastic disease (see also Neoplasm) D49.9 [G73.3]
pernicious anemia D51.0 [G73.3]
thyrotoxicosis E05.90 [G73.3]
with thyroid storm E05.91 [G73.3]

Myasthenic M62.81
Mycelium infection B49
Mycetismus — see Poisoning, food, noxious, mushroom
Mycetoma B47.9
actinomycotic B47.1
bone (mycotic) B47.9 [M90.80]
eumycotic B47.0
foot B47.9
actinomycotic B47.1
mycotic B47.0
madurae NEC B47.9
mycotic B47.0
maduromycotic B47.0
mycotic B47.0
nocardial B47.1
Mycobacteriosis — see Mycobacterium
Mycobacterium, mycobacterial (infection) A31.9
anonymous A31.9
atypical A31.9
cutaneous A31.1
pulmonary A31.0
tuberculous — see Tuberculosis, pulmonary
specified site NEC A31.8
avium (intracellulare complex) A31.0
balnei A31.1
Battey A31.0
chelonei A31.1
cutaneous A31.1
extrapulmonary systemic A31.8
fortuitum A31.8
intracellulare (Battey bacillus) A31.0
kakaferifu A31.8
kansasii (yellow bacillus) A31.0
kasongo A31.8
leprae (see also Leprosy) A30.9
luciflavum A31.8
marinum (M. balnei) A31.1
nonspecific — see Mycobacterium, atypical
pulmonary (atypical) A31.0
tuberculous — see Tuberculosis, pulmonary
scrofulaceum A31.8
simiae A31.8
systemic, extrapulmonary A31.8
szulgai A31.8
terrae A31.8
triviale A31.8
tuberculosis (human, bovine) — see Tuberculosis
ulcerans A31.1
xenopi A31.8
Mycoplasma (M.) pneumoniae, as cause of disease classified elsewhere B96.0
Mycosis, mycotic B49
cutaneous NEC B36.9
ear B36.9
fungoides (extranodal) (solid organ) C84.0-
mouth B37.0
nails B35.1
opportunistic B48.8
skin NEC B36.9
specified NEC B48.8
stomatitis B37.0
vagina, vaginitis (candidal) B37.3
Mydriasis (pupil) H57.04
Myelatelia Q06.1
Myelinolysis, pontine, central G37.2
Myelitis (acute) (ascending) (childhood) (chronic) (descending) (diffuse) (disseminated) (idiopathic) (pressure) (progressive) (spinal cord) (subacute) (see also Encephalitis) G04.91
herpes simplex B00.82
herpes zoster B02.24
in diseases classified elsewhere G05.4
necrotizing, subacute G37.4
optic neuritis in G36.0
postchickenpox B01.12
postherpetic B02.24
postimmunization G04.02
postinfectious NEC G04.89
postvaccinal G04.02
specified NEC G04.89
syphilitic (transverse) A52.14
toxic G92
transverse (in demyelinating diseases of central nervous system) G37.3
tuberculous A17.82
varicella B01.12
Myelo-osteo-musculodysplasia hereditaria Q79.8
Myeloblastic — see condition

Myeloblastoma
granular cell — see also Neoplasm, connective tissue
malignant — see Neoplasm, connective tissue, malignant
tongue D10.1
Myelocele — see Spina bifida
Myelocystocele — see Spina bifida
Myelocytic — see condition
Myelodysplasia D46.9
specified NEC D46.Z
spinal cord (congenital) Q06.1
Myelodysplastic syndrome D46.9
with
5q deletion D46.C
isolated del(5q) chromosomal abnormality D46.C
specified NEC D46.Z
Myeloencephalitis — see Encephalitis
Myelofibrosis D75.81
with myeloid metaplasia D47.4
acute C94.4-
idiopathic (chronic) D47.4
primary D47.1
secondary D75.81
in myeloproliferative disease D47.4
Myelogenous — see condition
Myeloid — see condition
Myelokathexis D70.9
Myeloleukodystrophy E75.29
Myelolipoma — see Lipoma
Myeloma (multiple) C90.0-
monostatic C90.3
plasma cell C90.0-
plasma cell C90.0-
solitary (see also Plasmacytoma, solitary) C90.3-
Myelomalacia G95.89
Myelomatosis C90.0-
Myelomeningitis — see Meningoencephalitis
Myelomeningocele (spinal cord) — see Spina bifida
Myelopathic
anemia D64.89
muscle atrophy — see Atrophy, muscle, spinal
pain syndrome G89.0
Myelopathy (spinal cord) G95.9
drug-induced G95.89
in (due to)
degeneration or displacement, intervertebral disc NEC — see Disorder, disc, with, myelopathy
infection — see Encephalitis
intervertebral disc disorder — see also Disorder, disc, with, myelopathy
mercury — see subcategory T56.1
neoplastic disease (see also Neoplasm) D49.9 [G99.2]
pernicious anemia D51.0 [G99.2]
spondylosis — see Spondylosis, with myelopathy NEC
necrotic (subacute) (vascular) G95.19
radiation-induced G95.89
spondylogenic NEC — see Spondylosis, with myelopathy NEC
toxic G95.89
transverse, acute G37.3
vascular G95.19
vitamin B12 E53.8 [G32.0]
Myelophthisis D61.82
Myeloradiculitis G04.91
Myeloradiculodysplasia (spinal) Q06.1
Myelosarcoma C92.3-
Myelosclerosis D75.89
with myeloid metaplasia D47.4
disseminated, of nervous system G35
megakaryocytic D47.4
with myeloid metaplasia D47.4
Myelosis
acute C92.0-
aleukemic C92.9-
chronic D47.1
erythremic (acute) C94.0-
megakaryocytic C94.2-
nonleukemic D72.828
subacute C92.9-
Myiasis (cavernous) B87.9
aural B87.4
creeping B87.0
cutaneous B87.0
dermal B87.0
ear (external) (middle) B87.4
eye B87.2
genitourinary B87.81
intestinal B87.82
laryngeal B87.3
nasopharyngeal B87.3
ocular B87.2
orbit B87.2

Myiasis (cavernous) B87.9 — *continued*
  skin B87.0
  specified site NEC B87.89
  traumatic B87.1
  wound B87.1
Myoadenoma, prostate — *see* Hyperplasia, prostate
Myoblastoma
  granular cell — *see also* Neoplasm, connective tissue, benign
    malignant — *see* Neoplasm, connective tissue, malignant
  tongue D10.1
Myocardial — *see* condition
Myocardiopathy (congestive) (constrictive) (familial) (hypertrophic nonobstructive) (idiopathic) (infiltrative) (obstructive) (primary) (restrictive) (sporadic) (*see also* Cardiomyopathy) I42.9
  alcoholic I42.6
  cobalt-beer I42.6
  glycogen storage E74.02 [I43]
  hypertrophic obstructive I42.1
  in (due to)
    beriberi E51.12
    cardiac glycogenosis E74.02 [I43]
    Friedreich's ataxia G11.1 [I43]
    myotonia atrophica G71.11 [I43]
    progressive muscular dystrophy G71.0 [I43]
  obscure (African) I42.8
  secondary I42.9
  thyrotoxic E05.90 [I43]
    with storm E05.91 [I43]
  toxic NEC I42.7
Myocarditis (with arteriosclerosis) (chronic) (fibroid) (interstitial) (old) (progressive) (senile) I51.4
  with
    rheumatic fever (conditions in I00) I09.0
      active — *see* Myocarditis, acute, rheumatic
      inactive or quiescent (with chorea) I09.0
  active I40.9
    rheumatic I01.2
      with chorea (acute) (rheumatic) (Sydenham's) I02.0
  acute or subacute (interstitial) I40.9
    due to
      streptococcus (beta-hemolytic) I01.2
    idiopathic I40.1
    rheumatic I01.2
      with chorea (acute) (rheumatic) (Sydenham's) I02.0
    specified NEC I40.8
  aseptic of newborn B33.22
  bacterial (acute) I40.0
  Coxsackie (virus) B33.22
  diphtheritic A36.81
  eosinophilic I40.1
  epidemic of newborn (Coxsackie) B33.22
  Fiedler's (acute) (isolated) I40.1
  giant cell (acute) (subacute) I40.1
  gonococcal A54.83
  granulomatous (idiopathic) (isolated) (nonspecific) I40.1
  hypertensive — *see* Hypertension, heart
  idiopathic (granulomatous) I40.1
  in (due to)
    diphtheria A36.81
    epidemic louse-borne typhus A75.0 [I41]
    Lyme disease A69.29
    sarcoidosis D86.85
    scarlet fever A38.1
    toxoplasmosis (acquired) B58.81
    typhoid A01.02
    typhus NEC A75.9 [I41]
  infective I40.0
  influenzal — *see* Influenza, with, myocarditis
  isolated (acute) I40.1
  meningococcal A39.52
  mumps B26.82
  nonrheumatic, active I40.9
  parenchymatous I40.9
  pneumococcal I40.0
  rheumatic (chronic) (inactive) (with chorea) I09.0
    active or acute I01.2
      with chorea (acute) (rheumatic) (Sydenham's) I02.0
  rheumatoid — *see* Rheumatoid, carditis
  septic I40.0
  staphylococcal I40.0
  suppurative I40.0
  syphilitic (chronic) A52.06

Myocarditis (with arteriosclerosis) (chronic) (fibroid) (interstitial) (old) (progressive) (senile) I51.4 — *continued*
  toxic I40.8
    rheumatic — *see* Myocarditis, acute, rheumatic
  tuberculous A18.84
  typhoid A01.02
  valvular — *see* Endocarditis
  virus, viral I40.0
    of newborn (Coxsackie) B33.22
Myocardium, myocardial — *see* condition
Myocardosis — *see* Cardiomyopathy
Myoclonus, myoclonic, myoclonia (familial) (essential) (multifocal) (simplex) G25.3
  drug-induced G25.3
  epilepsy (*see also* Epilepsy, generalized, specified NEC) G40.4-
    familial (progressive) G25.3
  epileptica G40.409
    with status epilepticus G40.401
  facial G51.3
  familial progressive G25.3
  Friedreich's G25.3
  jerks G25.3
  massive G25.3
  palatal G25.3
  pharyngeal G25.3
Myocytolysis I51.5
Myodiastasis — *see* Diastasis, muscle
Myoendocarditis — *see* Endocarditis
Myoepithelioma — *see* Neoplasm, benign, by site
Myofasciitis (acute) — *see* Myositis
Myofibroma — *see also* Neoplasm, connective tissue, benign
  uterus (cervix) (corpus) — *see* Leiomyoma
Myofibromatosis D48.1
  infantile Q89.8
Myofibrosis M62.89
  heart — *see* Myocarditis
  scapulohumeral — *see* Lesion, shoulder, specified NEC
Myofibrositis M79.7
  scapulohumeral — *see* Lesion, shoulder, specified NEC
Myoglobulinuria, myoglobinuria (primary) R82.1
Myokymia, facial G51.4
Myolipoma — *see* Lipoma
Myoma — *see also* Neoplasm, connective tissue, benign
  malignant — *see* Neoplasm, connective tissue, malignant
  prostate D29.1
  uterus (cervix) (corpus) — *see* Leiomyoma
Myomalacia M62.89
Myometritis — *see* Endometritis
Myometrium — *see* condition
Myonecrosis, clostridial A48.0
Myopathy G72.9
  acute
    necrotizing G72.81
    quadriplegic G72.81
  alcoholic G72.1
  benign congenital G71.2
  central core G71.2
  centronuclear G71.2
  congenital (benign) G71.2
  critical illness G72.81
  distal G71.0
  drug-induced G72.0
  endocrine NEC E34.9 [G73.7]
  extraocular muscles H05.82-
  facioscapulohumeral G71.0
  hereditary G71.9
    specified NEC G71.8
  immune NEC G72.49
  in (due to)
    Addison's disease E27.1 [G73.7]
    alcohol G72.1
    amyloidosis E85.0 [G73.7]
    cretinism E00.9 [G73.7]
    Cushing's syndrome E24.9 [G73.7]
    drugs G72.0
    endocrine disease NEC E34.9 [G73.7]
    giant cell arteritis M31.6 [G73.7]
    glycogen storage disease E74.00 [G73.7]
    hyperadrenocorticism E24.9 [G73.7]
    hyperparathyroidism NEC E21.3 [G73.7]
    hypoparathyroidism E20.9 [G73.7]
    hypopituitarism E23.0 [G73.7]
    hypothyroidism E03.9 [G73.7]
    infectious disease NEC B99 [G73.7]
    lipid storage disease E75.6 [G73.7]
    metabolic disease NEC E88.9 [G73.7]
    myxedema E03.9 [G73.7]
    parasitic disease NEC B89 [G73.7]
    polyarteritis nodosa M30.0 [G73.7]

Myopathy G72.9 — *continued*
  in (due to) — *continued*
    rheumatoid arthritis — *see* Rheumatoid, myopathy
    sarcoidosis D86.87
    scleroderma M34.82
    sicca syndrome M35.03
    Sjögren's syndrome M35.03
    systemic lupus erythematosus M32.19
    thyrotoxicosis (hyperthyroidism) E05.90 [G73.7]
      with thyroid storm E05.91 [G73.7]
    toxic agent NEC G72.2
  inflammatory NEC G72.49
  intensive care (ICU) G72.81
  limb-girdle G71.0
  mitochondrial NEC G71.3
  myotubular G71.2
  mytonic, proximal (PROMM) G71.11
  nemaline G71.2
  ocular G71.0
  oculopharyngeal G71.0
  of critical illness G72.81
  primary G71.9
    specified NEC G71.8
  progressive NEC G72.89
  proximal myotonic (PROMM) G71.11
  rod G71.2
  scapulohumeral G71.0
  specified NEC G72.89
  toxic G72.2
Myopericarditis — *see also* Pericarditis
  chronic rheumatic I09.2
Myopia (axial) (congenital) H52.1-
  degenerative (malignant) H44.2-
  malignant H44.2-
  pernicious H44.2-
  progressive high (degenerative) H44.2-
Myosarcoma — *see* Neoplasm, connective tissue, malignant
Myosis (pupil) H57.03
  stromal (endolymphatic) D39.0
Myositis M60.9
  clostridial A48.0
  due to posture — *see* Myositis, specified type NEC
  epidemic B33.0
  fibrosa or fibrous (chronic), Volkmann's T79.6
  foreign body granuloma — *see* Granuloma, foreign body
  in (due to)
    bilharziasis B65.9 [M63.8-]
    cysticercosis B69.81
    leprosy A30.9 [M63.8-]
    mycosis B49 [M63.8-]
    sarcoidosis D86.87
    schistosomiasis B65.9 [M63.8-]
    syphilis
      late A52.78
      secondary A51.49
    toxoplasmosis (acquired) B58.82
    trichinellosis B75 [M63.8-]
    tuberculosis A18.09
  inclusion body [IBM] G72.41
  infective M60.009
    arm M60.002
      left M60.001
      right M60.000
    leg M60.005
      left M60.004
      right M60.003
    lower limb M60.005
      ankle M60.07-
      foot M60.07-
      lower leg M60.06-
      thigh M60.05-
      toe M60.07-
    multiple sites M60.09
    specified site NEC M60.08
    upper limb M60.002
      finger M60.04-
      forearm M60.03-
      hand M60.04-
      shoulder region M60.01-
      upper arm M60.02-
  interstitial M60.10
    ankle M60.17-
    foot M60.17-
    forearm M60.13-
    hand M60.14-
    lower leg M60.16-
    multiple sites M60.19
    shoulder region M60.11-
    specified site NEC M60.18
    thigh M60.15-
    upper arm M60.12-
  mycotic B49 [M63.8-]
  orbital, chronic H05.12-

Myositis M60.9 — *continued*
  ossificans or ossifying (circumscripta) — *see also* Ossification, muscle, specified NEC
    in (due to)
      burns M61.30
        ankle M61.37-
        foot M61.37-
        forearm M61.33-
        hand M61.34-
        lower leg M61.36-
        multiple sites M61.39
        pelvic region M61.35-
        shoulder region M61.31-
        specified site NEC M61.38
        thigh M61.35-
        upper arm M61.32-
      quadriplegia or paraplegia M61.20
        ankle M61.27-
        foot M61.27-
        forearm M61.23-
        hand M61.24-
        lower leg M61.26-
        multiple sites M61.29
        pelvic region M61.25-
        shoulder region M61.21-
        specified site NEC M61.28
        thigh M61.25-
        upper arm M61.22-
  progressiva M61.10
    ankle M61.17-
    finger M61.14-
    foot M61.17-
    forearm M61.13-
    hand M61.14-
    lower leg M61.16-
    multiple sites M61.19
    pelvic region M61.15-
    shoulder region M61.11-
    specified site NEC M61.18
    thigh M61.15-
    toe M61.17-
    upper arm M61.12-
  traumatica M61.00
    ankle M61.07-
    foot M61.07-
    forearm M61.03-
    hand M61.04-
    lower leg M61.06-
    multiple sites M61.09
    pelvic region M61.05-
    shoulder region M61.01-
    specified site NEC M61.08
    thigh M61.05-
    upper arm M61.02-
  purulent — *see* Myositis, infective
  specified type NEC M60.80
    ankle M60.87-
    foot M60.87-
    forearm M60.83-
    hand M60.84-
    lower leg M60.86-
    multiple sites M60.89
    pelvic region M60.85-
    shoulder region M60.81-
    specified site NEC M60.88
    thigh M60.85-
    upper arm M60.82-
  suppurative — *see* Myositis, infective
  traumatic (old) — *see* Myositis, specified type NEC
Myospasia impulsiva F95.2
Myotonia (acquisita) (intermittens) M62.89
  atrophica G71.11
  chondrodystrophic G71.13
  congenita (acetazolamide responsive) (dominant) (recessive) G71.12
  drug-induced G71.14
  dystrophica G71.11
  fluctuans G71.19
  levior G71.12
  permanens G71.19
  symptomatic G71.19
Myotonic pupil — *see* Anomaly, pupil, function, tonic pupil
Myriapodiasis B88.2
Myringitis H73.2-
  with otitis media — *see* Otitis, media
  acute H73.00-
    bullous H73.01-
    specified NEC H73.09-
  bullous — *see* Myringitis, acute, bullous
  chronic H73.1-

Mysophobia F40.228
Mytilotoxism — *see* Poisoning, fish
Myxadenitis labialis K13.0
Myxedema (adult) (idiocy) (infantile) (juvenile) (*see also* Hypothyroidism) E03.9
  circumscribed E05.90
    with storm E05.91
  coma E03.5
  congenital E00.1
  cutis L98.5
  localized (pretibial) E05.90
    with storm E05.91
  papular L98.5
Myxochondrosarcoma — *see* Neoplasm, cartilage, malignant
Myxofibroma — *see* Neoplasm, connective tissue, benign
  odontogenic — *see* Cyst, calcifying odontogenic
Myxofibrosarcoma — *see* Neoplasm, connective tissue, malignant
Myxolipoma D17.9
Myxoliposarcoma — *see* Neoplasm, connective tissue, malignant
Myxoma — *see also* Neoplasm, connective tissue, benign
  nerve sheath — *see* Neoplasm, nerve, benign
  odontogenic — *see* Cyst, calcifying odontogenic
Myxosarcoma — *see* Neoplasm, connective tissue, malignant

N

Naegeli's
  disease Q82.8
  leukemia, monocytic C93.1-
Naegleriasis (with meningoencephalitis) B60.2
Naffziger's syndrome G54.0
Naga sore — *see* Ulcer, skin
Nägele's pelvis M95.5
  with disproportion (fetopelvic) O33.0
    causing obstructed labor O65.0
Nail — *see also* condition
  biting F98.8
  patella syndrome Q87.2
Nanism, nanosomia — *see* Dwarfism
Nanophyetiasis B66.8
Nanukayami A27.89
Napkin rash L22
Narcolepsy G47.419
  with cataplexy G47.411
  in conditions classified elsewhere G47.429
    with cataplexy G47.421
Narcosis R06.89
Narcotism — *see* Dependence
NARP (neuropathy, ataxia and retinitis pigmentosa) syndrome E88.49
Narrow
  anterior chamber angle H40.03-
  pelvis — *see* Contraction, pelvis
Narrowing — *see also* Stenosis
  artery I77.1
    auditory, internal I65.8
    basilar — *see* Occlusion, artery, basilar
    carotid — *see* Occlusion, artery, carotid
    cerebellar — *see* Occlusion, artery, cerebellar
    cerebral — *see* Occlusion artery, cerebral
    choroidal — *see* Occlusion, artery, cerebral, specified NEC
    communicating posterior — *see* Occlusion, artery, cerebral, specified NEC
    coronary — *see also* Disease, heart, ischemic, atherosclerotic
      congenital Q24.5
      syphilitic A50.54 [I52]
      due to syphilis NEC A52.06
    hypophyseal — *see* Occlusion, artery, cerebral, specified NEC
    pontine — *see* Occlusion, artery, cerebral, specified NEC
    precerebral — *see* Occlusion, artery, precerebral
    vertebral — *see* Occlusion, artery, vertebral
  auditory canal (external) — *see* Stenosis, external ear canal
  eustachian tube — *see* Obstruction, eustachian tube
  eyelid — *see* Disorder, eyelid function
  larynx J38.6
  mesenteric artery K55.0
  palate M26.89
  palpebral fissure — *see* Disorder, eyelid function
  ureter N13.5
    with infection N13.6
  urethra — *see* Stricture, urethra
Narrowness, abnormal, eyelid Q10.3
Nasal — *see* condition
Nasolachrymal, nasolacrimal — *see* condition
Nasopharyngeal — *see also* condition
  pituitary gland Q89.2
  torticollis M43.6
Nasopharyngitis (acute) (infective) (streptococcal) (subacute) J00
  chronic (suppurative) (ulcerative) J31.1
Nasopharynx, nasopharyngeal — *see* condition
Natal tooth, teeth K00.6
Nausea (without vomiting) R11.0
  with vomiting R11.2
  gravidarum — *see* Hyperemesis, gravidarum
  marina T75.3
  navalis T75.3
Navel — *see* condition
Neapolitan fever — *see* Brucellosis
Near drowning T75.1
Near-syncope R55

Nearsightedness — *see* Myopia
Nebula, cornea — *see* Opacity, cornea
Necator americanus infestation B76.1
Necatoriasis B76.1
Neck — *see* condition
Necrobiosis R68.89
  lipoidica NEC L92.1
    with diabetes — *see* E08-E13 with .620
Necrolysis, toxic epidermal L51.2
  due to drug
    correct substance properly administered — *see* Table of Drugs and Chemicals, by drug, adverse effect
    overdose or wrong substance given or taken — *see* Table of Drugs and Chemicals, by drug, poisoning
Necrophilia F65.89
Necrosis, necrotic (ischemic) — *see also* Gangrene
  adrenal (capsule) (gland) E27.49
  amputation stump (surgical) (late) T87.50
    arm T87.5-
    leg T87.5-
  antrum J32.0
  aorta (hyaline) — *see also* Aneurysm, aorta
    cystic medial — *see* Dissection, aorta
  artery I77.5
  bladder (aseptic) (sphincter) N32.89
  bone (*see also* Osteonecrosis) M87.9
    aseptic or avascular — *see* Osteonecrosis idiopathic M87.00
    ethmoid J32.2
    jaw M27.2
    tuberculous — *see* Tuberculosis, bone
  brain I67.89
  breast (aseptic) (fat) (segmental) N64.1
  bronchus J98.09
  central nervous system NEC I67.89
  cerebellar I67.89
  cerebral I67.89
  colon K55.0
  cornea H18.40
  cortical (acute) (renal) N17.1
  cystic medial (aorta) — *see* Dissection, aorta
  dental pulp K04.1
  esophagus K22.8
  ethmoid (bone) J32.2
  eyelid — *see* Disorder, eyelid, degenerative
  fat, fatty (generalized) — *see also* Disorder, soft tissue, specified type NEC
    abdominal wall K65.4
    breast (aseptic) (segmental) N64.1
    localized — *see* Degeneration, by site, fatty
    mesentery K65.4
    omentum K65.4
    pancreas K86.8
    peritoneum K65.4
    skin (subcutaneous), newborn P83.0
    subcutaneous, due to birth injury P15.6
  gallbladder — *see* Cholecystitis, acute
  heart — *see* Infarct, myocardium
  hip, aseptic or avascular — *see* Osteonecrosis, by type, femur
  intestine (acute) (hemorrhagic) (massive) K55.0
  jaw M27.2
  kidney (bilateral) N28.0
    acute N17.9
    cortical (acute) (bilateral) N17.1
      with ectopic or molar pregnancy O08.4
    medullary (bilateral) (in acute renal failure) (papillary) N17.2
    papillary (bilateral) (in acute renal failure) N17.2
    tubular N17.0
      with ectopic or molar pregnancy O08.4
      complicating
        abortion — *see* Abortion, by type, complicated by, tubular necrosis
        ectopic or molar pregnancy O08.4
        pregnancy — *see* Pregnancy, complicated by, diseases of, specified type or system NEC
      following ectopic or molar pregnancy O08.4
      traumatic T79.5
  larynx J38.7
  liver (with hepatic failure) (cell) — *see* Failure, hepatic
    hemorrhagic, central K76.2

Necrosis, necrotic (ischemic) — *see also* Gangrene — *continued*
  lung J85.0
  lymphatic gland — *see* Lymphadenitis, acute
  mammary gland (fat) (segmental) N64.1
  mastoid (chronic) — *see* Mastoiditis, chronic
  medullary (acute) (renal) N17.2
  mesentery K55.0
    fat K65.4
  mitral valve — *see* Insufficiency, mitral
  myocardium, myocardial — *see* Infarct, myocardium
  nose J34.0
  omentum (with mesenteric infarction) K55.0
    fat K65.4
  orbit, orbital — *see* Osteomyelitis, orbit
  ossicles, ear — *see* Abnormal, ear ossicles
  ovary N70.92
  pancreas (aseptic) (duct) (fat) K86.8
    acute (infective) — *see* Pancreatitis, acute
    infective — *see* Pancreatitis, acute
  papillary (acute) (renal) N17.2
  perineum N90.89
  peritoneum (with mesenteric infarction) K55.0
    fat K65.4
  pharynx J02.9
    in granulocytopenia — *see* Neutropenia Vincent's A69.1
  phosphorus — *see* subcategory T54.2
  pituitary (gland) (postpartum) (Sheehan) E23.0
  pressure — *see* Ulcer, pressure, by site
  pulmonary J85.0
  pulp (dental) K04.1
  radiation — *see* Necrosis, by site
  radium — *see* Necrosis, by site
  renal — *see* Necrosis, kidney
  sclera H15.89
  scrotum N50.8
  skin or subcutaneous tissue NEC I96
  spine, spinal (column) — *see also* Osteonecrosis, by type, vertebra
    cord G95.19
  spleen D73.5
  stomach K31.89
  stomatitis (ulcerative) A69.0
  subcutaneous fat, newborn P83.8
  subendocardial (acute) I21.4
    chronic I25.89
  suprarenal (capsule) (gland) E27.49
  testis N50.8
  thymus (gland) E32.8
  tonsil J35.8
  trachea J39.8
  tuberculous NEC — *see* Tuberculosis
  tubular (acute) (anoxic) (renal) (toxic) N17.0
    postprocedural N99.0
  vagina N89.8
  vertebra — *see also* Osteonecrosis, by type, vertebra
    tuberculous A18.01
  vulva N90.89
  X-ray — *see* Necrosis, by site
Necrospermia — *see* Infertility, male
Need (for)
  care provider because (of)
    assistance with personal care Z74.1
    continuous supervision required Z74.3
    impaired mobility Z74.09
    no other household member able to render care Z74.2
    specified reason NEC Z74.8
  immunization — *see* Vaccination
  vaccination — *see* Vaccination
Neglect
  adult
    confirmed T74.01
    history of Z91.412
    suspected T76.01
  child (childhood)
    confirmed T74.02
    history of Z62.812
    suspected T76.02
  emotional, in childhood Z62.898
  hemispatial R41.4
  left-sided R41.4
  sensory R41.4
  visuospatial R41.4

Neisserian infection NEC — *see*
    Gonococcus
Nelaton's syndrome G60.8
Nelson's syndrome E24.1
Nematodiasis (intestinal) B82.0
    Ancylostoma B76.0
Neonatal — *see also* Newborn
    acne L70.4
    bradycardia P29.12
    screening, abnormal findings on P09
    tachycardia P29.11
    tooth, teeth K00.6
Neonatorum — *see* condition
Neoplasia
    endocrine, multiple (MEN) E31.20
        type I E31.21
        type IIA E31.22
        type IIB E31.23
    intraepithelial (histologically confirmed)
        anal (AIN) (histologically confirmed)
            K62.82
            grade I K62.82
            grade II K62.82
            severe D01.3
        cervical glandular (histologically
            confirmed) D06.9
        cervix (uteri) (CIN) (histologically
            confirmed) N87.9
            glandular D06.9
            grade I N87.0
            grade II N87.1
            grade III (severe dysplasia) *(see also*
                Carcinoma, cervix uteri, in situ)
                D06.9
        prostate (histologically confirmed) (PIN
            I) (PIN II) N42.3
            grade I N42.3
            grade II N42.3
            severe D07.5
        vagina (histologically confirmed)
            (VAIN) N89.3
            grade I N89.0
            grade II N89.1
            grade III (severe dysplasia) D07.2
        vulva (histologically confirmed) (VIN)
            N90.3
            grade I N90.0
            grade II N90.1
            grade III (severe dysplasia) D07.1
Neoplasm, neoplastic — *see also* Table of
    Neoplasms
    lipomatous, benign — *see* Lipoma

NEOPLASM TABLE

Neoplasm Table	Malignant Primary	Malignant Secondary	Ca In situ	Benign	Uncertain Behavior	Unspecified Behavior

ICD-10-CM Table of Neoplasms

The list below gives the code numbers for neoplasms by anatomical site. For each site there are six possible code numbers according to whether the neoplasm in question is malignant, benign, in situ, of uncertain behavior, or of unspecified nature. The description of the neoplasm will often indicate which of the six columns is appropriate; e.g., malignant melanoma of skin, benign fibroadenoma of breast, carcinoma in situ of cervix uteri.

Where such descriptors are not present, the remainder of the Index should be consulted where guidance is given to the appropriate column for each morphological (histological) variety listed; e.g., Mesonephroma — *see* Neoplasm, malignant; Embryoma — *see also* Neoplasm, uncertain behavior; Disease, Bowen's — *see* Neoplasm, skin, in situ. However, the guidance in the Index can be overridden if one of the descriptors mentioned above is present; e.g., malignant adenoma of colon is coded to C18.9 and not to D12.6 as the adjective "malignant" overrides the Index entry "Adenoma — *see also* Neoplasm, benign."

Codes listed with a dash -, following the code have a required additional character for laterality. The tabular list must be reviewed for the complete code.

Neoplasm Table	Malignant Primary	Malignant Secondary	Ca In situ	Benign	Uncertain Behavior	Unspecified Behavior
Neoplasm, neoplastic	C80.1	C79.9	D09.9	D36.9	D48.9	D49.9
abdomen, abdominal	C76.2	C79.8-	D09.8	D36.7	D48.7	D49.89
cavity	C76.2	C79.8-	D09.8	D36.7	D48.7	D49.89
organ	C76.2	C79.8-	D09.8	D36.7	D48.7	D49.89
viscera	C76.2	C79.8-	D09.8	D36.7	D48.7	D49.89
wall — *see also* Neoplasm, abdomen, wall, skin	C44.509	C79.2-	D04.5	D23.5	D48.5	D49.2
connective tissue	C49.4	C79.8-	—	D21.4	D48.1	D49.2
skin	C44.509	—	—	—	—	—
basal cell carcinoma	C44.519	—	—	—	—	—
specified type NEC	C44.599	—	—	—	—	—
squamous cell carcinoma	C44.529	—	—	—	—	—
abdominopelvic	C76.8	C79.8-	—	D36.7	D48.7	D49.89
accessory sinus — *see* Neoplasm, sinus						
acoustic nerve	C72.4-	C79.49	—	D33.3	D43.3	D49.7
adenoid (pharynx) (tissue)	C11.1	C79.89	D00.08	D10.6	D37.05	D49.0
adipose tissue — *see also* Neoplasm, connective tissue	C49.4	C79.89	—	D21.9	D48.1	D49.2
adnexa (uterine)	C57.4	C79.89	D07.39	D28.7	D39.8	D49.5
adrenal	C74.9-	C79.7-	D09.3	D35.0-	D44.1-	D49.7
capsule	C74.9-	C79.7-	D09.3	D35.0-	D44.1-	D49.7
cortex	C74.0-	C79.7-	D09.3	D35.0-	D44.1-	D49.7
gland	C74.9-	C79.7-	D09.3	D35.0-	D44.1-	D49.7
medulla	C74.1-	C79.7-	D09.3	D35.0-	D44.1-	D49.7
ala nasi (external) — *see also* Neoplasm, skin, nose	C44.301	C79.2	D04.39	D23.39	D48.5	D49.2
alimentary canal or tract NEC	C26.9	C78.80	D01.9	D13.9	D37.9	D49.0
alveolar	C03.9	C79.89	D00.03	D10.39	D37.09	D49.0
mucosa	C03.9	C79.89	D00.03	D10.39	D37.09	D49.0
lower	C03.1	C79.89	D00.03	D10.39	D37.09	D49.0
upper	C03.0	C79.89	D00.03	D10.39	D37.09	D49.0
ridge or process	C41.1	C79.51	—	D16.5-	D48.0	D49.2
carcinoma	C03.9	C79.8-	—	—	—	—
lower	C03.1	C79.8-	—	—	—	—
upper	C03.0	C79.8-	—	—	—	—
lower	C41.1	C79.51	—	D16.5-	D48.0	D49.2
mucosa	C03.9	C79.89	D00.03	D10.39	D37.09	D49.0
lower	C03.1	C79.89	D00.03	D10.39	D37.09	D49.0
upper	C03.0	C79.89	D00.03	D10.39	D37.09	D49.0
upper	C41.0	C79.51	—	D16.4-	D48.0	D49.2
sulcus	C06.1	C79.89	D00.02	D10.39	D37.09	D49.0
alveolus	C03.9	C79.89	D00.03	D10.39	D37.09	D49.0
lower	C03.1	C79.89	D00.03	D10.39	D37.09	D49.0
upper	C03.0	C79.89	D00.03	D10.39	D37.09	D49.0
ampulla of Vater	C24.1	C78.89	D01.5	D13.5	D37.6	D49.0
ankle NEC	C76.5-	C79.89	D04.7-	D36.7	D48.7	D49.89
anorectum, anorectal (junction)	C21.8	C78.5	D01.3	D12.9	D37.8	D49.0
antecubital fossa or space	C76.4-	C79.89	D04.6-	D36.7	D48.7	D49.89
antrum (Highmore) (maxillary)	C31.0	C78.39	D02.3	D14.0	D38.5	D49.1
pyloric	C16.3	C78.89	D00.2	D13.1	D37.1	D49.0
tympanicum	C30.1	C78.39	D02.3	D14.0	D38.5	D49.1

Neoplasm Table	Malignant Primary	Malignant Secondary	Ca In situ	Benign	Uncertain Behavior	Unspecified Behavior
Neoplasm, neoplastic - *continued*						
anus, anal	C21.0	C78.5	D01.3	D12.9	D37.8	D49.0
canal	C21.1	C78.5	D01.3	D12.9	D37.8	D49.0
cloacogenic zone	C21.2	C78.5	D01.3	D12.9	D37.8	D49.0
margin — *see also* Neoplasm, anus, skin	C44.500	C79.2	D04.5	D23.5	D48.5	D49.2
overlapping lesion with rectosigmoid junction or rectum	C21.8	—	—	—	—	—
skin	C44.500	C79.2	D04.5	D23.5	D48.5	D49.2
basal cell carcinoma	C44.510	—	—	—	—	—
specified type NEC	C44.590	—	—	—	—	—
squamous cell carcinoma	C44.520	—	—	—	—	—
sphincter	C21.1	C78.5	D01.3	D12.9	D37.8	D49.0
aorta (thoracic)	C49.3	C79.89	—	D21.3	D48.1	D49.2
abdominal	C49.4	C79.89	—	D21.4	D48.1	D49.2
aortic body	C75.5	C79.89	—	D35.6	D44.7	D49.7
aponeurosis	C49.9	C79.89	—	D21.9	D48.1	D49.2
palmar	C49.1-	C79.89	—	D21.1-	D48.1	D49.2
plantar	C49.2-	C79.89	—	D21.2-	D48.1	D49.2
appendix	C18.1	C78.5	D01.0	D12.1	D37.3	D49.0
arachnoid	C70.9	C79.49	—	D32.9	D42.9	D49.7
cerebral	C70.0	C79.32	—	D32.0	D42.0	D49.7
spinal	C70.1	C79.49	—	D32.1	D42.1	D49.7
areola	C50.0-	C79.81	D05.-	D24.-	D48.6-	D49.3
arm NEC	C76.4-	C79.89	D04.6-	D36.7	D48.7	D49.89
artery — *see* Neoplasm, connective tissue						
aryepiglottic fold	C13.1	C79.89	D00.08	D10.7	D37.05	D49.0
hypopharyngeal aspect	C13.1	C79.89	D00.08	D10.7	D37.05	D49.0
laryngeal aspect	C32.1	C78.39	D02.0	D14.1	D38.0	D49.1
marginal zone	C13.1	C79.89	D00.08	D10.7	D37.05	D49.0
arytenoid (cartilage)	C32.3	C78.39	D02.0	D14.1	D38.0	D49.1
fold — *see* Neoplasm, aryepiglottic						
associated with transplanted organ	C80.2	—	—	—	—	D49.2
atlas	C41.2	C79.51	—	D16.6	D48.0	D49.2
atrium, cardiac	C38.0	C79.89	—	D15.1	D48.7	D49.89
auditory						
canal (external) (skin) A81	C44.20-	C79.2	D04.2-	D23.2-	D48.5	D49.2
internal	C30.1	C78.39	D02.3	D14.0	D38.5	D49.1
nerve	C72.4-	C79.49	—	D33.3	D43.3	D49.7
tube	C30.1	C78.39	D02.3	D14.0	D38.5	D49.1
opening	C11.2	C79.89	D00.08	D10.6	D37.05	D49.0
auricle, ear — *see also* Neoplasm, skin, ear	C44.20-	C79.2	D04.2-	D23.2-	D48.5	D49.2
auricular canal (external) — *see also* Neoplasm, skin, ear	C44.20-	C79.2	D04.2-	D23.2-	D48.5	D49.2
internal	C30.1	C78.39	D02.3	D14.0	D38.5	D49.2
autonomic nerve or nervous system NEC (*see* Neoplasm, nerve, peripheral)						
axilla, axillary	C76.1	C79.89	D09.8	D36.7	D48.7	D49.89
fold — *see also* Neoplasm, skin, trunk	C44.509	C79.2	D04.5	D23.5	D48.5	D49.2
back NEC	C76.8	C79.89	D04.5	D36.7	D48.7	D49.89
Bartholin's gland	C51.0	C79.82	D07.1	D28.0	D39.8	D49.5
basal ganglia	C71.0	C79.31	—	D33.0	D43.0	D49.6
basis pedunculi	C71.7	C79.31	—	D33.1	D43.1	D49.6
bile or biliary (tract)	C24.9	C78.89	D01.5	D13.5	D37.6	D49.0
canaliculi (biliferi) (intrahepatic)	C22.1	C78.7	D01.5	D13.4	D37.6	D49.0
canals, interlobular	C22.1	C78.89	D01.5	D13.4	D37.6	D49.0
duct or passage (common) (cystic) (extrahepatic)	C24.0	C78.89	D01.5	D13.5	D37.6	D49.0
interlobular	C22.1	C78.89	D01.5	D13.4	D37.6	D49.0
intrahepatic	C22.1	C78.7	D01.5	D13.4	D37.6	D49.0
and extrahepatic	C24.8	C78.89	D01.5	D13.5	D37.6	D49.0
bladder (urinary)	C67.9	C79.11	D09.0	D30.3	D41.4	D49.4
dome	C67.1	C79.11	D09.0	D30.3	D41.4	D49.4
neck	C67.5	C79.11	D09.0	D30.3	D41.4	D49.4
orifice	C67.9	C79.11	D09.0	D30.3	D41.4	D49.4
ureteric	C67.6	C79.11	D09.0	D30.3	D41.4	D49.4
urethral	C67.5	C79.11	D09.0	D30.3	D41.4	D49.4
overlapping lesion	C67.8	—	—	—	—	—
sphincter	C67.8	C79.11	D09.0	D30.3	D41.4	D49.4
trigone	C67.0	C79.11	D09.0	D30.3	D41.4	D49.4
urachus	C67.7	C79.11	D09.0	D30.3	D41.4	D49.4
wall	C67.9	C79.11	D09.0	D30.3	D41.4	D49.4
anterior	C67.3	C79.11	D09.0	D30.3	D41.4	D49.4
lateral	C67.2	C79.11	D09.0	D30.3	D41.4	D49.4
posterior	C67.4	C79.11	D09.0	D30.3	D41.4	D49.4
blood vessel — *see* Neoplasm, connective tissue						

N E O P L A S M   T A B L E

Neoplasm Table	Malignant Primary	Malignant Secondary	Ca In situ	Benign	Uncertain Behavior	Unspecified Behavior
Neoplasm, neoplastic - *continued*						
bone (periosteum) - *continued*	C41.9	C79.51	—	D16.9-	D48.0	D49.2
bone (periosteum)	C41.9	C79.51	—	D16.9-	D48.0	D49.2
acetabulum	C41.4	C79.51	—	D16.8-	D48.0	D49.2
ankle	C40.3-	C79.51	—	D16.3-	—	—
arm NEC	C40.0-	C79.51	—	D16.0-	—	—
astragalus	C40.3-	C79.51	—	D16.3-	—	—
atlas	C41.2	C79.51	—	D16.6-	D48.0	D49.2
axis	C41.2	C79.51	—	D16.6-	D48.0	D49.2
back NEC	C41.2	C79.51	—	D16.6-	D48.0	D49.2
calcaneus	C40.3-	C79.51	—	D16.3-	—	—
calvarium	C41.0	C79.51	—	D16.4-	D48.0	D49.2
carpus (any)	C40.1-	C79.51	—	D16.1-	—	—
cartilage NEC	C41.9	C79.51	—	D16.9-	D48.0	D49.2
clavicle	C41.3	C79.51	—	D16.7-	D48.0	D49.2
clivus	C41.0	C79.51	—	D16.4-	D48.0	D49.2
coccygeal vertebra	C41.4	C79.51	—	D16.8-	D48.0	D49.2
coccyx	C41.4	C79.51	—	D16.8-	D48.0	D49.2
costal cartilage	C41.3	C79.51	—	D16.7	D48.0	D49.2
costovertebral joint	C41.3	C79.51	—	D16.7-	D48.0	D49.2
cranial	C41.0	C79.51	—	D16.4-	D48.0	D49.2
cuboid	C40.3-	C79.51	—	D16.3-	—	—
cuneiform	C41.9	C79.51	—	D16.9-	D48.0	D49.2
elbow	C40.0-	C79.51	—	D16.0-	—	—
ethmoid (labyrinth)	C41.0	C79.51	—	D16.4-	D48.0	D49.2
face	C41.0	C79.51	—	D16.4-	D48.0	D49.2
femur (any part)	C40.2-	C79.51	—	D16.2-	—	—
fibula (any part)	C40.2-	C79.51	—	D16.2-	—	—
finger (any)	C40.1-	C79.51	—	D16.1-	—	—
foot	C40.3-	C79.51	—	D16.3-	—	—
forearm	C40.0-	C79.51	—	D16.0-	—	—
frontal	C41.0	C79.51	—	D16.4-	D48.0	D49.2
hand	C40.1-	C79.51	—	D16.1-	—	—
heel	C40.3-	C79.51	—	D16.3-	—	—
hip	C41.4	C79.51	—	D16.8-	D48.0	D49.2
humerus (any part)	C40.0-	C79.51	—	D16.0-	—	—
hyoid	C41.0	C79.51	—	D16.4-	D48.0	D49.2
ilium	C41.4	C79.51	—	D16.8-	D48.0	D49.2
innominate	C41.4	C79.51	—	D16.8-	D48.0	D49.2
intervertebral cartilage or disc	C41.2	C79.51	—	D16.6-	D48.0	D49.2
ischium	C41.4	C79.51	—	D16.8-	D48.0	D49.2
jaw (lower)	C41.1	C79.51	—	D16.5-	D48.0	D49.2
knee	C40.2-	C79.51	—	D16.2-	—	—
leg NEC	C40.2-	C79.51	—	D16.2-	—	—
limb NEC	C40.9-	C79.51	—	D16.9-	—	—
lower (long bones)	C40.2-	C79.51	—	D16.2-	—	—
short bones	C40.3-	C79.51	—	D16.3-	—	—
upper (long bones)	C40.0-	C79.51	—	D16.0-	—	—
short bones	C40.1-	C79.51	—	D16.1-	—	—
malar	C41.0	C79.51	—	D16.4-	D48.0	D49.2
mandible	C41.1	C79.51	—	D16.5-	D48.0	D49.2
marrow NEC (any bone)	C96.9	C79.52	—	—	D47.9	D49.89
mastoid	C41.0	C79.51	—	D16.4-	D48.0	D49.2
maxilla, maxillary (superior)	C41.0	C79.51	—	D16.4-	D48.0	D49.2
inferior	C41.1	C79.51	—	D16.5-	D48.0	D49.2
metacarpus (any)	C40.1-	C79.51	—	D16.1-	—	—
metatarsus (any)	C40.3-	C79.51	—	D16.3-	—	—
overlapping sites	C40.8-	—	—	—	—	—
navicular						
ankle	C40.3-	C79.51	—	—	—	—
hand	C40.1-	C79.51	—	—	—	—
nose, nasal	C41.0	C79.51	—	D16.4-	D48.0	D49.2
occipital	C41.0	C79.51	—	D16.4-	D48.0	D49.2
orbit	C41.0	C79.51	—	D16.4-	D48.0	D49.2
parietal	C41.0	C79.51	—	D16.4-	D48.0	D49.2
patella	C40.2-	C79.51	—	—	—	—
pelvic	C41.4	C79.51	—	D16.8	D48.0	D49.2
phalanges						
foot	C40.3-	C79.51	—	—	—	—
hand	C40.1-	C79.51	—	—	—	—
pubic	C41.4	C79.51	—	D16.8	D48.0	D49.2
radius (any part)	C40.0-	C79.51	—	D16.0-	—	—
rib	C41.3	C79.51	—	D16.7	D48.0	D49.2
sacral vertebra	C41.4	C79.51	—	D16.8	D48.0	D49.2
sacrum	C41.4	C79.51	—	D16.8	D48.0	D49.2
scaphoid	—	—		—	—	—
of ankle	C40.3-	C79.51	—	—	—	—
of hand	C40.1-	C79.51	—	—	—	—
scapula (any part)	C40.0-	C79.51	—	D16.0-	—	—
sella turcica	C41.0	C79.51	—	D16.4-	D48.0	D49.2
shoulder	C40.0-	C79.51	—	D16.0-	—	—
skull	C41.0	C79.51	—	D16.4-	D48.0	D49.2
sphenoid	C41.0	C79.51	—	D16.4-	D48.0	D49.2
spine, spinal (column)	C41.2	C79.51	—	D16.6	D48.0	D49.2
coccyx	C41.4	C79.51	—	D16.8	D48.0	D49.2
sacrum	C41.4	C79.51	—	D16.8	D48.0	D49.2
sternum	C41.3	C79.51	—	D16.7	D48.0	D49.2
tarsus (any)	C40.3-	C79.51	—	—	—	—
temporal	C41.0	C79.51	—	D16.4-	D48.0	D49.2
thumb	C40.1-	C79.51	—	—	—	—
Neoplasm, neoplastic - *continued*						
bone (periosteum) - *continued*	C41.9	C79.51	—	D16.9-	D48.0	D49.2
tibia (any part)	C40.2-	C79.51	—	—	—	—
toe (any)	C40.3-	C79.51	—	—	—	—
trapezium	C40.1-	C79.51	—	—	—	—
trapezoid	C40.1-	C79.51	—	—	—	—
turbinate	C41.0	C79.51	—	D16.4-	D48.0	D49.2
ulna (any part)	C40.0-	C79.51	—	D16.0-	—	—
unciform	C40.1-	C79.51	—	—	—	—
vertebra (column)	C41.2	C79.51	—	D16.6	D48.0	D49.2
coccyx	C41.4	C79.51	—	D16.8	D48.0	D49.2
sacrum	C41.4	C79.51	—	D16.8	D48.0	D49.2
vomer	C41.0	C79.51	—	D16.4-	D48.0	D49.2
wrist	C40.1-	C79.51	—	—	—	—
xiphoid process	C41.3	C79.51	—	D16.7	D48.0	D49.2
zygomatic	C41.0	C79.51	—	D16.4-	D48.0	D49.2
book-leaf (mouth) [ventral surface of tongue and floor of mouth]	C06.89	C79.89	D00.00	D10.39	D37.09	D49.0
bowel — *see* Neoplasm, intestine						
brachial plexus	C47.1-	C79.89	—	D36.12	D48.2	D49.2
brain NEC	C71.9	C79.31	—	D33.2	D43.2	D49.6
basal ganglia	C71.0	C79.31	—	D33.0	D43.0	D49.6
cerebellopontine angle	C71.6	C79.31	—	D33.1	D43.1	D49.6
cerebellum NOS	C71.6	C79.31	—	D33.1	D43.1	D49.6
cerebrum	C71.0	C79.31	—	D33.0	D43.0	D49.6
choroid plexus	C71.7	C79.31	—	D33.1	D43.1	D49.6
corpus callosum	C71.8	C79.31	—	D33.2	D43.2	D49.6
corpus striatum	C71.0	C79.31	—	D33.0	D43.0	D49.6
cortex (cerebral)	C71.0	C79.31	—	D33.0	D43.0	D49.6
frontal lobe	C71.1	C79.31	—	D33.0	D43.0	D49.6
globus pallidus	C71.0	C79.31	—	D33.0	D43.0	D49.6
hippocampus	C71.2	C79.31	—	D33.0	D43.0	D49.6
hypothalamus	C71.0	C79.31	—	D33.0	D43.0	D49.6
internal capsule	C71.0	C79.31	—	D33.0	D43.0	D49.6
medulla oblongata	C71.7	C79.31	—	D33.1	D43.1	D49.6
meninges	C70.0	C79.32	—	D32.0	D42.0	D49.7
midbrain	C71.7	C79.31	—	D33.1	D43.1	D49.6
occipital lobe	C71.4	C79.31	—	D33.0	D43.0	D49.6
overlapping lesion	C71.8	C79.31	—	—	—	—
parietal lobe	C71.3	C79.31	—	D33.0	D43.0	D49.6
peduncle	C71.7	C79.31	—	D33.1	D43.1	D49.6
pons	C71.7	C79.31	—	D33.1	D43.1	D49.6
stem	C71.7	C79.31	—	D33.1	D43.1	D49.6
tapetum	C71.8	C79.31	—	D33.2	D43.2	D49.6
temporal lobe	C71.2	C79.31	—	D33.0	D43.0	D49.6
thalamus	C71.0	C79.31	—	D33.0	D43.0	D49.6
uncus	C71.2	C79.31	—	D33.0	D43.0	D49.6
ventricle (floor)	C71.5	C79.31	—	D33.0	D43.0	D49.6
fourth	C71.7	C79.31	—	D33.1	D43.1	D49.6
branchial (cleft) (cyst) (vestiges)	C10.4	C79.89	D00.08	D10.5	D37.05	D49.0
breast (connective tissue) (glandular tissue) (soft parts)	C50.9-	C79.81	D05.-	D24.-	D48.6-	D49.3
areola	C50.0-	C79.81	D05.-	D24.-	D48.6-	D49.3
axillary tail	C50.6-	C79.81	D05.-	D24.-	D48.6-	D49.3
central portion	C50.1-	C79.81	D05.-	D24.-	D48.6-	D49.3
inner	C50.8-	C79.81	D05.-	D24.-	D48.6-	D49.3
lower	C50.8-	C79.81	D05.-	D24.-	D48.6-	D49.3
lower-inner quadrant	C50.3-	C79.81	D05.-	D24.-	D48.6-	D49.3
lower-outer quadrant	C50.5-	C79.81	D05.-	D24.-	D48.6-	D49.3
mastectomy site (skin) — *see also* Neoplasm, breast, skin	C44.501	C79.2		—	—	—
specified as breast tissue	C50.8-	C79.81	—	—	—	—
midline	C50.8-	C79.81	D05.-	D24.-	D48.6-	D49.3
nipple	C50.0-	C79.81	D05.-	D24.-	D48.6-	D49.3
outer	C50.8-	C79.81	D05.-	D24.-	D48.6-	D49.3
overlapping lesion	C50.8-	—				
skin	C44.501	C79.2	D04.5	D23.5	D48.5	D49.2
basal cell carcinoma	C44.511	—		—	—	—
specified type NEC	C44.591	—				
squamous cell carcinoma	C44.521	—		—	—	—
tail (axillary)	C50.6-	C79.81	D05.-	D24.-	D48.6-	D49.3
upper	C50.8-	C79.81	D05.-	D24.-	D48.6-	D49.3
upper-inner quadrant	C50.2-	C79.81	D05.-	D24.-	D48.6-	D49.3
upper-outer quadrant	C50.4-	C79.81	D05.-	D24.-	D48.6-	D49.3
broad ligament	C57.1	C79.82	D07.39	D28.2	D39.8	D49.5
bronchiogenic, bronchogenic (lung)	C34.9-	C78.0-	D02.2-	D14.3-	D38.1	D49.1
bronchiole	C34.9-	C78.0-	D02.2-	D14.3-	D38.1	D49.1
bronchus	C34.9-	C78.0-	D02.2-	D14.3-	D38.1	D49.1
carina	C34.0-	C78.0-	D02.2-	D14.3-	D38.1	D49.1
lower lobe of lung	C34.3-	C78.0-	D02.2-	D14.3-	D38.1	D49.1
main	C34.0-	C78.0-	D02.2-	D14.3-	D38.1	D49.1
middle lobe of lung	C34.2	C78.0-	D02.21	D14.31	D38.1	D49.1
overlapping lesion	C34.8-	—				
upper lobe of lung	C34.1-	C78.0-	D02.2-	D14.3-	D38.1	D49.1

NEOPLASM TABLE

Neoplasm Table	Malignant Primary	Malignant Secondary	Ca In situ	Benign	Uncertain Behavior	Unspecified Behavior
Neoplasm, neoplastic - *continued*						
brow	C44.309	C79.2	D04.39	D23.39	D48.5	D49.2
basal cell carcinoma	C44.319	—	—	—	—	—
specified type NEC	C44.399	—	—	—	—	—
squamous cell carcinoma	C44.329	—	—	—	—	—
buccal (cavity)	C06.9	C79.89	D00.00	D10.39	D37.09	D49.0
commissure	C06.0	C79.89	D00.02	D10.39	D37.09	D49.0
groove (lower) (upper)	C06.1	C79.89	D00.02	D10.39	D37.09	D49.0
mucosa	C06.0	C79.89	D00.02	D10.39	D37.09	D49.0
sulcus (lower) (upper)	C06.1	C79.89	D00.02	D10.39	D37.09	D49.0
bulbourethral gland	C68.0	C79.19	D09.19	D30.4	D41.3	D49.5
bursa — *see* Neoplasm, connective tissue						
buttock NEC	C76.3	C79.89	D04.5	D36.7	D48.7	D49.89
calf	C76.5-	C79.89	D04.7-	D36.7	D48.7	D49.89
calvarium	C41.0	C79.51	—	D16.4-	D48.0	D49.2
calyx, renal	C65.-	C79.0	D09.19	D30.1-	D41.1-	D49.5
canal						
anal	C21.1	C78.5	D01.3	D12.9	D37.8	D49.0
auditory (external) — *see also* Neoplasm, skin, ear	C44.20-	C79.2	D04.2-	D23.2-	D48.5	D49.2
auricular (external) — *see also* Neoplasm, skin, ear	C44.20-	C79.2	D04.2-	D23.2-	D48.5	D49.2
canaliculi, biliary (biliferi) (intrahepatic)	C22.1	C78.7	D01.5	D13.4	D37.6	D49.0
canthus (eye) (inner) (outer)	C44.10-	C79.2	D04.1-	D23.1-	D48.5	D49.2
basal cell carcinoma	C44.11-	—	—	—	—	—
specified type NEC	C44.19-	—	—	—	—	—
squamous cell carcinoma	C44.12-	—	—	—	—	—
capillary — *see* Neoplasm, connective tissue						
caput coli	C18.0	C78.5	D01.0	D12.0	D37.4	D49.0
carcinoid — *see* Tumor, carcinoid						
cardia (gastric)	C16.0	C78.89	D00.2	D13.1	D37.1	D49.0
cardiac orifice (stomach)	C16.0	C78.89	D00.2	D13.1	D37.1	D49.0
cardio-esophageal junction	C16.0	C78.89	D00.2	D13.1	D37.1	D49.0
cardio-esophagus	C16.0	C78.89	D00.2	D13.1	D37.1	D49.0
carina (bronchus)	C34.0-	C78.0-	D02.2-	D14.3-	D38.1	D49.1
carotid (artery)	C49.0	C79.89	—	D21.0	D48.1	D49.2
body	C75.4	C79.89	—	D35.5	D44.6	D49.7
carpus (any bone)	C40.1-	C79.51	—	D16.1-	—	—
cartilage (articular) (joint) NEC — *see also* Neoplasm, bone	C41.9	C79.51	—	D16.9-	D48.0	D49.2
arytenoid	C32.3	C78.39	D02.0	D14.1	D38.0	D49.1
auricular	C49.0	C79.89	—	D21.0	D48.1	D49.2
bronchi	C34.0-	C78.39	—	D14.3-	D38.1	D49.1
costal	C41.3	C79.51	—	D16.7	D48.0	D49.2
cricoid	C32.3	C78.39	D02.0	D14.1	D38.0	D49.1
cuneiform	C32.3	C78.39	D02.0	D14.1	D38.0	D49.1
ear (external)	C49.0	C79.89	—	D21.0	D48.1	D49.2
ensiform	C41.3	C79.51	—	D16.7	D48.0	D49.2
epiglottis	C32.1	C78.39	D02.0	D14.1	D38.0	D49.1
anterior surface	C10.1	C79.89	D00.08	D10.5	D37.05	D49.0
eyelid	C49.0	C79.89	—	D21.0	D48.1	D49.2
intervertebral	C41.2	C79.51	—	D16.6	D48.0	D49.2
larynx, laryngeal	C32.3	C78.39	D02.0	D14.1	D38.0	D49.1
nose, nasal	C30.0	C78.39	D02.3	D14.0	D38.5	D49.1
pinna	C49.0	C79.89	—	D21.0	D48.1	D49.2
rib	C41.3	C79.51	—	D16.7	D48.0	D49.2
semilunar (knee)	C40.2-	C79.51	—	D16.2-	D48.0	D49.2
thyroid	C32.3	C78.39	D02.0	D14.1	D38.0	D49.1
trachea	C33	C78.39	D02.1	D14.2	D38.1	D49.1
cauda equina	C72.1	C79.49	—	D33.4	D43.4	D49.7
cavity						
buccal	C06.9	C79.89	D00.00	D10.30	D37.09	D49.0
nasal	C30.0	C78.39	D02.3	D14.0	D38.5	D49.1
oral	C06.9	C79.89	D00.00	D10.30	D37.09	D49.0
peritoneal	C48.2	C78.6	—	D20.1	D48.4	D49.0
tympanic	C30.1	C78.39	D02.3	D14.0	D38.5	D49.1
cecum	C18.0	C78.5	D01.0	D12.0	D37.4	D49.0
central nervous system	C72.9	C79.40	—	—	—	—
cerebellopontine (angle)	C71.6	C79.31	—	D33.1	D43.1	D49.6
cerebellum, cerebellar	C71.6	C79.31	—	D33.1	D43.1	D49.6
cerebrum, cerebral (cortex) (hemisphere) (white matter)	C71.0	C79.31	—	D33.0	D43.0	D49.6
meninges	C70.0	C79.32	—	D32.0	D42.0	D49.7
peduncle	C71.7	C79.31	—	D33.1	D43.1	D49.6
ventricle	C71.5	C79.31	—	D33.0	D43.0	D49.6
fourth	C71.7	C79.31	—	D33.1	D43.1	D49.6
cervical region	C76.0	C79.89	D09.8	D36.7	D48.7	D49.89

Neoplasm Table	Malignant Primary	Malignant Secondary	Ca In situ	Benign	Uncertain Behavior	Unspecified Behavior
Neoplasm, neoplastic - *continued*						
cervix (cervical) (uteri) (uterus)	C53.9	C79.82	D06.9	D26.0	D39.0	D49.5
canal	C53.0	C79.82	D06.0	D26.0	D39.0	D49.5
endocervix (canal) (gland)	C53.0	C79.82	D06.0	D26.0	D39.0	D49.5
exocervix	C53.1	C79.82	D06.1	D26.0	D39.0	D49.5
external os	C53.1	C79.82	D06.1	D26.0	D39.0	D49.5
internal os	C53.0	C79.82	D06.0	D26.0	D39.0	D49.5
nabothian gland	C53.0	C79.82	D06.0	D26.0	D39.0	D49.5
overlapping lesion	C53.8					
squamocolumnar junction	C53.8	C79.82	D06.7	D26.0	D39.0	D49.5
stump	C53.8	C79.82	D06.7	D26.0	D39.0	D49.5
cheek	C76.0	C79.89	D09.8	D36.7	D48.7	D49.89
external	C44.309	C79.2	D04.39	D23.39	D48.5	D49.2
basal cell carcinoma	C44.319	—	—	—	—	—
specified type NEC	C44.399	—	—	—	—	—
squamous cell carcinoma	C44.329	—	—	—	—	—
inner aspect	C06.0	C79.89	D00.02	D10.39	D37.09	D49.0
internal	C06.0	C79.89	D00.02	D10.39	D37.09	D49.0
mucosa	C06.0	C79.89	D00.02	D10.39	D37.09	D49.0
chest (wall) NEC	C76.1	C79.89	D09.8	D36.7	D48.7	D49.89
chiasma opticum	C72.3-	C79.49	—	D33.3	D43.3	D49.7
chin	C44.309	C79.2	D04.39	D23.39	D48.5	D49.2
basal cell carcinoma	C44.319	—	—	—	—	—
specified type NEC	C44.399	—	—	—	—	—
squamous cell carcinoma	C44.329	—	—	—	—	—
choana	C11.3	C79.89	D00.08	D10.6	D37.05	D49.0
cholangiole	C22.1	C78.89	D01.5	D13.4	D37.6	D49.0
choledochal duct	C24.0	C78.89	D01.5	D13.5	D37.6	D49.0
choroid	C69.3-	C79.49	D09.2-	D31.3	D48.7	D49.81
plexus	C71.5	C79.31	—	D33.0	D43.0	D49.6
ciliary body	C69.4-	C79.49	D09.2-	D31.4-	D48.7	D49.89
clavicle	C41.3	C79.51	—	D16.7	D48.0	D49.2
clitoris	C51.2	C79.82	D07.1	D28.0	D39.8	D49.5
clivus	C41.0	C79.51	—	D16.4-	D48.0	D49.2
cloacogenic zone	C21.2	C78.5	D01.3	D12.9	D37.8	D49.0
coccygeal						
body or glomus	C49.5	C79.89	—	D21.5	D48.1	D49.2
vertebra	C41.4	C79.51	—	D16.8	D48.0	D49.2
coccyx	C41.4	C79.51	—	D16.8	D48.0	D49.2
colon — *see also* Neoplasm, intestine, large	C18.9	C78.5	—	—	—	—
with rectum	C19	C78.5	D01.1	D12.7	D37.5	D49.0
column, spinal — *see* Neoplasm, spine						
columnella — *see also* Neoplasm, skin, face	C44.390	C79.2	D04.39	D23.39	D48.5	D49.2
commissure						
labial, lip	C00.6	C79.89	D00.01	D10.39	D37.01	D49.0
laryngeal	C32.0	C78.39	D02.0	D14.1	D38.0	D49.1
common (bile) duct	C24.0	C78.89	D01.5	D13.5	D37.6	D49.0
concha — *see also* Neoplasm, skin, ear	C44.20-	C79.2	D04.2-	D23.2-	D48.5	D49.2
nose	C30.0	C78.39	D02.3	D14.0	D38.5	D49.1
conjunctiva	C69.0-	C79.49	D09.2-	D31.0-	D48.7	D49.89
connective tissue NEC	C49.9	C79.89	—	D21.9	D48.1	D49.2

Connective tissue Notes:

Note: For neoplasms of connective tissue (blood vessel, bursa, fascia, ligament, muscle, peripheral nerves, sympathetic and parasympathetic nerves and ganglia, synovia, tendon, etc.) or of morphological types that indicate connective tissue, code according to the list under "Neoplasm, connective tissue". For sites that do not appear in this list, code to neoplasm of that site; e.g., fibrosarcoma, pancreas (C25.9)

Note: Morphological types that indicate connective tissue appear in their proper place in the alphabetic index with the instruction "see Neoplasm, connective tissue ...."

abdomen	C49.4	C79.89	—	D21.4	D48.1	D49.2
abdominal wall	C49.4	C79.89	—	D21.4	D48.1	D49.2
ankle	C49.2-	C79.89	—	D21.2-	D48.1	D49.2
antecubital fossa or space	C49.1-	C79.89	—	D21.1-	D48.1	D49.2
arm	C49.1-	C79.89	—	D21.1-	D48.1	D49.2
auricle (ear)	C49.0	C79.89	—	D21.0	D48.1	D49.2
axilla	C49.3	C79.89	—	D21.3	D48.1	D49.2
back	C49.6	C79.89	—	D21.6	D48.1	D49.2
breast — *see* Neoplasm, breast						
buttock	C49.5	C79.89	—	D21.5	D48.1	D49.2
calf	C49.2-	C79.89	—	D21.2-	D48.1	D49.2
cervical region	C49.0	C79.89	—	D21.0	D48.1	D49.2
cheek	C49.0	C79.89	—	D21.0	D48.1	D49.2
chest (wall)	C49.3	C79.89	—	D21.3	D48.1	D49.2
chin	C49.0	C79.89	—	D21.0	D48.1	D49.2
diaphragm	C49.3	C79.89	—	D21.3	D48.1	D49.2

Neoplasm Table	Malignant Primary	Malignant Secondary	Ca In situ	Benign	Uncertain Behavior	Unspecified Behavior
Neoplasm, neoplastic - *continued*						
connective tissue NEC						
- *continued*	C49.9	C79.89	—	D21.9	D48.1	D49.2
ear (external)	C49.0	C79.89	—	D21.0	D48.1	D49.2
elbow	C49.1-	C79.89	—	D21.1-	D48.1	D49.2
extrarectal	C49.5	C79.89	—	D21.5	D48.1	D49.2
extremity	C49.9	C79.89	—	D21.9	D48.1	D49.2
lower	C49.2-	C79.89	—	D21.2-	D48.1	D49.2
upper	C49.1-	C79.89	—	D21.1-	D48.1	D49.2
eyelid	C49.0	C79.89	—	D21.0	D48.1	D49.2
face	C49.0	C79.89	—	D21.0	D48.1	D49.2
finger	C49.1-	C79.89	—	D21.1-	D48.1	D49.2
flank	C49.6	C79.89	—	D21.6	D48.1	D49.2
foot	C49.2-	C79.89	—	D21.2-	D48.1	D49.2
forearm	C49.1-	C79.89	—	D21.1-	D48.1	D49.2
forehead	C49.0	C79.89	—	D21.0	D48.1	D49.2
gastric	C49.4	C79.89	—	D21.4	D48.1	D49.2
gastrointestinal	C49.4	C79.89	—	D21.4	D48.1	D49.2
gluteal region	C49.5	C79.89	—	D21.5	D48.1	D49.2
great vessels NEC	C49.3	C79.89	—	D21.3	D48.1	D49.2
groin	C49.5	C79.89	—	D21.5	D48.1	D49.2
hand	C49.1-	C79.89	—	D21.1-	D48.1	D49.2
head	C49.0	C79.89	—	D21.0	D48.1	D49.2
heel	C49.2-	C79.89	—	D21.2-	D48.1	D49.2
hip	C49.2-	C79.89	—	D21.2-	D48.1	D49.2
hypochondrium	C49.4	C79.89	—	D21.4	D48.1	D49.2
iliopsoas muscle	C49.5	C79.89	—	D21.5	D48.1	D49.2
infraclavicular region	C49.3	C79.89	—	D21.3	D48.1	D49.2
inguinal (canal) (region)	C49.5	C79.89	—	D21.5	D48.1	D49.2
intestinal	C49.4	C79.89	—	D21.4	D48.1	D49.2
intrathoracic	C49.3	C79.89	—	D21.3	D48.1	D49.2
ischiorectal fossa	C49.5	C79.89	—	D21.5	D48.1	D49.2
jaw	C03.9	C79.89	D00.03	D10.39	D48.1	D49.0
knee	C49.2-	C79.89	—	D21.2-	D48.1	D49.2
leg	C49.2-	C79.89	—	D21.2-	D48.1	D49.2
limb NEC	C49.9	C79.89	—	D21.9	D48.1	D49.2
lower	C49.2-	C79.89	—	D21.2-	D48.1	D49.2
upper	C49.1-	C79.89	—	D21.1-	D48.1	D49.2
nates	C49.5	C79.89	—	D21.5	D48.1	D49.2
neck	C49.0	C79.89	—	D21.0	D48.1	D49.2
orbit	C69.6-	C79.49	D09.2-	D31.6-	D48.1	D49.89
overlapping lesion	C49.8	—	—	—	—	—
pararectal	C49.5	C79.89	—	D21.5	D48.1	D49.2
para-urethral	C49.5	C79.89	—	D21.5	D48.1	D49.2
paravaginal	C49.5	C79.89	—	D21.5	D48.1	D49.2
pelvis (floor)	C49.5	C79.89	—	D21.5	D48.1	D49.2
pelvo-abdominal	C49.8	C79.89	—	D21.6	D48.1	D49.2
perineum	C49.5	C79.89	—	D21.5	D48.1	D49.2
perirectal (tissue)	C49.5	C79.89	—	D21.5	D48.1	D49.2
periurethral (tissue)	C49.5	C79.89	—	D21.5	D48.1	D49.2
popliteal fossa or space	C49.2-	C79.89	—	D21.2-	D48.1	D49.2
presacral	C49.5	C79.89	—	D21.5	D48.1	D49.2
psoas muscle	C49.4	C79.89	—	D21.4	D48.1	D49.2
pterygoid fossa	C49.0	C79.89	—	D21.0	D48.1	D49.2
rectovaginal septum or wall	C49.5	C79.89	—	D21.5	D48.1	D49.2
rectovesical	C49.5	C79.89	—	D21.5	D48.1	D49.2
retroperitoneum	C48.0	C78.6	—	D20.0	D48.3	D49.0
sacrococcygeal region	C49.5	C79.89	—	D21.5	D48.1	D49.2
scalp	C49.0	C79.89	—	D21.0	D48.1	D49.2
scapular region	C49.3	C79.89	—	D21.3	D48.1	D49.2
shoulder	C49.1-	C79.89	—	D21.1-	D48.1	D49.2
skin (dermis) NEC — *see also* Neoplasm, skin, by site	C44.90	C79.2	D04.9	D23.9	D48.5	D49.2
stomach	C49.4	C79.89	—	D21.4	D48.1	D49.2
submental	C49.0	C79.89	—	D21.0	D48.1	D49.2
supraclavicular region	C49.0	C79.89	—	D21.0	D48.1	D49.2
temple	C49.0	C79.89	—	D21.0	D48.1	D49.2
temporal region	C49.0	C79.89	—	D21.0	D48.1	D49.2
thigh	C49.2-	C79.89	—	D21.2-	D48.1	D49.2
thoracic (duct) (wall)	C49.3	C79.89	—	D21.3	D48.1	D49.2
thorax	C49.3	C79.89	—	D21.3	D48.1	D49.2
thumb	C49.1-	C79.89	—	D21.1-	D48.1	D49.2
toe	C49.2-	C79.89	—	D21.2-	D48.1	D49.2
trunk	C49.6	C79.89	—	D21.6	D48.1	D49.2
umbilicus	C49.4	C79.89	—	D21.4	D48.1	D49.2
vesicorectal	C49.5	C79.89	—	D21.5	D48.1	D49.2
wrist	C49.1-	C79.89	—	D21.1-	D48.1	D49.2
conus medullaris	C72.0	C79.49	—	D33.4	D43.4	D49.7
cord (true) (vocal)	C32.0	C78.39	D02.0	D14.1	D38.0	D49.1
false	C32.1	C78.39	D02.0	D14.1	D38.0	D49.1
spermatic	C63.1-	C79.82	D07.69	D29.8	D40.8	D49.5
spinal (cervical) (lumbar) (thoracic)	C72.0	C79.49	—	D33.4	D43.4	D49.7
cornea (limbus)	C69.1-	C79.49	D09.2-	D31.1-	D48.7	D49.89
Neoplasm, neoplastic - *continued*						
corpus						
albicans	C56.-	C79.6-	D07.39	D27.-	D39.1-	D49.5
callosum, brain	C71.0	C79.31	—	D33.2	D43.2	D49.6
cavernosum	C60.2	C79.82	D07.4	D29.0	D40.8	D49.5
gastric	C16.2	C78.89	D00.2	D13.1	D37.1	D49.0
overlapping sites	C54.8	—	—	—	—	—
penis	C60.2	C79.82	D07.4	D29.0	D40.8	D49.5
striatum, cerebrum	C71.0	C79.31	—	D33.0	D43.0	D49.6
uteri	C54.9	C79.82	D07.0	D26.1	D39.0	D49.5
isthmus	C54.0	C79.82	D07.0	D26.1	D39.0	D49.5
cortex						
adrenal	C74.0-	C79.7-	D09.3	D35.0-	D44.1-	D49.7
cerebral	C71.0	C79.31	—	D33.0	D43.0	D49.6
costal cartilage	C41.3	C79.51	—	D16.7	D48.0	D49.2
costovertebral joint	C41.3	C79.51	—	D16.7	D48.0	D49.2
Cowper's gland	C68.0	C79.19	D09.19	D30.4	D41.3	D49.5
cranial (fossa, any)	C71.9	C79.31	—	D33.2	D43.2	D49.6
meninges	C70.0	C79.32	—	D32.0	D42.0	D49.7
nerve	C72.50	C79.49	—	D33.3	D43.3	D49.7
specified NEC	C72.59	C79.49	—	D33.3	D43.3	D49.7
craniobuccal pouch	C75.2	C79.89	D09.3	D35.2	D44.3	D49.7
craniopharyngeal (duct) (pouch)	C75.2	C79.89	D09.3	D35.3	D44.4	D49.7
cricoid	C13.0	C79.89	D00.08	D10.7	D37.05	D49.0
cartilage	C32.3	C78.39	D02.0	D14.1	D38.0	D49.1
cricopharynx	C13.0	C79.89	D00.08	D10.7	D37.05	D49.0
crypt of Morgagni	C21.8	C78.5	D01.3	D12.9	D37.8	D49.0
crystalline lens	C69.4-	C79.49	D09.2-	D31.4-	D48.7	D49.89
cul-de-sac (Douglas')	C48.1	C78.6	—	D20.1	D48.4	D49.0
cuneiform cartilage	C32.3	C78.39	D02.0	D14.1	D38.0	D49.1
cutaneous — *see* Neoplasm, skin						
cutis — *see* Neoplasm, skin						
cystic (bile) duct (common)	C24.0	C78.89	D01.5	D13.5	D37.6	D49.0
dermis — *see* Neoplasm, skin						
diaphragm	C49.3	C79.89	—	D21.3	D48.1-	D49.2
digestive organs, system, tube, or tract NEC	C26.9	C78.89	D01.9	D13.9	D37.9	D49.0
disc, intervertebral	C41.2	C79.51	—	D16.6	D48.0	D49.2
disease, generalized	C80.0	—	—	—	—	—
disseminated	C80.0	—	—	—	—	—
Douglas' cul-de-sac or pouch	C48.1	C78.6	—	D20.1	D48.4	D49.0
duodenojejunal junction	C17.8	C78.4	D01.49	D13.39	D37.2	D49.0
duodenum	C17.0	C78.4	D01.49	D13.2	D37.2	D49.0
dura (cranial) (mater)	C70.9	C79.49	—	D32.9	D42.9	D49.7
cerebral	C70.0	C79.32	—	D32.0	D42.0	D49.7
spinal	C70.1	C79.49	—	D32.1	D42.1	D49.7
ear (external) — *see also* Neoplasm, skin, ear	C44.20-	C79.2	D04.2-	D23.2-	D48.5	D49.2
auricle or auris — *see also* Neoplasm, skin, ear	C44.20-	C79.2	D04.2-	D23.2-	D48.5	D49.2
canal, external — *see also* Neoplasm, skin, ear	C44.20-	C79.2	D04.2-	D23.2-	D48.5	D49.2
cartilage	C49.0	C79.89	—	D21.0	D48.1	D49.2
external meatus — *see also* Neoplasm, skin, ear	C44.20-	C79.2	D04.2-	D23.2-	D48.5	D49.2
inner	C30.1	C78.39	D02.3	D14.0	D38.5	D49.1
lobule — *see also* Neoplasm, skin, ear	C44.20-	C79.2	D04.2-	D23.2-	D48.5	D49.2
middle	C30.1	C78.39	D02.3	D14.0	D38.5	D49.1
overlapping lesion with accessory sinuses	C31.8	—	—	—	—	—
skin	C44.20-	C79.2	D04.2-	D23.2-	D48.5	D49.2
basal cell carcinoma	C44.21-	—	—	—	—	—
specified type NEC	C44.29-	—	—	—	—	—
squamous cell carcinoma	C44.22-	—	—	—	—	—
earlobe	C44.20-	C79.2	D04.2-	D23.2-	D48.5	D49.2
basal cell carcinoma	C44.21-	—	—	—	—	—
specified type NEC	C44.29-	—	—	—	—	—
squamous cell carcinoma	C44.22-	—	—	—	—	—
ejaculatory duct	C63.7	C79.82	D07.69	D29.8	D40.8	D49.5
elbow NEC	C76.4-	C79.89	D04.6-	D36.7	D48.7	D49.89
endocardium	C38.0	C79.89	—	D15.1	D48.7	D49.89
endocervix (canal) (gland)	C53.0	C79.82	D06.0	D26.0	D39.0	D49.5
endocrine gland NEC	C75.9	C79.89	D09.3	D35.9	D44.9	D49.7
pluriglandular	C75.8	C79.89	D09.3	D35.7	D44.9	D49.7
endometrium (gland) (stroma)	C54.1	C79.82	D07.0	D26.1	D39.0	D49.5
ensiform cartilage	C41.3	C79.51	—	D16.7	D48.0	D49.2
enteric — *see* Neoplasm, intestine						
ependyma (brain)	C71.5	C79.31	—	D33.0	D43.0	D49.6
fourth ventricle	C71.7	C79.31	—	D33.1	D43.1	D49.6
epicardium	C38.0	C79.89	—	D15.1	D48.7	D49.89
epididymis	C63.0-	C79.82	D07.69	D29.3-	D40.8	D49.5
epidural	C72.9	C79.49	—	D33.9	D43.9	D49.7

Neoplasm Table	Malignant Primary	Malignant Secondary	Ca In situ	Benign	Uncertain Behavior	Unspecified Behavior
Neoplasm, neoplastic - *continued*						
epiglottis	C32.1	C78.39	D02.0	D14.1	D38.0	D49.1
anterior aspect or surface	C10.1	C79.89	D00.08	D10.5	D37.05	D49.0
cartilage	C32.3	C78.39	D02.0	D14.1	D38.0	D49.1
free border (margin)	C10.1	C79.89	D00.08	D10.5	D37.05	D49.0
junctional region	C10.8	C79.89	D00.08	D10.5	D37.05	D49.0
posterior (laryngeal) surface	C32.1	C78.39	D02.0	D14.1	D38.0	D49.1
suprahyoid portion	C32.1	C78.39	D02.0	D14.1	D38.0	D49.1
esophagogastric junction	C16.0	C78.89	D00.2	D13.1	D37.1	D49.0
esophagus	C15.9	C78.89	D00.1	D13.0	D37.8	D49.0
abdominal	C15.5	C78.89	D00.1	D13.0	D37.8	D49.0
cervical	C15.3	C78.89	D00.1	D13.0	D37.8	D49.0
distal (third)	C15.5	C78.89	D00.1	D13.0	D37.8	D49.0
lower (third)	C15.5	C78.89	D00.1	D13.0	D37.8	D49.0
middle (third)	C15.4	C78.89	D00.1	D13.0	D37.8	D49.0
overlapping lesion	C15.8	—	—	—	—	—
proximal (third)	C15.3	C78.89	D00.1	D13.0	D37.8	D49.0
thoracic	C15.4	C78.89	D00.1	D13.0	D37.8	D49.0
upper (third)	C15.3	C78.89	D00.1	D13.0	D37.8	D49.0
ethmoid (sinus)	C31.1	C78.39	D02.3	D14.0	D38.5	D49.1
bone or labyrinth	C41.0	C79.51	—	D16.4-	D48.0	D49.2
eustachian tube	C30.1	C78.39	D02.3	D14.0	D38.5	D49.1
exocervix	C53.1	C79.82	D06.1	D26.0	D39.0	D49.5
external						
meatus (ear) — *see also* Neoplasm, skin, ear	C44.20-	C79.2	D04.2-	D23.2-	D48.5	D49.2
os, cervix uteri	C53.1	C79.82	D06.1	D26.0	D39.0	D49.5
extradural	C72.9	C79.49	—	D33.9	D43.9	D49.7
extrahepatic (bile) duct	C24.0	C78.89	D01.5	D13.5	D37.6	D49.0
overlapping lesion with gallbladder	C24.8	—	—	—	—	—
extraocular muscle	C69.6-	C79.49	D09.2-	D31.6-	D48.7	D49.89
extrarectal	C76.3	C79.89	D09.8	D36.7	D48.7	D49.89
extremity	C76.8	C79.89	D04.8	D36.7	D48.7	D49.89
lower	C76.5-	C79.89	D04.7-	D36.7	D48.7	D49.89
upper	C76.4-	C79.89	D04.6-	D36.7	D48.7	D49.89
eye NEC	C69.9-	C79.49	D09.2	D31.9-	D48.7	D49.89
overlapping sites	C69.8	—	—	—	—	—
eyeball	C69.9-	C79.49	D09.2-	D31.9-	D48.7	D49.89
eyebrow	C44.309	C79.2	D04.39	D23.39	D48.5	D49.2
basal cell carcinoma	C44.319	—	—	—	—	—
specified type NEC	C44.399	—	—	—	—	—
squamous cell carcinoma	C44.329	—	—	—	—	—
eyelid (lower) (skin) (upper)	C44.10-	—	—	—	—	—
basal cell carcinoma	C44.11-	—	—	—	—	—
cartilage	C49.0	C79.89	—	D21.0	D48.1	D49.2
specified type NEC	C44.19-	—	—	—	—	—
squamous cell carcinoma	C44.12-	—	—	—	—	—
face NEC	C76.0	C79.89	D04.39	D36.7	D48.7	D49.89
fallopian tube (accessory)	C57.0-	C79.82	D07.39	D28.2	D39.8	D49.5
falx (cerebella) (cerebri)	C70.0	C79.32		D32.0	D42.0	D49.7
fascia — *see also* Neoplasm, connective tissue						
palmar	C49.1-	C79.89	—	D21.1-	D48.1	D49.2
plantar	C49.2-	C79.89	—	D21.2-	D48.1	D49.2
fatty tissue — *see* Neoplasm, connective tissue						
fauces, faucial NEC	C10.9	C79.89	D00.08	D10.5	D37.05	D49.0
pillars	C09.1	C79.89	D00.08	D10.5	D37.05	D49.0
tonsil	C09.9	C79.89	D00.08	D10.4	D37.05	D49.0
femur (any part)	C40.2-	—	—	D16.2-	—	—
fetal membrane	C58	C79.82	D07.0	D26.7	D39.2	D49.5
fibrous tissue — *see* Neoplasm, connective tissue						
fibula (any part)	C40.2-	C79.51	—	D16.2-	—	—
filum terminale	C72.0	C79.49	—	D33.4	D43.4	D49.7
finger NEC	C76.4-	C79.89	D04.6-	D36.7	D48.7	D49.89
flank NEC	C76.8	C79.89	D04.5	D36.7	D48.7	D49.89
follicle, nabothian	C53.0	C79.82	D06.0	D26.0	D39.0	D49.5
foot NEC	C76.5-	C79.89	D04.7-	D36.7	D48.7	D49.89
forearm NEC	C76.4-	C79.89	D04.6-	D36.7	D48.7	D49.89
forehead (skin)	C44.309	C79.2	D04.39	D23.39	D48.5	D49.2
basal cell carcinoma	C44.319	—	—	—	—	—
specified type NEC	C44.399	—	—	—	—	—
squamous cell carcinoma	C44.329	—	—	—	—	—
foreskin	C60.0	C79.82	D07.4	D29.0	D40.8	D49.5
fornix						
pharyngeal	C11.3	C79.89	D00.08	D10.6	D37.05	D49.0
vagina	C52	C79.82	D07.2	D28.1	D39.8	D49.5
fossa (of)						
anterior (cranial)	C71.9	C79.31	—	D33.2	D43.2	D49.6
cranial	C71.9	C79.31	—	D33.2	D43.2	D49.6
ischiorectal	C76.3	C79.89	D09.8	D36.7	D48.7	D49.89
middle (cranial)	C71.9	C79.31	—	D33.2	D43.2	D49.6
piriform	C12	C79.89	D00.08	D10.7	D37.05	D49.0
pituitary	C75.1	C79.89	D09.3	D35.2	D44.3	D49.7
posterior (cranial)	C71.9	C79.31	—	D33.2	D43.2	D49.6
pterygoid	C49.0	C79.89	—	D21.0	D48.1	D49.2
pyriform	C12	C79.89	D00.08	D10.7	D37.05	D49.0
Rosenmüller	C11.2	C79.89	D00.08	D10.6	D37.05	D49.0
tonsillar	C09.0	C79.89	D00.08	D10.5	D37.05	D49.0
Neoplasm, neoplastic - *continued*						
fourchette	C51.9	C79.82	D07.1	D28.0	D39.8	D49.5
frenulum						
labii — *see* Neoplasm, lip, internal						
linguae	C02.2	C79.89	D00.07	D10.1	D37.02	D49.0
frontal						
bone	C41.0	C79.51	—	D16.4-	D48.0	D49.2
lobe, brain	C71.1	C79.31	—	D33.0	D43.0	D49.6
pole	C71.1	C79.31	—	D33.0	D43.0	D49.6
sinus	C31.2	C78.39	D02.3	D14.0	D38.5	D49.1
fundus						
stomach	C16.1	C78.89	D00.2	D13.1	D37.1	D49.0
uterus	C54.3	C79.82	D07.0	D26.1	D39.0	D49.5
gall duct (extrahepatic)	C24.0	C78.89	D01.5	D13.5	D37.6	D49.0
intrahepatic	C22.1	C78.7	D01.5	D13.4	D37.6	D49.0
gallbladder	C23	C78.89	D01.5	D13.5	D37.6	D49.0
overlapping lesion with extrahepatic bile ducts	C24.8	—	—	—	—	—
ganglia — *see also* Neoplasm, nerve, peripheral	C47.9	C79.89	—	D36.10	D48.2	D49.2
basal	C71.0	C79.31	—	D33.0	D43.0	D49.6
cranial nerve	C72.50	C79.49	—	D33.3	D43.3	D49.7
Gartner's duct	C52	C79.82	D07.2	D28.1	D39.8	D49.5
gastric — *see also* Neoplasm, stomach						
gastrocolic	C26.9	C78.89	D01.9	D13.9	D37.9	D49.0
gastroesophageal junction	C16.0	C78.89	D00.2	D13.1	D37.1	D49.0
gastrointestinal (tract) NEC	C26.9	C78.89	D01.9	D13.9	D37.9	D49.0
generalized	C80.0	—	—	—	—	—
genital organ or tract						
female NEC	C57.9	C79.82	D07.30	D28.9	D39.9	D49.5
overlapping lesion	C57.8	—	—	—	—	—
specified site NEC	C57.7	C79.82	D07.39	D28.7	D39.8	D49.5
male NEC	C63.9	C79.82	D07.60	D29.9	D40.9	D49.5
overlapping lesion	C63.8	—	—	—	—	—
specified site NEC	C63.7	C79.82	D07.69	D29.8	D40.8	D49.5
genitourinary tract						
female	C57.9	C79.82	D07.30	D28.9	D39.9	D49.5
male	C63.9	C79.82	D07.60	D29.9	D40.9	D49.5
gingiva (alveolar) (marginal)	C03.9	C79.89	D00.03	D10.39	D37.09	D49.0
lower	C03.1	C79.89	D00.03	D10.39	D37.09	D49.0
mandibular	C03.1	C79.89	D00.03	D10.39	D37.09	D49.0
maxillary	C03.0	C79.89	D00.03	D10.39	D37.09	D49.0
upper	C03.0	C79.89	D00.03	D10.39	D37.09	D49.0
gland, glandular (lymphatic) (system) — *see also* Neoplasm, lymph gland						
endocrine NEC	C75.9	C79.89	D09.3	D35.9	D44.9	D49.7
salivary — *see* Neoplasm, salivary gland						
glans penis	C60.1	C79.82	D07.4	D29.0	D40.8	D49.5
globus pallidus	C71.0	C79.31	—	D33.0	D43.0	D49.6
glomus						
coccygeal	C49.5	C79.89	—	D21.5	D48.1	D49.2
jugularis	C75.5	C79.89	—	D35.6	D44.7	D49.7
glosso-epiglottic fold (s)	C10.1	C79.89	D00.08	D10.5	D37.05	D49.0
glossopalatine fold	C09.1	C79.89	D00.08	D10.5	D37.05	D49.0
glossopharyngeal sulcus	C09.0	C79.89	D00.08	D10.5	D37.05	D49.0
glottis	C32.0	C78.39	D02.0	D14.1	D38.0	D49.1
gluteal region	C76.3	C79.89	D04.5	D36.7	D48.7	D49.89
great vessels NEC	C49.3	C79.89	—	D21.3	D48.1	D49.2
groin NEC	C76.3	C79.89	D04.5	D36.7	D48.7	D49.89
gum	C03.9	C79.89	D00.03	D10.39	D37.09	D49.0
lower	C03.1	C79.89	D00.03	D10.39	D37.09	D49.0
upper	C03.0	C79.89	D00.03	D10.39	D37.09	D49.0
hand NEC	C76.4-	C79.89	D04.6-	D36.7	D48.7	D49.89
head NEC	C76.0	C79.89	D04.4	D36.7	D48.7	D49.89
heart	C38.0	C79.89	—	D15.1	D48.7	D49.89
heel NEC	C76.5-	C79.89	D04.7-	D36.7	D48.7	D49.89
helix — *see also* Neoplasm, skin, ear	C44.20-	C79.2	D04.2-	D23.2-	D48.5	D49.2
hematopoietic, hemopoietic tissue NEC	C96.9	—	—	—	—	—
specified NEC	C96.Z	—	—	—	—	—
hemisphere, cerebral	C71.0	C79.31	—	D33.0	D43.0	D49.6
hemorrhoidal zone	C21.1	C78.5	D01.3	D12.9	D37.8	D49.0
hepatic — *see also* Index to disease, by histology	C22.9	C78.7	D01.5	D13.4	D37.6	D49.0
duct (bile)	C24.0	C78.89	D01.5	D13.5	D37.6	D49.0
flexure (colon)	C18.3	C78.5	D01.0	D12.3	D37.4	D49.0
primary	C22.8	C78.7	D01.5	D13.4	D37.6	D49.0
hepatobiliary	C24.9	C78.89	D01.5	D13.5	D37.6	D49.0
hepatoblastoma	C22.2	C78.7	D01.5	D13.4	D37.6	D49.0
hepatoma	C22.0	C78.7	D01.5	D13.4	D37.6	D49.0
hilus of lung	C34.0-	C78.0-	D02.2-	D14.3-	D38.1	D49.1
hip NEC	C76.5-	C79.89	D04.7-	D36.7	D48.7	D49.89
hippocampus, brain	C71.2	C79.31	—	D33.0	D43.0	D49.6

NEOPLASM TABLE

NEOPLASM TABLE

Neoplasm, neoplastic - *continued*

Neoplasm Table	Malignant Primary	Malignant Secondary	Ca In situ	Benign	Uncertain Behavior	Unspecified Behavior
humerus (any part)	C40.0-	C79.51	—	D16.0-	—	—
hymen	C52	C79.82	D07.2	D28.1	D39.8	D49.5
hypopharynx, hypopharyngeal NEC	C13.9	C79.89	D00.08	D10.7	D37.05	D49.0
overlapping lesion	C13.8	—	—	—	—	—
postcricoid region	C13.0	C79.89	D00.08	D10.7	D37.05	D49.0
posterior wall	C13.2	C79.89	D00.08	D10.7	D37.05	D49.0
pyriform fossa (sinus)	C12	C79.89	D00.08	D10.7	D37.05	D49.0
hypophysis	C75.1	C79.3	D09.3	D35.2	D44.3	D49.7
hypothalamus	C71.0	C79.31	—	D33.0	D43.0	D49.6
ileocecum, ileocecal (coil) (junction) (valve)	C18.0	C78.5	D01.0	D12.0	D37.4	D49.0
ileum	C17.2	C78.4	D01.49	D13.39	D37.2	D49.0
ilium	C41.4	C79.51	—	D16.8	D48.0	D49.2
immunoproliferative NEC	C88.9					
infraclavicular (region)	C76.1	C79.89	D04.5	D36.7	D48.7	D49.89
inguinal (region)	C76.3	C79.89	D04.5	D36.7	D48.7	D49.89
insula	C71.0	C79.31	—	D33.0	D43.0	D49.6
insular tissue (pancreas)	C25.4	C78.89	D01.7	D13.7	D37.8	D49.0
brain	C71.0	C79.31	—	D33.0	D43.0	D49.6
interarytenoid fold	C13.1	C79.89	D00.08	D10.7	D37.05	D49.0
hypopharyngeal aspect	C13.1	C79.89	D00.08	D10.7	D37.05	D49.0
laryngeal aspect	C32.1	C78.39	D02.0	D14.1	D38.0	D49.1
marginal zone	C13.1	C79.89	D00.08	D10.7	D37.05	D49.0
interdental papillae	C03.9	C79.89	D00.03	D10.39	D37.09	D49.0
lower	C03.1	C79.89	D00.03	D10.39	D37.09	D49.0
upper	C03.0	C79.89	D00.03	D10.39	D37.09	D49.0
internal						
capsule	C71.0	C79.31	—	D33.0	D43.0	D49.6
os (cervix)	C53.0	C79.82	D06.0	D26.0	D39.0	D49.5
intervertebral cartilage or disc	C41.2	C79.51	—	D16.6	D48.0	D49.2
intestine, intestinal	C26.0	C78.80	D01.40	D13.9	D37.8	D49.0
large	C18.9	C78.5	D01.0	D12.6	D37.4	D49.0
appendix	C18.1	C78.5	D01.0	D12.1	D37.3	D49.0
caput coli	C18.0	C78.5	D01.0	D12.0	D37.4	D49.0
cecum	C18.0	C78.5	D01.0	D12.0	D37.4	D49.0
colon	C18.9	C78.5	D01.0	D12.6	D37.4	D49.0
and rectum	C19	C78.5	D01.1	D12.7	D37.5	D49.0
ascending	C18.2	C78.5	D01.0	D12.2	D37.4	D49.0
caput	C18.0	C78.5	D01.0	D12.0	D37.4	D49.0
descending	C18.6	C78.5	D01.0	D12.4	D37.4	D49.0
distal	C18.6	C78.5	D01.0	D12.4	D37.4	D49.0
left	C18.6	C78.5	D01.0	D12.4	D37.4	D49.0
overlapping lesion	C18.8	—	—	—	—	—
pelvic	C18.7	C78.5	D01.0	D12.5	D37.4	D49.0
right	C18.2	C78.5	D01.0	D12.2	D37.4	D49.0
sigmoid (flexure)	C18.7	C78.5	D01.0	D12.5	D37.4	D49.0
transverse	C18.4	C78.5	D01.0	D12.3	D37.4	D49.0
hepatic flexure	C18.3	C78.5	D01.0	D12.3	D37.4	D49.0
ileocecum, ileocecal (coil) (valve)	C18.0	C78.5	D01.0	D12.0	D37.4	D49.0
overlapping lesion	C18.8	—	—	—	—	—
sigmoid flexure (lower) (upper)	C18.7	C78.5	D01.0	D12.5	D37.4	D49.0
splenic flexure	C18.5	C78.5	D01.0	D12.3	D37.4	D49.0
small	C17.9	C78.4	D01.40	D13.30	D37.2	D49.0
duodenum	C17.0	C78.4	D01.49	D13.2	D37.2	D49.0
ileum	C17.2	C78.4	D01.49	D13.39	D37.2	D49.0
jejunum	C17.1	C78.4	D01.49	D13.39	D37.2	D49.0
overlapping lesion	C17.8					
tract NEC	C26.0	C78.89	D01.40	D13.9	D37.8	D49.0
intra-abdominal	C76.2	C79.89	D09.8	D36.7	D48.7	D49.89
intracranial NEC	C71.9	C79.31	—	D33.2	D43.2	D49.6
intrahepatic (bile) duct	C22.1	C78.7	D01.5	D13.4	D37.6	D49.0
intraocular	C69.9-	C79.49	D09.2-	D31.9-	D48.7	D49.89
intraorbital	C69.6-	C79.49	D09.2-	D31.6-	D48.7	D49.89
intrasellar	C75.1	C79.89	D09.3	D35.2	D44.3	D49.7
intrathoracic (cavity) (organs)	C76.1	C79.89	D09.8	D15.9	D48.7	D49.89
specified NEC	C76.1	C79.89	D09.8	D15.7		
iris	C69.4-	C79.49	D09.2-	D31.4-	D48.7	D49.89
ischiorectal (fossa)	C76.3	C79.89	D09.8	D36.7	D48.7	D49.89
ischium	C41.4	C79.51	—	D16.8	D48.0	D49.2
island of Reil	C71.0	C79.31	—	D33.0	D43.0	D49.6
islands or islets of Langerhans	C25.4	C78.89	D01.7	D13.7	D37.8	D49.0
isthmus uteri	C54.0	C79.82	D07.0	D26.1	D39.0	D49.5
jaw	C76.0	C79.89	D09.8	D36.7	D48.7	D49.89
bone	C41.1	C79.51	—	D16.5-	D48.0	D49.2
lower	C41.1	C79.51	—	D16.5-	—	—
upper	C41.0	C79.51	—	D16.4-	—	—
carcinoma (any type) (lower) (upper)	C76.0	C79.89	—	—	—	—
skin — *see also* Neoplasm, skin, face	C44.309	C79.2	D04.39	D23.39	D48.5	D49.2
soft tissues	C03.9	C79.89	D00.03	D10.39	D37.09	D49.0
lower	C03.1	C79.89	D00.03	D10.39	D37.09	D49.0
upper	C03.0	C79.89	D00.03	D10.39	D37.09	D49.0

Neoplasm, neoplastic - *continued*

Neoplasm Table	Malignant Primary	Malignant Secondary	Ca In situ	Benign	Uncertain Behavior	Unspecified Behavior
jejunum	C17.1	C78.4	D01.49	D13.39	D37.2	D49.0
joint NEC — *see also* Neoplasm, bone	C41.9	C79.51	—	D16.9-	D48.0	D49.2
acromioclavicular	C40.0-	C79.51	—	D16.0-	—	—
bursa or synovial membrane — *see* Neoplasm, connective tissue						
costovertebral	C41.3	C79.51	—	D16.7	D48.0	D49.2
sternocostal	C41.3	C79.51	—	D16.7	D48.0	D49.2
temporomandibular	C41.1	C79.51	—	D16.5-	D48.0	D49.2
junction						
anorectal	C21.8	C78.5	D01.3	D12.9	D37.8	D49.0
cardioesophageal	C16.0	C78.89	D00.2	D13.1	D37.1	D49.0
esophagogastric	C16.0	C78.89	D00.2	D13.1	D37.1	D49.0
gastroesophageal	C16.0	C78.89	D00.2	D13.1	D37.1	D49.0
hard and soft palate	C05.9	C79.89	D00.00	D10.39	D37.09	D49.0
ileocecal	C18.0	C78.5	D01.0	D12.0	D37.4	D49.0
pelvirectal	C19	C78.5	D01.1	D12.7	D37.5	D49.0
pelviureteric	C65.-	C79.0-	D09.19	D30.1-	D41.1-	D49.5
rectosigmoid	C19	C78.5	D01.1	D12.7	D37.5	D49.0
squamocolumnar, of cervix	C53.8	C79.82	D06.7	D26.0	D39.0	D49.5
Kaposi's sarcoma — *see* Kaposi's, sarcoma						
kidney (parenchymal)	C64.-	C79.0-	D09.19	D30.0-	D41.0-	D49.5
calyx	C65.-	C79.0-	D09.19	D30.1-	D41.1-	D49.5
hilus	C65.-	C79.0-	D09.19	D30.1-	D41.1-	D49.5
pelvis	C65.-	C79.0-	D09.19	D30.1-	D41.1-	D49.5
knee NEC	C76.5-	C79.89	D04.7-	D36.7	D48.7	D49.89
labia (skin)	C51.9	C79.82	D07.1	D28.0	D39.8	D49.5
majora	C51.0	C79.82	D07.1	D28.0	D39.8	D49.5
minora	C51.1	C79.82	D07.1	D28.0	D39.8	D49.5
labial — *see also* Neoplasm, lip	C00.9	C79.89	D00.01	D10.0	D37.01	D49.0
sulcus (lower) (upper)	C06.1	C79.89	D00.02	D10.39	D37.09	D49.0
labium (skin)	C51.9	C79.82	D07.1	D28.0	D39.8	D49.5
majus	C51.0	C79.82	D07.1	D28.0	D39.8	D49.5
minus	C51.1	C79.82	D07.1	D28.0	D39.8	D49.5
lacrimal						
canaliculi	C69.5-	C79.49	D09.2-	D31.5-	D48.7	D49.89
duct (nasal)	C69.5-	C79.49	D09.2-	D31.5-	D48.7	D49.89
gland	C69.5-	C79.49	D09.2-	D31.5-	D48.7	D49.89
punctum	C69.5-	C79.49	D09.2-	D31.5-	D48.7	D49.89
sac	C69.5-	C79.49	D09.2-	D31.5-	D48.7	D49.89
Langerhans, islands or islets	C25.4	C78.89	D01.7	D13.7	D37.8	D49.0
laryngopharynx	C13.9	C79.89	D00.08	D10.7	D37.05	D49.0
larynx, laryngeal NEC	C32.9	C78.39	D02.0	D14.1	D38.0	D49.1
aryepiglottic fold	C32.1	C78.39	D02.0	D14.1	D38.0	D49.1
cartilage (arytenoid) (cricoid) (cuneiform) (thyroid)	C32.3	C78.39	D02.0	D14.1	D38.0	D49.1
commissure (anterior) (posterior)	C32.0	C78.39	D02.0	D14.1	D38.0	D49.1
extrinsic NEC	C32.1	C78.39	D02.0	D14.1	D38.0	D49.1
meaning hypopharynx	C13.9	C79.89	D00.08	D10.7	D37.05	D49.0
interarytenoid fold	C32.1	C78.39	D02.0	D14.1	D38.0	D49.1
intrinsic	C32.0	C78.39	D02.0	D14.1	D38.0	D49.1
overlapping lesion	C32.8					
ventricular band	C32.1	C78.39	D02.0	D14.1	D38.0	D49.1
leg NEC	C76.5-	C79.89	D04.7-	D36.7	D48.7	D49.89
lens, crystalline	C69.4-	C79.49	D09.2-	D31.4-	D48.7	D49.89
lid (lower) (upper)	C44.10-	C79.2	D04.1-	D23.1-	D48.5	D49.2
basal cell carcinoma	C44.11-					
specified type NEC	C44.19-	—	—	—	—	—
squamous cell carcinoma	C44.12-					
ligament — *see also* Neoplasm, connective tissue						
broad	C57.1	C79.82	D07.39	D28.2	D39.8	D49.5
Mackenrodt's	C57.7	C79.82	D07.39	D28.7	D39.8	D49.5
non-uterine — *see* Neoplasm, connective tissue						
round	C57.2	C79.82	—	D28.2	D39.8	D49.5
sacro-uterine	C57.3	C79.82	—	D28.2	D39.8	D49.5
uterine	C57.3	C79.82	—	D28.2	D39.8	D49.5
utero-ovarian	C57.7	C79.82	D07.39	D28.2	D39.8	D49.5
uterosacral	C57.3	C79.82	—	D28.2	D39.8	D49.5
limb	C76.8	C79.89	D04.8	D36.7	D48.7	D49.89
lower	C76.5-	C79.89	D04.7-	D36.7	D48.7	D49.89
upper	C76.4-	C79.89	D04.6-	D36.7	D48.7	D49.89
limbus of cornea	C69.1-	C79.49	D09.2-	D31.1-	D48.7	D49.89
lingual NEC — *see also* Neoplasm, tongue	C02.9	C79.89	D00.07	D10.1	D37.02	D49.0
lingula, lung	C34.1-	C78.0-	D02.2-	D14.3-	D38.1	D49.1

NEOPLASM TABLE

Neoplasm Table	Malignant Primary	Malignant Secondary	Ca in situ	Benign	Uncertain Behavior	Unspecified Behavior
Neoplasm, neoplastic - *continued*						
lip	C00.9	C79.89	D00.01	D10.0	D37.01	D49.0
buccal aspect — *see* Neoplasm, lip, internal						
commissure	C00.6	C79.89	D00.01	D10.0	D37.01	D49.0
external	C00.2	C79.89	D00.01	D10.0	D37.01	D49.0
lower	C00.1	C79.89	D00.01	D10.0	D37.01	D49.0
upper	C00.0	C79.89	D00.01	D10.0	D37.01	D49.0
frenulum — *see* Neoplasm, lip, internal						
inner aspect — *see* Neoplasm, lip, internal						
internal	C00.5	C79.89	D00.01	D10.0	D37.01	D49.0
lower	C00.4	C79.89	D00.01	D10.0	D37.01	D49.0
upper	C00.3	C79.89	D00.01	D10.0	D37.01	D49.0
lipstick area	C00.2	C79.89	D00.01	D10.0	D37.01	D49.0
lower	C00.1	C79.89	D00.01	D10.0	D37.01	D49.0
upper	C00.0	C79.89	D00.01	D10.0	D37.01	D49.0
lower	C00.1	C79.89	D00.01	D10.0	D37.01	D49.0
internal	C00.4	C79.89	D00.01	D10.0	D37.01	D49.0
mucosa — *see* Neoplasm, lip, internal						
oral aspect — *see* Neoplasm, lip, internal						
overlapping lesion	C00.8	—	—	—	—	—
with oral cavity or pharynx	C14.8	—	—	—	—	—
skin (commissure) (lower) (upper)	C44.00	C79.2	D04.0	D23.0	D48.5	D49.2
basal cell carcinoma	C44.01	—	—	—	—	—
specified type NEC	C44.09	—	—	—	—	—
squamous cell carcinoma	C44.02	—	—	—	—	—
upper	C00.0	C79.89	D00.01	D10.0	D37.01	D49.0
internal	C00.3	C79.89	D00.01	D10.0	D37.01	D49.0
vermilion border	C00.2	C79.89	D00.01	D10.0	D37.01	D49.0
lower	C00.1	C79.89	D00.01	D10.0	D37.01	D49.0
upper	C00.0	C79.89	D00.01	D10.0	D37.01	D49.0
lipomatous — *see* Lipoma, by site						
liver — *see also* Index to disease, by histology	C22.9	C78.7	D01.5	D13.4	D37.6	D49.0
primary	C22.8	C78.7	D01.5	D13.4	D37.6	D49.0
lumbosacral plexus	C47.5	C79.89	—	D36.16	D48.2	D49.2
lung	C34.9-	C78.0-	D02.2-	D14.3-	D38.1	D49.1
azygos lobe	C34.1-	C78.0-	D02.2-	D14.3-	D38.1	D49.1
carina	C34.0-	C78.0-	D02.2-	D14.3-	D38.1	D49.1
hilus	C34.0-	C78.0-	D02.2-	D14.3-	D38.1	D49.1
lingula	C34.1-	C78.0-	D02.2-	D14.3-	D38.1	D49.1
lobe NEC	C34.9-	C78.0-	D02.2-	D14.3-	D38.1	D49.1
lower lobe	C34.3-	C78.0-	D02.2-	D14.3-	D38.1	D49.1
main bronchus	C34.0-	C78.0-	D02.2-	D14.3-	D38.1	D49.1
mesothelioma — *see* Mesothelioma						
middle lobe	C34.2	C78.0-	D02.21	D14.31	D38.1	D49.1
overlapping lesion	C34.8-	—	—	—	—	—
upper lobe	C34.1-	C78.0-	D02.2-	D14.3-	D38.1	D49.1
lymph, lymphatic channel NEC	C49.9	C79.89	—	D21.9	D48.1	D49.2
gland (secondary)	—	C77.9	—	D36.0	D48.7	D49.89
abdominal	—	C77.2	—	D36.0	D48.7	D49.89
aortic	—	C77.2	—	D36.0	D48.7	D49.89
arm	—	C77.3	—	D36.0	D48.7	D49.89
auricular (anterior) (posterior)	—	C77.0	—	D36.0	D48.7	D49.89
axilla, axillary	—	C77.3	—	D36.0	D48.7	D49.89
brachial	—	C77.3	—	D36.0	D48.7	D49.89
bronchial	—	C77.1	—	D36.0	D48.7	D49.89
bronchopulmonary	—	C77.1	—	D36.0	D48.7	D49.89
celiac	—	C77.2	—	D36.0	D48.7	D49.89
cervical	—	C77.0	—	D36.0	D48.7	D49.89
cervicofacial	—	C77.0	—	D36.0	D48.7	D49.89
Cloquet	—	C77.4	—	D36.0	D48.7	D49.89
colic	—	C77.2	—	D36.0	D48.7	D49.89
common duct	—	C77.2	—	D36.0	D48.7	D49.89
cubital	—	C77.3	—	D36.0	D48.7	D49.89
diaphragmatic	—	C77.1	—	D36.0	D48.7	D49.89
epigastric, inferior	—	C77.1	—	D36.0	D48.7	D49.89
epitrochlear	—	C77.3	—	D36.0	D48.7	D49.89
esophageal	—	C77.1	—	D36.0	D48.7	D49.89
face	—	C77.0	—	D36.0	D48.7	D49.89
femoral	—	C77.4	—	D36.0	D48.7	D49.89
gastric	—	C77.2	—	D36.0	D48.7	D49.89
groin	—	C77.4	—	D36.0	D48.7	D49.89
head	—	C77.0	—	D36.0	D48.7	D49.89
hepatic	—	C77.2	—	D36.0	D48.7	D49.89
hilar (pulmonary)	—	C77.1	—	D36.0	D48.7	D49.89
splenic	—	C77.2	—	D36.0	D48.7	D49.89
hypogastric	—	C77.5	—	D36.0	D48.7	D49.89
Neoplasm, neoplastic - *continued*						
lymph, lymphatic channel NEC - *continued*	C49.9	C79.89	—	D21.9	D48.1	D49.2
gland (secondary) - *continued*	—	C77.9	—	D36.0	D48.7	D49.89
ileocolic	—	C77.2	—	D36.0	D48.7	D49.89
iliac	—	C77.5	—	D36.0	D48.7	D49.89
infraclavicular	—	C77.3	—	D36.0	D48.7	D49.89
inguina, inguinal	—	C77.4	—	D36.0	D48.7	D49.89
innominate	—	C77.1	—	D36.0	D48.7	D49.89
intercostal	—	C77.1	—	D36.0	D48.7	D49.89
intestinal	—	C77.2	—	D36.0	D48.7	D49.89
intrabdominal	—	C77.2	—	D36.0	D48.7	D49.89
intrapelvic	—	C77.5	—	D36.0	D48.7	D49.89
intrathoracic	—	C77.1	—	D36.0	D48.7	D49.89
jugular	—	C77.0	—	D36.0	D48.7	D49.89
leg	—	C77.4	—	D36.0	D48.7	D49.89
limb						
lower	—	C77.4	—	D36.0	D48.7	D49.89
upper	—	C77.3	—	D36.0	D48.7	D49.89
lower limb	—	C77.4	—	D36.0	D48.7	D49.89
lumbar	—	C77.2	—	D36.0	D48.7	D49.89
mandibular	—	C77.0	—	D36.0	D48.7	D49.89
mediastinal	—	C77.1	—	D36.0	D48.7	D49.89
mesenteric (inferior) (superior)	—	C77.2	—	D36.0	D48.7	D49.89
midcolic	—	C77.2	—	D36.0	D48.7	D49.89
multiple sites in categories C77.0-C77.5	—	C77.8	—	D36.0	D48.7	D49.89
neck	—	C77.0	—	D36.0	D48.7	D49.89
obturator	—	C77.5	—	D36.0	D48.7	D49.89
occipital	—	C77.0	—	D36.0	D48.7	D49.89
pancreatic	—	C77.2	—	D36.0	D48.7	D49.89
para-aortic	—	C77.2	—	D36.0	D48.7	D49.89
paracervical	—	C77.5	—	D36.0	D48.7	D49.89
parametrial	—	C77.5	—	D36.0	D48.7	D49.89
parasternal	—	C77.1	—	D36.0	D48.7	D49.89
parotid	—	C77.0	—	D36.0	D48.7	D49.89
pectoral	—	C77.3	—	D36.0	D48.7	D49.89
pelvic	—	C77.5	—	D36.0	D48.7	D49.89
peri-aortic	—	C77.2	—	D36.0	D48.7	D49.89
peripancreatic	—	C77.2	—	D36.0	D48.7	D49.89
popliteal	—	C77.4	—	D36.0	D48.7	D49.89
porta hepatis	—	C77.2	—	D36.0	D48.7	D49.89
portal	—	C77.2	—	D36.0	D48.7	D49.89
preauricular	—	C77.0	—	D36.0	D48.7	D49.89
prelaryngeal	—	C77.0	—	D36.0	D48.7	D49.89
presymphysial	—	C77.5	—	D36.0	D48.7	D49.89
pretracheal	—	C77.0	—	D36.0	D48.7	D49.89
primary (any site) NEC	C96.9	—	—	—	—	—
pulmonary (hiler)	—	C77.1	—	D36.0	D48.7	D49.89
pyloric	—	C77.2	—	D36.0	D48.7	D49.89
retroperitoneal	—	C77.2	—	D36.0	D48.7	D49.89
retropharyngeal	—	C77.0	—	D36.0	D48.7	D49.89
Rosenmüller's	—	C77.4	—	D36.0	D48.7	D49.89
sacral	—	C77.5	—	D36.0	D48.7	D49.89
scalene	—	C77.0	—	D36.0	D48.7	D49.89
site NEC	—	C77.9	—	D36.0	D48.7	D49.89
splenic (hilar)	—	C77.2	—	D36.0	D48.7	D49.89
subclavicular	—	C77.3	—	D36.0	D48.7	D49.89
subinguinal	—	C77.4	—	D36.0	D48.7	D49.89
sublingual	—	C77.0	—	D36.0	D48.7	D49.89
submandibular	—	C77.0	—	D36.0	D48.7	D49.89
submaxillary	—	C77.0	—	D36.0	D48.7	D49.89
submental	—	C77.0	—	D36.0	D48.7	D49.89
subscapular	—	C77.3	—	D36.0	D48.7	D49.89
supraclavicular	—	C77.0	—	D36.0	D48.7	D49.89
thoracic	—	C77.1	—	D36.0	D48.7	D49.89
tibial	—	C77.4	—	D36.0	D48.7	D49.89
tracheal	—	C77.1	—	D36.0	D48.7	D49.89
tracheobronchial	—	C77.1	—	D36.0	D48.7	D49.89
upper limb	—	C77.3	—	D36.0	D48.7	D49.89
Virchow's	—	C77.0	—	D36.0	D48.7	D49.89
node — *see also* Neoplasm, lymph gland						
primary NEC	C96.9	—	—	—	—	—
vessel — *see also* Neoplasm, connective tissue	C49.9	C79.89	—	D21.9	D48.1	D49.2
Mackenrodt's ligament	C57.7	C79.82	D07.39	D28.7	D39.8	D49.5
malar	C41.0	C79.51	—	D16.4-	D48.0	D49.2
region — *see* Neoplasm, cheek						
mammary gland — *see* Neoplasm, breast						

NEOPLASM TABLE

Neoplasm Table	Malignant Primary	Malignant Secondary	Ca In situ	Benign	Uncertain Behavior	Unspecified Behavior
Neoplasm, neoplastic - *continued*						
mandible	C41.1	C79.51	—	D16.5-	D48.0	D49.2
alveolar						
mucosa (carcinoma)	C03.1	C79.89	D00.03	D10.39	D37.09	D49.0
ridge or process	C41.1	C79.51	—	D16.5-	D48.0	D49.2
marrow (bone) NEC	C96.9	C79.52	—	—	D47.9	D49.89
mastectomy site (skin) — *see also* Neoplasm, breast, skin	C44.501	C79.2	—	—	—	—
specified as breast tissue	C50.8	C79.81	—	—	—	—
mastoid (air cells) (antrum) (cavity)	C30.1	C78.39	D02.3	D14.0	D38.5	D49.1
bone or process	C41.0	C79.51	—	D16.4-	D48.0	D49.2
maxilla, maxillary (superior)	C41.0	C79.51	—	D16.4-	D48.0	D49.2
alveolar						
mucosa	C03.0	C79.89	D00.03	D10.39	D37.09	D49.0
ridge or process (carcinoma)	C41.0	C79.51	—	D16.4-	D48.0	D49.2
antrum	C31.0	C78.39	D02.3	D14.0	D38.5	D49.1
carcinoma	C03.0	C79.51	—	—		
inferior — *see* Neoplasm, mandible						
sinus	C31.0	C78.39	D02.3	D14.0	D38.5	D49.1
meatus external (ear) — *see also* Neoplasm, skin, ear	C44.20-	C79.2	D04.2-	D23.2-	D48.5	D49.2
Meckel diverticulum, malignant	C17.3	C78.4	D01.49	D13.39	D37.2	D49.0
mediastinum, mediastinal	C38.3	C78.1	—	D15.2	D38.3	D49.89
anterior	C38.1	C78.1	—	D15.2	D38.3	D49.89
posterior	C38.2	C78.1	—	D15.2	D38.3	D49.89
medulla						
adrenal	C74.1-	C79.7-	D09.3	D35.0-	D44.1-	D49.7
oblongata	C71.7	C79.31	—	D33.1	D43.1	D49.6
meibomian gland	C44.10-	C79.2	D04.1-	D23.1-	D48.5	D49.2
basal cell carcinoma	C44.11-	—	—	—	—	—
specified type NEC	C44.19-	—	—	—	—	—
squamous cell carcinoma	C44.12-	—	—	—	—	—
melanoma — *see* Melanoma						
meninges	C70.9	C79.49	—	D32.9	D42.9	D49.7
brain	C70.0	C79.32	—	D32.0	D42.0	D49.7
cerebral	C70.0	C79.32	—	D32.0	D42.0	D49.7
crainial	C70.0	C79.32	—	D32.0	D42.0	D49.7
intracranial	C70.0	C79.32	—	D32.0	D42.0	D49.7
spinal (cord)	C70.1	C79.49	—	D32.1	D42.1	D49.7
meniscus, knee joint (lateral) (medial)	C40.2-	C79.51	—	D16.2-	D48.0	D49.2
Merkel cell — *see* Carcinoma, Merkel cell						
mesentery, mesenteric	C48.1	C78.6	—	D20.1	D48.4	D49.0
mesoappendix	C48.1	C78.6	—	D20.1	D48.4	D49.0
mesocolon	C48.1	C78.6	—	D20.1	D48.4	D49.0
mesopharynx — *see* Neoplasm, oropharynx						
mesosalpinx	C57.1	C79.82	D07.39	D28.2	D39.8	D49.5
mesothelial tissue — *see* Mesothelioma						
mesothelioma — *see* Mesothelioma						
mesovarium	C57.1	C79.82	D07.39	D28.2	D39.8	D49.5
metacarpus (any bone)	C40.1-	C79.51	—	D16.1-	—	—
metastatic NEC — *see also* Neoplasm, by site, secondary	—	C79.9	—	—	—	—
metatarsus (any bone)	C40.3-	C79.51	—	D16.3-	—	—
midbrain	C71.7	C79.31	—	D33.1	D43.1	D49.6
milk duct — *see* Neoplasm, breast						
mons						
pubis	C51.9	C79.82	D07.1	D28.0	D39.8	D49.5
veneris	C51.9	C79.82	D07.1	D28.0	D39.8	D49.5
motor tract	C72.9	C79.49	—	D33.9	D43.9	D49.7
brain	C71.9	C79.31	—	D33.2	D43.2	D49.6
cauda equina	C72.1	C79.49	—	D33.4	D43.4	D49.7
spinal	C72.0	C79.49	—	D33.4	D43.4	D49.7
mouth	C06.9	C79.89	D00.00	D10.30	D37.09	D49.0
book-leaf	C06.89	C79.89	—	—	—	—
floor	C04.9	C79.89	D00.06	D10.2	D37.09	D49.0
anterior portion	C04.0	C79.89	D00.06	D10.2	D37.09	D49.0
lateral portion	C04.1	C79.89	D00.06	D10.2	D37.09	D49.0
overlapping lesion	C04.8	—	—	—	—	—
overlapping NEC	C06.80	—	—	—	—	—
roof	C05.9	C79.89	D00.00	D10.39	D37.09	D49.0
specified part NEC	C06.89	C79.89	D00.00	D10.39	D37.09	D49.0
vestibule	C06.1	C79.89	D00.00	D10.39	D37.09	D49.0
Neoplasm, neoplastic - *continued*						
mucosa						
alveolar (ridge or process)	C03.9	C79.89	D00.03	D10.39	D37.09	D49.0
lower	C03.1	C79.89	D00.03	D10.39	D37.09	D49.0
upper	C03.0	C79.89	D00.03	D10.39	D37.09	D49.0
buccal	C06.0	C79.89	D00.02	D10.39	D37.09	D49.0
cheek	C06.0	C79.89	D00.02	D10.39	D37.09	D49.0
lip — *see* Neoplasm, lip, internal						
nasal	C30.0	C78.39	D02.3	D14.0	D38.5	D49.1
oral	C06.0	C79.89	D00.02	D10.39	D37.09	D49.0
Müllerian duct						
female	C57.7	C79.82	D07.39	D28.7	D39.8	D49.5
male	C63.7	C79.82	D07.69	D29.8	D40.8	D49.5
muscle — *see also* Neoplasm, connective tissue						
extraocular	C69.6-	C79.49	D09.2-	D31.6-	D48.7	D49.89
myocardium	C38.0	C79.89	—	D15.1	D48.7	D49.89
myometrium	C54.2	C79.82	D07.0	D26.1	D39.0	D49.5
myopericardium	C38.0	C79.89	—	D15.1	D48.7	D49.89
nabothian gland (follicle)	C53.0	C79.82	D06.0	D26.0	D39.0	D49.5
nail — *see also* Neoplasm, skin, limb	C44.90	C79.2	D04.9	D23.9	D48.5	D49.2
finger — *see also* Neoplasm, skin, limb, upper	C44.60-	C79.2	D04.6-	D23.6-	D48.5	D49.2
toe — *see also* Neoplasm, skin, limb, lower	C44.70-	C79.2	D04.7-	D23.7-	D48.5	D49.2
nares, naris (anterior) (posterior)	C30.0	C78.39	D02.3	D14.0	D38.5	D49.1
nasal — *see* Neoplasm, nose						
nasolabial groove — *see also* Neoplasm, skin, face	C44.309	C79.2	D04.39	D23.39	D48.5	D49.2
nasolacrimal duct	C69.5-	C79.49	D09.2-	D31.5-	D48.7	D49.89
nasopharynx, nasopharyngeal	C11.9	C79.89	D00.08	D10.6	D37.05	D49.0
floor	C11.3	C79.89	D00.08	D10.6	D37.05	D49.0
overlapping lesion	C11.8	—	—	—	—	—
roof	C11.0	C79.89	D00.08	D10.6	D37.05	D49.0
wall	C11.9	C79.89	D00.08	D10.6	D37.05	D49.0
anterior	C11.3	C79.89	D00.08	D10.6	D37.05	D49.0
lateral	C11.2	C79.89	D00.08	D10.6	D37.05	D49.0
posterior	C11.1	C79.89	D00.08	D10.6	D37.05	D49.0
superior	C11.0	C79.89	D00.08	D10.6	D37.05	D49.0
nates — *see also* Neoplasm, skin, trunk	C44.509	C79.2	D04.5	D23.5	D48.5	D49.2
neck NEC	C76.0	C79.89	D09.8	D36.7	D48.7	D49.89
skin	C44.40	—	—	—	—	—
basal cell carcinoma	C44.41	—	—	—	—	—
specified type NEC	C44.49	—	—	—	—	—
squamous cell carcinoma	C44.42	—	—	—	—	—
nerve (ganglion)	C47.9	C79.89	—	D36.10	D48.2	D49.2
abducens	C72.59	C79.49	—	D33.3	D43.3	D49.7
accessory (spinal)	C72.59	C79.49	—	D33.3	D43.3	D49.7
acoustic	C72.4-	C79.49	—	D33.3	D43.3	D49.7
auditory	C72.4-	C79.49	—	D33.3	D43.3	D49.7
autonomic NEC — *see also* Neoplasm, nerve, peripheral	C47.9	C79.89	—	D36.10	D48.2	D49.2
brachial	C47.1-	C79.89	—	D36.12	D48.2	D49.2
cranial	C72.50	C79.49	—	D33.3	D43.3	D49.7
specified NEC	C72.59	C79.49	—	D33.3	D43.3	D49.7
facial	C72.59	C79.49	—	D33.3	D43.3	D49.7
femoral	C47.2-	C79.89	—	D36.13	D48.2	D49.2
ganglion NEC — *see also* Neoplasm, nerve, peripheral	C47.9	C79.89	—	D36.10	D48.2	D49.2
glossopharyngeal	C72.59	C79.49	—	D33.3	D43.3	D49.7
hypoglossal	C72.59	C79.49	—	D33.3	D43.3	D49.7
intercostal	C47.3	C79.89	—	D36.14	D48.2	D49.2
lumbar	C47.6	C79.89	—	D36.17	D48.2	D49.2
median	C47.1-	C79.89	—	D36.12	D48.2	D49.2
obturator	C47.2-	C79.89	—	D36.13	D48.2	D49.2
oculomotor	C72.59	C79.49	—	D33.3	D43.3	D49.7
olfactory	C47.2-	C79.49	—	D33.3	D43.3	D49.7
optic	C72.3-	C79.49	—	D33.3	D43.3	D49.7
parasympathetic NEC	C47.9	C79.89	—	D36.10	D48.2	D49.2
peripheral NEC	C47.9	C79.89	—	D36.10	D48.2	D49.2
abdomen	C47.4	C79.89	—	D36.15	D48.2	D49.2
abdominal wall	C47.4	C79.89	—	D36.15	D48.2	D49.2
ankle	C47.2-	C79.89	—	D36.13	D48.2	D49.2
antecubital fossa or space	C47.1-	C79.89	—	D36.12	D48.2	D49.2
arm	C47.1-	C79.89	—	D36.12	D48.2	D49.2
auricle (ear)	C47.0	C79.89	—	D36.11	D48.2	D49.2
axilla	C47.3	C79.89	—	D36.12	D48.2	D49.2
back	C47.6	C79.89	—	D36.17	D48.2	D49.2
buttock	C47.5	C79.89	—	D36.16	D48.2	D49.2
calf	C47.2-	C79.89	—	D36.13	D48.2	D49.2

Neoplasm Table	Malignant Primary	Malignant Secondary	Ca in situ	Benign	Uncertain Behavior	Unspecified Behavior
Neoplasm, neoplastic - *continued*						
nerve (ganglion) - *continued* ..	C47.9	C79.89	—	D36.10	D48.2	D49.2
peripheral NEC - *continued*	C47.9	C79.89	—	D36.10	D48.2	D49.2
cervical region	C47.0	C79.89	—	D36.11	D48.2	D49.2
cheek	C47.0	C79.89	—	D36.11	D48.2	D49.2
chest (wall)	C47.3	C79.89	—	D36.14	D48.2	D49.2
chin	C47.0	C79.89	—	D36.11	D48.2	D49.2
ear (external)	C47.0	C79.89	—	D36.11	D48.2	D49.2
elbow	C47.1-	C79.89	—	D36.12	D48.2	D49.2
extrarectal	C47.5	C79.89	—	D36.16	D48.2	D49.2
extremity	C47.9	C79.89	—	D36.10	D48.2	D49.2
lower	C47.2-	C79.89	—	D36.13	D48.2	D49.2
upper	C47.1-	C79.89	—	D36.12	D48.2	D49.2
eyelid	C47.0	C79.89	—	D36.11	D48.2	D49.2
face	C47.0	C79.89	—	D36.11	D48.2	D49.2
finger	C47.1-	C79.89	—	D36.12	D48.2	D49.2
flank	C47.6	C79.89	—	D36.17	D48.2	D49.2
foot	C47.2-	C79.89	—	D36.13	D48.2	D49.2
forearm	C47.1-	C79.89	—	D36.12	D48.2	D49.2
forehead	C47.0	C79.89	—	D36.11	D48.2	D49.2
gluteal region	C47.5	C79.89	—	D36.16	D48.2	D49.2
groin	C47.5	C79.89	—	D36.16	D48.2	D49.2
hand	C47.1-	C79.89	—	D36.12	D48.2	D49.2
head	C47.0	C79.89	—	D36.11	D48.2	D49.2
heel	C47.2-	C79.89	—	D36.13	D48.2	D49.2
hip	C47.2-	C79.89	—	D36.13	D48.2	D49.2
infraclavicular region	C47.3	C79.89	—	D36.14	D48.2	D49.2
inguinal (canal) (region)	C47.5	C79.89	—	D36.16	D48.2	D49.2
intrathoracic	C47.3	C79.89	—	D36.14	D48.2	D49.2
ischiorectal fossa	C47.5	C79.89	—	D36.16	D48.2	D49.2
knee	C47.2-	C79.89	—	D36.13	D48.2	D49.2
leg	C47.2-	C79.89	—	D36.13	D48.2	D49.2
limb NEC	C47.9	C79.89	—	D36.10	D48.2	D49.2
lower	C47.2	C79.89	—	D36.13	D48.2	D49.2
upper	C47.1	C79.89	—	D36.12	D48.2	D49.2
nates	C47.5	C79.89	—	D36.16	D48.2	D49.2
neck	C47.0	C79.89	—	D36.11	D48.2	D49.2
orbit	C69.6-	C79.49	—	D31.6-	D48.7	D49.2
pararectal	C47.5	C79.89	—	D36.16	D48.2	D49.2
paraurethral	C47.5	C79.89	—	D36.16	D48.2	D49.2
paravaginal	C47.5	C79.89	—	D36.16	D48.2	D49.2
pelvis (floor)	C47.5	C79.89	—	D36.16	D48.2	D49.2
pelvoabdominal	C47.8	C79.89	—	D36.17	D48.2	D49.2
perineum	C47.5	C79.89	—	D36.16	D48.2	D49.2
perirectal (tissue)	C47.5	C79.89	—	D36.16	D48.2	D49.2
periurethral (tissue)	C47.5	C79.89	—	D36.16	D48.2	D49.2
popliteal fossa or space	C47.2-	C79.89	—	D36.13	D48.2	D49.2
presacral	C47.5	C79.89	—	D36.16	D48.2	D49.2
pterygoid fossa	C47.0	C79.89	—	D36.11	D48.2	D49.2
rectovaginal septum or wall	C47.5	C79.89	—	D36.16	D48.2	D49.2
rectovesical	C47.5	C79.89	—	D36.16	D48.2	D49.2
sacrococcygeal region	C47.5	C79.89	—	D36.16	D48.2	D49.2
scalp	C47.0	C79.89	—	D36.11	D48.2	D49.2
scapular region	C47.3	C79.89	—	D36.14	D48.2	D49.2
shoulder	C47.1-	C79.89	—	D36.12	D48.2	D49.2
submental	C47.0	C79.89	—	D36.11	D48.2	D49.2
supraclavicular region	C47.0	C79.89	—	D36.11	D48.2	D49.2
temple	C47.0	C79.89	—	D36.11	D48.2	D49.2
temporal region	C47.0	C79.89	—	D36.11	D48.2	D49.2
thigh	C47.2-	C79.89	—	D36.13	D48.2	D49.2
thoracic (duct) (wall)	C47.3	C79.89	—	D36.14	D48.2	D49.2
thorax	C47.3	C79.89	—	D36.14	D48.2	D49.2
thumb	C47.1-	C79.89	—	D36.12	D48.2	D49.2
toe	C47.2-	C79.89	—	D36.13	D48.2	D49.2
trunk	C47.6	C79.89	—	D36.17	D48.2	D49.2
umbilicus	C47.4	C79.89	—	D36.15	D48.2	D49.2
vesicorectal	C47.5	C79.89	—	D36.16	D48.2	D49.2
wrist	C47.1-	C79.89	—	D36.12	D48.2	D49.2
radial	C47.1-	C79.89	—	D36.12	D48.2	D49.2
sacral	C47.5	C79.89	—	D36.16	D48.2	D49.2
sciatic	C47.2-	C79.89	—	D36.13	D48.2	D49.2
spinal NEC	C47.9	C79.89	—	D36.10	D48.2	D49.2
accessory	C72.59	C79.49	—	D33.3	D43.3	D49.7
sympathetic NEC — *see also* Neoplasm, nerve, peripheral	C47.9	C79.89	—	D36.10	D48.2	D49.2
trigeminal	C72.59	C79.49	—	D33.3	D43.3	D49.7
trochlear	C72.59	C79.49	—	D33.3	D43.3	D49.7
ulnar	C47.1-	C79.89	—	D36.12	D48.2	D49.2
vagus	C72.59	C79.49	—	D33.3	D43.3	D49.7
Neoplasm, neoplastic - *continued*						
nervous system (central)	C72.9	C79.40	—	D33.9	D43.9	D49.7
autonomic — *see* Neoplasm, nerve, peripheral						
parasympathetic — *see* Neoplasm, nerve, peripheral						
specified site NEC	—	C79.49	—	D33.7	D43.8	—
sympathetic — *see* Neoplasm, nerve, peripheral						
nevus — *see* Nevus						
nipple	C50.0-	C79.81	D05.-	D24.-	—	D49.89
nose, nasal	C76.0	C79.89	D09.8	D36.7	D48.7	D49.89
ala (external) (nasi) — *see also* Neoplasm, nose, skin						
skin	C44.301	C79.2	D04.39	D23.39	D48.5	D49.2
bone	C41.0	C79.51	—	D16.4-	D48.0	D49.2
cartilage	C30.0	C78.39	D02.3	D14.0	D38.5	D49.1
cavity	C30.0	C78.39	D02.3	D14.0	D38.5	D49.1
choana	C11.3	C79.89	D00.08	D10.6	D37.05	D49.0
external (skin) — *see also* Neoplasm, nose, skin	C44.301	C79.2	D04.39	D23.39	D48.5	D49.2
fossa	C30.0	C78.39	D02.3	D14.0	D38.5	D49.1
internal	C30.0	C78.39	D02.3	D14.0	D38.5	D49.1
mucosa	C30.0	C78.39	D02.3	D14.0	D38.5	D49.1
septum	C30.0	C78.39	D02.3	D14.0	D38.5	D49.1
posterior margin	C11.3	C79.89	D00.08	D10.6	D37.05	D49.0
sinus — *see* Neoplasm, sinus						
skin	C44.301	C79.2	D04.39	D23.39	D48.5	D49.2
basal cell carcinoma	C44.311	—	—	—	—	—
specified type NEC	C44.391	—	—	—	—	—
squamous cell carcinoma	C44.321	—	—	—	—	—
turbinate (mucosa)	C30.0	C78.39	D02.3	D14.0	D38.5	D49.1
bone	C41.0	C79.51	—	D16.4-	D48.0	D49.2
vestibule	C30.0	C78.39	D02.3	D14.0	D38.5	D49.1
nostril	C30.0	C78.39	D02.3	D14.0	D38.5	D49.1
nucleus pulposus	C41.2	C79.51	—	D16.6	D48.0	D49.2
occipital						
bone	C41.0	C79.51	—	D16.4-	D48.0	D49.2
lobe or pole, brain	C71.4	C79.31	—	D33.0	D43.0	D49.6
odontogenic — *see* Neoplasm, jaw bone						
olfactory nerve or bulb	C72.2-	C79.49	—	D33.3	D43.3	D49.7
olive (brain)	C71.7	C79.31	—	D33.1	D43.1	D49.6
omentum	C48.1	C78.6	—	D20.1	D48.4	D49.0
operculum (brain)	C71.0	C79.31	—	D33.0	D43.0	D49.6
optic nerve, chiasm, or tract	C72.3-	C79.49	—	D33.3	D43.3	D49.7
oral (cavity)	C06.9	C79.89	D00.00	D10.30	D37.09	D49.0
ill-defined	C14.8	C79.89	D00.00	D10.30	D37.09	D49.0
mucosa	C06.0	C79.89	D00.02	D10.39	D37.09	D49.0
orbit	C69.6-	C79.49	D09.2-	D31.6-	D48.7	D49.89
autonomic nerve	C69.6-	C79.49	—	D31.6-	D48.7	D49.2
bone	C41.0	C79.51	—	D16.4-	D48.0	D49.2
eye	C69.6-	C79.49	D09.2-	D31.6-	D48.7	D49.89
peripheral nerves	C69.6-	C79.49	—	D31.6-	D48.7	D49.2
soft parts	C69.6-	C79.49	D09.2-	D31.6-	D48.7	D49.89
organ of Zuckerkandl	C75.5	C79.89	—	D35.6	D44.7	D49.7
oropharynx	C10.9	C79.89	D00.08	D10.5	D37.05	D49.0
branchial cleft (vestige)	C10.4	C79.89	D00.08	D10.5	D37.05	D49.0
junctional region	C10.8	C79.89	D00.08	D10.5	D37.05	D49.0
lateral wall	C10.2	C79.89	D00.08	D10.5	D37.05	D49.0
overlapping lesion	C10.8	—	—	—	—	—
pillars or fauces	C09.1	C79.89	D00.08	D10.5	D37.05	D49.0
posterior wall	C10.3	C79.89	D00.08	D10.5	D37.05	D49.0
vallecula	C10.0	C79.89	D00.08	D10.5	D37.05	D49.0
os						
external	C53.1	C79.82	D06.1	D26.0	D39.0	D49.5
internal	C53.0	C79.82	D06.0	D26.0	D39.0	D49.5
ovary	C56.-	C79.6-	D07.39	D27.-	D39.1-	D49.5
oviduct	C57.0-	C79.82	D07.39	D28.2	D39.8	D49.5
palate	C05.9	C79.89	D00.00	D10.39	D37.09	D49.0
hard	C05.0	C79.89	D00.05	D10.39	D37.09	D49.0
junction of hard and soft palate	C05.9	C79.89	D00.00	D10.39	D37.09	D49.0
overlapping lesions	C05.8	—				
soft	C05.1	C79.89	D00.04	D10.39	D37.09	D49.0
nasopharyngeal surface	C11.3	C79.89	D00.08	D10.6	D37.05	D49.0
posterior surface	C11.3	C79.89	D00.08	D10.6	D37.05	D49.0
superior surface	C11.3	C79.89	D00.08	D10.6	D37.05	D49.0

NEOPLASM TABLE

Neoplasm Table	Malignant Primary	Malignant Secondary	Ca In situ	Benign	Uncertain Behavior	Unspecified Behavior
Neoplasm, neoplastic - *continued*						
palatoglossal arch	C09.1	C79.89	D00.00	D10.5	D37.09	D49.0
palatopharyngeal arch	C09.1	C79.89	D00.00	D10.5	D37.09	D49.0
pallium	C71.0	C79.31	—	D43.0	D49.6	
palpebra	C44.10-	C79.2	D04.1-	D23.1-	D48.5	D49.2
basal cell carcinoma	C44.11-	—	—	—	—	—
specified type NEC	C44.19-	—	—	—	—	—
squamous cell carcinoma	C44.12-	—	—	—	—	—
pancreas	C25.9	C78.89	D01.7	D13.6	D37.8	D49.0
body	C25.1	C78.89	D01.7	D13.6	D37.8	D49.0
duct (of Santorini) (of Wirsung)	C25.3	C78.89	D01.7	D13.6	D37.8	D49.0
ectopic tissue	C25.7			D13.6	D37.8	D49.0
head	C25.0	C78.89	D01.7	D13.6	D37.8	D49.0
islet cells	C25.4	C78.89	D01.7	D13.7	D37.8	D49.0
neck	C25.7	C78.89	D01.7	D13.6	D37.8	D49.0
overlapping lesion	C25.8					
tail	C25.2	C78.89	D01.7	D13.6	D37.8	D49.0
para-aortic body	C75.5	C79.89	—	D35.6	D44.7	D49.7
paraganglion NEC	C75.5	C79.89	—	D35.6	D44.7	D49.7
parametrium	C57.3	C79.82	—	D28.2	D39.8	D49.5
paranephric	C48.0	C78.6	—	D20.0	D48.3	D49.0
pararectal	C76.3		—	D36.7	D48.7	D49.89
parasagittal (region)	C76.0	C79.89	D09.8	D36.9	D48.7	D49.89
parasellar	C72.9	C79.49	—	D33.9	D43.2	D49.7
parathyroid (gland)	C75.0	C79.89	D09.3	D35.1	D44.2	D49.7
paraurethral	C76.3	C79.89		D36.7	D48.7	D49.89
gland	C68.1	C79.19	D09.19	D30.8	D41.8	D49.5
paravaginal	C76.3	C79.89		D36.7	D48.7	D49.89
parenchyma, kidney	C64.-	C79.0-	D09.19	D30.0-	D41.0-	D49.5
parietal						
bone	C41.0	C79.51	—	D16.4-	D48.0	D49.2
lobe, brain	C71.3	C79.31	—	D33.0	D43.0	D49.6
paroophoron	C57.1	C79.82	D07.39	D28.2	D39.8	D49.5
parotid (duct) (gland)	C07	C79.89	D00.00	D11.0	D37.030	D49.0
parovarium	C57.1	C79.82	D07.39	D28.2	D39.8	D49.5
patella	C40.20	C79.51	—	D16.-	—	—
peduncle, cerebral	C71.7	C79.31	—	D33.1	D43.1	D49.6
pelvirectal junction	C19	C78.5	D01.1	D12.7	D37.5	D49.0
pelvis, pelvic	C76.3	C79.89	D09.8	D36.7	D48.7	D49.89
bone	C41.4	C79.51	—	D16.8	D48.0	D49.2
floor	C76.3	C79.89	D09.8	D36.7	D48.7	D49.89
renal	C65.-	C79.0-	D09.19	D30.1-	D41.1-	D49.5
viscera	C76.3	C79.89	D09.8	D36.7	D48.7	D49.89
wall	C76.3	C79.89	D09.8	D36.7	D48.7	D49.89
pelvo-abdominal	C76.8	C79.89	D09.8	D36.7	D48.7	D49.89
penis	C60.9	C79.82	D07.4	D29.0	D40.8	D49.5
body	C60.2	C79.82	D07.4	D29.0	D40.8	D49.5
corpus (cavernosum)	C60.2	C79.82	D07.4	D29.0	D40.8	D49.5
glans	C60.1	C79.82	D07.4	D29.0	D40.8	D49.5
overlapping sites	C60.8	—	—	—	—	—
skin NEC	C60.9	C79.82	D07.4	D29.0	D40.8	D49.5
periadrenal (tissue)	C48.0	C78.6	—	D20.0	D48.3	D49.0
perianal (skin) — *see also* Neoplasm, anus, skin	C44.500	C79.2	D04.5	D23.5	D48.5	D49.2
pericardium	C38.0	C79.89		D15.1	D48.7	D49.89
perinephric	C48.0	C78.6	—	D20.0	D48.3	D49.0
perineum	C76.3	C79.89	D09.8	D36.7	D48.7	D49.89
periodontal tissue NEC	C03.9	C79.89	D00.03	D10.39	D37.09	D49.0
periosteum — *see* Neoplasm, bone						
peripancreatic	C48.0	C78.6	—	D20.0	D48.3	D49.0
peripheral nerve NEC	C47.9	C79.89	—	D36.10	D48.2	D49.2
perirectal (tissue)	C76.3	C79.89	—	D36.7	D48.7	D49.89
perirenal (tissue)	C48.0	C78.6	—	D20.0	D48.3	D49.0
peritoneum, peritoneal (cavity)	C48.2	C78.6		D20.1	D48.4	D49.0
benign mesothelial tissue — *see* Mesothelioma, benign						
overlapping lesion	C48.8	—		—	—	—
with digestive organs	C26.9					
parietal	C48.1	C78.6	—	D20.1	D48.4	D49.0
pelvic	C48.1	C78.6	—	D20.1	D48.4	D49.0
specified part NEC	C48.1	C78.6	—	D20.1	D48.4	D49.0
peritonsillar (tissue)	C76.0	C79.89	D09.8	D36.7	D48.7	D49.89
periurethral tissue	C76.3	C79.89		D36.7	D48.7	D49.89
phalanges						
foot	C40.3-	C79.51	—	D16.3-	—	—
hand	C40.1-	C79.51	—	D16.1-	—	—
pharynx, pharyngeal	C14.0	C79.89	D00.08	D10.9	D37.05	D49.0
bursa	C11.1	C79.89	D00.08	D10.6	D37.05	D49.0
fornix	C11.3	C79.89	D00.08	D10.6	D37.05	D49.0
recess	C11.2	C79.89	D00.08	D10.6	D37.05	D49.0
region	C14.0	C79.89	D00.08	D10.9	D37.05	D49.0
tonsil	C11.1	C79.89	D00.08	D10.6	D37.05	D49.0
wall (lateral) (posterior)	C14.0	C79.89	D00.08	D10.9	D37.05	D49.0
Neoplasm, neoplastic - *continued*						
pia mater	C70.9	C79.40	—	D32.9	D42.9	D49.7
cerebral	C70.0	C79.32	—	D32.0	D42.0	D49.7
cranial	C70.0	C79.32	—	D32.0	D42.0	D49.7
spinal	C70.1	C79.49	—	D32.1	D42.1	D49.7
pillars of fauces	C09.1	C79.89	D00.08	D10.5	D37.05	D49.0
pineal (body) (gland)	C75.3	C79.89	D09.3	D35.4	D44.5	D49.7
pinna (ear) NEC — *see also* Neoplasm, skin, ear	C44.20-	C79.2	D04.2-	D23.2-	D48.5	D49.2
piriform fossa or sinus	C12	C79.89	D00.08	D10.7	D37.05	D49.0
pituitary (body) (fossa) (gland) (lobe)	C75.1	C79.89	D09.3	D35.2	D44.3	D49.7
placenta	C58	C79.82	D07.0	D26.7	D39.2	D49.5
pleura, pleural (cavity)	C38.4	C78.2	—	D19.0	D38.2	D49.1
overlapping lesion with heart or mediastinum	C38.8					
parietal	C38.4	C78.2	—	D19.0	D38.2	D49.1
visceral	C38.4	C78.2	—	D19.0	D38.2	D49.1
plexus						
brachial	C47.1-	C79.89	—	D36.12	D48.2	D49.2
cervical	C47.0	C79.89	—	D36.11	D48.2	D49.2
choroid	C71.5	C79.31	—	D33.0	D43.0	D49.6
lumbosacral	C47.5	C79.89	—	D36.16	D48.2	D49.2
sacral	C47.5	C79.89	—	D36.16	D48.2	D49.2
pluriendocrine	C75.8	C79.89	D09.3	D35.7	D44.9	D49.7
pole						
frontal	C71.1	C79.31	—	D33.0	D43.0	D49.6
occipital	C71.4	C79.31	—	D33.0	D43.0	D49.6
pons (varolii)	C71.7	C79.31	—	D33.1	D43.1	D49.6
popliteal fossa or space	C76.5-	C79.89	D04.7-	D36.7	D48.7	D49.89
postcricoid (region)	C13.0	C79.89	D00.08	D10.7	D37.05	D49.0
posterior fossa (cranial)	C71.9	C79.31	—	D33.2	D43.2	D49.6
postnasal space	C11.9	C79.89	D00.08	D10.6	D37.05	D49.0
prepuce	C60.0	C79.82	D07.4	D29.0	D40.8	D49.5
prepylorus	C16.4	C78.89	D00.2	D13.1	D37.1	D49.0
presacral (region)	C76.3	C79.89		D36.7	D48.7	D49.89
prostate (gland)	C61	C79.82	D07.5	D29.1	D40.0	D49.5
utricle	C68.0	C79.19	D09.19	D30.4	D41.3	D49.5
pterygoid fossa	C49.0	C79.89		D21.0	D48.1	D49.2
pubic bone	C41.4	C79.51	—	D16.8	D48.0	D49.2
pudenda, pudendum (female)	C51.9	C79.82	D07.1	D28.0	D39.8	D49.5
pulmonary — *see also* Neoplasm, lung	C34.9-	C78.0-	D02.2-	D14.3-	D38.1	D49.1
putamen	C71.0	C79.31	—	D33.0	D43.0	D49.6
pyloric						
antrum	C16.3	C78.89	D00.2	D13.1	D37.1	D49.0
canal	C16.4	C78.89	D00.2	D13.1	D37.1	D49.0
pylorus	C16.4	C78.89	D00.2	D13.1	D37.1	D49.0
pyramid (brain)	C71.7	C79.31	—	D33.1	D43.1	D49.6
pyriform fossa or sinus	C12	C79.89	D00.08	D10.7	D37.05	D49.0
radius (any part)	C40.0-	C79.51	—	D16.0-	—	—
Rathke's pouch	C75.1	C79.89	D09.3	D35.2	D44.3	D49.7
rectosigmoid (junction)	C19	C78.5	D01.1	D12.7	D37.5	D49.0
overlapping lesion with anus or rectum	C21.8					
rectouterine pouch	C48.1	C78.6	—	D20.1	D48.4	D49.0
rectovaginal septum or wall	C76.3	C79.89	D09.8	D36.7	D48.7	D49.89
rectovesical septum	C76.3	C79.89	D09.8	D36.7	D48.7	D49.89
rectum (ampulla)	C20	C78.5	D01.2	D12.8	D37.5	D49.0
and colon	C19	C78.5	D01.1	D12.7	D37.5	D49.0
overlapping lesion with anus or rectosigmoid junction	C21.8					
renal	C64.-	C79.0-	D09.19	D30.0-	D41.0-	D49.5
calyx	C65.-	C79.0-	D09.19	D30.1-	D41.1-	D49.5
hilus	C65.-	C79.0-	D09.19	D30.1-	D41.1-	D49.5
parenchyma	C64.-	C79.0-	D09.19	D30.0-	D41.0-	D49.5
pelvis	C65.-	C79.0-	D09.19	D30.1-	D41.1-	D49.5
respiratory						
organs or system NEC	C39.9	C78.30	D02.4	D14.4	D38.6	D49.1
tract NEC	C39.9	C78.30	D02.4	D14.4	D38.5	D49.1
upper	C39.0	C78.30	D02.4	D14.4	D38.5	D49.1
retina	C69.2-	C79.49	D09.2-	D31.2-	D48.7	D49.81
retrobulbar	C69.6-	C79.49	—	D31.6-	D48.7	D49.89
retrocecal	C48.0	C78.6	—	D20.0	D48.3	D49.0
retromolar (area) (triangle) (trigone)	C06.2	C79.89	D00.00	D10.39	D37.09	D49.0
retro-orbital	C76.0	C79.89	D09.8	D36.7	D48.7	D49.89
retroperitoneal (space) (tissue)	C48.0	C78.6	—	D20.0	D48.3	D49.0
retroperitoneum	C48.0	C78.6	—	D20.0	D48.3	D49.0
retropharyngeal	C14.0	C79.89	D00.08	D10.9	D37.05	D49.0
retrovesical (septum)	C76.3	C79.89	D09.8	D36.7	D48.7	D49.89
rhinencephalon	C71.0	C79.31	—	D33.0	D43.0	D49.6
rib	C41.3	C79.51	—	D16.7	D48.0	D49.2
Rosenmüller's fossa	C11.2	C79.89	D00.08	D10.6	D37.05	D49.0
round ligament	C57.2	C79.82	—	D28.2	D39.8	D49.5

NEOPLASM TABLE

Neoplasm Table	Malignant Primary	Malignant Secondary	Ca In situ	Benign	Uncertain Behavior	Unspecified Behavior
Neoplasm, neoplastic - *continued*						
sacrococcyx, sacrococcygeal ..	C41.4	C79.51	—	D16.8	D48.0	D49.2
region	C76.3	C79.89	D09.8	D36.7	D48.7	D49.89
sacrouterine ligament	C57.3	C79.82	—	D28.2	D39.8	D49.5
sacrum, sacral (vertebra)	C41.4	C79.51	—	D16.8	D48.0	D49.2
salivary gland or duct (major)	C08.9	C79.89	D00.00	D11.9	D37.039	D49.0
minor NEC	C06.9	C79.89	D00.00	D10.39	D37.04	D49.0
overlapping lesion	C08.9					
parotid	C07	C79.89	D00.00	D11.0	D37.030	D49.0
pluriglandular	C08.9	C79.89	D00.00	D11.9	D37.039	D49.0
sublingual	C08.1	C79.89	D00.00	D11.7	D37.031	D49.0
submandibular	C08.0	C79.89	D00.00	D11.7	D37.032	D49.0
submaxillary	C08.0	C79.89	D00.00	D11.7	D37.032	D49.0
salpinx (uterine)	C57.0-	C79.82	D07.39	D28.2	D39.8	D49.5
Santorini's duct	C25.3	C78.89	D01.7	D13.6	D37.8	D49.0
scalp	C44.40	C79.2	D04.4	D23.4	D48.5	D49.2
basal cell carcinoma	C44.41	—	—	—	—	—
specified type NEC	C44.49	—	—	—	—	—
squamous cell carcinoma ...	C44.42	—	—	—	—	—
scapula (any part)	C40.0-	C79.51	—	D16.0-	—	—
scapular region	C76.1	C79.89	D09.8	D36.7	D48.7	D49.89
scar NEC — *see also* Neoplasm, skin, by site ..	C44.90	C79.2	D04.9	D23.9	D48.5	D49.2
sciatic nerve	C47.2-	C79.89	—	D36.13	D48.2	D49.2
sclera	C69.4-	C79.49	D09.2-	D31.4-	D48.7	D49.89
scrotum (skin)	C63.2	C79.82	D07.61	D29.4	D40.8	D49.5
sebaceous gland — *see* Neoplasm, skin						
sella turcica	C75.1	C79.89	D09.3	D35.2	D44.3	D49.7
bone	C41.0	C79.51	—	D16.4-	D48.0	D49.2
semilunar cartilage (knee)	C40.2-	C79.51	—	D16.2-	D48.0	D49.2
seminal vesicle	C63.7	C79.82	D07.69	D29.8	D40.8	D49.5
septum						
nasal	C30.0	C78.39	D02.3	D14.0	D38.5	D49.1
posterior margin	C11.3	C79.89	D00.08	D10.6	D37.05	D49.0
rectovaginal	C76.3	C79.89	D09.8	D36.7	D48.7	D49.89
rectovesical	C76.3	C79.89	D09.8	D36.7	D48.7	D49.89
urethrovaginal	C57.9	C79.82	D07.30	D28.9	D39.9	D49.5
vesicovaginal	C57.9	C79.82	D07.30	D28.9	D39.9	D49.5
shoulder NEC	C76.4-	C79.89	D04.6-	D36.7	D48.7	D49.89
sigmoid flexure (lower) (upper)	C18.7	C78.5	D01.0	D12.5	D37.4	D49.0
sinus (accessory)	C31.9	C78.39	D02.3	D14.0	D38.5	D49.1
bone (any)	C41.0	C79.51	—	D16.4-	D48.0	D49.2
ethmoidal	C31.1	C78.39	D02.3	D14.0	D38.5	D49.1
frontal	C31.2	C78.39	D02.3	D14.0	D38.5	D49.1
maxillary	C31.0	C78.39	D02.3	D14.0	D38.5	D49.1
nasal, paranasal NEC	C31.9	C78.39	D02.3	D14.0	D38.5	D49.1
overlapping lesion	C31.8					
pyriform	C12	C79.89	D00.08	D10.7	D37.05	D49.0
sphenoid	C31.3	C78.39	D02.3	D14.0	D38.5	D49.1
skeleton, skeletal NEC	C41.9	C79.51	—	D16.9-	D48.0	D49.2
Skene's gland	C68.1	C79.19	D09.19	D30.8	D41.8	D49.5
skin NOS	C44.90	C79.2	D04.9	D23.9	D48.5	D49.2
abdominal wall	C44.509	C79.2	D04.5	D23.5	D48.5	D49.2
basal cell carcinoma	C44.519	—	—	—	—	—
specified type NEC	C44.599	—	—	—	—	—
squamous cell carcinoma	C44.529	—	—	—	—	—
ala nasi — *see also* Neoplasm, nose, skin ..	C44.301	C79.2	D04.39	D23.39	D48.5	D49.2
ankle — *see also* Neoplasm, skin, limb, lower	C44.70-	C79.2	D04.7-	D23.7-	D48.5	D49.2
antecubital space — *see also* Neoplasm, skin, limb, upper	C44.60-	C79.2	D04.6-	D23.6-	D48.5	D49.2
anus	C44.500	C79.2	D04.5	D23.5	D48.5	D49.2
basal cell carcinoma	C44.510	—	—	—	—	—
specified type NEC	C44.590	—	—	—	—	—
squamous cell carcinoma	C44.520	—	—	—	—	—
arm — *see also* Neoplasm, skin, limb, upper	C44.60-	C79.2	D04.6-	D23.6-	D48.5	D49.2
auditory canal (external) — *see also* Neoplasm, skin, ear	C44.20-	C79.2	D04.2-	D23.2-	D48.5	D49.2
auricle (ear) — *see also* Neoplasm, skin, ear	C44.20-	C79.2	D04.2-	D23.2-	D48.5	D49.2
auricular canal (external) — *see also* Neoplasm, skin, ear	C44.20-	C79.2	D04.2-	D23.2-	D48.5	D49.2
axilla, axillary fold — *see also* Neoplasm, skin, trunk	C44.509	C79.2	D04.5	D23.5	D48.5	D49.2
back — *see also* Neoplasm, skin, trunk	C44.509	C79.2	D04.5	D23.5	D48.5	D49.2
basal cell carcinoma	C44.91	—	—	—	—	—
breast	C44.501	C79.2	D04.5	D23.5	D48.5	D49.2
basal cell carcinoma	C44.511	—	—	—	—	—
specified type NEC	C44.591	—	—	—	—	—
squamous cell carcinoma	C44.521	—	—	—	—	—
Neoplasm, neoplastic - *continued*						
skin NOS - *continued*	C44.90	C79.2	D04.9	D23.9	D48.5	D49.2
brow — *see also* Neoplasm, skin, face ..	C44.309	C79.2	D04.39	D23.39	D48.5	D49.2
buttock — *see also* Neoplasm, skin, trunk	C44.509	C79.2	D04.5	D23.5	D48.5	D49.2
calf — *see also* Neoplasm, skin, limb, lower	C44.70-	C79.2	D04.7-	D23.7-	D48.5	D49.2
canthus (eye) (inner) (outer)	C44.10-	C79.2	D04.1-	D23.1-	D48.5	D49.2
basal cell carcinoma	C44.11-	—	—	—	—	—
specified type NEC	C44.19-	—	—	—	—	—
squamous cell carcinoma	C44.12-	—	—	—	—	—
cervical region — *see also* Neoplasm, skin, neck ..	C44.40	C79.2	D04.4	D23.4	D48.5	D49.2
cheek (external) — *see also* Neoplasm, skin, face ..	C44.309	C79.2	D04.39	D23.39	D48.5	D49.2
chest (wall) — *see also* Neoplasm, trunk	C44.509	C79.2	D04.5	D23.5	D48.5	D49.2
chin — *see also* Neoplasm, skin, face	C44.309	C79.2	D04.39	D23.39	D48.5	D49.2
clavicular area — *see also* Neoplasm, skin, trunk	C44.509	C79.2	D04.5	D23.5	D48.5	D49.2
clitoris	C51.2	C79.82	D07.1	D28.0	D39.8	D49.5
columnella — *see also* Neoplasm, skin, face ..	C44.309	C79.2	D04.39	D23.39	D48.5	D49.2
concha — *see also* Neoplasm, skin, ear	C44.20-	C79.2	D04.2-	D23.2-	D48.5	D49.2
ear (external)	C44.20-	C79.2	D04.2-	D23.2-	D48.5	D49.2
basal cell carcinoma	C44.21-	—	—	—	—	—
specified type NEC	C44.29-	—	—	—	—	—
squamous cell carcinoma	C44.22-	—	—	—	—	—
elbow — *see also* Neoplasm, skin, limb, upper	C44.60-	C79.2	D04.6-	D23.6-	D48.5	D49.2
eyebrow — *see also* Neoplasm, skin, face ..	C44.309	C79.2	D04.39	D23.39	D48.5	D49.2
eyelid	C44.10-	C79.2	D04.1-	D23.1-	D48.5	D49.2
basal cell carcinoma	C44.11-	—	—	—	—	—
specified type NEC	C44.19-	—	—	—	—	—
squamous cell carcinoma	C44.12-	—	—	—	—	—
face NOS	C44.300	C79.2	D04.30	D23.30	D48.5	D49.2
basal cell carcinoma	C44.310	—	—	—	—	—
specified type NEC	C44.390	—	—	—	—	—
squamous cell carcinoma	C44.320	—	—	—	—	—
female genital organs (external)	C51.9	C79.82	D07.1	D28.0	D39.8	D49.5
clitoris	C51.2	C79.82	D07.1	D28.0	D39.8	D49.5
labium NEC	C51.9	C79.82	D07.1	D28.0	D39.8	D49.5
majus	C51.0	C79.82	D07.1	D28.0	D39.8	D49.5
minus	C51.1	C79.82	D07.1	D28.0	D39.8	D49.5
pudendum	C51.9	C79.82	D07.1	D28.0	D39.8	D49.5
vulva	C51.9	C79.82	D07.1	D28.0	D39.8	D49.5
finger — *see also* Neoplasm, skin, limb, upper	C44.60-	C79.2	D04.6-	D23.6-	D48.5	D49.2
flank — *see also* Neoplasm, skin, trunk	C44.509	C79.2	D04.5	D23.5	D48.5	D49.2
foot — *see also* Neoplasm, skin, limb, lower	C44.70-	C79.2	D04.7-	D23.7-	D48.5	D49.2
forearm — *see also* Neoplasm, skin, limb, upper	C44.60-	C79.2	D04.6-	D23.6-	D48.5	D49.2
forehead — *see also* Neoplasm, skin, face ..	C44.309	C79.2	D04.39	D23.39	D48.5	D49.2
glabella — *see also* Neoplasm, skin, face ..	C44.309	C79.2	D04.39	D23.39	D48.5	D49.2
gluteal region — *see also* Neoplasm, skin, trunk	C44.509	C79.2	D04.5	D23.5	D48.5	D49.2
groin — *see also* Neoplasm, skin, trunk	C44.509	C79.2	D04.5	D23.5	D48.5	D49.2
hand — *see also* Neoplasm, skin, limb, upper	C44.60-	C79.2	D04.6-	D23.6-	D48.5	D49.2
head NEC — *see also* Neoplasm, skin, scalp	C44.40	C79.2	D04.4	D23.4	D48.5	D49.2
heel — *see also* Neoplasm, skin, limb, lower	C44.70-	C79.2	D04.7-	D23.7-	D48.5	D49.2
helix — *see also* Neoplasm, skin, ear	C44.20-	C79.2	D04.2-	D23.2-	D48.5	D49.2
hip — *see also* Neoplasm, skin, limb, lower	C44.70-	C79.2	D04.7-	D23.7-	D48.5	D49.2
infraclavicular region — *see also* Neoplasm, skin, trunk	C44.509	C79.2	D04.5	D23.5	D48.5	D49.2
inguinal region — *see also* Neoplasm, skin, trunk	C44.509	C79.2	D04.5	D23.5	D48.5	D49.2
jaw — *see also* Neoplasm, skin, face ..	C44.309	C79.2	D04.39	D23.39	D48.5	D49.2

NEOPLASM TABLE

Neoplasm Table	Malignant Primary	Malignant Secondary	Ca In situ	Benign	Uncertain Behavior	Unspecified Behavior
Neoplasm, neoplastic - *continued*						
skin NOS - *continued*	C44.90	C79.2	D04.9	D23.9	D48.5	D49.2
Kaposi's sarcoma — *see* Kaposi's, sarcoma, skin						
knee — *see also* Neoplasm, skin, limb, lower	C44.70-	C79.2	D04.7-	D23.7-	D48.5	D49.2
labia						
majora	C51.0	C79.82	D07.1	D28.0	D39.8	D49.5
minora	C51.1	C79.82	D07.1	D28.0	D39.8	D49.5
leg — *see also* Neoplasm, skin, limb, lower	C44.70-	C79.2	D04.7-	D23.7-	D48.5	D49.2
lid (lower) (upper)	C44.10-	C79.2	D04.1-	D23.1-	D48.5	D49.2
basal cell carcinoma	C44.11-	—	—	—	—	—
specified type NEC	C44.19-	—	—	—	—	—
squamous cell carcinoma	C44.12-	—	—	—	—	—
limb NEC	C44.90	C79.2	D04.9	D23.9	D48.5	D49.2
basal cell carcinoma	C44.91	—	—	—	—	—
lower	C44.70-	C79.2	D04.7-	D23.7-	D48.5	D49.2
basal cell carcinoma	C44.71-	—	—	—	—	—
specified type NEC	C44.79-	—	—	—	—	—
squamous cell carcinoma	C44.72-	—	—	—	—	—
upper	C44.60-	C79.2	D04.6-	D23.6-	D48.5	D49.2
basal cell carcinoma	C44.61-	—	—	—	—	—
specified type NEC	C44.69-	—	—	—	—	—
squamous cell carcinoma	C44.62-	—	—	—	—	—
lip (lower) (upper)	C44.00	C79.2	D04.0	D23.0	D48.5	D49.2
basal cell carcinoma	C44.01	—	—	—	—	—
specified type NEC	C44.09	—	—	—	—	—
squamous cell carcinoma	C44.02	—	—	—	—	—
male genital organs	C63.9	C79.82	D07.60	D29.9	D40.8	D49.5
penis	C60.9	C79.82	D07.4	D29.0	D40.8	D49.5
prepuce	C60.0	C79.82	D07.4	D29.0	D40.8	D49.5
scrotum	C63.2	C79.82	D07.61	D29.4	D40.8	D49.5
mastectomy site (skin) — *see also* Neoplasm, skin, breast	C44.501	C79.2				
specified as breast tissue	C50.8-	C79.81				
meatus, acoustic (external) — *see also* Neoplasm, skin, ear	C44.20-	C79.2	D04.2-	D23.2-	D48.5	D49.2
melanotic — *see* Melanoma						
Merkel cell — *see* Carcinoma, Merkel cell						
nates — *see also* Neoplasm, skin, trunk	C44.509	C79.2	D04.5	D23.5	D48.5	D49.2
neck	C44.40	C79.2	D04.4	D23.4	D48.5	D49.2
basal cell carcinoma	C44.41	—	—	—	—	—
specified type NEC	C44.49	—	—	—	—	—
squamous cell carcinoma	C44.42	—	—	—	—	—
nevus — *see* Nevus, skin						
nose (external) — *see also* Neoplasm, nose, skin	C44.301	C79.2	D04.39	D23.39	D48.5	D49.2
overlapping lesion	C44.80	—	—	—	—	—
basal cell carcinoma	C44.81	—	—	—	—	—
specified type NEC	C44.89	—	—	—	—	—
squamous cell carcinoma	C44.82	—	—	—	—	—
palm — *see also* Neoplasm, skin, limb, upper	C44.60-	C79.2	D04.6-	D23.6-	D48.5	D49.2
palpebra	C44.10-	C79.2	D04.1-	D23.1-	D48.5	D49.2
basal cell carcinoma	C44.11-	—	—	—	—	—
specified type NEC	C44.19-	—	—	—	—	—
squamous cell carcinoma	C44.12-	—	—	—	—	—
penis NEC	C60.9	C79.82	D07.4	D29.0	D40.8	D49.5
perianal — *see also* Neoplasm, skin, anus	C44.500	C79.2	D04.5	D23.5	D48.5	D49.2
perineum — *see also* Neoplasm, skin, anus	C44.500	C79.2	D04.5	D23.5	D48.5	D49.2
pinna — *see also* Neoplasm, skin, ear	C44.20-	C79.2	D04.2-	D23.2-	D48.5	D49.2
plantar — *see also* Neoplasm, skin, limb, lower	C44.70-	C79.2	D04.7-	D23.7-	D48.5	D49.2
popliteal fossa or space — *see also* Neoplasm, skin, limb, lower	C44.70-	C79.2	D04.7-	D23.7-	D48.5	D49.2
prepuce	C60.0	C79.82	D07.4	D29.0	D40.8	D49.5
pubes — *see also* Neoplasm, skin, trunk	C44.509	C79.2	D04.5	D23.5	D48.5	D49.2
sacrococcygeal region — *see also* Neoplasm, skin, trunk	C44.509	C79.2	D04.5	D23.5	D48.5	D49.2
scalp	C44.40	C79.2	D04.4	D23.4	D48.5	D49.2
basal cell carcinoma	C44.41	—	—	—	—	—
specified type NEC	C44.49	—	—	—	—	—
squamous cell carcinoma	C44.42	—	—	—	—	—

Neoplasm Table	Malignant Primary	Malignant Secondary	Ca In situ	Benign	Uncertain Behavior	Unspecified Behavior
Neoplasm, neoplastic - *continued*						
skin NOS - *continued*	C44.90	C79.2	D04.9	D23.9	D48.5	D49.2
scapular region — *see also* Neoplasm, skin, trunk	C44.509	C79.2	D04.5	D23.5	D48.5	D49.2
scrotum	C63.2	C79.82	D07.61	D29.4	D40.8	D49.5
shoulder — *see also* Neoplasm, skin, limb, upper	C44.60-	C79.2	D04.6-	D23.6-	D48.5	D49.2
sole (foot) — *see also* Neoplasm, skin, limb, lower	C44.70-	C79.2	D04.7-	D23.7-	D48.5	D49.2
specified sites NEC	C44.80	C79.2	D04.8	D23.9	D48.5	D49.2
basal cell carcinoma	C44.81	—	—	—	—	—
specified type NEC	C44.89	—	—	—	—	—
squamous cell carcinoma	C44.82	—	—	—	—	—
specified type NEC	C44.99	—	—	—	—	—
squamous cell carcinoma	C44.92	—	—	—	—	—
submammary fold — *see also* Neoplasm, skin, trunk	C44.509	C79.2	D04.5	D23.5	D48.5	D49.2
supraclavicular region — *see also* Neoplasm, skin, neck	C44.40	C79.2	D04.4	D23.4	D48.5	D49.2
temple — *see also* Neoplasm, skin, face	C44.309	C79.2	D04.39	D23.39	D48.5	D49.2
thigh — *see also* Neoplasm, skin, limb, lower	C44.70-	C79.2	D04.7-	D23.7-	D48.5	D49.2
thoracic wall — *see also* Neoplasm, skin, trunk	C44.509	C79.2	D04.5	D23.5	D48.5	D49.2
thumb — *see also* Neoplasm, skin, limb, upper	C44.60-	C79.2	D04.6-	D23.6-	D48.5	D49.2
toe — *see also* Neoplasm, skin, limb, lower	C44.70-	C79.2	D04.7-	D23.7-	D48.5	D49.2
tragus — *see also* Neoplasm, skin, ear	C44.20-	C79.2	D04.2-	D23.2-	D48.5	D49.2
trunk	C44.509	C79.2	D04.5	D23.5	D48.5	D49.2
basal cell carcinoma	C44.519	—	—	—	—	—
specified type NEC	C44.599	—	—	—	—	—
squamous cell carcinoma	C44.529	—	—	—	—	—
umbilicus — *see also* Neoplasm, skin, trunk	C44.509	C79.2	D04.5	D23.5	D48.5	D49.2
vulva	C51.9	C79.82	D07.1	D28.0	D39.8	D49.5
overlapping lesion	C51.8	—	—	—	—	—
wrist — *see also* Neoplasm, skin, limb, upper	C44.60-	C79.2	D04.6-	D23.6-	D48.5	D49.2
skull	C41.0	C79.51	—	D16.4-	D48.0	D49.2
soft parts or tissues — *see* Neoplasm, connective tissue						
specified site NEC	C76.8	C79.89	D09.8	D36.7	D48.7	D49.89
spermatic cord	C63.1-	C79.82	D07.69	D29.8	D40.8	D49.5
sphenoid	C31.3	C78.39	D02.3	D14.0	D38.5	D49.1
bone	C41.0	C79.51	—	D16.4-	D48.0	D49.2
sinus	C31.3	C78.39	D02.3	D14.0	D38.5	D49.1
sphincter						
anal	C21.1	C78.5	D01.3	D12.9	D37.8	D49.0
of Oddi	C24.0	C78.89	D01.5	D13.5	D37.6	D49.0
spine, spinal (column)	C41.2	C79.51	—	D16.6	D48.0	D49.2
bulb	C71.7	C79.31	—	D33.1	D43.1	D49.6
coccyx	C41.4	C79.51	—	D16.8	D48.0	D49.2
cord (cervical) (lumbar) (sacral) (thoracic)	C72.0	C79.49	—	D33.4	D43.4	D49.7
dura mater	C70.1	C79.49	—	D32.1	D42.1	D49.7
lumbosacral	C41.2	C79.51	—	D16.6	D48.0	D49.2
marrow NEC	C96.9	C79.52	—	—	D47.9	D49.89
membrane	C70.1	C79.49	—	D32.1	D42.1	D49.7
meninges	C70.1	C79.49	—	D32.1	D42.1	D49.7
nerve (root)	C47.9	C79.89	—	D36.10	D48.2	D49.2
pia mater	C70.1	C79.49	—	D32.1	D42.1	D49.7
root	C47.9	C79.89	—	D36.10	D48.2	D49.2
sacrum	C41.4	C79.51	—	D16.8	D48.0	D49.2
spleen, splenic NEC	C26.1	C78.89	D01.7	D13.9	D37.8	D49.0
flexure (colon)	C18.5	C78.5	D01.0	D12.3	D37.4	D49.0
stem, brain	C71.7	C79.31	—	D33.1	D43.1	D49.6
Stensen's duct	C07	C79.89	D00.00	D11.0	D37.030	D49.0
sternum	C41.3	C79.51	—	D16.7	D48.0	D49.2
stomach	C16.9	C78.89	D00.2	D13.1	D37.1	D49.0
antrum (pyloric)	C16.3	C78.89	D00.2	D13.1	D37.1	D49.0
body	C16.2	C78.89	D00.2	D13.1	D37.1	D49.0
cardia	C16.0	C78.89	D00.2	D13.1	D37.1	D49.0
cardiac orifice	C16.0	C78.89	D00.2	D13.1	D37.1	D49.0
corpus	C16.2	C78.89	D00.2	D13.1	D37.1	D49.0
fundus	C16.1	C78.89	D00.2	D13.1	D37.1	D49.0
greater curvature NEC	C16.6	C78.89	D00.2	D13.1	D37.1	D49.0
lesser curvature NEC	C16.5	C78.89	D00.2	D13.1	D37.1	D49.0
overlapping lesion	C16.8	—	—	—	—	—
prepylorus	C16.4	C78.89	D00.2	D13.1	D37.1	D49.0
pylorus	C16.4	C78.89	D00.2	D13.1	D37.1	D49.0
wall NEC	C16.9	C78.89	D00.2	D13.1	D37.1	D49.0
anterior NEC	C16.8	C78.89	D00.2	D13.1	D37.1	D49.0
posterior NEC	C16.8	C78.89	D00.2	D13.1	D37.1	D49.0

Neoplasm Table	Malignant Primary	Malignant Secondary	Ca In situ	Benign	Uncertain Behavior	Unspecified Behavior
Neoplasm, neoplastic - *continued*						
stroma, endometrial	C54.1	C79.82	D07.0	D26.1	D39.0	D49.5
stump, cervical	C53.8	C79.82	D06.7	D26.0	D39.0	D49.5
subcutaneous (nodule) (tissue) NEC — *see* Neoplasm, connective tissue						
subdural	C70.9	C79.32	—	D32.9	D42.9	D49.7
subglottis, subglottic	C32.2	C78.39	D02.0	D14.1	D38.0	D49.1
sublingual	C04.9	C79.89	D00.06	D10.2	D37.09	D49.0
gland or duct	C08.1	C79.89	D00.00	D11.7	D37.031	D49.0
submandibular gland	C08.0	C79.89	D00.00	D11.7	D37.032	D49.0
submaxillary gland or duct	C08.0	C79.89	D00.00	D11.7	D37.032	D49.0
submental	C76.0	C79.89	D09.8	D36.7	D48.7	D49.89
subpleural	C34.9-	C78.0-	D02.2-	D14.3-	D38.1	D49.1
substernal	C38.1	C78.1	—	D15.2	D38.3	D49.89
sudoriferous, sudoriparous gland, site unspecified	C44.90	C79.2	D04.9	D23.9	D48.5	D49.2
specified site — *see* Neoplasm, skin						
supraclavicular region	C76.0	C79.89	D09.8	D36.7	D48.7	D49.89
supraglottis	C32.1	C78.39	D02.0	D14.1	D38.0	D49.1
suprarenal	C74.9-	C79.7-	D09.3	D35.0-	D44.1-	D49.7
capsule	C74.9-	C79.7-	D09.3	D35.0-	D44.1-	D49.7
cortex	C74.0-	C79.7-	D09.3	D35.0-	D44.1-	D49.7
gland	C74.9-	C79.7-	D09.3	D35.0-	D44.1-	D49.7
medulla	C74.1-	C79.7-	D09.3	D35.0-	D44.1-	D49.7
suprasellar (region)	C71.9	C79.31	—	D33.2	D43.2	D49.6
supratentorial (brain) NEC	C71.0	C79.31	—	D33.0	D43.0	D49.6
sweat gland (apocrine) (eccrine), site unspecified	C44.90	C79.2	D04.9	D23.9	D48.5	D49.2
specified site — *see* Neoplasm, skin						
sympathetic nerve or nervous system NEC	C47.9	C79.89	—	D36.10	D48.2	D49.2
symphysis pubis	C41.4	C79.51	—	D16.8	D48.0	D49.2
synovial membrane — *see* Neoplasm, connective tissue						
tapetum, brain	C71.8	C79.31	—	D33.2	D43.2	D49.6
tarsus (any bone)	C40.3-	C79.51	—	D16.3-	—	—
temple (skin) — *see also* Neoplasm, skin, face	C44.309	C79.2	D04.39	D23.39	D48.5	D49.2
temporal						
bone	C41.0	C79.51	—	D16.4-	D48.0	D49.2
lobe or pole	C71.2	C79.31	—	D33.0	D43.0	D49.6
region	C76.0	C79.89	D09.8	D36.7	D48.7	D49.89
skin — *see also* Neoplasm, skin, face	C44.309	C79.2	D04.39	D23.39	D48.5	D49.2
tendon (sheath) — *see* Neoplasm, connective tissue						
tentorium (cerebelli)	C70.0	C79.32	—	D32.0	D42.0	D49.7
testis, testes	C62.9-	C79.82	D07.69	D29.2-	D40.1-	D49.5
descended	C62.1-	C79.82	D07.69	D29.2-	D40.1-	D49.5
ectopic	C62.0-	C79.82	D07.69	D29.2-	D40.1-	D49.5
retained	C62.0-	C79.82	D07.69	D29.2-	D40.1-	D49.5
scrotal	C62.1-	C79.82	D07.69	D29.2-	D40.1-	D49.5
undescended	C62.0-	C79.82	D07.69	D29.2-	D40.1-	D49.5
unspecified whether descended or undescended	C62.9-	C79.82	D07.69	D29.2-	D40.1-	D49.5
thalamus	C71.0	C79.31	—	D33.0	D43.0	D49.6
thigh NEC	C76.5-	C79.89	D04.7-	D36.7	D48.7	D49.89
thorax, thoracic (cavity) (organs NEC)	C76.1	C79.89	D09.8	D36.7	D48.7	D49.89
duct	C49.3	C79.89	—	D21.3	D48.1	D49.2
wall NEC	C76.1	C79.89	D09.8	D36.7	D48.7	D49.89
throat	C14.0	C79.89	D00.08	D10.9	D37.05	D49.0
thumb NEC	C76.4-	C79.89	D04.6-	D36.7	D48.7	D49.89
thymus (gland)	C37	C79.89	D09.3	D15.0	D38.4	D49.89
thyroglossal duct	C73	C79.89	D09.3	D34	D44.0	D49.7
thyroid (gland)	C73	C79.89	D09.3	D34	D44.0	D49.7
cartilage	C32.3	C78.39	D02.0	D14.1	D38.0	D49.1
tibia (any part)	C40.2-	C79.51	—	D16.2-	—	—
toe NEC	C76.5-	C79.89	D04.7-	D36.7	D48.7	D49.89
Neoplasm, neoplastic - *continued*						
tongue	C02.9	C79.89	D00.07	D10.1	D37.02	D49.0
anterior (two-thirds) NEC	C02.3	C79.89	D00.07	D10.1	D37.02	D49.0
dorsal surface	C02.0	C79.89	D00.07	D10.1	D37.02	D49.0
ventral surface	C02.2	C79.89	D00.07	D10.1	D37.02	D49.0
base (dorsal surface)	C01	C79.89	D00.07	D10.1	D37.02	D49.0
border (lateral)	C02.1	C79.89	D00.07	D10.1	D37.02	D49.0
dorsal surface NEC	C02.0	C79.89	D00.07	D10.1	D37.02	D49.0
fixed part NEC	C01	C79.89	D00.07	D10.1	D37.02	D49.0
foreamen cecum	C02.0	C79.89	D00.07	D10.1	D37.02	D49.0
frenulum linguae	C02.2	C79.89	D00.07	D10.1	D37.02	D49.0
junctional zone	C02.8	C79.89	D00.07	D10.1	D37.02	D49.0
margin (lateral)	C02.1	C79.89	D00.07	D10.1	D37.02	D49.0
midline NEC	C02.0	C79.89	D00.07	D10.1	D37.02	D49.0
mobile part NEC	C02.3	C79.89	D00.07	D10.1	D37.02	D49.0
overlapping lesion	C02.8	—	—	—	—	—
posterior (third)	C01	C79.89	D00.07	D10.1	D37.02	D49.0
root	C01	C79.89	D00.07	D10.1	D37.02	D49.0
surface (dorsal)	C02.0	C79.89	D00.07	D10.1	D37.02	D49.0
base	C01	C79.89	D00.07	D10.1	D37.02	D49.0
ventral	C02.2	C79.89	D00.07	D10.1	D37.02	D49.0
tip	C02.1	C79.89	D00.07	D10.1	D37.02	D49.0
tonsil	C02.4	C79.89	D00.07	D10.1	D37.02	D49.0
tonsil	C09.9	C79.89	D00.08	D10.4	D37.05	D49.0
fauces, faucial	C09.9	C79.89	D00.08	D10.4	D37.05	D49.0
lingual	C02.4	C79.89	D00.07	D10.1	D37.02	D49.0
overlapping sites	C09.8	—	—	—	—	—
palatine	C09.9	C79.89	D00.08	D10.4	D37.05	D49.0
pharyngeal	C11.1	C79.89	D00.08	D10.6	D37.05	D49.0
pillar (anterior) (posterior)	C09.1	C79.89	D00.08	D10.5	D37.05	D49.0
tonsillar fossa	C09.0	C79.89	D00.08	D10.5	D37.05	D49.0
tooth socket NEC	C03.9	C79.89	D00.03	D10.39	D37.09	D49.0
trachea (cartilage) (mucosa)	C33	C78.39	D02.1	D14.2	D38.1	D49.1
overlapping lesion with bronchus or lung	C34.8-	—	—	—	—	—
tracheobronchial	C34.8-	C78.39	D02.1	D14.2	D38.1	D49.1
overlapping lesion with lung	C34.8-	—	—	—	—	—
tragus — *see also* Neoplasm, skin, ear	C44.20-	C79.2	D04.2-	D23.2-	D48.5	D49.2
trunk NEC	C76.8	C79.89	D04.5	D36.7	D48.7	D49.89
tubo-ovarian	C57.8	C79.82	D07.39	D28.7	D39.8	D49.5
tunica vaginalis	C63.7	C79.82	D07.69	D29.8	D40.8	D49.5
turbinate (bone)	C41.0	C79.51	—	D16.4-	D48.0	D49.2
nasal	C30.0	C78.39	D02.3	D14.0	D38.5	D49.1
tympanic cavity	C30.1	C78.39	D02.3	D14.0	D38.5	D49.1
ulna (any part)	C40.0-	C79.51	—	D16.0-	—	—
umbilicus, umbilical — *see also* Neoplasm, skin, trunk	C44.509	C79.2	D04.5	D23.5	D48.5	D49.2
uncus, brain	C71.2	C79.31	—	D33.0	D43.0	D49.6
unknown site or unspecified	C80.1	C79.9	D09.9	D36.9	D48.9	D49.9
urachus	C67.7	C79.11	D09.0	D30.3	D41.4	D49.4
ureter, ureteral	C66.-	C79.19	D09.19	D30.2-	D41.2-	D49.5
orifice (bladder)	C67.6	C79.11	D09.0	D30.3	D41.4	D49.4
ureter-bladder (junction)	C67.6	C79.11	D09.0	D30.3	D41.4	D49.4
urethra, urethral (gland)	C68.0	C79.19	D09.19	D30.4	D41.3	D49.5
orifice, internal	C67.5	C79.11	D09.0	D30.3	D41.4	D49.4
urethrovaginal (septum)	C57.9	C79.82	D07.30	D28.9	D39.8	D49.5
urinary organ or system	C68.9	C79.10	D09.10	D30.9	D41.9	D49.5
bladder — *see* Neoplasm, bladder						
overlapping lesion	C68.8	—	—	—	—	—
specified sites NEC	C68.8	C79.19	D09.19	D30.8	D41.8	D49.5
utero-ovarian	C57.8	C79.82	D07.39	D28.7	D39.8	D49.5
ligament	C57.1	C79.82	D07.39	D28.2	D39.8	D49.5
uterosacral ligament	C57.3	C79.82	—	D28.2	D39.8	D49.5
uterus, uteri, uterine	C55	C79.82	D07.0	D26.9	D39.0	D49.5
adnexa NEC	C57.4	C79.82	D07.39	D28.7	D39.8	D49.5
body	C54.9	C79.82	D07.0	D26.1	D39.0	D49.5
cervix	C53.9	C79.82	D06.9	D26.0	D39.0	D49.5
cornu	C54.9	C79.82	D07.0	D26.1	D39.0	D49.5
corpus	C54.9	C79.82	D07.0	D26.1	D39.0	D49.5
endocervix (canal) (gland)	C53.0	C79.82	D06.0	D26.0	D39.0	D49.5
endometrium	C54.1	C79.82	D07.0	D26.1	D39.0	D49.5
exocervix	C53.1	C79.82	D06.1	D26.0	D39.0	D49.5
external os	C53.1	C79.82	D06.1	D26.0	D39.0	D49.5
fundus	C54.3	C79.82	D07.0	D26.1	D39.0	D49.5
internal os	C53.0	C79.82	D06.0	D26.0	D39.0	D49.5
isthmus	C54.0	C79.82	D07.0	D26.1	D39.0	D49.5
ligament	C57.3	C79.82	—	D28.2	D39.8	D49.5
broad	C57.1	C79.82	D07.39	D28.2	D39.8	D49.5
round	C57.2	C79.82	—	D28.2	D39.8	D49.5
lower segment	C54.0	C79.82	D07.0	D26.1	D39.0	D49.5
myometrium	C54.2	C79.82	D07.0	D26.1	D39.0	D49.5
overlapping sites	C54.8	—	—	—	—	—
squamocolumnar junction	C53.8	C79.82	D06.7	D26.0	D39.0	D49.5
tube	C57.0-	C79.82	D07.39	D28.2	D39.8	D49.5
utricle, prostatic	C68.0	C79.19	D09.19	D30.4	D41.3	D49.5
uveal tract	C69.4-	C79.49	D09.2-	D31.4-	D48.7	D49.89
uvula	C05.2	C79.89	D00.04	D10.39	D37.09	D49.0

© 2013 Channel Publishing, Ltd.

NEOPLASM TABLE

Neoplasm Table	Malignant Primary	Malignant Secondary	Ca In situ	Benign	Uncertain Behavior	Unspecified Behavior
Neoplasm, neoplastic - *continued*						
vagina, vaginal (fornix)						
(vault) (wall)	C52	C79.82	D07.2	D28.1	D39.8	D49.5
vaginovesical	C57.9	C79.82	D07.30	D28.9	D39.9	D49.5
septum	C57.9	C79.82	D07.30	D28.9	D39.9	D49.5
vallecula (epigiottis)...........	C10.0	C79.89	D00.08	D10.5	D37.05	D49.0
vas deferens	C63.1-	C79.82	D07.69	D29.8	D40.8	D49.5
vascular — *see* Neoplasm, connective tissue						
Vater's ampulla....................	C24.1	C78.89	D01.5	D13.5	D37.6	D49.0
vein, venous — *see* Neoplasm, connective tissue						
vena cava (abdominal)						
(inferior).....................	C49.4	C79.89	—	D21.4	D48.1	D49.2
superior........................	C49.3	C79.89	—	D21.3	D48.1	D49.2
ventricle (cerebral) (floor)						
(lateral) (third)	C71.5	C79.31	—	D33.0	D43.0	D49.6
cardiac (left) (right)	C38.0	C79.89	—	D15.1	D48.7	D49.89
fourth	C71.7	C79.31	—	D33.1	D43.1	D49.6
ventricular band of larynx	C32.1	C78.39	D02.0	D14.1	D38.0	D49.1
ventriculus — *see* Neoplasm, stomach						
vermillion border — *see* Neoplasm, lip						
vermis, cerebellum	C71.6	C79.31	—	D33.1	D43.1	D49.6
vertebra (column)	C41.2	C79.51	—	D16.6	D48.0	D49.2
coccyx	C41.4	C79.51	—	D16.8-	D48.0	D49.2
marrow NEC	C96.9	C79.52	—	—	D47.9	D49.89
sacrum	C41.4	C79.51	—	D16.8-	D48.0	D49.2
vesical — *see* Neoplasm, bladder						
vesicle, seminal	C63.7	C79.82	D07.69	D29.8	D40.8	D49.5
vesicocervical tissue.............	C57.9	C79.82	D07.30	D28.9	D39.9	D49.5
vesicorectal......................	C76.3	C79.82	D09.8	D36.7	D48.7	D49.89
vesicovaginal	C57.9	C79.82	D07.30	D28.9	D39.9	D49.5
septum	C57.9	C79.82	D07.30	D28.9	D39.8	D49.5
vessel (blood) — *see* Neoplasm, connective tissue						
vestibular gland, greater	C51.0	C79.82	D07.1	D28.0	D39.8	D49.5
vestibule						
mouth	C06.1	C79.89	D00.00	D10.39	D37.09	D49.0
nose	C30.0	C78.39	D02.3	D14.0	D38.5	D49.1
Virchow's gland	C77.0	C77.0	—	D36.0	D48.7	D49.89
viscera NEC	C76.8	C79.89	D09.8	D36.7	D48.7	D49.89
vocal cords (true)	C32.0	C78.39	D02.0	D14.1	D38.0	D49.1
false	C32.1	C78.39	D02.0	D14.1	D38.0	D49.1
vomer	C41.0	C79.51	—	D16.4-	D48.0	D49.2
vulva.............................	C51.9	C79.82	D07.1	D28.0	D39.8	D49.5
vulvovaginal gland	C51.0	C79.82	D07.1	D28.0	D39.8	D49.5
Waldeyer's ring	C14.2	C79.89	D00.08	D10.9	D37.05	D49.0
Wharton's duct	C08.0	C79.89	D00.00	D11.7	D37.032	D49.0
white matter (central)						
(cerebral)	C71.0	C79.31	—	D33.0	D43.0	D49.6
windpipe..........................	C33	C78.39	D02.1	D14.2	D38.1	D49.1
Wirsung's duct	C25.3	C78.89	D01.7	D13.6	D37.8	D49.0
wolffian (body) (duct)						
female........................	C57.7	C79.82	D07.39	D28.7	D39.8	D49.5
male	C63.7	C79.82	D07.69	D29.8	D40.8	D49.5
womb — *see* Neoplasm, uterus						
wrist NEC.........................	C76.4-	C79.89	D04.6-	D36.7	D48.7	D49.89
xiphoid process...................	C41.3	C79.51	—	D16.7	D48.0	D49.2
Zuckerkandl organ	C75.5	C79.89	—	D35.6	D44.7	D49.7

DISEASE INDEX

Neovascularization
  ciliary body — *see* Disorder, iris, vascular
  cornea H16.40-
    deep H16.44-
    ghost vessels — *see* Ghost, vessels
    localized H16.43-
    pannus — *see* Pannus
  iris — *see* Disorder, iris, vascular
  retina H35.05-
Nephralgia N23
Nephritis, nephritic (albuminuric)
  (azotemic) (congenital) (disseminated)
  (epithelial) (familial) (focal)
  (granulomatous) (hemorrhagic)
  (infantile) (nonsuppurative, excretory)
  (uremic) N05.9
  with
    dense deposit disease N05.6
    diffuse
      crescentic glomerulonephritis N05.7
      endocapillary proliferative
        glomerulonephritis N05.4
      membranous glomerulonephritis
        N05.2
      mesangial proliferative
        glomerulonephritis N05.3
      mesangiocapillary glomerulonephritis
        N05.5
    edema — *see* Nephrosis
    focal and segmental glomerular lesions
      N05.1
    foot process disease N04.9
    glomerular lesion
      diffuse sclerosing N05.8
      hypocomplementemic — *see*
        Nephritis,
        membranoproliferative
      IgA — *see* Nephropathy, IgA
      lobular, lobulonodular — *see*
        Nephritis,
        membranoproliferative
      nodular — *see* Nephritis,
        membranoproliferative
    lesion of
      glomerulonephritis, proliferative
        N05.8
      renal necrosis N05.9
    minor glomerular abnormality N05.0
    specified morphological changes NEC
      N05.8
  acute N00.9
    with
      dense deposit disease N00.6
      diffuse
        crescentic glomerulonephritis
          N00.7
        endocapillary proliferative
          glomerulonephritis N00.4
        membranous glomerulonephritis
          N00.2
        mesangial proliferative
          glomerulonephritis N00.3
        mesangiocapillary
          glomerulonephritis N00.5
      focal and segmental glomerular
        lesions N00.1
      minor glomerular abnormality N00.0
      specified morphological changes NEC
        N00.8
  amyloid E85.4 [N08]
  antiglomerular basement membrane (anti-
    GBM) antibody NEC
    in Goodpasture's syndrome M31.0
  antitubular basement membrane (tubulo-
    interstitial) NEC N12
    toxic — *see* Nephropathy, toxic
  arteriolar — *see* Hypertension, kidney
  arteriosclerotic — *see* Hypertension,
    kidney
  ascending — *see* Nephritis, tubulo-
    interstitial
  atrophic N03.9
  Balkan (endemic) N15.0
  calculous, calculus — *see* Calculus, kidney
  cardiac — *see* Hypertension, kidney
  cardiovascular — *see* Hypertension, kidney

Nephritis, nephritic (albuminuric)
  (azotemic) (congenital) (disseminated)
  (epithelial) (familial) (focal)
  (granulomatous) (hemorrhagic)
  (infantile) (nonsuppurative, excretory)
  (uremic) N05.9 — *continued*
  chronic N03.9
    with
      dense deposit disease N03.6
      diffuse
        crescentic glomerulonephritis
          N03.7
        endocapillary proliferative
          glomerulonephritis N03.4
        membranous glomerulonephritis
          N03.2
        mesangial proliferative
          glomerulonephritis N03.3
        mesangiocapillary
          glomerulonephritis N03.5
      focal and segmental glomerular
        lesions N03.1
      minor glomerular abnormality N03.0
      specified morphological changes NEC
        N03.8
  arteriosclerotic — *see* Hypertension,
    kidney
  cirrhotic N26.9
  complicating pregnancy O26.83-
  croupous N00.9
  degenerative — *see* Nephrosis
  diffuse sclerosing N05.8
  due to
    diabetes mellitus — *see* E08-E13
      with .21
    subacute bacterial endocarditis I33.0
    systemic lupus erythematosus (chronic)
      M32.14
    typhoid fever A01.09
  gonococcal (acute) (chronic) A54.21
  hypocomplementemic — *see* Nephritis,
    membranoproliferative
  IgA — *see* Nephropathy, IgA
  immune complex (circulating) NEC N05.8
  infective — *see* Nephritis, tubulo-
    interstitial
  interstitial — *see* Nephritis, tubulo-
    interstitial
  lead N14.3
  membranoproliferative (diffuse) (type 1 or
    3) (*see also* N00-N07 with fourth
    character .5) N05.5
    type 2 (*see also* N00-N07 with fourth
      character .6) N05.6
  minimal change N05.0
  necrotic, necrotizing NEC (*see also* N00-
    N07 with fourth character .8) N05.8
  nephrotic — *see* Nephrosis
  nodular — *see* Nephritis,
    membranoproliferative
  polycystic Q61.3
    adult type Q61.2
    autosomal
      dominant Q61.2
      recessive NEC Q61.19
    childhood type NEC Q61.19
    infantile type NEC Q61.19
  poststreptococcal N05.9
    acute N00.9
    chronic N03.9
    rapidly progressive N01.9
  proliferative NEC (*see also* N00-N07 with
    fourth character .8) N05.8
  purulent — *see* Nephritis, tubulo-interstitial
  rapidly progressive N01.9
    with
      dense deposit disease N01.6
      diffuse
        crescentic glomerulonephritis
          N01.7
        endocapillary proliferative
          glomerulonephritis N01.4
        membranous glomerulonephritis
          N01.2
        mesangial proliferative
          glomerulonephritis N01.3
        mesangiocapillary
          glomerulonephritis N01.5
      focal and segmental glomerular
        lesions N01.1
      minor glomerular abnormality N01.0
      specified morphological changes NEC
        N01.8
  salt losing or wasting NEC N28.89
  saturnine N14.3
  sclerosing, diffuse N05.8
  septic — *see* Nephritis, tubulo-interstitial

Nephritis, nephritic (albuminuric)
  (azotemic) (congenital) (disseminated)
  (epithelial) (familial) (focal)
  (granulomatous) (hemorrhagic)
  (infantile) (nonsuppurative, excretory)
  (uremic) N05.9 — *continued*
  specified pathology NEC (*see also* N00-
    N07 with fourth character .8) N05.8
  subacute N01.9
  suppurative — *see* Nephritis, tubulo-
    interstitial
  syphilitic (late) A52.75
    congenital A50.59 [N08]
    early (secondary) A51.44
  toxic — *see* Nephropathy, toxic
  tubal, tubular — *see* Nephritis, tubulo-
    interstitial
  tuberculous A18.11
  tubulo-interstitial (in) N12
    acute (infectious) N10
    chronic (infectious) N11.9
      nonobstructive N11.8
        reflux-associated N11.0
      obstructive N11.1
      specified NEC N11.8
    due to
      brucellosis A23.9 [N16]
      cryoglobulinemia D89.1 [N16]
      glycogen storage disease E74.00
        [N16]
      Sjögren's syndrome M35.04
  vascular — *see* Hypertension, kidney
  war N00.9
Nephroblastoma (epithelial) (mesenchymal)
  C64-
Nephrocalcinosis E83.59 [N29]
Nephrocystitis, pustular — *see* Nephritis,
  tubulo-interstitial
Nephrolithiasis (congenital) (pelvis)
  (recurrent) — *see also* Calculus, kidney
Nephroma C64-
  mesoblastic D41.0-
Nephronephritis — *see* Nephrosis
Nephronophthisis Q61.5
Nephropathia epidemica A98.5
Nephropathy (*see also* Nephritis) N28.9
  with
    edema — *see* Nephrosis
    glomerular lesion — *see*
      Glomerulonephritis
  amyloid, hereditary E85.0
  analgesic N14.0
    with medullary necrosis, acute N17.2
  Balkan (endemic) N15.0
  chemical — *see* Nephropathy, toxic
  diabetic — *see* E08-E13 with .21
  drug-induced N14.2
    specified NEC N14.1
  focal and segmental hyalinosis or sclerosis
    N02.1
  heavy metal-induced N14.3
  hereditary NEC N07.9
    with
      dense deposit disease N07.6
      diffuse
        crescentic glomerulonephritis
          N07.7
        endocapillary proliferative
          glomerulonephritis N07.4
        membranous glomerulonephritis
          N07.2
        mesangial proliferative
          glomerulonephritis N07.3
        mesangiocapillary
          glomerulonephritis N07.5
      focal and segmental glomerular
        lesions N07.1
      minor glomerular abnormality N07.0
      specified morphological changes NEC
        N07.8
  hypercalcemic N25.89
  hypertensive — *see* Hypertension, kidney
  hypokalemic (vacuolar) N25.89
  IgA N02.8
    with glomerular lesion N02.9
      focal and segmental hyalinosis or
        sclerosis N02.1
      membranoproliferative (diffuse)
        N02.5
      membranous (diffuse) N02.2
      mesangial proliferative (diffuse)
        N02.3
      mesangiocapillary (diffuse) N02.5
      proliferative NEC N02.8
      specified pathology NEC N02.8

Nephropathy (*see also* Nephritis) N28.9 —
  continued
  lead N14.3
  membranoproliferative (diffuse) N02.5
  membranous (diffuse) N02.2
  mesangial (IgA/IgG) — *see* Nephropathy,
    IgA
    proliferative (diffuse) N02.3
  mesangiocapillary (diffuse) N02.5
  obstructive N13.8
  phenacetin N17.2
  phosphate-losing N25.0
  potassium depletion N25.89
  pregnancy-related O26.83-
  proliferative NEC (*see also* N00-N07 with
    fourth character .8) N05.8
  protein-losing N25.89
  saturnine N14.3
  sickle-cell D57-[N08]
  toxic NEC N14.4
    due to
      drugs N14.2
        analgesic N14.0
        specified NEC N14.1
      heavy metals N14.3
  vasomotor N17.0
  water-losing N25.89
Nephroptosis N28.83
Nephropyosis — *see* Abscess, kidney
Nephrorrhagia N28.89
Nephrosclerosis (arteriolar) (arteriosclerotic)
  (chronic) (hyaline) — *see also*
  Hypertension, kidney
  hyperplastic — *see* Hypertension, kidney
  senile N26.9
Nephrosis, nephrotic (Epstein's) (syndrome)
  (congenital) N04.9
  with
    foot process disease N04.9
    glomerular lesion N04.1
    hypocomplementemic N04.5
  acute N04.9
  anoxic — *see* Nephrosis, tubular
  chemical — *see* Nephrosis, tubular
  cholemic K76.7
  diabetic — *see* E08-E13 with .21
  Finnish type (congenital) Q89.8
  hemoglobin N10
  hemoglobinuric — *see* Nephrosis, tubular
  in
    amyloidosis E85.4 [N08]
    diabetes mellitus — *see* E08-E13
      with .21
    epidemic hemorrhagic fever A98.5
    malaria (malariae) B52.0
  ischemic — *see* Nephrosis, tubular
  lipoid N04.9
  lower nephron — *see* Nephrosis, tubular
  malarial (malariae) B52.0
  minimal change N04.0
  myoglobin N10
  necrotizing — *see* Nephrosis, tubular
  osmotic (sucrose) N25.89
  radiation N04.9
  syphilitic (late) A52.75
  toxic — *see* Nephrosis, tubular
  tubular (acute) N17.0
    postprocedural N99.0
    radiation N04.9
Nephrosonephritis, hemorrhagic (endemic)
  A98.5
Nephrostomy
  attention to Z43.6
  status Z93.6
Nerve — *see also* condition
  injury — *see* Injury, nerve, by body site
Nerves R45.0
Nervous (*see also* condition) R45.0
  heart F45.8
  stomach F45.8
  tension R45.0
Nervousness R45.0
Nesidioblastoma
  pancreas D13.7
  specified site NEC — *see* Neoplasm,
    benign, by site
  unspecified site D13.7
Nettleship's syndrome Q82.2
Neumann's disease or syndrome L10.1

D I S E A S E   I N D E X

Neuralgia, neuralgic (acute) M79.2
  accessory (nerve) G52.8
  acoustic (nerve) — see subcategory H93.3
  auditory (nerve) — see subcategory H93.3
  ciliary G44.009
    intractable G44.001
    not intractable G44.009
  cranial
    nerve — see also Disorder, nerve, cranial
      fifth or trigeminal — see Neuralgia, trigeminal
    postherpetic, postzoster B02.29
  ear — see subcategory H92.0
  facialis vera G51.1
  Fothergill's — see Neuralgia, trigeminal
  glossopharyngeal (nerve) G52.1
  Horton's G44.099
    intractable G44.091
    not intractable G44.099
  Hunt's B02.21
  hypoglossal (nerve) G52.3
  infraorbital — see Neuralgia, trigeminal
  malarial — see Malaria
  migrainous G44.009
    intractable G44.001
    not intractable G44.009
  Morton's G57.6-
  nerve, cranial — see Disorder, nerve, cranial
  nose G52.0
  occipital M54.81
  olfactory G52.0
  penis N48.9
  perineum R10.2
  postherpetic NEC B02.29
    trigeminal B02.22
  pubic region R10.2
  scrotum R10.2
  Sluder's G44.89
  specified nerve NEC G58.8
  spermatic cord R10.2
  sphenopalatine (ganglion) G90.09
  trifacial — see Neuralgia, trigeminal
  trigeminal G50.0
    postherpetic, postzoster B02.22
  vagus (nerve) G52.2
  writer's F48.8
    organic G25.89
Neurapraxia — see Injury, nerve
Neurasthenia F48.8
  cardiac F45.8
  gastric F45.8
  heart F45.8
Neurilemmoma — see also Neoplasm, nerve, benign
  acoustic (nerve) D33.3
  malignant — see also Neoplasm, nerve, malignant
    acoustic (nerve) C72.4-
Neurilemmosarcoma — see Neoplasm, nerve, malignant
Neurinoma — see Neoplasm, nerve, benign
Neurinomatosis — see Neoplasm, nerve, uncertain behavior
Neuritis (rheumatoid) M79.2
  abducens (nerve) — see Strabismus, paralytic, sixth nerve
  accessory (nerve) G52.8
  acoustic (nerve) (see also subcategory) H93.3
    in (due to)
      infectious disease NEC B99 [H94.-]
      parasitic disease NEC B89 [H94.-]
      syphilitic A52.15
  alcoholic G62.1
    with psychosis — see Psychosis, alcoholic
  amyloid, any site E85.4 [G63]
  auditory (nerve) — see subcategory H93.3
  brachial — see Radiculopathy
    due to displacement, intervertebral disc — see Disorder, disc, cervical, with neuritis
  cranial nerve
    due to Lyme disease A69.22
    eighth or acoustic or auditory — see subcategory H93.3
    eleventh or accessory G52.8
    fifth or trigeminal G51.0
    first or olfactory G52.0
    fourth or trochlear — see Strabismus, paralytic, fourth nerve
    second or optic — see Neuritis, optic
    seventh or facial G51.8
      newborn (birth injury) P11.3
    sixth or abducent — see Strabismus, paralytic, sixth nerve
    tenth or vagus G52.2
    third or oculomotor — see Strabismus, paralytic, third nerve
    twelfth or hypoglossal G52.3

Neuritis (rheumatoid) M79.2 — continued
  Déjérine-Sottas G60.0
  diabetic (mononeuropathy) — see E08-E13 with .41
    polyneuropathy — see E08-E13 with .42
  due to
    beriberi E51.11
    displacement, prolapse or rupture, intervertebral disc — see Disorder, disc, with, radiculopathy
    herniation, nucleus pulposus M51.9 [G55]
  endemic E51.11
  facial G51.8
    newborn (birth injury) P11.3
  general — see Polyneuropathy
  geniculate ganglion G51.1
    due to herpes (zoster) B02.21
  gouty M10.00 [G63]
  hypoglossal (nerve) G52.3
  ilioinguinal (nerve) G57.9-
  infectious (multiple) NEC G61.0
  interstitial hypertrophic progressive G60.0
  lumbar M54.16
  lumbosacral M54.17
  multiple — see also Polyneuropathy
    endemic E51.11
    infective, acute G61.0
  multiplex endemica E51.11
  nerve root — see Radiculopathy
  oculomotor (nerve) — see Strabismus, paralytic, third nerve
  olfactory nerve G52.0
  optic (nerve) (hereditary) (sympathetic) H46.9
    with demyelination G36.0
    in myelitis G36.0
    nutritional H46.2
    papillitis — see Papillitis, optic
    retrobulbar H46.1-
    specified type NEC H46.8
    toxic H46.3
  peripheral (nerve) G62.9
    multiple — see Polyneuropathy
    single — see Mononeuritis
  pneumogastric (nerve) G52.2
  postherpetic, postzoster B02.29
  progressive hypertrophic interstitial G60.0
  retrobulbar — see also Neuritis, optic, retrobulbar
    in (due to)
      late syphilis A52.15
      meningococcal infection A39.82
    meningococcal A39.82
    syphilitic A52.15
  sciatic (nerve) — see also Sciatica
    due to displacement of intervertebral disc — see Disorder, disc, with, radiculopathy
  serum (see also Reaction, serum) T80.69
  shoulder-girdle G54.5
  specified nerve NEC G58.8
  spinal (nerve) root — see Radiculopathy
  syphilitic A52.15
  thenar (median) G56.1-
  thoracic M54.14
  toxic NEC G62.2
  trochlear (nerve) — see Strabismus, paralytic, fourth nerve
  vagus (nerve) G52.2
Neuroastrocytoma — see Neoplasm, uncertain behavior, by site
Neuroavitaminosis E56.9 [G99.8]
Neuroblastoma
  olfactory C30.0
  specified site — see Neoplasm, malignant, by site
  unspecified site C74.90
Neurochorioretinitis — see Chorioretinitis
Neurocirculatory asthenia F45.8
Neurocysticercosis B69.0
Neurocytoma — see Neoplasm, benign, by site
Neurodermatitis (circumscribed) (circumscripta) (local) L28.0
  atopic L20.81
  diffuse (Brocq) L20.81
  disseminated L20.81
Neuroencephalomyelopathy, optic G36.0
Neuroepithelioma — see also Neoplasm, malignant, by site
  olfactory C30.0
Neurofibroma — see also Neoplasm, nerve, benign
  melanotic — see Neoplasm, nerve, benign
  multiple — see Neurofibromatosis
  plexiform — see Neoplasm, nerve, benign

Neurofibromatosis (multiple) (nonmalignant) Q85.00
  acoustic Q85.02
  malignant — see Neoplasm, nerve, malignant
  specified NEC Q85.09
  type 1 (von Recklinghausen) Q85.01
  type 2 Q85.02
Neurofibrosarcoma — see Neoplasm, nerve, malignant
Neurogenic — see also condition
  bladder (see also Dysfunction, bladder, neuromuscular) N31.9
    cauda equina syndrome G83.4
  bowel NEC K59.2
  heart F45.8
Neuroglioma — see Neoplasm, uncertain behavior, by site
Neurolabyrinthitis (of Dix and Hallpike) — see Neuronitis, vestibular
Neurolathyrism — see Poisoning, food, noxious, plant
Neuroleprosy A30.9
Neuroma — see also Neoplasm, nerve, benign
  acoustic (nerve) D33.3
  amputation (stump) (traumatic) (surgical complication) (late) T87.3-
    arm T87.3-
    leg T87.3-
  digital (toe) G57.6-
  interdigital (toe) G58.8
    lower limb G57.8-
    upper limb G56.8-
  intermetatarsal G57.8-
  Morton's G57.6-
  nonneoplastic
    arm G56.9-
    leg G57.9-
    lower extremity G57.9-
    upper extremity G56.9-
  optic (nerve) D33.3
  plantar G57.6-
  plexiform — see Neoplasm, nerve, benign
  surgical (nonneoplastic)
    arm G56.9-
    leg G57.9-
    lower extremity G57.9-
    upper extremity G56.9-
Neuromyalgia — see Neuralgia
Neuromyasthenia (epidemic) (postinfectious) G93.3
Neuromyelitis G36.9
  ascending G61.0
  optica G36.0
Neuromyopathy G70.9
  paraneoplastic D49.9 [G13.0]
Neuromyotonia (Isaacs) G71.19
Neuronevus — see Nevus
Neuronitis G58.9
  ascending (acute) G57.2-
  vestibular H81.2-
Neuroparalytic — see condition
Neuropathy, neuropathic G62.9
  acute motor G62.81
  alcoholic G62.1
    with psychosis — see Psychosis, alcoholic
  arm G56.9-
  autonomic, peripheral — see Neuropathy, peripheral, autonomic
  axillary G56.9-
  bladder N31.9
    atonic (motor) (sensory) N31.2
    autonomous N31.2
    flaccid N31.2
    nonreflex N31.2
    reflex N31.1
    uninhibited N31.0
  brachial plexus G54.0
  cervical plexus G54.2
  chronic
    progressive segmentally demyelinating G62.89
    relapsing demyelinating G62.89
  Déjérine-Sottas G60.0
  diabetic — see E08-E13 with .40
    mononeuropathy — see E08-E13 with .41
    polyneuropathy — see E08-E13 with .42

Neuropathy, neuropathic G62.9 — continued
  entrapment G58.9
    iliohypogastric nerve G57.8-
    ilioinguinal nerve G57.8-
    lateral cutaneous nerve of thigh G57.1-
    median nerve G56.0-
    obturator nerve G57.8-
    peroneal nerve G57.3-
    posterior tibial nerve G57.5-
    saphenous nerve G57.8-
    ulnar nerve G56.2-
  facial nerve G51.9
  hereditary G60.9
    motor and sensory (types I-IV) G60.0
    sensory G60.8
    specified NEC G60.8
  hypertrophic G60.0
    Charcot-Marie-Tooth G60.0
    Déjérine-Sottas G60.0
    interstitial progressive G60.0
    of infancy G60.0
    Refsum G60.1
  idiopathic G60.9
    progressive G60.3
    specified NEC G60.8
  in association with hereditary ataxia G60.2
  intercostal G58.0
  ischemic — see Disorder, nerve
  Jamaica (ginger) G62.2
  leg NEC G57.9-
  lower extremity G57.9-
  lumbar plexus G54.1
  median nerve G56.1-
  motor and sensory — see also Polyneuropathy
    hereditary (types I-IV) G60.0
  multiple (acute) (chronic) — see Polyneuropathy
  optic (nerve) — see also Neuritis, optic
    ischemic H47.01-
  paraneoplastic (sensorial) (Denny Brown) D49.9 [G13.0]
  peripheral (nerve) (see also Polyneuropathy) G62.9
    autonomic G90.9
      idiopathic G90.09
      in (due to)
        amyloidosis E85.4 [G99.0]
        diabetes mellitus — see E08-E13 with .43
        endocrine disease NEC E34.9 [G99.0]
        gout M10.00 [G99.0]
        hyperthyroidism E05.90 [G99.0]
          with thyroid storm E05.91 [G99.0]
        metabolic disease NEC E88.9 [G99.0]
      idiopathic G60.9
        progressive G60.3
      in (due to)
        antitetanus serum G62.0
        arsenic G62.2
        drugs NEC G62.0
        lead G62.2
        organophosphate compounds G62.2
        toxic agent NEC G62.2
  plantar nerves G57.6-
  progressive
    hypertrophic interstitial G60.0
    inflammatory G62.81
  radicular NEC — see Radiculopathy
  sacral plexus G54.1
  sciatic G57.0-
  serum G61.1
  toxic NEC G62.2
  trigeminal sensory G50.8
  ulnar nerve G56.2-
  uremic N18.9 [G63]
  vitamin B12 E53.8 [G63]
    with anemia (pernicious) D51.0 [G63]
    due to dietary deficiency D51.3 [G63]
Neurophthisis — see also Disorder, nerve
  peripheral, diabetic — see E08-E13 with .42
Neuroretinitis — see Chorioretinitis
Neuroretinopathy, hereditary optic H47.22
Neurosarcoma — see Neoplasm, nerve, malignant
Neurosclerosis — see Disorder, nerve
Neurosis, neurotic F48.9
  anankastic F42
  anxiety (state) F41.1
    panic type F41.0
  asthenic F48.8
  bladder F45.8

Neurosis, neurotic F48.9 — *continued*
cardiac (reflex) F45.8
cardiovascular F45.8
character F60.9
colon F45.8
compensation F68.1
compulsive, compulsion F42
conversion F44.9
craft F48.8
cutaneous F45.8
depersonalization F48.1
depressive (reaction) (type) F34.1
environmental F48.8
excoriation L98.1
fatigue F48.8
functional — *see* Disorder, somatoform
gastric F45.8
gastrointestinal F45.8
heart F45.8
hypochondriacal F45.21
hysterical F44.9
incoordination F45.8
larynx F45.8
vocal cord F45.8
intestine F45.8
larynx (sensory) F45.8
hysterical F44.4
mixed NEC F48.8
musculoskeletal F45.8
obsessional F42
obsessive-compulsive F42
occupational F48.8
ocular NEC F45.8
organ — *see* Disorder, somatoform
pharynx F45.8
phobic F40.9
posttraumatic (situational) F43.10
acute F43.11
chronic F43.12
psychasthenic (type) F48.8
railroad F48.8
rectum F45.8
respiratory F45.8
rumination F45.8
sexual F65.9
situational F48.8
social F40.10
generalized F40.11
specified type NEC F48.8
state F48.9
with depersonalization episode F48.1
stomach F45.8
traumatic F43.10
acute F43.11
chronic F43.12
vasomotor F45.8
visceral F45.8
war F48.8
Neurospongioblastosis diffusa Q85.1
Neurosyphilis (arrested) (early) (gumma)
(late) (latent) (recurrent) (relapse) A52.3
with ataxia (cerebellar) (locomotor)
(spastic) (spinal) A52.19
aneurysm (cerebral) A52.05
arachnoid (adhesive) A52.13
arteritis (any artery) (cerebral) A52.04
asymptomatic A52.2
congenital A50.40
dura (mater) A52.13
general paresis A52.17
hemorrhagic A52.05
juvenile (asymptomatic) (meningeal)
A50.40
leptomeninges (aseptic) A52.13
meningeal, meninges (adhesive) A52.13
meningitis A52.13
meningovascular (diffuse) A52.13
optic atrophy A52.15
parenchymatous (degenerative) A52.19
paresis, paretic A52.17
juvenile A50.45
remission in (sustained) A52.3
serological (without symptoms) A52.2
specified nature or site NEC A52.19
tabes, tabetic (dorsalis) A52.11
juvenile A50.45
taboparesis A52.17
juvenile A50.45
thrombosis (cerebral) A52.05
vascular (cerebral) NEC A52.05
Neurothekeoma — *see* Neoplasm, nerve,
benign
Neurotic — *see* Neurosis
Neurotoxemia — *see* Toxemia
Neutroclusion M26.211

Neutropenia, neutropenic (chronic)
(genetic) (idiopathic) (immune)
(infantile) (malignant) (pernicious)
(splenic) D70.9
congenital (primary) D70.0
cyclic D70.4
cytoreductive cancer chemotherapy sequela
D70.1
drug-induced D70.2
due to cytoreductive cancer
chemotherapy D70.1
due to infection D70.3
fever D70.9
neonatal, transitory (isoimmune) (maternal
transfer) P61.5
periodic D70.4
secondary (cyclic) (periodic) (splenic)
D70.4
drug-induced D70.2
due to cytoreductive cancer
chemotherapy D70.1
toxic D70.8
Neutrophilia, hereditary giant D72.0
Nevocarcinoma — *see* Melanoma
Nevus D22.9
achromic — *see* Neoplasm, skin, benign
amelanotic — *see* Neoplasm, skin, benign
angiomatous D18.00
intra-abdominal D18.03
intracranial D18.02
skin D18.01
specified site NEC D18.09
araneus I78.1
balloon cell — *see* Neoplasm, skin, benign
bathing trunk D48.5
blue — *see* Neoplasm, skin, benign
cellular — *see* Neoplasm, skin, benign
giant — *see* Neoplasm, skin, benign
Jadassohn's — *see* Neoplasm, skin,
benign
malignant — *see* Melanoma
capillary D18.00
intra-abdominal D18.03
intracranial D18.02
skin D18.01
specified site NEC D18.09
cavernous D18.00
intra-abdominal D18.03
intracranial D18.02
skin D18.01
specified site NEC D18.09
cellular — *see* Neoplasm, skin, benign
blue — *see* Neoplasm, skin, benign
choroid D31.3-
comedonicus Q82.5
conjunctiva D31.0-
dermal — *see* Neoplasm, skin, benign
with epidermal nevus — *see* Neoplasm,
skin, benign
dysplastic — *see* Neoplasm, skin, benign
eye D31.9-
flammeus Q82.5
hemangiomatous D18.00
intra-abdominal D18.03
intracranial D18.02
skin D18.01
specified site NEC D18.09
iris D31.4-
lacrimal gland D31.5-
lymphatic D18.1
magnocellular
specified site — *see* Neoplasm, benign,
by site
unspecified site D31.40
malignant — *see* Melanoma
meaning hemangioma D18.00
intra-abdominal D18.03
intracranial D18.02
skin D18.01
specified site NEC D18.09
mouth (mucosa) D10.30
specified site NEC D10.39
white sponge Q38.6
multiplex Q85.1
non-neoplastic I78.1
oral mucosa D10.30
specified site NEC D10.39
white sponge Q38.6
orbit D31.6-
pigmented
giant (*see also* Neoplasm, skin,
uncertain behavior) D48.5
malignant melanoma in — *see*
Melanoma
portwine Q82.5
retina D31.2-
retrobulbar D31.6-
sanguineous Q82.5
senile I78.1

Nevus D22.9 — *continued*
skin D22.9
abdominal wall D22.5
ala nasi D22.39
ankle D22.7-
anus, anal D22.5
arm D22.6-
auditory canal (external) D22.2-
auricle (ear) D22.2-
auricular canal (external) D22.2-
axilla, axillary fold D22.5
back D22.5
breast D22.5
brow D22.39
buttock D22.5
canthus (eye) D22.1-
cheek (external) D22.39
chest wall D22.5
chin D22.39
ear (external) D22.2-
external meatus (ear) D22.2-
eyebrow D22.39
eyelid (lower) (upper) D22.1-
face D22.30
specified NEC D22.39
female genital organ (external) NEC
D28.0
finger D22.6-
flank D22.5
foot D22.7-
forearm D22.6-
forehead D22.39
foreskin D29.0
genital organ (external) NEC
female D28.0
male D29.9
gluteal region D22.5
groin D22.5
hand D22.6-
heel D22.7-
helix D22.2-
hip D22.7-
interscapular region D22.5
jaw D22.39
knee D22.7-
labium (majus) (minus) D28.0
leg D22.7-
lip (lower) (upper) D22.0
lower limb D22.7-
male genital organ (external) D29.9
nail D22.9
finger D22.6-
toe D22.7-
nasolabial groove D22.39
nates D22.5
neck D22.4
nose (external) D22.39
palpebra D22.1-
penis D29.0
perianal skin D22.5
perineum D22.5
pinna D22.2-
popliteal fossa or space D22.7-
prepuce D29.0
pudendum D28.0
scalp D22.4
scrotum D29.4
shoulder D22.6-
submammary fold D22.5
temple D22.39
thigh D22.7-
toe D22.7-
trunk NEC D22.5
umbilicus D22.5
upper limb D22.6-
vulva D28.0
specified site NEC — *see* Neoplasm, by
site, benign
spider I78.1
stellar I78.1
strawberry Q82.5
Sutton's — *see* Neoplasm, skin, benign
unius lateris Q82.5
Unna's Q82.5
vascular Q82.5
verrucous Q82.5
Newborn (infant) (liveborn) (singleton)
Z38.2
abstinence syndrome P96.1
acne L70.4
affected by (suspected to be)
abnormalities of membranes P02.9
specified NEC P02.8
abruptio placenta P02.1
amino-acid metabolic disorder,
transitory P74.8

Newborn (infant) (liveborn) (singleton)
Z38.2 — *continued*
affected by (suspected to be) — *continued*
amniocentesis (while in utero) P00.6
amnionitis P02.7
apparent life threatening event (ALTE)
R68.13
bleeding (into)
cerebral cortex P52.22
germinal matrix P52.0
ventricles P52.1
breech delivery P03.0
cardiac arrest P29.81
cardiomyopathy I42.8
congenital I42.4
cerebral ischemia P91.0
cesarean delivery P03.4
chemotherapy agents P04.1
chorioamnionitis P02.7
cocaine (crack) P04.41
complications of labor and delivery
P03.9
specified NEC P03.89
compression of umbilical cord NEC
P02.5
contracted pelvis P03.1
delivery P03.9
cesarean P03.4
forceps P03.2
vacuum extractor P03.3
entanglement (knot) in umbilical cord
P02.5
environmental chemicals P04.6
fetal (intrauterine)
growth retardation P05.9
malnutrition not light or small for
gestational age P05.2
forceps delivery P03.2
heart rate abnormalities
bradycardia P29.12
intrauterine P03.819
before onset of labor P03.810
during labor P03.811
tachycardia P29.11
hemorrhage (antepartum) P02.1
cerebellar (nontraumatic) P52.6
intracerebral (nontraumatic) P52.4
intracranial (nontraumatic) P52.9
specified NEC P52.8
intraventricular (nontraumatic) P52.3
grade 1 P52.0
grade 2 P52.1
grade 3 P52.21
grade 4 P52.22
posterior fossa (nontraumatic) P52.6
subarachnoid (nontraumatic) P52.5
subependymal P52.0
with intracerebral extension P52.22
with intraventricular extension
P52.1
with enlargment of ventricles
P52.21
without intraventricular extension
P52.0
hypoxic ischemic encephalopathy [HIE]
P91.60
mild P91.61
moderate P91.62
severe P91.63
induction of labor P03.89
intestinal perforation P78.0
intrauterine (fetal) blood loss P50.9
due to (from)
cut end of co-twin cord P50.5
hemorrhage into
co-twin P50.3
maternal circulation P50.4
placenta P50.2
ruptured cord blood P50.1
vasa previa P50.0
specified NEC P50.8
intrauterine (fetal) hemorrhage P50.9
intrauterine (in utero) procedure P96.5
malpresentation (malposition) NEC
P03.1
maternal (complication of) (use of)
alcohol P04.3
analgesia (maternal) P04.0
anesthesia (maternal) P04.0
blood loss P02.1
circulatory disease P00.3
condition P00.9
specified NEC P00.89
delivery P03.9
Cesarean P03.4
forceps P03.2
vacuum extractor P03.3

DISEASE INDEX

Newborn (infant) (liveborn) (singleton)
Z38.2 — *continued*
affected by (suspected to be) — *continued*
maternal (complication of) (use of) — *continued*
diabetes mellitus (pre-existing) P70.1
disorder P00.9
specified NEC P00.89
drugs (addictive) (illegal) NEC P04.49
ectopic pregnancy P01.4
gestational diabetes P70.0
hemorrhage P02.1
hypertensive disorder P00.0
incompetent cervix P01.0
infectious disease P00.2
injury P00.5
labor and delivery P03.9
malpresentation before labor P01.7
maternal death P01.6
medical procedure P00.7
medication P04.1
multiple pregnancy P01.5
nutritional disorder P00.4
oligohydramnios P01.2
parasitic disease P00.2
periodontal disease P00.81
placenta previa P02.0
polyhydramnios P01.3
precipitate delivery P03.5
pregnancy P01.9
specified P01.8
premature rupture of membranes P01.1
renal disease P00.1
respiratory disease P00.3
surgical procedure P00.6
urinary tract disease P00.1
uterine contraction (abnormal) P03.6
meconium peritonitis P78.0
medication (legal) (maternal use) (prescribed) P04.1
membrane abnormalities P02.9
specified NEC P02.8
membranitis P02.7
methamphetamine(s) P04.49
mixed metabolic and respiratory acidosis P84
neonatal abstinence syndrome P96.1
noxious substances transmitted via placenta or breast milk P04.9
specified NEC P04.8
nutritional supplements P04.5
placenta previa P02.0
placental
abnormality (functional) (morphological) P02.20
specified NEC P02.29
dysfunction P02.29
infarction P02.29
insufficiency P02.29
separation NEC P02.1
transfusion syndromes P02.3
placentitis P02.7
precipitate delivery P03.5
prolapsed cord P02.4
respiratory arrest P28.81
slow intrauterine growth P05.9
tobacco P04.2
twin to twin transplacental transfusion P02.3
umbilical cord (tightly) around neck P02.5
umbilical cord condition P02.60
short cord P02.69
specified NEC P02.69
uterine contractions (abnormal) P03.6
vasa previa P02.69
from intrauterine blood loss P50.0
apnea P28.3
obstructive P28.4
primary P28.3
specified P28.4
born in hospital Z38.00
by cesarean Z38.01
born outside hospital Z38.1
breast buds P96.89
breast engorgement P83.4
check-up — *see* Newborn, examination
convulsion P90
dehydration P74.1
examination
8 to 28 days old Z00.111
under 8 days old Z00.110
fever P81.9
environmentally-induced P81.0
hyperbilirubinemia P59.9
of prematurity P59.0

Newborn (infant) (liveborn) (singleton)
Z38.2 — *continued*
hypernatremia P74.2
hyponatremia P74.2
infection P39.9
candidal P37.5
specified NEC P39.8
urinary tract P39.3
jaundice P59.8
due to
breast milk inhibitor P59.3
hepatocellular damage P59.20
specified NEC P59.29
preterm delivery P59.0
of prematurity P59.0
specified NEC P59.8
late metabolic acidosis P74.0
mastitis P39.0
infective P39.0
noninfective P83.4
multiple born NEC P38.8
born in hospital Z38.68
by cesarean Z38.69
born outside hospital Z38.7
omphalitis P38.9
with mild hemorrhage P38.1
without hemorrhage P38.9
post-term P08.21
prolonged gestation (over 42 completed weeks) P08.22
quadruplet Z38.8
born in hospital Z38.63
by cesarean Z38.64
born outside hospital Z38.7
quintuplet Z38.8
born in hospital Z38.65
by cesarean Z38.66
born outside hospital Z38.7
seizure P90
sepsis (congenital) P36.9
due to
anaerobes NEC P36.5
Escherichia coli P36.4
Staphylococcus P36.30
aureus P36.2
specified NEC P36.39
Streptococcus P36.10
group B P36.0
specified NEC P36.19
specified NEC P36.8
triplet Z38.8
born in hospital Z38.61
by cesarean Z38.62
born outside hospital Z38.7
twin Z38.5
born in hospital Z38.30
by cesarean Z38.31
born outside hospital Z38.4
vomiting P92.09
bilious P92.01
weight check Z00.111
Newcastle conjunctivitis or disease B30.8
Nezelof's syndrome (pure alymphocytosis) D81.4
Niacin(amide) deficiency E52
Nicolas(-Durand)-Favre disease A55
Nicotine — *see* Tobacco
Nicotinic acid deficiency E52
Niemann-Pick disease or syndrome E75.249
specified NEC E75.248
type
A E75.240
B E75.241
C E75.242
D E75.243
Night
blindness — *see* Blindness, night
sweats R61
terrors (child) F51.4
Nightmares (REM sleep type) F51.5
Nipple — *see* condition
Nisbet's chancre A57
Nishimoto (-Takeuchi) disease I67.5
Nitritoid crisis or reaction — *see* Crisis, nitritoid
Nitrosohemoglobinemia D74.8
Njovera A65
Nocardiosis, nocardiasis A43.9
cutaneous A43.1
lung A43.0
pneumonia A43.0
pulmonary A43.0
specified site NEC A43.8
Nocturia R35.1
psychogenic F45.8

Nocturnal — *see* condition
Nodal rhythm I49.8
Node(s) — *see also* Nodule
Bouchard's (with arthropathy) M15.2
Haygarth's M15.8
Heberden's (with arthropathy) M15.1
larynx J38.7
lymph — *see* condition
milker's B08.03
Osler's I33.0
Schmorl's — *see* Schmorl's disease
singer's J38.2
teacher's J38.2
tuberculous — *see* Tuberculosis, lymph gland
vocal cord J38.2
Nodule(s), nodular
actinomycotic — *see* Actinomycosis
breast NEC N63
colloid (cystic), thyroid E04.1
cutaneous — *see* Swelling, localized
endometrial (stromal) D26.1
Haygarth's M15.8
inflammatory — *see* Inflammation
juxta-articular
syphilitic A52.77
yaws A66.7
larynx J38.7
lung, solitary (subsegmental branch of the bronchial tree) R91.1
multiple R91.8
milker's B08.03
prostate N40.2
with lower urinary tract symptoms (LUTS) N40.3
without lower urinary tract symptoms (LUTS) N40.2
pulmonary, solitary (subsegmental branch of the bronchial tree) R91.1
retrocardiac R09.89
rheumatoid M06.30
ankle M06.37-
elbow M06.32-
foot joint M06.37-
hand joint M06.34-
hip M06.35-
knee M06.36-
multiple site M06.39
shoulder M06.31-
vertebra M06.38
wrist M06.33-
scrotum (inflammatory) N49.2
singer's J38.2
solitary, lung (subsegmental branch of the bronchial tree) R91.1
multiple R91.8
subcutaneous — *see* Swelling, localized
teacher's J38.2
thyroid (cold) (gland) (nontoxic) E04.1
with thyrotoxicosis E05.20
with thyroid storm E05.21
toxic or with hyperthyroidism E05.20
with thyroid storm E05.21
vocal cord J38.2
Noma (gangrenous) (hospital) (infective) A69.0
auricle I96
mouth A69.0
pudendi N76.89
vulvae N76.89
Nomad, nomadism Z59.0
Nonautoimmune hemolytic anemia D59.4
drug-induced D59.2
Nonclosure — *see also* Imperfect, closure
ductus arteriosus (Botallo's) Q25.0
foramen
botalli Q21.1
ovale Q21.1
Noncompliance Z91.19
with
dialysis Z91.15
dietary regimen Z91.11
medical treatment Z91.19
medication regimen NEC Z91.14
underdosing (*see also* Table of Drugs and Chemicals, categories T36-T50, with final character 6) Z91.14
intentional NEC Z91.128
due to financial hardship of patient Z91.120
unintentional NEC Z91.138
due to patient's age related debility Z91.130
renal dialysis Z91.15

Nondescent (congenital) — *see also* Malposition, congenital
cecum Q43.3
colon Q43.3
testicle Q53.9
bilateral Q53.20
abdominal Q53.21
perineal Q53.22
unilateral Q53.10
abdominal Q53.11
perineal Q53.12
Nondevelopment
brain Q02
part of Q04.3
heart Q24.8
organ or site, congenital NEC — *see* Hypoplasia
Nonengagement
head NEC O32.4
in labor, causing obstructed labor O64.8
Nonexanthematous tick fever A93.2
Nonexpansion, lung (newborn) P28.0
Nonfunctioning
cystic duct (*see also* Disease, gallbladder) K82.8
gallbladder (*see also* Disease, gallbladder) K82.8
kidney N28.9
labyrinth — *see* subcategory H83.2
Non-Hodgkin lymphoma NEC — *see* Lymphoma, non-Hodgkin
Nonimplantation, ovum N97.2
Noninsufflation, fallopian tube N97.1
Non-ketotic hyperglycinemia E72.51
Nonne-Milroy syndrome Q82.0
Nonovulation N97.0
Nonpatent fallopian tube N97.1
Nonpneumatization, lung NEC P28.0
Nonrotation — *see* Malrotation
Nonsecretion, urine — *see* Anuria
Nonunion
fracture — *see* Fracture, by site
organ or site, congenital NEC — *see* Imperfect, closure
symphysis pubis, congenital Q74.2
Nonvisualization, gallbladder R93.2
Nonvital, nonvitalized tooth K04.99
Non-working side interference M26.56
Noonan's syndrome Q87.1
Normocytic anemia (infectional) due to blood loss (chronic) D50.0
acute D62
Norrie's disease (congenital) Q15.8
North American blastomycosis B40.9
Norwegian itch B86
Nose, nasal — *see* condition
Nosebleed R04.0
Nosomania F45.21
Nosophobia F45.22
Nose-picking F98.8
Nostalgia F43.20
Notch of iris Q13.2
Notching nose, congenital (tip) Q30.2
Nothnagel's
syndrome — *see* Strabismus, paralytic, third nerve
vasomotor acroparesthesia I73.89
Novy's relapsing fever A68.9
louse-borne A68.0
tick-borne A68.1
Noxious
foodstuffs, poisoning by — *see* Poisoning, food, noxious, plant
substances transmitted through placenta or breast milk P04.9
Nucleus pulposus — *see* condition
Numbness R20.0
Nuns' knee — *see* Bursitis, prepatellar
Nursemaid's elbow S53.03-
Nutcracker esophagus K22.4
Nutmeg liver K76.1
Nutrient element deficiency E61.9
specified NEC E61.8
Nutrition deficient or insufficient (*see also* Malnutrition) E46
due to
insufficient food T73.0
lack of
care (child) T76.02
adult T76.01
food T73.0
Nutritional stunting E45
Nyctalopia (night blindness) — *see* Blindness, night
Nycturia R35.1
psychogenic F45.8
Nymphomania F52.8

Nystagmus H55.00
  benign paroxysmal — *see* Vertigo, benign
      paroxysmal
  central positional H81.4-
  congenital H55.01
  dissociated H55.04
  latent H55.02
  miners' H55.09
  positional
      benign paroxysmal H81.4-
      central H81.4-
  specified form NEC H55.09
  visual deprivation H55.03

O

Obermeyer's relapsing fever (European)
    A68.0
Obesity E66.9
  with alveolar hypoventilation E66.2
  adrenal E27.8
  complicating
      childbirth O99.214
      pregnancy O99.21-
      puerperium O99.215
  constitutional E66.8
  dietary counseling and surveillance Z71.3
  drug-induced E66.1
  due to
      drug E66.1
      excess calories E66.09
          morbid E66.01
          severe E66.01
  endocrine E66.8
  endogenous E66.8
  familial E66.8
  glandular E66.8
  hypothyroid — *see* Hypothyroidism
  morbid E66.01
      with alveolar hypoventilation E66.2
      due to excess calories E66.01
  nutritional E66.09
  pituitary E23.6
  severe E66.01
  specified type NEC E66.8
Oblique — *see* condition
Obliteration
  appendix (lumen) K38.8
  artery I77.1
  bile duct (noncalculous) K83.1
  common duct (noncalculous) K83.1
  cystic duct — *see* Obstruction, gallbladder
  disease, arteriolar I77.1
  endometrium N85.8
  eye, anterior chamber — *see* Disorder,
      globe, hypotony
  fallopian tube N97.1
  lymphatic vessel I89.0
      due to mastectomy I97.2
  organ or site, congenital NEC — *see*
      Atresia, by site
  ureter N13.5
      with infection N13.6
  urethra — *see* Stricture, urethra
  vein I87.8
  vestibule (oral) K08.8
Observation (following) (for) (without need
    for further medical care) Z04.9
  accident NEC Z04.3
      at work Z04.2
      transport Z04.1
  adverse effect of drug Z03.6
  alleged rape or sexual assault (victim),
      ruled out
      adult Z04.41
      child Z04.42
  criminal assault Z04.8
  development state
      adolescent Z00.3
      period of rapid growth in childhood
          Z00.2
      puberty Z00.3
  disease, specified NEC Z03.89
  following work accident Z04.2
  growth and development state — *see*
      Observation, development state
  injuries (accidental) NEC — *see also*
      Observation, accident
  newborn (for suspected condition, ruled
      out) — *see* Newborn, affected by
      (suspected to be), maternal
      (complication of) (use of)
  postpartum
      immediately after delivery Z39.0
      routine follow-up Z39.2
  pregnancy (normal) (without complication)
      Z34.9-
      high risk O09.9-
  suicide attempt, alleged NEC Z03.89
      self-poisoning Z03.6
  suspected, ruled out — *see also* Suspected
      condition, ruled out
      abuse, physical
          adult Z04.71
          child Z04.72
      accident at work Z04.2
      adult battering victim Z04.71
      child battering victim Z04.72

Observation (following) (for) (without need
    for further medical care) Z04.9 —
    continued
  suspected, ruled out *(see also* Suspected
      condition, ruled out) — *continued*
      condition NEC Z03.89
          newborn — *see* Newborn, affected by
              (suspected to be), maternal
              (complication of) (use of)
      drug poisoning or adverse effect Z03.6
      exposure (to)
          anthrax Z03.810
          biological agent NEC Z03.818
      inflicted injury NEC Z04.8
      suicide attempt, alleged Z03.89
          self-poisoning Z03.6
      toxic effects from ingested substance
          (drug) (poison) Z03.6
  toxic effects from ingested substance
      (drug) (poison) Z03.6
Obsession, obsessional state F42
Obsessive-compulsive neurosis or reaction
    F42
Obstetric embolism, septic — *see*
    Embolism, obstetric, septic
Obstetrical trauma (complicating delivery)
    O71.9
  with or following ectopic or molar
      pregnancy O08.6
  specified type NEC O71.89
Obstipation — *see* Constipation
Obstruction, obstructed, obstructive
  airway J98.8
      with
          allergic alveolitis J67.9
          asthma J45.909
              with
                  exacerbation (acute) J45.901
                  status asthmaticus J45.902
          bronchiectasis J47.9
              with
                  exacerbation (acute) J47.1
                  lower respiratory infection J47.0
          bronchitis (chronic) J44.9
          emphysema J43.9
      chronic J44.9
          with
              allergic alveolitis — *see*
                  Pneumonitis, hypersensitivity
              bronchiectasis J47.9
                  with
                      exacerbation (acute) J47.1
                      lower respiratory infection
                          J47.0
      due to
          foreign body — *see* Foreign body, by
              site, causing asphyxia
          inhalation of fumes or vapors J68.9
          laryngospasm J38.5
  ampulla of Vater K83.1
  aortic (heart) (valve) — *see* Stenosis, aortic
  aortoiliac I74.09
  aqueduct of Sylvius G91.1
      congenital Q03.0
          with spina bifida — *see* Spina bifida,
              by site, with hydrocephalus
      Arnold-Chiari — *see* Arnold-Chiari disease
  artery (*see also* Embolism, artery) I74.9
      basilar (complete) (partial) — *see*
          Occlusion, artery, basilar
      carotid (complete) (partial) — *see*
          Occlusion, artery, carotid
      cerebellar — *see* Occlusion, artery,
          cerebellar
      cerebral (anterior) (middle) (posterior)
          — *see* Occlusion, artery, cerebral
      precerebral — *see* Occlusion, artery,
          precerebral
      renal N28.0
      retinal NEC — *see* Occlusion, artery,
          retina
      vertebral (complete) (partial) — *see*
          Occlusion, artery, vertebral
  band (intestinal) K56.69
  bile duct or passage (common) (hepatic)
      (noncalculous) K83.1
      with calculus K80.51
      congenital (causing jaundice) Q44.3
  biliary (duct) (tract) K83.1
      gallbladder K82.0
  bladder-neck (acquired) N32.0
      congenital Q64.31
      due to hyperplasia (hypertrophy) of
          prostate — *see* Hyperplasia,
          prostate
  bowel — *see* Obstruction, intestine
  bronchus J98.09
  canal, ear — *see* Stenosis, external ear
      canal

Obstruction, obstructed, obstructive —
    continued
  cardia K22.2
  caval veins (inferior) (superior) I87.1
  cecum — *see* Obstruction, intestine
  circulatory I99.8
  colon — *see* Obstruction, intestine
  common duct (noncalculous) K83.1
  coronary (artery) — *see* Occlusion,
      coronary
  cystic duct — *see also* Obstruction,
      gallbladder
      with calculus K80.21
  device, implant or graft (*see also*
      Complications, by site and type,
      mechanical) T85.698
      arterial graft NEC — *see* Complication,
          cardiovascular device, mechanical,
          vascular
      catheter NEC T85.628
          cystostomy T83.090
          dialysis (renal) T82.49
              intraperitoneal T85.691
          infusion NEC T82.594
              spinal (epidural) (subdural)
                  T85.690
          urinary, indwelling T83.098
      due to infection T85.79
      gastrointestinal — *see* Complications,
          prosthetic device, mechanical,
          gastrointestinal device
      genital NEC T83.498
          intrauterine contraceptive device
              T83.39
          penile prosthesis T83.490
      heart NEC — *see* Complication,
          cardiovascular device, mechanical
      joint prosthesis — *see* Complications,
          joint prosthesis, mechanical,
          specified NEC, by site
      orthopedic NEC — *see* Complication,
          orthopedic, device, mechanical
      specified NEC T85.628
      urinary NEC — *see also* Complication,
          genitourinary, device, urinary,
          mechanical
          graft T83.29
      vascular NEC — *see* Complication,
          cardiovascular device, mechanical
      ventricular intracranial shunt T85.09
  due to foreign body accidentally left in
      operative wound T81.529
  duodenum K31.5
  ejaculatory duct N50.8
  esophagus K22.2
  eustachian tube (complete) (partial)
      H68.10-
      cartilagenous (extrinsic) H68.13-
          intrinsic H68.12-
      osseous H68.11-
  fallopian tube (bilateral) N97.1
  fecal K56.41
      with hernia — *see* Hernia, by site, with
          obstruction
  foramen of Monro (congenital) Q03.8
      with spina bifida — *see* Spina bifida, by
          site, with hydrocephalus
  foreign body — *see* Foreign body
  gallbladder K82.0
      with calculus, stones K80.21
      congenital Q44.1
  gastric outlet K31.1
  gastrointestinal — *see* Obstruction,
      intestine
  hepatic K76.89
      duct (noncalculous) K83.1
  hepatobiliary K83.1
  ileum — *see* Obstruction, intestine
  iliofemoral (artery) I74.5
  intestine K56.60
      with
          adhesions (intestinal) (peritoneal)
              K56.5
      adynamic K56.0
      by gallstone K56.3
      congenital (small) Q41.9
          large Q42.9
              specified part NEC Q42.8
      neurogenic K56.0
          Hirschsprung's disease or megacolon
              Q43.1
      newborn P76.9
          due to
              fecaliths P76.8
              inspissated milk P76.2
              meconium (plug) P76.0
                  in mucoviscidosis E84.11
          specified NEC P76.8

Obstruction, obstructed, obstructive — *continued*
  intestine K56.60 — *continued*
    postoperative K91.3
    reflex K56.0
    specified NEC K56.69
    volvulus K56.2
  intracardiac ball valve prosthesis T82.09
  jejunum — *see* Obstruction, intestine
  joint prosthesis — *see* Complications, joint prosthesis, mechanical, specified NEC, by site
  kidney (calices) N28.89
  labor — *see* Delivery
  lacrimal (passages) (duct)
    by
      dacryolith — *see* Dacryolith
      stenosis — *see* Stenosis, lacrimal
    congenital Q10.5
    neonatal H04.53-
  lacrimonasal duct — *see* Obstruction, lacrimal
  lacteal, with steatorrhea K90.2
  laryngitis — *see* Laryngitis
  larynx NEC J38.6
    congenital Q31.8
  lung J98.4
    disease, chronic J44.9
  lymphatic I89.0
  meconium (plug)
    newborn P76.0
      due to fecaliths P76.0
      in mucoviscidosis E84.11
  mitral — *see* Stenosis, mitral
  nasal J34.89
  nasolacrimal duct — *see also* Obstruction, lacrimal
    congenital Q10.5
  nasopharynx J39.2
  nose J34.89
  organ or site, congenital NEC — *see* Atresia, by site
  pancreatic duct K86.8
  parotid duct or gland K11.8
  pelviureteral junction N13.5
    congenital Q62.39
  pharynx J39.2
  portal (circulation) (vein) I81
  prostate — *see also* Hyperplasia, prostate
    valve (urinary) N32.0
  pulmonary valve (heart) I37.0
  pyelonephritis (chronic) N11.1
  pylorus
    adult K31.1
    congenital or infantile Q40.0
  rectosigmoid — *see* Obstruction, intestine
  rectum K62.4
  renal N28.89
    outflow N13.8
    pelvis, congenital Q62.39
  respiratory J98.8
    chronic J44.9
  retinal (vessels) H34.9
  salivary duct (any) K11.8
    with calculus K11.5
  sigmoid — *see* Obstruction, intestine
  sinus (accessory) (nasal) J34.89
  Stensen's duct K11.8
  stomach NEC K31.89
    acute K31.0
    congenital Q40.2
    due to pylorospasm K31.3
  submandibular duct K11.8
  submaxillary gland K11.8
    with calculus K11.5
  thoracic duct I89.0
  thrombotic — *see* Thrombosis
  trachea J39.8
  tracheostomy airway J95.03
  tricuspid (valve) — *see* Stenosis, tricuspid
  upper respiratory, congenital Q34.8
  ureter (functional) (pelvic junction) NEC N13.5
    with
      hydronephrosis N13.1
        with infection N13.6
      pyelonephritis (chronic) N11.1
    congenital Q62.39
    due to calculus — *see* Calculus, ureter
  urethra NEC N36.8
    congenital Q64.39
  urinary (moderate) N13.9
    due to hyperplasia (hypertrophy) of prostate — *see* Hyperplasia, prostate
    organ or tract (lower) N13.9
    prostatic valve N32.0
    specified NEC N13.8

Obstruction, obstructed, obstructive — *continued*
  uropathy N13.9
  uterus N85.8
  vagina N89.5
  valvular — *see* Endocarditis
  vein, venous I87.1
    caval (inferior) (superior) I87.1
    thrombotic — *see* Thrombosis
  vena cava (inferior) (superior) I87.1
  vesical NEC N32.0
  vesicourethral orifice N32.0
    congenital Q64.31
  vessel NEC I99.8
Obturator — *see* condition
Occlusal wear, teeth K03.0
Occlusio pupillae — *see* Membrane, pupillary
Occlusion, occluded
  anus K62.4
    congenital Q42.3
    with fistula Q42.2
  aortoiliac (chronic) I74.09
  aqueduct of Sylvius G91.1
    congenital Q03.0
    with spina bifida — *see* Spina bifida, by site, with hydrocephalus
  artery (*see also* Embolism, artery) I74.9
    auditory, internal I65.8
    basilar I65.1
      with
        infarction I63.22
          due to
            embolism I63.12
            thrombosis I63.02
    brain or cerebral I66.9
      with infarction (due to) I63.5
        embolism I63.4
        thrombosis I63.3
    carotid I65.2-
      with
        infarction I63.23-
          due to
            embolism I63.13-
            thrombosis I63.03-
    cerebellar (anterior inferior) (posterior inferior) (superior) I66.3
      with infarction I63.54-
        due to
          embolism I63.44-
          thrombosis I63.34-
    cerebral I66.9
      with infarction I63.50
        due to
          embolism I63.40
            specified NEC I63.49
          thrombosis I63.30
            specified NEC I63.39
    anterior I66.1-
      with infarction I63.52-
        due to
          embolism I63.42-
          thrombosis I63.32-
    middle I66.0-
      with infarction I63.51-
        due to
          embolism I63.41-
          thrombosis I63.31-
    posterior I66.2-
      with infarction I63.53-
        due to
          embolism I63.43-
          thrombosis I63.33-
    specified NEC I66.8
      with infarction I63.59
        due to
          embolism I63.4
          thrombosis I63.3
    choroidal (anterior) — *see* Occlusion, artery, precerebral, specified NEC
    communicating posterior — *see* Occlusion, artery, cerebral, specified NEC
    complete
      coronary I25.82
      extremities I70.92
    coronary (acute) (thrombotic) (without myocardial infarction) I24.0
      with myocardial infarction — *see* Infarction, myocardium
      chronic total I25.82
      complete I25.82
      healed or old I25.2
      total (chronic) I25.82

Occlusion, occluded — *continued*
  artery (*see also* Embolism, artery) I74.9 — *continued*
    hypophyseal — *see* Occlusion, artery, precerebral, specified NEC
    iliac I74.5
    lower extremities due to stenosis or stricture I77.1
    mesenteric (embolic) (thrombotic) K55.0
    perforating — *see* Occlusion, artery, cerebral, specified NEC
    peripheral I77.9
      thrombotic or embolic I74.4
    pontine — *see* Occlusion, artery, cerebral, specified NEC
    precerebral I65.9
      with infarction I63.20
        due to
          embolism I63.10
            specified NEC I63.19
          thrombosis I63.00
            specified NEC I63.09
        specified NEC I63.29
      basilar — *see* Occlusion, artery, basilar
      carotid — *see* Occlusion, artery, carotid
      puerperal O88.23
      specified NEC I65.8
        with infarction I63.29
          due to
            embolism I63.19
            thrombosis I63.00
      vertebral — *see* Occlusion, artery, vertebral
    renal N28.0
    retinal
      branch H34.23-
      central H34.1-
      partial H34.21-
      transient H34.0-
    spinal — *see* Occlusion, artery, precerebral, vertebral
    total (chronic)
      coronary I25.82
      extremities I70.92
    vertebral I65.0-
      with
        infarction I63.21-
          due to
            embolism I63.11-
            thrombosis I63.01-
  basilar artery — *see* Occlusion, artery, basilar
  bile duct (common) (hepatic) (noncalculous) K83.1
  bowel — *see* Obstruction, intestine
  carotid (artery) (common) (internal) — *see* Occlusion, artery, carotid
  centric (of teeth) M26.59
    maximum intercuspation discrepancy M26.55
  cerebellar (artery) — *see* Occlusion, artery, cerebellar
  cerebral (artery) — *see* Occlusion, artery, cerebral
  cerebrovascular — *see also* Occlusion, artery, cerebral
    with infarction I63.5
  cervical canal — *see* Stricture, cervix
  cervix (uteri) — *see* Stricture, cervix
  choanal Q30.0
  choroidal (artery) — *see* Occlusion, artery, precerebral, specified NEC
  colon — *see* Obstruction, intestine
  communicating posterior artery — *see* Occlusion, artery, precerebral, specified NEC
  coronary (artery) (vein) (thrombotic) — *see also* Infarct, myocardium
    chronic total I25.82
    healed or old I25.2
    not resulting in infarction I24.0
    total (chronic) I25.82
  cystic duct — *see* Obstruction, gallbladder
  embolic — *see* Embolism
  fallopian tube N97.1
    congenital Q50.6
  gallbladder — *see also* Obstruction, gallbladder
    congenital (causing jaundice) Q44.1
  gingiva, traumatic K06.2
  hymen N89.6
    congenital Q52.3

Occlusion, occluded — *continued*
  hypophyseal (artery) — *see* Occlusion, artery, precerebral, specified NEC
  iliac artery I74.5
  intestine — *see* Obstruction, intestine
  lacrimal passages — *see* Obstruction, lacrimal
  lung J98.4
  lymph or lymphatic channel I89.0
  mammary duct N64.89
  mesenteric artery (embolic) (thrombotic) K55.0
  nose J34.89
    congenital Q30.0
  organ or site, congenital NEC — *see* Atresia, by site
  oviduct N97.1
    congenital Q50.6
  peripheral arteries
    due to stricture or stenosis I77.1
    upper extremity I74.2
  pontine (artery) — *see* Occlusion, artery, precerebral, specified NEC
  posterior lingual, of mandibular teeth M26.29
  precerebral artery — *see* Occlusion, artery, precerebral
  punctum lacrimale — *see* Obstruction, lacrimal
  pupil — *see* Membrane, pupillary
  pylorus, adult (*see also* Stricture, pylorus) K31.1
  renal artery N28.0
  retina, retinal
    artery — *see* Occlusion, artery, retinal
    vein (central) H34.81-
      engorgement H34.82-
      tributary H34.83-
      vessels H34.9
  spinal artery — *see* Occlusion, artery, precerebral, vertebral
  teeth (mandibular) (posterior lingual) M26.29
  thoracic duct I89.0
  thrombotic — *see* Thrombosis, artery
  traumatic
    edentulous (alveolar) ridge K06.2
    gingiva K06.2
    periodontal K05.5
  tubal N97.1
  ureter (complete) (partial) N13.5
    congenital Q62.10
  ureteropelvic junction N13.5
    congenital Q62.11
  ureterovesical orifice N13.5
    congenital Q62.12
  urethra — *see* Stricture, urethra
  uterus N85.8
  vagina N89.5
  vascular NEC I99.8
  vein — *see* Thrombosis
    retinal — *see* Occlusion, retinal, vein
  vena cava (inferior) (superior) — *see* Embolism, vena cava
  ventricle (brain) NEC G91.1
  vertebral (artery) — *see* Occlusion, artery, vertebral
  vessel (blood) I99.8
  vulva N90.5
Occult
  blood in feces (stools) R19.5
Occupational
  problems NEC Z56.89
Ochlophobia — *see* Agoraphobia
Ochronosis (endogenous) E70.29
Ocular muscle — *see* condition
Oculogyric crisis or disturbance H51.8
  psychogenic F45.8
Oculomotor syndrome H51.9
Oculopathy
  syphilitic NEC A52.71
    congenital
      early A50.01
      late A50.30
    early (secondary) A51.43
    late A52.71
Oddi's sphincter spasm K83.4
Odontalgia K08.8
Odontoameloblastoma — *see* Cyst, calcifying odontogenic
Odontoclasia K03.89
Odontodysplasia, regional K00.4
Odontogenesis imperfecta K00.5
Odontoma (ameloblastic) (complex) (compound) (fibroameloblastic) — *see* Cyst, calcifying odontogenic

Odontomyelitis (closed) (open) K04.0
Odontorrhagia K08.8
Odontosarcoma, ameloblastic C41.1
  upper jaw (bone) C41.0
Oestriasis — see Myiasis
Oguchi's disease H53.63
Ohara's disease — see Tularemia
Oidiomycosis — see Candidiasis
Oidium albicans infection — see
  Candidiasis
Old age (without mention of debility) R54
  dementia F03
Old (previous) myocardial infarction I25.2
Olfactory — see condition
Oligemia — see Anemia
Oligoastrocytoma
  specified site — see Neoplasm, malignant,
    by site
  unspecified site C71.9
Oligocythemia D64.9
Oligodendroblastoma
  specified site — see Neoplasm, malignant
  unspecified site C71.9
Oligodendroglioma
  anaplastic type
    specified site — see Neoplasm,
      malignant, by site
    unspecified site C71.9
  specified site — see Neoplasm, malignant,
    by site
  unspecified site C71.9
Oligodontia — see Anodontia
Oligoencephalon Q02
Oligohidrosis L74.4
Oligohydramnios O41.0-
Oligohydrosis L74.4
Oligomenorrhea N91.5
  primary N91.3
  secondary N91.4
Oligophrenia — see also Disability,
  intellectual
  phenylpyruvic E70.0
Oligospermia N46.11
  due to
    drug therapy N46.121
    efferent duct obstruction N46.123
    infection N46.122
    radiation N46.124
    specified cause NEC N46.129
    systemic disease N46.125
Oligotrichia — see Alopecia
Oliguria R34
  postprocedural N99.0
  with, complicating or following ectopic or
    molar pregnancy O08.4
Ollier's disease Q78.4
Omenotocele — see Hernia, abdomen,
  specified site NEC
Omentitis — see Peritonitis
Omentum, omental — see condition
Omphalitis (congenital) (newborn) P38.9
  with mild hemorrhage P38.1
  not of newborn L08.82
  tetanus A33
  without hemorrhage P38.9
Omphalocele Q79.2
Omphalomesenteric duct, persistent Q43.0
Omphalorrhagia, newborn P51.9
Onanism (excessive) F98.8
Onchocerciasis, onchocercosis B73.1
  with
    eye disease B73.00
      endophthalmitis B73.01
      eyelid B73.09
      glaucoma B73.02
      specified NEC B73.09
    eye NEC B73.00
    eyelid B73.09
Oncocytoma — see Neoplasm, benign, by
  site
Oncovirus, as cause of disease classified
  elsewhere B97.32
Ondine's curse — see Apnea, sleep
Oneirophrenia F23
Onychauxis L60.2
  congenital Q84.5
Onychia — see also Cellulitis, digit
  with lymphangitis — see Lymphangitis,
    acute, digit
  candidal B37.2
  dermatophytic B35.1

Onychitis — see also Cellulitis, digit
  with lymphangitis — see Lymphangitis,
    acute, digit
Onychocryptosis L60.0
Onychodystrophy L60.3
  congenital Q84.6
Onychogryphosis, onychogryposis L60.2
Onycholysis L60.1
Onychomadesis L60.8
Onychomalacia L60.3
Onychomycosis (finger) (toe) B35.1
Onycho-osteodysplasia Q79.8
Onychophagia F98.8
Onychophosis L60.8
Onychoptosis L60.8
Onychorrhexis L60.3
  congenital Q84.6
Onychoschizia L60.3
Onyxis (finger) (toe) L60.0
Onyxitis — see also Cellulitis, digit
  with lymphangitis — see Lymphangitis,
    acute, digit
Oophoritis (cystic) (infectional) (interstitial)
  N70.92
  with salpingitis N70.93
  acute N70.02
    with salpingitis N70.03
  chronic N70.12
    with salpingitis N70.13
  complicating abortion — see Abortion, by
    type, complicated by, oophoritis
Oophorocele N83.4
Opacity, opacities
  cornea H17-
    central H17.1-
    congenital Q13.3
    degenerative — see Degeneration,
      cornea
    hereditary — see Dystrophy, cornea
    inflammatory — see Keratitis
    minor H17.81-
    peripheral H17.82-
    sequelae of trachoma (healed) B94.0
    specified NEC H17.89
  enamel (teeth) (fluoride) (nonfluoride)
    K00.3
  lens — see Cataract
  snowball — see Deposit, crystalline
  vitreous (humor) NEC H43.39-
    congenital Q14.0
    membranes and strands H43.31-
Opalescent dentin (hereditary) K00.5
Open, opening
  abnormal, organ or site, congenital — see
    Imperfect, closure
  angle with
    borderline
      findings
        high risk H40.02-
        low risk H40.01-
      intraocular pressure H40.00-
    cupping of discs H40.01-
    glaucoma (primary) — see Glaucoma,
      open angle
  bite
    anterior M26.220
    posterior M26.221
  false — see Imperfect, closure
  margin on tooth restoration K08.51
  restoration margins of tooth K08.51
  wound — see Wound, open
Operational fatigue F48.8
Operative — see condition
Operculitis — see Periodontitis
Operculum — see Break, retina
Ophiasis L63.2
Ophthalmia (see also Conjunctivitis) H10.9
  actinic rays — see Photokeratitis
  allergic (acute) — see Conjunctivitis, acute,
    atopic
  blennorrhagic (gonococcal) (neonatorum)
    A54.31
  diphtheritic A36.86
  Egyptian A71.1
  electrica — see Photokeratitis
  gonococcal (neonatorum) A54.31
  metastatic — see Endophthalmitis, purulent
  migraine — see Migraine, ophthalmoplegic
  neonatorum, newborn P39.1
    gonococcal A54.31
  nodosa H16.24-
  purulent — see Conjunctivitis, acute,
    mucopurulent
  spring — see Conjunctivitis, acute, atopic
  sympathetic — see Uveitis, sympathetic
Ophthalmitis — see Ophthalmia
Ophthalmocele (congenital) Q15.8
Ophthalmoneuromyelitis G36.0

Ophthalmoplegia — see also Strabismus,
  paralytic
  anterior internuclear — see
    Ophthalmoplegia, internuclear
  ataxia-areflexia G61.0
  diabetic — see E08-E13 with .39
  exophthalmic E05.00
    with thyroid storm E05.01
  external H49.88-
    progressive H49.4-
      with pigmentary retinopathy — see
        Kearns-Sayre syndrome
    total H49.3-
  internal (complete) (total) H52.51-
  internuclear H51.2-
  migraine — see Migraine, ophthalmoplegic
  Parinaud's H49.88-
  progressive external — see
    Ophthalmoplegia, external,
    progressive
  supranuclear, progressive G23.1
  total (external) — see Ophthalmoplegia,
    external, total
Opioid(s)
  abuse — see Abuse, drug, opioids
  dependence — see Dependence, drug,
    opioids
Opisthognathism M26.09
Opisthorchiasis (felineus) (viverrini) B66.0
Opitz' disease D73.2
Opium — see Dependence, drug, opioid
Opiumism — see Dependence, drug, opioid
Oppenheim's disease G70.2
Oppenheim-Urbach disease (necrobiosis
  lipoidica diabeticorum) — see E08-E13
  with .620
Optic nerve — see condition
Orbit — see condition
Orchioblastoma C62.9-
Orchitis (gangrenous) (nonspecific) (septic)
  (suppurative) N45.2
  blennorrhagic (gonococcal) (acute)
    (chronic) A54.23
  chlamydial A56.19
  filarial (see also Infestation, filarial) B74.9
    [N51]
  gonococcal (acute) (chronic) A54.23
  mumps B26.0
  syphilitic A52.76
  tuberculous A18.15
Orf (virus disease) B08.02
Organic — see also condition
  brain syndrome F09
  heart — see Disease, heart
  mental disorder F09
  psychosis F09
Orgasm
  anejaculatory N53.13
Oriental
  bilharziasis B65.2
  schistosomiasis B65.2
Orifice — see condition
Origin of both great vessels from right
  ventricle Q20.1
Ormond's disease (with ureteral obstruction)
  N13.5
  with infection N13.6
Ornithine metabolism disorder E72.4
Ornithinemia (Type I) (Type II) E72.4
Ornithosis A70
Orotaciduria, oroticaciduria (congenital)
  (hereditary) (pyrimidine deficiency)
  E79.8
  anemia D53.0
Orthodontics
  adjustment Z46.4
  fitting Z46.4
Orthopnea R06.01
Orthopoxvirus B08.09
  specified NEC B08.09
Os, uterus — see condition
Osgood-Schlatter disease or
  osteochondrosis — see
    Osteochondrosis, juvenile, tibia
Osler's nodes I33.0
Osler(-Weber)-Rendu disease I78.0
Osmidrosis L75.0
Osseous — see condition
Ossification
  artery — see Arteriosclerosis
  auricle (ear) — see Disorder, pinna,
    specified type NEC
  bronchial J98.09
  cardiac — see Degeneration, myocardial
  cartilage (senile) — see Disorder, cartilage,
    specified type NEC
  coronary (artery) — see Disease, heart,
    ischemic, atherosclerotic
  diaphragm J98.6
  ear, middle — see Otosclerosis
  falx cerebri G96.19

Ossification — continued
  fontanel, premature Q75.0
  heart — see also Degeneration, myocardial
    valve — see Endocarditis
  larynx J38.7
  ligament — see Disorder, tendon, specified
    type NEC
    posterior longitudinal — see
      Spondylopathy, specified NEC
  meninges (cerebral) (spinal) G96.19
  multiple, eccentric centers — see Disorder,
    bone, development or growth
  muscle — see also Calcification, muscle
    due to burns — see Myositis, ossificans,
      in, burns
    paralytic — see Myositis, ossificans, in,
      quadriplegia
    progressive — see Myositis, ossificans,
      progressiva
    specified NEC M61.50
      ankle M61.57-
      foot M61.57-
      forearm M61.53-
      hand M61.54-
      lower leg M61.56-
      multiple sites M61.59
      pelvic region M61.55-
      shoulder region M61.51-
      specified site NEC M61.58
      thigh M61.55-
      upper arm M61.52-
    traumatic — see Myositis, ossificans,
      traumatica
  myocardium, myocardial — see
    Degeneration, myocardial
  penis N48.89
  periarticular — see Disorder, joint,
    specified type NEC
  pinna — see Disorder, pinna, specified type
    NEC
  rider's bone — see Ossification, muscle,
    specified NEC
  sclera H15.89
  subperiosteal, post-traumatic M89.8x-
  tendon — see Disorder, tendon, specified
    type NEC
  trachea J39.8
  tympanic membrane — see Disorder,
    tympanic membrane, specified NEC
  vitreous (humor) — see Deposit, crystalline
Osteitis — see also Osteomyelitis
  alveolar M27.3
  condensans M85.30
    ankle M85.37-
    foot M85.37-
    forearm M85.33-
    hand M85.34-
    lower leg M85.36-
    multiple site M85.39
    neck M85.38
    rib M85.38
    shoulder M85.31-
    skull M85.38
    specified site NEC M85.38
    thigh M85.35-
    toe M85.37-
    upper arm M85.32-
    vertebra M85.38
  deformans M88.9
    in (due to)
      malignant neoplasm of bone C41.9
        [M90.60]
      neoplastic disease (see also
        Neoplasm) D49.9 [M90.60]
        carpus D49.9 [M90.6-]
        clavicle D49.9 [M90.6-]
        femur D49.9 [M90.6-]
        fibula D49.9 [M90.6-]
        finger D49.9 [M90.6-]
        humerus D49.9 [M90.6-]
        ilium D49.9 [M90.6-]
        ischium D49.9 [M90.6-]
        metacarpus D49.9 [M90.6-]
        metatarsus D49.9 [M90.6-]
        multiple sites D49.9 [M90.69]
        neck D49.9 [M90.68]
        radius D49.9 [M90.6-]
        rib D49.9 [M90.68]
        scapula D49.9 [M90.6-]
        skull D49.9 [M90.68]
        tarsus D49.9 [M90.6-]
        tibia D49.9 [M90.6-]
        toe D49.9 [M90.6-]
        ulna D49.9 [M90.6-]
        vertebra D49.9 [M90.68]
    skull M88.0
    specified NEC — see Paget's disease,
      bone, by site
    vertebra M88.1

DISEASE INDEX

Osteitis (see also Osteomyelitis) — continued
due to yaws A66.6
fibrosa NEC — see Cyst, bone, by site
circumscripta — see Dysplasia, fibrous, bone NEC
cystica (generalisata) E21.0
disseminata Q78.1
osteoplastica E21.0
fragilitans Q78.0
Garré's (sclerosing) — see Osteomyelitis, specified type NEC
jaw (acute) (chronic) (lower) (suppurative) (upper) M27.2
parathyroid E21.0
petrous bone (acute) (chronic) — see Petrositis
sclerotic, nonsuppurative — see Osteomyelitis, specified type NEC
tuberculosa A18.09
cystica D86.89
multiplex cystoides D86.89
Osteoarthritis M19.90
ankle M19.07-
elbow M19.02-
foot joint M19.07-
generalized M15.9
erosive M15.4
primary M15.0
specified NEC M15.8
hand joint M19.04-
first carpometacarpal joint M18.9
hip M16.1-
bilateral M16.0
due to hip dysplasia (unilateral) M16.3-
bilateral M16.2
interphalangeal
distal (Heberden) M15.1
proximal (Bouchard) M15.2
knee M17.9
bilateral M17.0
post-traumatic NEC M19.92
ankle M19.17-
elbow M19.12-
foot joint M19.17-
hand joint M19.14-
first carpometacarpal joint M18.3-
bilateral M18.2
hip M16.5-
bilateral M16.4
knee M17.3-
bilateral M17.2
shoulder M19.11-
wrist M19.13-
primary M19.91
ankle M19.07-
elbow M19.02-
foot joint M19.07-
hand joint M19.04-
first carpometacarpal joint M18.1-
bilateral M18.0
hip M16.1-
bilateral M16.0
knee M17.1-
bilateral M17.0
shoulder M19.01-
spine — see Spondylosis
wrist M19.03-
secondary M19.93
ankle M19.27-
elbow M19.22-
foot joint M19.27-
hand joint M19.24-
first carpometacarpal joint M18.5-
bilateral M18.4
hip M16.7
bilateral M16.6
knee M17.5
bilateral M17.4
multiple M15.3
shoulder M19.21-
spine — see Spondylosis
wrist M19.23-
shoulder M19.01-
spine — see Spondylosis
wrist M19.03-
Osteoarthropathy (hypertrophic) M19.90
ankle — see Osteoarthritis, primary, ankle
elbow — see Osteoarthritis, primary, elbow
foot joint — see Osteoarthritis, primary, foot
hand joint — see Osteoarthritis, primary, hand joint
knee joint — see Osteoarthritis, primary, knee

Osteoarthropathy (hypertrophic) M19.90 — continued
multiple site — see Osteoarthritis, primary, multiple joint
pulmonary — see also Osteoarthropathy, specified type NEC
hypertrophic — see Osteoarthropathy, hypertrophic, specified type NEC
secondary — see Osteoarthropathy, specified type NEC
secondary hypertrophic — see Osteoarthropathy, specified type NEC
shoulder — see Osteoarthritis, primary, shoulder
specified joint NEC — see Osteoarthritis, primary, specified joint NEC
specified type NEC M89.40
carpus M89.44-
clavicle M89.41-
femur M89.45-
fibula M89.46-
finger M89.44-
humerus M89.42-
ilium M89.459
ischium M89.459
metacarpus M89.44-
metatarsus M89.47-
multiple sites M89.49
neck M89.48
radius M89.43-
rib M89.48
scapula M89.41-
skull M89.48
tarsus M89.47-
tibia M89.46-
toe M89.47-
ulna M89.43-
vertebra M89.48
spine — see Spondylosis
wrist — see Osteoarthritis, primary, wrist
Osteoarthrosis (degenerative) (hypertrophic) (joint) — see also Osteoarthritis
deformans alkaptonurica E70.29 [M36.8]
erosive M15.4
generalized M15.9
primary M15.0
polyarticular M15.9
spine — see Spondylosis
Osteoblastoma — see Neoplasm, bone, benign
aggressive — see Neoplasm, bone, uncertain behavior
Osteochondritis — see also Osteochondropathy, by site
Brailsford's — see Osteochondrosis, juvenile, radius
dissecans M93.20
ankle M93.27-
elbow M93.22-
foot M93.27-
hand M93.24-
hip M93.25-
knee M93.26-
multiple sites M93.29
shoulder joint M93.21-
specified site NEC M93.28
wrist M93.23-
juvenile M92.9
patellar — see Osteochondrosis, juvenile, patella
syphilitic (congenital) (early) A50.02 [M90.80]
ankle A50.02 [M90.8-]
elbow A50.02 [M90.8-]
foot A50.02 [M90.8-]
forearm A50.02 [M90.8-]
hand A50.02 [M90.8-]
hip A50.02 [M90.8-]
knee A50.02 [M90.8-]
multiple sites A50.02 [M90.89]
shoulder joint A50.02 [M90.8-]
specified site NEC A50.02 [M90.88]
Osteochondroarthrosis deformans endemica — see Disease, Kaschin-Beck
Osteochondrodysplasia Q78.9
with defects of growth of tubular bones and spine Q77.9
specified NEC Q77.8
specified NEC Q78.8
Osteochondrodystrophy E78.9
Osteochondrolysis — see Osteochondritis, dissecans
Osteochondroma — see Neoplasm, bone, benign
Osteochondromatosis D48.0
syndrome Q78.4

Osteochondromyxosarcoma — see Neoplasm, bone, malignant
Osteochondropathy M93.90
ankle M93.97-
elbow M93.92-
foot M93.97-
hand M93.94-
hip M93.95-
Kienböck's disease of adults M93.1
knee M93.96-
multiple joints M93.99
osteochondritis dissecans — see Osteochondritis, dissecans
osteochondrosis — see Osteochondrosis
shoulder region M93.91-
slipped upper femoral epiphysis — see Slipped, epiphysis, upper femoral
specified joint NEC M93.98
specified type NEC M93.80
ankle M93.87-
elbow M93.82-
foot M93.87-
hand M93.84-
hip M93.85-
knee M93.86-
multiple joints M93.89
shoulder region M93.81-
specified joint NEC M93.88
wrist M93.83-
syphilitic, congenital
early A50.02 [M90.80]
late A50.56 [M90.80]
wrist M93.93-
Osteochondrosarcoma — see Neoplasm, bone, malignant
Osteochondrosis — see also Osteochondropathy, by site
acetabulum (juvenile) M91.0
adult — see Osteochondropathy, specified type NEC, by site
astragalus (juvenile) — see Osteochondrosis, juvenile, tarsus
Blount's — see Osteochondrosis, juvenile, tibia
Buchanan's M91.0
Burns' — see Osteochondrosis, juvenile, ulna
calcaneus (juvenile) — see Osteochondrosis, juvenile, tarsus
capitular epiphysis (femur) (juvenile) — see Legg-Calvé-Perthes disease
carpal (juvenile) (lunate) (scaphoid) — see Osteochondrosis, juvenile, hand, carpal lunate
adult M93.1
coxae juvenilis — see Legg-Calvé-Perthes disease
deformans juvenilis, coxae — see Legg-Calvé-Perthes disease
Diaz's — see Osteochondrosis, juvenile, tarsus
dissecans (knee) (shoulder) — see Osteochondritis, dissecans
femoral capital epiphysis (juvenile) — see Legg-Calvé-Perthes disease
femur (head), juvenile — see Legg-Calvé-Perthes disease
fibula (juvenile) — see Osteochondrosis, juvenile, fibula
foot NEC (juvenile) M92.8
Freiberg's — see Osteochondrosis, juvenile, metatarsus
Haas' (juvenile) — see Osteochondrosis, juvenile, humerus
Haglund's — see Osteochondrosis, juvenile, tarsus
hip (juvenile) — see Legg-Calvé-Perthes disease
humerus (capitulum) (head) (juvenile) — see Osteochondrosis, juvenile, humerus
ilium, iliac crest (juvenile) M91.0
ischiopubic synchondrosis M91.0
Iselin's — see Osteochondrosis, juvenile, metatarsus
juvenile, juvenilis M92.9
after congenital dislocation of hip reduction — see Osteochondrosis, juvenile, hip, specified NEC
arm — see Osteochondrosis, juvenile, upper limb NEC
capitular epiphysis (femur) — see Legg-Calvé-Perthes disease
clavicle, sternal epiphysis — see Osteochondrosis, juvenile, upper limb NEC

Osteochondrosis (see also Osteochondropathy, by site) — continued
juvenile, juvenilis M92.9 — continued
coxae — see Legg-Calvé-Perthes disease
deformans M92.9
fibula M92.5-
foot NEC M92.8
hand M92.20-
carpal lunate M92.21-
metacarpal head M92.22-
specified site NEC M92.29-
head of femur — see Legg-Calvé-Perthes disease
hip and pelvis M91.9-
coxa plana — see Coxa, plana
femoral head — see Legg-Calvé-Perthes disease
pelvis M91.0
pseudocoxalgia — see Pseudocoxalgia
specified NEC M91.8-
humerus M92.0-
limb
lower NEC M92.8
upper NEC — see Osteochondrosis, juvenile, upper limb NEC
medial cuneiform bone — see Osteochondrosis, juvenile, tarsus
metatarsus M92.7-
patella M92.4-
radius M92.1-
specified site NEC M92.8
spine M42.00
cervical region M42.02
cervicothoracic region M42.03
lumbar region M42.06
lumbosacral region M42.07
multiple sites M42.09
occipito-atlanto-axial region M42.01
sacrococcygeal region M42.08
thoracic region M42.04
thoracolumbar region M42.05
tarsus M92.6-
tibia M92.5-
ulna M92.1-
upper limb NEC M92.3-
vertebra (body) (epiphyseal plates) (Calvé's) (Scheuermann's) — see Osteochondrosis, juvenile, spine
Kienböck's — see Osteochondrosis, juvenile, hand, carpal lunate
adult M93.1
Köhler's
patellar — see Osteochondrosis, juvenile, patella
tarsal navicular — see Osteochondrosis, juvenile, tarsus
Legg-Perthes(-Calvé)(-Waldenström) — see Legg-Calvé-Perthes disease
limb
lower NEC (juvenile) M92.8
upper NEC (juvenile) — see Osteochondrosis, juvenile, upper limb NEC
lunate bone (carpal) (juvenile) — see also Osteochondrosis, juvenile, hand, carpal lunate
adult M93.1
Mauclaire's — see Osteochondrosis, juvenile, hand, metacarpal
metacarpal (head) (juvenile) — see Osteochondrosis, juvenile, hand, metacarpal
metatarsus (fifth) (head) (juvenile) (second) — see Osteochondrosis, juvenile, metatarsus
navicular (juvenile) — see Osteochondrosis, juvenile, tarsus
os
calcis (juvenile) — see Osteochondrosis, juvenile, tarsus
tibiale externum (juvenile) — see Osteochondrosis, juvenile, tarsus
Osgood-Schlatter — see Osteochondrosis, juvenile, tibia
Panner's — see Osteochondrosis, juvenile, humerus
patellar center (juvenile) (primary) (secondary) — see Osteochondrosis, juvenile, patella
pelvis (juvenile) M91.0
Pierson's M91.0
radius (head) (juvenile) — see Osteochondrosis, juvenile, radius
Scheuermann's — see Osteochondrosis, juvenile, spine
Sever's — see Osteochondrosis, juvenile, tarsus

© 2013 Channel Publishing Ltd

Osteochondrosis *(see also*
   Osteochondropathy, by site) —
   continued
  Sinding-Larsen — *see* Osteochondrosis,
    juvenile, patella
  spine M42.9
   adult M42.10
    cervical region M42.12
    cervicothoracic region M42.13
    lumbar region M42.16
    lumbosacral region M42.17
    multiple sites M42.19
    occipito-atlanto-axial region M42.11
    sacrococcygeal region M42.18
    thoracic region M42.14
    thoracolumbar region M42.15
   juvenile — *see* Osteochondrosis, .
    juvenile, spine
  symphysis pubis (juvenile) M91.0
  syphilitic (congenital) A50.02
  talus (juvenile) — *see* Osteochondrosis,
   juvenile, talus
  tarsus (navicular) (juvenile) — *see*
   Osteochondrosis, juvenile, tarsus
  tibia (proximal) (tubercle) (juvenile) — *see*
   Osteochondrosis, juvenile, tibia
  tuberculous — *see* Tuberculosis, bone
  ulna (lower) (juvenile) — *see*
   Osteochondrosis, juvenile, ulna
  van Neck's M91.0
  vertebral — *see* Osteochondrosis, spine
Osteoclastoma D48.0
  malignant — *see* Neoplasm, bone,
   malignant
Osteodynia — *see* Disorder, bone, specified
  type NEC
Osteodystrophy Q78.9
  azotemic N25.0
  congenital Q78.9
  parathyroid, secondary E21.1
  renal N25.0
Osteofibroma — *see* Neoplasm, bone, benign
Osteofibrosarcoma — *see* Neoplasm, bone,
  malignant
Osteogenesis imperfecta Q78.0
Osteogenic — *see* condition
Osteolysis M89.50
  carpus M89.54-
  clavicle M89.51-
  femur M89.55-
  fibula M89.56-
  finger M89.54-
  humerus M89.52-
  ilium M89.559
  ischium M89.559
  joint prosthesis (periprosthetic) — *see*
   Complications, joint prosthesis,
   mechanical, periprosthetic, osteolysis,
   by site
  metacarpus M89.54-
  metatarsus M89.57-
  multiple sites M89.59
  neck M89.58
  periprosthetic — *see* Complications, joint
   prosthesis, mechanical, periprosthetic,
   osteolysis, by site
  radius M89.53-
  rib M89.58
  scapula M89.51-
  skull M89.58
  tarsus M89.57-
  tibia M89.56-
  toe M89.57-
  ulna M89.53-
  vertebra M89.58
Osteoma — *see also* Neoplasm, bone, benign
  osteoid — *see also* Neoplasm, bone, benign
   giant — *see* Neoplasm, bone, benign
Osteomalacia M83.9
  adult M83.9
   drug-induced NEC M83.5
   due to
    malabsorption (postsurgical) M83.2
    malnutrition M83.3
   specified NEC M83.8
  aluminium-induced M83.4
  infantile — *see* Rickets
  juvenile — *see* Rickets
  oncogenic E83.89
  pelvis M83.8
  puerperal M83.0
  senile M83.1

Osteomalacia M83.9 — *continued*
  vitamin-D-resistant in adults E83.31
   [M90.-]
   carpus E83.31 [M90.8-]
   clavicle E83.31 [M90.8-]
   femur E83.31 [M90.8-]
   fibula E83.31 [M90.8-]
   finger E83.31 [M90.8-]
   humerus E83.31 [M90.8-]
   ilium E83.31 [M90.859]
   ischium E83.31 [M90.859]
   metacarpus E83.31 [M90.8-]
   metatarsus E83.31 [M90.8-]
   multiple sites E83.31 [M90.89]
   neck E83.31 [M90.88]
   radius E83.31 [M90.8-]
   rib E83.31 [M90.88]
   scapula E83.31 [M90.819]
   skull E83.31 [M90.88]
   tarsus E83.31 [M90.879]
   tibia E83.31 [M90.869]
   toe E83.31 [M90.879]
   ulna E83.31 [M90.839]
   vertebra E83.31 [M90.88]
Osteomyelitis (general) (infective)
  (localized) (neonatal) (purulent) (septic)
  (staphylococcal) (streptococcal)
  (suppurative) (with periostitis) M86.9
  acute M86.10
   carpus M86.14-
   clavicle M86.11-
   femur M86.15-
   fibula M86.16-
   finger M86.14-
   hematogenous M86.00
    carpus M86.04-
    clavicle M86.01-
    femur M86.05-
    fibula M86.06-
    finger M86.04-
    humerus M86.02-
    ilium M86.059
    ischium M86.059
    mandible M27.2
    metacarpus M86.04-
    metatarsus M86.07-
    multiple sites M86.09
    neck M86.08
    orbit H05.02-
    petrous bone — *see* Petrositis
    radius M86.03-
    rib M86.08
    scapula M86.01-
    skull M86.08
    tarsus M86.07-
    tibia M86.06-
    toe M86.07-
    ulna M86.03-
    vertebra — *see* Osteomyelitis,
     vertebra
   humerus M86.12-
   ilium M86.159
   ischium M86.159
   mandible M27.2
   metacarpus M86.14-
   metatarsus M86.17-
   multiple sites M86.19
   neck M86.18
   orbit H05.02-
   petrous bone — *see* Petrositis
   radius M86.13-
   rib M86.18
   scapula M86.11-
   skull M86.18
   tarsus M86.17-
   tibia M86.16-
   toe M86.17-
   ulna M86.13-
   vertebra — *see* Osteomyelitis, vertebra
  chronic (or old) M86.60
   with draining sinus M86.40
    carpus M86.44-
    clavicle M86.41-
    femur M86.45-
    fibula M86.46-
    finger M86.44-
    humerus M86.42-
    ilium M86.459
    ischium M86.459
    mandible M27.2
    metacarpus M86.44-
    metatarsus M86.47-
    multiple sites M86.49
    neck M86.48
    orbit H05.02-
    petrous bone — *see* Petrositis
    radius M86.43-

Osteomyelitis (general) (infective)
  (localized) (neonatal) (purulent) (septic)
  (staphylococcal) (streptococcal)
  (suppurative) (with periostitis) M86.9 —
  continued
  chronic (or old) M86.60 — *continued*
   with draining sinus M86.40 — *continued*
    rib M86.48
    scapula M86.41-
    skull M86.48
    tarsus M86.47-
    tibia M86.46-
    toe M86.47-
    ulna M86.43-
    vertebra — *see* Osteomyelitis,
     vertebra
   carpus M86.64-
   clavicle M86.61-
   femur M86.65-
   fibula M86.66-
   finger M86.64-
   hematogenous NEC M86.50
    carpus M86.54-
    clavicle M86.51-
    femur M86.55-
    fibula M86.56-
    finger M86.54-
    humerus M86.52-
    ilium M86.559
    ischium M86.559
    mandible M27.2
    metacarpus M86.54-
    metatarsus M86.57-
    multifocal M86.30
     carpus M86.34-
     clavicle M86.31-
     femur M86.35-
     fibula M86.36-
     finger M86.34-
     humerus M86.32-
     ilium M86.359
     ischium M86.359
     metacarpus M86.34-
     metatarsus M86.37-
     multiple sites M86.39
     neck M86.38
     radius M86.33-
     rib M86.38
     scapula M86.31-
     skull M86.38
     tarsus M86.37-
     tibia M86.36-
     toe M86.37-
     ulna M86.33-
     vertebra — *see* Osteomyelitis,
      vertebra
    multiple sites M86.59
    neck M86.58
    orbit H05.02-
    petrous bone — *see* Petrositis
    radius M86.53-
    rib M86.58
    scapula M86.51-
    skull M86.58
    tarsus M86.57-
    tibia M86.56-
    toe M86.57-
    ulna M86.53-
    vertebra — *see* Osteomyelitis,
     vertebra
   humerus M86.62-
   ilium M86.659
   ischium M86.659
   mandible M27.2
   metacarpus M86.64-
   metatarsus M86.67-
   multifocal — *see* Osteomyelitis, chronic,
    hematogenous, multifocal
   multiple sites M86.69
   neck M86.68
   orbit H05.02-
   petrous bone — *see* Petrositis
   radius M86.63-
   rib M86.68
   scapula M86.61-
   skull M86.68
   tarsus M86.67-
   tibia M86.66-
   toe M86.67-
   ulna M86.63-
   vertebra — *see* Osteomyelitis, vertebra
  echinococcal B67.2
  Garr's — *see* Osteomyelitis, specified type
   NEC
  jaw (acute) (chronic) (lower) (neonatal)
   (suppurative) (upper) M27.2
  nonsuppurating — *see* Osteomyelitis,
   specified type NEC

Osteomyelitis (general) (infective)
  (localized) (neonatal) (purulent) (septic)
  (staphylococcal) (streptococcal)
  (suppurative) (with periostitis) M86.9 —
  continued
  orbit H05.02-
  petrous bone — *see* Petrositis
  Salmonella (arizonae) (cholerae-suis)
   (enteritidis) (typhimurium) A02.24
  sclerosing, nonsuppurative — *see*
   Osteomyelitis, specified type NEC
  specified type NEC *(see also* subcategory)
   M86.8x-
   mandible M27.2
   orbit H05.02-
   petrous bone — *see* Petrositis
   vertebra — *see* Osteomyelitis, vertebra
  subacute M86.20
   carpus M86.24-
   clavicle M86.21-
   femur M86.25-
   fibula M86.26-
   finger M86.24-
   humerus M86.22-
   mandible M27.2
   metacarpus M86.24-
   metatarsus M86.27-
   multiple sites M86.29
   neck M86.28
   orbit H05.02-
   petrous bone — *see* Petrositis
   radius M86.23-
   rib M86.28
   scapula M86.21-
   skull M86.28
   tarsus M86.27-
   tibia M86.26-
   toe M86.27-
   ulna M86.23-
   vertebra — *see* Osteomyelitis, vertebra
  syphilitic A52.77
   congenital (early) A50.02 [M90.80]
  tuberculous — *see* Tuberculosis, bone
  typhoid A01.05
  vertebra M46.20
   cervical region M46.22
   cervicothoracic region M46.23
   lumbar region M46.26
   lumbosacral region M46.27
   occipito-atlanto-axial region M46.21
   sacrococcygeal region M46.28
   thoracic region M46.24
   thoracolumbar region M46.25
Osteomyelofibrosis D75.89
Osteomyelosclerosis D75.89
Osteonecrosis M87.9
  due to
   drugs — *see* Osteonecrosis, secondary,
    due to, drugs
   trauma — *see* Osteonecrosis, secondary,
    due to, trauma
  idiopathic aseptic M87.00
   ankle M87.07-
   carpus M87.03-
   clavicle M87.01-
   femur M87.05-
   fibula M87.06-
   finger M87.04-
   humerus M87.02-
   ilium M87.050
   ischium M87.050
   metacarpus M87.04-
   metatarsus M87.07-
   multiple sites M87.09
   neck M87.08
   pelvis M87.050
   radius M87.03-
   rib M87.08
   scapula M87.01-
   skull M87.08
   tarsus M87.07-
   tibia M87.06-
   toe M87.07-
   ulna M87.03-
   vertebra M87.08
  secondary NEC M87.30
   carpus M87.33-
   clavicle M87.31-
   due to
    drugs M87.10
     carpus M87.13-
     clavicle M87.11-
     femur M87.15-
     fibula M87.16-
     finger M87.14-
     humerus M87.12-
     ilium M87.159

DISEASE INDEX

Osteonecrosis M87.9 — *continued*
  secondary NEC M87.30 — *continued*
    due to — *continued*
      drugs M87.10
        ischium M87.159
        jaw M87.180
        metacarpus M87.14-
        metatarsus M87.17-
        multiple sites M87.19
        neck M87.18
        radius M87.13-
        rib M87.18
        scapula M87.11-
        skull M87.18
        tarsus M87.17-
        tibia M87.16-
        toe M87.17-
        ulna M87.13-
        vertebra M87.18
      hemoglobinopathy NEC D58.2 [M90.50]
        carpus D58.2 [M90.5-]
        clavicle D58.2 [M90.5-]
        femur D58.2 [M90.5-]
        fibula D58.2 [M90.5-]
        finger D58.2 [M90.5-]
        humerus D58.2 [M90.5-]
        ilium D58.2 [M90.5-]
        ischium D58.2 [M90.5-]
        metacarpus D58.2 [M90.5-]
        metatarsus D58.2 [M90.5-]
        multiple sites D58.2 [M90.58]
        neck D58.2 [M90.58]
        radius D58.2 [M90.5-]
        rib D58.2 [M90.58]
        scapula D58.2 [M90.5-]
        skull D58.2 [M90.58]
        tarsus D58.2 [M90.5-]
        tibia D58.2 [M90.5-]
        toe D58.2 [M90.5-]
        ulna D58.2 [M90.5-]
        vertebra D58.2 [M90.58]
      trauma (previous) M87.20
        carpus M87.23-
        clavicle M87.21-
        femur M87.25-
        fibula M87.26-
        finger M87.24-
        humerus M87.22-
        ilium M87.25-
        ischium M87.25-
        metacarpus M87.24-
        metatarsus M87.27-
        multiple sites M87.29
        neck M87.28
        radius M87.23-
        rib M87.28
        scapula M87.21-
        skull M87.28
        tarsus M87.27-
        tibia M87.26-
        toe M87.27-
        ulna M87.23-
        vertebra M87.28
      femur M87.35-
      fibula M87.36-
      finger M87.34-
      humerus M87.32-
      ilium M87.350
      in
        caisson disease T70.3 [M90.50]
          carpus T70.3 [M90.5-]
          clavicle T70.3 [M90.5-]
          femur T70.3 [M90.5-]
          fibula T70.3 [M90.5-]
          finger T70.3 [M90.5-]
          humerus T70.3 [M90.5-]
          ilium T70.3 [M90.5-]
          ischium T70.3 [M90.5-]
          metacarpus T70.3 [M90.5-]
          metatarsus T70.3 [M90.5-]
          multiple sites T70.3 [M90.59]
          neck T70.3 [M90.58]
          radius T70.3 [M90.5-]
          rib T70.3 [M90.58]
          scapula T70.3 [M90.5-]
          skull T70.3 [M90.58]
          tarsus T70.3 [M90.5-]
          tibia T70.3 [M90.5-]
          toe T70.3 [M90.5-]
          ulna T70.3 [M90.5-]
          vertebra T70.3 [M90.58]
      ischium M87.350
      metacarpus M87.34-
      metatarsus M87.37-

Osteonecrosis M87.9 — *continued*
  secondary NEC M87.30 — *continued*
    multiple site M87.39
    neck M87.38
    radius M87.33-
    rib M87.38
    scapula M87.319
    skull M87.38
    tarsus M87.379
    tibia M87.366
    toe M87.379
    ulna M87.33-
    vertebra M87.38
  specified type NEC M87.80
    carpus M87.83-
    clavicle M87.81-
    femur M87.85-
    fibula M87.86-
    finger M87.84-
    humerus M87.82-
    ilium M87.85-
    ischium M87.85-
    metacarpus M87.84-
    metatarsus M87.87-
    multiple sites M87.89
    neck M87.88
    radius M87.83-
    rib M87.88
    scapula M87.81-
    skull M87.88
    tarsus M87.87-
    tibia M87.86-
    toe M87.87-
    ulna M87.83-
    vertebra M87.88
Osteo-onycho-arthro-dysplasia Q79.8
Osteo-onychodysplasia, hereditary Q79.8
Osteopathia condensans disseminata Q78.8
Osteopathy — *see also* Osteomyelitis, Osteonecrosis, Osteoporosis
  after poliomyelitis M89.60
    carpus M89.64-
    clavicle M89.61-
    femur M89.65-
    fibula M89.66-
    finger M89.64-
    humerus M89.62-
    ilium M89.659
    ischium M89.659
    metacarpus M89.64-
    metatarsus M89.67-
    multiple sites M89.69
    neck M89.68
    radius M89.63-
    rib M89.68
    scapula M89.61-
    skull M89.68
    tarsus M89.67-
    tibia M89.66-
    toe M89.67-
    ulna M89.63-
    vertebra M89.68
  in (due to)
    renal osteodystrophy N25.0
    specified diseases classified elsewhere — *see subcategory* M90.8
Osteopenia M85.8-
  borderline M85.8-
Osteoperiostitis — *see* Osteomyelitis, specified type NEC
Osteopetrosis (familial) Q78.2
Osteophyte M25.70
  ankle M25.77-
  elbow M25.72-
  foot joint M25.77-
  hand joint M25.74-
  hip M25.75-
  knee M25.76-
  shoulder M25.71-
  spine M25.78
  vertebrae M25.78
  wrist M25.73-
Osteopoikilosis Q78.8
Osteoporosis (female) (male) M81.0
  with current pathological fracture M80.00
  age-related M81.0
    with current pathologic fracture M80.00
      carpus M80.04-
      clavicle M80.01-
      fibula M80.06-
      finger M80.04-
      humerus M80.02-
      ilium M80.05-
      ischium M80.05-
      metacarpus M80.04-
      metatarsus M80.07-

Osteoporosis (female) (male) M81.0 — *continued*
  age-related M81.0 — *continued*
    with current pathologic fracture M80.00 — *continued*
      pelvis M80.05-
      radius M80.03-
      scapula M80.01-
      tarsus M80.07-
      tibia M80.06-
      toe M80.07-
      ulna M80.03-
      vertebra M80.08
  disuse M81.8
    with current pathological fracture M80.80
      carpus M80.84-
      clavicle M80.81-
      fibula M80.86-
      finger M80.84-
      humerus M80.82-
      ilium M80.85-
      ischium M80.85-
      metacarpus M80.84-
      metatarsus M80.87-
      pelvis M80.85-
      radius M80.83-
      scapula M80.81-
      tarsus M80.87-
      tibia M80.86-
      toe M80.87-
      ulna M80.83-
      vertebra M80.88
  drug-induced — *see* Osteoporosis, specified type NEC
  idiopathic — *see* Osteoporosis, specified type NEC
  involutional — *see* Osteoporosis, age-related
  Lequesne M81.6
  localized M81.6
  post-traumatic — *see* Osteoporosis, specified type NEC
  postmenopausal M81.0
    with pathological fracture M80.00
      carpus M80.04-
      clavicle M80.01-
      fibula M80.06-
      finger M80.04-
      humerus M80.02-
      ilium M80.05-
      ischium M80.05-
      metacarpus M80.04-
      metatarsus M80.07-
      pelvis M80.05-
      radius M80.03-
      scapula M80.01-
      tarsus M80.07-
      tibia M80.06-
      toe M80.07-
      ulna M80.03-
      vertebra M80.08
  postoophorectomy — *see* Osteoporosis, specified type NEC
  postsurgical malabsorption — *see* Osteoporosis, specified type NEC
  senile — *see* Osteoporosis, age-related
  specified type NEC M81.8
    with pathological fracture M80.80
      carpus M80.84-
      clavicle M80.81-
      fibula M80.86-
      finger M80.84-
      humerus M80.82-
      ilium M80.85-
      ischium M80.85-
      metacarpus M80.84-
      metatarsus M80.87-
      pelvis M80.85-
      radius M80.83-
      scapula M80.81-
      tarsus M80.87-
      tibia M80.86-
      toe M80.87-
      ulna M80.83-
      vertebra M80.88
Osteopsathyrosis (idiopathica) Q78.0
Osteoradionecrosis, jaw (acute) (chronic) (lower) (suppurative) (upper) M27.2
Osteosarcoma (any form) — *see* Neoplasm, bone, malignant
Osteosclerosis Q78.2
  acquired M85.8-
  congenita Q77.4
  fragilitas (generalisata) Q78.2
  myelofibrosis D75.81
Osteosclerotic anemia D64.89

Osteosis
  cutis L94.2
  renal fibrocystic N25.0
Österreicher-Turner syndrome Q87.2
Ostium
  atrioventriculare commune Q21.2
  primum (arteriosum) (defect) (persistent) Q21.2
  secundum (arteriosum) (defect) (patent) (persistent) Q21.1
Ostrum-Furst syndrome Q75.8
Otalgia — *see subcategory* H92.0
Otitis (acute) H66.90
  with effusion — *see also* Otitis, media, nonsuppurative
    purulent — *see* Otitis, media, suppurative
  adhesive — *see subcategory* H74.1
  chronic — *see also* Otitis, media, chronic
    with effusion — *see also* Otitis, media, nonsuppurative, chronic
  externa H60.9-
    abscess — *see* Abscess, ear, external
    acute (noninfective) H60.50-
      actinic H60.51-
      chemical H60.52-
      contact H60.53-
      eczematoid H60.54-
      infective — *see* Otitis, externa, infective
      reactive H60.55-
      specified NEC H60.59-
    cellulitis — *see* Cellulitis, ear
    chronic H60.6-
    diffuse — *see* Otitis, externa, infective, diffuse
    hemorrhagic — *see* Otitis, externa, infective, hemorrhagic
    in (due to)
      aspergillosis B44.89
      candidiasis B37.84
      erysipelas A46 [H62.40]
      herpes (simplex) virus infection B00.1
        zoster B02.8
      impetigo L01.00 [H62.40]
      infectious disease NEC B99 [H62.-]
      mycosis NEC B36.9 [H62.40]
      parasitic disease NEC B89 [H62.40]
      viral disease NEC B34.9 [H62.40]
      zoster B02.8
    infective NEC H60.39-
      abscess — *see* Abscess, ear, external
      cellulitis — *see* Cellulitis, ear
      diffuse H60.31-
      hemorrhagic H60.32-
      swimmer's ear — *see* Swimmer's, ear
    malignant H60.2-
    mycotic B36.9 [H62.40]
    necrotizing — *see* Otitis, externa, malignant
    Pseudomonas aeruginosa — *see* Otitis, externa, malignant
    reactive — *see* Otitis, externa, acute, reactive
    specified NEC — *see subcategory* H60.8
    tropical B36.8
  insidiosa — *see* Otosclerosis
  interna — *see subcategory* H83.0
  media (hemorrhagic) (staphylococcal) (streptococcal) H66.9-
    with effusion (nonpurulent) — *see* Otitis, media, nonsuppurative
    acute, subacute H66.90
      allergic — *see* Otitis, media, nonsuppurative, acute, allergic
      exudative — *see* Otitis, media, nonsuppurative, acute
      mucoid — *see* Otitis, media, nonsuppurative, acute
      necrotizing — *see also* Otitis, media, suppurative, acute
      in
        measles B05.3
        scarlet fever A38.0
      nonsuppurative NEC — *see* Otitis, media, nonsuppurative, acute
      purulent — *see* Otitis, media, suppurative, acute
      sanguinous — *see* Otitis, media, nonsuppurative, acute
      secretory — *see* Otitis, media, nonsuppurative, acute, serous
      seromucinous — *see* Otitis, media, nonsuppurative, acute
      serous — *see* Otitis, media, nonsuppurative, acute, serous
      suppurative — *see* Otitis, media, suppurative, acute

Otitis (acute) H66.90 — *continued*
  media (hemorrhagic) (staphylococcal)
    (streptococcal) H66.9- — *continued*
    allergic — *see* Otitis, media,
      nonsuppurative
    catarrhal — *see* Otitis, media,
      nonsuppurative
    chronic H66.90
      with effusion (nonpurulent) — *see*
        Otitis, media, nonsuppurative,
        chronic
      allergic — *see* Otitis, media,
        nonsuppurative, chronic, allergic
      benign suppurative — *see* Otitis,
        media, suppurative, chronic,
        tubotympanic
      catarrhal — *see* Otitis, media,
        nonsuppurative, chronic, serous
      exudative — *see* Otitis, media,
        nonsuppurative, chronic
      mucinous — *see* Otitis, media,
        nonsuppurative, chronic, mucoid
      mucoid — *see* Otitis, media,
        nonsuppurative, chronic, mucoid
      nonsuppurative NEC — *see* Otitis,
        media, nonsuppurative, chronic
      purulent — *see* Otitis, media,
        suppurative, chronic
      secretory — *see* Otitis, media,
        nonsuppurative, chronic, mucoid
      seromucinous — *see* Otitis, media,
        nonsuppurative, chronic
      serous — *see* Otitis, media,
        nonsuppurative, chronic, serous
      suppurative — *see* Otitis, media,
        suppurative, chronic
      transudative — *see* Otitis, media,
        nonsuppurative, chronic, mucoid
    exudative — *see* Otitis, media,
      nonsuppurative
    in (due to) (with)
      influenza — *see* Influenza, with, otitis
        media
      measles B05.3
      scarlet fever A38.0
      tuberculosis A18.6
      viral disease NEC B34-[H67-]
    mucoid — *see* Otitis, media,
      nonsuppurative
    nonsuppurative H65.9-
      acute or subacute NEC H65.19-
        allergic H65.11-
          recurrent H65.11-
        recurrent H65.19-
        secretory — *see* Otitis, media,
          nonsuppurative, serous
        serous H65.0-
          recurrent H65.0-
      chronic H65.49-
        allergic H65.41-
        mucoid H65.3-
        serous H65.2-
      postmeasles B05.3
    purulent — *see* Otitis, media,
      suppurative
    secretory — *see* Otitis, media,
      nonsuppurative
    seromucinous — *see* Otitis, media,
      nonsuppurative
    serous — *see* Otitis, media,
      nonsuppurative
    suppurative H66.4-
      acute H66.00-
        with rupture of ear drum H66.01-
      recurrent H66.00-
        with rupture of ear drum
          H66.01-
      chronic (*see also* subcategory) H66.3
        atticoantral H66.2-
        benign — *see* Otitis, media,
          suppurative, chronic,
          tubotympanic
        tubotympanic H66.1-
      transudative — *see* Otitis, media,
        nonsuppurative
    tuberculous A18.6
Otocephaly Q18.2
Otolith syndrome — *see* subcategory H81.8
Otomycosis (diffuse) NEC B36.9 [H62.40]
  in
    aspergillosis B44.89
    candidiasis B37.84
    moniliasis B37.84
Otoporosis — *see* Otosclerosis
Otorrhagia (nontraumatic) H92.2-
  traumatic — *code by* Type of injury
Otorrhea H92.1-
  cerebrospinal G96.0

Otosclerosis (general) H80.9-
  cochlear (endosteal) H80.2-
  involving
    otic capsule — *see* Otosclerosis,
      cochlear
    oval window
      nonobliterative H80.0-
      obliterative H80.1-
    round window — *see* Otosclerosis,
      cochlear
  nonobliterative — *see* Otosclerosis,
    involving, oval window,
    nonobliterative
  obliterative — *see* Otosclerosis, involving,
    oval window, obliterative
  specified NEC H80.8-
Otospongiosis — *see* Otosclerosis
Otto's disease or pelvis M24.7
Outcome of delivery Z37.9
  multiple births Z37.9
    all liveborn Z37.50
      quadruplets Z37.52
      quintuplets Z37.53
      sextuplets Z37.54
      specified number NEC Z37.59
      triplets Z37.51
    all stillborn Z37.7
    some liveborn Z37.60
      quadruplets Z37.62
      quintuplets Z37.63
      sextuplets Z37.64
      specified number NEC Z37.69
      triplets Z37.61
  single NEC Z37.9
    liveborn Z37.0
    stillborn Z37.1
  twins NEC Z37.9
    both liveborn Z37.2
    both stillborn Z37.4
    one liveborn, one stillborn Z37.3
Outlet — *see* condition
Ovalocytosis (congenital) (hereditary) — *see*
  Elliptocytosis
Ovarian — *see* condition
Ovariocele N83.4
Ovaritis (cystic) — *see* Oophoritis
Ovary, ovarian — *see also* condition
  resistant syndrome E28.39
  vein syndrome N13.8
Overactive — *see also* Hyperfunction
  adrenal cortex NEC E27.0
  bladder N32.81
  hypothalamus E23.3
  thyroid — *see* Hyperthyroidism
Overactivity R46.3
  child — *see* Disorder, attention-deficit
    hyperactivity
Overbite (deep) (excessive) (horizontal)
  (vertical) M26.29
Overbreathing — *see* Hyperventilation
Overconscientious personality F60.5
Overdevelopment — *see* Hypertrophy
Overdistension — *see* Distension
Overdose, overdosage (drug) — *see* Table of
  Drugs and Chemicals, by drug,
  poisoning
Overeating R63.2
  nonorganic origin F50.8
  psychogenic F50.8
Overexertion (effects) (exhaustion) T73.3
Overexposure (effects) T73.9
  exhaustion T73.2
Overfeeding — *see* Overeating
  newborn P92.4
Overfill, endodontic M27.52
Overgrowth, bone — *see* Hypertrophy, bone
Overhanging of dental restorative material
  (unrepairable) K08.52
Overheated (places) (effects) — *see* Heat
Overjet (excessive horizontal) M26.23
Overlaid, overlying (suffocation) — *see*
  Asphyxia, traumatic, due to mechanical
  threat
Overlap, excessive horizontal (teeth)
  M26.23
Overlapping toe (acquired) — *see also*
  Deformity, toe, specified NEC
  congenital (fifth toe) Q66.89
Overload
  circulatory, due to transfusion (blood)
    (blood components) (TACO) E87.71
  fluid E87.70
    due to transfusion (blood) (blood
      components) E87.71
    specified NEC E87.79
  iron, due to repeated red blood cell
    transfusions E83.111
  potassium (K) E87.5
  sodium (Na) E87.0

Overnutrition — *see* Hyperalimentation
Overproduction — *see also* Hypersecretion
  ACTH E27.0
  catecholamine E27.5
  growth hormone E22.0
Overprotection, child by parent Z62.1
Overriding
  aorta Q25.4
  finger (acquired) — *see* Deformity, finger
    congenital Q68.1
  toe (acquired) — *see also* Deformity, toe,
    specified NEC
    congenital Q66.89
Overstrained R53.83
  heart — *see* Hypertrophy, cardiac
Overuse, muscle NEC M70.8-
Overweight E66.3
Overworked R53.83
Oviduct — *see* condition
Ovotestis Q56.0
Ovulation (cycle)
  failure or lack of N97.0
  pain N94.0
Ovum — *see* condition
Owren's disease or syndrome
  (parahemophilia) D68.2
Ox heart — *see* Hypertrophy, cardiac
Oxalosis E72.53
Oxaluria E72.53
Oxycephaly, oxycephalic Q75.0
  syphilitic, congenital A50.02
Oxyuriasis B80
Oxyuris vermicularis (infestation) B80
Ozena J31.0

P

Pachyderma, pachydermia L85.9
  larynx (verrucosa) J38.7
Pachydermatocele (congenital) Q82.8
Pachydermoperiostosis — *see also*
  Osteoarthropathy, hypertrophic,
  specified type NEC
  clubbed nail M89.40 [L62]
Pachygyria Q04.3
Pachymeningitis (adhesive) (basal) (brain)
  (cervical) (chronic) (circumscribed)
  (external) (fibrous) (hemorrhagic)
  (hypertrophic) (internal) (purulent)
  (spinal) (suppurative) — *see* Meningitis
Pachyonychia (congenital) Q84.5
Pacinian tumor — *see* Neoplasm, skin,
  benign
Pad, knuckle or Garrod's M72.1
Paget's disease
  with infiltrating duct carcinoma — *see*
    Neoplasm, breast, malignant
  bone M88.9
    carpus M88.84-
    clavicle M88.81-
    femur M88.85-
    fibula M88.86-
    finger M88.84-
    humerus M88.82-
    ilium M88.85-
    in neoplastic disease — *see* Osteitis,
      deformans, in neoplastic disease
    ischium M88.85-
    metacarpus M88.84-
    metatarsus M88.87-
    multiple sites M88.89
    neck M88.88
    radius M88.83-
    rib M88.88
    scapula M88.81-
    skull M88.0
    tarsus M88.87-
    tibia M88.86-
    toe M88.87-
    ulna M88.83-
    vertebra M88.88
  breast (female) C50.01-
    male C50.02-
  extramammary — *see also* Neoplasm, skin,
    malignant
    anus C21.0
      margin C44.590
      skin C44.590
  intraductal carcinoma — *see* Neoplasm,
    breast, malignant
  malignant — *see* Neoplasm, skin,
    malignant
    breast (female) C50.01-
      male C50.02-
      unspecified site (female) C50.01-
      male C50.02-
  mammary — *see* Paget's disease, breast
  nipple — *see* Paget's disease, breast
  osteitis deformans — *see* Paget's disease,
    bone
Paget-Schroetter syndrome I82.890
Pain(s) (*see also* Painful) R52
  abdominal R10.9
    colic R10.83
    generalized R10.84
      with acute abdomen R10.0
    lower R10.30
      left quadrant R10.32
      pelvic or perineal R10.2
      periumbilical R10.33
      right quadrant R10.31
    rebound — *see* Tenderness, abdominal,
      rebound
    severe with abdominal rigidity R10.0
    tenderness — *see* Tenderness, abdominal
    upper R10.10
      epigastric R10.13
      left quadrant R10.12
      right quadrant R10.11
  acute R52
    due to trauma G89.11
    neoplasm related G89.3
    post-thoracotomy G89.12
    postprocedural NEC G89.18
    specified by site — *code to* Pain, by site
  adnexa (uteri) R10.2
  anginoid — *see* Pain, precordial
  anus K62.89
  arm — *see* Pain, limb, upper

P

Pain(s) (see also Painful) R52 — continued
- axillary (axilla) M79.62-
- back (postural) M54.9
- bladder R39.89
  - associated with micturition — see Micturition, painful
- bone — see Disorder, bone, specified type NEC
- breast N64.4
- broad ligament R10.2
- cancer associated (acute) (chronic) G89.3
- cecum — see Pain, abdominal
- cervicobrachial M53.1
- chest (central) R07.9
  - anterior wall R07.89
  - atypical R07.89
  - ischemic I20.9
  - musculoskeletal R07.89
  - non-cardiac R07.89
  - on breathing R07.1
  - pleurodynia R07.81
  - precordial R07.2
  - wall (anterior) R07.89
- chronic G89.29
  - associated with significant psychosocial dysfunction G89.4
  - due to trauma G89.21
  - neoplasm related G89.3
  - post-thoracotomy G89.22
  - postoperative NEC G89.28
  - postprocedural NEC G89.28
  - specified NEC G89.29
- coccyx M53.3
- colon — see Pain, abdominal
- coronary — see Angina
- costochondral R07.1
- diaphragm R07.1
- due to cancer G89.3
- due to device, implant or graft (see also Complications, by site and type, specified NEC) T85.84
  - arterial graft NEC T82.848
  - breast (implant) T85.84
  - catheter NEC T85.84
    - dialysis (renal) T82.848
      - intraperitoneal T85.84
    - infusion NEC T82.848
      - spinal (epidural) (subdural) T85.84
    - urinary (indwelling) T83.84
  - electronic (electrode) (pulse generator) (stimulator)
    - bone T84.84
    - cardiac T82.847
    - nervous system (brain) (peripheral nerve) (spinal) T85.84
    - urinary T83.84
  - fixation, internal (orthopedic) NEC T84.84
  - gastrointestinal (bile duct) (esophagus) T85.84
  - genital NEC T83.84
  - heart NEC T82.847
  - infusion NEC T85.84
  - joint prosthesis T84.84
  - ocular (corneal graft) (orbital implant) NEC T85.84
  - orthopedic NEC T84.84
  - specified NEC T85.84
  - urinary NEC T83.84
  - vascular NEC T82.848
  - ventricular intracranial shunt T85.84
- due to malignancy (primary) (secondary) G89.3
- ear — see subcategory H92.0
- epigastric, epigastrium R10.13
- eye — see Pain, ocular
- face, facial R51
  - atypical G50.1
- female genital organs NEC N94.89
- finger — see Pain, limb, upper
- flank — see Pain, abdominal
- foot — see Pain, limb, lower
- gallbladder K82.9
- gas (intestinal) R14.1
- gastric — see Pain, abdominal
- generalized NOS R52
- genital organ
  - female N94.89
  - male N50.8
- groin — see Pain, abdominal, lower
- hand — see Pain, limb, upper
- head — see Headache
- heart — see Pain, precordial
- infra-orbital — see Neuralgia, trigeminal
- intercostal R07.82
- intermenstrual N94.0
- jaw R68.84

Pain(s) (see also Painful) R52 — continued
- joint M25.50
  - ankle M25.57-
  - elbow M25.52-
  - finger M79.64-
  - foot M25.57-
  - hand M79.64-
  - hip M25.55-
  - knee M25.56-
  - shoulder M25.51-
  - toe M25.57-
  - wrist M25.53-
- kidney N23
- laryngeal R07.0
- leg — see Pain, limb, lower
- limb M79.609
  - lower M79.60-
    - foot M79.67-
    - lower leg M79.66-
    - thigh M79.65-
    - toe M79.67-
  - upper M79.60-
    - axilla M79.62-
    - finger M79.64-
    - forearm M79.63-
    - hand M79.64-
    - upper arm M79.62-
- loin M54.5
- low back M54.5
- lumbar region M54.5
- mandibular R68.84
- mastoid — see subcategory H92.0
- maxilla R68.84
- menstrual (see also Dysmenorrhea) N94.6
- metacarpophalangeal (joint) — see Pain, joint, hand
- metatarsophalangeal (joint) — see Pain, joint, foot
- mouth K13.79
- muscle — see Myalgia
- musculoskeletal (see also Pain, by site) M79.1
  - myofascial M79.1
- nasal J34.89
- nasopharynx J39.2
- neck NEC M54.2
- nerve NEC — see Neuralgia
- neuromuscular — see Neuralgia
- nose J34.89
- ocular H57.1-
- ophthalmic — see Pain, ocular
- orbital region — see Pain, ocular
- ovary N94.89
- ovulation N94.0
- over heart — see Pain, precordial
- pelvic (female) R10.2
- penis N48.89
- pericardial — see Pain, precordial
- perineal, perineum R10.2
- pharynx J39.2
- pleura, pleural, pleuritic R07.81
- post-thoracotomy G89.12
- postoperative NOS G89.18
- postprocedural NOS G89.18
- precordial (region) R07.2
- premenstrual N94.3
- psychogenic (persistent) (any site) F45.41
- radicular (spinal) — see Radiculopathy
- rectum K62.89
- respiration R07.1
- retrosternal R07.2
- rheumatoid, muscular — see Myalgia
- rib R07.81
- root (spinal) — see Radiculopathy
- round ligament (stretch) R10.2
- sacroiliac M53.3
- sciatic — see Sciatica
- scrotum N50.8
- seminal vesicle N50.8
- shoulder M25.51-
- spermatic cord N50.8
- spinal root — see Radiculopathy
- spine M54.9
  - cervical M54.2
  - low back M54.5
    - with sciatica M54.4-
  - thoracic M54.6
- stomach — see Pain, abdominal
- substernal R07.2
- temporomandibular (joint) M26.62
- testis N50.8
- thoracic spine M54.6
  - with radicular and visceral pain M54.14
- throat R07.0
- tibia — see Pain, limb, lower
- toe — see Pain, limb, lower
- tongue K14.6
- tooth K08.8
- trigeminal — see Neuralgia, trigeminal

Pain(s) (see also Painful) R52 — continued
- tumor associated G89.3
- ureter N23
- urinary (organ) (system) N23
- uterus NEC N94.89
- vagina R10.2
- vertebrogenic (syndrome) M54.89
- vesical R39.89
  - associated with micturition — see Micturition, painful
- vulva R10.2

Painful — see also Pain
- coitus
  - female N94.1
  - male N53.12
  - psychogenic F52.6
- ejaculation (semen) N53.12
  - psychogenic F52.6
- erection — see Priapism
- feet syndrome E53.8
- joint replacement (hip) (knee) T84.84
- menstruation (see also Dysmenorrhea)
  - psychogenic F45.8
- micturition — see Micturition, painful
- respiration R07.1
- scar NEC L90.5
- wire sutures T81.89

Painter's colic — see subcategory T56.0
Palate — see condition
Palatoplegia K13.79
Palatoschisis — see Cleft, palate
Palilalia R48.8
Palliative care Z51.5
Pallor R23.1
- optic disc, temporal — see Atrophy, optic
Palmar — see also condition
- fascia — see condition
Palpable
- cecum K63.89
- kidney N28.89
- ovary N83.8
- prostate N42.9
- spleen — see Splenomegaly
Palpitations (heart) R00.2
- psychogenic F45.8
Palsy (see also Paralysis) G83.9
- atrophic diffuse (progressive) G12.22
- Bell's — see also Palsy, facial
  - newborn P11.3
- brachial plexus NEC G54.0
  - newborn (birth injury) P14.3
- brain — see Palsy, cerebral
- bulbar (progressive) (chronic) G12.22
  - of childhood (Fazio-Londe) G12.1
  - pseudo NEC G12.29
  - supranuclear (progressive) G23.1
- cerebral (congenital) G80.9
  - ataxic G80.4
  - athetoid G80.3
  - choreathetoid G80.3
  - diplegic G80.8
    - spastic G80.1
  - dyskinetic G80.3
    - athetoid G80.3
    - choreathetoid G80.3
    - distonic G80.3
    - dystonic G80.3
  - hemiplegic G80.8
    - spastic G80.2
  - mixed G80.8
  - monoplegic G80.8
    - spastic G80.1
  - paraplegic G80.8
    - spastic G80.1
  - quadriplegic G80.8
    - spastic G80.0
  - spastic G80.1
    - diplegic G80.1
    - hemiplegic G80.2
    - monoplegic G80.1
    - quadriplegic G80.0
    - specified NEC G80.1
    - tetrapelgic G80.0
  - specified NEC G80.8
  - syphilitic A52.12
    - congenital A50.49
  - tetraplegic G80.8
    - spastic G80.0
- cranial nerve — see also Disorder, nerve, cranial
  - multiple G52.7
    - in
      - infectious disease B99 [G53]
      - neoplastic disease (see also Neoplasm) D49.9 [G53]
      - parasitic disease B89 [G53]
      - sarcoidosis D86.82
- creeping G12.22
- diver's T70.3
- Erb's P14.0

Palsy (see also Paralysis) G83.9 — continued
- facial G51.0
  - newborn (birth injury) P11.3
- glossopharyngeal G52.1
- Klumpke(-Déjérine) P14.1
- lead — see subcategory T56.0
- median nerve (tardy) G56.1-
- nerve G58.9
  - specified NEC G58.8
- peroneal nerve (acute) (tardy) G57.3-
- progressive supranuclear G23.1
- pseudobulbar NEC G12.29
- radial nerve (acute) G56.3-
- seventh nerve — see also Palsy, facial
  - newborn P11.3
- shaking — see Parkinsonism
- spastic (cerebral) (spinal) G80.1
- ulnar nerve (tardy) G56.2-
- wasting G12.29
Paludism — see Malaria
Panangiitis M30.0
Panaris, panaritium — see also Cellulitis, digit
- with lymphangitis — see Lymphangitis, acute, digit
Panarteritis nodosa M30.0
- brain or cerebral I67.7
Pancake heart R93.1
- with cor pulmonale (chronic) I27.81
Pancarditis (acute) (chronic) I51.89
- rheumatic I09.89
  - active or acute I01.8
Pancoast's syndrome or tumor C34.1-
Pancolitis, ulcerative (chronic) K51.00
- with
  - abscess K51.014
  - complication K51.019
  - fistula K51.013
  - obstruction K51.012
  - rectal bleeding K51.011
  - specified complication NEC K51.018
Pancreas, pancreatic — see condition
Pancreatitis (annular) (apoplectic) (calcareous) (edematous) (hemorrhagic) (malignant) (recurrent) (subacute) (suppurative) K85.9
- acute K85.9
  - alcohol-induced K85.2
  - biliary K85.1
  - drug-induced K85.3
  - gallstone K85.1
  - idiopathic K85.0
  - specified NEC K85.8
- chronic (infectious) K86.1
  - alcohol-induced K86.0
  - recurrent K86.1
  - relapsing K86.1
- cystic (chronic) K86.1
- cytomegaloviral B25.2
- fibrous (chronic) K86.1
- gallstone K85.1
- gangrenous K85.8
- interstitial (chronic) K86.1
  - acute K85.8
- mumps B26.3
- recurrent (chronic) K86.1
- relapsing, chronic K86.1
- syphilitic A52.74
Pancreatoblastoma — see Neoplasm, pancreas, malignant
Pancreolithiasis K86.8
Pancytolysis D75.89
Pancytopenia (acquired) D61.818
- with
  - malformations D61.09
  - myelodysplastic syndrome — see Syndrome, myelodysplastic
- antineoplastic chemotherapy induced D61.810
- congenital D61.09
- drug-induced NEC D61.811
Panencephalitis, subacute, sclerosing A81.1
Panhematopenia D61.9
- congenital D61.09
- constitutional D61.09
- splenic, primary D73.1
Panhemocytopenia D61.9
- congenital D61.09
- constitutional D61.09
Panhypogonadism E29.1
Panhypopituitarism E23.0
- prepubertal E23.0
Panic (attack) (state) F41.0
- reaction to exceptional stress (transient) F43.0
Panmyelopathy, familial, constitutional D61.09
Panmyelophthisis D61.82
- congenital D61.09

Panmyelosis (acute) (with myelofibrosis) C94.4-
Panner's disease — see Osteochondrosis, juvenile, humerus
Panneuritis endemica E51.11
Panniculitis (nodular) (nonsuppurative) M79.3
　back M54.00
　　cervical region M54.02
　　cervicothoracic region M54.03
　　lumbar region M54.06
　　lumbosacral region M54.07
　　multiple sites M54.09
　　occipito-atlanto-axial region M54.01
　　sacrococcygeal region M54.08
　　thoracic region M54.04
　　thoracolumbar region M54.05
　lupus L93.2
　mesenteric K65.4
　neck M54.02
　　cervicothoracic region M54.03
　　occipito-atlanto-axial region M54.01
　relapsing M35.6
Panniculus adiposus (abdominal) E65
Pannus (allergic) (cornea) (degenerativus) (keratic) H16.42-
　abdominal (symptomatic) E65
　trachomatosus, trachomatous (active) A71.1
Panophthalmitis H44.01-
Pansinusitis (chronic) (hyperplastic) (nonpurulent) (purulent) J32.4
　acute J01.40
　　recurrent J01.41
　tuberculous A15.8
Panuveitis (sympathetic) H44.11-
Panvalvular disease I08.9
　specified NEC I08.8
Papanicolaou smear, cervix Z12.4
　as part of routine gynecological examination Z01.419
　　with abnormal findings Z01.411
　for suspected neoplasm Z12.4
　nonspecific abnormal finding R87.619
　routine Z01.419
　　with abnormal findings Z01.411
Papilledema (choked disc) H47.10
　associated with
　　decreased ocular pressure H47.12
　　increased intracranial pressure H47.11
　　retinal disorder H47.13
　Foster-Kennedy syndrome H47.14-
Papillitis H46.00
　anus K62.89
　chronic lingual K14.4
　necrotizing, kidney N17.2
　optic H46.0-
　rectum K62.89
　renal, necrotizing N17.2
　tongue K14.0
Papilloma — see also Neoplasm, benign, by site
　acuminatum (female) (male) (anogenital) A63.0
　benign pinta (primary) A67.0
　bladder (urinary) (transitional cell) D41.4
　choroid plexus (lateral ventricle) (third ventricle) D33.0
　　anaplastic C71.5
　　fourth ventricle D33.1
　　malignant C71.5
　renal pelvis (transitional cell) D41.1-
　　benign D30.1-
　Schneiderian
　　specified site — see Neoplasm, benign, by site
　　unspecified site D14.0
　serous surface
　　borderline malignancy
　　　specified site — see Neoplasm, uncertain behavior, by site
　　　unspecified site D39.10
　　specified site — see Neoplasm, benign, by site
　　unspecified site D27.9
　transitional (cell)
　　bladder (urinary) D41.4
　　inverted type — see Neoplasm, uncertain behavior, by site
　　renal pelvis D41.1-
　　ureter D41.2-
　ureter (transitional cell) D41.2-
　　benign D30.1-
　urothelial — see Neoplasm, uncertain behavior, by site
　villous — see Neoplasm, uncertain behavior, by site
　　adenocarcinoma in — see Neoplasm, malignant, by site
　　in situ — see Neoplasm, in situ
　yaws, plantar or palmar A66.1

Papillomata, multiple, of yaws A66.1
Papillomatosis — see also Neoplasm, benign, by site
　confluent and reticulated L83
　cystic, breast — see Mastopathy, cystic
　ductal, breast — see Mastopathy, cystic
　intraductal (diffuse) — see Neoplasm, benign, by site
　subareolar duct D24-
Papillomavirus, as cause of disease classified elsewhere B97.7
Papillon-Léage and Psaume syndrome Q87.0
Papule(s) R23.8
　carate (primary) A67.0
　fibrous, of nose D22.39
　Gottron's L94.4
　pinta (primary) A67.0
Papulosis
　lymphomatoid C86.6
　malignant I77.89
Papyraceous fetus O31.0-
Para-albuminemia E88.09
Paracephalus Q89.7
Parachute mitral valve Q23.2
Paracoccidioidomycosis B41.9
　disseminated B41.7
　generalized B41.7
　mucocutaneous-lymphangitic B41.8
　pulmonary B41.0
　specified NEC B41.8
　visceral B41.8
Paradentosis K05.4
Paraffinoma T88.8
Paraganglioma D44.7
　adrenal D35.0-
　　malignant C74.1-
　aortic body D44.7
　　malignant C75.5
　carotid body D44.6
　　malignant C75.4
　chromaffin — see also Neoplasm, benign, by site
　　malignant — see Neoplasm, malignant, by site
　extra-adrenal D44.7
　　malignant C75.5
　　　specified site — see Neoplasm, malignant, by site
　　　unspecified site C75.5
　　specified site — see Neoplasm, uncertain behavior, by site
　　unspecified site D44.7
　gangliocytic D13.2
　　specified site — see Neoplasm, benign, by site
　　unspecified site D13.2
　glomus jugulare D44.7
　　malignant C75.5
　jugular D44.7
　malignant C75.5
　　specified site — see Neoplasm, malignant, by site
　　unspecified site C75.5
　nonchromaffin D44.7
　　malignant C75.5
　　　specified site — see Neoplasm, malignant, by site
　　　unspecified site C75.5
　　specified site — see Neoplasm, uncertain behavior, by site
　　unspecified site D44.7
　parasympathetic D44.7
　　specified site — see Neoplasm, uncertain behavior, by site
　　unspecified site D44.7
　specified site — see Neoplasm, uncertain behavior, by site
　sympathetic D44.7
　　specified site — see Neoplasm, uncertain behavior, by site
　　unspecified site D44.7
　unspecified site D44.7
Parageusia R43.2
　psychogenic F45.8
Paragonimiasis B66.4
Paragranuloma, Hodgkin — see Lymphoma, Hodgkin, classical, specified type NEC
Parahemophilia (see also Defect, coagulation) D68.2
Parakeratosis R23.4
　variegata L41.0

Paralysis, paralytic (complete) (incomplete) G83.9
　with
　　syphilis A52.17
　abducens, abducent (nerve) — see Strabismus, paralytic, sixth nerve
　abductor, lower extremity G57.9-
　accessory nerve G52.8
　accommodation — see also Paresis, of accommodation
　　hysterical F44.89
　acoustic nerve (except Deafness) — see subcategory H93.3
　agitans (see also Parkinsonism) G20
　　arteriosclerotic G21.4
　alternating (oculomotor) G83.89
　amyotrophic G12.21
　ankle G57.9-
　anus (sphincter) K62.89
　arm — see Monoplegia, upper limb
　ascending (spinal), acute G61.0
　association G12.29
　asthenic bulbar G70.00
　　with exacerbation (acute) G70.01
　　in crisis G70.01
　ataxic (hereditary) G11.9
　　general (syphilitic) A52.17
　atrophic G58.9
　　infantile, acute — see Poliomyelitis, paralytic
　　progressive G12.22
　　spinal (acute) — see Poliomyelitis, paralytic
　axillary G54.0
　Babinski-Nageotte's G83.89
　Bell's G51.0
　　newborn P11.3
　Benedikt's G46.3
　birth injury P14.9
　　spinal cord P11.5
　bladder (neurogenic) (sphincter) N31.2
　bowel, colon or intestine K56.0
　brachial plexus G54.0
　　birth injury P14.3
　　newborn (birth injury) P14.3
　brain G83.9
　　diplegia G83.0
　　triplegia G83.89
　bronchial J98.09
　Brown-Séquard G83.81
　bulbar (chronic) (progressive) G12.22
　　infantile — see Poliomyelitis, paralytic
　　poliomyelitic — see Poliomyelitis, paralytic
　　pseudo G12.29
　bulbospinal G70.00
　　with exacerbation (acute) G70.01
　　in crisis G70.01
　cardiac (see also Failure, heart) I50.9
　cerebrocerebellar, diplegic G80.1
　cervical
　　plexus G54.2
　　sympathetic G90.09
　Cestan-Chenais G46.3
　Charcot-Marie-Tooth type G60.0
　Clark's G80.9
　colon K56.0
　compressed air T70.3
　compression
　　arm G56.9-
　　leg G57.9-
　　lower extremity G57.9-
　　upper extremity G56.9-
　congenital (cerebral) — see Palsy, cerebral
　conjugate movement (gaze) (of eye) H51.0
　　cortical (nuclear) (supranuclear) H51.0
　cordis — see Failure, heart
　cranial or cerebral nerve G52.9
　creeping G12.22
　crossed leg G83.89
　crutch — see Injury, brachial plexus
　deglutition R13.0
　　hysterical F44.4
　dementia A52.17
　descending (spinal) NEC G12.29
　diaphragm (flaccid) J98.6
　　due to accidental dissection of phrenic nerve during procedure — see Puncture, accidental complicating surgery
　digestive organs NEC K59.8
　diplegic — see Diplegia
　diver's T70.3
　divergence (nuclear) H51.8

Paralysis, paralytic (complete) (incomplete) G83.9 — continued
　Duchenne's
　　birth injury P14.0
　　due to or associated with
　　　motor neuron disease G12.22
　　　muscular dystrophy G71.0
　due to intracranial or spinal birth injury — see Palsy, cerebral
　embolic (current episode) I63.4
　Erb's syphilitic spastic spinal A52.17
　Erb(-Duchenne) (birth) (newborn) P14.0
　esophagus K22.8
　eye muscle (extrinsic) H49.9
　　intrinsic — see also Paresis, of accommodation
　facial (nerve) G51.0
　　birth injury P11.3
　　congenital P11.3
　　following operation NEC — see Puncture, accidental complicating surgery
　　newborn (birth injury) P11.3
　familial (recurrent) (periodic) G72.3
　　spastic G11.4
　fauces J39.2
　finger G56.9-
　gait R26.1
　gastric nerve (nondiabetic) G52.2
　gaze, conjugate H51.0
　general (progressive) (syphilitic) A52.17
　　juvenile A50.45
　glottis J38.00
　　bilateral J38.02
　　unilateral J38.01
　gluteal G54.1
　Gubler(-Millard) G46.3
　hand — see Monoplegia, upper limb
　heart — see Arrest, cardiac
　hemiplegic — see Hemiplegia
　hyperkalemic periodic (familial) G72.3
　hypoglossal (nerve) G52.3
　hypokalemic periodic G72.3
　hysterical F44.4
　ileus K56.0
　infantile (see also Poliomyelitis, paralytic) A80.30
　　bulbar — see Poliomyelitis, paralytic
　　cerebral — see Palsy, cerebral
　　spastic — see Palsy, cerebral, spastic
　infective — see Poliomyelitis, paralytic
　inferior nuclear G83.9
　internuclear — see Ophthalmoplegia, internuclear
　intestine K56.0
　iris H57.09
　　due to diphtheria (toxin) A36.89
　ischemic, Volkmann's (complicating trauma) T79.6
　Jackson's G83.89
　jake — see Poisoning, food, noxious, plant
　Jamaica ginger (jake) G62.2
　juvenile general A50.45
　Klumpke(-Déjérine) (birth) (newborn) P14.1
　labioglossal (laryngeal) (pharyngeal) G12.29
　Landry's G61.0
　laryngeal nerve (recurrent) (superior) (unilateral) J38.00
　　bilateral J38.02
　　unilateral J38.01
　larynx J38.00
　　bilateral J38.02
　　due to diphtheria (toxin) A36.2
　　unilateral J38.01
　lateral G12.21
　lead — see subcategory T56.0
　left side — see Hemiplegia
　leg G83.1-
　　both — see Paraplegia
　　crossed G83.89
　　hysterical F44.4
　　psychogenic F44.4
　　transient or transitory R29.818
　　　traumatic NEC — see Injury, nerve, leg
　levator palpebrae superioris — see Blepharoptosis, paralytic
　limb — see Monoplegia
　lip K13.0
　Lissauer's A52.17
　lower limb — see Monoplegia, lower limb
　　both — see Paraplegia
　lung J98.4
　median nerve G56.1-

Paralysis, paralytic (complete) (incomplete)
G83.9 — *continued*
  medullary (tegmental) G83.89
  mesencephalic NEC G83.89
    tegmental G83.89
  middle alternating G83.89
  Millard-Gubler-Foville G46.3
  monoplegic — *see* Monoplegia
  motor G83.9
  muscle, muscular NEC G72.89
    due to nerve lesion G58.9
    eye (extrinsic) H49.9
      intrinsic — *see* Paresis, of
        accommodation
      oblique — *see* Strabismus, paralytic,
        fourth nerve
    iris sphincter H21.9
    ischemic (Volkmann's) (complicating
      trauma) T79.6
    progressive G12.21
    pseudohypertrophic G71.0
  musculocutaneous nerve G56.9-
  musculospiral G56.9-
  nerve — *see also* Disorder, nerve
    abducent — *see* Strabismus, paralytic,
      sixth nerve
    accessory G52.8
    auditory (except Deafness) — *see*
      subcategory H93.3
    birth injury P14.9
    cranial or cerebral G52.9
    facial G51.0
      birth injury P11.3
      congenital P11.3
      newborn (birth injury) P11.3
    fourth or trochlear — *see* Strabismus,
      paralytic, fourth nerve
    newborn (birth injury) P14.9
    oculomotor — *see* Strabismus, paralytic,
      third nerve
    phrenic (birth injury) P14.2
    radial G56.3-
    seventh or facial G51.0
      newborn (birth injury) P11.3
    sixth or abducent — *see* Strabismus,
      paralytic, sixth nerve
    syphilitic A52.15
    third or oculomotor — *see* Strabismus,
      paralytic, third nerve
    trigeminal G50.9
    trochlear — *see* Strabismus, paralytic,
      fourth nerve
    ulnar G56.2-
  normokalemic periodic G72.3
  ocular H49.9
    alternating G83.89
  oculofacial, congenital (Moebius) Q87.0
  oculomotor (external bilateral) (nerve) —
    see Strabismus, paralytic, third nerve
  palate (soft) K13.79
  paratrigeminal G50.9
  periodic (familial) (hyperkalemic)
    (hypokalemic) (myotonic)
    (normokalemic) (potassium sensitive)
    (secondary) G72.3
  peripheral autonomic nervous system —
    see Neuropathy, peripheral,
    autonomic
  peroneal (nerve) G57.3-
  pharynx J39.2
  phrenic nerve G56.8-
  plantar nerve(s) G57.6-
  pneumogastric nerve G52.2
  poliomyelitis (current) — *see*
    Poliomyelitis, paralytic
  popliteal nerve G57.3-
  postepileptic transitory G83.84
  progressive (atrophic) (bulbar) (spinal)
    G12.22
    general A52.17
    infantile acute — *see* Poliomyelitis,
      paralytic
    supranuclear G23.1
  pseudobulbar G12.29
  pseudohypertrophic (muscle) G71.0
  psychogenic F44.4
  quadriceps G57.9-
  quadriplegic — *see* Tetraplegia
  radial nerve G56.3-
  rectus muscle (eye) H49.9
  recurrent isolated sleep G47.53
  respiratory (muscle) (system) (tract)
    R06.81
    center NEC G93.89
    congenital P28.89
    newborn P28.89
  right side — *see* Hemiplegia
  saturnine — *see* subcategory T56.0

Paralysis, paralytic (complete) (incomplete)
G83.9 — *continued*
  sciatic nerve G57.0-
  senile G83.9
  shaking — *see* Parkinsonism
  shoulder G56.9-
  sleep, recurrent isolated G47.53
  spastic G83.9
    cerebral — *see* Palsy, cerebral, spastic
    congenital (cerebral) — *see* Palsy,
      cerebral, spastic
    familial G11.4
    hereditary G11.4
    quadriplegic G80.0
    syphilitic (spinal) A52.17
  sphincter, bladder — *see* Paralysis, bladder
  spinal (cord) G83.9
    accessory nerve G52.8
    acute — *see* Poliomyelitis, paralytic
    ascending acute G61.0
    atrophic (acute) — *see also*
      Poliomyelitis, paralytic
      spastic, syphilitic A52.17
    congenital NEC — *see* Palsy, cerebral
    hereditary G95.89
    infantile — *see* Poliomyelitis, paralytic
    progressive G12.21
    sequelae NEC G83.89
  sternomastoid G52.8
  stomach K31.84
    diabetic — *see* Diabetes, by type, with
      gastroparesis
      nerve G52.2
        diabetic — *see* Diabetes, by type,
          with gastroparesis
  stroke — *see* Infarct, brain
  subcapsularis G56.8-
  supranuclear (progressive) G23.1
  sympathetic G90.8
    cervical G90.09
    nervous system — *see* Neuropathy,
      peripheral, autonomic
  syndrome G83.9
    specified NEC G83.89
  syphilitic spastic spinal (Erb's) A52.17
  thigh G57.9-
  throat J39.2
    diphtheritic A36.0
    muscle J39.2
  thrombotic (current episode) I63.3
  thumb G56.9-
  tick — *see* Toxicity, venom, arthropod,
    specified NEC
  Todd's (postepileptic transitory paralysis)
    G83.84
  toe G57.6-
  tongue K14.8
  transient R29.5
    arm or leg NEC R29.818
    traumatic NEC — *see* Injury, nerve
  trapezius G52.8
  traumatic, transient NEC — *see* Injury,
    nerve
  trembling — *see* Parkinsonism
  triceps brachii G56.9-
  trigeminal nerve G50.9
  trochlear (nerve) — *see* Strabismus,
    paralytic, fourth nerve
  ulnar nerve G56.2-
  upper limb — *see* Monoplegia, upper limb
  uremic N18.9 [G99.8]
  uveoparotitic D86.89
  uvula K13.79
    postdiphtheritic A36.0
  vagus nerve G52.2
  vasomotor NEC G90.8
  velum palati K13.79
  vesical — *see* Paralysis, bladder
  vestibular nerve (except Vertigo) — *see*
    subcategory H93.3
  vocal cords J38.00
    bilateral J38.02
    unilateral J38.01
  Volkmann's (complicating trauma) T79.6
  wasting G12.29
  Weber's G46.3
  wrist G56.9-
Paramedial urethrovesical orifice Q64.79
Paramenia N92.6
Parametritis (*see also* Disease, pelvis,
  inflammatory) N73.2
  acute N73.0
  complicating abortion — *see* Abortion, by
    type, complicated by, parametritis
Parametrium, parametric — *see* condition
Paramnesia — *see* Amnesia

Paramolar K00.1
Paramyloidosis E85.8
Paramyoclonus multiplex G25.3
Paramyotonia (congenita) G71.19
Parangi — *see* Yaws
Paranoia (querulans) F22
  senile F03
Paranoid
  dementia (senile) F03
    praecox — *see* Schizophrenia
  personality F60.0
  psychosis (climacteric) (involutional)
    (menopausal) F22
    psychogenic (acute) F23
    senile F03
  reaction (acute) F23
    chronic F22
  schizophrenia F20.0
  state (climacteric) (involutional)
    (menopausal) (simple) F22
    senile F03
  tendencies F60.0
  traits F60.0
  trends F60.0
  type, psychopathic personality F60.0
Paraparesis — *see* Paraplegia
Paraphasia R47.02
Paraphilia F65.9
Paraphimosis (congenital) N47.2
  chancroidal A57
Paraphrenia, paraphrenic (late) F22
  schizophrenia F20.0
Paraplegia (lower) G82.20
  ataxic — *see* Degeneration, combined,
    spinal cord
  complete G82.21
  congenital (cerebral) G80.8
    spastic G80.1
  familial spastic G11.4
  functional (hysterical) F44.4
  hereditary, spastic G11.4
  hysterical F44.4
  incomplete G82.22
  Pott's A18.01
  psychogenic F44.4
  spastic
    Erb's spinal, syphilitic A52.17
    hereditary G11.4
    tropical G04.1
  syphilitic (spastic) A52.17
  tropical spastic G04.1
Parapoxvirus B08.60
  specified NEC B08.69
Paraproteinemia D89.2
  benign (familial) D89.2
  monoclonal D47.2
  secondary to malignant disease D47.2
Parapsoriasis L41.9
  en plaques L41.4
  guttata L41.1
  large plaque L41.4
  retiform, retiformis L41.5
  small plaque L41.3
  specified NEC L41.8
  varioliformis (acuta) L41.0
Parasitic — *see also* condition
  disease NEC B89
  stomatitis B37.0
  sycosis (beard) (scalp) B35.0
  twin Q89.4
Parasitism B89
  intestinal B82.9
  skin B88.9
  specified — *see* Infestation
Parasitophobia F40.218
Parasomnia G47.50
  due to
    alcohol
      abuse F10.182
      dependence F10.282
      use F10.982
    amphetamines
      abuse F15.182
      dependence F15.282
      use F15.982
    caffeine
      abuse F15.182
      dependence F15.282
      use F15.982
    cocaine
      abuse F14.182
      dependence F14.282
      use F14.982
    drug NEC
      abuse F19.182
      dependence F19.282
      use F19.982

Parasomnia G47.50 — *continued*
  due to — *continued*
    opioid
      abuse F11.182
      dependence F11.282
      use F11.982
    psychoactive substance NEC
      abuse F19.182
      dependence F19.282
      use F19.982
    sedative, hypnotic, or anxiolytic
      abuse F13.182
      dependence F13.282
      use F13.982
    stimulant NEC
      abuse F15.182
      dependence F15.282
      use F15.982
  in conditions classified elsewhere G47.54
  nonorganic origin F51.8
  organic G47.50
  specified NEC G47.59
Paraspadias Q54.9
Paraspasmus facialis G51.8
Parasuicide (attempt)
  history of (personal) Z91.5
  in family Z81.8
Parathyroid gland — *see* condition
Parathyroid tetany E20.9
Paratrachoma A74.0
Paratyphilitis — *see* Appendicitis
Paratyphoid (fever) — *see* Fever,
  paratyphoid
Paratyphus — *see* Fever, paratyphoid
Paraurethral duct Q64.79
  nonorganic origin F51.5
Paraurethritis — *see also* Urethritis
  gonococcal (acute) (chronic) (with abscess)
    A54.1
Paravaccinia NEC B08.04
Paravaginitis — *see* Vaginitis
Parencephalitis — *see also* Encephalitis
  sequelae G09
Parent-child conflict — *see* Conflict, parent-
  child
  estrangement NEC Z62.890
Paresis — *see also* Paralysis
  accommodation — *see* Paresis, of
    accommodation
  Bernhardt's G57.1-
  bladder (sphincter) — *see also* Paralysis,
    bladder
    tabetic A52.17
  bowel, colon or intestine K56.0
  extrinsic muscle, eye H49.9
  general (progressive) (syphilitic) A52.17
    juvenile A50.45
  heart — *see* Failure, heart
  insane (syphilitic) A52.17
  juvenile (general) A50.45
  of accommodation H52.52-
  peripheral progressive (idiopathic) G60.3
  pseudohypertrophic G71.0
  senile G83.9
  syphilitic (general) A52.17
    congenital A50.45
  vesical NEC N31.2
Paresthesia — *see also* Disturbance,
  sensation
  Bernhardt G57.1-
Paretic — *see* condition
Parinaud's
  conjunctivitis H10.89
  oculoglandular syndrome H10.89
  ophthalmoplegia H49.88-
Parkinson's disease, syndrome or tremor
  — *see* Parkinsonism
Parkinsonism (idiopathic) (primary) G20
  with neurogenic orthostatic hypotension
    (symptomatic) G90.3
  arteriosclerotic G21.4
  dementia G31.83 [F02.80]
    with behavioral disturbance G31.83
      [F02.81]
  due to
    drugs NEC G21.19
      neuroleptic G21.11
  neuroleptic induced G21.11
  postencephalitic G21.3
  secondary G21.9
    due to
      arteriosclerosis G21.4
      drugs NEC G21.19
        neuroleptic G21.11
      encephalitis G21.3
      external agents NEC G21.2
      syphilis A52.19
    specified NEC G21.8

Parkinsonism (idiopathic) (primary) G20 — *continued*
  syphilitic A52.19
  treatment-induced NEC G21.19
  vascular G21.4
Parodontitis — *see* Periodontitis
Parodontosis K05.4
Paronychia — *see also* Cellulitis, digit
  with lymphangitis — *see* Lymphangitis, acute, digit
  candidal (chronic) B37.2
  tuberculous (primary) A18.4
Parorexia (psychogenic) F50.8
Parosmia R43.1
  psychogenic F45.8
Parotid gland — *see* condition
Parotitis, parotiditis (allergic) (nonspecific toxic) (purulent) (septic) (suppurative) — *see also* Sialoadenitis
  epidemic — *see* Mumps
  infectious — *see* Mumps
  postoperative K91.89
  surgical K91.89
Parrot fever A70
Parrot's disease (early congenital syphilitic pseudoparalysis) A50.02
Parry-Romberg syndrome G51.8
Parry's disease or syndrome E05.00
  with thyroid storm E05.01
Pars planitis — *see* Cyclitis
Parson's disease (exophthalmic goiter) E05.00
  with thyroid storm E05.01
Parsonage(-Aldren)-Turner syndrome G54.5
Particolored infant Q82.8
Parturition — *see* Delivery
Parulis K04.7
  with sinus K04.6
Parvovirus, as cause of disease classified elsewhere B97.6
Pasini and Pierini's atrophoderma L90.3
Passage
  false, urethra N36.5
  meconium (newborn) during delivery P03.82
  of sounds or bougies — *see* Attention to, artificial, opening
Passive — *see* condition
  smoking Z77.22
Pasteurella septica A28.0
Pasteurellosis — *see* Infection, Pasteurella
PAT (paroxysmal atrial tachycardia) I47.1
Patau's syndrome — *see* Trisomy, 13
Patches
  mucous (syphilitic) A51.39
    congenital A50.07
  smokers' (mouth) K13.24
Patellar — *see* condition
Patent — *see also* Imperfect, closure
  canal of Nuck Q52.4
  cervix N88.3
  ductus arteriosus or Botallo's Q25.0
  foramen
    botalli Q21.1
    ovale Q21.1
  interauricular septum Q21.1
  interventricular septum Q21.0
  omphalomesenteric duct Q43.0
  os (uteri) — *see* Patent, cervix
  ostium secundum Q21.1
  urachus Q64.4
  vitelline duct Q43.0
Paterson(-Brown)(-Kelly) syndrome or web D50.1
Pathologic, pathological — *see also* condition
  asphyxia R09.01
  fire-setting F63.1
  gambling F63.0
  ovum O02.0
  resorption, tooth K03.3
  stealing F63.2
Pathology (of) — *see* Disease
  periradicular, associated with previous endodontic treatment NEC M27.59
Pattern, sleep-wake, irregular G47.23
Patulous — *see also* Imperfect, closure
  (congenital)
  alimentary tract Q45.8
    lower Q43.8
    upper Q40.8
  eustachian tube H69.0-
Pause, sinoatrial I49.5
Paxton's disease B36.2

Pearl(s)
  enamel K00.2
  Epstein's K09.8
Pearl-worker's disease — *see* Osteomyelitis, specified type NEC
Pectenosis K62.4
Pectoral — *see* condition
Pectus
  carinatum (congenital) Q67.7
    acquired M95.4
    rachitic sequelae (late effect) E64.3
  excavatum (congenital) Q67.6
    acquired M95.4
    rachitic sequelae (late effect) E64.3
  recurvatum (congenital) Q67.6
Pedatrophia E41
Pederosis F65.4
Pediculosis (infestation) B85.2
  capitis (head-louse) (any site) B85.0
  corporis (body-louse) (any site) B85.1
  eyelid B85.0
  mixed (classifiable to more than one of the titles B85.0-B85.3) B85.4
  pubis (pubic louse) (any site) B85.3
  vestimenti B85.1
  vulvae B85.3
Pediculus (infestation) — *see* Pediculosis
Pedophilia F65.4
Peg-shaped teeth K00.2
Pelade — *see* Alopecia, areata
Pelger-Huët anomaly or syndrome D72.0
Peliosis (rheumatica) D69.0
  hepatis K76.4
  with toxic liver disease K71.8
Pelizaeus-Merzbacher disease E75.29
Pellagra (alcoholic) (with polyneuropathy) E52
Pellagra-cerebellar-ataxia-renal aminoaciduria syndrome E72.02
Pellegrini (-Stieda) disease or syndrome — *see* Bursitis, tibial collateral
Pellizzi's syndrome E34.8
Pel's crisis A52.11
Pelvic — *see also* condition
  examination (periodic) (routine) Z01.419
    with abnormal findings Z01.411
  kidney, congenital Q63.2
Pelviolithiasis — *see* Calculus, kidney
Pelviperitonitis — *see also* Peritonitis, pelvic
  gonococcal A54.24
  puerperal O85
Pelvis — *see* condition or type
Pemphigoid L12.9
  benign, mucous membrane L12.1
  bullous L12.0
  cicatricial L12.1
  juvenile L12.2
  ocular L12.1
  specified NEC L12.8
Pemphigus L10.9
  benign familial (chronic) Q82.8
  Brazilian L10.3
  circinatus L13.0
  conjunctiva L12.1
  drug-induced L10.5
  erythematosus L10.4
  foliaceous L10.2
  gangrenous — *see* Gangrene
  neonatorum L01.03
  ocular L12.1
  paraneoplastic L10.81
  specified NEC L10.89
  syphilitic (congenital) A50.06
  vegetans L10.1
  vulgaris L10.0
  wildfire L10.3
Pendred's syndrome E07.1
Pendulous
  abdomen, in pregnancy — *see* Pregnancy, complicated by, abnormal, pelvic organs or tissues NEC
  breast N64.89
Penetrating wound — *see also* Puncture
  with internal injury — *see* Injury, by site
  eyeball — *see* Puncture, eyeball
  orbit (with or without foreign body) — *see* Puncture, orbit
  uterus by instrument with or following ectopic or molar pregnancy O08.6
Penicillosis B48.4
Penis — *see* condition
Penitis N48.29
Pentalogy of Fallot Q21.8
Pentasomy X syndrome Q97.1
Pentosuria (essential) E74.8
Percreta placenta O43.23-
Peregrinating patient — *see* Disorder, factitious

Perforation, perforated (nontraumatic) (of)
  accidental during procedure (blood vessel) (nerve) (organ) — *see* Complication, accidental puncture or laceration
  antrum — *see* Sinusitis, maxillary
  appendix K35.2
  atrial septum, multiple Q21.1
  attic, ear — *see* Perforation, tympanum, attic
  bile duct (common) (hepatic) K83.2
    cystic K82.2
  bladder (urinary)
    with or following ectopic or molar pregnancy O08.6
    obstetrical trauma O71.5
    traumatic S37.29
      at delivery O71.5
  bowel K63.1
    with or following ectopic or molar pregnancy O08.6
    newborn P78.0
    obstetrical trauma O71.5
    traumatic — *see* Laceration, intestine
  broad ligament N83.8
    with or following ectopic or molar pregnancy O08.6
    obstetrical trauma O71.6
  by
    device, implant or graft (see also Complications, by site and type, mechanical) T85.628
      arterial graft NEC — *see* Complication, cardiovascular device, mechanical, vascular
      breast (implant) T85.49
      catheter NEC T85.698
        cystostomy T83.090
        dialysis (renal) T82.49
          intraperitoneal T85.691
        infusion NEC T82.594
          spinal (epidural) (subdural) T85.690
      electronic (electrode) (pulse generator) (stimulator)
        bone T84.390
        cardiac T82.199
          electrode T82.190
          pulse generator T82.191
          specified type NEC T82.198
        nervous system — *see* Complication, prosthetic device, mechanical, electronic nervous system stimulator
        urinary — *see* Complication, genitourinary, device, urinary, mechanical
      fixation, internal (orthopedic) NEC — *see* Complication, fixation device, mechanical
      gastrointestinal — *see* Complications, prosthetic device, mechanical, gastrointestinal device
      genital NEC T83.498
        intrauterine contraceptive device T83.39
        penile prosthesis T83.490
      heart NEC — *see* Complication, cardiovascular device, mechanical
      joint prosthesis — *see* Complications, joint prosthesis, mechanical, specified NEC, by site
      ocular NEC — *see* Complications, prosthetic device, mechanical, ocular device
      orthopedic NEC — *see* Complication, orthopedic, device, mechanical
      specified NEC T85.628
      urinary NEC — *see also* Complication, genitourinary, device, urinary, mechanical
        graft T83.29
        urinary, indwelling T83.098
      vascular NEC — *see* Complication, cardiovascular device, mechanical
      ventricular intracranial shunt T85.09
    foreign body left accidentally in operative wound T81.539
    instrument (any) during a procedure, accidental — *see* Puncture, accidental complicating surgery
  cecum K35.2
  cervix (uteri) N88.8
    with or following ectopic or molar pregnancy O08.6
    obstetrical trauma O71.3

Perforation, perforated (nontraumatic) (of) — *continued*
  colon K63.1
    newborn P78.0
    obstetrical trauma O71.5
    traumatic — *see* Laceration, intestine, large
  common duct (bile) K83.2
  cornea (due to ulceration) — *see* Ulcer, cornea, perforated
  cystic duct K82.2
  diverticulum (intestine) K57.80
    with bleeding K57.81
    large intestine K57.20
      with
        bleeding K57.21
        small intestine K57.40
          with bleeding K57.41
    small intestine K57.00
      with
        bleeding K57.01
        large intestine K57.40
          with bleeding K57.41
  ear drum — *see* Perforation, tympanum
  esophagus K22.3
  ethmoidal sinus — *see* Sinusitis, ethmoidal
  frontal sinus — *see* Sinusitis, frontal
  gallbladder K82.2
  heart valve — *see* Endocarditis
  ileum K63.1
    newborn P78.0
    obstetrical trauma O71.5
    traumatic — *see* Laceration, intestine, small
  instrumental, surgical (accidental) (blood vessel) (nerve) (organ) — *see* Puncture, accidental complicating surgery
  intestine NEC K63.1
    with ectopic or molar pregnancy O08.6
    newborn P78.0
    obstetrical trauma O71.5
    traumatic — *see* Laceration, intestine
    ulcerative NEC K63.1
      newborn P78.0
  jejunum, jejunal K63.1
    obstetrical trauma O71.5
    traumatic — *see* Laceration, intestine, small
    ulcer — *see* Ulcer, gastrojejunal, with perforation
  joint prosthesis — *see* Complications, joint prosthesis, mechanical, specified NEC, by site
  mastoid (antrum) (cell) — *see* Disorder, mastoid, specified NEC
  maxillary sinus — *see* Sinusitis, maxillary
  membrana tympani — *see* Perforation, tympanum
  nasal
    septum J34.89
      congenital Q30.3
      syphilitic A52.73
    sinus J34.89
      congenital Q30.8
      due to sinusitis — *see* Sinusitis
  palate (see also Cleft, palate) Q35.9
    syphilitic A52.79
    palatine vault (see also Cleft, palate, hard) Q35.1
      syphilitic A52.79
      congenital A50.59
  pars flaccida (ear drum) — *see* Perforation, tympanum, attic
  pelvic
    floor S31.030
      with
        ectopic or molar pregnancy O08.6
        penetration into retroperitoneal space S31.031
        retained foreign body S31.040
          with penetration into retroperitoneal space S31.041
      following ectopic or molar pregnancy O08.6
      obstetrical trauma O70.1
    organ S37.99
      adrenal gland S37.818
      bladder — *see* Perforation, bladder
      fallopian tube S37.599
        bilateral S37.592
        unilateral S37.591
      kidney S37.09-
        obstetrical trauma O71.5
      ovary S37.499
        bilateral S37.492
        unilateral S37.491

D I S E A S E   I N D E X

Perforation, perforated (nontraumatic) (of)
— continued
  pelvic — continued
    organ S37.99 — continued
      prostate S37.828
      specified organ NEC S37.898
      ureter — see Perforation, ureter
      urethra — see Perforation, urethra
      uterus — see Perforation, uterus
  perineum — see Laceration, perineum
  pharynx J39.2
  rectum K63.1
    newborn P78.0
    obstetrical trauma O71.5
    traumatic S36.63
  root canal space due to endodontic
    treatment M27.51
  sigmoid K63.1
    newborn P78.0
    obstetrical trauma O71.5
    traumatic S36.533
  sinus (accessory) (chronic) (nasal) J34.89
  sphenoidal sinus — see Sinusitis,
    sphenoidal
  surgical (accidental) (by instrument) (blood
    vessel) (nerve) (organ) — see
    Puncture, accidental complicating
    surgery
  traumatic
    external — see Puncture
    eye — see Puncture, eyeball
    internal organ — see Injury, by site
  tympanum, tympanic (membrane)
    (persistent post-traumatic)
    (postinflammatory) H72.9-
    attic H72.1-
      multiple — see Perforation,
        tympanum, multiple
      total — see Perforation, tympanum,
        total
    central H72.0-
      multiple — see Perforation,
        tympanum, multiple
      total — see Perforation, tympanum,
        total
    marginal NEC — see subcategory H72.2
    multiple H72.81-
    pars flaccida — see Perforation,
      tympanum, attic
    total H72.82-
    traumatic, current episode S09.2-
  typhoid, gastrointestinal — see Typhoid
  ulcer — see Ulcer, by site, with perforation
  ureter N28.89
    traumatic S37.19
  urethra N36.8
    with ectopic or molar pregnancy O08.6
    following ectopic or molar pregnancy
      O08.6
    obstetrical trauma O71.5
    traumatic S37.39
      at delivery O71.5
  uterus
    with ectopic or molar pregnancy O08.6
    by intrauterine contraceptive device
      T83.39
    following ectopic or molar pregnancy
      O08.6
    obstetrical trauma O71.1
    traumatic S37.69
      obstetric O71.1
  uvula K13.79
    syphilitic A52.79
  vagina
    obstetrical trauma O71.4
    other trauma — see Puncture, vagina
Periadenitis mucosa necrotica recurrens
  K12.0
Periappendicitis (acute) — see Appendicitis
Periarteritis nodosa (disseminated)
  (infectious) (necrotizing) M30.0
Periarthritis (joint) — see also Enthesopathy
  Duplay's M75.0-
  gonococcal A54.42
  humeroscapularis — see Capsulitis,
    adhesive
  scapulohumeral — see Capsulitis, adhesive
  shoulder — see Capsulitis, adhesive
  wrist M77.2-
Periarthrosis (angioneural) — see
  Enthesopathy
Pericapsulitis, adhesive (shoulder) — see
  Capsulitis, adhesive

Pericarditis (with decompensation) (with
  effusion) I31.9
  with rheumatic fever (conditions in I00)
    active — see Pericarditis, rheumatic
    inactive or quiescent I09.2
  acute (hemorrhagic) (nonrheumatic)
    (Sicca) I30.9
    with chorea (acute) (rheumatic)
      (Sydenham's) I02.0
    benign I30.8
    nonspecific I30.0
    rheumatic I01.0
      with chorea (acute) (Sydenham's)
        I02.0
  adhesive or adherent (chronic) (external)
    (internal) I31.0
    acute — see Pericarditis, acute
    rheumatic I09.2
  bacterial (acute) (subacute) (with serous or
    seropurulent effusion) I30.1
  calcareous I31.1
  cholesterol (chronic) I31.8
    acute I30.9
  chronic (nonrheumatic) I31.9
    rheumatic I09.2
  constrictive (chronic) I31.1
  coxsackie B33.23
  fibrinocaseous (tuberculous) A18.84
  fibrinopurulent I30.1
  fibrinous I30.8
  fibrous I31.0
  gonococcal A54.83
  idiopathic I30.0
  in systemic lupus erythematosus M32.12
  infective I30.1
  meningococcal A39.53
  neoplastic (chronic) I31.8
    acute I30.9
  obliterans, obliterating I31.0
  plastic I31.0
  pneumococcal I30.1
  postinfarction I24.1
  purulent I30.1
  rheumatic (active) (acute) (with effusion)
    (with pneumonia) I01.0
    with chorea (acute) (rheumatic)
      (Sydenham's) I02.0
    chronic or inactive (with chorea) I09.2
  rheumatoid — see Rheumatoid, carditis
  septic I30.1
  serofibrinous I30.8
  staphylococcal I30.1
  streptococcal I30.1
  suppurative I30.1
  syphilitic A52.06
  tuberculous A18.84
  uremic N18.9 [I32]
  viral I30.1
Pericardium, pericardial — see condition
Pericellulitis — see Cellulitis
Pericementitis (chronic) (suppurative) — see
  also Periodontitis
  acute K05.20
    generalized K05.22
    localized K05.21
Perichondritis
  auricle — see Perichondritis, ear
  bronchus J98.09
  ear (external) H61.00-
    acute H61.01-
    chronic H61.02-
  external auditory canal — see
    Perichondritis, ear
  larynx J38.7
    syphilitic A52.73
    typhoid A01.09
  nose J34.89
  pinna — see Perichondritis, ear
  trachea J39.8
Periclasia K05.4
Pericoronitis — see Periodontitis
Pericystitis N30.90
  with hematuria N30.91
Peridiverticulitis (intestine) K57.92
  cecum — see Diverticulitis, intestine, large
  colon — see Diverticulitis, intestine, large
  duodenum — see Diverticulitis, intestine,
    small
  intestine — see Diverticulitis, intestine
  jejunum — see Diverticulitis, intestine,
    small
  rectosigmoid — see Diverticulitis,
    intestine, large
  rectum — see Diverticulitis, intestine, large
  sigmoid — see Diverticulitis, intestine,
    large
Periendocarditis — see Endocarditis

Periepididymitis N45.1
Perifolliculitis L01.02
  abscedens, caput, scalp L66.3
  capitis, abscedens (et suffodiens) L66.3
  superficial pustular L01.02
Perihepatitis K65.8
Perilabyrinthitis (acute) — see subcategory
  H83.0
Perimeningitis — see Meningitis
Perimetritis — see Endometritis
Perimetrosalpingitis — see Salpingo-
  oophoritis
Perineocele N81.81
Perinephric, perinephritic — see condition
Perinephritis — see also Infection, kidney
  purulent — see Abscess, kidney
Perineum, perineal — see condition
Perineuritis NEC — see Neuralgia
Periodic — see condition
Periodontitis (chronic) (complex)
  (compound) (local) (simplex) K05.30
  acute K05.20
    generalized K05.22
    localized K05.21
  apical K04.5
    acute (pulpal origin) K04.4
  generalized K05.32
  localized K05.31
Periodontoclasia K05.4
Periodontosis (juvenile) K05.4
Periods — see also Menstruation
  heavy N92.0
  irregular N92.6
  shortened intervals (irregular) N92.1
Perionychia — see also Cellulitis, digit
  with lymphangitis — see Lymphangitis,
    acute, digit
Perioophoritis — see Salpingo-oophoritis
Periorchitis N45.2
Periosteum, periosteal — see condition
Periostitis (albuminosa) (circumscribed)
  (diffuse) (infective) (monomelic) — see
  also Osteomyelitis
  alveolar M27.3
  alveolodental M27.3
  dental M27.3
  gonorrheal A54.43
  jaw (lower) (upper) M27.2
  orbit H05.03-
  syphilitic A52.77
    congenital (early) A50.02 [M90.80]
    secondary A51.46
  tuberculous — see Tuberculosis, bone
  yaws (hypertrophic) (early) (late) A66.6
    [M90.80]
Periostosis (hyperplastic) — see also
  Disorder, bone, specified type NEC
  with osteomyelitis — see Osteomyelitis,
    specified type NEC
Peripartum
  cardiomyopathy O90.3
Periphlebitis — see Phlebitis
Periproctitis K62.89
Periprostatitis — see Prostatitis
Perirectal — see condition
Perirenal — see condition
Perisalpingitis — see Salpingo-oophoritis
Perisplenitis (infectional) D73.89
Peristalsis, visible or reversed R19.2
Peritendinitis — see Enthesopathy
Peritoneum, peritoneal — see condition
Peritonitis (adhesive) (bacterial) (fibrinous)
  (hemorrhagic) (idiopathic) (localized)
  (perforative) (primary) (with adhesions)
  (with effusion) K65.9
  with or following
    abscess K65.1
    appendicitis K35.2
      with perforation or rupture K35.2
      generalized K35.2
      localized K35.3
    diverticular disease (intestine) K57.80
      with bleeding K57.81
    ectopic or molar pregnancy O08.0
    large intestine K57.20
      with
        bleeding K57.21
        small intestine K57.40
          with bleeding K57.41
    small intestine K57.00
      with
        bleeding K57.01
        large intestine K57.40
          with bleeding K57.41
  acute (generalized) K65.0
  aseptic T81.61
  bile, biliary K65.3

Peritonitis (adhesive) (bacterial) (fibrinous)
  (hemorrhagic) (idiopathic) (localized)
  (perforative) (primary) (with adhesions)
  (with effusion) K65.9 — continued
  chemical T81.61
  chlamydial A74.81
  chronic proliferative K65.8
  complicating abortion — see Abortion, by
    type, complicated by, pelvic
    peritonitis
  congenital P78.1
  diaphragmatic K65.0
  diffuse K65.0
  diphtheritic A36.89
  disseminated K65.0
  due to
    bile K65.3
    foreign
      body or object accidentally left during
        a procedure (instrument)
        (sponge) (swab) T81.599
      substance accidentally left during a
        procedure (chemical) (powder)
        (talc) T81.61
    talc T81.61
    urine K65.8
  eosinophilic K65.8
    acute K65.0
  fibrocaseous (tuberculous) A18.31
  fibropurulent K65.0
  following ectopic or molar pregnancy
    O08.0
  general(ized) K65.0
  gonococcal A54.85
  meconium (newborn) P78.0
  neonatal P78.1
    meconium P78.0
  pancreatic K65.0
  paroxysmal, familial E85.0
    benign E85.0
  pelvic
    female N73.5
      acute N73.3
      chronic N73.4
        with adhesions N73.6
    male K65.0
  periodic, familial E85.0
  proliferative, chronic K65.8
  puerperal, postpartum, childbirth O85
  purulent K65.0
  septic K65.0
  specified NEC K65.8
  spontaneous bacterial K65.2
  subdiaphragmatic K65.0
  subphrenic K65.0
  suppurative K65.0
  syphilitic A52.74
    congenital (early) A50.08 [K67]
  talc T81.61
  tuberculous A18.31
  urine K65.8
Peritonsillar — see condition
Peritonsillitis J36
Perityphlitis K37
Periureteritis N28.89
Periurethral — see condition
Periurethritis (gangrenous) — see Urethritis
Periuterine — see condition
Perivaginitis — see Vaginitis
Perivasculitis, retinal H35.06-
Perivasitis (chronic) N49.1
Perivesiculitis (seminal) — see Vesiculitis
Perlèche NEC K13.0
  due to
    candidiasis B37.83
    moniliasis B37.83
    riboflavin deficiency E53.0
    vitamin B2 (riboflavin) deficiency E53.0
Pernicious — see condition
Pernio, perniosis T69.1
Perpetrator (of abuse) — see Index to
  External Causes of Injury, Perpetrator
Persecution
  delusion F22
  social Z60.5
Perseveration (tonic) R48.8
Persistence, persistent (congenital)
  anal membrane Q42.3
    with fistula Q42.2
  arteria stapedia Q16.3
  atrioventricular canal Q21.2
  branchial cleft Q18.0
  bulbus cordis in left ventricle Q21.8
  canal of Cloquet Q14.0
  capsule (opaque) Q12.8
  cilioretinal artery or vein Q14.8

Persistence, persistent (congenital) — *continued*
cloaca Q43.7
communication — *see* Fistula, congenital
convolutions
aortic arch Q25.4
fallopian tube Q50.6
oviduct Q50.6
uterine tube Q50.6
double aortic arch Q25.4
ductus arteriosus (Botalli) Q25.0
fetal
circulation P29.3
form of cervix (uteri) Q51.828
hemoglobin, hereditary (HPFH) D56.4
foramen
Botalli Q21.1
ovale Q21.1
Gartner's duct Q52.4
hemoglobin, fetal (hereditary) (HPFH) D56.4
hyaloid
artery (generally incomplete) Q14.0
system Q14.8
hymen, in pregnancy or childbirth — *see* Pregnancy, complicated by, abnormal, vulva
lanugo Q84.2
left
posterior cardinal vein Q26.8
root with right arch of aorta Q25.4
superior vena cava Q26.1
Meckel's diverticulum Q43.0
malignant — *see* Table of Neoplasms, small intestine, malignant
mucosal disease (middle ear) — *see* Otitis, media, suppurative, chronic, tubotympanic
nail(s), anomalous Q84.6
omphalomesenteric duct Q43.0
organ or site not listed — *see* Anomaly, by site
ostium
atrioventriculare commune Q21.2
primum Q21.2
secundum Q21.1
ovarian rests in fallopian tube Q50.6
pancreatic tissue in intestinal tract Q43.8
primary (deciduous)
teeth K00.6
vitreous hyperplasia Q14.0
pupillary membrane Q13.89
rhesus (Rh) titer — *see* Complication(s), transfusion, incompatibility reaction, Rh (factor)
right aortic arch Q25.4
sinus
urogenitalis
female Q52.8
male Q55.8
venosus with imperfect incorporation in right auricle Q26.8
thymus (gland) (hyperplasia) E32.0
thyroglossal duct Q89.2
thyrolingual duct Q89.2
truncus arteriosus or communis Q20.0
tunica vasculosa lentis Q12.2
umbilical sinus Q64.4
urachus Q64.4
vitelline duct Q43.0
Person (with)
admitted for clinical research, as a control subject (normal comparison) (participant) Z00.6
awaiting admission to adequate facility elsewhere Z75.1
concern (normal) about sick person in family Z63.6
consulting on behalf of another Z71.0
feigning illness Z76.5
living (in)
alone Z60.2
boarding school Z59.3
residential institution Z59.3
without
adequate housing (heating) (space) Z59.1
housing (permanent) (temporary) Z59.0
person able to render necessary care Z74.2
shelter Z59.0
on waiting list Z75.1
sick or handicapped in family Z63.6

Personality (disorder) F60.9
accentuation of traits (type A pattern) Z73.1
affective F34.0
aggressive F60.3
amoral F60.2
anacastic, anankastic F60.5
antisocial F60.2
anxious F60.6
asocial F60.2
asthenic F60.7
avoidant F60.6
borderline F60.3
change due to organic condition (enduring) F07.0
compulsive F60.5
cycloid F34.0
cyclothymic F34.0
dependent F60.7
depressive F34.1
dissocial F60.2
dual F44.81
eccentric F60.89
emotionally unstable F60.3
expansive paranoid F60.0
explosive F60.3
fanatic F60.0
haltlose type F60.89
histrionic F60.4
hyperthymic F34.0
hypothymic F34.1
hysterical F60.4
immature F60.89
inadequate F60.7
labile (emotional) F60.3
mixed (nonspecific) F60.81
morally defective F60.2
multiple F44.81
narcissistic F60.81
obsessional F60.5
obsessive(-compulsive) F60.5
organic F07.0
overconscientious F60.5
paranoid F60.0
passive-aggressive F60.89
passive(-dependent) F60.7
pathologic F60.9
pattern defect or disturbance F60.9
pseudopsychopathic (organic) F07.0
pseudoretarded (organic) F07.0
psychoinfantile F60.4
psychoneurotic NEC F60.89
psychopathic F60.2
querulant F60.0
sadistic F60.89
schizoid F60.1
self-defeating F60.7
sensitive paranoid F60.0
sociopathic (amoral) (antisocial) (asocial) (dissocial) F60.2
specified NEC F60.89
type A Z73.1
unstable (emotional) F60.3
Perthes' disease — *see* Legg-Calvé-Perthes disease
Pertussis (*see also* Whooping cough) A37.90
Perversion, perverted
appetite F50.8
psychogenic F50.8
function
pituitary gland E23.2
posterior lobe E22.2
sense of smell and taste R43.8
psychogenic F45.8
sexual — *see* Deviation, sexual
Pervious, congenital — *see also* Imperfect, closure
ductus arteriosus Q25.0
Pes (congenital) — *see also* Talipes
acquired — *see also* Deformity, limb, foot, specified NEC
planus — *see* Deformity, limb, flat foot
adductus Q66.89
cavus Q66.7
deformity NEC, acquired — *see* Deformity, limb, foot, specified NEC
planus (acquired) (any degree) — *see also* Deformity, limb, flat foot
rachitic sequelae (late effect) E64.3
valgus Q66.6
Pest, pestis — *see* Plague
Petechia, petechiae R23.3
newborn P54.5
Petechial typhus A75.9
Peter's anomaly Q13.4
Petit mal seizure — *see* Epilepsy, generalized, specified NEC

Petit's hernia — *see* Hernia, abdomen, specified site NEC
Petrellidosis B48.2
Petrositis H70.20-
acute H70.21-
chronic H70.22-
Peutz-Jeghers disease or syndrome Q85.8
Peyronie's disease N48.6
Pfeiffer's disease — *see* Mononucleosis, infectious
Phagedena (dry) (moist) (sloughing) — *see also* Gangrene
geometric L88
penis N48.29
tropical — *see* Ulcer, skin
vulva N76.6
Phagedenic — *see* condition
Phakoma H35.89
Phakomatosis (*see also* specific eponymous syndromes) Q85.9
Bourneville's Q85.1
specified NEC Q85.8
Phantom limb syndrome (without pain) G54.7
with pain G54.6
Pharyngeal pouch syndrome D82.1
Pharyngitis (acute) (catarrhal)(gangrenous) (infective) (malignant) (membranous) (phlegmonous) (pseudomembranous) (simple) (subacute) (suppurative) (ulcerative) (viral) J02.9
with influenza, flu, or grippe — *see* Influenza, with, pharyngitis
aphthous B08.5
atrophic J31.2
chlamydial A56.4
chronic (atrophic) (granular) (hypertrophic) J31.2
coxsackievirus B08.5
diphtheritic A36.0
enteroviral vesicular B08.5
follicular (chronic) J31.2
fusospirochetal A69.1
gonococcal A54.5
granular (chronic) J31.2
herpesviral B00.2
hypertrophic J31.2
infectional, chronic J31.2
influenzal — *see* Influenza, with, respiratory manifestations NEC
lymphonodular, acute (enteroviral) B08.8
pneumococcal J02.8
purulent J02.9
putrid J02.9
septic J02.0
sicca J31.2
specified organism NEC J02.8
staphylococcal J02.8
streptococcal J02.0
syphilitic, congenital (early) A50.03
tuberculous A15.8
vesicular, enteroviral B08.5
viral NEC J02.8
Pharyngoconjunctivitis, viral B30.2
Pharyngolaryngitis (acute) J06.0
chronic J37.0
Pharyngoplegia J39.2
Pharyngotonsillitis, herpesviral B00.2
Pharyngotracheitis, chronic J42
Pharynx, pharyngeal — *see* condition
Phenomenon
Arthus' — *see* Arthus' phenomenon
jaw-winking Q07.8
lupus erythematosus (LE) cell M32.9
Raynaud's (secondary) I73.00
with gangrene I73.01
vasomotor R55
vasospastic I73.9
vasovagal R55
Wenckebach's I44.1
Phenylketonuria E70.1
classical E70.0
maternal E70.1
Pheochromoblastoma
specified site — *see* Neoplasm, malignant, by site
unspecified site C74.10
Pheochromocytoma
malignant
specified site — *see* Neoplasm, malignant, by site
unspecified site C74.10
specified site — *see* Neoplasm, benign, by site
unspecified site D35.00
Pheohyphomycosis — *see* Chromomycosis
Pheomycosis — *see* Chromomycosis

Phimosis (congenital) (due to infection) N47.1
chancroidal A57
Phlebectasia — *see also* Varix
congenital Q27.4
Phlebitis (infective) (pyemic) (septic) (suppurative) I80.9
antepartum — *see* Thrombophlebitis, antepartum
blue — *see* Phlebitis, leg, deep
breast, superficial I80.8
cavernous (venous) sinus — *see* Phlebitis, intracranial (venous) sinus
cerebral (venous) sinus — *see* Phlebitis, intracranial (venous) sinus
chest wall, superficial I80.8
cranial (venous) sinus — *see* Phlebitis, intracranial (venous) sinus
deep (vessels) — *see* Phlebitis, leg, deep
due to implanted device — *see* Complications, by site and type, specified NEC
during or resulting from a procedure T81.72
femoral vein (superficial) I80.1-
femoropopliteal vein I80.0-
gestational — *see* Phlebopathy, gestational
hepatic veins I80.8
iliofemoral — *see* Phlebitis, femoral vein
intracranial (venous) sinus (any) G08
nonpyogenic I67.6
intraspinal venous sinuses and veins G08
nonpyogenic G95.19
lateral (venous) sinus — *see* Phlebitis, intracranial (venous) sinus
leg I80.3
antepartum — *see* Thrombophlebitis, antepartum
deep (vessels) NEC I80.20-
iliac I80.21-
popliteal vein I80.22-
specified vessel NEC I80.29-
tibial vein I80.23-
femoral vein (superficial) I80.1-
superficial (vessels) I80.0-
longitudinal sinus — *see* Phlebitis, intracranial (venous) sinus
lower limb — *see* Phlebitis, leg
migrans, migrating (superficial) I82.1
pelvic
with ectopic or molar pregnancy O08.0
following ectopic or molar pregnancy O08.0
puerperal, postpartum O87.1
popliteal vein — *see* Phlebitis, leg, deep, popliteal
portal (vein) K75.1
postoperative T81.72
pregnancy — *see* Thrombophlebitis, antepartum
puerperal, postpartum, childbirth O87.0
deep O87.1
pelvic O87.1
superficial O87.0
retina — *see* Vasculitis, retina
saphenous (accessory) (great) (long) (small) — *see* Phlebitis, leg, superficial
sinus (meninges) — *see* Phlebitis, intracranial (venous) sinus
specified site NEC I80.8
syphilitic A52.09
tibial vein — *see* Phlebitis, leg, deep, tibial
ulcerative I80.9
leg — *see* Phlebitis, leg
umbilicus I80.8
uterus (septic) — *see* Endometritis
varicose (leg) (lower limb) — *see* Varix, leg, with, inflammation
Phlebofibrosis I87.8
Phleboliths I87.8
Phlebopathy,
gestational O22.9-
puerperal O87.9
Phlebosclerosis I87.8
Phlebothrombosis — *see also* Thrombosis
antepartum — *see* Thrombophlebitis, antepartum
pregnancy — *see* Thrombophlebitis, antepartum
puerperal — *see* Thrombophlebitis, puerperal
Phlebotomus fever A93.1
Phlegmasia
alba dolens O87.1
nonpuerperal — *see* Phlebitis, femoral
cerulea dolens — *see* Phlebitis, leg, deep

Phlegmon — see Abscess
Phlegmonous — see condition
Phlyctenulosis (allergic)
   (keratoconjunctivitis) (nontuberculous)
   — see also Keratoconjunctivitis
  cornea — see Keratoconjunctivitis
  tuberculous A18.52
Phobia, phobic F40.9
  animal F40.218
    spiders F40.210
  examination F40.298
  reaction F40.9
  simple F40.298
  social F40.10
    generalized F40.11
  specific (isolated) F40.298
    animal F40.218
      spiders F40.210
    blood F40.230
    injection F40.231
    injury F40.233
    men F40.290
    natural environment F40.228
      thunderstorms F40.220
    situational F40.248
      bridges F40.242
      closed in spaces F40.240
      flying F40.243
      heights F40.241
    specified focus NEC F40.298
    transfusion F40.231
    women F40.291
  specified NEC F40.8
    medical care NEC F40.232
  state F40.9
Phocas' disease — see Mastopathy, cystic
Phocomelia Q73.1
  lower limb — see Agenesis, leg, with foot
    present
  upper limb — see Agenesis, arm, with hand
    present
Phoria H50.50
Phosphate-losing tubular disorder N25.0
Phosphatemia E83.39
Phosphaturia E83.39
Photodermatitis (sun) L56.8
  chronic L57.8
  due to drug L56.8
  light other than sun L59.8
Photokeratitis H16.13-
Photophobia H53.14
Photophthalmia — see Photokeratitis
Photopsia H53.19
Photoretinitis — see Retinopathy, solar
Photosensitivity, photosensitization (sun)
  skin L56.8
  light other than sun L59.8
Phrenitis — see Encephalitis
Phrynoderma (vitamin A deficiency) E50.8
Phthiriasis (pubis) B85.3
  with any infestation classifiable to B85.0-
    B85.2 B85.4
Phthirus infestation — see Phthiriasis
Phthisis — see also Tuberculosis
  bulbi (infectional) — see Disorder, globe,
    degenerated condition, atrophy
  eyeball (due to infection) — see Disorder,
    globe, degenerated condition, atrophy
Phycomycosis — see Zygomycosis
Physalopteriasis B81.8
Physical restraint status Z78.1
Phytobezoar T18.9
  intestine T18.3
  stomach T18.2
Pian — see Yaws
Pianoma A66.1
Pica F50.8
  in adults F50.8
  infant or child F98.3
Picking, nose F98.8
Pick-Niemann disease — see Niemann-Pick
  disease or syndrome
Pick's
  cerebral atrophy G31.01 [F02.80]
    with behavioral disturbance G31.01
      [F02.81]
  disease or syndrome (brain) G31.01
    [F02.80]
    with behavioral disturbance G31.01
      [F02.81]
Pickwickian syndrome E66.2
Piebaldism E70.39
Piedra (beard) (scalp) B36.8
  black B36.3
  white B36.2
Pierre Robin deformity or syndrome Q87.0
Pierson's disease or osteochondrosis M91.0
Pig-bel A05.2

Pigeon
  breast or chest (acquired) M95.4
    congenital Q67.7
    rachitic sequelae (late effect) E64.3
  breeder's disease or lung J67.2
  fancier's disease or lung J67.2
  toe — see Deformity, toe, specified NEC
Pigmentation (abnormal) (anomaly) L81.9
  conjunctiva H11.13-
  cornea (anterior) H18.01-
    posterior H18.05-
    stromal H18.06-
  diminished melanin formation NEC L81.6
  iron L81.8
  lids, congenital Q82.8
  limbus corneae — see Pigmentation,
    cornea
  metals L81.8
  optic papilla, congenital Q14.2
  retina, congenital (grouped) (nevoid)
    Q14.1
  scrotum, congenital Q82.8
  tattoo L81.8
Piles (see also Hemorrhoids) K64.9
Pili
  annulati or torti (congenital) Q84.1
  incarnati L73.1
Pill roller hand (intrinsic) — see
  Parkinsonism
Pilomatrixoma — see Neoplasm, skin,
  benign
  malignant — see Neoplasm, skin,
    malignant
Pilonidal — see condition
Pimple R23.8
Pinched nerve — see Neuropathy,
  entrapment
Pindborg tumor — see Cyst, calcifying
  odontogenic
Pineal body or gland — see condition
Pinealoblastoma C75.3
Pinealoma D44.5
  malignant C75.3
Pineoblastoma C75.3
Pineocytoma D44.5
Pinguecula H11.15-
Pingueculitis H10.81-
Pinhole meatus (see also Stricture, urethra)
  N35.9
Pink
  disease — see subcategory T56.1
  eye — see Conjunctivitis, acute,
    mucopurulent
Pinkus' disease (lichen nitidus) L44.1
Pinpoint
  meatus — see Stricture, urethra
  os (uteri) — see Stricture, cervix
Pins and needles R20.2
Pinta A67.9
  cardiovascular lesions A67.2
  chancre (primary) A67.0
  erythematous plaques A67.1
  hyperchromic lesions A67.1
  hyperkeratosis A67.1
  lesions A67.9
    cardiovascular A67.2
    hyperchromic A67.1
    intermediate A67.1
    late A67.2
    mixed A67.3
    primary A67.0
    skin (achromic) (cicatricial)
      (dyschromic) A67.2
      hyperchromic A67.1
      mixed (achromic and hyperchromic)
        A67.3
  papule (primary) A67.0
  skin lesions (achromic) (cicatricial)
    (dyschromic) A67.2
    hyperchromic A67.1
    mixed (achromic and hyperchromic)
      A67.3
  vitiligo A67.2
Pintids A67.1
Pinworm (disease) (infection) (infestation)
  B80
Piroplasmosis B60.0
Pistol wound — see Gunshot wound
Pitcher's elbow — see Derangement, joint,
  specified type NEC, elbow
Pithecoid pelvis Q74.2
  with disproportion (fetopelvic) O33.0
    causing obstructed labor O65.0
Pithiatism F48.8
Pitted — see Pitting
Pitting (see also Edema) R60.9
  lip R60.0
  nail L60.8
  teeth K00.4
Pituitary gland — see condition

Pituitary-snuff-taker's disease J67.8
Pityriasis (capitis) L21.0
  alba L30.5
  circinata (et maculata) L42
  furfuracea L21.0
  Hebra's L26
  lichenoides L41.0
    chronica L41.1
    et varioliformis (acuta) L41.0
  maculata (et circinata) L30.5
  nigra B36.1
  pilaris, Hebra's L44.0
  rosea L42
  rotunda L44.8
  rubra (Hebra) pilaris L44.0
  simplex L30.5
    specified type NEC L30.5
  streptogenes L30.5
  versicolor (scrotal) B36.0
Placenta, placental — see Pregnancy,
  complicated by (care of) (management
  affected by), specified condition
Placentitis O41.14-
Plagiocephaly Q67.3
Plague A20.9
  abortive A20.8
  ambulatory A20.8
  asymptomatic A20.8
  bubonic A20.0
  cellulocutaneous A20.1
  cutaneobubonic A20.1
  lymphatic gland A20.0
  meningitis A20.3
  pharyngeal A20.8
  pneumonic (primary) (secondary) A20.2
  pulmonary, pulmonic A20.2
  septicemic A20.7
  tonsillar A20.8
    septicemic A20.7
Planning, family
  contraception Z30.9
  procreation Z31.69
Plaque(s)
  artery, arterial — see Arteriosclerosis
  calcareous — see Calcification
  coronary, lipid rich I25.83
  epicardial I31.8
  erythematous, of pinta A67.1
  Hollenhorst's — see Occlusion, artery,
    retina
  lipid rich, coronary I25.83
  pleural (without asbestos) J92.9
    with asbestos J92.0
  tongue K13.29
Plasmacytoma C90.3-
  extramedullary C90.2-
  medullary C90.0-
  solitary C90.3-
Plasmacytopenia D72.818
Plasmacytosis D72.822
Plaster ulcer — see Ulcer, pressure, by site
Plateau iris syndrome (post-iridectomy)
  (postprocedural) (without glaucoma)
  H21.82
  with glaucoma H40.22-
Platybasia Q75.8
Platyonychia (congenital) Q84.6
  acquired L60.8
Platypelloid pelvis M95.5
  with disproportion (fetopelvic) O33.0
    causing obstructed labor O65.0
  congenital Q74.2
Platyspondylisis Q76.49
Platyspondylisis Q76.49
Plaut(-Vincent) disease (see also Vincent's)
  A69.1
Plethora R23.2
  newborn P61.1
Pleura, pleural — see condition
Pleuralgia R07.81
Pleurisy (acute) (adhesive) (chronic) (costal)
  (diaphragmatic) (double) (dry)
  (fibrinous) (fibrous) (interlobar) (latent)
  (plastic) (primary) (residual) (sicca)
  (sterile) (subacute) (unresolved) R09.1
  with
    adherent pleura J86.0
    effusion J90
      chylous, chyliform J94.0
      tuberculous (non primary) A15.6
        primary (progressive) A15.7
    tuberculosis — see Pleurisy, tuberculous
      (non primary)
  encysted — see Pleurisy, with effusion
  exudative — see Pleurisy, with effusion
  fibrinopurulent, fibropurulent — see
    Pyothorax
  hemorrhagic — see Hemothorax
  pneumococcal J90
  purulent — see Pyothorax
  septic — see Pyothorax

Pleurisy (acute) (adhesive) (chronic) (costal)
  (diaphragmatic) (double) (dry)
  (fibrinous) (fibrous) (interlobar) (latent)
  (plastic) (primary) (residual) (sicca)
  (sterile) (subacute) (unresolved) R09.1
  — continued
  serofibrinous — see Pleurisy, with effusion
  seropurulent — see Pyothorax
  serous — see Pleurisy, with effusion
  staphylococcal J86.9
  streptococcal J90
  suppurative — see Pyothorax
  traumatic (post) (current) — see Injury,
    intrathoracic, pleura
  tuberculous (with effusion) (non primary)
    A15.6
    primary (progressive) A15.7
Pleuritis sicca — see Pleurisy
Pleurobronchopneumonia — see
  Pneumonia, broncho-
Pleurodynia R07.81
  epidemic B33.0
  viral B33.0
Pleuropericarditis — see also Pericarditis
  acute I30.9
Pleuropneumonia (acute) (bilateral) (double)
  (septic) (see also Pneumonia) J18.8
  chronic — see Fibrosis, lung
Pleuro-pneumonia-like-organism (PPLO),
  as cause of disease classified elsewhere
  B96.0
Pleurorrhea — see Pleurisy, with effusion
Plexitis, brachial G54.0
Plica
  polonica B85.0
  syndrome, knee M67.5-
  tonsil J35.8
Plicated tongue K14.5
Plug
  bronchus NEC J98.09
  meconium (newborn) NEC syndrome P76.0
  mucus — see Asphyxia, mucus
Plumbism — see subcategory T56.0
Plummer's disease E05.20
  with thyroid storm E05.21
Plummer-Vinson syndrome D50.1
Pluricarential syndrome of infancy E40
Plus (and minus) hand (intrinsic) — see
  Deformity, limb, specified type NEC,
  forearm
Pneumathemia — see Air, embolism
Pneumatic hammer (drill) syndrome
  T75.21
Pneumatocele (lung) J98.4
  intracranial G93.89
  tension J44.9
Pneumatosis
  cystoides intestinalis K63.89
  intestinalis K63.89
  peritonei K66.8
Pneumaturia R39.89
Pneumoblastoma — see Neoplasm, lung,
  malignant
Pneumocephalus G93.89
Pneumococcemia A40.3
Pneumococcus, pneumococcal — see
  condition
Pneumoconiosis (due to) (inhalation of) J64
  with tuberculosis (any type in A15) J65
  aluminum J63.0
  asbestos J61
  bagasse, bagassosis J67.1
  bauxite J63.1
  beryllium J63.2
  coal miners' (simple) J60
  coalworkers' (simple) J60
  collier's J60
  cotton dust J66.0
  diatomite (diatomaceous earth) J62.8
  dust
    inorganic NEC J63.6
    lime J62.8
    marble J62.8
    organic NEC J66.8
  fumes or vapors (from silo) J68.9
  graphite J63.3
  grinder's J62.8
  kaolin J62.8
  mica J62.8
  millstone maker's J62.8
  miner's J60
  mineral fibers NEC J61
  moldy hay J67.0
  potter's J62.8
  rheumatoid — see Rheumatoid, lung
  sandblaster's J62.8
  silica, silicate NEC J62.8
    with carbon J60
  stonemason's J62.8
  talc (dust) J62.0

Pneumocystis carinii pneumonia B59
Pneumocystis jiroveci (pneumonia) B59
Pneumocystosis (with pneumonia) B59
Pneumohemopericardium I31.2
Pneumohemothorax J94.2
  traumatic S27.2
Pneumohydropericardium — *see*
  Pericarditis
Pneumohydrothorax — *see* Hydrothorax
Pneumomediastinum J98.2
  congenital or perinatal P25.2
Pneumomycosis B49 [J99]
Pneumonia (acute) (double) (migratory)
  (purulent) (septic) (unresolved) J18.9
  with
    influenza — *see* Influenza, with,
      pneumonia
    lung abscess J85.1
      due to specified organism — *see*
        Pneumonia, in (due to)
  adenoviral J12.0
  adynamic J18.2
  alba A50.04
  allergic (eosinophilic) J82
  alveolar — *see* Pneumonia, lobar
  anaerobes J15.8
  anthrax A22.1
  apex, apical — *see* Pneumonia, lobar
  Ascaris B77.81
  aspiration J69.0
    due to
      aspiration of microorganisms
        bacterial J15.9
        viral J12.9
      food (regurgitated) J69.0
      gastric secretions J69.0
      milk (regurgitated) J69.0
      oils, essences J69.1
      solids, liquids NEC J69.8
      vomitus J69.0
    newborn P24.81
      amniotic fluid (clear) P24.11
      blood P24.21
      food (regurgitated) P24.31
      liquor (amnii) P24.11
      meconium P24.01
      milk P24.31
      mucus P24.11
      specified NEC P24.81
      stomach contents P24.31
    postprocedural J95.4
  atypical NEC J18.9
  bacillus J15.9
    specified NEC J15.8
  bacterial J15.9
    specified NEC J15.8
  Bacteroides (fragilis) (oralis)
    (melaninogenicus) J15.8
  basal, basic, basilar — *see* Pneumonia, by
    type
  bronchiolitis obliterans organized (BOOP)
    J84.89
  broncho-, bronchial (confluent) (croupous)
    (diffuse) (disseminated)
    (hemorrhagic) (involving lobes)
    (lobar) (terminal) J18.0
    allergic (eosinophilic) J82
    aspiration — *see* Pneumonia, aspiration
    bacterial J15.9
      specified NEC J15.8
    chronic — *see* Fibrosis, lung
    diplococcal J13
    Eaton's agent J15.7
    Escherichia coli (E. coli) J15.5
    Friedländer's bacillus J15.0
    Hemophilus influenzae J14
    hypostatic J18.2
    inhalation — *see also* Pneumonia,
      aspiration
      due to fumes or vapors (chemical)
        J68.0
      of oils or essences J69.1
    Klebsiella (pneumoniae) J15.0
    lipid, lipoid J69.1
      endogenous J84.89
    Mycoplasma (pneumoniae) J15.7
    pleuro-pneumonia-like-organisms
      (PPLO) J15.7
    pneumococcal J13
    Proteus J15.6
    Pseudomonas J15.1
    Serratia marcescens J15.6
    specified organism NEC J16.8
    staphylococcal — *see* Pneumonia,
      staphylococcal
    streptococcal NEC J15.4
      group B J15.3
      pneumoniae J13
    viral, virus — *see* Pneumonia, viral

Pneumonia (acute) (double) (migratory)
  (purulent) (septic) (unresolved) J18.9 —
  continued
  Butyrivibrio (fibriosolvens) J15.8
  Candida B37.1
  caseous — *see* Tuberculosis, pulmonary
  catarrhal — *see* Pneumonia, broncho
  chlamydial J16.0
    congenital P23.1
  cholesterol J84.89
  cirrhotic (chronic) — *see* Fibrosis, lung
  Clostridium (haemolyticum) (novyi) J15.8
  confluent — *see* Pneumonia, broncho
  congenital (infective) P23.9
    due to
      bacterium NEC P23.6
      Chlamydia P23.1
      Escherichia coli P23.4
      Haemophilus influenzae P23.6
      infective organism NEC P23.8
      Klebsiella pneumoniae P23.6
      Mycoplasma P23.6
      Pseudomonas P23.5
      Staphylococcus P23.2
      Streptococcus (except group B) P23.6
        group B P23.3
      viral agent P23.0
      specified NEC P23.8
  croupous — *see* Pneumonia, lobar
  cryptogenic organizing J84.116
  cytomegalic inclusion B25.0
  cytomegaloviral B25.0
  deglutition — *see* Pneumonia, aspiration
  desquamative interstitial J84.117
  diffuse — *see* Pneumonia, broncho
  diplococcal, diplococcus (broncho-) (lobar)
    J13
  disseminated (focal) — *see* Pneumonia,
    broncho
  Eaton's agent J15.7
  embolic, embolism — *see* Embolism,
    pulmonary
  Enterobacter J15.6
  eosinophilic J82
  Escherichia coli (E. coli) J15.5
  Eubacterium J15.8
  fibrinous — *see* Pneumonia, lobar
  fibroid, fibrous (chronic) — *see* Fibrosis,
    lung
  Friedländer's bacillus J15.0
  Fusobacterium (nucleatum) J15.8
  gangrenous J85.0
  giant cell (measles) B05.2
  gonococcal A54.84
  gram-negative bacteria NEC J15.6
    anaerobic J15.8
  Hemophilus influenzae (broncho) (lobar)
    J14
  human metapneumovirus J12.3
  hypostatic (broncho) (lobar) J18.2
  in (due to)
    actinomycosis A42.0
    adenovirus J12.0
    anthrax A22.1
    ascariasis B77.81
    aspergillosis B44.9
    Bacillus anthracis A22.1
    Bacterium anitratum J15.6
    candidiasis B37.1
    chickenpox B01.2
    Chlamydia J16.0
      neonatal P23.1
    coccidioidomycosis B38.2
      acute B38.0
      chronic B38.1
    cytomegalovirus disease B25.0
    Diplococcus (pneumoniae) J13
    Eaton's agent J15.7
    Enterobacter J15.6
    Escherichia coli (E. coli) J15.5
    Friedländer's bacillus J15.0
    fumes and vapors (chemical)
      (inhalation) J68.0
    gonorrhea A54.84
    Hemophilus influenzae (H. influenzae)
      J14
    Herellea J15.6
    histoplasmosis B39.2
      acute B39.0
      chronic B39.1
    human metapneumovirus J12.3
    Klebsiella (pneumoniae) J15.0
    measles B05.2
    Mycoplasma (pneumoniae) J15.7
    nocardiosis, nocardiasis A43.0
    ornithosis A70
    parainfluenza virus J12.2
    pleuro-pneumonia-like-organism
      (PPLO) J15.7

Pneumonia (acute) (double) (migratory)
  (purulent) (septic) (unresolved) J18.9 —
  continued
  in (due to) — *continued*
    pneumococcus J13
    pneumocystosis (Pneumocystis carinii)
      (Pneumocystis jiroveci) B59
    Proteus J15.6
    Pseudomonas NEC J15.1
      pseudomallei A24.1
    psittacosis A70
    Q fever A78
    respiratory syncytial virus J12.1
    rheumatic fever I00 [J17]
    rubella B06.81
    Salmonella (infection) A02.22
      typhi A01.03
    schistosomiasis B65.9 [J17]
    Serratia marcescens J15.6
    specified
      bacterium NEC J15.8
      organism NEC J16.8
    spirochetal NEC A69.8
    Staphylococcus J15.20
      aureus (methicillin susceptible)
        (MSSA) J15.211
        methicillin resistant (MRSA)
          J15.212
      specified NEC J15.29
    Streptococcus J15.4
      group B J15.3
      pneumoniae J13
      specified NEC J15.4
    toxoplasmosis B58.3
    tularemia A21.2
    typhoid (fever) A01.03
    varicella B01.2
    virus — *see* Pneumonia, viral
    whooping cough A37.91
      due to
        Bordetella parapertussis A37.11
        Bordetella pertussis A37.01
        specified NEC A37.81
    Yersinia pestis A20.2
  inhalation of food or vomit — *see*
    Pneumonia, aspiration
  interstitial J84.9
    chronic J84.111
    desquamative J84.117
    due to
      collagen vascular disease J84.17
      known underlying cause J84.17
    idiopathic NOS J84.111
    in diseases classified elsewhere J84.17
    lymphocytic (due to collagen vacular
      disease) (in diseases classified
      elsewhere) J84.17
    lymphoid J84.2
    non-specific J84.89
      due to
        collagen vascular disease J84.17
        known underlying cause J84.17
      idiopathic J84.113
      in diseases classified elsewhere
        J84.17
    plasma cell B59
    pseudomonas J15.1
    usual J84.112
      due to collagen vascular disease
        J84.17
      idiopathic J84.112
      in diseases classified elsewhere
        J84.17
  Klebsiella (pneumoniae) J15.0
  lipid, lipoid (exogenous) J69.1
    endogenous J84.89
  lobar (disseminated) (double) (interstitial)
    J18.1
    bacterial J15.9
      specified NEC J15.8
    chronic — *see* Fibrosis, lung
    Escherichia coli (E. coli) J15.5
    Friedländer's bacillus J15.0
    Hemophilus influenzae J14
    hypostatic J18.2
    Klebsiella (pneumoniae) J15.0
    pneumococcal J13
    Proteus J15.6
    Pseudomonas J15.1
    specified organism NEC J16.8
    staphylococcal — *see* Pneumonia,
      staphylococcal
    streptococcal NEC J15.4
    Streptococcus pneumoniae J13
    viral, virus — *see* Pneumonia, viral
  lobular — *see* Pneumonia, broncho
  lymphoid interstitial J84.2
  Löffler's J82
  massive — *see* Pneumonia, lobar
  meconium P24.01

Pneumonia (acute) (double) (migratory)
  (purulent) (septic) (unresolved) J18.9 —
  continued
  MSSA (methicillin susceptible
    Staphylococcus aureus) J15.211
  Mycoplasma (pneumoniae) J15.7
  necrotic J85.0
  neonatal P23.9
    aspiration — *see* Aspiration, by
      substance, with pneumonia
  nitrogen dioxide J68.9
  organizing J84.89
    due to
      collagen vascular disease J84.17
      known underlying cause J84.17
    in diseases classified elsewhere J84.17
  orthostatic J18.2
  parainfluenza virus J12.2
  parenchymatous — *see* Fibrosis, lung
  passive J18.2
  patchy — *see* Pneumonia, broncho
  Peptococcus J15.8
  Peptostreptococcus J15.8
  plasma cell (of infants) B59
  pleurolobar — *see* Pneumonia, lobar
  pleuro-pneumonia-like organism (PPLO)
    J15.7
  pneumococcal (broncho) (lobar) J13
  Pneumocystis (carinii) (jiroveci) B59
  postinfectional NEC B99 [J17]
  postmeasles B05.2
  Proteus J15.6
  Pseudomonas J15.1
  psittacosis A70
  radiation J70.0
  respiratory syncytial virus J12.1
  resulting from a procedure J95.89
  rheumatic I00 [J17]
  Salmonella (arizonae) (cholerae-suis)
    (enteritidis) (typhimurium) A02.22
    typhi A01.03
    typhoid fever A01.03
  SARS-associated coronavirus J12.81
  segmented, segmental — *see* Pneumonia,
    broncho-
  Serratia marcescens J15.6
  specified NEC J18.8
    bacterium NEC J15.8
    organism NEC J16.8
    virus NEC J12.89
  spirochetal NEC A69.8
  staphylococcal (broncho) (lobar) J15.20
    aureus (methicillin susceptible) (MSSA)
      J15.211
      methicillin resistant (MRSA) J15.212
    specified NEC J15.29
  static, stasis J18.2
  streptococcal NEC (broncho) (lobar) J15.4
    group
      A J15.4
      B J15.3
      specified NEC J15.4
  Streptococcus pneumoniae J13
  syphilitic, congenital (early) A50.04
  traumatic (complication) (early)
    (secondary) T79.8
  tuberculous (any) — *see* Tuberculosis,
    pulmonary
  tularemic A21.2
  varicella B01.2
  Veillonella J15.8
  ventilator associated J95.851
  viral, virus (broncho) (interstitial) (lobar)
    J12.9
    adenoviral J12.0
    congenital P23.0
    human metapneumovirus J12.3
    parainfluenza J12.2
    respiratory syncytial J12.1
    SARS-associated coronavirus J12.81
    specified NEC J12.89
  white (congenital) A50.04

DISEASE INDEX

Pneumonic — *see* condition
Pneumonitis (acute) (primary) — *see also*
    Pneumonia
  air-conditioner J67.7
  allergic (due to) J67.9
    organic dust NEC J67.8
    red cedar dust J67.8
    sequoiosis J67.8
    wood dust J67.8
  aspiration J69.0
    due to
      anesthesia J95.4
        during
          labor and delivery O74.0
          pregnancy O29.01-
          puerperium O89.01
      fumes or gases J68.0
    obstetric O74.0
  chemical (due to gases, fumes or vapors)
    (inhalation) J68.0
    due to anesthesia J95.4
  cholesterol J84.89
  chronic — *see* Fibrosis, lung
  congenital rubella P35.0
  crack (cocaine) J68.0
  due to
    beryllium J68.0
    cadmium J68.0
    crack (cocaine) J68.0
    detergent J69.8
    fluorocarbon-polymer J68.0
    food, vomit (aspiration) J69.0
    fumes or vapors J68.0
    gases, fumes or vapors (inhalation) J68.0
    inhalation
      blood J69.8
      essences J69.1
      food (regurgitated), milk, vomit J69.0
      oils, essences J69.1
      saliva J69.0
      solids, liquids NEC J69.8
    manganese J68.0
    nitrogen dioxide J68.0
    oils, essences J69.1
    solids, liquids NEC J69.8
    toxoplasmosis (acquired) B58.3
      congenital P37.1
    vanadium J68.0
    ventilator J95.851
  eosinophilic J82
  hypersensitivity J67.9
    air conditioner lung J67.7
    bagassosis J67.1
    bird fancier's lung J67.2
    farmer's lung J67.0
    maltworker's lung J67.4
    maple bark-stripper's lung J67.6
    mushroom worker's lung J67.5
    specified organic dust NEC J67.8
    suberosis J67.3
  interstitial (chronic) J84.89
    acute J84.114
    lymphoid J84.2
    non-specific J84.89
      idiopathic J84.113
  lymphoid, interstitial J84.2
  meconium P24.01
  postanesthetic J95.4
    correct substance properly administered
      — *see* Table of Drugs and
      Chemcials, by drug, adverse effect
    in labor and delivery O74.0
    in pregnancy O29.01-
    obstetric O74.0
    overdose or wrong substance given or
      taken (by accident) — *see* Table of
      Drugs and Chemicals, by drug,
      poisoning
    postpartum, puerperal O89.01
  postoperative J95.4
    obstetric O74.0
  radiation J70.0
  rubella, congenital P35.0
  ventilation (air-conditioning) J67.7
  ventilator associated J95.851
  wood-dust J67.8
Pneumonoconiosis — *see* Pneumoconiosis
Pneumoparotid K11.8
Pneumopathy NEC J98.4
  alveolar J84.09
  due to organic dust NEC J66.8
  parietoalveolar J84.09
Pneumopericarditis — *see also* Pericarditis
  acute I30.9
Pneumopericardium — *see also* Pericarditis
  congenital P25.3
  newborn P25.3
  traumatic (post) — *see* Injury, heart

Pneumophagia (psychogenic) F45.8
Pneumopleurisy, pneumopleuritis (*see also*
  Pneumonia) J18.8
Pneumopyopericardium I30.1
Pneumopyothorax — *see* Pyopneumothorax
  with fistula J86.0
Pneumorrhagia — *see also* Hemorrhage,
  lung
  tuberculous — *see* Tuberculosis,
    pulmonary
Pneumothorax NOS J93.9
  acute J93.81
  chronic J93.81
  congenital P25.1
  perinatal period P25.1
  postprocedural J95.811
  specified NEC J93.83
  spontaneous NOS J93.83
    newborn P25.1
    primary J93.11
    secondary J93.12
    tension J93.0
  tense valvular, infectional J93.0
  tension (spontaneous) J93.0
  traumatic S27.0
    with hemothorax S27.2
  tuberculous — *see* Tuberculosis,
    pulmonary
Podagra (*see also* Gout) M10.9
Podencephalus Q01.9
Poikilocytosis R71.8
Poikiloderma L81.6
  Civatte's L57.3
  congenital Q82.8
  vasculare atrophicans L94.5
Poikilodermatomyositis M33.10
  with
    myopathy M33.12
    respiratory involvement M33.11
    specified organ involvement NEC
      M33.19
Pointed ear (congenital) Q17.3
Poison ivy, oak, sumac or other plant
  dermatitis (allergic) (contact) L23.7
Poisoning (acute) — *see also* Table of Drugs
  and Chemicals
  algae and toxins T65.82-
  Bacillus B (aertrycke) (cholerae (suis))
    (paratyphosus) (suipestifer) A02.9
  botulinus A05.1
  bacterial toxins A05.9
  berries, noxious — *see* Poisoning, food,
    noxious, berries
  botulism A05.1
  ciguatera fish T61.0-
  Clostridium botulinum A05.1
  death-cap (Amanita phalloides) (Amanita
    verna) — *see* Poisoning, food,
    noxious, mushrooms
  drug — *see* Table of Drugs and Chemicals,
    by drug, poisoning
  epidemic, fish (noxious) — *see* Poisoning,
    seafood
    bacterial A05.9
  fava bean D55.0
  fish (noxious) T61.9-
    bacterial — *see* Intoxication, foodborne,
      by agent
    ciguatera fish — *see* Poisoning,
      ciguatera fish
    scombroid fish — *see* Poisoning,
      scombroid fish
    specified type NEC T61.77-
  food (acute) (diseased) (infected) (noxious)
    NEC T62.9-
    bacterial — *see* Intoxication, foodborne,
      by agent
    due to
      Bacillus (aertrycke) (choleraesuis)
        (paratyphosus) (suipestifer)
        A02.9
      botulinus A05.1
      Clostridium (perfringens) (Welchii)
        A05.2
      salmonella (aertrycke) (callinarum)
        (choleraesuis) (enteritidis)
        (paratyphi) (suipestifer) A02.9
      with
        gastroenteritis A02.0
        sepsis A02.1
      staphylococcus A05.0
      Vibrio
        parahaemolyticus A05.3
        vulnificus A05.5

Poisoning (acute) (*see also* Table of Drugs
  and Chemicals) — *continued*
  food (acute) (diseased) (infected) (noxious)
    NEC T62.9- — *continued*
    noxious or naturally toxic T62.9-
      berries — *see* subcategory T62.1-
      fish — *see* Poisoning, seafood
      mushrooms — *see* subcategory
        T62.0x-
      plants NEC — *see* subcategory
        T62.2x-
      seafood — *see* Poisoning, seafood
      specified NEC — *see* subcategory
        T62.8x-
  ichthyotoxism — *see* Poisoning, seafood
  kreotoxism, food A05.9
  latex T65.81-
  lead T56.0-
  mushroom — *see* Poisoning, food, noxious,
    mushroom
  mussels — *see also* Poisoning, shellfish
    bacterial — *see* Intoxication, foodborne,
      by agent
  nicotine (tobacco) T65.2-
  noxious foodstuffs — *see* Poisoning, food,
    noxious
  plants, noxious — *see* Poisoning, food,
    noxious, plants NEC
  ptomaine — *see* Poisoning, food
  radiation J70.0
  Salmonella (arizonae) (cholerae-suis)
    (enteritidis) (typhimurium) A02.9
  scombroid fish T61.1-
  seafood (noxious) T61.9-
    bacterial — *see* Intoxication, foodborne,
      by agent
    fish — *see* Poisoning, fish
    shellfish — *see* Poisoning, shellfish
    specified NEC — *see* subcategory
      T61.8x-
    shellfish (amnesic) (azaspiracid) (diarrheic)
      (neurotoxic) (noxious) (paralytic)
      T61.78-
      bacterial — *see* Intoxication, foodborne,
        by agent
      ciguatera mollusk — *see* Poisoning,
        ciguatera fish
    specified substance NEC T65.891
  Staphylococcus, food A05.0
  tobacco (nicotine) T65.2-
  water E87.79
Poker spine — *see* Spondylitis, ankylosing
Poland syndrome Q79.8
Polioencephalitis (acute) (bulbar) A80.9
  inferior G12.22
  influenzal — *see* Influenza, with,
    encephalopathy
  superior hemorrhagic (acute) (Wernicke's)
    E51.2
  Wernicke's E51.2
Polioencephalomyelitis (acute) (anterior)
  A80.9
  with beriberi E51.2
Polioencephalopathy, superior
  hemorrhagic E51.2
  with
    beriberi E51.11
    pellagra E52
Poliomeningoencephalitis — *see*
  Meningoencephalitis
Poliomyelitis (acute) (anterior) (epidemic)
  A80.9
  with paralysis (bulbar) — *see*
    Poliomyelitis, paralytic
  abortive A80.4
  ascending (progressive) — *see*
    Poliomyelitis, paralytic
  bulbar (paralytic) — *see* Poliomyelitis,
    paralytic
  congenital P35.8
  nonepidemic A80.9
  nonparalytic A80.4
  paralytic A80.30
    specified NEC A80.39
    vaccine-associated A80.0
    wild virus
      imported A80.1
      indigenous A80.2
  spinal, acute A80.9
Poliosis (eyebrow) (eyelashes) L67.1
  circumscripta, acquired L67.1
Pollakiuria R35.0
  psychogenic F45.8
Pollinosis J30.1
Pollitzer's disease L73.2
Polyadenitis — *see also* Lymphadenitis
  malignant A20.0
Polyalgia M79.89

Polyangiitis M30.0
  microscopic M31.7
  overlap syndrome M30.8
Polyarteritis
  microscopic M31.7
  nodosa M30.0
    with lung involvement M30.1
    juvenile M30.2
    related condition NEC M30.8
Polyarthralgia — *see* Pain, joint
Polyarthritis, polyarthropathy (*see also*
  Arthritis) M13.0
  due to or associated with other specified
    conditions — *see* Arthritis
  epidemic (Australian) (with exanthema)
    B33.1
  infective — *see* Arthritis, pyogenic or
    pyemic
  inflammatory M06.4
  juvenile (chronic) (seronegative) M08.3
  migratory — *see* Fever, rheumatic
  rheumatic, acute — *see* Fever, rheumatic
Polyarthrosis M15.9
  post-traumatic M15.3
  primary M15.0
  specified NEC M15.8
Polycarential syndrome of infancy E40
Polychondritis (atrophic) (chronic) — *see*
  also Disorder, cartilage, specified type
  NEC
  relapsing M94.1
Polycoria Q13.2
Polycystic (disease)
  degeneration, kidney Q61.3
    autosomal dominant (adult type) Q61.2
    autosomal recessive (infantile type)
      NEC Q61.19
  kidney Q61.3
    autosomal
      dominant Q61.2
      recessive NEC Q61.19
    autosomal dominant (adult type) Q61.2
    autosomal recessive (childhood type)
      NEC Q61.19
    infantile type NEC Q61.19
  liver Q44.6
  lung J98.4
    congenital Q33.0
  ovary, ovaries E28.2
  spleen Q89.09
Polycythemia (secondary) D75.1
  acquired D75.1
  benign (familial) D75.0
  due to
    donor twin P61.1
    erythropoietin D75.1
    fall in plasma volume D75.1
    high altitude D75.1
    maternal-fetal transfusion P61.1
    stress D75.1
  emotional D75.1
  erythropoietin D75.1
  familial (benign) D75.0
  Gaisböck's (hypertonica) D75.1
  high altitude D75.1
  hypertonica D75.1
  hypoxemic D75.1
  neonatorum P61.1
  nephrogenous D75.1
  relative D75.1
  secondary D75.1
  spurious D75.1
  stress D75.1
  vera D45
Polycytosis cryptogenica D75.1
Polydactylism, polydactyly Q69.9
  toes Q69.2
Polydipsia R63.1
Polydystrophy, pseudo-Hurler E77.0
Polyembryoma — *see* Neoplasm, malignant,
  by site
Polyglandular
  deficiency E31.0
  dyscrasia E31.9
  dysfunction E31.9
  syndrome E31.8
Polyhydramnios O40-
Polymastia Q83.1
Polymenorrhea N92.0
Polymyalgia M35.3
  arteritica, giant cell M31.5
  rheumatica M35.3
    with giant cell arteritis M31.5

Polymyositis (acute) (chronic) (hemorrhagic) M33.20
  with
    myopathy M33.22
    respiratory involvement M33.21
    skin involvement — see
      Dermatopolymyositis
    specified organ involvement NEC
      M33.29
  ossificans (generalisata) (progressiva) —
    see Myositis, ossificans, progressiva
Polyneuritis, polyneuritic — see also
  Polyneuropathy
  acute (post-)infective G61.0
  alcoholic G62.1
  cranialis G52.7
  demyelinating, chronic inflammatory
    (CIDP) G61.81
  diabetic — see Diabetes, polyneuropathy
  diphtheritic A36.83
  due to lack of vitamin NEC E56.9 [G63]
  endemic E51.11
  erythredema — see subcategory T56.1
  febrile, acute G61.0
  hereditary ataxic G60.1
  idiopathic, acute G61.0
  infective (acute) G61.0
  inflammatory, chronic demyelinating
    (CIDP) G61.81
  nutritional E63.9 [G63]
  postinfective (acute) G61.0
  specified NEC G62.89
Polyneuropathy (peripheral) G62.9
  alcoholic G62.1
  amyloid (Portuguese) E85.1 [G63]
  arsenical G62.2
  critical illness G62.81
  demyelinating, chronic inflammatory
    (CIDP) G61.81
  diabetic — see Diabetes, polyneuropathy
  drug-induced G62.0
  hereditary G60.9
    specified NEC G60.8
  idiopathic G60.9
    progressive G60.3
  in (due to)
    alcohol G62.1
      sequelae G65.2
    amyloidosis, familial (Portuguese) E85.1
      [G63]
    antitetanus serum G61.1
    arsenic G62.2
      sequelae G65.2
    avitaminosis NEC E56.9 [G63]
    beriberi E51.11
    collagen vascular disease NEC M35.9
      [G63]
    deficiency (of)
      B(-complex) vitamins E53.9 [G63]
      vitamin B6 E53.1 [G63]
    diabetes — see Diabetes,
      polyneuropathy
    diphtheria A36.83
    drug or medicament G62.0
      correct substance properly
        administered — see Table of
        Drugs and Chemicals, by drug,
        adverse effect
      overdose or wrong substance given or
        taken — see Table of Drugs and
        Chemicals, by drug, poisoning
    endocrine disease NEC E34.9 [G63]
    herpes zoster B02.23
    hypoglycemia E16.2 [G63]
    infectious
      disease NEC B99 [G63]
      mononucleosis B27.91
    lack of vitamin NEC E56.9 [G63]
    lead G62.2
      sequelae G65.2
    leprosy A30.9 [G63]
    Lyme disease A69.22
    metabolic disease NEC E88.9 [G63]
    microscopic polyangiitis M31.7 [G63]
    mumps B26.84
    neoplastic disease (see also Neoplasm)
      D49.9 [G63]
    nutritional deficiency NEC E63.9 [G63]
    organophosphate compounds G62.2
      sequelae G65.2
    parasitic disease NEC B89 [G63]
    pellagra E52 [G63]
    polyarteritis nodosa M30.0
    porphyria E80.20 [G63]
    radiation G62.82
    rheumatoid arthritis — see Rheumatoid,
      polyneuropathy

Polyneuropathy (peripheral) G62.9 —
  continued
  in (due to) — continued
    sarcoidosis D86.89
    serum G61.1
    syphilis (late) A52.15
      congenital A50.43
    systemic
      connective tissue disorder M35.9
        [G63]
      lupus erythematosus M32.19
    toxic agent NEC G62.2
      sequelae G65.2
    triorthocresyl phosphate G62.2
      sequelae G65.2
    tuberculosis A17.89
    uremia N18.9 [G63]
    vitamin B12 deficiency E53.8 [G63]
      with anemia (pernicious) D51.0 [G63]
        due to dietary deficiency D51.3
          [G63]
    zoster B02.23
  inflammatory G61.9
    chronic demyelinating (CIDP) G61.81
    sequelae G65.1
    specified NEC G61.89
  lead G62.2
    sequelae G65.2
  nutritional NEC E63.9 [G63]
  postherpetic (zoster) B02.23
  progressive G60.3
  radiation-induced G62.82
  sensory (hereditary) (idiopathic) G60.8
  specified NEC G62.89
  syphilitic (late) A52.15
    congenital A50.43
Polyopia H53.8
Polyorchism, polyorchidism Q55.21
Polyosteoarthritis (see also Osteoarthritis,
  generalized) M15.9-
  post-traumatic M15.3
  specified NEC M15.8
Polyostotic fibrous dysplasia Q78.1
Polyotia Q17.0
Polyp, polypus
  accessory sinus J33.8
  adenocarcinoma in — see Neoplasm,
    malignant, by site
  adenocarcinoma in situ in — see
    Neoplasm, in situ, by site
  adenoid tissue J33.0
  adenomatous — see also Neoplasm,
    benign, by site
    adenocarcinoma in — see Neoplasm,
      malignant, by site
    adenocarcinoma in situ in — see
      Neoplasm, in situ, by site
    carcinoma in — see Neoplasm,
      malignant, by site
    carcinoma in situ in — see Neoplasm, in
      situ, by site
    multiple — see Neoplasm, benign
      adenocarcinoma in — see Neoplasm,
        malignant, by site
      adenocarcinoma in situ in — see
        Neoplasm, in situ, by site
  antrum J33.8
  anus, anal (canal) K62.0
  Bartholin's gland N84.3
  bladder D41.4
  carcinoma in — see Neoplasm, malignant,
    by site
  carcinoma in situ in — see Neoplasm, in
    situ, by site
  cecum K63.5
  cervix (uteri) N84.1
    in pregnancy or childbirth — see
      Pregnancy, complicated by,
      abnormal, cervix
    mucous N84.1
    nonneoplastic N84.1
  choanal J33.0
  cholesterol K82.4
  clitoris N84.3
  colon K63.5
    adenomatous D12.6
    ascending D12.2
    cecum D12.0
    descending D12.4
    inflammatory K51.40
      with
        abscess K51.414
        complication K51.419
          specified NEC K51.418
        fistula K51.413
        intestinal obstruction K51.412
        rectal bleeding K51.411
    sigmoid D12.5
    transverse D12.3

Polyp, polypus — continued
  corpus uteri N84.0
  dental K04.0
  duodenum K31.7
  ear (middle) H74.4-
  endometrium N84.0
  ethmoidal (sinus) J33.8
  fallopian tube N84.8
  female genital tract N84.9
    specified NEC N84.8
  frontal (sinus) J33.8
  gallbladder K82.4
  gingiva, gum K06.8
  labia, labium (majus) (minus) N84.3
  larynx (mucous) J38.1
    adenomatous D14.1
  malignant — see Neoplasm, malignant, by
    site
  maxillary (sinus) J33.8
  middle ear — see Polyp, ear (middle)
  myometrium N84.0
  nares
    anterior J33.9
    posterior J33.0
  nasal (mucous) J33.9
    cavity J33.0
    septum J33.0
  nasopharyngeal J33.0
  nose (mucous) J33.9
  oviduct N84.8
  pharynx J39.2
  placenta O90.89
  prostate — see Enlargement, enlarged,
    prostate
  pudenda, pudendum N84.3
  pulpal (dental) K04.0
  rectum (nonadenomatous) K62.1
    adenomatous — see Polyp, adenomatous
    septum (nasal) J33.0
  sinus (accessory) (ethmoidal) (frontal)
    (maxillary) (sphenoidal) J33.8
  sphenoidal (sinus) J33.8
  stomach K31.7
    adenomatous D13.1
  tube, fallopian N84.8
  turbinate, mucous membrane J33.8
  umbilical, newborn P83.6
  ureter N28.89
  urethra N36.2
  uterus (body) (corpus) (mucous) N84.0
    cervix N84.1
    in pregnancy or childbirth — see
      Pregnancy, complicated by, tumor,
      uterus
  vagina N84.2
  vocal cord (mucous) J38.1
  vulva N84.3
Polyphagia R63.2
Polyploidy Q92.7
Polypoid — see condition
Polyposis — see also Polyp
  coli (adenomatous) D12.6
    adenocarcinoma in C18.9
    adenocarcinoma in situ in — see
      Neoplasm, in situ, by site
    carcinoma in C18.9
  colon (adenomatous) D12.6
  familial D12.6
    adenocarcinoma in situ in — see
      Neoplasm, in situ, by site
  intestinal (adenomatous) D12.6
  malignant lymphomatous C83.1-
  multiple, adenomatous (see also Neoplasm,
    benign) D36.9
Polyradiculitis — see Polyneuropathy
Polyradiculoneuropathy (acute)
  (postinfective) (segmentally
  demyelinating) G61.0
Polyserositis
  due to pericarditis I31.1
  pericardial I31.1
  periodic, familial E85.0
  tuberculous A19.9
    acute A19.1
    chronic A19.8
Polysplenia syndrome Q89.09
Polysyndactyly (see also Syndactylism,
  syndactyly) Q70.4
Polytrichia L68.3
Polyunguia Q84.6
Polyuria R35.8
  nocturnal R35.1
  psychogenic F45.8
Pompe's disease (glycogen storage) E74.02
Pompholyx L30.1
Poncet's disease (tuberculous rheumatism)
  A18.09
Pond fracture — see Fracture, skull
Ponos B55.0

Pons, pontine — see condition
Poor
  aesthetic of existing restoration of tooth
    K08.56
  contractions, labor O62.2
  gingival margin to tooth restoration K08.51
  personal hygiene R46.0
  prenatal care, affecting management of
    pregnancy — see Pregnancy,
    complicated by, insufficient, prenatal
    care
  sucking reflex (newborn) R29.2
  urinary stream R39.12
  vision NEC H54.7
Poradenitis, nostras inguinalis or venerea
  A55
Porencephaly (congenital) (developmental)
  (true) Q04.6
  acquired G93.0
  nondevelopmental G93.0
  traumatic (post) F07.89
Porocephaliasis B88.8
Porokeratosis Q82.8
Poroma, eccrine — see Neoplasm, skin,
  benign
Porphyria (South African) E80.20
  acquired E80.20
  acute intermittent (hepatic) (Swedish)
    E80.21
  cutanea tarda (hereditary) (symptomatic)
    E80.1
  due to drugs E80.20
    correct substance properly administered
      — see Table of Drugs and
      Chemicals, by drug, adverse effect
    overdose or wrong substance given or
      taken — see Table of Drugs and
      Chemicals, by drug, poisoning
  erythropoietic (congenital) (hereditary)
    E80.0
  hepatocutaneous type E80.1
  secondary E80.20
  toxic NEC E80.20
  variegata E80.20
Porphyrinuria — see Porphyria
Porphyruria — see Porphyria
Port wine nevus, mark, or stain Q82.5
Portal — see condition
Posadas-Wernicke disease B38.9
Positive
  culture (nonspecific)
    blood R78.81
    bronchial washings R84.5
    cerebrospinal fluid R83.5
    cervix uteri R87.5
    nasal secretions R84.5
    nipple discharge R89.5
    nose R84.5
      staphylococcus (methicillin
        susceptible) Z22.321
        methicillin resistant Z22.322
    peritoneal fluid R85.5
    pleural fluid R84.5
    prostatic secretions R86.5
    saliva R85.5
    seminal fluid R86.5
    sputum R84.5
    synovial fluid R89.5
    throat scrapings R84.5
    urine R82.7
    vagina R87.5
    vulva R87.5
    wound secretions R89.5
  PPD (skin test) R76.11
  serology for syphilis A53.0
    with signs or symptoms — code as
      Syphilis, by site and stage
    false R76.8
  skin test, tuberculin (without active
    tuberculosis) R76.11
  test, human immunodeficiency virus (HIV)
    R75
  VDRL A53.0
    with signs or symptoms — code by
      site and stage under Syphilis
      A53.9
  Wassermann reaction A53.0
Postcardiotomy syndrome I97.0
Postcaval ureter Q62.62
Postcholecystectomy syndrome K91.5
Postclimacteric bleeding N95.0
Postcommissurotomy syndrome I97.0
Postconcussional syndrome F07.81
Postcontusional syndrome F07.81
Postcricoid region — see condition
Post-dates (40-42 weeks) (pregnancy)
  (mother) O48.0
  more than 42 weeks gestation O48.1
Postencephalitic syndrome F07.89
Posterior — see condition

Posterolateral sclerosis (spinal cord) — *see* Degeneration, combined
Postexanthematous — *see* condition
Postfebrile — *see* condition
Postgastrectomy dumping syndrome K91.1
Posthemiplegic chorea — *see* Monoplegia
Posthemorrhagic anemia (chronic) D50.0
  acute D62
  newborn P61.3
Postherpetic neuralgia (zoster) B02.29
  trigeminal B02.22
Posthitis N47.7
Postimmunization complication or reaction — *see* Complications, vaccination
Postinfectious — *see* condition
Postlaminectomy syndrome NEC M96.1
Postleukotomy syndrome F07.0
Postmastectomy lymphedema (syndrome) I97.2
Postmaturity, postmature (over 42 weeks)
  maternal (over 42 weeks gestation) O48.1
  newborn P08.22
Postmeasles complication NEC (*see also* condition) B05.89
Postmenopausal
  endometrium (atrophic) N95.8
    suppurative (*see also* Endometritis) N71.9
  osteoporosis — *see* Osteoporosis, postmenopausal
Postnasal drip R09.82
  due to
    allergic rhinitis — *see* Rhinitis, allergic
    common cold J00
    gastroesophageal reflux — *see* Reflux, gastroesophageal
    nasopharyngitis — *see* Nasopharyngitis
    other know condition — *code to* condition
    sinusitis — *see* Sinusitis
Postnatal — *see* condition
Postoperative (postprocedural) — *see* Complication, postoperative
  pneumothorax, therapeutic Z98.3
  state NEC Z98.89
Postpancreatectomy hyperglycemia E89.1
Postpartum — *see* Puerperal
Postphlebitic syndrome — *see* Syndrome, postthrombotic
Postpolio (myelitic) syndrome G14
Postpoliomyelitic — *see also* condition
  osteopathy — *see* Osteopathy, after poliomyelitis
Postprocedural — *see also* Postoperative
  hypoinsulinemia E89.1
Postschizophrenic depression F32.8
Postsurgery status — *see also* Status (post)
  pneumothorax, therapeutic Z98.3
Post-term (40-42 weeks) (pregnancy) (mother) O48.0
  infant P08.21
  more than 42 weeks gestation (mother) O48.1
Post-traumatic brain syndrome, nonpsychotic F07.81
Post-typhoid abscess A01.09
Postures, hysterical F44.2
Postvaccinal reaction or complication — *see* Complications, vaccination
Postvalvulotomy syndrome I97.0
Potain's
  disease (pulmonary edema) — *see* Edema, lung
  syndrome (gastrectasis with dyspepsia) K31.0
Potter's
  asthma J62.8
  facies Q60.6
  lung J62.8
  syndrome (with renal agenesis) Q60.6
Pott's
  curvature (spinal) A18.01
  disease or paraplegia A18.01
  spinal curvature A18.01
  tumor, puffy — *see* Osteomyelitis, specified type NEC
Pouch
  bronchus Q32.4
  Douglas' — *see* condition
  esophagus, esophageal, congenital Q39.6
    acquired K22.5
  gastric K31.4
  Hartmann's K82.8
  pharynx, pharyngeal (congenital) Q38.7
Pouchitis K91.850
Poultrymen's itch B88.0
Poverty NEC Z59.6
  extreme Z59.5

Poxvirus NEC B08.8
Prader-Willi syndrome Q87.1
Preauricular appendage or tag Q17.0
Prebetalipoproteinemia (acquired) (essential) (familial) (hereditary) (primary) (secondary) E78.1
  with chylomicronemia E78.3
Precipitate labor or delivery O62.3
Preclimacteric bleeding (menorrhagia) N92.4
Precocious
  adrenarche E30.1
  menarche E30.1
  menstruation E30.1
  pubarche E30.1
  puberty E30.1
    central E22.8
  sexual development NEC E30.1
  thelarche E30.8
Precocity, sexual (constitutional) (cryptogenic) (female) (idiopathic) (male) E30.1
  with adrenal hyperplasia E25.9
    congenital E25.0
Precordial pain R07.2
Predeciduous teeth K00.2
Prediabetes, prediabetic R73.09
  complicating
    pregnancy — *see* Pregnancy, complicated by, diseases of, specified type or system NEC
    puerperium O99.89
Predislocation status of hip at birth Q65.6
Pre-eclampsia O14.9-
  with pre-existing hypertension — *see* Hypertension, complicating pregnancy, pre-existing, with, pre-eclampsia
  mild O14.0-
  moderate O14.0-
  severe O14.1-
    with hemolysis, elevated liver enzymes and low platelet count (HELLP) O14.2-
Pre-eruptive color change, teeth, tooth K00.8
Pre-excitation atrioventricular conduction I45.6
Pre-glaucoma H40.00-
Pregnancy (childbirth) (labor) (puerperium) — *see also* Delivery and Puerperal
Note — *The tabular must be reviewed for assignment of the appropriate character indicating the trimester of the pregnancy*
Note — *The tabular must be reviewed for assignment of the appropriate seventh character for multiple gestation codes in Chapter 15*
  abdominal (ectopic) O00.0
    with viable fetus O36.7-
  ampullar O00.1
  biochemical O02.81
  broad ligament O00.8
  cervical O00.8
  chemical O02.81
  complicated by (care of) (management affected by)
    abnormal, abnormality
      cervix O34.4-
        causing obstructed labor O65.5
      cord (umbilical) O69.9
      findings on antenatal screening of mother O28.9
        biochemical O28.1
        chromosomal O28.5
        cytological O28.2
        genetic O28.5
        hematological O28.0
        radiological O28.4
        specified NEC O28.8
        ultrasonic O28.3
      glucose (tolerance) NEC O99.810
      pelvic organs O34.9-
        specified NEC O34.8-
          causing obstructed labor O65.5
      pelvis (bony) (major) NEC O33.0
      perineum O34.7-
      position
        placenta O44.1-
          without hemorrhage O44.0-
        uterus O34.59-
      uterus O34.59-
        causing obstructed labor O65.5
        congenital O34.0-
      vagina O34.6-
        causing obstructed labor O65.5
      vulva O34.7-
        causing obstructed labor O65.5
    abruptio placentae — *see* Abruptio placentae

Pregnancy (childbirth) (labor) (puerperium) (*see also* Delivery and Puerperal) — *continued*
  complicated by (care of) (management affected by) — *continued*
    abscess or cellulitis
      bladder O23.1-
      breast O91.11-
      genital organ or tract O23.9-
    abuse
      physical O9A.31-
      psychological O9A.51-
      sexual O9A.41-
    adverse effect anesthesia O29.9-
      aspiration pneumonitis O29.01-
      cardiac arrest O29.11-
      cardiac complication NEC O29.19-
      cardiac failure O29.12-
      central nervous system complication NEC O29.29-
      cerebral anoxia O29.21-
      failed or difficult intubation O29.6-
      inhalation of stomach contents or secretions NOS O29.01-
      local, toxic reaction O29.3x
      Mendelson's syndrome O29.01-
      pressure collapse of lung O29.02-
      pulmonary complications NEC O29.09-
      specified NEC O29.8x-
      spinal and epidural type NEC O29.5x
      induced headache O29.4-
    albuminuria O12.1-
    alcohol use O99.31-
    amnionitis O41.12-
    anaphylactoid syndrome of pregnancy O88.01-
    anemia (conditions in D50-D64) (pre-existing) O99.01-
      complicating the puerperium O99.03
    antepartum hemorrhage O46.9-
      with coagulation defect — *see* Hemorrhage, antepartum, with coagulation defect
      specified NEC O46.8x-
    appendicitis O99.61-
    atrophy (yellow) (acute) liver (subacute) O26.61-
    bariatric surgery status O99.84-
    bicornis or bicornuate uterus O34.59-
    biliary tract problems O26.61-
    breech presentation O32.1
    cardiovascular diseases (conditions in I00-I09, I20-I52, I70-I99) O99.41-
    cerebrovascular disorders (conditions in I60-I69) O99.41-
    cervical shortening O26.87-
    cervicitis O23.51-
    chloasma (gravidarum) O26.89-
    cholecystitis O99.61-
    cholestasis (intrahepatic) O26.61-
    chorioamnionitis O41.12-
    circulatory system disorder (conditions in I00-I09, I20-I99, O99.41-)
    compound presentation O32.6
    conjoined twins O30.02-
    connective system disorders (conditions in M00-M99) O99.89
    contracted pelvis (general) O33.1
      inlet O33.2
      outlet O33.3
    convulsions (eclamptic) (uremic) (*see also* Eclampsia) O15.9-
    cracked nipple O92.11-
    cystitis O23.1-
    cystocele O34.8-
    death of fetus (near term) O36.4
      early pregnancy O02.1
      of one fetus or more in multiple gestation O31.2-
    deciduitis O41.14-
    decreased fetal movement O36.81-
    dental problems O99.61-
    diabetes (mellitus) O24.91-
      gestational (pregnancy induced) — *see* Diabetes, gestational
      pre-existing O24.31-
        specified NEC O24.81-
        type 1 O24.01-
        type 2 O24.11-
    digestive system disorders (conditions in K00-K93) O99.61-
    diseases of — *see* Pregnancy, complicated by, specified body system disease
      biliary tract O26.61-
      blood NEC (conditions in D65-D77) O99.11-
      liver O26.61-
      specified NEC O99.89

Pregnancy (childbirth) (labor) (puerperium) (*see also* Delivery and Puerperal) — *continued*
  complicated by (care of) (management affected by) — *continued*
    disorders of — *see* Pregnancy, complicated by, specified body system disorder
    amniotic fluid and membranes O41.9-
      specified NEC O41.8x-
    biliary tract O26.61-
    ear and mastoid process (conditions in H60-H95) O99.89
    eye and adnexa (conditions in H00-H59) O99.89
    liver O26.61-
    skin (conditions in L00-L99) O99.71-
      specified NEC O99.89
    displacement, uterus NEC O34.59-
      causing obstructed labor O65.5
    disproportion (due to) O33.9
      fetal deformities NEC O33.7
      generally contracted pelvis O33.1
      hydrocephalic fetus O33.6
      inlet contraction of pelvis O33.2
      mixed maternal and fetal origin O33.4
      specified NEC O33.8
    double uterus O34.59-
      causing obstructed labor O65.5
    drug use (conditions in F11-F19) O99.32-
    eclampsia, eclamptic (coma) (convulsions) (delirium) (nephritis) (uremia) (*see also* Eclampsia) O15-
    ectopic pregnancy — *see* Pregnancy, ectopic
    edema O12.0-
      with
        gestational hypertension, mild (see also Pre-eclampsia) O14.0-
        proteinuria O12.2-
    effusion, amniotic fluid — *see* Pregnancy, complicated by, premature rupture of membranes
    elderly
      multigravida O09.52-
      primigravida O09.51-
    embolism (*see also* Embolism, obstetric, pregnancy) O88.-
    endocrine diseases NEC O99.28-
    endometritis O86.12
    excessive weight gain O26.0-
    exhaustion O26.81-
      during labor and delivery O75.81
    face presentation O32.3
    failed induction of labor O61.9
      instrumental O61.1
      mechanical O61.1
      medical O61.0
      specified NEC O61.8
      surgical O61.1
    failed or difficult intubation for anesthesia O29.6-
    false labor (pains) O47.9
      at or after 37 completed weeks of pregnancy O47.1
      before 37 completed weeks of pregnancy O47.0-
    fatigue O26.81-
      during labor and delivery O75.81
    fatty metamorphosis of liver O26.61-
    female genital mutilation O34.8-[N90.8-]
    fetal (maternal care for)
      abnormality or damage O35.9
        acid-base balance O68
        specified type NEC O35.8
      acidemia O68
      acidosis O68
      alkalosis O68
      anemia and thrombocytopenia O36.82-
      anencephaly O35.0
      chromosomal abnormality (conditions in Q90-Q99) O35.1
      conjoined twins O30.02-
      damage from
        amniocentesis O35.7
        biopsy procedures O35.7
        drug addiction O35.5
        hematological investigation O35.7
        intrauterine contraceptive device O35.7

Pregnancy (childbirth) (labor) (puerperium) *(see also* Delivery and Puerperal) — *continued*
  complicated by (care of) (management affected by) — *continued*
    fetal (maternal care for) — *continued*
      maternal
        alcohol addiction O35.4
        cytomegalovirus infection O35.3
        disease NEC O35.8
        drug addiction O35.5
        listeriosis O35.8
        rubella O35.3
        toxoplasmosis O35.8
        viral infection O35.3
        medical procedure NEC O35.7
        radiation O35.6
    death (near term) O36.4
      early pregnancy O02.1
    decreased movement O36.81-
    disproportion due to deformity (fetal) O33.7
    excessive growth (large for dates) O36.6-
    growth retardation O36.59-
      light for dates O36.59-
      small for dates O36.59-
    heart rate irregularity (bradycardia) (decelerations) (tachycardia) O76
    hereditary disease O35.2
    hydrocephalus O35.0
    intrauterine death O36.4
    poor growth O36.59-
      light for dates O36.59-
      small for dates O36.59-
    problem O36.9-
      specified NEC O36.89-
    reduction (elective) O31.3-
    selective termination O31.3-
    spina bifida O35.0
    thrombocytopenia O36.82-
  fibroid (tumor) (uterus) O34.1-
  fissure of nipple O92.11-
  gallstones O99.61-
  gastric banding status O99.84-
  gastric bypass status O99.84-
  genital herpes (asymptomatic) (history of) (inactive) O98.51-
  genital tract infection O23.9-
  glomerular diseases (conditions in N00-N07) O26.83-
    with hypertension, pre-existing — *see* Hypertension, complicating, pregnancy, pre-existing, with, renal disease
  gonorrhea O98.21-
  grand multiparity O09.4
  habitual aborter — *see* Pregnancy, complicated by, recurrent pregnancy loss
  HELLP syndrome (hemolysis, elevated liver enzymes and low platelet count) O14.2-
  hemorrhage
    antepartum — *see* Hemorrhage, antepartum
    before 20 completed weeks gestation O20.9
      specified NEC O20.8
    due to premature separation, placenta *(see also* Abruptio placentae) O45.9-
    early O20.9
      specified NEC O20.8
    threatened abortion O20.0
  hemorrhoids O22.4-
  hepatitis (viral) O98.41-
  herniation of uterus O34.59-
  high
    head at term O32.4
    risk — *see* Supervision (of) (for), high-risk
  history of in utero procedure during previous pregnancy O09.82-
  HIV O98.71-
  human immunodeficiency virus (HIV) disease O98.71-
  hydatidiform mole *(see also* Mole, hydatidiform) O01.9-
  hydramnios O40-
  hydrocephalic fetus (disproportion) O33.6
  hydrops
    amnii O40-
    fetalis O36.2-
      associated with isoimmunization *(see also* Pregnancy, complicated by, isoimmunization) O36.11-

Pregnancy (childbirth) (labor) (puerperium) *(see also* Delivery and Puerperal) — *continued*
  complicated by (care of) (management affected by) — *continued*
  hydrorrhea O42.90
  hyperemesis (gravidarum) (mild) *(see also* Hyperemesis, gravidarum) O21.0-
  hypertension — *see* Hypertension, complicating pregnancy
  hypertensive
    heart and renal disease, pre-existing — *see* Hypertension, complicating, pregnancy, pre-existing, with, heart disease,with renal disease
    heart disease, pre-existing — *see* Hypertension, complicating, pregnancy, pre-existing, with, heart disease
    renal disease, pre-existing — *see* Hypertension, complicating, pregnancy, pre-existing, with, renal disease
  hypotension O26.5-
  immune disorders NEC (conditions in D80-D89) O99.11-
  incarceration, uterus O34.51-
  incompetent cervix O34.3-
  inconclusive fetal viability O36.80
  infection(s) O98.91-
    amniotic fluid or sac O41.10-
    bladder O23.1-
    carrier state NEC O99.830
      streptococcus B O99.820
    genital organ or tract O23.9-
      specified NEC O23.59-
    genitourinary tract O23.9-
    gonorrhea O98.21-
    hepatitis (viral) O98.41-
    HIV O98.71-
    human immunodeficiency virus (HIV) O98.71-
    kidney O23.0-
    nipple O91.01-
    parasitic disease O98.91-
      specified NEC O98.81-
    protozoal disease O98.61-
    sexually transmitted NEC O98.31-
    specified type NEC O98.81-
    syphilis O98.11-
    tuberculosis O98.01-
    urethra O23.2-
    urinary (tract) O23.4-
      specified NEC O23.3-
    viral disease O98.51-
  injury or poisoning (conditions in S00-T88) O9A.21-
    due to abuse
      physical O9A.31-
      psychological O9A.51-
      sexual O9A.41-
  insufficient
    prenatal care O09.3-
    weight gain O26.1-
  insulin resistance O26.89-
  intrauterine fetal death (near term) O36.4
    early pregnancy O02.1
    multiple gestation (one fetus or more) O31.2-
  isoimmunization O36.11-
    anti-A sensitization O36.11-
    anti-B sensitization O36.19-
    Rh O36.09-
      anti-D antibody O36.01-
      specified NEC O36.19-
  laceration of uterus NEC O71.81
  malformation
    placenta, placental (vessel) O43.10-
      specified NEC O43.19-
    uterus (congenital) O34.0-
  malnutrition (conditions in E40-E46) O25.1-
  maternal hypotension syndrome O26.5-
  mental disorders (conditions in F01-F09, F20-F99) O99.34-
    alcohol use O99.31-
    drug use O99.32-
    smoking O99.33-
  mentum presentation O32.3
  metabolic disorders O99.28-
  missed
    abortion O02.1
    delivery O36.4

Pregnancy (childbirth) (labor) (puerperium) *(see also* Delivery and Puerperal) — *continued*
  complicated by (care of) (management affected by) — *continued*
  multiple gestations O30.9-
    conjoined twins O30.02-
    quadruplet — *see* Pregnancy, quadruplet
    specified complication NEC O31.8x-
    specified number of multiples NEC — *see* Pregnancy, multiple (gestation), specified NEC
    triplet — *see* Pregnancy, triplet
    twin — *see* Pregnancy, twin
  musculoskeletal condition (conditions is M00-M99) O99.89
  necrosis, liver (conditions in K72) O26.61-
  neoplasm
    benign
      cervix O34.4-
      corpus uteri O34.1-
      uterus O34.1-
    malignant O9A.11-
  nephropathy NEC O26.83-
  nervous system condition (conditions in G00-G99) O99.35-
  nutritional diseases NEC O99.28-
  obesity (pre-existing) O99.21-
  obesity surgery status O99.84-
  oblique lie or presentation O32.2
  older mother — *see* Pregnancy, complicated by, elderly
  oligohydramnios O41.0-
    with premature rupture of membranes *(see also* Pregnancy, complicated by, premature rupture of membranes) O42-
  onset (spontaneous) of labor after 37 completed weeks of gestation but before 39 completed weeks gestation, with delivery by (planned) cesarean section O75.82
  oophoritis O23.52-
  overdose, drug *(see also* Table of Drugs and Chemicals, by drug, poisoning) O9A.21-
  oversize fetus O33.5
  papyraceous fetus O31.0-
  pelvic inflammatory disease O99.89
  periodontal disease O99.61-
  peripheral neuritis O26.82-
  peritoneal (pelvic) adhesions O99.89
  phlebitis O22.9-
  phlebopathy O22.9-
  phlebothrombosis (superficial) O22.2-
    deep O22.3-
  placenta accreta O43.21-
  placenta increta O43.22-
  placenta percreta O43.23-
  placenta previa O44.1-
    without hemorrhage O44.0-
  placental disorder O43.9-
    specified NEC O43.89-
  placental dysfunction O43.89-
  placental infarction O43.81-
  placental insufficiency O36.51-
  placental transfusion syndromes
    fetomaternal O43.01-
    fetus to fetus O43.02-
    maternofetal O43.01-
  placentitis O41.14-
  pneumonia O99.51-
  poisoning *(see also* Table of Drugs and Chemicals) O9A.21-
  polyhydramnios O40-
  polymorphic eruption of pregnancy O26.86
  poor obstetric history NEC O09.29-
  postmaturity (post-term) (40 to 42 weeks) O48.0
    more than 42 completed weeks gestation (prolonged) O48.1
  pre-eclampsia O14.9-
    mild O14.0-
    moderate O14.0-
    severe O14.1-
      with hemolysis, elevated liver enzymes and low platelet count (HELLP) O14.2-
  premature labor — *see* Pregnancy, complicated by, preterm labor

Pregnancy (childbirth) (labor) (puerperium) *(see also* Delivery and Puerperal) — *continued*
  complicated by (care of) (management affected by) — *continued*
  premature rupture of membranes O42.90
    with onset of labor
      after 24 hours O42.10
        after 37 weeks gestation O42.12
        pre-term (before 37 completed weeks of gestation) O42.11-
      within 24 hours O42.00
        after 37 weeks gestation O42.02
        pre-term (before 37 completed weeks of gestation) O42.01-
    after 37 weeks gestation O42.92
    full-term O42.92
    pre-term (before 37 completed weeks of gestation) O42.91-
  premature separation of placenta *(see also* Abruptio placentae) O45.9-
  presentation, fetal — *see* Delivery, complicated by, malposition
  preterm delivery O60.10
  preterm labor
    with delivery O60.10
      preterm O60.10
      term O60.20
    without delivery O60.00
      second trimester O60.02
      third trimester O60.03
    second trimester
      with preterm delivery
        second trimester O60.12
        third trimester O60.13
      with term delivery O60.22
      without delivery O60.02
    third trimester
      with term delivery O60.23
      with third trimester preterm delivery O60.14
      without delivery O60.03
  previous history of — *see* Pregnancy, supervision of, high-risk
  prolapse, uterus O34.52-
  proteinuria (gestational) O12.1-
    with edema O12.2-
  pruritic urticarial papules and plaques of pregnancy (PUPPP) O26.86
  pruritus (neurogenic) O26.89-
  psychosis or psychoneurosis (puerperal) F53
  ptyalism O26.89-
  PUPPP (pruritic urticarial papules and plaques of pregnancy) O26.86
  pyelitis O23.0-
  recurrent pregnancy loss O26.2-
  renal disease or failure NEC O26.83-
    with secondary hypertension, pre-existing — *see* Hypertension, complicating, pregnancy, pre-existing, secondary
    hypertensive, pre-existing — *see* Hypertension, complicating, pregnancy, pre-existing, with, renal disease
  respiratory condition (conditions in J00-J99) O99.51-
  retained, retention
    dead ovum O02.0
    intrauterine contraceptive device O26.3-
  retroversion, uterus O34.53-
  Rh immunization, incompatibility or sensitization NEC O36.09-
    anti-D antibody O36.01-
  rupture
    amnion (premature) *(see also* Pregnancy, complicated by, premature rupture of membranes) O42-
    membranes (premature) *(see also* Pregnancy, complicated by, premature rupture of membranes) O42-
    uterus (during labor) O71.1
      before onset of labor O71.0-
  salivation (excessive) O26.89-
  salpingitis O23.52-
  salpingo-oophoritis O23.52-
  sepsis (conditions in A40, A41) O98.81-
  size date discrepancy (uterine) O26.84-
  skin condition (conditions in L00-L99) O99.71-
  smoking (tobacco) O99.33-
  social problem O09.7-
  specified condition NEC O26.89-
  spotting O26.85-

Premature (see also condition) — continued
 newborn
　extreme (less than 28 completed weeks)
　　— see Immaturity, extreme
　less than 37 completed weeks — see
　　Preterm, newborn
 puberty E30.1
 rupture membranes or amnion — see
　Pregnancy, complicated by, premature
　rupture of membranes
 senility E34.8
 thelarche E30.8
 ventricular systole I49.3
Prematurity NEC (less than 37 completed
　weeks) — see Preterm, newborn
 extreme (less than 28 completed weeks) —
　see Immaturity, extreme
Premenstrual
 dysphoric disorder (PMDD) N94.3
 tension (syndrome) N94.3
Premolarization, cuspids K00.2
Prenatal
 care, normal pregnancy — see Pregnancy,
　normal
 screening of mother Z36
 teeth K00.6
Preparatory care for subsequent treatment
 NEC
 for dialysis Z49.01
　peritoneal Z49.02
Prepartum — see condition
Preponderance, left or right ventricular
 I51.7
Prepuce — see condition
PRES (posterior reversible encephalopathy
　syndrome) I67.83
Presbycardia R54
Presbycusis, presbyacusia H91.1-
Presbyesophagus K22.8
Presbyophrenia F03
Presbyopia b
Prescription of contraceptives (initial)
 Z30.019
 emergency (postcoital) Z30.012
 implantable subdermal Z30.019
 injectable Z30.013
 intrauterine contraceptive device Z30.014
 pills Z30.011
 postcoital (emergency) Z30.012
 repeat Z30.40
　implantable subdermal Z30.49
　injectable Z30.42
　pills Z30.41
　specified type NEC Z30.49
 specified type NEC Z30.018
Presence (of)
 ankle-joint implant (functional)
　(prosthesis) Z96.66-
 aortocoronary (bypass) graft Z95.1
 arterial-venous shunt (dialysis) Z99.2
 artificial
　eye (globe) Z97.0
　heart (fully implantable) (mechanical)
　　Z95.812
　　valve Z95.2
　larynx Z96.3
　lens (intraocular) Z96.1
　limb (complete) (partial) Z97.1-
　　arm Z97.1-
　　　bilateral Z97.15
　　leg Z97.1-
　　　bilateral Z97.16
 audiological implant (functional) Z96.29
 bladder implant (functional) Z96.0
 bone
　conduction hearing device Z96.29
　implant (functional) NEC Z96.7
　joint (prosthesis) — see Presence, joint
　　implant
 cardiac
　defibrillator (functional) (with
　　synchronous cardiac pacemaker)
　　Z95.810
　implant or graft Z95.9
　　specified type NEC Z95.818
　pacemaker Z95.0
 cerebrospinal fluid drainage device Z98.2
 cochlear implant (functional) Z96.21
 contact lens(es) Z97.3
 coronary artery graft or prosthesis Z95.5
 CSF shunt Z98.2
 dental prosthesis device Z97.2
 dentures Z97.2
 device (external) NEC Z97.8
　cardiac NEC Z95.818
　heart assist Z95.811
　implanted (functional) Z96.9
　　specified NEC Z96.89
　prosthetic Z97.8

Presence (of) — continued
 ear implant Z96.20
　cochlear implant Z96.21
　myringotomy tube Z96.22
　specified type NEC Z96.29
 elbow-joint implant (functional)
　(prosthesis) Z96.62-
 endocrine implant (functional) NEC
　Z96.49
 eustachian tube stent or device (functional)
　Z96.29
 external hearing-aid or device Z97.4
 finger-joint implant (functional)
　(prosthetic) Z96.69-
 functional implant Z96.9
　specified NEC Z96.89
 graft
　cardiac NEC Z95.818
　vascular NEC Z95.828
 hearing-aid or device (external) Z97.4
　implant (bone) (cochlear) (functional)
　　Z96.21
 heart assist device Z95.811
 heart valve implant (functional) Z95.2
　prosthetic Z95.2
　specified type NEC Z95.4
　xenogenic Z95.3
 hip-joint implant (functional) (prosthesis)
　Z96.64-
 implanted device (artificial) (functional)
　(prosthetic) Z96.9
　automatic cardiac defibrillator (with
　　synchronous cardiac pacemaker)
　　Z95.810
　cardiac pacemaker Z95.0
　cochlear Z96.21
　dental Z96.5
　heart Z95.812
　heart valve Z95.2
　　prosthetic Z95.2
　　specified NEC Z95.4
　　xenogenic Z95.3
　insulin pump Z96.41
　intraocular lens Z96.1
　joint Z96.60
　　ankle Z96.66-
　　elbow Z96.62-
　　finger Z96.69-
　　hip Z96.64-
　　knee Z96.65-
　　shoulder Z96.61-
　　specified NEC Z96.698
　　wrist Z96.63-
　larynx Z96.3
　myringotomy tube Z96.22
　otological Z96.20
　　cochlear Z96.21
　　eustachian stent Z96.29
　　myringotomy Z96.22
　　specified NEC Z96.29
　　stapes Z96.29
　skin Z96.81
　skull plate Z96.7
　specified NEC Z96.89
　urogenital Z96.0
 insulin pump (functional) Z96.41
 intestinal bypass or anastomosis Z98.0
 intraocular lens (functional) Z96.1
 intrauterine contraceptive device (IUD)
　Z97.5
 intravascular implant (functional)
　(prosthetic) NEC Z95.9
　coronary artery Z95.5
　defibrillator (with synchronous cardiac
　　pacemaker) Z95.810
　peripheral vessel (with angioplasty)
　　Z95.820
 joint implant (prosthetic) (any) Z96.60
　ankle — see Presence, ankle joint
　　implant
　elbow — see Presence, elbow joint
　　implant
　finger — see Presence, finger joint
　　implant
　hip — see Presence, hip joint implant
　knee — see Presence, knee joint implant
　shoulder — see Presence, shoulder joint
　　implant
　specified joint NEC Z96.698
　wrist — see Presence, wrist joint implant
 knee-joint implant (functional) (prosthesis)
　Z96.65-
 laryngeal implant (functional) Z96.3
 mandibular implant (dental) Z96.5
 myringotomy tube(s) Z96.22
 orthopedic-joint implant (prosthetic) (any)
　— see Presence, joint implant
 otological implant (functional) Z96.29
 shoulder-joint implant (functional)
　(prosthesis) Z96.61-

Presence (of) — continued
 skull-plate implant Z96.7
 spectacles Z97.3
 stapes implant (functional) Z96.29
 systemic lupus erythematosus [SLE]
　inhibitor D68.62
 tendon implant (functional) (graft) Z96.7
 tooth root(s) implant Z96.5
 ureteral stent Z96.0
 urethral stent Z96.0
 urogenital implant (functional) Z96.0
 vascular implant or device Z95.9
　access port device Z95.828
　specified type NEC Z95.828
 wrist-joint implant (functional) (prosthesis)
　Z96.63-
Presenile — see also condition
 dementia F03
 premature aging E34.8
Presentation, fetal — see Delivery,
　complicated by, malposition
Prespondylolisthesis (congenital) Q76.2
Pressure
 area, skin — see Ulcer, pressure, by site
 brachial plexus G54.0
 brain G93.5
　injury at birth NEC P11.1
 cerebral — see Pressure, brain
 chest R07.89
 cone, tentorial G93.5
 hyposystolic — see also Hypotension
　incidental reading, without diagnosis of
　　hypotension R03.1
 increased
　intracranial (benign) G93.2
　　injury at birth P11.0
　intraocular H40.05-
 lumbosacral plexus G54.1
 mediastinum J98.5
 necrosis (chronic) — see Ulcer, pressure,
　by site
 parental, inappropriate (excessive) Z62.6
 sore (chronic) — see Ulcer, pressure, by
　site
 spinal cord G95.20
 ulcer (chronic) — see Ulcer, pressure, by
　site
 venous, increased I87.8
Pre-syncope R55
Preterm
 delivery (see also Pregnancy, complicated
　by, preterm labor) O60.10
 labor — see Pregnancy, complicated by,
　preterm labor
 newborn (infant) P07.30
　gestational age
　　28 completed weeks (28 weeks, 0
　　　days through 28 weeks, 6 days)
　　　P07.31
　　29 completed weeks (29 weeks, 0
　　　days through 29 weeks, 6 days)
　　　P07.32
　　30 completed weeks (30 weeks, 0
　　　days through 30 weeks, 6 days)
　　　P07.33
　　31 completed weeks (31 weeks, 0
　　　days through 31 weeks, 6 days)
　　　P07.34
　　32 completed weeks (32 weeks, 0
　　　days through 32 weeks, 6 days)
　　　P07.35
　　33 completed weeks (33 weeks, 0
　　　days through 33 weeks, 6 days)
　　　P07.36
　　34 completed weeks (34 weeks, 0
　　　days through 34 weeks, 6 days)
　　　P07.37
　　35 completed weeks (35 weeks, 0
　　　days through 35 weeks, 6 days)
　　　P07.38
　　36 completed weeks (36 weeks, 0
　　　days through 36 weeks, 6 days)
　　　P07.39
Previa
 placenta (low) (marginal) (partial) (total)
　(with hemorrhage) O44.1-
　without hemorrhage O44.0-
 vasa O69.4
Priapism N48.30
 due to
　disease classified elsewhere N48.32
　drug N48.33
　specified cause NEC N48.39
　trauma N48.31
Prickling sensation (skin) R20.2
Prickly heat L74.0
Primary — see condition

Primigravida
 elderly, affecting management of
　pregnancy, labor and delivery
　(supervision only) — see Pregnancy,
　complicated by, elderly, primigravida
 older, affecting management of pregnancy,
　labor and delivery (supervision only)
　— see Pregnancy, complicated by,
　elderly, primigravida
 very young, affecting management of
　pregnancy, labor and delivery
　(supervision only) — see Pregnancy,
　complicated by, young mother,
　primigravida
Primipara
 elderly, affecting management of
　pregnancy, labor and delivery
　(supervision only) — see Pregnancy,
　complicated by, elderly, primigravida
 older, affecting management of pregnancy,
　labor and delivery (supervision only)
　— see Pregnancy, complicated by,
　elderly, primigravida
 very young, affecting management of
　pregnancy, labor and delivery
　(supervision only) — see Pregnancy,
　complicated by, young mother,
　primigravida
Primus varus (bilateral) Q66.2
PRIND (prolonged reversible ischemic
　neurologic deficit) I63.9
Pringle's disease (tuberous sclerosis) Q85.1
Prinzmetal angina I20.1
Prizefighter ear — see Cauliflower ear
Problem (with) (related to)
 academic Z55.8
 acculturation Z60.3
 adjustment (to)
　change of job Z56.1
　life-cycle transition Z60.0
　pension Z60.0
　retirement Z60.0
 adopted child Z62.821
 alcoholism in family Z63.72
 atypical parenting situation Z62.9
 bankruptcy Z59.8
 behavioral (adult) F69
　drug seeking Z72.89
 birth of sibling affecting child Z62.898
 care (of)
　provider dependency Z74.9
　　specified NEC Z74.8
　sick or handicapped person in family or
　　household Z63.6
 child
　abuse (affecting the child) — see
　　Maltreatment, child
　custody or support proceedings Z65.3
　in care of non-parental family member
　　Z62.21
　in foster care Z62.21
　in welfare custody Z62.21
　living in orphanage or group home
　　Z62.22
 child-rearing Z62.9
　specified NEC Z62.898
 communication (developmental) F80.9
 conflict or discord (with)
　boss Z56.4
　classmates Z55.4
　counselor Z64.4
　employer Z56.4
　family Z63.9
　　specified NEC Z63.8
　probation officer Z64.4
　social worker Z64.4
　teachers Z55.4
　workmates Z56.4
 conviction in legal proceedings Z65.0
　with imprisonment Z65.1
 counselor Z64.4
 creditors Z59.8
 digestive K92.9
 drug addict in family Z63.72
 ear — see Disorder, ear
 economic Z59.9
　affecting care Z59.9
　specified NEC Z59.8
 education Z55.9
　specified NEC Z55.8
 employment Z56.9
　change of job Z56.1
　discord Z56.4
　environment Z56.5
　sexual harassment Z56.81
　specified NEC Z56.89
　stress NEC Z56.6
　stressful schedule Z56.3
　threat of job loss Z56.2
　unemployment Z56.0

DISEASE INDEX (side tab)

Prostration R53.83
heat — *see also* Heat, exhaustion
anhydrotic T67.3
due to
salt (and water) depletion T67.4
water depletion T67.3
nervous F48.8
senile R54
Protanomaly (anomalous trichromat) H53.54
Protanopia (complete) (incomplete) H53.54
Protection (against) (from) — *see* Prophylactic
Protein
deficiency NEC — *see* Malnutrition
malnutrition — *see* Malnutrition
sickness (*see also* Reaction, serum) T80.69
Proteinemia R77.9
Proteinosis
alveolar (pulmonary) J84.01
lipid or lipoid (of Urbach) E78.89
Proteinuria R80.9
Bence Jones R80.3
complicating pregnancy — *see* Proteinuria, gestational
gestational O12.1-
with edema O12.2-
idiopathic R80.0
isolated R80.0
with glomerular lesion N06.9
dense deposit disease N06.6
diffuse
crescentic glomerulonephritis N06.7
endocapillary proliferative glomerulonephritis N06.4
mesangiocapillary glomerulonephritis N06.5
focal and segmental hyalinosis or sclerosis N06.1
membranous (diffuse) N06.2
mesangial proliferative (diffuse) N06.3
minimal change N06.0
specified pathology NEC N06.8
orthostatic R80.2
with glomerular lesion — *see* Proteinuria, isolated, with glomerular lesion
persistent R80.1
with glomerular lesion — *see* Proteinuria, isolated, with glomerular lesion
postural R80.2
with glomerular lesion — *see* Proteinuria, isolated, with glomerular lesion
pre-eclamptic — *see* Pre-eclampsia
specified type NEC R80.8
Proteolysis, pathologic D65
Proteus (mirabilis) (morganii), as cause of disease classified elsewhere B96.4
Prothrombin gene mutation D68.52
Protoporphyria, erythropoietic E80.0
Protozoal — *see also* condition
disease B64
specified NEC B60.8
Protrusion, protrusio
acetabuli M24.7
acetabulum (into pelvis) M24.7
device, implant or graft (*see also* Complications, by site and type, mechanical) T85.698
arterial graft NEC — *see* Complication, cardiovascular device, mechanical, vascular
breast (implant) T85.49
catheter NEC T85.698
cystostomy T83.090
dialysis (renal) T82.49
intraperitoneal T85.691
infusion NEC T82.594
spinal (epidural) (subdural) T85.690
urinary, indwelling T83.098
electronic (electrode) (pulse generator) (stimulator)
bone T84.390
nervous system — *see* Complication, prosthetic device, mechanical, electronic nervous system stimulator
fixation, internal (orthopedic) NEC — *see* Complication, fixation device, mechanical
gastrointestinal — *see* Complications, prosthetic device, mechanical, gastrointestinal device

Protrusion, protrusio — *continued*
device, implant or graft (*see also* Complications, by site and type, mechanical) T85.698 — *continued*
genital NEC T83.498
intrauterine contraceptive device T83.39
penile prosthesis T83.490
heart NEC — *see* Complication, cardiovascular device, mechanical
joint prosthesis — *see* Complications, joint prosthesis, mechanical, specified NEC, by site
ocular NEC — *see* Complications, prosthetic device, mechanical, ocular device
orthopedic NEC — *see* Complication, orthopedic, device, mechanical
specified NEC T85.628
urinary NEC — *see also* Complication, genitourinary, device, urinary, mechanical
graft T83.29
vascular NEC — *see* Complication, cardiovascular device, mechanical
ventricular intracranial shunt T85.09
intervertebral disc — *see* Displacement, intervertebral disc
joint prosthesis — *see* Complications, joint prosthesis, mechanical, specified NEC, by site
nucleus pulposus — *see* Displacement, intervertebral disc
Prune belly (syndrome) Q79.4
Prurigo (ferox) (gravis) (Hebrae) (Hebra's) (mitis) (simplex) L28.2
Besnier's L20.0
estivalis L56.4
nodularis L28.1
psychogenic F45.8
Pruritus, pruritic (essential) L29.9
ani, anus L29.0
psychogenic F45.8
anogenital L29.3
psychogenic F45.8
due to onchocerca volvulus B73.1
gravidarum — *see* Pregnancy, complicated by, specified pregnancy-related condition NEC
hiemalis L29.8
neurogenic (any site) F45.8
perianal L29.0
psychogenic (any site) F45.8
scroti, scrotum L29.1
psychogenic F45.8
senile, senilis L29.8
specified NEC L29.8
psychogenic F45.8
Trichomonas A59.9
vulva, vulvae L29.2
psychogenic F45.8
Pseudarthrosis, pseudoarthrosis (bone) — *see* Nonunion, fracture
clavicle, congenital Q74.0
joint, following fusion or arthrodesis M96.0
Pseudoaneurysm — *see* Aneurysm
Pseudoangina (pectoris) — *see* Angina
Pseudoangioma I81
Pseudoarteriosus Q28.8
Pseudoarthrosis — *see* Pseudarthrosis
Pseudobulbar affect (PBA) F48.2
Pseudochromhidrosis L67.8
Pseudocirrhosis, liver, pericardial I31.1
Pseudocowpox B08.03
Pseudocoxalgia M91.3-
Pseudocroup J38.5
Pseudo-Cushing's syndrome, alcohol-induced E24.4
Pseudocyesis F45.8
Pseudocyst
lung J98.4
pancreas K86.3
retina — *see* Cyst, retina
Pseudoelephantiasis neuroarthritica Q82.0
Pseudoexfoliation, capsule (lens) — *see* Cataract, specified NEC
Pseudofolliculitis barbae L73.1
Pseudoglioma H44.89
Pseudohemophilia (Bernuth's) (hereditary) (type B) D68.0
Type A D69.8
vascular D69.8
Pseudohermaphroditism Q56.3
adrenal E25.8
female Q56.2
with adrenocortical disorder E25.8
without adrenocortical disorder Q56.2
adrenal, congenital E25.0

Pseudohermaphroditism Q56.3 — *continued*
male Q56.1
with
5-alpha-reductase deficiency E29.1
adrenocortical disorder E25.8
androgen resistance E34.51
cleft scrotum Q56.1
feminizing testis E34.51
without gonadal disorder Q56.1
adrenal E25.8
Pseudo-Hurler's polydystrophy E77.0
Pseudohydrocephalus G93.2
Pseudohypertrophic muscular dystrophy (Erb's) G71.0
Pseudohypertrophy, muscle G71.0
Pseudohypoparathyroidism E20.1
Pseudoinsomnia F51.03
Pseudoleukemia, infantile D64.89
Pseudo-obstruction intestine (acute) (chronic) (idiopathic) (intermittent secondary) (primary) K59.8
Pseudomembranous — *see* condition
Pseudomeningocele (cerebral) (infective) (post-traumatic) G96.19
postprocedural (spinal) G97.82
Pseudomenses (newborn) P54.6
Pseudomenstruation (newborn) P54.6
Pseudomonas
aeruginosa, as cause of disease classified elsewhere B96.5
mallei infection A24.0
as cause of disease classified elsewhere B96.5
pseudomallei, as cause of disease classified elsewhere B96.5
Pseudomyotonia G71.19
Pseudomyxoma peritonei C78.6
Pseudoneuritis, optic (nerve) (disc) (papilla), congenital Q14.2
Pseudopapilledema H47.33-
congenital Q14.2
Pseudoparalysis
arm or leg R29.818
atonic, congenital P94.2
Pseudopelade L66.0
Pseudophakia Z96.1
Pseudopolyarthritis, rhizomelic M35.3
Pseudopolycythemia D75.1
Pseudopseudohypoparathyroidism E20.1
Pseudopterygium H11.81-
Pseudoptosis (eyelid) — *see* Blepharochalasis
Pseudopuberty, precocious
female heterosexual E25.8
male isosexual E25.8
Pseudorickets (renal) N25.0
Pseudorubella B08.20
Pseudosclerema, newborn P83.8
Pseudosclerosis (brain)
Jakob's — *see* Creutzfeldt-Jakob disease or syndrome
of Westphal (Strümpell) E83.01
spastic — *see* Creutzfeldt-Jakob disease or syndrome
Pseudotetanus — *see* Convulsions
Pseudotetany R29.0
hysterical F44.5
Pseudotruncus arteriosus Q25.4
Pseudotuberculosis A28.2
enterocolitis A04.8
pasteurella (infection) A28.0
Pseudotumor
cerebri G93.2
orbital H05.11-
Pseudoxanthoma elasticum Q82.8
Psilosis (sprue) (tropical) K90.1
nontropical K90.0
Psittacosis A70
Psoitis M60.88
Psoriasis L40.9
arthropathic L40.50
arthritis mutilans L40.52
distal interphalangeal L40.51
juvenile L40.54
other specified L40.59
spondylitis L40.53
buccal K13.29
flexural L40.8
guttate L40.4
mouth K13.29
nummular L40.0
plaque L40.0
psychogenic F54
pustular (generalized) L40.1
palmaris et plantaris L40.3
specified NEC L40.8
vulgaris L40.0
Psychasthenia F48.8
Psychiatric disorder or problem F99

Psychogenic — *see also* condition
factors associated with physical conditions F54
Psychological and behavioral factors affecting medical condition F59
Psychoneurosis, psychoneurotic — *see also* Neurosis
anxiety (state) F41.1
depersonalization F48.1
hypochondriacal F45.21
hysteria F44.9
neurasthenic F48.8
personality NEC F60.89
Psychopathy, psychopathic
affectionless F94.2
autistic F84.5
constitution, post-traumatic F07.81
personality — *see* Disorder, personality
sexual — *see* Deviation, sexual
state F60.2
Psychosexual identity disorder of childhood F64.2
Psychosis, psychotic F29
acute (transient) F23
hysterical F44.9
affective — *see* Disorder, mood
alcoholic F10.959
with
abuse F10.159
anxiety disorder F10.980
with
abuse F10.180
dependence F10.280
delirium tremens F10.231
delusions F10.950
with
abuse F10.150
dependence F10.250
dementia F10.97
with dependence F10.27
dependence F10.259
hallucinosis F10.951
with
abuse F10.151
dependence F10.251
mood disorder F10.94
with
abuse F10.14
dependence F10.24
paranoia F10.950
with
abuse F10.150
dependence F10.250
persisting amnesia F10.96
with dependence F10.26
amnestic confabulatory F10.96
with dependence F10.26
delirium tremens F10.231
Korsakoff's, Korsakov's, Korsakow's F10.26
paranoid type F10.950
with
abuse F10.150
dependence F10.250
anergastic — *see* Psychosis, organic
arteriosclerotic (simple type) (uncomplicated) F01.50
with behavioral disturbance F01.51
childhood F84.0
atypical F84.8
climacteric — *see* Psychosis, involutional
confusional F29
acute or subacute F05
reactive F23
cycloid F23
depressive — *see* Disorder, depressive
disintegrative (childhood) F84.3
drug-induced — *see* F11-F19 with .x59
paranoid and hallucinatory states — *see* F11-F19 with .x50 or .x51
due to or associated with
addiction, drug — *see* F11-F19 with .x59
dependence
alcohol F10.259
drug — *see* F11-F19 with .x59
epilepsy F06.8
Huntington's chorea F06.8
ischemia, cerebrovascular (generalized) F06.8
multiple sclerosis F06.8
physical disease F06.8
presenile dementia F03
senile dementia F03
vascular disease (arteriosclerotic) (cerebral) F01.50
with behavioral disturbance F01.51
epileptic F06.8

Psychosis, psychotic F29 — *continued*
- episode F23
  - due to or associated with physical condition F06.8
  - exhaustive F43.0
  - hallucinatory, chronic F28
  - hypomanic F30.8
  - hysterical (acute) F44.9
  - induced F24
  - infantile F84.0
    - atypical F84.8
  - infective (acute) (subacute) F05
  - involutional F28
    - depressive — *see* Disorder, depressive
    - melancholic — *see* Disorder, depressive
    - paranoid (state) F22
  - Korsakoff's, Korsakov's, Korsakow's (nonalcoholic) F04
    - alcoholic F10.96
      - in dependence F10.26
    - induced by other psychoactive substance — *see* categories F11-F19 with .x5x
  - mania, manic (single episode) F30.2
    - recurrent type F31.89
  - manic-depressive — *see* Disorder, mood
  - menopausal — *see* Psychosis, involutional
  - mixed schizophrenic and affective F25.8
  - multi-infarct (cerebrovascular) F01.50
    - with behavioral disturbance F01.51
  - nonorganic F29
    - specified NEC F28
  - organic F09
    - due to or associated with
      - arteriosclerosis (cerebral) — *see* Psychosis, arteriosclerotic
      - cerebrovascular disease, arteriosclerotic — *see* Psychosis, arteriosclerotic
      - childbirth — *see* Psychosis, puerperal
      - Creutzfeldt-Jakob disease or syndrome — *see* Creutzfeldt-Jakob disease or syndrome
      - dependence, alcohol F10.259
      - disease
        - alcoholic liver F10.259
        - brain, arteriosclerotic — *see* Psychosis, arteriosclerotic
        - cerebrovascular F01.50
          - with behavioral disturbance F01.51
        - Creutzfeldt-Jakob — *see* Creutzfeldt-Jakob disease or syndrome
      - endocrine or metabolic F06.8
        - acute or subacute F05
      - epilepsy transient (acute) F05
      - infection
        - brain (intracranial) F06.8
          - acute or subacute F05
      - intoxication
        - alcoholic (acute) F10.259
        - drug F19 with .59 F11-
      - ischemia, cerebrovascular (generalized) — *see* Psychosis, arteriosclerotic
      - puerperium — *see* Psychosis, puerperal
      - trauma, brain (birth) (from electric current) (surgical) F06.8
        - acute or subacute F05
    - infective F06.8
      - acute or subacute F05
    - post-traumatic F06.8
      - acute or subacute F05
  - paranoiac F22
  - paranoid (climacteric) (involutional) (menopausal) F22
    - psychogenic (acute) F23
    - schizophrenic F20.0
    - senile F03
  - postpartum F53
  - presbyophrenic (type) F03
  - presenile F03
  - psychogenic (paranoid) F23
    - depressive F32.3
  - puerperal F53
    - specified type — *see* Psychosis, by type
  - reactive (brief) (transient) (emotional stress) (psychological trauma) F23
    - depressive F32.3
      - recurrent F33.3
    - excitative type F30.8
  - schizoaffective F25.9
    - depressive type F25.1
    - manic type F25.0
  - schizophrenia, schizophrenic — *see* Schizophrenia
  - schizophrenia-like, in epilepsy F06.2

Psychosis, psychotic F29 — *continued*
- schizophreniform F20.81
  - affective type F25.9
  - brief F23
  - confusional type F23
  - depressive type F25.1
  - manic type F25.0
  - mixed type F25.0
- senile NEC F03
  - depressed or paranoid type F03
  - simple deterioration F03
  - specified type — *code to* condition
- shared F24
- situational (reactive) F23
- symbiotic (childhood) F84.3
- symptomatic F09
Psychosomatic — *see* Disorder, psychosomatic
Psychosyndrome, organic F07.9
Psychotic episode due to or associated with physical condition F06.8
Pterygium (eye) H11.00-
- amyloid H11.01-
- central H11.02-
- colli Q18.3
- double H11.03-
- peripheral
  - progressive H11.05-
  - stationary H11.04-
- recurrent H11.06-
Ptilosis (eyelid) — *see* Madarosis
Ptomaine (poisoning) — *see* Poisoning, food
Ptosis — *see also* Blepharoptosis
- adiposa (false) — *see* Blepharoptosis
- breast N64.81
- cecum K63.4
- colon K63.4
- congenital (eyelid) Q10.0
  - specified site NEC — *see* Anomaly, by site
- eyelid — *see* Blepharoptosis
  - congenital Q10.0
- gastric K31.89
- intestine K63.4
- kidney N28.83
- liver K76.89
- renal N28.83
- splanchnic K63.4
- spleen D73.89
- stomach K31.89
- viscera K63.4
PTP D69.51
Ptyalism (periodic) K11.7
- hysterical F45.8
- pregnancy — *see* Pregnancy, complicated by, specified pregnancy-related condition NEC
- psychogenic F45.8
Ptyalolithiasis K11.5
Pubarche, precocious E30.1
Pubertas praecox E30.1
Puberty (development state) Z00.3
- bleeding (excessive) N92.2
- delayed E30.0
- precocious (constitutional) (cryptogenic) (idiopathic) E30.1
  - central E22.8
  - due to
    - ovarian hyperfunction E28.1
      - estrogen E28.0
    - testicular hyperfunction E29.0
- premature E30.1
  - due to
    - adrenal cortical hyperfunction E25.8
    - pineal tumor E34.8
    - pituitary (anterior) hyperfunction E22.8
Puckering, macula — *see* Degeneration, macula, puckering
Pudenda, pudendum — *see* condition
Puente's disease (simple glandular cheilitis) K13.0
Puerperal, puerperium (complicated by, complications)
- abnormal glucose (tolerance test) O99.815
- abscess
  - areola O91.02
    - associated with lactation O91.03
  - Bartholin's gland O86.19
  - breast O91.12
    - associated with lactation O91.13
  - cervix (uteri) O86.11
  - genital organ NEC O86.19
  - kidney O86.21
  - mammary O91.12
    - associated with lactation O91.13
  - nipple O91.02
    - associated with lactation O91.03
  - peritoneum O85

Puerperal, puerperium (complicated by, complications) — *continued*
- abscess — *continued*
  - subareolar O91.12
    - associated with lactation O91.13
  - urinary tract — *see* Puerperal, infection, urinary
  - uterus O86.12
  - vagina (wall) O86.13
  - vaginorectal O86.13
  - vulvovaginal gland O86.13
- adnexitis O86.19
- afibrinogenemia, or other coagulation defect O72.3
- albuminuria (acute) (subacute) — *see* Proteinuria, gestational
- alcohol use O99.315
- anemia O90.81
  - pre-existing (pre-pregnancy) O99.03
- anesthetic death O89.8
- apoplexy O99.43
- bariatric surgery status O99.845
- blood disorder NEC O99.13
- blood dyscrasia O72.3
- cardiomyopathy O90.3
- cerebrovascular disorder (conditions in I60-I69) O99.43
- cervicitis O86.11
- circulatory system disorder O99.43
- coagulopathy (any) O72.3
- complications O99.9
  - specified NEC O90.89
- convulsions — *see* Eclampsia
- cystitis O86.22
- cystopyelitis O86.29
- delirium NEC F05
- diabetes O24.93
  - gestational — *see* Puerperal, gestational diabetes
  - pre-existing O24.33
    - specified NEC O24.83
    - type 1 O24.03
    - type 2 O24.13
- digestive system disorder O99.63
- disease O90.9
  - breast NEC O92.29
  - cerebrovascular (acute) O99.43
  - nonobstetric NEC O99.89
  - tubo-ovarian O86.19
  - Valsuani's O99.03
- disorder O90.9
  - biliary tract O26.63
  - lactation O92.70
  - liver O26.63
  - nonobstetric NEC O99.89
- disruption
  - cesarean wound O90.0
  - episiotomy wound O90.1
  - perineal laceration wound O90.1
- drug use O99.325
- eclampsia (with pre-existing hypertension) O15.2
- embolism (pulmonary) (blood clot) — *see* Embolism, obstetric, puerperal
- endocrine, nutritional or metabolic disease NEC O99.285
- endophlebitis — *see* Puerperal, phlebitis
- endotrachelitis O86.11
- failure
  - lactation (complete) O92.3
    - partial O92.4
  - renal, acute O90.4
- fever (of unknown origin) O86.4
  - septic O85
- fissure, nipple O92.12
  - associated with lactation O92.13
- fistula
  - breast (due to mastitis) O91.12
    - associated with lactation O91.13
  - nipple O91.02
    - associated with lactation O91.03
- galactophoritis O91.22
  - associated with lactation O91.23
- galactorrhea O92.6
- gastric banding status O99.845
- gastric bypass status O99.845
- gastrointestinal disease NEC O99.63
- gestational diabetes O24.439
  - diet controlled O24.430
  - insulin (and diet) controlled O24.434
- gonorrhea O98.23
- hematoma, subdural O99.43
- hemiplegia, cerebral O99.355
  - due to cerebrovascular disorder O99.43

Puerperal, puerperium (complicated by, complications) — *continued*
- hemorrhage O72.1
  - brain O99.43
  - bulbar O99.43
  - cerebellar O99.43
  - cerebral O99.43
  - cortical O99.43
  - delayed or secondary O72.2
  - extradural O99.43
  - internal capsule O99.43
  - intracranial O99.43
  - intrapontine O99.43
  - meningeal O99.43
  - pontine O99.43
  - retained placenta O72.0
  - subarachnoid O99.43
  - subcortical O99.43
  - subdural O99.43
  - third stage O72.0
  - uterine, delayed O72.2
  - ventricular O99.43
- hemorrhoids O87.2
- hepatorenal syndrome O90.4
- hypertension — *see* Hypertension, complicating, puerperium
- hypertrophy, breast O92.29
- induration breast (fibrous) O92.29
- infection O86.4
  - cervix O86.11
  - generalized O85
  - genital tract NEC O86.19
    - obstetric surgical wound O86.0
  - kidney (bacillus coli) O86.21
  - maternal O98.93
    - carrier state NEC O99.835
    - gonorrhea O98.23
    - human immunodeficiency virus (HIV) O98.73
    - protozoal O98.63
    - sexually transmitted NEC O98.33
    - specified NEC O98.83
    - streptococcus B carrier state O99.825
    - syphilis O98.13
    - tuberculosis O98.03
    - viral hepatitis O98.43
    - viral NEC O98.53
  - nipple O91.02
    - associated with lactation O91.03
  - peritoneum O85
  - renal O86.21
  - specified NEC O86.89
  - urinary (asymptomatic) (tract) NEC O86.20
    - bladder O86.22
    - kidney O86.21
    - specified site NEC O86.29
    - urethra O86.22
  - vagina O86.13
  - vein — *see* Puerperal, phlebitis
- ischemia, cerebral O99.43
- lymphangitis O86.89
  - breast O91.22
    - associated with lactation O91.23
- malignancy O9A.13
- malnutrition O25.3
- mammillitis O91.02
  - associated with lactation O91.03
- mammitis O91.22
  - associated with lactation O91.23
- mania F30.8
- mastitis O91.22
  - associated with lactation O91.23
  - purulent O91.12
    - associated with lactation O91.13
- melancholia — *see* Disorder, depressive
- mental disorder NEC O99.345
- metroperitonitis O85
- metrorrhagia — *see* Hemorrhage, postpartum
- metrosalpingitis O86.19
- metrovaginitis O86.13
- milk leg O87.1
- monoplegia, cerebral O99.43
- mood disturbance O90.6
- necrosis, liver (acute) (subacute) (conditions in subcategory K72.0) O26.63
  - with renal failure O90.4
- nervous system disorder O99.355
- neuritis O90.89
- obesity (pre-existing prior to pregnancy) O99.215
- obesity surgery status O99.845
- occlusion, precerebral artery O99.43
- paralysis
  - bladder (sphincter) O90.89
  - cerebral O99.43
- paralytic stroke O99.43
- parametritis O85

Puerperal, puerperium (complicated by, complications) — *continued*
 paravaginitis O86.13
 pelviperitonitis O85
 perimetritis O86.12
 perimetrosalpingitis O86.19
 perinephritis O86.21
 periphlebitis — *see* Puerperal phlebitis
 peritoneal infection O85
 peritonitis (pelvic) O85
 perivaginitis O86.13
 phlebitis O87.0
  deep O87.1
  pelvic O87.1
  superficial O87.0
 phlebothrombosis, deep O87.1
 phlegmasia alba dolens O87.1
 placental polyp O90.89
 pneumonia, embolic — *see* Embolism, obstetric, puerperal
 pre-eclampsia — *see* Pre-eclampsia
 psychosis F53
 pyelitis O86.21
 pyelocystitis O86.29
 pyelonephritis O86.21
 pyelonephrosis O86.21
 pyemia O85
 pyocystitis O86.29
 pyohemia O85
 pyometra O86.12
 pyonephritis O86.21
 pyosalpingitis O86.19
 pyrexia (of unknown origin) O86.4
 renal
  disease NEC O90.89
  failure O90.4
 respiratory disease NEC O99.53
 retention
  decidua — *see* Retention, decidua
  placenta O72.0
  secundines — *see* Retention, secundines
 retrated nipple O92.02
 salpingo-ovaritis O86.19
 salpingoperitonitis O85
 secondary perineal tear O90.1
 sepsis O85
 sepsis (pelvic) O85
 septic thrombophlebitis O86.81
 skin disorder NEC O99.73
 specified condition NEC O99.89
 stroke O99.43
 subinvolution (uterus) O90.89
 subluxation of symphysis (pubis) O26.73
 suppuration — *see* Puerperal, abscess
 tetanus A34
 thelitis O91.02
  associated with lactation O91.03
 thrombocytopenia O72.3
 thrombophlebitis (superficial) O87.0
  deep O87.1
  pelvic O87.1
  septic O86.81
 thrombosis (venous) — *see* Thrombosis, puerperal
 thyroiditis O90.5
 toxemia (eclamptic) (pre-eclamptic) (with convulsions) O15.2
 trauma, non-obstetric O9A.23
  caused by abuse (physical) (suspected) O9A.33
   confirmed O9A.33
   psychological (suspected) O9A.53
    confirmed O9A.53
   sexual (suspected) O9A.43
    confirmed O9A.43
 uremia (due to renal failure) O90.4
 urethritis O86.22
 vaginitis O86.13
 varicose veins (legs) O87.4
  vulva or perineum O87.8
 venous O87.9
 vulvitis O86.19
 vulvovaginitis O86.13
 white leg O87.1
Puerperium — *see* Puerperal
Pulmolithiasis J98.4
Pulmonary — *see* condition
Pulpitis (acute) (anachoretic) (chronic) (hyperplastic) (irreversible) (putrescent) (reversible) (suppurative) (ulcerative) K04.0
Pulpless tooth K04.99
Pulse
 alternating R00.8
 bigeminal R00.8
 fast R00.0
 feeble, rapid due to shock following injury T79.4
 rapid R00.0
 weak R09.89

Pulsus alternans or trigeminus R00.8
Punch drunk F07.81
Punctum lacrimale occlusion — *see* Obstruction, lacrimal
Puncture
 abdomen, abdominal
  wall S31.139
   with
    foreign body S31.149
    penetration into peritoneal cavity S31.639
     with foreign body S31.649
   epigastric region S31.132
    with
     foreign body S31.142
     penetration into peritoneal cavity S31.632
      with foreign body S31.642
   left
    lower quadrant S31.134
     with
      foreign body S31.144
      penetration into peritoneal cavity S31.634
       with foreign body S31.644
    upper quadrant S31.131
     with
      foreign body S31.141
      penetration into peritoneal cavity S31.631
       with foreign body S31.641
   periumbilic region S31.135
    with
     foreign body S31.145
     penetration into peritoneal cavity S31.635
      with foreign body S31.645
   right
    lower quadrant S31.133
     with
      foreign body S31.143
      penetration into peritoneal cavity S31.633
       with foreign body S31.643
    upper quadrant S31.130
     with
      foreign body S31.140
      penetration into peritoneal cavity S31.630
       with foreign body S31.640
 accidental, complicating surgery — *see* Complication, accidental puncture or laceration
 alveolar (process) — *see* Puncture, oral cavity
 ankle S91.039
  with
   foreign body S91.049
  left S91.032
   with
    foreign body S91.042
  right S91.031
   with
    foreign body S91.041
 anus S31.833
  with foreign body S31.834
 arm (upper) S41.139
  with foreign body S41.149
  left S41.132
   with foreign body S41.142
  lower — *see* Puncture, forearm
  right S41.131
   with foreign body S41.141
 auditory canal (external) (meatus) — *see* Puncture, ear
 auricle, ear — *see* Puncture, ear
 axilla — *see* Puncture, arm
 back — *see also* Puncture, thorax, back
  lower S31.030
   with
    foreign body S31.040
    with penetration into retroperitoneal space S31.041
    penetration into retroperitoneal space S31.031
 bladder (traumatic) S37.29
  nontraumatic N32.89
 breast S21.039
  with foreign body S21.049
  left S21.032
   with foreign body S21.042
  right S21.031
   with foreign body S21.041
 buttock S31.803
  with foreign body S31.804
  left S31.823
   with foreign body S31.824
  right S31.813
   with foreign body S31.814

Puncture — *continued*
 by
  device, implant or graft — *see* Complications, by site and type, mechanical
  foreign body left accidentally in operative wound T81.539
  instrument (any) during a procedure, accidental — *see* Puncture, accidental complicating surgery
 calf — *see* Puncture, leg
 canaliculus lacrimalis — *see* Puncture, eyelid
 canthus, eye — *see* Puncture, eyelid
 cervical esophagus S11.23
  with foreign body S11.24
 cheek (external) S01.439
  with foreign body S01.449
  internal — *see* Puncture, oral cavity
  left S01.432
   with foreign body S01.442
  right S01.431
   with foreign body S01.441
 chest wall — *see* Puncture, thorax
 chin — *see* Puncture, head, specified site NEC
 clitoris — *see* Puncture, vulva
 costal region — *see* Puncture, thorax
 digit(s)
  foot — *see* Puncture, toe
  hand — *see* Puncture, finger
 ear (canal) (external) S01.339
  with foreign body S01.349
  drum S09.2-
  left S01.332
   with foreign body S01.342
  right S01.331
   with foreign body S01.341
 elbow S51.039
  with
   foreign body S51.049
  left S51.032
   with
    foreign body S51.042
  right S51.031
   with
    foreign body S51.041
 epididymis — *see* Puncture, testis
 epigastric region — *see* Puncture, abdomen, wall, epigastric
 epiglottis S11.83
  with foreign body S11.84
 esophagus
  cervical S11.23
   with foreign body S11.24
  thoracic S27.818
 eyeball S05.6-
  with foreign body S05.5-
 eyebrow — *see* Puncture, eyelid
 eyelid S01.13-
  with foreign body S01.14-
  left S01.132
   with foreign body S01.142
  right S01.131
   with foreign body S01.141
 face NEC — *see* Puncture, head, specified site NEC
 finger(s) S61.239
  with
   damage to nail S61.339
    with
     foreign body S61.349
   foreign body S61.249
  index S61.238
   with
    damage to nail S61.338
     with
      foreign body S61.348
    foreign body S61.248
   left S61.231
    with
     damage to nail S61.331
      with
       foreign body S61.341
     foreign body S61.241
   right S61.230
    with
     damage to nail S61.330
      with
       foreign body S61.340
     foreign body S61.240
  little S61.238
   with
    damage to nail S61.338
     with
      foreign body S61.348
    foreign body S61.248

Puncture — *continued*
 finger(s) S61.239 — *continued*
  little S61.238 — *continued*
   left S61.237
    with
     damage to nail S61.337
      with
       foreign body S61.347
     foreign body S61.247
   right S61.236
    with
     damage to nail S61.336
      with
       foreign body S61.346
     foreign body S61.246
  middle S61.238
   with
    damage to nail S61.338
     with
      foreign body S61.348
    foreign body S61.248
   left S61.233
    with
     damage to nail S61.333
      with
       foreign body S61.343
     foreign body S61.243
   right S61.232
    with
     damage to nail S61.332
      with
       foreign body S61.342
     foreign body S61.242
  ring S61.238
   with
    damage to nail S61.338
     with
      foreign body S61.348
    foreign body S61.248
   left S61.235
    with
     damage to nail S61.335
      with
       foreign body S61.345
     foreign body S61.245
   right S61.234
    with
     damage to nail S61.334
      with
       foreign body S61.344
     foreign body S61.244
 flank S31.139
  with foreign body S31.149
 foot (except toe(s) alone) S91.339
  with foreign body S91.349
  left S91.332
   with foreign body S91.342
  right S91.331
   with foreign body S91.341
  toe — *see* Puncture, toe
 forearm S51.839
  with
   foreign body S51.849
  elbow only — *see* Puncture, elbow
  left S51.832
   with
    foreign body S51.842
  right S51.831
   with
    foreign body S51.841
 forehead — *see* Puncture, head, specified site NEC
 genital organs, external
  female S31.532
   with foreign body S31.542
   vagina — *see* Puncture, vagina
   vulva — *see* Puncture, vulva
  male S31.531
   with foreign body S31.541
   penis — *see* Puncture, penis
   scrotum — *see* Puncture, scrotum
   testis — *see* Puncture, testis
 groin — *see* Puncture, abdomen, wall
 gum — *see* Puncture, oral cavity
 hand S61.439
  with
   foreign body S61.449
  finger — *see* Puncture, finger
  left S61.432
   with
    foreign body S61.442
  right S61.431
   with
    foreign body S61.441
  thumb — *see* Puncture, thumb

DISEASE INDEX

Puncture — *continued*
head S01.93
  with foreign body S01.94
  cheek — *see* Puncture, cheek
  ear — *see* Puncture, ear
  eyelid — *see* Puncture, eyelid
  lip — *see* Puncture, oral cavity
  nose — *see* Puncture, nose
  oral cavity — *see* Puncture, oral cavity
  scalp S01.03
    with foreign body S01.04
  specified site NEC S01.83
    with foreign body S01.84
  temporomandibular area — *see*
    Puncture, cheek
heart S26.99
  with hemopericardium S26.09
  without hemopericardium S26.19
heel — *see* Puncture, foot
hip S71.039
  with foreign body S71.049
  left S71.032
    with foreign body S71.042
  right S71.031
    with foreign body S71.041
hymen — *see* Puncture, vagina
hypochondrium — *see* Puncture, abdomen, wall
hypogastric region — *see* Puncture, abdomen, wall
inguinal region — *see* Puncture, abdomen, wall
instep — *see* Puncture, foot
internal organs — *see* Injury, by site
interscapular region — *see* Puncture, thorax, back
intestine
  large
    colon S36.599
      ascending S36.590
      descending S36.592
      sigmoid S36.593
      specified site NEC S36.598
      transverse S36.591
    rectum S36.69
  small S36.499
    duodenum S36.490
    specified site NEC S36.498
intra-abdominal organ S36.99
  gallbladder S36.128
  intestine — *see* Puncture, intestine
  liver S36.118
  pancreas — *see* Puncture, pancreas
  peritoneum S36.81
  specified site NEC S36.898
  spleen S36.09
  stomach S36.39
jaw — *see* Puncture, head, specified site NEC
knee S81.039
  with foreign body S81.049
  left S81.032
    with foreign body S81.042
  right S81.031
    with foreign body S81.041
labium (majus) (minus) — *see* Puncture, vulva
lacrimal duct — *see* Puncture, eyelid
larynx S11.013
  with foreign body S11.014
leg (lower) S81.839
  with foreign body S81.849
  foot — *see* Puncture, foot
  knee — *see* Puncture, knee
  left S81.832
    with foreign body S81.842
  right S81.831
    with foreign body S81.841
  upper — *see* Puncture, thigh
lip S01.531
  with foreign body S01.541
loin — *see* Puncture, abdomen, wall
lower back — *see* Puncture, back, lower
lumbar region — *see* Puncture, back, lower
malar region — *see* Puncture, head, specified site NEC
mammary — *see* Puncture, breast
mastoid region — *see* Puncture, head, specified site NEC
mouth — *see* Puncture, oral cavity
nail
  finger — *see* Puncture, finger, with damage to nail
  toe — *see* Puncture, toe, with damage to nail
nasal (septum) (sinus) — *see* Puncture, nose
nasopharynx — *see* Puncture, head, specified site NEC

Puncture — *continued*
neck S11.93
  with foreign body S11.94
  involving
    cervical esophagus — *see* Puncture, cervical esophagus
    larynx — *see* Puncture, larynx
    pharynx — *see* Puncture, pharynx
    thyroid gland — *see* Puncture, thyroid gland
    trachea — *see* Puncture, trachea
  specified site NEC S11.83
    with foreign body S11.84
nose (septum) (sinus) S01.23
  with foreign body S01.24
ocular — *see* Puncture, eyeball
oral cavity S01.532
  with foreign body S01.542
orbit S05.4-
palate — *see* Puncture, oral cavity
palm — *see* Puncture, hand
pancreas S36.299
  body S36.291
  head S36.290
  tail S36.292
pelvis — *see* Puncture, back, lower
penis S31.23
  with foreign body S31.24
perineum
  female S31.43
    with foreign body S31.44
  male S31.139
    with foreign body S31.149
periocular area (with or without lacrimal passages) — *see* Puncture, eyelid
phalanges
  finger — *see* Puncture, finger
  toe — *see* Puncture, toe
pharynx S11.23
  with foreign body S11.24
pinna — *see* Puncture, ear
popliteal space — *see* Puncture, knee
prepuce — *see* Puncture, penis
pubic region S31.139
  with foreign body S31.149
pudendum — *see* Puncture, genital organs, external
rectovaginal septum — *see* Puncture, vagina
sacral region — *see* Puncture, back, lower
sacroiliac region — *see* Puncture, back, lower
salivary gland — *see* Puncture, oral cavity
scalp S01.03
  with foreign body S01.04
scapular region — *see* Puncture, shoulder
scrotum S31.33
  with foreign body S31.34
shin — *see* Puncture, leg
shoulder S41.039
  with foreign body S41.049
  left S41.032
    with foreign body S41.042
  right S41.031
    with foreign body S41.041
spermatic cord — *see* Puncture, testis
sternal region — *see* Puncture, thorax, front
submaxillary region — *see* Puncture, head, specified site NEC
submental region — *see* Puncture, head, specified site NEC
subungual
  finger(s) — *see* Puncture, finger, with damage to nail
  toe — *see* Puncture, toe, with damage to nail
supraclavicular fossa — *see* Puncture, neck, specified site NEC
temple, temporal region — *see* Puncture, head, specified site NEC
temporomandibular area — *see* Puncture, cheek
testis S31.33
  with foreign body S31.34
thigh S71.139
  with foreign body S71.149
  left S71.132
    with foreign body S71.142
  right S71.131
    with foreign body S71.141
thorax, thoracic (wall) S21.93
  with foreign body S21.94
  back S21.23-
    with
      foreign body S21.24-
        with penetration S21.44
      penetration S21.43
  breast — *see* Puncture, breast

Puncture — *continued*
thorax, thoracic (wall) S21.93 — *continued*
  front S21.13-
    with
      foreign body S21.14-
        with penetration S21.34
      penetration S21.33
throat — *see* Puncture, neck
thumb S61.039
  with
    damage to nail S61.139
      with
        foreign body S61.149
    foreign body S61.049
  left S61.032
    with
      damage to nail S61.132
        with
          foreign body S61.142
      foreign body S61.042
  right S61.031
    with
      damage to nail S61.131
        with
          foreign body S61.141
      foreign body S61.041
thyroid gland S11.13
  with foreign body S11.14
toe(s) S91.139
  with
    damage to nail S91.239
      with
        foreign body S91.249
    foreign body S91.149
  great S91.133
    with
      damage to nail S91.233
        with
          foreign body S91.243
      foreign body S91.143
    left S91.132
      with
        damage to nail S91.232
          with
            foreign body S91.242
        foreign body S91.142
    right S91.131
      with
        damage to nail S91.231
          with
            foreign body S91.241
        foreign body S91.141
  lesser S91.136
    with
      damage to nail S91.236
        with
          foreign body S91.246
      foreign body S91.146
    left S91.135
      with
        damage to nail S91.235
          with
            foreign body S91.245
        foreign body S91.145
    right S91.134
      with
        damage to nail S91.234
          with
            foreign body S91.244
        foreign body S91.144
tongue — *see* Puncture, oral cavity
trachea S11.023
  with foreign body S11.024
tunica vaginalis — *see* Puncture, testis
tympanum, tympanic membrane S09.2-
umbilical region S31.135
  with foreign body S31.145
uvula — *see* Puncture, oral cavity
vagina S31.43
  with foreign body S31.44
vocal cords S11.033
  with foreign body S11.034
vulva S31.43
  with foreign body S31.44
wrist S61.539
  with
    foreign body S61.549
  left S61.532
    with
      foreign body S61.542
  right S61.531
    with
      foreign body S61.541
PUO (pyrexia of unknown origin) R50.9
Pupillary membrane (persistent) Q13.89
Pupillotonia — *see* Anomaly, pupil, function, tonic pupil

Purpura D69.2
abdominal D69.0
allergic D69.0
anaphylactoid D69.0
annularis telangiectodes L81.7
arthritic D69.0
autoerythrocyte sensitization D69.2
autoimmune D69.0
bacterial D69.0
Bateman's (senile) D69.2
capillary fragility (hereditary) (idiopathic) D69.8
cryoglobulinemic D89.1
Devil's pinches D69.2
fibrinolytic — *see* Fibrinolysis
fulminans, fulminous D65
gangrenous D65
hemorrhagic, hemorrhagica D69.3
  not due to thrombocytopenia D69.0
Henoch(-Schönlein) (allergic) D69.0
hypergammaglobulinemic (benign) (Waldenström) D89.0
idiopathic (thrombocytopenic) D69.3
  nonthrombocytopenic D69.0
immune thrombocytopenic D69.3
infectious D69.0
malignant D69.0
neonatorum P54.5
nervosa D69.0
newborn P54.5
nonthrombocytopenic D69.2
  hemorrhagic D69.0
  idiopathic D69.0
nonthrombopenic D69.2
peliosis rheumatica D69.0
posttransfusion (post-transfusion) (from (fresh) whole blood or blood products) D69.51
primary D69.49
red cell membrane sensitivity D69.2
rheumatica D69.0
Schönlein(-Henoch) (allergic) D69.0
scorbutic E54 [D77]
senile D69.2
simplex D69.2
symptomatica D69.0
telangiectasia annularis L81.7
thrombocytopenic D69.49
  congenital D69.42
  hemorrhagic D69.3
  hereditary D69.42
  idiopathic D69.3
  immune D69.3
  neonatal, transitory P61.0
  thrombotic M31.1
thrombohemolytic — *see* Fibrinolysis
thrombolytic — *see* Fibrinolysis
thrombopenic D69.49
thrombotic, thrombocytopenic M31.1
toxic D69.0
vascular D69.0
visceral symptoms D69.0
Purpuric spots R23.3
Purulent — *see* condition
Pus
in
  stool R19.5
  urine N39.0
tube (rupture) — *see* Salpingo-oophoritis
Pustular rash L08.0
Pustule (nonmalignant) L08.9
malignant A22.0
Pustulosis palmaris et plantaris L40.3
Putnam(-Dana) disease or syndrome — *see* Degeneration, combined
Putrescent pulp (dental) K04.1
Pyarthritis, pyarthrosis — *see* Arthritis, pyogenic or pyemic
tuberculous — *see* Tuberculosis, joint
Pyelectasis — *see* Hydronephrosis
Pyelitis (congenital) (uremic) — *see also* Pyelonephritis
with
  calculus — *see* category N20
    with hydronephrosis N13.2
  contracted kidney N11.9
acute N10
chronic N11.9
  with calculus — *see* category N20
    with hydronephrosis N13.2
cystica N28.84
puerperal (postpartum) O86.21
tuberculous A18.11
Pyelocystitis — *see* Pyelonephritis

Pyelonephritis — *see also* Nephritis, tubulo-interstitial
with
calculus — *see* category N20
with hydronephrosis N13.2
contracted kidney N11.9
acute N10
calculous — *see* category N20
with hydronephrosis N13.2
chronic N11.9
with calculus — *see* category N20
with hydronephrosis N13.2
associated with ureteral obstruction or stricture N11.1
nonobstructive N11.8
with reflux (vesicoureteral) N11.0
obstructive N11.1
specified NEC N11.8
in (due to)
brucellosis A23.9 [N16]
cryoglobulinemia (mixed) D89.1 [N16]
cystinosis E72.04
diphtheria A36.84
glycogen storage disease E74.09 [N16]
leukemia NEC C95.9-[N16]
lymphoma NEC C85.90 [N16]
multiple myeloma C90.0-[N16]
obstruction N11.1
Salmonella infection A02.25
sarcoidosis D86.84
sepsis A41.9 [N16]
Sjögren's disease M35.04
toxoplasmosis B58.83
transplant rejection T86.91 [N16]
Wilson's disease E83.01 [N16]
nonobstructive N12
with reflux (vesicoureteral) N11.0
chronic N11.8
syphilitic A52.75
Pyelonephrosis (obstructive) N11.1
chronic N11.9
Pyelophlebitis I80.8
Pyeloureteritis cystica N28.85
Pyemia, pyemic (fever) (infection) (purulent) — *see also* Sepsis
joint — *see* Arthritis, pyogenic or pyemic
liver K75.1
pneumococcal A40.3
portal K75.1
postvaccinal T88.0
puerperal, postpartum, childbirth O85
specified organism NEC A41.89
tuberculous — *see* Tuberculosis, miliary
Pygopagus Q89.4
Pyknoepilepsy (idiopathic) — *see* Pyknolepsy
Pyknolepsy
intractable G40.A19
with status epilepticus G40.A11
without status epilepticus G40.A19
not intractable G40.A09
with status epilepticus G40.A01
without status epilepticus G40.A09
Pylephlebitis K75.1
Pyle's syndrome Q78.5
Pylethrombophlebitis K75.1
Pylethrombosis K75.1
Pyloritis K29.90
with bleeding K29.91
Pylorospasm (reflex) NEC K31.3
congenital or infantile Q40.0
neurotic F45.8
newborn Q40.0
psychogenic F45.8
Pylorus, pyloric — *see* condition
Pyoarthrosis — *see* Arthritis, pyogenic or pyemic
Pyocele
mastoid — *see* Mastoiditis, acute
sinus (accessory) — *see* Sinusitis
turbinate (bone) J32.9
urethra (*see also* Urethritis) N34.0
Pyocolpos — *see* Vaginitis
Pyocystitis N30.80
with hematuria N30.81
Pyoderma, pyodermia L08.0
gangrenosum L88
newborn P39.4
phagedenic L88
vegetans L08.81
Pyodermatitis L08.0
vegetans L08.81
Pyogenic — *see* condition
Pyohydronephrosis N13.6
Pyometra, pyometrium, pyometritis — *see* Endometritis
Pyomyositis (tropical) — *see* Myositis, infective
Pyonephritis N12

Pyonephrosis N13.6
tuberculous A18.11
Pyo-oophoritis — *see* Salpingo-oophoritis
Pyo-ovarium — *see* Salpingo-oophoritis
Pyopericarditis, pyopericardium I30.1
Pyophlebitis — *see* Phlebitis
Pyopneumopericardium I30.1
Pyopneumothorax (infective) J86.9
with fistula J86.0
tuberculous NEC A15.6
Pyosalpinx, pyosalpingitis — *see also* Salpingo-oophoritis
Pyothorax J86.9
with fistula J86.0
tuberculous NEC A15.6
Pyoureter N28.89
tuberculous A18.11
Pyramidopallidonigral syndrome G20
Pyrexia (of unknown origin) R50.9
atmospheric T67.0
during labor NEC O75.2
heat T67.0
newborn P81.9
environmentally-induced P81.0
persistent R50.9
puerperal O86.4
Pyroglobulinemia NEC E88.09
Pyromania F63.1
Pyrosis R12
Pyuria (bacterial) N39.0

Q

Q fever A78
with pneumonia A78
Quadricuspid aortic valve Q23.8
Quadrilateral fever A78
Quadriparesis — *see* Quadriplegia
meaning muscle weakness M62.81
Quadriplegia G82.50
complete
C1-C4 level G82.51
C5-C7 level G82.53
congenital (cerebral) (spinal) G80.8
spastic G80.0
embolic (current episode) I63.4
incomplete
C1-C4 level G82.52
C5-C7 level G82.54
thrombotic (current episode) I63.3
traumatic — *code to* injury with seventh character S
current episode — *see* Injury, spinal (cord), cervical
Quadruplet, pregnancy — *see* Pregnancy, quadruplet
Quarrelsomeness F60.3
Queensland fever A77.3
Quervain's disease M65.4
thyroid E06.1
Queyrat's erythroplasia D07.4
penis D07.4
specified site — *see* Neoplasm, skin, in situ
unspecified site D07.4
Quincke's disease or edema T78.3
hereditary D84.1
Quinsy (gangrenous) J36
Quintan fever A79.0
Quintuplet, pregnancy — *see* Pregnancy, quintuplet

R

Rabbit fever — *see* Tularemia
Rabies A82.9
contact Z20.3
exposure to Z20.3
inoculation reaction — *see* Complications, vaccination
sylvatic A82.0
urban A82.1
Rachischisis — *see* Spina bifida
Rachitic — *see also* condition
deformities of spine (late effect) (sequelae) E64.3
pelvis (late effect) (sequelae) E64.3
with disproportion (fetopelvic) O33.0
causing obstructed labor O65.0
Rachitis, rachitism (acute) (tarda) — *see also* Rickets
renalis N25.0
sequelae E64.3
Radial nerve — *see* condition
Radiation
burn — *see* Burn
effects NOS T66
sickness NOS T66
therapy, encounter for Z51.0
Radiculitis (pressure) (vertebrogenic) — *see* Radiculopathy
Radiculomyelitis — *see also* Encephalitis
toxic, due to
Clostridium tetani A35
Corynebacterium diphtheriae A36.82
Radiculopathy M54.10
cervical region M54.12
cervicothoracic region M54.13
due to
disc disorder
C3 M50.11
C4 M50.11
C5 M50.12
C6 M50.12
C7 M50.12
C8 M50.13
displacement of intervertebral disc — *see* Disorder, disc, with, radiculopathy
leg M54.1-
lumbar region M54.16
lumbosacral region M54.17
occipito-atlanto-axial region M54.11
postherpetic B02.29
sacrococcygeal region M54.18
syphilitic A52.11
thoracic region (with visceral pain) M54.14
thoracolumbar region M54.15
Radiodermal burns (acute, chronic, or occupational) — *see* Burn
Radiodermatitis L58.9
acute L58.0
chronic L58.1
Radiotherapy session Z51.0
Rage, meaning rabies — *see* Rabies
Ragpicker's disease A22.1
Ragsorter's disease A22.1
Raillietiniasis B71.8
Railroad neurosis F48.8
Railway spine F48.8
Raised — *see also* Elevated
antibody titer R76.0
Rake teeth, tooth M26.39
Rales R09.89
Ramifying renal pelvis Q63.8
Ramsay-Hunt disease or syndrome (*see also* Hunt's disease) B02.21
meaning dyssynergia cerebellaris myoclonica G11.1
Ranula K11.6
congenital Q38.4
Rape
adult
confirmed T74.21
suspected T76.21
alleged, observation or examination, ruled out
adult Z04.41
child Z04.42
child
confirmed T74.22
suspected T76.22
Rapid
feeble pulse, due to shock, following injury T79.4
heart (beat) R00.0
psychogenic F45.8
second stage (delivery) O62.3

Rapid — *continued*
time-zone change syndrome — *see* Disorder, sleep, circadian rhythm, psychogenic
Rarefaction, bone — *see* Disorder, bone, density and structure, specified NEC
Rash (toxic) R21
canker A38.9
diaper L22
drug (internal use) L27.0
contact (*see also* Dermatitis, due to, drugs, external) L25.1
following immunization T88.1
food — *see* Dermatitis, due to, food
heat L74.0
napkin (psoriasiform) L22
nettle — *see* Urticaria
pustular L08.0
rose R21
epidemic B06.9
scarlet A38.9
serum (*see also* Reaction, serum) T80.69
wandering tongue K14.1
Rasmussen aneurysm — *see* Tuberculosis, pulmonary
Rasmussen encephalitis G04.81
Rat-bite fever A25.9
due to Streptobacillus moniliformis A25.1
spirochetal (morsus muris) A25.0
Rathke's pouch tumor D44.3
Raymond (-Céstan) syndrome I65.8
Raynaud's disease, phenomenon or syndrome (secondary) I73.00
with gangrene (symmetric) I73.01
RDS (newborn) (type I) P22.0
type II P22.1
Reaction — *see also* Disorder
adaptation — *see* Disorder, adjustment
adjustment (anxiety) (conduct disorder) (depressiveness) (distress) — *see* Disorder, adjustment
with
mutism, elective (child) (adolescent) F94.0
adverse
food (any) (ingested) NEC T78.1
anaphylactic — *see* Shock, anaphylactic, due to food
affective — *see* Disorder, mood
allergic — *see* Allergy
anaphylactic — *see* Shock, anaphylactic
anaphylactoid — *see* Shock, anaphylactic
anesthesia — *see* Anesthesia, complication
antitoxin (prophylactic) (therapeutic) — *see* Complications, vaccination
anxiety F41.1
Arthus — *see* Arthus' phenomenon
asthenic F48.8
combat and operational stress F43.0
compulsive F42
conversion F44.9
crisis, acute F43.0
deoxyribonuclease (DNA) (DNase) hypersensitivity D69.2
depressive (single episode) F32.9
affective (single episode) F31.4
recurrent episode F33.9
neurotic F34.1
psychoneurotic F34.1
psychotic F32.3
recurrent — *see* Disorder, depressive, recurrent
dissociative F44.9
drug NEC T88.7
addictive — *see* Dependence, drug
transmitted via placenta or breast milk — *see* Absorption, drug, addictive, through placenta
allergic — *see* Allergy, drug
lichenoid L43.2
newborn P93.8
gray baby syndrome P93.0
overdose or poisoning (by accident) — *see* Table of Drugs and Chemicals, by drug, poisoning
photoallergic L56.1
phototoxic L56.0
withdrawal — *see* Dependence, by drug, with, withdrawal
infant of dependent mother P96.1
newborn P96.1
wrong substance given or taken (by accident) — *see* Table of Drugs and Chemicals, by drug, poisoning
fear F40.9
child (abnormal) F93.8
febrile nonhemolytic transfusion (FNHTR) R50.84
fluid loss, cerebrospinal G97.1

Removal (from) (of) — continued
dressing (nonsurgical) Z48.00
  surgical Z48.01
external
  fixation device — code to fracture with
    seventh character D
  prosthesis, prosthetic device Z44.9
    breast Z44.3-
    specified NEC Z44.8
home in childhood (to foster home or
  institution) Z62.29
ileostomy Z43.2
insulin pump Z46.81
myringotomy device (stent) (tube) Z45.82
nervous system device NEC Z46.2
  brain neuropacemaker Z46.2
  visual substitution device Z46.2
    implanted Z45.31
non-vascular catheter Z46.82
organ, prophylactic (for neoplasia
  management) — see Prophylactic,
    organ removal
orthodontic device Z46.4
staples Z48.02
stent
  ureteral Z46.6
suture Z48.02
urinary device Z46.6
vascular access device or catheter Z45.2
Ren
arcuatus Q63.1
mobile, mobilis N28.89
  congenital Q63.8
unguliformis Q63.1
Renal — see condition
Rendu-Osler-Weber disease or syndrome
I78.0
Reninoma D41.0-
Renon-Delille syndrome E23.3
Reovirus, as cause of disease classified
  elsewhere B97.5
Repeated falls NEC R29.6
Replaced chromosome by dicentric ring
Q93.2
Replacement by artificial or mechanical
  device or prosthesis of
bladder Z96.0
blood vessel NEC Z95.828
bone NEC Z96.7
cochlea Z96.21
coronary artery Z95.5
eustachian tube Z96.29
eye globe Z97.0
heart Z95.812
  valve Z95.2
    prosthetic Z95.2
    specified NEC Z95.4
    xenogenic Z95.3
intestine Z96.89
joint Z96.60
  hip — see Presence, hip joint implant
  knee — see Presence, knee joint implant
  specified site NEC Z96.698
larynx Z96.3
lens Z96.1
limb(s) — see Presence, artificial, limb
mandible NEC (for tooth root implant(s))
  Z96.5
organ NEC Z96.89
peripheral vessel NEC Z95.828
stapes Z96.29
teeth Z97.2
tendon Z96.7
tissue NEC Z96.89
tooth root(s) Z96.5
vessel NEC Z95.828
  coronary (artery) Z95.5
Request for expert evidence Z04.8
Reserve, decreased or low
cardiac — see Disease, heart
kidney N28.89
Residual — see also condition
ovary syndrome N99.83
state, schizophrenic F20.5
urine R39.19

Resistance, resistant (to)
activated protein C D68.51
complicating pregnancy O26.89
insulin E88.81
organism(s)
  to
    drug
      aminoglycosides Z16.29
      amoxicillin Z16.11
      ampicillin Z16.11
      antibiotic(s) Z16.20
        multiple Z16.24
        specified NEC Z16.29
      antifungal Z16.32
      antimicrobial (single) Z16.30
        multiple Z16.35
        specified NEC Z16.39
      antimycobacterial (single) Z16.341
        multiple Z16.342
      antiparasitic Z16.31
      antiviral Z16.33
      beta lactam antibiotics Z16.10
        specified NEC Z16.19
      cephalosporins Z16.19
      extended beta lactamase (ESBL)
        Z16.12
      fluoroquinolones Z16.23
      macrolides Z16.29
      methicillin — see MRSA
      multiple drugs (MDRO)
        antibiotics Z16.24
      penicillins Z16.11
      quinine (and related compounds)
        Z16.31
      quinolones Z16.23
      sulfonamides Z16.29
      tetracyclines Z16.29
      tuberculostatics (single) Z16.341
        multiple Z16.342
      vancomycin Z16.21
        related antibiotics Z16.22
thyroid hormone E07.89
Resorption
dental (roots) K03.3
  alveoli M26.79
teeth (external) (internal) (pathological)
  (roots) K03.3
Respiration
Cheyne-Stokes R06.3
decreased due to shock, following injury
  T79.4
disorder of, psychogenic F45.8
insufficient, or poor R06.89
  newborn P28.5
painful R07.1
sighing, psychogenic F45.8
Respiratory — see also condition
distress syndrome (newborn) (type I) P22.0
  type II P22.1
syncytial virus, as cause of disease
  classified elsewhere B97.4
Respite care Z75.5
Response (drug)
photoallergic L56.1
phototoxic L56.0
Restless legs (syndrome) G25.81
Restlessness R45.1
Restoration (of)
dental
  aesthetically inadequate or displeasing
    K08.56
  defective K08.50
    specified NEC K08.59
  failure of marginal integrity K08.51
  failure of periodontal anatomical
    intergrity K08.54
  organ continuity from previous sterilization
    (tuboplasty) (vasoplasty) Z31.0
    aftercare Z31.42
  tooth (existing)
    contours biologically incompatible with
      oral health K08.54
    open margins K08.51
    overhanging K08.52
    poor aesthetic K08.56
    poor gingival margins K08.51
  unsatisfactory, of tooth K08.50
    specified NEC K08.59
Restorative material (dental)
allergy to K08.55
fractured K08.539
  with loss of material K08.531
  without loss of material K08.530
unrepairable overhanging of K08.52
Restriction of housing space Z59.1
Rests, ovarian, in fallopian tube Q50.6
Restzustand (schizophrenic) F20.5

Retained — see also Retention
cholelithiasis following cholecystectomy
  K91.86
foreign body fragments (type of) Z18.9
  acrylics Z18.2
  animal quill(s) or spines Z18.31
  cement Z18.83
  concrete Z18.83
  crystalline Z18.83
  depleted isotope Z18.09
  depleted uranium Z18.01
  diethylhexylphthalates Z18.2
  glass Z18.81
  isocyanate Z18.2
  magnetic metal Z18.11
  metal Z18.10
  nonmagnectic metal Z18.12
  nontherapeutic radioactive Z18.09
  organic NEC Z18.39
  plastic Z18.2
  quill(s) (animal) Z18.31
  radioactive (nontherapeutic) NEC
    Z18.09
  specified NEC Z18.89
  spine(s) (animal) Z18.31
  stone Z18.83
  tooth (teeth) Z18.32
  wood Z18.33
fragments (type of) Z18.9
  acrylics Z18.2
  animal quill(s) or spines Z18.31
  cement Z18.83
  concrete Z18.83
  crystalline Z18.83
  depleted isotope Z18.09
  depleted uranium Z18.01
  diethylhexylphthalates Z18.2
  glass Z18.81
  isocyanate Z18.2
  magnetic metal Z18.11
  metal Z18.10
  nonmagnectic metal Z18.12
  nontherapeutic radioactive Z18.09
  organic NEC Z18.39
  plastic Z18.2
  quill(s) (animal) Z18.31
  radioactive (nontherapeutic) NEC
    Z18.09
  specified NEC Z18.89
  spine(s) (animal) Z18.31
  stone Z18.83
  tooth (teeth) Z18.32
  wood Z18.33
gallstones, following cholecystectomy
  K91.86
Retardation
development, developmental, specific —
  see Disorder, developmental
endochondral bone growth — see Disorder,
  bone, development or growth
growth R62.50
  due to malnutrition E45
mental — see Disability, intellectual
motor function, specific F82
physical (child) R62.52
  due to malnutrition E45
reading (specific) F81.0
spelling (specific) (without reading
  disorder) F81.81
Retching — see Vomiting
Retention — see also Retained
bladder — see Retention, urine
carbon dioxide E87.2
cholelithiasis following cholecystectomy
  K91.86
cyst — see Cyst
dead
  fetus (at or near term) (mother) O36.4
    early fetal death O02.1
  ovum O02.0
decidua (fragments) (following delivery)
  (with hemorrhage) O72.2
  without hemorrhage O73.1
deciduous tooth K00.6
dental root K08.3
fecal — see Constipation
fetus
  dead O36.4
    early O02.1
fluid R60.9
foreign body — see also Foreign body,
  retained
  current trauma — code as Foreign body,
    by site or type
gallstones, following cholecystectomy
  K91.86
gastric K31.89

Retention (see also Retained) — continued
intrauterine contraceptive device, in
  pregnancy — see Pregnancy,
    complicated by, retention, intrauterine
    device
membranes (complicating delivery) (with
  hemorrhage) O72.2
  with abortion — see Abortion, by type
  without hemorrhage O73.1
meniscus — see Derangement, meniscus
menses N94.89
milk (puerperal, postpartum) O92.79
nitrogen, extrarenal R39.2
ovary syndrome N99.83
placenta (total) (with hemorrhage) O72.0
  portions or fragments (with hemorrhage)
    O72.2
    without hemorrhage O73.1
  without hemorrhage O73.0
products of conception
  early pregnancy (dead fetus) O02.1
  following
    delivery (with hemorrhage) O72.2
      without hemorrhage O73.1
  secundines (following delivery) (with
    hemorrhage) O72.0
  complicating puerperium (delayed
    hemorrhage) O72.2
  partial O72.2
    without hemorrhage O73.1
    without hemorrhage O73.0
smegma, clitoris N90.89
urine R33.9
  drug-induced R33.0
  due to hyperplasia (hypertrophy) of
    prostate — see Hyperplasia,
    prostate
  organic R33.8
    drug-induced R33.0
  psychogenic F45.8
  specified NEC R33.8
water (in tissues) — see Edema
Reticular erythematous mucinosis L98.5
Reticulation, dust — see Pneumoconiosis
Reticulocytosis R70.1
Reticuloendotheliosis
acute infantile C96.0
leukemic C91.4-
malignant C96.9
nonlipid C96.0
Reticulohistiocytoma (giant-cell) D76.3
Reticuloid, actinic L57.1
Reticulosis (skin)
acute of infancy C96.0
hemophagocytic, familial D76.1
histiocytic medullary C96.9
lipomelanotic I89.8
malignant (midline) C86.0
nonlipid C96.0
polymorphic C86.0
Sézary — see Sézary disease
Retina, retinal — see also condition
dark area D49.81
Retinitis — see also Inflammation,
  chorioretinal
albuminurica N18.9 [H32]
diabetic — see Diabetes, retinitis
disciformis — see Degeneration, macula
focal — see Inflammation, chorioretinal,
  focal
gravidarum — see Pregnancy, complicated
  by, specified pregnancy-related
    condition NEC
juxtapapillaris — see Inflammation,
  chorioretinal, focal, juxtapapillary
luetic — see Retinitis, syphilitic
pigmentosa H35.52
proliferans — see Disorder, globe,
  degenerative, specified type NEC
proliferating — see Disorder, globe,
  degenerative, specified type NEC
renal N18.9 [H32]
syphilitic (early) (secondary) A51.43
  central, recurrent A52.71
  congenital (early) A50.01 [H32]
  late A52.71
tuberculous A18.53
Retinoblastoma C69.2-
differentiated C69.2-
undifferentiated C69.2-
Retinochoroiditis — see also Inflammation,
  chorioretinal
disseminated — see Inflammation,
  chorioretinal, disseminated
  syphilitic A52.71
focal — see Inflammation, chorioretinal
juxtapapillaris — see Inflammation,
  chorioretinal, focal, juxtapapillary

DISEASE INDEX

Retinopathy (background) H35.00
  arteriosclerotic I70.8 [H35.0-]
  atherosclerotic I70.8 [H35.0-]
  central serous — see Chorioretinopathy, central serous
  Coats H35.02-
  diabetic — see Diabetes, retinopathy
  exudative H35.02-
  hypertensive H35.03-
  in (due to)
    diabetes — see Diabetes, retinopathy
    sickle-cell disorders D57-[H36]
  of prematurity H35.10-
    stage 0 H35.11-
    stage 1 H35.12-
    stage 2 H35.13-
    stage 3 H35.14-
    stage 4 H35.15-
    stage 5 H35.16-
  pigmentary, congenital — see Dystrophy, retina
  proliferative NEC H35.2-
    diabetic — see Diabetes, retinopathy, proliferative
    sickle-cell D57-[H36]
  solar H31.02-
Retinoschisis H33.10-
  congenital Q14.1
  specified type NEC H33.19-
Retortamoniasis A07.8
Retractile testis Q55.22
Retraction
  cervix — see Retroversion, uterus
  drum (membrane) — see Disorder, tympanic membrane, specified NEC
  finger — see Deformity, finger
  lid H02.539
    left H02.536
      lower H02.535
      upper H02.534
    right H02.533
      lower H02.532
      upper H02.531
  lung J98.4
  mediastinum J98.5
  nipple N64.53
    associated with
      lactation O92.03
      pregnancy O92.01-
      puerperium O92.02
    congenital Q83.8
  palmar fascia M72.0
  pleura — see Pleurisy
  ring, uterus (Bandl's) (pathological) O62.4
  sternum (congenital) Q76.7
    acquired M95.4
  uterus — see Retroversion, uterus
  valve (heart) — see Endocarditis
Retrobulbar — see condition
Retrocecal — see condition
Retrocession — see Retroversion
Retrodisplacement — see Retroversion
Retroflection, retroflexion — see Retroversion
Retrognathia, retrognathism (mandibular) (maxillary) M26.19
Retrograde menstruation N92.5
Retroperineal — see condition
Retroperitoneal — see condition
Retroperitonitis K68.9
Retropharyngeal — see condition
Retroplacental — see condition
Retroposition — see Retroversion
Retroprosthetic membrane T85.398
Retrosternal thyroid (congenital) Q89.2
Retroversion, retroverted
  cervix — see Retroversion, uterus
  female NEC — see Retroversion, uterus
  iris H21.89
  testis (congenital) Q55.29
  uterus (acquired) (acute) (any degree) (asymptomatic) (cervix) (postinfectional) (postpartal, old) N85.4
    congenital Q51.818
    in pregnancy O34.53-
Retrovirus, as cause of disease classified elsewhere B97.30
  human
    immunodeficiency, type 2 (HIV 2) B97.35
    T-cell lymphotropic
      type I (HTLV-I) B97.33
      type II (HTLV-II) B97.34
  lentivirus B97.31
  oncovirus B97.32
  specified NEC B97.39
Retrusion, premaxilla (developmental) M26.09
Rett's disease or syndrome F84.2

Reverse peristalsis R19.2
Reye's syndrome G93.7
Rh (factor)
  hemolytic disease (newborn) P55.0
  incompatibility, immunization or sensitization
    affecting management of pregnancy NEC O36.09-
      anti-D antibody O36.01-
    newborn P55.0
    transfusion reaction — see Complication(s), transfusion, incompatibility reaction, Rh (factor)
  negative mother affecting newborn P55.0
  titer elevated — see Complication(s), transfusion, incompatibility reaction, Rh (factor)
  transfusion reaction — see Complication(s), transfusion, incompatibility reaction, Rh (factor)
Rhabdomyolysis (idiopathic) NEC M62.82
  traumatic T79.6
Rhabdomyoma — see also Neoplasm, connective tissue, benign
  adult — see Neoplasm, connective tissue, benign
  fetal — see Neoplasm, connective tissue, benign
  glycogenic — see Neoplasm, connective tissue, benign
Rhabdomyosarcoma (any type) — see Neoplasm, connective tissue, malignant
Rhabdosarcoma — see Rhabdomyosarcoma
Rhesus (factor) incompatibility — see Rh, incompatibility
Rheumatic (acute) (subacute) (chronic)
  adherent pericardium I09.2
  coronary arteritis I01.9
  degeneration, myocardium I09.0
  fever (acute) — see Fever, rheumatic
  heart — see Disease, heart, rheumatic
  myocardial degeneration — see Degeneration, myocardium
  myocarditis (chronic) (inactive) (with chorea) I09.0
    with chorea (acute) (rheumatic) (Sydenham's) I02.0
    active or acute I01.2
  pancarditis, acute I01.8
    with chorea (acute (rheumatic) Sydenham's) I02.0
  pericarditis (active) (acute) (with effusion) (with pneumonia) I01.0
    with chorea (acute) (rheumatic) (Sydenham's) I02.0
    chronic or inactive I09.2
  pneumonia I00 [J17]
  torticollis M43.6
  typhoid fever A01.09
Rheumatism (articular) (neuralgic) (nonarticular) M79.0
  gout — see Arthritis, rheumatoid
  intercostal, meaning Tietze's disease M94.0
  palindromic (any site) M12.30
    ankle M12.37-
    elbow M12.32-
    foot joint M12.37-
    hand joint M12.34-
    hip M12.35-
    knee M12.36-
    multiple site M12.39
    shoulder M12.31-
    specified joint NEC M12.38
    vertebrae M12.38
    wrist M12.33-
  sciatic M54.4-
Rheumatoid — see also condition
  arthritis — see also Arthritis, rheumatoid
    with involvement of organs NEC M05.60
      ankle M05.67-
      elbow M05.62-
      foot joint M05.67-
      hand joint M05.64-
      hip M05.65-
      knee M05.66-
      multiple site M05.69
      shoulder M05.61-
      vertebra — see Spondylitis, ankylosing
      wrist M05.63-
    seronegative — see Arthritis, rheumatoid, seronegative
    seropositive — see Arthritis, rheumatoid, seropositive

Rheumatoid (see also condition) — continued
  carditis M05.30
    ankle M05.37-
    elbow M05.32-
    foot joint M05.37-
    hand joint M05.34-
    hip M05.35-
    knee M05.36-
    multiple site M05.39
    shoulder M05.31-
    vertebra — see Spondylitis, ankylosing
    wrist M05.33-
  endocarditis — see Rheumatoid, carditis
  lung (disease) M05.10
    ankle M05.17-
    elbow M05.12-
    foot joint M05.17-
    hand joint M05.14-
    hip M05.15-
    knee M05.16-
    multiple site M05.19
    shoulder M05.11-
    vertebra — see Spondylitis, ankylosing
    wrist M05.13-
  myocarditis — see Rheumatoid, carditis
  myopathy M05.40
    ankle M05.47-
    elbow M05.42-
    foot joint M05.47-
    hand joint M05.44-
    hip M05.45-
    knee M05.46-
    multiple site M05.49
    shoulder M05.41-
    vertebra — see Spondylitis, ankylosing
    wrist M05.43-
  pericarditis — see Rheumatoid, carditis
  polyarthritis — see Arthritis, rheumatoid
  polyneuropathy M05.50
    ankle M05.57-
    elbow M05.52-
    foot joint M05.57-
    hand joint M05.54-
    hip M05.55-
    knee M05.56-
    multiple site M05.59
    shoulder M05.51-
    vertebra — see Spondylitis, ankylosing
    wrist M05.53-
  vasculitis M05.20
    ankle M05.27-
    elbow M05.22-
    foot joint M05.27-
    hand joint M05.24-
    hip M05.25-
    knee M05.26-
    multiple site M05.29
    shoulder M05.21-
    vertebra — see Spondylitis, ankylosing
    wrist M05.23-
Rhinitis (atrophic) (catarrhal) (chronic) (croupous) (fibrinous) (granulomatous) (hyperplastic) (hypertrophic) (membranous) (obstructive) (purulent) (suppurative) (ulcerative) J31.0
  with
    sore throat — see Nasopharyngitis
  acute J00
  allergic J30.9
    with asthma J45.909
      with
        exacerbation (acute) J45.901
        status asthmaticus J45.902
    due to
      food J30.5
      pollen J30.1
    nonseasonal J30.89
    perennial J30.89
    seasonal NEC J30.2
    specified NEC J30.89
  infective J00
  pneumococcal J00
  syphilitic A52.73
    congenital A50.05 [J99]
  tuberculous A15.8
  vasomotor J30.0
Rhinoantritis (chronic) — see Sinusitis, maxillary
Rhinodacryolith — see Dacryolith
Rhinolith (nasal sinus) J34.89
Rhinomegaly J34.89
Rhinopharyngitis (acute) (subacute) — see also Nasopharyngitis
  chronic J31.1
  destructive ulcerating A66.5
  mutilans A66.5
Rhinophyma L71.1

Rhinorrhea J34.89
  cerebrospinal (fluid) G96.0
  paroxysmal — see Rhinitis, allergic
  spasmodic — see Rhinitis, allergic
Rhinosalpingitis — see Salpingitis, eustachian
Rhinoscleroma A48.8
Rhinosporidiosis B48.1
Rhinovirus infection NEC B34.8
Rhizomelic chondrodysplasia punctata E71.540
Rhythm
  atrioventricular nodal I49.8
  disorder I49.9
    coronary sinus I49.8
    ectopic I49.8
    nodal I49.8
  escape I49.9
  heart, abnormal I49.9
  idioventricular I44.2
  nodal I49.8
  sleep, inversion G47.2-
    nonorganic origin — see Disorder, sleep, circadian rhythm, psychogenic
Rhytidosis facialis L98.8
Rib — see also condition
  cervical Q76.5
Riboflavin deficiency E53.0
Rice bodies — see also Loose, body, joint
  knee M23.4-
Richter syndrome — see Leukemia, chronic lymphocytic, B-cell type
Richter's hernia — see Hernia, abdomen, with obstruction
Ricinism — see Poisoning, food, noxious, plant
Rickets (active) (acute) (adolescent) (chest wall) (congenital) (current) (infantile) (intestinal) E55.0
  adult — see Osteomalacia
  celiac K90.0
  hypophosphatemic with nephrotic-glycosuric dwarfism E72.09
  inactive E64.3
  kidney N25.0
  renal N25.0
  sequelae, any E64.3
  vitamin-D-resistant E83.31 [M90.80]
Rickettsial disease A79.9
  specified type NEC A79.89
Rickettsialpox (Rickettsia akari) A79.1
Rickettsiosis A79.9
  due to
    Ehrlichia sennetsu A79.81
    Rickettsia akari (rickettsialpox) A79.1
  specified type NEC A79.89
  tick-borne A77.9
  vesicular A79.1
Rider's bone — see Ossification, muscle, specified NEC
Ridge, alveolus — see also condition
  flabby K06.8
Ridged ear, congenital Q17.3
Riedel's
  lobe, liver Q44.7
  struma, thyroiditis or disease E06.5
Rieger's anomaly or syndrome Q13.81
Riehl's melanosis L81.4
Rietti-Greppi-Micheli anemia D56.9
Rieux's hernia — see Hernia, abdomen, specified site NEC
Riga (-Fede) disease K14.0
Riggs' disease — see Periodontitis
Right middle lobe syndrome J98.11
Rigid, rigidity — see also condition
  abdominal R19.30
    with severe abdominal pain R10.0
    epigastric R19.36
    generalized R19.37
    left lower quadrant R19.34
    left upper quadrant R19.32
    periumbilic R19.35
    right lower quadrant R19.33
    right upper quadrant R19.31
  articular, multiple, congenital Q68.8
  cervix (uteri) in pregnancy — see Pregnancy, complicated by, abnormal, cervix
  hymen (acquired) (congenital) N89.6
  nuchal R29.1
  pelvic floor in pregnancy — see Pregnancy, complicated by, abnormal, pelvic organs or tissues NEC
  perineum or vulva in pregnancy — see Pregnancy, complicated by, abnormal, vulva
  spine — see Dorsopathy, specified NEC
  vagina in pregnancy — see Pregnancy, complicated by, abnormal, vagina

DISEASE INDEX

Rigors R68.89
with fever R50.9
Riley-Day syndrome G90.1
RIND (reversible ischemic neurologic deficit) I63.9
Ring(s)
aorta (vascular) Q25.4
Bandl's O62.4
contraction, complicating delivery O62.4
esophageal, lower (muscular) K22.2
Fleischer's (cornea) H18.04-
hymenal, tight (acquired) (congenital) N89.6
Kayser-Fleischer (cornea) H18.04-
retraction, uterus, pathological O62.4
Schatzki's (esophagus) (lower) K22.2
congenital Q39.3
Soemmerring's — see Cataract, secondary
vascular (congenital) Q25.8
aorta Q25.4
Ringed hair (congenital) Q84.1
Ringworm B35.9
beard B35.0
black dot B35.0
body B35.4
Burmese B35.5
corporeal B35.4
foot B35.3
groin B35.6
hand B35.2
honeycomb B35.0
nails B35.1
perianal (area) B35.6
scalp B35.0
specified NEC B35.8
Tokelau B35.5
Rise, venous pressure I87.8
Risk, suicidal
meaning personal history of attempted suicide Z91.5
meaning suicidal ideation — see Ideation, suicidal
Ritter's disease L00
Rivalry, sibling Z62.891
Rivalta's disease A42.2
River blindness B73.01
Robert's pelvis Q74.2
with disproportion (fetopelvic) O33.0
causing obstructed labor O65.0
Robin(-Pierre) syndrome Q87.0
Robinow-Silvermann-Smith syndrome Q87.1
Robinson's (hidrotic) ectodermal dysplasia or syndrome Q82.4
Robles' disease B73.01
Rocky Mountain (spotted) fever A77.0
Roetheln — see Rubella
Roger's disease Q21.0
Rokitansky-Aschoff sinuses (gallbladder) K82.8
Rolando's fracture (displaced) S62.22-
nondisplaced S62.22-
Romano-Ward (prolonged QT interval) syndrome I45.81
Romberg's disease or syndrome G51.8
Roof, mouth — see condition
Rosacea L71.9
acne L71.9
keratitis L71.8
specified NEC L71.8
Rosary, rachitic E55.0
Rose
cold J30.1
fever J30.1
rash R21
epidemic B06.9
Rosenbach's erysipeloid A26.0
Rosenthal's disease or syndrome D68.1
Roseola B09
infantum B08.20
due to human herpesvirus 6 B08.21
due to human herpesvirus 7 B08.22
Ross River disease or fever B33.1
Rossbach's disease K31.89
psychogenic F45.8
Rostan's asthma (cardiac) — see Failure, ventricular, left
Rotation
anomalous, incomplete or insufficient, intestine Q43.3
cecum (congenital) Q43.3
colon (congenital) Q43.3
spine, incomplete or insufficient — see Dorsopathy, deforming, specified NEC
tooth, teeth, fully erupted M26.35
vertebra, incomplete or insufficient — see Dorsopathy, deforming, specified NEC

Rotes Quérol disease or syndrome — see Hyperostosis, ankylosing
Roth(-Bernhardt) disease or syndrome — see Meralgia paraesthetica
Rothmund(-Thomson) syndrome Q82.8
Rotor's disease or syndrome E80.6
Round
back (with wedging of vertebrae) — see Kyphosis
sequelae (late effect) of rickets E64.3
worms (large) (infestation) NEC B82.0
Ascariasis (see also Ascariasis) B77.9
Roussy-Lévy syndrome G60.0
Rubella (German measles) B06.9
complication NEC B06.09
neurological B06.00
congenital P35.0
contact Z20.4
exposure to Z20.4
maternal
care for (suspected) damage to fetus O35.3
manifest rubella in infant P35.0
suspected damage to fetus affecting management of pregnancy O35.3
specified complications NEC B06.89
Rubeola (meaning measles) — see Measles
meaning rubella — see Rubella
Rubeosis, iris — see Disorder, iris, vascular
Rubinstein-Taybi syndrome Q87.2
Rudimentary (congenital) — see also Agenesis
arm — see Defect, reduction, upper limb
bone Q79.9
cervix uteri Q51.828
eye Q11.2
lobule of ear Q17.3
patella Q74.1
respiratory organs in thoracopagus Q89.4
tracheal bronchus Q32.4
uterus Q51.818
in male Q56.1
vagina Q52.0
Ruled out condition — see Observation, suspected
Rumination R11.10
with nausea R11.2
disorder of infancy F98.21
neurotic F42
newborn P92.1
obsessional F42
psychogenic F42
Runeberg's disease D51.0
Runny nose R09.89
Rupia (syphilitic) A51.39
congenital A50.06
tertiary A52.79
Rupture, ruptured
abscess (spontaneous) — code by site under Abscess
aneurysm — see Aneurysm
anus (sphincter) — see Laceration, anus
aorta, aortic I71.8
abdominal I71.3
arch I71.1
ascending I71.1
descending I71.8
abdominal I71.3
thoracic I71.1
syphilitic A52.01
thoracoabdominal I71.5
thorax, thoracic I71.1
transverse I71.1
traumatic — see Injury, aorta, laceration, major
valve or cusp (see also Endocarditis, aortic) I35.8
appendix (with peritonitis) K35.2
arteriovenous fistula, brain I60.8
artery I77.2
brain — see Hemorrhage, intracranial, intracerebral
coronary — see Infarct, myocardium
heart — see Infarct, myocardium
pulmonary I28.8
traumatic (complication) — see Injury, blood vessel
bile duct (common) (hepatic) K83.2
cystic K82.2
bladder (sphincter) (nontraumatic) (spontaneous) N32.89
following ectopic or molar pregnancy O08.6
obstetrical trauma O71.5
traumatic S37.29

Rupture, ruptured — continued
blood vessel — see also Hemorrhage
brain — see Hemorrhage, intracranial, intracerebral
heart — see Infarct, myocardium
traumatic (complication) — see Injury, blood vessel, laceration, major, by site
bone — see Fracture
bowel (nontraumatic) K63.1
brain
aneurysm (congenital) — see also Hemorrhage, intracranial, subarachnoid
syphilitic A52.05
hemorrhagic — see Hemorrhage, intracranial, intracerebral
capillaries I78.8
cardiac (auricle) (ventricle) (wall) I23.3
with hemopericardium I23.0
infectional I40.9
traumatic — see Injury, heart
cartilage (articular) (current) — see also Sprain
knee S83.3-
semilunar — see Tear, meniscus
cecum (with peritonitis) K65.0
with peritoneal abscess K35.3
traumatic S36.598
celiac artery, traumatic — see Injury, blood vessel, celiac artery, laceration, major
cerebral aneurysm (congenital) (see Hemorrhage, intracranial, subarachnoid)
cervix (uteri)
with ectopic or molar pregnancy O08.6
following ectopic or molar pregnancy O08.6
obstetrical trauma O71.3
traumatic S37.69
chordae tendineae NEC I51.1
concurrent with acute myocardial infarction — see Infarct, myocardium
following acute myocardial infarction (current complication) I23.4
choroid (direct) (indirect) (traumatic) H31.32-
circle of Willis I60.6
colon (nontraumatic) K63.1
traumatic — see Injury, intestine, large
cornea (traumatic) — see Injury, eye, laceration
coronary (artery) (thrombotic) — see Infarct, myocardium
corpus luteum (infected) (ovary) N83.1
cyst — see Cyst
cystic duct K82.2
Descemet's membrane — see Change, corneal membrane, Descemet's, rupture
traumatic — see Injury, eye, laceration
diaphragm, traumatic — see Injury, intrathoracic, diaphragm
disc — see Rupture, intervertebral disc
diverticulum (intestine) K57.80
with bleeding K57.81
bladder N32.3
large intestine K57.20
with
bleeding K57.21
small intestine K57.40
with bleeding K57.41
small intestine K57.00
with
bleeding K57.01
large intestine K57.40
with bleeding K57.41
duodenal stump K31.89
ear drum (nontraumatic) — see also Perforation, tympanum
traumatic S09.2-
due to blast injury — see Injury, blast, ear
esophagus K22.3
eye (without prolapse or loss of intraocular tissue) — see Injury, eye, laceration
fallopian tube NEC (nonobstetric) (nontraumatic) N83.8
due to pregnancy O00.1
fontanel P13.1
gallbladder K82.2
traumatic S36.128
gastric — see also Rupture, stomach
vessel K92.2
globe (eye) (traumatic) — see Injury, eye, laceration
graafian follicle (hematoma) N83.0
heart — see Rupture, cardiac

Rupture, ruptured — continued
hymen (nontraumatic) (nonintentional) N89.8
internal organ, traumatic — see Injury, by site
intervertebral disc — see Displacement, intervertebral disc
traumatic — see Rupture, traumatic, intervertebral disc
intestine NEC (nontraumatic) K63.1
traumatic — see Injury, intestine
iris — see also Abnormality, pupillary
traumatic — see Injury, eye, laceration
joint capsule, traumatic — see Sprain
kidney (traumatic) S37.06-
birth injury P15.8
nontraumatic N28.89
lacrimal duct (traumatic) — see Injury, eye, specified site NEC
lens (cataract) (traumatic) — see Cataract, traumatic
ligament, traumatic — see Rupture, traumatic, ligament, by site
liver S36.116
birth injury P15.0
lymphatic vessel I89.8
marginal sinus (placental) (with hemorrhage) — see Hemorrhage, antepartum, specified cause NEC
membrana tympani (nontraumatic) — see Perforation, tympanum
membranes (spontaneous)
artificial
delayed delivery following O75.5
delayed delivery following — see Pregnancy, complicated by, premature rupture of membranes
meningeal artery I60.8
meniscus (knee) — see also Tear, meniscus
old — see Derangement, meniscus
site other than knee — code as Sprain
mesenteric artery, traumatic — see Injury, mesenteric, artery, laceration, major
mesentery (nontraumatic) K66.8
traumatic — see Injury, intra-abdominal, specified, site NEC
mitral (valve) I34.8
muscle (traumatic) — see also Strain
diastasis — see Diastasis, muscle
nontraumatic M62.10
ankle M62.17-
foot M62.17-
forearm M62.13-
hand M62.14-
lower leg M62.16-
pelvic region M62.15-
shoulder region M62.11-
specified site NEC M62.18
thigh M62.15-
upper arm M62.12-
traumatic — see Strain, by site
musculotendinous junction NEC, nontraumatic — see Rupture, tendon, spontaneous
mycotic aneurysm causing cerebral hemorrhage — see Hemorrhage, intracranial, subarachnoid
myocardium, myocardial — see Rupture, cardiac
traumatic — see Injury, heart
nontraumatic, meaning hernia — see Hernia
obstructed — see Hernia, by site, obstructed
operation wound — see Disruption, wound, operation
ovary, ovarian N83.8
corpus luteum cyst N83.1
follicle (graafian) N83.0
oviduct (nonobstetric) (nontraumatic) N83.8
due to pregnancy O00.1
pancreas (nontraumatic) K86.8
traumatic S36.299
papillary muscle NEC I51.2
following acute myocardial infarction (current complication) I23.5
pelvic
floor, complicating delivery O70.1
organ NEC, obstetrical trauma O71.5
perineum (nonobstetric) (nontraumatic) N90.89
complicating delivery — see Delivery, complicated, by, laceration, anus (sphincter)
postoperative wound — see Disruption, wound, operation
prostate (traumatic) S37.828

DISEASE INDEX

Rupture, ruptured — *continued*
pulmonary
  artery I28.8
  valve (heart) I37.8
  vein I28.8
  vessel I28.8
pus tube — *see* Salpingitis
pyosalpinx — *see* Salpingitis
rectum (nontraumatic) K63.1
  traumatic S36.69
retina, retinal (traumatic) (without detachment) — *see also* Break, retina
  with detachment — *see* Detachment, retina, with retinal, break
rotator cuff (nontraumatic) M75.10-
  complete M75.12-
  incomplete M75.11-
sclera — *see* Injury, eye, laceration
sigmoid (nontraumatic) K63.1
  traumatic S36.593
spinal cord — *see also* Injury, spinal cord, by region
  due to injury at birth P11.5
  newborn (birth injury) P11.5
spleen (traumatic) S36.09
  birth injury P15.1
  congenital (birth injury) P15.1
  due to P. vivax malaria B51.0
  nontraumatic D73.5
  spontaneous D73.5
splenic vein R58
  traumatic — *see* Injury, blood vessel, splenic vein
stomach (nontraumatic) (spontaneous) K31.89
  traumatic S36.39
supraspinatus (complete) (incomplete) (nontraumatic) — *see* Tear, rotator cuff
symphysis pubis
  obstetric O71.6
  traumatic S33.4
synovium (cyst) M66.10
  ankle M66.17-
  elbow M66.12-
  finger M66.14-
  foot M66.17-
  forearm M66.13-
  hand M66.14-
  pelvic region M66.15-
  shoulder region M66.11-
  specified site NEC M66.18
  thigh M66.15-
  toe M66.17-
  upper arm M66.12-
  wrist M66.13-
tendon (traumatic) — *see* Strain
  nontraumatic (spontaneous) M66.9
    ankle M66.87-
    extensor M66.20
      ankle M66.27-
      foot M66.27-
      forearm M66.23-
      hand M66.24-
      lower leg M66.26-
      multiple sites M66.29
      pelvic region M66.25-
      shoulder region M66.21-
      specified site NEC M66.28
      thigh M66.25-
      upper arm M66.22-
    flexor M66.30
      ankle M66.37-
      foot M66.37-
      forearm M66.33-
      hand M66.34-
      lower leg M66.36-
      multiple sites M66.39
      pelvic region M66.35-
      shoulder region M66.31-
      specified site NEC M66.38
      thigh M66.35-
      upper arm M66.32-
    foot M66.87-
    forearm M66.83-
    hand M66.84-
    lower leg M66.86-
    multiple sites M66.89
    pelvic region M66.85-
    shoulder region M66.81-
    specified
      site NEC M66.88
      tendon M66.80
    thigh M66.85-
    upper arm M66.82-
thoracic duct I89.8
tonsil J35.8

Rupture, ruptured — *continued*
traumatic
  aorta — *see* Injury, aorta, laceration, major
  diaphragm — *see* Injury, intrathoracic, diaphragm
  external site — *see* Wound, open, by site
  eye — *see* Injury, eye, laceration
  internal organ — *see* Injury, by site
  intervertebral disc
    cervical S13.0
    lumbar S33.0
    thoracic S23.0
  kidney S37.06-
  ligament — *see also* Sprain
    ankle — *see* Sprain, ankle
    carpus — *see* Rupture, traumatic, ligament, wrist
    collateral (hand) — *see* Rupture, traumatic, ligament, finger, collateral
    finger (metacarpophalangeal) (interphalangeal) S63.40-
      collateral S63.41-
        index S63.41-
        little S63.41-
        middle S63.41-
        ring S63.41-
      index S63.40-
      little S63.40-
      middle S63.40-
      palmar S63.42-
        index S63.42-
        little S63.42-
        middle S63.42-
        ring S63.42-
      ring S63.40-
      specified site NEC S63.499
        index S63.49-
        little S63.49-
        middle S63.49-
        ring S63.49-
      volar plate S63.43-
        index S63.43-
        little S63.43-
        middle S63.43-
        ring S63.43-
    foot — *see* Sprain, foot
    radial collateral S53.2-
    radiocarpal — *see* Rupture, traumatic, ligament, wrist, radiocarpal
    ulnar collateral S53.3-
    ulnocarpal — *see* Rupture, traumatic, ligament, wrist, ulnocarpal
    wrist S63.30-
      collateral S63.31-
      radiocarpal S63.32-
      specified site NEC S63.39-
      ulnocarpal (palmar) S63.33-
  liver S36.116
  membrana tympani — *see* Rupture, ear drum, traumatic
  muscle or tendon — *see* Strain
  myocardium — *see* Injury, heart
  pancreas S36.299
  rectum S36.69
  sigmoid S36.593
  spleen S36.09
  stomach S36.39
  symphysis pubis S33.4
  tympanum, tympanic (membrane) — *see* Rupture, ear drum, traumatic
  ureter S37.19
  uterus S37.69
  vagina — *see* Injury, vagina
  vena cava — *see* Injury, vena cava, laceration, major
tricuspid (heart) (valve) I07.8
tube, tubal (nonobstetric) (nontraumatic) N83.8
  abscess — *see* Salpingitis
  due to pregnancy O00.1
tympanum, tympanic (membrane) (nontraumatic) (*see also* Perforation, tympanic membrane) H72.9-
  traumatic — *see* Rupture, ear drum, traumatic
umbilical cord, complicating delivery O69.89
ureter (traumatic) S37.19
  nontraumatic N28.89
urethra (nontraumatic) N36.8
  with ectopic or molar pregnancy O08.6
  following ectopic or molar pregnancy O08.6
  obstetrical trauma O71.5
  traumatic S37.39
uterosacral ligament (nonobstetric) (nontraumatic) N83.8

Rupture, ruptured — *continued*
uterus (traumatic) S37.69
  before labor O71.0-
  during or after labor O71.1
  nonpuerperal, nontraumatic N85.8
  pregnant (during labor) O71.1
    before labor O71.0-
  vagina — *see* Injury, vagina
valve, valvular (heart) — *see* Endocarditis
varicose vein — *see* Varix
varix — *see* Varix
vena cava R58
  traumatic — *see* Injury, vena cava, laceration, major
vesical (urinary) N32.89
vessel (blood) R58
  pulmonary I28.8
  traumatic — *see* Injury, blood vessel
viscus R19.8
vulva complicating delivery O70.0
Russell-Silver syndrome Q87.1
Russian spring-summer type encephalitis A84.0
Rust's disease (tuberculous cervical spondylitis) A18.01
Ruvalcaba-Myhre-Smith syndrome E71.440
Rytand-Lipsitch syndrome I44.2

S

Saber, sabre shin or tibia (syphilitic) A50.56 [M90.-]
Sac lacrimal — *see* condition
Saccharomyces infection B37.9
Saccharopinuria E72.3
Saccular — *see* condition
Sacculation
  aorta (nonsyphilitic) — *see* Aneurysm, aorta
  bladder N32.3
  intralaryngeal (congenital) (ventricular) Q31.3
  larynx (congenital) (ventricular) Q31.3
  organ or site, congenital — *see* Distortion
  pregnant uterus — *see* Pregnancy, complicated by, abnormal, uterus
  ureter N28.89
  urethra N36.1
  vesical N32.3
Sachs' amaurotic familial idiocy or disease E75.02
Sachs-Tay disease E75.02
Sacks-Libman disease M32.11
Sacralgia M53.3
Sacralization Q76.49
Sacrodynia M53.3
Sacroiliac joint — *see* condition
Sacroiliitis NEC M46.1
Sacrum — *see* condition
Saddle
  back — *see* Lordosis
  embolus
    abdominal aorta I74.01
    pulmonary artery I26.92
      with acute cor pulmonale I26.02
  injury — *code to* condition
  nose M95.0
    due to syphilis A50.57
Sadism (sexual) F65.52
Sadness, postpartal O90.6
Sadomasochism F65.50
Saemisch's ulcer (cornea) — *see* Ulcer, cornea, central
Sahib disease B55.0
Sailors' skin L57.8
Saint
  Anthony's fire — *see* Erysipelas
  triad — *see* Hernia, diaphragm
  Vitus' dance — *see* Chorea, Sydenham's
Salaam
  attack(s) — *see* Epilepsy, spasms
  tic R25.8
Salicylism
  abuse F55.8
  overdose or wrong substance given — *see* Table of Drugs and Chemicals, by drug, poisoning
Salivary duct or gland — *see* condition
Salivation, excessive K11.7
Salmonella — *see* Infection, Salmonella
Salmonellosis A02.0
Salpingitis (catarrhal) (fallopian tube) (nodular) (pseudofollicular) (purulent) (septic) N70.91
  with oophoritis N70.93
  acute N70.01
    with oophoritis N70.03
  chlamydial A56.11
  chronic N70.11
    with oophoritis N70.13
  complicating abortion — *see* Abortion, by type, complicated by, salpingitis
  ear — *see* Salpingitis, eustachian
  eustachian (tube) H68.00-
    acute H68.01-
    chronic H68.02-
  follicularis N70.11
    with oophoritis N70.13
  gonococcal (acute) (chronic) A54.24
  interstitial, chronic N70.11
    with oophoritis N70.13
  isthmica nodosa N70.11
    with oophoritis N70.13
  specific (gonococcal) (acute) (chronic) A54.24
  tuberculous (acute) (chronic) A18.17
  venereal (gonococcal) (acute) (chronic) A54.24

Salpingocele N83.4
Salpingo-oophoritis (catarrhal) (purulent) (ruptured) (septic) (suppurative) N70.93
  acute N70.03
    with ectopic or molar pregnancy O08.0
    following ectopic or molar pregnancy O08.0
    gonococcal A54.24
  chronic N70.13
    following ectopic or molar pregnancy O08.0
    gonococcal (acute) (chronic) A54.24
  puerperal O86.19
  specific (gonococcal) (acute) (chronic) A54.24
  subacute N70.03
  tuberculous (acute) (chronic) A18.17
  venereal (gonococcal) (acute) (chronic) A54.24
Salpingo-ovaritis — see Salpingo-oophoritis
Salpingoperitonitis — see Salpingo-oophoritis
Salzmann's nodular dystrophy — see Degeneration, cornea, nodular
Sampson's cyst or tumor N80.1
San Joaquin (Valley) fever B38.0
Sandblaster's asthma, lung or pneumoconiosis J62.8
Sander's disease (paranoia) F22
Sandfly fever A93.1
Sandhoff's disease E75.01
Sanfilippo (Type B) (Type C) (Type D) syndrome E76.22
Sanger-Brown ataxia G11.2
Sao Paulo fever or typhus A77.0
Saponification, mesenteric K65.8
Sarcocele (benign)
  syphilitic A52.76
    congenital A50.59
Sarcocystosis A07.8
Sarcoepiplocele — see Hernia
Sarcoepiplomphalocele Q79.2
Sarcoid (of) — see also Sarcoidosis
  arthropathy D86.86
  Boeck's D86.9
  Darier-Roussy D86.3
  iridocyclitis D86.83
  meningitis D86.81
  myocarditis D86.85
  myositis D86.87
  pyelonephritis D86.84
  Spiegler-Fendt L08.89
Sarcoidosis D86.9
  with
    cranial nerve palsies D86.82
    hepatic granuloma D86.89
    polyarthritis D86.86
    tubulo-interstitial nephropathy D86.84
  combined sites NEC D86.89
  lung D86.0
    and lymph nodes D86.2
  lymph nodes D86.1
    and lung D86.2
  meninges D86.81
  skin D86.3
  specified type NEC D86.89
Sarcoma (of) — see also Neoplasm, connective tissue, malignant
  alveolar soft part — see Neoplasm, connective tissue, malignant
  ameloblastic C41.1
    upper jaw (bone) C41.0
  botryoid — see Neoplasm, connective tissue, malignant
  botryoides — see Neoplasm, connective tissue, malignant
  cerebellar C71.6
    circumscribed (arachnoidal) C71.6
  circumscribed (arachnoidal) cerebellar C71.6
  clear cell — see also Neoplasm, connective tissue, malignant
    kidney C64-
  dendritic cells (accessory cells) C96.4
  embryonal — see Neoplasm, connective tissue, malignant
  endometrial (stromal) C54.1
    isthmus C54.0
  epithelioid (cell) — see Neoplasm, connective tissue, malignant
  Ewing's — see Neoplasm, bone, malignant
  follicular dendritic cell C96.4
  germinoblastic (diffuse) — see Lymphoma, diffuse large cell
  follicular — see Lymphoma, follicular, specified NEC

Sarcoma (of) (see also Neoplasm, connective tissue, malignant) — continued
  giant cell (except of bone) — see also Neoplasm, connective tissue, malignant
    bone — see Neoplasm, bone, malignant
  glomoid — see Neoplasm, connective tissue, malignant
  granulocytic C92.3-
  hemangioendothelial — see Neoplasm, connective tissue, malignant
  hemorrhagic, multiple — see Sarcoma, Kaposi's
  histiocytic C96.A
  Hodgkin — see Lymphoma, Hodgkin
  immunoblastic (diffuse) — see Lymphoma, diffuse large cell
  interdigitating dendritic cell C96.4
  Kaposi's
    colon C46.4
    connective tissue C46.1
    gastrointestinal organ C46.4
    lung C46.5-
    lymph node(s) C46.3
    palate (hard) (soft) C46.2
    rectum C46.4
    skin C46.0
    specified site NEC C46.7
    stomach C46.4
    unspecified site C46.9
  Kupffer cell C22.3
  Langerhans cell C96.4
  leptomeningeal — see Neoplasm, meninges, malignant
  liver NEC C22.4
  lymphangioendothelial — see Neoplasm, connective tissue, malignant
  lymphoblastic — see Lymphoma, lymphoblastic (diffuse)
  lymphocytic — see Lymphoma, small cell B-cell
  mast cell C96.2
  melanotic — see Melanoma
  meningeal — see Neoplasm, meninges, malignant
  meningothelial — see Neoplasm, meninges, malignant
  mesenchymal — see also Neoplasm, connective tissue, malignant
    mixed — see Neoplasm, connective tissue, malignant
  mesothelial — see Mesothelioma
  monstrocellular
    specified site — see Neoplasm, malignant, by site
    unspecified site C71.9
  myeloid C92.3-
  neurogenic — see Neoplasm, nerve, malignant
  odontogenic C41.1
    upper jaw (bone) C41.0
  osteoblastic — see Neoplasm, bone, malignant
  osteogenic — see also Neoplasm, bone, malignant
    juxtacortical — see Neoplasm, bone, malignant
    periosteal — see Neoplasm, bone, malignant
  periosteal — see Neoplasm, bone, malignant
    osteogenic — see Neoplasm, bone, malignant
  pleomorphic cell — see Neoplasm, connective tissue, malignant
  reticulum cell (diffuse) — see Lymphoma, diffuse large cell
    nodular — see Lymphoma, follicular
    pleomorphic cell type — see Lymphoma, diffuse large cell
  rhabdoid — see Neoplasm, malignant, by site
  round cell — see Neoplasm, connective tissue, malignant
  small cell — see Neoplasm, connective tissue, malignant
  soft tissue — see Neoplasm, connective tissue, malignant
  spindle cell — see Neoplasm, connective tissue, malignant
  stromal (endometrial) C54.1
    isthmus C54.0
  synovial — see also Neoplasm, connective tissue, malignant
    biphasic — see Neoplasm, connective tissue, malignant
    epithelioid cell — see Neoplasm, connective tissue, malignant
    spindle cell — see Neoplasm, connective tissue, malignant

Sarcomatosis
  meningeal — see Neoplasm, meninges, malignant
  specified site NEC — see Neoplasm, connective tissue, malignant
  unspecified site C80.1
Sarcosinemia E72.59
Sarcosporidiosis (intestinal) A07.8
Satiety, early R68.81
Saturnine — see condition
Saturnism
  overdose or wrong substance given or taken — see Table of Drugs and Chemicals, by drug, poisoning
Satyriasis F52.8
Sauriasis — see Ichthyosis
SBE (subacute bacterial endocarditis) I33.0
Scabies (any site) B86
Scabs R23.4
Scaglietti-Dagnini syndrome E22.0
Scald — see Burn
Scalenus anticus (anterior) syndrome G54.0
Scales R23.4
Scaling, skin R23.4
Scalp — see condition
Scapegoating affecting child Z62.3
Scaphocephaly Q75.0
Scapulalgia M89.8x1
Scapulohumeral myopathy G71.0
Scar, scarring (see also Cicatrix) L90.5
  adherent L90.5
  atrophic L90.5
  cervix
    in pregnancy or childbirth — see Pregnancy, complicated by, abnormal cervix
  cheloid L91.0
  chorioretinal H31.00-
    posterior pole macula H31.01-
    postsurgical H59.81-
    solar retinopathy H31.02-
    specified type NEC H31.09-
  choroid — see Scar, chorioretinal
  conjunctiva H11.24-
  cornea H17.9
    xerophthalmic — see also Opacity, cornea
      vitamin A deficiency E50.6
  duodenum, obstructive K31.5
  hypertrophic L91.0
  keloid L91.0
  labia N90.89
  lung (base) J98.4
  macula — see Scar, chorioretinal, posterior pole
  muscle M62.89
  myocardium, myocardial I25.2
  painful L90.5
  posterior pole (eye) — see Scar, chorioretinal, posterior pole
  retina — see Scar, chorioretinal
  trachea J39.8
  uterus N85.8
    in pregnancy O34.29
  vagina N89.8
    postoperative N99.2
  vulva N90.89
Scarabiasis B88.2
Scarlatina (anginosa) (maligna) (ulcerosa) A38.9
  myocarditis (acute) A38.1
    old — see Myocarditis
  otitis media A38.0
Scarlet fever (albuminuria) (angina) A38.9
Schamberg's disease (progressive pigmentary dermatosis) L81.7
Schatzki's ring (acquired) (esophagus) (lower) K22.2
  congenital Q39.3
Schaufenster krankheit I20.8
Schaumann's
  benign lymphogranulomatosis D86.1
  disease or syndrome — see Sarcoidosis
Scheie's syndrome E76.03
Schenck's disease B42.1
Scheuermann's disease or osteochondrosis — see Osteochondrosis, juvenile, spine
Schilder(-Flatau) disease G37.0
Schilling-type monocytic leukemia C93.0-
Schimmelbusch's disease, cystic mastitis, or hyperplasia — see Mastopathy, cystic
Schistosoma infestation — see Infestation, Schistosoma

Schistosomiasis B65.9
  with muscle disorder B65.9 [M63.80]
    ankle B65.9 [M63.8-]
    foot B65.9 [M63.8-]
    forearm B65.9 [M63.8-]
    hand B65.9 [M63.8-]
    lower leg B65.9 [M63.8-]
    multiple sites B65.9 [M63.89]
    pelvic region B65.9 [M63.8-]
    shoulder region B65.9 [M63.8-]
    specified site NEC B65.9 [M63.88]
    thigh B65.9 [M63.8-]
    upper arm B65.9 [M63.8-]
  Asiatic B65.2
  bladder B65.0
  chestermani B65.8
  colon B65.1
  cutaneous B65.3
  due to
    S. haematobium B65.0
    S. japonicum B65.2
    S. mansoni B65.1
    S. mattheii B65.8
  Eastern B65.2
  genitourinary tract B65.0
  intestinal B65.1
  lung NEC B65.9 [J99]
    pneumonia B65.9 [J17]
  Manson's (intestinal) B65.1
  oriental B65.2
  pulmonary NEC B65.9 [J99]
    pneumonia B65.9
  Schistosoma
    haematobium B65.0
    japonicum B65.2
    mansoni B65.1
  specified type NEC B65.8
  urinary B65.0
  vesical B65.0
Schizencephaly Q04.6
Schizoaffective psychosis F25.9
Schizodontia K00.2
Schizoid personality F60.1
Schizophrenia, schizophrenic F20.9
  acute (brief) (undifferentiated) F23
  atypical (form) F20.3
  borderline F21
  catalepsy F20.2
  catatonic (type) (excited) (withdrawn) F20.2
  cenesthopathic, cenesthesiopathic F20.89
  childhood type F84.5
  chronic undifferentiated F20.5
  cyclic F25.0
  disorganized (type) F20.1
  flexibilitas cerea F20.2
  hebephrenic (type) F20.1
  incipient F21
  latent F21
  negative type F20.5
  paranoid (type) F20.0
  paraphrenic F20.0
  post-psychotic depression F32.8
  prepsychotic F21
  prodromal F21
  pseudoneurotic F21
  pseudopsychopathic F21
  reaction F23
  residual (state) (type) F20.5
  restzustand F20.5
  schizoaffective (type) — see Psychosis, schizoaffective
  simple (type) F20.89
  simplex F20.89
  specified type NEC F20.89
  stupor F20.2
  syndrome of childhood F84.5
  undifferentiated (type) F20.3
    chronic F20.5
Schizothymia (persistent) F60.1
Schlatter-Osgood disease or osteochondrosis — see Osteochondrosis, juvenile, tibia
Schlatter's tibia — see Osteochondrosis, juvenile, tibia
Schmidt's syndrome (polyglandular, autoimmune) E31.0
Schmincke's carcinoma or tumor — see Neoplasm, nasopharynx, malignant
Schmitz(-Stutzer) dysentery A03.0
Schmorl's disease or nodes
  lumbar region M51.46
  lumbosacral region M51.47
  sacrococcygeal region M53.3
  thoracic region M51.44
  thoracolumbar region M51.45

DISEASE INDEX

Schneiderian
  papilloma — see Neoplasm, nasopharynx, benign
    specified site — see Neoplasm, benign, by site
    unspecified site D14.0
  specified site — see Neoplasm, malignant, by site
    unspecified site C30.0
Scholte's syndrome (malignant carcinoid) E34.0
Scholz(-Bielchowsky-Henneberg) disease or syndrome E75.25
Schönlein(-Henoch) disease or purpura (primary) (rheumatic) D69.0
Schottmuller's disease A01.4
Schroeder's syndrome (endocrine hypertensive) E27.0
Schüller-Christian disease or syndrome C96.5
Schultze's type acroparesthesia, simple I73.89
Schultz's disease or syndrome — see Agranulocytosis
Schwalbe-Ziehen-Oppenheim disease G24.1
Schwannoma — see also Neoplasm, nerve, benign
  malignant — see also Neoplasm, nerve, malignant
    with rhabdomyoblastic differentiation — see Neoplasm, nerve, malignant
  melanocytic (9560/0) — see Neoplasm, nerve, benign
  pigmented — see Neoplasm, nerve, benign
Schwannomatosis Q85.03
Schwartz-Bartter syndrome E22.2
Schwartz(-Jampel) syndrome G71.13
Schweniger-Buzzi anetoderma L90.1
Sciatic — see condition
Sciatica (infective)
  with lumbago M54.4-
  due to intervertebral disc disorder — see Disorder, disc, with, radiculopathy
  due to displacement of intervertebral disc (with lumbago) — see Disorder, disc, with, radiculopathy
  wallet M54.3-
Scimitar syndrome Q26.8
Sclera — see condition
Sclerectasia H15.84-
Scleredema
  adultorum — see Sclerosis, systemic
  Buschke's — see Sclerosis, systemic
  newborn P83.0
Sclerema (adiposum) (edematosum) (neonatorum) (newborn) P83.0
  adultorum — see Sclerosis, systemic
Scleriasis — see Scleroderma
Scleritis H15.00-
  with corneal involvement H15.04-
  anterior H15.01-
  brawny H15.02-
  in (due to) zoster B02.34
  posterior H15.03-
  specified type NEC H15.09-
  syphilitic A52.71
  tuberculous (nodular) A18.51
Sclerochoroiditis H31.8
Scleroconjunctivitis — see Scleritis
Sclerocystic ovary syndrome E28.2
Sclerodactyly, sclerodactylia L94.3
Scleroderma, sclerodermia (acrosclerotic) (diffuse) (generalized) (progressive) (pulmonary) (see also Sclerosis, systemic) M34.9-
  circumscribed L94.0
  linear L94.1
  localized L94.0
  newborn P83.8
  systemic M34.9
Sclerokeratitis H16.8
  tuberculous A18.52
Scleroma nasi A48.8
Scleromalacia (perforans) H15.05-
Scleromyxedema L98.5
Sclérose en plaques G35
Sclerosis, sclerotic
  adrenal (gland) E27.8
  Alzheimer's — see Disease, Alzheimer's
  amyotrophic (lateral) G12.21
  aorta, aortic I70.0
  valve — see Endocarditis, aortic
  artery, arterial, arteriolar, arteriovascular — see Arteriosclerosis
  ascending multiple G35

Sclerosis, sclerotic — continued
  brain (generalized) (lobular) G37.9
    artery, arterial I67.2
    diffuse G37.0
    disseminated G35
    insular G35
    Krabbe's E75.23
    miliary G35
    multiple G35
    presenile (Alzheimer's) — see Disease, Alzheimer's, early onset
    senile (arteriosclerotic) I67.2
    stem, multiple G35
    tuberous Q85.1
  bulbar, multiple G35
  bundle of His I44.39
  cardiac — see Disease, heart, ischemic, atherosclerotic
  cardiorenal — see Hypertension, cardiorenal
  cardiovascular — see also Disease, cardiovascular
    renal — see Hypertension, cardiorenal
  cerebellar — see Sclerosis, brain
  cerebral — see Sclerosis, brain
  cerebrospinal (disseminated) (multiple) G35
  cerebrovascular I67.2
  choroid — see Degeneration, choroid
  combined (spinal cord) — see also Degeneration, combined
    multiple G35
  concentric (Balo) G37.5
  cornea — see Opacity, cornea
  coronary (artery) I25.10
    with angina pectoris — see Arteriosclerosis, coronary (artery),
  corpus cavernosum
    female N90.89
    male N48.6
  diffuse (brain) (spinal cord) G37.0
  disseminated G35
  dorsal G35
  dorsolateral (spinal cord) — see Degeneration, combined
  endometrium N85.5
  extrapyramidal G25.9
  eye, nuclear (senile) — see Cataract, senile, nuclear
  focal and segmental (glomerular) (see also N00-N07 with fourth character .1) N05.1
  Friedreich's (spinal cord) G11.1
  funicular (spermatic cord) N50.8
  general (vascular) — see Arteriosclerosis
  gland (lymphatic) I89.8
  hepatic K74.1
    alcoholic K70.2
  hereditary
    cerebellar G11.9
    spinal (Friedreich's ataxia) G11.1
  hippocampal G93.81
  insular G35
  kidney — see Sclerosis, renal
  larynx J38.7
  lateral (amyotrophic) (descending) (primary) (spinal) G12.21
  lens, senile nuclear — see Cataract, senile, nuclear
  liver K74.1
    with fibrosis K74.2
    alcoholic K70.2
    alcoholic K70.2
    cardiac K76.1
  lung — see Fibrosis, lung
  mastoid — see Mastoiditis, chronic
  mesial temporal G93.81
  mitral I05.8
  Mönckeberg's (medial) — see Arteriosclerosis, extremities
  multiple (brain stem) (cerebral) (generalized) (spinal cord) G35
  myocardium, myocardial — see Disease, heart, ischemic, atherosclerotic
  nuclear (senile), eye — see Cataract, senile, nuclear
  ovary N83.8
  pancreas K86.8
  penis N48.6
  peripheral arteries — see Arteriosclerosis, extremities
  plaques G35
  pluriglandular E31.8
  polyglandular E31.8
  posterolateral (spinal cord) — see Degeneration, combined

Sclerosis, sclerotic — continued
  presenile (Alzheimer's) — see Disease, Alzheimer's, early onset
  primary, lateral G12.29
  progressive, systemic M34.0
  pulmonary — see Fibrosis, lung
    artery I27.0
    valve (heart) — see Endocarditis, pulmonary
  renal N26.9
    with
      cystine storage disease E72.09
      hypertensive heart disease (conditions in I11) — see Hypertension, cardiorenal
    arteriolar (hyaline) (hyperplastic) — see Hypertension, kidney
  retina (senile) (vascular) H35.00
  senile (vascular) — see Arteriosclerosis
  spinal (cord) (progressive) G95.89
    ascending G61.0
    combined — see also Degeneration, combined
      multiple G35
      syphilitic A52.11
    disseminated G35
    dorsolateral — see Degeneration, combined
    hereditary (Friedreich's) (mixed form) G11.1
    lateral (amyotrophic) G12.21
    multiple G35
    posterior (syphilitic) A52.11
  stomach K31.89
  subendocardial, congenital I42.4
  systemic M34.9
    with
      lung involvement M34.81
      myopathy M34.82
      polyneuropathy M34.83
    drug-induced M34.2
    due to chemicals NEC M34.2
    progressive M34.0
    specified NEC M34.89
  temporal (mesial) G93.81
  tricuspid (heart) (valve) I07.8
  tuberous (brain) Q85.1
  tympanic membrane — see Disorder, tympanic membrane, specified NEC
  valve, valvular (heart) — see Endocarditis
  vascular — see Arteriosclerosis
  vein I87.8
Scoliosis (acquired) (postural) M41.9
  adolescent (idiopathic) — see Scoliosis, idiopathic, juvenile
  congenital Q67.5
    due to bony malformation Q76.3
    failure of segmentation (hemivertebra) Q76.3
    hemivertebra fusion Q76.3
    postural Q67.5
  idiopathic M41.20
    adolescent M41.129
      cervical region M41.122
      cervicothoracic region M41.123
      lumbar region M41.126
      lumbosacral region M41.127
      thoracic region M41.124
      thoracolumbar region M41.125
    cervical region M41.22
    cervicothoracic region M41.23
    infantile M41.00
      cervical region M41.02
      cervicothoracic region M41.03
      lumbar region M41.06
      lumbosacral region M41.07
      sacrococcygeal region M41.08
      thoracic region M41.04
      thoracolumbar region M41.05
    juvenile M41.119
      cervical region M41.112
      cervicothoracic region M41.113
      lumbar region M41.116
      lumbosacral region M41.117
      thoracic region M41.114
      thoracolumbar region M41.115
    lumbar region M41.26
    lumbosacral region M41.27
    thoracic region M41.24
    thoracolumbar region M41.25
  neuromuscular M41.40
    cervical region M41.42
    cervicothoracic region M41.43
    lumbar region M41.46
    lumbosacral region M41.47
    occipito-atlanto-axial region M41.41
    thoracic region M41.44
    thoracolumbar region M41.45

Scoliosis (acquired) (postural) M41.9 — continued
  paralytic — see Scoliosis, neuromuscular
  postradiation therapy M96.5
  rachitic (late effect or sequelae) E64.3 [M49.80]
    cervical region E64.3 [M49.82]
    cervicothoracic region E64.3 [M49.83]
    lumbar region E64.3 [M49.86]
    lumbosacral region E64.3 [M49.87]
    multiple sites E64.3 [M49.89]
    occipito-atlanto-axial region E64.3 [M49.81]
    sacrococcygeal region E64.3 [M49.88]
    thoracic region E64.3 [M49.84]
    thoracolumbar region E64.3 [M49.85]
  sciatic M54.4-
  secondary (to) NEC M41.50
    cerebral palsy, Friedreich's ataxia, poliomyelitis, neuromuscular disorders — see Scoliosis, neuromuscular
    cervical region M41.52
    cervicothoracic region M41.53
    lumbar region M41.56
    lumbosacral region M41.57
    thoracic region M41.54
    thoracolumbar region M41.55
  specified form NEC M41.80
    cervical region M41.82
    cervicothoracic region M41.83
    lumbar region M41.86
    lumbosacral region M41.87
    thoracic region M41.84
    thoracolumbar region M41.85
  thoracogenic M41.30
    thoracic region M41.34
    thoracolumbar region M41.35
  tuberculous A18.01
Scoliotic pelvis
  with disproportion (fetopelvic) O33.0
  causing obstructed labor O65.0
Scorbutus, scorbutic — see also Scurvy anemia D53.2
Scotoma (arcuate) (Bjerrum) (central) (ring) — see also Defect, visual field, localized, scotoma
  scintillating H53.19
Scratch — see Abrasion
Scratchy throat R09.89
Screening (for) Z13.9
  alcoholism Z13.89
  anemia Z13.0
  anomaly, congenital Z13.89
  antenatal, of mother Z36
  arterial hypertension Z13.6
  arthropod-borne viral disease NEC Z11.59
  bacteriuria, asymptomatic Z13.89
  behavioral disorder Z13.89
  brain injury, traumatic Z13.850
  bronchitis, chronic Z13.83
  brucellosis Z11.2
  cardiovascular disorder Z13.6
  cataract Z13.5
  chlamydial diseases Z11.8
  cholera Z11.0
  chromosomal abnormalities (nonprocreative) NEC Z13.79
  colonoscopy Z12.11
  congenital
    dislocation of hip Z13.89
    eye disorder Z13.5
    malformation or deformation Z13.89
  contamination NEC Z13.88
  cystic fibrosis Z13.228
  dengue fever Z11.59
  dental disorder Z13.84
  depression Z13.89
  developmental handicap Z13.4
    in early childhood Z13.4
  diabetes mellitus Z13.1
  diphtheria Z11.2
  disability, intellectual Z13.4
  disease or disorder Z13.9
    bacterial NEC Z11.2
      intestinal infectious Z11.0
      respiratory tuberculosis Z11.1
    blood or blood-forming organ Z13.0
    cardiovascular Z13.6
    Chagas' Z11.6
    chlamydial Z11.8
    dental Z13.89
    developmental Z13.4
    digestive tract NEC Z13.818
      lower GI Z13.811
      upper GI Z13.810
    ear Z13.5

Screening (for) Z13.9 — *continued*
  disease or disorder Z13.9 — *continued*
    endocrine Z13.29
    eye Z13.5
    genitourinary Z13.89
    heart Z13.6
    human immunodeficiency virus (HIV)
      infection Z11.4
    immunity Z13.0
    infection
      intestinal Z11.0
        specified NEC Z11.6
      infectious Z11.9
    mental Z13.89
    metabolic Z13.228
    neurological Z13.89
    nutritional Z13.21
      metabolic Z13.228
        lipoid disorders Z13.220
    protozoal Z11.6
      intestinal Z11.0
    respiratory Z13.83
    rheumatic Z13.828
    rickettsial Z11.8
    sexually-transmitted NEC Z11.3
      human immunodeficiency virus (HIV)
        Z11.4
    sickle-cell (trait) Z13.0
    skin Z13.89
    specified NEC Z13.89
    spirochetal Z11.8
    thyroid Z13.29
    vascular Z13.6
    venereal Z11.3
    viral NEC Z11.59
      human immunodeficiency virus (HIV)
        Z11.4
      intestinal Z11.0
  elevated titer Z13.89
  emphysema Z13.83
  encephalitis, viral (mosquito-or tick-borne)
    Z11.59
  exposure to contaminants (toxic) Z13.88
  fever
    dengue Z11.59
    hemorrhagic Z11.59
    yellow Z11.59
  filariasis Z11.6
  galactosemia Z13.228
  gastrointestinal condition Z13.818
  genetic (nonprocreative)
    disease carrier status (nonprocreative)
      Z13.71
    for procreative management — *see*
      Testing, genetic, for procreative
      management
    specified NEC (nonprocreative) Z13.79
  genitourinary condition Z13.89
  glaucoma Z13.5
  gonorrhea Z11.3
  gout Z13.89
  helminthiasis (intestinal) Z11.6
  hematopoietic malignancy Z12.89
  hemoglobinopathies NEC Z13.0
  hemorrhagic fever Z11.59
  Hodgkin disease Z12.89
  human immunodeficiency virus (HIV)
    Z11.4
  human papillomavirus Z11.51
  hypertension Z13.6
  immunity disorders Z13.0
  infection
    mycotic Z11.8
    parasitic Z11.8
  ingestion of radioactive substance Z13.88
  intellectual disability Z13.4
  intestinal
    helminthiasis Z11.6
    infectious disease Z11.0
  leishmaniasis Z11.6
  leprosy Z11.2
  leptospirosis Z11.8
  leukemia Z12.89
  lymphoma Z12.89
  malaria Z11.6
  malnutrition Z13.29
    metabolic Z13.228
    nutritional Z13.21
  measles Z11.59
  mental disorder Z13.89
  metabolic errors, inborn Z13.228
  multiphasic Z13.89
  musculoskeletal disorder Z13.828
    osteoporosis Z13.820

Screening (for) Z13.9 — *continued*
  mycoses Z11.8
  myocardial infarction (acute) Z13.6
  neoplasm (malignant) (of) Z12.9
    bladder Z12.6
    blood Z12.89
    breast Z12.39
      routine mammogram Z12.31
    cervix Z12.4
    colon Z12.11
    genitourinary organs NEC Z12.79
      bladder Z12.6
      cervix Z12.4
      ovary Z12.73
      prostate Z12.5
      testis Z12.71
      vagina Z12.72
    hematopoietic system Z12.89
    intestinal tract Z12.10
      colon Z12.11
      rectum Z12.12
      small intestine Z12.13
    lung Z12.2
    lymph (glands) Z12.89
    nervous system Z12.82
    oral cavity Z12.81
    prostate Z12.5
    rectum Z12.12
    respiratory organs Z12.2
    skin Z12.83
    small intestine Z12.13
    specified site NEC Z12.89
    stomach Z12.0
  nephropathy Z13.89
  nervous system disorders NEC Z13.858
  neurological condition Z13.89
  osteoporosis Z13.820
  parasitic infestation Z11.9
    specified NEC Z11.8
  phenylketonuria Z13.228
  plague Z11.2
  poisoning (chemical) (heavy metal) Z13.88
  poliomyelitis Z11.59
  postnatal, chromosomal abnormalities
    Z13.89
  prenatal, of mother Z36
  protozoal disease Z11.6
    intestinal Z11.0
  pulmonary tuberculosis Z11.1
  radiation exposure Z13.88
  respiratory condition Z13.83
  respiratory tuberculosis Z11.1
  rheumatoid arthritis Z13.828
  rubella Z11.59
  schistosomiasis Z11.6
  sexually-transmitted disease NEC Z11.3
    human immunodeficiency virus (HIV)
      Z11.4
  sickle-cell disease or trait Z13.0
  skin condition Z13.89
  sleeping sickness Z11.6
  special Z13.9
    specified NEC Z13.89
  syphilis Z11.3
  tetanus Z11.2
  trachoma Z11.8
  traumatic brain injury Z13.850
  trypanosomiasis Z11.6
  tuberculosis, respiratory Z11.1
  venereal disease Z11.3
  viral encephalitis (mosquito-or tick-borne)
    Z11.59
  whooping cough Z11.2
  worms, intestinal Z11.6
  yaws Z11.8
  yellow fever Z11.59
Scrofula, scrofulosis (tuberculosis of cervical
  lymph glands) A18.2
Scrofulide (primary) (tuberculous) A18.4
Scrofuloderma, scrofulodermia (any site)
  (primary) A18.4
Scrofulosus lichen (primary) (tuberculous)
  A18.4
Scrofulous — *see* condition
Scrotal tongue K14.5
Scrotum — *see* condition
Scurvy, scorbutic E54
  anemia D53.2
  gum E54
  infantile E54
  rickets E55.0 [M90.80]
Sealpox B08.62
Seasickness T75.3
Seatworm (infection) (infestation) B80
Sebaceous — *see also* condition
  cyst — *see* Cyst, sebaceous

Seborrhea, seborrheic L21.9
  capillitii R23.8
  capitis L21.0
  dermatitis L21.9
    infantile L21.1
  eczema L21.9
    infantile L21.1
  sicca L21.0
Seckel's syndrome Q87.1
Seclusion, pupil — *see* Membrane, pupillary
Second hand tobacco smoke exposure
  (acute) (chronic) Z77.22
  in the perinatal period P96.81
Secondary
  dentin (in pulp) K04.3
  neoplasm, secondaries — *see* Table of
    Neoplasms, secondary
Secretion
  antidiuretic hormone, inappropriate E22.2
  catecholamine, by pheochromocytoma
    E27.5
  hormone
    antidiuretic, inappropriate (syndrome)
      E22.2
    by
      carcinoid tumor E34.0
      pheochromocytoma E27.5
    ectopic NEC E34.2
  urinary
    excessive R35.8
    suppression R34
Section
  nerve, traumatic — *see* Injury, nerve
Segmentation, incomplete (congenital) —
  see also Fusion
  bone NEC Q78.8
  lumbosacral (joint) (vertebra) Q76.49
Seitelberger's syndrome (infantile
  neuraxonal dystrophy) G31.89
Seizure(s) (*see also* Convulsions) R56.9
  akinetic — *see* Epilepsy, generalized,
    specified NEC
  atonic — *see* Epilepsy, generalized,
    specified NEC
  autonomic (hysterical) F44.5
  convulsive — *see* Convulsions
  cortical (focal) (motor) — *see* Epilepsy,
    localization-related, symptomatic,
    with simple partial seizures
  disorder (*see also* Eplepsy) G40.909
  due to stroke — *see* Sequelae (of), disease,
    cerebrovascular, by type, specified
    NEC
  epileptic — *see* Epilepsy
  febrile (simple) R56.00
    with status epilepticus G40.901
    complex (atypical) (complicated)
      R56.01
      with status epilepticus G40.901
  grand mal G40.409
    intractable G40.419
      with status epilepticus G40.411
      without status epilepticus G40.419
    not intractable G40.409
      with status epilepticus G40.401
      without status epilepticus G40.409
  heart — *see* Disease, heart
  hysterical F44.5
  intractable G40.919
    with status epilepticus G40.911
  Jacksonian (focal) (motor type) (sensory
    type) — *see* Epilepsy, localization-
    related, symptomatic, with simple
    partial seizures
  newborn P90
  nonspecific epileptic
    atonic — *see* Epilepsy, generalized,
      specified NEC
    clonic — *see* Epilepsy, generalized,
      specified NEC
    myoclonic — *see* Epilepsy, generalized,
      specified NEC
    tonic — *see* Epilepsy, generalized,
      specified NEC
    tonic-clonic — *see* Epilepsy,
      generalized, specified NEC
  partial, developing into secondarily
    generalized seizures
    complex — *see* Epilepsy, localization-
      related, symptomatic, with complex
      partial seizures
    simple — *see* Epilepsy, localization-
      related, symptomatic, with simple
      partial seizures

Seizure(s) (*see also* Convulsions) R56.9 —
  continued
  petit mal G40.409
    intractable G40.419
      with status epilepticus G40.411
      without status epilepticus G40.419
    not intractable G40.409
      with status epilepticus G40.401
      without status epilepticus G40.409
  post traumatic R56.1
  recurrent G40.909
  specified NEC G40.89
  uncinate — *see* Epilepsy, localization-
    related, symptomatic, with complex
    partial seizures
Selenium deficiency, dietary E59
Self-damaging behavior (life-style) Z72.89
Self-harm (attempted)
  history (personal) Z91.5
    in family Z81.8
Self-mutilation (attempted)
  history (personal) Z91.5
    in family Z81.8
Self-poisoning
  history (personal) Z91.5
    in family Z81.8
  observation following (alleged) attempt
    Z03.6
Semicoma R40.1
Seminal vesiculitis N49.0
Seminoma C62.9-
  specified site — *see* Neoplasm, malignant,
    by site
Senear-Usher disease or syndrome L10.4
Senectus R54
Senescence (without mention of psychosis)
  R54
Senile, senility (*see also* condition) R41.81
  with
    acute confusional state F05
    mental changes NOS F03
    psychosis NEC — *see* Psychosis, senile
  asthenia R54
  cervix (atrophic) N88.8
  debility R54
  endometrium (atrophic) N85.8
  fallopian tube (atrophic) — *see* Atrophy,
    fallopian tube
  heart (failure) R54
  ovary (atrophic) — *see* Atrophy, ovary
  premature E34.8
  vagina, vaginitis (atrophic) N95.2
  wart L82.1
Sensation
  burning (skin) R20.8
    tongue K14.6
  loss of R20.8
  prickling (skin) R20.2
  tingling (skin) R20.2
Sense loss
  smell — *see* Disturbance, sensation, smell
  taste — *see* Disturbance, sensation, taste
  touch R20.8
Sensibility disturbance (cortical) (deep)
  (vibratory) R20.9
Sensitive, sensitivity — *see also* Allergy
  carotid sinus G90.01
  child (excessive) F93.8
  cold, autoimmune D59.1
  dentin K03.89
  latex Z91.040
  methemoglobin D74.8
  tuberculin, without clinical or radiological
    symptoms R76.11
  visual
    glare H53.71
    impaired contrast H53.72
Sensitiver Beziehungswahn F22
Sensitization, auto-erythrocytic D69.2
Separation
  anxiety, abnormal (of childhood) F93.0
  apophysis, traumatic — *code as* Fracture,
    by site
  choroid — *see* Detachment, choroid
  epiphysis, epiphyseal
    nontraumatic — *see also*
      Osteochondropathy, specified type
      NEC
      upper femoral — *see* Slipped,
        epiphysis, upper femoral
    traumatic — *code as* Fracture, by site
  fracture — *see* Fracture
  infundibulum cardiac from right ventricle
    by a partition Q24.3
  joint (traumatic) (current) — *code by* site
    under Dislocation
  pubic bone, obstetrical trauma O71.6
  retina, retinal — *see* Detachment, retina
  symphysis pubis, obstetrical trauma O71.6
  tracheal ring, incomplete, congenital Q32.1

Sepsis (generalized) (unspecified organism) A41.9
with
 organ dysfunction (acute) (multiple) R65.20
  with septic shock R65.21
 actinomycotic A42.7
 adrenal hemorrhage syndrome (meningococcal) A39.1
 anaerobic A41.4
 Bacillus anthracis A22.7
 Brucella (see also Brucellosis) A23.9
 candidal B37.7
 cryptogenic A41.9
 due to device, implant or graft T85.79
  arterial graft NEC T82.7
  breast (implant) T85.79
  catheter NEC T85.79
   dialysis (renal) T82.7
    intraperitoneal T85.71
   infusion NEC T82.7
    spinal (epidural) (subdural) T85.79
   urinary (indwelling) T83.51
 ectopic or molar pregnancy O08.82
 electronic (electrode) (pulse generator) (stimulator)
  bone T84.7
  cardiac T82.7
  nervous system (brain) (peripheral nerve) (spinal) T85.79
  urinary T83.59
 fixation, internal (orthopedic) — see Complication, fixation device, infection
 gastrointestinal (bile duct) (esophagus) T85.79
 genital T83.6
 heart NEC T82.7
  valve (prosthesis) T82.6
   graft T82.7
 joint prosthesis — see Complication, joint prosthesis, infection
 ocular (corneal graft) (orbital implant) T85.79
 orthopedic NEC T84.7
  fixation device, internal — see Complication, fixation device, infection
 specified NEC T85.79
 vascular T82.7
 ventricular intracranial shunt T85.79
 during labor O75.3
 Enterococcus A41.81
 Erysipelothrix (rhusiopathiae) (erysipeloid) A26.7
 Escherichia coli (E. coli) A41.5
 extraintestinal yersiniosis A28.2
 following
  abortion (subsequent episode) O08.0
   current episode — see Abortion
  ectopic or molar pregnancy O08.82
  immunization T88.0
  infusion, therapeutic injection or transfusion NEC T80.29
 gangrenous A41.9
 gonococcal A54.86
 Gram-negative (organism) A41.5
  anaerobic A41.4
 Haemophilus influenzae A41.3
 herpesviral B00.7
 intra-abdominal K65.1
 intraocular — see Endophthalmitis, purulent
 Listeria monocytogenes A32.7
 localized — code to specific localized infection
  in operation wound T81.4
  skin — see Abscess
 malleus A24.0
 melioidosis A24.1
 meningeal — see Meningitis
 meningococcal A39.4
  acute A39.2
  chronic A39.3
 MSSA (methicillin susceptible Staphylococcus aureus) A41.01
 newborn P36.9
  due to
   anaerobes NEC P36.5
   Escherichia coli P36.4
   Staphylococcus P36.30
    aureus P36.2
    specified NEC P36.39
   Streptococcus P36.10
    group B P36.0
    specified NEC P36.19
   specified NEC P36.8
 Pasteurella multocida A28.0
 pelvic, puerperal, postpartum, childbirth O85

Sepsis (generalized) (unspecified organism) A41.9 — continued
 pneumococcal A40.3
 postprocedural T81.4
 puerperal, postpartum, childbirth (pelvic) O85
 Salmonella (arizonae) (cholerae-suis) (enteritidis) (typhimurium) A02.1
 severe R65.20
  with septic shock R65.21
 Shigella (see also Dysentery, bacillary) A03.9
 skin, localized — see Abscess
 specified organism NEC A41.89
 Staphylococcus, staphylococcal A41.2
  aureus (methicillin susceptible) (MSSA) A41.01
   methicillin resistant (MRSA) A41.02
  coagulase-negative A41.1
  specified NEC A41.1
 Streptococcus, streptococcal A40.9
  agalactiae A40.1
  group
   A A40.0
   B A40.1
   D A41.81
  neonatal P36.10
   group B P36.0
   specified NEC P36.19
  pneumoniae A40.3
  pyogenes A40.0
  specified NEC A40.8
 tracheostomy stoma J95.02
 tularemic A21.7
 umbilical, umbilical cord (newborn) — see Sepsis, newborn
 Yersinia pestis A20.7
Septate — see Septum
Septic — see condition
 arm — see Cellulitis, upper limb
  with lymphangitis — see Lymphangitis, acute, upper limb
 embolus — see Embolism
 finger — see Cellulitis, digit
  with lymphangitis — see Lymphangitis, acute, digit
 foot — see Cellulitis, lower limb
  with lymphangitis — see Lymphangitis, acute, lower limb
 gallbladder (acute) K81.0
 hand — see Cellulitis, upper limb
  with lymphangitis — see Lymphangitis, acute, upper limb
 joint — see Arthritis, pyogenic or pyemic
 leg — see Cellulitis, lower limb
  with lymphangitis — see Lymphangitis, acute, lower limb
 nail — see also Cellulitis, digit
  with lymphangitis — see Lymphangitis, acute, digit
 sore — see also Abscess
  throat J02.0
   streptococcal J02.0
 spleen — see Abscess, spleen D73.89
 teeth, tooth (pulpal origin) K04.4
 throat — see Pharyngitis
 thrombus — see Thrombosis
 toe — see Cellulitis, digit
  with lymphangitis — see Lymphangitis, acute, digit
 tonsils, chronic J35.01
  with adenoiditis J35.03
 uterus — see Endometritis
Septicemia A41.9
 meaning sepsis — see Sepsis
Septum, septate (congenital) — see also Anomaly, by site
 anal Q42.3
  with fistula Q42.2
 aqueduct of Sylvius Q03.0
  with spina bifida — see Spina bifida, by site, with hydrocephalus
 uterus (complete) (partial) Q51.2
 vagina Q52.10
  in pregnancy — see Pregnancy, complicated by, abnormal vagina
   causing obstructed labor O65.5
  longitudinal (with or without obstruction) Q52.12
  transverse Q52.11
Sequelae (of) — see also condition
 abscess, intracranial or intraspinal (conditions in G06) G09
 amputation — code to injury with seventh character S
 burn and corrosion — code to injury with seventh character S
 calcium deficiency E64.8
 cerebrovascular disease — see Sequelae, disease, cerebrovascular

Sequelae (of) (see also condition) — continued
 childbirth O94
 contusion — code to injury with seventh character S
 corrosion — see Sequelae, burn and corrosion
 crushing injury — code to injury with seventh character S
 disease
  cerebrovascular I69.90
   alteration of sensation I69.998
   aphasia I69.920
   apraxia I69.990
   ataxia I69.993
   cognitive deficits I69.91
   disturbance of vision I69.998
   dysarthria I69.922
   dysphagia I69.991
   dysphasia I69.921
   facial droop I69.992
   facial weakness I69.992
   fluency disorder I69.923
   hemiplegia I69.95-
   hemorrhage
    intracerebral — see Sequelae, hemorrhage, intracerebral
    intracranial, nontraumatic NEC — see Sequelae, hemorrhage, intracranial, nontraumatic
    subarachnoid — see Sequelae, hemorrhage, subarachnoid
   language deficit I69.928
   monoplegia
    lower limb I69.84-
    upper limb I69.93-
   paralytic syndrome I69.96-
   specified effect NEC I69.998
  specified type NEC I69.80
   alteration of sensation I69.898
   aphasia I69.820
   apraxia I69.890
   ataxia I69.893
   cognitive deficits I69.81
   disturbance of vision I69.898
   dysarthria I69.822
   dysphagia I69.891
   dysphasia I69.821
   facial droop I69.892
   facial weakness I69.892
   fluency disorder I69.823
   hemiplegia I69.85-
   language deficit I69.828
   monoplegia
    lower limb I69.84-
    upper limb I69.83-
   paralytic syndrome I69.86-
   specified effect NEC I69.898
  speech deficit I69.928
   speech deficit I69.828
  stroke NOS — see Sequelae, stroke NOS
 dislocation — code to injury with seventh character S
 encephalitis or encephalomyelitis (conditions in G04) G09
  in infectious disease NEC B94.8
  viral B94.1
 external cause — code to injury with seventh character S
 foreign body entering natural orifice — code to injury with seventh character S
 fracture — code to injury with seventh character S
 frostbite — code to injury with seventh character S
 Hansen's disease B92
 hemorrhage
  intracerebral I69.10
   alteration of sensation I69.198
   aphasia I69.120
   apraxia I69.190
   ataxia I69.193
   cognitive deficits I69.11
   disturbance of vision I69.198
   dysarthria I69.122
   dysphagia I69.191
   dysphasia I69.121
   facial droop I69.192
   facial weakness I69.192
   fluency disorder I69.123
   hemiplegia I69.15-
   language deficit NEC I69.128
   monoplegia
    lower limb I69.14-
    upper limb I69.13-
   paralytic syndrome I69.16-
   specified effect NEC I69.198
   speech deficit NEC I69.128

Sequelae (of) (see also condition) — continued
 hemorrhage — continued
  intracranial, nontraumatic NEC I69.20
   alteration of sensation I69.298
   aphasia I69.220
   apraxia I69.290
   ataxia I69.293
   cognitive deficits I69.21
   disturbance of vision I69.298
   dysarthria I69.222
   dysphagia I69.291
   dysphasia I69.221
   facial droop I69.292
   facial weakness I69.292
   fluency disorder I69.223
   hemiplegia I69.25-
   language deficit NEC I69.228
   monoplegia
    lower limb I69.24-
    upper limb I69.23-
   paralytic syndrome I69.26-
   specified effect NEC I69.298
   speech deficit NEC I69.228
  subarachnoid I69.00
   alteration of sensation I69.098
   aphasia I69.020
   apraxia I69.090
   ataxia I69.093
   cognitive deficits I69.01
   disturbance of vision I69.098
   dysarthria I69.022
   dysphagia I69.091
   dysphasia I69.021
   facial droop I69.092
   facial weakness I69.092
   fluency disorder I69.023
   hemiplegia I69.05-
   language deficit NEC I69.028
   monoplegia
    lower limb I69.04-
    upper limb I69.03-
   paralytic syndrome I69.06-
   specified effect NEC I69.098
   speech deficit NEC I69.028
 hepatitis, viral B94.2
 hyperalimentation E68
 infarction
  cerebral I69.30
   alteration of sensation I69.398
   aphasia I69.320
   apraxia I69.390
   ataxia I69.393
   cognitive deficits I69.31
   disturbance of vision I69.398
   dysarthria I69.322
   dysphagia I69.391
   dysphasia I69.321
   facial droop I69.392
   facial weakness I69.392
   fluency disorder I69.323
   hemiplegia I69.35-
   language deficit NEC I69.328
   monoplegia
    lower limb I69.34-
    upper limb I69.33-
   paralytic syndrome I69.36-
   specified effect NEC I69.398
   speech deficit NEC I69.328
 infection, pyogenic, intracranial or intraspinal G09
 infectious disease B94.9
  specified NEC B94.8
 injury — code to injury with seventh character S
 leprosy B92
 meningitis
  bacterial (conditions in G00) G09
  other or unspecified cause (conditions in G03) G09
 muscle (and tendon) injury — code to injury with seventh character S
 myelitis — see Sequelae, encephalitis
 niacin deficiency E64.8
 nutritional deficiency E64.9
  specified NEC E64.8
 obstetrical condition O94
 parasitic disease B94.9
 phlebitis or thrombophlebitis of intracranial or intraspinal venous sinuses and veins (conditions in G08) G09
 poisoning — code to poisoning with seventh character S
  nonmedicinal substance — see Sequelae, toxic effect, nonmedicinal substance
 poliomyelitis (acute) B91
 pregnancy O94

Sequelae (of) *(see also* condition) — *continued*
  protein-energy malnutrition E64.0
  puerperium O94
  rickets E64.3
  selenium deficiency E64.8
  sprain and strain — *code to* injury with seventh character S
  stroke NOS I69.30
    alteration in sensation I69.398
    aphasia I69.320
    apraxia I69.390
    ataxia I69.393
    cognitive deficits I69.31
    disturbance of vision I69.398
    dysarthria I69.322
    dysphagia I69.391
    dysphasia I69.321
    facial droop I69.392
    facial weakness I69.392
    hemiplegia I69.35-
    language deficit NEC I69.328
    monoplegia
      lower limb I69.34-
      upper limb I69.33-
    paralytic syndrome I69.36-
    specified effect NEC I69.398
    speech deficit NEC I69.328
  tendon and muscle injury — *code to* injury with seventh character S
  thiamine deficiency E64.8
  trachoma B94.0
  tuberculosis B90.9
    bones and joints B90.2
    central nervous system B90.0
    genitourinary B90.1
    pulmonary (respiratory) B90.9
    specified organs NEC B90.8
  viral
    encephalitis B94.1
    hepatitis B94.2
  vitamin deficiency NEC E64.8
    A E64.1
    B E64.8
    C E64.2
  wound, open — *code to* injury with seventh character S
Sequestration — *see also* Sequestrum
  lung, congenital Q33.2
Sequestrum
  bone — *see* Osteomyelitis, chronic
  dental M27.2
  jaw bone M27.2
  orbit — *see* Osteomyelitis, orbit
  sinus (accessory) (nasal) — *see* Sinusitis
Sequoiosis lung or pneumonitis J67.8
Serology for syphilis
  doubtful
    with signs or symptoms — *code by* site and stage under Syphilis
    follow-up of latent syphilis — *see* Syphilis, latent
  negative, with signs or symptoms — *code by* site and stage under Syphilis
  positive A53.0
    with signs or symptoms — *code by* site and stage under Syphilis
    reactivated A53.0
Seroma — *see also* Hematoma
  traumatic, secondary and recurrent T79.2
Seropurulent — *see* condition
Serositis, multiple K65.8
  pericardial I31.1
  peritoneal K65.8
Serous — *see* condition
Sertoli cell
  adenoma
    specified site — *see* Neoplasm, benign, by site
    unspecified site
      female D27.9
      male D29.20
  carcinoma
    specified site — *see* Neoplasm, malignant, by site
    unspecified site (male) C62.9-
      female C56.9
  tumor
    with lipid storage
      specified site — *see* Neoplasm, benign, by site
      unspecified site
        female D27.9
        male D29.20
    specified site — *see* Neoplasm, benign, by site
    unspecified site
      female D27.9
      male D29.20

Sertoli-Leydig cell tumor — *see* Neoplasm, benign, by site
  specified site — *see* Neoplasm, benign, by site
  unspecified site
    female D27.9
    male D29.20
Serum
  allergy, allergic reaction *(see also* Reaction, serum) T80.69
    shock *(see also* Shock, anaphylactic) T80.59
  arthritis T80.6
  complication or reaction NEC *(see also* Reaction, serum) T80.69
  disease NEC *(see also* Reaction, serum) T80.69
  hepatitis — *see also* Hepatitis, viral, type B
    carrier (suspected) of Z22.51
  intoxication *(see also* Reaction, serum) T80.69
  neuritis *(see also* Reaction, serum) T80.69
  neuropathy G61.1
  poisoning NEC *(see also* Reaction, serum) T80.69
  rash NEC *(see also* Reaction, serum) T80.69
  reaction NEC *(see also* Reaction, serum) T80.69
  sickness NEC *(see also* Reaction, serum) T80.69
  urticaria *(see also* Reaction, serum) T80.69
Sesamoiditis M25.8-
Sever's disease or osteochondrosis — *see* Osteochondrosis, juvenile, tarsus
Severe sepsis R65.20
  with septic shock R65.21
Sex
  chromosome mosaics Q97.8
    lines with various numbers of X chromosomes Q97.2
  education Z70.8
  reassignment surgery status Z87.890
Sextuplet pregnancy — *see* Pregnancy, sextuplet
Sexual
  function, disorder of (psychogenic) F52.9
  immaturity (female) (male) E30.0
  impotence (psychogenic) organic origin NEC — *see* Dysfunction, sexual, male
  precocity (constitutional) (cryptogenic) (female) (idiopathic) (male) E30.1
Sexuality, pathologic — *see* Deviation, sexual
Sézary disease C84.1-
Shadow, lung R91.8
Shaking palsy or paralysis — *see* Parkinsonism
Shallowness, acetabulum — *see* Derangement, joint, specified type NEC, hip
Shaver's disease J63.1
Sheath (tendon) — *see* condition
Sheathing, retinal vessels H35.01
Shedding
  nail L60.8
  premature, primary (deciduous) teeth K00.6
Sheehan's disease or syndrome E23.0
Shelf, rectal K62.89
Shell teeth K00.5
Shellshock (current) F43.0
  lasting state — *see* Disorder, post-traumatic stress
Shield kidney Q63.1
Shift
  auditory threshold (temporary) H93.24-
  mediastinal R93.8
Shifting sleep-work schedule (affecting sleep) G47.26
Shiga(-Kruse) dysentery A03.0
Shiga's bacillus A03.0
Shigella (dysentery) — *see* Dysentery, bacillary
Shigellosis A03.9
  Group A A03.0
  Group B A03.1
  Group C A03.2
  Group D A03.3
Shin splints S86.89
Shingles — *see* Herpes, zoster
Shipyard disease or eye B30.0
Shirodkar suture, in pregnancy — *see* Pregnancy, complicated by, incompetent cervix

Shock R57.9
  with ectopic or molar pregnancy O08.3
  adrenal (cortical) (Addisonian) E27.2
  adverse food reaction (anaphylactic) — *see* Shock, anaphylactic, due to food
  allergic — *see* Shock, anaphylactic
  anaphylactic T78.2
    chemical — *see* Table of Drugs and Chemicals
    due to drug or medicinal substance
      correct substance properly administered T88.6
      overdose or wrong substance given or taken (by accident) — *see* Table of Drugs and Chemicals, by drug, poisoning
    due to food (nonpoisonous) T78.00
      additives T78.06
      dairy products T78.07
      eggs T78.08
      fish T78.03
        shellfish T78.02
      fruit T78.04
      milk T78.07
      nuts T78.05
        peanuts T78.01
      peanuts T78.01
      seeds T78.05
      specified type NEC T78.09
      vegetable T78.04
    following sting(s) — *see* Venom
    immunization T80.52
    serum T80.59
      blood and blood products T80.51
      immunization T80.52
      specified NEC T80.59
      vaccination T80.52
  anaphylactoid — *see* Shock, anaphylactic
  anesthetic
    correct substance properly administered T88.2
    overdose or wrong substance given or taken — *see* Table of Drugs and Chemicals, by drug, poisoning
    specified anesthetic — *see* Table of Drugs and Chemicals, by drug, poisoning
  cardiogenic R57.0
  chemical substance — *see* Table of Drugs and Chemicals
  complicating ectopic or molar pregnancy O08.3
  culture — *see* Disorder, adjustment
  drug
    due to correct substance properly administered T88.6
    overdose or wrong substance given or taken (by accident) — *see* Table of Drugs and Chemicals, by drug, poisoning
  during or after labor and delivery O75.1
  electric T75.4
    (taser) T75.4
  endotoxic R65.21
    postprocedural (during or resulting from a procedure, not elsewhere classified) T81.12
  following
    ectopic or molar pregnancy O08.3
    injury (immediate) (delayed) T79.4
    labor and delivery O75.1
  food (anaphylactic) — *see* Shock, anaphylactic, due to food
  from electroshock gun (taser) T75.4
  gram-negative R65.21
    postprocedural (during or resulting from a procedure, not elsewhere classified) T81.12
  hematologic R57.8
  hemorrhagic
    surgery (intraoperative) (postoperative) T81.19
    trauma T79.4
  hypovolemic R57.1
    surgical T81.19
    traumatic T79.4
  insulin E15
    therapeutic misadventure — *see* subcategory T38.3
  kidney N17.0
    traumatic (following crushing) T79.5
  lightning T75.01
  lung J80
  obstetric O75.1
    with ectopic or molar pregnancy O08.3
    following ectopic or molar pregnancy O08.3
  pleural (surgical) T81.19
    due to trauma T79.4

Shock R57.9 — *continued*
  postprocedural (postoperative) T81.10
    with ectopic or molar pregnancy O08.3
    cardiogenic T81.11
    endotoxic T81.12
    following ectopic or molar pregnancy O08.3
    gram-negative T81.12
    hypovolemic T81.19
    septic T81.12
    specified type NEC T81.19
  psychic F43.0
  septic (due to severe sepsis) R65.21
  specified NEC R57.8
  surgical T81.10
  taser gun (taser) T75.4
  therapeutic misadventure NEC T81.10
  thyroxin
    overdose or wrong substance given or taken — *see* Table of Drugs and Chemicals, by drug, poisoning
  toxic, syndrome A48.3
  transfusion — *see* Complications, transfusion
  traumatic (immediate) (delayed) T79.4
Shoemaker's chest M95.4
Short, shortening, shortness
  arm (acquired) — *see also* Deformity, limb, unequal length
    congenital Q71.81-
      forearm — *see* Deformity, limb, unequal length
  bowel syndrome K91.2
  breath R06.02
  cervical (complicating pregnancy) O26.87-
    non-gravid uterus N88.3
  common bile duct, congenital Q44.5
  cord (umbilical), complicating delivery O69.3
  cystic duct, congenital Q44.5
  esophagus (congenital) Q39.8
  femur (acquired) — *see also* Deformity, limb, unequal length, femur
    congenital — *see* Defect, reduction, lower limb, longitudinal, femur
  frenum, frenulum, linguae (congenital) Q38.1
  hip (acquired) — *see also* Deformity, limb, unequal length
    congenital Q65.89
  leg (acquired) — *see also* Deformity, limb, unequal length
    congenital Q72.81-
    lower leg — *see also* Deformity, limb, unequal length
  limbed stature, with immunodeficiency D82.2
  lower limb (acquired) — *see also* Deformity, limb, unequal length
    congenital Q72.81-
  organ or site, congenital NEC — *see* Distortion
  palate, congenital Q38.5
  radius (acquired) — *see also* Deformity, limb, unequal length
    congenital — *see* Defect, reduction, upper limb, longitudinal, radius
  rib syndrome Q77.2
  stature (child) (hereditary) (idiopathic) NEC R62.52
    constitutional E34.3
    due to endocrine disorder E34.3
    Laron-type E34.3
  tendon — *see also* Contraction, tendon
    with contracture of joint — *see* Contraction, joint
    Achilles (acquired) M67.0-
      congenital Q66.89
    congenital Q79.8
  thigh (acquired) — *see also* Deformity, limb, unequal length, femur
    congenital — *see* Defect, reduction, lower limb, longitudinal, femur
  tibialis anterior (tendon) — *see* Contraction, tendon
  umbilical cord
    complicating delivery O69.3
  upper limb, congenital — *see* Defect, reduction, upper limb, specified type NEC
  urethra N36.8
  uvula, congenital Q38.5
  vagina (congenital) Q52.4
Shortsightedness — *see* Myopia
Shoshin (acute fulminating beriberi) E51.11
Shoulder — *see* condition
Shovel-shaped incisors K00.2
Shower, thromboembolic — *see* Embolism

Shunt
- arterial-venous (dialysis) Z99.2
- arteriovenous, pulmonary (acquired) I28.0
  - congenital Q25.72
- cerebral ventricle (communicating) in situ Z98.2
- surgical, prosthetic, with complications — *see* Complications, cardiovascular, device or implant

Shutdown, renal N28.9
Shy-Drager syndrome G90.3
Sialadenitis, sialadenosis (any gland) (chronic) (periodic) (suppurative) — *see* Sialoadenitis
Sialectasia K11.8
Sialidosis E77.1
Sialitis, silitis (any gland) (chronic) (suppurative) — *see* Sialoadenitis
Sialoadenitis (any gland) (periodic) (suppurative) K11.20
- acute K11.21
- recurrent K11.22
- chronic K11.23

Sialoadenopathy K11.9
Sialoangitis — *see* Sialoadenitis
Sialodochitis (fibrinosa) — *see* Sialoadenitis
Sialodocholithiasis K11.5
Sialolithiasis K11.5
Sialometaplasia, necrotizing K11.8
Sialorrhea — *see also* Ptyalism
- periodic — *see* Sialoadenitis

Sialosis K11.7
Siamese twin Q89.4
Sibling rivalry Z62.891
Sicard's syndrome G52.7
Sicca syndrome M35.00
- with
  - keratoconjunctivitis M35.01
  - lung involvement M35.02
  - myopathy M35.03
  - renal tubulo-interstitial disorders M35.04
  - specified organ involvement NEC M35.09

Sick R69
- or handicapped person in family Z63.79
  - needing care at home Z63.6
- sinus (syndrome) I49.5

Sick-euthyroid syndrome E07.81
Sickle-cell
- anemia — *see* Disease, sickle-cell
- trait D57.3

Sicklemia — *see also* Disease, sickle-cell
- trait D57.3

Sickness
- air (travel) T75.3
- airplane T75.3
- alpine T70.29
- altitude T70.20
- Andes T70.29
- aviator's T70.29
- balloon T70.29
- car T75.3
- compressed air T70.3
- decompression T70.3
- green D50.8
- milk — *see* Poisoning, food, noxious
- motion T75.3
- mountain T70.29
  - acute D75.1
- protein (*see also* Reaction, serum) T80.69
- radiation T66
- roundabout (motion) T75.3
- sea T75.3
- serum NEC (*see also* Reaction, serum) T80.69
- sleeping (African) B56.9
  - by Trypanosoma B56.9
    - brucei
      - gambiense B56.0
      - rhodesiense B56.1
    - East African B56.1
    - Gambian B56.0
    - Rhodesian B56.1
    - West African B56.0
- swing (motion) T75.3
- train (railway) (travel) T75.3
- travel (any vehicle) T75.3

Sideropenia — *see* Anemia, iron deficiency
Siderosilicosis J62.8
Siderosis (lung) J63.4
- eye (globe) — *see* Disorder, globe, degenerative, siderosis

Siemens' syndrome (ectodermal dysplasia) Q82.8
Sighing R06.89
- psychogenic F45.8

Sigmoid — *see also* condition
- flexure — *see* condition
- kidney Q63.1

Sigmoiditis (*see also* Enteritis) K52.9
- infectious A09
- noninfectious K52.9

Silfverskiöld's syndrome Q78.9
Silicosiderosis J62.8
Silicosis, silicotic (simple) (complicated) J62.8
- with tuberculosis J65

Silicotuberculosis J65
Silo-fillers' disease J68.8
- bronchitis J68.0
- pneumonitis J68.0
- pulmonary edema J68.1

Silver's syndrome Q87.1
Simian malaria B53.1
Simmonds' cachexia or disease E23.0
Simons' disease or syndrome (progressive lipodystrophy) E88.1
Simple, simplex — *see* condition
Simulation, conscious (of illness) Z76.5
Simultanagnosia (asimultagnosia) R48.3
Sin Nombre virus disease (Hantavirus) (cardio)-pulmonary syndrome) B33.4
Sinding-Larsen disease or osteochondrosis — *see* Osteochondrosis, juvenile, patella
Singapore hemorrhagic fever A91
Singer's node or nodule J38.2
Single
- atrium Q21.2
- coronary artery Q24.5
- umbilical artery Q27.0
- ventricle Q20.4

Singultus R06.6
- epidemicus B33.0

Sinus — *see also* Fistula
- abdominal K63.89
- arrest I45.5
- arrhythmia I49.8
- bradycardia R00.1
- branchial cleft (internal) (external) Q18.0
- coccygeal — *see* Sinus, pilonidal
- dental K04.6
- dermal (congenital) Q06.8
  - with abscess Q06.8
  - coccygeal, pilonidal — *see* Sinus, coccygeal
- infected, skin NEC L08.89
- marginal, ruptured or bleeding — *see* Hemorrhage, antepartum, specified cause NEC
- medial, face and neck Q18.8
- pause I45.5
- pericranii Q01.9
- pilonidal (infected) (rectum) L05.92
  - with abscess L05.02
- preauricular Q18.1
- rectovaginal N82.3
- Rokitansky-Aschoff (gallbladder) K82.8
- sacrococcygeal (dermoid) (infected) — *see* Sinus, pilonidal
- tachycardia R00.0
  - paroxysmal I47.1
- tarsi syndrome M25.57-
- testis N50.8
- tract (postinfective) — *see* Fistula
- urachus Q64.4

Sinusitis (accessory) (chronic) (hyperplastic) (nasal) (nonpurulent) (purulent) J32.9
- acute J01.90
  - ethmoidal J01.20
    - recurrent J01.21
  - frontal J01.10
    - recurrent J01.11
  - involving more than one sinus, other than pansinusitis J01.80
    - recurrent J01.81
  - maxillary J01.00
    - recurrent J01.01
  - pansinusitis J01.40
    - recurrent J01.41
  - recurrent J01.91
  - specified NEC J01.80
    - recurrent J01.81
  - sphenoidal J01.30
    - recurrent J01.31
- allergic — *see* Rhinitis, allergic
- due to high altitude T70.1
- ethmoidal J32.2
  - acute J01.20
    - recurrent J01.21
- frontal J32.1
  - acute J01.10
    - recurrent J01.11
- influenzal — *see* Influenza, with, respiratory manifestations NEC
- involving more than one sinus but not pansinusitis J32.8
  - acute J01.80
    - recurrent J01.81

Sinusitis (accessory) (chronic) (hyperplastic) (nasal) (nonpurulent) (purulent) J32.9 — *continued*
- maxillary J32.0
  - acute J01.00
    - recurrent J01.01
  - sphenoidal J32.3
    - acute J01.30
    - recurrent J01.31
- tuberculous, any sinus A15.8

Sinusitis-bronchiectasis-situs inversus (syndrome) (triad) Q89.3
Sipple's syndrome E31.22
Sirenomelia (syndrome) Q87.2
Siriasis T67.0
Sirkari's disease B55.0
Siti A65
Situation, psychiatric F99
Situational
- disturbance (transient) — *see* Disorder, adjustment
  - acute F43.0
- maladjustment — *see* Disorder, adjustment
- reaction — *see* Disorder, adjustment
  - acute F43.0

Situs inversus or transversus (abdominalis) (thoracis) Q89.3
Sixth disease B08.20
- due to human herpesvirus 6 B08.21
- due to human herpesvirus 7 B08.22

Sjögren-Larsson syndrome Q87.1
Sjögren's syndrome or disease — *see* Sicca syndrome
Skeletal — *see* condition
Skene's gland — *see* condition
Skenitis — *see* Urethritis
Skerljevo A65
Skevas-Zerfus disease — *see* Toxicity, venom, marine animal, sea anemone
Skin — *see also* condition
- clammy R23.1
- donor — *see* Donor, skin
- hidebound M35.9

Slate-dressers' or slate-miners' lung J62.8
Sleep
- apnea — *see* Apnea, sleep
- deprivation Z72.820
- disorder or disturbance G47.9
  - child F51.9
  - nonorganic origin F51.9
  - specified NEC G47.8
- disturbance G47.9
  - nonorganic origin F51.9
- drunkenness F51.9
- rhythm inversion G47.2-
- terrors F51.4
- walking F51.3
  - hysterical F44.89

Sleep hygiene
- abuse Z72.821
- inadequate Z72.821
- poor Z72.821

Sleeping sickness — *see* Sickness, sleeping
Sleeplessness — *see* Insomnia
- menopausal N95.1

Sleep-wake schedule disorder G47.20
Slim disease (in HIV infection) B20
Slipped, slipping
- epiphysis (traumatic) — *see also* Osteochondropathy, specified type NEC
  - capital femoral (traumatic)
    - acute (on chronic) S79.01-
  - current traumatic — *code as* Fracture, by site
  - upper femoral (nontraumatic) M93.00-
    - acute M93.01-
    - on chronic M93.03-
    - chronic M93.02-
- intervertebral disc — *see* Displacement, intervertebral disc
- ligature, umbilical P51.8
- patella — *see* Disorder, patella, derangement NEC
- rib M89.8x8
- sacroiliac joint — *see* subcategory M53.2
- tendon — *see* Disorder, tendon
- ulnar nerve, nontraumatic — *see* Lesion, nerve, ulnar
- vertebra NEC — *see* Spondylolisthesis

Slocumb's syndrome E27.0

Sloughing (multiple) (phagedena) (skin) — *see also* Gangrene
- abscess — *see* Abscess
- appendix K38.8
- fascia — *see* Disorder, soft tissue, specified type NEC
- scrotum N50.8
- tendon — *see* Disorder, tendon
- transplanted organ — *see* Rejection, transplant
- ulcer — *see* Ulcer, skin

Slow
- feeding, newborn P92.2
- flow syndrome, coronary I20.8
- heart(beat) R00.1

Slowing, urinary stream R39.19
Sluder's neuralgia (syndrome) G44.89
Slurred, slurring speech R47.81
Small(ness)
- for gestational age — *see* Small for dates
- introitus, vagina N89.6
- kidney (unknown cause) N27.9
  - bilateral N27.1
  - unilateral N27.0
- ovary (congenital) Q50.39
- pelvis
  - with disproportion (fetopelvic) O33.1
    - causing obstructed labor O65.1
- uterus N85.8
- white kidney N03.9

Small-and-light-for-dates — *see* Small for dates
Small-for-dates (infant) P05.10
- with weight of
  - 1000-1249 grams P05.14
  - 1250-1499 grams P05.15
  - 1500-1749 grams P05.16
  - 1750-1999 grams P05.17
  - 2000-2499 grams P05.18
  - 499 grams or less P05.11
  - 500-749 grams P05.12
  - 750-999 grams P05.13

Smallpox B03
Smearing, fecal R15.1
Smith-Lemli-Opitz syndrome E78.72
Smith's fracture S52.54-
Smoker — *see* Dependence, drug, nicotine
Smoker's
- bronchitis J41.0
- cough J41.0
- palate K13.24
- throat J31.2
- tongue K13.24

Smoking
- passive Z77.22

Smothering spells R06.81
Snaggle teeth, tooth M26.39
Snapping
- finger — *see* Trigger finger
- hip — *see* Derangement, joint, specified type NEC, hip
  - involving the iliotibial band M76.3-
- knee — *see* Derangement, knee
  - involving the iliotiblial band M76.3-

Sneddon-Wilkinson disease or syndrome (sub-corneal pustular dermatosis) L13.1
Sneezing (intractable) R06.7
Sniffing
- cocaine
  - abuse — *see* Abuse, drug, cocaine
  - dependence — *see* Dependence, drug, cocaine
- gasoline
  - abuse — *see* Abuse, drug, inhalant
  - dependence — *see* Dependence, drug, inhalant
- glue (airplane)
  - abuse — *see* Abuse, drug, inhalant
  - drug dependence — *see* Dependence, drug, inhalant

Sniffles
- newborn P28.89

Snoring R06.83
Snow blindness — *see* Photokeratitis
Snuffles (non-syphilitic) R06.5
- newborn P28.89
- syphilitic (infant) A50.05 [J99]

Social
- exclusion Z60.4
  - due to discrimination or persecution (perceived) Z60.5
- migrant Z59.0
  - acculturation difficulty Z60.3
- rejection Z60.4
  - due to discrimination or persecution Z60.5
- role conflict NEC Z73.5
- skills inadequacy NEC Z73.4
- transplantation Z60.3

Sodoku A25.0

Soemmerring's ring — see Cataract, secondary
Soft — see also condition
　nails L60.3
Softening
　bone — see Osteomalacia
　brain (necrotic) (progressive) G93.89
　　congenital Q04.8
　　embolic I63.4
　　hemorrhagic — see Hemorrhage, intracranial, intracerebral
　　occlusive I63.5
　　thrombotic I63.3
　cartilage M94.2-
　　patella M22.4-
　cerebellar — see Softening, brain
　cerebral — see Softening, brain
　cerebrospinal — see Softening, brain
　myocardial, heart — see Degeneration, myocardial, myocardial
　spinal cord G95.89
　stomach K31.89
Soldier's
　heart F45.8
　patches I31.0
Solitary
　cyst, kidney N28.1
　kidney, congenital Q60.0
Solvent abuse — see Abuse, drug, inhalant
　dependence — see Dependence, drug, inhalant
Somatization reaction, somatic reaction — see Disorder, somatoform
Somnambulism F51.3
　hysterical F44.89
Somnolence R40.0
　nonorganic origin F51.11
Sonne dysentery A03.3
Soor B37.0
Sore
　bed — see Ulcer, pressure, by site
　chiclero B55.1
　Delhi B55.1
　desert — see Ulcer, skin
　eye H57.1-
　Lahore B55.1
　mouth K13.79
　　canker K12.0
　muscle M79.1
　Naga — see Ulcer, skin
　of skin — see Ulcer, skin
　oriental B55.1
　pressure — see Ulcer, pressure, by site
　skin L98.9
　soft A57
　throat (acute) — see also Pharyngitis
　　with influenza, flu, or grippe — see Influenza, with, respiratory manifestations NEC
　　chronic J31.2
　　coxsackie (virus) B08.5
　　diphtheritic A36.0
　　herpesviral B00.2
　　influenzal — see Influenza, with, respiratory manifestations NEC
　　septic J02.0
　　streptococcal (ulcerative) J02.0
　　viral NEC J02.8
　　　coxsackie B08.5
　　tropical — see Ulcer, skin
　　veldt — see Ulcer, skin
Soto's syndrome (cerebral gigantism) Q87.3
South African cardiomyopathy syndrome I42.8
Southeast Asian hemorrhagic fever A91
Spacing
　abnormal, tooth, teeth, fully erupted M26.30
　excessive, tooth, fully erupted M26.32
Spade-like hand (congenital) Q68.1
Spading nail L60.8
　congenital Q84.6
Spanish collar N47.1
Sparganosis B70.1
Spasm(s), spastic, spasticity (see also condition) R25.2
　accommodation — see Spasm, of accommodation
　ampulla of Vater K83.4
　anus, ani (sphincter) (reflex) K59.4
　　psychogenic F45.8
　artery I73.9
　　cerebral G45.9
　Bell's G51.3
　bladder (sphincter, external or internal) N32.89
　　psychogenic F45.8
　bronchus, bronchiole J98.01
　cardia K22.0
　cardiac I20.1

Spasm(s), spastic, spasticity (see also condition) R25.2 — continued
　carpopedal — see Tetany
　cerebral (arteries) (vascular) G45.9
　cervix, complicating delivery O62.4
　ciliary body (of accommodation) — see Spasm, of accommodation
　colon K58.9
　　with diarrhea K58.0
　　psychogenic F45.8
　common duct K83.8
　compulsive — see Tic
　conjugate H51.8
　coronary (artery) I20.1
　diaphragm (reflex) R06.6
　　epidemic B33.0
　　psychogenic F45.8
　duodenum K59.8
　epidemic diaphragmatic (transient) B33.0
　esophagus (diffuse) K22.4
　　psychogenic F45.8
　facial G51.3
　fallopian tube N83.8
　gastrointestinal (tract) K31.89
　　psychogenic F45.8
　glottis J38.5
　　hysterical F44.4
　　psychogenic F45.8
　　　conversion reaction F44.4
　　reflex through recurrent laryngeal nerve J38.5
　habit — see Tic
　heart I20.1
　hemifacial (clonic) G51.3
　hourglass — see Contraction, hourglass
　hysterical F44.4
　infantile — see Epilepsy, spasms
　inferior oblique, eye H51.8
　intestinal (see also Syndrome, irritable bowel) K58.9
　　psychogenic F45.8
　larynx, laryngeal J38.5
　　hysterical F44.4
　　psychogenic F45.8
　　　conversion reaction F44.4
　levator palpebrae superioris — see Disorder, eyelid function
　muscle NEC M62.838
　　back M62.830
　nerve, trigeminal G51.0
　nervous F45.8
　nodding F98.4
　occupational F48.8
　oculogyric H51.8
　　psychogenic F45.8
　of accommodation H52.53-
　ophthalmic artery — see Occlusion, artery, retina
　perineal, female N94.89
　peroneo-extensor — see also Deformity, limb, flat foot
　pharynx (reflex) J39.2
　　hysterical F45.8
　　psychogenic F45.8
　psychogenic F45.8
　pylorus NEC K31.3
　　adult hypertrophic K31.89
　　congenital or infantile Q40.0
　　psychogenic F45.8
　rectum (sphincter) K59.4
　　psychogenic F45.8
　retinal (artery) — see Occlusion, artery, retina
　sigmoid (see also Syndrome, irritable bowel) K58.9
　　psychogenic F45.8
　sphincter of Oddi K83.4
　stomach K31.89
　　neurotic F45.8
　throat J39.2
　　hysterical F45.8
　　psychogenic F45.8
　tic F95.9
　　chronic F95.1
　　transient of childhood F95.0
　tongue K14.8
　torsion (progressive) G24.1
　trigeminal nerve — see Neuralgia, trigeminal
　ureter N13.5
　urethra (sphincter) N35.9
　uterus N85.8
　　complicating labor O62.4
　vagina N94.2
　　psychogenic F52.5
　vascular I73.9
　vasomotor I73.9
　vein NEC I87.8
　viscera — see Pain, abdominal

Spasmodic — see condition
Spasmophilia — see Tetany
Spasmus nutans F98.4
Spastic, spasticity — see also Spasm
　child (cerebral) (congenital) (paralysis) G80.1
Speaker's throat R49.8
Specific, specified — see condition
Speech
　defect, disorder, disturbance, impediment R47.9
　　psychogenic, in childhood and adolescence F98.8
　slurring R47.81
　specified NEC R47.89
Spencer's disease A08.19
Spens' syndrome (syncope with heart block) I45.9
Sperm counts (fertility testing) Z31.41
　postvasectomy Z30.8
　reversal Z31.42
Spermatic cord — see condition
Spermatocele N43.40
　congenital Q55.4
　multiple N43.42
　single N43.41
Spermatocystitis N49.0
Spermatocytoma C62.9-
　specified site — see Neoplasm, malignant, by site
Spermatorrhea N50.8
Sphacelus — see Gangrene
Sphenoidal — see condition
Sphenoiditis (chronic) — see Sinusitis, sphenoidal
Sphenopalatine ganglion neuralgia G90.09
Sphericity, increased, lens (congenital) Q12.4
Spherocytosis (congenital) (familial) (hereditary) D58.0
　hemoglobin disease D58.0
　sickle-cell (disease) D57.8-
Spherophakia Q12.4
Sphincter — see condition
Sphincteritis, sphincter of Oddi — see Cholangitis
Sphingolipidosis E75.3
　specified NEC E75.29
Sphingomyelinosis E75.3
Spicule tooth K00.2
Spider
　bite — see Toxicity, venom, spider
　fingers — see Syndrome, Marfan's
　nevus I78.1
　toes — see Syndrome, Marfan's
　vascular I78.1
Spiegler-Fendt
　benign lymphocytoma L98.8
　sarcoid L08.89
Spielmeyer-Vogt disease E75.4
Spina bifida (aperta) Q05.9
　with hydrocephalus NEC Q05.4
　cervical Q05.5
　　with hydrocephalus Q05.0
　dorsal Q05.6
　　with hydrocephalus Q05.1
　lumbar Q05.7
　　with hydrocephalus Q05.2
　lumbosacral Q05.7
　　with hydrocephalus Q05.2
　occulta Q76.0
　sacral Q05.8
　　with hydrocephalus Q05.3
　thoracic Q05.6
　　with hydrocephalus Q05.1
　thoracolumbar Q05.6
　　with hydrocephalus Q05.1
Spindle, Krukenberg's — see Pigmentation, cornea, posterior
Spine, spinal — see condition
Spiradenoma (eccrine) — see Neoplasm, skin, benign
Spirillosis A25.0
Spirillum
　minus A25.0
　obermeieri infection A68.0
Spirochetal — see condition
Spirochetosis A69.9
　arthritic, arthritica A69.9
　bronchopulmonary A69.8
　icterohemorrhagic A27.0
　lung A69.8
Spirometrosis B70.1
Spitting blood — see Hemoptysis
Splanchnoptosis K63.4
Spleen, splenic — see condition
Splenectasis — see Splenomegaly

Splenitis (interstitial) (malignant) (nonspecific) D73.89
　malarial (see also Malaria) B54 [D77]
　tuberculous A18.85
Splenocele D73.89
Splenomegaly, splenomegalia (Bengal) (cryptogenic) (idiopathic) (tropical) R16.1
　with hepatomegaly R16.2
　cirrhotic D73.2
　congenital Q89.09
　congestive, chronic D73.2
　Egyptian B65.1
　Gaucher's E75.22
　malarial (see also Malaria) B54 [D77]
　neutropenic D73.81
　Niemann-Pick — see Niemann-Pick disease or syndrome
　sideritic D73.2
　syphilitic A52.79
　　congenital (early) A50.08 [D77]
Splenopathy D73.9
Splenoptosis D73.89
Splenosis D73.89
Splinter — see Foreign body, superficial, by site
Split, splitting
　foot Q72.7-
　heart sounds R01.2
　lip, congenital — see Cleft, lip
　nails L60.3
　urinary stream R39.13
Spondylarthrosis — see Spondylosis
Spondylitis (chronic) — see also Spondylopathy, inflammatory
　ankylopoietica — see Spondylitis, ankylosing
　ankylosing (chronic) M45.9
　　with lung involvement M45.9 [J99]
　　cervical region M45.2
　　cervicothoracic region M45.3
　　juvenile M08.1
　　lumbar region M45.6
　　lumbosacral region M45.7
　　multiple sites M45.0
　　occipito-atlanto-axial region M45.1
　　sacrococcygeal region M45.8
　　thoracic region M45.4
　　thoracolumbar region M45.5
　atrophic (ligamentous) — see Spondylitis, ankylosing
　deformans (chronic) — see Spondylosis
　gonococcal A54.41
　gouty M10.08
　in (due to)
　　brucellosis A23.9 [M49.80]
　　　cervical region A23.9 [M49.82]
　　　cervicothoracic region A23.9 [M49.83]
　　　lumbar region A23.9 [M49.86]
　　　lumbosacral region A23.9 [M49.87]
　　　multiple sites A23.9 [M49.89]
　　　occipito-atlanto-axial region A23.9 [M49.81]
　　　sacrococcygeal region A23.9 [M49.88]
　　　thoracic region A23.9 [M49.84]
　　　thoracolumbar region A23.9 [M49.85]
　　enterobacteria (see also subcategory M49.8) A04.9
　　tuberculosis A18.01
　infectious NEC — see Spondylopathy, infective
　juvenile ankylosing (chronic) M08.1
　Kümmell's — see Spondylopathy, traumatic
　Marie-Strümpell — see Spondylitis, ankylosing
　muscularis — see Spondylopathy, specified NEC
　psoriatic L40.53
　rheumatoid — see Spondylitis, ankylosing
　rhizomelica — see Spondylitis, ankylosing
　sacroiliac NEC M46.1
　senescent, senile — see Spondylosis
　traumatic (chronic) or post-traumatic — see Spondylopathy, traumatic
　tuberculous A18.01
　typhosa A01.05
Spondylolisthesis (acquired) (degenerative) M43.10
　with disproportion (fetopelvic) O33.0
　　causing obstructed labor O65.0
　cervical region M43.12
　cervicothoracic region M43.13
　congenital Q76.2
　lumbar region M43.16
　lumbosacral region M43.17
　multiple sites M43.19
　occipito-atlanto-axial region M43.11

Spondylolisthesis (acquired) (degenerative) M43.10 — *continued*
  sacrococcygeal region M43.18
  thoracic region M43.14
  thoracolumbar region M43.15
  traumatic (old) M43.10
    acute
      fifth cervical (displaced) S12.430
        nondisplaced S12.431
        specified type NEC (displaced) S12.450
          nondisplaced S12.451
        type III S12.44
      fourth cervical (displaced) S12.330
        nondisplaced S12.331
        specified type NEC (displaced) S12.350
          nondisplaced S12.351
        type III S12.34
      second cervical (displaced) S12.130
        nondisplaced S12.131
        specified type NEC (displaced) S12.150
          nondisplaced S12.151
        type III S12.14
      seventh cervical (displaced) S12.630
        nondisplaced S12.631
        specified type NEC (displaced) S12.650
          nondisplaced S12.651
        type III S12.64
      sixth cervical (displaced) S12.530
        nondisplaced S12.531
        specified type NEC (displaced) S12.550
          nondisplaced S12.551
        type III S12.54
      third cervical (displaced) S12.230
        nondisplaced S12.231
        specified type NEC (displaced) S12.250
          nondisplaced S12.251
        type III S12.24
Spondylolysis (acquired) M43.00
  cervical region M43.02
  cervicothoracic region M43.03
  congenital Q76.2
  lumbar region M43.06
  lumbosacral region M43.07
    with disproportion (fetopelvic) O33.0
      causing obstructed labor O65.8
  multiple sites M43.09
  occipito-atlanto-axial region M43.01
  sacrococcygeal region M43.08
  thoracic region M43.04
  thoracolumbar region M43.05
Spondylopathy M48.9
  infective NEC M46.50
    cervical region M46.52
    cervicothoracic region M46.53
    lumbar region M46.56
    lumbosacral region M46.57
    multiple sites M46.59
    occipito-atlanto-axial region M46.51
    sacrococcygeal region M46.58
    thoracic region M46.54
    thoracolumbar region M46.55
  inflammatory M46.90
    cervical region M46.92
    cervicothoracic region M46.93
    lumbar region M46.96
    lumbosacral region M46.97
    multiple sites M46.99
    occipito-atlanto-axial region M46.91
    sacrococcygeal region M46.98
    specified type NEC M46.80
      cervical region M46.82
      cervicothoracic region M46.83
      lumbar region M46.86
      lumbosacral region M46.87
      multiple sites M46.89
      occipito-atlanto-axial region M46.81
      sacrococcygeal region M46.88
      thoracic region M46.84
      thoracolumbar region M46.85
    thoracic region M46.94
    thoracolumbar region M46.95
  neuropathic, in
    syringomyelia and syringobulbia G95.0
    tabes dorsalis A52.11
  specified NEC — *see* subcategory M48.8
  traumatic M48.30
    cervical region M48.32
    cervicothoracic region M48.33
    lumbar region M48.36
    lumbosacral region M48.37
    occipito-atlanto-axial region M48.31
    sacrococcygeal region M48.38
    thoracic region M48.34
    thoracolumbar region M48.35

Spondylosis M47.9
  with
    disproportion (fetopelvic) O33.0
      causing obstructed labor O65.0
    myelopathy NEC M47.10
      cervical region M47.12
      cervicothoracic region M47.13
      lumbar region M47.16
      occipito-atlanto-axial region M47.11
      thoracic region M47.14
      thoracolumbar region M47.15
    radiculopathy M47.20
      cervical region M47.22
      cervicothoracic region M47.23
      lumbar region M47.26
      lumbosacral region M47.27
      occipito-atlanto-axial region M47.21
      sacrococcygeal region M47.28
      thoracic region M47.24
      thoracolumbar region M47.25
    specified NEC M47.899
      cervical region M47.892
      cervicothoracic region M47.893
      lumbar region M47.896
      lumbosacral region M47.897
      occipito-atlanto-axial region M47.891
      sacrococcygeal region M47.898
      thoracic region M47.894
      thoracolumbar region M47.895
  traumatic — *see* Spondylopathy, traumatic
  without myelopathy or radiculopathy M47.819
      cervical region M47.812
      cervicothoracic region M47.813
      lumbar region M47.816
      lumbosacral region M47.817
      occipito-atlanto-axial region M47.811
      sacrococcygeal region M47.818
      thoracic region M47.814
      thoracolumbar region M47.815
Sponge
  inadvertently left in operation wound — *see* Foreign body, accidentally left during a procedure
  kidney (medullary) Q61.5
Sponge-diver's disease — *see* Toxicity, venom, marine animal, sea anemone
Spongioblastoma (any type) — *see* Neoplasm, malignant, by site
  specified site — *see* Neoplasm, malignant, by site
  unspecified site C71.9
Spongioneuroblastoma — *see* Neoplasm, malignant, by site
Spontaneous — *see also* condition
  fracture (cause unknown) — *see* Fracture, pathological
Spoon nail L60.3
  congenital Q84.6
Sporadic — *see* condition
Sporothrix schenckii infection — *see* Sporotrichosis
Sporotrichosis B42.9
  arthritis B42.82
  disseminated B42.7
  generalized B42.7
  lymphocutaneous (fixed) (progressive) B42.1
  pulmonary B42.0
  specified NEC B42.89
Spots, spotting (in) (of)
  Bitot's — *see also* Pigmentation, conjunctiva
    in the young child E50.1
    vitamin A deficiency E50.1
  café, au lait L81.3
  Cayenne pepper I78.1
  cotton wool, retina — *see* Occlusion, artery, retina
  de Morgan's (senile angiomas) I78.1
  Fuchs' black (myopic) H44.2-
  intermenstrual (regular) N92.0
    irregular N92.1
  Koplik's B05.9
  liver L81.4
  pregnancy O26.85-
  purpuric R23.3
  ruby I78.1
Spotted fever — *see* Fever, spotted N92.3

Sprain (joint) (ligament)
  acromioclavicular joint or ligament S43.5-
  ankle S93.40-
    calcaneofibular ligament S93.41-
    deltoid ligament S93.42-
    internal collateral ligament — *see* Sprain, ankle, specified ligament NEC
    specified ligament NEC S93.49-
    talofibular ligament — *see* Sprain, ankle, specified ligament NEC
    tibiofibular ligament S93.43-
  anterior longitudinal, cervical S13.4
  atlas, atlanto-axial, atlanto-occipital S13.4
  breast bone — *see* Sprain, sternum
  calcaneofibular — *see* Sprain, ankle
  carpal — *see* Sprain, wrist
  carpometacarpal — *see* Sprain, hand, specified site NEC
  cartilage
    costal S23.41
    semilunar (knee) — *see* Sprain, knee, specified site NEC
      with current tear — *see* Tear, meniscus
    thyroid region S13.5
    xiphoid — *see* Sprain, sternum
  cervical, cervicodorsal, cervicothoracic S13.4
  chondrosternal S23.421
  coracoclavicular S43.8-
  coracohumeral S43.41-
  coronary, knee — *see* Sprain, knee, specified site NEC
  costal cartilage S23.41
  cricoarytenoid articulation or ligament S13.5
  cricothyroid articulation S13.5
  cruciate, knee — *see* Sprain, knee, cruciate
  deltoid, ankle — *see* Sprain, ankle
  dorsal (spine) S23.3
  elbow S53.40-
    radial collateral ligament S53.43-
    radiohumeral S53.41-
    rupture
      radial collateral ligament — *see* Rupture, traumatic, ligament, radial collateral
      ulnar collateral ligament — *see* Rupture, traumatic, ligament, ulnar collateral
    specified type NEC S53.49-
    ulnar collateral ligament S53.44-
    ulnohumeral S53.42-
  femur, head — *see* Sprain, hip
  fibular collateral, knee — *see* Sprain, knee, collateral
  fibulocalcaneal — *see* Sprain, ankle
  finger(s) S63.61-
    index S63.61-
    interphalangeal (joint) S63.63-
      index S63.63-
      little S63.63-
      middle S63.63-
      ring S63.63-
    little S63.61-
    metacarpophalangeal (joint) S63.65-
    middle S63.61-
    ring S63.61-
    specified site NEC S63.69-
      index S63.69-
      little S63.69-
      middle S63.69-
      ring S63.69-
  foot S93.60-
    specified ligament NEC S93.69-
    tarsal ligament S93.61-
    tarsometatarsal ligament S93.62-
    toe — *see* Sprain, toe
  hand S63.9-
    finger — *see* Sprain, finger
    specified site NEC — *see* subcategory S63.8
    thumb — *see* Sprain, thumb
  head S03.9
  hip S73.10-
    iliofemoral ligament S73.11-
    ischiocapsular (ligament) S73.12-
    specified NEC S73.19-
  iliofemoral — *see* Sprain, hip
  innominate
    acetabulum — *see* Sprain, hip
    sacral junction S33.6
  internal
    collateral, ankle — *see* Sprain, ankle
    semilunar cartilage — *see* Sprain, knee, specified site NEC

Sprain (joint) (ligament) — *continued*
  interphalangeal
    finger — *see* Sprain, finger, interphalangeal (joint)
    toe — *see* Sprain, toe, interphalangeal joint
  ischiocapsular — *see* Sprain, hip
  ischiofemoral — *see* Sprain, hip
  jaw (articular disc) (cartilage) (meniscus) S03.4
    old M26.69
  knee S83.9-
    collateral ligament S83.40-
      lateral (fibular) S83.42-
      medial (tibial) S83.41-
    cruciate ligament S83.50-
      anterior S83.51-
      posterior S83.52-
    lateral (fibular) collateral ligament S83.42-
    medial (tibial) collateral ligament S83.41-
    patellar ligament S76.11-
    specified site NEC S83.8x-
    superior tibiofibular joint (ligament) S83.6-
  lateral collateral, knee — *see* Sprain, knee, collateral
  lumbar (spine) S33.5
  lumbosacral S33.9
  mandible (articular disc) S03.4
    old M26.69
  medial collateral, knee — *see* Sprain, knee, collateral
  meniscus
    jaw S03.4
      old M26.69
    knee — *see* Sprain, knee, specified site NEC
      with current tear — *see* Tear, meniscus
      old — *see* Derangement, knee, meniscus, due to old tear
    mandible S03.4
      old M26.69
  metacarpal (distal) (proximal) — *see* Sprain, hand, specified site NEC
  metacarpophalangeal — *see* Sprain, finger, metacarpophalangeal (joint)
  metatarsophalangeal — *see* Sprain, toe, metatarsophalangeal joint
  midcarpal — *see* Sprain, hand, specified site NEC
  midtarsal — *see* Sprain, foot, specified site NEC
  neck S13.9
    anterior longitudinal cervical ligament S13.4
    atlanto-axial joint S13.4
    atlanto-occipital joint S13.4
    cervical spine S13.4
    cricoarytenoid ligament S13.5
    cricothyroid ligament S13.5
    specified site NEC S13.8
    thyroid region (cartilage) S13.5
  nose S03.8
  orbicular, hip — *see* Sprain, hip
  patella — *see* Sprain, knee, specified site NEC
  patellar ligament S76.11-
  pelvis NEC S33.8
  phalanx
    finger — *see* Sprain, finger
    toe — *see* Sprain, toe
  pubofemoral — *see* Sprain, hip
  radiocarpal — *see* Sprain, wrist
  radiohumeral — *see* Sprain, elbow
  radius, collateral — *see* Rupture, traumatic, ligament, radial collateral
  rib (cage) S23.41
  rotator cuff (capsule) S43.42-
  sacroiliac (region)
    chronic or old — *see* subcategory M53.2
    joint S33.6
  scaphoid (hand) — *see* Sprain, hand, specified site NEC
  scapula(r) — *see* Sprain, shoulder girdle, specified site NEC
  semilunar cartilage (knee) — *see* Sprain, knee, specified site NEC
    with current tear — *see* Tear, meniscus
    old — *see* Derangement, knee, meniscus, due to old tear

DISEASE INDEX

Sprain (joint) (ligament) — *continued*
  shoulder joint S43.40-
    acromioclavicular joint (ligament) — *see* Sprain, acromioclavicular joint
    blade — *see* Sprain, shoulder, girdle, specified site NEC
    coracoclavicular joint (ligament) — *see* Sprain, coracoclavicular joint
    coracohumeral ligament — *see* Sprain, coracohumeral joint
    girdle S43.9-
      specified site NEC S43.8-
    rotator cuff — *see* Sprain, rotator cuff
    specified site NEC S43.49-
    sternoclavicular joint (ligament) — *see* Sprain, sternoclavicular joint
  spine
    cervical S13.4
    lumbar S33.5
    thoracic S23.3
  sternoclavicular joint S43.6-
  sternum S23.429
    chondrosternal joint S23.421
    specified site NEC S23.428
    sternoclavicular (joint) (ligament) S23.420
  symphysis
    jaw S03.4
      old M26.69
    mandibular S03.4
      old M26.69
  talofibular — *see* Sprain, ankle
  tarsal — *see* Sprain, foot, specified site NEC
  tarsometatarsal — *see* Sprain, foot, specified site NEC
  temporomandibular S03.4
    old M26.69
  thorax S23.9
    ribs S23.41
    specified site NEC S23.8
    spine S23.3
    sternum — *see* Sprain, sternum
  thumb S63.60-
    interphalangeal (joint) S63.62-
    metacarpophalangeal (joint) S63.64-
    specified site NEC S63.68-
  thyroid cartilage or region S13.5
  tibia (proximal end) — *see* Sprain, knee, specified site NEC
  tibial collateral, knee — *see* Sprain, knee, collateral
  tibiofibular
    distal — *see* Sprain, ankle
    superior — *see* Sprain, knee, specified site NEC
  toe(s) S93.50-
    great S93.50-
    interphalangeal joint S93.51-
      great S93.51-
      lesser S93.51-
    lesser S93.50-
    metatarsophalangeal joint S93.52-
      great S93.52-
      lesser S93.52-
  ulna, collateral — *see* Rupture, traumatic, ligament, ulnar collateral
  ulnohumeral — *see* Sprain, elbow
  wrist S63.50-
    carpal S63.51-
    radiocarpal S63.52-
    specified site NEC S63.59-
  xiphoid cartilage — *see* Sprain, sternum
Sprengel's deformity (congenital) Q74.0
Sprue (tropical) K90.1
  celiac K90.0
  idiopathic K90.0
  meaning thrush B37.0
  nontropical K90.0
Spur, bone — *see also* Enthesopathy
  calcaneal M77.3-
  iliac crest M76.2-
  nose (septum) J34.89
Spurway's syndrome Q78.0
Sputum
  abnormal (amount) (color) (odor) (purulent) R09.3
  blood-stained R04.2
  excessive (cause unknown) R09.3
Squamous — *see also* condition
  epithelium in
    cervical canal (congenital) Q51.828
    uterine mucosa (congenital) Q51.818
Squashed nose M95.0
  congenital Q67.4
Squeeze, diver's T70.3
Squint — *see also* Strabismus
  accommodative — *see* Strabismus, convergent concomitant

St. Hubert's disease A82.9
Stab — *see also* Laceration
  internal organs — *see* Injury, by site
Stafne's cyst or cavity M27.0
Staggering gait R26.0
  hysterical F44.4
Staghorn calculus — *see* Calculus, kidney
Stain, staining
  meconium (newborn) P96.83
  port wine Q82.5
  tooth, teeth (hard tissues) (extrinsic) K03.6
    due to
      accretions K03.6
      deposits (betel) (black) (green) (materia alba) (orange) (soft) (tobacco) K03.6
      metals (copper) (silver) K03.7
      nicotine K03.6
      pulpal bleeding K03.7
      tobacco K03.6
    intrinsic K00.8
Stammering (*see also* Disorder, fluency) F80.81
Standstill
  auricular I45.5
  cardiac — *see* Arrest, cardiac
  sinoatrial I45.5
  ventricular — *see* Arrest, cardiac
Stannosis J63.5
Stanton's disease — *see* Melioidosis
Staphylitis (acute) (catarrhal) (chronic) (gangrenous) (membranous) (suppurative) (ulcerative) K12.2
Staphylococcal scalded skin syndrome L00
Staphylococcemia A41.2
Staphylococcus, staphylococcal — *see also* condition
  as cause of disease classified elsewhere B95.8
    aureus (methicillin susceptible) (MSSA) B95.61
      methicillin resistant (MRSA) B95.62
    specified NEC, as cause of disease classified elsewhere B95.7
Staphyloma (sclera)
  cornea H18.72-
  equatorial H15.81-
  localized (anterior) H15.82-
  posticum H15.83-
  ring H15.85-
Stargardt's disease — *see* Dystrophy, retina
Starvation (inanition) (due to lack of food) T73.0
  edema — *see* Malnutrition, severe
Stasis
  bile (noncalculous) K83.1
  bronchus J98.09
    with infection — *see* Bronchitis
  cardiac — *see* Failure, heart, congestive
  cecum K59.8
  colon K59.8
  dermatitis — *see* Varix, leg, with, inflammation
  duodenal K31.5
  eczema — *see* Varix, leg, with, inflammation
  edema — *see* Hypertension, venous (chronic), idiopathic
  foot T69.0-
  ileocecal coil K59.8
  ileum K59.8
  intestinal K59.8
  jejunum K59.8
  kidney N19
  liver (cirrhotic) K76.1
  lymphatic I89.8
  pneumonia J18.2
  pulmonary — *see* Edema, lung
  rectal K59.8
  renal N19
    tubular N17.0
  ulcer — *see* Varix, leg, with, ulcer
    without varicose veins I87.2
  urine — *see* Retention, urine
  venous I87.8
State (of)
  affective and paranoid, mixed, organic psychotic F06.8
  agitated R45.1
    acute reaction to stress F43.0
  anxiety (neurotic) F41.1
  apprehension F41.1
  burn-out Z73.0
  climacteric, female Z78.0
    symptomatic N95.1
  compulsive F42
    mixed with obsessional thoughts F42

State (of) — *continued*
  confusional (psychogenic) F44.89
    acute — *see also* Delirium
      with
        arteriosclerotic dementia F01.50
          with behavioral disturbance F01.51
        senility or dementia F05
      alcoholic F10.231
      epileptic F05
      reactive (from emotional stress, psychological trauma) F44.89
      subacute — *see* Delirium
  convulsive — *see* Convulsions
  crisis F43.0
  depressive F32.9
    neurotic F34.1
  dissociative F44.9
  emotional shock (stress) R45.7
  hypercoagulation — *see* Hypercoagulable
  locked-in G83.5
  menopausal Z78.0
    symptomatic N95.1
  neurotic F48.9
    with depersonalization F48.1
  obsessional F42
  oneiroid (schizophrenia-like) F23
  organic
    hallucinatory (nonalcoholic) F06.0
    paranoid(-hallucinatory) F06.2
  panic F41.0
  paranoid F22
    climacteric F22
    involutional F22
    menopausal F22
    organic F06.2
    senile F03
    simple F22
  persistent vegetative R40.3
  phobic F40.9
  postleukotomy F07.0
  pregnant, incidental Z33.1
  psychogenic, twilight F44.89
  psychopathic (constitutional) F60.2
  psychotic, organic — *see also* Psychosis, organic
    mixed paranoid and affective F06.8
    senile or presenile F03
    transient NEC F06.8
      with
        depression F06.31
        hallucinations F06.0
  residual schizophrenic F20.5
  restlessness R45.1
  stress (emotional) R45.7
  tension (mental) F48.9
    specified NEC F48.8
  transient organic psychotic NEC F06.8
    depressive type F06.31
    hallucinatory type F06.30
  twilight
    epileptic F05
    psychogenic F44.89
  vegetative, persistent R40.3
  vital exhaustion Z73.0
  withdrawal — *see* Withdrawal, state
Status (post) — *see also* Presence (of)
  absence, epileptic — *see* Epilepsy, by type, with status epilepticus
  administration of tPA (rtPA) in a different facility within the last 24 hours prior to admission to current facility Z92.82
  adrenalectomy (unilateral) (bilateral) E89.6
  anastomosis Z98.0
  anginosus I20.9
  angioplasty (peripheral) Z98.62
    with implant Z95.820
    coronary artery Z98.61
      with implant Z95.5
  aortocoronary bypass Z95.1
  arthrodesis Z98.1
  artificial opening (of) Z93.9
    gastrointestinal tract Z93.4
    specified NEC Z93.8
    urinary tract Z93.6
    vagina Z93.8
  asthmaticus — *see* Asthma, by type, with status asthmaticus
  awaiting organ transplant Z76.82
  bariatric surgery Z98.84
  bed confinement Z74.01
  bleb, filtering (vitreous), after glaucoma surgery Z98.83
  breast implant Z98.82
    removal Z98.86
  cataract extraction Z98.4-

Status (post) (*see also* Presence (of)) — *continued*
  cholecystectomy Z90.49
  clitorectomy N90.811
    with excision of labia minora N90.812
  colectomy (complete) (partial) Z90.49
  colonization — *see* Carrier (suspected) of
  colostomy Z93.3
  convulsivus idiopathicus — *see* Epilepsy, by type, with status epilepticus
  coronary artery angioplasty — *see* Status, angioplasty, coronary artery
  cystectomy (urinary bladder) Z90.6
  cystostomy Z93.50
    appendico-vesicostomy Z93.52
    cutaneous Z93.51
    specified NEC Z93.59
  delinquent immunization Z28.3
  dental Z98.818
    crown Z98.811
    fillings Z98.811
    restoration Z98.811
    sealant Z98.810
    specified NEC Z98.818
  deployment (current) (military) Z56.82
  dialysis (hemodialysis) (peritoneal) Z99.2
  do not resuscitate (DNR) Z66
  donor — *see* Donor
  embedded fragments — *see* Retained, foreign body fragments (type of)
  embedded splinter — *see* Retained, foreign body fragments (type of)
  enterostomy Z93.4
  epileptic, epilepticus (*see also* Epilepsy, by type, with status epilepticus) G40.901
  estrogen receptor
    negative Z17.1
    positive Z17.0
  female genital cutting — *see* Female genital mutilation status
  female genital mutilation — *see* Female genital mutilation status
  filtering (vitreous) bleb after glaucoma surgery Z98.83
  gastrectomy (complete) (partial) Z90.3
  gastric banding Z98.84
  gastric bypass for obesity Z98.84
  gastrostomy Z93.1
  human immunodeficiency virus (HIV) infection, asymptomatic Z21
  hysterectomy (complete) (total) Z90.710
    partial (with remaining cervial stump) Z90.711
  ileostomy Z93.2
  implant
    breast Z98.82
  infibulation N90.813
  intestinal bypass Z98.0
  jejunostomy Z93.4
  lapsed immunization schedule Z28.3
  laryngectomy Z90.02
  lymphaticus E32.8
  marmoratus G80.3
  mastectomy (unilateral) (bilateral) Z90.1-
  military deployment status (current) Z56.82
    in theater or in support of military war, peacekeeping and humanitarian operations Z56.82
  nephrectomy (unilateral) (bilateral) Z90.5
  nephrostomy Z93.6
  obesity surgery Z98.84
  oophorectomy
    bilateral Z90.722
    unilateral Z90.721
  organ replacement
    by artificial or mechanical device or prosthesis of
      artery Z95.828
      bladder Z96.0
      blood vessel Z95.828
      breast Z97.8
      eye globe Z97.0
      heart Z95.812
        valve Z95.2
      intestine Z97.8
      joint Z96.60
        hip — *see* Presence, hip joint implant
        knee — *see* Presence, knee joint implant
        specified site NEC Z96.698
      kidney Z97.8
      larynx Z96.3
      lens Z96.1
      limbs — *see* Presence, artificial, limb

DISEASE INDEX

Status (post) (see also Presence (of)) — continued
  organ replacement — continued
    by artificial or mechanical device or prosthesis of — continued
      liver Z97.8
      lung Z97.8
      pancreas Z97.8
    by organ transplant (heterologous) (homologous) — see Transplant
  pacemaker
    brain Z96.89
    cardiac Z95.0
    specified NEC Z96.89
  pancreatectomy Z90.410
    complete Z90.410
    partial Z90.411
    total Z90.410
  physical restraint Z78.1
  pneumonectomy (complete) (partial) Z90.2
  pneumothorax, therapeutic Z98.3
  postcommotio cerebri F07.81
  postoperative (postprocedural) NEC Z98.89
    breast implant Z98.82
    dental Z98.818
      crown Z98.811
      fillings Z98.811
      restoration Z98.811
      sealant Z98.810
      specified NEC Z98.818
    pneumothorax, therapeutic Z98.3
  postpartum (routine follow-up) Z39.2
    care immediately after delivery Z39.0
  postsurgical (postprocedural) NEC Z98.89
    pneumothorax, therapeutic Z98.3
  pregnancy, incidental Z33.1
  prosthesis coronary angioplasty Z95.5
  pseudophakia Z96.1
  renal dialysis (hemodialysis) (peritoneal) Z99.2
  retained foreign body — see Retained, foreign body fragments (type of)
  reversed jejunal transposition (for bypass) Z98.0
  salpingo-oophorectomy
    bilateral Z90.722
    unilateral Z90.721
  sex reassignment surgery status Z87.890
  shunt
    arteriovenous (for dialysis) Z99.2
    cerebrospinal fluid Z98.2
    ventricular (communicating) (for drainage) Z98.2
  splenectomy Z90.81
  thymicolymphaticus E32.8
  thymicus E32.8
  thymolymphaticus E32.8
  thyroidectomy (hypothyroidism) E89.0
  tooth (teeth) extraction (see also Absence, teeth, acquired) K08.409
  tPA (rtPA) administration in a different facility within the last 24 hours prior to admission to current facility Z92.82
  tracheostomy Z93.0
  transplant — see Transplant
    organ removed Z98.85
  tubal ligation Z98.51
  underimmunization Z28.3
  ureterostomy Z93.6
  urethrostomy Z93.6
  vagina, artificial Z93.8
  vasectomy Z98.52
  wheelchair confinement Z99.3
Stealing
  child problem F91.8
    in company with others Z72.810
  pathological (compulsive) F63.2
Steam burn — see Burn
Steatocystoma multiplex L72.2
Steatohepatitis (nonalcoholic) (NASH) K75.81
Steatoma L72.3
  eyelid (cystic) — see Dermatosis, eyelid
    infected — see Hordeolum
Steatorrhea (chronic) K90.4
  with lacteal obstruction K90.2
  idiopathic (adult) (infantile) K90.0
  pancreatic K90.3
  primary K90.0
  tropical K90.1
Steatosis E88.89
  heart — see Degeneration, myocardial
  kidney N28.89
  liver NEC K76.0
Steele-Richardson-Olszewski disease or syndrome G23.1

Stein-Leventhal syndrome E28.2
Stein's syndrome E28.2
Steinbrocker's syndrome G90.8
Steinert's disease G71.11
STEMI (see also Infarct, myocardium, ST elevation) I21.3
Stenocardia I20.8
Stenocephaly Q75.8
Stenosis, stenotic (cicatricial) — see also Stricture
  ampulla of Vater K83.1
  anus, anal (canal) (sphincter) K62.4
    and rectum K62.4
    congenital Q42.3
      with fistula Q42.2
  aorta (ascending) (supraventricular) (congenital) Q25.3
    arteriosclerotic I70.0
    calcified I70.0
  aortic (valve) I35.0
    with insufficiency I35.2
    congenital Q23.0
    rheumatic I06.0
      with
        incompetency, insufficiency or regurgitation I06.2
        with mitral (valve) disease I08.0
          with tricuspid (valve) disease I08.3
        mitral (valve) disease I08.0
          with tricuspid (valve) disease I08.3
        tricuspid (valve) disease I08.2
          with mitral (valve) disease I08.3
    specified cause NEC I35.0
    syphilitic A52.03
  aqueduct of Sylvius (congenital) Q03.0
    with spina bifida — see Spina bifida, by site, with hydrocephalus
    acquired G91.1
  artery NEC (see also Arteriosclerosis) I77.1
    celiac I77.4
    cerebral — see Occlusion, artery, cerebral
    extremities — see Arteriosclerosis, extremities
    precerebral — see Occlusion, artery, precerebral
    pulmonary (congenital) Q25.6
      acquired I28.8
    renal I70.1
  bile duct (common) (hepatic) K83.1
    congenital Q44.3
  bladder-neck (acquired) N32.0
    congenital Q64.31
  brain G93.89
  bronchus J98.09
    congenital Q32.3
    syphilitic A52.72
  cardia (stomach) K22.2
    congenital Q39.3
  cardiovascular — see Disease, cardiovascular
  caudal M48.08
  cervix, cervical (canal) N88.2
    congenital Q51.828
    in pregnancy or childbirth — see Pregnancy, complicated by, abnormal cervix
  colon — see also Obstruction, intestine
    congenital Q42.9
      specified NEC Q42.8
  colostomy K94.03
  common (bile) duct K83.1
    congenital Q44.3
  coronary (artery) — see Disease, heart, ischemic, atherosclerotic
  cystic duct — see Obstruction, gallbladder
  due to presence of device, implant or graft (see also Complications, by site and type, specified NEC) T85.85
    arterial graft NEC T82.858
    breast (implant) T85.85
    catheter T85.85
      dialysis (renal) T82.858
        intraperitoneal T85.85
      infusion NEC T82.858
        spinal (epidural) (subdural) T85.85
      urinary (indwelling) T83.85
    fixation, internal (orthopedic) NEC T84.85
    gastrointestinal (bile duct) (esophagus) T85.85
    genital NEC T83.85
    heart NEC T82.857

Stenosis, stenotic (cicatricial) (see also Stricture) — continued
  due to presence of device, implant or graft (see also Complications, by site and type, specified NEC) T85.85 — continued
    joint prosthesis T84.85
    ocular (corneal graft) (orbital implant) NEC T85.85
    orthopedic NEC T84.85
    specified NEC T85.85
    urinary NEC T83.85
    vascular NEC T82.858
    ventricular intracranial shunt T85.85
  duodenum K31.5
    congenital Q41.0
  ejaculatory duct NEC N50.8
  endocervical os — see Stenosis, cervix
  enterostomy K94.13
  esophagus K22.2
    congenital Q39.3
    syphilitic A52.79
      congenital A50.59 [K23]
  eustachian tube — see Obstruction, eustachian tube
  external ear canal (acquired) H61.30-
    congenital Q16.1
    due to
      inflammation H61.32-
      trauma H61.31-
    postprocedural H95.81-
    specified cause NEC H61.39-
  gallbladder — see Obstruction, gallbladder
  glottis J38.6
  heart valve (congenital) Q24.8
    aortic Q23.0
    mitral Q23.2
    pulmonary Q22.1
    tricuspid Q22.4
  hepatic duct K83.1
  hymen N89.6
  hypertrophic subaortic (idiopathic) I42.1
  ileum K56.69
    congenital Q41.2
  infundibulum cardia Q24.3
  intervertebral foramina — see also Lesion, biomechanical, specified NEC
    connective tissue M99.79
      abdomen M99.79
      cervical region M99.71
      cervicothoracic M99.71
      head region M99.70
      lumbar region M99.73
      lumbosacral M99.73
      occipitocervical M99.70
      sacral region M99.74
      sacrococcygeal M99.74
      sacroiliac M99.74
      specified NEC M99.79
      thoracic region M99.72
      thoracolumbar M99.72
    disc M99.79
      abdomen M99.79
      cervical region M99.71
      cervicothoracic M99.71
      head region M99.70
      lower extremity M99.76
      lumbar region M99.73
      lumbosacral M99.73
      occipitocervical M99.70
      pelvic M99.75
      rib cage M99.78
      sacral region M99.74
      sacrococcygeal M99.74
      sacroiliac M99.74
      specified NEC M99.79
      thoracic region M99.72
      thoracolumbar M99.72
      upper extremity M99.77
    osseous M99.69
      abdomen M99.69
      cervical region M99.61
      cervicothoracic M99.61
      head region M99.60
      lower extremity M99.66
      lumbar region M99.63
      lumbosacral M99.63
      occipitocervical M99.60
      pelvic M99.65
      rib cage M99.68
      sacral region M99.64
      sacrococcygeal M99.64
      sacroiliac M99.64
      specified NEC M99.69
      thoracic region M99.62
      thoracolumbar M99.62
      upper extremity M99.67
    subluxation — see Stenosis, intervertebral foramina, osseous

Stenosis, stenotic (cicatricial) (see also Stricture) — continued
  intestine — see also Obstruction, intestine
    congenital (small) Q41.9
      large Q42.9
        specified NEC Q42.8
      specified NEC Q41.8
  jejunum K56.69
    congenital Q41.1
  lacrimal (passage)
    canaliculi H04.54-
    congenital Q10.5
    duct H04.55-
      punctum H04.56-
      sac H04.57-
  lacrimonasal duct — see Stenosis, lacrimal, duct
    congenital Q10.5
  larynx J38.6
    congenital NEC Q31.8
      subglottic Q31.1
    syphilitic A52.73
      congenital A50.59 [J99]
  mitral (chronic) (inactive) (valve) I05.0
    with
      aortic valve disease I08.0
      incompetency, insufficiency or regurgitation I05.2
      active or acute I01.1
        with rheumatic or Sydenham's chorea I02.0
    congenital Q23.2
    specified cause, except rheumatic I34.2
    syphilitic A52.03
  myocardium, myocardial — see also Degeneration, myocardial
    hypertrophic subaortic (idiopathic) I42.1
  nares (anterior) (posterior) J34.89
    congenital Q30.0
  nasal duct — see also Stenosis, lacrimal, duct
    congenital Q10.5
  nasolacrimal duct — see also Stenosis, lacrimal, duct
    congenital Q10.5
  neural canal — see also Lesion, biomechanical, specified NEC
    connective tissue M99.49
      abdomen M99.49
      cervical region M99.41
      cervicothoracic M99.41
      head region M99.40
      lower extremity M99.46
      lumbar region M99.43
      lumbosacral M99.43
      occipitocervical M99.40
      pelvic M99.45
      rib cage M99.48
      sacral region M99.44
      sacrococcygeal M99.44
      sacroiliac M99.44
      specified NEC M99.49
      thoracic region M99.42
      thoracolumbar M99.42
      upper extremity M99.47
    intervertebral disc M99.59
      abdomen M99.59
      cervical region M99.51
      cervicothoracic M99.51
      head region M99.50
      lower extremity M99.56
      lumbar region M99.53
      lumbosacral M99.53
      occipitocervical M99.50
      pelvic M99.55
      rib cage M99.58
      sacral region M99.54
      sacrococcygeal M99.54
      sacroiliac M99.54
      specified NEC M99.59
      thoracic region M99.52
      thoracolumbar M99.52
      upper extremity M99.57
    osseous M99.39
      abdomen M99.39
      cervical region M99.31
      cervicothoracic M99.31
      head region M99.30
      lower extremity M99.36
      lumbar region M99.33
      lumbosacral M99.33
      occipitocervical M99.30
      pelvic M99.35
      rib cage M99.38
      sacral region M99.34
      sacrococcygeal M99.34

DISEASE INDEX

Stenosis, stenotic (cicatricial) *(see also* Stricture) — *continued*
neural canal — *see also* Lesion, biomechanical, specified NEC — *continued*
  osseous M99.39 — *continued*
    sacroiliac M99.34
    specified NEC M99.39
    thoracic region M99.32
    thoracolumbar M99.32
    upper extremity M99.37
  subluxation M99.29
    cervical region M99.21
    cervicothoracic M99.21
    head region M99.20
    lower extremity M99.26
    lumbar region M99.23
    lumbosacral M99.23
    occipitocervical M99.20
    pelvic M99.25
    rib cage M99.28
    sacral region M99.24
    sacrococcygeal M99.24
    sacroiliac M99.24
    specified NEC M99.29
    thoracic region M99.22
    thoracolumbar M99.22
    upper extremity M99.27
organ or site, congenital NEC — *see* Atresia, by site
papilla of Vater K83.1
pulmonary (artery) (congenital) Q25.6
  with ventricular septal defect, transposition of aorta, and hypertrophy of right ventricle Q21.3
  acquired I28.8
  in tetralogy of Fallot Q21.3
  infundibular Q24.3
  subvalvular Q24.3
  supravalvular Q25.6
  valve I37.0
    with insufficiency I37.2
    congenital Q22.1
    rheumatic I09.89
      with aortic, mitral or tricuspid (valve) disease I08.8
  vein, acquired I28.8
  vessel NEC I28.8
pulmonic (congenital) Q22.1
  infundibular Q24.3
  subvalvular Q24.3
pylorus (hypertrophic) (acquired) K31.1
  adult K31.1
  congenital Q40.0
  infantile Q40.0
rectum (sphincter) — *see* Stricture, rectum
renal artery I70.1
  congenital Q27.1
salivary duct (any) K11.8
sphincter of Oddi K83.1
spinal M48.00
  cervical region M48.02
  cervicothoracic region M48.03
  lumbar region M48.06
  lumbosacral region M48.07
  occipito-atlanto-axial region M48.01
  sacrococcygeal region M48.08
  thoracic region M48.04
  thoracolumbar region M48.05
stomach, hourglass K31.2
subaortic (congenital) Q24.4
  hypertrophic (idiopathic) I42.1
subglottic J38.6
  congenital Q31.1
  postprocedural J95.5
trachea J39.8
  congenital Q32.1
  syphilitic A52.73
  tuberculous NEC A15.5
tracheostomy J95.03
tricuspid (valve) I07.0
  with
    aortic (valve) disease I08.2
    incompetency, insufficiency or regurgitation I07.2
      with aortic (valve) disease I08.2
        with mitral (valve) disease I08.3
    mitral (valve) disease I08.1
      with aortic (valve) disease I08.3
  congenital Q22.4
  nonrheumatic I36.0
    with insufficiency I36.2
tubal N97.1
ureter — *see* Atresia, ureter
ureteropelvic junction, congenital Q62.11

Stenosis, stenotic (cicatricial) *(see also* Stricture) — *continued*
ureterovesical orifice, congenital Q62.12
urethra (valve) — *see also* Stricture, urethra
  congenital Q64.32
urinary meatus, congenital Q64.33
vagina N89.5
  congenital Q52.4
  in pregnancy — *see* Pregnancy, complicated by, abnormal vagina causing obstructed labor O65.5
valve (cardiac) (heart) *(see also* Endocarditis)* I38
  congenital Q24.8
    aortic Q23.0
    mitral Q23.2
    pulmonary Q22.1
    tricuspid Q22.4
vena cava (inferior) (superior) I87.1
  congenital Q26.0
vesicourethral orifice Q64.31
vulva N90.5
Stent jail T82.897
Stercolith (impaction) K56.41
  appendix K38.1
Stercoraceous, stercoral ulcer K63.3
  anus or rectum K62.6
Stereotypies NEC F98.4
Sterility — *see* Infertility
Sterilization — *see* Encounter (for), sterilization
Sternalgia — *see* Angina
Sternopagus Q89.4
Sternum bifidum Q76.7
Steroid
  effects (adverse) (adrenocortical) (iatrogenic)
    cushingoid E24.2
      correct substance properly administered — *see* Table of Drugs and Chemicals, by drug, adverse effect
      overdose or wrong substance given or taken — *see* Table of Drugs and Chemicals, by drug, poisoning
    diabetes — *see* category E09
      correct substance properly administered — *see* Table of Drugs and Chemicals, by drug, adverse effect
      overdose or wrong substance given or taken — *see* Table of Drugs and Chemicals, by drug, poisoning
    fever R50.2
    insufficiency E27.3
      correct substance properly administered — *see* Table of Drugs and Chemicals, by drug, adverse effect
      overdose or wrong substance given or taken — *see* Table of Drugs and Chemicals, by drug, poisoning
    responder H40.04-
Stevens-Johnson disease or syndrome L51.1
  toxic epidermal necrolysis overlap L51.3
Stewart-Morel syndrome M85.2
Sticker's disease B08.3
Sticky eye — *see* Conjunctivitis, acute, mucopurulent
Stieda's disease — *see* Bursitis, tibial collateral
Stiff neck — *see* Torticollis
Stiff-man syndrome G25.82
Stiffness, joint NEC M25.60-
  ankle M25.67-
  ankylosis — *see* Ankylosis, joint
  contracture — *see* Contraction, joint
  elbow M25.62-
  foot M25.67-
  hand M25.64-
  hip M25.65-
  knee M25.66-
  shoulder M25.61-
  wrist M25.63-
Stigmata congenital syphilis A50.59
Still's disease or syndrome (juvenile) M08.20
  adult-onset M06.1
  ankle M08.27-
  elbow M08.22-
  foot joint M08.27-
  hand joint M08.24-
  hip M08.25-
  knee M08.26-
  multiple site M08.29
  shoulder M08.21-
  vertebra M08.28
  wrist M08.23-

Still-Felty syndrome — *see* Felty's syndrome
Stillbirth P95
Stimulation, ovary E28.1
Sting (venomous) (with allergic or anaphylactic shock) — *see* Table of Drugs and Chemicals, by animal or substance, poisoning
Stippled epiphyses Q78.8
Stitch
  abscess T81.4
  burst (in operation wound) — *see* Disruption, wound, operation
Stokes' disease E05.00
  with thyroid storm E05.01
Stokes-Adams disease or syndrome I45.9
Stokvis(-Talma) disease D74.8
Stoma malfunction
  colostomy K94.03
  enterostomy K94.13
  gastrostomy K94.23
  ileostomy K94.13
  tracheostomy J95.03
Stomach — *see* condition
Stomatitis (denture) (ulcerative) K12.1
  angular K13.0
    due to dietary or vitamin deficiency E53.0
  aphthous K12.0
  bovine B08.61
  candidal B37.0
  catarrhal K12.1
  diphtheritic A36.89
  due to
    dietary deficiency E53.0
    thrush B37.0
    vitamin deficiency
      B group NEC E53.9
      B2 (riboflavin) E53.0
  epidemic B08.8
  epizootic B08.8
  follicular K12.1
  gangrenous A69.0
  Geotrichum B48.3
  herpesviral, herpetic B00.2
  herpetiformis K12.0
  malignant K12.1
  membranous acute K12.1
  monilial B37.0
  mycotic B37.0
  necrotizing ulcerative A69.0
  parasitic B37.0
  septic K12.1
  spirochetal A69.1
  suppurative (acute) K12.2
  ulceromembranous A69.1
  vesicular K12.1
    with exanthem (enteroviral) B08.4
    virus disease A93.8
  Vincent's A69.1
Stomatocytosis D58.8
Stomatomycosis B37.0
Stomatorrhagia K13.79
Stone(s) — *see also* Calculus
  bladder (diverticulum) N21.0
  cystine E72.09
  heart syndrome I50.1
  kidney N20.0
  prostate N42.0
  pulpal (dental) K04.2
  renal N20.0
  salivary gland or duct (any) K11.5
  urethra (impacted) N21.1
  urinary (duct) (impacted) (passage) N20.9
    bladder (diverticulum) N21.0
    lower tract N21.9
    specified NEC N21.8
  xanthine E79.8 [N22]
Stonecutter's lung J62.8
Stonemason's asthma, disease, lung or pneumoconiosis J62.8
Stoppage
  heart — *see* Arrest, cardiac
  urine — *see* Retention, urine
Storm, thyroid — *see* Thyrotoxicosis
Strabismus (congenital) (nonparalytic) H50.9
  concomitant H50.40
    convergent — *see* Strabismus, convergent concomitant
    divergent — *see* Strabismus, divergent concomitant

Strabismus (congenital) (nonparalytic) H50.9 — *continued*
convergent concomitant H50.00
  accommodative component H50.43
  alternating H50.05
    with
      A pattern H50.06
      specified nonconcomitances NEC H50.08
      V pattern H50.07
  monocular H50.01-
    with
      A pattern H50.02-
      specified nonconcomitances NEC H50.04-
      V pattern H50.03-
    intermittent H50.31-
      alternating H50.32
cyclotropia H50.1-
divergent concomitant H50.10
  alternating H50.15
    with
      A pattern H50.16
      specified nonconcomitances NEC H50.18
      V pattern H50.17
  monocular H50.11-
    with
      A pattern H50.12-
      specified nonconcomitances NEC H50.14-
      V pattern H50.13-
    intermittent H50.33
      alternating H50.34
Duane's syndrome H50.81-
due to adhesions, scars H50.69
heterophoria H50.50
  alternating H50.55
  cyclophoria H50.54
  esophoria H50.51
  exophoria H50.52
  vertical H50.53
heterotropia H50.40
  intermittent H50.30
hypertropia H50.2-
hypotropia — *see* Hypertropia
latent H50.50
mechanical H50.60
  Brown's sheath syndrome H50.61-
  specified type NEC H50.69
monofixation syndrome H50.42
paralytic H49.9
  abducens nerve H49.2-
  fourth nerve H49.1-
  Kearns-Sayre syndrome H49.81-
  ophthalmoplegia (external)
    progressive H49.4-
      with pigmentary retinopathy H49.81-
    total H49.3-
  sixth nerve H49.2-
  specified type NEC H49.88-
  third nerve H49.0-
  trochlear nerve H49.1-
specified type NEC H50.89
vertical H50.2-
Strain
back S39.012
cervical S16.1
eye NEC — *see* Disturbance, vision, subjective
heart — *see* Disease, heart
low back S39.012
mental NOS Z73.3
  work-related Z56.6
muscle (tendon) — *see* Injury, muscle, by site, strain
neck S16.1
physical NOS Z73.3
  work-related Z56.6
postural — *see also* Disorder, soft tissue, due to use
psychological NEC Z73.3
tendon — *see* Injury, muscle, by site, strain
Straining, on urination R39.16
Strand, vitreous — *see* Opacity, vitreous, membranes and strands
Strangulation, strangulated — *see also* Asphyxia, traumatic
appendix K38.8
bladder-neck N32.0
bowel or colon K56.2
food or foreign body — *see* Foreign body, by site
hemorrhoids — *see* Hemorrhoids, with complication

D I S E A S E   I N D E X

Strangulation, strangulated *(see also*
   Asphyxia, traumatic) — *continued*
   hernia — *see also* Hernia, by site, with
     obstruction
     with gangrene — *see* Hernia, by site,
      with gangrene
   intestine (large) (small) K56.2
     with hernia — *see also* Hernia, by site,
      with obstruction
      with gangrene — *see* Hernia, by site,
       with gangrene
   mesentery K56.2
   mucus — *see* Asphyxia, mucus
   omentum K56.2
   organ or site, congenital NEC — *see*
     Atresia, by site
   ovary — *see* Torsion, ovary
   penis N48.89
     foreign body T19.4
   rupture — *see* Hernia, by site, with
     obstruction
   stomach due to hernia — *see also* Hernia,
     by site, with obstruction
     with gangrene — *see* Hernia, by site,
      with gangrene
   vesicourethral orifice N32.0
Strangury R30.0
Straw itch B88.0
Strawberry
   gallbladder K82.4
   mark Q82.5
   tongue (red) (white) K14.3
Streak(s)
   macula, angioid H35.33
   ovarian Q50.32
Strephosymbolia F81.0
   secondary to organic lesion R48.8
Streptobacillary fever A25.1
Streptobacillosis A25.1
Streptobacillus moniliformis A25.1
Streptococcus, streptococcal — *see also*
   condition
   as cause of disease classified elsewhere
     B95.5
   group
     A, as cause of disease classified
      elsewhere B95.0
     B, as cause of disease classified
      elsewhere B95.1
     D, as cause of disease classified
      elsewhere B95.2
     pneumoniae, as cause of disease classified
      elsewhere B95.3
     specified NEC, as cause of disease
      classified elsewhere B95.4
Streptomycosis B47.1
Streptotrichosis A48.8
Stress F43.9
   family — *see* Disruption, family
   fetal P84
     complicating pregnancy O77.9
      due to drug administration O77.1
   mental NEC Z73.3
     work-related Z56.6
   physical NEC Z73.3
     work-related Z56.6
   polycythemia D75.1
   reaction (*see also* Reaction, stress) F43.9
   work schedule Z56.3
Stretching, nerve — *see* Injury, nerve
Striae albicantes, atrophicae or distensae
   (cutis) L90.6
Stricture — *see also* Stenosis
   ampulla of Vater K83.1
   anus (sphincter) K62.4
     congenital Q42.3
      with fistula Q42.2
     infantile Q42.3
      with fistula Q42.2
   aorta (ascending) (congenital) Q25.3
     arteriosclerotic I70.0
     calcified I70.0
     supravalvular, congenital Q25.3
   aortic (valve) — *see* Stenosis, aortic
   aqueduct of Sylvius (congenital) Q03.0
     with spina bifida — *see* Spina bifida, by
      site, with hydrocephalus
     acquired G91.1
   artery I77.1
     basilar — *see* Occlusion, artery, basilar
     carotid — *see* Occlusion, artery, carotid
     celiac I77.4

Stricture (*see also* Stenosis) — *continued*
   artery I77.1 — *continued*
     congenital (peripheral) Q27.8
      cerebral Q28.3
      coronary Q24.5
      digestive system Q27.8
      lower limb Q27.8
      retinal Q14.1
      specified site NEC Q27.8
      umbilical Q27.0
      upper limb Q27.8
     coronary Q24.5 — *see* Disease, heart, ischemic,
      atherosclerotic
      congenital Q24.5
     precerebral — *see* Occlusion, artery,
      precerebral
     pulmonary (congenital) Q25.6
      acquired I28.8
     renal I70.1
     vertebral — *see* Occlusion, artery,
      vertebral
   auditory canal (external) (congenital)
     acquired — *see* Stenosis, external ear
      canal
   bile duct (common) (hepatic) K83.1
     congenital Q44.3
     postoperative K91.89
   bladder N32.89
     neck N32.0
   bowel — *see* Obstruction, intestine
   brain G93.89
   bronchus J98.09
     congenital Q32.3
     syphilitic A52.72
   cardia (stomach) K22.2
     congenital Q39.3
   cardiac — *see also* Disease, heart
     orifice (stomach) K22.2
   cecum — *see* Obstruction, intestine
   cervix, cervical (canal) N88.2
     congenital Q51.828
     in pregnancy — *see* Pregnancy,
      complicated by, abnormal cervix
      causing obstructed labor O65.5
   colon — *see* Obstruction, intestine
     congenital Q42.9
      specified NEC Q42.8
   colostomy K94.03
   common (bile) duct K83.1
   coronary (artery) — *see* Disease, heart,
     ischemic, atherosclerotic
   cystic duct — *see* Obstruction, gallbladder
   digestive organs NEC, congenital Q45.8
   duodenum K31.5
     congenital Q41.0
   ear canal (external) (congenital) Q16.1
     acquired — *see* Stricture, auditory canal,
      acquired
   ejaculatory duct N50.8
   enterostomy K94.13
   esophagus K22.2
     congenital Q39.3
     syphilitic A52.79
      congenital A50.59 [K23]
   eustachian tube — *see also* Obstruction,
     eustachian tube
     congenital Q17.8
   fallopian tube N97.1
     gonococcal A54.24
     tuberculous A18.17
   gallbladder — *see* Obstruction, gallbladder
   glottis J38.6
   heart — *see also* Disease, heart
     valve (*see also* Endocarditis) I38
      aortic Q23.0
      mitral Q23.4
      pulmonary Q22.1
      tricuspid Q22.4
   hepatic duct K83.1
   hourglass, of stomach K31.2
   hymen N89.6
   hypopharynx J39.2
   ileum K56.69
     congenital Q41.2
   intestine — *see also* Obstruction, intestine
     congenital (small) Q41.9
      large Q42.9
       specified NEC Q42.8
      specified NEC Q41.8
     ischemic K55.1
   jejunum K56.69
     congenital Q41.1
   lacrimal passages — *see also* Stenosis,
     lacrimal
     congenital Q10.5

Stricture (*see also* Stenosis) — *continued*
   larynx J38.6
     congenital NEC Q31.8
      subglottic Q31.1
     syphilitic A52.73
      congenital A50.59 [J99]
   meatus
     ear (congenital) Q16.1
      acquired — *see* Stricture, auditory
       canal, acquired
     osseous (ear) (congenital) Q16.1
      acquired — *see* Stricture, auditory
       canal, acquired
     urinarius — *see also* Stricture, urethra
      congenital Q64.33
   mitral (valve) — *see* Stenosis, mitral
   myocardium, myocardial I51.5
     hypertrophic subaortic (idiopathic) I42.1
   nares (anterior) (posterior) J34.89
     congenital Q30.0
   nasal duct — *see also* Stenosis, lacrimal,
     duct
     congenital Q10.5
   nasolacrimal duct — *see also* Stenosis,
     lacrimal, duct
     congenital Q10.5
   nasopharynx J39.2
     syphilitic A52.73
   nose J34.89
     congenital Q30.0
   nostril (anterior) (posterior) J34.89
     congenital Q30.0
     syphilitic A52.73
      congenital A50.59 [J99]
   organ or site, congenital NEC — *see*
     Atresia, by site
   os uteri — *see* Stricture, cervix
   osseous meatus (ear) (congenital) Q16.1
     acquired — *see* Stricture, auditory canal,
      acquired
   oviduct — *see* Stricture, fallopian tube
   pelviureteric junction (congenital) Q62.11
   penis, by foreign body T19.4
   pharynx J39.2
   prostate N42.89
   pulmonary, pulmonic
     artery (congenital) Q25.6
      acquired I28.8
      noncongenital I28.8
     infundibulum (congenital) Q24.3
     valve I37.0
      congenital Q22.1
     vein, acquired I28.8
     vessel NEC I28.8
   punctum lacrimale — *see also* Stenosis,
     lacrimal, punctum
     congenital Q10.5
   pylorus (hypertrophic) K31.1
     adult K31.1
     congenital Q40.0
     infantile Q40.0
   rectosigmoid K56.69
   rectum (sphincter) K62.4
     congenital Q42.1
      with fistula Q42.0
     due to
      chlamydial lymphogranuloma A55
      irradiation K91.89
      lymphogranuloma venereum A55
     gonococcal A54.6
     inflammatory (chlamydial) A55
     syphilitic A52.74
     tuberculous A18.32
   renal artery I70.1
     congenital Q27.1
   salivary duct or gland (any) K11.8
   sigmoid (flexure) — *see* Obstruction,
     intestine
   spermatic cord N50.8
   stoma (following) (of)
     colostomy K94.03
     enterostomy K94.13
     gastrostomy K94.23
     ileostomy K94.13
     tracheostomy J95.03
   stomach K31.89
     congenital Q40.2
     hourglass K31.2
   subaortic Q24.4
     hypertrophic (acquired) (idiopathic)
      I42.1
   subglottic J38.6
   syphilitic NEC A52.79
   trachea J39.8
     congenital Q32.1
     syphilitic A52.73
     tuberculous NEC A15.5

Stricture (*see also* Stenosis) — *continued*
   tracheostomy J95.03
   tricuspid (valve) — *see* Stenosis, tricuspid
   tunica vaginalis N50.8
   ureter (postoperative) N13.5
     with
      hydronephrosis N13.1
       with infection N13.6
      pyelonephritis (chronic) N11.1
     congenital — *see* Atresia, ureter
     tuberculous A18.11
   ureteropelvic junction (congenital) Q62.11
   ureterovesical orifice N13.5
     with infection N13.6
   urethra (organic) (spasmodic) N35.9
     associated with schistosomiasis B65.0
      [N37]
     congenital Q64.39
      valvular (posterior) Q64.2
     due to
      infection — *see* Stricture, urethra,
       postinfective
      trauma — *see* Stricture, urethra, post-
       traumatic
     gonococcal, gonorrheal A54.01
     infective NEC — *see* Stricture, urethra,
      postinfective
     late effect (sequelae) of injury — *see*
      Stricture, urethra, post-traumatic
     post-traumatic
      female N35.028
       due to childbirth N35.021
      male N35.014
       anterior urethra N35.013
       bulbous urethra N35.011
       meatal N35.010
       membranous urethra N35.012
     postcatheterization — *see* Stricture,
      urethra, postprocedural
     postinfective NEC
      female N35.12
      male N35.119
       anterior urethra N35.114
       bulbous urethra N35.112
       meatal N35.111
       membranous urethra N35.113
     postobstetric N35.021
     postoperative — *see* Stricture, urethra,
      postprocedural
     postprocedural
      female N99.12
      male N99.114
       anterior urethra N99.113
       bulbous urethra N99.111
       meatal N99.110
       membranous urethra N99.112
     sequela (late effect) of
      childbirth N35.021
      injury — *see* Stricture, urethra, post-
       traumatic
     specified cause NEC N35.8
     syphilitic A52.76
     traumatic — *see* Stricture, urethra, post-
      traumatic
     valvular (posterior), congenital Q64.2
   urinary meatus — *see* Stricture, urethra
   uterus, uterine (synechiae) N85.6
     os (external) (internal) — *see* Stricture,
      cervix
   vagina (outlet) — *see* Stenosis, vagina
   valve (cardiac) (heart) — *see also*
     Endocarditis
     congenital
      aortic Q23.0
      mitral Q23.2
      pulmonary Q22.1
      tricuspid Q22.4
   vas deferens N50.8
     congenital Q55.4
   vein I87.1
   vena cava (inferior) (superior) NEC I87.1
     congenital Q26.0
   vesicourethral orifice N32.0
     congenital Q64.31
   vulva (acquired) N90.5
Stridor R06.1
   congenital (larynx) P28.89
Stridulous — *see* condition
Stroke (apoplectic) (brain) (embolic)
   (ischemic) (paralytic) (thrombotic) I63.9
   epileptic — *see* Epilepsy
   heat T67.0
   in evolution I63.9
   intraoperative
     during cardiac surgery I97.810
     during other surgery I97.811

Stroke (apoplectic) (brain) (embolic) (ischemic) (paralytic) (thrombotic) I63.9 — *continued*
  lightning — *see* Lightning
  meaning
    cerebral hemorrhage — *code to* Hemorrhage, intracranial
    cerebral infarction — *code to* Infarction, cerebral
  postprocedural
    following cardiac surgery I97.820
    following other surgery I97.821
  unspecified (NOS) I63.9
Stromatosis, endometrial D39.0
Strongyloidiasis, strongyloidosis B78.9
  cutaneous B78.1
  disseminated B78.7
  intestinal B78.0
Strophulus pruriginosus L28.2
Struck by lightning — *see* Lightning
Struma — *see also* Goiter
  Hashimoto E06.3
  lymphomatosa E06.3
  nodosa (simplex) E04.9
    endemic E01.2
      multinodular E01.1
    multinodular E04.2
      iodine-deficiency related E01.1
    toxic or with hyperthyroidism E05.20
      with thyroid storm E05.21
      multinodular E05.20
        with thyroid storm E05.21
      uninodular E05.10
        with thyroid storm E05.11
    toxicosa E05.20
      with thyroid storm E05.21
      multinodular E05.20
        with thyroid storm E05.21
      uninodular E05.10
        with thyroid storm E05.11
    uninodular E04.1
  ovarii D27.
  Riedel's E06.5
Strumipriva cachexia E03.4
Strümpell-Marie spine — *see* Spondylitis, ankylosing
Strümpell-Westphal pseudosclerosis E83.01
Stuart deficiency disease (factor X) D68.2
Stuart-Prower factor deficiency (factor X) D68.2
Student's elbow — *see* Bursitis, elbow, olecranon
Stump — *see* Amputation
Stunting, nutritional E45
Stupor (catatonic) R40.1
  depressive F32.8
  dissociative F44.2
  manic F30.2 '
  manic-depressive F31.89
  psychogenic (anergic) F44.2
  reaction to exceptional stress (transient) F43.0
Sturge (-Weber) (-Dimitri) (-Kalischer) **disease or syndrome** Q85.8
Stuttering F80.81
  adult onset F98.5
  childhood onset F80.81
  following cerebrovascular disease — *see* Disorder, fluency. following cerebrovascular disease
  in conditions classified elsewhere R47.82
Sty, stye (external) (internal) (meibomian) (zeisian) — *see* Hordeolum
Stähli's line (cornea) (pigment) — *see* Pigmentation, cornea, anterior
Subacidity, gastric K31.89
  psychogenic F45.8
Subacute — *see* condition
Subarachnoid — *see* condition
Subcortical — *see* condition
Subcostal syndrome, nerve compression — *see* Mononeuropathy, upper limb, specified site NEC
Subcutaneous, subcuticular — *see* condition
Subdural — *see* condition
Subendocardium — *see* condition
Subependymoma
  specified site — *see* Neoplasm, uncertain behavior, by site
  unspecified site D43.2
Suberosis J67.3
Subglossitis — *see* Glossitis
Subhemophilia D66

Subinvolution
  breast (postlactational) (postpuerperal) N64.89
  puerperal O90.89
  uterus (chronic) (nonpuerperal) N85.3
    puerperal O90.89
Sublingual — *see* condition
Sublinguitis — *see* Sialoadenitis
Subluxatable hip Q65.6
Subluxation — *see also* Dislocation
  acromioclavicular S43.11-
  ankle S93.0-
  atlantoaxial, recurrent M43.4
    with myelopathy M43.3
  carpometacarpal (joint) NEC S63.05-
    thumb S63.04-
  complex, vertebral — *see* Complex, subluxation
  congenital — *see also* Malposition, congenital
    hip — *see* Dislocation, hip, congenital, partial
    joint (excluding hip)
      lower limb Q68.8
      shoulder Q68.8
      upper limb Q68.8
  elbow (traumatic) S53.10-
    anterior S53.11-
    lateral S53.14-
    medial S53.13-
    posterior S53.12-
    specified type NEC S53.19-
  finger S63.20-
    index S63.20-
    interphalangeal S63.22-
      distal S63.24-
        index S63.24-
        little S63.24-
        middle S63.24-
        ring S63.24-
      index S63.22-
      little S63.22-
      middle S63.22-
      proximal S63.23-
        index S63.23-
        little S63.23-
        middle S63.23-
        ring S63.23-
      ring S63.22-
    little S63.20-
    metacarpophalangeal S63.21-
      index S63.21-
      little S63.21-
      middle S63.21-
      ring S63.21-
    middle S63.20-
    ring S63.20-
  foot S93.30-
    specified site NEC S93.33-
    tarsal joint S93.31-
    tarsometatarsal joint S93.32-
    toe — *see* Subluxation, toe
  hip S73.00-
    anterior S73.03-
      obturator S73.02-
    central S73.04-
    posterior S73.01-
  interphalangeal (joint)
    finger S63.22-
      distal joint S63.24-
        index S63.24-
        little S63.24-
        middle S63.24-
        ring S63.24-
      index S63.22-
      little S63.22-
      middle S63.22-
      proximal joint S63.23-
        index S63.23-
        little S63.23-
        middle S63.23-
        ring S63.23-
      ring S63.22-
    thumb S63.12-
      distal joint S63.14-
      proximal joint S63.13-
    toe S93.13-
      great S93.13-
      lesser S93.13-
  joint prosthesis — *see* Complications, joint prosthesis, mechanical, displacement, by site

Subluxation (*see also* Dislocation) — *continued*
  knee S83.10-
    cap — *see* Subluxation, patella
    patella — *see* Subluxation, patella
    proximal tibia
      anteriorly S83.11-
      laterally S83.14-
      medially S83.13-
      posteriorly S83.12-
    specified type NEC S83.19-
  lens — *see* Dislocation, lens, partial
  ligament, traumatic — *see* Sprain, by site
  metacarpal (bone)
    proximal end S63.06-
  metacarpophalangeal (joint)
    finger S63.21-
      index S63.21-
      little S63.21-
      middle S63.21-
      ring S63.21-
    thumb S63.11-
  metatarsophalangeal joint S93.14-
    great toe S93.14-
    lesser toe S93.14-
  midcarpal (joint) S63.03-
  patella S83.00-
    lateral S83.01-
    recurrent (nontraumatic) — *see* Dislocation, patella, recurrent, incomplete
    specified type NEC S83.09-
  pathological — *see* Dislocation, pathological
  radial head S53.00-
    anterior S53.01-
    nursemaid's elbow S53.03-
    posterior S53.02-
    specified type NEC S53.09-
  radiocarpal (joint) S63.02-
  radioulnar (joint)
    distal S63.01-
    proximal — *see* Subluxation, elbow
  shoulder
    congenital Q68.8
    girdle S43.30-
      scapula S43.31-
      specified site NEC S43.39-
    traumatic S43.00-
      anterior S43.01-
      inferior S43.03-
      posterior S43.02-
      specified type NEC S43.08-
  sternoclavicular (joint) S43.20-
    anterior S43.21-
    posterior S43.22-
  symphysis (pubis)
  thumb S63.103
    interphalangeal joint — *see* Subluxation, interphalangeal (joint), thumb
    metacarpophalangeal joint — *see* Subluxation, metacarpophalangeal (joint), thumb
  toe(s) S93.10-
    great S93.10-
      interphalangeal joint S93.13-
      metatarsophalangeal joint S93.14-
    interphalangeal joint S93.13-
    lesser S93.10-
      interphalangeal joint S93.13-
      metatarsophalangeal joint S93.14-
    metatarsophalangeal joint S93.149
  ulna
    distal end S63.07-
    proximal end — *see* Subluxation, elbow
  ulnohumeral joint — *see* Subluxation, elbow
  vertebral
    recurrent NEC — *see* subcategory M43.5
    traumatic
      cervical S13.100
        atlantoaxial joint S13.120
        atlantooccipital joint S13.110
        atloidooccipital joint S13.110
        joint between
          C0 and C1 S13.110
          C1 and C2 S13.120
          C2 and C3 S13.130
          C3 and C4 S13.140
          C4 and C5 S13.150
          C5and C6 S13.160
          C6and C7 S13.170
          C7and T1 S13.180
        occipitoatloid joint S13.110

Subluxation (*see also* Dislocation) — *continued*
  vertebral — *continued*
    traumatic — *continued*
      lumbar S33.100
        joint between
          L1and L2 S33.110
          L2and L3 S33.120
          L3 and L4 S33.130
          L4and L5 S33.140
      thoracic S23.100
        joint between
          T10 and T11 S23.160
          T11 and T12 S23.162
          T12 and L1 S23.170
          T1and T2 S23.110
          T2and T3 S23.120
          T3 and T4 S23.122
          T4 and T5 S23.130
          T5 and T6 S23.132
          T6 and T7 S23.140
          T7 and T8 S23.142
          T8 and T9 S23.150
          T9 and T10 S23.152
    wrist (carpal bone) S63.00-
      carpometacarpal joint — *see* Subluxation, carpometacarpal (joint)
      distal radioulnar joint — *see* Subluxation, radioulnar (joint), distal
      metacarpal bone, proximal — *see* Subluxation, metacarpal (bone), proximal end
      midcarpal — *see* Subluxation, midcarpal (joint)
      radiocarpal joint — *see* Subluxation, radiocarpal (joint)
      recurrent — *see* Dislocation, recurrent, wrist
      specified site NEC S63.09-
      ulna — *see* Subluxation, ulna, distal end
Submaxillary — *see* condition
Submersion (fatal) (nonfatal) T75.1
Submucous — *see* condition
Subnormal, subnormality
  accommodation (old age) H52.4
  mental — *see* Disability, intellectual
  temperature (accidental) T68
Subphrenic — *see* condition
Subscapular nerve — *see* condition
Subseptus uterus Q51.2
Subsiding appendicitis K36
Substernal thyroid E04.9
  congenital Q89.2
Substitution disorder F44.9
Subtentorial — *see* condition
Subthyroidism (acquired) — *see also* Hypothyroidism
  congenital E03.1
Succenturiate placenta O43.19-
Sucking thumb, child (excessive) F98.8
Sudamen, sudamina L74.1
Sudanese kala-azar B55.0
Sudden
  hearing loss — *see* Deafness, sudden
  heart failure — *see* Failure, heart
Sudeck's atrophy, disease, or syndrome — *see* Algoneurodystrophy
Suffocation — *see* Asphyxia, traumatic
Sugar
  blood
    high (transient) R73.9
    low (transient) E16.2
  in urine R81
Suicide, suicidal (attempted) T14.91
  by poisoning — *see* Table of Drugs and Chemicals
  history of (personal) Z91.5
    in family Z81.8
  ideation — *see* Ideation, suicidal
  risk
    meaning personal history of attempted suicide Z91.5
    meaning suicidal ideation — *see* Ideation, suicidal
  tendencies
    meaning personal history of attempted suicide Z91.5
    meaning suicidal ideation — *see* Ideation, suicidal
  trauma — *see* nature of injury by site

D I S E A S E   **I N D E X**

Suipestifer infection — *see* Infection, salmonella
Sulfhemoglobinemia, sulphemoglobinemia (acquired) (with methemoglobinemia) D74.8
Sumatran mite fever A75.3
Summer — *see* condition
Sunburn L55.9
  first degree L55.0
  second degree L55.1
  third degree L55.2
SUNCT (short lasting unilateral neuralgiform headache with conjunctival injection and tearing) G44.059
  intractable G44.051
  not intractable G44.059
Sunken acetabulum — *see* Derangement, joint, specified type NEC, hip
Sunstroke T67.0
Superfecundation — *see* Pregnancy, multiple
Superfetation — *see* Pregnancy, multiple
Superinvolution (uterus) N85.8
Supernumerary (congenital)
  aortic cusps Q23.8
  auditory ossicles Q16.3
  bone Q79.8
  breast Q83.1
  carpal bones Q74.0
  cusps, heart valve NEC Q24.8
    aortic Q23.8
    mitral Q23.2
    pulmonary Q22.3
  digit(s) Q69.9
  ear (lobule) Q17.0
  fallopian tube Q50.6
  finger Q69.0
  hymen Q52.4
  kidney Q63.0
  lacrimonasal duct Q10.6
  lobule (ear) Q17.0
  mitral cusps Q23.2
  muscle Q79.8
  nipple(s) Q83.3
  organ or site not listed — *see* Accessory
  ossicles, auditory Q16.3
  ovary Q50.31
  oviduct Q50.6
  pulmonary, pulmonic cusps Q22.3
  rib Q76.6
    cervical or first (syndrome) Q76.5
  roots (of teeth) K00.2
  spleen Q89.09
  tarsal bones Q74.2
  teeth K00.1
  testis Q55.29
  thumb Q69.1
  toe Q69.2
  uterus Q51.2
  vagina Q52.1
  vertebra Q76.49
Supervision (of)
  contraceptive — *see* Prescription, contraceptives
  dietary (for) Z71.3
    allergy (food) Z71.3
    colitis Z71.3
    diabetes mellitus Z71.3
    food allergy or intolerance Z71.3
    gastritis Z71.3
    hypercholesterolemia Z71.3
    hypoglycemia Z71.3
    intolerance (food) Z71.3
    obesity Z71.3
    specified NEC Z71.3
  healthy infant or child Z76.2
    foundling Z76.1
  high-risk pregnancy — *see* Pregnancy, complicated by, high, risk
  lactation Z39.1
  pregnancy — *see* Pregnancy, supervision of
Supplemental teeth K00.1
Suppression
  binocular vision H53.34
  lactation O92.5
  menstruation N94.89
  ovarian secretion E28.39
  renal N28.9
  urine, urinary secretion R34
Suppuration, suppurative — *see also* condition
  accessory sinus (chronic) — *see* Sinusitis
  adrenal gland
  antrum (chronic) — *see* Sinusitis, maxillary
  bladder — *see* Cystitis
  brain G06.0
    sequelae G09

Suppuration, suppurative (*see also* condition) — *continued*
  breast N61
    puerperal, postpartum or gestational — *see* Mastitis, obstetric, purulent
  dental periosteum M27.3
  ear (middle) — *see also* Otitis, media
    external NEC — *see* Otitis, externa, infective
    internal — *see* subcategory H83.0
  ethmoidal (chronic) (sinus) — *see* Sinusitis, ethmoidal
  fallopian tube — *see* Salpingo-oophoritis
  frontal (chronic) (sinus) — *see* Sinusitis, frontal
  gallbladder (acute) K81.0
  gum K05.20
    generalized K05.22
    localized K05.21
  intracranial G06.0
  joint — *see* Arthritis, pyogenic or pyemic
  labyrinthine — *see* subcategory H83.0
  lung — *see* Abscess, lung
  mammary gland N61
    puerperal, postpartum O91.12
      associated with lactation O91.13
  maxilla, maxillary M27.2
    sinus (chronic) — *see* Sinusitis, maxillary
  muscle — *see* Myositis, infective
  nasal sinus (chronic) — *see* Sinusitis
  pancreas, acute K85.8
  parotid gland — *see* Sialoadenitis
  pelvis, pelvic
    female — *see* Disease, pelvis, inflammatory
    male K65.0
  pericranial — *see* Osteomyelitis
  salivary duct or gland (any) — *see* Sialoadenitis
  sinus (accessory) (chronic) (nasal) — *see* Sinusitis
  sphenoidal sinus (chronic) — *see* Sinusitis, sphenoidal
  thymus (gland) E32.1
  thyroid (gland) E06.0
  tonsil — *see* Tonsillitis
  uterus — *see* Endometritis
Supraeruption of tooth (teeth) M26.34
Supraglottitis J04.30
  with obstruction J04.31
Suprarenal (gland) — *see* condition
Suprascapular nerve — *see* condition
Suprasellar — *see* condition
Surfer's knots or nodules S89.8-
Surgical
  emphysema T81.82
  procedures, complication or misadventure — *see* Complications, surgical procedures
  shock T81.10
Surveillance (of) (for) — *see also* Observation
  alcohol abuse Z71.41
  contraceptive — *see* Prescription, contraceptives
  dietary Z71.3
  drug abuse Z71.51
Susceptibility to disease, genetic Z15.89
  malignant neoplasm Z15.09
    breast Z15.01
    endometrium Z15.04
    ovary Z15.02
    prostate Z15.03
    specified NEC Z15.09
  multiple endocrine neoplasia Z15.81
Suspected condition, ruled out — *see also* Observation, suspected
  amniotic cavity and membrane Z03.71
  cervical shortening Z03.75
  fetal anomaly Z03.73
  fetal growth Z03.74
  maternal and fetal conditions NEC Z03.79
  oligohydramnios Z03.71
  placental problem Z03.72
  polyhydramnios Z03.71
Suspended uterus
  in pregnancy or childbirth — *see* Pregnancy, complicated by, abnormal uterus
Sutton's nevus D22.9

Suture
  burst (in operation wound) T81.31
    external operation wound T81.31
    internal operation wound T81.32
  inadvertently left in operation wound — *see* Foreign body, accidentally left during a procedure
  removal Z48.02
Swab inadvertently left in operation wound — *see* Foreign body, accidentally left during a procedure
Swallowed, swallowing
  difficulty — *see* Dysphagia
  foreign body — *see* Foreign body, alimentary tract
Swan-neck deformity (finger) — *see* Deformity, finger, swan-neck
Swearing, compulsive F42
  in Gilles de la Tourette's syndrome F95.2
Sweat, sweats
  fetid L75.0
  night R61
Sweating, excessive R61
Sweeley-Klionsky disease E75.21
Sweet's disease or dermatosis L98.2
Swelling (of) R60.9
  abdomen, abdominal (not referable to any particular organ) — *see* Mass, abdominal
  ankle — *see* Effusion, joint, ankle
  arm M79.89
    forearm M79.89
  breast N63
  Calabar B74.3
  cervical gland R59.0
  chest, localized R22.2
  ear H93.8-
  extremity (lower) (upper) — *see* Disorder, soft tissue, specified type NEC
  finger M79.89
  foot M79.89
  glands R59.9
    generalized R59.1
    localized R59.0
  hand M79.89
  head (localized) R22.0
  inflammatory — *see* Inflammation
  intra-abdominal — *see* Mass, abdominal
  joint — *see* Effusion, joint
  leg M79.89
    lower M79.89
  limb — *see* Disorder, soft tissue, specified type NEC
  localized (skin) R22.9
    chest R22.2
    head R22.0
    limb
      lower — *see* Mass, localized, limb, lower
      upper — *see* Mass, localized, limb, upper
    neck R22.1
    trunk R22.2
  neck (localized) R22.1
  pelvic — *see* Mass, abdominal
  scrotum N50.8
  splenic — *see* Splenomegaly
  testis N50.8
  toe M79.89
  umbilical R19.09
  wandering, due to Gnathostoma (spinigerum) B83.1
  white — *see* Tuberculosis, arthritis
Swift(-Feer) disease
  overdose or wrong substance given or taken — *see* Table of Drugs and Chemicals, by drug, poisoning
Swimmer's
  cramp T75.1
  ear H60.33-
  itch B65.3
Swimming in the head R42
Swollen — *see* Swelling
Swyer syndrome Q99.1
Sycosis L73.8
  barbae (not parasitic) L73.8
  contagiosa (mycotic) B35.0
  lupoides L73.8
  mycotic B35.0
  parasitic B35.0
  vulgaris L73.8
Sydenham's chorea — *see* Chorea, Sydenham's
Sylvatic yellow fever A95.0
Sylvest's disease B33.0
Symblepharon H11.23-
  congenital Q10.3

Symond's syndrome G93.2
Sympathetic — *see* condition
Sympatheticotonia G90.8
Sympathicoblastoma
  specified site — *see* Neoplasm, malignant, by site
  unspecified site C74.90
Sympathogonioma — *see* Sympathicoblastoma
Symphalangy (fingers) (toes) Q70.9
Symptoms NEC R68.89
  breast NEC N64.59
  development NEC R63.8
  factitious, self-induced — *see* Disorder, factitious
  genital organs, female R10.2
  involving
    abdomen NEC R19.8
    appearance NEC R46.89
    awareness R41.9
      altered mental status R41.82
      amnesia — *see* Amnesia
      borderline intellectual functioning R41.83
      coma — *see* Coma
      disorientation R41.0
      neurologic neglect syndrome R41.4
      senile cognitive decline R41.81
      specified symptom NEC R41.89
    behavior NEC R46.89
    cardiovascular system NEC R09.89
    chest NEC R09.89
    circulatory system NEC R09.89
    cognitive functions R41.9
      altered mental status R41.82
      amnesia — *see* Amnesia
      borderline intellectual functioning R41.83
      coma — *see* Coma
      disorientation R41.0
      neurologic neglect syndrome R41.4
      senile cognitive decline R41.81
      specified symptom NEC R41.89
    development NEC R62.50
    digestive system NEC R19.8
    emotional state NEC R45.89
      emotional lability R45.86
    food and fluid intake R63.8
    general perceptions and sensations R44.9
      specified NEC R44.8
    musculoskeletal system R29.91
      specified NEC R29.898
    nervous system R29.90
      specified NEC R29.818
    pelvis NEC R19.8
    respiratory system NEC R09.89
    skin and integument R23.9
    urinary system R39.9
  menopausal N95.1
  metabolism NEC R63.8
  neurotic F48.8
  of infancy R68.19
  pelvis NEC, female R10.2
  skin and integument NEC R23.9
  subcutaneous tissue NEC R23.9
Sympus Q74.2
Syncephalus Q89.4
Synchondrosis
  abnormal (congenital) Q78.8
  ischiopubic M91.0
Synchysis (scintillans) (senile) (vitreous body) H43.89
Syncope (near) (pre-) R55
  anginosa I20.8
  bradycardia R00.1
  cardiac R55
  carotid sinus G90.01
  due to spinal (lumbar) puncture G97.1
  heart R55
  heat T67.1
  laryngeal R05
  psychogenic F48.8
  tussive R05
  vasoconstriction R55
  vasodepressor R55
  vasomotor R55
  vasovagal R55
Syndactylism, syndactyly Q70.9
  complex (with synostosis)
    fingers Q70.0-
    toes Q70.2-
  simple (without synostosis)
    fingers Q70.1-
    toes Q70.3-

Syndrome — see also Disease
48,XXXX Q97.1
49,XXXXX Q97.1
5q minus NOS D46.C
abdominal
    acute R10.0
    muscle deficiency Q79.4
abnormal innervation H02.519
    left H02.516
        lower H02.515
        upper H02.514
    right H02.513
        lower H02.512
        upper H02.511
abstinence, neonatal P96.1
acid pulmonary aspiration, obstetric O74.0
acquired immunodeficiency — see Human,
    immunodeficiency virus (HIV)
    disease
acute abdominal R10.0
acute respiratory distress (adult) (child) J80
Adair-Dighton Q78.0
Adams-Stokes(-Morgagni) I45.9
adiposogenital E23.6
adrenal
    hemorrhage (meningococcal) A39.1
    meningococcic A39.1
adrenocortical — see Cushing's, syndrome
adrenogenital E25.9
    congenital, associated with enzyme
        deficiency E25.0
afferent loop NEC K91.89
Alagille's Q44.7
alcohol withdrawal (without convulsions)
    — see Dependence, alcohol, with,
    withdrawal
Alder's D72.0
Aldrich(-Wiskott) D82.0
alien hand R41.4
Alport Q87.81
alveolar hypoventilation E66.2
alveolocapillary block J84.10
amnesic, amnestic (confabulatory) (due to)
    — see Disorder, amnesic
amyostatic (Wilson's disease) E83.01
androgen insensitivity E34.50
    complete E34.51
    partial E34.52
androgen resistance (see also Syndrome,
    androgen insensitivity) E34.50
Angelman Q93.5
anginal — see Angina
ankyloglossia superior Q38.1
anterior
    chest wall R07.89
    cord G83.82
    spinal artery G95.19
        compression M47.019
            cervical region M47.012
            cervicothoracic region M47.013
            lumbar region M47.016
            occipito-atlanto-axial region
                M47.011
            thoracic region M47.014
            thoracolumbar region M47.015
    tibial M76.81-
antibody deficiency D80.9
    agammaglobulinemic D80.1
        hereditary D80.0
    congenital D80.0
    hypogammaglobulinemic D80.1
        hereditary D80.0
anticardiolipin (-antibody) D68.61
antiphospholipid (-antibody) D68.61
aortic
    arch M31.4
    bifurcation I74.09
aortomesenteric duodenum occlusion
    K31.5
apical ballooning (transient left ventricular)
    I51.81
arcuate ligament I77.4
argentaffin, argentaffinoma E34.0
Arnold-Chiari — see Arnold-Chiari disease
Arrillaga-Ayerza I27.0
Asherman's N85.6
aspiration, of newborn — see Aspiration,
    by substance, with pneumonia
    meconium P24.01
ataxia-telangiectasia G11.3
auriculotemporal G50.8
autoerythrocyte sensitization (Gardner-
    Diamond) D69.2
autoimmune lymphoproliferative [ALPS]
    D89.82
autoimmune polyglandular E31.0
autoimmune — see Abnormal, autosomes

Syndrome (see also Disease) — continued
Avellis' G46.8
Ayerza(-Arrillaga) I27.0
Babinski-Nageotte G83.89
Bakwin-Krida Q79.8
bare lymphocyte D81.6
Barrett's — see Barrett's, esophagus
Barré-Guillain G61.0
Barré-Liéou M53.0
Barsony-Polgar K22.4
Barsony-Teschendorf K22.4
Barth E78.71
Bartter's E26.81
basal cell nevus Q87.89
Basedow's E05.00
    with thyroid storm E05.01
basilar artery G45.0
Batten-Steinert G71.11
battered
    baby or child — see Maltreatment, child,
        physical abuse
    spouse — see Maltreatment, adult,
        physical abuse
Beals Q87.40
Beau's I51.5
Beck's I65.8
Benedikt's G46.3
Béquez César (-Steinbrinck-Chédiak-
    Higashi) E70.330
Bernhardt-Roth — see Meralgia
    paresthetica
Bernheim's I50.9
big spleen D73.1
bilateral polycystic ovarian E28.2
Bing-Horton's — see Horton's headache
Birt-Hogg-Dube syndrome Q87.89
Björck(-Thorsen) E34.0
black
    lung J60
        widow spider bite — see Toxicity,
            venom, spider, black widow
Blackfan-Diamond D61.01
blind loop K90.2
    congenital Q43.8
    postsurgical K91.2
blue sclera Q78.0
blue toe I75.02-
Boder-Sedgewick G11.3
Boerhaave's K22.3
Borjeson Forssman Lehmann Q89.8
Bouillaud's I01.9
Bourneville(-Pringle) Q85.1
Bouveret(-Hoffman) I47.9
brachial plexus G54.0
bradycardia-tachycardia I49.5
brain (nonpsychotic) F09
    with psychosis, psychotic reaction F09
    acute or subacute — see Delirium
    congenital — see Disability, intellectual
    organic F09
        post-traumatic (nonpsychotic) F07.81
        psychotic F09
    personality change F07.0
    post-traumatic, nonpsychotic F07.81
    postcontusional F07.81
    psycho-organic F09
    psychotic F06.8
brain stem stroke G46.3
Brandt's (acrodermatitis enteropathica)
    E83.2
broad ligament laceration N83.8
Brock's J98.11
bronze baby P83.8
Brown-Sequard G83.81
bubbly lung P27.0
Buchem's M85.2
Budd-Chiari I82.0
bulbar (progressive) G12.22
Bürger-Grütz E78.3
Burke's K86.8
Burnett's (milk-alkali) E83.52
burning feet E53.9
Bywaters' T79.5
Call-Fleming I67.841
carbohydrate-deficient glycoprotein
    (CDGS) E77.8
carcinogenic thrombophlebitis I82.1
carcinoid E34.0
cardiac asthma I50.1
cardiacos negros I27.0
cardiofaciocutaneous Q87.89
cardiopulmonary-obesity E66.2
cardiorenal — see Hypertension,
    cardiorenal
cardiorespiratory distress (idiopathic),
    newborn P22.0
cardiovascular renal — see Hypertension,
    cardiorenal

Syndrome (see also Disease) — continued
carotid
    artery (hemispheric) (internal) G45.1
    body G90.01
    sinus G90.01
carpal tunnel G56.0-
Cassidy(-Scholte) E34.0
cat cry Q93.4
cat eye Q92.8
cauda equina G83.4
causalgia — see Causalgia
celiac K90.0
    artery compression I77.4
    axis I77.4
central pain G89.0
cerebellar
    hereditary G11.9
    stroke G46.4
cerebellomedullary malformation — see
    Spina bifida
cerebral
    artery
        anterior G46.1
        middle G46.0
        posterior G46.2
    gigantism E22.0
cervical (root) M53.1
    disc — see Disorder, disc, cervical, with
        neuritis
    fusion Q76.1
    posterior, sympathicus M53.0
    rib Q76.5
    sympathetic paralysis G90.2
cervicobrachial (diffuse) M53.1
cervicocranial M53.0
cervicodorsal outlet G54.2
cervicothoracic outlet G54.0
Céstan(-Raymond) I65.8
Charcot's (angina cruris) (intermittent
    claudication) I73.9
Charcot-Weiss-Baker G90.09
CHARGE Q89.8
Chédiak-Higashi(-Steinbrinck) E70.330
chest wall R07.1
Chiari (hepatic vein thrombosis) I82.0
Chilaiditi's Q43.3
child maltreatment — see Maltreatment,
    child
chondrocostal junction M94.0
chondroectodermal dysplasia Q77.6
chromosome 4 short arm deletion Q93.3
chromosome 5 short arm deletion Q93.4
chronic
    pain G89.4
    personality F68.8
Clarke-Hadfield K86.8
Clerambault's automatism G93.89
Clouston's (hidrotic ectodermal dysplasia)
    Q82.4
clumsiness, clumsy child F82
cluster headache G44.009
    intractable G44.001
    not intractable G44.009
Coffin-Lowry Q89.8
cold injury (newborn) P80.0
combined immunity deficiency D81.9
compartment (deep) (posterior) (traumatic)
    T79.A0
    abdomen T79.A3
    lower extremity (hip, buttock, thigh, leg,
        foot, toes) T79.A2
    nontraumatic
        abdomen M79.A3
        lower extremity (hip, buttock, thigh,
            leg, foot, toes) M79.A2-
        specified site NEC M79.A9
        upper extremity (shoulder, arm,
            forearm, wrist, hand, fingers)
            M79.A1-
    postprocedural — see Syndrome,
        compartment, nontraumatic
    specified site NEC T79.A9
    upper extremity (shoulder, arm, forearm,
        wrist, hand, fingers) T79.A1
complex regional pain — see Syndrome,
    pain, complex regional
compression T79.5
    anterior spinal — see Syndrome,
        anterior, spinal artery, compression
    cauda equina G83.4
    celiac artery I77.4
    vertebral artery M47.029
        cervical region M47.022
        occipito-atlanto-axial region M47.021
concussion F07.81

Syndrome (see also Disease) — continued
congenital
    affecting multiple systems NEC Q87.89
    central alveolar hypoventilation G47.35
    facial diplegia Q87.0
    muscular hypertrophy-cerebral Q87.89
    oculo-auriculovertebral Q87.0
    oculofacial diplegia (Moebius) Q87.0
    rubella (manifest) P35.0
congestion-fibrosis (pelvic), female N94.89
congestive dysmenorrhea N94.6
Conn's E26.01
connective tissue M35.9
    overlap NEC M35.1
conus medullaris G95.81
cord
    anterior G83.82
    posterior G83.83
coronary
    acute NEC I24.9
    insufficiency or intermediate I20.0
    slow flow I20.8
Costen's (complex) M26.69
costochondral junction M94.0
costoclavicular G54.0
costovertebral E22.0
Cowden Q85.8
craniovertebral M53.0
Creutzfeldt-Jakob — see Creutzfeldt-Jakob
    disease or syndrome
crib death R99
cricopharyngeal — see Dysphagia
cri-du-chat Q93.4
croup J05.0
CRPS I — see Syndrome, pain, complex
    regional I
crush T79.5
cryptophthalmos Q87.0
cubital tunnel — see Lesion, nerve, ulnar
Curschmann (-Batten) (-Steinert) G71.11
Cushing's E24.9
    alcohol-induced E24.4
    drug-induced E24.2
    due to
        alcohol
        drugs E24.2
        ectopic ACTH E24.3
        overproduction of pituitary ACTH
            E24.0
        overdose or wrong substance given or
            taken — see Table of Drugs and
            Chemicals, by drug, poisoning
    pituitary-dependent E24.0
    specified type NEC E24.8
cystic duct stump K91.5
Dana-Putnam D51.0
Danbolt (-Cross) (acrodermatitis
    enteropathica) E83.2
Dandy-Walker Q03.1
    with spina bifida Q07.01
Danlos' Q79.8
De Quervain E34.51
de Toni-Fanconi (-Debré) E72.09
    with cystinosis E72.04
defibrination — see also Fibrinolysis
    with
        antepartum hemorrhage — see
            Hemorrhage, antepartum, with
            coagulation defect
        intrapartum hemorrhage — see
            Hemorrhage, complicating,
            delivery
    newborn P60
    postpartum O72.3
Degos' I77.89
Déjérine-Roussy G89.0
delayed sleep phase G47.21
demyelinating G37.9
dependence — see F10-F19 with fourth
    character .2
depersonalization(-derealization) F48.1
diabetes mellitus in newborn infant P70.2
diabetes mellitus-hypertension-nephrosis
    — see Diabetes, nephrosis
diabetes-nephrosis — see Diabetes,
    nephrosis
diabetic amyotrophy — see Diabetes,
    amyotrophy
Diamond-Blackfan D61.01
Diamond-Gardener D69.2
DIC (diffuse or disseminated intravascular
    coagulopathy) D65
di George's D82.1
Dighton's Q78.0
disequilibrium E87.8
Döhle body-panmyelopathic D72.0
dorsolateral medullary G46.4
double athetosis G80.3

me

Syndrome (see also Disease) — continued

...me (see also Disease) — continued
...wn (see also Down syndrome) Q90.9
...esbach's (elliptocytosis) D58.1
Dressler's (postmyocardial infarction) I24.1
postcardiotomy I97.0
drug withdrawal, infant of dependent mother P96.1
dry eye H04.12-
due to abnormality
chromosomal Q99.9
sex
female phenotype Q97.9
male phenotype Q98.9
specified NEC Q99.8
dumping (postgastrectomy) K91.1
nonsurgical K31.89
Dupré's (meningism) R29.1
dysmetabolic X E88.81
dyspraxia, developmental F82
Eagle-Barrett Q79.4
Eaton-Lambert — see Syndrome, Lambert-Eaton
Ebstein's Q22.5
ectopic ACTH E24.3
eczema-thrombocytopenia D82.0
Eddowes' Q78.0
effort (psychogenic) F45.8
Ehlers-Danlos Q79.6
Eisenmenger's I27.89
Ekman's Q78.0
electric feet E53.8
Ellis-van Creveld Q77.6
empty nest Z60.0
endocrine-hypertensive E27.0
entrapment — see Neuropathy, entrapment
eosinophilia-myalgia M35.8
epileptic — see also Epilepsy, by type
absence G40.A09
intractable G40.A19
with status epilepticus G40.A11
without status epilepticus G40.A19
not intractable G40.A09
with status epilepticus G40.A01
without status epilepticus G40.A09
Erdheim-Chester (ECD) E88.89
Erdheim's E22.0
erythrocyte fragmentation D59.4
Evans D69.41
exhaustion F48.8
extrapyramidal G25.9
specified NEC G25.89
eye retraction — see Strabismus
eyelid-malar-mandible Q87.0
Faber's D50.9
facial pain, paroxysmal G50.0
Fallot's Q21.3
familial eczema-thrombocytopenia (Wiskott-Aldrich) D82.0
Fanconi (-de Toni) (-Debré) E72.09
with cystinosis E72.04
Fanconi's (anemia) (congenital pancytopenia) D61.09
fatigue
chronic R53.82
psychogenic F48.8
faulty bowel habit K59.3
Feil-Klippel (brevicollis) Q76.1
Felty's — see Felty's syndrome
fertile eunuch E23.0
fetal
alcohol (dysmorphic) Q86.0
hydantoin Q86.1
Fiedler's I40.1
first arch Q87.0
fish odor E72.8
Fisher's G61.0
Fitz's K85.8
Fitzhugh-Curtis
due to
Chlamydia trachomatis A74.81
Neisseria gonorrhoea (gonococcal peritonitis) A54.85
Flajani (-Basedow) E05.00
with thyroid storm E05.01
flatback — see Flatback syndrome
floppy
baby P94.2
iris (intraoperative) (IFIS) H21.81
mitral valve I34.1
flush E34.0
Foix-Alajouanine G95.19
Fong's Q79.8
foramen magnum G93.5
Foster-Kennedy H47.14-
Foville's (peduncular) G46.3
fragile X Q99.2
Franceschetti Q75.4

Syndrome (see also Disease) — continued
Frey's
auriculotemporal G50.8
hyperhidrosis L74.52
Friderichsen-Waterhouse A39.1
Froin's G95.89
frontal lobe F07.0
Fukuhara E88.49
functional
bowel K59.9
prepubertal castrate E29.1
Gaisböck's D75.1
ganglion (basal ganglia brain) G25.9
geniculi G51.1
Gardner-Diamond D69.2
gastroesophageal
junction K22.0
laceration-hemorrhage K22.6
gastrojejunal loop obstruction K91.89
Gee-Herter-Heubner K90.0
Gelineau's G47.419
with cataplexy G47.411
genito-anorectal A55
Gerstmann-Sträussler-Scheinker (GSS) A81.82
Gianotti-Crosti L44.4
giant platelet (Bernard-Soulier) D69.1
Gilles de la Tourette's F95.2
goiter-deafness E07.1
Goldberg Q89.8
Goldberg-Maxwell E34.51
Good's D83.8
Gopalan' (burning feet) E53.8
Gorlin's Q87.89
Gougerot-Blum L81.7
Gouley's I31.1
Gower's R55
gray or grey (newborn) P93.0
platelet D69.1
Gubler-Millard G46.3
Guillain-Barré (-Strohl) G61.0
gustatory sweating G50.8
Hadfield-Clarke K86.8
hair tourniquet — see Constriction, external, by site
Hamman's J98.19
hand-foot L27.1
hand-shoulder G90.8
hantavirus (cardio)-pulmonary (HPS) (HCPS) B33.4
happy puppet Q93.5
Harada's H30.81-
Hayem-Faber D50.9
headache NEC G44.89
complicated NEC G44.59
Heberden's I20.8
Hedinger's E34.0
Hegglin's D72.0
HELLP (hemolysis, elevated liver enzymes and low platelet count) O14.2-
hemolytic-uremic D59.3
hemophagocytic, infection-associated D76.2
Henoch-Schönlein D69.0
hepatic flexure K59.8
hepatopulmonary K76.81
hepatorenal K76.7
following delivery O90.4
postoperative or postprocedural K91.83
postpartum, puerperal O90.4
hepatourologic K76.7
Herter (-Gee) (nontropical sprue) K90.0
Heubner-Herter K90.0
Heyd's K76.7
Hilger's G90.09
histamine-like (fish poisoning) — see Poisoning, fish
histiocytic D76.3
histiocytosis NEC D76.3
HIV infection, acute B20
Hoffmann-Werdnig G12.0
Hollander-Simons E88.1
Hoppe-Goldflam G70.00
with exacerbation (acute) G70.01
in crisis G70.01
Horner's G90.2
hungry bone E83.81
hunterian glossitis D51.0
Hutchinson's triad A50.53
hyperabduction G54.0
hyperammonemia-hyperornithinemia-homocitrullinemia E72.4
hypereosinophilic (idiopathic) D72.1
hyperimmunoglobulin E (IgE) D82.4
hyperkalemic E87.5
hyperkinetic — see Hyperkinesia
hypermobility M35.7
hypernatremia E87.0
hyperosmolarity E87.0
hyperperfusion G97.82

Syndrome (see also Disease) — continued
hypersplenic D73.1
hypertransfusion, newborn P61.1
hyperventilation F45.8
hyperviscosity (of serum)
polycythemic D75.1
sclerothymic D58.8
hypoglycemic (familial) (neonatal) E16.2
hypokalemic E87.6
hyponatremic E87.1
hypopituitarism E23.0
hypoplastic left-heart Q23.4
hypopotassemia E87.6
hyposmolality E87.1
hypotension, maternal O26.5-
hypothenar hammer I73.89
ICF (intravascular coagulation-fibrinolysis) D65
idiopathic
cardiorespiratory distress, newborn P22.0
nephrotic (infantile) N04.9
iliotibial band M76.3-
immobility, immobilization (paraplegic) M62.3
immune reconstitution D89.3
immune reconstitution inflammatory [IRIS] D89.3
immunity deficiency, combined D81.9
immunodeficiency
acquired — see Human, immunodeficiency virus (HIV) disease
combined D81.9
impending coronary I20.0
impingement, shoulder M75.4-
inappropriate secretion of antidiuretic hormone E22.2
infant
gestational diabetes P70.0
of diabetic mother P70.1
infantilism (pituitary) E23.0
inferior vena cava I87.1
inspissated bile (newborn) P59.1
institutional (childhood) F94.2
insufficient sleep F51.12
intermediate coronary (artery) I20.0
interspinous ligament — see Spondylopathy, specified NEC
intestinal
carcinoid E34.0
knot K56.2
intravascular coagulation-fibrinolysis (ICF) D65
iodine-deficiency, congenital E00.9
type
mixed E00.2
myxedematous E00.1
neurological E00.0
IRDS (idiopathic respiratory distress, newborn) P22.0
irritable
bowel K58.9
with diarrhea K58.0
psychogenic F45.8
heart (psychogenic) F45.8
weakness F48.8
ischemic bowel (transient) K55.9
chronic K55.1
due to mesenteric artery insufficiency K55.1
IVC (intravascular coagulopathy) D65
Ivemark's Q89.01
Jaccoud's — see Arthropathy, postrheumatic, chronic
Jackson's G83.89
Jakob-Creutzfeldt — see Creutzfeldt-Jakob disease or syndrome
jaw-winking Q07.8
Jervell-Lange-Nielsen I45.81
jet lag G47.25
Job's D71
Joseph-Diamond-Blackfan D61.01
jugular foramen G52.7
Kabuki Q89.8
Kanner's (autism) F84.0
Kartagener's Q89.3
Kelly's D50.1
Kimmelstiel-Wilson — see Diabetes, specified type, with Kimmelstiel-Wilson disease
Klein(e)-Levine G47.13
Klippel-Feil (brevicollis) Q76.1
Köhler-Pellegrini-Steida — see Bursitis, tibial collateral
König's K59.8
Korsakoff (-Wernicke) (nonalcoholic) F04
alcoholic F10.26
Kostmann's D70.0

Syndrome (see also Disease) — continued
Krabbe's congenital muscle hypoplasia Q79.8
labyrinthine — see subcategory H83.2
lacunar NEC G46.7
Lambert-Eaton G70.80
in
neoplastic disease G73.1
specified disease NEC G70.81
Landau-Kleffner — see Epilepsy, specified NEC
Larsen's Q74.8
lateral
cutaneous nerve of thigh G57.1-
medullary G46.4
Launois' E22.0
lazy
leukocyte D70.8
posture M62.3
Lemiere I80.8
Lennox-Gastaut G40.812
intractable G40.814
with status epilepticus G40.813
without status epilepticus G40.814
not intractable G40.812
with status epilepticus G40.811
without status epilepticus G40.812
lenticular, progressive E83.01
Leopold-Levi's E05.90
Lev's I44.2
Li-Fraumeni Z15.01
Lichtheim's D51.0
Lightwood's N25.89
Lignac (de Toni) (-Fanconi) (-Debré) E72.09
with cystinosis E72.04
Likoff's I20.8
limbic epilepsy personality F07.0
liver-kidney K76.7
lobotomy F07.0
Loffler's J82
long arm 18 or 21 deletion Q93.89
long QT I45.81
Louis-Barré G11.3
low
atmospheric pressure T70.29
back M54.5
output (cardiac) I50.9
lower radicular, newborn (birth injury) P14.8
Luetscher's (dehydration) E86.0
Lupus anticoagulant D68.62
Lutembacher's Q21.1
macrophage activation D76.1
due to infection D76.2
magnesium-deficiency R29.0
Mal de Debarquement R42
malformation, congenital, due to
alcohol Q86.0
exogenous cause NEC Q86.8
hydantoin Q86.1
warfarin Q86.2
malignant
carcinoid E34.0
neuroleptic G21.0
Mallory-Weiss K22.6
mandibulofacial dysostosis Q75.4
manic-depressive — see Disorder, bipolar, affective
maple-syrup-urine E71.0
Marable's I77.4
Marfan's Q87.40
with
cardiovascular manifestations Q87.418
aortic dilation Q87.410
ocular manifestations Q87.42
skeletal manifestations Q87.43
Marie's (acromegaly) E22.0
maternal hypotension — see Syndrome, hypotension, maternal
May (-Hegglin) D72.0
McArdle (-Schmidt) (-Pearson) E74.04
McQuarrie's E16.2
meconium plug (newborn) P76.0
median arcuate ligament I77.4
Meekeren-Ehlers-Danlos Q79.6
megavitamin-B6 E67.2
Meige G24.4
MELAS E88.41
Mendelson's O74.0
MERFF (myoclonic epilepsy associated with ragged-red fibers) E88.42
mesenteric
artery (superior) K55.1
vascular insufficiency K55.1
metabolic E88.81
metastatic carcinoid E34.0
micrognathia-glossoptosis Q87.0
midbrain NEC G93.89

Syndrome (see also Disease) — continued
middle lobe (lung) J98.19
middle radicular G54.0
migraine (see also Migraine) G43.909-
Mikulicz' K11.8
milk-alkali E83.52
Millard-Gubler G46.3
Miller-Dieker Q93.88
Miller-Fisher G61.0
Minkowski-Chauffard D58.0
Mirizzi's K83.1
MNGIE (mitochondrial
neurogastrointestinal encephalopathy)
E88.49
Möbius, ophthalmoplegic migraine — see
Migraine, ophthalmoplegic
monofixation H50.42
Morel-Moore M85.2
Morel-Morgagni M85.2
Morgagni (-Morel) (-Stewart) M85.2
Morgagni-Adams-Stokes I45.9
Mounier-Kuhn Q32.4
with bronchiectasis J47.9
with
exacerbation (acute) J47.1
lower respiratory infection J47.0
acquired J98.09
with bronchiectasis J47.9
with
exacerbation (acute) J47.1
lower respiratory infection J47.0
mucocutaneous lymph node (acute febrile)
(MCLS) M30.3
multiple endocrine neoplasia (MEN) — see
Neoplasia, endocrine, multiple (MEN)
multiple operations — see Disorder,
factitious
myasthenic G70.9
in
diabetes mellitus — see Diabetes,
amyotrophy
endocrine disease NEC E34.9 [G73.3]
neoplastic disease (see also
Neoplasm) D49.9 [G73.3]
thyrotoxicosis (hyperthyroidism)
E05.90 [G73.3]
with thyroid storm E05.91 [G73.3]
myelodysplastic D46.9
with
5q deletion D46.C
isolated del(5q) chromosomal
abnormality D46.C
lesions, low grade D46.20
specified NEC D46.Z
myelopathic pain G89.0
myeloproliferative (chronic) D47.1
myofascial pain M79.1
Naffziger's G54.0
nail patella Q87.2
NARP (Neuropathy, Ataxia and Retinitis
pigmentosa) E88.49
neonatal abstinence P96.1
nephritic (see also Nephritis)
with edema — see Nephrosis
acute N00.9
chronic N03.9
rapidly progressive N01.9
nephrotic (congenital) (see also Nephrosis)
N04.9
with
dense deposit disease N04.6
diffuse
crescentic glomerulonephritis
N04.7
endocapillary proliferative
glomerulonephritis N04.4
membranous glomerulonephritis
N04.2
mesangial proliferative
glomerulonephritis N04.3
mesangiocapillary
glomerulonephritis N04.5
focal and segmental glomerular
lesions N04.1
minor glomerular abnormality N04.0
specified morphological changes NEC
N04.8
diabetic — see Diabetes, nephrosis
neurologic neglect R41.4
Nezelof's D81.4
Nonne-Milroy-Meige Q82.0
Nothnagel's vasomotor acroparesthesia
I73.89
oculomotor H51.9
ophthalmoplegia-cerebellar ataxia — see
Strabismus, paralytic, third nerve
oral-facial-digital Q87.0

Syndrome (see also Disease) — continued
organic
affective F06.30
amnesic (not alcohol-or drug-induced)
F04
brain F09
depressive F06.31
hallucinosis F06.0
personality F07.0
Ormond's N13.5
oro-facial-digital Q87.0
os trigonum Q68.8
Osler-Weber-Rendu I78.0
osteoporosis-osteomalacia M83.8
Ostertreicher-Turner Q79.8
oto-palatal-digital Q87.0
otolith — see subcategory H81.8
outlet (thoracic) G54.0
ovary
polycystic E28.2
resistant E28.39
sclerocystic E28.2
Owren's D68.2
Paget-Schroetter I82.890
pain — see also Pain
complex regional I G90.50
lower limb G90.52-
specified site NEC G90.59
upper limb G90.51-
complex regional II — see Causalgia
painful
bruising D69.2
feet E53.8
prostate N42.81
paralysis agitans — see Parkinsonism
paralytic G83.9
specified NEC G83.89
Parinaud's H51.0
Parkinson's — see Parkinsonism
parkinsonian — see Parkinsonism
paroxysmal facial pain G50.0
Parry's E05.00
with thyroid storm E05.01
Parsonage(-Aldren)-Turner G54.5
patella clunk M25.86-
Paterson(-Brown) (-Kelly) D50.1
pectoral girdle I77.89
pectoralis minor I77.89
Pelger-Huet D72.0
pellagra-cerebellar ataxia-renal
aminoaciduria E72.02
pellagroid E52
Pellegrini-Stieda — see Bursitis, tibial
collateral
pelvic congestion-fibrosis, female N94.89
penta X Q97.1
peptic ulcer — see Ulcer, peptic
perabduction I77.89
periodic headache, in adults and children
— see Headache, periodic syndromes
in adults and children
periurethral fibrosis N13.5
phantom limb (without pain) G54.7
with pain G54.6
pharyngeal pouch D82.1
Pick's (heart) (liver) I31.1
Pickwickian E66.2
PIE (pulmonary infiltration with
eosinophilia) J82
pigmentary pallidal degeneration
(progressive) G23.0
pineal E34.8
pituitary E22.0
placental transfusion — see Pregnancy,
complicated by, placental transfusion
syndromes
plantar fascia M72.2
plateau iris (post-iridectomy)
(postprocedural) H21.82
Plummer-Vinson D50.1
pluricarential of infancy E40
plurideficiency E40
pluriglandular (compensatory) E31.8
autoimmune E31.0
pneumatic hammer T75.21
polyangiitis overlap M30.8
polycarential of infancy E40
polyglandular E31.8
autoimmune E31.0
polysplenia Q89.09
pontine NEC G93.89
popliteal
artery entrapment I77.89
web Q87.89
post chemoembolization — code to
associated conditions
postcardiac injury
postcardiotomy I97.0
postmyocardial infarction I24.1
postcardiotomy I97.0

Syndrome (see also Disease) — continued
postcholecystectomy K91.5
postcommissurotomy I97.0
postconcussional F07.81
postcontusional F07.81
postencephalitic F07.89
posterior
cervical sympathetic M53.0
cord G83.83
fossa compression G93.5
reversible encephalopathy (PRES)
I67.83
postgastrectomy (dumping) K91.1
postgastric surgery K91.1
postinfarction I24.1
postlaminectomy NEC M96.1
postleukotomy F07.0
postmastectomy lymphedema I97.2
postmyocardial infarction I24.1
postoperative NEC T81.9
blind loop K90.2
postpartum panhypopituitary (Sheehan)
E23.0
postpolio (myelitic) G14
postthrombotic I87.009
with
inflammation I87.02-
with ulcer I87.03-
specified complication NEC I87.09-
ulcer I87.01-
with inflammation I87.03-
asymptomatic I87.00-
postvagotomy K91.1
postvalvulotomy I97.0
postviral NEC G93.3
fatigue G93.3
Potain's K31.0
potassium intoxication E87.5
precerebral artery (multiple) (bilateral)
G45.2
preinfarction I20.0
preleukemic D46.9
premature senility E34.8
premenstrual dysphoric N94.3
premenstrual tension N94.3
Prinzmetal-Massumi R07.1
prune belly Q79.4
pseudocarpal tunnel (sublimis) — see
Syndrome, carpal tunnel
pseudoparalytica G70.00
with exacerbation (acute) G70.01
in crisis G70.01
pseudo-Turner's Q87.1
psycho-organic (nonpsychotic severity)
F07.9
acute or subacute F05
depressive type F06.31
hallucinatory type F06.0
nonpsychotic severity F07.0
specified NEC F07.89
pulmonary
arteriosclerosis I27.0
dysmaturity (Wilson-Mikity) P27.0
hypoperfusion (idiopathic) P22.0
renal (hemorrhagic) (Goodpasture's)
M31.0
pure
motor lacunar G46.5
sensory lacunar G46.6
Putnam-Dana D51.0
pyramidopallidonigral G20
pyriformis — see Lesion, nerve, sciatic
QT interval prolongation I45.81
radicular NEC — see Radiculopathy
upper limbs, newborn (birth injury)
P14.3
rapid time-zone change G47.25
Rasmussen G04.81
Raymond (-Céstan) I65.8
Raynaud's I73.00
with gangrene I73.01
RDS (respiratory distress syndrome,
newborn) P22.0
reactive airways dysfunction J68.3
Refsum's G60.1
Reifenstein E34.52
renal glomerulohyalinosis-diabetic — see
Diabetes, nephrosis
Rendu-Osler-Weber I78.0
residual ovary N99.83
resistant ovary E28.39
respiratory
distress
acute J80
adult J80
child J80
newborn (idiopathic) (type I) P22.0
type II P22.1

Syndrome (see also Disease) — continued
restless legs G25.81
retinoblastoma (familial) C69.2
retroperitoneal fibrosis N13.5
retroviral seroconversion (acute) Z21
Reye's G93.7
Richter — see Leukemia, chronic
lymphocytic, B-cell type
Ridley's I50.1
right
heart, hypoplastic Q22.6
ventricular obstruction — see Failure,
heart, congestive
Romano-Ward (prolonged QT interval)
I45.81
rotator cuff, shoulder (see also Tear, rotator
cuff) M75.10-
Rotes Quérol — see Hyperostosis,
ankylosing
Roth — see Meralgia paresthetica
rubella (congenital) P35.0
Ruvalcaba-Myhre-Smith E71.440
Rytand-Lipsitch I44.2
salt
depletion E87.1
due to heat NEC T67.8
causing heat exhaustion or
prostration T67.4
low E87.1
salt-losing N28.89
Scaglietti-Dagnini E22.0
scalenus anticus (anterior) G54.0
scapulocostal — see Mononeuropathy,
upper limb, specified site NEC
scapuloperoneal G71.0
schizophrenic, of childhood NEC F84.5
Schnitzler D47.2
Scholte's E34.0
Schroeder's E27.0
Schüller-Christian C96.5
Schwachman's — see Syndrome,
Shwachman's
Schwartz (-Jampel) G71.13
Schwartz-Bartter E22.2
scimitar Q26.8
sclerocystic ovary E28.2
Seitelberger's G31.89
septicemic adrenal hemorrhage A39.1
seroconversion, retroviral (acute) Z21
serous meningitis G93.2
severe acute respiratory (SARS) J12.81
shaken infant T74.4
shock (traumatic) T79.4
kidney N17.0
following crush injury T79.5
toxic A48.3
shock-lung J80
Shone's — code to specific anomalies
short
bowel K91.2
rib Q77.2
shoulder-hand — see Algoneurodystrophy
Shwachman's D70.4
sicca — see Sicca syndrome
sick
cell E87.1
sinus I49.5
sick-euthyroid E07.81
sideropenic D50.1
Siemens' ectodermal dysplasia Q82.4
Silfverskiöld's Q78.9
Simons' E88.1
sinus tarsi M25.57-
sinusitis-bronchiectasis-situs inversus
Q89.3
Sipple's E31.22
sirenomelia Q87.2
Slocumb's E27.0
slow flow, coronary I20.8
Sluder's G44.89
Smith-Magenis Q93.88
Sneddon-Wilkinson L13.1
Sotos' E22.0
South African cardiomyopathy I42.8
spasmodic
upward movement, eyes H51.8
winking F95.8
Spen's I45.9
splenic
agenesis Q89.01
flexure K59.8
neutropenia D73.81
Spurway's Q78.0
staphylococcal scalded skin L00
Stein-Leventhal E28.2
Stein's E28.2

DISEASE INDEX

drome (see also Disease) — continued
Stevens-Johnson syndrome L51.1
  toxic epidermal necrolysis overlap L51.3
Stewart-Morel M85.2
Stickler Q89.8
stiff baby Q89.8
stiff man G25.82
Still-Felty — see Felty's syndrome
Stokes (-Adams) I45.9
stone heart I50.1
straight back, congenital Q76.49
subclavian steal G45.8
subcoracoid-pectoralis minor G54.0
subcostal nerve compression I77.89
subphrenic interposition Q43.3
superior
  cerebellar artery I63.8
  mesenteric artery K55.1
  semi-circular canal dehiscence H83.8X-
  vena cava I87.1
supine hypotensive (maternal) — see
  Syndrome, hypotension, maternal
suprarenal cortical E27.0
supraspinatus (see also Tear, rotator cuff)
  M75.10-
Susac G93.49
swallowed blood P78.2
sweat retention L74.0
Swyer Q99.1
Symond's G93.2
sympathetic
  cervical paralysis G90.2
  pelvic, female N94.89
systemic inflammatory response (SIRS), of
  non-infectious origin (without organ
  dysfunction) R65.10
    with acute organ dysfunction R65.11
tachycardia-bradycardia I49.5
takotsubo I51.81
TAR (thrombocytopenia with absent
  radius) Q87.2
tarsal tunnel G57.5-
teething K00.7
tegmental G93.89
telangiectasic-pigmentation-cataract Q82.8
temporal pyramidal apex — see Otitis,
  media, suppurative, acute
temporomandibular joint-pain-dysfunction
  M26.62
Terry's H44.2-
testicular feminization (see also Syndrome,
  androgen insensitivity) E34.51
thalamic pain (hyperesthetic) G89.0
thoracic outlet (compression) G54.0
Thorson-Björck E34.0
thrombocytopenia with absent radius
  (TAR) Q87.2
thyroid-adrenocortical insufficiency E31.0
tibial
  anterior M76.81-
  posterior M76.82-
Tietze's M94.0
time-zone (rapid) G47.25
Toni-Fanconi E72.09
  with cystinosis E72.04
Touraine's Q79.8
tourniquet — see Constriction, external, by
  site
toxic shock A48.3
transient left ventricular apical ballooning
  I51.81
traumatic vasospastic T75.22
Treacher Collins Q75.4
triple X, female Q97.0
trisomy Q92.9
  13 Q91.7
    meiotic nondisjunction Q91.4
    mitotic nondisjunction Q91.5
    mosaicism Q91.5
    translocation Q91.6
  18 Q91.3
    meiotic nondisjunction Q91.0
    mitotic nondisjunction Q91.1
    mosaicism Q91.1
    translocation Q91.2
  20(q) (p) Q92.8
  21 Q90.9
    meiotic nondisjunction Q90.0
    mitotic nondisjunction Q90.1
    mosaicism Q90.1
    translocation Q90.2
  22 Q92.8
tropical wet feet T69.0-
Trousseau's I82.1
tumor lysis (following antineoplastic
  chemotherapy) (spontaneous) NEC
  E88.3

Syndrome (see also Disease) — continued
Twiddler's (due to)
  automatic implantable defibrillator
    T82.198
  cardiac pacemaker T82.198
Unverricht (-Lundborg) — see Epilepsy,
  generalized, idiopathic
upward gaze H51.8
uremia, chronic (see also Disease, kidney,
  chronic) N18.9
urethral N34.3
urethro-oculo-articular — see Reiter's
  disease
urohepatic K76.7
vago-hypoglossal G52.7
van Buchem's M85.2
van der Hoeve's Q78.0
vascular NEC in cerebrovascular disease
  G46.8
vasoconstriction, reversible
  cerebrovascular I67.841
vasomotor I73.9
vasospastic (traumatic) T75.22
vasovagal R55
VATER Q87.2
velo-cardio-facial Q93.81
vena cava (inferior) (superior)
  (obstruction) I87.1
vertebral
  artery G45.0
    compression — see Syndrome,
      anterior, spinal artery,
      compression
    steal G45.0
vertebro-basilar artery G45.0
vertebrogenic (pain) M54.89
vertiginous — see Disorder, vestibular
  function
Vinson-Plummer D50.1
virus B34.9
visceral larva migrans B83.0
visual disorientation H53.8
vitamin B6 deficiency E53.1
vitreal corneal H59.01-
vitreous (touch) H59.01-
Vogt-Koyanagi H20.82-
Volkmann's T79.6
von Schroetter's I82.890
von Willebrand (-Jürgen) D68.0
Waldenström-Kjellberg D50.1
Wallenberg's G46.3
water retention E87.79
Waterhouse (-Friderichsen) A39.1
Weber-Gubler G46.3
Weber-Leyden G46.3
Weber's G46.3
Wegener's M31.30
  with
    kidney involvement M31.31
    lung involvement M31.30
      with kidney involvement M31.31
Weingarten's (tropical eosinophilia) J82
Weiss-Baker G90.09
Werdnig-Hoffman G12.0
Werner's E31.21
Werner's E34.8
Wernicke-Korsakoff (nonalcoholic) F04
  alcoholic F10.26
West's — see Epilepsy, spasms
Westphal-Strümpell E83.01
wet
  feet (maceration) (tropical) T69.0-
  lung, newborn P22.1
whiplash S13.4
whistling face Q87.0
Wilkie's K55.1
Wilkinson-Sneddon L13.1
Willebrand (-Jürgens) D68.0
Wilson's (hepatolenticular degeneration)
  E83.01
Wiskott-Aldrich D82.0
withdrawal — see Withdrawal, state
  drug
    infant of dependent mother P96.1
    therapeutic use, newborn P96.2
Woakes' (ethmoiditis) J33.1
Wright's (hyperabduction) I77.89
X I20.9
XXXX Q97.1
XXXXX Q97.1
XXXXY Q98.1
XXY Q98.0
yellow nail L60.5
Zahorsky's B08.5
Zellweger syndrome E71.510
Zellweger-like syndrome E71.541

Synechia (anterior) (iris) (posterior) (pupil)
  — see also Adhesions, iris
  intra-uterine (traumatic) N85.6
Synesthesia R20.8
Syngamiasis, syngamosis B83.3
Synodontia K00.2
Synorchidism, synorchism Q55.1
Synostosis (congenital) Q78.8
  astragalo-scaphoid Q74.2
  radioulnar Q74.0
Synovial sarcoma — see Neoplasm,
  connective tissue, malignant
Synovioma (malignant) — see also
  Neoplasm, connective tissue, malignant
  benign — see Neoplasm, connective tissue,
    benign
Synoviosarcoma — see Neoplasm,
  connective tissue, malignant
Synovitis — see also Tenosynovitis
  crepitant
    hand M70.0-
      wrist M70.03-
  gonococcal A54.49
  gouty — see Gout, idiopathic
  in (due to)
    crystals M65.8-
    gonorrhea A54.49
    syphilis (late) A52.78
    use, overuse, pressure — see Disorder,
      soft tissue, due to use
  infective NEC — see Tenosynovitis,
    infective NEC
  specified NEC — see Tenosynovitis,
    specified type NEC
  syphilitic A52.78
    congenital (early) A50.02
  toxic — see Synovitis, transient
  transient M67.3-
    ankle M67.37-
    elbow M67.32-
    foot joint M67.37-
    hand joint M67.34-
    hip M67.35-
    knee M67.36-
    multiple site M67.39
    pelvic region M67.35-
    shoulder M67.31-
    specified joint NEC M67.38
    wrist M67.33-
  traumatic, current — see Sprain
  tuberculous — see Tuberculosis, synovitis
  villonodular (pigmented) M12.2-
    ankle M12.27-
    elbow M12.22-
    foot joint M12.27-
    hand joint M12.24-
    hip M12.25-
    knee M12.26-
    multiple site M12.29
    pelvic region M12.25-
    shoulder M12.21-
    specified joint NEC M12.28
    vertebrae M12.28
    wrist M12.23-
Syphilid A51.39
  congenital A50.06
  newborn A50.06
  tubercular (late) A52.79
Syphilis, syphilitic (acquired) A53.9
  abdomen (late) A52.79
  acoustic nerve A52.15
  adenopathy (secondary) A51.49
  adrenal (gland) (with cortical
    hypofunction) A52.79
  age under 2 years NOS — see also
    Syphilis, congenital, early
    acquired A51.9
  alopecia (secondary) A51.32
  anemia (late) A52.79 [D63.8]
  aneurysm (aorta) (ruptured) A52.01
    central nervous system A52.05
    congenital A50.54 [I79.0]
  anus (late) A52.74
    primary A51.1
    secondary A51.39
  aorta (arch) (abdominal) (thoracic) A52.02
    aneurysm A52.01
  aortic (insufficiency) (regurgitation)
    (stenosis) A52.03
    aneurysm A52.01
  arachnoid (adhesive) (cerebral) (spinal)
    A52.13
  asymptomatic — see Syphilis, latent
  ataxia (locomotor) A52.11
  atrophoderma maculatum A51.39
  auricular fibrillation A52.06
  bladder (late) A52.76

Syphilis, syphilitic (acquired) A53.9 —
  continued
  bone A52.77
    secondary A51.46
  brain A52.17
  breast (late) A52.79
  bronchus (late) A52.72
  bubo (primary) A51.0
  bulbar palsy A52.19
  bursa (late) A52.78
  cardiac decompensation A52.06
  cardiovascular A52.00
  central nervous system (late) (recurrent)
    (relapse) (tertiary) A52.3
  with
    ataxia A52.11
    general paralysis A52.17
      juvenile A50.45
    paresis (general) A52.17
      juvenile A50.45
    tabes (dorsalis) A52.11
      juvenile A50.45
    taboparesis A52.17
      juvenile A50.45
    aneurysm A52.05
    congenital A50.40
    juvenile A50.40
    remission in (sustained) A52.3
    serology doubtful, negative, or positive
      A52.3
    specified nature or site NEC A52.19
    vascular A52.05
  cerebral A52.17
    meningovascular A52.13
    nerves (multiple palsies) A52.15
    sclerosis A52.17
    thrombosis A52.05
  cerebrospinal (tabetic type) A52.12
  cerebrovascular A52.05
  cervix (late) A52.76
  chancre (multiple) A51.0
    extragenital A51.2
    Rollet's A51.0
  Charcôt's joint A52.16
  chorioretinitis A51.43
    congenital A50.01
    late A52.71
    prenatal A50.01
  choroiditis — see Syphilitic chorioretinitis
  choroidoretinitis — see Syphilitic
    chorioretinitis
  ciliary body (secondary) A51.43
    late A52.71
  colon (late) A52.74
  combined spinal sclerosis A52.11
  condyloma (latum) A51.31
  congenital A50.9
    with
      paresis (general) A50.45
      tabes (dorsalis) A50.45
      taboparesis A50.45
    chorioretinitis, choroiditis A50.01 [H32]
    early, or less than 2 years after birth
      NEC A50.2
      with manifestations — see Syphilis,
        congenital, early
      latent (without manifestations) A50.1
        negative spinal fluid test A50.1
        serology positive A50.1
      symptomatic A50.09
        cutaneous A50.06
        mucocutaneous A50.07
        oculopathy A50.01
        osteochondropathy A50.02
        pharyngitis A50.03
        pneumonia A50.04
        rhinitis A50.05
        visceral A50.08
    interstitial keratitis A50.31
    juvenile neurosyphilis A50.45
    late, or 2 years or more after birth NEC
      A50.7
      chorioretinitis, choroiditis A50.32
      interstitial keratitis A50.31
      juvenile neurosyphilis A50.45
      latent (without manifestations) A50.6
        negative spinal fluid test A50.6
        serology positive A50.6
      symptomatic or with manifestations
        NEC A50.59
        arthropathy A50.55
        cardiovascular A50.54
        Clutton's joints A50.51
        Hutchinson's teeth A50.52
        Hutchinson's triad A50.53
        osteochondropathy A50.56
        saddle nose A50.57

Syphilis, syphilitic (acquired) A53.9 — *continued*
- conjugal A53.9
  - tabes A52.11
- conjunctiva (late) A52.71
- contact Z20.2
- cord bladder A52.19
- cornea, late A52.71
- coronary (artery) (sclerosis) A52.06
- coryza, congenital A50.05
- cranial nerve A52.15
  - multiple palsies A52.15
- cutaneous — *see* Syphilis, skin
- dacryocystitis (late) A52.71
- degeneration, spinal cord A52.12
- dementia paralytica A52.17
  - juvenilis A50.45
- destruction of bone A52.77
- dilatation, aorta A52.01
- due to blood transfusion A53.9
- dura mater A52.13
- ear A52.79
  - inner A52.79
    - nerve (eighth) A52.15
    - neurorecurrence A52.15
- early A51.9
  - cardiovascular A52.00
  - central nervous system A52.3
  - latent (without manifestations) (less than 2 years after infection) A51.5
    - negative spinal fluid test A51.5
    - serological relapse after treatment A51.5
    - serology positive A51.5
  - relapse (treated, untreated) A51.9
  - skin A51.39
  - symptomatic A51.9
    - extragenital chancre A51.2
    - primary, except extragenital chancre A51.0
    - secondary (*see also* Syphilis, secondary) A51.39
      - relapse (treated, untreated) A51.49
    - ulcer A51.39
- eighth nerve (neuritis) A52.15
- endemic A65
- endocarditis A52.03
  - aortic A52.03
  - pulmonary A52.03
- epididymis (late) A52.76
- epiglottis (late) A52.73
- epiphysitis (congenital) (early) A50.02
- episcleritis (late) A52.71
- esophagus A52.79
- eustachian tube A52.73
- exposure to Z20.2
- eye A52.71
- eyelid (late) (with gumma) A52.71
- fallopian tube (late) A52.76
- fracture A52.77
- gallbladder (late) A52.74
- gastric (polyposis) (late) A52.74
- general A53.9
  - paralysis A52.17
    - juvenile A50.45
- genital (primary) A51.0
- glaucoma A52.71
- gumma NEC A52.79
  - cardiovascular system A52.00
  - central nervous system A52.3
  - congenital A50.59
- heart (block) (decompensation) (disease) (failure) A52.06 [I52]
  - valve NEC A52.03
- hemianesthesia A52.19
- hemianopsia A52.71
- hemiparesis A52.17
- hemiplegia A52.17
- hepatic artery A52.09
- hepatis A52.74
- hepatomegaly, congenital A50.08
- hereditaria tarda — *see* Syphilis, congenital, late
- hereditary — *see* Syphilis, congenital
- Hutchinson's teeth A50.52
- hyalitis A52.71
- inactive — *see* Syphilis, latent
- infantum — *see* Syphilis, congenital
- inherited — *see* Syphilis, congenital
- internal ear A52.79
- intestine (late) A52.74
- iris, iritis (secondary) A51.43
  - late A52.71
- joint (late) A52.77
- keratitis (congenital) (interstitial) (late) A50.31
- kidney A52.75
- lacrimal passages (late) A52.71
- larynx (late) A52.73

Syphilis, syphilitic (acquired) A53.9 — *continued*
- late A52.9
  - cardiovascular A52.00
  - central nervous system A52.3
  - kidney A52.75
  - latent or 2 years or more after infection (without manifestations) A52.8
    - negative spinal fluid test A52.8
    - serology positive A52.8
  - paresis A52.17
  - specified site NEC A52.79
  - symptomatic or with manifestations A52.79
  - tabes A52.11
- latent A53.0
  - with signs or symptoms — *code by* site and stage under Syphilis
  - central nervous system A52.2
  - date of infection unspecified A53.0
  - early, or less than 2 years after infection A51.5
  - follow-up of latent syphilis A53.0
    - date of infection unspecified A53.0
    - late, or 2 years or more after infection A52.8
  - late, or 2 years or more after infection A52.8
  - positive serology (only finding) A53.0
    - date of infection unspecified A53.0
    - early, or less than 2 years after infection A51.5
    - late, or 2 years or more after infection A52.8
- lens (late) A52.71
- leukoderma A51.39
  - late A52.79
- lienitis A52.79
- lip A51.39
  - chancre (primary) A51.2
  - late A52.79
- Lissauer's paralysis A52.17
- liver A52.74
- locomotor ataxia A52.11
- lung A52.72
- lymph gland (early) (secondary) A51.49
  - late A52.79
- lymphadenitis (secondary) A51.49
- macular atrophy of skin A51.39
  - striated A52.79
- mediastinum (late) A52.73
- meninges (adhesive) (brain) (spinal cord) A52.13
- meningitis A52.13
  - acute (secondary) A51.41
  - congenital A50.41
- meningoencephalitis A52.14
- meningovascular A52.13
  - congenital A50.41
- mesarteritis A52.09
  - brain A52.04
- middle ear A52.77
- mitral stenosis A52.03
- monoplegia A52.17
- mouth (secondary) A51.39
  - late A52.79
- mucocutaneous (secondary) A51.39
  - late A52.79
- mucous
  - membrane (secondary) A51.39
    - late A52.79
  - patches A51.39
    - congenital A50.07
- mulberry molars A50.52
- muscle A52.78
- myocardium A52.06
- nasal sinus (late) A52.73
- neonatorum — *see* Syphilis, congenital
- nephrotic syndrome (secondary) A51.44
- nerve palsy (any cranial nerve) A52.15
  - multiple A52.15
- nervous system, central A52.3
- neuritis A52.15
  - acoustic A52.15
- neurorecidive of retina A52.19
- neuroretinitis A52.19
- newborn — *see* Syphilis, congenital
- nodular superficial (late) A52.79
- nonvenereal A65
- nose (late) A52.73
  - saddle back deformity A50.57
- occlusive arterial disease A52.09
- oculopathy A52.71
- ophthalmic (late) A52.71
- optic nerve (atrophy) (neuritis) (papilla) A52.15
- orbit (late) A52.71
- organic A53.9
- osseous (late) A52.77

Syphilis, syphilitic (acquired) A53.9 — *continued*
- osteochondritis (congenital) (early) A50.02 [M90.80]
- osteoporosis A52.77
- ovary (late) A52.76
- oviduct (late) A52.76
- palate (late) A52.79
- pancreas (late) A52.74
- paralysis A52.17
  - general A52.17
    - juvenile A50.45
- paresis (general) A52.17
  - juvenile A50.45
- paresthesia A52.19
- Parkinson's disease or syndrome A52.19
- paroxysmal tachycardia A52.06
- pemphigus (congenital) A50.06
- penis (chancre) A51.0
  - late A52.76
- pericardium A52.06
- perichondritis, larynx (late) A52.73
- periosteum (late) A52.77
  - congenital (early) A50.02 [M90.80]
  - early (secondary) A51.46
- peripheral nerve A52.79
- petrous bone (late) A52.77
- pharynx (late) A52.73
  - secondary A51.39
- pituitary (gland) A52.79
- pleura (late) A52.73
- pneumonia, white A50.04
- pontine lesion A52.17
- portal vein A52.09
- primary A51.0
  - anal A51.1
  - and secondary — *see* Syphilis, secondary
  - central nervous system A52.3
  - extragenital chancre NEC A51.2
  - fingers A51.2
  - genital A51.0
  - lip A51.2
  - specified site NEC A51.2
  - tonsils A51.2
- prostate (late) A52.76
- ptosis (eyelid) A52.71
- pulmonary (late) A52.72
  - artery A52.09
- pyelonephritis (late) A52.75
- recently acquired, symptomatic A51.9
- rectum (late) A52.74
- respiratory tract (late) A52.73
- retina, late A52.71
- retrobulbar neuritis A52.15
- salpingitis A52.76
- sclera (late) A52.71
- sclerosis
  - cerebral A52.17
  - coronary A52.06
  - multiple A52.11
- scotoma (central) A52.71
- scrotum (late) A52.76
- secondary (and primary) A51.49
  - adenopathy A51.49
  - anus A51.39
  - bone A51.46
  - chorioretinitis, choroiditis A51.43
  - hepatitis A51.45
  - liver A51.45
  - lymphadenitis A51.49
  - meningitis (acute) A51.41
  - mouth A51.39
  - mucous membranes A51.39
  - periosteum, periostitis A51.46
  - pharynx A51.39
  - relapse (treated, untreated) A51.49
  - skin A51.39
  - specified form NEC A51.49
  - tonsil A51.39
  - ulcer A51.39
  - viscera NEC A51.49
  - vulva A51.39
- seminal vesicle (late) A52.76
- seronegative with signs or symptoms — *code by* site and stage under Syphilis
- seropositive
  - with signs or symptoms — *code by* site and stage under Syphilis
  - follow-up of latent syphilis — *see* Syphilis, latent
  - only finding — *see* Syphilis, latent
- seventh nerve (paralysis) A52.15
- sinus, sinusitis (late) A52.73
- skeletal system A52.77
- skin (with ulceration) (early) (secondary) A51.39
  - late or tertiary A52.79

Syphilis, syphilitic (acquired) A53.9 — *continued*
- small intestine A52.74
- spastic spinal paralysis A52.17
- spermatic cord (late) A52.76
- spinal (cord) A52.12
- spleen A52.79
- splenomegaly A52.79
- spondylitis A52.77
- staphyloma A52.71
- stigmata (congenital) A50.59
- stomach A52.74
- synovium A52.78
- tabes dorsalis (late) A52.11
  - juvenile A50.45
- tabetic type A52.11
  - juvenile A50.45
- taboparesis A52.17
  - juvenile A50.45
- tachycardia A52.06
- tendon (late) A52.78
- tertiary A52.9
  - with symptoms NEC A52.79
  - cardiovascular A52.00
  - central nervous system A52.3
  - multiple NEC A52.79
  - specified site NEC A52.79
- testis A52.76
- thorax A52.73
- throat A52.73
- thymus (gland) (late) A52.79
- thyroid (late) A52.79
- tongue (late) A52.79
- tonsil (lingual) (late) A52.73
  - primary A51.2
  - secondary A51.39
- trachea (late) A52.73
- tunica vaginalis (late) A52.76
- ulcer (any site) (early) (secondary) A51.39
  - late A52.79
  - perforating A52.79
    - foot A52.11
- urethra (late) A52.76
- urogenital (late) A52.76
- uterus (late) A52.76
- uveal tract (secondary) A51.43
  - late A52.71
- uveitis (secondary) A51.43
  - late A52.71
- uvula (late) (perforated) A52.79
- vagina A51.0
  - late A52.76
- valvulitis NEC A52.03
- vascular A52.00
  - brain (cerebral) A52.05
- ventriculi A52.74
- vesicae urinariae (late) A52.76
- viscera (abdominal) (late) A52.74
  - secondary A51.49
- vitreous (opacities) (late) A52.71
  - hemorrhage A52.71
- vulva A51.0
  - late A52.76
  - secondary A51.39

Syphiloma A52.79
- cardiovascular system A52.00
- central nervous system A52.3
- circulatory system A52.00
- congenital A50.59

Syphilophobia F45.29

Syringadenoma — *see also* Neoplasm, skin, benign
- papillary — *see* Neoplasm, skin, benign

Syringobulbia G95.0

Syringocystadenoma — *see* Neoplasm, skin, benign
- papillary — *see* Neoplasm, skin, benign

Syringoma — *see also* Neoplasm, skin, benign
- chondroid — *see* Neoplasm, skin, benign

Syringomyelia G95.0

Syringomyelitis — *see* Encephalitis

Syringomyelocele — *see* Spina bifida

Syringopontia G95.0

System, systemic — *see also* condition
- disease, combined — *see* Degeneration, combined
- inflammatory response syndrome (SIRS) of non-infectious origin (without organ dysfunction) R65.10
  - with acute organ dysfunction R65.11
- lupus erythematosus M32.9
  - inhibitor present D68.62

DISEASE INDEX

T

Tabacism, tabacosis, tabagism — *see also* Poisoning, tobacco
  meaning dependence (without remission) F17.200
  with
    disorder F17.299
      remission F17.211
      specified disorder NEC F17.298
      withdrawal F17.203
Tabardillo A75.9
  flea-borne A75.2
  louse-borne A75.0
Tabes, tabetic A52.10
  with
    central nervous system syphilis A52.10
    Charcot's joint A52.16
    cord bladder A52.19
    crisis, viscera (any) A52.19
    paralysis, general A52.17
    paresis (general) A52.17
    perforating ulcer (foot) A52.19
  arthropathy (Charcot) A52.16
  bladder A52.19
  bone A52.11
  cerebrospinal A52.12
  congenital A50.45
  conjugal A52.10
  dorsalis A52.11
    juvenile A50.49
  juvenile A50.49
  latent A52.19
  mesenterica A18.39
  paralysis, insane, general A52.17
  spasmodic A52.17
  syphilis (cerebrospinal) A52.12
Taboparalysis A52.17
Taboparesis (remission) A52.17
  juvenile A50.45
TAC (trigeminal autonomic cephalgia) NEC G44.099
  intractable G44.091
  not intractable G44.099
Tache noir S60.22-
Tachyalimentation K91.2
Tachyarrhythmia, tachyrhythmia — *see* Tachycardia
Tachycardia R00.0
  atrial (paroxysmal) I47.1
  auricular I47.1
  AV nodal re-entry (re-entrant) I47.1
  junctional (paroxysmal) I47.1
  newborn P29.11
  nodal (paroxysmal) I47.1
  non-paroxysmal AV nodal I45.89
  paroxysmal (sustained) (nonsustained) I47.9
    with sinus bradycardia I49.5
    atrial (PAT) I47.1
    atrioventricular (AV) (re-entrant) I47.1
      psychogenic F54
    junctional I47.1
      ectopic I47.1
    nodal I47.1
    psychogenic (atrial) (supraventricular) (ventricular) F54
    supraventricular (sustained) I47.1
      psychogenic F54
    ventricular I47.2
      psychogenic F54
  psychogenic F45.8
  sick sinus I49.5
  sinoauricular NOS R00.0
    paroxysmal I47.1
  sinus [sinusal] NOS R00.0
    paroxysmal I47.1
  supraventricular I47.1
  ventricular (paroxysmal) (sustained) I47.2
    psychogenic F54
Tachygastria K31.89
Tachypnea R06.82
  hysterical F45.8
  newborn (idiopathic) (transitory) P22.1
  psychogenic F45.8
  transitory, of newborn P22.1
TACO (transfusion associated circulatory overload) E87.71
Taenia (infection) (infestation) B68.9
  diminuta B71.0
  echinococcal infestation B67.90
  mediocanellata B68.1
  nana B71.0
  saginata B68.1
  solium (intestinal form) B68.0
    larval form — *see* Cysticercosis

Taeniasis (intestine) — *see* Taenia
Tag (hypertrophied skin) (infected) L91.8
  adenoid J35.8
  anus K64.4
  hemorrhoidal K64.4
  hymen N89.8
  perineal N90.89
  preauricular Q17.0
  sentinel K64.4
  skin L91.8
    accessory (congenital) Q82.8
    anus K64.4
    congenital Q82.8
    preauricular Q17.0
  tonsil J35.8
  urethra, urethral N36.8
  vulva N90.89
Tahyna fever B33.8
Takahara's disease E80.3
Takayasu's disease or syndrome M31.4
Talcosis (pulmonary) J62.0
Talipes (congenital) Q66.89
  acquired, planus — *see* Deformity, limb, flat foot
  asymmetric Q66.89
  calcaneovalgus Q66.4
  calcaneovarus Q66.1
  calcaneus Q66.89
  cavus Q66.7
  equinovalgus Q66.6
  equinovarus Q66.0
  equinus Q66.89
  percavus Q66.7
  planovalgus Q66.6
  planus (acquired) (any degree) — *see also* Deformity, limb, flat foot
    congenital Q66.5-
    due to rickets (sequelae) E64.3
  valgus Q66.6
  varus Q66.3
Tall stature, constitutional E34.4
Talma's disease M62.89
Talon noir S90.3-
  hand S60.22-
  heel S90.3-
  toe S90.1-
Tamponade, heart I31.4
Tanapox (virus disease) B08.71
Tangier disease E78.6
Tantrum, child problem F91.8
Tapeworm (infection) (infestation) — *see* Infestation, tapeworm
Tapia's syndrome G52.7
TAR (thrombocytopenia with absent radius) syndrome Q87.2
Tarral-Besnier disease L44.0
Tarsal tunnel syndrome — *see* Syndrome, tarsal tunnel
Tarsalgia — *see* Pain, limb, lower
Tarsitis (eyelid) H01.8
  syphilitic A52.71
  tuberculous A18.4
Tartar (teeth) (dental calculus) K03.6
Tattoo (mark) L81.8
Tauri's disease E74.09
Taurodontism K00.2
Taussig-Bing syndrome Q20.1
Taybi's syndrome Q87.2
Tay-Sachs amaurotic familial idiocy or disease E75.02
TBI (traumatic brain injury) — *see* category S06
Teacher's node or nodule J38.2
Tear, torn (traumatic) — *see also* Laceration
  with abortion — *see* Abortion
  annular fibrosis M51.35
  anus, anal (sphincter) S31.831
    complicating delivery
      with third degree perineal laceration O70.2
        with mucosa O70.3
      without third degree perineal laceration O70.4
    nontraumatic (healed) (old) K62.81
  articular cartilage, old — *see* Derangement, joint, articular cartilage, by site
  bladder
    with ectopic or molar pregnancy O08.6
    following ectopic or molar pregnancy O08.6
    obstetrical O71.5
    traumatic — *see* Injury, bladder
  bowel
    with ectopic or molar pregnancy O08.6
    following ectopic or molar pregnancy O08.6
    obstetrical trauma O71.5

Tear, torn (traumatic) (*see also* Laceration) — *continued*
  broad ligament
    with ectopic or molar pregnancy O08.6
    following ectopic or molar pregnancy O08.6
    obstetrical trauma O71.6
  bucket handle (knee) (meniscus) — *see* Tear, meniscus
  capsule, joint — *see* Sprain
  cartilage — *see also* Sprain
    articular, old — *see* Derangement, joint, articular cartilage, by site
  cervix
    with ectopic or molar pregnancy O08.6
    following ectopic or molar pregnancy O08.6
    obstetrical trauma (current) O71.3
    old N88.1
    traumatic — *see* Injury, uterus
  dural G97.41
    nontraumatic G96.11
  internal organ — *see* Injury, by site
  knee cartilage
    articular (current) S83.3-
    old — *see* Derangement, knee, meniscus, due to old tear
  ligament — *see* Sprain
  meniscus (knee) (current injury) S83.209
    bucket-handle S83.20-
    lateral
      bucket-handle S83.25-
      complex S83.27-
      peripheral S83.26-
      specified type NEC S83.28-
    medial
      bucket-handle S83.21-
      complex S83.23-
      peripheral S83.22-
      specified type NEC S83.24-
    old — *see* Derangement, knee, meniscus, due to old tear
    site other than knee — *code as* Sprain
    specified type NEC S83.20-
  muscle — *see* Strain
  pelvic
    floor, complicating delivery O70.1
    organ NEC, obstetrical trauma O71.5
      with ectopic or molar pregnancy O08.6
      following ectopic or molar pregnancy O08.6
  perineal, secondary O90.1
  periurethral tissue, obstetrical trauma O71.82
    with ectopic or molar pregnancy O08.6
    following ectopic or molar pregnancy O08.6
  rectovaginal septum — *see* Laceration, vagina
  retina, retinal (without detachment) (horseshoe) — *see also* Break, retina, horseshoe
    with detachment — *see* Detachment, retina, with retinal, break
  rotator cuff (nontraumatic) M75.10-
    complete M75.12-
    incomplete M75.11-
    traumatic S46.01-
      capsule S43.42-
  semilunar cartilage, knee — *see* Tear, meniscus
  supraspinatus (complete) (incomplete) (nontraumatic) (*see also* Tear, rotator cuff) M75.10-
  tendon — *see* Strain
  tentorial, at birth P10.4
  umbilical cord
    complicating delivery O69.89
  urethra
    with ectopic or molar pregnancy O08.6
    following ectopic or molar pregnancy O08.6
    obstetrical trauma O71.5
  uterus — *see* Injury, uterus
  vagina — *see* Laceration, vagina
  vessel, from catheter — *see* Puncture, accidental complicating surgery
  vulva, complicating delivery O70.0
Tear-stone — *see* Dacryolith
Teeth — *see also* condition
  grinding
    psychogenic F45.8
    sleep related G47.63
Teething (syndrome) K00.7

Telangiectasia, telangiectasis (verrucous) I78.1
  ataxic (cerebellar) (Louis-Bar) G11.3
  familial I78.0
  hemorrhagic, hereditary (congenital) (senile) I78.0
  hereditary, hemorrhagic (congenital) (senile) I78.0
  juxtafoveal H35.07-
  macular H35.07-
  parafoveal H35.07-
  retinal (idiopathic) (juxtafoveal) (macular) (parafoveal) H35.07-
  spider I78.1
Telephone scatologia F65.89
Telescoped bowel or intestine K56.1
  congenital Q43.8
Temperature
  body, high (of unknown origin) R50.9
  cold, trauma from T69.9
    newborn P80.0
    specified effect NEC T69.8
Temple — *see* condition
Temporal — *see* condition
Temporomandibular joint pain-dysfunction syndrome M26.62
Temporosphenoidal — *see* condition
Tendency
  bleeding — *see* Defect, coagulation
  suicide
    meaning personal history of attempted suicide Z91.5
    meaning suicidal ideation — *see* Ideation, suicidal
  to fall R29.6
Tenderness, abdominal R10.819
  epigastric R10.816
  generalized R10.817
  left lower quadrant R10.814
  left upper quadrant R10.812
  periumbilic R10.815
  rebound R10.829
    epigastric R10.826
    generalized R10.827
    left lower quadrant R10.824
    left upper quadrant R10.822
    periumbilic R10.825
    right lower quadrant R10.823
    right upper quadrant R10.821
  right lower quadrant R10.813
  right upper quadrant R10.811
Tendinitis, tendonitis — *see also* Enthesopathy
  Achilles M76.6-
  adhesive — *see* Tenosynovitis, specified type NEC
    shoulder — *see* Capsulitis, adhesive
  bicipital M75.2-
  calcific M65.2-
    ankle M65.27-
    foot M65.27-
    forearm M65.23-
    hand M65.24-
    lower leg M65.26-
    multiple sites M65.29
    pelvic region M65.25-
    shoulder M75.3-
    specified site NEC M65.28
    thigh M65.25-
    upper arm M65.22-
  due to use, overuse, pressure — *see also* Disorder, soft tissue, due to use
    specified NEC — *see* Disorder, soft tissue, due to use, specified NEC
  gluteal M76.0-
  patellar M76.5-
  peroneal M76.7-
  psoas M76.1-
  tibial (posterior) M76.82-
    anterior M76.81-
  trochanteric — *see* Bursitis, hip, trochanteric
Tendon — *see* condition
Tendosynovitis — *see* Tenosynovitis
Tenesmus (rectal) R19.8
  vesical R30.1
Tennis elbow — *see* Epicondylitis, lateral
Tenonitis — *see also* Tenosynovitis
  eye (capsule) H05.04-
Tenontosynovitis — *see* Tenosynovitis
Tenontothecitis — *see* Tenosynovitis
Tenophyte — *see* Disorder, synovium, specified type NEC

Tenosynovitis (see also Synovitis) M65.9
  adhesive — see Tenosynovitis, specified type NEC
    shoulder — see Capsulitis, adhesive
  bicipital (calcifying) — see Tendinitis, bicipital
  gonococcal A54.49
  in (due to)
    crystals M65.8-
    gonorrhea A54.49
    syphilis (late) A52.78
    use, overuse, pressure — see also Disorder, soft tissue, due to use
      specified NEC — see Disorder, soft tissue, due to use, specified NEC
  infective NEC M65.1-
    ankle M65.17-
    foot M65.17-
    forearm M65.13-
    hand M65.14-
    lower leg M65.16-
    multiple sites M65.19
    pelvic region M65.15-
    shoulder region M65.11-
    specified site NEC M65.18
    thigh M65.15-
    upper arm M65.12-
  radial styloid M65.4
  shoulder region M65.81-
    adhesive — see Capsulitis, adhesive
  specified type NEC M65.88
    ankle M65.87-
    foot M65.87-
    forearm M65.83-
    hand M65.84-
    lower leg M65.86-
    multiple sites M65.89
    pelvic region M65.85-
    shoulder region M65.81-
    specified site NEC M65.88
    thigh M65.85-
    upper arm M65.82-
  tuberculous — see also Tuberculosis, tenosynovitis
Tenovaginitis — see Tenosynovitis
Tension
  arterial, high — see also Hypertension
    without diagnosis of hypertension R03.0
  headache G44.209
    intractable G44.201
    not intractable G44.209
  nervous R45.0
  pneumothorax J93.0
  premenstrual N94.3
  state (mental) F48.9
Tentorium — see condition
Teratencephalus Q89.8
Teratism Q89.7
Teratoblastoma (malignant) — see Neoplasm, malignant, by site
Teratocarcinoma — see also Neoplasm, malignant, by site
  liver C22.7
Teratoma (solid) — see also Neoplasm, uncertain behavior, by site
  with embryonal carcinoma, mixed — see Neoplasm, malignant, by site
  with malignant transformation — see Neoplasm, malignant, by site
  adult (cystic) — see Neoplasm, benign, by site
  benign — see Neoplasm, benign, by site
  combined with choriocarcinoma — see Neoplasm, malignant, by site
  cystic (adult) — see Neoplasm, benign, by site
  differentiated — see Neoplasm, benign, by site
  embryonal — see also Neoplasm, malignant, by site
    liver C22.7
  immature — see Neoplasm, malignant, by site
  liver C22.7
    adult, benign, cystic, differentiated type or mature D13.4
  malignant — see also Neoplasm, malignant, by site
    anaplastic — see Neoplasm, malignant, by site
    intermediate — see Neoplasm, malignant, by site
      specified site — see Neoplasm, malignant, by site
      unspecified site C62.90
    undifferentiated — see Neoplasm, malignant, by site

Teratoma (solid) (see also Neoplasm, uncertain behavior, by site) — continued
  mature — see Neoplasm, uncertain behavior, by site
    malignant — see Neoplasm, by site, malignant, by site
  ovary D27-
    embryonal, immature or malignant C56-
  solid — see Neoplasm, uncertain behavior, by site
  testis C62.9-
    adult, benign, cystic, differentiated type or mature D29.2-
    scrotal C62.1-
    undescended C62.0-
Termination
  anomalous — see also Malposition, congenital
    right pulmonary vein Q26.3
  pregnancy, elective Z33.2
Ternidens diminutus infestation B81.8
Ternidensiasis B81.8
Terror(s) night (child) F51.4
Terrorism, victim of Z65.4
Terry's syndrome H44.2-
Tertiary — see condition
Test, tests, testing (for)
  adequacy (for dialysis)
    hemodialysis Z49.31
    peritoneal Z49.32
  blood pressure Z01.30
    abnormal reading — see Blood, pressure
  blood typing Z01.83
    Rh typing Z01.83
  blood-alcohol Z04.8
    positive — see Findings, abnormal, in blood
  blood-drug Z04.8
    positive — see Findings, abnormal, in blood
  cardiac pulse generator (battery) Z45.010
  fertility Z31.41
  genetic
    disease carrier status for procreative management
      female Z31.430
      male Z31.440
    male partner of patient with recurrent pregnancy loss Z31.441
    procreative management NEC
      female Z31.438
      male Z31.448
  hearing Z01.10
    with abnormal findings NEC Z01.118
  HIV (human immunodeficiency virus)
    nonconclusive (in infants) R75
    positive Z21
    seropositive Z21
  immunity status Z01.84
  intelligence NEC Z01.89
  laboratory (as part of a general medical examination) Z00.00
    with abnormal finding Z00.01
    for medicolegal reason NEC Z04.8
  male partner of patient with recurrent pregnancy loss Z31.441
  Mantoux (for tuberculosis) Z11.1
    abnormal result R76.11
  pregnancy, positive first pregnancy — see Pregnancy, normal, first
  procreative Z31.49
    fertility Z31.41
  skin, diagnostic
    allergy Z01.82
      special screening examination — see Screening, by name of disease
    Mantoux Z11.1
    tuberculin Z11.1
  specified NEC Z01.89
  tuberculin Z11.1
    abnormal result R76.11
  vision Z01.00
    with abnormal findings Z01.01
  Wassermann Z11.3
    positive — see Serology for syphilis, positive
Testicle, testicular, testis — see also condition
  feminization syndrome (see also Syndrome, androgen insensitivity) E34.51
  migrans Q55.29

Tetanus, tetanic (cephalic) (convulsions) A35
  with
    abortion A34
    ectopic or molar pregnancy O08.0
  following ectopic or molar pregnancy O08.0
  inoculation reaction (due to serum) — see Complications, vaccination
  neonatorum A33
  obstetrical A34
  puerperal, postpartum, childbirth A34
Tetany (due to) R29.0
  alkalosis E87.3
  associated with rickets E55.0
  convulsions R29.0
    hysterical F44.5
  functional (hysterical) F44.5
  hyperkinetic R29.0
    hysterical F44.5
  hyperpnea R06.4
    hysterical F44.5
    psychogenic F45.8
  hyperventilation (see also Hyperventilation) R06.4
    hysterical F44.5
  neonatal (without calcium or magnesium deficiency) P71.3
  parathyroid (gland) E20.9
  parathyroprival E89.2
  post- (para)thyroidectomy E89.2
  postoperative E89.2
  pseudotetany R29.0
  psychogenic (conversion reaction) F44.5
Tetralogy of Fallot Q21.3
Tetraplegia (chronic) (see also Quadriplegia) G82.50
Thailand hemorrhagic fever A91
Thalassanemia — see Thalassemia
Thalassemia (anemia) (disease) D56.9
  with other hemoglobinopathy D56.8
  alpha (major) (severe) (triple gene defect) D56.0
    minor D56.3
    silent carrier D56.3
    trait D56.3
  beta (severe) D56.1
    homozygous D56.1
    major D56.1
    minor D56.3
    trait D56.3
  delta-beta (homozygous) D56.2
    minor D56.3
    trait D56.3
  dominant D56.8
  hemoglobin
    C D56.8
    E-beta D56.5
  intermedia D56.1
    major D56.1
    minor D56.3
  mixed D56.8
  sickle-cell — see Disease, sickle-cell, thalassemia
  specified type NEC D56.8
  trait D56.3
  variants D56.8
Thanatophoric dwarfism or short stature Q77.1
Thaysen-Gee disease (nontropical sprue) K90.0
Thaysen's disease K90.0
Thecoma D27-
  luteinized D27-
  malignant C56-
Thelarche, premature E30.8
Thelaziasis B83.8
Thelitis N61
  puerperal, postpartum or gestational — see Infection, nipple
Therapeutic — see condition
Therapy
  drug, long-term (current) (prophylactic)
    agents affecting estrogen receptors and estrogen levels NEC Z79.818
    anastrozole (Arimidex) Z79.811
    anti-inflammatory Z79.1
    antibiotics Z79.2
      short-term use — omit code
    anticoagulants Z79.01
    antiplatelet Z79.02
    antithrombotics Z79.02
    aromatase inhibitors Z79.811
    aspirin Z79.82
    birth control pill or patch Z79.3
    bisphosphonates Z79.83
    contraceptive, oral Z79.3
    drug, specified NEC Z79.899
    estrogen receptor downregulators Z79.818

Therapy — continued
  drug, long-term (current) (prophylactic) — continued
    Evista Z79.810
    exemestane (Aromasin) Z79.811
    Fareston Z79.810
    fulvestrant (Faslodex) Z79.818
    gonadotropin-releasing hormone (GnRH) agonist Z79.818
    goserelin acetate (Zoladex) Z79.818
    hormone replacement (postmenopausal) Z79.890
    insulin Z79.4
    letrozole (Femara) Z79.811
    leuprolide acetate (leuprorelin) (Lupron) Z79.818
    megestrol acetate (Megace) Z79.818
    methadone
      for pain management Z79.891
      maintenance therapy F11.20
    Nolvadex Z79.810
    opiate analgesic Z79.891
    oral contraceptive Z79.3
    raloxifene (Evista) Z79.810
    selective estrogen receptor modulators (SERMs) Z79.810
    short term — omit code
    steroids
      inhaled Z79.51
      systemic Z79.52
    tamoxifen (Nolvadex) Z79.810
    toremifene (Fareston) Z79.810
Thermic — see condition
Thermography (abnormal) (see also Abnormal, diagnostic imaging) R93.8
  breast R92.8
Thermoplegia T67.0
Thesaurismosis, glycogen — see Disease, glycogen storage
Thiamin deficiency E51.9
  specified NEC E51.8
Thiaminic deficiency with beriberi E51.11
Thibierge-Weissenbach syndrome — see Sclerosis, systemic
Thickening
  bone — see Hypertrophy, bone
  breast N64.59
  endometrium R93.8
  epidermal L85.9
    specified NEC L85.8
  hymen N89.6
  larynx J38.7
  nail L60.2
    congenital Q84.5
  periosteal — see Hypertrophy, bone
  pleura J92.9
    with asbestos J92.0
  skin R23.4
  subepiglottic J38.7
  tongue K14.8
  valve, heart — see Endocarditis
Thigh — see condition
Thinning vertebra — see Spondylopathy, specified NEC
Thirst, excessive R63.1
  due to deprivation of water T73.1
Thomsen disease G71.12
Thoracic — see also condition
  kidney Q63.2
  outlet syndrome G54.0
Thoracogastroschisis (congenital) Q79.8
Thoracopagus Q89.4
Thorax — see condition
Thorn's syndrome N28.89
Thorson-Björck syndrome E34.0
Threadworm (infection) (infestation) B80
Threatened
  abortion O20.0
    with subsequent abortion O03.9
  job loss, anxiety concerning Z56.2
  labor (without delivery) O47.9
    after 37 completed weeks of gestation O47.1
    before 37 completed weeks of gestation O47.0-
  loss of job, anxiety concerning Z56.2
  miscarriage O20.0
  unemployment, anxiety concerning Z56.2
Three-day fever A93.1
Threshers' lung J67.0
Thrix annulata (congenital) Q84.1
Throat — see condition
Thrombasthenia (Glanzmann) (hemorrhagic) (hereditary) D69.1

DISEASE INDEX

Thromboangiitis I73.1
  obliterans (general) I73.1
    cerebral I67.89
    vessels
      brain I67.89
      spinal cord I67.89
Thromboarteritis — see Arteritis
Thromboasthenia (Glanzmann)
  (hemorrhagic) (hereditary) D69.1
Thrombocytasthenia (Glanzmann) D69.1
Thrombocythemia (essential) (hemorrhagic)
  (idiopathic) (primary) D47.3
Thrombocytopathy (dystrophic)
  (granulopenic) D69.1
Thrombocytopenia, thrombocytopenic
  D69.6
  with absent radius (TAR) Q87.2
  congenital D69.42
  dilutional D69.59
  due to
    drugs D69.59
    extracorporeal circulation of blood
      D69.59
    (massive) blood transfusion D69.59
    platelet alloimmunization D69.59
  essential D69.3
  heparin induced (HIT) D75.82
  hereditary D69.42
  idiopathic D69.3
  neonatal, transitory P61.0
    due to
      exchange transfusion P61.0
      idiopathic maternal thrombocytopenia
        P61.0
      isoimmunization P61.0
  primary NEC D69.49
    idiopathic D69.3
  puerperal, postpartum O72.3
  secondary D69.59
  transient neonatal P61.0
Thrombocytosis, essential D47.3
  primary D47.3
Thromboembolism — see Embolism
Thrombopathy (Bernard-Soulier) D69.1
  constitutional D68.0
  Willebrand-Jurgens D68.0
Thrombopenia — see Thrombocytopenia
Thrombophilia D68.59
  primary NEC D68.59
  secondary NEC D68.69
  specified NEC D68.69
Thrombophlebitis I80.9
  antepartum O22.2-
    deep O22.3-
    superficial O22.2-
  cavernous (venous) sinus G08
    complicating pregnancy O22.5-
    nonpyogenic I67.6
  cerebral (sinus) (vein) G08
    nonpyogenic I67.6
    sequelae G09
  due to implanted device — see
    Complications, by site and type,
    specified NEC
  during or resulting from a procedure NEC
    T81.72
  femoral vein (superficial) I80.1-
  femoropopliteal vein I80.0-
  hepatic (vein) I80.8
  idiopathic, recurrent I82.1
  iliofemoral I80.1-
  intracranial venous sinus (any) G08
    nonpyogenic I67.6
    sequelae G09
  intraspinal venous sinuses and veins G08
    nonpyogenic G95.19
  lateral (venous) sinus G08
    nonpyogenic I67.6
  leg I80.299
    superficial I80.0-
  longitudinal (venous) sinus G08
    nonpyogenic I67.6
  lower extremity I80.299
  migrans, migrating I82.1
  pelvic
    with ectopic or molar pregnancy O08.0
    following ectopic or molar pregnancy
      O08.0
    puerperal O87.1
  popliteal vein — see Phlebitis, leg, deep,
    popliteal
  portal (vein) K75.1
  postoperative T81.72
  pregnancy — see Thrombophlebitis,
    antepartum

Thrombophlebitis I80.9 — continued
  puerperal, postpartum, childbirth O87.0
    deep O87.1
    pelvic O87.1
    septic O86.81
    superficial O87.0
  saphenous (greater) (lesser) I80.0-
  sinus (intracranial) G08
    nonpyogenic I67.6
  specified site NEC I80.8
  tibial vein I80.23-
Thrombosis, thrombotic (bland) (multiple)
  (progressive) (silent) (vessel) I82.90
  anal K64.5
  antepartum — see Thrombophlebitis,
    antepartum
  aorta, aortic I74.10
    abdominal I74.09
      saddle I74.01
    bifurcation I74.09
    saddle I74.09
    specified site NEC I74.19
    terminal I74.09
    thoracic I74.11
    valve — see Endocarditis, aortic
  apoplexy I63.3
  artery, arteries (postinfectional) I74.9
    auditory, internal — see Occlusion,
      artery, precerebral, specified NEC
    basilar — see Occlusion, artery, basilar
    carotid (common) (internal) — see
      Occlusion, artery, carotid
    cerebellar (anterior inferior) (posterior
      inferior) (superior) — see
      Occlusion, artery, cerebellar
    cerebral — see Occlusion, artery,
      cerebral
    choroidal (anterior) — see Occlusion,
      artery, cerebral, specified NEC
    communicating, posterior — see
      Occlusion, artery, cerebral,
      specified NEC
    coronary — see also Infarct,
      myocardium
      not resulting in infarction I24.0
    hepatic I74.8
    hypophyseal — see Occlusion, artery,
      cerebral, specified NEC
    iliac I74.5
    limb I74.4
      lower I74.3
      upper I74.2
    meningeal, anterior or posterior — see
      Occlusion, artery, cerebral,
      specified NEC
    mesenteric (with gangrene) K55.0
    ophthalmic — see Occlusion, artery,
      retina
    pontine — see Occlusion, artery,
      cerebral, specified NEC
    precerebral — see Occlusion, artery,
      precerebral
    pulmonary (iatrogenic) — see
      Embolism, pulmonary
    renal N28.0
    retinal — see Occlusion, artery, retina
    spinal, anterior or posterior G95.11
    traumatic NEC T14.8
    vertebral — see Occlusion, artery,
      vertebral
  atrium, auricular — see also Infarct,
    myocardium
    following acute myocardial infarction
      (current complication) I23.6
    not resulting in infarction I24.0
  basilar (artery) — see Occlusion, artery,
    basilar
  brain (artery) (stem) — see also Occlusion,
    artery, cerebral
    due to syphilis A52.05
    puerperal O99.43
    sinus — see Thrombosis, intracranial
      venous sinus
  capillary I78.8
  cardiac — see also Infarct, myocardium
    not resulting in infarction I24.0
    valve — see Endocarditis
  carotid (artery) (common) (internal) — see
    Occlusion, artery, carotid
  cavernous (venous) sinus — see
    Thrombosis, intracranial venous sinus
  cerebellar artery (anterior inferior)
    (posterior inferior) (superior) I66.3
  cerebral (artery) — see Occlusion, artery,
    cerebral
  cerebrovenous sinus — see also
    Thrombosis, intracranial venous sinus
    puerperium O87.3

Thrombosis, thrombotic (bland) (multiple)
  (progressive) (silent) (vessel) I82.90 —
  continued
  chronic I82.91
  coronary (artery) (vein) — see also Infarct,
    myocardium
    not resulting in infarction I24.0
  corpus cavernosum N48.89
  cortical I66.9
  deep — see Embolism, vein, lower
    extremity
  due to device, implant or graft (see also
    Complications, by site and type,
    specified NEC) T85.86
    arterial graft NEC T82.868
    breast (implant) T85.86
    catheter NEC T85.86
      dialysis (renal) T82.868
        intraperitoneal T85.86
      infusion NEC T82.868
        spinal (epidural) (subdural) T85.86
      urinary (indwelling) T83.86
    electronic (electrode) (pulse generator)
      (stimulator)
      bone T84.86
      cardiac T82.867
      nervous system (brain) (peripheral
        nerve) (spinal) T85.86
      urinary T83.86
    fixation, internal (orthopedic) NEC
      T84.86
    gastrointestinal (bile duct) (esophagus)
      T85.86
    genital NEC T83.86
    heart T82.867
    joint prosthesis T84.86
    ocular (corneal graft) (orbital implant)
      NEC T85.86
    orthopedic NEC T84.86
    specified NEC T85.86
    urinary NEC T83.86
    vascular NEC T82.868
    ventricular intracranial shunt T85.86
  during the puerperium — see Thrombosis,
    puerperal
  endocardial — see also Infarct,
    myocardium
    not resulting in infarction I24.0
  eye — see Occlusion, retina
  genital organ
    female NEC N94.89
      pregnancy — see Thrombophlebitis,
        antepartum
    male N50.1
  gestational — see Phlebopathy, gestational
  heart (chamber) — see also Infarct,
    myocardium
    not resulting in infarction I24.0
  hepatic (vein) I82.0
    artery I74.8
  history (of) Z86.718
  intestine (with gangrene) K55.0
  intracardiac NEC (apical) (atrial)
    (auricular) (ventricular) (old) I51.3
  intracranial (arterial) I66.9
    venous sinus (any) G08
      nonpyogenic origin I67.6
      puerperium O87.3
  intramural — see also Infarct, myocardium
    not resulting in infarction I24.0
  intraspinal venous sinuses and veins G08
    nonpyogenic G95.19
  kidney (artery) N28.0
  lateral (venous) sinus — see Thrombosis,
    intracranial venous sinus
  leg — see Thrombosis, vein, lower
    extremity
    arterial I74.3
  liver (venous) I82.0
    artery I74.8
    portal vein I81
  longitudinal (venous) sinus — see
    Thrombosis, intracranial venous sinus
  lower limb — see Thrombosis, vein, lower
    extremity
  lung (iatrogenic) (postoperative) — see
    Embolism, pulmonary
  meninges (brain) (arterial) I66.8
  mesenteric (artery) (with gangrene) K55.0
    vein (inferior) (superior) I81
  mitral I34.8
  mural — see also Infarct, myocardium
    due to syphilis A52.06
    not resulting in infarction I24.0
  omentum (with gangrene) K55.0
  ophthalmic — see Occlusion, retina
  pampiniform plexus (male) N50.1
  parietal — see also Infarct, myocardium
    not resulting in infarction I24.0
  penis, superficial vein N48.81

Thrombosis, thrombotic (bland) (multiple)
  (progressive) (silent) (vessel) I82.90 —
  continued
  perianal venous K64.5
  peripheral arteries I74.4
    upper I74.2
  personal history (of) Z86.718
  portal I81
    due to syphilis A52.09
  precerebral artery — see Occlusion, artery,
    precerebral
  puerperal, postpartum O87.0
    brain (artery) O99.43
      venous (sinus) O87.3
    cardiac O99.43
    cerebral (artery) O99.43
      venous (sinus) O87.3
    superficial O87.0
  pulmonary (artery) (iatrogenic)
    (postoperative) (vein) — see
    Embolism, pulmonary
  renal (artery) N28.0
    vein I82.3
  resulting from presence of device, implant
    or graft — see Complications, by site
    and type, specified NEC
  retina, retinal — see Occlusion, retina
  scrotum N50.1
  seminal vesicle N50.1
  sigmoid (venous) sinus — see Thrombosis,
    intracranial venous sinus
  sinus, intracranial (any) — see Thrombosis,
    intracranial venous sinus
  specified site NEC I82.890
    chronic I82.891
  spermatic cord N50.1
  spinal cord (arterial) G95.11
    due to syphilis A52.09
    pyogenic origin G06.1
  spleen, splenic D73.5
    artery I74.8
  testis N50.1
  traumatic NEC T14.8
  tricuspid I07.8
  tumor — see Neoplasm, unspecified
    behavior, by site
  tunica vaginalis N50.1
  umbilical cord (vessels), complicating
    delivery O69.5
  vas deferens N50.1
  vein (acute) I82.90
    antecubital I82.61-
      chronic I82.61-
    axillary I82.A1-
      chronic I82.A2-
    basilic I82.61-
      chronic I82.71-
    brachial I82.62-
      chronic I82.72-
    brachiocephalic (innominate) I82.290
      chronic I82.291
    cephalic I82.61-
      chronic I82.71-
    cerebral, nonpyogenic I67.6
    chronic I82.91
    deep (DVT) I82.40-
      calf I82.4Z-
        chronic I82.5Z-
      lower leg I82.4Z-
        chronic I82.5Z-
      thigh I82.4Y-
        chronic I82.5Y-
      upper leg I82.4Y
        chronic I82.5Y-
    femoral I82.41-
      chronic I82.51-
    iliac (iliofemoral) I82.42-
      chronic I82.52-
    innominate I82.290
      chronic I82.291
    internal jugular I82.C1-
      chronic I82.C2-
    lower extremity
      deep I82.40-
        chronic I82.50-
        specified NEC I82.49-
          chronic NEC I82.59-
      distal
        deep I82.4Z-
      proximal
        deep I82.4Y-
          chronic I82.5Y-
      superficial I82.81-
    perianal K64.5
    popliteal I82.43-
      chronic I82.53-
    radial I82.62-
      chronic I82.72-
    renal I82.3
    saphenous (greater) (lesser) I82.81-

Thrombosis, thrombotic (bland) (multiple) (progressive) (silent) (vessel) I82.90 — *continued*
  vein (acute) I82.90 — *continued*
    specified NEC I82.890
      chronic NEC I82.891
    subclavian I82.B1-
      chronic I82.B2-
    thoracic NEC I82.290
      chronic I82.291
    tibial I82.44-
      chronic I82.54-
    ulnar I82.62-
      chronic I82.72-
    upper extremity I82.60-
      chronic I82.70-
      deep I82.62-
        chronic I82.72-
      superficial I82.61-
        chronic I82.71-
    vena cava
      inferior I82.220
        chronic I82.221
      superior I82.210
        chronic I82.211
  ventricle — *see also* Infarct, myocardium
    following acute myocardial infarction (current complication) I23.6
    not resulting in infarction I24.0
  venous, perianal K64.5
Thrombus — *see* Thrombosis
Thrush — *see also* Candidiasis
  newborn P37.5
  oral B37.0
  vaginal B37.3
Thumb — *see also* condition
  sucking (child problem) F98.8
Thymitis E32.8
Thymoma (benign) D15.0
  malignant C37
Thymus, thymic (gland) — *see* condition
Thyrocele — *see* Goiter
Thyroglossal — *see also* condition
  cyst Q89.2
  duct, persistent Q89.2
Thyroid (gland) (body) — *see also* condition
  hormone resistance E07.89
  lingual Q89.2
  nodule (cystic) (nontoxic) (single) E04.1
Thyroiditis E06.9
  acute (nonsuppurative) (pyogenic) (suppurative) E06.0
  autoimmune E06.3
  chronic (nonspecific) (sclerosing) E06.5
    with thyrotoxicosis, transient E06.2
    fibrous E06.5
    lymphadenoid E06.3
    lymphocytic E06.3
    lymphoid E06.3
  de Quervain's E06.1
  drug-induced E06.4
  fibrous (chronic) E06.5
  giant-cell (follicular) E06.1
  granulomatous (de Quervain) (subacute) E06.1
  Hashimoto's (struma lymphomatosa) E06.3
  iatrogenic E06.4
  ligneous E06.5
  lymphocytic (chronic) E06.3
  lymphoid E06.3
  lymphomatous E06.3
  nonsuppurative E06.1
  postpartum, puerperal O90.5
  pseudotuberculous E06.1
  pyogenic E06.0
  radiation E06.4
  Riedel's E06.5
  subacute (granulomatous) E06.1
  suppurative E06.0
  tuberculous A18.81
  viral E06.1
  woody E06.5
Thyrolingual duct, persistent Q89.2
Thyromegaly E01.0
Thyrotoxic
  crisis — *see* Thyrotoxicosis
  heart disease or failure (*see also* Thyrotoxicosis) E05.90 [I43]
    with thyroid storm E05.91 [I43]
  storm — *see* Thyrotoxicosis

Thyrotoxicosis (recurrent) E05.90
  with
    goiter (diffuse) E05.00
      with thyroid storm E05.01
      adenomatous uninodular E05.10
        with thyroid storm E05.11
      multinodular E05.20
        with thyroid storm E05.21
      nodular E05.20
        with thyroid storm E05.21
      uninodular E05.10
        with thyroid storm E05.11
    infiltrative
      dermopathy E05.00
        with thyroid storm E05.01
      ophthalmopathy E05.00
        with thyroid storm E05.01
    single thyroid nodule E05.10
      with thyroid storm E05.11
  due to
    ectopic thyroid nodule or tissue E05.30
      with thyroid storm E05.31
    ingestion of (excessive) thyroid material E05.40
      with thyroid storm E05.41
    overproduction of thyroid-stimulating hormone E05.80
      with thyroid storm E05.81
    specified cause NEC E05.80
      with thyroid storm E05.81
  factitia E05.40
    with thyroid storm E05.41
  heart E05.90 [I43]
    with thyroid storm E05.91 [I43]
    failure E05.90 [I43]
  neonatal (transient) P72.1
  transient with chronic thyroiditis E06.2
Tibia vara — *see* Osteochondrosis, juvenile, tibia
Tic (disorder) F95.9
  breathing F95.8
  child problem F95.0
  compulsive F95.1
  de la Tourette F95.2
  degenerative (generalized) (localized) G25.69
    facial G25.69
  disorder
    chronic
      motor F95.1
      vocal F95.1
    combined vocal and multiple motor F95.2
    transient F95.0
  douloureux G50.0
    atypical G50.1
    postherpetic, postzoster B02.22
  drug-induced G25.61
  eyelid F95.8
  habit F95.9
    chronic F95.1
    transient of childhood F95.0
  lid, transient of childhood F95.0
  motor-verbal F95.2
  occupational F48.8
  orbicularis F95.8
    transient of childhood F95.0
  organic origin G25.69
  postchoreic G25.69
  psychogenic, compulsive F95.1
  salaam R25.8
  spasm (motor or vocal) F95.9
    chronic F95.1
    transient of childhood F95.0
  specified NEC F95.8
Tick-borne — *see* condition
Tietze's disease or syndrome M94.0
Tight, tightness
  anus K62.89
  chest R07.89
  fascia (lata) M62.89
  foreskin (congenital) N47.1
  hymen, hymenal ring N89.6
  introitus (acquired) (congenital) N89.6
  rectal sphincter K62.89
  tendon — *see* Short, tendon
  urethral sphincter N35.9
Tilting vertebra — *see* Dorsopathy, deforming, specified NEC
Timidity, child F93.8
Tin-miner's lung J63.5
Tinea (intersecta) (tarsi) B35.9
  amiantacea L44.8
  asbestina B35.0
  barbae B35.0
  beard B35.0
  black dot B35.0
  blanca B36.2
  capitis B35.0
  corporis B35.4

Tinea (intersecta) (tarsi) B35.9 — *continued*
  cruris B35.6
  flava B36.0
  foot B35.3
  furfuracea B36.0
  imbricata (Tokelau) B35.5
  kerion B35.0
  manuum B35.2
  microsporic — *see* Dermatophytosis
  nigra B36.1
  nodosa — *see* Piedra
  pedis B35.3
  scalp B35.0
  specified site NEC B35.8
  sycosis B35.0
  tonsurans B35.0
  trichophytic — *see* Dermatophytosis
  unguium B35.1
  versicolor B36.0
Tingling sensation (skin) R20.2
Tinnitus (audible) (aurium) (subjective) — *see subcategory* H93.1
Tipped tooth (teeth) M26.33
Tipping
  pelvis M95.5
    with disproportion (fetopelvic) O33.0
      causing obstructed labor O65.0
  tooth (teeth), fully erupted M26.33
Tiredness R53.83
Tissue — *see* condition
Tobacco (nicotine)
  dependence — *see* Dependence, drug, nicotine
  harmful use Z72.0
  heart — *see* Tobacco, toxic effect
  maternal use, affecting newborn P04.2
  toxic effect — *see* Table of Drugs and Chemicals, by substance, poisoning
    chewing tobacco — *see* Table of Drugs and Chemicals, by substance, poisoning
    cigarettes — *see* Table of Drugs and Chemicals, by substance, poisoning
  use Z72.0
    complicating
      childbirth O99.334
      pregnancy O99.33-
      puerperium O99.335
    counseling and surveillance Z71.6
  withdrawal state — *see* Dependence, drug, nicotine
Tocopherol deficiency E56.0
Todd's
  cirrhosis K74.3
  paralysis (postepileptic) (transitory) G83.84
Toe — *see* condition
Toilet, artificial opening — *see* Attention to, artificial, opening
Tokelau (ringworm) B35.5
Tollwut — *see* Rabies
Tommaselli's disease R31.9
  correct substance properly administered — *see* Table of Drugs and Chemicals, by drug, adverse effect
  overdose or wrong substance given or taken — *see* Table of Drugs and Chemicals, by drug, poisoning
Tongue — *see also* condition
  tie Q38.1
Tonic pupil — *see* Anomaly, pupil, function, tonic pupil
Toni-Fanconi syndrome (cystinosis) E72.09
  with cystinosis E72.04
Tonsil — *see* condition
Tonsillitis (acute) (catarrhal) (croupous) (follicular) (gangrenous) (infective) (lacunar) (lingual) (malignant) (membranous) (parenchymatous) (phlegmonous) (pseudomembranous) (purulent) (septic) (subacute) (suppurative) (toxic) (ulcerative) (vesicular) (viral) J03.90
  chronic J35.01
    with adenoiditis J35.03
  diphtheritic A36.0
  hypertrophic J35.01
    with adenoiditis J35.03
  recurrent J03.91
  specified organism NEC J03.80
    recurrent J03.81
  staphylococcal J03.80
    recurrent J03.81
  streptococcal J03.00
    recurrent J03.01
  tuberculous A15.8
  Vincent's A69.1

Tooth, teeth — *see* condition
Toothache K08.8
Topagnosis R20.8
Tophi — *see* Gout, chronic
TORCH infection — *see* Infection, congenital
  without active infection P00.2
Torn — *see* Tear
Tornwaldt's cyst or disease J39.2
Torsion
  accessory tube — *see* Torsion, fallopian tube
  adnexa (female) — *see* Torsion, fallopian tube
  aorta, acquired I77.1
  appendix epididymis N44.04
  appendix testis N44.03
  bile duct (common) (hepatic) K83.8
    congenital Q44.5
  bowel, colon or intestine K56.2
  cervix — *see* Malposition, uterus
  cystic duct K82.8
  dystonia — *see* Dystonia, torsion
  epididymis (appendix) N44.04
  fallopian tube N83.52
    with ovary N83.53
  gallbladder K82.8
    congenital Q44.1
  hydatid of Morgagni
    female N83.52
    male N44.03
  kidney (pedicle) (leading to infarction) N28.0
  Meckel's diverticulum (congenital) Q43.0
    malignant — *see* Table of Neoplasms, small intestine, malignant
  mesentery K56.2
  omentum K56.2
  organ or site, congenital NEC — *see* Anomaly, by site
  ovary (pedicle) N83.51
    with fallopian tube N83.53
    congenital Q50.2
  oviduct — *see* Torsion, fallopian tube
  penis (acquired) N48.82
    congenital Q55.69
  spasm — *see* Dystonia, torsion
  spermatic cord N44.02
    extravaginal N44.01
    intravaginal N44.02
  spleen D73.5
  testis, testicle N44.00
    appendix N44.03
  tibia — *see* Deformity, limb, specified type NEC, lower leg
  uterus — *see* Malposition, uterus
Torticollis (intermittent) (spastic) M43.6
  congenital (sternomastoid) Q68.0
  due to birth injury P15.8
  hysterical F44.4
  ocular R29.891
  psychogenic F45.8
    conversion reaction F44.4
  rheumatic M43.6
  rheumatoid M06.88
  spasmodic G24.3
  traumatic, current S13.4
Tortipelvis G24.1
Tortuous
  artery I77.1
  organ or site, congenital NEC — *see* Distortion
  retinal vessel, congenital Q14.1
  ureter N13.8
  urethra N36.8
  vein — *see* Varix
Torture, victim of Z65.4
Torula, torular (histolytica) (infection) — *see* Cryptococcosis
Torulosis — *see* Cryptococcosis
Torus (mandibularis) (palatinus) M27.0
  fracture — *see* Fracture, by site, torus
Touraine's syndrome Q79.8
Tourette's syndrome F95.2
Tourniquet syndrome — *see* Constriction, external, by site
Tower skull Q75.0
  with exophthalmos Q87.0
Toxemia R68.89
  bacterial — *see* Sepsis
  burn — *see* Burn
  eclamptic (with pre-existing hypertension) — *see* Eclampsia
  erysipelatous — *see* Erysipelas
  fatigue R68.89
  food — *see* Poisoning, food
  gastrointestinal K52.1
  intestinal K52.1

...ia R68.89 — continued
kidney — see Uremia
malarial — see Malaria
myocardial — see Myocarditis, toxic
   of pregnancy — see Pre-eclampsia
pre-eclamptic — see Pre-eclampsia
small intestine K52.1
staphylococcal, due to food A05.0
stasis R68.89
uremic — see Uremia
urinary — see Uremia
Toxemica cerebropathia psychica
   (nonalcoholic) F04
alcoholic — see Alcohol, amnestic disorder
Toxic (poisoning) (see also condition) T65.91
effect — see Table of Drugs and
   Chemicals, by substance, poisoning
shock syndrome A48.3
thyroid (gland) — see Thyrotoxicosis
Toxicemia — see Toxemia
Toxicity — see Table of Drugs and
   Chemicals, by substance, poisoning
fava bean D55.0
food, noxious — see Poisoning, food
from drug or nonmedicinal substance
   see Table of Drugs and Chemicals, by
   drug
Toxicosis — see also Toxemia
capillary, hemorrhagic D69.0
Toxinfection, gastrointestinal K52.1
Toxocariasis B83.0
Toxoplasma, toxoplasmosis (acquired)
   B58.9
with
   hepatitis B58.1
   meningoencephalitis B58.2
   ocular involvement B58.00
   other organ involvement B58.89
   pneumonia, pneumonitis B58.3
congenital (acute) (subacute) (chronic)
   P37.1
maternal, manifest toxoplasmosis in infant
   (acute) (subacute) (chronic) P37.1
tPA (rtPA) administration in a different
   facility within the last 24 hours prior
   to admission to current facility Z92.82
Trabeculation, bladder N32.89
Trachea — see condition
Tracheitis (catarrhal) (infantile)
   (membranous) (plastic) (septal)
   (suppurative) (viral) J04.10
with
   bronchitis (15 years of age and above)
     J40
     acute or subacute — see Bronchitis,
       acute
     chronic J42
     tuberculous NEC A15.5
     under 15 years of age J20.9
   laryngitis (acute) J04.2
     chronic J37.1
     tuberculous NEC A15.5
acute J04.10
   with obstruction J04.11
chronic J42
   with
     bronchitis (chronic) J42
     laryngitis (chronic) J37.1
diphtheritic (membranous) A36.89
due to external agent — see Inflammation,
   respiratory, upper, due to
syphilitic A52.73
tuberculous A15.5
Trachelitis (nonvenereal) — see Cervicitis
Tracheobronchial — see condition
Tracheobronchitis (15 years of age and
   above) — see also Bronchitis
due to
   Bordetella bronchiseptica A37.80
     with pneumonia A37.81
   Francisella tularensis A21.8
Tracheobronchomegaly Q32.4
with bronchiectasis J47.9
   with
     exacerbation (acute) J47.1
     lower respiratory infection J47.0
acquired J98.09
   with bronchiectasis J47.9
     with
       exacerbation (acute) J47.1
       lower respiratory infection J47.0
Tracheobronchopneumonitis — see
   Pneumonia, broncho-
Tracheocele (external) (internal) J39.8
congenital Q32.1
Tracheomalacia J39.8
congenital Q32.0

Tracheopharyngitis (acute) J06.9
chronic J42
due to external agent — see Inflammation,
   respiratory, upper, due to
Tracheostenosis J39.8
Tracheostomy
complication — see Complication,
   tracheostomy
status Z93.0
   attention to Z43.0
   malfunctioning J95.03
Trachoma, trachomatous A71.9
active (stage) A71.1
contraction of conjunctiva A71.1
dubium A71.0
healed or sequelae B94.0
initial (stage) A71.0
pannus A71.1
Türck's J37.0
Traction, vitreomacular H43.82-
Train sickness T75.3
Trait(s)
Hb-S D57.3
hemoglobin
   abnormal NEC D58.2
     with thalassemia D56.3
   C — see Disease, hemoglobin C
   S (Hb-S) D57.3
Lepore D56.3
personality, accentuated Z73.1
sickle-cell D57.3
   with elliptocytosis or spherocytosis
     D57.3
type A personality Z73.1
Tramp Z59.0
Trance R41.89
hysterical F44.89
Transaminasemia R74.0
Transection
abdomen (partial) S38.3
aorta (incomplete) — see also Injury, aorta
   complete — see Injury, aorta, laceration,
     major
carotid artery (incomplete) — see also
   Injury, blood vessel, carotid,
   laceration
   complete — see Injury, blood vessel,
     carotid, laceration, major
celiac artery (incomplete) S35.211
   branch (incomplete) S35.291
     complete S35.292
   complete S35.212
innominate
   artery (incomplete) — see also Injury,
     blood vessel, thoracic, innominate,
     artery, laceration
     complete — see Injury, blood vessel,
       thoracic, innominate, artery,
       laceration, major
   vein (incomplete) — see also Injury,
     blood vessel, thoracic, innominate,
     vein, laceration
     complete — see Injury, blood vessel,
       thoracic, innominate, vein,
       laceration, major
jugular vein (external) (incomplete) —
   also Injury, blood vessel, jugular vein,
   laceration
   complete — see Injury, blood vessel,
     jugular vein, laceration, major
   internal (incomplete) — see also Injury,
     blood vessel, jugular vein, internal,
     laceration
     complete — see Injury, blood vessel,
       jugular vein, internal, laceration,
       major
mesenteric artery (incomplete) — see also
   Injury, mesenteric, artery, laceration
   complete — see Injury, mesenteric,
     artery, laceration, major
pulmonary vessel (incomplete) — see also
   Injury, blood vessel, thoracic,
   pulmonary, laceration
   complete — see Injury, blood vessel,
     thoracic, pulmonary, laceration,
     major
subclavian — see Transection, innominate
vena cava (incomplete) — see also Injury,
   vena cava
   complete — see Injury, vena cava,
     laceration, major
vertebral artery (incomplete) — see also
   Injury, blood vessel, vertebral,
   laceration
   complete — see Injury, blood vessel,
     vertebral, laceration, major

Transfusion
associated (red blood cell)
   hemochromatosis E83.111
blood
   ABO incompatible — see
     Complication(s), transfusion,
     incompatibility reaction, ABO
   minor blood group (Duffy) (E) (K(ell))
     (Kidd) (Lewis) (M) (N) (P) (S)
     T80.89
   reaction or complication — see
     Complications, transfusion
fetomaternal (mother) — see Pregnancy,
   complicated by, placenta, transfusion
   syndrome
maternofetal (mother) — see Pregnancy,
   complicated by, placenta, transfusion
   syndrome
placental (syndrome) (mother) — see
   Pregnancy, complicated by, placenta,
   transfusion syndrome
reaction (adverse) — see Complications,
   transfusion
related acute lung injury (TRALI) J95.84
twin-to-twin — see Pregnancy, complicated
   by, placenta, transfusion syndrome,
   fetus to fetus
Transient (meaning homeless) (see also
   condition) Z59.0
Translocation
balanced autosomal Q95.9
   in normal individual Q95.0
chromosomes NEC Q99.8
   balanced and insertion in normal
     individual Q95.0
Down syndrome Q90.2
trisomy
   13 Q91.6
   18 Q91.2
   21 Q90.2
Translucency, iris — see Degeneration, iris
Transmission of chemical substances
   through the placenta — see
   Absorption, chemical, through placenta
Transparency, lung, unilateral J43.0
Transplant(ed) (status) Z94.9
awaiting organ Z76.82
bone Z94.6
   marrow Z94.81
candidate Z76.82
complication — see Complication,
   transplant
cornea Z94.7
heart Z94.1
   and lung(s) Z94.3
   valve Z95.2
     prosthetic Z95.2
     specified NEC Z95.4
     xenogenic Z95.3
intestine Z94.82
kidney Z94.0
liver Z94.4
lung(s) Z94.2
   and heart Z94.3
organ (failure) (infection) (rejection) Z94.9
   removal status Z98.85
pancreas Z94.83
skin Z94.5
social Z60.3
specified organ or tissue NEC Z94.89
stem cells Z94.84
tissue Z94.9
Transplants, ovarian, endometrial N80.1
Transposed — see Transposition
Transposition (congenital) — see also
   Malposition, congenital
abdominal viscera Q89.3
aorta (dextra) Q20.3
appendix Q43.8
colon Q43.8
corrected Q20.5
great vessels (complete) (partial) Q20.3
heart Q24.0
   with complete transposition of viscera
     Q89.3
intestine (large) (small) Q43.8
reversed jejunal (for bypass) (status) Z98.0
scrotum Q55.23
stomach Q40.2
   with general transposition of viscera
     Q89.3
tooth, teeth, fully erupted M26.30
vessels, great (complete) (partial) Q20.3
viscera (abdominal) (thoracic) Q89.3

Transsexualism F64.1
Transverse — see also condition
arrest (deep), in labor O64.0
lie (mother) O32.2
   causing obstructed labor O64.8
Transvestism, transvestitism (dual-role)
   F64.1
fetishistic F65.1
Trapped placenta (with hemorrhage) O72.0
without hemorrhage O73.0
Trauma, traumatism — see also Injury
acoustic — see subcategory H83.3
birth — see Birth, injury
complicating ectopic or molar pregnancy
   O08.6
during delivery O71.9
following ectopic or molar pregnancy
   O08.6
obstetric O71.9
   specified NEC O71.89
Traumatic — see also condition
brain injury — see category S06
Treacher Collins syndrome Q75.4
Treitz's hernia — see Hernia, abdomen,
   specified site NEC
Trematode infestation — see Infestation,
   fluke
Trematodiasis — see Infestation, fluke
Trembling paralysis — see Parkinsonism
Tremor(s) R25.1
drug induced G25.1
essential (benign) G25.0
familial G25.0
hereditary G25.0
hysterical F44.4
intention G25.2
medication induced postural G25.1
mercurial — see subcategory T56.1
Parkinson's — see Parkinsonism
psychogenic (conversion reaction) F44.4
senilis R54
specified type NEC G25.2
Trench
fever A79.0
foot — see Immersion, foot
mouth A69.1
Treponema pallidum infection — see
   Syphilis
Treponematosis
due to
   T. pallidum — see Syphilis
   T. pertenue — see Yaws
Triad
Hutchinson's (congenital syphilis) A50.53
Kartagener's Q89.3
Saint's — see Hernia, diaphragm
Trichiasis (eyelid) H02.059
with entropion — see Entropion
left H02.056
   lower H02.055
   upper H02.054
right H02.053
   lower H02.052
   upper H02.051
Trichinella spiralis (infection) (infestation)
   B75
Trichinellosis, trichiniasis, trichinelliasis,
   trichinosis B75
with muscle disorder B75 [M63.80]
   ankle B75 [M63.8-]
   foot B75 [M63.8-]
   forearm B75 [M63.8-]
   hand B75 [M63.8-]
   lower leg B75 [M63.8-]
   multiple sites B75 [M63.89]
   pelvic region B75 [M63.8-]
   shoulder region B75 [M63.8-]
   specified site NEC B75 [M63.88]
   thigh B75 [M63.8-]
   upper arm B75 [M63.8-]
Trichobezoar T18.9
intestine T18.3
stomach T18.2
Trichocephaliasis, trichocephalosis B79
Trichocephalus infestation B79
Trichoclasis L67.8
Trichoepithelioma — see also Neoplasm,
   skin, benign
malignant — see Neoplasm, skin,
   malignant
Trichofolliculoma — see Neoplasm, skin,
   benign
Tricholemmoma — see Neoplasm, skin,
   benign

Trichomoniasis A59.9
  bladder A59.03
  cervix A59.09
  intestinal A07.8
  prostate A59.02
  seminal vesicles A59.09
  specified site NEC A59.8
  urethra A59.03
  urogenitalis A59.00
  vagina A59.01
  vulva A59.01
Trichomycosis
  axillaris A48.8
  nodosa, nodularis B36.8
Trichonodosis L67.8
Trichophytid, trichophyton infection — *see* Dermatophytosis
Trichophytobezoar T18.9
  intestine T18.3
  stomach T18.2
Trichophytosis — *see* Dermatophytosis
Trichoptilosis L67.8
Trichorrhexis (nodosa) (invaginata) L67.0
Trichosis axillaris A48.8
Trichosporosis nodosa B36.2
Trichostasis spinulosa (congenital) Q84.1
Trichostrongyliasis, trichostrongylosis (small intestine) B81.2
Trichostrongylus infection B81.2
Trichotillomania F63.3
Trichromat, trichromatopsia, anomalous (congenital) H53.55
Trichuriasis B79
Trichuris trichiura (infection) (infestation) (any site) B79
Tricuspid (valve) — *see* condition
Trifid — *see also* Accessory
  kidney (pelvis) Q63.8
  tongue Q38.3
Trigeminal neuralgia — *see* Neuralgia, trigeminal
Trigeminy R00.8
Trigger finger (acquired) M65.30
  congenital Q74.0
  index finger M65.32-
  little finger M65.35-
  middle finger M65.33-
  ring finger M65.34-
  thumb M65.31-
Trigonitis (bladder) (chronic) (pseudomembranous) N30.30
  with hematuria N30.31
Trigonocephaly Q75.0
Trilocular heart — *see* Cor triloculare
Trimethylaminuria E72.52
Triphalangeal thumb Q74.0
Tripartite placenta O43.19-
Triple — *see also* Accessory
  kidneys Q63.0
  uteri Q51.818
  X, female Q97.0
Triplegia G83.89
  congenital G80.8
Triplet (newborn) — *see also* Newborn, triplet
  complicating pregnancy — *see* Pregnancy, triplet
Triplication — *see* Accessory
Triploidy Q92.7
Trismus R25.2
  neonatorum A33
  newborn A33
Trisomy (syndrome) Q92.9
  13 (partial) Q91.7
    meiotic nondisjunction Q91.4
    mitotic nondisjunction Q91.5
    mosaicism Q91.5
    translocation Q91.6
  18 (partial) Q91.3
    meiotic nondisjunction Q91.0
    mitotic nondisjunction Q91.1
    mosaicism Q91.1
    translocation Q91.2
  20 Q92.8
  21 (partial) Q90.9
    meiotic nondisjunction Q90.0
    mitotic nondisjunction Q90.1
    mosaicism Q90.1
    translocation Q90.2
  22 Q92.8
  autosomes Q92.9
  chromosome specified NEC Q92.8
    partial Q92.2
      due to unbalanced translocation Q92.5
    specified NEC Q92.8
    whole (nonsex chromosome)
      meiotic nondisjunction Q92.0
      mitotic nondisjunction Q92.1
      mosaicism Q92.1

Trisomy (syndrome) Q92.9 — *continued*
  due to
    dicentrics — *see* Extra, marker chromosomes
    extra rings — *see* Extra, marker chromosomes
    isochromosomes — *see* Extra, marker chromosomes
  specified NEC Q92.8
  whole chromosome Q92.9
    meiotic nondisjunction Q92.0
    mitotic nondisjunction Q92.1
    mosaicism Q92.1
    partial Q92.9
    specified NEC Q92.8
Tritanomaly, tritanopia H53.55
Trombiculosis, trombiculiasis, trombidiosis B88.0
Trophedema (congenital) (hereditary) Q82.0
Trophoblastic disease (*see also* Mole, hydatidiform) O01.9
Tropholymphedema Q82.0
Trophoneurosis NEC G96.8
  disseminated M34.9
Tropical — *see* condition
Trouble — *see also* Disease
  heart — *see* Disease, heart
  kidney — *see* Disease, renal
  nervous R45.0
  sinus — *see* Sinusitis
Trousseau's syndrome (thrombophlebitis migrans) I82.1
Truancy, childhood
  from school Z72.810
Truncus
  arteriosus (persistent) Q20.0
  communis Q20.0
Trunk — *see* condition
Trypanosomiasis
  African B56.9
    by Trypanosoma brucei
      gambiense B56.0
      rhodesiense B56.1
  American — *see* Chagas' disease
  Brazilian — *see* Chagas' disease
  by Trypanosoma
    brucei gambiense B56.0
    brucei rhodesiense B56.1
    cruzi — *see* Chagas' disease
  gambiensis, Gambian B56.0
  rhodesiensis, Rhodesian B56.1
  South American — *see* Chagas' disease
  where
    African trypanosomiasis is prevalent B56.9
    Chagas' disease is prevalent B57.2
T-shaped incisors K00.2
Tsutsugamushi (disease) (fever) A75.3
Tube, tubal, tubular — *see* condition
Tubercle — *see also* Tuberculosis
  brain, solitary A17.81
  Darwin's Q17.8
  Ghon, primary infection A15.7
Tuberculid, tuberculide (indurating, subcutaneous) (lichenoid) (miliary) (papulonecrotic) (primary) (skin) A18.4
Tuberculoma — *see also* Tuberculosis
  brain A17.81
  meninges (cerebral) (spinal) A17.1
  spinal cord A17.81
Tuberculosis, tubercular, tuberculous (calcification) (calcified) (caseous) (chromogenic acid-fast bacilli) (degeneration) (fibrocaseous) (fistula) (interstitial) (isolated circumscribed lesions) (necrosis) (parenchymatous) (ulcerative) A15.9
  with pneumoconiosis (any condition in J60-J64) J65
  abdomen (lymph gland) A18.39
  abscess (respiratory) A15.9
    bone A18.03
      hip A18.02
      knee A18.02
      sacrum A18.01
      specified site NEC A18.03
      spinal A18.01
      vertebra A18.01
    brain A17.81
    breast A18.89
    Cowper's gland A18.15
    dura (mater) (cerebral) (spinal) A17.81
    epidural (cerebral) (spinal) A17.81
    female pelvis A18.17
    frontal sinus A15.8
    genital organs NEC A18.10
    genitourinary A18.10
    gland (lymphatic) — *see* Tuberculosis, lymph gland

Tuberculosis, tubercular, tuberculous (calcification) (calcified) (caseous) (chromogenic acid-fast bacilli) (degeneration) (fibrocaseous) (fistula) (interstitial) (isolated circumscribed lesions) (necrosis) (parenchymatous) (ulcerative) A15.9 — *continued*
  abscess (respiratory) A15.9 — *continued*
    hip A18.02
    intestine A18.32
    ischiorectal A18.32
    joint NEC A18.02
      hip A18.02
      knee A18.02
      specified NEC A18.02
      vertebral A18.01
    kidney A18.11
    knee A18.02
    latent R76.11
    lumbar (spine) A18.01
    lung — *see* Tuberculosis, pulmonary
    meninges (cerebral) (spinal) A17.0
    muscle A18.09
    perianal (fistula) A18.32
    perinephritic A18.11
    perirectal A18.32
    rectum A18.32
    retropharyngeal A15.8
    sacrum A18.01
    scrofulous A18.2
    scrotum A18.15
    skin (primary) A18.4
    spinal cord A17.81
    spine or vertebra (column) A18.01
    subdiaphragmatic A18.31
    testis A18.15
    urinary A18.13
    uterus A18.17
  accessory sinus — *see* Tuberculosis, sinus
  Addison's disease A18.7
  adenitis — *see* Tuberculosis, lymph gland
  adenoids A18.5
  adenopathy — *see* Tuberculosis, lymph gland
  adherent pericardium A18.84
  adnexa (uteri) A18.17
  adrenal (capsule) (gland) A18.7
  alimentary canal A18.32
  anemia A18.89
  ankle (joint) (bone) A18.02
  anus A18.32
  apex, apical — *see* Tuberculosis, pulmonary
  appendicitis, appendix A18.32
  arachnoid A17.0
  artery, arteritis A18.89
    cerebral A18.89
  arthritis (chronic) (synovial) A18.02
    spine or vertebra (column) A18.01
  articular — *see* Tuberculosis, joint
  ascites A18.31
  asthma — *see* Tuberculosis, pulmonary
  axilla, axillary (gland) A18.2
  bladder A18.12
  bone A18.03
    hip A18.02
    knee A18.02
    limb NEC A18.03
    sacrum A18.01
    spine or vertebral column A18.01
  bowel (miliary) A18.32
  brain A17.81
  breast A18.89
  broad ligament A18.17
  bronchi, bronchial, bronchus A15.5
    ectasia, ectasis (bronchiectasis) — *see* Tuberculosis, pulmonary
    fistula A15.5
      primary (progressive) A15.7
    gland or node A15.4
      primary (progressive) A15.7
    lymph gland or node A15.4
      primary (progressive) A15.7
  bronchiectasis — *see* Tuberculosis, pulmonary
  bronchitis A15.5
  bronchopleural A15.6
  bronchopneumonia, bronchopneumonic — *see* Tuberculosis, pulmonary
  bronchorrhagia A15.5
  bronchotracheal A15.5
  bronze disease A18.7
  buccal cavity A18.83
  bulbourethral gland A18.15
  bursa A18.09
  cachexia A15.9
  cardiomyopathy A18.84
  caries — *see* Tuberculosis, bone
  cartilage A18.02
    intervertebral A18.01

Tuberculosis, tubercular, tuberculous (calcification) (calcified) (caseous) (chromogenic acid-fast bacilli) (degeneration) (fibrocaseous) (fistula) (interstitial) (isolated circumscribed lesions) (necrosis) (parenchymatous) (ulcerative) A15.9 — *continued*
  catarrhal — *see* Tuberculosis, respiratory
  cecum A18.32
  cellulitis (primary) A18.4
  cerebellum A17.81
  cerebral, cerebrum A17.81
  cerebrospinal A17.81
    meninges A17.0
  cervical (lymph gland or node) A18.2
  cervicitis, cervix (uteri) A18.16
  chest — *see* Tuberculosis, respiratory
  chorioretinitis A18.53
  choroid, choroiditis A18.53
  ciliary body A18.54
  colitis A18.32
  collier's J65
  colliquativa (primary) A18.4
  colon A18.32
  complex, primary A15.7
  congenital P37.0
  conjunctiva A18.59
  connective tissue (systemic) A18.89
  contact Z20.1
  cornea (ulcer) A18.52
  Cowper's gland A18.15
  coxae A18.02
  coxalgia A18.02
  cul-de-sac of Douglas A18.17
  curvature, spine A18.01
  cutis (colliquativa) (primary) A18.4
  cyst, ovary A18.18
  cystitis A18.12
  dactylitis A18.03
  diarrhea A18.32
  diffuse — *see* Tuberculosis, miliary
  digestive tract A18.32
  disseminated — *see* Tuberculosis, miliary
  duodenum A18.32
  dura (mater) (cerebral) (spinal) A17.0
    abscess (cerebral) (spinal) A17.81
  dysentery A18.32
  ear (inner) (middle) A18.6
    bone A18.03
    external (primary) A18.4
    skin (primary) A18.4
  elbow A18.02
  emphysema — *see* Tuberculosis, pulmonary
  empyema A15.6
  encephalitis A17.82
  endarteritis A18.89
  endocarditis A18.84
    aortic A18.84
    mitral A18.84
    pulmonary A18.84
    tricuspid A18.84
  endocrine glands NEC A18.82
  endometrium A18.17
  enteric, enterica, enteritis A18.32
  enterocolitis A18.32
  epididymis, epididymitis A18.15
  epidural abscess (cerebral) (spinal) A17.81
  epiglottis A15.5
  episcleritis A18.51
  erythema (induratum) (nodosum) (primary) A18.4
  esophagus A18.83
  eustachian tube A18.6
  exposure (to) Z20.1
  exudative — *see* Tuberculosis, pulmonary
  eye A18.50
  eyelid (primary) (lupus) A18.4
  fallopian tube (acute) (chronic) A18.17
  fascia A18.09
  fauces A15.8
  female pelvic inflammatory disease A18.17
  finger A18.03
  first infection A15.7
  gallbladder A18.83
  ganglion A18.09
  gastritis A18.83
  gastrocolic fistula A18.32
  gastroenteritis A18.32
  gastrointestinal tract A18.32
  general, generalized — *see* Tuberculosis, miliary
  genital organs A18.10
  genitourinary A18.10
  genu A18.02
  glandula suprarenalis A18.7
  glandular, general A18.2
  glottis A15.5

D I S E A S E   I N D E X

Tuberculosis, tubercular, tuberculous
(calcification) (calcified) (caseous)
(chromogenic acid-fast bacilli)
(degeneration) (fibrocaseous) (fistula)
(interstitial) (isolated circumscribed
lesions) (necrosis) (parenchymatous)
(ulcerative) A15.9 — *continued*
grinder's J65
gum A18.83
hand A18.03
heart A18.84
hematogenous — *see* Tuberculosis, miliary
hemoptysis — *see* Tuberculosis, pulmonary
hemorrhage NEC — *see* Tuberculosis,
  pulmonary
hemothorax A15.6
hepatitis A18.83
hilar lymph nodes A15.4
  primary (progressive) A15.7
hip (joint) (disease) (bone) A18.02
hydropneumothorax A15.6
hydrothorax A15.6
hypoadrenalism A18.7
hypopharynx A15.8
ileocecal (hyperplastic) A18.32
ileocolitis A18.32
ileum A18.32
iliac spine (superior) A18.03
immunological findings only A15.7
indurativa (primary) A18.4
infantile A15.7
infection A15.9
  without clinical manifestations A15.7
infraclavicular gland A18.2
inguinal gland A18.2
inguinalis A18.2
intestine (any part) A18.32
iridocyclitis A18.54
iris, iritis A18.54
ischiorectal A18.32
jaw A18.03
jejunum A18.32
joint A18.02
  vertebral A18.01
keratitis (interstitial) A18.52
keratoconjunctivitis A18.52
kidney A18.11
knee (joint) A18.02
kyphosis, kyphoscoliosis A18.01
laryngitis A15.5
larynx A15.5
latent R76.11
leptomeninges, leptomeningitis (cerebral)
  (spinal) A17.0
lichenoides (primary) A18.4
linguae A18.83
lip A18.83
liver A18.83
lordosis A18.01
lung — *see* Tuberculosis, pulmonary
lupus vulgaris A18.4
lymph gland or node (peripheral) A18.2
  abdomen A18.39
  bronchial A15.4
    primary (progressive) A15.7
  cervical A18.2
  hilar A15.4
    primary (progressive) A15.7
  intrathoracic A15.4
    primary (progressive) A15.7
  mediastinal A15.4
    primary (progressive) A15.7
  mesenteric A18.39
  retroperitoneal A18.39
  tracheobronchial A15.4
    primary (progressive) A15.7
lymphadenitis — *see* Tuberculosis, lymph
  gland
lymphangitis — *see* Tuberculosis, lymph
  gland
lymphatic (gland) (vessel) — *see*
  Tuberculosis, lymph gland
mammary gland A18.89
marasmus A15.9
mastoiditis A18.03
mediastinal lymph gland or node A15.4
  primary (progressive) A15.7
mediastinitis A15.8
  primary (progressive) A15.7
mediastinum A15.8
  primary (progressive) A15.7
medulla A17.81
melanosis, Addisonian A18.7
meninges, meningitis (basilar) (cerebral)
  (cerebrospinal) (spinal) A17.0
meningoencephalitis A17.82
mesentery, mesenteric (gland or node)
  A18.39

Tuberculosis, tubercular, tuberculous
(calcification) (calcified) (caseous)
(chromogenic acid-fast bacilli)
(degeneration) (fibrocaseous) (fistula)
(interstitial) (isolated circumscribed
lesions) (necrosis) (parenchymatous)
(ulcerative) A15.9 — *continued*
miliary A19.9
  acute A19.2
    multiple sites A19.1
    single specified site A19.0
  chronic A19.8
  specified NEC A19.8
millstone makers' J65
miner's J65
molder's J65
mouth A18.83
multiple A19.9
  acute A19.1
  chronic A19.8
muscle A18.09
myelitis A17.82
myocardium, myocarditis A18.84
nasal (passage) (sinus) A15.8
nasopharynx A15.8
neck gland A18.2
nephritis A18.11
nerve (mononeuropathy) A17.83
nervous system A17.9
nose (septum) A15.8
ocular A18.50
omentum A18.31
oophoritis (acute) (chronic) A18.17
optic (nerve trunk) (papilla) A18.59
orbit A18.59
orchitis A18.15
organ, specified NEC A18.89
osseous — *see* Tuberculosis, bone
osteitis — *see* Tuberculosis, bone
osteomyelitis — *see* Tuberculosis, bone
otitis media A18.6
ovary, ovaritis (acute) (chronic) A18.17
oviduct (acute) (chronic) A18.17
pachymeningitis A17.0
palate (soft) A18.83
pancreas A18.83
papulonecrotic(a) (primary) A18.4
parathyroid glands A18.82
paronychia (primary) A18.4
parotid gland or region A18.83
pelvis (bony) A18.03
penis A18.15
peribronchitis A15.5
pericardium, pericarditis A18.84
perichondritis, larynx A15.5
periostitis — *see* Tuberculosis, bone
perirectal fistula A18.32
peritoneum NEC A18.31
peritonitis A18.31
pharynx, pharyngitis A15.8
phlyctenulosis (keratoconjunctivitis)
  A18.52
phthisis NEC — *see* Tuberculosis,
  pulmonary
pituitary gland A18.82
pleura, pleural, pleurisy, pleuritis
  (fibrinous) (obliterative) (purulent)
  (simple plastic) (with effusion) A15.6
  primary (progressive) A15.7
pneumonia, pneumonic — *see*
  Tuberculosis, pulmonary
pneumothorax (spontaneous) (tense
  valvular) — *see* Tuberculosis,
  pulmonary
polyneuropathy A17.89
polyserositis A19.9
  acute A19.1
  chronic A19.8
potter's J65
prepuce A18.15
primary (complex) A15.7
proctitis A18.32
prostate, prostatitis A18.14
pulmonalis — *see* Tuberculosis, pulmonary
pulmonary (cavitated) (fibrotic)
  (infiltrative) (nodular) A15.0
  childhood type or first infection A15.7
  primary (complex) A15.7
pyelitis A18.11
pyelonephritis A18.11
pyemia — *see* Tuberculosis, miliary
pyonephrosis A18.11
pyopneumothorax A15.6
pyothorax A15.6
rectum (fistula) (with abscess) A18.32
reinfection stage — *see* Tuberculosis,
  pulmonary
renal A18.11
renis A18.11

Tuberculosis, tubercular, tuberculous
(calcification) (calcified) (caseous)
(chromogenic acid-fast bacilli)
(degeneration) (fibrocaseous) (fistula)
(interstitial) (isolated circumscribed
lesions) (necrosis) (parenchymatous)
(ulcerative) A15.9 — *continued*
respiratory A15.9
  primary A15.7
  specified site NEC A15.8
retina, retinitis A18.53
retroperitoneal (lymph gland or node)
  A18.39
rheumatism NEC A18.09
rhinitis A15.8
sacroiliac (joint) A18.01
sacrum A18.01
salivary gland A18.83
salpingitis (acute) (chronic) A18.17
sandblaster's J65
sclera A18.51
scoliosis A18.01
scrofulous A18.2
scrotum A18.15
seminal tract or vesicle A18.15
senile A15.9
septic — *see* Tuberculosis, miliary
shoulder (joint) A18.02
  blade A18.03
sigmoid A18.32
sinus (any nasal) A15.8
  bone A18.03
  epididymis A18.15
skeletal NEC A18.03
skin (any site) (primary) A18.4
small intestine A18.32
soft palate A18.83
spermatic cord A18.15
spine, spinal (column) A18.01
  cord A17.81
    medulla A17.81
    membrane A17.0
    meninges A17.0
spleen, splenitis A18.85
spondylitis A18.01
sternoclavicular joint A18.02
stomach A18.83
stonemason's J65
subcutaneous tissue (cellular) (primary)
  A18.4
subcutis (primary) A18.4
subdeltoid bursa A18.83
submaxillary (region) A18.83
supraclavicular gland A18.2
suprarenal (capsule) (gland) A18.7
swelling, joint (*see also* category M01)
  (*see also* Tuberculosis, joint) A18.02
symphysis pubis A18.02
synovitis A18.09
  articular A18.02
  spine or vertebra A18.01
systemic — *see* Tuberculosis, miliary
tarsitis A18.4
tendon (sheath) — *see* Tuberculosis,
  tenosynovitis
tenosynovitis A18.09
  spine or vertebra A18.01
testis A18.15
throat A15.8
thymus gland A18.82
thyroid gland A18.81
tongue A18.83
tonsil, tonsillitis A15.8
trachea, tracheal A15.5
  lymph gland or node A15.4
    primary (progressive) A15.7
tracheobronchial A15.5
  lymph gland or node A15.4
    primary (progressive) A15.7
tubal (acute) (chronic) A18.17
tunica vaginalis A18.15
ulcer (skin) (primary) A18.4
  bowel or intestine A18.32
  specified NEC — *code under*
    Tuberculosis, by site
unspecified site A15.9
ureter A18.11
urethra, urethral (gland) A18.13
urinary organ or tract A18.13
uterus A18.17
uveal tract A18.54
uvula A18.83
vagina A18.18
vas deferens A18.15
verruca, verrucosa (cutis) (primary) A18.4
vertebra (column) A18.01
vesiculitis A18.15
vulva A18.18
wrist (joint) A18.02

Tuberculum
Carabelli — *see* Note at K00.2
occlusal — *see* Note at K00.2
paramolare K00.2
Tuberosity, enitre maxillary M26.07
Tuberous sclerosis (brain) Q85.1
Tubo-ovarian — *see* condition
Tuboplasty, after previous sterilization
  Z31.0
  aftercare Z31.42
Tubotympanitis, catarrhal (chronic) — *see*
  Otitis, media, nonsuppurative, chronic,
  serous
Tularemia A21.9
  with
    conjunctivitis A21.1
    pneumonia A21.2
  abdominal A21.3
  bronchopneumonic A21.2
  conjunctivitis A21.1
  cryptogenic A21.3
  enteric A21.3
  gastrointestinal A21.3
  generalized A21.7
  ingestion A21.3
  intestinal A21.3
  oculoglandular A21.1
  ophthalmic A21.1
  pneumonia (any), pneumonic A21.2
  pulmonary A21.2
  sepsis A21.7
  specified NEC A21.8
  typhoidal A21.7
  ulceroglandular A21.0
Tularensis conjunctivitis A21.1
Tumefaction — *see also* Swelling
  liver — *see* Hypertrophy, liver
Tumor — *see also* Neoplasm, unspecified
  behavior, by site
  acinar cell — *see* Neoplasm, uncertain
    behavior, by site
  acinic cell — *see* Neoplasm, uncertain
    behavior, by site
  adenocarcinoid — *see* Neoplasm,
    malignant, by site
  adenomatoid — *see also* Neoplasm,
    benign, by site
    odontogenic — *see* Cyst, calcifying
      odontogenic
  adnexal (skin) — *see* Neoplasm, skin,
    benign, by site
  adrenal
    cortical (benign) D35.0-
      malignant C74.0-
    rest — *see* Neoplasm, benign, by site
  alpha-cell
    malignant
      pancreas C25.4
      specified site NEC — *see* Neoplasm,
        malignant, by site
      unspecified site C25.4
    pancreas D13.7
    specified site NEC — *see* Neoplasm,
      benign, by site
    unspecified site D13.7
  aneurysmal — *see* Aneurysm
  aortic body D44.7
    malignant C75.5
  Askin's — *see* Neoplasm, connective
    tissue, malignant
  basal cell (*see also* Neoplasm, skin,
    uncertain behavior) D48.5
  Bednar — *see* Neoplasm, skin, malignant
  benign (unclassified) — *see* Neoplasm,
    benign, by site
  beta-cell
    malignant
      pancreas C25.4
      specified site NEC — *see* Neoplasm,
        malignant, by site
      unspecified site C25.4
    pancreas D13.7
    specified site NEC — *see* Neoplasm,
      benign, by site
    unspecified site D13.7
  Brenner D27.9
    borderline malignancy D39.1-
    malignant C56-
    proliferating D39.1-
  bronchial alveolar, intravascular D38.1
  Brooke's — *see* Neoplasm, skin, benign
  brown fat — *see* Lipoma
  Burkitt — *see* Lymphoma, Burkitt
  calcifying epithelial odontogenic — *see*
    Cyst, calcifying odontogenic

Tumor (see also Neoplasm, unspecified behavior, by site) — continued
carcinoid
  benign D3A.00
    appendix D3A.020
    ascending colon D3A.022
    bronchus (lung) D3A.090
    cecum D3A.021
    colon D3A.029
    descending colon D3A.024
    duodenum D3A.010
    foregut NOS D3A.094
    hindgut NOS D3A.096
    ileum D3A.012
    jejunum D3A.011
    kidney D3A.093
    large intestine D3A.029
    lung (bronchus) D3A.090
    midgut NOS D3A.095
    rectum D3A.026
    sigmoid colon D3A.025
    small intestine D3A.019
    specified NEC D3A.098
    stomach D3A.092
    thymus D3A.091
    transverse colon D3A.023
  malignant C7A.00
    appendix C7A.020
    ascending colon C7A.022
    bronchus (lung) C7A.090
    cecum C7A.021
    colon C7A.029
    descending colon C7A.024
    duodenum C7A.010
    foregut NOS C7A.094
    hindgut NOS C7A.096
    ileum C7A.012
    jejunum C7A.011
    kidney C7A.093
    large intestine C7A.029
    lung (bronchus) C7A.090
    midgut NOS C7A.095
    rectum C7A.026
    sigmoid colon C7A.025
    small intestine C7A.019
    specified NEC C7A.098
    stomach C7A.092
    thymus C7A.091
    transverse colon C7A.023
  mesentery metastasis C7B.04
  secondary C7B.00
    bone C7B.03
    distant lymph nodes C7B.01
    liver C7B.02
    peritoneum C7B.04
    specified NEC C7B.09
carotid body D44.6
  malignant C75.4
cells — see also Neoplasm, unspecified behavior, by site
  benign — see Neoplasm, benign, by site
  malignant — see Neoplasm, malignant, by site
  uncertain whether benign or malignant — see Neoplasm, uncertain behavior, by site
cervix, in pregnancy or childbirth — see Pregnancy, complicated by, tumor, cervix
chondromatous giant cell — see Neoplasm, bone, benign
chromaffin — see also Neoplasm, benign, by site
  malignant — see Neoplasm, malignant, by site
Cock's peculiar L72.3
Codman's — see Neoplasm, bone, benign
dentigerous, mixed — see Cyst, calcifying odontogenic
dermoid — see Neoplasm, benign, by site
  with malignant transformation C56-
desmoid (extra-abdominal) — see also Neoplasm, connective tissue, uncertain behavior
  abdominal — see Neoplasm, connective tissue, uncertain behavior
embolus — see Neoplasm, secondary, by site
embryonal (mixed) — see also Neoplasm, uncertain behavior, by site
  liver C22.7
endodermal sinus
  specified site — see Neoplasm, malignant, by site
  unspecified site
    female C56-
    male C62.90

Tumor (see also Neoplasm, unspecified behavior, by site) — continued
epithelial
  benign — see Neoplasm, benign, by site
  malignant — see Neoplasm, malignant, by site
Ewing's — see Neoplasm, bone, malignant, by site
fatty — see Lipoma
fibroid — see Leiomyoma
G cell
  malignant
    pancreas C25.4
    specified site NEC — see Neoplasm, malignant, by site
    unspecified site C25.4
  specified site — see Neoplasm, uncertain behavior, by site
  unspecified site D37.8
germ cell — see also Neoplasm, malignant, by site
  mixed — see Neoplasm, malignant, by site
ghost cell, odontogenic — see Cyst, calcifying odontogenic
giant cell — see also Neoplasm, uncertain behavior, by site
  bone D48.0
    malignant — see Neoplasm, bone, malignant
    chondromatous — see Neoplasm, bone, benign
    malignant — see Neoplasm, malignant, by site
  soft parts — see Neoplasm, connective tissue, uncertain behavior
    malignant — see Neoplasm, connective tissue, malignant
glomus D18.00
  intra-abdominal D18.03
  intracranial D18.02
  jugulare D44.7
    malignant C75.5
  skin D18.01
  specified site NEC D18.09
gonadal stromal — see Neoplasm, uncertain behavior, by site
granular cell — see also Neoplasm, connective tissue, benign
  malignant — see Neoplasm, connective tissue, malignant
granulosa cell D39.1-
  juvenile D39.1-
  malignant C56-
granulosa cell-theca cell D39.1-
  malignant C56-
Grawitz's C64-
hemorrhoidal — see Hemorrhoids
hilar cell D27-
hilus cell D27-
Hurthle cell (benign) D34
  malignant C73
hydatid — see Echinococcus
hypernephroid — see also Neoplasm, uncertain behavior, by site
interstitial cell — see also Neoplasm, uncertain behavior, by site
  benign — see Neoplasm, benign, by site
  malignant — see Neoplasm, malignant, by site
intravascular bronchial alveolar D38.1
islet cell — see Neoplasm, benign, by site
  malignant — see Neoplasm, malignant, by site
    pancreas C25.4
    specified site NEC — see Neoplasm, malignant, by site
    unspecified site C25.4
  pancreas D13.7
    specified site NEC — see Neoplasm, benign, by site
    unspecified site D13.7
juxtaglomerular D41.0-
Klatskin's C24.0
Krukenberg's C79.6-
Leydig cell — see Neoplasm, uncertain behavior, by site
  benign — see Neoplasm, benign, by site
    specified site — see Neoplasm, benign, by site
    unspecified site
      female D27.9
      male D29.20
  malignant — see Neoplasm, malignant, by site
    specified site — see Neoplasm, malignant, by site
    unspecified site
      female C56.9
      male C62.90

Tumor (see also Neoplasm, unspecified behavior, by site) — continued
Leydig cell (see Neoplasm, uncertain behavior, by site) — continued
    specified site — see Neoplasm, uncertain behavior, by site
    unspecified site
      female D39.10
      male D40.10
lipid cell, ovary D27-
lipoid cell, ovary D27-
malignant (see also Neoplasm, malignant, by site) C80.1
  fusiform cell (type) C80.1
  giant cell (type) C80.1
  localized, plasma cell — see Plasmacytoma, solitary
  mixed NEC C80.1
  small cell (type) C80.1
  spindle cell (type) C80.1
  unclassified C80.1
mast cell D47.0
  malignant C96.2
melanotic, neuroectodermal — see Neoplasm, benign, by site
Merkel cell — see Carcinoma, Merkel cell
mesenchymal
  malignant — see Neoplasm, connective tissue, malignant
  mixed — see Neoplasm, connective tissue, uncertain behavior
mesodermal, mixed — see also Neoplasm, malignant, by site
  liver C22.4
mesonephric — see also Neoplasm, uncertain behavior, by site
  malignant — see Neoplasm, malignant, by site
metastatic
  from specified site — see Neoplasm, malignant, by site
  of specified site — see Neoplasm, malignant, by site
  to specified site — see Neoplasm, secondary, by site
mixed NEC — see also Neoplasm, benign, by site
  malignant — see Neoplasm, malignant, by site
mucinous of low malignant potential
  specified site — see Neoplasm, malignant, by site
  unspecified site C56.9
mucocarcinoid
  specified site — see Neoplasm, malignant, by site
  unspecified site C18.1
mucoepidermoid — see Neoplasm, uncertain behavior, by site
Müllerian, mixed
  specified site — see Neoplasm, malignant, by site
  unspecified site C54.9
myoepithelial — see Neoplasm, benign, by site
neuroectodermal (peripheral) — see Neoplasm, malignant, by site
primitive
  specified site — see Neoplasm, malignant, by site
  unspecified site C71.9
neuroendocrine D3A.8
  malignant poorly differentiated C7A.1
  secondary NEC C7B.8
  specified NEC C7A.8
neurogenic olfactory C30.0
nonencapsulated sclerosing C73
odontogenic (adenomatoid) (benign) (calcifying epithelial) (keratocystic) (squamous) — see Cyst, calcifying odontogenic
  malignant C41.1
    upper jaw (bone) C41.0
ovarian stromal D39.1-
ovary, in pregnancy — see Pregnancy, complicated by
pacinian — see Neoplasm, skin, benign
Pancoast's — see Pancoast's syndrome
papillary — see also Papilloma
  cystic D37.9
  mucinous of low malignant potential C56-
    specified site — see Neoplasm, malignant, by site
    unspecified site C56.9
  serous of low malignant potential
    specified site — see Neoplasm, malignant, by site
    unspecified site C56.9

Tumor (see also Neoplasm, unspecified behavior, by site) — continued
pelvic, in pregnancy or childbirth — see Pregnancy, complicated by
phantom F45.8
phyllodes D48.6-
  benign D24-
  malignant — see Neoplasm, breast, malignant
Pindborg — see Cyst, calcifying odontogenic
placental site trophoblastic D39.2
plasma cell (malignant) (localized) — see Plasmacytoma, solitary
polyvesicular vitelline
  specified site — see Neoplasm, malignant, by site
  unspecified site
    female C56.9
    male C62.90
Pott's puffy — see Osteomyelitis, specified NEC
Rathke's pouch D44.3
retinal anlage — see Neoplasm, benign, by site
salivary gland type, mixed — see Neoplasm, salivary gland, benign
  malignant — see Neoplasm, salivary gland, malignant
Sampson's N80.1
Schmincke's — see Neoplasm, nasopharynx, malignant
sclerosing stromal D27-
sebaceous — see Cyst, sebaceous
secondary — see Neoplasm, secondary, by site
  carcinoid C7B.00
    bone C7B.03
    distant lymph nodes C7B.01
    liver C7B.02
    peritoneum C7B.04
    specified NEC C7B.09
  neuroendocrine NEC C7B.8
serous of low malignant potential
  specified site — see Neoplasm, malignant, by site
  unspecified site C56.9
Sertoli cell — see Neoplasm, benign, by site
  with lipid storage
    specified site — see Neoplasm, benign, by site
    unspecified site
      female D27.9
      male D29.20
  specified site — see Neoplasm, benign, by site
  unspecified site
    female D27.9
    male D29.20
Sertoli-Leydig cell — see Neoplasm, benign, by site
  specified site — see Neoplasm, benign, by site
  unspecified site
    female D27.9
    male D29.20
sex cord(-stromal) — see Neoplasm, uncertain behavior, by site
  with annular tubules D39.1-
skin appendage — see Neoplasm, skin, benign
smooth muscle — see Neoplasm, connective tissue, uncertain behavior
soft tissue
  benign — see Neoplasm, connective tissue, benign
  malignant — see Neoplasm, connective tissue, malignant
sternomastoid (congenital) Q68.0
stromal
  endometrial D39.0
  gastric D48.1
    benign D21.4
    malignant C16.9
    uncertain behavior D48.1
  gastrointestinal
    benign D21.4
    malignant C49.4
    uncertain behavior D48.1
  intestine
    benign D21.4
    malignant C49.4
    uncertain behavior D48.1
  ovarian D39.1-

Tumor *(see also* Neoplasm, unspecified behavior, by site) — *continued*
  stromal — *continued*
    stomach
      benign D21.4
      malignant C16.9
      uncertain behavior D48.1
    sweat gland — *see also* Neoplasm, skin, uncertain behavior
      benign — *see* Neoplasm, skin, benign
      malignant — *see* Neoplasm, skin, malignant
    syphilitic, brain A52.17
    testicular D40.10
    testicular stromal D40.1-
    theca cell D27-
    theca cell-granulosa cell D39.1-
    Triton, malignant — *see* Neoplasm, nerve, malignant
    trophoblastic, placental site D39.2
    turban D23.4
    uterus (body), in pregnancy or childbirth — *see* Pregnancy, complicated by, tumor, uterus
    vagina, in pregnancy or childbirth — *see* Pregnancy, complicated by
    varicose — *see* Varix
    von Recklinghausen's — *see* Neurofibromatosis
    vulva or perineum, in pregnancy or childbirth — *see* Pregnancy, complicated by
      causing obstructed labor O65.5
    Warthin's — *see* Neoplasm, salivary gland, benign
    Wilms' C64-
    yolk sac — *see* Neoplasm, malignant, by site
      specified site — *see* Neoplasm, malignant, by site
      unspecified site
        female C56.9
        male C62.90
Tumor lysis syndrome (following antineoplastic chemotherapy) (spontaneous) NEC E88.3
Tumorlet — *see* Neoplasm, uncertain behavior, by site
Tungiasis B88.1
Tunica vasculosa lentis Q12.2
Turban tumor D23.4
Türck's trachoma J37.0
Turner's
  hypoplasia (tooth) K00.4
  syndrome Q96.9
    specified NEC Q96.8
  tooth K00.4
Turner-Kieser syndrome Q79.8
Turner-like syndrome Q87.1
Turner-Ullrich syndrome Q96.9
Tussis convulsiva — *see* Whooping cough
Twiddler's syndrome (due to)
  automatic implantable defibrillator T82.198
  cardiac pacemaker T82.198
Twilight state
  epileptic F05
  psychogenic F44.89
Twin (newborn) — *see also* Newborn, twin
  conjoined Q89.4
  pregnancy — *see* Pregnancy, twin, conjoined
Twinning, teeth K00.2
Twist, twisted
  bowel, colon or intestine K56.2
  hair (congenital) Q84.1
  mesentery K56.2
  omentum K56.2
  organ or site, congenital NEC — *see* Anomaly, by site
  ovarian pedicle — *see* Torsion, ovary
Twitching R25.3
Tylosis (acquired) L84
  buccalis K13.29
  linguae K13.29
  palmaris et plantaris (congenital) (inherited) Q82.8
    acquired L85.1
Tympanism R14.0
Tympanites (abdominal) (intestinal) R14.0
Tympanitis — *see* Myringitis
Tympanosclerosis — *see* subcategory H74.0
Tympanum — *see* condition
Tympany
  abdomen R14.0
  chest R09.89

Type A behavior pattern Z73.1
Typhlitis — *see* Appendicitis
Typhoenteritis — *see* Typhoid
Typhoid (abortive) (ambulant) (any site) (clinical) (fever) (hemorrhagic) (infection) (intermittent) (malignant) (rheumatic) (Widal negative) A01.00
  with pneumonia A01.03
  abdominal A01.09
  arthritis A01.04
  carrier (suspected) of Z22.0
  cholecystitis (current) A01.09
  endocarditis A01.02
  heart involvement A01.02
  inoculation reaction — *see* Complications, vaccination
  meningitis A01.01
  mesenteric lymph nodes A01.09
  myocarditis A01.02
  osteomyelitis A01.05
  perichondritis, larynx A01.09
  pneumonia A01.03
  specified NEC A01.09
  spine A01.05
  ulcer (perforating) A01.09
Typhomalaria (fever) — *see* Malaria
Typhomania A01.00
Typhoperitonitis A01.09
Typhus (fever) A75.9
  abdominal, abdominalis — *see* Typhoid
  African tick A77.1
  amarillic A95.9
  brain A75.9 [G94]
  cerebral A75.9 [G94]
  classical A75.0
  due to Rickettsia
    prowazekii A75.0
      recrudescent A75.1
    tsutsugamushi A75.3
    typhi A75.2
  endemic (flea-borne) A75.2
  epidemic (louse-borne) A75.0
  exanthematic NEC A75.0
  exanthematicus SAI A75.0
    brillii SAI A75.1
    mexicanus SAI A75.2
    typhus murinus A75.2
  flea-borne A75.2
  India tick A77.1
  Kenya (tick) A77.1
  louse-borne A75.0
  Mexican A75.2
  mite-borne A75.3
  murine A75.2
  North Asian tick-borne A77.2
  petechial A75.9
  Queensland tick A77.3
  rat A75.2
  recrudescent A75.1
  recurrens — *see* Fever, relapsing
  Sao Paulo A77.0
  scrub (China) (India) (Malaysia) (New Guinea) A75.3
  shop (of Malaysia) A75.2
  Siberian tick A77.2
  tick-borne A77.9
  tropical (mite-borne) A75.3
Tyrosinemia E70.21
  newborn, transitory P74.5
Tyrosinosis E70.21
Tyrosinuria E70.29

U

Uhl's anomaly or disease Q24.8
Ulcer, ulcerated, ulcerating, ulceration, ulcerative
  alveolar process M27.3
  amebic (intestine) A06.1
    skin A06.7
  anastomotic — *see* Ulcer, gastrojejunal
  anorectal K62.6
  antral — *see* Ulcer, stomach
  anus (sphincter) (solitary) K62.6
  aorta — *see* Aneurysm
  aphthous (oral) (recurrent) K12.0
    genital organ(s)
      female N76.6
      male N50.8
  artery I77.2
  atrophic — *see* Ulcer, skin
    decubitus — *see* Ulcer, pressure, by site
  back L98.429
    with
      bone necrosis L98.424
      exposed fat layer L98.422
      muscle necrosis L98.423
      skin breakdown only L98.421
  Barrett's (esophagus) K22.10
    with bleeding K22.11
  bile duct (common) (hepatic) K83.8
  bladder (solitary) (sphincter) NEC N32.89
    bilharzial B65.9 [N33]
    in schistosomiasis (bilharzial) B65.9 [N33]
    submucosal — *see* Cystitis, interstitial
    tuberculous A18.12
  bleeding K27.4
  bone — *see* Osteomyelitis, specified type NEC
  bowel — *see* Ulcer, intestine
  breast N61
  bronchus J98.09
  buccal (cavity) (traumatic) K12.1
  Buruli A31.1
  buttock L98.419
    with
      bone necrosis L98.414
      exposed fat layer L98.412
      muscle necrosis L98.413
      skin breakdown only L98.411
  cancerous — *see* Neoplasm, malignant, by site
  cardia K22.10
    with bleeding K22.11
  cardioesophageal (peptic) K22.10
    with bleeding K22.11
  cecum — *see* Ulcer, intestine
  cervix (uteri) (decubitus) (trophic) N86
    with cervicitis N72
  chancroidal A57
  chiclero B55.1
  chronic (cause unknown) — *see* Ulcer, skin
  Cochin-China B55.1
  colon — *see* Ulcer, intestine
  conjunctiva H10.89
  cornea H16.00-
    with hypopyon H16.03-
    central H16.01-
    dendritic (herpes simplex) B00.52
    marginal H16.04-
    Mooren's H16.05-
    mycotic H16.06-
    perforated H16.07-
    ring H16.02-
    tuberculous (phlyctenular) A18.52
  corpus cavernosum (chronic) N48.5
  crural — *see* Ulcer, lower limb
  Curling's — *see* Ulcer, peptic, acute
  Cushing's — *see* Ulcer, peptic, acute
  cystic duct K82.8
  cystitis (interstitial) — *see* Cystitis, interstitial
  decubitus — *see* Ulcer, pressure, by site
  dendritic, cornea (herpes simplex) B00.52
  diabetes, diabetic — *see* Diabetes, ulcer
  Dieulafoy's K25.0
  due to
    infection NEC — *see* Ulcer, skin
    radiation NEC L59.8
    trophic disturbance (any region) — *see* Ulcer, skin
    X-ray L58.1

Ulcer, ulcerated, ulcerating, ulceration, ulcerative — *continued*
duodenum, duodenal (eroded) (peptic) K26.9
with
hemorrhage K26.4
and perforation K26.6
perforation K26.5
acute K26.3
with
hemorrhage K26.0
and perforation K26.2
perforation K26.1
chronic K26.7
with
hemorrhage K26.4
and perforation K26.6
perforation K26.5
dysenteric A09
elusive — *see* Cystitis, interstitial
endocarditis (acute) (chronic) (subacute) I28.8
epiglottis J38.7
esophagus (peptic) K22.10
with bleeding K22.11
due to
aspirin K22.10
with bleeding K22.11
gastrointestinal reflux disease K21.0
ingestion of chemical or medicament K22.10
with bleeding K22.11
fungal K22.10
with bleeding K22.11
infective K22.10
with bleeding K22.11
varicose — *see* Varix, esophagus
eyelid (region) H01.8
fauces J39.2
Fenwick (-Hunner) (solitary) — *see* Cystitis, interstitial
fistulous — *see* Ulcer, skin
foot (indolent) (trophic) — *see* Ulcer, lower limb
frambesial, initial A66.0
frenum (tongue) K14.0
gallbladder or duct K82.8
gangrenous — *see* Gangrene
gastric — *see* Ulcer, stomach
gastrocolic — *see* Ulcer, gastrojejunal
gastroduodenal — *see* Ulcer, peptic
gastroesophageal — *see* Ulcer, stomach
gastrointestinal — *see* Ulcer, gastrojejunal
gastrojejunal (peptic) K28.9
with
hemorrhage K28.4
and perforation K28.6
perforation K28.5
acute K28.3
with
hemorrhage K28.0
and perforation K28.2
perforation K28.1
chronic K28.7
with
hemorrhage K28.4
and perforation K28.6
perforation K28.5
gastrojejunocolic — *see* Ulcer, gastrojejunal
gingiva K06.8
gingivitis K05.10
nonplaque induced K05.11
plaque induced K05.10
glottis J38.7
granuloma of pudenda A58
gum K06.8
gumma, due to yaws A66.4
heel — *see* Ulcer, lower limb
hemorrhoid (see also Hemorrhoids, by degree) K64.8
Hunner's — *see* Cystitis, interstitial
hypopharynx J39.2
hypopyon (chronic) (subacute) — *see* Ulcer, cornea, with hypopyon
hypostaticum — *see* Ulcer, varicose
ileum — *see* Ulcer, intestine
intestine, intestinal K63.3
with perforation K63.1
amebic A06.1
duodenal — *see* Ulcer, duodenum
granulocytopenic (with hemorrhage) — *see* Neutropenia
marginal — *see* Ulcer, gastrojejunal
perforating K63.1
newborn P78.0
primary, small intestine K63.3
rectum K62.6

Ulcer, ulcerated, ulcerating, ulceration, ulcerative — *continued*
intestine, intestinal K63.3 — *continued*
stercoraceous, stercoral K63.3
tuberculous A18.32
typhoid (fever) — *see* Typhoid
varicose I86.8
jejunum, jejunal — *see* Ulcer, gastrojejunal
keratitis — *see* Ulcer, cornea
knee — *see* Ulcer, lower limb
labium (majus) (minus) N76.6
laryngitis — *see* Laryngitis
larynx (aphthous) (contact) J38.7
diphtheritic A36.2
leg — *see* Ulcer, lower limb
lip K13.0
Lipschütz's N76.6
lower limb (atrophic) (chronic) (neurogenic) (perforating) (pyogenic) (trophic) (tropical) L97.909
with
bone necrosis L97.904
exposed fat layer L97.902
muscle necrosis L97.903
skin breakdown only L97.901
ankle L97.309
with
bone necrosis L97.304
exposed fat layer L97.302
muscle necrosis L97.303
skin breakdown only L97.301
left L97.329
with
bone necrosis L97.324
exposed fat layer L97.322
muscle necrosis L97.323
skin breakdown only L97.321
right L97.319
with
bone necrosis L97.314
exposed fat layer L97.312
muscle necrosis L97.313
skin breakdown only L97.311
calf L97.209
with
bone necrosis L97.204
exposed fat layer L97.202
muscle necrosis L97.203
skin breakdown only L97.201
left L97.229
with
bone necrosis L97.224
exposed fat layer L97.222
muscle necrosis L97.223
skin breakdown only L97.221
right L97.219
with
bone necrosis L97.214
exposed fat layer L97.212
muscle necrosis L97.213
skin breakdown only L97.211
decubitus — *see* Ulcer, pressure, by site
foot specified NEC L97.509
with
bone necrosis L97.504
exposed fat layer L97.502
muscle necrosis L97.503
skin breakdown only L97.501
left L97.529
with
bone necrosis L97.524
exposed fat layer L97.522
muscle necrosis L97.523
skin breakdown only L97.521
right L97.519
with
bone necrosis L97.514
exposed fat layer L97.512
muscle necrosis L97.513
skin breakdown only L97.511
heel L97.409
with
bone necrosis L97.404
exposed fat layer L97.402
muscle necrosis L97.403
skin breakdown only L97.401
left L97.429
with
bone necrosis L97.424
exposed fat layer L97.422
muscle necrosis L97.423
skin breakdown only L97.421
right L97.419
with
bone necrosis L97.414
exposed fat layer L97.412
muscle necrosis L97.413
skin breakdown only L97.411

Ulcer, ulcerated, ulcerating, ulceration, ulcerative — *continued*
lower limb (atrophic) (chronic) (neurogenic) (perforating) (pyogenic) (trophic) (tropical) L97.909 — *continued*
left L97.929
with
bone necrosis L97.924
exposed fat layer L97.922
muscle necrosis L97.923
skin breakdown only L97.921
leprous A30.1
lower leg NOS L97.909
with
bone necrosis L97.904
exposed fat layer L97.902
muscle necrosis L97.903
skin breakdown only L97.901
left L97.929
with
bone necrosis L97.924
exposed fat layer L97.922
muscle necrosis L97.923
skin breakdown only L97.921
right L97.919
with
bone necrosis L97.914
exposed fat layer L97.912
muscle necrosis L97.913
skin breakdown only L97.911
specified site NEC L97.809
with
bone necrosis L97.804
exposed fat layer L97.802
muscle necrosis L97.803
skin breakdown only L97.801
left L97.829
with
bone necrosis L97.824
exposed fat layer L97.822
muscle necrosis L97.823
skin breakdown only L97.821
right L97.819
with
bone necrosis L97.814
exposed fat layer L97.812
muscle necrosis L97.813
skin breakdown only L97.811
midfoot L97.409
with
bone necrosis L97.404
exposed fat layer L97.402
muscle necrosis L97.403
skin breakdown only L97.401
left L97.429
with
bone necrosis L97.424
exposed fat layer L97.422
muscle necrosis L97.423
skin breakdown only L97.421
right L97.419
with
bone necrosis L97.414
exposed fat layer L97.412
muscle necrosis L97.413
skin breakdown only L97.411
right L97.919
with
bone necrosis L97.914
exposed fat layer L97.912
muscle necrosis L97.913
skin breakdown only L97.911
syphilitic A52.19
thigh L97.109
with
bone necrosis L97.104
exposed fat layer L97.102
muscle necrosis L97.103
skin breakdown only L97.101
left L97.129
with
bone necrosis L97.124
exposed fat layer L97.122
muscle necrosis L97.123
skin breakdown only L97.121
right L97.119
with
bone necrosis L97.114
exposed fat layer L97.112
muscle necrosis L97.113
skin breakdown only L97.111

Ulcer, ulcerated, ulcerating, ulceration, ulcerative — *continued*
lower limb (atrophic) (chronic) (neurogenic) (perforating) (pyogenic) (trophic) (tropical) L97.909 — *continued*
toe L97.509
with
bone necrosis L97.504
exposed fat layer L97.502
muscle necrosis L97.503
skin breakdown only L97.501
left L97.529
with
bone necrosis L97.524
exposed fat layer L97.522
muscle necrosis L97.523
skin breakdown only L97.521
right L97.519
with
bone necrosis L97.514
exposed fat layer L97.512
muscle necrosis L97.513
skin breakdown only L97.511
varicose — *see* Varix, leg, with, ulcer
luetic — *see* Ulcer, syphilitic
lung J98.4
tuberculous — *see* Tuberculosis, pulmonary
malignant — *see* Neoplasm, malignant, by site
marginal NEC — *see* Ulcer, gastrojejunal
meatus (urinarius) N34.2
Meckel's diverticulum Q43.0
malignant — *see* Table of Neoplasms, small intestine, malignant
Meleney's (chronic undermining) — *see* Ulcer, skin
Mooren's (cornea) — *see* Ulcer, cornea, Mooren's
mycobacterial (skin) A31.1
nasopharynx J39.2
neck, uterus N86
neurogenic NEC — *see* Ulcer, skin
nose, nasal (passage) (infective) (septum) J34.0
skin — *see* Ulcer, skin
spirochetal A69.8
varicose (bleeding) I86.8
oral mucosa (traumatic) K12.1
palate (soft) K12.1
penis (chronic) N48.5
peptic (site unspecified) K27.9
with
hemorrhage K27.4
and perforation K27.6
perforation K27.5
acute K27.3
with
hemorrhage K27.0
and perforation K27.2
perforation K27.1
chronic K27.7
with
hemorrhage K27.4
and perforation K27.6
perforation K27.5
esophagus K22.10
with bleeding K22.11
newborn P78.82
perforating K27.5
skin — *see* Ulcer, skin
peritonsillar J35.8
phagedenic (tropical) — *see* Ulcer, skin
pharynx J39.2
phlebitis — *see* Phlebitis
plaster — *see* Ulcer, pressure, by site
popliteal space — *see* Ulcer, lower limb
postpyloric — *see* Ulcer, duodenum
prepuce N47.7
prepyloric — *see* Ulcer, stomach
pressure (pressure area) L89.9-
ankle L89.5-
back L89.1-
buttock L89.3-
coccyx L89.15-
contiguous site of back, buttock, hip L89.4-
elbow L89.0-
face L89.81-
head L89.81-
heel L89.6-
hip L89.2-
sacral region (tailbone) L89.15-
specified site NEC L89.89-

D I S E A S E   I N D E X

Ulcer, ulcerated, ulcerating, ulceration, ulcerative — continued
pressure (pressure area) L89.9- — continued
  stage 1 (healing) (pre-ulcer skin changes limited to persistent focal edema)
    ankle L89.5-
    back L89.1-
    buttock L89.3-
    coccyx L89.15-
    contiguous site of back, buttock, hip L89.4-
    elbow L89.0-
    face L89.81-
    head L89.81-
    heel L89.6-
    hip L89.2-
    sacral region (tailbone) L89.15-
    specified site NEC L89.89-
  stage 2 (healing) (abrasion, blister, partial thickness skin loss involving epidermis and/or dermis)
    ankle L89.5-
    back L89.1-
    buttock L89.3-
    coccyx L89.15-
    contiguous site of back, buttock, hip L89.4-
    elbow L89.0-
    face L89.81-
    head L89.81-
    heel L89.6-
    hip L89.2-
    sacral region (tailbone) L89.15-
    specified site NEC L89.89-
  stage 3 (healing) (full thickness skin loss involving damage or necrosis of subcutaneous tissue)
    ankle L89.5-
    back L89.1-
    buttock L89.3-
    coccyx L89.15-
    contiguous site of back, buttock, hip L89.4-
    elbow L89.0-
    face L89.81-
    head L89.81-
    heel L89.6-
    hip L89.2-
    sacral region (tailbone) L89.15-
    specified site NEC L89.89-
  stage 4 (healing) (necrosis of soft tissues through to underlying muscle, tendon, or bone)
    ankle L89.5-
    back L89.1-
    buttock L89.3-
    coccyx L89.15-
    contiguous site of back, buttock, hip L89.4-
    elbow L89.0-
    face L89.81-
    head L89.81-
    heel L89.6-
    hip L89.2-
    sacral region (tailbone) L89.15-
    specified site NEC L89.89-
  unspecified stage
    ankle L89.5-
    back L89.1-
    buttock L89.3-
    coccyx L89.15-
    contiguous site of back, buttock, hip L89.4-
    elbow L89.0-
    face L89.81-
    head L89.81-
    heel L89.6-
    hip L89.2-
    sacral region (tailbone) L89.15-
    specified site NEC L89.89-
  unstageable
    ankle L89.5-
    back L89.1-
    buttock L89.3-
    coccyx L89.15-
    contiguous site of back, buttock, hip L89.4-
    elbow L89.0-
    face L89.81-
    head L89.81-
    heel L89.6-
    hip L89.2-
    sacral region (tailbone) L89.15-
    specified site NEC L89.89-
primary of intestine K63.3
  with perforation K63.1
prostate N41.9

Ulcer, ulcerated, ulcerating, ulceration, ulcerative — continued
pyloric — see Ulcer, stomach
rectosigmoid K63.3
  with perforation K63.1
rectum (sphincter) (solitary) K62.6
  stercoraceous, stercoral K62.6
retina — see Inflammation, chorioretinal
rodent — see also Neoplasm, skin, malignant
sclera — see Scleritis
scrofulous (tuberculous) A18.2
scrotum N50.8
  tuberculous A18.15
  varicose I86.1
seminal vesicle N50.8
sigmoid — see Ulcer, intestine
skin (atrophic) (chronic) (neurogenic) (non-healing) (perforating) (pyogenic) (trophic) (tropical) L98.499
  with gangrene — see Gangrene
  amebic A06.7
  back — see Ulcer, back
  buttock — see Ulcer, buttock
  decubitus — see Ulcer, pressure
  lower limb — see Ulcer, lower limb
  mycobacterial A31.1
  specified site NEC L98.499
    with
      bone necrosis L98.494
      exposed fat layer L98.492
      muscle necrosis L98.493
      skin breakdown only L98.491
  tuberculous (primary) A18.4
  varicose — see Ulcer, varicose
sloughing — see Ulcer, skin
solitary, anus or rectum (sphincter) K62.6
sore throat J02.9
  streptococcal J02.0
spermatic cord N50.8
spine (tuberculous) A18.01
stasis (venous) — see Varix, leg, with, ulcer
  without varicose veins I87.2
stercoraceous, stercoral K63.3
  with perforation K63.1
  anus or rectum K62.6
stoma, stomal — see Ulcer, gastrojejunal
stomach (eroded) (peptic) (round) K25.9
  with
    hemorrhage K25.4
      and perforation K25.6
    perforation K25.5
  acute K25.3
    with
      hemorrhage K25.0
        and perforation K25.2
      perforation K25.1
  chronic K25.7
    with
      hemorrhage K25.4
        and perforation K25.6
      perforation K25.5
stomal — see Ulcer, gastrojejunal
stomatitis K12.1
stress — see Ulcer, peptic
strumous (tuberculous) A18.2
submucosal, bladder — see Cystitis, interstitial
syphilitic (any site) (early) (secondary) A51.39
  late A52.79
  perforating A52.79
    foot A52.11
testis N50.8
thigh — see Ulcer, lower limb
throat J39.2
  diphtheritic A36.0
toe — see Ulcer, lower limb
tongue (traumatic) K14.0
tonsil J35.8
  diphtheritic A36.0
trachea J39.8
trophic — see Ulcer, skin
tropical — see Ulcer, skin
tuberculous — see Tuberculosis, ulcer
tunica vaginalis N50.8
turbinate J34.89
typhoid (perforating) — see Typhoid
unspecified site — see Ulcer, skin
urethra (meatus) — see Urethritis
uterus N85.8
  cervix N86
    with cervicitis N72
  neck N86
    with cervicitis N72
vagina N76.5
  in Behçet's disease M35.2 [N77.0]
  pessary N89.8
valve, heart I33.0

Ulcer, ulcerated, ulcerating, ulceration, ulcerative — continued
varicose (lower limb, any part) — see also Varix, leg, with, ulcer
  broad ligament I86.2
  esophagus — see Varix, esophagus
  inflamed or infected — see Varix, leg, with ulcer, with inflammation
  nasal septum I86.8
  perineum I86.3
  scrotum I86.1
  specified site NEC I86.8
  sublingual I86.0
  vulva I86.3
vas deferens N50.8
vulva (acute) (infectional) N76.6
  in (due to)
    Behçet's disease M35.2 [N77.0]
    herpesviral (herpes simplex) infection A60.04
    tuberculosis A18.18
vulvobuccal, recurring N76.6
X-ray L58.1
yaws A66.4
Ulcerosa scarlatina A38.8
Ulcus — see also Ulcer
cutis tuberculosum A18.4
duodeni — see Ulcer, duodenum
durum (syphilitic) A51.0
  extragenital A51.2
gastrojejunale — see Ulcer, gastrojejunal
hypostaticum — see Ulcer, varicose
molle (cutis) (skin) A57
serpens corneae — see Ulcer, cornea, central
ventriculi — see Ulcer, stomach
Ulegyria Q04.8
Ulerythema
ophryogenes, congenital Q84.2
sycosiforme L73.8
Ullrich(-Bonnevie)(-Turner) syndrome Q87.1
Ullrich-Feichtiger syndrome Q87.0
Ulnar — see condition
Ulorrhagia, ulorrhea K06.8
Umbilicus, umbilical — see condition
Unacceptable
contours of tooth K08.54
morphology of tooth K08.54
Unavailability (of)
bed at medical facility Z75.1
health service-related agencies Z75.4
medical facilities (at) Z75.3
  due to
    investigation by social service agency Z75.2
    lack of services at home Z75.0
    remoteness from facility Z75.3
    waiting list Z75.1
  home Z75.0
  outpatient clinic Z75.3
schooling Z55.1
social service agencies Z75.4
Uncinaria americana infestation B76.1
Uncinariasis B76.9
Uncongenial work Z56.5
Unconscious(ness) — see Coma
Under observation — see Observation
Underachievement in school Z55.3
Underdevelopment — see also Undeveloped
nose Q30.1
sexual E30.0
Underdosing (see also Table of Drugs and Chemicals, categories T36-T50, with final character 6) Z91.14
intentional NEC Z91.128
  due to financial hardship of patient Z91.120
unintentional NEC Z91.138
  due to patient's age related debility Z91.130
Underfeeding, newborn P92.3
Underfill, endodontic M27.53
Underimmunization status Z28.3
Undernourishment — see Malnutrition
Undernutrition — see Malnutrition
Underweight R63.6
for gestational age — see Light for dates
Underwood's disease P83.0
Undescended — see also Malposition, congenital
cecum Q43.3
colon Q43.3
testicle — see Cryptorchid

Undeveloped, undevelopment — see also Hypoplasia
brain (congenital) Q02
cerebral (congenital) Q02
heart Q24.8
lung Q33.6
testis E29.1
uterus E30.0
Undiagnosed (disease) R69
Undulant fever — see Brucellosis
Unemployment, anxiety concerning Z56.0
threatened Z56.2
Unequal length (acquired) (limb) — see also Deformity, limb, unequal length
leg — see also Deformity, limb, unequal length
congenital Q72.9-
Unextracted dental root K08.3
Unguis incarnatus L60.0
Unhappiness R45.2
Unicornate uterus Q51.4
Unilateral — see also condition
development, breast N64.89
organ or site, congenital NEC — see Agenesis, by site
Unilocular heart Q20.8
Union, abnormal — see also Fusion
larynx and trachea Q34.8
Universal mesentery Q43.3
Unrepairable overhanging of dental restorative materials K08.52
Unsatisfactory
restoration of tooth K08.50
  specified NEC K08.59
sample of cytologic smear
  anus R85.615
  cervix R87.615
  vagina R87.625
  surroundings Z59.1
  work Z56.5
Unsoundness of mind — see Psychosis
Unstable
back NEC — see Instability, joint, spine
hip (congenital) Q65.6
  acquired — see Derangement, joint, specified type NEC, hip
  joint — see Instability, joint
    secondary to removal of joint prosthesis M96.89
lie (mother) O32.0
lumbosacral joint (congenital)
  acquired — see subcategory M53.2
sacroiliac — see subcategory M53.2
spine NEC — see Instability, joint, spine
Unsteadiness on feet R26.81
Untruthfulness, child problem F91.8
Unverricht(-Lundborg) disease or epilepsy — see Epilepsy, generalized, idiopathic
Unwanted pregnancy Z64.0
Upbringing, institutional Z62.22
away from parents NEC Z62.29
in care of non-parental family member Z62.21
in foster care Z62.21
in orphanage or group home Z62.22
in welfare custody Z62.21
Upper respiratory — see condition
Upset
gastric K30
gastrointestinal K30
  psychogenic F45.8
intestinal (large) (small) K59.9
  psychogenic F45.8
menstruation N93.9
mental F48.9
stomach K30
  psychogenic F45.8
Urachus — see also condition
patent or persistent Q64.4
Urbach-Oppenheim disease (necrobiosis lipoidica diabeticorum) — see E08-E13 with .620
Urbach's lipoid proteinosis E78.89
Urbach-Wiethe disease E78.89
Urban yellow fever A95.1
Urea
blood, high — see Uremia
cycle metabolism disorder — see Disorder, urea cycle metabolism
Uremia, uremic N19
with
  ectopic or molar pregnancy O08.4
  polyneuropathy N18.9 [G63]
chronic (see also Disease, kidney, chronic) N18.9
  due to hypertension — see Hypertensive, kidney
complicating
  ectopic or molar pregnancy O08.4

Uremia, uremic N19 — *continued*
  congenital P96.0
  extrarenal R39.2
  following ectopic or molar pregnancy
    O08.4
  newborn P96.0
  prerenal R39.2
Ureter, ureteral — *see* condition
Ureteralgia N23
Ureterectasis — *see* Hydroureter
Ureteritis N28.89
  cystica N28.86
  due to calculus N20.1
    with calculus, kidney N20.2
      with hydronephrosis N13.2
  gonococcal (acute) (chronic) A54.21
  nonspecific N28.89
Ureterocele N28.89
  congenital (orthotopic) Q62.31
    ectopic Q62.32
Ureterolith, ureterolithiasis — *see* Calculus,
  ureter
Ureterostomy
  attention to Z43.6
  status Z93.6
Urethra, urethral — *see* condition
Urethralgia R39.89
Urethritis (anterior) (posterior) N34.2
  calculous N21.1
  candidal B37.41
  chlamydial A56.01
  diplococcal (gonococcal) A54.01
    with abscess (accessory gland)
      (periurethral) A54.1
  gonococcal A54.01
    with abscess (accessory gland)
      (periurethral) A54.1
  nongonococcal N34.1
    Reiter's — *see* Reiter's disease
  nonspecific N34.1
  nonvenereal N34.1
  postmenopausal N34.2
  puerperal O86.22
  Reiter's — *see* Reiter's disease
  specified NEC N34.2
  trichomonal or due to Trichomonas
    (vaginalis) A59.03
Urethrocele N81.0
  with
    cystocele — *see* Cystocele
    prolapse of uterus — *see* Prolapse,
      uterus
Urethrolithiasis (with colic or infection)
  N21.1
Urethrorectal — *see* condition
Urethrorrhagia N36.8
Urethrorrhea R36.9
Urethrostomy
  attention to Z43.6
  status Z93.6
Urethrotrigonitis — *see* Trigonitis
Urethrovaginal — *see* condition
Urgency
  fecal R15.2
  hypertensive — *see* Hypertension
  urinary N39.41
Urhidrosis, uridrosis L74.8
Uric acid in blood (increased) E79.0
Uricacidemia (asymptomatic) E79.0
Uricemia (asymptomatic) E79.0
Uricosuria R82.99
Urinary — *see* condition
Urination
  frequent R35.0
  painful R30.9
Urine
  blood in — *see* Hematuria
  discharge, excessive R35.8
  enuresis, nonorganic origin F98.0
  extravasation R39.0
  frequency R35.0
  incontinence R32
    nonorganic origin F98.0
  intermittent stream R39.19
  pus in N39.0
  retention or stasis R33.9
    organic R33.8
      drug-induced R33.0
    psychogenic F45.8
  secretion
    deficient R34
    excessive R35.8
    frequency R35.0
  stream
    intermittent R39.19
    slowing R39.19
    splitting R39.13
    weak R39.12

Urinemia — *see* Uremia
Urinoma, urethra N36.8
Uroarthritis, infectious (Reiter's) — *see*
  Reiter's disease
Urodialysis R34
Urolithiasis — *see* Calculus, urinary
Uronephrosis — *see* Hydronephrosis
Uropathy N39.9
  obstructive N13.9
    specified NEC N13.8
  reflux N13.9
    specified NEC N13.8
  vesicoureteral reflux-associated — *see*
    Reflux, vesicoureteral
Urosepsis — *code to* condition
Urticaria L50.9
  with angioneurotic edema T78.3
    hereditary D84.1
  allergic L50.0
  cholinergic L50.5
  chronic L50.8
  cold, familial L50.2
  contact L50.6
  dermatographic L50.3
  due to
    cold or heat L50.2
    drugs L50.0
    food L50.0
    inhalants L50.0
    plants L50.6
    serum (*see also* Reaction, serum) T80.69
  factitial L50.3
  giant T78.3
    hereditary D84.1
  gigantea T78.3
  idiopathic L50.1
  larynx T78.3
    hereditary D84.1
  neonatorum P83.8
  nonallergic L50.1
  papulosa (Hebra) L28.2
  pigmentosa Q82.2
  recurrent periodic L50.8
  serum (*see also* Reaction, serum) T80.69
  solar L56.3
  specified type NEC L50.8 ▪
  thermal (cold) (heat) L50.2
  vibratory L50.4
  xanthelasmoidea Q82.2
Use (of)
  alcohol F10.99
    with sleep disorder F10.982
    harmful — *see* Abuse, alcohol
  amphetamines — *see* Use, stimulant NEC
  caffeine — *see* Use, stimulant NEC
  cannabis F12.90
    with
      anxiety disorder F12.980
      intoxication F12.929
        with
          delirium F12.921
          perceptual disturbance F12.922
        uncomplicated F12.920
      other specified disorder F12.988
      psychosis F12.959
        delusions F12.950
        hallucinations F12.951
      unspecified disorder F12.99
  cocaine F14.90
    with
      anxiety disorder F14.980
      intoxication F14.929
        with
          delirium F14.921
          perceptual disturbance F14.922
        uncomplicated F14.920
      other specified disorder F14.988
      psychosis F14.959
        delusions F14.950
        hallucinations F14.951
      sexual dysfunction F14.981
      sleep disorder F14.982
      unspecified disorder F14.99
    harmful — *see* Abuse, drug, cocaine
  drug(s) NEC F19.90
    with sleep disorder F19.982
    harmful — *see* Abuse, drug, by type
  hallucinogen NEC F16.90
    with
      anxiety disorder F16.980
      intoxication F16.929
        with
          delirium F16.921
        uncomplicated F16.920
      mood disorder F16.94
      other specified disorder F16.988

Use (of) — *continued*
  hallucinogen NEC F16.90 — *continued*
    with — *continued*
      perception disorder (flashbacks)
        F16.983
      psychosis F16.959
        delusions F16.950
        hallucinations F16.951
      unspecified disorder F16.99
    harmful — *see* Abuse, drug,
      hallucinogen NEC
  inhalants F18.90
    with
      anxiety disorder F18.980
      intoxication F18.929
        with delirium F18.921
        uncomplicated F18.920
      mood disorder F18.94
      other specified disorder F18.988
      persisting dementia F18.97
      psychosis F18.959
        delusions F18.950
        hallucinations F18.951
      unspecified disorder F18.99
    harmful — *see* Abuse, drug, inhalant
  methadone F11.20
  nonprescribed drugs F19.90
    harmful — *see* Abuse, non-psychoactive
      substance
  opioid F11.90
    with
      disorder F11.99
        mood F11.94
        sleep F11.982
        specified type NEC F11.988
      intoxication F11.929
        with
          delirium F11.921
          perceptual disturbance F11.922
        uncomplicated F11.920
      withdrawal F11.93
    harmful — *see* Abuse, drug, opioid
  patent medicines F19.90
    harmful — *see* Abuse, non-psychoactive
      substance
  psychoactive drug NEC F19.90
    with
      anxiety disorder F19.980
      intoxication F19.929
        with
          delirium F19.921
          perceptual disturbance F19.922
        uncomplicated F19.920
      mood disorder F19.94
      other specified disorder F19.988
      persisting
        amnestic disorder F19.96
        dementia F19.97
      psychosis F19.959
        delusions F19.950
        hallucinations F19.951
      sexual dysfunction F19.981
      sleep disorder F19.982
      unspecified disorder F19.99
      withdrawal F19.939
        with
          delirium F19.931
          perceptual disturbance F19.932
        uncomplicated F19.930
    harmful — *see* Abuse, drug NEC,
      psychoactive NEC
  sedative, hypnotic, or anxiolytic F13.90
    with
      anxiety disorder F13.980
      intoxication F13.929
        with
          delirium F13.921
        uncomplicated F13.920
      other specified disorder F13.988
      persisting
        amnestic disorder F13.96
        dementia F13.97
      psychosis F13.959
        delusions F13.950
        hallucinations F13.951
      sexual dysfunction F13.981
      sleep disorder F13.982
      unspecified disorder F13.99
    harmful — *see* Abuse, drug, sedative,
      hypnotic, or anxiolytic
  stimulant NEC F15.90
    with
      anxiety disorder F15.980
      intoxication F15.929
        with
          delirium F15.921
          perceptual disturbance F15.922
        uncomplicated F15.920

Use (of) — *continued*
  stimulant NEC F15.90 — *continued*
    with — *continued*
      mood disorder F15.94
      other specified disorder F15.988
      psychosis F15.959
        delusions F15.950
        hallucinations F15.951
      sexual dysfunction F15.981
      sleep disorder F15.982
      unspecified disorder F15.99
      withdrawal F15.93
    harmful — *see* Abuse, drug, stimulant
      NEC
  tobacco Z72.0
    with dependence — *see* Dependence,
      drug, nicotine
  volatile solvents (*see also* Use, inhalant)
    F18.90
    harmful — *see* Abuse, drug, inhalant
Usher-Senear disease or syndrome L10.4
Uta B55.1
Uteromegaly N85.2
Uterovaginal — *see* condition
Uterovesical — *see* condition
Uveal — *see* condition
Uveitis (anterior) — *see also* Iridocyclitis
  acute — *see* Iridocyclitis, acute
  chronic — *see* Iridocyclitis, chronic
  due to toxoplasmosis (acquired) B58.09
    congenital P37.1
  granulomatous — *see* Iridocyclitis, chronic
  heterochromic — *see* Cyclitis, Fuchs'
    heterochromic
  lens-induced — *see* Iridocyclitis, lens-
    induced
  posterior — *see* Chorioretinitis
  sympathetic H44.13-
  syphilitic (secondary) A51.43
    congenital (early) A50.01
    late A52.71
  tuberculous A18.54
Uveoencephalitis — *see* Inflammation,
  chorioretinal
Uveokeratitis — *see* Iridocyclitis
Uveoparotitis D86.89
Uvula — *see* condition
Uvulitis (acute) (catarrhal) (chronic)
  (membranous) (suppurative) (ulcerative)
  K12.2

V

Vaccination (prophylactic)
  complication or reaction — *see*
    Complications, vaccination
  delayed Z28.9
  encounter for Z23
  not done — *see* Immunization, not done,
    because (of)
Vaccinia (generalized) (localized) T88.1
  congenital P35.8
  without vaccination B08.011
Vacuum, in sinus (accessory) (nasal) J34.89
Vagabond's disease B85.1
Vagabond, vagabondage Z59.0
Vagina, vaginal — *see* condition
Vaginitis (tunica) (testis) N49.1
Vaginismus (reflex) N94.2
  functional F52.5
  nonorganic F52.5
  psychogenic F52.5
  secondary N94.2
Vaginitis (acute) (circumscribed) (diffuse)
  (emphysematous) (nonvenereal)
  (ulcerative) N76.0
  with ectopic or molar pregnancy O08.0
  amebic A06.82
  atrophic, postmenopausal N95.2
  bacterial N76.0
  blennorrhagic (gonococcal) A54.02
  candidal B37.3
  chlamydial A56.02
  chronic N76.1
  due to Trichomonas (vaginalis) A59.01
  following ectopic or molar pregnancy
    O08.0
  gonococcal A54.02
    with abscess (accessory gland)
      (periurethral) A54.1
  granuloma A58
  in (due to)
    candidiasis B37.3
    herpesviral (herpes simplex) infection
      A60.04
    pinworm infection B80 [N77.1]
  monilial B37.3
  mycotic (candidal) B37.3
  postmenopausal atrophic N95.2
  puerperal (postpartum) O86.13
  senile (atrophic) N95.2
  subacute or chronic N76.1
  syphilitic (early) A51.0
    late A52.76
  trichomonal A59.01
  tuberculous A18.18
Vaginosis — *see* Vaginitis
Vagotonia G52.2
Vagrancy Z59.0
VAIN — *see* Neoplasia, intraepithelial,
  vagina
Vallecula — *see* condition
Valley fever B38.0
Valsuani's disease — *see* Anemia, obstetric
Valve, valvular (formation) — *see also*
  condition
  cerebral ventricle (communicating) in situ
    Z98.2
  cervix, internal os Q51.828
  congenital NEC — *see* Atresia, by site
  ureter (pelvic junction) (vesical orifice)
    Q62.39
  urethra (congenital) (posterior) Q64.2
Valvulitis (chronic) — *see* Endocarditis
Valvulopathy — *see* Endocarditis
Van Bogaert's leukoencephalopathy
  (sclerosing) (subacute) A81.1
Van Bogaert-Scherer-Epstein disease or
  syndrome E75.5
Van Buchem's syndrome M85.2
Van Creveld-von Gierke disease E74.01
Van der Hoeve(-de Kleyn) syndrome Q78.0
Van der Woude's syndrome Q38.0
Van Neck's disease or osteochondrosis
  M91.0
Vanishing lung J44.9
Vapor asphyxia or suffocation T59.9
  specified agent — *see* Table of Drugs and
    Chemicals
Variance, lethal ball, prosthetic heart valve
  T82.09
Variants, thalassemic D56.8
Variations in hair color L67.1

Varicella B01.9
  with
    complications NEC B01.89
    encephalitis B01.11
    encephalomyelitis B01.11
    meningitis B01.0
    myelitis B01.12
    pneumonia B01.2
  congenital P35.8
Varices — *see* Varix
Varicocele (scrotum) (thrombosed) I86.1
  ovary I86.2
  perineum I86.3
  spermatic cord (ulcerated) I86.1
Varicose
  aneurysm (ruptured) I77.0
  dermatitis — *see* Varix, leg, with,
    inflammation
  eczema — *see* Varix, leg, with,
    inflammation
  phlebitis — *see* Varix, with, inflammation
  tumor — *see* Varix
  ulcer (lower limb, any part) — *see also*
    Varix, leg, with, ulcer
    anus *(see also* Hemorrhoids) K64.8
    esophagus — *see* Varix, esophagus
    inflamed or infected — *see* Varix, leg,
      with ulcer, with inflammation
    nasal septum I86.8
    perineum I86.3
    scrotum I86.1
    specified site NEC I86.8
  vein — *see* Varix
  vessel — *see* Varix, leg
Varicosis, varicosities, varicosity — *see*
  Varix
Variola (major) (minor) B03
Varioloid B03
Varix (lower limb) (ruptured) I83.90
  with
    edema I83.899
    inflammation I83.10
      with ulcer (venous) I83.209
    pain I83.819
    specified complication NEC I83.899
    stasis dermatitis I83.10
      with ulcer (venous) I83.209
    swelling I83.899
    ulcer I83.009
      with inflammation I83.209
  aneurysmal I77.0
  asymptomatic I83.9-
  bladder I86.2
  broad ligament I86.2
  complicating
    childbirth (lower extremity) O87.4
      anus or rectum O87.2
      genital (vagina, vulva or perineum)
        O87.8
    pregnancy (lower extremity) O22.0-
      anus or rectum O22.4-
      genital (vagina, vulva or perineum)
        O22.1-
    puerperium (lower extremity) O87.4
      anus or rectum O87.2
      genital (vagina, vulva, perineum)
        O87.8
  congenital (any site) Q27.8
  esophagus (idiopathic) (primary)
    (ulcerated) I85.00
    bleeding I85.01
    congenital Q27.8
    in (due to)
      alcoholic liver disease I85.10
        bleeding I85.11
      cirrhosis of liver I85.10
        bleeding I85.11
      portal hypertension I85.10
        bleeding I85.11
      schistosomiasis I85.10
        bleeding I85.11
      toxic liver disease I85.10
        bleeding I85.11
    secondary I85.10
      bleeding I85.11
  gastric I86.4
  inflamed or infected I83.10
    ulcerated I83.209
  labia (majora) I86.3

Varix (lower limb) (ruptured) I83.90 —
  continued
  leg (asymptomatic) I83.90
    with
      edema I83.899
      inflammation I83.10
        with ulcer — *see* Varix, leg, with,
          ulcer, with inflammation by
          site
      pain I83.819
      specified complication NEC I83.899
      swelling I83.899
      ulcer I83.009
        with inflammation I83.209
        ankle I83.003
          with inflammation I83.203
        calf I83.002
          with inflammation I83.202
        foot NEC I83.005
          with inflammation I83.205
        heel I83.004
          with inflammation I83.204
        lower leg NEC I83.008
          with inflammation I83.208
        midfoot I83.004
          with inflammation I83.204
        thigh I83.001
          with inflammation I83.201
    bilateral (asymptomatic) I83.93
      with
        edema I83.893
        pain I83.813
        specified complication NEC
          I83.893
        swelling I83.893
        ulcer I83.009
          with inflammation I83.209
    left (asymptomatic) I83.92
      with
        edema I83.892
        inflammation I83.12
          with ulcer — *see* Varix, leg, with,
            ulcer, with inflammation by
            site
        pain I83.812
        specified complication NEC
          I83.892
        swelling I83.892
        ulcer I83.029
          with inflammation I83.229
          ankle I83.023
            with inflammation I83.223
          calf I83.022
            with inflammation I83.222
          foot NEC I83.025
            with inflammation I83.225
          heel I83.024
            with inflammation I83.224
          lower leg NEC I83.028
            with inflammation I83.228
          midfoot I83.024
            with inflammation I83.224
          thigh I83.021
            with inflammation I83.221
    right (asymptomatic) I83.91
      with
        edema I83.891
        inflammation I83.11
          with ulcer — *see* Varix, leg, with,
            ulcer, with inflammation by
            site
        pain I83.811
        specified complication NEC
          I83.891
        swelling I83.891
        ulcer I83.019
          with inflammation I83.219
          ankle I83.013
            with inflammation I83.213
          calf I83.012
            with inflammation I83.212
          foot NEC I83.015
            with inflammation I83.215
          heel I83.014
            with inflammation I83.214
          lower leg NEC I83.018
            with inflammation I83.218
          midfoot I83.014
            with inflammation I83.214
          thigh I83.011
            with inflammation I83.211
  nasal septum I86.8
  orbit I86.8
    congenital Q27.8
  ovary I86.2
  papillary I78.1

Varix (lower limb) (ruptured) I83.90 —
  continued
  pelvis I86.2
  perineum I86.3
  pharynx I86.8
  placenta O43.89-
  renal papilla I86.8
  retina H35.09
  scrotum (ulcerated) I86.1
  sigmoid colon I86.8
  specified site NEC I86.8
  spinal (cord) (vessels) I86.8
  spleen, splenic (vein) (with phlebolith)
    I86.8
  stomach I86.4
  sublingual I86.0
  ulcerated I83.009
    inflamed or infected I83.209
  uterine ligament I86.2
  vagina I86.8
  vocal cord I86.8
  vulva I86.3
Vas deferens — *see* condition
Vas deferentitis N49.1
Vasa previa O69.4
  hemorrhage from, affecting newborn P50.0
Vascular — *see also* condition
  loop on optic papilla Q14.2
  spasm I73.9
  spider I78.1
Vascularization, cornea — *see*
  Neovascularization, cornea
Vasculitis I77.6
  allergic D69.0
  cryoglobulinemic D89.1
  disseminated I77.6
  hypocomplementemic M31.8
  kidney I77.89
  livedoid L95.0
  nodular L95.8
  retina H35.06-
  rheumatic — *see* Fever, rheumatic
  rheumatoid — *see* Rheumatoid, vasculitis
  skin (limited to) L95.9
    specified NEC L95.8
Vasculopathy, necrotizing M31.9
  cardiac allograft T86.290
  specified NEC M31.8
Vasitis (nodosa) N49.1
  tuberculous A18.15
Vasodilation I73.9
Vasomotor — *see* condition
Vasoplasty, after previous sterilization
  Z31.0
  aftercare Z31.42
Vasospasm (vasoconstriction) I73.9
  cerebral (artery) (cerebrovascular) I67.848
    reversible I67.841
  coronary I20.1
  nerve
    arm — *see* Mononeuropathy, upper limb
    brachial plexus G54.0
    cervical plexus G54.2
    leg — *see* Mononeuropathy, lower limb
  peripheral NOS I73.9
  retina (artery) — *see* Occlusion, artery,
    retina
Vasospastic — *see* condition
Vasovagal attack (paroxysmal) R55
  psychogenic F45.8
VATER syndrome Q87.2
Vater's ampulla — *see* condition
Vegetation, vegetative
  adenoid (nasal fossa) J35.8
  endocarditis (acute) (any valve) (subacute)
    I33.0
  heart (mycotic) (valve) I33.0
Veil
  Jackson's Q43.3
Vein, venous — *see* condition
Veldt sore — *see* Ulcer, skin
Velpeau's hernia — *see* Hernia, femoral
Venereal
  bubo A55
  disease A64
  granuloma inguinale A58
  lymphogranuloma (Durand-Nicolas-Favre)
    A55
Venofibrosis I87.8
Venom, venomous — *see* Table of Drugs and
  Chemicals, by animal or substance,
  poisoning
Venous — *see* condition
Ventilator lung, newborn P27.8
Ventral — *see* condition

DISEASE INDEX

© 2013 Channel Publishing, Ltd.

W

D I S E A S E   I N D E X

Waiting list, person on Z75.1
  for organ transplant Z76.82
  undergoing social agency investigation Z75.2
Waldenström
  hypergammaglobulinemia D89.0
  syndrome or macroglobulinemia C88.0
Waldenström-Kjellberg syndrome D50.1
Walking
  difficulty R26.2
    psychogenic F44.4
  sleep F51.3
    hysterical F44.89
Wall, abdominal — *see* condition
Wallenberg's disease or syndrome G46.3
Wallgren's disease I87.8
Wandering
  gallbladder, congenital Q44.1
  in diseases classified elsewhere Z91.83
  kidney, congenital Q63.8
  organ or site, congenital NEC — *see* Malposition, congenital, by site
  pacemaker (heart) I49.8
  spleen D73.89
War neurosis F48.8
Wart (due to HPV) (filiform) (infectious) (viral) B07.9
  anogenital region (venereal) A63.0
  common B07.8
  external genital organs (venereal) A63.0
  flat B07.8
  Hassal-Henle's (of cornea) H18.49
  Peruvian A44.1
  plantar B07.0
  prosector (tuberculous) A18.4
  seborrheic L82.1
    inflamed L82.0
  senile (seborrheic) L82.1
    inflamed L82.0
  tuberculous A18.4
  venereal A63.0
Warthin's tumor — *see* Neoplasm, salivary gland, benign
Wassilieff's disease A27.0
Wasting
  disease R64
    due to malnutrition E41
  extreme (due to malnutrition) E41
  muscle NEC — *see* Atrophy, muscle
Water
  clefts (senile cataract) — *see* Cataract, senile, incipient
  deprivation of T73.1
  intoxication E87.79
  itch B76.9
  lack of T73.1
  loading E87.70
  on
    brain — *see* Hydrocephalus
    chest J94.8
  poisoning E87.79
Waterbrash R12
Water-losing nephritis N25.89
Waterhouse(-Friderichsen) syndrome or disease (meningococcal) A39.1
Watermelon stomach K31.819
  with hemorrhage K31.811
  without hemorrhage K31.819
Watsoniasis B66.8
Wax in ear — *see* Impaction, cerumen
Weak, weakening, weakness (generalized) R53.1
  arches (acquired) — *see also* Deformity, limb, flat foot
  bladder (sphincter) R32
  facial R29.810
    following
      cerebrovascular disease I69.992
        cerebral infarction I69.392
        intracerebral hemorrhage I69.192
        nontraumatic intracranial hemorrhage NEC I69.292
        specified disease NEC I69.892
        stroke I69.392
        subarachnoid hemorrhage I69.092
  foot (double) — *see* Weak, arches
  heart, cardiac — *see* Failure, heart
  mind F70
  muscle M62.81
  myocardium — *see* Failure, heart
  newborn P96.89

Weak, weakening, weakness (generalized) R53.1 — *continued*
  pelvic fundus N81.89
  pubocervical tissue N81.82
  rectovaginal tissue N81.83
  senile R54
  urinary stream R39.12
  valvular — *see* Endocarditis
Wear, worn (with normal or routine use)
  articular bearing surface of internal joint prosthesis — *see* Complications, joint prosthesis, mechanical, wear of articularbearing surfaces, by site
  device, implant or graft — *see* Complications, by site, mechanical complication
  tooth, teeth (approximal) (hard tissues) (interproximal) (occlusal) K03.0
Weather, weathered
  effects of
    cold T69.9
      specified effect NEC T69.8
    hot — *see* Heat
    skin L57.8
Weaver's syndrome Q87.3
Web, webbed (congenital)
  duodenal Q43.8
  esophagus Q39.4
  fingers Q70.1-
  larynx (glottic) (subglottic) Q31.0
  neck (pterygium colli) Q18.3
  Paterson-Kelly D50.1
  popliteal syndrome Q87.89
  toes Q70.3-
Weber-Christian disease M35.6
Weber-Cockayne syndrome (epidermolysis bullosa) Q81.8
Weber-Gubler syndrome G46.3
Weber-Leyden syndrome G46.3
Weber-Osler syndrome I78.0
Weber's paralysis or syndrome G46.3
Wedge-shaped or wedging vertebra — *see* Collapse, vertebra NEC
Wegener's granulomatosis or syndrome M31.30
  with
    kidney involvement M31.31
    lung involvement M31.30
      with kidney involvement M31.31
Wegner's disease A50.02
Weight
  1000-2499 grams at birth (low) — *see* Low, birthweight
  999 grams or less at birth (extremely low) — *see* Low, birthweight, extreme
  gain (abnormal) (excessive) R63.5
    in pregnancy — *see* Pregnancy, complicated by, excessive weight gain
    low — *see* Pregnancy, complicated by, insufficient, weight gain
  loss (abnormal) (cause unknown) R63.4
Weightlessness (effect of) T75.82
Weil (l)-Marchesani syndrome Q87.1
Weil's disease A27.0
Weingarten's syndrome J82
Weir Mitchell's disease I73.81
Weiss-Baker syndrome G90.09
Wells' disease L98.3
Wen — *see* Cyst, sebaceous
Wenckebach's block or phenomenon I44.1
Werdnig-Hoffmann syndrome (muscular atrophy) G12.0
Werlhof's disease D69.3
Wermer's disease or syndrome E31.21
Werner-His disease A79.0
Werner's disease or syndrome E34.8
Wernicke-Korsakoff's syndrome or psychosis (alcoholic) F10.96
  with dependence F10.26
  drug-induced
    due to drug abuse — *see* Abuse, drug, by type, with amnestic disorder
    due to drug dependence — *see* Dependence, drug, by type, with amnestic disorder
  nonalcoholic F04
Wernicke-Posadas disease B38.9
Wernicke's
  developmental aphasia F80.2
  disease or syndrome E51.2
  encephalopathy E51.2
  polioencephalitis, superior E51.2
West African fever B50.8
Westphal-Strümpell syndrome E83.01
West's syndrome — *see* Epilepsy, spasms

Wet
  feet, tropical (maceration) (syndrome) — *see* Immersion, foot
  lung (syndrome), newborn P22.1
Wharton's duct — *see* condition
Wheal — *see* Urticaria
Wheezing R06.2
Whiplash injury S13.4
Whipple's disease (*see also* subcategory M14.8-) K90.81
Whipworm (disease) (infection) (infestation) B79
Whistling face Q87.0
White — *see also* condition
  kidney, small N03.9
  leg, puerperal, postpartum, childbirth O87.1
  mouth B37.0
  patches of mouth K13.29
  spot lesions, teeth
    chewing surface K02.51
    pit and fissure surface K02.51
    smooth surface K02.61
Whitehead L70.0
Whitlow — *see also* Cellulitis, digit
  with lymphangitis — *see* Lymphangitis, acute, digit
  herpesviral B00.89
Whitmore's disease or fever — *see* Melioidosis
Whooping cough A37.90
  with pneumonia A37.91
    due to Bordetella
      bronchiseptica A37.81
      parapertussis A37.11
      pertussis A37.01
    specified organism NEC A37.81
  due to
    Bordetella
      bronchiseptica A37.80
        with pneumonia A37.81
      parapertussis A37.10
        with pneumonia A37.11
      pertussis A37.00
        with pneumonia A37.01
    specified NEC A37.80
      with pneumonia A37.81
Wichman's asthma J38.5
Wide cranial sutures, newborn P96.3
Widening aorta — *see* Ectasia, aorta
  with aneurysm — *see* Aneurysm, aorta
Wilkie's disease or syndrome K55.1
Wilkinson-Sneddon disease or syndrome L13.1
Willebrand (-Jürgens) thrombopathy D68.0
Willige-Hunt disease or syndrome G23.1
Wilms' tumor C64-
Wilson-Mikity syndrome P27.0
Wilson's
  disease or syndrome E83.01
  hepatolenticular degeneration E83.01
  lichen ruber L43.9
Window — *see also* Imperfect, closure
  aorticopulmonary Q21.4
Winter — *see* condition
Wiskott-Aldrich syndrome D82.0
Withdrawal state — *see also* Dependence, drug by type, with withdrawal
  newborn
    correct therapeutic substance properly administered P96.2
    infant of dependent mother P96.1
    therapeutic substance, neonatal P96.2
Witts' anemia D50.8
Witzelsucht F07.0
Woakes' ethmoiditis or syndrome J33.1
Wolff-Hirschorn syndrome Q93.3
Wolff-Parkinson-White syndrome I45.6
Wolhynian fever A79.0
Wolman's disease E75.5
Wood lung or pneumonitis J67.8
Woolly, wooly hair (congenital) (nevus) Q84.1
Woolsorter's disease A22.1
Word
  blindness (congenital) (developmental) F81.0
  deafness (congenital) (developmental) H93.25
Worm-eaten soles A66.3
Worm(s) (infection) (infestation) — *see also* Infestation, helminth
  guinea B72
  in intestine NEC B82.0

Worn out — *see* Exhaustion
  cardiac
    defibrillator (with synchronous cardiac pacemaker) Z45.02
    pacemaker
      battery Z45.010
      lead Z45.018
  device, implant or graft — *see* Complications, by site, mechanical
Worried well Z71.1
Worries R45.82
Wound, open
  abdomen, abdominal
    wall S31.109
      with penetration into peritoneal cavity S31.609
      bite — *see* Bite, abdomen, wall
      epigastric region S31.102
        with penetration into peritoneal cavity S31.602
        bite — *see* Bite, abdomen, wall, epigastric region
        laceration — *see* Laceration, abdomen, wall, epigastric region
        puncture — *see* Puncture, abdomen, wall, epigastric region
      laceration — *see* Laceration, abdomen, wall
      left
        lower quadrant S31.104
          with penetration into peritoneal cavity S31.604
          bite — *see* Bite, abdomen, wall, left, lower quadrant
          laceration — *see* Laceration, abdomen, wall, left, lower quadrant
          puncture — *see* Puncture, abdomen, wall, left, lower quadrant
        upper quadrant S31.101
          with penetration into peritoneal cavity S31.601
          bite — *see* Bite, abdomen, wall, left, upper quadrant
          laceration — *see* Laceration, abdomen, wall, left, upper quadrant
          puncture — *see* Puncture, abdomen, wall, left, upper quadrant
      periumbilic region S31.105
        with penetration into peritoneal cavity S31.605
        bite — *see* Bite, abdomen, wall, periumbilic region
        laceration — *see* Laceration, abdomen, wall, periumbilic region
        puncture — *see* Puncture, abdomen, wall, periumbilic region
      puncture — *see* Puncture, abdomen, wall
      right
        lower quadrant S31.103
          with penetration into peritoneal cavity S31.603
          bite — *see* Bite, abdomen, wall, right, lower quadrant
          laceration — *see* Laceration, abdomen, wall, right, lower quadrant
          puncture — *see* Puncture, abdomen, wall, right, lower quadrant
        upper quadrant S31.100
          with penetration into peritoneal cavity S31.600
          bite — *see* Bite, abdomen, wall, right, upper quadrant
          laceration — *see* Laceration, abdomen, wall, right, upper quadrant
          puncture — *see* Puncture, abdomen, wall, right, upper quadrant
  alveolar (process) — *see* Wound, open, oral cavity
  ankle S91.00-
    bite — *see* Bite, ankle
    laceration — *see* Laceration, ankle
    puncture — *see* Puncture, ankle
  antecubital space — *see* Wound, open, elbow
  anterior chamber, eye — *see* Wound, open, ocular

Wound, open — *continued*
anus S31.839
  bite S31.835
  laceration — *see* Laceration, anus
  puncture — *see* Puncture, anus
arm (upper) S41.10-
  with amputation — *see* Amputation, traumatic, arm
  bite — *see* Bite, arm
  forearm — *see* Wound, open, forearm
  laceration — *see* Laceration, arm
  puncture — *see* Puncture, arm
  auditory canal (external) (meatus) — *see* Wound, open, ear
  auricle, ear — *see* Wound, open, ear
  axilla — *see* Wound, open, arm
back — *see also* Wound, open, thorax, back
  lower S31.000
    with penetration into retroperitoneal space S31.001
    bite — *see* Bite, back, lower
    laceration — *see* Laceration, back, lower
    puncture — *see* Puncture, back, lower
  bite — *see* Bite
blood vessel — *see* Injury, blood vessel
breast S21.00-
  with amputation — *see* Amputation, traumatic, breast
  bite — *see* Bite, breast
  laceration — *see* Laceration, breast
  puncture — *see* Puncture, breast
buttock S31.809
  bite — *see* Bite, buttock
  laceration — *see* Laceration, buttock
  left S31.829
  puncture — *see* Puncture, buttock
  right S31.819
calf — *see* Wound, open, leg
canaliculus lacrimalis — *see* Wound, open, eyelid
canthus, eye — *see* Wound, open, eyelid
cervical esophagus S11.20
  bite S11.25
  laceration — *see* Laceration, esophagus, traumatic, cervical
  puncture — *see* Puncture, cervical esophagus
cheek (external) S01.40-
  bite — *see* Bite, cheek
  internal — *see* Wound, open, oral cavity
  laceration — *see* Laceration, cheek
  puncture — *see* Puncture, cheek
chest wall — *see* Wound, open, thorax
chin — *see* Wound, open, head, specified site NEC
choroid — *see* Wound, open, ocular
ciliary body (eye) — *see* Wound, open, ocular
clitoris S31.40
  with amputation — *see* Amputation, traumatic, clitoris
  bite S31.45
  laceration — *see* Laceration, vulva
  puncture — *see* Puncture, vulva
conjunctiva — *see* Wound, open, ocular
cornea — *see* Wound, open, ocular
costal region — *see* Wound, open, thorax
Descemet's membrane — *see* Wound, open, ocular
digit(s)
  foot — *see* Wound, open, toe
  hand — *see* Wound, open, finger
ear (canal) (external) S01.30-
  with amputation — *see* Amputation, traumatic, ear
  bite — *see* Bite, ear
  drum S09.2-
  laceration — *see* Laceration, ear
  puncture — *see* Puncture, ear
elbow S51.00-
  bite — *see* Bite, elbow
  laceration — *see* Laceration, elbow
  puncture — *see* Puncture, elbow
epididymis — *see* Wound, open, testis
epigastric region S31.102
  with penetration into peritoneal cavity S31.602
  bite — *see* Bite, abdomen, wall, epigastric region
  laceration — *see* Laceration, abdomen, wall, epigastric region
  puncture — *see* Puncture, abdomen, wall, epigastric region
epiglottis — *see* Wound, open, neck, specified site NEC

Wound, open — *continued*
esophagus (thoracic) S27.819
  cervical — *see* Wound, open, cervical esophagus
  laceration S27.813
  specified type NEC S27.818
eye — *see* Wound, open, ocular
eyeball — *see* Wound, open, ocular
eyebrow — *see* Wound, open, eyelid
eyelid S01.10-
  bite — *see* Bite, eyelid
  laceration — *see* Laceration, eyelid
  puncture — *see* Puncture, eyelid
face NEC — *see* Wound, open, head, specified site NEC
finger(s) S61.209
  with
    amputation — *see* Amputation, traumatic, finger
    damage to nail S61.309
  bite — *see* Bite, finger
  index S61.208
    with
      damage to nail S61.308
    left S61.201
      with
        damage to nail S61.301
    right S61.200
      with
        damage to nail S61.300
  laceration — *see* Laceration, finger
  little S61.208
    with
      damage to nail S61.308
    left S61.207
      with damage to nail S61.307
    right S61.206
      with damage to nail S61.306
  middle S61.208
    with
      damage to nail S61.308
    left S61.203
      with damage to nail S61.303
    right S61.202
      with damage to nail S61.302
  puncture — *see* Puncture, finger
  ring S61.208
    with
      damage to nail S61.308
    left S61.205
      with damage to nail S61.305
    right S61.204
      with damage to nail S61.304
flank — *see* Wound, open, abdomen, wall
foot (except toe(s) alone) S91.30-
  with amputation — *see* Amputation, traumatic, foot
  bite — *see* Bite, foot
  laceration — *see* Laceration, foot
  puncture — *see* Puncture, foot
  toe — *see* Wound, open, toe
forearm S51.80-
  with
    amputation — *see* Amputation, traumatic, forearm
  bite — *see* Bite, forearm
  elbow only — *see* Wound, open, elbow
  laceration — *see* Laceration, forearm
  puncture — *see* Puncture, forearm
forehead — *see* Wound, open, head, specified site NEC
genital organs, external
  with amputation — *see* Amputation, traumatic, genital organs
  bite — *see* Bite, genital organ
  female S31.502
    vagina S31.40
    vulva S31.40
  laceration — *see* Laceration, genital organ
  male S31.501
    penis S31.20
    scrotum S31.30
    testes S31.30
  puncture — *see* Puncture, genital organ
globe (eye) — *see* Wound, open, ocular
groin — *see* Wound, open, abdomen, wall
gum — *see* Wound, open, oral cavity
hand S61.40-
  with
    amputation — *see* Amputation, traumatic, hand
  bite — *see* Bite, hand
  finger(s) — *see* Wound, open, finger
  laceration — *see* Laceration, hand
  puncture — *see* Puncture, hand
  thumb — *see* Wound, open, thumb

Wound, open — *continued*
head S01.90
  bite — *see* Bite, head
  cheek — *see* Wound, open, cheek
  ear — *see* Wound, open, ear
  eyelid — *see* Wound, open, eyelid
  laceration — *see* Laceration, head
  lip — *see* Wound, open, lip
  nose S01.20
  oral cavity — *see* Wound, open, oral cavity
  puncture — *see* Puncture, head
  scalp — *see* Wound, open, scalp
  specified site NEC S01.80
  temporomandibular area — *see* Wound, open, cheek
heel — *see* Wound, open, foot
hip S71.00-
  with amputation — *see* Amputation, traumatic, hip
  bite — *see* Bite, hip
  laceration — *see* Laceration, hip
  puncture — *see* Puncture, hip
hymen S31.40
  bite — *see* Bite, vulva
  laceration — *see* Laceration, vagina
  puncture — *see* Puncture, vagina
hypochondrium S31.109
  bite — *see* Bite, hypochondrium
  laceration — *see* Laceration, hypochondrium
  puncture — *see* Puncture, hypochondrium
hypogastric region S31.109
  bite — *see* Bite, hypogastric region
  laceration — *see* Laceration, hypogastric region
  puncture — *see* Puncture, hypogastric region
iliac (region) — *see* Wound, open, inguinal region
inguinal region S31.109
  bite — *see* Bite, abdomen, wall, lower quadrant
  laceration — *see* Laceration, inguinal region
  puncture — *see* Puncture, inguinal region
instep — *see* Wound, open, foot
interscapular region — *see* Wound, open, thorax, back
intraocular — *see* Wound, open, ocular
iris — *see* Wound, open, ocular
jaw — *see* Wound, open, head, specified site NEC
knee S81.00-
  bite — *see* Bite, knee
  laceration — *see* Laceration, knee
  puncture — *see* Puncture, knee
labium (majus) (minus) — *see* Wound, open, vulva
laceration — *see* Laceration, by site
lacrimal duct — *see* Wound, open, eyelid
larynx S11.019
  bite — *see* Bite, larynx
  laceration — *see* Laceration, larynx
  puncture — *see* Puncture, larynx
left
  lower quadrant S31.104
    with penetration into peritoneal cavity S31.604
    bite — *see* Bite, abdomen, wall, left, lower quadrant
    laceration — *see* Laceration, abdomen, wall, left, lower quadrant
    puncture — *see* Puncture, abdomen, wall, left, lower quadrant
  upper quadrant S31.101
    with penetration into peritoneal cavity S31.601
    bite — *see* Bite, abdomen, wall, left, upper quadrant
    laceration — *see* Laceration, abdomen, wall, left, upper quadrant
    puncture — *see* Puncture, abdomen, wall, left, upper quadrant
leg (lower) S81.80-
  with amputation — *see* Amputation, traumatic, leg
  ankle — *see* Wound, open, ankle
  bite — *see* Bite, leg
  foot — *see* Wound, open, foot
  knee — *see* Wound, open, knee
  laceration — *see* Laceration, leg
  puncture — *see* Puncture, leg
  toe — *see* Wound, open, toe
  upper — *see* Wound, open, thigh

Wound, open — *continued*
lip S01.501
  bite — *see* Bite, lip
  laceration — *see* Laceration, lip
  puncture — *see* Puncture, lip
loin S31.109
  bite — *see* Bite, abdomen, wall
  laceration — *see* Laceration, loin
  puncture — *see* Puncture, loin
lower back — *see* Wound, open, back, lower
lumbar region — *see* Wound, open, back, lower
malar region — *see* Wound, open, head, specified site NEC
mammary — *see* Wound, open, breast
mastoid region — *see* Wound, open, head, specified site NEC
mouth — *see* Wound, open, oral cavity
nail
  finger — *see* Wound, open, finger, with damage to nail
  toe — *see* Wound, open, toe, with damage to nail
nape (neck) — *see* Wound, open, neck
nasal (septum) (sinus) — *see* Wound, open, nose
nasopharynx — *see* Wound, open, head, specified site NEC
neck S11.90
  bite — *see* Bite, neck
  involving
    cervical esophagus S11.20
    larynx — *see* Wound, open, larynx
    pharynx S11.20
    thyroid S11.10
    trachea (cervical) S11.029
      bite — *see* Bite, trachea
      laceration S11.021
        with foreign body S11.022
      puncture S11.023
        with foreign body S11.024
  laceration — *see* Laceration, neck
  puncture — *see* Puncture, neck
  specified site NEC S11.80
  specified type NEC S11.89
nose (septum) (sinus) S01.20
  with amputation — *see* Amputation, traumatic, nose
  bite — *see* Bite, nose
  laceration — *see* Laceration, nose
  puncture — *see* Puncture, nose
ocular S05.90
  avulsion (traumatic enucleation) S05.7-
  eyeball S05.6-
    with foreign body S05.5-
  eyelid — *see* Wound, open, eyelid
  laceration and rupture S05.3-
    with prolapse or loss of intraocular tissue S05.2-
  orbit (penetrating) (with or without foreign body) S05.4-
  periocular area — *see* Wound, open, eyelid
  specified NEC S05.8x-
oral cavity S01.502
  bite S01.552
  laceration — *see* Laceration, oral cavity
  puncture — *see* Puncture, oral cavity
orbit — *see* Wound, open, ocular, orbit
palate — *see* Wound, open, oral cavity
palm — *see* Wound, open, hand
pelvis, pelvic — *see also* Wound, open, back, lower
  girdle — *see* Wound, open, hip
  penetrating — *see* Puncture, by site
penis S31.20
  with amputation — *see* Amputation, traumatic, penis
  bite S31.25
  laceration — *see* Laceration, penis
  puncture — *see* Puncture, penis
perineum
  bite — *see* Bite, perineum
  female S31.502
  laceration — *see* Laceration, perineum
  male S31.501
  puncture — *see* Puncture, perineum
periocular area (with or without lacrimal passages) — *see* Wound, open, eyelid

Wound, open — *continued*
  periumbilic region S31.105
    with penetration into peritoneal cavity S31.605
    bite — *see* Bite, abdomen, wall, periumbilic region
    laceration — *see* Laceration, abdomen, wall, periumbilic region
    puncture — *see* Puncture, abdomen, wall, periumbilic region
  phalanges
    finger — *see* Wound, open, finger
    toe — *see* Wound, open, toe
  pharynx S11.20
  pinna — *see* Wound, open, ear
  popliteal space — *see* Wound, open, knee
  prepuce — *see* Wound, open, penis
  pubic region — *see* Wound, open, back, lower
  pudendum — *see* Wound, open, genital organs, external
  puncture wound — *see* Puncture
  rectovaginal septum — *see* Wound, open, vagina
  right
    lower quadrant S31.103
      with penetration into peritoneal cavity S31.603
      bite — *see* Bite, abdomen, wall, right, lower quadrant
      laceration — *see* Laceration, abdomen, wall, right, lower quadrant
      puncture — *see* Puncture, abdomen, wall, right, lower quadrant
    upper quadrant S31.100
      with penetration into peritoneal cavity S31.600
      bite — *see* Bite, abdomen, wall, right, upper quadrant
      laceration — *see* Laceration, abdomen, wall, right, upper quadrant
      puncture — *see* Puncture, abdomen, wall, right, upper quadrant
  sacral region — *see* Wound, open, back, lower
  sacroiliac region — *see* Wound, open, back, lower
  salivary gland — *see* Wound, open, oral cavity
  scalp S01.00
    bite S01.05
    laceration — *see* Laceration, scalp
    puncture — *see* Puncture, scalp
  scalpel, newborn (birth injury) P15.8
  scapular region — *see* Wound, open, shoulder
  sclera — *see* Wound, open, ocular
  scrotum S31.30
    with amputation — *see* Amputation, traumatic, scrotum
    bite S31.35
    laceration — *see* Laceration, scrotum
    puncture — *see* Puncture, scrotum
  shin — *see* Wound, open, leg
  shoulder S41.00-
    with amputation — *see* Amputation, traumatic, arm
    bite — *see* Bite, shoulder
    laceration — *see* Laceration, shoulder
    puncture — *see* Puncture, shoulder
  skin NOS T14.8
  spermatic cord — *see* Wound, open, testis
  sternal region — *see* Wound, open, thorax, front wall
  submaxillary region — *see* Wound, open, head, specified site NEC
  submental region — *see* Wound, open, head, specified site NEC
  subungual
    finger(s) — *see* Wound, open, finger
    toe(s) — *see* Wound, open, toe
  supraclavicular region — *see* Wound, open, neck, specified site NEC
  temple, temporal region — *see* Wound, open, head, specified site NEC
  temporomandibular area — *see* Wound, open, cheek
  testis S31.30
    with amputation — *see* Amputation, traumatic, testes
    bite S31.35
    laceration — *see* Laceration, testis
    puncture — *see* Puncture, testis

Wound, open — *continued*
  thigh S71.10-
    with amputation — *see* Amputation, traumatic, hip
    bite — *see* Bite, thigh
    laceration — *see* Laceration, thigh
    puncture — *see* Puncture, thigh
  thorax, thoracic (wall) S21.90
    back S21.20-
      with penetration S21.40
    bite — *see* Bite, thorax
    breast — *see* Wound, open, breast
    front S21.10-
      with penetration S21.30
    laceration — *see* Laceration, thorax
    puncture — *see* Puncture, thorax
  throat — *see* Wound, open, neck
  thumb S61.009
    with
      amputation — *see* Amputation, traumatic, thumb
      damage to nail S61.109
    bite — *see* Bite, thumb
    laceration — *see* Laceration, thumb
    left S61.002
      with
        damage to nail S61.102
      puncture — *see* Puncture, thumb
    right S61.001
      with
        damage to nail S61.101
  thyroid (gland) — *see* Wound, open, neck, thyroid
  toe(s) S91.109
    with
      amputation — *see* Amputation, traumatic, toe
      damage to nail S91.209
    bite — *see* Bite, toe
    great S91.103
      with
        damage to nail S91.203
      left S91.102
        with
          damage to nail S91.202
      right S91.101
        with
          damage to nail S91.201
      laceration — *see* Laceration, toe
    lesser S91.106
      with
        damage to nail S91.206
      left S91.105
        with
          damage to nail S91.205
      right S91.104
        with
          damage to nail S91.204
    puncture — *see* Puncture, toe
  tongue — *see* Wound, open, oral cavity
  trachea (cervical region) — *see* Wound, open, neck, trachea
  tunica vaginalis — *see* Wound, open, testis
  tympanum, tympanic membrane S09.2-
    laceration — *see* Laceration, ear, drum
    puncture — *see* Puncture, tympanum
  umbilical region — *see* Wound, open, abdomen, wall, periumbilic region
  uvula — *see* Wound, open, oral cavity
  vagina S31.40
    bite S31.45
    laceration — *see* Laceration, vagina
    puncture — *see* Puncture, vagina
  vitreous (humor) — *see* Wound, open, ocular
  vocal cord S11.039
    bite — *see* Bite, vocal cord
    laceration S11.031
      with foreign body S11.032
    puncture S11.033
      with foreign body S11.034
  vulva S31.40
    with amputation — *see* Amputation, traumatic, vulva
    bite S31.45
    laceration — *see* Laceration, vulva
    puncture — *see* Puncture, vulva
  wrist S61.50-
    bite — *see* Bite, wrist
    laceration — *see* Laceration, wrist
    puncture — *see* Puncture, wrist
Wound, superficial — *see* Injury — *see also* specified injury type
Wright's syndrome G54.0

Wrist — *see* condition
Wrong drug (by accident) (given in error) — *see* Table of Drugs and Chemicals, by drug, poisoning
Wry neck — *see* Torticollis
Wuchereria (bancrofti) infestation B74.0
Wuchereriasis B74.0
Wuchernde Struma Langhans C73

X

X-ray (of)
  abnormal findings — *see* Abnormal, diagnostic imaging
  breast (mammogram) (routine) Z12.31
  chest
    routine (as part of a general medical examination) Z00.00
      with abnormal findings Z00.01
  routine (as part of a general medical examination) Z00.00
    with abnormal findings Z00.01
Xanthelasma (eyelid) (palpebrarum) H02.60
  left H02.66
    lower H02.65
    upper H02.64
  right H02.63
    lower H02.62
    upper H02.61
Xanthelasmatosis (essential) E78.2
Xanthinuria, hereditary E79.8
Xanthoastrocytoma
  specified site — *see* Neoplasm, malignant, by site
  unspecified site C71.9
Xanthofibroma — *see* Neoplasm, connective tissue, benign
Xanthogranuloma D76.3
Xanthoma(s), xanthomatosis (primary) (familial) (hereditary) E75.5
  with
    hyperlipoproteinemia
      Type I E78.3
      Type III E78.2
      Type IV E78.1
      Type V E78.3
  bone (generalisata) C96.5
  cerebrotendinous E75.5
  cutaneotendinous E75.5
  disseminatum (skin) E78.2
  eruptive E78.2
  hypercholesterinemic E78.0
  hypercholesterolemic E78.0
  hyperlipidemic E78.5
  joint E75.5
  multiple (skin) E78.2
  tendon (sheath) E75.5
  tuberosum E78.2
  tuberous E78.2
  tubo-eruptive E78.2
  verrucous, oral mucosa K13.4
Xanthosis R23.8
Xenophobia F40.10
Xeroderma — *see also* Ichthyosis
  acquired L85.0
  eyelid H01.149
    left H01.146
      lower H01.145
      upper H01.144
    right H01.143
      lower H01.142
      upper H01.141
  pigmentosum Q82.1
  vitamin A deficiency E50.8
Xerophthalmia (vitamin A deficiency) E50.7
  unrelated to vitamin A deficiency — *see* Keratoconjunctivitis
Xerosis
  conjunctiva H11.14-
    with Bitot's spots — *see also* Pigmentation, conjunctiva
      vitamin A deficiency E50.1
    vitamin A deficiency E50.0
  cornea H18.89-
    with ulceration — *see* Ulcer, cornea
      vitamin A deficiency E50.3
    vitamin A deficiency E50.2
  cutis L85.3
  skin L85.3
Xerostomia K11.7
Xiphopagus Q89.4
XO syndrome Q96.9
XXXXY syndrome Q98.1
XXY syndrome Q98.0

Y

Yaba pox (virus disease) B08.72
Yatapoxvirus B08.70
  specified NEC B08.79
Yawning R06.89
  psychogenic F45.8
Yaws A66.9
  bone lesions A66.6
  butter A66.1
  chancre A66.0
  cutaneous, less than five years after infection A66.2
  early (cutaneous) (macular) (maculopapular) (micropapular) (papular) A66.2
    frambeside A66.2
    skin lesions NEC A66.2
  eyelid A66.2
  ganglion A66.6
  gangosis, gangosa A66.5
  gumma, gummata A66.4
    bone A66.6
  gummatous
    frambeside A66.4
    osteitis A66.6
    periostitis A66.6
  hydrarthrosis (*see also* subcategory M14.8-) A66.6
  hyperkeratosis (early) (late) A66.3
  initial lesions A66.0
  joint lesions (*see also* subcategory M14.8-) A66.6
  juxta-articular nodules A66.7
  late nodular (ulcerated) A66.4
  latent (without clinical manifestations) (with positive serology) A66.8
  mother A66.0
  mucosal A66.7
  multiple papillomata A66.1
  nodular, late (ulcerated) A66.4
  osteitis A66.6
  papilloma, plantar or palmar A66.1
  periostitis (hypertrophic) A66.6
  specified NEC A66.7
  ulcers A66.4
  wet crab A66.1
Yeast infection (*see also* Candidiasis) B37.9
Yellow
  atrophy (liver) — *see* Failure, hepatic
  fever — *see* Fever, yellow
  jack — *see* Fever, yellow
  jaundice — *see* Jaundice
  nail syndrome L60.5
Yersiniosis — *see also* Infection, Yersinia
  extraintestinal A28.2
  intestinal A04.6

Z

Zahorsky's syndrome (herpangina) B08.5
Zellweger's syndrome Q87.89
Zenker's diverticulum (esophagus) K22.5
Ziehen-Oppenheim disease G24.1
Zieve's syndrome K70.0
Zinc
  deficiency, dietary E60
  metabolism disorder E83.2
Zollinger-Ellison syndrome E16.4
Zona — *see* Herpes, zoster
Zoophobia F40.218
Zoster (herpes) — *see* Herpes, zoster
Zygomycosis B46.9
  specified NEC B46.8
Zymotic — *see* condition

Table of Drugs & Chemicals	POISONING Accidental (Unintentional)	Self-Harm (Intentional)	Assault	Undetermined	Adverse Effect	Underdosing
14-hydroxydihydro-morphinone	T40.2x1	T40.2x2	T40.2x3	T40.2x4	T40.2x5	T40.2x6
1-propanol	T51.3x1	T51.3x2	T51.3x3	T51.3x4	—	—
2,4,5-T (trichloro-phenoxyacetic acid)	T60.1x1	T60.1x2	T60.1x3	T60.1x4	—	—
2,4-D (dichlorophen-oxyacetic acid)	T60.3x1	T60.3x2	T60.3x3	T60.3x4	—	—
2,4-toluene diisocyanate	T65.0x1	T65.0x2	T65.0x3	T65.0x4	—	—
2-propanol	T51.2x1	T51.2x2	T51.2x3	T51.2x4	—	—
ABOB	T37.5x1	T37.5x2	T37.5x3	T37.5x4	T37.5x5	T37.5x6
Abrine	T62.2x1	T62.2x2	T62.2x3	T62.2x4	—	—
Abrus (seed)	T62.2x1	T62.2x2	T62.2x3	T62.2x4	—	—
Absinthe	T51.0x1	T51.0x2	T51.0x3	T51.0x4	—	—
beverage	T51.0x1	T51.0x2	T51.0x3	T51.0x4	—	—
Acaricide	T60.8x1	T60.8x2	T60.8x3	T60.8x4	—	—
Acebutolol	T44.7x1	T44.7x2	T44.7x3	T44.7x4	T44.7x5	T44.7x6
Acecarbromal	T42.6x1	T42.6x2	T42.6x3	T42.6x4	T42.6x5	T42.6x6
Aceclidine	T44.1x1	T44.1x2	T44.1x3	T44.1x4	T44.1x5	T44.1x6
Acedapsone	T37.0x1	T37.0x2	T37.0x3	T37.0x4	T37.0x5	T37.0x6
Acefylline piperazine	T48.6x1	T48.6x2	T48.6x3	T48.6x4	T48.6x5	T48.6x6
Acemorphan	T40.2x1	T40.2x2	T40.2x3	T40.2x4	T40.2x5	T40.2x6
Acenocoumarin	T45.511	T45.512	T45.513	T45.514	T45.515	T45.516
Acenocoumarol	T45.511	T45.512	T45.513	T45.514	T45.515	T45.516
Acepifylline	T48.6x1	T48.6x2	T48.6x3	T48.6x4	T48.6x5	T48.6x6
Acepromazine	T43.3x1	T43.3x2	T43.3x3	T43.3x4	T43.3x5	T43.3x6
Acesulfamethoxypyridazine	T37.0x1	T37.0x2	T37.0x3	T37.0x4	T37.0x5	T37.0x6
Acetal	T52.8x1	T52.8x2	T52.8x3	T52.8x4	—	—
Acetaldehyde (vapor)	T52.8x1	T52.8x2	T52.8x3	T52.8x4	—	—
liquid	T65.891	T65.892	T65.893	T65.894	—	—
P-Acetamidophenol	T39.1x1	T39.1x2	T39.1x3	T39.1x4	T39.1x5	T39.1x6
Acetaminophen	T39.1x1	T39.1x2	T39.1x3	T39.1x4	T39.1x5	T39.1x6
Acetaminosalol	T39.1x1	T39.1x2	T39.1x3	T39.1x4	T39.1x5	T39.1x6
Acetanilide	T39.1x1	T39.1x2	T39.1x3	T39.1x4	T39.1x5	T39.1x6
Acetarsol	T37.3x1	T37.3x2	T37.3x3	T37.3x4	T37.3x5	T37.3x6
Acetazolamide	T50.2x1	T50.2x2	T50.2x3	T50.2x4	T50.2x5	T50.2x6
Acetiamine	T45.2x1	T45.2x2	T45.2x3	T45.2x4	T45.2x5	T45.2x6
Acetic						
acid	T54.2x1	T54.2x2	T54.2x3	T54.2x4	—	—
with sodium acetate (ointment)	T49.3x1	T49.3x2	T49.3x3	T49.3x4	T49.3x5	T49.3x6
ester (solvent) (vapor)	T52.8x1	T52.8x2	T52.8x3	T52.8x4	—	—
irrigating solution	T50.3x1	T50.3x2	T50.3x3	T50.3x4	T50.3x5	T50.3x6
medicinal (lotion)	T49.2x1	T49.2x2	T49.2x3	T49.2x4	T49.2x5	T49.2x6
anhydride	T65.891	T65.892	T65.893	T65.894	—	—
ether (vapor)	T52.8x1	T52.8x2	T52.8x3	T52.8x4	—	—
Acetohexamide	T38.3x1	T38.3x2	T38.3x3	T38.3x4	T38.3x5	T38.3x6
Acetohydroxamic acid	T50.991	T50.992	T50.993	T50.994	T50.995	T50.996
Acetomenaphthone	T45.7x1	T45.7x2	T45.7x3	T45.7x4	T45.7x5	T45.7x6
Acetomorphine	T40.1x1	T40.1x2	T40.1x3	T40.1x4	—	—
Acetone (oils)	T52.4x1	T52.4x2	T52.4x3	T52.4x4	—	—
chlorinated	T52.4x1	T52.4x2	T52.4x3	T52.4x4	—	—
vapor	T52.4x1	T52.4x2	T52.4x3	T52.4x4	—	—
Acetonitrile	T52.8x1	T52.8x2	T52.8x3	T52.8x4	—	—
Acetophenazine	T43.3x1	T43.3x2	T43.3x3	T43.3x4	T43.3x5	T43.3x6
Acetophenetedin	T39.1x1	T39.1x2	T39.1x3	T39.1x4	T39.1x5	T39.1x6
Acetophenone	T52.4x1	T52.4x2	T52.4x3	T52.4x4	—	—
Acetorphine	T40.2x1	T40.2x2	T40.2x3	T40.2x4	—	—
Acetosulfone (sodium)	T37.1x1	T37.1x2	T37.1x3	T37.1x4	T37.1x5	T37.1x6
Acetrizoate (sodium)	T50.8x1	T50.8x2	T50.8x3	T50.8x4	T50.8x5	T50.8x6
Acetrizoic acid	T50.8x1	T50.8x2	T50.8x3	T50.8x4	T50.8x5	T50.8x6
Acetyl						
bromide	T53.6x1	T53.6x2	T53.6x3	T53.6x4	—	—
chloride	T53.6x1	T53.6x2	T53.6x3	T53.6x4	—	—
Acetylcarbromal	T42.6x1	T42.6x2	T42.6x3	T42.6x4	T42.6x5	T42.6x6
Acetylcholine						
chloride	T44.1x1	T44.1x2	T44.1x3	T44.1x4	T44.1x5	T44.1x6
derivative	T44.1x1	T44.1x2	T44.1x3	T44.1x4	T44.1x5	T44.1x6
Acetylcysteine	T48.4x1	T48.4x2	T48.4x3	T48.4x4	T48.4x5	T48.4x6
Acetyldigitoxin	T46.0x1	T46.0x2	T46.0x3	T46.0x4	T46.0x5	T46.0x6
Acetyldigoxin	T46.0x1	T46.0x2	T46.0x3	T46.0x4	T46.0x5	T46.0x6
Acetyldihydrocodeine	T40.2x1	T40.2x2	T40.2x3	T40.2x4	—	—
Acetyldihydrocodeinone	T40.2x1	T40.2x2	T40.2x3	T40.2x4	—	—

Table of Drugs & Chemicals	POISONING Accidental (Unintentional)	Self-Harm (Intentional)	Assault	Undetermined	Adverse Effect	Underdosing
Acetylene (gas)	T59.891	T59.892	T59.893	T59.894	—	—
dichloride	T53.6x1	T53.6x2	T53.6x3	T53.6x4	—	—
incomplete combustion of	T58.11	T58.12	T58.13	T58.14	—	—
industrial	T59.891	T59.892	T59.893	T59.894	—	—
tetrachloride	T53.6x1	T53.6x2	T53.6x3	T53.6x4	—	—
vapor	T53.6x1	T53.6x2	T53.6x3	T53.6x4	—	—
Acetylpheneturide	T42.6x1	T42.6x2	T42.6x3	T42.6x4	T42.6x5	T42.6x6
Acetylphenylhydrazine	T39.8x1	T39.8x2	T39.8x3	T39.8x4	T39.8x5	T39.8x6
Acetylsalicylic acid (salts)	T39.011	T39.012	T39.013	T39.014	T39.015	T39.016
enteric coated	T39.011	T39.012	T39.013	T39.014	T39.015	T39.016
Acetylsulfamethoxypyridazine	T37.0x1	T37.0x2	T37.0x3	T37.0x4	T37.0x5	T37.0x6
Achromycin	T36.4x1	T36.4x2	T36.4x3	T36.4x4	T36.4x5	T36.4x6
ophthalmic preparation	T49.5x1	T49.5x2	T49.5x3	T49.5x4	T49.5x5	T49.5x6
topical NEC	T49.0x1	T49.0x2	T49.0x3	T49.0x4	T49.0x5	T49.0x6
Aciclovir	T37.5x1	T37.5x2	T37.5x3	T37.5x4	T37.5x5	T37.5x6
Acid (corrosive) NEC	T54.2x1	T54.2x2	T54.2x3	T54.2x4	—	—
Acidifying agent NEC	T50.901	T50.902	T50.903	T50.904	T50.905	T50.906
Acipimox	T46.6x1	T46.6x2	T46.6x3	T46.6x4	T46.6x5	T46.6x6
Acitretin	T50.991	T50.992	T50.993	T50.994	T50.995	T50.996
Aclarubicin	T45.1x1	T45.1x2	T45.1x3	T45.1x4	T45.1x5	T45.1x6
Aclatonium napadisilate	T48.1x1	T48.1x2	T48.1x3	T48.1x4	T48.1x5	T48.1x6
Aconite (wild)	T46.991	T46.992	T46.993	T46.994	T46.995	T46.996
Aconitine	T46.991	T46.992	T46.993	T46.994	T46.995	T46.996
Aconitum ferox	T46.991	T46.992	T46.993	T46.994	T46.995	T46.996
Acridine	T65.6x1	T65.6x2	T65.6x3	T65.6x4	—	—
vapor	T59.891	T59.892	T59.893	T59.894	—	—
Acriflavine	T37.91	T37.92	T37.93	T37.94	T37.95	T37.96
Acriflavinium chloride	T49.0x1	T49.0x2	T49.0x3	T49.0x4	T49.0x5	T49.0x6
Acrinol	T49.0x1	T49.0x2	T49.0x3	T49.0x4	T49.0x5	T49.0x6
Acrisorcin	T49.0x1	T49.0x2	T49.0x3	T49.0x4	T49.0x5	T49.0x6
Acrivastine	T45.0x1	T45.0x2	T45.0x3	T45.0x4	T45.0x5	T45.0x6
Acrolein (gas)	T59.891	T59.892	T59.893	T59.894	—	—
liquid	T54.1x1	T54.1x2	T54.1x3	T54.1x4	—	—
Acrylamide	T65.891	T65.892	T65.893	T65.894	—	—
Acrylic resin	T49.3x1	T49.3x2	T49.3x3	T49.3x4	T49.3x5	T49.3x6
Acrylonitrile	T65.891	T65.892	T65.893	T65.894	—	—
Actaea spicata	T62.2x1	T62.2x2	T62.2x3	T62.2x4	—	—
berry	T62.1x1	T62.1x2	T62.1x3	T62.1x4	—	—
Acterol	T37.3x1	T37.3x2	T37.3x3	T37.3x4	T37.3x5	T37.3x6
ACTH	T38.811	T38.812	T38.813	T38.814	T38.815	T38.816
Actinomycin C	T45.1x1	T45.1x2	T45.1x3	T45.1x4	T45.1x5	T45.1x6
Actinomycin D	T45.1x1	T45.1x2	T45.1x3	T45.1x4	T45.1x5	T45.1x6
Activated charcoal — see also Charcoal, medicinal	T47.6x1	T47.6x2	T47.6x3	T47.6x4	T47.6x5	T47.6x6
Acyclovir	T37.5x1	T37.5x2	T37.5x3	T37.5x4	T37.5x5	T37.5x6
Adenine	T45.2x1	T45.2x2	T45.2x3	T45.2x4	T45.2x5	T45.2x6
arabinoside	T37.5x1	T37.5x2	T37.5x3	T37.5x4	T37.5x5	T37.5x6
Adenosine (phosphate)	T46.2x1	T46.2x2	T46.2x3	T46.2x4	T46.2x5	T46.2x6
ADH	T38.891	T38.892	T38.893	T38.894	T38.895	T38.896
Adhesive NEC	T65.891	T65.892	T65.893	T65.894	—	—
Adicillin	T36.0x1	T36.0x2	T36.0x3	T36.0x4	T36.0x5	T36.0x6
Adiphenine	T44.3x1	T44.3x2	T44.3x3	T44.3x4	T44.3x5	T44.3x6
Adipiodone	T50.8x1	T50.8x2	T50.8x3	T50.8x4	T50.8x5	T50.8x6
Adjunct, pharmaceutical	T50.901	T50.902	T50.903	T50.904	T50.905	T50.906
Adrenal (extract, cortex or medulla) (glucocorticoids) (hormones) (mineralocorticoids)	T38.0x1	T38.0x2	T38.0x3	T38.0x4	T38.0x5	T38.0x6
ENT agent	T49.6x1	T49.6x2	T49.6x3	T49.6x4	T49.6x5	T49.6x6
ophthalmic preparation	T49.5x1	T49.5x2	T49.5x3	T49.5x4	T49.5x5	T49.5x6
topical NEC	T49.0x1	T49.0x2	T49.0x3	T49.0x4	T49.0x5	T49.0x6
Adrenaline	T44.5x1	T44.5x2	T44.5x3	T44.5x4	T44.5x5	T44.5x6
Adrenalin — see Adrenaline						
Adrenergic NEC	T44.901	T44.902	T44.903	T44.904	T44.905	T44.906
blocking agent NEC	T44.8x1	T44.8x2	T44.8x3	T44.8x4	T44.8x5	T44.8x6
beta, heart	T44.7x1	T44.7x2	T44.7x3	T44.7x4	T44.7x5	T44.7x6
specified NEC	T44.991	T44.992	T44.993	T44.994	T44.995	T44.996

DRUGS&CHEMICALS

DRUGS&CHEMICALS

Table of Drugs & Chemicals	Accidental (Unintentional)	Self-Harm (Intentional)	Assault	Undetermined	Adverse Effect	Underdosing
Adrenochrome						
(mono) semicarbazone	T46.991	T46.992	T46.993	T46.994	T46.995	T46.996
derivative	T46.991	T46.992	T46.993	T46.994	T46.995	T46.996
Adrenocorticotrophic hormone	T38.811	T38.812	T38.813	T38.814	T38.815	T38.816
Adrenocorticotrophin	T38.811	T38.812	T38.813	T38.814	T38.815	T38.816
Adriamycin	T45.1x1	T45.1x2	T45.1x3	T45.1x4	T45.1x5	T45.1x6
Aerosol spray NEC	T65.91	T65.92	T65.93	T65.94		
Aerosporin	T36.8x1	T36.8x2	T36.8x3	T36.8x4	T36.8x5	T36.8x6
ENT agent	T49.6x1	T49.6x2	T49.6x3	T49.6x4	T49.6x5	T49.6x6
ophthalmic preparation	T49.5x1	T49.5x2	T49.5x3	T49.5x4	T49.5x5	T49.5x6
topical NEC	T49.0x1	T49.0x2	T49.0x3	T49.0x4	T49.0x5	T49.0x6
Aethusa cynapium	T62.2x1	T62.2x2	T62.2x3	T62.2x4	—	—
Afghanistan black	T40.7x1	T40.7x2	T40.7x3	T40.7x4	T40.7x5	T40.7x6
Aflatoxin	T64.01	T64.02	T64.03	T64.04		
Afloqualone	T42.8x1	T42.8x2	T42.8x3	T42.8x4	T42.8x5	T42.8x6
African boxwood	T62.2x1	T62.2x2	T62.2x3	T62.2x4		
Agar	T47.4x1	T47.4x2	T47.4x3	T47.4x4	T47.4x5	T47.4x6
Agonist						
predominantly						
alpha-adrenoreceptor	T44.4x1	T44.4x2	T44.4x3	T44.4x4	T44.4x5	T44.4x6
beta-adrenoreceptor	T44.5x1	T44.5x2	T44.5x3	T44.5x4	T44.5x5	T44.5x6
Agricultural agent NEC	T65.91	T65.92	T65.93	T65.94		
Agrypnal	T42.3x1	T42.3x2	T42.3x3	T42.3x4	T42.3x5	T42.3x6
AHLG	T50.Z11	T50.Z12	T50.Z13	T50.Z14	T50.Z15	T50.Z16
Air contaminant(s), source/type						
NOS	T65.91	T65.92	T65.93	T65.94	—	—
Ajmaline	T46.2x1	T46.2x2	T46.2x3	T46.2x4	T46.2x5	T46.2x6
Akee	T62.1x1	T62.1x2	T62.1x3	T62.1x4		
Akrinol	T49.0x1	T49.0x2	T49.0x3	T49.0x4	T49.0x5	T49.0x6
Akritoin	T37.8x1	T37.8x2	T37.8x3	T37.8x4	T37.8x5	T37.8x6
Alacepril	T46.4x1	T46.4x2	T46.4x3	T46.4x4	T46.4x5	T46.4x6
Alantolactone	T37.4x1	T37.4x2	T37.4x3	T37.4x4	T37.4x5	T37.4x6
Albamycin	T36.8x1	T36.8x2	T36.8x3	T36.8x4	T36.8x5	T36.8x6
Albendazole	T37.4x1	T37.4x2	T37.4x3	T37.4x4	T37.4x5	T37.4x6
Albumin						
bovine	T45.8x1	T45.8x2	T45.8x3	T45.8x4	T45.8x5	T45.8x6
human serum	T45.8x1	T45.8x2	T45.8x3	T45.8x4	T45.8x5	T45.8x6
salt-poor	T45.8x1	T45.8x2	T45.8x3	T45.8x4	T45.8x5	T45.8x6
normal human serum	T45.8x1	T45.8x2	T45.8x3	T45.8x4	T45.8x5	T45.8x6
Albuterol	T48.6x1	T48.6x2	T48.6x3	T48.6x4	T48.6x5	T48.6x6
Albutoin	T42.0x1	T42.0x2	T42.0x3	T42.0x4	T42.0x5	T42.0x6
Alclometasone	T49.0x1	T49.0x2	T49.0x3	T49.0x4	T49.0x5	T49.0x6
Alcohol	T51.91	T51.92	T51.93	T51.94	—	—
absolute	T51.0x1	T51.0x2	T51.0x3	T51.0x4	—	—
beverage	T51.0x1	T51.0x2	T51.0x3	T51.0x4	—	—
allyl	T51.8x1	T51.8x2	T51.8x3	T51.8x4	—	—
antifreeze	T51.1x1	T51.1x2	T51.1x3	T51.1x4	—	—
amyl	T51.3x1	T51.3x2	T51.3x3	T51.3x4	—	—
beverage	T51.0x1	T51.0x2	T51.0x3	T51.0x4	—	—
butyl	T51.3x1	T51.3x2	T51.3x3	T51.3x4	—	—
dehydrated	T51.0x1	T51.0x2	T51.0x3	T51.0x4	—	—
beverage	T51.0x1	T51.0x2	T51.0x3	T51.0x4	—	—
denatured	T51.0x1	T51.0x2	T51.0x3	T51.0x4	—	—
deterrent NEC	T50.6x1	T50.6x2	T50.6x3	T50.6x4	T50.6x5	T50.6x6
diagnostic (gastric function)	T50.8x1	T50.8x2	T50.8x3	T50.8x4	T50.8x5	T50.8x6
ethyl	T51.0x1	T51.0x2	T51.0x3	T51.0x4	—	—
beverage	T51.0x1	T51.0x2	T51.0x3	T51.0x4	—	—
grain	T51.0x1	T51.0x2	T51.0x3	T51.0x4	—	—
beverage	T51.0x1	T51.0x2	T51.0x3	T51.0x4	—	—
industrial	T51.0x1	T51.0x2	T51.0x3	T51.0x4	—	—
isopropyl	T51.2x1	T51.2x2	T51.2x3	T51.2x4	—	—
methyl	T51.1x1	T51.1x2	T51.1x3	T51.1x4	—	—
preparation for consumption	T51.0x1	T51.0x2	T51.0x3	T51.0x4	—	—
propyl	T51.3x1	T51.3x2	T51.3x3	T51.3x4	—	—
secondary	T51.2x1	T51.2x2	T51.2x3	T51.2x4	—	—
radiator	T51.1x1	T51.1x2	T51.1x3	T51.1x4	—	—
rubbing	T51.2x1	T51.2x2	T51.2x3	T51.2x4	—	—
specified type NEC	T51.8x1	T51.8x2	T51.8x3	T51.8x4	—	—
surgical	T51.0x1	T51.0x2	T51.0x3	T51.0x4	—	—
vapor (from any type of alcohol)	T59.891	T59.892	T59.893	T59.894	—	—
wood	T51.1x1	T51.1x2	T51.1x3	T51.1x4	—	—
Alcuronium (chloride)	T48.1x1	T48.1x2	T48.1x3	T48.1x4	T48.1x5	T48.1x6
Aldactone	T50.0x1	T50.0x2	T50.0x3	T50.0x4	T50.0x5	T50.0x6
Aldesulfone sodium	T37.1x1	T37.1x2	T37.1x3	T37.1x4	T37.1x5	T37.1x6
Aldicarb	T60.0x1	T60.0x2	T60.0x3	T60.0x4		
Aldomet	T46.5x1	T46.5x2	T46.5x3	T46.5x4	T46.5x5	T46.5x6
Aldosterone	T50.0x1	T50.0x2	T50.0x3	T50.0x4	T50.0x5	T50.0x6
Aldrin (dust)	T60.1x1	T60.1x2	T60.1x3	T60.1x4	—	—
Aleve — see Naproxen						
Alexitol sodium	T47.1x1	T47.1x2	T47.1x3	T47.1x4	T47.1x5	T47.1x6
Alfacalcidol	T45.2x1	T45.2x2	T45.2x3	T45.2x4	T45.2x5	T45.2x6
Alfadolone	T41.1x1	T41.1x2	T41.1x3	T41.1x4	T41.1x5	T41.1x6
Alfaxalone	T41.1x1	T41.1x2	T41.1x3	T41.1x4	T41.1x5	T41.1x6
Alfentanil	T40.4x1	T40.4x2	T40.4x3	T40.4x4	T40.4x5	T40.4x6
Alfuzosin (hydrochloride)	T44.8x1	T44.8x2	T44.8x3	T44.8x4	T44.8x5	T44.8x6
Algae (harmful) (toxin)	T65.821	T65.822	T65.823	T65.824	—	—
Algeldrate	T47.1x1	T47.1x2	T47.1x3	T47.1x4	T47.1x5	T47.1x6
Algin	T47.8x1	T47.8x2	T47.8x3	T47.8x4	T47.8x5	T47.8x6
Alglucerase	T45.3x1	T45.3x2	T45.3x3	T45.3x4	T45.3x5	T45.3x6
Alidase	T45.3x1	T45.3x2	T45.3x3	T45.3x4	T45.3x5	T45.3x6
Alimemazine	T43.3x1	T43.3x2	T43.3x3	T43.3x4	T43.3x5	T43.3x6
Aliphatic thiocyanates	T65.0x1	T65.0x2	T65.0x3	T65.0x4	—	—
Alizapride	T45.0x1	T45.0x2	T45.0x3	T45.0x4	T45.0x5	T45.0x6
Alkali (caustic)	T54.3x1	T54.3x2	T54.3x3	T54.3x4		
Alkaline antiseptic solution (aromatic)	T49.6x1	T49.6x2	T49.6x3	T49.6x4	T49.6x5	T49.6x6
Alkalinizing agents (medicinal)	T50.901	T50.902	T50.903	T50.904	T50.905	T50.906
Alkalizing agent NEC	T50.901	T50.902	T50.903	T50.904	T50.905	T50.906
Alka-seltzer	T39.011	T39.012	T39.013	T39.014	T39.015	T39.016
Alkavervir	T46.5x1	T46.5x2	T46.5x3	T46.5x4	T46.5x5	T46.5x6
Alkonium (bromide)	T49.0x1	T49.0x2	T49.0x3	T49.0x4	T49.0x5	T49.0x6
Alkylating drug NEC	T45.1x1	T45.1x2	T45.1x3	T45.1x4	T45.1x5	T45.1x6
antimyeloproliferative	T45.1x1	T45.1x2	T45.1x3	T45.1x4	T45.1x5	T45.1x6
lymphatic	T45.1x1	T45.1x2	T45.1x3	T45.1x4	T45.1x5	T45.1x6
Alkylisocyanate	T65.0x1	T65.0x2	T65.0x3	T65.0x4	—	—
Allantoin	T49.4x1	T49.4x2	T49.4x3	T49.4x4	T49.4x5	T49.4x6
Allegron	T43.011	T43.012	T43.013	T43.014	T43.015	T43.016
Allethrin	T49.0x1	T49.0x2	T49.0x3	T49.0x4	T49.0x5	T49.0x6
Allobarbital	T42.3x1	T42.3x2	T42.3x3	T42.3x4	T42.3x5	T42.3x6
Allopurinol	T50.4x1	T50.4x2	T50.4x3	T50.4x4	T50.4x5	T50.4x6
Allyl						
alcohol	T51.8x1	T51.8x2	T51.8x3	T51.8x4	—	—
disulfide	T46.6x1	T46.6x2	T46.6x3	T46.6x4	T46.6x5	T46.6x6
Allylestrenol	T38.5x1	T38.5x2	T38.5x3	T38.5x4	T38.5x5	T38.5x6
Allylisopropylacetylurea	T42.6x1	T42.6x2	T42.6x3	T42.6x4	T42.6x5	T42.6x6
Allylisopropylmalonylurea	T42.3x1	T42.3x2	T42.3x3	T42.3x4	T42.3x5	T42.3x6
Allylthiourea	T49.3x1	T49.3x2	T49.3x3	T49.3x4	T49.3x5	T49.3x6
Allyltribromide	T42.6x1	T42.6x2	T42.6x3	T42.6x4	T42.6x5	T42.6x6
Allypropymal	T42.3x1	T42.3x2	T42.3x3	T42.3x4	T42.3x5	T42.3x6
Almagate	T47.1x1	T47.1x2	T47.1x3	T47.1x4	T47.1x5	T47.1x6
Almasilate	T47.1x1	T47.1x2	T47.1x3	T47.1x4	T47.1x5	T47.1x6
Almitrine	T50.7x1	T50.7x2	T50.7x3	T50.7x4	T50.7x5	T50.7x6
Aloes	T47.2x1	T47.2x2	T47.2x3	T47.2x4	T47.2x5	T47.2x6
Aloglutamol	T47.1x1	T47.1x2	T47.1x3	T47.1x4	T47.1x5	T47.1x6
Aloin	T47.2x1	T47.2x2	T47.2x3	T47.2x4	T47.2x5	T47.2x6
Aloxidone	T42.2x1	T42.2x2	T42.2x3	T42.2x4	T42.2x5	T42.2x6
Alpha						
acetyldigoxin	T46.0x1	T46.0x2	T46.0x3	T46.0x4	T46.0x5	T46.0x6
adrenergic blocking drug	T44.6x1	T44.6x2	T44.6x3	T44.6x4	T44.6x5	T44.6x6
amylase	T45.3x1	T45.3x2	T45.3x3	T45.3x4	T45.3x5	T45.3x6
tocoferol (acetate)	T45.2x1	T45.2x2	T45.2x3	T45.2x4	T45.2x5	T45.2x6
Alphadolone	T41.1x1	T41.1x2	T41.1x3	T41.1x4	T41.1x5	T41.1x6
Alphaprodine	T40.4x1	T40.4x2	T40.4x3	T40.4x4	T40.4x5	T40.4x6
Alphaxalone	T41.1x1	T41.1x2	T41.1x3	T41.1x4	T41.1x5	T41.1x6
Alprazolam	T42.4x1	T42.4x2	T42.4x3	T42.4x4	T42.4x5	T42.4x6
Alprenolol	T44.7x1	T44.7x2	T44.7x3	T44.7x4	T44.7x5	T44.7x6
Alprostadil	T46.7x1	T46.7x2	T46.7x3	T46.7x4	T46.7x5	T46.7x6
Alsactide	T38.811	T38.812	T38.813	T38.814	T38.815	T38.816
Alseroxylon	T46.5x1	T46.5x2	T46.5x3	T46.5x4	T46.5x5	T46.5x6
Alteplase	T45.611	T45.612	T45.613	T45.614	T45.615	T45.616
Altizide	T50.2x1	T50.2x2	T50.2x3	T50.2x4	T50.2x5	T50.2x6
Altretamine	T45.1x1	T45.1x2	T45.1x3	T45.1x4	T45.1x5	T45.1x6

© 2013 Channel Publishing Ltd

Table of Drugs & Chemicals	POISONING Accidental (Unintentional)	Self-Harm (Intentional)	Assault	Undetermined	Adverse Effect	Underdosing
Alum (medicinal)	T49.4x1	T49.4x2	T49.4x3	T49.4x4	T49.4x5	T49.4x6
nonmedicinal (ammonium)						
(potassium)	T56.891	T56.892	T56.893	T56.894	—	—
Aluminium, aluminum						
acetate	T49.2x1	T49.2x2	T49.2x3	T49.2x4	T49.2x5	T49.2x6
solution	T49.0x1	T49.0x2	T49.0x3	T49.0x4	T49.0x5	T49.0x6
aspirin	T39.011	T39.012	T39.013	T39.014	T39.015	T39.016
bis (acetylsalicylate)	T39.011	T39.012	T39.013	T39.014	T39.015	T39.016
carbonate (gel, basic)	T47.1x1	T47.1x2	T47.1x3	T47.1x4	T47.1x5	T47.1x6
chlorhydroxide-complex	T47.1x1	T47.1x2	T47.1x3	T47.1x4	T47.1x5	T47.1x6
chloride	T49.2x1	T49.2x2	T49.2x3	T49.2x4	T49.2x5	T49.2x6
clofibrate	T46.6x1	T46.6x2	T46.6x3	T46.6x4	T46.6x5	T46.6x6
diacetate	T49.2x1	T49.2x2	T49.2x3	T49.2x4	T49.2x5	T49.2x6
glycinate	T47.1x1	T47.1x2	T47.1x3	T47.1x4	T47.1x5	T47.1x6
hydroxide (gel)						
hydroxide-magnesium						
carb. gel	T47.1x1	T47.1x2	T47.1x3	T47.1x4	T47.1x5	T47.1x6
magnesium silicate	T47.1x1	T47.1x2	T47.1x3	T47.1x4	T47.1x5	T47.1x6
nicotinate	T46.7x1	T46.7x2	T46.7x3	T46.7x4	T46.7x5	T46.7x6
ointment (surgical) (topical)	T49.3x1	T49.3x2	T49.3x3	T49.3x4	T49.3x5	T49.3x6
phosphate	T47.1x1	T47.1x2	T47.1x3	T47.1x4	T47.1x5	T47.1x6
salicylate	T39.091	T39.092	T39.093	T39.094	T39.095	T39.096
silicate	T47.1x1	T47.1x2	T47.1x3	T47.1x4	T47.1x5	T47.1x6
sodium silicate	T47.1x1	T47.1x2	T47.1x3	T47.1x4	T47.1x5	T47.1x6
subacetate	T49.2x1	T49.2x2	T49.2x3	T49.2x4	T49.2x5	T49.2x6
sulfate	T49.0x1	T49.0x2	T49.0x3	T49.0x4	T49.0x5	T49.0x6
tannate	T47.6x1	T47.6x2	T47.6x3	T47.6x4	T47.6x5	T47.6x6
topical NEC	T49.3x1	T49.3x2	T49.3x3	T49.3x4	T49.3x5	T49.3x6
Alurate	T42.3x1	T42.3x2	T42.3x3	T42.3x4	T42.3x5	T42.3x6
Alverine	T44.3x1	T44.3x2	T44.3x3	T44.3x4	T44.3x5	T44.3x6
Alvodine	T40.2x1	T40.2x2	T40.2x3	T40.2x4	T40.2x5	T40.2x6
Amanita phalloides	T62.0x1	T62.0x2	T62.0x3	T62.0x4	—	—
Amanitine	T62.0x1	T62.0x2	T62.0x3	T62.0x4	—	—
Amantadine	T42.8x1	T42.8x2	T42.8x3	T42.8x4	T42.8x5	T42.8x6
Ambazone	T49.6x1	T49.6x2	T49.6x3	T49.6x4	T49.6x5	T49.6x6
Ambenonium (chloride)	T44.0x1	T44.0x2	T44.0x3	T44.0x4	T44.0x5	T44.0x6
Ambroxol	T48.4x1	T48.4x2	T48.4x3	T48.4x4	T48.4x5	T48.4x6
Ambuphylline	T48.6x1	T48.6x2	T48.6x3	T48.6x4	T48.6x5	T48.6x6
Ambutonium bromide	T44.3x1	T44.3x2	T44.3x3	T44.3x4	T44.3x5	T44.3x6
Amcinonide	T49.0x1	T49.0x2	T49.0x3	T49.0x4	T49.0x5	T49.0x6
Amdinocilline	T36.0x1	T36.0x2	T36.0x3	T36.0x4	T36.0x5	T36.0x6
Ametazole	T50.8x1	T50.8x2	T50.8x3	T50.8x4	T50.8x5	T50.8x6
Amethocaine	T41.3x1	T41.3x2	T41.3x3	T41.3x4	T41.3x5	T41.3x6
regional	T41.3x1	T41.3x2	T41.3x3	T41.3x4	T41.3x5	T41.3x6
spinal	T41.3x1	T41.3x2	T41.3x3	T41.3x4	T41.3x5	T41.3x6
Amethopterin	T45.1x1	T45.1x2	T45.1x3	T45.1x4	T45.1x5	T45.1x6
Amezinium metilsulfate	T44.991	T44.992	T44.993	T44.994	T44.995	T44.996
Amfebutamone	T43.291	T43.292	T43.293	T43.294	T43.295	T43.296
Amfepramone	T50.5x1	T50.5x2	T50.5x3	T50.5x4	T50.5x5	T50.5x6
Amfetamine	T43.621	T43.622	T43.623	T43.624	T43.625	T43.626
Amfetaminil	T43.621	T43.622	T43.623	T43.624	T43.625	T43.626
Amfomycin	T36.8x1	T36.8x2	T36.8x3	T36.8x4	T36.8x5	T36.8x6
Amidefrine mesilate	T48.5x1	T48.5x2	T48.5x3	T48.5x4	T48.5x5	T48.5x6
Amidone	T40.3x1	T40.3x2	T40.3x3	T40.3x4	T40.3x5	T40.3x6
Amidopyrine	T39.2x1	T39.2x2	T39.2x3	T39.2x4	T39.2x5	T39.2x6
Amidotrizoate	T50.8x1	T50.8x2	T50.8x3	T50.8x4	T50.8x5	T50.8x6
Amiflamine	T43.1x1	T43.1x2	T43.1x3	T43.1x4	T43.1x5	T43.1x6
Amikacin	T36.5x1	T36.5x2	T36.5x3	T36.5x4	T36.5x5	T36.5x6
Amikhelline	T46.3x1	T46.3x2	T46.3x3	T46.3x4	T46.3x5	T46.3x6
Amiloride	T50.2x1	T50.2x2	T50.2x3	T50.2x4	T50.2x5	T50.2x6
Aminacrine	T49.0x1	T49.0x2	T49.0x3	T49.0x4	T49.0x5	T49.0x6
Amineptine	T43.011	T43.012	T43.013	T43.014	T43.015	T43.016
Aminitrozole	T37.3x1	T37.3x2	T37.3x3	T37.3x4	T37.3x5	T37.3x6
Amino acids	T50.3x1	T50.3x2	T50.3x3	T50.3x4	T50.3x5	T50.3x6
Aminoacetic acid (derivatives)	T50.3x1	T50.3x2	T50.3x3	T50.3x4	T50.3x5	T50.3x6
Aminoacridine	T49.0x1	T49.0x2	T49.0x3	T49.0x4	T49.0x5	T49.0x6
Aminobenzoic acid (-p)	T49.3x1	T49.3x2	T49.3x3	T49.3x4	T49.3x5	T49.3x6
4-Aminobutyric acid	T43.8x1	T43.8x2	T43.8x3	T43.8x4	T43.8x5	T43.8x6
Aminocaproic acid	T45.621	T45.622	T45.623	T45.624	T45.625	T45.626
Aminoethylisothiourium	T45.8x1	T45.8x2	T45.8x3	T45.8x4	T45.8x5	T45.8x6
Aminofenazone	T39.2x1	T39.2x2	T39.2x3	T39.2x4	T39.2x5	T39.2x6
Aminoglutethimide	T45.1x1	T45.1x2	T45.1x3	T45.1x4	T45.1x5	T45.1x6
Aminohippuric acid	T50.8x1	T50.8x2	T50.8x3	T50.8x4	T50.8x5	T50.8x6
Aminomethylbenzoic acid	T45.691	T45.692	T45.693	T45.694	T45.695	T45.696
Aminometradine	T50.2x1	T50.2x2	T50.2x3	T50.2x4	T50.2x5	T50.2x6
Aminopentamide	T44.3x1	T44.3x2	T44.3x3	T44.3x4	T44.3x5	T44.3x6
Aminophenazone	T39.2x1	T39.2x2	T39.2x3	T39.2x4	T39.2x5	T39.2x6
Aminophenol	T54.0x1	T54.0x2	T54.0x3	T54.0x4	—	—
4-Aminophenol derivatives	T39.1x1	T39.1x2	T39.1x3	T39.1x4	T39.1x5	T39.1x6
Aminophenylpyridone	T43.591	T43.592	T43.593	T43.594	T43.595	T43.596
Aminophylline	T48.6x1	T48.6x2	T48.6x3	T48.6x4	T48.6x5	T48.6x6
Aminopterin sodium	T45.1x1	T45.1x2	T45.1x3	T45.1x4	T45.1x5	T45.1x6
Aminopyrine	T39.2x1	T39.2x2	T39.2x3	T39.2x4	T39.2x5	T39.2x6
8-Aminoquinoline drugs	T37.2x1	T37.2x2	T37.2x3	T37.2x4	T37.2x5	T37.2x6
Aminorex	T50.5x1	T50.5x2	T50.5x3	T50.5x4	T50.5x5	T50.5x6
Aminosalicylic acid	T37.1x1	T37.1x2	T37.1x3	T37.1x4	T37.1x5	T37.1x6
Aminosalylum	T37.1x1	T37.1x2	T37.1x3	T37.1x4	T37.1x5	T37.1x6
Amiodarone	T46.2x1	T46.2x2	T46.2x3	T46.2x4	T46.2x5	T46.2x6
Amiphenazole	T50.7x1	T50.7x2	T50.7x3	T50.7x4	T50.7x5	T50.7x6
Amiquinsin	T46.5x1	T46.5x2	T46.5x3	T46.5x4	T46.5x5	T46.5x6
Amisometradine	T50.2x1	T50.2x2	T50.2x3	T50.2x4	T50.2x5	T50.2x6
Amisulpride	T43.591	T43.592	T43.593	T43.594	T43.595	T43.596
Amitriptyline	T43.011	T43.012	T43.013	T43.014	T43.015	T43.016
Amitriptylinoxide	T43.011	T43.012	T43.013	T43.014	T43.015	T43.016
Amlexanox	T48.6x1	T48.6x2	T48.6x3	T48.6x4	T48.6x5	T48.6x6
Ammonia (fumes) (gas) (vapor)	T59.891	T59.892	T59.893	T59.894	—	—
aromatic spirit	T48.991	T48.992	T48.993	T48.994	T48.995	T48.996
liquid (household)	T54.3x1	T54.3x2	T54.3x3	T54.3x4	—	—
Ammoniated mercury	T49.0x1	T49.0x2	T49.0x3	T49.0x4	T49.0x5	T49.0x6
Ammonium						
acid tartrate	T49.5x1	T49.5x2	T49.5x3	T49.5x4	T49.5x5	T49.5x6
bromide	T42.6x1	T42.6x2	T42.6x3	T42.6x4	T42.6x5	T42.6x6
carbonate	T54.3x1	T54.3x2	T54.3x3	T54.3x4	—	—
chloride	T50.991	T50.992	T50.993	T50.994	T50.995	T50.996
expectorant	T48.4x1	T48.4x2	T48.4x3	T48.4x4	T48.4x5	T48.4x6
compounds (household) NEC	T54.3x1	T54.3x2	T54.3x3	T54.3x4	—	—
fumes (any usage)	T59.891	T59.892	T59.893	T59.894	—	—
industrial	T54.3x1	T54.3x2	T54.3x3	T54.3x4	—	—
ichthyosulronate	T49.4x1	T49.4x2	T49.4x3	T49.4x4	T49.4x5	T49.4x6
mandelate	T37.91	T37.92	T37.93	T37.94	T37.95	T37.96
sulfamate	T60.3x1	T60.3x2	T60.3x3	T60.3x4	—	—
sulfonate resin	T47.8x1	T47.8x2	T47.8x3	T47.8x4	T47.8x5	T47.8x6
Amobarbital (sodium)	T42.3x1	T42.3x2	T42.3x3	T42.3x4	T42.3x5	T42.3x6
Amodiaquine	T37.2x1	T37.2x2	T37.2x3	T37.2x4	T37.2x5	T37.2x6
Amopyroquin (e)	T37.2x1	T37.2x2	T37.2x3	T37.2x4	T37.2x5	T37.2x6
Amoxapine	T43.011	T43.012	T43.013	T43.014	T43.015	T43.016
Amoxicillin	T36.0x1	T36.0x2	T36.0x3	T36.0x4	T36.0x5	T36.0x6
Amperozide	T43.591	T43.592	T43.593	T43.594	T43.595	T43.596
Amphenidone	T43.591	T43.592	T43.593	T43.594	T43.595	T43.596
Amphetamine NEC	T43.621	T43.622	T43.623	T43.624	T43.625	T43.626
Amphomycin	T36.8x1	T36.8x2	T36.8x3	T36.8x4	T36.8x5	T36.8x6
Amphotalide	T37.4x1	T37.4x2	T37.4x3	T37.4x4	T37.4x5	T37.4x6
Amphotericin B	T36.7x1	T36.7x2	T36.7x3	T36.7x4	T36.7x5	T36.7x6
topical	T49.0x1	T49.0x2	T49.0x3	T49.0x4	T49.0x5	T49.0x6
Ampicillin	T36.0x1	T36.0x2	T36.0x3	T36.0x4	T36.0x5	T36.0x6
Amprotropine	T44.3x1	T44.3x2	T44.3x3	T44.3x4	T44.3x5	T44.3x6
Amsacrine	T45.1x1	T45.1x2	T45.1x3	T45.1x4	T45.1x5	T45.1x6
Amygdaline	T62.2x1	T62.2x2	T62.2x3	T62.2x4	—	—
Amyl						
acetate	T52.8x1	T52.8x2	T52.8x3	T52.8x4	—	—
vapor	T59.891	T59.892	T59.893	T59.894	—	—
alcohol	T51.3x1	T51.3x2	T51.3x3	T51.3x4	—	—
chloride	T53.6x1	T53.6x2	T53.6x3	T53.6x4	—	—
formate	T52.8x1	T52.8x2	T52.8x3	T52.8x4	—	—
nitrite	T46.3x1	T46.3x2	T46.3x3	T46.3x4	T46.3x5	T46.3x6
propionate	T65.891	T65.892	T65.893	T65.894	—	—
Amylase	T47.5x1	T47.5x2	T47.5x3	T47.5x4	T47.5x5	T47.5x6
Amyleine, regional	T41.3x1	T41.3x2	T41.3x3	T41.3x4	T41.3x5	T41.3x6
Amylene						
dichloride	T53.6x1	T53.6x2	T53.6x3	T53.6x4	—	—
hydrate	T51.3x1	T51.3x2	T51.3x3	T51.3x4	—	—

DRUGS&CHEMICALS

DRUGS & CHEMICALS

Table of Drugs & Chemicals	POISONING Accidental (Unintentional)	POISONING Self-Harm (Intentional)	POISONING Assault	POISONING Undetermined	Adverse Effect	Underdosing
Amylmetacresol	T49.6x1	T49.6x2	T49.6x3	T49.6x4	T49.6x5	T49.6x6
Amylobarbitone	T42.3x1	T42.3x2	T42.3x3	T42.3x4	T42.3x5	T42.3x6
Amylocaine, regional	T41.3x1	T41.3x2	T41.3x3	T41.3x4	T41.3x5	T41.3x6
infiltration (subcutaneous)	T41.3x1	T41.3x2	T41.3x3	T41.3x4	T41.3x5	T41.3x6
nerve block (peripheral)						
(plexus)	T41.3x1	T41.3x2	T41.3x3	T41.3x4	T41.3x5	T41.3x6
spinal	T41.3x1	T41.3x2	T41.3x3	T41.3x4	T41.3x5	T41.3x6
topical (surface)	T41.3x1	T41.3x2	T41.3x3	T41.3x4	T41.3x5	T41.3x6
Amylopectin	T47.6x1	T47.6x2	T47.6x3	T47.6x4	T47.6x5	T47.6x6
Amytal (sodium)	T42.3x1	T42.3x2	T42.3x3	T42.3x4	T42.3x5	T42.3x6
Anabolic steroid	T38.7x1	T38.7x2	T38.7x3	T38.7x4	T38.7x5	T38.7x6
Analeptic NEC	T50.7x1	T50.7x2	T50.7x3	T50.7x4	T50.7x5	T50.7x6
Analgesic	T39.91	T39.92	T39.93	T39.94	T39.95	T39.96
anti-inflammatory NEC	T39.91	T39.92	T39.93	T39.94	T39.95	T39.96
propionic acid derivative	T39.311	T39.312	T39.313	T39.314	T39.315	T39.316
antirheumatic NEC	T39.4x1	T39.4x2	T39.4x3	T39.4x4	T39.4x5	T39.4x6
aromatic NEC	T39.1x1	T39.1x2	T39.1x3	T39.1x4	T39.1x5	T39.1x6
narcotic NEC	T40.601	T40.602	T40.603	T40.604	T40.605	T40.606
combination	T40.601	T40.602	T40.603	T40.604	T40.605	T40.606
obstetric	T40.601	T40.602	T40.603	T40.604	T40.605	T40.606
non-narcotic NEC	T39.91	T39.93	T39.93	T39.94	T39.95	T39.96
combination	T39.91	T39.92	T39.93	T39.94	T39.95	T39.96
pyrazole	T39.2x1	T39.2x2	T39.2x3	T39.2x4	T39.2x5	T39.2x6
specified NEC	T39.8x1	T39.8x2	T39.8x3	T39.8x4	T39.8x5	T39.8x6
Analgin	T39.2x1	T39.2x2	T39.2x3	T39.2x4	T39.2x5	T39.2x6
Anamirta cocculus	T62.1x1	T62.1x2	T62.1x3	T62.1x4	—	—
Ancillin	T36.0x1	T36.0x2	T36.0x3	T36.0x4	T36.0x5	T36.0x6
Ancrod	T45.691	T45.692	T45.693	T45.694	T45.695	T45.696
Androgen	T38.7x1	T38.7x2	T38.7x3	T38.7x4	T38.7x5	T38.7x6
Androgen-estrogen mixture	T38.7x1	T38.7x2	T38.7x3	T38.7x4	T38.7x5	T38.7x6
Androstalone	T38.7x1	T38.7x2	T38.7x3	T38.7x4	T38.7x5	T38.7x6
Androstanolone	T38.7x1	T38.7x2	T38.7x3	T38.7x4	T38.7x5	T38.7x6
Androsterone	T38.7x1	T38.7x2	T38.7x3	T38.7x4	T38.7x5	T38.7x6
Anemone pulsatilla	T62.2x1	T62.2x2	T62.2x3	T62.2x4	—	—
Anesthesia						
caudal	T41.3x1	T41.3x2	T41.3x3	T41.3x4	T41.3x5	T41.3x6
endotracheal	T41.0x1	T41.0x2	T41.0x3	T41.0x4	T41.0x5	T41.0x6
epidural	T41.3x1	T41.3x2	T41.3x3	T41.3x4	T41.3x5	T41.3x6
inhalation	T41.0x1	T41.0x2	T41.0x3	T41.0x4	T41.0x5	T41.0x6
local	T41.3x1	T41.3x2	T41.3x3	T41.3x4	T41.3x5	T41.3x6
mucosal	T41.3x1	T41.3x2	T41.3x3	T41.3x4	T41.3x5	T41.3x6
muscle relaxation	T48.1x1	T48.1x2	T48.1x3	T48.1x4	T48.1x5	T48.1x6
nerve blocking	T41.3x1	T41.3x2	T41.3x3	T41.3x4	T41.3x5	T41.3x6
plexus blocking	T41.3x1	T41.3x2	T41.3x3	T41.3x4	T41.3x5	T41.3x6
potentiated	T41.201	T41.202	T41.203	T41.204	T41.205	T41.206
rectal	T41.201	T41.202	T41.203	T41.204	T41.205	T41.206
general	T41.201	T41.202	T41.203	T41.204	T41.205	T41.206
local	T41.3x1	T41.3x2	T41.3x3	T41.3x4	T41.3x5	T41.3x6
regional	T41.3x1	T41.3x2	T41.3x3	T41.3x4	T41.3x5	T41.3x6
surface	T41.3x1	T41.3x2	T41.3x3	T41.3x4	T41.3x5	T41.3x6
Anesthetic NEC — *see also*						
Anesthesia	T41.41	T41.42	T41.43	T41.44	T41.45	T41.46
with muscle relaxant	T41.201	T41.202	T41.203	T41.204	T41.205	T41.206
general	T41.201	T41.202	T41.203	T41.204	T41.205	T41.206
local	T41.3x1	T41.3x2	T41.3x3	T41.3x4	T41.3x5	T41.3x6
gaseous NEC	T41.0x1	T41.0x2	T41.0x3	T41.0x4	T41.0x5	T41.0x6
general NEC	T41.201	T41.202	T41.203	T41.204	T41.205	T41.206
halogenated hydrocarbon						
derivatives NEC	T41.0x1	T41.0x2	T41.0x3	T41.0x4	T41.0x5	T41.0x6
infiltration NEC	T41.3x1	T41.3x2	T41.3x3	T41.3x4	T41.3x5	T41.3x6
intravenous NEC	T41.1x1	T41.1x2	T41.1x3	T41.1x4	T41.1x5	T41.1x6
local NEC	T41.3x1	T41.3x2	T41.3x3	T41.3x4	T41.3x5	T41.3x6
rectal	T41.201	T41.202	T41.203	T41.204	T41.205	T41.206
general	T41.201	T41.202	T41.203	T41.204	T41.205	T41.206
local	T41.3x1	T41.3x2	T41.3x3	T41.3x4	T41.3x5	T41.3x6
regional NEC	T41.3x1	T41.3x2	T41.3x3	T41.3x4	T41.3x5	T41.3x6
spinal NEC	T41.3x1	T41.3x2	T41.3x3	T41.3x4	T41.3x5	T41.3x6
thiobarbiturate	T41.1x1	T41.1x2	T41.1x3	T41.1x4	T41.1x5	T41.1x6
topical	T41.3x1	T41.3x2	T41.3x3	T41.3x4	T41.3x5	T41.3x6
Aneurine	T45.2x1	T45.2x2	T45.2x3	T45.2x4	T45.2x5	T45.2x6
Angio-Conray	T50.8x1	T50.8x2	T50.8x3	T50.8x4	T50.8x5	T50.8x6
Angiotensin	T44.5x1	T44.5x2	T44.5x3	T44.5x4	T44.5x5	T44.5x6
Angiotensinamide	T44.991	T44.992	T44.993	T44.994	T44.995	T44.996
Anhydrohydroxy-progesterone	T38.5x1	T38.5x2	T38.5x3	T38.5x4	T38.5x5	T38.5x6
Anhydron	T50.2x1	T50.2x2	T50.2x3	T50.2x4	T50.2x5	T50.2x6
Anileridine	T40.4x1	T40.4x2	T40.4x3	T40.4x4	T40.4x5	T40.4x6
Aniline (dye) (liquid)	T65.3x1	T65.3x2	T65.3x3	T65.3x4	—	—
analgesic	T39.1x1	T39.1x2	T39.1x3	T39.1x4	T39.1x5	T39.1x6
derivatives, therapeutic NEC	T39.1x1	T39.1x2	T39.1x3	T39.1x4	T39.1x5	T39.1x6
vapor	T65.3x1	T65.3x2	T65.3x3	T65.3x4	—	—
Aniscoropine	T44.3x1	T44.3x2	T44.3x3	T44.3x4	T44.3x5	T44.3x6
Anise oil	T47.5x1	T47.5x2	T47.5x3	T47.5x4	T47.5x5	T47.5x6
Anisidine	T65.3x1	T65.3x2	T65.3x3	T65.3x4	—	—
Anisindione	T45.511	T45.512	T45.513	T45.514	T45.515	T45.516
Anisotropine methyl-bromide	T44.3x1	T44.3x2	T44.3x3	T44.3x4	T44.3x5	T44.3x6
Anistreplase	T45.611	T45.612	T45.613	T45.614	T45.615	T45.616
Anorexiant (central)	T50.5x1	T50.5x2	T50.5x3	T50.5x4	T50.5x5	T50.5x6
Anorexic agents	T50.5x1	T50.5x2	T50.5x3	T50.5x4	T50.5x5	T50.5x6
Ansamycin	T36.6x1	T36.6x2	T36.6x3	T36.6x4	T36.6x5	T36.6x6
Ant (bite) (sting) Insecticide	T63.421	T63.422	T63.423	T63.424	—	—
Ant poison — *see* Insecticide						
Antabuse	T50.6x1	T50.6x2	T50.6x3	T50.6x4	T50.6x5	T50.6x6
Antacid NEC	T47.1x1	T47.1x2	T47.1x3	T47.1x4	T47.1x5	T47.1x6
Antagonist						
aldosterone	T50.0x1	T50.0x2	T50.0x3	T50.0x4	T50.0x5	T50.0x6
alpha-adrenoreceptor	T44.6x1	T44.6x2	T44.6x3	T44.6x4	T44.6x5	T44.6x6
anticoagulant	T45.7x1	T45.7x2	T45.7x3	T45.7x4	T45.7x5	T45.7x6
beta-adrenoreceptor	T44.7x1	T44.7x2	T44.7x3	T44.7x4	T44.7x5	T44.7x6
extrapyramidal NEC	T44.3x1	T44.3x2	T44.3x3	T44.3x4	T44.3x5	T44.3x6
folic acid	T45.1x1	T45.1x2	T45.1x3	T45.1x4	T45.1x5	T45.1x6
heavy metal	T45.8x1	T45.8x2	T45.8x3	T45.8x4	T45.8x5	T45.8x6
H2 receptor	T47.0x1	T47.0x2	T47.0x3	T47.0x4	T47.0x5	T47.0x6
narcotic analgesic	T50.7x1	T50.7x2	T50.7x3	T50.7x4	T50.7x5	T50.7x6
opiate	T50.7x1	T50.7x2	T50.7x3	T50.7x4	T50.7x5	T50.7x6
pyrimidine	T45.1x1	T45.1x2	T45.1x3	T45.1x4	T45.1x5	T45.1x6
serotonin	T46.5x1	T46.5x2	T46.5x3	T46.5x4	T46.5x5	T46.5x6
Antazolin(e)	T45.0x1	T45.0x2	T45.0x3	T45.0x4	T45.0x5	T45.0x6
Anterior pituitary hormone NEC	T38.811	T38.812	T38.813	T38.814	T38.815	T38.816
Anthelmintic NEC	T37.4x1	T37.4x2	T37.4x3	T37.4x4	T37.4x5	T37.4x6
Anthiolimine	T37.4x1	T37.4x2	T37.4x3	T37.4x4	T37.4x5	T37.4x6
Anthralin	T49.4x1	T49.4x2	T49.4x3	T49.4x4	T49.4x5	T49.4x6
Anthramycin	T45.1x1	T45.1x2	T45.1x3	T45.1x4	T45.1x5	T45.1x6
Antiadrenergic NEC	T44.8x1	T44.8x2	T44.8x3	T44.8x4	T44.8x5	T44.8x6
Antiallergic NEC	T45.0x1	T45.0x2	T45.0x3	T45.0x4	T45.0x5	T45.0x6
Antiandrogen NEC	T38.6x1	T38.6x2	T38.6x3	T38.6x4	T38.6x5	T38.6x6
Anti-anemic (drug) (preparation)	T45.8x1	T45.8x2	T45.8x3	T45.8x4	T45.8x5	T45.8x6
Antianxiety drug NEC	T43.501	T43.502	T43.503	T43.504	T43.505	T43.506
Antiaris toxicaria	T65.891	T65.892	T65.893	T65.894	—	—
Antiarteriosclerotic drug	T46.6x1	T46.6x2	T46.6x3	T46.6x4	T46.6x5	T46.6x6
Antiasthmatic drug NEC	T48.6x1	T48.6x2	T48.6x3	T48.6x4	T48.6x5	T48.6x6
Antibiotic NEC	T36.91	T36.92	T36.93	T36.94	T36.95	T36.96
aminoglycoside	T36.5x1	T36.5x2	T36.5x3	T36.5x4	T36.5x5	T36.5x6
anticancer	T45.1x1	T45.1x2	T45.1x3	T45.1x4	T45.1x5	T45.1x6
antifungal	T36.7x1	T36.7x2	T36.7x3	T36.7x4	T36.7x5	T36.7x6
antimycobacterial	T36.5x1	T36.5x2	T36.5x3	T36.5x4	T36.5x5	T36.5x6
antineoplastic	T45.1x1	T45.1x2	T45.1x3	T45.1x4	T45.1x5	T45.1x6
cephalosporin (group)	T36.1x1	T36.1x2	T36.1x3	T36.1x4	T36.1x5	T36.1x6
chloramphenicol (group)	T36.2x1	T36.2x2	T36.2x3	T36.2x4	T36.2x5	T36.2x6
ENT	T49.6x1	T49.6x2	T49.6x3	T49.6x4	T49.6x5	T49.6x6
eye	T49.5x1	T49.5x2	T49.5x3	T49.5x4	T49.5x5	T49.5x6
fungicidal (local)	T49.0x1	T49.0x2	T49.0x3	T49.0x4	T49.0x5	T49.0x6
intestinal	T36.8x1	T36.8x2	T36.8x3	T36.8x4	T36.8x5	T36.8x6
b-lactam NEC	T36.1x1	T36.1x2	T36.1x3	T36.1x4	T36.1x5	T36.1x6
local	T49.0x1	T49.0x2	T49.0x3	T49.0x4	T49.0x5	T49.0x6
macrolides	T36.3x1	T36.3x2	T36.3x3	T36.3x4	T36.3x5	T36.3x6
polypeptide	T36.8x1	T36.8x2	T36.8x3	T36.8x4	T36.8x5	T36.8x6
specified NEC	T36.8x1	T36.8x2	T36.8x3	T36.8x4	T36.8x5	T36.8x6
tetracycline (group)	T36.4x1	T36.4x2	T36.4x3	T36.4x4	T36.4x5	T36.4x6
throat	T49.6x1	T49.6x2	T49.6x3	T49.6x4	T49.6x5	T49.6x6
Anticancer agents NEC	T45.1x1	T45.1x2	T45.1x3	T45.1x4	T45.1x5	T45.1x6
Anticholesterolemic drug NEC	T46.6x1	T46.6x2	T46.6x3	T46.6x4	T46.6x5	T46.6x6
Anticholinergic NEC	T44.3x1	T44.3x2	T44.3x3	T44.3x4	T44.3x5	T44.3x6

DRUGS&CHEMICALS

Table of Drugs & Chemicals	POISONING Accidental (Unintentional)	Self-Harm (Intentional)	Assault	Undetermined	Adverse Effect	Underdosing
Anticholinesterase	T44.0x1	T44.0x2	T44.0x3	T44.0x4	T44.0x5	T44.0x6
organophosphorus	T44.0x1	T44.0x2	T44.0x3	T44.0x4	T44.0x5	T44.0x6
insecticide	T60.0x1	T60.0x2	T60.0x3	T60.0x4	—	—
nerve gas	T59.891	T59.892	T59.893	T59.894	—	—
reversible	T44.0x1	T44.0x2	T44.0x3	T44.0x4	T44.0x5	T44.0x6
ophthalmological	T49.5x1	T49.5x2	T49.5x3	T49.5x4	T49.5x5	T49.5x6
Anticoagulant NEC	T45.511	T45.512	T45.513	T45.514	T45.515	T45.516
antagonist	T45.7x1	T45.7x2	T45.7x3	T45.7x4	T45.7x5	T45.7x6
Anti-common-cold drug NEC	T48.5x1	T48.5x2	T48.5x3	T48.5x4	T48.5x5	T48.5x6
Anticonvulsant	T42.71	T42.72	T42.73	T42.74	T42.75	T42.76
barbiturate	T42.3x1	T42.3x2	T42.3x3	T42.3x4	T42.3x5	T42.3x6
combination (with barbiturate)	T42.3x1	T42.3x2	T42.3x3	T42.3x4	T42.3x5	T42.3x6
hydantoin	T42.0x1	T42.0x2	T42.0x3	T42.0x4	T42.0x5	T42.0x6
hypnotic NEC	T42.6x1	T42.6x2	T42.6x3	T42.6x4	T42.6x5	T42.6x6
oxazolidinedione	T42.2x1	T42.2x2	T42.2x3	T42.2x4	T42.2x5	T42.2x6
pyrimidinedione	T42.6x1	T42.6x2	T42.6x3	T42.6x4	T42.6x5	T42.6x6
specified NEC	T42.6x1	T42.6x2	T42.6x3	T42.6x4	T42.6x5	T42.6x6
succinimide	T42.2x1	T42.2x2	T42.2x3	T42.2x4	T42.2x5	T42.2x6
Anti-D immunoglobulin (human)	T50.Z11	T50.Z12	T50.Z13	T50.Z14	T50.Z15	T50.Z16
Antidepressant	T43.201	T43.202	T43.203	T43.204	T43.205	T43.206
monoamine oxidase inhibitor	T43.1x1	T43.1x2	T43.1x3	T43.1x4	T43.1x5	T43.1x6
selective serotonin norepinephrine reuptake inhibitor	T43.211	T43.212	T43.213	T43.214	T43.215	T43.216
selective serotonin reuptake inhibitor	T43.221	T43.222	T43.223	T43.224	T43.225	T43.226
specified NEC	T43.291	T43.292	T43.293	T43.294	T43.295	T43.296
triazolopyridine	T43.211	T43.212	T43.213	T43.214	T43.215	T43.216
tetracyclic	T43.021	T43.022	T43.023	T43.024	T43.025	T43.026
tricyclic	T43.011	T43.012	T43.013	T43.014	T43.015	T43.016
Antidiabetic NEC	T38.3x1	T38.3x2	T38.3x3	T38.3x4	T38.3x5	T38.3x6
biguanide	T38.3x1	T38.3x2	T38.3x3	T38.3x4	T38.3x5	T38.3x6
and sulfonyl combined	T38.3x1	T38.3x2	T38.3x3	T38.3x4	T38.3x5	T38.3x6
combined	T38.3x1	T38.3x2	T38.3x3	T38.3x4	T38.3x5	T38.3x6
sulfonylurea	T38.3x1	T38.3x2	T38.3x3	T38.3x4	T38.3x5	T38.3x6
Antidiarrheal drug NEC	T47.6x1	T47.6x2	T47.6x3	T47.6x4	T47.6x5	T47.6x6
absorbent	T47.6x1	T47.6x2	T47.6x3	T47.6x4	T47.6x5	T47.6x6
Antidiphtheria serum	T50.Z11	T50.Z12	T50.Z13	T50.Z14	T50.Z15	T50.Z16
Antidiuretic hormone	T38.891	T38.892	T38.893	T38.894	T38.895	T38.896
Antidote NEC	T50.6x1	T50.6x2	T50.6x3	T50.6x4	T50.6x5	T50.6x6
heavy metal	T45.8x1	T45.8x2	T45.8x3	T45.8x4	T45.8x5	T45.8x6
Antidysrhythmic NEC	T46.2x1	T46.2x2	T46.2x3	T46.2x4	T46.2x5	T46.2x6
Antiemetic drug	T45.0x1	T45.0x2	T45.0x3	T45.0x4	T45.0x5	T45.0x6
Antiepilepsy agent	T42.71	T42.72	T42.73	T42.74	T42.75	T42.76
combination	T42.5x1	T42.5x2	T42.5x3	T42.5x4	T42.5x5	T42.5x6
mixed	T42.5x1	T42.5x2	T42.5x3	T42.5x4	T42.5x5	T42.5x6
specified, NEC	T42.6x1	T42.6x2	T42.6x3	T42.6x4	T42.6x5	T42.6x6
Antiestrogen NEC	T38.6x1	T38.6x2	T38.6x3	T38.6x4	T38.6x5	T38.6x6
Antifertility pill	T38.4x1	T38.4x2	T38.4x3	T38.4x4	T38.4x5	T38.4x6
Antifibrinolytic drug	T45.621	T45.622	T45.623	T45.624	T45.625	T45.626
Antifilarial drug	T37.4x1	T37.4x2	T37.4x3	T37.4x4	T37.4x5	T37.4x6
Antiflatulent	T47.5x1	T47.5x2	T47.5x3	T47.5x4	T47.5x5	T47.5x6
Antifreeze	T65.91	T65.92	T65.93	T65.94	—	—
alcohol	T51.1x1	T51.1x2	T51.1x3	T51.1x4	—	—
ethylene glycol	T51.8x1	T51.8x2	T51.8x3	T51.8x4	—	—
Antifungal						
antibiotic (systemic)	T36.7x1	T36.7x2	T36.7x3	T36.7x4	T36.7x5	T36.7x6
anti-infective NEC	T37.91	T37.92	T37.93	T37.94	T37.95	T37.96
disinfectant, local	T49.0x1	T49.0x2	T49.0x3	T49.0x4	T49.0x5	T49.0x6
nonmedicinal (spray)	T60.3x1	T60.3x2	T60.3x3	T60.3x4	—	—
topical	T49.0x1	T49.0x2	T49.0x3	T49.0x4	T49.0x5	T49.0x6
Anti-gastric-secretion drug NEC	T47.1x1	T47.1x2	T47.1x3	T47.1x4	T47.1x5	T47.1x6
Antigonadotrophin NEC	T38.6x1	T38.6x2	T38.6x3	T38.6x4	T38.6x5	T38.6x6
Antihallucinogen	T43.501	T43.502	T43.503	T43.504	T43.505	T43.506
Antihelmintics	T37.4x1	T37.4x2	T37.4x3	T37.4x4	T37.4x5	T37.4x6
Antihemophilic						
factor	T45.8x1	T45.8x2	T45.8x3	T45.8x4	T45.8x5	T45.8x6
fraction	T45.8x1	T45.8x2	T45.8x3	T45.8x4	T45.8x5	T45.8x6
globulin concentrate	T45.7x1	T45.7x2	T45.7x3	T45.7x4	T45.7x5	T45.7x6
human plasma	T45.8x1	T45.8x2	T45.8x3	T45.8x4	T45.8x5	T45.8x6
plasma, dried	T45.7x1	T45.7x2	T45.7x3	T45.7x4	T45.7x5	T45.7x6
Antihemorrhoidal preparation	T49.2x1	T49.2x2	T49.2x3	T49.2x4	T49.2x5	T49.2x6
Antiheparin drug	T45.7x1	T45.7x2	T45.7x3	T45.7x4	T45.7x5	T45.7x6
Antihistamine	T45.0x1	T45.0x2	T45.0x3	T45.0x4	T45.0x5	T45.0x6
Antihookworm drug	T37.4x1	T37.4x2	T37.4x3	T37.4x4	T37.4x5	T37.4x6
Anti-human lymphocytic globulin	T50.Z11	T50.Z12	T50.Z13	T50.Z14	T50.Z15	T50.Z16
Antihyperlipidemic drug	T46.6x1	T46.6x2	T46.6x3	T46.6x4	T46.6x5	T46.6x6
Antihypertensive drug NEC	T46.5x1	T46.5x2	T46.5x3	T46.5x4	T46.5x5	T46.5x6
Anti-infective NEC	T37.91	T37.92	T37.93	T37.94	T37.95	T37.96
antibiotics	T36.91	T36.92	T36.93	T36.94	T36.95	T36.96
specified NEC	T36.8x1	T36.8x2	T36.8x3	T36.8x4	T36.8x5	T36.8x6
anthelmintic	T37.4x1	T37.4x2	T37.4x3	T37.4x4	T37.4x5	T37.4x6
antimalarial	T37.2x1	T37.2x2	T37.2x3	T37.2x4	T37.2x5	T37.2x6
antimycobacterial NEC	T37.1x1	T37.1x2	T37.1x3	T37.1x4	T37.1x5	T37.1x6
antibiotics	T36.5x1	T36.5x2	T36.5x3	T36.5x4	T36.5x5	T36.5x6
antiprotozoal NEC	T37.3x1	T37.3x2	T37.3x3	T37.3x4	T37.3x5	T37.3x6
blood	T37.2x1	T37.2x2	T37.2x3	T37.2x4	T37.2x5	T37.2x6
antiviral	T37.5x1	T37.5x2	T37.5x3	T37.5x4	T37.5x5	T37.5x6
arsenical	T37.8x1	T37.8x2	T37.8x3	T37.8x4	T37.8x5	T37.8x6
bismuth, local	T49.0x1	T49.0x2	T49.0x3	T49.0x4	T49.0x5	T49.0x6
ENT	T49.6x1	T49.6x2	T49.6x3	T49.6x4	T49.6x5	T49.6x6
eye NEC	T49.5x1	T49.5x2	T49.5x3	T49.5x4	T49.5x5	T49.5x6
heavy metals NEC	T37.8x1	T37.8x2	T37.8x3	T37.8x4	T37.8x5	T37.8x6
local NEC	T49.0x1	T49.0x2	T49.0x3	T49.0x4	T49.0x5	T49.0x6
specified NEC	T49.0x1	T49.0x2	T49.0x3	T49.0x4	T49.0x5	T49.0x6
mixed	T37.91	T37.92	T37.93	T37.94	T37.95	T37.96
ophthalmic preparation	T49.5x1	T49.5x2	T49.5x3	T49.5x4	T49.5x5	T49.5x6
topical NEC	T49.0x1	T49.0x2	T49.0x3	T49.0x4	T49.0x5	T49.0x6
Anti-inflammatory drug NEC	T39.391	T39.392	T39.393	T39.394	T39.395	T39.396
local	T49.0x1	T49.0x2	T49.0x3	T49.0x4	T49.0x5	T49.0x6
nonsteroidal NEC	T39.391	T39.392	T39.393	T39.394	T39.395	T39.396
propionic acid derivative	T39.311	T39.312	T39.313	T39.314	T39.315	T39.316
specified NEC	T39.391	T39.392	T39.393	T39.394	T39.395	T39.396
Antikaluretic	T50.3x1	T50.3x2	T50.3x3	T50.3x4	T50.3x5	T50.3x6
Antiknock (tetraethyl lead)	T56.0x1	T56.0x2	T56.0x3	T56.0x4	—	—
Antilipemic drug NEC	T46.6x1	T46.6x2	T46.6x3	T46.6x4	T46.6x5	T46.6x6
Antimalarial	T37.2x1	T37.2x2	T37.2x3	T37.2x4	T37.2x5	T37.2x6
prophylactic NEC	T37.2x1	T37.2x2	T37.2x3	T37.2x4	T37.2x5	T37.2x6
pyrimidine derivative	T37.2x1	T37.2x2	T37.2x3	T37.2x4	T37.2x5	T37.2x6
Antimetabolite	T45.1x1	T45.1x2	T45.1x3	T45.1x4	T45.1x5	T45.1x6
Antimitotic agent	T45.1x1	T45.1x2	T45.1x3	T45.1x4	T45.1x5	T45.1x6
Antimony (compounds) (vapor) NEC	T56.891	T56.892	T56.893	T56.894	—	—
anti-infectives	T37.8x1	T37.8x2	T37.8x3	T37.8x4	T37.8x5	T37.8x6
dimercaptosuccinate	T37.3x1	T37.3x2	T37.3x3	T37.3x4	T37.3x5	T37.3x6
hydride	T56.891	T56.892	T56.893	T56.894	—	—
pesticide (vapor)	T60.8x1	T60.8x2	T60.8x3	T60.8x4	—	—
potassium (sodium) tartrate	T37.8x1	T37.8x2	T37.8x3	T37.8x4	T37.8x5	T37.8x6
tartrated	T37.8x1	T37.8x2	T37.8x3	T37.8x4	T37.8x5	T37.8x6
sodium dimercaptosuccinate	T37.3x1	T37.3x2	T37.3x3	T37.3x4	T37.3x5	T37.3x6
Antimuscarinic NEC	T44.3x1	T44.3x2	T44.3x3	T44.3x4	T44.3x5	T44.3x6
Antimycobacterial drug NEC	T37.1x1	T37.1x2	T37.1x3	T37.1x4	T37.1x5	T37.1x6
antibiotics	T36.5x1	T36.5x2	T36.5x3	T36.5x4	T36.5x5	T36.5x6
combination	T37.1x1	T37.1x2	T37.1x3	T37.1x4	T37.1x5	T37.1x6
Antinausea drug	T45.0x1	T45.0x2	T45.0x3	T45.0x4	T45.0x5	T45.0x6
Antinematode drug	T37.4x1	T37.4x2	T37.4x3	T37.4x4	T37.4x5	T37.4x6
Antineoplastic NEC	T45.1x1	T45.1x2	T45.1x3	T45.1x4	T45.1x5	T45.1x6
antibiotics	T45.1x1	T45.1x2	T45.1x3	T45.1x4	T45.1x5	T45.1x6
alkaloidal	T45.1x1	T45.1x2	T45.1x3	T45.1x4	T45.1x5	T45.1x6
combination	T45.1x1	T45.1x2	T45.1x3	T45.1x4	T45.1x5	T45.1x6
estrogen	T38.5x1	T38.5x2	T38.5x3	T38.5x4	T38.5x5	T38.5x6
steroid	T38.7x1	T38.7x2	T38.7x3	T38.7x4	T38.7x5	T38.7x6
Antiparasitic drug (systemic)	T37.91	T37.92	T37.93	T37.94	T37.95	T37.96
local	T49.0x1	T49.0x2	T49.0x3	T49.0x4	T49.0x5	T49.0x6
specified NEC	T37.8x1	T37.8x2	T37.8x3	T37.8x4	T37.8x5	T37.8x6
Antiparkinsonism drug NEC	T42.8x1	T42.8x2	T42.8x3	T42.8x4	T42.8x5	T42.8x6
Antiperspirant NEC	T49.2x1	T49.2x2	T49.2x3	T49.2x4	T49.2x5	T49.2x6
Antiphlogistic NEC	T39.4x1	T39.4x2	T39.4x3	T39.4x4	T39.4x5	T39.4x6
Antiplatyhelmintic drug	T37.4x1	T37.4x2	T37.4x3	T37.4x4	T37.4x5	T37.4x6

DRUGS&CHEMICALS

Table of Drugs & Chemicals	POISONING Accidental (Unintentional)	Self-Harm (Intentional)	Assault	Undetermined	Adverse Effect	Underdosing
Antiprotozoal drug NEC	T37.3x1	T37.3x2	T37.3x3	T37.3x4	T37.3x5	T37.3x6
blood	T37.2x1	T37.2x2	T37.2x3	T37.2x4	T37.2x5	T37.2x6
local	T49.0x1	T49.0x2	T49.0x3	T49.0x4	T49.0x5	T49.0x6
Antipruritic drug NEC	T49.1x1	T49.1x2	T49.1x3	T49.1x4	T49.1x5	T49.1x6
Antipsychotic drug	T43.501	T43.502	T43.503	T43.504	T43.505	T43.506
specified NEC	T43.591	T43.592	T43.593	T43.594	T43.595	T43.596
Antipyretic	T39.91	T39.92	T39.93	T39.94	T39.95	T39.96
specified NEC	T39.8x1	T39.8x2	T39.8x3	T39.8x4	T39.8x5	T39.8x6
Antipyrine	T39.2x1	T39.2x2	T39.2x3	T39.2x4	T39.2x5	T39.2x6
Antirabies hyperimmune serum	T50.Z11	T50.Z12	T50.Z13	T50.Z14	T50.Z15	T50.Z16
Antirheumatic NEC	T39.4x1	T39.4x2	T39.4x3	T39.4x4	T39.4x5	T39.4x6
Antirigidity drug NEC	T42.8x1	T42.8x2	T42.8x3	T42.8x4	T42.8x5	T42.8x6
Antischistosomal drug	T37.4x1	T37.4x2	T37.4x3	T37.4x4	T37.4x5	T37.4x6
Antiscorpion sera	T50.Z11	T50.Z12	T50.Z13	T50.Z14	T50.Z15	T50.Z16
Antiseborrheics	T49.4x1	T49.4x2	T49.4x3	T49.4x4	T49.4x5	T49.4x6
Antiseptics (external) (medicinal)	T49.0x1	T49.0x2	T49.0x3	T49.0x4	T49.0x5	T49.0x6
Antistine	T45.0x1	T45.0x2	T45.0x3	T45.0x4	T45.0x5	T45.0x6
Antitapeworm drug	T37.4x1	T37.4x2	T37.4x3	T37.4x4	T37.4x5	T37.4x6
Antitetanus immunoglobulin	T50.Z11	T50.Z12	T50.Z13	T50.Z14	T50.Z15	T50.Z16
Antithyroid drug NEC	T38.2x1	T38.2x2	T38.2x3	T38.2x4	T38.2x5	T38.2x6
Antitoxin	T50.Z11	T50.Z12	T50.Z13	T50.Z14	T50.Z15	T50.Z16
diphtheria	T50.Z11	T50.Z12	T50.Z13	T50.Z14	T50.Z15	T50.Z16
gas gangrene	T50.Z11	T50.Z12	T50.Z13	T50.Z14	T50.Z15	T50.Z16
tetanus	T50.Z11	T50.Z12	T50.Z13	T50.Z14	T50.Z15	T50.Z16
Antitrichomonal drug	T37.3x1	T37.3x2	T37.3x3	T37.3x4	T37.3x5	T37.3x6
Antituberculars	T37.1x1	T37.1x2	T37.1x3	T37.1x4	T37.1x5	T37.1x6
antibiotics	T36.5x1	T36.5x2	T36.5x3	T36.5x4	T36.5x5	T36.5x6
Antitussive NEC	T48.3x1	T48.3x2	T48.3x3	T48.3x4	T48.3x5	T48.3x6
codeine mixture	T40.2x1	T40.2x2	T40.2x3	T40.2x4	T40.2x5	T40.2x6
opiate	T40.2x1	T40.2x2	T40.2x3	T40.2x4	T40.2x5	T40.2x6
Antivaricose drug	T46.8x1	T46.8x2	T46.8x3	T46.8x4	T46.8x5	T46.8x6
Antivenin, antivenom (sera)	T50.Z11	T50.Z12	T50.Z13	T50.Z14	T50.Z15	T50.Z16
crotaline	T50.Z11	T50.Z12	T50.Z13	T50.Z14	T50.Z15	T50.Z16
spider bite	T50.Z11	T50.Z12	T50.Z13	T50.Z14	T50.Z15	T50.Z16
Antivertigo drug	T45.0x1	T45.0x2	T45.0x3	T45.0x4	T45.0x5	T45.0x6
Antiviral drug NEC	T37.5x1	T37.5x2	T37.5x3	T37.5x4	T37.5x5	T37.5x6
eye	T49.5x1	T49.5x2	T49.5x3	T49.5x4	T49.5x5	T49.5x6
Antiwhipworm drug	T37.4x1	T37.4x2	T37.4x3	T37.4x4	T37.4x5	T37.4x6
Antrol — see also by specific chemical substance	T60.91	T60.92	T60.93	T60.94	—	—
fungicide	T60.91	T60.92	T60.93	T60.94	—	—
ANTU (alpha naphthylthiourea)	T60.4x1	T60.4x2	T60.4x3	T60.4x4	—	—
Apalcillin	T36.0x1	T36.0x2	T36.0x3	T36.0x4	T36.0x5	T36.0x6
APC	T48.5x1	T48.5x2	T48.5x3	T48.5x4	T48.5x5	T48.5x6
Aplonidine	T44.4x1	T44.4x2	T44.4x3	T44.4x4	T44.4x5	T44.4x6
Apomorphine	T47.7x1	T47.7x2	T47.7x3	T47.7x4	T47.7x5	T47.7x6
Appetite depressants, central	T50.5x1	T50.5x2	T50.5x3	T50.5x4	T50.5x5	T50.5x6
Apraclonidine (hydrochloride)	T44.4x1	T44.4x2	T44.4x3	T44.4x4	T44.4x5	T44.4x6
Apresoline	T46.5x1	T46.5x2	T46.5x3	T46.5x4	T46.5x5	T46.5x6
Aprindine	T46.2x1	T46.2x2	T46.2x3	T46.2x4	T46.2x5	T46.2x6
Aprobarbital	T42.3x1	T42.3x2	T42.3x3	T42.3x4	T42.3x5	T42.3x6
Apronalide	T42.6x1	T42.6x2	T42.6x3	T42.6x4	T42.6x5	T42.6x6
Aprotinin	T45.621	T45.622	T45.623	T45.624	T45.625	T45.626
Aptocaine	T41.3x1	T41.3x2	T41.3x3	T41.3x4	T41.3x5	T41.3x6
Aqua fortis	T54.2x1	T54.2x2	T54.2x3	T54.2x4	—	—
Ara-A	T37.5x1	T37.5x2	T37.5x3	T37.5x4	T37.5x5	T37.5x6
Ara-C	T45.1x1	T45.1x2	T45.1x3	T45.1x4	T45.1x5	T45.1x6
Arachis oil	T49.3x1	T49.3x2	T49.3x3	T49.3x4	T49.3x5	T49.3x6
cathartic	T47.4x1	T47.4x2	T47.4x3	T47.4x4	T47.4x5	T47.4x6
Aralen	T37.2x1	T37.2x2	T37.2x3	T37.2x4	T37.2x5	T37.2x6
Arecoline	T44.1x1	T44.1x2	T44.1x3	T44.1x4	T44.1x5	T44.1x6
Arginine	T50.991	T50.992	T50.993	T50.994	T50.995	T50.996
glutamate	T50.991	T50.992	T50.993	T50.994	T50.995	T50.996
Argyrol	T49.0x1	T49.0x2	T49.0x3	T49.0x4	T49.0x5	T49.0x6
ENT agent	T49.6x1	T49.6x2	T49.6x3	T49.6x4	T49.6x5	T49.6x6
ophthalmic preparation	T49.5x1	T49.5x2	T49.5x3	T49.5x4	T49.5x5	T49.5x6
Aristocort	T38.0x1	T38.0x2	T38.0x3	T38.0x4	T38.0x5	T38.0x6
ENT agent	T49.6x1	T49.6x2	T49.6x3	T49.6x4	T49.6x5	T49.6x6
ophthalmic preparation	T49.5x1	T49.5x2	T49.5x3	T49.5x4	T49.5x5	T49.5x6
topical NEC	T49.0x1	T49.0x2	T49.0x3	T49.0x4	T49.0x5	T49.0x6
Aromatics, corrosive	T54.1x1	T54.1x2	T54.1x3	T54.1x4	—	—
disinfectants	T54.1x1	T54.1x2	T54.1x3	T54.1x4	—	—
Arsenate of lead	T57.0x1	T57.0x2	T57.0x3	T57.0x4	—	—
herbicide	T57.0x1	T57.0x2	T57.0x3	T57.0x4	—	—
Arsenic, arsenicals (compounds) (dust) (vapor) NEC	T57.0x1	T57.0x2	T57.0x3	T57.0x4	—	—
anti-infectives	T37.8x1	T37.8x2	T37.8x3	T37.8x4	T37.8x5	T37.8x6
pesticide (dust) (fumes)	T57.0x1	T57.0x2	T57.0x3	T57.0x4	—	—
Arsine (gas)	T57.0x1	T57.0x2	T57.0x3	T57.0x4	—	—
Arsphenamine (silver)	T37.8x1	T37.8x2	T37.8x3	T37.8x4	T37.8x5	T37.8x6
Arsthinol	T37.3x1	T37.3x2	T37.3x3	T37.3x4	T37.3x5	T37.3x6
Artane	T44.3x1	T44.3x2	T44.3x3	T44.3x4	T44.3x5	T44.3x6
Arthropod (venomous) NEC	T63.481	T63.482	T63.483	T63.484	—	—
Articaine	T41.3x1	T41.3x2	T41.3x3	T41.3x4	T41.3x5	T41.3x6
Asbestos	T57.8x1	T57.8x2	T57.8x3	T57.8x4	—	—
Ascaridole	T37.4x1	T37.4x2	T37.4x3	T37.4x4	T37.4x5	T37.4x6
Ascorbic acid	T45.2x1	T45.2x2	T45.2x3	T45.2x4	T45.2x5	T45.2x6
Asiaticoside	T49.0x1	T49.0x2	T49.0x3	T49.0x4	T49.0x5	T49.0x6
Asparaginase	T45.1x1	T45.1x2	T45.1x3	T45.1x4	T45.1x5	T45.1x6
Aspidium (oleoresin)	T37.4x1	T37.4x2	T37.4x3	T37.4x4	T37.4x5	T37.4x6
Aspirin (aluminum) (soluble)	T39.011	T39.012	T39.013	T39.014	T39.015	T39.016
Aspoxicillin	T36.0x1	T36.0x2	T36.0x3	T36.0x4	T36.0x5	T36.0x6
Astemizole	T45.0x1	T45.0x2	T45.0x3	T45.0x4	T45.0x5	T45.0x6
Astringent (local)	T49.2x1	T49.2x2	T49.2x3	T49.2x4	T49.2x5	T49.2x6
specified NEC	T49.2x1	T49.2x2	T49.2x3	T49.2x4	T49.2x5	T49.2x6
Astromicin	T36.5x1	T36.5x2	T36.5x3	T36.5x4	T36.5x5	T36.5x6
Ataractic drug NEC	T43.501	T43.502	T43.503	T43.504	T43.505	T43.506
Atenolol	T44.7x1	T44.7x2	T44.7x3	T44.7x4	T44.7x5	T44.7x6
Atonia drug, intestinal	T47.4x1	T47.4x2	T47.4x3	T47.4x4	T47.4x5	T47.4x6
Atophan	T50.4x1	T50.4x2	T50.4x3	T50.4x4	T50.4x5	T50.4x6
Atracurium besilate	T48.1x1	T48.1x2	T48.1x3	T48.1x4	T48.1x5	T48.1x6
Atropine	T44.3x1	T44.3x2	T44.3x3	T44.3x4	T44.3x5	T44.3x6
derivative	T44.3x1	T44.3x2	T44.3x3	T44.3x4	T44.3x5	T44.3x6
methonitrate	T44.3x1	T44.3x2	T44.3x3	T44.3x4	T44.3x5	T44.3x6
Attapulgite	T47.6x1	T47.6x2	T47.6x3	T47.6x4	T47.6x5	T47.6x6
Auramine	T65.891	T65.892	T65.893	T65.894	—	—
dye	T65.6x1	T65.6x2	T65.6x3	T65.6x4	—	—
fungicide	T60.3x1	T60.3x2	T60.3x3	T60.3x4	—	—
Auranofin	T39.4x1	T39.4x2	T39.4x3	T39.4x4	T39.4x5	T39.4x6
Aurantiin	T46.991	T46.992	T46.993	T46.994	T46.995	T46.996
Aureomycin	T36.4x1	T36.4x2	T36.4x3	T36.4x4	T36.4x5	T36.4x6
ophthalmic preparation	T49.5x1	T49.5x2	T49.5x3	T49.5x4	T49.5x5	T49.5x6
topical NEC	T49.0x1	T49.0x2	T49.0x3	T49.0x4	T49.0x5	T49.0x6
Aurothioglucose	T39.4x1	T39.4x2	T39.4x3	T39.4x4	T39.4x5	T39.4x6
Aurothioglycanide	T39.4x1	T39.4x2	T39.4x3	T39.4x4	T39.4x5	T39.4x6
Aurothiomalate sodium	T39.4x1	T39.4x2	T39.4x3	T39.4x4	T39.4x5	T39.4x6
Aurotioprol	T39.4x1	T39.4x2	T39.4x3	T39.4x4	T39.4x5	T39.4x6
Automobile fuel	T52.0x1	T52.0x2	T52.0x3	T52.0x4	—	—
Autonomic nervous system agent NEC	T44.901	T44.902	T44.903	T44.904	T44.905	T44.906
Avlosulfon	T37.1x1	T37.1x2	T37.1x3	T37.1x4	T37.1x5	T37.1x6
Avomine	T42.6x1	T42.6x2	T42.6x3	T42.6x4	T42.6x5	T42.6x6
Axerophthol	T45.2x1	T45.2x2	T45.2x3	T45.2x4	T45.2x5	T45.2x6
Azacitidine	T45.1x1	T45.1x2	T45.1x3	T45.1x4	T45.1x5	T45.1x6
Azacyclonol	T43.591	T43.592	T43.593	T43.594	T43.595	T43.596
Azadirachta	T60.2x1	T60.2x2	T60.2x3	T60.2x4	—	—
Azanidazole	T37.3x1	T37.3x2	T37.3x3	T37.3x4	T37.3x5	T37.3x6
Azapetine	T46.7x1	T46.7x2	T46.7x3	T46.7x4	T46.7x5	T46.7x6
Azapropazone	T39.2x1	T39.2x2	T39.2x3	T39.2x4	T39.2x5	T39.2x6
Azaribine	T45.1x1	T45.1x2	T45.1x3	T45.1x4	T45.1x5	T45.1x6
Azaserine	T45.1x1	T45.1x2	T45.1x3	T45.1x4	T45.1x5	T45.1x6
Azatadine	T45.0x1	T45.0x2	T45.0x3	T45.0x4	T45.0x5	T45.0x6
Azatepa	T45.1x1	T45.1x2	T45.1x3	T45.1x4	T45.1x5	T45.1x6
Azathioprine	T45.1x1	T45.1x2	T45.1x3	T45.1x4	T45.1x5	T45.1x6
Azelaic acid	T49.0x1	T49.0x2	T49.0x3	T49.0x4	T49.0x5	T49.0x6
Azelastine	T45.0x1	T45.0x2	T45.0x3	T45.0x4	T45.0x5	T45.0x6
Azidocillin	T36.0x1	T36.0x2	T36.0x3	T36.0x4	T36.0x5	T36.0x6
Azidothymidine	T37.5x1	T37.5x2	T37.5x3	T37.5x4	T37.5x5	T37.5x6
Azinphos (ethyl) (methyl)	T60.0x1	T60.0x2	T60.0x3	T60.0x4	—	—
Aziridine (chelating)	T54.1x1	T54.1x2	T54.1x3	T54.1x4	—	—
Azithromycin	T36.3x1	T36.3x2	T36.3x3	T36.3x4	T36.3x5	T36.3x6

Table of Drugs & Chemicals	POISONING Accidental (Unintentional)	Self-Harm (Intentional)	Assault	Undetermined	Adverse Effect	Underdosing
Azlocillin	T36.0x1	T36.0x2	T36.0x3	T36.0x4	T36.0x5	T36.0x6
Azobenzene smoke	T65.3x1	T65.3x2	T65.3x3	T65.3x4	—	—
acaricide	T60.8x1	T60.8x2	T60.8x3	T60.8x4	—	—
Azosulfamide	T37.0x1	T37.0x2	T37.0x3	T37.0x4	T37.0x5	T37.0x6
AZT	T37.5x1	T37.5x2	T37.5x3	T37.5x4	T37.5x5	T37.5x6
Aztreonam	T36.1x1	T36.1x2	T36.1x3	T36.1x4	T36.1x5	T36.1x6
Azulfidine	T37.0x1	T37.0x2	T37.0x3	T37.0x4	T37.0x5	T37.0x6
Azuresin	T50.8x1	T50.8x2	T50.8x3	T50.8x4	T50.8x5	T50.8x6
Bacampicillin	T36.0x1	T36.0x2	T36.0x3	T36.0x4	T36.0x5	T36.0x6
b-acetyldigoxin	T46.0x1	T46.0x2	T46.0x3	T46.0x4	T46.0x5	T46.0x6
Bacillus						
lactobacillus	T47.8x1	T47.8x2	T47.8x3	T47.8x4	T47.8x5	T47.8x6
subtilis	T47.6x1	T47.6x2	T47.6x3	T47.6x4	T47.6x5	T47.6x6
Bacimycin	T49.0x1	T49.0x2	T49.0x3	T49.0x4	T49.0x5	T49.0x6
ophthalmic preparation	T49.5x1	T49.5x2	T49.5x3	T49.5x4	T49.5x5	T49.5x6
Bacitracin zinc	T49.0x1	T49.0x2	T49.0x3	T49.0x4	T49.0x5	T49.0x6
with neomycin	T49.0x1	T49.0x2	T49.0x3	T49.0x4	T49.0x5	T49.0x6
ENT agent	T49.6x1	T49.6x2	T49.6x3	T49.6x4	T49.6x5	T49.6x6
ophthalmic preparation	T49.5x1	T49.5x2	T49.5x3	T49.5x4	T49.5x5	T49.5x6
topical NEC	T49.0x1	T49.0x2	T49.0x3	T49.0x4	T49.0x5	T49.0x6
Baclofen	T42.8x1	T42.8x2	T42.8x3	T42.8x4	T42.8x5	T42.8x6
Baking soda	T50.991	T50.992	T50.993	T50.994	T50.995	T50.996
BAL	T45.8x1	T45.8x2	T45.8x3	T45.8x4	T45.8x5	T45.8x6
Bambuterol	T48.6x1	T48.6x2	T48.6x3	T48.6x4	T48.6x5	T48.6x6
Bamethan (sulfate)	T46.7x1	T46.7x2	T46.7x3	T46.7x4	T46.7x5	T46.7x6
Bamifylline	T48.6x1	T48.6x2	T48.6x3	T48.6x4	T48.6x5	T48.6x6
Bamipine	T45.0x1	T45.0x2	T45.0x3	T45.0x4	T45.0x5	T45.0x6
Baneberry — see Actaea spicata						
Banewort — see Belladonna						
Barbenyl	T42.3x1	T42.3x2	T42.3x3	T42.3x4	T42.3x5	T42.3x6
Barbexaclone	T42.6x1	T42.6x2	T42.6x3	T42.6x4	T42.6x5	T42.6x6
Barbital	T42.3x1	T42.3x2	T42.3x3	T42.3x4	T42.3x5	T42.3x6
sodium	T42.3x1	T42.3x2	T42.3x3	T42.3x4	T42.3x5	T42.3x6
Barbitone	T42.3x1	T42.3x2	T42.3x3	T42.3x4	T42.3x5	T42.3x6
Barbiturate NEC	T42.3x1	T42.3x2	T42.3x3	T42.3x4	T42.3x5	T42.3x6
with tranquilizer	T42.3x1	T42.3x2	T42.3x3	T42.3x4	T42.3x5	T42.3x6
anesthetic (intravenous)	T41.1x1	T41.1x2	T41.1x3	T41.1x4	T41.1x5	T41.1x6
Barium (carbonate) (chloride) (sulfite)	T57.8x1	T57.8x2	T57.8x3	T57.8x4	—	—
diagnostic agent	T50.8x1	T50.8x2	T50.8x3	T50.8x4	T50.8x5	T50.8x6
pesticide	T60.4x1	T60.4x2	T60.4x3	T60.4x4	—	—
rodenticide	T60.4x1	T60.4x2	T60.4x3	T60.4x4	—	—
sulfate (medicinal)	T50.8x1	T50.8x2	T50.8x3	T50.8x4	T50.8x5	T50.8x6
Barrier cream	T49.3x1	T49.3x2	T49.3x3	T49.3x4	T49.3x5	T49.3x6
Basic fuchsin	T49.0x1	T49.0x2	T49.0x3	T49.0x4	T49.0x5	T49.0x6
Battery acid or fluid	T54.2x1	T54.2x2	T54.2x3	T54.2x4	—	—
Bay rum	T51.8x1	T51.8x2	T51.8x3	T51.8x4	—	—
b-benzalbutyramide	T46.6x1	T46.6x2	T46.6x3	T46.6x4	T46.6x5	T46.6x6
BCG (vaccine)	T50.A91	T50.A92	T50.A93	T50.A94	T50.A95	T50.A96
BCNU	T45.1x1	T45.1x2	T45.1x3	T45.1x4	T45.1x5	T45.1x6
Bearsfoot	T62.2x1	T62.2x2	T62.2x3	T62.2x4		
Beclamide	T42.6x1	T42.6x2	T42.6x3	T42.6x4	T42.6x5	T42.6x6
Beclomethasone	T44.5x1	T44.5x2	T44.5x3	T44.5x4	T44.5x5	T44.5x6
Bee (sting) (venom)	T63.441	T63.442	T63.443	T63.444		
Befunolol	T49.5x1	T49.5x2	T49.5x3	T49.5x4	T49.5x5	T49.5x6
Bekanamycin	T36.5x1	T36.5x2	T36.5x3	T36.5x4	T36.5x5	T36.5x6
Belladonna — see also Nightshade						
alkaloids	T44.3x1	T44.3x2	T44.3x3	T44.3x4	T44.3x5	T44.3x6
extract	T44.3x1	T44.3x2	T44.3x3	T44.3x4	T44.3x5	T44.3x6
herb	T44.3x1	T44.3x2	T44.3x3	T44.3x4	T44.3x5	T44.3x6
Bemegride	T50.7x1	T50.7x2	T50.7x3	T50.7x4	T50.7x5	T50.7x6
Benactyzine	T44.3x1	T44.3x2	T44.3x3	T44.3x4	T44.3x5	T44.3x6
Benadryl	T45.0x1	T45.0x2	T45.0x3	T45.0x4	T45.0x5	T45.0x6
Benaprizine	T44.3x1	T44.3x2	T44.3x3	T44.3x4	T44.3x5	T44.3x6
Benazepril	T46.4x1	T46.4x2	T46.4x3	T46.4x4	T46.4x5	T46.4x6
Bencyclane	T46.7x1	T46.7x2	T46.7x3	T46.7x4	T46.7x5	T46.7x6
Bendazol	T46.3x1	T46.3x2	T46.3x3	T46.3x4	T46.3x5	T46.3x6
Bendrofluazide	T50.2x1	T50.2x2	T50.2x3	T50.2x4	T50.2x5	T50.2x6
Bendroflumethiazide	T50.2x1	T50.2x2	T50.2x3	T50.2x4	T50.2x5	T50.2x6
Benemid	T50.4x1	T50.4x2	T50.4x3	T50.4x4	T50.4x5	T50.4x6
Benethamine penicillin	T36.0x1	T36.0x2	T36.0x3	T36.0x4	T36.0x5	T36.0x6
Benexate	T47.1x1	T47.1x2	T47.1x3	T47.1x4	T47.1x5	T47.1x6
Benfluorex	T46.6x1	T46.6x2	T46.6x3	T46.6x4	T46.6x5	T46.6x6
Benfotiamine	T45.2x1	T45.2x2	T45.2x3	T45.2x4	T45.2x5	T45.2x6
Benisone	T49.0x1	T49.0x2	T49.0x3	T49.0x4	T49.0x5	T49.0x6
Benomyl	T60.0x1	T60.0x2	T60.0x3	T60.0x4	—	—
Benoquin	T49.8x1	T49.8x2	T49.8x3	T49.8x4	T49.8x5	T49.8x6
Benoxinate	T41.3x1	T41.3x2	T41.3x3	T41.3x4	T41.3x5	T41.3x6
Benperidol	T43.4x1	T43.4x2	T43.4x3	T43.4x4	T43.4x5	T43.4x6
Benproperine	T48.3x1	T48.3x2	T48.3x3	T48.3x4	T48.3x5	T48.3x6
Benserazide	T42.8x1	T42.8x2	T42.8x3	T42.8x4	T42.8x5	T42.8x6
Bentazepam	T42.4x1	T42.4x2	T42.4x3	T42.4x4	T42.4x5	T42.4x6
Bentiromide	T50.8x1	T50.8x2	T50.8x3	T50.8x4	T50.8x5	T50.8x6
Bentonite	T49.3x1	T49.3x2	T49.3x3	T49.3x4	T49.3x5	T49.3x6
Benzalbutyramide	T46.6x1	T46.6x2	T46.6x3	T46.6x4	T46.6x5	T46.6x6
Benzalkonium (chloride)	T49.0x1	T49.0x2	T49.0x3	T49.0x4	T49.0x5	T49.0x6
ophthalmic preparation	T49.5x1	T49.5x2	T49.5x3	T49.5x4	T49.5x5	T49.5x6
Benzamidosalicylate (calcium)	T37.1x1	T37.1x2	T37.1x3	T37.1x4	T37.1x5	T37.1x6
Benzamine	T41.3x1	T41.3x2	T41.3x3	T41.3x4	T41.3x5	T41.3x6
lactate	T49.1x1	T49.1x2	T49.1x3	T49.1x4	T49.1x5	T49.1x6
Benzamphetamine	T50.5x1	T50.5x2	T50.5x3	T50.5x4	T50.5x5	T50.5x6
Benzapril hydrochloride	T46.5x1	T46.5x2	T46.5x3	T46.5x4	T46.5x5	T46.5x6
Benzathine benzylpenicillin	T36.0x1	T36.0x2	T36.0x3	T36.0x4	T36.0x5	T36.0x6
Benzathine penicillin	T36.0x1	T36.0x2	T36.0x3	T36.0x4	T36.0x5	T36.0x6
Benzatropine	T42.8x1	T42.8x2	T42.8x3	T42.8x4	T42.8x5	T42.8x6
Benzbromarone	T50.4x1	T50.4x2	T50.4x3	T50.4x4	T50.4x5	T50.4x6
Benzcarbimine	T45.1x1	T45.1x2	T45.1x3	T45.1x4	T45.1x5	T45.1x6
Benzdrex	T44.991	T44.992	T44.993	T44.994	T44.995	T44.996
Benzedrine (amphetamine)	T43.621	T43.622	T43.623	T43.624	T43.625	T43.626
Benzenamine	T65.3x1	T65.3x2	T65.3x3	T65.3x4	—	—
Benzene	T52.1x1	T52.1x2	T52.1x3	T52.1x4	—	—
homologues (acetyl) (dimethyl) (methyl) (solvent)	T52.2x1	T52.2x2	T52.2x3	T52.2x4	—	—
Benzethonium (chloride)	T49.0x1	T49.0x2	T49.0x3	T49.0x4	T49.0x5	T49.0x6
Benzetamine	T50.5x1	T50.5x2	T50.5x3	T50.5x4	T50.5x5	T50.5x6
Benzhexol	T44.3x1	T44.3x2	T44.3x3	T44.3x4	T44.3x5	T44.3x6
Benzhydramine (chloride)	T45.0x1	T45.0x2	T45.0x3	T45.0x4	T45.0x5	T45.0x6
Benzidine	T65.891	T65.892	T65.893	T65.894	—	—
Benzilonium bromide	T44.3x1	T44.3x2	T44.3x3	T44.3x4	T44.3x5	T44.3x6
Benzimidazole	T60.3x1	T60.3x2	T60.3x3	T60.3x4	—	—
Benzin (e) — see Ligroin						
Benziodarone	T46.3x1	T46.3x2	T46.3x3	T46.3x4	T46.3x5	T46.3x6
Benznidazole	T37.3x1	T37.3x2	T37.3x3	T37.3x4	T37.3x5	T37.3x6
Benzocaine	T41.3x1	T41.3x2	T41.3x3	T41.3x4	T41.3x5	T41.3x6
Benzodiapin	T42.4x1	T42.4x2	T42.4x3	T42.4x4	T42.4x5	T42.4x6
Benzodiazepine NEC	T42.4x1	T42.4x2	T42.4x3	T42.4x4	T42.4x5	T42.4x6
Benzoic acid	T49.0x1	T49.0x2	T49.0x3	T49.0x4	T49.0x5	T49.0x6
with salicylic acid	T49.0x1	T49.0x2	T49.0x3	T49.0x4	T49.0x5	T49.0x6
Benzoin (tincture)	T48.5x1	T48.5x2	T48.5x3	T48.5x4	T48.5x5	T48.5x6
Benzol (benzene)	T52.1x1	T52.1x2	T52.1x3	T52.1x4	—	—
vapor	T52.0x1	T52.0x2	T52.0x3	T52.0x4	—	—
Benzomorphan	T40.2x1	T40.2x2	T40.2x3	T40.2x4	T40.2x5	T40.2x6
Benzonatate	T48.3x1	T48.3x2	T48.3x3	T48.3x4	T48.3x5	T48.3x6
Benzophenones	T49.3x1	T49.3x2	T49.3x3	T49.3x4	T49.3x5	T49.3x6
Benzopyrone	T46.991	T46.992	T46.993	T46.994	T46.995	T46.996
Benzothiadiazides	T50.2x1	T50.2x2	T50.2x3	T50.2x4	T50.2x5	T50.2x6
Benzoxonium chloride	T49.0x1	T49.0x2	T49.0x3	T49.0x4	T49.0x5	T49.0x6
Benzoyl peroxide	T49.0x1	T49.0x2	T49.0x3	T49.0x4	T49.0x5	T49.0x6
Benzoylpas calcium	T37.1x1	T37.1x2	T37.1x3	T37.1x4	T37.1x5	T37.1x6
Benzperidin	T43.591	T43.592	T43.593	T43.594	T43.595	T43.596
Benzperidol	T43.591	T43.592	T43.593	T43.594	T43.595	T43.596
Benzphetamine	T50.5x1	T50.5x2	T50.5x3	T50.5x4	T50.5x5	T50.5x6
Benzpyrinium bromide	T44.1x1	T44.1x2	T44.1x3	T44.1x4	T44.1x5	T44.1x6
Benzquinamide	T45.0x1	T45.0x2	T45.0x3	T45.0x4	T45.0x5	T45.0x6
Benzthiazide	T50.2x1	T50.2x2	T50.2x3	T50.2x4	T50.2x5	T50.2x6
Benztropine						
anticholinergic	T44.3x1	T44.3x2	T44.3x3	T44.3x4	T44.3x5	T44.3x6
antiparkinson	T42.8x1	T42.8x2	T42.8x3	T42.8x4	T42.8x5	T42.8x6
Benzydamine	T49.0x1	T49.0x2	T49.0x3	T49.0x4	T49.0x5	T49.0x6

DRUGS&CHEMICALS

Table of Drugs & Chemicals	POISONING Accidental (Unintentional)	Self-Harm (Intentional)	Assault	Undetermined	Adverse Effect	Underdosing
Benzyl						
acetate	T52.8x1	T52.8x2	T52.8x3	T52.8x4	—	—
alcohol	T49.0x1	T49.0x2	T49.0x3	T49.0x4	T49.0x5	T49.0x6
benzoate	T49.0x1	T49.0x2	T49.0x3	T49.0x4	T49.0x5	T49.0x6
Benzoic acid	T49.0x1	T49.0x2	T49.0x3	T49.0x4	T49.0x5	T49.0x6
morphine	T40.2x1	T40.2x2	T40.2x3	T40.2x4		
nicotinate	T46.6x1	T46.6x2	T46.6x3	T46.6x4	T46.6x5	T46.6x6
penicillin	T36.0x1	T36.0x2	T36.0x3	T36.0x4	T36.0x5	T36.0x6
Benzylhydrochlorthia-zide	T50.2x1	T50.2x2	T50.2x3	T50.2x4	T50.2x5	T50.2x6
Benzylpenicillin	T36.0x1	T36.0x2	T36.0x3	T36.0x4	T36.0x5	T36.0x6
Benzylthiouracil	T38.2x1	T38.2x2	T38.2x3	T38.2x4	T38.2x5	T38.2x6
Bephenium hydroxy-naphthoate	T37.4x1	T37.4x2	T37.4x3	T37.4x4	T37.4x5	T37.4x6
Bepridil	T46.1x1	T46.1x2	T46.1x3	T46.1x4	T46.1x5	T46.1x6
Bergamot oil	T65.891	T65.892	T65.893	T65.894		
Bergapten	T50.991	T50.992	T50.993	T50.994	T50.995	T50.996
Berries, poisonous	T62.1x1	T62.1x2	T62.1x3	T62.1x4		
Beryllium (compounds)	T56.7x1	T56.7x2	T56.7x3	T56.7x4	—	—
Beta adrenergic blocking agent, heart	T44.7x1	T44.7x2	T44.7x3	T44.7x4	T44.7x5	T44.7x6
Betacarotene	T45.2x1	T45.2x2	T45.2x3	T45.2x4	T45.2x5	T45.2x6
Beta-Chlor	T42.6x1	T42.6x2	T42.6x3	T42.6x4	T42.6x5	T42.6x6
Betahistine	T46.7x1	T46.7x2	T46.7x3	T46.7x4	T46.7x5	T46.7x6
Betaine	T47.5x1	T47.5x2	T47.5x3	T47.5x4	T47.5x5	T47.5x6
Betamethasone	T49.0x1	T49.0x2	T49.0x3	T49.0x4	T49.0x5	T49.0x6
topical	T49.0x1	T49.0x2	T49.0x3	T49.0x4	T49.0x5	T49.0x6
Betamicin	T36.8x1	T36.8x2	T36.8x3	T36.8x4	T36.8x5	T36.8x6
Betanidine	T46.5x1	T46.5x2	T46.5x3	T46.5x4	T46.5x5	T46.5x6
Betaxolol	T44.7x1	T44.7x2	T44.7x3	T44.7x4	T44.7x5	T44.7x6
Betazole	T50.8x1	T50.8x2	T50.8x3	T50.8x4	T50.8x5	T50.8x6
Bethanechol	T44.1x1	T44.1x2	T44.1x3	T44.1x4	T44.1x5	T44.1x6
chloride	T44.1x1	T44.1x2	T44.1x3	T44.1x4	T44.1x5	T44.1x6
Bethanidine	T46.5x1	T46.5x2	T46.5x3	T46.5x4	T46.5x5	T46.5x6
Betoxycaine	T41.3x1	T41.3x2	T41.3x3	T41.3x4	T41.3x5	T41.3x6
Betula oil	T49.3x1	T49.3x2	T49.3x3	T49.3x4	T49.3x5	T49.3x6
b-eucaine	T49.1x1	T49.1x2	T49.1x3	T49.1x4	T49.1x5	T49.1x6
Bevantolol	T44.7x1	T44.7x2	T44.7x3	T44.7x4	T44.7x5	T44.7x6
Bevonium metilsulfate	T44.3x1	T44.3x2	T44.3x3	T44.3x4	T44.3x5	T44.3x6
Bezafibrate	T46.6x1	T46.6x2	T46.6x3	T46.6x4	T46.6x5	T46.6x6
Bezitramide	T40.4x1	T40.4x2	T40.4x3	T40.4x4	T40.4x5	T40.4x6
b-galactosidase	T47.5x1	T47.5x2	T47.5x3	T47.5x4	T47.5x5	T47.5x6
BHA	T50.991	T50.992	T50.993	T50.994	T50.995	T50.996
Bhang	T40.7x1	T40.7x2	T40.7x3	T40.7x4	T40.7x5	T40.7x6
BHC (medicinal)	T49.0x1	T49.0x2	T49.0x3	T49.0x4	T49.0x5	T49.0x6
nonmedicinal (vapor)	T53.6x1	T53.6x2	T53.6x3	T53.6x4	—	—
Bialamicol	T37.3x1	T37.3x2	T37.3x3	T37.3x4	T37.3x5	T37.3x6
Bibenzonium bromide	T48.3x1	T48.3x2	T48.3x3	T48.3x4	T48.3x5	T48.3x6
Bibrocathol	T49.5x1	T49.5x2	T49.5x3	T49.5x4	T49.5x5	T49.5x6
Bichloride of mercury — see Mercury, chloride						
Bichromates (calcium) (potassium) (sodium) (crystals)	T57.8x1	T57.8x2	T57.8x3	T57.8x4	—	—
fumes	T56.2x1	T56.2x2	T56.2x3	T56.2x4	—	—
Biclotymol	T49.6x1	T49.6x2	T49.6x3	T49.6x4	T49.6x5	T49.6x6
Bicuculline	T50.7x1	T50.7x2	T50.7x3	T50.7x4	T50.7x5	T50.7x6
Bifemelane	T43.291	T43.292	T43.293	T43.294	T43.295	T43.296
Biguanide derivatives, oral	T38.3x1	T38.3x2	T38.3x3	T38.3x4	T38.3x5	T38.3x6
Bile salts	T47.5x1	T47.5x2	T47.5x3	T47.5x4	T47.5x5	T47.5x6
Biligrafin	T50.8x1	T50.8x2	T50.8x3	T50.8x4	T50.8x5	T50.8x6
Bilopaque	T50.8x1	T50.8x2	T50.8x3	T50.8x4	T50.8x5	T50.8x6
Binifibrate	T46.6x1	T46.6x2	T46.6x3	T46.6x4	T46.6x5	T46.6x6
Binitrobenzol	T65.3x1	T65.3x2	T65.3x3	T65.3x4	—	—
Bioflavonoid(s)	T46.991	T46.992	T46.993	T46.994	T46.995	T46.996
Biological substance NEC	T50.901	T50.902	T50.903	T50.904	T50.905	T50.906
Biotin	T45.2x1	T45.2x2	T45.2x3	T45.2x4	T45.2x5	T45.2x6
Biperiden	T44.3x1	T44.3x2	T44.3x3	T44.3x4	T44.3x5	T44.3x6
Bisacodyl	T47.2x1	T47.2x2	T47.2x3	T47.2x4	T47.2x5	T47.2x6
Bisbentiamine	T45.2x1	T45.2x2	T45.2x3	T45.2x4	T45.2x5	T45.2x6
Bisbutiamine	T45.2x1	T45.2x2	T45.2x3	T45.2x4	T45.2x5	T45.2x6
Bisdequalinium (salts) (diacetate)	T49.6x1	T49.6x2	T49.6x3	T49.6x4	T49.6x5	T49.6x6

Table of Drugs & Chemicals	POISONING Accidental (Unintentional)	Self-Harm (Intentional)	Assault	Undetermined	Adverse Effect	Underdosing
Bishydroxycoumarin	T45.511	T45.512	T45.513	T45.514	T45.515	T45.516
Bismarsen	T37.8x1	T37.8x2	T37.8x3	T37.8x4	T37.8x5	T37.8x6
Bismuth salts	T47.6x1	T47.6x2	T47.6x3	T47.6x4	T47.6x5	T47.6x6
aluminate	T47.1x1	T47.1x2	T47.1x3	T47.1x4	T47.1x5	T47.1x6
anti-infectives	T37.8x1	T37.8x2	T37.8x3	T37.8x4	T37.8x5	T37.8x6
formic iodide	T49.0x1	T49.0x2	T49.0x3	T49.0x4	T49.0x5	T49.0x6
glycolylarsenate	T49.0x1	T49.0x2	T49.0x3	T49.0x4	T49.0x5	T49.0x6
nonmedicinal (compounds) NEC	T65.91	T65.92	T65.93	T65.94	—	—
subcarbonate	T47.6x1	T47.6x2	T47.6x3	T47.6x4	T47.6x5	T47.6x6
subsalicylate	T37.8x1	T37.8x2	T37.8x3	T37.8x4	T37.8x5	T37.8x6
sulfarsphenamine	T37.8x1	T37.8x2	T37.8x3	T37.8x4	T37.8x5	T37.8x6
Bisoprolol	T44.7x1	T44.7x2	T44.7x3	T44.7x4	T44.7x5	T44.7x6
Bisoxatin	T47.2x1	T47.2x2	T47.2x3	T47.2x4	T47.2x5	T47.2x6
Bisulepin (hydrochloride)	T45.0x1	T45.0x2	T45.0x3	T45.0x4	T45.0x5	T45.0x6
Bithionol	T37.8x1	T37.8x2	T37.8x3	T37.8x4	T37.8x5	T37.8x6
anthelminthic	T37.4x1	T37.4x2	T37.4x3	T37.4x4	T37.4x5	T37.4x6
Bitolterol	T48.6x1	T48.6x2	T48.6x3	T48.6x4	T48.6x5	T48.6x6
Bitoscanate	T37.4x1	T37.4x2	T37.4x3	T37.4x4	T37.4x5	T37.4x6
Bitter almond oil	T62.8x1	T62.8x2	T62.8x3	T62.8x4	—	—
Bittersweet	T62.2x1	T62.2x2	T62.2x3	T62.2x4	—	—
Black						
flag	T60.91	T60.92	T60.93	T60.94	—	—
henbane	T62.2x1	T62.2x2	T62.2x3	T62.2x4	—	—
leaf (40)	T60.91	T60.92	T60.93	T60.94	—	—
widow spider (bite)	T63.311	T63.312	T63.313	T63.314	—	—
antivenin	T50.Z11	T50.Z12	T50.Z13	T50.Z14	T50.Z15	T50.Z16
Blast furnace gas (carbon monoxide from)	T58.8x1	T58.8x2	T58.8x3	T58.8x4		
Bleach	T54.91	T54.92	T54.93	T54.94	—	—
Bleaching agent (medicinal)	T49.4x1	T49.4x2	T49.4x3	T49.4x4	T49.4x5	T49.4x6
Bleomycin	T45.1x1	T45.1x2	T45.1x3	T45.1x4	T45.1x5	T45.1x6
Blockain	T41.3x1	T41.3x2	T41.3x3	T41.3x4	T41.3x5	T41.3x6
infiltration (subcutaneous)	T41.3x1	T41.3x2	T41.3x3	T41.3x4	T41.3x5	T41.3x6
nerve block (peripheral) (plexus)	T41.3x1	T41.3x2	T41.3x3	T41.3x4	T41.3x5	T41.3x6
topical (surface)	T41.3x1	T41.3x2	T41.3x3	T41.3x4	T41.3x5	T41.3x6
Blockers, calcium channel	T46.1x1	T46.1x2	T46.1x3	T46.1x4	T46.1x5	T46.1x6
Blood (derivatives) (natural) (plasma) (whole)	T45.8x1	T45.8x2	T45.8x3	T45.8x4	T45.8x5	T45.8x6
dried	T45.8x1	T45.8x2	T45.8x3	T45.8x4	T45.8x5	T45.8x6
drug affecting NEC	T45.91	T45.92	T45.93	T45.94	T45.95	T45.96
expander NEC	T45.8x1	T45.8x2	T45.8x3	T45.8x4	T45.8x5	T45.8x6
fraction NEC	T45.8x1	T45.8x2	T45.8x3	T45.8x4	T45.8x5	T45.8x6
substitute (macromolecular)	T45.8x1	T45.8x2	T45.8x3	T45.8x4	T45.8x5	T45.8x6
Blue velvet	T40.2x1	T40.2x2	T40.2x3	T40.2x4	—	—
Bone meal	T62.8x1	T62.8x2	T62.8x3	T62.8x4	—	—
Bonine	T45.0x1	T45.0x2	T45.0x3	T45.0x4	T45.0x5	T45.0x6
Bopindolol	T44.7x1	T44.7x2	T44.7x3	T44.7x4	T44.7x5	T44.7x6
Boracic acid	T49.0x1	T49.0x2	T49.0x3	T49.0x4	T49.0x5	T49.0x6
ENT agent	T49.6x1	T49.6x2	T49.6x3	T49.6x4	T49.6x5	T49.6x6
ophthalmic preparation	T49.5x1	T49.5x2	T49.5x3	T49.5x4	T49.5x5	T49.5x6
Borane complex	T57.8x1	T57.8x2	T57.8x3	T57.8x4	—	—
Borate (s)	T57.8x1	T57.8x2	T57.8x3	T57.8x4	—	—
buffer	T50.991	T50.992	T50.993	T50.994	T50.995	T50.996
cleanser	T54.91	T54.92	T54.93	T54.94		
sodium	T57.8x1	T57.8x2	T57.8x3	T57.8x4		
Borax (cleanser)	T54.91	T54.92	T54.93	T54.94		
Bordeaux mixture	T60.3x1	T60.3x2	T60.3x3	T60.3x4	—	
Boric acid	T49.0x1	T49.0x2	T49.0x3	T49.0x4	T49.0x5	T49.0x6
ENT agent	T49.6x1	T49.6x2	T49.6x3	T49.6x4	T49.6x5	T49.6x6
ophthalmic preparation	T49.5x1	T49.5x2	T49.5x3	T49.5x4	T49.5x5	T49.5x6
Bornaprine	T44.3x1	T44.3x2	T44.3x3	T44.3x4	T44.3x5	T44.3x6
Boron	T57.8x1	T57.8x2	T57.8x3	T57.8x4	—	—
hydride NEC	T57.8x1	T57.8x2	T57.8x3	T57.8x4	—	
fumes or gas	T57.8x1	T57.8x2	T57.8x3	T57.8x4	—	—
trifluoride	T59.891	T59.892	T59.893	T59.894	—	
Botox	T48.291	T48.292	T48.293	T48.294	T48.295	T48.296
Botulinus anti-toxin (type A, B)	T50.Z11	T50.Z12	T50.Z13	T50.Z14	T50.Z15	T50.Z16
Brake fluid vapor	T59.891	T59.892	T59.893	T59.894	—	—
Brallobarbital	T42.3x1	T42.3x2	T42.3x3	T42.3x4	T42.3x5	T42.3x6

Table of Drugs & Chemicals	Accidental (Unintentional)	Self-Harm (Intentional)	Assault	Undetermined	Adverse Effect	Underdosing
Bran (wheat)	T47.4x1	T47.4x2	T47.4x3	T47.4x4	T47.4x5	T47.4x6
Brass (fumes)	T56.891	T56.892	T56.893	T56.894	—	—
Brasso	T52.0x1	T52.0x2	T52.0x3	T52.0x4	—	—
Bretylium tosilate	T46.2x1	T46.2x2	T46.2x3	T46.2x4	T46.2x5	T46.2x6
Brevital (sodium)	T41.1x1	T41.1x2	T41.1x3	T41.1x4	T41.1x5	T41.1x6
Brinase	T45.3x1	T45.3x2	T45.3x3	T45.3x4	T45.3x5	T45.3x6
British antilewisite	T45.8x1	T45.8x2	T45.8x3	T45.8x4	T45.8x5	T45.8x6
Brodifacoum	T60.4x1	T60.4x2	T60.4x3	T60.4x4	—	—
Bromal (hydrate)	T42.6x1	T42.6x2	T42.6x3	T42.6x4	T42.6x5	T42.6x6
Bromazepam	T42.4x1	T42.4x2	T42.4x3	T42.4x4	T42.4x5	T42.4x6
Bromazine	T45.0x1	T45.0x2	T45.0x3	T45.0x4	T45.0x5	T45.0x6
Brombenzylcyanide	T59.3x1	T59.3x2	T59.3x3	T59.3x4	—	—
Bromelains	T45.3x1	T45.3x2	T45.3x3	T45.3x4	T45.3x5	T45.3x6
Bromethalin	T60.4x1	T60.4x2	T60.4x3	T60.4x4	—	—
Bromhexine	T48.4x1	T48.4x2	T48.4x3	T48.4x4	T48.4x5	T48.4x6
Bromide salts	T42.6x1	T42.6x2	T42.6x3	T42.6x4	T42.6x5	T42.6x6
Bromindione	T45.511	T45.512	T45.513	T45.514	T45.515	T45.516
Bromine compounds (medicinal)	T42.6x1	T42.6x2	T42.6x3	T42.6x4	T42.6x5	T42.6x6
sedative	T42.6x1	T42.6x2	T42.6x3	T42.6x4	T42.6x5	T42.6x6
vapor	T59.891	T59.892	T59.893	T59.894	—	—
Bromisoval	T42.6x1	T42.6x2	T42.6x3	T42.6x4	T42.6x5	T42.6x6
Bromisovalum	T42.6x1	T42.6x2	T42.6x3	T42.6x4	T42.6x5	T42.6x6
Bromobenzylcyanide	T59.3x1	T59.3x2	T59.3x3	T59.3x4	—	—
Bromochlorosalicylani-lide	T49.0x1	T49.0x2	T49.0x3	T49.0x4	T49.0x5	T49.0x6
Bromocriptine	T42.8x1	T42.8x2	T42.8x3	T42.8x4	T42.8x5	T42.8x6
Bromodiphenhydramine	T45.0x1	T45.0x2	T45.0x3	T45.0x4	T45.0x5	T45.0x6
Bromoform	T42.6x1	T42.6x2	T42.6x3	T42.6x4	T42.6x5	T42.6x6
Bromophenol blue reagent	T50.991	T50.992	T50.993	T50.994	T50.995	T50.996
Bromopride	T47.8x1	T47.8x2	T47.8x3	T47.8x4	T47.8x5	T47.8x6
Bromosalicylchloranitide	T49.0x1	T49.0x2	T49.0x3	T49.0x4	T49.0x5	T49.0x6
Bromosalicylhydroxamic acid	T37.1x1	T37.1x2	T37.1x3	T37.1x4	T37.1x5	T37.1x6
Bromo-seltzer	T39.1x1	T39.1x2	T39.1x3	T39.1x4	T39.1x5	T39.1x6
Bromoxynil	T60.3x1	T60.3x2	T60.3x3	T60.3x4	—	—
Bromperidol	T43.4x1	T43.4x2	T43.4x3	T43.4x4	T43.4x5	T43.4x6
Brompheniramine	T45.0x1	T45.0x2	T45.0x3	T45.0x4	T45.0x5	T45.0x6
Bromsulfophthalein	T50.8x1	T50.8x2	T50.8x3	T50.8x4	T50.8x5	T50.8x6
Bromural	T42.6x1	T42.6x2	T42.6x3	T42.6x4	T42.6x5	T42.6x6
Bromvaletone	T42.6x1	T42.6x2	T42.6x3	T42.6x4	T42.6x5	T42.6x6
Bronchodilator NEC	T48.6x1	T48.6x2	T48.6x3	T48.6x4	T48.6x5	T48.6x6
Brotizolam	T42.4x1	T42.4x2	T42.4x3	T42.4x4	T42.4x5	T42.4x6
Brovincamine	T46.7x1	T46.7x2	T46.7x3	T46.7x4	T46.7x5	T46.7x6
Brown recluse spider (bite) (venom)	T63.331	T63.332	T63.333	T63.334	—	—
Brown spider (bite) (venom)	T63.391	T63.392	T63.393	T63.394	—	—
Broxaterol	T48.6x1	T48.6x2	T48.6x3	T48.6x4	T48.6x5	T48.6x6
Broxuridine	T45.1x1	T45.1x2	T45.1x3	T45.1x4	T45.1x5	T45.1x6
Broxyquinoline	T37.8x1	T37.8x2	T37.8x3	T37.8x4	T37.8x5	T37.8x6
Bruceine	T48.291	T48.292	T48.293	T48.294	T48.295	T48.296
Brucia	T62.2x1	T62.2x2	T62.2x3	T62.2x4	—	—
Brucine	T65.1x1	T65.1x2	T65.1x3	T65.1x4	—	—
Brunswick green — see Copper						
Bruten — see Ibuprofen						
Bryonia	T47.2x1	T47.2x2	T47.2x3	T47.2x4	T47.2x5	T47.2x6
b-sitosterol(s)	T46.6x1	T46.6x2	T46.6x3	T46.6x4	T46.6x5	T46.6x6
Buclizine	T45.0x1	T45.0x2	T45.0x3	T45.0x4	T45.0x5	T45.0x6
Buclosamide	T49.0x1	T49.0x2	T49.0x3	T49.0x4	T49.0x5	T49.0x6
Budesonide	T44.5x1	T44.5x2	T44.5x3	T44.5x4	T44.5x5	T44.5x6
Budralazine	T46.5x1	T46.5x2	T46.5x3	T46.5x4	T46.5x5	T46.5x6
Bufferin	T39.011	T39.012	T39.013	T39.014	T39.015	T39.016
Buflomedil	T46.7x1	T46.7x2	T46.7x3	T46.7x4	T46.7x5	T46.7x6
Buformin	T38.3x1	T38.3x2	T38.3x3	T38.3x4	T38.3x5	T38.3x6
Bufotenine	T40.991	T40.992	T40.993	T40.994	—	—
Bufrolin	T48.6x1	T48.6x2	T48.6x3	T48.6x4	T48.6x5	T48.6x6
Bufylline	T48.6x1	T48.6x2	T48.6x3	T48.6x4	T48.6x5	T48.6x6
Bulk filler	T50.5x1	T50.5x2	T50.5x3	T50.5x4	T50.5x5	T50.5x6
cathartic	T47.4x1	T47.4x2	T47.4x3	T47.4x4	T47.4x5	T47.4x6
Bumetanide	T50.1x1	T50.1x2	T50.1x3	T50.1x4	T50.1x5	T50.1x6
Bunaftine	T46.2x1	T46.2x2	T46.2x3	T46.2x4	T46.2x5	T46.2x6
Bunamiodyl	T50.8x1	T50.8x2	T50.8x3	T50.8x4	T50.8x5	T50.8x6
Bunazosin	T44.6x1	T44.6x2	T44.6x3	T44.6x4	T44.6x5	T44.6x6
Bunitrolol	T44.7x1	T44.7x2	T44.7x3	T44.7x4	T44.7x5	T44.7x6
Buphenine	T46.7x1	T46.7x2	T46.7x3	T46.7x4	T46.7x5	T46.7x6
Bupivacaine	T41.3x1	T41.3x2	T41.3x3	T41.3x4	T41.3x5	T41.3x6
infiltration (subcutaneous)	T41.3x1	T41.3x2	T41.3x3	T41.3x4	T41.3x5	T41.3x6
nerve block (peripheral) (plexus)	T41.3x1	T41.3x2	T41.3x3	T41.3x4	T41.3x5	T41.3x6
spinal	T41.3x1	T41.3x2	T41.3x3	T41.3x4	T41.3x5	T41.3x6
Bupranolol	T44.7x1	T44.7x2	T44.7x3	T44.7x4	T44.7x5	T44.7x6
Buprenorphine	T40.4x1	T40.4x2	T40.4x3	T40.4x4	T40.4x5	T40.4x6
Bupropion	T43.291	T43.292	T43.293	T43.294	T43.295	T43.296
Burimamide	T47.1x1	T47.1x2	T47.1x3	T47.1x4	T47.1x5	T47.1x6
Buserelin	T38.891	T38.892	T38.893	T38.894	T38.895	T38.896
Buspirone	T43.591	T43.592	T43.593	T43.594	T43.595	T43.596
Busulfan, busulphan	T45.1x1	T45.1x2	T45.1x3	T45.1x4	T45.1x5	T45.1x6
Butabarbital (sodium)	T42.3x1	T42.3x2	T42.3x3	T42.3x4	T42.3x5	T42.3x6
Butabarbitone	T42.3x1	T42.3x2	T42.3x3	T42.3x4	T42.3x5	T42.3x6
Butabarpal	T42.3x1	T42.3x2	T42.3x3	T42.3x4	T42.3x5	T42.3x6
Butacaine	T41.3x1	T41.3x2	T41.3x3	T41.3x4	T41.3x5	T41.3x6
Butalamine	T46.7x1	T46.7x2	T46.7x3	T46.7x4	T46.7x5	T46.7x6
Butalbital	T42.3x1	T42.3x2	T42.3x3	T42.3x4	T42.3x5	T42.3x6
Butallylonal	T42.3x1	T42.3x2	T42.3x3	T42.3x4	T42.3x5	T42.3x6
Butamben	T41.3x1	T41.3x2	T41.3x3	T41.3x4	T41.3x5	T41.3x6
Butamirate	T48.3x1	T48.3x2	T48.3x3	T48.3x4	T48.3x5	T48.3x6
Butane (distributed in mobile container)	T59.891	T59.892	T59.893	T59.894	—	—
distributed through pipes	T59.891	T59.892	T59.893	T59.894	—	—
incomplete combustion	T58.11	T58.12	T58.13	T58.14	—	—
Butanilicaine	T41.3x1	T41.3x2	T41.3x3	T41.3x4	T41.3x5	T41.3x6
Butanol	T51.3x1	T51.3x2	T51.3x3	T51.3x4	—	—
Butanone, 2-butanone	T52.4x1	T52.4x2	T52.4x3	T52.4x4	—	—
Butantrone	T49.4x1	T49.4x2	T49.4x3	T49.4x4	T49.4x5	T49.4x6
Butaperazine	T43.3x1	T43.3x2	T43.3x3	T43.3x4	T43.3x5	T43.3x6
Butazolidin	T39.2x1	T39.2x2	T39.2x3	T39.2x4	T39.2x5	T39.2x6
Butetamate	T48.6x1	T48.6x2	T48.6x3	T48.6x4	T48.6x5	T48.6x6
Butethal	T42.3x1	T42.3x2	T42.3x3	T42.3x4	T42.3x5	T42.3x6
Butethamate	T44.3x1	T44.3x2	T44.3x3	T44.3x4	T44.3x5	T44.3x6
Buthalitone (sodium)	T41.1x1	T41.1x2	T41.1x3	T41.1x4	T41.1x5	T41.1x6
Butisol (sodium)	T42.3x1	T42.3x2	T42.3x3	T42.3x4	T42.3x5	T42.3x6
Butizide	T50.2x1	T50.2x2	T50.2x3	T50.2x4	T50.2x5	T50.2x6
Butobarbital	T42.3x1	T42.3x2	T42.3x3	T42.3x4	T42.3x5	T42.3x6
sodium	T42.3x1	T42.3x2	T42.3x3	T42.3x4	T42.3x5	T42.3x6
Butobarbitone	T42.3x1	T42.3x2	T42.3x3	T42.3x4	T42.3x5	T42.3x6
Butoconazole (nitrate)	T49.0x1	T49.0x2	T49.0x3	T49.0x4	T49.0x5	T49.0x6
Butorphanol	T40.4x1	T40.4x2	T40.4x3	T40.4x4	T40.4x5	T40.4x6
Butriptyline	T43.011	T43.012	T43.013	T43.014	T43.015	T43.016
Butropium bromide	T44.3x1	T44.3x2	T44.3x3	T44.3x4	T44.3x5	T44.3x6
Butter of antimony — see Antimony						
Buttercups	T62.2x1	T62.2x2	T62.2x3	T62.2x4	—	—
Butyl acetate (secondary)	T52.8x1	T52.8x2	T52.8x3	T52.8x4	—	—
alcohol	T51.3x1	T51.3x2	T51.3x3	T51.3x4	—	—
aminobenzoate	T41.3x1	T41.3x2	T41.3x3	T41.3x4	T41.3x5	T41.3x6
butyrate	T52.8x1	T52.8x2	T52.8x3	T52.8x4	—	—
carbinol	T51.3x1	T51.3x2	T51.3x3	T51.3x4	—	—
carbitol	T52.3x1	T52.3x2	T52.3x3	T52.3x4	—	—
cellosolve	T52.3x1	T52.3x2	T52.3x3	T52.3x4	—	—
chloral (hydrate)	T42.6x1	T42.6x2	T42.6x3	T42.6x4	T42.6x5	T42.6x6
formate	T52.8x1	T52.8x2	T52.8x3	T52.8x4	—	—
lactate	T52.8x1	T52.8x2	T52.8x3	T52.8x4	—	—
propionate	T52.8x1	T52.8x2	T52.8x3	T52.8x4	—	—
scopolamine bromide	T44.3x1	T44.3x2	T44.3x3	T44.3x4	T44.3x5	T44.3x6
thiobarbital sodium	T41.1x1	T41.1x2	T41.1x3	T41.1x4	T41.1x5	T41.1x6
Butylated hydroxy-anisole	T50.991	T50.992	T50.993	T50.994	T50.995	T50.996
Butylchloral hydrate	T42.6x1	T42.6x2	T42.6x3	T42.6x4	T42.6x5	T42.6x6
Butyltoluene	T52.2x1	T52.2x2	T52.2x3	T52.2x4	—	—
Butyn	T41.3x1	T41.3x2	T41.3x3	T41.3x4	T41.3x5	T41.3x6
Butyrophenone (-based tranquilizers)	T43.4x1	T43.4x2	T43.4x3	T43.4x4	T43.4x5	T43.4x6

DRUGS&CHEMICALS

Table of Drugs & Chemicals	Poisoning Accidental (Unintentional)	Self-Harm (Intentional)	Assault	Undetermined	Adverse Effect	Underdosing
Cabergoline	T42.8x1	T42.8x2	T42.8x3	T42.8x4	T42.8x5	T42.8x6
Cacodyl, cacodylic acid	T57.0x1	T57.0x2	T57.0x3	T57.0x4	—	—
Cactinomycin	T45.1x1	T45.1x2	T45.1x3	T45.1x4	T45.1x5	T45.1x6
Cade oil	T49.4x1	T49.4x2	T49.4x3	T49.4x4	T49.4x5	T49.4x6
Cadexomer iodine	T49.0x1	T49.0x2	T49.0x3	T49.0x4	T49.0x5	T49.0x6
Cadmium (chloride) (fumes) (oxide)	T56.3x1	T56.3x2	T56.3x3	T56.3x4	—	—
sulfide (medicinal) NEC	T49.4x1	T49.4x2	T49.4x3	T49.4x4	T49.4x5	T49.4x6
Cadralazine	T46.5x1	T46.5x2	T46.5x3	T46.5x4	T46.5x5	T46.5x6
Caffeine	T43.611	T43.612	T43.613	T43.614	T43.615	T43.616
Calabar bean	T62.2x1	T62.2x2	T62.2x3	T62.2x4	—	—
Caladium seguinum	T62.2x1	T62.2x2	T62.2x3	T62.2x4	—	—
Calamine (lotion)	T49.3x1	T49.3x2	T49.3x3	T49.3x4	T49.3x5	T49.3x6
Calcifediol	T45.2x1	T45.2x2	T45.2x3	T45.2x4	T45.2x5	T45.2x6
Calciferol	T45.2x1	T45.2x2	T45.2x3	T45.2x4	T45.2x5	T45.2x6
Calcitonin	T50.991	T50.992	T50.993	T50.994	T50.995	T50.996
Calcitriol	T45.2x1	T45.2x2	T45.2x3	T45.2x4	T45.2x5	T45.2x6
Calcium	T50.3x1	T50.3x2	T50.3x3	T50.3x4	T50.3x5	T50.3x6
actylsalicylate	T39.011	T39.012	T39.013	T39.014	T39.015	T39.016
benzamidosalicylate	T37.1x1	T37.1x2	T37.1x3	T37.1x4	T37.1x5	T37.1x6
bromide	T42.6x1	T42.6x2	T42.6x3	T42.6x4	T42.6x5	T42.6x6
bromolactobionate	T42.6x1	T42.6x2	T42.6x3	T42.6x4	T42.6x5	T42.6x6
carbaspirin	T39.011	T39.012	T39.013	T39.014	T39.015	T39.016
carbimide	T50.6x1	T50.6x2	T50.6x3	T50.6x4	T50.6x5	T50.6x6
carbonate	T47.1x1	T47.1x2	T47.1x3	T47.1x4	T47.1x5	T47.1x6
chloride	T50.991	T50.992	T50.993	T50.994	T50.995	T50.996
anhydrous	T50.991	T50.992	T50.993	T50.994	T50.995	T50.996
cyanide	T57.8x1	T57.8x2	T57.8x3	T57.8x4	—	—
dioctyl sulfosuccinate	T47.4x1	T47.4x2	T47.4x3	T47.4x4	T47.4x5	T47.4x6
disodium edathamil	T45.8x1	T45.8x2	T45.8x3	T45.8x4	T45.8x5	T45.8x6
disodium edetate	T45.8x1	T45.8x2	T45.8x3	T45.8x4	T45.8x5	T45.8x6
dobesilate	T46.991	T46.992	T46.993	T46.994	T46.995	T46.996
EDTA	T45.8x1	T45.8x2	T45.8x3	T45.8x4	T45.8x5	T45.8x6
ferrous citrate	T45.4x1	T45.4x2	T45.4x3	T45.4x4	T45.4x5	T45.4x6
folinate	T45.8x1	T45.8x2	T45.8x3	T45.8x4	T45.8x5	T45.8x6
glubionate	T50.3x1	T50.3x2	T50.3x3	T50.3x4	T50.3x5	T50.3x6
gluconate	T50.3x1	T50.3x2	T50.3x3	T50.3x4	T50.3x5	T50.3x6
gluconogalactogluc-onate	T50.3x1	T50.3x2	T50.3x3	T50.3x4	T50.3x5	T50.3x6
hydrate, hydroxide	T54.3x1	T54.3x2	T54.3x3	T54.3x4	—	—
hypochlorite	T54.3x1	T54.3x2	T54.3x3	T54.3x4	—	—
iodide	T48.4x1	T48.4x2	T48.4x3	T48.4x4	T48.4x5	T48.4x6
ipodate	T50.8x1	T50.8x2	T50.8x3	T50.8x4	T50.8x5	T50.8x6
lactate	T50.3x1	T50.3x2	T50.3x3	T50.3x4	T50.3x5	T50.3x6
leucovorin	T45.8x1	T45.8x2	T45.8x3	T45.8x4	T45.8x5	T45.8x6
mandelate	T37.91	T37.92	T37.93	T37.94	T37.95	T37.96
oxide	T54.3x1	T54.3x2	T54.3x3	T54.3x4	—	—
pantothenate	T45.2x1	T45.2x2	T45.2x3	T45.2x4	T45.2x5	T45.2x6
phosphate	T50.3x1	T50.3x2	T50.3x3	T50.3x4	T50.3x5	T50.3x6
salicylate	T39.091	T39.092	T39.093	T39.094	T39.095	T39.096
salts	T50.3x1	T50.3x2	T50.3x3	T50.3x4	T50.3x5	T50.3x6
Calculus-dissolving drug	T50.991	T50.992	T50.993	T50.994	T50.995	T50.996
Calomel	T49.0x1	T49.0x2	T49.0x3	T49.0x4	T49.0x5	T49.0x6
Caloric agent	T50.3x1	T50.3x2	T50.3x3	T50.3x4	T50.3x5	T50.3x6
Calusterone	T38.7x1	T38.7x2	T38.7x3	T38.7x4	T38.7x5	T38.7x6
Camazepam	T42.4x1	T42.4x2	T42.4x3	T42.4x4	T42.4x5	T42.4x6
Camomile	T49.0x1	T49.0x2	T49.0x3	T49.0x4	T49.0x5	T49.0x6
Camoquin	T37.2x1	T37.2x2	T37.2x3	T37.2x4	T37.2x5	T37.2x6
Camphor insecticide	T60.2x1	T60.2x2	T60.2x3	T60.2x4	—	—
medicinal	T49.8x1	T49.8x2	T49.8x3	T49.8x4	T49.8x5	T49.8x6
Camylofin	T44.3x1	T44.3x2	T44.3x3	T44.3x4	T44.3x5	T44.3x6
Cancer chemotherapy drug regimen	T45.1x1	T45.1x2	T45.1x3	T45.1x4	T45.1x5	T45.1x6
Candeptin	T49.0x1	T49.0x2	T49.0x3	T49.0x4	T49.0x5	T49.0x6
Candicidin	T49.0x1	T49.0x2	T49.0x3	T49.0x4	T49.0x5	T49.0x6
Cannabinol	T40.7x1	T40.7x2	T40.7x3	T40.7x4	T40.7x5	T40.7x6
Cannabis (derivatives)	T40.7x1	T40.7x2	T40.7x3	T40.7x4	T40.7x5	T40.7x6
Canned heat	T51.1x1	T51.1x2	T51.1x3	T51.1x4	—	—
Canrenoic acid	T50.0x1	T50.0x2	T50.0x3	T50.0x4	T50.0x5	T50.0x6
Canrenone	T50.0x1	T50.0x2	T50.0x3	T50.0x4	T50.0x5	T50.0x6
Cantharides, cantharidin, cantharis	T49.8x1	T49.8x2	T49.8x3	T49.8x4	T49.8x5	T49.8x6
Canthaxanthin	T50.991	T50.992	T50.993	T50.994	T50.995	T50.996
Capillary-active drug NEC	T46.901	T46.902	T46.903	T46.904	T46.905	T46.906
Capreomycin	T36.8x1	T36.8x2	T36.8x3	T36.8x4	T36.8x5	T36.8x6
Capsicum	T49.4x1	T49.4x2	T49.4x3	T49.4x4	T49.4x5	T49.4x6
Captafol	T60.3x1	T60.3x2	T60.3x3	T60.3x4	—	—
Captan	T60.3x1	T60.3x2	T60.3x3	T60.3x4	—	—
Captodiame, captodiamine	T43.591	T43.592	T43.593	T43.594	T43.595	T43.596
Captopril	T46.4x1	T46.4x2	T46.4x3	T46.4x4	T46.4x5	T46.4x6
Caramiphen	T44.3x1	T44.3x2	T44.3x3	T44.3x4	T44.3x5	T44.3x6
Carazolol	T44.7x1	T44.7x2	T44.7x3	T44.7x4	T44.7x5	T44.7x6
Carbachol	T44.1x1	T44.1x2	T44.1x3	T44.1x4	T44.1x5	T44.1x6
Carbacrylamine (resin)	T50.3x1	T50.3x2	T50.3x3	T50.3x4	T50.3x5	T50.3x6
Carbamate (insecticide)	T60.0x1	T60.0x2	T60.0x3	T60.0x4	—	—
Carbamate (sedative)	T42.6x1	T42.6x2	T42.6x3	T42.6x4	T42.6x5	T42.6x6
herbicide	T60.0x1	T60.0x2	T60.0x3	T60.0x4	—	—
insecticide	T60.0x1	T60.0x2	T60.0x3	T60.0x4	—	—
Carbamazepine	T42.1x1	T42.1x2	T42.1x3	T42.1x4	T42.1x5	T42.1x6
Carbamide	T47.3x1	T47.3x2	T47.3x3	T47.3x4	T47.3x5	T47.3x6
peroxide	T49.0x1	T49.0x2	T49.0x3	T49.0x4	T49.0x5	T49.0x6
topical	T49.8x1	T49.8x2	T49.8x3	T49.8x4	T49.8x5	T49.8x6
Carbamylcholine chloride	T44.1x1	T44.1x2	T44.1x3	T44.1x4	T44.1x5	T44.1x6
Carbaril	T60.0x1	T60.0x2	T60.0x3	T60.0x4	—	—
Carbarsone	T37.3x1	T37.3x2	T37.3x3	T37.3x4	T37.3x5	T37.3x6
Carbaryl	T60.0x1	T60.0x2	T60.0x3	T60.0x4	—	—
Carbaspirin	T39.011	T39.012	T39.013	T39.014	T39.015	T39.016
Carbazochrome (salicylate) (sodium sulfonate)	T49.4x1	T49.4x2	T49.4x3	T49.4x4	T49.4x5	T49.4x6
Carbenicillin	T36.0x1	T36.0x2	T36.0x3	T36.0x4	T36.0x5	T36.0x6
Carbenoxolone	T47.1x1	T47.1x2	T47.1x3	T47.1x4	T47.1x5	T47.1x6
Carbetapentane	T48.3x1	T48.3x2	T48.3x3	T48.3x4	T48.3x5	T48.3x6
Carbethyl salicylate	T39.091	T39.092	T39.093	T39.094	T39.095	T39.096
Carbidopa (with levodopa)	T42.8x1	T42.8x2	T42.8x3	T42.8x4	T42.8x5	T42.8x6
Carbimazole	T38.2x1	T38.2x2	T38.2x3	T38.2x4	T38.2x5	T38.2x6
Carbinol	T51.1x1	T51.1x2	T51.1x3	T51.1x4	—	—
Carbinoxamine	T45.0x1	T45.0x2	T45.0x3	T45.0x4	T45.0x5	T45.0x6
Carbiphene	T39.8x1	T39.8x2	T39.8x3	T39.8x4	T39.8x5	T39.8x6
Carbitol	T52.3x1	T52.3x2	T52.3x3	T52.3x4	—	—
Carbo medicinalis	T47.6x1	T47.6x2	T47.6x3	T47.6x4	T47.6x5	T47.6x6
Carbocaine	T41.3x1	T41.3x2	T41.3x3	T41.3x4	T41.3x5	T41.3x6
infiltration (subcutaneous)	T41.3x1	T41.3x2	T41.3x3	T41.3x4	T41.3x5	T41.3x6
nerve block (peripheral) (plexus)	T41.3x1	T41.3x2	T41.3x3	T41.3x4	T41.3x5	T41.3x6
topical (surface)	T41.3x1	T41.3x2	T41.3x3	T41.3x4	T41.3x5	T41.3x6
Carbocisteine	T48.4x1	T48.4x2	T48.4x3	T48.4x4	T48.4x5	T48.4x6
Carbocromen	T46.3x1	T46.3x2	T46.3x3	T46.3x4	T46.3x5	T46.3x6
Carbol fuchsin	T49.0x1	T49.0x2	T49.0x3	T49.0x4	T49.0x5	T49.0x6
Carbolic acid — see also Phenol	T54.0x1	T54.0x2	T54.0x3	T54.0x4	—	—
Carbolonium (bromide)	T48.1x1	T48.1x2	T48.1x3	T48.1x4	T48.1x5	T48.1x6
Carbomycin	T36.8x1	T36.8x2	T36.8x3	T36.8x4	T36.8x5	T36.8x6
Carbon bisulfide (liquid)	T65.4x1	T65.4x2	T65.4x3	T65.4x4	—	—
vapor	T65.4x1	T65.4x2	T65.4x3	T65.4x4	—	—
dioxide (gas)	T59.7x1	T59.7x2	T59.7x3	T59.7x4	—	—
medicinal	T41.5x1	T41.5x2	T41.5x3	T41.5x4	T41.5x5	T41.5x6
nonmedicinal	T59.7x1	T59.7x2	T59.7x3	T59.7x4	—	—
snow	T49.4x1	T49.4x2	T49.4x3	T49.4x4	T49.4x5	T49.4x6
disulfide (liquid)	T65.4x1	T65.4x2	T65.4x3	T65.4x4	—	—
vapor	T65.4x1	T65.4x2	T65.4x3	T65.4x4	—	—

Table of Drugs & Chemicals	Poisoning Accidental (Unintentional)	Poisoning Self-Harm (Intentional)	Poisoning Assault	Poisoning Undetermined	Adverse Effect	Underdosing
Carbon – *continued*						
monoxide (from incomplete combustion)	T58.91	T58.92	T58.93	T58.94	—	—
blast furnace gas	T58.8x1	T58.8x2	T58.8x3	T58.8x4	—	—
butane (distributed in mobile container)	T58.11	T58.12	T58.13	T58.14	—	—
distributed through pipes	T58.11	T58.12	T58.13	T58.14	—	—
charcoal fumes	T58.2x1	T58.2x2	T58.2x3	T58.2x4	—	—
coal	T58.2x1	T58.2x2	T58.2x3	T58.2x4	—	—
gas (piped)	T58.11	T58.12	T58.13	T58.14	—	—
solid (in domestic stoves, fireplaces)	T58.2x1	T58.2x2	T58.2x3	T58.2x4	—	—
coke (in domestic stoves, fireplaces)	T58.2x1	T58.2x2	T58.2x3	T58.2x4	—	—
exhaust gas (motor) not in transit	T58.01	T58.02	T58.03	T58.04	—	—
combustion engine, any not in watercraft	T58.01	T58.02	T58.03	T58.04	—	—
farm tractor, not in transit	T58.01	T58.02	T58.03	T58.04	—	—
gas engine	T58.01	T58.02	T58.03	T58.04	—	—
motor pump	T58.01	T58.02	T58.03	T58.04	—	—
motor vehicle, not in transit	T58.01	T58.02	T58.03	T58.04	—	—
fuel (in domestic use)	T58.2x1	T58.2x2	T58.2x3	T58.2x4	—	—
gas (piped)	T58.11	T58.12	T58.13	T58.14	—	—
in mobile container	T58.11	T58.12	T58.13	T58.14	—	—
utility	T58.11	T58.12	T58.13	T58.14	—	—
in mobile container	T58.11	T58.12	T58.13	T58.14	—	—
piped (natural)	T58.11	T58.12	T58.13	T58.14	—	—
illuminating gas	T58.11	T58.12	T58.13	T58.14	—	—
industrial fuels or gases, any	T58.8x1	T58.8x2	T58.8x3	T58.8x4	—	—
kerosene (in domestic stoves, fireplaces)	T58.2x1	T58.2x2	T58.2x3	T58.2x4	—	—
kiln gas or vapor	T58.8x1	T58.8x2	T58.8x3	T58.8x4	—	—
motor exhaust gas, not in transit	T58.01	T58.02	T58.03	T58.04	—	—
piped gas (manufactured) (natural)	T58.11	T58.12	T58.13	T58.14	—	—
producer gas	T58.8x1	T58.8x2	T58.8x3	T58.8x4	—	—
propane (distributed in mobile container)	T58.11	T58.12	T58.13	T58.14	—	—
distributed through pipes	T58.11	T58.12	T58.13	T58.14	—	—
specified source NEC	T58.8x1	T58.8x2	T58.8x3	T58.8x4	—	—
stove gas	T58.11	T58.12	T58.13	T58.14	—	—
piped	T58.11	T58.12	T58.13	T58.14	—	—
utility gas	T58.11	T58.12	T58.13	T58.14	—	—
piped	T58.11	T58.12	T58.13	T58.14	—	—
water gas	T58.11	T58.12	T58.13	T58.14	—	—
wood (in domestic stoves, fireplaces)	T58.2x1	T58.2x2	T58.2x3	T58.2x4	—	—
tetrachloride (vapor) NEC	T53.0x1	T53.0x2	T53.0x3	T53.0x4	—	—
liquid (cleansing agent) NEC	T53.0x1	T53.0x2	T53.0x3	T53.0x4	—	—
solvent	T53.0x1	T53.0x2	T53.0x3	T53.0x4	—	—
Carbonic acid gas	T59.7x1	T59.7x2	T59.7x3	T59.7x4	—	—
anhydrase inhibitor NEC	T50.2x1	T50.2x2	T50.2x3	T50.2x4	T50.2x5	T50.2x6
Carbophenothion	T60.0x1	T60.0x2	T60.0x3	T60.0x4	—	—
Carboplatin	T45.1x1	T45.1x2	T45.1x3	T45.1x4	T45.1x5	T45.1x6
Carboprost	T48.0x1	T48.0x2	T48.0x3	T48.0x4	T48.0x5	T48.0x6
Carboquone	T45.1x1	T45.1x2	T45.1x3	T45.1x4	T45.1x5	T45.1x6
Carbowax	T49.3x1	T49.3x2	T49.3x3	T49.3x4	T49.3x5	T49.3x6
Carboxymethyl-cellulose	T47.4x1	T47.4x2	T47.4x3	T47.4x4	T47.4x5	T47.4x6
S-Carboxymethyl-cysteine	T48.4x1	T48.4x2	T48.4x3	T48.4x4	T48.4x5	T48.4x6
Carbrital	T42.3x1	T42.3x2	T42.3x3	T42.3x4	T42.3x5	T42.3x6
Carbromal	T42.6x1	T42.6x2	T42.6x3	T42.6x4	T42.6x5	T42.6x6
Carbutamide	T38.3x1	T38.3x2	T38.3x3	T38.3x4	T38.3x5	T38.3x6
Carbuterol	T48.6x1	T48.6x2	T48.6x3	T48.6x4	T48.6x5	T48.6x6
Cardiac						
depressants	T46.2x1	T46.2x2	T46.2x3	T46.2x4	T46.2x5	T46.2x6
rhythm regulator	T46.2x1	T46.2x2	T46.2x3	T46.2x4	T46.2x5	T46.2x6
specified NEC	T46.2x1	T46.2x2	T46.2x3	T46.2x4	T46.2x5	T46.2x6
Cardiografin	T50.8x1	T50.8x2	T50.8x3	T50.8x4	T50.8x5	T50.8x6
Cardio-green	T50.8x1	T50.8x2	T50.8x3	T50.8x4	T50.8x5	T50.8x6
Cardiotonic (glycoside) NEC	T46.0x1	T46.0x2	T46.0x3	T46.0x4	T46.0x5	T46.0x6
Cardiovascular drug NEC	T46.901	T46.902	T46.903	T46.904	T46.905	T46.906
Cardrase	T50.2x1	T50.2x2	T50.2x3	T50.2x4	T50.2x5	T50.2x6
Carfecillin	T36.0x1	T36.0x2	T36.0x3	T36.0x4	T36.0x5	T36.0x6
Carfenazine	T43.3x1	T43.3x2	T43.3x3	T43.3x4	T43.3x5	T43.3x6
Carfusin	T49.0x1	T49.0x2	T49.0x3	T49.0x4	T49.0x5	T49.0x6
Carindacillin	T36.0x1	T36.0x2	T36.0x3	T36.0x4	T36.0x5	T36.0x6
Carisoprodol	T42.8x1	T42.8x2	T42.8x3	T42.8x4	T42.8x5	T42.8x6
Carmellose	T47.4x1	T47.4x2	T47.4x3	T47.4x4	T47.4x5	T47.4x6
Carminative	T47.5x1	T47.5x2	T47.5x3	T47.5x4	T47.5x5	T47.5x6
Carmofur	T45.1x1	T45.1x2	T45.1x3	T45.1x4	T45.1x5	T45.1x6
Carmustine	T45.1x1	T45.1x2	T45.1x3	T45.1x4	T45.1x5	T45.1x6
Carotene	T45.2x1	T45.2x2	T45.2x3	T45.2x4	T45.2x5	T45.2x6
Carphenazine	T43.3x1	T43.3x2	T43.3x3	T43.3x4	T43.3x5	T43.3x6
Carpipramine	T42.4x1	T42.4x2	T42.4x3	T42.4x4	T42.4x5	T42.4x6
Carprofen	T39.311	T39.312	T39.313	T39.314	T39.315	T39.316
Carpronium chloride	T44.3x1	T44.3x2	T44.3x3	T44.3x4	T44.3x5	T44.3x6
Carrageenan	T47.8x1	T47.8x2	T47.8x3	T47.8x4	T47.8x5	T47.8x6
Carteolol	T44.7x1	T44.7x2	T44.7x3	T44.7x4	T44.7x5	T44.7x6
Carter's Little Pills	T47.2x1	T47.2x2	T47.2x3	T47.2x4	T47.2x5	T47.2x6
Cascara (sagrada)	T47.2x1	T47.2x2	T47.2x3	T47.2x4	T47.2x5	T47.2x6
Cassava	T62.2x1	T62.2x2	T62.2x3	T62.2x4	—	—
Castellani's paint	T49.0x1	T49.0x2	T49.0x3	T49.0x4	T49.0x5	T49.0x6
Castor						
bean	T62.2x1	T62.2x2	T62.2x3	T62.2x4	—	—
oil	T47.2x1	T47.2x2	T47.2x3	T47.2x4	T47.2x5	T47.2x6
Catalase	T45.3x1	T45.3x2	T45.3x3	T45.3x4	T45.3x5	T45.3x6
Caterpillar (sting)	T63.431	T63.432	T63.433	T63.434	—	—
Catha (edulis) (tea)	T43.691	T43.692	T43.693	T43.694	—	—
Cathartic NEC	T47.4x1	T47.4x2	T47.4x3	T47.4x4	T47.4x5	T47.4x6
anthacene derivative	T47.2x1	T47.2x2	T47.2x3	T47.2x4	T47.2x5	T47.2x6
bulk	T47.4x1	T47.4x2	T47.4x3	T47.4x4	T47.4x5	T47.4x6
contact	T47.2x1	T47.2x2	T47.2x3	T47.2x4	T47.2x5	T47.2x6
emollient NEC	T47.4x1	T47.4x2	T47.4x3	T47.4x4	T47.4x5	T47.4x6
irritant NEC	T47.2x1	T47.2x2	T47.2x3	T47.2x4	T47.2x5	T47.2x6
mucilage	T47.4x1	T47.4x2	T47.4x3	T47.4x4	T47.4x5	T47.4x6
saline	T47.3x1	T47.3x2	T47.3x3	T47.3x4	T47.3x5	T47.3x6
vegetable	T47.2x1	T47.2x2	T47.2x3	T47.2x4	T47.2x5	T47.2x6
Cathine	T50.5x1	T50.5x2	T50.5x3	T50.5x4	T50.5x5	T50.5x6
Cathomycin	T36.8x1	T36.8x2	T36.8x3	T36.8x4	T36.8x5	T36.8x6
Cation exchange resin	T50.3x1	T50.3x2	T50.3x3	T50.3x4	T50.3x5	T50.3x6
Caustic(s) NEC	T54.91	T54.92	T54.93	T54.94	—	—
alkali	T54.3x1	T54.3x2	T54.3x3	T54.3x4	—	—
hydroxide	T54.3x1	T54.3x2	T54.3x3	T54.3x4	—	—
potash	T54.3x1	T54.3x2	T54.3x3	T54.3x4	—	—
specified NEC	T54.91	T54.92	T54.93	T54.94	—	—
soda	T54.3x1	T54.3x2	T54.3x3	T54.3x4	—	—
Ceepryn	T49.0x1	T49.0x2	T49.0x3	T49.0x4	T49.0x5	T49.0x6
ENT agent	T49.6x1	T49.6x2	T49.6x3	T49.6x4	T49.6x5	T49.6x6
lozenges	T49.6x1	T49.6x2	T49.6x3	T49.6x4	T49.6x5	T49.6x6
Cefacetrile	T36.1x1	T36.1x2	T36.1x3	T36.1x4	T36.1x5	T36.1x6
Cefaclor	T36.1x1	T36.1x2	T36.1x3	T36.1x4	T36.1x5	T36.1x6
Cefadroxil	T36.1x1	T36.1x2	T36.1x3	T36.1x4	T36.1x5	T36.1x6
Cefalexin	T36.1x1	T36.1x2	T36.1x3	T36.1x4	T36.1x5	T36.1x6
Cefaloglycin	T36.1x1	T36.1x2	T36.1x3	T36.1x4	T36.1x5	T36.1x6
Cefaloridine	T36.1x1	T36.1x2	T36.1x3	T36.1x4	T36.1x5	T36.1x6
Cefalosporins	T36.1x1	T36.1x2	T36.1x3	T36.1x4	T36.1x5	T36.1x6
Cefalotin	T36.1x1	T36.1x2	T36.1x3	T36.1x4	T36.1x5	T36.1x6
Cefamandole	T36.1x1	T36.1x2	T36.1x3	T36.1x4	T36.1x5	T36.1x6
Cefamycin antibiotic	T36.1x1	T36.1x2	T36.1x3	T36.1x4	T36.1x5	T36.1x6
Cefapirin	T36.1x1	T36.1x2	T36.1x3	T36.1x4	T36.1x5	T36.1x6
Cefatrizine	T36.1x1	T36.1x2	T36.1x3	T36.1x4	T36.1x5	T36.1x6
Cefazedone	T36.1x1	T36.1x2	T36.1x3	T36.1x4	T36.1x5	T36.1x6
Cefazolin	T36.1x1	T36.1x2	T36.1x3	T36.1x4	T36.1x5	T36.1x6
Cefbuperazone	T36.1x1	T36.1x2	T36.1x3	T36.1x4	T36.1x5	T36.1x6
Cefetamet	T36.1x1	T36.1x2	T36.1x3	T36.1x4	T36.1x5	T36.1x6
Cefixime	T36.1x1	T36.1x2	T36.1x3	T36.1x4	T36.1x5	T36.1x6
Cefmenoxime	T36.1x1	T36.1x2	T36.1x3	T36.1x4	T36.1x5	T36.1x6

DRUGS&CHEMICALS

DRUGS&CHEMICALS

Table of Drugs & Chemicals	POISONING Accidental (Unintentional)	Self-Harm (Intentional)	Assault	Undetermined	Adverse Effect	Underdosing
Cefmetazole	T36.1x1	T36.1x2	T36.1x3	T36.1x4	T36.1x5	T36.1x6
Cefminox	T36.1x1	T36.1x2	T36.1x3	T36.1x4	T36.1x5	T36.1x6
Cefonicid	T36.1x1	T36.1x2	T36.1x3	T36.1x4	T36.1x5	T36.1x6
Cefoperazone	T36.1x1	T36.1x2	T36.1x3	T36.1x4	T36.1x5	T36.1x6
Ceforanide	T36.1x1	T36.1x2	T36.1x3	T36.1x4	T36.1x5	T36.1x6
Cefotaxime	T36.1x1	T36.1x2	T36.1x3	T36.1x4	T36.1x5	T36.1x6
Cefotetan	T36.1x1	T36.1x2	T36.1x3	T36.1x4	T36.1x5	T36.1x6
Cefotiam	T36.1x1	T36.1x2	T36.1x3	T36.1x4	T36.1x5	T36.1x6
Cefoxitin	T36.1x1	T36.1x2	T36.1x3	T36.1x4	T36.1x5	T36.1x6
Cefpimizole	T36.1x1	T36.1x2	T36.1x3	T36.1x4	T36.1x5	T36.1x6
Cefpiramide	T36.1x1	T36.1x2	T36.1x3	T36.1x4	T36.1x5	T36.1x6
Cefradine	T36.1x1	T36.1x2	T36.1x3	T36.1x4	T36.1x5	T36.1x6
Cefroxadine	T36.1x1	T36.1x2	T36.1x3	T36.1x4	T36.1x5	T36.1x6
Cefsulodin	T36.1x1	T36.1x2	T36.1x3	T36.1x4	T36.1x5	T36.1x6
Ceftazidime	T36.1x1	T36.1x2	T36.1x3	T36.1x4	T36.1x5	T36.1x6
Cefteram	T36.1x1	T36.1x2	T36.1x3	T36.1x4	T36.1x5	T36.1x6
Ceftezole	T36.1x1	T36.1x2	T36.1x3	T36.1x4	T36.1x5	T36.1x6
Ceftizoxime	T36.1x1	T36.1x2	T36.1x3	T36.1x4	T36.1x5	T36.1x6
Ceftriaxone	T36.1x1	T36.1x2	T36.1x3	T36.1x4	T36.1x5	T36.1x6
Cefuroxime	T36.1x1	T36.1x2	T36.1x3	T36.1x4	T36.1x5	T36.1x6
Cefuzonam	T36.1x1	T36.1x2	T36.1x3	T36.1x4	T36.1x5	T36.1x6
Celestone	T38.0x1	T38.0x2	T38.0x3	T38.0x4	T38.0x5	T38.0x6
topical	T49.0x1	T49.0x2	T49.0x3	T49.0x4	T49.0x5	T49.0x6
Celiprolol	T44.7x1	T44.7x2	T44.7x3	T44.7x4	T44.7x5	T44.7x6
Cell stimulants and proliferants	T49.8x1	T49.8x2	T49.8x3	T49.8x4	T49.8x5	T49.8x6
Cellosolve	T52.91	T52.92	T52.93	T52.94	—	—
Cellulose						
cathartic	T47.4x1	T47.4x2	T47.4x3	T47.4x4	T47.4x5	T47.4x6
hydroxyethyl	T47.4x1	T47.4x2	T47.4x3	T47.4x4	T47.4x5	T47.4x6
nitrates (topical)	T49.3x1	T49.3x2	T49.3x3	T49.3x4	T49.3x5	T49.3x6
oxidized	T49.4x1	T49.4x2	T49.4x3	T49.4x4	T49.4x5	T49.4x6
Centipede (bite)	T63.411	T63.412	T63.413	T63.414	—	—
Central nervous system						
depressants	T42.71	T42.72	T42.73	T42.74	T42.75	T42.76
anesthetic (general) NEC	T41.201	T41.202	T41.203	T41.204	T41.205	T41.206
gases NEC	T41.0x1	T41.0x2	T41.0x3	T41.0x4	T41.0x5	T41.0x6
intravenous	T41.1x1	T41.1x2	T41.1x3	T41.1x4	T41.1x5	T41.1x6
barbiturates	T42.3x1	T42.3x2	T42.3x3	T42.3x4	T42.3x5	T42.3x6
benzodiazepines	T42.4x1	T42.4x2	T42.4x3	T42.4x4	T42.4x5	T42.4x6
bromides	T42.6x1	T42.6x2	T42.6x3	T42.6x4	T42.6x5	T42.6x6
cannabis sativa	T40.7x1	T40.7x2	T40.7x3	T40.7x4	T40.7x5	T40.7x6
chloral hydrate	T42.6x1	T42.6x2	T42.6x3	T42.6x4	T42.6x5	T42.6x6
ethanol	T51.0x1	T51.0x2	T51.0x3	T51.0x4	—	—
hallucinogenics	T40.901	T40.902	T40.903	T40.904	T40.905	T40.906
hypnotics	T42.71	T42.72	T42.73	T42.74	T42.75	T42.76
specified NEC	T42.6x1	T42.6x2	T42.6x3	T42.6x4	T42.6x5	T42.6x6
muscle relaxants	T42.8x1	T42.8x2	T42.8x3	T42.8x4	T42.8x5	T42.8x6
paraldehyde	T42.6x1	T42.6x2	T42.6x3	T42.6x4	T42.6x5	T42.6x6
sedatives; sedative-hypnotics	T42.71	T42.72	T42.73	T42.74	T42.75	T42.76
mixed NEC	T42.6x1	T42.6x2	T42.6x3	T42.6x4	T42.6x5	T42.6x6
specified NEC	T42.6x1	T42.6x2	T42.6x3	T42.6x4	T42.6x5	T42.6x6
muscle-tone depressants	T42.8x1	T42.8x2	T42.8x3	T42.8x4	T42.8x5	T42.8x6
stimulants	T43.601	T43.602	T43.603	T43.604	T43.605	T43.606
amphetamines	T43.621	T43.622	T43.623	T43.624	T43.625	T43.626
analeptics	T50.7x1	T50.7x2	T50.7x3	T50.7x4	T50.7x5	T50.7x6
antidepressants	T43.201	T43.202	T43.203	T43.204	T43.205	T43.206
opiate antagonists	T50.7x1	T50.7x2	T50.7x3	T50.7x4	T50.7x5	T50.7x6
specified NEC	T43.691	T43.692	T43.693	T43.694	T43.695	T43.696
Cephalexin	T36.1x1	T36.1x2	T36.1x3	T36.1x4	T36.1x5	T36.1x6
Cephaloglycin	T36.1x1	T36.1x2	T36.1x3	T36.1x4	T36.1x5	T36.1x6
Cephaloridine	T36.1x1	T36.1x2	T36.1x3	T36.1x4	T36.1x5	T36.1x6
Cephalosporins	T36.1x1	T36.1x2	T36.1x3	T36.1x4	T36.1x5	T36.1x6
N (adicillin)	T36.0x1	T36.0x2	T36.0x3	T36.0x4	T36.0x5	T36.0x6
Cephalothin	T36.1x1	T36.1x2	T36.1x3	T36.1x4	T36.1x5	T36.1x6
Cephalotin	T36.1x1	T36.1x2	T36.1x3	T36.1x4	T36.1x5	T36.1x6
Cephradine	T36.1x1	T36.1x2	T36.1x3	T36.1x4	T36.1x5	T36.1x6
Cerbera (odallam)	T62.2x1	T62.2x2	T62.2x3	T62.2x4	—	—
Cerberin	T46.0x1	T46.0x2	T46.0x3	T46.0x4	T46.0x5	T46.0x6
Cerebral stimulants	T43.601	T43.602	T43.603	T43.604	T43.605	T43.606
psychotherapeutic	T43.601	T43.602	T43.603	T43.604	T43.605	T43.606
specified NEC	T43.691	T43.692	T43.693	T43.694	T43.695	T43.696

Table of Drugs & Chemicals	POISONING Accidental (Unintentional)	Self-Harm (Intentional)	Assault	Undetermined	Adverse Effect	Underdosing
Cerium oxalate	T45.0x1	T45.0x2	T45.0x3	T45.0x4	T45.0x5	T45.0x6
Cerous oxalate	T45.0x1	T45.0x2	T45.0x3	T45.0x4	T45.0x5	T45.0x6
Ceruletide	T50.8x1	T50.8x2	T50.8x3	T50.8x4	T50.8x5	T50.8x6
Cetalkonium (chloride)	T49.0x1	T49.0x2	T49.0x3	T49.0x4	T49.0x5	T49.0x6
Cethexonium chloride	T49.0x1	T49.0x2	T49.0x3	T49.0x4	T49.0x5	T49.0x6
Cetiedil	T46.7x1	T46.7x2	T46.7x3	T46.7x4	T46.7x5	T46.7x6
Cetirizine	T45.0x1	T45.0x2	T45.0x3	T45.0x4	T45.0x5	T45.0x6
Cetomacrogol	T50.991	T50.992	T50.993	T50.994	T50.995	T50.996
Cetotiamine	T45.2x1	T45.2x2	T45.2x3	T45.2x4	T45.2x5	T45.2x6
Cetoxime	T45.0x1	T45.0x2	T45.0x3	T45.0x4	T45.0x5	T45.0x6
Cetraxate	T47.1x1	T47.1x2	T47.1x3	T47.1x4	T47.1x5	T47.1x6
Cetrimide	T49.0x1	T49.0x2	T49.0x3	T49.0x4	T49.0x5	T49.0x6
Cetrimonium (bromide)	T49.0x1	T49.0x2	T49.0x3	T49.0x4	T49.0x5	T49.0x6
Cetylpyridinium chloride	T49.0x1	T49.0x2	T49.0x3	T49.0x4	T49.0x5	T49.0x6
ENT agent	T49.6x1	T49.6x2	T49.6x3	T49.6x4	T49.6x5	T49.6x6
lozenges	T49.6x1	T49.6x2	T49.6x3	T49.6x4	T49.6x5	T49.6x6
Cevadilla — *see* Sabadilla						
Cevitamic acid	T45.2x1	T45.2x2	T45.2x3	T45.2x4	T45.2x5	T45.2x6
Ch'an su	T46.0x1	T46.0x2	T46.0x3	T46.0x4	T46.0x5	T46.0x6
Chalk, precipitated	T47.1x1	T47.1x2	T47.1x3	T47.1x4	T47.1x5	T47.1x6
Chamomile	T49.0x1	T49.0x2	T49.0x3	T49.0x4	T49.0x5	T49.0x6
Charcoal	T47.6x1	T47.6x2	T47.6x3	T47.6x4	T47.6x5	T47.6x6
activated — *see also* Charcoal, medicinal	T47.6x1	T47.6x2	T47.6x3	T47.6x4	T47.6x5	T47.6x6
fumes (carbon monoxide)	T58.2x1	T58.2x2	T58.2x3	T58.2x4	—	—
industrial	T58.8x1	T58.8x2	T58.8x3	T58.8x4	—	—
medicinal (activated)	T47.6x1	T47.6x2	T47.6x3	T47.6x4	T47.6x5	T47.6x6
antidiarrheal	T47.6x1	T47.6x2	T47.6x3	T47.6x4	T47.6x5	T47.6x6
poison control	T47.8x1	T47.8x2	T47.8x3	T47.8x4	T47.8x5	T47.8x6
specified use other than for diarrhea	T47.8x1	T47.8x2	T47.8x3	T47.8x4	T47.8x5	T47.8x6
topical	T49.8x1	T49.8x2	T49.8x3	T49.8x4	T49.8x5	T49.8x6
Chaulmosulfone	T37.1x1	T37.1x2	T37.1x3	T37.1x4	T37.1x5	T37.1x6
Chelating agent NEC	T50.6x1	T50.6x2	T50.6x3	T50.6x4	T50.6x5	T50.6x6
Chelidonium majus	T62.2x1	T62.2x2	T62.2x3	T62.2x4	—	—
Chemical substance NEC	T65.91	T65.92	T65.93	T65.94	—	—
Chenodeoxycholic acid	T47.5x1	T47.5x2	T47.5x3	T47.5x4	T47.5x5	T47.5x6
Chenodiol	T47.5x1	T47.5x2	T47.5x3	T47.5x4	T47.5x5	T47.5x6
Chenopodium	T37.4x1	T37.4x2	T37.4x3	T37.4x4	T37.4x5	T37.4x6
Cherry laurel	T62.2x1	T62.2x2	T62.2x3	T62.2x4	—	—
Chinidin(e)	T46.2x1	T46.2x2	T46.2x3	T46.2x4	T46.2x5	T46.2x6
Chiniofon	T37.8x1	T37.8x2	T37.8x3	T37.8x4	T37.8x5	T37.8x6
Chlophedianol	T48.3x1	T48.3x2	T48.3x3	T48.3x4	T48.3x5	T48.3x6
Chloral	T42.6x1	T42.6x2	T42.6x3	T42.6x4	T42.6x5	T42.6x6
derivative	T42.6x1	T42.6x2	T42.6x3	T42.6x4	T42.6x5	T42.6x6
hydrate	T42.6x1	T42.6x2	T42.6x3	T42.6x4	T42.6x5	T42.6x6
Chloralamide	T42.6x1	T42.6x2	T42.6x3	T42.6x4	T42.6x5	T42.6x6
Chloralodol	T42.6x1	T42.6x2	T42.6x3	T42.6x4	T42.6x5	T42.6x6
Chloralose	T60.4x1	T60.4x2	T60.4x3	T60.4x4	—	—
Chlorambucil	T45.1x1	T45.1x2	T45.1x3	T45.1x4	T45.1x5	T45.1x6
Chloramine	T57.8x1	T57.8x2	T57.8x3	T57.8x4	—	—
T	T49.0x1	T49.0x2	T49.0x3	T49.0x4	T49.0x5	T49.0x6
topical	T49.0x1	T49.0x2	T49.0x3	T49.0x4	T49.0x5	T49.0x6
Chloramphenicol	T36.2x1	T36.2x2	T36.2x3	T36.2x4	T36.2x5	T36.2x6
ENT agent	T49.6x1	T49.6x2	T49.6x3	T49.6x4	T49.6x5	T49.6x6
ophthalmic preparation	T49.5x1	T49.5x2	T49.5x3	T49.5x4	T49.5x5	T49.5x6
topical NEC	T49.0x1	T49.0x2	T49.0x3	T49.0x4	T49.0x5	T49.0x6
Chlorate (potassium) (sodium)						
NEC	T60.3x1	T60.3x2	T60.3x3	T60.3x4	—	—
herbicide	T60.3x1	T60.3x2	T60.3x3	T60.3x4	—	—
Chlorazanil	T50.2x1	T50.2x2	T50.2x3	T50.2x4	T50.2x5	T50.2x6
Chlorbenzene, chlorbenzol	T53.7x1	T53.7x2	T53.7x3	T53.7x4	—	—
Chlorbenzoxamine	T44.3x1	T44.3x2	T44.3x3	T44.3x4	T44.3x5	T44.3x6
Chlorbutol	T42.6x1	T42.6x2	T42.6x3	T42.6x4	T42.6x5	T42.6x6
Chlorcyclizine	T45.0x1	T45.0x2	T45.0x3	T45.0x4	T45.0x5	T45.0x6
Chlordan(e) (dust)	T60.1x1	T60.1x2	T60.1x3	T60.1x4	—	—
Chlordantoin	T49.0x1	T49.0x2	T49.0x3	T49.0x4	T49.0x5	T49.0x6
Chlordiazepoxide	T42.4x1	T42.4x2	T42.4x3	T42.4x4	T42.4x5	T42.4x6
Chlordiethyl benzamide	T49.3x1	T49.3x2	T49.3x3	T49.3x4	T49.3x5	T49.3x6
Chloresium	T49.8x1	T49.8x2	T49.8x3	T49.8x4	T49.8x5	T49.8x6

DRUGS&CHEMICALS

Table of Drugs & Chemicals	Accidental (Unintentional)	Self-Harm (Intentional)	Assault	Undetermined	Adverse Effect	Underdosing
Chlorethiazol	T42.6x1	T42.6x2	T42.6x3	T42.6x4	T42.6x5	T42.6x6
Chlorethyl — see Ethyl chloride						
Chloretone	T42.6x1	T42.6x2	T42.6x3	T42.6x4	T42.6x5	T42.6x6
Chlorex	T53.6x1	T53.6x2	T53.6x3	T53.6x4	—	—
insecticide	T60.1x1	T60.1x2	T60.1x3	T60.1x4	—	—
Chlorfenvinphos	T60.0x1	T60.0x2	T60.0x3	T60.0x4	—	—
Chlorhexadol	T42.6x1	T42.6x2	T42.6x3	T42.6x4	T42.6x5	T42.6x6
Chlorhexamide	T45.1x1	T45.1x2	T45.1x3	T45.1x4	T45.1x5	T45.1x6
Chlorhexidine	T49.0x1	T49.0x2	T49.0x3	T49.0x4	T49.0x5	T49.0x6
Chlorhydroxyquinolin	T49.0x1	T49.0x2	T49.0x3	T49.0x4	T49.0x5	T49.0x6
Chloride of lime (bleach)	T54.3x1	T54.3x2	T54.3x3	T54.3x4	—	—
Chlorimipramine	T43.011	T43.012	T43.013	T43.014	T43.015	T43.016
Chlorinated						
camphene	T53.6x1	T53.6x2	T53.6x3	T53.6x4	—	—
diphenyl	T53.7x1	T53.7x2	T53.7x3	T53.7x4	—	—
hydrocarbons NEC	T53.91	T53.92	T53.93	T53.94	—	—
solvents	T53.91	T53.92	T53.93	T53.94	—	—
lime (bleach)	T54.3x1	T54.3x2	T54.3x3	T54.3x4	—	—
and boric acid solution	T49.0x1	T49.0x2	T49.0x3	T49.0x4	T49.0x5	T49.0x6
naphthalene (insecticide)	T60.1x1	T60.1x2	T60.1x3	T60.1x4	—	—
industrial (non-pesticide)	T53.7x1	T53.7x2	T53.7x3	T53.7x4	—	—
pesticide NEC	T60.8x1	T60.8x2	T60.8x3	T60.8x4	—	—
soda — see also sodium hypochlorite						
solution	T49.0x1	T49.0x2	T49.0x3	T49.0x4	T49.0x5	T49.0x6
Chlorine (fumes) (gas)	T59.4x1	T59.4x2	T59.4x3	T59.4x4	—	—
bleach	T54.3x1	T54.3x2	T54.3x3	T54.3x4	—	—
compound gas NEC	T59.4x1	T59.4x2	T59.4x3	T59.4x4	—	—
disinfectant	T59.4x1	T59.4x2	T59.4x3	T59.4x4	—	—
releasing agents NEC	T59.4x1	T59.4x2	T59.4x3	T59.4x4	—	—
Chlorisondamine chloride	T46.991	T46.992	T46.993	T46.994	T46.995	T46.996
Chlormadinone	T38.5x1	T38.5x2	T38.5x3	T38.5x4	T38.5x5	T38.5x6
Chlormephos	T60.0x1	T60.0x2	T60.0x3	T60.0x4	—	—
Chlormerodrin	T50.2x1	T50.2x2	T50.2x3	T50.2x4	T50.2x5	T50.2x6
Chlormethiazole	T42.6x1	T42.6x2	T42.6x3	T42.6x4	T42.6x5	T42.6x6
Chlormethine	T45.1x1	T45.1x2	T45.1x3	T45.1x4	T45.1x5	T45.1x6
Chlormethylenecycline	T36.4x1	T36.4x2	T36.4x3	T36.4x4	T36.4x5	T36.4x6
Chlormezanone	T42.6x1	T42.6x2	T42.6x3	T42.6x4	T42.6x5	T42.6x6
Chloroacetic acid	T60.3x1	T60.3x2	T60.3x3	T60.3x4	—	—
Chloroacetone	T59.3x1	T59.3x2	T59.3x3	T59.3x4	—	—
Chloroacetophenone	T59.3x1	T59.3x2	T59.3x3	T59.3x4	—	—
Chloroaniline	T53.7x1	T53.7x2	T53.7x3	T53.7x4	—	—
Chlorobenzene, chlorobenzol	T53.7x1	T53.7x2	T53.7x3	T53.7x4	—	—
Chlorobromomethane (fire extinguisher)	T53.6x1	T53.6x2	T53.6x3	T53.6x4	—	—
Chlorobutanol	T49.0x1	T49.0x2	T49.0x3	T49.0x4	T49.0x5	T49.0x6
Chlorocresol	T49.0x1	T49.0x2	T49.0x3	T49.0x4	T49.0x5	T49.0x6
Chlorodehydro-methyltestosterone	T38.7x1	T38.7x2	T38.7x3	T38.7x4	T38.7x5	T38.7x6
Chlorodinitrobenzene	T53.7x1	T53.7x2	T53.7x3	T53.7x4	—	—
dust or vapor	T53.7x1	T53.7x2	T53.7x3	T53.7x4	—	—
Chlorodiphenyl	T53.7x1	T53.7x2	T53.7x3	T53.7x4	—	—
Chloroethane — see Ethyl chloride						
Chloroethylene	T53.6x1	T53.6x2	T53.6x3	T53.6x4	—	—
Chlorofluorocarbons	T53.5x1	T53.5x2	T53.5x3	T53.5x4	—	—
Chloroform (fumes) (vapor)	T53.1x1	T53.1x2	T53.1x3	T53.1x4	—	—
anesthetic	T41.0x1	T41.0x2	T41.0x3	T41.0x4	T41.0x5	T41.0x6
solvent	T53.1x1	T53.1x2	T53.1x3	T53.1x4	—	—
water, concentrated	T41.0x1	T41.0x2	T41.0x3	T41.0x4	T41.0x5	T41.0x6
Chloroguanide	T37.2x1	T37.2x2	T37.2x3	T37.2x4	T37.2x5	T37.2x6
Chloromycetin	T36.2x1	T36.2x2	T36.2x3	T36.2x4	T36.2x5	T36.2x6
ENT agent	T49.6x1	T49.6x2	T49.6x3	T49.6x4	T49.6x5	T49.6x6
ophthalmic preparation	T49.5x1	T49.5x2	T49.5x3	T49.5x4	T49.5x5	T49.5x6
otic solution	T49.6x1	T49.6x2	T49.6x3	T49.6x4	T49.6x5	T49.6x6
topical NEC	T49.0x1	T49.0x2	T49.0x3	T49.0x4	T49.0x5	T49.0x6
Chloronitrobenzene	T53.7x1	T53.7x2	T53.7x3	T53.7x4	—	—
dust or vapor	T53.7x1	T53.7x2	T53.7x3	T53.7x4	—	—
Chlorophacinone	T60.4x1	T60.4x2	T60.4x3	T60.4x4	—	—
Chlorophenol	T53.7x1	T53.7x2	T53.7x3	T53.7x4	—	—
Chlorophenothane	T60.1x1	T60.1x2	T60.1x3	T60.1x4	—	—
Chlorophyll	T50.991	T50.992	T50.993	T50.994	T50.995	T50.996

Table of Drugs & Chemicals	Accidental (Unintentional)	Self-Harm (Intentional)	Assault	Undetermined	Adverse Effect	Underdosing
Chloropicrin (fumes)	T53.6x1	T53.6x2	T53.6x3	T53.6x4	—	—
fumigant	T60.8x1	T60.8x2	T60.8x3	T60.8x4	—	—
fungicide	T60.3x1	T60.3x2	T60.3x3	T60.3x4	—	—
pesticide	T60.8x1	T60.8x2	T60.8x3	T60.8x4	—	—
Chloroprocaine	T41.3x1	T41.3x2	T41.3x3	T41.3x4	T41.3x5	T41.3x6
infiltration (subcutaneous)	T41.3x1	T41.3x2	T41.3x3	T41.3x4	T41.3x5	T41.3x6
nerve block (peripheral) (plexus)	T41.3x1	T41.3x2	T41.3x3	T41.3x4	T41.3x5	T41.3x6
spinal	T41.3x1	T41.3x2	T41.3x3	T41.3x4	T41.3x5	T41.3x6
Chloroptic	T49.5x1	T49.5x2	T49.5x3	T49.5x4	T49.5x5	T49.5x6
Chloropurine	T45.1x1	T45.1x2	T45.1x3	T45.1x4	T45.1x5	T45.1x6
Chloropyramine	T45.0x1	T45.0x2	T45.0x3	T45.0x4	T45.0x5	T45.0x6
Chloropyrifos	T60.0x1	T60.0x2	T60.0x3	T60.0x4		
Chloropyrilene	T45.0x1	T45.0x2	T45.0x3	T45.0x4	T45.0x5	T45.0x6
Chloroquine	T37.2x1	T37.2x2	T37.2x3	T37.2x4	T37.2x5	T37.2x6
Chlorothalonil	T60.3x1	T60.3x2	T60.3x3	T60.3x4		
Chlorothen	T45.0x1	T45.0x2	T45.0x3	T45.0x4	T45.0x5	T45.0x6
Chlorothiazide	T50.2x1	T50.2x2	T50.2x3	T50.2x4	T50.2x5	T50.2x6
Chlorothymol	T49.4x1	T49.4x2	T49.4x3	T49.4x4	T49.4x5	T49.4x6
Chlorotrianisene	T38.5x1	T38.5x2	T38.5x3	T38.5x4	T38.5x5	T38.5x6
Chlorovinyldichloro-arsine, not in war	T57.0x1	T57.0x2	T57.0x3	T57.0x4	—	—
Chloroxine	T49.4x1	T49.4x2	T49.4x3	T49.4x4	T49.4x5	T49.4x6
Chloroxylenol	T49.0x1	T49.0x2	T49.0x3	T49.0x4	T49.0x5	T49.0x6
Chlorphenamine	T45.0x1	T45.0x2	T45.0x3	T45.0x4	T45.0x5	T45.0x6
Chlorphenesin	T42.8x1	T42.8x2	T42.8x3	T42.8x4	T42.8x5	T42.8x6
topical (antifungal)	T49.0x1	T49.0x2	T49.0x3	T49.0x4	T49.0x5	T49.0x6
Chlorpheniramine	T45.0x1	T45.0x2	T45.0x3	T45.0x4	T45.0x5	T45.0x6
Chlorphenoxamine	T45.0x1	T45.0x2	T45.0x3	T45.0x4	T45.0x5	T45.0x6
Chlorphentermine	T50.5x1	T50.5x2	T50.5x3	T50.5x4	T50.5x5	T50.5x6
Chlorprocaine — see Chloroprocaine						
Chlorproguanil	T37.2x1	T37.2x2	T37.2x3	T37.2x4	T37.2x5	T37.2x6
Chlorpromazine	T43.3x1	T43.3x2	T43.3x3	T43.3x4	T43.3x5	T43.3x6
Chlorpropamide	T38.3x1	T38.3x2	T38.3x3	T38.3x4	T38.3x5	T38.3x6
Chlorprothixene	T43.4x1	T43.4x2	T43.4x3	T43.4x4	T43.4x5	T43.4x6
Chlorquinaldol	T49.0x1	T49.0x2	T49.0x3	T49.0x4	T49.0x5	T49.0x6
Chlorquinol	T49.0x1	T49.0x2	T49.0x3	T49.0x4	T49.0x5	T49.0x6
Chlortalidone	T50.2x1	T50.2x2	T50.2x3	T50.2x4	T50.2x5	T50.2x6
Chlortetracycline	T36.4x1	T36.4x2	T36.4x3	T36.4x4	T36.4x5	T36.4x6
Chlorthalidone	T50.2x1	T50.2x2	T50.2x3	T50.2x4	T50.2x5	T50.2x6
Chlorthion	T60.0x1	T60.0x2	T60.0x3	T60.0x4		
Chlorthiophos	T60.0x1	T60.0x2	T60.0x3	T60.0x4		
Chlortrianisene	T38.5x1	T38.5x2	T38.5x3	T38.5x4	T38.5x5	T38.5x6
Chlor-Trimeton	T45.0x1	T45.0x2	T45.0x3	T45.0x4	T45.0x5	T45.0x6
Chlorzoxazone	T42.8x1	T42.8x2	T42.8x3	T42.8x4	T42.8x5	T42.8x6
Choke damp	T59.7x1	T59.7x2	T59.7x3	T59.7x4	—	—
Cholagogues	T47.5x1	T47.5x2	T47.5x3	T47.5x4	T47.5x5	T47.5x6
Cholebrine	T50.8x1	T50.8x2	T50.8x3	T50.8x4	T50.8x5	T50.8x6
Cholecalciferol	T45.2x1	T45.2x2	T45.2x3	T45.2x4	T45.2x5	T45.2x6
Cholecystokinin	T50.8x1	T50.8x2	T50.8x3	T50.8x4	T50.8x5	T50.8x6
Cholera vaccine	T50.A91	T50.A92	T50.A93	T50.A94	T50.A95	T50.A96
Choleretic	T47.5x1	T47.5x2	T47.5x3	T47.5x4	T47.5x5	T47.5x6
Cholesterol-lowering agents	T46.6x1	T46.6x2	T46.6x3	T46.6x4	T46.6x5	T46.6x6
Cholestyramine (resin)	T46.6x1	T46.6x2	T46.6x3	T46.6x4	T46.6x5	T46.6x6
Cholic acid	T47.5x1	T47.5x2	T47.5x3	T47.5x4	T47.5x5	T47.5x6
Choline	T48.6x1	T48.6x2	T48.6x3	T48.6x4	T48.6x5	T48.6x6
chloride	T50.991	T50.992	T50.993	T50.994	T50.995	T50.996
dihydrogen citrate	T50.991	T50.992	T50.993	T50.994	T50.995	T50.996
salicylate	T39.091	T39.092	T39.093	T39.094	T39.095	T39.096
theophyllinate	T48.6x1	T48.6x2	T48.6x3	T48.6x4	T48.6x5	T48.6x6
Cholinergic (drug) NEC	T44.1x1	T44.1x2	T44.1x3	T44.1x4	T44.1x5	T44.1x6
muscle tone enhancer	T44.1x1	T44.1x2	T44.1x3	T44.1x4	T44.1x5	T44.1x6
organophosphorus	T44.0x1	T44.0x2	T44.0x3	T44.0x4	T44.0x5	
insecticide	T60.0x1	T60.0x2	T60.0x3	T60.0x4	—	—
nerve gas	T59.891	T59.892	T59.893	T59.894	—	—
trimethyl ammonium propanediol	T44.1x1	T44.1x2	T44.1x3	T44.1x4	T44.1x5	T44.1x6
Cholinesterase reactivator	T50.6x1	T50.6x2	T50.6x3	T50.6x4	T50.6x5	T50.6x6
Cholografin	T50.8x1	T50.8x2	T50.8x3	T50.8x4	T50.8x5	T50.8x6

DRUGS&CHEMICALS

Table of Drugs & Chemicals	POISONING Accidental (Unintentional)	Self-Harm (Intentional)	Assault	Undetermined	Adverse Effect	Underdosing
Chorionic gonadotropin	T38.891	T38.892	T38.893	T38.894	T38.895	T38.896
Chromate	T56.2x1	T56.2x2	T56.2x3	T56.2x4	—	—
dust or mist	T56.2x1	T56.2x2	T56.2x3	T56.2x4	—	—
lead — see also lead	T56.0x1	T56.0x2	T56.0x3	T56.0x4	—	—
paint	T56.0x1	T56.0x2	T56.0x3	T56.0x4	—	—
Chromic						
acid	T56.2x1	T56.2x2	T56.2x3	T56.2x4	—	—
dust or mist	T56.2x1	T56.2x2	T56.2x3	T56.2x4	—	—
phosphate 32P	T45.1x1	T45.1x2	T45.1x3	T45.1x4	T45.1x5	T45.1x6
Chromium	T56.2x1	T56.2x2	T56.2x3	T56.2x4	—	—
compounds — see Chromate						
sesquioxide	T50.8x1	T50.8x2	T50.8x3	T50.8x4	T50.8x5	T50.8x6
Chromomycin A3	T45.1x1	T45.1x2	T45.1x3	T45.1x4	T45.1x5	T45.1x6
Chromonar	T46.3x1	T46.3x2	T46.3x3	T46.3x4	T46.3x5	T46.3x6
Chromyl chloride	T56.2x1	T56.2x2	T56.2x3	T56.2x4		
Chrysarobin	T49.4x1	T49.4x2	T49.4x3	T49.4x4	T49.4x5	T49.4x6
Chrysazin	T47.2x1	T47.2x2	T47.2x3	T47.2x4	T47.2x5	T47.2x6
Chymar	T45.3x1	T45.3x2	T45.3x3	T45.3x4	T45.3x5	T45.3x6
ophthalmic preparation	T49.5x1	T49.5x2	T49.5x3	T49.5x4	T49.5x5	T49.5x6
Chymopapain	T45.3x1	T45.3x2	T45.3x3	T45.3x4	T45.3x5	T45.3x6
Chymotrypsin	T45.3x1	T45.3x2	T45.3x3	T45.3x4	T45.3x5	T45.3x6
ophthalmic preparation	T49.5x1	T49.5x2	T49.5x3	T49.5x4	T49.5x5	T49.5x6
Cianidanol	T50.991	T50.992	T50.993	T50.994	T50.995	T50.996
Cianopramine	T43.011	T43.012	T43.013	T43.014	T43.015	T43.016
Cibenzoline	T46.2x1	T46.2x2	T46.2x3	T46.2x4	T46.2x5	T46.2x6
Ciclacillin	T36.0x1	T36.0x2	T36.0x3	T36.0x4	T36.0x5	T36.0x6
Ciclobarbital — see Hexobarbital						
Ciclonicate	T46.7x1	T46.7x2	T46.7x3	T46.7x4	T46.7x5	T46.7x6
Ciclopirox (olamine)	T49.0x1	T49.0x2	T49.0x3	T49.0x4	T49.0x5	T49.0x6
Ciclosporin	T45.1x1	T45.1x2	T45.1x3	T45.1x4	T45.1x5	T45.1x6
Cicuta maculata or virosa	T62.2x1	T62.2x2	T62.2x3	T62.2x4	—	—
Cicutoxin	T62.2x1	T62.2x2	T62.2x3	T62.2x4	—	—
Cigarette lighter fluid	T52.0x1	T52.0x2	T52.0x3	T52.0x4	—	—
Cigarettes (tobacco)	T65.221	T65.222	T65.223	T65.224	—	—
Ciguatoxin	T61.01	T61.02	T61.03	T61.04	—	—
Cilazapril	T46.4x1	T46.4x2	T46.4x3	T46.4x4	T46.4x5	T46.4x6
Cimetidine	T47.0x1	T47.0x2	T47.0x3	T47.0x4	T47.0x5	T47.0x6
Cimetropium bromide	T44.3x1	T44.3x2	T44.3x3	T44.3x4	T44.3x5	T44.3x6
Cinchocaine	T41.3x1	T41.3x2	T41.3x3	T41.3x4	T41.3x5	T41.3x6
topical (surface)	T41.3x1	T41.3x2	T41.3x3	T41.3x4	T41.3x5	T41.3x6
Cinchona	T37.2x1	T37.2x2	T37.2x3	T37.2x4	T37.2x5	T37.2x6
Cinchonine alkaloids	T37.2x1	T37.2x2	T37.2x3	T37.2x4	T37.2x5	T37.2x6
Cinchophen	T50.4x1	T50.4x2	T50.4x3	T50.4x4	T50.4x5	T50.4x6
Cinepazide	T46.7x1	T46.7x2	T46.7x3	T46.7x4	T46.7x5	T46.7x6
Cinnamedrine	T48.5x1	T48.5x2	T48.5x3	T48.5x4	T48.5x5	T48.5x6
Cinnarizine	T45.0x1	T45.0x2	T45.0x3	T45.0x4	T45.0x5	T45.0x6
Cinoxacin	T37.8x1	T37.8x2	T37.8x3	T37.8x4	T37.8x5	T37.8x6
Ciprofibrate	T46.6x1	T46.6x2	T46.6x3	T46.6x4	T46.6x5	T46.6x6
Ciprofloxacin	T36.8x1	T36.8x2	T36.8x3	T36.8x4	T36.8x5	T36.8x6
Cisapride	T47.8x1	T47.8x2	T47.8x3	T47.8x4	T47.8x5	T47.8x6
Cisplatin	T45.1x1	T45.1x2	T45.1x3	T45.1x4	T45.1x5	T45.1x6
Citalopram	T43.221	T43.222	T43.223	T43.224	T43.225	T43.226
Citanest	T41.3x1	T41.3x2	T41.3x3	T41.3x4	T41.3x5	T41.3x6
infiltration (subcutaneous)	T41.3x1	T41.3x2	T41.3x3	T41.3x4	T41.3x5	T41.3x6
nerve block (peripheral) (plexus)	T41.3x1	T41.3x2	T41.3x3	T41.3x4	T41.3x5	T41.3x6
Citric acid	T47.5x1	T47.5x2	T47.5x3	T47.5x4	T47.5x5	T47.5x6
Citrovorum (factor)	T45.8x1	T45.8x2	T45.8x3	T45.8x4	T45.8x5	T45.8x6
Claviceps purpurea	T62.2x1	T62.2x2	T62.2x3	T62.2x4	—	—
Clavulanic acid	T36.1x1	T36.1x2	T36.1x3	T36.1x4	T36.1x5	T36.1x6
Cleaner, cleansing agent, type						
not specified	T65.891	T65.892	T65.893	T65.894	—	—
of paint or varnish	T52.91	T52.92	T52.93	T52.94	—	—
specified type NEC	T65.891	T65.892	T65.893	T65.894	—	—
Clebopride	T47.8x1	T47.8x2	T47.8x3	T47.8x4	T47.8x5	T47.8x6
Clefamide	T37.3x1	T37.3x2	T37.3x3	T37.3x4	T37.3x5	T37.3x6
Clemastine	T45.0x1	T45.0x2	T45.0x3	T45.0x4	T45.0x5	T45.0x6
Clematis vitalba	T62.2x1	T62.2x2	T62.2x3	T62.2x4	—	—
Clemizole	T45.0x1	T45.0x2	T45.0x3	T45.0x4	T45.0x5	T45.0x6
penicillin	T36.0x1	T36.0x2	T36.0x3	T36.0x4	T36.0x5	T36.0x6
Clenbuterol	T48.6x1	T48.6x2	T48.6x3	T48.6x4	T48.6x5	T48.6x6
Clidinium bromide	T44.3x1	T44.3x2	T44.3x3	T44.3x4	T44.3x5	T44.3x6
Clindamycin	T36.8x1	T36.8x2	T36.8x3	T36.8x4	T36.8x5	T36.8x6
Clinofibrate	T46.6x1	T46.6x2	T46.6x3	T46.6x4	T46.6x5	T46.6x6
Clioquinol	T37.8x1	T37.8x2	T37.8x3	T37.8x4	T37.8x5	T37.8x6
Cliradon	T40.2x1	T40.2x2	T40.2x3	T40.2x4	—	—
Clobazam	T42.4x1	T42.4x2	T42.4x3	T42.4x4	T42.4x5	T42.4x6
Clobenzorex	T50.5x1	T50.5x2	T50.5x3	T50.5x4	T50.5x5	T50.5x6
Clobetasol	T49.0x1	T49.0x2	T49.0x3	T49.0x4	T49.0x5	T49.0x6
Clobetasone	T49.0x1	T49.0x2	T49.0x3	T49.0x4	T49.0x5	T49.0x6
Clobutinol	T48.3x1	T48.3x2	T48.3x3	T48.3x4	T48.3x5	T48.3x6
Clocortolone	T38.0x1	T38.0x2	T38.0x3	T38.0x4	T38.0x5	T38.0x6
Clodantoin	T49.0x1	T49.0x2	T49.0x3	T49.0x4	T49.0x5	T49.0x6
Clodronic acid	T50.991	T50.992	T50.993	T50.994	T50.995	T50.996
Clofazimine	T37.1x1	T37.1x2	T37.1x3	T37.1x4	T37.1x5	T37.1x6
Clofedanol	T48.3x1	T48.3x2	T48.3x3	T48.3x4	T48.3x5	T48.3x6
Clofenamide	T50.2x1	T50.2x2	T50.2x3	T50.2x4	T50.2x5	T50.2x6
Clofenotane	T49.0x1	T49.0x2	T49.0x3	T49.0x4	T49.0x5	T49.0x6
Clofezone	T39.2x1	T39.2x2	T39.2x3	T39.2x4	T39.2x5	T39.2x6
Clofibrate	T46.6x1	T46.6x2	T46.6x3	T46.6x4	T46.6x5	T46.6x6
Clofibride	T46.6x1	T46.6x2	T46.6x3	T46.6x4	T46.6x5	T46.6x6
Cloforex	T50.5x1	T50.5x2	T50.5x3	T50.5x4	T50.5x5	T50.5x6
Clomethiazole	T42.6x1	T42.6x2	T42.6x3	T42.6x4	T42.6x5	T42.6x6
Clometocillin	T36.0x1	T36.0x2	T36.0x3	T36.0x4	T36.0x5	T36.0x6
Clomifene	T38.5x1	T38.5x2	T38.5x3	T38.5x4	T38.5x5	T38.5x6
Clomiphene	T38.5x1	T38.5x2	T38.5x3	T38.5x4	T38.5x5	T38.5x6
Clomipramine	T43.011	T43.012	T43.013	T43.014	T43.015	T43.016
Clomocycline	T36.4x1	T36.4x2	T36.4x3	T36.4x4	T36.4x5	T36.4x6
Clonazepam	T42.4x1	T42.4x2	T42.4x3	T42.4x4	T42.4x5	T42.4x6
Clonidine	T46.5x1	T46.5x2	T46.5x3	T46.5x4	T46.5x5	T46.5x6
Clonixin	T39.8x1	T39.8x2	T39.8x3	T39.8x4	T39.8x5	T39.8x6
Clopamide	T50.2x1	T50.2x2	T50.2x3	T50.2x4	T50.2x5	T50.2x6
Clopenthixol	T43.4x1	T43.4x2	T43.4x3	T43.4x4	T43.4x5	T43.4x6
Cloperastine	T48.3x1	T48.3x2	T48.3x3	T48.3x4	T48.3x5	T48.3x6
Clophedianol	T48.3x1	T48.3x2	T48.3x3	T48.3x4	T48.3x5	T48.3x6
Cloponone	T36.2x1	T36.2x2	T36.2x3	T36.2x4	T36.2x5	T36.2x6
Cloprednol	T38.0x1	T38.0x2	T38.0x3	T38.0x4	T38.0x5	T38.0x6
Cloral betaine	T42.6x1	T42.6x2	T42.6x3	T42.6x4	T42.6x5	T42.6x6
Cloramfenicol	T36.2x1	T36.2x2	T36.2x3	T36.2x4	T36.2x5	T36.2x6
Clorazepate (dipotassium)	T42.4x1	T42.4x2	T42.4x3	T42.4x4	T42.4x5	T42.4x6
Clorexolone	T50.2x1	T50.2x2	T50.2x3	T50.2x4	T50.2x5	T50.2x6
Clorfenamine	T45.0x1	T45.0x2	T45.0x3	T45.0x4	T45.0x5	T45.0x6
Clorgiline	T43.1x1	T43.1x2	T43.1x3	T43.1x4	T43.1x5	T43.1x6
Clorotepine	T44.3x1	T44.3x2	T44.3x3	T44.3x4	T44.3x5	T44.3x6
Clorox (bleach)	T54.91	T54.92	T54.93	T54.94	—	—
Clorprenaline	T48.6x1	T48.6x2	T48.6x3	T48.6x4	T48.6x5	T48.6x6
Clortermine	T50.5x1	T50.5x2	T50.5x3	T50.5x4	T50.5x5	T50.5x6
Clotiapine	T43.591	T43.592	T43.593	T43.594	T43.595	T43.596
Clotiazepam	T42.4x1	T42.4x2	T42.4x3	T42.4x4	T42.4x5	T42.4x6
Clotibric acid	T46.6x1	T46.6x2	T46.6x3	T46.6x4	T46.6x5	T46.6x6
Clotrimazole	T49.0x1	T49.0x2	T49.0x3	T49.0x4	T49.0x5	T49.0x6
Cloxacillin	T36.0x1	T36.0x2	T36.0x3	T36.0x4	T36.0x5	T36.0x6
Cloxazolam	T42.4x1	T42.4x2	T42.4x3	T42.4x4	T42.4x5	T42.4x6
Cloxiquine	T49.0x1	T49.0x2	T49.0x3	T49.0x4	T49.0x5	T49.0x6
Clozapine	T42.4x1	T42.4x2	T42.4x3	T42.4x4	T42.4x5	T42.4x6
Coagulant NEC	T45.7x1	T45.7x2	T45.7x3	T45.7x4	T45.7x5	T45.7x6
Coal (carbon monoxide from) — see also Carbon, monoxide, coal	T58.2x1	T58.2x2	T58.2x3	T58.2x4	—	—
oil — see Kerosene						
tar	T49.1x1	T49.1x2	T49.1x3	T49.1x4	T49.1x5	T49.1x6
fumes	T59.891	T59.892	T59.893	T59.894	—	—
medicinal (ointment)	T49.4x1	T49.4x2	T49.4x3	T49.4x4	T49.4x5	T49.4x6
analgesics NEC	T39.2x1	T39.2x2	T39.2x3	T39.2x4	T39.2x5	T39.2x6
naphtha (solvent)	T52.0x1	T52.0x2	T52.0x3	T52.0x4	—	—
Cobalamine	T45.2x1	T45.2x2	T45.2x3	T45.2x4	T45.2x5	T45.2x6
Cobalt (nonmedicinal) (fumes) (industrial)	T56.891	T56.892	T56.893	T56.894	—	—
medicinal (trace) (chloride)	T45.8x1	T45.8x2	T45.8x3	T45.8x4	T45.8x5	T45.8x6
Cobra (venom)	T63.041	T63.042	T63.043	T63.044	—	—

DRUGS&CHEMICALS

Table of Drugs & Chemicals	POISONING Accidental (Unintentional)	Self-Harm (Intentional)	Assault	Undetermined	Adverse Effect	Underdosing
Coca (leaf)	T40.5x1	T40.5x2	T40.5x3	T40.5x4	T40.5x5	T40.5x6
Cocaine	T40.5x1	T40.5x2	T40.5x3	T40.5x4	T40.5x5	T40.5x6
topical anesthetic	T41.3x1	T41.3x2	T41.3x3	T41.3x4	T41.3x5	T41.3x6
Cocarboxylase	T45.3x1	T45.3x2	T45.3x3	T45.3x4	T45.3x5	T45.3x6
Coccidioidin	T50.8x1	T50.8x2	T50.8x3	T50.8x4	T50.8x5	T50.8x6
Cocculus indicus	T62.1x1	T62.1x2	T62.1x3	T62.1x4	—	—
Cochineal	T65.6x1	T65.6x2	T65.6x3	T65.6x4	—	—
medicinal products	T50.991	T50.992	T50.993	T50.994	T50.995	T50.996
Codeine	T40.2x1	T40.2x2	T40.2x3	T40.2x4	T40.2x5	T40.2x6
Cod-liver oil	T45.2x1	T45.2x2	T45.2x3	T45.2x4	T45.2x5	T45.2x6
Coenzyme A	T50.991	T50.992	T50.993	T50.994	T50.995	T50.996
Coffee	T62.8x1	T62.8x2	T62.8x3	T62.8x4	—	—
Cogalactoiso-merase	T50.991	T50.992	T50.993	T50.994	T50.995	T50.996
Cogentin	T44.3x1	T44.3x2	T44.3x3	T44.3x4	T44.3x5	T44.3x6
Coke fumes or gas (carbon monoxide)	T58.2x1	T58.2x2	T58.2x3	T58.2x4	—	—
industrial use	T58.8x1	T58.8x2	T58.8x3	T58.8x4	—	—
Colace	T47.4x1	T47.4x2	T47.4x3	T47.4x4	T47.4x5	T47.4x6
Colaspase	T45.1x1	T45.1x2	T45.1x3	T45.1x4	T45.1x5	T45.1x6
Colchicine	T50.4x1	T50.4x2	T50.4x3	T50.4x4	T50.4x5	T50.4x6
Colchicum	T62.2x1	T62.2x2	T62.2x3	T62.2x4	—	—
Cold cream	T49.3x1	T49.3x2	T49.3x3	T49.3x4	T49.3x5	T49.3x6
Colecalciferol	T45.2x1	T45.2x2	T45.2x3	T45.2x4	T45.2x5	T45.2x6
Colestipol	T46.6x1	T46.6x2	T46.6x3	T46.6x4	T46.6x5	T46.6x6
Colestyramine	T46.6x1	T46.6x2	T46.6x3	T46.6x4	T46.6x5	T46.6x6
Colimycin	T36.8x1	T36.8x2	T36.8x3	T36.8x4	T36.8x5	T36.8x6
Colistimethate	T36.8x1	T36.8x2	T36.8x3	T36.8x4	T36.8x5	T36.8x6
Colistin	T36.8x1	T36.8x2	T36.8x3	T36.8x4	T36.8x5	T36.8x6
sulfate (eye preparation)	T49.5x1	T49.5x2	T49.5x3	T49.5x4	T49.5x5	T49.5x6
Collagen	T50.991	T50.992	T50.993	T50.994	T50.995	T50.996
Collagenase	T49.4x1	T49.4x2	T49.4x3	T49.4x4	T49.4x5	T49.4x6
Collodion	T49.3x1	T49.3x2	T49.3x3	T49.3x4	T49.3x5	T49.3x6
Colocynth	T47.2x1	T47.2x2	T47.2x3	T47.2x4	T47.2x5	T47.2x6
Colophony adhesive	T49.3x1	T49.3x2	T49.3x3	T49.3x4	T49.3x5	T49.3x6
Colorant — see also Dye	T50.991	T50.992	T50.993	T50.994	T50.995	T50.996
Coloring matter — see Dye(s)						
Combustion gas (after combustion) — see Carbon, monoxide						
prior to combustion	T59.891	T59.892	T59.893	T59.894	—	—
Compazine	T43.3x1	T43.3x2	T43.3x3	T43.3x4	T43.3x5	T43.3x6
Compound						
1080 (sodium fluoroacetate)	T60.4x1	T60.4x2	T60.4x3	T60.4x4	—	—
269 (endrin)	T60.1x1	T60.1x2	T60.1x3	T60.1x4	—	—
497 (dieldrin)	T60.1x1	T60.1x2	T60.1x3	T60.1x4	—	—
3422 (parathion)	T60.0x1	T60.0x2	T60.0x3	T60.0x4	—	—
3911 (phorate)	T60.0x1	T60.0x2	T60.0x3	T60.0x4	—	—
3956 (toxaphene)	T60.1x1	T60.1x2	T60.1x3	T60.1x4	—	—
4049 (malathion)	T60.0x1	T60.0x2	T60.0x3	T60.0x4	—	—
4069 (malathion)	T60.0x1	T60.0x2	T60.0x3	T60.0x4	—	—
4124 (dicapthon)	T60.0x1	T60.0x2	T60.0x3	T60.0x4	—	—
E (cortisone)	T38.0x1	T38.0x2	T38.0x3	T38.0x4	T38.0x5	T38.0x6
F (hydrocortisone)	T38.0x1	T38.0x2	T38.0x3	T38.0x4	T38.0x5	T38.0x6
Congener, anabolic	T38.7x1	T38.7x2	T38.7x3	T38.7x4	T38.7x5	T38.7x6
Congo red	T50.8x1	T50.8x2	T50.8x3	T50.8x4	T50.8x5	T50.8x6
Coniine, conine	T62.2x1	T62.2x2	T62.2x3	T62.2x4	—	—
Conium (maculatum)	T62.2x1	T62.2x2	T62.2x3	T62.2x4	—	—
Conjugated estrogenic substances	T38.5x1	T38.5x2	T38.5x3	T38.5x4	T38.5x5	T38.5x6
Contac	T48.5x1	T48.5x2	T48.5x3	T48.5x4	T48.5x5	T48.5x6
Contact lens solution	T49.5x1	T49.5x2	T49.5x3	T49.5x4	T49.5x5	T49.5x6
Contraceptive (oral)	T38.4x1	T38.4x2	T38.4x3	T38.4x4	T38.4x5	T38.4x6
vaginal	T49.8x1	T49.8x2	T49.8x3	T49.8x4	T49.8x5	T49.8x6
Contrast medium, radiography	T50.8x1	T50.8x2	T50.8x3	T50.8x4	T50.8x5	T50.8x6
Convallaria glycosides	T46.0x1	T46.0x2	T46.0x3	T46.0x4	T46.0x5	T46.0x6
Convallaria majalis	T62.2x1	T62.2x2	T62.2x3	T62.2x4	—	—
berry	T62.1x1	T62.1x2	T62.1x3	T62.1x4	—	—
Copper (dust) (fumes) (nonmedicinal) NEC	T56.4x1	T56.4x2	T56.4x3	T56.4x4	—	—
arsenate, arsenite	T57.0x1	T57.0x2	T57.0x3	T57.0x4	—	—
insecticide	T60.2x1	T60.2x2	T60.2x3	T60.2x4	—	—
emetic	T47.7x1	T47.7x2	T47.7x3	T47.7x4	T47.7x5	T47.7x6
fungicide	T60.3x1	T60.3x2	T60.3x3	T60.3x4	—	—
gluconate	T49.0x1	T49.0x2	T49.0x3	T49.0x4	T49.0x5	T49.0x6
insecticide	T60.2x1	T60.2x2	T60.2x3	T60.2x4	—	—
medicinal (trace)	T45.8x1	T45.8x2	T45.8x3	T45.8x4	T45.8x5	T45.8x6
oleate	T49.0x1	T49.0x2	T49.0x3	T49.0x4	T49.0x5	T49.0x6
sulfate	T56.4x1	T56.4x2	T56.4x3	T56.4x4	—	—
cupric	T56.4x1	T56.4x2	T56.4x3	T56.4x4	—	—
fungicide	T60.3x1	T60.3x2	T60.3x3	T60.3x4	—	—
medicinal ear	T49.6x1	T49.6x2	T49.6x3	T49.6x4	T49.6x5	T49.6x6
emetic	T47.7x1	T47.7x2	T47.7x3	T47.7x4	T47.7x5	T47.7x6
eye	T49.5x1	T49.5x2	T49.5x3	T49.5x4	T49.5x5	T49.5x6
cuprous	T56.4x1	T56.4x2	T56.4x3	T56.4x4	—	—
fungicide	T60.3x1	T60.3x2	T60.3x3	T60.3x4	—	—
medicinal ear	T49.6x1	T49.6x2	T49.6x3	T49.6x4	T49.6x5	T49.6x6
emetic	T47.7x1	T47.7x2	T47.7x3	T47.7x4	T47.7x5	T47.7x6
eye	T49.5x1	T49.5x2	T49.5x3	T49.5x4	T49.5x5	T49.5x6
Copperhead snake (bite) (venom)	T63.061	T63.062	T63.063	T63.064		
Coral (sting)	T63.691	T63.692	T63.693	T63.694	—	—
snake (bite) (venom)	T63.021	T63.022	T63.023	T63.024		
Corbadrine	T49.6x1	T49.6x2	T49.6x3	T49.6x4	T49.6x5	T49.6x6
Cordite	T65.891	T65.892	T65.893	T65.894	—	—
vapor	T59.891	T59.892	T59.893	T59.894		
Cordran	T49.0x1	T49.0x2	T49.0x3	T49.0x4	T49.0x5	T49.0x6
Corn cures	T49.4x1	T49.4x2	T49.4x3	T49.4x4	T49.4x5	T49.4x6
Corn starch	T49.3x1	T49.3x2	T49.3x3	T49.3x4	T49.3x5	T49.3x6
Cornhusker's lotion	T49.3x1	T49.3x2	T49.3x3	T49.3x4	T49.3x5	T49.3x6
Coronary vasodilator NEC	T46.3x1	T46.3x2	T46.3.93	T46.3x4	T46.3x5	T46.3x6
Corrosive NEC	T54.91	T54.92	T54.93	T54.94	—	—
acid NEC	T54.2x1	T54.2x2	T54.2x3	T54.2x4	—	—
aromatics	T54.1x1	T54.1x2	T54.1x3	T54.1x4	—	—
disinfectant	T54.1x1	T54.1x2	T54.1x3	T54.1x4	—	—
fumes NEC	T54.91	T54.92	T54.93	T54.94	—	—
specified NEC	T54.91	T54.92	T54.93	T54.94	—	—
sublimate	T56.1x1	T56.1x2	T56.1x3	T56.1x4	—	—
Cortate	T38.0x1	T38.0x2	T38.0x3	T38.0x4	T38.0x5	T38.0x6
Cort-Dome	T38.0x1	T38.0x2	T38.0x3	T38.0x4	T38.0x5	T38.0x6
ENT agent	T49.6x1	T49.6x2	T49.6x3	T49.6x4	T49.6x5	T49.6x6
ophthalmic preparation	T49.5x1	T49.5x2	T49.5x3	T49.5x4	T49.5x5	T49.5x6
topical NEC	T49.0x1	T49.0x2	T49.0x3	T49.0x4	T49.0x5	T49.0x6
Cortef	T38.0x1	T38.0x2	T38.0x3	T38.0x4	T38.0x5	T38.0x6
ENT agent	T49.6x1	T49.6x2	T49.6x3	T49.6x4	T49.6x5	T49.6x6
ophthalmic preparation	T49.5x1	T49.5x2	T49.5x3	T49.5x4	T49.5x5	T49.5x6
topical NEC	T49.0x1	T49.0x2	T49.0x3	T49.0x4	T49.0x5	T49.0x6
Corticosteroid	T38.0x1	T38.0x2	T38.0x3	T38.0x4	T38.0x5	T38.0x6
ENT agent	T49.6x1	T49.6x2	T49.6x3	T49.6x4	T49.6x5	T49.6x6
mineral	T50.0x1	T50.0x2	T50.0x3	T50.0x4	T50.0x5	T50.0x6
ophthalmic	T49.5x1	T49.5x2	T49.5x3	T49.5x4	T49.5x5	T49.5x6
topical NEC	T49.0x1	T49.0x2	T49.0x3	T49.0x4	T49.0x5	T49.0x6
Corticotropin	T38.811	T38.812	T38.813	T38.814	T38.815	T38.816
Cortisol	T38.0x1	T38.0x2	T38.0x3	T38.0x4	T38.0x5	T38.0x6
ENT agent	T49.6x1	T49.6x2	T49.6x3	T49.6x4	T49.6x5	T49.6x6
ophthalmic preparation	T49.5x1	T49.5x2	T49.5x3	T49.5x4	T49.5x5	T49.5x6
topical NEC	T49.0x1	T49.0x2	T49.0x3	T49.0x4	T49.0x5	T49.0x6
Cortisone (acetate)	T38.0x1	T38.0x2	T38.0x3	T38.0x4	T38.0x5	T38.0x6
ENT agent	T49.6x1	T49.6x2	T49.6x3	T49.6x4	T49.6x5	T49.6x6
ophthalmic preparation	T49.5x1	T49.5x2	T49.5x3	T49.5x4	T49.5x5	T49.5x6
topical NEC	T49.0x1	T49.0x2	T49.0x3	T49.0x4	T49.0x5	T49.0x6
Cortivazol	T38.0x1	T38.0x2	T38.0x3	T38.0x4	T38.0x5	T38.0x6
Cortogen	T38.0x1	T38.0x2	T38.0x3	T38.0x4	T38.0x5	T38.0x6
ENT agent	T49.6x1	T49.6x2	T49.6x3	T49.6x4	T49.6x5	T49.6x6
ophthalmic preparation	T49.5x1	T49.5x2	T49.5x3	T49.5x4	T49.5x5	T49.5x6

DRUGS & CHEMICALS

Table of Drugs & Chemicals	POISONING Accidental (Unintentional)	Self-Harm (Intentional)	Assault	Undetermined	Adverse Effect	Underdosing
Cortone	T38.0x1	T38.0x2	T38.0x3	T38.0x4	T38.0x5	T38.0x6
ENT agent	T49.6x1	T49.6x2	T49.6x3	T49.6x4	T49.6x5	T49.6x6
ophthalmic preparation	T49.5x1	T49.5x2	T49.5x3	T49.5x4	T49.5x5	T49.5x6
Cortril	T38.0x1	T38.0x2	T38.0x3	T38.0x4	T38.0x5	T38.0x6
ENT agent	T49.6x1	T49.6x2	T49.6x3	T49.6x4	T49.6x5	T49.6x6
ophthalmic preparation	T49.5x1	T49.5x2	T49.5x3	T49.5x4	T49.5x5	T49.5x6
topical NEC	T49.0x1	T49.0x2	T49.0x3	T49.0x4	T49.0x5	T49.0x6
Corynebacterium parvum	T45.1x1	T45.1x2	T45.1x3	T45.1x4	T45.1x5	T45.1x6
Cosmetic preparation	T49.8x1	T49.8x2	T49.8x3	T49.8x4	T49.8x5	T49.8x6
Cosmetics	T49.8x1	T49.8x2	T49.8x3	T49.8x4	T49.8x5	T49.8x6
Cosyntropin	T38.811	T38.812	T38.813	T38.814	T38.815	T38.816
Cotarnine	T45.7x1	T45.7x2	T45.7x3	T45.7x4	T45.7x5	T45.7x6
Co-trimoxazole	T36.8x1	T36.8x2	T36.8x3	T36.8x4	T36.8x5	T36.8x6
Cottonseed oil	T49.3x1	T49.3x2	T49.3x3	T49.3x4	T49.3x5	T49.3x6
Cough mixture (syrup)	T48.4x1	T48.4x2	T48.4x3	T48.4x4	T48.4x5	T48.4x6
containing opiates	T40.2x1	T40.2x2	T40.2x3	T40.2x4	T40.2x5	T40.2x6
expectorants	T48.4x1	T48.4x2	T48.4x3	T48.4x4	T48.4x5	T48.4x6
Coumadin	T45.511	T45.512	T45.513	T45.514	T45.515	T45.516
rodenticide	T60.4x1	T60.4x2	T60.4x3	T60.4x4	—	—
Coumaphos	T60.0x1	T60.0x2	T60.0x3	T60.0x4	—	—
Coumarin	T45.511	T45.512	T45.513	T45.514	T45.515	T45.516
Coumetarol	T45.511	T45.512	T45.513	T45.514	T45.515	T45.516
Cowbane	T62.2x1	T62.2x2	T62.2x3	T62.2x4	—	—
Cozyme	T45.2x1	T45.2x2	T45.2x3	T45.2x4	T45.2x5	T45.2x6
Crack	T40.5x1	T40.5x2	T40.5x3	T40.5x4	—	—
Crataegus extract	T46.0x1	T46.0x2	T46.0x3	T46.0x4	T46.0x5	T46.0x6
Creolin	T54.1x1	T54.1x2	T54.1x3	T54.1x4	—	—
disinfectant	T54.1x1	T54.1x2	T54.1x3	T54.1x4	—	—
Creosol (compound)	T49.0x1	T49.0x2	T49.0x3	T49.0x4	T49.0x5	T49.0x6
Creosote (coal tar) (beechwood)	T49.0x1	T49.0x2	T49.0x3	T49.0x4	T49.0x5	T49.0x6
medicinal (expectorant)	T48.4x1	T48.4x2	T48.4x3	T48.4x4	T48.4x5	T48.4x6
syrup	T48.4x1	T48.4x2	T48.4x3	T48.4x4	T48.4x5	T48.4x6
Cresol(s)	T49.0x1	T49.0x2	T49.0x3	T49.0x4	T49.0x5	T49.0x6
and soap solution	T49.0x1	T49.0x2	T49.0x3	T49.0x4	T49.0x5	T49.0x6
Cresyl acetate	T49.0x1	T49.0x2	T49.0x3	T49.0x4	T49.0x5	T49.0x6
Cresylic acid	T49.0x1	T49.0x2	T49.0x3	T49.0x4	T49.0x5	T49.0x6
Crimidine	T60.4x1	T60.4x2	T60.4x3	T60.4x4	—	—
Croconazole	T37.8x1	T37.8x2	T37.8x3	T37.8x4	T37.8x5	T37.8x6
Cromoglicic acid	T48.6x1	T48.6x2	T48.6x3	T48.6x4	T48.6x5	T48.6x6
Cromolyn	T48.6x1	T48.6x2	T48.6x3	T48.6x4	T48.6x5	T48.6x6
Cromonar	T46.3x1	T46.3x2	T46.3x3	T46.3x4	T46.3x5	T46.3x6
Cropropamide	T39.8x1	T39.8x2	T39.8x3	T39.8x4	T39.8x5	T39.8x6
with crotethamide	T50.7x1	T50.7x2	T50.7x3	T50.7x4	T50.7x5	T50.7x6
Crotamiton	T49.0x1	T49.0x2	T49.0x3	T49.0x4	T49.0x5	T49.0x6
Crotethamide	T39.8x1	T39.8x2	T39.8x3	T39.8x4	T39.8x5	T39.8x6
with cropropamide	T50.7x1	T50.7x2	T50.7x3	T50.7x4	T50.7x5	T50.7x6
Croton (oil)	T47.2x1	T47.2x2	T47.2x3	T47.2x4	T47.2x5	T47.2x6
chloral	T42.6x1	T42.6x2	T42.6x3	T42.6x4	T42.6x5	T42.6x6
Crude oil	T52.0x1	T52.0x2	T52.0x3	T52.0x4	—	—
Cryogenine	T39.8x1	T39.8x2	T39.8x3	T39.8x4	T39.8x5	T39.8x6
Cryolite (vapor)	T60.1x1	T60.1x2	T60.1x3	T60.1x4	—	—
insecticide	T60.1x1	T60.1x2	T60.1x3	T60.1x4	—	—
Cryptenamine (tannates)	T46.5x1	T46.5x2	T46.5x3	T46.5x4	T46.5x5	T46.5x6
Crystal violet	T49.0x1	T49.0x2	T49.0x3	T49.0x4	T49.0x5	T49.0x6
Cuckoopint	T62.2x1	T62.2x2	T62.2x3	T62.2x4	—	—
Cumetharol	T45.511	T45.512	T45.513	T45.514	T45.515	T45.516
Cupric						
acetate	T60.3x1	T60.3x2	T60.3x3	T60.3x4	—	—
acetoarsenite	T57.0x1	T57.0x2	T57.0x3	T57.0x4	—	—
arsenate	T57.0x1	T57.0x2	T57.0x3	T57.0x4	—	—
gluconate	T49.0x1	T49.0x2	T49.0x3	T49.0x4	T49.0x5	T49.0x6
oleate	T49.0x1	T49.0x2	T49.0x3	T49.0x4	T49.0x5	T49.0x6
sulfate	T56.4x1	T56.4x2	T56.4x3	T56.4x4	—	—
Cuprous sulfate — see also						
Copper sulfate	T56.4x1	T56.4x2	T56.4x3	T56.4x4	—	—
Curare, curarine	T48.1x1	T48.1x2	T48.1x3	T48.1x4	T48.1x5	T48.1x6
Cyamemazine	T43.3x1	T43.3x2	T43.3x3	T43.3x4	T43.3x5	T43.3x6
Cyamopsis tetragono-loba	T46.6x1	T46.6x2	T46.6x3	T46.6x4	T46.6x5	T46.6x6

Table of Drugs & Chemicals	POISONING Accidental (Unintentional)	Self-Harm (Intentional)	Assault	Undetermined	Adverse Effect	Underdosing
Cyanacetyl hydrazide	T37.1x1	T37.1x2	T37.1x3	T37.1x4	T37.1x5	T37.1x6
Cyanic acid (gas)	T59.891	T59.892	T59.893	T59.894	—	—
Cyanide (s) (compounds)						
(potassium) (sodium) NEC	T65.0x1	T65.0x2	T65.0x3	T65.0x4	—	—
dust or gas (inhalation) NEC	T57.3x1	T57.3x2	T57.3x3	T57.3x4	—	—
fumigant	T65.0x1	T65.0x2	T65.0x3	T65.0x4	—	—
hydrogen	T57.3x1	T57.3x2	T57.3x3	T57.3x4	—	—
mercuric — see Mercury						
pesticide (dust) (fumes)	T65.0x1	T65.0x2	T65.0x3	T65.0x4	—	—
Cyanoacrylate adhesive	T49.3x1	T49.3x2	T49.3x3	T49.3x4	T49.3x5	T49.3x6
Cyanocobalamin	T45.8x1	T45.8x2	T45.8x3	T45.8x4	T45.8x5	T45.8x6
Cyanogen (chloride) (gas) NEC	T59.891	T59.892	T59.893	T59.894	—	—
Cyclacillin	T36.0x1	T36.0x2	T36.0x3	T36.0x4	T36.0x5	T36.0x6
Cyclaine	T41.3x1	T41.3x2	T41.3x3	T41.3x4	T41.3x5	T41.3x6
Cyclamate	T50.991	T50.992	T50.993	T50.994	T50.995	T50.996
Cyclamen europaeum	T62.2x1	T62.2x2	T62.2x3	T62.2x4	—	—
Cyclandelate	T46.7x1	T46.7x2	T46.7x3	T46.7x4	T46.7x5	T46.7x6
Cyclazocine	T50.7x1	T50.7x2	T50.7x3	T50.7x4	T50.7x5	T50.7x6
Cyclizine	T45.0x1	T45.0x2	T45.0x3	T45.0x4	T45.0x5	T45.0x6
Cyclobarbital	T42.3x1	T42.3x2	T42.3x3	T42.3x4	T42.3x5	T42.3x6
Cyclobarbitone	T42.3x1	T42.3x2	T42.3x3	T42.3x4	T42.3x5	T42.3x6
Cyclobenzaprine	T48.1x1	T48.1x2	T48.1x3	T48.1x4	T48.1x5	T48.1x6
Cyclodrine	T44.3x1	T44.3x2	T44.3x3	T44.3x4	T44.3x5	T44.3x6
Cycloguanil embonate	T37.2x1	T37.2x2	T37.2x3	T37.2x4	T37.2x5	T37.2x6
Cyclohexane	T52.8x1	T52.8x2	T52.8x3	T52.8x4	—	—
Cyclohexanol	T51.8x1	T51.8x2	T51.8x3	T51.8x4	—	—
Cyclohexanone	T52.4x1	T52.4x2	T52.4x3	T52.4x4	—	—
Cycloheximide	T60.3x1	T60.3x2	T60.3x3	T60.3x4	—	—
Cyclohexyl acetate	T52.8x1	T52.8x2	T52.8x3	T52.8x4	—	—
Cycloleucin	T45.1x1	T45.1x2	T45.1x3	T45.1x4	T45.1x5	T45.1x6
Cyclomethycaine	T41.3x1	T41.3x2	T41.3x3	T41.3x4	T41.3x5	T41.3x6
Cyclopentamine	T44.4x1	T44.4x2	T44.4x3	T44.4x4	T44.4x5	T44.4x6
Cyclopenthiazide	T50.2x1	T50.2x2	T50.2x3	T50.2x4	T50.2x5	T50.2x6
Cyclopentolate	T44.3x1	T44.3x2	T44.3x3	T44.3x4	T44.3x5	T44.3x6
Cyclophosphamide	T45.1x1	T45.1x2	T45.1x3	T45.1x4	T45.1x5	T45.1x6
Cycloplegic drug	T49.5x1	T49.5x2	T49.5x3	T49.5x4	T49.5x5	T49.5x6
Cyclopropane	T41.291	T41.292	T41.293	T41.294	T41.295	T41.296
Cyclopyrabital	T39.8x1	T39.8x2	T39.8x3	T39.8x4	T39.8x5	T39.8x6
Cycloserine	T37.1x1	T37.1x2	T37.1x3	T37.1x4	T37.1x5	T37.1x6
Cyclosporin	T45.1x1	T45.1x2	T45.1x3	T45.1x4	T45.1x5	T45.1x6
Cyclothiazide	T50.2x1	T50.2x2	T50.2x3	T50.2x4	T50.2x5	T50.2x6
Cycrimine	T44.3x1	T44.3x2	T44.3x3	T44.3x4	T44.3x5	T44.3x6
Cyhalothrin	T60.1x1	T60.1x2	T60.1x3	T60.1x4	—	—
Cymarin	T46.0x1	T46.0x2	T46.0x3	T46.0x4	T46.0x5	T46.0x6
Cypermethrin	T60.1x1	T60.1x2	T60.1x3	T60.1x4	—	—
Cyphenothrin	T60.2x1	T60.2x2	T60.2x3	T60.2x4	—	—
Cyproheptadine	T45.0x1	T45.0x2	T45.0x3	T45.0x4	T45.0x5	T45.0x6
Cyproterone	T38.6x1	T38.6x2	T38.6x3	T38.6x4	T38.6x5	T38.6x6
Cysteamine	T50.6x1	T50.6x2	T50.6x3	T50.6x4	T50.6x5	T50.6x6
Cytarabine	T45.1x1	T45.1x2	T45.1x3	T45.1x4	T45.1x5	T45.1x6
Cytisus						
laburnum	T62.2x1	T62.2x2	T62.2x3	T62.2x4	—	—
scoparius	T62.2x1	T62.2x2	T62.2x3	T62.2x4	—	—
Cytochrome C	T47.5x1	T47.5x2	T47.5x3	T47.5x4	T47.5x5	T47.5x6
Cytomel	T38.1x1	T38.1x2	T38.1x3	T38.1x4	T38.1x5	T38.1x6
Cytosine arabinoside	T45.1x1	T45.1x2	T45.1x3	T45.1x4	T45.1x5	T45.1x6
Cytoxan	T45.1x1	T45.1x2	T45.1x3	T45.1x4	T45.1x5	T45.1x6
Cytozyme	T45.7x1	T45.7x2	T45.7x3	T45.7x4	T45.7x5	T45.7x6
2,4-D	T60.3x1	T60.3x2	T60.3x3	T60.3x4	—	—
Dacarbazine	T45.1x1	T45.1x2	T45.1x3	T45.1x4	T45.1x5	T45.1x6
Dactinomycin	T45.1x1	T45.1x2	T45.1x3	T45.1x4	T45.1x5	T45.1x6
DADPS	T37.1x1	T37.1x2	T37.1x3	T37.1x4	T37.1x5	T37.1x6
Dakin's solution	T49.0x1	T49.0x2	T49.0x3	T49.0x4	T49.0x5	T49.0x6
Dalapon (sodium)	T60.3x1	T60.3x2	T60.3x3	T60.3x4	—	—
Dalmane	T42.4x1	T42.4x2	T42.4x3	T42.4x4	T42.4x5	T42.4x6
Danazol	T38.6x1	T38.6x2	T38.6x3	T38.6x4	T38.6x5	T38.6x6
Danilone	T45.511	T45.512	T45.513	T45.514	T45.515	T45.516
Danthron	T47.2x1	T47.2x2	T47.2x3	T47.2x4	T47.2x5	T47.2x6

DRUGS&CHEMICALS

Table of Drugs & Chemicals	POISONING Accidental (Unintentional)	POISONING Self-Harm (Intentional)	POISONING Assault	POISONING Undetermined	Adverse Effect	Underdosing
Dantrolene	T42.8x1	T42.8x2	T42.8x3	T42.8x4	T42.8x5	T42.8x6
Dantron	T47.2x1	T47.2x2	T47.2x3	T47.2x4	T47.2x5	T47.2x6
Daphne (gnidium) (mezereum)	T62.2x1	T62.2x2	T62.2x3	T62.2x4	—	—
berry	T62.1x1	T62.1x2	T62.1x3	T62.1x4	—	—
Dapsone	T37.1x1	T37.1x2	T37.1x3	T37.1x4	T37.1x5	T37.1x6
Daraprim	T37.2x1	T37.2x2	T37.2x3	T37.2x4	T37.2x5	T37.2x6
Darnel	T62.2x1	T62.2x2	T62.2x3	T62.2x4		
Darvon	T39.8x1	T39.8x2	T39.8x3	T39.8x4	T39.8x5	T39.8x6
Daunomycin	T45.1x1	T45.1x2	T45.1x3	T45.1x4	T45.1x5	T45.1x6
Daunorubicin	T45.1x1	T45.1x2	T45.1x3	T45.1x4	T45.1x5	T45.1x6
DBI	T38.3x1	T38.3x2	T38.3x3	T38.3x4	T38.3x5	T38.3x6
D-Con	T60.91	T60.92	T60.93	T60.94	—	—
insecticide	T60.2x1	T60.2x2	T60.2x3	T60.2x4	—	—
rodenticide	T60.4x1	T60.4x2	T60.4x3	T60.4x4	—	—
DDAVP	T38.891	T38.892	T38.893	T38.894	T38.895	T38.896
DDE (bis(chlorophenyl)-dichloroethylene)	T60.2x1	T60.2x2	T60.2x3	T60.2x4	—	—
DDS	T37.1x1	T37.1x2	T37.1x3	T37.1x4	T37.1x5	T37.1x6
DDT (dust)	T60.1x1	T60.1x2	T60.1x3	T60.1x4		
Deadly nightshade — see also Belladonna	T62.2x1	T62.2x2	T62.2x3	T62.2x4		
berry	T62.1x1	T62.1x2	T62.1x3	T62.1x4		
Deamino-D-arginine vasopressin	T38.891	T38.892	T38.893	T38.894	T38.895	T38.896
Deanol (aceglumate)	T50.991	T50.992	T50.993	T50.994	T50.995	T50.996
Debrisoquine	T46.5x1	T46.5x2	T46.5x3	T46.5x4	T46.5x5	T46.5x6
Decaborane	T57.8x1	T57.8x2	T57.8x3	T57.8x4		
fumes	T59.891	T59.892	T59.893	T59.894		
Decadron	T38.0x1	T38.0x2	T38.0x3	T38.0x4	T38.0x5	T38.0x6
ENT agent	T49.6x1	T49.6x2	T49.6x3	T49.6x4	T49.6x5	T49.6x6
ophthalmic preparation	T49.5x1	T49.5x2	T49.5x3	T49.5x4	T49.5x5	T49.5x6
topical NEC	T49.0x1	T49.0x2	T49.0x3	T49.0x4	T49.0x5	T49.0x6
Decahydronaphthalene	T52.8x1	T52.8x2	T52.8x3	T52.8x4	—	—
Decalin	T52.8x1	T52.8x2	T52.8x3	T52.8x4	—	
Decamethonium (bromide)	T48.1x1	T48.1x2	T48.1x3	T48.1x4	T48.1x5	T48.1x6
Decholin	T47.5x1	T47.5x2	T47.5x3	T47.5x4	T47.5x5	T47.5x6
Declomycin	T36.4x1	T36.4x2	T36.4x3	T36.4x4	T36.4x5	T36.4x6
Decongestant, nasal (mucosa)	T48.5x1	T48.5x2	T48.5x3	T48.5x4	T48.5x5	T48.5x6
combination	T48.5x1	T48.5x2	T48.5x3	T48.5x4	T48.5x5	T48.5x6
Deet	T60.8x1	T60.8x2	T60.8x3	T60.8x4	—	—
Deferoxamine	T45.8x1	T45.8x2	T45.8x3	T45.8x4	T45.8x5	T45.8x6
Deflazacort	T38.0x1	T38.0x2	T38.0x3	T38.0x4	T38.0x5	T38.0x6
Deglycyrrhizinized extract of licorice	T48.4x1	T48.4x2	T48.4x3	T48.4x4	T48.4x5	T48.4x6
Dehydrocholic acid	T47.5x1	T47.5x2	T47.5x3	T47.5x4	T47.5x5	T47.5x6
Dehydroemetine	T37.3x1	T37.3x2	T37.3x3	T37.3x4	T37.3x5	T37.3x6
Dekalin	T52.8x1	T52.8x2	T52.8x3	T52.8x4	—	—
Delalutin	T38.5x1	T38.5x2	T38.5x3	T38.5x4	T38.5x5	T38.5x6
Delorazepam	T42.4x1	T42.4x2	T42.4x3	T42.4x4	T42.4x5	T42.4x6
Delphinium	T62.2x1	T62.2x2	T62.2x3	T62.2x4	—	—
Deltamethrin	T60.1x1	T60.1x2	T60.1x3	T60.1x4		
Deltasone	T38.0x1	T38.0x2	T38.0x3	T38.0x4	T38.0x5	T38.0x6
Deltra	T38.0x1	T38.0x2	T38.0x3	T38.0x4	T38.0x5	T38.0x6
Delvinal	T42.3x1	T42.3x2	T42.3x3	T42.3x4	T42.3x5	T42.3x6
Demecarium (bromide)	T49.5x1	T49.5x2	T49.5x3	T49.5x4	T49.5x5	T49.5x6
Demeclocycline	T36.4x1	T36.4x2	T36.4x3	T36.4x4	T36.4x5	T36.4x6
Demecolcine	T45.1x1	T45.1x2	T45.1x3	T45.1x4	T45.1x5	T45.1x6
Demegestone	T38.5x1	T38.5x2	T38.5x3	T38.5x4	T38.5x5	T38.5x6
Demelanizing agents	T49.8x1	T49.8x2	T49.8x3	T49.8x4	T49.8x5	T49.8x6
Demephion -O and -S	T60.0x1	T60.0x2	T60.0x3	T60.0x4	—	—
Demerol	T40.2x1	T40.2x2	T40.2x3	T40.2x4	T40.2x5	T40.2x6
Demethylchlortetracycline	T36.4x1	T36.4x2	T36.4x3	T36.4x4	T36.4x5	T36.4x6
Demethyltetracycline	T36.4x1	T36.4x2	T36.4x3	T36.4x4	T36.4x5	T36.4x6
Demeton -O and -S	T60.0x1	T60.0x2	T60.0x3	T60.0x4		
Demulcent (external)	T49.3x1	T49.3x2	T49.3x3	T49.3x4	T49.3x5	T49.3x6
specified NEC	T49.3x1	T49.3x2	T49.3x3	T49.3x4	T49.3x5	T49.3x6
Demulen	T38.4x1	T38.4x2	T38.4x3	T38.4x4	T38.4x5	T38.4x6
Denatured alcohol	T51.0x1	T51.0x2	T51.0x3	T51.0x4	—	

Table of Drugs & Chemicals	POISONING Accidental (Unintentional)	POISONING Self-Harm (Intentional)	POISONING Assault	POISONING Undetermined	Adverse Effect	Underdosing
Dendrid	T49.5x1	T49.5x2	T49.5x3	T49.5x4	T49.5x5	T49.5x6
Dental drug, topical application NEC	T49.7x1	T49.7x2	T49.7x3	T49.7x4	T49.7x5	T49.7x6
Dentifrice	T49.7x1	T49.7x2	T49.7x3	T49.7x4	T49.7x5	T49.7x6
Deodorant spray (feminine hygiene)	T49.8x1	T49.8x2	T49.8x3	T49.8x4	T49.8x5	T49.8x6
Deoxycortone	T50.0x1	T50.0x2	T50.0x3	T50.0x4	T50.0x5	T50.0x6
2-Deoxy-5-fluorouridine	T45.1x1	T45.1x2	T45.1x3	T45.1x4	T45.1x5	T45.1x6
5-Deoxy-5-fluorouridine	T45.1x1	T45.1x2	T45.1x3	T45.1x4	T45.1x5	T45.1x6
Deoxyribonuclease (pancreatic)	T45.3x1	T45.3x2	T45.3x3	T45.3x4	T45.3x5	T45.3x6
Depilatory	T49.4x1	T49.4x2	T49.4x3	T49.4x4	T49.4x5	T49.4x6
Deprenalin	T42.8x1	T42.8x2	T42.8x3	T42.8x4	T42.8x5	T42.8x6
Deprenyl	T42.8x1	T42.8x2	T42.8x3	T42.8x4	T42.8x5	T42.8x6
Depressant, appetite	T50.5x1	T50.5x2	T50.5x3	T50.5x4	T50.5x5	T50.5x6
Depressant appetite, central	T50.5x1	T50.5x2	T50.5x3	T50.5x4	T50.5x5	T50.5x6
cardiac	T46.2x1	T46.2x2	T46.2x3	T46.2x4	T46.2x5	T46.2x6
central nervous system (anesthetic) — see also Central nervous system, depressants	T42.71	T42.72	T42.73	T42.74	T42.75	T42.76
general anesthetic	T41.201	T41.202	T41.203	T41.204	T41.205	T41.206
muscle tone	T42.8x1	T42.8x2	T42.8x3	T42.8x4	T42.8x5	T42.8x6
muscle tone, central	T42.8x1	T42.8x2	T42.8x3	T42.8x4	T42.8x5	T42.8x6
psychotherapeutic	T43.501	T43.502	T43.503	T43.504	T43.505	T43.506
Deptropine	T45.0x1	T45.0x2	T45.0x3	T45.0x4	T45.0x5	T45.0x6
Dequalinium (chloride)	T49.0x1	T49.0x2	T49.0x3	T49.0x4	T49.0x5	T49.0x6
Derris root	T60.2x1	T60.2x2	T60.2x3	T60.2x4	—	—
Deserpidine	T46.5x1	T46.5x2	T46.5x3	T46.5x4	T46.5x5	T46.5x6
Desferrioxamine	T45.8x1	T45.8x2	T45.8x3	T45.8x4	T45.8x5	T45.8x6
Desipramine	T43.011	T43.012	T43.013	T43.014	T43.015	T43.016
Deslanoside	T46.0x1	T46.0x2	T46.0x3	T46.0x4	T46.0x5	T46.0x6
Desloughing agent	T49.4x1	T49.4x2	T49.4x3	T49.4x4	T49.4x5	T49.4x6
Desmethylimipramine	T43.011	T43.012	T43.013	T43.014	T43.015	T43.016
Desmopressin	T38.891	T38.892	T38.893	T38.894	T38.895	T38.896
Desocodeine	T40.2x1	T40.2x2	T40.2x3	T40.2x4	T40.2x5	T40.2x6
Desogestrel	T38.5x1	T38.5x2	T38.5x3	T38.5x4	T38.5x5	T38.5x6
Desomorphine	T40.2x1	T40.2x2	T40.2x3	T40.2x4	—	
Desonide	T49.0x1	T49.0x2	T49.0x3	T49.0x4	T49.0x5	T49.0x6
Desoximetasone	T49.0x1	T49.0x2	T49.0x3	T49.0x4	T49.0x5	T49.0x6
Desoxycorticosteroid	T50.0x1	T50.0x2	T50.0x3	T50.0x4	T50.0x5	T50.0x6
Desoxycortone	T50.0x1	T50.0x2	T50.0x3	T50.0x4	T50.0x5	T50.0x6
Desoxyephedrine	T43.621	T43.622	T43.623	T43.624	T43.625	T43.626
Detaxtran	T46.6x1	T46.6x2	T46.6x3	T46.6x4	T46.6x5	T46.6x6
Detergent	T49.2x1	T49.2x2	T49.2x3	T49.2x4	T49.2x5	T49.2x6
external medication	T49.2x1	T49.2x2	T49.2x3	T49.2x4	T49.2x5	T49.2x6
local	T49.2x1	T49.2x2	T49.2x3	T49.2x4	T49.2x5	T49.2x6
medicinal	T49.2x1	T49.2x2	T49.2x3	T49.2x4	T49.2x5	T49.2x6
nonmedicinal	T55.1x1	T55.1x2	T55.1x3	T55.1x4	—	—
specified NEC	T55.1x1	T55.1x2	T55.1x3	T55.1x4	—	—
Deterrent, alcohol	T50.6x1	T50.6x2	T50.6x3	T50.6x4	T50.6x5	T50.6x6
Detoxifying agent	T50.6x1	T50.6x2	T50.6x3	T50.6x4	T50.6x5	T50.6x6
Detrothyronine	T38.1x1	T38.1x2	T38.1x3	T38.1x4	T38.1x5	T38.1x6
Dettol (external medication)	T49.0x1	T49.0x2	T49.0x3	T49.0x4	T49.0x5	T49.0x6
Dexamethasone	T38.0x1	T38.0x2	T38.0x3	T38.0x4	T38.0x5	T38.0x6
ENT agent	T49.6x1	T49.6x2	T49.6x3	T49.6x4	T49.6x5	T49.6x6
ophthalmic preparation	T49.5x1	T49.5x2	T49.5x3	T49.5x4	T49.5x5	T49.5x6
topical NEC	T49.0x1	T49.0x2	T49.0x3	T49.0x4	T49.0x5	T49.0x6
Dexamfetamine	T43.621	T43.622	T43.623	T43.624	T43.625	T43.626
Dexamphetamine	T43.621	T43.622	T43.623	T43.624	T43.625	T43.626
Dexbrompheniramine	T45.0x1	T45.0x2	T45.0x3	T45.0x4	T45.0x5	T45.0x6
Dexchlorpheniramine	T45.0x1	T45.0x2	T45.0x3	T45.0x4	T45.0x5	T45.0x6
Dexedrine	T43.621	T43.622	T43.623	T43.624	T43.625	T43.626
Dexetimide	T44.3x1	T44.3x2	T44.3x3	T44.3x4	T44.3x5	T44.3x6
Dexfenfluramine	T50.5x1	T50.5x2	T50.5x3	T50.5x4	T50.5x5	T50.5x6
Dexpanthenol	T45.2x1	T45.2x2	T45.2x3	T45.2x4	T45.2x5	T45.2x6
Dextran (40) (70) (150)	T45.8x1	T45.8x2	T45.8x3	T45.8x4	T45.8x5	T45.8x6

DRUGS & CHEMICALS

Table of Drugs & Chemicals	POISONING				Adverse Effect	Underdosing
	Accidental (Unintentional)	Self-Harm (Intentional)	Assault	Undetermined		
Dextriferron	T45.4x1	T45.4x2	T45.4x3	T45.4x4	T45.4x5	T45.4x6
Dextro calcium pantothenate	T45.2x1	T45.2x2	T45.2x3	T45.2x4	T45.2x5	T45.2x6
Dextro pantothenyl alcohol	T45.2x1	T45.2x2	T45.2x3	T45.2x4	T45.2x5	T45.2x6
Dextroamphetamine	T43.621	T43.622	T43.623	T43.624	T43.625	T43.626
Dextromethorphan	T48.3x1	T48.3x2	T48.3x3	T48.3x4	T48.3x5	T48.3x6
Dextromoramide	T40.4x1	T40.4x2	T40.4x3	T40.4x4	—	—
topical	T49.8x1	T49.8x2	T49.8x3	T49.8x4	T49.8x5	T49.8x6
Dextropropoxyphene	T40.4x1	T40.4x2	T40.4x3	T40.4x4	T40.4x5	T40.4x6
Dextrorphan	T40.2x1	T40.2x2	T40.2x3	T40.2x4	T40.2x5	T40.2x6
Dextrose	T50.3x1	T50.3x2	T50.3x3	T50.3x4	T50.3x5	T50.3x6
concentrated solution, intravenous	T46.8x1	T46.8x2	T46.8x3	T46.8x4	T46.8x5	T46.8x6
Dextrothyroxin	T38.1x1	T38.1x2	T38.1x3	T38.1x4	T38.1x5	T38.1x6
Dextrothyroxine sodium	T38.1x1	T38.1x2	T38.1x3	T38.1x4	T38.1x5	T38.1x6
DFP	T44.0x1	T44.0x2	T44.0x3	T44.0x4	T44.0x5	T44.0x6
DHE	T37.3x1	T37.3x2	T37.3x3	T37.3x4	T37.3x5	T37.3x6
45	T46.5x1	T46.5x2	T46.5x3	T46.5x4	T46.5x5	T46.5x6
Diabinese	T38.3x1	T38.3x2	T38.3x3	T38.3x4	T38.3x5	T38.3x6
Diacetone alcohol	T52.4x1	T52.4x2	T52.4x3	T52.4x4	—	—
Diacetyl monoxime	T50.991	T50.992	T50.993	T50.994	—	—
Diacetylmorphine	T40.1x1	T40.1x2	T40.1x3	T40.1x4	—	—
Diachylon plaster	T49.4x1	T49.4x2	T49.4x3	T49.4x4	T49.4x5	T49.4x6
Diaethylstilboestrolum	T38.5x1	T38.5x2	T38.5x3	T38.5x4	T38.5x5	T38.5x6
Diagnostic agent NEC	T50.8x1	T50.8x2	T50.8x3	T50.8x4	T50.8x5	T50.8x6
Dial (soap)	T49.2x1	T49.2x2	T49.2x3	T49.2x4	T49.2x5	T49.2x6
sedative	T42.3x1	T42.3x2	T42.3x3	T42.3x4	T42.3x5	T42.3x6
Dialkyl carbonate	T52.91	T52.92	T52.93	T52.94		
Diallylbarbituric acid	T42.3x1	T42.3x2	T42.3x3	T42.3x4	T42.3x5	T42.3x6
Diallymal	T42.3x1	T42.3x2	T42.3x3	T42.3x4	T42.3x5	T42.3x6
Dialysis solution (intraperitoneal)	T50.3x1	T50.3x2	T50.3x3	T50.3x4	T50.3x5	T50.3x6
Diaminodiphenylsulfone	T37.1x1	T37.1x2	T37.1x3	T37.1x4	T37.1x5	T37.1x6
Diamorphine	T40.1x1	T40.1x2	T40.1x3	T40.1x4		
Diamox	T50.2x1	T50.2x2	T50.2x3	T50.2x4	T50.2x5	T50.2x6
Diamthazole	T49.0x1	T49.0x2	T49.0x3	T49.0x4	T49.0x5	T49.0x6
Dianthone	T47.2x1	T47.2x2	T47.2x3	T47.2x4	T47.2x5	T47.2x6
Diaphenylsulfone	T37.0x1	T37.0x2	T37.0x3	T37.0x4	T37.0x5	T37.0x6
Diasone (sodium)	T37.1x1	T37.1x2	T37.1x3	T37.1x4	T37.1x5	T37.1x6
Diastase	T47.5x1	T47.5x2	T47.5x3	T47.5x4	T47.5x5	T47.5x6
Diatrizoate	T50.8x1	T50.8x2	T50.8x3	T50.8x4	T50.8x5	T50.8x6
Diazepam	T42.4x1	T42.4x2	T42.4x3	T42.4x4	T42.4x5	T42.4x6
Diazinon	T60.0x1	T60.0x2	T60.0x3	T60.0x4	—	—
Diazomethane (gas)	T59.891	T59.892	T59.893	T59.894	—	—
Diazoxide	T46.5x1	T46.5x2	T46.5x3	T46.5x4	T46.5x5	T46.5x6
Dibekacin	T36.5x1	T36.5x2	T36.5x3	T36.5x4	T36.5x5	T36.5x6
Dibenamine	T44.6x1	T44.6x2	T44.6x3	T44.6x4	T44.6x5	T44.6x6
Dibenzepin	T43.011	T43.012	T43.013	T43.014	T43.015	T43.016
Dibenzheptropine	T45.0x1	T45.0x2	T45.0x3	T45.0x4	T45.0x5	T45.0x6
Dibenzyline	T44.6x1	T44.6x2	T44.6x3	T44.6x4	T44.6x5	T44.6x6
Diborane (gas)	T59.891	T59.892	T59.893	T59.894	—	—
Dibromochloropropane	T60.8x1	T60.8x2	T60.8x3	T60.8x4	—	—
Dibromodulcitol	T45.1x1	T45.1x2	T45.1x3	T45.1x4	T45.1x5	T45.1x6
Dibromoethane	T53.6x1	T53.6x2	T53.6x3	T53.6x4		
Dibromomannitol	T45.1x1	T45.1x2	T45.1x3	T45.1x4	T45.1x5	T45.1x6
Dibromopropamidine isethionate	T49.0x1	T49.0x2	T49.0x3	T49.0x4	T49.0x5	T49.0x6
Dibrompropamidine	T49.0x1	T49.0x2	T49.0x3	T49.0x4	T49.0x5	T49.0x6
Dibucaine	T41.3x1	T41.3x2	T41.3x3	T41.3x4	T41.3x5	T41.3x6
topical (surface)	T41.3x1	T41.3x2	T41.3x3	T41.3x4	T41.3x5	T41.3x6
Dibunate sodium	T48.3x1	T48.3x2	T48.3x3	T48.3x4	T48.3x5	T48.3x6
Dibutoline sulfate	T44.3x1	T44.3x2	T44.3x3	T44.3x4	T44.3x5	T44.3x6
Dicamba	T60.3x1	T60.3x2	T60.3x3	T60.3x4	—	—
Dicapthon	T60.0x1	T60.0x2	T60.0x3	T60.0x4	—	—
Dichlobenil	T60.3x1	T60.3x2	T60.3x3	T60.3x4	—	—
Dichlone	T60.3x1	T60.3x2	T60.3x3	T60.3x4	—	—
Dichloralphenazone	T42.6x1	T42.6x2	T42.6x3	T42.6x4	T42.6x5	T42.6x6
Dichlorbenzidine	T65.3x1	T65.3x2	T65.3x3	T65.3x4	—	—
Dichlorhydrin	T52.8x1	T52.8x2	T52.8x3	T52.8x4	—	—
Dichlorhydroxyquinoline	T37.8x1	T37.8x2	T37.8x3	T37.8x4	T37.8x5	T37.8x6
Dichlorobenzene	T53.7x1	T53.7x2	T53.7x3	T53.7x4	—	—

Table of Drugs & Chemicals	POISONING				Adverse Effect	Underdosing
	Accidental (Unintentional)	Self-Harm (Intentional)	Assault	Undetermined		
Dichlorobenzyl alcohol	T49.6x1	T49.6x2	T49.6x3	T49.6x4	T49.6x5	T49.6x6
Dichlorodifluoromethane	T53.5x1	T53.5x2	T53.5x3	T53.5x4	—	—
Dichloroethane	T52.8x1	T52.8x2	T52.8x3	T52.8x4	—	—
Sym-Dichloroethyl ether	T53.6x1	T53.6x2	T53.6x3	T53.6x4	—	—
Dichloroethyl sulfide, not in war	T59.891	T59.892	T59.893	T59.894	—	—
Dichloroethylene	T53.6x1	T53.6x2	T53.6x3	T53.6x4	—	—
Dichloroformoxine, not in war	T59.891	T59.892	T59.893	T59.894	—	—
Dichlorohydrin, alpha-dichlorohydrin	T52.8x1	T52.8x2	T52.8x3	T52.8x4	—	—
Dichloromethane (solvent)	T53.4x1	T53.4x2	T53.4x3	T53.4x4	—	—
vapor	T53.4x1	T53.4x2	T53.4x3	T53.4x4	—	—
Dichloronaphthoquinone	T60.3x1	T60.3x2	T60.3x3	T60.3x4	—	—
Dichlorophen	T37.4x1	T37.4x2	T37.4x3	T37.4x4	T37.4x5	T37.4x6
2,4-Dichlorophenoxyacetic acid	T60.3x1	T60.3x2	T60.3x3	T60.3x4	—	—
Dichloropropene	T60.3x1	T60.3x2	T60.3x3	T60.3x4	—	—
Dichloropropionic acid	T60.3x1	T60.3x2	T60.3x3	T60.3x4	—	—
Dichlorphenamide	T50.2x1	T50.2x2	T50.2x3	T50.2x4	T50.2x5	T50.2x6
Dichlorvos	T60.0x1	T60.0x2	T60.0x3	T60.0x4	—	—
Diclofenac	T39.391	T39.392	T39.393	T39.394	T39.395	T39.396
Diclofenamide	T50.2x1	T50.2x2	T50.2x3	T50.2x4	T50.2x5	T50.2x6
Diclofensine	T43.291	T43.292	T43.293	T43.294	T43.295	T43.296
Diclonixine	T39.8x1	T39.8x2	T39.8x3	T39.8x4	T39.8x5	T39.8x6
Dicloxacillin	T36.0x1	T36.0x2	T36.0x3	T36.0x4	T36.0x5	T36.0x6
Dicophane	T49.0x1	T49.0x2	T49.0x3	T49.0x4	T49.0x5	T49.0x6
Dicoumarol, dicoumarin, dicumarol	T45.511	T45.512	T45.513	T45.514	T45.515	T45.516
Dicrotophos	T60.0x1	T60.0x2	T60.0x3	T60.0x4	—	—
Dicyanogen (gas)	T65.0x1	T65.0x2	T65.0x3	T65.0x4	—	—
Dicyclomine	T44.3x1	T44.3x2	T44.3x3	T44.3x4	T44.3x5	T44.3x6
Dicycloverine	T44.3x1	T44.3x2	T44.3x3	T44.3x4	T44.3x5	T44.3x6
Dideoxycytidine	T37.5x1	T37.5x2	T37.5x3	T37.5x4	T37.5x5	T37.5x6
Dideoxyinosine	T37.5x1	T37.5x2	T37.5x3	T37.5x4	T37.5x5	T37.5x6
Dieldrin (vapor)	T60.1x1	T60.1x2	T60.1x3	T60.1x4	—	—
Diemal	T42.3x1	T42.3x2	T42.3x3	T42.3x4	T42.3x5	T42.3x6
Dienestrol	T38.5x1	T38.5x2	T38.5x3	T38.5x4	T38.5x5	T38.5x6
Dienoestrol	T38.5x1	T38.5x2	T38.5x3	T38.5x4	T38.5x5	T38.5x6
Dietetic drug NEC	T50.901	T50.902	T50.903	T50.904	T50.905	T50.906
Diethazine	T42.8x1	T42.8x2	T42.8x3	T42.8x4	T42.8x5	T42.8x6
Diethyl						
barbituric acid	T42.3x1	T42.3x2	T42.3x3	T42.3x4	T42.3x5	T42.3x6
carbamazine	T37.4x1	T37.4x2	T37.4x3	T37.4x4	T37.4x5	T37.4x6
carbinol	T51.3x1	T51.3x2	T51.3x3	T51.3x4	—	—
carbonate	T52.8x1	T52.8x2	T52.8x3	T52.8x4	—	—
ether (vapor) — see also Ether	T41.0x1	T41.0x2	T41.0x3	T41.0x4	T41.0x5	T41.0x6
oxide	T52.8x1	T52.8x2	T52.8x3	T52.8x4	—	—
propion	T50.5x1	T50.5x2	T50.5x3	T50.5x4	T50.5x5	T50.5x6
stilbestrol	T38.5x1	T38.5x2	T38.5x3	T38.5x4	T38.5x5	T38.5x6
toluamide (nonmedicinal)	T60.8x1	T60.8x2	T60.8x3	T60.8x4	—	—
medicinal	T49.3x1	T49.3x2	T49.3x3	T49.3x4	T49.3x5	T49.3x6
Diethylcarbamazine	T37.4x1	T37.4x2	T37.4x3	T37.4x4	T37.4x5	T37.4x6
Diethylene						
dioxide	T52.8x1	T52.8x2	T52.8x3	T52.8x4	—	—
glycol (monoacetate) (monobutyl ether) (monoethyl ether)	T52.3x1	T52.3x2	T52.3x3	T52.3x4	—	—
Diethylhexylphthalate	T65.891	T65.892	T65.893	T65.894	—	—
Diethylpropion	T50.5x1	T50.5x2	T50.5x3	T50.5x4	T50.5x5	T50.5x6
Diethylstilbestrol	T38.5x1	T38.5x2	T38.5x3	T38.5x4	T38.5x5	T38.5x6
Diethylstilboestrol	T38.5x1	T38.5x2	T38.5x3	T38.5x4	T38.5x5	T38.5x6
Diethylsulfone-diethylmethane	T42.6x1	T42.6x2	T42.6x3	T42.6x4	T42.6x5	T42.6x6
Diethyltoluamide	T49.0x1	T49.0x2	T49.0x3	T49.0x4	T49.0x5	T49.0x6
Diethyltryptamine (DET)	T40.991	T40.992	T40.993	T40.994	—	—
Difebarbamate	T42.3x1	T42.3x2	T42.3x3	T42.3x4	T42.3x5	T42.3x6
Difencloxazine	T40.2x1	T40.2x2	T40.2x3	T40.2x4	T40.2x5	T40.2x6
Difenidol	T45.0x1	T45.0x2	T45.0x3	T45.0x4	T45.0x5	T45.0x6
Difenoxin	T47.6x1	T47.6x2	T47.6x3	T47.6x4	T47.6x5	T47.6x6
Difetarsone	T37.3x1	T37.3x2	T37.3x3	T37.3x4	T37.3x5	T37.3x6
Diffusin	T45.3x1	T45.3x2	T45.3x3	T45.3x4	T45.3x5	T45.3x6

Table of Drugs & Chemicals	POISONING				Adverse Effect	Underdosing
	Accidental (Unintentional)	Self-Harm (Intentional)	Assault	Undetermined		
Diflorasone	T49.0x1	T49.0x2	T49.0x3	T49.0x4	T49.0x5	T49.0x6
Diflos	T44.0x1	T44.0x2	T44.0x3	T44.0x4	T44.0x5	T44.0x6
Diflubenzuron	T60.1x1	T60.1x2	T60.1x3	T60.1x4	—	—
Diflucortolone	T49.0x1	T49.0x2	T49.0x3	T49.0x4	T49.0x5	T49.0x6
Diflunisal	T39.091	T39.092	T39.093	T39.094	T39.095	T39.096
Difluoromethyldopa	T42.8x1	T42.8x2	T42.8x3	T42.8x4	T42.8x5	T42.8x6
Difluorophate	T44.0x1	T44.0x2	T44.0x3	T44.0x4	T44.0x5	T44.0x6
Digestant NEC	T47.5x1	T47.5x2	T47.5x3	T47.5x4	T47.5x5	T47.5x6
Digitalin(e)	T46.0x1	T46.0x2	T46.0x3	T46.0x4	T46.0x5	T46.0x6
Digitalis (leaf) (glycoside)	T46.0x1	T46.0x2	T46.0x3	T46.0x4	T46.0x5	T46.0x6
lanata	T46.0x1	T46.0x2	T46.0x3	T46.0x4	T46.0x5	T46.0x6
purpurea	T46.0x1	T46.0x2	T46.0x3	T46.0x4	T46.0x5	T46.0x6
Digitoxin	T46.0x1	T46.0x2	T46.0x3	T46.0x4	T46.0x5	T46.0x6
Digitoxose	T46.0x1	T46.0x2	T46.0x3	T46.0x4	T46.0x5	T46.0x6
Digoxin	T46.0x1	T46.0x2	T46.0x3	T46.0x4	T46.0x5	T46.0x6
Digoxine	T46.0x1	T46.0x2	T46.0x3	T46.0x4	T46.0x5	T46.0x6
Dihydralazine	T46.5x1	T46.5x2	T46.5x3	T46.5x4	T46.5x5	T46.5x6
Dihydrazine	T46.5x1	T46.5x2	T46.5x3	T46.5x4	T46.5x5	T46.5x6
Dihydrocodeine	T40.2x1	T40.2x2	T40.2x3	T40.2x4	T40.2x5	T40.2x6
Dihydrocodein-one	T40.2x1	T40.2x2	T40.2x3	T40.2x4	T40.2x5	T40.2x6
Dihydroergocornine	T46.7x1	T46.7x2	T46.7x3	T46.7x4	T46.7x5	T46.7x6
Dihydroergocristine (mesilate)	T46.7x1	T46.7x2	T46.7x3	T46.7x4	T46.7x5	T46.7x6
Dihydroergokryptine	T46.7x1	T46.7x2	T46.7x3	T46.7x4	T46.7x5	T46.7x6
Dihydroergotamine	T46.5x1	T46.5x2	T46.5x3	T46.5x4	T46.5x5	T46.5x6
Dihydroergotoxine	T46.7x1	T46.7x2	T46.7x3	T46.7x4	T46.7x5	T46.7x6
mesilate	T46.7x1	T46.7x2	T46.7x3	T46.7x4	T46.7x5	T46.7x6
Dihydrohydroxycodein-one	T40.2x1	T40.2x2	T40.2x3	T40.2x4	T40.2x5	T40.2x6
Dihydrohydroxymorphinone	T40.2x1	T40.2x2	T40.2x3	T40.2x4	T40.2x5	T40.2x6
Dihydroisocodeine	T40.2x1	T40.2x2	T40.2x3	T40.2x4	T40.2x5	T40.2x6
Dihydromorphine	T40.2x1	T40.2x2	T40.2x3	T40.2x4	—	—
Dihydromorphinone	T40.2x1	T40.2x2	T40.2x3	T40.2x4	T40.2x5	T40.2x6
Dihydrostreptomycin	T36.5x1	T36.5x2	T36.5x3	T36.5x4	T36.5x5	T36.5x6
Dihydrotachysterol	T45.2x1	T45.2x2	T45.2x3	T45.2x4	T45.2x5	T45.2x6
Dihydroxyaluminum aminoacetate	T47.1x1	T47.1x2	T47.1x3	T47.1x4	T47.1x5	T47.1x6
Dihydroxyaluminum sodium carbonate	T47.1x1	T47.1x2	T47.1x3	T47.1x4	T47.1x5	T47.1x6
Dihydroxyanthraquinone	T47.2x1	T47.2x2	T47.2x3	T47.2x4	T47.2x5	T47.2x6
Dihydroxycodeinone	T40.2x1	T40.2x2	T40.2x3	T40.2x4	T40.2x5	T40.2x6
Dihydroxypropyl theophylline	T50.2x1	T50.2x2	T50.2x3	T50.2x4	T50.2x5	T50.2x6
Diiodohydroxyquin	T37.8x1	T37.8x2	T37.8x3	T37.8x4	T37.8x5	T37.8x6
topical	T49.0x1	T49.0x2	T49.0x3	T49.0x4	T49.0x5	T49.0x6
Diiodohydroxyquinoline	T37.8x1	T37.8x2	T37.8x3	T37.8x4	T37.8x5	T37.8x6
Diiodotyrosine	T38.2x1	T38.2x2	T38.2x3	T38.2x4	T38.2x5	T38.2x6
Diisopromine	T44.3x1	T44.3x2	T44.3x3	T44.3x4	T44.3x5	T44.3x6
Diisopropylamine	T46.3x1	T46.3x2	T46.3x3	T46.3x4	T46.3x5	T46.3x6
Diisopropylfluorophos-phonate	T44.0x1	T44.0x2	T44.0x3	T44.0x4	T44.0x5	T44.0x6
Dilantin	T42.0x1	T42.0x2	T42.0x3	T42.0x4	T42.0x5	T42.0x6
Dilaudid	T40.2x1	T40.2x2	T40.2x3	T40.2x4	T40.2x5	T40.2x6
Dilazep	T46.3x1	T46.3x2	T46.3x3	T46.3x4	T46.3x5	T46.3x6
Dill	T47.5x1	T47.5x2	T47.5x3	T47.5x4	T47.5x5	T47.5x6
Diloxanide	T37.3x1	T37.3x2	T37.3x3	T37.3x4	T37.3x5	T37.3x6
Diltiazem	T46.1x1	T46.1x2	T46.1x3	T46.1x4	T46.1x5	T46.1x6
Dimazole	T49.0x1	T49.0x2	T49.0x3	T49.0x4	T49.0x5	T49.0x6
Dimefline	T50.7x1	T50.7x2	T50.7x3	T50.7x4	T50.7x5	T50.7x6
Dimefox	T60.0x1	T60.0x2	T60.0x3	T60.0x4	—	—
Dimemorfan	T48.3x1	T48.3x2	T48.3x3	T48.3x4	T48.3x5	T48.3x6
Dimenhydrinate	T45.0x1	T45.0x2	T45.0x3	T45.0x4	T45.0x5	T45.0x6
Dimercaprol (British anti-lewisite)	T45.8x1	T45.8x2	T45.8x3	T45.8x4	T45.8x5	T45.8x6
Dimercaptopropanol	T45.8x1	T45.8x2	T45.8x3	T45.8x4	T45.8x5	T45.8x6
Dimestrol	T38.5x1	T38.5x2	T38.5x3	T38.5x4	T38.5x5	T38.5x6
Dimetane	T45.0x1	T45.0x2	T45.0x3	T45.0x4	T45.0x5	T45.0x6
Dimethicone	T47.1x1	T47.1x2	T47.1x3	T47.1x4	T47.1x5	T47.1x6
Dimethindene	T45.0x1	T45.0x2	T45.0x3	T45.0x4	T45.0x5	T45.0x6
Dimethisoquin	T49.1x1	T49.1x2	T49.1x3	T49.1x4	T49.1x5	T49.1x6
Dimethisterone	T38.5x1	T38.5x2	T38.5x3	T38.5x4	T38.5x5	T38.5x6
Dimethoate	T60.0x1	T60.0x2	T60.0x3	T60.0x4	—	—
Dimethocaine	T41.3x1	T41.3x2	T41.3x3	T41.3x4	T41.3x5	T41.3x6
Dimethoxanate	T48.3x1	T48.3x2	T48.3x3	T48.3x4	T48.3x5	T48.3x6

Table of Drugs & Chemicals	POISONING				Adverse Effect	Underdosing
	Accidental (Unintentional)	Self-Harm (Intentional)	Assault	Undetermined		
Dimethyl						
arsine, arsinic acid	T57.0x1	T57.0x2	T57.0x3	T57.0x4	—	—
carbinol	T51.2x1	T51.2x2	T51.2x3	T51.2x4	—	—
carbonate	T52.8x1	T52.8x2	T52.8x3	T52.8x4	—	—
diguanide	T38.3x1	T38.3x2	T38.3x3	T38.3x4	T38.3x5	T38.3x6
ketone	T52.4x1	T52.4x2	T52.4x3	T52.4x4	—	—
vapor	T52.4x1	T52.4x2	T52.4x3	T52.4x4	—	—
meperidine	T40.2x1	T40.2x2	T40.2x3	T40.2x4	T40.2x5	T40.2x6
parathion	T60.0x1	T60.0x2	T60.0x3	T60.0x4	—	—
phthlate	T49.3x1	T49.3x2	T49.3x3	T49.3x4	T49.3x5	T49.3x6
polysiloxane	T47.8x1	T47.8x2	T47.8x3	T47.8x4	T47.8x5	T47.8x6
sulfate (fumes)	T59.891	T59.892	T59.893	T59.894	—	—
liquid	T65.891	T65.892	T65.893	T65.894	—	—
sulfoxide (nonmedicinal)	T52.8x1	T52.8x2	T52.8x3	T52.8x4	—	—
medicinal	T49.4x1	T49.4x2	T49.4x3	T49.4x4	T49.4x5	T49.4x6
tryptamine	T40.991	T40.992	T40.993	T40.994	—	—
tubocurarine	T48.1x1	T48.1x2	T48.1x3	T48.1x4	T48.1x5	T48.1x6
Dimethylamine sulfate	T49.4x1	T49.4x2	T49.4x3	T49.4x4	T49.4x5	T49.4x6
Dimethylformamide	T52.8x1	T52.8x2	T52.8x3	T52.8x4	—	—
Dimethyltubocurarinium chloride	T48.1x1	T48.1x2	T48.1x3	T48.1x4	T48.1x5	T48.1x6
Dimeticone	T47.1x1	T47.1x2	T47.1x3	T47.1x4	T47.1x5	T47.1x6
Dimetilan	T60.0x1	T60.0x2	T60.0x3	T60.0x4	—	—
Dimetindene	T45.0x1	T45.0x2	T45.0x3	T45.0x4	T45.0x5	T45.0x6
Dimetotiazine	T43.3x1	T43.3x2	T43.3x3	T43.3x4	T43.3x5	T43.3x6
Dimorpholamine	T50.7x1	T50.7x2	T50.7x3	T50.7x4	T50.7x5	T50.7x6
Dimoxyline	T46.3x1	T46.3x2	T46.3x3	T46.3x4	T46.3x5	T46.3x6
Dinitro (-ortho-)cresol (pesticide) (spray)	T65.3x1	T65.3x2	T65.3x3	T65.3x4	—	—
Dinitrobenzene	T65.3x1	T65.3x2	T65.3x3	T65.3x4	—	—
vapor	T59.891	T59.892	T59.893	T59.894	—	—
Dinitrobenzol	T65.3x1	T65.3x2	T65.3x3	T65.3x4	—	—
vapor	T59.891	T59.892	T59.893	T59.894	—	—
Dinitrobutylphenol	T65.3x1	T65.3x2	T65.3x3	T65.3x4	—	—
Dinitrocyclohexylphenol	T65.3x1	T65.3x2	T65.3x3	T65.3x4	—	—
Dinitrophenol	T65.3x1	T65.3x2	T65.3x3	T65.3x4	—	—
Dinoprost	T48.0x1	T48.0x2	T48.0x3	T48.0x4	T48.0x5	T48.0x6
Dinoprostone	T48.0x1	T48.0x2	T48.0x3	T48.0x4	T48.0x5	T48.0x6
Dinoseb	T60.3x1	T60.3x2	T60.3x3	T60.3x4	—	—
Dioctyl sulfosuccinate (calcium) (sodium)	T47.4x1	T47.4x2	T47.4x3	T47.4x4	T47.4x5	T47.4x6
Diodone	T50.8x1	T50.8x2	T50.8x3	T50.8x4	T50.8x5	T50.8x6
Diodoquin	T37.8x1	T37.8x2	T37.8x3	T37.8x4	T37.8x5	T37.8x6
Dionin	T40.2x1	T40.2x2	T40.2x3	T40.2x4	T40.2x5	T40.2x6
Diosmin	T46.991	T46.992	T46.993	T46.994	T46.995	T46.996
Dioxane	T52.8x1	T52.8x2	T52.8x3	T52.8x4	—	—
Dioxathion	T60.0x1	T60.0x2	T60.0x3	T60.0x4	—	—
Dioxin	T53.7x1	T53.7x2	T53.7x3	T53.7x4	—	—
Dioxopromethazine	T43.3x1	T43.3x2	T43.3x3	T43.3x4	T43.3x5	T43.3x6
Dioxyline	T46.3x1	T46.3x2	T46.3x3	T46.3x4	T46.3x5	T46.3x6
Dipentene	T52.8x1	T52.8x2	T52.8x3	T52.8x4	—	—
Diperodon	T41.3x1	T41.3x2	T41.3x3	T41.3x4	T41.3x5	T41.3x6
Diphacinone	T60.4x1	T60.4x2	T60.4x3	T60.4x4	—	—
Diphemanil	T44.3x1	T44.3x2	T44.3x3	T44.3x4	T44.3x5	T44.3x6
metilsulfate	T44.3x1	T44.3x2	T44.3x3	T44.3x4	T44.3x5	T44.3x6
Diphenadione	T45.511	T45.512	T45.513	T45.514	T45.515	T45.516
rodenticide	T60.4x1	T60.4x2	T60.4x3	T60.4x4	—	—
Diphenhydramine	T45.0x1	T45.0x2	T45.0x3	T45.0x4	T45.0x5	T45.0x6
Diphenidol	T45.0x1	T45.0x2	T45.0x3	T45.0x4	T45.0x5	T45.0x6
Diphenoxylate	T47.6x1	T47.6x2	T47.6x3	T47.6x4	T47.6x5	T47.6x6
Diphenylamine	T65.3x1	T65.3x2	T65.3x3	T65.3x4	—	—
Diphenylbutazone	T39.2x1	T39.2x2	T39.2x3	T39.2x4	T39.2x5	T39.2x6
Diphenylchloroarsine, not in war	T57.0x1	T57.0x2	T57.0x3	T57.0x4	—	—
Diphenylhydantoin	T42.0x1	T42.0x2	T42.0x3	T42.0x4	T42.0x5	T42.0x6
Diphenylmethane dye	T52.1x1	T52.1x2	T52.1x3	T52.1x4	—	—
Diphenylpyraline	T45.0x1	T45.0x2	T45.0x3	T45.0x4	T45.0x5	T45.0x6

DRUGS&CHEMICALS

Table of Drugs & Chemicals	POISONING Accidental (Unintentional)	Self-Harm (Intentional)	Assault	Undetermined	Adverse Effect	Underdosing
Diphtheria						
antitoxin	T50.Z11	T50.Z12	T50.Z13	T50.Z14	T50.Z15	T50.Z16
toxoid	T50.A91	T50.A92	T50.A93	T50.A94	T50.A95	T50.A96
with tetanus toxoid	T50.A21	T50.A22	T50.A23	T50.A24	T50.A25	T50.A26
with pertussis component	T50.A11	T50.A12	T50.A13	T50.A14	T50.A15	T50.A16
vaccine	T50.A91	T50.A92	T50.A93	T50.A94	T50.A95	T50.A96
combination						
including pertussis	T50.A11	T50.A12	T50.A13	T50.A14	T50.A15	T50.A16
without pertussis	T50.A21	T50.A22	T50.A23	T50.A24	T50.A25	T50.A26
Diphylline	T50.2x1	T50.2x2	T50.2x3	T50.2x4	T50.2x5	T50.2x6
Dipipanone	T40.4x1	T40.4x2	T40.4x3	T40.4x4	—	—
Dipivefrine	T49.5x1	T49.5x2	T49.5x3	T49.5x4	T49.5x5	T49.5x6
Diplovax	T50.B91	T50.B92	T50.B93	T50.B94	T50.B95	T50.B96
Diprophylline	T50.2x1	T50.2x2	T50.2x3	T50.2x4	T50.2x5	T50.2x6
Dipropyline	T48.291	T48.292	T48.293	T48.294	T48.295	T48.296
Dipyridamole	T46.3x1	T46.3x2	T46.3x3	T46.3x4	T46.3x5	T46.3x6
Dipyrone	T39.2x1	T39.2x2	T39.2x3	T39.2x4	T39.2x5	T39.2x6
Diquat (dibromide)	T60.3x1	T60.3x2	T60.3x3	T60.3x4	—	—
Disinfectant	T65.891	T65.892	T65.893	T65.894	—	—
alkaline	T54.3x1	T54.3x2	T54.3x3	T54.3x4	—	—
aromatic	T54.1x1	T54.1x2	T54.1x3	T54.1x4	—	—
intestinal	T37.8x1	T37.8x2	T37.8x3	T37.8x4	T37.8x5	T37.8x6
Disipal	T42.8x1	T42.8x2	T42.8x3	T42.8x4	T42.8x5	T42.8x6
Disodium edetate	T50.6x1	T50.6x2	T50.6x3	T50.6x4	T50.6x5	T50.6x6
Disoprofol	T41.291	T41.292	T41.293	T41.294	T41.295	T41.296
Distigmine (bromide)	T44.0x1	T44.0x2	T44.0x3	T44.0x4	T44.0x5	T44.0x6
Disulfamide	T50.2x1	T50.2x2	T50.2x3	T50.2x4	T50.2x5	T50.2x6
Disulfanilamide	T37.0x1	T37.0x2	T37.0x3	T37.0x4	T37.0x5	T37.0x6
Disulfiram	T50.6x1	T50.6x2	T50.6x3	T50.6x4	T50.6x5	T50.6x6
Disulfoton	T60.0x1	T60.0x2	T60.0x3	T60.0x4	—	—
Dithiazanine iodide	T37.4x1	T37.4x2	T37.4x3	T37.4x4	T37.4x5	T37.4x6
Dithiocarbamate	T60.0x1	T60.0x2	T60.0x3	T60.0x4	—	—
Dithranol	T49.4x1	T49.4x2	T49.4x3	T49.4x4	T49.4x5	T49.4x6
Diucardin	T50.2x1	T50.2x2	T50.2x3	T50.2x4	T50.2x5	T50.2x6
Diupres	T50.2x1	T50.2x2	T50.2x3	T50.2x4	T50.2x5	T50.2x6
Diuretic NEC	T50.2x1	T50.2x2	T50.2x3	T50.2x4	T50.2x5	T50.2x6
benzothiadiazine	T50.2x1	T50.2x2	T50.2x3	T50.2x4	T50.2x5	T50.2x6
carbonic acid anhydrase inhibitors	T50.2x1	T50.2x2	T50.2x3	T50.2x4	T50.2x5	T50.2x6
furfuryl NEC	T50.2x1	T50.2x2	T50.2x3	T50.2x4	T50.2x5	T50.2x6
loop (high-ceiling)	T50.1x1	T50.1x2	T50:1x3	T50.1x4	T50.1x5	T50.1x6
mercurial NEC	T50.2x1	T50.2x2	T50.2x3	T50.2x4	T50.2x5	T50.2x6
osmotic	T50.2x1	T50.2x2	T50.2x3	T50.2x4	T50.2x5	T50.2x6
purine NEC	T50.2x1	T50.2x2	T50.2x3	T50.2x4	T50.2x5	T50.2x6
saluretic NEC	T50.2x1	T50.2x2	T50.2x3	T50.2x4	T50.2x5	T50.2x6
sulfonamide	T50.2x1	T50.2x2	T50.2x3	T50.2x4	T50.2x5	T50.2x6
thiazide NEC	T50.2x1	T50.2x2	T50.2x3	T50.2x4	T50.2x5	T50.2x6
xanthine	T50.2x1	T50.2x2	T50.2x3	T50.2x4	T50.2x5	T50.2x6
Diurgin	T50.2x1	T50.2x2	T50.2x3	T50.2x4	T50.2x5	T50.2x6
Diuril	T50.2x1	T50.2x2	T50.2x3	T50.2x4	T50.2x5	T50.2x6
Diuron	T60.3x1	T60.3x2	T60.3x3	T60.3x4	—	—
Divalproex	T42.6x1	T42.6x2	T42.6x3	T42.6x4	T42.6x5	T42.6x6
Divinyl ether	T41.0x1	T41.0x2	T41.0x3	T41.0x4	T41.0x5	T41.0x6
Dixanthogen	T49.0x1	T49.0x2	T49.0x3	T49.0x4	T49.0x5	T49.0x6
Dixyrazine	T43.3x1	T43.3x2	T43.3x3	T43.3x4	T43.3x5	T43.3x6
D-lysergic acid diethylamide	T40.8x1	T40.8x2	T40.8x3	T40.8x4	—	—
DMCT	T36.4x1	T36.4x2	T36.4x3	T36.4x4	T36.4x5	T36.4x6
DMSO — see Dimethyl sulfoxide						
DNBP	T60.3x1	T60.3x2	T60.3x3	T60.3x4	—	—
DNOC	T65.3x1	T65.3x2	T65.3x3	T65.3x4	—	—
Dobutamine	T44.5x1	T44.5x2	T44.5x3	T44.5x4	T44.5x5	T44.5x6
DOCA	T38.0x1	T38.0x2	T38.0x3	T38.0x4	T38.0x5	T38.0x6
Docusate sodium	T47.4x1	T47.4x2	T47.4x3	T47.4x4	T47.4x5	T47.4x6
Dodicin	T49.0x1	T49.0x2	T49.0x3	T49.0x4	T49.0x5	T49.0x6
Dofamium chloride	T49.0x1	T49.0x2	T49.0x3	T49.0x4	T49.0x5	T49.0x6
Dolophine	T40.3x1	T40.3x2	T40.3x3	T40.3x4	T40.3x5	T40.3x6
Doloxene	T39.8x1	T39.8x2	T39.8x3	T39.8x4	T39.8x5	T39.8x6

Table of Drugs & Chemicals	POISONING Accidental (Unintentional)	Self-Harm (Intentional)	Assault	Undetermined	Adverse Effect	Underdosing
Domestic gas (after combustion)						
— see Gas, utility						
prior to combustion	T59.891	T59.892	T59.893	T59.894		
Domiodol	T48.4x1	T48.4x2	T48.4x3	T48.4x4	T48.4x5	T48.4x6
Domiphen (bromide)	T49.0x1	T49.0x2	T49.0x3	T49.0x4	T49.0x5	T49.0x6
Domperidone	T45.0x1	T45.0x2	T45.0x3	T45.0x4	T45.0x5	T45.0x6
Dopa	T42.8x1	T42.8x2	T42.8x3	T42.8x4	T42.8x5	T42.8x6
Dopamine	T44.991	T44.992	T44.993	T44.994	T44.995	T44.996
Doriden	T42.6x1	T42.6x2	T42.6x3	T42.6x4	T42.6x5	T42.6x6
Dormiral	T42.3x1	T42.3x2	T42.3x3	T42.3x4	T42.3x5	T42.3x6
Dormison	T42.6x1	T42.6x2	T42.6x3	T42.6x4	T42.6x5	T42.6x6
Dornase	T48.4x1	T48.4x2	T48.4x3	T48.4x4	T48.4x5	T48.4x6
Dorsacaine	T41.3x1	T41.3x2	T41.3x3	T41.3x4	T41.3x5	T41.3x6
Dosulepin	T43.011	T43.012	T43.013	T43.014	T43.015	T43.016
Dothiepin	T43.011	T43.012	T43.013	T43.014	T43.015	T43.016
Doxantrazole	T48.6x1	T48.6x2	T48.6x3	T48.6x4	T48.6x5	T48.6x6
Doxapram	T50.7x1	T50.7x2	T50.7x3	T50.7x4	T50.7x5	T50.7x6
Doxazosin	T44.6x1	T44.6x2	T44.6x3	T44.6x4	T44.6x5	T44.6x6
Doxepin	T43.011	T43.012	T43.013	T43.014	T43.015	T43.016
Doxifluridine	T45.1x1	T45.1x2	T45.1x3	T45.1x4	T45.1x5	T45.1x6
Doxorubicin	T45.1x1	T45.1x2	T45.1x3	T45.1x4	T45.1x5	T45.1x6
Doxycycline	T36.4x1	T36.4x2	T36.4x3	T36.4x4	T36.4x5	T36.4x6
Doxylamine	T45.0x1	T45.0x2	T45.0x3	T45.0x4	T45.0x5	T45.0x6
Dramamine	T45.0x1	T45.0x2	T45.0x3	T45.0x4	T45.0x5	T45.0x6
Drano (drain cleaner)	T54.3x1	T54.3x2	T54.3x3	T54.3x4	—	—
Dressing, live pulp	T49.7x1	T49.7x2	T49.7x3	T49.7x4	T49.7x5	T49.7x6
Drocode	T40.2x1	T40.2x2	T40.2x3	T40.2x4	T40.2x5	T40.2x6
Dromoran	T40.2x1	T40.2x2	T40.2x3	T40.2x4	T40.2x5	T40.2x6
Dromostanolone	T38.7x1	T38.7x2	T38.7x3	T38.7x4	T38.7x5	T38.7x6
Dronabinol	T40.7x1	T40.7x2	T40.7x3	T40.7x4	T40.7x5	T40.7x6
Droperidol	T43.591	T43.592	T43.593	T43.594	T43.595	T43.596
Dropropizine	T48.3x1	T48.3x2	T48.3x3	T48.3x4	T48.3x5	T48.3x6
Drostanolone	T38.7x1	T38.7x2	T38.7x3	T38.7x4	T38.7x5	T38.7x6
Drotaverine	T44.3x1	T44.3x2	T44.3x3	T44.3x4	T44.3x5	T44.3x6
Drotrecogin alfa	T45.511	T45.512	T45.513	T45.514	T45.515	T45.516
Drug NEC	T50.901	T50.902	T50.903	T50.904	T50.905	T50.906
specified NEC	T50.991	T50.992	T50.993	T50.994	T50.995	T50.996
DTIC	T45.1x1	T45.1x2	T45.1x3	T45.1x4	T45.1x5	T45.1x6
Duboisine	T44.3x1	T44.3x2	T44.3x3	T44.3x4	T44.3x5	T44.3x6
Dulcolax	T47.2x1	T47.2x2	T47.2x3	T47.2x4	T47.2x5	T47.2x6
Duponol (C) (EP)	T49.2x1	T49.2x2	T49.2x3	T49.2x4	T49.2x5	T49.2x6
Durabolin	T38.7x1	T38.7x2	T38.7x3	T38.7x4	T38.7x5	T38.7x6
Dyclone	T41.3x1	T41.3x2	T41.3x3	T41.3x4	T41.3x5	T41.3x6
Dyclonine	T41.3x1	T41.3x2	T41.3x3	T41.3x4	T41.3x5	T41.3x6
Dydrogesterone	T38.5x1	T38.5x2	T38.5x3	T38.5x4	T38.5x5	T38.5x6
Dye NEC	T65.6x1	T65.6x2	T65.6x3	T65.6x4	—	—
antiseptic	T49.0x1	T49.0x2	T49.0x3	T49.0x4	T49.0x5	T49.0x6
diagnostic agents	T50.8x1	T50.8x2	T50.8x3	T50.8x4	T50.8x5	T50.8x6
pharmaceutical NEC	T50.901	T50.902	T50.903	T50.904	T50.905	T50.906
Dyflos	T44.0x1	T44.0x2	T44.0x3	T44.0x4	T44.0x5	T44.0x6
Dymelor	T38.3x1	T38.3x2	T38.3x3	T38.3x4	T38.3x5	T38.3x6
Dynamite	T65.3x1	T65.3x2	T65.3x3	T65.3x4	—	—
fumes	T59.891	T59.892	T59.893	T59.894	—	—
Dyphylline	T44.3x1	T44.3x2	T44.3x3	T44.3x4	T44.3x5	T44.3x6
Ear drug NEC	T49.6x1	T49.6x2	T49.6x3	T49.6x4	T49.6x5	T49.6x6
Ear preparations	T49.6x1	T49.6x2	T49.6x3	T49.6x4	T49.6x5	T49.6x6
Echothiophate, echothiopate, ecothiopate	T49.5x1	T49.5x2	T49.5x3	T49.5x4	T49.5x5	T49.5x6
Econazole	T49.0x1	T49.0x2	T49.0x3	T49.0x4	T49.0x5	T49.0x6
Ecothiopate iodide	T49.5x1	T49.5x2	T49.5x3	T49.5x4	T49.5x5	T49.5x6
Ecstasy	T43.621	T43.622	T43.623	T43.624	T43.625	T43.626
Ectylurea	T42.6x1	T42.6x2	T42.6x3	T42.6x4	T42.6x5	T42.6x6
Edathamil disodium	T45.8x1	T45.8x2	T45.8x3	T45.8x4	T45.8x5	T45.8x6
Edecrin	T50.1x1	T50.1x2	T50.1x3	T50.1x4	T50.1x5	T50.1x6
Edetate, disodium (calcium)	T45.8x1	T45.8x2	T45.8x3	T45.8x4	T45.8x5	T45.8x6
Edoxudine	T49.5x1	T49.5x2	T49.5x3	T49.5x4	T49.5x5	T49.5x6
Edrophonium	T44.0x1	T44.0x2	T44.0x3	T44.0x4	T44.0x5	T44.0x6
chloride	T44.0x1	T44.0x2	T44.0x3	T44.0x4	T44.0x5	T44.0x6

Table of Drugs & Chemicals	POISONING				Adverse Effect	Underdosing
	Accidental (Unintentional)	Self-Harm (Intentional)	Assault	Undetermined		
EDTA	T50.6x1	T50.6x2	T50.6x3	T50.6x4	T50.6x5	T50.6x6
Eflornithine	T37.2x1	T37.2x2	T37.2x3	T37.2x4	T37.2x5	T37.2x6
Efloxate	T46.3x1	T46.3x2	T46.3x3	T46.3x4	T46.3x5	T46.3x6
Elase	T49.8x1	T49.8x2	T49.8x3	T49.8x4	T49.8x5	T49.8x6
Elastase	T47.5x1	T47.5x2	T47.5x3	T47.5x4	T47.5x5	T47.5x6
Elaterium	T47.2x1	T47.2x2	T47.2x3	T47.2x4	T47.2x5	T47.2x6
Elcatonin	T50.991	T50.992	T50.993	T50.994	T50.995	T50.996
Elder	T62.2x1	T62.2x2	T62.2x3	T62.2x4	—	—
berry, (unripe)	T62.1x1	T62.1x2	T62.1x3	T62.1x4	—	—
Electrolyte balance drug	T50.3x1	T50.3x2	T50.3x3	T50.3x4	T50.3x5	T50.3x6
Electrolytes NEC	T50.3x1	T50.3x2	T50.3x3	T50.3x4	T50.3x5	T50.3x6
Electrolytic agent NEC	T50.3x1	T50.3x2	T50.3x3	T50.3x4	T50.3x5	T50.3x6
Elemental diet	T50.901	T50.902	T50.903	T50.904	T50.905	T50.906
Elliptinium acetate	T45.1x1	T45.1x2	T45.1x3	T45.1x4	T45.1x5	T45.1x6
Embramine	T45.0x1	T45.0x2	T45.0x3	T45.0x4	T45.0x5	T45.0x6
Emepronium (salts)	T44.3x1	T44.3x2	T44.3x3	T44.3x4	T44.3x5	T44.3x6
bromide	T44.3x1	T44.3x2	T44.3x3	T44.3x4	T44.3x5	T44.3x6
Emetic NEC	T47.7x1	T47.7x2	T47.7x3	T47.7x4	T47.7x5	T47.7x6
Emetine	T37.3x1	T37.3x2	T37.3x3	T37.3x4	T37.3x5	T37.3x6
Emollient NEC	T49.3x1	T49.3x2	T49.3x3	T49.3x4	T49.3x5	T49.3x6
Emorfazone	T39.8x1	T39.8x2	T39.8x3	T39.8x4	T39.8x5	T39.8x6
Emylcamate	T43.591	T43.592	T43.593	T43.594	T43.595	T43.596
Enalapril	T46.4x1	T46.4x2	T46.4x3	T46.4x4	T46.4x5	T46.4x6
Enalaprilat	T46.4x1	T46.4x2	T46.4x3	T46.4x4	T46.4x5	T46.4x6
Encainide	T46.2x1	T46.2x2	T46.2x3	T46.2x4	T46.2x5	T46.2x6
Endocaine	T41.3x1	T41.3x2	T41.3x3	T41.3x4	T41.3x5	T41.3x6
Endosulfan	T60.2x1	T60.2x2	T60.2x3	T60.2x4	—	—
Endothall	T60.3x1	T60.3x2	T60.3x3	T60.3x4	—	—
Endralazine	T46.5x1	T46.5x2	T46.5x3	T46.5x4	T46.5x5	T46.5x6
Endrin	T60.1x1	T60.1x2	T60.1x3	T60.1x4	—	—
Enflurane	T41.0x1	T41.0x2	T41.0x3	T41.0x4	T41.0x5	T41.0x6
Enhexymal	T42.3x1	T42.3x2	T42.3x3	T42.3x4	T42.3x5	T42.3x6
Enocitabine	T45.1x1	T45.1x2	T45.1x3	T45.1x4	T45.1x5	T45.1x6
Enovid	T38.4x1	T38.4x2	T38.4x3	T38.4x4	T38.4x5	T38.4x6
Enoxacin	T36.8x1	T36.8x2	T36.8x3	T36.8x4	T36.8x5	T36.8x6
Enoxaparin (sodium)	T45.511	T45.512	T45.513	T45.514	T45.515	T45.516
Enpiprazole	T43.591	T43.592	T43.593	T43.594	T43.595	T43.596
Enprofylline	T48.6x1	T48.6x2	T48.6x3	T48.6x4	T48.6x5	T48.6x6
Enprostil	T47.1x1	T47.1x2	T47.1x3	T47.1x4	T47.1x5	T47.1x6
ENT preparations (anti-infectives)	T49.6x1	T49.6x2	T49.6x3	T49.6x4	T49.6x5	T49.6x6
Enterogastrone	T38.891	T38.892	T38.893	T38.894	T38.895	T38.896
Enviomycin	T36.8x1	T36.8x2	T36.8x3	T36.8x4	T36.8x5	T36.8x6
Enzodase	T45.3x1	T45.3x2	T45.3x3	T45.3x4	T45.3x5	T45.3x6
Enzyme NEC	T45.3x1	T45.3x2	T45.3x3	T45.3x4	T45.3x5	T45.3x6
depolymerizing	T49.8x1	T49.8x2	T49.8x3	T49.8x4	T49.8x5	T49.8x6
fibrolytic	T45.3x1	T45.3x2	T45.3x3	T45.3x4	T45.3x5	T45.3x6
gastric	T47.5x1	T47.5x2	T47.5x3	T47.5x4	T47.5x5	T47.5x6
intestinal	T47.5x1	T47.5x2	T47.5x3	T47.5x4	T47.5x5	T47.5x6
local action	T49.4x1	T49.4x2	T49.4x3	T49.4x4	T49.4x5	T49.4x6
proteolytic	T49.4x1	T49.4x2	T49.4x3	T49.4x4	T49.4x5	T49.4x6
thrombolytic	T45.3x1	T45.3x2	T45.3x3	T45.3x4	T45.3x5	T45.3x6
EPAB	T41.3x1	T41.3x2	T41.3x3	T41.3x4	T41.3x5	T41.3x6
Epanutin	T42.0x1	T42.0x2	T42.0x3	T42.0x4	T42.0x5	T42.0x6
Ephedra	T44.991	T44.992	T44.993	T44.994	T44.995	T44.996
Ephedrine	T44.991	T44.992	T44.993	T44.994	T44.995	T44.996
Epichlorhydrin, epichlorohydrin	T52.8x1	T52.8x2	T52.8x3	T52.8x4	—	—
Epicillin	T36.0x1	T36.0x2	T36.0x3	T36.0x4	T36.0x5	T36.0x6
Epiestriol	T38.5x1	T38.5x2	T38.5x3	T38.5x4	T38.5x5	T38.5x6
Epilim — see Sodium valproate						
Epimestrol	T38.5x1	T38.5x2	T38.5x3	T38.5x4	T38.5x5	T38.5x6
Epinephrine	T44.5x1	T44.5x2	T44.5x3	T44.5x4	T44.5x5	T44.5x6
Epirubicin	T45.1x1	T45.1x2	T45.1x3	T45.1x4	T45.1x5	T45.1x6
Epitiostanol	T38.7x1	T38.7x2	T38.7x3	T38.7x4	T38.7x5	T38.7x6
Epitizide	T50.2x1	T50.2x2	T50.2x3	T50.2x4	T50.2x5	T50.2x6
EPN	T60.0x1	T60.0x2	T60.0x3	T60.0x4	—	—
EPO	T45.8x1	T45.8x2	T45.8x3	T45.8x4	T45.8x5	T45.8x6
Epoetin alpha	T45.8x1	T45.8x2	T45.8x3	T45.8x4	T45.8x5	T45.8x6
Epomediol	T50.991	T50.992	T50.993	T50.994	T50.995	T50.996
Epoprostenol	T45.521	T45.522	T45.523	T45.524	T45.525	T45.526
Epoxy resin	T65.891	T65.892	T65.893	T65.894	—	—
Eprazinone	T48.4x1	T48.4x2	T48.4x3	T48.4x4	T48.4x5	T48.4x6
Epsilon amino-caproic acid	T45.621	T45.622	T45.623	T45.624	T45.625	T45.626
Epsom salt	T47.3x1	T47.3x2	T47.3x3	T47.3x4	T47.3x5	T47.3x6
Eptazocine	T40.4x1	T40.4x2	T40.4x3	T40.4x4	T40.4x5	T40.4x6
Equanil	T43.591	T43.592	T43.593	T43.594	T43.595	T43.596
Equisetum	T62.2x1	T62.2x2	T62.2x3	T62.2x4	—	—
diuretic	T50.2x1	T50.2x2	T50.2x3	T50.2x4	T50.2x5	T50.2x6
Ergobasine	T48.0x1	T48.0x2	T48.0x3	T48.0x4	T48.0x5	T48.0x6
Ergocalciferol	T45.2x1	T45.2x2	T45.2x3	T45.2x4	T45.2x5	T45.2x6
Ergoloid mesylates	T46.7x1	T46.7x2	T46.7x3	T46.7x4	T46.7x5	T46.7x6
Ergometrine	T48.0x1	T48.0x2	T48.0x3	T48.0x4	T48.0x5	T48.0x6
Ergonovine	T48.0x1	T48.0x2	T48.0x3	T48.0x4	T48.0x5	T48.0x6
Ergot NEC	T64.81	T64.82	T64.83	T64.84	—	—
derivative	T48.0x1	T48.0x2	T48.0x3	T48.0x4	T48.0x5	T48.0x6
medicinal (alkaloids)	T48.0x1	T48.0x2	T48.0x3	T48.0x4	T48.0x5	T48.0x6
prepared	T48.0x1	T48.0x2	T48.0x3	T48.0x4	T48.0x5	T48.0x6
Ergotamine	T46.5x1	T46.5x2	T46.5x3	T46.5x4	T46.5x5	T46.5x6
Ergotocine	T48.0x1	T48.0x2	T48.0x3	T48.0x4	T48.0x5	T48.0x6
Ergotrate	T48.0x1	T48.0x2	T48.0x3	T48.0x4	T48.0x5	T48.0x6
Eritrityl tetranitrate	T46.3x1	T46.3x2	T46.3x3	T46.3x4	T46.3x5	T46.3x6
Erythrityl tetranitrate	T46.3x1	T46.3x2	T46.3x3	T46.3x4	T46.3x5	T46.3x6
Erythrol tetranitrate	T46.3x1	T46.3x2	T46.3x3	T46.3x4	T46.3x5	T46.3x6
Erythromycin (salts)	T36.3x1	T36.3x2	T36.3x3	T36.3x4	T36.3x5	T36.3x6
ophthalmic preparation	T49.5x1	T49.5x2	T49.5x3	T49.5x4	T49.5x5	T49.5x6
topical NEC	T49.0x1	T49.0x2	T49.0x3	T49.0x4	T49.0x5	T49.0x6
Erythropoietin	T45.8x1	T45.8x2	T45.8x3	T45.8x4	T45.8x5	T45.8x6
human	T45.8x1	T45.8x2	T45.8x3	T45.8x4	T45.8x5	T45.8x6
Escin	T46.991	T46.992	T46.993	T46.994	T46.995	T46.996
Esculin	T45.2x1	T45.2x2	T45.2x3	T45.2x4	T45.2x5	T45.2x6
Esculoside	T45.2x1	T45.2x2	T45.2x3	T45.2x4	T45.2x5	T45.2x6
ESDT (ether-soluble tar distillate)	T49.1x1	T49.1x2	T49.1x3	T49.1x4	T49.1x5	T49.1x6
Eserine	T49.5x1	T49.5x2	T49.5x3	T49.5x4	T49.5x5	T49.5x6
Esflurbiprofen	T39.311	T39.312	T39.313	T39.314	T39.315	T39.316
Eskabarb	T42.3x1	T42.3x2	T42.3x3	T42.3x4	T42.3x5	T42.3x6
Eskalith	T43.8x1	T43.8x2	T43.8x3	T43.8x4	T43.8x5	T43.8x6
Esmolol	T44.7x1	T44.7x2	T44.7x3	T44.7x4	T44.7x5	T44.7x6
Estanozolol	T38.7x1	T38.7x2	T38.7x3	T38.7x4	T38.7x5	T38.7x6
Estazolam	T42.4x1	T42.4x2	T42.4x3	T42.4x4	T42.4x5	T42.4x6
Estradiol	T38.5x1	T38.5x2	T38.5x3	T38.5x4	T38.5x5	T38.5x6
with testosterone	T38.7x1	T38.7x2	T38.7x3	T38.7x4	T38.7x5	T38.7x6
benzoate	T38.5x1	T38.5x2	T38.5x3	T38.5x4	T38.5x5	T38.5x6
Estramustine	T45.1x1	T45.1x2	T45.1x3	T45.1x4	T45.1x5	T45.1x6
Estriol	T38.5x1	T38.5x2	T38.5x3	T38.5x4	T38.5x5	T38.5x6
Estrogen	T38.5x1	T38.5x2	T38.5x3	T38.5x4	T38.5x5	T38.5x6
with progesterone	T38.5x1	T38.5x2	T38.5x3	T38.5x4	T38.5x5	T38.5x6
conjugated	T38.5x1	T38.5x2	T38.5x3	T38.5x4	T38.5x5	T38.5x6
Estrone	T38.5x1	T38.5x2	T38.5x3	T38.5x4	T38.5x5	T38.5x6
Estropipate	T38.5x1	T38.5x2	T38.5x3	T38.5x4	T38.5x5	T38.5x6
Etacrynate sodium	T50.1x1	T50.1x2	T50.1x3	T50.1x4	T50.1x5	T50.1x6
Etacrynic acid	T50.1x1	T50.1x2	T50.1x3	T50.1x4	T50.1x5	T50.1x6
Etafedrine	T48.6x1	T48.6x2	T48.6x3	T48.6x4	T48.6x5	T48.6x6
Etafenone	T46.3x1	T46.3x2	T46.3x3	T46.3x4	T46.3x5	T46.3x6
Etambutol	T37.1x1	T37.1x2	T37.1x3	T37.1x4	T37.1x5	T37.1x6
Etamiphylline	T48.6x1	T48.6x2	T48.6x3	T48.6x4	T48.6x5	T48.6x6
Etamivan	T50.7x1	T50.7x2	T50.7x3	T50.7x4	T50.7x5	T50.7x6
Etamsylate	T45.7x1	T45.7x2	T45.7x3	T45.7x4	T45.7x5	T45.7x6
Etebenecid	T50.4x1	T50.4x2	T50.4x3	T50.4x4	T50.4x5	T50.4x6
Ethacridine	T49.0x1	T49.0x2	T49.0x3	T49.0x4	T49.0x5	T49.0x6
Ethacrynic acid	T50.1x1	T50.1x2	T50.1x3	T50.1x4	T50.1x5	T50.1x6
Ethadione	T42.2x1	T42.2x2	T42.2x3	T42.2x4	T42.2x5	T42.2x6
Ethambutol	T37.1x1	T37.1x2	T37.1x3	T37.1x4	T37.1x5	T37.1x6
Ethamide	T50.2x1	T50.2x2	T50.2x3	T50.2x4	T50.2x5	T50.2x6
Ethamivan	T50.7x1	T50.7x2	T50.7x3	T50.7x4	T50.7x5	T50.7x6
Ethamsylate	T45.7x1	T45.7x2	T45.7x3	T45.7x4	T45.7x5	T45.7x6
Ethanol	T51.0x1	T51.0x2	T51.0x3	T51.0x4	—	—
beverage	T51.0x1	T51.0x2	T51.0x3	T51.0x4	—	—

DRUGS&CHEMICALS

DRUGS & CHEMICALS

Table of Drugs & Chemicals	POISONING Accidental (Unintentional)	Self-Harm (Intentional)	Assault	Undetermined	Adverse Effect	Underdosing
Ethanolamine oleate	T46.8x1	T46.8x2	T46.8x3	T46.8x4	T46.8x5	T46.8x6
Ethaverine	T44.3x1	T44.3x2	T44.3x3	T44.3x4	T44.3x5	T44.3x6
Ethchlorvynol	T42.6x1	T42.6x2	T42.6x3	T42.6x4	T42.6x5	T42.6x6
Ethebenecid	T50.4x1	T50.4x2	T50.4x3	T50.4x4	T50.4x5	T50.4x6
Ether (vapor)	T41.0x1	T41.0x2	T41.0x3	T41.0x4	T41.0x5	T41.0x6
anesthetic	T41.0x1	T41.0x2	T41.0x3	T41.0x4	T41.0x5	T41.0x6
divinyl	T41.0x1	T41.0x2	T41.0x3	T41.0x4	T41.0x5	T41.0x6
ethyl (medicinal)	T41.0x1	T41.0x2	T41.0x3	T41.0x4	T41.0x5	T41.0x6
nonmedicinal	T52.8x1	T52.8x2	T52.8x3	T52.8x4	—	—
petroleum — see Ligroin						
solvent	T52.8x1	T52.8x2	T52.8x3	T52.8x4	—	—
Ethiazide	T50.2x1	T50.2x2	T50.2x3	T50.2x4	T50.2x5	T50.2x6
Ethidium chloride (vapor)	T59.891	T59.892	T59.893	T59.894	—	—
Ethinamate	T42.6x1	T42.6x2	T42.6x3	T42.6x4	T42.6x5	T42.6x6
Ethinylestradiol, ethinyloestradiol	T38.5x1	T38.5x2	T38.5x3	T38.5x4	T38.5x5	T38.5x6
with						
levonorgestrel	T38.4x1	T38.4x2	T38.4x3	T38.4x4	T38.4x5	T38.4x6
norethisterone	T38.4x1	T38.4x2	T38.4x3	T38.4x4	T38.4x5	T38.4x6
Ethiodized oil (131 I)	T50.8x1	T50.8x2	T50.8x3	T50.8x4	T50.8x5	T50.8x6
Ethion	T60.0x1	T60.0x2	T60.0x3	T60.0x4	—	—
Ethionamide	T37.1x1	T37.1x2	T37.1x3	T37.1x4	T37.1x5	T37.1x6
Ethioniamide	T37.1x1	T37.1x2	T37.1x3	T37.1x4	T37.1x5	T37.1x6
Ethisterone	T38.5x1	T38.5x2	T38.5x3	T38.5x4	T38.5x5	T38.5x6
Ethobral	T42.3x1	T42.3x2	T42.3x3	T42.3x4	T42.3x5	T42.3x6
Ethocaine (infiltration) (topical)	T41.3x1	T41.3x2	T41.3x3	T41.3x4	T41.3x5	T41.3x6
nerve block (peripheral)						
(plexus)	T41.3x1	T41.3x2	T41.3x3	T41.3x4	T41.3x5	T41.3x6
spinal	T41.3x1	T41.3x2	T41.3x3	T41.3x4	T41.3x5	T41.3x6
Ethoheptazine	T40.4x1	T40.4x2	T40.4x3	T40.4x4	T40.4x5	T40.4x6
Ethopropazine	T44.3x1	T44.3x2	T44.3x3	T44.3x4	T44.3x5	T44.3x6
Ethosuximide	T42.2x1	T42.2x2	T42.2x3	T42.2x4	T42.2x5	T42.2x6
Ethotoin	T42.0x1	T42.0x2	T42.0x3	T42.0x4	T42.0x5	T42.0x6
Ethoxazene	T37.91	T37.92	T37.93	T37.94	T37.95	T37.96
Ethoxazorutoside	T46.991	T46.992	T46.993	T46.994	T46.995	T46.996
2-Ethoxyethanol	T52.3x1	T52.3x2	T52.3x3	T52.3x4	—	—
Ethoxzolamide	T50.2x1	T50.2x2	T50.2x3	T50.2x4	T50.2x5	T50.2x6
Ethyl						
acetate	T52.8x1	T52.8x2	T52.8x3	T52.8x4	—	—
alcohol	T51.0x1	T51.0x2	T51.0x3	T51.0x4	—	—
beverage	T51.0x1	T51.0x2	T51.0x3	T51.0x4	—	—
aldehyde (vapor)	T59.891	T59.892	T59.893	T59.894	—	—
liquid	T52.8x1	T52.8x2	T52.8x3	T52.8x4	—	—
aminobenzoate	T41.3x1	T41.3x2	T41.3x3	T41.3x4	T41.3x5	T41.3x6
aminophenothiazine	T43.3x1	T43.3x2	T43.3x3	T43.3x4	T43.3x5	T43.3x6
benzoate	T52.8x1	T52.8x2	T52.8x3	T52.8x4	—	—
biscoumacetate	T45.511	T45.512	T45.513	T45.514	T45.515	T45.516
bromide (anesthetic)	T41.0x1	T41.0x2	T41.0x3	T41.0x4	T41.0x5	T41.0x6
carbamate	T45.1x1	T45.1x2	T45.1x3	T45.1x4	T45.1x5	T45.1x6
carbinol	T51.3x1	T51.3x2	T51.3x3	T51.3x4	—	—
carbonate	T52.8x1	T52.8x2	T52.8x3	T52.8x4	—	—
chaulmoograte	T37.1x1	T37.1x2	T37.1x3	T37.1x4	T37.1x5	T37.1x6
chloride (anesthetic)	T41.0x1	T41.0x2	T41.0x3	T41.0x4	T41.0x5	T41.0x6
anesthetic (local)	T41.3x1	T41.3x2	T41.3x3	T41.3x4	T41.3x5	T41.3x6
inhaled	T41.0x1	T41.0x2	T41.0x3	T41.0x4	T41.0x5	T41.0x6
local	T49.4x1	T49.4x2	T49.4x3	T49.4x4	T49.4x5	T49.4x6
solvent	T53.6x1	T53.6x2	T53.6x3	T53.6x4	—	—
dibunate	T48.3x1	T48.3x2	T48.3x3	T48.3x4	T48.3x5	T48.3x6
dichloroarsine (vapor)	T57.0x1	T57.0x2	T57.0x3	T57.0x4	—	—
estranol	T38.7x1	T38.7x2	T38.7x3	T38.7x4	T38.7x5	T38.7x6
ether — see also ether	T52.8x1	T52.8x2	T52.8x3	T52.8x4	—	—
formate NEC (solvent)	T52.0x1	T52.0x2	T52.0x3	T52.0x4	—	—
fumarate	T49.4x1	T49.4x2	T49.4x3	T49.4x4	T49.4x5	T49.4x6
hydroxyisobutyrate NEC						
(solvent)	T52.8x1	T52.8x2	T52.8x3	T52.8x4	—	—
iodoacetate	T59.3x1	T59.3x2	T59.3x3	T59.3x4	—	—
lactate NEC (solvent)	T52.8x1	T52.8x2	T52.8x3	T52.8x4	—	—
loflazepate	T42.4x1	T42.4x2	T42.4x3	T42.4x4	T42.4x5	T42.4x6

Table of Drugs & Chemicals	POISONING Accidental (Unintentional)	Self-Harm (Intentional)	Assault	Undetermined	Adverse Effect	Underdosing
Ethyl – continued						
mercuric chloride	T56.1x1	T56.1x2	T56.1x3	T56.1x4	—	—
methylcarbinol	T51.8x1	T51.8x2	T51.8x3	T51.8x4	—	—
morphine	T40.2x1	T40.2x2	T40.2x3	T40.2x4	T40.2x5	T40.2x6
noradrenaline	T48.6x1	T48.6x2	T48.6x3	T48.6x4	T48.6x5	T48.6x6
oxybutyrate NEC (solvent)	T52.8x1	T52.8x2	T52.8x3	T52.8x4	—	—
Ethylene (gas)	T59.891	T59.892	T59.893	T59.894	—	—
anesthetic (general)	T41.0x1	T41.0x2	T41.0x3	T41.0x4	T41.0x5	T41.0x6
chlorohydrin	T52.8x1	T52.8x2	T52.8x3	T52.8x4	—	—
vapor	T53.6x1	T53.6x2	T53.6x3	T53.6x4	—	—
dichloride	T52.8x1	T52.8x2	T52.8x3	T52.8x4	—	—
vapor	T53.6x1	T53.6x2	T53.6x3	T53.6x4	—	—
dinitrate	T52.3x1	T52.3x2	T52.3x3	T52.3x4	—	—
glycol(s)	T52.8x1	T52.8x2	T52.8x3	T52.8x4	—	—
dinitrate	T52.3x1	T52.3x2	T52.3x3	T52.3x4	—	—
monobutyl ether	T52.3x1	T52.3x2	T52.3x3	T52.3x4	—	—
imine	T54.1x1	T54.1x2	T54.1x3	T54.1x4	—	—
oxide (fumigant)						
(nonmedicinal)	T59.891	T59.892	T59.893	T59.894	—	—
medicinal	T49.0x1	T49.0x2	T49.0x3	T49.0x4	T49.0x5	T49.0x6
Ethylenediamine theophylline	T48.6x1	T48.6x2	T48.6x3	T48.6x4	T48.6x5	T48.6x6
Ethylenediaminetetra-acetic acid	T50.6x1	T50.6x2	T50.6x3	T50.6x4	T50.6x5	T50.6x6
Ethylenedinitrilotetra-acetate	T50.6x1	T50.6x2	T50.6x3	T50.6x4	T50.6x5	T50.6x6
Ethylestrenol	T38.7x1	T38.7x2	T38.7x3	T38.7x4	T38.7x5	T38.7x6
Ethylhydroxycellulose	T47.4x1	T47.4x2	T47.4x3	T47.4x4	T47.4x5	T47.4x6
Ethylidene						
chloride NEC	T53.6x1	T53.6x2	T53.6x3	T53.6x4	—	—
diacetate	T60.3x1	T60.3x2	T60.3x3	T60.3x4	—	—
dicoumarin	T45.511	T45.512	T45.513	T45.514	T45.515	T45.516
dicoumarol	T45.511	T45.512	T45.513	T45.514	T45.515	T45.516
diethyl ether	T52.0x1	T52.0x2	T52.0x3	T52.0x4	—	—
Ethylmorphine	T40.2x1	T40.2x2	T40.2x3	T40.2x4	T40.2x5	T40.2x6
Ethylnorepinephrine	T48.6x1	T48.6x2	T48.6x3	T48.6x4	T48.6x5	T48.6x6
Ethylparachlorophen-oxyisobutyrate	T46.6x1	T46.6x2	T46.6x3	T46.6x4	T46.6x5	T46.6x6
Ethynodiol	T38.4x1	T38.4x2	T38.4x3	T38.4x4	T38.4x5	T38.4x6
with mestranol diacetate	T38.4x1	T38.4x2	T38.4x3	T38.4x4	T38.4x5	T38.4x6
Etidocaine	T41.3x1	T41.3x2	T41.3x3	T41.3x4	T41.3x5	T41.3x6
infiltration (subcutaneous)	T41.3x1	T41.3x2	T41.3x3	T41.3x4	T41.3x5	T41.3x6
nerve (peripheral) (plexus)	T41.3x1	T41.3x2	T41.3x3	T41.3x4	T41.3x5	T41.3x6
Etidronate	T50.991	T50.992	T50.993	T50.994	T50.995	T50.996
Etidronic acid (disodium salt)	T50.991	T50.992	T50.993	T50.994	T50.995	T50.996
Etifoxine	T42.6x1	T42.6x2	T42.6x3	T42.6x4	T42.6x5	T42.6x6
Etilefrine	T44.4x1	T44.4x2	T44.4x3	T44.4x4	T44.4x5	T44.4x6
Etilfen	T42.3x1	T42.3x2	T42.3x3	T42.3x4	T42.3x5	T42.3x6
Etinodiol	T38.4x1	T38.4x2	T38.4x3	T38.4x4	T38.4x5	T38.4x6
Etiroxate	T46.6x1	T46.6x2	T46.6x3	T46.6x4	T46.6x5	T46.6x6
Etizolam	T42.4x1	T42.4x2	T42.4x3	T42.4x4	T42.4x5	T42.4x6
Etodolac	T39.391	T39.392	T39.393	T39.394	T39.395	T39.396
Etofamide	T37.3x1	T37.3x2	T37.3x3	T37.3x4	T37.3x5	T37.3x6
Etofibrate	T46.6x1	T46.6x2	T46.6x3	T46.6x4	T46.6x5	T46.6x6
Etofylline	T46.7x1	T46.7x2	T46.7x3	T46.7x4	T46.7x5	T46.7x6
clofibrate	T46.6x1	T46.6x2	T46.6x3	T46.6x4	T46.6x5	T46.6x6
Etoglucid	T45.1x1	T45.1x2	T45.1x3	T45.1x4	T45.1x5	T45.1x6
Etomidate	T41.1x1	T41.1x2	T41.1x3	T41.1x4	T41.1x5	T41.1x6
Etomide	T39.8x1	T39.8x2	T39.8x3	T39.8x4	T39.8x5	T39.8x6
Etomidoline	T44.3x1	T44.3x2	T44.3x3	T44.3x4	T44.3x5	T44.3x6
Etoposide	T45.1x1	T45.1x2	T45.1x3	T45.1x4	T45.1x5	T45.1x6
Etorphine	T40.2x1	T40.2x2	T40.2x3	T40.2x4	T40.2x5	T40.2x6
Etoval	T42.3x1	T42.3x2	T42.3x3	T42.3x4	T42.3x5	T42.3x6
Etozolin	T50.1x1	T50.1x2	T50.1x3	T50.1x4	T50.1x5	T50.1x6
Etretinate	T50.991	T50.992	T50.993	T50.994	T50.995	T50.996
Etryptamine	T43.691	T43.692	T43.693	T43.694	T43.695	T43.696
Etybenzatropine	T44.3x1	T44.3x2	T44.3x3	T44.3x4	T44.3x5	T44.3x6
Etynodiol	T38.4x1	T38.4x2	T38.4x3	T38.4x4	T38.4x5	T38.4x6
Eucaine	T41.3x1	T41.3x2	T41.3x3	T41.3x4	T41.3x5	T41.3x6
Eucalyptus oil	T49.7x1	T49.7x2	T49.7x3	T49.7x4	T49.7x5	T49.7x6

DRUGS&CHEMICALS

Table of Drugs & Chemicals	POISONING Accidental (Unintentional)	Self-Harm (Intentional)	Assault	Undetermined	Adverse Effect	Underdosing
Eucatropine	T49.5x1	T49.5x2	T49.5x3	T49.5x4	T49.5x5	T49.5x6
Eucodal	T40.2x1	T40.2x2	T40.2x3	T40.2x4	T40.2x5	T40.2x6
Euneryl	T42.3x1	T42.3x2	T42.3x3	T42.3x4	T42.3x5	T42.3x6
Euphthalmine	T44.3x1	T44.3x2	T44.3x3	T44.3x4	T44.3x5	T44.3x6
Eurax	T49.0x1	T49.0x2	T49.0x3	T49.0x4	T49.0x5	T49.0x6
Euresol	T49.4x1	T49.4x2	T49.4x3	T49.4x4	T49.4x5	T49.4x6
Euthroid	T38.1x1	T38.1x2	T38.1x3	T38.1x4	T38.1x5	T38.1x6
Evans blue	T50.8x1	T50.8x2	T50.8x3	T50.8x4	T50.8x5	T50.8x6
Evipal	T42.3x1	T42.3x2	T42.3x3	T42.3x4	T42.3x5	T42.3x6
sodium	T41.1x1	T41.1x2	T41.1x3	T41.1x4	T41.1x5	T41.1x6
Evipan	T42.3x1	T42.3x2	T42.3x3	T42.3x4	T42.3x5	T42.3x6
sodium	T41.1x1	T41.1x2	T41.1x3	T41.1x4	T41.1x5	T41.1x6
Exalamide	T49.0x1	T49.0x2	T49.0x3	T49.0x4	T49.0x5	T49.0x6
Exalgin	T39.1x1	T39.1x2	T39.1x3	T39.1x4	T39.1x5	T39.1x6
Excipients, pharmaceutical	T50.901	T50.902	T50.903	T50.904	T50.905	T50.906
Exhaust gas (engine)						
(motor vehicle)	T58.01	T58.02	T58.03	T58.04	—	—
Ex-Lax (phenolphthalein)	T47.2x1	T47.2x2	T47.2x3	T47.2x4	T47.2x5	T47.2x6
Expectorant NEC	T48.4x1	T48.4x2	T48.4x3	T48.4x4	T48.4x5	T48.4x6
Extended insulin zinc suspension	T38.3x1	T38.3x2	T38.3x3	T38.3x4	T38.3x5	T38.3x6
External medications (skin)						
(mucous membrane)	T49.91	T49.92	T49.93	T49.94	T49.95	T49.96
dental agent	T49.7x1	T49.7x2	T49.7x3	T49.7x4	T49.7x5	T49.7x6
ENT agent	T49.6x1	T49.6x2	T49.6x3	T49.6x4	T49.6x5	T49.6x6
ophthalmic preparation	T49.5x1	T49.5x2	T49.5x3	T49.5x4	T49.5x5	T49.5x6
specified NEC	T49.8x1	T49.8x2	T49.8x3	T49.8x4	T49.8x5	T49.8x6
Extrapyramidal antagonist NEC	T44.3x1	T44.3x2	T44.3x3	T44.3x4	T44.3x5	T44.3x6
Eye agents (anti-infective)	T49.5x1	T49.5x2	T49.5x3	T49.5x4	T49.5x5	T49.5x6
Eye drug NEC	T49.5x1	T49.5x2	T49.5x3	T49.5x4	T49.5x5	T49.5x6
FAC (fluorouracil + doxorubicin + cyclophosphamide)	T45.1x1	T45.1x2	T45.1x3	T45.1x4	T45.1x5	T45.1x6
Factor						
I (fibrinogen)	T45.8x1	T45.8x2	T45.8x3	T45.8x4	T45.8x5	T45.8x6
III (thromboplastin)	T45.8x1	T45.8x2	T45.8x3	T45.8x4	T45.8x5	T45.8x6
VIII (antihemophilic Factor)						
(concentrate)	T45.8x1	T45.8x2	T45.8x3	T45.8x4	T45.8x5	T45.8x6
IX complex	T45.7x1	T45.7x2	T45.7x3	T45.7x4	T45.7x5	T45.7x6
human	T45.8x1	T45.8x2	T45.8x3	T45.8x4	T45.8x5	T45.8x6
Famotidine	T47.0x1	T47.0x2	T47.0x3	T47.0x4	T47.0x5	T47.0x6
Fat suspension, intravenous	T50.991	T50.992	T50.993	T50.994	T50.995	T50.996
Fazadinium bromide	T48.1x1	T48.1x2	T48.1x3	T48.1x4	T48.1x5	T48.1x6
Febarbamate	T42.3x1	T42.3x2	T42.3x3	T42.3x4	T42.3x5	T42.3x6
Fecal softener	T47.4x1	T47.4x2	T47.4x3	T47.4x4	T47.4x5	T47.4x6
Fedrilate	T48.3x1	T48.3x2	T48.3x3	T48.3x4	T48.3x5	T48.3x6
Felodipine	T46.1x1	T46.1x2	T46.1x3	T46.1x4	T46.1x5	T46.1x6
Felypressin	T38.891	T38.892	T38.893	T38.894	T38.895	T38.896
Femoxetine	T43.221	T43.222	T43.223	T43.224	T43.225	T43.226
Fenalcomine	T46.3x1	T46.3x2	T46.3x3	T46.3x4	T46.3x5	T46.3x6
Fenamisal	T37.1x1	T37.1x2	T37.1x3	T37.1x4	T37.1x5	T37.1x6
Fenazone	T39.2x1	T39.2x2	T39.2x3	T39.2x4	T39.2x5	T39.2x6
Fenbendazole	T37.4x1	T37.4x2	T37.4x3	T37.4x4	T37.4x5	T37.4x6
Fenbutrazate	T50.5x1	T50.5x2	T50.5x3	T50.5x4	T50.5x5	T50.5x6
Fencamfamine	T43.691	T43.692	T43.693	T43.694	T43.695	T43.696
Fendiline	T46.1x1	T46.1x2	T46.1x3	T46.1x4	T46.1x5	T46.1x6
Fenetylline	T43.691	T43.692	T43.693	T43.694	T43.695	T43.696
Fenflumizole	T39.391	T39.392	T39.393	T39.394	T39.395	T39.396
Fenfluramine	T50.5x1	T50.5x2	T50.5x3	T50.5x4	T50.5x5	T50.5x6
Fenobarbital	T42.3x1	T42.3x2	T42.3x3	T42.3x4	T42.3x5	T42.3x6
Fenofibrate	T46.6x1	T46.6x2	T46.6x3	T46.6x4	T46.6x5	T46.6x6
Fenoprofen	T39.311	T39.312	T39.313	T39.314	T39.315	T39.316
Fenoterol	T48.6x1	T48.6x2	T48.6x3	T48.6x4	T48.6x5	T48.6x6
Fenoverine	T44.3x1	T44.3x2	T44.3x3	T44.3x4	T44.3x5	T44.3x6
Fenoxazoline	T48.5x1	T48.5x2	T48.5x3	T48.5x4	T48.5x5	T48.5x6
Fenproporex	T50.5x1	T50.5x2	T50.5x3	T50.5x4	T50.5x5	T50.5x6
Fenquizone	T50.2x1	T50.2x2	T50.2x3	T50.2x4	T50.2x5	T50.2x6
Fentanyl	T40.4x1	T40.4x2	T40.4x3	T40.4x4	T40.4x5	T40.4x6
Fentazin	T43.3x1	T43.3x2	T43.3x3	T43.3x4	T43.3x5	T43.3x6
Fenthion	T60.0x1	T60.0x2	T60.0x3	T60.0x4	—	—

Table of Drugs & Chemicals	POISONING Accidental (Unintentional)	Self-Harm (Intentional)	Assault	Undetermined	Adverse Effect	Underdosing
Fenticlor	T49.0x1	T49.0x2	T49.0x3	T49.0x4	T49.0x5	T49.0x6
Fenylbutazone	T39.2x1	T39.2x2	T39.2x3	T39.2x4	T39.2x5	T39.2x6
Feprazone	T39.2x1	T39.2x2	T39.2x3	T39.2x4	T39.2x5	T39.2x6
Fer de lance (bite) (venom)	T63.061	T63.062	T63.063	T63.064	—	—
Ferric — see also Iron						
chloride	T45.4x1	T45.4x2	T45.4x3	T45.4x4	T45.4x5	T45.4x6
citrate	T45.4x1	T45.4x2	T45.4x3	T45.4x4	T45.4x5	T45.4x6
hydroxide						
colloidal	T45.4x1	T45.4x2	T45.4x3	T45.4x4	T45.4x5	T45.4x6
polymaltose	T45.4x1	T45.4x2	T45.4x3	T45.4x4	T45.4x5	T45.4x6
pyrophosphate	T45.4x1	T45.4x2	T45.4x3	T45.4x4	T45.4x5	T45.4x6
Ferritin	T45.4x1	T45.4x2	T45.4x3	T45.4x4	T45.4x5	T45.4x6
Ferrocholinate	T45.4x1	T45.4x2	T45.4x3	T45.4x4	T45.4x5	T45.4x6
Ferrodextrane	T45.4x1	T45.4x2	T45.4x3	T45.4x4	T45.4x5	T45.4x6
Ferropolimaler	T45.4x1	T45.4x2	T45.4x3	T45.4x4	T45.4x5	T45.4x6
Ferrous — see also Iron						
phosphate	T45.4x1	T45.4x2	T45.4x3	T45.4x4	T45.4x5	T45.4x6
salt	T45.4x1	T45.4x2	T45.4x3	T45.4x4	T45.4x5	T45.4x6
with folic acid	T45.4x1	T45.4x2	T45.4x3	T45.4x4	T45.4x5	T45.4x6
Ferrous fumarate, gluconate, lactate, salt NEC, sulfate (medicinal)	T45.4x1	T45.4x2	T45.4x3	T45.4x4	T45.4x5	T45.4x6
Ferrovanadium (fumes)	T59.891	T59.892	T59.893	T59.894	—	—
Ferrum — see Iron						
Fertilizers NEC	T65.891	T65.892	T65.893	T65.894	—	—
with herbicide mixture	T60.3x1	T60.3x2	T60.3x3	T60.3x4	—	—
Fetoxilate	T47.6x1	T47.6x2	T47.6x3	T47.6x4	T47.6x5	T47.6x6
Fiber, dietary	T47.4x1	T47.4x2	T47.4x3	T47.4x4	T47.4x5	T47.4x6
Fiberglass	T65.831	T65.832	T65.833	T65.834	—	—
Fibrinogen (human)	T45.8x1	T45.8x2	T45.8x3	T45.8x4	T45.8x5	T45.8x6
Fibrinolysin (human)	T45.691	T45.692	T45.693	T45.694	T45.695	T45.696
Fibrinolysis						
affecting drug	T45.601	T45.602	T45.603	T45.604	T45.605	T45.606
inhibitor NEC	T45.621	T45.622	T45.623	T45.624	T45.625	T45.626
Fibrinolytic drug	T45.611	T45.612	T45.613	T45.614	T45.615	T45.616
Filix mas	T37.4x1	T37.4x2	T37.4x3	T37.4x4	T37.4x5	T37.4x6
Filtering cream	T49.3x1	T49.3x2	T49.3x3	T49.3x4	T49.3x5	T49.3x6
Fiorinal	T39.011	T39.012	T39.013	T39.014	T39.015	T39.016
Firedamp	T59.891	T59.892	T59.893	T59.894	—	—
Fish, noxious, nonbacterial	T61.91	T61.92	T61.93	T61.94	—	—
ciguatera	T61.01	T61.02	T61.03	T61.04	—	—
scombroid	T61.11	T61.12	T61.13	T61.14	—	—
shell	T61.781	T61.782	T61.783	T61.784	—	—
specified NEC	T61.771	T61.772	T61.773	T61.774	—	—
Flagyl	T37.3x1	T37.3x2	T37.3x3	T37.3x4	T37.3x5	T37.3x6
Flavine adenine dinucleotide	T45.2x1	T45.2x2	T45.2x3	T45.2x4	T45.2x5	T45.2x6
Flavodic acid	T46.991	T46.992	T46.993	T46.994	T46.995	T46.996
Flavoxate	T44.3x1	T44.3x2	T44.3x3	T44.3x4	T44.3x5	T44.3x6
Flaxedil	T48.1x1	T48.1x2	T48.1x3	T48.1x4	T48.1x5	T48.1x6
Flaxseed (medicinal)	T49.3x1	T49.3x2	T49.3x3	T49.3x4	T49.3x5	T49.3x6
Flecainide	T46.2x1	T46.2x2	T46.2x3	T46.2x4	T46.2x5	T46.2x6
Fleroxacin	T36.8x1	T36.8x2	T36.8x3	T36.8x4	T36.8x5	T36.8x6
Floctafenine	T39.8x1	T39.8x2	T39.8x3	T39.8x4	T39.8x5	T39.8x6
Flomax	T44.6x1	T44.6x2	T44.6x3	T44.6x4	T44.6x5	T44.6x6
Flomoxef	T36.1x1	T36.1x2	T36.1x3	T36.1x4	T36.1x5	T36.1x6
Flopropione	T44.3x1	T44.3x2	T44.3x3	T44.3x4	T44.3x5	T44.3x6
Florantyrone	T47.5x1	T47.5x2	T47.5x3	T47.5x4	T47.5x5	T47.5x6
Floraquin	T37.8x1	T37.8x2	T37.8x3	T37.8x4	T37.8x5	T37.8x6
Florinef	T38.0x1	T38.0x2	T38.0x3	T38.0x4	T38.0x5	T38.0x6
ENT agent	T49.6x1	T49.6x2	T49.6x3	T49.6x4	T49.6x5	T49.6x6
ophthalmic preparation	T49.5x1	T49.5x2	T49.5x3	T49.5x4	T49.5x5	T49.5x6
topical NEC	T49.0x1	T49.0x2	T49.0x3	T49.0x4	T49.0x5	T49.0x6
Flowers of sulfur	T49.4x1	T49.4x2	T49.4x3	T49.4x4	T49.4x5	T49.4x6
Floxuridine	T45.1x1	T45.1x2	T45.1x3	T45.1x4	T45.1x5	T45.1x6
Fluanisone	T43.4x1	T43.4x2	T43.4x3	T43.4x4	T43.4x5	T43.4x6
Flubendazole	T37.4x1	T37.4x2	T37.4x3	T37.4x4	T37.4x5	T37.4x6
Fluclorolone acetonide	T49.0x1	T49.0x2	T49.0x3	T49.0x4	T49.0x5	T49.0x6
Flucloxacillin	T36.0x1	T36.0x2	T36.0x3	T36.0x4	T36.0x5	T36.0x6

DRUGS & CHEMICALS

Table of Drugs & Chemicals	Poisoning — Accidental (Unintentional)	Poisoning — Self-Harm (Intentional)	Poisoning — Assault	Poisoning — Undetermined	Adverse Effect	Underdosing
Fluconazole	T37.8x1	T37.8x2	T37.8x3	T37.8x4	T37.8x5	T37.8x6
Flucytosine	T37.8x1	T37.8x2	T37.8x3	T37.8x4	T37.8x5	T37.8x6
Fludeoxyglucose (18F)	T50.8x1	T50.8x2	T50.8x3	T50.8x4	T50.8x5	T50.8x6
Fludiazepam	T42.4x1	T42.4x2	T42.4x3	T42.4x4	T42.4x5	T42.4x6
Fludrocortisone	T50.0x1	T50.0x2	T50.0x3	T50.0x4	T50.0x5	T50.0x6
ENT agent	T49.6x1	T49.6x2	T49.6x3	T49.6x4	T49.6x5	T49.6x6
ophthalmic preparation	T49.5x1	T49.5x2	T49.5x3	T49.5x4	T49.5x5	T49.5x6
topical NEC	T49.0x1	T49.0x2	T49.0x3	T49.0x4	T49.0x5	T49.0x6
Fludroxycortide	T49.0x1	T49.0x2	T49.0x3	T49.0x4	T49.0x5	T49.0x6
Flufenamic acid	T39.391	T39.392	T39.393	T39.394	T39.395	T39.396
Fluindione	T45.511	T45.512	T45.513	T45.514	T45.515	T45.516
Flumequine	T37.8x1	T37.8x2	T37.8x3	T37.8x4	T37.8x5	T37.8x6
Flumethasone	T49.0x1	T49.0x2	T49.0x3	T49.0x4	T49.0x5	T49.0x6
Flumethiazide	T50.2x1	T50.2x2	T50.2x3	T50.2x4	T50.2x5	T50.2x6
Flumidin	T37.5x1	T37.5x2	T37.5x3	T37.5x4	T37.5x5	T37.5x6
Flunarizine	T46.7x1	T46.7x2	T46.7x3	T46.7x4	T46.7x5	T46.7x6
Flunidazole	T37.8x1	T37.8x2	T37.8x3	T37.8x4	T37.8x5	T37.8x6
Flunisolide	T48.6x1	T48.6x2	T48.6x3	T48.6x4	T48.6x5	T48.6x6
Flunitrazepam	T42.4x1	T42.4x2	T42.4x3	T42.4x4	T42.4x5	T42.4x6
Fluocinolone (acetonide)	T49.0x1	T49.0x2	T49.0x3	T49.0x4	T49.0x5	T49.0x6
Fluocinonide	T49.0x1	T49.0x2	T49.0x3	T49.0x4	T49.0x5	T49.0x6
Fluocortin (butyl)	T49.0x1	T49.0x2	T49.0x3	T49.0x4	T49.0x5	T49.0x6
Fluocortolone	T49.0x1	T49.0x2	T49.0x3	T49.0x4	T49.0x5	T49.0x6
Fluohydrocortisone	T38.0x1	T38.0x2	T38.0x3	T38.0x4	T38.0x5	T38.0x6
ENT agent	T49.6x1	T49.6x2	T49.6x3	T49.6x4	T49.6x5	T49.6x6
ophthalmic preparation	T49.5x1	T49.5x2	T49.5x3	T49.5x4	T49.5x5	T49.5x6
topical NEC	T49.0x1	T49.0x2	T49.0x3	T49.0x4	T49.0x5	T49.0x6
Fluonid	T49.0x1	T49.0x2	T49.0x3	T49.0x4	T49.0x5	T49.0x6
Fluopromazine	T43.3x1	T43.3x2	T43.3x3	T43.3x4	T43.3x5	T43.3x6
Fluoracetate	T60.8x1	T60.8x2	T60.8x3	T60.8x4	—	—
Fluorescein	T50.8x1	T50.8x2	T50.8x3	T50.8x4	T50.8x5	T50.8x6
Fluorhydrocortisone	T50.0x1	T50.0x2	T50.0x3	T50.0x4	T50.0x5	T50.0x6
Fluoride (nonmedicinal) (pesticide) (sodium) NEC	T60.8x1	T60.8x2	T60.8x3	T60.8x4	—	—
hydrogen — see Hydrofluoric acid						
medicinal NEC	T50.991	T50.992	T50.993	T50.994	T50.995	T50.996
dental use	T49.7x1	T49.7x2	T49.7x3	T49.7x4	T49.7x5	T49.7x6
not pesticide NEC	T54.91	T54.92	T54.93	T54.94	—	—
stannous	T49.7x1	T49.7x2	T49.7x3	T49.7x4	T49.7x5	T49.7x6
Fluorinated corticosteroids	T38.0x1	T38.0x2	T38.0x3	T38.0x4	T38.0x5	T38.0x6
Fluorine (gas)	T59.5x1	T59.5x2	T59.5x3	T59.5x4	—	—
salt — see Fluoride(s)						
Fluoristan	T49.7x1	T49.7x2	T49.7x3	T49.7x4	T49.7x5	T49.7x6
Fluormetholone	T49.0x1	T49.0x2	T49.0x3	T49.0x4	T49.0x5	T49.0x6
Fluoroacetate	T60.8x1	T60.8x2	T60.8x3	T60.8x4	—	—
Fluorocarbon monomer	T53.6x1	T53.6x2	T53.6x3	T53.6x4	—	—
Fluorocytosine	T37.8x1	T37.8x2	T37.8x3	T37.8x4	T37.8x5	T37.8x6
Fluorodeoxyuridine	T45.1x1	T45.1x2	T45.1x3	T45.1x4	T45.1x5	T45.1x6
Fluorometholone	T49.0x1	T49.0x2	T49.0x3	T49.0x4	T49.0x5	T49.0x6
ophthalmic preparation	T49.5x1	T49.5x2	T49.5x3	T49.5x4	T49.5x5	T49.5x6
Fluorophosphate insecticide	T60.0x1	T60.0x2	T60.0x3	T60.0x4	—	—
Fluorosol	T46.3x1	T46.3x2	T46.3x3	T46.3x4	T46.3x5	T46.3x6
Fluorouracil	T45.1x1	T45.1x2	T45.1x3	T45.1x4	T45.1x5	T45.1x6
Fluorphenylalanine	T49.5x1	T49.5x2	T49.5x3	T49.5x4	T49.5x5	T49.5x6
Fluothane	T41.0x1	T41.0x2	T41.0x3	T41.0x4	T41.0x5	T41.0x6
Fluoxetine	T43.221	T43.222	T43.223	T43.224	T43.225	T43.226
Fluoxymesterone	T38.7x1	T38.7x2	T38.7x3	T38.7x4	T38.7x5	T38.7x6
Flupenthixol	T43.4x1	T43.4x2	T43.4x3	T43.4x4	T43.4x5	T43.4x6
Flupentixol	T43.4x1	T43.4x2	T43.4x3	T43.4x4	T43.4x5	T43.4x6
Fluphenazine	T43.3x1	T43.3x2	T43.3x3	T43.3x4	T43.3x5	T43.3x6
Fluprednidene	T49.0x1	T49.0x2	T49.0x3	T49.0x4	T49.0x5	T49.0x6
Fluprednisolone	T38.0x1	T38.0x2	T38.0x3	T38.0x4	T38.0x5	T38.0x6
Fluradoline	T39.8x1	T39.8x2	T39.8x3	T39.8x4	T39.8x5	T39.8x6
Flurandrenolide	T49.0x1	T49.0x2	T49.0x3	T49.0x4	T49.0x5	T49.0x6
Flurandrenolone	T49.0x1	T49.0x2	T49.0x3	T49.0x4	T49.0x5	T49.0x6
Flurazepam	T42.4x1	T42.4x2	T42.4x3	T42.4x4	T42.4x5	T42.4x6
Flurbiprofen	T39.311	T39.312	T39.313	T39.314	T39.315	T39.316

Table of Drugs & Chemicals	Poisoning — Accidental (Unintentional)	Poisoning — Self-Harm (Intentional)	Poisoning — Assault	Poisoning — Undetermined	Adverse Effect	Underdosing
Flurobate	T49.0x1	T49.0x2	T49.0x3	T49.0x4	T49.0x5	T49.0x6
Fluroxene	T41.0x1	T41.0x2	T41.0x3	T41.0x4	T41.0x5	T41.0x6
Fluspirilene	T43.591	T43.592	T43.593	T43.594	T43.595	T43.596
Flutamide	T38.6x1	T38.6x2	T38.6x3	T38.6x4	T38.6x5	T38.6x6
Flutazolam	T42.4x1	T42.4x2	T42.4x3	T42.4x4	T42.4x5	T42.4x6
Fluticasone propionate	T49.1x1	T49.1x2	T49.1x3	T49.1x4	T49.1x5	T49.1x6
Flutoprazepam	T42.4x1	T42.4x2	T42.4x3	T42.4x4	T42.4x5	T42.4x6
Flutropium bromide	T48.6x1	T48.6x2	T48.6x3	T48.6x4	T48.6x5	T48.6x6
Fluvoxamine	T43.221	T43.222	T43.223	T43.224	T43.225	T43.226
Folacin	T45.8x1	T45.8x2	T45.8x3	T45.8x4	T45.8x5	T45.8x6
Folic acid	T45.8x1	T45.8x2	T45.8x3	T45.8x4	T45.8x5	T45.8x6
with ferrous salt	T45.2x1	T45.2x2	T45.2x3	T45.2x4	T45.2x5	T45.2x6
antagonist	T45.1x1	T45.1x2	T45.1x3	T45.1x4	T45.1x5	T45.1x6
Folinic acid	T45.8x1	T45.8x2	T45.8x3	T45.8x4	T45.8x5	T45.8x6
Folium stramoniae	T48.6x1	T48.6x2	T48.6x3	T48.6x4	T48.6x5	T48.6x6
Follicle-stimulating hormone, human	T38.811	T38.812	T38.813	T38.814	T38.815	T38.816
Folpet	T60.3x1	T60.3x2	T60.3x3	T60.3x4	—	—
Fominoben	T48.3x1	T48.3x2	T48.3x3	T48.3x4	T48.3x5	T48.3x6
Food, foodstuffs, noxious, nonbacterial, NEC	T62.91	T62.92	T62.93	T62.94	—	—
berries	T62.1x1	T62.1x2	T62.1x3	T62.1x4	—	—
fish — see also Fish	T61.91	T61.92	T61.93	T61.94	—	—
mushrooms	T62.0x1	T62.0x2	T62.0x3	T62.0x4	—	—
plants	T62.2x1	T62.2x2	T62.2x3	T62.2x4	—	—
seafood	T61.91	T61.92	T61.93	T61.94	—	—
specified NEC	T61.8x1	T61.8x2	T61.8x3	T61.8x4	—	—
seeds	T62.2x1	T62.2x2	T62.2x3	T62.2x4	—	—
shellfish	T61.781	T61.782	T61.783	T61.784	—	—
specified NEC	T62.8x1	T62.8x2	T62.8x3	T62.8x4	—	—
Fool's parsley	T62.2x1	T62.2x2	T62.2x3	T62.2x4	—	—
Formaldehyde (solution), gas or vapor	T59.2x1	T59.2x2	T59.2x3	T59.2x4	—	—
fungicide	T60.3x1	T60.3x2	T60.3x3	T60.3x4	—	—
Formalin	T59.2x1	T59.2x2	T59.2x3	T59.2x4	—	—
fungicide	T60.3x1	T60.3x2	T60.3x3	T60.3x4	—	—
vapor	T59.2x1	T59.2x2	T59.2x3	T59.2x4	—	—
Formic acid	T54.2x1	T54.2x2	T54.2x3	T54.2x4	—	—
vapor	T59.891	T59.892	T59.893	T59.894	—	—
Foscarnet sodium	T37.5x1	T37.5x2	T37.5x3	T37.5x4	T37.5x5	T37.5x6
Fosfestrol	T38.5x1	T38.5x2	T38.5x3	T38.5x4	T38.5x5	T38.5x6
Fosfomycin	T36.8x1	T36.8x2	T36.8x3	T36.8x4	T36.8x5	T36.8x6
Fosfonet sodium	T37.5x1	T37.5x2	T37.5x3	T37.5x4	T37.5x5	T37.5x6
Fosinopril	T46.4x1	T46.4x2	T46.4x3	T46.4x4	T46.4x5	T46.4x6
sodium	T46.4x1	T46.4x2	T46.4x3	T46.4x4	T46.4x5	T46.4x6
Fowler's solution	T57.0x1	T57.0x2	T57.0x3	T57.0x4	—	—
Foxglove	T62.2x1	T62.2x2	T62.2x3	T62.2x4	—	—
Framycetin	T36.5x1	T36.5x2	T36.5x3	T36.5x4	T36.5x5	T36.5x6
Frangula	T47.2x1	T47.2x2	T47.2x3	T47.2x4	T47.2x5	T47.2x6
extract	T47.2x1	T47.2x2	T47.2x3	T47.2x4	T47.2x5	T47.2x6
Frei antigen	T50.8x1	T50.8x2	T50.8x3	T50.8x4	T50.8x5	T50.8x6
Freon	T53.5x1	T53.5x2	T53.5x3	T53.5x4	—	—
Fructose	T50.3x1	T50.3x2	T50.3x3	T50.3x4	T50.3x5	T50.3x6
Frusemide	T50.1x1	T50.1x2	T50.1x3	T50.1x4	T50.1x5	T50.1x6
FSH	T38.811	T38.812	T38.813	T38.814	T38.815	T38.816
Ftorafur	T45.1x1	T45.1x2	T45.1x3	T45.1x4	T45.1x5	T45.1x6
Fuel						
automobile	T52.0x1	T52.0x2	T52.0x3	T52.0x4	—	—
exhaust gas, not in transit	T58.01	T58.02	T58.03	T58.04	—	—
vapor NEC	T52.0x1	T52.0x2	T52.0x3	T52.0x4	—	—
gas (domestic use) — see also Carbon, monoxide, fuel, utility	T59.891	T59.892	T59.893	T59.894	—	—
utility	T59.891	T59.892	T59.893	T59.894	—	—
incomplete combustion of — see Carbon, monoxide, fuel, utility						
in mobile container	T59.891	T59.892	T59.893	T59.894	—	—
piped (natural)	T59.891	T59.892	T59.893	T59.894	—	—

DRUGS&CHEMICALS

Table of Drugs & Chemicals	POISONING Accidental (Unintentional)	Self-Harm (Intentional)	Assault	Undetermined	Adverse Effect	Underdosing
Fuel – *continued*						
industrial, incomplete combustion	T58.8x1	T58.8x2	T58.8x3	T58.8x4	—	—
Fugillin	T36.8x1	T36.8x2	T36.8x3	T36.8x4	T36.8x5	T36.8x6
Fulminate of mercury	T56.1x1	T56.1x2	T56.1x3	T56.1x4	—	—
Fulvicin	T36.7x1	T36.7x2	T36.7x3	T36.7x4	T36.7x5	T36.7x6
Fumadil	T36.8x1	T36.8x2	T36.8x3	T36.8x4	T36.8x5	T36.8x6
Fumagillin	T36.8x1	T36.8x2	T36.8x3	T36.8x4	T36.8x5	T36.8x6
Fumaric acid	T49.4x1	T49.4x2	T49.4x3	T49.4x4	T49.4x5	T49.4x6
Fumes (from)	T59.91	T59.92	T59.93	T59.94	—	—
carbon monoxide — *see* Carbon, monoxide						
charcoal (domestic use) — *see* Charcoal, fumes						
chloroform — *see* Chloroform						
coke (in domestic stoves, fireplaces) — *see* Coke fumes						
corrosive NEC	T54.91	T54.92	T54.93	T54.94	—	—
ether — *see* ether						
freons	T53.5x1	T53.5x2	T53.5x3	T53.5x4	—	—
hydrocarbons	T59.891	T59.892	T59.893	T59.894	—	—
petroleum (liquefied)	T59.891	T59.892	T59.893	T59.894	—	—
distributed through pipes (pure or mixed with air)	T59.891	T59.892	T59.893	T59.894	—	—
lead — *see* lead						
metal — *see* Metals, or the specified metal						
nitrogen dioxide	T59.0x1	T59.0x2	T59.0x3	T59.0x4	—	—
pesticides — *see* Pesticides						
petroleum (liquefied)	T59.891	T59.892	T59.893	T59.894	—	—
distributed through pipes (pure or mixed with air)	T59.891	T59.892	T59.893	T59.894	—	—
polyester	T59.891	T59.892	T59.893	T59.894	—	—
specified source NEC — *see also* substance, specified	T59.891	T59.892	T59.893	T59.894	—	—
sulfur dioxide	T59.1x1	T59.1x2	T59.1x3	T59.1x4	—	—
Fumigant NEC	T60.91	T60.92	T60.93	T60.94	—	—
Fungi, noxious, used as food	T62.0x1	T62.0x2	T62.0x3	T62.0x4	—	—
Fungicide NEC (nonmedicinal)	T60.3x1	T60.3x2	T60.3x3	T60.3x4	—	—
Fungizone	T36.7x1	T36.7x2	T36.7x3	T36.7x4	T36.7x5	T36.7x6
topical	T49.0x1	T49.0x2	T49.0x3	T49.0x4	T49.0x5	T49.0x6
Furacin	T49.0x1	T49.0x2	T49.0x3	T49.0x4	T49.0x5	T49.0x6
Furadantin	T37.91	T37.92	T37.93	T37.94	T37.95	T37.96
Furazolidone	T37.8x1	T37.8x2	T37.8x3	T37.8x4	T37.8x5	T37.8x6
Furazolium chloride	T49.0x1	T49.0x2	T49.0x3	T49.0x4	T49.0x5	T49.0x6
Furfural	T52.8x1	T52.8x2	T52.8x3	T52.8x4	—	—
Furnace (coal burning) (domestic), gas from	T58.2x1	T58.2x2	T58.2x3	T58.2x4	—	—
industrial	T58.8x1	T58.8x2	T58.8x3	T58.8x4	—	—
Furniture polish	T65.891	T65.892	T65.893	T65.894	—	—
Furosemide	T50.1x1	T50.1x2	T50.1x3	T50.1x4	T50.1x5	T50.1x6
Furoxone	T37.91	T37.92	T37.93	T37.94	T37.95	T37.96
Fursultiamine	T45.2x1	T45.2x2	T45.2x3	T45.2x4	T45.2x5	T45.2x6
Fusafungine	T36.8x1	T36.8x2	T36.8x3	T36.8x4	T36.8x5	T36.8x6
Fusel oil (any) (amyl) (butyl) (propyl), vapor	T51.3x1	T51.3x2	T51.3x3	T51.3x4	—	—
Fusidate (ethanolamine) (sodium)	T36.8x1	T36.8x2	T36.8x3	T36.8x4	T36.8x5	T36.8x6
Fusidic acid	T36.8x1	T36.8x2	T36.8x3	T36.8x4	T36.8x5	T36.8x6
Fytic acid, nonasodium	T50.6x1	T50.6x2	T50.6x3	T50.6x4	T50.6x5	T50.6x6
GABA	T43.8x1	T43.8x2	T43.8x3	T43.8x4	T43.8x5	T43.8x6
Gadopentetic acid	T50.8x1	T50.8x2	T50.8x3	T50.8x4	T50.8x5	T50.8x6
Galactose	T50.3x1	T50.3x2	T50.3x3	T50.3x4	T50.3x5	T50.3x6
b-Galactosidase	T47.5x1	T47.5x2	T47.5x3	T47.5x4	T47.5x5	T47.5x6
Galantamine	T44.0x1	T44.0x2	T44.0x3	T44.0x4	T44.0x5	T44.0x6
Gallamine (triethiodide)	T48.1x1	T48.1x2	T48.1x3	T48.1x4	T48.1x5	T48.1x6
Gallium citrate	T50.991	T50.992	T50.993	T50.994	T50.995	T50.996
Gallopamil	T46.1x1	T46.1x2	T46.1x3	T46.1x4	T46.1x5	T46.1x6
Gamboge	T47.2x1	T47.2x2	T47.2x3	T47.2x4	T47.2x5	T47.2x6
Gamimune	T50.Z11	T50.Z12	T50.Z13	T50.Z14	T50.Z15	T50.Z16
Gamma globulin	T50.Z11	T50.Z12	T50.Z13	T50.Z14	T50.Z15	T50.Z16
Gamma-aminobutyric acid	T43.8x1	T43.8x2	T43.8x3	T43.8x4	T43.8x5	T43.8x6
Gamma-benzene hexachloride (medicinal)	T49.0x1	T49.0x2	T49.0x3	T49.0x4	T49.0x5	T49.0x6
nonmedicinal, vapor	T53.6x1	T53.6x2	T53.6x3	T53.6x4	—	—
Gamma-BHC (medicinal) — *see also* Gamma-benzene hexachloride	T49.0x1	T49.0x2	T49.0x3	T49.0x4	T49.0x5	T49.0x6
Gamulin	T50.Z11	T50.Z12	T50.Z13	T50.Z14	T50.Z15	T50.Z16
Ganciclovir (sodium)	T37.5x1	T37.5x2	T37.5x3	T37.5x4	T37.5x5	T37.5x6
Ganglionic blocking drug NEC	T44.2x1	T44.2x2	T44.2x3	T44.2x4	T44.2x5	T44.2x6
specified NEC	T44.2x1	T44.2x2	T44.2x3	T44.2x4	T44.2x5	T44.2x6
Ganja	T40.7x1	T40.7x2	T40.7x3	T40.7x4	T40.7x5	T40.7x6
Garamycin	T36.5x1	T36.5x2	T36.5x3	T36.5x4	T36.5x5	T36.5x6
ophthalmic preparation	T49.5x1	T49.5x2	T49.5x3	T49.5x4	T49.5x5	T49.5x6
topical NEC	T49.0x1	T49.0x2	T49.0x3	T49.0x4	T49.0x5	T49.0x6
Gardenal	T42.3x1	T42.3x2	T42.3x3	T42.3x4	T42.3x5	T42.3x6
Gardepanyl	T42.3x1	T42.3x2	T42.3x3	T42.3x4	T42.3x5	T42.3x6
Gas	T59.91	T59.92	T59.93	T59.94	—	—
acetylene	T59.891	T59.892	T59.893	T59.894	—	—
incomplete combustion of	T58.11	T58.12	T58.13	T58.14	—	—
air contaminants, source or type not specified	T59.91	T59.92	T59.93	T59.94	—	—
anesthetic	T41.0x1	T41.0x2	T41.0x3	T41.0x4	T41.0x5	T41.0x6
blast furnace	T58.8x1	T58.8x2	T58.8x3	T58.8x4	—	—
butane — *see* butane						
carbon monoxide — *see* Carbon, monoxide						
chlorine	T59.4x1	T59.4x2	T59.4x3	T59.4x4	—	—
coal	T58.2x1	T58.2x2	T58.2x3	T58.2x4	—	—
cyanide	T57.3x1	T57.3x2	T57.3x3	T57.3x4	—	—
dicyanogen	T65.0x1	T65.0x2	T65.0x3	T65.0x4	—	—
domestic — *see* Domestic gas						
exhaust	T58.01	T58.02	T58.03	T58.04	—	—
from utility (for cooking, heating, or lighting) (after combustion) — *see* Carbon, monoxide, fuel, utility						
prior to combustion	T59.891	T59.892	T59.893	T59.894	—	—
from wood- or coal-burning stove or fireplace	T58.2x1	T58.2x2	T58.2x3	T58.2x4	—	—
fuel (domestic use) (after combustion) — *see also* Carbon, monoxide, fuel						
industrial use	T58.8x1	T58.8x2	T58.8x3	T58.8x4	—	—
prior to combustion	T59.891	T59.892	T59.893	T59.894	—	—
utility	T59.891	T59.892	T59.893	T59.894	—	—
incomplete combustion of — *see* Carbon, monoxide, fuel, utility						
in mobile container	T59.891	T59.892	T59.893	T59.894	—	—
piped (natural)	T59.891	T59.892	T59.893	T59.894	—	—
garage	T58.01	T58.02	T58.03	T58.04	—	—
hydrocarbon NEC	T59.891	T59.892	T59.893	T59.894	—	—
incomplete combustion of — *see* Carbon, monoxide, fuel, utility						
liquefied — *see* Butane						
piped	T59.891	T59.892	T59.893	T59.894	—	—

DRUGS & CHEMICALS

Table of Drugs & Chemicals	Accidental (Unintentional)	Self-Harm (Intentional)	Assault	Undetermined	Adverse Effect	Underdosing
Gas – continued	T59.91	T59.92	T59.93	T59.94	—	—
hydrocyanic acid	T65.0x1	T65.0x2	T65.0x3	T65.0x4	—	—
illuminating (after combustion)	T58.11	T58.12	T58.13	T58.14	—	—
prior to combustion	T59.891	T59.892	T59.893	T59.894	—	—
incomplete combustion, any — see Carbon, monoxide						
kiln	T58.8x1	T58.8x2	T58.8x3	T58.8x4	—	—
lacrimogenic	T59.3x1	T59.3x2	T59.3x3	T59.3x4	—	—
liquefied petroleum — see Butane						
marsh	T59.891	T59.892	T59.893	T59.894	—	—
motor exhaust, not in transit	T58.01	T58.02	T58.03	T58.04	—	—
mustard, not in war	T59.891	T59.892	T59.893	T59.894	—	—
natural	T59.891	T59.892	T59.893	T59.894	—	—
nerve, not in war	T59.91	T59.92	T59.93	T59.94	—	—
oil	T52.0x1	T52.0x2	T52.0x3	T52.0x4	—	—
petroleum (liquefied) (distributed in mobile containers)	T59.891	T59.892	T59.893	T59.894	—	—
piped (pure or mixed with air)	T59.891	T59.892	T59.893	T59.894	—	—
piped (manufactured) (natural) NEC	T59.891	T59.892	T59.893	T59.894	—	—
producer	T58.8x1	T58.8x2	T58.8x3	T58.8x4	—	—
propane — see Propane						
refrigerant (chlorofluoro-carbon)	T53.5x1	T53.5x2	T53.5x3	T53.5x4	—	—
not chlorofluoro-carbon	T59.891	T59.892	T59.893	T59.894	—	—
sewer	T59.91	T59.92	T59.93	T59.94	—	—
specified source NEC	T59.91	T59.92	T59.93	T59.94	—	—
stove (after combustion)	T58.11	T58.12	T58.13	T58.14	—	—
prior to combustion	T59.891	T59.892	T59.893	T59.894	—	—
tear	T59.3x1	T59.3x2	T59.3x3	T59.3x4	—	—
therapeutic	T41.5x1	T41.5x2	T41.5x3	T41.5x4	T41.5x5	T41.5x6
utility (for cooking, heating, or lighting) (piped) NEC	T59.891	T59.892	T59.893	T59.894	—	—
incomplete combustion of — see Carbon, monoxide, fuel, utilty						
in mobile container	T59.891	T59.892	T59.893	T59.894	—	—
piped (natural)	T59.891	T59.892	T59.893	T59.894	—	—
water	T58.11	T58.12	T58.13	T58.14	—	—
incomplete combustion of — see Carbon, monoxide, fuel, utility						
Gaseous substance — see Gas						
Gasoline	T52.0x1	T52.0x2	T52.0x3	T52.0x4	—	—
vapor	T52.0x1	T52.0x2	T52.0x3	T52.0x4	—	—
Gastric enzymes	T47.5x1	T47.5x2	T47.5x3	T47.5x4	T47.5x5	T47.5x6
Gastrografin	T50.8x1	T50.8x2	T50.8x3	T50.8x4	T50.8x5	T50.8x6
Gastrointestinal drug	T47.91	T47.92	T47.93	T47.94	T47.95	T47.96
biological	T47.8x1	T47.8x2	T47.8x3	T47.8x4	T47.8x5	T47.8x6
specified NEC	T47.8x1	T47.8x2	T47.8x3	T47.8x4	T47.8x5	T47.8x6
Gaultheria procumbens	T62.2x1	T62.2x2	T62.2x3	T62.2x4	—	—
Gefarnate	T44.3x1	T44.3x2	T44.3x3	T44.3x4	T44.3x5	T44.3x6
Gelatin (intravenous)	T45.8x1	T45.8x2	T45.8x3	T45.8x4	T45.8x5	T45.8x6
absorbable (sponge)	T45.7x1	T45.7x2	T45.7x3	T45.7x4	T45.7x5	T45.7x6
Gelfilm	T49.8x1	T49.8x2	T49.8x3	T49.8x4	T49.8x5	T49.8x6
Gelfoam	T45.7x1	T45.7x2	T45.7x3	T45.7x4	T45.7x5	T45.7x6
Gelsemine	T50.991	T50.992	T50.993	T50.994	T50.995	T50.996
Gelsemium (sempervirens)	T62.2x1	T62.2x2	T62.2x3	T62.2x4	—	—
Gemeprost	T48.0x1	T48.0x2	T48.0x3	T48.0x4	T48.0x5	T48.0x6
Gemfibrozil	T46.6x1	T46.6x2	T46.6x3	T46.6x4	T46.6x5	T46.6x6
Gemonil	T42.3x1	T42.3x2	T42.3x3	T42.3x4	T42.3x5	T42.3x6
Gentamicin	T36.5x1	T36.5x2	T36.5x3	T36.5x4	T36.5x5	T36.5x6
ophthalmic preparation	T49.5x1	T49.5x2	T49.5x3	T49.5x4	T49.5x5	T49.5x6
topical NEC	T49.0x1	T49.0x2	T49.0x3	T49.0x4	T49.0x5	T49.0x6
Gentian	T47.5x1	T47.5x2	T47.5x3	T47.5x4	T47.5x5	T47.5x6
violet	T49.0x1	T49.0x2	T49.0x3	T49.0x4	T49.0x5	T49.0x6

Table of Drugs & Chemicals	Accidental (Unintentional)	Self-Harm (Intentional)	Assault	Undetermined	Adverse Effect	Underdosing
Gepefrine	T44.4x1	T44.4x2	T44.4x3	T44.4x4	T44.4x5	T44.4x6
Gestonorone caproate	T38.5x1	T38.5x2	T38.5x3	T38.5x4	T38.5x5	T38.5x6
Gexane	T49.0x1	T49.0x2	T49.0x3	T49.0x4	T49.0x5	T49.0x6
Gila monster (venom)	T63.111	T63.112	T63.113	T63.114		
Ginger	T47.5x1	T47.5x2	T47.5x3	T47.5x4	T47.5x5	T47.5x6
Jamaica — see Jamaica, ginger						
Gitalin	T46.0x1	T46.0x2	T46.0x3	T46.0x4	T46.0x5	T46.0x6
amorphous	T46.0x1	T46.0x2	T46.0x3	T46.0x4	T46.0x5	T46.0x6
Gitaloxin	T46.0x1	T46.0x2	T46.0x3	T46.0x4	T46.0x5	T46.0x6
Gitoxin	T46.0x1	T46.0x2	T46.0x3	T46.0x4	T46.0x5	T46.0x6
Glafenine	T39.8x1	T39.8x2	T39.8x3	T39.8x4	T39.8x5	T39.8x6
Glandular extract (medicinal) NEC	T50.Z91	T50.Z92	T50.Z93	T50.Z94	T50.Z95	T50.Z96
Glaucarubin	T37.3x1	T37.3x2	T37.3x3	T37.3x4	T37.3x5	T37.3x6
Glibenclamide	T38.3x1	T38.3x2	T38.3x3	T38.3x4	T38.3x5	T38.3x6
Glibornuride	T38.3x1	T38.3x2	T38.3x3	T38.3x4	T38.3x5	T38.3x6
Gliclazide	T38.3x1	T38.3x2	T38.3x3	T38.3x4	T38.3x5	T38.3x6
Glimidine	T38.3x1	T38.3x2	T38.3x3	T38.3x4	T38.3x5	T38.3x6
Glipizide	T38.3x1	T38.3x2	T38.3x3	T38.3x4	T38.3x5	T38.3x6
Gliquidone	T38.3x1	T38.3x2	T38.3x3	T38.3x4	T38.3x5	T38.3x6
Glisolamide	T38.3x1	T38.3x2	T38.3x3	T38.3x4	T38.3x5	T38.3x6
Glisoxepide	T38.3x1	T38.3x2	T38.3x3	T38.3x4	T38.3x5	T38.3x6
Globin zinc insulin	T38.3x1	T38.3x2	T38.3x3	T38.3x4	T38.3x5	T38.3x6
Globulin						
antilymphocytic	T50.Z11	T50.Z12	T50.Z13	T50.Z14	T50.Z15	T50.Z16
antirhesus	T50.Z11	T50.Z12	T50.Z13	T50.Z14	T50.Z15	T50.Z16
antivenin	T50.Z11	T50.Z12	T50.Z13	T50.Z14	T50.Z15	T50.Z16
antiviral	T50.Z11	T50.Z12	T50.Z13	T50.Z14	T50.Z15	T50.Z16
Glucagon	T38.3x1	T38.3x2	T38.3x3	T38.3x4	T38.3x5	T38.3x6
Glucocorticoids	T38.0x1	T38.0x2	T38.0x3	T38.0x4	T38.0x5	T38.0x6
Glucocorticosteroid	T38.0x1	T38.0x2	T38.0x3	T38.0x4	T38.0x5	T38.0x6
Gluconic acid	T50.991	T50.992	T50.993	T50.994	T50.995	T50.996
Glucosamine sulfate	T39.4x1	T39.4x2	T39.4x3	T39.4x4	T39.4x5	T39.4x6
Glucose	T50.3x1	T50.3x2	T50.3x3	T50.3x4	T50.3x5	T50.3x6
with sodium chloride	T50.3x1	T50.3x2	T50.3x3	T50.3x4	T50.3x5	T50.3x6
Glucosulfone sodium	T37.1x1	T37.1x2	T37.1x3	T37.1x4	T37.1x5	T37.1x6
Glucurolactone	T47.8x1	T47.8x2	T47.8x3	T47.8x4	T47.8x5	T47.8x6
Glue NEC	T52.8x1	T52.8x2	T52.8x3	T52.8x4	—	—
Glutamic acid	T47.5x1	T47.5x2	T47.5x3	T47.5x4	T47.5x5	T47.5x6
Glutaral (medicinal)	T49.0x1	T49.0x2	T49.0x3	T49.0x4	T49.0x5	T49.0x6
nonmedicinal	T65.891	T65.892	T65.893	T65.894	—	—
Glutaraldehyde (nonmedicinal)	T65.891	T65.892	T65.893	T65.894	—	—
medicinal	T49.0x1	T49.0x2	T49.0x3	T49.0x4	T49.0x5	T49.0x6
Glutathione	T50.6x1	T50.6x2	T50.6x3	T50.6x4	T50.6x5	T50.6x6
Glutethimide	T42.6x1	T42.6x2	T42.6x3	T42.6x4	T42.6x5	T42.6x6
Glyburide	T38.3x1	T38.3x2	T38.3x3	T38.3x4	T38.3x5	T38.3x6
Glycerin	T47.4x1	T47.4x2	T47.4x3	T47.4x4	T47.4x5	T47.4x6
Glycerol	T47.4x1	T47.4x2	T47.4x3	T47.4x4	T47.4x5	T47.4x6
borax	T49.6x1	T49.6x2	T49.6x3	T49.6x4	T49.6x5	T49.6x6
intravenous	T50.3x1	T50.3x2	T50.3x3	T50.3x4	T50.3x5	T50.3x6
iodinated	T48.4x1	T48.4x2	T48.4x3	T48.4x4	T48.4x5	T48.4x6
Glycerophosphate	T50.991	T50.992	T50.993	T50.994	T50.995	T50.996
Glyceryl						
gualacolate	T48.4x1	T48.4x2	T48.4x3	T48.4x4	T48.4x5	T48.4x6
nitrate	T46.3x1	T46.3x2	T46.3x3	T46.3x4	T46.3x5	T46.3x6
triacetate (topical)	T49.0x1	T49.0x2	T49.0x3	T49.0x4	T49.0x5	T49.0x6
trinitrate	T46.3x1	T46.3x2	T46.3x3	T46.3x4	T46.3x5	T46.3x6
Glycine	T50.3x1	T50.3x2	T50.3x3	T50.3x4	T50.3x5	T50.3x6
Glyclopyramide	T38.3x1	T38.3x2	T38.3x3	T38.3x4	T38.3x5	T38.3x6
Glycobiarsol	T37.3x1	T37.3x2	T37.3x3	T37.3x4	T37.3x5	T37.3x6
Glycols (ether)	T52.3x1	T52.3x2	T52.3x3	T52.3x4	—	—
Glyconiazide	T37.1x1	T37.1x2	T37.1x3	T37.1x4	T37.1x5	T37.1x6
Glycopyrrolate	T44.3x1	T44.3x2	T44.3x3	T44.3x4	T44.3x5	T44.3x6
Glycopyrronium	T44.3x1	T44.3x2	T44.3x3	T44.3x4	T44.3x5	T44.3x6
bromide	T44.3x1	T44.3x2	T44.3x3	T44.3x4	T44.3x5	T44.3x6
Glycoside, cardiac (stimulant)	T46.0x1	T46.0x2	T46.0x3	T46.0x4	T46.0x5	T46.0x6
Glycyclamide	T38.3x1	T38.3x2	T38.3x3	T38.3x4	T38.3x5	T38.3x6
Glycyrrhiza extract	T48.4x1	T48.4x2	T48.4x3	T48.4x4	T48.4x5	T48.4x6
Glycyrrhizic acid	T48.4x1	T48.4x2	T48.4x3	T48.4x4	T48.4x5	T48.4x6

Table of Drugs & Chemicals	POISONING Accidental (Unintentional)	Self-Harm (Intentional)	Assault	Undetermined	Adverse Effect	Underdosing
Glycyrrhizinate potassium	T48.4x1	T48.4x2	T48.4x3	T48.4x4	T48.4x5	T48.4x6
Glymidine sodium	T38.3x1	T38.3x2	T38.3x3	T38.3x4	T38.3x5	T38.3x6
Glyphosate	T60.3x1	T60.3x2	T60.3x3	T60.3x4	—	—
Glyphylline	T48.6x1	T48.6x2	T48.6x3	T48.6x4	T48.6x5	T48.6x6
Gold						
colloidal (l98Au)	T45.1x1	T45.1x2	T45.1x3	T45.1x4	T45.1x5	T45.1x6
salts	T39.4x1	T39.4x2	T39.4x3	T39.4x4	T39.4x5	T39.4x6
Golden sulfide of antimony	T56.891	T56.892	T56.893	T56.894	—	—
Goldylocks	T62.2x1	T62.2x2	T62.2x3	T62.2x4	—	—
Gonadal tissue extract	T38.901	T38.902	T38.903	T38.904	T38.905	T38.906
female	T38.5x1	T38.5x2	T38.5x3	T38.5x4	T38.5x5	T38.5x6
male	T38.7x1	T38.7x2	T38.7x3	T38.7x4	T38.7x5	T38.7x6
Gonadorelin	T38.891	T38.892	T38.893	T38.894	T38.895	T38.896
Gonadotropin	T38.891	T38.892	T38.893	T38.894	T38.895	T38.896
chorionic	T38.891	T38.892	T38.893	T38.894	T38.895	T38.896
pituitary	T38.811	T38.812	T38.813	T38.814	T38.815	T38.816
Goserelin	T45.1x1	T45.1x2	T45.1x3	T45.1x4	T45.1x5	T45.1x6
Grain alcohol	T51.0x1	T51.0x2	T51.0x3	T51.0x4	—	—
Gramicidin	T49.0x1	T49.0x2	T49.0x3	T49.0x4	T49.0x5	T49.0x6
Granisetron	T45.0x1	T45.0x2	T45.0x3	T45.0x4	T45.0x5	T45.0x6
Gratiola officinalis	T62.2x1	T62.2x2	T62.2x3	T62.2x4	—	—
Grease	T65.891	T65.892	T65.893	T65.894	—	—
Green hellebore	T62.2x1	T62.2x2	T62.2x3	T62.2x4	—	—
Green soap	T49.2x1	T49.2x2	T49.2x3	T49.2x4	T49.2x5	T49.2x6
Grifulvin	T36.7x1	T36.7x2	T36.7x3	T36.7x4	T36.7x5	T36.7x6
Griseofulvin	T36.7x1	T36.7x2	T36.7x3	T36.7x4	T36.7x5	T36.7x6
Growth hormone	T38.811	T38.812	T38.813	T38.814	T38.815	T38.816
Guaiac reagent	T50.991	T50.992	T50.993	T50.994	T50.995	T50.996
Guaiacol derivatives	T48.4x1	T48.4x2	T48.4x3	T48.4x4	T48.4x5	T48.4x6
Guaifenesin	T48.4x1	T48.4x2	T48.4x3	T48.4x4	T48.4x5	T48.4x6
Guaimesal	T48.4x1	T48.4x2	T48.4x3	T48.4x4	T48.4x5	T48.4x6
Guaiphenesin	T48.4x1	T48.4x2	T48.4x3	T48.4x4	T48.4x5	T48.4x6
Guamecycline	T36.4x1	T36.4x2	T36.4x3	T36.4x4	T36.4x5	T36.4x6
Guanabenz	T46.5x1	T46.5x2	T46.5x3	T46.5x4	T46.5x5	T46.5x6
Guanacline	T46.5x1	T46.5x2	T46.5x3	T46.5x4	T46.5x5	T46.5x6
Guanadrel	T46.5x1	T46.5x2	T46.5x3	T46.5x4	T46.5x5	T46.5x6
Guanatol	T37.2x1	T37.2x2	T37.2x3	T37.2x4	T37.2x5	T37.2x6
Guanethidine	T46.5x1	T46.5x2	T46.5x3	T46.5x4	T46.5x5	T46.5x6
Guanfacine	T46.5x1	T46.5x2	T46.5x3	T46.5x4	T46.5x5	T46.5x6
Guano	T65.891	T65.892	T65.893	T65.894	—	—
Guanochlor	T46.5x1	T46.5x2	T46.5x3	T46.5x4	T46.5x5	T46.5x6
Guanoclor	T46.5x1	T46.5x2	T46.5x3	T46.5x4	T46.5x5	T46.5x6
Guanoctine	T46.5x1	T46.5x2	T46.5x3	T46.5x4	T46.5x5	T46.5x6
Guanoxabenz	T46.5x1	T46.5x2	T46.5x3	T46.5x4	T46.5x5	T46.5x6
Guanoxan	T46.5x1	T46.5x2	T46.5x3	T46.5x4	T46.5x5	T46.5x6
Guar gum (medicinal)	T46.6x1	T46.6x2	T46.6x3	T46.6x4	T46.6x5	T46.6x6
Hachimycin	T36.7x1	T36.7x2	T36.7x3	T36.7x4	T36.7x5	T36.7x6
Hair						
dye	T49.4x1	T49.4x2	T49.4x3	T49.4x4	T49.4x5	T49.4x6
preparation NEC	T49.4x1	T49.4x2	T49.4x3	T49.4x4	T49.4x5	T49.4x6
Halazepam	T42.4x1	T42.4x2	T42.4x3	T42.4x4	T42.4x5	T42.4x6
Halcinolone	T49.0x1	T49.0x2	T49.0x3	T49.0x4	T49.0x5	T49.0x6
Halcinonide	T49.0x1	T49.0x2	T49.0x3	T49.0x4	T49.0x5	T49.0x6
Halethazole	T49.0x1	T49.0x2	T49.0x3	T49.0x4	T49.0x5	T49.0x6
Hallucinogen NEC	T40.901	T40.902	T40.903	T40.904	T40.905	T40.906
Halofantrine	T37.2x1	T37.2x2	T37.2x3	T37.2x4	T37.2x5	T37.2x6
Halofenate	T46.6x1	T46.6x2	T46.6x3	T46.6x4	T46.6x5	T46.6x6
Halometasone	T49.0x1	T49.0x2	T49.0x3	T49.0x4	T49.0x5	T49.0x6
Haloperidol	T43.4x1	T43.4x2	T43.4x3	T43.4x4	T43.4x5	T43.4x6
Haloprogin	T49.0x1	T49.0x2	T49.0x3	T49.0x4	T49.0x5	T49.0x6
Halotex	T49.0x1	T49.0x2	T49.0x3	T49.0x4	T49.0x5	T49.0x6
Halothane	T41.0x1	T41.0x2	T41.0x3	T41.0x4	T41.0x5	T41.0x6
Haloxazolam	T42.4x1	T42.4x2	T42.4x3	T42.4x4	T42.4x5	T42.4x6
Halquinols	T49.0x1	T49.0x2	T49.0x3	T49.0x4	T49.0x5	T49.0x6
Hamamelis	T49.2x1	T49.2x2	T49.2x3	T49.2x4	T49.2x5	T49.2x6
Haptendextran	T45.8x1	T45.8x2	T45.8x3	T45.8x4	T45.8x5	T45.8x6
Harmonyl	T46.5x1	T46.5x2	T46.5x3	T46.5x4	T46.5x5	T46.5x6
Hartmann's solution	T50.3x1	T50.3x2	T50.3x3	T50.3x4	T50.3x5	T50.3x6

Table of Drugs & Chemicals	POISONING Accidental (Unintentional)	Self-Harm (Intentional)	Assault	Undetermined	Adverse Effect	Underdosing
Hashish	T40.7x1	T40.7x2	T40.7x3	T40.7x4	T40.7x5	T40.7x6
Hawaiian Woodrose seeds	T40.991	T40.992	T40.993	T40.994	—	—
HCB	T60.3x1	T60.3x2	T60.3x3	T60.3x4	—	—
HCH	T53.6x1	T53.6x2	T53.6x3	T53.6x4	—	—
medicinal	T49.0x1	T49.0x2	T49.0x3	T49.0x4	T49.0x5	T49.0x6
HCN	T57.3x1	T57.3x2	T57.3x3	T57.3x4	—	—
Headache cures, drugs, powders NEC	T50.901	T50.902	T50.903	T50.904	T50.905	T50.906
Heavenly Blue (morning glory)	T40.991	T40.992	T40.993	T40.994	—	—
Heavy metal antidote	T45.8x1	T45.8x2	T45.8x3	T45.8x4	T45.8x5	T45.8x6
Hedaquinium	T49.0x1	T49.0x2	T49.0x3	T49.0x4	T49.0x5	T49.0x6
Hedge hyssop	T62.2x1	T62.2x2	T62.2x3	T62.2x4	—	—
Heet	T49.8x1	T49.8x2	T49.8x3	T49.8x4	T49.8x5	T49.8x6
Helenin	T37.4x1	T37.4x2	T37.4x3	T37.4x4	T37.4x5	T37.4x6
Helium (nonmedicinal) NEC	T59.891	T59.892	T59.893	T59.894	—	—
medicinal	T48.991	T48.992	T48.993	T48.994	T48.995	T48.996
Hellebore (black) (green) (white)	T62.2x1	T62.2x2	T62.2x3	T62.2x4	—	—
Hematin	T45.8x1	T45.8x2	T45.8x3	T45.8x4	T45.8x5	T45.8x6
Hematinic preparation	T45.8x1	T45.8x2	T45.8x3	T45.8x4	T45.8x5	T45.8x6
Hematological agent	T45.91	T45.92	T45.93	T45.94	T45.95	T45.96
specified NEC	T45.8x1	T45.8x2	T45.8x3	T45.8x4	T45.8x5	T45.8x6
Hemlock	T62.2x1	T62.2x2	T62.2x3	T62.2x4	—	—
Hemostatic	T45.621	T45.622	T45.623	T45.624	T45.625	T45.626
drug, systemic	T45.621	T45.622	T45.623	T45.624	T45.625	T45.626
Hemostyptic	T49.4x1	T49.4x2	T49.4x3	T49.4x4	T49.4x5	T49.4x6
Henbane	T62.2x1	T62.2x2	T62.2x3	T62.2x4	—	—
Heparin (sodium)	T45.511	T45.512	T45.513	T45.514	T45.515	T45.516
action reverser	T45.7x1	T45.7x2	T45.7x3	T45.7x4	T45.7x5	T45.7x6
Heparin-fraction	T45.511	T45.512	T45.513	T45.514	T45.515	T45.516
Heparinoid (systemic)	T45.511	T45.512	T45.513	T45.514	T45.515	T45.516
Hepatic secretion stimulant	T47.8x1	T47.8x2	T47.8x3	T47.8x4	T47.8x5	T47.8x6
Hepatitis B						
immune globulin	T50.Z11	T50.Z12	T50.Z13	T50.Z14	T50.Z15	T50.Z16
vaccine	T50.B91	T50.B92	T50.B93	T50.B94	T50.B95	T50.B96
Hepronicate	T46.7x1	T46.7x2	T46.7x3	T46.7x4	T46.7x5	T46.7x6
Heptabarb	T42.3x1	T42.3x2	T42.3x3	T42.3x4	T42.3x5	T42.3x6
Heptabarbital	T42.3x1	T42.3x2	T42.3x3	T42.3x4	T42.3x5	T42.3x6
Heptabarbitone	T42.3x1	T42.3x2	T42.3x3	T42.3x4	T42.3x5	T42.3x6
Heptachlor	T60.1x1	T60.1x2	T60.1x3	T60.1x4	—	—
Heptalgin	T40.2x1	T40.2x2	T40.2x3	T40.2x4	T40.2x5	T40.2x6
Heptaminol	T46.3x1	T46.3x2	T46.3x3	T46.3x4	T46.3x5	T46.3x6
Herbicide NEC	T60.3x1	T60.3x2	T60.3x3	T60.3x4	—	—
Heroin	T40.1x1	T40.1x2	T40.1x3	T40.1x4	—	—
Herplex	T49.5x1	T49.5x2	T49.5x3	T49.5x4	T49.5x5	T49.5x6
HES	T45.8x1	T45.8x2	T45.8x3	T45.8x4	T45.8x5	T45.8x6
Hesperidin	T46.991	T46.992	T46.993	T46.994	T46.995	T46.996
Hetacillin	T36.0x1	T36.0x2	T36.0x3	T36.0x4	T36.0x5	T36.0x6
Hetastarch	T45.8x1	T45.8x2	T45.8x3	T45.8x4	T45.8x5	T45.8x6
HETP	T60.0x1	T60.0x2	T60.0x3	T60.0x4	—	—
Hexachlorobenzene (vapor)	T60.3x1	T60.3x2	T60.3x3	T60.3x4	—	—
Hexachlorocyclohexane	T53.6x1	T53.6x2	T53.6x3	T53.6x4	—	—
Hexachlorophene	T49.0x1	T49.0x2	T49.0x3	T49.0x4	T49.0x5	T49.0x6
Hexadiline	T46.3x1	T46.3x2	T46.3x3	T46.3x4	T46.3x5	T46.3x6
Hexadimethrine (bromide)	T45.7x1	T45.7x2	T45.7x3	T45.7x4	T45.7x5	T45.7x6
Hexadylamine	T46.3x1	T46.3x2	T46.3x3	T46.3x4	T46.3x5	T46.3x6
Hexaethyl tetraphos-phate	T60.0x1	T60.0x2	T60.0x3	T60.0x4	—	—
Hexafluorenium bromide	T48.1x1	T48.1x2	T48.1x3	T48.1x4	T48.1x5	T48.1x6
Hexafluronium (bromide)	T48.1x1	T48.1x2	T48.1x3	T48.1x4	T48.1x5	T48.1x6
Hexa-germ	T49.2x1	T49.2x2	T49.2x3	T49.2x4	T49.2x5	T49.2x6
Hexahydrobenzol	T52.8x1	T52.8x2	T52.8x3	T52.8x4	—	—
Hexahydrocresol(s)	T51.8x1	T51.8x2	T51.8x3	T51.8x4	—	—
arsenide	T57.0x1	T57.0x2	T57.0x3	T57.0x4	—	—
arseniurated	T57.0x1	T57.0x2	T57.0x3	T57.0x4	—	—
cyanide	T57.3x1	T57.3x2	T57.3x3	T57.3x4	—	—
gas	T59.891	T59.892	T59.893	T59.894	—	—
Fluoride (liquid)	T57.8x1	T57.8x2	T57.8x3	T57.8x4	—	—
vapor	T59.891	T59.892	T59.893	T59.894	—	—
phophorated	T60.0x1	T60.0x2	T60.0x3	T60.0x4	—	—
sulfate	T57.8x1	T57.8x2	T57.8x3	T57.8x4	—	—
sulfide (gas)	T59.6x1	T59.6x2	T59.6x3	T59.6x4	—	—
arseniurated	T57.0x1	T57.0x2	T57.0x3	T57.0x4	—	—
sulfurated	T57.8x1	T57.8x2	T57.8x3	T57.8x4	—	—

DRUGS&CHEMICALS

DRUGS&CHEMICALS

Table of Drugs & Chemicals	POISONING Accidental (Unintentional)	Self-Harm (Intentional)	Assault	Undetermined	Adverse Effect	Underdosing
Hexahydrophenol	T51.8x1	T51.8x2	T51.8x3	T51.8x4	—	—
Hexalen	T51.8x1	T51.8x2	T51.8x3	T51.8x4	—	—
Hexamethonium bromide	T44.2x1	T44.2x2	T44.2x3	T44.2x4	T44.2x5	T44.2x6
Hexamethylene	T52.8x1	T52.8x2	T52.8x3	T52.8x4	—	—
Hexamethylmelamine	T45.1x1	T45.1x2	T45.1x3	T45.1x4	T45.1x5	T45.1x6
Hexamidine	T49.0x1	T49.0x2	T49.0x3	T49.0x4	T49.0x5	T49.0x6
Hexamine (mandelate)	T37.8x1	T37.8x2	T37.8x3	T37.8x4	T37.8x5	T37.8x6
Hexanone, 2-hexanone	T52.4x1	T52.4x2	T52.4x3	T52.4x4	—	—
Hexanuorenium	T48.1x1	T48.1x2	T48.1x3	T48.1x4	T48.1x5	T48.1x6
Hexapropymate	T42.6x1	T42.6x2	T42.6x3	T42.6x4	T42.6x5	T42.6x6
Hexasonium iodide	T44.3x1	T44.3x2	T44.3x3	T44.3x4	T44.3x5	T44.3x6
Hexcarbacholine bromide	T48.1x1	T48.1x2	T48.1x3	T48.1x4	T48.1x5	T48.1x6
Hexemal	T42.3x1	T42.3x2	T42.3x3	T42.3x4	T42.3x5	T42.3x6
Hexestrol	T38.5x1	T38.5x2	T38.5x3	T38.5x4	T38.5x5	T38.5x6
Hexethal (sodium)	T42.3x1	T42.3x2	T42.3x3	T42.3x4	T42.3x5	T42.3x6
Hexetidine	T37.8x1	T37.8x2	T37.8x3	T37.8x4	T37.8x5	T37.8x6
Hexobarbital	T42.3x1	T42.3x2	T42.3x3	T42.3x4	T42.3x5	T42.3x6
rectal	T41.291	T41.292	T41.293	T41.294	T41.295	T41.296
sodium	T41.1x1	T41.1x2	T41.1x3	T41.1x4	T41.1x5	T41.1x6
Hexobendine	T46.3x1	T46.3x2	T46.3x3	T46.3x4	T46.3x5	T46.3x6
Hexocyclium	T44.3x1	T44.3x2	T44.3x3	T44.3x4	T44.3x5	T44.3x6
metilsulfate	T44.3x1	T44.3x2	T44.3x3	T44.3x4	T44.3x5	T44.3x6
Hexoestrol	T38.5x1	T38.5x2	T38.5x3	T38.5x4	T38.5x5	T38.5x6
Hexone	T52.4x1	T52.4x2	T52.4x3	T52.4x4	—	—
Hexoprenaline	T48.6x1	T48.6x2	T48.6x3	T48.6x4	T48.6x5	T48.6x6
Hexylcaine	T41.3x1	T41.3x2	T41.3x3	T41.3x4	T41.3x5	T41.3x6
Hexylresorcinol	T52.2x1	T52.2x2	T52.2x3	T52.2x4	—	—
HGH (human growth hormone)	T38.811	T38.812	T38.813	T38.814	T38.815	T38.816
Hinkle's pills	T47.2x1	T47.2x2	T47.2x3	T47.2x4	T47.2x5	T47.2x6
Histalog	T50.8x1	T50.8x2	T50.8x3	T50.8x4	T50.8x5	T50.8x6
Histamine (phosphate)	T50.8x1	T50.8x2	T50.8x3	T50.8x4	T50.8x5	T50.8x6
Histoplasmin	T50.8x1	T50.8x2	T50.8x3	T50.8x4	T50.8x5	T50.8x6
Holly berries	T62.2x1	T62.2x2	T62.2x3	T62.2x4	—	—
Homatropine	T44.3x1	T44.3x2	T44.3x3	T44.3x4	T44.3x5	T44.3x6
methylbromide	T44.3x1	T44.3x2	T44.3x3	T44.3x4	T44.3x5	T44.3x6
Homochlorcyclizine	T45.0x1	T45.0x2	T45.0x3	T45.0x4	T45.0x5	T45.0x6
Homosalate	T49.3x1	T49.3x2	T49.3x3	T49.3x4	T49.3x5	T49.3x6
Homo-tet	T50.Z11	T50.Z12	T50.Z13	T50.Z14	T50.Z15	T50.Z16
Hormone	T38.801	T38.802	T38.803	T38.804	T38.805	T38.806
adrenal cortical steroids	T38.0x1	T38.0x2	T38.0x3	T38.0x4	T38.0x5	T38.0x6
androgenic	T38.7x1	T38.7x2	T38.7x3	T38.7x4	T38.7x5	T38.7x6
anterior pituitary NEC	T38.811	T38.812	T38.813	T38.814	T38.815	T38.816
antidiabetic agents	T38.3x1	T38.3x2	T38.3x3	T38.3x4	T38.3x5	T38.3x6
antidiuretic	T38.891	T38.892	T38.893	T38.894	T38.895	T38.896
cancer therapy	T45.1x1	T45.1x2	T45.1x3	T45.1x4	T45.1x5	T45.1x6
follicle stimulating	T38.811	T38.812	T38.813	T38.814	T38.815	T38.816
gonadotropic	T38.891	T38.892	T38.893	T38.894	T38.895	T38.896
pituitary	T38.811	T38.812	T38.813	T38.814	T38.815	T38.816
growth	T38.811	T38.812	T38.813	T38.814	T38.815	T38.816
luteinizing	T38.811	T38.812	T38.813	T38.814	T38.815	T38.816
ovarian	T38.5x1	T38.5x2	T38.5x3	T38.5x4	T38.5x5	T38.5x6
oxytocic	T48.0x1	T48.0x2	T48.0x3	T48.0x4	T48.0x5	T48.0x6
parathyroid (derivatives)	T50.991	T50.992	T50.993	T50.994	T50.995	T50.996
pituitary (posterior) NEC	T38.891	T38.892	T38.893	T38.894	T38.895	T38.896
anterior	T38.811	T38.812	T38.813	T38.814	T38.815	T38.816
specified, NEC	T38.891	T38.892	T38.893	T38.894	T38.895	T38.896
thyroid	T38.1x1	T38.1x2	T38.1x3	T38.1x4	T38.1x5	T38.1x6
Hornet (sting)	T63.451	T63.452	T63.453	T63.454	—	—
Horse anti-human lymphocytic serum	T50.Z11	T50.Z12	T50.Z13	T50.Z14	T50.Z15	T50.Z16
Horticulture agent NEC	T65.91	T65.92	T65.93	T65.94	—	—
with pesticide	T60.91	T60.92	T60.93	T60.94	—	—
Human albumin	T45.8x1	T45.8x2	T45.8x3	T45.8x4	T45.8x5	T45.8x6
growth hormone (HGH)	T38.811	T38.812	T38.813	T38.814	T38.815	T38.816
immune serum	T50.Z11	T50.Z12	T50.Z13	T50.Z14	T50.Z15	T50.Z16
Hyaluronidase	T45.3x1	T45.3x2	T45.3x3	T45.3x4	T45.3x5	T45.3x6
Hyazyme	T45.3x1	T45.3x2	T45.3x3	T45.3x4	T45.3x5	T45.3x6

Table of Drugs & Chemicals	POISONING Accidental (Unintentional)	Self-Harm (Intentional)	Assault	Undetermined	Adverse Effect	Underdosing
Hycodan	T40.2x1	T40.2x2	T40.2x3	T40.2x4	T40.2x5	T40.2x6
Hydantoin derivative NEC	T42.0x1	T42.0x2	T42.0x3	T42.0x4	T42.0x5	T42.0x6
Hydeltra	T38.0x1	T38.0x2	T38.0x3	T38.0x4	T38.0x5	T38.0x6
Hydergine	T44.6x1	T44.6x2	T44.6x3	T44.6x4	T44.6x5	T44.6x6
Hydrabamine penicillin	T36.0x1	T36.0x2	T36.0x3	T36.0x4	T36.0x5	T36.0x6
Hydralazine	T46.5x1	T46.5x2	T46.5x3	T46.5x4	T46.5x5	T46.5x6
Hydrargaphen	T49.0x1	T49.0x2	T49.0x3	T49.0x4	T49.0x5	T49.0x6
Hydrargyri amino-chloridum	T49.0x1	T49.0x2	T49.0x3	T49.0x4	T49.0x5	T49.0x6
Hydrastine	T48.291	T48.292	T48.293	T48.294	T48.295	T48.296
Hydrazine	T54.1x1	T54.1x2	T54.1x3	T54.1x4	—	—
monoamine oxidase inhibitors	T43.1x1	T43.1x2	T43.1x3	T43.1x4	T43.1x5	T43.1x6
Hydrazoic acid, azides	T54.2x1	T54.2x2	T54.2x3	T54.2x4	—	—
Hydriodic acid	T48.4x1	T48.4x2	T48.4x3	T48.4x4	T48.4x5	T48.4x6
Hydrocarbon gas	T59.891	T59.892	T59.893	T59.894	—	—
incomplete combustion of — see Carbon, monoxide, fuel, utility						
liquefied (mobile container)	T59.891	T59.892	T59.893	T59.894	—	—
piped (natural)	T59.891	T59.892	T59.893	T59.894	—	—
Hydrochloric acid (liquid)	T54.2x1	T54.2x2	T54.2x3	T54.2x4	—	—
medicinal (digestant)	T47.5x1	T47.5x2	T47.5x3	T47.5x4	T47.5x5	T47.5x6
vapor	T59.891	T59.892	T59.893	T59.894	—	—
Hydrochlorothiazide	T50.2x1	T50.2x2	T50.2x3	T50.2x4	T50.2x5	T50.2x6
Hydrocodone	T40.2x1	T40.2x2	T40.2x3	T40.2x4	T40.2x5	T40.2x6
Hydrocortisone (derivatives)	T49.0x1	T49.0x2	T49.0x3	T49.0x4	T49.0x5	T49.0x6
aceponate	T49.0x1	T49.0x2	T49.0x3	T49.0x4	T49.0x5	T49.0x6
ENT agent	T49.6x1	T49.6x2	T49.6x3	T49.6x4	T49.6x5	T49.6x6
ophthalmic preparation	T49.5x1	T49.5x2	T49.5x3	T49.5x4	T49.5x5	T49.5x6
topical NEC	T49.0x1	T49.0x2	T49.0x3	T49.0x4	T49.0x5	T49.0x6
Hydrocortone	T38.0x1	T38.0x2	T38.0x3	T38.0x4	T38.0x5	T38.0x6
ENT agent	T49.6x1	T49.6x2	T49.6x3	T49.6x4	T49.6x5	T49.6x6
ophthalmic preparation	T49.5x1	T49.5x2	T49.5x3	T49.5x4	T49.5x5	T49.5x6
topical NEC	T49.0x1	T49.0x2	T49.0x3	T49.0x4	T49.0x5	T49.0x6
Hydrocyanic acid (liquid)	T57.3x1	T57.3x2	T57.3x3	T57.3x4	—	—
gas	T65.0x1	T65.0x2	T65.0x3	T65.0x4	—	—
Hydroflumethiazide	T50.2x1	T50.2x2	T50.2x3	T50.2x4	T50.2x5	T50.2x6
Hydrofluoric acid (liquid)	T54.2x1	T54.2x2	T54.2x3	T54.2x4	—	—
vapor	T59.891	T59.892	T59.893	T59.894	—	—
Hydrogen	T59.891	T59.892	T59.893	T59.894	—	—
arsenide	T57.0x1	T57.0x2	T57.0x3	T57.0x4	—	—
arseniureted	T57.0x1	T57.0x2	T57.0x3	T57.0x4	—	—
chloride	T57.8x1	T57.8x2	T57.8x3	T57.8x4	—	—
cyanide (salts)	T57.3x1	T57.3x2	T57.3x3	T57.3x4	—	—
gas	T57.3x1	T57.3x2	T57.3x3	T57.3x4	—	—
fluoride	T59.5x1	T59.5x2	T59.5x3	T59.5x4	—	—
vapor	T59.5x1	T59.5x2	T59.5x3	T59.5x4	—	—
peroxide	T49.0x1	T49.0x2	T49.0x3	T49.0x4	T49.0x5	T49.0x6
phosphureted	T57.1x1	T57.1x2	T57.1x3	T57.1x4	—	—
sulfide	T59.6x1	T59.6x2	T59.6x3	T59.6x4	—	—
arseniureted	T57.0x1	T57.0x2	T57.0x3	T57.0x4	—	—
sulfureted	T59.6x1	T59.6x2	T59.6x3	T59.6x4	—	—
Hydromethylpyridine	T46.7x1	T46.7x2	T46.7x3	T46.7x4	T46.7x5	T46.7x6
Hydromorphinol	T40.2x1	T40.2x2	T40.2x3	T40.2x4	—	—
Hydromorphinone	T40.2x1	T40.2x2	T40.2x3	T40.2x4	T40.2x5	T40.2x6
Hydromorphone	T40.2x1	T40.2x2	T40.2x3	T40.2x4	T40.2x5	T40.2x6
Hydromox	T50.2x1	T50.2x2	T50.2x3	T50.2x4	T50.2x5	T50.2x6
Hydrophilic lotion	T49.3x1	T49.3x2	T49.3x3	T49.3x4	T49.3x5	T49.3x6
Hydroquinidine	T46.2x1	T46.2x2	T46.2x3	T46.2x4	T46.2x5	T46.2x6
Hydroquinone	T52.2x1	T52.2x2	T52.2x3	T52.2x4	—	—
vapor	T59.891	T59.892	T59.893	T59.894	—	—
Hydrosulfuric acid (gas)	T59.6x1	T59.6x2	T59.6x3	T59.6x4	—	—
Hydrotalcite	T47.1x1	T47.1x2	T47.1x3	T47.1x4	T47.1x5	T47.1x6
Hydrous wool fat	T49.3x1	T49.3x2	T49.3x3	T49.3x4	T49.3x5	T49.3x6
Hydroxide, caustic	T54.3x1	T54.3x2	T54.3x3	T54.3x4	—	—
Hydroxocobalamin	T45.8x1	T45.8x2	T45.8x3	T45.8x4	T45.8x5	T45.8x6
Hydroxyamphetamine	T49.5x1	T49.5x2	T49.5x3	T49.5x4	T49.5x5	T49.5x6
Hydroxycarbamide	T45.1x1	T45.1x2	T45.1x3	T45.1x4	T45.1x5	T45.1x6

DRUGS&CHEMICALS

Table of Drugs & Chemicals	POISONING Accidental (Unintentional)	POISONING Self-Harm (Intentional)	POISONING Assault	POISONING Undetermined	Adverse Effect	Underdosing
Hydroxychloroquine	T37.8x1	T37.8x2	T37.8x3	T37.8x4	T37.8x5	T37.8x6
Hydroxydihydrocodeinone	T40.2x1	T40.2x2	T40.2x3	T40.2x4	T40.2x5	T40.2x6
Hydroxyestrone	T38.5x1	T38.5x2	T38.5x3	T38.5x4	T38.5x5	T38.5x6
Hydroxyethyl starch	T45.8x1	T45.8x2	T45.8x3	T45.8x4	T45.8x5	T45.8x6
Hydroxymethylpenta-none	T52.4x1	T52.4x2	T52.4x3	T52.4x4	—	—
Hydroxyphenamate	T43.591	T43.592	T43.593	T43.594	T43.595	T43.596
Hydroxyphenylbutazone	T39.2x1	T39.2x2	T39.2x3	T39.2x4	T39.2x5	T39.2x6
Hydroxyprogesterone	T38.5x1	T38.5x2	T38.5x3	T38.5x4	T38.5x5	T38.5x6
caproate	T38.5x1	T38.5x2	T38.5x3	T38.5x4	T38.5x5	T38.5x6
Hydroxyquinoline (derivatives) NEC	T37.8x1	T37.8x2	T37.8x3	T37.8x4	T37.8x5	T37.8x6
Hydroxystilbamidine	T37.3x1	T37.3x2	T37.3x3	T37.3x4	T37.3x5	T37.3x6
Hydroxytoluene (nonmedicinal)	T54.0x1	T54.0x2	T54.0x3	T54.0x4	—	—
medicinal	T49.0x1	T49.0x2	T49.0x3	T49.0x4	T49.0x5	T49.0x6
Hydroxyurea	T45.1x1	T45.1x2	T45.1x3	T45.1x4	T45.1x5	T45.1x6
Hydroxyzine	T43.591	T43.592	T43.593	T43.594	T43.595	T43.596
Hyoscine	T44.3x1	T44.3x2	T44.3x3	T44.3x4	T44.3x5	T44.3x6
Hyoscyamine	T44.3x1	T44.3x2	T44.3x3	T44.3x4	T44.3x5	T44.3x6
Hyoscyamus	T44.3x1	T44.3x2	T44.3x3	T44.3x4	T44.3x5	T44.3x6
dry extract	T44.3x1	T44.3x2	T44.3x3	T44.3x4	T44.3x5	T44.3x6
Hypaque	T50.8x1	T50.8x2	T50.8x3	T50.8x4	T50.8x5	T50.8x6
Hypertussis	T50.Z12	T50.Z12	T50.Z13	T50.Z14	T50.Z15	T50.Z16
Hypnotic	T42.71	T42.72	T42.73	T42.74	T42.75	T42.76
anticonvulsant	T42.71	T42.72	T42.73	T42.74	T42.75	T42.76
specified NEC	T42.6x1	T42.6x2	T42.6x3	T42.6x4	T42.6x5	T42.6x6
Hypochlorite	T49.0x1	T49.0x2	T49.0x3	T49.0x4	T49.0x5	T49.0x6
Hypophysis, posterior	T38.891	T38.892	T38.893	T38.894	T38.895	T38.896
Hypotensive NEC	T46.5x1	T46.5x2	T46.5x3	T46.5x4	T46.5x5	T46.5x6
Hypromellose	T49.5x1	T49.5x2	T49.5x3	T49.5x4	T49.5x5	T49.5x6
Ibacitabine	T37.5x1	T37.5x2	T37.5x3	T37.5x4	T37.5x5	T37.5x6
Ibopamine	T44.991	T44.992	T44.993	T44.994	T44.995	T44.996
Ibufenac	T39.311	T39.312	T39.313	T39.314	T39.315	T39.316
Ibuprofen	T39.311	T39.312	T39.313	T39.314	T39.315	T39.316
Ibuproxam	T39.311	T39.312	T39.313	T39.314	T39.315	T39.316
Ibuterol	T48.6x1	T48.6x2	T48.6x3	T48.6x4	T48.6x5	T48.6x6
Ichthammol	T49.0x1	T49.0x2	T49.0x3	T49.0x4	T49.0x5	T49.0x6
Ichthyol	T49.4x1	T49.4x2	T49.4x3	T49.4x4	T49.4x5	T49.4x6
Idarubicin	T45.1x1	T45.1x2	T45.1x3	T45.1x4	T45.1x5	T45.1x6
Idrocilamide	T42.8x1	T42.8x2	T42.8x3	T42.8x4	T42.8x5	T42.8x6
Ifenprodil	T46.7x1	T46.7x2	T46.7x3	T46.7x4	T46.7x5	T46.7x6
Ifosfamide	T45.1x1	T45.1x2	T45.1x3	T45.1x4	T45.1x5	T45.1x6
Iletin	T38.3x1	T38.3x2	T38.3x3	T38.3x4	T38.3x5	T38.3x6
Ilex	T62.2x1	T62.2x2	T62.2x3	T62.2x4	—	—
Illuminating gas (after combustion)	T58.11	T58.12	T58.13	T58.14	—	—
prior to combustion	T59.891	T59.892	T59.893	T59.894	—	—
Ilopan	T45.2x1	T45.2x2	T45.2x3	T45.2x4	T45.2x5	T45.2x6
Iloprost	T46.7x1	T46.7x2	T46.7x3	T46.7x4	T46.7x5	T46.7x6
Ilotycin	T36.3x1	T36.3x2	T36.3x3	T36.3x4	T36.3x5	T36.3x6
ophthalmic preparation	T49.5x1	T49.5x2	T49.5x3	T49.5x4	T49.5x5	T49.5x6
topical NEC	T49.0x1	T49.0x2	T49.0x3	T49.0x4	T49.0x5	T49.0x6
Imidazole-4-carboxamide	T45.1x1	T45.1x2	T45.1x3	T45.1x4	T45.1x5	T45.1x6
Iminostilbene	T42.1x1	T42.1x2	T42.1x3	T42.1x4	T42.1x5	T42.1x6
Imipenem	T36.0x1	T36.0x2	T36.0x3	T36.0x4	T36.0x5	T36.0x6
Imipramine	T43.011	T43.012	T43.013	T43.014	T43.015	T43.016
Immu-G	T50.Z11	T50.Z12	T50.Z13	T50.Z14	T50.Z15	T50.Z16
Immuglobin	T50.Z11	T50.Z12	T50.Z13	T50.Z14	T50.Z15	T50.Z16
Immune						
globulin	T50.Z11	T50.Z12	T50.Z13	T50.Z14	T50.Z15	T50.Z16
serum globulin	T50.Z11	T50.Z12	T50.Z13	T50.Z14	T50.Z15	T50.Z16
Immunoglobin human (intravenous) (normal)	T50.Z11	T50.Z12	T50.Z13	T50.Z14	T50.Z15	T50.Z16
unmodified	T50.Z11	T50.Z12	T50.Z13	T50.Z14	T50.Z15	T50.Z16
Immunosuppressive drug	T45.1x1	T45.1x2	T45.1x3	T45.1x4	T45.1x5	T45.1x6
Immu-tetanus	T50.Z11	T50.Z12	T50.Z13	T50.Z14	T50.Z15	T50.Z16
Indalpine	T43.221	T43.222	T43.223	T43.224	T43.225	T43.226
Indanazoline	T48.5x1	T48.5x2	T48.5x3	T48.5x4	T48.5x5	T48.5x6
Indandione (derivatives)	T45.511	T45.512	T45.513	T45.514	T45.515	T45.516
Indapamide	T46.5x1	T46.5x2	T46.5x3	T46.5x4	T46.5x5	T46.5x6
Indendione (derivatives)	T45.511	T45.512	T45.513	T45.514	T45.515	T45.516
Indenolol	T44.7x1	T44.7x2	T44.7x3	T44.7x4	T44.7x5	T44.7x6
Inderal	T44.7x1	T44.7x2	T44.7x3	T44.7x4	T44.7x5	T44.7x6
Indian						
hemp	T40.7x1	T40.7x2	T40.7x3	T40.7x4	T40.7x5	T40.7x6
tobacco	T62.2x1	T62.2x2	T62.2x3	T62.2x4	—	—
Indigo carmine	T50.8x1	T50.8x2	T50.8x3	T50.8x4	T50.8x5	T50.8x6
Indobufen	T45.521	T45.522	T45.523	T45.524	T45.525	T45.526
Indocin	T39.2x1	T39.2x2	T39.2x3	T39.2x4	T39.2x5	T39.2x6
Indocyanine green	T50.8x1	T50.8x2	T50.8x3	T50.8x4	T50.8x5	T50.8x6
Indometacin	T39.391	T39.392	T39.393	T39.394	T39.395	T39.396
Indomethacin	T39.391	T39.392	T39.393	T39.394	T39.395	T39.396
farnesil	T39.4x1	T39.4x2	T39.4x3	T39.4x4	T39.4x5	T39.4x6
Indoramin	T44.6x1	T44.6x2	T44.6x3	T44.6x4	T44.6x5	T44.6x6
Industrial						
alcohol	T51.0x1	T51.0x2	T51.0x3	T51.0x4	—	—
fumes	T59.891	T59.892	T59.893	T59.894	—	—
solvents (fumes) (vapors)	T52.91	T52.92	T52.93	T52.94	—	—
Influenza vaccine	T50.B91	T50.B92	T50.B93	T50.B94	T50.B95	T50.B96
Ingested substance NEC	T65.91	T65.92	T65.93	T65.94	—	—
INH	T37.1x1	T37.1x2	T37.1x3	T37.1x4	T37.1x5	T37.1x6
Inhalation, gas (noxious) — see Gas						
Inhibitor						
angiotensin-converting enzyme	T46.4x1	T46.4x2	T46.4x3	T46.4x4	T46.4x5	T46.4x6
carbonic anhydrase	T50.2x1	T50.2x2	T50.2x3	T50.2x4	T50.2x5	T50.2x6
fibrinolysis	T45.621	T45.622	T45.623	T45.624	T45.625	T45.626
monoamine oxidase NEC	T43.1x1	T43.1x2	T43.1x3	T43.1x4	T43.1x5	T43.1x6
hydrazine	T43.1x1	T43.1x2	T43.1x3	T43.1x4	T43.1x5	T43.1x6
postsynaptic	T43.8x1	T43.8x2	T43.8x3	T43.8x4	T43.8x5	T43.8x6
prothrombin synthesis	T45.511	T45.512	T45.513	T45.514	T45.515	T45.516
Ink	T65.891	T65.892	T65.893	T65.894	—	—
Inorganic substance	T57.91	T57.92	T57.93	T57.94	—	—
Inosine pranobex	T37.5x1	T37.5x2	T37.5x3	T37.5x4	T37.5x5	T37.5x6
Inositol	T50.991	T50.992	T50.993	T50.994	T50.995	T50.996
nicotinate	T46.7x1	T46.7x2	T46.7x3	T46.7x4	T46.7x5	T46.7x6
Inproquone	T45.1x1	T45.1x2	T45.1x3	T45.1x4	T45.1x5	T45.1x6
Insect (sting), venomous	T63.481	T63.482	T63.483	T63.484	—	—
ant	T63.421	T63.422	T63.423	T63.424	—	—
bee	T63.441	T63.442	T63.443	T63.444	—	—
caterpillar	T63.431	T63.432	T63.433	T63.434	—	—
hornet	T63.451	T63.452	T63.453	T63.454	—	—
wasp	T63.461	T63.462	T63.463	T63.464	—	—
Insecticide NEC	T60.91	T60.92	T60.93	T60.94	—	—
carbamate	T60.0x1	T60.0x2	T60.0x3	T60.0x4	—	—
chlorinated	T60.1x1	T60.1x2	T60.1x3	T60.1x4	—	—
mixed	T60.91	T60.92	T60.93	T60.94	—	—
organochlorine	T60.1x1	T60.1x2	T60.1x3	T60.1x4	—	—
organophosphorus	T60.0x1	T60.0x2	T60.0x3	T60.0x4	—	—
Insular tissue extract	T38.3x1	T38.3x2	T38.3x3	T38.3x4	T38.3x5	T38.3x6
Insulin (amorphous) (globin) (isophane) (Lente) (NPH) (Semilente) (Ultralente) (zinc)	T38.3x1	T38.3x2	T38.3x3	T38.3x4	T38.3x5	T38.3x6
defalan	T38.3x1	T38.3x2	T38.3x3	T38.3x4	T38.3x5	T38.3x6
human	T38.3x1	T38.3x2	T38.3x3	T38.3x4	T38.3x5	T38.3x6
injection, soluble	T38.3x1	T38.3x2	T38.3x3	T38.3x4	T38.3x5	T38.3x6
biphasic	T38.3x1	T38.3x2	T38.3x3	T38.3x4	T38.3x5	T38.3x6
intermediate acting	T38.3x1	T38.3x2	T38.3x3	T38.3x4	T38.3x5	T38.3x6
protamine zinc	T38.3x1	T38.3x2	T38.3x3	T38.3x4	T38.3x5	T38.3x6
slow acting	T38.3x1	T38.3x2	T38.3x3	T38.3x4	T38.3x5	T38.3x6
zinc						
protamine injection	T38.3x1	T38.3x2	T38.3x3	T38.3x4	T38.3x5	T38.3x6
suspension (amorphous) (crystalline)	T38.3x1	T38.3x2	T38.3x3	T38.3x4	T38.3x5	T38.3x6
Interferon (alpha) (beta) (gamma)	T37.5x1	T37.5x2	T37.5x3	T37.5x4	T37.5x5	T37.5x6
Intestinal motility control drug	T47.6x1	T47.6x2	T47.6x3	T47.6x4	T47.6x5	T47.6x6
biological	T47.8x1	T47.8x2	T47.8x3	T47.8x4	T47.8x5	T47.8x6

DRUGS&CHEMICALS

Table of Drugs & Chemicals	POISONING Accidental (Unintentional)	Self-Harm (Intentional)	Assault	Undetermined	Adverse Effect	Underdosing
Intranarcon	T41.1x1	T41.1x2	T41.1x3	T41.1x4	T41.1x5	T41.1x6
Intravenous						
amino acids	T50.991	T50.992	T50.993	T50.994	T50.995	T50.996
fat suspension	T50.991	T50.992	T50.993	T50.994	T50.995	T50.996
Inulin	T50.8x1	T50.8x2	T50.8x3	T50.8x4	T50.8x5	T50.8x6
Invert sugar	T50.3x1	T50.3x2	T50.3x3	T50.3x4	T50.3x5	T50.3x6
Inza — *see* Naproxen						
Iobenzamic acid	T50.8x1	T50.8x2	T50.8x3	T50.8x4	T50.8x5	T50.8x6
Iocarmic acid	T50.8x1	T50.8x2	T50.8x3	T50.8x4	T50.8x5	T50.8x6
Iocetamic acid	T50.8x1	T50.8x2	T50.8x3	T50.8x4	T50.8x5	T50.8x6
Iodamide	T50.8x1	T50.8x2	T50.8x3	T50.8x4	T50.8x5	T50.8x6
Iodide NEC — *see also* Iodine	T49.0x1	T49.0x2	T49.0x3	T49.0x4	T49.0x5	T49.0x6
mercury (ointment)	T49.0x1	T49.0x2	T49.0x3	T49.0x4	T49.0x5	T49.0x6
methylate	T49.0x1	T49.0x2	T49.0x3	T49.0x4	T49.0x5	T49.0x6
potassium (expectorant) NEC	T48.4x1	T48.4x2	T48.4x3	T48.4x4	T48.4x5	T48.4x6
Iodinated						
contrast medium	T50.8x1	T50.8x2	T50.8x3	T50.8x4	T50.8x5	T50.8x6
glycerol	T48.4x1	T48.4x2	T48.4x3	T48.4x4	T48.4x5	T48.4x6
human serum albumin (131I)	T50.8x1	T50.8x2	T50.8x3	T50.8x4	T50.8x5	T50.8x6
Iodine (antiseptic, external)						
(tincture) NEC	T49.0x1	T49.0x2	T49.0x3	T49.0x4	T49.0x5	T49.0x6
125 — *see also* Radiation sickness, and Exposure to radioactivce isotopes	T50.8x1	T50.8x2	T50.8x3	T50.8x4	T50.8x5	T50.8x6
therapeutic	T50.991	T50.992	T50.993	T50.994	T50.995	T50.996
131 — *see also* Radiation sickness, and Exposure to radioactivce isotopes	T50.8x1	T50.8x2	T50.8x3	T50.8x4	T50.8x5	T50.8x6
therapeutic	T38.2x1	T38.2x2	T38.2x3	T38.2x4	T38.2x5	T38.2x6
diagnostic	T50.8x1	T50.8x2	T50.8x3	T50.8x4	T50.8x5	T50.8x6
for thyroid conditions (antithyroid)	T38.2x1	T38.2x2	T38.2x3	T38.2x4	T38.2x5	T38.2x6
solution	T49.0x1	T49.0x2	T49.0x3	T49.0x4	T49.0x5	T49.0x6
vapor	T59.891	T59.892	T59.893	T59.894	—	—
Iodipamide	T50.8x1	T50.8x2	T50.8x3	T50.8x4	T50.8x5	T50.8x6
Iodized (poppy seed) oil	T50.8x1	T50.8x2	T50.8x3	T50.8x4	T50.8x5	T50.8x6
Iodobismitol	T37.8x1	T37.8x2	T37.8x3	T37.8x4	T37.8x5	T37.8x6
Iodochlorhydroxyquin	T37.8x1	T37.8x2	T37.8x3	T37.8x4	T37.8x5	T37.8x6
topical	T49.0x1	T49.0x2	T49.0x3	T49.0x4	T49.0x5	T49.0x6
Iodochlorhydroxyquinoline	T37.8x1	T37.8x2	T37.8x3	T37.8x4	T37.8x5	T37.8x6
Iodocholesterol (131I)	T50.8x1	T50.8x2	T50.8x3	T50.8x4	T50.8x5	T50.8x6
Iodoform	T49.0x1	T49.0x2	T49.0x3	T49.0x4	T49.0x5	T49.0x6
Iodohippuric acid	T50.8x1	T50.8x2	T50.8x3	T50.8x4	T50.8x5	T50.8x6
Iodopanoic acid	T50.8x1	T50.8x2	T50.8x3	T50.8x4	T50.8x5	T50.8x6
Iodophthalein (sodium)	T50.8x1	T50.8x2	T50.8x3	T50.8x4	T50.8x5	T50.8x6
Iodopyracet	T50.8x1	T50.8x2	T50.8x3	T50.8x4	T50.8x5	T50.8x6
Iodoquinol	T37.8x1	T37.8x2	T37.8x3	T37.8x4	T37.8x5	T37.8x6
Iodoxamic acid	T50.8x1	T50.8x2	T50.8x3	T50.8x4	T50.8x5	T50.8x6
Iofendylate	T50.8x1	T50.8x2	T50.8x3	T50.8x4	T50.8x5	T50.8x6
Ioglycamic acid	T50.8x1	T50.8x2	T50.8x3	T50.8x4	T50.8x5	T50.8x6
Iohexol	T50.8x1	T50.8x2	T50.8x3	T50.8x4	T50.8x5	T50.8x6
Ion exchange resin						
anion	T47.8x1	T47.8x2	T47.8x3	T47.8x4	T47.8x5	T47.8x6
cation	T50.3x1	T50.3x2	T50.3x3	T50.3x4	T50.3x5	T50.3x6
cholestyramine	T46.6x1	T46.6x2	T46.6x3	T46.6x4	T46.6x5	T46.6x6
intestinal	T47.8x1	T47.8x2	T47.8x3	T47.8x4	T47.8x5	T47.8x6
Iopamidol	T50.8x1	T50.8x2	T50.8x3	T50.8x4	T50.8x5	T50.8x6
Iopanoic acid	T50.8x1	T50.8x2	T50.8x3	T50.8x4	T50.8x5	T50.8x6
Iophenoic acid	T50.8x1	T50.8x2	T50.8x3	T50.8x4	T50.8x5	T50.8x6
Iopodate, sodium	T50.8x1	T50.8x2	T50.8x3	T50.8x4	T50.8x5	T50.8x6
Iopodic acid	T50.8x1	T50.8x2	T50.8x3	T50.8x4	T50.8x5	T50.8x6
Iopromide	T50.8x1	T50.8x2	T50.8x3	T50.8x4	T50.8x5	T50.8x6
Iopydol	T50.8x1	T50.8x2	T50.8x3	T50.8x4	T50.8x5	T50.8x6
Iotalamic acid	T50.8x1	T50.8x2	T50.8x3	T50.8x4	T50.8x5	T50.8x6
Iothalamate	T50.8x1	T50.8x2	T50.8x3	T50.8x4	T50.8x5	T50.8x6
Iothiouracil	T38.2x1	T38.2x2	T38.2x3	T38.2x4	T38.2x5	T38.2x6
Iotrol	T50.8x1	T50.8x2	T50.8x3	T50.8x4	T50.8x5	T50.8x6

Table of Drugs & Chemicals	POISONING Accidental (Unintentional)	Self-Harm (Intentional)	Assault	Undetermined	Adverse Effect	Underdosing
Iotrolan	T50.8x1	T50.8x2	T50.8x3	T50.8x4	T50.8x5	T50.8x6
Iotroxate	T50.8x1	T50.8x2	T50.8x3	T50.8x4	T50.8x5	T50.8x6
Iotroxic acid	T50.8x1	T50.8x2	T50.8x3	T50.8x4	T50.8x5	T50.8x6
Ioversol	T50.8x1	T50.8x2	T50.8x3	T50.8x4	T50.8x5	T50.8x6
Ioxaglate	T50.8x1	T50.8x2	T50.8x3	T50.8x4	T50.8x5	T50.8x6
Ioxaglic acid	T50.8x1	T50.8x2	T50.8x3	T50.8x4	T50.8x5	T50.8x6
Ioxitalamic acid	T50.8x1	T50.8x2	T50.8x3	T50.8x4	T50.8x5	T50.8x6
Ipecac	T47.7x1	T47.7x2	T47.7x3	T47.7x4	T47.7x5	T47.7x6
Ipecacuanha	T48.4x1	T48.4x2	T48.4x3	T48.4x4	T48.4x5	T48.4x6
Ipodate, calcium	T50.8x1	T50.8x2	T50.8x3	T50.8x4	T50.8x5	T50.8x6
Ipral	T42.3x1	T42.3x2	T42.3x3	T42.3x4	T42.3x5	T42.3x6
Ipratropium (bromide)	T48.6x1	T48.6x2	T48.6x3	T48.6x4	T48.6x5	T48.6x6
Ipriflavone	T46.3x1	T46.3x2	T46.3x3	T46.3x4	T46.3x5	T46.3x6
Iprindole	T43.011	T43.012	T43.013	T43.014	T43.015	T43.016
Iproclozide	T43.1x1	T43.1x2	T43.1x3	T43.1x4	T43.1x5	T43.1x6
Iprofenin	T50.8x1	T50.8x2	T50.8x3	T50.8x4	T50.8x5	T50.8x6
Iproheptine	T49.2x1	T49.2x2	T49.2x3	T49.2x4	T49.2x5	T49.2x6
Iproniazid	T43.1x1	T43.1x2	T43.1x3	T43.1x4	T43.1x5	T43.1x6
Iproplatin	T45.1x1	T45.1x2	T45.1x3	T45.1x4	T45.1x5	T45.1x6
Iproveratril	T46.1x1	T46.1x2	T46.1x3	T46.1x4	T46.1x5	T46.1x6
Iron (compounds) (medicinal)						
NEC	T45.4x1	T45.4x2	T45.4x3	T45.4x4	T45.4x5	T45.4x6
ammonium	T45.4x1	T45.4x2	T45.4x3	T45.4x4	T45.4x5	T45.4x6
dextran injection	T45.4x1	T45.4x2	T45.4x3	T45.4x4	T45.4x5	T45.4x6
nonmedicinal	T56.891	T56.892	T56.893	T56.894	—	—
salts	T45.4x1	T45.4x2	T45.4x3	T45.4x4	T45.4x5	T45.4x6
sorbitex	T45.4x1	T45.4x2	T45.4x3	T45.4x4	T45.4x5	T45.4x6
sorbitol citric acid complex	T45.4x1	T45.4x2	T45.4x3	T45.4x4	T45.4x5	T45.4x6
Irrigating fluid (vaginal)	T49.8x1	T49.8x2	T49.8x3	T49.8x4	T49.8x5	T49.8x6
eye	T49.5x1	T49.5x2	T49.5x3	T49.5x4	T49.5x5	T49.5x6
Isepamicin	T36.5x1	T36.5x2	T36.5x3	T36.5x4	T36.5x5	T36.5x6
Isoaminile (citrate)	T48.3x1	T48.3x2	T48.3x3	T48.3x4	T48.3x5	T48.3x6
Isoamyl nitrite	T46.3x1	T46.3x2	T46.3x3	T46.3x4	T46.3x5	T46.3x6
Isobenzan	T60.1x1	T60.1x2	T60.1x3	T60.1x4	—	—
Isobutyl acetate	T52.8x1	T52.8x2	T52.8x3	T52.8x4	—	—
Isocarboxazid	T43.1x1	T43.1x2	T43.1x3	T43.1x4	T43.1x5	T43.1x6
Isoconazole	T49.0x1	T49.0x2	T49.0x3	T49.0x4	T49.0x5	T49.0x6
Isocyanate	T65.0x1	T65.0x2	T65.0x3	T65.0x4	—	—
Isoephedrine	T44.991	T44.992	T44.993	T44.994	T44.995	T44.996
Isoetarine	T48.6x1	T48.6x2	T48.6x3	T48.6x4	T48.6x5	T48.6x6
Isoethadione	T42.2x1	T42.2x2	T42.2x3	T42.2x4	T42.2x5	T42.2x6
Isoetharine	T44.5x1	T44.5x2	T44.5x3	T44.5x4	T44.5x5	T44.5x6
Isoflurane	T41.0x1	T41.0x2	T41.0x3	T41.0x4	T41.0x5	T41.0x6
Isoflurophate	T44.0x1	T44.0x2	T44.0x3	T44.0x4	T44.0x5	T44.0x6
Isomaltose, ferric complex	T45.4x1	T45.4x2	T45.4x3	T45.4x4	T45.4x5	T45.4x6
Isometheptene	T44.3x1	T44.3x2	T44.3x3	T44.3x4	T44.3x5	T44.3x6
Isoniazid	T37.1x1	T37.1x2	T37.1x3	T37.1x4	T37.1x5	T37.1x6
with						
rifampicin	T36.6x1	T36.6x2	T36.6x3	T36.6x4	T36.6x5	T36.6x6
thioacetazone	T37.1x1	T37.1x2	T37.1x3	T37.1x4	T37.1x5	T37.1x6
Isonicotinic acid hydrazide	T37.1x1	T37.1x2	T37.1x3	T37.1x4	T37.1x5	T37.1x6
Isonipecaine	T40.4x1	T40.4x2	T40.4x3	T40.4x4	T40.4x5	T40.4x6
Isopentaquine	T37.2x1	T37.2x2	T37.2x3	T37.2x4	T37.2x5	T37.2x6
Isophane insulin	T38.3x1	T38.3x2	T38.3x3	T38.3x4	T38.3x5	T38.3x6
Isophorone	T65.891	T65.892	T65.893	T65.894	—	—
Isophosphamide	T45.1x1	T45.1x2	T45.1x3	T45.1x4	T45.1x5	T45.1x6
Isopregnenone	T38.5x1	T38.5x2	T38.5x3	T38.5x4	T38.5x5	T38.5x6
Isoprenaline	T48.6x1	T48.6x2	T48.6x3	T48.6x4	T48.6x5	T48.6x6
Isopromethazine	T43.3x1	T43.3x2	T43.3x3	T43.3x4	T43.3x5	T43.3x6
Isopropamide	T44.3x1	T44.3x2	T44.3x3	T44.3x4	T44.3x5	T44.3x6
iodide	T44.3x1	T44.3x2	T44.3x3	T44.3x4	T44.3x5	T44.3x6
Isopropanol	T51.2x1	T51.2x2	T51.2x3	T51.2x4	—	—
Isopropyl						
acetate	T52.8x1	T52.8x2	T52.8x3	T52.8x4	—	—
alcohol	T51.2x1	T51.2x2	T51.2x3	T51.2x4	—	—
medicinal	T49.4x1	T49.4x2	T49.4x3	T49.4x4	T49.4x5	T49.4x6
ether	T52.8x1	T52.8x2	T52.8x3	T52.8x4	—	—
Isopropylaminophenazone	T39.2x1	T39.2x2	T39.2x3	T39.2x4	T39.2x5	T39.2x6

DRUGS&CHEMICALS

Table of Drugs & Chemicals	POISONING Accidental (Unintentional)	Self-Harm (Intentional)	Assault	Undetermined	Adverse Effect	Underdosing
Isoproterenol	T48.6x1	T48.6x2	T48.6x3	T48.6x4	T48.6x5	T48.6x6
Isosorbide dinitrate	T46.3x1	T46.3x2	T46.3x3	T46.3x4	T46.3x5	T46.3x6
Isothipendyl	T45.0x1	T45.0x2	T45.0x3	T45.0x4	T45.0x5	T45.0x6
Isotretinoin	T50.991	T50.992	T50.993	T50.994	T50.995	T50.996
Isoxazolyl penicillin	T36.0x1	T36.0x2	T36.0x3	T36.0x4	T36.0x5	T36.0x6
Isoxicam	T39.391	T39.392	T39.393	T39.394	T39.395	T39.396
Isoxsuprine	T46.7x1	T46.7x2	T46.7x3	T46.7x4	T46.7x5	T46.7x6
Ispagula	T47.4x1	T47.4x2	T47.4x3	T47.4x4	T47.4x5	T47.4x6
husk	T47.4x1	T47.4x2	T47.4x3	T47.4x4	T47.4x5	T47.4x6
Isradipine	T46.1x1	T46.1x2	T46.1x3	T46.1x4	T46.1x5	T46.1x6
I-thyroxine sodium	T38.1x1	T38.1x2	T38.1x3	T38.1x4	T38.1x5	T38.1x6
Itraconazole	T37.8x1	T37.8x2	T37.8x3	T37.8x4	T37.8x5	T37.8x6
Itramin tosilate	T46.3x1	T46.3x2	T46.3x3	T46.3x4	T46.3x5	T46.3x6
Ivermectin	T37.4x1	T37.4x2	T37.4x3	T37.4x4	T37.4x5	T37.4x6
Izoniazid	T37.1x1	T37.1x2	T37.1x3	T37.1x4	T37.1x5	T37.1x6
with thioacetazone	T37.1x1	T37.1x2	T37.1x3	T37.1x4	T37.1x5	T37.1x6
Jalap	T47.2x1	T47.2x2	T47.2x3	T47.2x4	T47.2x5	T47.2x6
Jamaica						
dogwood (bark)	T39.8x1	T39.8x2	T39.8x3	T39.8x4	T39.8x5	T39.8x6
ginger	T65.891	T65.892	T65.893	T65.894	—	—
root	T62.2x1	T62.2x2	T62.2x3	T62.2x4	—	—
Jatropha	T62.2x1	T62.2x2	T62.2x3	T62.2x4	—	—
curcas	T62.2x1	T62.2x2	T62.2x3	T62.2x4	—	—
Jectofer	T45.4x1	T45.4x2	T45.4x3	T45.4x4	T45.4x5	T45.4x6
Jellyfish (sting)	T63.621	T63.622	T63.623	T63.624	—	—
Jequirity (bean)	T62.2x1	T62.2x2	T62.2x3	T62.2x4	—	—
Jimson weed (stramonium)	T62.2x1	T62.2x2	T62.2x3	T62.2x4	—	—
seeds	T62.2x1	T62.2x2	T62.2x3	T62.2x4	—	—
Josamycin	T36.3x1	T36.3x2	T36.3x3	T36.3x4	T36.3x5	T36.3x6
Juniper tar	T49.1x1	T49.1x2	T49.1x3	T49.1x4	T49.1x5	T49.1x6
Kallidinogenase	T46.7x1	T46.7x2	T46.7x3	T46.7x4	T46.7x5	T46.7x6
Kallikrein	T46.7x1	T46.7x2	T46.7x3	T46.7x4	T46.7x5	T46.7x6
Kanamycin	T36.5x1	T36.5x2	T36.5x3	T36.5x4	T36.5x5	T36.5x6
Kantrex	T36.5x1	T36.5x2	T36.5x3	T36.5x4	T36.5x5	T36.5x6
Kaolin	T47.6x1	T47.6x2	T47.6x3	T47.6x4	T47.6x5	T47.6x6
light	T47.6x1	T47.6x2	T47.6x3	T47.6x4	T47.6x5	T47.6x6
Karaya (gum)	T47.4x1	T47.4x2	T47.4x3	T47.4x4	T47.4x5	T47.4x6
Kebuzone	T39.2x1	T39.2x2	T39.2x3	T39.2x4	T39.2x5	T39.2x6
Kelevan	T60.1x1	T60.1x2	T60.1x3	T60.1x4	—	—
Kemithal	T41.1x1	T41.1x2	T41.1x3	T41.1x4	T41.1x5	T41.1x6
Kenacort	T38.0x1	T38.0x2	T38.0x3	T38.0x4	T38.0x5	T38.0x6
Keratolytic drug NEC	T49.4x1	T49.4x2	T49.4x3	T49.4x4	T49.4x5	T49.4x6
anthracene	T49.4x1	T49.4x2	T49.4x3	T49.4x4	T49.4x5	T49.4x6
Keratoplastic NEC	T49.4x1	T49.4x2	T49.4x3	T49.4x4	T49.4x5	T49.4x6
Kerosene, kerosine (fuel)						
(solvent) NEC	T52.0x1	T52.0x2	T52.0x3	T52.0x4	—	—
insecticide	T52.0x1	T52.0x2	T52.0x3	T52.0x4	—	—
vapor	T52.0x1	T52.0x2	T52.0x3	T52.0x4	—	—
Ketamine	T41.291	T41.292	T41.293	T41.294	T41.295	T41.296
Ketazolam	T42.4x1	T42.4x2	T42.4x3	T42.4x4	T42.4x5	T42.4x6
Ketazon	T39.2x1	T39.2x2	T39.2x3	T39.2x4	T39.2x5	T39.2x6
Ketobemidone	T40.4x1	T40.4x2	T40.4x3	T40.4x4	—	—
Ketoconazole	T49.0x1	T49.0x2	T49.0x3	T49.0x4	T49.0x5	T49.0x6
Ketols	T52.4x1	T52.4x2	T52.4x3	T52.4x4	—	—
Ketone oils	T52.4x1	T52.4x2	T52.4x3	T52.4x4	—	—
Ketoprofen	T39.311	T39.312	T39.313	T39.314	T39.315	T39.316
Ketorolac	T39.8x1	T39.8x2	T39.8x3	T39.8x4	T39.8x5	T39.8x6
Ketotifen	T45.0x1	T45.0x2	T45.0x3	T45.0x4	T45.0x5	T45.0x6
Khat	T43.691	T43.692	T43.693	T43.694	—	—
Khellin	T46.3x1	T46.3x2	T46.3x3	T46.3x4	T46.3x5	T46.3x6
Khelloside	T46.3x1	T46.3x2	T46.3x3	T46.3x4	T46.3x5	T46.3x6
Kiln gas or vapor (carbon monoxide)	T58.8x1	T58.8x2	T58.8x3	T58.8x4	—	—
Kitasamycin	T36.3x1	T36.3x2	T36.3x3	T36.3x4	T36.3x5	T36.3x6
Konsyl	T47.4x1	T47.4x2	T47.4x3	T47.4x4	T47.4x5	T47.4x6
Kosam seed	T62.2x1	T62.2x2	T62.2x3	T62.2x4	—	—
Krait (venom)	T63.091	T63.092	T63.093	T63.094	—	—
Kwell (insecticide)	T60.1x1	T60.1x2	T60.1x3	T60.1x4	—	—
anti-infective (topical)	T49.0x1	T49.0x2	T49.0x3	T49.0x4	T49.0x5	T49.0x6

Table of Drugs & Chemicals	POISONING Accidental (Unintentional)	Self-Harm (Intentional)	Assault	Undetermined	Adverse Effect	Underdosing
Labetalol	T44.8x1	T44.8x2	T44.8x3	T44.8x4	T44.8x5	T44.8x6
Laburnum (seeds)	T62.2x1	T62.2x2	T62.2x3	T62.2x4	—	—
leaves	T62.2x1	T62.2x2	T62.2x3	T62.2x4	—	—
Lachesine	T49.5x1	T49.5x2	T49.5x3	T49.5x4	T49.5x5	T49.5x6
Lacidipine	T46.5x1	T46.5x2	T46.5x3	T46.5x4	T46.5x5	T46.5x6
Lacquer	T65.6x1	T65.6x2	T65.6x3	T65.6x4	—	—
Lacrimogenic gas	T59.3x1	T59.3x2	T59.3x3	T59.3x4	—	—
Lactated potassic saline	T50.3x1	T50.3x2	T50.3x3	T50.3x4	T50.3x5	T50.3x6
Lactic acid	T49.8x1	T49.8x2	T49.8x3	T49.8x4	T49.8x5	T49.8x6
Lactobacillus						
acidophilus	T47.6x1	T47.6x2	T47.6x3	T47.6x4	T47.6x5	T47.6x6
compound	T47.6x1	T47.6x2	T47.6x3	T47.6x4	T47.6x5	T47.6x6
bifidus, lyophilized	T47.6x1	T47.6x2	T47.6x3	T47.6x4	T47.6x5	T47.6x6
bulgaricus	T47.6x1	T47.6x2	T47.6x3	T47.6x4	T47.6x5	T47.6x6
sporogenes	T47.6x1	T47.6x2	T47.6x3	T47.6x4	T47.6x5	T47.6x6
Lactoflavin	T45.2x1	T45.2x2	T45.2x3	T45.2x4	T45.2x5	T45.2x6
Lactose (as excipient)	T50.901	T50.902	T50.903	T50.904	T50.905	T50.906
Lactuca (virosa) (extract)	T42.6x1	T42.6x2	T42.6x3	T42.6x4	T42.6x5	T42.6x6
Lactucarium	T42.6x1	T42.6x2	T42.6x3	T42.6x4	T42.6x5	T42.6x6
Lactulose	T47.3x1	T47.3x2	T47.3x3	T47.3x4	T47.3x5	T47.3x6
Laevo — see Levo-						
Lanatosides	T46.0x1	T46.0x2	T46.0x3	T46.0x4	T46.0x5	T46.0x6
Lanolin	T49.3x1	T49.3x2	T49.3x3	T49.3x4	T49.3x5	T49.3x6
Largactil	T43.3x1	T43.3x2	T43.3x3	T43.3x4	T43.3x5	T43.3x6
Larkspur	T62.2x1	T62.2x2	T62.2x3	T62.2x4	—	—
Laroxyl	T43.011	T43.012	T43.013	T43.014	T43.015	T43.016
Lasix	T50.1x1	T50.1x2	T50.1x3	T50.1x4	T50.1x5	T50.1x6
Lassar's paste	T49.4x1	T49.4x2	T49.4x3	T49.4x4	T49.4x5	T49.4x6
Latamoxef	T36.1x1	T36.1x2	T36.1x3	T36.1x4	T36.1x5	T36.1x6
Latex	T65.811	T65.812	T65.813	T65.814	—	—
Lathyrus (seed)	T62.2x1	T62.2x2	T62.2x3	T62.2x4	—	—
Laudanum	T40.0x1	T40.0x2	T40.0x3	T40.0x4	T40.0x5	T40.0x6
Laudexium	T48.1x1	T48.1x2	T48.1x3	T48.1x4	T48.1x5	T48.1x6
Laughing gas	T41.0x1	T41.0x2	T41.0x3	T41.0x4	T41.0x5	T41.0x6
Laurel, black or cherry	T62.2x1	T62.2x2	T62.2x3	T62.2x4	—	—
Laurolinium	T49.0x1	T49.0x2	T49.0x3	T49.0x4	T49.0x5	T49.0x6
Lauryl sulfoacetate	T49.2x1	T49.2x2	T49.2x3	T49.2x4	T49.2x5	T49.2x6
Laxative NEC	T47.4x1	T47.4x2	T47.4x3	T47.4x4	T47.4x5	T47.4x6
osmotic	T47.3x1	T47.3x2	T47.3x3	T47.3x4	T47.3x5	T47.3x6
saline	T47.3x1	T47.3x2	T47.3x3	T47.3x4	T47.3x5	T47.3x6
stimulant	T47.2x1	T47.2x2	T47.2x3	T47.2x4	T47.2x5	T47.2x6
L-dopa	T42.8x1	T42.8x2	T42.8x3	T42.8x4	T42.8x5	T42.8x6
Lead (dust) (fumes) (vapor) NEC	T56.0x1	T56.0x2	T56.0x3	T56.0x4	—	—
acetate	T56.0x1	T56.0x2	T56.0x3	T56.0x4	—	—
alkyl (fuel additive)	T56.0x1	T56.0x2	T56.0x3	T56.0x4	—	—
anti-infectives	T37.8x1	T37.8x2	T37.8x3	T37.8x4	T37.8x5	T37.8x6
antiknock compound (tetraethyl)	T56.0x1	T56.0x2	T56.0x3	T56.0x4	—	—
arsenate, arsenite (dust) (herbicide) (insecticide) (vapor)	T57.0x1	T57.0x2	T57.0x3	T57.0x4	—	—
carbonate	T56.0x1	T56.0x2	T56.0x3	T56.0x4	—	—
paint	T56.0x1	T56.0x2	T56.0x3	T56.0x4	—	—
chromate	T56.0x1	T56.0x2	T56.0x3	T56.0x4	—	—
paint	T56.0x1	T56.0x2	T56.0x3	T56.0x4	—	—
dioxide	T56.0x1	T56.0x2	T56.0x3	T56.0x4	—	—
inorganic	T56.0x1	T56.0x2	T56.0x3	T56.0x4	—	—
iodide	T56.0x1	T56.0x2	T56.0x3	T56.0x4	—	—
pigment (paint)	T56.0x1	T56.0x2	T56.0x3	T56.0x4	—	—
monoxide (dust)	T56.0x1	T56.0x2	T56.0x3	T56.0x4	—	—
paint	T56.0x1	T56.0x2	T56.0x3	T56.0x4	—	—
organic	T56.0x1	T56.0x2	T56.0x3	T56.0x4	—	—
oxide	T56.0x1	T56.0x2	T56.0x3	T56.0x4	—	—
paint	T56.0x1	T56.0x2	T56.0x3	T56.0x4	—	—
paint	T56.0x1	T56.0x2	T56.0x3	T56.0x4	—	—
salts	T56.0x1	T56.0x2	T56.0x3	T56.0x4	—	—
specified compound NEC	T56.0x1	T56.0x2	T56.0x3	T56.0x4	—	—
tetra-ethyl	T56.0x1	T56.0x2	T56.0x3	T56.0x4	—	—
Lebanese red	T40.7x1	T40.7x2	T40.7x3	T40.7x4	T40.7x5	T40.7x6
Lefetamine	T39.8x1	T39.8x2	T39.8x3	T39.8x4	T39.8x5	T39.8x6
Lenperone	T43.4x1	T43.4x2	T43.4x3	T43.4x4	T43.4x5	T43.4x6

DRUGS&CHEMICALS

Table of Drugs & Chemicals	POISONING Accidental (Unintentional)	Self-Harm (Intentional)	Assault	Undetermined	Adverse Effect	Underdosing
Lente lietin (insulin)	T38.3x1	T38.3x2	T38.3x3	T38.3x4	T38.3x5	T38.3x6
Leptazol	T50.7x1	T50.7x2	T50.7x3	T50.7x4	T50.7x5	T50.7x6
Leptophos	T60.0x1	T60.0x2	T60.0x3	T60.0x4	—	—
Leritine	T40.2x1	T40.2x2	T40.2x3	T40.2x4	T40.2x5	T40.2x6
Letosteine	T48.4x1	T48.4x2	T48.4x3	T48.4x4	T48.4x5	T48.4x6
Letter	T38.1x1	T38.1x2	T38.1x3	T38.1x4	T38.1x5	T38.1x6
Lettuce opium	T42.6x1	T42.6x2	T42.6x3	T42.6x4	T42.6x5	T42.6x6
Leucinocaine	T41.3x1	T41.3x2	T41.3x3	T41.3x4	T41.3x5	T41.3x6
Leucocianidol	T46.991	T46.992	T46.993	T46.994	T46.995	T46.996
Leucovorin (factor)	T45.8x1	T45.8x2	T45.8x3	T45.8x4	T45.8x5	T45.8x6
Leukeran	T45.1x1	T45.1x2	T45.1x3	T45.1x4	T45.1x5	T45.1x6
Leuprolide	T38.891	T38.892	T38.893	T38.894	T38.895	T38.896
Levalbuterol	T48.6x1	T48.6x2	T48.6x3	T48.6x4	T48.6x5	T48.6x6
Levallorphan	T50.7x1	T50.7x2	T50.7x3	T50.7x4	T50.7x5	T50.7x6
Levamisole	T37.4x1	T37.4x2	T37.4x3	T37.4x4	T37.4x5	T37.4x6
Levanil	T42.6x1	T42.6x2	T42.6x3	T42.6x4	T42.6x5	T42.6x6
Levarterenol	T44.4x1	T44.4x2	T44.4x3	T44.4x4	T44.4x5	T44.4x6
Levdropropizine	T48.3x1	T48.3x2	T48.3x3	T48.3x4	T48.3x5	T48.3x6
Levobunolol	T49.5x1	T49.5x2	T49.5x3	T49.5x4	T49.5x5	T49.5x6
Levocabastine (hydrochloride)	T45.0x1	T45.0x2	T45.0x3	T45.0x4	T45.0x5	T45.0x6
Levocarnitine	T50.991	T50.992	T50.993	T50.994	T50.995	T50.996
Levodopa	T42.8x1	T42.8x2	T42.8x3	T42.8x4	T42.8x5	T42.8x6
with carbidopa	T42.8x1	T42.8x2	T42.8x3	T42.8x4	T42.8x5	T42.8x6
Levo-dromoran	T40.2x1	T40.2x2	T40.2x3	T40.2x4	T40.2x5	T40.2x6
Levoglutamide	T50.991	T50.992	T50.993	T50.994	T50.995	T50.996
Levoid	T38.1x1	T38.1x2	T38.1x3	T38.1x4	T38.1x5	T38.1x6
Levo-iso-methadone	T40.3x1	T40.3x2	T40.3x3	T40.3x4	T40.3x5	T40.3x6
Levomepromazine	T43.3x1	T43.3x2	T43.3x3	T43.3x4	T43.3x5	T43.3x6
Levonordefrin	T49.6x1	T49.6x2	T49.6x3	T49.6x4	T49.6x5	T49.6x6
Levonorgestrel	T38.4x1	T38.4x2	T38.4x3	T38.4x4	T38.4x5	T38.4x6
with ethinylestradiol	T38.5x1	T38.5x2	T38.5x3	T38.5x4	T38.5x5	T38.5x6
Levopromazine	T43.3x1	T43.3x2	T43.3x3	T43.3x4	T43.3x5	T43.3x6
Levoprome	T42.6x1	T42.6x2	T42.6x3	T42.6x4	T42.6x5	T42.6x6
Levopropoxyphene	T40.4x1	T40.4x2	T40.4x3	T40.4x4	T40.4x5	T40.4x6
Levopropylhexedrine	T50.5x1	T50.5x2	T50.5x3	T50.5x4	T50.5x5	T50.5x6
Levoproxyphylline	T48.6x1	T48.6x2	T48.6x3	T48.6x4	T48.6x5	T48.6x6
Levorphanol	T40.4x1	T40.4x2	T40.4x3	T40.4x4	T40.4x5	T40.4x6
Levothyroxine	T38.1x1	T38.1x2	T38.1x3	T38.1x4	T38.1x5	T38.1x6
sodium	T38.1x1	T38.1x2	T38.1x3	T38.1x4	T38.1x5	T38.1x6
Levsin	T44.3x1	T44.3x2	T44.3x3	T44.3x4	T44.3x5	T44.3x6
Levulose	T50.3x1	T50.3x2	T50.3x3	T50.3x4	T50.3x5	T50.3x6
Lewisite (gas), not in war	T57.0x1	T57.0x2	T57.0x3	T57.0x4	—	—
Librium	T42.4x1	T42.4x2	T42.4x3	T42.4x4	T42.4x5	T42.4x6
Lidex	T49.0x1	T49.0x2	T49.0x3	T49.0x4	T49.0x5	T49.0x6
Lidocaine	T41.3x1	T41.3x2	T41.3x3	T41.3x4	T41.3x5	T41.3x6
regional	T41.3x1	T41.3x2	T41.3x3	T41.3x4	T41.3x5	T41.3x6
spinal	T41.3x1	T41.3x2	T41.3x3	T41.3x4	T41.3x5	T41.3x6
Lidofenin	T50.8x1	T50.8x2	T50.8x3	T50.8x4	T50.8x5	T50.8x6
Lidoflazine	T46.1x1	T46.1x2	T46.1x3	T46.1x4	T46.1x5	T46.1x6
Lighter fluid	T52.0x1	T52.0x2	T52.0x3	T52.0x4	—	—
Lignin hemicellulose	T47.6x1	T47.6x2	T47.6x3	T47.6x4	T47.6x5	T47.6x6
Lignocaine	T41.3x1	T41.3x2	T41.3x3	T41.3x4	T41.3x5	T41.3x6
regional	T41.3x1	T41.3x2	T41.3x3	T41.3x4	T41.3x5	T41.3x6
spinal	T41.3x1	T41.3x2	T41.3x3	T41.3x4	T41.3x5	T41.3x6
Ligroin(e) (solvent)	T52.0x1	T52.0x2	T52.0x3	T52.0x4	—	—
vapor	T59.891	T59.892	T59.893	T59.894	—	—
Ligustrum vulgare	T62.2x1	T62.2x2	T62.2x3	T62.2x4	—	—
Lily of the valley	T62.2x1	T62.2x2	T62.2x3	T62.2x4	—	—
Lime (chloride)	T54.3x1	T54.3x2	T54.3x3	T54.3x4	—	—
Limonene	T52.8x1	T52.8x2	T52.8x3	T52.8x4	—	—
Lincomycin	T36.8x1	T36.8x2	T36.8x3	T36.8x4	T36.8x5	T36.8x6
Lindane (insecticide) (nonmedicinal) (vapor)	T53.6x1	T53.6x2	T53.6x3	T53.6x4	—	—
medicinal	T49.0x1	T49.0x2	T49.0x3	T49.0x4	T49.0x5	T49.0x6
Liniments NEC	T49.91	T49.92	T49.93	T49.94	T49.95	T49.96
Linoleic acid	T46.6x1	T46.6x2	T46.6x3	T46.6x4	T46.6x5	T46.6x6
Linolenic acid	T46.6x1	T46.6x2	T46.6x3	T46.6x4	T46.6x5	T46.6x6
Linseed	T47.4x1	T47.4x2	T47.4x3	T47.4x4	T47.4x5	T47.4x6

Table of Drugs & Chemicals	POISONING Accidental (Unintentional)	Self-Harm (Intentional)	Assault	Undetermined	Adverse Effect	Underdosing
Liothyronine	T38.1x1	T38.1x2	T38.1x3	T38.1x4	T38.1x5	T38.1x6
Liotrix	T38.1x1	T38.1x2	T38.1x3	T38.1x4	T38.1x5	T38.1x6
Lipancreatin	T47.5x1	T47.5x2	T47.5x3	T47.5x4	T47.5x5	T47.5x6
Lipo-alprostadil	T46.7x1	T46.7x2	T46.7x3	T46.7x4	T46.7x5	T46.7x6
Lipo-Lutin	T38.5x1	T38.5x2	T38.5x3	T38.5x4	T38.5x5	T38.5x6
Lipotropic drug NEC	T50.901	T50.902	T50.903	T50.904	T50.905	T50.906
Liquefied petroleum gases	T59.891	T59.892	T59.893	T59.894	—	—
piped (pure or mixed with air)	T59.891	T59.892	T59.893	T59.894	—	—
Liquid						
paraffin	T47.4x1	T47.4x2	T47.4x3	T47.4x4	T47.4x5	T47.4x6
petrolatum	T47.4x1	T47.4x2	T47.4x3	T47.4x4	T47.4x5	T47.4x6
topical	T49.3x1	T49.3x2	T49.3x3	T49.3x4	T49.3x5	T49.3x6
specified NEC	T65.891	T65.892	T65.893	T65.894	—	—
substance	T65.91	T65.92	T65.93	T65.94	—	—
Liquor creosolis compositus	T65.891	T65.892	T65.893	T65.894		
Liquorice	T48.4x1	T48.4x2	T48.4x3	T48.4x4	T48.4x5	T48.4x6
extract	T47.8x1	T47.8x2	T47.8x3	T47.8x4	T47.8x5	T47.8x6
Lisinopril	T46.4x1	T46.4x2	T46.4x3	T46.4x4	T46.4x5	T46.4x6
Lisuride	T42.8x1	T42.8x2	T42.8x3	T42.8x4	T42.8x5	T42.8x6
Lithane	T43.8x1	T43.8x2	T43.8x3	T43.8x4	T43.8x5	T43.8x6
Lithium	T56.891	T56.892	T56.893	T56.894	—	—
gluconate	T43.591	T43.592	T43.593	T43.594	T43.595	T43.596
salts (carbonate)	T43.591	T43.592	T43.593	T43.594	T43.595	T43.596
Lithonate	T43.8x1	T43.8x2	T43.8x3	T43.8x4	T43.8x5	T43.8x6
Liver						
extract	T45.8x1	T45.8x2	T45.8x3	T45.8x4	T45.8x5	T45.8x6
for parenteral use	T45.8x1	T45.8x2	T45.8x3	T45.8x4	T45.8x5	T45.8x6
fraction 1	T45.8x1	T45.8x2	T45.8x3	T45.8x4	T45.8x5	T45.8x6
hydrolysate	T45.8x1	T45.8x2	T45.8x3	T45.8x4	T45.8x5	T45.8x6
Lizard (bite) (venom)	T63.121	T63.122	T63.123	T63.124	—	—
LMD	T45.8x1	T45.8x2	T45.8x3	T45.8x4	T45.8x5	T45.8x6
Lobelia	T62.2x1	T62.2x2	T62.2x3	T62.2x4	—	—
Lobeline	T50.7x1	T50.7x2	T50.7x3	T50.7x4	T50.7x5	T50.7x6
Local action drug NEC	T49.8x1	T49.8x2	T49.8x3	T49.8x4	T49.8x5	T49.8x6
Locorten	T49.0x1	T49.0x2	T49.0x3	T49.0x4	T49.0x5	T49.0x6
Lofepramine	T43.011	T43.012	T43.013	T43.014	T43.015	T43.016
Lolium temulentum	T62.2x1	T62.2x2	T62.2x3	T62.2x4	—	—
Lomotil	T47.6x1	T47.6x2	T47.6x3	T47.6x4	T47.6x5	T47.6x6
Lomustine	T45.1x1	T45.1x2	T45.1x3	T45.1x4	T45.1x5	T45.1x6
Lonidamine	T45.1x1	T45.1x2	T45.1x3	T45.1x4	T45.1x5	T45.1x6
Loperamide	T47.6x1	T47.6x2	T47.6x3	T47.6x4	T47.6x5	T47.6x6
Loprazolam	T42.4x1	T42.4x2	T42.4x3	T42.4x4	T42.4x5	T42.4x6
Lorajmine	T46.2x1	T46.2x2	T46.2x3	T46.2x4	T46.2x5	T46.2x6
Loratidine	T45.0x1	T45.0x2	T45.0x3	T45.0x4	T45.0x5	T45.0x6
Lorazepam	T42.4x1	T42.4x2	T42.4x3	T42.4x4	T42.4x5	T42.4x6
Lorcainide	T46.2x1	T46.2x2	T46.2x3	T46.2x4	T46.2x5	T46.2x6
Lormetazepam	T42.4x1	T42.4x2	T42.4x3	T42.4x4	T42.4x5	T42.4x6
Lotions NEC	T49.91	T49.92	T49.93	T49.94	T49.95	T49.96
Lotusate	T42.3x1	T42.3x2	T42.3x3	T42.3x4	T42.3x5	T42.3x6
Lovastatin	T46.6x1	T46.6x2	T46.6x3	T46.6x4	T46.6x5	T46.6x6
Lowila	T49.2x1	T49.2x2	T49.2x3	T49.2x4	T49.2x5	T49.2x6
Loxapine	T43.591	T43.592	T43.593	T43.594	T43.595	T43.596
Lozenges (throat)	T49.6x1	T49.6x2	T49.6x3	T49.6x4	T49.6x5	T49.6x6
LSD	T40.8x1	T40.8x2	T40.8x3	T40.8x4		
L-Tryptophan — see amino acid						
Lubricant, eye	T49.5x1	T49.5x2	T49.5x3	T49.5x4	T49.5x5	T49.5x6
Lubricating oil NEC	T52.0x1	T52.0x2	T52.0x3	T52.0x4	—	—
Lucanthone	T37.4x1	T37.4x2	T37.4x3	T37.4x4	T37.4x5	T37.4x6
Luminal	T42.3x1	T42.3x2	T42.3x3	T42.3x4	T42.3x5	T42.3x6
Lung irritant (gas) NEC	T59.91	T59.92	T59.93	T59.94	—	—
Luteinizing hormone	T38.811	T38.812	T38.813	T38.814	T38.815	T38.816
Lutocylol	T38.5x1	T38.5x2	T38.5x3	T38.5x4	T38.5x5	T38.5x6
Lutromone	T38.5x1	T38.5x2	T38.5x3	T38.5x4	T38.5x5	T38.5x6
Lututrin	T48.291	T48.292	T48.293	T48.294	T48.295	T48.296
Lye (concentrated)	T54.3x1	T54.3x2	T54.3x3	T54.3x4	—	—
Lygranum (skin test)	T50.8x1	T50.8x2	T50.8x3	T50.8x4	T50.8x5	T50.8x6
Lymecycline	T36.4x1	T36.4x2	T36.4x3	T36.4x4	T36.4x5	T36.4x6

Table of Drugs & Chemicals	Poisoning — Accidental (Unintentional)	Poisoning — Self-Harm (Intentional)	Poisoning — Assault	Poisoning — Undetermined	Adverse Effect	Underdosing
Lymphogranuloma venereum antigen	T50.8x1	T50.8x2	T50.8x3	T50.8x4	T50.8x5	T50.8x6
Lynestrenol	T38.4x1	T38.4x2	T38.4x3	T38.4x4	T38.4x5	T38.4x6
Lyovac Sodium Edecrin	T50.1x1	T50.1x2	T50.1x3	T50.1x4	T50.1x5	T50.1x6
Lypressin	T38.891	T38.892	T38.893	T38.894	T38.895	T38.896
Lysergic acid diethylamide	T40.8x1	T40.8x2	T40.8x3	T40.8x4	—	—
Lysergide	T40.8x1	T40.8x2	T40.8x3	T40.8x4	—	—
Lysine vasopressin	T38.891	T38.892	T38.893	T38.894	T38.895	T38.896
Lysol	T54.1x1	T54.1x2	T54.1x3	T54.1x4	—	—
Lysozyme	T49.0x1	T49.0x2	T49.0x3	T49.0x4	T49.0x5	T49.0x6
Lytta (vitatta)	T49.8x1	T49.8x2	T49.8x3	T49.8x4	T49.8x5	T49.8x6
Mace	T59.3x1	T59.3x2	T59.3x3	T59.3x4	—	—
Macrogol	T50.991	T50.992	T50.993	T50.994	T50.995	T50.996
Macrolide						
anabolic drug	T38.7x1	T38.7x2	T38.7x3	T38.7x4	T38.7x5	T38.7x6
antibiotic	T36.3x1	T36.3x2	T36.3x3	T36.3x4	T36.3x5	T36.3x6
Mafenide	T49.0x1	T49.0x2	T49.0x3	T49.0x4	T49.0x5	T49.0x6
Magaldrate	T47.1x1	T47.1x2	T47.1x3	T47.1x4	T47.1x5	T47.1x6
Magic mushroom	T40.991	T40.992	T40.993	T40.994	—	—
Magnamycin	T36.8x1	T36.8x2	T36.8x3	T36.8x4	T36.8x5	T36.8x6
Magnesia magma	T47.1x1	T47.1x2	T47.1x3	T47.1x4	T47.1x5	T47.1x6
Magnesium NEC	T56.891	T56.892	T56.893	T56.894	—	—
carbonate	T47.1x1	T47.1x2	T47.1x3	T47.1x4	T47.1x5	T47.1x6
citrate	T47.4x1	T47.4x2	T47.4x3	T47.4x4	T47.4x5	T47.4x6
hydroxide	T47.1x1	T47.1x2	T47.1x3	T47.1x4	T47.1x5	T47.1x6
oxide	T47.1x1	T47.1x2	T47.1x3	T47.1x4	T47.1x5	T47.1x6
peroxide	T49.0x1	T49.0x2	T49.0x3	T49.0x4	T49.0x5	T49.0x6
salicylate	T39.091	T39.092	T39.093	T39.094	T39.095	T39.096
silicofluoride	T50.3x1	T50.3x2	T50.3x3	T50.3x4	T50.3x5	T50.3x6
sulfate	T47.4x1	T47.4x2	T47.4x3	T47.4x4	T47.4x5	T47.4x6
thiosulfate	T45.0x1	T45.0x2	T45.0x3	T45.0x4	T45.0x5	T45.0x6
trisilicate	T47.1x1	T47.1x2	T47.1x3	T47.1x4	T47.1x5	T47.1x6
Malathion (medicinal)	T49.0x1	T49.0x2	T49.0x3	T49.0x4	T49.0x5	T49.0x6
insecticide	T60.0x1	T60.0x2	T60.0x3	T60.0x4	—	—
Male fern extract	T37.4x1	T37.4x2	T37.4x3	T37.4x4	T37.4x5	T37.4x6
M-AMSA	T45.1x1	T45.1x2	T45.1x3	T45.1x4	T45.1x5	T45.1x6
Mandelic acid	T37.8x1	T37.8x2	T37.8x3	T37.8x4	T37.8x5	T37.8x6
Manganese (dioxide) (salts)	T57.2x1	T57.2x2	T57.2x3	T57.2x4	—	—
medicinal	T50.991	T50.992	T50.993	T50.994	T50.995	T50.996
Mannitol	T47.3x1	T47.3x2	T47.3x3	T47.3x4	T47.3x5	T47.3x6
hexanitrate	T46.3x1	T46.3x2	T46.3x3	T46.3x4	T46.3x5	T46.3x6
Mannomustine	T45.1x1	T45.1x2	T45.1x3	T45.1x4	T45.1x5	T45.1x6
MAO inhibitors	T43.1x1	T43.1x2	T43.1x3	T43.1x4	T43.1x5	T43.1x6
Mapharsen	T37.8x1	T37.8x2	T37.8x3	T37.8x4	T37.8x5	T37.8x6
Maphenide	T49.0x1	T49.0x2	T49.0x3	T49.0x4	T49.0x5	T49.0x6
Maprotiline	T43.021	T43.022	T43.023	T43.024	T43.025	T43.026
Marcaine	T41.3x1	T41.3x2	T41.3x3	T41.3x4	T41.3x5	T41.3x6
infiltration (subcutaneous)	T41.3x1	T41.3x2	T41.3x3	T41.3x4	T41.3x5	T41.3x6
nerve block (peripheral) (plexus)	T41.3x1	T41.3x2	T41.3x3	T41.3x4	T41.3x5	T41.3x6
Marezine	T45.0x1	T45.0x2	T45.0x3	T45.0x4	T45.0x5	T45.0x6
Marihuana	T40.7x1	T40.7x2	T40.7x3	T40.7x4	T40.7x5	T40.7x6
Marijuana	T40.7x1	T40.7x2	T40.7x3	T40.7x4	T40.7x5	T40.7x6
Marine (sting)	T63.691	T63.692	T63.693	T63.694	—	—
animals (sting)	T63.691	T63.692	T63.693	T63.694	—	—
plants (sting)	T63.711	T63.712	T63.713	T63.714	—	—
Marplan	T43.1x1	T43.1x2	T43.1x3	T43.1x4	T43.1x5	T43.1x6
Marsh gas	T59.891	T59.892	T59.893	T59.894	—	—
Marsilid	T43.1x1	T43.1x2	T43.1x3	T43.1x4	T43.1x5	T43.1x6
Matulane	T45.1x1	T45.1x2	T45.1x3	T45.1x4	T45.1x5	T45.1x6
Mazindol	T50.5x1	T50.5x2	T50.5x3	T50.5x4	T50.5x5	T50.5x6
MCPA	T60.3x1	T60.3x2	T60.3x3	T60.3x4	—	—
MDMA	T43.621	T43.622	T43.623	T43.624	T43.625	T43.626
Meadow saffron	T62.2x1	T62.2x2	T62.2x3	T62.2x4	—	—
Measles virus vaccine (attenuated)	T50.B91	T50.B92	T50.B93	T50.B94	T50.B95	T50.B96
Meat, noxious	T62.8x1	T62.8x2	T62.8x3	T62.8x4	—	—
Meballymal	T42.3x1	T42.3x2	T42.3x3	T42.3x4	T42.3x5	T42.3x6
Mebanazine	T43.1x1	T43.1x2	T43.1x3	T43.1x4	T43.1x5	T43.1x6
Mebaral	T42.3x1	T42.3x2	T42.3x3	T42.3x4	T42.3x5	T42.3x6
Mebendazole	T37.4x1	T37.4x2	T37.4x3	T37.4x4	T37.4x5	T37.4x6
Mebeverine	T44.3x1	T44.3x2	T44.3x3	T44.3x4	T44.3x5	T44.3x6
Mebhydrolin	T45.0x1	T45.0x2	T45.0x3	T45.0x4	T45.0x5	T45.0x6
Mebumal	T42.3x1	T42.3x2	T42.3x3	T42.3x4	T42.3x5	T42.3x6
Mebutamate	T43.591	T43.592	T43.593	T43.594	T43.595	T43.596
Mecamylamine	T44.2x1	T44.2x2	T44.2x3	T44.2x4	T44.2x5	T44.2x6
Mechlorethamine	T45.1x1	T45.1x2	T45.1x3	T45.1x4	T45.1x5	T45.1x6
Mecillinam	T36.0x1	T36.0x2	T36.0x3	T36.0x4	T36.0x5	T36.0x6
Meclizine (hydrochloride)	T45.0x1	T45.0x2	T45.0x3	T45.0x4	T45.0x5	T45.0x6
Meclocycline	T36.4x1	T36.4x2	T36.4x3	T36.4x4	T36.4x5	T36.4x6
Meclofenamate	T39.391	T39.392	T39.393	T39.394	T39.395	T39.396
Meclofenamic acid	T39.391	T39.392	T39.393	T39.394	T39.395	T39.396
Meclofenoxate	T43.691	T43.692	T43.693	T43.694	T43.695	T43.696
Meclozine	T45.0x1	T45.0x2	T45.0x3	T45.0x4	T45.0x5	T45.0x6
Mecobalamin	T45.8x1	T45.8x2	T45.8x3	T45.8x4	T45.8x5	T45.8x6
Mecoprop	T60.3x1	T60.3x2	T60.3x3	T60.3x4	—	—
Mecrilate	T49.3x1	T49.3x2	T49.3x3	T49.3x4	T49.3x5	T49.3x6
Mecysteine	T48.4x1	T48.4x2	T48.4x3	T48.4x4	T48.4x5	T48.4x6
Medazepam	T42.4x1	T42.4x2	T42.4x3	T42.4x4	T42.4x5	T42.4x6
Medicament NEC	T50.901	T50.902	T50.903	T50.904	T50.905	T50.906
Medinal	T42.3x1	T42.3x2	T42.3x3	T42.3x4	T42.3x5	T42.3x6
Medomin	T42.3x1	T42.3x2	T42.3x3	T42.3x4	T42.3x5	T42.3x6
Medrogestone	T38.5x1	T38.5x2	T38.5x3	T38.5x4	T38.5x5	T38.5x6
Medroxalol	T44.8x1	T44.8x2	T44.8x3	T44.8x4	T44.8x5	T44.8x6
Medroxyprogesterone acetate (depot)	T38.5x1	T38.5x2	T38.5x3	T38.5x4	T38.5x5	T38.5x6
Medrysone	T49.0x1	T49.0x2	T49.0x3	T49.0x4	T49.0x5	T49.0x6
Mefenamic acid	T39.391	T39.392	T39.393	T39.394	T39.395	T39.396
Mefenorex	T50.5x1	T50.5x2	T50.5x3	T50.5x4	T50.5x5	T50.5x6
Mefloquine	T37.2x1	T37.2x2	T37.2x3	T37.2x4	T37.2x5	T37.2x6
Mefruside	T50.2x1	T50.2x2	T50.2x3	T50.2x4	T50.2x5	T50.2x6
Megahallucinogen	T40.901	T40.902	T40.903	T40.904	T40.905	T40.906
Megestrol	T38.5x1	T38.5x2	T38.5x3	T38.5x4	T38.5x5	T38.5x6
Meglumine						
antimoniate	T37.8x1	T37.8x2	T37.8x3	T37.8x4	T37.8x5	T37.8x6
diatrizoate	T50.8x1	T50.8x2	T50.8x3	T50.8x4	T50.8x5	T50.8x6
iodipamide	T50.8x1	T50.8x2	T50.8x3	T50.8x4	T50.8x5	T50.8x6
iotroxate	T50.8x1	T50.8x2	T50.8x3	T50.8x4	T50.8x5	T50.8x6
MEK (methyl ethyl ketone)	T52.4x1	T52.4x2	T52.4x3	T52.4x4	—	—
Meladinin	T49.3x1	T49.3x2	T49.3x3	T49.3x4	T49.3x5	T49.3x6
Meladrazine	T44.3x1	T44.3x2	T44.3x3	T44.3x4	T44.3x5	T44.3x6
Melaleuca alternifolia oil	T49.0x1	T49.0x2	T49.0x3	T49.0x4	T49.0x5	T49.0x6
Melanizing agents	T49.3x1	T49.3x2	T49.3x3	T49.3x4	T49.3x5	T49.3x6
Melanocyte-stimulating hormone	T38.891	T38.892	T38.893	T38.894	T38.895	T38.896
Melarsonyl potassium	T37.3x1	T37.3x2	T37.3x3	T37.3x4	T37.3x5	T37.3x6
Melarsoprol	T37.3x1	T37.3x2	T37.3x3	T37.3x4	T37.3x5	T37.3x6
Melia azedarach	T62.2x1	T62.2x2	T62.2x3	T62.2x4	—	—
Melitracen	T43.011	T43.012	T43.013	T43.014	T43.015	T43.016
Mellaril	T43.3x1	T43.3x2	T43.3x3	T43.3x4	T43.3x5	T43.3x6
Meloxine	T49.3x1	T49.3x2	T49.3x3	T49.3x4	T49.3x5	T49.3x6
Melperone	T43.4x1	T43.4x2	T43.4x3	T43.4x4	T43.4x5	T43.4x6
Melphalan	T45.1x1	T45.1x2	T45.1x3	T45.1x4	T45.1x5	T45.1x6
Memantine	T43.8x1	T43.8x2	T43.8x3	T43.8x4	T43.8x5	T43.8x6
Menadiol	T45.7x1	T45.7x2	T45.7x3	T45.7x4	T45.7x5	T45.7x6
sodium sulfate	T45.7x1	T45.7x2	T45.7x3	T45.7x4	T45.7x5	T45.7x6
Menadione	T45.7x1	T45.7x2	T45.7x3	T45.7x4	T45.7x5	T45.7x6
sodium bisulfite	T45.7x1	T45.7x2	T45.7x3	T45.7x4	T45.7x5	T45.7x6
Menaphthone	T45.7x1	T45.7x2	T45.7x3	T45.7x4	T45.7x5	T45.7x6
Menaquinone	T45.7x1	T45.7x2	T45.7x3	T45.7x4	T45.7x5	T45.7x6
Menatetrenone	T45.7x1	T45.7x2	T45.7x3	T45.7x4	T45.7x5	T45.7x6
Meningococcal vaccine	T50.A91	T50.A92	T50.A93	T50.A94	T50.A95	T50.A96
Menningovax (-AC) (-C)	T50.A91	T50.A92	T50.A93	T50.A94	T50.A95	T50.A96
Menotropins	T38.811	T38.812	T38.813	T38.814	T38.815	T38.816
Menthol	T48.5x1	T48.5x2	T48.5x3	T48.5x4	T48.5x5	T48.5x6
Mepacrine	T37.2x1	T37.2x2	T37.2x3	T37.2x4	T37.2x5	T37.2x6
Meparfynol	T42.6x1	T42.6x2	T42.6x3	T42.6x4	T42.6x5	T42.6x6
Mepartricin	T36.7x1	T36.7x2	T36.7x3	T36.7x4	T36.7x5	T36.7x6

DRUGS&CHEMICALS

DRUGS & CHEMICALS

Table of Drugs & Chemicals	Accidental (Unintentional)	Self-Harm (Intentional)	Assault	Undetermined	Adverse Effect	Underdosing
Mepazine	T43.3x1	T43.3x2	T43.3x3	T43.3x4	T43.3x5	T43.3x6
Mepenzolate	T44.3x1	T44.3x2	T44.3x3	T44.3x4	T44.3x5	T44.3x6
bromide	T44.3x1	T44.3x2	T44.3x3	T44.3x4	T44.3x5	T44.3x6
Meperidine	T40.4x1	T40.4x2	T40.4x3	T40.4x4	T40.4x5	T40.4x6
Mephebarbital	T42.3x1	T42.3x2	T42.3x3	T42.3x4	T42.3x5	T42.3x6
Mephenamin(e)	T42.8x1	T42.8x2	T42.8x3	T42.8x4	T42.8x5	T42.8x6
Mephenesin	T42.8x1	T42.8x2	T42.8x3	T42.8x4	T42.8x5	T42.8x6
Mephenhydramine	T45.0x1	T45.0x2	T45.0x3	T45.0x4	T45.0x5	T45.0x6
Mephenoxalone	T42.8x1	T42.8x2	T42.8x3	T42.8x4	T42.8x5	T42.8x6
Mephentermine	T44.991	T44.992	T44.993	T44.994	T44.995	T44.996
Mephenytoin	T42.0x1	T42.0x2	T42.0x3	T42.0x4	T42.0x5	T42.0x6
with phenobarbital	T42.3x1	T42.3x2	T42.3x3	T42.3x4	T42.3x5	T42.3x6
Mephobarbital	T42.3x1	T42.3x2	T42.3x3	T42.3x4	T42.3x5	T42.3x6
Mephosfolan	T60.0x1	T60.0x2	T60.0x3	T60.0x4	—	—
Mepindolol	T44.7x1	T44.7x2	T44.7x3	T44.7x4	T44.7x5	T44.7x6
Mepiperphenidol	T44.3x1	T44.3x2	T44.3x3	T44.3x4	T44.3x5	T44.3x6
Mepitiostane	T38.7x1	T38.7x2	T38.7x3	T38.7x4	T38.7x5	T38.7x6
Mepivacaine	T41.3x1	T41.3x2	T41.3x3	T41.3x4	T41.3x5	T41.3x6
epidural	T41.3x1	T41.3x2	T41.3x3	T41.3x4	T41.3x5	T41.3x6
Meprednisone	T38.0x1	T38.0x2	T38.0x3	T38.0x4	T38.0x5	T38.0x6
Meprobam	T43.591	T43.592	T43.593	T43.594	T43.595	T43.596
Meprobamate	T43.591	T43.592	T43.593	T43.594	T43.595	T43.596
Meproscillarin	T46.0x1	T46.0x2	T46.0x3	T46.0x4	T46.0x5	T46.0x6
Meprylcaine	T41.3x1	T41.3x2	T41.3x3	T41.3x4	T41.3x5	T41.3x6
Meptazinol	T39.8x1	T39.8x2	T39.8x3	T39.8x4	T39.8x5	T39.8x6
Mepyramine	T45.0x1	T45.0x2	T45.0x3	T45.0x4	T45.0x5	T45.0x6
Mequitazine	T43.3x1	T43.3x2	T43.3x3	T43.3x4	T43.3x5	T43.3x6
Meralluride	T50.2x1	T50.2x2	T50.2x3	T50.2x4	T50.2x5	T50.2x6
Merbaphen	T50.2x1	T50.2x2	T50.2x3	T50.2x4	T50.2x5	T50.2x6
Merbromin	T49.0x1	T49.0x2	T49.0x3	T49.0x4	T49.0x5	T49.0x6
Mercaptobenzothiazole salts	T49.0x1	T49.0x2	T49.0x3	T49.0x4	T49.0x5	T49.0x6
Mercaptomerin	T50.2x1	T50.2x2	T50.2x3	T50.2x4	T50.2x5	T50.2x6
Mercaptopurine	T45.1x1	T45.1x2	T45.1x3	T45.1x4	T45.1x5	T45.1x6
Mercumatilin	T50.2x1	T50.2x2	T50.2x3	T50.2x4	T50.2x5	T50.2x6
Mercuramide	T50.2x1	T50.2x2	T50.2x3	T50.2x4	T50.2x5	T50.2x6
Mercurochrome	T49.0x1	T49.0x2	T49.0x3	T49.0x4	T49.0x5	T49.0x6
Mercurophylline	T50.2x1	T50.2x2	T50.2x3	T50.2x4	T50.2x5	T50.2x6
Mercury, mercurial, mercuric, mercurous (compounds) (cyanide) (fumes) (nonmedicinal) (vapor) NEC	T56.1x1	T56.1x2	T56.1x3	T56.1x4	—	—
ammoniated	T49.0x1	T49.0x2	T49.0x3	T49.0x4	T49.0x5	T49.0x6
anti-infective						
local	T49.0x1	T49.0x2	T49.0x3	T49.0x4	T49.0x5	T49.0x6
systemic	T37.8x1	T37.8x2	T37.8x3	T37.8x4	T37.8x5	T37.8x6
topical	T49.0x1	T49.0x2	T49.0x3	T49.0x4	T49.0x5	T49.0x6
chloride (ammoniated)	T49.0x1	T49.0x2	T49.0x3	T49.0x4	T49.0x5	T49.0x6
fungicide	T56.1x1	T56.1x2	T56.1x3	T56.1x4	—	—
diuretic NEC	T50.2x1	T50.2x2	T50.2x3	T50.2x4	T50.2x5	T50.2x6
fungicide	T56.1x1	T56.1x2	T56.1x3	T56.1x4		
organic (fungicide)	T56.1x1	T56.1x2	T56.1x3	T56.1x4		
oxide, yellow	T49.0x1	T49.0x2	T49.0x3	T49.0x4	T49.0x5	T49.0x6
Mersalyl	T50.2x1	T50.2x2	T50.2x3	T50.2x4	T50.2x5	T50.2x6
Merthiolate	T49.0x1	T49.0x2	T49.0x3	T49.0x4	T49.0x5	T49.0x6
ophthalmic preparation	T49.5x1	T49.5x2	T49.5x3	T49.5x4	T49.5x5	T49.5x6
Meruvax	T50.B91	T50.B92	T50.B93	T50.B94	T50.B95	T50.B96
Mesalazine	T47.8x1	T47.8x2	T47.8x3	T47.8x4	T47.8x5	T47.8x6
Mescal buttons	T40.991	T40.992	T40.993	T40.994	—	—
Mescaline	T40.991	T40.992	T40.993	T40.994		
Mesna	T48.4x1	T48.4x2	T48.4x3	T48.4x4	T48.4x5	T48.4x6
Mesoglycan	T46.6x1	T46.6x2	T46.6x3	T46.6x4	T46.6x5	T46.6x6
Mesoridazine	T43.3x1	T43.3x2	T43.3x3	T43.3x4	T43.3x5	T43.3x6
Mestanolone	T38.7x1	T38.7x2	T38.7x3	T38.7x4	T38.7x5	T38.7x6
Mesterolone	T38.7x1	T38.7x2	T38.7x3	T38.7x4	T38.7x5	T38.7x6
Mestranol	T38.5x1	T38.5x2	T38.5x3	T38.5x4	T38.5x5	T38.5x6
Mesulergine	T42.8x1	T42.8x2	T42.8x3	T42.8x4	T42.8x5	T42.8x6
Mesulfen	T49.0x1	T49.0x2	T49.0x3	T49.0x4	T49.0x5	T49.0x6
Mesuximide	T42.2x1	T42.2x2	T42.2x3	T42.2x4	T42.2x5	T42.2x6
Metabutethamine	T41.3x1	T41.3x2	T41.3x3	T41.3x4	T41.3x5	T41.3x6
Metactesylacetate	T49.0x1	T49.0x2	T49.0x3	T49.0x4	T49.0x5	T49.0x6
Metacycline	T36.4x1	T36.4x2	T36.4x3	T36.4x4	T36.4x5	T36.4x6
Metaldehyde (snail killer) NEC	T60.8x1	T60.8x2	T60.8x3	T60.8x4	—	—
Metals (heavy) (nonmedicinal)	T56.91	T56.92	T56.93	T56.94	—	—
dust, fumes, or vapor NEC	T56.91	T56.92	T56.93	T56.94	—	—
light NEC	T56.91	T56.92	T56.93	T56.94	—	—
dust, fumes, or vapor NEC	T56.91	T56.92	T56.93	T56.94	—	—
specified NEC	T56.891	T56.892	T56.893	T56.894	—	—
thallium	T56.811	T56.812	T56.813	T56.814	—	—
Metamfetamine	T43.621	T43.622	T43.623	T43.624	T43.625	T43.626
Metamizole sodium	T39.2x1	T39.2x2	T39.2x3	T39.2x4	T39.2x5	T39.2x6
Metampicillin	T36.0x1	T36.0x2	T36.0x3	T36.0x4	T36.0x5	T36.0x6
Metamucil	T47.4x1	T47.4x2	T47.4x3	T47.4x4	T47.4x5	T47.4x6
Metandienone	T38.7x1	T38.7x2	T38.7x3	T38.7x4	T38.7x5	T38.7x6
Metandrostenolone	T38.7x1	T38.7x2	T38.7x3	T38.7x4	T38.7x5	T38.7x6
Metaphen	T49.0x1	T49.0x2	T49.0x3	T49.0x4	T49.0x5	T49.0x6
Metaphos	T60.0x1	T60.0x2	T60.0x3	T60.0x4	—	—
Metapramine	T43.011	T43.012	T43.013	T43.014	T43.015	T43.016
Metaproterenol	T48.291	T48.292	T48.293	T48.294	T48.295	T48.296
Metaraminol	T44.4x1	T44.4x2	T44.4x3	T44.4x4	T44.4x5	T44.4x6
Metaxalone	T42.8x1	T42.8x2	T42.8x3	T42.8x4	T42.8x5	T42.8x6
Metenolone	T38.7x1	T38.7x2	T38.7x3	T38.7x4	T38.7x5	T38.7x6
Metergoline	T42.8x1	T42.8x2	T42.8x3	T42.8x4	T42.8x5	T42.8x6
Metescufylline	T46.991	T46.992	T46.993	T46.994	T46.995	T46.996
Metetoin	T42.0x1	T42.0x2	T42.0x3	T42.0x4	T42.0x5	T42.0x6
Metformin	T38.3x1	T38.3x2	T38.3x3	T38.3x4	T38.3x5	T38.3x6
Methacholine	T44.1x1	T44.1x2	T44.1x3	T44.1x4	T44.1x5	T44.1x6
Methacycline	T36.4x1	T36.4x2	T36.4x3	T36.4x4	T36.4x5	T36.4x6
Methadone	T40.3x1	T40.3x2	T40.3x3	T40.3x4	T40.3x5	T40.3x6
Methallenestril	T38.5x1	T38.5x2	T38.5x3	T38.5x4	T38.5x5	T38.5x6
Methallenoestril	T38.5x1	T38.5x2	T38.5x3	T38.5x4	T38.5x5	T38.5x6
Methamphetamine	T43.621	T43.622	T43.623	T43.624	T43.625	T43.626
Methampyrone	T39.2x1	T39.2x2	T39.2x3	T39.2x4	T39.2x5	T39.2x6
Methandienone	T38.7x1	T38.7x2	T38.7x3	T38.7x4	T38.7x5	T38.7x6
Methandriol	T38.7x1	T38.7x2	T38.7x3	T38.7x4	T38.7x5	T38.7x6
Methandrostenolone	T38.7x1	T38.7x2	T38.7x3	T38.7x4	T38.7x5	T38.7x6
Methane	T59.891	T59.892	T59.893	T59.894	—	—
Methanethiol	T59.891	T59.892	T59.893	T59.894	—	—
Methaniazide	T37.1x1	T37.1x2	T37.1x3	T37.1x4	T37.1x5	T37.1x6
Methanol (vapor)	T51.1x1	T51.1x2	T51.1x3	T51.1x4	—	—
Methantheline	T44.3x1	T44.3x2	T44.3x3	T44.3x4	T44.3x5	T44.3x6
Methanthelinium bromide	T44.3x1	T44.3x2	T44.3x3	T44.3x4	T44.3x5	T44.3x6
Methaphenilene	T45.0x1	T45.0x2	T45.0x3	T45.0x4	T45.0x5	T45.0x6
Methapyrilene	T45.0x1	T45.0x2	T45.0x3	T45.0x4	T45.0x5	T45.0x6
Methaqualone (compound)	T42.6x1	T42.6x2	T42.6x3	T42.6x4	T42.6x5	T42.6x6
Metharbital	T42.3x1	T42.3x2	T42.3x3	T42.3x4	T42.3x5	T42.3x6
Methazolamide	T50.2x1	T50.2x2	T50.2x3	T50.2x4	T50.2x5	T50.2x6
Methdilazine	T43.3x1	T43.3x2	T43.3x3	T43.3x4	T43.3x5	T43.3x6
Methedrine	T43.621	T43.622	T43.623	T43.624	T43.625	T43.626
Methenamine (mandelate)	T37.8x1	T37.8x2	T37.8x3	T37.8x4	T37.8x5	T37.8x6
Methenolone	T38.7x1	T38.7x2	T38.7x3	T38.7x4	T38.7x5	T38.7x6
Methergine	T48.0x1	T48.0x2	T48.0x3	T48.0x4	T48.0x5	T48.0x6
Methetoin	T42.0x1	T42.0x2	T42.0x3	T42.0x4	T42.0x5	T42.0x6
Methiacil	T38.2x1	T38.2x2	T38.2x3	T38.2x4	T38.2x5	T38.2x6
Methicillin	T36.0x1	T36.0x2	T36.0x3	T36.0x4	T36.0x5	T36.0x6
Methimazole	T38.2x1	T38.2x2	T38.2x3	T38.2x4	T38.2x5	T38.2x6
Methiodal sodium	T50.8x1	T50.8x2	T50.8x3	T50.8x4	T50.8x5	T50.8x6
Methionine	T50.991	T50.992	T50.993	T50.994	T50.995	T50.996
Methisazone	T37.5x1	T37.5x2	T37.5x3	T37.5x4	T37.5x5	T37.5x6
Methisoprinol	T37.5x1	T37.5x2	T37.5x3	T37.5x4	T37.5x5	T37.5x6
Methitural	T42.3x1	T42.3x2	T42.3x3	T42.3x4	T42.3x5	T42.3x6
Methixene	T44.3x1	T44.3x2	T44.3x3	T44.3x4	T44.3x5	T44.3x6
Methobarbital, methobarbitone	T42.3x1	T42.3x2	T42.3x3	T42.3x4	T42.3x5	T42.3x6
Methocarbamol	T42.8x1	T42.8x2	T42.8x3	T42.8x4	T42.8x5	T42.8x6
skeletal muscle relaxant	T48.1x1	T48.1x2	T48.1x3	T48.1x4	T48.1x5	T48.1x6
Methohexital	T41.1x1	T41.1x2	T41.1x3	T41.1x4	T41.1x5	T41.1x6
Methohexitone	T41.1x1	T41.1x2	T41.1x3	T41.1x4	T41.1x5	T41.1x6

DRUGS&CHEMICALS

Table of Drugs & Chemicals	Accidental (Unintentional)	Self-Harm (Intentional)	Assault	Undetermined	Adverse Effect	Underdosing
Methoin	T42.0x1	T42.0x2	T42.0x3	T42.0x4	T42.0x5	T42.0x6
Methopholine	T39.8x1	T39.8x2	T39.8x3	T39.8x4	T39.8x5	T39.8x6
Methopromazine	T43.3x1	T43.3x2	T43.3x3	T43.3x4	T43.3x5	T43.3x6
Methorate	T48.3x1	T48.3x2	T48.3x3	T48.3x4	T48.3x5	T48.3x6
Methoserpidine	T46.5x1	T46.5x2	T46.5x3	T46.5x4	T46.5x5	T46.5x6
Methotrexate	T45.1x1	T45.1x2	T45.1x3	T45.1x4	T45.1x5	T45.1x6
Methotrimeprazine	T43.3x1	T43.3x2	T43.3x3	T43.3x4	T43.3x5	T43.3x6
Methoxa-Dome	T49.3x1	T49.3x2	T49.3x3	T49.3x4	T49.3x5	T49.3x6
Methoxamine	T44.4x1	T44.4x2	T44.4x3	T44.4x4	T44.4x5	T44.4x6
Methoxsalen	T50.991	T50.992	T50.993	T50.994	T50.995	T50.996
Methoxyaniline	T65.3x1	T65.3x2	T65.3x3	T65.3x4	—	—
Methoxybenzyl penicillin	T36.0x1	T36.0x2	T36.0x3	T36.0x4	T36.0x5	T36.0x6
Methoxychlor	T53.7x1	T53.7x2	T53.7x3	T53.7x4	—	—
Methoxy-DDT	T53.7x1	T53.7x2	T53.7x3	T53.7x4	—	—
2-Methoxyethanol	T52.3x1	T52.3x2	T52.3x3	T52.3x4	—	—
Methoxyflurane	T41.0x1	T41.0x2	T41.0x3	T41.0x4	T41.0x5	T41.0x6
Methoxyphenamine	T48.6x1	T48.6x2	T48.6x3	T48.6x4	T48.6x5	T48.6x6
Methoxypromazine	T43.3x1	T43.3x2	T43.3x3	T43.3x4	T43.3x5	T43.3x6
5-Methoxypsoralen (5-MOP)	T50.991	T50.992	T50.993	T50.994	T50.995	T50.996
8-Methoxypsoralen (8-MOP)	T50.991	T50.992	T50.993	T50.994	T50.995	T50.996
Methscopolamine bromide	T44.3x1	T44.3x2	T44.3x3	T44.3x4	T44.3x5	T44.3x6
Methsuximide	T42.2x1	T42.2x2	T42.2x3	T42.2x4	T42.2x5	T42.2x6
Methyclothiazide	T50.2x1	T50.2x2	T50.2x3	T50.2x4	T50.2x5	T50.2x6
Methyl						
acetate	T52.4x1	T52.4x2	T52.4x3	T52.4x4	—	—
acetone	T52.4x1	T52.4x2	T52.4x3	T52.4x4	—	—
acrylate	T65.891	T65.892	T65.893	T65.894	—	—
alcohol	T51.1x1	T51.1x2	T51.1x3	T51.1x4	—	—
aminophenol	T65.3x1	T65.3x2	T65.3x3	T65.3x4	—	—
amphetamine	T43.621	T43.622	T43.623	T43.624	T43.625	T43.626
androstanolone	T38.7x1	T38.7x2	T38.7x3	T38.7x4	T38.7x5	T38.7x6
atropine	T44.3x1	T44.3x2	T44.3x3	T44.3x4	T44.3x5	T44.3x6
benzene	T52.2x1	T52.2x2	T52.2x3	T52.2x4	—	—
benzoate	T52.8x1	T52.8x2	T52.8x3	T52.8x4	—	—
benzol	T52.2x1	T52.2x2	T52.2x3	T52.2x4	—	—
bromide (gas)	T59.891	T59.892	T59.893	T59.894	—	—
fumigant	T60.8x1	T60.8x2	T60.8x3	T60.8x4	—	—
butanol	T51.3x1	T51.3x2	T51.3x3	T51.3x4	—	—
carbonate	T52.8x1	T52.8x2	T52.8x3	T52.8x4	—	—
carbinol	T51.1x1	T51.1x2	T51.1x3	T51.1x4	—	—
CCNU	T45.1x1	T45.1x2	T45.1x3	T45.1x4	T45.1x5	T45.1x6
cellosolve	T52.91	T52.92	T52.93	T52.94	—	—
cellulose	T47.4x1	T47.4x2	T47.4x3	T47.4x4	T47.4x5	T47.4x6
chloride (gas)	T59.891	T59.892	T59.893	T59.894	—	—
chloroformate	T59.3x1	T59.3x2	T59.3x3	T59.3x4	—	—
cyclohexane	T52.8x1	T52.8x2	T52.8x3	T52.8x4	—	—
cyclohexanol	T51.8x1	T51.8x2	T51.8x3	T51.8x4	—	—
cyclohexanone	T52.8x1	T52.8x2	T52.8x3	T52.8x4	—	—
cyclohexyl acetate	T52.8x1	T52.8x2	T52.8x3	T52.8x4	—	—
demeton	T60.0x1	T60.0x2	T60.0x3	T60.0x4	—	—
dihydromorphinone	T40.2x1	T40.2x2	T40.2x3	T40.2x4	T40.2x5	T40.2x6
ergometrine	T48.0x1	T48.0x2	T48.0x3	T48.0x4	T48.0x5	T48.0x6
ergonovine	T48.0x1	T48.0x2	T48.0x3	T48.0x4	T48.0x5	T48.0x6
ethyl ketone	T52.4x1	T52.4x2	T52.4x3	T52.4x4	—	—
glucamine antimonate	T37.8x1	T37.8x2	T37.8x3	T37.8x4	T37.8x5	T37.8x6
hydrazine	T65.891	T65.892	T65.893	T65.894	—	—
iodide	T65.891	T65.892	T65.893	T65.894	—	—
isobutyl ketone	T52.4x1	T52.4x2	T52.4x3	T52.4x4	—	—
isothiocyanate	T60.3x1	T60.3x2	T60.3x3	T60.3x4	—	—
mercaptan	T59.891	T59.892	T59.893	T59.894	—	—
morphine NEC	T40.2x1	T40.2x2	T40.2x3	T40.2x4	T40.2x5	T40.2x6
nicotinate	T49.4x1	T49.4x2	T49.4x3	T49.4x4	T49.4x5	T49.4x6
paraben	T49.0x1	T49.0x2	T49.0x3	T49.0x4	T49.0x5	T49.0x6
parafynol	T42.6x1	T42.6x2	T42.6x3	T42.6x4	T42.6x5	T42.6x6
parathion	T60.0x1	T60.0x2	T60.0x3	T60.0x4	—	—
propylcarbinol	T51.3x1	T51.3x2	T51.3x3	T51.3x4	—	—
peridol	T43.4x1	T43.4x2	T43.4x3	T43.4x4	T43.4x5	T43.4x6
phenidate	T43.631	T43.632	T43.633	T43.634	T43.635	T43.636
prednisolone	T38.0x1	T38.0x2	T38.0x3	T38.0x4	T38.0x5	T38.0x6
ENT agent	T49.6x1	T49.6x2	T49.6x3	T49.6x4	T49.6x5	T49.6x6
ophthalmic preparation	T49.5x1	T49.5x2	T49.5x3	T49.5x4	T49.5x5	T49.5x6
topical NEC	T49.0x1	T49.0x2	T49.0x3	T49.0x4	T49.0x5	T49.0x6

Table of Drugs & Chemicals	Accidental (Unintentional)	Self-Harm (Intentional)	Assault	Undetermined	Adverse Effect	Underdosing
Methyl – continued						
rosaniline NEC	T49.0x1	T49.0x2	T49.0x3	T49.0x4	T49.0x5	T49.0x6
salicylate	T49.2x1	T49.2x2	T49.2x3	T49.2x4	T49.2x5	T49.2x6
sulfate (fumes)	T59.891	T59.892	T59.893	T59.894	—	—
liquid	T52.8x1	T52.8x2	T52.8x3	T52.8x4	—	—
sulfonal	T42.6x1	T42.6x2	T42.6x3	T42.6x4	T42.6x5	T42.6x6
testosterone	T38.7x1	T38.7x2	T38.7x3	T38.7x4	T38.7x5	T38.7x6
thiouracil	T38.2x1	T38.2x2	T38.2x3	T38.2x4	T38.2x5	T38.2x6
Methylamphetamine	T43.621	T43.622	T43.623	T43.624	T43.625	T43.626
Methylated spirit	T51.1x1	T51.1x2	T51.1x3	T51.1x4	—	—
Methylatropine nitrate	T44.3x1	T44.3x2	T44.3x3	T44.3x4	T44.3x5	T44.3x6
Methylbenactyzium bromide	T44.3x1	T44.3x2	T44.3x3	T44.3x4	T44.3x5	T44.3x6
Methylbenzethonium chloride	T49.0x1	T49.0x2	T49.0x3	T49.0x4	T49.0x5	T49.0x6
Methylcellulose	T47.4x1	T47.4x2	T47.4x3	T47.4x4	T47.4x5	T47.4x6
laxative	T47.4x1	T47.4x2	T47.4x3	T47.4x4	T47.4x5	T47.4x6
Methylchlorophenoxy-acetic acid	T60.3x1	T60.3x2	T60.3x3	T60.3x4	—	—
Methyldopa	T46.5x1	T46.5x2	T46.5x3	T46.5x4	T46.5x5	T46.5x6
Methyldopate	T46.5x1	T46.5x2	T46.5x3	T46.5x4	T46.5x5	T46.5x6
Methylene						
blue	T50.6x1	T50.6x2	T50.6x3	T50.6x4	T50.6x5	T50.6x6
chloride or dichloride (solvent) NEC	T53.4x1	T53.4x2	T53.4x3	T53.4x4	—	—
Methylenedioxyamphetamine	T43.621	T43.622	T43.623	T43.624	T43.625	T43.626
Methylenedioxymethamphetamine	T43.621	T43.622	T43.623	T43.624	T43.625	T43.626
Methylergometrine	T48.0x1	T48.0x2	T48.0x3	T48.0x4	T48.0x5	T48.0x6
Methylergonovine	T48.0x1	T48.0x2	T48.0x3	T48.0x4	T48.0x5	T48.0x6
Methylestrenolone	T38.5x1	T38.5x2	T38.5x3	T38.5x4	T38.5x5	T38.5x6
Methylethyl cellulose	T50.991	T50.992	T50.993	T50.994	T50.995	T50.996
Methylhexabital	T42.3x1	T42.3x2	T42.3x3	T42.3x4	T42.3x5	T42.3x6
Methylmorphine	T40.2x1	T40.2x2	T40.2x3	T40.2x4	T40.2x5	T40.2x6
Methylparaben (ophthalmic)	T49.5x1	T49.5x2	T49.5x3	T49.5x4	T49.5x5	T49.5x6
Methylparafynol	T42.6x1	T42.6x2	T42.6x3	T42.6x4	T42.6x5	T42.6x6
Methylpentynol, methylpenthynol	T42.6x1	T42.6x2	T42.6x3	T42.6x4	T42.6x5	T42.6x6
Methylphenidate	T43.631	T43.632	T43.633	T43.634	T43.635	T43.636
Methylphenobarbital	T42.3x1	T42.3x2	T42.3x3	T42.3x4	T42.3x5	T42.3x6
Methylpolysiloxane	T47.1x1	T47.1x2	T47.1x3	T47.1x4	T47.1x5	T47.1x6
Methylprednisolone — see Methyl, prednisolone						
Methylrosaniline	T49.0x1	T49.0x2	T49.0x3	T49.0x4	T49.0x5	T49.0x6
Methylrosanilinium chloride	T49.0x1	T49.0x2	T49.0x3	T49.0x4	T49.0x5	T49.0x6
Methyltestosterone	T38.7x1	T38.7x2	T38.7x3	T38.7x4	T38.7x5	T38.7x6
Methylthionine chloride	T50.6x1	T50.6x2	T50.6x3	T50.6x4	T50.6x5	T50.6x6
Methylthioninium chloride	T50.6x1	T50.6x2	T50.6x3	T50.6x4	T50.6x5	T50.6x6
Methylthiouracil	T38.2x1	T38.2x2	T38.2x3	T38.2x4	T38.2x5	T38.2x6
Methyprylon	T42.6x1	T42.6x2	T42.6x3	T42.6x4	T42.6x5	T42.6x6
Methysergide	T46.5x1	T46.5x2	T46.5x3	T46.5x4	T46.5x5	T46.5x6
Metiamide	T47.1x1	T47.1x2	T47.1x3	T47.1x4	T47.1x5	T47.1x6
Meticillin	T36.0x1	T36.0x2	T36.0x3	T36.0x4	T36.0x5	T36.0x6
Meticrane	T50.2x1	T50.2x2	T50.2x3	T50.2x4	T50.2x5	T50.2x6
Metildigoxin	T46.0x1	T46.0x2	T46.0x3	T46.0x4	T46.0x5	T46.0x6
Metipranolol	T49.5x1	T49.5x2	T49.5x3	T49.5x4	T49.5x5	T49.5x6
Metirosine	T46.5x1	T46.5x2	T46.5x3	T46.5x4	T46.5x5	T46.5x6
Metisazone	T37.5x1	T37.5x2	T37.5x3	T37.5x4	T37.5x5	T37.5x6
Metixene	T44.3x1	T44.3x2	T44.3x3	T44.3x4	T44.3x5	T44.3x6
Metizoline	T48.5x1	T48.5x2	T48.5x3	T48.5x4	T48.5x5	T48.5x6
Metoclopramide	T45.0x1	T45.0x2	T45.0x3	T45.0x4	T45.0x5	T45.0x6
Metofenazate	T43.3x1	T43.3x2	T43.3x3	T43.3x4	T43.3x5	T43.3x6
Metofoline	T39.8x1	T39.8x2	T39.8x3	T39.8x4	T39.8x5	T39.8x6
Metolazone	T50.2x1	T50.2x2	T50.2x3	T50.2x4	T50.2x5	T50.2x6
Metopon	T40.2x1	T40.2x2	T40.2x3	T40.2x4	T40.2x5	T40.2x6
Metoprine	T45.1x1	T45.1x2	T45.1x3	T45.1x4	T45.1x5	T45.1x6
Metoprolol	T44.7x1	T44.7x2	T44.7x3	T44.7x4	T44.7x5	T44.7x6
Metrifonate	T60.0x1	T60.0x2	T60.0x3	T60.0x4	—	—
Metrizamide	T50.8x1	T50.8x2	T50.8x3	T50.8x4	T50.8x5	T50.8x6
Metrizoic acid	T50.8x1	T50.8x2	T50.8x3	T50.8x4	T50.8x5	T50.8x6
Metronidazole	T37.8x1	T37.8x2	T37.8x3	T37.8x4	T37.8x5	T37.8x6
Metycaine	T41.3x1	T41.3x2	T41.3x3	T41.3x4	T41.3x5	T41.3x6
infiltration (subcutaneous)	T41.3x1	T41.3x2	T41.3x3	T41.3x4	T41.3x5	T41.3x6
nerve block (peripheral) (plexus)	T41.3x1	T41.3x2	T41.3x3	T41.3x4	T41.3x5	T41.3x6
topical (surface)	T41.3x1	T41.3x2	T41.3x3	T41.3x4	T41.3x5	T41.3x6

DRUGS&CHEMICALS

Table of Drugs & Chemicals	POISONING Accidental (Unintentional)	POISONING Self-Harm (Intentional)	POISONING Assault	POISONING Undetermined	Adverse Effect	Underdosing
Metyrapone	T50.8x1	T50.8x2	T50.8x3	T50.8x4	T50.8x5	T50.8x6
Mevinphos	T60.0x1	T60.0x2	T60.0x3	T60.0x4	—	—
Mexazolam	T42.4x1	T42.4x2	T42.4x3	T42.4x4	T42.4x5	T42.4x6
Mexenone	T49.3x1	T49.3x2	T49.3x3	T49.3x4	T49.3x5	T49.3x6
Mexiletine	T46.2x1	T46.2x2	T46.2x3	T46.2x4	T46.2x5	T46.2x6
Mezereon	T62.2x1	T62.2x2	T62.2x3	T62.2x4	—	—
berries	T62.1x1	T62.1x2	T62.1x3	T62.1x4	—	—
Mezlocillin	T36.0x1	T36.0x2	T36.0x3	T36.0x4	T36.0x5	T36.0x6
Mianserin	T43.021	T43.022	T43.023	T43.024	T43.025	T43.026
Micatin	T49.0x1	T49.0x2	T49.0x3	T49.0x4	T49.0x5	T49.0x6
Miconazole	T49.0x1	T49.0x2	T49.0x3	T49.0x4	T49.0x5	T49.0x6
Micronomicin	T36.5x1	T36.5x2	T36.5x3	T36.5x4	T36.5x5	T36.5x6
Midazolam	T42.4x1	T42.4x2	T42.4x3	T42.4x4	T42.4x5	T42.4x6
Midecamycin	T36.3x1	T36.3x2	T36.3x3	T36.3x4	T36.3x5	T36.3x6
Mifepristone	T38.6x1	T38.6x2	T38.6x3	T38.6x4	T38.6x5	T38.6x6
Milk of magnesia	T47.1x1	T47.1x2	T47.1x3	T47.1x4	T47.1x5	T47.1x6
Millipede (tropical) (venomous)	T63.411	T63.412	T63.413	T63.414	—	—
Miltown	T43.591	T43.592	T43.593	T43.594	T43.595	T43.596
Milverine	T44.3x1	T44.3x2	T44.3x3	T44.3x4	T44.3x5	T44.3x6
Minaprine	T43.291	T43.292	T43.293	T43.294	T43.295	T43.296
Minaxolone	T41.291	T41.292	T41.293	T41.294	T41.295	T41.296
Mineral						
acids	T54.2x1	T54.2x2	T54.2x3	T54.2x4	—	—
oil (laxative) (medicinal)	T47.4x1	T47.4x2	T47.4x3	T47.4x4	T47.4x5	T47.4x6
emulsion	T47.2x1	T47.2x2	T47.2x3	T47.2x4	T47.2x5	T47.2x6
nonmedicinal	T52.0x1	T52.0x2	T52.0x3	T52.0x4	—	—
topical	T49.3x1	T49.3x2	T49.3x3	T49.3x4	T49.3x5	T49.3x6
salt NEC	T50.3x1	T50.3x2	T50.3x3	T50.3x4	T50.3x5	T50.3x6
spirits	T52.0x1	T52.0x2	T52.0x3	T52.0x4	—	—
Mineralocorticosteroid	T50.0x1	T50.0x2	T50.0x3	T50.0x4	T50.0x5	T50.0x6
Minocycline	T36.4x1	T36.4x2	T36.4x3	T36.4x4	T36.4x5	T36.4x6
Minoxidil	T46.7x1	T46.7x2	T46.7x3	T46.7x4	T46.7x5	T46.7x6
Miokamycin	T36.3x1	T36.3x2	T36.3x3	T36.3x4	T36.3x5	T36.3x6
Miotic drug	T49.5x1	T49.5x2	T49.5x3	T49.5x4	T49.5x5	T49.5x6
Mipafox	T60.0x1	T60.0x2	T60.0x3	T60.0x4	—	—
Mirex	T60.1x1	T60.1x2	T60.1x3	T60.1x4	—	—
Mirtazapine	T43.021	T43.022	T43.023	T43.024	T43.025	T43.026
Misonidazole	T37.3x1	T37.3x2	T37.3x3	T37.3x4	T37.3x5	T37.3x6
Misoprostol	T47.1x1	T47.1x2	T47.1x3	T47.1x4	T47.1x5	T47.1x6
Mithramycin	T45.1x1	T45.1x2	T45.1x3	T45.1x4	T45.1x5	T45.1x6
Mitobronitol	T45.1x1	T45.1x2	T45.1x3	T45.1x4	T45.1x5	T45.1x6
Mitoguazone	T45.1x1	T45.1x2	T45.1x3	T45.1x4	T45.1x5	T45.1x6
Mitolactol	T45.1x1	T45.1x2	T45.1x3	T45.1x4	T45.1x5	T45.1x6
Mitomycin	T45.1x1	T45.1x2	T45.1x3	T45.1x4	T45.1x5	T45.1x6
Mitopodozide	T45.1x1	T45.1x2	T45.1x3	T45.1x4	T45.1x5	T45.1x6
Mitotane	T45.1x1	T45.1x2	T45.1x3	T45.1x4	T45.1x5	T45.1x6
Mitoxantrone	T45.1x1	T45.1x2	T45.1x3	T45.1x4	T45.1x5	T45.1x6
Mivacurium chloride	T48.1x1	T48.1x2	T48.1x3	T48.1x4	T48.1x5	T48.1x6
Miyari bacteria	T47.6x1	T47.6x2	T47.6x3	T47.6x4	T47.6x5	T47.6x6
Moclobemide	T43.1x1	T43.1x2	T43.1x3	T43.1x4	T43.1x5	T43.1x6
Moderil	T46.5x1	T46.5x2	T46.5x3	T46.5x4	T46.5x5	T46.5x6
Mofebutazone	T39.2x1	T39.2x2	T39.2x3	T39.2x4	T39.2x5	T39.2x6
Mogadon — see Nitrazepam						
Molindone	T43.591	T43.592	T43.593	T43.594	T43.595	T43.596
Molsidomine	T46.3x1	T46.3x2	T46.3x3	T46.3x4	T46.3x5	T46.3x6
Mometasone	T49.0x1	T49.0x2	T49.0x3	T49.0x4	T49.0x5	T49.0x6
Monistat	T49.0x1	T49.0x2	T49.0x3	T49.0x4	T49.0x5	T49.0x6
Monkshood	T62.2x1	T62.2x2	T62.2x3	T62.2x4	—	—
Monoamine oxidase inhibitor						
NEC	T43.1x1	T43.1x2	T43.1x3	T43.1x4	T43.1x5	T43.1x6
hydrazine	T43.1x1	T43.1x2	T43.1x3	T43.1x4	T43.1x5	T43.1x6
Monobenzone	T49.4x1	T49.4x2	T49.4x3	T49.4x4	T49.4x5	T49.4x6
Monochloroacetic acid	T60.3x1	T60.3x2	T60.3x3	T60.3x4	—	—
Monochlorobenzene	T53.7x1	T53.7x2	T53.7x3	T53.7x4	—	—
Monoethanolamine	T46.8x1	T46.8x2	T46.8x3	T46.8x4	T46.8x5	T46.8x6
oleate	T46.8x1	T46.8x2	T46.8x3	T46.8x4	T46.8x5	T46.8x6
Monooctanoin	T50.991	T50.992	T50.993	T50.994	T50.995	T50.996
Monophenylbutazone	T39.2x1	T39.2x2	T39.2x3	T39.2x4	T39.2x5	T39.2x6
Monosodium glutamate	T65.891	T65.892	T65.893	T65.894	—	—
Monosulfiram	T49.0x1	T49.0x2	T49.0x3	T49.0x4	T49.0x5	T49.0x6
Monoxide, carbon— see Carbon, monoxide						
Monoxidine hydrochloride	T46.1x1	T46.1x2	T46.1x3	T46.1x4	T46.1x5	T46.1x6
Monuron	T60.3x1	T60.3x2	T60.3x3	T60.3x4	—	—
Moperone	T43.4x1	T43.4x2	T43.4x3	T43.4x4	T43.4x5	T43.4x6
Mopidamol	T45.1x1	T45.1x2	T45.1x3	T45.1x4	T45.1x5	T45.1x6
MOPP (mechloreth-amine + vincristine + prednisone + procarba-zine)	T45.1x1	T45.1x2	T45.1x3	T45.1x4	T45.1x5	T45.1x6
Morfin	T40.2x1	T40.2x2	T40.2x3	T40.2x4	T40.2x5	T40.2x6
Morinamide	T37.1x1	T37.1x2	T37.1x3	T37.1x4	T37.1x5	T37.1x6
Morning glory seeds	T40.991	T40.992	T40.993	T40.994	—	—
Moroxydine	T37.5x1	T37.5x2	T37.5x3	T37.5x4	T37.5x5	T37.5x6
Morphazinamide	T37.1x1	T37.1x2	T37.1x3	T37.1x4	T37.1x5	T37.1x6
Morphine	T40.2x1	T40.2x2	T40.2x3	T40.2x4	T40.2x5	T40.2x6
antagonist	T50.7x1	T50.7x2	T50.7x3	T50.7x4	T50.7x5	T50.7x6
Morpholinylethylmorphine	T40.2x1	T40.2x2	T40.2x3	T40.2x4	—	—
Morsuximide	T42.2x1	T42.2x2	T42.2x3	T42.2x4	T42.2x5	T42.2x6
Mosapramine	T43.591	T43.592	T43.593	T43.594	T43.595	T43.596
Moth balls — see also Pesticides	T60.2x1	T60.2x2	T60.2x3	T60.2x4	—	—
naphthalene	T60.2x1	T60.2x2	T60.2x3	T60.2x4	—	—
paradichlorobenzene	T60.1x1	T60.1x2	T60.1x3	T60.1x4	—	—
Motor exhaust gas	T58.01	T58.02	T58.03	T58.04	—	—
Mouthwash (antiseptic) (zinc chloride)	T49.6x1	T49.6x2	T49.6x3	T49.6x4	T49.6x5	T49.6x6
Moxastine	T45.0x1	T45.0x2	T45.0x3	T45.0x4	T45.0x5	T45.0x6
Moxaverine	T44.3x1	T44.3x2	T44.3x3	T44.3x4	T44.3x5	T44.3x6
Moxisylyte	T46.7x1	T46.7x2	T46.7x3	T46.7x4	T46.7x5	T46.7x6
Mucilage, plant	T47.4x1	T47.4x2	T47.4x3	T47.4x4	T47.4x5	T47.4x6
Mucolytic drug	T48.4x1	T48.4x2	T48.4x3	T48.4x4	T48.4x5	T48.4x6
Mucomyst	T48.4x1	T48.4x2	T48.4x3	T48.4x4	T48.4x5	T48.4x6
Mucous membrane agents						
(external)	T49.91	T49.92	T49.93	T49.94	T49.95	T49.96
specified NEC	T49.8x1	T49.8x2	T49.8x3	T49.8x4	T49.8x5	T49.8x6
Mumps						
immune globulin (human)	T50.Z11	T50.Z12	T50.Z13	T50.Z14	T50.Z15	T50.Z16
skin test antigen	T50.8x1	T50.8x2	T50.8x3	T50.8x4	T50.8x5	T50.8x6
vaccine	T50.B91	T50.B92	T50.B93	T50.B94	T50.B95	T50.B96
Mumpsvax	T50.B91	T50.B92	T50.B93	T50.B94	T50.B95	T50.B96
Mupirocin	T49.0x1	T49.0x2	T49.0x3	T49.0x4	T49.0x5	T49.0x6
Muriatic acid — see Hydrochloric acid						
Muromonab-CD3	T45.1x1	T45.1x2	T45.1x3	T45.1x4	T45.1x5	T45.1x6
Muscle affecting agents NEC	T48.201	T48.202	T48.203	T48.204	T48.205	T48.206
oxytocic	T48.0x1	T48.0x2	T48.0x3	T48.0x4	T48.0x5	T48.0x6
relaxants	T48.201	T48.202	T48.203	T48.204	T48.205	T48.206
central nervous system	T42.8x1	T42.8x2	T42.8x3	T42.8x4	T42.8x5	T42.8x6
skeletal	T48.1x1	T48.1x2	T48.1x3	T48.1x4	T48.1x5	T48.1x6
smooth	T44.3x1	T44.3x2	T44.3x3	T44.3x4	T44.3x5	T44.3x6
Muscle relaxant — see Relaxant, muscle						
Muscle-action drug NEC	T48.201	T48.202	T48.203	T48.204	T48.205	T48.206
Muscle-tone depressant, central						
NEC	T42.8x1	T42.8x2	T42.8x3	T42.8x4	T42.8x5	T42.8x6
specified NEC	T42.8x1	T42.8x2	T42.8x3	T42.8x4	T42.8x5	T42.8x6
Mushroom, noxious	T62.0x1	T62.0x2	T62.0x3	T62.0x4	—	—
Mussel, noxious	T61.781	T61.782	T61.783	T61.784	—	—
Mustard (emetic)	T47.7x1	T47.7x2	T47.7x3	T47.7x4	T47.7x5	T47.7x6
black	T47.7x1	T47.7x2	T47.7x3	T47.7x4	T47.7x5	T47.7x6
gas, not in war	T59.91	T59.92	T59.93	T59.94	—	—
nitrogen	T45.1x1	T45.1x2	T45.1x3	T45.1x4	T45.1x5	T45.1x6
Mustine	T45.1x1	T45.1x2	T45.1x3	T45.1x4	T45.1x5	T45.1x6
M-vac	T45.1x1	T45.1x2	T45.1x3	T45.1x4	T45.1x5	T45.1x6
Mycifradin	T36.5x1	T36.5x2	T36.5x3	T36.5x4	T36.5x5	T36.5x6
topical	T49.0x1	T49.0x2	T49.0x3	T49.0x4	T49.0x5	T49.0x6
Mycitracin	T36.8x1	T36.8x2	T36.8x3	T36.8x4	T36.8x5	T36.8x6
ophthalmic preparation	T49.5x1	T49.5x2	T49.5x3	T49.5x4	T49.5x5	T49.5x6

Table of Drugs & Chemicals	POISONING Accidental (Unintentional)	Self-Harm (Intentional)	Assault	Undetermined	Adverse Effect	Underdosing
Mycostatin	T36.7x1	T36.7x2	T36.7x3	T36.7x4	T36.7x5	T36.7x6
topical	T49.0x1	T49.0x2	T49.0x3	T49.0x4	T49.0x5	T49.0x6
Mycotoxins	T64.81	T64.82	T64.83	T64.84	—	—
aflatoxin	T64.01	T64.02	T64.03	T64.04	—	—
specified NEC	T64.81	T64.82	T64.83	T64.84	—	—
Mydriacyl	T44.3x1	T44.3x2	T44.3x3	T44.3x4	T44.3x5	T44.3x6
Mydriatic drug	T49.5x1	T49.5x2	T49.5x3	T49.5x4	T49.5x5	T49.5x6
Myelobromal	T45.1x1	T45.1x2	T45.1x3	T45.1x4	T45.1x5	T45.1x6
Myleran	T45.1x1	T45.1x2	T45.1x3	T45.1x4	T45.1x5	T45.1x6
Myochrysin(e)	T39.2x1	T39.2x2	T39.2x3	T39.2x4	T39.2x5	T39.2x6
Myoneural blocking agents	T48.1x1	T48.1x2	T48.1x3	T48.1x4	T48.1x5	T48.1x6
Myralact	T49.0x1	T49.0x2	T49.0x3	T49.0x4	T49.0x5	T49.0x6
Myristica fragrans	T62.2x1	T62.2x2	T62.2x3	T62.2x4	—	—
Myristicin	T65.891	T65.892	T65.893	T65.894	—	—
Mysoline	T42.3x1	T42.3x2	T42.3x3	T42.3x4	T42.3x5	T42.3x6
Nabilone	T40.7x1	T40.7x2	T40.7x3	T40.7x4	T40.7x5	T40.7x6
Nabumetone	T39.391	T39.392	T39.393	T39.394	T39.395	T39.396
Nadolol	T44.7x1	T44.7x2	T44.7x3	T44.7x4	T44.7x5	T44.7x6
Nafcillin	T36.0x1	T36.0x2	T36.0x3	T36.0x4	T36.0x5	T36.0x6
Nafoxidine	T38.6x1	T38.6x2	T38.6x3	T38.6x4	T38.6x5	T38.6x6
Naftidrofuryl (oxalate)	T46.7x1	T46.7x2	T46.7x3	T46.7x4	T46.7x5	T46.7x6
Naftifine	T49.0x1	T49.0x2	T49.0x3	T49.0x4	T49.0x5	T49.0x6
Nail polish remover	T52.91	T52.92	T52.93	T52.94	—	—
Nalbuphine	T40.4x1	T40.4x2	T40.4x3	T40.4x4	T40.4x5	T40.4x6
Naled	T60.0x1	T60.0x2	T60.0x3	T60.0x4	—	—
Nalidixic acid	T37.8x1	T37.8x2	T37.8x3	T37.8x4	T37.8x5	T37.8x6
Nalorphine	T50.7x1	T50.7x2	T50.7x3	T50.7x4	T50.7x5	T50.7x6
Naloxone	T50.7x1	T50.7x2	T50.7x3	T50.7x4	T50.7x5	T50.7x6
Naltrexone	T50.7x1	T50.7x2	T50.7x3	T50.7x4	T50.7x5	T50.7x6
Namenda	T43.8x1	T43.8x2	T43.8x3	T43.8x4	T43.8x5	T43.8x6
Nandrolone	T38.7x1	T38.7x2	T38.7x3	T38.7x4	T38.7x5	T38.7x6
Naphazoline	T48.5x1	T48.5x2	T48.5x3	T48.5x4	T48.5x5	T48.5x6
Naphtha (painters') (petroleum)	T52.0x1	T52.0x2	T52.0x3	T52.0x4	—	—
solvent	T52.0x1	T52.0x2	T52.0x3	T52.0x4	—	—
vapor	T52.0x1	T52.0x2	T52.0x3	T52.0x4	—	—
Naphthalene (non-chlorinated)	T60.2x1	T60.2x2	T60.2x3	T60.2x4	—	—
chlorinated	T60.1x1	T60.1x2	T60.1x3	T60.1x4	—	—
vapor	T60.1x1	T60.1x2	T60.1x3	T60.1x4	—	—
insecticide or moth repellent	T60.2x1	T60.2x2	T60.2x3	T60.2x4	—	—
chlorinated	T60.1x1	T60.1x2	T60.1x3	T60.1x4	—	—
vapor	T60.2x1	T60.2x2	T60.2x3	T60.2x4	—	—
chlorinated	T60.1x1	T60.1x2	T60.1x3	T60.1x4	—	—
Naphthol	T65.891	T65.892	T65.893	T65.894	—	—
Naphthylamine	T65.891	T65.892	T65.893	T65.894	—	—
Naphthylthiourea (ANTU)	T60.4x1	T60.4x2	T60.4x3	T60.4x4	—	—
Naprosyn — see Naproxen						
Naproxen	T39.311	T39.312	T39.313	T39.314	T39.315	T39.316
Narcotic (drug)	T40.601	T40.602	T40.603	T40.604	T40.605	T40.606
analgesic NEC	T40.601	T40.602	T40.603	T40.604	T40.605	T40.606
antagonist	T50.7x1	T50.7x2	T50.7x3	T50.7x4	T50.7x5	T50.7x6
specified NEC	T40.691	T40.692	T40.693	T40.694	T40.695	T40.696
synthetic	T40.4x1	T40.4x2	T40.4x3	T40.4x4	T40.4x5	T40.4x6
Narcotine	T48.3x1	T48.3x2	T48.3x3	T48.3x4	T48.3x5	T48.3x6
Nardil	T43.1x1	T43.1x2	T43.1x3	T43.1x4	T43.1x5	T43.1x6
Nasal drug NEC	T49.6x1	T49.6x2	T49.6x3	T49.6x4	T49.6x5	T49.6x6
Natamycin	T49.0x1	T49.0x2	T49.0x3	T49.0x4	T49.0x5	T49.0x6
Natrium cyanide — see Cyanide(s)						
Natural						
blood (product)	T45.8x1	T45.8x2	T45.8x3	T45.8x4	T45.8x5	T45.8x6
gas (piped)	T59.891	T59.892	T59.893	T59.894	—	—
incomplete combustion	T58.11	T58.12	T58.13	T58.14	—	—
Nealbarbital	T42.3x1	T42.3x2	T42.3x3	T42.3x4	T42.3x5	T42.3x6
Nectadon	T48.3x1	T48.3x2	T48.3x3	T48.3x4	T48.3x5	T48.3x6
Nedocromil	T48.6x1	T48.6x2	T48.6x3	T48.6x4	T48.6x5	T48.6x6
Nefopam	T39.8x1	T39.8x2	T39.8x3	T39.8x4	T39.8x5	T39.8x6
Nematocyst (sting)	T63.691	T63.692	T63.693	T63.694	—	—
Nembutal	T42.3x1	T42.3x2	T42.3x3	T42.3x4	T42.3x5	T42.3x6
Nemonapride	T43.591	T43.592	T43.593	T43.594	T43.595	T43.596
Neoarsphenamine	T37.8x1	T37.8x2	T37.8x3	T37.8x4	T37.8x5	T37.8x6
Neocinchophen	T50.4x1	T50.4x2	T50.4x3	T50.4x4	T50.4x5	T50.4x6
Neomycin (derivatives)	T36.5x1	T36.5x2	T36.5x3	T36.5x4	T36.5x5	T36.5x6
with						
bacitracin	T49.0x1	T49.0x2	T49.0x3	T49.0x4	T49.0x5	T49.0x6
neostigmine	T44.0x1	T44.0x2	T44.0x3	T44.0x4	T44.0x5	T44.0x6
ENT agent	T49.6x1	T49.6x2	T49.6x3	T49.6x4	T49.6x5	T49.6x6
ophthalmic preparation	T49.5x1	T49.5x2	T49.5x3	T49.5x4	T49.5x5	T49.5x6
topical NEC	T49.0x1	T49.0x2	T49.0x3	T49.0x4	T49.0x5	T49.0x6
Neonal	T42.3x1	T42.3x2	T42.3x3	T42.3x4	T42.3x5	T42.3x6
Neoprontosil	T37.0x1	T37.0x2	T37.0x3	T37.0x4	T37.0x5	T37.0x6
Neosalvarsan	T37.8x1	T37.8x2	T37.8x3	T37.8x4	T37.8x5	T37.8x6
Neosilversalvarsan	T37.8x1	T37.8x2	T37.8x3	T37.8x4	T37.8x5	T37.8x6
Neosporin	T36.8x1	T36.8x2	T36.8x3	T36.8x4	T36.8x5	T36.8x6
ENT agent	T49.6x1	T49.6x2	T49.6x3	T49.6x4	T49.6x5	T49.6x6
ophthalmic preparation	T49.5x1	T49.5x2	T49.5x3	T49.5x4	T49.5x5	T49.5x6
topical NEC	T49.0x1	T49.0x2	T49.0x3	T49.0x4	T49.0x5	T49.0x6
Neostigmine bromide	T44.0x1	T44.0x2	T44.0x3	T44.0x4	T44.0x5	T44.0x6
Neraval	T42.3x1	T42.3x2	T42.3x3	T42.3x4	T42.3x5	T42.3x6
Neravan	T42.3x1	T42.3x2	T42.3x3	T42.3x4	T42.3x5	T42.3x6
Nerium oleander	T62.2x1	T62.2x2	T62.2x3	T62.2x4	—	—
Nerve gas, not in war	T59.91	T59.92	T59.93	T59.94	—	—
Nesacaine	T41.3x1	T41.3x2	T41.3x3	T41.3x4	T41.3x5	T41.3x6
infiltration (subcutaneous)	T41.3x1	T41.3x2	T41.3x3	T41.3x4	T41.3x5	T41.3x6
nerve block (peripheral) (plexus)	T41.3x1	T41.3x2	T41.3x3	T41.3x4	T41.3x5	T41.3x6
Netilmicin	T36.5x1	T36.5x2	T36.5x3	T36.5x4	T36.5x5	T36.5x6
Neurobarb	T42.3x1	T42.3x2	T42.3x3	T42.3x4	T42.3x5	T42.3x6
Neuroleptic drug NEC	T43.501	T43.502	T43.503	T43.504	T43.505	T43.506
Neuromuscular blocking drug	T48.1x1	T48.1x2	T48.1x3	T48.1x4	T48.1x5	T48.1x6
Neutral insulin injection	T38.3x1	T38.3x2	T38.3x3	T38.3x4	T38.3x5	T38.3x6
Neutral spirits	T51.0x1	T51.0x2	T51.0x3	T51.0x4	—	—
beverage	T51.0x1	T51.0x2	T51.0x3	T51.0x4	—	—
Niacin	T46.7x1	T46.7x2	T46.7x3	T46.7x4	T46.7x5	T46.7x6
Niacinamide	T45.2x1	T45.2x2	T45.2x3	T45.2x4	T45.2x5	T45.2x6
Nialamide	T43.1x1	T43.1x2	T43.1x3	T43.1x4	T43.1x5	T43.1x6
Niaprazine	T42.6x1	T42.6x2	T42.6x3	T42.6x4	T42.6x5	T42.6x6
Nicametate	T46.7x1	T46.7x2	T46.7x3	T46.7x4	T46.7x5	T46.7x6
Nicardipine	T46.1x1	T46.1x2	T46.1x3	T46.1x4	T46.1x5	T46.1x6
Nicergoline	T46.7x1	T46.7x2	T46.7x3	T46.7x4	T46.7x5	T46.7x6
Nickel (carbonyl) (tetra-carbonyl) (fumes) (vapor)	T56.891	T56.892	T56.893	T56.894	—	—
Nickelocene	T56.891	T56.892	T56.893	T56.894	—	—
Niclosamide	T37.4x1	T37.4x2	T37.4x3	T37.4x4	T37.4x5	T37.4x6
Nicofuranose	T46.7x1	T46.7x2	T46.7x3	T46.7x4	T46.7x5	T46.7x6
Nicomorphine	T40.2x1	T40.2x2	T40.2x3	T40.2x4	—	—
Nicorandil	T46.3x1	T46.3x2	T46.3x3	T46.3x4	T46.3x5	T46.3x6
Nicotiana (plant)	T62.2x1	T62.2x2	T62.2x3	T62.2x4	—	—
Nicotinamide	T45.2x1	T45.2x2	T45.2x3	T45.2x4	T45.2x5	T45.2x6
Nicotine (insecticide) (spray) (sulfate) NEC	T60.2x1	T60.2x2	T60.2x3	T60.2x4	—	—
from tobacco	T65.291	T65.292	T65.293	T65.294	—	—
cigarettes	T65.221	T65.222	T65.223	T65.224	—	—
not insecticide	T65.291	T65.292	T65.293	T65.294	—	—
Nicotinic acid	T46.7x1	T46.7x2	T46.7x3	T46.7x4	T46.7x5	T46.7x6
Nicotinyl alcohol	T46.7x1	T46.7x2	T46.7x3	T46.7x4	T46.7x5	T46.7x6
Nicoumalone	T45.511	T45.512	T45.513	T45.514	T45.515	T45.516
Nifedipine	T46.1x1	T46.1x2	T46.1x3	T46.1x4	T46.1x5	T46.1x6
Nifenazone	T39.2x1	T39.2x2	T39.2x3	T39.2x4	T39.2x5	T39.2x6
Nifuraldezone	T37.91	T37.92	T37.93	T37.94	T37.95	T37.96
Nifuratel	T37.8x1	T37.8x2	T37.8x3	T37.8x4	T37.8x5	T37.8x6
Nifurtimox	T37.3x1	T37.3x2	T37.3x3	T37.3x4	T37.3x5	T37.3x6
Nifurtoinol	T37.8x1	T37.8x2	T37.8x3	T37.8x4	T37.8x5	T37.8x6
Nightshade, deadly (solanum) — see also Belladonna	T62.2x1	T62.2x2	T62.2x3	T62.2x4	—	—
berry	T62.1x1	T62.1x2	T62.1x3	T62.1x4	—	—
Nikethamide	T50.7x1	T50.7x2	T50.7x3	T50.7x4	T50.7x5	T50.7x6
Nilstat	T36.7x1	T36.7x2	T36.7x3	T36.7x4	T36.7x5	T36.7x6
topical	T49.0x1	T49.0x2	T49.0x3	T49.0x4	T49.0x5	T49.0x6
Nilutamide	T38.6x1	T38.6x2	T38.6x3	T38.6x4	T38.6x5	T38.6x6
Nimesulide	T39.391	T39.392	T39.393	T39.394	T39.395	T39.396

DRUGS&CHEMICALS

Table of Drugs & Chemicals	Accidental (Unintentional)	Self-Harm (Intentional)	Assault	Undetermined	Adverse Effect	Underdosing
Nimetazepam	T42.4x1	T42.4x2	T42.4x3	T42.4x4	T42.4x5	T42.4x6
Nimodipine	T46.1x1	T46.1x2	T46.1x3	T46.1x4	T46.1x5	T46.1x6
Nimorazole	T37.3x1	T37.3x2	T37.3x3	T37.3x4	T37.3x5	T37.3x6
Nimustine	T45.1x1	T45.1x2	T45.1x3	T45.1x4	T45.1x5	T45.1x6
Niridazole	T37.4x1	T37.4x2	T37.4x3	T37.4x4	T37.4x5	T37.4x6
Nisentil	T40.2x1	T40.2x2	T40.2x3	T40.2x4	T40.2x5	T40.2x6
Nisoldipine	T46.1x1	T46.1x2	T46.1x3	T46.1x4	T46.1x5	T46.1x6
Nitramine	T65.3x1	T65.3x2	T65.3x3	T65.3x4	—	—
Nitrate, organic	T46.3x1	T46.3x2	T46.3x3	T46.3x4	T46.3x5	T46.3x6
Nitrazepam	T42.4x1	T42.4x2	T42.4x3	T42.4x4	T42.4x5	T42.4x6
Nitrefazole	T50.6x1	T50.6x2	T50.6x3	T50.6x4	T50.6x5	T50.6x6
Nitrendipine	T46.1x1	T46.1x2	T46.1x3	T46.1x4	T46.1x5	T46.1x6
Nitric						
acid (liquid)	T54.2x1	T54.2x2	T54.2x3	T54.2x4	—	—
vapor	T59.891	T59.892	T59.893	T59.894	—	—
oxide (gas)	T59.0x1	T59.0x2	T59.0x3	T59.0x4	—	—
Nitrimidazine	T37.3x1	T37.3x2	T37.3x3	T37.3x4	T37.3x5	T37.3x6
Nitrite, amyl (medicinal) (vapor)	T46.3x1	T46.3x2	T46.3x3	T46.3x4	T46.3x5	T46.3x6
Nitroaniline	T65.3x1	T65.3x2	T65.3x3	T65.3x4	—	—
vapor	T59.891	T59.892	T59.893	T59.894	—	—
Nitrobenzene, nitrobenzol	T65.3x1	T65.3x2	T65.3x3	T65.3x4	—	—
vapor	T65.3x1	T65.3x2	T65.3x3	T65.3x4	—	—
Nitrocellulose	T65.891	T65.892	T65.893	T65.894	—	—
lacquer	T65.891	T65.892	T65.893	T65.894	—	—
Nitrodiphenyl	T65.3x1	T65.3x2	T65.3x3	T65.3x4	—	—
Nitrofural	T49.0x1	T49.0x2	T49.0x3	T49.0x4	T49.0x5	T49.0x6
Nitrofurantoin	T37.8x1	T37.8x2	T37.8x3	T37.8x4	T37.8x5	T37.8x6
Nitrofurazone	T49.0x1	T49.0x2	T49.0x3	T49.0x4	T49.0x5	T49.0x6
Nitrogen	T59.0x1	T59.0x2	T59.0x3	T59.0x4	—	—
mustard	T45.1x1	T45.1x2	T45.1x3	T45.1x4	T45.1x5	T45.1x6
Nitroglycerin, nitro-glycerol (medicinal)	T46.3x1	T46.3x2	T46.3x3	T46.3x4	T46.3x5	T46.3x6
nonmedicinal	T65.5x1	T65.5x2	T65.5x3	T65.5x4	—	—
fumes	T65.5x1	T65.5x2	T65.5x3	T65.5x4	—	—
Nitroglycol	T52.3x1	T52.3x2	T52.3x3	T52.3x4	—	—
Nitrohydrochloric acid	T54.2x1	T54.2x2	T54.2x3	T54.2x4	—	—
Nitromersol	T49.0x1	T49.0x2	T49.0x3	T49.0x4	T49.0x5	T49.0x6
Nitronaphthalene	T65.891	T65.892	T65.893	T65.894	—	—
Nitrophenol	T54.0x1	T54.0x2	T54.0x3	T54.0x4	—	—
Nitropropane	T52.8x1	T52.8x2	T52.8x3	T52.8x4	—	—
Nitroprusside	T46.5x1	T46.5x2	T46.5x3	T46.5x4	T46.5x5	T46.5x6
Nitrosodimethylamine	T65.3x1	T65.3x2	T65.3x3	T65.3x4	—	—
Nitrothiazol	T37.4x1	T37.4x2	T37.4x3	T37.4x4	T37.4x5	T37.4x6
Nitrotoluene, nitrotoluol	T65.3x1	T65.3x2	T65.3x3	T65.3x4	—	—
vapor	T65.3x1	T65.3x2	T65.3x3	T65.3x4	—	—
Nitrous						
acid (liquid)	T54.2x1	T54.2x2	T54.2x3	T54.2x4	—	—
fumes	T59.891	T59.892	T59.893	T59.894	—	—
ether spirit	T46.3x1	T46.3x2	T46.3x3	T46.3x4	T46.3x5	T46.3x6
oxide	T41.0x1	T41.0x2	T41.0x3	T41.0x4	T41.0x5	T41.0x6
Nitroxoline	T37.8x1	T37.8x2	T37.8x3	T37.8x4	T37.8x5	T37.8x6
Nitrozone	T49.0x1	T49.0x2	T49.0x3	T49.0x4	T49.0x5	T49.0x6
Nizatidine	T47.0x1	T47.0x2	T47.0x3	T47.0x4	T47.0x5	T47.0x6
Nizofenone	T43.8x1	T43.8x2	T43.8x3	T43.8x4	T43.8x5	T43.8x6
Noctec	T42.6x1	T42.6x2	T42.6x3	T42.6x4	T42.6x5	T42.6x6
Noludar	T42.6x1	T42.6x2	T42.6x3	T42.6x4	T42.6x5	T42.6x6
Nomegestrol	T38.5x1	T38.5x2	T38.5x3	T38.5x4	T38.5x5	T38.5x6
Nomifensine	T43.291	T43.292	T43.293	T43.294	T43.295	T43.296
Nonoxinol	T49.8x1	T49.8x2	T49.8x3	T49.8x4	T49.8x5	T49.8x6
Nonylphenoxy (polyethoxy-ethanol)	T49.8x1	T49.8x2	T49.8x3	T49.8x4	T49.8x5	T49.8x6
Noptil	T42.3x1	T42.3x2	T42.3x3	T42.3x4	T42.3x5	T42.3x6
Noradrenaline	T44.4x1	T44.4x2	T44.4x3	T44.4x4	T44.4x5	T44.4x6
Noramidopyrine	T39.2x1	T39.2x2	T39.2x3	T39.2x4	T39.2x5	T39.2x6
methanesulfonate sodium	T39.2x1	T39.2x2	T39.2x3	T39.2x4	T39.2x5	T39.2x6
Norbormide	T60.4x1	T60.4x2	T60.4x3	T60.4x4	—	—
Nordazepam	T42.4x1	T42.4x2	T42.4x3	T42.4x4	T42.4x5	T42.4x6
Norepinephrine	T44.4x1	T44.4x2	T44.4x3	T44.4x4	T44.4x5	T44.4x6

Table of Drugs & Chemicals	Accidental (Unintentional)	Self-Harm (Intentional)	Assault	Undetermined	Adverse Effect	Underdosing
Norethandrolone	T38.7x1	T38.7x2	T38.7x3	T38.7x4	T38.7x5	T38.7x6
Norethindrone	T38.4x1	T38.4x2	T38.4x3	T38.4x4	T38.4x5	T38.4x6
Norethisterone (acetate) (enantate)	T38.4x1	T38.4x2	T38.4x3	T38.4x4	T38.4x5	T38.4x6
with ethinylestradiol	T38.5x1	T38.5x2	T38.5x3	T38.5x4	T38.5x5	T38.5x6
Noretynodrel	T38.5x1	T38.5x2	T38.5x3	T38.5x4	T38.5x5	T38.5x6
Norfenefrine	T44.4x1	T44.4x2	T44.4x3	T44.4x4	T44.4x5	T44.4x6
Norfloxacin	T36.8x1	T36.8x2	T36.8x3	T36.8x4	T36.8x5	T36.8x6
Norgestrel	T38.4x1	T38.4x2	T38.4x3	T38.4x4	T38.4x5	T38.4x6
Norgestrienone	T38.4x1	T38.4x2	T38.4x3	T38.4x4	T38.4x5	T38.4x6
Norlestrin	T38.4x1	T38.4x2	T38.4x3	T38.4x4	T38.4x5	T38.4x6
Norlutin	T38.4x1	T38.4x2	T38.4x3	T38.4x4	T38.4x5	T38.4x6
Normal serum albumin (human), salt-poor	T45.8x1	T45.8x2	T45.8x3	T45.8x4	T45.8x5	T45.8x6
Normethandrone	T38.5x1	T38.5x2	T38.5x3	T38.5x4	T38.5x5	T38.5x6
Normison — see Benzodiazepines						
Normorphine	T40.2x1	T40.2x2	T40.2x3	T40.2x4	—	—
Norpseudoephedrine	T50.5x1	T50.5x2	T50.5x3	T50.5x4	T50.5x5	T50.5x6
Nortestosterone (furanpropionate)	T38.7x1	T38.7x2	T38.7x3	T38.7x4	T38.7x5	T38.7x6
Nortriptyline	T43.011	T43.012	T43.013	T43.014	T43.015	T43.016
Noscapine	T48.3x1	T48.3x2	T48.3x3	T48.3x4	T48.3x5	T48.3x6
Nose preparations	T49.6x1	T49.6x2	T49.6x3	T49.6x4	T49.6x5	T49.6x6
Novobiocin	T36.5x1	T36.5x2	T36.5x3	T36.5x4	T36.5x5	T36.5x6
Novocain (infiltration) (topical)	T41.3x1	T41.3x2	T41.3x3	T41.3x4	T41.3x5	T41.3x6
nerve block (peripheral) (plexus)	T41.3x1	T41.3x2	T41.3x3	T41.3x4	T41.3x5	T41.3x6
spinal	T41.3x1	T41.3x2	T41.3x3	T41.3x4	T41.3x5	T41.3x6
Noxious foodstuff	T62.91	T62.92	T62.93	T62.94	—	—
specified NEC	T62.8x1	T62.8x2	T62.8x3	T62.8x4	—	—
Noxiptiline	T43.011	T43.012	T43.013	T43.014	T43.015	T43.016
Noxytiolin	T49.0x1	T49.0x2	T49.0x3	T49.0x4	T49.0x5	T49.0x6
NPH Iletin (insulin)	T38.3x1	T38.3x2	T38.3x3	T38.3x4	T38.3x5	T38.3x6
Numorphan	T40.2x1	T40.2x2	T40.2x3	T40.2x4	T40.2x5	T40.2x6
Nunol	T42.3x1	T42.3x2	T42.3x3	T42.3x4	T42.3x5	T42.3x6
Nupercaine (spinal anesthetic)	T41.3x1	T41.3x2	T41.3x3	T41.3x4	T41.3x5	T41.3x6
topical (surface)	T41.3x1	T41.3x2	T41.3x3	T41.3x4	T41.3x5	T41.3x6
Nutmeg oil (liniment)	T49.3x1	T49.3x2	T49.3x3	T49.3x4	T49.3x5	T49.3x6
Nutritional supplement	T50.901	T50.902	T50.903	T50.904	T50.905	T50.906
Nux vomica	T65.1x1	T65.1x2	T65.1x3	T65.1x4	—	—
Nydrazid	T37.1x1	T37.1x2	T37.1x3	T37.1x4	T37.1x5	T37.1x6
Nylidrin	T46.7x1	T46.7x2	T46.7x3	T46.7x4	T46.7x5	T46.7x6
Nystatin	T36.7x1	T36.7x2	T36.7x3	T36.7x4	T36.7x5	T36.7x6
topical	T49.0x1	T49.0x2	T49.0x3	T49.0x4	T49.0x5	T49.0x6
Nytol	T45.0x1	T45.0x2	T45.0x3	T45.0x4	T45.0x5	T45.0x6
Obidoxime chloride	T50.6x1	T50.6x2	T50.6x3	T50.6x4	T50.6x5	T50.6x6
Octafonium (chloride)	T49.3x1	T49.3x2	T49.3x3	T49.3x4	T49.3x5	T49.3x6
Octamethyl pyrophos-phoramide	T60.0x1	T60.0x2	T60.0x3	T60.0x4	—	—
Octanoin	T50.991	T50.992	T50.993	T50.994	T50.995	T50.996
Octatropine methyl-bromide	T44.3x1	T44.3x2	T44.3x3	T44.3x4	T44.3x5	T44.3x6
Octotiamine	T45.2x1	T45.2x2	T45.2x3	T45.2x4	T45.2x5	T45.2x6
Octoxinol (9)	T49.8x1	T49.8x2	T49.8x3	T49.8x4	T49.8x5	T49.8x6
Octreotide	T38.991	T38.992	T38.993	T38.994	T38.995	T38.996
Octyl nitrite	T46.3x1	T46.3x2	T46.3x3	T46.3x4	T46.3x5	T46.3x6
Oestradiol	T38.5x1	T38.5x2	T38.5x3	T38.5x4	T38.5x5	T38.5x6
Oestriol	T38.5x1	T38.5x2	T38.5x3	T38.5x4	T38.5x5	T38.5x6
Oestrogen	T38.5x1	T38.5x2	T38.5x3	T38.5x4	T38.5x5	T38.5x6
Oestrone	T38.5x1	T38.5x2	T38.5x3	T38.5x4	T38.5x5	T38.5x6
Ofloxacin	T36.8x1	T36.8x2	T36.8x3	T36.8x4	T36.8x5	T36.8x6
Oil (of)	T65.891	T65.892	T65.893	T65.894	—	—
bitter almond	T62.8x1	T62.8x2	T62.8x3	T62.8x4	—	—
cloves	T49.7x1	T49.7x2	T49.7x3	T49.7x4	T49.7x5	T49.7x6
colors	T65.6x1	T65.6x2	T65.6x3	T65.6x4	—	—
fumes	T59.891	T59.892	T59.893	T59.894	—	—
lubricating	T52.0x1	T52.0x2	T52.0x3	T52.0x4	—	—
Niobe	T52.8x1	T52.8x2	T52.8x3	T52.8x4	—	—
vitriol (liquid)	T54.2x1	T54.2x2	T54.2x3	T54.2x4	—	—
fumes	T54.2x1	T54.2x2	T54.2x3	T54.2x4	—	—
wintergreen (bitter) NEC	T49.3x1	T49.3x2	T49.3x3	T49.3x4	T49.3x5	T49.3x6
Oily preparation (for skin)	T49.3x1	T49.3x2	T49.3x3	T49.3x4	T49.3x5	T49.3x6

DRUGS&CHEMICALS

Table of Drugs & Chemicals	Poisoning Accidental (Unintentional)	Poisoning Self-Harm (Intentional)	Poisoning Assault	Poisoning Undetermined	Adverse Effect	Underdosing
Ointment NEC	T49.3x1	T49.3x2	T49.3x3	T49.3x4	T49.3x5	T49.3x6
Olanzapine	T43.591	T43.592	T43.593	T43.594	T43.595	T43.596
Oleander	T62.2x1	T62.2x2	T62.2x3	T62.2x4	—	—
Oleandomycin	T36.3x1	T36.3x2	T36.3x3	T36.3x4	T36.3x5	T36.3x6
Oleandrin	T46.0x1	T46.0x2	T46.0x3	T46.0x4	T46.0x5	T46.0x6
Oleic acid	T46.6x1	T46.6x2	T46.6x3	T46.6x4	T46.6x5	T46.6x6
Oleovitamin A	T45.2x1	T45.2x2	T45.2x3	T45.2x4	T45.2x5	T45.2x6
Oleum ricini	T47.2x1	T47.2x2	T47.2x3	T47.2x4	T47.2x5	T47.2x6
Olive oil (medicinal) NEC	T47.4x1	T47.4x2	T47.4x3	T47.4x4	T47.4x5	T47.4x6
Olivomycin	T45.1x1	T45.1x2	T45.1x3	T45.1x4	T45.1x5	T45.1x6
Olsalazine	T47.8x1	T47.8x2	T47.8x3	T47.8x4	T47.8x5	T47.8x6
Omeprazole	T47.1x1	T47.1x2	T47.1x3	T47.1x4	T47.1x5	T47.1x6
OMPA	T60.0x1	T60.0x2	T60.0x3	T60.0x4	—	—
Oncovin	T45.1x1	T45.1x2	T45.1x3	T45.1x4	T45.1x5	T45.1x6
Ondansetron	T45.0x1	T45.0x2	T45.0x3	T45.0x4	T45.0x5	T45.0x6
Ophthaine	T41.3x1	T41.3x2	T41.3x3	T41.3x4	T41.3x5	T41.3x6
Ophthetic	T41.3x1	T41.3x2	T41.3x3	T41.3x4	T41.3x5	T41.3x6
Opiate NEC	T40.601	T40.602	T40.603	T40.604	T40.605	T40.606
antagonists	T50.7x1	T50.7x2	T50.7x3	T50.7x4	T50.7x5	T50.7x6
Opioid NEC	T40.2x1	T40.2x2	T40.2x3	T40.2x4	T40.2x5	T40.2x6
Opipramol	T43.011	T43.012	T43.013	T43.014	T43.015	T43.016
Opium alkaloids (total)	T40.0x1	T40.0x2	T40.0x3	T40.0x4	T40.0x5	T40.0x6
standardized powdered	T40.0x1	T40.0x2	T40.0x3	T40.0x4	T40.0x5	T40.0x6
tincture (camphorated)	T40.0x1	T40.0x2	T40.0x3	T40.0x4	T40.0x5	T40.0x6
Oracon	T38.4x1	T38.4x2	T38.4x3	T38.4x4	T38.4x5	T38.4x6
Oragrafin	T50.8x1	T50.8x2	T50.8x3	T50.8x4	T50.8x5	T50.8x6
Oral contraceptives	T38.4x1	T38.4x2	T38.4x3	T38.4x4	T38.4x5	T38.4x6
Oral rehydration salts	T50.3x1	T50.3x2	T50.3x3	T50.3x4	T50.3x5	T50.3x6
Orazamide	T50.991	T50.992	T50.993	T50.994	T50.995	T50.996
Orciprenaline	T48.291	T48.292	T48.293	T48.294	T48.295	T48.296
Organidin	T48.4x1	T48.4x2	T48.4x3	T48.4x4	T48.4x5	T48.4x6
Organonitrate NEC	T46.3x1	T46.3x2	T46.3x3	T46.3x4	T46.3x5	T46.3x6
Organophosphates	T60.0x1	T60.0x2	T60.0x3	T60.0x4	—	—
Orimune	T50.B91	T50.B92	T50.B93	T50.B94	T50.B95	T50.B96
Orinase	T38.3x1	T38.3x2	T38.3x3	T38.3x4	T38.3x5	T38.3x6
Ormeloxifene	T38.6x1	T38.6x2	T38.6x3	T38.6x4	T38.6x5	T38.6x6
Ornidazole	T37.3x1	T37.3x2	T37.3x3	T37.3x4	T37.3x5	T37.3x6
Ornithine aspartate	T50.991	T50.992	T50.993	T50.994	T50.995	T50.996
Ornoprostil	T47.1x1	T47.1x2	T47.1x3	T47.1x4	T47.1x5	T47.1x6
Orphenadrine (hydrochloride)	T42.8x1	T42.8x2	T42.8x3	T42.8x4	T42.8x5	T42.8x6
Ortal (sodium)	T42.3x1	T42.3x2	T42.3x3	T42.3x4	T42.3x5	T42.3x6
Orthoboric acid	T49.0x1	T49.0x2	T49.0x3	T49.0x4	T49.0x5	T49.0x6
ENT agent	T49.6x1	T49.6x2	T49.6x3	T49.6x4	T49.6x5	T49.6x6
ophthalmic preparation	T49.5x1	T49.5x2	T49.5x3	T49.5x4	T49.5x5	T49.5x6
Orthocaine	T41.3x1	T41.3x2	T41.3x3	T41.3x4	T41.3x5	T41.3x6
Orthodichlorobenzene	T53.7x1	T53.7x2	T53.7x3	T53.7x4	—	—
Ortho-Novum	T38.4x1	T38.4x2	T38.4x3	T38.4x4	T38.4x5	T38.4x6
Orthotolidine (reagent)	T54.2x1	T54.2x2	T54.2x3	T54.2x4	—	—
Osmic acid (liquid)	T54.2x1	T54.2x2	T54.2x3	T54.2x4	—	—
fumes	T54.2x1	T54.2x2	T54.2x3	T54.2x4	—	—
Osmotic diuretics	T50.2x1	T50.2x2	T50.2x3	T50.2x4	T50.2x5	T50.2x6
Otilonium bromide	T44.3x1	T44.3x2	T44.3x3	T44.3x4	T44.3x5	T44.3x6
Otorhinolaryngological drug NEC	T49.6x1	T49.6x2	T49.6x3	T49.6x4	T49.6x5	T49.6x6
Ouabain(e)	T46.0x1	T46.0x2	T46.0x3	T46.0x4	T46.0x5	T46.0x6
Ovarian						
hormone	T38.5x1	T38.5x2	T38.5x3	T38.5x4	T38.5x5	T38.5x6
stimulant	T38.5x1	T38.5x2	T38.5x3	T38.5x4	T38.5x5	T38.5x6
Ovral	T38.4x1	T38.4x2	T38.4x3	T38.4x4	T38.4x5	T38.4x6
Ovulen	T38.4x1	T38.4x2	T38.4x3	T38.4x4	T38.4x5	T38.4x6
Ox bile extract	T47.5x1	T47.5x2	T47.5x3	T47.5x4	T47.5x5	T47.5x6
Oxacillin	T36.0x1	T36.0x2	T36.0x3	T36.0x4	T36.0x5	T36.0x6
Oxalic acid	T54.2x1	T54.2x2	T54.2x3	T54.2x4	—	—
ammonium salt	T50.991	T50.992	T50.993	T50.994	T50.995	T50.996
Oxamniquine	T37.4x1	T37.4x2	T37.4x3	T37.4x4	T37.4x5	T37.4x6
Oxanamide	T43.591	T43.592	T43.593	T43.594	T43.595	T43.596
Oxandrolone	T38.7x1	T38.7x2	T38.7x3	T38.7x4	T38.7x5	T38.7x6
Oxantel	T37.4x1	T37.4x2	T37.4x3	T37.4x4	T37.4x5	T37.4x6
Oxapium iodide	T44.3x1	T44.3x2	T44.3x3	T44.3x4	T44.3x5	T44.3x6
Oxaprotiline	T43.021	T43.022	T43.023	T43.024	T43.025	T43.026
Oxaprozin	T39.311	T39.312	T39.313	T39.314	T39.315	T39.316
Oxatomide	T45.0x1	T45.0x2	T45.0x3	T45.0x4	T45.0x5	T45.0x6
Oxazepam	T42.4x1	T42.4x2	T42.4x3	T42.4x4	T42.4x5	T42.4x6
Oxazimedrine	T50.5x1	T50.5x2	T50.5x3	T50.5x4	T50.5x5	T50.5x6
Oxazolam	T42.4x1	T42.4x2	T42.4x3	T42.4x4	T42.4x5	T42.4x6
Oxazolidine derivatives	T42.2x1	T42.2x2	T42.2x3	T42.2x4	T42.2x5	T42.2x6
Oxazolidinedione (derivative)	T42.2x1	T42.2x2	T42.2x3	T42.2x4	T42.2x5	T42.2x6
Oxcarbazepine	T42.1x1	T42.1x2	T42.1x3	T42.1x4	T42.1x5	T42.1x6
Oxedrine	T44.4x1	T44.4x2	T44.4x3	T44.4x4	T44.4x5	T44.4x6
Oxeladin (citrate)	T48.3x1	T48.3x2	T48.3x3	T48.3x4	T48.3x5	T48.3x6
Oxendolone	T38.5x1	T38.5x2	T38.5x3	T38.5x4	T38.5x5	T38.5x6
Oxetacaine	T41.3x1	T41.3x2	T41.3x3	T41.3x4	T41.3x5	T41.3x6
Oxethazine	T41.3x1	T41.3x2	T41.3x3	T41.3x4	T41.3x5	T41.3x6
Oxetorone	T39.8x1	T39.8x2	T39.8x3	T39.8x4	T39.8x5	T39.8x6
Oxiconazole	T49.0x1	T49.0x2	T49.0x3	T49.0x4	T49.0x5	T49.0x6
Oxidizing agent NEC	T54.91	T54.92	T54.93	T54.94	—	—
Oxipurinol	T50.4x1	T50.4x2	T50.4x3	T50.4x4	T50.4x5	T50.4x6
Oxitriptan	T43.291	T43.292	T43.293	T43.294	T43.295	T43.296
Oxitropium bromide	T48.6x1	T48.6x2	T48.6x3	T48.6x4	T48.6x5	T48.6x6
Oxodipine	T46.1x1	T46.1x2	T46.1x3	T46.1x4	T46.1x5	T46.1x6
Oxolamine	T48.3x1	T48.3x2	T48.3x3	T48.3x4	T48.3x5	T48.3x6
Oxolinic acid	T37.8x1	T37.8x2	T37.8x3	T37.8x4	T37.8x5	T37.8x6
Oxomemazine	T43.3x1	T43.3x2	T43.3x3	T43.3x4	T43.3x5	T43.3x6
Oxophenarsine	T37.3x1	T37.3x2	T37.3x3	T37.3x4	T37.3x5	T37.3x6
Oxprenolol	T44.7x1	T44.7x2	T44.7x3	T44.7x4	T44.7x5	T44.7x6
Oxsoralen	T49.3x1	T49.3x2	T49.3x3	T49.3x4	T49.3x5	T49.3x6
Oxtriphylline	T48.6x1	T48.6x2	T48.6x3	T48.6x4	T48.6x5	T48.6x6
Oxybate sodium	T41.291	T41.292	T41.293	T41.294	T41.295	T41.296
Oxybuprocaine	T41.3x1	T41.3x2	T41.3x3	T41.3x4	T41.3x5	T41.3x6
Oxybutynin	T44.3x1	T44.3x2	T44.3x3	T44.3x4	T44.3x5	T44.3x6
Oxychlorosene	T49.0x1	T49.0x2	T49.0x3	T49.0x4	T49.0x5	T49.0x6
Oxycodone	T40.2x1	T40.2x2	T40.2x3	T40.2x4	T40.2x5	T40.2x6
Oxyfedrine	T46.3x1	T46.3x2	T46.3x3	T46.3x4	T46.3x5	T46.3x6
Oxygen	T41.5x1	T41.5x2	T41.5x3	T41.5x4	T41.5x5	T41.5x6
Oxylone	T49.0x1	T49.0x2	T49.0x3	T49.0x4	T49.0x5	T49.0x6
ophthalmic preparation	T49.5x1	T49.5x2	T49.5x3	T49.5x4	T49.5x5	T49.5x6
Oxymesterone	T38.7x1	T38.7x2	T38.7x3	T38.7x4	T38.7x5	T38.7x6
Oxymetazoline	T48.5x1	T48.5x2	T48.5x3	T48.5x4	T48.5x5	T48.5x6
Oxymetholone	T38.7x1	T38.7x2	T38.7x3	T38.7x4	T38.7x5	T38.7x6
Oxymorphone	T40.2x1	T40.2x2	T40.2x3	T40.2x4	T40.2x5	T40.2x6
Oxypertine	T43.591	T43.592	T43.593	T43.594	T43.595	T43.596
Oxyphenbutazone	T39.2x1	T39.2x2	T39.2x3	T39.2x4	T39.2x5	T39.2x6
Oxyphencyclimine	T44.3x1	T44.3x2	T44.3x3	T44.3x4	T44.3x5	T44.3x6
Oxyphenisatine	T47.2x1	T47.2x2	T47.2x3	T47.2x4	T47.2x5	T47.2x6
Oxyphenonium bromide	T44.3x1	T44.3x2	T44.3x3	T44.3x4	T44.3x5	T44.3x6
Oxypolygelatin	T45.8x1	T45.8x2	T45.8x3	T45.8x4	T45.8x5	T45.8x6
Oxyquinoline (derivatives)	T37.8x1	T37.8x2	T37.8x3	T37.8x4	T37.8x5	T37.8x6
Oxytetracycline	T36.4x1	T36.4x2	T36.4x3	T36.4x4	T36.4x5	T36.4x6
Oxytocic drug NEC	T48.0x1	T48.0x2	T48.0x3	T48.0x4	T48.0x5	T48.0x6
Oxytocin (synthetic)	T48.0x1	T48.0x2	T48.0x3	T48.0x4	T48.0x5	T48.0x6
Ozone	T59.891	T59.892	T59.893	T59.894	—	—
PABA	T49.3x1	T49.3x2	T49.3x3	T49.3x4	T49.3x5	T49.3x6
Packed red cells	T45.8x1	T45.8x2	T45.8x3	T45.8x4	T45.8x5	T45.8x6
Padimate	T49.3x1	T49.3x2	T49.3x3	T49.3x4	T49.3x5	T49.3x6
Paint NEC	T65.6x1	T65.6x2	T65.6x3	T65.6x4	—	—
cleaner	T52.91	T52.92	T52.93	T52.94	—	—
fumes NEC	T59.891	T59.892	T59.893	T59.894	—	—
lead (fumes)	T56.0x1	T56.0x2	T56.0x3	T56.0x4	—	—
solvent NEC	T52.8x1	T52.8x2	T52.8x3	T52.8x4	—	—
stripper	T52.8x1	T52.8x2	T52.8x3	T52.8x4	—	—
Palfium	T40.2x1	T40.2x2	T40.2x3	T40.2x4	—	—
Palm kernel oil	T50.991	T50.992	T50.993	T50.994	T50.995	T50.996
Paludrine	T37.2x1	T37.2x2	T37.2x3	T37.2x4	T37.2x5	T37.2x6
PAM (pralidoxime)	T50.6x1	T50.6x2	T50.6x3	T50.6x4	T50.6x5	T50.6x6
Pamaquine (naphthoute)	T37.2x1	T37.2x2	T37.2x3	T37.2x4	T37.2x5	T37.2x6
Panadol	T39.1x1	T39.1x2	T39.1x3	T39.1x4	T39.1x5	T39.1x6
Pancreatic						
digestive secretion stimulant	T47.8x1	T47.8x2	T47.8x3	T47.8x4	T47.8x5	T47.8x6
dornase	T45.3x1	T45.3x2	T45.3x3	T45.3x4	T45.3x5	T45.3x6

DRUGS & CHEMICALS

Table of Drugs & Chemicals	POISONING Accidental (Unintentional)	Self-Harm (Intentional)	Assault	Undetermined	Adverse Effect	Underdosing
Pancreatin	T47.5x1	T47.5x2	T47.5x3	T47.5x4	T47.5x5	T47.5x6
Pancrelipase	T47.5x1	T47.5x2	T47.5x3	T47.5x4	T47.5x5	T47.5x6
Pancuronium (bromide)	T48.1x1	T48.1x2	T48.1x3	T48.1x4	T48.1x5	T48.1x6
Pangamic acid	T45.2x1	T45.2x2	T45.2x3	T45.2x4	T45.2x5	T45.2x6
Panthenol	T45.2x1	T45.2x2	T45.2x3	T45.2x4	T45.2x5	T45.2x6
topical	T49.8x1	T49.8x2	T49.8x3	T49.8x4	T49.8x5	T49.8x6
Pantopon	T40.0x1	T40.0x2	T40.0x3	T40.0x4	T40.0x5	T40.0x6
Pantothenic acid	T45.2x1	T45.2x2	T45.2x3	T45.2x4	T45.2x5	T45.2x6
Panwarfin	T45.511	T45.512	T45.513	T45.514	T45.515	T45.516
Papain	T47.5x1	T47.5x2	T47.5x3	T47.5x4	T47.5x5	T47.5x6
digestant	T47.5x1	T47.5x2	T47.5x3	T47.5x4	T47.5x5	T47.5x6
Papaveretum	T40.0x1	T40.0x2	T40.0x3	T40.0x4	T40.0x5	T40.0x6
Papaverine	T44.3x1	T44.3x2	T44.3x3	T44.3x4	T44.3x5	T44.3x6
Para-acetamidophenol	T39.1x1	T39.1x2	T39.1x3	T39.1x4	T39.1x5	T39.1x6
Para-aminobenzoic acid	T49.3x1	T49.3x2	T49.3x3	T49.3x4	T49.3x5	T49.3x6
Para-aminophenol derivatives	T39.1x1	T39.1x2	T39.1x3	T39.1x4	T39.1x5	T39.1x6
Para-aminosalicylic acid	T37.1x1	T37.1x2	T37.1x3	T37.1x4	T37.1x5	T37.1x6
Paracetaldehyde	T42.6x1	T42.6x2	T42.6x3	T42.6x4	T42.6x5	T42.6x6
Paracetamol	T39.1x1	T39.1x2	T39.1x3	T39.1x4	T39.1x5	T39.1x6
Parachlorophenol (camphorated)	T49.0x1	T49.0x2	T49.0x3	T49.0x4	T49.0x5	T49.0x6
Paracodin	T40.2x1	T40.2x2	T40.2x3	T40.2x4	T40.2x5	T40.2x6
Paradione	T42.2x1	T42.2x2	T42.2x3	T42.2x4	T42.2x5	T42.2x6
Paraffin(s) (wax)	T52.0x1	T52.0x2	T52.0x3	T52.0x4	—	—
liquid (medicinal)	T47.4x1	T47.4x2	T47.4x3	T47.4x4	T47.4x5	T47.4x6
nonmedicinal	T52.0x1	T52.0x2	T52.0x3	T52.0x4	—	—
Paraformaldehyde	T60.3x1	T60.3x2	T60.3x3	T60.3x4	—	—
Paraldehyde	T42.6x1	T42.6x2	T42.6x3	T42.6x4	T42.6x5	T42.6x6
Paramethadione	T42.2x1	T42.2x2	T42.2x3	T42.2x4	T42.2x5	T42.2x6
Paramethasone	T38.0x1	T38.0x2	T38.0x3	T38.0x4	T38.0x5	T38.0x6
acetate	T49.0x1	T49.0x2	T49.0x3	T49.0x4	T49.0x5	T49.0x6
Paraoxon	T60.0x1	T60.0x2	T60.0x3	T60.0x4	—	—
Paraquat	T60.3x1	T60.3x2	T60.3x3	T60.3x4	—	—
Parasympatholytic NEC	T44.3x1	T44.3x2	T44.3x3	T44.3x4	T44.3x5	T44.3x6
Parasympathomimetic drug NEC	T44.1x1	T44.1x2	T44.1x3	T44.1x4	T44.1x5	T44.1x6
Parathion	T60.0x1	T60.0x2	T60.0x3	T60.0x4	—	—
Parathormone	T50.991	T50.992	T50.993	T50.994	T50.995	T50.996
Parathyroid extract	T50.991	T50.992	T50.993	T50.994	T50.995	T50.996
Paratyphoid vaccine	T50.A91	T50.A92	T50.A93	T50.A94	T50.A95	T50.A96
Paredrine	T44.4x1	T44.4x2	T44.4x3	T44.4x4	T44.4x5	T44.4x6
Paregoric	T40.0x1	T40.0x2	T40.0x3	T40.0x4	T40.0x5	T40.0x6
Pargyline	T46.5x1	T46.5x2	T46.5x3	T46.5x4	T46.5x5	T46.5x6
Paris green	T57.0x1	T57.0x2	T57.0x3	T57.0x4	—	—
insecticide	T57.0x1	T57.0x2	T57.0x3	T57.0x4	—	—
Parnate	T43.1x1	T43.1x2	T43.1x3	T43.1x4	T43.1x5	T43.1x6
Paromomycin	T36.5x1	T36.5x2	T36.5x3	T36.5x4	T36.5x5	T36.5x6
Paroxypropione	T45.1x1	T45.1x2	T45.1x3	T45.1x4	T45.1x5	T45.1x6
Parzone	T40.2x1	T40.2x2	T40.2x3	T40.2x4	T40.2x5	T40.2x6
PAS	T37.1x1	T37.1x2	T37.1x3	T37.1x4	T37.1x5	T37.1x6
Pasiniazid	T37.1x1	T37.1x2	T37.1x3	T37.1x4	T37.1x5	T37.1x6
PBB (polybrominated biphenyls)	T65.891	T65.892	T65.893	T65.894	—	—
PCB	T65.891	T65.892	T65.893	T65.894	—	—
PCP						
meaning pentachlorophenol	T60.1x1	T60.1x2	T60.1x3	T60.1x4	—	—
fungicide	T60.3x1	T60.3x2	T60.3x3	T60.3x4	—	—
herbicide	T60.3x1	T60.3x2	T60.3x3	T60.3x4	—	—
insecticide	T60.1x1	T60.1x2	T60.1x3	T60.1x4	—	—
meaning phencyclidine	T40.991	T40.992	T40.993	T40.994	—	—
Peach kernel oil (emulsion)	T47.4x1	T47.4x2	T47.4x3	T47.4x4	T47.4x5	T47.4x6
Peanut oil (emulsion) NEC	T47.4x1	T47.4x2	T47.4x3	T47.4x4	T47.4x5	T47.4x6
topical	T49.3x1	T49.3x2	T49.3x3	T49.3x4	T49.3x5	T49.3x6
Pearly Gates (morning glory seeds)	T40.991	T40.992	T40.993	T40.994	—	—
Pecazine	T43.3x1	T43.3x2	T43.3x3	T43.3x4	T43.3x5	T43.3x6
Pectin	T47.6x1	T47.6x2	T47.6x3	T47.6x4	T47.6x5	T47.6x6
Pefloxacin	T37.8x1	T37.8x2	T37.8x3	T37.8x4	T37.8x5	T37.8x6
Pegademase, bovine	T50.Z91	T50.Z92	T50.Z93	T50.Z94	T50.Z95	T50.Z96
Pelletierine tannate	T37.4x1	T37.4x2	T37.4x3	T37.4x4	T37.4x5	T37.4x6
Pemirolast (potassium)	T48.6x1	T48.6x2	T48.6x3	T48.6x4	T48.6x5	T48.6x6
Pemoline	T50.7x1	T50.7x2	T50.7x3	T50.7x4	T50.7x5	T50.7x6
Pempidine	T44.2x1	T44.2x2	T44.2x3	T44.2x4	T44.2x5	T44.2x6
Penamecillin	T36.0x1	T36.0x2	T36.0x3	T36.0x4	T36.0x5	T36.0x6
Penbutolol	T44.7x1	T44.7x2	T44.7x3	T44.7x4	T44.7x5	T44.7x6
Penethamate	T36.0x1	T36.0x2	T36.0x3	T36.0x4	T36.0x5	T36.0x6
Penfluridol	T43.591	T43.592	T43.593	T43.594	T43.595	T43.596
Penflutizide	T50.2x1	T50.2x2	T50.2x3	T50.2x4	T50.2x5	T50.2x6
Pengitoxin	T46.0x1	T46.0x2	T46.0x3	T46.0x4	T46.0x5	T46.0x6
Penicillamine	T50.6x1	T50.6x2	T50.6x3	T50.6x4	T50.6x5	T50.6x6
Penicillin (any)	T36.0x1	T36.0x2	T36.0x3	T36.0x4	T36.0x5	T36.0x6
Penicillinase	T45.3x1	T45.3x2	T45.3x3	T45.3x4	T45.3x5	T45.3x6
Penicilloyl polylysine	T50.8x1	T50.8x2	T50.8x3	T50.8x4	T50.8x5	T50.8x6
Penimepicycline	T36.4x1	T36.4x2	T36.4x3	T36.4x4	T36.4x5	T36.4x6
Pentachloroethane	T53.6x1	T53.6x2	T53.6x3	T53.6x4	—	—
Pentachloronaphthalene	T53.7x1	T53.7x2	T53.7x3	T53.7x4	—	—
Pentachlorophenol (pesticide)	T60.1x1	T60.1x2	T60.1x3	T60.1x4	—	—
fungicide	T60.3x1	T60.3x2	T60.3x3	T60.3x4	—	—
herbicide	T60.3x1	T60.3x2	T60.3x3	T60.3x4	—	—
insecticide	T60.1x1	T60.1x2	T60.1x3	T60.1x4	—	—
Pentaerythritol	T46.3x1	T46.3x2	T46.3x3	T46.3x4	T46.3x5	T46.3x6
chloral	T42.6x1	T42.6x2	T42.6x3	T42.6x4	T42.6x5	T42.6x6
tetranitrate NEC	T46.3x1	T46.3x2	T46.3x3	T46.3x4	T46.3x5	T46.3x6
Pentaerythrityl tetranitrate	T46.3x1	T46.3x2	T46.3x3	T46.3x4	T46.3x5	T46.3x6
Pentagastrin	T50.8x1	T50.8x2	T50.8x3	T50.8x4	T50.8x5	T50.8x6
Pentalin	T53.6x1	T53.6x2	T53.6x3	T53.6x4	—	—
Pentamethonium bromide	T44.2x1	T44.2x2	T44.2x3	T44.2x4	T44.2x5	T44.2x6
Pentamidine	T37.3x1	T37.3x2	T37.3x3	T37.3x4	T37.3x5	T37.3x6
Pentanol	T51.3x1	T51.3x2	T51.3x3	T51.3x4	—	—
Pentapyrrolinium (bitartrate)	T44.2x1	T44.2x2	T44.2x3	T44.2x4	T44.2x5	T44.2x6
Pentaquine	T37.2x1	T37.2x2	T37.2x3	T37.2x4	T37.2x5	T37.2x6
Pentazocine	T40.4x1	T40.4x2	T40.4x3	T40.4x4	T40.4x5	T40.4x6
Pentetrazole	T50.7x1	T50.7x2	T50.7x3	T50.7x4	T50.7x5	T50.7x6
Penthienate bromide	T44.3x1	T44.3x2	T44.3x3	T44.3x4	T44.3x5	T44.3x6
Pentifylline	T46.7x1	T46.7x2	T46.7x3	T46.7x4	T46.7x5	T46.7x6
Pentobarbital	T42.3x1	T42.3x2	T42.3x3	T42.3x4	T42.3x5	T42.3x6
sodium	T42.3x1	T42.3x2	T42.3x3	T42.3x4	T42.3x5	T42.3x6
Pentobarbitone	T42.3x1	T42.3x2	T42.3x3	T42.3x4	T42.3x5	T42.3x6
Pentolonium tartrate	T44.2x1	T44.2x2	T44.2x3	T44.2x4	T44.2x5	T44.2x6
Pentosan polysulfate (sodium)	T39.8x1	T39.8x2	T39.8x3	T39.8x4	T39.8x5	T39.8x6
Pentostatin	T45.1x1	T45.1x2	T45.1x3	T45.1x4	T45.1x5	T45.1x6
Pentothal	T41.1x1	T41.1x2	T41.1x3	T41.1x4	T41.1x5	T41.1x6
Pentoxifylline	T46.7x1	T46.7x2	T46.7x3	T46.7x4	T46.7x5	T46.7x6
Pentoxyverine	T48.3x1	T48.3x2	T48.3x3	T48.3x4	T48.3x5	T48.3x6
Pentrinat	T46.3x1	T46.3x2	T46.3x3	T46.3x4	T46.3x5	T46.3x6
Pentylenetetrazole	T50.7x1	T50.7x2	T50.7x3	T50.7x4	T50.7x5	T50.7x6
Pentylsalicylamide	T37.1x1	T37.1x2	T37.1x3	T37.1x4	T37.1x5	T37.1x6
Pentymal	T42.3x1	T42.3x2	T42.3x3	T42.3x4	T42.3x5	T42.3x6
Peplomycin	T45.1x1	T45.1x2	T45.1x3	T45.1x4	T45.1x5	T45.1x6
Peppermint (oil)	T47.5x1	T47.5x2	T47.5x3	T47.5x4	T47.5x5	T47.5x6
Pepsin	T47.5x1	T47.5x2	T47.5x3	T47.5x4	T47.5x5	T47.5x6
digestant	T47.5x1	T47.5x2	T47.5x3	T47.5x4	T47.5x5	T47.5x6
Pepstatin	T47.1x1	T47.1x2	T47.1x3	T47.1x4	T47.1x5	T47.1x6
Peptavlon	T50.8x1	T50.8x2	T50.8x3	T50.8x4	T50.8x5	T50.8x6
Perazine	T43.3x1	T43.3x2	T43.3x3	T43.3x4	T43.3x5	T43.3x6
Percaine (spinal)	T41.3x1	T41.3x2	T41.3x3	T41.3x4	T41.3x5	T41.3x6
topical (surface)	T41.3x1	T41.3x2	T41.3x3	T41.3x4	T41.3x5	T41.3x6
Perchloroethylene	T53.3x1	T53.3x2	T53.3x3	T53.3x4	—	—
vapor	T53.3x1	T53.3x2	T53.3x3	T53.3x4	—	—
medicinal	T37.4x1	T37.4x2	T37.4x3	T37.4x4	T37.4x5	T37.4x6
Percodan	T40.2x1	T40.2x2	T40.2x3	T40.2x4	T40.2x5	T40.2x6
Percogesic — see also Acetaminophen	T45.0x1	T45.0x2	T45.0x3	T45.0x4	T45.0x5	T45.0x6
Percorten	T38.0x1	T38.0x2	T38.0x3	T38.0x4	T38.0x5	T38.0x6
Pergolide	T42.8x1	T42.8x2	T42.8x3	T42.8x4	T42.8x5	T42.8x6
Pergonal	T38.811	T38.812	T38.813	T38.814	T38.815	T38.816
Perhexilene	T46.3x1	T46.3x2	T46.3x3	T46.3x4	T46.3x5	T46.3x6
Perhexiline (maleate)	T46.3x1	T46.3x2	T46.3x3	T46.3x4	T46.3x5	T46.3x6
Periactin	T45.0x1	T45.0x2	T45.0x3	T45.0x4	T45.0x5	T45.0x6
Periciazine	T43.3x1	T43.3x2	T43.3x3	T43.3x4	T43.3x5	T43.3x6
Periclor	T42.6x1	T42.6x2	T42.6x3	T42.6x4	T42.6x5	T42.6x6

DRUGS&CHEMICALS

Table of Drugs & Chemicals	POISONING Accidental (Unintentional)	Self-Harm (Intentional)	Assault	Undetermined	Adverse Effect	Underdosing
Perindopril	T46.4x1	T46.4x2	T46.4x3	T46.4x4	T46.4x5	T46.4x6
Perisoxal	T39.8x1	T39.8x2	T39.8x3	T39.8x4	T39.8x5	T39.8x6
Peritoneal dialysis solution	T50.3x1	T50.3x2	T50.3x3	T50.3x4	T50.3x5	T50.3x6
Peritrate	T46.3x1	T46.3x2	T46.3x3	T46.3x4	T46.3x5	T46.3x6
Perlapine	T42.4x1	T42.4x2	T42.4x3	T42.4x4	T42.4x5	T42.4x6
Permanganate	T65.891	T65.892	T65.893	T65.894	—	—
Permethrin	T60.1x1	T60.1x2	T60.1x3	T60.1x4	—	—
Pernocton	T42.3x1	T42.3x2	T42.3x3	T42.3x4	T42.3x5	T42.3x6
Pernoston	T42.3x1	T42.3x2	T42.3x3	T42.3x4	T42.3x5	T42.3x6
Peronine	T40.2x1	T40.2x2	T40.2x3	T40.2x4	—	—
Perphenazine	T43.3x1	T43.3x2	T43.3x3	T43.3x4	T43.3x5	T43.3x6
Pertofrane	T43.011	T43.012	T43.013	T43.014	T43.015	T43.016
Pertussis						
immune serum (human)	T50.Z11	T50.Z12	T50.Z13	T50.Z14	T50.Z15	T50.Z16
vaccine (with diphtheria toxoid)						
(with tetanus toxoid)	T50.A11	T50.A12	T50.A13	T50.A14	T50.A15	T50.A16
Peruvian balsam	T49.0x1	T49.0x2	T49.0x3	T49.0x4	T49.0x5	T49.0x6
Peruvoside	T46.0x1	T46.0x2	T46.0x3	T46.0x4	T46.0x5	T46.0x6
Pesticide (dust) (fumes) (vapor) ..						
NEC	T60.91	T60.92	T60.93	T60.94	—	—
arsenic	T57.0x1	T57.0x2	T57.0x3	T57.0x4	—	—
chlorinated	T60.1x1	T60.1x2	T60.1x3	T60.1x4	—	—
cyanide	T65.0x1	T65.0x2	T65.0x3	T65.0x4	—	—
kerosene	T52.0x1	T52.0x2	T52.0x3	T52.0x4	—	—
mixture (of compounds)	T60.91	T60.92	T60.93	T60.94	—	—
naphthalene	T60.2x1	T60.2x2	T60.2x3	T60.2x4	—	—
organochlorine (compounds)	T60.1x1	T60.1x2	T60.1x3	T60.1x4	—	—
petroleum (distillate) (products)						
NEC	T60.8x1	T60.8x2	T60.8x3	T60.8x4	—	—
specified ingredient NEC	T60.8x1	T60.8x2	T60.8x3	T60.8x4	—	—
strychnine	T65.1x1	T65.1x2	T65.1x3	T65.1x4	—	—
thallium	T60.4x1	T60.4x2	T60.4x3	T60.4x4	—	—
Pethidine	T40.4x1	T40.4x2	T40.4x3	T40.4x4	T40.4x5	T40.4x6
Petrichloral	T42.6x1	T42.6x2	T42.6x3	T42.6x4	T42.6x5	T42.6x6
Petrol	T52.0x1	T52.0x2	T52.0x3	T52.0x4	—	—
vapor	T52.0x1	T52.0x2	T52.0x3	T52.0x4	—	—
Petrolatum	T49.3x1	T49.3x2	T49.3x3	T49.3x4	T49.3x5	T49.3x6
hydrophilic	T49.3x1	T49.3x2	T49.3x3	T49.3x4	T49.3x5	T49.3x6
liquid	T47.4x1	T47.4x2	T47.4x3	T47.4x4	T47.4x5	T47.4x6
topical	T49.3x1	T49.3x2	T49.3x3	T49.3x4	T49.3x5	T49.3x6
nonmedicinal	T52.0x1	T52.0x2	T52.0x3	T52.0x4	—	—
red veterinary	T49.3x1	T49.3x2	T49.3x3	T49.3x4	T49.3x5	T49.3x6
white	T49.3x1	T49.3x2	T49.3x3	T49.3x4	T49.3x5	T49.3x6
Petroleum (products) NEC	T52.0x1	T52.0x2	T52.0x3	T52.0x4	—	—
benzine (s) — see Ligroin						
ether — see Ligroin						
jelly — see Petrolatum						
naphtha — see Ligroin						
pesticide	T60.8x1	T60.8x2	T60.8x3	T60.8x4	—	—
solids	T52.0x1	T52.0x2	T52.0x3	T52.0x4	—	—
solvents	T52.0x1	T52.0x2	T52.0x3	T52.0x4	—	—
vapor	T52.0x1	T52.0x2	T52.0x3	T52.0x4	—	—
Peyote	T40.991	T40.992	T40.993	T40.994	—	—
Phanodorm, phanodorn	T42.3x1	T42.3x2	T42.3x3	T42.3x4	T42.3x5	T42.3x6
Phanquinone	T37.3x1	T37.3x2	T37.3x3	T37.3x4	T37.3x5	T37.3x6
Phanquone	T37.3x1	T37.3x2	T37.3x3	T37.3x4	T37.3x5	T37.3x6
Pharmaceutical						
adjunct NEC	T50.901	T50.902	T50.903	T50.904	T50.905	T50.906
excipient NEC	T50.901	T50.902	T50.903	T50.904	T50.905	T50.906
sweetener	T50.901	T50.902	T50.903	T50.904	T50.905	T50.906
viscous agent	T50.901	T50.902	T50.903	T50.904	T50.905	T50.906
Phemitone	T42.3x1	T42.3x2	T42.3x3	T42.3x4	T42.3x5	T42.3x6
Phenacaine	T41.3x1	T41.3x2	T41.3x3	T41.3x4	T41.3x5	T41.3x6
Phenacemide	T42.6x1	T42.6x2	T42.6x3	T42.6x4	T42.6x5	T42.6x6
Phenacetin	T39.1x1	T39.1x2	T39.1x3	T39.1x4	T39.1x5	T39.1x6
Phenadoxone	T40.2x1	T40.2x2	T40.2x3	T40.2x4	—	—
Phenaglycodol	T43.591	T43.592	T43.593	T43.594	T43.595	T43.596

Table of Drugs & Chemicals	POISONING Accidental (Unintentional)	Self-Harm (Intentional)	Assault	Undetermined	Adverse Effect	Underdosing
Phenantoin	T42.0x1	T42.0x2	T42.0x3	T42.0x4	T42.0x5	T42.0x6
Phenaphthazine reagent	T50.991	T50.992	T50.993	T50.994	T50.995	T50.996
Phenazocine	T40.4x1	T40.4x2	T40.4x3	T40.4x4	T40.4x5	T40.4x6
Phenazone	T39.2x1	T39.2x2	T39.2x3	T39.2x4	T39.2x5	T39.2x6
Phenazopyridine	T39.8x1	T39.8x2	T39.8x3	T39.8x4	T39.8x5	T39.8x6
Phenbenicillin	T36.0x1	T36.0x2	T36.0x3	T36.0x4	T36.0x5	T36.0x6
Phenbutrazate	T50.5x1	T50.5x2	T50.5x3	T50.5x4	T50.5x5	T50.5x6
Phencyclidine	T40.991	T40.992	T40.993	T40.994	T40.995	T40.996
Phendimetrazine	T50.5x1	T50.5x2	T50.5x3	T50.5x4	T50.5x5	T50.5x6
Phenelzine	T43.1x1	T43.1x2	T43.1x3	T43.1x4	T43.1x5	T43.1x6
Phenemal	T42.3x1	T42.3x2	T42.3x3	T42.3x4	T42.3x5	T42.3x6
Phenergan	T42.6x1	T42.6x2	T42.6x3	T42.6x4	T42.6x5	T42.6x6
Pheneticillin	T36.0x1	T36.0x2	T36.0x3	T36.0x4	T36.0x5	T36.0x6
Pheneturide	T42.6x1	T42.6x2	T42.6x3	T42.6x4	T42.6x5	T42.6x6
Phenformin	T38.3x1	T38.3x2	T38.3x3	T38.3x4	T38.3x5	T38.3x6
Phenglutarimide	T44.3x1	T44.3x2	T44.3x3	T44.3x4	T44.3x5	T44.3x6
Phenicarbazide	T39.8x1	T39.8x2	T39.8x3	T39.8x4	T39.8x5	T39.8x6
Phenindamine	T45.0x1	T45.0x2	T45.0x3	T45.0x4	T45.0x5	T45.0x6
Phenindione	T45.511	T45.512	T45.513	T45.514	T45.515	T45.516
Pheniprazine	T43.1x1	T43.1x2	T43.1x3	T43.1x4	T43.1x5	T43.1x6
Pheniramine	T45.0x1	T45.0x2	T45.0x3	T45.0x4	T45.0x5	T45.0x6
Phenisatin	T47.2x1	T47.2x2	T47.2x3	T47.2x4	T47.2x5	T47.2x6
Phenmetrazine	T50.5x1	T50.5x2	T50.5x3	T50.5x4	T50.5x5	T50.5x6
Phenobal	T42.3x1	T42.3x2	T42.3x3	T42.3x4	T42.3x5	T42.3x6
Phenobarbital	T42.3x1	T42.3x2	T42.3x3	T42.3x4	T42.3x5	T42.3x6
with						
mephenytoin	T42.3x1	T42.3x2	T42.3x3	T42.3x4	T42.3x5	T42.3x6
phenytoin	T42.3x1	T42.3x2	T42.3x3	T42.3x4	T42.3x5	T42.3x6
sodium	T42.3x1	T42.3x2	T42.3x3	T42.3x4	T42.3x5	T42.3x6
Phenobarbitone	T42.3x1	T42.3x2	T42.3x3	T42.3x4	T42.3x5	T42.3x6
Phenobutiodil	T50.8x1	T50.8x2	T50.8x3	T50.8x4	T50.8x5	T50.8x6
Phenoctide	T49.0x1	T49.0x2	T49.0x3	T49.0x4	T49.0x5	T49.0x6
Phenol	T49.0x1	T49.0x2	T49.0x3	T49.0x4	T49.0x5	T49.0x6
disinfectant	T54.0x1	T54.0x2	T54.0x3	T54.0x4	—	—
in oil injection	T46.8x1	T46.8x2	T46.8x3	T46.8x4	T46.8x5	T46.8x6
medicinal	T49.1x1	T49.1x2	T49.1x3	T49.1x4	T49.1x5	T49.1x6
nonmedicinal NEC	T54.0x1	T54.0x2	T54.0x3	T54.0x4	—	—
pesticide	T60.8x1	T60.8x2	T60.8x3	T60.8x4	—	—
red	T50.8x1	T50.8x2	T50.8x3	T50.8x4	T50.8x5	T50.8x6
Phenolic preparation	T49.1x1	T49.1x2	T49.1x3	T49.1x4	T49.1x5	T49.1x6
Phenolphthalein	T47.2x1	T47.2x2	T47.2x3	T47.2x4	T47.2x5	T47.2x6
Phenolsulfonphthalein	T50.8x1	T50.8x2	T50.8x3	T50.8x4	T50.8x5	T50.8x6
Phenomorphan	T40.2x1	T40.2x2	T40.2x3	T40.2x4	—	—
Phenonyl	T42.3x1	T42.3x2	T42.3x3	T42.3x4	T42.3x5	T42.3x6
Phenoperidine	T40.4x1	T40.4x2	T40.4x3	T40.4x4	—	—
Phenopyrazone	T46.991	T46.992	T46.993	T46.994	T46.995	T46.996
Phenoquin	T50.4x1	T50.4x2	T50.4x3	T50.4x4	T50.4x5	T50.4x6
Phenothiazine (psychotropic) NEC	T43.3x1	T43.3x2	T43.3x3	T43.3x4	T43.3x5	T43.3x6
insecticide	T60.2x1	T60.2x2	T60.2x3	T60.2x4	—	—
Phenothrin	T49.0x1	T49.0x2	T49.0x3	T49.0x4	T49.0x5	T49.0x6
Phenoxybenzamine	T46.7x1	T46.7x2	T46.7x3	T46.7x4	T46.7x5	T46.7x6
Phenoxyethanol	T49.0x1	T49.0x2	T49.0x3	T49.0x4	T49.0x5	T49.0x6
Phenoxymethyl penicillin	T36.0x1	T36.0x2	T36.0x3	T36.0x4	T36.0x5	T36.0x6
Phenprobamate	T42.8x1	T42.8x2	T42.8x3	T42.8x4	T42.8x5	T42.8x6
Phenprocoumon	T45.511	T45.512	T45.513	T45.514	T45.515	T45.516
Phensuximide	T42.2x1	T42.2x2	T42.2x3	T42.2x4	T42.2x5	T42.2x6
Phentermine	T50.5x1	T50.5x2	T50.5x3	T50.5x4	T50.5x5	T50.5x6
Phenthicillin	T36.0x1	T36.0x2	T36.0x3	T36.0x4	T36.0x5	T36.0x6
Phentolamine	T46.7x1	T46.7x2	T46.7x3	T46.7x4	T46.7x5	T46.7x6
Phenyl						
butazone	T39.2x1	T39.2x2	T39.2x3	T39.2x4	T39.2x5	T39.2x6
enediamine	T65.3x1	T65.3x2	T65.3x3	T65.3x4	—	—
hydrazine	T65.3x1	T65.3x2	T65.3x3	T65.3x4	—	—
antineoplastic	T45.1x1	T45.1x2	T45.1x3	T45.1x4	T45.1x5	T45.1x6
mercuric compounds — see Mercury						
salicylate	T49.3x1	T49.3x2	T49.3x3	T49.3x4	T49.3x5	T49.3x6
Phenylalanine mustard	T45.1x1	T45.1x2	T45.1x3	T45.1x4	T45.1x5	T45.1x6

DRUGS&CHEMICALS

Table of Drugs & Chemicals	POISONING Accidental (Unintentional)	Self-Harm (Intentional)	Assault	Undetermined	Adverse Effect	Underdosing
Phenylbutazone	T39.2x1	T39.2x2	T39.2x3	T39.2x4	T39.2x5	T39.2x6
Phenylenediamine	T65.3x1	T65.3x2	T65.3x3	T65.3x4	—	—
Phenylephrine	T44.4x1	T44.4x2	T44.4x3	T44.4x4	T44.4x5	T44.4x6
Phenylethylbiguanide	T38.3x1	T38.3x2	T38.3x3	T38.3x4	T38.3x5	T38.3x6
Phenylmercuric						
acetate	T49.0x1	T49.0x2	T49.0x3	T49.0x4	T49.0x5	T49.0x6
borate	T49.0x1	T49.0x2	T49.0x3	T49.0x4	T49.0x5	T49.0x6
nitrate	T49.0x1	T49.0x2	T49.0x3	T49.0x4	T49.0x5	T49.0x6
Phenylmethylbarbitone	T42.3x1	T42.3x2	T42.3x3	T42.3x4	T42.3x5	T42.3x6
Phenylpropanol	T47.5x1	T47.5x2	T47.5x3	T47.5x4	T47.5x5	T47.5x6
Phenylpropanolamine	T44.991	T44.992	T44.993	T44.994	T44.995	T44.996
Phenylsulfthion	T60.0x1	T60.0x2	T60.0x3	T60.0x4	—	—
Phenyltoloxamine	T45.0x1	T45.0x2	T45.0x3	T45.0x4	T45.0x5	T45.0x6
Phenyramidol, phenyramidon	T39.8x1	T39.8x2	T39.8x3	T39.8x4	T39.8x5	T39.8x6
Phenytoin	T42.0x1	T42.0x2	T42.0x3	T42.0x4	T42.0x5	T42.0x6
with phenobarbital	T42.3x1	T42.3x2	T42.3x3	T42.3x4	T42.3x5	T42.3x6
pHisoHex	T49.2x1	T49.2x2	T49.2x3	T49.2x4	T49.2x5	T49.2x6
Pholcodine	T48.3x1	T48.3x2	T48.3x3	T48.3x4	T48.3x5	T48.3x6
Pholedrine	T46.991	T46.992	T46.993	T46.994	T46.995	T46.996
Phorate	T60.0x1	T60.0x2	T60.0x3	T60.0x4	—	—
Phosdrin	T60.0x1	T60.0x2	T60.0x3	T60.0x4	—	—
Phosfolan	T60.0x1	T60.0x2	T60.0x3	T60.0x4	—	—
Phosgene (gas)	T59.891	T59.892	T59.893	T59.894	—	—
Phosphamidon	T60.0x1	T60.0x2	T60.0x3	T60.0x4	—	—
Phosphate	T65.891	T65.892	T65.893	T65.894	—	—
laxative	T47.4x1	T47.4x2	T47.4x3	T47.4x4	T47.4x5	T47.4x6
organic	T60.0x1	T60.0x2	T60.0x3	T60.0x4	—	—
solvent	T52.91	T52.92	T52.93	T52.94	—	—
tricresyl	T65.891	T65.892	T65.893	T65.894	—	—
Phosphine	T57.1x1	T57.1x2	T57.1x3	T57.1x4	—	—
fumigant	T57.1x1	T57.1x2	T57.1x3	T57.1x4	—	—
Phospholine	T49.5x1	T49.5x2	T49.5x3	T49.5x4	T49.5x5	T49.5x6
Phosphoric acid	T54.2x1	T54.2x2	T54.2x3	T54.2x4	—	—
Phosphorus (compound) NEC	T57.1x1	T57.1x2	T57.1x3	T57.1x4	—	—
pesticide	T60.0x1	T60.0x2	T60.0x3	T60.0x4	—	—
Phthalates	T65.891	T65.892	T65.893	T65.894	—	—
Phthalic anhydride	T65.891	T65.892	T65.893	T65.894	—	—
Phthalimidoglutarimide	T42.6x1	T42.6x2	T42.6x3	T42.6x4	T42.6x5	T42.6x6
Phthalylsulfathiazole	T37.0x1	T37.0x2	T37.0x3	T37.0x4	T37.0x5	T37.0x6
Phylloquinone	T45.7x1	T45.7x2	T45.7x3	T45.7x4	T45.7x5	T45.7x6
Physeptone	T40.3x1	T40.3x2	T40.3x3	T40.3x4	T40.3x5	T40.3x6
Physostigma venenosum	T62.2x1	T62.2x2	T62.2x3	T62.2x4	—	—
Physostigmine	T49.5x1	T49.5x2	T49.5x3	T49.5x4	T49.5x5	T49.5x6
Phytolacca decandra	T62.2x1	T62.2x2	T62.2x3	T62.2x4	—	—
berries	T62.1x1	T62.1x2	T62.1x3	T62.1x4	—	—
Phytomenadione	T45.7x1	T45.7x2	T45.7x3	T45.7x4	T45.7x5	T45.7x6
Phytonadione	T45.7x1	T45.7x2	T45.7x3	T45.7x4	T45.7x5	T45.7x6
Picoperine	T48.3x1	T48.3x2	T48.3x3	T48.3x4	T48.3x5	T48.3x6
Picosulfate (sodium)	T47.2x1	T47.2x2	T47.2x3	T47.2x4	T47.2x5	T47.2x6
Picric (acid)	T54.2x1	T54.2x2	T54.2x3	T54.2x4	—	—
Picrotoxin	T50.7x1	T50.7x2	T50.7x3	T50.7x4	T50.7x5	T50.7x6
Piketoprofen	T49.0x1	T49.0x2	T49.0x3	T49.0x4	T49.0x5	T49.0x6
Pilocarpine	T44.1x1	T44.1x2	T44.1x3	T44.1x4	T44.1x5	T44.1x6
Pilocarpus (jaborandi) extract	T44.1x1	T44.1x2	T44.1x3	T44.1x4	T44.1x5	T44.1x6
Pilsicainide (hydrochloride)	T46.2x1	T46.2x2	T46.2x3	T46.2x4	T46.2x5	T46.2x6
Pimaricin	T36.7x1	T36.7x2	T36.7x3	T36.7x4	T36.7x5	T36.7x6
Pimeclone	T50.7x1	T50.7x2	T50.7x3	T50.7x4	T50.7x5	T50.7x6
Pimelic ketone	T52.8x1	T52.8x2	T52.8x3	T52.8x4	—	—
Pimethixene	T45.0x1	T45.0x2	T45.0x3	T45.0x4	T45.0x5	T45.0x6
Piminodine	T40.2x1	T40.2x2	T40.2x3	T40.2x4	T40.2x5	T40.2x6
Pimozide	T43.591	T43.592	T43.593	T43.594	T43.595	T43.596
Pinacidil	T46.5x1	T46.5x2	T46.5x3	T46.5x4	T46.5x5	T46.5x6
Pinaverium bromide	T44.3x1	T44.3x2	T44.3x3	T44.3x4	T44.3x5	T44.3x6
Pinazepam	T42.4x1	T42.4x2	T42.4x3	T42.4x4	T42.4x5	T42.4x6
Pindolol	T44.7x1	T44.7x2	T44.7x3	T44.7x4	T44.7x5	T44.7x6
Pindone	T60.4x1	T60.4x2	T60.4x3	T60.4x4	—	—
Pine oil (disinfectant)	T65.891	T65.892	T65.893	T65.894	—	—
Pinkroot	T37.4x1	T37.4x2	T37.4x3	T37.4x4	T37.4x5	T37.4x6

Table of Drugs & Chemicals	POISONING Accidental (Unintentional)	Self-Harm (Intentional)	Assault	Undetermined	Adverse Effect	Underdosing
Pipadone	T40.2x1	T40.2x2	T40.2x3	T40.2x4	—	—
Pipamazine	T45.0x1	T45.0x2	T45.0x3	T45.0x4	T45.0x5	T45.0x6
Pipamperone	T43.4x1	T43.4x2	T43.4x3	T43.4x4	T43.4x5	T43.4x6
Pipazetate	T48.3x1	T48.3x2	T48.3x3	T48.3x4	T48.3x5	T48.3x6
Pipemidic acid	T37.8x1	T37.8x2	T37.8x3	T37.8x4	T37.8x5	T37.8x6
Pipenzolate bromide	T44.3x1	T44.3x2	T44.3x3	T44.3x4	T44.3x5	T44.3x6
Piper cubeba	T62.2x1	T62.2x2	T62.2x3	T62.2x4	—	—
Piperacetazine	T43.3x1	T43.3x2	T43.3x3	T43.3x4	T43.3x5	T43.3x6
Piperacillin	T36.0x1	T36.0x2	T36.0x3	T36.0x4	T36.0x5	T36.0x6
Piperazine	T37.4x1	T37.4x2	T37.4x3	T37.4x4	T37.4x5	T37.4x6
estrone sulfate	T38.5x1	T38.5x2	T38.5x3	T38.5x4	T38.5x5	T38.5x6
Piperidione	T48.3x1	T48.3x2	T48.3x3	T48.3x4	T48.3x5	T48.3x6
Piperidolate	T44.3x1	T44.3x2	T44.3x3	T44.3x4	T44.3x5	T44.3x6
Piperocaine	T41.3x1	T41.3x2	T41.3x3	T41.3x4	T41.3x5	T41.3x6
infiltration (subcutaneous)	T41.3x1	T41.3x2	T41.3x3	T41.3x4	T41.3x5	T41.3x6
nerve block (peripheral) (plexus)	T41.3x1	T41.3x2	T41.3x3	T41.3x4	T41.3x5	T41.3x6
topical (surface)	T41.3x1	T41.3x2	T41.3x3	T41.3x4	T41.3x5	T41.3x6
Piperonyl butoxide	T60.8x1	T60.8x2	T60.8x3	T60.8x4	—	—
Pipethanate	T44.3x1	T44.3x2	T44.3x3	T44.3x4	T44.3x5	T44.3x6
Pipobroman	T45.1x1	T45.1x2	T45.1x3	T45.1x4	T45.1x5	T45.1x6
Pipotiazine	T43.3x1	T43.3x2	T43.3x3	T43.3x4	T43.3x5	T43.3x6
Pipoxizine	T45.0x1	T45.0x2	T45.0x3	T45.0x4	T45.0x5	T45.0x6
Pipradrol	T43.691	T43.692	T43.693	T43.694	T43.695	T43.696
Piprinhydrinate	T45.0x1	T45.0x2	T45.0x3	T45.0x4	T45.0x5	T45.0x6
Pirarubicin	T45.1x1	T45.1x2	T45.1x3	T45.1x4	T45.1x5	T45.1x6
Pirazinamide	T37.1x1	T37.1x2	T37.1x3	T37.1x4	T37.1x5	T37.1x6
Pirbuterol	T48.6x1	T48.6x2	T48.6x3	T48.6x4	T48.6x5	T48.6x6
Pirenzepine	T47.1x1	T47.1x2	T47.1x3	T47.1x4	T47.1x5	T47.1x6
Piretanide	T50.1x1	T50.1x2	T50.1x3	T50.1x4	T50.1x5	T50.1x6
Piribedil	T42.8x1	T42.8x2	T42.8x3	T42.8x4	T42.8x5	T42.8x6
Piridoxilate	T46.3x1	T46.3x2	T46.3x3	T46.3x4	T46.3x5	T46.3x6
Piritramide	T40.4x1	T40.4x2	T40.4x3	T40.4x4	—	—
Piromidic acid	T37.8x1	T37.8x2	T37.8x3	T37.8x4	T37.8x5	T37.8x6
Piroxicam	T39.391	T39.392	T39.393	T39.394	T39.395	T39.396
beta-cyclodextrin complex	T39.8x1	T39.8x2	T39.8x3	T39.8x4	T39.8x5	T39.8x6
Pirozadil	T46.6x1	T46.6x2	T46.6x3	T46.6x4	T46.6x5	T46.6x6
Piscidia (bark) (erythrina)	T39.8x1	T39.8x2	T39.8x3	T39.8x4	T39.8x5	T39.8x6
Pitch	T65.891	T65.892	T65.893	T65.894	—	—
Pitkin's solution	T41.3x1	T41.3x2	T41.3x3	T41.3x4	T41.3x5	T41.3x6
Pitocin	T48.0x1	T48.0x2	T48.0x3	T48.0x4	T48.0x5	T48.0x6
Pitressin (tannate)	T38.891	T38.892	T38.893	T38.894	T38.895	T38.896
Pituitary extracts (posterior)	T38.891	T38.892	T38.893	T38.894	T38.895	T38.896
anterior	T38.811	T38.812	T38.813	T38.814	T38.815	T38.816
Pituitrin	T38.891	T38.892	T38.893	T38.894	T38.895	T38.896
Pivampicillin	T36.0x1	T36.0x2	T36.0x3	T36.0x4	T36.0x5	T36.0x6
Pivmecillinam	T36.0x1	T36.0x2	T36.0x3	T36.0x4	T36.0x5	T36.0x6
Placental hormone	T38.891	T38.892	T38.893	T38.894	T38.895	T38.896
Placidyl	T42.6x1	T42.6x2	T42.6x3	T42.6x4	T42.6x5	T42.6x6
Plague vaccine	T50.A91	T50.A92	T50.A93	T50.A94	T50.A95	T50.A96
Plant						
food or fertilizer NEC	T65.891	T65.892	T65.893	T65.894	—	—
containing herbicide	T60.3x1	T60.3x2	T60.3x3	T60.3x4	—	—
noxious, used as food	T62.2x1	T62.2x2	T62.2x3	T62.2x4	—	—
berries	T62.1x1	T62.1x2	T62.1x3	T62.1x4	—	—
seeds	T62.2x1	T62.2x2	T62.2x3	T62.2x4	—	—
specified type NEC	T62.2x1	T62.2x2	T62.2x3	T62.2x4	—	—
Plasma	T45.8x1	T45.8x2	T45.8x3	T45.8x4	T45.8x5	T45.8x6
expander NEC	T45.8x1	T45.8x2	T45.8x3	T45.8x4	T45.8x5	T45.8x6
protein fraction (human)	T45.8x1	T45.8x2	T45.8x3	T45.8x4	T45.8x5	T45.8x6
Plasmanate	T45.8x1	T45.8x2	T45.8x3	T45.8x4	T45.8x5	T45.8x6
Plasminogen (tissue) activator	T45.611	T45.612	T45.613	T45.614	T45.615	T45.616
Plaster dressing	T49.3x1	T49.3x2	T49.3x3	T49.3x4	T49.3x5	T49.3x6
Plastic dressing	T49.3x1	T49.3x2	T49.3x3	T49.3x4	T49.3x5	T49.3x6
Plegicil	T43.3x1	T43.3x2	T43.3x3	T43.3x4	T43.3x5	T43.3x6
Plicamycin	T45.1x1	T45.1x2	T45.1x3	T45.1x4	T45.1x5	T45.1x6
Podophyllotoxin	T49.8x1	T49.8x2	T49.8x3	T49.8x4	T49.8x5	T49.8x6
Podophyllum (resin)	T49.4x1	T49.4x2	T49.4x3	T49.4x4	T49.4x5	T49.4x6

Table of Drugs & Chemicals	Accidental (Unintentional)	Self-Harm (Intentional)	Assault	Undetermined	Adverse Effect	Underdosing
Poison NEC	T65.91	T65.92	T65.93	T65.94	—	—
Poisonous berries	T62.1x1	T62.1x2	T62.1x3	T62.1x4	—	—
Pokeweed (any part)	T62.2x1	T62.2x2	T62.2x3	T62.2x4	—	—
Poldine metilsulfate	T44.3x1	T44.3x2	T44.3x3	T44.3x4	T44.3x5	T44.3x6
Polidexide (sulfate)	T46.6x1	T46.6x2	T46.6x3	T46.6x4	T46.6x5	T46.6x6
Polidocanol	T46.8x1	T46.8x2	T46.8x3	T46.8x4	T46.8x5	T46.8x6
Poliomyelitis vaccine	T50.B91	T50.B92	T50.B93	T50.B94	T50.B95	T50.B96
Polish (car) (floor) (furni-ture) (metal) (porcelain) (silver)	T65.891	T65.892	T65.893	T65.894	—	—
abrasive	T65.891	T65.892	T65.893	T65.894	—	—
porcelain	T65.891	T65.892	T65.893	T65.894	—	—
Poloxalkol	T47.4x1	T47.4x2	T47.4x3	T47.4x4	T47.4x5	T47.4x6
Poloxamer	T47.4x1	T47.4x2	T47.4x3	T47.4x4	T47.4x5	T47.4x6
Polyaminostyrene resins	T50.3x1	T50.3x2	T50.3x3	T50.3x4	T50.3x5	T50.3x6
Polycarbophil	T47.4x1	T47.4x2	T47.4x3	T47.4x4	T47.4x5	T47.4x6
Polychlorinated biphenyl	T65.892	T65.892	T65.893	T65.894	—	—
Polycycline	T36.4x1	T36.4x2	T36.4x3	T36.4x4	T36.4x5	T36.4x6
Polyester fumes	T59.891	T59.892	T59.893	T59.894	—	—
Polyester resin hardener	T52.91	T52.92	T52.93	T52.94	—	—
fumes	T59.891	T59.892	T59.893	T59.894	—	—
Polyestradiol phosphate	T38.5x1	T38.5x2	T38.5x3	T38.5x4	T38.5x5	T38.5x6
Polyethanolamine alkyl sulfate	T49.2x1	T49.2x2	T49.2x3	T49.2x4	T49.2x5	T49.2x6
Polyethylene adhesive	T49.3x1	T49.3x2	T49.3x3	T49.3x4	T49.3x5	T49.3x6
Polyferose	T45.4x1	T45.4x2	T45.4x3	T45.4x4	T45.4x5	T45.4x6
Polygeline	T45.8x1	T45.8x2	T45.8x3	T45.8x4	T45.8x5	T45.8x6
Polymyxin	T36.8x1	T36.8x2	T36.8x3	T36.8x4	T36.8x5	T36.8x6
B	T36.8x1	T36.8x2	T36.8x3	T36.8x4	T36.8x5	T36.8x6
ENT agent	T49.6x1	T49.6x2	T49.6x3	T49.6x4	T49.6x5	T49.6x6
ophthalmic preparation	T49.5x1	T49.5x2	T49.5x3	T49.5x4	T49.5x5	T49.5x6
topical NEC	T49.0x1	T49.0x2	T49.0x3	T49.0x4	T49.0x5	T49.0x6
E sulfate (eye preparation)	T49.5x1	T49.5x2	T49.5x3	T49.5x4	T49.5x5	T49.5x6
Polynoxylin	T49.0x1	T49.0x2	T49.0x3	T49.0x4	T49.0x5	T49.0x6
Polyoestradiol phosphate	T38.5x1	T38.5x2	T38.5x3	T38.5x4	T38.5x5	T38.5x6
Polyoxymethyleneurea	T49.0x1	T49.0x2	T49.0x3	T49.0x4	T49.0x5	T49.0x6
Polysilane	T47.8x1	T47.8x2	T47.8x3	T47.8x4	T47.8x5	T47.8x6
Polytetrafluoroethylene (inhaled)	T59.891	T59.892	T59.893	T59.894	—	—
Polythiazide	T50.2x1	T50.2x2	T50.2x3	T50.2x4	T50.2x5	T50.2x6
Polyvidone	T45.8x1	T45.8x2	T45.8x3	T45.8x4	T45.8x5	T45.8x6
Polyvinylpyrrolidone	T45.8x1	T45.8x2	T45.8x3	T45.8x4	T45.8x5	T45.8x6
Pontocaine (hydrochloride) (infiltration) (topical)	T41.3x1	T41.3x2	T41.3x3	T41.3x4	T41.3x5	T41.3x6
nerve block (peripheral) (plexus)	T41.3x1	T41.3x2	T41.3x3	T41.3x4	T41.3x5	T41.3x6
spinal	T41.3x1	T41.3x2	T41.3x3	T41.3x4	T41.3x5	T41.3x6
Porfiromycin	T45.1x1	T45.1x2	T45.1x3	T45.1x4	T45.1x5	T45.1x6
Posterior pituitary hormone NEC	T38.891	T38.892	T38.893	T38.894	T38.895	T38.896
Pot	T40.7x1	T40.7x2	T40.7x3	T40.7x4	T40.7x5	T40.7x6
Potash (caustic)	T54.3x1	T54.3x2	T54.3x3	T54.3x4	—	—
Potassic saline injection (lactated)	T50.3x1	T50.3x2	T50.3x3	T50.3x4	T50.3x5	T50.3x6
Potassium (salts) NEC	T50.3x1	T50.3x2	T50.3x3	T50.3x4	T50.3x5	T50.3x6
aminobenzoate	T45.8x1	T45.8x2	T45.8x3	T45.8x4	T45.8x5	T45.8x6
aminosalicylate	T37.1x1	T37.1x2	T37.1x3	T37.1x4	T37.1x5	T37.1x6
antimony 'tartrate'	T37.8x1	T37.8x2	T37.8x3	T37.8x4	T37.8x5	T37.8x6
arsenite (solution)	T57.0x1	T57.0x2	T57.0x3	T57.0x4	—	—
bichromate	T56.2x1	T56.2x2	T56.2x3	T56.2x4	—	—
bisulfate	T47.3x1	T47.3x2	T47.3x3	T47.3x4	T47.3x5	T47.3x6
bromide	T42.6x1	T42.6x2	T42.6x3	T42.6x4	T42.6x5	T42.6x6
canrenoate	T50.0x1	T50.0x2	T50.0x3	T50.0x4	T50.0x5	T50.0x6
carbonate	T54.3x1	T54.3x2	T54.3x3	T54.3x4	—	—
chlorate NEC	T65.891	T65.892	T65.893	T65.894	—	—
chloride	T50.3x1	T50.3x2	T50.3x3	T50.3x4	T50.3x5	T50.3x6
citrate	T50.991	T50.992	T50.993	T50.994	T50.995	T50.996
cyanide	T65.0x1	T65.0x2	T65.0x3	T65.0x4	—	—
ferric hexacyanoferrate (medicinal)	T50.6x1	T50.6x2	T50.6x3	T50.6x4	T50.6x5	T50.6x6
nonmedicinal	T65.891	T65.892	T65.893	T65.894	—	—
fluoride	T57.8x1	T57.8x2	T57.8x3	T57.8x4	—	—
glucaldrate	T47.1x1	T47.1x2	T47.1x3	T47.1x4	T47.1x5	T47.1x6
Potassium (salts)						
NEC – continued	T50.3x1	T50.3x2	T50.3x3	T50.3x4	T50.3x5	T50.3x6
hydroxide	T54.3x1	T54.3x2	T54.3x3	T54.3x4	—	—
iodate	T49.0x1	T49.0x2	T49.0x3	T49.0x4	T49.0x5	T49.0x6
iodide	T48.4x1	T48.4x2	T48.4x3	T48.4x4	T48.4x5	T48.4x6
nitrate	T57.8x1	T57.8x2	T57.8x3	T57.8x4	—	—
oxalate	T65.891	T65.892	T65.893	T65.894	—	—
perchlorate (nonmedicinal) NEC	T65.891	T65.892	T65.893	T65.894	—	—
antithyroid	T38.2x1	T38.2x2	T38.2x3	T38.2x4	T38.2x5	T38.2x6
medicinal	T38.2x1	T38.2x2	T38.2x3	T38.2x4	T38.2x5	T38.2x6
permanganate (nonmedicinal)	T65.891	T65.892	T65.893	T65.894	—	—
medicinal	T49.0x1	T49.0x2	T49.0x3	T49.0x4	T49.0x5	T49.0x6
sulfate	T47.2x1	T47.2x2	T47.2x3	T47.2x4	T47.2x5	T47.2x6
Potassium-removing resin	T50.3x1	T50.3x2	T50.3x3	T50.3x4	T50.3x5	T50.3x6
Potassium-retaining drug	T50.3x1	T50.3x2	T50.3x3	T50.3x4	T50.3x5	T50.3x6
Povidone	T45.8x1	T45.8x2	T45.8x3	T45.8x4	T45.8x5	T45.8x6
iodine	T49.0x1	T49.0x2	T49.0x3	T49.0x4	T49.0x5	T49.0x6
Practolol	T44.7x1	T44.7x2	T44.7x3	T44.7x4	T44.7x5	T44.7x6
Prajmalium bitartrate	T46.2x1	T46.2x2	T46.2x3	T46.2x4	T46.2x5	T46.2x6
Pralidoxime (iodide)	T50.6x1	T50.6x2	T50.6x3	T50.6x4	T50.6x5	T50.6x6
chloride	T50.6x1	T50.6x2	T50.6x3	T50.6x4	T50.6x5	T50.6x6
Pramiverine	T44.3x1	T44.3x2	T44.3x3	T44.3x4	T44.3x5	T44.3x6
Pramocaine	T49.1x1	T49.1x2	T49.1x3	T49.1x4	T49.1x5	T49.1x6
Pramoxine	T49.1x1	T49.1x2	T49.1x3	T49.1x4	T49.1x5	T49.1x6
Prasterone	T38.7x1	T38.7x2	T38.7x3	T38.7x4	T38.7x5	T38.7x6
Pravastatin	T46.6x1	T46.6x2	T46.6x3	T46.6x4	T46.6x5	T46.6x6
Prazepam	T42.4x1	T42.4x2	T42.4x3	T42.4x4	T42.4x5	T42.4x6
Praziquantel	T37.4x1	T37.4x2	T37.4x3	T37.4x4	T37.4x5	T37.4x6
Prazitone	T43.291	T43.292	T43.293	T43.294	T43.295	T43.296
Prazosin	T44.6x1	T44.6x2	T44.6x3	T44.6x4	T44.6x5	T44.6x6
Prednicarbate	T49.0x1	T49.0x2	T49.0x3	T49.0x4	T49.0x5	T49.0x6
Prednimustine	T45.1x1	T45.1x2	T45.1x3	T45.1x4	T45.1x5	T45.1x6
Prednisolone	T38.0x1	T38.0x2	T38.0x3	T38.0x4	T38.0x5	T38.0x6
ENT agent	T49.6x1	T49.6x2	T49.6x3	T49.6x4	T49.6x5	T49.6x6
ophthalmic preparation	T49.5x1	T49.5x2	T49.5x3	T49.5x4	T49.5x5	T49.5x6
steaglate	T38.0x1	T38.0x2	T38.0x3	T38.0x4	T38.0x5	T38.0x6
topical NEC	T49.0x1	T49.0x2	T49.0x3	T49.0x4	T49.0x5	T49.0x6
Prednisone	T38.0x1	T38.0x2	T38.0x3	T38.0x4	T38.0x5	T38.0x6
Prednylidene	T38.0x1	T38.0x2	T38.0x3	T38.0x4	T38.0x5	T38.0x6
Pregnandiol	T38.5x1	T38.5x2	T38.5x3	T38.5x4	T38.5x5	T38.5x6
Pregneninolone	T38.5x1	T38.5x2	T38.5x3	T38.5x4	T38.5x5	T38.5x6
Preludin	T43.691	T43.692	T43.693	T43.694	T43.695	T43.696
Premarin	T38.5x1	T38.5x2	T38.5x3	T38.5x4	T38.5x5	T38.5x6
Premedication anesthetic	T41.201	T41.202	T41.203	T41.204	T41.205	T41.206
Prenalterol	T44.5x1	T44.5x2	T44.5x3	T44.5x4	T44.5x5	T44.5x6
Prenoxdiazine	T48.3x1	T48.3x2	T48.3x3	T48.3x4	T48.3x5	T48.3x6
Prenylamine	T46.3x1	T46.3x2	T46.3x3	T46.3x4	T46.3x5	T46.3x6
Preparation, local	T49.4x1	T49.4x2	T49.4x3	T49.4x4	T49.4x5	T49.4x6
Preparation H	T49.8x1	T49.8x2	T49.8x3	T49.8x4	T49.8x5	T49.8x6
Preservative (nonmedicinal)	T65.891	T65.892	T65.893	T65.894	—	—
medicinal	T50.901	T50.902	T50.903	T50.904	T50.905	T50.906
wood	T60.91	T60.92	T60.93	T60.94	—	—
Prethcamide	T50.7x1	T50.7x2	T50.7x3	T50.7x4	T50.7x5	T50.7x6
Pride of China	T62.2x1	T62.2x2	T62.2x3	T62.2x4	—	—
Pridinol	T44.3x1	T44.3x2	T44.3x3	T44.3x4	T44.3x5	T44.3x6
Prifinium bromide	T44.3x1	T44.3x2	T44.3x3	T44.3x4	T44.3x5	T44.3x6
Prilocaine	T41.3x1	T41.3x2	T41.3x3	T41.3x4	T41.3x5	T41.3x6
infiltration (subcutaneous)	T41.3x1	T41.3x2	T41.3x3	T41.3x4	T41.3x5	T41.3x6
nerve block (peripheral) (plexus)	T41.3x1	T41.3x2	T41.3x3	T41.3x4	T41.3x5	T41.3x6
regional	T41.3x1	T41.3x2	T41.3x3	T41.3x4	T41.3x5	T41.3x6
Primaquine	T37.2x1	T37.2x2	T37.2x3	T37.2x4	T37.2x5	T37.2x6
Primidone	T42.6x1	T42.6x2	T42.6x3	T42.6x4	T42.6x5	T42.6x6
Primula (veris)	T62.2x1	T62.2x2	T62.2x3	T62.2x4	—	—
Prinadol	T40.2x1	T40.2x2	T40.2x3	T40.2x4	T40.2x5	T40.2x6
Priscol, Priscoline	T44.6x1	T44.6x2	T44.6x3	T44.6x4	T44.6x5	T44.6x6
Pristinamycin	T36.3x1	T36.3x2	T36.3x3	T36.3x4	T36.3x5	T36.3x6
Privet	T62.2x1	T62.2x2	T62.2x3	T62.2x4	—	—
berries	T62.1x1	T62.1x2	T62.1x3	T62.1x4	—	—

DRUGS&CHEMICALS

DRUGS&CHEMICALS

Table of Drugs & Chemicals	Accidental (Unintentional)	Self-Harm (Intentional)	Assault	Undetermined	Adverse Effect	Underdosing
Privine	T44.4x1	T44.4x2	T44.4x3	T44.4x4	T44.4x5	T44.4x6
Pro-Banthine	T44.3x1	T44.3x2	T44.3x3	T44.3x4	T44.3x5	T44.3x6
Probarbital	T42.3x1	T42.3x2	T42.3x3	T42.3x4	T42.3x5	T42.3x6
Probenecid	T50.4x1	T50.4x2	T50.4x3	T50.4x4	T50.4x5	T50.4x6
Probucol	T46.6x1	T46.6x2	T46.6x3	T46.6x4	T46.6x5	T46.6x6
Procainamide	T46.2x1	T46.2x2	T46.2x3	T46.2x4	T46.2x5	T46.2x6
Procaine	T41.3x1	T41.3x2	T41.3x3	T41.3x4	T41.3x5	T41.3x6
benzylpenicillin	T36.0x1	T36.0x2	T36.0x3	T36.0x4	T36.0x5	T36.0x6
nerve block (periphreal) (plexus)	T41.3x1	T41.3x2	T41.3x3	T41.3x4	T41.3x5	T41.3x6
penicillin G	T36.0x1	T36.0x2	T36.0x3	T36.0x4	T36.0x5	T36.0x6
regional	T41.3x1	T41.3x2	T41.3x3	T41.3x4	T41.3x5	T41.3x6
spinal	T41.3x1	T41.3x2	T41.3x3	T41.3x4	T41.3x5	T41.3x6
Procalmidol	T43.591	T43.592	T43.593	T43.594	T43.595	T43.596
Procarbazine	T45.1x1	T45.1x2	T45.1x3	T45.1x4	T45.1x5	T45.1x6
Procaterol	T44.5x1	T44.5x2	T44.5x3	T44.5x4	T44.5x5	T44.5x6
Prochlorperazine	T43.3x1	T43.3x2	T43.3x3	T43.3x4	T43.3x5	T43.3x6
Procyclidine	T44.3x1	T44.3x2	T44.3x3	T44.3x4	T44.3x5	T44.3x6
Producer gas	T58.8x1	T58.8x2	T58.8x3	T58.8x4	—	—
Profadol	T40.4x1	T40.4x2	T40.4x3	T40.4x4	T40.4x5	T40.4x6
Profenamine	T44.3x1	T44.3x2	T44.3x3	T44.3x4	T44.3x5	T44.3x6
Profenil	T44.3x1	T44.3x2	T44.3x3	T44.3x4	T44.3x5	T44.3x6
Proflavine	T49.0x1	T49.0x2	T49.0x3	T49.0x4	T49.0x5	T49.0x6
Progabide	T42.6x1	T42.6x2	T42.6x3	T42.6x4	T42.6x5	T42.6x6
Progesterone	T38.5x1	T38.5x2	T38.5x3	T38.5x4	T38.5x5	T38.5x6
Progestin	T38.5x1	T38.5x2	T38.5x3	T38.5x4	T38.5x5	T38.5x6
oral contraceptive	T38.4x1	T38.4x2	T38.4x3	T38.4x4	T38.4x5	T38.4x6
Progestogen NEC	T38.5x1	T38.5x2	T38.5x3	T38.5x4	T38.5x5	T38.5x6
Progestone	T38.5x1	T38.5x2	T38.5x3	T38.5x4	T38.5x5	T38.5x6
Proglumide	T47.1x1	T47.1x2	T47.1x3	T47.1x4	T47.1x5	T47.1x6
Proguanil	T37.2x1	T37.2x2	T37.2x3	T37.2x4	T37.2x5	T37.2x6
Prolactin	T38.811	T38.812	T38.813	T38.814	T38.815	T38.816
Prolintane	T43.691	T43.692	T43.693	T43.694	T43.695	T43.696
Proloid	T38.1x1	T38.1x2	T38.1x3	T38.1x4	T38.1x5	T38.1x6
Proluton	T38.5x1	T38.5x2	T38.5x3	T38.5x4	T38.5x5	T38.5x6
Promacetin	T37.1x1	T37.1x2	T37.1x3	T37.1x4	T37.1x5	T37.1x6
Promazine	T43.3x1	T43.3x2	T43.3x3	T43.3x4	T43.3x5	T43.3x6
Promedol	T40.2x1	T40.2x2	T40.2x3	T40.2x4	—	—
Promegestone	T38.5x1	T38.5x2	T38.5x3	T38.5x4	T38.5x5	T38.5x6
Promethazine (teoclate)	T43.3x1	T43.3x2	T43.3x3	T43.3x4	T43.3x5	T43.3x6
Promin	T37.1x1	T37.1x2	T37.1x3	T37.1x4	T37.1x5	T37.1x6
Pronase	T45.3x1	T45.3x2	T45.3x3	T45.3x4	T45.3x5	T45.3x6
Pronestyl (hydrochloride)	T46.2x1	T46.2x2	T46.2x3	T46.2x4	T46.2x5	T46.2x6
Pronetalol	T44.7x1	T44.7x2	T44.7x3	T44.7x4	T44.7x5	T44.7x6
Prontosil	T37.0x1	T37.0x2	T37.0x3	T37.0x4	T37.0x5	T37.0x6
Propachlor	T60.3x1	T60.3x2	T60.3x3	T60.3x4	—	—
Propafenone	T46.2x1	T46.2x2	T46.2x3	T46.2x4	T46.2x5	T46.2x6
Propallylonal	T42.3x1	T42.3x2	T42.3x3	T42.3x4	T42.3x5	T42.3x6
Propamidine	T49.0x1	T49.0x2	T49.0x3	T49.0x4	T49.0x5	T49.0x6
Propane (distributed in mobile container)	T59.891	T59.892	T59.893	T59.894	—	—
distributed through pipes	T59.891	T59.892	T59.893	T59.894	—	—
incomplete combustion	T58.11	T58.12	T58.13	T58.14	—	—
Propanidid	T41.291	T41.292	T41.293	T41.294	T41.295	T41.296
Propanil	T60.3x1	T60.3x2	T60.3x3	T60.3x4	—	—
1-Propanol	T51.3x1	T51.3x2	T51.3x3	T51.3x4	—	—
2-Propanol	T51.2x1	T51.2x2	T51.2x3	T51.2x4	—	—
Propantheline	T44.3x1	T44.3x2	T44.3x3	T44.3x4	T44.3x5	T44.3x6
bromide	T44.3x1	T44.3x2	T44.3x3	T44.3x4	T44.3x5	T44.3x6
Proparacaine	T41.3x1	T41.3x2	T41.3x3	T41.3x4	T41.3x5	T41.3x6
Propatylnitrate	T46.3x1	T46.3x2	T46.3x3	T46.3x4	T46.3x5	T46.3x6
Propicillin	T36.0x1	T36.0x2	T36.0x3	T36.0x4	T36.0x5	T36.0x6
Propiolactone	T49.0x1	T49.0x2	T49.0x3	T49.0x4	T49.0x5	T49.0x6
Propiomazine	T45.0x1	T45.0x2	T45.0x3	T45.0x4	T45.0x5	T45.0x6
Propion gel	T49.0x1	T49.0x2	T49.0x3	T49.0x4	T49.0x5	T49.0x6
Propionaidehyde (medicinal)	T42.6x1	T42.6x2	T42.6x3	T42.6x4	T42.6x5	T42.6x6
Propionate (calcium) (sodium)	T49.0x1	T49.0x2	T49.0x3	T49.0x4	T49.0x5	T49.0x6
Propitocaine	T41.3x1	T41.3x2	T41.3x3	T41.3x4	T41.3x5	T41.3x6
infiltration (subcutaneous)	T41.3x1	T41.3x2	T41.3x3	T41.3x4	T41.3x5	T41.3x6
nerve block (peripheral) (plexus)	T41.3x1	T41.3x2	T41.3x3	T41.3x4	T41.3x5	T41.3x6

Table of Drugs & Chemicals	Accidental (Unintentional)	Self-Harm (Intentional)	Assault	Undetermined	Adverse Effect	Underdosing
Propofol	T41.291	T41.292	T41.293	T41.294	T41.295	T41.296
Propoxur	T60.0x1	T60.0x2	T60.0x3	T60.0x4	—	—
Propoxycaine	T41.3x1	T41.3x2	T41.3x3	T41.3x4	T41.3x5	T41.3x6
infiltration (subcutaneous) nerve block (peripheral) (plexus)	T41.3x1	T41.3x2	T41.3x3	T41.3x4	T41.3x5	T41.3x6
topical (surface)	T41.3x1	T41.3x2	T41.3x3	T41.3x4	T41.3x5	T41.3x6
Propoxyphene	T40.4x1	T40.4x2	T40.4x3	T40.4x4	T40.4x5	T40.4x6
Propranolol	T44.7x1	T44.7x2	T44.7x3	T44.7x4	T44.7x5	T44.7x6
Propyl						
alcohol	T51.3x1	T51.3x2	T51.3x3	T51.3x4	—	—
carbinol	T51.3x1	T51.3x2	T51.3x3	T51.3x4	—	—
hexadrine	T44.4x1	T44.4x2	T44.4x3	T44.4x4	T44.4x5	T44.4x6
iodone	T50.8x1	T50.8x2	T50.8x3	T50.8x4	T50.8x5	T50.8x6
thiouracil	T38.2x1	T38.2x2	T38.2x3	T38.2x4	T38.2x5	T38.2x6
Propylaminopheno-thiazine	T43.3x1	T43.3x2	T43.3x3	T43.3x4	T43.3x5	T43.3x6
Propylene	T59.891	T59.892	T59.893	T59.894	—	—
Propylhexedrine	T48.5x1	T48.5x2	T48.5x3	T48.5x4	T48.5x5	T48.5x6
Propyliodone	T50.8x1	T50.8x2	T50.8x3	T50.8x4	T50.8x5	T50.8x6
Propylparaben (ophthalmic)	T49.5x1	T49.5x2	T49.5x3	T49.5x4	T49.5x5	T49.5x6
Propylthiouracil	T38.2x1	T38.2x2	T38.2x3	T38.2x4	T38.2x5	T38.2x6
Propyphenazone	T39.2x1	T39.2x2	T39.2x3	T39.2x4	T39.2x5	T39.2x6
Proquazone	T39.391	T39.392	T39.393	T39.394	T39.395	T39.396
Proscillaridin	T46.0x1	T46.0x2	T46.0x3	T46.0x4	T46.0x5	T46.0x6
Prostacyclin	T45.521	T45.522	T45.523	T45.524	T45.525	T45.526
Prostaglandin (I2)	T45.521	T45.522	T45.523	T45.524	T45.525	T45.526
E1	T46.7x1	T46.7x2	T46.7x3	T46.7x4	T46.7x5	T46.7x6
E2	T48.0x1	T48.0x2	T48.0x3	T48.0x4	T48.0x5	T48.0x6
F2 alpha	T48.0x1	T48.0x2	T48.0x3	T48.0x4	T48.0x5	T48.0x6
Prostigmin	T44.0x1	T44.0x2	T44.0x3	T44.0x4	T44.0x5	T44.0x6
Prosultiamine	T45.2x1	T45.2x2	T45.2x3	T45.2x4	T45.2x5	T45.2x6
Protamine sulfate	T45.7x1	T45.7x2	T45.7x3	T45.7x4	T45.7x5	T45.7x6
zinc insulin	T38.3x1	T38.3x2	T38.3x3	T38.3x4	T38.3x5	T38.3x6
Protease	T47.5x1	T47.5x2	T47.5x3	T47.5x4	T47.5x5	T47.5x6
Protectant, skin NEC	T49.3x1	T49.3x2	T49.3x3	T49.3x4	T49.3x5	T49.3x6
Protein hydrolysate	T50.991	T50.992	T50.993	T50.994	T50.995	T50.996
Prothiaden — see Dothiepin hydrochloride						
Prothionamide	T37.1x1	T37.1x2	T37.1x3	T37.1x4	T37.1x5	T37.1x6
Prothipendyl	T43.591	T43.592	T43.593	T43.594	T43.595	T43.596
Prothoate	T60.0x1	T60.0x2	T60.0x3	T60.0x4	—	—
Prothrombin						
activator	T45.7x1	T45.7x2	T45.7x3	T45.7x4	T45.7x5	T45.7x6
synthesis inhibitor	T45.511	T45.512	T45.513	T45.514	T45.515	T45.516
Protionamide	T37.1x1	T37.1x2	T37.1x3	T37.1x4	T37.1x5	T37.1x6
Protirelin	T38.891	T38.892	T38.893	T38.894	T38.895	T38.896
Protokylol	T48.6x1	T48.6x2	T48.6x3	T48.6x4	T48.6x5	T48.6x6
Protopam	T50.6x1	T50.6x2	T50.6x3	T50.6x4	T50.6x5	T50.6x6
Protoveratrine(s) (A) (B)	T46.5x1	T46.5x2	T46.5x3	T46.5x4	T46.5x5	T46.5x6
Protriptyline	T43.011	T43.012	T43.013	T43.014	T43.015	T43.016
Provera	T38.5x1	T38.5x2	T38.5x3	T38.5x4	T38.5x5	T38.5x6
Provitamin A	T45.2x1	T45.2x2	T45.2x3	T45.2x4	T45.2x5	T45.2x6
Proxibarbal	T42.3x1	T42.3x2	T42.3x3	T42.3x4	T42.3x5	T42.3x6
Proxymetacaine	T41.3x1	T41.3x2	T41.3x3	T41.3x4	T41.3x5	T41.3x6
Proxyphylline	T48.6x1	T48.6x2	T48.6x3	T48.6x4	T48.6x5	T48.6x6
Prozac — see Fluoxetine hydrochloride						
Prunus						
laurocerasus	T62.2x1	T62.2x2	T62.2x3	T62.2x4	—	—
virginiana	T62.2x1	T62.2x2	T62.2x3	T62.2x4	—	—
Prussian blue						
commercial	T65.891	T65.892	T65.893	T65.894	—	—
therapeutic	T50.6x1	T50.6x2	T50.6x3	T50.6x4	T50.6x5	T50.6x6
Prussic acid	T65.0x1	T65.0x2	T65.0x3	T65.0x4	—	—
vapor	T57.3x1	T57.3x2	T57.3x3	T57.3x4	—	—
Pseudoephedrine	T44.991	T44.992	T44.993	T44.994	T44.995	T44.996
Psilocin	T40.991	T40.992	T40.993	T40.994	—	—
Psilocybin	T40.991	T40.992	T40.993	T40.994	—	—

DRUGS&CHEMICALS

Table of Drugs & Chemicals	Poisoning Accidental (Unintentional)	Poisoning Self-Harm (Intentional)	Poisoning Assault	Poisoning Undetermined	Adverse Effect	Underdosing
Psilocybine	T40.991	T40.992	T40.993	T40.994	—	—
Psoralene (nonmedicinal)	T65.891	T65.892	T65.893	T65.894	—	—
Psoralens (medicinal)	T50.991	T50.992	T50.993	T50.994	T50.995	T50.996
PSP (phenolsulfonphthalein)	T50.8x1	T50.8x2	T50.8x3	T50.8x4	T50.8x5	T50.8x6
Psychodysleptic drug NEC	T40.901	T40.902	T40.903	T40.904	T40.905	T40.906
Psychostimulant	T43.601	T43.602	T43.603	T43.604	T43.605	T43.606
amphetamine	T43.621	T43.622	T43.623	T43.624	T43.625	T43.626
caffeine	T43.611	T43.612	T43.613	T43.614	T43.615	T43.616
methylphenidate	T43.631	T43.632	T43.633	T43.634	T43.635	T43.636
specified NEC	T43.691	T43.692	T43.693	T43.694	T43.695	T43.696
Psychotherapeutic drug NEC	T43.91	T43.92	T43.93	T43.94	T43.95	T43.96
antidepressants — see also						
Antidepressant	T43.201	T43.202	T43.203	T43.204	T43.205	T43.206
specified NEC	T43.8x1	T43.8x2	T43.8x3	T43.8x4	T43.8x5	T43.8x6
tranquilizers NEC	T43.501	T43.502	T43.503	T43.504	T43.505	T43.506
Psychotomimetic agents	T40.901	T40.902	T40.903	T40.904	T40.905	T40.906
Psychotropic drug NEC	T43.91	T43.92	T43.93	T43.94	T43.95	T43.96
specified NEC	T43.8x1	T43.8x2	T43.8x3	T43.8x4	T43.8x5	T43.8x6
Psyllium hydrophilic mucilloid	T47.4x1	T47.4x2	T47.4x3	T47.4x4	T47.4x5	T47.4x6
Pteroylglutamic acid	T45.8x1	T45.8x2	T45.8x3	T45.8x4	T45.8x5	T45.8x6
Pteroyltriglutamate	T45.1x1	T45.1x2	T45.1x3	T45.1x4	T45.1x5	T45.1x6
PTFE — see						
Polytetrafluoroethylene						
Pulp						
devitalizing paste	T49.7x1	T49.7x2	T49.7x3	T49.7x4	T49.7x5	T49.7x6
dressing	T49.7x1	T49.7x2	T49.7x3	T49.7x4	T49.7x5	T49.7x6
Pulsatilla	T62.2x1	T62.2x2	T62.2x3	T62.2x4	—	—
Pumpkin seed extract	T37.4x1	T37.4x2	T37.4x3	T37.4x4	T37.4x5	T37.4x6
Purex (bleach)	T54.91	T54.92	T54.93	T54.94	—	—
Purgative NEC — see also						
Cathartic	T47.4x1	T47.4x2	T47.4x3	T47.4x4	T47.4x5	T47.4x6
Purine analogue (antineoplastic)	T45.1x1	T45.1x2	T45.1x3	T45.1x4	T45.1x5	T45.1x6
Purine diuretics	T50.2x1	T50.2x2	T50.2x3	T50.2x4	T50.2x5	T50.2x6
Purinethol	T45.1x1	T45.1x2	T45.1x3	T45.1x4	T45.1x5	T45.1x6
PVP	T45.8x1	T45.8x2	T45.8x3	T45.8x4	T45.8x5	T45.8x6
Pyrabital	T39.8x1	T39.8x2	T39.8x3	T39.8x4	T39.8x5	T39.8x6
Pyramidon	T39.2x1	T39.2x2	T39.2x3	T39.2x4	T39.2x5	T39.2x6
Pyrantel	T37.4x1	T37.4x2	T37.4x3	T37.4x4	T37.4x5	T37.4x6
Pyrathiazine	T45.0x1	T45.0x2	T45.0x3	T45.0x4	T45.0x5	T45.0x6
Pyrazinamide	T37.1x1	T37.1x2	T37.1x3	T37.1x4	T37.1x5	T37.1x6
Pyrazinoic acid (amide)	T37.1x1	T37.1x2	T37.1x3	T37.1x4	T37.1x5	T37.1x6
Pyrazole (derivatives)	T39.2x1	T39.2x2	T39.2x3	T39.2x4	T39.2x5	T39.2x6
Pyrazolone analgesic NEC	T39.2x1	T39.2x2	T39.2x3	T39.2x4	T39.2x5	T39.2x6
Pyrethrin, pyrethrum (nonmedicinal)	T60.2x1	T60.2x2	T60.2x3	T60.2x4	—	—
Pyrethrum extract	T49.0x1	T49.0x2	T49.0x3	T49.0x4	T49.0x5	T49.0x6
Pyribenzamine	T45.0x1	T45.0x2	T45.0x3	T45.0x4	T45.0x5	T45.0x6
Pyridine	T52.8x1	T52.8x2	T52.8x3	T52.8x4	—	—
aldoxime methiodide	T50.6x1	T50.6x2	T50.6x3	T50.6x4	T50.6x5	T50.6x6
aldoxime methyl chloride	T50.6x1	T50.6x2	T50.6x3	T50.6x4	T50.6x5	T50.6x6
vapor	T59.891	T59.892	T59.893	T59.894	—	—
Pyridium	T39.8x1	T39.8x2	T39.8x3	T39.8x4	T39.8x5	T39.8x6
Pyridostigmine bromide	T44.0x1	T44.0x2	T44.0x3	T44.0x4	T44.0x5	T44.0x6
Pyridoxal phosphate	T45.2x1	T45.2x2	T45.2x3	T45.2x4	T45.2x5	T45.2x6
Pyridoxine	T45.2x1	T45.2x2	T45.2x3	T45.2x4	T45.2x5	T45.2x6
Pyrilamine	T45.0x1	T45.0x2	T45.0x3	T45.0x4	T45.0x5	T45.0x6
Pyrimethamine	T37.2x1	T37.2x2	T37.2x3	T37.2x4	T37.2x5	T37.2x6
with sulfadoxine	T37.2x1	T37.2x2	T37.2x3	T37.2x4	T37.2x5	T37.2x6
Pyrimidine antagonist	T45.1x1	T45.1x2	T45.1x3	T45.1x4	T45.1x5	T45.1x6
Pyriminil	T60.4x1	T60.4x2	T60.4x3	T60.4x4	—	—
Pyrithione zinc	T49.4x1	T49.4x2	T49.4x3	T49.4x4	T49.4x5	T49.4x6
Pyrithyldione	T42.6x1	T42.6x2	T42.6x3	T42.6x4	T42.6x5	T42.6x6
Pyrogallic acid	T49.0x1	T49.0x2	T49.0x3	T49.0x4	T49.0x5	T49.0x6
Pyrogallol	T49.0x1	T49.0x2	T49.0x3	T49.0x4	T49.0x5	T49.0x6
Pyroxylin	T49.3x1	T49.3x2	T49.3x3	T49.3x4	T49.3x5	T49.3x6
Pyrrobutamine	T45.0x1	T45.0x2	T45.0x3	T45.0x4	T45.0x5	T45.0x6
Pyrrolizidine alkaloids	T62.8x1	T62.8x2	T62.8x3	T62.8x4	—	—
Pyrvinium chloride	T37.4x1	T37.4x2	T37.4x3	T37.4x4	T37.4x5	T37.4x6
PZI	T38.3x1	T38.3x2	T38.3x3	T38.3x4	T38.3x5	T38.3x6

Table of Drugs & Chemicals	Poisoning Accidental (Unintentional)	Poisoning Self-Harm (Intentional)	Poisoning Assault	Poisoning Undetermined	Adverse Effect	Underdosing
Quaalude	T42.6x1	T42.6x2	T42.6x3	T42.6x4	T42.6x5	T42.6x6
Quarternary ammonium						
anti-infective	T49.0x1	T49.0x2	T49.0x3	T49.0x4	T49.0x5	T49.0x6
ganglion blocking	T44.2x1	T44.2x2	T44.2x3	T44.2x4	T44.2x5	T44.2x6
parasympatholytic	T44.3x1	T44.3x2	T44.3x3	T44.3x4	T44.3x5	T44.3x6
Quazepam	T42.4x1	T42.4x2	T42.4x3	T42.4x4	T42.4x5	T42.4x6
Quicklime	T54.3x1	T54.3x2	T54.3x3	T54.3x4	—	—
Quillaja extract	T48.4x1	T48.4x2	T48.4x3	T48.4x4	T48.4x5	T48.4x6
Quinacrine	T37.2x1	T37.2x2	T37.2x3	T37.2x4	T37.2x5	T37.2x6
Quinaglute	T46.2x1	T46.2x2	T46.2x3	T46.2x4	T46.2x5	T46.2x6
Quinalbarbital	T42.3x1	T42.3x2	T42.3x3	T42.3x4	T42.3x5	T42.3x6
Quinalbarbitone sodium	T42.3x1	T42.3x2	T42.3x3	T42.3x4	T42.3x5	T42.3x6
Quinalphos	T60.0x1	T60.0x2	T60.0x3	T60.0x4	—	—
Quinapril	T46.4x1	T46.4x2	T46.4x3	T46.4x4	T46.4x5	T46.4x6
Quinestradiol	T38.5x1	T38.5x2	T38.5x3	T38.5x4	T38.5x5	T38.5x6
Quinestradol	T38.5x1	T38.5x2	T38.5x3	T38.5x4	T38.5x5	T38.5x6
Quinestrol	T38.5x1	T38.5x2	T38.5x3	T38.5x4	T38.5x5	T38.5x6
Quinethazone	T50.2x1	T50.2x2	T50.2x3	T50.2x4	T50.2x5	T50.2x6
Quingestanol	T38.4x1	T38.4x2	T38.4x3	T38.4x4	T38.4x5	T38.4x6
Quinidine	T46.2x1	T46.2x2	T46.2x3	T46.2x4	T46.2x5	T46.2x6
Quinine	T37.2x1	T37.2x2	T37.2x3	T37.2x4	T37.2x5	T37.2x6
Quiniobine	T37.8x1	T37.8x2	T37.8x3	T37.8x4	T37.8x5	T37.8x6
Quinisocaine	T49.1x1	T49.1x2	T49.1x3	T49.1x4	T49.1x5	T49.1x6
Quinocide	T37.2x1	T37.2x2	T37.2x3	T37.2x4	T37.2x5	T37.2x6
Quinoline (derivatives) NEC	T37.8x1	T37.8x2	T37.8x3	T37.8x4	T37.8x5	T37.8x6
Quinupramine	T43.011	T43.012	T43.013	T43.014	T43.015	T43.016
Quotane	T41.3x1	T41.3x2	T41.3x3	T41.3x4	T41.3x5	T41.3x6
Rabies						
immune globulin (human)	T50.Z11	T50.Z12	T50.Z13	T50.Z14	T50.Z15	T50.Z16
vaccine	T50.B91	T50.B92	T50.B93	T50.B94	T50.B95	T50.B96
Racemoramide	T40.2x1	T40.2x2	T40.2x3	T40.2x4	—	—
Racemorphan	T40.2x1	T40.2x2	T40.2x3	T40.2x4	T40.2x5	T40.2x6
Racepinefrin	T44.5x1	T44.5x2	T44.5x3	T44.5x4	T44.5x5	T44.5x6
Raclopride	T43.591	T43.592	T43.593	T43.594	T43.595	T43.596
Radiator alcohol	T51.1x1	T51.1x2	T51.1x3	T51.1x4	—	—
Radioactive drug NEC	T50.8x1	T50.8x2	T50.8x3	T50.8x4	T50.8x5	T50.8x6
Radio-opaque (drugs) (materials)	T50.8x1	T50.8x2	T50.8x3	T50.8x4	T50.8x5	T50.8x6
Ramifenazone	T39.2x1	T39.2x2	T39.2x3	T39.2x4	T39.2x5	T39.2x6
Ramipril	T46.4x1	T46.4x2	T46.4x3	T46.4x4	T46.4x5	T46.4x6
Ranitidine	T47.0x1	T47.0x2	T47.0x3	T47.0x4	T47.0x5	T47.0x6
Ranunculus	T62.2x1	T62.2x2	T62.2x3	T62.2x4	—	—
Rat poison NEC	T60.4x1	T60.4x2	T60.4x3	T60.4x4	—	—
Rattlesnake (venom)	T63.011	T63.012	T63.013	T63.014	—	—
Raubasine	T46.7x1	T46.7x2	T46.7x3	T46.7x4	T46.7x5	T46.7x6
Raudixin	T46.5x1	T46.5x2	T46.5x3	T46.5x4	T46.5x5	T46.5x6
Rautensin	T46.5x1	T46.5x2	T46.5x3	T46.5x4	T46.5x5	T46.5x6
Rautina	T46.5x1	T46.5x2	T46.5x3	T46.5x4	T46.5x5	T46.5x6
Rautotal	T46.5x1	T46.5x2	T46.5x3	T46.5x4	T46.5x5	T46.5x6
Rauwiloid	T46.5x1	T46.5x2	T46.5x3	T46.5x4	T46.5x5	T46.5x6
Rauwoldin	T46.5x1	T46.5x2	T46.5x3	T46.5x4	T46.5x5	T46.5x6
Rauwolfia (alkaloids)	T46.5x1	T46.5x2	T46.5x3	T46.5x4	T46.5x5	T46.5x6
Razoxane	T45.1x1	T45.1x2	T45.1x3	T45.1x4	T45.1x5	T45.1x6
Realgar	T57.0x1	T57.0x2	T57.0x3	T57.0x4	—	—
Recombinant (R) — see specific						
protein						
Red blood cells, packed	T45.8x1	T45.8x2	T45.8x3	T45.8x4	T45.8x5	T45.8x6
Red squill (scilliroside)	T60.4x1	T60.4x2	T60.4x3	T60.4x4	—	—
Reducing agent, industrial NEC	T65.891	T65.892	T65.893	T65.894	—	—
Refrigerant gas						
(chlorofluoro-carbon)	T53.5x1	T53.5x2	T53.5x3	T53.5x4	—	—
not chlorofluoro-carbon	T59.891	T59.892	T59.893	T59.894	—	—
Regroton	T50.2x1	T50.2x2	T50.2x3	T50.2x4	T50.2x5	T50.2x6
Rehydration salts (oral)	T50.3x1	T50.3x2	T50.3x3	T50.3x4	T50.3x5	T50.3x6
Rela	T42.8x1	T42.8x2	T42.8x3	T42.8x4	T42.8x5	T42.8x6
Relaxant, muscle						
anesthetic	T48.1x1	T48.1x2	T48.1x3	T48.1x4	T48.1x5	T48.1x6
central nervous system	T42.8x1	T42.8x2	T42.8x3	T42.8x4	T42.8x5	T42.8x6
skeletal NEC	T48.1x1	T48.1x2	T48.1x3	T48.1x4	T48.1x5	T48.1x6
smooth NEC	T44.3x1	T44.3x2	T44.3x3	T44.3x4	T44.3x5	T44.3x6

DRUGS&CHEMICALS

Table of Drugs & Chemicals	Poisoning Accidental (Unintentional)	Poisoning Self-Harm (Intentional)	Poisoning Assault	Poisoning Undetermined	Adverse Effect	Underdosing
Remoxipride	T43.591	T43.592	T43.593	T43.594	T43.595	T43.596
Renese	T50.2x1	T50.2x2	T50.2x3	T50.2x4	T50.2x5	T50.2x6
Renografin	T50.8x1	T50.8x2	T50.8x3	T50.8x4	T50.8x5	T50.8x6
Replacement solution	T50.3x1	T50.3x2	T50.3x3	T50.3x4	T50.3x5	T50.3x6
Reproterol	T48.6x1	T48.6x2	T48.6x3	T48.6x4	T48.6x5	T48.6x6
Rescinnamine	T46.5x1	T46.5x2	T46.5x3	T46.5x4	T46.5x5	T46.5x6
Reserpin(e)	T46.5x1	T46.5x2	T46.5x3	T46.5x4	T46.5x5	T46.5x6
Resorcin, resorcinol (nonmedicinal)	T65.891	T65.892	T65.893	T65.894	—	—
medicinal	T49.4x1	T49.4x2	T49.4x3	T49.4x4	T49.4x5	T49.4x6
Respaire	T48.4x1	T48.4x2	T48.4x3	T48.4x4	T48.4x5	T48.4x6
Respiratory drug NEC	T48.901	T48.902	T48.903	T48.904	T48.905	T48.906
antiasthmatic NEC	T48.6x1	T48.6x2	T48.6x3	T48.6x4	T48.6x5	T48.6x6
anti-common-cold NEC	T48.5x1	T48.5x2	T48.5x3	T48.5x4	T48.5x5	T48.5x6
expectorant NEC	T48.4x1	T48.4x2	T48.4x3	T48.4x4	T48.4x5	T48.4x6
stimulant	T48.901	T48.902	T48.903	T48.904	T48.905	T48.906
Retinoic acid	T49.0x1	T49.0x2	T49.0x3	T49.0x4	T49.0x5	T49.0x6
Retinol	T45.2x1	T45.2x2	T45.2x3	T45.2x4	T45.2x5	T45.2x6
Rh (D) immune globulin (human)	T50.Z11	T50.Z12	T50.Z13	T50.Z14	T50.Z15	T50.Z16
Rhodine	T39.011	T39.012	T39.013	T39.014	T39.015	T39.016
RhoGAM	T50.Z11	T50.Z12	T50.Z13	T50.Z14	T50.Z15	T50.Z16
Rhubarb						
dry extract	T47.2x1	T47.2x2	T47.2x3	T47.2x4	T47.2x5	T47.2x6
tincture, compound	T47.2x1	T47.2x2	T47.2x3	T47.2x4	T47.2x5	T47.2x6
Ribavirin	T37.5x1	T37.5x2	T37.5x3	T37.5x4	T37.5x5	T37.5x6
Riboflavin	T45.2x1	T45.2x2	T45.2x3	T45.2x4	T45.2x5	T45.2x6
Ribostamycin	T36.5x1	T36.5x2	T36.5x3	T36.5x4	T36.5x5	T36.5x6
Ricin	T62.2x1	T62.2x2	T62.2x3	T62.2x4	—	—
Ricinus communis	T62.2x1	T62.2x2	T62.2x3	T62.2x4	—	—
Rickettsial vaccine NEC	T50.A91	T50.A92	T50.A93	T50.A94	T50.A95	T50.A96
Rifabutin	T36.6x1	T36.6x2	T36.6x3	T36.6x4	T36.6x5	T36.6x6
Rifamide	T36.6x1	T36.6x2	T36.6x3	T36.6x4	T36.6x5	T36.6x6
Rifampicin	T36.6x1	T36.6x2	T36.6x3	T36.6x4	T36.6x5	T36.6x6
with isoniazid	T37.1x1	T37.1x2	T37.1x3	T37.1x4	T37.1x5	T37.1x6
Rifampin	T36.6x1	T36.6x2	T36.6x3	T36.6x4	T36.6x5	T36.6x6
Rifamycin	T36.6x1	T36.6x2	T36.6x3	T36.6x4	T36.6x5	T36.6x6
Rifaximin	T36.6x1	T36.6x2	T36.6x3	T36.6x4	T36.6x5	T36.6x6
Rimantadine	T37.5x1	T37.5x2	T37.5x3	T37.5x4	T37.5x5	T37.5x6
Rimazolium metilsulfate	T39.8x1	T39.8x2	T39.8x3	T39.8x4	T39.8x5	T39.8x6
Rimifon	T37.1x1	T37.1x2	T37.1x3	T37.1x4	T37.1x5	T37.1x6
Rimiterol	T48.6x1	T48.6x2	T48.6x3	T48.6x4	T48.6x5	T48.6x6
Ringer (lactate) solution	T50.3x1	T50.3x2	T50.3x3	T50.3x4	T50.3x5	T50.3x6
Ristocetin	T36.8x1	T36.8x2	T36.8x3	T36.8x4	T36.8x5	T36.8x6
Ritalin	T43.631	T43.632	T43.633	T43.634	T43.635	T43.636
Ritodrine	T44.5x1	T44.5x2	T44.5x3	T44.5x4	T44.5x5	T44.5x6
Roach killer — see Insecticide						
Rociverine	T44.3x1	T44.3x2	T44.3x3	T44.3x4	T44.3x5	T44.3x6
Rocky Mountain spotted fever vaccine	T50.A91	T50.A92	T50.A93	T50.A94	T50.A95	T50.A96
Rodenticide NEC	T60.4x1	T60.4x2	T60.4x3	T60.4x4	—	—
Rohypnol	T42.4x1	T42.4x2	T42.4x3	T42.4x4	T42.4x5	T42.4x6
Rokitamycin	T36.3x1	T36.3x2	T36.3x3	T36.3x4	T36.3x5	T36.3x6
Rolaids	T47.1x1	T47.1x2	T47.1x3	T47.1x4	T47.1x5	T47.1x6
Rolitetracycline	T36.4x1	T36.4x2	T36.4x3	T36.4x4	T36.4x5	T36.4x6
Romilar	T48.3x1	T48.3x2	T48.3x3	T48.3x4	T48.3x5	T48.3x6
Ronifibrate	T46.6x1	T46.6x2	T46.6x3	T46.6x4	T46.6x5	T46.6x6
Rosaprostol	T47.1x1	T47.1x2	T47.1x3	T47.1x4	T47.1x5	T47.1x6
Rose bengal sodium (131I)	T50.8x1	T50.8x2	T50.8x3	T50.8x4	T50.8x5	T50.8x6
Rose water ointment	T49.3x1	T49.3x2	T49.3x3	T49.3x4	T49.3x5	T49.3x6
Rosoxacin	T37.8x1	T37.8x2	T37.8x3	T37.8x4	T37.8x5	T37.8x6
Rotenone	T60.2x1	T60.2x2	T60.2x3	T60.2x4	—	—
Rotoxamine	T45.0x1	T45.0x2	T45.0x3	T45.0x4	T45.0x5	T45.0x6
Rough-on-rats	T60.4x1	T60.4x2	T60.4x3	T60.4x4	—	—
Roxatidine	T47.0x1	T47.0x2	T47.0x3	T47.0x4	T47.0x5	T47.0x6
Roxithromycin	T36.3x1	T36.3x2	T36.3x3	T36.3x4	T36.3x5	T36.3x6
Rt-PA	T45.611	T45.612	T45.613	T45.614	T45.615	T45.616
Rubbing alcohol	T51.2x1	T51.2x2	T51.2x3	T51.2x4	—	—
Rubefacient	T49.4x1	T49.4x2	T49.4x3	T49.4x4	T49.4x5	T49.4x6
Rubella vaccine	T50.B91	T50.B92	T50.B93	T50.B94	T50.B95	T50.B96
Rubeola vaccine	T50.B91	T50.B92	T50.B93	T50.B94	T50.B95	T50.B96
Rubidium chloride Rb82	T50.8x1	T50.8x2	T50.8x3	T50.8x4	T50.8x5	T50.8x6
Rubidomycin	T45.1x1	T45.1x2	T45.1x3	T45.1x4	T45.1x5	T45.1x6
Rue	T62.2x1	T62.2x2	T62.2x3	T62.2x4	—	—
Rufocromomycin	T45.1x1	T45.1x2	T45.1x3	T45.1x4	T45.1x5	T45.1x6
Russel's viper venin	T45.7x1	T45.7x2	T45.7x3	T45.7x4	T45.7x5	T45.7x6
Ruta (graveolens)	T62.2x1	T62.2x2	T62.2x3	T62.2x4	—	—
Rutinum	T46.991	T46.992	T46.993	T46.994	T46.995	T46.996
Rutoside	T46.991	T46.992	T46.993	T46.994	T46.995	T46.996
Sabadilla (plant)	T62.2x1	T62.2x2	T62.2x3	T62.2x4	—	—
pesticide	T60.2x1	T60.2x2	T60.2x3	T60.2x4	—	—
Saccharated iron oxide	T45.8x1	T45.8x2	T45.8x3	T45.8x4	T45.8x5	T45.8x6
Saccharin	T50.901	T50.902	T50.903	T50.904	T50.905	T50.906
Saccharomyces boulardii	T47.6x1	T47.6x2	T47.6x3	T47.6x4	T47.6x5	T47.6x6
Safflower oil	T46.6x1	T46.6x2	T46.6x3	T46.6x4	T46.6x5	T46.6x6
Safrazine	T43.1x1	T43.1x2	T43.1x3	T43.1x4	T43.1x5	T43.1x6
Salazosulfapyridine	T37.0x1	T37.0x2	T37.0x3	T37.0x4	T37.0x5	T37.0x6
Salbutamol	T48.6x1	T48.6x2	T48.6x3	T48.6x4	T48.6x5	T48.6x6
Salicylamide	T39.091	T39.092	T39.093	T39.094	T39.095	T39.096
Salicylate NEC	T39.091	T39.092	T39.093	T39.094	T39.095	T39.096
methyl	T49.3x1	T49.3x2	T49.3x3	T49.3x4	T49.3x5	T49.3x6
theobromine calcium	T50.2x1	T50.2x2	T50.2x3	T50.2x4	T50.2x5	T50.2x6
Salicylazosulfapyridine	T37.0x1	T37.0x2	T37.0x3	T37.0x4	T37.0x5	T37.0x6
Salicylhydroxamic acid	T49.0x1	T49.0x2	T49.0x3	T49.0x4	T49.0x5	T49.0x6
Salicylic acid	T49.4x1	T49.4x2	T49.4x3	T49.4x4	T49.4x5	T49.4x6
with benzoic acid	T49.4x1	T49.4x2	T49.4x3	T49.4x4	T49.4x5	T49.4x6
congeners	T39.091	T39.092	T39.093	T39.094	T39.095	T39.096
derivative	T39.091	T39.092	T39.093	T39.094	T39.095	T39.096
salts	T39.091	T39.092	T39.093	T39.094	T39.095	T39.096
Salinazid	T37.1x1	T37.1x2	T37.1x3	T37.1x4	T37.1x5	T37.1x6
Salmeterol	T48.6x1	T48.6x2	T48.6x3	T48.6x4	T48.6x5	T48.6x6
Salol	T49.3x1	T49.3x2	T49.3x3	T49.3x4	T49.3x5	T49.3x6
Salsalate	T39.091	T39.092	T39.093	T39.094	T39.095	T39.096
Salt substitute	T50.901	T50.902	T50.903	T50.904	T50.905	T50.906
Salt-replacing drug	T50.901	T50.902	T50.903	T50.904	T50.905	T50.906
Salt-retaining mineralocorticoid	T50.0x1	T50.0x2	T50.0x3	T50.0x4	T50.0x5	T50.0x6
Saluretic NEC	T50.2x1	T50.2x2	T50.2x3	T50.2x4	T50.2x5	T50.2x6
Saluron	T50.2x1	T50.2x2	T50.2x3	T50.2x4	T50.2x5	T50.2x6
Salvarsan 606 (neosilver) (silver)	T37.8x1	T37.8x2	T37.8x3	T37.8x4	T37.8x5	T37.8x6
Sambucus canadensis	T62.2x1	T62.2x2	T62.2x3	T62.2x4	—	—
berry	T62.1x1	T62.1x2	T62.1x3	T62.1x4	—	—
Sandril	T46.5x1	T46.5x2	T46.5x3	T46.5x4	T46.5x5	T46.5x6
Sanguinaria canadensis	T62.2x1	T62.2x2	T62.2x3	T62.2x4	—	—
Saniflush (cleaner)	T54.2x1	T54.2x2	T54.2x3	T54.2x4	—	—
Santonin	T37.4x1	T37.4x2	T37.4x3	T37.4x4	T37.4x5	T37.4x6
Santyl	T49.8x1	T49.8x2	T49.8x3	T49.8x4	T49.8x5	T49.8x6
Saralasin	T46.5x1	T46.5x2	T46.5x3	T46.5x4	T46.5x5	T46.5x6
Sarcolysin	T45.1x1	T45.1x2	T45.1x3	T45.1x4	T45.1x5	T45.1x6
Sarkomycin	T45.1x1	T45.1x2	T45.1x3	T45.1x4	T45.1x5	T45.1x6
Saroten	T43.011	T43.012	T43.013	T43.014	T43.015	T43.016
Saturnine — see Lead						
Savin (oil)	T49.4x1	T49.4x2	T49.4x3	T49.4x4	T49.4x5	T49.4x6
Scammony	T47.2x1	T47.2x2	T47.2x3	T47.2x4	T47.2x5	T47.2x6
Scarlet red	T49.8x1	T49.8x2	T49.8x3	T49.8x4	T49.8x5	T49.8x6
Scheele's green	T57.0x1	T57.0x2	T57.0x3	T57.0x4	—	—
insecticide	T57.0x1	T57.0x2	T57.0x3	T57.0x4	—	—
Schizontozide (blood) (tissue)	T37.2x1	T37.2x2	T37.2x3	T37.2x4	T37.2x5	T37.2x6
Schradan	T60.0x1	T60.0x2	T60.0x3	T60.0x4	—	—
Schweinfurth green	T57.0x1	T57.0x2	T57.0x3	T57.0x4	—	—
insecticide	T57.0x1	T57.0x2	T57.0x3	T57.0x4	—	—
Scilla, rat poison	T60.4x1	T60.4x2	T60.4x3	T60.4x4	—	—
Scillaren	T60.4x1	T60.4x2	T60.4x3	T60.4x4	—	—
Sclerosing agent	T46.8x1	T46.8x2	T46.8x3	T46.8x4	T46.8x5	T46.8x6
Scombrotoxin	T61.11	T61.12	T61.13	T61.14	—	—
Scopolamine	T44.3x1	T44.3x2	T44.3x3	T44.3x4	T44.3x5	T44.3x6
Scopolia extract	T44.3x1	T44.3x2	T44.3x3	T44.3x4	T44.3x5	T44.3x6

DRUGS&CHEMICALS

Table of Drugs & Chemicals	POISONING Accidental (Unintentional)	Self-Harm (Intentional)	Assault	Undetermined	Adverse Effect	Underdosing
Scouring powder	T65.891	T65.892	T65.893	T65.894	—	—
Sea						
anemone (sting)	T63.631	T63.632	T63.633	T63.634	—	—
cucumber (sting)	T63.691	T63.692	T63.693	T63.694	—	—
snake (bite) (venom)	T63.091	T63.092	T63.093	T63.094	—	—
urchin spine (puncture)	T63.691	T63.692	T63.693	T63.694	—	—
Seafood	T61.91	T61.92	T61.93	T61.94	—	—
specified NEC	T61.8x1	T61.8x2	T61.8x3	T61.8x4	—	—
Secbutabarbital	T42.3x1	T42.3x2	T42.3x3	T42.3x4	T42.3x5	T42.3x6
Secbutabarbitone	T42.3x1	T42.3x2	T42.3x3	T42.3x4	T42.3x5	T42.3x6
Secnidazole	T37.3x1	T37.3x2	T37.3x3	T37.3x4	T37.3x5	T37.3x6
Secobarbital	T42.3x1	T42.3x2	T42.3x3	T42.3x4	T42.3x5	T42.3x6
Seconal	T42.3x1	T42.3x2	T42.3x3	T42.3x4	T42.3x5	T42.3x6
Secretin	T50.8x1	T50.8x2	T50.8x3	T50.8x4	T50.8x5	T50.8x6
Sedative NEC	T42.71	T42.72	T42.73	T42.74	T42.75	T42.76
mixed NEC	T42.6x1	T42.6x2	T42.6x3	T42.6x4	T42.6x5	T42.6x6
Sedormid	T42.6x1	T42.6x2	T42.6x3	T42.6x4	T42.6x5	T42.6x6
Seed disinfectant or dressing	T60.8x1	T60.8x2	T60.8x3	T60.8x4	—	—
Seeds (poisonous)	T62.2x1	T62.2x2	T62.2x3	T62.2x4	—	—
Selegiline	T42.8x1	T42.8x2	T42.8x3	T42.8x4	T42.8x5	T42.8x6
Selenium NEC	T56.891	T56.892	T56.893	T56.894	—	—
disulfide or sulfide	T49.4x1	T49.4x2	T49.4x3	T49.4x4	T49.4x5	T49.4x6
fumes	T59.891	T59.892	T59.893	T59.894	—	—
sulfide	T49.4x1	T49.4x2	T49.4x3	T49.4x4	T49.4x5	T49.4x6
Selenomethionine (75Se)	T50.8x1	T50.8x2	T50.8x3	T50.8x4	T50.8x5	T50.8x6
Selsun	T49.4x1	T49.4x2	T49.4x3	T49.4x4	T49.4x5	T49.4x6
Semustine	T45.1x1	T45.1x2	T45.1x3	T45.1x4	T45.1x5	T45.1x6
Senega syrup	T48.4x1	T48.4x2	T48.4x3	T48.4x4	T48.4x5	T48.4x6
Senna	T47.2x1	T47.2x2	T47.2x3	T47.2x4	T47.2x5	T47.2x6
Sennoside A+B	T47.2x1	T47.2x2	T47.2x3	T47.2x4	T47.2x5	T47.2x6
Septisol	T49.2x1	T49.2x2	T49.2x3	T49.2x4	T49.2x5	T49.2x6
Seractide	T38.811	T38.812	T38.813	T38.814	T38.815	T38.816
Serax	T42.4x1	T42.4x2	T42.4x3	T42.4x4	T42.4x5	T42.4x6
Serenesil	T42.6x1	T42.6x2	T42.6x3	T42.6x4	T42.6x5	T42.6x6
Serenium (hydrochloride)	T37.91	T37.92	T37.93	T37.94	T37.95	T37.96
Serepax — see Oxazepam						
Sermorelin	T38.891	T38.892	T38.893	T38.894	T38.895	T38.896
Sernyl	T41.1x1	T41.1x2	T41.1x3	T41.1x4	T41.1x5	T41.1x6
Serotonin	T50.991	T50.992	T50.993	T50.994	T50.995	T50.996
Serpasil	T46.5x1	T46.5x2	T46.5x3	T46.5x4	T46.5x5	T46.5x6
Serrapeptase	T45.3x1	T45.3x2	T45.3x3	T45.3x4	T45.3x5	T45.3x6
Serum						
antibotulinus	T50.Z11	T50.Z12	T50.Z13	T50.Z14	T50.Z15	T50.Z16
anticytotoxic	T50.Z11	T50.Z12	T50.Z13	T50.Z14	T50.Z15	T50.Z16
antidiphtheria	T50.Z11	T50.Z12	T50.Z13	T50.Z14	T50.Z15	T50.Z16
antimeningococcus	T50.Z11	T50.Z12	T50.Z13	T50.Z14	T50.Z15	T50.Z16
anti-Rh	T50.Z11	T50.Z12	T50.Z13	T50.Z14	T50.Z15	T50.Z16
anti-snake-bite	T50.Z11	T50.Z12	T50.Z13	T50.Z14	T50.Z15	T50.Z16
antitetanic	T50.Z11	T50.Z12	T50.Z13	T50.Z14	T50.Z15	T50.Z16
antitoxic	T50.Z11	T50.Z12	T50.Z13	T50.Z14	T50.Z15	T50.Z16
complement (inhibitor)	T45.8x1	T45.8x2	T45.8x3	T45.8x4	T45.8x5	T45.8x6
convalescent	T50.Z11	T50.Z12	T50.Z13	T50.Z14	T50.Z15	T50.Z16
hemolytic complement	T45.8x1	T45.8x2	T45.8x3	T45.8x4	T45.8x5	T45.8x6
immune (human)	T50.Z11	T50.Z12	T50.Z13	T50.Z14	T50.Z15	T50.Z16
protective NEC	T50.Z11	T50.Z12	T50.Z13	T50.Z14	T50.Z15	T50.Z16
Setastine	T45.0x1	T45.0x2	T45.0x3	T45.0x4	T45.0x5	T45.0x6
Setoperone	T43.591	T43.592	T43.593	T43.594	T43.595	T43.596
Sewer gas	T59.91	T59.92	T59.93	T59.94	—	—
Shampoo	T55.0x1	T55.0x2	T55.0x3	T55.0x4	—	—
Shellfish, noxious, nonbacterial	T61.781	T61.782	T61.783	T61.784	—	—
Sildenafil	T46.7x1	T46.7x2	T46.7x3	T46.7x4	T46.7x5	T46.7x6
Silibinin	T50.991	T50.992	T50.993	T50.994	T50.995	T50.996
Silicone NEC	T65.891	T65.892	T65.893	T65.894	—	—
medicinal	T49.3x1	T49.3x2	T49.3x3	T49.3x4	T49.3x5	T49.3x6
Silvadene	T49.0x1	T49.0x2	T49.0x3	T49.0x4	T49.0x5	T49.0x6
Silver	T49.0x1	T49.0x2	T49.0x3	T49.0x4	T49.0x5	T49.0x6
anti-infectives	T49.0x1	T49.0x2	T49.0x3	T49.0x4	T49.0x5	T49.0x6
arsphenamine	T37.8x1	T37.8x2	T37.8x3	T37.8x4	T37.8x5	T37.8x6
colloidal	T49.0x1	T49.0x2	T49.0x3	T49.0x4	T49.0x5	T49.0x6
nitrate	T49.0x1	T49.0x2	T49.0x3	T49.0x4	T49.0x5	T49.0x6
ophthalmic preparation	T49.5x1	T49.5x2	T49.5x3	T49.5x4	T49.5x5	T49.5x6
toughened (keratolytic)	T49.4x1	T49.4x2	T49.4x3	T49.4x4	T49.4x5	T49.4x6
nonmedicinal (dust)	T56.891	T56.892	T56.893	T56.894	—	—
protein	T49.5x1	T49.5x2	T49.5x3	T49.5x4	T49.5x5	T49.5x6
salvarsan	T37.8x1	T37.8x2	T37.8x3	T37.8x4	T37.8x5	T37.8x6
sulfadiazine	T49.4x1	T49.4x2	T49.4x3	T49.4x4	T49.4x5	T49.4x6
Silymarin	T50.991	T50.992	T50.993	T50.994	T50.995	T50.996
Simaldrate	T47.1x1	T47.1x2	T47.1x3	T47.1x4	T47.1x5	T47.1x6
Simazine	T60.3x1	T60.3x2	T60.3x3	T60.3x4	—	—
Simethicone	T47.1x1	T47.1x2	T47.1x3	T47.1x4	T47.1x5	T47.1x6
Simfibrate	T46.6x1	T46.6x2	T46.6x3	T46.6x4	T46.6x5	T46.6x6
Simvastatin	T46.6x1	T46.6x2	T46.6x3	T46.6x4	T46.6x5	T46.6x6
Sincalide	T50.8x1	T50.8x2	T50.8x3	T50.8x4	T50.8x5	T50.8x6
Sinequan	T43.011	T43.012	T43.013	T43.014	T43.015	T43.016
Singoserp	T46.5x1	T46.5x2	T46.5x3	T46.5x4	T46.5x5	T46.5x6
Sintrom	T45.511	T45.512	T45.513	T45.514	T45.515	T45.516
Sisomicin	T36.5x1	T36.5x2	T36.5x3	T36.5x4	T36.5x5	T36.5x6
Sitosterols	T46.6x1	T46.6x2	T46.6x3	T46.6x4	T46.6x5	T46.6x6
Skeletal muscle relaxants	T48.1x1	T48.1x2	T48.1x3	T48.1x4	T48.1x5	T48.1x6
Skin						
agents (external)	T49.91	T49.92	T49.93	T49.94	T49.95	T49.96
specified NEC	T49.8x1	T49.8x2	T49.8x3	T49.8x4	T49.8x5	T49.8x6
test antigen	T50.8x1	T50.8x2	T50.8x3	T50.8x4	T50.8x5	T50.8x6
Sleep-eze	T45.0x1	T45.0x2	T45.0x3	T45.0x4	T45.0x5	T45.0x6
Sleeping draught, pill	T42.71	T42.72	T42.73	T42.74	T42.75	T42.76
Smallpox vaccine	T50.B11	T50.B12	T50.B13	T50.B14	T50.B15	T50.B16
Smelter fumes NEC	T56.91	T56.92	T56.93	T56.94	—	—
Smog	T59.1x1	T59.1x2	T59.1x3	T59.1x4	—	—
Smoke NEC	T59.811	T59.812	T59.813	T59.814	—	—
Smooth muscle relaxant	T44.3x1	T44.3x2	T44.3x3	T44.3x4	T44.3x5	T44.3x6
Snail killer NEC	T60.8x1	T60.8x2	T60.8x3	T60.8x4	—	—
Snake venom or bite	T63.001	T63.002	T63.003	T63.004	—	—
hemocoagulase	T45.7x1	T45.7x2	T45.7x3	T45.7x4	T45.7x5	T45.7x6
Snuff	T65.211	T65.212	T65.213	T65.214	—	—
Soap (powder) (product)	T55.0x1	T55.0x2	T55.0x3	T55.0x4	—	—
enema	T47.4x1	T47.4x2	T47.4x3	T47.4x4	T47.4x5	T47.4x6
medicinal, soft	T49.2x1	T49.2x2	T49.2x3	T49.2x4	T49.2x5	T49.2x6
superfatted	T49.2x1	T49.2x2	T49.2x3	T49.2x4	T49.2x5	T49.2x6
Sobrerol	T48.4x1	T48.4x2	T48.4x3	T48.4x4	T48.4x5	T48.4x6
Soda (caustic)	T54.3x1	T54.3x2	T54.3x3	T54.3x4	—	—
bicarb	T47.1x1	T47.1x2	T47.1x3	T47.1x4	T47.1x5	T47.1x6
chlorinated — see Sodium, hypochlorite						
Sodium						
l-triiodothyronine	T38.1x1	T38.1x2	T38.1x3	T38.1x4	T38.1x5	T38.1x6
acetosulfone	T37.1x1	T37.1x2	T37.1x3	T37.1x4	T37.1x5	T37.1x6
acetrizoate	T50.8x1	T50.8x2	T50.8x3	T50.8x4	T50.8x5	T50.8x6
acid phosphate	T50.3x1	T50.3x2	T50.3x3	T50.3x4	T50.3x5	T50.3x6
alginate	T47.8x1	T47.8x2	T47.8x3	T47.8x4	T47.8x5	T47.8x6
amidotrizoate	T50.8x1	T50.8x2	T50.8x3	T50.8x4	T50.8x5	T50.8x6
aminopterin	T45.1x1	T45.1x2	T45.1x3	T45.1x4	T45.1x5	T45.1x6
amylosulfate	T47.8x1	T47.8x2	T47.8x3	T47.8x4	T47.8x5	T47.8x6
amytal	T42.3x1	T42.3x2	T42.3x3	T42.3x4	T42.3x5	T42.3x6
antimony gluconate	T37.3x1	T37.3x2	T37.3x3	T37.3x4	T37.3x5	T37.3x6
arsenate	T57.0x1	T57.0x2	T57.0x3	T57.0x4	—	—
aurothiomalate	T39.4x1	T39.4x2	T39.4x3	T39.4x4	T39.4x5	T39.4x6
aurothiosulfate	T39.4x1	T39.4x2	T39.4x3	T39.4x4	T39.4x5	T39.4x6
barbiturate	T42.3x1	T42.3x2	T42.3x3	T42.3x4	T42.3x5	T42.3x6
basic phosphate	T47.4x1	T47.4x2	T47.4x3	T47.4x4	T47.4x5	T47.4x6
bicarbonate	T47.1x1	T47.1x2	T47.1x3	T47.1x4	T47.1x5	T47.1x6
bichromate	T57.8x1	T57.8x2	T57.8x3	T57.8x4	—	—
biphosphate	T50.3x1	T50.3x2	T50.3x3	T50.3x4	T50.3x5	T50.3x6
bisulfate	T65.891	T65.892	T65.893	T65.894	—	—

DRUGS&CHEMICALS

Table of Drugs & Chemicals	Accidental (Unintentional)	Self-Harm (Intentional)	Assault	Undetermined	Adverse Effect	Underdosing
Sodium – *continued*						
borate						
cleanser	T57.8x1	T57.8x2	T57.8x3	T57.8x4	—	—
eye	T49.5x1	T49.5x2	T49.5x3	T49.5x4	T49.5x5	T49.5x6
therapeutic	T49.8x1	T49.8x2	T49.8x3	T49.8x4	T49.8x5	T49.8x6
bromide	T42.6x1	T42.6x2	T42.6x3	T42.6x4	T42.6x5	T42.6x6
cacodylate (nonmedicinal) NEC	T50.8x1	T50.8x2	T50.8x3	T50.8x4	T50.8x5	T50.8x6
anti-infective	T37.8x1	T37.8x2	T37.8x3	T37.8x4	T37.8x5	T37.8x6
herbicide	T60.3x1	T60.3x2	T60.3x3	T60.3x4		
calcium edetate	T45.8x1	T45.8x2	T45.8x3	T45.8x4	T45.8x5	
carbonate NEC	T54.3x1	T54.3x2	T54.3x3	T54.3x4	—	—
chlorate NEC	T65.891	T65.892	T65.893	T65.894	—	—
herbicide	T54.91	T54.92	T54.93	T54.94	—	—
chloride	T50.3x1	T50.3x2	T50.3x3	T50.3x4	T50.3x5	T50.3x6
with glucose	T50.3x1	T50.3x2	T50.3x3	T50.3x4	T50.3x5	T50.3x6
chromate	T65.891	T65.892	T65.893	T65.894	—	—
citrate	T50.991	T50.992	T50.993	T50.994	T50.995	T50.996
cromoglicate	T48.6x1	T48.6x2	T48.6x3	T48.6x4	T48.6x5	T48.6x6
cyanide	T65.0x1	T65.0x2	T65.0x3	T65.0x4	—	—
cyclamate	T50.3x1	T50.3x2	T50.3x3	T50.3x4	T50.3x5	T50.3x6
dehydrocholate	T45.8x1	T45.8x2	T45.8x3	T45.8x4	T45.8x5	T45.8x6
diatrizoate	T50.8x1	T50.8x2	T50.8x3	T50.8x4	T50.8x5	T50.8x6
dibunate	T48.4x1	T48.4x2	T48.4x3	T48.4x4	T48.4x5	T48.4x6
dioctyl sulfosuccinate	T47.4x1	T47.4x2	T47.4x3	T47.4x4	T47.4x5	T47.4x6
dipantoyl ferrate	T45.8x1	T45.8x2	T45.8x3	T45.8x4	T45.8x5	T45.8x6
edetate	T45.8x1	T45.8x2	T45.8x3	T45.8x4	T45.8x5	T45.8x6
ethacrynate	T50.1x1	T50.1x2	T50.1x3	T50.1x4	T50.1x5	T50.1x6
feredetate	T45.8x1	T45.8x2	T45.8x3	T45.8x4	T45.8x5	T45.8x6
fluoride — *see* Fluoride						
fluoroacetate (dust) (pesticide)	T60.4x1	T60.4x2	T60.4x3	T60.4x4	—	—
free salt	T50.3x1	T50.3x2	T50.3x3	T50.3x4	T50.3x5	T50.3x6
fusidate	T36.8x1	T36.8x2	T36.8x3	T36.8x4	T36.8x5	T36.8x6
glucaldrate	T47.1x1	T47.1x2	T47.1x3	T47.1x4	T47.1x5	T47.1x6
glucosulfone	T37.1x1	T37.1x2	T37.1x3	T37.1x4	T37.1x5	T37.1x6
glutamate	T45.8x1	T45.8x2	T45.8x3	T45.8x4	T45.8x5	T45.8x6
hydrogen carbonate	T50.3x1	T50.3x2	T50.3x3	T50.3x4	T50.3x5	T50.3x6
hydroxide	T54.3x1	T54.3x2	T54.3x3	T54.3x4	—	—
hypochlorite (bleach) NEC	T54.3x1	T54.3x2	T54.3x3	T54.3x4	—	—
disinfectant	T54.3x1	T54.3x2	T54.3x3	T54.3x4	—	—
medicinal (anti-infective) (external)	T49.0x1	T49.0x2	T49.0x3	T49.0x4	T49.0x5	T49.0x6
vapor	T54.3x1	T54.3x2	T54.3x3	T54.3x4	—	—
hyposulfite	T49.0x1	T49.0x2	T49.0x3	T49.0x4	T49.0x5	T49.0x6
indigotin disulfonate	T50.8x1	T50.8x2	T50.8x3	T50.8x4	T50.8x5	T50.8x6
iodide	T50.991	T50.992	T50.993	T50.994	T50.995	T50.996
I-131	T50.8x1	T50.8x2	T50.8x3	T50.8x4	T50.8x5	T50.8x6
therapeutic	T38.2x1	T38.2x2	T38.2x3	T38.2x4	T38.2x5	T38.2x6
iodohippurate (131I)	T50.8x1	T50.8x2	T50.8x3	T50.8x4	T50.8x5	T50.8x6
iopodate	T50.8x1	T50.8x2	T50.8x3	T50.8x4	T50.8x5	T50.8x6
iothalamate	T50.8x1	T50.8x2	T50.8x3	T50.8x4	T50.8x5	T50.8x6
iron edetate	T45.4x1	T45.4x2	T45.4x3	T45.4x4	T45.4x5	T45.4x6
lactate (compound solution)	T45.8x1	T45.8x2	T45.8x3	T45.8x4	T45.8x5	T45.8x6
lauryl (sulfate)	T49.2x1	T49.2x2	T49.2x3	T49.2x4	T49.2x5	T49.2x6
(L)-triiodothyronine	T38.1x1	T38.1x2	T38.1x3	T38.1x4	T38.1x5	T38.1x6
magnesium citrate	T50.991	T50.992	T50.993	T50.994	T50.995	T50.996
mersalate	T50.2x1	T50.2x2	T50.2x3	T50.2x4	T50.2x5	T50.2x6
metasilicate	T65.891	T65.892	T65.893	T65.894	—	—
metrizoate	T50.8x1	T50.8x2	T50.8x3	T50.8x4	T50.8x5	T50.8x6
monofluoroacetate (pesticide)	T60.1x1	T60.1x2	T60.1x3	T60.1x4	—	—
morrhuate	T46.8x1	T46.8x2	T46.8x3	T46.8x4	T46.8x5	T46.8x6
nafcillin	T36.0x1	T36.0x2	T36.0x3	T36.0x4	T36.0x5	T36.0x6
nitrate (oxidizing agent)	T65.891	T65.892	T65.893	T65.894	—	—
nitrite	T50.6x1	T50.6x2	T50.6x3	T50.6x4	T50.6x5	T50.6x6
nitroferricyanide	T46.5x1	T46.5x2	T46.5x3	T46.5x4	T46.5x5	T46.5x6
nitroprusside	T46.5x1	T46.5x2	T46.5x3	T46.5x4	T46.5x5	T46.5x6
oxalate	T65.891	T65.892	T65.893	T65.894	—	—
oxide/peroxide	T65.891	T65.892	T65.893	T65.894	—	—
oxybate	T41.291	T41.292	T41.293	T41.294	T41.295	T41.296
Sodium – *continued*						
para-aminohippurate	T50.8x1	T50.8x2	T50.8x3	T50.8x4	T50.8x5	T50.8x6
perborate (nonmedicinal) NEC	T65.891	T65.892	T65.893	T65.894		
medicinal	T49.0x1	T49.0x2	T49.0x3	T49.0x4	T49.0x5	T49.0x6
soap	T55.0x1	T55.0x2	T55.0x3	T55.0x4	—	
percarbonate — *see* Sodium, perborate						
pertechnetate Tc99m	T50.8x1	T50.8x2	T50.8x3	T50.8x4	T50.8x5	T50.8x6
phosphate						
cellulose	T45.8x1	T45.8x2	T45.8x3	T45.8x4	T45.8x5	T45.8x6
dibasic	T47.2x1	T47.2x2	T47.2x3	T47.2x4	T47.2x5	T47.2x6
monobasic	T47.2x1	T47.2x2	T47.2x3	T47.2x4	T47.2x5	T47.2x6
phytate	T50.6x1	T50.6x2	T50.6x3	T50.6x4	T50.6x5	T50.6x6
picosulfate	T47.2x1	T47.2x2	T47.2x3	T47.2x4	T47.2x5	T47.2x6
polyhydroxyaluminium monocarbonate	T47.1x1	T47.1x2	T47.1x3	T47.1x4	T47.1x5	T47.1x6
polystyrene sulfonate	T50.3x1	T50.3x2	T50.3x3	T50.3x4	T50.3x5	T50.3x6
propionate	T49.0x1	T49.0x2	T49.0x3	T49.0x4	T49.0x5	T49.0x6
propyl hydroxybenzoate	T50.991	T50.992	T50.993	T50.994	T50.995	T50.996
psylliate	T46.8x1	T46.8x2	T46.8x3	T46.8x4	T46.8x5	T46.8x6
removing resins	T50.3x1	T50.3x2	T50.3x3	T50.3x4	T50.3x5	T50.3x6
salicylate	T39.091	T39.092	T39.093	T39.094	T39.095	T39.096
salt NEC	T50.3x1	T50.3x2	T50.3x3	T50.3x4	T50.3x5	T50.3x6
selenate	T60.2x1	T60.2x2	T60.2x3	T60.2x4		
stibogluconate	T37.3x1	T37.3x2	T37.3x3	T37.3x4	T37.3x5	T37.3x6
sulfate	T47.4x1	T47.4x2	T47.4x3	T47.4x4	T47.4x5	T47.4x6
sulfoxone	T37.1x1	T37.1x2	T37.1x3	T37.1x4	T37.1x5	T37.1x6
tetradecyl sulfate	T46.8x1	T46.8x2	T46.8x3	T46.8x4	T46.8x5	T46.8x6
thiopental	T41.1x1	T41.1x2	T41.1x3	T41.1x4	T41.1x5	T41.1x6
thiosalicylate	T39.091	T39.092	T39.093	T39.094	T39.095	T39.096
thiosulfate	T50.6x1	T50.6x2	T50.6x3	T50.6x4	T50.6x5	T50.6x6
tolbutamide	T38.3x1	T38.3x2	T38.3x3	T38.3x4	T38.3x5	T38.3x6
tyropanoate	T50.8x1	T50.8x2	T50.8x3	T50.8x4	T50.8x5	T50.8x6
valproate	T42.6x1	T42.6x2	T42.6x3	T42.6x4	T42.6x5	T42.6x6
versenate	T50.6x1	T50.6x2	T50.6x3	T50.6x4	T50.6x5	T50.6x6
Sodium-free salt	T50.901	T50.902	T50.903	T50.904	T50.905	T50.906
Sodium-removing resin	T50.3x1	T50.3x2	T50.3x3	T50.3x4	T50.3x5	T50.3x6
Soft soap	T55.0x1	T55.0x2	T55.0x3	T55.0x4	—	—
Solanine	T62.2x1	T62.2x2	T62.2x3	T62.2x4		
berries	T62.1x1	T62.1x2	T62.1x3	T62.1x4	—	
Solanum dulcamara	T62.2x1	T62.2x2	T62.2x3	T62.2x4	—	
berries	T62.1x1	T62.1x2	T62.1x3	T62.1x4	—	
Solapsone	T37.1x1	T37.1x2	T37.1x3	T37.1x4	T37.1x5	T37.1x6
Solar lotion	T49.3x1	T49.3x2	T49.3x3	T49.3x4	T49.3x5	T49.3x6
Solasulfone	T37.1x1	T37.1x2	T37.1x3	T37.1x4	T37.1x5	T37.1x6
Soldering fluid	T65.891	T65.892	T65.893	T65.894	—	
Solid substance	T65.91	T65.92	T65.93	T65.94	—	
specified NEC	T65.891	T65.892	T65.893	T65.894	—	
Solvent, industrial NEC	T52.91	T52.92	T52.93	T52.94	—	
naphtha	T52.0x1	T52.0x2	T52.0x3	T52.0x4	—	
petroleum	T52.0x1	T52.0x2	T52.0x3	T52.0x4	—	
specified NEC	T52.8x1	T52.8x2	T52.8x3	T52.8x4	—	
Soma	T42.8x1	T42.8x2	T42.8x3	T42.8x4	T42.8x5	T42.8x6
Somatorelin	T38.891	T38.892	T38.893	T38.894	T38.895	T38.896
Somatostatin	T38.991	T38.992	T38.993	T38.994	T38.995	T38.996
Somatotropin	T38.811	T38.812	T38.813	T38.814	T38.815	T38.816
Somatrem	T38.811	T38.812	T38.813	T38.814	T38.815	T38.816
Somatropin	T38.811	T38.812	T38.813	T38.814	T38.815	T38.816
Sominex	T45.0x1	T45.0x2	T45.0x3	T45.0x4	T45.0x5	T45.0x6
Somnos	T42.6x1	T42.6x2	T42.6x3	T42.6x4	T42.6x5	T42.6x6
Somonal	T42.3x1	T42.3x2	T42.3x3	T42.3x4	T42.3x5	T42.3x6
Soneryl	T42.3x1	T42.3x2	T42.3x3	T42.3x4	T42.3x5	T42.3x6
Soothing syrup	T50.901	T50.902	T50.903	T50.904	T50.905	T50.906
Sopor	T42.6x1	T42.6x2	T42.6x3	T42.6x4	T42.6x5	T42.6x6
Soporific	T42.71	T42.72	T42.73	T42.74	T42.75	T42.76
Soporific drug	T42.71	T42.72	T42.73	T42.74	T42.75	T42.76
specified type NEC	T42.6x1	T42.6x2	T42.6x3	T42.6x4	T42.6x5	T42.6x6
Sorbide nitrate	T46.3x1	T46.3x2	T46.3x3	T46.3x4	T46.3x5	T46.3x6

DRUGS&CHEMICALS

Table of Drugs & Chemicals	Accidental (Unintentional)	Self-Harm (Intentional)	Assault	Undetermined	Adverse Effect	Underdosing
Sorbitol	T47.4x1	T47.4x2	T47.4x3	T47.4x4	T47.4x5	T47.4x6
Sotalol	T44.7x1	T44.7x2	T44.7x3	T44.7x4	T44.7x5	T44.7x6
Sotradecol	T46.8x1	T46.8x2	T46.8x3	T46.8x4	T46.8x5	T46.8x6
Soysterol	T46.6x1	T46.6x2	T46.6x3	T46.6x4	T46.6x5	T46.6x6
Spacoline	T44.3x1	T44.3x2	T44.3x3	T44.3x4	T44.3x5	T44.3x6
Spanish fly	T49.8x1	T49.8x2	T49.8x3	T49.8x4	T49.8x5	T49.8x6
Sparine	T43.3x1	T43.3x2	T43.3x3	T43.3x4	T43.3x5	T43.3x6
Sparteine	T48.0x1	T48.0x2	T48.0x3	T48.0x4	T48.0x5	T48.0x6
Spasmolytic						
anticholinergics	T44.3x1	T44.3x2	T44.3x3	T44.3x4	T44.3x5	T44.3x6
autonomic	T44.3x1	T44.3x2	T44.3x3	T44.3x4	T44.3x5	T44.3x6
bronchial NEC	T48.6x1	T48.6x2	T48.6x3	T48.6x4	T48.6x5	T48.6x6
quaternary ammonium	T44.3x1	T44.3x2	T44.3x3	T44.3x4	T44.3x5	T44.3x6
skeletal muscle NEC	T48.1x1	T48.1x2	T48.1x3	T48.1x4	T48.1x5	T48.1x6
Spectinomycin	T36.5x1	T36.5x2	T36.5x3	T36.5x4	T36.5x5	T36.5x6
Speed	T43.621	T43.622	T43.623	T43.624	T43.625	T43.626
Spermicide	T49.8x1	T49.8x2	T49.8x3	T49.8x4	T49.8x5	T49.8x6
Spider (bite) (venom)	T63.391	T63.392	T63.393	T63.394	—	—
antivenin	T50.Z11	T50.Z12	T50.Z13	T50.Z14	T50.Z15	T50.Z16
Spigelia (root)	T37.4x1	T37.4x2	T37.4x3	T37.4x4	T37.4x5	T37.4x6
Spindle inactivator	T50.4x1	T50.4x2	T50.4x3	T50.4x4	T50.4x5	T50.4x6
Spiperone	T43.4x1	T43.4x2	T43.4x3	T43.4x4	T43.4x5	T43.4x6
Spiramycin	T36.3x1	T36.3x2	T36.3x3	T36.3x4	T36.3x5	T36.3x6
Spirapril	T46.4x1	T46.4x2	T46.4x3	T46.4x4	T46.4x5	T46.4x6
Spirilene	T43.591	T43.592	T43.593	T43.594	T43.595	T43.596
Spirit (s) (neutral) NEC	T51.0x1	T51.0x2	T51.0x3	T51.0x4	—	—
beverage	T51.0x1	T51.0x2	T51.0x3	T51.0x4	—	—
industrial	T51.0x1	T51.0x2	T51.0x3	T51.0x4	—	—
mineral	T52.0x1	T52.0x2	T52.0x3	T52.0x4	—	—
of salt — see Hydrochloric acid						
surgical	T51.0x1	T51.0x2	T51.0x3	T51.0x4	—	—
Spironolactone	T50.0x1	T50.0x2	T50.0x3	T50.0x4	T50.0x5	T50.0x6
Spiroperidol	T43.4x1	T43.4x2	T43.4x3	T43.4x4	T43.4x5	T43.4x6
Sponge, absorbable (gelatin)	T45.7x1	T45.7x2	T45.7x3	T45.7x4	T45.7x5	T45.7x6
Sporostacin	T49.0x1	T49.0x2	T49.0x3	T49.0x4	T49.0x5	T49.0x6
Spray (aerosol)	T65.91	T65.92	T65.93	T65.94		
cosmetic	T65.891	T65.892	T65.893	T65.894		
medicinal NEC	T50.901	T50.902	T50.903	T50.904	T50.905	T50.906
pesticides — see Pesticides						
specified content — see specific substance						
Spurge flax	T62.2x1	T62.2x2	T62.2x3	T62.2x4	—	—
Spurges	T62.2x1	T62.2x2	T62.2x3	T62.2x4	—	—
Sputum viscosity-lowering drug	T48.4x1	T48.4x2	T48.4x3	T48.4x4	T48.4x5	T48.4x6
Squill	T46.0x1	T46.0x2	T46.0x3	T46.0x4	T46.0x5	T46.0x6
rat poison	T60.4x1	T60.4x2	T60.4x3	T60.4x4	—	—
Squirting cucumber (cathartic)	T47.2x1	T47.2x2	T47.2x3	T47.2x4	T47.2x5	T47.2x6
Stains	T65.6x1	T65.6x2	T65.6x3	T65.6x4	—	—
Stannous fluoride	T49.7x1	T49.7x2	T49.7x3	T49.7x4	T49.7x5	T49.7x6
Stanolone	T38.7x1	T38.7x2	T38.7x3	T38.7x4	T38.7x5	T38.7x6
Stanozolol	T38.7x1	T38.7x2	T38.7x3	T38.7x4	T38.7x5	T38.7x6
Staphisagria or stavesacre (pediculicide)	T49.0x1	T49.0x2	T49.0x3	T49.0x4	T49.0x5	T49.0x6
Starch	T50.901	T50.902	T50.903	T50.904	T50.905	T50.906
Stelazine	T43.3x1	T43.3x2	T43.3x3	T43.3x4	T43.3x5	T43.3x6
Stemetil	T43.3x1	T43.3x2	T43.3x3	T43.3x4	T43.3x5	T43.3x6
Stepronin	T48.4x1	T48.4x2	T48.4x3	T48.4x4	T48.4x5	T48.4x6
Sterculia	T47.4x1	T47.4x2	T47.4x3	T47.4x4	T47.4x5	T47.4x6
Sternutator gas	T59.891	T59.892	T59.893	T59.894		
Steroid	T38.0x1	T38.0x2	T38.0x3	T38.0x4	T38.0x5	T38.0x6
anabolic	T38.7x1	T38.7x2	T38.7x3	T38.7x4	T38.7x5	T38.7x6
androgenic	T38.7x1	T38.7x2	T38.7x3	T38.7x4	T38.7x5	T38.7x6
antineoplastic, hormone	T38.7x1	T38.7x2	T38.7x3	T38.7x4	T38.7x5	T38.7x6
estrogen	T38.5x1	T38.5x2	T38.5x3	T38.5x4	T38.5x5	T38.5x6
ENT agent	T49.6x1	T49.6x2	T49.6x3	T49.6x4	T49.6x5	T49.6x6
ophthalmic preparation	T49.5x1	T49.5x2	T49.5x3	T49.5x4	T49.5x5	T49.5x6
topical NEC	T49.0x1	T49.0x2	T49.0x3	T49.0x4	T49.0x5	T49.0x6
Stibine	T56.891	T56.892	T56.893	T56.894	—	—
Stibogluconate	T37.3x1	T37.3x2	T37.3x3	T37.3x4	T37.3x5	T37.3x6
Stibophen	T37.4x1	T37.4x2	T37.4x3	T37.4x4	T37.4x5	T37.4x6
Stilbamidine (isetionate)	T37.3x1	T37.3x2	T37.3x3	T37.3x4	T37.3x5	T37.3x6
Stilbestrol	T38.5x1	T38.5x2	T38.5x3	T38.5x4	T38.5x5	T38.5x6
Stilboestrol	T38.5x1	T38.5x2	T38.5x3	T38.5x4	T38.5x5	T38.5x6
Stimulant						
central nervous system — see also Psychostimulant	T43.601	T43.602	T43.603	T43.604	T43.605	T43.606
analeptics	T50.7x1	T50.7x2	T50.7x3	T50.7x4	T50.7x5	T50.7x6
opiate antagonist	T50.7x1	T50.7x2	T50.7x3	T50.7x4	T50.7x5	T50.7x6
psychotherapeutic NEC — see also Psychotherapeutic drug	T43.601	T43.602	T43.603	T43.604	T43.605	T43.606
specified NEC	T43.691	T43.692	T43.693	T43.694	T43.695	T43.696
respiratory	T48.901	T48.902	T48.903	T48.904	T48.905	T48.906
Stone-dissolving drug	T50.901	T50.902	T50.903	T50.904	T50.905	T50.906
Storage battery (cells) (acid)	T54.2x1	T54.2x2	T54.2x3	T54.2x4	—	—
Stovaine	T41.3x1	T41.3x2	T41.3x3	T41.3x4	T41.3x5	T41.3x6
infiltration (subcutaneous)	T41.3x1	T41.3x2	T41.3x3	T41.3x4	T41.3x5	T41.3x6
nerve block (peripheral) (plexus)	T41.3x1	T41.3x2	T41.3x3	T41.3x4	T41.3x5	T41.3x6
spinal	T41.3x1	T41.3x2	T41.3x3	T41.3x4	T41.3x5	T41.3x6
topical (surface)	T41.3x1	T41.3x2	T41.3x3	T41.3x4	T41.3x5	T41.3x6
Stovarsal	T37.8x1	T37.8x2	T37.8x3	T37.8x4	T37.8x5	T37.8x6
Stove gas — see Gas, stove						
Stoxil	T49.5x1	T49.5x2	T49.5x3	T49.5x4	T49.5x5	T49.5x6
Stramonium	T48.6x1	T48.6x2	T48.6x3	T48.6x4	T48.6x5	T48.6x6
natural state	T62.2x1	T62.2x2	T62.2x3	T62.2x4	—	—
Streptodornase	T45.3x1	T45.3x2	T45.3x3	T45.3x4	T45.3x5	T45.3x6
Streptoduocin	T36.5x1	T36.5x2	T36.5x3	T36.5x4	T36.5x5	T36.5x6
Streptokinase	T45.611	T45.612	T45.613	T45.614	T45.615	T45.616
Streptomycin (derivative)	T36.5x1	T36.5x2	T36.5x3	T36.5x4	T36.5x5	T36.5x6
Streptonivicin	T36.5x1	T36.5x2	T36.5x3	T36.5x4	T36.5x5	T36.5x6
Streptovarycin	T36.5x1	T36.5x2	T36.5x3	T36.5x4	T36.5x5	T36.5x6
Streptozocin	T45.1x1	T45.1x2	T45.1x3	T45.1x4	T45.1x5	T45.1x6
Streptozotocin	T45.1x1	T45.1x2	T45.1x3	T45.1x4	T45.1x5	T45.1x6
Stripper (paint) (solvent)	T52.8x1	T52.8x2	T52.8x3	T52.8x4	—	—
Strobane	T60.1x1	T60.1x2	T60.1x3	T60.1x4	—	—
Strofantina	T46.0x1	T46.0x2	T46.0x3	T46.0x4	T46.0x5	T46.0x6
Strophanthin (g) (k)	T46.0x1	T46.0x2	T46.0x3	T46.0x4	T46.0x5	T46.0x6
Strophanthus	T46.0x1	T46.0x2	T46.0x3	T46.0x4	T46.0x5	T46.0x6
Strophantin	T46.0x1	T46.0x2	T46.0x3	T46.0x4	T46.0x5	T46.0x6
Strophantin-g	T46.0x1	T46.0x2	T46.0x3	T46.0x4	T46.0x5	T46.0x6
Strychnine (nonmedicinal) (pesticide) (salts)	T65.1x1	T65.1x2	T65.1x3	T65.1x4	—	—
medicinal	T48.291	T48.292	T48.293	T48.294	T48.295	T48.296
Strychnos (ignatii) — see Strychnine						
Styramate	T42.8x1	T42.8x2	T42.8x3	T42.8x4	T42.8x5	T42.8x6
Styrene	T65.891	T65.892	T65.893	T65.894		
Succinimide, antiepileptic or anticonvulsant	T42.2x1	T42.2x2	T42.2x3	T42.2x4	T42.2x5	T42.2x6
mercuric — see Mercury						
Succinylcholine	T48.1x1	T48.1x2	T48.1x3	T48.1x4	T48.1x5	T48.1x6
Succinylsulfathiazole	T37.0x1	T37.0x2	T37.0x3	T37.0x4	T37.0x5	T37.0x6
Sucralfate	T47.1x1	T47.1x2	T47.1x3	T47.1x4	T47.1x5	T47.1x6
Sucrose	T50.3x1	T50.3x2	T50.3x3	T50.3x4	T50.3x5	T50.3x6
Sufentanil	T40.4x1	T40.4x2	T40.4x3	T40.4x4	T40.4x5	T40.4x6
Sulbactam	T36.0x1	T36.0x2	T36.0x3	T36.0x4	T36.0x5	T36.0x6
Sulbenicillin	T36.0x1	T36.0x2	T36.0x3	T36.0x4	T36.0x5	T36.0x6
Sulbentine	T49.0x1	T49.0x2	T49.0x3	T49.0x4	T49.0x5	T49.0x6
Sulfacetamide	T49.0x1	T49.0x2	T49.0x3	T49.0x4	T49.0x5	T49.0x6
ophthalmic preparation	T49.5x1	T49.5x2	T49.5x3	T49.5x4	T49.5x5	T49.5x6
Sulfachlorpyridazine	T37.0x1	T37.0x2	T37.0x3	T37.0x4	T37.0x5	T37.0x6
Sulfacitine	T37.0x1	T37.0x2	T37.0x3	T37.0x4	T37.0x5	T37.0x6
Sulfadiasulfone sodium	T37.0x1	T37.0x2	T37.0x3	T37.0x4	T37.0x5	T37.0x6
Sulfadiazine	T37.0x1	T37.0x2	T37.0x3	T37.0x4	T37.0x5	T37.0x6
silver (topical)	T49.0x1	T49.0x2	T49.0x3	T49.0x4	T49.0x5	T49.0x6
Sulfadimethoxine	T37.0x1	T37.0x2	T37.0x3	T37.0x4	T37.0x5	T37.0x6
Sulfadimidine	T37.0x1	T37.0x2	T37.0x3	T37.0x4	T37.0x5	T37.0x6

DRUGS&CHEMICALS

Table of Drugs & Chemicals	POISONING Accidental (Unintentional)	Self-Harm (Intentional)	Assault	Undetermined	Adverse Effect	Underdosing
Sulfadoxine	T37.0x1	T37.0x2	T37.0x3	T37.0x4	T37.0x5	T37.0x6
with pyrimethamine	T37.2x1	T37.2x2	T37.2x3	T37.2x4	T37.2x5	T37.2x6
Sulfaethidole	T37.0x1	T37.0x2	T37.0x3	T37.0x4	T37.0x5	T37.0x6
Sulfafurazole	T37.0x1	T37.0x2	T37.0x3	T37.0x4	T37.0x5	T37.0x6
Sulfaguanidine	T37.0x1	T37.0x2	T37.0x3	T37.0x4	T37.0x5	T37.0x6
Sulfalene	T37.0x1	T37.0x2	T37.0x3	T37.0x4	T37.0x5	T37.0x6
Sulfaloxate	T37.0x1	T37.0x2	T37.0x3	T37.0x4	T37.0x5	T37.0x6
Sulfaloxic acid	T37.0x1	T37.0x2	T37.0x3	T37.0x4	T37.0x5	T37.0x6
Sulfamazone	T39.2x1	T39.2x2	T39.2x3	T39.2x4	T39.2x5	T39.2x6
Sulfamerazine	T37.0x1	T37.0x2	T37.0x3	T37.0x4	T37.0x5	T37.0x6
Sulfameter	T37.0x1	T37.0x2	T37.0x3	T37.0x4	T37.0x5	T37.0x6
Sulfamethazine	T37.0x1	T37.0x2	T37.0x3	T37.0x4	T37.0x5	T37.0x6
Sulfamethizole	T37.0x1	T37.0x2	T37.0x3	T37.0x4	T37.0x5	T37.0x6
Sulfamethoxazole	T37.0x1	T37.0x2	T37.0x3	T37.0x4	T37.0x5	T37.0x6
with trimethoprim	T36.8x1	T36.8x2	T36.8x3	T36.8x4	T36.8x5	T36.8x6
Sulfamethoxydiazine	T37.0x1	T37.0x2	T37.0x3	T37.0x4	T37.0x5	T37.0x6
Sulfamethoxypyridazine	T37.0x1	T37.0x2	T37.0x3	T37.0x4	T37.0x5	T37.0x6
Sulfamethylthiazole	T37.0x1	T37.0x2	T37.0x3	T37.0x4	T37.0x5	T37.0x6
Sulfametoxydiazine	T37.0x1	T37.0x2	T37.0x3	T37.0x4	T37.0x5	T37.0x6
Sulfamidopyrine	T39.2x1	T39.2x2	T39.2x3	T39.2x4	T39.2x5	T39.2x6
Sulfamonomethoxine	T37.0x1	T37.0x2	T37.0x3	T37.0x4	T37.0x5	T37.0x6
Sulfamoxole	T37.0x1	T37.0x2	T37.0x3	T37.0x4	T37.0x5	T37.0x6
Sulfamylon	T49.0x1	T49.0x2	T49.0x3	T49.0x4	T49.0x5	T49.0x6
Sulfan blue (diagnostic dye)	T50.8x1	T50.8x2	T50.8x3	T50.8x4	T50.8x5	T50.8x6
Sulfanilamide	T37.0x1	T37.0x2	T37.0x3	T37.0x4	T37.0x5	T37.0x6
Sulfanilylguanidine	T37.0x1	T37.0x2	T37.0x3	T37.0x4	T37.0x5	T37.0x6
Sulfaperin	T37.0x1	T37.0x2	T37.0x3	T37.0x4	T37.0x5	T37.0x6
Sulfaphenazole	T37.0x1	T37.0x2	T37.0x3	T37.0x4	T37.0x5	T37.0x6
Sulfaphenylthiazole	T37.0x1	T37.0x2	T37.0x3	T37.0x4	T37.0x5	T37.0x6
Sulfaproxyline	T37.0x1	T37.0x2	T37.0x3	T37.0x4	T37.0x5	T37.0x6
Sulfapyridine	T37.0x1	T37.0x2	T37.0x3	T37.0x4	T37.0x5	T37.0x6
Sulfapyrimidine	T37.0x1	T37.0x2	T37.0x3	T37.0x4	T37.0x5	T37.0x6
Sulfarsphenamine	T37.8x1	T37.8x2	T37.8x3	T37.8x4	T37.8x5	T37.8x6
Sulfasalazine	T37.0x1	T37.0x2	T37.0x3	T37.0x4	T37.0x5	T37.0x6
Sulfasuxidine	T37.0x1	T37.0x2	T37.0x3	T37.0x4	T37.0x5	T37.0x6
Sulfasymazine	T37.0x1	T37.0x2	T37.0x3	T37.0x4	T37.0x5	T37.0x6
Sulfated amylopectin	T47.8x1	T47.8x2	T47.8x3	T47.8x4	T47.8x5	T47.8x6
Sulfathiazole	T37.0x1	T37.0x2	T37.0x3	T37.0x4	T37.0x5	T37.0x6
Sulfatostearate	T49.2x1	T49.2x2	T49.2x3	T49.2x4	T49.2x5	T49.2x6
Sulfinpyrazone	T50.4x1	T50.4x2	T50.4x3	T50.4x4	T50.4x5	T50.4x6
Sulfiram	T49.0x1	T49.0x2	T49.0x3	T49.0x4	T49.0x5	T49.0x6
Sulfisomidine	T37.0x1	T37.0x2	T37.0x3	T37.0x4	T37.0x5	T37.0x6
Sulfisoxazole	T37.0x1	T37.0x2	T37.0x3	T37.0x4	T37.0x5	T37.0x6
ophthalmic preparation	T49.5x1	T49.5x2	T49.5x3	T49.5x4	T49.5x5	T49.5x6
Sulfobromophthalein (sodium)	T50.8x1	T50.8x2	T50.8x3	T50.8x4	T50.8x5	T50.8x6
Sulfobromphthalein	T50.8x1	T50.8x2	T50.8x3	T50.8x4	T50.8x5	T50.8x6
Sulfogaiacol	T48.4x1	T48.4x2	T48.4x3	T48.4x4	T48.4x5	T48.4x6
Sulfomyxin	T36.8x1	T36.8x2	T36.8x3	T36.8x4	T36.8x5	T36.8x6
Sulfonal	T42.6x1	T42.6x2	T42.6x3	T42.6x4	T42.6x5	T42.6x6
Sulfonamide NEC	T37.0x1	T37.0x2	T37.0x3	T37.0x4	T37.0x5	T37.0x6
eye	T49.5x1	T49.5x2	T49.5x3	T49.5x4	T49.5x5	T49.5x6
Sulfonazide	T37.1x1	T37.1x2	T37.1x3	T37.1x4	T37.1x5	T37.1x6
Sulfones	T37.1x1	T37.1x2	T37.1x3	T37.1x4	T37.1x5	T37.1x6
Sulfonethylmethane	T42.6x1	T42.6x2	T42.6x3	T42.6x4	T42.6x5	T42.6x6
Sulfonmethane	T42.6x1	T42.6x2	T42.6x3	T42.6x4	T42.6x5	T42.6x6
Sulfonphthal, sulfonphthol	T50.8x1	T50.8x2	T50.8x3	T50.8x4	T50.8x5	T50.8x6
Sulfonylurea derivatives, oral	T38.3x1	T38.3x2	T38.3x3	T38.3x4	T38.3x5	T38.3x6
Sulforidazine	T43.3x1	T43.3x2	T43.3x3	T43.3x4	T43.3x5	T43.3x6
Sulfoxone	T37.1x1	T37.1x2	T37.1x3	T37.1x4	T37.1x5	T37.1x6
Sulfur, sulfurated, sulfuric, sulfurous, sulfuryl (compounds NEC) (medicinal)	T49.4x1	T49.4x2	T49.4x3	T49.4x4	T49.4x5	T49.4x6
acid	T54.2x1	T54.2x2	T54.2x3	T54.2x4	—	—
dioxide (gas)	T59.1x1	T59.1x2	T59.1x3	T59.1x4	—	—
ether — see Ether(s)						
hydrogen	T59.6x1	T59.6x2	T59.6x3	T59.6x4	—	—
medicinal (keratolytic) (ointment) NEC	T49.4x1	T49.4x2	T49.4x3	T49.4x4	T49.4x5	T49.4x6
ointment	T49.0x1	T49.0x2	T49.0x3	T49.0x4	T49.0x5	T49.0x6
pesticide (vapor)	T60.91	T60.92	T60.93	T60.94	—	—
vapor NEC	T59.891	T59.892	T59.893	T59.894		

Table of Drugs & Chemicals	POISONING Accidental (Unintentional)	Self-Harm (Intentional)	Assault	Undetermined	Adverse Effect	Underdosing
Sulfuric acid	T54.2x1	T54.2x2	T54.2x3	T54.2x4		
Sulglicotide	T47.1x1	T47.1x2	T47.1x3	T47.1x4	T47.1x5	T47.1x6
Sulindac	T39.391	T39.392	T39.393	T39.394	T39.395	T39.396
Sulisatin	T47.2x1	T47.2x2	T47.2x3	T47.2x4	T47.2x5	T47.2x6
Sulisobenzone	T49.3x1	T49.3x2	T49.3x3	T49.3x4	T49.3x5	T49.3x6
Sulkowitch's reagent	T50.8x1	T50.8x2	T50.8x3	T50.8x4	T50.8x5	T50.8x6
Sulmetozine	T44.3x1	T44.3x2	T44.3x3	T44.3x4	T44.3x5	T44.3x6
Suloctidil	T46.7x1	T46.7x2	T46.7x3	T46.7x4	T46.7x5	T46.7x6
Sulph- — see also Sulf-						
Sulphadiazine	T37.0x1	T37.0x2	T37.0x3	T37.0x4	T37.0x5	T37.0x6
Sulphadimethoxine	T37.0x1	T37.0x2	T37.0x3	T37.0x4	T37.0x5	T37.0x6
Sulphadimidine	T37.0x1	T37.0x2	T37.0x3	T37.0x4	T37.0x5	T37.0x6
Sulphadione	T37.1x1	T37.1x2	T37.1x3	T37.1x4	T37.1x5	T37.1x6
Sulphafurazole	T37.0x1	T37.0x2	T37.0x3	T37.0x4	T37.0x5	T37.0x6
Sulphamethizole	T37.0x1	T37.0x2	T37.0x3	T37.0x4	T37.0x5	T37.0x6
Sulphamethoxazole	T37.0x1	T37.0x2	T37.0x3	T37.0x4	T37.0x5	T37.0x6
Sulphan blue	T50.8x1	T50.8x2	T50.8x3	T50.8x4	T50.8x5	T50.8x6
Sulphaphenazole	T37.0x1	T37.0x2	T37.0x3	T37.0x4	T37.0x5	T37.0x6
Sulphapyridine	T37.0x1	T37.0x2	T37.0x3	T37.0x4	T37.0x5	T37.0x6
Sulphasalazine	T37.0x1	T37.0x2	T37.0x3	T37.0x4	T37.0x5	T37.0x6
Sulphinpyrazone	T50.4x1	T50.4x2	T50.4x3	T50.4x4	T50.4x5	T50.4x6
Sulpiride	T43.591	T43.592	T43.593	T43.594	T43.595	T43.596
Sulprostone	T48.0x1	T48.0x2	T48.0x3	T48.0x4	T48.0x5	T48.0x6
Sulpyrine	T39.2x1	T39.2x2	T39.2x3	T39.2x4	T39.2x5	T39.2x6
Sultamicillin	T36.0x1	T36.0x2	T36.0x3	T36.0x4	T36.0x5	T36.0x6
Sulthiame	T42.6x1	T42.6x2	T42.6x3	T42.6x4	T42.6x5	T42.6x6
Sultiame	T42.6x1	T42.6x2	T42.6x3	T42.6x4	T42.6x5	T42.6x6
Sultopride	T43.591	T43.592	T43.593	T43.594	T43.595	T43.596
Sumatriptan	T39.8x1	T39.8x2	T39.8x3	T39.8x4	T39.8x5	T39.8x6
Sunflower seed oil	T46.6x1	T46.6x2	T46.6x3	T46.6x4	T46.6x5	T46.6x6
Superinone	T48.4x1	T48.4x2	T48.4x3	T48.4x4	T48.4x5	T48.4x6
Suprofen	T39.311	T39.312	T39.313	T39.314	T39.315	T39.316
Suramin (sodium)	T37.4x1	T37.4x2	T37.4x3	T37.4x4	T37.4x5	T37.4x6
Surfacaine	T41.3x1	T41.3x2	T41.3x3	T41.3x4	T41.3x5	T41.3x6
Surital	T41.1x1	T41.1x2	T41.1x3	T41.1x4	T41.1x5	T41.1x6
Sutilains	T45.3x1	T45.3x2	T45.3x3	T45.3x4	T45.3x5	T45.3x6
Suxamethonium (chloride)	T48.1x1	T48.1x2	T48.1x3	T48.1x4	T48.1x5	T48.1x6
Suxethonium (chloride)	T48.1x1	T48.1x2	T48.1x3	T48.1x4	T48.1x5	T48.1x6
Suxibuzone	T39.2x1	T39.2x2	T39.2x3	T39.2x4	T39.2x5	T39.2x6
Sweet niter spirit	T46.3x1	T46.3x2	T46.3x3	T46.3x4	T46.3x5	T46.3x6
Sweet oil (birch)	T49.3x1	T49.3x2	T49.3x3	T49.3x4	T49.3x5	T49.3x6
Sweetener	T50.901	T50.902	T50.903	T50.904	T50.905	T50.906
Sym-dichloroethyl ether	T53.6x1	T53.6x2	T53.6x3	T53.6x4		
Sympatholytic NEC	T44.8x1	T44.8x2	T44.8x3	T44.8x4	T44.8x5	T44.8x6
haloalkylamine	T44.8x1	T44.8x2	T44.8x3	T44.8x4	T44.8x5	T44.8x6
Sympathomimetic NEC	T44.901	T44.902	T44.903	T44.904	T44.905	T44.906
anti-common-cold	T48.5x1	T48.5x2	T48.5x3	T48.5x4	T48.5x5	T48.5x6
bronchodilator	T48.6x1	T48.6x2	T48.6x3	T48.6x4	T48.6x5	T48.6x6
specified NEC	T44.991	T44.992	T44.993	T44.994	T44.995	T44.996
Synagis	T50.B91	T50.B92	T50.B93	T50.B94	T50.B95	T50.B96
Synalar	T49.0x1	T49.0x2	T49.0x3	T49.0x4	T49.0x5	T49.0x6
Synthroid	T38.1x1	T38.1x2	T38.1x3	T38.1x4	T38.1x5	T38.1x6
Syntocinon	T48.0x1	T48.0x2	T48.0x3	T48.0x4	T48.0x5	T48.0x6
Syrosingopine	T46.5x1	T46.5x2	T46.5x3	T46.5x4	T46.5x5	T46.5x6
Systemic drug	T45.91	T45.92	T45.93	T45.94	T45.95	T45.96
specified NEC	T45.8x1	T45.8x2	T45.8x3	T45.8x4	T45.8x5	T45.8x6
2,4,5-T	T60.3x1	T60.3x2	T60.3x3	T60.3x4	—	—
Tablets — see also specified substance	T50.901	T50.902	T50.903	T50.904	T50.905	T50.906
Tace	T38.5x1	T38.5x2	T38.5x3	T38.5x4	T38.5x5	T38.5x6
Tacrine	T44.0x1	T44.0x2	T44.0x3	T44.0x4	T44.0x5	T44.0x6
Tadalafil	T46.7x1	T46.7x2	T46.7x3	T46.7x4	T46.7x5	T46.7x6
Talampicillin	T36.0x1	T36.0x2	T36.0x3	T36.0x4	T36.0x5	T36.0x6
Talbutal	T42.3x1	T42.3x2	T42.3x3	T42.3x4	T42.3x5	T42.3x6
Talc powder	T49.3x1	T49.3x2	T49.3x3	T49.3x4	T49.3x5	T49.3x6
Talcum	T49.3x1	T49.3x2	T49.3x3	T49.3x4	T49.3x5	T49.3x6
Taleranol	T38.6x1	T38.6x2	T38.6x3	T38.6x4	T38.6x5	T38.6x6
Tamoxifen	T38.6x1	T38.6x2	T38.6x3	T38.6x4	T38.6x5	T38.6x6
Tamsulosin	T44.6x1	T44.6x2	T44.6x3	T44.6x4	T44.6x5	T44.6x6

DRUGS&CHEMICALS

Table of Drugs & Chemicals	Accidental (Unintentional)	Self-Harm (Intentional)	Assault	Undetermined	Adverse Effect	Underdosing
Tandearil, tanderil	T39.2x1	T39.2x2	T39.2x3	T39.2x4	T39.2x5	T39.2x6
Tannic acid	T49.2x1	T49.2x2	T49.2x3	T49.2x4	T49.2x5	T49.2x6
medicinal (astringent)	T49.2x1	T49.2x2	T49.2x3	T49.2x4	T49.2x5	T49.2x6
Tannin — see Tannic acid						
Tansy	T62.2x1	T62.2x2	T62.2x3	T62.2x4	—	—
TAO	T36.3x1	T36.3x2	T36.3x3	T36.3x4	T36.3x5	T36.3x6
Tapazole	T38.2x1	T38.2x2	T38.2x3	T38.2x4	T38.2x5	T38.2x6
Tar NEC	T52.0x1	T52.0x2	T52.0x3	T52.0x4	—	—
camphor	T60.1x1	T60.1x2	T60.1x3	T60.1x4	—	—
distillate	T49.1x1	T49.1x2	T49.1x3	T49.1x4	T49.1x5	T49.1x6
fumes	T59.891	T59.892	T59.893	T59.894	—	—
medicinal	T49.1x1	T49.1x2	T49.1x3	T49.1x4	T49.1x5	T49.1x6
ointment	T49.1x1	T49.1x2	T49.1x3	T49.1x4	T49.1x5	T49.1x6
Taractan	T43.591	T43.592	T43.593	T43.594	T43.595	T43.596
Tarantula (venomous)	T63.321	T63.322	T63.323	T63.324	—	—
Tartar emetic	T37.8x1	T37.8x2	T37.8x3	T37.8x4	T37.8x5	T37.8x6
Tartaric acid	T65.891	T65.892	T65.893	T65.894	—	—
Tartrate, laxative	T47.4x1	T47.4x2	T47.4x3	T47.4x4	T47.4x5	T47.4x6
Tartrated antimony (anti-infective)	T37.8x1	T37.8x2	T37.8x3	T37.8x4	T37.8x5	T37.8x6
Tauromustine	T45.1x1	T45.1x2	T45.1x3	T45.1x4	T45.1x5	T45.1x6
TCA — see Trichloroacetic acid						
TCDD	T53.7x1	T53.7x2	T53.7x3	T53.7x4	—	—
TDI (vapor)	T65.0x1	T65.0x2	T65.0x3	T65.0x4	—	—
Tear						
gas	T59.3x1	T59.3x2	T59.3x3	T59.3x4	—	—
solution	T49.5x1	T49.5x2	T49.5x3	T49.5x4	T49.5x5	T49.5x6
Teclothiazide	T50.2x1	T50.2x2	T50.2x3	T50.2x4	T50.2x5	T50.2x6
Teclozan	T37.3x1	T37.3x2	T37.3x3	T37.3x4	T37.3x5	T37.3x6
Tegafur	T45.1x1	T45.1x2	T45.1x3	T45.1x4	T45.1x5	T45.1x6
Tegretol	T42.1x1	T42.1x2	T42.1x3	T42.1x4	T42.1x5	T42.1x6
Teicoplanin	T36.8x1	T36.8x2	T36.8x3	T36.8x4	T36.8x5	T36.8x6
Telepaque	T50.8x1	T50.8x2	T50.8x3	T50.8x4	T50.8x5	T50.8x6
Tellurium	T56.891	T56.892	T56.893	T56.894	—	—
fumes	T56.891	T56.892	T56.893	T56.894	—	—
TEM	T45.1x1	T45.1x2	T45.1x3	T45.1x4	T45.1x5	T45.1x6
Temazepam	T42.4x1	T42.4x2	T42.4x3	T42.4x4	T42.4x5	T42.4x6
Temocillin	T36.0x1	T36.0x2	T36.0x3	T36.0x4	T36.0x5	T36.0x6
Tenamfetamine	T43.621	T43.622	T43.623	T43.624	T43.625	T43.626
Teniposide	T45.1x1	T45.1x2	T45.1x3	T45.1x4	T45.1x5	T45.1x6
Tenitramine	T46.3x1	T46.3x2	T46.3x3	T46.3x4	T46.3x5	T46.3x6
Tenoglicin	T48.4x1	T48.4x2	T48.4x3	T48.4x4	T48.4x5	T48.4x6
Tenonitrozole	T37.3x1	T37.3x2	T37.3x3	T37.3x4	T37.3x5	T37.3x6
Tenoxicam	T39.391	T39.392	T39.393	T39.394	T39.395	T39.396
TEPA	T45.1x1	T45.1x2	T45.1x3	T45.1x4	T45.1x5	T45.1x6
TEPP	T60.0x1	T60.0x2	T60.0x3	T60.0x4	—	—
Teprotide	T46.5x1	T46.5x2	T46.5x3	T46.5x4	T46.5x5	T46.5x6
Terazosin	T44.6x1	T44.6x2	T44.6x3	T44.6x4	T44.6x5	T44.6x6
Terbufos	T60.0x1	T60.0x2	T60.0x3	T60.0x4	—	—
Terbutaline	T48.6x1	T48.6x2	T48.6x3	T48.6x4	T48.6x5	T48.6x6
Terconazole	T49.0x1	T49.0x2	T49.0x3	T49.0x4	T49.0x5	T49.0x6
Terfenadine	T45.0x1	T45.0x2	T45.0x3	T45.0x4	T45.0x5	T45.0x6
Teriparatide (acetate)	T50.991	T50.992	T50.993	T50.994	T50.995	T50.996
Terizidone	T37.1x1	T37.1x2	T37.1x3	T37.1x4	T37.1x5	T37.1x6
Terlipressin	T38.891	T38.892	T38.893	T38.894	T38.895	T38.896
Terodiline	T46.3x1	T46.3x2	T46.3x3	T46.3x4	T46.3x5	T46.3x6
Teroxalene	T37.4x1	T37.4x2	T37.4x3	T37.4x4	T37.4x5	T37.4x6
Terpin (cis) hydrate	T48.4x1	T48.4x2	T48.4x3	T48.4x4	T48.4x5	T48.4x6
Terramycin	T36.4x1	T36.4x2	T36.4x3	T36.4x4	T36.4x5	T36.4x6
Tertatolol	T44.7x1	T44.7x2	T44.7x3	T44.7x4	T44.7x5	T44.7x6
Tessalon	T48.3x1	T48.3x2	T48.3x3	T48.3x4	T48.3x5	T48.3x6
Testolactone	T38.7x1	T38.7x2	T38.7x3	T38.7x4	T38.7x5	T38.7x6
Testosterone	T38.7x1	T38.7x2	T38.7x3	T38.7x4	T38.7x5	T38.7x6
Tetanus toxoid or vaccine	T50.A91	T50.A92	T50.A93	T50.A94	T50.A95	T50.A96
antitoxin	T50.Z11	T50.Z12	T50.Z13	T50.Z14	T50.Z15	T50.Z16
immune globulin (human)	T50.Z11	T50.Z12	T50.Z13	T50.Z14	T50.Z15	T50.Z16
toxoid	T50.A91	T50.A92	T50.A93	T50.A94	T50.A95	T50.A96
with diphtheria toxoid	T50.A21	T50.A22	T50.A23	T50.A24	T50.A25	T50.A26
with pertussis	T50.A11	T50.A12	T50.A13	T50.A14	T50.A15	T50.A16
Tetrabenazine	T43.591	T43.592	T43.593	T43.594	T43.595	T43.596
Tetracaine	T41.3x1	T41.3x2	T41.3x3	T41.3x4	T41.3x5	T41.3x6
nerve block (peripheral) (plexus)	T41.3x1	T41.3x2	T41.3x3	T41.3x4	T41.3x5	T41.3x6
regional	T41.3x1	T41.3x2	T41.3x3	T41.3x4	T41.3x5	T41.3x6
spinal	T41.3x1	T41.3x2	T41.3x3	T41.3x4	T41.3x5	T41.3x6
Tetrachlorethylene — see Tetrachloroethylene						
Tetrachlormethiazide	T50.2x1	T50.2x2	T50.2x3	T50.2x4	T50.2x5	T50.2x6
2,3,7,8-Tetrachlorodibenzo-p-dioxin	T53.7x1	T53.7x2	T53.7x3	T53.7x4	—	—
Tetrachloroethane	T53.6x1	T53.6x2	T53.6x3	T53.6x4	—	—
vapor	T53.6x1	T53.6x2	T53.6x3	T53.6x4	—	—
paint or varnish	T53.6x1	T53.6x2	T53.6x3	T53.6x4	—	—
Tetrachloroethylene (liquid)	T53.3x1	T53.3x2	T53.3x3	T53.3x4	—	—
medicinal	T37.4x1	T37.4x2	T37.4x3	T37.4x4	T37.4x5	T37.4x6
vapor	T53.3x1	T53.3x2	T53.3x3	T53.3x4	—	—
Tetrachloromethane — see Carbon tetrachloride						
Tetracosactide	T38.811	T38.812	T38.813	T38.814	T38.815	T38.816
Tetracosactrin	T38.811	T38.812	T38.813	T38.814	T38.815	T38.816
Tetracycline	T36.4x1	T36.4x2	T36.4x3	T36.4x4	T36.4x5	T36.4x6
ophthalmic preparation	T49.5x1	T49.5x2	T49.5x3	T49.5x4	T49.5x5	T49.5x6
topical NEC	T49.0x1	T49.0x2	T49.0x3	T49.0x4	T49.0x5	T49.0x6
Tetradifon	T60.8x1	T60.8x2	T60.8x3	T60.8x4	—	—
Tetradotoxin	T61.771	T61.772	T61.773	T61.774	—	—
Tetraethyl						
lead	T56.0x1	T56.0x2	T56.0x3	T56.0x4	—	—
pyrophosphate	T60.0x1	T60.0x2	T60.0x3	T60.0x4	—	—
Tetraethylammonium chloride	T44.2x1	T44.2x2	T44.2x3	T44.2x4	T44.2x5	T44.2x6
Tetraethylthiuram disulfide	T50.6x1	T50.6x2	T50.6x3	T50.6x4	T50.6x5	T50.6x6
Tetrahydroaminoacridine	T44.0x1	T44.0x2	T44.0x3	T44.0x4	T44.0x5	T44.0x6
Tetrahydrocannabinol	T40.7x1	T40.7x2	T40.7x3	T40.7x4	T40.7x5	T40.7x6
Tetrahydrofuran	T52.8x1	T52.8x2	T52.8x3	T52.8x4	—	—
Tetrahydronaphthalene	T52.8x1	T52.8x2	T52.8x3	T52.8x4	—	—
Tetrahydrozoline	T49.5x1	T49.5x2	T49.5x3	T49.5x4	T49.5x5	—
Tetralin	T52.8x1	T52.8x2	T52.8x3	T52.8x4	—	—
Tetramethrin	T60.2x1	T60.2x2	T60.2x3	T60.2x4	—	—
Tetramethylthiuram (disulfide)						
NEC	T60.3x1	T60.3x2	T60.3x3	T60.3x4	—	—
medicinal	T49.0x1	T49.0x2	T49.0x3	T49.0x4	T49.0x5	T49.0x6
Tetramisole	T37.4x1	T37.4x2	T37.4x3	T37.4x4	T37.4x5	T37.4x6
Tetranicotinoyl fructose	T46.7x1	T46.7x2	T46.7x3	T46.7x4	T46.7x5	T46.7x6
Tetrazepam	T42.4x1	T42.4x2	T42.4x3	T42.4x4	T42.4x5	T42.4x6
Tetronal	T42.6x1	T42.6x2	T42.6x3	T42.6x4	T42.6x5	T42.6x6
Tetryl	T65.3x1	T65.3x2	T65.3x3	T65.3x4	—	—
Tetrylammonium chloride	T44.2x1	T44.2x2	T44.2x3	T44.2x4	T44.2x5	T44.2x6
Tetryzoline	T49.5x1	T49.5x2	T49.5x3	T49.5x4	T49.5x5	T49.5x6
Thalidomide	T45.1x1	T45.1x2	T45.1x3	T45.1x4	T45.1x5	T45.1x6
Thallium (compounds) (dust)						
NEC	T56.811	T56.812	T56.813	T56.814	—	—
pesticide	T60.4x1	T60.4x2	T60.4x3	T60.4x4	—	—
THC	T40.7x1	T40.7x2	T40.7x3	T40.7x4	T40.7x5	T40.7x6
Thebacon	T48.3x1	T48.3x2	T48.3x3	T48.3x4	T48.3x5	T48.3x6
Thebaine	T40.2x1	T40.2x2	T40.2x3	T40.2x4	T40.2x5	T40.2x6
Thenoic acid	T49.6x1	T49.6x2	T49.6x3	T49.6x4	T49.6x5	T49.6x6
Thenyldiamine	T45.0x1	T45.0x2	T45.0x3	T45.0x4	T45.0x5	T45.0x6
Theobromine (calcium salicylate)	T48.6x1	T48.6x2	T48.6x3	T48.6x4	T48.6x5	T48.6x6
sodium salicylate	T48.6x1	T48.6x2	T48.6x3	T48.6x4	T48.6x5	T48.6x6
Theophyllamine	T48.6x1	T48.6x2	T48.6x3	T48.6x4	T48.6x5	T48.6x6
Theophylline	T48.6x1	T48.6x2	T48.6x3	T48.6x4	T48.6x5	T48.6x6
aminobenzoic acid	T48.6x1	T48.6x2	T48.6x3	T48.6x4	T48.6x5	T48.6x6
ethylenediamine	T48.6x1	T48.6x2	T48.6x3	T48.6x4	T48.6x5	T48.6x6
piperazine p-amino-benzoate	T48.6x1	T48.6x2	T48.6x3	T48.6x4	T48.6x5	T48.6x6
Thiabendazole	T37.4x1	T37.4x2	T37.4x3	T37.4x4	T37.4x5	T37.4x6
Thialbarbital	T41.1x1	T41.1x2	T41.1x3	T41.1x4	T41.1x5	T41.1x6
Thiamazole	T38.2x1	T38.2x2	T38.2x3	T38.2x4	T38.2x5	T38.2x6
Thiambutosine	T37.1x1	T37.1x2	T37.1x3	T37.1x4	T37.1x5	T37.1x6
Thiamine	T45.2x1	T45.2x2	T45.2x3	T45.2x4	T45.2x5	T45.2x6
Thiamphenicol	T36.2x1	T36.2x2	T36.2x3	T36.2x4	T36.2x5	T36.2x6

DRUGS&CHEMICALS

Table of Drugs & Chemicals	POISONING Accidental (Unintentional)	Self-Harm (Intentional)	Assault	Undetermined	Adverse Effect	Underdosing
Thiamylal	T41.1x1	T41.1x2	T41.1x3	T41.1x4	T41.1x5	T41.1x6
sodium	T41.1x1	T41.1x2	T41.1x3	T41.1x4	T41.1x5	T41.1x6
Thiazesim	T43.291	T43.292	T43.293	T43.294	T43.295	T43.296
Thiazides (diuretics)	T50.2x1	T50.2x2	T50.2x3	T50.2x4	T50.2x5	T50.2x6
Thiazinamium metilsulfate	T43.3x1	T43.3x2	T43.3x3	T43.3x4	T43.3x5	T43.3x6
Thiethylperazine	T43.3x1	T43.3x2	T43.3x3	T43.3x4	T43.3x5	T43.3x6
Thimerosal	T49.0x1	T49.0x2	T49.0x3	T49.0x4	T49.0x5	T49.0x6
ophthalmic preparation	T49.5x1	T49.5x2	T49.5x3	T49.5x4	T49.5x5	T49.5x6
Thioacetazone	T37.1x1	T37.1x2	T37.1x3	T37.1x4	T37.1x5	T37.1x6
with isoniazid	T37.1x1	T37.1x2	T37.1x3	T37.1x4	T37.1x5	T37.1x6
Thiobarbital sodium	T41.1x1	T41.1x2	T41.1x3	T41.1x4	T41.1x5	T41.1x6
Thiobarbiturate anesthetic	T41.1x1	T41.1x2	T41.1x3	T41.1x4	T41.1x5	T41.1x6
Thiobismol	T37.8x1	T37.8x2	T37.8x3	T37.8x4	T37.8x5	T37.8x6
Thiobutabarbital sodium	T41.1x1	T41.1x2	T41.1x3	T41.1x4	T41.1x5	T41.1x6
Thiocarbamate (insecticide)	T60.0x1	T60.0x2	T60.0x3	T60.0x4	—	—
Thiocarbamide	T38.2x1	T38.2x2	T38.2x3	T38.2x4	T38.2x5	T38.2x6
Thiocarbarsone	T37.8x1	T37.8x2	T37.8x3	T37.8x4	T37.8x5	T37.8x6
Thiocarlide	T37.1x1	T37.1x2	T37.1x3	T37.1x4	T37.1x5	T37.1x6
Thioctamide	T50.991	T50.992	T50.993	T50.994	T50.995	T50.996
Thioctic acid	T50.991	T50.992	T50.993	T50.994	T50.995	T50.996
Thiofos	T60.0x1	T60.0x2	T60.0x3	T60.0x4	—	—
Thioglycolate	T49.4x1	T49.4x2	T49.4x3	T49.4x4	T49.4x5	T49.4x6
Thioglycolic acid	T65.891	T65.892	T65.893	T65.894	—	—
Thioguanine	T45.1x1	T45.1x2	T45.1x3	T45.1x4	T45.1x5	T45.1x6
Thiomercaptomerin	T50.2x1	T50.2x2	T50.2x3	T50.2x4	T50.2x5	T50.2x6
Thiomerin	T50.2x1	T50.2x2	T50.2x3	T50.2x4	T50.2x5	T50.2x6
Thiomersal	T49.0x1	T49.0x2	T49.0x3	T49.0x4	T49.0x5	T49.0x6
Thionazin	T60.0x1	T60.0x2	T60.0x3	T60.0x4	—	—
Thiopental (sodium)	T41.1x1	T41.1x2	T41.1x3	T41.1x4	T41.1x5	T41.1x6
Thiopentone (sodium)	T41.1x1	T41.1x2	T41.1x3	T41.1x4	T41.1x5	T41.1x6
Thiopropazate	T43.3x1	T43.3x2	T43.3x3	T43.3x4	T43.3x5	T43.3x6
Thioproperazine	T43.3x1	T43.3x2	T43.3x3	T43.3x4	T43.3x5	T43.3x6
Thioridazine	T43.3x1	T43.3x2	T43.3x3	T43.3x4	T43.3x5	T43.3x6
Thiosinamine	T49.3x1	T49.3x2	T49.3x3	T49.3x4	T49.3x5	T49.3x6
Thiotepa	T45.1x1	T45.1x2	T45.1x3	T45.1x4	T45.1x5	T45.1x6
Thiothixene	T43.4x1	T43.4x2	T43.4x3	T43.4x4	T43.4x5	T43.4x6
Thiouracil (benzyl) (methyl) (propyl)	T38.2x1	T38.2x2	T38.2x3	T38.2x4	T38.2x5	T38.2x6
Thiourea	T38.2x1	T38.2x2	T38.2x3	T38.2x4	T38.2x5	T38.2x6
Thiphenamil	T44.3x1	T44.3x2	T44.3x3	T44.3x4	T44.3x5	T44.3x6
Thiram	T60.3x1	T60.3x2	T60.3x3	T60.3x4	—	—
medicinal	T49.2x1	T49.2x2	T49.2x3	T49.2x4	T49.2x5	T49.2x6
Thonzylamine (systemic)	T45.0x1	T45.0x2	T45.0x3	T45.0x4	T45.0x5	T45.0x6
mucosal decongestant	T48.5x1	T48.5x2	T48.5x3	T48.5x4	T48.5x5	T48.5x6
Thorazine	T43.3x1	T43.3x2	T43.3x3	T43.3x4	T43.3x5	T43.3x6
Thorium dioxide suspension	T50.8x1	T50.8x2	T50.8x3	T50.8x4	T50.8x5	T50.8x6
Thornapple	T62.2x1	T62.2x2	T62.2x3	T62.2x4	—	—
Throat drug NEC	T49.6x1	T49.6x2	T49.6x3	T49.6x4	T49.6x5	T49.6x6
Thrombin	T45.7x1	T45.7x2	T45.7x3	T45.7x4	T45.7x5	T45.7x6
Thrombolysin	T45.611	T45.612	T45.613	T45.614	T45.615	T45.616
Thromboplastin	T45.7x1	T45.7x2	T45.7x3	T45.7x4	T45.7x5	T45.7x6
Thurfyl nicotinate	T46.7x1	T46.7x2	T46.7x3	T46.7x4	T46.7x5	T46.7x6
Thymol	T49.0x1	T49.0x2	T49.0x3	T49.0x4	T49.0x5	T49.0x6
Thymopentin	T37.5x1	T37.5x2	T37.5x3	T37.5x4	T37.5x5	T37.5x6
Thymoxamine	T46.7x1	T46.7x2	T46.7x3	T46.7x4	T46.7x5	T46.7x6
Thymus extract	T38.891	T38.892	T38.893	T38.894	T38.895	T38.896
Thyreotrophic hormone	T38.811	T38.812	T38.813	T38.814	T38.815	T38.816
Thyroglobulin	T38.1x1	T38.1x2	T38.1x3	T38.1x4	T38.1x5	T38.1x6
Thyroid (hormone)	T38.1x1	T38.1x2	T38.1x3	T38.1x4	T38.1x5	T38.1x6
Thyrolar	T38.1x1	T38.1x2	T38.1x3	T38.1x4	T38.1x5	T38.1x6
Thyrotrophin	T38.811	T38.812	T38.813	T38.814	T38.815	T38.816
Thyrotropic hormone	T38.811	T38.812	T38.813	T38.814	T38.815	T38.816
Thyroxine	T38.1x1	T38.1x2	T38.1x3	T38.1x4	T38.1x5	T38.1x6
Tiabendazole	T37.4x1	T37.4x2	T37.4x3	T37.4x4	T37.4x5	T37.4x6
Tiamizide	T50.2x1	T50.2x2	T50.2x3	T50.2x4	T50.2x5	T50.2x6
Tianeptine	T43.291	T43.292	T43.293	T43.294	T43.295	T43.296
Tiapamil	T46.1x1	T46.1x2	T46.1x3	T46.1x4	T46.1x5	T46.1x6
Tiapride	T43.591	T43.592	T43.593	T43.594	T43.595	T43.596

Table of Drugs & Chemicals	POISONING Accidental (Unintentional)	Self-Harm (Intentional)	Assault	Undetermined	Adverse Effect	Underdosing
Tiaprofenic acid	T39.311	T39.312	T39.313	T39.314	T39.315	T39.316
Tiaramide	T39.8x1	T39.8x2	T39.8x3	T39.8x4	T39.8x5	T39.8x6
Ticarcillin	T36.0x1	T36.0x2	T36.0x3	T36.0x4	T36.0x5	T36.0x6
Ticlatone	T49.0x1	T49.0x2	T49.0x3	T49.0x4	T49.0x5	T49.0x6
Ticlopidine	T45.521	T45.522	T45.523	T45.524	T45.525	T45.526
Ticrynafen	T50.1x1	T50.1x2	T50.1x3	T50.1x4	T50.1x5	T50.1x6
Tidiacic	T50.991	T50.992	T50.993	T50.994	T50.995	T50.996
Tiemonium	T44.3x1	T44.3x2	T44.3x3	T44.3x4	T44.3x5	T44.3x6
iodide	T44.3x1	T44.3x2	T44.3x3	T44.3x4	T44.3x5	T44.3x6
Tienilic acid	T50.1x1	T50.1x2	T50.1x3	T50.1x4	T50.1x5	T50.1x6
Tifenamil	T44.3x1	T44.3x2	T44.3x3	T44.3x4	T44.3x5	T44.3x6
Tigan	T45.0x1	T45.0x2	T45.0x3	T45.0x4	T45.0x5	T45.0x6
Tigloidine	T44.3x1	T44.3x2	T44.3x3	T44.3x4	T44.3x5	T44.3x6
Tilactase	T47.5x1	T47.5x2	T47.5x3	T47.5x4	T47.5x5	T47.5x6
Tiletamine	T41.291	T41.292	T41.293	T41.294	T41.295	T41.296
Tilidine	T40.4x1	T40.4x2	T40.4x3	T40.4x4	—	—
Timepidium bromide	T44.3x1	T44.3x2	T44.3x3	T44.3x4	T44.3x5	T44.3x6
Timiperone	T43.4x1	T43.4x2	T43.4x3	T43.4x4	T43.4x5	T43.4x6
Timolol	T44.7x1	T44.7x2	T44.7x3	T44.7x4	T44.7x5	T44.7x6
Tin (chloride) (dust) (oxide) NEC	T56.6x1	T56.6x2	T56.6x3	T56.6x4	—	—
anti-infectives	T37.8x1	T37.8x2	T37.8x3	T37.8x4	T37.8x5	T37.8x6
Tincture, iodine — see Iodine						
Tindal	T43.3x1	T43.3x2	T43.3x3	T43.3x4	T43.3x5	T43.3x6
Tinidazole	T37.3x1	T37.3x2	T37.3x3	T37.3x4	T37.3x5	T37.3x6
Tinoridine	T39.8x1	T39.8x2	T39.8x3	T39.8x4	T39.8x5	T39.8x6
Tiocarlide	T37.1x1	T37.1x2	T37.1x3	T37.1x4	T37.1x5	T37.1x6
Tioclomarol	T45.511	T45.512	T45.513	T45.514	T45.515	T45.516
Tioconazole	T49.0x1	T49.0x2	T49.0x3	T49.0x4	T49.0x5	T49.0x6
Tioguanine	T45.1x1	T45.1x2	T45.1x3	T45.1x4	T45.1x5	T45.1x6
Tiopronin	T50.991	T50.992	T50.993	T50.994	T50.995	T50.996
Tiotixene	T43.4x1	T43.4x2	T43.4x3	T43.4x4	T43.4x5	T43.4x6
Tioxolone	T49.4x1	T49.4x2	T49.4x3	T49.4x4	T49.4x5	T49.4x6
Tipepidine	T48.3x1	T48.3x2	T48.3x3	T48.3x4	T48.3x5	T48.3x6
Tiquizium bromide	T44.3x1	T44.3x2	T44.3x3	T44.3x4	T44.3x5	T44.3x6
Tiratricol	T38.1x1	T38.1x2	T38.1x3	T38.1x4	T38.1x5	T38.1x6
Tisopurine	T50.4x1	T50.4x2	T50.4x3	T50.4x4	T50.4x5	T50.4x6
Titanium (compounds) (vapor)	T56.891	T56.892	T56.893	T56.894	—	—
dioxide	T49.3x1	T49.3x2	T49.3x3	T49.3x4	T49.3x5	T49.3x6
ointment	T49.3x1	T49.3x2	T49.3x3	T49.3x4	T49.3x5	T49.3x6
oxide	T49.3x1	T49.3x2	T49.3x3	T49.3x4	T49.3x5	T49.3x6
tetrachloride	T56.891	T56.892	T56.893	T56.894	—	—
Titanocene	T56.891	T56.892	T56.893	T56.894	—	—
Titroid	T38.1x1	T38.1x2	T38.1x3	T38.1x4	T38.1x5	T38.1x6
Tizanidine	T42.8x1	T42.8x2	T42.8x3	T42.8x4	T42.8x5	T42.8x6
TMTD	T60.3x1	T60.3x2	T60.3x3	T60.3x4	—	—
TNT (fumes)	T65.3x1	T65.3x2	T65.3x3	T65.3x4	—	—
Toadstool	T62.0x1	T62.0x2	T62.0x3	T62.0x4	—	—
Tobacco NEC	T65.291	T65.292	T65.293	T65.294	—	—
cigarettes	T65.221	T65.222	T65.223	T65.224	—	—
Indian	T62.2x1	T62.2x2	T62.2x3	T62.2x4	—	—
smoke, second-hand	T65.221	T65.222	T65.223	T65.224	—	—
Tobramycin	T36.5x1	T36.5x2	T36.5x3	T36.5x4	T36.5x5	T36.5x6
Tocainide	T46.2x1	T46.2x2	T46.2x3	T46.2x4	T46.2x5	T46.2x6
Tocoferol	T45.2x1	T45.2x2	T45.2x3	T45.2x4	T45.2x5	T45.2x6
Tocopherol	T45.2x1	T45.2x2	T45.2x3	T45.2x4	T45.2x5	T45.2x6
acetate	T45.2x1	T45.2x2	T45.2x3	T45.2x4	T45.2x5	T45.2x6
Tocosamine	T48.0x1	T48.0x2	T48.0x3	T48.0x4	T48.0x5	T48.0x6
Todralazine	T46.5x1	T46.5x2	T46.5x3	T46.5x4	T46.5x5	T46.5x6
Tofisopam	T42.4x1	T42.4x2	T42.4x3	T42.4x4	T42.4x5	T42.4x6
Tofranil	T43.011	T43.012	T43.013	T43.014	T43.015	T43.016
Toilet deodorizer	T65.891	T65.892	T65.893	T65.894	—	—
Tolamolol	T44.7x1	T44.7x2	T44.7x3	T44.7x4	T44.7x5	T44.7x6
Tolazamide	T38.3x1	T38.3x2	T38.3x3	T38.3x4	T38.3x5	T38.3x6
Tolazoline	T46.7x1	T46.7x2	T46.7x3	T46.7x4	T46.7x5	T46.7x6
Tolbutamide (sodium)	T38.3x1	T38.3x2	T38.3x3	T38.3x4	T38.3x5	T38.3x6
Tolciclate	T49.0x1	T49.0x2	T49.0x3	T49.0x4	T49.0x5	T49.0x6

DRUGS&CHEMICALS

Table of Drugs & Chemicals	Accidental (Unintentional)	Self-Harm (Intentional)	Assault	Undetermined	Adverse Effect	Underdosing
Tolmetin	T39.391	T39.392	T39.393	T39.394	T39.395	T39.396
Tolnaftate	T49.0x1	T49.0x2	T49.0x3	T49.0x4	T49.0x5	T49.0x6
Tolonidine	T46.5x1	T46.5x2	T46.5x3	T46.5x4	T46.5x5	T46.5x6
Toloxatone	T42.6x1	T42.6x2	T42.6x3	T42.6x4	T42.6x5	T42.6x6
Tolperisone	T44.3x1	T44.3x2	T44.3x3	T44.3x4	T44.3x5	T44.3x6
Tolserol	T42.8x1	T42.8x2	T42.8x3	T42.8x4	T42.8x5	T42.8x6
Toluene (liquid)	T52.2x1	T52.2x2	T52.2x3	T52.2x4	—	—
diisocyanate	T65.0x1	T65.0x2	T65.0x3	T65.0x4	—	—
Toluidine	T65.891	T65.892	T65.893	T65.894	—	—
vapor	T59.891	T59.892	T59.893	T59.894	—	—
Toluol (liquid)	T52.2x1	T52.2x2	T52.2x3	T52.2x4	—	—
vapor	T52.2x1	T52.2x2	T52.2x3	T52.2x4	—	—
Toluylenediamine	T65.3x1	T65.3x2	T65.3x3	T65.3x4	—	—
Tolylene-2,4-diisocyanate	T65.0x1	T65.0x2	T65.0x3	T65.0x4	—	—
Tonic NEC	T50.901	T50.902	T50.903	T50.904	T50.905	T50.906
Topical action drug NEC	T49.91	T49.92	T49.93	T49.94	T49.95	T49.96
ear, nose or throat	T49.6x1	T49.6x2	T49.6x3	T49.6x4	T49.6x5	T49.6x6
eye	T49.5x1	T49.5x2	T49.5x3	T49.5x4	T49.5x5	T49.5x6
skin	T49.91	T49.92	T49.93	T49.94	T49.95	T49.96
specified NEC	T49.8x1	T49.8x2	T49.8x3	T49.8x4	T49.8x5	T49.8x6
Toquizine	T44.3x1	T44.3x2	T44.3x3	T44.3x4	T44.3x5	T44.3x6
Toremifene	T38.6x1	T38.6x2	T38.6x3	T38.6x4	T38.6x5	T38.6x6
Tosylchloramide sodium	T49.8x1	T49.8x2	T49.8x3	T49.8x4	T49.8x5	T49.8x6
Toxaphene (dust) (spray)	T60.1x1	T60.1x2	T60.1x3	T60.1x4	—	—
Toxin, diphtheria (Schick Test)	T50.8x1	T50.8x2	T50.8x3	T50.8x4	T50.8x5	T50.8x6
Toxoid						
combined	T50.A21	T50.A22	T50.A23	T50.A24	T50.A25	T50.A26
diphtheria	T50.A91	T50.A92	T50.A93	T50.A94	T50.A95	T50.A96
tetanus	T50.A91	T50.A92	T50.A93	T50.A94	T50.A95	T50.A96
Trace element NEC	T45.8x1	T45.8x2	T45.8x3	T45.8x4	T45.8x5	T45.8x6
Tractor fuel NEC	T52.0x1	T52.0x2	T52.0x3	T52.0x4	—	—
Tragacanth	T50.991	T50.992	T50.993	T50.994	T50.995	T50.996
Tramadol	T40.4x1	T40.4x2	T40.4x3	T40.4x4	T40.4x5	T40.4x6
Tramazoline	T48.5x1	T48.5x2	T48.5x3	T48.5x4	T48.5x5	T48.5x6
Tranexamic acid	T45.621	T45.622	T45.623	T45.624	T45.625	T45.626
Tranilast	T45.0x1	T45.0x2	T45.0x3	T45.0x4	T45.0x5	T45.0x6
Tranquilizer NEC	T43.501	T43.502	T43.503	T43.504	T43.505	T43.506
with hypnotic or sedative	T42.6x1	T42.6x2	T42.6x3	T42.6x4	T42.6x5	T42.6x6
benzodiazepine NEC	T42.4x1	T42.4x2	T42.4x3	T42.4x4	T42.4x5	T42.4x6
butyrophenone NEC	T43.4x1	T43.4x2	T43.4x3	T43.4x4	T43.4x5	T43.4x6
carbamate	T43.591	T43.592	T43.593	T43.594	T43.595	T43.596
dimethylamine	T43.3x1	T43.3x2	T43.3x3	T43.3x4	T43.3x5	T43.3x6
ethylamine	T43.3x1	T43.3x2	T43.3x3	T43.3x4	T43.3x5	T43.3x6
hydroxyzine	T43.591	T43.592	T43.593	T43.594	T43.595	T43.596
major NEC	T43.501	T43.502	T43.503	T43.504	T43.505	T43.506
penothiazine NEC	T43.3x1	T43.3x2	T43.3x3	T43.3x4	T43.3x5	T43.3x6
phenothiazine-based	T43.3x1	T43.3x2	T43.3x3	T43.3x4	T43.3x5	T43.3x6
piperazine NEC	T43.3x1	T43.3x2	T43.3x3	T43.3x4	T43.3x5	T43.3x6
piperidine	T43.3x1	T43.3x2	T43.3x3	T43.3x4	T43.3x5	T43.3x6
propylamine	T43.3x1	T43.3x2	T43.3x3	T43.3x4	T43.3x5	T43.3x6
specified NEC	T43.591	T43.592	T43.593	T43.594	T43.595	T43.596
thioxanthene NEC	T43.591	T43.592	T43.593	T43.594	T43.595	T43.596
Tranxene	T42.4x1	T42.4x2	T42.4x3	T42.4x4	T42.4x5	T42.4x6
Tranylcypromine	T43.1x1	T43.1x2	T43.1x3	T43.1x4	T43.1x5	T43.1x6
Trapidil	T46.3x1	T46.3x2	T46.3x3	T46.3x4	T46.3x5	T46.3x6
Trasentine	T44.3x1	T44.3x2	T44.3x3	T44.3x4	T44.3x5	T44.3x6
Travert	T50.3x1	T50.3x2	T50.3x3	T50.3x4	T50.3x5	T50.3x6
Trazodone	T43.211	T43.212	T43.213	T43.214	T43.215	T43.216
Trecator	T37.1x1	T37.1x2	T37.1x3	T37.1x4	T37.1x5	T37.1x6
Treosulfan	T45.1x1	T45.1x2	T45.1x3	T45.1x4	T45.1x5	T45.1x6
Tretamine	T45.1x1	T45.1x2	T45.1x3	T45.1x4	T45.1x5	T45.1x6
Tretinoin	T49.0x1	T49.0x2	T49.0x3	T49.0x4	T49.0x5	T49.0x6
Tretoquinol	T48.6x1	T48.6x2	T48.6x3	T48.6x4	T48.6x5	T48.6x6
Triacetin	T49.0x1	T49.0x2	T49.0x3	T49.0x4	T49.0x5	T49.0x6
Triacetoxyanthracene	T49.4x1	T49.4x2	T49.4x3	T49.4x4	T49.4x5	T49.4x6
Triacetyloleandomycin	T36.3x1	T36.3x2	T36.3x3	T36.3x4	T36.3x5	T36.3x6

Table of Drugs & Chemicals	Accidental (Unintentional)	Self-Harm (Intentional)	Assault	Undetermined	Adverse Effect	Underdosing
Triamcinolone	T49.0x1	T49.0x2	T49.0x3	T49.0x4	T49.0x5	T49.0x6
ENT agent	T49.6x1	T49.6x2	T49.6x3	T49.6x4	T49.6x5	T49.6x6
hexacetonide	T49.0x1	T49.0x2	T49.0x3	T49.0x4	T49.0x5	T49.0x6
ophthalmic preparation	T49.5x1	T49.5x2	T49.5x3	T49.5x4	T49.5x5	T49.5x6
topical NEC	T49.0x1	T49.0x2	T49.0x3	T49.0x4	T49.0x5	T49.0x6
Triampyzine	T44.3x1	T44.3x2	T44.3x3	T44.3x4	T44.3x5	T44.3x6
Triamterene	T50.2x1	T50.2x2	T50.2x3	T50.2x4	T50.2x5	T50.2x6
Triazine (herbicide)	T60.3x1	T60.3x2	T60.3x3	T60.3x4	—	—
Triaziquone	T45.1x1	T45.1x2	T45.1x3	T45.1x4	T45.1x5	T45.1x6
Triazolam	T42.4x1	T42.4x2	T42.4x3	T42.4x4	T42.4x5	T42.4x6
Triazole (herbicide)	T60.3x1	T60.3x2	T60.3x3	T60.3x4	—	—
Tribenoside	T46.991	T46.992	T46.993	T46.994	T46.995	T46.996
Tribromacetaldehyde	T42.6x1	T42.6x2	T42.6x3	T42.6x4	T42.6x5	T42.6x6
Tribromoethanol, rectal	T41.291	T41.292	T41.293	T41.294	T41.295	T41.296
Tribromomethane	T42.6x1	T42.6x2	T42.6x3	T42.6x4	T42.6x5	T42.6x6
Trichlorethane	T53.2x1	T53.2x2	T53.2x3	T53.2x4	—	—
Trichlorethylene	T53.2x1	T53.2x2	T53.2x3	T53.2x4	—	—
Trichlorfon	T60.0x1	T60.0x2	T60.0x3	T60.0x4	—	—
Trichlormethiazide	T50.2x1	T50.2x2	T50.2x3	T50.2x4	T50.2x5	T50.2x6
Trichlormethine	T45.1x1	T45.1x2	T45.1x3	T45.1x4	T45.1x5	T45.1x6
Trichloroacetic acid, trichloracetic acid	T54.2x1	T54.2x2	T54.2x3	T54.2x4	—	—
medicinal	T49.4x1	T49.4x2	T49.4x3	T49.4x4	T49.4x5	T49.4x6
Trichloroethane	T53.2x1	T53.2x2	T53.2x3	T53.2x4	—	—
Trichloroethanol	T42.6x1	T42.6x2	T42.6x3	T42.6x4	T42.6x5	T42.6x6
Trichloroethyl phosphate	T42.6x1	T42.6x2	T42.6x3	T42.6x4	T42.6x5	T42.6x6
Trichloroethylene (liquid) (vapor)	T53.2x1	T53.2x2	T53.2x3	T53.2x4	—	—
anesthetic (gas)	T41.0x1	T41.0x2	T41.0x3	T41.0x4	T41.0x5	—
vapor NEC	T53.2x1	T53.2x2	T53.2x3	T53.2x4	—	—
Trichlorofluoromethane NEC	T53.5x1	T53.5x2	T53.5x3	T53.5x4	—	—
Trichloronate	T60.0x1	T60.0x2	T60.0x3	T60.0x4	—	—
2,4,5-Trichlorophen-oxyacetic acid	T60.3x1	T60.3x2	T60.3x3	T60.3x4	—	—
Trichloropropane	T53.6x1	T53.6x2	T53.6x3	T53.6x4	—	—
Trichlorotriethylamine	T45.1x1	T45.1x2	T45.1x3	T45.1x4	T45.1x5	T45.1x6
Trichomonacides NEC	T37.3x1	T37.3x2	T37.3x3	T37.3x4	T37.3x5	T37.3x6
Trichomycin	T36.7x1	T36.7x2	T36.7x3	T36.7x4	T36.7x5	T36.7x6
Triclobisonium chloride	T49.0x1	T49.0x2	T49.0x3	T49.0x4	T49.0x5	T49.0x6
Triclocarban	T49.0x1	T49.0x2	T49.0x3	T49.0x4	T49.0x5	T49.0x6
Triclofos	T42.6x1	T42.6x2	T42.6x3	T42.6x4	T42.6x5	T42.6x6
Triclosan	T49.0x1	T49.0x2	T49.0x3	T49.0x4	T49.0x5	T49.0x6
Tricresyl phosphate	T65.891	T65.892	T65.893	T65.894	—	—
solvent	T52.91	T52.92	T52.93	T52.94	—	—
Tricyclamol chloride	T44.3x1	T44.3x2	T44.3x3	T44.3x4	T44.3x5	T44.3x6
Tridesilon	T49.0x1	T49.0x2	T49.0x3	T49.0x4	T49.0x5	T49.0x6
Tridihexethyl iodide	T44.3x1	T44.3x2	T44.3x3	T44.3x4	T44.3x5	T44.3x6
Tridione	T42.2x1	T42.2x2	T42.2x3	T42.2x4	T42.2x5	T42.2x6
Trientine	T45.8x1	T45.8x2	T45.8x3	T45.8x4	T45.8x5	T45.8x6
Triethanolamine NEC	T54.3x1	T54.3x2	T54.3x3	T54.3x4	—	—
detergent	T54.3x1	T54.3x2	T54.3x3	T54.3x4	—	—
trinitrate (biphosphate)	T46.3x1	T46.3x2	T46.3x3	T46.3x4	T46.3x5	T46.3x6
Triethanomelamine	T45.1x1	T45.1x2	T45.1x3	T45.1x4	T45.1x5	T45.1x6
Triethylenemelamine	T45.1x1	T45.1x2	T45.1x3	T45.1x4	T45.1x5	T45.1x6
Triethylenephosphoramide	T45.1x1	T45.1x2	T45.1x3	T45.1x4	T45.1x5	T45.1x6
Triethylenethiophosphoramide	T45.1x1	T45.1x2	T45.1x3	T45.1x4	T45.1x5	T45.1x6
Trifluoperazine	T43.3x1	T43.3x2	T43.3x3	T43.3x4	T43.3x5	T43.3x6
Trifluoroethyl vinyl ether	T41.0x1	T41.0x2	T41.0x3	T41.0x4	T41.0x5	T41.0x6
Trifluperidol	T43.4x1	T43.4x2	T43.4x3	T43.4x4	T43.4x5	T43.4x6
Triflupromazine	T43.3x1	T43.3x2	T43.3x3	T43.3x4	T43.3x5	T43.3x6
Trifluridine	T37.5x1	T37.5x2	T37.5x3	T37.5x4	T37.5x5	T37.5x6
Triflusal	T45.521	T45.522	T45.523	T45.524	T45.525	T45.526
Trihexyphenidyl	T44.3x1	T44.3x2	T44.3x3	T44.3x4	T44.3x5	T44.3x6
Triiodothyronine	T38.1x1	T38.1x2	T38.1x3	T38.1x4	T38.1x5	T38.1x6
Trilene	T41.0x1	T41.0x2	T41.0x3	T41.0x4	T41.0x5	T41.0x6
Trilostane	T38.991	T38.992	T38.993	T38.994	T38.995	T38.996
Trimebutine	T44.3x1	T44.3x2	T44.3x3	T44.3x4	T44.3x5	T44.3x6
Trimecaine	T41.3x1	T41.3x2	T41.3x3	T41.3x4	T41.3x5	T41.3x6
Trimeprazine (tartrate)	T44.3x1	T44.3x2	T44.3x3	T44.3x4	T44.3x5	T44.3x6
Trimetaphan camsilate	T44.2x1	T44.2x2	T44.2x3	T44.2x4	T44.2x5	T44.2x6
Trimetazidine	T46.7x1	T46.7x2	T46.7x3	T46.7x4	T46.7x5	T46.7x6

DRUGS&CHEMICALS

Table of Drugs & Chemicals	POISONING Accidental (Unintentional)	Self-Harm (Intentional)	Assault	Undetermined	Adverse Effect	Underdosing
Trimethadione	T42.2x1	T42.2x2	T42.2x3	T42.2x4	T42.2x5	T42.2x6
Trimethaphan	T44.2x1	T44.2x2	T44.2x3	T44.2x4	T44.2x5	T44.2x6
Trimethidinium	T44.2x1	T44.2x2	T44.2x3	T44.2x4	T44.2x5	T44.2x6
Trimethobenzamide	T45.0x1	T45.0x2	T45.0x3	T45.0x4	T45.0x5	T45.0x6
Trimethoprim	T37.8x1	T37.8x2	T37.8x3	T37.8x4	T37.8x5	T37.8x6
with sulfamethoxazole	T36.8x1	T36.8x2	T36.8x3	T36.8x4	T36.8x5	T36.8x6
Trimethylcarbinol	T51.3x1	T51.3x2	T51.3x3	T51.3x4	—	—
Trimethylpsoralen	T49.3x1	T49.3x2	T49.3x3	T49.3x4	T49.3x5	T49.3x6
Trimeton	T45.0x1	T45.0x2	T45.0x3	T45.0x4	T45.0x5	T45.0x6
Trimetrexate	T45.1x1	T45.1x2	T45.1x3	T45.1x4	T45.1x5	T45.1x6
Trimipramine	T43.011	T43.012	T43.013	T43.014	T43.015	T43.016
Trimustine	T45.1x1	T45.1x2	T45.1x3	T45.1x4	T45.1x5	T45.1x6
Trinitrine	T46.3x1	T46.3x2	T46.3x3	T46.3x4	T46.3x5	T46.3x6
Trinitrobenzol	T65.3x1	T65.3x2	T65.3x3	T65.3x4	—	—
Trinitrophenol	T65.3x1	T65.3x2	T65.3x3	T65.3x4	—	—
Trinitrotoluene (fumes)	T65.3x1	T65.3x2	T65.3x3	T65.3x4	—	—
Trional	T42.6x1	T42.6x2	T42.6x3	T42.6x4	T42.6x5	T42.6x6
Triorthocresyl phosphate	T65.891	T65.892	T65.893	T65.894	—	—
Trioxide of arsenic	T57.0x1	T57.0x2	T57.0x3	T57.0x4	—	—
Trioxysalen	T49.4x1	T49.4x2	T49.4x3	T49.4x4	T49.4x5	T49.4x6
Tripamide	T50.2x1	T50.2x2	T50.2x3	T50.2x4	T50.2x5	T50.2x6
Triparanol	T46.6x1	T46.6x2	T46.6x3	T46.6x4	T46.6x5	T46.6x6
Tripelennamine	T45.0x1	T45.0x2	T45.0x3	T45.0x4	T45.0x5	T45.0x6
Triperiden	T44.3x1	T44.3x2	T44.3x3	T44.3x4	T44.3x5	T44.3x6
Triperidol	T43.4x1	T43.4x2	T43.4x3	T43.4x4	T43.4x5	T43.4x6
Triphenylphosphate	T65.891	T65.892	T65.893	T65.894	—	—
Triple						
bromides	T42.6x1	T42.6x2	T42.6x3	T42.6x4	T42.6x5	T42.6x6
carbonate	T47.1x1	T47.1x2	T47.1x3	T47.1x4	T47.1x5	T47.1x6
vaccine						
DPT	T50.A11	T50.A12	T50.A13	T50.A14	T50.A15	T50.A16
including pertussis	T50.A11	T50.A12	T50.A13	T50.A14	T50.A15	T50.A16
MMR	T50.B91	T50.B92	T50.B93	T50.B94	T50.B95	T50.B96
Triprolidine	T45.0x1	T45.0x2	T45.0x3	T45.0x4	T45.0x5	T45.0x6
Trisodium hydrogen edetate	T50.6x1	T50.6x2	T50.6x3	T50.6x4	T50.6x5	T50.6x6
Trisoralen	T49.3x1	T49.3x2	T49.3x3	T49.3x4	T49.3x5	T49.3x6
Trisulfapyrimidines	T37.0x1	T37.0x2	T37.0x3	T37.0x4	T37.0x5	T37.0x6
Trithiozine	T44.3x1	T44.3x2	T44.3x3	T44.3x4	T44.3x5	T44.3x6
Tritiozine	T44.3x1	T44.3x2	T44.3x3	T44.3x4	T44.3x5	T44.3x6
Tritoqualine	T45.0x1	T45.0x2	T45.0x3	T45.0x4	T45.0x5	T45.0x6
Trofosfamide	T45.1x1	T45.1x2	T45.1x3	T45.1x4	T45.1x5	T45.1x6
Troleandomycin	T36.3x1	T36.3x2	T36.3x3	T36.3x4	T36.3x5	T36.3x6
Trolnitrate (phosphate)	T46.3x1	T46.3x2	T46.3x3	T46.3x4	T46.3x5	T46.3x6
Tromantadine	T37.5x1	T37.5x2	T37.5x3	T37.5x4	T37.5x5	T37.5x6
Trometamol	T50.2x1	T50.2x2	T50.2x3	T50.2x4	T50.2x5	T50.2x6
Tromethamine	T50.2x1	T50.2x2	T50.2x3	T50.2x4	T50.2x5	T50.2x6
Tronothane	T41.3x1	T41.3x2	T41.3x3	T41.3x4	T41.3x5	T41.3x6
Tropacine	T44.3x1	T44.3x2	T44.3x3	T44.3x4	T44.3x5	T44.3x6
Tropatepine	T44.3x1	T44.3x2	T44.3x3	T44.3x4	T44.3x5	T44.3x6
Tropicamide	T44.3x1	T44.3x2	T44.3x3	T44.3x4	T44.3x5	T44.3x6
Trospium chloride	T44.3x1	T44.3x2	T44.3x3	T44.3x4	T44.3x5	T44.3x6
Troxerutin	T46.991	T46.992	T46.993	T46.994	T46.995	T46.996
Troxidone	T42.2x1	T42.2x2	T42.2x3	T42.2x4	T42.2x5	T42.2x6
Tryparsamide	T37.3x1	T37.3x2	T37.3x3	T37.3x4	T37.3x5	T37.3x6
Trypsin	T45.3x1	T45.3x2	T45.3x3	T45.3x4	T45.3x5	T45.3x6
Tryptizol	T43.011	T43.012	T43.013	T43.014	T43.015	T43.016
TSH	T38.811	T38.812	T38.813	T38.814	T38.815	T38.816
Tuaminoheptane	T48.5x1	T48.5x2	T48.5x3	T48.5x4	T48.5x5	T48.5x6
Tuberculin, purified protein derivative (PPD)	T50.8x1	T50.8x2	T50.8x3	T50.8x4	T50.8x5	T50.8x6
Tubocurare	T48.1x1	T48.1x2	T48.1x3	T48.1x4	T48.1x5	T48.1x6
Tubocurarine (chloride)	T48.1x1	T48.1x2	T48.1x3	T48.1x4	T48.1x5	T48.1x6
Tulobuterol	T48.6x1	T48.6x2	T48.6x3	T48.6x4	T48.6x5	T48.6x6
Turpentine (spirits of)	T52.8x1	T52.8x2	T52.8x3	T52.8x4	—	—
vapor	T52.8x1	T52.8x2	T52.8x3	T52.8x4	—	—
Tybamate	T43.591	T43.592	T43.593	T43.594	T43.595	T43.596
Tyloxapol	T48.4x1	T48.4x2	T48.4x3	T48.4x4	T48.4x5	T48.4x6
Tymazoline	T48.5x1	T48.5x2	T48.5x3	T48.5x4	T48.5x5	T48.5x6
Typhoid-paratyphoid vaccine	T50.A91	T50.A92	T50.A93	T50.A94	T50.A95	T50.A96
Typhus vaccine	T50.A91	T50.A92	T50.A93	T50.A94	T50.A95	T50.A96
Tyropanoate	T50.8x1	T50.8x2	T50.8x3	T50.8x4	T50.8x5	T50.8x6
Tyrothricin	T49.6x1	T49.6x2	T49.6x3	T49.6x4	T49.6x5	T49.6x6
ENT agent	T49.6x1	T49.6x2	T49.6x3	T49.6x4	T49.6x5	T49.6x6
ophthalmic preparation	T49.5x1	T49.5x2	T49.5x3	T49.5x4	T49.5x5	T49.5x6
Ufenamate	T39.391	T39.392	T39.393	T39.394	T39.395	T39.396
Ultraviolet light protectant	T49.3x1	T49.3x2	T49.3x3	T49.3x4	T49.3x5	T49.3x6
Undecenoic acid	T49.0x1	T49.0x2	T49.0x3	T49.0x4	T49.0x5	T49.0x6
Undecoylium	T49.0x1	T49.0x2	T49.0x3	T49.0x4	T49.0x5	T49.0x6
Undecylenic acid (derivatives)	T49.0x1	T49.0x2	T49.0x3	T49.0x4	T49.0x5	T49.0x6
Unna's boot	T49.3x1	T49.3x2	T49.3x3	T49.3x4	T49.3x5	T49.3x6
Unsaturated fatty acid	T46.6x1	T46.6x2	T46.6x3	T46.6x4	T46.6x5	T46.6x6
Uracil mustard	T45.1x1	T45.1x2	T45.1x3	T45.1x4	T45.1x5	T45.1x6
Uramustine	T45.1x1	T45.1x2	T45.1x3	T45.1x4	T45.1x5	T45.1x6
Urapidil	T46.5x1	T46.5x2	T46.5x3	T46.5x4	T46.5x5	T46.5x6
Urari	T48.1x1	T48.1x2	T48.1x3	T48.1x4	T48.1x5	T48.1x6
Urate oxidase	T50.4x1	T50.4x2	T50.4x3	T50.4x4	T50.4x5	T50.4x6
Urea	T47.3x1	T47.3x2	T47.3x3	T47.3x4	T47.3x5	T47.3x6
peroxide	T49.0x1	T49.0x2	T49.0x3	T49.0x4	T49.0x5	T49.0x6
stibamine	T37.4x1	T37.4x2	T37.4x3	T37.4x4	T37.4x5	T37.4x6
topical	T49.8x1	T49.8x2	T49.8x3	T49.8x4	T49.8x5	T49.8x6
Urethane	T45.1x1	T45.1x2	T45.1x3	T45.1x4	T45.1x5	T45.1x6
Urginea (maritima) (scilla) — see Squill						
Uric acid metabolism drug NEC	T50.4x1	T50.4x2	T50.4x3	T50.4x4	T50.4x5	T50.4x6
Uricosuric agent	T50.4x1	T50.4x2	T50.4x3	T50.4x4	T50.4x5	T50.4x6
Urinary anti-infective	T37.8x1	T37.8x2	T37.8x3	T37.8x4	T37.8x5	T37.8x6
Urofollitropin	T38.811	T38.812	T38.813	T38.814	T38.815	T38.816
Urokinase	T45.611	T45.612	T45.613	T45.614	T45.615	T45.616
Urokon	T50.8x1	T50.8x2	T50.8x3	T50.8x4	T50.8x5	T50.8x6
Ursodeoxycholic acid	T50.991	T50.992	T50.993	T50.994	T50.995	T50.996
Ursodiol	T50.991	T50.992	T50.993	T50.994	T50.995	T50.996
Urtica	T62.2x1	T62.2x2	T62.2x3	T62.2x4	—	—
Utility gas — see Gas, utility						
Vaccine NEC	T50.Z91	T50.Z92	T50.Z93	T50.Z94	T50.Z95	T50.Z96
antineoplastic	T50.Z91	T50.Z92	T50.Z93	T50.Z94	T50.Z95	T50.Z96
bacterial NEC	T50.A91	T50.A92	T50.A93	T50.A94	T50.A95	T50.A96
with						
other bacterial component	T50.A21	T50.A22	T50.A23	T50.A24	T50.A25	T50.A26
pertussis component	T50.A11	T50.A12	T50.A13	T50.A14	T50.A15	T50.A16
viral-rickettsial component	T50.A21	T50.A22	T50.A23	T50.A24	T50.A25	T50.A26
mixed NEC	T50.A21	T50.A22	T50.A23	T50.A24	T50.A25	T50.A26
BCG	T50.A91	T50.A92	T50.A93	T50.A94	T50.A95	T50.A96
cholera	T50.A91	T50.A92	T50.A93	T50.A94	T50.A95	T50.A96
diphtheria	T50.A91	T50.A92	T50.A93	T50.A94	T50.A95	T50.A96
with tetanus	T50.A21	T50.A22	T50.A23	T50.A24	T50.A25	T50.A26
and pertussis	T50.A11	T50.A12	T50.A13	T50.A14	T50.A15	T50.A16
influenza	T50.B91	T50.B92	T50.B93	T50.B94	T50.B95	T50.B96
measles	T50.B91	T50.B92	T50.B93	T50.B94	T50.B95	T50.B96
with mumps and rubella	T50.B91	T50.B92	T50.B93	T50.B94	T50.B95	T50.B96
meningococcal	T50.A91	T50.A92	T50.A93	T50.A94	T50.A95	T50.A96
mumps	T50.B91	T50.B92	T50.B93	T50.B94	T50.B95	T50.B96
paratyphoid	T50.A91	T50.A92	T50.A93	T50.A94	T50.A95	T50.A96
pertussis	T50.A11	T50.A12	T50.A13	T50.A14	T50.A15	T50.A16
with diphtheria	T50.A11	T50.A12	T50.A13	T50.A14	T50.A15	T50.A16
and tetanus	T50.A11	T50.A12	T50.A13	T50.A14	T50.A15	T50.A16
with other component	T50.A11	T50.A12	T50.A13	T50.A14	T50.A15	T50.A16
plague	T50.A91	T50.A92	T50.A93	T50.A94	T50.A95	T50.A96
poliomyelitis	T50.B91	T50.B92	T50.B93	T50.B94	T50.B95	T50.B96
poliovirus	T50.B91	T50.B92	T50.B93	T50.B94	T50.B95	T50.B96
rabies	T50.B91	T50.B92	T50.B93	T50.B94	T50.B95	T50.B96
respiratory syncytial virus	T50.B91	T50.B92	T50.B93	T50.B94	T50.B95	T50.B96
rickettsial NEC	T50.A91	T50.A92	T50.A93	T50.A94	T50.A95	T50.A96
with						
bacterial component	T50.A21	T50.A22	T50.A23	T50.A24	T50.A25	T50.A26
Rocky Mountain spotted fever	T50.A91	T50.A92	T50.A93	T50.A94	T50.A95	T50.A96
rubella	T50.B91	T50.B92	T50.B93	T50.B94	T50.B95	T50.B96

DRUGS&CHEMICALS

Table of Drugs & Chemicals	POISONING Accidental (Unintentional)	Self-Harm (Intentional)	Assault	Undetermined	Adverse Effect	Underdosing
Vaccine NEC – continued	T50.Z91	T50.Z92	T50.Z93	T50.Z94	T50.Z95	T50.Z96
sabin oral	T50.B91	T50.B92	T50.B93	T50.B94	T50.B95	T50.B96
smallpox	T50.B11	T50.B12	T50.B13	T50.B14	T50.B15	T50.B16
TAB	T50.A91	T50.A92	T50.A93	T50.A94	T50.A95	T50.A96
tetanus	T50.A91	T50.A92	T50.A93	T50.A94	T50.A95	T50.A96
typhoid	T50.A91	T50.A92	T50.A93	T50.A94	T50.A95	T50.A96
typhus	T50.A91	T50.A92	T50.A93	T50.A94	T50.A95	T50.A96
viral NEC	T50.B91	T50.B92	T50.B93	T50.B94	T50.B95	T50.B96
yellow fever	T50.B91	T50.B92	T50.B93	T50.B94	T50.B95	T50.B96
Vaccinia immune globulin	T50.Z11	T50.Z12	T50.Z13	T50.Z14	T50.Z15	T50.Z16
Vaginal contraceptives	T49.8x1	T49.8x2	T49.8x3	T49.8x4	T49.8x5	T49.8x6
Valerian						
root	T42.6x1	T42.6x2	T42.6x3	T42.6x4	T42.6x5	T42.6x6
tincture	T42.6x1	T42.6x2	T42.6x3	T42.6x4	T42.6x5	T42.6x6
Valethamate bromide	T44.3x1	T44.3x2	T44.3x3	T44.3x4	T44.3x5	T44.3x6
Valisone	T49.0x1	T49.0x2	T49.0x3	T49.0x4	T49.0x5	T49.0x6
Valium	T42.4x1	T42.4x2	T42.4x3	T42.4x4	T42.4x5	T42.4x6
Valmid	T42.6x1	T42.6x2	T42.6x3	T42.6x4	T42.6x5	T42.6x6
Valnoctamide	T42.6x1	T42.6x2	T42.6x3	T42.6x4	T42.6x5	T42.6x6
Valproate (sodium)	T42.6x1	T42.6x2	T42.6x3	T42.6x4	T42.6x5	T42.6x6
Valproic acid	T42.6x1	T42.6x2	T42.6x3	T42.6x4	T42.6x5	T42.6x6
Valpromide	T42.6x1	T42.6x2	T42.6x3	T42.6x4	T42.6x5	T42.6x6
Vanadium	T56.891	T56.892	T56.893	T56.894	—	—
Vancomycin	T36.8x1	T36.8x2	T36.8x3	T36.8x4	T36.8x5	T36.8x6
Vapor — see also Gas	T59.91	T59.92	T59.93	T59.94	—	—
kiln (carbon monoxide)	T58.8x1	T58.8x2	T58.8x3	T58.8x4	—	—
lead — see lead						
specified source NEC	T59.891	T59.892	T59.893	T59.894	—	—
Vardenafil	T46.7x1	T46.7x2	T46.7x3	T46.7x4	T46.7x5	T46.7x6
Varicose reduction drug	T46.8x1	T46.8x2	T46.8x3	T46.8x4	T46.8x5	T46.8x6
Varnish	T65.4x1	T65.4x2	T65.4x3	T65.4x4	—	—
cleaner	T52.91	T52.92	T52.93	T52.94	—	—
Vaseline	T49.3x1	T49.3x2	T49.3x3	T49.3x4	T49.3x5	T49.3x6
Vasodilan	T46.7x1	T46.7x2	T46.7x3	T46.7x4	T46.7x5	T46.7x6
Vasodilator						
coronary NEC	T46.3x1	T46.3x2	T46.3x3	T46.3x4	T46.3x5	T46.3x6
peripheral NEC	T46.7x1	T46.7x2	T46.7x3	T46.7x4	T46.7x5	T46.7x6
Vasopressin	T38.891	T38.892	T38.893	T38.894	T38.895	T38.896
Vasopressor drugs	T38.891	T38.892	T38.893	T38.894	T38.895	T38.896
Vecuronium bromide	T48.1x1	T48.1x2	T48.1x3	T48.1x4	T48.1x5	T48.1x6
Vegetable extract, astringent	T49.2x1	T49.2x2	T49.2x3	T49.2x4	T49.2x5	T49.2x6
Venlafaxine	T43.211	T43.212	T43.213	T43.214	T43.215	T43.216
Venom, venomous (bite) (sting)	T63.91	T63.92	T63.93	T63.94	—	—
ant	T63.421	T63.422	T63.423	T63.424	—	—
amphibian NEC	T63.831	T63.832	T63.833	T63.834	—	—
animal NEC	T63.891	T63.892	T63.893	T63.894	—	—
arthropod NEC	T63.481	T63.482	T63.483	T63.484	—	—
bee	T63.441	T63.442	T63.443	T63.444	—	—
centipede	T63.411	T63.412	T63.413	T63.414	—	—
fish	T63.591	T63.592	T63.593	T63.594	—	—
frog	T63.811	T63.812	T63.813	T63.814	—	—
hornet	T63.451	T63.452	T63.453	T63.454	—	—
insect NEC	T63.481	T63.482	T63.483	T63.484	—	—
lizard	T63.121	T63.122	T63.123	T63.124	—	—
marine						
animals	T63.691	T63.692	T63.693	T63.694	—	—
bluebottle	T63.611	T63.612	T63.613	T63.614	—	—
jellyfish NEC	T63.621	T63.622	T63.623	T63.624	—	—
Portugese Man-o-war	T63.611	T63.612	T63.613	T63.614	—	—
sea anemone	T63.631	T63.632	T63.633	T63.634	—	—
specified NEC	T63.691	T63.692	T63.693	T63.694	—	—
fish	T63.591	T63.592	T63.593	T63.594	—	—
sting ray	T63.511	T63.512	T63.513	T63.514	—	—
plants	T63.711	T63.712	T63.713	T63.714	—	—
millipede (tropical)	T63.411	T63.412	T63.413	T63.414	—	—
plant NEC	T63.791	T63.792	T63.793	T63.794	—	—
marine	T63.711	T63.712	T63.713	T63.714	—	—
reptile	T63.191	T63.192	T63.193	T63.194	—	—
gila monster	T63.111	T63.112	T63.113	T63.114	—	—
lizard NEC	T63.121	T63.122	T63.123	T63.124	—	—
scorpion	T63.2x1	T63.2x2	T63.2x3	T63.2x4	—	—

Table of Drugs & Chemicals	POISONING Accidental (Unintentional)	Self-Harm (Intentional)	Assault	Undetermined	Adverse Effect	Underdosing
Venom, venomous (bite) (sting)						
– continued	T63.91	T63.92	T63.93	T63.94	—	—
snake	T63.001	T63.002	T63.003	T63.004	—	—
African NEC	T63.081	T63.082	T63.083	T63.084	—	—
American (North) (South) NEC	T63.061	T63.062	T63.063	T63.064	—	—
Asian	T63.081	T63.082	T63.083	T63.084	—	—
Australian	T63.071	T63.072	T63.073	T63.074	—	—
cobra	T63.041	T63.042	T63.043	T63.044	—	—
coral snake	T63.021	T63.022	T63.023	T63.024	—	—
rattlesnake	T63.011	T63.012	T63.013	T63.014	—	—
specified NEC	T63.091	T63.092	T63.093	T63.094	—	—
taipan	T63.031	T63.032	T63.033	T63.034	—	—
specified NEC	T63.891	T63.892	T63.893	T63.894	—	—
spider	T63.301	T63.302	T63.303	T63.304	—	—
black widow	T63.311	T63.312	T63.313	T63.314	—	—
brown recluse	T63.331	T63.332	T63.333	T63.334	—	—
specified NEC	T63.391	T63.392	T63.393	T63.394	—	—
tarantula	T63.321	T63.322	T63.323	T63.324	—	—
sting ray	T63.511	T63.512	T63.513	T63.514	—	—
toad	T63.821	T63.822	T63.823	T63.824	—	—
wasp	T63.461	T63.462	T63.463	T63.464	—	—
Venous sclerosing drug NEC	T46.8x1	T46.8x2	T46.8x3	T46.8x4	T46.8x5	T46.8x6
Ventolin — see Albuterol						
Veramon	T42.3x1	T42.3x2	T42.3x3	T42.3x4	T42.3x5	T42.3x6
Verapamil	T46.1x1	T46.1x2	T46.1x3	T46.1x4	T46.1x5	T46.1x6
Veratrine	T46.5x1	T46.5x2	T46.5x3	T46.5x4	T46.5x5	T46.5x6
Veratrum						
album	T62.2x1	T62.2x2	T62.2x3	T62.2x4	—	—
alkaloids	T46.5x1	T46.5x2	T46.5x3	T46.5x4	T46.5x5	T46.5x6
viride	T62.2x1	T62.2x2	T62.2x3	T62.2x4	—	—
Verdigris	T60.3x1	T60.3x2	T60.3x3	T60.3x4	—	—
Veronal	T42.3x1	T42.3x2	T42.3x3	T42.3x4	T42.3x5	T42.3x6
Veroxil	T37.4x1	T37.4x2	T37.4x3	T37.4x4	T37.4x5	T37.4x6
Versenate	T50.6x1	T50.6x2	T50.6x3	T50.6x4	T50.6x5	T50.6x6
Versidyne	T39.8x1	T39.8x2	T39.8x3	T39.8x4	T39.8x5	T39.8x6
Vetrabutine	T48.0x1	T48.0x2	T48.0x3	T48.0x4	T48.0x5	T48.0x6
Vidarabine	T37.5x1	T37.5x2	T37.5x3	T37.5x4	T37.5x5	T37.5x6
Vienna						
green	T57.0x1	T57.0x2	T57.0x3	T57.0x4	—	—
insecticide	T60.2x1	T60.2x2	T60.2x3	T60.2x4	—	—
red	T57.0x1	T57.0x2	T57.0x3	T57.0x4	—	—
pharmaceutical dye	T50.991	T50.992	T50.993	T50.994	T50.995	T50.996
Vigabatrin	T42.6x1	T42.6x2	T42.6x3	T42.6x4	T42.6x5	T42.6x6
Viloxazine	T43.291	T43.292	T43.293	T43.294	T43.295	T43.296
Viminol	T39.8x1	T39.8x2	T39.8x3	T39.8x4	T39.8x5	T39.8x6
Vinbarbital, vinbarbitone	T42.3x1	T42.3x2	T42.3x3	T42.3x4	T42.3x5	T42.3x6
Vinblastine	T45.1x1	T45.1x2	T45.1x3	T45.1x4	T45.1x5	T45.1x6
Vinburnine	T46.7x1	T46.7x2	T46.7x3	T46.7x4	T46.7x5	T46.7x6
Vincamine	T45.1x1	T45.1x2	T45.1x3	T45.1x4	T45.1x5	T45.1x6
Vincristine	T45.1x1	T45.1x2	T45.1x3	T45.1x4	T45.1x5	T45.1x6
Vindesine	T45.1x1	T45.1x2	T45.1x3	T45.1x4	T45.1x5	T45.1x6
Vinesthene, vinethene	T41.0x1	T41.0x2	T41.0x3	T41.0x4	T41.0x5	T41.0x6
Vinorelbine tartrate	T45.1x1	T45.1x2	T45.1x3	T45.1x4	T45.1x5	T45.1x6
Vinpocetine	T46.7x1	T46.7x2	T46.7x3	T46.7x4	T46.7x5	T46.7x6
Vinyl						
acetate	T65.891	T65.892	T65.893	T65.894	—	—
bital	T42.3x1	T42.3x2	T42.3x3	T42.3x4	T42.3x5	T42.3x6
bromide	T65.891	T65.892	T65.893	T65.894	—	—
chloride	T59.891	T59.892	T59.893	T59.894	—	—
ether	T41.0x1	T41.0x2	T41.0x3	T41.0x4	T41.0x5	T41.0x6
Vinylbital	T42.3x1	T42.3x2	T42.3x3	T42.3x4	T42.3x5	T42.3x6
Vinylidene chloride	T65.891	T65.892	T65.893	T65.894	—	—
Vioform	T37.8x1	T37.8x2	T37.8x3	T37.8x4	T37.8x5	T37.8x6
topical	T49.0x1	T49.0x2	T49.0x3	T49.0x4	T49.0x5	T49.0x6
Viomycin	T36.8x1	T36.8x2	T36.8x3	T36.8x4	T36.8x5	T36.8x6
Viosterol	T45.2x1	T45.2x2	T45.2x3	T45.2x4	T45.2x5	T45.2x6
Viper (venom)	T63.091	T63.092	T63.093	T63.094	—	—

305

DRUGS & CHEMICALS

Table of Drugs & Chemicals	POISONING				Adverse Effect	Underdosing
	Accidental (Unintentional)	Self-Harm (Intentional)	Assault	Undetermined		
Viprynium	T37.4x1	T37.4x2	T37.4x3	T37.4x4	T37.4x5	T37.4x6
Viquidil	T46.7x1	T46.7x2	T46.7x3	T46.7x4	T46.7x5	T46.7x6
Viral vaccine NEC	T50.B91	T50.B92	T50.B93	T50.B94	T50.B95	T50.B96
Virginiamycin	T36.8x1	T36.8x2	T36.8x3	T36.8x4	T36.8x5	T36.8x6
Virugon	T37.5x1	T37.5x2	T37.5x3	T37.5x4	T37.5x5	T37.5x6
Viscous agent	T50.901	T50.902	T50.903	T50.904	T50.905	T50.906
Visine	T49.5x1	T49.5x2	T49.5x3	T49.5x4	T49.5x5	T49.5x6
Visnadine	T46.3x1	T46.3x2	T46.3x3	T46.3x4	T46.3x5	T46.3x6
Vitamin NEC	T45.2x1	T45.2x2	T45.2x3	T45.2x4	T45.2x5	T45.2x6
A	T45.2x1	T45.2x2	T45.2x3	T45.2x4	T45.2x5	T45.2x6
B NEC	T45.2x1	T45.2x2	T45.2x3	T45.2x4	T45.2x5	T45.2x6
nicotinic acid	T46.7x1	T46.7x2	T46.7x3	T46.7x4	T46.7x5	T46.7x6
B1	T45.2x1	T45.2x2	T45.2x3	T45.2x4	T45.2x5	T45.2x6
B2	T45.2x1	T45.2x2	T45.2x3	T45.2x4	T45.2x5	T45.2x6
B6	T45.2x1	T45.2x2	T45.2x3	T45.2x4	T45.2x5	T45.2x6
B12	T45.2x1	T45.2x2	T45.2x3	T45.2x4	T45.2x5	T45.2x6
B15	T45.2x1	T45.2x2	T45.2x3	T45.2x4	T45.2x5	T45.2x6
C	T45.2x1	T45.2x2	T45.2x3	T45.2x4	T45.2x5	T45.2x6
D	T45.2x1	T45.2x2	T45.2x3	T45.2x4	T45.2x5	T45.2x6
D2	T45.2x1	T45.2x2	T45.2x3	T45.2x4	T45.2x5	T45.2x6
D3	T45.2x1	T45.2x2	T45.2x3	T45.2x4	T45.2x5	T45.2x6
E	T45.2x1	T45.2x2	T45.2x3	T45.2x4	T45.2x5	T45.2x6
E acetate	T45.2x1	T45.2x2	T45.2x3	T45.2x4	T45.2x5	T45.2x6
hematopoietic	T45.8x1	T45.8x2	T45.8x3	T45.8x4	T45.8x5	T45.8x6
K NEC	T45.7x1	T45.7x2	T45.7x3	T45.7x4	T45.7x5	T45.7x6
K1	T45.7x1	T45.7x2	T45.7x3	T45.7x4	T45.7x5	T45.7x6
K2	T45.7x1	T45.7x2	T45.7x3	T45.7x4	T45.7x5	T45.7x6
PP	T45.2x1	T45.2x2	T45.2x3	T45.2x4	T45.2x5	T45.2x6
ulceroprotectant	T47.1x1	T47.1x2	T47.1x3	T47.1x4	T47.1x5	T47.1x6
Vleminckx's solution	T49.4x1	T49.4x2	T49.4x3	T49.4x4	T49.4x5	T49.4x6
Voltaren — see Diclofenac sodium						
Warfarin	T45.511	T45.512	T45.513	T45.514	T45.515	T45.516
rodenticide	T60.4x1	T60.4x2	T60.4x3	T60.4x4	—	—
sodium	T60.4x1	T60.4x2	T60.4x3	T60.4x4	—	—
Wasp (sting)	T63.461	T63.462	T63.463	T63.464	—	—
Water						
balance drug	T50.3x1	T50.3x2	T50.3x3	T50.3x4	T50.3x5	T50.3x6
distilled	T50.3x1	T50.3x2	T50.3x3	T50.3x4	T50.3x5	T50.3x6
gas — see Gas, water						
incomplete combustion of						
— see Carbon, monoxide,						
fuel, utility						
hemlock	T62.2x1	T62.2x2	T62.2x3	T62.2x4	—	—
moccasin (venom)	T63.061	T63.062	T63.063	T63.064	—	—
purified	T50.3x1	T50.3x2	T50.3x3	T50.3x4	T50.3x5	T50.3x6
Wax (paraffin) (petroleum)	T52.0x1	T52.0x2	T52.0x3	T52.0x4	—	—
automobile	T65.891	T65.892	T65.893	T65.894	—	—
floor	T52.0x1	T52.0x2	T52.0x3	T52.0x4	—	—
Weed killers NEC	T60.3x1	T60.3x2	T60.3x3	T60.3x4	—	—
Welldorm	T42.6x1	T42.6x2	T42.6x3	T42.6x4	T42.6x5	T42.6x6
White						
arsenic	T57.0x1	T57.0x2	T57.0x3	T57.0x4	—	—
hellebore	T62.2x1	T62.2x2	T62.2x3	T62.2x4	—	—
lotion (keratolytic)	T49.4x1	T49.4x2	T49.4x3	T49.4x4	T49.4x5	T49.4x6
spirit	T52.0x1	T52.0x2	T52.0x3	T52.0x4	—	—
Whitewash	T65.891	T65.892	T65.893	T65.894	—	—
Whole blood (human)	T45.8x1	T45.8x2	T45.8x3	T45.8x4	T45.8x5	T45.8x6
Wild						
black cherry	T62.2x1	T62.2x2	T62.2x3	T62.2x4	—	—
poisonous plants NEC	T62.2x1	T62.2x2	T62.2x3	T62.2x4	—	—
Window cleaning fluid	T65.891	T65.892	T65.893	T65.894	—	—
Wintergreen (oil)	T49.3x1	T49.3x2	T49.3x3	T49.3x4	T49.3x5	T49.3x6
Wisterine	T62.2x1	T62.2x2	T62.2x3	T62.2x4	—	—
Witch hazel	T49.2x1	T49.2x2	T49.2x3	T49.2x4	T49.2x5	T49.2x6
Wood alcohol or spirit	T51.1x1	T51.1x2	T51.1x3	T51.1x4	—	—
Wool fat (hydrous)	T49.3x1	T49.3x2	T49.3x3	T49.3x4	T49.3x5	T49.3x6
Woorali	T48.1x1	T48.1x2	T48.1x3	T48.1x4	T48.1x5	T48.1x6
Wormseed, American	T37.4x1	T37.4x2	T37.4x3	T37.4x4	T37.4x5	T37.4x6
Xamoterol	T44.5x1	T44.5x2	T44.5x3	T44.5x4	T44.5x5	T44.5x6
Xanthine diuretics	T50.2x1	T50.2x2	T50.2x3	T50.2x4	T50.2x5	T50.2x6
Xanthinol nicotinate	T46.7x1	T46.7x2	T46.7x3	T46.7x4	T46.7x5	T46.7x6
Xanthotoxin	T49.3x1	T49.3x2	T49.3x3	T49.3x4	T49.3x5	T49.3x6
Xantinol nicotinate	T46.7x1	T46.7x2	T46.7x3	T46.7x4	T46.7x5	T46.7x6
Xantocillin	T36.0x1	T36.0x2	T36.0x3	T36.0x4	T36.0x5	T36.0x6
Xenon (127Xe) (133Xe)	T50.8x1	T50.8x2	T50.8x3	T50.8x4	T50.8x5	T50.8x6
Xenysalate	T49.4x1	T49.4x2	T49.4x3	T49.4x4	T49.4x5	T49.4x6
Xibornol	T37.8x1	T37.8x2	T37.8x3	T37.8x4	T37.8x5	T37.8x6
Xigris	T45.511	T45.512	T45.513	T45.514	T45.515	T45.516
Xipamide	T50.2x1	T50.2x2	T50.2x3	T50.2x4	T50.2x5	T50.2x6
Xylene (vapor)	T52.2x1	T52.2x2	T52.2x3	T52.2x4	—	—
Xylocaine (infiltration) (topical)	T41.3x1	T41.3x2	T41.3x3	T41.3x4	T41.3x5	T41.3x6
nerve block (peripheral)						
(plexus)	T41.3x1	T41.3x2	T41.3x3	T41.3x4	T41.3x5	T41.3x6
spinal	T41.3x1	T41.3x2	T41.3x3	T41.3x4	T41.3x5	T41.3x6
Xylol (vapor)	T52.2x1	T52.2x2	T52.2x3	T52.2x4	—	—
Xylometazoline	T48.5x1	T48.5x2	T48.5x3	T48.5x4	T48.5x5	T48.5x6
Yeast	T45.2x1	T45.2x2	T45.2x3	T45.2x4	T45.2x5	T45.2x6
dried	T45.2x1	T45.2x2	T45.2x3	T45.2x4	T45.2x5	T45.2x6
Yellow						
fever vaccine	T50.B91	T50.B92	T50.B93	T50.B94	T50.B95	T50.B96
jasmine	T62.2x1	T62.2x2	T62.2x3	T62.2x4	—	—
phenolphthalein	T47.2x1	T47.2x2	T47.2x3	T47.2x4	T47.2x5	T47.2x6
Yew	T62.2x1	T62.2x2	T62.2x3	T62.2x4	—	—
Yohimbic acid	T40.991	T40.992	T40.993	T40.994	T40.995	T40.996
Zactane	T39.8x1	T39.8x2	T39.8x3	T39.8x4	T39.8x5	T39.8x6
Zalcitabine	T37.5x1	T37.5x2	T37.5x3	T37.5x4	T37.5x5	T37.5x6
Zaroxolyn	T50.2x1	T50.2x2	T50.2x3	T50.2x4	T50.2x5	T50.2x6
Zephiran (topical)	T49.0x1	T49.0x2	T49.0x3	T49.0x4	T49.0x5	T49.0x6
ophthalmic preparation	T49.5x1	T49.5x2	T49.5x3	T49.5x4	T49.5x5	T49.5x6
Zeranol	T38.7x1	T38.7x2	T38.7x3	T38.7x4	T38.7x5	T38.7x6
Zerone	T51.1x1	T51.1x2	T51.1x3	T51.1x4	—	—
Zidovudine	T37.5x1	T37.5x2	T37.5x3	T37.5x4	T37.5x5	T37.5x6
Zimeldine	T43.221	T43.222	T43.223	T43.224	T43.225	T43.226
Zinc (compounds) (fumes) (vapor) NEC	T56.5x1	T56.5x2	T56.5x3	T56.5x4	—	—
anti-infectives	T49.0x1	T49.0x2	T49.0x3	T49.0x4	T49.0x5	T49.0x6
antivaricose	T46.8x1	T46.8x2	T46.8x3	T46.8x4	T46.8x5	T46.8x6
bacitracin	T49.0x1	T49.0x2	T49.0x3	T49.0x4	T49.0x5	T49.0x6
chloride (mouthwash)	T49.6x1	T49.6x2	T49.6x3	T49.6x4	T49.6x5	T49.6x6
chromate	T56.5x1	T56.5x2	T56.5x3	T56.5x4	—	—
gelatin	T49.3x1	T49.3x2	T49.3x3	T49.3x4	T49.3x5	T49.3x6
oxide	T49.3x1	T49.3x2	T49.3x3	T49.3x4	T49.3x5	T49.3x6
plaster	T49.3x1	T49.3x2	T49.3x3	T49.3x4	T49.3x5	T49.3x6
peroxide	T49.0x1	T49.0x2	T49.0x3	T49.0x4	T49.0x5	T49.0x6
pesticides	T56.5x1	T56.5x2	T56.5x3	T56.5x4	—	—
phosphide	T60.4x1	T60.4x2	T60.4x3	T60.4x4	—	—
pyrithionate	T49.4x1	T49.4x2	T49.4x3	T49.4x4	T49.4x5	T49.4x6
stearate	T49.3x1	T49.3x2	T49.3x3	T49.3x4	T49.3x5	T49.3x6
sulfate	T49.5x1	T49.5x2	T49.5x3	T49.5x4	T49.5x5	T49.5x6
ENT agent	T49.6x1	T49.6x2	T49.6x3	T49.6x4	T49.6x5	T49.6x6
ophthalmic solution	T49.5x1	T49.5x2	T49.5x3	T49.5x4	T49.5x5	T49.5x6
topical NEC	T49.0x1	T49.0x2	T49.0x3	T49.0x4	T49.0x5	T49.0x6
undecylenate	T49.0x1	T49.0x2	T49.0x3	T49.0x4	T49.0x5	T49.0x6
Zineb	T60.0x1	T60.0x2	T60.0x3	T60.0x4	—	—
Zinostatin	T45.1x1	T45.1x2	T45.1x3	T45.1x4	T45.1x5	T45.1x6
Zipeprol	T48.3x1	T48.3x2	T48.3x3	T48.3x4	T48.3x5	T48.3x6
Zofenopril	T46.4x1	T46.4x2	T46.4x3	T46.4x4	T46.4x5	T46.4x6
Zolpidem	T42.6x1	T42.6x2	T42.6x3	T42.6x4	T42.6x5	T42.6x6
Zomepirac	T39.391	T39.392	T39.393	T39.394	T39.395	T39.396
Zopiclone	T42.6x1	T42.6x2	T42.6x3	T42.6x4	T42.6x5	T42.6x6
Zorubicin	T45.1x1	T45.1x2	T45.1x3	T45.1x4	T45.1x5	T45.1x6
Zotepine	T43.591	T43.592	T43.593	T43.594	T43.595	T43.596
Zovant	T45.511	T45.512	T45.513	T45.514	T45.515	T45.516
Zoxazolamine	T42.8x1	T42.8x2	T42.8x3	T42.8x4	T42.8x5	T42.8x6
Zuclopenthixol	T43.4x1	T43.4x2	T43.4x3	T43.4x4	T43.4x5	T43.4x6
Zygadenus (venenosus)	T62.2x1	T62.2x2	T62.2x3	T62.2x4	—	—
Zyprexa	T43.591	T43.592	T43.593	T43.594	T43.595	T43.596

A

Abandonment (causing exposure to weather conditions) (with intent to injure or kill) NEC X58
Abuse (adult) (child) (mental) (physical) (sexual) X58
Accident (to) X58
  aircraft (in transit) (powered) — *see also* Accident, transport, aircraft
    due to, caused by cataclysm — *see* Forces of nature, by type
  animal-drawn vehicle — *see* Accident, transport, animal-drawn vehicle occupant
  animal-rider — *see* Accident, transport, animal-rider
  automobile — *see* Accident, transport, car occupant
  bare foot water skier V94.4
  boat, boating — *see also* Accident, watercraft
    striking swimmer
      powered V94.11
      unpowered V94.12
  bus — *see* Accident, transport, bus occupant
  cable car, not on rails V98.0
    on rails — *see* Accident, transport, streetcar occupant
  car — *see* Accident, transport, car occupant
  caused by, due to
    animal NEC W64
    chain hoist W24.0
    cold (excessive) — *see* Exposure, cold
    corrosive liquid, substance — *see* Table of Drugs and Chemicals
    cutting or piercing instrument — *see* Contact, with, by type of instrument
    drive belt W24.0
    electric
      current — *see* Exposure, electric current
      motor (*see also* Contact, with, by type of machine) W31.3
      current (of) W86.8
    environmental factor NEC X58
    explosive material — *see* Explosion
    fire, flames — *see* Exposure, fire
    firearm missile — *see* Discharge, firearm by type
    heat (excessive) — *see* Heat
    hot — *see* Contact, with, hot
    ignition — *see* Ignition
    lifting device W24.0
    lightning — *see* subcategory T75.0
      causing fire — *see* Exposure, fire
    machine, machinery — *see* Contact, with, by type of machine
    natural factor NEC X58
    pulley (block) W24.0
    radiation — *see* Radiation
    steam X13.1
      inhalation X13.0
      pipe X16
    thunderbolt — *see* subcategory T75.0
      causing fire — *see* Exposure, fire
    transmission device W24.1
  coach — *see* Accident, transport, bus occupant
  coal car — *see* Accident, transport, industrial vehicle occupant
  diving — *see also* Fall, into, water
    with
      drowning or submersion — *see* Drowning
  forklift — *see* Accident, transport, industrial vehicle occupant
  heavy transport vehicle NOS — *see* Accident, transport, truck occupant
  ice yacht V98.2
  in
    medical, surgical procedure
      as, or due to misadventure — *see* Misadventure
      causing an abnormal reaction or later complication without mention of misadventure (*see also* Complication of or following, by type of procedure) Y84.9
  land yacht V98.1
  late effect of — *see* W00-X58 with 7th character S
  logging car — *see* Accident, transport, industrial vehicle occupant

Accident (to) — *continued*
  machine, machinery — *see also* Contact, with, by type of machine
    on board watercraft V93.69
      explosion — *see* Explosion, in, watercraft
      fire — *see* Burn, on board watercraft
      powered craft V93.63
        ferry boat V93.61
        fishing boat V93.62
        jetskis V93.63
        liner V93.61
        merchant ship V93.60
        passenger ship V93.61
        sailboat V93.64
  mine tram — *see* Accident, transport, industrial vehicle occupant
  mobility scooter (motorized) — *see* Accident, transport, pedestrian, conveyance, specified type NEC
  motor scooter — *see* Accident, transport, motorcyclist
  motor vehicle NOS (traffic) (*see also* Accident, transport) V89.2
    nontraffic V89.0
    three-wheeled NOS — *see* Accident, transport, three-wheeled motor vehicle occupant
  motorcycle NOS — *see* Accident, transport, motorcyclist
  nonmotor vehicle NOS (nontraffic) (*see also* Accident, transport) V89.1
    traffic NOS V89.3
  nontraffic (victim's mode of transport NOS) V88.9
    collision (between) V88.7
      bus and truck V88.5
      car and:
        bus V88.3
        pickup V88.2
        three-wheeled motor vehicle V88.0
        train V88.6
        truck V88.4
        two-wheeled motor vehicle V88.0
        van V88.2
      specified vehicle NEC and:
        three-wheeled motor vehicle V88.1
        two-wheeled motor vehicle V88.1
    known mode of transport — *see* Accident, transport, by type of vehicle
    noncollision V88.8
  on board watercraft V93.89
    powered craft V93.83
      ferry boat V93.81
      fishing boat V93.82
      jetskis V93.83
      liner V93.81
      merchant ship V93.80
      passenger ship V93.81
    unpowered craft V93.88
      canoe V93.85
      inflatable V93.86
        in tow
          recreational V94.31
          specified NEC V94.32
      kayak V93.85
      sailboat V93.84
      surfboard V93.88
      water skis V93.87
      windsurfer V93.88
  parachutist V97.29
    entangled in object V97.21
    injured on landing V97.22
  pedal cycle — *see* Accident, transport, pedal cyclist
  pedestrian (on foot)
    with
      another pedestrian W51
        with fall W03
          due to ice or snow W00.0
      on pedestrian conveyance NEC V00.09
      roller skater (in-line) V00.01
      skate boarder V00.02
      transport vehicle — *see* Accident, transport
    on pedestrian conveyance — *see* Accident, transport, pedestrian, conveyance
  pickup truck or van — *see* Accident, transport, pickup truck occupant
  quarry truck — *see* Accident, transport, industrial vehicle occupant
  railway vehicle (any) (in motion) — *see* Accident, transport, railway vehicle occupant
    due to cataclysm — *see* Forces of nature, by type

Accident (to) — *continued*
  scooter (non-motorized) — *see* Accident, transport, pedestrian, conveyance, scooter
  sequelae of — *see* W00-X58 with 7th character S
  skateboard — *see* Accident, transport, pedestrian, conveyance, skateboard
  ski(ing) — *see* Accident, transport, pedestrian, conveyance
    lift V98.3
  specified cause NEC X58
  streetcar — *see* Accident, transport, streetcar occupant
  traffic (victim's mode of transport NOS) V87.9
    collision (between) V87.7
      bus and truck V87.5
      car and:
        bus V87.3
        pickup V87.2
        three-wheeled motor vehicle V87.0
        train V87.6
        truck V87.4
        two-wheeled motor vehicle V87.0
        van V87.2
      specified vehicle NEC and:
        three-wheeled motor vehicle V87.1
        two-wheeled motor vehicle V87.1
    known mode of transport — *see* Accident, transport, by type of vehicle
    noncollision V87.8
  transport (involving injury to) V99
    18 wheeler — *see* Accident, transport, truck occupant
    agricultural vehicle occupant (nontraffic) V84.9
      driver V84.5
      hanger-on V84.7
      passenger V84.6
      traffic V84.3
        driver V84.0
        hanger-on V84.2
        passenger V84.1
      while boarding or alighting V84.4
    aircraft NEC V97.89
      military NEC V97.818
        with civlian aircraft V97.810
        civilian injured by V97.811
      occupant injured (in)
        nonpowered craft accident V96.9
          balloon V96.00
            collision V96.03
            crash V96.01
            explosion V96.05
            fire V96.04
            forced landing V96.02
            specified type NEC V96.09
          glider V96.20
            collision V96.23
            crash V96.21
            explosion V96.25
            fire V96.24
            forced landing V96.22
            specified type NEC V96.29
          hang glider V96.10
            collision V96.13
            crash V96.11
            explosion V96.15
            fire V96.14
            forced landing V96.12
            specified type NEC V96.19
          specified craft NEC V96.8
        powered craft accident V95.9
          fixed wing NEC
            commercial V95.30
              collision V95.33
              crash V95.31
              explosion V95.35
              fire V95.34
              forced landing V95.32
              specified type NEC V95.39
            private V95.20
              collision V95.23
              crash V95.21
              explosion V95.25
              fire V95.24
              forced landing V95.22
              specified type NEC V95.29
          glider V95.10
            collision V95.13
            crash V95.11
            explosion V95.15
            fire V95.14
            forced landing V95.12
            specified type NEC V95.19

Accident (to) — *continued*
  transport (involving injury to) — *continued*
    aircraft NEC — *continued*
      occupant injured (in) — *continued*
        powered craft accident — *continued*
          helicopter V95.00
            collision V95.03
            crash V95.01
            explosion V95.05
            fire V95.04
            forced landing V95.02
            specified type NEC V95.09
          spacecraft V95.40
            collision V95.43
            crash V95.41
            explosion V95.45
            fire V95.44
            forced landing V95.42
            specified type NEC V95.49
          specified craft NEC V95.8
          ultralight V95.10
            collision V95.13
            crash V95.11
            explosion V95.15
            fire V95.14
            forced landing V95.12
            specified type NEC V95.19
        specified accident NEC V97.0
        while boarding or alighting V97.1
      person (injured by)
        falling from, in or on aircraft V97.0
        machinery on aircraft V97.89
        on ground with aircraft involvement V97.39
        rotating propeller V97.32
        struck by object falling from aircraft V97.31
        sucked into aircraft jet V97.33
        while boarding or alighting aircraft V97.1
    airport (battery-powered) passenger vehicle — *see* Accident, transport, industrial vehicle occupant
    all-terrain vehicle occupant (nontraffic) V86.99
      driver V86.59
      dune buggy — *see* Accident, transport, dune buggy occupant
      hanger-on V86.79
      passenger V86.69
      snowmobile — *see* Accident, transport, snowmobile occupant
      traffic V86.39
        driver V86.09
        hanger-on V86.29
        passenger V86.19
      while boarding or alighting V86.49
    ambulance occupant (traffic) V86.31
      driver V86.01
      hanger-on V86.21
      nontraffic V86.91
        driver V86.51
      passenger V86.11
      while boarding or alighting V86.41
    animal-drawn vehicle occupant (in) V80.929
      collision (with)
        animal V80.12
          being ridden V80.711
        animal-drawn vehicle V80.721
        bus V80.42
        car V80.42
        fixed or stationary object V80.82
        military vehicle V80.920
        nonmotor vehicle V80.791
        pedal cycle V80.22
        pedestrian V80.12
        pickup V80.42
        railway train or vehicle V80.62
        specified motor vehicle NEC V80.52
        streetcar V80.731
        truck V80.42
        two-or three-wheeled motor vehicle V80.32
        van V80.42
      noncollision V80.02
      specified circumstance NEC V80.928
    animal-rider V80.919
      collision (with)
        animal V80.11
          being ridden V80.710
        animal-drawn vehicle V80.720
        bus V80.41
        car V80.41
        fixed or stationary object V80.81
        military vehicle V80.910

Accident (to) — *continued*
transport (involving injury to) — *continued*
animal-rider — *continued*
collision (with) — *continued*
nonmotor vehicle V80.790
pedal cycle V80.21
pedestrian V80.11
pickup V80.41
railway train or vehicle V80.61
specified motor vehicle NEC V80.51
streetcar V80.730
truck V80.41
two-or three-wheeled motor vehicle V80.31
van V80.41
noncollision V80.018
specified as horse rider V80.010
specified circumstance NEC V80.918
armored car — *see* Accident, transport, truck occupant
battery-powered truck (baggage) (mail) — *see* Accident, transport, industrial vehicle occupant
bus occupant V79.9
collision (with)
animal (traffic) V70.9
being ridden (traffic) V76.9
nontraffic V76.3
while boarding or alighting V76.4
nontraffic V70.3
while boarding or alighting V70.4
animal-drawn vehicle (traffic) V76.9
nontraffic V76.3
while boarding or alighting V76.4
bus (traffic) V74.9
nontraffic V74.3
while boarding or alighting V74.4
car (traffic) V73.9
nontraffic V73.3
while boarding or alighting V73.4
motor vehicle NOS (traffic) V79.60
nontraffic V79.20
specified type NEC (traffic) V79.69
nontraffic V79.29
pedal cycle (traffic) V71.9
nontraffic V71.3
while boarding or alighting V71.4
pickup truck (traffic) V73.9
nontraffic V73.3
while boarding or alighting V73.4
railway vehicle (traffic) V75.9
nontraffic V75.3
while boarding or alighting V75.4
specified vehicle NEC (traffic) V76.9
nontraffic V76.3
while boarding or alighting V76.4
stationary object (traffic) V77.9
nontraffic V77.3
while boarding or alighting V77.4
streetcar (traffic) V76.9
nontraffic V76.3
while boarding or alighting V76.4
three wheeled motor vehicle (traffic) V72.9
nontraffic V72.3
while boarding or alighting V72.4
truck (traffic) V74.9
nontraffic V74.3
while boarding or alighting V74.4
two wheeled motor vehicle (traffic) V72.9
nontraffic V72.3
while boarding or alighting V72.4
van (traffic) V73.9
nontraffic V73.3
while boarding or alighting V73.4

Accident (to) — *continued*
transport (involving injury to) — *continued*
bus occupant — *continued*
driver
collision (with)
animal (traffic) V70.5
being ridden (traffic) V76.5
nontraffic V76.0
nontraffic V70.0
animal-drawn vehicle (traffic) V76.5
nontraffic V76.0
bus (traffic) V74.5
nontraffic V74.0
car (traffic) V73.5
nontraffic V73.0
motor vehicle NOS (traffic) V79.40
nontraffic V79.00
specified type NEC (traffic) V79.49
nontraffic V79.09
pedal cycle (traffic) V71.5
nontraffic V71.0
pickup truck (traffic) V73.5
nontraffic V73.0
railway vehicle (traffic) V75.5
nontraffic V75.0
specified vehicle NEC (traffic) V76.5
nontraffic V76.0
stationary object (traffic) V77.5
nontraffic V77.0
streetcar (traffic) V76.5
nontraffic V76.0
three wheeled motor vehicle (traffic) V72.5
nontraffic V72.0
truck (traffic) V74.5
nontraffic V74.0
two wheeled motor vehicle (traffic) V72.5
nontraffic V72.0
van (traffic) V73.5
nontraffic V73.0
noncollision accident (traffic) V78.5
nontraffic V78.0
hanger-on
collision (with)
animal (traffic) V70.7
being ridden (traffic) V76.7
nontraffic V76.2
nontraffic V70.2
animal-drawn vehicle (traffic) V76.7
nontraffic V76.2
bus (traffic) V74.7
nontraffic V74.2
car (traffic) V73.7
nontraffic V73.2
pedal cycle (traffic) V71.7
nontraffic V71.2
pickup truck (traffic) V73.7
nontraffic V73.2
railway vehicle (traffic) V75.7
nontraffic V75.2
specified vehicle NEC (traffic) V76.7
nontraffic V76.2
stationary object (traffic) V77.7
nontraffic V77.2
streetcar (traffic) V76.7
nontraffic V76.2
three wheeled motor vehicle (traffic) V72.7
nontraffic V72.2
truck (traffic) V74.7
nontraffic V74.2
two wheeled motor vehicle (traffic) V72.7
nontraffic V72.2
van (traffic) V73.7
nontraffic V73.2
noncollision accident (traffic) V78.7
nontraffic V78.2
noncollision accident (traffic) V78.9
nontraffic V78.3
while boarding or alighting V78.4
nontraffic V79.3

Accident (to) — *continued*
transport (involving injury to) — *continued*
bus occupant — *continued*
passenger
collision (with)
animal (traffic) V70.6
being ridden (traffic) V76.6
nontraffic V76.1
nontraffic V70.1
animal-drawn vehicle (traffic) V76.6
nontraffic V76.1
bus (traffic) V74.6
nontraffic V74.1
car (traffic) V73.6
nontraffic V73.1
motor vehicle NOS (traffic) V79.50
nontraffic V79.10
specified type NEC (traffic) V79.59
nontraffic V79.19
pedal cycle (traffic) V71.6
nontraffic V71.1
pickup truck (traffic) V73.6
nontraffic V73.1
railway vehicle (traffic) V75.6
nontraffic V75.1
specified vehicle NEC (traffic) V76.6
nontraffic V76.1
stationary object (traffic) V77.6
nontraffic V77.1
streetcar (traffic) V76.6
nontraffic V76.1
three wheeled motor vehicle (traffic) V72.6
nontraffic V72.1
truck (traffic) V74.6
nontraffic V74.1
two wheeled motor vehicle (traffic) V72.6
nontraffic V72.1
van (traffic) V73.6
nontraffic V73.1
noncollision accident (traffic) V78.6
nontraffic V78.1
specified type NEC V79.88
military vehicle V79.81
cable car, not on rails V98.0
on rails — *see* Accident, transport, streetcar occupant
car occupant V49.9
ambulance occupant — *see* Accident, transport, ambulance occupant
collision (with)
animal (traffic) V40.9
being ridden (traffic) V46.9
nontraffic V46.3
while boarding or alighting V46.4
nontraffic V40.3
while boarding or alighting V40.4
animal-drawn vehicle (traffic) V46.9
nontraffic V46.3
while boarding or alighting V46.4
bus (traffic) V44.9
nontraffic V44.3
while boarding or alighting V44.4
car (traffic) V43.92
nontraffic V43.32
while boarding or alighting V43.42
motor vehicle NOS (traffic) V49.60
nontraffic V49.20
specified type NEC (traffic) V49.69
nontraffic V49.29
pedal cycle (traffic) V41.9
nontraffic V41.3
while boarding or alighting V41.4
pickup truck (traffic) V43.93
nontraffic V43.33
while boarding or alighting V43.43
railway vehicle (traffic) V45.9
nontraffic V45.3
while boarding or alighting V45.4
specified vehicle NEC (traffic) V46.9
nontraffic V46.3
while boarding or alighting V46.4

Accident (to) — *continued*
transport (involving injury to) — *continued*
car occupant — *continued*
collision (with) — *continued*
sport utility vehicle (traffic) V43.91
nontraffic V43.31
while boarding or alighting V43.41
stationary object (traffic) V47.92
nontraffic V47.32
while boarding or alighting V47.4
streetcar (traffic) V46.9
nontraffic V46.3
while boarding or alighting V46.4
three wheeled motor vehicle (traffic) V42.9
nontraffic V42.3
while boarding or alighting V42.4
truck (traffic) V44.9
nontraffic V44.3
while boarding or alighting V44.4
two wheeled motor vehicle (traffic) V42.9
nontraffic V42.3
while boarding or alighting V42.4
van (traffic) V43.94
nontraffic V43.34
while boarding or alighting V43.44
driver
collision (with)
animal (traffic) V40.5
being ridden (traffic) V46.5
nontraffic V46.0
nontraffic V40.0
animal-drawn vehicle (traffic) V46.5
nontraffic V46.0
bus (traffic) V44.5
nontraffic V44.0
car (traffic) V43.52
nontraffic V43.02
motor vehicle NOS (traffic) V49.40
nontraffic V49.00
specified type NEC (traffic) V49.49
nontraffic V49.09
pedal cycle (traffic) V41.5
nontraffic V41.0
pickup truck (traffic) V43.53
nontraffic V43.03
railway vehicle (traffic) V45.5
nontraffic V45.0
specified vehicle NEC (traffic) V46.5
nontraffic V46.0
sport utility vehicle (traffic) V43.51
nontraffic V43.01
stationary object (traffic) V47.52
nontraffic V47.02
streetcar (traffic) V46.5
nontraffic V46.0
three wheeled motor vehicle (traffic) V42.5
nontraffic V42.0
truck (traffic) V44.5
nontraffic V44.0
two wheeled motor vehicle (traffic) V42.5
nontraffic V42.0
van (traffic) V43.54
nontraffic V43.04
noncollision accident (traffic) V48.5
nontraffic V48.0
hanger-on
collision (with)
animal (traffic) V40.7
being ridden (traffic) V46.7
nontraffic V46.2
nontraffic V40.2
animal-drawn vehicle (traffic) V46.7
nontraffic V46.2
bus (traffic) V44.7
nontraffic V44.2
car (traffic) V43.72
nontraffic V43.22
pedal cycle (traffic) V41.7
nontraffic V41.2
pickup truck (traffic) V43.73
nontraffic V43.23

Accident (to) — *continued*
transport (involving injury to) — *continued*
car occupant — *continued*
hanger-on — *continued*
collision (with) — *continued*
railway vehicle (traffic) V45.7
nontraffic V45.2
specified vehicle NEC (traffic)
V46.7
nontraffic V46.2
sport utility vehicle (traffic)
V43.71
nontraffic V43.21
stationary object (traffic) V47.7
nontraffic V47.2
streetcar (traffic) V46.7
nontraffic V46.2
three wheeled motor vehicle
(traffic) V42.7
nontraffic V42.2
truck (traffic) V44.7
nontraffic V44.2
two wheeled motor vehicle
(traffic) V42.7
nontraffic V42.2
van (traffic) V43.74
nontraffic V43.24
noncollision accident (traffic)
V48.7
nontraffic V48.2
noncollision accident (traffic) V48.9
nontraffic V48.3
while boarding or alighting V48.4
nontraffic V49.3
passenger
collision (with)
animal (traffic) V40.6
being ridden (traffic) V46.6
nontraffic V46.1
nontraffic V40.1
animal-drawn vehicle (traffic)
V46.6
nontraffic V46.1
bus (traffic) V44.6
nontraffic V44.1
car (traffic) V43.62
nontraffic V43.12
motor vehicle NOS (traffic)
V49.50
nontraffic V49.10
specified type NEC (traffic)
V49.59
nontraffic V49.19
pedal cycle (traffic) V41.6
nontraffic V41.1
pickup truck (traffic) V43.63
nontraffic V43.13
railway vehicle (traffic) V45.6
nontraffic V45.1
specified vehicle NEC (traffic)
V46.6
nontraffic V46.1
sport utility vehicle (traffic)
V43.61
nontraffic V43.11
stationary object (traffic) V47.62
nontraffic V47.12
streetcar (traffic) V46.6
nontraffic V46.1
three wheeled motor vehicle
(traffic) V42.6
nontraffic V42.1
truck (traffic) V44.6
nontraffic V44.1
two wheeled motor vehicle
(traffic) V42.6
nontraffic V42.1
van (traffic) V43.64
nontraffic V43.14
noncollision accident (traffic)
V48.6
nontraffic V48.1
specified type NEC V49.88
military vehicle V49.81
coal car — *see* Accident, transport,
industrial vehicle occupant
construction vehicle occupant
(nontraffic) V85.9
driver V85.5
hanger-on V85.7
passenger V85.6
traffic V85.3
driver V85.0
hanger-on V85.2
passenger V85.1
while boarding or alighting V85.4
dirt bike rider — *see* Accident, transport,
all-terrain vehicle occupant
due to cataclysm — *see* Forces of nature,
by type

Accident (to) — *continued*
transport (involving injury to) — *continued*
dune buggy occupant (nontraffic)
V86.93
driver V86.53
hanger-on V86.73
passenger V86.63
traffic V86.33
driver V86.03
hanger-on V86.23
passenger V86.13
while boarding or alighting V86.43
forklift — *see* Accident, transport,
industrial vehicle occupant
go cart — *see* Accident, transport, all-
terrain vehicle occupant
golf cart — *see* Accident, transport, all-
terrain vehicle occupant
heavy transport vehicle occupant — *see*
Accident, transport, truck occupant
ice yacht V98.2
industrial vehicle occupant (nontraffic)
V83.9
driver V83.5
hanger-on V83.7
passenger V83.6
traffic V83.3
driver V83.0
hanger-on V83.2
passenger V83.1
while boarding or alighting V83.4
interurban electric car — *see* Accident,
transport, streetcar
land yacht V98.1
logging car — *see* Accident, transport,
industrial vehicle occupant
military vehicle occupant (traffic)
V86.34
driver V86.04
hanger-on V86.24
nontraffic V86.94
driver V86.54
hanger-on V86.74
passenger V86.64
passenger V86.14
while boarding or alighting V86.44
mine tram — *see* Accident, transport,
industrial vehicle occupant
motor vehicle NEC occupant (traffic)
V86.39
driver V86.09
hanger-on V86.29
nontraffic V86.99
driver V86.59
hanger-on V86.79
passenger V86.69
passenger V86.19
while boarding or alighting V86.49
motorcoach — *see* Accident, transport,
bus occupant
motorcyclist V29.9
collision (with)
animal (traffic) V20.9
being ridden (traffic) V26.9
nontraffic V26.2
while boarding or alighting
V26.3
nontraffic V20.2
while boarding or alighting
V20.3
animal-drawn vehicle (traffic)
V26.9
nontraffic V26.2
while boarding or alighting
V26.3
bus (traffic) V24.9
nontraffic V24.2
while boarding or alighting
V24.3
car (traffic) V23.9
nontraffic V23.2
while boarding or alighting
V23.3
motor vehicle NOS (traffic) V29.60
nontraffic V29.20
specified type NEC (traffic)
V29.69
nontraffic V29.29
pedal cycle (traffic) V21.9
nontraffic V21.2
while boarding or alighting
V21.3
pickup truck (traffic) V23.9
nontraffic V23.2
while boarding or alighting
V23.3
railway vehicle (traffic) V25.9
nontraffic V25.2
while boarding or alighting
V25.3

Accident (to) — *continued*
transport (involving injury to) — *continued*
motorcyclist — *continued*
collision (with) — *continued*
specified vehicle NEC (traffic)
V26.9
nontraffic V26.2
while boarding or alighting
V26.3
stationary object (traffic) V27.9
nontraffic V27.2
while boarding or alighting
V27.3
streetcar (traffic) V26.9
nontraffic V26.2
while boarding or alighting
V26.3
three wheeled motor vehicle
(traffic) V22.9
nontraffic V22.2
while boarding or alighting
V22.3
truck (traffic) V24.9
nontraffic V24.2
while boarding or alighting
V24.3
two wheeled motor vehicle (traffic)
V22.9
nontraffic V22.2
while boarding or alighting
V22.3
van (traffic) V23.9
nontraffic V23.2
while boarding or alighting
V23.3
driver
collision (with)
animal (traffic) V20.4
being ridden (traffic) V26.4
nontraffic V26.0
nontraffic V20.0
animal-drawn vehicle (traffic)
V26.4
nontraffic V26.0
bus (traffic) V24.4
nontraffic V24.0
car (traffic) V23.4
nontraffic V23.0
motor vehicle NOS (traffic)
V29.40
nontraffic V29.00
specified type NEC (traffic)
V29.49
nontraffic V29.09
pedal cycle (traffic) V21.4
nontraffic V21.0
pickup truck (traffic) V23.4
nontraffic V23.0
railway vehicle (traffic) V25.4
nontraffic V25.0
specified vehicle NEC (traffic)
V26.4
nontraffic V26.0
stationary object (traffic) V27.4
nontraffic V27.0
streetcar (traffic) V26.4
nontraffic V26.0
three wheeled motor vehicle
(traffic) V22.4
nontraffic V22.0
truck (traffic) V24.4
nontraffic V24.0
two wheeled motor vehicle
(traffic) V22.4
nontraffic V22.0
van (traffic) V23.4
nontraffic V23.0
noncollision accident (traffic)
V28.4
nontraffic V28.0
noncollision accident (traffic) V28.9
nontraffic V28.2
while boarding or alighting V28.3
nontraffic V29.3
passenger
collision (with)
animal (traffic) V20.5
being ridden (traffic) V26.5
nontraffic V26.1
nontraffic V20.1
animal-drawn vehicle (traffic)
V26.5
nontraffic V26.1
bus (traffic) V24.5
nontraffic V24.1
car (traffic) V23.5
nontraffic V23.1

Accident (to) — *continued*
transport (involving injury to) — *continued*
motorcyclist — *continued*
passenger — *continued*
collision (with) — *continued*
motor vehicle NOS (traffic)
V29.50
nontraffic V29.10
specified type NEC (traffic)
V29.59
nontraffic V29.19
pedal cycle (traffic) V21.5
nontraffic V21.1
pickup truck (traffic) V23.5
nontraffic V23.1
railway vehicle (traffic) V25.5
nontraffic V25.1
specified vehicle NEC (traffic)
V26.5
nontraffic V26.1
stationary object (traffic) V27.5
nontraffic V27.1
streetcar (traffic) V26.5
nontraffic V26.1
three wheeled motor vehicle
(traffic) V22.5
nontraffic V22.1
truck (traffic) V24.5
nontraffic V24.1
two wheeled motor vehicle
(traffic) V22.5
nontraffic V22.1
van (traffic) V23.5
nontraffic V23.1
noncollision accident (traffic)
V28.5
nontraffic V28.1
specified type NEC V29.88
military vehicle V29.81
occupant (of)
aircraft (powered) V95.9
fixed wing
commercial — *see* Accident,
transport, aircraft, occupant,
powered, fixed wing,
commercial
private — *see* Accident,
transport, aircraft, occupant,
powered, fixed wing,
private
nonpowered V96.9
specified NEC V95.8
airport battery-powered vehicle — *see*
Accident, transport, industrial
vehicle occupant
all-terrain vehicle (ATV) — *see*
Accident, transport, all-terrain
vehicle occupant
animal-drawn vehicle — *see* Accident,
transport, animal-drawn vehicle
occupant
automobile — *see* Accident, transport,
car occupant
balloon V96.00
battery-powered vehicle — *see*
Accident, transport, industrial
vehicle occupant
bicycle — *see* Accident, transport,
pedal cyclist
motorized — *see* Accident,
transport, motorcycle rider
boat NEC — *see* Accident, watercraft
bulldozer — *see* Accident, transport,
construction vehicle occupant
bus — *see* Accident, transport, bus
occupant
cable car (on rails) — *see also*
Accident, transport, streetcar
occupant
not on rails V98.0
car — *see also* Accident, transport, car
occupant
cable (on rails) — *see also*
Accident, transport, streetcar
occupant
not on rails V98.0
coach — *see* Accident, transport, bus
occupant
coal-car — *see* Accident, transport,
industrial vehicle occupant
digger — *see* Accident, transport,
construction vehicle occupant
dump truck — *see* Accident, transport,
construction vehicle occupant
earth-leveler — *see* Accident,
transport, construction vehicle
occupant
farm machinery (self-propelled) —
see Accident, transport,
agricultural vehicle occupant

EXTERNAL CAUSES

Accident (to) — *continued*
  transport (involving injury to) — *continued*
    occupant (of) — *continued*
      forklift — *see* Accident, transport, industrial vehicle occupant
      glider (unpowered) V96.20
        hang V96.10
        powered (microlight) (ultralight) — *see* Accident, transport, aircraft, occupant, powered, glider
      glider (unpowered) NEC V96.20
      hang-glider V96.10
      harvester — *see* Accident, transport, agricultural vehicle occupant
      heavy (transport) vehicle — *see* Accident, transport, truck occupant
      helicopter — *see* Accident, transport, aircraft, occupant, helicopter
      ice-yacht V98.2
      kite (carrying person) V96.8
      land-yacht V98.1
      logging car — *see* Accident, transport, industrial vehicle occupant
      mechanical shovel — *see* Accident, transport, construction vehicle occupant
      microlight — *see* Accident, transport, aircraft, occupant, powered, glider
      minibus — *see* Accident, transport, car occupant
      minivan — *see* Accident, transport, car occupant
      moped — *see* Accident, transport, motorcycle
      motor scooter — *see* Accident, transport, motorcycle
      motorcycle (with sidecar) — *see* Accident, transport, motorcycle
      pedal cycle — *see also* Accident, transport, pedal cyclist
      pickup (truck) — *see* Accident, transport, pickup truck occupant
      railway (train) (vehicle) (subterranean) (elevated) — *see* Accident, transport, railway vehicle occupant
      rickshaw — *see* Accident, transport, pedal cycle
        motorized — *see* Accident, transport, three-wheeled motor vehicle
      pedal driven — *see* Accident, transport, pedal cyclist
      road-roller — *see* Accident, transport, construction vehicle occupant
      ship NOS V94.9
      ski-lift (chair) (gondola) V98.3
      snowmobile — *see* Accident, transport, snowmobile occupant
      spacecraft, spaceship — *see* Accident, transport, aircraft, occupant, spacecraft
      sport utility vehicle — *see* Accident, transport, car occupant
      streetcar (interurban) (operating on public street or highway) — *see* Accident, transport, streetcar occupant
      SUV — *see* Accident, transport, car occupant
      téléférique V98.0
      three-wheeled vehicle (motorized) — *see also* Accident, transport, three-wheeled motor vehicle occupant
        nonmotorized — *see* Accident, transport, pedal cycle
      tractor (farm) (and trailer) — *see* Accident, transport, agricultural vehicle occupant
      train — *see* Accident, transport, railway vehicle occupant
      tram — *see* Accident, transport, streetcar occupant
        in mine or quarry — *see* Accident, transport, industrial vehicle occupant
      tricycle — *see* Accident, transport, pedal cycle
        motorized — *see* Accident, transport, three-wheeled motor vehicle
      trolley — *see* Accident, transport, streetcar occupant
        in mine or quarry — *see* Accident, transport, industrial vehicle occupant

Accident (to) — *continued*
  transport (involving injury to) — *continued*
    occupant (of) — *continued*
      tub, in mine or quarry — *see* Accident, transport, industrial vehicle occupant
      ultralight — *see* Accident, transport, aircraft, occupant, powered, glider
      van — *see* Accident, transport, van occupant
      vehicle NEC V89.9
        heavy transport — *see* Accident, transport, truck occupant
        motor (traffic) NEC V89.2
        nontraffic NEC V89.0
      watercraft NOS V94.9
        causing drowning — *see* Drowning, resulting from accident to boat
    parachutist V97.29
      after accident to aircraft — *see* Accident, transport, aircraft
      entangled in object V97.21
      injured on landing V97.22
    pedal cyclist V19.9
      collision (with)
        animal (traffic) V10.9
          being ridden (traffic) V16.9
            nontraffic V16.2
            while boarding or alighting V16.3
          nontraffic V10.2
          while boarding or alighting V10.3
        animal-drawn vehicle (traffic) V16.9
          nontraffic V16.2
          while boarding or alighting V16.3
        bus (traffic) V14.9
          nontraffic V14.2
          while boarding or alighting V14.3
        car (traffic) V13.9
          nontraffic V13.2
          while boarding or alighting V13.3
        motor vehicle NOS (traffic) V19.60
          nontraffic V19.20
          specified type NEC (traffic) V19.69
            nontraffic V19.29
        pedal cycle (traffic) V11.9
          nontraffic V11.2
          while boarding or alighting V11.3
        pickup truck (traffic) V13.9
          nontraffic V13.2
          while boarding or alighting V13.3
        railway vehicle (traffic) V15.9
          nontraffic V15.2
          while boarding or alighting V15.3
        specified vehicle NEC (traffic) V16.9
          nontraffic V16.2
          while boarding or alighting V16.3
        stationary object (traffic) V17.9
          nontraffic V17.2
          while boarding or alighting V17.3
        streetcar (traffic) V16.9
          nontraffic V16.2
          while boarding or alighting V16.3
        three wheeled motor vehicle (traffic) V12.9
          nontraffic V12.2
          while boarding or alighting V12.3
        truck (traffic) V14.9
          nontraffic V14.2
          while boarding or alighting V14.3
        two wheeled motor vehicle (traffic) V12.9
          nontraffic V12.2
          while boarding or alighting V12.3
        van (traffic) V13.9
          nontraffic V13.2
          while boarding or alighting V13.3

Accident (to) — *continued*
  transport (involving injury to) — *continued*
    pedal cyclist — *continued*
      driver
        collision (with)
          animal (traffic) V10.4
            being ridden (traffic) V16.4
            nontraffic V16.0
            nontraffic V10.0
          animal-drawn vehicle (traffic) V16.4
            nontraffic V16.0
          bus (traffic) V14.4
            nontraffic V14.0
          car (traffic) V13.4
            nontraffic V13.0
          motor vehicle NOS (traffic) V19.40
            nontraffic V19.00
            specified type NEC (traffic) V19.49
              nontraffic V19.09
          pedal cycle (traffic) V11.4
            nontraffic V11.0
          pickup truck (traffic) V13.4
            nontraffic V13.0
          railway vehicle (traffic) V15.4
            nontraffic V15.0
          specified vehicle NEC (traffic) V16.4
            nontraffic V16.0
          stationary object (traffic) V17.4
            nontraffic V17.0
          streetcar (traffic) V16.4
            nontraffic V16.0
          three wheeled motor vehicle (traffic) V12.4
            nontraffic V12.0
          truck (traffic) V14.4
            nontraffic V14.0
          two wheeled motor vehicle (traffic) V12.4
            nontraffic V12.0
          van (traffic) V13.4
            nontraffic V13.0
        noncollision accident (traffic) V18.4
          nontraffic V18.0
      noncollision accident (traffic) V18.9
        nontraffic V18.2
        while boarding or alighting V18.3
      nontraffic V18.3
      passenger
        collision (with)
          animal (traffic) V10.5
            being ridden (traffic) V16.5
            nontraffic V16.1
            nontraffic V10.1
          animal-drawn vehicle (traffic) V16.5
            nontraffic V16.1
          bus (traffic) V14.5
            nontraffic V14.1
          car (traffic) V13.5
            nontraffic V13.1
          motor vehicle NOS (traffic) V19.50
            nontraffic V19.10
            specified type NEC (traffic) V19.59
              nontraffic V19.19
          pedal cycle (traffic) V11.5
            nontraffic V11.1
          pickup truck (traffic) V13.5
            nontraffic V13.1
          railway vehicle (traffic) V15.5
            nontraffic V15.1
          specified vehicle NEC (traffic) V16.5
            nontraffic V16.1
          stationary object (traffic) V17.5
            nontraffic V17.1
          streetcar (traffic) V16.5
            nontraffic V16.1
          three wheeled motor vehicle (traffic) V12.5
            nontraffic V12.1
          truck (traffic) V14.5
            nontraffic V14.1
          two wheeled motor vehicle (traffic) V12.5
            nontraffic V12.1
          van (traffic) V13.5
            nontraffic V13.1
        noncollision accident (traffic) V18.5
          nontraffic V18.1
      specified type NEC V19.88
      military vehicle V19.81

Accident (to) — *continued*
  transport (involving injury to) — *continued*
    pedestrian
      conveyance (occupant) V09.9
        babystroller V00.828
          collision (with) V09.9
            animal being ridden or animal drawn vehicle V06.99
              nontraffic V06.09
              traffic V06.19
            bus or heavy transport V04.99
              nontraffic V04.09
              traffic V04.19
            car V03.99
              nontraffic V03.09
              traffic V03.19
            pedal cycle V01.99
              nontraffic V01.09
              traffic V01.19
            pickup truck or van V03.99
              nontraffic V03.09
              traffic V03.19
            railway (train) (vehicle) V05.99
              nontraffic V05.09
              traffic V05.19
            stationary object V00.822
            streetcar V06.99
              nontraffic V06.09
              traffic V06.19
            two-or three-wheeled motor vehicle V02.99
              nontraffic V02.09
              traffic V02.19
            vehicle V09.9
              animal-drawn V06.99
                nontraffic V06.09
                traffic V06.19
              motor
                nontraffic V09.00
                traffic V09.20
        fall V00.821
        nontraffic V09.1
          involving motor vehicle NEC V09.00
        traffic V09.3
          involving motor vehicle NEC V09.20
      flat-bottomed NEC V00.388
        collision (with) V09.9
          animal being ridden or animal drawn vehicle V06.99
            nontraffic V06.09
            traffic V06.19
          bus or heavy transport V04.99
            nontraffic V04.09
            traffic V04.19
          car V03.99
            nontraffic V03.09
            traffic V03.19
          pedal cycle V01.99
            nontraffic V01.09
            traffic V01.19
          pickup truck or van V03.99
            nontraffic V03.09
            traffic V03.19
          railway (train) (vehicle) V05.99
            nontraffic V05.09
            traffic V05.19
          stationary object V00.382
          streetcar V06.99
            nontraffic V06.09
            traffic V06.19
          two-or three-wheeled motor vehicle V02.99
            nontraffic V02.09
            traffic V02.19
          vehicle V09.9
            animal-drawn V06.99
              nontraffic V06.09
              traffic V06.19
            motor
              nontraffic V09.00
              traffic V09.20
      fall V00.381
      nontraffic V09.1
        involving motor vehicle NEC V09.00
      snow
        board — *see* Accident, transport, pedestrian, conveyance, snow board
        ski — *see* Accident, transport, pedestrian, conveyance, skis (snow)
      traffic V09.3
        involving motor vehicle NEC V09.20

Accident (to) — *continued*
  transport (involving injury to) — *continued*
    pedestrian — *continued*
      conveyance (occupant) — *continued*
        gliding type NEC V00.288
          collision (with) V09.9
            animal being ridden or animal drawn vehicle V06.99
              nontraffic V06.09
              traffic V06.19
            bus or heavy transport V04.99
              nontraffic V04.09
              traffic V04.19
            car V03.99
              nontraffic V03.09
              traffic V03.19
            pedal cycle V01.99
              nontraffic V01.09
              traffic V01.19
            pick-up truck or van V03.99
              nontraffic V03.09
              traffic V03.19
            railway (train) (vehicle) V05.99
              nontraffic V05.09
              traffic V05.19
            stationary object V00.282
            streetcar V06.99
              nontraffic V06.09
              traffic V06.19
            two-or three-wheeled motor vehicle V02.99
              nontraffic V02.09
              traffic V02.19
            vehicle V09.9
              animal-drawn V06.99
                nontraffic V06.09
                traffic V06.19
              motor
                nontraffic V09.00
                traffic V09.20
          fall V00.281
        heelies — *see* Accident, transport, pedestrian, conveyance, heelies
        ice skate — *see* Accident, transport, pedestrian, conveyance, ice skate
        nontraffic V09.1
          involving motor vehicle NEC V09.00
        sled — *see* Accident, transport, pedestrian, conveyance, sled
        traffic V09.3
          involving motor vehicle NEC V09.20
        wheelies — *see* Accident, transport, pedestrian, conveyance, heelies
      heelies V00.158
        colliding with stationary object V00.152
        fall V00.151
      ice skates V00.218
        collision (with) V09.9
          animal being ridden or animal drawn vehicle V06.99
            nontraffic V06.09
            traffic V06.19
          bus or heavy transport V04.99
            nontraffic V04.09
            traffic V04.19
          car V03.99
            nontraffic V03.09
            traffic V03.19
          pedal cycle V01.99
            nontraffic V01.09
            traffic V01.19
          pick-up truck or van V03.99
            nontraffic V03.09
            traffic V03.19
          railway (train) (vehicle) V05.99
            nontraffic V05.09
            traffic V05.19
          stationary object V00.212
          streetcar V06.99
            nontraffic V06.09
            traffic V06.19
          two-or three-wheeled motor vehicle V02.99
            nontraffic V02.09
            traffic V02.19

Accident (to) — *continued*
  transport (involving injury to) — *continued*
    pedestrian — *continued*
      conveyance (occupant) — *continued*
        ice skates — *continued*
          collision (with) — *continued*
            vehicle V09.9
              animal-drawn V06.99
                nontraffic V06.09
                traffic V06.19
              motor
                nontraffic V09.00
                traffic V09.20
          fall V00.211
        nontraffic V09.1
          involving motor vehicle NEC V09.00
        traffic V09.3
          involving motor vehicle NEC V09.20
        motorized mobility scooter V00.838
          collision with stationary object V00.832
          fall from V00.831
        nontraffic V09.1
          involving motor vehicle V09.00
            military V09.01
            specified type NEC V09.09
        roller skates (non in-line) V00.128
          collision (with) V09.9
            animal being ridden or animal drawn vehicle V06.91
              nontraffic V06.01
              traffic V06.11
            bus or heavy transport V04.91
              nontraffic V04.01
              traffic V04.11
            car V03.91
              nontraffic V03.01
              traffic V03.11
            pedal cycle V01.91
              nontraffic V01.01
              traffic V01.11
            pickup truck or van V03.91
              nontraffic V03.01
              traffic V03.11
            railway (train) (vehicle) V05.91
              nontraffic V05.01
              traffic V05.11
            stationary object V00.122
            streetcar V06.91
              nontraffic V06.01
              traffic V06.11
            two-or three-wheeled motor vehicle V02.91
              nontraffic V02.01
              traffic V02.11
            vehicle V09.9
              animal-drawn V06.91
                nontraffic V06.01
                traffic V06.11
              motor
                nontraffic V09.00
                traffic V09.20
          fall V00.121
          in-line V00.118
            collision — *see also* Accident, transport, pedestrian, conveyance occupant, roller skates, collision with stationary object V00.112
            fall V00.111
            nontraffic V09.1
              involving motor vehicle NEC V09.00
            traffic V09.3
              involving motor vehicle NEC V09.20
        rolling shoes V00.158
          colliding with stationary object V00.152
          fall V00.151
        rolling type NEC V00.188
          collision (with) V09.9
            animal being ridden or animal drawn vehicle V06.99
              nontraffic V06.09
              traffic V06.19
            bus or heavy transport V04.99
              nontraffic V04.09
              traffic V04.19
            car V03.99
              nontraffic V03.09
              traffic V03.19
            pedal cycle V01.99
              nontraffic V01.09
              traffic V01.19

Accident (to) — *continued*
  transport (involving injury to) — *continued*
    pedestrian — *continued*
      conveyance (occupant) — *continued*
        rolling type NEC — *continued*
          collision (with) — *continued*
            pickup truck or van V03.99
              nontraffic V03.09
              traffic V03.19
            railway (train) (vehicle) V05.99
              nontraffic V05.09
              traffic V05.19
            stationary object V00.182
            streetcar V06.99
              nontraffic V06.09
              traffic V06.19
            two-or three-wheeled motor vehicle V02.99
              nontraffic V02.09
              traffic V02.19
            vehicle V09.9
              animal-drawn V06.99
                nontraffic V06.09
                traffic V06.19
              motor
                nontraffic V09.00
                traffic V09.20
          fall V00.181
        in-line roller skate — *see* Accident, transport, pedestrian, conveyance, roller skate, in-line
        nontraffic V09.1
          involving motor vehicle NEC V09.00
        roller skate — *see* Accident, transport, pedestrian, conveyance, roller skate
        scooter (non-motorized) — *see* Accident, transport, pedestrian, conveyance, scooter
        skateboard — *see* Accident, transport, pedestrian, conveyance, skateboard
        traffic V09.3
          involving motor vehicle NEC V09.20
        scooter (non-motorized) V00.148
          collision (with) V09.9
            animal being ridden or animal drawn vehicle V06.99
              nontraffic V06.09
              traffic V06.19
            bus or heavy transport V04.99
              nontraffic V04.09
              traffic V04.19
            car V03.99
              nontraffic V03.09
              traffic V03.19
            pedal cycle V01.99
              nontraffic V01.09
              traffic V01.19
            pickup truck or van V03.99
              nontraffic V03.09
              traffic V03.19
            railway (train) (vehicle) V05.99
              nontraffic V05.09
              traffic V05.19
            stationary object V00.142
            streetcar V06.99
              nontraffic V06.09
              traffic V06.19
            two-or three-wheeled motor vehicle V02.99
              nontraffic V02.09
              traffic V02.19
            vehicle V09.9
              animal-drawn V06.99
                nontraffic V06.09
                traffic V06.19
              motor
                nontraffic V09.00
                traffic V09.20
          fall V00.141
        nontraffic V09.1
          involving motor vehicle NEC V09.00
        traffic V09.3
          involving motor vehicle NEC V09.20

Accident (to) — *continued*
  transport (involving injury to) — *continued*
    pedestrian — *continued*
      conveyance (occupant) — *continued*
        skate board V00.138
          collision (with) V09.9
            animal being ridden or animal drawn vehicle V06.92
              nontraffic V06.02
              traffic V06.12
            bus or heavy transport V04.92
              nontraffic V04.02
              traffic V04.12
            car V03.92
              nontraffic V03.02
              traffic V03.12
            pedal cycle V01.92
              nontraffic V01.02
              traffic V01.12
            pickup truck or van V03.92
              nontraffic V03.02
              traffic V03.12
            railway (train) (vehicle) V05.92
              nontraffic V05.02
              traffic V05.12
            stationary object V00.132
            streetcar V06.92
              nontraffic V06.02
              traffic V06.12
            two-or three-wheeled motor vehicle V02.92
              nontraffic V02.02
              traffic V02.12
            vehicle V09.9
              animal-drawn V06.92
                nontraffic V06.02
                traffic V06.12
              motor
                nontraffic V09.00
                traffic V09.20
          fall V00.131
        nontraffic V09.1
          involving motor vehicle NEC V09.00
        traffic V09.3
          involving motor vehicle NEC V09.20
        skis (snow) V00.328
          collision (with) V09.9
            animal being ridden or animal drawn vehicle V06.99
              nontraffic V06.09
              traffic V06.19
            bus or heavy transport V04.99
              nontraffic V04.09
              traffic V04.19
            car V03.99
              nontraffic V03.09
              traffic V03.19
            pedal cycle V01.99
              nontraffic V01.09
              traffic V01.19
            pickup truck or van V03.99
              nontraffic V03.09
              traffic V03.19
            railway (train) (vehicle) V05.99
              nontraffic V05.09
              traffic V05.19
            stationary object V00.322
            streetcar V06.99
              nontraffic V06.09
              traffic V06.19
            two-or three-wheeled motor vehicle V02.99
              nontraffic V02.09
              traffic V02.19
            vehicle V09.9
              animal-drawn V06.99
                nontraffic V06.09
                traffic V06.19
              motor
                nontraffic V09.00
                traffic V09.20
          fall V00.321
        nontraffic V09.1
          involving motor vehicle NEC V09.00
        traffic V09.3
          involving motor vehicle NEC V09.20

EXTERNAL CAUSES

Accident (to) — continued
transport (involving injury to) — continued
  pedestrian — continued
    conveyance (occupant) — continued
      sled V00.228
        collision (with) V09.9
          animal being ridden or animal
            drawn vehicle V06.99
            nontraffic V06.09
            traffic V06.19
          bus or heavy transport V04.99
            nontraffic V04.09
            traffic V04.19
          car V03.99
            nontraffic V03.09
            traffic V03.19
          pedal cycle V01.99
            nontraffic V01.09
            traffic V01.19
          pickup truck or van V03.99
            nontraffic V03.09
            traffic V03.19
          railway (train) (vehicle)
            V05.99
            nontraffic V05.09
            traffic V05.19
          stationary object V00.222
          streetcar V06.99
            nontraffic V06.09
            traffic V06.19
          two-or three-wheeled motor
            vehicle V02.99
            nontraffic V02.09
            traffic V02.19
          vehicle V09.9
            animal-drawn V06.99
              nontraffic V06.09
              traffic V06.19
            motor
              nontraffic V09.00
              traffic V09.20
        fall V00.221
        nontraffic V09.1
          involving motor vehicle NEC
            V09.00
        traffic V09.3
          involving motor vehicle NEC
            V09.20
      snow board V00.318
        collision (with) V09.9
          animal being ridden or animal
            drawn vehicle V06.99
            nontraffic V06.09
            traffic V06.19
          bus or heavy transport V04.99
            nontraffic V04.09
            traffic V04.19
          car V03.99
            nontraffic V03.09
            traffic V03.19
          pedal cycle V01.99
            nontraffic V01.09
            traffic V01.19
          pickup truck or van V03.99
            nontraffic V03.09
            traffic V03.19
          railway (train) (vehicle)
            V05.99
            nontraffic V05.09
            traffic V05.19
          stationary object V00.312
          streetcar V06.99
            nontraffic V06.09
            traffic V06.19
          two-or three-wheeled motor
            vehicle V02.99
            nontraffic V02.09
            traffic V02.19
          vehicle V09.9
            animal-drawn V06.99
              nontraffic V06.09
              traffic V06.19
            motor
              nontraffic V09.00
              traffic V09.20
        fall V00.311
        nontraffic V09.1
          involving motor vehicle NEC
            V09.00
        traffic V09.3
          involving motor vehicle NEC
            V09.20

Accident (to) — continued
transport (involving injury to) — continued
  pedestrian — continued
    conveyance (occupant) — continued
      specified type NEC V00.898
        collision (with) V09.9
          animal being ridden or animal
            drawn vehicle V06.99
            nontraffic V06.09
            traffic V06.19
          bus or heavy transport V04.99
            nontraffic V04.09
            traffic V04.19
          car V03.99
            nontraffic V03.09
            traffic V03.19
          pedal cycle V01.99
            nontraffic V01.09
            traffic V01.19
          pickup truck or van V03.99
            nontraffic V03.09
            traffic V03.19
          railway (train) (vehicle)
            V05.99
            nontraffic V05.09
            traffic V05.19
          stationary object V00.892
          streetcar V06.99
            nontraffic V06.09
            traffic V06.19
          two-or three-wheeled motor
            vehicle V02.99
            nontraffic V02.09
            traffic V02.19
          vehicle V09.9
            animal-drawn V06.99
              nontraffic V06.09
              traffic V06.19
            motor
              nontraffic V09.00
              traffic V09.20
        fall V00.891
        nontraffic V09.1
          involving motor vehicle NEC
            V09.00
        traffic V09.3
          involving motor vehicle NEC
            V09.20
      wheelchair (powered) V00.818
        collision (with) V09.9
          animal being ridden or animal
            drawn vehicle V06.99
            nontraffic V06.09
            traffic V06.19
          bus or heavy transport V04.99
            nontraffic V04.09
            traffic V04.19
          car V03.99
            nontraffic V03.09
            traffic V03.19
          pedal cycle V01.99
            nontraffic V01.09
            traffic V01.19
          pickup truck or van V03.99
            nontraffic V03.09
            traffic V03.19
          railway (train) (vehicle)
            V05.99
            nontraffic V05.09
            traffic V05.19
          stationary object V00.812
          streetcar V06.99
            nontraffic V06.09
            traffic V06.19
          two-or three-wheeled motor
            vehicle V02.99
            nontraffic V02.09
            traffic V02.19
          vehicle V09.9
            animal-drawn V06.99
              nontraffic V06.09
              traffic V06.19
            motor
              nontraffic V09.00
              traffic V09.20
        fall V00.811
        nontraffic V09.1
          involving motor vehicle NEC
            V09.00
        traffic V09.3
          involving motor vehicle NEC
            V09.20

Accident (to) — continued
transport (involving injury to) — continued
  pedestrian — continued
    conveyance (occupant) — continued
      wheeled shoe V00.158
        colliding with stationary object
          V00.152
        fall V00.151
  on foot — see also Accident,
    pedestrian
    collision (with)
      animal being ridden or animal
        drawn vehicle V06.90
        nontraffic V06.00
        traffic V06.10
      bus or heavy transport V04.90
        nontraffic V04.00
        traffic V04.10
      car V03.90
        nontraffic V03.00
        traffic V03.10
      pedal cycle V01.90
        nontraffic V01.00
        traffic V01.10
      pickup truck or van V03.90
        nontraffic V03.00
        traffic V03.10
      railway (train) (vehicle) V05.90
        nontraffic V05.00
        traffic V05.10
      streetcar V06.90
        nontraffic V06.00
        traffic V06.10
      two-or three-wheeled motor
        vehicle V02.90
        nontraffic V02.00
        traffic V02.10
      vehicle V09.9
        animal-drawn V06.90
          nontraffic V06.00
          traffic V06.10
        motor
          nontraffic V09.00
          traffic V09.20
    nontraffic V09.1
      involving motor vehicle V09.00
        military V09.01
        specified type NEC V09.09
    traffic V09.3
      involving motor vehicle V09.20
        military V09.21
        specified type NEC V09.29
  person NEC (unknown way or
    transportation) V99
  collision (between)
    bus (with)
      heavy transport vehicle (traffic)
        V87.5
        nontraffic V88.5
    car (with)
      bus (traffic) V87.3
        nontraffic V88.3
      heavy transport vehicle (traffic)
        V87.4
        nontraffic V88.4
      nontraffic V88.5
      pickup truck or van (traffic)
        V87.2
        nontraffic V88.2
      train or railway vehicle (traffic)
        V87.6
        nontraffic V88.6
      two-or three-wheeled motor
        vehicle (traffic) V87.0
        nontraffic V88.0
      motor vehicle (traffic) NEC V87.7
        nontraffic V88.7
      two-or three-wheeled vehicle
        (with) (traffic)
        motor vehicle NEC V87.1
          nontraffic V88.1
    nonmotor vehicle (collision)
      (noncollision) (traffic) V87.9
      nontraffic V88.9
  pickup truck occupant V59.9
    collision (with)
      animal (traffic) V50.9
        being ridden (traffic) V56.9
          nontraffic V56.3
          while boarding or alighting
            V56.4
        nontraffic V50.3
        while boarding or alighting
          V50.4
      animal-drawn vehicle (traffic)
        V56.9
        nontraffic V56.3
        while boarding or alighting
          V56.4

Accident (to) — continued
transport (involving injury to) — continued
  pickup truck occupant — continued
    collision (with) — continued
      bus (traffic) V54.9
        nontraffic V54.3
        while boarding or alighting
          V54.4
      car (traffic) V53.9
        nontraffic V53.3
        while boarding or alighting
          V53.4
      motor vehicle NOS (traffic) V59.60
        nontraffic V59.20
        specified type NEC (traffic)
          V59.69
        nontraffic V59.29
      pedal cycle (traffic) V51.9
        nontraffic V51.3
        while boarding or alighting
          V51.4
      pickup truck (traffic) V53.9
        nontraffic V53.3
        while boarding or alighting
          V53.4
      railway vehicle (traffic) V55.9
        nontraffic V55.3
        while boarding or alighting
          V55.4
      specified vehicle NEC (traffic)
        V56.9
        nontraffic V56.3
        while boarding or alighting
          V56.4
      stationary object (traffic) V57.9
        nontraffic V57.3
        while boarding or alighting
          V57.4
      streetcar (traffic) V56.9
        nontraffic V56.3
        while boarding or alighting
          V56.4
      three wheeled motor vehicle
        (traffic) V52.9
        nontraffic V52.3
        while boarding or alighting
          V52.4
      truck (traffic) V54.9
        nontraffic V54.3
        while boarding or alighting
          V54.4
      two wheeled motor vehicle (traffic)
        V52.9
        nontraffic V52.3
        while boarding or alighting
          V52.4
      van (traffic) V53.9
        nontraffic V53.3
        while boarding or alighting
          V53.4
    driver
      collision (with)
        animal (traffic) V50.5
          being ridden (traffic) V56.5
           nontraffic V56.0
          nontraffic V50.0
        animal-drawn vehicle (traffic)
          V56.5
          nontraffic V56.0
        bus (traffic) V54.5
          nontraffic V54.0
        car (traffic) V53.5
          nontraffic V53.0
        motor vehicle NOS (traffic)
          V59.40
          nontraffic V59.00
          specified type NEC (traffic)
           V59.49
          nontraffic V59.09
        pedal cycle (traffic) V51.5
          nontraffic V51.0
        pickup truck (traffic) V53.5
          nontraffic V53.0
        railway vehicle (traffic) V55.5
          nontraffic V55.0
        specified vehicle NEC (traffic)
          V56.5
          nontraffic V56.0
        stationary object (traffic) V57.5
          nontraffic V57.0
        streetcar (traffic) V56.5
          nontraffic V56.0
        three wheeled motor vehicle
          (traffic) V52.5
          nontraffic V52.0
        truck (traffic) V54.5
          nontraffic V54.0
        two wheeled motor vehicle
          (traffic) V52.5
          nontraffic V52.0

EXTERNAL CAUSES

Accident (to) — *continued*
  transport (involving injury to) — *continued*
    pickup truck occupant — *continued*
      driver — *continued*
        collision (with) — *continued*
          van (traffic) V53.5
            nontraffic V53.0
          noncollision accident (traffic) V58.5
            nontraffic V58.0
      hanger-on
        collision (with)
          animal (traffic) V50.7
            being ridden (traffic) V56.7
              nontraffic V56.2
            nontraffic V50.2
          animal-drawn vehicle (traffic) V56.7
            nontraffic V56.2
          bus (traffic) V54.7
            nontraffic V54.2
          car (traffic) V53.7
            nontraffic V53.2
          pedal cycle (traffic) V51.7
            nontraffic V51.2
          pickup truck (traffic) V53.7
            nontraffic V53.2
          railway vehicle (traffic) V55.7
            nontraffic V55.2
          specified vehicle NEC (traffic) V56.7
            nontraffic V56.2
          stationary object (traffic) V57.7
            nontraffic V57.2
          streetcar (traffic) V56.7
            nontraffic V56.2
          three wheeled motor vehicle (traffic) V52.7
            nontraffic V52.2
          truck (traffic) V54.7
            nontraffic V54.2
          two wheeled motor vehicle (traffic) V52.7
            nontraffic V52.2
          van (traffic) V53.7
            nontraffic V53.2
        noncollision accident (traffic) V58.7
          nontraffic V58.2
      noncollision accident (traffic) V58.9
        nontraffic V58.3
        while boarding or alighting V58.4
      nontraffic V59.3
      passenger
        collision (with)
          animal (traffic) V50.6
            being ridden (traffic) V56.6
              nontraffic V56.1
            nontraffic V50.1
          animal-drawn vehicle (traffic) V56.6
            nontraffic V56.1
          bus (traffic) V54.6
            nontraffic V54.1
          car (traffic) V53.6
            nontraffic V53.1
          motor vehicle NOS (traffic) V59.50
            nontraffic V59.10
            specified type NEC (traffic) V59.59
              nontraffic V59.19
          pedal cycle (traffic) V51.6
            nontraffic V51.1
          pickup truck (traffic) V53.6
            nontraffic V53.1
          railway vehicle (traffic) V55.6
            nontraffic V55.1
          specified vehicle NEC (traffic) V56.6
            nontraffic V56.1
          stationary object (traffic) V57.6
            nontraffic V57.1
          streetcar (traffic) V56.6
            nontraffic V56.1
          three wheeled motor vehicle (traffic) V52.6
            nontraffic V52.1
          truck (traffic) V54.6
            nontraffic V54.1
          two wheeled motor vehicle (traffic) V52.6
            nontraffic V52.1

Accident (to) — *continued*
  transport (involving injury to) — *continued*
    pickup truck occupant — *continued*
      passenger — *continued*
        collision (with) — *continued*
          van (traffic) V53.6
            nontraffic V53.1
          noncollision accident (traffic) V58.6
            nontraffic V58.1
        specified type NEC V59.88
          military vehicle V59.81
    quarry truck — *see* Accident, transport, industrial vehicle occupant
    race car — *see* Accident, transport, motor vehicle NEC occupant
    railway vehicle occupant V81.9
      collision (with) V81.3
        motor vehicle (non-military) (traffic) V81.1
          military V81.83
          nontraffic V81.0
        rolling stock V81.2
        specified object NEC V81.3
      during derailment V81.7
        with antecedent collision — *see* Accident, transport, railway vehicle occupant, collision
      explosion V81.81
      fall (in railway vehicle) V81.5
        during derailment V81.7
          with antecedent collision — *see* Accident, transport, railway vehicle occupant, collision
        from railway vehicle V81.6
          during derailment V81.7
            with antecedent collision — *see* Accident, transport, railway vehicle occupant, collision
        while boarding or alighting V81.4
      fire V81.81
      object falling onto train V81.82
      specified type NEC V81.89
      while boarding or alighting V81.4
    ski lift V98.3
    snowmobile occupant (nontraffic) V86.92
      driver V86.52
      hanger-on V86.72
      passenger V86.62
      traffic V86.32
        driver V86.02
        hanger-on V86.22
        passenger V86.12
      while boarding or alighting V86.42
    specified NEC V98.8
    sport utility vehicle occupant — *see also* Accident, transport, car occupant
      collision (with)
        stationary object (traffic) V47.91
          nontraffic V47.31
      driver
        collision (with)
          stationary object (traffic) V47.51
            nontraffic V47.01
      passenger
        collision (with)
          stationary object (traffic) V47.61
            nontraffic V47.11
    streetcar occupant V82.9
      collision (with) V82.3
        motor vehicle (traffic) V82.1
          nontraffic V82.0
        rolling stock V82.2
      during derailment V82.7
        with antecedent collision — *see* Accident, transport, streetcar occupant, collision
      fall (in streetcar) V82.5
        during derailment V82.7
          with antecedent collision — *see* Accident, transport, streetcar occupant, collision
        from streetcar V82.6
          during derailment V82.7
            with antecedent collision — *see* Accident, transport, streetcar occupant, collision
        while boarding or alighting V82.4
      while boarding or alighting V82.4
    specified type NEC V82.8
      while boarding or alighting V82.4

Accident (to) — *continued*
  transport (involving injury to) — *continued*
    three-wheeled motor vehicle occupant V39.9
      collision (with)
        animal (traffic) V30.9
          being ridden (traffic) V36.9
            nontraffic V36.3
            while boarding or alighting V36.4
          nontraffic V30.3
          while boarding or alighting V30.4
        animal-drawn vehicle (traffic) V36.9
          nontraffic V36.3
          while boarding or alighting V36.4
        bus (traffic) V34.9
          nontraffic V34.3
          while boarding or alighting V34.4
        car (traffic) V33.9
          nontraffic V33.3
          while boarding or alighting V33.4
        motor vehicle NOS (traffic) V39.60
          nontraffic V39.20
          specified type NEC (traffic) V39.69
            nontraffic V39.29
        pedal cycle (traffic) V31.9
          nontraffic V31.3
          while boarding or alighting V31.4
        pickup truck (traffic) V33.9
          nontraffic V33.3
          while boarding or alighting V33.4
        railway vehicle (traffic) V35.9
          nontraffic V35.3
          while boarding or alighting V35.4
        specified vehicle NEC (traffic) V36.9
          nontraffic V36.3
          while boarding or alighting V36.4
        stationary object (traffic) V37.9
          nontraffic V37.3
          while boarding or alighting V37.4
        streetcar (traffic) V36.9
          nontraffic V36.3
          while boarding or alighting V36.4
        three wheeled motor vehicle (traffic) V32.9
          nontraffic V32.3
          while boarding or alighting V32.4
        truck (traffic) V34.9
          nontraffic V34.3
          while boarding or alighting V34.4
        two wheeled motor vehicle (traffic) V32.9
          nontraffic V32.3
          while boarding or alighting V32.4
        van (traffic) V33.9
          nontraffic V33.3
          while boarding or alighting V33.4
      driver
        collision (with)
          animal (traffic) V30.5
            being ridden (traffic) V36.5
              nontraffic V36.0
            nontraffic V30.0
          animal-drawn vehicle (traffic) V36.5
            nontraffic V36.0
          bus (traffic) V34.5
            nontraffic V34.0
          car (traffic) V33.5
            nontraffic V33.0
          motor vehicle NOS (traffic) V39.40
            nontraffic V39.00
            specified type NEC (traffic) V39.49
              nontraffic V39.09
          pedal cycle (traffic) V31.5
            nontraffic V31.0
          pickup truck (traffic) V33.5
            nontraffic V33.0
          railway vehicle (traffic) V35.5
            nontraffic V35.0

Accident (to) — *continued*
  transport (involving injury to) — *continued*
    three-wheeled motor vehicle occupant — *continued*
      driver — *continued*
        collision (with) — *continued*
          specified vehicle NEC (traffic) V36.5
            nontraffic V36.0
          stationary object (traffic) V37.5
            nontraffic V37.0
          streetcar (traffic) V36.5
            nontraffic V36.0
          three wheeled motor vehicle (traffic) V32.5
            nontraffic V32.0
          truck (traffic) V34.5
            nontraffic V34.0
          two wheeled motor vehicle (traffic) V32.5
            nontraffic V32.0
          van (traffic) V33.5
            nontraffic V33.0
          noncollision accident (traffic) V38.5
            nontraffic V38.0
      hanger-on
        collision (with)
          animal (traffic) V30.7
            being ridden (traffic) V36.7
              nontraffic V36.2
            nontraffic V30.2
          animal-drawn vehicle (traffic) V36.7
            nontraffic V36.2
          bus (traffic) V34.7
            nontraffic V34.2
          car (traffic) V33.7
            nontraffic V33.2
          pedal cycle (traffic) V31.7
            nontraffic V31.2
          pickup truck (traffic) V33.7
            nontraffic V33.2
          railway vehicle (traffic) V35.7
            nontraffic V35.2
          specified vehicle NEC (traffic) V36.7
            nontraffic V36.2
          stationary object (traffic) V37.7
            nontraffic V37.2
          streetcar (traffic) V36.7
            nontraffic V36.2
          three wheeled motor vehicle (traffic) V32.7
            nontraffic V32.2
          truck (traffic) V34.7
            nontraffic V34.2
          two wheeled motor vehicle (traffic) V32.7
            nontraffic V32.2
          van (traffic) V33.7
            nontraffic V33.2
          noncollision accident (traffic) V38.7
            nontraffic V38.2
        noncollision accident (traffic) V38.9
          nontraffic V38.3
          while boarding or alighting V38.4
      nontraffic V39.3
      passenger
        collision (with)
          animal (traffic) V30.6
            being ridden (traffic) V36.6
              nontraffic V36.1
            nontraffic V30.1
          animal-drawn vehicle (traffic) V36.6
            nontraffic V36.1
          bus (traffic) V34.6
            nontraffic V34.1
          car (traffic) V33.6
            nontraffic V33.1
          motor vehicle NOS (traffic) V39.50
            nontraffic V39.10
            specified type NEC (traffic) V39.59
              nontraffic V39.19
          pedal cycle (traffic) V31.6
            nontraffic V31.1
          pickup truck (traffic) V33.6
            nontraffic V33.1
          railway vehicle (traffic) V35.6
            nontraffic V35.1
          specified vehicle NEC (traffic) V36.6
            nontraffic V36.1
          stationary object (traffic) V37.6
            nontraffic V37.1

Accident (to) — *continued*
transport (involving injury to) — *continued*
three-wheeled motor vehicle occupant — *continued*
passenger — *continued*
collision (with) — *continued*
streetcar (traffic) V36.6
nontraffic V36.1
three wheeled motor vehicle (traffic) V32.6
nontraffic V32.1
truck (traffic) V34.6
nontraffic V34.1
two wheeled motor vehicle (traffic) V32.6
nontraffic V32.1
van (traffic) V33.6
nontraffic V33.1
noncollision accident (traffic) V38.6
nontraffic V38.1
specified type NEC V39.89
military vehicle V39.81
tractor (farm) (and trailer) — *see* Accident, transport, agricultural vehicle occupant
tram — *see* Accident, transport, streetcar
in mine or quarry — *see* Accident, transport, industrial vehicle occupant
trolley — *see* Accident, transport, streetcar
in mine or quarry — *see* Accident, transport, industrial vehicle occupant
truck (heavy) occupant V69.9
collision (with)
animal (traffic) V60.9
being ridden (traffic) V66.9
nontraffic V66.3
while boarding or alighting V66.4
nontraffic V60.3
while boarding or alighting V60.4
animal-drawn vehicle (traffic) V66.9
nontraffic V66.3
while boarding or alighting V66.4
bus (traffic) V64.9
nontraffic V64.3
while boarding or alighting V64.4
car (traffic) V63.9
nontraffic V63.3
while boarding or alighting V63.4
motor vehicle NOS (traffic) V69.60
nontraffic V69.20
specified type NEC (traffic) V69.69
nontraffic V69.29
pedal cycle (traffic) V61.9
nontraffic V61.3
while boarding or alighting V61.4
pickup truck (traffic) V63.9
nontraffic V63.3
while boarding or alighting V63.4
railway vehicle (traffic) V65.9
nontraffic V65.3
while boarding or alighting V65.4
specified vehicle NEC (traffic) V66.9
nontraffic V66.3
while boarding or alighting V66.4
stationary object (traffic) V67.9
nontraffic V67.3
while boarding or alighting V67.4
streetcar (traffic) V66.9
nontraffic V66.3
while boarding or alighting V66.4
three wheeled motor vehicle (traffic) V62.9
nontraffic V62.3
while boarding or alighting V62.4
truck (traffic) V64.9
nontraffic V64.3
while boarding or alighting V64.4

Accident (to) — *continued*
transport (involving injury to) — *continued*
truck (heavy) occupant — *continued*
collision (with) — *continued*
two wheeled motor vehicle (traffic) V62.9
nontraffic V62.3
while boarding or alighting V62.4
van (traffic) V63.9
nontraffic V63.3
while boarding or alighting V63.4
driver
collision (with)
animal (traffic) V60.5
being ridden (traffic) V66.5
nontraffic V66.0
nontraffic V60.0
animal-drawn vehicle (traffic) V66.5
nontraffic V66.0
bus (traffic) V64.5
nontraffic V64.0
car (traffic) V63.5
nontraffic V63.0
motor vehicle NOS (traffic) V69.40
nontraffic V69.00
specified type NEC (traffic) V69.49
nontraffic V69.09
pedal cycle (traffic) V61.5
nontraffic V61.0
pickup truck (traffic) V63.5
nontraffic V63.0
railway vehicle (traffic) V65.5
nontraffic V65.0
specified vehicle NEC (traffic) V66.5
nontraffic V66.0
stationary object (traffic) V67.5
nontraffic V67.0
streetcar (traffic) V66.5
nontraffic V66.0
three wheeled motor vehicle (traffic) V62.5
nontraffic V62.0
truck (traffic) V64.5
nontraffic V64.0
two wheeled motor vehicle (traffic) V62.5
nontraffic V62.0
van (traffic) V63.5
nontraffic V63.0
noncollision accident (traffic) V68.5
nontraffic V68.0
dump — *see* Accident, transport, construction vehicle occupant
hanger-on
collision (with)
animal (traffic) V60.7
being ridden (traffic) V66.7
nontraffic V66.2
nontraffic V60.2
animal-drawn vehicle (traffic) V66.7
nontraffic V66.2
bus (traffic) V64.7
nontraffic V64.2
car (traffic) V63.7
nontraffic V63.2
pedal cycle (traffic) V61.7
nontraffic V61.2
pickup truck (traffic) V63.7
nontraffic V63.2
railway vehicle (traffic) V65.7
nontraffic V65.2
specified vehicle NEC (traffic) V66.7
nontraffic V66.2
stationary object (traffic) V67.7
nontraffic V67.2
streetcar (traffic) V66.7
nontraffic V66.2
three wheeled motor vehicle (traffic) V62.7
nontraffic V62.2
truck (traffic) V64.7
nontraffic V64.2
two wheeled motor vehicle (traffic) V62.7
nontraffic V62.2
van (traffic) V63.7
nontraffic V63.2
noncollision accident (traffic) V68.7
nontraffic V68.2

Accident (to) — *continued*
transport (involving injury to) — *continued*
truck (heavy) occupant — *continued*
noncollision accident (traffic) V68.9
nontraffic V68.3
while boarding or alighting V68.4
nontraffic V69.3
passenger
collision (with)
animal (traffic) V60.6
being ridden (traffic) V66.6
nontraffic V66.1
nontraffic V60.1
animal-drawn vehicle (traffic) V66.6
nontraffic V66.1
bus (traffic) V64.6
nontraffic V64.1
car (traffic) V63.6
nontraffic V63.1
motor vehicle NOS (traffic) V69.50
nontraffic V69.10
specified type NEC (traffic) V69.59
nontraffic V69.19
pedal cycle (traffic) V61.6
nontraffic V61.1
pickup truck (traffic) V63.6
nontraffic V63.1
railway vehicle (traffic) V65.6
nontraffic V65.1
specified vehicle NEC (traffic) V66.6
nontraffic V66.1
stationary object (traffic) V67.6
nontraffic V67.1
streetcar (traffic) V66.6
nontraffic V66.1
three wheeled motor vehicle (traffic) V62.6
nontraffic V62.1
truck (traffic) V64.6
nontraffic V64.1
two wheeled motor vehicle (traffic) V62.6
nontraffic V62.1
van (traffic) V63.6
nontraffic V63.1
noncollision accident (traffic) V68.6
nontraffic V68.1
pickup — *see* Accident, transport, pickup truck occupant
specified type NEC V69.88
military vehicle V69.81
van occupant V59.9
collision (with)
animal (traffic) V50.9
being ridden (traffic) V56.9
nontraffic V56.3
while boarding or alighting V56.4
nontraffic V50.3
while boarding or alighting V50.4
animal-drawn vehicle (traffic) V56.9
nontraffic V56.3
while boarding or alighting V56.4
bus (traffic) V54.9
nontraffic V54.3
while boarding or alighting V54.4
car (traffic) V53.9
nontraffic V53.3
while boarding or alighting V53.4
motor vehicle NOS (traffic) V59.60
nontraffic V59.20
specified type NEC (traffic) V59.69
nontraffic V59.29
pedal cycle (traffic) V51.9
nontraffic V51.3
while boarding or alighting V51.4
pickup truck (traffic) V53.9
nontraffic V53.3
while boarding or alighting V53.4
railway vehicle (traffic) V55.9
nontraffic V55.3
while boarding or alighting V55.4

Accident (to) — *continued*
transport (involving injury to) — *continued*
van occupant — *continued*
collision (with) — *continued*
specified vehicle NEC (traffic) V56.9
nontraffic V56.3
while boarding or alighting V56.4
stationary object (traffic) V57.9
nontraffic V57.3
while boarding or alighting V57.4
streetcar (traffic) V56.9
nontraffic V56.3
while boarding or alighting V56.4
three wheeled motor vehicle (traffic) V52.9
nontraffic V52.3
while boarding or alighting V52.4
truck (traffic) V54.9
nontraffic V54.3
while boarding or alighting V54.4
two wheeled motor vehicle (traffic) V52.9
nontraffic V52.3
while boarding or alighting V52.4
van (traffic) V53.9
nontraffic V53.3
while boarding or alighting V53.4
driver
collision (with)
animal (traffic) V50.5
being ridden (traffic) V56.5
nontraffic V56.0
nontraffic V50.0
animal-drawn vehicle (traffic) V56.5
nontraffic V56.0
bus (traffic) V54.5
nontraffic V54.0
car (traffic) V53.5
nontraffic V53.0
motor vehicle NOS (traffic) V59.40
nontraffic V59.00
specified type NEC (traffic) V59.49
nontraffic V59.09
pedal cycle (traffic) V51.5
nontraffic V51.0
pickup truck (traffic) V53.5
nontraffic V53.0
railway vehicle (traffic) V55.5
nontraffic V55.0
specified vehicle NEC (traffic) V56.5
nontraffic V56.0
stationary object (traffic) V57.5
nontraffic V57.0
streetcar (traffic) V56.5
nontraffic V56.0
three wheeled motor vehicle (traffic) V52.5
nontraffic V52.0
truck (traffic) V54.5
nontraffic V54.0
two wheeled motor vehicle (traffic) V52.5
nontraffic V52.0
van (traffic) V53.5
nontraffic V53.0
noncollision accident (traffic) V58.5
nontraffic V58.0
hanger-on
collision (with)
animal (traffic) V50.7
being ridden (traffic) V56.7
nontraffic V56.2
nontraffic V50.2
animal-drawn vehicle (traffic) V56.7
nontraffic V56.2
bus (traffic) V54.7
nontraffic V54.2
car (traffic) V53.7
nontraffic V53.2
pedal cycle (traffic) V51.7
nontraffic V51.2
pickup truck (traffic) V53.7
nontraffic V53.2
railway vehicle (traffic) V55.7
nontraffic V55.2

EXTERNAL CAUSES

© 2013 Channel Publishing Ltd

Blood alcohol level Y90.9
  100-119mg/100ml Y90.5
  120-199mg/100ml Y90.6
  20-39mg/100ml Y90.1
  200-239mg/100ml Y90.7
  40-59mg/100ml Y90.2
  60-79mg/100ml Y90.3
  80-99mg/100ml Y90.4
  less than 20mg/100ml Y90.0
  presence in blood, level not specified
    Y90.9
Blow X58
  by law-enforcing agent, police (on duty) —
    see Legal, intervention, manhandling
  blunt object — *see* Legal, intervention,
    blunt object
Blowing up — *see* Explosion
Brawl (hand) (fists) (foot) Y04.0
Breakage (accidental) (part of)
  ladder (causing fall) W11
  scaffolding (causing fall) W12
Broken
  glass, contact with — *see* Contact, with,
    glass
  power line (causing electric shock) W85
Bumping against, into (accidentally)
  object NEC W22.8
    with fall — *see* Fall, due to, bumping
      against, object
    caused by crowd or human stampede
      (with fall) W52
    sports equipment W21.9
  person(s) W51
    with fall W03
      due to ice or snow W00.0
    assault Y04.2
    caused by a crowd or human stampede
      (with fall) W52
    homicide (attempt) Y04.2
    sports equipment W21.9
Burn, burned, burning (accidental) (by)
  (from) (on)
  acid NEC — *see* Table of Drugs and
    Chemicals
  bed linen — *see* Exposure, fire,
    uncontrolled, in building, bed
  blowtorch X08.8
    with ignition of clothing NEC X06.2
      nightwear X05
  bonfire, campfire (controlled) — *see also*
    Exposure, fire, controlled, not in
    building
    uncontrolled — *see* Exposure, fire,
      uncontrolled, not in building
  candle X08.8
    with ignition of clothing NEC X06.2
      nightwear X05
  caustic liquid, substance (external)
    (internal) NEC — *see* Table of Drugs
    and Chemicals
  chemical (external) (internal) — *see also*
    Table of Drugs and Chemicals
    in war operations — *see* War operations.
      fire
  cigar(s) or cigarette(s) X08.8
    with ignition of clothing NEC X06.2
      nightwear X05
  clothes, clothing NEC (from controlled
    fire) X06.2
    with conflagration — *see* Exposure, fire,
      uncontrolled, building
      not in building or structure — *see*
        Exposure, fire, uncontrolled, not
        in building
  cooker (hot) X15.8
    stated as undetermined whether
      accidental or intentional Y27.3
    suicide (attempt) X77.3
  electric blanket X16
  engine (hot) X17
  fire, flames — *see* Exposure, fire
  flare, Very pistol — *see* Discharge, firearm
    NEC
  heat
    from appliance (electrical) (household)
      X15.8
      cooker X15.8
      hotplate X15.2
      kettle X15.8
      light bulb X15.8
      saucepan X15.3
      skillet X15.3
      stated as undetermined whether
        accidental or intentional Y27.3
      stove X15.0
      suicide (attempt) X77.3
      toaster X15.1
    in local application or packing during
      medical or surgical procedure
      Y63.5

Burn, burned, burning (accidental) (by)
  (from) (on) — *continued*
  heating
    appliance, radiator or pipe X16
  homicide (attempt) — *see* Assault, burning
  hot
    air X14.1
    cooker X15.8
    drink X10.0
    engine X17
    fat X10.2
    fluid NEC X12
    food X10.1
    gases X14.1
    heating appliance X16
    household appliance NEC X15.8
    kettle X15.8
    liquid NEC X12
    machinery X17
    metal (molten) (liquid) NEC X18
    object (not producing fire or flames)
      NEC X19
    oil (cooking) X10.2
    pipe(s) X16
    radiator X16
    saucepan (glass) (metal) X15.3
    stove (kitchen) X15.0
    substance NEC X19
      caustic or corrosive NEC — *see* Table
        of Drugs and Chemicals
    toaster X15.1
    tool X17
    vapor X13.1
    water (tap) — *see* Contact, with, hot, tap
      water
  hotplate X15.2
    suicide (attempt) X77.3
  ignition — *see* Ignition
  in war operations — *see* War operations,
    fire
  inflicted by other person X97
    by hot objects, hot vapor, and steam —
      see Assault, burning, hot object
  internal, from swallowed caustic, corrosive
    liquid, substance — *see* Table of
    Drugs and Chemicals
  iron (hot) X15.8
    stated as undetermined whether
      accidental or intentional Y27.3
    suicide (attempt) X77.3
  kettle (hot) X15.8
    stated as undetermined whether
      accidental or intentional Y27.3
    suicide (attempt) X77.3
  lamp (flame) X08.8
    with ignition of clothing NEC X06.2
      nightwear X05
  lighter (cigar) (cigarette) X08.8
    with ignition of clothing NEC X06.2
      nightwear X05
  lightning — *see* subcategory T75.0
    causing fire — *see* Exposure, fire
  liquid (boiling) (hot) NEC X12
    stated as undetermined whether
      accidental or intentional Y27.2
    suicide (attempt) X77.2
  local application of externally applied
    substance in medical or surgical care
    Y63.5
  machinery (hot) X17
  matches X08.8
    with ignition of clothing NEC X06.2
      nightwear X05
  mattress — *see* Exposure, fire,
    uncontrolled, building, bed
  medicament, externally applied Y63.5
  metal (hot) (liquid) (molten) NEC X18
  nightwear (nightclothes, nightdress, gown,
    pajamas, robe) X05
  object (hot) NEC X19
  on board watercraft
    due to
      accident to watercraft V91.09
        powered craft V91.03
          ferry boat V91.01
          fishing boat V91.02
          jetskis V91.03
          liner V91.01
          merchant ship V91.00
          passenger ship V91.01
        unpowered craft V91.08
          canoe V91.05
          inflatable V91.06
          kayak V91.05
          sailboat V91.04
          surfboard V91.08
          water skis V91.07
          windsurfer V91.08

Burn, burned, burning (accidental) (by)
  (from) (on) — *continued*
  on board watercraft — *continued*
    due to — *continued*
      fire on board V93.09
        ferry boat V93.01
        fishing boat V93.02
        jetskis V93.03
        liner V93.01
        merchant ship V93.00
        passenger ship V93.01
        powered craft NEC V93.03
        sailboat V93.04
      specified heat source NEC on board
        V93.19
        ferry boat V93.11
        fishing boat V93.12
        jetskis V93.13
        liner V93.11
        merchant ship V93.10
        passenger ship V93.11
        powered craft NEC V93.13
        sailboat V93.14
  pipe (hot) X16
    smoking X08.8
      with ignition of clothing NEC X06.2
        nightwear X05
  powder — *see* Powder burn
  radiator (hot) X16
  saucepan (hot) (glass) (metal) X15.3
    stated as undetermined whether
      accidental or intentional Y27.3
    suicide (attempt) X77.3
  self-inflicted X76
    stated as undetermined whether
      accidental or intentional Y26
  stated as undetermined whether accidental
    or intentional Y27.0
  steam X13.1
    pipe X16
      stated as undetermined whether
        accidental or intentional Y27.8
    stated as undetermined whether
      accidental or intentional Y27.0
    suicide (attempt) X77.0
  stove (hot) (kitchen) X15.0
    stated as undetermined whether
      accidental or intentional Y27.3
    suicide (attempt) X77.3
  substance (hot) NEC X19
    boiling X12
      stated as undetermined whether
        accidental or intentional Y27.2
      suicide (attempt) X77.2
    molten (metal) X18
  suicide (attempt) NEC X76
    hot
      household appliance X77.3
      object X77.9
  therapeutic misadventure
    heat in local application or packing
      during medical or surgical
      procedure Y63.5
    overdose of radiation Y63.2
  toaster (hot) X15.1
    stated as undetermined whether
      accidental or intentional Y27.3
    suicide (attempt) X77.3
  tool (hot) X17
  torch, welding X08.8
    with ignition of clothing NEC X06.2
      nightwear X05
  trash fire (controlled) — *see* Exposure, fire,
    controlled, not in building
    uncontrolled — *see* Exposure, fire,
      uncontrolled, not in building
  vapor (hot) X13.1
    stated as undetermined whether
      accidental or intentional Y27.0
    suicide (attempt) X77.0
  Very pistol — *see* Discharge, firearm NEC
Butted by animal W55.82
  bull W55.22
  cow W55.22
  goat W55.32
  horse W55.12
  pig W55.42
  sheep W55.32

C

Caisson disease — *see* Air, pressure, change
Campfire (exposure to) (controlled) — *see
  also* Exposure, fire, controlled, not in
  building
  uncontrolled — *see* Exposure, fire,
    uncontrolled, not in building
Capital punishment (any means) — *see*
  Legal, intervention
Car sickness T75.3
Casualty (not due to war) NEC X58
  war — *see* War operations
Cat
  bite W55.01
  scratch W55.03
Cataclysm, cataclysmic (any injury) NEC
  — *see* Forces of nature
Catching fire — *see* Exposure, fire
Caught
  between
    folding object W23.0
    objects (moving) (stationary and
      moving) W23.0
      and machinery — *see* Contact, with,
        by type of machine
    stationary W23.1
    sliding door and door frame W23.0
  by, in
    machinery (moving parts of) — *see*
      Contact, with, by type of machine
    washing-machine wringer W23.0
  under packing crate (due to losing grip)
    W23.1
**Cave-in caused by cataclysmic earth
  surface movement or eruption** — *see*
  Landslide
Change(s) in air pressure — *see* Air,
  pressure, change
Choked, choking (on) (any object except
  food or vomitus)
  food (bone) (seed) — *see* categories T17
    and T18
  vomitus T17.81-
Civil insurrection — *see* War operations
Cloudburst (any injury) X37.8
Cold, exposure to (accidental) (excessive)
  (extreme) (natural) (place) NEC — *see*
  Exposure, cold
Collapse
  building W20.1
    burning (uncontrolled fire) X00.2
  dam or man-made structure (causing earth
    movement) X36.0
  machinery — *see* Contact, with, by type of
    machine
  structure W20.1
    burning (uncontrolled fire) X00.2
Collision (accidental) NEC (*see also*
  Accident, transport) V89.9
  pedestrian W51
    with fall W03
      due to ice or snow W00.0
      involving pedestrian conveyance —
        see Accident, transport,
        pedestrian, conveyance
    and
      crowd or human stampede (with fall)
        W52
      object W22.8
        with fall — *see* Fall, due to,
          bumping against, object
    person(s) — *see* Collision, pedestrian
  transport vehicle NEC V89.9
    and
      avalanche, fallen or not moving — *see*
        Accident, transport
      falling or moving — *see* Landslide
      landslide, fallen or not moving — *see*
        Accident, transport
        falling or moving — *see* Landslide
      due to cataclysm — *see* Forces of nature,
        by type
      intentional, purposeful suicide (attempt)
        — *see* Suicide, collision
Combustion, spontaneous — *see* Ignition
Complication (delayed) of or following
  (medical or surgical procedure) Y84.9
  with misadventure — *see* Misadventure
  amputation of limb(s) Y83.5
  anastomosis (arteriovenous) (blood vessel)
    (gastrojejunal) (tendon) (natural or
    artificial material) Y83.2
  aspiration (of fluid) Y84.4
    tissue Y84.8
  biopsy Y84.8

EXTERNAL CAUSES

Complication (delayed) of or following
(medical or surgical procedure) Y84.9
blood
  sampling Y84.7
  transfusion
    procedure Y84.8
bypass Y83.2
catheterization (urinary) Y84.6
  cardiac Y84.0
colostomy Y83.3
cystostomy Y83.3
dialysis (kidney) Y84.1
drug — see Table of Drugs and Chemicals
due to misadventure — see Misadventure
duodenostomy Y83.3
electroshock therapy Y84.3
external stoma, creation of Y83.3
formation of external stoma Y83.3
gastrostomy Y83.3
graft Y83.2
hypothermia (medically-induced) Y84.8
implant, implantation (of)
  artificial
    internal device (cardiac pacemaker)
      (electrodes in brain) (heart valve
      prosthesis) (orthopedic) Y83.1
    material or tissue (for anastomosis or
      bypass) Y83.2
      with creation of external stoma
        Y83.3
    natural tissues (for anastomosis or
      bypass) Y83.2
      with creation of external stoma Y83.3
infusion
  procedure Y84.8
injection — see Table of Drugs and
    Chemicals
  procedure Y84.8
insertion of gastric or duodenal sound
    Y84.5
insulin-shock therapy Y84.3
paracentesis (abdominal) (thoracic)
    (aspirative) Y84.4
procedures other than surgical operation —
    see Complication of or following, by
    type of procedure
radiological procedure or therapy Y84.2
removal of organ (partial) (total) NEC
    Y83.6
sampling
  blood Y84.7
  fluid NEC Y84.4
  tissue Y84.8
shock therapy Y84.3
surgical operation NEC (see also
    Complication of or following, by type
    of operation) Y83.9
  reconstructive NEC Y83.4
    with
      anastomosis, bypass or graft Y83.2
      formation of external stoma Y83.3
  specified NEC Y83.8
transfusion — see also Table of Drugs and
    Chemicals
  procedure Y84.8
transplant, transplantation (heart) (kidney)
    (liver) (whole organ, any) Y83.0
  partial organ Y83.4
ureterostomy Y83.3
vaccination — see also Table of Drugs and
    Chemicals
  procedure Y84.8

Compression
divers' squeeze — see Air, pressure,
    change
trachea by
  food (lodged in esophagus) — see
    categories T17 and T18
  vomitus (lodged in esophagus) T17.81-

Conflagration — see Exposure, fire,
    uncontrolled

Constriction (external)
hair W49.01
jewelry W49.04
ring W49.04
rubber band W49.03
specified item NEC W49.09
string W49.02
thread W49.02

Contact (accidental)
with
  abrasive wheel (metalworking) W31.1
  alligator W58.09
    bite W58.01
    crushing W58.03
    strike W58.02
  amphibian W62.9
    frog W62.0
    toad W62.1

Contact (accidental) — continued
with — continued
  animal (nonvenomous) NEC W64
    marine W56.89
      bite W56.81
      dolphin — see Contact, with,
        dolphin
      fish NEC — see Contact, with, fish
      mammal — see Contact, with,
        mammal, marine
      orca — see Contact, with, orca
      sea lion — see Contact, with, sea
        lion
      shark — see Contact, with, shark
      strike W56.82
  animate mechanical force NEC W64
  arrow W21.89
    not thrown, projected or falling
      W45.8
  arthropods (nonvenomous) W57
  axe W27.0
  band-saw (industrial) W31.2
  bayonet — see Bayonet wound
  bee(s) X58
  bench-saw (industrial) W31.2
  bird W61.99
    bite W61.91
    chicken — see Contact, with, chicken
    duck — see Contact, with, duck
    goose — see Contact, with, goose
    macaw — see Contact, with, macaw
    parrot — see Contact, with, parrot
    psittacine — see Contact, with,
      psittacine
    strike W61.92
    turkey — see Contact, with, turkey
  blender W29.0
  boiling water X12
    stated as undetermined whether
      accidental or intentional Y27.2
    suicide (attempt) X77.2
  bore, earth-drilling or mining (land)
    (seabed) W31.0
  buffalo — see Contact, with, hoof stock
    NEC
  bull W55.29
    bite W55.21
    gored W55.22
    strike W55.22
  bumper cars W31.81
  camel — see Contact, with, hoof stock
    NEC
  can
    lid W45.2
    opener W27.4
      powered W29.0
  cat W55.09
    bite W55.01
    scratch W55.03
  caterpillar (venomous) X58
  centipede (venomous) X58
  chain
    hoist W24.0
      agricultural operations W30.89
    saw W29.3
  chicken W61.39
    peck W61.33
    strike W61.32
  chisel W27.0
  circular saw W31.2
  cobra X58
  combine (harvester) W30.0
  conveyer belt W24.1
  cooker (hot) X15.8
    stated as undetermined whether
      accidental or intentional Y27.3
    suicide (attempt) X77.3
  coral X58
  cotton gin W31.82
  cow W55.29
    bite W55.21
    strike W55.22
  crane W24.0
    agricultural operations W30.89
  crocodile W58.19
    bite W58.11
    crushing W58.13
    strike W58.12
  dagger W26.1
    stated as undetermined whether
      accidental or intentional Y28.2
    suicide (attempt) X78.2
  dairy equipment W31.82
  dart W21.89
    not thrown, projected or falling
      W45.8
  deer — see Contact, with, hoof stock
    NEC

Contact (accidental) — continued
with — continued
  derrick W24.0
    agricultural operations W30.89
      hay W30.2
  dog W54.8
    bite W54.0
    strike W54.1
  dolphin W56.09
    bite W56.01
    strike W56.02
  donkey — see Contact, with, hoof stock
    NEC
  drill (powered) W29.8
    earth (land) (seabed) W31.0
    nonpowered W27.8
  drive belt W24.0
    agricultural operations W30.89
  dry ice — see Exposure, cold, man-made
  dryer (clothes) (powered) (spin) W29.2
  duck W61.69
    bite W61.61
    strike W61.62
  earth(-)
    drilling machine (industrial) W31.0
    scraping machine in stationary use
      W31.83
  edge of stiff paper W45.1
  electric
    beater W29.0
    blanket X16
    fan W29.2
      commercial W31.82
    knife W29.1
    mixer W29.0
  elevator (building) W24.0
    agricultural operations W30.89
      grain W30.3
  engine(s), hot NEC X17
  excavating machine W31.0
  farm machine W30.9
  feces — see Contact, with, by type of
    animal
  fer de lance X58
  fish W56.59
    bite W56.51
    shark — see Contact, with, shark
    strike W56.52
  flying horses W31.81
  forging (metalworking) machine W31.1
  fork W27.4
  forklift (truck) W24.0
    agricultural operations W30.89
  frog W62.0
  garden
    cultivator (powered) W29.3
      riding W30.89
    fork W27.1
  gas turbine W31.3
  Gila monster X58
  giraffe — see Contact, with, hoof stock
    NEC
  glass (sharp) (broken) W25
    with subsequent fall W18.02
    assault X99.0
    due to fall — see Fall, by type
    stated as undetermined whether
      accidental or intentional Y28.0
    suicide (attempt) X78.0
  goat W55.39
    bite W55.31
    strike W55.32
  goose W61.59
    bite W61.51
    strike W61.52
  hand
    saw W27.0
    tool (not powered) NEC W27.8
      powered W29.8
  harvester W30.0
  hay-derrick W30.2
  heat NEC X19
    from appliance (electrical)
      (household) — see Contact, with,
      hot, household appliance
    heating appliance X16
  heating
    appliance (hot) X16
    pad (electric) X16
  hedge-trimmer (powered) W29.3
  hoe W27.1
  hoist (chain) (shaft) NEC W24.0
    agricultural W30.89
  hoof stock NEC W55.39
    bite W55.31
    strike W55.32
  hornet(s) X58
  horse W55.19
    bite W55.11
    strike W55.12

Contact (accidental) — continued
with — continued
  hot
    air X14.1
      inhalation X14.0
    cooker X15.8
    drinks X10.0
    engine X17
    fats X10.2
    fluids NEC X12
      assault X98.2
      suicide (attempt) X77.2
      undetermined whether accidental or
        intentional Y27.2
    food X10.1
    gases X14.1
      inhalation X14.0
    heating appliance X16
    household appliance X15.8
      assault X98.3
      cooker X15.8
      hotplate X15.2
      kettle X15.8
      light bulb X15.8
      object NEC X19
        assault X98.8
        stated as undetermined whether
          accidental or intentional
          Y27.9
        suicide (attempt) X77.8
      saucepan X15.3
      skillet X15.3
      stated as undetermined whether
        accidental or intentional
        Y27.3
      stove X15.0
      suicide (attempt) X77.3
      toaster X15.1
    kettle X15.8
    light bulb X15.8
    liquid NEC (see also Burn) X12
      drinks X10.0
      stated as undetermined whether
        accidental or intentional
        Y27.2
      suicide (attempt) X77.2
      tap water X11.8
        stated as undetermined whether
          accidental or intentional
          Y27.1
        suicide (attempt) X77.1
    machinery X17
    metal (molten) (liquid) NEC X18
    object (not producing fire or flames)
      NEC X19
    oil (cooking) X10.2
    pipe X16
    plate X15.2
    radiator X16
    saucepan (glass) (metal) X15.3
    skillet X15.3
    stove (kitchen) X15.0
    substance NEC X19
    tap-water X11.8
      assault X98.1
      heated on stove X12
        stated as undetermined whether
          accidental or intentional
          Y27.2
        suicide (attempt) X77.2
      in bathtub X11.0
      running X11.1
      stated as undetermined whether
        accidental or intentional
        Y27.1
      suicide (attempt) X77.1
    toaster X15.1
    tool X17
    vapors X13.1
      inhalation X13.0
    water (tap) X11.8
      boiling X12
        stated as undetermined whether
          accidental or intentional
          Y27.2
        suicide (attempt) X77.2
      heated on stove X12
        stated as undetermined whether
          accidental or intentional
          Y27.2
        suicide (attempt) X77.2
      in bathtub X11.0
      running X11.1
      stated as undetermined whether
        accidental or intentional
        Y27.1
      suicide (attempt) X77.1

EXTERNAL CAUSES

EXTERNAL CAUSES

Contact (accidental) — *continued*
  with — *continued*
    venomous
      animal X58
      arthropods X58
      lizard X58
      marine animal NEC X58
      marine plant NEC X58
      millipedes (tropical) X58
      plant(s) X58
      snake X58
      spider X58
      viper X58
    washing-machine (powered) W29.2
    wasp X58
    weaving-machine W31.89
    winch W24.0
      agricultural operations W30.89
    wire NEC W24.0
      agricultural operations W30.89
    wood slivers W45.8
    yellow jacket X58
    zebra — *see* Contact, with, hoof stock NEC
Coup de soleil X32
Crash
  aircraft (in transit) (powered) V95.9
    balloon V96.01
    fixed wing NEC (private) V95.21
      commercial V95.31
    glider V96.21
      hang V96.11
      powered V95.11
    helicopter V95.01
    in war operations — *see* War operations, destruction of aircraft
    microlight V95.11
    nonpowered V96.9
      specified NEC V96.8
    powered NEC V95.8
    stated as
      homicide (attempt) Y08.81
      suicide (attempt) X83.0
    ultralight V95.11
  spacecraft V95.41
  transport vehicle NEC (*see also* Accident, transport) V89.9
    homicide (attempt) Y03.8
    motor NEC (traffic) V89.2
      homicide (attempt) Y03.8
      suicide (attempt) — *see* Suicide, collision
Cruelty (mental) (physical) (sexual) X58
Crushed (accidentally) X58
  between objects (moving) (stationary and moving) W23.0
    stationary W23.1
  by
    alligator W58.03
    avalanche NEC — *see* Landslide
    cave-in W20.0
      caused by cataclysmic earth surface movement — *see* Landslide
    crocodile W58.13
    crowd or human stampede W52
    falling
      aircraft V97.39
        in war operations — *see* War operations, destruction of aircraft
      earth, material W20.0
        caused by cataclysmic earth surface movement — *see* Landslide
      object NEC W20.8
    landslide NEC — *see* Landslide
    lizard (nonvenomous) W59.09
    machinery — *see* Contact, with, by type of machine
    reptile NEC W59.89
    snake (nonvenomous) W59.13
  in
    machinery — *see* Contact, with, by type of machine
Cut, cutting (any part of body) (accidental) — *see also* Contact, with, by object or machine
  during medical or surgical treatment as misadventure — *see* Index to Diseases and Injuries, Complications
  homicide (attempt) — *see* Assault, cutting or piercing instrument
  inflicted by other person — *see* Assault, cutting or piercing instrument
  legal
    execution — *see* Legal, intervention
    intervention — *see* Legal, intervention, sharp object
  machine NEC (*see also* Contact, with, by type of machine) W31.9

Cut, cutting (any part of body) (accidental) — *continued*
  self-inflicted — *see* Suicide, cutting or piercing instrument
  suicide (attempt) — *see* Suicide, cutting or piercing instrument
Cyclone (any injury) X37.1

D

Decapitation (accidental circumstances) NEC X58
  homicide X99.9
  legal execution — *see* Legal, intervention
Dehydration from lack of water X58
Deprivation X58
Derailment (accidental)
  railway (rolling stock) (train) (vehicle) (without antecedent collision) V81.7
    with antecedent collision — *see* Accident, transport, railway vehicle occupant
  streetcar (without antecedent collision) V82.7
    with antecedent collision — *see* Accident, transport, streetcar occupant
Descent
  parachute (voluntary) (without accident to aircraft) V97.29
    due to accident to aircraft — *see* Accident, transport, aircraft
Desertion X58
Destitution X58
Disability, late effect or sequela of injury — *see* Sequelae
Discharge (accidental)
  airgun W34.010
    assault X95.01
    homicide (attempt) X95.01
    stated as undetermined whether accidental or intentional Y24.0
    suicide (attempt) X74.01
  BB gun — *see* Discharge, airgun
  firearm (accidental) W34.00
    assault X95.9
    handgun (pistol) (revolver) W32.0
      assault X93
      homicide (attempt) X93
      legal intervention — *see* Legal, intervention, firearm, handgun
      stated as undetermined whether accidental or intentional Y22
      suicide (attempt) X72
    homicide (attempt) X95.9
    hunting rifle W33.02
      assault X94.1
      homicide (attempt) X94.1
      legal intervention
        injuring
          bystander Y35.032
          law enforcement personnel Y35.031
          suspect Y35.033
      stated as undetermined whether accidental or intentional Y23.1
      suicide (attempt) X73.1
    larger W33.00
      assault X94.9
      homicide (attempt) X94.9
      hunting rifle — *see* Discharge, firearm, hunting rifle
      legal intervention — *see* Legal, intervention, firearm by type of firearm
      machine gun — *see* Discharge, firearm, machine gun
      shotgun — *see* Discharge, firearm, shotgun
      specified NEC W33.09
        assault X94.8
        homicide (attempt) X94.8
        legal intervention
          injuring
            bystander Y35.092
            law enforcement personnel Y35.091
            suspect Y35.093
        stated as undetermined whether accidental or intentional Y23.8
        suicide (attempt) X73.8
      stated as undetermined whether accidental or intentional Y23.9
      suicide (attempt) X73.9

Discharge (accidental) — *continued*
  firearm (accidental) — *continued*
    legal intervention
      injuring
        bystander Y35.002
        law enforcement personnel Y35.001
        suspect Y35.03
      using rubber bullet
        injuring
          bystander Y35.042
          law enforcement personnel Y35.041
          suspect Y35.043
    machine gun W33.03
      assault X94.2
      homicide (attempt) X94.2
      legal intervention — *see* Legal, intervention, firearm, machine gun
      stated as undetermined whether accidental or intentional Y23.3
      suicide (attempt) X73.2
    pellet gun — *see* Discharge, airgun
    shotgun W33.01
      assault X94.0
      homicide (attempt) X94.0
      legal intervention — *see* Legal, intervention, firearm, specified NEC
      stated as undetermined whether accidental or intentional Y23.0
      suicide (attempt) X73.0
    specified NEC W34.09
      assault X95.8
      homicide (attempt) X95.8
      legal intervention — *see* Legal, intervention, firearm, specified NEC
      stated as undetermined whether accidental or intentional Y24.8
      suicide (attempt) X74.8
    stated as undetermined whether accidental or intentional Y24.9
    suicide (attempt) X74.9
    Very pistol W34.09
      assault X95.8
      homicide (attempt) X95.8
      stated as undetermined whether accidental or intentional Y24.8
      suicide (attempt) X74.8
  firework(s) W39
    stated as undetermined whether accidental or intentional Y25
  gas-operated gun NEC W34.018
    airgun — *see* Discharge, airgun
    assault X95.09
    homicide (attempt) X95.09
    paintball gun — *see* Discharge, paintball gun
    stated as undetermined whether accidental or intentional Y24.8
    suicide (attempt) X74.09
  gun NEC — *see also* Discharge, firearm NEC
    air — *see* Discharge, airgun
    BB — *see* Discharge, airgun
    for single hand use — *see* Discharge, firearm, handgun
    hand — *see* Discharge, firearm, handgun
    machine — *see* Discharge, firearm, machine gun
    other specified — *see* Discharge, firearm NEC
    paintball — *see* Discharge, paintball gun
    pellet — *see* Discharge, airgun
  handgun — *see* Discharge, firearm, handgun
  machine gun — *see* Discharge, firearm, machine gun
  paintball gun W34.011
    assault X95.02
    homicide (attempt) X95.02
    stated as undetermined whether accidental or intentional Y24.8
    suicide (attempt) X74.02
  pistol — *see* Discharge, firearm, handgun
    flare — *see* Discharge, firearm, Very pistol
    pellet — *see* Discharge, airgun
    Very — *see* Discharge, firearm, Very pistol
  revolver — *see* Discharge, firearm, handgun
  rifle (hunting) — *see* Discharge, firearm, hunting rifle
  shotgun — *see* Discharge, firearm, shotgun

Discharge (accidental) — *continued*
  spring-operated gun NEC W34.018
    assault X95.09
    homicide (attempt) X95.09
    stated as undetermined whether accidental or intentional Y24.8
    suicide (attempt) X74.09
Disease
  Andes W94.11
  aviator's — *see* Air, pressure
  range W94.11
Diver's disease, palsy, paralysis, squeeze — *see* Air, pressure
Diving (into water) — *see* Accident, diving
Dog bite W54.0
Dragged by transport vehicle NEC (*see also* Accident, transport) V09.9
Drinking poison (accidental) — *see* Table of Drugs and Chemicals
Dropped (accidentally) while being carried or supported by other person W04
Drowning (accidental) W74
  assault X92.9
  due to
    accident (to)
      machinery — *see* Contact, with, by type of machine
      watercraft V90.89
        burning V90.29
          powered V90.23
            fishing boat V90.22
            jetskis V90.23
            merchant ship V90.20
            passenger ship V90.21
          unpowered V90.28
            canoe V90.25
            inflatable V90.26
            kayak V90.25
            sailboat V90.24
            water skis V90.27
        crushed V90.39
          powered V90.33
            fishing boat V90.32
            jetskis V90.33
            merchant ship V90.30
            passenger ship V90.31
          unpowered V90.38
            canoe V90.35
            inflatable V90.36
            kayak V90.35
            sailboat V90.34
            water skis V90.37
        overturning V90.09
          powered V90.03
            fishing boat V90.02
            jetskis V90.03
            merchant ship V90.00
            passenger ship V90.01
          unpowered V90.08
            canoe V90.05
            inflatable V90.06
            kayak V90.05
            sailboat V90.04
        sinking V90.19
          powered V90.13
            fishing boat V90.12
            jetskis V90.13
            merchant ship V90.10
            passenger ship V90.11
          unpowered V90.18
            canoe V90.15
            inflatable V90.16
            kayak V90.15
            sailboat V90.14
        specified type NEC V90.89
          powered V90.83
            fishing boat V90.82
            jetskis V90.83
            merchant ship V90.80
            passenger ship V90.81
          unpowered V90.88
            canoe V90.85
            inflatable V90.86
            kayak V90.85
            sailboat V90.84
            water skis V90.87
    avalanche — *see* Landslide
    cataclysmic
      earth surface movement NEC — *see* Forces of nature, earth movement
      storm — *see* Forces of nature, cataclysmic storm
    cloudburst X37.8
    cyclone X37.1

Drowning (accidental) — *continued*
  due to — *continued*
    fall overboard (from) V92.09
      powered craft V92.03
        ferry boat V92.01
        fishing boat V92.02
        jetskis V92.03
        liner V92.01
        merchant ship V92.00
        passenger ship V92.01
      resulting from
        accident to watercraft — *see*
          Drowning, due to, accident to,
          watercraft
        being washed overboard (from)
          V92.29
          powered craft V92.23
            ferry boat V92.21
            fishing boat V92.22
            jetskis V92.23
            liner V92.21
            merchant ship V92.20
            passenger ship V92.21
          unpowered craft V92.28
            canoe V92.25
            inflatable V92.26
            kayak V92.25
            sailboat V92.24
            surfboard V92.28
            water skis V92.27
            windsurfer V92.28
        motion of watercraft V92.19
          powered craft V92.13
            ferry boat V92.11
            fishing boat V92.12
            jetskis V92.13
            liner V92.11
            merchant ship V92.10
            passenger ship V92.11
          unpowered craft
            canoe V92.15
            inflatable V92.16
            kayak V92.15
            sailboat V92.14
      unpowered craft V92.08
        canoe V92.05
        inflatable V92.06
        kayak V92.05
        sailboat V92.04
        surfboard V92.08
        water skis V92.07
        windsurfer V92.08
    hurricane X37.0
    jumping into water from watercraft
      (involved in accident) — *see also*
      Drowning, due to, accident to,
      watercraft
      without accident to or on watercraft
        W16.711
    tidal wave NEC — *see* Forces of nature,
      tidal wave
    torrential rain X37.8
  following
    fall
      into
        bathtub W16.211
        bucket W16.221
        fountain — *see* Drowning,
          following, fall, into, water,
          specified NEC
        quarry — *see* Drowning, following,
          fall, into, water, specified
          NEC
        reservoir — *see* Drowning,
          following, fall, into, water,
          specified NEC
        swimming pool W16.011
          stated as undetermined whether
            accidental or intentional
            Y21.3
          striking
            bottom W16.021
            wall W16.031
          suicide (attempt) X71.2
        water NOS W16.41
          natural (lake) (open sea) (pond)
            (river) (stream) W16.111
            striking
              bottom W16.121
              side W16.131
          specified NEC W16.311
            striking
              bottom W16.321
              wall W16.331
    overboard NEC — *see* Drowning, due
      to, fall overboard

Drowning (accidental) — *continued*
  due to — *continued*
    jump or dive
      from boat W16.711
        striking bottom W16.721
        into
          fountain — *see* Drowning,
            following, jump or dive, into,
            water, specified NEC
          quarry — *see* Drowning, following,
            jump or dive, into, water,
            specified NEC
          reservoir — *see* Drowning,
            following, jump or dive, into,
            water, specified NEC
          swimming pool W16.511
            striking
              bottom W16.521
              wall W16.531
            suicide (attempt) X71.2
          water NOS W16.91
            natural (lake) (open sea) (pond)
              (river) (stream) W16.611
            specified NEC W16.811
              striking
                bottom W16.821
                wall W16.831
              striking bottom W16.621
  homicide (attempt) X92.9
  in
    bathtub (accidental) W65
      assault X92.0
      following fall W16.211
        stated as undetermined whether
          accidental or intentional
          Y21.1
      stated as undetermined whether
        accidental or intentional Y21.0
      suicide (attempt) X71.0
    lake — *see* Drowning, in, natural water
    natural water (lake) (open sea) (pond)
      (river) (stream) W69
      assault X92.3
      following
        dive or jump W16.611
          striking bottom W16.621
        fall W16.111
          striking
            bottom W16.121
            side W16.131
      stated as undetermined whether
        accidental or intentional Y21.4
      suicide (attempt) X71.3
    quarry — *see* Drowning, in, specified
      place NEC
    quenching tank — *see* Drowning, in,
      specified place NEC
    reservoir — *see* Drowning, in, specified
      place NEC
    river — *see* Drowning, in, natural water
    sea — *see* Drowning, in, natural water
    specified place NEC W73
      assault X92.8
      following
        dive or jump W16.811
          striking
            bottom W16.821
            wall W16.831
        fall W16.311
          striking
            bottom W16.321
            wall W16.331
      stated as undetermined whether
        accidental or intentional Y21.8
      suicide (attempt) X71.8
    stream — *see* Drowning, in, natural
      water
    swimming pool W67
      assault X92.1
      following fall X92.2
      following
        dive or jump W16.511
          striking
            bottom W16.521
            wall W16.531
        fall W16.011
          striking
            bottom W16.021
            wall W16.031
      stated as undetermined whether
        accidental or intentional Y21.2
      following fall Y21.3
      suicide (attempt) X71.1
      following fall X71.2
    war operations — *see* War operations,
      restriction of airway
  resulting from accident to watercraftCsee
    Drowning, due to, accident, watercraft

Drowning (accidental) — *continued*
  self-inflicted X71.9
  stated as undetermined whether accidental
    or intentional Y21.9
  suicide (attempt) X71.9

E

Earth falling (on) W20.0
  caused by cataclysmic earth surface
    movement or eruption — *see*
    Landslide
Earth (surface) movement NEC — *see*
  Forces of nature, earth movement
Earthquake (any injury) X34
Effect(s) (adverse) of
  air pressure (any) — *see* Air, pressure
  cold, excessive (exposure to) — *see*
    Exposure, cold
  heat (excessive) — *see* Heat
  hot place (weather) — *see* Heat
  insolation X30
  late — *see* Sequelae
  motion — *see* Motion
  nuclear explosion or weapon in war
    operations — *see* War operations,
    nuclear weapon
  radiation — *see* Radiation
  travel — *see* Travel
Electric shock (accidental) (by) (in) — *see*
  Exposure, electric current
Electrocution (accidental) — *see* Exposure,
  electric current
**Endotracheal tube wrongly placed during
  anesthetic procedure**
Entanglement
  in
    bed linen, causing suffocation — *see*
      category T71
    wheel of pedal cycle V19.88
Entry of foreign body or material — *see*
  Foreign body
Environmental pollution related condition
  — *see* Z57
Execution, legal (any method) — *see* Legal,
  intervention
Exhaustion
  cold — *see* Exposure, cold
  due to excessive exertion — *see* category
    Y93
  heat — *see* Heat
Explosion (accidental) (of) (with secondary
  fire) W40.9
  acetylene W40.1
  aerosol can W36.1
  air tank (compressed) (in machinery)
    W36.2
  aircraft (in transit) (powered) NEC V95.9
    balloon V96.05
    fixed wing NEC (private) V95.25
      commercial V95.35
    glider V96.25
      hang V96.15
      powered V95.15
    helicopter V95.05
    in war operations — *see* War operations,
      destruction of aircraft
    microlight V95.15
    nonpowered V96.9
      specified NEC V96.8
    powered NEC V95.8
    stated as
      homicide (attempt) Y03.8
      suicide (attempt) X83.0
    ultralight V95.15
  anesthetic gas in operating room W40.1
  antipersonnel bomb W40.8
    assault X96.0
    homicide (attempt) X96.0
    suicide (attempt) X75
  assault X96.9
  bicycle tire W37.0
  blasting (cap) (materials) W40.0
  boiler (machinery), not on transport vehicle
    W35
    on watercraft — *see* Explosion, in,
      watercraft
  butane W40.1
  caused by other person X96.9
  coal gas W40.1
  detonator W40.0
  dump (munitions) W40.8

Explosion (accidental) (of) (with secondary
  fire) — *continued*
  dynamite W40.0
    in
      assault X96.8
      homicide (attempt) X96.8
      legal intervention
        injuring
          bystander Y35.112
          law enforcement personnel
            Y35.111
          suspect Y35.113
      suicide (attempt) X75
  explosive (material) W40.9
    gas W40.1
    in blasting operation W40.0
    specified NEC W40.8
      in
        assault X96.8
        homicide (attempt) X96.8
        legal intervention
          injuring
            bystander Y35.192
            law enforcement personnel
              Y35.191
            suspect Y35.193
        suicide (attempt) X75
  factory (munitions) W40.8
  fertilizer bomb W40.8
    assault X96.3
    homicide (attempt) X96.3
    suicide (attempt) X75
  fire-damp W40.1
  firearm (parts) NEC W34.19
    airgun W34.110
    BB gun W34.110
    gas, air or spring-operated gun NEC
      W34.118
    hangun W32.1
    hunting rifle W33.12
    larger firearm W33.10
      specified NEC W33.19
    machine gun W33.13
    paintball gun W34.111
    pellet gun W34.110
    shotgun W33.11
    Very pistol [flare] W34.19
  fireworks W39
  gas (coal) (explosive) W40.1
    cylinder W36.9
      aerosol can W36.1
      air tank W36.2
      pressurized W36.3
      specified NEC W36.8
    gasoline (fumes) (tank) not in moving
      motor vehicle W40.1
      bomb W40.8
        assault X96.1
        homicide (attempt) X96.1
        suicide (attempt) X75
      in motor vehicle — *see* Accident,
        transport, by type of vehicle
  grain store W40.8
  grenade W40.8
    in
      assault X96.8
      homicide (attempt) X96.8
      legal intervention
        injuring
          bystander Y35.192
          law enforcement personnel
            Y35.191
          suspect Y35.193
      suicide (attempt) X75
  handgun (parts) — *see* Explosion, firearm,
    hangun (parts)
  homicide (attempt) X96.9
    antipersonnel bomb — *see* Explosion,
      antipersonnel bomb
    fertilizer bomb — *see* Explosion,
      fertilizer bomb
    gasoline bomb — *see* Explosion,
      gasoline bomb
    letter bomb — *see* Explosion, letter
      bomb
    pipe bomb — *see* Explosion, pipe bomb
    specified NEC X96.8
  hose, pressurized W37.8
  hot water heater, tank (in machinery) W35
    on watercraft — *see* Explosion, in,
      watercraft

EXTERNAL CAUSES

Explosion (accidental) (of) (with secondary fire) — *continued*
  in, on
    dump W40.8
    factory W40.8
    mine (of explosive gases) NEC W40.1
    watercraft V93.59
      powered craft V93.53
        ferry boat V93.51
        fishing boat V93.52
        jetskis V93.53
        liner V93.51
        merchant ship V93.50
        passenger ship V93.51
        sailboat V93.54
  letter bomb W40.8
    assault X96.2
    homicide (attempt) X96.2
    suicide (attempt) X75
  machinery — *see also* Contact, with, by type of machine
    on board watercraft — *see* Explosion, in, watercraft
    pressure vessel — *see* Explosion, by type of vessel
  methane W40.1
  mine W40.1
  missile NEC W40.8
  mortar bomb W40.8
    in
      assault X96.8
      homicide (attempt) X96.8
      legal intervention
        injuring
          bystander Y35.192
          law enforcement personnel Y35.191
          suspect Y35.193
      suicide (attempt) X75
  munitions (dump) (factory) W40.8
  pipe, pressurized W37.8
    bomb W40.8
      assault X96.4
      homicide (attempt) X96.4
      suicide (attempt) X75
  pressure, pressurized
    cooker W38
    gas tank (in machinery) W36.3
    hose W37.8
    pipe W37.8
    specified device NEC W38
    tire W37.8
      bicycle W37.0
    vessel (in machinery) W38
  propane W40.1
  self-inflicted X75
  shell (artillery) NEC W40.8
    during war operations — *see* War operations, explosion
    in
      legal intervention
        injuring
          bystander Y35.122
          law enforcement personnel Y35.121
          suspect Y35.123
      war — *see* War operations, explosion
  spacecraft V95.45
  stated as undetermined whether accidental or intentional Y25
  steam or water lines (in machinery) W37.8
  stove W40.9
  suicide (attempt) X75
  tire, pressurized W37.8
    bicycle W37.0
  undetermined whether accidental or intentional Y25
  vehicle tire NEC W37.8
    bicycle W37.0
  war operations — *see* War operations, explosion

Exposure (to) X58
  air pressure change — *see* Air, pressure
  cold (accidental) (excessive) (extreme) (natural) (place) X31
    assault Y08.89
    due to
      man-made conditions W93.8
        dry ice (contact) W93.01
          inhalation W93.02
        liquid air (contact) (hydrogen) (nitrogen) W93.11
          inhalation W93.12
        refrigeration unit (deep freeze) W93.2
      suicide (attempt) X83.2
    weather (conditions) X31
    homicide (attempt) Y08.89
    self-inflicted X83.2

Exposure (to) — *continued*
  due to abandonment or neglect X58
  electric current W86.8
    appliance (faulty) W86.8
      domestic W86.0
    caused by other person Y08.89
    conductor (faulty) W86.1
    control apparatus (faulty) W86.1
    electric power generating plant, distribution station W86.1
    electroshock gun — *see* Exposure, electric current, taser
    high-voltage cable W85
    homicide (attempt) Y08.89
    legal execution — *see* Legal, intervention, specified means NEC
    lightning — *see* subcategory T75.0
    live rail W86.8
    misadventure in medical or surgical procedure in electroshock therapy Y63.4
    motor (electric) (faulty) W86.8
      domestic W86.0
    self-inflicted X83.1
    specified NEC W86.8
      domestic W86.0
    stun gun — *see* Exposure, electric current, taser
    suicide (attempt) X83.1
    taser W86.8
      assault Y08.89
      legal intervention — *see* category Y35
      self-harm (intentional) X83.8
      undetermined intent Y33
    third rail W86.8
    transformer (faulty) W86.1
    transmission lines W85
  environmental tobacco smoke X58
  excessive
    cold — *see* Exposure, cold
    heat (natural) NEC X30
      man-made W92
  factor(s) NOS X58
    environmental NEC X58
      man-made NEC W99
    natural NEC — *see* Forces of nature
    specified NEC X58
  fire, flames (accidental) X08.8
    assault X97
    campfire — *see* Exposure, fire, controlled, not in building
    controlled (in)
      with ignition (of) clothing (*see also* Ignition, clothes) X06.2
        nightwear X05
      bonfire — *see* Exposure, fire, controlled, not in building
      brazier (in building or structure) — *see also* Exposure, fire, controlled, building
        not in building or structure — *see* Exposure, fire, controlled, not in building
      building or structure X02.0
        with
          fall from building X02.3
          from building X02.5
          injury due to building collapse X02.2
          smoke inhalation X02.1
          hit by object from building X02.4
          specified mode of injury NEC X02.8
      fireplace, furnace or stove — *see* Exposure, fire, controlled, building
      not in building or structure X03.0
        with
          fall X03.3
          smoke inhalation X03.1
        hit by object X03.4
        specified mode of injury NEC X03.8
      trash — *see* Exposure, fire, controlled, not in building
    fireplace — *see* Exposure, fire, controlled, building
    fittings or furniture (in building or structure) (uncontrolled) — *see* Exposure, fire, uncontrolled, building
    forest (uncontrolled) — *see* Exposure, fire, uncontrolled, not in building
    grass (uncontrolled) — *see* Exposure, fire, uncontrolled, not in building
    hay (uncontrolled) — *see* Exposure, fire, uncontrolled, not in building
    homicide (attempt) X97

Exposure (to) — *continued*
  fire, flames (accidental) — *continued*
    ignition of highly flammable material X04
    in, of, on, starting in
      machinery — *see* Contact, with, by type of machine
      motor vehicle (in motion) (*see also* Accident, transport, occupant by type of vehicle) V87.8
        with collision — *see* Collision
      railway rolling stock, train, vehicle V81.81
        with collision — *see* Accident, transport, railway vehicle occupant
      street car (in motion) V82.8
        with collision — *see* Accident, transport, streetcar occupant
      transport vehicle NEC — *see also* Accident, transport
        with collision — *see* Collision
      war operations — *see also* War operations, fire
        from nuclear explosion — *see* War operations, nuclear weapons
      watercraft (in transit) (not in transit) V91.09
        localized — *see* Burn, on board watercraft, due to, fire on board
        powered craft V91.03
          ferry boat V91.01
          fishing boat V91.02
          jet skis V91.03
          liner V91.01
          merchant ship V91.00
          passenger ship V91.01
        unpowered craft V91.08
          canoe V91.05
          inflatable V91.06
          kayak V91.05
          sailboat V91.04
          surfboard V91.08
          waterskis V91.07
          windsurfer V91.08
    lumber (uncontrolled) — *see* Exposure, fire, uncontrolled, not in building
    mine (uncontrolled) — *see* Exposure, fire, uncontrolled, not in building
    prairie (uncontrolled) — *see* Exposure, fire, uncontrolled, not in building
    resulting from
      explosion — *see* Explosion
      lightning X08.8
    self-inflicted X76
    specified NEC X08.8
    started by other person X97
    stated as undetermined whether accidental or intentional Y26
    stove — *see* Exposure, fire, controlled, building
    suicide (attempt) X76
    tunnel (uncontrolled) — *see* Exposure, fire, uncontrolled, not in building
    uncontrolled
      in building or structure X00.0
        with
          fall from building X00.3
          injury due to building collapse X00.2
          jump from building X00.5
          smoke inhalation X00.1
        bed X08.00
          due to
            cigarette X08.01
            specified material NEC X08.09
        furniture NEC X08.20
          due to
            cigarette X08.21
            specified material NEC X08.29
        hit by object from building X00.4
        sofa X08.10
          due to
            cigarette X08.11
            specified material NEC X08.19
        specified mode of injury NEC X00.8
      not in building or structure (any) X01.0
        with
          fall X01.3
          smoke inhalation X01.1
        hit by object X01.4
        specified mode of injury NEC X01.8

Exposure (to) — *continued*
  fire, flames (accidental) — *continued*
    undetermined whether accidental or intentional Y26
  forces of nature NEC — *see* Forces of nature
  G-forces (abnormal) W49.9
  gravitational forces (abnormal) W49.9
  heat (natural) NEC — *see* Heat
  high-pressure jet (hydraulic) (pneumatic) W49.9
  hydraulic jet W49.9
  inanimate mechanical force W49.9
  jet, high-pressure (hydraulic) (pneumatic) W49.9
  lightning — *see* subcategory T75.0
    causing fire — *see* Exposure, fire
  mechanical forces NEC W49.9
    animate NEC W64
    inanimate NEC W49.9
  noise W42.9
    supersonic W42.0
  noxious substance — *see* Table of Drugs and Chemicals
  pneumatic jet W49.9
  prolonged in deep-freeze unit or refrigerator W93.2
  radiation — *see* Radiation
  smoke — *see also* Exposure, fire
    tobacco, second hand Z77.22
  specified factors NEC X58
  sunlight X32
    man-made (sun lamp) W89.8
    tanning bed W89.1
  supersonic waves W42.0
  transmission line(s), electric W85
  vibration W49.9
  waves
    infrasound W49.9
    sound W42.9
    supersonic W42.0
  weather NEC — *see* Forces of nature

External cause status Y99.9
  child assisting in compensated work for family Y99.8
  civilian activity done for financial or other compensation Y99.0
  civilian activity done for income or pay Y99.0
  family member assisting in compensated work for other family member Y99.8
  hobby not done for income Y99.8
  leisure activity Y99.8
  military activity Y99.1
  off-duty activity of military personnel Y99.8
  recreation or sport not for income or while a student Y99.8
  specified NEC Y99.8
  student activity Y99.8
  volunteer activity Y99.2

F

Factors, supplemental
  alcohol
    blood level
      100-119mg/100ml Y90.5
      120-199mg/100ml Y90.6
      20-39mg/100ml Y90.1
      200-239mg/100ml Y90.7
      240mg/100ml or more Y90.8
      40-59mg/100ml Y90.2
      60-79mg/100ml Y90.3
      80-99mg/100ml Y90.4
      less than 20mg/100ml Y90.0
    presence in blood, level not specified
      Y90.9
    presence in blood, but level not specified
      Y90.9
  environmental-pollution-related condition
    — see Z57
  nosocomial condition Y95
  work-related condition Y99.0
Failure
  in suture or ligature during surgical
    procedure Y65.2
  mechanical, of instrument or apparatus
    (any) (during any medical or surgical
    procedure) Y65.8
  sterile precautions (during medical and
    surgical care) — see Misadventure,
    failure, sterile precautions, by type
    ofprocedure
  to
    introduce tube or instrument Y65.4
      endotracheal tube during anesthesia
        Y65.3
    make curve (transport vehicle) NEC —
      see Accident, transport
    remove tube or instrument Y65.4
Fall, falling (accidental) W19
  building W20.1
    burning (uncontrolled fire) X00.3
  down
    embankment W17.81
    escalator W10.0
    hill W17.81
    ladder W11
    ramp W10.2
    stairs, steps W10.9
  due to
    bumping against
      object W18.00
        sharp glass W18.02
        specified NEC W18.09
        sports equipment W18.01
      person W03
        due to ice or snow W00.0
        on pedestrian conveyance — see
          Accident, transport,
          pedestrian, conveyance
    collision with another person W03
      due to ice or snow W00.0
      involving pedestrian conveyance —
        see Accident, transport,
        pedestrian, conveyance
    grocery cart tipping over W17.82
    ice or snow W00.9
      from one level to another W00.2
      on stairs or steps W00.1
      involving pedestrian conveyance —
        see Accident, transport,
        pedestrian, conveyance
      on same level W00.0
    slipping (on moving sidewalk) W01.0
      with subsequent striking against
        object W01.10
        furniture W01.190
        sharp object W01.119
          glass W01.110
          power tool or machine W01.111
          specified NEC W01.118
        specified NEC W01.198
    striking against
      object W18.00
        sharp glass W18.02
        specified NEC W18.09
        sports equipment W18.01
      person W03
        due to ice or snow W00.0
        on pedestrian conveyance — see
          Accident, transport,
          pedestrian, conveyance
  earth (with asphyxia or suffocation (by
    pressure)) — see Earth, falling

Fall, falling (accidental) — *continued*
  from, off, out of
    aircraft NEC (with accident to aircraft
      NEC) V97.0
      while boarding or alighting V97.1
    balcony W13.0
    bed W06
    boat, ship, watercraft NEC (with
      drowning or submersion) — see
      Drowning, due to, fall overboard
      with hitting bottom or object V94.0
    bridge W13.1
    building W13.9
      burning (uncontrolled fire) X00.3
    cavity W17.2
    chair W07
    cherry picker W17.89
    cliff W15
    dock W17.4
    embankment W17.81
    escalator W10.0
    flagpole W13.8
    furniture NEC W08
    grocery cart W17.82
    haystack W17.89
    high place NEC W17.89
      stated as undetermined whether
        accidental or intentional Y30
    hole W17.2
    incline W10.2
    ladder W11
    lifting device W17.89
    machine, machinery — see also Contact,
      with, by type of machine
      not in operation W17.89
    manhole W17.1
    mobile elevated work platform [MEWP]
      W17.89
    motorized mobility scooter W05.2
    one level to another NEC W17.89
      intentional, purposeful, suicide
        (attempt) X80
      stated as undetermined whether
        accidental or intentional Y30
    pit W17.2
    playground equipment W09.8
      jungle gym W09.2
      slide W09.0
      swing W09.1
    quarry W17.89
    railing W13.9
    ramp W10.2
    roof W13.2
    scaffolding W12
    scooter (nonmotorized) W05.1
      motorized mobility W05.2
    sky lift W17.89
    stairs, steps W10.9
      curb W10.1
      due to ice or snow W00.1
      escalator W10.0
      incline W10.2
      ramp W10.2
      sidewalk curb W10.1
      specified NEC W10.8
    stepladder W11
    storm drain W17.1
    streetcar NEC V82.6
      with antecedent collision — see
        Accident, transport, streetcar
        occupant
      while boarding or alighting V82.4
    structure NEC W13.8
      burning (uncontrolled fire) X00.3
    table W08
    toilet W18.11
      with subsequent striking against
        object W18.12
    train NEC V81.6
      during derailment (without antecedent
        collision) V81.7
      with antecedent collision — see
        Accident, transport, railway
        vehicle occupant
      while boarding or alighting V81.4
    transport vehicle after collision — see
      Accident, transport, by type of
      vehicle, collision
    tree W14
    vehicle (in motion) NEC (see also
      Accident, transport) V89.9
      motor NEC (see also Accident,
        transport, occupant, by type of
        vehicle) V87.8
      stationary) W17.89
        while boarding or alighting — see
          Accident, transport, by type of
          vehicle, while boarding or
          alighting
    viaduct W13.8

Fall, falling (accidental) — *continued*
  from, off, out of — *continued*
    wall W13.8
    watercraft — see also Drowning, due to,
      fall overboard
      with hitting bottom or object V94.0
    well W17.0
    wheelchair, non-moving W05.0
      powered — see Accident, transport,
        pedestrian, conveyance
        occupant, specified type NEC
    window W13.4
  in, on
    aircraft NEC V97.0
      with accident to aircraft V97.0
      while boarding or alighting V97.1
    bathtub (empty) W18.2
      filled W16.212
        causing drowning W16.211
    escalator W10.0
    incline W10.2
    ladder W11
    machine, machinery — see Contact,
      with, by type of machine
    object, edged, pointed or sharp (with
      cut) — see Fall, by type
    playground equipment W09.8
      jungle gym W09.2
      slide W09.0
      swing W09.1
    ramp W10.2
    scaffolding W12
    shower W18.2
      causing drowning W16.211
    staircase, stairs, steps W10.9
      curb W10.1
      due to ice or snow W00.1
      escalator W10.0
      incline W10.2
      specified NEC W10.8
    streetcar (without antecedent collision)
      V82.5
      with antecedent collision — see
        Accident, transport, streetcar
        occupant
      while boarding or alighting V82.4
    train (without antecedent collision)
      V81.5
      with antecedent collision — see
        Accident, transport, railway
        vehicle occupant
      during derailment (without antecedent
        collision) V81.7
        with antecedent collision — see
          Accident, transport, railway
          vehicle occupant
      while boarding or alighting V81.4
    transport vehicle after collision — see
      Accident, transport, by type of
      vehicle, collision
    watercraft V93.39
      due to
        accident to craft V91.29
          powered craft V91.23
            ferry boat V91.21
            fishing boat V91.22
            jetskis V91.23
            liner V91.21
            merchant ship V91.20
            passenger ship V91.21
          unpowered craft
            canoe V91.25
            inflatable V91.26
            kayak V91.25
            sailboat V91.24
        powered craft V93.33
          ferry boat V93.31
          fishing boat V93.32
          jetskis V93.33
          liner V93.31
          merchant ship V93.30
          passenger ship V93.31
        unpowered craft V93.38
          canoe V93.35
          inflatable V93.36
          kayak V93.35
          sailboat V93.34
          surfboard V93.38
          windsurfer V93.38
  into
    cavity W17.2
    dock W17.4
    fire — see Exposure, fire, by type
    haystack W17.89
    hole W17.2
    manhole W17.1
    moving part of machinery — see
      Contact, with, by type of machine
    ocean — see Fall, into, water
    opening in surface NEC W17.89

Fall, falling (accidental) — *continued*
  into — *continued*
    pit W17.2
    pond — see Fall, into, water
    quarry W17.89
    river — see Fall, into, water
    shaft W17.89
    storm drain W17.1
    stream — see Fall, into, water
    swimming pool — see also Fall, into,
      water, in, swimming pool
      empty W17.3
    tank W17.89
    water W16.42
      causing drowning W16.41
      from watercraft — see Drowning, due
        to, fall overboard
      hitting diving board W21.4
      in
        bathtub W16.212
          causing drowning W16.211
        bucket W16.222
          causing drowning W16.221
        natural body of water W16.112
          causing drowning W16.111
          striking
            bottom W16.122
              causing drowning W16.121
            side W16.132
              causing drowning W16.131
        specified water NEC W16.312
          causing drowning W16.311
          striking
            bottom W16.322
              causing drowning W16.321
            wall W16.332
              causing drowning W16.331
        swimming pool W16.012
          causing drowning W16.011
          striking
            bottom W16.022
              causing drowning W16.021
            wall W16.032
              causing drowning W16.031
        utility bucket W16.222
          causing drowning W16.221
    well W17.0
  involving
    bed W06
    chair W07
    furniture NEC W08
    glass — see Fall, by type
    playground equipment W09.8
      jungle gym W09.2
      slide W09.0
      swing W09.1
    roller blades — see Accident, transport,
      pedestrian, conveyance
    skateboard(s) — see Accident, transport,
      pedestrian, conveyance
    skates (ice) (in line) (roller) —
      see Accident, transport, pedestrian,
      conveyance
    skis — see Accident, transport,
      pedestrian, conveyance
    table W08
    wheelchair, non-moving W05.0
      powered — see Accident, transport,
        pedestrian, conveyance,
        specified type NEC
  object — see Struck by, object, falling
  off
    toilet W18.11
      with subsequent striking against
        object W18.12
  on same level W18.30
    due to
      specified NEC W18.39
      stepping on an object W18.31
  out of
    bed W06
    building NEC W13.8
    chair W07
    furniture NEC W08
    wheelchair, non-moving W05.0
      powered — see Accident, transport,
        pedestrian, conveyance,
        specified type NEC
    window W13.4
  over
    animal W01.0
    cliff W15
    embankment W17.81
    small object W01.0
  rock W20.8

EXTERNAL CAUSES

EXTERNAL CAUSES

EXTERNAL CAUSES

Incident, adverse — *continued*
device — *continued*
radiological Y78.8
accessory Y78.2
diagnostic Y78.0
miscellaneous Y78.8
monitoring Y78.0
prosthetic Y78.2
rehabilitative Y78.1
surgical Y78.3
therapeutic Y78.1
urology Y73.8
accessory Y73.2
diagnostic Y73.0
miscellaneous Y73.8
monitoring Y73.0
prosthetic Y73.2
rehabilitative Y73.1
surgical Y73.3
therapeutic Y73.1
Incineration (accidental) — *see* Exposure, fire
Infanticide — *see* Assault
Infrasound waves (causing injury) W49.9
Ingestion
foreign body (causing injury) (with obstruction) — *see* Foreign body, alimentary canal
poisonous
plant(s) X58
substance NEC — *see* Table of Drugs and Chemicals
Inhalation
excessively cold substance, man-made — *see* Exposure, cold, man-made
food (any type) (into respiratory tract) (with asphyxia, obstruction respiratory tract, suffocation) — *see* categories T17 and T18
foreign body — *see* Foreign body, aspiration
gastric contents (with asphyxia, obstruction respiratory passage, suffocation) T17.81-
hot air or gases X14.0
liquid air, hydrogen, nitrogen W93.12
suicide (attempt) X83.2
steam X13.0
assault X98.0
stated as undetermined whether accidental or intentional Y27.0
suicide (attempt) X77.0
toxic gas — *see* Table of Drugs and Chemicals
vomitus (with asphyxia, obstruction respiratory passage, suffocation) T17.81-
Injury, injured (accidental(ly)) NOS X58
by, caused by, from
assault — *see* Assault
law-enforcing agent, police, in course of legal intervention — *see* Legal intervention
suicide (attempt) X83.8
due to, in
civil insurrection — *see* War operations
fight (*see also* Assault, fight) Y04.0
war operations — *see* War operations
homicide (*see also* Assault) Y09
inflicted (by)
in course of arrest (attempted), suppression of disturbance, maintenance of order, by law-enforcing agents — *see* Legal intervention
other person
stated as
accidental X58
intentional, homicide (attempt) — *see* Assault
undetermined whether accidental or intentional Y33
purposely (inflicted) by other person(s) — *see* Assault
self-inflicted X83.8
stated as accidental X58
specified cause NEC X58
undetermined whether accidental or intentional Y33
Insolation, effects X30
Insufficient nourishment X58
Interruption of respiration (by)
food (lodged in esophagus) — *see* categories T17 and T18
vomitus (lodged in esophagus) T17.81-
Intervention, legal — *see* Legal intervention

Intoxication
drug — *see* Table of Drugs and Chemicals
poison — *see* Table of Drugs and Chemicals

J

Jammed (accidentally)
between objects (moving) (stationary and moving) W23.0
stationary W23.1
Jumped, jumping
before moving object NEC X81.8
motor vehicle X81.0
subway train X81.1
train X81.1
undetermined whether accidental or intentional Y31
from
boat (into water) voluntarily, without accident (to or on boat) W16.712
with
accident to or on boat — *see* Accident, watercraft
drowning or submersion W16.711
suicide (attempt) X71.3
striking bottom W16.722
causing drowning W16.721
building (*see also* Jumped, from, high place) W13.9
burning (uncontrolled fire) X00.5
high place NEC W17.89
suicide (attempt) X80
undetermined whether accidental or intentional Y30
structure (*see also* Jumped, from, high place) W13.9
burning (uncontrolled fire) X00.5
into water W16.92
causing drowning W16.91
from, off watercraft — *see* Jumped, from, boat
in
natural body W16.612
causing drowning W16.611
striking bottom W16.622
causing drowning W16.621
specified place NEC W16.812
causing drowning W16.811
striking
bottom W16.822
causing drowning W16.821
wall W16.832
causing drowning W16.831
swimming pool W16.512
causing drowning W16.511
striking
bottom W16.522
causing drowning W16.521
wall W16.532
causing drowning W16.531
suicide (attempt) X71.3

K

Kicked by
animal NEC W55.82
person(s) (accidentally) W50.1
with intent to injure or kill Y04.0
as, or caused by, a crowd or human stampede (with fall) W52
assault Y04.0
homicide (attempt) Y04.0
in
fight Y04.0
legal intervention
injuring
bystander Y35.812
law enforcement personnel Y35.811
suspect Y35.813
Kicking against
object W22.8
sports equipment W21.9
stationary wW22.09
sports equipment W21.89
person — *see* Striking against, person
sports equipment W21.9

Killed, killing (accidentally) NOS (*see also* Injury) X58
in
action — *see* War operations
brawl, fight (hand) (fists) (foot) Y04.0
by weapon — *see also* Assault
cutting, piercing — *see* Assault, cutting or piercing instrument
firearm — *see* Discharge, firearm, by type, homicide
self
stated as
accident NOS X58
suicide — *see* Suicide
undetermined whether accidental or intentional Y33
Knocked down (accidentally) (by) NOS X58
animal (not being ridden) NEC — *see also* Struck by, by type of animal
crowd or human stampede W52
person W51
in brawl, fight Y04.0
transport vehicle NEC (*see also* Accident, transport) V09.9

L

Laceration NEC — *see* Injury
Lack of
care (helpless person) (infant) (newborn) X58
food except as result of abandonment or neglect X58
due to abandonment or neglect X58
water except as result of transport accident X58
due to transport accident — *see* Accident, transport, by type
helpless person, infant, newborn X58
Landslide (falling on transport vehicle) X36.1
caused by collapse of man-made structure X36.0
Late effect — *see* Sequelae
Legal
execution (any method) — *see* Legal, intervention
intervention (by)
baton — *see* Legal, intervention, blunt object, baton
bayonet — *see* Legal, intervention, sharp object, bayonet
blow — *see* Legal, intervention, manhandling
blunt object
baton
injuring
bystander Y35.312
law enforcement personnel Y35.311
suspect Y35.313
injuring
bystander Y35.302
law enforcement personnel Y35.301
suspect Y35.303
specified NEC
injuring
bystander Y35.392
law enforcement personnel Y35.391
suspect Y35.393
stave
injuring
bystander Y35.392
law enforcement personnel Y35.391
suspect Y35.393
bomb — *see* Legal, intervention, explosive
cutting or piercing instrument — *see* Legal, intervention, sharp object
dynamite — *see* Legal, intervention, explosive, dynamite
explosive(s)
dynamite
injuring
bystander Y35.112
law enforcement personnel Y35.111
suspect Y35.113

Legal — *continued*
intervention (by) — *continued*
explosive(s) — *continued*
grenade
injuring
bystander Y35.192
law enforcement personnel Y35.191
suspect Y35.193
injuring
bystander Y35.102
law enforcement personnel Y35.101
suspect Y35.103
mortar bomb
injuring
bystander Y35.192
law enforcement personnel Y35.191
suspect Y35.193
shell
injuring
bystander Y35.122
law enforcement personnel Y35.121
suspect Y35.123
specified NEC
injuring
bystander Y35.192
law enforcement personnel Y35.191
suspect Y35.193
firearm(s) (discharge)
handgun
injuring
bystander Y35.022
law enforcement personnel Y35.021
suspect Y35.023
injuring
bystander Y35.002
law enforcement personnel Y35.001
suspect Y35.003
machine gun
injuring
bystander Y35.012
law enforcement personnel Y35.011
suspect Y35.013
rifle pellet
injuring
bystander Y35.032
law enforcement personnel Y35.031
suspect Y35.033
rubber bullet
injuring
bystander Y35.042
law enforcement personnel Y35.041
suspect Y35.043
shotgun — *see* Legal, intervention, firearm, specified NEC
specified NEC
injuring
bystander Y35.092
law enforcement personnel Y35.091
suspect Y35.093
gas (asphyxiation) (poisoning)
injuring
bystander Y35.202
law enforcement personnel Y35.201
suspect Y35.203
specified NEC
injuring
bystander Y35.292
law enforcement personnel Y35.291
suspect Y35.293
tear gas
injuring
bystander Y35.212
law enforcement personnel Y35.211
suspect Y35.213
grenade — *see* Legal, intervention, explosive, grenade
injuring
bystander Y35.92
law enforcement personnel Y35.91
suspect Y35.93
late effect (of) — *see* with 7th character S Y35

EXTERNAL CAUSES

Legal — *continued*
  intervention (by) — *continued*
    manhandling
      injuring
        bystander Y35.812
        law enforcement personnel Y35.811
        suspect Y35.813
    sequelae (of) — *see* with 7th character S Y35
    sharp objects
      bayonet
        injuring
          bystander Y35.412
          law enforcement personnel Y35.411
          suspect Y35.413
      injuring
        bystander Y35.402
        law enforcement personnel Y35.401
        suspect Y35.403
      specified NEC
        injuring
          bystander Y35.492
          law enforcement personnel Y35.491
          suspect Y35.493
    specified means NEC
      injuring
        bystander Y35.892
        law enforcement personnel Y35.891
        suspect Y35.893
    stabbing — *see* Legal, intervention, sharp object
    stave — *see* Legal, intervention, blunt object, stave
    tear gas — *see* Legal, intervention, gas, tear gas
    truncheon — *see* Legal, intervention, blunt object, stave
Lightning (shock) (stroke) (struck by) — *see* subcategory T75.0
  causing fire — *see* Exposure, fire
Loss of control (transport vehicle) NEC — *see* Accident, transport
Lost at sea NOS — *see* Drowning, due to, fall overboard
Low
  pressure (effects) — *see* Air, pressure, low
  temperature (effects) — *see* Exposure, cold
Lying before train, vehicle or other moving object X81.8
  subway train X81.1
  train X81.1
  undetermined whether accidental or intentional Y31
Lynching — *see* Assault

M

Malfunction (mechanism or component) (of)
  firearm W34.10
    airgun W34.110
    BB gun W34.110
    gas, air or spring-operated gun NEC W34.118
    handgun W32.1
    hunting rifle W33.12
    larger firearm W33.10
      specified NEC W33.19
    machine gun W33.13
    paintball gun W34.111
    pellet gun W34.110
    shotgun W33.11
    specified NEC W34.19
    Very pistol [flare] W34.19
  handgun — *see* Malfunction, firearm, handgun
Maltreatment — *see* Perpetrator
Mangled (accidentally) NOS X58
Manhandling (in brawl, fight) Y04.0
  legal intervention — *see* Legal, intervention, manhandling
Manslaughter (nonaccidental) — *see* Assault
Mauled by animal NEC W55.89
Medical procedure, complication of (delayed or as an abnormal reaction without mention of misadventure) — *see* Complication of or following, by specified type of procedure
  due to or as a result of misadventure — *see* Misadventure

Melting (due to fire) — *see also* Exposure, fire
  apparel NEC X06.3
  clothes, clothing NEC X06.3
    nightwear X05
  fittings or furniture (burning building) (uncontrolled fire) X00.8
  nightwear X05
  plastic jewelry X06.1
Mental cruelty X58
Military operations (injuries to military and civilians occuring during peacetime on military property and during routine military exercises and operations) (by) (from) (involving) Y37.90-
  air blast Y37.20-
  aircraft
    destruction — *see* Military operations, destruction of aircraft
    airway restriction — *see* Military operations, restriction of airways
    asphyxiation — *see* Military operations, restriction of airways
  biological weapons Y37.6x-
  blast Y37.20-
  blast fragments Y37.20-
  blast wave Y37.20-
  blast wind Y37.20-
  bomb Y37.20-
    dirty Y37.50-
    gasoline Y37.31-
    incendiary Y37.31-
    petrol Y37.31-
  bullet Y37.43-
    incendiary Y37.32-
    rubber Y37.41-
  chemical weapons Y37.7x-
  combat
    hand to hand (unarmed) combat Y37.44-
    using blunt or piercing object Y37.45-
  conflagration — *see* Military operations, fire
  conventional warfare NEC Y37.49-
  depth-charge Y37.01-
  destruction of aircraft Y37.10-
    due to
      air to air missile Y37.11-
      collision with other aircraft Y37.12-
      detonation (accidental) of onboard munitions and explosives Y37.14-
      enemy fire or explosives Y37.11-
      explosive placed on aircraft Y37.11-
      onboard fire Y37.13-
      rocket propelled grenade [RPG] Y37.11-
      small arms fire Y37.11-
      surface to air missile Y37.11-
    specified NEC Y37.19-
  detonation (accidental) of onboard marine weapons Y37.05-
    own munitions or munitions launch device Y37.24-
  dirty bomb Y37.50-
  explosion (of) Y37.20-
    aerial bomb Y37.21-
    bomb NOS (*see also* Military operations, bomb(s)) Y37.20-
    fragments Y37.20-
    grenade Y37.29-
    guided missile Y37.22-
    improvised explosive device [IED] (person-borne) (roadside) (vehicle-borne) Y37.23-
    land mine Y37.29-
    marine mine (at sea) (in harbor) Y37.02-
    marine weapon Y37.00-
      specified NEC Y37.09-
    own munitions or munitions launch device (accidental) Y37.24-
    sea-based artillery shell Y37.03-
    specified NEC Y37.29-
    torpedo Y37.04-
  fire Y37.30-
    specified NEC Y37.39-
  firearms
    discharge Y37.43-
    pellets Y37.42-
  flamethrower Y37.33-
  fragments (from) (of)
    improvised explosive device [IED] (person-borne) (roadside) (vehicle-borne) Y37.26-
    munitions Y37.25-
    specified NEC Y37.29-
    weapons Y37.27-
  friendly fire Y37.92-
  hand to hand (unarmed) combat Y37.44-

Military operations (injuries to military and civilians occuring during peacetime on military property and during routine military exercises and operations) (by) (from) (involving) — *continued*
  hot substances — *see* Military operations, fire
  incendiary bullet Y37.32-
  nuclear weapon (effects of) Y37.50-
    acute radiation exposure Y37.54-
    blast pressure Y37.51-
    direct blast Y37.51-
    direct heat Y37.53-
    fallout exposure Y37.54-
    fireball Y37.53-
    indirect blast (struck or crushed by blast debris) (being thrown by blast) Y37.52-
    ionizing radiation (immediate exposure) Y37.54-
    nuclear radiation Y37.54-
    radiation
      ionizing (immediate exposure) Y37.54-
      nuclear Y37.54-
      thermal Y37.53-
    secondary effects Y37.54-
    specified NEC Y37.59-
    thermal radiation Y37.53-
  restriction of air (airway)
    intentional Y37.46-
    unintentional Y37.47-
  rubber bullets Y37.41-
  shrapnel NOS Y37.29-
  suffocation — *see* Military operations, restriction of airways
  unconventional warfare NEC Y37.7x-
  underwater blast NOS Y37.00-
  warfare
    conventional NEC Y37.49-
    unconventional NEC Y37.7x-
  weapon of mass destruction [WMD] Y37.91-
  weapons
    biological weapons Y37.6x-
    chemical Y37.7x-
    nuclear (effects of) Y37.50-
      acute radiation exposure Y37.54-
      blast pressure Y37.51-
      direct blast Y37.51-
      direct heat Y37.53-
      fallout exposure Y37.54-
      fireball Y37.53-
      radiation
        ionizing (immediate exposure) Y37.54-
        nuclear Y37.54-
        thermal Y37.53-
      secondary effects Y37.54-
      specified NEC Y37.59-
    of mass destruction [WMD] Y37.91-
Misadventure(s) to patient(s) during surgical or medical care Y69
  contaminated medical or biological substance (blood, drug, fluid) Y64.9
    administered (by) NEC Y64.9
      immunization Y64.1
      infusion Y64.0
      injection Y64.1
      specified means NEC Y64.8
      transfusion Y64.0
      vaccination Y64.1
  excessive amount of blood or other fluid during transfusion or infusion Y63.0
  failure
    in dosage Y63.9
      electroshock therapy Y63.4
      inappropriate temperature (too hot or too cold) in local application and packing Y63.5
      infusion
        excessive amount of fluid Y63.0
        incorrect dilution of fluid Y63.1
      insulin-shock therapy Y63.4
      nonadministration of necessary drug or biological substance Y63.6
      overdose — *see* Table of Drugs and Chemicals
      radiation, in therapy Y63.2
      radiation
        overdose Y63.2
      specified procedure NEC Y63.8
      transfusion
        excessive amount of blood Y63.0

Misadventure(s) to patient(s) during surgical or medical care — *continued*
  failure — *continued*
    mechanical, of instrument or apparatus (any) (during any procedure) Y65.8
    sterile precautions (during procedure) Y62.9
      aspiration of fluid or tissue (by puncture or catheterization, except heart) Y62.6
      biopsy (except needle aspiration) Y62.8
        needle (aspirating) Y62.6
      blood sampling Y62.6
      catheterization Y62.6
        heart Y62.5
      dialysis (kidney) Y62.2
      endoscopic examination Y62.4
      enema Y62.8
      immunization Y62.3
      infusion Y62.1
      injection Y62.3
      needle biopsy Y62.6
      paracentesis (abdominal) (thoracic) Y62.6
      perfusion Y62.2
      puncture (lumbar) Y62.6
      removal of catheter or packing Y62.8
      specified procedure NEC Y62.8
      surgical operation Y62.0
      transfusion Y62.1
      vaccination Y62.3
    suture or ligature during surgical procedure Y65.2
    to introduce or to remove tube or instrument — *see* Failure, to
  hemorrhage — *see* Index to Diseases and Injuries, Complication(s)
  inadvertent exposure of patient to radiation Y63.3
  inappropriate
    operation performed — *see* Inappropriate operation performed
    temperature (too hot or too cold) in local application or packing Y63.5
  infusion (*see also* Misadventure, by type, infusion) Y69
    excessive amount of fluid Y63.0
    incorrect dilution of fluid Y63.1
    wrong fluid Y65.1
  mismatched blood in transfusion Y65.0
  nonadministration of necessary drug or biological substance Y63.6
  overdose — *see* Table of Drugs and Chemicals
  radiation (in therapy) Y63.2
  perforation — *see* Index to Diseases and Injuries, Complication(s)
  performance of inappropriate operation — *see* Inappropriate operation performed
  puncture — *see* Index to Diseases and Injuries, Complication(s)
  specified type NEC Y65.8
    failure
      suture or ligature during surgical operation Y65.2
      to introduce or to remove tube or instrument — *see* Failure, to
    infusion of wrong fluid Y65.1
    performance of inappropriate operation — *see* Inappropriate operation performed
    transfusion of mismatched blood Y65.0
    wrong
      fluid in infusion Y65.1
      placement of endotracheal tube during anesthetic procedure Y65.3
  transfusion — *see* Misadventure, by type, transfusion
    excessive amount of blood Y63.0
    mismatched blood Y65.0
  wrong
    drug given in error — *see* Table of Drugs and Chemicals
    fluid in infusion Y65.1
    placement of endotracheal tube during anesthetic procedure Y65.3
Mismatched blood in transfusion Y65.0
Motion sickness T75.3
Mountain sickness W94.11
Mudslide (of cataclysmic nature) — *see* Landslide
Murder (attempt) — *see* Assault

© 2013 Channel Publishing Ltd

N

Nail, contact with W45.0
  gun W29.4
Neglect (criminal) (homicidal intent) X58
Noise (causing injury) (pollution) W42.9
  supersonic W42.0
Nonadministration (of)
  drug or biological substance (necessary) Y63.6
  surgical and medical care Y66
Nosocomial condition Y95

O

Object
  falling
    from, in, on, hitting
      machinery — *see* Contact, with, by type of machine
  set in motion by
    accidental explosion or rupture of pressure vessel W38
    firearm — *see* Discharge, firearm, by type
    machine(ry) — *see* Contact, with, by type of machine
Overdose (drug) — *see* Table of Drugs and Chemicals
  radiation Y63.2
Overexertion — *see* category Y93
Overexposure (accidental) (to)
  cold (*see also* Exposure, cold) X31
    due to man-made conditions — *see* Exposure, cold, man-made
  heat (*see also* Heat) X30
  radiation — *see* Radiation
  radioactivity W88.0
  sun (sunburn) X32
  weather NEC — *see* Forces of nature
  wind NEC — *see* Forces of nature
Overheated — *see* Heat
Overturning (accidental)
  machinery — *see* Contact, with, by type of machine
  transport vehicle NEC (*see also* Accident, transport) V89.9
  watercraft (causing drowning, submersion) — *see also* Drowning, due to, accident to, watercraft, overturning
    causing injury except drowning or submersion — *see* Accident, watercraft, causing, injury NEC

P

Parachute descent (voluntary) (without accident to aircraft) V97.29
  due to accident to aircraft — *see* Accident, transport, aircraft
Pecked by bird W61.99
Perforation during medical or surgical treatment as misadventure — *see* Index to Diseases and Injuries, Complication(s)
Perpetrator, perpetration, of assault, maltreatment and neglect (by) Y07.9
  boyfriend Y07.03
  brother Y07.410
    stepbrother Y07.435
  coach Y07.53
  cousin
    female Y07.491
    male Y07.490
  daycare provider Y07.519
    at-home
      adult care Y07.512
      childcare Y07.510
    care center
      adult care Y07.513
      childcare Y07.511
  family member NEC Y07.499
  father Y07.11
    adoptive Y07.13
    foster Y07.420
    stepfather Y07.430
    foster father Y07.420
    foster mother Y07.421

Perpetrator, perpetration, of assault, maltreatment and neglect — *continued*
  girl friend Y07.04
  healthcare provider Y07.529
    mental health Y07.521
    specified NEC Y07.528
  husband Y07.01
  instructor Y07.53
  mother Y07.12
    adoptive Y07.14
    foster Y07.421
    stepmother Y07.433
  nonfamily member Y07.50
    specified NEC Y07.59
  nurse Y07.528
  occupational therapist Y07.528
  partner of parent
    female Y07.434
    male Y07.432
  physical therapist Y07.528
  sister Y07.411
  speech therapist Y07.528
  stepbrother Y07.435
  stepfather Y07.430
  stepmother Y07.433
  stepsister Y07.436
  teacher Y07.53
  wife Y07.02
Piercing — *see* Contact, with, by type of object or machine
Pinched
  between objects (moving) (stationary and moving) W23.0
  stationary W23.1
Pinned under machine(ry) — *see* Contact, with, by type of machine
Place of occurrence Y92.9
  abandoned house Y92.89
  airplane Y92.813
  airport Y92.520
  ambulatory health services establishment NEC Y92.538
  ambulatory surgery center Y92.530
  amusement park Y92.831
  apartment (co-op) — *see* Place of occurrence, residence, apartment
  assembly hall Y92.29
  bank Y92.510
  barn Y92.71
  baseball field Y92.320
  basketball court Y92.310
  beach Y92.832
  boarding house — *see* Place of occurrence, residence, boarding house
  boat Y92.814
  bowling alley Y92.39
  bridge Y92.89
  building under construction Y92.61
  bus Y92.811
    station Y92.521
  cafe Y92.511
  campsite Y92.833
  campus — *see* Place of occurrence, school
  canal Y92.89
  car Y92.810
  casino Y92.59
  children's home — *see* Place of occurrence, residence, institutional, orphanage
  church Y92.22
  cinema Y92.26
  clubhouse Y92.29
  coal pit Y92.64
  college (community) Y92.214
  condominium — *see* Place of occurrence, residence, apartment
  construction area — *see* Place of occurrence, industrial and construction area
  convalescent home — *see* Place of occurrence, residence, institutional, nursing home
  court-house Y92.240
  cricket ground Y92.328
  cultural building Y92.258
    art gallery Y92.250
    museum Y92.251
    music hall Y92.252
    opera house Y92.253
    specified NEC Y92.258
    theater Y92.254
  dancehall Y92.252
  day nursery Y92.210
  dentist office Y92.531
  derelict house Y92.89
  desert Y92.820
  dock NOS Y92.89
  dockyard Y92.62
  doctor's office Y92.531

Place of occurrence — *continued*
  dormitory — *see* Place of occurrence, residence, institutional, school dormitory
  dry dock Y92.62
  factory (building) (premises) Y92.63
  farm (land under cultivation) (outbuildings) Y92.79
    barn Y92.71
    chicken coop Y92.72
    field Y92.73
    hen house Y92.72
    house — *see* Place of occurrence, residence, house
    orchard Y92.74
    specified NEC Y92.79
  football field Y92.321
  forest Y92.821
  freeway Y92.411
  gallery Y92.250
  garage (commercial) Y92.59
    boarding house Y92.044
    military base Y92.135
    mobile home Y92.025
    nursing home Y92.124
    orphanage Y92.114
    private house Y92.015
    reform school Y92.155
  gas station Y92.524
  gasworks Y92.69
  golf course Y92.39
  gravel pit Y92.64
  grocery Y92.512
  gymnasium Y92.39
  handball court Y92.318
  harbor Y92.89
  harness racing course Y92.39
  healthcare provider office Y92.531
  highway (interstate) Y92.411
  hill Y92.828
  hockey rink Y92.330
  home — *see* Place of occurrence, residence
  hospice — *see* Place of occurrence, residence, institutional, nursing home
  hospital Y92.239
    cafeteria Y92.233
    corridor Y92.232
    operating room Y92.234
    patient
      bathroom Y92.231
      room Y92.230
    specified NEC Y92.238
  hotel Y92.59
  house — *see also* Place of occurrence, residence
    abandoned Y92.89
    under construction Y92.61
  industrial and construction area (yard) Y92.69
    building under construction Y92.61
    dock Y92.62
    dry dock Y92.62
    factory Y92.63
    gasworks Y92.69
    mine Y92.64
    oil rig Y92.65
    pit Y92.64
    power station Y92.69
    shipyard Y92.62
    specified NEC Y92.69
    tunnel under construction Y92.69
    workshop Y92.69
  kindergarten Y92.211
  lacrosse field Y92.328
  lake Y92.828
  library Y92.241
  mall Y92.59
  market Y92.512
  marsh Y92.828
  military
    base — *see* Place of occurrence, residence, institutional, military base
    training ground Y92.84
  mine Y92.64
  mosque Y92.22
  motel Y92.59
  motorway (interstate) Y92.411
  mountain Y92.828
  movie-house Y92.26
  museum Y92.251
  music-hall Y92.252
  not applicable Y92.9
  nuclear power station Y92.69
  nursing home — *see* Place of occurrence, residence, institutional, nursing home
  office building Y92.59
  offshore installation Y92.65
  oil rig Y92.65

Place of occurrence — *continued*
  old people's home — *see* Place of occurrence, residence, institutional, specified NEC
  opera-house Y92.253
  orphanage — *see* Place of occurrence, residence, institutional, orphanage
  outpatient surgery center Y92.530
  park (public) Y92.830
    amusement Y92.831
  parking garage Y92.89
    lot Y92.481
  pavement Y92.480
  physician office Y92.531
  polo field Y92.328
  pond Y92.828
  post office Y92.242
  power station Y92.69
  prairie Y92.828
  prison — *see* Place of occurrence, residence, institutional, prison
  public
    administration building Y92.248
      city hall Y92.243
      courthouse Y92.240
      library Y92.241
      post office Y92.242
      specified NEC Y92.248
    building NEC Y92.29
    hall Y92.29
    place NOS Y92.89
  race course Y92.39
  radio station Y92.59
  railway line (bridge) Y92.85
  ranch (outbuildings) — *see* Place of occurrence, farm
  recreation area Y92.838
    amusement park Y92.831
    beach Y92.832
    campsite Y92.833
    park (public) Y92.830
    seashore Y92.832
    specified NEC Y92.838
  reform school — *see* Place of occurrence, residence, institutional, reform school
  religious institution Y92.22
  residence (non-institutional) (private) Y92.009
    apartment Y92.039
      bathroom Y92.031
      bedroom Y92.032
      kitchen Y92.030
      specified NEC Y92.038
    bathroom Y92.002
    bedroom Y92.003
    boarding house Y92.049
      bathroom Y92.041
      bedroom Y92.042
      driveway Y92.043
      garage Y92.044
      garden Y92.046
      kitchen Y92.040
      specified NEC Y92.048
      swimming pool Y92.045
      yard Y92.046
    dining room Y92.001
    garden Y92.007
    home Y92.009
    house, single family Y92.019
      bathroom Y92.012
      bedroom Y92.013
      dining room Y92.011
      driveway Y92.014
      garage Y92.015
      garden Y92.017
      kitchen Y92.010
      specified NEC Y92.018
      swimming pool Y92.016
      yard Y92.017
    institutional Y92.10
      children's home — *see* Place of occurrence, residence, institutional, orphanage
      hospice — *see* Place of occurrence, residence, institutional, nursing home
      military base Y92.139
        barracks Y92.133
        garage Y92.135
        garden Y92.137
        kitchen Y92.130
        mess hall Y92.131
        specified NEC Y92.138
        swimming pool Y92.136
        yard Y92.137

EXTERNAL CAUSES

Place of occurrence — *continued*
  residence (non-institutional) (private) —
    continued
    institutional — *continued*
      nursing home Y92.129
        bathroom Y92.121
        bedroom Y92.122
        driveway Y92.123
        garage Y92.124
        garden Y92.126
        kitchen Y92.120
        specified NEC Y92.128
        swimming pool Y92.125
        yard Y92.126
      orphanage Y92.119
        bathroom Y92.111
        bedroom Y92.112
        driveway Y92.113
        garage Y92.114
        garden Y92.116
        kitchen Y92.110
        specified NEC Y92.118
        swimming pool Y92.115
        yard Y92.116
      prison Y92.149
        bathroom Y92.142
        cell Y92.143
        courtyard Y92.147
        dining room Y92.141
        kitchen Y92.140
        specified NEC Y92.148
        swimming pool Y92.146
      reform school Y92.159
        bathroom Y92.152
        bedroom Y92.153
        dining room Y92.151
        driveway Y92.154
        garage Y92.155
        garden Y92.157
        kitchen Y92.150
        specified NEC Y92.158
        swimming pool Y92.156
        yard Y92.157
      school dormitory Y92.169
        bathroom Y92.162
        bedroom Y92.163
        dining room Y92.161
        kitchen Y92.160
        specified NEC Y92.168
      specified NEC Y92.199
        bathroom Y92.192
        bedroom Y92.193
        dining room Y92.191
        driveway Y92.194
        garage Y92.195
        garden Y92.197
        kitchen Y92.190
        specified NEC Y92.198
        swimming pool Y92.196
        yard Y92.197
    kitchen Y92.000
    mobile home Y92.029
      bathroom Y92.022
      bedroom Y92.023
      dining room Y92.021
      driveway Y92.024
      garage Y92.025
      garden Y92.027
      kitchen Y92.020
      specified NEC Y92.028
      swimming pool Y92.026
      yard Y92.027
    specified place in residence NEC
      Y92.008
    specified residence type NEC Y92.099
      bathroom Y92.091
      bedroom Y92.092
      driveway Y92.093
      garage Y92.094
      garden Y92.096
      kitchen Y92.090
      specified NEC Y92.098
      swimming pool Y92.095
      yard Y92.096
  restaurant Y92.511
  riding school Y92.39
  river Y92.828
  road Y92.488
  rodeo ring Y92.39
  rugby field Y92.328
  same day surgery center Y92.530
  sand pit Y92.64

Place of occurrence — *continued*
  school (private) (public) (state) Y92.219
    college Y92.214
    daycare center Y92.210
    elementary school Y92.211
    high school Y92.213
    kindergarten Y92.211
    middle school Y92.212
    specified NEC Y92.218
    trace school Y92.215
    university Y92.214
    vocational school Y92.215
  sea (shore) Y92.832
  senior citizen center Y92.29
  service area
    airport Y92.520
    bus station Y92.521
    gas station Y92.524
    highway rest stop Y92.523
    railway station Y92.522
  shipyard Y92.62
  shop (commercial) Y92.513
  sidewalk Y92.480
  silo Y92.79
  skating rink (roller) Y92.331
    ice Y92.330
  slaughter house Y92.86
  soccer field Y92.322
  specified place NEC Y92.89
  sports area Y92.39
    athletic
      court Y92.318
        basketball Y92.310
        specified NEC Y92.318
        squash Y92.311
        tennis Y92.312
      field Y92.328
        baseball Y92.320
        cricket ground Y92.328
        football Y92.321
        hockey Y92.328
        soccer Y92.322
        specified NEC Y92.328
    golf course Y92.39
    gymnasium Y92.39
    riding school Y92.39
    skating rink (roller) Y92.331
      ice Y92.330
    stadium Y92.39
    swimming pool Y92.34
  squash court Y92.311
  stadium Y92.39
  steeplechasing course Y92.39
  store Y92.512
  stream Y92.828
  street and highway Y92.410
    bike path Y92.482
    freeway Y92.411
    highway ramp Y92.415
    interstate highway Y92.411
    local residential or business street
      Y92.414
    motorway Y92.411
    parking lot Y92.481
    parkway Y92.412
    sidewalk Y92.480
    specified NEC Y92.488
    state road Y92.413
  subway car Y92.816
  supermarket Y92.512
  swamp Y92.828
  swimming pool (public) Y92.34
    private (at) Y92.095
      boarding house Y92.045
      military base Y92.136
      mobile home Y92.026
      nursing home Y92.125
      orphanage Y92.115
      prison Y92.146
      reform school Y92.156
      single family residence Y92.016
  synagogue Y92.22
  television station Y92.59
  tennis court Y92.312
  theater Y92.254
  trade area Y92.59
    bank Y92.510
    cafe Y92.511
    casino Y92.59
    garage Y92.59
    hotel Y92.59
    market Y92.512
    office building Y92.59
    radio station Y92.59
    restaurant Y92.511
    shop Y92.513
    shopping mall Y92.59
    store Y92.512
    supermarket Y92.512
    television station Y92.59

Place of occurrence — *continued*
  trade area Y92.59 — *continued*
    warehouse Y92.59
  trailer park, residential — *see* Place of
    occurrence, residence, mobile home
  trailer site NOS Y92.89
  train Y92.815
    station Y92.522
  truck Y92.812
  tunnel under construction Y92.69
  university Y92.214
  urgent (health) care center Y92.532
  vehicle (transport) Y92.818
    airplane Y92.813
    boat Y92.814
    bus Y92.811
    car Y92.810
    specified NEC Y92.818
    subway car Y92.816
    train Y92.815
    truck Y92.812
  warehouse Y92.59
  water reservoir Y92.89
  wilderness area Y92.828
    desert Y92.820
    forest Y92.821
    marsh Y92.828
    mountain Y92.828
    prairie Y92.828
    specified NEC Y92.828
    swamp Y92.828
  workshop Y92.69
  yard, private Y92.096
    boarding house Y92.046
    mobile home Y92.027
    single family house Y92.017
  youth center Y92.29
  zoo (zoological garden) Y92.834
Plumbism — *see* Table of Drugs and
  Chemicals, lead
Poisoning (accidental) (by) — *see also* Table
  of Drugs and Chemicals
  by plant, thorns, spines, sharp leaves or
    other mechanisms NEC X58
  carbon monoxide
    generated by
      motor vehicle — *see* Accident,
        transport
      watercraft (in transit) (not in transit)
        V93.89
        ferry boat V93.81
        fishing boat V93.82
        jet skis V93.83
        liner V93.81
        merchant ship V93.80
        passenger ship V93.81
        powered craft NEC V93.83
  caused by injection of poisons into skin by
    plant thorns, spines, sharp leaves X58
    marine or sea plants (venomous) X58
  exhaust gas
    generated by
      motor vehicle — *see* Accident,
        transport
      watercraft (in transit) (not in transit)
        V93.89
        ferry boat V93.81
        fishing boat V93.82
        jet skis V93.83
        liner V93.81
        merchant ship V93.80
        passenger ship V93.81
        powered craft NEC V93.83
  fumes or smoke due to
    explosion (*see also* Explosion) W40.9
    fire — *see* Exposure, fire
    ignition — *see* Ignition
  gas
    in legal intervention — *see* Legal,
      intervention, gas
    legal execution — *see* Legal,
      intervention, gas
  in war operations — *see* War operations
  legal execution — *see* Legal, intervention
  intervention
    by gas — *see* Legal, intervention, gas
    by other specified means — *see* Legal,
      intervention, specified means
      NEC
Powder burn (by) (from)
  airgun W34.110
  BB gun W34.110
  firearm NEC W34.19
  gas, air or spring-operated gun NEC
    W34.118
  handgun W32.1
  hunting rifle W33.12
  larger firearm W33.10
    specified NEC W33.19
  machine gun W33.13

Powder burn (by) (from) — *continued*
  paintball gun W34.111
  pellet gun W34.110
  shotgun W33.11
  Very pistol [flare] W34.19
**Premature cessation (of) surgical and
  medical care** Y66
Privation (food) (water) X58
Procedure (operation)
  correct, on wrong side or body part (wrong
    side) (wrong site) Y65.53
  intended for another patient done on wrong
    patient Y65.52
  performed on patient not scheduled for
    surgery Y65.52
  performed on wrong patient Y65.52
  wrong, performed on correct patient
    Y65.51
Prolonged
  sitting in transport vehicle — *see* Travel, by
    type of vehicle
  stay in
    high altitude as cause of anoxia,
      barodontalgia, barotitis or hypoxia
      W94.11
    weightless environment X52
Pulling, excessive — *see* category Y93
Puncture, puncturing — *see also* Contact,
  with, by type of object or machine
  by
    plant thorns, spines, sharp leaves or
      other mechanisms NEC W60
  during medical or surgical treatment as
    misadventure — *see* Index to Diseases
    and Injuries, Complication(s)
Pushed, pushing (accidental) (injury in)
  (overexertion) — *see* category Y93
  by other person(s) (accidental) W51
    with fall W03
      due to ice or snow W00.0
    as, or caused by, a crowd or human
      stampede (with fall) W52
    before moving object NEC Y02.8
      motor vehicle Y02.0
      subway train Y02.1
      train Y02.1
    from
      high place NEC
        in accidental circumstances
          W17.89
        stated as
          intentional, homicide (attempt)
            Y01
          undetermined whether accidental
            or intentional Y30
      transport vehicle NEC (*see also*
        Accident, transport) V89.9
        stated as
          intentional, homicide (attempt)
            Y08.89

Q

R

Radiation (exposure to)
arc lamps W89.0
atomic power plant (malfunction) NEC W88.1
complication of or abnormal reaction to medical radiotherapy Y84.2
electromagnetic, ionizing W88.0
gamma rays W88.1
in
    war operations (from or following nuclear explosion) — *see* War operations
    inadvertent exposure of patient (receiving test or therapy) Y63.3
infrared (heaters and lamps) W90.1
    excessive heat from W92
ionized, ionizing (particles, artificially accelerated)
    radioisotopes W88.1
    specified NEC W88.8
    x-rays W88.0
isotopes, radioactive — *see* Radiation, radioactive isotopes
laser(s) W90.2
    in war operations — *see* War operations
    misadventure in medical care Y63.2
light sources (man-made visible and ultraviolet) W89.9
    natural X32
    specified NEC W89.8
    tanning bed W89.1
    welding light W89.0
man-made visible light W89.9
    specified NEC W89.8
    tanning bed W89.1
    welding light W89.0
microwave W90.8
misadventure in medical or surgical procedure Y63.2
natural NEC X39.08
    radon X39.01
overdose (in medical or surgical procedure) Y63.2
radar W90.0
radioactive isotopes (any) W88.1
    atomic power plant malfunction W88.1
    misadventure in medical or surgical treatment Y63.2
radiofrequency W90.0
radium NEC W88.1
sun X32
ultraviolet (light) (man-made) W89.9
    natural X32
    specified NEC W89.8
    tanning bed W89.1
    welding light W89.0
welding arc, torch, or light W89.0
    excessive heat from W92
x-rays (hard) (soft) W88.0
Range disease W94.11
Rape (attempted) T74.2-
Rat bite W53.11
Reaction, abnormal to medical procedure (*see also* Complication of or following, by type of procedure) Y84.9
with misadventure — *see* Misadventure
biologicals — *see* Table of Drugs and Chemicals
drugs — *see* Table of Drugs and Chemicals
vaccine — *see* Table of Drugs and Chemicals
Recoil
airgun W34.110
BB gun W34.110
firearm NEC W34.19
gas, air or spring-operated gun NEC W34.118
handgun W32.1
hunting rifle W33.12
larger firearm W33.10
    specified NEC W33.19
machine gun W33.13
paintball gun W34.111
pellet W34.110
shotgun W33.11
Very pistol [flare] W34.19
Reduction in
atmospheric pressure — *see* Air, pressure, change
Rock falling on or hitting (accidentally) (person) W20.8
in cave-in W20.0

Run over (accidentally) (by)
animal (not being ridden) NEC W55.89
machinery — *see* Contact, with, by specified type of machine
transport vehicle NEC (*see also* Accident, transport) V09.9
    intentional homicide (attempt) Y03.0
    motor NEC V09.20
        intentional homicide (attempt) Y03.0
Running
before moving object X81.8
    motor vehicle X81.0
Running off, away
animal (being ridden) (*see also* Accident, transport) V80.918
    not being ridden W55.89
animal-drawn vehicle NEC (*see also* Accident, transport) V80.928
highway, road(way), street
    transport vehicle NEC (*see also* Accident, transport) V89.9
Rupture pressurized devices — *see* Explosion, by type of device

S

Saturnism — *see* Table of Drugs and Chemicals, lead
Scald, scalding (accidental) (by) (from) (in) X19
air (hot) X14.1
gases (hot) X14.1
homicide (attempt) — *see* Assault, burning, hot object
inflicted by other person
    stated as intentional, homicide (attempt) — *see* Assault, burning, hot object
liquid (boiling) (hot) NEC X12
    stated as undetermined whether accidental or intentional Y27.2
    suicide (attempt) X77.2
local application of externally applied substance in medical or surgical care Y63.5
metal (molten) (liquid) (hot) NEC X18
self-inflicted X77.9
stated as undetermined whether accidental or intentional Y27.8
steam X13.1
    assault X98.0
    stated as undetermined whether accidental or intentional Y27.0
    suicide (attempt) X77.0
suicide (attempt) X77.9
vapor (hot) X13.1
    assault X98.0
    stated as undetermined whether accidental or intentional Y27.0
    suicide (attempt) X77.0
Scratched by
cat W55.03
person(s) (accidentally) W50.4
    with intent to injure or kill Y04.0
    as, or caused by, a crowd or human stampede (with fall) W52
    assault Y04.0
    homicide (attempt) Y04.0
    in
        fight Y04.0
        legal intervention
            injuring
                bystander Y35.892
                law enforcement personnel Y35.891
                suspect Y35.893
Seasickness T75.3
Self-harm NEC — *see also* External cause by type, undetermined whether accidental or intentional
intentional — *see* Suicide
poisoning NEC — *see* Table of Drugs and Chemicals, accident
Self-inflicted (injury) NEC — *see also* External cause by type, undetermined whether accidental or intentional
intentional — *see* Suicide
poisoning NEC — *see* Table of Drugs and Chemicals, accident
Sequelae (of)
accident NEC — *see* W00-X58 with 7th character S
assault (homicidal) (any means) — *see* X92-Y08 with 7th character S
homicide, attempt (any means) — *see* X92-Y08 with 7th character S

Sequelae (of) — *continued*
injury undetermined whether accidentally or purposely inflicted — *see* Y21-Y33 with 7th character S
intentional self-harm (classifiable to X71-X83) — *see* X71-X83 with 7th character S
legal intervention — *see* with 7th character S Y35
motor vehicle accident — *see* V00-V99 with 7th character S
suicide, attempt (any means) — *see* X71-X83 with 7th character S
transport accident — *see* V00-V99 with 7th character S
war operations — *see* War operations
Shock
electric — *see* Exposure, electric current
from electric appliance (any) (faulty) W86.8
    domestic W86.0
    suicide (attempt) X83.1
Shooting, shot (accidental(ly)) — *see also* Discharge, firearm, by type
herself or himself — *see* Discharge, firearm by type, self-inflicted
homicide (attempt) — *see* Discharge, firearm by type, homicide
in war operations — *see* War operations
inflicted by other person — *see* Discharge, firearm by type, homicide
    accidental — *see* Discharge, firearm, by type of firearm
legal
    execution — *see* Legal, intervention, firearm
    intervention — *see* Legal, intervention, firearm
self-inflicted — *see* Discharge, firearm by type, suicide
    accidental — *see* Discharge, firearm, by type of firearm
suicide (attempt) — *see* Discharge, firearm by type, suicide
Shoving (accidentally) by other person — *see* Pushed, by other person
Sickness
alpine W94.11
motion — *see* Motion
mountain W94.11
Sinking (accidental)
watercraft (causing drowning, submersion) — *see also* Drowning, due to, accident to, watercraft, sinking
causing injury except drowning or submersion — *see* Accident, watercraft, causing, injury NEC
Siriasis X32
Slashed wrists — *see* Cut, self-inflicted
Slipping (accidental) (on same level) (with fall) W01.0
on
    ice W00.0
        with skates — *see* Accident, transport, pedestrian, conveyance
    mud W01.0
    oil W01.0
    snow W00.0
        with skis — *see* Accident, transport, pedestrian, conveyance
    surface (slippery) (wet) NEC W01.0
without fall W18.40
    due to
        specified NEC W18.49
        stepping from one level to another W18.43
        stepping into hole or opening W18.42
        stepping on object W18.41
Sliver, wood, contact with W45.8
Smoldering (due to fire) — *see* Exposure, fire
Sodomy (attempted) by force T74.2-
Sound waves (causing injury) W42.9
supersonic W42.0
Splinter, contact with W45.8
Stab, stabbing — *see* Cut
Starvation X58
Status of external cause Y99.9
child assisting in compensated work for family Y99.8
civilian activity done for financial or other compensation Y99.0
civilian activity done for income or pay Y99.0
family member assisting in compensated work for other family member Y99.8
hobby not done for income Y99.8
leisure activity Y99.8
military activity Y99.1

Status of external cause — *continued*
off-duty activity of military personnel Y99.8
recreation or sport not for income or while a student Y99.8
specified NEC Y99.8
student activity Y99.8
volunteer activity Y99.2
Stepped on
by
    animal (not being ridden) NEC W55.89
    crowd or human stampede W52
    person W50.0
Stepping on
object W22.8
    with fall W18.31
    sports equipment W21.9
    stationary W22.09
        sports equipment W21.89
person W51
    by crowd or human stampede W52
    sports equipment W21.9
Sting
arthropod, nonvenomous W57
insect, nonvenomous W57
Storm (cataclysmic) — *see* Forces of nature, cataclysmic storm
Straining, excessive — *see* category Y93
Strangling — *see* Strangulation
Strangulation (accidental) — *see* category T71
Strenuous movements — *see* category Y93
Striking against
airbag (automobile) W22.10
    driver side W22.11
    front passenger side W22.12
    specified NEC W22.19
bottom when
    diving or jumping into water (in) W16.822
        causing drowning W16.821
    from boat W16.722
        causing drowning W16.721
    natural body W16.622
        causing drowning W16.821
    swimming pool W16.522
        causing drowning W16.521
    falling into water (in) W16.322
        causing drowning W16.321
    fountain — *see* Striking against, bottom when, falling into water, specified NEC
    natural body W16.122
        causing drowning W16.121
    reservoir — *see* Striking against, bottom when, falling into water, specified NEC
    specified NEC W16.322
        causing drowning W16.321
    swimming pool W16.022
        causing drowning W16.021
diving board (swimming pool) W21.4
object W22.8
    with
        drowning or submersion — *see* Drowning
        fall — *see* Fall, due to, bumping against, object
    caused by crowd or human stampede (with fall) W52
    furniture W22.03
    lamppost W22.02
    sports equipment W21.9
    stationary W22.09
        sports equipment W21.89
    wall W22.01
person(s) W51
    with fall W03
        due to ice or snow W00.0
    as, or caused by, a crowd or human stampede (with fall) W52
    assault Y04.2
    homicide (attempt) Y04.2
    sports equipment W21.9
wall (when) W22.01
    diving or jumping into water (in) W16.832
        causing drowning W16.831
        swimming pool W16.532
            causing drowning W16.531
    falling into water (in) W16.332
        causing drowning W16.331
    fountain — *see* Striking against, wall when, falling into water, specified NEC
    natural body W16.132
        causing drowning W16.131

EXTERNAL CAUSES

Striking against — *continued*
  wall (when) — *continued*
    falling into water (in) — *continued*
      reservoir — *see* Striking against, wall
        when, falling into water,
        specified NEC
      specified NEC W16.332
        causing drowning W16.331
      swimming pool W16.032
        causing drowning W16.031
    swimming pool (when) W22.042
      causing drowning W22.041
      diving or jumping into water W16.532
        causing drowning W16.531
      falling into water W16.032
        causing drowning W16.031
Struck (accidentally) by
  airbag (automobile) W22.10
    driver side W22.11
    front passenger side W22.12
    specified NEC W22.19
  alligator W58.02
  animal (not being ridden) NEC W55.89
  avalanche — *see* Landslide
  ball (hit) (thrown) W21.00
    assault Y08.09
    baseball W21.03
    basketball W21.05
    football W21.01
    golf ball W21.04
    soccer W21.02
    softball W21.07
    specified NEC W21.09
    volleyball W21.06
  bat or racquet
    baseball bat W21.11
      assault Y08.02
    golf club W21.13
      assault Y08.09
    specified NEC W21.19
      assault Y08.09
    tennis racquet W21.12
      assault Y08.09
  bullet — *see also* Discharge, firearm by
    type
    in war operations — *see* War operations
  crocodile W58.12
  dog W54.1
  flare, Very pistol — *see* Discharge, firearm
    NEC
  hailstones X39.8
  hockey (ice)
    field
      puck W21.221
      stick W21.211
    puck W21.220
    stick W21.210
      assault Y08.01
  landslide — *see* Landslide
  law-enforcement agent (on duty) — *see*
    Legal, intervention, manhandling
    with blunt object — *see* Legal,
      intervention, blunt object
  lightning — *see* subcategory T75.0
    causing fire — *see* Exposure, fire
  machine — *see* Contact, with, by type of
    machine
  mammal NEC W55.89
    marine W56.32
  marine animal W56.82
  missile
    firearm — *see* Discharge, firearm by
      type
    in war operations — *see* War operations,
      missile
  object W22.8
    blunt W22.8
      assault Y00
      suicide (attempt) X79
      undetermined whether accidental or
        intentional Y29
    falling W20.8
      from, in, on
        building W20.1
          burning (uncontrolled fire)
            X00.4
        cataclysmic
          earth surface movement NEC —
            see Landslide
          storm — *see* Forces of nature,
            cataclysmic storm
        cave-in W20.0
        earthquake X34
        machine (in operation) — *see*
          Contact, with, by type of
          machine
        structure W20.1
          burning X00.4

Struck (accidentally) by — *continued*
  object — *continued*
    falling — *continued*
      from, in, on — *continued*
        transport vehicle (in motion) — *see*
          Accident, transport, by type of
          vehicle
        watercraft V93.49
          due to
            accident to craft V91.39
              powered craft V91.33
                ferry boat V91.31
                fishing boat V91.32
                jetskis V91.33
                liner V91.31
                merchant ship V91.30
                passenger ship V91.31
             unpowered craft V91.38
                canoe V91.35
                inflatable V91.36
                kayak V91.35
                sailboat V91.34
                surfboard V91.38
                windsurfer V91.38
            powered craft V93.43
              ferry boat V93.41
              fishing boat V93.42
              jetskis V93.43
              liner V93.41
              merchant ship V93.40
              passenger ship V93.41
            unpowered craft V93.48
              sailboat V93.44
              surfboard V93.48
              windsurfer V93.48
    moving NEC W20.8
    projected W20.8
      assault Y00
      in sports W21.9
        assault Y08.09
      ball W21.00
        baseball W21.03
        basketball W21.05
        football W21.01
        golf ball W21.04
        soccer W21.02
        softball W21.07
        specified NEC W21.09
        volleyball W21.06
      bat or racquet
        baseball bat W21.11
          assault Y08.02
        golf club W21.13
          assault Y08.09
        specified NEC W21.19
          assault Y08.09
        tennis racquet W21.12
          assault Y08.09
      hockey (ice)
        field
          puck W21.221
          stick W21.211
        puck W21.220
        stick W21.210
          assault Y08.01
      specified NEC W21.89
    set in motion by explosion — *see*
      Explosion
    thrown W20.8
      assault Y00
      in sports W21.9
        assault Y08.09
      ball W21.00
        baseball W21.03
        basketball W21.05
        football W21.01
        golf ball W21.04
        soccer W21.02
        soft ball W21.07
        specified NEC W21.09
        volleyball W21.06
      bat or racquet
        baseball bat W21.11
          assault Y08.02
        golf club W21.13
          assault Y08.09
        specified NEC W21.19
          assault Y08.09
        tennis racquet W21.12
          assault Y08.09
      hockey (ice)
        field
          puck W21.221
          stick W21.211
        puck W21.220
        stick W21.210
          assault Y08.01
      specified NEC W21.89

Struck (accidentally) by — *continued*
  other person(s) W50.0
    with
      blunt object W22.8
        intentional, homicide (attempt) Y00
        sports equipment W21.9
        undetermined whether accidental or
          intentional Y29
    fall W03
      due to ice or snow W00.0
    as, or caused by, a crowd or human
      stampede (with fall) W52
    assault Y04.2
    homicide (attempt) Y04.2
    in legal intervention
      injuring
        bystander Y35.812
        law enforcement personnel
          Y35.811
        suspect Y35.813
  police (on duty) — *see* Legal, intervention,
    manhandling
    with blunt object — *see* Legal,
      intervention, blunt object
  sports equipment W21.9
    assault Y08.09
    ball W21.00
      baseball W21.03
      basketball W21.05
      football W21.01
      golf ball W21.04
      soccer W21.02
      soft ball W21.07
      specified NEC W21.09
      volleyball W21.06
    bat or racquet
      baseball bat W21.11
        assault Y08.02
      golf club W21.13
        assault Y08.09
      specified NEC W21.19
        assault Y08.09
      tennis racquet W21.12
        assault Y08.09
    cleats (shoe) W21.31
    foot wear NEC W21.39
    football helmet W21.81
    hockey (ice)
      field
        puck W21.221
        stick W21.211
      puck W21.220
      stick W21.210
        assault Y08.01
    skate blades W21.32
    specified NEC W21.89
      assault Y08.09
  thunderbolt — *see* subcategory T75.0
    causing fire — *see* Exposure, fire
  transport vehicle NEC (*see also* Accident,
    transport) V09.9
    intentional, homicide (attempt) Y03.0
    motor NEC (*see also* Accident,
      transport) V09.20
      homicide V03.0
  vehicle (transport) NEC — *see* Accident,
    transport, by type of vehicle
    stationary (falling from jack, hydraulic
      lift, ramp) W20.8
Stumbling
  over
    animal NEC W01.0
      with fall W18.09
    carpet, rug or (small) object W22.8
      with fall W18.09
    person W51
      with fall W03
        due to ice or snow W00.0
  without fall W18.40
    due to
      specified NEC W18.49
      stepping from one level to another
        W18.43
      stepping into hole or opening W18.42
      stepping on object W18.41
Submersion (accidental) — *see* Drowning
Suffocation (accidental) (by external means)
  (by pressure) (mechanical) (*see also*
  category) T71
  due to, by
    avalanche — *see* Landslide
    explosion — *see* Explosion
    fire — *see* Exposure, fire
    food, any type (aspiration) (ingestion)
      (inhalation) — *see* categories T17
      and T18
    ignition — *see* Ignition
    landslide — *see* Landslide

Suffocation (accidental) (by external means)
  (by pressure) (mechanical) (*see also*
  category) — *continued*
  due to, by — *continued*
    machine(ry) — *see* Contact, with, by
      type of machine
    vomitus (aspiration) (inhalation) T17.81-
      in
      burning building X00.8
Suicide, suicidal (attempted) (by) X83.8
  blunt object X79
  burning, burns X76
    hot object X77.9
      fluid NEC X77.2
      household appliance X77.3
      specified NEC X77.8
      steam X77.0
      tap water X77.1
      vapors X77.0
  caustic substance — *see* Table of Drugs
    and Chemicals
  cold, extreme X83.2
  collision of motor vehicle with
    motor vehicle X82.0
    specified NEC X82.8
    train X82.1
    tree X82.2
  crashing of aircraft X83.0
  cut (any part of body) X78.9
  cutting or piercing instrument X78.9
    dagger X78.2
    glass X78.0
    knife X78.1
    specified NEC X78.8
    sword X78.2
  drowning (in) X71.9
    bathtub X71.0
    natural water X71.3
    specified NEC X71.8
    swimming pool X71.1
      following fall X71.2
  electrocution X83.1
  explosive(s) (material) X75
  fire, flames X76
  firearm X74.9
    airgun X74.01
    handgun X72
    hunting rifle X73.1
    larger X73.9
      specified NEC X73.8
    machine gun X73.2
    shotgun X73.0
    specified NEC X74.8
  hanging X83.8
  hot object — *see* Suicide, burning, hot
    object
  jumping
    before moving object X81.8
      motor vehicle X81.0
      subway train X81.1
      train X81.1
    from high place X80
  late effect of attempt — *see* X71-X83 with
    7th character S
  lying before moving object, train, vehicle
    X81.8
  poisoning — *see* Table of Drugs and
    Chemicals
  puncture (any part of body) — *see* Suicide,
    cutting or piercing instrument
  scald — *see* Suicide, burning, hot object
  sequelae of attempt — *see* X71-X83 with
    7th character S
  sharp object (any) — *see* Suicide, cutting
    or piercing instrument
  shooting — *see* Suicide, firearm
  specified means NEC X83.8
  stab (any part of body) — *see* Suicide,
    cutting or piercing instrument
  steam, hot vapors X77.0
  strangulation X83.8
  submersion — *see* Suicide, drowning
  suffocation X83.8
  wound NEC X83.8
Sunstroke X32
Supersonic waves (causing injury) W42.0
Surgical procedure, complication of
  (delayed or as an abnormal reaction
    without mention of misadventure) — *see*
    also Complication of or following, by
    type of procedure
  due to or as a result of misadventure — *see*
    Misadventure

Swallowed, swallowing
  foreign body — *see* Foreign body,
    alimentary canal
  poison — *see* Table of Drugs and
    Chemicals
  substance
    caustic or corrosive — *see* Table of
      Drugs and Chemicals
    poisonous — *see* Table of Drugs and
      Chemicals

T

Tackle in sport W03
Terrorism (involving) Y38.80
  biological weapons Y38.6x-
  chemical weapons Y38.7x-
  conflagration Y38.3x-
  drowning and submersion Y38.89-
  explosion Y38.2x-
    destruction of aircraft Y38.1x-
    marine weapons Y38.0x-
  fire Y38.3x-
  firearms Y38.4x-
  hot substances Y38.5x-
  lasers Y38.89-
  nuclear weapons Y38.5x-
  piercing or stabbing instruments Y38.89-
  secondary effects Y38.9x-
  specified method NEC Y38.89-
  suicide bomber Y38.81-
Thirst X58
Threat to breathing
  aspiration — *see* Aspiration
  due to cave-in, falling earth or substance
    NEC — *see* category T71
Thrown (accidentally)
  against part (any) of or object in transport
    vehicle (in motion) NEC — *see also*
    Accident, transport
  from
    high place, homicide (attempt) Y01
    machinery — *see* Contact, with, by type
      of machine
    transport vehicle NEC (*see also*
      Accident, transport) V89.9
  off — *see* Thrown, from
Thunderbolt — *see* subcategory T75.0
  causing fire — *see* Exposure, fire
Tidal wave (any injury) NEC — *see* Forces
  of nature, tidal wave
Took
  overdose (drug) — *see* Table of Drugs and
    Chemicals
  poison — *see* Table of Drugs and
    Chemicals
Tornado (any injury) X37.1
Torrential rain (any injury) X37.8
Torture X58
Trampled by animal NEC W55.89
Trapped (accidentally)
  between objects (moving) (stationary and
    moving) — *see* Caught
  by part (any) of
    motorcycle V29.88
    pedal cycle V19.88
    transport vehicle NEC (*see also*
      Accident, transport) V89.9
Travel (effects) (sickness) T75.3
Tree falling on or hitting (accidentally)
  (person) W20.8
Tripping
  over
    animal W01.0
      with fall W01.0
    carpet, rug or (small) object W22.8
      with fall W18.09
    person W51
      with fall W03
        due to ice or snow W00.0
    without fall W18.40
      due to
        specified NEC W18.49
        stepping from one level to another
          W18.43
        stepping into hole or opening W18.42
        stepping on object W18.41
Twisted by person(s) (accidentally) W50.2
  with intent to injure or kill Y04.0
  as, or caused by, a crowd or human
    stampede (with fall) W52
  assault Y04.0
  homicide (attempt) Y04.0
  in
    fight Y04.0
    legal intervention — *see* Legal,
      intervention, manhandling
Twisting, excessive — *see* category Y93

U

Underdosing of necessary drugs,
  medicaments or biological substances
  Y63.6
Undetermined intent (contact) (exposure)
  automobile collision Y32
  blunt object Y29
  drowning (submersion) (in) Y21.9
    bathtub Y21.0
      after fall Y21.1
    natural water (lake) (ocean) (pond)
      (river) (stream) Y21.4
    specified place NEC Y21.8
    swimming pool Y21.2
      after fall Y21.3
  explosive material Y25
  fall, jump or push from high place Y30
  falling, lying or running before moving
    object Y31
  fire Y26
  firearm discharge Y24.9
    airgun (BB) (pellet) Y24.0
    handgun (pistol) (revolver) Y22
    hunting rifle Y23.1
    larger Y23.9
      hunting rifle Y23.1
      machine gun Y23.3
      military Y23.2
      shotgun Y23.0
      specified type NEC Y23.8
    machine gun Y23.3
    military Y23.2
    shotgun Y23.0
    specified type NEC Y24.8
    Very pistol Y24.8
  hot object Y27.9
    fluid NEC Y27.2
    household appliance Y27.3
    specified object NEC Y27.8
    steam Y27.0
    tap water Y27.1
    vapor Y27.0
  jump, fall or push from high place Y30
  lying, falling or running before moving
    object Y31
  motor vehicle crash Y32
  push, fall or jump from high place Y30
  running, falling or lying before moving
    object Y31
  sharp object Y28.9
    dagger Y28.2
    glass Y28.0
    knife Y28.1
    specified object NEC Y28.8
    sword Y28.2
  smoke Y26
  specified event NEC Y33

V

Vibration (causing injury) W49.9
Victim (of)
  avalanche — *see* Landslide
  earth movements NEC — *see* Forces of
    nature, earth movement
  earthquake X34
  flood — *see* Flood
  landslide — *see* Landslide
  lightning — *see* subcategory T75.0
    causing fire — *see* Exposure, fire
  storm (cataclysmic) NEC — *see* Forces of
    nature, cataclysmic storm
  volcanic eruption X35
Volcanic eruption (any injury) X35
Vomitus, gastric contents in air passages
  (with asphyxia, obstruction or
  suffocation) T17.81-

EXTERNAL CAUSES

W

EXTERNAL CAUSES

Walked into stationary object (any) W22.09
  furniture W22.03
  lamppost W22.02
  wall W22.01
War operations (injuries to military
    personnel and civilians during war, civil
    insurrection and peacekeeping missions)
    (by) (from) (involving) Y36.90
  after cessation of hostilities Y36.89-
    explosion (of)
      bomb placed during war operations
        Y36.82-
      mine placed during war operations
        Y36.81-
    specified NEC Y36.88-
  air blast Y36.20-
  aircraft
    destruction — *see* War operations,
        destruction of aircraft
  airway restriction — *see* War operations,
        restriction of airways
  asphyxiation — *see* War operations,
        restriction of airways
  biological weapons Y36.6x-
  blast Y36.20-
  blast fragments Y36.20-
  blast wave Y36.20-
  blast wind Y36.20-
  bomb Y36.20-
    dirty Y36.50-
    gasoline Y36.31-
    incendiary Y36.31-
    petrol Y36.31-
  bullet Y36.43-
    incendiary Y36.32-
    rubber Y36.41-
  chemical weapons Y36.7x-
  combat
    hand to hand (unarmed) combat Y36.44-
    using blunt or piercing object Y36.45-
  conflagration — *see* War operations, fire
  conventional warfare NEC Y36.49-
  depth-charge Y36.01-
  destruction of aircraft Y36.10-
    due to
      air to air missile Y36.11-
      collision with other aircraft Y36.12-
      detonation (accidental) of onboard
          munitions and explosives
          Y36.14-
      enemy fire or explosives Y36.11-
      explosive placed on aircraft Y36.11-
      onboard fire Y36.13-
      rocket propelled grenade [RPG]
          Y36.11-
      small arms fire Y36.11-
      surface to air missile Y36.11-
    specified NEC Y36.19-
  detonation (accidental) of
    onboard marine weapons Y36.05-
    own munitions or munitions launch
        device Y36.24-
  dirty bomb Y36.50-
  explosion (of) Y36.20-
    aerial bomb Y36.21-
    after cessation of hostilities
      bomb placed during war operations
        Y36.82-
      mine placed during war operations
        Y36.81-
    bomb NOS (*see also* War operations,
        bomb(s)) Y36.20-
    fragments Y36.20-
    grenade Y36.29-
    guided missile Y36.22-
    improvised explosive device [IED]
        (person-borne) (roadside) (vehicle-
        borne) Y36.23-
    land mine Y36.29-
    marine mine (at sea) (in harbor) Y36.02-
    marine weapon Y36.00-
      specified NEC Y36.09-
    own munitions or munitions launch
        device (accidental) Y36.24-
    sea-based artillery shell Y36.03-
    specified NEC Y36.29-
    torpedo Y36.04-

War operations (injuries to military
    personnel and civilians during war, civil
    insurrection and peacekeeping missions)
    (by) (from) (involving) — *continued*
  fire Y36.30-
    specified NEC Y36.39-
  firearms
    discharge Y36.43-
    pellets Y36.42-
  flamethrower Y36.33-
  fragments (from) (of)
    improvised explosive device [IED]
        (person-borne) (roadside) (vehicle-
        borne) Y36.26-
    munitions Y36.25-
    specified NEC Y36.29-
    weapons Y36.27-
  friendly fire Y36.92
  hand to hand (unarmed) combat Y36.44-
  hot substances — *see* War operations, fire
  incendiary bullet Y36.32-
  nuclear weapon (effects of) Y36.50-
    acute radiation exposure Y36.54-
    blast pressure Y36.51-
    direct blast Y36.51-
    direct heat Y36.53-
    fallout exposure Y36.54-
    fireball Y36.53-
    indirect blast (struck or crushed by blast
        debris) (being thrown by blast)
        Y36.52-
    ionizing radiation (immediate exposure)
        Y36.54-
    nuclear radiation Y36.54-
    radiation
      ionizing (immediate exposure)
          Y36.54-
      nuclear Y36.54-
      thermal Y36.53-
    secondary effects Y36.54-
    specified NEC Y36.59-
    thermal radiation Y36.53-
  restriction of air (airway)
    intentional Y36.46-
    unintentional Y36.47-
  rubber bullets Y36.41-
  shrapnel NOS Y36.29-
  suffocation — *see* War operations,
      restriction of airways
  unconventional warfare NEC Y36.7x-
  underwater blast NOS Y36.00-
  warfare
    conventional NEC Y36.49-
    unconventional NEC Y36.7x-
  weapon of mass destruction [WMD]
      Y36.91
  weapons
    biological weapons Y36.6x-
    chemical Y36.7x-
    nuclear (effects of) Y36.50-
      acute radiation exposure Y36.54-
      blast pressure Y36.51-
      direct blast Y36.51-
      direct heat Y36.53-
      fallout exposure Y36.54-
      fireball Y36.53-
      radiation
        ionizing (immediate exposure)
            Y36.54-
        nuclear Y36.54-
        thermal Y36.53-
      secondary effects Y36.54-
      specified NEC Y36.59-
    of mass destruction [WMD] Y36.91
Washed
  away by flood — *see* Flood
  off road by storm (transport vehicle) — *see*
      Forces of nature, cataclysmic storm
Weather exposure NEC — *see* Forces of
    nature
Weightlessness (causing injury) (effects of)
    (in spacecraft, real or simulated) X52
Work related condition Y99.0
Wound (accidental) NEC (*see also* Injury)
    X58
  battle (*see also* War operations) Y36.90
  gunshot — *see* Discharge, firearm by type
Wreck transport vehicle NEC (*see also*
    Accident, transport) V89.9
Wrong
  device implanted into correct surgical site
      Y65.51
  fluid in infusion Y65.1
  patient, procedure performed on Y65.52
  procedure (operation) on correct patient
      Y65.51

X

Y

Z

Chapter 1 – Certain infectious and parasitic diseases (A00-B99)

Includes: Diseases generally recognized as communicable or transmissible

Use additional code to identify resistance to antimicrobial drugs (Z16.-)

Excludes 1: *certain localized infections — see body system, related chapters*

Excludes ❷: *carrier or suspected carrier of infectious disease (Z22-)*
infectious and parasitic diseases complicating pregnancy, childbirth and the puerperium (O98.-)
infectious and parasitic diseases specific to the perinatal period (P35-P39)
influenza and other acute respiratory infections (J00-J22)

This chapter contains the following blocks:

A00-A09	Intestinal infectious diseases
A15-A19	Tuberculosis
A20-A28	Certain zoonotic bacterial diseases
A30-A49	Other bacterial diseases
A50-A64	Infections with a predominantly sexual mode of transmission
A65-A69	Other spirochetal diseases
A70-A74	Other diseases caused by chlamydiae
A75-A79	Rickettsioses
A80-A89	Viral and prion infections of the central nervous system
A90-A99	Arthropod-borne viral fevers and viral hemorrhagic fevers
B00-B09	Viral infections characterized by skin and mucous membrane lesions
B10	Other human herpesviruses
B15-B19	Viral hepatitis
B20	Human immunodeficiency virus [HIV] disease
B25-B34	Other viral diseases
B35-B49	Mycoses
B50-B64	Protozoal diseases
B65-B83	Helminthiases
B85-B89	Pediculosis, acariasis and other infestations
B90-B94	Sequelae of infectious and parasitic diseases
B95-B97	Bacterial and viral infectious agents
B99	Other infectious diseases

Intestinal infectious diseases (A00-A09)

A00- Cholera
A00.0   **Cholera due to Vibrio cholerae 01, biovar cholerae**
Classical cholera
A00.1   **Cholera due to Vibrio cholerae 01, biovar el tor**
Cholera el tor
A00.9   **Cholera, unspecified**

A01- Typhoid and paratyphoid fevers
A01.0- Typhoid fever
Infection due to Salmonella typhi
A01.00 **Typhoid fever, unspecified**
A01.01 **Typhoid meningitis**
A01.02 **Typhoid fever with heart involvement**
Typhoid endocarditis
Typhoid myocarditis
A01.03 **Typhoid pneumonia**
A01.04 **Typhoid arthritis**
A01.05 **Typhoid osteomyelitis**
A01.09 **Typhoid fever with other complications**
A01.1   **Paratyphoid fever A**
A01.2   **Paratyphoid fever B**
A01.3   **Paratyphoid fever C**
A01.4   **Paratyphoid fever, unspecified**
Infection due to Salmonella paratyphi NOS

A02- Other salmonella infections
Includes: Infection or foodborne intoxication due to any Salmonella species other than S. typhi and S. paratyphi
A02.0   **Salmonella enteritis**
Salmonellosis
A02.1   **Salmonella sepsis**
A02.2- Localized salmonella infections
A02.20 **Localized salmonella infection, unspecified**
A02.21 **Salmonella meningitis**
A02.22 **Salmonella pneumonia**
A02.23 **Salmonella arthritis**
A02.24 **Salmonella osteomyelitis**

A02.25 **Salmonella pyelonephritis**
Salmonella tubulo-interstitial nephropathy
A02.29 **Salmonella with other localized infection**
A02.8   **Other specified salmonella infections**
A02.9   **Salmonella infection, unspecified**

A03- Shigellosis
A03.0   **Shigellosis due to Shigella dysenteriae**
Group A shigellosis [Shiga-Kruse dysentery]
A03.1   **Shigellosis due to Shigella flexneri**
Group B shigellosis
A03.2   **Shigellosis due to Shigella boydii**
Group C shigellosis
A03.3   **Shigellosis due to Shigella sonnei**
Group D shigellosis
A03.8   **Other shigellosis**
A03.9   **Shigellosis, unspecified**
Bacillary dysentery NOS

A04- Other bacterial intestinal infections
Excludes 1: *bacterial foodborne intoxications, NEC (A05.-)*
tuberculous enteritis (A18.32)
A04.0   **Enteropathogenic Escherichia coli infection**
A04.1   **Enterotoxigenic Escherichia coli infection**
A04.2   **Enteroinvasive Escherichia coli infection**
A04.3   **Enterohemorrhagic Escherichia coli infection**
A04.4   **Other intestinal Escherichia coli infections**
Escherichia coli enteritis NOS
A04.5   **Campylobacter enteritis**
A04.6   **Enteritis due to Yersinia enterocolitica**
Excludes 1: *extraintestinal yersiniosis (A28.2)*
A04.7   **Enterocolitis due to Clostridium difficile**
Foodborne intoxication by Clostridium difficile
Pseudomembraneous colitis
A04.8   **Other specified bacterial intestinal infections**
A04.9   **Bacterial intestinal infection, unspecified**
Bacterial enteritis NOS

A05- Other bacterial foodborne intoxications, not elsewhere classified
Excludes 1: *Clostridium difficile foodborne intoxication and infection (A04.7)*
Escherichia coli infection (A04.0-A04.4)
listeriosis (A32.-)
salmonella foodborne intoxication and infection (A02.-)
toxic effect of noxious foodstuffs (T61-T62)
A05.0   **Foodborne staphylococcal intoxication**
A05.1   **Botulism food poisoning**
Botulism NOS
Classical foodborne intoxication due to Clostridium botulinum
Excludes 1: *infant botulism (A48.51)*
wound botulism (A48.52)
A05.2   **Foodborne Clostridium perfringens [Clostridium welchii] intoxication**
Enteritis necroticans
Pig-bel
A05.3   **Foodborne Vibrio parahaemolyticus intoxication**
A05.4   **Foodborne Bacillus cereus intoxication**
A05.5   **Foodborne Vibrio vulnificus intoxication**
A05.8   **Other specified bacterial foodborne intoxications**
A05.9   **Bacterial foodborne intoxication, unspecified**

Excludes 1: = NOT CODED HERE! (Do not code both)

Excludes ❷: = Not Included Here

A06-   Amebiasis
Includes: Infection due to Entamoeba histolytica
Excludes 1:   other protozoal intestinal diseases (A07.-)
Excludes ❷: acanthamebiasis (B60.1-)
Naegleriasis (B60.2)

A06.0   Acute amebic dysentery
Acute amebiasis
Intestinal amebiasis NOS

A06.1   Chronic intestinal amebiasis

A06.2   Amebic nondysenteric colitis

A06.3   Ameboma of intestine
Ameboma NOS

A06.4   Amebic liver abscess
Hepatic amebiasis

A06.5   Amebic lung abscess
Amebic abscess of lung (and liver)

A06.6   Amebic brain abscess
Amebic abscess of brain (and liver) (and lung)

A06.7   Cutaneous amebiasis

A06.8-   Amebic infection of other sites

A06.81   Amebic cystitis

A06.82   Other amebic genitourinary infections
Amebic balanitis
Amebic vesiculitis
Amebic vulvovaginitis

A06.89   Other amebic infections
Amebic appendicitis
Amebic splenic abscess

A06.9   Amebiasis, unspecified

A07-   Other protozoal intestinal diseases

A07.0   Balantidiasis
Balantidial dysentery

A07.1   Giardiasis [lambliasis]

A07.2   Cryptosporidiosis

A07.3   Isosporiasis
Infection due to Isospora belli and Isospora hominis
Intestinal coccidiosis
Isosporosis

A07.4   Cyclosporiasis

A07.8   Other specified protozoal intestinal diseases
Intestinal microsporidiosis
Intestinal trichomoniasis
Sarcocystosis
Sarcosporidiosis

A07.9   Protozoal intestinal disease, unspecified
Flagellate diarrhea
Protozoal colitis
Protozoal diarrhea
Protozoal dysentery

A08-   Viral and other specified intestinal infections
Excludes 1:   influenza with involvement of gastrointestinal tract (J09.X3, J10.2, J11.2)

A08.0   Rotaviral enteritis

A08.1-   Acute gastroenteropathy due to Norwalk agent and other small round viruses

A08.11   Acute gastroenteropathy due to Norwalk agent
Acute gastroenteropathy due to Norovirus
Acute gastroenteropathy due to Norwalk-like agent

A08.19   Acute gastroenteropathy due to other small round viruses
Acute gastroenteropathy due to small round virus [SRV] NOS

A08.2   Adenoviral enteritis

A08.3-   Other viral enteritis

A08.31   Calicivirus enteritis

A08.32   Astrovirus enteritis

A08.39   Other viral enteritis
Coxsackie virus enteritis
Echovirus enteritis
Enterovirus enteritis NEC
Torovirus enteritis

A08.4   Viral intestinal infection, unspecified
Viral enteritis NOS
Viral gastroenteritis NOS
Viral gastroenteropathy NOS

A08.8   Other specified intestinal infections

A09   Infectious gastroenteritis and colitis, unspecified
Infectious colitis NOS
Infectious enteritis NOS
Infectious gastroenteritis NOS
Excludes 1:   colitis NOS (K52.9)
diarrhea NOS (R19.7)
enteritis NOS (K52.9)
gastroenteritis NOS (K52.9)
noninfective gastroenteritis and colitis, unspecified (K52.9)

Tuberculosis (A15-A19)

Includes: Infections due to Mycobacterium tuberculosis and
Mycobacterium bovis
Excludes 1:   congenital tuberculosis (P37.0)
nonspecific reaction to test for tuberculosis without active tuberculosis (R76.1-)
pneumoconiosis associated with tuberculosis, any type in A15 (J65)
positive PPD (R76.11)
positive tuberculin skin test without active tuberculosis (R76.11)
sequelae of tuberculosis (B90.-)
silicotuberculosis (J65)

A15-   Respiratory tuberculosis

A15.0   Tuberculosis of lung
Tuberculous bronchiectasis
Tuberculous fibrosis of lung
Tuberculous pneumonia
Tuberculous pneumothorax

A15.4   Tuberculosis of intrathoracic lymph nodes
Tuberculosis of hilar lymph nodes
Tuberculosis of mediastinal lymph nodes
Tuberculosis of tracheobronchial lymph nodes
Excludes 1:   tuberculosis specified as primary (A15.7)

A15.5   Tuberculosis of larynx, trachea and bronchus
Tuberculosis of bronchus
Tuberculosis of glottis
Tuberculosis of larynx
Tuberculosis of trachea

A15.6   Tuberculous pleurisy
Tuberculosis of pleura Tuberculous empyema
Excludes 1:   primary respiratory tuberculosis (A15.7)

A15.7   Primary respiratory tuberculosis

A15.8   Other respiratory tuberculosis
Mediastinal tuberculosis
Nasopharyngeal tuberculosis
Tuberculosis of nose
Tuberculosis of sinus [any nasal]

A15.9   Respiratory tuberculosis unspecified

A17-   Tuberculosis of nervous system

A17.0   Tuberculous meningitis
Tuberculosis of meninges (cerebral) (spinal)
Tuberculous leptomeningitis
Excludes 1:   tuberculous meningoencephalitis (A17.82)

A17.1   Meningeal tuberculoma
Tuberculoma of meninges (cerebral) (spinal)
Excludes ❷: tuberculoma of brain and spinal cord (A17.81)

A17.8-   Other tuberculosis of nervous system

A17.81   Tuberculoma of brain and spinal cord
Tuberculous abscess of brain and spinal cord

A17.82   Tuberculous meningoencephalitis
Tuberculous myelitis

A17.83   Tuberculous neuritis
Tuberculous mononeuropathy

A17.89   Other tuberculosis of nervous system
Tuberculous polyneuropathy

A17.9   Tuberculosis of nervous system, unspecified

A18-   Tuberculosis of other organs

A18.0-   Tuberculosis of bones and joints

A18.01   Tuberculosis of spine
Pott's disease or curvature of spine
Tuberculous arthritis
Tuberculous osteomyelitis of spine
Tuberculous spondylitis

A18.02   Tuberculous arthritis of other joints
Tuberculosis of hip (joint)
Tuberculosis of knee (joint)

A18.03   Tuberculosis of other bones
Tuberculous mastoiditis
Tuberculous osteomyelitis

A 0 6 - A 2 4

A18.09   Other musculoskeletal tuberculosis
  Tuberculous myositis
  Tuberculous synovitis
  Tuberculous tenosynovitis

A18.1- Tuberculosis of <u>genitourinary</u> system

  A18.10   Tuberculosis of genitourinary system, unspecified

  A18.11   Tuberculosis of kidney and ureter

  A18.12   Tuberculosis of bladder

  A18.13   Tuberculosis of other urinary organs
    Tuberculous urethritis

  A18.14   Tuberculosis of prostate

  A18.15   Tuberculosis of other male genital organs

  A18.16   Tuberculosis of cervix

  A18.17   Tuberculous female pelvic inflammatory disease
    Tuberculous endometritis
    Tuberculous oophoritis and salpingitis

  A18.18   Tuberculosis of other female genital organs
    Tuberculous ulceration of vulva

A18.2   Tuberculous peripheral <u>lymphadenopathy</u>
  Tuberculous adenitis
  Excludes❷: tuberculosis of bronchial and mediastinal lymph nodes
          (A15.4)
       tuberculosis of mesenteric and retroperitoneal lymph
          nodes (A18.39)
       tuberculous tracheobronchial adenopathy (A15.4)

A18.3- Tuberculosis of <u>intestines</u>, peritoneum and mesenteric glands

  A18.31   Tuberculous peritonitis
    Tuberculous ascites

  A18.32   Tuberculous enteritis
    Tuberculosis of anus and rectum
    Tuberculosis of intestine (large) (small)

  A18.39   Retroperitoneal tuberculosis
    Tuberculosis of mesenteric glands
    Tuberculosis of retroperitoneal (lymph glands)

A18.4   Tuberculosis of <u>skin</u> and subcutaneous tissue
  Erythema induratum, tuberculous
  Lupus excedens
  Lupus vulgaris NOS
  Lupus vulgaris of eyelid
  Scrofuloderma
  Tuberculosis of external ear
  Excludes❷: lupus erythematosus (L93.-)
       lupus NOS (M32.9)
       systemic (M32.-)

A18.5- Tuberculosis of <u>eye</u>
  Excludes❷: lupus vulgaris of eyelid (A18.4)

  A18.50   Tuberculosis of eye, unspecified

  A18.51   Tuberculous episcleritis

  A18.52   Tuberculous keratitis
    Tuberculous interstitial keratitis
    Tuberculous keratoconjunctivitis (interstitial) (phlyctenular)

  A18.53   Tuberculous chorioretinitis

  A18.54   Tuberculous iridocyclitis

  A18.59   Other tuberculosis of eye
    Tuberculous conjunctivitis

A18.6   Tuberculosis of (inner) (middle) <u>ear</u>
  Tuberculous otitis media
  Excludes❷: tuberculosis of external ear (A18.4)
       tuberculous mastoiditis (A18.03)

A18.7   Tuberculosis of <u>adrenal</u> glands
  Tuberculous Addison's disease

A18.8- Tuberculosis of <u>other specified</u> organs

  A18.81   Tuberculosis of thyroid gland

  A18.82   Tuberculosis of other endocrine glands
    Tuberculosis of pituitary gland
    Tuberculosis of thymus gland

  A18.83   Tuberculosis of digestive tract organs, not elsewhere classified
    Excludes 1: tuberculosis of intestine (A18.32)

  A18.84   Tuberculosis of heart
    Tuberculous cardiomyopathy
    Tuberculous endocarditis
    Tuberculous myocarditis
    Tuberculous pericarditis

  A18.85   Tuberculosis of spleen

  A18.89   Tuberculosis of other sites
    Tuberculosis of muscle
    Tuberculous cerebral arteritis

A19- <u>Miliary</u> tuberculosis
  Includes: Disseminated tuberculosis
         Generalized tuberculosis
         Tuberculous polyserositis

  A19.0   Acute miliary tuberculosis of a single specified site

  A19.1   Acute miliary tuberculosis of multiple sites

  A19.2   Acute miliary tuberculosis, unspecified

  A19.8   Other miliary tuberculosis

  A19.9   Miliary tuberculosis, unspecified

Certain zoonotic bacterial diseases (A20-A28)

A20- <u>Plague</u>
  Includes: Infection due to Yersinia pestis

  A20.0   Bubonic plague

  A20.1   Cellulocutaneous plague

  A20.2   Pneumonic plague

  A20.3   Plague meningitis

  A20.7   Septicemic plague

  A20.8   Other forms of plague
    Abortive plague
    Asymptomatic plague
    Pestis minor

  A20.9   Plague, unspecified

A21- <u>Tularemia</u>
  Includes: Deer-fly fever
         Infection due to Francisella tularensis
         Rabbit fever

  A21.0   Ulceroglandular tularemia

  A21.1   Oculoglandular tularemia
    Ophthalmic tularemia

  A21.2   Pulmonary tularemia

  A21.3   Gastrointestinal tularemia
    Abdominal tularemia

  A21.7   Generalized tularemia

  A21.8   Other forms of tularemia

  A21.9   Tularemia, unspecified

A22- <u>Anthrax</u>
  Includes: Infection due to Bacillus anthracis

  A22.0   Cutaneous anthrax
    Malignant carbuncle
    Malignant pustule

  A22.1   Pulmonary anthrax
    Inhalation anthrax
    Ragpicker's disease
    Woolsorter's disease

  A22.2   Gastrointestinal anthrax

  A22.7   Anthrax sepsis

  A22.8   Other forms of anthrax
    Anthrax meningitis

  A22.9   Anthrax, unspecified

A23- <u>Brucellosis</u>
  Includes: Malta fever
         Mediterranean fever
         Undulant fever

  A23.0   Brucellosis due to Brucella melitensis

  A23.1   Brucellosis due to Brucella abortus

  A23.2   Brucellosis due to Brucella suis

  A23.3   Brucellosis due to Brucella canis

  A23.8   Other brucellosis

  A23.9   Brucellosis, unspecified

A24- Glanders and melioidosis

  A24.0   Glanders
    Infection due to Pseudomonas mallei
    Malleus

  A24.1   Acute and fulminating melioidosis
    Melioidosis pneumonia
    Melioidosis sepsis

  A24.2   Subacute and chronic melioidosis

  A24.3   Other melioidosis

  A24.9   Melioidosis, unspecified
    Infection due to Pseudomonas pseudomallei NOS
    Whitmore's disease

A
0
6
I
A
2
4

Excludes 1: = NOT CODED HERE! (Do not code both)   **335**   *Excludes❷:* = Not Included Here

A25- Rat-bite fevers

A25.0 Spirillosis
Sodoku

A25.1 Streptobacillosis
Epidemic arthritic erythema
Haverhill fever
Streptobacillary rat-bite fever

A25.9 Rat-bite fever, unspecified

A26- Erysipeloid

A26.0 Cutaneous erysipeloid
Erythema migrans

A26.7 Erysipelothrix sepsis

A26.8 Other forms of erysipeloid

A26.9 Erysipeloid, unspecified

A27- Leptospirosis

A27.0 Leptospirosis icterohemorrhagica
Leptospiral or spirochetal jaundice (hemorrhagic)
Weil's disease

A27.8- Other forms of leptospirosis

A27.81 Aseptic meningitis in leptospirosis

A27.89 Other forms of leptospirosis

A27.9 Leptospirosis, unspecified

A28- Other zoonotic bacterial diseases, not elsewhere classified

A28.0 Pasteurellosis

A28.1 Cat-scratch disease
Cat-scratch fever

A28.2 Extraintestinal yersiniosis
Excludes 1: *enteritis due to Yersinia enterocolitica (A04.6)*
plague (A20.-)

A28.8 Other specified zoonotic bacterial diseases, not elsewhere classified

A28.9 Zoonotic bacterial disease, unspecified

Other bacterial diseases (A30-A49)

A30- Leprosy [Hansen's disease]
Includes: Infection due to Mycobacterium leprae
Excludes 1: *sequelae of leprosy (B92)*

A30.0 Indeterminate leprosy
I leprosy

A30.1 Tuberculoid leprosy
TT leprosy

A30.2 Borderline tuberculoid leprosy
BT leprosy

A30.3 Borderline leprosy
BB leprosy

A30.4 Borderline lepromatous leprosy
BL leprosy

A30.5 Lepromatous leprosy
LL leprosy

A30.8 Other forms of leprosy

A30.9 Leprosy, unspecified

A31- Infection due to other mycobacteria
Excludes❷: *leprosy (A30.-)*
tuberculosis (A15-A19)

A31.0 Pulmonary mycobacterial infection
Infection due to Mycobacterium avium
Infection due to Mycobacterium intracellulare [Battey bacillus]
Infection due to Mycobacterium kansasii

A31.1 Cutaneous mycobacterial infection
Buruli ulcer
Infection due to Mycobacterium marinum
Infection due to Mycobacterium ulcerans

A31.2 Disseminated mycobacterium avium-intracellulare complex (DMAC)
MAC sepsis

A31.8 Other mycobacterial infections

A31.9 Mycobacterial infection, unspecified
Atypical mycobacterial infection NOS
Mycobacteriosis NOS

A32- Listeriosis
Includes: Listerial foodborne infection
Excludes 1: *neonatal (disseminated) listeriosis (P37.2)*

A32.0 Cutaneous listeriosis

A32.1- Listerial meningitis and meningoencephalitis

A32.11 Listerial meningitis

A32.12 Listerial meningoencephalitis

A32.7 Listerial sepsis

A32.8- Other forms of listeriosis

A32.81 Oculoglandular listeriosis

A32.82 Listerial endocarditis

A32.89 Other forms of listeriosis
Listerial cerebral arteritis

A32.9 Listeriosis, unspecified

A33 Tetanus neonatorum

A34 Obstetrical tetanus

A35 Other tetanus
Tetanus NOS
Excludes 1: *obstetrical tetanus (A34)*
tetanus neonatorum (A33)

A36- Diphtheria

A36.0 Pharyngeal diphtheria
Diphtheritic membranous angina
Tonsillar diphtheria

A36.1 Nasopharyngeal diphtheria

A36.2 Laryngeal diphtheria
Diphtheritic laryngotracheitis

A36.3 Cutaneous diphtheria
Excludes❷: *erythrasma (L08.1)*

A36.8- Other diphtheria

A36.81 Diphtheritic cardiomyopathy
Diphtheritic myocarditis

A36.82 Diphtheritic radiculomyelitis

A36.83 Diphtheritic polyneuritis

A36.84 Diphtheritic tubulo-interstitial nephropathy

A36.85 Diphtheritic cystitis

A36.86 Diphtheritic conjunctivitis

A36.89 Other diphtheritic complications
Diphtheritic peritonitis

A36.9 Diphtheria, unspecified

A37- Whooping cough

A37.0- Whooping cough due to Bordetella pertussis

A37.00 Whooping cough due to Bordetella pertussis without pneumonia

A37.01 Whooping cough due to Bordetella pertussis with pneumonia

A37.1- Whooping cough due to Bordetella parapertussis

A37.10 Whooping cough due to Bordetella parapertussis without pneumonia

A37.11 Whooping cough due to Bordetella parapertussis with pneumonia

A37.8- Whooping cough due to other Bordetella species

A37.80 Whooping cough due to other Bordetella species without pneumonia

A37.81 Whooping cough due to other Bordetella species with pneumonia

A37.9- Whooping cough, unspecified species

A37.90 Whooping cough, unspecified species without pneumonia

A37.91 Whooping cough, unspecified species with pneumonia

A38- Scarlet fever
Includes: scarlatina
Excludes❷: *streptococcal sore throat (J02.0)*

A38.0 Scarlet fever with otitis media

A38.1 Scarlet fever with myocarditis

A38.8 Scarlet fever with other complications

A38.9 Scarlet fever, uncomplicated
Scarlet fever, NOS

A39- Meningococcal infection

A39.0 Meningococcal meningitis

A39.1 Waterhouse-Friderichsen syndrome
Meningococcal hemorrhagic adrenalitis
Meningococcic adrenal syndrome

A39.2 Acute meningococcemia

A39.3 Chronic meningococcemia

A39.4 Meningococcemia, unspecified

A39.5- Meningococcal heart disease

A39.50 Meningococcal carditis, unspecified

A39.51 Meningococcal endocarditis

A39.52 Meningococcal myocarditis

A39.53 Meningococcal pericarditis

A
2
5
-
A
4
9

A39.8- Other meningococcal infections
    A39.81 Meningococcal encephalitis
    A39.82 Meningococcal retrobulbar neuritis
    A39.83 Meningococcal arthritis
    A39.84 Postmeningococcal arthritis
    A39.89 Other meningococcal infections
        Meningococcal conjunctivitis
A39.9 Meningococcal infection, unspecified
    Meningococcal disease NOS

A40- Streptococcal sepsis
    Code first: Postprocedural streptococcal sepsis (T81.4)
        Streptococcal sepsis during labor (O75.3)
        Streptococcal sepsis following abortion or ectopic or molar
          pregnancy (O03-O07, O08.0)
        Streptococcal sepsis following immunization (T88.0)
        Streptococcal sepsis following infusion, transfusion or
          therapeutic injection (T80.2-)
    Excludes 1: neonatal (P36.0-P36.1)
             puerperal sepsis (O85)
             sepsis due to Streptococcus, group D (A41.81)
A40.0 Sepsis due to streptococcus, group A
A40.1 Sepsis due to streptococcus, group B
A40.3 Sepsis due to Streptococcus pneumoniae
    Pneumococcal sepsis
A40.8 Other streptococcal sepsis
A40.9 Streptococcal sepsis, unspecified

A41- Other sepsis
    Code first: Postprocedural sepsis (T81.4)
        Sepsis during labor (O75.3)
        Sepsis following abortion, ectopic or molar pregnancy (O03-
          O07, O08.0)
        Sepsis following immunization (T88.0)
        Sepsis following infusion, transfusion or therapeutic injection
          (T80.2-)
    Excludes 1: bacteremia NOS (R78.81)
             neonatal (P36.-)
             puerperal sepsis (O85)
             sepsis NOS (A41.9)
             streptococcal sepsis (A40.-)
    Excludes ❷: sepsis (due to) (in) actinomycotic (A42.7)
             sepsis (due to) (in) anthrax (A22.7)
             sepsis (due to) (in) candidal (B37.7)
             sepsis (due to) (in) Erysipelothrix (A26.7)
             sepsis (due to) (in) extraintestinal yersiniosis (A28.2)
             sepsis (due to) (in) gonococcal (A54.86)
             sepsis (due to) (in) herpesviral (B00.7)
             sepsis (due to) (in) listerial (A32.7)
             sepsis (due to) (in) melioidosis (A24.1)
             sepsis (due to) (in) meningococcal (A39.2-A39.4)
             sepsis (due to) (in) plague (A20.7)
             sepsis (due to) (in) tularemia (A21.7)
             toxic shock syndrome (A48.3)
  A41.0- Sepsis due to Staphylococcus aureus
    A41.01 Sepsis due to methicillin susceptible Staphylococcus aureus
        MSSA sepsis
        Staphylococcus aureus sepsis NOS
    A41.02 Sepsis due to methicillin resistant Staphylococcus aureus
  A41.1 Sepsis due to other specified staphylococcus
    Coagulase negative staphylococcus sepsis
  A41.2 Sepsis due to unspecified staphylococcus
  A41.3 Sepsis due to Hemophilus influenzae
  A41.4 Sepsis due to anaerobes
    Excludes 1: gas gangrene (A48.0)
  A41.5- Sepsis due to other Gram-negative organisms
    A41.50 Gram-negative sepsis, unspecified
        Gram-negative sepsis NOS
    A41.51 Sepsis due to Escherichia coli [E. coli]
    A41.52 Sepsis due to Pseudomonas
        Pseudomonas aeroginosa
    A41.53 Sepsis due to Serratia
    A41.59 Other Gram-negative sepsis
  A41.8- Other specified sepsis
    A41.81 Sepsis due to Enterococcus
    A41.89 Other specified sepsis
  A41.9 Sepsis, unspecified organism
    Septicemia NOS

A42- Actinomycosis
    Excludes 1: actinomycetoma (B47.1)
  A42.0 Pulmonary actinomycosis
  A42.1 Abdominal actinomycosis
  A42.2 Cervicofacial actinomycosis
  A42.7 Actinomycotic sepsis
  A42.8- Other forms of actinomycosis
    A42.81 Actinomycotic meningitis
    A42.82 Actinomycotic encephalitis
    A42.89 Other forms of actinomycosis
  A42.9 Actinomycosis, unspecified

A43- Nocardiosis
  A43.0 Pulmonary nocardiosis
  A43.1 Cutaneous nocardiosis
  A43.8 Other forms of nocardiosis
  A43.9 Nocardiosis, unspecified

A44- Bartonellosis
  A44.0 Systemic bartonellosis
    Oroya fever
  A44.1 Cutaneous and mucocutaneous bartonellosis
    Verruga peruana
  A44.8 Other forms of bartonellosis
  A44.9 Bartonellosis, unspecified

A46 Erysipelas
    Excludes 1: postpartum or puerperal erysipelas (O86.89)

A48- Other bacterial diseases, not elsewhere classified
    Excludes 1: actinomycetoma (B47.1)
  A48.0 Gas gangrene
    Clostridial cellulitis
    Clostridial myonecrosis
  A48.1 Legionnaires' disease
  A48.2 Nonpneumonic Legionnaires' disease [Pontiac fever]
  A48.3 Toxic shock syndrome
    Use additional code to identify the organism (B95, B96)
    Excludes 1: endotoxic shock NOS (R57.8)
             sepsis NOS (A41.9)
  A48.4 Brazilian purpuric fever
    Systemic Hemophilus aegyptius infection
  A48.5- Other specified botulism
    Non-foodborne intoxication due to toxins of Clostridium
        botulinum [C. botulinum]
    Excludes 1: food poisoning due to toxins of Clostridium botulinum
             (A05.1)
    A48.51 Infant botulism
    A48.52 Wound botulism
        Non-foodborne botulism NOS
        Use additional code for associated wound
  A48.8 Other specified bacterial diseases

A49- Bacterial infection of unspecified site
    Excludes 1: bacterial agents as the cause of diseases classified elsewhere
             (B95-B96)
             chlamydial infection NOS (A74.9)
             meningococcal infection NOS (A39.9)
             rickettsial infection NOS (A79.9)
             spirochetal infection NOS (A69.9)
  A49.0- Staphylococcal infection, unspecified site
    A49.01 Methicillin susceptible Staphylococcus aureus infection, unspecified site
        Methicillin susceptible Staphylococcus aureus (MSSA)
          infection
        Staphylococcus aureus infection NOS
    A49.02 Methicillin resistant Staphylococcus aureus infection, unspecified site
        Methicillin resistant Staphylococcus aureus (MRSA) infection
  A49.1 Streptococcal infection, unspecified site
  A49.2 Hemophilus influenzae infection, unspecified site
  A49.3 Mycoplasma infection, unspecified site
  A49.8 Other bacterial infections of unspecified site
  A49.9 Bacterial infection, unspecified
    Excludes 1: bacteremia NOS (R78.81)

A
2
5
-
A
4
9

Infections with a <u>predominantly sexual mode</u> of transmission (A50-A64)

Excludes 1:   human immunodeficiency virus [HIV] disease (B20)
nonspecific and nongonococcal urethritis (N34.1)
Reiter's disease (M02.3-)

A50-   <u>Congenital</u> syphilis

  A50.0-   **Early congenital syphilis, symptomatic**
      Any congenital syphilitic condition specified as early or manifest less than two years after birth.

    A50.01   **Early congenital syphilitic oculopathy**

    A50.02   **Early congenital syphilitic osteochondropathy**

    A50.03   **Early congenital syphilitic pharyngitis**
        Early congenital syphilitic laryngitis

    A50.04   **Early congenital syphilitic pneumonia**

    A50.05   **Early congenital syphilitic rhinitis**

    A50.06   **Early cutaneous congenital syphilis**

    A50.07   **Early mucocutaneous congenital syphilis**

    A50.08   **Early visceral congenital syphilis**

    A50.09   **Other early congenital syphilis, symptomatic**

  A50.1   **Early congenital syphilis, latent**
      Congenital syphilis without clinical manifestations, with positive serological reaction and negative spinal fluid test, less than two years after birth

  A50.2   **Early congenital syphilis, unspecified**
      Congenital syphilis NOS less than two years after birth

  A50.3-   **Late congenital syphilitic oculopathy**
      Excludes 1:   Hutchinson's triad (A50.53)

    A50.30   **Late congenital syphilitic oculopathy, unspecified**

    A50.31   **Late congenital syphilitic interstitial keratitis**

    A50.32   **Late congenital syphilitic chorioretinitis**

    A50.39   **Other late congenital syphilitic oculopathy**

  A50.4-   **Late congenital neurosyphilis [juvenile neurosyphilis]**
      Use additional code to identify any associated mental disorder
      Excludes 1:   Hutchinson's triad (A50.53)

    A50.40   **Late congenital neurosyphilis, unspecified**
        Juvenile neurosyphilis NOS

    A50.41   **Late congenital syphilitic meningitis**

    A50.42   **Late congenital syphilitic encephalitis**

    A50.43   **Late congenital syphilitic polyneuropathy**

    A50.44   **Late congenital syphilitic optic nerve atrophy**

    A50.45   **Juvenile general paresis**
        Dementia paralytica juvenilis
        Juvenile tabetoparetic neurosyphilis

    A50.49   **Other late congenital neurosyphilis**
        Juvenile tabes dorsalis

  A50.5-   **Other late congenital syphilis, symptomatic**
      Any congenital syphilitic condition specified as late or manifest two years or more after birth

    A50.51   **Clutton's joints**

    A50.52   **Hutchinson's teeth**

    A50.53   **Hutchinson's triad**

    A50.54   **Late congenital cardiovascular syphilis**

    A50.55   **Late congenital syphilitic arthropathy**

    A50.56   **Late congenital syphilitic osteochondropathy**

    A50.57   **Syphilitic saddle nose**

    A50.59   **Other late congenital syphilis, symptomatic**

  A50.6   **Late congenital syphilis, latent**
      Congenital syphilis without clinical manifestations, with positive serological reaction and negative spinal fluid test, two years or more after birth

  A50.7   **Late congenital syphilis, unspecified**
      Congenital syphilis NOS two years or more after birth

  A50.9   **Congenital syphilis, unspecified**

A51-   <u>Early</u> syphilis

  A51.0   **Primary genital syphilis**
      Syphilitic chancre NOS

  A51.1   **Primary anal syphilis**

  A51.2   **Primary syphilis of other sites**

  A51.3-   **Secondary syphilis of skin and mucous membranes**

    A51.31   **Condyloma latum**

    A51.32   **Syphilitic alopecia**

    A51.39   **Other secondary syphilis of skin**
        Syphilitic leukoderma
        Syphilitic mucous patch
        Excludes 1:   late syphilitic leukoderma (A52.79)

  A51.4-   **Other secondary syphilis**

    A51.41   **Secondary syphilitic meningitis**

    A51.42   **Secondary syphilitic female pelvic disease**

    A51.43   **Secondary syphilitic oculopathy**
        Secondary syphilitic chorioretinitis
        Secondary syphilitic iridocyclitis, iritis
        Secondary syphilitic uveitis

    A51.44   **Secondary syphilitic nephritis**

    A51.45   **Secondary syphilitic hepatitis**

    A51.46   **Secondary syphilitic osteopathy**

    A51.49   **Other secondary syphilitic conditions**
        Secondary syphilitic lymphadenopathy
        Secondary syphilitic myositis

  A51.5   **Early syphilis, latent**
      Syphilis (acquired) without clinical manifestations, with positive serological reaction and negative spinal fluid test, less than two years after infection

  A51.9   **Early syphilis, unspecified**

A52-   <u>Late</u> syphilis

  A52.0-   **Cardiovascular and cerebrovascular syphilis**

    A52.00   **Cardiovascular syphilis, unspecified**

    A52.01   **Syphilitic aneurysm of aorta**

    A52.02   **Syphilitic aortitis**

    A52.03   **Syphilitic endocarditis**
        Syphilitic aortic valve incompetence or stenosis
        Syphilitic mitral valve stenosis
        Syphilitic pulmonary valve regurgitation

    A52.04   **Syphilitic cerebral arteritis**

    A52.05   **Other cerebrovascular syphilis**
        Syphilitic cerebral aneurysm (ruptured) (non-ruptured)
        Syphilitic cerebral thrombosis

    A52.06   **Other syphilitic heart involvement**
        Syphilitic coronary artery disease
        Syphilitic myocarditis
        Syphilitic pericarditis

    A52.09   **Other cardiovascular syphilis**

  A52.1-   **Symptomatic neurosyphilis**

    A52.10   **Symptomatic neurosyphilis, unspecified**

    A52.11   **Tabes dorsalis**
        Locomotor ataxia (progressive)
        Tabetic neurosyphilis

    A52.12   **Other cerebrospinal syphilis**

    A52.13   **Late syphilitic meningitis**

    A52.14   **Late syphilitic encephalitis**

    A52.15   **Late syphilitic neuropathy**
        Late syphilitic acoustic neuritis
        Late syphilitic optic (nerve) atrophy
        Late syphilitic polyneuropathy
        Late syphilitic retrobulbar neuritis

    A52.16   **Charcôt's arthropathy (tabetic)**

    A52.17   **General paresis**
        Dementia paralytica

    A52.19   **Other symptomatic neurosyphilis**
        Syphilitic parkinsonism

  A52.2   **Asymptomatic neurosyphilis**

  A52.3   **Neurosyphilis, unspecified**
      Gumma (syphilitic)
      Syphilis (late)
      Syphiloma

  A52.7-   **Other symptomatic late syphilis**

    A52.71   **Late syphilitic oculopathy**
        Late syphilitic chorioretinitis
        Late syphilitic episcleritis

    A52.72   **Syphilis of lung and bronchus**

    A52.73   **Symptomatic late syphilis of other respiratory organs**

    A52.74   **Syphilis of liver and other viscera**
        Late syphilitic peritonitis

    A52.75   **Syphilis of kidney and ureter**
        Syphilitic glomerular disease

    A52.76   **Other genitourinary symptomatic late syphilis**
        Late syphilitic female pelvic inflammatory disease

    A52.77   **Syphilis of bone and joint**

    A52.78   **Syphilis of other musculoskeletal tissue**
        Late syphilitic bursitis
        Syphilis [stage unspecified] of bursa
        Syphilis [stage unspecified] of muscle
        Syphilis [stage unspecified] of synovium
        Syphilis [stage unspecified] of tendon

A52.79   Other symptomatic late syphilis
Late syphilitic leukoderma
Syphilis of adrenal gland
Syphilis of pituitary gland
Syphilis of thyroid gland
Syphilitic splenomegaly
Excludes 1: syphilitic leukoderma (secondary) (A51.39)

A52.8   Late syphilis, latent
Syphilis (acquired) without clinical manifestations, with positive serological reaction and negative spinal fluid test, two years or more after infection

A52.9   Late syphilis, unspecified

A53- Other and unspecified syphilis

A53.0   Latent syphilis, unspecified as early or late
Latent syphilis NOS
Positive serological reaction for syphilis

A53.9   Syphilis, unspecified
Infection due to Treponema pallidum NOS
Syphilis (acquired) NOS
Excludes 1: syphilis NOS under two years of age (A50.2)

A54- Gonococcal infection

A54.0-   Gonococcal infection of lower genitourinary tract <u>without</u> periurethral or accessory gland abscess
Excludes 1: gonococcal infection with genitourinary gland abscess (A54.1)
gonococcal infection with periurethral abscess (A54.1)

A54.00   Gonococcal infection of lower genitourinary tract, unspecified

A54.01   Gonococcal cystitis and urethritis, unspecified

A54.02   Gonococcal vulvovaginitis, unspecified

A54.03   Gonococcal cervicitis, unspecified

A54.09   Other gonococcal infection of lower genitourinary tract

A54.1   Gonococcal infection of lower genitourinary tract <u>with</u> periurethral and accessory gland abscess
Gonococcal Bartholin's gland abscess

A54.2-   Gonococcal pelviperitonitis and other gonococcal genitourinary infection

A54.21   Gonococcal infection of kidney and ureter

A54.22   Gonococcal prostatitis

A54.23   Gonococcal infection of other male genital organs
Gonococcal epididymitis
Gonococcal orchitis

A54.24   Gonococcal female pelvic inflammatory disease
Gonococcal pelviperitonitis
Excludes 1: gonococcal peritonitis (A54.85)

A54.29   Other gonococcal genitourinary infections

A54.3-   Gonococcal infection of eye

A54.30   Gonococcal infection of eye, unspecified

A54.31   Gonococcal conjunctivitis
Ophthalmia neonatorum due to gonococcus

A54.32   Gonococcal iridocyclitis

A54.33   Gonococcal keratitis

A54.39   Other gonococcal eye infection
Gonococcal endophthalmia

A54.4-   Gonococcal infection of musculoskeletal system

A54.40   Gonococcal infection of musculoskeletal system, unspecified

A54.41   Gonococcal spondylopathy

A54.42   Gonococcal arthritis
Excludes❷: gonococcal infection of spine (A54.41)

A54.43   Gonococcal osteomyelitis
Excludes❷: gonococcal infection of spine (A54.41)

A54.49   Gonococcal infection of other musculoskeletal tissue
Gonococcal bursitis
Gonococcal myositis
Gonococcal synovitis
Gonococcal tenosynovitis

A54.5   Gonococcal pharyngitis

A54.6   Gonococcal infection of anus and rectum

A54.8-   Other gonococcal infections

A54.81   Gonococcal meningitis

A54.82   Gonococcal brain abscess

A54.83   Gonococcal heart infection
Gonococcal endocarditis
Gonococcal myocarditis
Gonococcal pericarditis

A54.84   Gonococcal pneumonia

A54.85   Gonococcal peritonitis
Excludes 1: gonococcal pelviperitonitis (A54.24)

A54.86   Gonococcal sepsis

A54.89   Other gonococcal infections
Gonococcal keratoderma
Gonococcal lymphadenitis

A54.9   Gonococcal infection, unspecified

A55   <u>Chlamydial lymphogranuloma (venereum)</u>
Climatic or tropical bubo
Durand-Nicolas-Favre disease
Esthiomene
Lymphogranuloma inguinale

A56-   <u>Other sexually transmitted chlamydial diseases</u>
Includes: Sexually transmitted diseases due to Chlamydia Trachomatis
Excludes 1: neonatal chlamydial conjunctivitis (P39.1)
neonatal chlamydial pneumonia (P23.1)
Excludes❷: chlamydial lymphogranuloma (A55)
conditions classified to A74.-

A56.0-   Chlamydial infection of lower genitourinary tract

A56.00   Chlamydial infection of lower genitourinary tract, unspecified

A56.01   Chlamydial cystitis and urethritis

A56.02   Chlamydial vulvovaginitis

A56.09   Other chlamydial infection of lower genitourinary tract
Chlamydial cervicitis

A56.1-   Chlamydial infection of pelviperitoneum and other genitourinary organs

A56.11   Chlamydial female pelvic inflammatory disease

A56.19   Other chlamydial genitourinary infection
Chlamydial epididymitis
Chlamydial orchitis

A56.2   Chlamydial infection of genitourinary tract, unspecified

A56.3   Chlamydial infection of anus and rectum

A56.4   Chlamydial infection of pharynx

A56.8   Sexually transmitted chlamydial infection of other sites

A57   <u>Chancroid</u>
Ulcus molle

A58   <u>Granuloma inguinale</u>
Donovanosis

A59-   <u>Trichomoniasis</u>
Excludes❷: intestinal trichomoniasis (A07.8)

A59.0-   Urogenital trichomoniasis

A59.00   Urogenital trichomoniasis, unspecified
Fluor (vaginalis) due to Trichomonas
Leukorrhea (vaginalis) due to Trichomonas

A59.01   Trichomonal vulvovaginitis

A59.02   Trichomonal prostatitis

A59.03   Trichomonal cystitis and urethritis

A59.09   Other urogenital trichomoniasis
Trichomonas cervicitis

A59.8   Trichomoniasis of other sites

A59.9   Trichomoniasis, unspecified

A60-   <u>Anogenital herpesviral [herpes simplex] infections</u>

A60.0-   Herpesviral infection of genitalia and urogenital tract

A60.00   Herpesviral infection of urogenital system, unspecified

A60.01   Herpesviral infection of penis

A60.02   Herpesviral infection of other male genital organs

A60.03   Herpesviral cervicitis

A60.04   Herpesviral vulvovaginitis
Herpesviral [herpes simplex] ulceration
Herpesviral [herpes simplex] vaginitis
Herpesviral [herpes simplex] vulvitis

A60.09   Herpesviral infection of other urogenital tract

A60.1   Herpesviral infection of perianal skin and rectum

A60.9   Anogenital herpesviral infection, unspecified

A63-   Other predominantly sexually transmitted diseases, not elsewhere classified
Excludes❷: molluscum contagiosum (B08.1)
papilloma of cervix (D26.0)

A63.0   Anogenital (venereal) warts
Anogenital warts due to (human) papillomavirus [HPV]
Condyloma acuminatum

A63.8   Other specified predominantly sexually transmitted diseases

A64   Unspecified sexually transmitted disease

A
5
0
-
A
6
4

Excludes 1: = NOT CODED HERE! (Do not code both)

Excludes❷: = Not Included Here

Other spirochetal diseases (A65-A69)

Excludes❷: leptospirosis (A27.-)
         syphilis (A50-A53)

A65   Nonvenereal syphilis
         Bejel
         Endemic syphilis
         Njovera

A66- Yaws
         Includes: Bouba
                     Frambesia (tropica)
                     Pian

   A66.0   Initial lesions of yaws
           Chancre of yaws
           Frambesia, initial or primary
           Initial frambesial ulcer
           Mother yaw

   A66.1   Multiple papillomata and wet crab yaws
           Frambesioma
           Pianoma
           Plantar or palmar papilloma of yaws

   A66.2   Other early skin lesions of yaws
           Cutaneous yaws, less than five years after infection
           Early yaws (cutaneous) (macular) (maculopapular) (micropapular)
                 (papular)
           Frambeside of early yaws

   A66.3   Hyperkeratosis of yaws
           Ghoul hand
           Hyperkeratosis, palmar or plantar (early) (late) due to yaws
           Worm-eaten soles

   A66.4   Gummata and ulcers of yaws
           Gummatous frambeside
           Nodular late yaws (ulcerated)

   A66.5   Gangosa
           Rhinopharyngitis mutilans

   A66.6   Bone and joint lesions of yaws
           Yaws ganglion
           Yaws goundou
           Yaws gumma, bone
           Yaws gummatous osteitis or periostitis
           Yaws hydrarthrosis
           Yaws osteitis
           Yaws periostitis (hypertrophic)

   A66.7   Other manifestations of yaws
           Juxta-articular nodules of yaws
           Mucosal yaws

   A66.8   Latent yaws
           Yaws without clinical manifestations, with positive serology

   A66.9   Yaws, unspecified

A67- Pinta [carate]
   A67.0   Primary lesions of pinta
           Chancre (primary) of pinta
           Papule (primary) of pinta

   A67.1   Intermediate lesions of pinta
           Erythematous plaques of pinta
           Hyperchromic lesions of pinta
           Hyperkeratosis of pinta
           Pintids

   A67.2   Late lesions of pinta
           Achromic skin lesions of pinta
           Cicatricial skin lesions of pinta
           Dyschromic skin lesions of pinta

   A67.3   Mixed lesions of pinta
           Achromic with hyperchromic skin lesions of pinta [carate]

   A67.9   Pinta, unspecified

A68- Relapsing fevers
         Includes: Recurrent fever
         Excludes❷: Lyme disease (A69.2-)

   A68.0   Louse-borne relapsing fever
           Relapsing fever due to Borrelia recurrentis

   A68.1   Tick-borne relapsing fever
           Relapsing fever due to any Borrelia species other than Borrelia
                 recurrentis

   A68.9   Relapsing fever, unspecified

A69- Other spirochetal infections
   A69.0   Necrotizing ulcerative stomatitis
           Cancrum oris
           Fusospirochetal gangrene
           Noma
           Stomatitis gangrenosa

   A69.1   Other Vincent's infections
           Fusospirochetal pharyngitis
           Necrotizing ulcerative (acute) gingivitis
           Necrotizing ulcerative (acute) gingivostomatitis
           Spirochetal stomatitis
           Trench mouth
           Vincent's angina
           Vincent's gingivitis

   A69.2- Lyme disease
           Erythema chronicum migrans due to Borrelia burgdorferi

       A69.20   Lyme disease, unspecified
       A69.21   Meningitis due to Lyme disease
       A69.22   Other neurologic disorders in Lyme disease
               Cranial neuritis
               Meningoencephalitis
               Polyneuropathy
       A69.23   Arthritis due to Lyme disease
       A69.29   Other conditions associated with Lyme disease
               Myopericarditis due to Lyme disease

   A69.8   Other specified spirochetal infections
   A69.9   Spirochetal infection, unspecified

Other diseases caused by chlamydiae (A70-A74)

Excludes 1: sexually transmitted chlamydial diseases (A55-A56)

A70   Chlamydia psittaci infections
         Ornithosis
         Parrot fever
         Psittacosis

A71- Trachoma
         Excludes 1: sequelae of trachoma (B94.0)
   A71.0   Initial stage of trachoma
           Trachoma dubium

   A71.1   Active stage of trachoma
           Granular conjunctivitis (trachomatous)
           Trachomatous follicular conjunctivitis
           Trachomatous pannus

   A71.9   Trachoma, unspecified

A74- Other diseases caused by chlamydiae
         Excludes 1: neonatal chlamydial conjunctivitis (P39.1)
                  neonatal chlamydial pneumonia (P23.1)
                  Reiter's disease (M02.3-)
                  sexually transmitted chlamydial diseases (A55-A56)
         Excludes❷: chlamydial pneumonia (J16.0)
   A74.0   Chlamydial conjunctivitis
           Paratrachoma

   A74.8- Other chlamydial diseases
       A74.81   Chlamydial peritonitis
       A74.89   Other chlamydial diseases

   A74.9   Chlamydial infection, unspecified
           Chlamydiosis NOS

Rickettsioses (A75-A79)

A75- Typhus fever
         Excludes 1: rickettsiosis due to Ehrlichia sennetsu (A79.81)
   A75.0   Epidemic louse-borne typhus fever due to Rickettsia prowazekii
           Classical typhus (fever)
           Epidemic (louse-borne) typhus

   A75.1   Recrudescent typhus [Brill's disease]
           Brill-Zinsser disease

   A75.2   Typhus fever due to Rickettsia typhi
           Murine (flea-borne) typhus

   A75.3   Typhus fever due to Rickettsia tsutsugamushi
           Scrub (mite-borne) typhus
           Tsutsugamushi fever

   A75.9   Typhus fever, unspecified
           Typhus (fever) NOS

A77- Spotted fever [tick-borne rickettsioses]

    A77.0 **Spotted fever due to Rickettsia rickettsii**
        Rocky Mountain spotted fever
        Sao Paulo fever

    A77.1 **Spotted fever due to Rickettsia conorii**
        African tick typhus
        Boutonneuse fever
        India tick typhus
        Kenya tick typhus
        Marseilles fever
        Mediterranean tick fever

    A77.2 **Spotted fever due to Rickettsia siberica**
        North Asian tick fever
        Siberian tick typhus

    A77.3 **Spotted fever due to Rickettsia australis**
        Queensland tick typhus

    A77.4- **Ehrlichiosis**
        Excludes 1: Rickettsiosis due to Ehrlichia sennetsu (A79.81)
     A77.40 **Ehrlichiosis, unspecified**
     A77.41 **Ehrlichiosis chafeensis [E. chafeensis]**
     A77.49 **Other ehrlichiosis**

    A77.8 **Other spotted fevers**
    A77.9 **Spotted fever, unspecified**
        Tick-borne typhus NOS

A78 Q fever
    Infection due to Coxiella burnetii
    Nine Mile fever
    Quadrilateral fever

A79- Other rickettsioses
    A79.0 **Trench fever**
        Quintan fever
        Wolhynian fever

    A79.1 **Rickettsialpox due to Rickettsia akari**
        Kew Garden fever
        Vesicular rickettsiosis

    A79.8- **Other specified rickettsioses**
     A79.81 **Rickettsiosis due to Ehrlichia sennetsu**
     A79.89 **Other specified rickettsioses**

    A79.9 **Rickettsiosis, unspecified**
        Rickettsial infection NOS

Viral and prion infections of the central nervous system
(A80-A89)

    Excludes 1: postpolio syndrome (G14)
            sequelae of poliomyelitis (B91)
            sequelae of viral encephalitis (B94.1)

A80- Acute poliomyelitis
    A80.0 **Acute paralytic poliomyelitis, vaccine-associated**
    A80.1 **Acute paralytic poliomyelitis, wild virus, imported**
    A80.2 **Acute paralytic poliomyelitis, wild virus, indigenous**
    A80.3- **Acute paralytic poliomyelitis, other and unspecified**
     A80.30 **Acute paralytic poliomyelitis, unspecified**
     A80.39 **Other acute paralytic poliomyelitis**
    A80.4 **Acute nonparalytic poliomyelitis**
    A80.9 **Acute poliomyelitis, unspecified**

A81- Atypical virus infections of central nervous system
    Includes: Diseases of the central nervous system caused by prions
    Use additional code to identify:
    Dementia with behavioral disturbance (F02.81)
    Dementia without behavioral disturbance (F02.80)
    A81.0- **Creutzfeldt-Jakob disease**
     A81.00 **Creutzfeldt-Jakob disease, unspecified**
        Jakob-Creutzfeldt disease, unspecified
     A81.01 **Variant Creutzfeldt-Jakob disease**
        vCJD
     A81.09 **Other Creutzfeldt-Jakob disease**
        CJD
        Familial Creutzfeldt-Jakob disease
        Iatrogenic Creutzfeldt-Jakob disease
        Sporadic Creutzfeldt-Jakob disease
        Subacute spongiform encephalopathy (with dementia)
    A81.1 **Subacute sclerosing panencephalitis**
        Dawson's inclusion body encephalitis
        Van Bogaert's sclerosing leukoencephalopathy
    A81.2 **Progressive multifocal leukoencephalopathy**
        Multifocal leukoencephalopathy NOS

    A81.8- **Other atypical virus infections of central nervous system**
     A81.81 **Kuru**
     A81.82 **Gerstmann-Sträussler-Scheinker syndrome**
        GSS syndrome
     A81.83 **Fatal familial insomnia**
        FFI
     A81.89 **Other atypical virus infections of central nervous system**
    A81.9 **Atypical virus infection of central nervous system, unspecified**
        Prion diseases of the central nervous system NOS

A82- Rabies
    A82.0 **Sylvatic rabies**
    A82.1 **Urban rabies**
    A82.9 **Rabies, unspecified**

A83- Mosquito-borne viral encephalitis
    Includes: Mosquito-borne viral meningoencephalitis
    Excludes ❷: Venezuelan equine encephalitis (A92.2)
            West Nile fever (A92.3-)
            West Nile virus (A92.3-)
    A83.0 **Japanese encephalitis**
    A83.1 **Western equine encephalitis**
    A83.2 **Eastern equine encephalitis**
    A83.3 **St. Louis encephalitis**
    A83.4 **Australian encephalitis**
        Kunjin virus disease
    A83.5 **California encephalitis**
        California meningoencephalitis
        La Crosse encephalitis
    A83.6 **Rocio virus disease**
    A83.8 **Other mosquito-borne viral encephalitis**
    A83.9 **Mosquito-borne viral encephalitis, unspecified**

A84- Tick-borne viral encephalitis
    Includes: Tick-borne viral meningoencephalitis
    A84.0 **Far Eastern tick-borne encephalitis [Russian spring-summer encephalitis]**
    A84.1 **Central European tick-borne encephalitis**
    A84.8 **Other tick-borne viral encephalitis**
        Louping ill
        Powassan virus disease
    A84.9 **Tick-borne viral encephalitis, unspecified**

A85- Other viral encephalitis, not elsewhere classified
    Includes: Specified viral encephalomyelitis NEC
             Specified viral meningoencephalitis NEC
    Excludes 1: benign myalgic encephalomyelitis (G93.3)
            encephalitis due to cytomegalovirus (B25.8)
            encephalitis due to herpesvirus NEC (B10.0-)
            encephalitis due to herpesvirus [herpes simplex] (B00.4)
            encephalitis due to measles virus (B05.0)
            encephalitis due to mumps virus (B26.2)
            encephalitis due to poliomyelitis virus (A80.-)
            encephalitis due to zoster (B02.0)
            lymphocytic choriomeningitis (A87.2)
    A85.0 **Enteroviral encephalitis**
        Enteroviral encephalomyelitis
    A85.1 **Adenoviral encephalitis**
        Adenoviral meningoencephalitis
    A85.2 **Arthropod-borne viral encephalitis, unspecified**
        Excludes 1: West Nile virus with encephalitis (A92.31)
    A85.8 **Other specified viral encephalitis**
        Encephalitis lethargica
        Von Economo-Cruchet disease

A86 Unspecified viral encephalitis
    Viral encephalomyelitis NOS
    Viral meningoencephalitis NOS

A87- Viral meningitis
    Excludes 1: meningitis due to herpesvirus [herpes simplex] (B00.3)
            meningitis due to measles virus (B05.1)
            meningitis due to mumps virus (B26.1)
            meningitis due to poliomyelitis virus (A80.-)
            meningitis due to zoster (B02.1)
    A87.0 **Enteroviral meningitis**
        Coxsackievirus meningitis
        Echovirus meningitis
    A87.1 **Adenoviral meningitis**
    A87.2 **Lymphocytic choriomeningitis**
        Lymphocytic meningoencephalitis
    A87.8 **Other viral meningitis**
    A87.9 **Viral meningitis, unspecified**

A
6
5
–
A
8
7

Excludes 1: = NOT CODED HERE! (Do not code both)   *Excludes ❷:* = Not Included Here

A88- **Other viral infections of central nervous system, not elsewhere classified**
Excludes 1: viral encephalitis NOS (A86)
viral meningitis NOS (A87.9)

A88.0   **Enteroviral exanthematous fever [Boston exanthem]**
A88.1   **Epidemic vertigo**
A88.8   **Other specified viral infections of central nervous system**

A89   **Unspecified viral infection of central nervous system**

Arthropod-borne viral fevers and viral hemorrhagic fevers (A90-A99)

A90   **Dengue fever [classical dengue]**
Excludes 1: dengue hemorrhagic fever (A91)

A91   **Dengue hemorrhagic fever**

A92-   **Other mosquito-borne viral fevers**
Excludes 1: Ross River disease (B33.1)

A92.0   **Chikungunya virus disease**
Chikungunya (hemorrhagic) fever

A92.1   **O'nyong-nyong fever**

A92.2   **Venezuelan equine fever**
Venezuelan equine encephalitis
Venezuelan equine encephalomyelitis virus disease

A92.3-   **West Nile virus infection**
West Nile fever

A92.30   **West Nile virus infection, unspecified**
West Nile fever NOS
West Nile fever without complications
West Nile virus NOS

A92.31   **West Nile virus infection with encephalitis**
West Nile encephalitis
West Nile encephalomyelitis

A92.32   **West Nile virus infection with other neurologic manifestation**
Use additional code to specify the neurologic manifestation

A92.39   **West Nile virus infection with other complications**
Use additional code to specify the other conditions

A92.4   **Rift Valley fever**
A92.8   **Other specified mosquito-borne viral fevers**
A92.9   **Mosquito-borne viral fever, unspecified**

A93-   **Other arthropod-borne viral fevers, not elsewhere classified**

A93.0   **Oropouche virus disease**
Oropouche fever

A93.1   **Sandfly fever**
Pappataci fever
Phlebotomus fever

A93.2   **Colorado tick fever**

A93.8   **Other specified arthropod-borne viral fevers**
Piry virus disease
Vesicular stomatitis virus disease [Indiana fever]

A94   **Unspecified arthropod-borne viral fever**
Arboviral fever NOS
Arbovirus infection NOS

A95-   **Yellow fever**

A95.0   **Sylvatic yellow fever**
Jungle yellow fever

A95.1   **Urban yellow fever**
A95.9   **Yellow fever, unspecified**

A96-   **Arenaviral hemorrhagic fever**

A96.0   **Junin hemorrhagic fever**
Argentinian hemorrhagic fever

A96.1   **Machupo hemorrhagic fever**
Bolivian hemorrhagic fever

A96.2   **Lassa fever**
A96.8   **Other arenaviral hemorrhagic fevers**
A96.9   **Arenaviral hemorrhagic fever, unspecified**

A98-   **Other viral hemorrhagic fevers, not elsewhere classified**
Excludes 1: chikungunya hemorrhagic fever (A92.0)
dengue hemorrhagic fever (A91)

A98.0   **Crimean-Congo hemorrhagic fever**
Central Asian hemorrhagic fever

A98.1   **Omsk hemorrhagic fever**
A98.2   **Kyasanur Forest disease**
A98.3   **Marburg virus disease**
A98.4   **Ebola virus disease**

A98.5   **Hemorrhagic fever with renal syndrome**
Epidemic hemorrhagic fever
Korean hemorrhagic fever
Russian hemorrhagic fever
Hantaan virus disease
Hantavirus disease with renal manifestations
Nephropathia epidemica
Songo fever
Excludes 1: hantavirus (cardio)-pulmonary syndrome (B33.4)

A98.8   **Other specified viral hemorrhagic fevers**

A99   **Unspecified viral hemorrhagic fever**

Viral infections characterized by skin and mucous membrane lesions (B00-B09)

B00-   **Herpesviral [herpes simplex] infections**
Excludes 1: congenital herpesviral infections (P35.2)
Excludes ❷: anogenital herpesviral infection (A60.-)
gammaherpesviral mononucleosis (B27.0-)
herpangina (B08.5)

B00.0   **Eczema herpeticum**
Kaposi's varicelliform eruption

B00.1   **Herpesviral vesicular dermatitis**
Herpes simplex facialis
Herpes simplex labialis
Herpes simplex otitis externa
Vesicular dermatitis of ear
Vesicular dermatitis of lip

B00.2   **Herpesviral gingivostomatitis and pharyngotonsillitis**
Herpesviral pharyngitis

B00.3   **Herpesviral meningitis**

B00.4   **Herpesviral encephalitis**
Herpesviral meningoencephalitis
Simian B disease
Excludes 1: herpesviral encephalitis due to herpesvirus 6 and 7 (B10.01, B10.09)
non-simplex herpesviral encephalitis (B10.0-)

B00.5-   **Herpesviral ocular disease**

B00.50   **Herpesviral ocular disease, unspecified**

B00.51   **Herpesviral iridocyclitis**
Herpesviral iritis
Herpesviral uveitis, anterior

B00.52   **Herpesviral keratitis**
Herpesviral keratoconjunctivitis

B00.53   **Herpesviral conjunctivitis**

B00.59   **Other herpesviral disease of eye**
Herpesviral dermatitis of eyelid

B00.7   **Disseminated herpesviral disease**
Herpesviral sepsis

B00.8-   **Other forms of herpesviral infections**

B00.81   **Herpesviral hepatitis**

B00.82   **Herpes simplex myelitis**

B00.89   **Other herpesviral infection**
Herpesviral whitlow

B00.9   **Herpesviral infection, unspecified**
Herpes simplex infection NOS

B01-   **Varicella [chickenpox]**

B01.0   **Varicella meningitis**

B01.1-   **Varicella encephalitis, myelitis and encephalomyelitis**
Postchickenpox encephalitis, myelitis and encephalomyelitis

B01.11   **Varicella encephalitis and encephalomyelitis**
Postchickenpox encephalitis and encephalomyelitis

B01.12   **Varicella myelitis**
Postchickenpox myelitis

B01.2   **Varicella pneumonia**

B01.8-   **Varicella with other complications**

B01.81   **Varicella keratitis**

B01.89   **Other varicella complications**

B01.9   **Varicella without complication**
Varicella NOS

B02- Zoster [herpes zoster]
  Includes: Shingles
         Zona
  B02.0   Zoster encephalitis
       Zoster meningoencephalitis
  B02.1   Zoster meningitis
  B02.2- Zoster with other nervous system involvement
    B02.21 Postherpetic geniculate ganglionitis
    B02.22 Postherpetic trigeminal neuralgia
    B02.23 Postherpetic polyneuropathy
    B02.24 Postherpetic myelitis
         Herpes zoster myelitis
    B02.29 Other postherpetic nervous system involvement
         Postherpetic radiculopathy
  B02.3- Zoster ocular disease
    B02.30 Zoster ocular disease, unspecified
    B02.31 Zoster conjunctivitis
    B02.32 Zoster iridocyclitis
    B02.33 Zoster keratitis
         Herpes zoster keratoconjunctivitis
    B02.34 Zoster scleritis
    B02.39 Other herpes zoster eye disease
         Zoster blepharitis
  B02.7   Disseminated zoster
  B02.8   Zoster with other complications
       Herpes zoster otitis externa
  B02.9   Zoster without complications
       Zoster NOS

B03   Smallpox
    Note: In 1980 the 33rd World Health Assembly declared that smallpox had
         been eradicated. The classification is maintained for surveillance
         purposes.

B04   Monkeypox

B05- Measles
    Includes: Morbilli
    Excludes 1: subacute sclerosing panencephalitis (A81.1)
  B05.0   Measles complicated by encephalitis
       Postmeasles encephalitis
  B05.1   Measles complicated by meningitis
       Postmeasles meningitis
  B05.2   Measles complicated by pneumonia
       Postmeasles pneumonia
  B05.3   Measles complicated by otitis media
       Postmeasles otitis media
  B05.4   Measles with intestinal complications
  B05.8- Measles with other complications
    B05.81 Measles keratitis and keratoconjunctivitis
    B05.89 Other measles complications
  B05.9   Measles without complication
       Measles NOS

B06- Rubella [German measles]
    Excludes 1: congenital rubella (P35.0)
  B06.0- Rubella with neurological complications
    B06.00 Rubella with neurological complication, unspecified
    B06.01 Rubella encephalitis
         Rubella meningoencephalitis
    B06.02 Rubella meningitis
    B06.09 Other neurological complications of rubella
  B06.8- Rubella with other complications
    B06.81 Rubella pneumonia
    B06.82 Rubella arthritis
    B06.89 Other rubella complications
  B06.9   Rubella without complication
       Rubella NOS

B07- Viral warts
    Includes: Verruca simplex
         Verruca vulgaris
         Viral warts due to human papillomavirus
    Excludes ❷: anogenital (venereal) warts (A63.0)
         papilloma of bladder (D41.4)
         papilloma of cervix (D26.0)
         papilloma larynx (D14.1)
  B07.0   Plantar wart
       Verruca plantaris
  B07.8   Other viral warts
       Common wart
       Flat wart
       Verruca plana
  B07.9   Viral wart, unspecified

B08- Other viral infections characterized by skin and mucous membrane lesions, not elsewhere classified
    Excludes 1: vesicular stomatitis virus disease (A93.8)
  B08.0- Other orthopoxvirus infections
      Excludes ❷: monkeypox (B04)
    B08.01- Cowpox and vaccinia not from vaccine
      B08.010   Cowpox
      B08.011   Vaccinia not from vaccine
           Excludes 1: vaccinia (from vaccination) (generalized)
                    (T88.1)
    B08.02 Orf virus disease
         Contagious pustular dermatitis
         Ecthyma contagiosum
    B08.03 Pseudocowpox [milker's node]
    B08.04 Paravaccinia, unspecified
    B08.09 Other orthopoxvirus infections
         Orthopoxvirus infection NOS
  B08.1   Molluscum contagiosum
  B08.2- Exanthema subitum [sixth disease]
       Roseola infantum
    B08.20 Exanthema subitum [sixth disease], unspecified
         Roseola infantum, unspecified
    B08.21 Exanthema subitum [sixth disease] due to human herpesvirus 6
         Roseola infantum due to human herpesvirus 6
    B08.22 Exanthema subitum [sixth disease] due to human herpesvirus 7
         Roseola infantum due to human herpesvirus 7
  B08.3   Erythema infectiosum [fifth disease]
  B08.4   Enteroviral vesicular stomatitis with exanthem
       Hand, foot and mouth disease
  B08.5   Enteroviral vesicular pharyngitis
       Herpangina
  B08.6- Parapoxvirus infections
    B08.60 Parapoxvirus infection, unspecified
    B08.61 Bovine stomatitis
    B08.62 Sealpox
    B08.69 Other parapoxvirus infections
  B08.7- Yatapoxvirus infections
    B08.70 Yatapoxvirus infection, unspecified
    B08.71 Tanapox virus disease
    B08.72 Yaba pox virus disease
         Yaba monkey tumor disease
    B08.79 Other yatapoxvirus infections
  B08.8   Other specified viral infections characterized by skin and mucous membrane lesions
       Enteroviral lymphonodular pharyngitis
       Foot-and-mouth disease
       Poxvirus NEC

B09   Unspecified viral infection characterized by skin and mucous membrane lesions
    Viral enanthema NOS
    Viral exanthema NOS

Excludes 1: = NOT CODED HERE! (Do not code both)   *Excludes ❷:* = Not Included Here

Other human herpesviruses (B10)

B10-   <u>Other human herpesviruses</u>
    Excludes❷: cytomegalovirus (B25.9)
         Epstein-Barr virus (B27.0-)
         herpes NOS (B00.9)
         herpes simplex (B00-)
         herpes zoster (B02-)
         human herpesvirus NOS (B00-)
         human herpesvirus 1 and 2 (B00-)
         human herpesvirus 3 (B01.-, B02.-)
         human herpesvirus 4 (B27.0-)
         human herpesvirus 5 (B25-)
         varicella (B01-)
         zoster (B02-)

B10.0-   **Other human herpesvirus encephalitis**
    Excludes❷: herpes encephalitis NOS (B00.4)
         herpes simplex encephalitis (B00.4)
         human herpesvirus encephalitis (B00.4)
         simian B herpes virus encephalitis (B00.4)

    B10.01   **Human herpesvirus 6 encephalitis**
    B10.09   **Other human herpesvirus encephalitis**
        Human herpesvirus 7 encephalitis

B10.8-   **Other human herpesvirus infection**
    B10.81   **Human herpesvirus 6 infection**
    B10.82   **Human herpesvirus 7 infection**
    B10.89   **Other human herpesvirus infection**
        Human herpesvirus 8 infection
        Kaposi's sarcoma-associated herpesvirus infection

Viral hepatitis (B15-B19)

  Excludes 1: sequelae of viral hepatitis (B94.2)
  Excludes❷: cytomegaloviral hepatitis (B25.1)
       herpesviral [herpes simplex] hepatitis (B00.81)

B15-   <u>Acute hepatitis A</u>
  B15.0   **Hepatitis A with hepatic coma**
  B15.9   **Hepatitis A without hepatic coma**
      Hepatitis A (acute) (viral) NOS

B16-   <u>Acute hepatitis B</u>
  B16.0   **Acute hepatitis B with delta-agent with hepatic coma**
  B16.1   **Acute hepatitis B with delta-agent without hepatic coma**
  B16.2   **Acute hepatitis B without delta-agent with hepatic coma**
  B16.9   **Acute hepatitis B without delta-agent and without hepatic coma**
      Hepatitis B (acute) (viral) NOS

B17-   <u>Other acute</u> viral hepatitis
  B17.0   **Acute delta-(super) infection of hepatitis B carrier**
  B17.1-   **Acute hepatitis C**
    B17.10   **Acute hepatitis C without hepatic coma**
        Acute hepatitis C NOS
    B17.11   **Acute hepatitis C with hepatic coma**
  B17.2   **Acute hepatitis E**
  B17.8   **Other specified acute viral hepatitis**
      Hepatitis non-A non-B (acute) (viral) NEC
  B17.9   **Acute viral hepatitis, unspecified**
      Acute hepatitis NOS

B18-   <u>Chronic viral hepatitis</u>
  B18.0   **Chronic viral hepatitis B with delta-agent**
  B18.1   **Chronic viral hepatitis B without delta-agent**
      Chronic (viral) hepatitis B
  B18.2   **Chronic viral hepatitis C**
  B18.8   **Other chronic viral hepatitis**
  B18.9   **Chronic viral hepatitis, unspecified**

B19-   <u>Unspecified</u> viral hepatitis
  B19.0   **Unspecified viral hepatitis with hepatic coma**
  B19.1-   **Unspecified viral hepatitis B**
    B19.10   **Unspecified viral hepatitis B without hepatic coma**
        Unspecified viral hepatitis B NOS
    B19.11   **Unspecified viral hepatitis B with hepatic coma**
  B19.2-   **Unspecified viral hepatitis C**
    B19.20   **Unspecified viral hepatitis C without hepatic coma**
        Viral hepatitis C NOS
    B19.21   **Unspecified viral hepatitis C with hepatic coma**
  B19.9   **Unspecified viral hepatitis without hepatic coma**
      Viral hepatitis NOS

Human immunodeficiency virus [HIV] disease (B20)

B20   **Human immunodeficiency virus [<u>HIV</u>] disease**
  Includes: Acquired immune deficiency syndrome [AIDS]
         AIDS-related complex [ARC]
         HIV infection, symptomatic
  Code first Human immunodeficiency virus [HIV] disease complicating
    pregnancy, childbirth and the puerperium, if applicable (O98.7-)
  Use additional code(s) to identify all manifestations of HIV infection
  Excludes 1: asymptomatic human immunodeficiency virus [HIV] infection
         status (Z21)
        exposure to HIV virus (Z20.6)
        inconclusive serologic evidence of HIV (R75)

Other viral diseases (B25-B34)

B25-   <u>Cytomegaloviral disease</u>
  Excludes 1: congenital cytomegalovirus infection (P35.1)
       cytomegaloviral mononucleosis (B27.1-)
  B25.0   **Cytomegaloviral pneumonitis**
  B25.1   **Cytomegaloviral hepatitis**
  B25.2   **Cytomegaloviral pancreatitis**
  B25.8   **Other cytomegaloviral diseases**
      Cytomegaloviral encephalitis
  B25.9   **Cytomegaloviral disease, unspecified**

B26-   <u>Mumps</u>
  Includes: Epidemic parotitis
         Infectious parotitis
  B26.0   **Mumps orchitis**
  B26.1   **Mumps meningitis**
  B26.2   **Mumps encephalitis**
  B26.3   **Mumps pancreatitis**
  B26.8-   **Mumps with other complications**
    B26.81   **Mumps hepatitis**
    B26.82   **Mumps myocarditis**
    B26.83   **Mumps nephritis**
    B26.84   **Mumps polyneuropathy**
    B26.85   **Mumps arthritis**
    B26.89   **Other mumps complications**
  B26.9   **Mumps without complication**
      Mumps NOS
      Mumps parotitis NOS

B27-   <u>Infectious mononucleosis</u>
  Includes: Glandular fever
         Monocytic angina
         Pfeiffer's disease
  B27.0-   **Gammaherpesviral mononucleosis**
      Mononucleosis due to Epstein-Barr virus
    B27.00   **Gammaherpesviral mononucleosis without complication**
    B27.01   **Gammaherpesviral mononucleosis with polyneuropathy**
    B27.02   **Gammaherpesviral mononucleosis with meningitis**
    B27.09   **Gammaherpesviral mononucleosis with other complications**
        Hepatomegaly in gammaherpesviral mononucleosis
  B27.1-   **Cytomegaloviral mononucleosis**
    B27.10   **Cytomegaloviral mononucleosis without complications**
    B27.11   **Cytomegaloviral mononucleosis with polyneuropathy**
    B27.12   **Cytomegaloviral mononucleosis with meningitis**
    B27.19   **Cytomegaloviral mononucleosis with other complication**
        Hepatomegaly in cytomegaloviral mononucleosis
  B27.8-   **Other infectious mononucleosis**
    B27.80   **Other infectious mononucleosis without complication**
    B27.81   **Other infectious mononucleosis with polyneuropathy**
    B27.82   **Other infectious mononucleosis with meningitis**
    B27.89   **Other infectious mononucleosis with other complication**
        Hepatomegaly in other infectious mononucleosis
  B27.9-   **Infectious mononucleosis, unspecified**
    B27.90   **Infectious mononucleosis, unspecified without complication**
    B27.91   **Infectious mononucleosis, unspecified with polyneuropathy**
    B27.92   **Infectious mononucleosis, unspecified with meningitis**
    B27.99   **Infectious mononucleosis, unspecified with other complication**
        Hepatomegaly in unspecified infectious mononucleosis

B10 - B37

B30- Viral conjunctivitis
    Excludes 1: herpesviral [herpes simplex] ocular disease (B00.5)
              ocular zoster (B02.3)

  B30.0 **Keratoconjunctivitis due to adenovirus**
      Epidemic keratoconjunctivitis
      Shipyard eye

  B30.1 **Conjunctivitis due to adenovirus**
      Acute adenoviral follicular conjunctivitis
      Swimming-pool conjunctivitis

  B30.2 **Viral pharyngoconjunctivitis**

  B30.3 **Acute epidemic hemorrhagic conjunctivitis (enteroviral)**
      Conjunctivitis due to coxsackievirus 24
      Conjunctivitis due to enterovirus 70
      Hemorrhagic conjunctivitis (acute) (epidemic)

  B30.8 **Other viral conjunctivitis**
      Newcastle conjunctivitis

  B30.9 **Viral conjunctivitis, unspecified**

B33- Other viral diseases, not elsewhere classified

  B33.0 **Epidemic myalgia**
      Bornholm disease

  B33.1 **Ross River disease**
      Epidemic polyarthritis and exanthema
      Ross River fever

  B33.2- Viral carditis
      Coxsackie (virus) carditis

    B33.20 **Viral carditis, unspecified**
    B33.21 **Viral endocarditis**
    B33.22 **Viral myocarditis**
    B33.23 **Viral pericarditis**
    B33.24 **Viral cardiomyopathy**

  B33.3 **Retrovirus infections, not elsewhere classified**
      Retrovirus infection NOS

  B33.4 **Hantavirus (cardio)-pulmonary syndrome [HPS] [HCPS]**
      Hantavirus disease with pulmonary manifestations
      Sin nombre virus disease
    Use additional code to identify any associated acute kidney failure
      (N17.9)
    Excludes 1: hantavirus disease with renal manifestations (A98.5)
              hemorrhagic fever with renal manifestations (A98.5)

  B33.8 **Other specified viral diseases**
    Excludes 1: anogenital human papillomavirus infection (A63.0)
              viral warts due to human papillomavirus infection
                 (B07)

B34- Viral infection of unspecified site
    Excludes 1: anogenital human papillomavirus infection (A63.0)
              cytomegaloviral disease NOS (B25.9)
              herpesvirus [herpes simplex] infection NOS (B00.9)
              retrovirus infection NOS (B33.3)
              viral agents as the cause of diseases classified elsewhere
                 (B97-)
              viral warts due to human papillomavirus infection (B07)

  B34.0 **Adenovirus infection, unspecified**

  B34.1 **Enterovirus infection, unspecified**
      Coxsackievirus infection NOS
      Echovirus infection NOS

  B34.2 **Coronavirus infection, unspecified**
    Excludes 1: pneumonia due to SARS-associated coronavirus
              (J12.81)

  B34.3 **Parvovirus infection, unspecified**
  B34.4 **Papovavirus infection, unspecified**
  B34.8 **Other viral infections of unspecified site**
  B34.9 **Viral infection, unspecified**
      Viremia NOS

Mycoses (B35-B49)

    Excludes ❷: hypersensitivity pneumonitis due to organic dust (J67.-)
              mycosis fungoides (C84.0-)

B35- Dermatophytosis
    Includes: Favus
          Infections due to species of Epidermophyton, Micro-sporum and
             Trichophyton
          Tinea, any type except those in B36.-

  B35.0 **Tinea barbae and tinea capitis**
      Beard ringworm
      Kerion
      Scalp ringworm
      Sycosis, mycotic

  B35.1 **Tinea unguium**
      Dermatophytic onychia
      Dermatophytosis of nail
      Onychomycosis
      Ringworm of nails

  B35.2 **Tinea manuum**
      Dermatophytosis of hand
      Hand ringworm

  B35.3 **Tinea pedis**
      Athlete's foot
      Dermatophytosis of foot
      Foot ringworm

  B35.4 **Tinea corporis**
      Ringworm of the body

  B35.5 **Tinea imbricata**
      Tokelau

  B35.6 **Tinea cruris**
      Dhobi itch
      Groin ringworm
      Jock itch

  B35.8 **Other dermatophytoses**
      Disseminated dermatophytosis
      Granulomatous dermatophytosis

  B35.9 **Dermatophytosis, unspecified**
      Ringworm NOS

B36- Other superficial mycoses

  B36.0 **Pityriasis versicolor**
      Tinea flava
      Tinea versicolor

  B36.1 **Tinea nigra**
      Keratomycosis nigricans palmaris
      Microsporosis nigra
      Pityriasis nigra

  B36.2 **White piedra**
      Tinea blanca

  B36.3 **Black piedra**
  B36.8 **Other specified superficial mycoses**
  B36.9 **Superficial mycosis, unspecified**

B37- Candidiasis
    Includes: Candidosis
          Moniliasis
    Excludes 1: neonatal candidiasis (P37.5)

  B37.0 **Candidal stomatitis**
      Oral thrush

  B37.1 **Pulmonary candidiasis**
      Candidal bronchitis
      Candidal pneumonia

  B37.2 **Candidiasis of skin and nail**
      Candidal onychia
      Candidal paronychia
    Excludes ❷: diaper dermatitis (L22)

  B37.3 **Candidiasis of vulva and vagina**
      Candidal vulvovaginitis
      Monilial vulvovaginitis
      Vaginal thrush

  B37.4- Candidiasis of other urogenital sites
    B37.41 **Candidal cystitis and urethritis**
    B37.42 **Candidal balanitis**
    B37.49 **Other urogenital candidiasis**
        Candidal pyelonephritis

  B37.5 **Candidal meningitis**
  B37.6 **Candidal endocarditis**
  B37.7 **Candidal sepsis**
      Disseminated candidiasis
      Systemic candidiasis

B
1
0
-
B
3
7

Excludes 1: = NOT CODED HERE! (Do not code both)   **345**   *Excludes ❷:* = Not Included Here

B37.8- **Candidiasis of other sites**
   B37.81 **Candidal esophagitis**
   B37.82 **Candidal enteritis**
         Candidal proctitis
   B37.83 **Candidal cheilitis**
   B37.84 **Candidal otitis externa**
   B37.89 **Other sites of candidiasis**
         Candidal osteomyelitis
B37.9 **Candidiasis, unspecified**
      Thrush NOS

B38- **Coccidioidomycosis**
B38.0 **Acute pulmonary coccidioidomycosis**
B38.1 **Chronic pulmonary coccidioidomycosis**
B38.2 **Pulmonary coccidioidomycosis, unspecified**
B38.3 **Cutaneous coccidioidomycosis**
B38.4 **Coccidioidomycosis meningitis**
B38.7 **Disseminated coccidioidomycosis**
      Generalized coccidioidomycosis
B38.8- **Other forms of coccidioidomycosis**
   B38.81 **Prostatic coccidioidomycosis**
   B38.89 **Other forms of coccidioidomycosis**
B38.9 **Coccidioidomycosis, unspecified**

B39- **Histoplasmosis**
      Code first associated AIDS (B20)
      Use additional code for any associated manifestations, such as:
      Eendocarditis (I39)
      Meningitis (G02)
      Pericarditis (I32)
      Retinitits (H32)
B39.0 **Acute pulmonary histoplasmosis capsulati**
B39.1 **Chronic pulmonary histoplasmosis capsulati**
B39.2 **Pulmonary histoplasmosis capsulati, unspecified**
B39.3 **Disseminated histoplasmosis capsulati**
      Generalized histoplasmosis capsulati
B39.4 **Histoplasmosis capsulati, unspecified**
      American histoplasmosis
B39.5 **Histoplasmosis duboisii**
      African histoplasmosis
B39.9 **Histoplasmosis, unspecified**

B40- **Blastomycosis**
      Excludes 1: Brazilian blastomycosis (B41.-)
             keloidal blastomycosis (B48.0)
B40.0 **Acute pulmonary blastomycosis**
B40.1 **Chronic pulmonary blastomycosis**
B40.2 **Pulmonary blastomycosis, unspecified**
B40.3 **Cutaneous blastomycosis**
B40.7 **Disseminated blastomycosis**
      Generalized blastomycosis
B40.8- **Other forms of blastomycosis**
   B40.81 **Blastomycotic meningoencephalitis**
         Meningomyelitis due to blastomycosis
   B40.89 **Other forms of blastomycosis**
B40.9 **Blastomycosis, unspecified**

B41- **Paracoccidioidomycosis**
      Includes: Brazilian blastomycosis
              Lutz' disease
B41.0 **Pulmonary paracoccidioidomycosis**
B41.7 **Disseminated paracoccidioidomycosis**
      Generalized paracoccidioidomycosis
B41.8 **Other forms of paracoccidioidomycosis**
B41.9 **Paracoccidioidomycosis, unspecified**

B42- **Sporotrichosis**
B42.0 **Pulmonary sporotrichosis**
B42.1 **Lymphocutaneous sporotrichosis**
B42.7 **Disseminated sporotrichosis**
      Generalized sporotrichosis
B42.8- **Other forms of sporotrichosis**
   B42.81 **Cerebral sporotrichosis**
         Meningitis due to sporotrichosis
   B42.82 **Sporotrichosis arthritis**
   B42.89 **Other forms of sporotrichosis**
B42.9 **Sporotrichosis, unspecified**

B43- **Chromomycosis and pheomycotic abscess**
B43.0 **Cutaneous chromomycosis**
      Dermatitis verrucosa
B43.1 **Pheomycotic brain abscess**
      Cerebral chromomycosis
B43.2 **Subcutaneous pheomycotic abscess and cyst**
B43.8 **Other forms of chromomycosis**
B43.9 **Chromomycosis, unspecified**

B44- **Aspergillosis**
      Includes: Aspergilloma
B44.0 **Invasive pulmonary aspergillosis**
B44.1 **Other pulmonary aspergillosis**
B44.2 **Tonsillar aspergillosis**
B44.7 **Disseminated aspergillosis**
      Generalized aspergillosis
B44.8- **Other forms of aspergillosis**
   B44.81 **Allergic bronchopulmonary aspergillosis**
   B44.89 **Other forms of aspergillosis**
B44.9 **Aspergillosis, unspecified**

B45- **Cryptococcosis**
B45.0 **Pulmonary cryptococcosis**
B45.1 **Cerebral cryptococcosis**
      Cryptococcal meningitis
      Cryptococcosis meningocerebralis
B45.2 **Cutaneous cryptococcosis**
B45.3 **Osseous cryptococcosis**
B45.7 **Disseminated cryptococcosis**
      Generalized cryptococcosis
B45.8 **Other forms of cryptococcosis**
B45.9 **Cryptococcosis, unspecified**

B46- **Zygomycosis**
B46.0 **Pulmonary mucormycosis**
B46.1 **Rhinocerebral mucormycosis**
B46.2 **Gastrointestinal mucormycosis**
B46.3 **Cutaneous mucormycosis**
      Subcutaneous mucormycosis
B46.4 **Disseminated mucormycosis**
      Generalized mucormycosis
B46.5 **Mucormycosis, unspecified**
B46.8 **Other zygomycoses**
      Entomophthoromycosis
B46.9 **Zygomycosis, unspecified**
      Phycomycosis NOS

B47- **Mycetoma**
B47.0 **Eumycetoma**
      Madura foot, mycotic
      Maduromycosis
B47.1 **Actinomycetoma**
B47.9 **Mycetoma, unspecified**
      Madura foot NOS

B48- **Other mycoses, not elsewhere classified**
B48.0 **Lobomycosis**
      Keloidal blastomycosis
      Lobo's disease
B48.1 **Rhinosporidiosis**
B48.2 **Allescheriasis**
      Infection due to Pseudallescheria boydii
      Excludes 1: eumycetoma (B47.0)
B48.3 **Geotrichosis**
      Geotrichum stomatitis
B48.4 **Penicillosis**
B48.8 **Other specified mycoses**
      Adiaspiromycosis
      Infection of tissue and organs by Alternaria
      Infection of tissue and organs by Drechslera
      Infection of tissue and organs by Fusarium
      Infection of tissue and organs by saprophytic fungi NEC

B49 **Unspecified mycosis**
      Fungemia NOS

B
3
7
–
B
6
6

© 2013 Channel Publishing, Ltd

Protozoal diseases (B50-B64)

Excludes 1: amebiasis (A06.-)
other protozoal intestinal diseases (A07.-)

B50- Plasmodium <u>falciparum</u> malaria
Includes: Mixed infections of Plasmodium falciparum with any other Plasmodium species

B50.0 Plasmodium falciparum malaria with cerebral complications
Cerebral malaria NOS

B50.8 Other severe and complicated Plasmodium falciparum malaria
Severe or complicated Plasmodium falciparum malaria NOS

B50.9 Plasmodium falciparum malaria, unspecified

B51- Plasmodium <u>vivax</u> malaria
Includes: Mixed infections of Plasmodium vivax with other Plasmodium species, except Plasmodium falciparum
Excludes 1: Plasmodium vivav with Plasmodium falciparum (B50.-)

B51.0 Plasmodium vivax malaria with rupture of spleen

B51.8 Plasmodium vivax malaria with other complications

B51.9 Plasmodium vivax malaria without complication
Plasmodium vivax malaria NOS

B52- Plasmodium malariae malaria
Includes: Mixed infections of Plasmodium malariae with other Plasmodium species, except Plasmodium falciparum and Plasmodium vivax
Excludes 1: Plasmodium falciparum (B50.-)
Plasmodium vivax (B51.-)

B52.0 Plasmodium malariae malaria with nephropathy

B52.8 Plasmodium malariae malaria with other complications

B52.9 Plasmodium malariae malaria without complication
Plasmodium malariae malaria NOS

B53- Other specified malaria
B53.0 Plasmodium <u>ovale</u> malaria
Excludes 1: Plasmodium ovale with Plasmodium falciparum (B50.-)
Plasmodium ovale with Plasmodium malariae (B52.-)
Plasmodium ovale with Plasmodium vivax (B51.-)

B53.1 Malaria due to <u>simian</u> plasmodia
Excludes 1: malaria due to simian plasmodia with Plasmodium falciparum (B50.-)
malaria due to simian plasmodia with Plasmodium malariae (B52.-)
malaria due to simian plasmodia with Plasmodium ovale (B53.0)
malaria due to simian plasmodia with Plasmodium vivax (B51.-)

B53.8 Other malaria, not elsewhere classified

B54 Unspecified malaria

B55- Leishmaniasis
B55.0 Visceral leishmaniasis
Kala-azar
Post-kala-azar dermal leishmaniasis

B55.1 Cutaneous leishmaniasis

B55.2 Mucocutaneous leishmaniasis

B55.9 Leishmaniasis, unspecified

B56- African trypanosomiasis
B56.0 Gambiense trypanosomiasis
Infection due to Trypanosoma brucei gambiense
West African sleeping sickness

B56.1 Rhodesiense trypanosomiasis
East African sleeping sickness
Infection due to Trypanosoma brucei rhodesiense

B56.9 African trypanosomiasis, unspecified
Sleeping sickness NOS

B57- Chagas' disease
Includes: American trypanosomiasis
Infection due to Trypanosoma cruzi

B57.0 Acute Chagas' disease with heart involvement
Acute Chagas' disease with myocarditis

B57.1 Acute Chagas' disease without heart involvement
Acute Chagas' disease NOS

B57.2 Chagas' disease (chronic) with heart involvement
American trypanosomiasis NOS
Chagas' disease (chronic) NOS
Chagas' disease (chronic) with myocarditis
Trypanosomiasis NOS

B57.3- Chagas' disease (chronic) with digestive system involvement
B57.30 Chagas' disease with digestive system involvement, unspecified
B57.31 Megaesophagus in Chagas' disease
B57.32 Megacolon in Chagas' disease
B57.39 Other digestive system involvement in Chagas' disease

B57.4- Chagas' disease (chronic) with nervous system involvement
B57.40 Chagas' disease with nervous system involvement, unspecified
B57.41 Meningitis in Chagas' disease
B57.42 Meningoencephalitis in Chagas' disease
B57.49 Other nervous system involvement in Chagas' disease

B57.5 Chagas' disease (chronic) with other organ involvement

B58- Toxoplasmosis
Includes: Infection due to Toxoplasma gondii
Excludes 1: congenital toxoplasmosis (P37.1)

B58.0- Toxoplasma oculopathy
B58.00 Toxoplasma oculopathy, unspecified
B58.01 Toxoplasma chorioretinitis
B58.09 Other toxoplasma oculopathy
Toxoplasma uveitis

B58.1 Toxoplasma hepatitis

B58.2 Toxoplasma meningoencephalitis

B58.3 Pulmonary toxoplasmosis

B58.8- Toxoplasmosis with other organ involvement
B58.81 Toxoplasma myocarditis
B58.82 Toxoplasma myositis
B58.83 Toxoplasma tubulo-interstitial nephropathy
Toxoplasma pyelonephritis
B58.89 Toxoplasmosis with other organ involvement

B58.9 Toxoplasmosis, unspecified

B59 Pneumocystosis
Pneumonia due to Pneumocystis carinii
Pneumonia due to Pneumocystis jiroveci

B60- Other protozoal diseases, not elsewhere classified
Excludes 1: cryptosporidiosis (A07.2)
intestinal microsporidiosis (A07.8)
isosporiasis (A07.3)

B60.0 Babesiosis
Piroplasmosis

B60.1- Acanthamebiasis
B60.10 Acanthamebiasis, unspecified
B60.11 Meningoencephalitis due to Acanthamoeba (culbertsoni)
B60.12 Conjunctivitis due to Acanthamoeba
B60.13 Keratoconjunctivitis due to Acanthamoeba
B60.19 Other acanthamebic disease

B60.2 Naegleriasis
Primary amebic meningoencephalitis

B60.8 Other specified protozoal diseases
Microsporidiosis

B64 Unspecified protozoal disease

Helminthiases (B65-B83)

B65- Schistosomiasis [bilharziasis]
Includes: Snail fever

B65.0 Schistosomiasis due to Schistosoma haematobium [urinary schistosomiasis]

B65.1 Schistosomiasis due to Schistosoma mansoni [intestinal schistosomiasis]

B65.2 Schistosomiasis due to Schistosoma japonicum
Asiatic schistosomiasis

B65.3 Cercarial dermatitis
Swimmer's itch

B65.8 Other schistosomiasis
Infection due to Schistosoma intercalatum
Infection due to Schistosoma mattheei
Infection due to Schistosoma mekongi

B65.9 Schistosomiasis, unspecified

B66- Other fluke infections
B66.0 Opisthorchiasis
Infection due to cat liver fluke
Infection due to Opisthorchis (felineus) (viverrini)

B66.1 Clonorchiasis
Chinese liver fluke disease
Infection due to Clonorchis sinensis
Oriental liver fluke disease

B 3 7 - B 6 6

B66.2   Dicroceliasis
    Infection due to Dicrocoelium dendriticum
    Lancet fluke infection

B66.3   Fascioliasis
    Infection due to Fasciola gigantica
    Infection due to Fasciola hepatica
    Infection due to Fasciola indica
    Sheep liver fluke disease

B66.4   Paragonimiasis
    Infection due to Paragonimus species
    Lung fluke disease
    Pulmonary distomiasis

B66.5   Fasciolopsiasis
    Infection due to Fasciolopsis buski
    Intestinal distomiasis

B66.8   Other specified fluke infections
    Echinostomiasis
    Heterophyiasis
    Metagonimiasis
    Nanophyetiasis
    Watsoniasis

B66.9   Fluke infection, unspecified

B67-   Echinococcosis
    Includes: Hydatidosis

B67.0   Echinococcus granulosus infection of liver

B67.1   Echinococcus granulosus infection of lung

B67.2   Echinococcus granulosus infection of bone

B67.3-   Echinococcus granulosus infection, other and multiple sites

    B67.31   Echinococcus granulosus infection, thyroid gland

    B67.32   Echinococcus granulosus infection, multiple sites

    B67.39   Echinococcus granulosus infection, other sites

B67.4   Echinococcus granulosus infection, unspecified
    Dog tapeworm (infection)

B67.5   Echinococcus multilocularis infection of liver

B67.6-   Echinococcus multilocularis infection, other and multiple sites

    B67.61   Echinococcus multilocularis infection, multiple sites

    B67.69   Echinococcus multilocularis infection, other sites

B67.7   Echinococcus multilocularis infection, unspecified

B67.8   Echinococcosis, unspecified, of liver

B67.9-   Echinococcosis, other and unspecified

    B67.90   Echinococcosis, unspecified
        Echinococcosis NOS

    B67.99   Other echinococcosis

B68-   Taeniasis
    Excludes 1: cysticercosis (B69.-)

B68.0   Taenia solium taeniasis
    Pork tapeworm (infection)

B68.1   Taenia saginata taeniasis
    Beef tapeworm (infection)
    Infection due to adult tapeworm Taenia saginata

B68.9   Taeniasis, unspecified

B69-   Cysticercosis
    Includes: Cysticerciasis infection due to larval form of Taenia solium

B69.0   Cysticercosis of central nervous system

B69.1   Cysticercosis of eye

B69.8-   Cysticercosis of other sites

    B69.81   Myositis in cysticercosis

    B69.89   Cysticercosis of other sites

B69.9   Cysticercosis, unspecified

B70-   Diphyllobothriasis and sparganosis

B70.0   Diphyllobothriasis
    Diphyllobothrium (adult) (latum) (pacificum) infection
    Fish tapeworm (infection)
    Excludes❷: larval diphyllobothriasis (B70.1)

B70.1   Sparganosis
    Infection due to Sparganum (mansoni) (proliferum)
    Infection due to Spirometra larva
    Larval diphyllobothriasis
    Spirometrosis

B71-   Other cestode infections

B71.0   Hymenolepiasis
    Dwarf tapeworm infection
    Rat tapeworm (infection)

B71.1   Dipylidiasis

B71.8   Other specified cestode infections
    Coenurosis

B71.9   Cestode infection, unspecified
    Tapeworm (infection) NOS

B72   Dracunculiasis
    Includes: Guinea worm infection
            Infection due to Dracunculus medinensis

B73-   Onchocerciasis
    Includes: Onchocerca volvulus infection
            Onchocercosis
            River blindness

    B73.0-   Onchocerciasis with eye disease

      B73.00   Onchocerciasis with eye involvement, unspecified

      B73.01   Onchocerciasis with endophthalmitis

      B73.02   Onchocerciasis with glaucoma

      B73.09   Onchocerciasis with other eye involvement
          Infestation of eyelid due to onchocerciasis

    B73.1   Onchocerciasis without eye disease

B74-   Filariasis
    Excludes❷: onchocerciasis (B73)
            tropical (pulmonary) eosinophilia NOS (J82)

B74.0   Filariasis due to Wuchereria bancrofti
    Bancroftian elephantiasis
    Bancroftian filariasis

B74.1   Filariasis due to Brugia malayi

B74.2   Filariasis due to Brugia timori

B74.3   Loiasis
    Calabar swelling
    Eyeworm disease of Africa
    Loa loa infection

B74.4   Mansonelliasis
    Infection due to Mansonella ozzardi
    Infection due to Mansonella perstans
    Infection due to Mansonella streptocerca

B74.8   Other filariases
    Dirofilariasis

B74.9   Filariasis, unspecified

B75   Trichinellosis
    Includes: Infection due to Trichinella species
            Trichiniasis

B76-   Hookworm diseases
    Includes: Uncinariasis

B76.0   Ancylostomiasis
    Infection due to Ancylostoma species

B76.1   Necatoriasis
    Infection due to Necator americanus

B76.8   Other hookworm diseases

B76.9   Hookworm disease, unspecified
    Cutaneous larva migrans NOS

B77-   Ascariasis
    Includes: Ascaridiasis
           Roundworm infection

B77.0   Ascariasis with intestinal complications

B77.8-   Ascariasis with other complications

    B77.81   Ascariasis pneumonia

    B77.89   Ascariasis with other complications

B77.9   Ascariasis, unspecified

B78-   Strongyloidiasis
    Excludes 1: trichostrongyliasis (B81.2)

B78.0   Intestinal strongyloidiasis

B78.1   Cutaneous strongyloidiasis

B78.7   Disseminated strongyloidiasis

B78.9   Strongyloidiasis, unspecified

B79   Trichuriasis
    Includes: Trichocephaliasis
           Whipworm (disease) (infection)

B80   Enterobiasis
    Includes: Oxyuriasis
           Pinworm infection
           Threadworm infection

B81-   Other intestinal helminthiases, not elsewhere classified
    Excludes 1: angiostrongyliasis due to Parastrongylus cantonensis (B83.2)

B81.0   Anisakiasis
    Infection due to Anisakis larva

B81.1   Intestinal capillariasis
    Capillariasis NOS
    Infection due to Capillaria philippinensis
    Excludes❷: hepatic capillariasis (B83.8)

B81.2   Trichostrongyliasis

B81.3   Intestinal angiostrongyliasis
    Angiostrongyliasis due to Parastrongylus costaricensis

Excludes 1: = NOT CODED HERE! (Do not code both)

Excludes❷: = Not Included Here

B 6 6 – B 9 4

B81.4   Mixed intestinal helminthiases
Infection due to intestinal helminths classified to more than one of the categories B65.0-B81.3 and B81.8
Mixed helminthiasis NOS

B81.8   Other specified intestinal helminthiases
Infection due to Oesophagostomum species [esophagostomiasis]
Infection due to Ternidens diminutus [ternidensiasis]

B82- Unspecified intestinal parasitism

B82.0   Intestinal helminthiasis, unspecified

B82.9   Intestinal parasitism, unspecified

B83- Other helminthiases
Excludes 1: capillariasis NOS (B81.1)
Excludes❷: intestinal capillariasis (B81.1)

B83.0   Visceral larva migrans
Toxocariasis

B83.1   Gnathostomiasis
Wandering swelling

B83.2   Angiostrongyliasis due to Parastrongylus cantonensis
Eosinophilic meningoencephalitis due to Parastrongylus cantonensis
Excludes❷: intestinal angiostrongyliasis (B81.3)

B83.3   Syngamiasis
Syngamosis

B83.4   Internal hirudiniasis
Excludes❷: external hirudiniasis (B88.3)

B83.8   Other specified helminthiases
Acanthocephaliasis
Gongylonemiasis
Hepatic capillariasis
Metastrongyliasis
Thelaziasis

B83.9   Helminthiasis, unspecified
Worms NOS
Excludes 1: intestinal helminthiasis NOS (B82.0)

Pediculosis, acariasis and other infestations (B85-B89)

B85- Pediculosis and phthiriasis

B85.0   Pediculosis due to Pediculus humanus capitis
Head-louse infestation

B85.1   Pediculosis due to Pediculus humanus corporis
Body-louse infestation

B85.2   Pediculosis, unspecified

B85.3   Phthiriasis
Infestation by crab-louse
Infestation by Phthirus pubis

B85.4   Mixed pediculosis and phthiriasis
Infestation classifiable to more than one of the categories B85.0-B85.3

B86   Scabies
Sarcoptic itch

B87- Myiasis
Includes: Infestation by larva of flies

B87.0   Cutaneous myiasis
Creeping myiasis

B87.1   Wound myiasis
Traumatic myiasis

B87.2   Ocular myiasis

B87.3   Nasopharyngeal myiasis
Laryngeal myiasis

B87.4   Aural myiasis

B87.8- Myiasis of other sites

B87.81   Genitourinary myiasis

B87.82   Intestinal myiasis

B87.89   Myiasis of other sites

B87.9   Myiasis, unspecified

B88- Other infestations

B88.0   Other acariasis
Acarine dermatitis
Dermatitis due to Demodex species
Dermatitis due to Dermanyssus gallinae
Dermatitis due to Liponyssoides sanguineus
Trombiculosis
Excludes❷: scabies (B86)

B88.1   Tungiasis [sandflea infestation]

B88.2   Other arthropod infestations
Scarabiasis

B88.3   External hirudiniasis
Leech infestation NOS
Excludes❷: internal hirudiniasis (B83.4)

B88.8   Other specified infestations
Ichthyoparasitism due to Vandellia cirrhosa
Linguatulosis
Porocephaliasis

B88.9   Infestation, unspecified
Infestation (skin) NOS
Infestation by mites NOS
Skin parasites NOS

B89   Unspecified parasitic disease

Sequelae of infectious and parasitic diseases (B90-B94)

Note: Categories B90-B94 are to be used to indicate conditions in categories A00-B89 as the cause of sequelae, which are themselves classified elsewhere. The "sequelae" include conditions specified as such; they also include residuals of diseases classifiable to the above categories if there is evidence that the disease itself is no longer present. Codes from these categories are not to be used for chronic infections. Code chronic current infections to active infectious disease as appropriate.
Code first condition resulting from (sequela) the infectious or parasitic disease

B90- Sequelae of tuberculosis

B90.0   Sequelae of central nervous system tuberculosis

B90.1   Sequelae of genitourinary tuberculosis

B90.2   Sequelae of tuberculosis of bones and joints

B90.8   Sequelae of tuberculosis of other organs
Excludes❷: sequelae of respiratory tuberculosis (B90.9)

B90.9   Sequelae of respiratory and unspecified tuberculosis
Sequelae of tuberculosis NOS

B91   Sequelae of poliomyelitis
Excludes 1: postpolio syndrome (G14)

B92   Sequelae of leprosy

B94- Sequelae of other and unspecified infectious and parasitic diseases

B94.0   Sequelae of trachoma

B94.1   Sequelae of viral encephalitis

B94.2   Sequelae of viral hepatitis

B94.8   Sequelae of other specified infectious and parasitic diseases

B94.9   Sequelae of unspecified infectious and parasitic disease

B66 - B94

Excludes 1: = NOT CODED HERE! (Do not code both)

Excludes❷: = Not Included Here

Bacterial and viral infectious agents (B95-B97)

Note: These categories are provided for use as supplementary or additional codes to identify the infectious agent(s) in diseases classified elsewhere.

B95- Streptococcus, Staphylococcus, and Enterococcus as the cause of diseases classified elsewhere

B95.0 Streptococcus, group A, as the cause of diseases classified elsewhere

B95.1 Streptococcus, group B, as the cause of diseases classified elsewhere

B95.2 Enterococcus as the cause of diseases classified elsewhere

B95.3 Streptococcus pneumoniae as the cause of diseases classified elsewhere

B95.4 Other streptococcus as the cause of diseases classified elsewhere

B95.5 Unspecified streptococcus as the cause of diseases classified elsewhere

B95.6- Staphylococcus aureus as the cause of diseases classified elsewhere

B95.61 Methicillin susceptible Staphylococcus aureus infection as the cause of diseases classified elsewhere
Methicillin susceptible Staphylococcus aureus (MSSA) infection as the cause of diseases classified elsewhere
Staphylococcus aureus infection NOS as the cause of diseases classified elsewhere

B95.62 Methicillin resistant Staphylococcus aureus infection as the cause of diseases classified elsewhere
Methicillin resistant Staphylococcus aureus (MRSA) infection as the cause of diseases classified elsewhere

B95.7 Other staphylococcus as the cause of diseases classified elsewhere

B95.8 Unspecified staphylococcus as the cause of diseases classified elsewhere

B96- Other bacterial agents as the cause of diseases classified elsewhere

B96.0 Mycoplasma pneumoniae [M. pneumoniae] as the cause of diseases classified elsewhere
Pleuro-pneumonia-like-organism [PPLO]

B96.1 Klebsiella pneumoniae [K. pneumoniae] as the cause of diseases classified elsewhere

B96.2- Escherichia coli [E. coli] as the cause of diseases classified elsewhere

B96.20 Unspecified Escherichia coli [E. coli] as the cause of diseases classified elsewhere
Escherichia coli [E. coli] NOS

B96.21 Shiga toxin-producing Escherichia coli [E. coli] (STEC) O157 as the cause of diseases classified elsewhere
E. coli O157:H- (nonmotile) with confirmation of Shiga toxin
E. coli O157 with confirmation of Shiga toxin when H antigen is unknown, or is not H7
O157:H7 Escherichia coli [E. coli] with or without confirmation of Shiga toxin-production
Shiga toxin-producing Escherichia coli [E. coli] O157:H7 with or without confirmation of Shiga toxin-production
STEC O157:H7 with or without confirmation of Shiga toxin-production

B96.22 Other specified Shiga toxin-producing Escherichia coli [E. coli] (STEC) as the cause of diseases classified elsewhere
Non-O157 Shiga toxin-producing Escherichia coli [E. coli]
Non-O157 Shiga toxin-producing Escherichia coli [E. coli] with known O group

B96.23 Unspecified Shiga toxin-producing Escherichia coli [E. coli] (STEC) as the cause of diseases classified elsewhere
Shiga toxin-producing Escherichia coli [E. coli] with specified O group
STEC NOS

B96.29 Other Escherichia coli [E. coli] as the cause of diseases classified elsewhere
Non-Shiga toxin-producing [E. coli]

B96.3 Hemophilus influenzae [H. influenzae] as the cause of diseases classified elsewhere

B96.4 Proteus (mirabilis) (morganii) as the cause of diseases classified elsewhere

B96.5 Pseudomonas (aeruginosa) (mallei) (pseudomallei) as the cause of diseases classified elsewhere

B96.6 Bacteroides fragilis [B. fragilis] as the cause of diseases classified elsewhere

B96.7 Clostridium perfringens [C. perfringens] as the cause of diseases classified elsewhere

B96.8- Other specified bacterial agents as the cause of diseases classified elsewhere

B96.81 Helicobacter pylori [H. pylori] as the cause of diseases classified elsewhere

B96.82 Vibrio vulnificus as the cause of diseases classified elsewhere

B96.89 Other specified bacterial agents as the cause of diseases classified elsewhere

B97- Viral agents as the cause of diseases classified elsewhere

B97.0 Adenovirus as the cause of diseases classified elsewhere

B97.1- Enterovirus as the cause of diseases classified elsewhere

B97.10 Unspecified enterovirus as the cause of diseases classified elsewhere

B97.11 Coxsackievirus as the cause of diseases classified elsewhere

B97.12 Echovirus as the cause of diseases classified elsewhere

B97.19 Other enterovirus as the cause of diseases classified elsewhere

B97.2- Coronavirus as the cause of diseases classified elsewhere

B97.21 SARS-associated coronavirus as the cause of diseases classified elsewhere
Excludes 1: pneumonia due to SARS-associated coronavirus (J12.81)

B97.29 Other coronavirus as the cause of diseases classified elsewhere

B97.3- Retrovirus as the cause of diseases classified elsewhere
Excludes 1: Human immunodeficiency virus [HIV] disease (B20)

B97.30 Unspecified retrovirus as the cause of diseases classified elsewhere

B97.31 Lentivirus as the cause of diseases classified elsewhere

B97.32 Oncovirus as the cause of diseases classified elsewhere

B97.33 Human T-cell lymphotrophic virus, type I [HTLV-I] as the cause of diseases classified elsewhere

B97.34 Human T-cell lymphotrophic virus, type II [HTLV-II] as the cause of diseases classified elsewhere

B97.35 Human immunodeficiency virus, type 2 [HIV 2] as the cause of diseases classified elsewhere

B97.39 Other retrovirus as the cause of diseases classified elsewhere

B97.4 Respiratory syncytial virus as the cause of diseases classified elsewhere

B97.5 Reovirus as the cause of diseases classified elsewhere

B97.6 Parvovirus as the cause of diseases classified elsewhere

B97.7 Papillomavirus as the cause of diseases classified elsewhere

B97.8- Other viral agents as the cause of diseases classified elsewhere

B97.81 Human metapneumovirus as the cause of diseases classified elsewhere

B97.89 Other viral agents as the cause of diseases classified elsewhere

Other infectious diseases (B99)

B99- Other and unspecified infectious diseases

B99.8 Other infectious disease

B99.9 Unspecified infectious disease

B 9 5 - C 0 2

Excludes 1: = NOT CODED HERE! (Do not code both)

350

Excludes❷: = Not Included Here

Chapter 2 – Neoplasms (C00-D49)

Note: Functional activity

All neoplasms are classified in this chapter, whether they are functionally active or not. An additional code from Chapter 4 may be used, to identify functional activity associated with any neoplasm.

Morphology [Histology]

Chapter 2 classifies neoplasms primarily by site (topography), with broad groupings for behavior, malignant, in situ, benign, etc. The Table of Neoplasms should be used to identify the correct topography code. In a few cases, such as for malignant melanoma and certain neuroendocrine tumors, the morphology (histologic type) is included in the category and codes.

Primary malignant neoplasms overlapping site boundaries

A primary malignant neoplasm that overlaps two or more contiguous (next to each other) sites should be classified to the subcategory/code .8 ("overlapping lesion"), unless the combination is specifically indexed elsewhere. For multiple neoplasms of the same site that are not contiguous, such as tumors in different quadrants of the same breast, codes for each site should be assigned.

Malignant neoplasm of ectopic tissue

Malignant neoplasms of ectopic tissue are to be coded to the site mentioned, e.g., ectopic pancreatic malignant neoplasms are coded to pancreas, unspecified (C25.9).

This chapter contains the following blocks:

C00-C14	Malignant neoplasm of lip, oral cavity and pharynx
C15-C26	Malignant neoplasm of digestive organs
C30-C39	Malignant neoplasm of respiratory and intrathoracic organs
C40-C41	Malignant neoplasm of bone and articular cartilage
C43-C44	Melanoma and other malignant neoplasms of skin
C45-C49	Malignant neoplasms of mesothelial and soft tissue
C50	Malignant neoplasm of breast
C51-C58	Malignant neoplasm of female genital organs
C60-C63	Malignant neoplasms of male genital organs
C64-C68	Malignant neoplasm of urinary tract
C69-C72	Malignant neoplasms of eye, brain and other parts of central nervous system
C73-C75	Malignant neoplasm of thyroid and other endocrine glands
C7A	Malignant neuroendocrine tumors
C7B	Secondary neuroendocrine tumors
C76-C80	Malignant neoplasms of ill-defined, other secondary and unspecified sites
C81-C96	Malignant neoplasms of lymphoid, hematopoietic and related tissue
D00-D09	In situ neoplasms
D10-D36	Benign neoplasms, except benign neuroendocrine tumors
D3A	Benign neuroendocrine tumors
D37-D48	Neoplasms of uncertain behavior, polycythemia vera and myelodysplastic syndromes
D49	Neoplasms of unspecified behavior

Malignant neoplasms (C00-C96)

Malignant neoplasms, stated or presumed to be primary (of specified sites), and certain specified histologies, except neuroendocrine, and of lymphoid, hematopoietic and related tissue (C00-C75)

Malignant neoplasms of lip, oral cavity and pharynx (C00-C14)

C00- Malignant neoplasm of lip
Use additional code to identify:
Alcohol abuse and dependence (F10.-)
History of tobacco use (Z87.891)
Tobacco dependence (F17.-)
Tobacco use (Z72.0)
Excludes 1: malignant melanoma of lip (C43.0)
                Merkel cell carcinoma of lip (C4A.0)
                other and unspecified malignant neoplasm of skin of lip (C44.0-)

    C00.0   **Malignant neoplasm of <u>external upper</u> lip**
            Malignant neoplasm of lipstick area of upper lip
            Malignant neoplasm of upper lip NOS
            Malignant neoplasm of vermilion border of upper lip

    C00.1   **Malignant neoplasm of <u>external lower</u> lip**
            Malignant neoplasm of lower lip NOS
            Malignant neoplasm of lipstick area of lower lip
            Malignant neoplasm of vermilion border of lower lip

    C00.2   **Malignant neoplasm of external lip, unspecified**
            Malignant neoplasm of vermilion border of lip NOS

    C00.3   **Malignant neoplasm of <u>upper</u> lip, <u>inner</u> aspect**
            Malignant neoplasm of buccal aspect of upper lip
            Malignant neoplasm of frenulum of upper lip
            Malignant neoplasm of mucosa of upper lip
            Malignant neoplasm of oral aspect of upper lip

    C00.4   **Malignant neoplasm of <u>lower</u> lip, <u>inner</u> aspect**
            Malignant neoplasm of buccal aspect of lower lip
            Malignant neoplasm of frenulum of lower lip
            Malignant neoplasm of mucosa of lower lip
            Malignant neoplasm of oral aspect of lower lip

    C00.5   **Malignant neoplasm of lip, unspecified, inner aspect**
            Malignant neoplasm of buccal aspect of lip, unspecified
            Malignant neoplasm of frenulum of lip, unspecified
            Malignant neoplasm of mucosa of lip, unspecified
            Malignant neoplasm of oral aspect of lip, unspecified

    C00.6   **Malignant neoplasm of <u>commissure</u> of lip, unspecified**

    C00.8   **Malignant neoplasm of <u>overlapping</u> sites of lip**

    C00.9   **Malignant neoplasm of lip, unspecified**

C01 Malignant neoplasm of <u>base of tongue</u>
    Malignant neoplasm of dorsal surface of base of tongue
    Malignant neoplasm of fixed part of tongue NOS
    Malignant neoplasm of posterior third of tongue
    Use additional code to identify:
    Alcohol abuse and dependence (F10.-)
    History of tobacco use (Z87.891)
    Tobacco dependence (F17.-)
    Tobacco use (Z72.0)

C02- Malignant neoplasm of other and unspecified parts of tongue
    Use additional code to identify:
    Alcohol abuse and dependence (F10.-)
    History of tobacco use (Z87.891)
    Tobacco dependence (F17.-)
    Tobacco use (Z72.0)

    C02.0   **Malignant neoplasm of <u>dorsal surface</u> of tongue**
            Malignant neoplasm of anterior two-thirds of tongue, dorsal surface
            Excludes❷: malignant neoplasm of dorsal surface of base of tongue (C01)

    C02.1   **Malignant neoplasm of <u>border</u> of tongue**
            Malignant neoplasm of tip of tongue

    C02.2   **Malignant neoplasm of <u>ventral</u> surface of tongue**
            Malignant neoplasm of anterior two-thirds of tongue, ventral surface
            Malignant neoplasm of frenulum linguae

    C02.3   **Malignant neoplasm of <u>anterior two-thirds</u> of tongue, part unspecified**
            Malignant neoplasm of middle third of tongue NOS
            Malignant neoplasm of mobile part of tongue NOS

B 9 5 - C 0 2

C02.4   **Malignant neoplasm of <u>lingual</u> tonsil**
     Excludes❷: malignant neoplasm of tonsil NOS (C09.9)

C02.8   **Malignant neoplasm of <u>overlapping</u> sites of tongue**
     Malignant neoplasm of two or more contiguous sites of tongue

C02.9   **Malignant neoplasm of tongue, unspecified**

C03-   **Malignant neoplasm of <u>gum</u>**
     Includes: Malignant neoplasm of alveolar (ridge) mucosa
                Malignant neoplasm of gingiva
     Use additional code to identify:
       Alcohol abuse and dependence (F10.-)
       History of tobacco use (Z87.891)
       Tobacco dependence (F17.-)
       Tobacco use (Z72.0)
     Excludes❷: malignant odontogenic neoplasms (C41.0-C41.1)

C03.0   **Malignant neoplasm of <u>upper</u> gum**

C03.1   **Malignant neoplasm of <u>lower</u> gum**

C03.9   **Malignant neoplasm of gum, unspecified**

C04-   **Malignant neoplasm of <u>floor of mouth</u>**
     Use additional code to identify:
       Alcohol abuse and dependence (F10.-)
       History of tobacco use (Z87.891)
       Tobacco dependence (F17.-)
       Tobacco use (Z72.0)

C04.0   **Malignant neoplasm of <u>anterior</u> floor of mouth**
     Malignant neoplasm of anterior to the premolar-canine junction

C04.1   **Malignant neoplasm of <u>lateral</u> floor of mouth**

C04.8   **Malignant neoplasm of <u>overlapping</u> sites of floor of mouth**

C04.9   **Malignant neoplasm of floor of mouth, unspecified**

C05-   **Malignant neoplasm of <u>palate</u>**
     Use additional code to identify:
       Alcohol abuse and dependence (F10.-)
       History of tobacco use (Z87.891)
       Tobacco dependence (F17.-)
       Tobacco use (Z72.0)
     Excludes 1: Kaposi's sarcoma of palate (C46.2)

C05.0   **Malignant neoplasm of <u>hard</u> palate**

C05.1   **Malignant neoplasm of <u>soft</u> palate**
     Excludes❷: malignant neoplasm of nasopharyngeal surface of soft
            palate (C11.3)

C05.2   **Malignant neoplasm of <u>uvula</u>**

C05.8   **Malignant neoplasm of <u>overlapping</u> sites of palate**

C05.9   **Malignant neoplasm of palate, unspecified**
     Malignant neoplasm of roof of mouth

C06-   **Malignant neoplasm of other and unspecified parts of mouth**
     Use additional code to identify:
       Alcohol abuse and dependence (F10.-)
       History of tobacco use (Z87.891)
       Tobacco dependence (F17.-)
       Tobacco use (Z72.0)

C06.0   **Malignant neoplasm of <u>cheek mucosa</u>**
     Malignant neoplasm of buccal mucosa NOS
     Malignant neoplasm of internal cheek

C06.1   **Malignant neoplasm of <u>vestibule</u> of mouth**
     Malignant neoplasm of buccal sulcus (upper) (lower)
     Malignant neoplasm of labial sulcus (upper) (lower)

C06.2   **Malignant neoplasm of <u>retromolar area</u>**

C06.8-   **Malignant neoplasm of overlapping sites of other and unspecified parts of mouth**

   C06.80   **Malignant neoplasm of overlapping sites of unspecified parts of mouth**

   C06.89   **Malignant neoplasm of overlapping sites of other parts of mouth**
       "Book leaf" neoplasm [ventral surface of tongue and floor of mouth]

C06.9   **Malignant neoplasm of mouth, unspecified**
     Malignant neoplasm of minor salivary gland, unspecified site
     Malignant neoplasm of oral cavity NOS

C07   **Malignant neoplasm of <u>parotid gland</u>**
     Use additional code to identify:
       Alcohol abuse and dependence (F10.-)
       Exposure to environmental tobacco smoke (Z77.22)
       Exposure to tobacco smoke in the perinatal period (P96.81)
       History of tobacco use (Z87.891)
       Occupational exposure to environmental tobacco smoke (Z57.31)
       Tobacco dependence (F17.-)
       Tobacco use (Z72.0)

C08-   **Malignant neoplasm of other and unspecified major salivary glands**
     Includes: malignant neoplasm of salivary ducts
     Use additional code to identify:
       Alcohol abuse and dependence (F10.-)
       Exposure to environmental tobacco smoke (Z77.22)
       Exposure to tobacco smoke in the perinatal period (P96.81)
       History of tobacco use (Z87.891)
       Occupational exposure to environmental tobacco smoke (Z57.31)
       Tobacco dependence (F17.-)
       Tobacco use (Z72.0)
     Excludes 1: malignant neoplasms of specified minor salivary glands which
                  are classified according to their anatomical location
     Excludes❷: malignant neoplasms of minor salivary glands NOS (C06.9)
              malignant neoplasm of parotid gland (C07)

   C08.0   **Malignant neoplasm of <u>submandibular gland</u>**
     Malignant neoplasm of submaxillary gland

   C08.1   **Malignant neoplasm of <u>sublingual gland</u>**

   C08.9   **Malignant neoplasm of major salivary gland, unspecified**
     Malignant neoplasm of salivary gland (major) NOS

C09-   **Malignant neoplasm of <u>tonsil</u>**
     Use additional code to identify:
       Alcohol abuse and dependence (F10.-)
       Exposure to environmental tobacco smoke (Z77.22)
       Exposure to tobacco smoke in the perinatal period (P96.81)
       History of tobacco use (Z87.891)
       Occupational exposure to environmental tobacco smoke (Z57.31)
       Tobacco dependence (F17.-)
       Tobacco use (Z72.0)
     Excludes❷: malignant neoplasm of lingual tonsil (C02.4)
              malignant neoplasm of pharyngeal tonsil (C11.1)

   C09.0   **Malignant neoplasm of tonsillar <u>fossa</u>**

   C09.1   **Malignant neoplasm of tonsillar <u>pillar</u> (anterior) (posterior)**

   C09.8   **Malignant neoplasm of <u>overlapping</u> sites of tonsil**

   C09.9   **Malignant neoplasm of tonsil, unspecified**
     Malignant neoplasm of tonsil NOS
     Malignant neoplasm of faucial tonsils
     Malignant neoplasm of palatine tonsils

C10-   **Malignant neoplasm of <u>oropharynx</u>**
     Use additional code to identify:
       Alcohol abuse and dependence (F10.-)
       Exposure to environmental tobacco smoke (Z77.22)
       Exposure to tobacco smoke in the perinatal period (P96.81)
       History of tobacco use (Z87.891)
       Occupational exposure to environmental tobacco smoke (Z57.31)
       Tobacco dependence (F17.-)
       Tobacco use (Z72.0)
     Excludes❷: malignant neoplasm of tonsil (C09.-)

   C10.0   **Malignant neoplasm of <u>vallecula</u>**

   C10.1   **Malignant neoplasm of anterior surface of <u>epiglottis</u>**
     Malignant neoplasm of epiglottis, free border [margin]
     Malignant neoplasm of glossoepiglottic fold(s)
     Excludes❷: malignant neoplasm of epiglottis (suprahyoid portion)
              NOS (C32.1)

   C10.2   **Malignant neoplasm of <u>lateral wall</u> of oropharynx**

   C10.3   **Malignant neoplasm of <u>posterior wall</u> of oropharynx**

   C10.4   **Malignant neoplasm of <u>branchial cleft</u>**
     Malignant neoplasm of branchial cyst [site of neoplasm]

   C10.8   **Malignant neoplasm of <u>overlapping</u> sites of oropharynx**
     Malignant neoplasm of junctional region of oropharynx

   C10.9   **Malignant neoplasm of oropharynx, unspecified**

C11-   **Malignant neoplasm of <u>nasopharynx</u>**
     Use additional code to identify:
       Exposure to environmental tobacco smoke (Z77.22)
       Exposure to tobacco smoke in the perinatal period (P96.81)
       History of tobacco use (Z87.891)
       Occupational exposure to environmental tobacco smoke (Z57.31)
       Tobacco dependence (F17.-)
       Tobacco use (Z72.0)

   C11.0   **Malignant neoplasm of <u>superior wall</u> of nasopharynx**
     Malignant neoplasm of roof of nasopharynx

   C11.1   **Malignant neoplasm of <u>posterior wall</u> of nasopharynx**
     Malignant neoplasm of adenoid
     Malignant neoplasm of pharyngeal tonsil

   C11.2   **Malignant neoplasm of <u>lateral wall</u> of nasopharynx**
     Malignant neoplasm of fossa of Rosenmüller
     Malignant neoplasm of opening of auditory tube
     Malignant neoplasm of pharyngeal recess

C02-C21 *(side tab)*

C11.3   Malignant neoplasm of <u>anterior wall</u> of nasopharynx
   Malignant neoplasm of floor of nasopharynx
   Malignant neoplasm of nasopharyngeal (anterior) (posterior)
      surface of soft palate
   Malignant neoplasm of posterior margin of nasal choana
   Malignant neoplasm of posterior margin of nasal septum
C11.8   Malignant neoplasm of <u>overlapping</u> sites of nasopharynx
C11.9   Malignant neoplasm of nasopharynx, unspecified
   Malignant neoplasm of nasopharyngeal wall NOS

C12   Malignant neoplasm of <u>pyriform sinus</u>
   Malignant neoplasm of pyriform fossa
   Use additional code to identify:
   Exposure to environmental tobacco smoke (Z77.22)
   Exposure to tobacco smoke in the perinatal period (P96.81)
   History of tobacco use (Z87.891)
   Occupational exposure to environmental tobacco smoke (Z57.31)
   Tobacco dependence (F17.-)
   Tobacco use (Z72.0)

C13-   Malignant neoplasm of <u>hypopharynx</u>
   Use additional code to identify:
   Exposure to environmental tobacco smoke (Z77.22)
   Exposure to tobacco smoke in the perinatal period (P96.81)
   History of tobacco use (Z87.891)
   Occupational exposure to environmental tobacco smoke (Z57.31)
   Tobacco dependence (F17.-)
   Tobacco use (Z72.0)
   Excludes❷: malignant neoplasm of pyriform sinus (C12)
C13.0   Malignant neoplasm of <u>postcricoid region</u>
C13.1   Malignant neoplasm of <u>aryepiglottic fold</u>, hypopharyngeal aspect
   Malignant neoplasm of aryepiglottic fold NOS
   Malignant neoplasm of interarytenoid fold NOS
   Malignant neoplasm of aryepiglottic fold, marginal zone
   Malignant neoplasm of interarytenoid fold, marginal zone
   *Excludes❷: malignant neoplasm of aryepiglottic fold or
      interarytenoid fold, laryngeal aspect (C32.1)*
C13.2   Malignant neoplasm of <u>posterior wall</u> of hypopharynx
C13.8   Malignant neoplasm of <u>overlapping</u> sites of hypopharynx
C13.9   Malignant neoplasm of hypopharynx, unspecified
   Malignant neoplasm of hypopharyngeal wall NOS

C14-   Malignant neoplasm of other and ill-defined sites in the lip, oral cavity
   and pharynx
   Use additional code to identify:
   Alcohol abuse and dependence (F10.-)
   Exposure to environmental tobacco smoke (Z77.22)
   Exposure to tobacco smoke in the perinatal period (P96.81)
   History of tobacco use (Z87.891)
   Occupational exposure to environmental tobacco smoke (Z57.31)
   Tobacco dependence (F17.-)
   Tobacco use (Z72.0)
   Excludes 1: malignant neoplasm of oral cavity NOS (C06.9)
C14.0   Malignant neoplasm of pharynx, unspecified
C14.2   Malignant neoplasm of Waldeyer's ring
C14.8   Malignant neoplasm of overlapping sites of lip, oral cavity and
   pharynx
   Primary malignant neoplasm of two or more contiguous sites of
      lip, oral cavity and pharynx
   *Excludes 1: "book leaf" neoplasm [ventral surface of tongue and
      floor of mouth] (C06.89)*

Malignant neoplasms of digestive organs (C15-C26)

Excludes 1: Kaposi's sarcoma of gastrointestinal sites (C46.4)

C15-   Malignant neoplasm of <u>esophagus</u>
   Use additional code to identify:
   Alcohol abuse and dependence (F10.-)
C15.3   Malignant neoplasm of <u>upper third</u> of esophagus
C15.4   Malignant neoplasm of <u>middle third</u> of esophagus
C15.5   Malignant neoplasm of <u>lower third</u> of esophagus
   *Excludes 1: malignant neoplasm of cardio-esophageal junction
      (C16.0)*
C15.8   Malignant neoplasm of <u>overlapping</u> sites of esophagus
C15.9   Malignant neoplasm of esophagus, unspecified

C16-   Malignant neoplasm of <u>stomach</u>
   Use additional code to identify:
   Alcohol abuse and dependence (F10.-)
   Excludes❷: malignant carcinoid tumor of the stomach (C7A.092)
C16.0   Malignant neoplasm of <u>cardia</u>
   Malignant neoplasm of cardiac orifice
   Malignant neoplasm of cardio-esophageal junction
   Malignant neoplasm of esophagus and stomach
   Malignant neoplasm of gastro-esophageal junction
C16.1   Malignant neoplasm of <u>fundus</u> of stomach
C16.2   Malignant neoplasm of <u>body</u> of stomach
C16.3   Malignant neoplasm of <u>pyloric antrum</u>
   Malignant neoplasm of gastric antrum
C16.4   Malignant neoplasm of <u>pylorus</u>
   Malignant neoplasm of prepylorus
   Malignant neoplasm of pyloric canal
C16.5   Malignant neoplasm of lesser curvature of stomach, unspecified
   Malignant neoplasm of lesser curvature of stomach, not
      classifiable to C16.1-C16.4
C16.6   Malignant neoplasm of greater curvature of stomach, unspecified
   Malignant neoplasm of greater curvature of stomach, not
      classifiable to C16.0-C16.4
C16.8   Malignant neoplasm of <u>overlapping</u> sites of stomach
C16.9   Malignant neoplasm of stomach, unspecified
   Gastric cancer NOS

C17-   Malignant neoplasm of <u>small intestine</u>
   Excludes 1: malignant carcinoid tumors of the small intestine (C7A.01)
C17.0   Malignant neoplasm of <u>duodenum</u>
C17.1   Malignant neoplasm of <u>jejunum</u>
C17.2   Malignant neoplasm of <u>ileum</u>
   Excludes 1: malignant neoplasm of ileocecal valve (C18.0)
C17.3   <u>Meckel's</u> diverticulum, malignant
   Excludes 1: Meckel's diverticulum, congenital (Q43.0)
C17.8   Malignant neoplasm of <u>overlapping</u> sites of small intestine
C17.9   Malignant neoplasm of small intestine, unspecified

C18-   Malignant neoplasm of <u>colon</u>
   Excludes 1: malignant carcinoid tumors of the colon (C7A.02-)
C18.0   Malignant neoplasm of <u>cecum</u>
   Malignant neoplasm of ileocecal valve
C18.1   Malignant neoplasm of <u>appendix</u>
C18.2   Malignant neoplasm of <u>ascending colon</u>
C18.3   Malignant neoplasm of <u>hepatic flexure</u>
C18.4   Malignant neoplasm of <u>transverse colon</u>
C18.5   Malignant neoplasm of <u>splenic flexure</u>
C18.6   Malignant neoplasm of <u>descending colon</u>
C18.7   Malignant neoplasm of <u>sigmoid colon</u>
   Malignant neoplasm of sigmoid (flexure)
   Excludes 1: malignant neoplasm of rectosigmoid junction (C19)
C18.8   Malignant neoplasm of <u>overlapping</u> sites of colon
C18.9   Malignant neoplasm of colon, unspecified
   Malignant neoplasm of large intestine NOS

C19   Malignant neoplasm of <u>rectosigmoid junction</u>
   Malignant neoplasm of colon with rectum
   Malignant neoplasm of rectosigmoid (colon)
   Excludes 1: malignant carcinoid tumors of the colon (C7A.02-)

C20   Malignant neoplasm of <u>rectum</u>
   Malignant neoplasm of rectal ampulla
   Excludes 1: malignant carcinoid tumor of the rectum (C7A.026)

C21-   Malignant neoplasm of <u>anus and anal canal</u>
   *Excludes❷: malignant carcinoid tumors of the colon (C7A.02-)
      other and unspecified malignant neoplasm of anal margin
         (C44.500, C44.510, C44.520, C44.590)
      other and unspecified malignant neoplasm of anal skin
         (C44.500, C44.510, C44.520, C44.590)
      other and unspecified malignant neoplasm of perianal skin
         (C44.500, C44.510, C44.520, C44.590)*
C21.0   Malignant neoplasm of anus, unspecified
C21.1   Malignant neoplasm of <u>anal canal</u>
   Malignant neoplasm of anal sphincter
C21.2   Malignant neoplasm of <u>cloacogenic zone</u>
C21.8   Malignant neoplasm of <u>overlapping</u> sites of rectum, anus and
   anal canal
   Malignant neoplasm of anorectal junction
   Malignant neoplasm of anorectum
   Primary malignant neoplasm of two or more contiguous sites of
      rectum, anus and anal canal

C
0
2
-
C
2
1

Excludes 1: = NOT CODED HERE! (Do not code both)

353

Excludes❷: = Not Included Here

C22- **Malignant neoplasm of <u>liver</u> and intrahepatic bile ducts**
Use additional code to identify:
  Alcohol abuse and dependence (F10.-)
  Hepatitis B (B16.-, B18.0-B18.1)
  Hepatitis C (B17.1-, B18.2)
  Excludes 1: malignant neoplasm of biliary tract NOS (C24.9)
              secondary malignant neoplasm of liver and intrahepatic bile
              duct (C78.7)

C22.0 **<u>Liver cell</u> carcinoma**
  Hepatocellular carcinoma
  Hepatoma

C22.1 **<u>Intrahepatic bile duct</u> carcinoma**
  Cholangiocarcinoma
  Excludes 1: malignant neoplasm of hepatic duct (C24.0)

C22.2 **<u>Hepatoblastoma</u>**

C22.3 **<u>Angiosarcoma</u> of liver**
  Kupffer cell sarcoma

C22.4 **Other sarcomas of liver**

C22.7 **Other specified carcinomas of liver**

C22.8 **Malignant neoplasm of liver, primary, unspecified as to type**

C22.9 **Malignant neoplasm of liver, not specified as primary or secondary**

C23 **Malignant neoplasm of <u>gallbladder</u>**

C24- **Malignant neoplasm of other and unspecified parts of biliary tract**
  Excludes 1: malignant neoplasm of intrahepatic bile duct (C22.1)

C24.0 **Malignant neoplasm of <u>extrahepatic bile duct</u>**
  Malignant neoplasm of biliary duct or passage NOS
  Malignant neoplasm of common bile duct
  Malignant neoplasm of cystic duct
  Malignant neoplasm of hepatic duct

C24.1 **Malignant neoplasm of <u>ampulla of Vater</u>**

C24.8 **Malignant neoplasm of <u>overlapping</u> sites of biliary tract**
  Malignant neoplasm involving both intrahepatic and extrahepatic bile ducts
  Primary malignant neoplasm of two or more contiguous sites of biliary tract

C24.9 **Malignant neoplasm of biliary tract, unspecified**

C25- **Malignant neoplasm of <u>pancreas</u>**
Use additional code to identify:
  Alcohol abuse and dependence (F10.-)

C25.0 **Malignant neoplasm of <u>head</u> of pancreas**

C25.1 **Malignant neoplasm of <u>body</u> of pancreas**

C25.2 **Malignant neoplasm of <u>tail</u> of pancreas**

C25.3 **Malignant neoplasm of <u>pancreatic duct</u>**

C25.4 **Malignant neoplasm of <u>endocrine</u> pancreas**
  Malignant neoplasm of islets of Langerhans
  Use additional code to identify any functional activity

C25.7 **Malignant neoplasm of other parts of pancreas**
  Malignant neoplasm of neck of pancreas

C25.8 **Malignant neoplasm of <u>overlapping</u> sites of pancreas**

C25.9 **Malignant neoplasm of pancreas, unspecified**

C26- **Malignant neoplasm of other and ill-defined digestive organs**
  Excludes 1: malignant neoplasm of peritoneum and retroperitoneum
              (C48.-)

C26.0 **Malignant neoplasm of intestinal tract, part unspecified**
  Malignant neoplasm of intestine NOS

C26.1 **Malignant neoplasm of <u>spleen</u>**
  Excludes 1: Hodgkin lymphoma (C81.-)
              non-Hodgkin lymphoma (C82-C85)

C26.9 **Malignant neoplasm of ill-defined sites within the digestive system**
  Malignant neoplasm of alimentary canal or tract NOS
  Malignant neoplasm of gastrointestinal tract NOS
  Excludes 1: malignant neoplasm of abdominal NOS (C76.2)
              malignant neoplasm of intra-abdominal NOS (C76.2)

Malignant neoplasms of respiratory and intrathoracic organs (C30-C39)

  Includes: Malignant neoplasm of middle ear
  Excludes 1: mesothelioma (C45.-)

C30- **Malignant neoplasm of nasal cavity and middle ear**

C30.0 **Malignant neoplasm of <u>nasal cavity</u>**
  Malignant neoplasm of cartilage of nose
  Malignant neoplasm of nasal concha
  Malignant neoplasm of internal nose
  Malignant neoplasm of septum of nose
  Malignant neoplasm of vestibule of nose
  Excludes 1: malignant melanoma of skin of nose (C43.31)
              malignant neoplasm of nasal bone (C41.0)
              malignant neoplasm of nose NOS (C76.0)
              malignant neoplasm of olfactory bulb (C72.2-)
              malignant neoplasm of posterior margin of nasal
              septum and choana (C11.3)
              malignant neoplasm of turbinates (C41.0)
              other and unspecified malignant neoplasm of skin of
              nose (C44.301, C44.311, C44.321, C44.391)

C30.1 **Malignant neoplasm of <u>middle ear</u>**
  Malignant neoplasm of antrum tympanicum
  Malignant neoplasm of auditory tube
  Malignant neoplasm of eustachian tube
  Malignant neoplasm of inner ear
  Malignant neoplasm of mastoid air cells
  Malignant neoplasm of tympanic cavity
  Excludes 1: malignant melanoma of skin of (external) ear (C43.2-)
              malignant neoplasm of auricular canal (external)
              (C43.2-,C44.2-)
              malignant neoplasm of bone of ear (meatus) (C41.0)
              malignant neoplasm of cartilage of ear (C49.0)
              other and unspecified malignant neoplasm of skin of
              (external) ear (C44.2-)

C31- **Malignant neoplasm of accessory <u>sinuses</u>**

C31.0 **Malignant neoplasm of <u>maxillary</u> sinus**
  Malignant neoplasm of antrum (Highmore) (maxillary)

C31.1 **Malignant neoplasm of <u>ethmoidal</u> sinus**

C31.2 **Malignant neoplasm of <u>frontal</u> sinus**

C31.3 **Malignant neoplasm of <u>sphenoid</u> sinus**

C31.8 **Malignant neoplasm of <u>overlapping</u> sites of accessory sinuses**

C31.9 **Malignant neoplasm of accessory sinus, unspecified**

C32- **Malignant neoplasm of <u>larynx</u>**
Use additional code to identify:
  Alcohol abuse and dependence (F10.-)
  Exposure to environmental tobacco smoke (Z77.22)
  Exposure to tobacco smoke in the perinatal period (P96.81)
  History of tobacco use (Z87.891)
  Occupational exposure to environmental tobacco smoke (Z57.31)
  Tobacco dependence (F17.-)
  Tobacco use (Z72.0)

C32.0 **Malignant neoplasm of <u>glottis</u>**
  Malignant neoplasm of intrinsic larynx
  Malignant neoplasm of laryngeal commissure (anterior)(posterior)
  Malignant neoplasm of vocal cord (true) NOS

C32.1 **Malignant neoplasm of <u>supraglottis</u>**
  Malignant neoplasm of aryepiglottic fold or interarytenoid fold, laryngeal aspect
  Malignant neoplasm of epiglottis (suprahyoid portion) NOS
  Malignant neoplasm of extrinsic larynx
  Malignant neoplasm of false vocal cord
  Malignant neoplasm of posterior (laryngeal) surface of epiglottis
  Malignant neoplasm of ventricular bands
  Excludes❷: malignant neoplasm of anterior surface of epiglottis
              (C10.1)
              malignant neoplasm of aryepiglottic fold or
              interarytenoid fold, hypopharyngeal aspect (C13.1)
              malignant neoplasm of aryepiglottic fold or
              interarytenoid fold, marginal zone (C13.1)
              malignant neoplasm of aryepiglottic fold or
              interarytenoid fold NOS (C13.1)

C32.2 **Malignant neoplasm of <u>subglottis</u>**

C32.3 **Malignant neoplasm of <u>laryngeal cartilage</u>**

C32.8 **Malignant neoplasm of <u>overlapping</u> sites of larynx**

C32.9 **Malignant neoplasm of larynx, unspecified**

C
2
2
-
C
4
1

Excludes 1: = NOT CODED HERE! (Do not code both)

Excludes❷: = Not Included Here

C33　Malignant neoplasm of underline trachea
Use additional code to identify:
　Exposure to environmental tobacco smoke (Z77.22)
　Exposure to tobacco smoke in the perinatal period (P96.81)
　History of tobacco use (Z87.891)
　Occupational exposure to environmental tobacco smoke (Z57.31)
　Tobacco dependence (F17.-)
　Tobacco use (Z72.0)

C34-　Malignant neoplasm of bronchus and lung
Use additional code to identify:
　Exposure to environmental tobacco smoke (Z77.22)
　Exposure to tobacco smoke in the perinatal period (P96.81)
　History of tobacco use (Z87.891)
　Occupational exposure to environmental tobacco smoke (Z57.31)
　Tobacco dependence (F17.-)
　Tobacco use (Z72.0)
　Excludes 1:　Kaposi's sarcoma of lung (C46.5-)
　　　　　　malignant carcinoid tumor of the bronchus and lung
　　　　　　(C7A.090)
　C34.0-　Malignant neoplasm of main bronchus
　　　Malignant neoplasm of carina
　　　Malignant neoplasm of hilus (of lung)
　　C34.00　Malignant neoplasm of unspecified main bronchus
　　C34.01　Malignant neoplasm of right main bronchus
　　C34.02　Malignant neoplasm of left main bronchus
　C34.1-　Malignant neoplasm of upper lobe, bronchus or lung
　　C34.10　Malignant neoplasm of upper lobe, unspecified bronchus or lung
　　C34.11　Malignant neoplasm of upper lobe, right bronchus or lung
　　C34.12　Malignant neoplasm of upper lobe, left bronchus or lung
　C34.2　Malignant neoplasm of middle lobe, bronchus or lung
　C34.3-　Malignant neoplasm of lower lobe, bronchus or lung
　　C34.30　Malignant neoplasm of lower lobe, unspecified bronchus or lung
　　C34.31　Malignant neoplasm of lower lobe, right bronchus or lung
　　C34.32　Malignant neoplasm of lower lobe, left bronchus or lung
　C34.8-　Malignant neoplasm of overlapping sites of bronchus and lung
　　C34.80　Malignant neoplasm of overlapping sites of unspecified bronchus and lung
　　C34.81　Malignant neoplasm of overlapping sites of right bronchus and lung
　　C34.82　Malignant neoplasm of overlapping sites of left bronchus and lung
　C34.9-　Malignant neoplasm of unspecified part of bronchus or lung
　　C34.90　Malignant neoplasm of unspecified part of unspecified bronchus or lung
　　　　Lung cancer NOS
　　C34.91　Malignant neoplasm of unspecified part of right bronchus or lung
　　C34.92　Malignant neoplasm of unspecified part of left bronchus or lung

C37　Malignant neoplasm of underline thymus
　Excludes 1:　malignant carcinoid tumor of the thymus (C7A.091)

C38-　Malignant neoplasm of heart, mediastinum and pleura
　Excludes 1:　mesothelioma (C45.-)
　C38.0　Malignant neoplasm of heart
　　　Malignant neoplasm of pericardium
　　　Excludes 1:　malignant neoplasm of great vessels (C49.3)
　C38.1　Malignant neoplasm of anterior mediastinum
　C38.2　Malignant neoplasm of posterior mediastinum
　C38.3　Malignant neoplasm of mediastinum, part unspecified
　C38.4　Malignant neoplasm of pleura
　C38.8　Malignant neoplasm of overlapping sites of heart, mediastinum and pleura

C39-　Malignant neoplasm of other and ill-defined sites in the respiratory system and intrathoracic organs
Use additional code to identify:
　Exposure to environmental tobacco smoke (Z77.22)
　Exposure to tobacco smoke in the perinatal period (P96.81)
　History of tobacco use (Z87.891)
　Occupational exposure to environmental tobacco smoke (Z57.31)
　Tobacco dependence (F17.-)
　Tobacco use (Z72.0)
　Excludes 1:　intrathoracic malignant neoplasm NOS (C76.1)
　　　　　　thoracic malignant neoplasm NOS (C76.1)
　C39.0　Malignant neoplasm of upper respiratory tract, part unspecified
　C39.9　Malignant neoplasm of lower respiratory tract, part unspecified
　　　Malignant neoplasm of respiratory tract NOS

Malignant neoplasms of bone and articular cartilage (C40-C41)

Includes:　Malignant neoplasm of cartilage (articular) (joint)
　　　　Malignant neoplasm of periosteum
Excludes 1:　malignant neoplasm of bone marrow NOS (C96.9)
　　　　　malignant neoplasm of synovia (C49.-)

C40-　Malignant neoplasm of bone and articular cartilage of limbs
Use additional code to identify major osseous defect, if applicable (M89.7-)
　C40.0-　Malignant neoplasm of scapula and long bones of upper limb
　　C40.00　Malignant neoplasm of scapula and long bones of unspecified upper limb
　　C40.01　Malignant neoplasm of scapula and long bones of right upper limb
　　C40.02　Malignant neoplasm of scapula and long bones of left upper limb
　C40.1-　Malignant neoplasm of short bones of upper limb
　　C40.10　Malignant neoplasm of short bones of unspecified upper limb
　　C40.11　Malignant neoplasm of short bones of right upper limb
　　C40.12　Malignant neoplasm of short bones of left upper limb
　C40.2-　Malignant neoplasm of long bones of lower limb
　　C40.20　Malignant neoplasm of long bones of unspecified lower limb
　　C40.21　Malignant neoplasm of long bones of right lower limb
　　C40.22　Malignant neoplasm of long bones of left lower limb
　C40.3-　Malignant neoplasm of short bones of lower limb
　　C40.30　Malignant neoplasm of short bones of unspecified lower limb
　　C40.31　Malignant neoplasm of short bones of right lower limb
　　C40.32　Malignant neoplasm of short bones of left lower limb
　C40.8-　Malignant neoplasm of overlapping sites of bone and articular cartilage of limb
　　C40.80　Malignant neoplasm of overlapping sites of bone and articular cartilage of unspecified limb
　　C40.81　Malignant neoplasm of overlapping sites of bone and articular cartilage of right limb
　　C40.82　Malignant neoplasm of overlapping sites of bone and articular cartilage of left limb
　C40.9-　Malignant neoplasm of unspecified bones and articular cartilage of limb
　　C40.90　Malignant neoplasm of unspecified bones and articular cartilage of unspecified limb
　　C40.91　Malignant neoplasm of unspecified bones and articular cartilage of right limb
　　C40.92　Malignant neoplasm of unspecified bones and articular cartilage of left limb

C41-　Malignant neoplasm of bone and articular cartilage of other and unspecified sites
　Excludes 1:　malignant neoplasm of bones of limbs (C40.-)
　　　　　malignant neoplasm of cartilage of ear (C49.0)
　　　　　malignant neoplasm of cartilage of eyelid (C49.0)
　　　　　malignant neoplasm of cartilage of larynx (C32.3)
　　　　　malignant neoplasm of cartilage of limbs (C40.-)
　　　　　malignant neoplasm of cartilage of nose (C30.0)
　C41.0　Malignant neoplasm of bones of skull and face
　　　Malignant neoplasm of maxilla (superior)
　　　Malignant neoplasm of orbital bone
　　　Excludes❷:　carcinoma, any type except intraosseous or
　　　　　　odontogenic of:
　　　　　　maxillary sinus (C31.0)
　　　　　　upper jaw (C03.0)
　　　　　malignant neoplasm of jaw bone (lower) (C41.1)
　C41.1　Malignant neoplasm of mandible
　　　Malignant neoplasm of inferior maxilla
　　　Malignant neoplasm of lower jaw bone
　　　Excludes❷:　carcinoma, any type except intraosseous or
　　　　　　odontogenic of:
　　　　　　jaw NOS (C03.9)
　　　　　　lower (C03.1)
　　　　　malignant neoplasm of upper jaw bone (C41.0)
　C41.2　Malignant neoplasm of vertebral column
　　　Excludes 1:　malignant neoplasm of sacrum and coccyx (C41.4)
　C41.3　Malignant neoplasm of ribs, sternum and clavicle
　C41.4　Malignant neoplasm of pelvic bones, sacrum and coccyx
　C41.9　Malignant neoplasm of bone and articular cartilage, unspecified

C 2 2 - C 4 1

Excludes 1: = NOT CODED HERE! (Do not code both)　　**355**　　*Excludes❷:* = Not Included Here

Melanoma and other malignant neoplasms of skin (C43-C44)

C43- Malignant <u>melanoma</u> of skin
  Excludes 1: melanoma in situ (D03.-)
  Excludes❷: malignant melanoma of skin of genital organs (C51-C52, C60.-, C63.-)
    Merkel cell carcinoma (C4A.-)
    sites other than skin — code to malignant neoplasm of the site
  C43.0   Malignant melanoma of <u>lip</u>
    Excludes 1: malignant neoplasm of vermilion border of lip (C00.0-C00.2)
  C43.1- Malignant melanoma of <u>eyelid, including canthus</u>
    C43.10   Malignant melanoma of unspecified eyelid, including canthus
    C43.11   Malignant melanoma of <u>right</u> eyelid, including canthus
    C43.12   Malignant melanoma of <u>left</u> eyelid, including canthus
  C43.2- Malignant melanoma of <u>ear and external auricular canal</u>
    C43.20   Malignant melanoma of unspecified ear and external auricular canal
    C43.21   Malignant melanoma of <u>right</u> ear and external auricular canal
    C43.22   Malignant melanoma of <u>left</u> ear and external auricular canal
  C43.3- Malignant melanoma of other and unspecified parts of face
    C43.30   Malignant melanoma of unspecified part of face
    C43.31   Malignant melanoma of <u>nose</u>
    C43.39   Malignant melanoma of other parts of face
  C43.4   Malignant melanoma of <u>scalp and neck</u>
  C43.5- Malignant melanoma of <u>trunk</u>
    Excludes❷: malignant neoplasm of anus NOS (C21.0)
      malignant neoplasm of scrotum (C63.2)
    C43.51   Malignant melanoma of <u>anal skin</u>
      Malignant melanoma of anal margin
      Malignant melanoma of perianal skin
    C43.52   Malignant melanoma of <u>skin of breast</u>
    C43.59   Malignant melanoma of other part of <u>trunk</u>
  C43.6- Malignant melanoma of <u>upper limb</u>, including shoulder
    C43.60   Malignant melanoma of unspecified upper limb, including shoulder
    C43.61   Malignant melanoma of <u>right</u> upper limb, including shoulder
    C43.62   Malignant melanoma of <u>left</u> upper limb, including shoulder
  C43.7- Malignant melanoma of <u>lower limb</u>, including hip
    C43.70   Malignant melanoma of unspecified lower limb, including hip
    C43.71   Malignant melanoma of <u>right</u> lower limb, including hip
    C43.72   Malignant melanoma of <u>left</u> lower limb, including hip
  C43.8   Malignant melanoma of <u>overlapping sites</u> of skin
  C43.9   Malignant melanoma of skin, unspecified
      Malignant melanoma of unspecified site of skin
      Melanoma (malignant) NOS

C4A- Merkel cell carcinoma
  C4A.0   Merkel cell carcinoma of <u>lip</u>
    Excludes 1: malignant neoplasm of vermilion border of lip (C00.0-C00.2)
  C4A.1- Merkel cell carcinoma of <u>eyelid, including canthus</u>
    C4A.10   Merkel cell carcinoma of unspecified eyelid, including canthus
    C4A.11   Merkel cell carcinoma of <u>right</u> eyelid, including canthus
    C4A.12   Merkel cell carcinoma of <u>left</u> eyelid, including canthus
  C4A.2- Merkel cell carcinoma of <u>ear and external auricular canal</u>
    C4A.20   Merkel cell carcinoma of unspecified ear and external auricular canal
    C4A.21   Merkel cell carcinoma of <u>right</u> ear and external auricular canal
    C4A.22   Merkel cell carcinoma of <u>left</u> ear and external auricular canal
  C4A.3- Merkel cell carcinoma of other and unspecified parts of face
    C4A.30   Merkel cell carcinoma of unspecified part of face
    C4A.31   Merkel cell carcinoma of <u>nose</u>
    C4A.39   Merkel cell carcinoma of other parts of face
  C4A.4   Merkel cell carcinoma of <u>scalp and neck</u>
  C4A.5- Merkel cell carcinoma of trunk
    Excludes❷: malignant neoplasm of anus NOS (C21.0)
      malignant neoplasm of scrotum (C63.2)
    C4A.51   Merkel cell carcinoma of <u>anal skin</u>
      Merkel cell carcinoma of anal margin
      Merkel cell carcinoma of perianal skin
    C4A.52   Merkel cell carcinoma of <u>skin of breast</u>
    C4A.59   Merkel cell carcinoma of other part of trunk

  C4A.6- Merkel cell carcinoma of <u>upper limb</u>, including shoulder
    C4A.60   Merkel cell carcinoma of unspecified upper limb, including shoulder
    C4A.61   Merkel cell carcinoma of <u>right</u> upper limb, including shoulder
    C4A.62   Merkel cell carcinoma of <u>left</u> upper limb, including shoulder
  C4A.7- Merkel cell carcinoma of <u>lower limb</u>, including hip
    C4A.70   Merkel cell carcinoma of unspecified lower limb, including hip
    C4A.71   Merkel cell carcinoma of <u>right</u> lower limb, including hip
    C4A.72   Merkel cell carcinoma of <u>left</u> lower limb, including hip
  C4A.8   Merkel cell carcinoma of <u>overlapping sites</u>
  C4A.9   Merkel cell carcinoma, unspecified
      Merkel cell carcinoma of unspecified site
      Merkel cell carcinoma NOS

C44- <u>Other and unspecified malignant</u> neoplasm of <u>skin</u>
  Includes: Malignant neoplasm of sebaceous glands
      Malignant neoplasm of sweat glands
  Excludes 1: Kaposi's sarcoma of skin (C46.0)
      malignant melanoma of skin (C43.-)
      malignant neoplasm of skin of genital organs (C51-C52, C60.-, C63.2)
      Merkel cell carcinoma (C4A.-)
  C44.0- Other and unspecified malignant neoplasm of skin of <u>lip</u>
    Excludes 1: malignant neoplasm of lip (C00.-)
    C44.00   <u>Unspecified</u> malignant neoplasm of skin of lip
    C44.01   <u>Basal cell</u> carcinoma of skin of lip
    C44.02   <u>Squamous cell</u> carcinoma of skin of lip
    C44.09   <u>Other specified</u> malignant neoplasm of skin of lip
  C44.1- Other and unspecified malignant neoplasm of skin of <u>eyelid, including canthus</u>
    Excludes 1: connective tissue of eyelid (C49.0)
    C44.10- <u>Unspecified</u> malignant neoplasm of skin of eyelid, including canthus
      C44.101   Unspecified malignant neoplasm of skin of unspecified eyelid, including canthus
      C44.102   Unspecified malignant neoplasm of skin of <u>right</u> eyelid, including canthus
      C44.109   Unspecified malignant neoplasm of skin of <u>left</u> eyelid, including canthus
    C44.11- <u>Basal cell</u> carcinoma of skin of eyelid, including canthus
      C44.111   Basal cell carcinoma of skin of unspecified eyelid, including canthus
      C44.112   Basal cell carcinoma of skin of <u>right</u> eyelid, including canthus
      C44.119   Basal cell carcinoma of skin of <u>left</u> eyelid, including canthus
    C44.12- <u>Squamous cell</u> carcinoma of skin of eyelid, including canthus
      C44.121   Squamous cell carcinoma of skin of unspecified eyelid, including canthus
      C44.122   Squamous cell carcinoma of skin of <u>right</u> eyelid, including canthus
      C44.129   Squamous cell carcinoma of skin of <u>left</u> eyelid, including canthus
    C44.19- <u>Other specified</u> malignant neoplasm of skin of eyelid, including canthus
      C44.191   Other specified malignant neoplasm of skin of unspecified eyelid, including canthus
      C44.192   Other specified malignant neoplasm of skin of <u>right</u> eyelid, including canthus
      C44.199   Other specified malignant neoplasm of skin of <u>left</u> eyelid, including canthus
  C44.2- Other and unspecified malignant neoplasm of skin of <u>ear and external auricular canal</u>
    Excludes 1: connective tissue of ear (C49.0)
    C44.20- <u>Unspecified</u> malignant neoplasm of skin of ear and external auricular canal
      C44.201   Unspecified malignant neoplasm of skin of unspecified ear and external auricular canal
      C44.202   Unspecified malignant neoplasm of skin of <u>right</u> ear and external auricular canal
      C44.209   Unspecified malignant neoplasm of skin of <u>left</u> ear and external auricular canal
    C44.21- <u>Basal cell</u> carcinoma of skin of ear and external auricular canal
      C44.211   Basal cell carcinoma of skin of unspecified ear and external auricular canal
      C44.212   Basal cell carcinoma of skin of <u>right</u> ear and external auricular canal

C
4
3
-
C
4
4

Excludes 1: = NOT CODED HERE! (Do not code both)   **356**   *Excludes❷: = Not Included Here*

C44.219   Basal cell carcinoma of skin of <u>left</u> ear and external auricular canal

C44.22- <u>Squamous cell</u> carcinoma of skin of ear and external auricular canal

    C44.221   Squamous cell carcinoma of skin of unspecified ear and external auricular canal

    C44.222   Squamous cell carcinoma of skin of <u>right</u> ear and external auricular canal

    C44.229   Squamous cell carcinoma of skin of <u>left</u> ear and external auricular canal

C44.29- <u>Other specified</u> malignant neoplasm of skin of ear and external auricular canal

    C44.291   Other specified malignant neoplasm of skin of unspecified ear and external auricular canal

    C44.292   Other specified malignant neoplasm of skin of <u>right</u> ear and external auricular canal

    C44.299   Other specified malignant neoplasm of skin of <u>left</u> ear and external auricular canal

C44.3- Other and unspecified malignant neoplasm of skin of <u>other and unspecified parts of face</u>

C44.30- <u>Unspecified</u> malignant neoplasm of skin of other and unspecified parts of face

    C44.300   Unspecified malignant neoplasm of skin of unspecified part of face

    C44.301   Unspecified malignant neoplasm of skin of <u>nose</u>

    C44.309   Unspecified malignant neoplasm of skin of <u>other parts</u> of face

C44.31- <u>Basal cell</u> carcinoma of skin of other and unspecified parts of face

    C44.310   Basal cell carcinoma of skin of unspecified parts of face

    C44.311   Basal cell carcinoma of skin of <u>nose</u>

    C44.319   Basal cell carcinoma of skin of <u>other parts</u> of face

C44.32- <u>Squamous cell</u> carcinoma of skin of other and unspecified parts of face

    C44.320   Squamous cell carcinoma of skin of unspecified parts of face

    C44.321   Squamous cell carcinoma of skin of <u>nose</u>

    C44.329   Squamous cell carcinoma of skin of <u>other parts</u> of face

C44.39- <u>Other specified</u> malignant neoplasm of skin of other and unspecified parts of face

    C44.390   Other specified malignant neoplasm of skin of unspecified parts of face

    C44.391   Other specified malignant neoplasm of skin of <u>nose</u>

    C44.399   Other specified malignant neoplasm of skin of <u>other parts</u> of face

C44.4- Other and unspecified malignant neoplasm of skin of <u>scalp and neck</u>

    C44.40   <u>Unspecified</u> malignant neoplasm of skin of scalp and neck

    C44.41   <u>Basal cell</u> carcinoma of skin of scalp and neck

    C44.42   <u>Squamous cell</u> carcinoma of skin of scalp and neck

    C44.49   <u>Other specified</u> malignant neoplasm of skin of scalp and neck

C44.5- Other and unspecified malignant neoplasm of skin of <u>trunk</u>

    Excludes 1: anus NOS (C21.0)
                   scrotum (C63.2)

C44.50- <u>Unspecified</u> malignant neoplasm of skin of trunk

    C44.500   Unspecified malignant neoplasm of <u>anal skin</u>
        Unspecified malignant neoplasm of anal margin
        Unspecified malignant neoplasm of perianal skin

    C44.501   Unspecified malignant neoplasm of skin of <u>breast</u>

    C44.509   Unspecified malignant neoplasm of skin of other part of trunk

C44.51- <u>Basal cell</u> carcinoma of skin of trunk

    C44.510   Basal cell carcinoma of <u>anal skin</u>
        Basal cell carcinoma of anal margin
        Basal cell carcinoma of perianal skin

    C44.511   Basal cell carcinoma of skin of <u>breast</u>

    C44.519   Basal cell carcinoma of skin of other part of trunk

C44.52- <u>Squamous cell</u> carcinoma of skin of trunk

    C44.520   Squamous cell carcinoma of <u>anal skin</u>
        Squamous cell carcinoma of anal margin
        Squamous cell carcinoma of perianal skin

    C44.521   Squamous cell carcinoma of skin of <u>breast</u>

    C44.529   Squamous cell carcinoma of skin of other part of trunk

C44.59- <u>Other specified</u> malignant neoplasm of skin of trunk

    C44.590   Other specified malignant neoplasm of <u>anal skin</u>
        Other specified malignant neoplasm of anal margin
        Other specified malignant neoplasm of perianal skin

    C44.591   Other specified malignant neoplasm of skin of <u>breast</u>

    C44.599   Other specified malignant neoplasm of skin of other part of trunk

C44.6- Other and unspecified malignant neoplasm of skin of <u>upper limb</u>, including shoulder

C44.60- <u>Unspecified</u> malignant neoplasm of skin of upper limb, including shoulder

    C44.601   Unspecified malignant neoplasm of skin of unspecified upper limb, including shoulder

    C44.602   Unspecified malignant neoplasm of skin of <u>right</u> upper limb, including shoulder

    C44.609   Unspecified malignant neoplasm of skin of <u>left</u> upper limb, including shoulder

C44.61- <u>Basal cell</u> carcinoma of skin of upper limb, including shoulder

    C44.611   Basal cell carcinoma of skin of unspecified upper limb, including shoulder

    C44.612   Basal cell carcinoma of skin of <u>right</u> upper limb, including shoulder

    C44.619   Basal cell carcinoma of skin of <u>left</u> upper limb, including shoulder

C44.62- <u>Squamous cell</u> carcinoma of skin of upper limb, including shoulder

    C44.621   Squamous cell carcinoma of skin of unspecified upper limb, including shoulder

    C44.622   Squamous cell carcinoma of skin of <u>right</u> upper limb, including shoulder

    C44.629   Squamous cell carcinoma of skin of <u>left</u> upper limb, including shoulder

C44.69- <u>Other specified</u> malignant neoplasm of skin of upper limb, including shoulder

    C44.691   Other specified malignant neoplasm of skin of unspecified upper limb, including shoulder

    C44.692   Other specified malignant neoplasm of skin of <u>right</u> upper limb, including shoulder

    C44.699   Other specified malignant neoplasm of skin of <u>left</u> upper limb, including shoulder

C44.7- Other and unspecified malignant neoplasm of skin of <u>lower limb</u>, including hip

C44.70- <u>Unspecified</u> malignant neoplasm of skin of lower limb, including hip

    C44.701   Unspecified malignant neoplasm of skin of unspecified lower limb, including hip

    C44.702   Unspecified malignant neoplasm of skin of <u>right</u> lower limb, including hip

    C44.709   Unspecified malignant neoplasm of skin of <u>left</u> lower limb, including hip

C44.71- <u>Basal cell</u> carcinoma of skin of lower limb, including hip

    C44.711   Basal cell carcinoma of skin of unspecified lower limb, including hip

    C44.712   Basal cell carcinoma of skin of <u>right</u> lower limb, including hip

    C44.719   Basal cell carcinoma of skin of <u>left</u> lower limb, including hip

C44.72- <u>Squamous cell</u> carcinoma of skin of lower limb, including hip

    C44.721   Squamous cell carcinoma of skin of unspecified lower limb, including hip

    C44.722   Squamous cell carcinoma of skin of <u>right</u> lower limb, including hip

    C44.729   Squamous cell carcinoma of skin of <u>left</u> lower limb, including hip

C44.79- <u>Other specified</u> malignant neoplasm of skin of lower limb, including hip

    C44.791   Other specified malignant neoplasm of skin of unspecified lower limb, including hip

    C44.792   Other specified malignant neoplasm of skin of <u>right</u> lower limb, including hip

    C44.799   Other specified malignant neoplasm of skin of <u>left</u> lower limb, including hip

C43 - C44

C44.8- **Other and unspecified malignant neoplasm of <u>overlapping sites</u> of skin**

    C44.80 <u>Unspecified</u> malignant neoplasm of overlapping sites of skin

    C44.81 <u>Basal cell</u> carcinoma of overlapping sites of skin

    C44.82 <u>Squamous cell</u> carcinoma of overlapping sites of skin

    C44.89 <u>Other specified</u> malignant neoplasm of overlapping sites of skin

C44.9- **Other and unspecified malignant neoplasm of skin, unspecified**

    C44.90 <u>Unspecified</u> malignant neoplasm of skin, unspecified
        Malignant neoplasm of unspecified site of skin

    C44.91 <u>Basal cell</u> carcinoma of skin, unspecified

    C44.92 <u>Squamous cell</u> carcinoma of skin, unspecified

    C44.99 <u>Other specified</u> malignant neoplasm of skin, unspecified

Malignant neoplasms of mesothelial and soft tissue (C45-C49)

C45- <u>Mesothelioma</u>

    C45.0 **Mesothelioma of <u>pleura</u>**
        Excludes 1: other malignant neoplasm of pleura (C38.4)

    C45.1 **Mesothelioma of <u>peritoneum</u>**
        Mesothelioma of cul-de-sac
        Mesothelioma of mesentery
        Mesothelioma of mesocolon
        Mesothelioma of omentum
        Mesothelioma of peritoneum (parietal) (pelvic)
        Excludes 1: other malignant neoplasm of soft tissue of peritoneum (C48.-)

    C45.2 **Mesothelioma of <u>pericardium</u>**
        Excludes 1: other malignant neoplasm of pericardium (C38.0)

    C45.7 **Mesothelioma of other sites**

    C45.9 **Mesothelioma, unspecified**

C46- <u>Kaposi's sarcoma</u>
    Code first any human immunodeficiency virus [HIV] disease (B20)

    C46.0 **Kaposi's sarcoma of <u>skin</u>**

    C46.1 **Kaposi's sarcoma of <u>soft tissue</u>**
        Kaposi's sarcoma of blood vessel
        Kaposi's sarcoma of connective tissue
        Kaposi's sarcoma of fascia
        Kaposi's sarcoma of ligament
        Kaposi's sarcoma of lymphatic(s) NEC
        Kaposi's sarcoma of muscle
        Excludes❷: Kaposi's sarcoma of lymph glands and nodes (C46.3)

    C46.2 **Kaposi's sarcoma of <u>palate</u>**

    C46.3 **Kaposi's sarcoma of <u>lymph nodes</u>**

    C46.4 **Kaposi's sarcoma of <u>gastrointestinal</u> sites**

    C46.5- **Kaposi's sarcoma of <u>lung</u>**

        C46.50 Kaposi's sarcoma of unspecified lung

        C46.51 Kaposi's sarcoma of <u>right</u> lung

        C46.52 Kaposi's sarcoma of <u>left</u> lung

    C46.7 **Kaposi's sarcoma of other sites**

    C46.9 **Kaposi's sarcoma, unspecified**
        Kaposi's sarcoma of unspecified site

C47- **Malignant neoplasm of <u>peripheral nerves</u> and <u>autonomic nervous system</u>**
    Includes: Malignant neoplasm of sympathetic and parasympathetic nerves and ganglia
    Excludes 1: Kaposi's sarcoma of soft tissue (C46.1)

    C47.0 **Malignant neoplasm of peripheral nerves of head, face and neck**
        Excludes 1: malignant neoplasm of peripheral nerves of orbit (C69.6-)

    C47.1- **Malignant neoplasm of peripheral nerves of <u>upper limb</u>, including shoulder**

        C47.10 Malignant neoplasm of peripheral nerves of unspecified upper limb, including shoulder

        C47.11 Malignant neoplasm of peripheral nerves of <u>right</u> upper limb, including shoulder

        C47.12 Malignant neoplasm of peripheral nerves of <u>left</u> upper limb, including shoulder

    C47.2- **Malignant neoplasm of peripheral nerves of <u>lower limb</u>, including hip**

        C47.20 Malignant neoplasm of peripheral nerves of unspecified lower limb, including hip

        C47.21 Malignant neoplasm of peripheral nerves of <u>right</u> lower limb, including hip

        C47.22 Malignant neoplasm of peripheral nerves of <u>left</u> lower limb, including hip

    C47.3 **Malignant neoplasm of peripheral nerves of <u>thorax</u>**

    C47.4 **Malignant neoplasm of peripheral nerves of <u>abdomen</u>**

    C47.5 **Malignant neoplasm of peripheral nerves of <u>pelvis</u>**

    C47.6 **Malignant neoplasm of peripheral nerves of trunk, unspecified**
        Malignant neoplasm of peripheral nerves of unspecified part of trunk

    C47.8 **Malignant neoplasm of <u>overlapping sites</u> of peripheral nerves and autonomic nervous system**

    C47.9 **Malignant neoplasm of peripheral nerves and autonomic nervous system, unspecified**
        Malignant neoplasm of unspecified site of peripheral nerves and autonomic nervous system

C48- **Malignant neoplasm of retroperitoneum and peritoneum**
    Excludes 1: Kaposi's sarcoma of connective tissue (C46.1)
               mesothelioma (C45.-)

    C48.0 **Malignant neoplasm of <u>retroperitoneum</u>**

    C48.1 **Malignant neoplasm of specified parts of <u>peritoneum</u>**
        Malignant neoplasm of cul-de-sac
        Malignant neoplasm of mesentery
        Malignant neoplasm of mesocolon
        Malignant neoplasm of omentum
        Malignant neoplasm of parietal peritoneum
        Malignant neoplasm of pelvic peritoneum

    C48.2 **Malignant neoplasm of peritoneum, unspecified**

    C48.8 **Malignant neoplasm of <u>overlapping sites</u> of retroperitoneum and peritoneum**

C49- **Malignant neoplasm of <u>other connective and soft tissue</u>**
    Includes: Malignant neoplasm of blood vessel
             Malignant neoplasm of bursa
             Malignant neoplasm of cartilage
             Malignant neoplasm of fascia
             Malignant neoplasm of fat
             Malignant neoplasm of ligament, except uterine
             Malignant neoplasm of lymphatic vessel
             Malignant neoplasm of muscle
             Malignant neoplasm of synovia
             Malignant neoplasm of tendon (sheath)
    Excludes 1: malignant neoplasm of cartilage (of):
               articular (C40-C41)
               larynx (C32.3)
               nose (C30.0)
             malignant neoplasm of connective tissue of breast (C50.-)
    Excludes❷: Kaposi's sarcoma of soft tissue (C46.1)
             malignant neoplasm of heart (C38.0)
             malignant neoplasm of peripheral nerves and autonomic nervous system (C47.-)
             malignant neoplasm of peritoneum (C48.2)
             malignant neoplasm of retroperitoneum (C48.0)
             malignant neoplasm of uterine ligament (C57.3)
             mesothelioma (C45.-)

    C49.0 **Malignant neoplasm of connective and soft tissue of <u>head, face and neck</u>**
        Malignant neoplasm of connective tissue of ear
        Malignant neoplasm of connective tissue of eyelid
        Excludes 1: connective tissue of orbit (C69.6-)

    C49.1- **Malignant neoplasm of connective and soft tissue of <u>upper limb</u>, including shoulder**

        C49.10 Malignant neoplasm of connective and soft tissue of unspecified upper limb, including shoulder

        C49.11 Malignant neoplasm of connective and soft tissue of <u>right</u> upper limb, including shoulder

        C49.12 Malignant neoplasm of connective and soft tissue of <u>left</u> upper limb, including shoulder

    C49.2- **Malignant neoplasm of connective and soft tissue of <u>lower limb</u>, including hip**

        C49.20 Malignant neoplasm of connective and soft tissue of unspecified lower limb, including hip

        C49.21 Malignant neoplasm of connective and soft tissue of <u>right</u> lower limb, including hip

        C49.22 Malignant neoplasm of connective and soft tissue of <u>left</u> lower limb, including hip

    C49.3 **Malignant neoplasm of connective and soft tissue of <u>thorax</u>**
        Malignant neoplasm of axilla
        Malignant neoplasm of diaphragm
        Malignant neoplasm of great vessels
        Excludes 1: malignant neoplasm of breast (C50.-)
               malignant neoplasm of heart (C38.0)
               malignant neoplasm of mediastinum (C38.1-C38.3)
               malignant neoplasm of thymus (C37)

    C49.4 **Malignant neoplasm of connective and soft tissue of <u>abdomen</u>**
        Malignant neoplasm of abdominal wall
        Malignant neoplasm of hypochondrium

    C49.5 **Malignant neoplasm of connective and soft tissue of <u>pelvis</u>**
        Malignant neoplasm of buttock
        Malignant neoplasm of groin
        Malignant neoplasm of perineum

C44-C50

Excludes 1: = NOT CODED HERE! (Do not code both)

358

Excludes❷: = Not Included Here

C49.6   **Malignant neoplasm of connective and soft tissue of trunk, unspecified**
     Malignant neoplasm of back NOS

C49.8   **Malignant neoplasm of <u>overlapping sites</u> of connective and soft tissue**
     Primary malignant neoplasm of two or more contiguous sites of connective and soft tissue

C49.9   **Malignant neoplasm of connective and soft tissue, unspecified**

Malignant neoplasms of breast (C50)

C50-   **Malignant neoplasm of <u>breast</u>**
     Includes: Connective tissue of breast
            Paget's disease of breast
            Paget's disease of nipple
     Use additional code to identify estrogen receptor status (Z17.0, Z17.1)
     Excludes 1:   *skin of breast (C44.501, C44.511, C44.521, C44.591)*

C50.0-   **Malignant neoplasm of <u>nipple and areola</u>**
   C50.01- **Malignant neoplasm of nipple and areola, <u>female</u>**
     C50.011   Malignant neoplasm of nipple and areola, <u>right</u> female breast
     C50.012   Malignant neoplasm of nipple and areola, <u>left</u> female breast
     C50.019   Malignant neoplasm of nipple and areola, unspecified female breast
   C50.02- **Malignant neoplasm of nipple and areola, <u>male</u>**
     C50.021   Malignant neoplasm of nipple and areola, <u>right</u> male breast
     C50.022   Malignant neoplasm of nipple and areola, <u>left</u> male breast
     C50.029   Malignant neoplasm of nipple and areola, unspecified male breast

C50.1-   **Malignant neoplasm of <u>central portion</u> of breast**
   C50.11- **Malignant neoplasm of central portion of breast, <u>female</u>**
     C50.111   Malignant neoplasm of central portion of <u>right</u> female breast
     C50.112   Malignant neoplasm of central portion of <u>left</u> female breast
     C50.119   Malignant neoplasm of central portion of unspecified female breast
   C50.12- **Malignant neoplasm of central portion of breast, <u>male</u>**
     C50.121   Malignant neoplasm of central portion of <u>right</u> male breast
     C50.122   Malignant neoplasm of central portion of <u>left</u> male breast
     C50.129   Malignant neoplasm of central portion of unspecified male breast

C50.2-   **Malignant neoplasm of <u>upper-inner quadrant</u> of breast**
   C50.21- **Malignant neoplasm of upper-inner quadrant of breast, <u>female</u>**
     C50.211   Malignant neoplasm of upper-inner quadrant of <u>right</u> female breast
     C50.212   Malignant neoplasm of upper-inner quadrant of <u>left</u> female breast
     C50.219   Malignant neoplasm of upper-inner quadrant of unspecified female breast
   C50.22- **Malignant neoplasm of upper-inner quadrant of breast, <u>male</u>**
     C50.221   Malignant neoplasm of upper-inner quadrant of <u>right</u> male breast
     C50.222   Malignant neoplasm of upper-inner quadrant of <u>left</u> male breast
     C50.229   Malignant neoplasm of upper-inner quadrant of unspecified male breast

C50.3-   **Malignant neoplasm of <u>lower-inner quadrant</u> of breast**
   C50.31- **Malignant neoplasm of lower-inner quadrant of breast, <u>female</u>**
     C50.311   Malignant neoplasm of lower-inner quadrant of <u>right</u> female breast
     C50.312   Malignant neoplasm of lower-inner quadrant of <u>left</u> female breast
     C50.319   Malignant neoplasm of lower-inner quadrant of unspecified female breast
   C50.32- **Malignant neoplasm of lower-inner quadrant of breast, <u>male</u>**
     C50.321   Malignant neoplasm of lower-inner quadrant of <u>right</u> male breast
     C50.322   Malignant neoplasm of lower-inner quadrant of <u>left</u> male breast
     C50.329   Malignant neoplasm of lower-inner quadrant of unspecified male breast

C50.4-   **Malignant neoplasm of <u>upper-outer quadrant</u> of breast**
   C50.41- **Malignant neoplasm of upper-outer quadrant of breast, <u>female</u>**
     C50.411   Malignant neoplasm of upper-outer quadrant of <u>right</u> female breast
     C50.412   Malignant neoplasm of upper-outer quadrant of <u>left</u> female breast
     C50.419   Malignant neoplasm of upper-outer quadrant of unspecified female breast
   C50.42- **Malignant neoplasm of upper-outer quadrant of breast, <u>male</u>**
     C50.421   Malignant neoplasm of upper-outer quadrant of <u>right</u> male breast
     C50.422   Malignant neoplasm of upper-outer quadrant of <u>left</u> male breast
     C50.429   Malignant neoplasm of upper-outer quadrant of unspecified male breast

C50.5-   **Malignant neoplasm of <u>lower-outer quadrant</u> of breast**
   C50.51- **Malignant neoplasm of lower-outer quadrant of breast, <u>female</u>**
     C50.511   Malignant neoplasm of lower-outer quadrant of <u>right</u> female breast
     C50.512   Malignant neoplasm of lower-outer quadrant of <u>left</u> female breast
     C50.519   Malignant neoplasm of lower-outer quadrant of unspecified female breast
   C50.52- **Malignant neoplasm of lower-outer quadrant of breast, <u>male</u>**
     C50.521   Malignant neoplasm of lower-outer quadrant of <u>right</u> male breast
     C50.522   Malignant neoplasm of lower-outer quadrant of <u>left</u> male breast
     C50.529   Malignant neoplasm of lower-outer quadrant of unspecified male breast

C50.6-   **Malignant neoplasm of <u>axillary tail</u> of breast**
   C50.61- **Malignant neoplasm of axillary tail of breast, <u>female</u>**
     C50.611   Malignant neoplasm of axillary tail of <u>right</u> female breast
     C50.612   Malignant neoplasm of axillary tail of <u>left</u> female breast
     C50.619   Malignant neoplasm of axillary tail of unspecified female breast
   C50.62- **Malignant neoplasm of axillary tail of breast, <u>male</u>**
     C50.621   Malignant neoplasm of axillary tail of <u>right</u> male breast
     C50.622   Malignant neoplasm of axillary tail of <u>left</u> male breast
     C50.629   Malignant neoplasm of axillary tail of unspecified male breast

C50.8-   **Malignant neoplasm of <u>overlapping sites</u> of breast**
   C50.81- **Malignant neoplasm of overlapping sites of breast, <u>female</u>**
     C50.811   Malignant neoplasm of overlapping sites of <u>right</u> female breast
     C50.812   Malignant neoplasm of overlapping sites of <u>left</u> female breast
     C50.819   Malignant neoplasm of overlapping sites of unspecified female breast
   C50.82- **Malignant neoplasm of overlapping sites of breast, <u>male</u>**
     C50.821   Malignant neoplasm of overlapping sites of <u>right</u> male breast
     C50.822   Malignant neoplasm of overlapping sites of <u>left</u> male breast
     C50.829   Malignant neoplasm of overlapping sites of unspecified male breast

C50.9-   **Malignant neoplasm of breast of unspecified site**
   C50.91- **Malignant neoplasm of breast of unspecified site, <u>female</u>**
     C50.911   Malignant neoplasm of unspecified site of <u>right</u> female breast
     C50.912   Malignant neoplasm of unspecified site of <u>left</u> female breast
     C50.919   Malignant neoplasm of unspecified site of unspecified female breast
   C50.92- **Malignant neoplasm of breast of unspecified site, <u>male</u>**
     C50.921   Malignant neoplasm of unspecified site of <u>right</u> male breast
     C50.922   Malignant neoplasm of unspecified site of <u>left</u> male breast
     C50.929   Malignant neoplasm of unspecified site of unspecified male breast

C
4
4
-
C
5
0

Excludes 1: = NOT CODED HERE! (Do not code both)   **359**   *Excludes❷:* = Not Included Here

Malignant neoplasms of female genital organs (C51-C58)

Includes: Malignant neoplasm of skin of female genital organs

C51- Malignant neoplasm of <u>vulva</u>
Excludes 1: carcinoma in situ of vulva (D07.1)

C51.0   Malignant neoplasm of <u>labium majus</u>
Malignant neoplasm of Bartholin's [greater vestibular] gland

C51.1   Malignant neoplasm of <u>labium minus</u>

C51.2   Malignant neoplasm of <u>clitoris</u>

C51.8   Malignant neoplasm of <u>overlapping sites</u> of vulva

C51.9   Malignant neoplasm of vulva, unspecified
Malignant neoplasm of external female genitalia NOS
Malignant neoplasm of pudendum

C52   Malignant neoplasm of <u>vagina</u>
Excludes 1: carcinoma in situ of vagina (D07.2)

C53- Malignant neoplasm of <u>cervix</u> uteri
Excludes 1: carcinoma in situ of cervix uteri (D06.-)

C53.0   Malignant neoplasm of <u>endocervix</u>

C53.1   Malignant neoplasm of <u>exocervix</u>

C53.8   Malignant neoplasm of <u>overlapping sites</u> of cervix uteri

C53.9   Malignant neoplasm of cervix uteri, unspecified

C54- Malignant neoplasm of <u>corpus</u> uteri

C54.0   Malignant neoplasm of <u>isthmus</u> uteri
Malignant neoplasm of lower uterine segment

C54.1   Malignant neoplasm of <u>endometrium</u>

C54.2   Malignant neoplasm of <u>myometrium</u>

C54.3   Malignant neoplasm of <u>fundus</u> uteri

C54.8   Malignant neoplasm of <u>overlapping sites</u> of corpus uteri

C54.9   Malignant neoplasm of corpus uteri, unspecified

C55   Malignant neoplasm of uterus, part unspecified

C56- Malignant neoplasm of <u>ovary</u>
Use additional code to identify any functional activity

C56.1   Malignant neoplasm of <u>right</u> ovary

C56.2   Malignant neoplasm of <u>left</u> ovary

C56.9   Malignant neoplasm of unspecified ovary

C57- Malignant neoplasm of other and unspecified female genital organs

C57.0-   Malignant neoplasm of <u>fallopian tube</u>
Malignant neoplasm of oviduct
Malignant neoplasm of uterine tube

C57.00   Malignant neoplasm of unspecified fallopian tube

C57.01   Malignant neoplasm of <u>right</u> fallopian tube

C57.02   Malignant neoplasm of <u>left</u> fallopian tube

C57.1-   Malignant neoplasm of <u>broad ligament</u>

C57.10   Malignant neoplasm of unspecified broad ligament

C57.11   Malignant neoplasm of <u>right</u> broad ligament

C57.12   Malignant neoplasm of <u>left</u> broad ligament

C57.2-   Malignant neoplasm of <u>round ligament</u>

C57.20   Malignant neoplasm of unspecified round ligament

C57.21   Malignant neoplasm of <u>right</u> round ligament

C57.22   Malignant neoplasm of <u>left</u> round ligament

C57.3   Malignant neoplasm of <u>parametrium</u>
Malignant neoplasm of uterine ligament NOS

C57.4   Malignant neoplasm of uterine adnexa, unspecified

C57.7   Malignant neoplasm of other specified female genital organs
Malignant neoplasm of wolffian body or duct

C57.8   Malignant neoplasm of <u>overlapping sites</u> of female genital organs
Primary malignant neoplasm of two or more contiguous sites of the
female genital organs whose point of origin cannot be
determined
Primary tubo-ovarian malignant neoplasm whose point of origin
cannot be determined
Primary utero-ovarian malignant neoplasm whose point of origin
cannot be determined

C57.9   Malignant neoplasm of female genital organ, unspecified
Malignant neoplasm of female genitourinary tract NOS

C58   Malignant neoplasm of <u>placenta</u>
Includes: Choriocarcinoma NOS
Chorionepithelioma NOS
Excludes 1: chorioadenoma (destruens) (D39.2)
hydatidiform mole NOS (O01.9)
invasive hydatidiform mole (D39.2)
male choriocarcinoma NOS (C62.9-)
malignant hydatidiform mole (D39.2)

Malignant neoplasms of male genital organs (C60-C63)

Includes: Malignant neoplasm of skin of male genital organs

C60- Malignant neoplasm of <u>penis</u>

C60.0   Malignant neoplasm of <u>prepuce</u>
Malignant neoplasm of foreskin

C60.1   Malignant neoplasm of <u>glans</u> penis

C60.2   Malignant neoplasm of <u>body</u> of penis
Malignant neoplasm of corpus cavernosum

C60.8   Malignant neoplasm of <u>overlapping sites</u> of penis

C60.9   Malignant neoplasm of penis, unspecified
Malignant neoplasm of skin of penis NOS

C61   Malignant neoplasm of <u>prostate</u>
Excludes 1: malignant neoplasm of seminal vesicle (C63.7)

C62- Malignant neoplasm of <u>testis</u>
Use additional code to identify any functional activity

C62.0-   Malignant neoplasm of <u>undescended</u> testis
Malignant neoplasm of ectopic testis
Malignant neoplasm of retained testis

C62.00   Malignant neoplasm of unspecified undescended testis

C62.01   Malignant neoplasm of undescended <u>right</u> testis

C62.02   Malignant neoplasm of undescended <u>left</u> testis

C62.1-   Malignant neoplasm of <u>descended</u> testis
Malignant neoplasm of scrotal testis

C62.10   Malignant neoplasm of unspecified descended testis

C62.11   Malignant neoplasm of descended <u>right</u> testis

C62.12   Malignant neoplasm of descended <u>left</u> testis

C62.9-   Malignant neoplasm of testis, <u>unspecified whether descended or undescended</u>

**C62.90   Malignant neoplasm of unspecified testis, unspecified
whether descended or undescended**
Malignant neoplasm of testis NOS

**C62.91   Malignant neoplasm of <u>right</u> testis, unspecified whether
descended or undescended**

**C62.92   Malignant neoplasm of <u>left</u> testis, unspecified whether
descended or undescended**

C63- Malignant neoplasm of other and unspecified male genital organs

C63.0-   Malignant neoplasm of <u>epididymis</u>

C63.00   Malignant neoplasm of unspecified epididymis

C63.01   Malignant neoplasm of <u>right</u> epididymis

C63.02   Malignant neoplasm of <u>left</u> epididymis

C63.1-   Malignant neoplasm of <u>spermatic cord</u>

C63.10   Malignant neoplasm of unspecified spermatic cord

C63.11   Malignant neoplasm of <u>right</u> spermatic cord

C63.12   Malignant neoplasm of <u>left</u> spermatic cord

C63.2   Malignant neoplasm of <u>scrotum</u>
Malignant neoplasm of skin of scrotum

C63.7   Malignant neoplasm of other specified male genital organs
Malignant neoplasm of seminal vesicle
Malignant neoplasm of tunica vaginalis

C63.8   Malignant neoplasm of <u>overlapping sites</u> of male genital organs
Primary malignant neoplasm of two or more contiguous sites of
male genital organs whose point of origin cannot be
determined

C63.9   Malignant neoplasm of male genital organ, unspecified
Malignant neoplasm of male genitourinary tract NOS

C
5
1
-
C
7
2

Malignant neoplasms of urinary tract (C64-C68)

C64- **Malignant neoplasm of <u>kidney</u>, except renal pelvis**
     Excludes 1: malignant carcinoid tumor of the kidney (C7A.093)
                 malignant neoplasm of renal calyces (C65.-)
                 malignant neoplasm of renal pelvis (C65.-)
   C64.1 **Malignant neoplasm of <u>right</u> kidney, except renal pelvis**
   C64.2 **Malignant neoplasm of <u>left</u> kidney, except renal pelvis**
   C64.9 **Malignant neoplasm of unspecified kidney, except renal pelvis**

C65- **Malignant neoplasm of <u>renal pelvis</u>**
     Includes: Malignant neoplasm of pelviureteric junction
                Malignant neoplasm of renal calyces
   C65.1 **Malignant neoplasm of <u>right</u> renal pelvis**
   C65.2 **Malignant neoplasm of <u>left</u> renal pelvis**
   C65.9 **Malignant neoplasm of unspecified renal pelvis**

C66- **Malignant neoplasm of <u>ureter</u>**
     Excludes 1: malignant neoplasm of ureteric orifice of bladder (C67.6)
   C66.1 **Malignant neoplasm of <u>right</u> ureter**
   C66.2 **Malignant neoplasm of <u>left</u> ureter**
   C66.9 **Malignant neoplasm of unspecified ureter**

C67- **Malignant neoplasm of <u>bladder</u>**
   C67.0 **Malignant neoplasm of <u>trigone</u> of bladder**
   C67.1 **Malignant neoplasm of <u>dome</u> of bladder**
   C67.2 **Malignant neoplasm of <u>lateral wall</u> of bladder**
   C67.3 **Malignant neoplasm of <u>anterior wall</u> of bladder**
   C67.4 **Malignant neoplasm of <u>posterior wall</u> of bladder**
   C67.5 **Malignant neoplasm of bladder <u>neck</u>**
          Malignant neoplasm of internal urethral orifice
   C67.6 **Malignant neoplasm of <u>ureteric orifice</u>**
   C67.7 **Malignant neoplasm of <u>urachus</u>**
   C67.8 **Malignant neoplasm of <u>overlapping sites</u> of bladder**
   C67.9 **Malignant neoplasm of bladder, unspecified**

C68- **Malignant neoplasm of other and unspecified urinary organs**
     Excludes 1: malignant neoplasm of female genitourinary tract NOS
                (C57.9)
                malignant neoplasm of male genitourinary tract NOS (C63.9)
   C68.0 **Malignant neoplasm of <u>urethra</u>**
       Excludes 1: malignant neoplasm of urethral orifice of bladder
                  (C67.5)
   C68.1 **Malignant neoplasm of <u>paraurethral glands</u>**
   C68.8 **Malignant neoplasm of overlapping sites of urinary organs**
          Primary malignant neoplasm of two or more contiguous sites of
            urinary organs whose point of origin cannot be determined
   C68.9 **Malignant neoplasm of urinary organ, unspecified**
          Malignant neoplasm of urinary system NOS

Malignant neoplasms of eye, brain and other parts of central nervous system (C69-C72)

C69- **Malignant neoplasm of <u>eye and adnexa</u>**
     Excludes 1: malignant neoplasm of connective tissue of eyelid (C49.0)
                malignant neoplasm of eyelid (skin) (C43.1-, C44.1-)
                malignant neoplasm of optic nerve (C72.3-)
   C69.0- **Malignant neoplasm of <u>conjunctiva</u>**
     C69.00 **Malignant neoplasm of unspecified conjunctiva**
     C69.01 **Malignant neoplasm of <u>right</u> conjunctiva**
     C69.02 **Malignant neoplasm of <u>left</u> conjunctiva**
   C69.1- **Malignant neoplasm of <u>cornea</u>**
     C69.10 **Malignant neoplasm of unspecified cornea**
     C69.11 **Malignant neoplasm of <u>right</u> cornea**
     C69.12 **Malignant neoplasm of <u>left</u> cornea**
   C69.2- **Malignant neoplasm of <u>retina</u>**
       Excludes 1: dark area on retina (D49.81)
               neoplasm of unspecified behavior of retina and choroid
                 (D49.81)
               retinal freckle (D49.81)
     C69.20 **Malignant neoplasm of unspecified retina**
     C69.21 **Malignant neoplasm of <u>right</u> retina**
     C69.22 **Malignant neoplasm of <u>left</u> retina**
   C69.3- **Malignant neoplasm of <u>choroid</u>**
     C69.30 **Malignant neoplasm of unspecified choroid**
     C69.31 **Malignant neoplasm of <u>right</u> choroid**
     C69.32 **Malignant neoplasm of <u>left</u> choroid**

C69.4- **Malignant neoplasm of <u>ciliary body</u>**
     C69.40 **Malignant neoplasm of unspecified ciliary body**
     C69.41 **Malignant neoplasm of <u>right</u> ciliary body**
     C69.42 **Malignant neoplasm of <u>left</u> ciliary body**
C69.5- **Malignant neoplasm of <u>lacrimal gland and duct</u>**
       Malignant neoplasm of lacrimal sac
       Malignant neoplasm of nasolacrimal duct
     C69.50 **Malignant neoplasm of unspecified lacrimal gland and duct**
     C69.51 **Malignant neoplasm of <u>right</u> lacrimal gland and duct**
     C69.52 **Malignant neoplasm of <u>left</u> lacrimal gland and duct**
C69.6- **Malignant neoplasm of <u>orbit</u>**
       Malignant neoplasm of connective tissue of orbit
       Malignant neoplasm of extraocular muscle
       Malignant neoplasm of peripheral nerves of orbit
       Malignant neoplasm of retrobulbar tissue
       Malignant neoplasm of retro-ocular tissue
       Excludes 1: malignant neoplasm of orbital bone (C41.0)
     C69.60 **Malignant neoplasm of unspecified orbit**
     C69.61 **Malignant neoplasm of <u>right</u> orbit**
     C69.62 **Malignant neoplasm of <u>left</u> orbit**
C69.8- **Malignant neoplasm of <u>overlapping sites</u> of eye and adnexa**
     C69.80 **Malignant neoplasm of overlapping sites of unspecified eye and adnexa**
     C69.81 **Malignant neoplasm of overlapping sites of <u>right</u> eye and adnexa**
     C69.82 **Malignant neoplasm of overlapping sites of <u>left</u> eye and adnexa**
C69.9- **Malignant neoplasm of unspecified site of eye**
       Malignant neoplasm of eyeball
     C69.90 **Malignant neoplasm of unspecified site of unspecified eye**
     C69.91 **Malignant neoplasm of unspecified site of <u>right</u> eye**
     C69.92 **Malignant neoplasm of unspecified site of <u>left</u> eye**

C70- **Malignant neoplasm of <u>meninges</u>**
   C70.0 **Malignant neoplasm of <u>cerebral</u> meninges**
   C70.1 **Malignant neoplasm of <u>spinal</u> meninges**
   C70.9 **Malignant neoplasm of meninges, unspecified**

C71- **Malignant neoplasm of <u>brain</u>**
     Excludes 1: malignant neoplasm of cranial nerves (C72.2-C72.5)
                retrobulbar malignant neoplasm (C69.6-)
   C71.0 **Malignant neoplasm of <u>cerebrum</u>, except lobes and ventricles**
       Malignant neoplasm of supratentorial NOS
   C71.1 **Malignant neoplasm of <u>frontal lobe</u>**
   C71.2 **Malignant neoplasm of <u>temporal lobe</u>**
   C71.3 **Malignant neoplasm of <u>parietal lobe</u>**
   C71.4 **Malignant neoplasm of <u>occipital lobe</u>**
   C71.5 **Malignant neoplasm of <u>cerebral ventricle</u>**
       Excludes 1: malignant neoplasm of fourth cerebral ventricle
                 (C71.7)
   C71.6 **Malignant neoplasm of <u>cerebellum</u>**
   C71.7 **Malignant neoplasm of <u>brain stem</u>**
       Malignant neoplasm of fourth cerebral ventricle
       Infratentorial malignant neoplasm NOS
   C71.8 **Malignant neoplasm of <u>overlapping sites</u> of brain**
   C71.9 **Malignant neoplasm of brain, unspecified**

C72- **Malignant neoplasm of spinal cord, cranial nerves and other parts of central nervous system**
     Excludes 1: malignant neoplasm of meninges (C70.-)
                malignant neoplasm of peripheral nerves and autonomic
                 nervous system (C47.-)
   C72.0 **Malignant neoplasm of <u>spinal cord</u>**
   C72.1 **Malignant neoplasm of <u>cauda equina</u>**
   C72.2- **Malignant neoplasm of <u>olfactory nerve</u>**
       Malignant neoplasm of olfactory bulb
     C72.20 **Malignant neoplasm of unspecified olfactory nerve**
     C72.21 **Malignant neoplasm of <u>right</u> olfactory nerve**
     C72.22 **Malignant neoplasm of <u>left</u> olfactory nerve**
   C72.3- **Malignant neoplasm of <u>optic nerve</u>**
     C72.30 **Malignant neoplasm of unspecified optic nerve**
     C72.31 **Malignant neoplasm of <u>right</u> optic nerve**
     C72.32 **Malignant neoplasm of <u>left</u> optic nerve**
   C72.4- **Malignant neoplasm of <u>acoustic nerve</u>**
     C72.40 **Malignant neoplasm of unspecified acoustic nerve**
     C72.41 **Malignant neoplasm of <u>right</u> acoustic nerve**
     C72.42 **Malignant neoplasm of <u>left</u> acoustic nerve**

C51 - C72

Excludes 1: = NOT CODED HERE! (Do not code both)   **361**   *Excludes ❷:* = Not Included Here

C72.5- Malignant neoplasm of <u>other and unspecified cranial nerves</u>
     C72.50 Malignant neoplasm of unspecified cranial nerve
         Malignant neoplasm of cranial nerve NOS
     C72.59 Malignant neoplasm of other cranial nerves
C72.9- Malignant neoplasm of central nervous system, unspecified
     Malignant neoplasm of unspecified site of central nervous system
     Malignant neoplasm of nervous system NOS

Malignant neoplasms of thyroid and other endocrine glands (C73-C75)

C73   **Malignant neoplasm of <u>thyroid</u> gland**
     Use additional code to identify any functional activity
C74- **Malignant neoplasm of <u>adrenal</u> gland**
   C74.0- **Malignant neoplasm of <u>cortex</u> of adrenal gland**
     C74.00 **Malignant neoplasm of cortex of unspecified adrenal gland**
     C74.01 **Malignant neoplasm of cortex of <u>right</u> adrenal gland**
     C74.02 **Malignant neoplasm of cortex of <u>left</u> adrenal gland**
   C74.1- **Malignant neoplasm of <u>medulla</u> of adrenal gland**
     C74.10 **Malignant neoplasm of medulla of unspecified adrenal gland**
     C74.11 **Malignant neoplasm of medulla of <u>right</u> adrenal gland**
     C74.12 **Malignant neoplasm of medulla of <u>left</u> adrenal gland**
   C74.9- **Malignant neoplasm of unspecified part of adrenal gland**
     C74.90 **Malignant neoplasm of unspecified part of unspecified adrenal gland**
     C74.91 **Malignant neoplasm of unspecified part of <u>right</u> adrenal gland**
     C74.92 **Malignant neoplasm of unspecified part of <u>left</u> adrenal gland**
C75- **Malignant neoplasms of other <u>endocrine glands</u> and related structures**
     Excludes 1: malignant carcinoid tumors (C7A.0-)
         malignant neoplasm of adrenal gland (C74.-)
         malignant neoplasm of endocrine pancreas (C25.4)
         malignant neoplasm of islets of Langerhans (C25.4)
         malignant neoplasm of ovary (C56.-)
         malignant neoplasm of testis (C62.-)
         malignant neoplasm of thymus (C37)
         malignant neoplasm of thyroid gland (C73)
         malignant neuroendocrine tumors (C7A.-)
   C75.0 **Malignant neoplasm of <u>parathyroid gland</u>**
   C75.1 **Malignant neoplasm of <u>pituitary gland</u>**
   C75.2 **Malignant neoplasm of <u>craniopharyngeal duct</u>**
   C75.3 **Malignant neoplasm of <u>pineal gland</u>**
   C75.4 **Malignant neoplasm of <u>carotid body</u>**
   C75.5 **Malignant neoplasm of <u>aortic body</u> and other paraganglia**
   C75.8 **Malignant neoplasm with <u>pluriglandular involvement</u>, unspecified**
   C75.9 **Malignant neoplasm of endocrine gland, unspecified**

Malignant neuroendocrine tumors (C7A)

C7A- **Malignant <u>neuroendocrine tumors</u>**
     Use additional code to identify any associated endocrine syndrome, such as:
     Carcinoid syndrome (E34.0)
     Excludes❷: malignant pancreatic islet cell tumors (C25.4)
         Merkel cell carcinoma (C4A.-)
     Code also any associated multiple endocrine neoplasia [MEN] syndromes (E31.2-)
   C7A.0- **Malignant <u>carcinoid</u> tumors**
     C7A.00 **Malignant carcinoid tumor of unspecified site**
     C7A.01- **Malignant carcinoid tumors of the <u>small intestine</u>**
       C7A.010 **Malignant carcinoid tumor of the <u>duodenum</u>**
       C7A.011 **Malignant carcinoid tumor of the <u>jejunum</u>**
       C7A.012 **Malignant carcinoid tumor of the <u>ileum</u>**
       C7A.019 **Malignant carcinoid tumor of the small intestine, unspecified portion**
     C7A.02- **Malignant carcinoid tumors of the <u>appendix, large intestine, and rectum</u>**
       C7A.020 **Malignant carcinoid tumor of the <u>appendix</u>**
       C7A.021 **Malignant carcinoid tumor of the <u>cecum</u>**
       C7A.022 **Malignant carcinoid tumor of the <u>ascending colon</u>**
       C7A.023 **Malignant carcinoid tumor of the <u>transverse colon</u>**
       C7A.024 **Malignant carcinoid tumor of the <u>descending colon</u>**
       C7A.025 **Malignant carcinoid tumor of the <u>sigmoid colon</u>**
       C7A.026 **Malignant carcinoid tumor of the <u>rectum</u>**
       C7A.029 **Malignant carcinoid tumor of the large intestine, unspecified portion**
         Malignant carcinoid tumor of the colon NOS

C7A.09- **Malignant <u>carcinoid</u> tumors of other sites**
     C7A.090 **Malignant carcinoid tumor of the <u>bronchus and lung</u>**
     C7A.091 **Malignant carcinoid tumor of the <u>thymus</u>**
     C7A.092 **Malignant carcinoid tumor of the <u>stomach</u>**
     C7A.093 **Malignant carcinoid tumor of the <u>kidney</u>**
     C7A.094 **Malignant carcinoid tumor of the foregut NOS**
     C7A.095 **Malignant carcinoid tumor of the midgut NOS**
     C7A.096 **Malignant carcinoid tumor of the hindgut NOS**
     C7A.098 **Malignant carcinoid tumors of other sites**
   C7A.1 **Malignant <u>poorly differentiated</u> neuroendocrine tumors**
     High grade neuroendocrine carcinoma, any site
     Malignant poorly differentiated neuroendocrine carcinoma, any site
     Malignant poorly differentiated neuroendocrine tumor NOS
   C7A.8 **Other malignant neuroendocrine tumors**

Secondary neuroendocrine tumors (C7B)

C7B- **Secondary <u>neuroendocrine</u> tumors**
     Use additional code to identify any functional activity
   C7B.0- **Secondary <u>carcinoid</u> tumors**
     C7B.00 **Secondary carcinoid tumors, unspecified site**
     C7B.01 **Secondary carcinoid tumors of <u>distant lymph nodes</u>**
     C7B.02 **Secondary carcinoid tumors of <u>liver</u>**
     C7B.03 **Secondary carcinoid tumors of <u>bone</u>**
     C7B.04 **Secondary carcinoid tumors of <u>peritoneum</u>**
         Mesentary metastasis of carcinoid tumor
     C7B.09 **Secondary carcinoid tumors of other sites**
   C7B.1 **Secondary <u>Merkel cell</u> carcinoma**
     Merkel cell carcinoma nodal presentation
     Merkel cell carcinoma visceral metastatic presentation
   C7B.8 **Other secondary neuroendocrine tumors**

Malignant neoplasms of ill-defined, other secondary and unspecified sites (C76-C80)

C76- **Malignant neoplasm of other and ill-defined sites**
     Excludes 1: malignant neoplasm of female genitourinary tract NOS (C57.9)
         malignant neoplasm of male genitourinary tract NOS (C63.9)
         malignant neoplasm of lymphoid, hematopoietic and related tissue (C81-C96)
         malignant neoplasm of skin (C44.-)
         malignant neoplasm of unspecified site NOS (C80.1)
   C76.0 **Malignant neoplasm of head, face and neck**
     Malignant neoplasm of cheek NOS
     Malignant neoplasm of nose NOS
   C76.1 **Malignant neoplasm of thorax**
     Intrathoracic malignant neoplasm NOS
     Malignant neoplasm of axilla NOS
     Thoracic malignant neoplasm NOS
   C76.2 **Malignant neoplasm of abdomen**
   C76.3 **Malignant neoplasm of pelvis**
     Malignant neoplasm of groin NOS
     Malignant neoplasm of sites overlapping systems within the pelvis
     Rectovaginal (septum) malignant neoplasm
     Rectovesical (septum) malignant neoplasm
   C76.4- **Malignant neoplasm of <u>upper limb</u>**
     C76.40 **Malignant neoplasm of unspecified upper limb**
     C76.41 **Malignant neoplasm of <u>right</u> upper limb**
     C76.42 **Malignant neoplasm of <u>left</u> upper limb**
   C76.5- **Malignant neoplasm of <u>lower limb</u>**
     C76.50 **Malignant neoplasm of unspecified lower limb**
     C76.51 **Malignant neoplasm of <u>right</u> lower limb**
     C76.52 **Malignant neoplasm of <u>left</u> lower limb**
   C76.8 **Malignant neoplasm of other specified ill-defined sites**
     Malignant neoplasm of overlapping ill-defined sites

Excludes 1: = NOT CODED HERE! (Do not code both)

Excludes❷: = Not Included Here

C77- Secondary and unspecified malignant neoplasm of lymph nodes
  Excludes 1: *malignant neoplasm of lymph nodes, specified as primary*
          (C81-C86, C88, C96.-)
          mesentary metastasis of carcinoid tumor (C7B.04)
          secondary carcinoid tumors of distant lymph nodes (C7B.01)

  **C77.0 Secondary and unspecified malignant neoplasm of lymph nodes
        of head, face and neck**
        Secondary and unspecified malignant neoplasm of supraclavicular
        lymph nodes
  **C77.1 Secondary and unspecified malignant neoplasm of intrathoracic
        lymph nodes**
  **C77.2 Secondary and unspecified malignant neoplasm of intra-
        abdominal lymph nodes**
  **C77.3 Secondary and unspecified malignant neoplasm of axilla and
        upper limb lymph nodes**
        Secondary and unspecified malignant neoplasm of pectoral lymph
        nodes
  **C77.4 Secondary and unspecified malignant neoplasm of inguinal and
        lower limb lymph nodes**
  **C77.5 Secondary and unspecified malignant neoplasm of intrapelvic
        lymph nodes**
  **C77.8 Secondary and unspecified malignant neoplasm of lymph nodes
        of multiple regions**
  **C77.9 Secondary and unspecified malignant neoplasm of lymph node,
        unspecified**

C78- Secondary malignant neoplasm of respiratory and digestive organs
  Excludes 1: *lymph node metastases (C77.0)*
          secondary carcinoid tumors of liver (C7B.02)
          secondary carcinoid tumors of peritoneum (C7B.04)

  C78.0- Secondary malignant neoplasm of lung
    C78.00 Secondary malignant neoplasm of unspecified lung
    C78.01 Secondary malignant neoplasm of right lung
    C78.02 Secondary malignant neoplasm of left lung
  C78.1 Secondary malignant neoplasm of mediastinum
  C78.2 Secondary malignant neoplasm of pleura
  **C78.3- Secondary malignant neoplasm of other and unspecified
        respiratory organs**
    **C78.30 Secondary malignant neoplasm of unspecified respiratory
          organ**
    C78.39 Secondary malignant neoplasm of other respiratory organs
  C78.4 Secondary malignant neoplasm of small intestine
  C78.5 Secondary malignant neoplasm of large intestine and rectum
  **C78.6 Secondary malignant neoplasm of retroperitoneum and
        peritoneum**
  **C78.7 Secondary malignant neoplasm of liver and intrahepatic bile
        duct**
  **C78.8- Secondary malignant neoplasm of other and unspecified digestive
        organs**
    **C78.80 Secondary malignant neoplasm of unspecified digestive
          organ**
    C78.89 Secondary malignant neoplasm of other digestive organs

C79- Secondary malignant neoplasm of other and unspecified sites
  Excludes 1: *lymph node metastases (C77.0)*
          secondary carcinoid tumors (C7B.-)
          secondary neuroendocrine tumors (C7B.-)

  C79.0- Secondary malignant neoplasm of kidney and renal pelvis
    **C79.00 Secondary malignant neoplasm of unspecified kidney and
          renal pelvis**
    **C79.01 Secondary malignant neoplasm of right kidney and renal
          pelvis**
    **C79.02 Secondary malignant neoplasm of left kidney and renal
          pelvis**
  **C79.1- Secondary malignant neoplasm of bladder and other and
        unspecified urinary organs**
    **C79.10 Secondary malignant neoplasm of unspecified urinary
          organs**
    C79.11 Secondary malignant neoplasm of bladder
    C79.19 Secondary malignant neoplasm of other urinary organs
  C79.2 Secondary malignant neoplasm of skin
        Excludes 1: *secondary Merkel cell carcinoma (C7B.1)*
  C79.3- Secondary malignant neoplasm of brain and cerebral meninges
    C79.31 Secondary malignant neoplasm of brain
    C79.32 Secondary malignant neoplasm of cerebral meninges
  **C79.4- Secondary malignant neoplasm of other and unspecified parts of
        nervous system**
    **C79.40 Secondary malignant neoplasm of unspecified part of
          nervous system**
    **C79.49 Secondary malignant neoplasm of other parts of nervous
          system**

C79.5- Secondary malignant neoplasm of bone and bone marrow
    Excludes 1: *secondary carcinoid tumors of bone (C7B.03)*
  C79.51 Secondary malignant neoplasm of bone
  C79.52 Secondary malignant neoplasm of bone marrow
C79.6- Secondary malignant neoplasm of ovary
  C79.60 Secondary malignant neoplasm of unspecified ovary
  C79.61 Secondary malignant neoplasm of right ovary
  C79.62 Secondary malignant neoplasm of left ovary
C79.7- Secondary malignant neoplasm of adrenal gland
  C79.70 Secondary malignant neoplasm of unspecified adrenal gland
  C79.71 Secondary malignant neoplasm of right adrenal gland
  C79.72 Secondary malignant neoplasm of left adrenal gland
C79.8- Secondary malignant neoplasm of other specified sites
  C79.81 Secondary malignant neoplasm of breast
  C79.82 Secondary malignant neoplasm of genital organs
  C79.89 Secondary malignant neoplasm of other specified sites
C79.9 Secondary malignant neoplasm of unspecified site
    Metastatic cancer NOS
    Metastatic disease NOS
    Excludes 1: *carcinomatosis NOS (C80.0)*
            generalized cancer NOS (C80.0)
            malignant (primary) neoplasm of unspecified site
            (C80.1)

C80- Malignant neoplasm without specification of site
    Excludes 1: *malignant carcinoid tumor of unspecified site (C7A.00)*
            malignant neoplasm of specified multiple sites — code to each
            site
  C80.0 Disseminated malignant neoplasm, unspecified
    Carcinomatosis NOS
    Generalized cancer, unspecified site (primary) (secondary)
    Generalized malignancy, unspecified site (primary) (secondary)
  C80.1 Malignant (primary) neoplasm, unspecified
    Cancer NOS
    Cancer unspecified site (primary)
    Carcinoma unspecified site (primary)
    Malignancy unspecified site (primary)
    Excludes 1: *secondary malignant neoplasm of unspecified site*
            (C79.9)
  C80.2 Malignant neoplasm associated with transplanted organ
    Code first complication of transplanted organ (T86.-)
    Use additional code to identify the specific malignancy

C7 2 - C8 0

© 2013 Channel Publishing, Ltd.

Malignant neoplasms of lymphoid, hematopoietic and related tissue (C81-C96)

*Excludes❷: Kaposi's sarcoma of lymph nodes (C46.3)
secondary and unspecified neoplasm of lymph nodes (C77.-)
secondary neoplasm of bone marrow (C79.52)
secondary neoplasm of spleen (C78.89)*

C81- Hodgkin lymphoma
Excludes 1: personal history of Hodgkin lymphoma (Z85.71)

C81.0- Nodular lymphocyte predominant Hodgkin lymphoma
- **C81.00** Nodular lymphocyte predominant Hodgkin lymphoma, unspecified site
- **C81.01** Nodular lymphocyte predominant Hodgkin lymphoma, lymph nodes of head, face, and neck
- **C81.02** Nodular lymphocyte predominant Hodgkin lymphoma, intrathoracic lymph nodes
- **C81.03** Nodular lymphocyte predominant Hodgkin lymphoma, intra-abdominal lymph nodes
- **C81.04** Nodular lymphocyte predominant Hodgkin lymphoma, lymph nodes of axilla and upper limb
- **C81.05** Nodular lymphocyte predominant Hodgkin lymphoma, lymph nodes of inguinal region and lower limb
- **C81.06** Nodular lymphocyte predominant Hodgkin lymphoma, intrapelvic lymph nodes
- **C81.07** Nodular lymphocyte predominant Hodgkin lymphoma, spleen
- **C81.08** Nodular lymphocyte predominant Hodgkin lymphoma, lymph nodes of multiple sites
- **C81.09** Nodular lymphocyte predominant Hodgkin lymphoma, extranodal and solid organ sites

C81.1- Nodular sclerosis classical Hodgkin lymphoma
- **C81.10** Nodular sclerosis classical Hodgkin lymphoma, unspecified site
- **C81.11** Nodular sclerosis classical Hodgkin lymphoma, lymph nodes of head, face, and neck
- **C81.12** Nodular sclerosis classical Hodgkin lymphoma, intrathoracic lymph nodes
- **C81.13** Nodular sclerosis classical Hodgkin lymphoma, intra-abdominal lymph nodes
- **C81.14** Nodular sclerosis classical Hodgkin lymphoma, lymph nodes of axilla and upper limb
- **C81.15** Nodular sclerosis classical Hodgkin lymphoma, lymph nodes of inguinal region and lower limb
- **C81.16** Nodular sclerosis classical Hodgkin lymphoma, intrapelvic lymph nodes
- **C81.17** Nodular sclerosis classical Hodgkin lymphoma, spleen
- **C81.18** Nodular sclerosis classical Hodgkin lymphoma, lymph nodes of multiple sites
- **C81.19** Nodular sclerosis classical Hodgkin lymphoma, extranodal and solid organ sites

C81.2- Mixed cellularity classical Hodgkin lymphoma
- **C81.20** Mixed cellularity classical Hodgkin lymphoma, unspecified site
- **C81.21** Mixed cellularity classical Hodgkin lymphoma, lymph nodes of head, face, and neck
- **C81.22** Mixed cellularity classical Hodgkin lymphoma, intrathoracic lymph nodes
- **C81.23** Mixed cellularity classical Hodgkin lymphoma, intra-abdominal lymph nodes
- **C81.24** Mixed cellularity classical Hodgkin lymphoma, lymph nodes of axilla and upper limb
- **C81.25** Mixed cellularity classical Hodgkin lymphoma, lymph nodes of inguinal region and lower limb
- **C81.26** Mixed cellularity classical Hodgkin lymphoma, intrapelvic lymph nodes
- **C81.27** Mixed cellularity classical Hodgkin lymphoma, spleen
- **C81.28** Mixed cellularity classical Hodgkin lymphoma, lymph nodes of multiple sites
- **C81.29** Mixed cellularity classical Hodgkin lymphoma, extranodal and solid organ sites

C81.3- Lymphocyte depleted classical Hodgkin lymphoma
- **C81.30** Lymphocyte depleted classical Hodgkin lymphoma, unspecified site
- **C81.31** Lymphocyte depleted classical Hodgkin lymphoma, lymph nodes of head, face, and neck
- **C81.32** Lymphocyte depleted classical Hodgkin lymphoma, intrathoracic lymph nodes
- **C81.33** Lymphocyte depleted classical Hodgkin lymphoma, intra-abdominal lymph nodes
- **C81.34** Lymphocyte depleted classical Hodgkin lymphoma, lymph nodes of axilla and upper limb
- **C81.35** Lymphocyte depleted classical Hodgkin lymphoma, lymph nodes of inguinal region and lower limb
- **C81.36** Lymphocyte depleted classical Hodgkin lymphoma, intrapelvic lymph nodes
- **C81.37** Lymphocyte depleted classical Hodgkin lymphoma, spleen
- **C81.38** Lymphocyte depleted classical Hodgkin lymphoma, lymph nodes of multiple sites
- **C81.39** Lymphocyte depleted classical Hodgkin lymphoma, extranodal and solid organ sites

C81.4- Lymphocyte-rich classical Hodgkin lymphoma
Excludes 1: nodular lymphocyte predominant Hodgkin lymphoma (C81.0-)
- **C81.40** Lymphocyte-rich classical Hodgkin lymphoma, unspecified site
- **C81.41** Lymphocyte-rich classical Hodgkin lymphoma, lymph nodes of head, face, and neck
- **C81.42** Lymphocyte-rich classical Hodgkin lymphoma, intrathoracic lymph nodes
- **C81.43** Lymphocyte-rich classical Hodgkin lymphoma, intra-abdominal lymph nodes
- **C81.44** Lymphocyte-rich classical Hodgkin lymphoma, lymph nodes of axilla and upper limb
- **C81.45** Lymphocyte-rich classical Hodgkin lymphoma, lymph nodes of inguinal region and lower limb
- **C81.46** Lymphocyte-rich classical Hodgkin lymphoma, intrapelvic lymph nodes
- **C81.47** Lymphocyte-rich classical Hodgkin lymphoma, spleen
- **C81.48** Lymphocyte-rich classical Hodgkin lymphoma, lymph nodes of multiple sites
- **C81.49** Lymphocyte-rich classical Hodgkin lymphoma, extranodal and solid organ sites

C81.7- Other classical Hodgkin lymphoma
Classical Hodgkin lymphoma NOS
- **C81.70** Other classical Hodgkin lymphoma, unspecified site
- **C81.71** Other classical Hodgkin lymphoma, lymph nodes of head, face, and neck
- **C81.72** Other classical Hodgkin lymphoma, intrathoracic lymph nodes
- **C81.73** Other classical Hodgkin lymphoma, intra-abdominal lymph nodes
- **C81.74** Other classical Hodgkin lymphoma, lymph nodes of axilla and upper limb
- **C81.75** Other classical Hodgkin lymphoma, lymph nodes of inguinal region and lower limb
- **C81.76** Other classical Hodgkin lymphoma, intrapelvic lymph nodes
- **C81.77** Other classical Hodgkin lymphoma, spleen
- **C81.78** Other classical Hodgkin lymphoma, lymph nodes of multiple sites
- **C81.79** Other classical Hodgkin lymphoma, extranodal and solid organ sites

C81.9- Hodgkin lymphoma, unspecified
- **C81.90** Hodgkin lymphoma, unspecified, unspecified site
- **C81.91** Hodgkin lymphoma, unspecified, lymph nodes of head, face, and neck
- **C81.92** Hodgkin lymphoma, unspecified, intrathoracic lymph nodes
- **C81.93** Hodgkin lymphoma, unspecified, intra-abdominal lymph nodes
- **C81.94** Hodgkin lymphoma, unspecified, lymph nodes of axilla and upper limb
- **C81.95** Hodgkin lymphoma, unspecified, lymph nodes of inguinal region and lower limb
- **C81.96** Hodgkin lymphoma, unspecified, intrapelvic lymph nodes
- **C81.97** Hodgkin lymphoma, unspecified, spleen
- **C81.98** Hodgkin lymphoma, unspecified, lymph nodes of multiple sites
- **C81.99** Hodgkin lymphoma, unspecified, extranodal and solid organ sites

C
8
1
–
C
8
2

C82- Follicular lymphoma
  Includes: Follicular lymphoma with or without diffuse areas
  Excludes 1: mature T/NK-cell lymphomas (C84.-)
                personal history of non-Hodgkin lymphoma (Z85.72)

  C82.0- Follicular lymphoma grade I
    C82.00 Follicular lymphoma grade I, unspecified site
    C82.01 Follicular lymphoma grade I, lymph nodes of <u>head, face, and neck</u>
    C82.02 Follicular lymphoma grade I, <u>intrathoracic</u> lymph nodes
    C82.03 Follicular lymphoma grade I, <u>intra-abdominal</u> lymph nodes
    C82.04 Follicular lymphoma grade I, lymph nodes of <u>axilla and upper limb</u>
    C82.05 Follicular lymphoma grade I, lymph nodes of <u>inguinal region and lower limb</u>
    C82.06 Follicular lymphoma grade I, <u>intrapelvic</u> lymph nodes
    C82.07 Follicular lymphoma grade I, <u>spleen</u>
    C82.08 Follicular lymphoma grade I, lymph nodes of <u>multiple sites</u>
    C82.09 Follicular lymphoma grade I, <u>extranodal and solid organ sites</u>

  C82.1- Follicular lymphoma grade II
    C82.10 Follicular lymphoma grade II, unspecified site
    C82.11 Follicular lymphoma grade II, lymph nodes of <u>head, face, and neck</u>
    C82.12 Follicular lymphoma grade II, <u>intrathoracic</u> lymph nodes
    C82.13 Follicular lymphoma grade II, <u>intra-abdominal</u> lymph nodes
    C82.14 Follicular lymphoma grade II, lymph nodes of <u>axilla and upper limb</u>
    C82.15 Follicular lymphoma grade II, lymph nodes of <u>inguinal region and lower limb</u>
    C82.16 Follicular lymphoma grade II, <u>intrapelvic</u> lymph nodes
    C82.17 Follicular lymphoma grade II, <u>spleen</u>
    C82.18 Follicular lymphoma grade II, lymph nodes of <u>multiple sites</u>
    C82.19 Follicular lymphoma grade II, <u>extranodal and solid organ sites</u>

  C82.2- Follicular lymphoma grade III, unspecified
    C82.20 Follicular lymphoma grade III, unspecified, unspecified site
    C82.21 Follicular lymphoma grade III, unspecified, lymph nodes of <u>head, face, and neck</u>
    C82.22 Follicular lymphoma grade III, unspecified, <u>intrathoracic</u> lymph nodes
    C82.23 Follicular lymphoma grade III, unspecified, <u>intra-abdominal</u> lymph nodes
    C82.24 Follicular lymphoma grade III, unspecified, lymph nodes of <u>axilla and upper limb</u>
    C82.25 Follicular lymphoma grade III, unspecified, lymph nodes of <u>inguinal region and lower limb</u>
    C82.26 Follicular lymphoma grade III, unspecified, <u>intrapelvic</u> lymph nodes
    C82.27 Follicular lymphoma grade III, unspecified, <u>spleen</u>
    C82.28 Follicular lymphoma grade III, unspecified, lymph nodes of <u>multiple sites</u>
    C82.29 Follicular lymphoma grade III, unspecified, <u>extranodal and solid organ sites</u>

  C82.3- Follicular lymphoma grade IIIa
    C82.30 Follicular lymphoma grade IIIa, unspecified site
    C82.31 Follicular lymphoma grade IIIa, lymph nodes of <u>head, face, and neck</u>
    C82.32 Follicular lymphoma grade IIIa, <u>intrathoracic</u> lymph nodes
    C82.33 Follicular lymphoma grade IIIa, <u>intra-abdominal</u> lymph nodes
    C82.34 Follicular lymphoma grade IIIa, lymph nodes of <u>axilla and upper limb</u>
    C82.35 Follicular lymphoma grade IIIa, lymph nodes of <u>inguinal region and lower limb</u>
    C82.36 Follicular lymphoma grade IIIa, <u>intrapelvic</u> lymph nodes
    C82.37 Follicular lymphoma grade IIIa, <u>spleen</u>
    C82.38 Follicular lymphoma grade IIIa, lymph nodes of <u>multiple sites</u>
    C82.39 Follicular lymphoma grade IIIa, <u>extranodal and solid organ sites</u>

  C82.4- Follicular lymphoma grade IIIb
    C82.40 Follicular lymphoma grade IIIb, unspecified site
    C82.41 Follicular lymphoma grade IIIb, lymph nodes of <u>head, face, and neck</u>
    C82.42 Follicular lymphoma grade IIIb, <u>intrathoracic</u> lymph nodes
    C82.43 Follicular lymphoma grade IIIb, <u>intra-abdominal</u> lymph nodes

C82.44 Follicular lymphoma grade IIIb, lymph nodes of <u>axilla and upper limb</u>
C82.45 Follicular lymphoma grade IIIb, lymph nodes of <u>inguinal region and lower limb</u>
C82.46 Follicular lymphoma grade IIIb, <u>intrapelvic</u> lymph nodes
C82.47 Follicular lymphoma grade IIIb, <u>spleen</u>
C82.48 Follicular lymphoma grade IIIb, lymph nodes of <u>multiple sites</u>
C82.49 Follicular lymphoma grade IIIb, <u>extranodal and solid organ sites</u>

  C82.5- Diffuse follicle center lymphoma
    C82.50 Diffuse follicle center lymphoma, unspecified site
    C82.51 Diffuse follicle center lymphoma, lymph nodes of <u>head, face, and neck</u>
    C82.52 Diffuse follicle center lymphoma, <u>intrathoracic</u> lymph nodes
    C82.53 Diffuse follicle center lymphoma, <u>intra-abdominal</u> lymph nodes
    C82.54 Diffuse follicle center lymphoma, lymph nodes of <u>axilla and upper limb</u>
    C82.55 Diffuse follicle center lymphoma, lymph nodes of <u>inguinal region and lower limb</u>
    C82.56 Diffuse follicle center lymphoma, <u>intrapelvic</u> lymph nodes
    C82.57 Diffuse follicle center lymphoma, <u>spleen</u>
    C82.58 Diffuse follicle center lymphoma, lymph nodes of <u>multiple sites</u>
    C82.59 Diffuse follicle center lymphoma, <u>extranodal and solid organ sites</u>

  C82.6- Cutaneous follicle center lymphoma
    C82.60 Cutaneous follicle center lymphoma, unspecified site
    C82.61 Cutaneous follicle center lymphoma, lymph nodes of <u>head, face, and neck</u>
    C82.62 Cutaneous follicle center lymphoma, <u>intrathoracic</u> lymph nodes
    C82.63 Cutaneous follicle center lymphoma, <u>intra-abdominal</u> lymph nodes
    C82.64 Cutaneous follicle center lymphoma, lymph nodes of <u>axilla and upper limb</u>
    C82.65 Cutaneous follicle center lymphoma, lymph nodes of <u>inguinal region and lower limb</u>
    C82.66 Cutaneous follicle center lymphoma, intrapelvic lymph nodes
    C82.67 Cutaneous follicle center lymphoma, <u>spleen</u>
    C82.68 Cutaneous follicle center lymphoma, lymph nodes of <u>multiple sites</u>
    C82.69 Cutaneous follicle center lymphoma, <u>extranodal and solid organ sites</u>

  C82.8- Other types of follicular lymphoma
    C82.80 Other types of follicular lymphoma, unspecified site
    C82.81 Other types of follicular lymphoma, lymph nodes of <u>head, face, and neck</u>
    C82.82 Other types of follicular lymphoma, <u>intrathoracic</u> lymph nodes
    C82.83 Other types of follicular lymphoma, <u>intra-abdominal</u> lymph nodes
    C82.84 Other types of follicular lymphoma, lymph nodes of <u>axilla and upper limb</u>
    C82.85 Other types of follicular lymphoma, lymph nodes of <u>inguinal region and lower limb</u>
    C82.86 Other types of follicular lymphoma, <u>intrapelvic</u> lymph nodes
    C82.87 Other types of follicular lymphoma, <u>spleen</u>
    C82.88 Other types of follicular lymphoma, lymph nodes of <u>multiple sites</u>
    C82.89 Other types of follicular lymphoma, <u>extranodal and solid organ sites</u>

  C82.9- Follicular lymphoma, unspecified
    C82.90 Follicular lymphoma, unspecified, unspecified site
    C82.91 Follicular lymphoma, unspecified, lymph nodes of <u>head, face, and neck</u>
    C82.92 Follicular lymphoma, unspecified, <u>intrathoracic</u> lymph nodes
    C82.93 Follicular lymphoma, unspecified, <u>intra-abdominal</u> lymph nodes
    C82.94 Follicular lymphoma, unspecified, lymph nodes of <u>axilla and upper limb</u>
    C82.95 Follicular lymphoma, unspecified, lymph nodes of <u>inguinal region and lower limb</u>
    C82.96 Follicular lymphoma, unspecified, <u>intrapelvic</u> lymph nodes
    C82.97 Follicular lymphoma, unspecified, <u>spleen</u>
    C82.98 Follicular lymphoma, unspecified, lymph nodes of <u>multiple sites</u>

C
8
1
–
C
8
2

Excludes 1: = NOT CODED HERE! (Do not code both)   365   *Excludes ❷:* = Not Included Here

C82.99 Follicular lymphoma, unspecified, <u>extranodal and solid organ sites</u>

C83- Non-follicular lymphoma
    Excludes 1: personal history of non-Hodgkin lymphoma (Z85.72)

C83.0- <u>Small cell</u> B-cell lymphoma
    Lymphoplasmacytic lymphoma
    Nodal marginal zone lymphoma
    Non-leukemic variant of B-CLL
    Splenic marginal zone lymphoma
    Excludes 1: chronic lymphocytic leukemia (C91.1)
                mature T/NK-cell lymphomas (C84.-)
                Waldenström macroglobulinemia (C88.0)

C83.00 Small cell B-cell lymphoma, unspecified site
C83.01 Small cell B-cell lymphoma, lymph nodes of <u>head, face, and neck</u>
C83.02 Small cell B-cell lymphoma, <u>intrathoracic</u> lymph nodes
C83.03 Small cell B-cell lymphoma, <u>intra-abdominal</u> lymph nodes
C83.04 Small cell B-cell lymphoma, lymph nodes of <u>axilla and upper limb</u>
C83.05 Small cell B-cell lymphoma, lymph nodes of <u>inguinal region and lower limb</u>
C83.06 Small cell B-cell lymphoma, intrapelvic lymph nodes
C83.07 Small cell B-cell lymphoma, <u>spleen</u>
C83.08 Small cell B-cell lymphoma, lymph nodes of <u>multiple sites</u>
C83.09 Small cell B-cell lymphoma, <u>extranodal and solid organ sites</u>

C83.1- <u>Mantle cell</u> lymphoma
    Centrocytic lymphoma
    Malignant lymphomatous polyposis

C83.10 Mantle cell lymphoma, unspecified site
C83.11 Mantle cell lymphoma, lymph nodes of <u>head, face, and neck</u>
C83.12 Mantle cell lymphoma, <u>intrathoracic</u> lymph nodes
C83.13 Mantle cell lymphoma, <u>intra-abdominal</u> lymph nodes
C83.14 Mantle cell lymphoma, lymph nodes of <u>axilla and upper limb</u>
C83.15 Mantle cell lymphoma, lymph nodes of <u>inguinal region and lower limb</u>
C83.16 Mantle cell lymphoma, <u>intrapelvic</u> lymph nodes
C83.17 Mantle cell lymphoma, <u>spleen</u>
C83.18 Mantle cell lymphoma, lymph nodes of <u>multiple sites</u>
C83.19 Mantle cell lymphoma, <u>extranodal and solid organ sites</u>

C83.3- <u>Diffuse large</u> B-cell lymphoma
    Anaplastic diffuse large B-cell lymphoma
    CD30-positive diffuse large B-cell lymphoma
    Centroblastic diffuse large B-cell lymphoma
    Diffuse large B-cell lymphoma, subtype not specified
    Immunoblastic diffuse large B-cell lymphoma
    Plasmablastic diffuse large B-cell lymphoma
    Diffuse large B-cell lymphoma, subtype not specified
    T-cell rich diffuse large B-cell lymphoma
    Excludes 1: mediastinal (thymic) large B-cell lymphoma (C85.2-)
                mature T/NK-cell lymphomas (C84.-)

C83.30 Diffuse large B-cell lymphoma, unspecified site
C83.31 Diffuse large B-cell lymphoma, lymph nodes of <u>head, face, and neck</u>
C83.32 Diffuse large B-cell lymphoma, <u>intrathoracic</u> lymph nodes
C83.33 Diffuse large B-cell lymphoma, <u>intra-abdominal</u> lymph nodes
C83.34 Diffuse large B-cell lymphoma, lymph nodes of <u>axilla and upper limb</u>
C83.35 Diffuse large B-cell lymphoma, lymph nodes of <u>inguinal region and lower limb</u>
C83.36 Diffuse large B-cell lymphoma, <u>intrapelvic</u> lymph nodes
C83.37 Diffuse large B-cell lymphoma, <u>spleen</u>
C83.38 Diffuse large B-cell lymphoma, lymph nodes of <u>multiple sites</u>
C83.39 Diffuse large B-cell lymphoma, <u>extranodal and solid organ sites</u>

C83.5- <u>Lymphoblastic (diffuse)</u> lymphoma
    B-precursor lymphoma
    Lymphoblastic B-cell lymphoma
    Lymphoblastic lymphoma NOS
    Lymphoblastic T-cell lymphoma
    T-precursor lymphoma

C83.50 Lymphoblastic (diffuse) lymphoma, unspecified site
C83.51 Lymphoblastic (diffuse) lymphoma, lymph nodes of <u>head, face, and neck</u>
C83.52 Lymphoblastic (diffuse) lymphoma, <u>intrathoracic</u> lymph nodes
C83.53 Lymphoblastic (diffuse) lymphoma, <u>intra-abdominal</u> lymph nodes
C83.54 Lymphoblastic (diffuse) lymphoma, lymph nodes of <u>axilla and upper limb</u>

C83.55 Lymphoblastic (diffuse) lymphoma, lymph nodes of <u>inguinal region and lower limb</u>
C83.56 Lymphoblastic (diffuse) lymphoma, <u>intrapelvic</u> lymph nodes
C83.57 Lymphoblastic (diffuse) lymphoma, <u>spleen</u>
C83.58 Lymphoblastic (diffuse) lymphoma, lymph nodes of <u>multiple sites</u>
C83.59 Lymphoblastic (diffuse) lymphoma, <u>extranodal and solid organ sites</u>

C83.7- <u>Burkitt</u> lymphoma
    Atypical Burkitt lymphoma
    Burkitt-like lymphoma
    Excludes 1: mature B-cell leukemia Burkitt type (C91.A-)

C83.70 Burkitt lymphoma, unspecified site
C83.71 Burkitt lymphoma, lymph nodes of <u>head, face, and neck</u>
C83.72 Burkitt lymphoma, <u>intrathoracic</u> lymph nodes
C83.73 Burkitt lymphoma, <u>intra-abdominal</u> lymph nodes
C83.74 Burkitt lymphoma, lymph nodes of <u>axilla and upper limb</u>
C83.75 Burkitt lymphoma, lymph nodes of <u>inguinal region and lower limb</u>
C83.76 Burkitt lymphoma, <u>intrapelvic</u> lymph nodes
C83.77 Burkitt lymphoma, <u>spleen</u>
C83.78 Burkitt lymphoma, lymph nodes of <u>multiple sites</u>
C83.79 Burkitt lymphoma, <u>extranodal and solid organ sites</u>

C83.8- <u>Other non-follicular</u> lymphoma
    Intravascular large B-cell lymphoma
    Lymphoid granulomatosis
    Primary effusion B-cell lymphoma
    Excludes 1: mediastinal (thymic) large B-cell lymphoma (C85.2-)
                T-cell rich B-cell lymphoma (C83.3-)

C83.80 Other non-follicular lymphoma, unspecified site
C83.81 Other non-follicular lymphoma, lymph nodes of <u>head, face, and neck</u>
C83.82 Other non-follicular lymphoma, <u>intrathoracic</u> lymph nodes
C83.83 Other non-follicular lymphoma, <u>intra-abdominal</u> lymph nodes
C83.84 Other non-follicular lymphoma, lymph nodes of <u>axilla and upper limb</u>
C83.85 Other non-follicular lymphoma, lymph nodes of <u>inguinal region and lower limb</u>
C83.86 Other non-follicular lymphoma, <u>intrapelvic</u> lymph nodes
C83.87 Other non-follicular lymphoma, <u>spleen</u>
C83.88 Other non-follicular lymphoma, lymph nodes of <u>multiple sites</u>
C83.89 Other non-follicular lymphoma, <u>extranodal and solid organ sites</u>

C83.9- Non-follicular (diffuse) lymphoma, <u>unspecified</u>
C83.90 Non-follicular (diffuse) lymphoma, unspecified, unspecified site
C83.91 Non-follicular (diffuse) lymphoma, unspecified, lymph nodes of <u>head, face, and neck</u>
C83.92 Non-follicular (diffuse) lymphoma, unspecified, <u>intrathoracic</u> lymph nodes
C83.93 Non-follicular (diffuse) lymphoma, unspecified, <u>intra-abdominal</u> lymph nodes
C83.94 Non-follicular (diffuse) lymphoma, unspecified, lymph nodes of <u>axilla and upper limb</u>
C83.95 Non-follicular (diffuse) lymphoma, unspecified, lymph nodes of <u>inguinal region and lower limb</u>
C83.96 Non-follicular (diffuse) lymphoma, unspecified, <u>intrapelvic</u> lymph nodes
C83.97 Non-follicular (diffuse) lymphoma, unspecified, <u>spleen</u>
C83.98 Non-follicular (diffuse) lymphoma, unspecified, lymph nodes of <u>multiple sites</u>
C83.99 Non-follicular (diffuse) lymphoma, unspecified, <u>extranodal and solid organ sites</u>

C82
-
C84

Excludes 1: = NOT CODED HERE! (Do not code both)

Excludes ❷: = Not Included Here

C84- Mature T/NK-cell lymphomas
　　Excludes 1: personal history of non-Hodgkin lymphoma (Z85.72)
　C84.0- Mycosis fungoides
　　　Excludes 1: peripheral T-cell lymphoma, not classified (C84.4-)
　　C84.00 Mycosis fungoides, unspecified site
　　C84.01 Mycosis fungoides, lymph nodes of head, face, and neck
　　C84.02 Mycosis fungoides, intrathoracic lymph nodes
　　C84.03 Mycosis fungoides, intra-abdominal lymph nodes
　　C84.04 Mycosis fungoides, lymph nodes of axilla and upper limb
　　C84.05 Mycosis fungoides, lymph nodes of inguinal region and lower limb
　　C84.06 Mycosis fungoides, intrapelvic lymph nodes
　　C84.07 Mycosis fungoides, spleen
　　C84.08 Mycosis fungoides, lymph nodes of multiple sites
　　C84.09 Mycosis fungoides, extranodal and solid organ sites
　C84.1- Sézary disease
　　C84.10 Sézary disease, unspecified site
　　C84.11 Sézary disease, lymph nodes of head, face, and neck
　　C84.12 Sézary disease, intrathoracic lymph nodes
　　C84.13 Sézary disease, intra-abdominal lymph nodes
　　C84.14 Sézary disease, lymph nodes of axilla and upper limb
　　C84.15 Sézary disease, lymph nodes of inguinal region and lower limb
　　C84.16 Sézary disease, intrapelvic lymph nodes
　　C84.17 Sézary disease, spleen
　　C84.18 Sézary disease, lymph nodes of multiple sites
　　C84.19 Sézary disease, extranodal and solid organ sites
　C84.4- Peripheral T-cell lymphoma, not classified
　　　Lennert's lymphoma
　　　Lymphoepithelioid lymphoma
　　　Mature T-cell lymphoma, not elsewhere classified
　　C84.40 Peripheral T-cell lymphoma, not classified, unspecified site
　　C84.41 Peripheral T-cell lymphoma, not classified, lymph nodes of head, face, and neck
　　C84.42 Peripheral T-cell lymphoma, not classified, intrathoracic lymph nodes
　　C84.43 Peripheral T-cell lymphoma, not classified, intra-abdominal lymph nodes
　　C84.44 Peripheral T-cell lymphoma, not classified, lymph nodes of axilla and upper limb
　　C84.45 Peripheral T-cell lymphoma, not classified, lymph nodes of inguinal region and lower limb
　　C84.46 Peripheral T-cell lymphoma, not classified, intrapelvic lymph nodes
　　C84.47 Peripheral T-cell lymphoma, not classified, spleen
　　C84.48 Peripheral T-cell lymphoma, not classified, lymph nodes of multiple sites
　　C84.49 Peripheral T-cell lymphoma, not classified, extranodal and solid organ sites
　C84.6- Anaplastic large cell lymphoma, ALK-positive
　　　Anaplastic large cell lymphoma, CD30-positive
　　C84.60 Anaplastic large cell lymphoma, ALK-positive, unspecified site
　　C84.61 Anaplastic large cell lymphoma, ALK-positive, lymph nodes of head, face, and neck
　　C84.62 Anaplastic large cell lymphoma, ALK-positive, intrathoracic lymph nodes
　　C84.63 Anaplastic large cell lymphoma, ALK-positive, intra-abdominal lymph nodes
　　C84.64 Anaplastic large cell lymphoma, ALK-positive, lymph nodes of axilla and upper limb
　　C84.65 Anaplastic large cell lymphoma, ALK-positive, lymph nodes of inguinal region and lower limb
　　C84.66 Anaplastic large cell lymphoma, ALK-positive, intrapelvic lymph nodes
　　C84.67 Anaplastic large cell lymphoma, ALK-positive, spleen
　　C84.68 Anaplastic large cell lymphoma, ALK-positive, lymph nodes of multiple sites
　　C84.69 Anaplastic large cell lymphoma, ALK-positive, extranodal and solid organ sites
　C84.7- Anaplastic large cell lymphoma, ALK-negative
　　　Excludes 1: primary cutaneous CD30-positive T-cell proliferations (C86.6-)
　　C84.70 Anaplastic large cell lymphoma, ALK-negative, unspecified site
　　C84.71 Anaplastic large cell lymphoma, ALK-negative, lymph nodes of head, face, and neck
　　C84.72 Anaplastic large cell lymphoma, ALK-negative, intrathoracic lymph nodes

　　C84.73 Anaplastic large cell lymphoma, ALK-negative, intra-abdominal lymph nodes
　　C84.74 Anaplastic large cell lymphoma, ALK-negative, lymph nodes of axilla and upper limb
　　C84.75 Anaplastic large cell lymphoma, ALK-negative, lymph nodes of inguinal region and lower limb
　　C84.76 Anaplastic large cell lymphoma, ALK-negative, intrapelvic lymph nodes
　　C84.77 Anaplastic large cell lymphoma, ALK-negative, spleen
　　C84.78 Anaplastic large cell lymphoma, ALK-negative, lymph nodes of multiple sites
　　C84.79 Anaplastic large cell lymphoma, ALK-negative, extranodal and solid organ sites
　C84.A- Cutaneous T-cell lymphoma, unspecified
　　C84.A0 Cutaneous T-cell lymphoma, unspecified, unspecified site
　　C84.A1 Cutaneous T-cell lymphoma, unspecified lymph nodes of head, face, and neck
　　C84.A2 Cutaneous T-cell lymphoma, unspecified, intrathoracic lymph nodes
　　C84.A3 Cutaneous T-cell lymphoma, unspecified, intra-abdominal lymph nodes
　　C84.A4 Cutaneous T-cell lymphoma, unspecified, lymph nodes of axilla and upper limb
　　C84.A5 Cutaneous T-cell lymphoma, unspecified, lymph nodes of inguinal region and lower limb
　　C84.A6 Cutaneous T-cell lymphoma, unspecified, intrapelvic lymph nodes
　　C84.A7 Cutaneous T-cell lymphoma, unspecified, spleen
　　C84.A8 Cutaneous T-cell lymphoma, unspecified, lymph nodes of multiple sites
　　C84.A9 Cutaneous T-cell lymphoma, unspecified, extranodal and solid organ sites
　C84.Z- Other mature T/NK-cell lymphomas
　　　Note: If T-cell lineage or involvement is mentioned in conjunction with a specific lymphoma, code to the more specific description.
　　　Excludes 1: angioimmunoblastic T-cell lymphoma (C86.5)
　　　　blastic NK-cell lymphoma (C86.4)
　　　　enteropathy-type T-cell lymphoma (C86.2)
　　　　extranodal NK-cell lymphoma, nasal type (C86.0)
　　　　hepatosplenic T-cell lymphoma (C86.1)
　　　　primary cutaneous CD30-positive T-cell proliferations (C86.6)
　　　　subcutaneous panniculitis-like T-cell lymphoma (C86.3)
　　　　T-cell leukemia (C91.1-)
　　C84.Z0 Other mature T/NK-cell lymphomas, unspecified site
　　C84.Z1 Other mature T/NK-cell lymphomas, lymph nodes of head, face, and neck
　　C84.Z2 Other mature T/NK-cell lymphomas, intrathoracic lymph nodes
　　C84.Z3 Other mature T/NK-cell lymphomas, intra-abdominal lymph nodes
　　C84.Z4 Other mature T/NK-cell lymphomas, lymph nodes of axilla and upper limb
　　C84.Z5 Other mature T/NK-cell lymphomas, lymph nodes of inguinal region and lower limb
　　C84.Z6 Other mature T/NK-cell lymphomas, intrapelvic lymph nodes
　　C84.Z7 Other mature T/NK-cell lymphomas, spleen
　　C84.Z8 Other mature T/NK-cell lymphomas, lymph nodes of multiple sites
　　C84.Z9 Other mature T/NK-cell lymphomas, extranodal and solid organ sites
　C84.9- Mature T/NK-cell lymphomas, unspecified
　　　NK/T cell lymphoma NOS
　　　Excludes 1: mature T-cell lymphoma, not elsewhere classified (C84.4-)
　　C84.90 Mature T/NK-cell lymphomas, unspecified, unspecified site
　　C84.91 Mature T/NK-cell lymphomas, unspecified, lymph nodes of head, face, and neck
　　C84.92 Mature T/NK-cell lymphomas, unspecified, intrathoracic lymph nodes
　　C84.93 Mature T/NK-cell lymphomas, unspecified, intra-abdominal lymph nodes
　　C84.94 Mature T/NK-cell lymphomas, unspecified, lymph nodes of axilla and upper limb
　　C84.95 Mature T/NK-cell lymphomas, unspecified, lymph nodes of inguinal region and lower limb
　　C84.96 Mature T/NK-cell lymphomas, unspecified, intrapelvic lymph nodes
　　C84.97 Mature T/NK-cell lymphomas, unspecified, spleen

C82 - C84

C84.98 Mature T/NK-cell lymphomas, unspecified, lymph nodes of <u>multiple sites</u>

C84.99 Mature T/NK-cell lymphomas, unspecified, <u>extranodal and solid organ sites</u>

C85- <u>Other specified and unspecified types of non-Hodgkin</u> lymphoma

Excludes 1: *other specified types of T/NK-cell lymphoma (C86.-)*
personal history of non-Hodgkin lymphoma (Z85.72)

C85.1- <u>Unspecified B-cell</u> lymphoma

Note: If B-cell lineage or involvement is mentioned in conjunction with a specific lymphoma, code to the more specific description.

C85.10 Unspecified B-cell lymphoma, unspecified site

C85.11 Unspecified B-cell lymphoma, lymph nodes of <u>head, face, and neck</u>

C85.12 Unspecified B-cell lymphoma, <u>intrathoracic</u> lymph nodes

C85.13 Unspecified B-cell lymphoma, <u>intra-abdominal</u> lymph nodes

C85.14 Unspecified B-cell lymphoma, lymph nodes of <u>axilla and upper limb</u>

C85.15 Unspecified B-cell lymphoma, lymph nodes of <u>inguinal region and lower limb</u>

C85.16 Unspecified B-cell lymphoma, <u>intrapelvic</u> lymph nodes

C85.17 Unspecified B-cell lymphoma, <u>spleen</u>

C85.18 Unspecified B-cell lymphoma, lymph nodes of <u>multiple sites</u>

C85.19 Unspecified B-cell lymphoma, <u>extranodal and solid organ sites</u>

C85.2- <u>Mediastinal (thymic) large B-cell</u> lymphoma

C85.20 Mediastinal (thymic) large B-cell lymphoma, unspecified site

C85.21 Mediastinal (thymic) large B-cell lymphoma, lymph nodes of <u>head, face, and neck</u>

C85.22 Mediastinal (thymic) large B-cell lymphoma, <u>intrathoracic</u> lymph nodes

C85.23 Mediastinal (thymic) large B-cell lymphoma, <u>intra-abdominal</u> lymph nodes

C85.24 Mediastinal (thymic) large B-cell lymphoma, lymph nodes of <u>axilla and upper limb</u>

C85.25 Mediastinal (thymic) large B-cell lymphoma, lymph nodes of <u>inguinal region and lower limb</u>

C85.26 Mediastinal (thymic) large B-cell lymphoma, <u>intrapelvic</u> lymph nodes

C85.27 Mediastinal (thymic) large B-cell lymphoma, <u>spleen</u>

C85.28 Mediastinal (thymic) large B-cell lymphoma, lymph nodes of <u>multiple sites</u>

C85.29 Mediastinal (thymic) large B-cell lymphoma, <u>extranodal and solid organ sites</u>

C85.8- <u>Other specified types of non-Hodgkin</u> lymphoma

C85.80 Other specified types of non-Hodgkin lymphoma, unspecified site

C85.81 Other specified types of non-Hodgkin lymphoma, lymph nodes of <u>head, face, and neck</u>

C85.82 Other specified types of non-Hodgkin lymphoma, <u>intrathoracic</u> lymph nodes

C85.83 Other specified types of non-Hodgkin lymphoma, <u>intra-abdominal</u> lymph nodes

C85.84 Other specified types of non-Hodgkin lymphoma, lymph nodes of <u>axilla and upper limb</u>

C85.85 Other specified types of non-Hodgkin lymphoma, lymph nodes of <u>inguinal region and lower limb</u>

C85.86 Other specified types of non-Hodgkin lymphoma, <u>intrapelvic</u> lymph nodes

C85.87 Other specified types of non-Hodgkin lymphoma, <u>spleen</u>

C85.88 Other specified types of non-Hodgkin lymphoma, lymph nodes of <u>multiple sites</u>

C85.89 Other specified types of non-Hodgkin lymphoma, <u>extranodal and solid organ sites</u>

C85.9- Non-Hodgkin lymphoma, <u>unspecified</u>

Lymphoma NOS
Malignant lymphoma NOS
Non-Hodgkin lymphoma NOS

C85.90 Non-Hodgkin lymphoma, unspecified, unspecified site

C85.91 Non-Hodgkin lymphoma, unspecified, lymph nodes of <u>head, face, and neck</u>

C85.92 Non-Hodgkin lymphoma, unspecified, <u>intrathoracic</u> lymph nodes

C85.93 Non-Hodgkin lymphoma, unspecified, <u>intra-abdominal</u> lymph nodes

C85.94 Non-Hodgkin lymphoma, unspecified, lymph nodes of <u>axilla and upper limb</u>

C85.95 Non-Hodgkin lymphoma, unspecified, lymph nodes of <u>inguinal region and lower limb</u>

C85.96 Non-Hodgkin lymphoma, unspecified, <u>intrapelvic</u> lymph nodes

C85.97 Non-Hodgkin lymphoma, unspecified, <u>spleen</u>

C85.98 Non-Hodgkin lymphoma, unspecified, lymph nodes of <u>multiple sites</u>

C85.99 Non-Hodgkin lymphoma, unspecified, <u>extranodal and solid organ sites</u>

C86- <u>Other specified types of T/NK-cell</u> lymphoma

Excludes 1: *anaplastic large cell lymphoma, ALK negative (C84.7-)*
anaplastic large cell lymphoma, ALK positive (C84.6-)
mature T/NK-cell lymphomas (C84.-)
other specified types of non-Hodgkin lymphoma (C85.8-)

C86.0 <u>Extranodal NK/T-cell lymphoma, nasal type</u>

C86.1 <u>Hepatosplenic T-cell lymphoma</u>

Alpha-beta and gamma delta types

C86.2 <u>Enteropathy-type (intestinal) T-cell lymphoma</u>

Enteropathy associated T-cell lymphoma

C86.3 <u>Subcutaneous panniculitis-like</u> T-cell lymphoma

C86.4 <u>Blastic NK-cell</u> lymphoma

C86.5 <u>Angioimmunoblastic</u> T-cell lymphoma

Angioimmunoblastic lymphadenopathy with dysproteinemia (AILD)

C86.6 <u>Primary cutaneous CD30-positive</u> T-cell proliferations

Lymphomatoid papulosis
Primary cutaneous anaplastic large cell lymphoma
Primary cutaneous CD30-positive large T-cell lymphoma

C88- <u>Malignant immunoproliferative diseases and certain other B-cell lymphomas</u>

Excludes 1: *B-cell lymphoma, unspecified (C85.1-)*
personal history of other malignant neoplasms of lymphoid, hematopoietic and related tissues (Z85.79)

C88.0 <u>Waldenström macroglobulinemia</u>

Lymphoplasmacytic lymphoma with IgM-production
Macroglobulinemia (idiopathic) (primary)
Excludes 1: *small cell B-cell lymphoma (C83.0)*

C88.2 <u>Heavy chain disease</u>

Franklin disease
Gamma heavy chain disease
Mu heavy chain disease

C88.3 <u>Immunoproliferative small intestinal disease</u>

Alpha heavy chain disease
Mediterranean lymphoma

C88.4 <u>Extranodal marginal zone B-cell lymphoma of mucosa-associated lymphoid tissue [MALT-lymphoma]</u>

Lymphoma of skin-associated lymphoid tissue [SALT-lymphoma]
Lymphoma of bronchial-associated lymphoid tissue [BALT-lymphoma]
Excludes 1: *high malignant (diffuse large B-cell) lymphoma (C83.3-)*

C88.8 <u>Other malignant immunoproliferative diseases</u>

C88.9 <u>Malignant immunoproliferative disease, unspecified</u>

Immunoproliferative disease NOS

C90- <u>Multiple myeloma and malignant plasma cell neoplasms</u>

Excludes 1: *personal history of other malignant neoplasms of lymphoid, hematopoietic and related tissues (Z85.79)*

C90.0- <u>Multiple myeloma</u>

Kahler's disease
Medullary plasmacytoma
Myelomatosis
Plasma cell myeloma
Excludes 1: *solitary myeloma (C90.3-)*
solitary plasmactyoma (C90.3-)

C90.00 Multiple myeloma <u>not</u> having achieved remission

Multiple myeloma with failed remission
Multiple myeloma NOS

C90.01 Multiple myeloma <u>in remission</u>

C90.02 Multiple myeloma <u>in relapse</u>

C90.1- <u>Plasma cell leukemia</u>

Plasmacytic leukemia

C90.10 Plasma cell leukemia <u>not</u> having achieved remission

Plasma cell leukemia with failed remission
Plasma cell leukemia NOS

C90.11 Plasma cell leukemia <u>in remission</u>

C90.12 Plasma cell leukemia <u>in relapse</u>

C90.2- <u>Extramedullary plasmacytoma</u>

C90.20 Extramedullary plasmacytoma <u>not</u> having achieved remission

Extramedullary plasmacytoma with failed remission
Extramedullary plasmacytoma NOS

C90.21 Extramedullary plasmacytoma <u>in remission</u>

C90.22 Extramedullary plasmacytoma <u>in relapse</u>

Excludes 1: = NOT CODED HERE! (Do not code both)

Excludes ❷: = Not Included Here

C 8 4 - C 9 2

C90.3- <u>Solitary plasmacytoma</u>
    Localized malignant plasma cell tumor NOS
    Plasmacytoma NOS
    Solitary myeloma

    C90.30 Solitary plasmacytoma <u>not</u> having achieved remission
        Solitary plasmacytoma with failed remission
        Solitary plasmacytoma NOS

    C90.31 Solitary plasmacytoma <u>in remission</u>

    C90.32 Solitary plasmacytoma <u>in relapse</u>

C91- <u>Lymphoid leukemia</u>
    Excludes 1: personal history of leukemia (Z85.6)

C91.0- <u>Acute lymphoblastic</u> leukemia [ALL]
    Note: Code C91.0 should only be used for T-cell and B-cell
        precursor leukemia

    C91.00 Acute lymphoblastic leukemia <u>not</u> having achieved remission
        Acute lymphoblastic leukemia with failed remission
        Acute lymphoblastic leukemia NOS

    C91.01 Acute lymphoblastic leukemia, <u>in remission</u>

    C91.02 Acute lymphoblastic leukemia, <u>in relapse</u>

C91.1- <u>Chronic lymphocytic</u> leukemia of B-cell type
    Lymphoplasmacytic leukemia
    Richter syndrome
    Excludes 1: lymphoplasmacytic lymphoma (C83.0-)

    C91.10 Chronic lymphocytic leukemia of B-cell type <u>not</u> having achieved remission
        Chronic lymphocytic leukemia of B-cell type with failed remission
        Chronic lymphocytic leukemia of B-cell type NOS

    C91.11 Chronic lymphocytic leukemia of B-cell type <u>in remission</u>

    C91.12 Chronic lymphocytic leukemia of B-cell type <u>in relapse</u>

C91.3- <u>Prolymphocytic</u> leukemia of <u>B-cell type</u>

    C91.30 Prolymphocytic leukemia of B-cell type <u>not</u> having achieved remission
        Prolymphocytic leukemia of B-cell type with failed remission
        Prolymphocytic leukemia of B-cell type NOS

    C91.31 Prolymphocytic leukemia of B-cell type, <u>in remission</u>

    C91.32 Prolymphocytic leukemia of B-cell type, <u>in relapse</u>

C91.4- <u>Hairy cell</u> leukemia
    Leukemic reticuloendotheliosis

    C91.40 Hairy cell leukemia <u>not</u> having achieved remission
        Hairy cell leukemia with failed remission
        Hairy cell leukemia NOS

    C91.41 Hairy cell leukemia, <u>in remission</u>

    C91.42 Hairy cell leukemia, <u>in relapse</u>

C91.5- <u>Adult T-cell</u> lymphoma/leukemia (HTLV-1-associated)
    Acute variant of adult T-cell lymphoma/leukemia (HTLV-1-associated)
    Chronic variant of adult T-cell lymphoma/leukemia (HTLV-1-associated)
    Lymphomatoid variant of adult T-cell lymphoma/leukemia (HTLV-1-associated)
    Smouldering variant of adult T-cell lymphoma/leukemia (HTLV-1-associated)

    C91.50 Adult T-cell lymphoma/leukemia (HTLV-1-associated) <u>not</u> having achieved remission
        Adult T-cell lymphoma/leukemia (HTLV-1-associated) with failed remission
        Adult T-cell lymphoma/leukemia (HTLV-1-associated) NOS

    C91.51 Adult T-cell lymphoma/leukemia (HTLV-1-associated), <u>in remission</u>

    C91.52 Adult T-cell lymphoma/leukemia (HTLV-1-associated), <u>in relapse</u>

C91.6- <u>Prolymphocytic</u> leukemia of <u>T-cell type</u>

    C91.60 Prolymphocytic leukemia of T-cell type <u>not</u> having achieved remission
        Prolymphocytic leukemia of T-cell type with failed remission
        Prolymphocytic leukemia of T-cell type NOS

    C91.61 Prolymphocytic leukemia of T-cell type, <u>in remission</u>

    C91.62 Prolymphocytic leukemia of T-cell type, <u>in relapse</u>

C91.A- <u>Mature B-cell</u> leukemia <u>Burkitt-type</u>
    Excludes 1: Burkitt lymphoma (C83.7-)

    C91.A0 Mature B-cell leukemia Burkitt-type <u>not</u> having achieved remission
        Mature B-cell leukemia Burkitt-type with failed remission
        Mature B-cell leukemia Burkitt-type NOS

    C91.A1 Mature B-cell leukemia Burkitt-type, <u>in remission</u>

    C91.A2 Mature B-cell leukemia Burkitt-type, <u>in relapse</u>

C91.Z- <u>Other lymphoid</u> leukemia
    T-cell large granular lymphocytic leukemia (associated with rheumatoid arthritis)

    C91.Z0 Other lymphoid leukemia <u>not</u> having achieved remission
        Other lymphoid leukemia with failed remission
        Other lymphoid leukemia NOS

    C91.Z1 Other lymphoid leukemia, <u>in remission</u>

    C91.Z2 Other lymphoid leukemia, <u>in relapse</u>

C91.9- Lymphoid leukemia, <u>unspecified</u>

    C91.90 Lymphoid leukemia, unspecified <u>not</u> having achieved remission
        Lymphoid leukemia with failed remission
        Lymphoid leukemia NOS

    C91.91 Lymphoid leukemia, unspecified, <u>in remission</u>

    C91.92 Lymphoid leukemia, unspecified, <u>in relapse</u>

C92 <u>Myeloid leukemia</u>
    Includes: Granulocytic leukemia
              Myelogenous leukemia
    Excludes 1: personal history of leukemia (Z85.6)

C92.0- <u>Acute myeloblastic</u> leukemia
    Acute myeloblastic leukemia, minimal differentiation
    Acute myeloblastic leukemia (with maturation)
    Acute myeloblastic leukemia 1/ETO
    Acute myeloblastic leukemia M0
    Acute myeloblastic leukemia M1
    Acute myeloblastic leukemia M2
    Acute myeloblastic leukemia with t(8;21)
    Acute myeloblastic leukemia (without a FAB classification) NOS
    Refractory anemia with excess blasts in transformation [RAEB T]
    Excludes 1: acute exacerbation of chronic myeloid leukemia (C92.10)
                refractory anemia with excess of blasts not in transformation (D46.2-)

    C92.00 Acute myeloblastic leukemia, <u>not</u> having achieved remission
        Acute myeloblastic leukemia with failed remission
        Acute myeloblastic leukemia NOS

    C92.01 Acute myeloblastic leukemia, <u>in remission</u>

    C92.02 Acute myeloblastic leukemia, <u>in relapse</u>

C92.1- <u>Chronic</u> myeloid leukemia, <u>BCR/ABL-positive</u>
    Chronic myelogenous leukemia, Philadelphia chromosome (Ph1) positive
    Chronic myelogenous leukemia, t(9;22) (q34;q11)
    Chronic myelogenous leukemia with crisis of blast cells
    Excludes 1: atypical chronic myeloid leukemia BCR/ABL-negative (C92.2-)
                chronic myelomonocytic leukemia (C93.1-)
                chronic myeloproliferative disease (D47.1)

    C92.10 Chronic myeloid leukemia, BCR/ABL-positive, <u>not</u> having achieved remission
        Chronic myeloid leukemia, BCR/ABL-positive with failed remission
        Chronic myeloid leukemia, BCR/ABL-positive NOS

    C92.11 Chronic myeloid leukemia, BCR/ABL-positive, <u>in remission</u>

    C92.12 Chronic myeloid leukemia, BCR/ABL-positive, <u>in relapse</u>

C92.2- <u>Atypical chronic</u> myeloid leukemia, <u>BCR/ABL-negative</u>

    C92.20 Atypical chronic myeloid leukemia, BCR/ABL-negative, <u>not</u> having achieved remission
        Atypical chronic myeloid leukemia, BCR/ABL-negative with failed remission
        Atypical chronic myeloid leukemia, BCR/ABL-negative NOS

    C92.21 Atypical chronic myeloid leukemia, BCR/ABL-negative, <u>in remission</u>

    C92.22 Atypical chronic myeloid leukemia, BCR/ABL-negative, <u>in relapse</u>

C92.3- <u>Myeloid sarcoma</u>
    A malignant tumor of immature myeloid cells
    Chloroma
    Granulocytic sarcoma

    C92.30 Myeloid sarcoma, <u>not</u> having achieved remission
        Myeloid sarcoma with failed remission
        Myeloid sarcoma NOS

    C92.31 Myeloid sarcoma, <u>in remission</u>

    C92.32 Myeloid sarcoma, <u>in relapse</u>

C92.4- <u>Acute promyelocytic</u> leukemia
    AML M3
    AML Me with t(15;17) and variants

    C92.40 Acute promyelocytic leukemia, <u>not</u> having achieved remission
        Acute promyelocytic leukemia with failed remission
        Acute promyelocytic leukemia NOS

    C92.41 Acute promyelocytic leukemia, <u>in remission</u>

    C92.42 Acute promyelocytic leukemia, <u>in relapse</u>

C84 – C92

Excludes 1: = NOT CODED HERE! (Do not code both)   **369**   *Excludes ❷:* = Not Included Here

C92.5- <u>Acute myelomonocytic</u> leukemia
AML M4
AML M4 Eo with inv(16) or t(16;16)

C92.50 Acute myelomonocytic leukemia, <u>not</u> having achieved remission
Acute myelomonocytic leukemia with failed remission
Acute myelomonocytic leukemia NOS

C92.51 Acute myelomonocytic leukemia, <u>in remission</u>

C92.52 Acute myelomonocytic leukemia, <u>in relapse</u>

C92.6- <u>Acute myeloid</u> leukemia <u>with 11q23-abnormality</u>
Acute myeloid leukemia with variation of MLL-gene

C92.60 Acute myeloid leukemia with 11q23-abnormality <u>not</u> having achieved remission
Acute myeloid leukemia with 11q23-abnormality with failed remission
Acute myeloid leukemia with 11q23-abnormality NOS

C92.61 Acute myeloid leukemia with 11q23-abnormality <u>in remission</u>

C92.62 Acute myeloid leukemia with 11q23-abnormality <u>in relapse</u>

C92.A- <u>Acute myeloid</u> leukemia <u>with multilineage dysplasia</u>
Acute myeloid leukemia with dysplasia of remaining hematopoesis and/or myelodysplastic disease in its history

C92.A0 Acute myeloid leukemia with multilineage dysplasia, <u>not</u> having achieved remission
Acute myeloid leukemia with multilineage dysplasia with failed remission
Acute myeloid leukemia with multilineage dysplasia NOS

C92.A1 Acute myeloid leukemia with multilineage dysplasia, <u>in remission</u>

C92.A2 Acute myeloid leukemia with multilineage dysplasia, <u>in relapse</u>

C92.Z- <u>Other</u> myeloid leukemia

C92.Z0 Other myeloid leukemia <u>not</u> having achieved remission
Myeloid leukemia NEC with failed remission
Myeloid leukemia NEC

C92.Z1 Other myeloid leukemia, <u>in remission</u>

C92.Z2 Other myeloid leukemia, <u>in relapse</u>

C92.9- Myeloid leukemia, <u>unspecified</u>

C92.90 Myeloid leukemia, unspecified, <u>not</u> having achieved remission
Myeloid leukemia, unspecified with failed remission
Myeloid leukemia, unspecified NOS

C92.91 Myeloid leukemia, unspecified <u>in remission</u>

C92.92 Myeloid leukemia, unspecified <u>in relapse</u>

C93- <u>Monocytic</u> leukemia
Includes: Monocytoid leukemia
Excludes 1: personal history of leukemia (Z85.6)

C93.0- <u>Acute monoblastic/monocytic</u> leukemia
AML M5
AML M5a
AML M5b

C93.00 Acute monoblastic/monocytic leukemia, <u>not</u> having achieved remission
Acute monoblastic/monocytic leukemia with failed remission
Acute monoblastic/monocytic leukemia NOS

C93.01 Acute monoblastic/monocytic leukemia, <u>in remission</u>

C93.02 Acute monoblastic/monocytic leukemia, <u>in relapse</u>

C93.1- <u>Chronic myelomonocytic</u> leukemia
Chronic monocytic leukemia
CMML-1
CMML-2
CMML with eosinophilia

C93.10 Chronic myelomonocytic leukemia <u>not</u> having achieved remission
Chronic myelomonocytic leukemia with failed remission
Chronic myelomonocytic leukemia NOS

C93.11 Chronic myelomonocytic leukemia, <u>in remission</u>

C93.12 Chronic myelomonocytic leukemia, <u>in relapse</u>

C93.3- <u>Juvenile myelomonocytic</u> leukemia

C93.30 Juvenile myelomonocytic leukemia, <u>not</u> having achieved remission
Juvenile myelomonocytic leukemia with failed remission
Juvenile myelomonocytic leukemia NOS

C93.31 Juvenile myelomonocytic leukemia, <u>in remission</u>

C93.32 Juvenile myelomonocytic leukemia, <u>in relapse</u>

C93.Z- <u>Other monocytic</u> leukemia

C93.Z0 Other monocytic leukemia, <u>not</u> having achieved remission
Other monocytic leukemia NOS

C93.Z1 Other monocytic leukemia, <u>in remission</u>

C93.Z2 Other monocytic leukemia, <u>in relapse</u>

C93.9- <u>Monocytic</u> leukemia, <u>unspecified</u>

C93.90 Monocytic leukemia, unspecified, <u>not</u> having achieved remission
Monocytic leukemia, unspecified with failed remission
Monocytic leukemia, unspecified NOS

C93.91 Monocytic leukemia, unspecified <u>in remission</u>

C93.92 Monocytic leukemia, unspecified <u>in relapse</u>

C94- **Other leukemias of specified cell type**
Excludes 1: leukemic reticuloendotheliosis (C91.4-)
myelodysplastic syndromes (D46.-)
personal history of leukemia (Z85.6)
plasma cell leukemia (C90.1-)

C94.0- <u>Acute erythroid</u> leukemia
Acute myeloid leukemia M6(a)(b)
Erythroleukemia

C94.00 Acute erythroid leukemia, <u>not</u> having achieved remission
Acute erythroid leukemia with failed remission
Acute erythroid leukemia NOS

C94.01 Acute erythroid leukemia, <u>in remission</u>

C94.02 Acute erythroid leukemia, <u>in relapse</u>

C94.2- <u>Acute megakaryoblastic</u> leukemia
Acute myeloid leukemia M7
Acute megakaryocytic leukemia

C94.20 Acute megakaryoblastic leukemia <u>not</u> having achieved remission
Acute megakaryoblastic leukemia with failed remission
Acute megakaryoblastic leukemia NOS

C94.21 Acute megakaryoblastic leukemia, <u>in remission</u>

C94.22 Acute megakaryoblastic leukemia, <u>in relapse</u>

C94.3- <u>Mast cell</u> leukemia

C94.30 Mast cell leukemia <u>not</u> having achieved remission
Mast cell leukemia with failed remission
Mast cell leukemia NOS

C94.31 Mast cell leukemia, <u>in remission</u>

C94.32 Mast cell leukemia, <u>in relapse</u>

C94.4- <u>Acute panmyelosis</u> with myelofibrosis
Acute myelofibrosis
Excludes 1: myelofibrosis NOS (D75.81)
secondary myelofibrosis NOS (D75.81)

C94.40 Acute panmyelosis with myelofibrosis <u>not</u> having achieved remission
Acute myelofibrosis NOS
Acute panmyelosis with myelofibrosis with failed remission
Acute panmyelosis NOS

C94.41 Acute panmyelosis with myelofibrosis, <u>in remission</u>

C94.42 Acute panmyelosis with myelofibrosis, <u>in relapse</u>

C94.6 Myelodysplastic disease, not classified
Myeloproliferative disease, not classified

C94.8- <u>Other specified</u> leukemias
Aggressive NK-cell leukemia
Acute basophilic leukemia

C94.80 Other specified leukemias <u>not</u> having achieved remission
Other specified leukemia with failed remission
Other specified leukemias NOS

C94.81 Other specified leukemias, <u>in remission</u>

C94.82 Other specified leukemias, <u>in relapse</u>

C95- **Leukemia of <u>unspecified cell type</u>**
Excludes 1: personal history of leukemia (Z85.6)

C95.0- <u>Acute</u> leukemia of unspecified cell type
Acute bilineal leukemia
Acute mixed lineage leukemia
Biphenotypic acute leukemia
Stem cell leukemia of unclear lineage
Excludes 1: acute exacerbation of unspecified chronic leukemia (C95.10)

C95.00 Acute leukemia of unspecified cell type <u>not</u> having achieved remission
Acute leukemia of unspecified cell type with failed remission
Acute leukemia NOS

C95.01 Acute leukemia of unspecified cell type, <u>in remission</u>

C95.02 Acute leukemia of unspecified cell type, <u>in relapse</u>

C95.1- <u>Chronic</u> leukemia of unspecified cell type

C95.10 Chronic leukemia of unspecified cell type <u>not</u> having achieved remission
Chronic leukemia of unspecified cell type with failed remission
Chronic leukemia NOS

C95.11 Chronic leukemia of unspecified cell type, <u>in remission</u>

C95.12 Chronic leukemia of unspecified cell type, <u>in relapse</u>

Excludes 1: = NOT CODED HERE! (Do not code both)   370   *Excludes ❷:* = Not Included Here

C92 - D03

C95.9- Leukemia, <u>unspecified</u>
    C95.90 Leukemia, unspecified <u>not</u> having achieved remission
        Leukemia, unspecified with failed remission
        Leukemia NOS
    C95.91 Leukemia, unspecified, <u>in remission</u>
    C95.92 Leukemia, unspecified, <u>in relapse</u>

C96- Other and unspecified malignant neoplasms of lymphoid, hematopoietic and related tissue
    Excludes 1: personal history of other malignant neoplasms of lymphoid, hematopoietic and related tissues (Z85.79)

C96.0 Multifocal and <u>multisystemic</u> (disseminated) Langerhans-cell histiocytosis
    Histiocytosis X, multisystemic
    Letterer-Siwe disease
    Excludes 1: adult pulmonary Langerhans-cell histiocytosis (J84.82)
           multifocal and unisystemic Langerhans-cell histiocytosis (C96.5)
           unifocal Langerhans-cell histiocytosis (C96.6)

C96.2 Malignant <u>mast cell</u> tumor
    Aggressive systemic mastocytosis
    Mast cell sarcoma
    Excludes 1: indolent mastocytosis (D47.0)
           mast cell leukemia (C94.30)
           mastocytosis (congenital) (cutaneous) (Q82.2)

C96.4 Sarcoma of <u>dendritic cells</u> (accessory cells)
    Follicular dendritic cell sarcoma
    Interdigitating dendritic cell sarcoma
    Langerhans cell sarcoma

C96.5 Multifocal and <u>unisystemic</u> Langerhans-cell histiocytosis
    Hand-Schüller-Christian disease
    Histiocytosis X, multifocal
    Excludes 1: multifocal and multisystemic (disseminated) Langerhans-cell histiocytosis (C96.0)
           unifocal Langerhans-cell histiocytosis (C96.6)

C96.6 <u>Unifocal</u> Langerhans-cell histiocytosis
    Eosinophilic granuloma
    Histiocytosis X, unifocal
    Histiocytosis X NOS
    Langerhans-cell histiocytosis NOS
    Excludes 1: multifocal and multisysemic (disseminated) Langerhans-cell histiocytosis (C96.0)
           multifocal and unisystemic Langerhans-cell histiocytosis (C96.5)

C96.A Histiocytic sarcoma
    Malignant histiocytosis

C96.Z Other specified malignant neoplasms of lymphoid, hematopoietic and related tissue

C96.9 Malignant neoplasm of lymphoid, hematopoietic and related tissue, unspecified

In situ neoplasms (D00-D09)

Includes: Bowen's disease
           Erythroplasia
           Grade III intraepithelial neoplasia
           Queyrat's erythroplasia

D00- <u>Carcinoma in situ</u> of oral cavity, esophagus and stomach
    Excludes 1: melanoma in situ (D03.-)

    D00.0- Carcinoma in situ of <u>lip, oral cavity and pharynx</u>
        Use additional code to identify:
        Exposure to environmental tobacco smoke (Z77.22)
        Exposure to tobacco smoke in the perinatal period (P96.81)
        History of tobacco use (Z87.891)
        Occupational exposure to environmental tobacco smoke (Z57.31)
        Tobacco dependence (F17.-)
        Tobacco use (Z72.0)
        Excludes 1: carcinoma in situ of aryepiglottic fold or interarytenoid fold, laryngeal aspect (D02.0)
           carcinoma in situ of epiglottis NOS (D02.0)
           carcinoma in situ of epiglottis suprahyoid portion (D02.0)
           carcinoma in situ of skin of lip (D03.0, D04.0)

      D00.00 Carcinoma in situ of oral cavity, unspecified site
      D00.01 Carcinoma in situ of <u>labial mucosa and vermilion border</u>
      D00.02 Carcinoma in situ of <u>buccal</u> mucosa
      D00.03 Carcinoma in situ of <u>gingiva</u> and edentulous alveolar ridge
      D00.04 Carcinoma in situ of <u>soft</u> palate
      D00.05 Carcinoma in situ of <u>hard</u> palate
      D00.06 Carcinoma in situ of <u>floor</u> of mouth
      D00.07 Carcinoma in situ of <u>tongue</u>

      D00.08 Carcinoma in situ of <u>pharynx</u>
        Carcinoma in situ of aryepiglottic fold NOS
        Carcinoma in situ of hypopharyngeal aspect of aryepiglottic fold
        Carcinoma in situ of marginal zone of aryepiglottic fold

    D00.1 Carcinoma in situ of <u>esophagus</u>
    D00.2 Carcinoma in situ of <u>stomach</u>

D01- <u>Carcinoma in situ</u> of other and unspecified digestive organs
    Excludes 1: melanoma in situ (D03.-)

    D01.0 Carcinoma in situ of <u>colon</u>
        Excludes 1: carcinoma in situ of rectosigmoid junction (D01.1)
    D01.1 Carcinoma in situ of <u>rectosigmoid</u> junction
    D01.2 Carcinoma in situ of <u>rectum</u>
    D01.3 Carcinoma in situ of <u>anus and anal canal</u>
        Excludes 1: carcinoma in situ of anal margin (D04.5)
           carcinoma in situ of anal skin (D04.5)
           carcinoma in situ of perianal skin (D04.5)

    D01.4- Carcinoma in situ of other and unspecified parts of intestine
        Excludes 1: carcinoma in situ of ampulla of Vater (D01.5)
      D01.40 Carcinoma in situ of unspecified part of intestine
      D01.49 Carcinoma in situ of other parts of intestine

    D01.5 Carcinoma in situ of <u>liver, gallbladder and bile ducts</u>
        Carcinoma in situ of ampulla of Vater
    D01.7 Carcinoma in situ of other specified digestive organs
        Carcinoma in situ of pancreas
    D01.9 Carcinoma in situ of digestive organ, unspecified

D02- <u>Carcinoma in situ</u> of middle ear and respiratory system
    Use additional code to identify:
    Exposure to environmental tobacco smoke (Z77.22)
    Exposure to tobacco smoke in the perinatal period (P96.81)
    History of tobacco use (Z87.891)
    Occupational exposure to environmental tobacco smoke (Z57.31)
    Tobacco dependence (F17.-)
    Tobacco use (Z72.0)
    Excludes 1: melanoma in situ (D03.-)

    D02.0 Carcinoma in situ of <u>larynx</u>
        Carcinoma in situ of aryepiglottic fold or interarytenoid fold, laryngeal aspect
        Carcinoma in situ of epiglottis (suprahyoid portion)
        Excludes 1: carcinoma in situ of aryepiglottic fold or interarytenoid fold NOS (D00.08)
           carcinoma in situ of hypopharyngeal aspect (D00.08)
           carcinoma in situ of marginal zone (D00.08)

    D02.1 Carcinoma in situ of <u>trachea</u>
    D02.2- Carcinoma in situ of <u>bronchus and lung</u>
      D02.20 Carcinoma in situ of unspecified bronchus and lung
      D02.21 Carcinoma in situ of <u>right</u> bronchus and lung
      D02.22 Carcinoma in situ of <u>left</u> bronchus and lung
    D02.3 Carcinoma in situ of other parts of respiratory system
        Carcinoma in situ of accessory sinuses
        Carcinoma in situ of middle ear
        Carcinoma in situ of nasal cavities
        Excludes 1: carcinoma in situ of ear (external) (skin) (D04.2-)
           carcinoma in situ of nose NOS (D09.8)
           carcinoma in situ of skin of nose (D04.3)

    D02.4 Carcinoma in situ of respiratory system, unspecified

D03- <u>Melanoma in situ</u>
    D03.0 Melanoma in situ of <u>lip</u>
    D03.1- Melanoma in situ of <u>eyelid, including canthus</u>
      D03.10 Melanoma in situ of unspecified eyelid, including canthus
      D03.11 Melanoma in situ of <u>right</u> eyelid, including canthus
      D03.12 Melanoma in situ of <u>left</u> eyelid, including canthus
    D03.2- Melanoma in situ of ear and external auricular canal
      D03.20 Melanoma in situ of unspecified <u>ear and external auricular canal</u>
      D03.21 Melanoma in situ of <u>right</u> ear and external auricular canal
      D03.22 Melanoma in situ of <u>left</u> ear and external auricular canal
    D03.3- Melanoma in situ of other and unspecified parts of face
      D03.30 Melanoma in situ of unspecified part of face
      D03.39 Melanoma in situ of other parts of face
    D03.4 Melanoma in situ of <u>scalp and neck</u>
    D03.5- Melanoma in situ of trunk
      D03.51 Melanoma in situ of <u>anal skin</u>
        Melanoma in situ of anal margin
        Melanoma in situ of perianal skin
      D03.52 Melanoma in situ of <u>breast</u> (skin) (soft tissue)
      D03.59 Melanoma in situ of other part of trunk

C
9
2
-
D
0
3

D03.6- Melanoma in situ of <u>upper limb</u>, including shoulder

  D03.60 Melanoma in situ of unspecified upper limb, including shoulder

  D03.61 Melanoma in situ of <u>right</u> upper limb, including shoulder

  D03.62 Melanoma in situ of <u>left</u> upper limb, including shoulder

D03.7- Melanoma in situ of <u>lower limb</u>, including hip

  D03.70 Melanoma in situ of unspecified lower limb, including hip

  D03.71 Melanoma in situ of <u>right</u> lower limb, including hip

  D03.72 Melanoma in situ of <u>left</u> lower limb, including hip

D03.8 Melanoma in situ of other sites

  Melanoma in situ of scrotum

  Excludes 1: carcinoma in situ of scrotum (D07.61)

D03.9 Melanoma in situ, unspecified

D04- <u>Carcinoma in situ</u> of <u>skin</u>

  Excludes 1: erythroplasia of Queyrat (penis) NOS (D07.4)
           melanoma in situ (D03.-)

D04.0 Carcinoma in situ of <u>skin</u> of <u>lip</u>

  Excludes 1: carcinoma in situ of vermilion border of lip (D00.01)

D04.1- Carcinoma in situ of <u>skin</u> of <u>eyelid, including canthus</u>

  D04.10 Carcinoma in situ of skin of unspecified eyelid, including canthus

  D04.11 Carcinoma in situ of skin of <u>right</u> eyelid, including canthus

  D04.12 Carcinoma in situ of skin of <u>left</u> eyelid, including canthus

D04.2- Carcinoma in situ of <u>skin</u> of <u>ear and external auricular canal</u>

  D04.20 Carcinoma in situ of skin of unspecified ear and external auricular canal

  D04.21 Carcinoma in situ of skin of <u>right</u> ear and external auricular canal

  D04.22 Carcinoma in situ of skin of <u>left</u> ear and external auricular canal

D04.3- Carcinoma in situ of <u>skin</u> of other and unspecified parts of face

  D04.30 Carcinoma in situ of skin of unspecified part of face

  D04.39 Carcinoma in situ of skin of other parts of face

D04.4 Carcinoma in situ of <u>skin</u> of <u>scalp and neck</u>

D04.5 Carcinoma in situ of <u>skin</u> of <u>trunk</u>

  Carcinoma in situ of anal margin

  Carcinoma in situ of anal skin

  Carcinoma in situ of perianal skin

  Carcinoma in situ of skin of breast

  Excludes 1: carcinoma in situ of anus NOS (D01.3)
           carcinoma in situ of scrotum (D07.61)
           carcinoma in situ of skin of genital organs (D07.-)

D04.6- Carcinoma in situ of <u>skin</u> of <u>upper limb</u>, including shoulder

  D04.60 Carcinoma in situ of skin of unspecified upper limb, including shoulder

  D04.61 Carcinoma in situ of skin of <u>right</u> upper limb, including shoulder

  D04.62 Carcinoma in situ of skin of <u>left</u> upper limb, including shoulder

D04.7- Carcinoma in situ of <u>skin</u> of <u>lower limb</u>, including hip

  D04.70 Carcinoma in situ of skin of unspecified lower limb, including hip

  D04.71 Carcinoma in situ of skin of <u>right</u> lower limb, including hip

  D04.72 Carcinoma in situ of skin of <u>left</u> lower limb, including hip

D04.8 Carcinoma in situ of <u>skin</u> of other sites

D04.9 Carcinoma in situ of <u>skin</u>, unspecified

D05- <u>Carcinoma in situ</u> of breast

  Excludes 1: carcinoma in situ of skin of breast (D04.5)
           melanoma in situ of breast (skin) (D03.5)
           Paget's disease of breast or nipple (C50.-)

D05.0- <u>Lobular</u> carcinoma in situ of breast

  D05.00 Lobular carcinoma in situ of unspecified breast

  D05.01 Lobular carcinoma in situ of <u>right</u> breast

  D05.02 Lobular carcinoma in situ of <u>left</u> breast

D05.1- <u>Intraductal</u> carcinoma in situ of breast

  D05.10 Intraductal carcinoma in situ of unspecified breast

  D05.11 Intraductal carcinoma in situ of <u>right</u> breast

  D05.12 Intraductal carcinoma in situ of <u>left</u> breast

D05.8- <u>Other specified type</u> of carcinoma in situ of breast

  D05.80 Other specified type of carcinoma in situ of unspecified breast

  D05.81 Other specified type of carcinoma in situ of <u>right</u> breast

  D05.82 Other specified type of carcinoma in situ of <u>left</u> breast

D05.9- <u>Unspecified</u> type of carcinoma in situ of breast

  D05.90 Unspecified type of carcinoma in situ of unspecified breast

  D05.91 Unspecified type of carcinoma in situ of <u>right</u> breast

  D05.92 Unspecified type of carcinoma in situ of <u>left</u> breast

D06- <u>Carcinoma in situ</u> of cervix uteri

  Includes: Cervical adenocarcinoma in situ
          Cervical intraepithelial glandular neoplasia
          Cervical intraepithelial neoplasia III [CIN III]
          Severe dysplasia of cervix uteri

  Excludes 1: cervical intraepithelial neoplasia II [CIN II] (N87.1)
           cytologic evidence of malignancy of cervix without histologic confirmation (R87.614)
           high grade squamous intraepithelial lesion (HGSIL) of cervix (R87.613)
           melanoma in situ of cervix (D03.5)
           moderate cervical dysplasia (N87.1)

D06.0 Carcinoma in situ of <u>endocervix</u>

D06.1 Carcinoma in situ of <u>exocervix</u>

D06.7 Carcinoma in situ of other parts of cervix

D06.9 Carcinoma in situ of cervix, unspecified

D07- <u>Carcinoma in situ</u> of other and unspecified genital organs

  Excludes 1: melanoma in situ of trunk (D03.5)

D07.0 Carcinoma in situ of <u>endometrium</u>

D07.1 Carcinoma in situ of <u>vulva</u>

  Severe dysplasia of vulva

  Vulvar intraepithelial neoplasia III [VIN III]

  Excludes 1: moderate dysplasia of vulva (N90.1)
           vulvar intraepithelial neoplasia II [VIN II] (N90.1)

D07.2 Carcinoma in situ of <u>vagina</u>

  Severe dysplasia of vagina

  Vaginal intraepithelial neoplasia III [VAIN III]

  Excludes 1: moderate dysplasia of vagina (N89.1)
           vaginal intraepithelial neoplasia II [VIN II] (N89.1)

D07.3- Carcinoma in situ of other and unspecified female genital organs

  D07.30 Carcinoma in situ of unspecified female genital organs

  D07.39 Carcinoma in situ of other female genital organs

D07.4 Carcinoma in situ of <u>penis</u>

  Erythroplasia of Queyrat NOS

D07.5 Carcinoma in situ of <u>prostate</u>

  Prostatic intraepithelial neoplasia III (PIN III)

  Severe dysplasia of prostate

  Excludes 1: dysplasia (mild) (moderate) of prostate (N42.3)

D07.6- Carcinoma in situ of other and unspecified male genital organs

  D07.60 Carcinoma in situ of unspecified male genital organs

  D07.61 Carcinoma in situ of <u>scrotum</u>

  D07.69 Carcinoma in situ of other male genital organs

D09- <u>Carcinoma in situ</u> of other and unspecified sites

  Excludes 1: melanoma in situ (D03.-)

D09.0 Carcinoma in situ of <u>bladder</u>

D09.1- Carcinoma in situ of other and unspecified urinary organs

  D09.10 Carcinoma in situ of unspecified urinary organ

  D09.19 Carcinoma in situ of other urinary organs

D09.2- Carcinoma in situ of <u>eye</u>

  Excludes 1: carcinoma in situ of skin of eyelid (D04.1-)

  D09.20 Carcinoma in situ of unspecified eye

  D09.21 Carcinoma in situ of <u>right</u> eye

  D09.22 Carcinoma in situ of <u>left</u> eye

D09.3 Carcinoma in situ of <u>thyroid</u> and other endocrine glands

  Excludes 1: carcinoma in situ of endocrine pancreas (D01.7)
           carcinoma in situ of ovary (D07.39)
           carcinoma in situ of testis (D07.69)

D09.8 Carcinoma in situ of other specified sites

D09.9 Carcinoma in situ, unspecified

D 0 3 – D 1 6

Benign neoplasms, except benign neuroendocrine tumors (D10-D36)

D10- Benign neoplasm of mouth and pharynx

D10.0 **Benign neoplasm of lip**
Benign neoplasm of lip (frenulum) (inner aspect) (mucosa) (vermilion border)
Excludes 1: benign neoplasm of skin of lip (D22.0, D23.0)

D10.1 **Benign neoplasm of tongue**
Benign neoplasm of lingual tonsil

D10.2 **Benign neoplasm of floor of mouth**

D10.3- **Other and unspecified parts of mouth**

D10.30 Benign neoplasm of unspecified part of mouth

D10.39 Benign neoplasm of other parts of mouth
Benign neoplasm of minor salivary gland NOS
Excludes 1: benign odontogenic neoplasms (D16.4-D16.5)
benign neoplasm of mucosa of lip (D10.0)
benign neoplasm of nasopharyngeal surface of soft palate (D10.6)

D10.4 **Benign neoplasm of tonsil**
Benign neoplasm of tonsil (faucial) (palatine)
Excludes 1: benign neoplasm of lingual tonsil (D10.1)
benign neoplasm of pharyngeal tonsil (D10.6)
benign neoplasm of tonsillar fossa (D10.5)
benign neoplasm of tonsillar pillars (D10.5)

D10.5 **Benign neoplasm of other parts of oropharynx**
Benign neoplasm of epiglottis, anterior aspect
Benign neoplasm of tonsillar fossa
Benign neoplasm of tonsillar pillars
Benign neoplasm of vallecula
Excludes 1: benign neoplasm of epiglottis NOS (D14.1)
benign neoplasm of epiglottis, suprahyoid portion (D14.1)

D10.6 **Benign neoplasm of nasopharynx**
Benign neoplasm of pharyngeal tonsil
Benign neoplasm of posterior margin of septum and choanae

D10.7 **Benign neoplasm of hypopharynx**

D10.9 **Benign neoplasm of pharynx, unspecified**

D11- Benign neoplasm of major salivary glands
Excludes 1: benign neoplasms of specified minor salivary glands which are classified according to their anatomic allocation
benign neoplasms of minor salivary glands NOS (D10.39)

D11.0 **Benign neoplasm of parotid gland**

D11.7 **Benign neoplasm of other major salivary glands**
Benign neoplasm of sublingual salivary gland
Benign neoplasm of submandibular salivary gland

D11.9 **Benign neoplasm of major salivary gland, unspecified**

D12- Benign neoplasm of colon, rectum, anus and anal canal
Excludes 1: benign carcinoid tumors of the large intestine, and rectum (D3A.02-)

D12.0 **Benign neoplasm of cecum**
Benign neoplasm of ileocecal valve

D12.1 **Benign neoplasm of appendix**
Excludes 1: benign carcinoid tumor of the appendix (D3A.020)

D12.2 **Benign neoplasm of ascending colon**

D12.3 **Benign neoplasm of transverse colon**
Benign neoplasm of hepatic flexure
Benign neoplasm of splenic flexure

D12.4 **Benign neoplasm of descending colon**

D12.5 **Benign neoplasm of sigmoid colon**

D12.6 **Benign neoplasm of colon, unspecified**
Adenomatosis of colon
Benign neoplasm of large intestine NOS
Polyposis (hereditary) of colon
Excludes 1: inflammatory polyp of colon (K51.4-)
polyp of colon NOS (K63.5)

D12.7 **Benign neoplasm of rectosigmoid junction**

D12.8 **Benign neoplasm of rectum**
Excludes 1: benign carcinoid tumor of the rectum (D3A.026)

D12.9 **Benign neoplasm of anus and anal canal**
Benign neoplasm of anus NOS
Excludes 1: benign neoplasm of anal margin (D22.5, D23.5)
benign neoplasm of anal skin (D22.5, D23.5)
benign neoplasm of perianal skin (D22.5, D23.5)

D13- Benign neoplasm of other and ill-defined parts of digestive system
Excludes 1: benign stromal tumors of digestive system (D21.4)

D13.0 **Benign neoplasm of esophagus**

D13.1 **Benign neoplasm of stomach**
Excludes 1: benign carcinoid tumor of the stomach (D3A.092)

D13.2 **Benign neoplasm of duodenum**
Excludes 1: benign carcinoid tumor of the duodenum (D3A.010)

D13.3- **Benign neoplasm of other and unspecified parts of small intestine**
Excludes 1: benign carcinoid tumors of the small intestine(D3A.01-)
benign neoplasm of ileocecal valve (D12.0)

D13.30 Benign neoplasm of unspecified part of small intestine

D13.39 Benign neoplasm of other parts of small intestine

D13.4 **Benign neoplasm of liver**
Benign neoplasm of intrahepatic bile ducts

D13.5 **Benign neoplasm of extrahepatic bile ducts**

D13.6 **Benign neoplasm of pancreas**
Excludes 1: benign neoplasm of endocrine pancreas (D13.7)

D13.7 **Benign neoplasm of endocrine pancreas**
Islet cell tumor
Benign neoplasm of islets of Langerhans
Use additional code to identify any functional activity.

D13.9 **Benign neoplasm of ill-defined sites within the digestive system**
Benign neoplasm of digestive system NOS
Benign neoplasm of intestine NOS
Benign neoplasm of spleen

D14- Benign neoplasm of middle ear and respiratory system

D14.0 **Benign neoplasm of middle ear, nasal cavity and accessory sinuses**
Benign neoplasm of cartilage of nose
Excludes 1: benign neoplasm of auricular canal (external) (D22.2-, D23.2-)
benign neoplasm of bone of ear (D16.4)
benign neoplasm of bone of nose (D16.4)
benign neoplasm of cartilage of ear (D21.0)
benign neoplasm of ear (external)(skin) (D22.2-, D23.2-)
benign neoplasm of nose NOS (D36.7)
benign neoplasm of skin of nose (D22.39, D23.39)
benign neoplasm of olfactory bulb (D33.3)
benign neoplasm of posterior margin of septum and choanae (D10.6)
polyp of accessory sinus (J33.8)
polyp of ear (middle) (H74.4)
polyp of nasal (cavity) (J33.-)

D14.1 **Benign neoplasm of larynx**
Adenomatous polyp of larynx
Benign neoplasm of epiglottis (suprahyoid portion)
Excludes 1: benign neoplasm of epiglottis, anterior aspect (D10.5)
polyp (nonadenomatous) of vocal cord or larynx (J38.1)

D14.2 **Benign neoplasm of trachea**

D14.3- **Benign neoplasm of bronchus and lung**
Excludes 1: benign carcinoid tumor of the bronchus and lung (D3A.090)

D14.30 Benign neoplasm of unspecified bronchus and lung

D14.31 Benign neoplasm of right bronchus and lung

D14.32 Benign neoplasm of left bronchus and lung

D14.4 **Benign neoplasm of respiratory system, unspecified**

D15- Benign neoplasm of other and unspecified intrathoracic organs
Excludes 1: benign neoplasm of mesothelial tissue (D19.-)

D15.0 **Benign neoplasm of thymus**
Excludes 1: benign carcinoid tumor of the thymus (D3A.091)

D15.1 **Benign neoplasm of heart**
Excludes 1: benign neoplasm of great vessels (D21.3)

D15.2 **Benign neoplasm of mediastinum**

D15.7 **Benign neoplasm of other specified intrathoracic organs**

D15.9 **Benign neoplasm of intrathoracic organ, unspecified**

D16- Benign neoplasm of bone and articular cartilage
Excludes 1: benign neoplasm of connective tissue of ear (D21.0)
benign neoplasm of connective tissue of eyelid (D21.0)
benign neoplasm of connective tissue of larynx (D14.1)
benign neoplasm of connective tissue of nose (D14.0)
benign neoplasm of synovia (D21.-)

D16.0- **Benign neoplasm of scapula and long bones of upper limb**

D16.00 Benign neoplasm of scapula and long bones of unspecified upper limb

D16.01 Benign neoplasm of scapula and long bones of right upper limb

D16.02 Benign neoplasm of scapula and long bones of left upper limb

D
0
3
|
D
1
6

Excludes 1: = NOT CODED HERE! (Do not code both)

Excludes❷: = Not Included Here

D16.1- Benign neoplasm of <u>short bones of upper limb</u>
    D16.10 Benign neoplasm of short bones of unspecified upper limb
    D16.11 Benign neoplasm of short bones of <u>right</u> upper limb
    D16.12 Benign neoplasm of short bones of <u>left</u> upper limb
D16.2- Benign neoplasm of <u>long bones of lower limb</u>
    D16.20 Benign neoplasm of long bones of unspecified lower limb
    D16.21 Benign neoplasm of long bones of <u>right</u> lower limb
    D16.22 Benign neoplasm of long bones of <u>left</u> lower limb
D16.3- Benign neoplasm of <u>short bones of lower limb</u>
    D16.30 Benign neoplasm of short bones of unspecified lower limb
    D16.31 Benign neoplasm of short bones of <u>right</u> lower limb
    D16.32 Benign neoplasm of short bones of <u>left</u> lower limb
D16.4 Benign neoplasm of <u>bones of skull and face</u>
    Benign neoplasm of maxilla (superior)
    Benign neoplasm of orbital bone
    Keratocyst of maxilla
    Keratocystic odontogenic tumor of maxilla
    Excludes 1: benign neoplasm of lower jaw bone (D16.5)
D16.5 Benign neoplasm of <u>lower jaw</u> bone
    Keratocyst of mandible
    Keratocystic odontogenic tumor of mandible
D16.6 Benign neoplasm of <u>vertebral</u> column
    Excludes 1: benign neoplasm of sacrum and coccyx (D16.8)
D16.7 Benign neoplasm of <u>ribs, sternum and clavicle</u>
D16.8 Benign neoplasm of <u>pelvic bones, sacrum and coccyx</u>
D16.9 Benign neoplasm of bone and articular cartilage, unspecified

D17- <u>Benign lipomatous</u> neoplasm
D17.0 Benign lipomatous neoplasm of <u>skin</u> and subcutaneous tissue of <u>head, face and neck</u>
D17.1 Benign lipomatous neoplasm of <u>skin</u> and subcutaneous tissue of <u>trunk</u>
D17.2- Benign lipomatous neoplasm of <u>skin</u> and subcutaneous tissue of <u>limb</u>
    D17.20 Benign lipomatous neoplasm of skin and subcutaneous tissue of unspecified limb
    D17.21 Benign lipomatous neoplasm of skin and subcutaneous tissue of <u>right</u> arm
    D17.22 Benign lipomatous neoplasm of skin and subcutaneous tissue of <u>left</u> arm
    D17.23 Benign lipomatous neoplasm of skin and subcutaneous tissue of <u>right</u> leg
    D17.24 Benign lipomatous neoplasm of skin and subcutaneous tissue of <u>left</u> leg
D17.3- Benign lipomatous neoplasm of <u>skin</u> and subcutaneous tissue of other and unspecified sites
    D17.30 Benign lipomatous neoplasm of skin and subcutaneous tissue of unspecified sites
    D17.39 Benign lipomatous neoplasm of skin and subcutaneous tissue of other sites
D17.4 Benign lipomatous neoplasm of <u>intrathoracic organs</u>
D17.5 Benign lipomatous neoplasm of <u>intra-abdominal organs</u>
    Excludes 1: benign lipomatous neoplasm of peritoneum and retroperitoneum (D17.79)
D17.6 Benign lipomatous neoplasm of <u>spermatic cord</u>
D17.7- Benign lipomatous neoplasm of other sites
    D17.71 Benign lipomatous neoplasm of <u>kidney</u>
    D17.72 Benign lipomatous neoplasm of <u>other genitourinary organ</u>
    D17.79 Benign lipomatous neoplasm of <u>other sites</u>
      Benign lipomatous neoplasm of peritoneum
      Benign lipomatous neoplasm of retroperitoneum
D17.9 Benign lipomatous neoplasm, unspecified
    Lipoma NOS

D18- Hemangioma and lymphangioma, any site
    Excludes 1: benign neoplasm of glomus jugulare (D35.6)
           blue or pigmented nevus (D22.-)
           nevus NOS (D22.-)
           vascular nevus (Q82.5)
D18.0- <u>Hemangioma</u>
    Angioma NOS
    Cavernous nevus
    D18.00 Hemangioma unspecified site
    D18.01 Hemangioma of <u>skin</u> and subcutaneous tissue
    D18.02 Hemangioma of <u>intracranial</u> structures
    D18.03 Hemangioma of <u>intra-abdominal</u> structures
    D18.09 Hemangioma of other sites
D18.1 <u>Lymphangioma</u>, any site

D19- <u>Benign neoplasm</u> of <u>mesothelial tissue</u>
    D19.0 Benign neoplasm of mesothelial tissue of <u>pleura</u>
    D19.1 Benign neoplasm of mesothelial tissue of <u>peritoneum</u>
    D19.7 Benign neoplasm of mesothelial tissue of other sites
    D19.9 Benign neoplasm of mesothelial tissue, unspecified
      Benign mesothelioma NOS
D20- <u>Benign neoplasm</u> of <u>soft tissue</u> of retroperitoneum and peritoneum
    Excludes 1: benign lipomatous neoplasm of peritoneum and retroperitoneum (D17.79)
           benign neoplasm of mesothelial tissue (D19.-)
    D20.0 Benign neoplasm of soft tissue of <u>retroperitoneum</u>
    D20.1 Benign neoplasm of soft tissue of <u>peritoneum</u>
D21- <u>Other benign neoplasms</u> of <u>connective</u> and other soft tissue
    Includes: Benign neoplasm of blood vessel
          Benign neoplasm of bursa
          Benign neoplasm of cartilage
          Benign neoplasm of fascia
          Benign neoplasm of fat
          Benign neoplasm of ligament, except uterine
          Benign neoplasm of lymphatic channel
          Benign neoplasm of muscle
          Benign neoplasm of synovia
          Benign neoplasm of tendon (sheath)
          Benign stromal tumors
    Excludes 1: benign neoplasm of articular cartilage (D16.-)
           benign neoplasm of cartilage of larynx (D14.1)
           benign neoplasm of cartilage of nose (D14.0)
           benign neoplasm of connective tissue of breast (D24.-)
           benign neoplasm of peripheral nerves and autonomic nervous system (D36.1-)
           benign neoplasm of peritoneum (D20.1)
           benign neoplasm of retroperitoneum (D20.0)
           benign neoplasm of uterine ligament, any (D28.2)
           benign neoplasm of vascular tissue (D18.-)
           hemangioma (D18.0-)
           lipomatous neoplasm (D17.-)
           lymphangioma (D18.1)
           uterine leiomyoma (D25.-)
    D21.0 Benign neoplasm of connective and other soft tissue of <u>head, face and neck</u>
      Benign neoplasm of connective tissue of ear
      Benign neoplasm of connective tissue of eyelid
      Excludes 1: benign neoplasm of connective tissue of orbit (D31.6-)
    D21.1- Benign neoplasm of connective and other soft tissue of <u>upper limb</u>, including shoulder
      D21.10 Benign neoplasm of connective and other soft tissue of unspecified upper limb, including shoulder
      D21.11 Benign neoplasm of connective and other soft tissue of <u>right</u> upper limb, including shoulder
      D21.12 Benign neoplasm of connective and other soft tissue of <u>left</u> upper limb, including shoulder
    D21.2- Benign neoplasm of connective and other soft tissue of <u>lower limb</u>, including hip
      D21.20 Benign neoplasm of connective and other soft tissue of unspecified lower limb, including hip
      D21.21 Benign neoplasm of connective and other soft tissue of <u>right</u> lower limb, including hip
      D21.22 Benign neoplasm of connective and other soft tissue of <u>left</u> lower limb, including hip
    D21.3 Benign neoplasm of connective and other soft tissue of <u>thorax</u>
      Benign neoplasm of axilla
      Benign neoplasm of diaphragm
      Benign neoplasm of great vessels
      Excludes 1: benign neoplasm of heart (D15.1)
           benign neoplasm of mediastinum (D15.2)
           benign neoplasm of thymus (D15.0)
    D21.4 Benign neoplasm of connective and other soft tissue of <u>abdomen</u>
      Benign stromal tumors of abdomen
    D21.5 Benign neoplasm of connective and other soft tissue of <u>pelvis</u>
      Excludes 1: benign neoplasm of any uterine ligament (D28.2)
           uterine leiomyoma (D25.-)
    D21.6 Benign neoplasm of connective and other soft tissue of trunk, unspecified
      Benign neoplasm of back NOS
    D21.9 Benign neoplasm of connective and other soft tissue, unspecified

D16 - D29

D22- **Melanocytic nevi**
    Includes: Atypical nevus
                   Blue hairy pigmented nevus
                   Nevus NOS

D22.0 Melanocytic nevi of <u>lip</u>

D22.1- Melanocytic nevi of <u>eyelid, including canthus</u>
    D22.10 Melanocytic nevi of unspecified eyelid, including canthus
    D22.11 Melanocytic nevi of <u>right</u> eyelid, including canthus
    D22.12 Melanocytic nevi of <u>left</u> eyelid, including canthus

D22.2- Melanocytic nevi of <u>ear and external auricular canal</u>
    D22.20 Melanocytic nevi of unspecified ear and external auricular canal
    D22.21 Melanocytic nevi of <u>right</u> ear and external auricular canal
    D22.22 Melanocytic nevi of <u>left</u> ear and external auricular canal

D22.3- Melanocytic nevi of other and unspecified parts of face
    D22.30 Melanocytic nevi of unspecified part of face
    D22.39 Melanocytic nevi of other parts of face

D22.4 Melanocytic nevi of <u>scalp and neck</u>

D22.5 Melanocytic nevi of <u>trunk</u>
    Melanocytic nevi of anal margin
    Melanocytic nevi of anal skin
    Melanocytic nevi of perianal skin
    Melanocytic nevi of skin of breast

D22.6- Melanocytic nevi of <u>upper limb</u>, including shoulder
    D22.60 Melanocytic nevi of unspecified upper limb, including shoulder
    D22.61 Melanocytic nevi of <u>right</u> upper limb, including shoulder
    D22.62 Melanocytic nevi of <u>left</u> upper limb, including shoulder

D22.7- Melanocytic nevi of <u>lower limb</u>, including hip
    D22.70 Melanocytic nevi of unspecified lower limb, including hip
    D22.71 Melanocytic nevi of <u>right</u> lower limb, including hip
    D22.72 Melanocytic nevi of <u>left</u> lower limb, including hip

D22.9 Melanocytic nevi, unspecified

D23- <u>Other benign neoplasms</u> of <u>skin</u>
    Includes: Benign neoplasm of hair follicles
                   Benign neoplasm of sebaceous glands
                   Benign neoplasm of sweat glands
    Excludes 1: benign lipomatous neoplasms of skin (D17.0-D17.3)
                  melanocytic nevi (D22.-)

D23.0 <u>Other</u> benign neoplasm of <u>skin</u> of <u>lip</u>
    Excludes 1: benign neoplasm of vermilion border of lip (D10.0)

D23.1- <u>Other</u> benign neoplasm of <u>skin</u> of <u>eyelid, including canthus</u>
    D23.10 Other benign neoplasm of skin of unspecified eyelid, including canthus
    D23.11 Other benign neoplasm of skin of <u>right</u> eyelid, including canthus
    D23.12 Other benign neoplasm of skin of <u>left</u> eyelid, including canthus

D23.2- <u>Other</u> benign neoplasm of <u>skin</u> of <u>ear and external auricular canal</u>
    D23.20 Other benign neoplasm of skin of unspecified ear and external auricular canal
    D23.21 Other benign neoplasm of skin of <u>right</u> ear and external auricular canal
    D23.22 Other benign neoplasm of skin of <u>left</u> ear and external auricular canal

D23.3- <u>Other</u> benign neoplasm of <u>skin</u> of other and unspecified parts of face
    D23.30 Other benign neoplasm of skin of unspecified part of face
    D23.39 Other benign neoplasm of skin of other parts of face

D23.4 <u>Other</u> benign neoplasm of <u>skin</u> of <u>scalp and neck</u>

D23.5 <u>Other</u> benign neoplasm of <u>skin</u> of <u>trunk</u>
    Other benign neoplasm of anal margin
    Other benign neoplasm of anal skin
    Other benign neoplasm of perianal skin
    Other benign neoplasm of skin of breast
    Excludes 1: benign neoplasm of anus NOS (D12.9)

D23.6- <u>Other</u> benign neoplasm of <u>skin</u> of <u>upper limb</u>, including shoulder
    D23.60 Other benign neoplasm of skin of unspecified upper limb, including shoulder
    D23.61 Other benign neoplasm of skin of <u>right</u> upper limb, including shoulder
    D23.62 Other benign neoplasm of skin of <u>left</u> upper limb, including shoulder

D23.7- <u>Other</u> benign neoplasm of <u>skin</u> of <u>lower limb</u>, including hip
    D23.70 Other benign neoplasm of skin of unspecified lower limb, including hip
    D23.71 Other benign neoplasm of skin of <u>right</u> lower limb, including hip
    D23.72 Other benign neoplasm of skin of <u>left</u> lower limb, including hip

D23.9 <u>Other</u> benign neoplasm of <u>skin</u>, unspecified

D24- <u>Benign neoplasm</u> of breast
    Includes: Benign neoplasm of connective tissue of breast
                   Benign neoplasm of soft parts of breast
                   Fibroadenoma of breast
    Excludes❷: adenofibrosis of breast (N60.2)
              benign cyst of breast (N60.-)
              benign mammary dysplasia (N60.-)
              benign neoplasm of skin of breast (D22.5, D23.5)
              fibrocystic disease of breast (N60.-)

D24.1 Benign neoplasm of <u>right</u> breast

D24.2 Benign neoplasm of <u>left</u> breast

D24.9 Benign neoplasm of unspecified breast

D25- <u>Leiomyoma</u> of uterus
    Includes: Uterine fibroid
                   Uterine fibromyoma
                   Uterine myoma

D25.0 <u>Submucous</u> leiomyoma of uterus

D25.1 <u>Intramural</u> leiomyoma of uterus
    Interstitial leiomyoma of uterus

D25.2 <u>Subserosal</u> leiomyoma of uterus
    Subperitoneal leiomyoma of uterus

D25.9 Leiomyoma of uterus, unspecified

D26- <u>Other</u> benign neoplasms of <u>uterus</u>
    D26.0 Other benign neoplasm of <u>cervix</u> uteri
    D26.1 Other benign neoplasm of <u>corpus</u> uteri
    D26.7 Other benign neoplasm of other parts of uterus
    D26.9 Other benign neoplasm of uterus, unspecified

D27- <u>Benign neoplasm</u> of ovary
    Use additional code to identify any functional activity.
    Excludes❷: corpus albicans cyst (N83.2)
              corpus luteum cyst (N83.1)
              endometrial cyst (N80.1)
              follicular (atretic) cyst (N83.0)
              graafian follicle cyst (N83.0)
              ovarian cyst NEC (N83.2)
              ovarian retention cyst (N83.2)

D27.0 Benign neoplasm of <u>right</u> ovary

D27.1 Benign neoplasm of <u>left</u> ovary

D27.9 Benign neoplasm of unspecified ovary

D28- <u>Benign neoplasm</u> of other and unspecified female genital organs
    Includes: Adenomatous polyp
                   Benign neoplasm of skin of female genital organs
                   Benign teratoma
    Excludes 1: epoophoron cyst (Q50.5)
              fimbrial cyst (Q50.4)
              Gartner's duct cyst (Q52.4)
              parovarian cyst (Q50.5)

D28.0 Benign neoplasm of <u>vulva</u>

D28.1 Benign neoplasm of <u>vagina</u>

D28.2 Benign neoplasm of <u>uterine tubes and ligaments</u>
    Benign neoplasm of fallopian tube
    Benign neoplasm of uterine ligament (broad) (round)

D28.7 Benign neoplasm of other specified female genital organs

D28.9 Benign neoplasm of female genital organ, unspecified

D29- <u>Benign neoplasm</u> of male genital organs
    Includes: Benign neoplasm of skin of male genital organs

D29.0 Benign neoplasm of <u>penis</u>

D29.1 Benign neoplasm of <u>prostate</u>
    Excludes 1: enlarged prostate (N40.-)

D29.2- Benign neoplasm of <u>testis</u>
    Use additional code to identify any functional activity.
    D29.20 Benign neoplasm of unspecified testis
    D29.21 Benign neoplasm of <u>right</u> testis
    D29.22 Benign neoplasm of <u>left</u> testis

D29.3- Benign neoplasm of <u>epididymis</u>
    D29.30 Benign neoplasm of unspecified epididymis
    D29.31 Benign neoplasm of <u>right</u> epididymis
    D29.32 Benign neoplasm of <u>left</u> epididymis

D29.4 Benign neoplasm of <u>scrotum</u>
    Benign neoplasm of skin of scrotum

D29.8   Benign neoplasm of other specified male genital organs
Benign neoplasm of seminal vesicle
Benign neoplasm of spermatic cord
Benign neoplasm of tunica vaginalis

D29.9   Benign neoplasm of male genital organ, unspecified

D30-   Benign neoplasm of urinary organs

D30.0-   Benign neoplasm of kidney
Excludes 1:   benign carcinoid tumor of the kidney (D3A.093)
benign neoplasm of renal calyces (D30.1-)
benign neoplasm of renal pelvis (D30.1-)

D30.00   Benign neoplasm of unspecified kidney

D30.01   Benign neoplasm of right kidney

D30.02   Benign neoplasm of left kidney

D30.1-   Benign neoplasm of renal pelvis

D30.10   Benign neoplasm of unspecified renal pelvis

D30.11   Benign neoplasm of right renal pelvis

D30.12   Benign neoplasm of left renal pelvis

D30.2-   Benign neoplasm of ureter
Excludes 1:   benign neoplasm of ureteric orifice of bladder (D30.3)

D30.20   Benign neoplasm of unspecified ureter

D30.21   Benign neoplasm of right ureter

D30.22   Benign neoplasm of left ureter

D30.3   Benign neoplasm of bladder
Benign neoplasm of ureteric orifice of bladder
Benign neoplasm of urethral orifice of bladder

D30.4   Benign neoplasm of urethra
Excludes 1:   benign neoplasm of urethral orifice of bladder (D30.3)

D30.8   Benign neoplasm of other specified urinary organs
Benign neoplasm of paraurethral glands

D30.9   Benign neoplasm of urinary organ, unspecified
Benign neoplasm of urinary system NOS

D31-   Benign neoplasm of eye and adnexa
Excludes 1:   benign neoplasm of connective tissue of eyelid (D21.0)
benign neoplasm of optic nerve (D33.3)
benign neoplasm of skin of eyelid (D22.1-, D23.1-)

D31.0-   Benign neoplasm of conjunctiva

D31.00   Benign neoplasm of unspecified conjunctiva

D31.01   Benign neoplasm of right conjunctiva

D31.02   Benign neoplasm of left conjunctiva

D31.1-   Benign neoplasm of cornea

D31.10   Benign neoplasm of unspecified cornea

D31.11   Benign neoplasm of right cornea

D31.12   Benign neoplasm of left cornea

D31.2-   Benign neoplasm of retina
Excludes 1:   dark area on retina (D49.81)
hemangioma of retina (D49.81)
neoplasm of unspecified behavior of retina and choroid (D49.81)
retinal freckle (D49.81)

D31.20   Benign neoplasm of unspecified retina

D31.21   Benign neoplasm of right retina

D31.22   Benign neoplasm of left retina

D31.3-   Benign neoplasm of choroid

D31.30   Benign neoplasm of unspecified choroid

D31.31   Benign neoplasm of right choroid

D31.32   Benign neoplasm of left choroid

D31.4-   Benign neoplasm of ciliary body

D31.40   Benign neoplasm of unspecified ciliary body

D31.41   Benign neoplasm of right ciliary body

D31.42   Benign neoplasm of left ciliary body

D31.5-   Benign neoplasm of lacrimal gland and duct
Benign neoplasm of lacrimal sac
Benign neoplasm of nasolacrimal duct

D31.50   Benign neoplasm of unspecified lacrimal gland and duct

D31.51   Benign neoplasm of right lacrimal gland and duct

D31.52   Benign neoplasm of left lacrimal gland and duct

D31.6-   Benign neoplasm of unspecified site of orbit
Benign neoplasm of connective tissue of orbit
Benign neoplasm of extraocular muscle
Benign neoplasm of peripheral nerves of orbit
Benign neoplasm of retrobulbar tissue
Benign neoplasm of retro-ocular tissue
Excludes 1:   benign neoplasm of orbital bone (D16.4)

D31.60   Benign neoplasm of unspecified site of unspecified orbit

D31.61   Benign neoplasm of unspecified site of right orbit

D31.62   Benign neoplasm of unspecified site of left orbit

D31.9-   Benign neoplasm of unspecified part of eye
Benign neoplasm of eyeball

D31.90   Benign neoplasm of unspecified part of unspecified eye

D31.91   Benign neoplasm of unspecified part of right eye

D31.92   Benign neoplasm of unspecified part of left eye

D32-   Benign neoplasm of meninges

D32.0   Benign neoplasm of cerebral meninges

D32.1   Benign neoplasm of spinal meninges

D32.9   Benign neoplasm of meninges, unspecified
Meningioma NOS

D33-   Benign neoplasm of brain and other parts of central nervous system
Excludes 1:   angioma (D18.0-)
benign neoplasm of meninges (D32.-)
benign neoplasm of peripheral nerves and autonomic nervous system (D36.1-)
hemangioma (D18.0-)
neurofibromatosis (Q85.0-)
retro-ocular benign neoplasm (D31.6-)

D33.0   Benign neoplasm of brain, supratentorial
Benign neoplasm of cerebral ventricle
Benign neoplasm of cerebrum
Benign neoplasm of frontal lobe
Benign neoplasm of occipital lobe
Benign neoplasm of parietal lobe
Benign neoplasm of temporal lobe
Excludes 1:   benign neoplasm of fourth ventricle (D33.1)

D33.1   Benign neoplasm of brain, infratentorial
Benign neoplasm of brain stem
Benign neoplasm of cerebellum
Benign neoplasm of fourth ventricle

D33.2   Benign neoplasm of brain, unspecified

D33.3   Benign neoplasm of cranial nerves
Benign neoplasm of olfactory bulb

D33.4   Benign neoplasm of spinal cord

D33.7   Benign neoplasm of other specified parts of central nervous system

D33.9   Benign neoplasm of central nervous system, unspecified
Benign neoplasm of nervous system (central) NOS

D34   Benign neoplasm of thyroid gland
Use additional code to identify any functional activity

D35-   Benign neoplasm of other and unspecified endocrine glands
Use additional code to identify any functional activity
Excludes 1:   benign neoplasm of endocrine pancreas (D13.7)
benign neoplasm of ovary (D27.-)
benign neoplasm of testis (D29.2.-)
benign neoplasm of thymus (D15.0)

D35.0-   Benign neoplasm of adrenal gland

D35.00   Benign neoplasm of unspecified adrenal gland

D35.01   Benign neoplasm of right adrenal gland

D35.02   Benign neoplasm of left adrenal gland

D35.1   Benign neoplasm of parathyroid gland

D35.2   Benign neoplasm of pituitary gland

D35.3   Benign neoplasm of craniopharyngeal duct

D35.4   Benign neoplasm of pineal gland

D35.5   Benign neoplasm of carotid body

D35.6   Benign neoplasm of aortic body and other paraganglia
Benign tumor of glomus jugulare

D35.7   Benign neoplasm of other specified endocrine glands

D35.9   Benign neoplasm of endocrine gland, unspecified
Benign neoplasm of unspecified endocrine gland

D36-   Benign neoplasm of other and unspecified sites

D36.0   Benign neoplasm of lymph nodes
Excludes 1:   lymphangioma (D18.1)

D36.1-   Benign neoplasm of peripheral nerves and autonomic nervous system
Excludes 1:   benign neoplasm of peripheral nerves of orbit (D31.6-)
neurofibromatosis (Q85.0-)

D36.10   Benign neoplasm of peripheral nerves and autonomic nervous system, unspecified

D36.11   Benign neoplasm of peripheral nerves and autonomic nervous system of face, head, and neck

D36.12   Benign neoplasm of peripheral nerves and autonomic nervous system, upper limb, including shoulder

D36.13   Benign neoplasm of peripheral nerves and autonomic nervous system of lower limb, including hip

D36.14   Benign neoplasm of peripheral nerves and autonomic nervous system of thorax

D36.15   Benign neoplasm of peripheral nerves and autonomic nervous system of abdomen

D29 - D37

D36.16 **Benign neoplasm of peripheral nerves and autonomic nervous system of <u>pelvis</u>**

D36.17 **Benign neoplasm of peripheral nerves and autonomic nervous system of trunk, unspecified**

D36.7 **Benign neoplasm of other specified sites**
Benign neoplasm of nose NOS

D36.9 **Benign neoplasm, unspecified site**

Benign neuroendocrine tumors (D3A)

D3A- **<u>Benign neuroendocrine</u> tumors**
Use additional code to identify any associated endocrine syndrome, such as:
Carcinoid syndrome (E34.0)
Excludes❷: benign pancreatic islet cell tumors (D13.7)
Code also any associated multiple endocrine neoplasia [MEN] syndromes (E31.2-)

D3A.0- **<u>Benign carcinoid</u> tumors**

D3A.00 **<u>Benign carcinoid</u> tumor of unspecified site**
Carcinoid tumor NOS

D3A.01-**<u>Benign carcinoid</u> tumors of the small intestine**

D3A.010 **Benign carcinoid tumor of the <u>duodenum</u>**

D3A.011 **Benign carcinoid tumor of the <u>jejunum</u>**

D3A.012 **Benign carcinoid tumor of the <u>ileum</u>**

D3A.019 **Benign carcinoid tumor of the small intestine, unspecified portion**

D3A.02-**<u>Benign carcinoid</u> tumors of the appendix, large intestine, and rectum**

D3A.020 **Benign carcinoid tumor of the <u>appendix</u>**

D3A.021 **Benign carcinoid tumor of the <u>cecum</u>**

D3A.022 **Benign carcinoid tumor of the <u>ascending colon</u>**

D3A.023 **Benign carcinoid tumor of the <u>transverse colon</u>**

D3A.024 **Benign carcinoid tumor of the <u>descending colon</u>**

D3A.025 **Benign carcinoid tumor of the <u>sigmoid colon</u>**

D3A.026 **Benign carcinoid tumor of the <u>rectum</u>**

D3A.029 **Benign carcinoid tumor of the large intestine, unspecified portion**
Benign carcinoid tumor of the colon NOS

D3A.09-**<u>Benign carcinoid</u> tumors of other sites**

D3A.090 **Benign carcinoid tumor of the <u>bronchus and lung</u>**

D3A.091 **Benign carcinoid tumor of the <u>thymus</u>**

D3A.092 **Benign carcinoid tumor of the <u>stomach</u>**

D3A.093 **Benign carcinoid tumor of the <u>kidney</u>**

D3A.094 **Benign carcinoid tumor of the foregut NOS**

D3A.095 **Benign carcinoid tumor of the midgut NOS**

D3A.096 **Benign carcinoid tumor of the hindgut NOS**

D3A.098 **Benign carcinoid tumors of other sites**

D3A.8 **<u>Other benign neuroendocrine</u> tumors**
Neuroendocrine tumor NOS

Neoplasms of uncertain behavior, polycythemia vera and myelodysplastic syndromes (D37-D48)

Note: Categories D37-D44, and D48 classify by site neoplasms of uncertain behavior, i.e., histologic confirmation whether the neoplasm is malignant or benign cannot be made.
Excludes 1: neoplasms of unspecified behavior (D49.-)

D37- **Neoplasm of <u>uncertain behavior</u> of oral cavity and digestive organs**
Excludes 1: stromal tumors of uncertain behavior of digestive system (D48.1)

D37.0- **Neoplasm of uncertain behavior of lip, oral cavity and pharynx**
Excludes 1: neoplasm of uncertain behavior of aryepiglottic fold or interarytenoid fold, laryngeal aspect (D38.0)
neoplasm of uncertain behavior of epiglottis NOS (D38.0)
neoplasm of uncertain behavior of skin of lip (D48.5)
neoplasm of uncertain behavior of suprahyoid portion of epiglottis (D38.0)

D37.01 **Neoplasm of uncertain behavior of <u>lip</u>**
Neoplasm of uncertain behavior of vermilion border of lip

D37.02 **Neoplasm of uncertain behavior of <u>tongue</u>**

D37.03- **Neoplasm of uncertain behavior of the <u>major</u> salivary glands**

D37.030 **Neoplasm of uncertain behavior of the <u>parotid</u> salivary glands**

D37.031 **Neoplasm of uncertain behavior of the <u>sublingual</u> salivary glands**

D37.032 **Neoplasm of uncertain behavior of the <u>submandibular</u> salivary glands**

D37.039 **Neoplasm of uncertain behavior of the major salivary glands, unspecified**

D37.04 **Neoplasm of uncertain behavior of the <u>minor</u> salivary glands**
Neoplasm of uncertain behavior of submucosal salivary glands of lip
Neoplasm of uncertain behavior of submucosal salivary glands of cheek
Neoplasm of uncertain behavior of submucosal salivary glands of hard palate
Neoplasm of uncertain behavior of submucosal salivary glands of soft palate

D37.05 **Neoplasm of uncertain behavior of <u>pharynx</u>**
Neoplasm of uncertain behavior of aryepiglottic fold of pharynx NOS
Neoplasm of uncertain behavior of hypopharyngeal aspect of aryepiglottic fold of pharynx
Neoplasm of uncertain behavior of marginal zone of aryepiglottic fold of pharynx

D37.09 **Neoplasm of uncertain behavior of other specified sites of the oral cavity**

D37.1 **Neoplasm of uncertain behavior of <u>stomach</u>**

D37.2 **Neoplasm of uncertain behavior of <u>small intestine</u>**

D37.3 **Neoplasm of uncertain behavior of <u>appendix</u>**

D37.4 **Neoplasm of uncertain behavior of <u>colon</u>**

D37.5 **Neoplasm of uncertain behavior of <u>rectum</u>**
Neoplasm of uncertain behavior of rectosigmoid junction

D37.6 **Neoplasm of uncertain behavior of <u>liver, gallbladder and bile ducts</u>**
Neoplasm of uncertain behavior of ampulla of Vater

D37.8 **Neoplasm of uncertain behavior of other specified digestive organs**
Neoplasm of uncertain behavior of anal canal
Neoplasm of uncertain behavior of anal sphincter
Neoplasm of uncertain behavior of anus NOS
Neoplasm of uncertain behavior of esophagus
Neoplasm of uncertain behavior of intestine NOS
Neoplasm of uncertain behavior of pancreas
Excludes 1: neoplasm of uncertain behavior of anal margin (D48.5)
neoplasm of uncertain behavior of anal skin (D48.5)
neoplasm of uncertain behavior of perianal skin (D48.5)

D37.9 **Neoplasm of uncertain behavior of digestive organ, unspecified**

D 2 9 - D 3 7

D38- Neoplasm of <u>uncertain behavior</u> of middle ear and respiratory and intrathoracic organs
   Excludes 1:   neoplasm of uncertain behavior of heart (D48.7)
  D38.0 Neoplasm of uncertain behavior of <u>larynx</u>
     Neoplasm of uncertain behavior of aryepiglottic fold or interarytenoid fold, laryngeal aspect
     Neoplasm of uncertain behavior of epiglottis (suprahyoid portion)
     Excludes 1:   neoplasm of uncertain behavior of aryepiglottic fold or interarytenoid fold NOS (D37.05)
     neoplasm of uncertain behavior of hypopharyngeal aspect of aryepiglottic fold (D37.05)
     neoplasm of uncertain behavior of marginal zone of aryepiglottic fold (D37.05)
  D38.1 Neoplasm of uncertain behavior of <u>trachea, bronchus and lung</u>
  D38.2 Neoplasm of uncertain behavior of <u>pleura</u>
  D38.3 Neoplasm of uncertain behavior of <u>mediastinum</u>
  D38.4 Neoplasm of uncertain behavior of <u>thymus</u>
  D38.5 Neoplasm of uncertain behavior of other respiratory organs
     Neoplasm of uncertain behavior of accessory sinuses
     Neoplasm of uncertain behavior of cartilage of nose
     Neoplasm of uncertain behavior of middle ear
     Neoplasm of uncertain behavior of nasal cavities
     Excludes 1:   neoplasm of uncertain behavior of ear (external) (skin) (D48.5)
     neoplasm of uncertain behavior of nose NOS (D48.7)
     neoplasm of uncertain behavior of skin of nose (D48.5)
  D38.6 Neoplasm of uncertain behavior of respiratory organ, unspecified

D39- Neoplasm of <u>uncertain behavior</u> of female genital organs
  D39.0 Neoplasm of uncertain behavior of <u>uterus</u>
  D39.1- Neoplasm of uncertain behavior of <u>ovary</u>
     Use additional code to identify any functional activity.
    D39.10 Neoplasm of uncertain behavior of unspecified ovary
    D39.11 Neoplasm of uncertain behavior of <u>right</u> ovary
    D39.12 Neoplasm of uncertain behavior of <u>left</u> ovary
  D39.2 Neoplasm of uncertain behavior of <u>placenta</u>
     Chorioadenoma destruens
     Invasive hydatidiform mole
     Malignant hydatidiform mole
     Excludes 1:   hydatidiform mole NOS (O01.9)
  D39.8 Neoplasm of uncertain behavior of other specified female genital organs
     Neoplasm of uncertain behavior of skin of female genital organs
  D39.9 Neoplasm of uncertain behavior of female genital organ, unspecified

D40- Neoplasm of <u>uncertain behavior</u> of male genital organs
  D40.0 Neoplasm of uncertain behavior of <u>prostate</u>
  D40.1- Neoplasm of uncertain behavior of <u>testis</u>
    D40.10 Neoplasm of uncertain behavior of unspecified testis
    D40.11 Neoplasm of uncertain behavior of <u>right</u> testis
    D40.12 Neoplasm of uncertain behavior of <u>left</u> testis
  D40.8 Neoplasm of uncertain behavior of other specified male genital organs
     Neoplasm of uncertain behavior of skin of male genital organs
  D40.9 Neoplasm of uncertain behavior of male genital organ, unspecified

D41- Neoplasm of <u>uncertain behavior</u> of urinary organs
  D41.0- Neoplasm of uncertain behavior of <u>kidney</u>
     Excludes 1:   neoplasm of uncertain behavior of renal pelvis (D41.1-)
    D41.00 Neoplasm of uncertain behavior of unspecified kidney
    D41.01 Neoplasm of uncertain behavior of <u>right</u> kidney
    D41.02 Neoplasm of uncertain behavior of <u>left</u> kidney
  D41.1- Neoplasm of uncertain behavior of <u>renal pelvis</u>
    D41.10 Neoplasm of uncertain behavior of unspecified renal pelvis
    D41.11 Neoplasm of uncertain behavior of <u>right</u> renal pelvis
    D41.12 Neoplasm of uncertain behavior of <u>left</u> renal pelvis
  D41.2- Neoplasm of uncertain behavior of <u>ureter</u>
    D41.20 Neoplasm of uncertain behavior of unspecified ureter
    D41.21 Neoplasm of uncertain behavior of <u>right</u> ureter
    D41.22 Neoplasm of uncertain behavior of <u>left</u> ureter
  D41.3 Neoplasm of uncertain behavior of <u>urethra</u>
  D41.4 Neoplasm of uncertain behavior of <u>bladder</u>
  D41.8 Neoplasm of uncertain behavior of other specified urinary organs
  D41.9 Neoplasm of uncertain behavior of unspecified urinary organ

D42- Neoplasm of <u>uncertain behavior</u> of meninges
  D42.0 Neoplasm of uncertain behavior of <u>cerebral meninges</u>
  D42.1 Neoplasm of uncertain behavior of <u>spinal meninges</u>
  D42.9 Neoplasm of uncertain behavior of meninges, unspecified

D43- Neoplasm of <u>uncertain behavior</u> of brain and central nervous system
   Excludes 1:   neoplasm of uncertain behavior of peripheral nerves and autonomic nervous system (D48.2)
  D43.0 Neoplasm of uncertain behavior of <u>brain, supratentorial</u>
     Neoplasm of uncertain behavior of cerebral ventricle
     Neoplasm of uncertain behavior of cerebrum
     Neoplasm of uncertain behavior of frontal lobe
     Neoplasm of uncertain behavior of occipital lobe
     Neoplasm of uncertain behavior of parietal lobe
     Neoplasm of uncertain behavior of temporal lobe
     Excludes 1:   neoplasm of uncertain behavior of fourth ventricle (D43.1)
  D43.1 Neoplasm of uncertain behavior of <u>brain, infratentorial</u>
     Neoplasm of uncertain behavior of brain stem
     Neoplasm of uncertain behavior of cerebellum
     Neoplasm of uncertain behavior of fourth ventricle
  D43.2 Neoplasm of uncertain behavior of brain, unspecified
  D43.3 Neoplasm of uncertain behavior of <u>cranial nerves</u>
  D43.4 Neoplasm of uncertain behavior of <u>spinal cord</u>
  D43.8 Neoplasm of uncertain behavior of other specified parts of central nervous system
  D43.9 Neoplasm of uncertain behavior of central nervous system, unspecified
     Neoplasm of uncertain behavior of nervous system (central) NOS

D44- Neoplasm of <u>uncertain behavior</u> of endocrine glands
   Excludes 1:   multiple endocrine adenomatosis (E31.2-)
   multiple endocrine neoplasia (E31.2-)
   neoplasm of uncertain behavior of endocrine pancreas (D37.8)
   neoplasm of uncertain behavior of ovary (D39.1-)
   neoplasm of uncertain behavior of testis (D40.1-)
   neoplasm of uncertain behavior of thymus (D38.4)
  D44.0 Neoplasm of uncertain behavior of <u>thyroid gland</u>
  D44.1- Neoplasm of uncertain behavior of <u>adrenal gland</u>
     Use additional code to identify any functional activity.
    D44.10 Neoplasm of uncertain behavior of unspecified adrenal gland
    D44.11 Neoplasm of uncertain behavior of <u>right</u> adrenal gland
    D44.12 Neoplasm of uncertain behavior of <u>left</u> adrenal gland
  D44.2 Neoplasm of uncertain behavior of <u>parathyroid gland</u>
  D44.3 Neoplasm of uncertain behavior of <u>pituitary gland</u>
     Use additional code to identify any functional activity.
  D44.4 Neoplasm of uncertain behavior of <u>craniopharyngeal duct</u>
  D44.5 Neoplasm of uncertain behavior of <u>pineal gland</u>
  D44.6 Neoplasm of uncertain behavior of <u>carotid body</u>
  D44.7 Neoplasm of uncertain behavior of <u>aortic body</u> and other <u>paraganglia</u>
  D44.9 Neoplasm of uncertain behavior of unspecified endocrine gland

D45 <u>Polycythemia vera</u>
   Excludes 1:   familial polycythemia (D75.0)
   secondary polycythemia (D75.1)

D46- <u>Myelodysplastic syndromes</u>
   Use additional code for adverse effect, if applicable, to identify drug (T36-T50 with fifth or sixth character 5)
   Excludes ❷: drug-induced aplastic anemia (D61.1)
  D46.0 Refractory anemia <u>without</u> ring sideroblasts, so stated
     Refractory anemia without sideroblasts, without excess of blasts
  D46.1 Refractory anemia <u>with</u> ring sideroblasts
     RARS
  D46.2- Refractory anemia <u>with excess of blasts</u>
    D46.20 Refractory anemia with excess of blasts, unspecified
     RAEB NOS
    D46.21 Refractory anemia with excess of <u>blasts 1</u>
     RAEB 1
    D46.22 Refractory anemia with excess of <u>blasts 2</u>
     RAEB 2
  D46.A Refractory cytopenia with multilineage dysplasia
  D46.B Refractory cytopenia with multilineage dysplasia <u>and ring sideroblasts</u>
     RCMD RS
  D46.C Myelodysplastic syndrome with isolated del(5q) chromosomal abnormality
     Myelodysplastic syndrome with 5q deletion
     5q minus syndrome NOS
  D46.4 Refractory anemia, unspecified
  D46.Z Other myelodysplastic syndromes
     Excludes 1:   chronic myelomonocytic leukemia (C93.1-)
  D46.9 Myelodysplastic syndrome, unspecified
     Myelodysplasia NOS

Excludes 1: = NOT CODED HERE! (Do not code both)

Excludes ❷: = Not Included Here

D38 - D49

D47- Other neoplasms of <u>uncertain behavior</u> of lymphoid, hematopoietic and related tissue

D47.0 <u>Histiocytic and mast cell tumors</u> of uncertain behavior
Indolent systemic mastocytosis
Mast cell tumor NOS
Mastocytoma NOS
Excludes 1:   malignant mast cell tumor (C96.2)
mastocytosis (congenital) (cutaneous) (Q82.2)

D47.1 <u>Chronic myeloproliferative disease</u>
Chronic neutrophilic leukemia
Myeloproliferative disease, unspecified
Excludes 1:   atypical chronic myeloid leukemia BCR/ABL-negative
(C92.2-)
chronic myeloid leukemia BCR/ABL-positive (C92.1-)
myelofibrosis NOS (D75.81)
myelophthisic anemia (D61.82)
myelophthisis (D61.82)
secondary myelofibrosis NOS (D75.81)

D47.2 <u>Monoclonal gammopathy</u>
Monoclonal gammopathy of undetermined significance [MGUS]

D47.3 <u>Essential (hemorrhagic) thrombocythemia</u>
Essential thrombocytosis
Idiopathic hemorrhagic thrombocythemia

D47.4 <u>Osteomyelofibrosis</u>
Chronic idiopathic myelofibrosis
Myelofibrosis (idiopathic) (with myeloid metaplasia)
Myelosclerosis (megakaryocytic) with myeloid metaplasia
Secondary myelofibrosis in myeloproliferative disease
Excludes 1:   acute myelofibrosis (C94.4-)

D47.Z- Other specified neoplasms of uncertain behavior of lymphoid, hematopoietic and related tissue

D47.Z1 **Post-transplant lymphoproliferative disorder (PTLD)**
Code first complications of transplanted organs and tissue (T86.-)

D47.Z9 **Other specified neoplasms of uncertain behavior of lymphoid, hematopoietic and related tissue**
Histiocytic tumors of uncertain behavior

D47.9 Neoplasm of uncertain behavior of lymphoid, hematopoietic and related tissue, unspecified
Lymphoproliferative disease NOS

D48- Neoplasm of <u>uncertain behavior</u> of other and unspecified sites
Excludes 1:   neurofibromatosis (nonmalignant) (Q85.0-)

D48.0 Neoplasm of uncertain behavior of <u>bone and articular cartilage</u>
Excludes 1:   neoplasm of uncertain behavior of cartilage of ear
(D48.1)
neoplasm of uncertain behavior of cartilage of larynx
(D38.0)
neoplasm of uncertain behavior of cartilage of nose
(D38.5)
neoplasm of uncertain behavior of connective tissue of
eyelid (D48.1)
neoplasm of uncertain behavior of synovia (D48.1)

D48.1 Neoplasm of uncertain behavior of <u>connective and other soft tissue</u>
Neoplasm of uncertain behavior of connective tissue of ear
Neoplasm of uncertain behavior of connective tissue of eyelid
Stromal tumors of uncertain behavior of digestive system
Excludes 1:   neoplasm of uncertain behavior of articular cartilage
(D48.0)
neoplasm of uncertain behavior of cartilage of larynx
(D38.0)
neoplasm of uncertain behavior of cartilage of nose
(D38.5)
neoplasm of uncertain behavior of connective tissue of
breast (D48.6-)

D48.2 Neoplasm of uncertain behavior of <u>peripheral nerves and autonomic nervous system</u>
Excludes 1:   neoplasm of uncertain behavior of peripheral nerves of
orbit (D48.7)

D48.3 Neoplasm of uncertain behavior of <u>retroperitoneum</u>

D48.4 Neoplasm of uncertain behavior of <u>peritoneum</u>

D48.5 Neoplasm of uncertain behavior of <u>skin</u>
Neoplasm of uncertain behavior of anal margin
Neoplasm of uncertain behavior of anal skin
Neoplasm of uncertain behavior of perianal skin
Neoplasm of uncertain behavior of skin of breast
Excludes 1:   neoplasm of uncertain behavior of anus NOS (D37.8)
neoplasm of uncertain behavior of skin of genital
organs (D39.8, D40.8)
neoplasm of uncertain behavior of vermilion border of
lip (D37.0)

D48.6- Neoplasm of uncertain behavior of <u>breast</u>
Neoplasm of uncertain behavior of connective tissue of breast
Cystosarcoma phyllodes
Excludes 1:   neoplasm of uncertain behavior of skin of breast
(D48.5)

D48.60 Neoplasm of uncertain behavior of unspecified breast

D48.61 Neoplasm of uncertain behavior of <u>right</u> breast

D48.62 Neoplasm of uncertain behavior of <u>left</u> breast

D48.7 Neoplasm of uncertain behavior of other specified sites
Neoplasm of uncertain behavior of eye
Neoplasm of uncertain behavior of heart
Neoplasm of uncertain behavior of peripheral nerves of orbit
Excludes 1:   neoplasm of uncertain behavior of connective tissue
(D48.1)
neoplasm of uncertain behavior of skin of eyelid
(D48.5)

D48.9 Neoplasm of uncertain behavior, unspecified

Neoplasms of unspecified behavior (D49)

D49- Neoplasms of <u>unspecified</u> <u>behavior</u>
Note: Category D49 classifies by site neoplasms of unspecified morphology and behavior. The term "mass", unless otherwise stated, is not to be regarded as a neoplastic growth.
Includes: "Growth" NOS
Neoplasm NOS
New growth NOS
Tumor NOS
Excludes 1:   neoplasms of uncertain behavior (D37-D44, D48)

D49.0 Neoplasm of unspecified behavior of <u>digestive system</u>
Excludes 1:   neoplasm of unspecified behavior of margin of anus
(D49.2)
neoplasm of unspecified behavior of perianal skin
(D49.2)
neoplasm of unspecified behavior of skin of anus
(D49.2)

D49.1 Neoplasm of unspecified behavior of <u>respiratory system</u>

D49.2 Neoplasm of unspecified behavior of <u>bone, soft tissue, and skin</u>
Excludes 1:   neoplasm of unspecified behavior of anal canal (D49.0)
neoplasm of unspecified behavior of anus NOS (D49.0)
neoplasm of unspecified behavior of bone marrow
(D49.89)
neoplasm of unspecified behavior of cartilage of larynx
(D49.1)
neoplasm of unspecified behavior of cartilage of nose
(D49.1)
neoplasm of unspecified behavior of connective tissue
of breast (D49.3)
neoplasm of unspecified behavior of skin of genital
organs (D49.5)
neoplasm of unspecified behavior of vermilion border
of lip (D49.0)

D49.3 Neoplasm of unspecified behavior of <u>breast</u>
Excludes 1:   neoplasm of unspecified behavior of skin of breast
(D49.2)

D49.4 Neoplasm of unspecified behavior of <u>bladder</u>

D49.5 Neoplasm of unspecified behavior of <u>other genitourinary organs</u>

D49.6 Neoplasm of unspecified behavior of <u>brain</u>
Excludes 1:   neoplasm of unspecified behavior of cerebral meninges
(D49.7)
neoplasm of unspecified behavior of cranial nerves
(D49.7)

D49.7 Neoplasm of unspecified behavior of <u>endocrine glands and other parts of nervous system</u>
Excludes 1:   neoplasm of unspecified behavior of peripheral,
sympathetic, and parasympathetic nerves and
ganglia (D49.2)

D49.8- Neoplasm of unspecified behavior of other specified sites
Excludes 1:   neoplasm of unspecified behavior of eyelid (skin)
(D49.2)
neoplasm of unspecified behavior of eyelid cartilage
(D49.2)
neoplasm of unspecified behavior of great vessels
(D49.2)
neoplasm of unspecified behavior of optic nerve
(D49.7)

D49.81 Neoplasm of unspecified behavior of retina and choroid
Dark area on retina
Retinal freckle

D49.89 Neoplasm of unspecified behavior of other specified sites

D49.9 Neoplasm of unspecified behavior of unspecified site

D 3 8 - D 4 9

Chapter 3 – Diseases of the blood and blood-forming organs and certain disorders involving the immune mechanism (D50-D89)

Excludes❷: *autoimmune disease (systemic) NOS (M35.9)*
certain conditions originating in the perinatal period (P00-P96)
complications of pregnancy, childbirth and the puerperium (O00-O9A)
congenital malformations, deformations and chromosomal abnormalities (Q00-Q99)
endocrine, nutritional and metabolic diseases (E00-E88)
human immunodeficiency virus [HIV] disease (B20)
injury, poisoning and certain other consequences of external causes (S00-T88)
neoplasms (C00-D49)
symptoms, signs and abnormal clinical and laboratory findings, not elsewhere classified (R00-R94)

This chapter contains the following blocks:
D50-D53	Nutritional anemias
D55-D59	Hemolytic anemias
D60-D64	Aplastic and other anemias and other bone marrow failure syndromes
D65-D69	Coagulation defects, purpura and other hemorrhagic conditions
D70-D77	Other disorders of blood and blood-forming organs
D78	Intraoperative and postprocedural complications of the spleen
D80-D89	Certain disorders involving the immune mechanism

Nutritional anemias (D50-D53)

D50-   <u>Iron deficiency</u> **anemia**
Includes: Asiderotic anemia
          Hypochromic anemia

D50.0   **Iron deficiency anemia secondary to <u>blood loss</u> (chronic)**
Posthemorrhagic anemia (chronic)
Excludes 1:   acute posthemorrhagic anemia (D62)
                congenital anemia from fetal blood loss (P61.3)

D50.1   **Sideropenic dysphagia**
Kelly-Paterson syndrome
Plummer-Vinson syndrome

D50.8   **Other iron deficiency anemias**
Iron deficiency anemia due to inadequate dietary iron intake

D50.9   **Iron deficiency anemia, unspecified**

D51-   <u>Vitamin B12 deficiency</u> **anemia**
Excludes 1:   vitamin B12 deficiency (E53.8)

D51.0   **Vitamin B12 deficiency anemia due to <u>intrinsic factor</u> deficiency**
Addison anemia
Biermer anemia
Pernicious (congenital) anemia
Congenital intrinsic factor deficiency

D51.1   **Vitamin B12 deficiency anemia due to <u>selective vitamin B12</u> malabsorption with proteinuria**
Imerslund (Gräsbeck) syndrome
Megaloblastic hereditary anemia

D51.2   <u>**Transcobalamin II**</u> **deficiency**

D51.3   **Other dietary vitamin B12 deficiency anemia**
Vegan anemia

D51.8   **Other vitamin B12 deficiency anemias**

D51.9   **Vitamin B12 deficiency anemia, unspecified**

D52-   <u>Folate deficiency</u> **anemia**
Excludes 1:   folate deficiency without anemia (E53.8)

D52.0   <u>**Dietary**</u> **folate deficiency anemia**
Nutritional megaloblastic anemia

D52.1   <u>**Drug-induced**</u> **folate deficiency anemia**
Use additional code for adverse effect, if applicable, to identify drug (T36-T50 with fifth or sixth character 5)

D52.8   **Other folate deficiency anemias**

D52.9   **Folate deficiency anemia, unspecified**
Folic acid deficiency anemia NOS

D53-   <u>Other nutritional</u> **anemias**
Includes: Megaloblastic anemia unresponsive to vitamin B12 or folate therapy

D53.0   <u>**Protein**</u> **deficiency anemia**
Amino-acid deficiency anemia
Orotaciduric anemia
Excludes 1:   Lesch-Nyhan syndrome (E79.1)

D53.1   **Other megaloblastic anemias, not elsewhere classified**
Megaloblastic anemia NOS
Excludes 1:   Di Guglielmo's disease (C94.0)

D53.2   <u>**Scorbutic**</u> **anemia**
Excludes 1:   scurvy (E54)

D53.8   **Other specified nutritional anemias**
Anemia associated with deficiency of copper
Anemia associated with deficiency of molybdenum
Anemia associated with deficiency of zinc
Excludes 1:   nutritional deficiencies without anemia, such as:
         copper deficiency NOS (E61.0)
         molybdenum deficiency NOS (E61.5)
         zinc deficiency NOS (E60)

D53.9   **Nutritional anemia, unspecified**
Simple chronic anemia
Excludes 1:   anemia NOS (D64.9)

Hemolytic anemias (D55-D59)

D55-   **Anemia due to <u>enzyme disorders</u>**
Excludes 1:   drug-induced enzyme deficiency anemia (D59.2)

D55.0   **Anemia due to glucose-6-phosphate dehydrogenase [G6PD] deficiency**
Favism
G6PD deficiency anemia

D55.1   **Anemia due to other disorders of glutathione metabolism**
Anemia (due to) enzyme deficiencies, except G6PD, related to the hexose monophosphate [HMP] shunt pathway
Anemia (due to) hemolytic nonspherocytic (hereditary), type I

D55.2   **Anemia due to disorders of glycolytic enzymes**
Hemolytic nonspherocytic (hereditary) anemia, type II
Hexokinase deficiency anemia
Pyruvate kinase [PK] deficiency anemia
Triose-phosphate isomerase deficiency anemia
Excludes 1:   disorders of glycolysis not associated with anemia (E74.8)

D55.3   **Anemia due to disorders of nucleotide metabolism**

D55.8   **Other anemias due to enzyme disorders**

D55.9   **Anemia due to enzyme disorder, unspecified**

D56-   <u>Thalassemia</u>
Excludes 1:   sickle-cell thalassemia (D57.4-)

D56.0   <u>Alpha</u> **thalassemia**
Alpha thalassemia major
Hemoglobin H Constant Spring
Hemoglobin H disease
Hydrops fetalis due to alpha thalassemia
Severe alpha thalassemia
Triple gene defect alpha thalassemia
Use additional code, if applicable, for hydrops fetalis due to alpha thalassemia (P56.99)
Excludes 1:   alpha thalassemia trait or minor (D56.3)
              asymptomatic alpha thalassemia (D56.3)
              hydrops fetalis due to isoimmunization (P56.0)
              hydrops fetalis not due to immune hemolysis (P83.2)

D56.1   <u>Beta</u> **thalassemia**
Beta thalassemia major
Cooley's anemia
Homozygous beta thalassemia
Severe beta thalassemia
Thalassemia intermedia
Thalassemia major
Excludes 1:   beta thalassemia minor (D56.3)
              beta thalassemia trait (D56.3)
              delta-beta thalassemia (D56.2)
              hemoglobin E-beta thalassemia (D56.5)
              sickle-cell beta thalassemia (D57.4-)

D56.2   <u>Delta-beta</u> **thalassemia**
Homozygous delta-beta thalassemia
Excludes 1:   delta-beta thalassemia minor (D56.3)
              delta-beta thalassemia trait (D56.3)

D56.3   **Thalassemia <u>minor</u>**
Alpha thalassemia minor
Alpha thalassemia silent carrier
Alpha thalassemia trait
Beta thalassemia minor
Beta thalassemia trait
Delta-beta thalassemia minor
Delta-beta thalassemia trait
Thalassemia trait NOS
Excludes 1:   alpha thalassemia (D56.0)
              beta thalassemia (D56.1)
              delta-beta thalassemia (D56.2)
              hemoglobin E-beta thalassemia (D56.5)
              sickle-cell trait (D57.3)

D56.4   **Hereditary persistence of fetal hemoglobin [HPFH]**

D56.5   Hemoglobin E-beta thalassemia
Excludes 1: beta thalassemia (D56.1)
                    beta thalassemia minor (D56.3)
                    beta thalassemia trait (D56.3)
                    delta-beta thalassemia (D56.2)
                    delta-beta thalassemia trait (D56.3)
                    hemoglobin E disease (D58.2)
                    other hemoglobinopathies (D58.2)
                    sickle-cell beta thalassemia (D57.4-)

D56.8   Other thalassemias
Dominant thalassemia
Hemoglobin C thalassemia
Mixed thalassemia
Thalassemia with other hemoglobinopathy
Excludes 1: hemoglobin C disease (D58.2)
                    hemoglobin E disease (D58.2)
                    other hemoglobinopathies (D58.2)
                    sickle-cell anemia (D57.-)

D56.9   Thalassemia, unspecified
Mediterranean anemia (with other hemoglobinopathy)

D57-   Sickle-cell disorders
Use additional code for any associated fever (R50.81)
Excludes 1: other hemoglobinopathies (D58.-)

D57.0-   Hb-SS disease with crisis
Sickle-cell disease NOS with crisis
Hb-SS disease with vasoocclusive pain

D57.00   Hb-SS disease with crisis, unspecified
D57.01   Hb-SS disease with acute chest syndrome
D57.02   Hb-SS disease with splenic sequestration

D57.1   Sickle-cell disease without crisis
Hb-SS disease without crisis
Sickle-cell anemia NOS
Sickle-cell disease NOS
Sickle-cell disorder NOS

D57.2-   Sickle-cell/Hb-C disease
Hb-SC disease
Hb-S/Hb-C disease

D57.20   Sickle-cell/Hb-C disease without crisis
D57.21- Sickle-cell/Hb-C disease with crisis
D57.211   Sickle-cell/Hb-C disease with acute chest syndrome
D57.212   Sickle-cell/Hb-C disease with splenic sequestration
D57.219   Sickle-cell/Hb-C disease with crisis, unspecified
Sickle-cell/Hb-C disease with crisis NOS

D57.3   Sickle-cell trait
Hb-S trait
Heterozygous hemoglobin S

D57.4-   Sickle-cell thalassemia
Sickle-cell beta thalassemia
Thalassemia Hb-S disease

D57.40   Sickle-cell thalassemia without crisis
Microdrepanocytosis
Sickle-cell thalassemia NOS
D57.41- Sickle-cell thalassemia with crisis
Sickle-cell thalassemia with vasoocclusive pain
D57.411   Sickle-cell thalassemia with acute chest syndrome
D57.412   Sickle-cell thalassemia with splenic sequestration
D57.419   Sickle-cell thalassemia with crisis, unspecified
Sickle-cell thalassemia with crisis NOS

D57.8-   Other sickle-cell disorders
Hb-SD disease
Hb-SE disease
D57.80   Other sickle-cell disorders without crisis
D57.81- Other sickle-cell disorders with crisis
D57.811   Other sickle-cell disorders with acute chest syndrome
D57.812   Other sickle-cell disorders with splenic sequestration
D57.819   Other sickle-cell disorders with crisis, unspecified
Other sickle-cell disorders with crisis NOS

D58-   Other hereditary hemolytic anemias
Excludes 1: hemolytic anemia of the newborn (P55.-)

D58.0   Hereditary spherocytosis
Acholuric (familial) jaundice
Congenital (spherocytic) hemolytic icterus
Minkowski-Chauffard syndrome

D58.1   Hereditary elliptocytosis
Elliptocytosis (congenital)
Ovalocytosis (congenital) (hereditary)

D58.2   Other hemoglobinopathies
Abnormal hemoglobin NOS
Congenital Heinz body anemia
Hb-C disease
Hb-D disease
Hb-E disease
Hemoglobinopathy NOS
Unstable hemoglobin hemolytic disease
Excludes 1: familial polycythemia (D75.0)
                    Hb-M disease (D74.0)
                    hemoglobin E-beta thalassemia (D56.5)
                    hereditary persistence of fetal hemoglobin [HPFH]
                        (D56.4)
                    high-altitude polycythemia (D75.1)
                    methemoglobinemia (D74.-)
                    other hemoglobinopathies with thalassemia (D56.8)

D58.8   Other specified hereditary hemolytic anemias
Stomatocytosis

D58.9   Hereditary hemolytic anemia, unspecified

D59-   Acquired hemolytic anemia

D59.0   Drug-induced autoimmune hemolytic anemia
Use additional code for adverse effect, if applicable, to identify drug
(T36-T50 with fifth or sixth character 5)

D59.1   Other autoimmune hemolytic anemias
Autoimmune hemolytic disease (cold type) (warm type)
Chronic cold hemagglutinin disease
Cold agglutinin disease
Cold agglutinin hemoglobinuria
Cold type (secondary) (symptomatic) hemolytic anemia
Warm type (secondary) (symptomatic) hemolytic anemia
Excludes 1: Evans syndrome (D69.41)
                    hemolytic disease of newborn (P55.-)
                    paroxysmal cold hemoglobinuria (D59.6)

D59.2   Drug-induced nonautoimmune hemolytic anemia
Drug-induced enzyme deficiency anemia
Use additional code for adverse effect, if applicable, to identify drug
(T36-T50 with fifth or sixth character 5)

D59.3   Hemolytic-uremic syndrome
Use additional code to identify associated:
E. coli infection (B96.2-)
Pneumococcal pneumonia (J13)
Shigella dysenteriae (A03.9)

D59.4   Other nonautoimmune hemolytic anemias
Mechanical hemolytic anemia
Microangiopathic hemolytic anemia
Toxic hemolytic anemia

D59.5   Paroxysmal nocturnal hemoglobinuria [Marchiafava-Micheli]
Excludes 1: hemoglobinuria NOS (R82.3)

D59.6   Hemoglobinuria due to hemolysis from other external causes
Hemoglobinuria from exertion
March hemoglobinuria
Paroxysmal cold hemoglobinuria
Use additional code (Chapter 20) to identify external cause
Excludes 1: hemoglobinuria NOS (R82.3)

D59.8   Other acquired hemolytic anemias

D59.9   Acquired hemolytic anemia, unspecified
Idiopathic hemolytic anemia, chronic

Aplastic and other anemias and other bone marrow failure syndromes (D60-D64)

D60-   Acquired pure red cell aplasia [erythroblastopenia]
Includes: Red cell aplasia (acquired) (adult) (with thymoma)
Excludes 1: congenital red cell aplasia (D61.01)

D60.0   Chronic acquired pure red cell aplasia
D60.1   Transient acquired pure red cell aplasia
D60.8   Other acquired pure red cell aplasia
D60.9   Acquired pure red cell aplasia, unspecified

D61-   Other aplastic anemias and other bone marrow failure syndromes
Excludes 1: neutropenia (D70.-)

D61.0-   Constitutional aplastic anemia
D61.01   Constitutional (pure) red blood cell aplasia
Blackfan-Diamond syndrome
Congenital (pure) red cell aplasia
Familial hypoplastic anemia
Primary (pure) red cell aplasia
Red cell (pure) aplasia of infants
Excludes 1: acquired red cell aplasia (D60.9)

D61.09   Other constitutional aplastic anemia
Fanconi's anemia
Pancytopenia with malformations

D
5
0
-
D
6
1

D61.1   <u>Drug-induced</u> aplastic anemia
Use additional code for adverse effect, if applicable, to identify drug (T36-T50 with fifth or sixth character 5)

D61.2   Aplastic anemia <u>due to other</u> external agents
Code first, if applicable, toxic effects of substances chiefly nonmedicinal as to source (T51-T65)

D61.3   <u>Idiopathic</u> aplastic anemia

D61.8-   Other specified aplastic anemias and other bone marrow failure syndromes

    D61.81-   <u>Pancytopenia</u>
Excludes 1:   pancytopenia (due to) (with) aplastic anemia (D61.-)
pancytopenia (due to) (with) bone marrow infiltration (D61.82)
pancytopenia (due to) (with) congenital (pure) red cell aplasia (D61.01)
pancytopenia (due to) (with) hairy cell leukemia (C91.4-)
pancytopenia (due to) (with) human immunodeficiency virus disease (B20.-)
pancytopenia (due to) (with) leukoerythroblastic anemia (D61.82)
pancytopenia (due to) (with) myelodysplastic syndromes (D46.-)
pancytopenia (due to) (with) myeloproliferative disease (D47.1)

       D61.810   Antineoplastic <u>chemotherapy induced</u> pancytopenia
Excludes ❷: aplastic anemia due to antineoplastic chemotherapy (D61.1)

       D61.811   Other <u>drug-induced</u> pancytopenia
Excludes ❷: aplastic anemia due to drugs (D61.1)

       D61.818   Other pancytopenia

    D61.82   Myelophthisis
Leukoerythroblastic anemia
Myelophthisic anemia
Panmyelophthisis
Excludes 1:   idiopathic myelofibrosis (D47.1)
myelofibrosis NOS (D75.81)
myelofibrosis with myeloid metaplasia (D47.4)
primary myelofibrosis (D47.1)
secondary myelofibrosis (D75.81)
Code also the underlying disorder, such as:
Malignant neoplasm of breast (C50.-)
Tuberculosis (A15.-)

    D61.89   Other specified aplastic anemias and other bone marrow failure syndromes

D61.9   Aplastic anemia, unspecified
Hypoplastic anemia NOS
Medullary hypoplasia

D62   <u>Acute posthemorrhagic</u> anemia
Excludes 1:   anemia due to chronic blood loss (D50.0)
blood loss anemia NOS (D50.0)
congenital anemia from fetal blood loss (P61.3)

D63-   <u>Anemia in chronic diseases</u> classified elsewhere

    D63.0   Anemia in <u>neoplastic</u> disease
Code first neoplasm (C00-D49)
Excludes 1:   anemia due to antineoplastic chemotherapy (D64.81)
aplastic anemia due to antineoplastic chemotherapy (D61.1)

    D63.1   Anemia in <u>chronic kidney</u> disease
Erythropoietin resistant anemia (EPO resistant anemia)
Code first underlying chronic kidney disease (CKD) (N18.-)

    D63.8   Anemia in <u>other chronic</u> diseases classified elsewhere
Code first underlying disease, such as:
Diphyllobothriasis (B70.0)
Hookworm disease (B76.0-B76.9)
Hypothyroidism (E00.0-E03.9)
Malaria (B50.0-B54)
Symptomatic late syphilis (A52.79)
Tuberculosis (A18.89)

D64-   <u>Other</u> anemias
Excludes 1:   refractory anemia (D46.-)
refractory anemia with excess blasts in transformation [RAEB T] (C92.0-)

    D64.0   <u>Hereditary</u> sideroblastic anemia
Sex-linked hypochromic sideroblastic anemia

    D64.1   <u>Secondary</u> sideroblastic anemia <u>due to disease</u>
Code first underlying disease

    D64.2   <u>Secondary</u> sideroblastic anemia <u>due to drugs and toxins</u>
Code first poisoning due to drug or toxin, if applicable (T36-T65 with fifth or sixth character 1-4 or 6)
Use additional code for adverse effect, if applicable, to identify drug (T36-T50 with fifth or sixth character 5)

    D64.3   Other sideroblastic anemias
Sideroblastic anemia NOS
Pyridoxine-responsive sideroblastic anemia NEC

    D64.4   Congenital dyserythropoietic anemia
Dyshematopoietic anemia (congenital)
Excludes 1:   Blackfan-Diamond syndrome (D61.01)
Di Guglielmo's disease (C94.0)

    D64.8-   Other specified anemias

       D64.81   Anemia <u>due to antineoplastic chemotherapy</u>
Antineoplastic chemotherapy induced anemia
Excludes 1:   anemia in neoplastic disease (D63.0)
aplastic anemia due to antineoplastic chemotherapy (D61.1)

       D64.89   Other specified anemias
Infantile pseudoleukemia

    D64.9   Anemia, unspecified

Coagulation defects, purpura and other hemorrhagic conditions (D65-D69)

D65   Disseminated intravascular coagulation [defibrination syndrome]
Afibrinogenemia, acquired
Consumption coagulopathy
Diffuse or disseminated intravascular coagulation [DIC]
Fibrinolytic hemorrhage, acquired
Fibrinolytic purpura
Purpura fulminans
Excludes 1:   disseminated intravascular coagulation (complicating):
abortion or ectopic or molar pregnancy (O00-O07, O08.1)
in newborn (P60)
pregnancy, childbirth and the puerperium (O45.0, O46.0, O67.0, O72.3)

D66   Hereditary factor <u>VIII</u> deficiency
Classical hemophilia
Deficiency factor VIII (with functional defect)
Hemophilia NOS
Hemophilia A
Excludes 1:   factor VIII deficiency with vascular defect (D68.0)

D67   Hereditary factor <u>IX</u> deficiency
Christmas disease
Factor IX deficiency (with functional defect)
Hemophilia B
Plasma thromboplastin component [PTC] deficiency

D68-   Other coagulation defects
Excludes 1:   abnormal coagulation profile (R79.1)
coagulation defects complicating abortion or ectopic or molar pregnancy (O00-O07, O08.1)
coagulation defects complicating pregnancy, childbirth and the puerperium (O45.0, O46.0, O67.0, O72.3)

    D68.0   Von Willebrand's disease
Angiohemophilia
Factor VIII deficiency with vascular defect
Vascular hemophilia
Excludes 1:   capillary fragility (hereditary) (D69.8)
factor VIII deficiency NOS (D66)
factor VIII deficiency with functional defect (D66)

    D68.1   Hereditary factor <u>XI</u> deficiency
Hemophilia C
Plasma thromboplastin antecedent [PTA] deficiency
Rosenthal's disease

D
6
1
I
D
6
9

Excludes 1: = NOT CODED HERE! (Do not code both)   **382**   *Excludes ❷: = Not Included Here*

D68.2 Hereditary deficiency of other clotting factors
AC globulin deficiency
Congenital afibrinogenemia
Deficiency of factor I [fibrinogen]
Deficiency of factor II [prothrombin]
Deficiency of factor V [labile]
Deficiency of factor VII [stable]
Deficiency of factor X [Stuart-Prower]
Deficiency of factor XII [Hageman]
Deficiency of factor XIII [fibrin stabilizing]
Dysfibrinogenemia (congenital)
Hypoproconvertinemia
Owren's disease
Proaccelerin deficiency

D68.3- Hemorrhagic disorder due to circulating anticoagulants
D68.31- Hemorrhagic disorder due to intrinsic circulating anticoagulants, antibodies, or inhibitors
D68.311 Acquired hemophilia
Autoimmune hemophilia
Autoimmune inhibitors to clotting factors
Secondary hemophilia

D68.312 Antiphospholipid antibody with hemorrhagic disorder
Lupus anticoagulant (LAC) with hemorrhagic disorder
Systemic lupus erythematosus [SLE] inhibitor with hemorrhagic disorder
Excludes 1: antiphospholipid antibody finding without diagnosis (R76.0)
antiphospholipid antibody syndrome (D68.61)
antiphospholipid antibody with hypercoagulable state (D68.61)
lupus anticoagulant (LAC) finding without diagnosis (R76.0)
lupus anticoagulant (LAC) with hypercoagulable state (D68.62)
systemic lupus erythematosus [SLE] inhibitor finding without diagnosis (R76.0)
systemic lupus erythematosus [SLE] inhibitor with hypercoagulable state (D68.62)

D68.318 Other hemorrhagic disorder due to intrinsic circulating anticoagulants, antibodies, or inhibitors
Antithromboplastinemia
Antithromboplastinogenemia
Hemorrhagic disorder due to intrinsic increase in antithrombin
Hemorrhagic disorder due to intrinsic increase in anti-VIIIa
Hemorrhagic disorder due to intrinsic increase in anti-IXa
Hemorrhagic disorder due to intrinsic increase in anti-XIa

D68.32 Hemorrhagic disorder due to extrinsic circulating anticoagulants
Drug-induced hemorrhagic disorder
Hemorrhagic disorder due to increase in anti-IIa
Hemorrhagic disorder due to increase in anti-Xa
Hyperheparinemia
Use additional code for adverse effect, if applicable, to identify drug (T45.515-, T45.525-)

D68.4 Acquired coagulation factor deficiency
Deficiency of coagulation factor due to liver disease
Deficiency of coagulation factor due to vitamin K deficiency
Excludes 1: vitamin K deficiency of newborn (P53)

D68.5- Primary thrombophilia
Primary hypercoagulable states
Excludes 1: antiphospholipid syndrome (D68.61)
lupus anticoagulant (D68.62)
secondary activated protein C resistance (D68.69)
secondary antiphospholipid antibody syndrome (D68.69)
secondary lupus anticoagulant with hypercoagulable state (D68.69)
secondary systemic lupus erythematosus [SLE] inhibitor with hypercoagulable state (D68.69)
systemic lupus erythematosus [SLE] inhibitor finding without diagnosis (R76.0)
systemic lupus erythematosus [SLE] inhibitor with hemorrhagic disorder (D68.312)
thrombotic thrombocytopenic purpura (M31.1)

D68.51 Activated protein C resistance
Factor V Leiden mutation

D68.52 Prothrombin gene mutation

D68.59 Other primary thrombophilia
Antithrombin III deficiency
Hypercoagulable state NOS
Primary hypercoagulable state NEC
Primary thrombophilia NEC
Protein C deficiency
Protein S deficiency
Thrombophilia NOS

D68.6- Other thrombophilia
Other hypercoagulable states
Excludes 1: diffuse or disseminated intravascular coagulation [DIC] (D65)
heparin induced thrombocytopenia (HIT) (D75.82)
hyperhomocysteinemia (E72.11)

D68.61 Antiphospholipid syndrome
Anticardiolipin syndrome
Antiphospholipid antibody syndrome
Excludes 1: antiphospholipid antibody finding without diagnosis (R76.0)
antiphospholipid antibody with hemorrhagic disorder (D68.312)
lupus anticoagulant syndrome (D68.62)

D68.62 Lupus anticoagulant syndrome
Lupus anticoagulant
Presence of systemic lupus erythematosus [SLE] inhibitor
Excludes 1: anticardiolipin syndrome (D68.61)
antiphospholipid syndrome (D68.61)
lupus anticoagulant (LAC) finding without diagnosis (R79.0)
lupus anticoagulant (LAC) with hemorrhagic disorder (D68.312)

D68.69 Other thrombophilia
Hypercoagulable states NEC
Secondary hypercoagulable state NOS

D68.8 Other specified coagulation defects
Excludes 1: hemorrhagic disease of newborn (P53)

D68.9 Coagulation defect, unspecified

D69- Purpura and other hemorrhagic conditions
Excludes 1: benign hypergammaglobulinemic purpura (D89.0)
cryoglobulinemic purpura (D89.1)
essential (hemorrhagic) thrombocythemia (D47.3)
hemorrhagic thrombocythemia (D47.3)
purpura fulminans (D65)
thrombotic thrombocytopenic purpura (M31.1)
Waldenström hypergammaglobulinemic purpura (D89.0)

D69.0 Allergic purpura
Allergic vasculitis
Nonthrombocytopenic hemorrhagic purpura
Nonthrombocytopenic idiopathic purpura
Purpura anaphylactoid
Purpura Henoch(-Schönlein)
Purpura rheumatica
Vascular purpura
Excludes 1: thrombocytopenic hemorrhagic purpura (D69.3)

D69.1 Qualitative platelet defects
Bernard-Soulier [giant platelet] syndrome
Glanzmann's disease
Grey platelet syndrome
Thromboasthenia (hemorrhagic) (hereditary)
Thrombocytopathy
Excludes 1: von Willebrand's disease (D68.0)

D69.2 Other nonthrombocytopenic purpura
Purpura NOS
Purpura simplex
Senile purpura

D69.3 Immune thrombocytopenic purpura
Hemorrhagic (thrombocytopenic) purpura
Idiopathic thrombocytopenic purpura
Tidal platelet dysgenesis

D69.4- Other primary thrombocytopenia
Excludes 1: transient neonatal thrombocytopenia (P61.0)
Wiskott-Aldrich syndrome (D82.0)

D69.41 Evans syndrome

D69.42 Congenital and hereditary thrombocytopenia purpura
Congenital thrombocytopenia
Hereditary thrombocytopenia
Code first congenital or hereditary disorder, such as:
Thrombocytopenia with absent radius (TAR syndrome) (Q87.2)

D69.49 Other primary thrombocytopenia
Megakaryocytic hypoplasia
Primary thrombocytopenia NOS

D61 - D69

D69.5- <u>Secondary</u> thrombocytopenia
   Excludes 1: *heparin induced thrombocytopenia (HIT) (D75.82)*
                     transient thrombocytopenia of newborn (P61.0)
   D69.51 <u>Posttransfusion</u> purpura
      Posttransfusion purpura from whole blood (fresh) or blood
         products
      PTP
   D69.59 **Other secondary thrombocytopenia**
D69.6 **Thrombocytopenia, unspecified**
D69.8 **Other specified hemorrhagic conditions**
      Capillary fragility (hereditary)
      Vascular pseudohemophilia
D69.9 **Hemorrhagic condition, unspecified**

Other disorders of blood and blood-forming organs (D70-D77)

D70- <u>Neutropenia</u>
   Includes: Agranulocytosis
                  Decreased absolute neurophile count (ANC)
   Use additional code for any associated:
      Fever (R50.81)
      Mucositis (J34.81, K12.3-, K92.81, N76.81)
   Excludes 1: *neutropenic splenomegaly (D73.81)*
                     transient neonatal neutropenia (P61.5)
   D70.0 <u>Congenital</u> agranulocytosis
      Congenital neutropenia
      Infantile genetic agranulocytosis
      Kostmann's disease
   D70.1 **Agranulocytosis <u>secondary</u> to cancer <u>chemotherapy</u>**
      Use additional code for adverse effect, if applicable, to identify drug
         (T45.1X5-)
      Code also underlying neoplasm
   D70.2 **Other <u>drug-induced</u> agranulocytosis**
      Use additional code for adverse effect, if applicable, to identify drug
         (T36-T50 with fifth or sixth character 5)
   D70.3 **Neutropenia due to <u>infection</u>**
   D70.4 <u>Cyclic</u> neutropenia
      Cyclic hematopoiesis
      Periodic neutropenia
   D70.8 **Other neutropenia**
   D70.9 **Neutropenia, unspecified**
D71 **Functional disorders of polymorphonuclear neutrophils**
      Cell membrane receptor complex [CR3] defect
      Chronic (childhood) granulomatous disease
      Congenital dysphagocytosis
      Progressive septic granulomatosis
D72- **Other disorders of <u>white blood cells</u>**
   Excludes 1: *basophilia (D72.824)*
                     immunity disorders (D80-D89)
                     neutropenia (D70)
                     preleukemia (syndrome) (D46.9)
   D72.0 **Genetic anomalies of leukocytes**
      Alder (granulation) (granulocyte) anomaly
      Alder syndrome
      Hereditary leukocytic hypersegmentation
      Hereditary leukocytic hyposegmentation
      Hereditary leukomelanopathy
      May-Hegglin (granulation) (granulocyte) anomaly
      May-Hegglin syndrome
      Pelger-Huët (granulation) (granulocyte) anomaly
      Pelger-Huët syndrome
   Excludes 1: *Chédiak (-Steinbrinck)-Higashi syndrome (E70.330)*
   D72.1 <u>Eosinophilia</u>
      Allergic eosinophilia
      Hereditary eosinophilia
   Excludes 1: *Löffler's syndrome (J82)*
                     pulmonary eosinophilia (J82)
   D72.8- Other specified disorders of white blood cells
   Excludes 1: *leukemia (C91-C95)*
      D72.81- Decreased white blood cell count
         Excludes 1: *neutropenia (D70.-)*
         D72.810 <u>Lymphocytopenia</u>
            Decreased lymphocytes
         D72.818 **Other decreased white blood cell count**
            Basophilic leukopenia
            Eosinophilic leukopenia
            Monocytopenia
            Other decreased leukocytes
            Plasmacytopenia

D72.819 **Decreased white blood cell count, unspecified**
      Decreased leukocytes, unspecified
      Leukocytopenia, unspecified
      Leukopenia
   Excludes 1: *malignant leukopenia (D70.9)*
D72.82- Elevated white blood cell count
   Excludes 1: *eosinophilia (D72.1)*
   D72.820 <u>Lymphocytosis</u> (symptomatic)
      Elevated lymphocytes
   D72.821 <u>Monocytosis</u> (symptomatic)
      Excludes 1: *infectious mononucleosis (B27.-)*
   D72.822 <u>Plasmacytosis</u>
   D72.823 <u>Leukemoid reaction</u>
      Basophilic leukemoid reaction
      Leukemoid reaction NOS
      Lymphocytic leukemoid reaction
      Monocytic leukemoid reaction
      Myelocytic leukemoid reaction
      Neutrophilic leukemoid reaction
   D72.824 <u>Basophilia</u>
   D72.825 <u>Bandemia</u>
      Bandemia without diagnosis of specific infection
      Excludes 1: *confirmed infection — code to infection*
                        leukemia (C91.-, C92.-, C93.-, C94.-, C95.-)
   D72.828 **Other elevated white blood cell count**
   D72.829 **Elevated white blood cell count, unspecified**
      Elevated leukocytes, unspecified
      Leukocytosis, unspecified
   D72.89 **Other specified disorders of white blood cells**
      Abnormality of white blood cells NEC
D72.9 **Disorder of white blood cells, unspecified**
      Abnormal leukocyte differential NOS
D73- **Diseases of <u>spleen</u>**
   D73.0 <u>Hyposplenism</u>
      Atrophy of spleen
      Excludes 1: *asplenia (congenital) (Q89.01)*
                        postsurgical absence of spleen (Z90.81)
   D73.1 <u>Hypersplenism</u>
      Excludes 1: *neutropenic splenomegaly (D73.81)*
                        primary splenic neutropenia (D73.81)
                        splenitis, splenomegaly in late syphilis (A52.79)
                        splenitis, splenomegaly in tuberculosis (A18.85)
                        splenomegaly NOS (R16.1)
                        splenomegaly congenital (Q89.0)
   D73.2 **Chronic <u>congestive</u> splenomegaly**
   D73.3 <u>Abscess</u> of spleen
   D73.4 <u>Cyst</u> of spleen
   D73.5 <u>Infarction</u> of spleen
      Splenic rupture, nontraumatic
      Torsion of spleen
      Excludes 1: *rupture of spleen due to Plasmodium vivax malaria*
                        (B51.0)
                        traumatic rupture of spleen (S36.03-)
   D73.8- Other diseases of spleen
      D73.81 **Neutropenic splenomegaly**
         Werner-Schultz disease
      D73.89 **Other diseases of spleen**
         Fibrosis of spleen NOS
         Perisplenitis
         Splenitis NOS
   D73.9 **Disease of spleen, unspecified**
D74- **Methemoglobinemia**
   D74.0 **Congenital methemoglobinemia**
      Congenital NADH-methemoglobin reductase deficiency
      Hemoglobin-M [Hb-M] disease
      Methemoglobinemia, hereditary
   D74.8 **Other methemoglobinemias**
      Acquired methemoglobinemia (with sulfhemoglobinemia)
      Toxic methemoglobinemia
   D74.9 **Methemoglobinemia, unspecified**

Excludes 1: = NOT CODED HERE! (Do not code both)

Excludes ❷: = Not Included Here

D75- Other and unspecified diseases of blood and blood-forming organs
   Excludes ❷: acute lymphadenitis (L04.-)
          chronic lymphadenitis (I88.1)
          enlarged lymph nodes (R59.-)
          hypergammaglobulinemia NOS (D89.2)
          lymphadenitis NOS (I88.9)
          mesenteric lymphadenitis (acute) (chronic) (I88.0)

   D75.0   Familial erythrocytosis
          Benign polycythemia
          Familial polycythemia
          Excludes 1: hereditary ovalocytosis (D58.1)

   D75.1   Secondary polycythemia
          Acquired polycythemia
          Emotional polycythemia
          Erythrocytosis NOS
          Hypoxemic polycythemia
          Nephrogenous polycythemia
          Polycythemia due to erythropoietin
          Polycythemia due to fall in plasma volume
          Polycythemia due to high altitude
          Polycythemia due to stress
          Polycythemia NOS
          Relative polycythemia
          Excludes 1: polycythemia neonatorum (P61.1)
                   polycythemia vera (D45)

   D75.8- Other specified diseases of blood and blood-forming organs
      D75.81 Myelofibrosis
             Myelofibrosis NOS
             Secondary myelofibrosis NOS
             Code first the underlying disorder, such as:
                Malignant neoplasm of breast (C50.-)
             Use additional code, if applicable, for associated therapy-related
                myelodysplastic syndrome (D46.-)
             Use additional code for adverse effect, if applicable, to identify
                drug (T45.1X5-)
             Excludes 1: acute myelofibrosis (C94.4-)
                      idiopathic myelofibrosis (D47.1)
                      leukoerythroblastic anemia (D61.82)
                      myelofibrosis with myeloid metaplasia (D47.4)
                      myelophthisic anemia (D61.82)
                      myelophthisis (D61.82)
                      primary myelofibrosis (D47.1)
      D75.82 Heparin induced thrombocytopenia (HIT)
      D75.89 Other specified diseases of blood and blood-forming organs
   D75.9   Disease of blood and blood-forming organs, unspecified

**D76- Other specified diseases with participation of lymphoreticular and
   reticulohistiocytic tissue**
   Excludes 1: (Abt-) Letterer-Siwe disease (C96.0)
          eosinophilic granuloma (C96.6)
          Hand-Schüller-Christian disease (C96.5)
          histiocytic sarcoma (C96.A)
          histiocytosis X, multifocal (C96.5)
          histiocytosis X, unifocal (C96.6)
          malignant histiocytosis (C96.A)
          Langerhans-cell histiocytosis, multifocal (C96.5)
          Langerhans-cell histiocytosis NOS (C96.6)
          Langerhans-cell histiocytosis, unifocal (C96.6)
          leukemic reticuloendotheliosis or reticulosis (C91.4-)
          lipomelanotic reticuloendotheliosis or reticulosis (I89.8)

   D76.1   Hemophagocytic lymphohistiocytosis
          Familial hemophagocytic reticulosis
          Histiocytoses of mononuclear phagocytes

   D76.2   Hemophagocytic syndrome, infection-associated
          Use additional code to identify infectious agent or disease.

   D76.3   Other histiocytosis syndromes
          Reticulohistiocytoma (giant-cell)
          Sinus histiocytosis with massive lymphadenopathy
          Xanthogranuloma

**D77   Other disorders of blood and blood-forming organs in diseases
   classified elsewhere**
          Code first underlying disease, such as:
             Amyloidosis (E85.-)
             Congenital early syphilis (A50.0)
             Echinococcosis (B67.0-B67.9)
             Malaria (B50.0-B54)
             Schistosomiasis [bilharziasis] (B65.0-B65.9)
             Vitamin C deficiency (E54)
          Excludes 1: rupture of spleen due to Plasmodium vivax malaria (B51.0)
                   splenitis, splenomegaly in late syphilis (A52.79)
                   splenitis, splenomegaly in tuberculosis (A18.85)

Intraoperative and postprocedural complications of the spleen (D78)

D78- Intraoperative and postprocedural complications of the spleen
   **D78.0- Intraoperative hemorrhage and hematoma of the spleen
      complicating a procedure**
          *Excludes 1: intraoperative hemorrhage and hematoma of the spleen
                   due to accidental puncture or laceration during a
                   procedure (D78.1-)*
      **D78.01 Intraoperative hemorrhage and hematoma of the spleen
             complicating a procedure on the spleen**
      **D78.02 Intraoperative hemorrhage and hematoma of the spleen
             complicating other procedure**
   **D78.1- Accidental puncture and laceration of the spleen during a
      procedure**
      **D78.11 Accidental puncture and laceration of the spleen during a
             procedure on the spleen**
      **D78.12 Accidental puncture and laceration of the spleen during
             other procedure**
   **D78.2- Postprocedural hemorrhage and hematoma of the spleen
      following a procedure**
      **D78.21 Postprocedural hemorrhage and hematoma of the spleen
             following a procedure on the spleen**
      **D78.22 Postprocedural hemorrhage and hematoma of the spleen
             following other procedure**
   **D78.8- Other intraoperative and postprocedural complications of the
      spleen**
          Use additional code, if applicable, to further specify disorder
      D78.81 Other intraoperative complications of the spleen
      D78.89 Other postprocedural complications of the spleen

Certain disorders involving the immune mechanism (D80-D89)

   Includes: Defects in the complement system
          Immunodeficiency disorders, except human immunodeficiency
             virus [HIV] disease
          Sarcoidosis
   Excludes 1: autoimmune disease (systemic) NOS (M35.9)
          functional disorders of polymorphonuclear neutrophils (D71)
          human immunodeficiency virus [HIV] disease (B20)

D80- Immunodeficiency with predominantly antibody defects
   D80.0   Hereditary hypogammaglobulinemia
          Autosomal recessive agammaglobulinemia (Swiss type)
          X-linked agammaglobulinemia [Bruton] (with growth hormone
             deficiency)
   D80.1   Nonfamilial hypogammaglobulinemia
          Agammaglobulinemia with immunoglobulin-bearing B-
             lymphocytes
          Common variable agammaglobulinemia [CVAgamma]
          Hypogammaglobulinemia NOS
   D80.2   Selective deficiency of immunoglobulin A [IgA]
   D80.3   Selective deficiency of immunoglobulin G [IgG] subclasses
   D80.4   Selective deficiency of immunoglobulin M [IgM]
   D80.5   Immunodeficiency with increased immunoglobulin M [IgM]
   **D80.6   Antibody deficiency with near-normal immunoglobulins or with
      hyperimmunoglobulinemia**
   D80.7   Transient hypogammaglobulinemia of infancy
   D80.8   Other immunodeficiencies with predominantly antibody defects
          Kappa light chain deficiency
   **D80.9   Immunodeficiency with predominantly antibody defects,
      unspecified**

D81- Combined immunodeficiencies
   *Excludes 1: autosomal recessive agammaglobulinemia (Swiss type)
             (D80.0)*
   **D81.0   Severe combined immunodeficiency [SCID] with reticular
      dysgenesis**
   **D81.1   Severe combined immunodeficiency [SCID] with low T- and B-
      cell numbers**
   **D81.2   Severe combined immunodeficiency [SCID] with low or normal
      B-cell numbers**
   D81.3   Adenosine deaminase [ADA] deficiency
   D81.4   Nezelof's syndrome
   D81.5   Purine nucleoside phosphorylase [PNP] deficiency
   D81.6   Major histocompatibility complex class I deficiency
          Bare lymphocyte syndrome
   D81.7   Major histocompatibility complex class II deficiency

**D
6
9
–
D
8
1**

© 2013 Channel Publishing, Ltd.

D81.8- **Other combined immunodeficiencies**
    D81.81- **Biotin-dependent carboxylase deficiency**
        Multiple carboxylase deficiency
        Excludes 1: biotin-dependent carboxylase deficiency due to
                dietary deficiency of biotin (E53.8)
        D81.810   **Biotinidase deficiency**
        D81.818   **Other biotin-dependent carboxylase deficiency**
                 Holocarboxylase synthetase deficiency
                 Other multiple carboxylase deficiency
        D81.819   **Biotin-dependent carboxylase deficiency, unspecified**
                 Multiple carboxylase deficiency, unspecified
    D81.89 **Other combined immunodeficiencies**
D81.9   **Combined immunodeficiency, unspecified**
      Severe combined immunodeficiency disorder [SCID] NOS

D82- **Immunodeficiency** associated with other **major defects**
    Excludes 1: ataxia telangiectasia [Louis-Bar] (G11.3)
    D82.0 **Wiskott-Aldrich syndrome**
        Immunodeficiency with thrombocytopenia and eczema
    D82.1 **Di George's syndrome**
        Pharyngeal pouch syndrome
        Thymic alymphoplasia
        Thymic aplasia or hypoplasia with immunodeficiency
    D82.2 **Immunodeficiency with short-limbed stature**
    D82.3 **Immunodeficiency following hereditary defective response to Epstein-Barr virus**
        X-linked lymphoproliferative disease
    D82.4 **Hyperimmunoglobulin E [IgE] syndrome**
    D82.8 **Immunodeficiency associated with other specified major defects**
    D82.9 **Immunodeficiency associated with major defect, unspecified**

D83- **Common variable** immunodeficiency
    D83.0 **Common variable immunodeficiency with predominant abnormalities of B-cell numbers and function**
    D83.1 **Common variable immunodeficiency with predominant immunoregulatory T-cell disorders**
    D83.2 **Common variable immunodeficiency with autoantibodies to B- or T-cells**
    D83.8 **Other common variable immunodeficiencies**
    D83.9 **Common variable immunodeficiency, unspecified**

D84- **Other** immunodeficiencies
    D84.0 **Lymphocyte function antigen-1 [LFA-1] defect**
    D84.1 **Defects in the complement system**
        C1 esterase inhibitor [C1-INH] deficiency
    D84.8 **Other specified immunodeficiencies**
    D84.9 **Immunodeficiency, unspecified**

D86- **Sarcoidosis**
    D86.0 **Sarcoidosis of lung**
    D86.1 **Sarcoidosis of lymph nodes**
    D86.2 **Sarcoidosis of lung with sarcoidosis of lymph nodes**
    D86.3 **Sarcoidosis of skin**
    D86.8- **Sarcoidosis of other sites**
        D86.81 **Sarcoid meningitis**
        D86.82 **Multiple cranial nerve palsies in sarcoidosis**
        D86.83 **Sarcoid iridocyclitis**
        D86.84 **Sarcoid pyelonephritis**
            Tubulo-interstitial nephropathy in sarcoidosis
        D86.85 **Sarcoid myocarditis**
        D86.86 **Sarcoid arthropathy**
            Polyarthritis in sarcoidosis
        D86.87 **Sarcoid myositis**
        D86.89 **Sarcoidosis of other sites**
            Hepatic granuloma
            Uveoparotid fever [Heerfordt]
    D86.9 **Sarcoidosis, unspecified**

D89- **Other disorders involving the immune mechanism, not elsewhere classified**
    Excludes 1: hyperglobulinemia NOS (R77.1)
                    monoclonal gammopathy (of undetermined significance)
                      (D47.2)
    Excludes ❷: transplant failure and rejection (T86.-)
    D89.0 **Polyclonal hypergammaglobulinemia**
        Benign hypergammaglobulinemic purpura
        Polyclonal gammopathy NOS
    D89.1 **Cryoglobulinemia**
        Cryoglobulinemic purpura
        Cryoglobulinemic vasculitis
        Essential cryoglobulinemia
        Idiopathic cryoglobulinemia
        Mixed cryoglobulinemia
        Primary cryoglobulinemia
        Secondary cryoglobulinemia
    D89.2 **Hypergammaglobulinemia, unspecified**
    D89.3 **Immune reconstitution syndrome**
        Immune reconstitution inflammatory syndrome [IRIS]
        Use additional code for adverse effect, if applicable, to identify drug (T36-T50 with fifth or sixth character 5)
    D89.8- **Other specified disorders involving the immune mechanism, not elsewhere classified**
        D89.81- **Graft-versus-host disease**
            Code first underlying cause, such as:
                Complications of transplanted organs and tissue (T86.-)
                Complications of blood transfusion (T80.89)
            Use additional code to identify associated manifestations, such as:
                Desquamative dermatitis (L30.8)
                Diarrhea (R19.7)
                Elevated bilirubin (R17)
                Hair loss (L65.9)
            D89.810   **Acute** graft-versus-host disease
            D89.811   **Chronic** graft-versus-host disease
            D89.812   **Acute on chronic** graft-versus-host disease
            D89.813   **Graft-versus-host disease, unspecified**
        D89.82 **Autoimmune lymphoproliferative syndrome [ALPS]**
        D89.89 **Other specified disorders involving the immune mechanism, not elsewhere classified**
            Excludes 1: human immunodeficiency virus disease (B20)
    D89.9 **Disorder involving the immune mechanism, unspecified**
        Immune disease NOS

D 8 1 ▪ E 0 6

Chapter 4 – Endocrine, nutritional and metabolic diseases (E00-E89)

Note: All neoplasms, whether functionally active or not, are classified in Chapter 2. Appropriate codes in this chapter (i.e. E05.8, E07.0, E16-E31, E34.-) may be used as additional codes to indicate either functional activity by neoplasms and ectopic endocrine tissue or hyperfunction and hypofunction of endocrine glands associated with neoplasms and other conditions classified elsewhere.

Excludes 1: transitory endocrine and metabolic disorders specific to newborn (P70-P74)

This chapter contains the following blocks:

E00-E07	Disorders of thyroid gland
E08-E13	Diabetes mellitus
E15-E16	Other disorders of glucose regulation and pancreatic internal secretion
E20-E35	Disorders of other endocrine glands
E36	Intraoperative complications of endocrine system
E40-E46	Malnutrition
E50-E64	Other nutritional deficiencies
E65-E68	Overweight, obesity and other hyperalimentation
E70-E88	Metabolic disorders
E89	Postprocedural endocrine and metabolic complications and disorders, not elsewhere classified

Disorders of thyroid gland (E00-E07)

E00- Congenital iodine-deficiency syndrome
Use additional code (F70-F79) to identify associated intellectual disabilities.
Excludes 1: subclinical iodine-deficiency hypothyroidism (E02)

E00.0 Congenital iodine-deficiency syndrome, neurological type
Endemic cretinism, neurological type

E00.1 Congenital iodine-deficiency syndrome, myxedematous type
Endemic hypothyroid cretinism
Endemic cretinism, myxedematous type

E00.2 Congenital iodine-deficiency syndrome, mixed type
Endemic cretinism, mixed type

E00.9 Congenital iodine-deficiency syndrome, unspecified
Congenital iodine-deficiency hypothyroidism NOS
Endemic cretinism NOS

E01- Iodine-deficiency related thyroid disorders and allied conditions
Excludes 1: congenital iodine-deficiency syndrome (E00.-)
subclinical iodine-deficiency hypothyroidism (E02)

E01.0 Iodine-deficiency related diffuse (endemic) goiter

E01.1 Iodine-deficiency related multinodular (endemic) goiter
Iodine-deficiency related nodular goiter

E01.2 Iodine-deficiency related (endemic) goiter, unspecified
Endemic goiter NOS

E01.8 Other iodine-deficiency related thyroid disorders and allied conditions
Acquired iodine-deficiency hypothyroidism NOS

E02 Subclinical iodine-deficiency hypothyroidism

E03- Other hypothyroidism
Excludes 1: iodine-deficiency related hypothyroidism (E00-E02)
postprocedural hypothyroidism (E89.0)

E03.0 Congenital hypothyroidism with diffuse goiter
Congenital parenchymatous goiter (nontoxic)
Congenital goiter (nontoxic) NOS
Excludes 1: transitory congenital goiter with normal function (P72.0)

E03.1 Congenital hypothyroidism without goiter
Aplasia of thyroid (with myxedema)
Congenital atrophy of thyroid
Congenital hypothyroidism NOS

E03.2 Hypothyroidism due to medicaments and other exogenous substances
Code first poisoning due to drug or toxin, if applicable (T36-T65 with fifth or sixth character 1-4 or 6)
Use additional code for adverse effect, if applicable, to identify drug (T36-T50 with fifth or sixth character 5)

E03.3 Postinfectious hypothyroidism

E03.4 Atrophy of thyroid (acquired)
Excludes 1: congenital atrophy of thyroid (E03.1)

E03.5 Myxedema coma

E03.8 Other specified hypothyroidism

E03.9 Hypothyroidism, unspecified
Myxedema NOS

E04- Other nontoxic goiter
Excludes 1: congenital goiter (NOS) (diffuse) (parenchymatous) (E03.0)
iodine-deficiency related goiter (E00-E02)

E04.0 Nontoxic diffuse goiter
Diffuse (colloid) nontoxic goiter
Simple nontoxic goiter

E04.1 Nontoxic single thyroid nodule
Colloid nodule (cystic) (thyroid)
Nontoxic uninodular goiter
Thyroid (cystic) nodule NOS

E04.2 Nontoxic multinodular goiter
Cystic goiter NOS
Multinodular (cystic) goiter NOS

E04.8 Other specified nontoxic goiter

E04.9 Nontoxic goiter, unspecified
Goiter NOS
Nodular goiter (nontoxic) NOS

E05- Thyrotoxicosis [hyperthyroidism]
Excludes 1: chronic thyroiditis with transient thyrotoxicosis (E06.2)
neonatal thyrotoxicosis (P72.1)

E05.0- Thyrotoxicosis with diffuse goiter
Exophthalmic or toxic goiter NOS
Graves' disease
Toxic diffuse goiter

E05.00 Thyrotoxicosis with diffuse goiter without thyrotoxic crisis or storm

E05.01 Thyrotoxicosis with diffuse goiter with thyrotoxic crisis or storm

E05.1- Thyrotoxicosis with toxic single thyroid nodule
Thyrotoxicosis with toxic uninodular goiter

E05.10 Thyrotoxicosis with toxic single thyroid nodule without thyrotoxic crisis or storm

E05.11 Thyrotoxicosis with toxic single thyroid nodule with thyrotoxic crisis or storm

E05.2- Thyrotoxicosis with toxic multinodular goiter
Toxic nodular goiter NOS

E05.20 Thyrotoxicosis with toxic multinodular goiter without thyrotoxic crisis or storm

E05.21 Thyrotoxicosis with toxic multinodular goiter with thyrotoxic crisis or storm

E05.3- Thyrotoxicosis from ectopic thyroid tissue

E05.30 Thyrotoxicosis from ectopic thyroid tissue without thyrotoxic crisis or storm

E05.31 Thyrotoxicosis from ectopic thyroid tissue with thyrotoxic crisis or storm

E05.4- Thyrotoxicosis factitia

E05.40 Thyrotoxicosis factitia without thyrotoxic crisis or storm

E05.41 Thyrotoxicosis factitia with thyrotoxic crisis or storm

E05.8- Other thyrotoxicosis
Overproduction of thyroid-stimulating hormone

E05.80 Other thyrotoxicosis without thyrotoxic crisis or storm

E05.81 Other thyrotoxicosis with thyrotoxic crisis or storm

E05.9- Thyrotoxicosis, unspecified
Hyperthyroidism NOS

E05.90 Thyrotoxicosis, unspecified without thyrotoxic crisis or storm

E05.91 Thyrotoxicosis, unspecified with thyrotoxic crisis or storm

E06- Thyroiditis
Excludes 1: postpartum thyroiditis (O90.5)

E06.0 Acute thyroiditis
Abscess of thyroid
Pyogenic thyroiditis
Suppurative thyroiditis
Use additional code (B95-B97) to identify infectious agent.

E06.1 Subacute thyroiditis
de Quervain thyroiditis
Giant-cell thyroiditis
Granulomatous thyroiditis
Nonsuppurative thyroiditis
Viral thyroiditis
Excludes 1: autoimmune thyroiditis (E06.3)

E06.2 Chronic thyroiditis with transient thyrotoxicosis
Excludes 1: autoimmune thyroiditis (E06.3)

E06.3 Autoimmune thyroiditis
Hashimoto's thyroiditis
Hashitoxicosis (transient)
Lymphadenoid goiter
Lymphocytic thyroiditis
Struma lymphatosa

D 8 1 - E 0 6

E06.4 **Drug-induced** thyroiditis
Use additional code for adverse effect, if applicable, to identify drug (T36-T50 with fifth or sixth character 5)

E06.5 **Other chronic thyroiditis**
Chronic fibrous thyroiditis
Chronic thyroiditis NOS
Ligneous thyroiditis
Riedel thyroiditis

E06.9 **Thyroiditis, unspecified**

E07- Other disorders of thyroid
E07.0 **Hypersecretion of calcitonin**
C-cell hyperplasia of thyroid
Hypersecretion of thyrocalcitonin

E07.1 **Dyshormogenetic goiter**
Familial dyshormogenetic goiter
Pendred's syndrome
Excludes 1: transitory congenital goiter with normal function (P72.0)

E07.8- **Other specified disorders of thyroid**
E07.81 **Sick-euthyroid syndrome**
Euthyroid sick-syndrome

E07.89 **Other specified disorders of thyroid**
Abnormality of thyroid-binding globulin
Hemorrhage of thyroid
Infarction of thyroid

E07.9 **Disorder of thyroid, unspecified**

Diabetes mellitus (E08-E13)

E08- **Diabetes mellitus due to underlying condition**
Code first the underlying condition, such as:
Congenital rubella (P35.0)
Cushing's syndrome (E24.-)
Cystic fibrosis (E84.-)
Malignant neoplasm (C00-C96)
Malnutrition (E40-E46)
Pancreatitis and other diseases of the pancreas (K85-, K86-)
Use additional code to identify any insulin use (Z79.4)
Excludes 1: drug or chemical induced diabetes mellitus (E09-)
gestational diabetes (O24.4-)
neonatal diabetes mellitus (P70.2)
postpancreatectomy diabetes mellitus (E13-)
postprocedural diabetes mellitus (E13-)
secondary diabetes mellitus NEC (E13-)
type 1 diabetes mellitus (E10-)
type 2 diabetes mellitus (E11-)

E08.0- **Diabetes mellitus due to underlying condition with hyperosmolarity**
E08.00 **Diabetes mellitus due to underlying condition with hyperosmolarity without nonketotic hyperglycemic-hyperosmolar coma (NKHHC)**
E08.01 **Diabetes mellitus due to underlying condition with hyperosmolarity with coma**

E08.1- **Diabetes mellitus due to underlying condition with ketoacidosis**
E08.10 **Diabetes mellitus due to underlying condition with ketoacidosis without coma**
E08.11 **Diabetes mellitus due to underlying condition with ketoacidosis with coma**

E08.2- **Diabetes mellitus due to underlying condition with kidney complications**
E08.21 **Diabetes mellitus due to underlying condition with diabetic nephropathy**
Diabetes mellitus due to underlying condition with intercapillary glomerulosclerosis
Diabetes mellitus due to underlying condition with intracapillary glomerulonephrosis
Diabetes mellitus due to underlying condition with Kimmelstiel-Wilson disease
E08.22 **Diabetes mellitus due to underlying condition with diabetic chronic kidney disease**
Use additional code to identify stage of chronic kidney disease (N18.1-N18.6)
E08.29 **Diabetes mellitus due to underlying condition with other diabetic kidney complication**
Renal tubular degeneration in diabetes mellitus due to underlying condition

E08.3- **Diabetes mellitus due to underlying condition with ophthalmic complications**
E08.31- Diabetes mellitus due to underlying condition with unspecified diabetic retinopathy
E08.311 Diabetes mellitus due to underlying condition with unspecified diabetic retinopathy with macular edema
E08.319 Diabetes mellitus due to underlying condition with unspecified diabetic retinopathy without macular edema
E08.32- Diabetes mellitus due to underlying condition with mild nonproliferative diabetic retinopathy
Diabetes mellitus due to underlying condition with nonproliferative diabetic retinopathy NOS
E08.321 Diabetes mellitus due to underlying condition with mild nonproliferative diabetic retinopathy with macular edema
E08.329 Diabetes mellitus due to underlying condition with mild nonproliferative diabetic retinopathy without macular edema
E08.33- Diabetes mellitus due to underlying condition with moderate nonproliferative diabetic retinopathy
E08.331 Diabetes mellitus due to underlying condition with moderate nonproliferative diabetic retinopathy with macular edema
E08.339 Diabetes mellitus due to underlying condition with moderate nonproliferative diabetic retinopathy without macular edema
E08.34- Diabetes mellitus due to underlying condition with severe nonproliferative diabetic retinopathy
E08.341 Diabetes mellitus due to underlying condition with severe nonproliferative diabetic retinopathy with macular edema
E08.349 Diabetes mellitus due to underlying condition with severe nonproliferative diabetic retinopathy without macular edema
E08.35- Diabetes mellitus due to underlying condition with proliferative diabetic retinopathy
E08.351 Diabetes mellitus due to underlying condition with proliferative diabetic retinopathy with macular edema
E08.359 Diabetes mellitus due to underlying condition with proliferative diabetic retinopathy without macular edema
E08.36 Diabetes mellitus due to underlying condition with diabetic cataract
E08.39 Diabetes mellitus due to underlying condition with other diabetic ophthalmic complication
Use additional code to identify manifestation, such as:
Diabetic glaucoma (H40-H42)

E08.4- **Diabetes mellitus due to underlying condition with neurological complications**
E08.40 Diabetes mellitus due to underlying condition with diabetic neuropathy, unspecified
E08.41 Diabetes mellitus due to underlying condition with diabetic mononeuropathy
E08.42 Diabetes mellitus due to underlying condition with diabetic polyneuropathy
Diabetes mellitus due to underlying condition with diabetic neuralgia
E08.43 Diabetes mellitus due to underlying condition with diabetic autonomic (poly)neuropathy
Diabetes mellitus due to underlying condition with diabetic gastroparesis
E08.44 Diabetes mellitus due to underlying condition with diabetic amyotrophy
E08.49 Diabetes mellitus due to underlying condition with other diabetic neurological complication

E08.5- **Diabetes mellitus due to underlying condition with circulatory complications**
E08.51 Diabetes mellitus due to underlying condition with diabetic peripheral angiopathy without gangrene
E08.52 Diabetes mellitus due to underlying condition with diabetic peripheral angiopathy with gangrene
Diabetes mellitus due to underlying condition with diabetic gangrene
E08.59 Diabetes mellitus due to underlying condition with other circulatory complications

E
0
6
-
E
0
9

E08.6- **Diabetes mellitus due to <u>underlying condition</u> with other specified complications**

    E08.61- Diabetes mellitus due to underlying condition with diabetic <u>arthropathy</u>

        E08.610 **Diabetes mellitus due to underlying condition with diabetic <u>neuropathic</u> arthropathy**
            Diabetes mellitus due to underlying condition with Charcôt's joints

        E08.618 **Diabetes mellitus due to underlying condition with other diabetic arthropathy**

    E08.62- Diabetes mellitus due to underlying condition with <u>skin</u> complications

        E08.620 **Diabetes mellitus due to underlying condition with diabetic <u>dermatitis</u>**
            Diabetes mellitus due to underlying condition with diabetic necrobiosis lipoidica

        E08.621 **Diabetes mellitus due to underlying condition with <u>foot ulcer</u>**
            Use additional code to identify site of ulcer (L97.4-, L97.5-)

        E08.622 **Diabetes mellitus due to underlying condition with <u>other skin ulcer</u>**
            Use additional code to identify site of ulcer (L97.1-L97.9, L98.41-L98.49)

        E08.628 **Diabetes mellitus due to underlying condition with other skin complications**

    E08.63- Diabetes mellitus due to underlying condition with <u>oral</u> complications

        E08.630 **Diabetes mellitus due to underlying condition with periodontal disease**

        E08.638 **Diabetes mellitus due to underlying condition with other oral complications**

    E08.64- Diabetes mellitus due to underlying condition with <u>hypoglycemia</u>

        E08.641 **Diabetes mellitus due to underlying condition with hypoglycemia <u>with coma</u>**

        E08.649 **Diabetes mellitus due to underlying condition with hypoglycemia <u>without</u> coma**

    E08.65 **Diabetes mellitus due to underlying condition with <u>hyperglycemia</u>**

    E08.69 **Diabetes mellitus due to underlying condition with <u>other specified</u> complication**
        Use additional code to identify complication

E08.8 **Diabetes mellitus due to <u>underlying condition</u> with <u>unspecified</u> complications**

E08.9 **Diabetes mellitus due to <u>underlying condition</u> <u>without</u> complications**

E09- **<u>Drug or chemical induced</u> diabetes mellitus**
    Code first poisoning due to drug or toxin, if applicable (T36-T65 with fifth or sixth character 1-4 or 6)
    Use additional code for adverse effect, if applicable, to identify drug (T36-T50 with fifth or sixth character 5)
    Use additional code to identify any insulin use (Z79.4)
    Excludes 1: diabetes mellitus due to underlying condition (E08.-)
            gestational diabetes (O24.4-)
            neonatal diabetes mellitus (P70.2)
            postpancreatectomy diabetes mellitus (E13.-)
            postprocedural diabetes mellitus (E13.-)
            secondary diabetes mellitus NEC (E13.-)
            type 1 diabetes mellitus (E10.-)
            type 2 diabetes mellitus (E11.-)

    E09.0- **<u>Drug or chemical induced</u> diabetes mellitus with <u>hyperosmolarity</u>**

        E09.00 **Drug or chemical induced diabetes mellitus with hyperosmolarity <u>without</u> nonketotic hyperglycemic-hyperosmolar coma (NKHHC)**

        E09.01 **Drug or chemical induced diabetes mellitus with hyperosmolarity <u>with coma</u>**

    E09.1- **<u>Drug or chemical induced</u> diabetes mellitus with <u>ketoacidosis</u>**

        E09.10 **Drug or chemical induced diabetes mellitus with ketoacidosis <u>without</u> coma**

        E09.11 **Drug or chemical induced diabetes mellitus with ketoacidosis <u>with coma</u>**

    E09.2- **<u>Drug or chemical induced</u> diabetes mellitus with <u>kidney</u> complications**

        E09.21 **Drug or chemical induced diabetes mellitus with diabetic <u>nephropathy</u>**
            Drug or chemical induced diabetes mellitus with intercapillary glomerulosclerosis
            Drug or chemical induced diabetes mellitus with intracapillary glomerulonephrosis
            Drug or chemical induced diabetes mellitus with Kimmelstiel-Wilson disease

        E09.22 **Drug or chemical induced diabetes mellitus with diabetic <u>chronic kidney disease</u>**
            Use additional code to identify stage of chronic kidney disease (N18.1-N18.6)

        E09.29 **Drug or chemical induced diabetes mellitus with other diabetic kidney complication**
            Drug or chemical induced diabetes mellitus with renal tubular degeneration

E09.3- **<u>Drug or chemical induced</u> diabetes mellitus with ophthalmic complications**

    E09.31- Drug or chemical induced diabetes mellitus with <u>unspecified</u> diabetic retinopathy

        E09.311 **Drug or chemical induced diabetes mellitus with unspecified diabetic retinopathy <u>with macular edema</u>**

        E09.319 **Drug or chemical induced diabetes mellitus with unspecified diabetic retinopathy <u>without</u> macular edema**

    E09.32- Drug or chemical induced diabetes mellitus with <u>mild nonproliferative</u> diabetic retinopathy
        Drug or chemical induced diabetes mellitus with nonproliferative diabetic retinopathy NOS

        E09.321 **Drug or chemical induced diabetes mellitus with mild nonproliferative diabetic retinopathy <u>with macular edema</u>**

        E09.329 **Drug or chemical induced diabetes mellitus with mild nonproliferative diabetic retinopathy <u>without</u> macular edema**

    E09.33- Drug or chemical induced diabetes mellitus with <u>moderate nonproliferative</u> diabetic retinopathy

        E09.331 **Drug or chemical induced diabetes mellitus with moderate nonproliferative diabetic retinopathy <u>with macular edema</u>**

        E09.339 **Drug or chemical induced diabetes mellitus with moderate nonproliferative diabetic retinopathy <u>without</u> macular edema**

    E09.34- Drug or chemical induced diabetes mellitus with <u>severe nonproliferative</u> diabetic retinopathy

        E09.341 **Drug or chemical induced diabetes mellitus with severe nonproliferative diabetic retinopathy <u>with macular edema</u>**

        E09.349 **Drug or chemical induced diabetes mellitus with severe nonproliferative diabetic retinopathy <u>without</u> macular edema**

    E09.35- Drug or chemical induced diabetes mellitus with <u>proliferative</u> diabetic retinopathy

        E09.351 **Drug or chemical induced diabetes mellitus with proliferative diabetic retinopathy <u>with macular edema</u>**

        E09.359 **Drug or chemical induced diabetes mellitus with proliferative diabetic retinopathy <u>without</u> macular edema**

    E09.36 **Drug or chemical induced diabetes mellitus with diabetic <u>cataract</u>**

    E09.39 **Drug or chemical induced diabetes mellitus with other diabetic <u>ophthalmic complication</u>**
        Use additional code to identify manifestation, such as:
        Diabetic glaucoma (H40-H42)

E09.4- **<u>Drug or chemical induced</u> diabetes mellitus with <u>neurological</u> complications**

    E09.40 **Drug or chemical induced diabetes mellitus with neurological complications with diabetic <u>neuropathy, unspecified</u>**

    E09.41 **Drug or chemical induced diabetes mellitus with neurological complications with diabetic mononeuropathy**

    E09.42 **Drug or chemical induced diabetes mellitus with neurological complications with diabetic polyneuropathy**
        Drug or chemical induced diabetes mellitus with diabetic neuralgia

    E09.43 **Drug or chemical induced diabetes mellitus with neurological complications with diabetic <u>autonomic</u> (poly)neuropathy**
        Drug or chemical induced diabetes mellitus with diabetic gastroparesis

    E09.44 **Drug or chemical induced diabetes mellitus with neurological complications with diabetic <u>amyotrophy</u>**

    E09.49 **Drug or chemical induced diabetes mellitus with neurological complications with other diabetic neurological complication**

E 0 6 – E 0 9

Excludes 1: = NOT CODED HERE! (Do not code both)

Excludes ❷: = Not Included Here

E09.5- <u>Drug or chemical induced</u> diabetes mellitus with <u>circulatory</u> complications

  E09.51 Drug or chemical induced diabetes mellitus with <u>diabetic peripheral angiopathy without</u> gangrene

  E09.52 Drug or chemical induced diabetes mellitus with <u>diabetic peripheral angiopathy with gangrene</u>
    Drug or chemical induced diabetes mellitus with diabetic gangrene

  E09.59 Drug or chemical induced diabetes mellitus with other circulatory complications

E09.6- <u>Drug or chemical induced</u> diabetes mellitus with other specified complications

  E09.61- Drug or chemical induced diabetes mellitus with diabetic <u>arthropathy</u>

    E09.610 Drug or chemical induced diabetes mellitus with diabetic <u>neuropathic</u> arthropathy
      Drug or chemical induced diabetes mellitus with Charcôt's joints

    E09.618 Drug or chemical induced diabetes mellitus with other diabetic arthropathy

  E09.62- Drug or chemical induced diabetes mellitus with <u>skin</u> complications

    E09.620 Drug or chemical induced diabetes mellitus with diabetic <u>dermatitis</u>
      Drug or chemical induced diabetes mellitus with diabetic necrobiosis lipoidica

    E09.621 Drug or chemical induced diabetes mellitus with <u>foot ulcer</u>
      Use additional code to identify site of ulcer (L97.4-, L97.5-)

    E09.622 Drug or chemical induced diabetes mellitus with <u>other skin ulcer</u>
      Use additional code to identify site of ulcer (L97.1-L97.9, L98.41-L98.49)

    E09.628 Drug or chemical induced diabetes mellitus with other skin complications

  E09.63- Drug or chemical induced diabetes mellitus with <u>oral</u> complications

    E09.630 Drug or chemical induced diabetes mellitus with periodontal disease

    E09.638 Drug or chemical induced diabetes mellitus with other oral complications

  E09.64- Drug or chemical induced diabetes mellitus with <u>hypoglycemia</u>

    E09.641 Drug or chemical induced diabetes mellitus with hypoglycemia <u>with coma</u>

    E09.649 Drug or chemical induced diabetes mellitus with hypoglycemia <u>without</u> coma

  E09.65 Drug or chemical induced diabetes mellitus with <u>hyperglycemia</u>

  E09.69 Drug or chemical induced diabetes mellitus with <u>other specified</u> complication
    Use additional code to identify complication

E09.8 <u>Drug or chemical induced</u> diabetes mellitus with <u>unspecified</u> complications

E09.9 <u>Drug or chemical induced</u> diabetes mellitus <u>without</u> complications

E10- <u>Type 1</u> diabetes mellitus
  Includes: Brittle diabetes (mellitus)
    Diabetes (mellitus) due to autoimmune process
    Diabetes (mellitus) due to immune mediated pancreatic islet beta-cell destruction
    Idiopathic diabetes (mellitus)
    Juvenile onset diabetes (mellitus)
    Ketosis-prone diabetes (mellitus)
  Excludes 1: diabetes mellitus due to underlying condition (E08.-)
    drug or chemical induced diabetes mellitus (E09.-)
    gestational diabetes (O24.4-)
    hyperglycemia NOS (R73.9)
    neonatal diabetes mellitus (P70.2)
    postpancreatectomy diabetes mellitus (E13.-)
    postprocedural diabetes mellitus (E13.-)
    secondary diabetes mellitus NEC (E13.-)
    type 2 diabetes mellitus (E11.-)

E10.1- <u>Type 1</u> diabetes mellitus with <u>ketoacidosis</u>

  E10.10 <u>Type 1</u> diabetes mellitus with ketoacidosis <u>without</u> coma

  E10.11 <u>Type 1</u> diabetes mellitus with ketoacidosis <u>with coma</u>

E10.2- <u>Type 1</u> diabetes mellitus with <u>kidney</u> complications

  E10.21 <u>Type 1</u> diabetes mellitus with diabetic <u>nephropathy</u>
    Type 1 diabetes mellitus with intercapillary glomerulosclerosis
    Type 1 diabetes mellitus with intracapillary glomerulonephrosis
    Type 1 diabetes mellitus with Kimmelstiel-Wilson disease

  E10.22 <u>Type 1</u> diabetes mellitus with diabetic <u>chronic kidney disease</u>
    Use additional code to identify stage of chronic kidney disease (N18.1-N18.6)

  E10.29 <u>Type 1</u> diabetes mellitus with other diabetic kidney complication
    Type 1 diabetes mellitus with renal tubular degeneration

E10.3- <u>Type 1</u> diabetes mellitus with <u>ophthalmic</u> complications

  E10.31- <u>Type 1</u> diabetes mellitus with <u>unspecified</u> diabetic retinopathy

    E10.311 <u>Type 1</u> diabetes mellitus with unspecified diabetic retinopathy <u>with macular edema</u>

    E10.319 <u>Type 1</u> diabetes mellitus with unspecified diabetic retinopathy <u>without</u> macular edema

  E10.32- <u>Type 1</u> diabetes mellitus with <u>mild nonproliferative</u> diabetic retinopathy
    Type 1 diabetes mellitus with nonproliferative diabetic retinopathy NOS

    E10.321 <u>Type 1</u> diabetes mellitus with mild nonproliferative diabetic retinopathy <u>with macular edema</u>

    E10.329 <u>Type 1</u> diabetes mellitus with mild nonproliferative diabetic retinopathy <u>without</u> macular edema

  E10.33- <u>Type 1</u> diabetes mellitus with <u>moderate nonproliferative</u> diabetic retinopathy

    E10.331 <u>Type 1</u> diabetes mellitus with moderate nonproliferative diabetic retinopathy <u>with macular edema</u>

    E10.339 <u>Type 1</u> diabetes mellitus with moderate nonproliferative diabetic retinopathy <u>without</u> macular edema

  E10.34- <u>Type 1</u> diabetes mellitus with <u>severe nonproliferative</u> diabetic retinopathy

    E10.341 <u>Type 1</u> diabetes mellitus with severe nonproliferative diabetic retinopathy <u>with macular edema</u>

    E10.349 <u>Type 1</u> diabetes mellitus with severe nonproliferative diabetic retinopathy <u>without</u> macular edema

  E10.35- <u>Type 1</u> diabetes mellitus with <u>proliferative</u> diabetic retinopathy

    E10.351 <u>Type 1</u> diabetes mellitus with proliferative diabetic retinopathy <u>with macular edema</u>

    E10.359 <u>Type 1</u> diabetes mellitus with proliferative diabetic retinopathy <u>without</u> macular edema

  E10.36 <u>Type 1</u> diabetes mellitus with diabetic <u>cataract</u>

  E10.39 <u>Type 1</u> diabetes mellitus with other diabetic <u>ophthalmic complication</u>
    Use additional code to identify manifestation, such as:
    Diabetic glaucoma (H40-H42)

E10.4- <u>Type 1</u> diabetes mellitus with <u>neurological</u> complications

  E10.40 <u>Type 1</u> diabetes mellitus with diabetic <u>neuropathy, unspecified</u>

  E10.41 <u>Type 1</u> diabetes mellitus with diabetic <u>mononeuropathy</u>

  E10.42 <u>Type 1</u> diabetes mellitus with diabetic <u>polyneuropathy</u>
    Type 1 diabetes mellitus with diabetic neuralgia

  E10.43 <u>Type 1</u> diabetes mellitus with diabetic <u>autonomic (poly)neuropathy</u>
    Type 1 diabetes mellitus with diabetic gastroparesis

E09 - E11

© 2013 Channel Publishing Ltd

E10.44   <u>Type 1</u> diabetes mellitus with diabetic <u>amyotrophy</u>
E10.49   <u>Type 1</u> diabetes mellitus with other diabetic neurological complication
E10.5-   <u>Type 1</u> diabetes mellitus with <u>circulatory</u> complications
E10.51   <u>Type 1</u> diabetes mellitus with diabetic <u>peripheral angiopathy without</u> gangrene
E10.52   <u>Type 1</u> diabetes mellitus with diabetic <u>peripheral angiopathy with gangrene</u>
       Type 1 diabetes mellitus with diabetic gangrene
E10.59   <u>Type 1</u> diabetes mellitus with other circulatory complications
E10.6-   <u>Type 1</u> diabetes mellitus with <u>other specified</u> complications
E10.61-   <u>Type 1</u> diabetes mellitus with diabetic <u>arthropathy</u>
E10.610   <u>Type 1</u> diabetes mellitus with diabetic <u>neuropathic</u> arthropathy
       Type 1 diabetes mellitus with Charcôt's joints
E10.618   <u>Type 1</u> diabetes mellitus with other diabetic arthropathy
E10.62-   <u>Type 1</u> diabetes mellitus with <u>skin</u> complications
E10.620   <u>Type 1</u> diabetes mellitus with diabetic <u>dermatitis</u>
       Type 1 diabetes mellitus with diabetic necrobiosis lipoidica
E10.621   <u>Type 1</u> diabetes mellitus with <u>foot ulcer</u>
       Use additional code to identify site of ulcer (L97.4-, L97.5-)
E10.622   <u>Type 1</u> diabetes mellitus with <u>other skin ulcer</u>
       Use additional code to identify site of ulcer (L97.1-L97.9, L98.41-L98.49)
E10.628   Type 1 diabetes mellitus with other skin complications
E10.63-   <u>Type 1</u> diabetes mellitus with <u>oral</u> complications
E10.630   <u>Type 1</u> diabetes mellitus with periodontal disease
E10.638   <u>Type 1</u> diabetes mellitus with other oral complications
E10.64-   <u>Type 1</u> diabetes mellitus with <u>hypoglycemia</u>
E10.641   <u>Type 1</u> diabetes mellitus with hypoglycemia <u>with coma</u>
E10.649   <u>Type 1</u> diabetes mellitus with hypoglycemia <u>without</u> coma
E10.65   <u>Type 1</u> diabetes mellitus with <u>hyperglycemia</u>
E10.69   <u>Type 1</u> diabetes mellitus with <u>other specified</u> complication
       Use additional code to identify complication
E10.8   <u>Type 1</u> diabetes mellitus with <u>unspecified</u> complications
E10.9   <u>Type 1</u> diabetes mellitus <u>without</u> complications

E11-   <u>Type 2 diabetes mellitus</u>
    Includes: Diabetes (mellitus) due to insulin secretory defect
          Diabetes NOS
          Insulin resistant diabetes (mellitus)
    Use additional code to identify any insulin use (Z79.4)
    Excludes 1: diabetes mellitus due to underlying condition (E08.-)
             drug or chemical induced diabetes mellitus (E09.-)
             gestational diabetes (O24.4-)
             neonatal diabetes mellitus (P70.2)
             postpancreatectomy diabetes mellitus (E13.-)
             postprocedural diabetes mellitus (E13.-)
             secondary diabetes mellitus NEC (E13.-)
             type 1 diabetes mellitus (E10.-)
E11.0-   <u>Type 2</u> diabetes mellitus with <u>hyperosmolarity</u>
E11.00   <u>Type 2</u> diabetes mellitus with hyperosmolarity <u>without</u> nonketotic hyperglycemic-hyperosmolar coma (NKHHC)
E11.01   <u>Type 2</u> diabetes mellitus with hyperosmolarity <u>with coma</u>
E11.2-   <u>Type 2</u> diabetes mellitus with <u>kidney</u> complications
E11.21   <u>Type 2</u> diabetes mellitus with diabetic <u>nephropathy</u>
       Type 2 diabetes mellitus with intercapillary glomerulosclerosis
       Type 2 diabetes mellitus with intracapillary glomerulonephrosis
       Type 2 diabetes mellitus with Kimmelstiel-Wilson disease
E11.22   <u>Type 2</u> diabetes mellitus with diabetic <u>chronic kidney disease</u>
       Use additional code to identify stage of chronic kidney disease (N18.1-N18.6)
E11.29   <u>Type 2</u> diabetes mellitus with other diabetic kidney complication
       Type 2 diabetes mellitus with renal tubular degeneration
E11.3-   <u>Type 2</u> diabetes mellitus with <u>ophthalmic</u> complications
E11.31-   <u>Type 2</u> diabetes mellitus with <u>unspecified</u> diabetic retinopathy
E11.311   <u>Type 2</u> diabetes mellitus with unspecified diabetic retinopathy <u>with macular edema</u>
E11.319   <u>Type 2</u> diabetes mellitus with unspecified diabetic retinopathy <u>without</u> macular edema

E11.32-   <u>Type 2</u> diabetes mellitus with <u>mild</u> <u>non</u>proliferative diabetic retinopathy
       Type 2 diabetes mellitus with nonproliferative diabetic retinopathy NOS
E11.321   <u>Type 2</u> diabetes mellitus with mild nonproliferative diabetic retinopathy <u>with macular edema</u>
E11.329   <u>Type 2</u> diabetes mellitus with mild nonproliferative diabetic retinopathy <u>without</u> macular edema
E11.33-   <u>Type 2</u> diabetes mellitus with <u>moderate nonproliferative</u> diabetic retinopathy
E11.331   <u>Type 2</u> diabetes mellitus with moderate nonproliferative diabetic retinopathy <u>with macular edema</u>
E11.339   <u>Type 2</u> diabetes mellitus with moderate nonproliferative diabetic retinopathy <u>without</u> macular edema
E11.34-   <u>Type 2</u> diabetes mellitus with <u>severe</u> <u>non</u>proliferative diabetic retinopathy
E11.341   <u>Type 2</u> diabetes mellitus with severe nonproliferative diabetic retinopathy <u>with macular edema</u>
E11.349   <u>Type 2</u> diabetes mellitus with severe nonproliferative diabetic retinopathy <u>without</u> macular edema
E11.35-   <u>Type 2</u> diabetes mellitus with <u>proliferative</u> diabetic retinopathy
E11.351   <u>Type 2</u> diabetes mellitus with proliferative diabetic retinopathy <u>with macular edema</u>
E11.359   <u>Type 2</u> diabetes mellitus with proliferative diabetic retinopathy <u>without</u> macular edema
E11.36   <u>Type 2</u> diabetes mellitus with diabetic <u>cataract</u>
E11.39   <u>Type 2</u> diabetes mellitus with other diabetic <u>ophthalmic complication</u>
       Use additional code to identify manifestation, such as: Diabetic glaucoma (H40-H42)
E11.4-   <u>Type 2</u> diabetes mellitus with <u>neurological</u> complications
E11.40   <u>Type 2</u> diabetes mellitus with diabetic <u>neuropathy, unspecified</u>
E11.41   <u>Type 2</u> diabetes mellitus with diabetic <u>mononeuropathy</u>
E11.42   <u>Type 2</u> diabetes mellitus with diabetic <u>polyneuropathy</u>
       Type 2 diabetes mellitus with diabetic neuralgia
E11.43   <u>Type 2</u> diabetes mellitus with diabetic <u>autonomic (poly)neuropathy</u>
       Type 2 diabetes mellitus with diabetic gastroparesis
E11.44   <u>Type 2</u> diabetes mellitus with diabetic <u>amyotrophy</u>
E11.49   <u>Type 2</u> diabetes mellitus with other diabetic neurological complication
E11.5-   <u>Type 2</u> diabetes mellitus with <u>circulatory</u> complications
E11.51   <u>Type 2</u> diabetes mellitus with diabetic <u>peripheral angiopathy without</u> gangrene
E11.52   <u>Type 2</u> diabetes mellitus with diabetic <u>peripheral angiopathy with gangrene</u>
       Type 2 diabetes mellitus with diabetic gangrene
E11.59   <u>Type 2</u> diabetes mellitus with other circulatory complications
E11.6-   <u>Type 2</u> diabetes mellitus with <u>other specified</u> complications
E11.61-   <u>Type 2</u> diabetes mellitus with diabetic <u>arthropathy</u>
E11.610   <u>Type 2</u> diabetes mellitus with diabetic <u>neuropathic</u> arthropathy
       Type 2 diabetes mellitus with Charcôt's joints
E11.618   <u>Type 2</u> diabetes mellitus with other diabetic arthropathy
E11.62-   <u>Type 2</u> diabetes mellitus with <u>skin</u> complications
E11.620   <u>Type 2</u> diabetes mellitus with diabetic <u>dermatitis</u>
       Type 2 diabetes mellitus with diabetic necrobiosis lipoidica
E11.621   <u>Type 2</u> diabetes mellitus with <u>foot ulcer</u>
       Use additional code to identify site of ulcer (L97.4-, L97.5-)
E11.622   <u>Type 2</u> diabetes mellitus with <u>other skin ulcer</u>
       Use additional code to identify site of ulcer (L97.1-L97.9, L98.41-L98.49)
E11.628   <u>Type 2</u> diabetes mellitus with other skin complications
E11.63-   <u>Type 2</u> diabetes mellitus with <u>oral</u> complications
E11.630   <u>Type 2</u> diabetes mellitus with periodontal disease
E11.638   <u>Type 2</u> diabetes mellitus with other oral complications
E11.64-   <u>Type 2</u> diabetes mellitus with <u>hypoglycemia</u>
E11.641   <u>Type 2</u> diabetes mellitus with hypoglycemia <u>with coma</u>
E11.649   <u>Type 2</u> diabetes mellitus with hypoglycemia <u>without</u> coma
E11.65   <u>Type 2</u> diabetes mellitus with <u>hyperglycemia</u>
E11.69   <u>Type 2</u> diabetes mellitus with <u>other specified</u> complication
       Use additional code to identify complication

E
0
9
–
E
1
1

E11.8   <u>Type 2</u> diabetes mellitus with <u>unspecified</u> complications

E11.9   <u>Type 2</u> diabetes mellitus <u>without</u> complications

E13-   <u>Other specified</u> diabetes mellitus

     Includes: Diabetes mellitus due to genetic defects of beta-cell function
               Diabetes mellitus due to genetic defects in insulin action
               Postpancreatectomy diabetes mellitus
               Postprocedural diabetes mellitus
               Secondary diabetes mellitus NEC

     Use additional code to identify any insulin use (Z79.4)

     Excludes 1:   *diabetes (mellitus) due to autoimmune process (E10.-)*
                 diabetes (mellitus) due to immune mediated pancreatic islet
                   beta-cell destruction (E10.-)
                 diabetes mellitus due to underlying condition (E08.-)
                 drug or chemical induced diabetes mellitus (E09.-)
                 gestational diabetes (O24.4-)
                 neonatal diabetes mellitus (P70.2)
                 type 2 diabetes mellitus (E11.-)

E13.0-   <u>Other specified</u> diabetes mellitus with <u>hyperosmolarity</u>

     E13.00   Other specified diabetes mellitus with hyperosmolarity <u>without</u> nonketotic hyperglycemic-hyperosmolar coma (NKHHC)

     E13.01   Other specified diabetes mellitus with hyperosmolarity <u>with</u> <u>coma</u>

E13.1-   <u>Other specified</u> diabetes mellitus with <u>ketoacidosis</u>

     E13.10   Other specified diabetes mellitus with ketoacidosis <u>without</u> coma

     E13.11   Other specified diabetes mellitus with ketoacidosis <u>with</u> <u>coma</u>

E13.2-   <u>Other specified</u> diabetes mellitus with <u>kidney</u> complications

     E13.21   Other specified diabetes mellitus with diabetic <u>nephropathy</u>
         Other specified diabetes mellitus with intercapillary glomerulosclerosis
         Other specified diabetes mellitus with intracapillary glomerulonephrosis
         Other specified diabetes mellitus with Kimmelstiel-Wilson disease

     E13.22   Other specified diabetes mellitus with diabetic <u>chronic</u> <u>kidney disease</u>
         Use additional code to identify stage of chronic kidney disease (N18.1-N18.6)

     E13.29   Other specified diabetes mellitus with other diabetic kidney complication
         Other specified diabetes mellitus with renal tubular degeneration

E13.3-   <u>Other specified</u> diabetes mellitus with ophthalmic complications

     E13.31-   Other specified diabetes mellitus with <u>unspecified diabetic retinopathy</u>

         E13.311   Other specified diabetes mellitus with unspecified diabetic retinopathy <u>with macular edema</u>

         E13.319   Other specified diabetes mellitus with unspecified diabetic retinopathy <u>without</u> macular edema

     E13.32-   Other specified diabetes mellitus with <u>mild non</u>proliferative diabetic retinopathy
         Other specified diabetes mellitus with nonproliferative diabetic retinopathy NOS

         E13.321   Other specified diabetes mellitus with mild nonproliferative diabetic retinopathy <u>with macular edema</u>

         E13.329   Other specified diabetes mellitus with mild nonproliferative diabetic retinopathy <u>without</u> macular edema

     E13.33-   Other specified diabetes mellitus with <u>moderate non</u>proliferative diabetic retinopathy

         E13.331   Other specified diabetes mellitus with moderate nonproliferative diabetic retinopathy <u>with macular edema</u>

         E13.339   Other specified diabetes mellitus with moderate nonproliferative diabetic retinopathy <u>without</u> macular edema

     E13.34-   Other specified diabetes mellitus with <u>severe non</u>proliferative diabetic retinopathy

         E13.341   Other specified diabetes mellitus with severe nonproliferative diabetic retinopathy <u>with macular edema</u>

         E13.349   Other specified diabetes mellitus with severe nonproliferative diabetic retinopathy <u>without</u> macular edema

     E13.35-   Other specified diabetes mellitus with <u>proliferative</u> diabetic retinopathy

         E13.351   Other specified diabetes mellitus with proliferative diabetic retinopathy <u>with macular edema</u>

         E13.359   Other specified diabetes mellitus with proliferative diabetic retinopathy <u>without</u> macular edema

     E13.36   Other specified diabetes mellitus with diabetic <u>cataract</u>

     E13.39   Other specified diabetes mellitus with other diabetic <u>ophthalmic complication</u>
         Use additional code to identify manifestation, such as: Diabetic glaucoma (H40-H42)

E13.4-   <u>Other specified</u> diabetes mellitus with <u>neurological</u> complications

     E13.40   Other specified diabetes mellitus with diabetic <u>neuropathy, unspecified</u>

     E13.41   Other specified diabetes mellitus with diabetic <u>mononeuropathy</u>

     E13.42   Other specified diabetes mellitus with diabetic <u>polyneuropathy</u>
         Other specified diabetes mellitus with diabetic neuralgia

     E13.43   Other specified diabetes mellitus with diabetic <u>autonomic</u> (poly)neuropathy
         Other specified diabetes mellitus with diabetic gastroparesis

     E13.44   Other specified diabetes mellitus with diabetic <u>amyotrophy</u>

     E13.49   Other specified diabetes mellitus with other diabetic neurological complication

E13.5-   <u>Other specified</u> diabetes mellitus with <u>circulatory</u> complications

     E13.51   Other specified diabetes mellitus with diabetic <u>peripheral angiopathy without</u> gangrene

     E13.52   Other specified diabetes mellitus with diabetic <u>peripheral angiopathy with gangrene</u>
         Other specified diabetes mellitus with diabetic gangrene

     E13.59   Other specified diabetes mellitus with other circulatory complications

E13.6-   <u>Other specified</u> diabetes mellitus with other specified complications

     E13.61-   Other specified diabetes mellitus with diabetic <u>arthropathy</u>

         E13.610   Other specified diabetes mellitus with diabetic <u>neuropathic</u> arthropathy
             Other specified diabetes mellitus with Charcôt's joints

         E13.618   Other specified diabetes mellitus with other diabetic arthropathy

     E13.62-   Other specified diabetes mellitus with <u>skin</u> complications

         E13.620   Other specified diabetes mellitus with diabetic <u>dermatitis</u>
             Other specified diabetes mellitus with diabetic necrobiosis lipoidica

         E13.621   Other specified diabetes mellitus with <u>foot ulcer</u>
             Use additional code to identify site of ulcer (L97.4-, L97.5-)

         E13.622   Other specified diabetes mellitus with <u>other skin ulcer</u>
             Use additional code to identify site of ulcer (L97.1-L97.9, L98.41-L98.49)

         E13.628   Other specified diabetes mellitus with other skin complications

     E13.63-   Other specified diabetes mellitus with <u>oral</u> complications

         E13.630   Other specified diabetes mellitus with periodontal disease

         E13.638   Other specified diabetes mellitus with other oral complications

     E13.64-   Other specified diabetes mellitus with <u>hypoglycemia</u>

         E13.641   Other specified diabetes mellitus with hypoglycemia <u>with coma</u>

         E13.649   Other specified diabetes mellitus with hypoglycemia <u>without</u> coma

     E13.65   Other specified diabetes mellitus with <u>hyperglycemia</u>

     E13.69   Other specified diabetes mellitus with <u>other specified</u> <u>complication</u>
         Use additional code to identify complication

E13.8   <u>Other specified</u> diabetes mellitus with <u>unspecified</u> complications

E13.9   <u>Other specified</u> diabetes mellitus <u>without</u> complications

Other disorders of glucose regulation and pancreatic internal secretion (E15-E16)

E15   <u>Nondiabetic</u> hypoglycemic coma
     Includes: Drug-induced insulin coma in nondiabetic
               Hyperinsulinism with hypoglycemic coma
               Hypoglycemic coma NOS

E16-   Other disorders of pancreatic internal secretion

     E16.0   <u>Drug-induced hypoglycemia</u> without coma
         Use additional code for adverse effect, if applicable, to identify drug (T36-T50 with fifth or sixth character 5)

Sidebar: E11 - E26

E16.1   Other hypoglycemia
  Functional hyperinsulinism
  Functional nonhyperinsulinemic hypoglycemia
  Hyperinsulinism NOS
  Hyperplasia of pancreatic islet beta cells NOS
  Excludes 1: hypoglycemia in infant of diabetic mother (P70.1)
        neonatal hypoglycemia (P70.4)

E16.2   Hypoglycemia, unspecified
E16.3   Increased secretion of glucagon
  Hyperplasia of pancreatic endocrine cells with glucagon excess

E16.4   Increased secretion of gastrin
  Hypergastrinemia
  Hyperplasia of pancreatic endocrine cells with gastrin excess
  Zollinger-Ellison syndrome

E16.8   Other specified disorders of pancreatic internal secretion
  Increased secretion from endocrine pancreas of growth hormone-
    releasing hormone
  Increased secretion from endocrine pancreas of pancreatic
    polypeptide
  Increased secretion from endocrine pancreas of somatostatin
  Increased secretion from endocrine pancreas of vasoactive-
    intestinal polypeptide

E16.9   Disorder of pancreatic internal secretion, unspecified
  Islet-cell hyperplasia NOS
  Pancreatic endocrine cell hyperplasia NOS

Disorders of other endocrine glands (E20-E35)

Excludes 1: galactorrhea (N64.3)
      gynecomastia (N62)

E20- Hypoparathyroidism
  Excludes 1: Di George's syndrome (D82.1)
        postprocedural hypoparathyroidism (E89.2)
        tetany NOS (R29.0)
        transitory neonatal hypoparathyroidism (P71.4)

E20.0   Idiopathic hypoparathyroidism
E20.1   Pseudohypoparathyroidism
E20.8   Other hypoparathyroidism
E20.9   Hypoparathyroidism, unspecified
  Parathyroid tetany

E21- Hyperparathyroidism and other disorders of parathyroid gland
  Excludes 1: adult osteomalacia (M83.-)
        ectopic hyperparathyroidism (E34.2)
        familial hypocalciuric hypercalcemia (E83.52)
        hungry bone syndrome (E83.81)
        infantile and juvenile osteomalacia (E55.0)

E21.0   Primary hyperparathyroidism
  Hyperplasia of parathyroid
  Osteitis fibrosa cystica generalisata [von Recklinghausen's disease
    of bone]

E21.1   Secondary hyperparathyroidism, not elsewhere classified
  Excludes 1: secondary hyperparathyroidism of renal origin
        (N25.81)

E21.2   Other hyperparathyroidism
  Tertiary hyperparathyroidism
  Excludes 1: familial hypocalciuric hypercalcemia (E83.52)

E21.3   Hyperparathyroidism, unspecified
E21.4   Other specified disorders of parathyroid gland
E21.5   Disorder of parathyroid gland, unspecified

E22- Hyperfunction of pituitary gland
  Excludes 1: Cushing's syndrome (E24.-)
        Nelson's syndrome (E24.1)
        overproduction of ACTH not associated with Cushing's
          disease (E27.0)
        overproduction of pituitary ACTH (E24.0)
        overproduction of thyroid-stimulating hormone (E05.8-)

E22.0   Acromegaly and pituitary gigantism
  Overproduction of growth hormone
  Excludes 1: constitutional gigantism (E34.4)
        constitutional tall stature (E34.4)
        increased secretion from endocrine pancreas of growth
          hormone-releasing hormone (E16.8)

E22.1   Hyperprolactinemia
  Use additional code for adverse effect, if applicable, to identify drug
    (T36-T50 with fifth or sixth character 5)

E22.2   Syndrome of inappropriate secretion of antidiuretic hormone
E22.8   Other hyperfunction of pituitary gland
  Central precocious puberty
E22.9   Hyperfunction of pituitary gland, unspecified

E23- Hypofunction and other disorders of the pituitary gland
  Includes: The listed conditions whether the disorder is in the pituitary or
        the hypothalamus
  Excludes 1: postprocedural hypopituitarism (E89.3)

E23.0   Hypopituitarism
  Fertile eunuch syndrome
  Hypogonadotropic hypogonadism
  Idiopathic growth hormone deficiency
  Isolated deficiency of gonadotropin
  Isolated deficiency of growth hormone
  Isolated deficiency of pituitary hormone
  Kallmann's syndrome
  Lorain-Levi short stature
  Necrosis of pituitary gland (postpartum)
  Panhypopituitarism
  Pituitary cachexia
  Pituitary insufficiency NOS
  Pituitary short stature
  Sheehan's syndrome
  Simmonds' disease

E23.1   Drug-induced hypopituitarism
  Use additional code for adverse effect, if applicable, to identify drug
    (T36-T50 with fifth or sixth character 5)

E23.2   Diabetes insipidus
  Excludes 1: nephrogenic diabetes insipidus (N25.1)

E23.3   Hypothalamic dysfunction, not elsewhere classified
  Excludes 1: Prader-Willi syndrome (Q87.1)
        Russell-Silver syndrome (Q87.1)

E23.6   Other disorders of pituitary gland
  Abscess of pituitary
  Adiposogenital dystrophy

E23.7   Disorder of pituitary gland, unspecified

E24- Cushing's syndrome
  Excludes 1: congenital adrenal hyperplasia (E25.0)

E24.0   Pituitary-dependent Cushing's disease
  Overproduction of pituitary ACTH
  Pituitary-dependent hypercorticalism

E24.1   Nelson's syndrome
E24.2   Drug-induced Cushing's syndrome
  Use additional code for adverse effect, if applicable, to identify drug
    (T36-T50 with fifth or sixth character 5)

E24.3   Ectopic ACTH syndrome
E24.4   Alcohol-induced pseudo-Cushing's syndrome
E24.8   Other Cushing's syndrome
E24.9   Cushing's syndrome, unspecified

E25- Adrenogenital disorders
  Includes: Adrenogenital syndromes, virilizing or feminizing, whether
        acquired or due to adrenal hyperplasia consequent on inborn
        enzyme defects in hormone synthesis
  Female adrenal pseudohermaphroditism
  Female heterosexual precocious pseudopuberty
  Male isosexual precocious pseudopuberty
  Male macrogenitosomia praecox
  Male sexual precocity with adrenal hyperplasia
  Male virilization (female)
  Excludes 1: indeterminate sex and pseudohermaphroditism (Q56)
        chromosomal abnormalities (Q90-Q99)

**E25.0   Congenital adrenogenital disorders associated with enzyme
        deficiency**
  Congenital adrenal hyperplasia
  21-Hydroxylase deficiency
  Salt-losing congenital adrenal hyperplasia

E25.8   Other adrenogenital disorders
  Idiopathic adrenogenital disorder
  Use additional code for adverse effect, if applicable, to identify drug
    (T36-T50 with fifth or sixth character 5)

E25.9   Adrenogenital disorder, unspecified
  Adrenogenital syndrome NOS

E26- Hyperaldosteronism
E26.0- Primary hyperaldosteronism
  E26.01 Conn's syndrome
    Code also adrenal adenoma (D35.0-)
  E26.02 Glucocorticoid-remediable aldosteronism
    Familial aldosteronism type I
  E26.09 Other primary hyperaldosteronism
    Primary aldosteronism due to adrenal hyperplasia (bilateral)

E26.1   Secondary hyperaldosteronism
E26.8- Other hyperaldosteronism
  E26.81 Bartter's syndrome
  E26.89 Other hyperaldosteronism

E
1
1
-
E
2
6

E26.9 **Hyperaldosteronism, unspecified**
Aldosteronism NOS
Hyperaldosteronism NOS

E27- <u>Other disorders of adrenal gland</u>
E27.0 **Other adrenocortical overactivity**
Overproduction of ACTH, not associated with Cushing's disease
Premature adrenarche
Excludes 1: Cushing's syndrome (E24.-)

E27.1 **Primary adrenocortical insufficiency**
Addison's disease
Autoimmune adrenalitis
Excludes 1: Addison only phenotype adrenoleukodystrophy
(E71.528)
amyloidosis (E85.-)
tuberculous Addison's disease (A18.7)
Waterhouse-Friderichsen syndrome (A39.1)

E27.2 **Addisonian crisis**
Adrenal crisis
Adrenocortical crisis

E27.3 **Drug-induced adrenocortical insufficiency**
Use additional code for adverse effect, if applicable, to identify drug
(T36-T50 with fifth or sixth character 5)

E27.4- **Other and unspecified adrenocortical insufficiency**
Excludes 1: adrenoleukodystrophy [Addison-Schilder] (E71.528)
Waterhouse-Friderichsen syndrome (A39.1)

E27.40 **Unspecified adrenocortical insufficiency**
Adrenocortical insufficiency NOS
Hypoaldosteronism

E27.49 **Other adrenocortical insufficiency**
Adrenal hemorrhage
Adrenal infarction

E27.5 **Adrenomedullary hyperfunction**
Adrenomedullary hyperplasia
Catecholamine hypersecretion

E27.8 **Other specified disorders of adrenal gland**
Abnormality of cortisol-binding globulin

E27.9 **Disorder of adrenal gland, unspecified**

E28- <u>Ovarian dysfunction</u>
Excludes 1: isolated gonadotropin deficiency (E23.0)
postprocedural ovarian failure (E89.4-)

E28.0 **Estrogen excess**
Use additional code for adverse effect, if applicable, to identify drug
(T36-T50 with fifth or sixth character 5)

E28.1 **Androgen excess**
Hypersecretion of ovarian androgens
Use additional code for adverse effect, if applicable, to identify drug
(T36-T50 with fifth or sixth character 5)

E28.2 **Polycystic ovarian syndrome**
Sclerocystic ovary syndrome
Stein-Leventhal syndrome

E28.3- **Primary ovarian failure**
Excludes 1: pure gonadal dysgenesis (Q99.1)
Turner's syndrome (Q96.-)

E28.31- **Premature menopause**
E28.310 **Symptomatic premature menopause**
Symptoms such as flushing, sleeplessness, headache,
lack of concentration, associated with premature
menopause

E28.319 **Asymptomatic premature menopause**
Premature menopause NOS

E28.39 **Other primary ovarian failure**
Decreased estrogen
Resistant ovary syndrome

E28.8 **Other ovarian dysfunction**
Ovarian hyperfunction NOS
Excludes 1: postprocedural ovarian failure (E89.4-)

E28.9 **Ovarian dysfunction, unspecified**

E29- <u>Testicular dysfunction</u>
Excludes 1: androgen insensitivity syndrome (E34.5-)
azoospermia or oligospermia NOS (N46.0-N46.1)
isolated gonadotropin deficiency (E23.0)
Klinefelter's syndrome (Q98.0-Q98.2, Q98.4)

E29.0 **Testicular <u>hyperfunction</u>**
Hypersecretion of testicular hormones

E29.1 **Testicular <u>hypofunction</u>**
Defective biosynthesis of testicular androgen NOS
5-delta-Reductase deficiency (with male pseudohermaphroditism)
Testicular hypogonadism NOS
Use additional code for adverse effect, if applicable, to identify drug
(T36-T50 with fifth or sixth character 5)
Excludes 1: postprocedural testicular hypofunction (E89.5)

E29.8 **Other testicular dysfunction**
E29.9 **Testicular dysfunction, unspecified**

E30- <u>Disorders of puberty</u>, not elsewhere classified
E30.0 <u>Delayed</u> **puberty**
Constitutional delay of puberty
Delayed sexual development

E30.1 <u>Precocious</u> **puberty**
Precocious menstruation
Excludes 1: Albright (-McCune) (-Sternberg) syndrome (Q78.1)
central precocious puberty (E22.8)
congenital adrenal hyperplasia (E25.0)
female heterosexual precocious pseudopuberty (E25.-)
male isosexual precocious pseudopuberty (E25.-)

E30.8 **Other disorders of puberty**
Premature thelarche

E30.9 **Disorder of puberty, unspecified**

E31- <u>Polyglandular dysfunction</u>
Excludes 1: ataxia telangiectasia [Louis-Bar] (G11.3)
dystrophia myotonica [Steinert] (G71.11)
pseudohypoparathyroidism (E20.1)

E31.0 <u>Autoimmune</u> **polyglandular failure**
Schmidt's syndrome

E31.1 **Polyglandular <u>hyperfunction</u>**
Excludes 1: multiple endocrine adenomatosis (E31.2-)
multiple endocrine neoplasia (E31.2-)

E31.2- <u>Multiple endocrine neoplasia [MEN] syndromes</u>
Multiple endocrine adenomatosis
Code also any associated malignancies and other conditions
associated with the syndromes

E31.20 **Multiple endocrine neoplasia [MEN] syndrome, unspecified**
Multiple endocrine adenomatosis NOS
Multiple endocrine neoplasia [MEN] syndrome NOS

E31.21 **Multiple endocrine neoplasia [MEN] <u>type I</u>**
Wermer's syndrome

E31.22 **Multiple endocrine neoplasia [MEN] <u>type IIA</u>**
Sipple's syndrome

E31.23 **Multiple endocrine neoplasia [MEN] <u>type IIB</u>**

E31.8 **Other polyglandular dysfunction**
E31.9 **Polyglandular dysfunction, unspecified**

E32- <u>Diseases of thymus</u>
Excludes 1: aplasia or hypoplasia of thymus with immunodeficiency
(D82.1)
myasthenia gravis (G70.0)

E32.0 **Persistent <u>hyperplasia</u> of thymus**
Hypertrophy of thymus

E32.1 **<u>Abscess</u> of thymus**

E32.8 **Other diseases of thymus**
Excludes 1: aplasia or hypoplasia with immunodeficiency (D82.1)
thymoma (D15.0)

E32.9 **Disease of thymus, unspecified**

E34- <u>Other endocrine disorders</u>
Excludes 1: pseudohypoparathyroidism (E20.1)
E34.0 **Carcinoid syndrome**
Note: May be used as an additional code to identify functional
activity associated with a carcinoid tumor.

E34.1 **Other hypersecretion of intestinal hormones**
E34.2 **Ectopic hormone secretion, not elsewhere classified**
Excludes 1: ectopic ACTH syndrome (E24.3)

E34.3 **Short stature due to endocrine disorder**
Constitutional short stature
Laron-type short stature
Excludes 1: achondroplastic short stature (Q77.4)
hypochondroplastic short stature (Q77.4)
nutritional short stature (E45)
pituitary short stature (E23.0)
progeria (E34.8)
renal short stature (N25.0)
Russell-Silver syndrome (Q87.1)
short-limbed stature with immunodeficiency (D82.2)
short stature in specific dysmorphic syndromes — code
to syndrome – see Alphabetical Index
short stature NOS (R62.52)

E34.4 **Constitutional tall stature**
Constitutional gigantism

E34.5- <u>Androgen insensitivity syndrome</u>
E34.50 **Androgen insensitivity syndrome, unspecified**
Androgen insensitivity NOS

E34.51 **<u>Complete</u> androgen insensitivity syndrome**
Complete androgen insensitivity
de Quervain syndrome
Goldberg-Maxwell syndrome

E26 | E55 *(side margin)*

Excludes ❷: = Not Included Here

© 2013 Channel Publishing, Ltd

E34.52 **Partial** androgen insensitivity syndrome
Partial androgen insensitivity
Reifenstein syndrome

E34.8   **Other specified endocrine disorders**
Pineal gland dysfunction
Progeria
Excludes❷: pseudohypoparathyroidism (E20.1)

E34.9   **Endocrine disorder, unspecified**
Endocrine disturbance NOS
Hormone disturbance NOS

E35   **Disorders of endocrine glands in diseases classified elsewhere**
Code first underlying disease, such as:
Late congenital syphilis of thymus gland [Dubois disease] (A50.5)
Use additional code, if applicable, to identify:
Sequelae of tuberculosis of other organs (B90.8)
Excludes 1: Echinococcus granulosus infection of thyroid gland (B67.3)
meningococcal hemorrhagic adrenalitis (A39.1)
syphilis of endocrine gland (A52.79)
tuberculosis of adrenal gland, except calcification (A18.7)
tuberculosis of endocrine gland NEC (A18.82)
tuberculosis of thyroid gland (A18.81)
Waterhouse-Friderichsen syndrome (A39.1)

Intraoperative complications of endocrine system (E36)

E36-   **Intraoperative complications** of endocrine system
Excludes❷: postprocedural endocrine and metabolic complications and disorders, not elsewhere classified (E89.-)

E36.0-   **Intraoperative hemorrhage and hematoma of an endocrine system organ or structure complicating a procedure**
Excludes 1: intraoperative hemorrhage and hematoma of an endocrine system organ or structure due to accidental puncture or laceration during a procedure (E36.1-)

E36.01   **Intraoperative hemorrhage and hematoma of an endocrine system organ or structure complicating an endocrine system procedure**

E36.02   **Intraoperative hemorrhage and hematoma of an endocrine system organ or structure complicating other procedure**

E36.1-   **Accidental puncture** and laceration of an endocrine system organ or structure during a procedure

E36.11   **Accidental puncture and laceration of an endocrine system organ or structure during an endocrine system procedure**

E36.12   **Accidental puncture and laceration of an endocrine system organ or structure during other procedure**

E36.8   **Other intraoperative complications** of endocrine system
Use additional code, if applicable, to further specify disorder

Malnutrition (E40-E46)

Excludes 1: intestinal malabsorption (K90.-)
sequelae of protein-calorie malnutrition (E64.0)
Excludes❷: nutritional anemias (D50-D53)
starvation (T73.0)

E40   **Kwashiorkor**
Severe malnutrition with nutritional edema with dyspigmentation of skin and hair
Excludes 1: marasmic kwashiorkor (E42)

E41   **Nutritional marasmus**
Severe malnutrition with marasmus
Excludes 1: marasmic kwashiorkor (E42)

E42   **Marasmic kwashiorkor**
Intermediate form severe protein-calorie malnutrition
Severe protein-calorie malnutrition with signs of both kwashiorkor and marasmus

E43   **Unspecified severe protein-calorie malnutrition**
Starvation edema

E44-   **Protein-calorie malnutrition of moderate and mild degree**
E44.0   **Moderate protein-calorie malnutrition**
E44.1   **Mild protein-calorie malnutrition**

E45   **Retarded development following protein-calorie malnutrition**
Nutritional short stature
Nutritional stunting
Physical retardation due to malnutrition

E46   **Unspecified protein-calorie malnutrition**
Malnutrition NOS
Protein-calorie imbalance NOS
Excludes 1: nutritional deficiency NOS (E63.9)

Other nutritional deficiencies (E50-E64)

Excludes❷: nutritional anemias (D50-D53)

E50-   **Vitamin A deficiency**
Excludes 1: sequelae of vitamin A deficiency (E64.1)

E50.0   **Vitamin A deficiency with conjunctival xerosis**

E50.1   **Vitamin A deficiency with Bitot's spot and conjunctival xerosis**
Bitot's spot in the young child

E50.2   **Vitamin A deficiency with corneal xerosis**

E50.3   **Vitamin A deficiency with corneal ulceration and xerosis**

E50.4   **Vitamin A deficiency with keratomalacia**

E50.5   **Vitamin A deficiency with night blindness**

E50.6   **Vitamin A deficiency with xerophthalmic scars of cornea**

E50.7   **Other ocular manifestations of vitamin A deficiency**
Xerophthalmia NOS

E50.8   **Other manifestations of vitamin A deficiency**
Follicular keratosis
Xeroderma

E50.9   **Vitamin A deficiency, unspecified**
Hypovitaminosis A NOS

E51-   **Thiamine deficiency**
Excludes 1: sequelae of thiamine deficiency (E64.8)

E51.1-   **Beriberi**
E51.11   **Dry beriberi**
Beriberi NOS
Beriberi with polyneuropathy

E51.12   **Wet beriberi**
Beriberi with cardiovascular manifestations
Cardiovascular beriberi
Shoshin disease

E51.2   **Wernicke's encephalopathy**

E51.8   **Other manifestations of thiamine deficiency**

E51.9   **Thiamine deficiency, unspecified**

E52   **Niacin deficiency [pellagra]**
Niacin (-tryptophan) deficiency
Nicotinamide deficiency
Pellagra (alcoholic)
Excludes 1: sequelae of niacin deficiency (E64.8)

E53-   **Deficiency of other B group vitamins**
Excludes 1: sequelae of vitamin B deficiency (E64.8)

E53.0   **Riboflavin deficiency**
Ariboflavinosis
Vitamin B2 deficiency

E53.1   **Pyridoxine deficiency**
Vitamin B6 deficiency
Excludes 1: pyridoxine-responsive sideroblastic anemia (D64.3)

E53.8   **Deficiency of other specified B group vitamins**
Biotin deficiency
Cyanocobalamin deficiency
Folate deficiency
Folic acid deficiency
Pantothenic acid deficiency
Vitamin B12 deficiency
Excludes 1: folate deficiency anemia (D52.-)
vitamin B12 deficiency anemia (D51.-)

E53.9   **Vitamin B deficiency, unspecified**

E54   **Ascorbic acid deficiency**
Deficiency of vitamin C
Scurvy
Excludes 1: scorbutic anemia (D53.2)
sequelae of vitamin C deficiency (E64.2)

E55-   **Vitamin D deficiency**
Excludes 1: adult osteomalacia (M83.-)
osteoporosis (M80.-)
sequelae of rickets (E64.3)

E55.0   **Rickets, active**
Infantile osteomalacia
Juvenile osteomalacia
Excludes 1: celiac rickets (K90.0)
Crohn's rickets (K50.-)
hereditary vitamin D-dependent rickets (E83.32)
inactive rickets (E64.3)
renal rickets (N25.0)
sequelae of rickets (E64.3)
vitamin D-resistant rickets (E83.31)

E55.9   **Vitamin D deficiency, unspecified**
Avitaminosis D

E
2
6
|
E
5
5

Excludes 1: = NOT CODED HERE! (Do not code both)

Excludes❷: = Not Included Here

E56-   Other vitamin deficiencies
    Excludes 1:   sequelae of other vitamin deficiencies (E64.8)
   E56.0   **Deficiency of vitamin E**
   E56.1   **Deficiency of vitamin K**
      Excludes 1:   deficiency of coagulation factor due to vitamin K
             deficiency (D68.4)
             vitamin K deficiency of newborn (P53)
   E56.8   **Deficiency of other vitamins**
   E56.9   **Vitamin deficiency, unspecified**

E58   Dietary calcium deficiency
    Excludes 1:   disorders of calcium metabolism (E83.5-)
              sequelae of calcium deficiency (E64.8)

E59   Dietary selenium deficiency
    Keshan disease
    Excludes 1:   sequelae of selenium deficiency (E64.8)

E60   Dietary zinc deficiency

E61-   Deficiency of other nutrient elements
    Use additional code for adverse effect, if applicable, to identify drug
    (T36-T50 with fifth or sixth character 5)
    Excludes 1:   disorders of mineral metabolism (E83.-)
              iodine deficiency related thyroid disorders (E00-E02)
              sequelae of malnutrition and other nutritional deficiencies
                (E64.-)
   E61.0   **Copper deficiency**
   E61.1   **Iron deficiency**
      Excludes 1:   iron deficiency anemia (D50.-)
   E61.2   **Magnesium deficiency**
   E61.3   **Manganese deficiency**
   E61.4   **Chromium deficiency**
   E61.5   **Molybdenum deficiency**
   E61.6   **Vanadium deficiency**
   E61.7   **Deficiency of multiple nutrient elements**
   E61.8   **Deficiency of other specified nutrient elements**
   E61.9   **Deficiency of nutrient element, unspecified**

E63-   Other nutritional deficiencies
    Excludes 1:   dehydration (E86.0)
              failure to thrive, adult (R62.7)
              failure to thrive, child (R62.51)
              feeding problems in newborn (P92.-)
              sequelae of malnutrition and other nutritional deficiencies
                (E64.-)
   E63.0   **Essential fatty acid [EFA] deficiency**
   E63.1   **Imbalance of constituents of food intake**
   E63.8   **Other specified nutritional deficiencies**
   E63.9   **Nutritional deficiency, unspecified**

E64-   Sequelae of malnutrition and other nutritional deficiencies
    Note: This category is to be used to indicate conditions in categories E43,
          E44, E46, E50-E63 as the cause of sequelae, which are themselves
          classified elsewhere. The "sequelae" include conditions specified as
          such; they also include the late effects of diseases classifiable to the
          above categories if the disease itself is no longer present
    Code first condition resulting from (sequela) of malnutrition and other
    nutritional deficiencies
   E64.0   **Sequelae of protein-calorie malnutrition**
      Excludes ❷: retarded development following protein-calorie
                  malnutrition (E45)
   E64.1   **Sequelae of vitamin A deficiency**
   E64.2   **Sequelae of vitamin C deficiency**
   E64.3   **Sequelae of rickets**
   E64.8   **Sequelae of other nutritional deficiencies**
   E64.9   **Sequelae of unspecified nutritional deficiency**

Overweight, obesity and other hyperalimentation (E65-E68)

E65   Localized adiposity
    Fat pad

E66-   Overweight and obesity
    Code first obesity complicating pregnancy, childbirth and the puerperium, if
    applicable (O99.21-)
    Use additional code to identify body mass index (BMI), if known (Z68.-)
    Excludes 1:   adiposogenital dystrophy (E23.6)
              lipomatosis NOS (E88.2)
              lipomatosis dolorosa [Dercum] (E88.2)
              Prader-Willi syndrome (Q87.1)
   E66.0-   Obesity due to excess calories
     E66.01   Morbid (severe) obesity due to excess calories
        Excludes 1:   morbid (severe) obesity with alveolar
                 hypoventilation (E66.2)
     E66.09   **Other obesity due to excess calories**

   E66.1   Drug-induced obesity
      Use additional code for adverse effect, if applicable, to identify drug
      (T36-T50 with fifth or sixth character 5)
   E66.2   Morbid (severe) obesity with alveolar hypoventilation
      Pickwickian syndrome
   E66.3   Overweight
   E66.8   **Other obesity**
   E66.9   **Obesity, unspecified**
      Obesity NOS

E67-   Other hyperalimentation
    Excludes 1:   hyperalimentation NOS (R63.2)
              sequelae of hyperalimentation (E68)
   E67.0   **Hypervitaminosis A**
   E67.1   **Hypercarotinemia**
   E67.2   **Megavitamin-B6 syndrome**
   E67.3   **Hypervitaminosis D**
   E67.8   **Other specified hyperalimentation**

E68   Sequelae of hyperalimentation
    Code first condition resulting from (sequela) of hyperalimentation

Metabolic disorders (E70-E88)

    Excludes 1:   androgen insensitivity syndrome (E34.5-)
              congenital adrenal hyperplasia (E25.0)
              Ehlers-Danlos syndrome (Q79.6)
              hemolytic anemias attributable to enzyme disorders (D55.-)
              Marfan's syndrome (Q87.4)
              5-alpha-reductase deficiency (E29.1)

E70-   Disorders of aromatic amino-acid metabolism
   E70.0   **Classical phenylketonuria**
   E70.1   **Other hyperphenylalaninemias**
   E70.2-   Disorders of tyrosine metabolism
      Excludes 1:   transitory tyrosinemia of newborn (P74.5)
     E70.20   **Disorder of tyrosine metabolism, unspecified**
     E70.21   Tyrosinemia
        Hypertyrosinemia
     E70.29   **Other disorders of tyrosine metabolism**
        Alkaptonuria
        Ochronosis
   E70.3-   Albinism
     E70.30   **Albinism, unspecified**
     E70.31-   Ocular albinism
       E70.310   X-linked ocular albinism
       E70.311   Autosomal recessive ocular albinism
       E70.318   **Other ocular albinism**
       E70.319   **Ocular albinism, unspecified**
     E70.32-   Oculocutaneous albinism
        Excludes 1:   Chediak-Higashi syndrome (E70.330)
                 Hermansky-Pudlak syndrome (E70.331)
       E70.320   Tyrosinase negative oculocutaneous albinism
          Albinism I
          Oculocutaneous albinism ty-neg
       E70.321   Tyrosinase positive oculocutaneous albinism
          Albinism II
          Oculocutaneous albinism ty-pos
       E70.328   **Other oculocutaneous albinism**
          Cross syndrome
       E70.329   **Oculocutaneous albinism, unspecified**
     E70.33-   Albinism with hematologic abnormality
       E70.330   **Chediak-Higashi syndrome**
       E70.331   **Hermansky-Pudlak syndrome**
       E70.338   **Other albinism with hematologic abnormality**
       E70.339   **Albinism with hematologic abnormality, unspecified**
     E70.39   **Other specified albinism**
        Piebaldism
   E70.4-   Disorders of histidine metabolism
     E70.40   **Disorders of histidine metabolism, unspecified**
     E70.41   **Histidinemia**
     E70.49   **Other disorders of histidine metabolism**
   E70.5   Disorders of tryptophan metabolism
   E70.8   **Other disorders of aromatic amino-acid metabolism**
   E70.9   **Disorder of aromatic amino-acid metabolism, unspecified**

E 5 6 – E 7 3

E71- Disorders of branched-chain amino-acid metabolism and fatty-acid metabolism

E71.0   Maple-syrup-urine disease

E71.1-   Other disorders of <u>branched-chain amino-acid metabolism</u>

E71.11- Branched-chain organic acidurias

E71.110   Isovaleric acidemia

E71.111   3-methylglutaconic aciduria

E71.118   Other branched-chain organic acidurias

E71.12- Disorders of propionate metabolism

E71.120   Methylmalonic acidemia

E71.121   Propionic acidemia

E71.128   Other disorders of propionate metabolism

E71.19   Other disorders of branched-chain amino-acid metabolism
Hyperleucine-isoleucinemia
Hypervalinemia

E71.2   Disorder of branched-chain amino-acid metabolism, unspecified

E71.3-   Disorders of <u>fatty-acid metabolism</u>
Excludes 1: peroxisomal disorders (E71.5)
Refsum's disease (G60.1)
Schilder's disease (G37.0)
Excludes ❷: carnitine deficiency due to inborn error of metabolism (E71.42)

E71.30   Disorder of fatty-acid metabolism, unspecified

E71.31- Disorders of <u>fatty-acid oxidation</u>

E71.310   Long chain/very long chain acyl CoA dehydrogenase deficiency
LCAD
VLCAD

E71.311   Medium chain acyl CoA dehydrogenase deficiency
MCAD

E71.312   Short chain acyl CoA dehydrogenase deficiency
SCAD

E71.313   Glutaric aciduria type II
Glutaric aciduria type II A
Glutaric aciduria type II B
Glutaric aciduria type II C
Excludes 1: glutaric aciduria (type 1) NOS (E72.3)

E71.314   Muscle carnitine palmitoyltransferase deficiency

E71.318   Other disorders of fatty-acid oxidation

E71.32   Disorders of <u>ketone metabolism</u>

E71.39   Other disorders of fatty-acid metabolism

E71.4-   Disorders of <u>carnitine metabolism</u>
Excludes 1:muscle carnitine palmitoyltransferase deficiency (E71.314)

E71.40   Disorder of carnitine metabolism, unspecified

E71.41   Primary carnitine deficiency

E71.42   Carnitine deficiency due to inborn errors of metabolism
Code also associated inborn error or metabolism

E71.43   Iatrogenic carnitine deficiency
Carnitine deficiency due to hemodialysis
Carnitine deficiency due to valproic acid therapy

E71.44- Other secondary carnitine deficiency

E71.440   Ruvalcaba-Myhre-Smith syndrome

E71.448   Other secondary carnitine deficiency

E71.5-   <u>Peroxisomal</u> disorders
Excludes 1: Schilder's disease (G37.0)

E71.50   Peroxisomal disorder, unspecified

E71.51- Disorders of peroxisome biogenesis
Group 1 peroxisomal disorders
Excludes 1: Refsum's disease (G60.1)

E71.510   Zellweger syndrome

E71.511   Neonatal adrenoleukodystrophy
Excludes 1: X-linked adrenoleukodystrophy (E71.42-)

E71.518   Other disorders of peroxisome biogenesis

E71.52- X-linked adrenoleukodystrophy

E71.520   Childhood cerebral X-linked adrenoleukodystrophy

E71.521   Adolescent X-linked adrenoleukodystrophy

E71.522   Adrenomyeloneuropathy

E71.528   Other X-linked adrenoleukodystrophy
Addison only phenotype adrenoleukodystrophy
Addison-Schilder adrenoleukodystrophy

E71.529   X-linked adrenoleukodystrophy, unspecified type

E71.53   Other group 2 peroxisomal disorders

E71.54- Other peroxisomal disorders

E71.540   Rhizomelic chondrodysplasia punctata
Excludes 1: chondrodysplasia punctata NOS (Q77.3)

E71.541   Zellweger-like syndrome

E71.542   Other group 3 peroxisomal disorders

E71.548   Other peroxisomal disorders

E72- Other disorders of amino-acid metabolism
Excludes 1: disorders of:
aromatic amino-acid metabolism (E70.-)
branched-chain amino-acid metabolism (E71.0-E71.2)
fatty-acid metabolism (E71.3)
purine and pyrimidine metabolism (E79.-)
gout (M1A.-, M10.-)

E72.0-   Disorders of <u>amino-acid transport</u>
Excludes 1: disorders of tryptophan metabolism (E70.5)

E72.00   Disorders of amino-acid transport, unspecified

E72.01   Cystinuria

E72.02   Hartnup's disease

E72.03   Lowe's syndrome
Use additional code for associated glaucoma (H42)

E72.04   Cystinosis
Fanconi (-de Toni) (-Debré) syndrome with cystinosis
Excludes 1: Fanconi (-de Toni) (-Debré) syndrome without cystinosis (E72.09)

E72.09   Other disorders of amino-acid transport
Fanconi (-de Toni) (-Debré) syndrome, unspecified

E72.1-   Disorders of <u>sulfur-bearing amino-acid metabolism</u>
Excludes 1: cystinosis (E72.04)
cystinuria (E72.01)
transcobalamin II deficiency (D51.2)

E72.10   Disorders of sulfur-bearing amino-acid metabolism, unspecified

E72.11   Homocystinuria
Cystathionine synthase deficiency

E72.12   Methylenetetrahydrofolate reductase deficiency

E72.19   Other disorders of sulfur-bearing amino-acid metabolism
Cystathioninuria
Methioninemia
Sulfite oxidase deficiency

E72.2-   Disorders of <u>urea cycle metabolism</u>
Excludes 1: disorders of ornithine metabolism (E72.4)

E72.20   Disorder of urea cycle metabolism, unspecified
Hyperammonemia
Excludes 1: hyperammonemia-hyperornithinemia-homocitrullinemia syndrome E72.4
transient hyperammonemia of newborn (P74.6)

E72.21   Argininemia

E72.22   Arginosuccinic aciduria

E72.23   Citrullinemia

E72.29   Other disorders of urea cycle metabolism

E72.3   Disorders of <u>lysine and hydroxylysine metabolism</u>
Glutaric aciduria NOS
Glutaric aciduria (type I)
Hydroxylysinemia
Hyperlysinemia
Excludes 1: glutaric aciduria type II (E71.313)
Refsum's dsease (G60.1)
Zellweger syndrome (E71.510)

E72.4   Disorders of <u>ornithine metabolism</u>
Hyperammonemia-Hyperornithinemia-Homocitrullinemia syndrome
Ornithinemia (types I, II)
Ornithine transcarbamylase deficiency
Excludes 1: hereditary choroidal dystrophy (H31.2-)

E72.5-   Disorders of <u>glycine metabolism</u>

E72.50   Disorder of glycine metabolism, unspecified

E72.51   Non-ketotic hyperglycinemia

E72.52   Trimethylaminuria

E72.53   Hyperoxaluria
Oxalosis
Oxaluria

E72.59   Other disorders of glycine metabolism
D-glycericacidemia
Hyperhydroxyprolinemia
Hyperprolinemia (types I, II)
Sarcosinemia

E72.8   Other specified disorders of amino-acid metabolism
Disorders of beta-amino-acid metabolism
Disorders of gamma-glutamyl cycle

E72.9   Disorder of amino-acid metabolism, unspecified

E73- <u>Lactose intolerance</u>

E73.0   Congenital lactase deficiency

E73.1   Secondary lactase deficiency

E73.8   Other lactose intolerance

E73.9   Lactose intolerance, unspecified

E 5 6 I E 7 3

Excludes 1: = NOT CODED HERE! (Do not code both)

Excludes ❷: = Not Included Here

E74- **Other disorders of** <u>carbohydrate metabolism</u>
  Excludes 1:   diabetes mellitus (E08-E13)
  hypoglycemia NOS (E16.2)
  increased secretion of glucagon (E16.3)
  mucopolysaccharidosis (E76.0-E76.3)

  E74.0- <u>Glycogen storage</u> disease
    E74.00 **Glycogen storage disease, unspecified**
    E74.01 **von Gierke disease**
        Type I glycogen storage disease
    E74.02 **Pompe disease**
        Cardiac glycogenosis
        Type II glycogen storage disease
    E74.03 **Cori disease**
        Forbes disease
        Type III glycogen storage disease
    E74.04 **McArdle disease**
        Type V glycogen storage disease
    E74.09 **Other glycogen storage disease**
        Andersen disease
        Hers disease
        Tauri disease
        Glycogen storage disease, types 0, IV, VI-XI
        Liver phosphorylase deficiency
        Muscle phosphofructokinase deficiency

  E74.1- **Disorders of** <u>fructose metabolism</u>
    Excludes 1:   muscle phosphofructokinase deficiency (E74.09)
    E74.10 **Disorder of fructose metabolism, unspecified**
    E74.11 **Essential fructosuria**
        Fructokinase deficiency
    E74.12 **Hereditary fructose intolerance**
        Fructosemia
    E74.19 **Other disorders of fructose metabolism**
        Fructose-1, 6-diphosphatase deficiency

  E74.2- **Disorders of** <u>galactose metabolism</u>
    E74.20 **Disorders of galactose metabolism, unspecified**
    E74.21 **Galactosemia**
    E74.29 **Other disorders of galactose metabolism**
        Galactokinase deficiency

  E74.3- **Other disorders of intestinal carbohydrate absorption**
    Excludes ❷: lactose intolerance (E73.-)
    E74.31 **Sucrase-isomaltase deficiency**
    E74.39 **Other disorders of intestinal carbohydrate absorption**
        Disorder of intestinal carbohydrate absorption NOS
        Glucose-galactose malabsorption
        Sucrase deficiency

  E74.4 **Disorders of** <u>pyruvate metabolism and gluconeogenesis</u>
        Deficiency of phosphoenolpyruvate carboxykinase
        Deficiency of pyruvate carboxylase
        Deficiency of pyruvate dehydrogenase
    Excludes 1:   disorders of pyruvate metabolism and gluconeogenesis
    with anemia (D55.-)
    Leigh's syndrome (G31.82)

  E74.8 **Other specified disorders of carbohydrate metabolism**
        Essential pentosuria
        Renal glycosuria
  E74.9 **Disorder of carbohydrate metabolism, unspecified**

E75- **Disorders of** <u>sphingolipid metabolism</u> and <u>other lipid storage disorders</u>
  Excludes 1:   mucolipidosis, types I-III (E77.0-E77.1)
  Refsum's disease (G60.1)

  E75.0- **GM2 gangliosidosis**
    E75.00 **GM2 gangliosidosis, unspecified**
    E75.01 **Sandhoff disease**
    E75.02 **Tay-Sachs disease**
    E75.09 **Other GM2 gangliosidosis**
        Adult GM2 gangliosidosis
        Juvenile GM2 gangliosidosis

  E75.1- **Other and unspecified gangliosidosis**
    E75.10 **Unspecified gangliosidosis**
        Gangliosidosis NOS
    E75.11 **Mucolipidosis IV**
    E75.19 **Other gangliosidosis**
        GM1 gangliosidosis
        GM3 gangliosidosis

  E75.2- **Other sphingolipidosis**
    Excludes 1:   adrenoleukodystrophy [Addison-Schilder] (E71.528)
    E75.21 **Fabry (-Anderson) disease**
    E75.22 **Gaucher disease**
    E75.23 **Krabbe disease**
    E75.24- **Niemann-Pick disease**
        E75.240 **Niemann-Pick disease type A**
        E75.241 **Niemann-Pick disease type B**
        E75.242 **Niemann-Pick disease type C**
        E75.243 **Niemann-Pick disease type D**
        E75.248 **Other Niemann-Pick disease**
        E75.249 **Niemann-Pick disease, unspecified**
    E75.25 **Metachromatic leukodystrophy**
    E75.29 **Other sphingolipidosis**
        Farber's syndrome
        Sulfatase deficiency
        Sulfatide lipidosis

  E75.3 **Sphingolipidosis, unspecified**
  E75.4 **Neuronal ceroid lipofuscinosis**
        Batten disease
        Bielschowsky-Jansky disease
        Kufs disease
        Spielmeyer-Vogt disease
  E75.5 **Other lipid storage disorders**
        Cerebrotendinous cholesterosis [van Bogaert-Scherer-Epstein]
        Wolman's disease
  E75.6 **Lipid storage disorder, unspecified**

E76- **Disorders of** <u>glycosaminoglycan metabolism</u>
  E76.0- **Mucopolysaccharidosis,** <u>type I</u>
    E76.01 **Hurler's syndrome**
    E76.02 **Hurler-Scheie syndrome**
    E76.03 **Scheie's syndrome**
  E76.1 **Mucopolysaccharidosis,** <u>type II</u>
        Hunter's syndrome
  E76.2- **Other mucopolysaccharidoses**
    E76.21- **Morquio mucopolysaccharidoses**
        E76.210 **Morquio A mucopolysaccharidoses**
            Classic Morquio syndrome
            Morquio syndrome A
            Mucopolysaccharidosis, type IVA
        E76.211 **Morquio B mucopolysaccharidoses**
            Morquio-like mucopolysaccharidoses
            Morquio-like syndrome
            Morquio syndrome B
            Mucopolysaccharidosis, type IVB
        E76.219 **Morquio mucopolysaccharidoses, unspecified**
            Morquio syndrome
            Mucopolysaccharidosis, type IV
    E76.22 **Sanfilippo mucopolysaccharidoses**
        Mucopolysaccharidosis, type III (A) (B) (C) (D)
        Sanfilippo A syndrome
        Sanfilippo B syndrome
        Sanfilippo C syndrome
        Sanfilippo D syndrome
    E76.29 **Other mucopolysaccharidoses**
        beta-Glucuronidase deficiency
        Maroteaux-Lamy (mild) (severe) syndrome
        Mucopolysaccharidosis, types VI, VII

  E76.3 **Mucopolysaccharidosis, unspecified**
  E76.8 **Other disorders of glucosaminoglycan metabolism**
  E76.9 **Glucosaminoglycan metabolism disorder, unspecified**

E77- **Disorders of** <u>glycoprotein metabolism</u>
  E77.0 **Defects in post-translational modification of lysosomal enzymes**
        Mucolipidosis II [I-cell disease]
        Mucolipidosis III [pseudo-Hurler polydystrophy]
  E77.1 **Defects in glycoprotein degradation**
        Aspartylglucosaminuria
        Fucosidosis
        Mannosidosis
        Sialidosis [mucolipidosis I]
  E77.8 **Other disorders of glycoprotein metabolism**
  E77.9 **Disorder of glycoprotein metabolism, unspecified**

E78- **Disorders of** <u>lipoprotein metabolism</u> and other lipidemias
  Excludes 1:   sphingolipidosis (E75.0-E75.3)
  E78.0 **Pure hypercholesterolemia**
        Familial hypercholesterolemia
        Fredrickson's hyperlipoproteinemia, type IIa
        Hyperbetalipoproteinemia
        Hyperlipidemia, Group A
        Low-density-lipoprotein-type [LDL] hyperlipoproteinemia
  E78.1 **Pure hyperglyceridemia**
        Elevated fasting triglycerides
        Endogenous hyperglyceridemia
        Fredrickson's hyperlipoproteinemia, type IV
        Hyperlipidemia, group B
        Hyperprebetalipoproteinemia
        Very-low-density-lipoprotein-type [VLDL] hyperlipoproteinemia

E74-E84 (side tab)

Excludes 1: = NOT CODED HERE! (Do not code both)   **398**   *Excludes ❷:* = Not Included Here

E78.2   Mixed hyperlipidemia
Broad- or floating-betalipoproteinemia
Combined hyperlipidemia NOS
Elevated cholesterol with elevated triglycerides NEC
Fredrickson's hyperlipoproteinemia, type IIb or III
Hyperbetalipoproteinemia with prebetalipoproteinemia
Hypercholesteremia with endogenous hyperglyceridemia
Hyperlipidemia, group C
Tubo-eruptive xanthoma
Xanthoma tuberosum
Excludes 1:   cerebrotendinous cholesterosis [van Bogaert-Scherer-Epstein] (E75.5)
familial combined hyperlipidemia (E78.4)

E78.3   Hyperchylomicronemia
Chylomicron retention disease
Fredrickson's hyperlipoproteinemia, type I or V
Hyperlipidemia, group D
Mixed hyperglyceridemia

E78.4   Other hyperlipidemia
Familial combined hyperlipidemia

E78.5   Hyperlipidemia, unspecified

E78.6   Lipoprotein deficiency
Abetalipoproteinemia
Depressed HDL cholesterol
High-density lipoprotein deficiency
Hypoalphalipoproteinemia
Hypobetalipoproteinemia (familial)
Lecithin cholesterol acyltransferase deficiency
Tangier disease

E78.7- Disorders of bile acid and cholesterol metabolism
Excludes 1: Niemann-Pick disease type C (E75.242)

   E78.70   Disorder of bile acid and cholesterol metabolism, unspecified
   E78.71   Barth syndrome
   E78.72   Smith-Lemli-Opitz syndrome
   E78.79   Other disorders of bile acid and cholesterol metabolism

E78.8- Other disorders of lipoprotein metabolism
   E78.81   Lipoid dermatoarthritis
   E78.89   Other lipoprotein metabolism disorders

E78.9   Disorder of lipoprotein metabolism, unspecified

E79- Disorders of purine and pyrimidine metabolism
Excludes 1: Ataxia-telangiectasia (Q87.1)
Bloom's syndrome (Q82.8)
Cockayne's syndrome (Q87.1)
calculus of kidney (N20.0)
combined immunodeficiency disorders (D81.-)
Fanconi's anemia (D61.09)
gout (M1A.-, M10.-)
orotaciduric anemia (D53.0)
progeria (E34.8)
Werner's syndrome (E34.8)
xeroderma pigmentosum (Q82.1)

E79.0   Hyperuricemia without signs of inflammatory arthritis and tophaceous disease
Asymptomatic hyperuricemia

E79.1   Lesch-Nyhan syndrome
HGPRT deficiency

E79.2   Myoadenylate deaminase deficiency

E79.8   Other disorders of purine and pyrimidine metabolism
Hereditary xanthinuria

E79.9   Disorder of purine and pyrimidine metabolism, unspecified

E80- Disorders of porphyrin and bilirubin metabolism
Includes: Defects of catalase and peroxidase

E80.0   Hereditary erythropoietic porphyria
Congenital erythropoietic porphyria
Erythropoietic protoporphyria

E80.1   Porphyria cutanea tarda

E80.2- Other and unspecified porphyria
   E80.20   Unspecified porphyria
Porphyria NOS
   E80.21   Acute intermittent (hepatic) porphyria
   E80.29   Other porphyria
Hereditary coproporphyria

E80.3   Defects of catalase and peroxidase
Acatalasia [Takahara]

E80.4   Gilbert syndrome

E80.5   Crigler-Najjar syndrome

E80.6   Other disorders of bilirubin metabolism
Dubin-Johnson syndrome
Rotor's syndrome

E80.7   Disorder of bilirubin metabolism, unspecified

E83- Disorders of mineral metabolism
Excludes 1:   dietary mineral deficiency (E58-E61)
parathyroid disorders (E20-E21)
vitamin D deficiency (E55.-)

E83.0- Disorders of copper metabolism
   E83.00   Disorder of copper metabolism, unspecified
   E83.01   Wilson's disease
Code also associated Kayser Fleischer ring (H18.04-)
   E83.09   Other disorders of copper metabolism
Menkes' (kinky hair) (steely hair) disease

E83.1- Disorders of iron metabolism
Excludes 1: iron deficiency anemia (D50.-)
sideroblastic anemia (D64.0-D64.3)
   E83.10   Disorder of iron metabolism, unspecified
   E83.11- Hemochromatosis
     E83.110   Hereditary hemochromatosis
Bronzed diabetes
Pigmentary cirrhosis (of liver)
Primary (hereditary) hemochromatosis
     E83.111   Hemochromatosis due to repeated red blood cell transfusions
Iron overload due to repeated red blood cell transfusions
Transfusion (red blood cell) associated hemochromatosis
     E83.118   Other hemochromatosis
     E83.119   Hemochromatosis, unspecified
   E83.19   Other disorders of iron metabolism
Use additional code, if applicable, for idiopathic pulmonary hemosiderosis (J84.03)

E83.2   Disorders of zinc metabolism
Acrodermatitis enteropathica

E83.3- Disorders of phosphorus metabolism and phosphatases
Excludes 1: adult osteomalacia (M83.-)
osteoporosis (M80.-)
   E83.30   Disorder of phosphorus metabolism, unspecified
   E83.31   Familial hypophosphatemia
Vitamin D-resistant osteomalacia
Vitamin D-resistant rickets
Excludes 1: vitamin D-deficiency rickets (E55.0)
   E83.32   Hereditary vitamin D-dependent rickets (type 1) (type 2)
25-hydroxyvitamin D 1-alpha-hydroxylase deficiency
Pseudovitamin D deficiency
Vitamin D receptor defect
   E83.39   Other disorders of phosphorus metabolism
Acid phosphatase deficiency
Hypophosphatasia

E83.4- Disorders of magnesium metabolism
   E83.40   Disorders of magnesium metabolism, unspecified
   E83.41   Hypermagnesemia
   E83.42   Hypomagnesemia
   E83.49   Other disorders of magnesium metabolism

E83.5- Disorders of calcium metabolism
Excludes 1: chondrocalcinosis (M11.1-M11.2)
hungry bone syndrome (E83.81)
hyperparathyroidism (E21.0-E21.3)
   E83.50   Unspecified disorder of calcium metabolism
   E83.51   Hypocalcemia
   E83.52   Hypercalcemia
Familial hypocalciuric hypercalcemia
   E83.59   Other disorders of calcium metabolism
Idiopathic hypercalciuria

E83.8- Other disorders of mineral metabolism
   E83.81   Hungry bone syndrome
   E83.89   Other disorders of mineral metabolism

E83.9   Disorder of mineral metabolism, unspecified

E84- Cystic fibrosis
Includes: Mucoviscidosis

E84.0   Cystic fibrosis with pulmonary manifestations
Use additional code to identify any infectious organism present, such as:
Pseudomonas (B96.5)

E84.1- Cystic fibrosis with intestinal manifestations
   E84.11   Meconium ileus in cystic fibrosis
Excludes 1: meconium ileus not due to cystic fibrosis (P76.0)
   E84.19   Cystic fibrosis with other intestinal manifestations
Distal intestinal obstruction syndrome

E84.8   Cystic fibrosis with other manifestations

E84.9   Cystic fibrosis, unspecified

E
7
4
–
E
8
4

Excludes 1: = NOT CODED HERE! (Do not code both)

Excludes ❷: = Not Included Here

E 8 5 - F 0 6

E85-   <u>Amyloidosis</u>
    Excludes 1: Alzheimer's disease (G30.0-)

E85.0   <u>Non-neuropathic</u> heredofamilial amyloidosis
    Familial Mediterranean fever
    Hereditary amyloid nephropathy

E85.1   <u>Neuropathic</u> heredofamilial amyloidosis
    Amyloid polyneuropathy (Portuguese)

E85.2   **Heredofamilial amyloidosis, unspecified**

E85.3   <u>Secondary</u> systemic amyloidosis
    Hemodialysis-associated amyloidosis

E85.4   **Organ-limited amyloidosis**
    Localized amyloidosis

E85.8   **Other amyloidosis**

E85.9   **Amyloidosis, unspecified**

E86-   <u>Volume depletion</u>
    Excludes 1: dehydration of newborn (P74.1)
         hypovolemic shock NOS (R57.1)
         postprocedural hypovolemic shock (T81.19)
         traumatic hypovolemic shock (T79.4)

E86.0   **Dehydration**

E86.1   **Hypovolemia**
    Depletion of volume of plasma

E86.9   **Volume depletion, unspecified**

E87-   <u>Other disorders of fluid, electrolyte and acid-base balance</u>
    Excludes 1: diabetes insipidus (E23.2)
         electrolyte imbalance associated with hyperemesis gravidarum (O21.1)
         electrolyte imbalance following ectopic or molar pregnancy (O08.5)
         familial periodic paralysis (G72.3)

E87.0   <u>Hyperosmolality</u> and <u>hypernatremia</u>
    Sodium [Na] excess
    Sodium [Na] overload

E87.1   <u>Hypo-osmolality</u> and <u>hyponatremia</u>
    Sodium [Na] deficiency
    Excludes 1: syndrome of inappropriate secretion of antidiuretic hormone (E22.2)

E87.2   **Acidosis**
    Acidosis NOS
    Lactic acidosis
    Metabolic acidosis
    Respiratory acidosis
    Excludes 1: diabetic acidosis — see categories E08-E10, E13 with ketoacidosis

E87.3   **Alkalosis**
    Alkalosis NOS
    Metabolic alkalosis
    Respiratory alkalosis

E87.4   **Mixed disorder of acid-base balance**

E87.5   <u>Hyperkalemia</u>
    Potassium [K] excess
    Potassium [K] overload

E87.6   <u>Hypokalemia</u>
    Potassium [K] deficiency

E87.7-   **Fluid overload**
    Excludes 1: edema NOS (R60.9)
         fluid retention (R60.9)

    E87.70   **Fluid overload, unspecified**

    E87.71   <u>Transfusion associated circulatory overload</u>
         Fluid overload due to transfusion (blood) (blood components)
         TACO

    E87.79   **Other fluid overload**

E87.8   **Other disorders of electrolyte and fluid balance, not elsewhere classified**
    Electrolyte imbalance NOS
    Hyperchloremia
    Hypochloremia

E88-   **Other and unspecified metabolic disorders**
    Use additional codes for associated conditions
    Excludes 1: histiocytosis X (chronic) (C96.6)

E88.0-   **Disorders of plasma-protein metabolism, not elsewhere classified**
    Excludes 1: disorder of lipoprotein metabolism (E78.-)
         monoclonal gammopathy (of undetermined significance) (D47.2)
         polyclonal hypergammaglobulinemia (D89.0)
         Waldenström macroglobulinemia (C88.0)

    E88.01   **Alpha-1-antitrypsin deficiency**
         AAT deficiency

    E88.09   **Other disorders of plasma-protein metabolism, not elsewhere classified**
         Bisalbuminemia

E88.1   **Lipodystrophy, not elsewhere classified**
    Lipodystrophy NOS
    Excludes 1: Whipple's disease (K90.81)

E88.2   **Lipomatosis, not elsewhere classified**
    Lipomatosis NOS
    Lipomatosis (Check) dolorosa [Dercum]

E88.3   **Tumor lysis syndrome**
    Tumor lysis syndrome (spontaneous)
    Tumor lysis syndrome following antineoplastic drug chemotherapy
    Use additional code for adverse effect, if applicable, to identify drug (T45.1X5-)

E88.4-   <u>Mitochondrial metabolism</u> disorders
    Excludes 1: disorders of pyruvate metabolism (E74.4)
         Kearns-Sayre syndrome (H49.81)
         Leber's disease (H47.22)
         Leigh's encephalopathy (G31.82)
         Mitochondrial myopathy, NEC (G71.3)
         Reye's syndrome (G93.7)

    E88.40   **Mitochondrial metabolism disorder, unspecified**

    E88.41   <u>MELAS</u> syndrome
         Mitochondrial myopathy, encephalopathy, lactic acidosis and stroke-like episodes

    E88.42   <u>MERRF</u> syndrome
         Myoclonic epilepsy associated with ragged-red fibers
         Code also myoclonic epilepsy (G40.3-)

    E88.49   **Other mitochondrial metabolism disorders**

E88.8-   **Other specified metabolic disorders**

    E88.81   **Metabolic syndrome**
         Dysmetabolic syndrome X
         Use additional codes for associated manifestations, such as:
         Obesity (E66.-)

    E88.89   **Other specified metabolic disorders**
         Launois-Bensaude adenolipomatosis
         Excludes 1: adult pulmonary Langerhans cell histiocytosis (J84.82)

E88.9   **Metabolic disorder, unspecified**

Postprocedural endocrine and metabolic complications and disorders, not elsewhere classified (E89)

E89-   <u>Postprocedural</u> endocrine and metabolic complications and disorders, not elsewhere classified
    Excludes ❷: intraoperative complications of endocrine system organ or structure (E36.0-, E36.1-, E36.8)

E89.0   **Postprocedural hypothyroidism**
    Postirradiation hypothyroidism
    Postsurgical hypothyroidism

E89.1   **Postprocedural hypoinsulinemia**
    Postpancreatectomy hyperglycemia
    Postsurgical hypoinsulinemia
    Use additional code, if applicable, to identify:
    Acquired absence of pancreas (Z90.41-)
    Diabetes mellitus (postpancreatectomy) (postprocedural) (E13.-)
    Insulin use (Z79.4)
    Excludes 1: transient postprocedural hyperglycemia (R73.9)
         transient postprocedural hypoglycemia (E16.2)

E89.2   **Postprocedural hypoparathyroidism**
    Parathyroprival tetany

E89.3   **Postprocedural hypopituitarism**
    Postirradiation hypopituitarism

E89.4-   **Postprocedural <u>ovarian failure</u>**

    E89.40   **Asymptomatic postprocedural ovarian failure**
         Postprocedural ovarian failure NOS

    E89.41   **Symptomatic postprocedural ovarian failure**
         Symptoms such as flushing, sleeplessness, headache, lack of concentration, associated with postprocedural menopause

E89.5   **Postprocedural testicular hypofunction**

E89.6   **Postprocedural adrenocortical (-medullary) hypofunction**

E89.8-   **Other postprocedural endocrine and metabolic complications and disorders**

    E89.81-   <u>Postprocedural hemorrhage</u> and hematoma of an endocrine system organ or structure following a procedure

         E89.810   **Postprocedural hemorrhage and hematoma of an endocrine system organ or structure following an endocrine system procedure**

         E89.811   **Postprocedural hemorrhage and hematoma of an endocrine system organ or structure following other procedure**

    E89.89   **Other postprocedural endocrine and metabolic complications and disorders**
         Use additional code, if applicable, to further specify disorder

---

Chapter – 5 Mental, behavioral and neurodevelopmental disorders (F01-F99)

Includes: Disorders of psychological development
*Excludes❷: symptoms, signs and abnormal clinical laboratory findings,
        not elsewhere classified (R00-R99)*

This chapter contains the following blocks:

F01-F09	Mental disorders due to known physiological conditions
F10-F19	Mental and behavioral disorders due to psychoactive substance use
F20-F29	Schizophrenia, schizotypal, delusional, and other non-mood psychotic disorders
F30-F39	Mood [affective] disorders
F40-F48	Anxiety, dissociative, stress-related, somatoform and other nonpsychotic mental disorders
F50-F59	Behavioral syndromes associated with physiological disturbances and physical factors
F60-F69	Disorders of adult personality and behavior
F70-F79	Intellectual disabilities
F80-F89	Pervasive and specific developmental disorders
F90-F98	Behavioral and emotional disorders with onset usually occurring in childhood and adolescence
F99	Unspecified mental disorder

Mental disorders due to known physiological conditions (F01-F09)

Note: This block comprises a range of mental disorders grouped together
        on the basis of their having in common a demonstrable etiology in
        cerebral disease, brain injury, or other insult leading to cerebral
        dysfunction. The dysfunction may be primary, as in diseases, injuries,
        and insults that affect the brain directly and selectively; or secondary,
        as in systemic diseases and disorders that attack the brain only as one
        of the multiple organs or systems of the body that are involved.

F01-   Vascular dementia
Vascular dementia as a result of infarction of the brain due to vascular
        disease, including hypertensive cerebrovascular disease
Includes: Arteriosclerotic dementia
Code first the underlying physiological condition or sequelae of
        cerebrovascular disease

F01.5-   Vascular dementia

   F01.50   Vascular dementia without behavioral disturbance

   F01.51   Vascular dementia with behavioral disturbance
        Vascular dementia with aggressive behavior
        Vascular dementia with combative behavior
        Vascular dementia with violent behavior
        Use additional code, if applicable, to identify wandering in
            vascular dementia (Z91.83)

F02-   Dementia in other diseases classified elsewhere
Code first the underlying physiological condition, such as:
   Alzheimer's (G30.-)
   Cerebral lipidosis (E75.4)
   Creutzfeldt-Jakob disease (A81.0-)
   Dementia with Lewy bodies (G31.83)
   Epilepsy and recurrent seizures (G40.-)
   Frontotemporal dementia (G31.09)
   Hepatolenticular degeneration (E83.0)
   Human immunodeficiency virus [HIV] disease (B20)
   Hypercalcemia (E83.52)
   Hypothyroidism, acquired (E00-E03.-)
   Intoxications (T36-T65)
   Jakob-Creutzfeldt disease (A81.0-)
   Multiple sclerosis (G35)
   Neurosyphilis (A52.17)
   Niacin deficiency [pellagra] (E52)
   Parkinson's disease (G20)
   Pick's disease (G31.01)
   Polyarteritis nodosa (M30.0)
   Systemic lupus erythematosus (M32.-)
   Trypanosomiasis (B56.-, B57.-)
   Vitamin B deficiency (E53.8)
Excludes 1: dementia with Parkinsonism (G31.83)
*Excludes❷: dementia in alcohol and psychoactive substance disorders
        (F10-F19, with .17, .27, .97)
        vascular dementia (F01.5-)*

F02.8-   Dementia in other diseases classified elsewhere
   **F02.80   Dementia in other diseases classified elsewhere without
        behavioral disturbance**
        Dementia in other diseases classified elsewhere NOS

   **F02.81   Dementia in other diseases classified elsewhere with
        behavioral disturbance**
        Dementia in other diseases classified elsewhere with
            aggressive behavior
        Dementia in other diseases classified elsewhere with
            combative behavior
        Dementia in other diseases classified elsewhere with violent
            behavior
        Use additional code, if applicable, to identify wandering in
            dementia in conditions classified elsewhere (Z91.83)

F03-   Unspecified dementia
   Presenile dementia NOS
   Presenile psychosis NOS
   Primary degenerative dementia NOS
   Senile dementia NOS
   Senile dementia depressed or paranoid type
   Senile psychosis NOS
Excludes 1: senility NOS (R41.81)
*Excludes❷: mild memory disturbance due to known physiological
        condition (F06.8)
        senile dementia with delirium or acute confusional state (F05)*

F03.9-   Unspecified dementia
   F03.90   Unspecified dementia without behavioral disturbance
        Dementia NOS

   F03.91   Unspecified dementia with behavioral disturbance
        Unspecified dementia with aggressive behavior
        Unspecified dementia with combative behavior
        Unspecified dementia with violent behavior
        Use additional code, if applicable, to identify wandering in
            unspecified dementia (Z91.83)

F04   Amnestic disorder due to known physiological condition
   Korsakov's psychosis or syndrome, nonalcoholic
   Code first the underlying physiological condition
*Excludes 1: amnesia NOS (R41.3)
        anterograde amnesia (R41.1)
        dissociative amnesia (F44.0)
        retrograde amnesia (R41.2)*
*Excludes❷: alcohol-induced or unspecified Korsakov's syndrome (F10.26,
        F10.96)
        Korsakov's syndrome induced by other psychoactive
            substances (F13.26, F13.96, F19.16, F19.26, F19.96)*

F05   Delirium due to known physiological condition
   Acute or subacute brain syndrome
   Acute or subacute confusional state (nonalcoholic)
   Acute or subacute infective psychosis
   Acute or subacute organic reaction
   Acute or subacute psycho-organic syndrome
   Delirium of mixed etiology
   Delirium superimposed on dementia
   Sundowning
   Code first the underlying physiological condition
Excludes 1: delirium NOS (R41.0)
*Excludes❷: delirium tremens alcohol-induced or unspecified (F10.231,
        F10.921)*

F06-   Other mental disorders due to known physiological condition
   Includes: Mental disorders due to endocrine disorder
        Mental disorders due to exogenous hormone
        Mental disorders due to exogenous toxic substance
        Mental disorders due to primary cerebral disease
        Mental disorders due to somatic illness
        Mental disorders due to systemic disease affecting the brain
   Code first the underlying physiological condition
Excludes 1: unspecified dementia (F03)
*Excludes❷: delirium due to known physiological condition (F05)
        dementia as classified in F01-F02
        other mental disorders associated with alcohol and other
            psychoactive substances (F10-F19)*

   **F06.0   Psychotic disorder with hallucinations due to known
        physiological condition**
        Organic hallucinatory state (nonalcoholic)
        *Excludes❷: hallucinations and perceptual disturbance induced by
            alcohol and other psychoactive substances (F10-
            F19 with .151, .251, .951)
            schizophrenia (F20.-)*

   F06.1   Catatonic disorder due to known physiological condition
        *Excludes 1: catatonic stupor (R40.1)
            stupor NOS (R40.1)*
        *Excludes❷: catatonic schizophrenia (F20.2)
            dissociative stupor (F44.2)*

E85-F06

F06.2   <u>Psychotic</u> disorder with <u>delusions</u> due to known physiological condition

> Paranoid and paranoid-hallucinatory organic states
> Schizophrenia-like psychosis in epilepsy
> *Excludes❷: alcohol and drug-induced psychotic disorder (F10-F19 with .150, .250, .950)*
> > *brief psychotic disorder (F23)*
> > *delusional disorder (F22)*
> > *schizophrenia (F20.-)*

F06.3-   <u>Mood disorder due to known physiological condition</u>

> *Excludes❷: mood disorders due to alcohol and other psychoactive substances (F10-F19 with .14, .24, .94)*
> > *mood disorders, not due to known physiological condition or unspecified (F30-F39)*

> **F06.30**   Mood disorder due to known physiological condition, **unspecified**

> **F06.31**   Mood disorder due to known physiological condition with <u>depressive features</u>

> **F06.32**   Mood disorder due to known physiological condition with <u>major depressive-like</u> episode

> **F06.33**   Mood disorder due to known physiological condition with <u>manic</u> features

> **F06.34**   Mood disorder due to known physiological condition with <u>mixed</u> features

F06.4   <u>Anxiety</u> disorder <u>due to known physiological condition</u>

> *Excludes❷: anxiety disorders due to alcohol and other psychoactive substances (F10-F19 with .180, .280, .980)*
> > *anxiety disorders, not due to known physiological condition or unspecified (F40.-, F41.-)*

F06.8   <u>Other specified</u> mental disorders <u>due to known physiological condition</u>

> Epileptic psychosis NOS
> Organic dissociative disorder
> Organic emotionally labile [asthenic] disorder

F07-   <u>Personality and behavioral</u> disorders <u>due to known physiological condition</u>

> Code first the underlying physiological condition

F07.0   <u>Personality change</u> due to known physiological condition

> Frontal lobe syndrome
> Limbic epilepsy personality syndrome
> Lobotomy syndrome
> Organic personality disorder
> Organic pseudopsychopathic personality
> Organic pseudoretarded personality
> Postleucotomy syndrome
> Code first underlying physiological condition
> *Excludes 1: mild cognitive impairment (G31.84)*
> > *postconcussional syndrome (F07.81)*
> > *postencephalitic syndrome (F07.89)*
> > *signs and symptoms involving emotional state (R45.-)*
> *Excludes❷: specific personality disorder (F60.-)*

F07.8-   Other personality and behavioral disorders due to known physiological condition

> **F07.81**   <u>Postconcussional syndrome</u>
> > Postcontusional syndrome (encephalopathy)
> > Post-traumatic brain syndrome, nonpsychotic
> > Use additional code to identify associated post-traumatic headache, if applicable (G44.3-)
> > *Excludes 1: current concussion (brain) (S06.0-)*
> > > *postencephalitic syndrome (F07.89)*

> **F07.89**   Other personality and behavioral disorders due to known physiological condition
> > Postencephalitic syndrome
> > Right hemispheric organic affective disorder

F07.9   Unspecified personality and behavioral disorder due to known physiological condition

> Organic psychosyndrome

F09   <u>Unspecified</u> mental disorder <u>due to known physiological condition</u>

> Mental disorder NOS due to known physiological condition
> Organic brain syndrome NOS
> Organic mental disorder NOS
> Organic psychosis NOS
> Symptomatic psychosis NOS
> Code first the underlying physiological condition
> *Excludes 1: psychosis NOS (F29)*

Mental and behavioral disorders due to psychoactive substance use (F10-F19)

F10-   <u>Alcohol related disorders</u>

> Use additional code for blood alcohol level, if applicable (Y90.-)

F10.1-   <u>Alcohol abuse</u>

> *Excludes 1: alcohol dependence (F10.2-)*
> > *alcohol use, unspecified (F10.9-)*

> **F10.10**   Alcohol abuse, **uncomplicated**

> **F10.12-**   Alcohol abuse <u>with intoxication</u>
> > **F10.120**   Alcohol abuse with intoxication, <u>uncomplicated</u>
> > **F10.121**   Alcohol abuse with intoxication <u>delirium</u>
> > **F10.129**   Alcohol abuse with intoxication, <u>unspecified</u>

> **F10.14**   Alcohol abuse <u>with</u> alcohol-induced <u>mood</u> disorder

> **F10.15-**   Alcohol abuse <u>with</u> alcohol-induced <u>psychotic</u> disorder
> > **F10.150**   Alcohol abuse with alcohol-induced psychotic disorder <u>with delusions</u>
> > **F10.151**   Alcohol abuse with alcohol-induced psychotic disorder <u>with hallucinations</u>
> > **F10.159**   Alcohol abuse with alcohol-induced psychotic disorder, unspecified

> **F10.18-**   Alcohol abuse <u>with other</u> alcohol-induced disorders
> > **F10.180**   Alcohol abuse <u>with</u> alcohol-induced <u>anxiety</u> disorder
> > **F10.181**   Alcohol abuse <u>with</u> alcohol-induced <u>sexual dysfunction</u>
> > **F10.182**   Alcohol abuse <u>with</u> alcohol-induced <u>sleep</u> disorder
> > **F10.188**   Alcohol abuse <u>with other</u> alcohol-induced disorder

> **F10.19**   Alcohol abuse <u>with</u> unspecified alcohol-induced disorder

F10.2-   Alcohol <u>dependence</u>

> *Excludes 1: alcohol abuse (F10.1-)*
> > *alcohol use, unspecified (F10.9-)*
> *Excludes❷: toxic effect of alcohol (T51.0-)*

> **F10.20**   Alcohol dependence, <u>uncomplicated</u>

> **F10.21**   Alcohol dependence, <u>in remission</u>

> **F10.22-**   Alcohol dependence <u>with intoxication</u>
> > Acute drunkenness (in alcoholism)
> > *Excludes 1: alcohol dependence with withdrawal (F10.23-)*
> > **F10.220**   Alcohol dependence with intoxication, <u>uncomplicated</u>
> > **F10.221**   Alcohol dependence with intoxication delirium
> > **F10.229**   Alcohol dependence with intoxication, <u>unspecified</u>

> **F10.23-**   Alcohol dependence <u>with withdrawal</u>
> > *Excludes 1: Alcohol dependence with intoxication (F10.22-)*
> > **F10.230**   Alcohol dependence with withdrawal, <u>uncomplicated</u>
> > **F10.231**   Alcohol dependence with withdrawal <u>delirium</u>
> > **F10.232**   Alcohol dependence with withdrawal <u>with perceptual disturbance</u>
> > **F10.239**   Alcohol dependence with withdrawal, <u>unspecified</u>

> **F10.24**   Alcohol dependence <u>with</u> alcohol-induced <u>mood</u> disorder

> **F10.25-**   Alcohol dependence <u>with</u> alcohol-induced <u>psychotic</u> disorder
> > **F10.250**   Alcohol dependence <u>with</u> alcohol-induced psychotic disorder <u>with delusions</u>
> > **F10.251**   Alcohol dependence <u>with</u> alcohol-induced psychotic disorder <u>with hallucinations</u>
> > **F10.259**   Alcohol dependence with alcohol-induced psychotic disorder, unspecified

> **F10.26**   Alcohol dependence <u>with</u> alcohol-induced <u>persisting amnestic disorder</u>

> **F10.27**   Alcohol dependence <u>with</u> alcohol-induced <u>persisting dementia</u>

> **F10.28-**   Alcohol dependence <u>with other</u> alcohol-induced disorders
> > **F10.280**   Alcohol dependence with alcohol-induced <u>anxiety</u> disorder
> > **F10.281**   Alcohol dependence with alcohol-induced <u>sexual dysfunction</u>
> > **F10.282**   Alcohol dependence with alcohol-induced <u>sleep</u> disorder
> > **F10.288**   Alcohol dependence with other alcohol-induced disorder

> **F10.29**   Alcohol dependence with unspecified alcohol-induced disorder

F10.9-   <u>Alcohol use, unspecified</u>

> *Excludes 1: alcohol abuse (F10.1-)*
> > *alcohol dependence (F10.2-)*

> **F10.92-**   Alcohol use, unspecified <u>with intoxication</u>
> > **F10.920**   Alcohol use, unspecified with intoxication, <u>uncomplicated</u>
> > **F10.921**   Alcohol use, unspecified with intoxication <u>delirium</u>
> > **F10.929**   Alcohol use, unspecified with intoxication, <u>unspecified</u>

> **F10.94**   Alcohol use, unspecified <u>with</u> alcohol-induced <u>mood</u> disorder

---

F10.95- Alcohol use, unspecified <u>with</u> alcohol-induced <u>psychotic</u> disorder
- **F10.950** Alcohol use, unspecified with alcohol-induced psychotic disorder <u>with delusions</u>
- **F10.951** Alcohol use, unspecified with alcohol-induced psychotic disorder <u>with hallucinations</u>
- **F10.959** Alcohol use, unspecified with alcohol-induced psychotic disorder, unspecified

F10.96 Alcohol use, unspecified <u>with</u> alcohol-induced <u>persisting amnestic disorder</u>

F10.97 Alcohol use, unspecified <u>with</u> alcohol-induced <u>persisting dementia</u>

F10.98- Alcohol use, unspecified <u>with</u> <u>other</u> alcohol-induced disorders
- **F10.980** Alcohol use, unspecified with alcohol-induced <u>anxiety</u> disorder
- **F10.981** Alcohol use, unspecified with alcohol-induced <u>sexual dysfunction</u>
- **F10.982** Alcohol use, unspecified with alcohol-induced <u>sleep</u> disorder
- **F10.988** Alcohol use, unspecified with other alcohol-induced disorder

F10.99 Alcohol use, unspecified with unspecified alcohol-induced disorder

F11- Opioid related disorders
F11.1- Opioid abuse
Excludes 1: opioid dependence (F11.2-)
opioid use, unspecified (F11.9-)
- **F11.10** Opioid abuse, <u>uncomplicated</u>
- **F11.12-** Opioid abuse <u>with intoxication</u>
  - **F11.120** Opioid abuse with intoxication, <u>uncomplicated</u>
  - **F11.121** Opioid abuse with intoxication <u>delirium</u>
  - **F11.122** Opioid abuse with intoxication <u>with perceptual disturbance</u>
  - **F11.129** Opioid abuse with intoxication, <u>unspecified</u>
- **F11.14** Opioid abuse <u>with</u> opioid-induced <u>mood</u> disorder
- **F11.15-** Opioid abuse <u>with</u> opioid-induced <u>psychotic</u> disorder
  - **F11.150** Opioid abuse with opioid-induced psychotic disorder <u>with delusions</u>
  - **F11.151** Opioid abuse with opioid-induced psychotic disorder <u>with hallucinations</u>
  - **F11.159** Opioid abuse with opioid-induced psychotic disorder, unspecified
- **F11.18-** Opioid abuse <u>with</u> <u>other</u> opioid-induced disorder
  - **F11.181** Opioid abuse with opioid-induced <u>sexual dysfunction</u>
  - **F11.182** Opioid abuse with opioid-induced <u>sleep</u> disorder
  - **F11.188** Opioid abuse with other opioid-induced disorder
- **F11.19** Opioid abuse with unspecified opioid-induced disorder
F11.2- Opioid dependence
Excludes 1: opioid abuse (F11.1-)
opioid use, unspecified (F11.9-)
Excludes❷: opioid poisoning (T40.0-T40.2-)
- **F11.20** Opioid dependence, <u>uncomplicated</u>
- **F11.21** Opioid dependence, <u>in remission</u>
- **F11.22-** Opioid dependence <u>with intoxication</u>
  Excludes 1: opioid dependence with withdrawal (F11.23)
  - **F11.220** Opioid dependence with intoxication, <u>uncomplicated</u>
  - **F11.221** Opioid dependence with intoxication <u>delirium</u>
  - **F11.222** Opioid dependence with intoxication <u>with perceptual disturbance</u>
  - **F11.229** Opioid dependence with intoxication, <u>unspecified</u>
- **F11.23** Opioid dependence with withdrawal
  Excludes 1: opioid dependence with intoxication (F11.22-)
- **F11.24** Opioid dependence <u>with</u> opioid-induced <u>mood</u> disorder
- **F11.25-** Opioid dependence <u>with</u> opioid-induced <u>psychotic</u> disorder
  - **F11.250** Opioid dependence with opioid-induced psychotic disorder <u>with delusions</u>
  - **F11.251** Opioid dependence with opioid-induced psychotic disorder <u>with hallucinations</u>
  - **F11.259** Opioid dependence with opioid-induced psychotic disorder, unspecified
- **F11.28-** Opioid dependence <u>with</u> <u>other</u> opioid-induced disorder
  - **F11.281** Opioid dependence <u>with</u> opioid-induced <u>sexual dysfunction</u>
  - **F11.282** Opioid dependence with opioid-induced <u>sleep</u> disorder
  - **F11.288** Opioid dependence with other opioid-induced disorder
- **F11.29** Opioid dependence with unspecified opioid-induced disorder

F11.9- Opioid use, unspecified
Excludes 1: opioid abuse (F11.1-)
opioid dependence (F11.2-)
- **F11.90** Opioid use, unspecified, <u>uncomplicated</u>
- **F11.92-** Opioid use, unspecified <u>with intoxication</u>
  Excludes 1: opioid use, unspecified with withdrawal (F11.93)
  - **F11.920** Opioid use, unspecified with intoxication, <u>uncomplicated</u>
  - **F11.921** Opioid use, unspecified with intoxication <u>delirium</u>
  - **F11.922** Opioid use, unspecified with intoxication <u>with perceptual disturbance</u>
  - **F11.929** Opioid use, unspecified with intoxication, unspecified
- **F11.93** Opioid use, unspecified <u>with withdrawal</u>
  Excludes 1: opioid use, unspecified with intoxication (F11.92-)
- **F11.94** Opioid use, unspecified <u>with</u> opioid-induced <u>mood</u> disorder
- **F11.95-** Opioid use, unspecified <u>with</u> opioid-induced <u>psychotic</u> disorder
  - **F11.950** Opioid use, unspecified with opioid-induced psychotic disorder <u>with delusions</u>
  - **F11.951** Opioid use, unspecified with opioid-induced psychotic disorder <u>with hallucinations</u>
  - **F11.959** Opioid use, unspecified with opioid-induced psychotic disorder, unspecified
- **F11.98-** Opioid use, unspecified <u>with</u> <u>other</u> specified opioid-induced disorder
  - **F11.981** Opioid use, unspecified <u>with</u> opioid-induced <u>sexual dysfunction</u>
  - **F11.982** Opioid use, unspecified <u>with</u> opioid-induced <u>sleep</u> disorder
  - **F11.988** Opioid use, unspecified <u>with</u> <u>other</u> opioid-induced disorder
- **F11.99** Opioid use, unspecified with unspecified opioid-induced disorder

F12- Cannabis related disorders
Includes: Marijuana
F12.1- Cannabis <u>abuse</u>
Excludes 1: cannabis dependence (F12.2-)
cannabis use, unspecified (F12.9-)
- **F12.10** Cannabis abuse, <u>uncomplicated</u>
- **F12.12-** Cannabis abuse <u>with intoxication</u>
  - **F12.120** Cannabis abuse with intoxication, <u>uncomplicated</u>
  - **F12.121** Cannabis abuse with intoxication <u>delirium</u>
  - **F12.122** Cannabis abuse with intoxication <u>with perceptual disturbance</u>
  - **F12.129** Cannabis abuse with intoxication, <u>unspecified</u>
- **F12.15-** Cannabis abuse <u>with psychotic</u> disorder
  - **F12.150** Cannabis abuse with psychotic disorder <u>with delusions</u>
  - **F12.151** Cannabis abuse with psychotic disorder <u>with hallucinations</u>
  - **F12.159** Cannabis abuse with psychotic disorder, unspecified
- **F12.18-** Cannabis abuse <u>with</u> <u>other</u> cannabis-induced disorder
  - **F12.180** Cannabis abuse with cannabis-induced <u>anxiety</u> disorder
  - **F12.188** Cannabis abuse with other cannabis-induced disorder
- **F12.19** Cannabis abuse with unspecified cannabis-induced disorder
F12.2- Cannabis <u>dependence</u>
Excludes 1: cannabis abuse (F12.1-)
cannabis use, unspecified (F12.9-)
Excludes❷: cannabis poisoning (T40.7-)
- **F12.20** Cannabis dependence, <u>uncomplicated</u>
- **F12.21** Cannabis dependence, <u>in remission</u>
- **F12.22-** Cannabis dependence <u>with intoxication</u>
  - **F12.220** Cannabis dependence with intoxication, <u>uncomplicated</u>
  - **F12.221** Cannabis dependence with intoxication <u>delirium</u>
  - **F12.222** Cannabis dependence with intoxication <u>with perceptual disturbance</u>
  - **F12.229** Cannabis dependence with intoxication, unspecified
- **F12.25-** Cannabis dependence <u>with psychotic</u> disorder
  - **F12.250** Cannabis dependence with psychotic disorder <u>with delusions</u>
  - **F12.251** Cannabis dependence with psychotic disorder <u>with hallucinations</u>
  - **F12.259** Cannabis dependence with psychotic disorder, unspecified

F06-F12

© 2013 Channel Publishing, Ltd.

F12.28- Cannabis dependence <u>with</u> <u>other</u> cannabis-induced disorder
  F12.280 Cannabis dependence with cannabis-induced <u>anxiety</u> disorder
  F12.288 Cannabis dependence with other cannabis-induced disorder
F12.29 Cannabis dependence with unspecified cannabis-induced disorder
F12.9- <u>Cannabis use, unspecified</u>
  Excludes 1: cannabis abuse (F12.1-)
            cannabis dependence (F12.2-)
F12.90 Cannabis use, unspecified, <u>uncomplicated</u>
F12.92- Cannabis use, unspecified <u>with intoxication</u>
  F12.920 Cannabis use, unspecified with intoxication, <u>uncomplicated</u>
  F12.921 Cannabis use, unspecified with intoxication <u>delirium</u>
  F12.922 Cannabis use, unspecified with intoxication <u>with perceptual disturbance</u>
  F12.929 Cannabis use, unspecified with intoxication, <u>unspecified</u>
F12.95- Cannabis use, unspecified <u>with</u> <u>psychotic</u> disorder
  F12.950 Cannabis use, unspecified with psychotic disorder <u>with delusions</u>
  F12.951 Cannabis use, unspecified with psychotic disorder <u>with hallucinations</u>
  F12.959 Cannabis use, unspecified with psychotic disorder, unspecified
F12.98- Cannabis use, unspecified <u>with</u> <u>other</u> cannabis-induced disorder
  F12.980 Cannabis use, unspecified with <u>anxiety</u> disorder
  F12.988 Cannabis use, unspecified with other cannabis-induced disorder
F12.99 Cannabis use, unspecified with unspecified cannabis-induced disorder

F13- <u>Sedative, hypnotic, or anxiolytic related disorders</u>
F13.1- Sedative, hypnotic or anxiolytic-related <u>abuse</u>
  Excludes 1: sedative, hypnotic or anxiolytic-related dependence (F13.2-)
            sedative, hypnotic, or anxiolytic use, unspecified (F13.9-)
F13.10 Sedative, hypnotic or anxiolytic abuse, <u>uncomplicated</u>
F13.12- Sedative, hypnotic or anxiolytic abuse <u>with intoxication</u>
  F13.120 Sedative, hypnotic or anxiolytic abuse with intoxication, <u>uncomplicated</u>
  F13.121 Sedative, hypnotic or anxiolytic abuse with intoxication <u>delirium</u>
  F13.129 Sedative, hypnotic or anxiolytic abuse with intoxication, <u>unspecified</u>
F13.14 Sedative, hypnotic or anxiolytic abuse <u>with</u> sedative, hypnotic or anxiolytic-induced <u>mood</u> disorder
F13.15- Sedative, hypnotic or anxiolytic abuse <u>with</u> sedative, hypnotic or anxiolytic-induced <u>psychotic</u> disorder
  F13.150 Sedative, hypnotic or anxiolytic abuse with sedative, hypnotic or anxiolytic-induced psychotic disorder <u>with delusions</u>
  F13.151 Sedative, hypnotic or anxiolytic abuse with sedative, hypnotic or anxiolytic-induced psychotic disorder <u>with hallucinations</u>
  F13.159 Sedative, hypnotic or anxiolytic abuse with sedative, hypnotic or anxiolytic-induced psychotic disorder, unspecified
F13.18- Sedative, hypnotic or anxiolytic abuse <u>with</u> <u>other</u> sedative, hypnotic or anxiolytic-induced disorders
  F13.180 Sedative, hypnotic or anxiolytic abuse <u>with</u> sedative, hypnotic or anxiolytic-induced <u>anxiety</u> disorder
  F13.181 Sedative, hypnotic or anxiolytic abuse <u>with</u> sedative, hypnotic or anxiolytic-induced <u>sexual dysfunction</u>
  F13.182 Sedative, hypnotic or anxiolytic abuse <u>with</u> sedative, hypnotic or anxiolytic-induced <u>sleep</u> disorder
  F13.188 Sedative, hypnotic or anxiolytic abuse with other sedative, hypnotic or anxiolytic-induced disorder
F13.19 Sedative, hypnotic or anxiolytic abuse with unspecified sedative, hypnotic or anxiolytic-induced disorder

F13.2- Sedative, hypnotic or anxiolytic-related <u>dependence</u>
  Excludes 1: sedative, hypnotic or anxiolytic-related abuse (F13.1-)
            sedative, hypnotic, or anxiolytic use, unspecified (F13.9-)
  Excludes ❷: sedative, hypnotic, or anxiolytic poisoning (T42.-)
F13.20 Sedative, hypnotic or anxiolytic dependence, <u>uncomplicated</u>
F13.21 Sedative, hypnotic or anxiolytic dependence, <u>in remission</u>
F13.22- Sedative, hypnotic or anxiolytic dependence <u>with</u> <u>intoxication</u>
  Excludes 1: sedative, hypnotic or anxiolytic dependence with withdrawal (F13.23-)
  F13.220 Sedative, hypnotic or anxiolytic dependence with intoxication, <u>uncomplicated</u>
  F13.221 Sedative, hypnotic or anxiolytic dependence with intoxication <u>delirium</u>
  F13.229 Sedative, hypnotic or anxiolytic dependence with intoxication, <u>unspecified</u>
F13.23- Sedative, hypnotic or anxiolytic dependence <u>with withdrawal</u>
  Excludes 1: sedative, hypnotic or anxiolytic dependence with intoxication (F13.22-)
  F13.230 Sedative, hypnotic or anxiolytic dependence with withdrawal, <u>uncomplicated</u>
  F13.231 Sedative, hypnotic or anxiolytic dependence with withdrawal <u>delirium</u>
  F13.232 Sedative, hypnotic or anxiolytic dependence with withdrawal <u>with perceptual disturbance</u>
  F13.239 Sedative, hypnotic or anxiolytic dependence with withdrawal, unspecified
F13.24 Sedative, hypnotic or anxiolytic dependence <u>with</u> sedative, hypnotic or anxiolytic-induced <u>mood</u> disorder
F13.25- Sedative, hypnotic or anxiolytic dependence <u>with</u> sedative, hypnotic or anxiolytic-induced <u>psychotic</u> disorder
  F13.250 Sedative, hypnotic or anxiolytic dependence with sedative, hypnotic or anxiolytic-induced psychotic disorder <u>with delusions</u>
  F13.251 Sedative, hypnotic or anxiolytic dependence with sedative, hypnotic or anxiolytic-induced psychotic disorder <u>with hallucinations</u>
  F13.259 Sedative, hypnotic or anxiolytic dependence with sedative, hypnotic or anxiolytic-induced psychotic disorder, unspecified
F13.26 Sedative, hypnotic or anxiolytic dependence <u>with</u> sedative, hypnotic or anxiolytic-induced <u>persisting amnestic</u> disorder
F13.27 Sedative, hypnotic or anxiolytic dependence <u>with</u> sedative, hypnotic or anxiolytic-induced <u>persisting dementia</u>
F13.28- Sedative, hypnotic or anxiolytic dependence <u>with</u> <u>other</u> sedative, hypnotic or anxiolytic-induced disorders
  F13.280 Sedative, hypnotic or anxiolytic dependence <u>with</u> sedative, hypnotic or anxiolytic-induced <u>anxiety</u> disorder
  F13.281 Sedative, hypnotic or anxiolytic dependence <u>with</u> sedative, hypnotic or anxiolytic-induced <u>sexual dysfunction</u>
  F13.282 Sedative, hypnotic or anxiolytic dependence <u>with</u> sedative, hypnotic or anxiolytic-induced <u>sleep</u> disorder
  F13.288 Sedative, hypnotic or anxiolytic dependence with other sedative, hypnotic or anxiolytic-induced disorder
F13.29 Sedative, hypnotic or anxiolytic dependence with unspecified sedative, hypnotic or anxiolytic-induced disorder
F13.9- <u>Sedative, hypnotic or anxiolytic-related use, unspecified</u>
  Excludes 1: sedative, hypnotic or anxiolytic-related abuse (F13.1-)
            sedative, hypnotic or anxiolytic-related dependence (F13.2-)
F13.90 Sedative, hypnotic, or anxiolytic use, unspecified, <u>uncomplicated</u>
F13.92- Sedative, hypnotic or anxiolytic use, unspecified <u>with intoxication</u>
  Excludes 1: sedative, hypnotic or anxiolytic use, unspecified with withdrawal (F13.93-)
  F13.920 Sedative, hypnotic or anxiolytic use, unspecified with intoxication, <u>uncomplicated</u>
  F13.921 Sedative, hypnotic or anxiolytic use, unspecified with intoxication <u>delirium</u>
  F13.929 Sedative, hypnotic or anxiolytic use, unspecified with intoxication, <u>unspecified</u>

F 1 2 - F 1 5

F13.93- Sedative, hypnotic or anxiolytic use, unspecified <u>with withdrawal</u>
Excludes 1: sedative, hypnotic or anxiolytic use, unspecified with intoxication (F13.92-)

    F13.930 Sedative, hypnotic or anxiolytic use, unspecified with withdrawal, <u>uncomplicated</u>

    F13.931 Sedative, hypnotic or anxiolytic use, unspecified with withdrawal <u>delirium</u>

    F13.932 Sedative, hypnotic or anxiolytic use, unspecified with withdrawal <u>with perceptual disturbances</u>

    F13.939 Sedative, hypnotic or anxiolytic use, unspecified with withdrawal, unspecified

F13.94 Sedative, hypnotic or anxiolytic use, unspecified <u>with</u> sedative, hypnotic or anxiolytic-induced <u>mood</u> disorder

F13.95- Sedative, hypnotic or anxiolytic use, unspecified <u>with</u> sedative, hypnotic or anxiolytic-induced <u>psychotic</u> disorder

    F13.950 Sedative, hypnotic or anxiolytic use, unspecified with sedative, hypnotic or anxiolytic-induced psychotic disorder <u>with delusions</u>

    F13.951 Sedative, hypnotic or anxiolytic use, unspecified with sedative, hypnotic or anxiolytic-induced psychotic disorder <u>with hallucinations</u>

    F13.959 Sedative, hypnotic or anxiolytic use, unspecified with sedative, hypnotic or anxiolytic-induced psychotic disorder, unspecified

F13.96 Sedative, hypnotic or anxiolytic use, unspecified <u>with</u> sedative, hypnotic or anxiolytic-induced <u>persisting amnestic</u> disorder

F13.97 Sedative, hypnotic or anxiolytic use, unspecified <u>with</u> sedative, hypnotic or anxiolytic-induced <u>persisting dementia</u>

F13.98- Sedative, hypnotic or anxiolytic use, unspecified <u>with other</u> sedative, hypnotic or anxiolytic-induced disorders

    F13.980 Sedative, hypnotic or anxiolytic use, unspecified <u>with</u> sedative, hypnotic or anxiolytic-induced <u>anxiety</u> disorder

    F13.981 Sedative, hypnotic or anxiolytic use, unspecified <u>with</u> sedative, hypnotic or anxiolytic-induced <u>sexual</u> <u>dysfunction</u>

    F13.982 Sedative, hypnotic or anxiolytic use, unspecified <u>with</u> sedative, hypnotic or anxiolytic-induced <u>sleep</u> disorder

    F13.988 Sedative, hypnotic or anxiolytic use, unspecified with other sedative, hypnotic or anxiolytic-induced disorder

F13.99 Sedative, hypnotic or anxiolytic use, unspecified with unspecified sedative, hypnotic or anxiolytic-induced disorder

F14- <u>Cocaine related disorders</u>
Excludes❷: other stimulant-related disorders (F15.-)

F14.1- Cocaine <u>abuse</u>
Excludes 1: cocaine dependence (F14.2-)
cocaine use, unspecified (F14.9-)

F14.10 Cocaine abuse, <u>uncomplicated</u>

F14.12- Cocaine abuse <u>with intoxication</u>

    F14.120 Cocaine abuse with intoxication, <u>uncomplicated</u>

    F14.121 Cocaine abuse with intoxication <u>with delirium</u>

    F14.122 Cocaine abuse with intoxication <u>with perceptual disturbance</u>

    F14.129 Cocaine abuse with intoxication, <u>unspecified</u>

F14.14 Cocaine abuse <u>with</u> cocaine-induced <u>mood</u> disorder

F14.15- Cocaine abuse <u>with</u> cocaine-induced <u>psychotic</u> disorder

    F14.150 Cocaine abuse with cocaine-induced psychotic disorder <u>with delusions</u>

    F14.151 Cocaine abuse with cocaine-induced psychotic disorder <u>with hallucinations</u>

    F14.159 Cocaine abuse with cocaine-induced psychotic disorder, unspecified

F14.18 Cocaine abuse <u>with other</u> cocaine-induced disorder

    F14.180 Cocaine abuse <u>with</u> cocaine-induced <u>anxiety</u> disorder

    F14.181 Cocaine abuse <u>with</u> cocaine-induced <u>sexual</u> <u>dysfunction</u>

    F14.182 Cocaine abuse <u>with</u> cocaine-induced <u>sleep</u> disorder

    F14.188 Cocaine abuse with other cocaine-induced disorder

F14.19 Cocaine abuse with unspecified cocaine-induced disorder

F14.2- Cocaine <u>dependence</u>
Excludes 1: cocaine abuse (F14.1-)
cocaine use, unspecified (F14.9-)
Excludes❷: cocaine poisoning (T40.5-)

F14.20 Cocaine dependence, <u>uncomplicated</u>

F14.21 Cocaine dependence, <u>in remission</u>

F14.22- Cocaine dependence <u>with intoxication</u>
Excludes 1: cocaine dependence with withdrawal (F14.23)

    F14.220 Cocaine dependence with intoxication, <u>uncomplicated</u>

    F14.221 Cocaine dependence with intoxication <u>delirium</u>

    F14.222 Cocaine dependence with intoxication <u>with perceptual disturbance</u>

    F14.229 Cocaine dependence with intoxication, <u>unspecified</u>

F14.23 Cocaine dependence <u>with withdrawal</u>
Excludes 1: cocaine dependence with intoxication (F14.22-)

F14.24 Cocaine dependence <u>with</u> cocaine-induced <u>mood</u> disorder

F14.25- Cocaine dependence <u>with</u> cocaine-induced <u>psychotic</u> disorder

    F14.250 Cocaine dependence with cocaine-induced psychotic disorder <u>with delusions</u>

    F14.251 Cocaine dependence with cocaine-induced psychotic disorder <u>with hallucinations</u>

    F14.259 Cocaine dependence with cocaine-induced psychotic disorder, unspecified

F14.28- Cocaine dependence <u>with other</u> cocaine-induced disorder

    F14.280 Cocaine dependence with cocaine-induced <u>anxiety</u> disorder

    F14.281 Cocaine dependence with cocaine-induced <u>sexual</u> <u>dysfunction</u>

    F14.282 Cocaine dependence with cocaine-induced <u>sleep</u> disorder

    F14.288 Cocaine dependence with other cocaine-induced disorder

F14.29 Cocaine dependence with unspecified cocaine-induced disorder

F14.9- Cocaine <u>use, unspecified</u>
Excludes 1: cocaine abuse (F14.1-)
cocaine dependence (F14.2-)

F14.90 Cocaine use, unspecified, <u>uncomplicated</u>

F14.92- Cocaine use, unspecified <u>with intoxication</u>

    F14.920 Cocaine use, unspecified with intoxication, <u>uncomplicated</u>

    F14.921 Cocaine use, unspecified with intoxication <u>delirium</u>

    F14.922 Cocaine use, unspecified with intoxication <u>with perceptual disturbance</u>

    F14.929 Cocaine use, unspecified with intoxication, <u>unspecified</u>

F14.94 Cocaine use, unspecified <u>with</u> cocaine-induced <u>mood</u> disorder

F14.95- Cocaine use, unspecified <u>with</u> cocaine-induced <u>psychotic</u> disorder

    F14.950 Cocaine use, unspecified with cocaine-induced psychotic disorder <u>with delusions</u>

    F14.951 Cocaine use, unspecified with cocaine-induced psychotic disorder <u>with hallucinations</u>

    F14.959 Cocaine use, unspecified with cocaine-induced psychotic disorder, unspecified

F14.98- Cocaine use, unspecified <u>with other</u> specified cocaine-induced disorder

    F14.980 Cocaine use, unspecified with cocaine-induced <u>anxiety</u> disorder

    F14.981 Cocaine use, unspecified with cocaine-induced <u>sexual</u> <u>dysfunction</u>

    F14.982 Cocaine use, unspecified with cocaine-induced <u>sleep</u> disorder

    F14.988 Cocaine use, unspecified with other cocaine-induced disorder

F14.99 Cocaine use, unspecified with unspecified cocaine-induced disorder

F15- <u>Other stimulant related disorders</u>
Includes: Amphetamine-related disorders
          Caffeine
Excludes❷: cocaine-related disorders (F14.-)

F15.1- Other stimulant <u>abuse</u>
Excludes 1: other stimulant dependence (F15.2-)
other stimulant use, unspecified (F15.9-)

F15.10 Other stimulant abuse, <u>uncomplicated</u>

F15.12- Other stimulant abuse <u>with intoxication</u>

    F15.120 Other stimulant abuse with intoxication, <u>uncomplicated</u>

    F15.121 Other stimulant abuse with intoxication <u>delirium</u>

    F15.122 Other stimulant abuse with intoxication <u>with perceptual disturbance</u>

    F15.129 Other stimulant abuse with intoxication, <u>unspecified</u>

F15.14 Other stimulant abuse <u>with</u> stimulant-induced <u>mood</u> disorder

F
1
2
-
F
1
5

Excludes 1: = NOT CODED HERE! (Do not code both)

Excludes❷: = Not Included Here

F15.15- Other stimulant abuse <u>with</u> stimulant-induced <u>psychotic</u> disorder

  F15.150 Other stimulant abuse with stimulant-induced psychotic disorder <u>with delusions</u>

  F15.151 Other stimulant abuse with stimulant-induced psychotic disorder <u>with hallucinations</u>

  F15.159 Other stimulant abuse with stimulant-induced psychotic disorder, unspecified

F15.18- Other stimulant abuse <u>with</u> <u>other</u> stimulant-induced disorder

  F15.180 Other stimulant abuse with stimulant-induced <u>anxiety</u> disorder

  F15.181 Other stimulant abuse with stimulant-induced <u>sexual dysfunction</u>

  F15.182 Other stimulant abuse with stimulant-induced <u>sleep</u> disorder

  F15.188 Other stimulant abuse with other stimulant-induced disorder

F15.19 Other stimulant abuse with unspecified stimulant-induced disorder

F15.2- Other stimulant <u>dependence</u>
Excludes 1: other stimulant abuse (F15.1-)
other stimulant use, unspecified (F15.9-)

F15.20 Other stimulant dependence, <u>uncomplicated</u>

F15.21 Other stimulant dependence, <u>in remission</u>

F15.22- Other stimulant dependence <u>with intoxication</u>
Excludes 1: other stimulant dependence with withdrawal (F15.23)

  F15.220 Other stimulant dependence with intoxication, <u>uncomplicated</u>

  F15.221 Other stimulant dependence with intoxication <u>delirium</u>

  F15.222 Other stimulant dependence with intoxication <u>with perceptual disturbance</u>

  F15.229 Other stimulant dependence with intoxication, <u>unspecified</u>

F15.23 Other stimulant dependence <u>with withdrawal</u>
Excludes 1: other stimulant dependence with intoxication (F15.22-)

F15.24 Other stimulant dependence <u>with</u> stimulant-induced <u>mood</u> disorder

F15.25- Other stimulant dependence <u>with</u> stimulant-induced <u>psychotic</u> disorder

  F15.250 Other stimulant dependence with stimulant-induced psychotic disorder <u>with delusions</u>

  F15.251 Other stimulant dependence with stimulant-induced psychotic disorder <u>with hallucinations</u>

  F15.259 Other stimulant dependence with stimulant-induced psychotic disorder, unspecified

F15.28- Other stimulant dependence <u>with</u> <u>other</u> stimulant-induced disorder

  F15.280 Other stimulant dependence <u>with</u> stimulant-induced <u>anxiety</u> disorder

  F15.281 Other stimulant dependence <u>with</u> stimulant-induced <u>sexual dysfunction</u>

  F15.282 Other stimulant dependence <u>with</u> stimulant-induced <u>sleep</u> disorder

  F15.288 Other stimulant dependence with other stimulant-induced disorder

F15.29 Other stimulant dependence with unspecified stimulant-induced disorder

F15.9- Other stimulant <u>use, unspecified</u>
Excludes 1: other stimulant abuse (F15.1-)
other stimulant dependence (F15.2-)

F15.90 Other stimulant use, unspecified, <u>uncomplicated</u>

F15.92- Other stimulant use, unspecified <u>with intoxication</u>
Excludes 1: other stimulant use, unspecified with withdrawal (F15.93)

  F15.920 Other stimulant use, unspecified with intoxication, <u>uncomplicated</u>

  F15.921 Other stimulant use, unspecified with intoxication <u>delirium</u>

  F15.922 Other stimulant use, unspecified with intoxication <u>with perceptual disturbance</u>

  F15.929 Other stimulant use, unspecified with intoxication, <u>unspecified</u>

F15.93 Other stimulant use, unspecified U
Excludes 1: other stimulant use, unspecified with intoxication (F15.92-)

F15.94 Other stimulant use, unspecified <u>with</u> stimulant-induced <u>mood</u> disorder

F15.95- Other stimulant use, unspecified <u>with</u> stimulant-induced <u>psychotic</u> disorder

  F15.950 Other stimulant use, unspecified with stimulant-induced psychotic disorder <u>with delusions</u>

  F15.951 Other stimulant use, unspecified with stimulant-induced psychotic disorder <u>with hallucinations</u>

  F15.959 Other stimulant use, unspecified with stimulant-induced psychotic disorder, unspecified

F15.98- Other stimulant use, unspecified <u>with</u> <u>other</u> stimulant-induced disorder

  F15.980 Other stimulant use, unspecified with stimulant-induced <u>anxiety</u> disorder

  F15.981 Other stimulant use, unspecified with stimulant-induced <u>sexual dysfunction</u>

  F15.982 Other stimulant use, unspecified with stimulant-induced <u>sleep</u> disorder

  F15.988 Other stimulant use, unspecified with other stimulant-induced disorder

F15.99 Other stimulant use, unspecified with unspecified stimulant-induced disorder

F16- <u>Hallucinogen related disorders</u>
Includes: Ecstasy
    PCP
    Phencyclidine

F16.1- Hallucinogen <u>abuse</u>
Excludes 1: hallucinogen dependence (F16.2-)
hallucinogen use, unspecified (F16.9-)

F16.10 Hallucinogen abuse, <u>uncomplicated</u>

F16.12- Hallucinogen abuse <u>with intoxication</u>

  F16.120 Hallucinogen abuse with intoxication, <u>uncomplicated</u>

  F16.121 Hallucinogen abuse with intoxication with <u>delirium</u>

  F16.122 Hallucinogen abuse with intoxication <u>with perceptual disturbance</u>

  F16.129 Hallucinogen abuse with intoxication, <u>unspecified</u>

F16.14 Hallucinogen abuse <u>with</u> hallucinogen-induced <u>mood</u> disorder

F16.15- Hallucinogen abuse <u>with</u> hallucinogen-induced <u>psychotic</u> disorder

  F16.150 Hallucinogen abuse with hallucinogen-induced psychotic disorder <u>with delusions</u>

  F16.151 Hallucinogen abuse with hallucinogen-induced psychotic disorder <u>with hallucinations</u>

  F16.159 Hallucinogen abuse with hallucinogen-induced psychotic disorder, unspecified

F16.18- Hallucinogen abuse <u>with</u> <u>other</u> hallucinogen-induced disorder

  F16.180 Hallucinogen abuse with hallucinogen-induced <u>anxiety</u> disorder

  F16.183 Hallucinogen abuse with hallucinogen <u>persisting perception disorder (flashbacks)</u>

  F16.188 Hallucinogen abuse with other hallucinogen-induced disorder

F16.19 Hallucinogen abuse with unspecified hallucinogen-induced disorder

F16.2- Hallucinogen <u>dependence</u>
Excludes 1: hallucinogen abuse (F16.1-)
hallucinogen use, unspecified (F16.9-)

F16.20 Hallucinogen dependence, <u>uncomplicated</u>

F16.21 Hallucinogen dependence, <u>in remission</u>

F16.22- Hallucinogen dependence <u>with intoxication</u>

  F16.220 Hallucinogen dependence with intoxication, <u>uncomplicated</u>

  F16.221 Hallucinogen dependence with intoxication with <u>delirium</u>

  F16.229 Hallucinogen dependence with intoxication, <u>unspecified</u>

F16.24 Hallucinogen dependence <u>with</u> hallucinogen-induced <u>mood</u> disorder

F16.25- Hallucinogen dependence <u>with</u> hallucinogen-induced <u>psychotic</u> disorder

  F16.250 Hallucinogen dependence with hallucinogen-induced psychotic disorder <u>with delusions</u>

  F16.251 Hallucinogen dependence with hallucinogen-induced psychotic disorder <u>with hallucinations</u>

  F16.259 Hallucinogen dependence with hallucinogen-induced psychotic disorder, unspecified

F16.28- Hallucinogen dependence <u>with</u> <u>other</u> hallucinogen-induced disorder
    F16.280 Hallucinogen dependence <u>with</u> hallucinogen-induced <u>anxiety</u> disorder
    F16.283 Hallucinogen dependence <u>with</u> hallucinogen <u>persisting perception disorder (flashbacks)</u>
    F16.288 Hallucinogen dependence with other hallucinogen-induced disorder
F16.29 Hallucinogen dependence with unspecified hallucinogen-induced disorder
F16.9- Hallucinogen <u>use, unspecified</u>
    Excludes 1: hallucinogen abuse (F16.1-)
                   hallucinogen dependence (F16.2-)
    F16.90 Hallucinogen use, unspecified, <u>uncomplicated</u>
    F16.92- Hallucinogen use, unspecified <u>with intoxication</u>
        F16.920 Hallucinogen use, unspecified with intoxication, <u>uncomplicated</u>
        F16.921 Hallucinogen use, unspecified with intoxication with <u>delirium</u>
        F16.929 Hallucinogen use, unspecified with intoxication, <u>unspecified</u>
    F16.94 Hallucinogen use, unspecified <u>with</u> hallucinogen-induced <u>mood</u> disorder
    F16.95- Hallucinogen use, unspecified <u>with</u> hallucinogen-induced <u>psychotic</u> disorder
        F16.950 Hallucinogen use, unspecified with hallucinogen-induced psychotic disorder <u>with delusions</u>
        F16.951 Hallucinogen use, unspecified with hallucinogen-induced psychotic disorder <u>with hallucinations</u>
        F16.959 Hallucinogen use, unspecified with hallucinogen-induced psychotic disorder, unspecified
    F16.98- Hallucinogen use, unspecified <u>with</u> <u>other</u> specified hallucinogen-induced disorder
        F16.980 Hallucinogen use, unspecified with hallucinogen-induced <u>anxiety</u> disorder
        F16.983 Hallucinogen use, unspecified <u>with</u> hallucinogen <u>persisting perception disorder (flashbacks)</u>
        F16.988 Hallucinogen use, unspecified with other hallucinogen-induced disorder
    F16.99 Hallucinogen use, unspecified with unspecified hallucinogen-induced disorder

F17- <u>Nicotine dependence</u>
    Excludes 1: history of tobacco dependence (Z87.891)
                 tobacco use NOS (Z72.0)
    Excludes❷: tobacco use (smoking) during pregnancy, childbirth and the puerperium (O99.33-)
                 toxic effect of nicotine (T65.2-)
  F17.2- Nicotine <u>dependence</u>
    F17.20- Nicotine <u>dependence, unspecified</u>
        F17.200 Nicotine dependence, unspecified, <u>uncomplicated</u>
        F17.201 Nicotine dependence, unspecified, <u>in remission</u>
        F17.203 Nicotine dependence unspecified, <u>with withdrawal</u>
        F17.208 Nicotine dependence, unspecified, with other nicotine-induced disorders
        F17.209 Nicotine dependence, unspecified, with unspecified nicotine-induced disorders
    F17.21- Nicotine dependence, <u>cigarettes</u>
        F17.210 Nicotine dependence, cigarettes, <u>uncomplicated</u>
        F17.211 Nicotine dependence, cigarettes, <u>in remission</u>
        F17.213 Nicotine dependence, cigarettes, <u>with withdrawal</u>
        F17.218 Nicotine dependence, cigarettes, with other nicotine-induced disorders
        F17.219 Nicotine dependence, cigarettes, with unspecified nicotine-induced disorders
    F17.22- Nicotine dependence, <u>chewing tobacco</u>
        F17.220 Nicotine dependence, chewing tobacco, <u>uncomplicated</u>
        F17.221 Nicotine dependence, chewing tobacco, <u>in remission</u>
        F17.223 Nicotine dependence, chewing tobacco, <u>with withdrawal</u>
        F17.228 Nicotine dependence, chewing tobacco, with other nicotine-induced disorders
        F17.229 Nicotine dependence, chewing tobacco, with unspecified nicotine-induced disorders

F17.29- Nicotine dependence, <u>other tobacco product</u>
    F17.290 Nicotine dependence, other tobacco product, <u>uncomplicated</u>
    F17.291 Nicotine dependence, other tobacco product, <u>in remission</u>
    F17.293 Nicotine dependence, other tobacco product, <u>with withdrawal</u>
    F17.298 Nicotine dependence, other tobacco product, with other nicotine-induced disorders
    F17.299 Nicotine dependence, other tobacco product, with unspecified nicotine-induced disorders

F18- <u>Inhalant related disorders</u>
    Includes: Volatile solvents
  F18.1- Inhalant <u>abuse</u>
    Excludes 1: inhalant dependence (F18.2-)
                 inhalant use, unspecified (F18.9-)
    F18.10 Inhalant abuse, <u>uncomplicated</u>
    F18.12- Inhalant abuse <u>with intoxication</u>
        F18.120 Inhalant abuse with intoxication, <u>uncomplicated</u>
        F18.121 Inhalant abuse with intoxication <u>delirium</u>
        F18.129 Inhalant abuse with intoxication, <u>unspecified</u>
    F18.14 Inhalant abuse <u>with</u> inhalant-induced <u>mood</u> disorder
    F18.15- Inhalant abuse <u>with</u> inhalant-induced <u>psychotic</u> disorder
        F18.150 Inhalant abuse with inhalant-induced psychotic disorder <u>with delusions</u>
        F18.151 Inhalant abuse with inhalant-induced psychotic disorder <u>with hallucinations</u>
        F18.159 Inhalant abuse with inhalant-induced psychotic disorder, unspecified
    F18.17 Inhalant abuse <u>with</u> inhalant-induced <u>dementia</u>
    F18.18- Inhalant abuse <u>with</u> <u>other</u> inhalant-induced disorders
        F18.180 Inhalant abuse with inhalant-induced <u>anxiety</u> disorder
        F18.188 Inhalant abuse with other inhalant-induced disorder
    F18.19 Inhalant abuse with unspecified inhalant-induced disorder
  F18.2- Inhalant <u>dependence</u>
    Excludes 1: inhalant abuse (F18.1-)
                 inhalant use, unspecified (F18.9-)
    F18.20 Inhalant dependence, <u>uncomplicated</u>
    F18.21 Inhalant dependence, <u>in remission</u>
    F18.22- Inhalant dependence <u>with intoxication</u>
        F18.220 Inhalant dependence with intoxication, <u>uncomplicated</u>
        F18.221 Inhalant dependence with intoxication <u>delirium</u>
        F18.229 Inhalant dependence with intoxication, <u>unspecified</u>
    F18.24 Inhalant dependence <u>with</u> inhalant-induced <u>mood</u> disorder
    F18.25- Inhalant dependence <u>with</u> inhalant-induced <u>psychotic</u> disorder
        F18.250 Inhalant dependence with inhalant-induced psychotic disorder <u>with delusions</u>
        F18.251 Inhalant dependence with inhalant-induced psychotic disorder <u>with hallucinations</u>
        F18.259 Inhalant dependence with inhalant-induced psychotic disorder, unspecified
    F18.27 Inhalant dependence <u>with</u> inhalant-induced <u>dementia</u>
    F18.28- Inhalant dependence <u>with</u> <u>other</u> inhalant-induced disorders
        F18.280 Inhalant dependence with inhalant-induced <u>anxiety</u> disorder
        F18.288 Inhalant dependence with other inhalant-induced disorder
    F18.29 Inhalant dependence with unspecified inhalant-induced disorder
  F18.9- Inhalant <u>use, unspecified</u>
    Excludes 1: inhalant abuse (F18.1-)
                 inhalant dependence (F18.2-)
    F18.90 Inhalant use, unspecified, <u>uncomplicated</u>
    F18.92- Inhalant use, unspecified <u>with intoxication</u>
        F18.920 Inhalant use, unspecified with intoxication, <u>uncomplicated</u>
        F18.921 Inhalant use, unspecified with intoxication with <u>delirium</u>
        F18.929 Inhalant use, unspecified with intoxication, <u>unspecified</u>
    F18.94 Inhalant use, unspecified <u>with</u> inhalant-induced <u>mood</u> disorder

F 1 5 - F 1 8

F18.95- **Inhalant use, unspecified <u>with</u> inhalant-induced <u>psychotic</u> disorder**
 F18.950 Inhalant use, unspecified with inhalant-induced psychotic disorder <u>with delusions</u>
 F18.951 Inhalant use, unspecified with inhalant-induced psychotic disorder <u>with hallucinations</u>
 F18.959 Inhalant use, unspecified with inhalant-induced psychotic disorder, unspecified

F18.97 Inhalant use, unspecified <u>with</u> inhalant-induced <u>persisting dementia</u>

F18.98- **Inhalant use, unspecified <u>with</u> <u>other</u> inhalant-induced disorders**
 F18.980 Inhalant use, unspecified with inhalant-induced <u>anxiety</u> disorder
 F18.988 Inhalant use, unspecified with other inhalant-induced disorder

F18.99 Inhalant use, unspecified with unspecified inhalant-induced disorder

F19- <u>Other psychoactive substance related disorders</u>
 Includes: Polysubstance drug use (indiscriminate drug use)

F19.1- **Other psychoactive substance <u>abuse</u>**
 Excludes 1: other psychoactive substance dependence (F19.2-)
    other psychoactive substance use, unspecified (F19.9-)

F19.10 Other psychoactive substance abuse, <u>uncomplicated</u>

F19.12- Other psychoactive substance abuse <u>with intoxication</u>
 F19.120 Other psychoactive substance abuse with intoxication, <u>uncomplicated</u>
 F19.121 Other psychoactive substance abuse with intoxication <u>delirium</u>
 F19.122 Other psychoactive substance abuse with intoxication <u>with perceptual disturbances</u>
 F19.129 Other psychoactive substance abuse with intoxication, unspecified

F19.14 Other psychoactive substance abuse <u>with</u> psychoactive substance-induced mood disorder

F19.15- Other psychoactive substance abuse <u>with</u> psychoactive substance-induced <u>psychotic</u> disorder
 F19.150 Other psychoactive substance abuse with psychoactive substance-induced psychotic disorder <u>with delusions</u>
 F19.151 Other psychoactive substance abuse with psychoactive substance-induced psychotic disorder <u>with hallucinations</u>
 F19.159 Other psychoactive substance abuse with psychoactive substance-induced psychotic disorder, unspecified

F19.16 Other psychoactive substance abuse <u>with</u> psychoactive substance-induced <u>persisting amnestic</u> disorder

F19.17 Other psychoactive substance abuse <u>with</u> psychoactive substance-induced <u>persisting dementia</u>

F19.18- Other psychoactive substance abuse <u>with</u> <u>other</u> psychoactive substance-induced disorders
 F19.180 Other psychoactive substance abuse with psychoactive substance-induced <u>anxiety</u> disorder
 F19.181 Other psychoactive substance abuse <u>with</u> psychoactive substance-induced <u>sexual dysfunction</u>
 F19.182 Other psychoactive substance abuse <u>with</u> psychoactive substance-induced <u>sleep</u> disorder
 F19.188 Other psychoactive substance abuse with other psychoactive substance-induced disorder

F19.19 Other psychoactive substance abuse with unspecified psychoactive substance-induced disorder

F19.2- **Other psychoactive substance <u>dependence</u>**
 Excludes 1: other psychoactive substance abuse (F19.1-)
    other psychoactive substance use, unspecified (F19.9-)

F19.20 Other psychoactive substance dependence, <u>uncomplicated</u>

F19.21 Other psychoactive substance dependence, <u>in remission</u>

F19.22- Other psychoactive substance dependence <u>with intoxication</u>
 Excludes 1: other psychoactive substance dependence with withdrawal (F19.23-)
 F19.220 Other psychoactive substance dependence with intoxication, <u>uncomplicated</u>
 F19.221 Other psychoactive substance dependence with intoxication <u>delirium</u>
 F19.222 Other psychoactive substance dependence with intoxication <u>with perceptual disturbance</u>
 F19.229 Other psychoactive substance dependence with intoxication, <u>unspecified</u>

F19.23- Other psychoactive substance dependence <u>with withdrawal</u>
 Excludes 1: other psychoactive substance dependence with intoxication (F19.22-)
 F19.230 Other psychoactive substance dependence with withdrawal, <u>uncomplicated</u>
 F19.231 Other psychoactive substance dependence with withdrawal <u>delirium</u>
 F19.232 Other psychoactive substance dependence with withdrawal <u>with perceptual disturbance</u>
 F19.239 Other psychoactive substance dependence with withdrawal, <u>unspecified</u>

F19.24 Other psychoactive substance dependence <u>with</u> psychoactive substance-induced <u>mood</u> disorder

F19.25- Other psychoactive substance dependence <u>with</u> psychoactive substance-induced <u>psychotic</u> disorder
 F19.250 Other psychoactive substance dependence with psychoactive substance-induced psychotic disorder <u>with delusions</u>
 F19.251 Other psychoactive substance dependence with psychoactive substance-induced psychotic disorder <u>with hallucinations</u>
 F19.259 Other psychoactive substance dependence with psychoactive substance-induced psychotic disorder, unspecified

F19.26 Other psychoactive substance dependence <u>with</u> psychoactive substance-induced <u>persisting amnestic</u> disorder

F19.27 Other psychoactive substance dependence <u>with</u> psychoactive substance-induced <u>persisting dementia</u>

F19.28- Other psychoactive substance dependence <u>with</u> <u>other</u> psychoactive substance-induced disorders
 F19.280 Other psychoactive substance dependence with psychoactive substance-induced <u>anxiety</u> disorder
 F19.281 Other psychoactive substance dependence with psychoactive substance-induced <u>sexual dysfunction</u>
 F19.282 Other psychoactive substance dependence with psychoactive substance-induced <u>sleep</u> disorder
 F19.288 Other psychoactive substance dependence with other psychoactive substance-induced disorder

F19.29 Other psychoactive substance dependence with unspecified psychoactive substance-induced disorder

F19.9- **Other psychoactive substance <u>use, unspecified</u>**
 Excludes 1: other psychoactive substance abuse (F19.1-)
    other psychoactive substance dependence (F19.2-)

F19.90 Other psychoactive substance use, unspecified, <u>uncomplicated</u>

F19.92- Other psychoactive substance use, unspecified <u>with intoxication</u>
 Excludes 1: other psychoactive substance use, unspecified with withdrawal (F19.93)
 F19.920 Other psychoactive substance use, unspecified with intoxication, <u>uncomplicated</u>
 F19.921 Other psychoactive substance use, unspecified with intoxication <u>with delirium</u>
 F19.922 Other psychoactive substance use, unspecified with intoxication <u>with perceptual disturbance</u>
 F19.929 Other psychoactive substance use, unspecified with intoxication, <u>unspecified</u>

F19.93- Other psychoactive substance use, unspecified <u>with withdrawal</u>
 Excludes 1: other psychoactive substance use, unspecified with intoxication (F19.92-)
 F19.930 Other psychoactive substance use, unspecified with withdrawal, <u>uncomplicated</u>
 F19.931 Other psychoactive substance use, unspecified with withdrawal <u>delirium</u>
 F19.932 Other psychoactive substance use, unspecified with withdrawal <u>with perceptual disturbance</u>
 F19.939 Other psychoactive substance use, unspecified with withdrawal, <u>unspecified</u>

F19.94 Other psychoactive substance use, unspecified <u>with</u> psychoactive substance-induced <u>mood</u> disorder

F18 - F30

F19.95- Other psychoactive substance use, unspecified <u>with</u> psychoactive substance-induced <u>psychotic</u> disorder

    F19.950 Other psychoactive substance use, unspecified with psychoactive substance-induced psychotic disorder <u>with delusions</u>

    F19.951 Other psychoactive substance use, unspecified with psychoactive substance-induced psychotic disorder <u>with hallucinations</u>

    F19.959 Other psychoactive substance use, unspecified with psychoactive substance-induced psychotic disorder, unspecified

F19.96 Other psychoactive substance use, unspecified <u>with</u> psychoactive substance-induced <u>persisting amnestic</u> disorder

F19.97 Other psychoactive substance use, unspecified <u>with</u> psychoactive substance-induced <u>persisting dementia</u>

F19.98- Other psychoactive substance use, unspecified <u>with other</u> psychoactive substance-induced disorders

    F19.980 Other psychoactive substance use, unspecified <u>with</u> psychoactive substance-induced <u>anxiety</u> disorder

    F19.981 Other psychoactive substance use, unspecified <u>with</u> psychoactive substance-induced <u>sexual dysfunction</u>

    F19.982 Other psychoactive substance use, unspecified <u>with</u> psychoactive substance-induced <u>sleep</u> disorder

    F19.988 Other psychoactive substance use, unspecified with other psychoactive substance-induced disorder

F19.99 Other psychoactive substance use, unspecified with unspecified psychoactive substance-induced disorder

Schizophrenia, schizotypal, delusional, and other non-mood psychotic disorders (F20-F29)

F20- <u>Schizophrenia</u>

Excludes 1: brief psychotic disorder (F23)
cyclic schizophrenia (F25.0)
mood [affective] disorders with psychotic symptoms (F30.2, F31.2, F31.5, F31.64, F32.3, F33.3)
schizoaffective disorder (F25.-)
schizophrenic reaction NOS (F23)

Excludes❷: schizophrenic reaction in:
alcoholism (F10.15-, F10.25-, F10.95-)
brain disease (F06.2)
epilepsy (F06.2)
psychoactive drug use (F11-F19 with .15, .25, .95)
schizotypal disorder (F21)

F20.0 Paranoid schizophrenia
    Paraphrenic schizophrenia
    Excludes 1: involutional paranoid state (F22)
               paranoia (F22)

F20.1 Disorganized schizophrenia
    Hebephrenic schizophrenia
    Hebephrenia

F20.2 Catatonic schizophrenia
    Schizophrenic catalepsy
    Schizophrenic catatonia
    Schizophrenic flexibilitas cerea
    Excludes 1: catatonic stupor (R40.1)

F20.3 Undifferentiated schizophrenia
    Atypical schizophrenia
    Excludes 1: acute schizophrenia-like psychotic disorder (F23)
    Excludes❷: post-schizophrenic depression (F32.8)

F20.5 Residual schizophrenia
    Restzustand (schizophrenic)
    Schizophrenic residual state

F20.8- Other schizophrenia
    F20.81 Schizophreniform disorder
        Schizophreniform psychosis NOS
    F20.89 Other schizophrenia
        Cenesthopathic schizophrenia
        Simple schizophrenia

F20.9 Schizophrenia, unspecified

F21 <u>Schizotypal</u> disorder
    Borderline schizophrenia
    Latent schizophrenia
    Latent schizophrenic reaction
    Prepsychotic schizophrenia
    Prodromal schizophrenia
    Pseudoneurotic schizophrenia
    Pseudopsychopathic schizophrenia
    Schizotypal personality disorder
    Excludes❷: Asperger's syndrome (F84.5)
          schizoid personality disorder (F60.1)

F22 Delusional disorders
    Delusional dysmorphophobia
    Involutional paranoid state
    Paranoia
    Paranoia querulans
    Paranoid psychosis
    Paranoid state
    Paraphrenia (late)
    Sensitiver Beziehungswahn
    Excludes 1: mood [affective] disorders with psychotic symptoms (F30.2, F31.2, F31.5, F31.64, F32.3, F33.3)
          paranoid schizophrenia (F20.0)
    Excludes❷: paranoid personality disorder (F60.0)
          paranoid psychosis, psychogenic (F23)
          paranoid reaction (F23)

F23 <u>Brief</u> psychotic disorder
    Paranoid reaction
    Psychogenic paranoid psychosis
    Excludes❷: mood [affective] disorders with psychotic symptoms (F30.2, F31.2, F31.5, F31.64, F32.3, F33.3)

F24 <u>Shared</u> psychotic disorder
    Folie à deux
    Induced paranoid disorder
    Induced psychotic disorder

F25- <u>Schizoaffective</u> disorders
    Excludes 1: mood [affective] disorders with psychotic symptoms (F30.2, F31.2, F31.5, F31.64, F32.3, F33.3)
          schizophrenia (F20.-)

    F25.0 Schizoaffective disorder, <u>bipolar</u> type
        Cyclic schizophrenia
        Schizoaffective disorder, manic type
        Schizoaffective disorder, mixed type
        Schizoaffective psychosis, bipolar type
        Schizophreniform psychosis, manic type

    F25.1 Schizoaffective disorder, <u>depressive</u> type
        Schizoaffective psychosis, depressive type
        Schizophreniform psychosis, depressive type

    F25.8 Other schizoaffective disorders

    F25.9 Schizoaffective disorder, unspecified
        Schizoaffective psychosis NOS

F28 Other psychotic disorder <u>not</u> due to a substance or known physiological condition
    Chronic hallucinatory psychosis

F29 Unspecified psychosis <u>not</u> due to a substance or known physiological condition
    Psychosis NOS
    Excludes 1: mental disorder NOS (F99)
          unspecified mental disorder due to known physiological condition (F09)

Mood [affective] disorders (F30-F39)

F30- <u>Manic episode</u>
    Includes: Bipolar disorder, single manic episode
              Mixed affective episode
    Excludes 1: bipolar disorder (F31.-)
          major depressive disorder, single episode (F32.-)
          major depressive disorder, recurrent (F33.-)

    F30.1- Manic episode <u>without psychotic symptoms</u>
        F30.10 Manic episode without psychotic symptoms, unspecified
        F30.11 Manic episode without psychotic symptoms, <u>mild</u>
        F30.12 Manic episode without psychotic symptoms, <u>moderate</u>
        F30.13 Manic episode, severe, without psychotic symptoms

    F30.2 Manic episode, severe <u>with psychotic symptoms</u>
        Manic stupor
        Mania with mood-congruent psychotic symptoms
        Mania with mood-incongruent psychotic symptoms

    F30.3 Manic episode in <u>partial</u> remission

    F30.4 Manic episode in <u>full</u> remission

    F30.8 Other manic episodes
        Hypomania

    F30.9 Manic episode, unspecified
        Mania NOS

F
1
8
I
F
3
0

Excludes 1: = NOT CODED HERE! (Do not code both)

Excludes❷: = Not Included Here

F31-   Bipolar disorder
     Includes: Manic-depressive illness
              Manic-depressive psychosis
              Manic-depressive reaction
     Excludes 1:   *bipolar disorder, single manic episode (F30.-)*
               major depressive disorder, single episode (F32.-)
               major depressive disorder, recurrent (F33.-)
     Excludes❷: *cyclothymia (F34.0)*

F31.0   **Bipolar disorder, current episode <u>hypomanic</u>**
F31.1-   **Bipolar disorder, current episode <u>manic</u> <u>without</u> psychotic features**
     F31.10   **Bipolar disorder, current episode manic without psychotic features, <u>unspecified</u>**
     F31.11   **Bipolar disorder, current episode manic without psychotic features, <u>mild</u>**
     F31.12   **Bipolar disorder, current episode manic without psychotic features, <u>moderate</u>**
     F31.13   **Bipolar disorder, current episode manic without psychotic features, <u>severe</u>**
F31.2   **Bipolar disorder, current episode <u>manic</u> <u>severe</u> <u>with psychotic features</u>**
     Bipolar disorder, current episode manic with mood-congruent psychotic symptoms
     Bipolar disorder, current episode manic with mood-incongruent psychotic symptoms
F31.3-   **Bipolar disorder, current episode <u>depressed</u>, mild or moderate severity**
     F31.30   **Bipolar disorder, current episode depressed, mild or moderate severity, unspecified**
     F31.31   **Bipolar disorder, current episode depressed, <u>mild</u>**
     F31.32   **Bipolar disorder, current episode depressed, <u>moderate</u>**
F31.4   **Bipolar disorder, current episode depressed, <u>severe</u>, without psychotic features**
F31.5   **Bipolar disorder, current episode depressed, severe, <u>with psychotic features</u>**
     Bipolar disorder, current episode depressed with mood-incongruent psychotic symptoms
     Bipolar disorder, current episode depressed with mood-congruent psychotic symptoms
F31.6-   **Bipolar disorder, current episode <u>mixed</u>**
     F31.60   **Bipolar disorder, current episode mixed, <u>unspecified</u>**
     F31.61   **Bipolar disorder, current episode mixed, <u>mild</u>**
     F31.62   **Bipolar disorder, current episode mixed, <u>moderate</u>**
     F31.63   **Bipolar disorder, current episode mixed, <u>severe</u>, without psychotic features**
     F31.64   **Bipolar disorder, current episode mixed, <u>severe</u>, <u>with psychotic features</u>**
         Bipolar disorder, current episode mixed with mood-congruent psychotic symptoms
         Bipolar disorder, current episode mixed with mood-incongruent psychotic symptoms
F31.7-   **Bipolar disorder, currently <u>in remission</u>**
     F31.70   **Bipolar disorder, currently in remission, <u>most recent episode unspecified</u>**
     F31.71   **Bipolar disorder, in <u>partial</u> remission, most recent episode <u>hypomanic</u>**
     F31.72   **Bipolar disorder, in <u>full</u> remission, most recent episode <u>hypomanic</u>**
     F31.73   **Bipolar disorder, in <u>partial</u> remission, most recent episode <u>manic</u>**
     F31.74   **Bipolar disorder, in <u>full</u> remission, most recent episode <u>manic</u>**
     F31.75   **Bipolar disorder, in <u>partial</u> remission, most recent episode <u>depressed</u>**
     F31.76   **Bipolar disorder, in <u>full</u> remission, most recent episode <u>depressed</u>**
     F31.77   **Bipolar disorder, in <u>partial</u> remission, most recent episode <u>mixed</u>**
     F31.78   **Bipolar disorder, in <u>full</u> remission, most recent episode <u>mixed</u>**
F31.8-   **Other bipolar disorders**
     F31.81   **<u>Bipolar II</u> disorder**
     F31.89   **Other bipolar disorder**
         Recurrent manic episodes NOS
F31.9   **Bipolar disorder, unspecified**

F32-   Major depressive disorder, single episode
     Includes: Single episode of agitated depression
              Single episode of depressive reaction
              Single episode of major depression
              Single episode of psychogenic depression
              Single episode of reactive depression
              Single episode of vital depression
     Excludes 1:   *bipolar disorder (F31.-)*
               manic episode (F30.-)
               recurrent depressive disorder (F33.-)
     Excludes❷: *adjustment disorder (F43.2)*

F32.0   **Major depressive disorder, single episode, <u>mild</u>**
F32.1   **Major depressive disorder, single episode, <u>moderate</u>**
F32.2   **Major depressive disorder, single episode, <u>severe</u> <u>without</u> psychotic features**
F32.3   **Major depressive disorder, single episode, <u>severe</u> <u>with psychotic features</u>**
     Single episode of major depression with mood-congruent psychotic symptoms
     Single episode of major depression with mood-incongruent psychotic symptoms
     Single episode of major depression with psychotic symptoms
     Single episode of psychogenic depressive psychosis
     Single episode of psychotic depression
     Single episode of reactive depressive psychosis
F32.4   **Major depressive disorder, single episode, in <u>partial</u> remission**
F32.5   **Major depressive disorder, single episode, in <u>full</u> remission**
F32.8   **Other depressive episodes**
     Atypical depression
     Post-schizophrenic depression
     Single episode of "masked" depression NOS
F32.9   **Major depressive disorder, single episode, <u>unspecified</u>**
     Depression NOS
     Depressive disorder NOS
     Major depression NOS

F33-   Major depressive disorder, recurrent
     Includes: Recurrent episodes of depressive reaction
              Recurrent episodes of endogenous depression
              Recurrent episodes of major depression
              Recurrent episodes of psychogenic depression
              Recurrent episodes of reactive depression
              Recurrent episodes of seasonal depressive disorder
              Recurrent episodes of vital depression
     Excludes 1:   *bipolar disorder (F31.-)*
               manic episode (F30.-)

F33.0   **Major depressive disorder, recurrent, <u>mild</u>**
F33.1   **Major depressive disorder, recurrent, <u>moderate</u>**
F33.2   **Major depressive disorder, recurrent <u>severe</u> <u>without</u> psychotic features**
F33.3   **Major depressive disorder, recurrent, <u>severe</u> <u>with psychotic symptoms</u>**
     Endogenous depression with psychotic symptoms
     Recurrent severe episodes of major depression with mood-congruent psychotic symptoms
     Recurrent severe episodes of major depression with mood-incongruent psychotic symptoms
     Recurrent severe episodes of major depression with psychotic symptoms
     Recurrent severe episodes of psychogenic depressive psychosis
     Recurrent severe episodes of psychotic depression
     Recurrent severe episodes of reactive depressive psychosis
F33.4-   **Major depressive disorder, recurrent, in remission**
     F33.40   **Major depressive disorder, recurrent, in remission, unspecified**
     F33.41   **Major depressive disorder, recurrent, in <u>partial</u> remission**
     F33.42   **Major depressive disorder, recurrent, in <u>full</u> remission**
F33.8   **Other recurrent depressive disorders**
     Recurrent brief depressive episodes
F33.9   **Major depressive disorder, recurrent, unspecified**
     Monopolar depression NOS

F
3
1
-
F
4
4

F34- **Persistent mood [affective] disorders**

    F34.0 **Cyclothymic disorder**
        Affective personality disorder
        Cycloid personality
        Cyclothymia
        Cyclothymic personality

    F34.1 **Dysthymic disorder**
        Depressive neurosis
        Depressive personality disorder
        Dysthymia
        Neurotic depression
        Persistent anxiety depression
        Excludes❷: anxiety depression (mild or not persistent) (F41.8)

    F34.8 **Other persistent mood [affective] disorders**
    F34.9 **Persistent mood [affective] disorder, unspecified**

F39 **Unspecified mood [affective] disorder**
    Affective psychosis NOS

Anxiety, dissociative, stress-related, somatoform and other nonpsychotic mental disorders (F40-F48)

F40- **Phobic anxiety disorders**

    F40.0- **Agoraphobia**
        F40.00 **Agoraphobia, unspecified**
        F40.01 **Agoraphobia with panic disorder**
            Panic disorder with agoraphobia
            Excludes 1: panic disorder without agoraphobia (F41.0)
        F40.02 **Agoraphobia without panic disorder**

    F40.1- **Social phobias**
        Anthropophobia
        Social anxiety disorder of childhood
        Social neurosis
        F40.10 **Social phobia, unspecified**
        F40.11 **Social phobia, generalized**

    F40.2- **Specific (isolated) phobias**
        Excludes❷: dysmorphophobia (nondelusional) (F45.22)
                nosophobia (F45.22)
        F40.21- **Animal type phobia**
            F40.210 **Arachnophobia**
                Fear of spiders
            F40.218 **Other animal type phobia**
        F40.22- **Natural environment type phobia**
            F40.220 **Fear of thunderstorms**
            F40.228 **Other natural environment type phobia**
        F40.23- **Blood, injection, injury type phobia**
            F40.230 **Fear of blood**
            F40.231 **Fear of injections and transfusions**
            F40.232 **Fear of other medical care**
            F40.233 **Fear of injury**
        F40.24- **Situational type phobia**
            F40.240 **Claustrophobia**
            F40.241 **Acrophobia**
            F40.242 **Fear of bridges**
            F40.243 **Fear of flying**
            F40.248 **Other situational type phobia**
        F40.29- **Other specified phobia**
            F40.290 **Androphobia**
                Fear of men
            F40.291 **Gynephobia**
                Fear of women
            F40.298 **Other specified phobia**

    F40.8 **Other phobic anxiety disorders**
        Phobic anxiety disorder of childhood
    F40.9 **Phobia anxiety disorder, unspecified**
        Phobia NOS
        Phobic state NOS

F41- **Other anxiety disorders**
    Excludes❷: anxiety in:
        acute stress reaction (F43.0)
        transient adjustment reaction (F43.2)
        neurasthenia (F48.8)
        psychophysiologic disorders (F45.-)
        separation anxiety (F93.0)

    F41.0 **Panic disorder [episodic paroxysmal anxiety] without agoraphobia**
        Panic attack
        Panic state
        Excludes 1: panic disorder with agoraphobia (F40.01)

    F41.1 **Generalized anxiety disorder**
        Anxiety neurosis
        Anxiety reaction
        Anxiety state
        Overanxious disorder
        Excludes❷: neurasthenia (F48.8)

    F41.3 **Other mixed anxiety disorders**
    F41.8 **Other specified anxiety disorders**
        Anxiety depression (mild or not persistent)
        Anxiety hysteria
        Mixed anxiety and depressive disorder
    F41.9 **Anxiety disorder, unspecified**
        Anxiety NOS

F42 **Obsessive-compulsive disorder**
    Anancastic neurosis
    Obsessive-compulsive neurosis
    Excludes❷: obsessive-compulsive personality (disorder) (F60.5)
        obsessive-compulsive symptoms occurring in depression (F32-F33)
        obsessive-compulsive symptoms occurring in schizophrenia (F20.-)

F43- **Reaction to severe stress, and adjustment disorders**
    F43.0 **Acute stress reaction**
        Acute crisis reaction
        Acute reaction to stress
        Combat and operational stress reaction
        Combat fatigue
        Crisis state
        Psychic shock

    F43.1- **Post-traumatic stress disorder (PTSD)**
        Traumatic neurosis
        F43.10 **Post-traumatic stress disorder, unspecified**
        F43.11 **Post-traumatic stress disorder, acute**
        F43.12 **Post-traumatic stress disorder, chronic**

    F43.2- **Adjustment disorders**
        Culture shock
        Grief reaction
        Hospitalism in children
        Excludes❷: separation anxiety disorder of childhood (F93.0)
        F43.20 **Adjustment disorder, unspecified**
        F43.21 **Adjustment disorder with depressed mood**
        F43.22 **Adjustment disorder with anxiety**
        F43.23 **Adjustment disorder with mixed anxiety and depressed mood**
        F43.24 **Adjustment disorder with disturbance of conduct**
        F43.25 **Adjustment disorder with mixed disturbance of emotions and conduct**
        F43.29 **Adjustment disorder with other symptoms**

    F43.8 **Other reactions to severe stress**
    F43.9 **Reaction to severe stress, unspecified**

F44- **Dissociative and conversion disorders**
    Includes: Conversion hysteria
        Conversion reaction
        Hysteria
        Hysterical psychosis
    Excludes❷: malingering [conscious simulation] (Z76.5)

    F44.0 **Dissociative amnesia**
        Excludes 1: amnesia NOS (R41.3)
            anterograde amnesia (R41.1)
            retrograde amnesia (R41.2)
        Excludes❷: alcohol-or other psychoactive substance-induced amnestic disorder (F10, F13, F19 with .26, .96)
            amnestic disorder due to known physiological condition (F04)
            postictal amnesia in epilepsy (G40.-)

    F44.1 **Dissociative fugue**
        Excludes❷: postictal fugue in epilepsy (G40.-)

F 3 1 – F 4 4

F44.2   Dissociative <u>stupor</u>
Excludes 1:   catatonic stupor (R40.1)
*   stupor NOS (R40.1)*
Excludes❷: catatonic disorder due to known physiological
*   condition (F06.1)*
*   depressive stupor (F32, F33)*
*   manic stupor (F30, F31)*

F44.4   <u>Conversion disorder</u> <u>with motor symptom or deficit</u>
Dissociative motor disorders
Psychogenic aphonia
Psychogenic dysphonia

F44.5   <u>Conversion disorder</u> <u>with seizures or convulsions</u>
Dissociative convulsions

F44.6   <u>Conversion disorder</u> <u>with sensory symptom or deficit</u>
Dissociative anesthesia and sensory loss
Psychogenic deafness

F44.7   <u>Conversion disorder</u> <u>with mixed symptom presentation</u>

F44.8-   Other dissociative and conversion disorders

   F44.81   Dissociative identity disorder
      Multiple personality disorder

   F44.89   Other dissociative and conversion disorders
      Ganser's syndrome
      Psychogenic confusion
      Psychogenic twilight state
      Trance and possession disorders

F44.9   Dissociative and conversion disorder, unspecified
Dissociative disorder NOS

F45-   <u>Somatoform disorders</u>
Excludes❷: dissociative and conversion disorders (F44.-)
*   factitious disorders (F68.1-)*
*   hair-plucking (F63.3)*
*   lalling (F80.0)*
*   lisping (F80.0)*
*   malingering [conscious simulation] (Z76.5)*
*   nail-biting (F98.8)*
*   psychological or behavioral factors associated with disorders*
*   or diseases classified elsewhere (F54)*
*   sexual dysfunction, not due to a substance or known*
*   physiological condition (F52.-)*
*   thumb-sucking (F98.8)*
*   tic disorders (in childhood and adolescence) (F95.-)*
*   Tourette's syndrome (F95.2)*
*   trichotillomania (F63.3)*

F45.0   Somatization disorder
Briquet's disorder
Multiple psychosomatic disorder

F45.1   Undifferentiated somatoform disorder
Undifferentiated psychosomatic disorder

F45.2-   <u>Hypochondriacal</u> disorders
Excludes❷: delusional dysmorphophobia (F22)
*   fixed delusions about bodily functions or shape (F22)*

   F45.20   Hypochondriacal disorder, unspecified

   F45.21   Hypochondriasis
      Hypochondriacal neurosis

   F45.22   Body dysmorphic disorder
      Dysmorphophobia (nondelusional)
      Nosophobia

   F45.29   Other hypochondriacal disorders

F45.4-   <u>Pain disorders related to psychological factors</u>
Excludes 1:   pain NOS (R52)

   F45.41   Pain disorder exclusively related to psychological factors
      Somatoform pain disorder (persistent)

   F45.42   Pain disorder with related psychological factors
      Code also associated acute or chronic pain (G89.-)

F45.8   Other somatoform disorders
Psychogenic dysmenorrhea
Psychogenic dysphagia, including "globus hystericus"
Psychogenic pruritus
Psychogenic torticollis
Somatoform autonomic dysfunction
Teeth grinding
Excludes 1:   sleep related teeth grinding (G47.63)

F45.9   Somatoform disorder, unspecified
Psychosomatic disorder NOS

F48-   Other nonpsychotic mental disorders

   F48.1   Depersonalization-derealization syndrome

   F48.2   Pseudobulbar affect
      Involuntary emotional expression disorder
      Code first underlying cause, if known, such as:
      Amyotrophic lateral sclerosis (G12.21)
      Multiple sclerosis (G35)
      Sequelae of cerebrovascular disease (I69-)
      Sequelae of traumatic intracranial injury (S06-)

F48.8   Other specified nonpsychotic mental disorders
Dhat syndrome
Neurasthenia
Occupational neurosis, including writer's cramp
Psychasthenia
Psychasthenic neurosis
Psychogenic syncope

F48.9   Nonpsychotic mental disorder, unspecified
Neurosis NOS

Behavioral syndromes associated with physiological disturbances and physical factors (F50-F59)

F50-   <u>Eating disorders</u>
Excludes 1:   anorexia NOS (R63.0)
*   feeding difficulties (R63.3)*
*   polyphagia (R63.2)*
Excludes❷: feeding disorder in infancy or childhood (F98.2-)

F50.0-   <u>Anorexia nervosa</u>
Excludes 1:   loss of appetite (R63.0)
*   psychogenic loss of appetite (F50.8)*

   F50.00   Anorexia nervosa, unspecified

   F50.01   Anorexia nervosa, restricting type

   F50.02   Anorexia nervosa, binge eating/purging type
      Excludes 1:   bulimia nervosa (F50.2)

F50.2   <u>Bulimia nervosa</u>
Bulimia NOS
Hyperorexia nervosa
Excludes 1:   anorexia nervosa, binge eating/purging type (F50.02)

F50.8   Other eating disorders
Pica in adults
Psychogenic loss of appetite
Excludes❷: pica of infancy and childhood (F98.3)

F50.9   Eating disorder, unspecified
Atypical anorexia nervosa
Atypical bulimia nervosa

F51-   <u>Sleep disorders not</u> due to a substance or known physiological condition
Excludes❷: organic sleep disorders (G47.-)

F51.0-   <u>Insomnia</u> not due to a substance or known physiological condition
Excludes❷: alcohol related insomnia (F10.182, F10.282, F10.982)
*   drug-related insomnia (F11.182, F11.282, F11.982,*
*   F13.182, F13.282, F13.982, F14.182, F14.282,*
*   F14.982, F15.182, F15.282, F15.982, F19.182,*
*   F19.282, F19.982)*
*   insomnia NOS (G47.0-)*
*   insomnia due to known physiological condition*
*   (G47.0-)*
*   organic insomnia (G47.0-)*
*   sleep deprivation (Z72.820)*

   F51.01   <u>Primary</u> insomnia
      Idiopathic insomnia

   F51.02   <u>Adjustment</u> insomnia

   F51.03   <u>Paradoxical</u> insomnia

   F51.04   <u>Psychophysiologic</u> insomnia

   F51.05   Insomnia due to other mental disorder
      Code also associated mental disorder

   F51.09   Other insomnia not due to a substance or known physiological condition

F51.1-   <u>Hypersomnia</u> not due to a substance or known physiological condition
Excludes❷: alcohol related hypersomnia (F10.182, F10.282, F10.982)
*   drug-related hypersomnia (F11.182, F11.282, F11.982,*
*   F13.182, F13.282, F13.982, F14.182, F14.282,*
*   F14.982, F15.182, F15.282, F15.982, F19.182,*
*   F19.282, F19.982)*
*   hypersomnia NOS (G47.10)*
*   hypersomnia due to known physiological condition*
*   (G47.10)*
*   idiopathic hypersomnia (G47.11, G47.12)*
*   narcolepsy (G47.4-)*

   F51.11   <u>Primary</u> hypersomnia

   F51.12   <u>Insufficient</u> sleep syndrome
      Excludes 1:   sleep deprivation (Z72.820)

   F51.13   Hypersomnia due to other mental disorder
      Code also associated mental disorder

   F51.19   Other hypersomnia not due to a substance or known physiological condition

F51.3   Sleepwalking [somnambulism]

F51.4   Sleep terrors [night terrors]

F
4
4
-
F
6
3

Excludes 1: = NOT CODED HERE! (Do not code both)

Excludes❷: = Not Included Here

F51.5   **Nightmare disorder**
  Dream anxiety disorder

F51.8   **Other sleep disorders not due to a substance or known physiological condition**

F51.9   **Sleep disorder not due to a substance or known physiological condition, unspecified**
  Emotional sleep disorder NOS

F52-   **Sexual dysfunction** not due to a substance or known physiological condition
  Excludes❷: Dhat syndrome (F48.8)

F52.0   **Hypoactive sexual desire disorder**
  Anhedonia (sexual)
  Lack or loss of sexual desire
  Excludes 1: decreased libido (R68.82)

F52.1   **Sexual aversion disorder**
  Sexual aversion and lack of sexual enjoyment

F52.2-   **Sexual arousal disorders**
  Failure of genital response

  F52.21   **Male erectile disorder**
    Psychogenic impotence
    Excludes 1: impotence of organic origin (N52.-)
        impotence NOS (N52.-)

  F52.22   **Female sexual arousal disorder**
    Frigidity

F52.3-   **Orgasmic disorder**
  Inhibited orgasm
  Psychogenic anorgasmy

  F52.31   **Female orgasmic disorder**

  F52.32   **Male orgasmic disorder**

F52.4   **Premature ejaculation**

F52.5   **Vaginismus not due to a substance or known physiological condition**
  Psychogenic vaginismus
  Excludes❷: vaginismus (due to a known physiological condition) (N94.2)

F52.6   **Dyspareunia not due to a substance or known physiological condition**
  Psychogenic dyspareunia
  Excludes❷: dyspareunia (due to a known physiological condition) (N94.1)

F52.8   **Other sexual dysfunction not due to a substance or known physiological condition**
  Excessive sexual drive
  Nymphomania
  Satyriasis

F52.9   **Unspecified sexual dysfunction not due to a substance or known physiological condition**
  Sexual dysfunction NOS

F53   **Puerperal psychosis**
  Postpartum depression
  Excludes 1: mood disorders with psychotic features (F30.2, F31.2, F31.5, F31.64, F32.3, F33.3)
      postpartum dysphoria (O90.6)
      psychosis in schizophrenia, schizotypal, delusional, and other psychotic disorders (F20-F29)

F54   **Psychological and behavioral factors associated with disorders or diseases classified elsewhere**
  Psychological factors affecting physical conditions
  Code first the associated physical disorder, such as:
  Asthma (J45.-)
  Dermatitis (L23-L25)
  Gastric ulcer (K25.-)
  Mucous colitis (K58.-)
  Ulcerative colitis (K51.-)
  Urticaria (L50.-)
  Excludes❷: tension-type headache (G44.2)

F55-   **Abuse of non-psychoactive substances**
  Excludes❷: abuse of psychoactive substances (F10-F19)

F55.0   **Abuse of antacids**

F55.1   **Abuse of herbal or folk remedies**

F55.2   **Abuse of laxatives**

F55.3   **Abuse of steroids or hormones**

F55.4   **Abuse of vitamins**

F55.8   **Abuse of other non-psychoactive substances**

F59   **Unspecified behavioral syndromes associated with physiological disturbances and physical factors**
  Psychogenic physiological dysfunction NOS

Disorders of adult personality and behavior (F60-F69)

F60-   Specific personality disorders

F60.0   **Paranoid personality disorder**
  Expansive paranoid personality (disorder)
  Fanatic personality (disorder)
  Querulant personality (disorder)
  Paranoid personality (disorder)
  Sensitive paranoid personality (disorder)
  Excludes❷: paranoia (F22)
      paranoia querulans (F22)
      paranoid psychosis (F22)
      paranoid schizophrenia (F20.0)
      paranoid state (F22)

F60.1   **Schizoid personality disorder**
  Excludes❷: Asperger's syndrome (F84.5)
      delusional disorder (F22)
      schizoid disorder of childhood (F84.5)
      schizophrenia (F20.-)
      schizotypal disorder (F21)

F60.2   **Antisocial personality disorder**
  Amoral personality (disorder)
  Asocial personality (disorder)
  Dissocial personality disorder
  Psychopathic personality (disorder)
  Sociopathic personality (disorder)
  Excludes 1: conduct disorders (F91.-)
  Excludes❷: borderline personality disorder (F60.3)

F60.3   **Borderline personality disorder**
  Aggressive personality (disorder)
  Emotionally unstable personality disorder
  Explosive personality (disorder)
  Excludes❷: antisocial personality disorder (F60.2)

F60.4   **Histrionic personality disorder**
  Hysterical personality (disorder)
  Psychoinfantile personality (disorder)

F60.5   **Obsessive-compulsive personality disorder**
  Anankastic personality (disorder)
  Compulsive personality (disorder)
  Obsessional personality (disorder)
  Excludes❷: obsessive-compulsive disorder (F42)

F60.6   **Avoidant personality disorder**
  Anxious personality disorder

F60.7   **Dependent personality disorder**
  Asthenic personality (disorder)
  Inadequate personality (disorder)
  Passive personality (disorder)

F60.8-   **Other specific personality disorders**

  F60.81   **Narcissistic personality disorder**

  F60.89   **Other specific personality disorders**
    Eccentric personality disorder
    "Haltlose" type personality disorder
    Immature personality disorder
    Passive-aggressive personality disorder
    Psychoneurotic personality disorder
    Self-defeating personality disorder

F60.9   **Personality disorder, unspecified**
  Character disorder NOS
  Character neurosis NOS
  Pathological personality NOS

F63-   **Impulse disorders**
  Excludes❷: habitual excessive use of alcohol or psychoactive substances (F10-F19)
      impulse disorders involving sexual behavior (F65.-)

F63.0   **Pathological gambling**
  Compulsive gambling
  Excludes 1: gambling and betting NOS (Z72.6)
  Excludes❷: excessive gambling by manic patients (F30, F31)
      gambling in antisocial personality disorder (F60.2)

F63.1   **Pyromania**
  Pathological fire-setting
  Excludes❷: fire-setting (by) (in):
      adult with antisocial personality disorder (F60.2)
      alcohol or psychoactive substance intoxication (F10-F19)
      conduct disorders (F91.-)
      mental disorders due to known physiological condition (F01-F09)
      schizophrenia (F20.-)

F 4 4 – F 6 3

F63.2   Kleptomania
Pathological stealing
Excludes 1:   shoplifting as the reason for observation for suspected mental disorder (Z03.8)
Excludes❷: depressive disorder with stealing (F31-F33)
stealing due to underlying mental condition-code to mental condition
stealing in mental disorders due to known physiological condition (F01-F09)

F63.3   Trichotillomania
Hair plucking
Excludes❷: other stereotyped movement disorder (F98.4)

F63.8-   Other impulse disorders
   F63.81   Intermittent explosive disorder
   F63.89   Other impulse disorders

F63.9   Impulse disorder, unspecified
Impulse control disorder NOS

F64-   Gender identity disorders
   F64.1   Gender identity disorder <u>in adolescence and adulthood</u>
Dual role transvestism
Transsexualism
Use additional code to identify sex reassignment status (Z87.890)
Excludes 1:   gender identity disorder in childhood (F64.2)
Excludes❷: fetishistic transvestism (F65.1)

   F64.2   Gender identity disorder <u>of childhood</u>
Excludes 1:   gender identity disorder in adolescence and adulthood (F64.1)
Excludes❷: sexual maturation disorder (F66)

   F64.8   Other gender identity disorders

   F64.9   Gender identity disorder, unspecified
Gender-role disorder NOS

F65-   Paraphilias
   F65.0   Fetishism

   F65.1   Transvestic fetishism
Fetishistic transvestism

   F65.2   Exhibitionism

   F65.3   Voyeurism

   F65.4   Pedophilia

   F65.5-   Sadomasochism
      F65.50   Sadomasochism, unspecified
      F65.51   Sexual masochism
      F65.52   Sexual sadism

   F65.8-   Other paraphilias
      F65.81   Frotteurism
      F65.89   Other paraphilias
Necrophilia

   F65.9   Paraphilia, unspecified
Sexual deviation NOS

F66   Other sexual disorders
Sexual maturation disorder
Sexual relationship disorder

F68-   Other disorders of adult personality and behavior
   F68.1-   <u>Factitious disorder</u>
Compensation neurosis
Elaboration of physical symptoms for psychological reasons
Hospital hopper syndrome
Münchausen's syndrome
Peregrinating patient
Excludes❷: factitial dermatitis (L98.1)
person feigning illness (with obvious motivation) (Z76.5)

      F68.10   Factitious disorder, unspecified
      F68.11   Factitious disorder with predominantly <u>psychological</u> signs and symptoms
      F68.12   Factitious disorder with predominantly <u>physical</u> signs and symptoms
      F68.13   Factitious disorder with <u>combined</u> psychological and physical signs and symptoms

   F68.8   Other specified disorders of adult personality and behavior

F69   Unspecified disorder of adult personality and behavior

Intellectual disabilities (F70-F79)

Code first any associated physical or developmental disorders
Excludes 1:   borderline intellectual functioning, IQ above 70 to 84 (R41.83)

F70   Mild intellectual disabilities
IQ level 50-55 to approximately 70
Mild mental subnormality

F71   Moderate intellectual disabilities
IQ level 35-40 to 50-55
Moderate mental subnormality

F72   Severe intellectual disabilities
IQ 20-25 to 35-40
Severe mental subnormality

F73   Profound intellectual disabilities
IQ level below 20-25
Profound mental subnormality

F78   Other intellectual disabilities

F79   Unspecified intellectual disabilities
Mental deficiency NOS
Mental subnormality NOS

Pervasive and specific developmental disorders (F80-F89)

F80-   Specific developmental disorders of speech and language
   F80.0   Phonological disorder
Dyslalia
Functional speech articulation disorder
Lalling
Lisping
Phonological developmental disorder
Speech articulation developmental disorder
Excludes 1:   speech articulation impairment due to aphasia NOS (R47.01)
speech articulation impairment due to apraxia (R48.2)
Excludes❷: speech articulation impairment due to hearing loss (F80.4)
speech articulation impairment due to intellectual disabilities (F70-F79)
speech articulation impairment with expressive language developmental disorder (F80.1)
speech articulation impairment with mixed receptive expressive language developmental disorder (F80.2)

   F80.1   Expressive language disorder
Developmental dysphasia or aphasia, expressive type
Excludes 1:   mixed receptive-expressive language disorder (F80.2)
dysphasia and aphasia NOS (R47.-)
Excludes❷: acquired aphasia with epilepsy [Landau-Kleffner] (G40.80-)
intellectual disabilities (F70-F79)
pervasive developmental disorders (F84.-)
selective mutism (F94.0)

   F80.2   Mixed receptive-expressive language disorder
Developmental dysphasia or aphasia, receptive type
Developmental Wernicke's aphasia
Excludes 1:   central auditory processing disorder (H93.25)
dysphasia or aphasia NOS (R47.-)
expressive language disorder (F80.1)
expressive type dysphasia or aphasia (F80.1)
word deafness (H93.25)
Excludes❷: acquired aphasia with epilepsy [Landau-Kleffner] (G40.80-)
intellectual disabilities (F70-F79)
pervasive developmental disorders (F84.-)
selective mutism (F94.0)

   F80.4   Speech and language development delay due to hearing loss
Code also type of hearing loss (H90.-, H91.-)

   F80.8-   Other developmental disorders of speech and language
      F80.81   Childhood onset fluency disorder
Cluttering NOS
Stuttering NOS
Excludes 1:   adult onset fluency disorder (F98.5)
fluency disorder in conditions classified elsewhere (R47.82)
fluency disorder (stuttering) following cerebrovascular disease (I69. with final characters -23)

      F80.89   Other developmental disorders of speech and language

   F80.9   Developmental disorder of speech and language, unspecified
Communication disorder NOS
Language disorder NOS

F
6
3
-
F
9
4

F81- **Specific developmental disorders of scholastic skills**
  F81.0 **Specific reading disorder**
      "Backward reading"
      Developmental dyslexia
      Specific reading retardation
      Excludes 1: alexia NOS (R48.0)
                dyslexia NOS (R48.0)
  F81.2 **Mathematics disorder**
      Developmental acalculia
      Developmental arithmetical disorder
      Developmental Gerstmann's syndrome
      Excludes 1: acalculia NOS (R48.8)
      Excludes❷: arithmetical difficulties associated with a reading
               disorder (F81.0)
               arithmetical difficulties associated with a spelling
                 disorder (F81.81)
               arithmetical difficulties due to inadequate teaching
                 (Z55.8)
  F81.8- **Other developmental disorders of scholastic skills**
    F81.81 **Disorder of written expression**
        Specific spelling disorder
    F81.89 **Other developmental disorders of scholastic skills**
  F81.9 **Developmental disorder of scholastic skills, unspecified**
      Knowledge acquisition disability NOS
      Learning disability NOS
      Learning disorder NOS
F82 **Specific developmental disorder of motor function**
    Clumsy child syndrome
    Developmental coordination disorder
    Developmental dyspraxia
    Excludes 1: abnormalities of gait and mobility (R26.-)
             lack of coordination (R27.-)
    Excludes❷: lack of coordination secondary to intellectual disabilities
             (F70-F79)
F84- **Pervasive developmental disorders**
    Use additional code to identify any associated medical condition and
      intellectual disabilities
  F84.0 **Autistic disorder**
      Infantile autism
      Infantile psychosis
      Kanner's syndrome
      Excludes 1: Asperger's syndrome (F84.5)
  F84.2 **Rett's syndrome**
      Excludes 1: Asperger's syndrome (F84.5)
             autistic disorder (F84.0)
             other childhood disintegrative disorder (F84.3)
  F84.3 **Other childhood disintegrative disorder**
      Dementia infantilis
      Disintegrative psychosis
      Heller's syndrome
      Symbiotic psychosis
      Use additional code to identify any associated neurological condition
      Excludes 1: Asperger's syndrome (F84.5)
             autistic disorder (F84.0)
             Rett's syndrome (F84.2)
  F84.5 **Asperger's syndrome**
      Asperger's disorder
      Autistic psychopathy
      Schizoid disorder of childhood
  F84.8 **Other pervasive developmental disorders**
      Overactive disorder associated with intellectual disabilities and
        stereotyped movements
  F84.9 **Pervasive developmental disorder, unspecified**
      Atypical autism
F88 **Other disorders of psychological development**
    Developmental agnosia
F89 **Unspecified disorder of psychological development**
    Developmental disorder NOS

Behavioral and emotional disorders with onset usually occurring in childhood and adolescence (F90-F98)

Note: Codes within categories F90-F98 may be used regardless of the age
     of a patient. These disorders generally have onset within the
     childhood or adolescent years, but may continue throughout life or
     not be diagnosed until adulthood.

F90- **Attention-deficit hyperactivity disorders**
    Includes: Attention deficit disorder with hyperactivity
             Attention deficit syndrome with hyperactivity
    Excludes❷: anxiety disorders (F40.-, F41.-)
             mood [affective] disorders (F30-F39)
             pervasive developmental disorders (F84.-)
             schizophrenia (F20.-)
  F90.0 **Attention-deficit hyperactivity disorder, predominantly inattentive type**
  F90.1 **Attention-deficit hyperactivity disorder, predominantly hyperactive type**
  F90.2 **Attention-deficit hyperactivity disorder, combined type**
  F90.8 **Attention-deficit hyperactivity disorder, other type**
  F90.9 **Attention-deficit hyperactivity disorder, unspecified type**
      Attention-deficit hyperactivity disorder of childhood or
        adolescence NOS
      Attention-deficit hyperactivity disorder NOS
F91- **Conduct disorders**
    Excludes 1: antisocial behavior (Z72.81-)
             antisocial personality disorder (F60.2)
    Excludes❷: conduct problems associated with attention-deficit
              hyperactivity disorder (F90.-)
             mood [affective] disorders (F30-F39)
             pervasive developmental disorders (F84.-)
             schizophrenia (F20.-)
  F91.0 **Conduct disorder confined to family context**
  F91.1 **Conduct disorder, childhood-onset type**
      Unsocialized conduct disorder
      Conduct disorder, solitary aggressive type
      Unsocialized aggressive disorder
  F91.2 **Conduct disorder, adolescent-onset type**
      Socialized conduct disorder
      Conduct disorder, group type
  F91.3 **Oppositional defiant disorder**
  F91.8 **Other conduct disorders**
  F91.9 **Conduct disorder, unspecified**
      Behavioral disorder NOS
      Conduct disorder NOS
      Disruptive behavior disorder NOS
F93- **Emotional disorders with onset specific to childhood**
  F93.0 **Separation anxiety disorder of childhood**
      Excludes❷: mood [affective] disorders (F30-F39)
              nonpsychotic mental disorders (F40-F48)
              phobic anxiety disorder of childhood (F40.8)
              social phobia (F40.1)
  F93.8 **Other childhood emotional disorders**
      Identity disorder
      Excludes❷: gender identity disorder of childhood (F64.2)
  F93.9 **Childhood emotional disorder, unspecified**
F94- **Disorders of social functioning with onset specific to childhood and adolescence**
  F94.0 **Selective mutism**
      Elective mutism
      Excludes❷: pervasive developmental disorders (F84.-)
              schizophrenia (F20.-)
              specific developmental disorders of speech and
                language (F80.-)
              transient mutism as part of separation anxiety in young
                children (F93.0)
  F94.1 **Reactive attachment disorder of childhood**
      Use additional code to identify any associated failure to thrive or
        growth retardation
      Excludes 1: disinhibited attachment disorder of childhood (F94.2)
             normal variation in pattern of selective attachment
      Excludes❷: Asperger's syndrome (F84.5)
             maltreatment syndromes (T74.-)
             sexual or physical abuse in childhood, resulting in
               psychosocial problems (Z62.81-)
  F94.2 **Disinhibited attachment disorder of childhood**
      Affectionless psychopathy
      Institutional syndrome
      Excludes 1: reactive attachment disorder of childhood (F94.1)
      Excludes❷: Asperger's syndrome (F84.5)
             attention-deficit hyperactivity disorders (F90.-)
             hospitalism in children (F43.2-)

F 6 3 - F 9 4

Excludes 1: = NOT CODED HERE! (Do not code both)   **415**   *Excludes❷: = Not Included Here*

F94.8   Other childhood disorders of social functioning
F94.9   Childhood disorder of social functioning, unspecified

F95-   Tic disorder

F95.0   Transient tic disorder

F95.1   Chronic motor or vocal tic disorder

F95.2   Tourette's disorder
         Combined vocal and multiple motor tic disorder [de la Tourette]
         Tourette's syndrome

F95.8   Other tic disorders

F95.9   Tic disorder, unspecified
         Tic NOS

F98-   Other behavioral and emotional disorders with onset usually occurring
        in childhood and adolescence
        Excludes❷: breath-holding spells (R06.89)
                    gender identity disorder of childhood (F64.2)
                    Kleine-Levin syndrome (G47.13)
                    obsessive-compulsive disorder (F42)
                    sleep disorders not due to a substance or known physiological
                        condition (F51.-)

F98.0   Enuresis **not** due to a substance or known physiological condition
         Enuresis (primary) (secondary) of nonorganic origin
         Functional enuresis
         Psychogenic enuresis
         Urinary incontinence of nonorganic origin
         Excludes 1: enuresis NOS (R32)

F98.1   Encopresis **not** due to a substance or known physiological
         condition
         Functional encopresis
         Incontinence of feces of nonorganic origin
         Psychogenic encopresis
         Use additional code to identify the cause of any coexisting
            constipation
         Excludes 1: encopresis NOS (R15.-)

F98.2-   Other feeding disorders of infancy and childhood
         Excludes 1: feeding difficulties (R63.3)
         Excludes❷: anorexia nervosa and other eating disorders (F50.-)
                    feeding problems of newborn (P92.-)
                    pica of infancy or childhood (F98.3)

   F98.21   Rumination disorder of infancy
   F98.29   Other feeding disorders of infancy and early childhood

F98.3   Pica of infancy and childhood

F98.4   Stereotyped movement disorders
         Stereotype/habit disorder
         Excludes 1: abnormal involuntary movements (R25.-)
         Excludes❷: compulsions in obsessive-compulsive disorder (F42)
                    hair plucking (F63.3)
                    movement disorders of organic origin (G20-G25)
                    nail-biting (F98.8)
                    nose-picking (F98.8)
                    stereotypies that are part of a broader psychiatric
                        condition (F01-F95)
                    thumb-sucking (F98.8)
                    tic disorders (F95.-)
                    trichotillomania (F63.3)

F98.5   Adult onset fluency disorder
         Excludes 1: childhood onset fluency disorder (F80.81)
                    dysphasia (R47.02)
                    fluency disorder in conditions classified elsewhere
                        (R47.82)
                    fluency disorder (stuttering) following cerebrovascular
                        disease (I69. with final characters -23)
                    tic disorders (F95.-)

F98.8   Other specified behavioral and emotional disorders with onset
         usually occurring in childhood and adolescence
         Excessive masturbation
         Nail-biting
         Nose-picking
         Thumb-sucking

F98.9   Unspecified behavioral and emotional disorders with onset
         usually occurring in childhood and adolescence

Unspecified mental disorder (F99)

F99   **Mental disorder, not otherwise specified**
       Mental illness NOS
       Excludes 1: unspecified mental disorder due to known physiological
                    condition (F09)

F
9
4
-
G
0
4

Chapter 6 – Diseases of the nervous system (G00-G99)

Excludes❷: certain conditions originating in the perinatal period (P04-P96)
certain infectious and parasitic diseases (A00-B99)
complications of pregnancy, childbirth and the puerperium (O00-O9A)
congenital malformations, deformations, and chromosomal abnormalities (Q00-Q99)
endocrine, nutritional and metabolic diseases (E00-E88)
injury, poisoning and certain other consequences of external causes (S00-T88)
neoplasms (C00-D49)
symptoms, signs and abnormal clinical and laboratory findings, not elsewhere classified (R00-R94)

This chapter contains the following blocks:
G00-G09   Inflammatory diseases of the central nervous system
G10-G14   Systemic atrophies primarily affecting the central nervous system
G20-G26   Extrapyramidal and movement disorders
G30-G32   Other degenerative diseases of the nervous system
G35-G37   Demyelinating diseases of the central nervous system
G40-G47   Episodic and paroxysmal disorders
G50-G59   Nerve, nerve root and plexus disorders
G60-G65   Polyneuropathies and other disorders of the peripheral nervous system
G70-G73   Diseases of myoneural junction and muscle
G80-G83   Cerebral palsy and other paralytic syndromes
G89-G99   Other disorders of the nervous system

Inflammatory diseases of the central nervous system (G00-G09)

G00-   Bacterial meningitis, not elsewhere classified
Includes: Bacterial arachnoiditis
Bacterial leptomeningitis
Bacterial meningitis
Bacterial pachymeningitis
Excludes 1: bacterial:
meningoencephalitis (G04.2)
meningomyelitis (G04.2)

G00.0   Hemophilus meningitis
Meningitis due to Hemophilus influenzae

G00.1   Pneumococcal meningitis

G00.2   Streptococcal meningitis
Use additional code to further identify organism (B95.0-B95.5)

G00.3   Staphylococcal meningitis
Use additional code to further identify organism (B95.61-B95.8)

G00.8   Other bacterial meningitis
Meningitis due to Escherichia coli
Meningitis due to Friedländer's bacillus
Meningitis due to Klebsiella
Use additional code to further identify organism (B96.-)

G00.9   Bacterial meningitis, unspecified
Meningitis due to gram-negative bacteria, unspecified
Purulent meningitis NOS
Pyogenic meningitis NOS
Suppurative meningitis NOS

G01   Meningitis in bacterial diseases classified elsewhere
Code first underlying disease
Excludes 1: meningitis (in):
gonococcal (A54.81)
leptospirosis (A27.81)
listeriosis (A32.11)
Lyme disease (A69.21)
meningococcal (A39.0)
neurosyphilis (A52.13)
tuberculosis (A17.0)
meningoencephalitis and meningomyelitis in bacterial diseases classified elsewhere (G05)

G02   Meningitis in other infectious and parasitic diseases classified elsewhere
Code first underlying disease, such as:
African trypanosomiasis (B56-)
Poliovirus infection (A80-)
Excludes 1: candidal meningitis (B37.5)
coccidioidomycosis meningitis (B38.4)
cryptococcal meningitis (B45.1)
herpesviral [herpes simplex] meningitis (B00.3)
infectious mononucleosis complicated by meningitis (B27- with fifth character 2)
measles complicated by meningitis (B05.1)
meningoencephalitis and meningomyelitis in other infectious and parasitic diseases classified elsewhere (G05)
mumps meningitis (B26.1)
rubella meningitis (B06.02)
varicella [chickenpox] meningitis (B01.0)
zoster meningitis (B02.1)

G03-   Meningitis due to other and unspecified causes
Includes: Arachnoiditis NOS
Leptomeningitis NOS
Meningitis NOS
Pachymeningitis NOS
Excludes 1: meningoencephalitis (G04.-)
meningomyelitis (G04.-)

G03.0   Nonpyogenic meningitis
Aseptic meningitis
Nonbacterial meningitis

G03.1   Chronic meningitis

G03.2   Benign recurrent meningitis [Mollaret]

G03.8   Meningitis due to other specified causes

G03.9   Meningitis, unspecified
Arachnoiditis (spinal) NOS

G04-   Encephalitis, myelitis and encephalomyelitis
Includes: Acute ascending myelitis
Meningoencephalitis
Meningomyelitis
Excludes 1: encephalopathy NOS (G93.40)
Excludes❷: acute transverse myelitis (G37.3-)
alcoholic encephalopathy (G31.2)
benign myalgic encephalomyelitis (G93.3)
multiple sclerosis (G35)
subacute necrotizing myelitis (G37.4)
toxic encephalitis (G92)
toxic encephalopathy (G92)

G04.0-   Acute disseminated encephalitis and encephalomyelitis (ADEM)
Excludes 1: acute necrotizing hemorrhagic encephalopathy (G04.3-)
other noninfectious acute disseminated encephalomyelitis (noninfectious ADEM) (G04.81)

G04.00   Acute disseminated encephalitis and encephalomyelitis, unspecified

G04.01   Postinfectious acute disseminated encephalitis and encephalomyelitis (postinfectious ADEM)
Excludes 1: post chickenpox encephalitis (B01.1)
post measles encephalitis (B05.0)
post measles myelitis (B05.1)

G04.02   Postimmunization acute disseminated encephalitis, myelitis and encephalomyelitis
Encephalitis, post immunization
Encephalomyelitis, post immunization
Use additional code to identify the vaccine (T50.A-, T50.B-, T50.Z-)

G04.1   Tropical spastic paraplegia

G04.2   Bacterial meningoencephalitis and meningomyelitis, not elsewhere classified

G04.3-   Acute necrotizing hemorrhagic encephalopathy
Excludes 1: acute disseminated encephalitis and encephalomyelitis (G04.0-)

G04.30   Acute necrotizing hemorrhagic encephalopathy, unspecified

G04.31   Postinfectious acute necrotizing hemorrhagic encephalopathy

G04.32   Postimmunization acute necrotizing hemorrhagic encephalopathy
Use additional code to identify the vaccine (T50.A-, T50.B-, T50.Z-)

G04.39   Other acute necrotizing hemorrhagic encephalopathy
Code also underlying etiology, if applicable

F
9
4
-
G
0
4

G04.8- Other encephalitis, myelitis and encephalomyelitis
Code also any associated seizure (G40.-, R56.9)

G04.81 Other encephalitis and encephalomyelitis
Noninfectious acute disseminated encephalomyelitis (noninfectious ADEM)

G04.89 Other myelitis

G04.9- Encephalitis, myelitis and encephalomyelitis, unspecified

G04.90 Encephalitis and encephalomyelitis, unspecified
Ventriculitis (cerebral) NOS

G04.91 Myelitis, unspecified

G05- Encephalitis, myelitis and encephalomyelitis <u>in diseases classified elsewhere</u>
Code first underlying disease, such as:
Human immunodeficiency virus [HIV] disease (B20)
Poliovirus (A80.-)
Suppurative otitis media (H66.01-H66.4)
Trichinellosis (B75)
Excludes 1: adenoviral encephalitis, myelitis and encephalomyelitis (A85.1)
congenital toxoplasmosis encephalitis, myelitis and encephalomyelitis (P37.1)
cytomegaloviral encephalitis, myelitis and encephalomyelitis (B25.8)
encephalitis, myelitis and encephalomyelitis (in) measles (B05.0)
encephalitis, myelitis and encephalomyelitis (in) systemic lupus erythematosus (M32.19)
enteroviral encephalitis, myelitis and encephalomyelitis (A85.0)
eosinophilic meningoencephalitis (B83.2)
herpesviral [herpes simplex] encephalitis, myelitis and encephalomyelitis (B00.4)
listerial encephalitis, myelitis and encephalomyelitis (A32.12)
meningococcal encephalitis, myelitis and encephalomyelitis (A39.81)
mumps encephalitis, myelitis and encephalomyelitis (B26.2)
postchickenpox encephalitis, myelitis and encephalomyelitis (B01.1-)
rubella encephalitis, myelitis and encephalomyelitis (B06.01)
toxoplasmosis encephalitis, myelitis and encephalomyelitis (B58.2)
zoster encephalitis, myelitis and encephalomyelitis (B02.0)

G05.3 Encephalitis and encephalomyelitis in diseases classified elsewhere
Meningoencephalitis in diseases classified elsewhere

G05.4 Myelitis in diseases classified elsewhere
Meningomyelitis in diseases classified elsewhere

G06- Intracranial and intraspinal abscess and granuloma
Use additional code (B95-B97) to identify infectious agent.

G06.0 Intracranial abscess and granuloma
Brain [any part] abscess (embolic)
Cerebellar abscess (embolic)
Cerebral abscess (embolic)
Intracranial epidural abscess or granuloma
Intracranial extradural abscess or granuloma
Intracranial subdural abscess or granuloma
Otogenic abscess (embolic)
Excludes 1: tuberculous intracranial abscess and granuloma (A17.81)

G06.1 Intraspinal abscess and granuloma
Abscess (embolic) of spinal cord [any part]
Intraspinal epidural abscess or granuloma
Intraspinal extradural abscess or granuloma
Intraspinal subdural abscess or granuloma
Excludes 1: tuberculous intraspinal abscess and granuloma (A17.81)

G06.2 Extradural and subdural abscess, unspecified

G07 Intracranial and intraspinal abscess and granuloma in diseases classified elsewhere
Code first underlying disease, such as:
Schistosomiasis granuloma of brain (B65.-)
Excludes 1: abscess of brain:
amebic (A06.6)
chromomycotic (B43.1)
gonococcal (A54.82)
tuberculous (A17.81)
tuberculoma of meninges (A17.1)

G08 Intracranial and intraspinal phlebitis and thrombophlebitis
Septic embolism of intracranial or intraspinal venous sinuses and veins
Septic endophlebitis of intracranial or intraspinal venous sinuses and veins
Septic phlebitis of intracranial or intraspinal venous sinuses and veins
Septic thrombophlebitis of intracranial or intraspinal venous sinuses and veins
Septic thrombosis of intracranial or intraspinal venous sinuses and veins
Excludes 1: intracranial phlebitis and thrombophlebitis complicating:
abortion, ectopic or molar pregnancy (O00-O07, O08.7)
nonpyogenic intracranial phlebitis and thrombophlebitis (I67.6)
pregnancy, childbirth and the puerperium (O22.5, O87.3)
Excludes❷: intracranial phlebitis and thrombophlebitis complicating nonpyogenic intraspinal phlebitis and thrombophlebitis (G95.1)

G09 <u>Sequelae of inflammatory diseases of central nervous system</u>
Note: Category G09 is to be used to indicate conditions whose primary classification is to G00-G08 as the cause of sequelae, themselves classifiable elsewhere. The "sequelae" include conditions specified as residuals.
Code first condition resulting from (sequela) of inflammatory diseases of central nervous system

Systemic atrophies primarily affecting the central nervous system (G10-G14)

G10 Huntington's disease
Huntington's chorea
Huntington's dementia

G11- <u>Hereditary ataxia</u>
Excludes❷: cerebral palsy (G80.-)
hereditary and idiopathic neuropathy (G60.-)
metabolic disorders (E70-E88)

G11.0 <u>Congenital</u> nonprogressive ataxia

G11.1 <u>Early-onset</u> cerebellar ataxia
Early-onset cerebellar ataxia with essential tremor
Early-onset cerebellar ataxia with myoclonus [Hunt's ataxia]
Early-onset cerebellar ataxia with retained tendon reflexes
Friedreich's ataxia (autosomal recessive)
X-linked recessive spinocerebellar ataxia

G11.2 <u>Late-onset</u> cerebellar ataxia

G11.3 Cerebellar ataxia <u>with defective DNA repair</u>
Ataxia telangiectasia [Louis-Bar]
Excludes❷: Cockayne's syndrome (Q87.1)
other disorders of purine and pyrimidine metabolism (E79.-)
xeroderma pigmentosum (Q82.1)

G11.4 Hereditary <u>spastic paraplegia</u>

G11.8 Other hereditary ataxias

G11.9 Hereditary ataxia, unspecified
Hereditary cerebellar ataxia NOS
Hereditary cerebellar degeneration
Hereditary cerebellar disease
Hereditary cerebellar syndrome

G12- Spinal muscular atrophy and related syndromes

G12.0 Infantile spinal muscular atrophy, type I [Werdnig-Hoffman]

G12.1 Other inherited spinal muscular atrophy
Adult form spinal muscular atrophy
Childhood form, type II spinal muscular atrophy
Distal spinal muscular atrophy
Juvenile form, type III spinal muscular atrophy [Kugelberg-Welander]
Progressive bulbar palsy of childhood [Fazio-Londe]
Scapuloperoneal form spinal muscular atrophy

G12.2- Motor neuron disease

G12.20 Motor neuron disease, unspecified

G12.21 Amyotrophic lateral sclerosis
Progressive spinal muscle atrophy

G12.22 Progressive bulbar palsy

G12.29 Other motor neuron disease
Familial motor neuron disease
Primary lateral sclerosis

G12.8 Other spinal muscular atrophies and related syndromes

G12.9 Spinal muscular atrophy, unspecified

G13- Systemic atrophies primarily affecting central nervous system in diseases classified elsewhere

G13.0 Paraneoplastic neuromyopathy and neuropathy
Carcinomatous neuromyopathy
Sensorial paraneoplastic neuropathy [Denny Brown]
Code first underlying neoplasm (C00-D49)

G
0
4
-
G
2
6

Excludes 1: = NOT CODED HERE! (Do not code both)

Excludes❷: = Not Included Here

© 2013 Channel Publishing Ltd

G13.1   **Other systemic atrophy primarily affecting central nervous system in neoplastic disease**
Paraneoplastic limbic encephalopathy
Code first underlying neoplasm (C00-D49)

G13.2   **Systemic atrophy primarily affecting central nervous system in myxedema**
Code first underlying disease, such as:
Hypothyroidism (E03-)
Myxedematous congenital iodine deficiency (E00.1)

G13.8   **Systemic atrophy primarily affecting central nervous system in other diseases classified elsewhere**
Code first underlying disease

G14   **Postpolio syndrome**
Includes: Postpolio myelitic syndrome
Excludes 1:   sequelae of poliomyelitis (B91)

Extrapyramidal and movement disorders (G20-G26)

G20   **Parkinson's disease**
Hemiparkinsonism
Idiopathic Parkinsonism or Parkinson's disease
Paralysis agitans
Parkinsonism or Parkinson's disease NOS
Primary Parkinsonism or Parkinson's disease
Excludes 1:   dementia with Parkinsonism (G31.83)

G21-   **Secondary parkinsonism**
Excludes 1:   dementia with Parkinsonism (G31.83)
Huntington's disease (G10)
Shy-Drager syndrome (G90.3)
syphilitic Parkinsonism (A52.19)

G21.0   **Malignant neuroleptic syndrome**
Use additional code for adverse effect, if applicable, to identify drug (T43.3X5, T43.4X5, T43.505, T43.595)
Excludes 1:   neuroleptic induced parkinsonism (G21.11)

G21.1-   **Other drug-induced secondary parkinsonism**

G21.11   **Neuroleptic induced parkinsonism**
Use additional code for adverse effect, if applicable, to identify drug (T43.3X5, T43.4X5, T43.505, T43.595)
Excludes 1:   malignant neuroleptic syndrome (G21.0)

G21.19   **Other drug-induced secondary parkinsonism**
Use additional code for adverse effect, if applicable, to identify drug (T36-T50 with fifth or sixth character 5)

G21.2   **Secondary parkinsonism due to other external agents**
Code first (T51-T65) to identify external agent

G21.3   **Postencephalitic parkinsonism**

G21.4   **Vascular parkinsonism**

G21.8   **Other secondary parkinsonism**

G21.9   **Secondary parkinsonism, unspecified**

G23-   **Other degenerative diseases of basal ganglia**
Excludes❷: multi-system degeneration of the autonomic nervous system (G90.3)

G23.0   **Hallervorden-Spatz disease**
Pigmentary pallidal degeneration

G23.1   **Progressive supranuclear ophthalmoplegia [Steele-Richardson-Olszewski]**
Progressive supranuclear palsy

G23.2   **Striatonigral degeneration**

G23.8   **Other specified degenerative diseases of basal ganglia**
Calcification of basal ganglia

G23.9   **Degenerative disease of basal ganglia, unspecified**

G24-   **Dystonia**
Includes: Dyskinesia
Excludes❷: athetoid cerebral palsy (G80.3)

G24.0-   **Drug-induced dystonia**
Use additional code for adverse effect, if applicable, to identify drug (T36-T50 with fifth or sixth character 5)

G24.01   **Drug-induced subacute dyskinesia**
Drug induced blepharospasm
Drug induced orofacial dyskinesia
Neuroleptic induced tardive dyskinesia
Tardive dyskinesia

G24.02   **Drug-induced acute dystonia**
Acute dystonic reaction to drugs
Neuroleptic induced acute dystonia

G24.09   **Other drug-induced dystonia**

G24.1   **Genetic torsion dystonia**
Dystonia deformans progressiva
Dystonia musculorum deformans
Familial torsion dystonia
Idiopathic familial dystonia
Idiopathic (torsion) dystonia NOS
(Schwalbe-) Ziehen-Oppenheim disease

G24.2   **Idiopathic nonfamilial dystonia**

G24.3   **Spasmodic torticollis**
Excludes 1:   congenital torticollis (Q68.0)
hysterical torticollis (F44.4)
ocular torticollis (R29.891)
psychogenic torticollis (F45.8)
torticollis NOS (M43.6)
traumatic recurrent torticollis (S13.4)

G24.4   **Idiopathic orofacial dystonia**
Orofacial dyskinesia
Excludes 1:   drug induced orofacial dyskinesia (G24.01)

G24.5   **Blepharospasm**
Excludes 1:   drug induced blepharospasm (G24.01)

G24.8   **Other dystonia**
Acquired torsion dystonia NOS

G24.9   **Dystonia, unspecified**
Dyskinesia NOS

G25-   **Other extrapyramidal and movement disorders**
Excludes❷: sleep related movement disorders (G47.6-)

G25.0   **Essential tremor**
Familial tremor
Excludes 1:   tremor NOS (R25.1)

G25.1   **Drug-induced tremor**
Use additional code for adverse effect, if applicable, to identify drug (T36-T50 with fifth or sixth character 5)

G25.2   **Other specified forms of tremor**
Intention tremor

G25.3   **Myoclonus**
Drug-induced myoclonus
Palatal myoclonus
Use additional code for adverse effect, if applicable, to identify drug (T36-T50 with fifth or sixth character 5)
Excludes 1:   facial myokymia (G51.4)
myoclonic epilepsy (G40.-)

G25.4   **Drug-induced chorea**
Use additional code for adverse effect, if applicable, to identify drug (T36-T50 with fifth or sixth character 5)

G25.5   **Other chorea**
Chorea NOS
Excludes 1:   chorea NOS with heart involvement (I02.0)
Huntington's chorea (G10)
rheumatic chorea (I02.-)
Sydenham's chorea (I02.-)

G25.6-   **Drug-induced tics and other tics of organic origin**

G25.61   **Drug-induced tics**
Use additional code for adverse effect, if applicable, to identify drug (T36-T50 with fifth or sixth character 5)

G25.69   **Other tics of organic origin**
Excludes 1:   habit spasm (F95.9)
tic NOS (F95.9)
Tourette's syndrome (F95.2)

G25.7-   **Other and unspecified drug induced movement disorders**
Use additional code for adverse effect, if applicable, to identify drug (T36-T50 with fifth or sixth character 5)

G25.70   **Drug-induced movement disorder, unspecified**

G25.71   **Drug-induced akathisia**
Drug induced acathisia
Neuroleptic induced acute akathisia

G25.79   **Other drug-induced movement disorders**

G25.8-   **Other specified extrapyramidal and movement disorders**

G25.81   **Restless legs syndrome**

G25.82   **Stiff-man syndrome**

G25.83   **Benign shuddering attacks**

G25.89   **Other specified extrapyramidal and movement disorders**

G25.9   **Extrapyramidal and movement disorder, unspecified**

G26   **Extrapyramidal and movement disorders in diseases classified elsewhere**
Code first underlying disease

G04-G26

Excludes 1: = NOT CODED HERE! (Do not code both)   **419**   *Excludes❷:* = Not Included Here

Other degenerative diseases of the nervous system (G30-G32)

G30- **Alzheimer's disease**
Includes: Alzheimer's dementia senile and presenile forms
Use additional code to identify:
  Delirium, if applicable (F05)
  Dementia with behavioral disturbance (F02.81)
  Dementia without behavioral disturbance (F02.80)
  Excludes 1: senile degeneration of brain NEC (G31.1)
          senile dementia NOS (F03)
          senility NOS (R41.81)

G30.0 **Alzheimer's disease with <u>early</u> onset**

G30.1 **Alzheimer's disease with <u>late</u> onset**

G30.8 **Other Alzheimer's disease**

G30.9 **Alzheimer's disease, unspecified**

G31- **Other degenerative diseases of nervous system, not elsewhere classified**
Use additional code to identify:
  Dementia with behavioral disturbance (F02.81)
  Dementia without behavioral disturbance (F02.80)
  Excludes❷: Reye's syndrome (G93.7)

G31.0- **Frontotemporal dementia**

G31.01 **Pick's disease**
      Primary progressive aphasia
      Progressive isolated aphasia

G31.09 **Other frontotemporal dementia**
      Frontal dementia

G31.1 **Senile degeneration of brain, not elsewhere classified**
      Excludes 1: Alzheimer's disease (G30.-)
            senility NOS (R41.81)

G31.2 **Degeneration of nervous system due to alcohol**
      Alcoholic cerebellar ataxia
      Alcoholic cerebellar degeneration
      Alcoholic cerebral degeneration
      Alcoholic encephalopathy
      Dysfunction of the autonomic nervous system due to alcohol
      Code also associated alcoholism (F10-)

G31.8- **Other specified degenerative diseases of nervous system**

G31.81 **Alpers disease**
      Grey-matter degeneration

G31.82 **Leigh's disease**
      Subacute necrotizing encephalopathy

G31.83 **Dementia with Lewy bodies**
      Dementia with Parkinsonism
      Lewy body dementia
      Lewy body disease

G31.84 **Mild cognitive impairment, so stated**
      Excludes 1: age related cognitive decline (R41.81)
            altered mental status (R41.82)
            cerebral degeneration (G31.9)
            change in mental status (R41.82)
            cognitive deficits following (sequelae of) cerebral
              hemorrhage or infarction (I69.01, I69.11,
              I69.21, I69.31, I69.81, I69.91)
            cognitive impairment due to intracranial or head
              injury (S06.-)
            dementia (F01-, F02-, F03)
            mild memory disturbance (F06.8)
            neurologic neglect syndrome (R41.4)
            personality change, nonpsychotic (F68.8)

G31.85 **Corticobasal degeneration**

G31.89 **Other specified degenerative diseases of nervous system**

G31.9 **Degenerative disease of nervous system, unspecified**

G32- **Other degenerative disorders of nervous system in diseases classified elsewhere**

G32.0 **Subacute combined degeneration of spinal cord in diseases classified elsewhere**
      Dana-Putnam syndrome
      Sclerosis of spinal cord (combined) (dorsolateral) (posterolateral)
      Code first underlying disease, such as:
        Anemia (D51.9)
        Dietary (D51.3)
        Pernicious (D51.0)
        Vitamin B12 deficiency (E53.8)
      Excludes 1: syphilitic combined degeneration of spinal cord
            (A52.11)

G32.8- **Other specified degenerative disorders of nervous system in diseases classified elsewhere**
      Code first underlying disease, such as:
        Amyloidosis cerebral degeneration (E85.-)
        Cerebral degeneration (due to) hypothyroidism (E00.0-E03.9)
        Cerebral degeneration (due to) neoplasm (C00-D49)
        Cerebral degeneration (due to) vitamin B deficiency, except thiamine (E52-E53-)
      Excludes 1: superior hemorrhagic polioencephalitis [Wernicke's encephalopathy] (E51.2)

G32.81 **Cerebellar ataxia in diseases classified elsewhere**
      Code first underlying disease, such as:
        Celiac disease (with gluten ataxia) (K90.0)
        Cerebellar ataxia (in) neoplastic disease (paraneoplastic cerebellar degeneration) (C00-D49)
        Non-celiac gluten ataxia (M35.9)
      Excludes 1: systemic atrophy primarily affecting the central nervous system in alcoholic cerebellar ataxia (G13.2)
            systemic atrophy primarily affecting the central nervous system in myxedema (G13.2)

G32.89 **Other specified degenerative disorders of nervous system in diseases classified elsewhere**
      Degenerative encephalopathy in diseases classified elsewhere

Demyelinating diseases of the central nervous system (G35-G37)

G35 **Multiple sclerosis**
      Disseminated multiple sclerosis
      Generalized multiple sclerosis
      Multiple sclerosis NOS
      Multiple sclerosis of brain stem
      Multiple sclerosis of cord

G36- **Other acute disseminated demyelination**
      Excludes 1: postinfectious encephalitis and encephalomyelitis NOS (G04.01)

G36.0 **Neuromyelitis optica [Devic]**
      Demyelination in optic neuritis
      Excludes 1: optic neuritis NOS (H46)

G36.1 **Acute and subacute hemorrhagic leukoencephalitis [Hurst]**

G36.8 **Other specified acute disseminated demyelination**

G36.9 **Acute disseminated demyelination, unspecified**

G37- **Other demyelinating diseases of central nervous system**

G37.0 **Diffuse sclerosis of central nervous system**
      Periaxial encephalitis
      Schilder's disease
      Excludes 1: X linked adrenoleukodystrophy (E71.52-)

G37.1 **Central demyelination of corpus callosum**

G37.2 **Central pontine myelinolysis**

G37.3 **Acute transverse myelitis in demyelinating disease of central nervous system**
      Acute transverse myelitis NOS
      Acute transverse myelopathy
      Excludes 1: multiple sclerosis (G35)
            neuromyelitis optica [Devic] (G36.0)

G37.4 **Subacute necrotizing myelitis of central nervous system**

G37.5 **Concentric sclerosis [Balo] of central nervous system**

G37.8 **Other specified demyelinating diseases of central nervous system**

G37.9 **Demyelinating disease of central nervous system, unspecified**

G
3
0
-
G
4
0

Excludes 1: = NOT CODED HERE! (Do not code both)   **420**   *Excludes❷:* = Not Included Here

Episodic and paroxysmal disorders (G40-G47)

G40- **Epilepsy and recurrent seizures**
  Note: The following terms are to be considered equivalent to intractable: pharmacoresistant (pharmacologically resistant), treatment resistant, refractory (medically) and poorly controlled.
  Excludes 1: *conversion disorder with seizures (F44.5)*
        convulsions NOS (R56.9)
        hippocampal sclerosis (G93.81)
        mesial temporal sclerosis (G93.81)
        post traumatic seizures (R56.1)
        seizure (convulsive) NOS (R56.9)
        seizure of newborn (P90)
        temporal sclerosis (G93.81)
        Todd's paralysis (G83.8)

G40.0- **Localization-related** (focal) (partial) idiopathic epilepsy and epileptic syndromes with seizures of localized onset
  Benign childhood epilepsy with centrotemporal EEG spikes
  Childhood epilepsy with occipital EEG paroxysms
  Excludes 1: *adult onset localization-related epilepsy (G40.1-, G40.2-)*

  G40.00- Localization-related (focal) (partial) idiopathic epilepsy and epileptic syndromes with seizures of localized onset, **not intractable**
    Localization-related (focal) (partial) idiopathic epilepsy and epileptic syndromes with seizures of localized onset without intractability

    G40.001 Localization-related (focal) (partial) idiopathic epilepsy and epileptic syndromes with seizures of localized onset, **not** intractable, **with status epilepticus**

    G40.009 Localization-related (focal) (partial) idiopathic epilepsy and epileptic syndromes with seizures of localized onset, **not** intractable, **without** status epilepticus
        Localization-related (focal) (partial) idiopathic epilepsy and epileptic syndromes with seizures of localized onset NOS

  G40.01- Localization-related (focal) (partial) idiopathic epilepsy and epileptic syndromes with seizures of localized onset, **intractable**

    G40.011 Localization-related (focal) (partial) idiopathic epilepsy and epileptic syndromes with seizures of localized onset, intractable, **with status epilepticus**

    G40.019 Localization-related (focal) (partial) idiopathic epilepsy and epileptic syndromes with seizures of localized onset, intractable, **without** status epilepticus

G40.1- **Localization-related** (focal) (partial) symptomatic epilepsy and epileptic syndromes with simple partial seizures
  Attacks without alteration of consciousness
  Epilepsia partialis continua [Kozhevnikof]
  Simple partial seizures developing into secondarily generalized seizures

  G40.10- Localization-related (focal) (partial) symptomatic epilepsy and epileptic syndromes with simple partial seizures, **not intractable**
    Localization-related (focal) (partial) symptomatic epilepsy and epileptic syndromes with simple partial seizures without intractability

    G40.101 Localization-related (focal) (partial) symptomatic epilepsy and epileptic syndromes with simple partial seizures, **not** intractable, **with status epilepticus**

    G40.109 Localization-related (focal) (partial) symptomatic epilepsy and epileptic syndromes with simple partial seizures, **not** intractable, **without** status epilepticus
        Localization-related (focal) (partial) symptomatic epilepsy and epileptic syndromes with simple partial seizures NOS

  G40.11- Localization-related (focal) (partial) symptomatic epilepsy and epileptic syndromes with simple partial seizures, **intractable**

    G40.111 Localization-related (focal) (partial) symptomatic epilepsy and epileptic syndromes with simple partial seizures, intractable, **with status epilepticus**

    G40.119 Localization-related (focal) (partial) symptomatic epilepsy and epileptic syndromes with simple partial seizures, intractable, **without** status epilepticus

G40.2- **Localization-related** (focal) (partial) symptomatic epilepsy and epileptic syndromes with complex partial seizures
  Attacks with alteration of consciousness, often with automatisms
  Complex partial seizures developing into secondarily generalized seizures

  G40.20- Localization-related (focal) (partial) symptomatic epilepsy and epileptic syndromes with complex partial seizures, **not intractable**
    Localization-related (focal) (partial) symptomatic epilepsy and epileptic syndromes with complex partial seizures without intractability

    G40.201 Localization-related (focal) (partial) symptomatic epilepsy and epileptic syndromes with complex partial seizures, **not** intractable, **with status epilepticus**

    G40.209 Localization-related (focal) (partial) symptomatic epilepsy and epileptic syndromes with complex partial seizures, **not** intractable, **without** status epilepticus
        Localization-related (focal) (partial) symptomatic epilepsy and epileptic syndromes with complex partial seizures NOS

  G40.21- Localization-related (focal) (partial) symptomatic epilepsy and epileptic syndromes with complex partial seizures, **intractable**

    G40.211 Localization-related (focal) (partial) symptomatic epilepsy and epileptic syndromes with complex partial seizures, intractable, **with status epilepticus**

    G40.219 Localization-related (focal) (partial) symptomatic epilepsy and epileptic syndromes with complex partial seizures, intractable, **without** status epilepticus

G40.3- **Generalized** idiopathic epilepsy and epileptic syndromes
  Code also MERRF syndrome, if applicable (E88.42)

  G40.30- Generalized idiopathic epilepsy and epileptic syndromes, **not intractable**
    Generalized idiopathic epilepsy and epileptic syndromes without intractability

    G40.301 Generalized idiopathic epilepsy and epileptic syndromes, **not** intractable, **with status epilepticus**

    G40.309 Generalized idiopathic epilepsy and epileptic syndromes, **not** intractable, **without** status epilepticus
        Generalized idiopathic epilepsy and epileptic syndromes NOS

  G40.31- Generalized idiopathic epilepsy and epileptic syndromes, **intractable**

    G40.311 Generalized idiopathic epilepsy and epileptic syndromes, intractable, **with status epilepticus**

    G40.319 Generalized idiopathic epilepsy and epileptic syndromes, intractable, **without** status epilepticus

G40.A- **Absence epileptic** syndrome
  Absence epileptic syndrome NOS
  Childhood absence epilepsy [pyknolepsy]
  Juvenile absence epilepsy

  G40.A0- Absence epileptic syndrome, **not** intractable
    G40.A01 Absence epileptic syndrome, not intractable, **with status epilepticus**
    G40.A09 Absence epileptic syndrome, not intractable, **without status epilepticus**

  G40.A1- Absence epileptic syndrome, **intractable**
    G40.A11 Absence epileptic syndrome, intractable, **with status epilepticus**
    G40.A19 Absence epileptic syndrome, intractable, **without status epilepticus**

G40.B- **Juvenile myoclonic** epilepsy [impulsive petit mal]
  G40.B0- Juvenile myoclonic epilepsy, **not** intractable
    G40.B01 Juvenile myoclonic epilepsy, not intractable, **with status epilepticus**
    G40.B09 Juvenile myoclonic epilepsy, not intractable, **without status epilepticus**

  G40.B1- Juvenile myoclonic epilepsy, **intractable**
    G40.B11 Juvenile myoclonic epilepsy, intractable, **with status epilepticus**
    G40.B19 Juvenile myoclonic epilepsy, intractable, **without status epilepticus**

G
3
0
–
G
4
0

Excludes 1: = NOT CODED HERE! (Do not code both)   **421**   *Excludes ❷:* = Not Included Here

G40.4- <u>Other generalized</u> epilepsy and epileptic syndromes
    Epilepsy with grand mal seizures on awakening
    Epilepsy with myoclonic absences
    Epilepsy with myoclonic-astatic seizures
    Grand mal seizure NOS
    Nonspecific atonic epileptic seizures
    Nonspecific clonic epileptic seizures
    Nonspecific myoclonic epileptic seizures
    Nonspecific tonic epileptic seizures
    Nonspecific tonic-clonic epileptic seizures
    Symptomatic early myoclonic encephalopathy

G40.40- Other <u>generalized</u> epilepsy and epileptic syndromes, <u>not</u> intractable
    Other generalized epilepsy and epileptic syndromes without intractability
    Other generalized epilepsy and epileptic syndromes NOS

    G40.401 Other <u>generalized</u> epilepsy and epileptic syndromes, <u>not</u> intractable, <u>with status epilepticus</u>
    G40.409 Other <u>generalized</u> epilepsy and epileptic syndromes, <u>not</u> intractable, <u>without</u> status epilepticus

G40.41- Other <u>generalized</u> epilepsy and epileptic syndromes, <u>intractable</u>
    G40.411 Other <u>generalized</u> epilepsy and epileptic syndromes, intractable, <u>with status epilepticus</u>
    G40.419 Other <u>generalized</u> epilepsy and epileptic syndromes, intractable, <u>without</u> status epilepticus

G40.5- Epileptic seizures <u>related to external causes</u>
    Epileptic seizures related to alcohol
    Epileptic seizures related to drugs
    Epileptic seizures related to hormonal changes
    Epileptic seizures related to sleep deprivation
    Epileptic seizures related to stress
    Use additional code for adverse effect, if applicable, to identify drug (T36-T50 with fifth or sixth digit 5)
    Code also, if applicable, associated epilepsy and recurrent seizures (G40-)

G40.50- Epileptic seizures related to external causes, <u>not</u> intractable
    G40.501 Epileptic seizures related to external causes, <u>not</u> intractable, <u>with status epilepticus</u>
    G40.509 Epileptic seizures related to external causes, <u>not</u> intractable, <u>without</u> status epilepticus
        Epileptic seizures related to external causes NOS

G40.8- <u>Other epilepsy</u> and recurrent seizures
    Epilepsies and epileptic syndromes undetermined as to whether they are focal or generalized
    Landau-Kleffner syndrome

G40.80- Other epilepsy
    G40.801 Other epilepsy, <u>not</u> intractable, <u>with status epilepticus</u>
        Other epilepsy without intractability with status epilepticus
    G40.802 Other epilepsy, <u>not</u> intractable, <u>without</u> status epilepticus
        Other epilepsy NOS
        Other epilepsy without intractability without status epilepticus
    G40.803 Other epilepsy, <u>intractable</u>, <u>with status epilepticus</u>
    G40.804 Other epilepsy, <u>intractable</u>, <u>without</u> status epilepticus

G40.81- Lennox-Gastaut syndrome
    G40.811 Lennox-Gastaut syndrome, <u>not</u> intractable, <u>with status epilepticus</u>
    G40.812 Lennox-Gastaut syndrome, <u>not</u> intractable, <u>without</u> status epilepticus
    G40.813 Lennox-Gastaut syndrome, <u>intractable</u>, <u>with status epilepticus</u>
    G40.814 Lennox-Gastaut syndrome, <u>intractable</u>, <u>without</u> status epilepticus

G40.82- Epileptic spasms
    Infantile spasms
    Salaam attacks
    West's syndrome
    G40.821 Epileptic spasms, <u>not</u> intractable, <u>with status epilepticus</u>
    G40.822 Epileptic spasms, <u>not</u> intractable, <u>without</u> status epilepticus
    G40.823 Epileptic spasms, <u>intractable</u>, <u>with status epilepticus</u>
    G40.824 Epileptic spasms, <u>intractable</u>, <u>without</u> status epilepticus

G40.89 Other seizures
    Excludes 1: post traumatic seizures (R56.1)
    recurrent seizures NOS (G40.909)
    seizure NOS (R56.9)

G40.9- <u>Epilepsy, unspecified</u>
G40.90- Epilepsy, unspecified, <u>not</u> intractable
    Epilepsy, unspecified, without intractability
    G40.901 Epilepsy, unspecified, <u>not</u> intractable, <u>with status epilepticus</u>
    G40.909 Epilepsy, unspecified, <u>not</u> intractable, <u>without</u> status epilepticus
        Epilepsy NOS
        Epileptic convulsions NOS
        Epileptic fits NOS
        Epileptic seizures NOS
        Recurrent seizures NOS
        Seizure disorder NOS

G40.91- Epilepsy, unspecified, <u>intractable</u>
    Intractable seizure disorder NOS
    G40.911 Epilepsy, unspecified, intractable, <u>with status epilepticus</u>
    G40.919 Epilepsy, unspecified, intractable, <u>without</u> status epilepticus

G43 **Migraine**
Note: The following terms are to be considered equivalent to intractable: pharmacoresistant (pharmacologically resistant), treatment resistant, refractory (medically) and poorly controlled.
Use additional code for adverse effect, if applicable, to identify drug (T36-T50 with fifth or sixth character 5)
Excludes 1: headache NOS (R51)
    lower half migraine (G44.00)
Excludes ❷: headache syndromes (G44.-)

G43.0- <u>Migraine without aura</u>
    Common migraine
    Excludes 1: chronic migraine without aura (G43.7-)
G43.00- Migraine without aura, <u>not</u> intractable
    Migraine without aura without mention of refractory migraine
    G43.001 Migraine without aura, <u>not</u> intractable, <u>with status migrainosus</u>
    G43.009 Migraine without aura, <u>not</u> intractable, <u>without</u> status migrainosus
        Migraine without aura NOS
G43.01- Migraine without aura, <u>intractable</u>
    Migraine without aura with refractory migraine
    G43.011 Migraine without aura, intractable, <u>with status migrainosus</u>
    G43.019 Migraine without aura, intractable, <u>without</u> status migrainosus

G43.1- <u>Migraine with aura</u>
    Basilar migraine
    Classical migraine
    Migraine equivalents
    Migraine preceded or accompanied by transient focal neurological phenomena
    Migraine triggered seizures
    Migraine with acute-onset aura
    Migraine with aura without headache (migraine equivalents)
    Migraine with prolonged aura
    Migraine with typical aura
    Retinal migraine
    Code also any associated seizure (G40.-, R56.9)
    Excludes 1: persistent migraine aura (G43.5-, G43.6-)
G43.10- Migraine with aura, <u>not</u> intractable
    Migraine with aura without mention of refractory migraine
    G43.101 Migraine with aura, <u>not</u> intractable, <u>with status migrainosus</u>
    G43.109 Migraine with aura, <u>not</u> intractable, <u>without</u> status migrainosus
        Migraine with aura NOS
G43.11- Migraine with aura, <u>intractable</u>
    Migraine with aura with refractory migraine
    G43.111 Migraine with aura, intractable, <u>with status migrainosus</u>
    G43.119 Migraine with aura, intractable, <u>without</u> status migrainosus

G 4 0 - G 4 3

G43.4- <u>Hemiplegic</u> migraine
    Familial migraine
    Sporadic migraine
  G43.40- Hemiplegic migraine, <u>not</u> intractable
    Hemiplegic migraine without refractory migraine
    G43.401 **Hemiplegic migraine, <u>not</u> intractable, <u>with status migrainosus</u>**
    G43.409 **Hemiplegic migraine, <u>not</u> intractable, <u>without</u> status migrainosus**
      Hemiplegic migraine NOS
  G43.41- Hemiplegic migraine, <u>intractable</u>
    Hemiplegic migraine with refractory migraine
    G43.411 **Hemiplegic migraine, intractable, <u>with status migrainosus</u>**
    G43.419 **Hemiplegic migraine, intractable, <u>without</u> status migrainosus**

G43.5- <u>Persistent</u> migraine aura <u>without</u> cerebral infarction
  G43.50- Persistent migraine aura without cerebral infarction, <u>not</u> intractable
    Persistent migraine aura without cerebral infarction, without refractory migraine
    G43.501 **Persistent migraine aura without cerebral infarction, not intractable, <u>with status migrainosus</u>**
    G43.509 **Persistent migraine aura without cerebral infarction, not intractable, <u>without</u> status migrainosus**
      Persistent migraine aura NOS
  G43.51- Persistent migraine aura without cerebral infarction, <u>intractable</u>
    Persistent migraine aura without cerebral infarction, with refractory migraine
    G43.511 **Persistent migraine aura without cerebral infarction, intractable, <u>with status migrainosus</u>**
    G43.519 **Persistent migraine aura without cerebral infarction, intractable, <u>without</u> status migrainosus**

G43.6- <u>Persistent</u> migraine aura <u>with cerebral infarction</u>
  Code also the type of cerebral infarction (I63.-)
  G43.60- Persistent migraine aura with cerebral infarction, <u>not</u> intractable
    Persistent migraine aura with cerebral infarction, without refractory migraine
    G43.601 **Persistent migraine aura with cerebral infarction, <u>not</u> intractable, <u>with status migrainosus</u>**
    G43.609 **Persistent migraine aura with cerebral infarction, <u>not</u> intractable, <u>without</u> status migrainosus**
  G43.61- Persistent migraine aura with cerebral infarction, <u>intractable</u>
    Persistent migraine aura with cerebral infarction, with refractory migraine
    G43.611 **Persistent migraine aura with cerebral infarction, intractable, <u>with status migrainosus</u>**
    G43.619 **Persistent migraine aura with cerebral infarction, intractable, <u>without</u> status migrainosus**

G43.7 <u>Chronic</u> migraine <u>without</u> aura
  Transformed migraine
  Excludes 1: migraine without aura (G43.0-)
  G43.70- Chronic migraine without aura, <u>not</u> intractable
    Chronic migraine without aura, without refractory migraine
    G43.701 **Chronic migraine without aura, <u>not</u> intractable, <u>with</u> status migrainosus**
    G43.709 **Chronic migraine without aura, <u>not</u> intractable, <u>without</u> status migrainosus**
      Chronic migraine without aura NOS
  G43.71- Chronic migraine without aura, <u>intractable</u>
    Chronic migraine without aura, with refractory migraine
    G43.711 **Chronic migraine without aura, intractable, <u>with status migrainosus</u>**
    G43.719 **Chronic migraine without aura, intractable, <u>without</u> status migrainosus**

G43.A- <u>Cyclical vomiting</u>
  G43.A0 Cyclical vomiting, <u>not</u> intractable
    Cyclical vomiting, without refractory migraine
  G43.A1 Cyclical vomiting, <u>intractable</u>
    Cyclical vomiting, with refractory migraine

G43.B- <u>Ophthalmoplegic migraine</u>
  G43.B0 Ophthalmoplegic migraine, <u>not</u> intractable
    Ophthalmoplegic migraine, without refractory migraine
  G43.B1 Ophthalmoplegic migraine, <u>intractable</u>
    Ophthalmoplegic migraine, with refractory migraine

G43.C- <u>Periodic headache syndromes in child or adult</u>
  G43.C0 Periodic headache syndromes in child or adult, <u>not</u> intractable
    Periodic headache syndromes in child or adult, without refractory migraine
  G43.C1 Periodic headache syndromes in child or adult, <u>intractable</u>
    Periodic headache syndromes in child or adult, with refractory migraine

G43.D- <u>Abdominal migraine</u>
  G43.D0 Abdominal migraine, <u>not</u> intractable
    Abdominal migraine, without refractory migraine
  G43.D1 Abdominal migraine, <u>intractable</u>
    Abdominal migraine, with refractory migraine

G43.8- <u>Other migraine</u>
  G43.80- Other migraine, <u>not</u> intractable
    Other migraine, without refractory migraine
    G43.801 **Other migraine, <u>not</u> intractable, <u>with status migrainosus</u>**
    G43.809 **Other migraine, <u>not</u> intractable, <u>without</u> status migrainosus**
  G43.81- Other migraine, <u>intractable</u>
    Other migraine, with refractory migraine
    G43.811 **Other migraine, intractable, <u>with status migrainosus</u>**
    G43.819 **Other migraine, intractable, <u>without</u> status migrainosus**
  G43.82- Menstrual migraine, <u>not</u> intractable
    Menstrual headache, not intractable
    Menstrual migraine, without refractory migraine
    Menstrually related migraine, not intractable
    Pre-menstrual headache, not intractable
    Pre-menstrual migraine, not intractable
    Pure menstrual migraine, not intractable
    Code also associated premenstrual tension syndrome (N94.3)
    G43.821 **Menstrual migraine, <u>not</u> intractable, <u>with status migrainosus</u>**
    G43.829 **Menstrual migraine, <u>not</u> intractable, <u>without</u> status migrainosus**
      Menstrual migraine NOS
  G43.83- Menstrual migraine, <u>intractable</u>
    Menstrual headache, intractable
    Menstrual migraine, with refractory migraine
    Menstrually related migraine, intractable
    Pre-menstrual headache, intractable
    Pre-menstrual migraine, intractable
    Pure menstrual migraine, intractable
    Code also associated premenstrual tension syndrome (N94.3)
    G43.831 **Menstrual migraine, <u>intractable</u>, <u>with status migrainosus</u>**
    G43.839 **Menstrual migraine, <u>intractable</u>, <u>without</u> status migrainosus**

G43.9- <u>Migraine, unspecified</u>
  G43.90- Migraine, unspecified, <u>not</u> intractable
    Migraine, unspecified, without refractory migraine
    G43.901 **Migraine, unspecified, <u>not</u> intractable, <u>with status migrainosus</u>**
      Status migrainosus NOS
    G43.909 **Migraine, unspecified, <u>not</u> intractable, <u>without</u> status migrainosus**
      Migraine NOS
  G43.91- Migraine, unspecified, <u>intractable</u>
    Migraine, unspecified, with refractory migraine
    G43.911 **Migraine, unspecified, intractable, <u>with status migrainosus</u>**
    G43.919 **Migraine, unspecified, intractable, <u>without</u> status migrainosus**

G
4
0
-
G
4
3

Excludes 1: = NOT CODED HERE! (Do not code both)   **423**   *Excludes ❷: = Not Included Here*

G44- Other headache syndromes
Excludes 1: headache NOS (R51)
Excludes ❷: atypical facial pain (G50.1)
  headache due to lumbar puncture (G97.1)
  migraines (G43.-)
  trigeminal neuralgia (G50.0)

G44.0- Cluster headaches and other trigeminal autonomic cephalgias (TAC)

G44.00- Cluster headache syndrome, unspecified
Ciliary neuralgia
Cluster headache NOS
Histamine cephalgia
Lower half migraine
Migrainous neuralgia

G44.001 Cluster headache syndrome, unspecified, intractable
G44.009 Cluster headache syndrome, unspecified, not intractable
Cluster headache syndrome NOS

G44.01- Episodic cluster headache
G44.011 Episodic cluster headache, intractable
G44.019 Episodic cluster headache, not intractable
Episodic cluster headache NOS

G44.02- Chronic cluster headache
G44.021 Chronic cluster headache, intractable
G44.029 Chronic cluster headache, not intractable
Chronic cluster headache NOS

G44.03- Episodic paroxysmal hemicrania
Paroxysmal hemicrania NOS
G44.031 Episodic paroxysmal hemicrania, intractable
G44.039 Episodic paroxysmal hemicrania, not intractable
Episodic paroxysmal hemicrania NOS

G44.04- Chronic paroxysmal hemicrania
G44.041 Chronic paroxysmal hemicrania, intractable
G44.049 Chronic paroxysmal hemicrania, not intractable
Chronic paroxysmal hemicrania NOS

G44.05- Short lasting unilateral neuralgiform headache with conjunctival injection and tearing (SUNCT)
G44.051 Short lasting unilateral neuralgiform headache with conjunctival injection and tearing (SUNCT), intractable
G44.059 Short lasting unilateral neuralgiform headache with conjunctival injection and tearing (SUNCT), not intractable
Short lasting unilateral neuralgiform headache with conjunctival injection and tearing (SUNCT) NOS

G44.09- Other trigeminal autonomic cephalgias (TAC)
G44.091 Other trigeminal autonomic cephalgias (TAC), intractable
G44.099 Other trigeminal autonomic cephalgias (TAC), not intractable

G44.1 Vascular headache, not elsewhere classified
Excludes ❷: cluster headache (G44.0)
  complicated headache syndromes (G44.5-)
  drug-induced headache (G44.4-)
  migraine (G43-)
  other specified headache syndromes (G44.8-)
  post-traumatic headache (G44.3-)
  tension-type headache (G44.2-)

G44.2- Tension-type headache

G44.20- Tension-type headache, unspecified
G44.201 Tension-type headache, unspecified, intractable
G44.209 Tension-type headache, unspecified, not intractable
Tension headache NOS

G44.21- Episodic tension-type headache
G44.211 Episodic tension-type headache, intractable
G44.219 Episodic tension-type headache, not intractable
Episodic tension-type headache NOS

G44.22- Chronic tension-type headache
G44.221 Chronic tension-type headache, intractable
G44.229 Chronic tension-type headache, not intractable
Chronic tension-type headache NOS

G44.3- Post-traumatic headache

G44.30- Post-traumatic headache, unspecified
G44.301 Post-traumatic headache, unspecified, intractable
G44.309 Post-traumatic headache, unspecified, not intractable
Post-traumatic headache NOS

G44.31- Acute post-traumatic headache
G44.311 Acute post-traumatic headache, intractable
G44.319 Acute post-traumatic headache, not intractable
Acute post-traumatic headache NOS

G44.32- Chronic post-traumatic headache
G44.321 Chronic post-traumatic headache, intractable
G44.329 Chronic post-traumatic headache, not intractable
Chronic post-traumatic headache NOS

G44.4- Drug-induced headache, not elsewhere classified
Medication overuse headache
Use additional code for adverse effect, if applicable, to identify drug (T36-T50 with fifth or sixth character 5)

G44.40 Drug-induced headache, not elsewhere classified, not intractable
G44.41 Drug-induced headache, not elsewhere classified, intractable

G44.5- Complicated headache syndromes
G44.51 Hemicrania continua
G44.52 New daily persistent headache (NDPH)
G44.53 Primary thunderclap headache
G44.59 Other complicated headache syndrome

G44.8- Other specified headache syndromes
G44.81 Hypnic headache
G44.82 Headache associated with sexual activity
Orgasmic headache
Preorgasmic headache
G44.83 Primary cough headache
G44.84 Primary exertional headache
G44.85 Primary stabbing headache
G44.89 Other headache syndrome

G45- Transient cerebral ischemic attacks and related syndromes
Excludes 1: neonatal cerebral ischemia (P91.0)
  transient retinal artery occlusion (H34.0-)

G45.0 Vertebro-basilar artery syndrome
G45.1 Carotid artery syndrome (hemispheric)
G45.2 Multiple and bilateral precerebral artery syndromes
G45.3 Amaurosis fugax
G45.4 Transient global amnesia
Excludes 1: amnesia NOS (R41.3)
G45.8 Other transient cerebral ischemic attacks and related syndromes
G45.9 Transient cerebral ischemic attack, unspecified
Spasm of cerebral artery
TIA
Transient cerebral ischemia NOS

G46- Vascular syndromes of brain in cerebrovascular diseases
Code first underlying cerebrovascular disease (I60-I69)
G46.0 Middle cerebral artery syndrome
G46.1 Anterior cerebral artery syndrome
G46.2 Posterior cerebral artery syndrome
G46.3 Brain stem stroke syndrome
Benedikt syndrome
Claude syndrome
Foville syndrome
Millard-Gubler syndrome
Wallenberg syndrome
Weber syndrome
G46.4 Cerebellar stroke syndrome
G46.5 Pure motor lacunar syndrome
G46.6 Pure sensory lacunar syndrome
G46.7 Other lacunar syndromes
G46.8 Other vascular syndromes of brain in cerebrovascular diseases

G47- Sleep disorders
Excludes ❷: nightmares (F51.5)
  nonorganic sleep disorders (F51.-)
  sleep terrors (F51.4)
  sleepwalking (F51.3)

G47.0- Insomnia
Excludes ❷: alcohol related insomnia (F10.182, F10.282, F10.982)
  drug-related insomnia F11.182, F11.282, F11.982, F13.182, F13.282, F13.982, F14.182, F14.282, F14.982, F15.182, F15.282, F15.982, F19.182, F19.282, F19.982
  idiopathic insomnia (F51.01)
  insomnia due to a mental disorder (F51.05)
  insomnia not due to a substance or known physiological condition (F51.0-)
  nonorganic insomnia (F51.0-)
  primary insomnia (F51.01)
  sleep apnea (G47.3-)

G47.00 Insomnia, unspecified
Insomnia NOS
G47.01 Insomnia due to medical condition
Code also associated medical condition
G47.09 Other insomnia

G44-G52

Excludes 1: = NOT CODED HERE! (Do not code both)

Excludes ❷: = Not Included Here

G47.1- Hypersomnia
Excludes❷: alcohol-related hypersomnia (F10.182, F10.282,
F10.982)
drug-related hypersomnia F11.182, F11.282, F11.982,
F13.182, F13.282, F13.982, F14.182, F14.282,
F14.982, F15.182, F15.282, F15.982, F19.182,
F19.282, F19.982
hypersomnia due to a mental disorder (F51.13)
hypersomnia not due to a substance or known
physiological condition (F51.1-)
primary hypersomnia (F51.11)
sleep apnea (G47.3-)

G47.10 Hypersomnia, unspecified
Hypersomnia NOS

G47.11 Idiopathic hypersomnia with long sleep time
Idiopathic hypersomnia NOS

G47.12 Idiopathic hypersomnia without long sleep time

G47.13 Recurrent hypersomnia
Kleine-Levin syndrome
Menstrual related hypersomnia

G47.14 Hypersomnia due to medical condition
Code also associated medical condition

G47.19 Other hypersomnia

G47.2- Circadian rhythm sleep disorders
Disorders of the sleep wake schedule
Inversion of nyctohemeral rhythm
Inversion of sleep rhythm

G47.20 Circadian rhythm sleep disorder, unspecified type
Sleep wake schedule disorder NOS

G47.21 Circadian rhythm sleep disorder, delayed sleep phase type
Delayed sleep phase syndrome

G47.22 Circadian rhythm sleep disorder, advanced sleep phase type

G47.23 Circadian rhythm sleep disorder, irregular sleep wake type
Irregular sleep-wake pattern

G47.24 Circadian rhythm sleep disorder, free running type

G47.25 Circadian rhythm sleep disorder, jet lag type

G47.26 Circadian rhythm sleep disorder, shift work type

G47.27 Circadian rhythm sleep disorder in conditions classified elsewhere
Code first underlying condition

G47.29 Other circadian rhythm sleep disorder

G47.3- Sleep apnea
Code also any associated underlying condition
Excludes 1: apnea NOS (R06.81)
Cheyne-Stokes breathing (R06.3)
pickwickian syndrome (E66.2)
sleep apnea of newborn (P28.3)

G47.30 Sleep apnea, unspecified
Sleep apnea NOS

G47.31 Primary central sleep apnea

G47.32 High altitude periodic breathing

G47.33 Obstructive sleep apnea (adult) (pediatric)
Excludes 1: obstructive sleep apnea of newborn (P28.3)

G47.34 Idiopathic sleep related nonobstructive alveolar hypoventilation
Sleep related hypoxia

G47.35 Congenital central alveolar hypoventilation syndrome

G47.36 Sleep related hypoventilation in conditions classified elsewhere
Sleep related hypoxemia in conditions classified elsewhere
Code first underlying condition

G47.37 Central sleep apnea in conditions classified elsewhere
Code first underlying condition

G47.39 Other sleep apnea

G47.4- Narcolepsy and cataplexy

G47.41- Narcolepsy

G47.411 Narcolepsy with cataplexy

G47.419 Narcolepsy without cataplexy
Narcolepsy NOS

G47.42- Narcolepsy in conditions classified elsewhere
Code first underlying condition

G47.421 Narcolepsy in conditions classified elsewhere with cataplexy

G47.429 Narcolepsy in conditions classified elsewhere without cataplexy

G47.5- Parasomnia
Excludes 1: alcohol induced parasomnia (F10.182, F10.282,
F10.982)
drug induced parasomnia (F11.182, F11.282, F11.982,
F13.182, F13.282, F13.982, F14.182, F14.282,
F14.982, F15.182, F15.282, F15.982, F19.182,
F19.282, F19.982)
parasomnia not due to a substance or known
physiological condition (F51.8)

G47.50 Parasomnia, unspecified
Parasomnia NOS

G47.51 Confusional arousals

G47.52 REM sleep behavior disorder

G47.53 Recurrent isolated sleep paralysis

G47.54 Parasomnia in conditions classified elsewhere
Code first underlying condition

G47.59 Other parasomnia

G47.6- Sleep related movement disorders
Excludes❷: restless legs syndrome (G25.81)

G47.61 Periodic limb movement disorder
Periodic limb movement disorder

G47.62 Sleep related leg cramps

G47.63 Sleep related bruxism
Excludes 1: psychogenic bruxism (F45.8)

G47.69 Other sleep related movement disorders

G47.8 Other sleep disorders

G47.9 Sleep disorder, unspecified
Sleep disorder NOS

Nerve, nerve root and plexus disorders (G50-G59)

Excludes 1: current traumatic nerve, nerve root and plexus disorders —
see Injury, nerve by body region
neuralgia NOS (M79.2)
neuritis NOS (M79.2)
peripheral neuritis in pregnancy (O26.82-)
radiculitis NOS (M54.1-)

G50- Disorders of trigeminal nerve
Includes: Disorders of 5th cranial nerve

G50.0 Trigeminal neuralgia
Syndrome of paroxysmal facial pain
Tic douloureux

G50.1 Atypical facial pain

G50.8 Other disorders of trigeminal nerve

G50.9 Disorder of trigeminal nerve, unspecified

G51- Facial nerve disorders
Includes: Disorders of 7th cranial nerve

G51.0 Bell's palsy
Facial palsy

G51.1 Geniculate ganglionitis
Excludes 1: postherpetic geniculate ganglionitis (B02.21)

G51.2 Melkersson's syndrome
Melkersson-Rosenthal syndrome

G51.3 Clonic hemifacial spasm

G51.4 Facial myokymia

G51.8 Other disorders of facial nerve

G51.9 Disorder of facial nerve, unspecified

G52- Disorders of other cranial nerves
Excludes❷: disorders of acoustic [8th] nerve (H93.3)
disorders of optic [2nd] nerve (H46, H47.0)
paralytic strabismus due to nerve palsy (H49.0-H49.2)

G52.0 Disorders of olfactory nerve
Disorders of 1st cranial nerve

G52.1 Disorders of glossopharyngeal nerve
Disorder of 9th cranial nerve
Glossopharyngeal neuralgia

G52.2 Disorders of vagus nerve
Disorders of pneumogastric [10th] nerve

G52.3 Disorders of hypoglossal nerve
Disorders of 12th cranial nerve

G52.7 Disorders of multiple cranial nerves
Polyneuritis cranialis

G52.8 Disorders of other specified cranial nerves

G52.9 Cranial nerve disorder, unspecified

G44 - G52

G53   **Cranial nerve disorders in diseases classified elsewhere**
Code first underlying disease, such as:
   Neoplasm (C00-D49)
Excludes 1:   multiple cranial nerve palsy in sarcoidosis (D86.82)
*   multiple cranial nerve palsy in syphilis (A52.15)*
*   postherpetic geniculate ganglionitis (B02.21)*
*   postherpetic trigeminal neuralgia (B02.22)*

G54-   **Nerve root and plexus disorders**
Excludes 1:   current traumatic nerve root and plexus disorders — see nerve
*   injury by body region*
*   intervertebral disc disorders (M50-M51)*
*   neuralgia or neuritis NOS (M79.2)*
*   neuritis or radiculitis brachial NOS (M54.13)*
*   neuritis or radiculitis lumbar NOS (M54.16)*
*   neuritis or radiculitis lumbosacral NOS (M54.17)*
*   neuritis or radiculitis thoracic NOS (M54.14)*
*   radiculitis NOS (M54.10)*
*   radiculopathy NOS (M54.10)*
*   spondylosis (M47.-)*
  G54.0   **Brachial plexus disorders**
    Thoracic outlet syndrome
  G54.1   **Lumbosacral plexus disorders**
  G54.2   **Cervical root disorders, not elsewhere classified**
  G54.3   **Thoracic root disorders, not elsewhere classified**
  G54.4   **Lumbosacral root disorders, not elsewhere classified**
  G54.5   **Neuralgic amyotrophy**
    Parsonage-Aldren-Turner syndrome
    Shoulder-girdle neuritis
    Excludes 1:   neuralgic amyotrophy in diabetes mellitus (E08-E13
     with .44)
  G54.6   **Phantom limb syndrome with pain**
  G54.7   **Phantom limb syndrome without pain**
    Phantom limb syndrome NOS
  G54.8   **Other nerve root and plexus disorders**
  G54.9   **Nerve root and plexus disorder, unspecified**

G55   **Nerve root and plexus compressions in diseases classified elsewhere**
Code first underlying disease, such as:
   Neoplasm (C00-D49)
Excludes 1:   nerve root compression (due to) (in) ankylosing spondylitis
*   (M45.-)*
*   nerve root compression (due to) (in) ankylosing spondylitis*
*   (M45.-)*
*   nerve root compression (due to) (in) dorsopathies (M53.-,*
*   M54.-)*
*   nerve root compression (due to) (in) intervertebral disc*
*   disorders (M50.1-, M51.1-)*
*   nerve root compression (due to) (in) spondylopathies (M46.-,*
*   M48.-)*

G56-   **Mononeuropathies of upper limb**
Excludes 1:   current traumatic nerve disorder — see nerve injury by body
*   region*
  G56.0-   **Carpal tunnel syndrome**
    G56.00   **Carpal tunnel syndrome, unspecified upper limb**
    G56.01   **Carpal tunnel syndrome, right upper limb**
    G56.02   **Carpal tunnel syndrome, left upper limb**
  G56.1-   **Other lesions of median nerve**
    G56.10   **Other lesions of median nerve, unspecified upper limb**
    G56.11   **Other lesions of median nerve, right upper limb**
    G56.12   **Other lesions of median nerve, left upper limb**
  G56.2-   **Lesion of ulnar nerve**
    Tardy ulnar nerve palsy
    G56.20   **Lesion of ulnar nerve, unspecified upper limb**
    G56.21   **Lesion of ulnar nerve, right upper limb**
    G56.22   **Lesion of ulnar nerve, left upper limb**
  G56.3-   **Lesion of radial nerve**
    G56.30   **Lesion of radial nerve, unspecified upper limb**
    G56.31   **Lesion of radial nerve, right upper limb**
    G56.32   **Lesion of radial nerve, left upper limb**

  G56.4-   **Causalgia of upper limb**
    Complex regional pain syndrome II of upper limb
    Excludes 1:   complex regional pain syndrome I of lower limb
*   (G90.52-)*
*   complex regional pain syndrome I of upper limb*
*   (G90.51-)*
*   complex regional pain syndrome II of lower limb*
*   (G57.7-)*
*   reflex sympathetic dystrophy of lower limb (G90.52-)*
*   reflex sympathetic dystrophy of upper limb (G90.51-)*
    G56.40   **Causalgia of unspecified upper limb**
    G56.41   **Causalgia of right upper limb**
    G56.42   **Causalgia of left upper limb**
  G56.8-   **Other specified mononeuropathies of upper limb**
    Interdigital neuroma of upper limb
    G56.80   **Other specified mononeuropathies of unspecified upper limb**
    G56.81   **Other specified mononeuropathies of right upper limb**
    G56.82   **Other specified mononeuropathies of left upper limb**
  G56.9-   **Unspecified mononeuropathy of upper limb**
    G56.90   **Unspecified mononeuropathy of unspecified upper limb**
    G56.91   **Unspecified mononeuropathy of right upper limb**
    G56.92   **Unspecified mononeuropathy of left upper limb**

G57-   **Mononeuropathies of lower limb**
Excludes 1:   current traumatic nerve disorder — see nerve injury by body
*   region*
  G57.0-   **Lesion of sciatic nerve**
    Excludes 1:   sciatica NOS (M54.3-)
    Excludes ❷: sciatica attributed to intervertebral disc disorder
*   (M51.1.-)*
    G57.00   **Lesion of sciatic nerve, unspecified lower limb**
    G57.01   **Lesion of sciatic nerve, right lower limb**
    G57.02   **Lesion of sciatic nerve, left lower limb**
  G57.1-   **Meralgia paresthetica**
    Lateral cutaneous nerve of thigh syndrome
    G57.10   **Meralgia paresthetica, unspecified lower limb**
    G57.11   **Meralgia paresthetica, right lower limb**
    G57.12   **Meralgia paresthetica, left lower limb**
  G57.2-   **Lesion of femoral nerve**
    G57.20   **Lesion of femoral nerve, unspecified lower limb**
    G57.21   **Lesion of femoral nerve, right lower limb**
    G57.22   **Lesion of femoral nerve, left lower limb**
  G57.3-   **Lesion of lateral popliteal nerve**
    Peroneal nerve palsy
    G57.30   **Lesion of lateral popliteal nerve, unspecified lower limb**
    G57.31   **Lesion of lateral popliteal nerve, right lower limb**
    G57.32   **Lesion of lateral popliteal nerve, left lower limb**
  G57.4-   **Lesion of medial popliteal nerve**
    G57.40   **Lesion of medial popliteal nerve, unspecified lower limb**
    G57.41   **Lesion of medial popliteal nerve, right lower limb**
    G57.42   **Lesion of medial popliteal nerve, left lower limb**
  G57.5-   **Tarsal tunnel syndrome**
    G57.50   **Tarsal tunnel syndrome, unspecified lower limb**
    G57.51   **Tarsal tunnel syndrome, right lower limb**
    G57.52   **Tarsal tunnel syndrome, left lower limb**
  G57.6-   **Lesion of plantar nerve**
    Morton's metatarsalgia
    G57.60   **Lesion of plantar nerve, unspecified lower limb**
    G57.61   **Lesion of plantar nerve, right lower limb**
    G57.62   **Lesion of plantar nerve, left lower limb**
  G57.7-   **Causalgia of lower limb**
    Complex regional pain syndrome II of lower limb
    Excludes 1:   complex regional pain syndrome I of lower limb
*   (G90.52-)*
*   complex regional pain syndrome I of upper limb*
*   (G90.51-)*
*   complex regional pain syndrome II of upper limb*
*   (G56.4-)*
*   reflex sympathetic dystrophy of lower limb (G90.52-)*
*   reflex sympathetic dystrophy of upper limb (G90.51-)*
    G57.70   **Causalgia of unspecified lower limb**
    G57.71   **Causalgia of right lower limb**
    G57.72   **Causalgia of left lower limb**
  G57.8-   **Other specified mononeuropathies of lower limb**
    Interdigital neuroma of lower limb
    G57.80   **Other specified mononeuropathies of unspecified lower limb**
    G57.81   **Other specified mononeuropathies of right lower limb**
    G57.82   **Other specified mononeuropathies of left lower limb**

G53 - G71

Excludes 1: = NOT CODED HERE! (Do not code both)

Excludes ❷: = Not Included Here

G57.9- Unspecified mononeuropathy of lower limb
   G57.90 Unspecified mononeuropathy of unspecified lower limb
   G57.91 Unspecified mononeuropathy of right lower limb
   G57.92 Unspecified mononeuropathy of left lower limb
G58- Other mononeuropathies
   G58.0 Intercostal neuropathy
   G58.7 Mononeuritis multiplex
   G58.8 Other specified mononeuropathies
   G58.9 Mononeuropathy, unspecified
G59 Mononeuropathy in diseases classified elsewhere
   Code first underlying disease
   Excludes 1: diabetic mononeuropathy (E08-E13 with .41)
      syphilitic nerve paralysis (A52.19)
      syphilitic neuritis (A52.15)
      tuberculous mononeuropathy (A17.83)

Polyneuropathies and other disorders of the peripheral nervous system (G60-G65)

Excludes 1: neuralgia NOS (M79.2)
      neuritis NOS (M79.2)
      peripheral neuritis in pregnancy (O26.82-)
      radiculitis NOS (M54.10)

G60- Hereditary and idiopathic neuropathy
   G60.0 Hereditary motor and sensory neuropathy
      Charcot-Marie-Tooth disease
      Déjérine-Sottas disease
      Hereditary motor and sensory neuropathy, types I-IV
      Hypertrophic neuropathy of infancy
      Peroneal muscular atrophy (axonal type) (hypertrophic type)
      Roussy-Levy syndrome
   G60.1 Refsum's disease
      Infantile Refsum disease
   G60.2 Neuropathy in association with hereditary ataxia
   G60.3 Idiopathic progressive neuropathy
   G60.8 Other hereditary and idiopathic neuropathies
      Dominantly inherited sensory neuropathy
      Morvan's disease
      Nelaton's syndrome
      Recessively inherited sensory neuropathy
   G60.9 Hereditary and idiopathic neuropathy, unspecified
G61- Inflammatory polyneuropathy
   G61.0 Guillain-Barre syndrome
      Acute (post-)infective polyneuritis
      Miller Fisher Syndrome
   G61.1 Serum neuropathy
      Use additional code for adverse effect, if applicable, to identify serum (T50-)
   G61.8- Other inflammatory polyneuropathies
      G61.81 Chronic inflammatory demyelinating polyneuritis
      G61.89 Other inflammatory polyneuropathies
   G61.9 Inflammatory polyneuropathy, unspecified
G62- Other and unspecified polyneuropathies
   G62.0 Drug-induced polyneuropathy
      Use additional code for adverse effect, if applicable, to identify drug (T36-T50 with fifth or sixth character 5)
   G62.1 Alcoholic polyneuropathy
   G62.2 Polyneuropathy due to other toxic agents
      Code first (T51-T65) to identify toxic agent
   G62.8- Other specified polyneuropathies
      G62.81 Critical illness polyneuropathy
        Acute motor neuropathy
      G62.82 Radiation-induced polyneuropathy
        Use additional external cause code (W88-W90, X39.0-) to identify cause
      G62.89 Other specified polyneuropathies
   G62.9 Polyneuropathy, unspecified
      Neuropathy NOS

G63 Polyneuropathy in diseases classified elsewhere
   Code first underlying disease, such as:
      Amyloidosis (E85.-)
      Endocrine disease, except diabetes (E00-E07, E15-E16, E20-E34)
      Metabolic diseases (E70-E88)
      Neoplasm (C00-D49)
      Nutritional deficiency (E40-E64)
   Excludes 1: polyneuropathy (in):
      diabetes mellitus (E08-E13 with .42)
      diphtheria (A36.83)
      infectious mononucleosis (B27.0-B27.9 with 1)
      Lyme disease (A69.22)
      mumps (B26.84)
      postherpetic (B02.23)
      rheumatoid arthritis (M05.33)
      scleroderma (M34.83)
      systemic lupus erythematosus (M32.19)
G64 Other disorders of peripheral nervous system
   Disorder of peripheral nervous system NOS
G65- Sequelae of inflammatory and toxic polyneuropathies
   Code first condition resulting from (sequela) of inflammatory and toxic polyneuropathies
   G65.0 Sequelae of Guillain-Barré syndrome
   G65.1 Sequelae of other inflammatory polyneuropathy
   G65.2 Sequelae of toxic polyneuropathy

Diseases of myoneural junction and muscle (G70-G73)

G70- Myasthenia gravis and other myoneural disorders
   Excludes 1: botulism (A05.1, A48.51-A48.52)
      transient neonatal myasthenia gravis (P94.0)
   G70.0- Myasthenia gravis
      G70.00 Myasthenia gravis without (acute) exacerbation
        Myasthenia gravis NOS
      G70.01 Myasthenia gravis with (acute) exacerbation
        Myasthenia gravis in crisis
   G70.1 Toxic myoneural disorders
      Code first (T51-T65) to identify toxic agent
   G70.2 Congenital and developmental myasthenia
   G70.8- Other specified myoneural disorders
      G70.80 Lambert-Eaton syndrome, unspecified
        Lambert-Eaton syndrome NOS
      G70.81 Lambert-Eaton syndrome in disease classified elsewhere
        Code first underlying disease
        Excludes 1: Lambert-Eaton syndrome in neoplastic disease (G73.1)
      G70.89 Other specified myoneural disorders
   G70.9 Myoneural disorder, unspecified
G71- Primary disorders of muscles
   Excludes❷: arthrogryposis multiplex congenita (Q74.3)
      metabolic disorders (E70-E88)
      myositis (M60.-)
   G71.0 Muscular dystrophy
      Autosomal recessive, childhood type, muscular dystrophy resembling Duchenne or Becker muscular dystrophy
      Benign [Becker] muscular dystrophy
      Benign scapuloperoneal muscular dystrophy with early contractures [Emery-Dreifuss]
      Congenital muscular dystrophy NOS
      Congenital muscular dystrophy with specific morphological abnormalities of the muscle fiber
      Distal muscular dystrophy
      Facioscapulohumeral muscular dystrophy
      Limb-girdle muscular dystrophy
      Ocular muscular dystrophy
      Oculopharyngeal muscular dystrophy
      Scapuloperoneal muscular dystrophy
      Severe [Duchenne] muscular dystrophy
   G71.1- Myotonic disorders
      G71.11 Myotonic muscular dystrophy
        Dystrophia myotonica [Steinert]
        Myotonia atrophica
        Myotonic dystrophy
        Proximal myotonic myopathy (PROMM)
        Steinert disease
      G71.12 Myotonia congenita
        Acetazolamide responsive myotonia congenita
        Dominant myotonia congenita [Thomsen disease]
        Myotonia levior
        Recessive myotonia congenita [Becker disease]

G
5
3
-
G
7
1

Excludes 1: = NOT CODED HERE! (Do not code both)

Excludes❷: = Not Included Here

G71.13 Myotonic chondrodystrophy
　　　Chondrodystrophic myotonia
　　　Congenital myotonic chondrodystrophy
　　　Schwartz-Jampel disease

G71.14 Drug-induced myotonia
　　　Use additional code for adverse effect, if applicable, to identify
　　　　drug (T36-T50 with fifth or sixth character 5)

G71.19 Other specified myotonic disorders
　　　Myotonia fluctuans
　　　Myotonia permanens
　　　Neuromyotonia [Isaacs]
　　　Paramyotonia congenita (of von Eulenburg)
　　　Pseudomyotonia
　　　Symptomatic myotonia

G71.2 Congenital myopathies
　　　Central core disease
　　　Fiber-type disproportion
　　　Minicore disease
　　　Multicore disease
　　　Myotubular (centronuclear) myopathy
　　　Nemaline myopathy
　　　Excludes 1: arthrogryposis multiplex congenita (Q74.3)

G71.3 Mitochondrial myopathy, not elsewhere classified
　　　Excludes 1: Kearns-Sayre syndrome (H49.81)
　　　　　Leber's disease (H47.21)
　　　　　Leigh's encephalopathy (G31.82)
　　　　　mitochondrial metabolism disorders (E88.4.-)
　　　　　Reye's syndrome (G93.7)

G71.8 Other primary disorders of muscles

G71.9 Primary disorder of muscle, unspecified
　　　Hereditary myopathy NOS

G72- Other and unspecified myopathies
　　　Excludes 1: arthrogryposis multiplex congenita (Q74.3)
　　　　　dermatopolymyositis (M33.-)
　　　　　ischemic infarction of muscle (M62.2-)
　　　　　myositis (M60.-)
　　　　　polymyositis (M33.2.-)

G72.0 Drug-induced myopathy
　　　Use additional code for adverse effect, if applicable, to identify drug
　　　　(T36-T50 with fifth or sixth character 5)

G72.1 Alcoholic myopathy
　　　Use additional code to identify alcoholism (F10.-)

G72.2 Myopathy due to other toxic agents
　　　Code first (T51-T65) to identify toxic agent

G72.3 Periodic paralysis
　　　Familial periodic paralysis
　　　Hyperkalemic periodic paralysis (familial)
　　　Hypokalemic periodic paralysis (familial)
　　　Myotonic periodic paralysis (familial)
　　　Normokalemic paralysis (familial)
　　　Potassium sensitive periodic paralysis
　　　Excludes 1: paramyotonia congenita (of von Eulenburg) (G71.19)

G72.4- Inflammatory and immune myopathies, not elsewhere classified

G72.41 Inclusion body myositis [IBM]

G72.49 Other inflammatory and immune myopathies, not elsewhere classified
　　　Inflammatory myopathy NOS

G72.8- Other specified myopathies

G72.81 Critical illness myopathy
　　　Acute necrotizing myopathy
　　　Acute quadriplegic myopathy
　　　Intensive care (ICU) myopathy
　　　Myopathy of critical illness

G72.89 Other specified myopathies

G72.9 Myopathy, unspecified

G73- Disorders of myoneural junction and muscle in diseases classified elsewhere

G73.1 Lambert-Eaton syndrome in neoplastic disease
　　　Code first underlying neoplasm (C00-D49)
　　　Excludes 1: Lambert-Eaton syndrome not associated with neoplasm
　　　　　(G70.80-G70.81)

G73.3 Myasthenic syndromes in other diseases classified elsewhere
　　　Code first underlying neoplasm (C00-D49)

G73.7 Myopathy in diseases classified elsewhere
　　　Code first underlying disease, such as:
　　　　Glycogen storage disease (E74.0)
　　　　Hyperparathyroidism (E21.0, E21.3)
　　　　Hypoparathyroidism (E20.-)
　　　　Lipid storage disorders (E75.-)
　　　Excludes 1: myopathy in:
　　　　　rheumatoid arthritis (M05.32)
　　　　　sarcoidosis (D86.87)
　　　　　scleroderma (M34.82)
　　　　　sicca syndrome [Sjögren] (M35.03)
　　　　　systemic lupus erythematosus (M32.19)

G71-G83 (margin tab)

Cerebral palsy and other paralytic syndromes (G80-G83)

G80- Cerebral palsy
Excludes 1: hereditary spastic paraplegia (G11.4)

G80.0 Spastic quadriplegic cerebral palsy
Congenital spastic paralysis (cerebral)

G80.1 Spastic diplegic cerebral palsy
Spastic cerebral palsy NOS

G80.2 Spastic hemiplegic cerebral palsy

G80.3 Athetoid cerebral palsy
Double athetosis (syndrome)
Dyskinetic cerebral palsy
Dystonic cerebral palsy
Vogt disease

G80.4 Ataxic cerebral palsy

G80.8 Other cerebral palsy
Mixed cerebral palsy syndromes

G80.9 Cerebral palsy, unspecified
Cerebral palsy NOS

G81- Hemiplegia and hemiparesis
Note: This category is to be used only when hemiplegia (complete) (incomplete) is reported without further specification, or is stated to be old or longstanding but of unspecified cause. The category is also for use in multiple coding to identify these types of hemiplegia resulting from any cause.
Excludes 1: congenital cerebral palsy (G80.-)
hemiplegia and hemiparesis due to sequela of cerebrovascular disease (I69.05-, I69.15-, I69.25-, I69.35-, I69.85-, I69.95-)

G81.0- Flaccid hemiplegia
G81.00 Flaccid hemiplegia affecting unspecified side
G81.01 Flaccid hemiplegia affecting <u>right dominant</u> side
G81.02 Flaccid hemiplegia affecting <u>left dominant</u> side
G81.03 Flaccid hemiplegia affecting <u>right nondominant</u> side
G81.04 Flaccid hemiplegia affecting <u>left nondominant</u> side

G81.1- Spastic hemiplegia
G81.10 Spastic hemiplegia affecting unspecified side
G81.11 Spastic hemiplegia affecting <u>right dominant</u> side
G81.12 Spastic hemiplegia affecting <u>left dominant</u> side
G81.13 Spastic hemiplegia affecting <u>right nondominant</u> side
G81.14 Spastic hemiplegia affecting <u>left nondominant</u> side

G81.9- Hemiplegia, unspecified
G81.90 Hemiplegia, unspecified affecting unspecified side
G81.91 Hemiplegia, unspecified affecting <u>right dominant</u> side
G81.92 Hemiplegia, unspecified affecting <u>left dominant</u> side
G81.93 Hemiplegia, unspecified affecting <u>right nondominant</u> side
G81.94 Hemiplegia, unspecified affecting <u>left nondominant</u> side

G82- Paraplegia (paraparesis) and quadriplegia (quadriparesis)
Note: This category is to be used only when the listed conditions are reported without further specification, or are stated to be old or longstanding but of unspecified cause. The category is also for use in multiple coding to identify these conditions resulting from any cause.
Excludes 1: congenital cerebral palsy (G80.-)
functional quadriplegia (R53.2)
hysterical paralysis (F44.4)

G82.2- Paraplegia
Paralysis of both lower limbs NOS
Paraparesis (lower) NOS
Paraplegia (lower) NOS

G82.20 Paraplegia, unspecified
G82.21 Paraplegia, complete
G82.22 Paraplegia, incomplete

G82.5- Quadriplegia
G82.50 Quadriplegia, unspecified
G82.51 Quadriplegia, C1-C4 complete
G82.52 Quadriplegia, C1-C4 incomplete
G82.53 Quadriplegia, C5-C7 complete
G82.54 Quadriplegia, C5-C7 incomplete

G83- Other paralytic syndromes
Note: This category is to be used only when the listed conditions are reported without further specification, or are stated to be old or longstanding but of unspecified cause. The category is also for use in multiple coding to identify these conditions resulting from any cause.
Includes: Paralysis (complete) (incomplete), except as in G80-G82

G83.0 Diplegia of upper limbs
Diplegia (upper)
Paralysis of both upper limbs

G83.1- Monoplegia of <u>lower</u> limb
Paralysis of lower limb
Excludes 1: monoplegia of lower limbs due to sequela of cerebrovascular disease (I69.04-, I69.14-, I69.24-, I69.34-, I69.84-, I69.94-)

G83.10 Monoplegia of lower limb affecting unspecified side
G83.11 Monoplegia of lower limb affecting <u>right dominant</u> side
G83.12 Monoplegia of lower limb affecting <u>left dominant</u> side
G83.13 Monoplegia of lower limb affecting <u>right nondominant</u> side
G83.14 Monoplegia of lower limb affecting <u>left nondominant</u> side

G83.2- Monoplegia of <u>upper</u> limb
Paralysis of upper limb
Excludes 1: monoplegia of upper limbs due to sequela of cerebrovascular disease (I69.03-, I69.13-, I69.23-, I69.33-, I69.83-, I69.93-)

G83.20 Monoplegia of upper limb affecting unspecified side
G83.21 Monoplegia of upper limb affecting <u>right dominant</u> side
G83.22 Monoplegia of upper limb affecting <u>left dominant</u> side
G83.23 Monoplegia of upper limb affecting <u>right nondominant</u> side
G83.24 Monoplegia of upper limb affecting <u>left nondominant</u> side

G83.3- Monoplegia, <u>unspecified</u>
G83.30 Monoplegia, unspecified affecting unspecified side
G83.31 Monoplegia, unspecified affecting <u>right dominant</u> side
G83.32 Monoplegia, unspecified affecting <u>left dominant</u> side
G83.33 Monoplegia, unspecified affecting <u>right nondominant</u> side
G83.34 Monoplegia, unspecified affecting <u>left nondominant</u> side

G83.4 Cauda equina syndrome
Neurogenic bladder due to cauda equina syndrome
Excludes 1: cord bladder NOS (G95.89)
neurogenic bladder NOS (N31.9)

G83.5 Locked-in state

G83.8- Other specified paralytic syndromes
Excludes 1: paralytic syndromes due to current spinal cord injury- code to spinal cord injury (S14, S24, S34)

G83.81 Brown-Séquard syndrome
G83.82 Anterior cord syndrome
G83.83 Posterior cord syndrome
G83.84 Todd's paralysis (postepileptic)
G83.89 Other specified paralytic syndromes

G83.9 Paralytic syndrome, unspecified

G
7
1
-
G
8
3

Excludes 1: = NOT CODED HERE! (Do not code both)

Excludes ❷: = Not Included Here

Other disorders of the nervous system (G89-G99)

G89- Pain, not elsewhere classified
Code also related psychological factors associated with pain (F45.42)
Excludes 1: *generalized pain NOS (R52)*
pain disorders exclusively related to psychological factors (F45.41)
pain NOS (R52)
Excludes ❷ *atypical face pain (G50.1)*
headache syndromes (G44.-)
localized pain, unspecified type — code to pain by site, such as:
abdomen pain (R10.-)
back pain (M54.9)
breast pain (N64.4)
chest pain (R07.1-R07.9)
ear pain (H92.0-)
eye pain (H57.1)
headache (R51)
joint pain (M25.5-)
limb pain (M79.6-)
lumbar region pain (M54.5)
painful urination (R30.9)
pelvic and perineal pain (R10.2)
shoulder pain (M25.51-)
spine pain (M54.-)
throat pain (R07.0)
tongue pain (K14.6)
tooth pain (K08.8)
migraines (G43.-)
myalgia (M79.1)
pain from prosthetic devices, implants, and grafts (T82.84, T83.84, T84.84, T85.84)
phantom limb syndrome with pain (G54.6)
renal colic (N23)
vulvar vestibulitis (N94.810)
vulvodynia (N94.81-)

G89.0 Central pain syndrome
Déjérine-Roussy syndrome
Myelopathic pain syndrome
Thalamic pain syndrome (hyperesthetic)

G89.1- Acute pain, not elsewhere classified

G89.11 Acute pain due to trauma

G89.12 Acute post-thoracotomy pain
Post-thoracotomy pain NOS

G89.18 Other acute postprocedural pain
Postoperative pain NOS
Postprocedural pain NOS

G89.2- Chronic pain, not elsewhere classified
Excludes 1: *causalgia, lower limb (G57.7-)*
causalgia, upper limb (G56.4-)
central pain syndrome (G89.0)
chronic pain syndrome (G89.4)
complex regional pain syndrome II, lower limb (G57.7-)
complex regional pain syndrome II, upper limb (G56.4-)
neoplasm related chronic pain (G89.3)
reflex sympathetic dystrophy (G90.5-)

G89.21 Chronic pain due to trauma

G89.22 Chronic post-thoracotomy pain

G89.28 Other chronic postprocedural pain
Other chronic postoperative pain

G89.29 Other chronic pain

G89.3 Neoplasm related pain (acute) (chronic)
Cancer associated pain
Pain due to malignancy (primary) (secondary)
Tumor associated pain

G89.4 Chronic pain syndrome
Chronic pain associated with significant psychosocial dysfunction

G90- Disorders of autonomic nervous system
Excludes 1: *dysfunction of the autonomic nervous system due to alcohol (G31.2)*

G90.0- Idiopathic peripheral autonomic neuropathy

G90.01 Carotid sinus syncope
Carotid sinus syndrome

G90.09 Other idiopathic peripheral autonomic neuropathy
Idiopathic peripheral autonomic neuropathy NOS

G90.1 Familial dysautonomia [Riley-Day]

G90.2 Horner's syndrome
Bernard(-Horner) syndrome
Cervical sympathetic dystrophy or paralysis

G90.3 Multi-system degeneration of the autonomic nervous system
Neurogenic orthostatic hypotension [Shy-Drager]
Excludes 1: *orthostatic hypotension NOS (I95.1)*

G90.4 Autonomic dysreflexia
Use additional code to identify the cause, such as:
Fecal impaction (K56.41)
Pressure ulcer (pressure area) (L89.-)
Urinary tract infection (N39.0)

G90.5- Complex regional pain syndrome I (CRPS I)
Reflex sympathetic dystrophy
Excludes 1: *causalgia of lower limb (G57.7-)*
causalgia of upper limb (G56.4-)
complex regional pain syndrome II of lower limb (G57.7-)
complex regional pain syndrome II of upper limb (G56.4-)

G90.50 Complex regional pain syndrome I, unspecified

G90.51- Complex regional pain syndrome I of upper limb

G90.511 Complex regional pain syndrome I of right upper limb

G90.512 Complex regional pain syndrome I of left upper limb

G90.513 Complex regional pain syndrome I of upper limb, bilateral

G90.519 Complex regional pain syndrome I of unspecified upper limb

G90.52- Complex regional pain syndrome I of lower limb

G90.521 Complex regional pain syndrome I of right lower limb

G90.522 Complex regional pain syndrome I of left lower limb

G90.523 Complex regional pain syndrome I of lower limb, bilateral

G90.529 Complex regional pain syndrome I of unspecified lower limb

G90.59 Complex regional pain syndrome I of other specified site

G90.8 Other disorders of autonomic nervous system

G90.9 Disorder of the autonomic nervous system, unspecified

G91- Hydrocephalus
Includes: Acquired hydrocephalus
Excludes 1: *Arnold-Chiari syndrome with hydrocephalus (Q07.-)*
congenital hydrocephalus (Q03.-)
spina bifida with hydrocephalus (Q05.-)

G91.0 Communicating hydrocephalus
Secondary normal pressure hydrocephalus

G91.1 Obstructive hydrocephalus

G91.2 (Idiopathic) normal pressure hydrocephalus
Normal pressure hydrocephalus NOS

G91.3 Post-traumatic hydrocephalus, unspecified

G91.4 Hydrocephalus in diseases classified elsewhere
Code first underlying condition, such as:
Congenital syphilis (A50.4-)
Neoplasm (C00-D49)
Excludes 1: *hydrocephalus due to congenital toxoplasmosis (P37.1)*

G91.8 Other hydrocephalus

G91.9 Hydrocephalus, unspecified

G92 Toxic encephalopathy
Toxic encephalitis
Toxic metabolic encephalopathy
Code first (T51-T65) to identify toxic agent

G
8
9
–
G
9
8

G93- Other disorders of brain

G93.0   Cerebral cysts
Arachnoid cyst
Porencephalic cyst, acquired
Excludes 1:   acquired periventricular cysts of newborn (P91.1)
congenital cerebral cysts (Q04.6)

G93.1   Anoxic brain damage, not elsewhere classified
Excludes 1:   cerebral anoxia due to anesthesia during labor and
delivery (O74.3)
cerebral anoxia due to anesthesia during the
puerperium (O89.2)
neonatal anoxia (P84)

G93.2   Benign intracranial hypertension
Excludes 1:   hypertensive encephalopathy (I67.4)

G93.3   Postviral fatigue syndrome
Benign myalgic encephalomyelitis
Excludes 1:   chronic fatigue syndrome NOS (R53.82)

G93.4-   Other and unspecified encephalopathy
Excludes 1:   alcoholic encephalopathy (G31.2)
encephalopathy in diseases classified elsewhere (G94)
hypertensive encephalopathy (I67.4)
toxic (metabolic) encephalopathy (G92)

  G93.40   Encephalopathy, unspecified

  G93.41   Metabolic encephalopathy
Septic encephalopathy

  G93.49   Other encephalopathy
Encephalopathy NEC

G93.5   Compression of brain
Arnold-Chiari type 1 compression of brain
Compression of brain (stem)
Herniation of brain (stem)
Excludes 1:   diffuse traumatic compression of brain (S06.2-)
focal traumatic compression of brain (S06.3-)

G93.6   Cerebral edema
Excludes 1:   cerebral edema due to birth injury (P11.0)
traumatic cerebral edema (S06.1-)

G93.7   Reye's syndrome
Code first (T39.0-), if salicylates-induced

G93.8-   Other specified disorders of brain

  G93.81   Temporal sclerosis
Hippocampal sclerosis
Mesial temporal sclerosis

  G93.82   Brain death

  G93.89   Other specified disorders of brain
Postradiation encephalopathy

G93.9   Disorder of brain, unspecified

G94   Other disorders of brain in diseases classified elsewhere
Code first underlying disease
Excludes 1:   encephalopathy in congenital syphilis (A50.49)
encephalopathy in influenza (J09.X9, J10.81, J11.81)
encephalopathy in syphilis (A52.19)
hydrocephalus in diseases classified elsewhere (G91.4)

G95- Other and unspecified diseases of spinal cord
Excludes❷: myelitis (G04.-)

G95.0   Syringomyelia and syringobulbia

G95.1-   Vascular myelopathies
Excludes❷: intraspinal phlebitis and thrombophlebitis, except non-
pyogenic (G08)

  G95.11   Acute infarction of spinal cord (embolic) (nonembolic)
Anoxia of spinal cord
Arterial thrombosis of spinal cord

  G95.19   Other vascular myelopathies
Edema of spinal cord
Hematomyelia
Nonpyogenic intraspinal phlebitis and thrombophlebitis
Subacute necrotic myelopathy

G95.2-   Other and unspecified cord compression

  G95.20   Unspecified cord compression

  G95.29   Other cord compression

G95.8-   Other specified diseases of spinal cord
Excludes 1:   neurogenic bladder NOS (N31.9)
neurogenic bladder due to cauda equina syndrome
(G83.4)
neuromuscular dysfunction of bladder without spinal
cord lesion (N31.-)

  G95.81   Conus medullaris syndrome

  G95.89   Other specified diseases of spinal cord
Cord bladder NOS
Drug-induced myelopathy
Radiation-induced myelopathy
Excludes 1:   myelopathy NOS (G95.9)

G95.9   Disease of spinal cord, unspecified
Myelopathy NOS

G96- Other disorders of central nervous system

G96.0   Cerebrospinal fluid leak
Excludes 1:   cerebrospinal fluid leak from spinal puncture (G97.0)

G96.1-   Disorders of meninges, not elsewhere classified

  G96.11   Dural tear
Excludes 1:   accidental puncture or laceration of dura during a
procedure (G97.41)

  G96.12   Meningeal adhesions (cerebral) (spinal)

  G96.19   Other disorders of meninges, not elsewhere classified

G96.8   Other specified disorders of central nervous system

G96.9   Disorder of central nervous system, unspecified

G97-   Intraoperative and postprocedural complications and disorders of nervous system, not elsewhere classified
Excludes❷: intraoperative and postprocedural cerebrovascular infarction
(I97.81-, I97.82-)

G97.0   Cerebrospinal fluid leak from spinal puncture

G97.1   Other reaction to spinal and lumbar puncture
Headache due to lumbar puncture

G97.2   Intracranial hypotension following ventricular shunting

G97.3-   Intraoperative hemorrhage and hematoma of a nervous system organ or structure complicating a procedure
Excludes 1:   intraoperative hemorrhage and hematoma of a nervous
system organ or structure due to accidental
puncture and laceration during a procedure
(G97.4-)

  G97.31   Intraoperative hemorrhage and hematoma of a nervous system organ or structure complicating a nervous system procedure

  G97.32   Intraoperative hemorrhage and hematoma of a nervous system organ or structure complicating other procedure

G97.4-   Accidental puncture and laceration of a nervous system organ or structure during a procedure

  G97.41   Accidental puncture or laceration of dura during a procedure
Incidental (inadvertent) durotomy

  G97.48   Accidental puncture and laceration of other nervous system organ or structure during a nervous system procedure

  G97.49   Accidental puncture and laceration of other nervous system organ or structure during other procedure

G97.5-   Postprocedural hemorrhage and hematoma of a nervous system organ or structure following a procedure

  G97.51   Postprocedural hemorrhage and hematoma of a nervous system organ or structure following a nervous system procedure

  G97.52   Postprocedural hemorrhage and hematoma of a nervous system organ or structure following other procedure

G97.8-   Other intraoperative and postprocedural complications and disorders of nervous system
Use additional code to further specify disorder

  G97.81   Other intraoperative complications of nervous system

  G97.82   Other postprocedural complications and disorders of nervous system

G98- Other disorders of nervous system not elsewhere classified
Includes: Nervous system disorder NOS

G98.0   Neurogenic arthritis, not elsewhere classified
Nonsyphilitic neurogenic arthropathy NEC
Nonsyphilitic neurogenic spondylopathy NEC
Excludes 1:   spondylopathy (in):
syringomyelia and syringobulbia (G95.0)
tabes dorsalis (A52.11)

G98.8   Other disorders of nervous system
Nervous system disorder NOS

G89 – G98

Excludes 1: = NOT CODED HERE! (Do not code both)   *Excludes❷: = Not Included Here*

G99- Other disorders of nervous system <u>in diseases classified elsewhere</u>

G99.0   Autonomic neuropathy in diseases classified elsewhere
Code first underlying disease, such as:
Amyloidosis (E85.-)
Gout (M1A.-, M10.-)
Hyperthyroidism (E05.-)
Excludes 1: *diabetic autonomic neuropathy (E08-E14 with .43)*

G99.2   Myelopathy in diseases classified elsewhere
Code first underlying disease, such as:
Neoplasm (C00-D49)
Excludes 1: *myelopathy in:*
intervertebral disease (M50.0-, M51.0-)
spondylosis (M47.0-, M47.1-)

G99.8   Other specified disorders of nervous system in diseases classified elsewhere
Code first underlying disorder, such as:
Amyloidosis (E85.-)
Avitaminosis (E56.9)
Excludes 1: *nervous system involvement in:*
cysticercosis (B69.0)
rubella (B06.0-)
syphilis (A52.1-)

G
9
9
-
H
0
1

Chapter 7 – Diseases of the eye and adnexa (H00-H59)

Note: Use an external cause code following the code for the eye condition, if applicable, to identify the cause of the eye condition

Excludes❷: certain conditions originating in the perinatal period
(P04-P96)
certain infectious and parasitic diseases (A00-B99)
complications of pregnancy, childbirth and the puerperium
(O00-O9A)
congenital malformations, deformations, and chromosomal
abnormalities (Q00-Q99)
diabetes mellitus related eye conditions (E09.3-, E10.3-,
E11.3-, E13.3-)
endocrine, nutritional and metabolic diseases (E00-E88)
injury (trauma) of eye and orbit (S05.-)
injury, poisoning and certain other consequences of external
causes (S00-T88)
neoplasms (C00-D49)
symptoms, signs and abnormal clinical and laboratory
findings, not elsewhere classified (R00-R94)
syphilis related eye disorders (A50.01, A50.3-, A51.43,
A52.71)

This chapter contains the following blocks:

H00-H05	Disorders of eyelid, lacrimal system and orbit
H10-H11	Disorders of conjunctiva
H15-H22	Disorders of sclera, cornea, iris and ciliary body
H25-H28	Disorders of lens
H30-H36	Disorders of choroid and retina
H40-H42	Glaucoma
H43-H44	Disorders of vitreous body and globe
H46-H47	Disorders of optic nerve and visual pathways
H49-H52	Disorders of ocular muscles, binocular movement, accommodation and refraction
H53-H54	Visual disturbances and blindness
H55-H57	Other disorders of eye and adnexa
H59	Intraoperative and postprocedural complications and disorders of eye and adnexa, not elsewhere classified

Disorders of eyelid, lacrimal system and orbit (H00-H05)

Excludes❷: open wound of eyelid (S01.1-)
superficial injury of eyelid (S00.1-, S00.2-)

H00-   **Hordeolum and chalazion**

    H00.0-   <u>Hordeolum</u> (externum) (internum) of eyelid

       H00.01- Hordeolum <u>externum</u>
          Hordeolum NOS
          Stye
          H00.011   Hordeolum externum <u>right</u> <u>upper</u> eyelid
          H00.012   Hordeolum externum <u>right</u> <u>lower</u> eyelid
          H00.013   Hordeolum externum <u>right</u> eye, <u>unspecified</u> eyelid
          H00.014   Hordeolum externum <u>left</u> <u>upper</u> eyelid
          H00.015   Hordeolum externum <u>left</u> <u>lower</u> eyelid
          H00.016   Hordeolum externum <u>left</u> eye, <u>unspecified</u> eyelid
          H00.019   Hordeolum externum <u>unspecified</u> eye, <u>unspecified</u> eyelid

       H00.02- Hordeolum <u>internum</u>
          Infection of meibomian gland
          H00.021   Hordeolum internum <u>right</u> <u>upper</u> eyelid
          H00.022   Hordeolum internum <u>right</u> <u>lower</u> eyelid
          H00.023   Hordeolum internum <u>right</u> eye, <u>unspecified</u> eyelid
          H00.024   Hordeolum internum <u>left</u> <u>upper</u> eyelid
          H00.025   Hordeolum internum <u>left</u> <u>lower</u> eyelid
          H00.026   Hordeolum internum <u>left</u> eye, <u>unspecified</u> eyelid
          H00.029   Hordeolum internum <u>unspecified</u> eye, <u>unspecified</u> eyelid

       H00.03- <u>Abscess</u> of eyelid
          Furuncle of eyelid
          H00.031   Abscess of <u>right</u> <u>upper</u> eyelid
          H00.032   Abscess of <u>right</u> <u>lower</u> eyelid
          H00.033   Abscess of eyelid <u>right</u> eye, <u>unspecified</u> eyelid
          H00.034   Abscess of <u>left</u> <u>upper</u> eyelid
          H00.035   Abscess of <u>left</u> <u>lower</u> eyelid
          H00.036   Abscess of eyelid <u>left</u> eye, <u>unspecified</u> eyelid
          H00.039   Abscess of eyelid <u>unspecified</u> eye, <u>unspecified</u> eyelid

    H00.1-   <u>Chalazion</u>
       Meibomian (gland) cyst
       Excludes❷: infected meibomian gland (H00.02-)
       H00.11   Chalazion <u>right</u> <u>upper</u> eyelid
       H00.12   Chalazion <u>right</u> <u>lower</u> eyelid
       H00.13   Chalazion <u>right</u> eye, <u>unspecified</u> eyelid

       H00.14   Chalazion <u>left</u> <u>upper</u> eyelid
       H00.15   Chalazion <u>left</u> <u>lower</u> eyelid
       H00.16   Chalazion <u>left</u> eye, <u>unspecified</u> eyelid
       H00.19   Chalazion <u>unspecified</u> eye, <u>unspecified</u> eyelid

H01-   **Other inflammation of eyelid**

    H01.0-   <u>Blepharitis</u>
       Excludes 1: blepharoconjunctivitis (H10.5-)
       H01.00- <u>Unspecified</u> blepharitis
          H01.001   Unspecified blepharitis <u>right</u> <u>upper</u> eyelid
          H01.002   Unspecified blepharitis <u>right</u> <u>lower</u> eyelid
          H01.003   Unspecified blepharitis <u>right</u> eye, <u>unspecified</u> eyelid
          H01.004   Unspecified blepharitis <u>left</u> <u>upper</u> eyelid
          H01.005   Unspecified blepharitis <u>left</u> <u>lower</u> eyelid
          H01.006   Unspecified blepharitis <u>left</u> eye, <u>unspecified</u> eyelid
          H01.009   Unspecified blepharitis <u>unspecified</u> eye, <u>unspecified</u> eyelid

       H01.01- <u>Ulcerative</u> blepharitis
          H01.011   Ulcerative blepharitis <u>right</u> <u>upper</u> eyelid
          H01.012   Ulcerative blepharitis <u>right</u> <u>lower</u> eyelid
          H01.013   Ulcerative blepharitis <u>right</u> eye, <u>unspecified</u> eyelid
          H01.014   Ulcerative blepharitis <u>left</u> <u>upper</u> eyelid
          H01.015   Ulcerative blepharitis <u>left</u> <u>lower</u> eyelid
          H01.016   Ulcerative blepharitis <u>left</u> eye, <u>unspecified</u> eyelid
          H01.019   Ulcerative blepharitis <u>unspecified</u> eye, <u>unspecified</u> eyelid

       H01.02- <u>Squamous</u> blepharitis
          H01.021   Squamous blepharitis <u>right</u> <u>upper</u> eyelid
          H01.022   Squamous blepharitis <u>right</u> <u>lower</u> eyelid
          H01.023   Squamous blepharitis <u>right</u> eye, <u>unspecified</u> eyelid
          H01.024   Squamous blepharitis <u>left</u> <u>upper</u> eyelid
          H01.025   Squamous blepharitis <u>left</u> <u>lower</u> eyelid
          H01.026   Squamous blepharitis <u>left</u> eye, <u>unspecified</u> eyelid
          H01.029   Squamous blepharitis <u>unspecified</u> eye, <u>unspecified</u> eyelid

    H01.1-   <u>Noninfectious dermatoses</u> of eyelid
       H01.11- <u>Allergic dermatitis</u> of eyelid
          Contact dermatitis of eyelid
          H01.111   Allergic dermatitis of <u>right</u> <u>upper</u> eyelid
          H01.112   Allergic dermatitis of <u>right</u> <u>lower</u> eyelid
          H01.113   Allergic dermatitis of <u>right</u> eye, <u>unspecified</u> eyelid
          H01.114   Allergic dermatitis of <u>left</u> <u>upper</u> eyelid
          H01.115   Allergic dermatitis of <u>left</u> <u>lower</u> eyelid
          H01.116   Allergic dermatitis of <u>left</u> eye, <u>unspecified</u> eyelid
          H01.119   Allergic dermatitis of <u>unspecified</u> eye, <u>unspecified</u> eyelid

       H01.12- <u>Discoid lupus erythematosus</u> of eyelid
          H01.121   Discoid lupus erythematosus of <u>right</u> <u>upper</u> eyelid
          H01.122   Discoid lupus erythematosus of <u>right</u> <u>lower</u> eyelid
          H01.123   Discoid lupus erythematosus of <u>right</u> eye, <u>unspecified</u> eyelid
          H01.124   Discoid lupus erythematosus of <u>left</u> <u>upper</u> eyelid
          H01.125   Discoid lupus erythematosus of <u>left</u> <u>lower</u> eyelid
          H01.126   Discoid lupus erythematosus of <u>left</u> eye, <u>unspecified</u> eyelid
          H01.129   Discoid lupus erythematosus of <u>unspecified</u> eye, <u>unspecified</u> eyelid

       H01.13- <u>Eczematous dermatitis</u> of eyelid
          H01.131   Eczematous dermatitis of <u>right</u> <u>upper</u> eyelid
          H01.132   Eczematous dermatitis of <u>right</u> <u>lower</u> eyelid
          H01.133   Eczematous dermatitis of <u>right</u> eye, <u>unspecified</u> eyelid
          H01.134   Eczematous dermatitis of <u>left</u> <u>upper</u> eyelid
          H01.135   Eczematous dermatitis of <u>left</u> <u>lower</u> eyelid
          H01.136   Eczematous dermatitis of <u>left</u> eye, <u>unspecified</u> eyelid
          H01.139   Eczematous dermatitis of <u>unspecified</u> eye, <u>unspecified</u> eyelid

       H01.14- <u>Xeroderma</u> of eyelid
          H01.141   Xeroderma of <u>right</u> <u>upper</u> eyelid
          H01.142   Xeroderma of <u>right</u> <u>lower</u> eyelid
          H01.143   Xeroderma of <u>right</u> eye, <u>unspecified</u> eyelid
          H01.144   Xeroderma of <u>left</u> <u>upper</u> eyelid
          H01.145   Xeroderma of <u>left</u> <u>lower</u> eyelid
          H01.146   Xeroderma of <u>left</u> eye, <u>unspecified</u> eyelid
          H01.149   Xeroderma of <u>unspecified</u> eye, <u>unspecified</u> eyelid

    H01.8   **Other specified inflammations of eyelid**
    H01.9   **Unspecified inflammation of eyelid**
       Inflammation of eyelid NOS

Excludes 1: = NOT CODED HERE! (Do not code both)   **433**   *Excludes❷: = Not Included Here*

G 9 9 - H 0 1

H02- Other disorders of eyelid

    Excludes 1: congenital malformations of eyelid (Q10.0-Q10.3)

  H02.0- Entropion and trichiasis of eyelid

    H02.00- Unspecified entropion of eyelid

      H02.001   Unspecified entropion of right upper eyelid
      H02.002   Unspecified entropion of right lower eyelid
      H02.003   Unspecified entropion of right eye, unspecified eyelid
      H02.004   Unspecified entropion of left upper eyelid
      H02.005   Unspecified entropion of left lower eyelid
      H02.006   Unspecified entropion of left eye, unspecified eyelid
      H02.009   Unspecified entropion of unspecified eye, unspecified eyelid

    H02.01- Cicatricial entropion of eyelid

      H02.011   Cicatricial entropion of right upper eyelid
      H02.012   Cicatricial entropion of right lower eyelid
      H02.013   Cicatricial entropion of right eye, unspecified eyelid
      H02.014   Cicatricial entropion of left upper eyelid
      H02.015   Cicatricial entropion of left lower eyelid
      H02.016   Cicatricial entropion of left eye, unspecified eyelid
      H02.019   Cicatricial entropion of unspecified eye, unspecified eyelid

    H02.02- Mechanical entropion of eyelid

      H02.021   Mechanical entropion of right upper eyelid
      H02.022   Mechanical entropion of right lower eyelid
      H02.023   Mechanical entropion of right eye, unspecified eyelid
      H02.024   Mechanical entropion of left upper eyelid
      H02.025   Mechanical entropion of left lower eyelid
      H02.026   Mechanical entropion of left eye, unspecified eyelid
      H02.029   Mechanical entropion of unspecified eye, unspecified eyelid

    H02.03- Senile entropion of eyelid

      H02.031   Senile entropion of right upper eyelid
      H02.032   Senile entropion of right lower eyelid
      H02.033   Senile entropion of right eye, unspecified eyelid
      H02.034   Senile entropion of left upper eyelid
      H02.035   Senile entropion of left lower eyelid
      H02.036   Senile entropion of left eye, unspecified eyelid
      H02.039   Senile entropion of unspecified eye, unspecified eyelid

    H02.04- Spastic entropion of eyelid

      H02.041   Spastic entropion of right upper eyelid
      H02.042   Spastic entropion of right lower eyelid
      H02.043   Spastic entropion of right eye, unspecified eyelid
      H02.044   Spastic entropion of left upper eyelid
      H02.045   Spastic entropion of left lower eyelid
      H02.046   Spastic entropion of left eye, unspecified eyelid
      H02.049   Spastic entropion of unspecified eye, unspecified eyelid

    H02.05- Trichiasis without entropian

      H02.051   Trichiasis without entropian right upper eyelid
      H02.052   Trichiasis without entropian right lower eyelid
      H02.053   Trichiasis without entropian right eye, unspecified eyelid
      H02.054   Trichiasis without entropian left upper eyelid
      H02.055   Trichiasis without entropian left lower eyelid
      H02.056   Trichiasis without entropian left eye, unspecified eyelid
      H02.059   Trichiasis without entropian unspecified eye, unspecified eyelid

  H02.1- Ectropion of eyelid

    H02.10- Unspecified ectropion of eyelid

      H02.101   Unspecified ectropion of right upper eyelid
      H02.102   Unspecified ectropion of right lower eyelid
      H02.103   Unspecified ectropion of right eye, unspecified eyelid
      H02.104   Unspecified ectropion of left upper eyelid
      H02.105   Unspecified ectropion of left lower eyelid
      H02.106   Unspecified ectropion of left eye, unspecified eyelid
      H02.109   Unspecified ectropion of unspecified eye, unspecified eyelid

    H02.11- Cicatricial ectropion of eyelid

      H02.111   Cicatricial ectropion of right upper eyelid
      H02.112   Cicatricial ectropion of right lower eyelid
      H02.113   Cicatricial ectropion of right eye, unspecified eyelid
      H02.114   Cicatricial ectropion of left upper eyelid
      H02.115   Cicatricial ectropion of left lower eyelid
      H02.116   Cicatricial ectropion of left eye, unspecified eyelid
      H02.119   Cicatricial ectropion of unspecified eye, unspecified eyelid

    H02.12- Mechanical ectropion of eyelid

      H02.121   Mechanical ectropion of right upper eyelid
      H02.122   Mechanical ectropion of right lower eyelid
      H02.123   Mechanical ectropion of right eye, unspecified eyelid
      H02.124   Mechanical ectropion of left upper eyelid
      H02.125   Mechanical ectropion of left lower eyelid
      H02.126   Mechanical ectropion of left eye, unspecified eyelid
      H02.129   Mechanical ectropion of unspecified eye, unspecified eyelid

    H02.13- Senile ectropion of eyelid

      H02.131   Senile ectropion of right upper eyelid
      H02.132   Senile ectropion of right lower eyelid
      H02.133   Senile ectropion of right eye, unspecified eyelid
      H02.134   Senile ectropion of left upper eyelid
      H02.135   Senile ectropion of left lower eyelid
      H02.136   Senile ectropion of left eye, unspecified eyelid
      H02.139   Senile ectropion of unspecified eye, unspecified eyelid

    H02.14- Spastic ectropion of eyelid

      H02.141   Spastic ectropion of right upper eyelid
      H02.142   Spastic ectropion of right lower eyelid
      H02.143   Spastic ectropion of right eye, unspecified eyelid
      H02.144   Spastic ectropion of left upper eyelid
      H02.145   Spastic ectropion of left lower eyelid
      H02.146   Spastic ectropion of left eye, unspecified eyelid
      H02.149   Spastic ectropion of unspecified eye, unspecified eyelid

  H02.2- Lagophthalmos

    H02.20- Unspecified lagophthalmos

      H02.201   Unspecified lagophthalmos right upper eyelid
      H02.202   Unspecified lagophthalmos right lower eyelid
      H02.203   Unspecified lagophthalmos right eye, unspecified eyelid
      H02.204   Unspecified lagophthalmos left upper eyelid
      H02.205   Unspecified lagophthalmos left lower eyelid
      H02.206   Unspecified lagophthalmos left eye, unspecified eyelid
      H02.209   Unspecified lagophthalmos unspecified eye, unspecified eyelid

    H02.21- Cicatricial lagophthalmos

      H02.211   Cicatricial lagophthalmos right upper eyelid
      H02.212   Cicatricial lagophthalmos right lower eyelid
      H02.213   Cicatricial lagophthalmos right eye, unspecified eyelid
      H02.214   Cicatricial lagophthalmos left upper eyelid
      H02.215   Cicatricial lagophthalmos left lower eyelid
      H02.216   Cicatricial lagophthalmos left eye, unspecified eyelid
      H02.219   Cicatricial lagophthalmos unspecified eye, unspecified eyelid

    H02.22- Mechanical lagophthalmos

      H02.221   Mechanical lagophthalmos right upper eyelid
      H02.222   Mechanical lagophthalmos right lower eyelid
      H02.223   Mechanical lagophthalmos right eye, unspecified eyelid
      H02.224   Mechanical lagophthalmos left upper eyelid
      H02.225   Mechanical lagophthalmos left lower eyelid
      H02.226   Mechanical lagophthalmos left eye, unspecified eyelid
      H02.229   Mechanical lagophthalmos unspecified eye, unspecified eyelid

    H02.23- Paralytic lagophthalmos

      H02.231   Paralytic lagophthalmos right upper eyelid
      H02.232   Paralytic lagophthalmos right lower eyelid
      H02.233   Paralytic lagophthalmos right eye, unspecified eyelid
      H02.234   Paralytic lagophthalmos left upper eyelid
      H02.235   Paralytic lagophthalmos left lower eyelid
      H02.236   Paralytic lagophthalmos left eye, unspecified eyelid
      H02.239   Paralytic lagophthalmos unspecified eye, unspecified eyelid

  H02.3- Blepharochalasis

    Pseudoptosis

    H02.30   Blepharochalasis unspecified eye, unspecified eyelid
    H02.31   Blepharochalasis right upper eyelid
    H02.32   Blepharochalasis right lower eyelid
    H02.33   Blepharochalasis right eye, unspecified eyelid
    H02.34   Blepharochalasis left upper eyelid
    H02.35   Blepharochalasis left lower eyelid
    H02.36   Blepharochalasis left eye, unspecified eyelid

H02 - H02

H02.4-   Ptosis of eyelid
   H02.40- Unspecified ptosis of eyelid
      H02.401   Unspecified ptosis of right eyelid
      H02.402   Unspecified ptosis of left eyelid
      H02.403   Unspecified ptosis of bilateral eyelids
      H02.409   Unspecified ptosis of unspecified eyelid
   H02.41- Mechanical ptosis of eyelid
      H02.411   Mechanical ptosis of right eyelid
      H02.412   Mechanical ptosis of left eyelid
      H02.413   Mechanical ptosis of bilateral eyelids
      H02.419   Mechanical ptosis of unspecified eyelid
   H02.42- Myogenic ptosis of eyelid
      H02.421   Myogenic ptosis of right eyelid
      H02.422   Myogenic ptosis of left eyelid
      H02.423   Myogenic ptosis of bilateral eyelids
      H02.429   Myogenic ptosis of unspecified eyelid
   H02.43- Paralytic ptosis of eyelid
          Neurogenic ptosis of eyelid
      H02.431   Paralytic ptosis of right eyelid
      H02.432   Paralytic ptosis of left eyelid
      H02.433   Paralytic ptosis of bilateral eyelids
      H02.439   Paralytic ptosis unspecified eyelid
H02.5-   Other disorders affecting eyelid function
     Excludes❷: blepharospasm (G24.5)
            organic tic (G25.69)
            psychogenic tic (F95.-)
   H02.51- Abnormal innervation syndrome
      H02.511   Abnormal innervation syndrome right upper eyelid
      H02.512   Abnormal innervation syndrome right lower eyelid
      H02.513   Abnormal innervation syndrome right eye, unspecified eyelid
      H02.514   Abnormal innervation syndrome left upper eyelid
      H02.515   Abnormal innervation syndrome left lower eyelid
      H02.516   Abnormal innervation syndrome left eye, unspecified eyelid
      H02.519   Abnormal innervation syndrome unspecified eye, unspecified eyelid
   H02.52- Blepharophimosis
          Ankyloblepharon
      H02.521   Blepharophimosis right upper eyelid
      H02.522   Blepharophimosis right lower eyelid
      H02.523   Blepharophimosis right eye, unspecified eyelid
      H02.524   Blepharophimosis left upper eyelid
      H02.525   Blepharophimosis left lower eyelid
      H02.526   Blepharophimosis left eye, unspecified eyelid
      H02.529   Blepharophimosis unspecified eye, unspecified lid
   H02.53- Eyelid retraction
          Eyelid lag
      H02.531   Eyelid retraction right upper eyelid
      H02.532   Eyelid retraction right lower eyelid
      H02.533   Eyelid retraction right eye, unspecified eyelid
      H02.534   Eyelid retraction left upper eyelid
      H02.535   Eyelid retraction left lower eyelid
      H02.536   Eyelid retraction left eye, unspecified eyelid
      H02.539   Eyelid retraction unspecified eye, unspecified lid
   H02.59- Other disorders affecting eyelid function
          Deficient blink reflex
          Sensory disorders
H02.6-   Xanthelasma of eyelid
   H02.60   Xanthelasma of unspecified eye, unspecified eyelid
   H02.61   Xanthelasma of right upper eyelid
   H02.62   Xanthelasma of right lower eyelid
   H02.63   Xanthelasma of right eye, unspecified eyelid
   H02.64   Xanthelasma of left upper eyelid
   H02.65   Xanthelasma of left lower eyelid
   H02.66   Xanthelasma of left eye, unspecified eyelid
H02.7-   Other and unspecified degenerative disorders of eyelid and periocular area
   H02.70   Unspecified degenerative disorders of eyelid and periocular area
   H02.71- Chloasma of eyelid and periocular area
          Dyspigmentation of eyelid
          Hyperpigmentation of eyelid
      H02.711   Chloasma of right upper eyelid and periocular area
      H02.712   Chloasma of right lower eyelid and periocular area
      H02.713   Chloasma of right eye, unspecified eyelid and periocular area

      H02.714   Chloasma of left upper eyelid and periocular area
      H02.715   Chloasma of left lower eyelid and periocular area
      H02.716   Chloasma of left eye, unspecified eyelid and periocular area
      H02.719   Chloasma of unspecified eye, unspecified eyelid and periocular area
   H02.72- Madarosis of eyelid and periocular area
          Hypotrichosis of eyelid
      H02.721   Madarosis of right upper eyelid and periocular area
      H02.722   Madarosis of right lower eyelid and periocular area
      H02.723   Madarosis of right eye, unspecified eyelid and periocular area
      H02.724   Madarosis of left upper eyelid and periocular area
      H02.725   Madarosis of left lower eyelid and periocular area
      H02.726   Madarosis of left eye, unspecified eyelid and periocular area
      H02.729   Madarosis of unspecified eye, unspecified eyelid and periocular area
   H02.73- Vitiligo of eyelid and periocular area
          Hypopigmentation of eyelid
      H02.731   Vitiligo of right upper eyelid and periocular area
      H02.732   Vitiligo of right lower eyelid and periocular area
      H02.733   Vitiligo of right eye, unspecified eyelid and periocular area
      H02.734   Vitiligo of left upper eyelid and periocular area
      H02.735   Vitiligo of left lower eyelid and periocular area
      H02.736   Vitiligo of left eye, unspecified eyelid and periocular area
      H02.739   Vitiligo of unspecified eye, unspecified eyelid and periocular area
   H02.79   Other degenerative disorders of eyelid and periocular area
H02.8-   Other specified disorders of eyelid
   H02.81- Retained foreign body in eyelid
          Use additional code to identify the type of retained foreign body (Z18.-)
          Excludes 1: laceration of eyelid with foreign body (S01.12-)
              retained intraocular foreign body (H44.6-, H44.7-)
              superficial foreign body of eyelid and periocular area (S00.25-)
      H02.811   Retained foreign body in right upper eyelid
      H02.812   Retained foreign body in right lower eyelid
      H02.813   Retained foreign body in right eye, unspecified eyelid
      H02.814   Retained foreign body in left upper eyelid
      H02.815   Retained foreign body in left lower eyelid
      H02.816   Retained foreign body in left eye, unspecified eyelid
      H02.819   Retained foreign body in unspecified eye, unspecified eyelid
   H02.82- Cysts of eyelid
          Sebaceous cyst of eyelid
      H02.821   Cysts of right upper eyelid
      H02.822   Cysts of right lower eyelid
      H02.823   Cysts of right eye, unspecified eyelid
      H02.824   Cysts of left upper eyelid
      H02.825   Cysts of left lower eyelid
      H02.826   Cysts of left eye, unspecified eyelid
      H02.829   Cysts of unspecified eye, unspecified eyelid
   H02.83- Dermatochalasis of eyelid
      H02.831   Dermatochalasis of right upper eyelid
      H02.832   Dermatochalasis of right lower eyelid
      H02.833   Dermatochalasis of right eye, unspecified eyelid
      H02.834   Dermatochalasis of left upper eyelid
      H02.835   Dermatochalasis of left lower eyelid
      H02.836   Dermatochalasis of left eye, unspecified eyelid
      H02.839   Dermatochalasis of unspecified eye, unspecified eyelid
   H02.84- Edema of eyelid
          Hyperemia of eyelid
      H02.841   Edema of right upper eyelid
      H02.842   Edema of right lower eyelid
      H02.843   Edema of right eye, unspecified eyelid
      H02.844   Edema of left upper eyelid
      H02.845   Edema of left lower eyelid
      H02.846   Edema of left eye, unspecified eyelid
      H02.849   Edema of unspecified eye, unspecified eyelid

H02 - H02

Excludes 1: = NOT CODED HERE! (Do not code both)   **435**   *Excludes❷: = Not Included Here*

H
0
2
-
H
0
5

H02.85- <u>Elephantiasis</u> of eyelid
  H02.851 Elephantiasis of <u>right</u> <u>upper</u> eyelid
  H02.852 Elephantiasis of <u>right</u> <u>lower</u> eyelid
  H02.853 Elephantiasis of <u>right</u> eye, <u>unspecified</u> eyelid
  H02.854 Elephantiasis of <u>left</u> <u>upper</u> eyelid
  H02.855 Elephantiasis of <u>left</u> <u>lower</u> eyelid
  H02.856 Elephantiasis of <u>left</u> eye, <u>unspecified</u> eyelid
  H02.859 Elephantiasis of <u>unspecified</u> eye, <u>unspecified</u> eyelid
H02.86- <u>Hypertrichosis</u> of eyelid
  H02.861 Hypertrichosis of <u>right</u> <u>upper</u> eyelid
  H02.862 Hypertrichosis of <u>right</u> <u>lower</u> eyelid
  H02.863 Hypertrichosis of <u>right</u> eye, <u>unspecified</u> eyelid
  H02.864 Hypertrichosis of <u>left</u> <u>upper</u> eyelid
  H02.865 Hypertrichosis of <u>left</u> <u>lower</u> eyelid
  H02.866 Hypertrichosis of <u>left</u> eye, <u>unspecified</u> eyelid
  H02.869 Hypertrichosis of <u>unspecified</u> eye, <u>unspecified</u> eyelid
H02.87- <u>Vascular anomalies</u> of eyelid
  H02.871 Vascular anomalies of <u>right</u> <u>upper</u> eyelid
  H02.872 Vascular anomalies of <u>right</u> <u>lower</u> eyelid
  H02.873 Vascular anomalies of <u>right</u> eye, <u>unspecified</u> eyelid
  H02.874 Vascular anomalies of <u>left</u> <u>upper</u> eyelid
  H02.875 Vascular anomalies of <u>left</u> <u>lower</u> eyelid
  H02.876 Vascular anomalies of <u>left</u> eye, <u>unspecified</u> eyelid
  H02.879 Vascular anomalies of <u>unspecified</u> eye, <u>unspecified</u> eyelid
H02.89 Other specified disorders of eyelid
        Hemorrhage of eyelid
H02.9   Unspecified disorder of eyelid
        Disorder of eyelid NOS

H04- Disorders of <u>lacrimal system</u>
    Excludes 1: congenital malformations of lacrimal system (Q10.4-Q10.6)
  H04.0- <u>Dacryoadenitis</u>
    H04.00- <u>Unspecified</u> dacryoadenitis
      H04.001 Unspecified dacryoadenitis, <u>right</u> lacrimal gland
      H04.002 Unspecified dacryoadenitis, <u>left</u> lacrimal gland
      H04.003 Unspecified dacryoadenitis, <u>bilateral</u> lacrimal glands
      H04.009 Unspecified dacryoadenitis, <u>unspecified</u> lacrimal gland
    H04.01- <u>Acute</u> dacryoadenitis
      H04.011 Acute dacryoadenitis, <u>right</u> lacrimal gland
      H04.012 Acute dacryoadenitis, <u>left</u> lacrimal gland
      H04.013 Acute dacryoadenitis, <u>bilateral</u> lacrimal glands
      H04.019 Acute dacryoadenitis, <u>unspecified</u> lacrimal gland
    H04.02- <u>Chronic</u> dacryoadenitis
      H04.021 Chronic dacryoadenitis, <u>right</u> lacrimal gland
      H04.022 Chronic dacryoadenitis, <u>left</u> lacrimal gland
      H04.023 Chronic dacryoadenitis, <u>bilateral</u> lacrimal gland
      H04.029 Chronic dacryoadenitis, <u>unspecified</u> lacrimal gland
    H04.03- <u>Chronic enlargement</u> of lacrimal gland
      H04.031 Chronic enlargement of <u>right</u> lacrimal gland
      H04.032 Chronic enlargement of <u>left</u> lacrimal gland
      H04.033 Chronic enlargement of <u>bilateral</u> lacrimal glands
      H04.039 Chronic enlargement of <u>unspecified</u> lacrimal gland
  H04.1- Other disorders of <u>lacrimal gland</u>
    H04.11- <u>Dacryops</u>
      H04.111 Dacryops of <u>right</u> lacrimal gland
      H04.112 Dacryops of <u>left</u> lacrimal gland
      H04.113 Dacryops of <u>bilateral</u> lacrimal glands
      H04.119 Dacryops of <u>unspecified</u> lacrimal gland
    H04.12- <u>Dry eye</u> syndrome
          Tear film insufficiency, NOS
      H04.121 Dry eye syndrome of <u>right</u> lacrimal gland
      H04.122 Dry eye syndrome of <u>left</u> lacrimal gland
      H04.123 Dry eye syndrome of <u>bilateral</u> lacrimal glands
      H04.129 Dry eye syndrome of <u>unspecified</u> lacrimal gland
    H04.13- Lacrimal <u>cyst</u>
          Lacrimal cystic degeneration
      H04.131 Lacrimal cyst, <u>right</u> lacrimal gland
      H04.132 Lacrimal cyst, <u>left</u> lacrimal gland
      H04.133 Lacrimal cyst, <u>bilateral</u> lacrimal glands
      H04.139 Lacrimal cyst, <u>unspecified</u> lacrimal gland
    H04.14- <u>Primary</u> lacrimal <u>gland atrophy</u>
      H04.141 Primary lacrimal gland atrophy, <u>right</u> lacrimal gland
      H04.142 Primary lacrimal gland atrophy, <u>left</u> lacrimal gland
      H04.143 Primary lacrimal gland atrophy, <u>bilateral</u> lacrimal glands

H04.149 Primary lacrimal gland atrophy, <u>unspecified</u> lacrimal gland
H04.15- <u>Secondary</u> lacrimal <u>gland atrophy</u>
  H04.151 Secondary lacrimal gland atrophy, <u>right</u> lacrimal gland
  H04.152 Secondary lacrimal gland atrophy, <u>left</u> lacrimal gland
  H04.153 Secondary lacrimal gland atrophy, <u>bilateral</u> lacrimal glands
  H04.159 Secondary lacrimal gland atrophy, <u>unspecified</u> lacrimal gland
H04.16- Lacrimal gland <u>dislocation</u>
  H04.161 Lacrimal gland dislocation, <u>right</u> lacrimal gland
  H04.162 Lacrimal gland dislocation, <u>left</u> lacrimal gland
  H04.163 Lacrimal gland dislocation, <u>bilateral</u> lacrimal glands
  H04.169 Lacrimal gland dislocation, <u>unspecified</u> lacrimal gland
H04.19 Other specified disorders of lacrimal gland
H04.2- <u>Epiphora</u>
  H04.20- <u>Unspecified</u> epiphora
    H04.201 Unspecified epiphora, <u>right</u> lacrimal gland
    H04.202 Unspecified epiphora, <u>left</u> lacrimal gland
    H04.203 Unspecified epiphora, <u>bilateral</u> lacrimal glands
    H04.209 Unspecified epiphora, <u>unspecified</u> lacrimal gland
  H04.21- Epiphora due to <u>excess lacrimation</u>
    H04.211 Epiphora due to excess lacrimation, <u>right</u> lacrimal gland
    H04.212 Epiphora due to excess lacrimation, <u>left</u> lacrimal gland
    H04.213 Epiphora due to excess lacrimation, <u>bilateral</u> lacrimal glands
    H04.219 Epiphora due to excess lacrimation, <u>unspecified</u> lacrimal gland
  H04.22- Epiphora due to <u>insufficient drainage</u>
    H04.221 Epiphora due to insufficient drainage, <u>right</u> lacrimal gland
    H04.222 Epiphora due to insufficient drainage, <u>left</u> lacrimal gland
    H04.223 Epiphora due to insufficient drainage, <u>bilateral</u> lacrimal glands
    H04.229 Epiphora due to insufficient drainage, <u>unspecified</u> lacrimal gland
H04.3- <u>Acute</u> and unspecified <u>inflammation of lacrimal passages</u>
    Excludes 1: neonatal dacryocystitis (P39.1)
  H04.30- <u>Unspecified dacryocystitis</u>
    H04.301 Unspecified dacryocystitis of <u>right</u> lacrimal passage
    H04.302 Unspecified dacryocystitis of <u>left</u> lacrimal passage
    H04.303 Unspecified dacryocystitis of <u>bilateral</u> lacrimal passages
    H04.309 Unspecified dacryocystitis of <u>unspecified</u> lacrimal passage
  H04.31- <u>Phlegmonous</u> <u>dacryocystitis</u>
    H04.311 Phlegmonous dacryocystitis of <u>right</u> lacrimal passage
    H04.312 Phlegmonous dacryocystitis of <u>left</u> lacrimal passage
    H04.313 Phlegmonous dacryocystitis of <u>bilateral</u> lacrimal passages
    H04.319 Phlegmonous dacryocystitis of <u>unspecified</u> lacrimal passage
  H04.32- <u>Acute</u> <u>dacryocystitis</u>
        Acute dacryopericystitis
    H04.321 Acute dacryocystitis of <u>right</u> lacrimal passage
    H04.322 Acute dacryocystitis of <u>left</u> lacrimal passage
    H04.323 Acute dacryocystitis of <u>bilateral</u> lacrimal passages
    H04.329 Acute dacryocystitis of <u>unspecified</u> lacrimal passage
  H04.33- <u>Acute lacrimal canaliculitis</u>
    H04.331 Acute lacrimal canaliculitis of <u>right</u> lacrimal passage
    H04.332 Acute lacrimal canaliculitis of <u>left</u> lacrimal passage
    H04.333 Acute lacrimal canaliculitis of <u>bilateral</u> lacrimal passages
    H04.339 Acute lacrimal canaliculitis of <u>unspecified</u> lacrimal passage
H04.4- <u>Chronic</u> inflammation of lacrimal passages
  H04.41- <u>Chronic dacryocystitis</u>
    H04.411 Chronic dacryocystitis of <u>right</u> lacrimal passage
    H04.412 Chronic dacryocystitis of <u>left</u> lacrimal passage
    H04.413 Chronic dacryocystitis of <u>bilateral</u> lacrimal passages
    H04.419 Chronic dacryocystitis of <u>unspecified</u> lacrimal passage

H04.42- Chronic lacrimal <u>canaliculitis</u>
    H04.421   Chronic lacrimal canaliculitis of <u>right</u> lacrimal passage
    H04.422   Chronic lacrimal canaliculitis of <u>left</u> lacrimal passage
    H04.423   Chronic lacrimal canaliculitis of <u>bilateral</u> lacrimal passages
    H04.429   Chronic lacrimal canaliculitis of <u>unspecified</u> lacrimal passage
H04.43- Chronic lacrimal <u>mucocele</u>
    H04.431   Chronic lacrimal mucocele of <u>right</u> lacrimal passage
    H04.432   Chronic lacrimal mucocele of <u>left</u> lacrimal passage
    H04.433   Chronic lacrimal mucocele of <u>bilateral</u> lacrimal passages
    H04.439   Chronic lacrimal mucocele of <u>unspecified</u> lacrimal passage
H04.5- <u>Stenosis and insufficiency</u> of lacrimal passages
  H04.51- <u>Dacryolith</u>
    H04.511   Dacryolith of <u>right</u> lacrimal passage
    H04.512   Dacryolith of <u>left</u> lacrimal passage
    H04.513   Dacryolith of <u>bilateral</u> lacrimal passages
    H04.519   Dacryolith of <u>unspecified</u> lacrimal passage
  H04.52- <u>Eversion</u> of lacrimal <u>punctum</u>
    H04.521   Eversion of <u>right</u> lacrimal punctum
    H04.522   Eversion of <u>left</u> lacrimal punctum
    H04.523   Eversion of <u>bilateral</u> lacrimal punctum
    H04.529   Eversion of <u>unspecified</u> lacrimal punctum
  H04.53- <u>Neonatal obstruction</u> of <u>nasolacrimal duct</u>
      Excludes 1: congenital stenosis and stricture of lacrimal duct (Q10.5)
    H04.531   Neonatal obstruction of <u>right</u> nasolacrimal duct
    H04.532   Neonatal obstruction of <u>left</u> nasolacrimal duct
    H04.533   Neonatal obstruction of <u>bilateral</u> nasolacrimal duct
    H04.539   Neonatal obstruction of <u>unspecified</u> nasolacrimal duct
  H04.54- <u>Stenosis</u> of lacrimal <u>canaliculi</u>
    H04.541   Stenosis of <u>right</u> lacrimal canaliculi
    H04.542   Stenosis of <u>left</u> lacrimal canaliculi
    H04.543   Stenosis of <u>bilateral</u> lacrimal canaliculi
    H04.549   Stenosis of <u>unspecified</u> lacrimal canaliculi
  H04.55- <u>Acquired stenosis</u> of <u>nasolacrimal duct</u>
    H04.551   Acquired stenosis of <u>right</u> nasolacrimal duct
    H04.552   Acquired stenosis of <u>left</u> nasolacrimal duct
    H04.553   Acquired stenosis of <u>bilateral</u> nasolacrimal duct
    H04.559   Acquired stenosis of <u>unspecified</u> nasolacrimal duct
  H04.56- <u>Stenosis</u> of lacrimal <u>punctum</u>
    H04.561   Stenosis of <u>right</u> lacrimal punctum
    H04.562   Stenosis of <u>left</u> lacrimal punctum
    H04.563   Stenosis of <u>bilateral</u> lacrimal punctum
    H04.569   Stenosis of <u>unspecified</u> lacrimal punctum
  H04.57- <u>Stenosis</u> of lacrimal <u>sac</u>
    H04.571   Stenosis of <u>right</u> lacrimal sac
    H04.572   Stenosis of <u>left</u> lacrimal sac
    H04.573   Stenosis of <u>bilateral</u> lacrimal sac
    H04.579   Stenosis of <u>unspecified</u> lacrimal sac
H04.6- Other changes of lacrimal passages
  H04.61- Lacrimal <u>fistula</u>
    H04.611   Lacrimal fistula <u>right</u> lacrimal passage
    H04.612   Lacrimal fistula <u>left</u> lacrimal passage
    H04.613   Lacrimal fistula <u>bilateral</u> lacrimal passages
    H04.619   Lacrimal fistula <u>unspecified</u> lacrimal passage
  H04.69 Other changes of lacrimal passages
H04.8- Other disorders of lacrimal system
  H04.81- <u>Granuloma</u> of lacrimal passages
    H04.811   Granuloma of <u>right</u> lacrimal passage
    H04.812   Granuloma of <u>left</u> lacrimal passage
    H04.813   Granuloma of <u>bilateral</u> lacrimal passages
    H04.819   Granuloma of <u>unspecified</u> lacrimal passage
  H04.89 Other disorders of lacrimal system
H04.9   Disorder of lacrimal system, unspecified

H05- Disorders of <u>orbit</u>
    Excludes 1: congenital malformation of orbit (Q10.7)
  H05.0- <u>Acute inflammation</u> of orbit
    H05.00 <u>Unspecified</u> acute inflammation of orbit
    H05.01- <u>Cellulitis</u> of orbit
        Abscess of orbit
      H05.011   Cellulitis of <u>right</u> orbit
      H05.012   Cellulitis of <u>left</u> orbit
      H05.013   Cellulitis of <u>bilateral</u> orbits
      H05.019   Cellulitis of <u>unspecified</u> orbit
    H05.02- <u>Osteomyelitis</u> of orbit
      H05.021   Osteomyelitis of <u>right</u> orbit
      H05.022   Osteomyelitis of <u>left</u> orbit
      H05.023   Osteomyelitis of <u>bilateral</u> orbits
      H05.029   Osteomyelitis of <u>unspecified</u> orbit
    H05.03- <u>Periostitis</u> of orbit
      H05.031   Periostitis of <u>right</u> orbit
      H05.032   Periostitis of <u>left</u> orbit
      H05.033   Periostitis of <u>bilateral</u> orbits
      H05.039   Periostitis of <u>unspecified</u> orbit
    H05.04- <u>Tenonitis</u> of orbit
      H05.041   Tenonitis of <u>right</u> orbit
      H05.042   Tenonitis of <u>left</u> orbit
      H05.043   Tenonitis of <u>bilateral</u> orbits
      H05.049   Tenonitis of <u>unspecified</u> orbit
  H05.1- <u>Chronic inflammatory disorders</u> of orbit
    H05.10 <u>Unspecified</u> chronic inflammatory disorders of orbit
    H05.11- <u>Granuloma</u> of orbit
        Pseudotumor (inflammatory) of orbit
      H05.111   Granuloma of <u>right</u> orbit
      H05.112   Granuloma of <u>left</u> orbit
      H05.113   Granuloma of <u>bilateral</u> orbits
      H05.119   Granuloma of <u>unspecified</u> orbit
    H05.12- Orbital <u>myositis</u>
      H05.121   Orbital myositis, <u>right</u> orbit
      H05.122   Orbital myositis, <u>left</u> orbit
      H05.123   Orbital myositis, <u>bilateral</u>
      H05.129   Orbital myositis, <u>unspecified</u> orbit
  H05.2- <u>Exophthalmic conditions</u>
    H05.20 Unspecified exophthalmos
    H05.21- <u>Displacement</u> (lateral) of <u>globe</u>
      H05.211   Displacement (lateral) of globe, <u>right</u> eye
      H05.212   Displacement (lateral) of globe, <u>left</u> eye
      H05.213   Displacement (lateral) of globe, <u>bilateral</u>
      H05.219   Displacement (lateral) of globe, <u>unspecified</u> eye
    H05.22- <u>Edema</u> of orbit
        Orbital congestion
      H05.221   Edema of <u>right</u> orbit
      H05.222   Edema of <u>left</u> orbit
      H05.223   Edema of <u>bilateral</u> orbit
      H05.229   Edema of <u>unspecified</u> orbit
    H05.23- <u>Hemorrhage</u> of orbit
      H05.231   Hemorrhage of <u>right</u> orbit
      H05.232   Hemorrhage of <u>left</u> orbit
      H05.233   Hemorrhage of <u>bilateral</u> orbit
      H05.239   Hemorrhage of <u>unspecified</u> orbit
    H05.24- <u>Constant</u> exophthalmos
      H05.241   Constant exophthalmos, <u>right</u> eye
      H05.242   Constant exophthalmos, <u>left</u> eye
      H05.243   Constant exophthalmos, <u>bilateral</u>
      H05.249   Constant exophthalmos, <u>unspecified</u> eye
    H05.25- <u>Intermittent</u> exophthalmos
      H05.251   Intermittent exophthalmos, <u>right</u> eye
      H05.252   Intermittent exophthalmos, <u>left</u> eye
      H05.253   Intermittent exophthalmos, <u>bilateral</u>
      H05.259   Intermittent exophthalmos, <u>unspecified</u> eye
    H05.26- <u>Pulsating</u> exophthalmos
      H05.261   Pulsating exophthalmos, <u>right</u> eye
      H05.262   Pulsating exophthalmos, <u>left</u> eye
      H05.263   Pulsating exophthalmos, <u>bilateral</u>
      H05.269   Pulsating exophthalmos, <u>unspecified</u> eye

H02 - H05

H05.3- Deformity of orbit
Excludes 1: congenital deformity of orbit (Q10.7)
hypertelorism (Q75.2)
H05.30 Unspecified deformity of orbit
H05.31- Atrophy of orbit
  H05.311 Atrophy of right orbit
  H05.312 Atrophy of left orbit
  H05.313 Atrophy of bilateral orbit
  H05.319 Atrophy of unspecified orbit
H05.32- Deformity of orbit due to bone disease
Code also associated bone disease
  H05.321 Deformity of right orbit due to bone disease
  H05.322 Deformity of left orbit due to bone disease
  H05.323 Deformity of bilateral orbits due to bone disease
  H05.329 Deformity of unspecified orbit due to bone disease
H05.33- Deformity of orbit due to trauma or surgery
  H05.331 Deformity of right orbit due to trauma or surgery
  H05.332 Deformity of left orbit due to trauma or surgery
  H05.333 Deformity of bilateral orbits due to trauma or surgery
  H05.339 Deformity of unspecified orbit due to trauma or surgery
H05.34- Enlargement of orbit
  H05.341 Enlargement of right orbit
  H05.342 Enlargement of left orbit
  H05.343 Enlargement of bilateral orbits
  H05.349 Enlargement of unspecified orbit
H05.35- Exostosis of orbit
  H05.351 Exostosis of right orbit
  H05.352 Exostosis of left orbit
  H05.353 Exostosis of bilateral orbits
  H05.359 Exostosis of unspecified orbit
H05.4- Enophthalmos
H05.40- Unspecified enophthalmos
  H05.401 Unspecified enophthalmos, right eye
  H05.402 Unspecified enophthalmos, left eye
  H05.403 Unspecified enophthalmos, bilateral
  H05.409 Unspecified enophthalmos, unspecified eye
H05.41- Enophthalmos due to atrophy of orbital tissue
  H05.411 Enophthalmos due to atrophy of orbital tissue, right eye
  H05.412 Enophthalmos due to atrophy of orbital tissue, left eye
  H05.413 Enophthalmos due to atrophy of orbital tissue, bilateral
  H05.419 Enophthalmos due to atrophy of orbital tissue, unspecified eye
H05.42- Enophthalmos due to trauma or surgery
  H05.421 Enophthalmos due to trauma or surgery, right eye
  H05.422 Enophthalmos due to trauma or surgery, left eye
  H05.423 Enophthalmos due to trauma or surgery, bilateral
  H05.429 Enophthalmos due to trauma or surgery, unspecified eye
H05.5- Retained (old) foreign body following penetrating wound of orbit
Retrobulbar foreign body
Use additional code to identify the type of retained foreign body (Z18.-)
Excludes 1: current penetrating wound of orbit (S05.4-)
Excludes ❷: retained foreign body of eyelid (H02.81-)
retained intraocular foreign body (H44.6-, H44.7-)
H05.50 Retained (old) foreign body following penetrating wound of unspecified orbit
H05.51 Retained (old) foreign body following penetrating wound of right orbit
H05.52 Retained (old) foreign body following penetrating wound of left orbit
H05.53 Retained (old) foreign body following penetrating wound of bilateral orbits
H05.8- Other disorders of orbit
H05.81- Cyst of orbit
Encephalocele of orbit
  H05.811 Cyst of right orbit
  H05.812 Cyst of left orbit
  H05.813 Cyst of bilateral orbits
  H05.819 Cyst of unspecified orbit
H05.82- Myopathy of extraocular muscles
  H05.821 Myopathy of extraocular muscles, right orbit
  H05.822 Myopathy of extraocular muscles, left orbit
  H05.823 Myopathy of extraocular muscles, bilateral

H05.829 Myopathy of extraocular muscles, unspecified orbit
H05.89 Other disorders of orbit
H05.9 Unspecified disorder of orbit

Disorders of conjunctiva (H10-H11)

H10- Conjunctivitis
Excludes 1: keratoconjunctivitis (H16.2-)
H10.0- Mucopurulent conjunctivitis
H10.01- Acute follicular conjunctivitis
  H10.011 Acute follicular conjunctivitis, right eye
  H10.012 Acute follicular conjunctivitis, left eye
  H10.013 Acute follicular conjunctivitis, bilateral
  H10.019 Acute follicular conjunctivitis, unspecified eye
H10.02- Other mucopurulent conjunctivitis
  H10.021 Other mucopurulent conjunctivitis, right eye
  H10.022 Other mucopurulent conjunctivitis, left eye
  H10.023 Other mucopurulent conjunctivitis, bilateral
  H10.029 Other mucopurulent conjunctivitis, unspecified eye
H10.1- Acute atopic conjunctivitis
Acute papillary conjunctivitis
H10.10 Acute atopic conjunctivitis, unspecified eye
H10.11 Acute atopic conjunctivitis, right eye
H10.12 Acute atopic conjunctivitis, left eye
H10.13 Acute atopic conjunctivitis, bilateral
H10.2- Other acute conjunctivitis
H10.21- Acute toxic conjunctivitis
Acute chemical conjunctivitis
Code first (T51-T65) to identify chemical and intent
Excludes 1: burn and corrosion of eye and adnexa (T26.-)
  H10.211 Acute toxic conjunctivitis, right eye
  H10.212 Acute toxic conjunctivitis, left eye
  H10.213 Acute toxic conjunctivitis, bilateral
  H10.219 Acute toxic conjunctivitis, unspecified eye
H10.22- Pseudomembranous conjunctivitis
  H10.221 Pseudomembranous conjunctivitis, right eye
  H10.222 Pseudomembranous conjunctivitis, left eye
  H10.223 Pseudomembranous conjunctivitis, bilateral
  H10.229 Pseudomembranous conjunctivitis, unspecified eye
H10.23- Serous conjunctivitis, except viral
Excludes 1: viral conjunctivitis (B30.-)
  H10.231 Serous conjunctivitis, except viral, right eye
  H10.232 Serous conjunctivitis, except viral, left eye
  H10.233 Serous conjunctivitis, except viral, bilateral
  H10.239 Serous conjunctivitis, except viral, unspecified eye
H10.3- Unspecified acute conjunctivitis
Excludes 1: ophthalmia neonatorum NOS (P39.1)
H10.30 Unspecified acute conjunctivitis, unspecified eye
H10.31 Unspecified acute conjunctivitis, right eye
H10.32 Unspecified acute conjunctivitis, left eye
H10.33 Unspecified acute conjunctivitis, bilateral
H10.4- Chronic conjunctivitis
H10.40- Unspecified chronic conjunctivitis
  H10.401 Unspecified chronic conjunctivitis, right eye
  H10.402 Unspecified chronic conjunctivitis, left eye
  H10.403 Unspecified chronic conjunctivitis, bilateral
  H10.409 Unspecified chronic conjunctivitis, unspecified eye
H10.41- Chronic giant papillary conjunctivitis
  H10.411 Chronic giant papillary conjunctivitis, right eye
  H10.412 Chronic giant papillary conjunctivitis, left eye
  H10.413 Chronic giant papillary conjunctivitis, bilateral
  H10.419 Chronic giant papillary conjunctivitis, unspecified eye
H10.42- Simple chronic conjunctivitis
  H10.421 Simple chronic conjunctivitis, right eye
  H10.422 Simple chronic conjunctivitis, left eye
  H10.423 Simple chronic conjunctivitis, bilateral
  H10.429 Simple chronic conjunctivitis, unspecified eye
H10.43- Chronic follicular conjunctivitis
  H10.431 Chronic follicular conjunctivitis, right eye
  H10.432 Chronic follicular conjunctivitis, left eye
  H10.433 Chronic follicular conjunctivitis, bilateral
  H10.439 Chronic follicular conjunctivitis, unspecified eye
H10.44 Vernal conjunctivitis
Excludes 1: vernal keratoconjunctivitis with limbar and corneal involvement (H16.26-)
H10.45 Other chronic allergic conjunctivitis

H05 - H11

© 2013 Channel Publishing, Ltd.

H10.5-   Blepharoconjunctivitis
   H10.50- Unspecified blepharoconjunctivitis
     H10.501   Unspecified blepharoconjunctivitis, right eye
     H10.502   Unspecified blepharoconjunctivitis, left eye
     H10.503   Unspecified blepharoconjunctivitis, bilateral
     H10.509   Unspecified blepharoconjunctivitis, unspecified eye
   H10.51- Ligneous conjunctivitis
     H10.511   Ligneous conjunctivitis, right eye
     H10.512   Ligneous conjunctivitis, left eye
     H10.513   Ligneous conjunctivitis, bilateral
     H10.519   Ligneous conjunctivitis, unspecified eye
   H10.52- Angular blepharoconjunctivitis
     H10.521   Angular blepharoconjunctivitis, right eye
     H10.522   Angular blepharoconjunctivitis, left eye
     H10.523   Angular blepharoconjunctivitis, bilateral
     H10.529   Angular blepharoconjunctivitis, unspecified eye
   H10.53- Contact blepharoconjunctivitis
     H10.531   Contact blepharoconjunctivitis, right eye
     H10.532   Contact blepharoconjunctivitis, left eye
     H10.533   Contact blepharoconjunctivitis, bilateral
     H10.539   Contact blepharoconjunctivitis, unspecified eye
H10.8-   Other conjunctivitis
   H10.81- Pingueculitis
     Excludes 1: pinguecula (H11.15-)
     H10.811   Pingueculitis, right eye
     H10.812   Pingueculitis, left eye
     H10.813   Pingueculitis, bilateral
     H10.819   Pingueculitis, unspecified eye
   H10.89   Other conjunctivitis
H10.9   Unspecified conjunctivitis
H11-   Other disorders of conjunctiva
   Excludes 1: keratoconjunctivitis (H16.2-)
   H11.0-   Pterygium of eye
     Excludes 1: pseudopterygium (H11.81-)
   H11.00- Unspecified pterygium of eye
     H11.001   Unspecified pterygium of right eye
     H11.002   Unspecified pterygium of left eye
     H11.003   Unspecified pterygium of eye, bilateral
     H11.009   Unspecified pterygium of unspecified eye
   H11.01- Amyloid pterygium
     H11.011   Amyloid pterygium of right eye
     H11.012   Amyloid pterygium of left eye
     H11.013   Amyloid pterygium of eye, bilateral
     H11.019   Amyloid pterygium of unspecified eye
   H11.02- Central pterygium of eye
     H11.021   Central pterygium of right eye
     H11.022   Central pterygium of left eye
     H11.023   Central pterygium of eye, bilateral
     H11.029   Central pterygium of unspecified eye
   H11.03- Double pterygium of eye
     H11.031   Double pterygium of right eye
     H11.032   Double pterygium of left eye
     H11.033   Double pterygium of eye, bilateral
     H11.039   Double pterygium of unspecified eye
   H11.04- Peripheral pterygium of eye, stationary
     H11.041   Peripheral pterygium, stationary, right eye
     H11.042   Peripheral pterygium, stationary, left eye
     H11.043   Peripheral pterygium, stationary, bilateral
     H11.049   Peripheral pterygium, stationary, unspecified eye
   H11.05- Peripheral pterygium of eye, progressive
     H11.051   Peripheral pterygium, progressive, right eye
     H11.052   Peripheral pterygium, progressive, left eye
     H11.053   Peripheral pterygium, progressive, bilateral
     H11.059   Peripheral pterygium, progressive, unspecified eye
   H11.06- Recurrent pterygium of eye
     H11.061   Recurrent pterygium of right eye
     H11.062   Recurrent pterygium of left eye
     H11.063   Recurrent pterygium of eye, bilateral
     H11.069   Recurrent pterygium of unspecified eye
   H11.1-   Conjunctival degenerations and deposits
     Excludes ❷: pseudopterygium (H11.81)
   H11.10   Unspecified conjunctival degenerations
   H11.11- Conjunctival deposits
     H11.111   Conjunctival deposits, right eye
     H11.112   Conjunctival deposits, left eye

     H11.113   Conjunctival deposits, bilateral
     H11.119   Conjunctival deposits, unspecified eye
   H11.12- Conjunctival concretions
     H11.121   Conjunctival concretions, right eye
     H11.122   Conjunctival concretions, left eye
     H11.123   Conjunctival concretions, bilateral
     H11.129   Conjunctival concretions, unspecified eye
   H11.13- Conjunctival pigmentations
     Conjunctival argyrosis [argyria]
     H11.131   Conjunctival pigmentations, right eye
     H11.132   Conjunctival pigmentations, left eye
     H11.133   Conjunctival pigmentations, bilateral
     H11.139   Conjunctival pigmentations, unspecified eye
   H11.14- Conjunctival xerosis, unspecified
     Excludes 1: xerosis of conjunctiva due to vitamin A deficiency
          (E50.0, E50.1)
     H11.141   Conjunctival xerosis, unspecified, right eye
     H11.142   Conjunctival xerosis, unspecified, left eye
     H11.143   Conjunctival xerosis, unspecified, bilateral
     H11.149   Conjunctival xerosis, unspecified, unspecified eye
   H11.15- Pinguecula
     Excludes 1: pingueculitis (H10.81-)
     H11.151   Pinguecula, right eye
     H11.152   Pinguecula, left eye
     H11.153   Pinguecula, bilateral
     H11.159   Pinguecula, unspecified eye
H11.2-   Conjunctival scars
   H11.21- Conjunctival adhesions and strands (localized)
     H11.211   Conjunctival adhesions and strands (localized), right eye
     H11.212   Conjunctival adhesions and strands (localized), left eye
     H11.213   Conjunctival adhesions and strands (localized), bilateral
     H11.219   Conjunctival adhesions and strands (localized), unspecified eye
   H11.22- Conjunctival granuloma
     H11.221   Conjunctival granuloma, right eye
     H11.222   Conjunctival granuloma, left eye
     H11.223   Conjunctival granuloma, bilateral
     H11.229   Conjunctival granuloma, unspecified
   H11.23- Symblepharon
     H11.231   Symblepharon, right eye
     H11.232   Symblepharon, left eye
     H11.233   Symblepharon, bilateral
     H11.239   Symblepharon, unspecified eye
   H11.24- Scarring of conjunctiva
     H11.241   Scarring of conjunctiva, right eye
     H11.242   Scarring of conjunctiva, left eye
     H11.243   Scarring of conjunctiva, bilateral
     H11.249   Scarring of conjunctiva, unspecified eye
H11.3-   Conjunctival hemorrhage
   Subconjunctival hemorrhage
   H11.30   Conjunctival hemorrhage, unspecified eye
   H11.31   Conjunctival hemorrhage, right eye
   H11.32   Conjunctival hemorrhage, left eye
   H11.33   Conjunctival hemorrhage, bilateral
H11.4-   Other conjunctival vascular disorders and cysts
   H11.41- Vascular abnormalities of conjunctiva
     Conjunctival aneurysm
     H11.411   Vascular abnormalities of conjunctiva, right eye
     H11.412   Vascular abnormalities of conjunctiva, left eye
     H11.413   Vascular abnormalities of conjunctiva, bilateral
     H11.419   Vascular abnormalities of conjunctiva, unspecified eye
   H11.42- Conjunctival edema
     H11.421   Conjunctival edema, right eye
     H11.422   Conjunctival edema, left eye
     H11.423   Conjunctival edema, bilateral
     H11.429   Conjunctival edema, unspecified eye
   H11.43- Conjunctival hyperemia
     H11.431   Conjunctival hyperemia, right eye
     H11.432   Conjunctival hyperemia, left eye
     H11.433   Conjunctival hyperemia, bilateral
     H11.439   Conjunctival hyperemia, unspecified eye

H05 - H11

H11.44- Conjunctival <u>cysts</u>
  H11.441 Conjunctival cysts, <u>right</u> eye
  H11.442 Conjunctival cysts, <u>left</u> eye
  H11.443 Conjunctival cysts, <u>bilateral</u>
  H11.449 Conjunctival cysts, <u>unspecified</u> eye
H11.8- Other specified disorders of conjunctiva
  H11.81- <u>Pseudopterygium</u> of conjunctiva
    H11.811 Pseudopterygium of conjunctiva, <u>right</u> eye
    H11.812 Pseudopterygium of conjunctiva, <u>left</u> eye
    H11.813 Pseudopterygium of conjunctiva, <u>bilateral</u>
    H11.819 Pseudopterygium of conjunctiva, <u>unspecified</u> eye
  H11.82- <u>Conjunctivochalasis</u>
    H11.821 Conjunctivochalasis, <u>right</u> eye
    H11.822 Conjunctivochalasis, <u>left</u> eye
    H11.823 Conjunctivochalasis, <u>bilateral</u>
    H11.829 Conjunctivochalasis, <u>unspecified</u> eye
  H11.89 Other specified disorders of conjunctiva
H11.9 Unspecified disorder of conjunctiva

Disorders of sclera, cornea, iris and ciliary body (H15-H22)

H15- <u>Disorders of sclera</u>
  H15.0- <u>Scleritis</u>
    H15.00- <u>Unspecified</u> scleritis
      H15.001 Unspecified scleritis, <u>right</u> eye
      H15.002 Unspecified scleritis, <u>left</u> eye
      H15.003 Unspecified scleritis, <u>bilateral</u>
      H15.009 Unspecified scleritis, <u>unspecified</u> eye
    H15.01- <u>Anterior</u> scleritis
      H15.011 Anterior scleritis, <u>right</u> eye
      H15.012 Anterior scleritis, <u>left</u> eye
      H15.013 Anterior scleritis, <u>bilateral</u>
      H15.019 Anterior scleritis, <u>unspecified</u> eye
    H15.02- <u>Brawny</u> scleritis
      H15.021 Brawny scleritis, <u>right</u> eye
      H15.022 Brawny scleritis, <u>left</u> eye
      H15.023 Brawny scleritis, <u>bilateral</u>
      H15.029 Brawny scleritis, <u>unspecified</u> eye
    H15.03- <u>Posterior</u> scleritis
        Sclerotenonitis
      H15.031 Posterior scleritis, <u>right</u> eye
      H15.032 Posterior scleritis, <u>left</u> eye
      H15.033 Posterior scleritis, <u>bilateral</u>
      H15.039 Posterior scleritis, <u>unspecified</u> eye
    H15.04- <u>Scleritis with corneal involvement</u>
      H15.041 Scleritis with corneal involvement, <u>right</u> eye
      H15.042 Scleritis with corneal involvement, <u>left</u> eye
      H15.043 Scleritis with corneal involvement, <u>bilateral</u>
      H15.049 Scleritis with corneal involvement, <u>unspecified</u> eye
    H15.05- <u>Scleromalacia perforans</u>
      H15.051 Scleromalacia perforans, <u>right</u> eye
      H15.052 Scleromalacia perforans, <u>left</u> eye
      H15.053 Scleromalacia perforans, <u>bilateral</u>
      H15.059 Scleromalacia perforans, <u>unspecified</u> eye
    H15.09- <u>Other</u> scleritis
        Scleral abscess
      H15.091 Other scleritis, <u>right</u> eye
      H15.092 Other scleritis, <u>left</u> eye
      H15.093 Other scleritis, <u>bilateral</u>
      H15.099 Other scleritis, <u>unspecified</u> eye
  H15.1- <u>Episcleritis</u>
    H15.10- <u>Unspecified</u> episcleritis
      H15.101 Unspecified episcleritis, <u>right</u> eye
      H15.102 Unspecified episcleritis, <u>left</u> eye
      H15.103 Unspecified episcleritis, <u>bilateral</u>
      H15.109 Unspecified episcleritis, <u>unspecified</u> eye
    H15.11- Episcleritis <u>periodica fugax</u>
      H15.111 Episcleritis periodica fugax, <u>right</u> eye
      H15.112 Episcleritis periodica fugax, <u>left</u> eye
      H15.113 Episcleritis periodica fugax, <u>bilateral</u>
      H15.119 Episcleritis periodica fugax, <u>unspecified</u> eye
    H15.12- <u>Nodular</u> episcleritis
      H15.121 Nodular episcleritis, <u>right</u> eye
      H15.122 Nodular episcleritis, <u>left</u> eye
      H15.123 Nodular episcleritis, <u>bilateral</u>

      H15.129 Nodular episcleritis, <u>unspecified</u> eye
H15.8- <u>Other disorders</u> of sclera
    Excludes❷: blue sclera (Q13.5)
              degenerative myopia (H44.2-)
  H15.81- <u>Equatorial staphyloma</u>
    H15.811 Equatorial staphyloma, <u>right</u> eye
    H15.812 Equatorial staphyloma, <u>left</u> eye
    H15.813 Equatorial staphyloma, <u>bilateral</u>
    H15.819 Equatorial staphyloma, <u>unspecified</u> eye
  H15.82- <u>Localized anterior staphyloma</u>
    H15.821 Localized anterior staphyloma, <u>right</u> eye
    H15.822 Localized anterior staphyloma, <u>left</u> eye
    H15.823 Localized anterior staphyloma, <u>bilateral</u>
    H15.829 Localized anterior staphyloma, <u>unspecified</u> eye
  H15.83- <u>Staphyloma posticum</u>
    H15.831 Staphyloma posticum, <u>right</u> eye
    H15.832 Staphyloma posticum, <u>left</u> eye
    H15.833 Staphyloma posticum, <u>bilateral</u>
    H15.839 Staphyloma posticum, <u>unspecified</u> eye
  H15.84- Scleral <u>ectasia</u>
    H15.841 Scleral ectasia, <u>right</u> eye
    H15.842 Scleral ectasia, <u>left</u> eye
    H15.843 Scleral ectasia, <u>bilateral</u>
    H15.849 Scleral ectasia, <u>unspecified</u> eye
  H15.85- <u>Ring staphyloma</u>
    H15.851 Ring staphyloma, <u>right</u> eye
    H15.852 Ring staphyloma, <u>left</u> eye
    H15.853 Ring staphyloma, <u>bilateral</u>
    H15.859 Ring staphyloma, <u>unspecified</u> eye
  H15.89 Other disorders of sclera
H15.9 Unspecified disorder of sclera
H16- <u>Keratitis</u>
  H16.0- <u>Corneal ulcer</u>
    H16.00- <u>Unspecified</u> corneal ulcer
      H16.001 Unspecified corneal ulcer, <u>right</u> eye
      H16.002 Unspecified corneal ulcer, <u>left</u> eye
      H16.003 Unspecified corneal ulcer, <u>bilateral</u>
      H16.009 Unspecified corneal ulcer, <u>unspecified</u> eye
    H16.01- <u>Central</u> corneal ulcer
      H16.011 Central corneal ulcer, <u>right</u> eye
      H16.012 Central corneal ulcer, <u>left</u> eye
      H16.013 Central corneal ulcer, <u>bilateral</u>
      H16.019 Central corneal ulcer, <u>unspecified</u> eye
    H16.02- <u>Ring</u> corneal ulcer
      H16.021 Ring corneal ulcer, <u>right</u> eye
      H16.022 Ring corneal ulcer, <u>left</u> eye
      H16.023 Ring corneal ulcer, <u>bilateral</u>
      H16.029 Ring corneal ulcer, <u>unspecified</u> eye
    H16.03- Corneal ulcer <u>with hypopyon</u>
      H16.031 Corneal ulcer with hypopyon, <u>right</u> eye
      H16.032 Corneal ulcer with hypopyon, <u>left</u> eye
      H16.033 Corneal ulcer with hypopyon, <u>bilateral</u>
      H16.039 Corneal ulcer with hypopyon, <u>unspecified</u> eye
    H16.04- <u>Marginal</u> corneal ulcer
      H16.041 Marginal corneal ulcer, <u>right</u> eye
      H16.042 Marginal corneal ulcer, <u>left</u> eye
      H16.043 Marginal corneal ulcer, <u>bilateral</u>
      H16.049 Marginal corneal ulcer, <u>unspecified</u> eye
    H16.05- <u>Mooren's</u> corneal ulcer
      H16.051 Mooren's corneal ulcer, <u>right</u> eye
      H16.052 Mooren's corneal ulcer, <u>left</u> eye
      H16.053 Mooren's corneal ulcer, <u>bilateral</u>
      H16.059 Mooren's corneal ulcer, <u>unspecified</u> eye
    H16.06- <u>Mycotic</u> corneal ulcer
      H16.061 Mycotic corneal ulcer, <u>right</u> eye
      H16.062 Mycotic corneal ulcer, <u>left</u> eye
      H16.063 Mycotic corneal ulcer, <u>bilateral</u>
      H16.069 Mycotic corneal ulcer, <u>unspecified</u> eye
    H16.07- <u>Perforated</u> corneal ulcer
      H16.071 Perforated corneal ulcer, <u>right</u> eye
      H16.072 Perforated corneal ulcer, <u>left</u> eye
      H16.073 Perforated corneal ulcer, <u>bilateral</u>
      H16.079 Perforated corneal ulcer, <u>unspecified</u> eye

Excludes 1: = NOT CODED HERE! (Do not code both)   **440**   *Excludes❷:* = Not Included Here

© 2013 Channel Publishing, Ltd.

H16.1- Other and <u>unspecified</u> superficial keratitis without conjunctivitis
  H16.10- <u>Unspecified superficial</u> keratitis
    H16.101 Unspecified superficial keratitis, <u>right</u> eye
    H16.102 Unspecified superficial keratitis, <u>left</u> eye
    H16.103 Unspecified superficial keratitis, <u>bilateral</u>
    H16.109 Unspecified superficial keratitis, <u>unspecified</u> eye
  H16.11- <u>Macular</u> keratitis
    Areolar keratitis
    Nummular keratitis
    Stellate keratitis
    Striate keratitis
    H16.111 Macular keratitis, <u>right</u> eye
    H16.112 Macular keratitis, <u>left</u> eye
    H16.113 Macular keratitis, <u>bilateral</u>
    H16.119 Macular keratitis, <u>unspecified</u> eye
  H16.12- <u>Filamentary</u> keratitis
    H16.121 Filamentary keratitis, <u>right</u> eye
    H16.122 Filamentary keratitis, <u>left</u> eye
    H16.123 Filamentary keratitis, <u>bilateral</u>
    H16.129 Filamentary keratitis, <u>unspecified</u> eye
  H16.13- <u>Photokeratitis</u>
    Snow blindness
    Welders keratitis
    H16.131 Photokeratitis, <u>right</u> eye
    H16.132 Photokeratitis, <u>left</u> eye
    H16.133 Photokeratitis, <u>bilateral</u>
    H16.139 Photokeratitis, <u>unspecified</u> eye
  H16.14- <u>Punctate</u> keratitis
    H16.141 Punctate keratitis, <u>right</u> eye
    H16.142 Punctate keratitis, <u>left</u> eye
    H16.143 Punctate keratitis, <u>bilateral</u>
    H16.149 Punctate keratitis, <u>unspecified</u> eye
H16.2- <u>Keratoconjunctivitis</u>
  H16.20- <u>Unspecified</u> keratoconjunctivitis
    Superficial keratitis with conjunctivitis NOS
    H16.201 Unspecified keratoconjunctivitis, <u>right</u> eye
    H16.202 Unspecified keratoconjunctivitis, <u>left</u> eye
    H16.203 Unspecified keratoconjunctivitis, <u>bilateral</u>
    H16.209 Unspecified keratoconjunctivitis, <u>unspecified</u> eye
  H16.21- <u>Exposure</u> keratoconjunctivitis
    H16.211 Exposure keratoconjunctivitis, <u>right</u> eye
    H16.212 Exposure keratoconjunctivitis, <u>left</u> eye
    H16.213 Exposure keratoconjunctivitis, <u>bilateral</u>
    H16.219 Exposure keratoconjunctivitis, <u>unspecified</u> eye
  H16.22- Keratoconjunctivitis <u>sicca, not specified as Sjögren's</u>
    Excludes 1: Sjögren's syndrome (M35.01)
    H16.221 Keratoconjunctivitis sicca, not specified as Sjögren's, <u>right</u> eye
    H16.222 Keratoconjunctivitis sicca, not specified as Sjögren's, <u>left</u> eye
    H16.223 Keratoconjunctivitis sicca, not specified as Sjögren's, <u>bilateral</u>
    H16.229 Keratoconjunctivitis sicca, not specified as Sjögren's, <u>unspecified</u> eye
  H16.23- <u>Neurotrophic</u> keratoconjunctivitis
    H16.231 Neurotrophic keratoconjunctivitis, <u>right</u> eye
    H16.232 Neurotrophic keratoconjunctivitis, <u>left</u> eye
    H16.233 Neurotrophic keratoconjunctivitis, <u>bilateral</u>
    H16.239 Neurotrophic keratoconjunctivitis, <u>unspecified</u> eye
  H16.24- <u>Ophthalmia nodosa</u>
    H16.241 Ophthalmia nodosa, <u>right</u> eye
    H16.242 Ophthalmia nodosa, <u>left</u> eye
    H16.243 Ophthalmia nodosa, <u>bilateral</u>
    H16.249 Ophthalmia nodosa, <u>unspecified</u> eye
  H16.25- <u>Phlyctenular</u> keratoconjunctivitis
    H16.251 Phlyctenular keratoconjunctivitis, <u>right</u> eye
    H16.252 Phlyctenular keratoconjunctivitis, <u>left</u> eye
    H16.253 Phlyctenular keratoconjunctivitis, <u>bilateral</u>
    H16.259 Phlyctenular keratoconjunctivitis, <u>unspecified</u> eye

  H16.26- <u>Vernal</u> keratoconjunctivitis, <u>with limbar and corneal involvement</u>
    Excludes 1: vernal conjunctivitis without limbar and corneal involvement (H10.44)
    H16.261 Vernal keratoconjunctivitis, with limbar and corneal involvement, <u>right</u> eye
    H16.262 Vernal keratoconjunctivitis, with limbar and corneal involvement, <u>left</u> eye
    H16.263 Vernal keratoconjunctivitis, with limbar and corneal involvement, <u>bilateral</u>
    H16.269 Vernal keratoconjunctivitis, with limbar and corneal involvement, <u>unspecified</u> eye
  H16.29- <u>Other</u> keratoconjunctivitis
    H16.291 Other keratoconjunctivitis, <u>right</u> eye
    H16.292 Other keratoconjunctivitis, <u>left</u> eye
    H16.293 Other keratoconjunctivitis, <u>bilateral</u>
    H16.299 Other keratoconjunctivitis, <u>unspecified</u> eye
H16.3- <u>Interstitial and deep</u> keratitis
  H16.30- <u>Unspecified interstitial</u> keratitis
    H16.301 Unspecified interstitial keratitis, <u>right</u> eye
    H16.302 Unspecified interstitial keratitis, <u>left</u> eye
    H16.303 Unspecified interstitial keratitis, <u>bilateral</u>
    H16.309 Unspecified interstitial keratitis, <u>unspecified</u> eye
  H16.31- <u>Corneal abscess</u>
    H16.311 Corneal abscess, <u>right</u> eye
    H16.312 Corneal abscess, <u>left</u> eye
    H16.313 Corneal abscess, <u>bilateral</u>
    H16.319 Corneal abscess, <u>unspecified</u> eye
  H16.32- <u>Diffuse interstitial</u> keratitis
    Cogan's syndrome
    H16.321 Diffuse interstitial keratitis, <u>right</u> eye
    H16.322 Diffuse interstitial keratitis, <u>left</u> eye
    H16.323 Diffuse interstitial keratitis, <u>bilateral</u>
    H16.329 Diffuse interstitial keratitis, <u>unspecified</u> eye
  H16.33- <u>Sclerosing</u> keratitis
    H16.331 Sclerosing keratitis, <u>right</u> eye
    H16.332 Sclerosing keratitis, <u>left</u> eye
    H16.333 Sclerosing keratitis, <u>bilateral</u>
    H16.339 Sclerosing keratitis, <u>unspecified</u> eye
  H16.39- <u>Other interstitial</u> and deep keratitis
    H16.391 Other interstitial and deep keratitis, <u>right</u> eye
    H16.392 Other interstitial and deep keratitis, <u>left</u> eye
    H16.393 Other interstitial and deep keratitis, <u>bilateral</u>
    H16.399 Other interstitial and deep keratitis, <u>unspecified</u> eye
H16.4- <u>Corneal neovascularization</u>
  H16.40- <u>Unspecified</u> corneal neovascularization
    H16.401 Unspecified corneal neovascularization, <u>right</u> eye
    H16.402 Unspecified corneal neovascularization, <u>left</u> eye
    H16.403 Unspecified corneal neovascularization, <u>bilateral</u>
    H16.409 Unspecified corneal neovascularization, <u>unspecified</u> eye
  H16.41- <u>Ghost vessels</u> (corneal)
    H16.411 Ghost vessels (corneal), <u>right</u> eye
    H16.412 Ghost vessels (corneal), <u>left</u> eye
    H16.413 Ghost vessels (corneal), <u>bilateral</u>
    H16.419 Ghost vessels (corneal), <u>unspecified</u> eye
  H16.42- <u>Pannus</u> (corneal)
    H16.421 Pannus (corneal), <u>right</u> eye
    H16.422 Pannus (corneal), <u>left</u> eye
    H16.423 Pannus (corneal), <u>bilateral</u>
    H16.429 Pannus (corneal), <u>unspecified</u> eye
  H16.43- <u>Localized vascularization</u> of cornea
    H16.431 Localized vascularization of cornea, <u>right</u> eye
    H16.432 Localized vascularization of cornea, <u>left</u> eye
    H16.433 Localized vascularization of cornea, <u>bilateral</u>
    H16.439 Localized vascularization of cornea, <u>unspecified</u> eye
  H16.44- <u>Deep vascularization</u> of cornea
    H16.441 Deep vascularization of cornea, <u>right</u> eye
    H16.442 Deep vascularization of cornea, <u>left</u> eye
    H16.443 Deep vascularization of cornea, <u>bilateral</u>
    H16.449 Deep vascularization of cornea, <u>unspecified</u> eye
H16.8   Other keratitis
H16.9   Unspecified keratitis

H1 1 - H 1 6

H17- Corneal scars and opacities
   H17.0- Adherent leukoma
      H17.00 Adherent leukoma, unspecified eye
      H17.01 Adherent leukoma, right eye
      H17.02 Adherent leukoma, left eye
      H17.03 Adherent leukoma, bilateral
   H17.1- Central corneal opacity
      H17.10 Central corneal opacity, unspecified eye
      H17.11 Central corneal opacity, right eye
      H17.12 Central corneal opacity, left eye
      H17.13 Central corneal opacity, bilateral
   H17.8- Other corneal scars and opacities
      H17.81- Minor opacity of cornea
         Corneal nebula
      H17.811 Minor opacity of cornea, right eye
      H17.812 Minor opacity of cornea, left eye
      H17.813 Minor opacity of cornea, bilateral
      H17.819 Minor opacity of cornea, unspecified eye
      H17.82- Peripheral opacity of cornea
      H17.821 Peripheral opacity of cornea, right eye
      H17.822 Peripheral opacity of cornea, left eye
      H17.823 Peripheral opacity of cornea, bilateral
      H17.829 Peripheral opacity of cornea, unspecified eye
      H17.89 Other corneal scars and opacities
   H17.9 Unspecified corneal scar and opacity

H18- Other disorders of cornea
   H18.0- Corneal pigmentations and deposits
      H18.00- Unspecified corneal deposit
      H18.001 Unspecified corneal deposit, right eye
      H18.002 Unspecified corneal deposit, left eye
      H18.003 Unspecified corneal deposit, bilateral
      H18.009 Unspecified corneal deposit, unspecified eye
      H18.01- Anterior corneal pigmentations
         Staehli's line
      H18.011 Anterior corneal pigmentations, right eye
      H18.012 Anterior corneal pigmentations, left eye
      H18.013 Anterior corneal pigmentations, bilateral
      H18.019 Anterior corneal pigmentations, unspecified eye
      H18.02- Argentous corneal deposits
      H18.021 Argentous corneal deposits, right eye
      H18.022 Argentous corneal deposits, left eye
      H18.023 Argentous corneal deposits, bilateral
      H18.029 Argentous corneal deposits, unspecified eye
      H18.03- Corneal deposits in metabolic disorders
         Code also associated metabolic disorder
      H18.031 Corneal deposits in metabolic disorders, right eye
      H18.032 Corneal deposits in metabolic disorders, left eye
      H18.033 Corneal deposits in metabolic disorders, bilateral
      H18.039 Corneal deposits in metabolic disorders, unspecified eye
      H18.04- Kayser-Fleischer ring
         Code also associated Wilson's disease (E83.01)
      H18.041 Kayser-Fleischer ring, right eye
      H18.042 Kayser-Fleischer ring, left eye
      H18.043 Kayser-Fleischer ring, bilateral
      H18.049 Kayser-Fleischer ring, unspecified eye
      H18.05- Posterior corneal pigmentations
         Krukenberg's spindle
      H18.051 Posterior corneal pigmentations, right eye
      H18.052 Posterior corneal pigmentations, left eye
      H18.053 Posterior corneal pigmentations, bilateral
      H18.059 Posterior corneal pigmentations, unspecified eye
      H18.06- Stromal corneal pigmentations
         Hematocornea
      H18.061 Stromal corneal pigmentations, right eye
      H18.062 Stromal corneal pigmentations, left eye
      H18.063 Stromal corneal pigmentations, bilateral
      H18.069 Stromal corneal pigmentations, unspecified eye
   H18.1- Bullous keratopathy
      H18.10 Bullous keratopathy, unspecified eye
      H18.11 Bullous keratopathy, right eye
      H18.12 Bullous keratopathy, left eye
      H18.13 Bullous keratopathy, bilateral

H18.2- Other and unspecified corneal edema
   H18.20 Unspecified corneal edema
   H18.21- Corneal edema secondary to contact lens
      Excludes❷: other corneal disorders due to contact lens (H18.82-)
      H18.211 Corneal edema secondary to contact lens, right eye
      H18.212 Corneal edema secondary to contact lens, left eye
      H18.213 Corneal edema secondary to contact lens, bilateral
      H18.219 Corneal edema secondary to contact lens, unspecified eye
   H18.22- Idiopathic corneal edema
      H18.221 Idiopathic corneal edema, right eye
      H18.222 Idiopathic corneal edema, left eye
      H18.223 Idiopathic corneal edema, bilateral
      H18.229 Idiopathic corneal edema, unspecified eye
   H18.23- Secondary corneal edema
      H18.231 Secondary corneal edema, right eye
      H18.232 Secondary corneal edema, left eye
      H18.233 Secondary corneal edema, bilateral
      H18.239 Secondary corneal edema, unspecified eye
   H18.3- Changes of corneal membranes
      H18.30 Unspecified corneal membrane change
      H18.31- Folds and rupture in Bowman's membrane
      H18.311 Folds and rupture in Bowman's membrane, right eye
      H18.312 Folds and rupture in Bowman's membrane, left eye
      H18.313 Folds and rupture in Bowman's membrane, bilateral
      H18.319 Folds and rupture in Bowman's membrane, unspecified eye
      H18.32- Folds in Descemet's membrane
      H18.321 Folds in Descemet's membrane, right eye
      H18.322 Folds in Descemet's membrane, left eye
      H18.323 Folds in Descemet's membrane, bilateral
      H18.329 Folds in Descemet's membrane, unspecified eye
      H18.33- Rupture in Descemet's membrane
      H18.331 Rupture in Descemet's membrane, right eye
      H18.332 Rupture in Descemet's membrane, left eye
      H18.333 Rupture in Descemet's membrane, bilateral
      H18.339 Rupture in Descemet's membrane, unspecified eye
   H18.4- Corneal degeneration
      Excludes 1: Mooren's ulcer (H16.0-)
      recurrent erosion of cornea (H18.83-)
      H18.40 Unspecified corneal degeneration
      H18.41- Arcus senilis
         Senile corneal changes
      H18.411 Arcus senilis, right eye
      H18.412 Arcus senilis, left eye
      H18.413 Arcus senilis, bilateral
      H18.419 Arcus senilis, unspecified eye
      H18.42- Band keratopathy
      H18.421 Band keratopathy, right eye
      H18.422 Band keratopathy, left eye
      H18.423 Band keratopathy, bilateral
      H18.429 Band keratopathy, unspecified eye
      H18.43 Other calcerous corneal degeneration
      H18.44- Keratomalacia
         Excludes 1: keratomalacia due to vitamin A deficiency (E50.4)
      H18.441 Keratomalacia, right eye
      H18.442 Keratomalacia, left eye
      H18.443 Keratomalacia, bilateral
      H18.449 Keratomalacia, unspecified eye
      H18.45- Nodular corneal degeneration
      H18.451 Nodular corneal degeneration, right eye
      H18.452 Nodular corneal degeneration, left eye
      H18.453 Nodular corneal degeneration, bilateral
      H18.459 Nodular corneal degeneration, unspecified eye
      H18.46- Peripheral corneal degeneration
      H18.461 Peripheral corneal degeneration, right eye
      H18.462 Peripheral corneal degeneration, left eye
      H18.463 Peripheral corneal degeneration, bilateral
      H18.469 Peripheral corneal degeneration, unspecified eye
      H18.49 Other corneal degeneration

H
1
7
-
H
2
0

H18.5- Hereditary corneal dystrophies
  H18.50 Unspecified hereditary corneal dystrophies
  H18.51 Endothelial corneal dystrophy
    Fuchs' dystrophy
  H18.52 Epithelial (juvenile) corneal dystrophy
  H18.53 Granular corneal dystrophy
  H18.54 Lattice corneal dystrophy
  H18.55 Macular corneal dystrophy
  H18.59 Other hereditary corneal dystrophies
H18.6- Keratoconus
  H18.60- Keratoconus, unspecified
    H18.601 Keratoconus, unspecified, right eye
    H18.602 Keratoconus, unspecified, left eye
    H18.603 Keratoconus, unspecified, bilateral
    H18.609 Keratoconus, unspecified, unspecified eye
  H18.61- Keratoconus, stable
    H18.611 Keratoconus, stable, right eye
    H18.612 Keratoconus, stable, left eye
    H18.613 Keratoconus, stable, bilateral
    H18.619 Keratoconus, stable, unspecified eye
  H18.62- Keratoconus, unstable
    Acute hydrops
    H18.621 Keratoconus, unstable, right eye
    H18.622 Keratoconus, unstable, left eye
    H18.623 Keratoconus, unstable, bilateral
    H18.629 Keratoconus, unstable, unspecified eye
H18.7- Other and unspecified corneal deformities
  Excludes 1: congenital malformations of cornea (Q13.3-Q13.4)
  H18.70 Unspecified corneal deformity
  H18.71- Corneal ectasia
    H18.711 Corneal ectasia, right eye
    H18.712 Corneal ectasia, left eye
    H18.713 Corneal ectasia, bilateral
    H18.719 Corneal ectasia, unspecified eye
  H18.72- Corneal staphyloma
    H18.721 Corneal staphyloma, right eye
    H18.722 Corneal staphyloma, left eye
    H18.723 Corneal staphyloma, bilateral
    H18.729 Corneal staphyloma, unspecified eye
  H18.73- Descemetocele
    H18.731 Descemetocele, right eye
    H18.732 Descemetocele, left eye
    H18.733 Descemetocele, bilateral
    H18.739 Descemetocele, unspecified eye
  H18.79- Other corneal deformities
    H18.791 Other corneal deformities, right eye
    H18.792 Other corneal deformities, left eye
    H18.793 Other corneal deformities, bilateral
    H18.799 Other corneal deformities, unspecified eye
H18.8- Other specified disorders of cornea
  H18.81- Anesthesia and hypoesthesia of cornea
    H18.811 Anesthesia and hypoesthesia of cornea, right eye
    H18.812 Anesthesia and hypoesthesia of cornea, left eye
    H18.813 Anesthesia and hypoesthesia of cornea, bilateral
    H18.819 Anesthesia and hypoesthesia of cornea, unspecified eye
  H18.82- Corneal disorder due to contact lens
    Excludes❷: corneal edema due to contact lens (H18.21-)
    H18.821 Corneal disorder due to contact lens, right eye
    H18.822 Corneal disorder due to contact lens, left eye
    H18.823 Corneal disorder due to contact lens, bilateral
    H18.829 Corneal disorder due to contact lens, unspecified eye
  H18.83- Recurrent erosion of cornea
    H18.831 Recurrent erosion of cornea, right eye
    H18.832 Recurrent erosion of cornea, left eye
    H18.833 Recurrent erosion of cornea, bilateral
    H18.839 Recurrent erosion of cornea, unspecified eye
  H18.89- Other specified disorders of cornea
    H18.891 Other specified disorders of cornea, right eye
    H18.892 Other specified disorders of cornea, left eye
    H18.893 Other specified disorders of cornea, bilateral
    H18.899 Other specified disorders of cornea, unspecified eye
H18.9 Unspecified disorder of cornea

H20- Iridocyclitis
  H20.0- Acute and subacute iridocyclitis
    Acute anterior uveitis
    Acute cyclitis
    Acute iritis
    Subacute anterior uveitis
    Subacute cyclitis
    Subacute iritis
    Excludes 1: iridocyclitis, iritis, uveitis (due to) (in) diabetes mellitus (E08-E13 with .39)
    iridocyclitis, iritis, uveitis (due to) (in) diphtheria (A36.89)
    iridocyclitis, iritis, uveitis (due to) (in) gonococcal (A54.32)
    iridocyclitis, iritis, uveitis (due to) (in) herpes (simplex) (B00.51)
    iridocyclitis, iritis, uveitis (due to) (in) herpes zoster (B02.32)
    iridocyclitis, iritis, uveitis (due to) (in) late congenital syphilis (A50.39)
    iridocyclitis, iritis, uveitis (due to) (in) late syphilis (A52.71)
    iridocyclitis, iritis, uveitis (due to) (in) sarcoidosis (D86.83)
    iridocyclitis, iritis, uveitis (due to) (in) syphilis (A51.43)
    iridocyclitis, iritis, uveitis (due to) (in) toxoplasmosis (B58.09)
    iridocyclitis, iritis, uveitis (due to) (in) tuberculosis (A18.54)
  H20.00 Unspecified acute and subacute iridocyclitis
  H20.01- Primary iridocyclitis
    H20.011 Primary iridocyclitis, right eye
    H20.012 Primary iridocyclitis, left eye
    H20.013 Primary iridocyclitis, bilateral
    H20.019 Primary iridocyclitis, unspecified eye
  H20.02- Recurrent acute iridocyclitis
    H20.021 Recurrent acute iridocyclitis, right eye
    H20.022 Recurrent acute iridocyclitis, left eye
    H20.023 Recurrent acute iridocyclitis, bilateral
    H20.029 Recurrent acute iridocyclitis, unspecified eye
  H20.03- Secondary infectious iridocyclitis
    H20.031 Secondary infectious iridocyclitis, right eye
    H20.032 Secondary infectious iridocyclitis, left eye
    H20.033 Secondary infectious iridocyclitis, bilateral
    H20.039 Secondary infectious iridocyclitis, unspecified eye
  H20.04- Secondary noninfectious iridocyclitis
    H20.041 Secondary noninfectious iridocyclitis, right eye
    H20.042 Secondary noninfectious iridocyclitis, left eye
    H20.043 Secondary noninfectious iridocyclitis, bilateral
    H20.049 Secondary noninfectious iridocyclitis, unspecified eye
  H20.05- Hypopyon
    H20.051 Hypopyon, right eye
    H20.052 Hypopyon, left eye
    H20.053 Hypopyon, bilateral
    H20.059 Hypopyon, unspecified eye
  H20.1- Chronic iridocyclitis
    Use additional code for any associated cataract (H26.21-)
    Excludes❷: posterior cyclitis (H30.2-)
  H20.10 Chronic iridocyclitis, unspecified eye
  H20.11 Chronic iridocyclitis, right eye
  H20.12 Chronic iridocyclitis, left eye
  H20.13 Chronic iridocyclitis, bilateral
  H20.2- Lens-induced iridocyclitis
  H20.20 Lens-induced iridocyclitis, unspecified eye
  H20.21 Lens-induced iridocyclitis, right eye
  H20.22 Lens-induced iridocyclitis, left eye
  H20.23 Lens-induced iridocyclitis, bilateral
  H20.8- Other iridocyclitis
    Excludes❷: glaucomatocyclitis crises (H40.4-)
    posterior cyclitis (H30.2-)
    sympathetic uveitis (H44.13-)
  H20.81- Fuchs' heterochromic cyclitis
    H20.811 Fuchs' heterochromic cyclitis, right eye
    H20.812 Fuchs' heterochromic cyclitis, left eye
    H20.813 Fuchs' heterochromic cyclitis, bilateral
    H20.819 Fuchs' heterochromic cyclitis, unspecified eye

H17 - H20

H20.82- Vogt-Koyanagi syndrome
  H20.821 Vogt-Koyanagi syndrome, <u>right</u> eye
  H20.822 Vogt-Koyanagi syndrome, <u>left</u> eye
  H20.823 Vogt-Koyanagi syndrome, <u>bilateral</u>
  H20.829 Vogt-Koyanagi syndrome, <u>unspecified</u> eye
H20.9 Unspecified iridocyclitis
  Uveitis NOS

H21- Other disorders of iris and ciliary body
  Excludes❷: sympathetic uveitis (H44.1-)
H21.0- Hyphema
  Excludes 1: traumatic hyphema (S05.1-)
  H21.00 Hyphema, <u>unspecified</u> eye
  H21.01 Hyphema, <u>right</u> eye
  H21.02 Hyphema, <u>left</u> eye
  H21.03 Hyphema, <u>bilateral</u>
H21.1- Other vascular disorders of iris and ciliary body
  Neovascularization of iris or ciliary body
  Rubeosis iridis
  Rubeosis of iris
H21.1x- Other vascular disorders of iris and ciliary body
  H21.1x1 Other vascular disorders of iris and ciliary body, <u>right</u> eye
  H21.1x2 Other vascular disorders of iris and ciliary body, <u>left</u> eye
  H21.1x3 Other vascular disorders of iris and ciliary body, <u>bilateral</u>
  H21.1x9 Other vascular disorders of iris and ciliary body, <u>unspecified</u> eye
H21.2- Degeneration of iris and ciliary body
H21.21- Degeneration of chamber angle
  H21.211 Degeneration of chamber angle, <u>right</u> eye
  H21.212 Degeneration of chamber angle, <u>left</u> eye
  H21.213 Degeneration of chamber angle, <u>bilateral</u>
  H21.219 Degeneration of chamber angle, <u>unspecified</u> eye
H21.22- Degeneration of ciliary body
  H21.221 Degeneration of ciliary body, <u>right</u> eye
  H21.222 Degeneration of ciliary body, <u>left</u> eye
  H21.223 Degeneration of ciliary body, <u>bilateral</u>
  H21.229 Degeneration of ciliary body, <u>unspecified</u> eye
H21.23- Degeneration of iris (pigmentary)
  Translucency of iris
  H21.231 Degeneration of iris (pigmentary), <u>right</u> eye
  H21.232 Degeneration of iris (pigmentary), <u>left</u> eye
  H21.233 Degeneration of iris (pigmentary), <u>bilateral</u>
  H21.239 Degeneration of iris (pigmentary), <u>unspecified</u> eye
H21.24- Degeneration of pupillary margin
  H21.241 Degeneration of pupillary margin, <u>right</u> eye
  H21.242 Degeneration of pupillary margin, <u>left</u> eye
  H21.243 Degeneration of pupillary margin, <u>bilateral</u>
  H21.249 Degeneration of pupillary margin, <u>unspecified</u> eye
H21.25- Iridoschisis
  H21.251 Iridoschisis, <u>right</u> eye
  H21.252 Iridoschisis, <u>left</u> eye
  H21.253 Iridoschisis, <u>bilateral</u>
  H21.259 Iridoschisis, <u>unspecified</u> eye
H21.26- Iris atrophy (essential) (progressive)
  H21.261 Iris atrophy (essential) (progressive), <u>right</u> eye
  H21.262 Iris atrophy (essential) (progressive), <u>left</u> eye
  H21.263 Iris atrophy (essential) (progressive), <u>bilateral</u>
  H21.269 Iris atrophy (essential) (progressive), <u>unspecified</u> eye
H21.27- Miotic pupillary cyst
  H21.271 Miotic pupillary cyst, <u>right</u> eye
  H21.272 Miotic pupillary cyst, <u>left</u> eye
  H21.273 Miotic pupillary cyst, <u>bilateral</u>
  H21.279 Miotic pupillary cyst, <u>unspecified</u> eye
H21.29 Other iris atrophy
H21.3- Cyst of iris, ciliary body and anterior chamber
  Excludes❷: miotic pupillary cyst (H21.27-)
H21.30- Idiopathic cysts of iris, ciliary body or anterior chamber
  Cyst of iris, ciliary body or anterior chamber NOS
  H21.301 Idiopathic cysts of iris, ciliary body or anterior chamber, <u>right</u> eye
  H21.302 Idiopathic cysts of iris, ciliary body or anterior chamber, <u>left</u> eye
  H21.303 Idiopathic cysts of iris, ciliary body or anterior chamber, <u>bilateral</u>

  H21.309 Idiopathic cysts of iris, ciliary body or anterior chamber, <u>unspecified</u> eye
H21.31- Exudative cysts of iris or anterior chamber
  H21.311 Exudative cysts of iris or anterior chamber, <u>right</u> eye
  H21.312 Exudative cysts of iris or anterior chamber, <u>left</u> eye
  H21.313 Exudative cysts of iris or anterior chamber, <u>bilateral</u>
  H21.319 Exudative cysts of iris or anterior chamber, <u>unspecified</u> eye
H21.32- Implantation cysts of iris, ciliary body or anterior chamber
  H21.321 Implantation cysts of iris, ciliary body or anterior chamber, <u>right</u> eye
  H21.322 Implantation cysts of iris, ciliary body or anterior chamber, <u>left</u> eye
  H21.323 Implantation cysts of iris, ciliary body or anterior chamber, <u>bilateral</u>
  H21.329 Implantation cysts of iris, ciliary body or anterior chamber, <u>unspecified</u> eye
H21.33- Parasitic cyst of iris, ciliary body or anterior chamber
  H21.331 Parasitic cyst of iris, ciliary body or anterior chamber, <u>right</u> eye
  H21.332 Parasitic cyst of iris, ciliary body or anterior chamber, <u>left</u> eye
  H21.333 Parasitic cyst of iris, ciliary body or anterior chamber, <u>bilateral</u>
  H21.339 Parasitic cyst of iris, ciliary body or anterior chamber, <u>unspecified</u> eye
H21.34- Primary cyst of pars plana
  H21.341 Primary cyst of pars plana, <u>right</u> eye
  H21.342 Primary cyst of pars plana, <u>left</u> eye
  H21.343 Primary cyst of pars plana, <u>bilateral</u>
  H21.349 Primary cyst of pars plana, <u>unspecified</u> eye
H21.35- Exudative cyst of pars plana
  H21.351 Exudative cyst of pars plana, <u>right</u> eye
  H21.352 Exudative cyst of pars plana, <u>left</u> eye
  H21.353 Exudative cyst of pars plana, <u>bilateral</u>
  H21.359 Exudative cyst of pars plana, <u>unspecified</u> eye
H21.4- Pupillary membranes
  Iris bombé
  Pupillary occlusion
  Pupillary seclusion
  Excludes 1: congenital pupillary membranes (Q13.8)
  H21.40 Pupillary membranes, <u>unspecified</u> eye
  H21.41 Pupillary membranes, <u>right</u> eye
  H21.42 Pupillary membranes, <u>left</u> eye
  H21.43 Pupillary membranes, <u>bilateral</u>
H21.5- Other and unspecified adhesions and disruptions of iris and ciliary body
  Excludes 1: corectopia (Q13.2)
H21.50- Unspecified adhesions of iris
  Synechia (iris) NOS
  H21.501 Unspecified adhesions of iris, <u>right</u> eye
  H21.502 Unspecified adhesions of iris, <u>left</u> eye
  H21.503 Unspecified adhesions of iris, <u>bilateral</u>
  H21.509 Unspecified adhesions of iris and ciliary body, <u>unspecified</u> eye
H21.51- Anterior synechiae (iris)
  H21.511 Anterior synechiae (iris), <u>right</u> eye
  H21.512 Anterior synechiae (iris), <u>left</u> eye
  H21.513 Anterior synechiae (iris), <u>bilateral</u>
  H21.519 Anterior synechiae (iris), <u>unspecified</u> eye
H21.52- Goniosynechiae
  H21.521 Goniosynechiae, <u>right</u> eye
  H21.522 Goniosynechiae, <u>left</u> eye
  H21.523 Goniosynechiae, <u>bilateral</u>
  H21.529 Goniosynechiae, <u>unspecified</u> eye
H21.53- Iridodialysis
  H21.531 Iridodialysis, <u>right</u> eye
  H21.532 Iridodialysis, <u>left</u> eye
  H21.533 Iridodialysis, <u>bilateral</u>
  H21.539 Iridodialysis, <u>unspecified</u> eye
H21.54- Posterior synechiae (iris)
  H21.541 Posterior synechiae (iris), <u>right</u> eye
  H21.542 Posterior synechiae (iris), <u>left</u> eye
  H21.543 Posterior synechiae (iris), <u>bilateral</u>
  H21.549 Posterior synechiae (iris), <u>unspecified</u> eye

H20-H26

H21.55- **Recession of chamber angle**
  H21.551   Recession of chamber angle, <u>right</u> eye
  H21.552   Recession of chamber angle, <u>left</u> eye
  H21.553   Recession of chamber angle, <u>bilateral</u>
  H21.559   Recession of chamber angle, <u>unspecified</u> eye
H21.56- **Pupillary abnormalities**
  Deformed pupil
  Ectopic pupil
  Rupture of sphincter, pupil
  Excludes 1: congenital deformity of pupil (Q13.2-)
  H21.561   Pupillary abnormality, <u>right</u> eye
  H21.562   Pupillary abnormality, <u>left</u> eye
  H21.563   Pupillary abnormality, <u>bilateral</u>
  H21.569   Pupillary abnormality, <u>unspecified</u> eye
H21.8- **Other specified disorders of iris and ciliary body**
  H21.81   Floppy iris syndrome
    Intraoperative floppy iris syndrome (IFIS)
    Use additional code for adverse effect, if applicable, to identify drug (T36-T50 with fifth or sixth character 5)
  H21.82   Plateau iris syndrome (post-iridectomy) (postprocedural)
  H21.89   Other specified disorders of iris and ciliary body
H21.9   Unspecified disorder of iris and ciliary body
H22   **Disorders of iris and ciliary body in diseases classified elsewhere**
  Code first underlying disease, such as:
  Gout (M1A.-, M10.-)
  Leprosy (A30.-)
  Parasitic disease (B89)

Disorders of lens (H25-H28)

H25- **Age-related cataract**
  Senile cataract
  Excludes❷: capsular glaucoma with pseudoexfoliation of lens (H40.1-)
H25.0- **Age-related incipient cataract**
  H25.01- Cortical age-related cataract
    H25.011   Cortical age-related cataract, <u>right</u> eye
    H25.012   Cortical age-related cataract, <u>left</u> eye
    H25.013   Cortical age-related cataract, <u>bilateral</u>
    H25.019   Cortical age-related cataract, <u>unspecified</u> eye
  H25.03- Anterior subcapsular polar age-related cataract
    H25.031   Anterior subcapsular polar age-related cataract, <u>right</u> eye
    H25.032   Anterior subcapsular polar age-related cataract, <u>left</u> eye
    H25.033   Anterior subcapsular polar age-related cataract, <u>bilateral</u>
    H25.039   Anterior subcapsular polar age-related cataract, <u>unspecified</u> eye
  H25.04- Posterior subcapsular polar age-related cataract
    H25.041   Posterior subcapsular polar age-related cataract, <u>right</u> eye
    H25.042   Posterior subcapsular polar age-related cataract, <u>left</u> eye
    H25.043   Posterior subcapsular polar age-related cataract, <u>bilateral</u>
    H25.049   Posterior subcapsular polar age-related cataract, <u>unspecified</u> eye
  H25.09- Other age-related incipient cataract
    Coronary age-related cataract
    Punctate age-related cataract
    Water clefts
    H25.091   Other age-related incipient cataract, <u>right</u> eye
    H25.092   Other age-related incipient cataract, <u>left</u> eye
    H25.093   Other age-related incipient cataract, <u>bilateral</u>
    H25.099   Other age-related incipient cataract, <u>unspecified</u> eye
H25.1- **Age-related nuclear cataract**
  Cataracta brunescens
  Nuclear sclerosis cataract
  H25.10   Age-related nuclear cataract, <u>unspecified</u> eye
  H25.11   Age-related nuclear cataract, <u>right</u> eye
  H25.12   Age-related nuclear cataract, <u>left</u> eye
  H25.13   Age-related nuclear cataract, <u>bilateral</u>
H25.2- **Age-related cataract, morgagnian type**
  Age-related hypermature cataract
  H25.20   Age-related cataract, morgagnian type, <u>unspecified</u> eye
  H25.21   Age-related cataract, morgagnian type, <u>right</u> eye
  H25.22   Age-related cataract, morgagnian type, <u>left</u> eye
  H25.23   Age-related cataract, morgagnian type, <u>bilateral</u>

H25.8- **Other age-related cataract**
  H25.81- Combined forms of age-related cataract
    H25.811   Combined forms of age-related cataract, <u>right</u> eye
    H25.812   Combined forms of age-related cataract, <u>left</u> eye
    H25.813   Combined forms of age-related cataract, <u>bilateral</u>
    H25.819   Combined forms of age-related cataract, <u>unspecified</u> eye
  H25.89   Other age-related cataract
H25.9   Unspecified age-related cataract
H26- **Other cataract**
  Excludes 1: congenital cataract (Q12.0)
H26.0- **Infantile and juvenile cataract**
  H26.00- Unspecified infantile and juvenile cataract
    H26.001   Unspecified infantile and juvenile cataract, <u>right</u> eye
    H26.002   Unspecified infantile and juvenile cataract, <u>left</u> eye
    H26.003   Unspecified infantile and juvenile cataract, <u>bilateral</u>
    H26.009   Unspecified infantile and juvenile cataract, <u>unspecified</u> eye
  H26.01- Infantile and juvenile cortical, lamellar, or zonular cataract
    H26.011   Infantile and juvenile cortical, lamellar, or zonular cataract, <u>right</u> eye
    H26.012   Infantile and juvenile cortical, lamellar, or zonular cataract, <u>left</u> eye
    H26.013   Infantile and juvenile cortical, lamellar, or zonular cataract, <u>bilateral</u>
    H26.019   Infantile and juvenile cortical, lamellar, or zonular cataract, <u>unspecified</u> eye
  H26.03- Infantile and juvenile nuclear cataract
    H26.031   Infantile and juvenile nuclear cataract, <u>right</u> eye
    H26.032   Infantile and juvenile nuclear cataract, <u>left</u> eye
    H26.033   Infantile and juvenile nuclear cataract, <u>bilateral</u>
    H26.039   Infantile and juvenile nuclear cataract, <u>unspecified</u> eye
  H26.04- Anterior subcapsular polar infantile and juvenile cataract
    H26.041   Anterior subcapsular polar infantile and juvenile cataract, <u>right</u> eye
    H26.042   Anterior subcapsular polar infantile and juvenile cataract, <u>left</u> eye
    H26.043   Anterior subcapsular polar infantile and juvenile cataract, <u>bilateral</u>
    H26.049   Anterior subcapsular polar infantile and juvenile cataract, <u>unspecified</u> eye
  H26.05- Posterior subcapsular polar infantile and juvenile cataract
    H26.051   Posterior subcapsular polar infantile and juvenile cataract, <u>right</u> eye
    H26.052   Posterior subcapsular polar infantile and juvenile cataract, <u>left</u> eye
    H26.053   Posterior subcapsular polar infantile and juvenile cataract, <u>bilateral</u>
    H26.059   Posterior subcapsular polar infantile and juvenile cataract, <u>unspecified</u> eye
  H26.06- Combined forms of infantile and juvenile cataract
    H26.061   Combined forms of infantile and juvenile cataract, <u>right</u> eye
    H26.062   Combined forms of infantile and juvenile cataract, <u>left</u> eye
    H26.063   Combined forms of infantile and juvenile cataract, <u>bilateral</u>
    H26.069   Combined forms of infantile and juvenile cataract, <u>unspecified</u> eye
  H26.09   Other infantile and juvenile cataract
H26.1- **Traumatic cataract**
  Use additional code (Chapter 20) to identify external cause
  H26.10- Unspecified traumatic cataract
    H26.101   Unspecified traumatic cataract, <u>right</u> eye
    H26.102   Unspecified traumatic cataract, <u>left</u> eye
    H26.103   Unspecified traumatic cataract, <u>bilateral</u>
    H26.109   Unspecified traumatic cataract, <u>unspecified</u> eye
  H26.11- Localized traumatic opacities
    H26.111   Localized traumatic opacities, <u>right</u> eye
    H26.112   Localized traumatic opacities, <u>left</u> eye
    H26.113   Localized traumatic opacities, <u>bilateral</u>
    H26.119   Localized traumatic opacities, <u>unspecified</u> eye
  H26.12- Partially resolved traumatic cataract
    H26.121   Partially resolved traumatic cataract, <u>right</u> eye
    H26.122   Partially resolved traumatic cataract, <u>left</u> eye
    H26.123   Partially resolved traumatic cataract, <u>bilateral</u>
    H26.129   Partially resolved traumatic cataract, <u>unspecified</u> eye

H26.13- <u>Total</u> traumatic cataract
    H26.131   Total traumatic cataract, <u>right</u> eye
    H26.132   Total traumatic cataract, <u>left</u> eye
    H26.133   Total traumatic cataract, <u>bilateral</u>
    H26.139   Total traumatic cataract, <u>unspecified</u> eye
H26.2-   <u>Complicated</u> cataract
    H26.20   <u>Unspecified</u> complicated cataract
            Cataracta complicata NOS
    H26.21- Cataract <u>with neovascularization</u>
            Code also associated condition, such as:
            Chronic iridocyclitis (H20.1-)
        H26.211   Cataract with neovascularization, <u>right</u> eye
        H26.212   Cataract with neovascularization, <u>left</u> eye
        H26.213   Cataract with neovascularization, <u>bilateral</u>
        H26.219   Cataract with neovascularization, <u>unspecified</u> eye
    H26.22- Cataract <u>secondary to ocular disorders</u> (degenerative) (inflammatory)
            Code also associated ocular disorder
        H26.221   Cataract secondary to ocular disorders (degenerative) (inflammatory), <u>right</u> eye
        H26.222   Cataract secondary to ocular disorders (degenerative) (inflammatory), <u>left</u> eye
        H26.223   Cataract secondary to ocular disorders (degenerative) (inflammatory), <u>bilateral</u>
        H26.229   Cataract secondary to ocular disorders (degenerative) (inflammatory), <u>unspecified</u> eye
    H26.23- <u>Glaucomatous flecks</u> (subcapsular)
            Code first underlying glaucoma (H40-H42)
        H26.231   Glaucomatous flecks (subcapsular), <u>right</u> eye
        H26.232   Glaucomatous flecks (subcapsular), <u>left</u> eye
        H26.233   Glaucomatous flecks (subcapsular), <u>bilateral</u>
        H26.239   Glaucomatous flecks (subcapsular), <u>unspecified</u> eye
H26.3-   <u>Drug-induced</u> cataract
        Toxic cataract
        Use additional code for adverse effect, if applicable, to identify drug (T36-T50 with fifth or sixth character 5)
    H26.30   Drug-induced cataract, <u>unspecified</u> eye
    H26.31   Drug-induced cataract, <u>right</u> eye
    H26.32   Drug-induced cataract, <u>left</u> eye
    H26.33   Drug-induced cataract, <u>bilateral</u>
H26.4-   <u>Secondary</u> cataract
    H26.40   <u>Unspecified</u> secondary cataract
    H26.41- <u>Soemmering's ring</u>
        H26.411   Soemmering's ring, <u>right</u> eye
        H26.412   Soemmering's ring, <u>left</u> eye
        H26.413   Soemmering's ring, <u>bilateral</u>
        H26.419   Soemmering's ring, <u>unspecified</u> eye
    H26.49- <u>Other</u> secondary cataract
        H26.491   Other secondary cataract, <u>right</u> eye
        H26.492   Other secondary cataract, <u>left</u> eye
        H26.493   Other secondary cataract, <u>bilateral</u>
        H26.499   Other secondary cataract, <u>unspecified</u> eye
H26.8   Other specified cataract
H26.9   Unspecified cataract
H27-   Other disorders of lens
        Excludes 1: congenital lens malformations (Q12.-)
                mechanical complications of intraocular lens implant (T85.2)
                pseudophakia (Z96.1)
    H27.0-   <u>Aphakia</u>
            Acquired absence of lens
            Acquired aphakia
            Aphakia due to trauma
            Excludes 1: cataract extraction status (Z98.4-)
                    congenital absence of lens (Q12.3)
                    congenital aphakia (Q12.3)
        H27.00   Aphakia, <u>unspecified</u> eye
        H27.01   Aphakia, <u>right</u> eye
        H27.02   Aphakia, <u>left</u> eye
        H27.03   Aphakia, <u>bilateral</u>

H27.1-   <u>Dislocation</u> of lens
    H27.10   <u>Unspecified</u> dislocation of lens
    H27.11- <u>Subluxation</u> of lens
        H27.111   Subluxation of lens, <u>right</u> eye
        H27.112   Subluxation of lens, <u>left</u> eye
        H27.113   Subluxation of lens, <u>bilateral</u>
        H27.119   Subluxation of lens, <u>unspecified</u> eye
    H27.12- <u>Anterior</u> dislocation of lens
        H27.121   Anterior dislocation of lens, <u>right</u> eye
        H27.122   Anterior dislocation of lens, <u>left</u> eye
        H27.123   Anterior dislocation of lens, <u>bilateral</u>
        H27.129   Anterior dislocation of lens, <u>unspecified</u> eye
    H27.13- <u>Posterior</u> dislocation of lens
        H27.131   Posterior dislocation of lens, <u>right</u> eye
        H27.132   Posterior dislocation of lens, <u>left</u> eye
        H27.133   Posterior dislocation of lens, <u>bilateral</u>
        H27.139   Posterior dislocation of lens, <u>unspecified</u> eye
H27.8   Other specified disorders of lens
H27.9   Unspecified disorder of lens
H28   Cataract <u>in diseases classified elsewhere</u>
        Code first underlying disease, such as:
            Hypoparathyroidism (E20.-)
            Myotonia (G71.1-)
            Myxedema (E03.-)
            Protein-calorie malnutrition (E40-E46)
        Excludes 1: cataract in diabetes mellitus (E08.36, E09.36, E10.36, E11.36, E13.36)

Disorders of choroid and retina (H30-H36)

H30-   <u>Chorioretinal inflammation</u>
    H30.0-   <u>Focal</u> chorioretinal inflammation
            Focal chorioretinitis
            Focal choroiditis
            Focal retinitis
            Focal retinochoroiditis
        H30.00- <u>Unspecified</u> focal chorioretinal inflammation
                Focal chorioretinitis NOS
                Focal choroiditis NOS
                Focal retinitis NOS
                Focal retinochoroiditis NOS
            H30.001   Unspecified focal chorioretinal inflammation, <u>right</u> eye
            H30.002   Unspecified focal chorioretinal inflammation, <u>left</u> eye
            H30.003   Unspecified focal chorioretinal inflammation, <u>bilateral</u>
            H30.009   Unspecified focal chorioretinal inflammation, <u>unspecified</u> eye
        H30.01- Focal chorioretinal inflammation, <u>juxtapapillary</u>
            H30.011   Focal chorioretinal inflammation, juxtapapillary, <u>right</u> eye
            H30.012   Focal chorioretinal inflammation, juxtapapillary, <u>left</u> eye
            H30.013   Focal chorioretinal inflammation, juxtapapillary, <u>bilateral</u>
            H30.019   Focal chorioretinal inflammation, juxtapapillary, <u>unspecified</u> eye
        H30.02- Focal chorioretinal inflammation of <u>posterior pole</u>
            H30.021   Focal chorioretinal inflammation of posterior pole, <u>right</u> eye
            H30.022   Focal chorioretinal inflammation of posterior pole, <u>left</u> eye
            H30.023   Focal chorioretinal inflammation of posterior pole, <u>bilateral</u>
            H30.029   Focal chorioretinal inflammation of posterior pole, <u>unspecified</u> eye
        H30.03- Focal chorioretinal inflammation, <u>peripheral</u>
            H30.031   Focal chorioretinal inflammation, peripheral, <u>right</u> eye
            H30.032   Focal chorioretinal inflammation, peripheral, <u>left</u> eye
            H30.033   Focal chorioretinal inflammation, peripheral, <u>bilateral</u>
            H30.039   Focal chorioretinal inflammation, peripheral, <u>unspecified</u> eye
        H30.04- Focal chorioretinal inflammation, <u>macular or paramacular</u>
            H30.041   Focal chorioretinal inflammation, macular or paramacular, <u>right</u> eye
            H30.042   Focal chorioretinal inflammation, macular or paramacular, <u>left</u> eye
            H30.043   Focal chorioretinal inflammation, macular or paramacular, <u>bilateral</u>
            H30.049   Focal chorioretinal inflammation, macular or paramacular, <u>unspecified</u> eye

H
2
6
-
H
3
1

H30.1- **Disseminated** choriretinal inflammation
    Disseminated chorioretinitis
    Disseminated choroiditis
    Disseminated retinitis
    Disseminated retinochoroiditis
    Excludes❷: exudative retinopathy (H35.02-)

H30.10- **Unspecified** disseminated choriretinal inflammation
    Disseminated chorioretinitis NOS
    Disseminated choroiditis NOS
    Disseminated retinitis NOS
    Disseminated retinochoroiditis NOS
    H30.101 Unspecified disseminated chorioretinal inflammation, **right** eye
    H30.102 Unspecified disseminated chorioretinal inflammation, **left** eye
    H30.103 Unspecified disseminated chorioretinal inflammation, **bilateral**
    H30.109 Unspecified disseminated chorioretinal inflammation, **unspecified** eye

H30.11- Disseminated chorioretinal inflammation of **posterior pole**
    H30.111 Disseminated chorioretinal inflammation of posterior pole, **right** eye
    H30.112 Disseminated chorioretinal inflammation of posterior pole, **left** eye
    H30.113 Disseminated chorioretinal inflammation of posterior pole, **bilateral**
    H30.119 Disseminated chorioretinal inflammation of posterior pole, **unspecified** eye

H30.12- Disseminated chorioretinal inflammation, **peripheral**
    H30.121 Disseminated chorioretinal inflammation, peripheral **right** eye
    H30.122 Disseminated chorioretinal inflammation, peripheral, **left** eye
    H30.123 Disseminated chorioretinal inflammation, peripheral, **bilateral**
    H30.129 Disseminated chorioretinal inflammation, peripheral, **unspecified** eye

H30.13- Disseminated chorioretinal inflammation, **generalized**
    H30.131 Disseminated chorioretinal inflammation, generalized, **right** eye
    H30.132 Disseminated chorioretinal inflammation, generalized, **left** eye
    H30.133 Disseminated chorioretinal inflammation, generalized, **bilateral**
    H30.139 Disseminated chorioretinal inflammation, generalized, **unspecified** eye

H30.14- **Acute posterior multifocal placoid pigment epitheliopathy**
    H30.141 Acute posterior multifocal placoid pigment epitheliopathy, **right** eye
    H30.142 Acute posterior multifocal placoid pigment epitheliopathy, **left** eye
    H30.143 Acute posterior multifocal placoid pigment epitheliopathy, **bilateral**
    H30.149 Acute posterior multifocal placoid pigment epitheliopathy, **unspecified** eye

H30.2- **Posterior cyclitis**
    Pars planitis
    H30.20 Posterior cyclitis, **unspecified** eye
    H30.21 Posterior cyclitis, **right** eye
    H30.22 Posterior cyclitis, **left** eye
    H30.23 Posterior cyclitis, **bilateral**

H30.8- **Other** chorioretinal inflammations
H30.81- **Harada's disease**
    H30.811 Harada's disease, **right** eye
    H30.812 Harada's disease, **left** eye
    H30.813 Harada's disease, **bilateral**
    H30.819 Harada's disease, **unspecified** eye

H30.89- **Other** chorioretinal inflammations
    H30.891 Other chorioretinal inflammations, **right** eye
    H30.892 Other chorioretinal inflammations, **left** eye
    H30.893 Other chorioretinal inflammations, **bilateral**
    H30.899 Other chorioretinal inflammations, **unspecified** eye

H30.9- **Unspecified** chorioretinal inflammation
    Chorioretinitis NOS
    Choroiditis NOS
    Neuroretinitis NOS
    Retinitis NOS
    Retinochoroiditis NOS
    H30.90 Unspecified chorioretinal inflammation, **unspecified** eye
    H30.91 Unspecified chorioretinal inflammation, **right** eye
    H30.92 Unspecified chorioretinal inflammation, **left** eye
    H30.93 Unspecified chorioretinal inflammation, **bilateral**

H31- **Other disorders of choroid**
H31.0- **Chorioretinal scars**
    Excludes❷: postsurgical chorioretinal scars (H59.81-)

H31.00- **Unspecified** chorioretinal scars
    H31.001 Unspecified chorioretinal scars, **right** eye
    H31.002 Unspecified chorioretinal scars, **left** eye
    H31.003 Unspecified chorioretinal scars, **bilateral**
    H31.009 Unspecified chorioretinal scars, **unspecified** eye

H31.01- **Macula scars** of posterior pole (postinflammatory) (post-traumatic)
    Excludes 1: postprocedural choriorentinal scar (H59.81-)
    H31.011 Macula scars of posterior pole (postinflammatory) (post-traumatic), **right** eye
    H31.012 Macula scars of posterior pole (postinflammatory) (post-traumatic), **left** eye
    H31.013 Macula scars of posterior pole (postinflammatory) (post-traumatic), **bilateral**
    H31.019 Macula scars of posterior pole (postinflammatory) (post-traumatic), **unspecified** eye

H31.02- **Solar retinopathy**
    H31.021 Solar retinopathy, **right** eye
    H31.022 Solar retinopathy, **left** eye
    H31.023 Solar retinopathy, **bilateral**
    H31.029 Solar retinopathy, **unspecified** eye

H31.09- **Other** chorioretinal scars
    H31.091 Other chorioretinal scars, **right** eye
    H31.092 Other chorioretinal scars, **left** eye
    H31.093 Other chorioretinal scars, **bilateral**
    H31.099 Other chorioretinal scars, **unspecified** eye

H31.1- **Choroidal degeneration**
    Excludes❷: angioid streaks of macula (H35.33)

H31.10- **Unspecified** choroidal degeneration
    Choroidal sclerosis NOS
    H31.101 Choroidal degeneration, unspecified, **right** eye
    H31.102 Choroidal degeneration, unspecified, **left** eye
    H31.103 Choroidal degeneration, unspecified, **bilateral**
    H31.109 Choroidal degeneration, unspecified, **unspecified** eye

H31.11- **Age-related choroidal atrophy**
    H31.111 Age-related choroidal atrophy, **right** eye
    H31.112 Age-related choroidal atrophy, **left** eye
    H31.113 Age-related choroidal atrophy, **bilateral**
    H31.119 Age-related choroidal atrophy, **unspecified** eye

H31.12- **Diffuse secondary atrophy** of choroid
    H31.121 Diffuse secondary atrophy of choroid, **right** eye
    H31.122 Diffuse secondary atrophy of choroid, **left** eye
    H31.123 Diffuse secondary atrophy of choroid, **bilateral**
    H31.129 Diffuse secondary atrophy of choroid, **unspecified** eye

H31.2- **Hereditary choroidal dystrophy**
    Excludes❷: hyperornithinemia (E72.4)
    ornithinemia (E72.4)
    H31.20 Hereditary choroidal dystrophy, unspecified
    H31.21 Choroideremia
    H31.22 Choroidal dystrophy (central areolar) (generalized) (peripapillary)
    H31.23 Gyrate atrophy, choroid
    H31.29 Other hereditary choroidal dystrophy

H31.3- **Choroidal hemorrhage and rupture**
H31.30- **Unspecified** choroidal hemorrhage
    H31.301 Unspecified choroidal hemorrhage, **right** eye
    H31.302 Unspecified choroidal hemorrhage, **left** eye
    H31.303 Unspecified choroidal hemorrhage, **bilateral**
    H31.309 Unspecified choroidal hemorrhage, **unspecified** eye

H31.31- **Expulsive** choroidal hemorrhage
    H31.311 Expulsive choroidal hemorrhage, **right** eye
    H31.312 Expulsive choroidal hemorrhage, **left** eye
    H31.313 Expulsive choroidal hemorrhage, **bilateral**
    H31.319 Expulsive choroidal hemorrhage, **unspecified** eye

H
2
6
–
H
3
1

Excludes 1: = NOT CODED HERE! (Do not code both)

Excludes❷: = Not Included Here

H31.32- Choroidal <u>rupture</u>
    H31.321   Choroidal rupture, <u>right</u> eye
    H31.322   Choroidal rupture, <u>left</u> eye
    H31.323   Choroidal rupture, <u>bilateral</u>
    H31.329   Choroidal rupture, <u>unspecified</u> eye
H31.4- Choroidal <u>detachment</u>
  H31.40- <u>Unspecified</u> choroidal detachment
    H31.401   Unspecified choroidal detachment, <u>right</u> eye
    H31.402   Unspecified choroidal detachment, <u>left</u> eye
    H31.403   Unspecified choroidal detachment, <u>bilateral</u>
    H31.409   Unspecified choroidal detachment, <u>unspecified</u> eye
  H31.41- <u>Hemorrhagic</u> choroidal detachment
    H31.411   Hemorrhagic choroidal detachment, <u>right</u> eye
    H31.412   Hemorrhagic choroidal detachment, <u>left</u> eye
    H31.413   Hemorrhagic choroidal detachment, <u>bilateral</u>
    H31.419   Hemorrhagic choroidal detachment, <u>unspecified</u> eye
  H31.42- <u>Serous</u> choroidal detachment
    H31.421   Serous choroidal detachment, <u>right</u> eye
    H31.422   Serous choroidal detachment, <u>left</u> eye
    H31.423   Serous choroidal detachment, <u>bilateral</u>
    H31.429   Serous choroidal detachment, <u>unspecified</u> eye
H31.8   Other specified disorders of choroid
H31.9   Unspecified disorder of choroid
H32 Chorioretinal disorders <u>in diseases classified elsewhere</u>
   Code first underlying disease, such as:
    Congenital toxoplasmosis (P37.1)
    Histoplasmosis (B39.-)
    Leprosy (A30.-)
   Excludes 1: chorioretinitis (in):
      toxoplasmosis (acquired) (B58.01)
      tuberculosis (A18.53)
H33- Retinal detachments and breaks
   Excludes 1: detachment of retinal pigment epithelium (H35.72-, H35.73-)
  H33.0- <u>Retinal detachment with retinal break</u>
    Rhegmatogenous retinal detachment
   Excludes 1: serous retinal detachment (without retinal break) (H33.2-)
  H33.00- <u>Unspecified</u> retinal detachment with retinal break
    H33.001   Unspecified retinal detachment with retinal break, <u>right</u> eye
    H33.002   Unspecified retinal detachment with retinal break, <u>left</u> eye
    H33.003   Unspecified retinal detachment with retinal break, <u>bilateral</u>
    H33.009   Unspecified retinal detachment with retinal break, <u>unspecified</u> eye
  H33.01- Retinal detachment with <u>single break</u>
    H33.011   Retinal detachment with single break, <u>right</u> eye
    H33.012   Retinal detachment with single break, <u>left</u> eye
    H33.013   Retinal detachment with single break, <u>bilateral</u>
    H33.019   Retinal detachment with single break, <u>unspecified</u> eye
  H33.02- Retinal detachment with <u>multiple</u> breaks
    H33.021   Retinal detachment with multiple breaks, <u>right</u> eye
    H33.022   Retinal detachment with multiple breaks, <u>left</u> eye
    H33.023   Retinal detachment with multiple breaks, <u>bilateral</u>
    H33.029   Retinal detachment with multiple breaks, <u>unspecified</u> eye
  H33.03- Retinal detachment with <u>giant retinal tear</u>
    H33.031   Retinal detachment with giant retinal tear, <u>right</u> eye
    H33.032   Retinal detachment with giant retinal tear, <u>left</u> eye
    H33.033   Retinal detachment with giant retinal tear, <u>bilateral</u>
    H33.039   Retinal detachment with giant retinal tear, <u>unspecified</u> eye
  H33.04- Retinal detachment with <u>retinal dialysis</u>
    H33.041   Retinal detachment with retinal dialysis, <u>right</u> eye
    H33.042   Retinal detachment with retinal dialysis, <u>left</u> eye
    H33.043   Retinal detachment with retinal dialysis, <u>bilateral</u>
    H33.049   Retinal detachment with retinal dialysis, <u>unspecified</u> eye
  H33.05- <u>Total</u> retinal detachment
    H33.051   Total retinal detachment, <u>right</u> eye
    H33.052   Total retinal detachment, <u>left</u> eye
    H33.053   Total retinal detachment, <u>bilateral</u>
    H33.059   Total retinal detachment, <u>unspecified</u> eye

H33.1- <u>Retinoschisis</u> and retinal cysts
   Excludes 1: congenital retinoschisis (Q14.1)
      microcystoid degeneration of retina (H35.42-)
  H33.10- <u>Unspecified</u> retinoschisis
    H33.101   Unspecified retinoschisis, <u>right</u> eye
    H33.102   Unspecified retinoschisis, <u>left</u> eye
    H33.103   Unspecified retinoschisis, <u>bilateral</u>
    H33.109   Unspecified retinoschisis, <u>unspecified</u> eye
  H33.11- <u>C</u>yst of ora serrata
    H33.111   Cyst of ora serrata, <u>right</u> eye
    H33.112   Cyst of ora serrata, <u>left</u> eye
    H33.113   Cyst of ora serrata, <u>bilateral</u>
    H33.119   Cyst of ora serrata, <u>unspecified</u> eye
  H33.12- Parasitic cyst of retina
    H33.121   Parasitic cyst of retina, <u>right</u> eye
    H33.122   Parasitic cyst of retina, <u>left</u> eye
    H33.123   Parasitic cyst of retina, <u>bilateral</u>
    H33.129   Parasitic cyst of retina, <u>unspecified</u> eye
  H33.19- <u>Other</u> retinoschisis and retinal cysts
    Pseudocyst of retina
    H33.191   Other retinoschisis and retinal cysts, <u>right</u> eye
    H33.192   Other retinoschisis and retinal cysts, <u>left</u> eye
    H33.193   Other retinoschisis and retinal cysts, <u>bilateral</u>
    H33.199   Other retinoschisis and retinal cysts, <u>unspecified</u> eye
H33.2- <u>Serous retinal detachment</u>
    Retinal detachment NOS
    Retinal detachment without retinal break
   Excludes 1: central serous chorioretinopathy (H35.71-)
  H33.20 Serous retinal detachment, <u>unspecified</u> eye
  H33.21 Serous retinal detachment, <u>right</u> eye
  H33.22 Serous retinal detachment, <u>left</u> eye
  H33.23 Serous retinal detachment, <u>bilateral</u>
H33.3- <u>Retinal breaks without detachment</u>
   Excludes 1: chorioretinal scars after surgery for detachment (H59.81-)
      peripheral retinal degeneration without break (H35.4-)
  H33.30- <u>Unspecified</u> retinal break
    H33.301   Unspecified retinal break, <u>right</u> eye
    H33.302   Unspecified retinal break, <u>left</u> eye
    H33.303   Unspecified retinal break, <u>bilateral</u>
    H33.309   Unspecified retinal break, <u>unspecified</u> eye
  H33.31- <u>Horseshoe tear</u> of retina without detachment
    Operculum of retina without detachment
    H33.311   Horseshoe tear of retina without detachment, <u>right</u> eye
    H33.312   Horseshoe tear of retina without detachment, <u>left</u> eye
    H33.313   Horseshoe tear of retina without detachment, <u>bilateral</u>
    H33.319   Horseshoe tear of retina without detachment, <u>unspecified</u> eye
  H33.32- <u>Round hole</u> of retina without detachment
    H33.321   Round hole, <u>right</u> eye
    H33.322   Round hole, <u>left</u> eye
    H33.323   Round hole, <u>bilateral</u>
    H33.329   Round hole, <u>unspecified</u> eye
  H33.33- <u>Multiple defects</u> of retina without detachment
    H33.331   Multiple defects of retina without detachment, <u>right</u> eye
    H33.332   Multiple defects of retina without detachment, <u>left</u> eye
    H33.333   Multiple defects of retina without detachment, <u>bilateral</u>
    H33.339   Multiple defects of retina without detachment, <u>unspecified</u> eye
H33.4- <u>Traction</u> detachment of retina
    Proliferative vitreo-retinopathy with retinal detachment
  H33.40 Traction detachment of retina, <u>unspecified</u> eye
  H33.41 Traction detachment of retina, <u>right</u> eye
  H33.42 Traction detachment of retina, <u>left</u> eye
  H33.43 Traction detachment of retina, <u>bilateral</u>
H33.8   Other retinal detachments
H34- Retinal vascular occlusions
   Excludes 1: amaurosis fugax (G45.3)
  H34.0- <u>Transient retinal artery occlusion</u>
  H34.00 Transient retinal artery occlusion, <u>unspecified</u> eye
  H34.01 Transient retinal artery occlusion, <u>right</u> eye
  H34.02 Transient retinal artery occlusion, <u>left</u> eye
  H34.03 Transient retinal artery occlusion, <u>bilateral</u>

H31 - H35

© 2013 Channel Publishing Ltd

H34.1- Central retinal artery occlusion
  H34.10 Central retinal artery occlusion, unspecified eye
  H34.11 Central retinal artery occlusion, right eye
  H34.12 Central retinal artery occlusion, left eye
  H34.13 Central retinal artery occlusion, bilateral
H34.2- Other retinal artery occlusions
  H34.21- Partial retinal artery occlusion
    Hollenhorst's plaque
    Retinal microembolism
    H34.211 Partial retinal artery occlusion, right eye
    H34.212 Partial retinal artery occlusion, left eye
    H34.213 Partial retinal artery occlusion, bilateral
    H34.219 Partial retinal artery occlusion, unspecified eye
  H34.23- Retinal artery branch occlusion
    H34.231 Retinal artery branch occlusion, right eye
    H34.232 Retinal artery branch occlusion, left eye
    H34.233 Retinal artery branch occlusion, bilateral
    H34.239 Retinal artery branch occlusion, unspecified eye
H34.8- Other retinal vascular occlusions
  H34.81- Central retinal vein occlusion
    H34.811 Central retinal vein occlusion, right eye
    H34.812 Central retinal vein occlusion, left eye
    H34.813 Central retinal vein occlusion, bilateral
    H34.819 Central retinal vein occlusion, unspecified eye
  H34.82- Venous engorgement
    Incipient retinal vein occlusion
    Partial retinal vein occlusion
    H34.821 Venous engorgement, right eye
    H34.822 Venous engorgement, left eye
    H34.823 Venous engorgement, bilateral
    H34.829 Venous engorgement, unspecified eye
  H34.83- Tributary (branch) retinal vein occlusion
    H34.831 Tributary (branch) retinal vein occlusion, right eye
    H34.832 Tributary (branch) retinal vein occlusion, left eye
    H34.833 Tributary (branch) retinal vein occlusion, bilateral
    H34.839 Tributary (branch) retinal vein occlusion, unspecified eye
H34.9 Unspecified retinal vascular occlusion
H35- Other retinal disorders
  Excludes❷: diabetic retinal disorders (E08.311- E08.359, E09.311- E09.359, E10.311- E10.359, E11.311- E11.359, E13.311- E13.359)
H35.0- Background retinopathy and retinal vascular changes
  Code also any associated hypertension (I10.-)
  H35.00 Unspecified background retinopathy
  H35.01- Changes in retinal vascular appearance
    Retinal vascular sheathing
    H35.011 Changes in retinal vascular appearance, right eye
    H35.012 Changes in retinal vascular appearance, left eye
    H35.013 Changes in retinal vascular appearance, bilateral
    H35.019 Changes in retinal vascular appearance, unspecified eye
  H35.02- Exudative retinopathy
    Coats retinopathy
    H35.021 Exudative retinopathy, right eye
    H35.022 Exudative retinopathy, left eye
    H35.023 Exudative retinopathy, bilateral
    H35.029 Exudative retinopathy, unspecified eye
  H35.03- Hypertensive retinopathy
    H35.031 Hypertensive retinopathy, right eye
    H35.032 Hypertensive retinopathy, left eye
    H35.033 Hypertensive retinopathy, bilateral
    H35.039 Hypertensive retinopathy, unspecified eye
  H35.04- Retinal micro-aneurysms, unspecified
    H35.041 Retinal micro-aneurysms, unspecified, right eye
    H35.042 Retinal micro-aneurysms, unspecified, left eye
    H35.043 Retinal micro-aneurysms, unspecified, bilateral
    H35.049 Retinal micro-aneurysms, unspecified, unspecified eye
  H35.05- Retinal neovascularization, unspecified
    H35.051 Retinal neovascularization, unspecified, right eye
    H35.052 Retinal neovascularization, unspecified, left eye
    H35.053 Retinal neovascularization, unspecified, bilateral
    H35.059 Retinal neovascularization, unspecified, unspecified eye

H35.06- Retinal vasculitis
  Eales disease
  Retinal perivasculitis
  H35.061 Retinal vasculitis, right eye
  H35.062 Retinal vasculitis, left eye
  H35.063 Retinal vasculitis, bilateral
  H35.069 Retinal vasculitis, unspecified eye
H35.07- Retinal telangiectasis
  H35.071 Retinal telangiectasis, right eye
  H35.072 Retinal telangiectasis, left eye
  H35.073 Retinal telangiectasis, bilateral
  H35.079 Retinal telangiectasis, unspecified eye
H35.09 Other intraretinal microvascular abnormalities
  Retinal varices
H35.1- Retinopathy of prematurity
  H35.10- Retinopathy of prematurity, unspecified
    Retinopathy of prematurity NOS
    H35.101 Retinopathy of prematurity, unspecified, right eye
    H35.102 Retinopathy of prematurity, unspecified, left eye
    H35.103 Retinopathy of prematurity, unspecified, bilateral
    H35.109 Retinopathy of prematurity, unspecified, unspecified eye
  H35.11- Retinopathy of prematurity, stage 0
    H35.111 Retinopathy of prematurity, stage 0, right eye
    H35.112 Retinopathy of prematurity, stage 0, left eye
    H35.113 Retinopathy of prematurity, stage 0, bilateral
    H35.119 Retinopathy of prematurity, stage 0, unspecified eye
  H35.12- Retinopathy of prematurity, stage 1
    H35.121 Retinopathy of prematurity, stage 1, right eye
    H35.122 Retinopathy of prematurity, stage 1, left eye
    H35.123 Retinopathy of prematurity, stage 1, bilateral
    H35.129 Retinopathy of prematurity, stage 1, unspecified eye
  H35.13- Retinopathy of prematurity, stage 2
    H35.131 Retinopathy of prematurity, stage 2, right eye
    H35.132 Retinopathy of prematurity, stage 2, left eye
    H35.133 Retinopathy of prematurity, stage 2, bilateral
    H35.139 Retinopathy of prematurity, stage 2, unspecified eye
  H35.14- Retinopathy of prematurity, stage 3
    H35.141 Retinopathy of prematurity, stage 3, right eye
    H35.142 Retinopathy of prematurity, stage 3, left eye
    H35.143 Retinopathy of prematurity, stage 3, bilateral
    H35.149 Retinopathy of prematurity, stage 3, unspecified eye
  H35.15- Retinopathy of prematurity, stage 4
    H35.151 Retinopathy of prematurity, stage 4, right eye
    H35.152 Retinopathy of prematurity, stage 4, left eye
    H35.153 Retinopathy of prematurity, stage 4, bilateral
    H35.159 Retinopathy of prematurity, stage 4, unspecified eye
  H35.16- Retinopathy of prematurity, stage 5
    H35.161 Retinopathy of prematurity, stage 5, right eye
    H35.162 Retinopathy of prematurity, stage 5, left eye
    H35.163 Retinopathy of prematurity, stage 5, bilateral
    H35.169 Retinopathy of prematurity, stage 5, unspecified eye
  H35.17- Retrolental fibroplasia
    H35.171 Retrolental fibroplasia, right eye
    H35.172 Retrolental fibroplasia, left eye
    H35.173 Retrolental fibroplasia, bilateral
    H35.179 Retrolental fibroplasia, unspecified eye
H35.2- Other non-diabetic proliferative retinopathy
  Proliferative vitreo-retinopathy
  Excludes 1: proliferative vitreo-retinopathy with retinal detachment (H33.4-)
  H35.20 Other non-diabetic proliferative retinopathy, unspecified eye
  H35.21 Other non-diabetic proliferative retinopathy, right eye
  H35.22 Other non-diabetic proliferative retinopathy, left eye
  H35.23 Other non-diabetic proliferative retinopathy, bilateral
H35.3- Degeneration of macula and posterior pole
  H35.30 Unspecified macular degeneration
    Age-related macular degeneration
  H35.31 Nonexudative age-related macular degeneration
    Atrophic age-related macular degeneration
  H35.32 Exudative age-related macular degeneration
  H35.33 Angioid streaks of macula
  H35.34- Macular cyst, hole, or pseudohole
    H35.341 Macular cyst, hole, or pseudohole, right eye
    H35.342 Macular cyst, hole, or pseudohole, left eye
    H35.343 Macular cyst, hole, or pseudohole, bilateral

H3 1 - H3 5

H35.349   Macular cyst, hole, or pseudohole, <u>unspecified</u> eye
H35.35- <u>Cystoid macular degeneration</u>
    Excludes 1: cystoid macular edema following cataract surgery
        (H59.03-)
    H35.351   Cystoid macular degeneration, <u>right</u> eye
    H35.352   Cystoid macular degeneration, <u>left</u> eye
    H35.353   Cystoid macular degeneration, <u>bilateral</u>
    H35.359   Cystoid macular degeneration, <u>unspecified</u> eye
H35.36- <u>Drusen (degenerative) of macula</u>
    H35.361   Drusen (degenerative) of macula, <u>right</u> eye
    H35.362   Drusen (degenerative) of macula, <u>left</u> eye
    H35.363   Drusen (degenerative) of macula, <u>bilateral</u>
    H35.369   Drusen (degenerative) of macula, <u>unspecified</u> eye
H35.37- Puckering of macula
    H35.371   Puckering of macula, <u>right</u> eye
    H35.372   Puckering of macula, <u>left</u> eye
    H35.373   Puckering of macula, <u>bilateral</u>
    H35.379   Puckering of macula, <u>unspecified</u> eye
H35.38- <u>Toxic maculopathy</u>
    Code first poisoning due to drug or toxin, if applicable (T36-T65
      with fifth or sixth character 1-4 or 6)
    Use additional code for adverse effect, if applicable, to identify
      drug (T36-T50 with fifth or sixth character 5)
    H35.381   Toxic maculopathy, <u>right</u> eye
    H35.382   Toxic maculopathy, <u>left</u> eye
    H35.383   Toxic maculopathy, <u>bilateral</u>
    H35.389   Toxic maculopathy, <u>unspecified</u> eye
H35.4- <u>Peripheral retinal degeneration</u>
    Excludes 1: hereditary retinal degeneration (dystrophy) (H35.5-)
        peripheral retinal degeneration with retinal break
        (H33.3-)
H35.40   <u>Unspecified</u> peripheral retinal degeneration
H35.41- <u>Lattice</u> degeneration of retina
    Palisade degeneration of retina
    H35.411   Lattice degeneration of retina, <u>right</u> eye
    H35.412   Lattice degeneration of retina, <u>left</u> eye
    H35.413   Lattice degeneration of retina, <u>bilateral</u>
    H35.419   Lattice degeneration of retina, <u>unspecified</u> eye
H35.42- <u>Microcystoid</u> degeneration of retina
    H35.421   Microcystoid degeneration of retina, <u>right</u> eye
    H35.422   Microcystoid degeneration of retina, <u>left</u> eye
    H35.423   Microcystoid degeneration of retina, <u>bilateral</u>
    H35.429   Microcystoid degeneration of retina, <u>unspecified</u> eye
H35.43- <u>Paving stone</u> degeneration of retina
    H35.431   Paving stone degeneration of retina, <u>right</u> eye
    H35.432   Paving stone degeneration of retina, <u>left</u> eye
    H35.433   Paving stone degeneration of retina, <u>bilateral</u>
    H35.439   Paving stone degeneration of retina, <u>unspecified</u> eye
H35.44- Age-related reticular degeneration of retina
    H35.441   Age-related reticular degeneration of retina, <u>right</u> eye
    H35.442   Age-related reticular degeneration of retina, <u>left</u> eye
    H35.443   Age-related reticular degeneration of retina, <u>bilateral</u>
    H35.449   Age-related reticular degeneration of retina,
         <u>unspecified</u> eye
H35.45- <u>Secondary pigmentary</u> degeneration
    H35.451   Secondary pigmentary degeneration, <u>right</u> eye
    H35.452   Secondary pigmentary degeneration, <u>left</u> eye
    H35.453   Secondary pigmentary degeneration, <u>bilateral</u>
    H35.459   Secondary pigmentary degeneration, <u>unspecified</u> eye
H35.46- <u>Secondary vitreoretinal</u> degeneration
    H35.461   Secondary vitreoretinal degeneration, <u>right</u> eye
    H35.462   Secondary vitreoretinal degeneration, <u>left</u> eye
    H35.463   Secondary vitreoretinal degeneration, <u>bilateral</u>
    H35.469   Secondary vitreoretinal degeneration, <u>unspecified</u> eye
H35.5- <u>Hereditary retinal dystrophy</u>
    Excludes 1: dystrophies primarily involving Bruch's membrane
        (H31.1-)
H35.50   Unspecified hereditary retinal dystrophy
H35.51   Vitreoretinal dystrophy
H35.52   Pigmentary retinal dystrophy
    Albipunctate retinal dystrophy
    Retinitis pigmentosa
    Tapetoretinal dystrophy
H35.53   Other dystrophies primarily involving the sensory retina
    Stargardt's disease

H35.54   Dystrophies primarily involving the retinal pigment
       epithelium
    Vitelliform retinal dystrophy
H35.6- <u>Retinal hemorrhage</u>
    H35.60   Retinal hemorrhage, <u>unspecified</u> eye
    H35.61   Retinal hemorrhage, <u>right</u> eye
    H35.62   Retinal hemorrhage, <u>left</u> eye
    H35.63   Retinal hemorrhage, <u>bilateral</u>
H35.7- <u>Separation of retinal layers</u>
    Excludes 1: retinal detachment (serous) (H33.2-)
        rhegmatogenous retinal detachment (H33.0-)
    H35.70   Unspecified separation of retinal layers
H35.71- <u>Central</u> serous chorioretinopathy
    H35.711   Central serous chorioretinopathy, <u>right</u> eye
    H35.712   Central serous chorioretinopathy, <u>left</u> eye
    H35.713   Central serous chorioretinopathy, <u>bilateral</u>
    H35.719   Central serous chorioretinopathy, <u>unspecified</u> eye
H35.72- <u>Serous</u> detachment of retinal pigment epithelium
    H35.721   Serous detachment of retinal pigment epithelium,
         <u>right</u> eye
    H35.722   Serous detachment of retinal pigment epithelium, <u>left</u>
         eye
    H35.723   Serous detachment of retinal pigment epithelium,
         <u>bilateral</u>
    H35.729   Serous detachment of retinal pigment epithelium,
         <u>unspecified</u> eye
H35.73- <u>Hemorrhagic</u> detachment of retinal pigment epithelium
    H35.731   Hemorrhagic detachment of retinal pigment
         epithelium, <u>right</u> eye
    H35.732   Hemorrhagic detachment of retinal pigment
         epithelium, <u>left</u> eye
    H35.733   Hemorrhagic detachment of retinal pigment
         epithelium, <u>bilateral</u>
    H35.739   Hemorrhagic detachment of retinal pigment
         epithelium, <u>unspecified</u> eye
H35.8- Other specified retinal disorders
    Excludes❷: retinal hemorrhage (H35.6-)
    H35.81   Retinal edema
        Retinal cotton wool spots
    H35.82   Retinal ischemia
    H35.89   Other specified retinal disorders
H35.9   Unspecified retinal disorder
H36   Retinal disorders in diseases classified elsewhere
    Code first underlying disease, such as:
    Lipid storage disorders (E75.-)
    Sickle-cell disorders (D57.-)
    Excludes 1: arteriosclerotic retinopathy (H35.0-)
        diabetic retinopathy (E08.3-, E09.3-, E10.3-, E11.3-, E13.3-)

Glaucoma (H40-H42)

H40- <u>Glaucoma</u>
    Excludes 1: absolute glaucoma (H44.51-)
        congenital glaucoma (Q15.0)
        traumatic glaucoma due to birth injury (P15.3)
H40.0- Glaucoma suspect
    H40.00- <u>Preglaucoma</u>, unspecified
        H40.001   Preglaucoma, unspecified, <u>right</u> eye
        H40.002   Preglaucoma, unspecified, <u>left</u> eye
        H40.003   Preglaucoma, unspecified, <u>bilateral</u>
        H40.009   Preglaucoma, unspecified, <u>unspecified</u> eye
    H40.01- <u>Open angle</u> with borderline findings, <u>low risk</u>
        Open angle, low risk
        H40.011   Open angle with borderline findings, low risk, <u>right</u>
            eye
        H40.012   Open angle with borderline findings, low risk, <u>left</u> eye
        H40.013   Open angle with borderline findings, low risk,
            <u>bilateral</u>
        H40.019   Open angle with borderline findings, low risk,
            <u>unspecified</u> eye
    H40.02- <u>Open angle</u> with borderline findings, <u>high risk</u>
        Open angle, high risk
        H40.021   Open angle with borderline findings, high risk, <u>right</u>
            eye
        H40.022   Open angle with borderline findings, high risk, <u>left</u> eye
        H40.023   Open angle with borderline findings, high risk,
            <u>bilateral</u>
        H40.029   Open angle with borderline findings, high risk,
            <u>unspecified</u> eye

H35 - H40

© 2013 Channel Publishing Ltd

H40.03- Anatomical <u>narrow angle</u>
        Primary angle closure suspect
    H40.031   Anatomical narrow angle, <u>right</u> eye
    H40.032   Anatomical narrow angle, <u>left</u> eye
    H40.033   Anatomical narrow angle, <u>bilateral</u>
    H40.039   Anatomical narrow angle, <u>unspecified</u> eye
H40.04- <u>Steroid responder</u>
    H40.041   Steroid responder, <u>right</u> eye
    H40.042   Steroid responder, <u>left</u> eye
    H40.043   Steroid responder, <u>bilateral</u>
    H40.049   Steroid responder, <u>unspecified</u> eye
H40.05- Ocular hypertension
    H40.051   Ocular hypertension, <u>right</u> eye
    H40.052   Ocular hypertension, <u>left</u> eye
    H40.053   Ocular hypertension, <u>bilateral</u>
    H40.059   Ocular hypertension, <u>unspecified</u> eye
H40.06- Primary angle closure without glaucoma damage
    H40.061   Primary angle closure without glaucoma damage, <u>right</u> eye
    H40.062   Primary angle closure without glaucoma damage, <u>left</u> eye
    H40.063   Primary angle closure without glaucoma damage, <u>bilateral</u>
    H40.069   Primary angle closure without glaucoma damage, <u>unspecified</u> eye
H40.1- <u>Open-angle glaucoma</u>
H40.10x- <u>Unspecified</u> open-angle glaucoma
        One of the following 7th characters is to be assigned to
        code H40.10x- to designate the stage of glaucoma:
        0   Stage unspecified
        1   Mild stage
        2   Moderate stage
        3   Severe stage
        4   Indeterminate stage
H40.11x- <u>Primary</u> open-angle glaucoma
        Chronic simple glaucoma
        One of the following 7th characters is to be assigned to
        code H40.11x- to designate the stage of glaucoma:
        0   Stage unspecified
        1   Mild stage
        2   Moderate stage
        3   Severe stage
        4   Indeterminate stage
H40.12- <u>Low-tension</u> glaucoma
        One of the following 7th characters is to be assigned to code
        H40.12- to designate the stage of glaucoma:
        0   Stage unspecified
        1   Mild stage
        2   Moderate stage
        3   Severe stage
        4   Indeterminate stage
    H40.121- Low-tension glaucoma, <u>right</u> eye
    H40.122- Low-tension glaucoma, <u>left</u> eye
    H40.123- Low-tension glaucoma, <u>bilateral</u>
    H40.129- Low-tension glaucoma, <u>unspecified</u> eye
H40.13- <u>Pigmentary</u> glaucoma
        One of the following 7th characters is to be assigned to code
        H40.13- to designate the stage of glaucoma:
        0   Stage unspecified
        1   Mild stage
        2   Moderate stage
        3   Severe stage
        4   Indeterminate stage
    H40.131- Pigmentary glaucoma, <u>right</u> eye
    H40.132- Pigmentary glaucoma, <u>left</u> eye
    H40.133- Pigmentary glaucoma, <u>bilateral</u>
    H40.139- Pigmentary glaucoma, <u>unspecified</u> eye
H40.14- <u>Capsular</u> glaucoma with pseudoexfoliation of lens
        One of the following 7th characters is to be assigned to code
        H40.14- to designate the stage of glaucoma:
        0   Stage unspecified
        1   Mild stage
        2   Moderate stage
        3   Severe stage
        4   Indeterminate stage
    H40.141- Capsular glaucoma with pseudoexfoliation of lens, <u>right</u> eye
    H40.142- Capsular glaucoma with pseudoexfoliation of lens, <u>left</u> eye
    H40.143- Capsular glaucoma with pseudoexfoliation of lens, <u>bilateral</u>

    H40.149- Capsular glaucoma with pseudoexfoliation of lens, <u>unspecified</u> eye
H40.15- <u>Residual stage</u> of open-angle glaucoma
    H40.151   Residual stage of open-angle glaucoma, <u>right</u> eye
    H40.152   Residual stage of open-angle glaucoma, <u>left</u> eye
    H40.153   Residual stage of open-angle glaucoma, <u>bilateral</u>
    H40.159   Residual stage of open-angle glaucoma, <u>unspecified</u> eye
H40.2- <u>Primary angle-closure</u> glaucoma
        Excludes 1: aqueous misdirection (H40.83-)
                      malignant glaucoma (H40.83-)
    H40.20x- <u>Unspecified</u> primary angle-closure glaucoma
            One of the following 7th characters is to be assigned to
            code H40.20x- to designate the stage of glaucoma:
            0   Stage unspecified
            1   Mild stage
            2   Moderate stage
            3   Severe stage
            4   Indeterminate stage
    H40.21- <u>Acute</u> angle-closure glaucoma
            Acute angle-closure glaucoma attack
            Acute angle-closure glaucoma crisis
        H40.211   Acute angle-closure glaucoma, <u>right</u> eye
        H40.212   Acute angle-closure glaucoma, <u>left</u> eye
        H40.213   Acute angle-closure glaucoma, <u>bilateral</u>
        H40.219   Acute angle-closure glaucoma, <u>unspecified</u> eye
    H40.22- <u>Chronic</u> angle-closure glaucoma
            Chronic primary angle-closure glaucoma
            One of the following 7th characters is to be assigned to code
            H40.22- to designate the stage of glaucoma:
            0   Stage unspecified
            1   Mild stage
            2   Moderate stage
            3   Severe stage
            4   Indeterminate stage
        H40.221- Chronic angle-closure glaucoma, <u>right</u> eye
        H40.222- Chronic angle-closure glaucoma, <u>left</u> eye
        H40.223- Chronic angle-closure glaucoma, <u>bilateral</u>
        H40.229- Chronic angle-closure glaucoma, <u>unspecified</u> eye
    H40.23- <u>Intermittent</u> angle-closure glaucoma
        H40.231   Intermittent angle-closure glaucoma, <u>right</u> eye
        H40.232   Intermittent angle-closure glaucoma, <u>left</u> eye
        H40.233   Intermittent angle-closure glaucoma, <u>bilateral</u>
        H40.239   Intermittent angle-closure glaucoma, <u>unspecified</u> eye
    H40.24- <u>Residual stage</u> of angle-closure glaucoma
        H40.241   Residual stage of angle-closure glaucoma, <u>right</u> eye
        H40.242   Residual stage of angle-closure glaucoma, <u>left</u> eye
        H40.243   Residual stage of angle-closure glaucoma, <u>bilateral</u>
        H40.249   Residual stage of angle-closure glaucoma, <u>unspecified</u> eye
H40.3- Glaucoma <u>secondary to eye trauma</u>
        Code also underlying condition
        One of the following 7th characters is to be assigned to code
        H40.3- to designate the stage of glaucoma:
        0   Stage unspecified
        1   Mild stage
        2   Moderate stage
        3   Severe stage
        4   Indeterminate stage
    H40.30x- Glaucoma secondary to eye trauma, <u>unspecified</u> eye
    H40.31x- Glaucoma secondary to eye trauma, <u>right</u> eye
    H40.32x- Glaucoma secondary to eye trauma, <u>left</u> eye
    H40.33x- Glaucoma secondary to eye trauma, <u>bilateral</u>
H40.4- Glaucoma <u>secondary to eye inflammation</u>
        Code also underlying condition
        One of the following 7th characters is to be assigned to code
        H40.4- to designate the stage of glaucoma:
        0   Stage unspecified
        1   Mild stage
        2   Moderate stage
        3   Severe stage
        4   Indeterminate stage
    H40.40x- Glaucoma secondary to eye inflammation, <u>unspecified</u> eye
    H40.41x- Glaucoma secondary to eye inflammation, <u>right</u> eye
    H40.42x- Glaucoma secondary to eye inflammation, <u>left</u> eye
    H40.43x- Glaucoma secondary to eye inflammation, <u>bilateral</u>

H35-H40

H40.5- Glaucoma secondary to other eye disorders
Code also underlying eye disorder
One of the following 7th characters is to be assigned to code H40.5- to designate the stage of glaucoma:
0   Stage unspecified
1   Mild stage
2   Moderate stage
3   Severe stage
4   Indeterminate stage
H40.50x- Glaucoma secondary to other eye disorders, unspecified eye
H40.51x- Glaucoma secondary to other eye disorders, right eye
H40.52x- Glaucoma secondary to other eye disorders, left eye
H40.53x- Glaucoma secondary to other eye disorders, bilateral
H40.6- Glaucoma secondary to drugs
Use additional code for adverse effect, if applicable, to identify drug (T36-T50 with fifth or sixth character 5)
One of the following 7th characters is to be assigned to code H40.6- to designate the stage of glaucoma:
0   Stage unspecified
1   Mild stage
2   Moderate stage
3   Severe stage
4   Indeterminate stage
H40.60x- Glaucoma secondary to drugs, unspecified eye
H40.61x- Glaucoma secondary to drugs, right eye
H40.62x- Glaucoma secondary to drugs, left eye
H40.63x- Glaucoma secondary to drugs, bilateral
H40.8- Other glaucoma
H40.81- Glaucoma with increased episcleral venous pressure
H40.811   Glaucoma with increased episcleral venous pressure, right eye
H40.812   Glaucoma with increased episcleral venous pressure, left eye
H40.813   Glaucoma with increased episcleral venous pressure, bilateral
H40.819   Glaucoma with increased episcleral venous pressure, unspecified eye
H40.82- Hypersecretion glaucoma
H40.821   Hypersecretion glaucoma, right eye
H40.822   Hypersecretion glaucoma, left eye
H40.823   Hypersecretion glaucoma, bilateral
H40.829   Hypersecretion glaucoma, unspecified eye
H40.83- Aqueous misdirection
Malignant glaucoma
H40.831   Aqueous misdirection, right eye
H40.832   Aqueous misdirection, left eye
H40.833   Aqueous misdirection, bilateral
H40.839   Aqueous misdirection, unspecified eye
H40.89 Other specified glaucoma
H40.9 Unspecified glaucoma
H42   Glaucoma in diseases classified elsewhere
Code first underlying condition, such as:
Amyloidosis (E85.-)
Aniridia (Q13.1)
Lowe's syndrome (E72.03)
Reiger's anomaly (Q13.81)
Specified metabolic disorder (E70-E88)
Excludes 1: glaucoma (in):
diabetes mellitus (E08.39, E09.39, E10.39, E11.39, E13.39)
onchocerciasis (B73.02)
syphilis (A52.71)
tuberculous (A18.59)

Disorders of vitreous body and globe (H43-H44)

H43- Disorders of vitreous body
H43.0- Vitreous prolapse
Excludes 1: vitreous syndrome following cataract surgery (H59.0-)
traumatic vitreous prolapse (S05.2-)
H43.00 Vitreous prolapse, unspecified eye
H43.01 Vitreous prolapse, right eye
H43.02 Vitreous prolapse, left eye
H43.03 Vitreous prolapse, bilateral
H43.1- Vitreous hemorrhage
H43.10 Vitreous hemorrhage, unspecified eye
H43.11 Vitreous hemorrhage, right eye
H43.12 Vitreous hemorrhage, left eye
H43.13 Vitreous hemorrhage, bilateral

H43.2- Crystalline deposits in vitreous body
H43.20 Crystalline deposits in vitreous body, unspecified eye
H43.21 Crystalline deposits in vitreous body, right eye
H43.22 Crystalline deposits in vitreous body, left eye
H43.23 Crystalline deposits in vitreous body, bilateral
H43.3- Other vitreous opacities
H43.31- Vitreous membranes and strands
H43.311   Vitreous membranes and strands, right eye
H43.312   Vitreous membranes and strands, left eye
H43.313   Vitreous membranes and strands, bilateral
H43.319   Vitreous membranes and strands, unspecified eye
H43.39- Other vitreous opacities
Vitreous floaters
H43.391   Other vitreous opacities, right eye
H43.392   Other vitreous opacities, left eye
H43.393   Other vitreous opacities, bilateral
H43.399   Other vitreous opacities, unspecified eye
H43.8- Other disorders of vitreous body
Excludes 1: proliferative vitreo-retinopathy with retinal detachment (H33.4-)
Excludes❷: vitreous abscess (H44.02-)
H43.81- Vitreous degeneration
Vitreous detachment
H43.811   Vitreous degeneration, right eye
H43.812   Vitreous degeneration, left eye
H43.813   Vitreous degeneration, bilateral
H43.819   Vitreous degeneration, unspecified eye
H43.82- Vitreomacular adhesion
Vitreomacular traction
H43.821   Vitreomacular adhesion, right eye
H43.822   Vitreomacular adhesion, left eye
H43.823   Vitreomacular adhesion, bilateral
H43.829   Vitreomacular adhesion, unspecified eye
H43.89 Other disorders of vitreous body
H43.9 Unspecified disorder of vitreous body
H44- Disorders of globe
Includes: Disorders affecting multiple structures of eye
H44.0- Purulent endophthalmitis
Use additional code to identify organism
Excludes 1: bleb associated endophthalmitis (H59.4-)
H44.00- Unspecified purulent endophthalmitis
H44.001   Unspecified purulent endophthalmitis, right eye
H44.002   Unspecified purulent endophthalmitis, left eye
H44.003   Unspecified purulent endophthalmitis, bilateral
H44.009   Unspecified purulent endophthalmitis, unspecified eye
H44.01- Panophthalmitis (acute)
H44.011   Panophthalmitis (acute), right eye
H44.012   Panophthalmitis (acute), left eye
H44.013   Panophthalmitis (acute), bilateral
H44.019   Panophthalmitis (acute), unspecified eye
H44.02- Vitreous abscess (chronic)
H44.021   Vitreous abscess (chronic), right eye
H44.022   Vitreous abscess (chronic), left eye
H44.023   Vitreous abscess (chronic), bilateral
H44.029   Vitreous abscess (chronic), unspecified eye
H44.1- Other endophthalmitis
Excludes 1: bleb associated endophthalmitis (H59.4-)
Excludes❷: ophthalmia nodosa (H16.2-)
H44.11- Panuveitis
H44.111   Panuveitis, right eye
H44.112   Panuveitis, left eye
H44.113   Panuveitis, bilateral
H44.119   Panuveitis, unspecified eye
H44.12- Parasitic endophthalmitis, unspecified
H44.121   Parasitic endophthalmitis, unspecified, right eye
H44.122   Parasitic endophthalmitis, unspecified, left eye
H44.123   Parasitic endophthalmitis, unspecified, bilateral
H44.129   Parasitic endophthalmitis, unspecified, unspecified eye
H44.13- Sympathetic uveitis
H44.131   Sympathetic uveitis, right eye
H44.132   Sympathetic uveitis, left eye
H44.133   Sympathetic uveitis, bilateral
H44.139   Sympathetic uveitis, unspecified eye
H44.19 Other endophthalmitis

H
4
0
-
H
4
4

H44.2- Degenerative myopia
    Malignant myopia
  H44.20 Degenerative myopia, <u>unspecified</u> eye
  H44.21 Degenerative myopia, <u>right</u> eye
  H44.22 Degenerative myopia, <u>left</u> eye
  H44.23 Degenerative myopia, <u>bilateral</u>
H44.3- Other and unspecified degenerative disorders of globe
  H44.30 Unspecified degenerative disorder of globe
  H44.31- <u>Chalcosis</u>
    H44.311 Chalcosis, <u>right</u> eye
    H44.312 Chalcosis, <u>left</u> eye
    H44.313 Chalcosis, <u>bilateral</u>
    H44.319 Chalcosis, <u>unspecified</u> eye
  H44.32- <u>Siderosis</u> of eye
    H44.321 Siderosis of eye, <u>right</u> eye
    H44.322 Siderosis of eye, <u>left</u> eye
    H44.323 Siderosis of eye, <u>bilateral</u>
    H44.329 Siderosis of eye, <u>unspecified</u> eye
  H44.39- <u>Other</u> degenerative disorders of globe
    H44.391 Other degenerative disorders of globe, <u>right</u> eye
    H44.392 Other degenerative disorders of globe, <u>left</u> eye
    H44.393 Other degenerative disorders of globe, <u>bilateral</u>
    H44.399 Other degenerative disorders of globe, <u>unspecified</u> eye
H44.4- <u>Hypotony</u> of eye
  H44.40 <u>Unspecified</u> hypotony of eye
  H44.41- <u>Flat anterior chamber</u> hypotony of eye
    H44.411 Flat anterior chamber hypotony of <u>right</u> eye
    H44.412 Flat anterior chamber hypotony of <u>left</u> eye
    H44.413 Flat anterior chamber hypotony of eye, <u>bilateral</u>
    H44.419 Flat anterior chamber hypotony of <u>unspecified</u> eye
  H44.42- Hypotony of eye <u>due to ocular fistula</u>
    H44.421 Hypotony of <u>right</u> eye due to ocular fistula
    H44.422 Hypotony of <u>left</u> eye due to ocular fistula
    H44.423 Hypotony of eye due to ocular fistula, <u>bilateral</u>
    H44.429 Hypotony of <u>unspecified</u> eye due to ocular fistula
  H44.43- Hypotony of eye <u>due to other ocular disorders</u>
    H44.431 Hypotony of eye due to other ocular disorders, <u>right</u> eye
    H44.432 Hypotony of eye due to other ocular disorders, <u>left</u> eye
    H44.433 Hypotony of eye due to other ocular disorders, <u>bilateral</u>
    H44.439 Hypotony of eye due to other ocular disorders, <u>unspecified</u> eye
  H44.44- <u>Primary</u> hypotony of eye
    H44.441 Primary hypotony of <u>right</u> eye
    H44.442 Primary hypotony of <u>left</u> eye
    H44.443 Primary hypotony of eye, <u>bilateral</u>
    H44.449 Primary hypotony of <u>unspecified</u> eye
H44.5- <u>Degenerated conditions of globe</u>
  H44.50 <u>Unspecified</u> degenerated conditions of globe
  H44.51- <u>Absolute glaucoma</u>
    H44.511 Absolute glaucoma, <u>right</u> eye
    H44.512 Absolute glaucoma, <u>left</u> eye
    H44.513 Absolute glaucoma, <u>bilateral</u>
    H44.519 Absolute glaucoma, <u>unspecified</u> eye
  H44.52- <u>Atrophy</u> of globe
    Phthisis bulbi
    H44.521 Atrophy of globe, <u>right</u> eye
    H44.522 Atrophy of globe, <u>left</u> eye
    H44.523 Atrophy of globe, <u>bilateral</u>
    H44.529 Atrophy of globe, <u>unspecified</u> eye
  H44.53- <u>Leucocoria</u>
    H44.531 Leucocoria, <u>right</u> eye
    H44.532 Leucocoria, <u>left</u> eye
    H44.533 Leucocoria, <u>bilateral</u>
    H44.539 Leucocoria, <u>unspecified</u> eye

H44.6- Retained (old) intraocular foreign body, magnetic
Use additional code to identify magnetic foreign body (Z18.11)
Excludes 1: current intraocular foreign body (S05.-)
Excludes ❷: retained foreign body in eyelid (H02.81-)
*   retained (old) foreign body following penetrating*
*   wound of orbit (H05.5-)*
*   retained (old) intraocular foreign body, nonmagnetic*
*   (H44.7-)*
  H44.60- <u>Unspecified</u> retained (old) intraocular foreign body, <u>magnetic</u>
    H44.601 Unspecified retained (old) intraocular foreign body, magnetic, <u>right</u> eye
    H44.602 Unspecified retained (old) intraocular foreign body, magnetic, <u>left</u> eye
    H44.603 Unspecified retained (old) intraocular foreign body, magnetic, <u>bilateral</u>
    H44.609 Unspecified retained (old) intraocular foreign body, magnetic, <u>unspecified</u> eye
  H44.61- Retained (old) <u>magnetic</u> foreign body <u>in anterior chamber</u>
    H44.611 Retained (old) magnetic foreign body in anterior chamber, <u>right</u> eye
    H44.612 Retained (old) magnetic foreign body in anterior chamber, <u>left</u> eye
    H44.613 Retained (old) magnetic foreign body in anterior chamber, <u>bilateral</u>
    H44.619 Retained (old) magnetic foreign body in anterior chamber, <u>unspecified</u> eye
  H44.62- Retained (old) <u>magnetic</u> foreign body <u>in iris or ciliary body</u>
    H44.621 Retained (old) magnetic foreign body in iris or ciliary body, <u>right</u> eye
    H44.622 Retained (old) magnetic foreign body in iris or ciliary body, <u>left</u> eye
    H44.623 Retained (old) magnetic foreign body in iris or ciliary body, <u>bilateral</u>
    H44.629 Retained (old) magnetic foreign body in iris or ciliary body, <u>unspecified</u> eye
  H44.63- Retained (old) <u>magnetic</u> foreign body <u>in lens</u>
    H44.631 Retained (old) magnetic foreign body in lens, <u>right</u> eye
    H44.632 Retained (old) magnetic foreign body in lens, <u>left</u> eye
    H44.633 Retained (old) magnetic foreign body in lens, <u>bilateral</u>
    H44.639 Retained (old) magnetic foreign body in lens, <u>unspecified</u> eye
  H44.64- Retained (old) <u>magnetic</u> foreign body <u>in posterior wall of globe</u>
    H44.641 Retained (old) magnetic foreign body in posterior wall of globe, <u>right</u> eye
    H44.642 Retained (old) magnetic foreign body in posterior wall of globe, <u>left</u> eye
    H44.643 Retained (old) magnetic foreign body in posterior wall of globe, <u>bilateral</u>
    H44.649 Retained (old) magnetic foreign body in posterior wall of globe, <u>unspecified</u> eye
  H44.65- Retained (old) <u>magnetic</u> foreign body <u>in vitreous body</u>
    H44.651 Retained (old) magnetic foreign body in vitreous body, <u>right</u> eye
    H44.652 Retained (old) magnetic foreign body in vitreous body, <u>left</u> eye
    H44.653 Retained (old) magnetic foreign body in vitreous body, <u>bilateral</u>
    H44.659 Retained (old) magnetic foreign body in vitreous body, <u>unspecified</u> eye
  H44.69- Retained (old) intraocular foreign body, <u>magnetic, in other or multiple sites</u>
    H44.691 Retained (old) intraocular foreign body, magnetic, in other or multiple sites, <u>right</u> eye
    H44.692 Retained (old) intraocular foreign body, magnetic, in other or multiple sites, <u>left</u> eye
    H44.693 Retained (old) intraocular foreign body, magnetic, in other or multiple sites, <u>bilateral</u>
    H44.699 Retained (old) intraocular foreign body, magnetic, in other or multiple sites, <u>unspecified</u> eye

H40 - H44

H44.7-   Retained (old) intraocular foreign body, nonmagnetic
Use additional code to identify nonmagnetic foreign body (Z18.01-Z18.10, Z18.12, Z18.2-Z18.9)
Excludes 1:   current intraocular foreign body (S05.-)
Excludes❷: retained foreign body in eyelid (H02.81-)
retained (old) foreign body following penetrating wound of orbit (H05.5-)
retained (old) intraocular foreign body, magnetic (H44.6-)

H44.70- Unspecified retained (old) intraocular foreign body, nonmagnetic
   H44.701   Unspecified retained (old) intraocular foreign body, nonmagnetic, right eye
   H44.702   Unspecified retained (old) intraocular foreign body, nonmagnetic, left eye
   H44.703   Unspecified retained (old) intraocular foreign body, nonmagnetic, bilateral
   H44.709   Unspecified retained (old) intraocular foreign body, nonmagnetic, unspecified eye
         Retained (old) intraocular foreign body NOS

H44.71- Retained (nonmagnetic) (old) foreign body in anterior chamber
   H44.711   Retained (nonmagnetic) (old) foreign body in anterior chamber, right eye
   H44.712   Retained (nonmagnetic) (old) foreign body in anterior chamber, left eye
   H44.713   Retained (nonmagnetic) (old) foreign body in anterior chamber, bilateral
   H44.719   Retained (nonmagnetic) (old) foreign body in anterior chamber, unspecified eye

H44.72- Retained (nonmagnetic) (old) foreign body in iris or ciliary body
   H44.721   Retained (nonmagnetic) (old) foreign body in iris or ciliary body, right eye
   H44.722   Retained (nonmagnetic) (old) foreign body in iris or ciliary body, left eye
   H44.723   Retained (nonmagnetic) (old) foreign body in iris or ciliary body, bilateral
   H44.729   Retained (nonmagnetic) (old) foreign body in iris or ciliary body, unspecified eye

H44.73- Retained (nonmagnetic) (old) foreign body in lens
   H44.731   Retained (nonmagnetic) (old) foreign body in lens, right eye
   H44.732   Retained (nonmagnetic) (old) foreign body in lens, left eye
   H44.733   Retained (nonmagnetic) (old) foreign body in lens, bilateral
   H44.739   Retained (nonmagnetic) (old) foreign body in lens, unspecified eye

H44.74- Retained (nonmagnetic) (old) foreign body in posterior wall of globe
   H44.741   Retained (nonmagnetic) (old) foreign body in posterior wall of globe, right eye
   H44.742   Retained (nonmagnetic) (old) foreign body in posterior wall of globe, left eye
   H44.743   Retained (nonmagnetic) (old) foreign body in posterior wall of globe, bilateral
   H44.749   Retained (nonmagnetic) (old) foreign body in posterior wall of globe, unspecified eye

H44.75- Retained (nonmagnetic) (old) foreign body in vitreous body
   H44.751   Retained (nonmagnetic) (old) foreign body in vitreous body, right eye
   H44.752   Retained (nonmagnetic) (old) foreign body in vitreous body, left eye
   H44.753   Retained (nonmagnetic) (old) foreign body in vitreous body, bilateral
   H44.759   Retained (nonmagnetic) (old) foreign body in vitreous body, unspecified eye

H44.79- Retained (old) intraocular foreign body, nonmagnetic, in other or multiple sites
   H44.791   Retained (old) intraocular foreign body, nonmagnetic, in other or multiple sites, right eye
   H44.792   Retained (old) intraocular foreign body, nonmagnetic, in other or multiple sites, left eye
   H44.793   Retained (old) intraocular foreign body, nonmagnetic, in other or multiple sites, bilateral
   H44.799   Retained (old) intraocular foreign body, nonmagnetic, in other or multiple sites, unspecified eye

H44.8-   Other disorders of globe
   H44.81- Hemophthalmos
      H44.811   Hemophthalmos, right eye
      H44.812   Hemophthalmos, left eye
      H44.813   Hemophthalmos, bilateral
      H44.819   Hemophthalmos, unspecified eye
   H44.82- Luxation of globe
      H44.821   Luxation of globe, right eye
      H44.822   Luxation of globe, left eye
      H44.823   Luxation of globe, bilateral
      H44.829   Luxation of globe, unspecified eye
   H44.89   Other disorders of globe
H44.9   Unspecified disorder of globe

Disorders of optic nerve and visual pathways (H46-H47)

H46-   Optic neuritis
Excludes❷: ischemic optic neuropathy (H47.01-)
neuromyelitis optica [Devic] (G36.0)
   H46.0- Optic papillitis
      H46.00 Optic papillitis, unspecified eye
      H46.01 Optic papillitis, right eye
      H46.02 Optic papillitis, left eye
      H46.03 Optic papillitis, bilateral
   H46.1- Retrobulbar neuritis
         Retrobulbar neuritis NOS
      Excludes 1:   syphilitic retrobulbar neuritis (A52.15)
      H46.10 Retrobulbar neuritis, unspecified eye
      H46.11 Retrobulbar neuritis, right eye
      H46.12 Retrobulbar neuritis, left eye
      H46.13 Retrobulbar neuritis, bilateral
   H46.2   Nutritional optic neuropathy
   H46.3   Toxic optic neuropathy
         Code first (T51-T65) to identify cause
   H46.8   Other optic neuritis
   H46.9   Unspecified optic neuritis

H47-   Other disorders of optic [2nd] nerve and visual pathways
   H47.0- Disorders of optic nerve, not elsewhere classified
      H47.01- Ischemic optic neuropathy
         H47.011   Ischemic optic neuropathy, right eye
         H47.012   Ischemic optic neuropathy, left eye
         H47.013   Ischemic optic neuropathy, bilateral
         H47.019   Ischemic optic neuropathy, unspecified eye
      H47.02- Hemorrhage in optic nerve sheath
         H47.021   Hemorrhage in optic nerve sheath, right eye
         H47.022   Hemorrhage in optic nerve sheath, left eye
         H47.023   Hemorrhage in optic nerve sheath, bilateral
         H47.029   Hemorrhage in optic nerve sheath, unspecified eye
      H47.03- Optic nerve hypoplasia
         H47.031   Optic nerve hypoplasia, right eye
         H47.032   Optic nerve hypoplasia, left eye
         H47.033   Optic nerve hypoplasia, bilateral
         H47.039   Optic nerve hypoplasia, unspecified eye
      H47.09- Other disorders of optic nerve, not elsewhere classified
            Compression of optic nerve
         H47.091   Other disorders of optic nerve, not elsewhere classified, right eye
         H47.092   Other disorders of optic nerve, not elsewhere classified, left eye
         H47.093   Other disorders of optic nerve, not elsewhere classified, bilateral
         H47.099   Other disorders of optic nerve, not elsewhere classified, unspecified eye
   H47.1- Papilledema
      H47.10 Unspecified papilledema
      H47.11 Papilledema associated with increased intracranial pressure
      H47.12 Papilledema associated with decreased ocular pressure
      H47.13 Papilledema associated with retinal disorder
      H47.14- Foster-Kennedy syndrome
         H47.141   Foster-Kennedy syndrome, right eye
         H47.142   Foster-Kennedy syndrome, left eye
         H47.143   Foster-Kennedy syndrome, bilateral
         H47.149   Foster-Kennedy syndrome, unspecified eye

H
4
4
-
H
4
9

H47.2- Optic atrophy
  H47.20 <u>Unspecified</u> optic atrophy
  H47.21- <u>Primary</u> optic atrophy
    H47.211 Primary optic atrophy, <u>right</u> eye
    H47.212 Primary optic atrophy, <u>left</u> eye
    H47.213 Primary optic atrophy, <u>bilateral</u>
    H47.219 Primary optic atrophy, <u>unspecified</u> eye
  H47.22 <u>Hereditary</u> optic atrophy
    Leber's optic atrophy
  H47.23- <u>Glaucomatous</u> optic atrophy
    H47.231 Glaucomatous optic atrophy, <u>right</u> eye
    H47.232 Glaucomatous optic atrophy, <u>left</u> eye
    H47.233 Glaucomatous optic atrophy, <u>bilateral</u>
    H47.239 Glaucomatous optic atrophy, <u>unspecified</u> eye
  H47.29- <u>Other</u> optic atrophy
    Temporal pallor of optic disc
    H47.291 Other optic atrophy, <u>right</u> eye
    H47.292 Other optic atrophy, <u>left</u> eye
    H47.293 Other optic atrophy, <u>bilateral</u>
    H47.299 Other optic atrophy, <u>unspecified</u> eye
H47.3- <u>Other disorders of optic disc</u>
  H47.31- <u>Coloboma</u> of optic disc
    H47.311 Coloboma of optic disc, <u>right</u> eye
    H47.312 Coloboma of optic disc, <u>left</u> eye
    H47.313 Coloboma of optic disc, <u>bilateral</u>
    H47.319 Coloboma of optic disc, <u>unspecified</u> eye
  H47.32- <u>Drusen</u> of optic disc
    H47.321 Drusen of optic disc, <u>right</u> eye
    H47.322 Drusen of optic disc, <u>left</u> eye
    H47.323 Drusen of optic disc, <u>bilateral</u>
    H47.329 Drusen of optic disc, <u>unspecified</u> eye
  H47.33- <u>Pseudopapilledema</u> of optic disc
    H47.331 Pseudopapilledema of optic disc, <u>right</u> eye
    H47.332 Pseudopapilledema of optic disc, <u>left</u> eye
    H47.333 Pseudopapilledema of optic disc, <u>bilateral</u>
    H47.339 Pseudopapilledema of optic disc, <u>unspecified</u> eye
  H47.39- <u>Other</u> disorders of optic disc
    H47.391 Other disorders of optic disc, <u>right</u> eye
    H47.392 Other disorders of optic disc, <u>left</u> eye
    H47.393 Other disorders of optic disc, <u>bilateral</u>
    H47.399 Other disorders of optic disc, <u>unspecified</u> eye
H47.4- Disorders of optic chiasm
    Code also underlying condition
    H47.41 Disorders of optic chiasm in (due to) inflammatory disorders
    H47.42 Disorders of optic chiasm in (due to) neoplasm
    H47.43 Disorders of optic chiasm in (due to) vascular disorders
    H47.49 Disorders of optic chiasm in (due to) other disorders
H47.5- <u>Disorders of other visual pathways</u>
    Disorders of optic tracts, geniculate nuclei and optic radiations
    Code also underlying condition
  H47.51- Disorders of visual pathways <u>in (due to) inflammatory</u> <u>disorders</u>
    H47.511 Disorders of visual pathways in (due to) inflammatory disorders, <u>right</u> side
    H47.512 Disorders of visual pathways in (due to) inflammatory disorders, <u>left</u> side
    H47.519 Disorders of visual pathways in (due to) inflammatory disorders, <u>unspecified</u> side
  H47.52- Disorders of visual pathways <u>in (due to) neoplasm</u>
    H47.521 Disorders of visual pathways in (due to) neoplasm, <u>right</u> side
    H47.522 Disorders of visual pathways in (due to) neoplasm, <u>left</u> side
    H47.529 Disorders of visual pathways in (due to) neoplasm, <u>unspecified</u> side
  H47.53- Disorders of visual pathways <u>in (due to) vascular disorders</u>
    H47.531 Disorders of visual pathways in (due to) vascular disorders, <u>right</u> side
    H47.532 Disorders of visual pathways in (due to) vascular disorders, <u>left</u> side
    H47.539 Disorders of visual pathways in (due to) vascular disorders, <u>unspecified</u> side

H47.6- <u>Disorders of visual cortex</u>
    Code also underlying condition
    Excludes 1: injury to visual cortex S04.04
  H47.61- <u>Cortical blindness</u>
    H47.611 Cortical blindness, <u>right</u> side of brain
    H47.612 Cortical blindness, <u>left</u> side of brain
    H47.619 Cortical blindness, <u>unspecified</u> side of brain
  H47.62- Disorders of visual cortex <u>in (due to) inflammatory disorders</u>
    H47.621 Disorders of visual cortex in (due to) inflammatory disorders, <u>right</u> side of brain
    H47.622 Disorders of visual cortex in (due to) inflammatory disorders, <u>left</u> side of brain
    H47.629 Disorders of visual cortex in (due to) inflammatory disorders, <u>unspecified</u> side of brain
  H47.63- Disorders of visual cortex <u>in (due to) neoplasm</u>
    H47.631 Disorders of visual cortex in (due to) neoplasm, <u>right</u> side of brain
    H47.632 Disorders of visual cortex in (due to) neoplasm, <u>left</u> side of brain
    H47.639 Disorders of visual cortex in (due to) neoplasm, <u>unspecified</u> side of brain
  H47.64- Disorders of visual cortex <u>in (due to) vascular disorders</u>
    H47.641 Disorders of visual cortex in (due to) vascular disorders, <u>right</u> side of brain
    H47.642 Disorders of visual cortex in (due to) vascular disorders, <u>left</u> side of brain
    H47.649 Disorders of visual cortex in (due to) vascular disorders, <u>unspecified</u> side of brain
H47.9   Unspecified disorder of visual pathways

Disorders of ocular muscles, binocular movement, accommodation and refraction (H49-H52)

  Excludes❷: nystagmus and other irregular eye movements (H55)
H49- <u>Paralytic strabismus</u>
    Excludes❷: internal ophthalmoplegia (H52.51-)
        internuclear ophthalmoplegia (H51.2-)
        progressive supranuclear ophthalmoplegia (G23.1)
  H49.0- <u>Third</u> [oculomotor] nerve palsy
    H49.00 Third [oculomotor] nerve palsy, <u>unspecified</u> eye
    H49.01 Third [oculomotor] nerve palsy, <u>right</u> eye
    H49.02 Third [oculomotor] nerve palsy, <u>left</u> eye
    H49.03 Third [oculomotor] nerve palsy, <u>bilateral</u>
  H49.1- <u>Fourth</u> [trochlear] nerve palsy
    H49.10 Fourth [trochlear] nerve palsy, <u>unspecified</u> eye
    H49.11 Fourth [trochlear] nerve palsy, <u>right</u> eye
    H49.12 Fourth [trochlear] nerve palsy, <u>left</u> eye
    H49.13 Fourth [trochlear] nerve palsy, <u>bilateral</u>
  H49.2- <u>Sixth</u> [abducent] nerve palsy
    H49.20 Sixth [abducent] nerve palsy, <u>unspecified</u> eye
    H49.21 Sixth [abducent] nerve palsy, <u>right</u> eye
    H49.22 Sixth [abducent] nerve palsy, <u>left</u> eye
    H49.23 Sixth [abducent] nerve palsy, <u>bilateral</u>
  H49.3- <u>Total</u> (external) ophthalmoplegia
    H49.30 Total (external) ophthalmoplegia, <u>unspecified</u> eye
    H49.31 Total (external) ophthalmoplegia, <u>right</u> eye
    H49.32 Total (external) ophthalmoplegia, <u>left</u> eye
    H49.33 Total (external) ophthalmoplegia, <u>bilateral</u>
  H49.4- <u>Progressive</u> external ophthalmoplegia
    Excludes 1: Kearns-Sayre syndrome (H49.81-)
    H49.40 Progressive external ophthalmoplegia, <u>unspecified</u> eye
    H49.41 Progressive external ophthalmoplegia, <u>right</u> eye
    H49.42 Progressive external ophthalmoplegia, <u>left</u> eye
    H49.43 Progressive external ophthalmoplegia, <u>bilateral</u>

**H
4
4
-
H
4
9**

H49.8- Other paralytic strabismus
  H49.81- <u>Kearns-Sayre syndrome</u>
       Progressive external ophthalmoplegia with pigmentary retinopathy
       Use additional code for other manifestation, such as:
       Heart block (I45.9)
     H49.811 Kearns-Sayre syndrome, <u>right</u> eye
     H49.812 Kearns-Sayre syndrome, <u>left</u> eye
     H49.813 Kearns-Sayre syndrome, <u>bilateral</u>
     H49.819 Kearns-Sayre syndrome, <u>unspecified</u> eye
  H49.88- <u>Other</u> paralytic strabismus
       External ophthalmoplegia NOS
     H49.881 Other paralytic strabismus, <u>right</u> eye
     H49.882 Other paralytic strabismus, <u>left</u> eye
     H49.883 Other paralytic strabismus, <u>bilateral</u>
     H49.889 Other paralytic strabismus, <u>unspecified</u> eye
  H49.9 Unspecified paralytic strabismus
H50- Other strabismus
  H50.0- <u>Esotropia</u>
       Convergent concomitant strabismus
       Excludes 1: intermittent esotropia (H50.31-, H50.32)
     H50.00 <u>Unspecified</u> esotropia
     H50.01- <u>Monocular</u> esotropia
       H50.011 Monocular esotropia, <u>right</u> eye
       H50.012 Monocular esotropia, <u>left</u> eye
     H50.02- Monocular esotropia <u>with A pattern</u>
       H50.021 Monocular esotropia with A pattern, <u>right</u> eye
       H50.022 Monocular esotropia with A pattern, <u>left</u> eye
     H50.03- Monocular esotropia <u>with V pattern</u>
       H50.031 Monocular esotropia with V pattern, <u>right</u> eye
       H50.032 Monocular esotropia with V pattern, <u>left</u> eye
     H50.04- Monocular esotropia <u>with other noncomitancies</u>
       H50.041 Monocular esotropia with other noncomitancies, <u>right</u> eye
       H50.042 Monocular esotropia with other noncomitancies, <u>left</u> eye
     H50.05 Alternating esotropia
     H50.06 Alternating esotropia with A pattern
     H50.07 Alternating esotropia with V pattern
     H50.08 Alternating esotropia with other noncomitancies
  H50.1- <u>Exotropia</u>
       Divergent concomitant strabismus
       Excludes 1: intermittent exotropia (H50.33-, H50.34)
     H50.10 <u>Unspecified</u> exotropia
     H50.11- <u>Monocular</u> exotropia
       H50.111 Monocular exotropia, <u>right</u> eye
       H50.112 Monocular exotropia, <u>left</u> eye
     H50.12- Monocular exotropia <u>with A pattern</u>
       H50.121 Monocular exotropia with A pattern, <u>right</u> eye
       H50.122 Monocular exotropia with A pattern, <u>left</u> eye
     H50.13- Monocular exotropia <u>with V pattern</u>
       H50.131 Monocular exotropia with V pattern, <u>right</u> eye
       H50.132 Monocular exotropia with V pattern, <u>left</u> eye
     H50.14- Monocular exotropia <u>with other noncomitancies</u>
       H50.141 Monocular exotropia with other noncomitancies, <u>right</u> eye
       H50.142 Monocular exotropia with other noncomitancies, <u>left</u> eye
     H50.15 Alternating exotropia
     H50.16 Alternating exotropia with A pattern
     H50.17 Alternating exotropia with V pattern
     H50.18 Alternating exotropia with other noncomitancies
  H50.2- <u>Vertical strabismus</u>
       Hypertropia
     H50.21 Vertical strabismus, <u>right</u> eye
     H50.22 Vertical strabismus, <u>left</u> eye
  H50.3- <u>Intermittent heterotropia</u>
     H50.30 <u>Unspecified</u> intermittent heterotropia
     H50.31- Intermittent <u>monocular</u> esotropia
       H50.311 Intermittent monocular esotropia, <u>right</u> eye
       H50.312 Intermittent monocular esotropia, <u>left</u> eye
     H50.32 Intermittent alternating esotropia
     H50.33- Intermittent <u>monocular</u> exotropia
       H50.331 Intermittent monocular exotropia, <u>right</u> eye
       H50.332 Intermittent monocular exotropia, <u>left</u> eye
     H50.34 Intermittent alternating <u>exotropia</u>

H50.4- Other and unspecified heterotropia
  H50.40 Unspecified heterotropia
  H50.41- <u>Cyclotropia</u>
     H50.411 Cyclotropia, right eye
     H50.412 Cyclotropia, left eye
  H50.42 Monofixation syndrome
  H50.43 Accommodative component in esotropia
H50.5- Heterophoria
  H50.50 Unspecified heterophoria
  H50.51 Esophoria
  H50.52 Exophoria
  H50.53 Vertical heterophoria
  H50.54 Cyclophoria
  H50.55 Alternating heterophoria
H50.6- Mechanical strabismus
  H50.60 Mechanical strabismus, unspecified
  H50.61- Brown's sheath syndrome
     H50.611 Brown's sheath syndrome, <u>right</u> eye
     H50.612 Brown's sheath syndrome, <u>left</u> eye
  H50.69 Other mechanical strabismus
       Strabismus due to adhesions
       Traumatic limitation of duction of eye muscle
H50.8- Other specified strabismus
  H50.81- Duane's syndrome
     H50.811 Duane's syndrome, <u>right</u> eye
     H50.812 Duane's syndrome, <u>left</u> eye
  H50.89 Other specified strabismus
H50.9 Unspecified strabismus
H51- Other disorders of binocular movement
  H51.0 Palsy (spasm) of conjugate gaze
  H51.1- Convergence insufficiency and excess
     H51.11 Convergence insufficiency
     H51.12 Convergence excess
  H51.2- <u>Internuclear ophthalmoplegia</u>
     H51.20 Internuclear ophthalmoplegia, <u>unspecified</u> eye
     H51.21 Internuclear ophthalmoplegia, <u>right</u> eye
     H51.22 Internuclear ophthalmoplegia, <u>left</u> eye
     H51.23 Internuclear ophthalmoplegia, <u>bilateral</u>
  H51.8 Other specified disorders of binocular movement
  H51.9 Unspecified disorder of binocular movement
H52- Disorders of refraction and accommodation
  H52.0- <u>Hypermetropia</u>
     H52.00 Hypermetropia, <u>unspecified</u> eye
     H52.01 Hypermetropia, <u>right</u> eye
     H52.02 Hypermetropia, <u>left</u> eye
     H52.03 Hypermetropia, <u>bilateral</u>
  H52.1- <u>Myopia</u>
       Excludes 1: degenerative myopia (H44.2-)
     H52.10 Myopia, <u>unspecified</u> eye
     H52.11 Myopia, <u>right</u> eye
     H52.12 Myopia, <u>left</u> eye
     H52.13 Myopia, <u>bilateral</u>
  H52.2- <u>Astigmatism</u>
     H52.20- <u>Unspecified</u> astigmatism
       H52.201 Unspecified astigmatism, <u>right</u> eye
       H52.202 Unspecified astigmatism, <u>left</u> eye
       H52.203 Unspecified astigmatism, <u>bilateral</u>
       H52.209 Unspecified astigmatism, <u>unspecified</u> eye
     H52.21- <u>Irregular</u> astigmatism
       H52.211 Irregular astigmatism, <u>right</u> eye
       H52.212 Irregular astigmatism, <u>left</u> eye
       H52.213 Irregular astigmatism, <u>bilateral</u>
       H52.219 Irregular astigmatism, <u>unspecified</u> eye
     H52.22- <u>Regular</u> astigmatism
       H52.221 Regular astigmatism, <u>right</u> eye
       H52.222 Regular astigmatism, <u>left</u> eye
       H52.223 Regular astigmatism, <u>bilateral</u>
       H52.229 Regular astigmatism, <u>unspecified</u> eye
  H52.3- Anisometropia and aniseikonia
     H52.31 Anisometropia
     H52.32 Aniseikonia
  H52.4 Presbyopia

H52.5-   Disorders of accommodation
   H52.51-   Internal ophthalmoplegia (complete) (total)
      H52.511   Internal ophthalmoplegia (complete) (total), right eye
      H52.512   Internal ophthalmoplegia (complete) (total), left eye
      H52.513   Internal ophthalmoplegia (complete) (total), bilateral
      H52.519   Internal ophthalmoplegia (complete) (total), unspecified eye
   H52.52-   Paresis of accommodation
      H52.521   Paresis of accommodation, right eye
      H52.522   Paresis of accommodation, left eye
      H52.523   Paresis of accommodation, bilateral
      H52.529   Paresis of accommodation, unspecified eye
   H52.53-   Spasm of accommodation
      H52.531   Spasm of accommodation, right eye
      H52.532   Spasm of accommodation, left eye
      H52.533   Spasm of accommodation, bilateral
      H52.539   Spasm of accommodation, unspecified eye
H52.6   Other disorders of refraction
H52.7   Unspecified disorder of refraction

Visual disturbances and blindness (H53-H54)

H53-   Visual disturbances
   H53.0-   Amblyopia ex anopsia
      Excludes 1:   amblyopia due to vitamin A deficiency (E50.5)
   H53.00-   Unspecified amblyopia
      H53.001   Unspecified amblyopia, right eye
      H53.002   Unspecified amblyopia, left eye
      H53.003   Unspecified amblyopia, bilateral
      H53.009   Unspecified amblyopia, unspecified eye
   H53.01-   Deprivation amblyopia
      H53.011   Deprivation amblyopia, right eye
      H53.012   Deprivation amblyopia, left eye
      H53.013   Deprivation amblyopia, bilateral
      H53.019   Deprivation amblyopia, unspecified eye
   H53.02-   Refractive amblyopia
      H53.021   Refractive amblyopia, right eye
      H53.022   Refractive amblyopia, left eye
      H53.023   Refractive amblyopia, bilateral
      H53.029   Refractive amblyopia, unspecified eye
   H53.03-   Strabismic amblyopia
      Excludes 1:   strabismus (H50.-)
      H53.031   Strabismic amblyopia, right eye
      H53.032   Strabismic amblyopia, left eye
      H53.033   Strabismic amblyopia, bilateral
      H53.039   Strabismic amblyopia, unspecified eye
   H53.1-   Subjective visual disturbances
      Excludes 1:   subjective visual disturbances due to vitamin A deficiency (E50.5)
               visual hallucinations (R44.1)
   H53.10   Unspecified subjective visual disturbances
   H53.11   Day blindness
      Hemeralopia
   H53.12-   Transient visual loss
      Scintillating scotoma
      Excludes 1:   amaurosis fugax (G45.3-)
               transient retinal artery occlusion (H34.0-)
      H53.121   Transient visual loss, right eye
      H53.122   Transient visual loss, left eye
      H53.123   Transient visual loss, bilateral
      H53.129   Transient visual loss, unspecified eye
   H53.13-   Sudden visual loss
      H53.131   Sudden visual loss, right eye
      H53.132   Sudden visual loss, left eye
      H53.133   Sudden visual loss, bilateral
      H53.139   Sudden visual loss, unspecified eye
   H53.14-   Visual discomfort
      Asthenopia
      Photophobia
      H53.141   Visual discomfort, right eye
      H53.142   Visual discomfort, left eye
      H53.143   Visual discomfort, bilateral
      H53.149   Visual discomfort, unspecified
   H53.15   Visual distortions of shape and size
      Metamorphopsia

H53.16   Psychophysical visual disturbances
H53.19   Other subjective visual disturbances
      Visual halos
H53.2   Diplopia
      Double vision
H53.3-   Other and unspecified disorders of binocular vision
   H53.30   Unspecified disorder of binocular vision
   H53.31   Abnormal retinal correspondence
   H53.32   Fusion with defective stereopsis
   H53.33   Simultaneous visual perception without fusion
   H53.34   Suppression of binocular vision
H53.4-   Visual field defects
   H53.40   Unspecified visual field defects
   H53.41-   Scotoma involving central area
      Central scotoma
      H53.411   Scotoma involving central area, right eye
      H53.412   Scotoma involving central area, left eye
      H53.413   Scotoma involving central area, bilateral
      H53.419   Scotoma involving central area, unspecified eye
   H53.42-   Scotoma of blind spot area
      Enlarged blind spot
      H53.421   Scotoma of blind spot area, right eye
      H53.422   Scotoma of blind spot area, left eye
      H53.423   Scotoma of blind spot area, bilateral
      H53.429   Scotoma of blind spot area, unspecified eye
   H53.43-   Sector or arcuate defects
      Arcuate scotoma
      Bjerrum scotoma
      H53.431   Sector or arcuate defects, right eye
      H53.432   Sector or arcuate defects, left eye
      H53.433   Sector or arcuate defects, bilateral
      H53.439   Sector or arcuate defects, unspecified eye
   H53.45-   Other localized visual field defect
      Peripheral visual field defect
      Ring scotoma NOS
      Scotoma NOS
      H53.451   Other localized visual field defect, right eye
      H53.452   Other localized visual field defect, left eye
      H53.453   Other localized visual field defect, bilateral
      H53.459   Other localized visual field defect, unspecified eye
   H53.46-   Homonymous bilateral field defects
      Homonymous hemianopia
      Homonymous hemianopsia
      Quadrant anopia
      Quadrant anopsia
      H53.461   Homonymous bilateral field defects, right side
      H53.462   Homonymous bilateral field defects, left side
      H53.469   Homonymous bilateral field defects, unspecified side
           Homonymous bilateral field defects NOS
   H53.47   Heteronymous bilateral field defects
      Heteronymous hemianop(s)ia
   H53.48-   Generalized contraction of visual field
      H53.481   Generalized contraction of visual field, right eye
      H53.482   Generalized contraction of visual field, left eye
      H53.483   Generalized contraction of visual field, bilateral
      H53.489   Generalized contraction of visual field, unspecified eye
H53.5-   Color vision deficiencies
      Color blindness
      Excludes❷: day blindness (H53.11)
   H53.50   Unspecified color vision deficiencies
      Color blindness NOS
   H53.51   Achromatopsia
   H53.52   Acquired color vision deficiency
   H53.53   Deuteranomaly
      Deuteranopia
   H53.54   Protanomaly
      Protanopia
   H53.55   Tritanomaly
      Tritanopia
   H53.59   Other color vision deficiencies
H53.6-   Night blindness
      Excludes 1:   night blindness due to vitamin A deficiency (E50.5)
   H53.60   Unspecified night blindness
   H53.61   Abnormal dark adaptation curve
   H53.62   Acquired night blindness
   H53.63   Congenital night blindness
   H53.69   Other night blindness

H
4
9
–
H
5
3

© 2013 Channer Publishing, Ltd.

H53.7- **Vision sensitivity deficiencies**
    H53.71 **Glare sensitivity**
    H53.72 **Impaired contrast sensitivity**
H53.8 **Other visual disturbances**
H53.9 **Unspecified visual disturbance**
H54- **Blindness and low vision**
    Note: For definition of visual impairment categories see table below
    Code first any associated underlying cause of the blindness
    Excludes 1: *amaurosis fugax (G45.3)*
    H54.0 <u>Blindness, both eyes</u>
        Visual impairment categories 3, 4, 5 in both eyes.
    H54.1- <u>Blindness, one eye, low vision other eye</u>
        Visual impairment categories 3, 4, 5 in one eye, with categories 1
        or 2 in the other eye
        H54.10 **Blindness, one eye, low vision other eye, <u>unspecified</u> eyes**
        H54.11 **Blindness, <u>right</u> eye, low vision <u>left</u> eye**
        H54.12 **Blindness, <u>left</u> eye, low vision <u>right</u> eye**
    H54.2 **Low vision, both eyes**
        Visual impairment categories 1 or 2 in both eyes.
    H54.3 **Unqualified visual loss, both eyes**
        Visual impairment category 9 in both eyes.
    H54.4- <u>Blindness, one eye</u>
        Visual impairment categories 3, 4, 5 in one eye [normal vision in
        other eye]
        H54.40 **Blindness, one eye, <u>unspecified</u> eye**
        H54.41 **Blindness, <u>right</u> eye, normal vision <u>left</u> eye**
        H54.42 **Blindness, <u>left</u> eye, normal vision <u>right</u> eye**
    H54.5- <u>Low vision, one eye</u>
        Visual impairment categories 1 or 2 in one eye [normal vision in
        other eye]
        H54.50 **Low vision, one eye, <u>unspecified</u> eye**
        H54.51 **Low vision, <u>right</u> eye, normal vision <u>left</u> eye**
        H54.52 **Low vision, <u>left</u> eye, normal vision <u>right</u> eye**
    H54.6- <u>Unqualified visual loss, one eye</u>
        Visual impairment category 9 in one eye [normal vision in other
        eye]
        H54.60 **Unqualified visual loss, one eye, <u>unspecified</u>**
        H54.61 **Unqualified visual loss, <u>right</u> eye, normal vision <u>left</u> eye**
        H54.62 **Unqualified visual loss, <u>left</u> eye, normal vision <u>right</u> eye**
    H54.7 **Unspecified visual loss**
        Visual impairment category 9 NOS
    H54.8 **Legal blindness, as defined in USA**
        Blindness NOS according to USA definition
        Excludes 1: *legal blindness with specification of impairment level*
            (H54.0-H54.7)
        Note: The table below gives a classification of severity of visual
            impairment recommended by a WHO Study Group on the
            Prevention of Blindness, Geneva, 6-10 November 1972.
        The term "low vision" in category H54 comprises categories 1 and 2
            of the table, the term "blindness" categories 3, 4 and 5, and the
            term "unqualified visual loss" category 9.
        If the extent of the visual field is taken into account, patients with a
            field no greater than 10 but greater than 5 around central fixation
            should be placed in category 3 and patients with a field no
            greater than 5 around central fixation should be placed in
            category 4, even if the central acuity is not impaired.

Category of Visual Impairment	Visual Acuity With Best Possible Correction	
	Maximum less than:	Minimum equal to or better than:
1	6/18 3/10 (0.3) 20/70	6/60 1/10 (0.1) 20/200
2	6/60 1/10 (0.1) 20/200	3/60 1/20 (0.5) 20/400
3	3/60 1/20 (0.05) 20/400	1/60 (finger counting at one meter) 1/50 (0.02) 5/300 (20/1200)
4	1/60 (finger counting at one meter) 1/50 (0.02) 5/300	Light perception
5	No light perception	—
9	Undetermined or unspecified	—

Other disorders of eye and adnexa (H55-H57)

H55- **Nystagmus and other irregular eye movements**
    H55.0- **Nystagmus**
        H55.00 **Unspecified nystagmus**
        H55.01 **Congenital nystagmus**
        H55.02 **Latent nystagmus**
        H55.03 **Visual deprivation nystagmus**
        H55.04 **Dissociated nystagmus**
        H55.09 **Other forms of nystagmus**
    H55.8- **Other irregular eye movements**
        H55.81 **Saccadic eye movements**
        H55.89 **Other irregular eye movements**
H57- **Other disorders of eye and adnexa**
    H57.0- **Anomalies of pupillary function**
        H57.00 **Unspecified anomaly of pupillary function**
        H57.01 **Argyll Robertson pupil, atypical**
            Excludes 1: *syphilitic Argyll Robertson pupil (A52.19)*
        H57.02 **Anisocoria**
        H57.03 **Miosis**
        H57.04 **Mydriasis**
        H57.05- <u>Tonic pupil</u>
            H57.051 **Tonic pupil, <u>right</u> eye**
            H57.052 **Tonic pupil, <u>left</u> eye**
            H57.053 **Tonic pupil, <u>bilateral</u>**
            H57.059 **Tonic pupil, <u>unspecified</u> eye**
        H57.09 **Other anomalies of pupillary function**
    H57.1- <u>Ocular pain</u>
        H57.10 **Ocular pain, <u>unspecified</u> eye**
        H57.11 **Ocular pain, <u>right</u> eye**
        H57.12 **Ocular pain, <u>left</u> eye**
        H57.13 **Ocular pain, <u>bilateral</u>**
    H57.8 **Other specified disorders of eye and adnexa**
    H57.9 **Unspecified disorder of eye and adnexa**

Intraoperative and postprocedural complications and disorders of eye and adnexa, not elsewhere classified (H59)

H59- **Intraoperative and postprocedural complications and disorders of eye and adnexa, not elsewhere classified**
    Excludes 1: *mechanical complication of intraocular lens (T85.2)*
        mechanical complication of other ocular prosthetic devices,
            implants and grafts (T85.3)
        pseudophakia (Z96.1)
        secondary cataracts (H26.4-)
    H59.0- **Disorders of the eye <u>following cataract surgery</u>**
        H59.01- <u>Keratopathy (bullous aphakic)</u> **following cataract surgery**
            Vitreal corneal syndrome
            Vitreous (touch) syndrome
            H59.011 **Keratopathy (bullous aphakic) following cataract surgery, <u>right</u> eye**
            H59.012 **Keratopathy (bullous aphakic) following cataract surgery, <u>left</u> eye**
            H59.013 **Keratopathy (bullous aphakic) following cataract surgery, <u>bilateral</u>**
            H59.019 **Keratopathy (bullous aphakic) following cataract surgery, <u>unspecified</u> eye**
        H59.02- <u>Cataract (lens) fragments in eye</u> **following cataract surgery**
            H59.021 **Cataract (lens) fragments in eye following cataract surgery, <u>right</u> eye**
            H59.022 **Cataract (lens) fragments in eye following cataract surgery, <u>left</u> eye**
            H59.023 **Cataract (lens) fragments in eye following cataract surgery, <u>bilateral</u>**
            H59.029 **Cataract (lens) fragments in eye following cataract surgery, <u>unspecified</u> eye**
        H59.03- <u>Cystoid macular edema</u> **following cataract surgery**
            H59.031 **Cystoid macular edema following cataract surgery, <u>right</u> eye**
            H59.032 **Cystoid macular edema following cataract surgery, <u>left</u> eye**
            H59.033 **Cystoid macular edema following cataract surgery, <u>bilateral</u>**
            H59.039 **Cystoid macular edema following cataract surgery, <u>unspecified</u> eye**

Excludes 1: = NOT CODED HERE! (Do not code both)   *Excludes ❷: =* Not Included Here

H59.09- <u>Other disorders of the eye</u> following cataract surgery
    H59.091   Other disorders of the <u>right</u> eye following cataract surgery
    H59.092   Other disorders of the <u>left</u> eye following cataract surgery
    H59.093   Other disorders of the eye following cataract surgery, <u>bilateral</u>
    H59.099   Other disorders of <u>unspecified</u> eye following cataract surgery

H59.1- <u>Intraoperative hemorrhage and hematoma of eye and adnexa complicating a procedure</u>
    Excludes 1: intraoperative hemorrhage and hematoma of eye and adnexa due to accidental puncture or laceration during a procedure (H59.2-)

H59.11- <u>Intraoperative hemorrhage and hematoma</u> of eye and adnexa complicating <u>an ophthalmic procedure</u>
    H59.111   Intraoperative hemorrhage and hematoma of <u>right</u> eye and adnexa complicating an ophthalmic procedure
    H59.112   Intraoperative hemorrhage and hematoma of <u>left</u> eye and adnexa complicating an ophthalmic procedure
    H59.113   Intraoperative hemorrhage and hematoma of eye and adnexa complicating an ophthalmic procedure, <u>bilateral</u>
    H59.119   Intraoperative hemorrhage and hematoma of <u>unspecified</u> eye and adnexa complicating an ophthalmic procedure

H59.12- <u>Intraoperative hemorrhage and hematoma</u> of eye and adnexa complicating <u>other procedure</u>
    H59.121   Intraoperative hemorrhage and hematoma of <u>right</u> eye and adnexa complicating other procedure
    H59.122   Intraoperative hemorrhage and hematoma of <u>left</u> eye and adnexa complicating other procedure
    H59.123   Intraoperative hemorrhage and hematoma of eye and adnexa complicating other procedure, <u>bilateral</u>
    H59.129   Intraoperative hemorrhage and hematoma of <u>unspecified</u> eye and adnexa complicating other procedure

H59.2- <u>Accidental puncture and laceration</u> of eye and adnexa during a procedure
H59.21- Accidental puncture and laceration of eye and adnexa during an <u>ophthalmic procedure</u>
    H59.211   Accidental puncture and laceration of <u>right</u> eye and adnexa during an ophthalmic procedure
    H59.212   Accidental puncture and laceration of <u>left</u> eye and adnexa during an ophthalmic procedure
    H59.213   Accidental puncture and laceration of eye and adnexa during an ophthalmic procedure, <u>bilateral</u>
    H59.219   Accidental puncture and laceration of <u>unspecified</u> eye and adnexa during an ophthalmic procedure

H59.22- Accidental puncture and laceration of eye and adnexa during <u>other procedure</u>
    H59.221   Accidental puncture and laceration of <u>right</u> eye and adnexa during other procedure
    H59.222   Accidental puncture and laceration of <u>left</u> eye and adnexa during other procedure
    H59.223   Accidental puncture and laceration of eye and adnexa during other procedure, <u>bilateral</u>
    H59.229   Accidental puncture and laceration of <u>unspecified</u> eye and adnexa during other procedure

H59.3- <u>Postprocedural hemorrhage and hematoma</u> of eye and adnexa following a procedure
H59.31- Postprocedural hemorrhage and hematoma of eye and adnexa following an <u>ophthalmic procedure</u>
    H59.311   Postprocedural hemorrhage and hematoma of <u>right</u> eye and adnexa following an ophthalmic procedure
    H59.312   Postprocedural hemorrhage and hematoma of <u>left</u> eye and adnexa following an ophthalmic procedure
    H59.313   Postprocedural hemorrhage and hematoma of eye and adnexa following an ophthalmic procedure, <u>bilateral</u>
    H59.319   Postprocedural hemorrhage and hematoma of <u>unspecified</u> eye and adnexa following an ophthalmic procedure

H59.32- Postprocedural hemorrhage and hematoma of eye and adnexa following <u>other procedure</u>
    H59.321   Postprocedural hemorrhage and hematoma of <u>right</u> eye and adnexa following other procedure
    H59.322   Postprocedural hemorrhage and hematoma of <u>left</u> eye and adnexa following other procedure
    H59.323   Postprocedural hemorrhage and hematoma of eye and adnexa following other procedure, <u>bilateral</u>
    H59.329   Postprocedural hemorrhage and hematoma of <u>unspecified</u> eye and adnexa following other procedure

H59.4- <u>Inflammation (infection) of postprocedural bleb</u>
    Postprocedural blebitis
    Excludes 1: filtering (vitreous) bleb after glaucoma surgery status (Z98.83)
    H59.40   Inflammation (infection) of postprocedural bleb, unspecified
    H59.41   Inflammation (infection) of postprocedural bleb, stage 1
    H59.42   Inflammation (infection) of postprocedural bleb, stage 2
    H59.43   Inflammation (infection) of postprocedural bleb, stage 3
       Bleb endophthalmitis

H59.8- Other intraoperative and postprocedural complications and disorders of eye and adnexa, not elsewhere classified
H59.81- <u>Chorioretinal scars after surgery for detachment</u>
    H59.811   Chorioretinal scars after surgery for detachment, <u>right</u> eye
    H59.812   Chorioretinal scars after surgery for detachment, <u>left</u> eye
    H59.813   Chorioretinal scars after surgery for detachment, <u>bilateral</u>
    H59.819   Chorioretinal scars after surgery for detachment, <u>unspecified</u> eye

H59.88 Other intraoperative complications of eye and adnexa, not elsewhere classified
H59.89 Other postprocedural complications and disorders of eye and adnexa, not elsewhere classified

H
5
3
-
H
5
9

This page is intentionally blank.

H
5
9
–
H
6
0

Chapter 8 – Diseases of the ear and mastoid process
(H60-H95)

Note: Use an external cause code following the code for the ear condition, if applicable, to identify the cause of the ear condition
Excludes❷: certain conditions originating in the perinatal period (P04-P96)
certain infectious and parasitic diseases (A00-B99)
complications of pregnancy, childbirth and the puerperium (O00-O9A)
congenital malformations, deformations and chromosomal abnormalities (Q00-Q99)
endocrine, nutritional and metabolic diseases (E00-E88)
injury, poisoning and certain other consequences of external causes (S00-T88)
neoplasms (C00-D49)
symptoms, signs and abnormal clinical and laboratory findings, not elsewhere classified (R00-R94)

This chapter contains the following blocks:
H60-H62   Diseases of external ear
H65-H75   Diseases of middle ear and mastoid
H80-H83   Diseases of inner ear
H90-H94   Other disorders of ear
H95   Intraoperative and postprocedural complications and disorders of ear and mastoid process, not elsewhere classified

Diseases of external ear (H60-H62)

H60- Otitis externa
H60.0- Abscess of external ear
    Boil of external ear
    Carbuncle of auricle or external auditory canal
    Furuncle of external ear
  H60.00 Abscess of external ear, unspecified ear
  H60.01 Abscess of right external ear
  H60.02 Abscess of left external ear
  H60.03 Abscess of external ear, bilateral
H60.1- Cellulitis of external ear
    Cellulitis of auricle
    Cellulitis of external auditory canal
  H60.10 Cellulitis of external ear, unspecified ear
  H60.11 Cellulitis of right external ear
  H60.12 Cellulitis of left external ear
  H60.13 Cellulitis of external ear, bilateral
H60.2- Malignant otitis externa
  H60.20 Malignant otitis externa, unspecified ear
  H60.21 Malignant otitis externa, right ear
  H60.22 Malignant otitis externa, left ear
  H60.23 Malignant otitis externa, bilateral
H60.3- Other infective otitis externa
  H60.31- Diffuse otitis externa
    H60.311 Diffuse otitis externa, right ear
    H60.312 Diffuse otitis externa, left ear
    H60.313 Diffuse otitis externa, bilateral
    H60.319 Diffuse otitis externa, unspecified ear
  H60.32- Hemorrhagic otitis externa
    H60.321 Hemorrhagic otitis externa, right ear
    H60.322 Hemorrhagic otitis externa, left ear
    H60.323 Hemorrhagic otitis externa, bilateral
    H60.329 Hemorrhagic otitis externa, unspecified ear
  H60.33- Swimmer's ear
    H60.331 Swimmer's ear, right ear
    H60.332 Swimmer's ear, left ear
    H60.333 Swimmer's ear, bilateral
    H60.339 Swimmer's ear, unspecified ear
  H60.39- Other infective otitis externa
    H60.391 Other infective otitis externa, right ear
    H60.392 Other infective otitis externa, left ear
    H60.393 Other infective otitis externa, bilateral
    H60.399 Other infective otitis externa, unspecified ear

H60.4- Cholesteatoma of external ear
    Keratosis obturans of external ear (canal)
    Excludes❷: cholesteatoma of middle ear (H71.-)
    recurrent cholesteatoma of postmastoidectomy cavity (H95.0-)
  H60.40 Cholesteatoma of external ear, unspecified ear
  H60.41 Cholesteatoma of right external ear
  H60.42 Cholesteatoma of left external ear
  H60.43 Cholesteatoma of external ear, bilateral
H60.5- Acute noninfective otitis externa
  H60.50- Unspecified acute noninfective otitis externa
    Acute otitis externa NOS
    H60.501 Unspecified acute noninfective otitis externa, right ear
    H60.502 Unspecified acute noninfective otitis externa, left ear
    H60.503 Unspecified acute noninfective otitis externa, bilateral
    H60.509 Unspecified acute noninfective otitis externa, unspecified ear
  H60.51- Acute actinic otitis externa
    H60.511 Acute actinic otitis externa, right ear
    H60.512 Acute actinic otitis externa, left ear
    H60.513 Acute actinic otitis externa, bilateral
    H60.519 Acute actinic otitis externa, unspecified ear
  H60.52- Acute chemical otitis externa
    H60.521 Acute chemical otitis externa, right ear
    H60.522 Acute chemical otitis externa, left ear
    H60.523 Acute chemical otitis externa, bilateral
    H60.529 Acute chemical otitis externa, unspecified ear
  H60.53- Acute contact otitis externa
    H60.531 Acute contact otitis externa, right ear
    H60.532 Acute contact otitis externa, left ear
    H60.533 Acute contact otitis externa, bilateral
    H60.539 Acute contact otitis externa, unspecified ear
  H60.54- Acute eczematoid otitis externa
    H60.541 Acute eczematoid otitis externa, right ear
    H60.542 Acute eczematoid otitis externa, left ear
    H60.543 Acute eczematoid otitis externa, bilateral
    H60.549 Acute eczematoid otitis externa, unspecified ear
  H60.55- Acute reactive otitis externa
    H60.551 Acute reactive otitis externa, right ear
    H60.552 Acute reactive otitis externa, left ear
    H60.553 Acute reactive otitis externa, bilateral
    H60.559 Acute reactive otitis externa, unspecified ear
  H60.59- Other noninfective acute otitis externa
    H60.591 Other noninfective acute otitis externa, right ear
    H60.592 Other noninfective acute otitis externa, left ear
    H60.593 Other noninfective acute otitis externa, bilateral
    H60.599 Other noninfective acute otitis externa, unspecified ear
H60.6- Unspecified chronic otitis externa
  H60.60 Unspecified chronic otitis externa, unspecified ear
  H60.61 Unspecified chronic otitis externa, right ear
  H60.62 Unspecified chronic otitis externa, left ear
  H60.63 Unspecified chronic otitis externa, bilateral
H60.8- Other otitis externa
  H60.8x- Other otitis externa
    H60.8x1 Other otitis externa, right ear
    H60.8x2 Other otitis externa, left ear
    H60.8x3 Other otitis externa, bilateral
    H60.8x9 Other otitis externa, unspecified ear
H60.9- Unspecified otitis externa
  H60.90 Unspecified otitis externa, unspecified ear
  H60.91 Unspecified otitis externa, right ear
  H60.92 Unspecified otitis externa, left ear
  H60.93 Unspecified otitis externa, bilateral

H 5 9 - H 6 0

Excludes 1: = NOT CODED HERE! (Do not code both)   *Excludes❷: = Not Included Here*

H61- Other disorders of external ear

H61.0- Chondritis and perichondritis of external ear
Chondrodermatitis nodularis chronica helicis
Perichondritis of auricle
Perichondritis of pinna

H61.00- Unspecified perichondritis of external ear
H61.001   Unspecified perichondritis of <u>right</u> external ear
H61.002   Unspecified perichondritis of <u>left</u> external ear
H61.003   Unspecified perichondritis of external ear, <u>bilateral</u>
H61.009   Unspecified perichondritis of external ear, <u>unspecified</u> ear

H61.01- Acute perichondritis of external ear
H61.011   Acute perichondritis of <u>right</u> external ear
H61.012   Acute perichondritis of <u>left</u> external ear
H61.013   Acute perichondritis of external ear, <u>bilateral</u>
H61.019   Acute perichondritis of external ear, <u>unspecified</u> ear

H61.02- Chronic perichondritis of external ear
H61.021   Chronic perichondritis of <u>right</u> external ear
H61.022   Chronic perichondritis of <u>left</u> external ear
H61.023   Chronic perichondritis of external ear, <u>bilateral</u>
H61.029   Chronic perichondritis of external ear, <u>unspecified</u> ear

H61.03- Chondritis of external ear
Chondritis of auricle
Chondritis of pinna
H61.031   Chondritis of <u>right</u> external ear
H61.032   Chondritis of <u>left</u> external ear
H61.033   Chondritis of external ear, <u>bilateral</u>
H61.039   Chondritis of external ear, <u>unspecified</u> ear

H61.1- Noninfective disorders of pinna
Excludes❷: cauliflower ear (M95.1-)
gouty tophi of ear (M1A.-)

H61.10- Unspecified noninfective disorders of pinna
Disorder of pinna NOS
H61.101   Unspecified noninfective disorders of pinna, <u>right</u> ear
H61.102   Unspecified noninfective disorders of pinna, <u>left</u> ear
H61.103   Unspecified noninfective disorders of pinna, <u>bilateral</u>
H61.109   Unspecified noninfective disorders of pinna, <u>unspecified</u> ear

H61.11- Acquired deformity of pinna
Acquired deformity of auricle
Excludes❷: cauliflower ear (M95.1-)
H61.111   Acquired deformity of pinna, <u>right</u> ear
H61.112   Acquired deformity of pinna, <u>left</u> ear
H61.113   Acquired deformity of pinna, <u>bilateral</u>
H61.119   Acquired deformity of pinna, <u>unspecified</u> ear

H61.12- Hematoma of pinna
Hematoma of auricle
H61.121   Hematoma of pinna, <u>right</u> ear
H61.122   Hematoma of pinna, <u>left</u> ear
H61.123   Hematoma of pinna, <u>bilateral</u>
H61.129   Hematoma of pinna, <u>unspecified</u> ear

H61.19- Other noninfective disorders of pinna
H61.191   Noninfective disorders of pinna, <u>right</u> ear
H61.192   Noninfective disorders of pinna, <u>left</u> ear
H61.193   Noninfective disorders of pinna, <u>bilateral</u>
H61.199   Noninfective disorders of pinna, <u>unspecified</u> ear

H61.2- Impacted cerumen
Wax in ear
H61.20   Impacted cerumen, <u>unspecified</u> ear
H61.21   Impacted cerumen, <u>right</u> ear
H61.22   Impacted cerumen, <u>left</u> ear
H61.23   Impacted cerumen, <u>bilateral</u>

H61.3- Acquired stenosis of external ear canal
Collapse of external ear canal
Excludes 1: postprocedural stenosis of external ear canal (H95.81-)

H61.30- Acquired stenosis of external ear canal, <u>unspecified</u>
H61.301   Acquired stenosis of <u>right</u> external ear canal, unspecified
H61.302   Acquired stenosis of <u>left</u> external ear canal, unspecified
H61.303   Acquired stenosis of external ear canal, unspecified, <u>bilateral</u>
H61.309   Acquired stenosis of external ear canal, unspecified, <u>unspecified</u> ear

H61.31- <u>Acquired stenosis</u> of external ear canal <u>secondary to trauma</u>
H61.311   Acquired stenosis of <u>right</u> external ear canal secondary to trauma
H61.312   Acquired stenosis of <u>left</u> external ear canal secondary to trauma
H61.313   Acquired stenosis of external ear canal secondary to trauma, <u>bilateral</u>
H61.319   Acquired stenosis of external ear canal secondary to trauma, <u>unspecified</u> ear

H61.32- <u>Acquired stenosis</u> of external ear canal <u>secondary to inflammation and infection</u>
H61.321   Acquired stenosis of <u>right</u> external ear canal secondary to inflammation and infection
H61.322   Acquired stenosis of <u>left</u> external ear canal secondary to inflammation and infection
H61.323   Acquired stenosis of external ear canal secondary to inflammation and infection, <u>bilateral</u>
H61.329   Acquired stenosis of external ear canal secondary to inflammation and infection, <u>unspecified</u> ear

H61.39- Other acquired stenosis of external ear canal
H61.391   Other acquired stenosis of <u>right</u> external ear canal
H61.392   Other acquired stenosis of <u>left</u> external ear canal
H61.393   Other acquired stenosis of external ear canal, <u>bilateral</u>
H61.399   Other acquired stenosis of external ear canal, <u>unspecified</u> ear

H61.8- Other specified disorders of external ear

H61.81- <u>Exostosis</u> of external canal
H61.811   Exostosis of <u>right</u> external canal
H61.812   Exostosis of <u>left</u> external canal
H61.813   Exostosis of external canal, <u>bilateral</u>
H61.819   Exostosis of external canal, <u>unspecified</u> ear

H61.89- <u>Other specified disorders</u> of external ear
H61.891   Other specified disorders of <u>right</u> external ear
H61.892   Other specified disorders of <u>left</u> external ear
H61.893   Other specified disorders of external ear, <u>bilateral</u>
H61.899   Other specified disorders of external ear, <u>unspecified</u> ear

H61.9- Disorder of external ear, unspecified
H61.90   Disorder of external ear, unspecified, <u>unspecified</u> ear
H61.91   Disorder of <u>right</u> external ear, unspecified
H61.92   Disorder of <u>left</u> external ear, unspecified
H61.93   Disorder of external ear, unspecified, <u>bilateral</u>

H62- Disorders of external ear <u>in diseases classified elsewhere</u>

H62.4- Otitis externa <u>in other diseases classified elsewhere</u>
Code first underlying disease, such as:
Erysipelas (A46)
Impetigo (L01.0)
Excludes 1: otitis externa (in):
candidiasis (B37.84)
herpes viral [herpes simplex] (B00.1)
herpes zoster (B02.8)
H62.40   Otitis externa in other diseases classified elsewhere, <u>unspecified</u> ear
H62.41   Otitis externa in other diseases classified elsewhere, <u>right</u> ear
H62.42   Otitis externa in other diseases classified elsewhere, <u>left</u> ear
H62.43   Otitis externa in other diseases classified elsewhere, <u>bilateral</u>

H62.8- Other disorders of external ear <u>in diseases classified elsewhere</u>
Code first underlying disease, such as:
Gout (M1A.-, M10.-)
H62.8x- Other disorders of external ear in diseases classified elsewhere
H62.8x1   Other disorders of <u>right</u> external ear in diseases classified elsewhere
H62.8x2   Other disorders of <u>left</u> external ear in diseases classified elsewhere
H62.8x3   Other disorders of external ear in diseases classified elsewhere, <u>bilateral</u>
H62.8x9   Other disorders of external ear in diseases classified elsewhere, <u>unspecified</u> ear

H
6
1
–
H
6
6

Diseases of middle ear and mastoid (H65-H75)

H65- **Nonsuppurative** otitis media
Includes: Nonsuppurative otitis media with myringitis
Use additional code for any associated perforated tympanic membrane
(H72.-)
Use additional code to identify:
Exposure to environmental tobacco smoke (Z77.22)
Exposure to tobacco smoke in the perinatal period (P96.81)
History of tobacco use (Z87.891)
Occupational exposure to environmental tobacco smoke (Z57.31)
Tobacco dependence (F17.-)
Tobacco use (Z72.0)

H65.0- **Acute serous** otitis media
Acute and subacute secretory otitis
H65.00 Acute serous otitis media, **unspecified** ear
H65.01 Acute serous otitis media, **right** ear
H65.02 Acute serous otitis media, **left** ear
H65.03 Acute serous otitis media, **bilateral**
H65.04 Acute serous otitis media, **recurrent, right** ear
H65.05 Acute serous otitis media, **recurrent, left** ear
H65.06 Acute serous otitis media, **recurrent, bilateral**
H65.07 Acute serous otitis media, **recurrent, unspecified** ear

H65.1- **Other acute** nonsuppurative otitis media
Excludes 1: otitic barotrauma (T70.0)
otitis media (acute) NOS (H66.9)
H65.11- Acute and subacute **allergic** otitis media (mucoid)
(sanguinous) (serous)
H65.111 Acute and subacute allergic otitis media (mucoid)
(sanguinous) (serous), **right** ear
H65.112 Acute and subacute allergic otitis media (mucoid)
(sanguinous) (serous), **left** ear
H65.113 Acute and subacute allergic otitis media (mucoid)
(sanguinous) (serous), **bilateral**
H65.114 Acute and subacute allergic otitis media (mucoid)
(sanguinous) (serous), **recurrent, right** ear
H65.115 Acute and subacute allergic otitis media (mucoid)
(sanguinous) (serous), **recurrent, left** ear
H65.116 Acute and subacute allergic otitis media (mucoid)
(sanguinous) (serous), **recurrent, bilateral**
H65.117 Acute and subacute allergic otitis media (mucoid)
(sanguinous) (serous), **recurrent, unspecified** ear
H65.119 Acute and subacute allergic otitis media (mucoid)
(sanguinous) (serous), **unspecified** ear

H65.19- Other acute nonsuppurative otitis media
Acute and subacute mucoid otitis media
Acute and subacute nonsuppurative otitis media NOS
Acute and subacute sanguinous otitis media
Acute and subacute seromucinous otitis media
H65.191 Other acute nonsuppurative otitis media, **right** ear
H65.192 Other acute nonsuppurative otitis media, **left** ear
H65.193 Other acute nonsuppurative otitis media, **bilateral**
H65.194 Other acute nonsuppurative otitis media, **recurrent,
right** ear
H65.195 Other acute nonsuppurative otitis media, **recurrent,
left** ear
H65.196 Other acute nonsuppurative otitis media, **recurrent,
bilateral**
H65.197 Other acute nonsuppurative otitis media **recurrent,
unspecified** ear
H65.199 Other acute nonsuppurative otitis media, **unspecified**
ear

H65.2- **Chronic serous** otitis media
Chronic tubotympanal catarrh
H65.20 Chronic serous otitis media, **unspecified** ear
H65.21 Chronic serous otitis media, **right** ear
H65.22 Chronic serous otitis media, **left** ear
H65.23 Chronic serous otitis media, **bilateral**

H65.3- **Chronic mucoid** otitis media
Chronic mucinous otitis media
Chronic secretory otitis media
Chronic transudative otitis media
Glue ear
Excludes 1: adhesive middle ear disease (H74.1)
H65.30 Chronic mucoid otitis media, **unspecified** ear
H65.31 Chronic mucoid otitis media, **right** ear
H65.32 Chronic mucoid otitis media, **left** ear
H65.33 Chronic mucoid otitis media, **bilateral**

H65.4- **Other chronic nonsuppurative** otitis media
H65.41- Chronic **allergic** otitis media
H65.411 Chronic allergic otitis media, **right** ear
H65.412 Chronic allergic otitis media, **left** ear
H65.413 Chronic allergic otitis media, **bilateral**
H65.419 Chronic allergic otitis media, **unspecified** ear
H65.49- **Other chronic** nonsuppurative otitis media
Chronic exudative otitis media
Chronic nonsuppurative otitis media NOS
Chronic otitis media with effusion (nonpurulent)
Chronic seromucinous otitis media
H65.491 Other chronic nonsuppurative otitis media, **right** ear
H65.492 Other chronic nonsuppurative otitis media, **left** ear
H65.493 Other chronic nonsuppurative otitis media, **bilateral**
H65.499 Other chronic nonsuppurative otitis media,
unspecified ear

H65.9- **Unspecified** nonsuppurative otitis media
Allergic otitis media NOS
Catarrhal otitis media NOS
Exudative otitis media NOS
Mucoid otitis media NOS
Otitis media with effusion (nonpurulent) NOS
Secretory otitis media NOS
Seromucinous otitis media NOS
Serous otitis media NOS
Transudative otitis media NOS
H65.90 Unspecified nonsuppurative otitis media, **unspecified** ear
H65.91 Unspecified nonsuppurative otitis media, **right** ear
H65.92 Unspecified nonsuppurative otitis media, **left** ear
H65.93 Unspecified nonsuppurative otitis media, **bilateral**

H66- **Suppurative and unspecified** otitis media
Includes: Suppurative and unspecified otitis media with myringitis
Use additional code to identify:
Exposure to environmental tobacco smoke (Z77.22)
Exposure to tobacco smoke in the perinatal period (P96.81)
History of tobacco use (Z87.891)
Occupational exposure to environmental tobacco smoke (Z57.31)
Tobacco dependence (F17.-)
Tobacco use (Z72.0)

H66.0- **Acute suppurative** otitis media
H66.00- Acute suppurative otitis media **without** spontaneous rupture
of ear drum
H66.001 Acute suppurative otitis media without spontaneous
rupture of ear drum, **right** ear
H66.002 Acute suppurative otitis media without spontaneous
rupture of ear drum, **left** ear
H66.003 Acute suppurative otitis media without spontaneous
rupture of ear drum, **bilateral**
H66.004 Acute suppurative otitis media without spontaneous
rupture of ear drum, **recurrent, right** ear
H66.005 Acute suppurative otitis media without spontaneous
rupture of ear drum, **recurrent, left** ear
H66.006 Acute suppurative otitis media without spontaneous
rupture of ear drum, **recurrent, bilateral**
H66.007 Acute suppurative otitis media without spontaneous
rupture of ear drum, **recurrent, unspecified** ear
H66.009 Acute suppurative otitis media without spontaneous
rupture of ear drum, **unspecified** ear

H66.01- Acute suppurative otitis media **with spontaneous rupture of
ear drum**
H66.011 Acute suppurative otitis media with spontaneous
rupture of ear drum, **right** ear
H66.012 Acute suppurative otitis media with spontaneous
rupture of ear drum, **left** ear
H66.013 Acute suppurative otitis media with spontaneous
rupture of ear drum, **bilateral**
H66.014 Acute suppurative otitis media with spontaneous
rupture of ear drum, **recurrent, right** ear
H66.015 Acute suppurative otitis media with spontaneous
rupture of ear drum, **recurrent, left** ear
H66.016 Acute suppurative otitis media with spontaneous
rupture of ear drum, **recurrent, bilateral**
H66.017 Acute suppurative otitis media with spontaneous
rupture of ear drum, **recurrent, unspecified** ear
H66.019 Acute suppurative otitis media with spontaneous
rupture of ear drum, **unspecified** ear

H
6
1
-
H
6
6

H66.1- <u>Chronic tubotympanic</u> suppurative otitis media
    Benign chronic suppurative otitis media
    Chronic tubotympanic disease
    Use additional code for any associated perforated tympanic
      membrane (H72.-)
  H66.10 Chronic tubotympanic suppurative otitis media, <u>unspecified</u>
  H66.11 Chronic tubotympanic suppurative otitis media, <u>right</u> ear
  H66.12 Chronic tubotympanic suppurative otitis media, <u>left</u> ear
  H66.13 Chronic tubotympanic suppurative otitis media, <u>bilateral</u>

H66.2- <u>Chronic atticoantral</u> suppurative otitis media
    Chronic atticoantral disease
    Use additional code for any associated perforated tympanic
      membrane (H72.-)
  H66.20 Chronic atticoantral suppurative otitis media, <u>unspecified</u>
       ear
  H66.21 Chronic atticoantral suppurative otitis media, <u>right</u> ear
  H66.22 Chronic atticoantral suppurative otitis media, <u>left</u> ear
  H66.23 Chronic atticoantral suppurative otitis media, <u>bilateral</u>

H66.3- <u>Other chronic</u> suppurative otitis media
    Chronic suppurative otitis media NOS
    Use additional code for any associated perforated tympanic
      membrane (H72.-)
    Excludes 1: *tuberculous otitis media (A18.6)*
  H66.3x- <u>Other chronic</u> suppurative otitis media
    H66.3x1 Other chronic suppurative otitis media, <u>right</u> ear
    H66.3x2 Other chronic suppurative otitis media, <u>left</u> ear
    H66.3x3 Other chronic suppurative otitis media, <u>bilateral</u>
    H66.3x9 Other chronic suppurative otitis media, <u>unspecified</u>
         ear

H66.4- <u>Suppurative</u> otitis media, <u>unspecified</u>
    Purulent otitis media NOS
    Use additional code for any associated perforated tympanic
      membrane (H72.-)
  H66.40 Suppurative otitis media, unspecified, <u>unspecified</u> ear
  H66.41 Suppurative otitis media, unspecified, <u>right</u> ear
  H66.42 Suppurative otitis media, unspecified, <u>left</u> ear
  H66.43 Suppurative otitis media, unspecified, <u>bilateral</u>

H66.9- Otitis media, <u>unspecified</u>
    Otitis media NOS
    Acute otitis media NOS
    Chronic otitis media NOS
    Use additional code for any associated perforated tympanic
      membrane (H72.-)
  H66.90 Otitis media, unspecified, <u>unspecified</u> ear
  H66.91 Otitis media, unspecified, <u>right</u> ear
  H66.92 Otitis media, unspecified, <u>left</u> ear
  H66.93 Otitis media, unspecified, <u>bilateral</u>

H67- Otitis media <u>in diseases classified elsewhere</u>
    Code first underlying disease, such as:
      Viral disease NEC (B00-B34)
    Use additional code for any associated perforated tympanic membrane
      (H72.-)
    Excludes 1: *otitis media in:*
        influenza (J09.X9, J10.83, J11.83)
        measles (B05.3)
        scarlet fever (A38.0)
        tuberculosis (A18.6)
  H67.1 Otitis media in diseases classified elsewhere, <u>right</u> ear
  H67.2 Otitis media in diseases classified elsewhere, <u>left</u> ear
  H67.3 Otitis media in diseases classified elsewhere, <u>bilateral</u>
  H67.9 Otitis media in diseases classified elsewhere, <u>unspecified</u> ear

H68- Eustachian salpingitis and obstruction
  H68.0- <u>Eustachian salpingitis</u>
    H68.00- <u>Unspecified</u> Eustachian salpingitis
      H68.001 Unspecified Eustachian salpingitis, <u>right</u> ear
      H68.002 Unspecified Eustachian salpingitis, <u>left</u> ear
      H68.003 Unspecified Eustachian salpingitis, <u>bilateral</u>
      H68.009 Unspecified Eustachian salpingitis, <u>unspecified</u> ear
    H68.01- <u>Acute</u> Eustachian salpingitis
      H68.011 Acute Eustachian salpingitis, <u>right</u> ear
      H68.012 Acute Eustachian salpingitis, <u>left</u> ear
      H68.013 Acute Eustachian salpingitis, <u>bilateral</u>
      H68.019 Acute Eustachian salpingitis, <u>unspecified</u> ear
    H68.02- <u>Chronic</u> Eustachian salpingitis
      H68.021 Chronic Eustachian salpingitis, <u>right</u> ear
      H68.022 Chronic Eustachian salpingitis, <u>left</u> ear
      H68.023 Chronic Eustachian salpingitis, <u>bilateral</u>
      H68.029 Chronic Eustachian salpingitis, <u>unspecified</u> ear

H68.1- <u>Obstruction</u> of Eustachian tube
    Stenosis of Eustachian tube
    Stricture of Eustachian tube
  H68.10- <u>Unspecified</u> obstruction of Eustachian tube
    H68.101 Unspecified obstruction of Eustachian tube, <u>right</u> ear
    H68.102 Unspecified obstruction of Eustachian tube, <u>left</u> ear
    H68.103 Unspecified obstruction of Eustachian tube, <u>bilateral</u>
    H68.109 Unspecified obstruction of Eustachian tube,
         <u>unspecified</u> ear
  H68.11- <u>Osseous</u> obstruction of Eustachian tube
    H68.111 Osseous obstruction of Eustachian tube, <u>right</u> ear
    H68.112 Osseous obstruction of Eustachian tube, <u>left</u> ear
    H68.113 Osseous obstruction of Eustachian tube, <u>bilateral</u>
    H68.119 Osseous obstruction of Eustachian tube, <u>unspecified</u>
         ear
  H68.12- <u>Intrinsic cartilagenous</u> obstruction of Eustachian tube
    H68.121 Intrinsic cartilagenous obstruction of Eustachian tube,
         <u>right</u> ear
    H68.122 Intrinsic cartilagenous obstruction of Eustachian tube,
         <u>left</u> ear
    H68.123 Intrinsic cartilagenous obstruction of Eustachian tube,
         <u>bilateral</u>
    H68.129 Intrinsic cartilagenous obstruction of Eustachian tube,
         <u>unspecified</u> ear
  H68.13- <u>Extrinsic cartilagenous</u> obstruction of Eustachian tube
    Compression of Eustachian tube
    H68.131 Extrinsic cartilagenous obstruction of Eustachian
         tube, <u>right</u> ear
    H68.132 Extrinsic cartilagenous obstruction of Eustachian
         tube, <u>left</u> ear
    H68.133 Extrinsic cartilagenous obstruction of Eustachian
         tube, <u>bilateral</u>
    H68.139 Extrinsic cartilagenous obstruction of Eustachian
         tube, <u>unspecified</u> ear

H69- Other and unspecified disorders of Eustachian tube
  H69.0- <u>Patulous</u> Eustachian tube
    H69.00 Patulous Eustachian tube, <u>unspecified</u> ear
    H69.01 Patulous Eustachian tube, <u>right</u> ear
    H69.02 Patulous Eustachian tube, <u>left</u> ear
    H69.03 Patulous Eustachian tube, <u>bilateral</u>
  H69.8- <u>Other specified</u> disorders of Eustachian tube
    H69.80 Other specified disorders of Eustachian tube, <u>unspecified</u> ear
    H69.81 Other specified disorders of Eustachian tube, <u>right</u> ear
    H69.82 Other specified disorders of Eustachian tube, <u>left</u> ear
    H69.83 Other specified disorders of Eustachian tube, <u>bilateral</u>
  H69.9- <u>Unspecified</u> Eustachian tube disorder
    H69.90 Unspecified Eustachian tube disorder, <u>unspecified</u> ear
    H69.91 Unspecified Eustachian tube disorder, <u>right</u> ear
    H69.92 Unspecified Eustachian tube disorder, <u>left</u> ear
    H69.93 Unspecified Eustachian tube disorder, <u>bilateral</u>

H70- Mastoiditis and related conditions
  H70.0- <u>Acute mastoiditis</u>
    Abscess of mastoid
    Empyema of mastoid
  H70.00- Acute mastoiditis <u>without</u> complications
    H70.001 Acute mastoiditis without complications, <u>right</u> ear
    H70.002 Acute mastoiditis without complications, <u>left</u> ear
    H70.003 Acute mastoiditis without complications, <u>bilateral</u>
    H70.009 Acute mastoiditis without complications, <u>unspecified</u>
         ear
  H70.01- <u>Subperiosteal abscess</u> of mastoid
    H70.011 Subperiosteal abscess of mastoid, <u>right</u> ear
    H70.012 Subperiosteal abscess of mastoid, <u>left</u> ear
    H70.013 Subperiosteal abscess of mastoid, <u>bilateral</u>
    H70.019 Subperiosteal abscess of mastoid, <u>unspecified</u> ear
  H70.09- Acute mastoiditis <u>with other complications</u>
    H70.091 Acute mastoiditis with other complications, <u>right</u> ear
    H70.092 Acute mastoiditis with other complications, <u>left</u> ear
    H70.093 Acute mastoiditis with other complications, <u>bilateral</u>
    H70.099 Acute mastoiditis with other complications,
         <u>unspecified</u> ear

H 6 6 - H 7 3

H70.1- Chronic mastoiditis
Caries of mastoid
Fistula of mastoid
Excludes 1: tuberculous mastoiditis (A18.03)
 H70.10 Chronic mastoiditis, <u>unspecified</u> ear
 H70.11 Chronic mastoiditis, <u>right</u> ear
 H70.12 Chronic mastoiditis, <u>left</u> ear
 H70.13 Chronic mastoiditis, <u>bilateral</u>
H70.2- Petrositis
Inflammation of petrous bone
 H70.20- <u>Unspecified</u> petrositis
 H70.201 Unspecified petrositis, <u>right</u> ear
 H70.202 Unspecified petrositis, <u>left</u> ear
 H70.203 Unspecified petrositis, <u>bilateral</u>
 H70.209 Unspecified petrositis, <u>unspecified</u> ear
 H70.21- <u>Acute</u> petrositis
 H70.211 Acute petrositis, <u>right</u> ear
 H70.212 Acute petrositis, <u>left</u> ear
 H70.213 Acute petrositis, <u>bilateral</u>
 H70.219 Acute petrositis, <u>unspecified</u> ear
 H70.22- Chronic petrositis
 H70.221 Chronic petrositis, <u>right</u> ear
 H70.222 Chronic petrositis, <u>left</u> ear
 H70.223 Chronic petrositis, <u>bilateral</u>
 H70.229 Chronic petrositis, <u>unspecified</u> ear
H70.8- Other mastoiditis and related conditions
Excludes 1: preauricular sinus and cyst (Q18.1)
sinus, fistula, and cyst of branchial cleft (Q18.0)
 H70.81- <u>Postauricular fistula</u>
 H70.811 Postauricular fistula, <u>right</u> ear
 H70.812 Postauricular fistula, <u>left</u> ear
 H70.813 Postauricular fistula, <u>bilateral</u>
 H70.819 Postauricular fistula, <u>unspecified</u> ear
 H70.89- <u>Other mastoiditis and related conditions</u>
 H70.891 Other mastoiditis and related conditions, <u>right</u> ear
 H70.892 Other mastoiditis and related conditions, <u>left</u> ear
 H70.893 Other mastoiditis and related conditions, <u>bilateral</u>
 H70.899 Other mastoiditis and related conditions, <u>unspecified</u> ear
H70.9- <u>Unspecified</u> mastoiditis
 H70.90 Unspecified mastoiditis, <u>unspecified</u> ear
 H70.91 Unspecified mastoiditis, <u>right</u> ear
 H70.92 Unspecified mastoiditis, <u>left</u> ear
 H70.93 Unspecified mastoiditis, <u>bilateral</u>
H71- Cholesteatoma of <u>middle ear</u>
Excludes❷: cholesteatoma of external ear (H60.4-)
recurrent cholesteatoma of postmastoidectomy cavity (H95.0-)
H71.0- Cholesteatoma of <u>attic</u>
 H71.00 Cholesteatoma of attic, <u>unspecified</u> ear
 H71.01 Cholesteatoma of attic, <u>right</u> ear
 H71.02 Cholesteatoma of attic, <u>left</u> ear
 H71.03 Cholesteatoma of attic, <u>bilateral</u>
H71.1- Cholesteatoma of <u>tympanum</u>
 H71.10 Cholesteatoma of tympanum, <u>unspecified</u> ear
 H71.11 Cholesteatoma of tympanum, <u>right</u> ear
 H71.12 Cholesteatoma of tympanum, <u>left</u> ear
 H71.13 Cholesteatoma of tympanum, <u>bilateral</u>
H71.2- Cholesteatoma of <u>mastoid</u>
 H71.20 Cholesteatoma of mastoid, <u>unspecified</u> ear
 H71.21 Cholesteatoma of mastoid, <u>right</u> ear
 H71.22 Cholesteatoma of mastoid, <u>left</u> ear
 H71.23 Cholesteatoma of mastoid, <u>bilateral</u>
H71.3- <u>Diffuse</u> cholesteatosis
 H71.30 Diffuse cholesteatosis, <u>unspecified</u> ear
 H71.31 Diffuse cholesteatosis, <u>right</u> ear
 H71.32 Diffuse cholesteatosis, <u>left</u> ear
 H71.33 Diffuse cholesteatosis, <u>bilateral</u>
H71.9- <u>Unspecified</u> cholesteatoma
 H71.90 Unspecified cholesteatoma, <u>unspecified</u> ear
 H71.91 Unspecified cholesteatoma, <u>right</u> ear
 H71.92 Unspecified cholesteatoma, <u>left</u> ear
 H71.93 Unspecified cholesteatoma, <u>bilateral</u>

H72- Perforation of tympanic membrane
Includes: Persistent post-traumatic perforation of ear drum
Postinflammatory perforation of ear drum
Code first any associated otitis media (H65.-, H66.1-, H66.2-, H66.3-, H66.4-, H66.9-, H67.-)
Excludes 1: acute suppurative otitis media with rupture of the tympanic membrane (H66.01-)
traumatic rupture of ear drum (S09.2-)
H72.0- <u>Central</u> perforation of tympanic membrane
 H72.00 Central perforation of tympanic membrane, <u>unspecified</u> ear
 H72.01 Central perforation of tympanic membrane, <u>right</u> ear
 H72.02 Central perforation of tympanic membrane, <u>left</u> ear
 H72.03 Central perforation of tympanic membrane, <u>bilateral</u>
H72.1- <u>Attic</u> perforation of tympanic membrane
Perforation of pars flaccida
 H72.10 Attic perforation of tympanic membrane, <u>unspecified</u> ear
 H72.11 Attic perforation of tympanic membrane, <u>right</u> ear
 H72.12 Attic perforation of tympanic membrane, <u>left</u> ear
 H72.13 Attic perforation of tympanic membrane, <u>bilateral</u>
H72.2- Other marginal perforations of tympanic membrane
 H72.2x- <u>Other marginal perforations</u> of tympanic membrane
 H72.2x1 Other marginal perforations of tympanic membrane, <u>right</u> ear
 H72.2x2 Other marginal perforations of tympanic membrane, <u>left</u> ear
 H72.2x3 Other marginal perforations of tympanic membrane, <u>bilateral</u>
 H72.2x9 Other marginal perforations of tympanic membrane, <u>unspecified</u> ear
H72.8- Other perforations of tympanic membrane
 H72.81- <u>Multiple</u> perforations of tympanic membrane
 H72.811 Multiple perforations of tympanic membrane, <u>right</u> ear
 H72.812 Multiple perforations of tympanic membrane, <u>left</u> ear
 H72.813 Multiple perforations of tympanic membrane, <u>bilateral</u>
 H72.819 Multiple perforations of tympanic membrane, <u>unspecified</u> ear
 H72.82- <u>Total</u> perforations of tympanic membrane
 H72.821 Total perforations of tympanic membrane, <u>right</u> ear
 H72.822 Total perforations of tympanic membrane, <u>left</u> ear
 H72.823 Total perforations of tympanic membrane, <u>bilateral</u>
 H72.829 Total perforations of tympanic membrane, <u>unspecified</u> ear
H72.9- <u>Unspecified</u> perforation of tympanic membrane
 H72.90 Unspecified perforation of tympanic membrane, <u>unspecified</u> ear
 H72.91 Unspecified perforation of tympanic membrane, <u>right</u> ear
 H72.92 Unspecified perforation of tympanic membrane, <u>left</u> ear
 H72.93 Unspecified perforation of tympanic membrane, <u>bilateral</u>
H73- Other disorders of tympanic membrane
H73.0- <u>Acute myringitis</u>
Excludes 1: acute myringitis with otitis media (H65, H66)
 H73.00- <u>Unspecified</u> acute myringitis
Acute tympanitis NOS
 H73.001 Acute myringitis, <u>right</u> ear
 H73.002 Acute myringitis, <u>left</u> ear
 H73.003 Acute myringitis, <u>bilateral</u>
 H73.009 Acute myringitis, <u>unspecified</u> ear
 H73.01- <u>Bullous</u> myringitis
 H73.011 Bullous myringitis, <u>right</u> ear
 H73.012 Bullous myringitis, <u>left</u> ear
 H73.013 Bullous myringitis, <u>bilateral</u>
 H73.019 Bullous myringitis, <u>unspecified</u> ear
 H73.09- <u>Other</u> acute myringitis
 H73.091 Other acute myringitis, <u>right</u> ear
 H73.092 Other acute myringitis, <u>left</u> ear
 H73.093 Other acute myringitis, <u>bilateral</u>
 H73.099 Other acute myringitis, <u>unspecified</u> ear

H66 - H73

© 2013 Channel Publishing, Ltd.

H73.1- Chronic myringitis
    Chronic tympanitis
    Excludes 1: chronic myringitis with otitis media (H65, H66)
  H73.10 Chronic myringitis, unspecified ear
  H73.11 Chronic myringitis, right ear
  H73.12 Chronic myringitis, left ear
  H73.13 Chronic myringitis, bilateral
H73.2- Unspecified myringitis
  H73.20 Unspecified myringitis, unspecified ear
  H73.21 Unspecified myringitis, right ear
  H73.22 Unspecified myringitis, left ear
  H73.23 Unspecified myringitis, bilateral
H73.8- Other specified disorders of tympanic membrane
  H73.81- Atrophic flaccid tympanic membrane
    H73.811 Atrophic flaccid tympanic membrane, right ear
    H73.812 Atrophic flaccid tympanic membrane, left ear
    H73.813 Atrophic flaccid tympanic membrane, bilateral
    H73.819 Atrophic flaccid tympanic membrane, unspecified ear
  H73.82- Atrophic nonflaccid tympanic membrane
    H73.821 Atrophic nonflaccid tympanic membrane, right ear
    H73.822 Atrophic nonflaccid tympanic membrane, left ear
    H73.823 Atrophic nonflaccid tympanic membrane, bilateral
    H73.829 Atrophic nonflaccid tympanic membrane, unspecified ear
  H73.89- Other specified disorders of tympanic membrane
    H73.891 Other specified disorders of tympanic membrane, right ear
    H73.892 Other specified disorders of tympanic membrane, left ear
    H73.893 Other specified disorders of tympanic membrane, bilateral
    H73.899 Other specified disorders of tympanic membrane, unspecified ear
H73.9- Unspecified disorder of tympanic membrane
  H73.90 Unspecified disorder of tympanic membrane, unspecified ear
  H73.91 Unspecified disorder of tympanic membrane, right ear
  H73.92 Unspecified disorder of tympanic membrane, left ear
  H73.93 Unspecified disorder of tympanic membrane, bilateral
H74- Other disorders of middle ear mastoid
  Excludes❷: mastoiditis (H70.-)
H74.0- Tympanosclerosis
  H74.01 Tympanosclerosis, right ear
  H74.02 Tympanosclerosis, left ear
  H74.03 Tympanosclerosis, bilateral
  H74.09 Tympanosclerosis, unspecified ear
H74.1- Adhesive middle ear disease
    Adhesive otitis
    Excludes 1: glue ear (H65.3-)
  H74.11 Adhesive right middle ear disease
  H74.12 Adhesive left middle ear disease
  H74.13 Adhesive middle ear disease, bilateral
  H74.19 Adhesive middle ear disease, unspecified ear
H74.2- Discontinuity and dislocation of ear ossicles
  H74.20 Discontinuity and dislocation of ear ossicles, unspecified ear
  H74.21 Discontinuity and dislocation of right ear ossicles
  H74.22 Discontinuity and dislocation of left ear ossicles
  H74.23 Discontinuity and dislocation of ear ossicles, bilateral
H74.3- Other acquired abnormalities of ear ossicles
  H74.31- Ankylosis of ear ossicles
    H74.311 Ankylosis of ear ossicles, right ear
    H74.312 Ankylosis of ear ossicles, left ear
    H74.313 Ankylosis of ear ossicles, bilateral
    H74.319 Ankylosis of ear ossicles, unspecified ear
  H74.32- Partial loss of ear ossicles
    H74.321 Partial loss of ear ossicles, right ear
    H74.322 Partial loss of ear ossicles, left ear
    H74.323 Partial loss of ear ossicles, bilateral
    H74.329 Partial loss of ear ossicles, unspecified ear
  H74.39- Other acquired abnormalities of ear ossicles
    H74.391 Other acquired abnormalities of right ear ossicles
    H74.392 Other acquired abnormalities of left ear ossicles
    H74.393 Other acquired abnormalities of ear ossicles, bilateral
    H74.399 Other acquired abnormalities of ear ossicles, unspecified ear

H74.4- Polyp of middle ear
  H74.40 Polyp of middle ear, unspecified ear
  H74.41 Polyp of right middle ear
  H74.42 Polyp of left middle ear
  H74.43 Polyp of middle ear, bilateral
H74.8- Other specified disorders of middle ear and mastoid
  H74.8x- Other specified disorders of middle ear and mastoid
    H74.8x1 Other specified disorders of right middle ear and mastoid
    H74.8x2 Other specified disorders of left middle ear and mastoid
    H74.8x3 Other specified disorders of middle ear and mastoid, bilateral
    H74.8x9 Other specified disorders of middle ear and mastoid, unspecified ear
H74.9- Unspecified disorder of middle ear and mastoid
  H74.90 Unspecified disorder of middle ear and mastoid, unspecified ear
  H74.91 Unspecified disorder of right middle ear and mastoid
  H74.92 Unspecified disorder of left middle ear and mastoid
  H74.93 Unspecified disorder of middle ear and mastoid, bilateral
H75- Other disorders of middle ear and mastoid in diseases classified elsewhere
  Code first underlying disease
H75.0- Mastoiditis in infectious and parasitic diseases classified elsewhere
    Excludes 1: mastoiditis (in):
        syphilis (A52.77)
        tuberculosis (A18.03)
  H75.00 Mastoiditis in infectious and parasitic diseases classified elsewhere, unspecified ear
  H75.01 Mastoiditis in infectious and parasitic diseases classified elsewhere, right ear
  H75.02 Mastoiditis in infectious and parasitic diseases classified elsewhere, left ear
  H75.03 Mastoiditis in infectious and parasitic diseases classified elsewhere, bilateral
H75.8- Other specified disorders of middle ear and mastoid in diseases classified elsewhere
  H75.80 Other specified disorders of middle ear and mastoid in diseases classified elsewhere, unspecified ear
  H75.81 Other specified disorders of right middle ear and mastoid in diseases classified elsewhere
  H75.82 Other specified disorders of left middle ear and mastoid in diseases classified elsewhere
  H75.83 Other specified disorders of middle ear and mastoid in diseases classified elsewhere, bilateral

H73 - H83

© 2013 Channel Publishing, Ltd

Diseases of inner ear (H80-H83)

H80- Otosclerosis
Includes: Otospongiosis
H80.0- Otosclerosis involving oval window, nonobliterative
 H80.00 Otosclerosis involving oval window, nonobliterative, unspecified ear
 H80.01 Otosclerosis involving oval window, nonobliterative, right ear
 H80.02 Otosclerosis involving oval window, nonobliterative, left ear
 H80.03 Otosclerosis involving oval window, nonobliterative, bilateral
H80.1- Otosclerosis involving oval window, obliterative
 H80.10 Otosclerosis involving oval window, obliterative, unspecified ear
 H80.11 Otosclerosis involving oval window, obliterative, right ear
 H80.12 Otosclerosis involving oval window, obliterative, left ear
 H80.13 Otosclerosis involving oval window, obliterative, bilateral
H80.2- Cochlear otosclerosis
 Otosclerosis involving otic capsule
 Otosclerosis involving round window
 H80.20 Cochlear otosclerosis, unspecified ear
 H80.21 Cochlear otosclerosis, right ear
 H80.22 Cochlear otosclerosis, left ear
 H80.23 Cochlear otosclerosis, bilateral
H80.8- Other otosclerosis
 H80.80 Other otosclerosis, unspecified ear
 H80.81 Other otosclerosis, right ear
 H80.82 Other otosclerosis, left ear
 H80.83 Other otosclerosis, bilateral
H80.9- Unspecified otosclerosis
 H80.90 Unspecified otosclerosis, unspecified ear
 H80.91 Unspecified otosclerosis, right ear
 H80.92 Unspecified otosclerosis, left ear
 H80.93 Unspecified otosclerosis, bilateral
H81- Disorders of vestibular function
 Excludes 1: epidemic vertigo (A88.1)
  vertigo NOS (R42)
H81.0- Ménière's disease
 Labyrinthine hydrops
 Ménière's syndrome or vertigo
 H81.01 Ménière's disease, right ear
 H81.02 Ménière's disease, left ear
 H81.03 Ménière's disease, bilateral
 H81.09 Ménière's disease, unspecified ear
H81.1- Benign paroxysmal vertigo
 H81.10 Benign paroxysmal vertigo, unspecified ear
 H81.11 Benign paroxysmal vertigo, right ear
 H81.12 Benign paroxysmal vertigo, left ear
 H81.13 Benign paroxysmal vertigo, bilateral
H81.2- Vestibular neuronitis
 H81.20 Vestibular neuronitis, unspecified ear
 H81.21 Vestibular neuronitis, right ear
 H81.22 Vestibular neuronitis, left ear
 H81.23 Vestibular neuronitis, bilateral
H81.3- Other peripheral vertigo
 H81.31- Aural vertigo
  H81.311 Aural vertigo, right ear
  H81.312 Aural vertigo, left ear
  H81.313 Aural vertigo, bilateral
  H81.319 Aural vertigo, unspecified ear
 H81.39- Other peripheral vertigo
  Lermoyez' syndrome
  Otogenic vertigo
  Peripheral vertigo NOS
  H81.391 Other peripheral vertigo, right ear
  H81.392 Other peripheral vertigo, left ear
  H81.393 Other peripheral vertigo, bilateral
  H81.399 Other peripheral vertigo, unspecified ear

H81.4- Vertigo of central origin
 Central positional nystagmus
 H81.41 Vertigo of central origin, right ear
 H81.42 Vertigo of central origin, left ear
 H81.43 Vertigo of central origin, bilateral
 H81.49 Vertigo of central origin, unspecified ear
H81.8- Other disorders of vestibular function
 H81.8x- Other disorders of vestibular function
  H81.8x1 Other disorders of vestibular function, right ear
  H81.8x2 Other disorders of vestibular function, left ear
  H81.8x3 Other disorders of vestibular function, bilateral
  H81.8x9 Other disorders of vestibular function, unspecified ear
H81.9- Unspecified disorder of vestibular function
 Vertiginous syndrome NOS
 H81.90 Unspecified disorder of vestibular function, unspecified ear
 H81.91 Unspecified disorder of vestibular function, right ear
 H81.92 Unspecified disorder of vestibular function, left ear
 H81.93 Unspecified disorder of vestibular function, bilateral
H82- Vertiginous syndromes in diseases classified elsewhere
 Code first underlying disease
 Excludes 1: epidemic vertigo (A88.1)
 H82.1 Vertiginous syndromes in diseases classified elsewhere, right ear
 H82.2 Vertiginous syndromes in diseases classified elsewhere, left ear
 H82.3 Vertiginous syndromes in diseases classified elsewhere, bilateral
 H82.9 Vertiginous syndromes in diseases classified elsewhere, unspecified ear
H83- Other diseases of inner ear
 H83.0- Labyrinthitis
  H83.01 Labyrinthitis, right ear
  H83.02 Labyrinthitis, left ear
  H83.03 Labyrinthitis, bilateral
  H83.09 Labyrinthitis, unspecified ear
 H83.1- Labyrinthine fistula
  H83.11 Labyrinthine fistula, right ear
  H83.12 Labyrinthine fistula, left ear
  H83.13 Labyrinthine fistula, bilateral
  H83.19 Labyrinthine fistula, unspecified ear
 H83.2- Labyrinthine dysfunction
  Labyrinthine hypersensitivity
  Labyrinthine hypofunction
  Labyrinthine loss of function
  H83.2x- Labyrinthine dysfunction
   H83.2x1 Labyrinthine dysfunction, right ear
   H83.2x2 Labyrinthine dysfunction, left ear
   H83.2x3 Labyrinthine dysfunction, bilateral
   H83.2x9 Labyrinthine dysfunction, unspecified ear
 H83.3- Noise effects on inner ear
  Acoustic trauma of inner ear
  Noise-induced hearing loss of inner ear
  H83.3x- Noise effects on inner ear
   H83.3x1 Noise effects on right inner ear
   H83.3x2 Noise effects on left inner ear
   H83.3x3 Noise effects on inner ear, bilateral
   H83.3x9 Noise effects on inner ear, unspecified ear
 H83.8- Other specified diseases of inner ear
  H83.8x- Other specified diseases of inner ear
   H83.8x1 Other specified diseases of right inner ear
   H83.8x2 Other specified diseases of left inner ear
   H83.8x3 Other specified diseases of inner ear, bilateral
   H83.8x9 Other specified diseases of inner ear, unspecified ear
 H83.9- Unspecified disease of inner ear
  H83.90 Unspecified disease of inner ear, unspecified ear
  H83.91 Unspecified disease of right inner ear
  H83.92 Unspecified disease of left inner ear
  H83.93 Unspecified disease of inner ear, bilateral

H73 - H83

Other disorders of ear (H90-H94)

H90- Conductive and sensorineural hearing loss
  Excludes 1:   deaf nonspeaking NEC (H91.3)
  deafness NOS (H91.9-)
  hearing loss NOS (H91.9-)
  noise-induced hearing loss (H83.3-)
  ototoxic hearing loss (H91.0-)
  sudden (idiopathic) hearing loss (H91.2-)

H90.0 Conductive hearing loss, bilateral

H90.1- Conductive hearing loss, unilateral with unrestricted hearing on the contralateral side

  H90.11 Conductive hearing loss, unilateral, right ear, with unrestricted hearing on the contralateral side

  H90.12 Conductive hearing loss, unilateral, left ear, with unrestricted hearing on the contralateral side

H90.2 Conductive hearing loss, unspecified
  Conductive deafness NOS

H90.3 Sensorineural hearing loss, bilateral

H90.4- Sensorineural hearing loss, unilateral with unrestricted hearing on the contralateral side

  H90.41 Sensorineural hearing loss, unilateral, right ear, with unrestricted hearing on the contralateral side

  H90.42 Sensorineural hearing loss, unilateral, left ear, with unrestricted hearing on the contralateral side

H90.5 Unspecified sensorineural hearing loss
  Central hearing loss NOS
  Congenital deafness NOS
  Neural hearing loss NOS
  Perceptive hearing loss NOS
  Sensorineural deafness NOS
  Sensory hearing loss NOS
  Excludes 1:   abnormal auditory perception (H93.2-)
  psychogenic deafness (F44.6)

H90.6 Mixed conductive and sensorineural hearing loss, bilateral

H90.7- Mixed conductive and sensorineural hearing loss, unilateral with unrestricted hearing on the contralateral side

  H90.71 Mixed conductive and sensorineural hearing loss, unilateral, right ear, with unrestricted hearing on the contralateral side

  H90.72 Mixed conductive and sensorineural hearing loss, unilateral, left ear, with unrestricted hearing on the contralateral side

H90.8 Mixed conductive and sensorineural hearing loss, unspecified

H91- Other and unspecified hearing loss
  Excludes 1:   abnormal auditory perception (H93.2-)
  hearing loss as classified in H90.-
  impacted cerumen (H61.2-)
  noise-induced hearing loss (H83.3-)
  psychogenic deafness (F44.6)
  transient ischemic deafness (H93.01-)

H91.0- Ototoxic hearing loss
  Code first poisoning due to drug or toxin, if applicable (T36-T65 with fifth or sixth character 1-4 or 6)
  Use additional code for adverse effect, if applicable, to identify drug (T36-T50 with fift or sixth character 5)

  H91.01 Ototoxic hearing loss, right ear
  H91.02 Ototoxic hearing loss, left ear
  H91.03 Ototoxic hearing loss, bilateral
  H91.09 Ototoxic hearing loss, unspecified ear

H91.1- Presbycusis
  Presbyacusis
  H91.10 Presbycusis, unspecified ear
  H91.11 Presbycusis, right ear
  H91.12 Presbycusis, left ear
  H91.13 Presbycusis, bilateral

H91.2- Sudden idiopathic hearing loss
  Sudden hearing loss NOS
  H91.20 Sudden idiopathic hearing loss, unspecified ear
  H91.21 Sudden idiopathic hearing loss, right ear
  H91.22 Sudden idiopathic hearing loss, left ear
  H91.23 Sudden idiopathic hearing loss, bilateral

H91.3 Deaf nonspeaking, not elsewhere classified

H91.8- Other specified hearing loss
  H91.8x- Other specified hearing loss
    H91.8x1 Other specified hearing loss, right ear
    H91.8x2 Other specified hearing loss, left ear
    H91.8x3 Other specified hearing loss, bilateral
    H91.8x9 Other specified hearing loss, unspecified ear

H91.9- Unspecified hearing loss
  Deafness NOS
  High frequency deafness
  Low frequency deafness
  H91.90 Unspecified hearing loss, unspecified ear
  H91.91 Unspecified hearing loss, right ear
  H91.92 Unspecified hearing loss, left ear
  H91.93 Unspecified hearing loss, bilateral

H92- Otalgia and effusion of ear
  H92.0- Otalgia
    H92.01 Otalgia, right ear
    H92.02 Otalgia, left ear
    H92.03 Otalgia, bilateral
    H92.09 Otalgia, unspecified ear
  H92.1- Otorrhea
    Excludes 1:   leakage of cerebrospinal fluid through ear (G96.0)
    H92.10 Otorrhea, unspecified ear
    H92.11 Otorrhea, right ear
    H92.12 Otorrhea, left ear
    H92.13 Otorrhea, bilateral
  H92.2- Otorrhagia
    Excludes 1:   traumatic otorrhagia — code to injury
    H92.20 Otorrhagia, unspecified ear
    H92.21 Otorrhagia, right ear
    H92.22 Otorrhagia, left ear
    H92.23 Otorrhagia, bilateral

H93- Other disorders of ear, not elsewhere classified
  H93.0- Degenerative and vascular disorders of ear
    Excludes 1:   presbycusis (H91.1)
    H93.01- Transient ischemic deafness
      H93.011 Transient ischemic deafness, right ear
      H93.012 Transient ischemic deafness, left ear
      H93.013 Transient ischemic deafness, bilateral
      H93.019 Transient ischemic deafness, unspecified ear
    H93.09- Unspecified degenerative and vascular disorders of ear
      H93.091 Unspecified degenerative and vascular disorders of right ear
      H93.092 Unspecified degenerative and vascular disorders of left ear
      H93.093 Unspecified degenerative and vascular disorders of ear, bilateral
      H93.099 Unspecified degenerative and vascular disorders of unspecified ear
  H93.1- Tinnitus
    H93.11 Tinnitus, right ear
    H93.12 Tinnitus, left ear
    H93.13 Tinnitus, bilateral
    H93.19 Tinnitus, unspecified ear
  H93.2- Other abnormal auditory perceptions
    Excludes ❷: auditory hallucinations (R44.0)
    H93.21- Auditory recruitment
      H93.211 Auditory recruitment, right ear
      H93.212 Auditory recruitment, left ear
      H93.213 Auditory recruitment, bilateral
      H93.219 Auditory recruitment, unspecified ear
    H93.22- Diplacusis
      H93.221 Diplacusis, right ear
      H93.222 Diplacusis, left ear
      H93.223 Diplacusis, bilateral
      H93.229 Diplacusis, unspecified ear
    H93.23- Hyperacusis
      H93.231 Hyperacusis, right ear
      H93.232 Hyperacusis, left ear
      H93.233 Hyperacusis, bilateral
      H93.239 Hyperacusis, unspecified ear
    H93.24- Temporary auditory threshold shift
      H93.241 Temporary auditory threshold shift, right ear
      H93.242 Temporary auditory threshold shift, left ear
      H93.243 Temporary auditory threshold shift, bilateral
      H93.249 Temporary auditory threshold shift, unspecified ear

H90-H95

© 2013 Channel Publishing, Ltd.

H93.25 Central auditory processing disorder
Congenital auditory imperception
Word deafness
Excludes 1: mixed receptive-expressive language disorder
(F80.2)

H93.29- <u>Other</u> abnormal auditory perceptions
H93.291 Other abnormal auditory perceptions, <u>right</u> ear
H93.292 Other abnormal auditory perceptions, <u>left</u> ear
H93.293 Other abnormal auditory perceptions, <u>bilateral</u>
H93.299 Other abnormal auditory perceptions, <u>unspecified</u> ear

H93.3- Disorders of acoustic nerve
Disorder of 8th cranial nerve
Excludes 1: acoustic neuroma (D33.3)
syphilitic acoustic neuritis (A52.15)

H93.3x- <u>Disorders of acoustic nerve</u>
H93.3x1 Disorders of <u>right</u> acoustic nerve
H93.3x2 Disorders of <u>left</u> acoustic nerve
H93.3x3 Disorders of <u>bilateral</u> acoustic nerves
H93.3x9 Disorders of <u>unspecified</u> acoustic nerve

H93.8- Other specified disorders of ear
H93.8x- <u>Other specified disorders of ear</u>
H93.8x1 Other specified disorders of <u>right</u> ear
H93.8x2 Other specified disorders of <u>left</u> ear
H93.8x3 Other specified disorders of ear, <u>bilateral</u>
H93.8x9 Other specified disorders of ear, <u>unspecified</u> ear

H93.9- <u>Unspecified</u> disorder of ear
H93.90 Unspecified disorder of ear, <u>unspecified</u> ear
H93.91 Unspecified disorder of <u>right</u> ear
H93.92 Unspecified disorder of <u>left</u> ear
H93.93 Unspecified disorder of ear, <u>bilateral</u>

H94- Other disorders of ear <u>in diseases classified elsewhere</u>
H94.0- Acoustic neuritis <u>in infectious and parasitic diseases classified</u>
<u>elsewhere</u>
Code first underlying disease, such as:
Parasitic disease (B65-B89)
Excludes 1: acoustic neuritis (in):
herpes zoster (B02.29)
syphilis (A52.15)

H94.00 Acoustic neuritis in infectious and parasitic diseases
classified elsewhere, <u>unspecified</u> ear
H94.01 Acoustic neuritis in infectious and parasitic diseases
classified elsewhere, <u>right</u> ear
H94.02 Acoustic neuritis in infectious and parasitic diseases
classified elsewhere, <u>left</u> ear
H94.03 Acoustic neuritis in infectious and parasitic diseases
classified elsewhere, <u>bilateral</u>

H94.8- Other specified disorders of ear <u>in diseases classified elsewhere</u>
Code first underlying disease, such as:
Congenital syphilis (A50.0)
Excludes 1: aural myiasis (B87.4)
syphilitic labyrinthitis (A52.79)

H94.80 Other specified disorders of ear in diseases classified
elsewhere, <u>unspecified</u> ear
H94.81 Other specified disorders of <u>right</u> ear in diseases classified
elsewhere
H94.82 Other specified disorders of <u>left</u> ear in diseases classified
elsewhere
H94.83 Other specified disorders of ear in diseases classified
elsewhere, <u>bilateral</u>

Intraoperative and postprocedural complications and disorders of ear and mastoid process, not elsewhere classified (H95)

H95- <u>Intraoperative and postprocedural complications</u> and disorders of ear
and mastoid process, not elsewhere classified
H95.0- <u>Recurrent cholesteatoma of postmastoidectomy cavity</u>
H95.00 Recurrent cholesteatoma of postmastoidectomy cavity,
<u>unspecified</u> ear
H95.01 Recurrent cholesteatoma of postmastoidectomy cavity, <u>right</u>
ear
H95.02 Recurrent cholesteatoma of postmastoidectomy cavity, <u>left</u>
ear
H95.03 Recurrent cholesteatoma of postmastoidectomy cavity,
<u>bilateral</u> ears

H95.1- <u>Other</u> disorders of ear and mastoid process <u>following</u>
<u>mastoidectomy</u>
H95.11- Chronic inflammation of postmastoidectomy cavity
H95.111 Chronic inflammation of postmastoidectomy cavity,
<u>right</u> ear
H95.112 Chronic inflammation of postmastoidectomy cavity,
<u>left</u> ear
H95.113 Chronic inflammation of postmastoidectomy cavity,
<u>bilateral</u> ears
H95.119 Chronic inflammation of postmastoidectomy cavity,
<u>unspecified</u> ear

H95.12- <u>Granulation</u> of <u>postmastoidectomy cavity</u>
H95.121 Granulation of postmastoidectomy cavity, <u>right</u> ear
H95.122 Granulation of postmastoidectomy cavity, <u>left</u> ear
H95.123 Granulation of postmastoidectomy cavity, <u>bilateral</u>
ears
H95.129 Granulation of postmastoidectomy cavity, <u>unspecified</u>
ear

H95.13- <u>Mucosal cyst</u> of <u>postmastoidectomy cavity</u>
H95.131 Mucosal cyst of postmastoidectomy cavity, <u>right</u> ear
H95.132 Mucosal cyst of postmastoidectomy cavity, <u>left</u> ear
H95.133 Mucosal cyst of postmastoidectomy cavity, <u>bilateral</u>
ears
H95.139 Mucosal cyst of postmastoidectomy cavity, <u>unspecified</u>
ear

H95.19- <u>Other</u> disorders <u>following mastoidectomy</u>
H95.191 Other disorders following mastoidectomy, <u>right</u> ear
H95.192 Other disorders following mastoidectomy, <u>left</u> ear
H95.193 Other disorders following mastoidectomy, <u>bilateral</u>
ears
H95.199 Other disorders following mastoidectomy, <u>unspecified</u>
ear

H95.2- <u>Intraoperative hemorrhage and hematoma</u> of ear and mastoid
process complicating a procedure
Excludes 1: intraoperative hemorrhage and hematoma of ear and
mastoid process due to accidental puncture or
laceration during a procedure (H95.3-)

H95.21 Intraoperative hemorrhage and hematoma of ear and
mastoid process complicating a <u>procedure on the ear and</u>
<u>mastoid process</u>
H95.22 Intraoperative hemorrhage and hematoma of ear and
mastoid process complicating <u>other procedure</u>

H95.3- <u>Accidental puncture and laceration</u> of ear and mastoid process
during a procedure
H95.31 Accidental puncture and laceration of the ear and mastoid
process during a <u>procedure on the ear and mastoid process</u>
H95.32 Accidental puncture and laceration of the ear and mastoid
process during <u>other procedure</u>

H95.4- <u>Postprocedural</u> <u>hemorrhage and hematoma</u> of ear and mastoid
process following a procedure
H95.41 Postprocedural hemorrhage and hematoma of ear and
mastoid process following a <u>procedure on the ear and</u>
<u>mastoid process</u>
H95.42 Postprocedural hemorrhage and hematoma of ear and
mastoid process following <u>other procedure</u>

H90 – H95

H95.8- **Other intraoperative and postprocedural complications and disorders of the ear and mastoid process, not elsewhere classified**
Excludes❷: postprocedural complications and disorders following mastoidectomy (H95.0-, H95.1-)

H95.81- <u>Postprocedural stenosis</u> of external ear canal

    H95.811 Postprocedural stenosis of <u>right</u> external ear canal

    H95.812 Postprocedural stenosis of <u>left</u> external ear canal

    H95.813 Postprocedural stenosis of external ear canal, <u>bilateral</u>

    H95.819 Postprocedural stenosis of <u>unspecified</u> external ear canal

H95.88 **Other intraoperative complications and disorders of the ear and mastoid process, no telsewhere classified**
Use additional code , if applicable, to further specify disorder

H95.89 **Other postprocedural complications and disorders of the ear and mastoid process, not elsewhere classified**
Use additional code, if applicable, to further specify disorder

H 9 5 - I 0 9

Chapter 9 – Diseases of the circulatory system (I00-I99)

Excludes❷: *certain conditions originating in the perinatal period (P04-P96)*
certain infectious and parasitic diseases (A00-B99)
complications of pregnancy, childbirth and the puerperium (O00-O9A)
congenital malformations, deformations, and chromosomal abnormalities (Q00-Q99)
endocrine, nutritional and metabolic diseases (E00-E88)
injury, poisoning and certain other consequences of external causes (S00-T88)
neoplasms (C00-D49)
symptoms, signs and abnormal clinical and laboratory findings, not elsewhere classified (R00-R94)
systemic connective tissue disorders (M30-M36)
transient cerebral ischemic attacks and related syndromes (G45-)

This chapter contains the following blocks:

I00-I02	Acute rheumatic fever
I05-I09	Chronic rheumatic heart diseases
I10-I15	Hypertensive diseases
I20-I25	Ischemic heart diseases
I26-I28	Pulmonary heart disease and diseases of pulmonary circulation
I30-I52	Other forms of heart disease
I60-I69	Cerebrovascular diseases
I70-I79	Diseases of arteries, arterioles and capillaries
I80-I89	Diseases of veins, lymphatic vessels and lymph nodes, not elsewhere classified
I95-I99	Other and unspecified disorders of the circulatory system

Acute rheumatic fever (I00-I02)

I00   **Rheumatic fever <u>without</u> heart involvement**
Includes: Arthritis, rheumatic, acute or subacute
Excludes 1:   rheumatic fever with heart involvement (I01.0 - I01.9)

I01-   **Rheumatic fever <u>with heart involvement</u>**
Excludes 1:   chronic diseases of rheumatic origin (I05-I09) unless rheumatic fever is also present or there is evidence of reactivation or activity of the rheumatic process

   I01.0   **Acute rheumatic pericarditis**
Any condition in I00 with pericarditis
Rheumatic pericarditis (acute)
Excludes 1:   acute pericarditis not specified as rheumatic (I30.-)

   I01.1   **Acute rheumatic endocarditis**
Any condition in I00 with endocarditis or valvulitis
Acute rheumatic valvulitis

   I01.2   **Acute rheumatic myocarditis**
Any condition in I00 with myocarditis

   I01.8   **Other acute rheumatic heart disease**
Any condition in I00 with other or multiple types of heart involvement
Acute rheumatic pancarditis

   I01.9   **Acute rheumatic heart disease, unspecified**
Any condition in I00 with unspecified type of heart involvement
Rheumatic carditis, acute
Rheumatic heart disease, active or acute

I02-   **Rheumatic <u>chorea</u>**
Includes: Sydenham's chorea
Excludes 1:   chorea NOS (G25.5)
Huntington's chorea (G10)

   I02.0   **Rheumatic chorea with heart involvement**
Chorea NOS with heart involvement
Rheumatic chorea with heart involvement of any type classifiable under I01.-

   I02.9   **Rheumatic chorea without heart involvement**
Rheumatic chorea NOS

Chronic rheumatic heart diseases (I05-I09)

I05-   **Rheumatic <u>mitral valve diseases</u>**
Includes: Conditions classifiable to both I05.0 and I05.2-I05.9, whether specified as rheumatic or not
Excludes 1:   mitral valve disease specified as nonrheumatic (I34.-)
mitral valve disease with aortic and/or tricuspid valve involvement (I08.-)

   I05.0   **Rheumatic mitral stenosis**
Mitral (valve) obstruction (rheumatic)

   I05.1   **Rheumatic mitral insufficiency**
Rheumatic mitral incompetence
Rheumatic mitral regurgitation
Excludes 1:   mitral insufficiency not specified as rheumatic (I34.0)

   I05.2   **Rheumatic mitral stenosis <u>with insufficiency</u>**
Rheumatic mitral stenosis with incompetence or regurgitation

   I05.8   **Other rheumatic mitral valve diseases**
Rheumatic mitral (valve) failure

   I05.9   **Rheumatic mitral valve disease, unspecified**
Rheumatic mitral (valve) disorder (chronic) NOS

I06-   **Rheumatic aortic valve diseases**
Excludes 1:   aortic valve disease not specified as rheumatic (I35.-)
aortic valve disease with mitral and/or tricuspid valve involvement (I08.-)

   I06.0   **Rheumatic aortic stenosis**
Rheumatic aortic (valve) obstruction

   I06.1   **Rheumatic aortic insufficiency**
Rheumatic aortic incompetence
Rheumatic aortic regurgitation

   I06.2   **Rheumatic aortic stenosis <u>with insufficiency</u>**
Rheumatic aortic stenosis with incompetence or regurgitation

   I06.8   **Other rheumatic aortic valve diseases**

   I06.9   **Rheumatic aortic valve disease, unspecified**
Rheumatic aortic (valve) disease NOS

I07-   **Rheumatic tricuspid valve diseases**
Includes: Rheumatic tricuspid valve diseases specified as rheumatic or unspecified
Excludes 1:   tricuspid valve disease specified as nonrheumatic (I36.-)
tricuspid valve disease with aortic and/or mitral valve involvement (I08.-)

   I07.0   **Rheumatic tricuspid stenosis**
Tricuspid (valve) stenosis (rheumatic)

   I07.1   **Rheumatic tricuspid insufficiency**
Tricuspid (valve) insufficiency (rheumatic)

   I07.2   **Rheumatic tricuspid stenosis and insufficiency**

   I07.8   **Other rheumatic tricuspid valve diseases**

   I07.9   **Rheumatic tricuspid valve disease, unspecified**
Rheumatic tricuspid valve disorder NOS

I08-   **Multiple valve diseases**
Includes: Multiple valve diseases specified as rheumatic or unspecified
Excludes 1:   endocarditis, valve unspecified (I38)
multiple valve disease specified a nonrheumatic (I34.-, I35.-, I36.-, I37.-, I38.-, Q22.-, Q23.-, Q24.8-)
rheumatic valve disease NOS (I09.1)

   I08.0   **Rheumatic disorders of both mitral and aortic valves**
Involvement of both mitral and aortic valves specified as rheumatic or unspecified

   I08.1   **Rheumatic disorders of both mitral and tricuspid valves**

   I08.2   **Rheumatic disorders of both aortic and tricuspid valves**

   I08.3   **Combined rheumatic disorders of mitral, aortic and tricuspid valves**

   I08.8   **Other rheumatic multiple valve diseases**

   I08.9   **Rheumatic multiple valve disease, unspecified**

I09-   **Other rheumatic heart diseases**

   I09.0   **Rheumatic myocarditis**
Excludes 1:   myocarditis not specified as rheumatic (I51.4)

   I09.1   **Rheumatic diseases of endocardium, valve unspecified**
Rheumatic endocarditis (chronic)
Rheumatic valvulitis (chronic)
Excludes 1:   endocarditis, valve unspecified (I38)

   I09.2   **Chronic rheumatic pericarditis**
Adherent pericardium, rheumatic
Chronic rheumatic mediastinopericarditis
Chronic rheumatic myopericarditis
Excludes 1:   chronic pericarditis not specified as rheumatic (I31.-)

   I09.8-   **Other specified rheumatic heart diseases**

     I09.81   **Rheumatic heart failure**
Use additional code to identify type of heart failure (I50.-)

     I09.89   **Other specified rheumatic heart diseases**
Rheumatic disease of pulmonary valve

   I09.9   **Rheumatic heart disease, unspecified**
Rheumatic carditis
Excludes 1:   rheumatoid carditis (M05.31)

H95-I09

Excludes 1: = NOT CODED HERE! (Do not code both)   **471**   *Excludes❷:* = Not Included Here

Hypertensive diseases (I10-I15)

Use additional code to identify:
   Exposure to environmental tobacco smoke (Z77.22)
   History of tobacco use (Z87.891)
   Occupational exposure to environmental tobacco smoke (Z57.31)
   Tobacco dependence (F17.-)
   Tobacco use (Z72.0)
   Excludes 1: hypertensive disease complicating pregnancy, childbirth and
   *   the puerperium (O10-O11, O13-O16)*
   *   neonatal hypertension (P29.2)*
   *   primary pulmonary hypertension (I27.0)*

I10   Essential (primary) hypertension
   Includes: High blood pressure
            Hypertension (arterial) (benign) (essential) (malignant)
               (primary) (systemic)
   Excludes 1: hypertensive disease complicating pregnancy, childbirth and
   *   the puerperium (O10-O11, O13-O16)*
   Excludes❷: essential (primary) hypertension involving vessels of brain
   *   (I60-I69)*
   *   essential (primary) hypertension involving vessels of eye*
   *   (H35.0-)*

I11-   Hypertensive heart disease
   Includes: Any condition in I51.4-I51.9 due to hypertension

   I11.0   Hypertensive heart disease with heart failure
            Hypertensive heart failure
            Use additional code to identify type of heart failure (I50.-)

   I11.9   Hypertensive heart disease without heart failure
            Hypertensive heart disease NOS

I12-   Hypertensive chronic kidney disease
   Includes: Any condition in N18 and N26 due to hypertension
            Arteriosclerosis of kidney
            Arteriosclerotic nephritis (chronic) (interstitial)
            Hypertensive nephropathy
            Nephrosclerosis
   Excludes 1: hypertension due to kidney disease (I15.0, I15.1)
   *   renovascular hypertension (I15.0)*
   *   secondary hypertension (I15.-)*
   Excludes❷: acute kidney failure (N17.-)

   I12.0   Hypertensive chronic kidney disease with stage 5 chronic kidney
            disease or end stage renal disease
            Use additional code to identify the stage of chronic kidney disease
               (N18.5, N18.6)

   I12.9   Hypertensive chronic kidney disease with stage 1 through stage 4
            chronic kidney disease, or unspecified chronic kidney disease
            Hypertensive chronic kidney disease NOS
            Hypertensive renal disease NOS
            Use additional code to identify the stage of chronic kidney disease
               (N18.1-N18.4, N18.9)

I13-   Hypertensive heart and chronic kidney disease
   Includes: Any condition in I11.- with any condition in I12.-
            Cardiorenal disease
            Cardiovascular renal disease

   I13.0   Hypertensive heart and chronic kidney disease with heart failure
            and stage 1 through stage 4 chronic kidney disease, or
            unspecified chronic kidney disease
            Use additional code to identify type of heart failure (I50.-)
            Use additional code to identify stage of chronic kidney disease
               (N18.1-N18.4, N18.9)

   I13.1-   Hypertensive heart and chronic kidney disease without heart
            failure

      I13.10   Hypertensive heart and chronic kidney disease without heart
               failure, with stage 1 through stage 4 chronic kidney disease,
               or unspecified chronic kidney disease
               Hypertensive heart disease and hypertensive chronic kidney
                  disease NOS
               Use additional code to identify the stage of chronic kidney
                  disease (N18.1-N18.4, N18.9)

      I13.11   Hypertensive heart and chronic kidney disease without heart
               failure, with stage 5 chronic kidney disease, or end stage
               renal disease
               Use additional code to identify the stage of chronic kidney
                  disease (N18.5, N18.6)

   I13.2   Hypertensive heart and chronic kidney disease with heart failure
            and with stage 5 chronic kidney disease, or end stage renal
            disease
            Use additional code to identify type of heart failure (I50.-)
            Use additional code to identify the stage of chronic kidney disease
               (N18.5, N18.6)

I15-   Secondary hypertension
   Code also underlying condition
   Excludes 1: postprocedural hypertension (I97.3)
   Excludes❷: secondary hypertension involving vessels of brain (I60-I69)
   *   secondary hypertension involving vessels of eye (H35.0-)*

I15.0   Renovascular hypertension
I15.1   Hypertension secondary to other renal disorders
I15.2   Hypertension secondary to endocrine disorders
I15.8   Other secondary hypertension
I15.9   Secondary hypertension, unspecified

I
1
0
-
I
2
2

Ischemic heart diseases (I20-I25)

Use additional code to identify presence of hypertension (I10-I15)

I20- <u>Angina pectoris</u>
Use additional code to identify:
Exposure to environmental tobacco smoke (Z77.22)
History of tobacco use (Z87.891)
Occupational exposure to environmental tobacco smoke (Z57.31)
Tobacco dependence (F17.-)
Tobacco use (Z72.0)
Excludes 1: angina pectoris with atherosclerotic heart disease of native
coronary arteries (I25.1-)
atherosclerosis of coronary artery bypass graft(s) and
coronary artery of transplanted heart with angina
pectoris (I25.7-)
postinfarction angina (I23.7)

I20.0 <u>Unstable</u> angina
Accelerated angina
Crescendo angina
De novo effort angina
Intermediate coronary syndrome
Preinfarction syndrome
Worsening effort angina

I20.1 Angina pectoris <u>with documented spasm</u>
Angiospastic angina
Prinzmetal angina
Spasm-induced angina
Variant angina

I20.8 <u>Other forms</u> of angina pectoris
Angina equivalent
Angina of effort
Coronary slow flow syndrome
Stenocardia
Use additioal code(s) for symptoms associated with angina
equivalent

I20.9 Angina pectoris, <u>unspecified</u>
Angina NOS
Anginal syndrome
Cardiac angina
Ischemic chest pain

I21- ST elevation (STEMI) and non-ST elevation (NSTEMI) <u>myocardial infarction</u>
Includes: Cardiac infarction
Coronary (artery) embolism
Coronary (artery) occlusion
Coronary (artery) rupture
Coronary (artery) thrombosis
Infarction of heart, myocardium, or ventricle
Myocardial infarction specified as acute or with a stated duration
of 4 weeks (28 days) or less from onset
Use additional code, if applicable, to identify:
Exposure to environmental tobacco smoke (Z77.22)
History of tobacco use (Z87.891)
Occupational exposure to environmental tobacco smoke (Z57.31)
Status post administration of tPA (rtPA) in a different facility within the
last 24 hours prior to admission to current facility (Z92.82)
Tobacco dependence (F17.-)
Tobacco use (Z72.0)
Excludes❷: old myocardial infarction (I25.2)
postmyocardial infarction syndrome (I24.1)
subsequent myocardial infarction (I22.-)

I21.0- ST elevation (STEMI) myocardial infarction of <u>anterior wall</u>
I21.01 ST elevation (STEMI) myocardial infarction involving <u>left main</u> coronary artery
I21.02 ST elevation (STEMI) myocardial infarction involving <u>left anterior descending</u> coronary artery
ST elevation (STEMI) myocardial infarction involving
diagonal coronary artery
I21.09 ST elevation (STEMI) myocardial infarction involving <u>other coronary artery</u> of anterior wall
Acute transmural myocardial infarction of anterior wall
Anteroapical transmural (Q wave) infarction (acute)
Anterolateral transmural (Q wave) infarction (acute)
Anteroseptal transmural (Q wave) infarction (acute)
Transmural (Q wave) infarction (acute) (of) anterior (wall)
NOS

I21.1- ST elevation (STEMI) myocardial infarction of <u>inferior wall</u>
I21.11 ST elevation (STEMI) myocardial infarction involving <u>right coronary</u> artery
Inferoposterior transmural (Q wave) infarction (acute)
I21.19 ST elevation (STEMI) myocardial infarction involving <u>other coronary</u> artery of inferior wall
Acute transmural myocardial infarction of inferior wall
Inferolateral transmural (Q wave) infarction (acute)
Transmural (Q wave) infarction (acute) (of) diaphragmatic
wall
Transmural (Q wave) infarction (acute) (of) inferior (wall)
NOS
Excludes❷: ST elevation (STEMI) myocardial infarction
involving left circumflex coronary artery
(I21.21)

I21.2- ST elevation (STEMI) myocardial infarction of <u>other sites</u>
I21.21 ST elevation (STEMI) myocardial infarction involving <u>left circumflex</u> coronary artery
ST elevation (STEMI) myocardial infarction involving oblique
marginal coronary artery
I21.29 ST elevation (STEMI) myocardial infarction involving <u>other sites</u>
Acute transmural myocardial infarction of other sites
Apical-lateral transmural (Q wave) infarction (acute)
Basal-lateral transmural (Q wave) infarction (acute)
High lateral transmural (Q wave) infarction (acute)
Lateral (wall) NOS transmural (Q wave) infarction (acute)
Posterior (true) transmural (Q wave) infarction (acute)
Posterobasal transmural (Q wave) infarction (acute)
Posterolateral transmural (Q wave) infarction (acute)
Posteroseptal transmural (Q wave) infarction (acute)
Septal transmural (Q wave) infarction (acute) NOS

I21.3 ST elevation (STEMI) myocardial infarction of <u>unspecified site</u>
Acute transmural myocardial infarction of unspecified site
Myocardial infarction (acute) NOS
Transmural (Q wave) myocardial infarction NOS

I21.4 Non-ST elevation (NSTEMI) myocardial infarction
Acute subendocardial myocardial infarction
Non-Q wave myocardial infarction NOS
Nontransmural myocardial infarction NOS

I22- Subsequent ST elevation (STEMI) and non-ST elevation (NSTEMI) myocardial infarction
Includes: Acute myocardial infarction occurring within four weeks (28 days)
of a previous acute myocardial infarction, regardless of site
Cardiac infarction
Coronary (artery) embolism
Coronary (artery) occlusion
Coronary (artery) rupture
Coronary (artery) thrombosis
Infarction of heart, myocardium, or ventricle
Recurrent myocardial infarction
Reinfarction of myocardium
Rupture of heart, myocardium, or ventricle
Use additional code, if applicable, to identify:
Exposure to environmental tobacco smoke (Z77.22)
History of tobacco use (Z87.891)
Occupational exposure to environmental tobacco smoke (Z57.31)
Status post administration of tPA (rtPA) in a different facility within the
last 24 hours prior to admission to current facility (Z92.82)
Tobacco dependence (F17.-)
Tobacco use (Z72.0)

I22.0 Subsequent ST elevation (STEMI) myocardial infarction of anterior wall
Subsequent acute transmural myocardial infarction of anterior wall
Subsequent transmural (Q wave) infarction (acute)(of) anterior
(wall) NOS
Subsequent anteroapical transmural (Q wave) infarction (acute)
Subsequent anterolateral transmural (Q wave) infarction (acute)
Subsequent anteroseptal transmural (Q wave) infarction (acute)

I22.1 Subsequent ST elevation (STEMI) myocardial infarction of inferior wall
Subsequent acute transmural myocardial infarction of inferior wall
Subsequent transmural (Q wave) infarction (acute)(of)
diaphragmatic wall
Subsequent transmural (Q wave) infarction (acute)(of) inferior
(wall) NOS
Subsequent inferolateral transmural (Q wave) infarction (acute)
Subsequent inferoposterior transmural (Q wave) infarction (acute)

I22.2 Subsequent non-ST elevation (NSTEMI) myocardial infarction
Subsequent acute subendocardial myocardial infarction
Subsequent non-Q wave myocardial infarction NOS
Subsequent nontransmural myocardial infarction NOS

I10-I22

Excludes 1: = NOT CODED HERE! (Do not code both)   473   *Excludes❷:* = Not Included Here

I22.8   **Subsequent** <u>ST elevation</u> **(STEMI) myocardial infarction of** <u>other</u>
<u>sites</u>
Subsequent acute transmural myocardial infarction of other sites
Subsequent apical-lateral transmural (Q wave) myocardial
infarction (acute)
Subsequent basal-lateral transmural (Q wave) myocardial
infarction (acute)
Subsequent high lateral transmural (Q wave) myocardial infarction
(acute)
Subsequent transmural (Q wave) myocardial infarction (acute)(of)
lateral (wall) NOS
Subsequent posterior (true)transmural (Q wave) myocardial
infarction (acute)
Subsequent posterobasal transmural (Q wave) myocardial
infarction (acute)
Subsequent posterolateral transmural (Q wave) myocardial
infarction (acute)
Subsequent posteroseptal transmural (Q wave) myocardial
infarction (acute)
Subsequent septal NOS transmural (Q wave) myocardial infarction
(acute)

I22.9   **Subsequent** <u>ST elevation</u> **(STEMI) myocardial infarction of**
<u>unspecified site</u>
Subsequent acute myocardial infarction of unspecified site
Subsequent myocardial infarction (acute) NOS

I23-   **Certain current complications** <u>following</u> **ST elevation (STEMI) and**
non-ST elevation (NSTEMI) <u>myocardial infarction</u> **(within the 28 day**
period)
I23.0   <u>Hemopericardium</u> **as current complication following acute**
myocardial infarction
Excludes 1:   hemopericardium not specified as current complication
following acute myocardial infarction (I31.2)
I23.1   <u>Atrial septal defect</u> **as current complication following acute**
myocardial infarction
Excludes 1:   acquired atrial septal defect not specified as current
complication following acute myocardial infarction
(I51.0)
I23.2   <u>Ventricular septal defect</u> **as current complication following acute**
myocardial infarction
Excludes 1:   acquired ventricular septal defect not specified as
current complication following acute myocardial
infarction (I51.0)
I23.3   <u>Rupture of cardiac wall</u> **without hemopericardium as current**
complication following acute myocardial infarction
I23.4   <u>Rupture of chordae tendineae</u> **as current complication following**
acute myocardial infarction
Excludes 1:   rupture of chordae tendineae not specified as current
complication following acute myocardial infarction
(I51.1)
I23.5   <u>Rupture of papillary muscle</u> **as current complication following**
acute myocardial infarction
Excludes 1:   rupture of papillary muscle not specified as current
complication following acute myocardial infarction
(I51.2)
I23.6   <u>Thrombosis of atrium, auricular appendage, and ventricle</u> **as**
current complications following acute myocardial infarction
Excludes 1:   thrombosis of atrium, auricular appendage, and
ventricle not specified as current complication
following acute myocardial infarction (I51.3)
I23.7   <u>Postinfarction angina</u>
I23.8   <u>Other current complications</u> **following acute myocardial**
infarction

I24-   <u>Other acute ischemic heart diseases</u>
Excludes 1:   angina pectoris (I20.-)
transient myocardial ischemia in newborn (P29.4)
I24.0   <u>Acute coronary thrombosis</u> <u>not</u> **resulting in myocardial infarction**
Acute coronary (artery) (vein) embolism not resulting in
myocardial infarction
Acute coronary (artery) (vein) occlusion not resulting in
myocardial infarction
Acute coronary (artery) (vein) thromboembolism not resulting in
myocardial infarction
Excludes 1:   atherosclerotic heart disease (I25.1-)
I24.1   **Dressler's syndrome**
Postmyocardial infarction syndrome
Excludes 1:   postinfarction angina (I23.7)
I24.8   **Other forms of acute ischemic heart disease**
I24.9   **Acute ischemic heart disease, unspecified**
Excludes 1:   ischemic heart disease (chronic) NOS (I25.9)

I25-   **Chronic ischemic heart disease**
Use additional code to identify:
Chronic total occlusion of coronary artery (I25.82)
Exposure to environmental tobacco smoke (Z77.22)
History of tobacco use (Z87.891)
Occupational exposure to environmental tobacco smoke (Z57.31)
Tobacco dependence (F17.-)
Tobacco use (Z72.0)
I25.1-   <u>Atherosclerotic heart disease</u> <u>of native</u> **coronary artery**
Atherosclerotic cardiovascular disease
Coronary (artery) atheroma
Coronary (artery) atherosclerosis
Coronary (artery) disease
Coronary (artery) sclerosis
Use additional code, if applicable, to identify:
Coronary atherosclerosis due to calcified coronary lesion (I25.84)
Coronary atherosclerosis due to lipid rich plaque (I25.83)
Excludes❷: atheroembolism (I75.-)
atherosclerosis of coronary artery bypass graft(s) and
transplanted heart (I25.7-)
I25.10   **Atherosclerotic heart disease of native coronary artery**
<u>without</u> **angina pectoris**
Atherosclerotic heart disease NOS
I25.11-   **Atherosclerotic heart disease of native coronary artery** <u>with</u>
angina pectoris
I25.110   **Atherosclerotic heart disease of native coronary artery**
with <u>unstable</u> **angina pectoris**
Excludes 1:   unstable angina without atherosclerotic
heart disease (I20.0)
I25.111   **Atherosclerotic heart disease of native coronary artery**
with angina pectoris <u>with documented spasm</u>
Excludes 1:   angina pectoris with documented spasm
without atherosclerotic heart disease
(I20.1)
I25.118   **Atherosclerotic heart disease of native coronary artery**
with <u>other forms</u> **of angina pectoris**
Excludes 1:   other forms of angina pectoris without
atherosclerotic heart disease (I20.8)
I25.119   **Atherosclerotic heart disease of native coronary artery**
with <u>unspecified</u> **angina pectoris**
Atherosclerotic heart disease with angina NOS
Atherosclerotic heart disease with ischemic chest pain
Excludes 1:   unspecified angina pectoris without
atherosclerotic heart disease (I20.9)
I25.2   <u>Old</u> **myocardial infarction**
Healed myocardial infarction
Past myocardial infarction diagnosed by ECG or other
investigation, but currently presenting no symptoms
I25.3   <u>Aneurysm</u> **of heart**
Mural aneurysm
Ventricular aneurysm
I25.4-   **Coronary artery aneurysm and dissection**
I25.41   **Coronary artery aneurysm**
Coronary arteriovenous fistula, acquired
Excludes 1:   congenital coronary (artery) aneurysm (Q24.5)
I25.42   **Coronary artery dissection**
I25.5   **Ischemic cardiomyopathy**
Excludes❷: coronary atherosclerosis (I25.1-, I25.7-)
I25.6   **Silent myocardial ischemia**

I22 - I25

I25.7-   <u>Atherosclerosis</u> of coronary artery bypass graft(s) and coronary artery of transplanted heart <u>with angina pectoris</u>
Use additional code, if applicable, to identify:
Coronary atherosclerosis due to calcified coronary lesion (I25.84)
Coronary atherosclerosis due to lipid rich plaque (I25.83)
Excludes 1:   atherosclerosis of bypass graft(s) of transplanted heart without angina pectoris (I25.812)
atherosclerosis of coronary artery bypass graft(s) without angina pectoris (I25.810)
atherosclerosis of native coronary artery of transplanted heart without angina pectoris (I25.811)
embolism or thrombus of coronary artery bypass graft(s) (T82.8-)

I25.70- Atherosclerosis of <u>coronary artery bypass graft(s), unspecified, with angina pectoris</u>
  I25.700   Atherosclerosis of coronary artery bypass graft(s), unspecified, <u>with unstable</u> angina pectoris
             Excludes 1:   unstable angina pectoris without atherosclerosis of coronary artery bypass graft (I20.0)
  I25.701   Atherosclerosis of coronary artery bypass graft(s), unspecified, with angina pectoris <u>with documented spasm</u>
             Excludes 1:   angina pectoris with documented spasm without atherosclerosis of coronary artery bypass graft (I20.1)
  I25.708   Atherosclerosis of coronary artery bypass graft(s), unspecified, <u>with other forms</u> of angina pectoris
             Excludes 1:   other forms of angina pectoris without atherosclerosis of coronary artery bypass graft (I20.8)
  I25.709   Atherosclerosis of coronary artery bypass graft(s), unspecified, <u>with unspecified</u> angina pectoris
             Excludes 1:   unspecified angina pectoris without atherosclerosis of coronary artery bypass graft (I20.9)

I25.71- Atherosclerosis of <u>autologous vein coronary artery bypass graft(s)</u> with angina pectoris
  I25.710   Atherosclerosis of autologous <u>vein</u> coronary artery bypass graft(s) <u>with unstable</u> angina pectoris
             Excludes 1:   unstable angina without atherosclerosis of autologous vein coronary artery bypass graft(s) (I20.0)
  I25.711   Atherosclerosis of autologous <u>vein</u> coronary artery bypass graft(s) with angina pectoris <u>with documented spasm</u>
             Excludes 1:   angina pectoris with documented spasm without atherosclerosis of autologous vein coronary artery bypass graft(s) (I20.1)
  I25.718   Atherosclerosis of autologous <u>vein</u> coronary artery bypass graft(s) <u>with other forms</u> of angina pectoris
             Excludes 1:   other forms of angina pectoris without atherosclerosis of autologous vein coronary artery bypass graft(s) (I20.8)
  I25.719   Atherosclerosis of autologous <u>vein</u> coronary artery bypass graft(s) <u>with unspecified</u> angina pectoris
             Excludes 1:   unspecified angina pectoris without atherosclerosis of autologous vein coronary artery bypass graft(s) (I20.9)

I25.72- Atherosclerosis of autologous <u>artery</u> coronary artery bypass graft(s) <u>with angina pectoris</u>
Atherosclerosis of internal mammary artery graft with angina pectoris
  I25.720   Atherosclerosis of autologous <u>artery</u> coronary artery bypass graft(s) <u>with unstable</u> angina pectoris
             Excludes 1:   unstable angina without atherosclerosis of autologous artery coronary artery bypass graft(s) (I20.0)
  I25.721   Atherosclerosis of autologous <u>artery</u> coronary artery bypass graft(s) with angina pectoris <u>with documented spasm</u>
             Excludes 1:   angina pectoris with documented spasm without atherosclerosis of autologous artery coronary artery bypass graft(s) (I20.1)
  I25.728   Atherosclerosis of autologous <u>artery</u> coronary artery bypass graft(s) <u>with other forms</u> of angina pectoris
             Excludes 1:   other forms of angina pectoris without atherosclerosis of autologous artery coronary artery bypass graft(s) (I20.8)

  I25.729   Atherosclerosis of autologous <u>artery</u> coronary artery bypass graft(s) <u>with unspecified</u> angina pectoris
             Excludes 1:   unspecified angina pectoris without atherosclerosis of autologous artery coronary artery bypass graft(s) (I20.9)

I25.73- Atherosclerosis of <u>nonautologous biological</u> coronary artery bypass graft(s) <u>with angina pectoris</u>
  I25.730   Atherosclerosis of <u>nonautologous biological</u> coronary artery bypass graft(s) <u>with unstable</u> angina pectoris
             Excludes 1:   unstable angina without atherosclerosis of nonautologous biological coronary artery bypass graft(s) (I20.0)
  I25.731   Atherosclerosis of <u>nonautologous biological</u> coronary artery bypass graft(s) with angina pectoris <u>with documented spasm</u>
             Excludes 1:   angina pectoris with documented spasm without atherosclerosis of nonautologous biological coronary artery bypass graft(s) (I20.1)
  I25.738   Atherosclerosis of <u>nonautologous biological</u> coronary artery bypass graft(s) <u>with other forms</u> of angina pectoris
             Excludes 1:   other forms of angina pectoris without atherosclerosis of nonautologous biological coronary artery bypass graft(s) (I20.8)
  I25.739   Atherosclerosis of <u>nonautologous biological</u> coronary artery bypass graft(s) <u>with unspecified</u> angina pectoris
             Excludes 1:   unspecified angina pectoris without atherosclerosis of nonautologous biological coronary artery bypass graft(s) (I20.9)

I25.75- Atherosclerosis of <u>native coronary artery of transplanted heart</u> <u>with angina pectoris</u>
             Excludes 1:   atherosclerosis of native coronary artery of transplanted heart without angina pectoris (I25.811)
  I25.750   Atherosclerosis of native coronary artery of transplanted heart <u>with unstable</u> angina
  I25.751   Atherosclerosis of native coronary artery of transplanted heart with angina pectoris <u>with documented spasm</u>
  I25.758   Atherosclerosis of native coronary artery of transplanted heart <u>with other forms</u> of angina pectoris
  I25.759   Atherosclerosis of native coronary artery of transplanted heart <u>with unspecified</u> angina pectoris

I25.76- Atherosclerosis of <u>bypass graft</u> of coronary artery of <u>transplanted heart</u> <u>with angina pectoris</u>
             Excludes 1:   atherosclerosis of bypass graft of coronary artery of transplanted heart without angina pectoris (I25.812)
  I25.760   Atherosclerosis of bypass graft of coronary artery of transplanted heart <u>with unstable angina</u>
  I25.761   Atherosclerosis of bypass graft of coronary artery of transplanted heart with angina pectoris <u>with documented spasm</u>
  I25.768   Atherosclerosis of bypass graft of coronary artery of transplanted heart <u>with other forms</u> of angina pectoris
  I25.769   Atherosclerosis of bypass graft of coronary artery of transplanted heart <u>with unspecified</u> angina pectoris

I25.79- Atherosclerosis of <u>other</u> coronary artery bypass graft(s) <u>with angina pectoris</u>
  I25.790   Atherosclerosis of other coronary artery bypass graft(s) <u>with unstable</u> angina pectoris
             Excludes 1:   unstable angina without atherosclerosis of other coronary artery bypass graft(s) (I20.0)
  I25.791   Atherosclerosis of other coronary artery bypass graft(s) with angina pectoris <u>with documented spasm</u>
             Excludes 1:   angina pectoris with documented spasm without atherosclerosis of other coronary artery bypass graft(s) (I20.1)
  I25.798   Atherosclerosis of other coronary artery bypass graft(s) <u>with other forms</u> of angina pectoris
             Excludes 1:   other forms of angina pectoris without atherosclerosis of other coronary artery bypass graft(s) (I20.8)
  I25.799   Atherosclerosis of other coronary artery bypass graft(s) <u>with unspecified</u> angina pectoris
             Excludes 1:   unspecified angina pectoris without atherosclerosis of other coronary artery bypass graft(s) (I20.9)

I22 - I25

I25.8- **Other forms of chronic ischemic heart disease**
  I25.81- <u>Atherosclerosis of other coronary vessels</u> <u>without</u> angina pectoris
    Use additional code, if applicable, to identify:
    Coronary atherosclerosis due to calcified coronary lesion (I25.84)
    Coronary atherosclerosis due to lipid rich plaque (I25.83)
    Excludes 1: atherosclerotic heart disease of native coronary artery without angina pectoris (I25.10)

    I25.810 **Atherosclerosis of <u>coronary artery bypass graft(s)</u> <u>without</u> angina pectoris**
      Atherosclerosis of coronary artery bypass graft NOS
      Excludes 1: atherosclerosis of coronary bypass graft(s) with angina pectoris (I25.70-I25.73-, I25.79-)

    I25.811 **Atherosclerosis of <u>native coronary artery of transplanted heart</u> <u>without</u> angina pectoris**
      Atherosclerosis of native coronary artery of transplanted heart NOS
      Excludes 1: atherosclerosis of native coronary artery of transplanted heart with angina pectoris (I25.75-)

    I25.812 **Atherosclerosis of <u>bypass graft of coronary artery of transplanted heart</u> <u>without</u> angina pectoris**
      Atherosclerosis of bypass graft of transplanted heart NOS
      Excludes 1: atherosclerosis of bypass graft of transplanted heart with angina pectoris (I25.76)

  I25.82 <u>Chronic total occlusion of coronary artery</u>
    Complete occlusion of coronary artery
    Total occlusion of coronary artery
    Code first coronary atherosclerosis (I25.1-, I25.7-, I25.81-)
    Excludes 1: acute coronary occulsion with myocardial infarction (I21.-, I22.-)
    acute coronary occulsion without myocardial infarction (I24.0)

  I25.83 **Coronary atherosclerosis <u>due to lipid rich plaque</u>**
    Code first coronary atherosclerosis (I25.1-, I25.7-, I25.81-)

  I25.84 **Coronary atherosclerosis <u>due to calcified coronary lesion</u>**
    Coronary atherosclerosis due to severely calcified coronary lesion
    Code first coronary atherosclerosis (I25.1-, I25.7-, I25.81-)

  I25.89 **Other forms of chronic ischemic heart disease**

I25.9 **Chronic ischemic heart disease, unspecified**
  Ischemic heart disease (chronic) NOS

Pulmonary heart disease and diseases of pulmonary circulation (I26-I28)

I26- **Pulmonary embolism**
  Includes: Pulmonary (acute) (artery) (vein) infarction
    Pulmonary (acute) (artery) (vein) thromboembolism
    Pulmonary (acute) (artery) (vein) thrombosis
  Excludes❷: chronic pulmonary embolism (I27.82)
    personal history of pulmonary embolism (Z86.711)
    pulmonary embolism complicating abortion, ectopic or molar pregnancy (O00-O07, O08.2)
    pulmonary embolism complicating pregnancy, childbirth and the puerperium (O88.-)
    pulmonary embolism due to complications of surgical and medical care (T80.0, T81.7-, T82.8-)
    pulmonary embolism due to trauma (T79.0, T79.1)
    septic (non-pulmonary) arterial embolism (I76)

  I26.0- **Pulmonary embolism <u>with acute cor pulmonale</u>**
    I26.01 **<u>Septic</u> pulmonary embolism with acute cor pulmonale**
      Code first underlying infection
    I26.02 **<u>Saddle</u> embolus of pulmonary artery with acute cor pulmonale**
    I26.09 **<u>Other</u> pulmonary embolism with acute cor pulmonale**
      Acute cor pulmonale NOS

  I26.9- **Pulmonary embolism <u>without</u> acute cor pulmonale**
    I26.90 **<u>Septic</u> pulmonary embolism without acute cor pulmonale**
      Code first underlying infection
    I26.92 **<u>Saddle</u> embolus of pulmonary artery without acute cor pulmonale**
    I26.99 **<u>Other</u> pulmonary embolism without acute cor pulmonale**
      Acute pulmonary embolism NOS
      Pulmonary embolism NOS

I27- **Other pulmonary heart diseases**
  I27.0 **Primary pulmonary hypertension**
    Excludes 1: pulmonary hypertension NOS (I27.2)
    secondary pulmonary hypertension (I27.2)

I27.1 **Kyphoscoliotic heart disease**
I27.2 **Other secondary pulmonary hypertension**
  Pulmonary hypertension NOS
  Code also associated underlying condition
I27.8- **Other specified pulmonary heart diseases**
  I27.81 **Cor pulmonale (chronic)**
    Cor pulmonale NOS
    Excludes 1: acute cor pulmonale (I26.0-)
  I27.82 **Chronic pulmonary embolism**
    Use additional code, if applicable, for associated long-term (current) use of anticoagulants (Z79.01)
    Excludes 1: personal history of pulmonary embolism (Z86.711)
  I27.89 **Other specified pulmonary heart diseases**
    Eisenmenger's complex
    Eisenmenger's syndrome
    Excludes 1: Eisenmenger's defect (Q21.8)
I27.9 **Pulmonary heart disease, unspecified**
  Chronic cardiopulmonary disease

I28- **Other diseases of pulmonary vessels**
  I28.0 **Arteriovenous fistula of pulmonary vessels**
    Excludes 1: congenital arteriovenous fistula (Q25.72)
  I28.1 **Aneurysm of pulmonary artery**
    Excludes 1: congenital aneurysm (Q25.79)
    congenital arteriovenous aneurysm (Q25.72)
  I28.8 **Other diseases of pulmonary vessels**
    Pulmonary arteritis
    Pulmonary endarteritis
    Rupture of pulmonary vessels
    Stenosis of pulmonary vessels
    Stricture of pulmonary vessels
  I28.9 **Disease of pulmonary vessels, unspecified**

Other forms of heart disease (I30-I52)

I30- <u>Acute pericarditis</u>
  Includes: Acute mediastinopericarditis
    Acute myopericarditis
    Acute pericardial effusion
    Acute pleuropericarditis
    Acute pneumopericarditis
  Excludes 1: Dressler's syndrome (I24.1)
    rheumatic pericarditis (acute) (I01.0)
  I30.0 **Acute nonspecific idiopathic pericarditis**
  I30.1 **Infective pericarditis**
    Pneumococcal pericarditis
    Pneumopyopericardium
    Purulent pericarditis
    Pyopericarditis
    Pyopericardium
    Pyopneumopericardium
    Staphylococcal pericarditis
    Streptococcal pericarditis
    Suppurative pericarditis
    Viral pericarditis
    Use additional code (B95-B97) to identify infectious agent
  I30.8 **Other forms of acute pericarditis**
  I30.9 **Acute pericarditis, unspecified**

I31- **Other diseases of pericardium**
  Excludes 1: diseases of pericardium specified as rheumatic (I09.2)
    postcardiotomy syndrome (I97.0)
    traumatic injury to pericardium (S26.-)
  I31.0 **Chronic <u>adhesive</u> pericarditis**
    Accretio cordis
    Adherent pericardium
    Adhesive mediastinopericarditis
  I31.1 **Chronic <u>constrictive</u> pericarditis**
    Concretio cordis
    Pericardial calcification
  I31.2 **Hemopericardium, not elsewhere classified**
    Excludes 1: hemopericardium as current complication following acute myocardial infarction (I23.0)
  I31.3 **Pericardial effusion (noninflammatory)**
    Chylopericardium
    Excludes 1: acute pericardial effusion (I30.9)
  I31.4 **Cardiac tamponade**
    Code first underlying cause
  I31.8 **Other specified diseases of pericardium**
    Epicardial plaques
    Focal pericardial adhesions
  I31.9 **Disease of pericardium, unspecified**
    Pericarditis (chronic) NOS

I 2 5 - I 4 2

I32   Pericarditis in diseases classified elsewhere
Code first underlying disease
Excludes 1:   pericarditis (in):
coxsackie (virus) (B33.23)
gonococcal (A54.83)
meningococcal (A39.53)
rheumatoid (arthritis) (M05.31)
syphilitic (A52.06)
systemic lupus erythematosus (M32.12)
tuberculosis (A18.84)

I33-   Acute and subacute endocarditis
Excludes 1:   acute rheumatic endocarditis (I01.1)
endocarditis NOS (I38)

I33.0   Acute and subacute infective endocarditis
Bacterial endocarditis (acute) (subacute)
Infective endocarditis (acute) (subacute) NOS
Endocarditis lenta (acute) (subacute)
Malignant endocarditis (acute) (subacute)
Purulent endocarditis (acute) (subacute)
Septic endocarditis (acute) (subacute)
Ulcerative endocarditis (acute) (subacute)
Vegetative endocarditis (acute) (subacute)
Use additional code (B95-B97) to identify infectious agent

I33.9   Acute and subacute endocarditis, unspecified
Acute endocarditis NOS
Acute myoendocarditis NOS
Acute periendocarditis NOS
Subacute endocarditis NOS
Subacute myoendocarditis NOS
Subacute periendocarditis NOS

I34-   Nonrheumatic mitral valve disorders
Excludes 1:   mitral valve disease (I05.9)
mitral valve failure (I05.8)
mitral valve stenosis (I05.0)
mitral valve disorder of unspecified cause with diseases of
aortic and/or tricuspid valve(s) (I08.-)
mitral valve disorder of unspecified cause with mitral stenosis
or obstruction (I05.0)
mitral valve disorder specified as congenital (Q23.2, Q23.3)
mitral valve disorder specified as rheumatic (I05.-)

I34.0   Nonrheumatic mitral (valve) insufficiency
Nonrheumatic mitral (valve) incompetence NOS
Nonrheumatic mitral (valve) regurgitation NOS

I34.1   Nonrheumatic mitral (valve) prolapse
Floppy nonrheumatic mitral valve syndrome
Excludes 1:   Marfan's syndrome (Q87.4-)

I34.2   Nonrheumatic mitral (valve) stenosis

I34.8   Other nonrheumatic mitral valve disorders

I34.9   Nonrheumatic mitral valve disorder, unspecified

I35-   Nonrheumatic aortic valve disorders
Excludes 1:   aortic valve disorder of unspecified cause but with diseases of
mitral and/or tricuspid valve(s) (I08.-)
aortic valve disorder specified as congenital (Q23.0, Q23.1)
aortic valve disorder specified as rheumatic (I06.-)
hypertrophic subaortic stenosis (I42.1)

I35.0   Nonrheumatic aortic (valve) stenosis

I35.1   Nonrheumatic aortic (valve) insufficiency
Nonrheumatic aortic (valve) incompetence NOS
Nonrheumatic aortic (valve) regurgitation NOS

I35.2   Nonrheumatic aortic (valve) stenosis with insufficiency

I35.8   Other nonrheumatic aortic valve disorders

I35.9   Nonrheumatic aortic valve disorder, unspecified

I36-   Nonrheumatic tricuspid valve disorders
Excludes 1:   tricuspid valve disorders of unspecified cause (I07.-)
tricuspid valve disorders specified as congenital (Q22.4,
Q22.8, Q22.9)
tricuspid valve disorders specified as rheumatic (I07.-)
tricuspid valve disorders with aortic and/or mitral valve
involvement (I08.-)

I36.0   Nonrheumatic tricuspid (valve) stenosis

I36.1   Nonrheumatic tricuspid (valve) insufficiency
Nonrheumatic tricuspid (valve) incompetence
Nonrheumatic tricuspid (valve) regurgitation

I36.2   Nonrheumatic tricuspid (valve) stenosis with insufficiency

I36.8   Other nonrheumatic tricuspid valve disorders

I36.9   Nonrheumatic tricuspid valve disorder, unspecified

I37-   Nonrheumatic pulmonary valve disorders
Excludes 1:   pulmonary valve disorder specified as congenital (Q22.1,
Q22.2, Q22.3)
pulmonary valve disorder specified as rheumatic (I09.89)

I37.0   Nonrheumatic pulmonary valve stenosis

I37.1   Nonrheumatic pulmonary valve insufficiency
Nonrheumatic pulmonary valve incompetence
Nonrheumatic pulmonary valve regurgitation

I37.2   Nonrheumatic pulmonary valve stenosis with insufficiency

I37.8   Other nonrheumatic pulmonary valve disorders

I37.9   Nonrheumatic pulmonary valve disorder, unspecified

I38   Endocarditis, valve unspecified
Includes: Endocarditis (chronic) NOS
Valvular incompetence NOS
Valvular insufficiency NOS
Valvular regurgitation NOS
Valvular stenosis NOS
Valvulitis (chronic) NOS
Excludes 1:   congenital insufficiency of cardiac valve NOS (Q24.8)
congenital stenosis of cardiac valve NOS (Q24.8)
endocardial fibroelastosis (I42.4)
endocarditis specified as rheumatic (I09.1)

I39   Endocarditis and heart valve disorders in diseases classified elsewhere
Code first underlying disease, such as:
Q fever (A78)
Excludes 1:   endocardial involvement in:
candidiasis (B37.6)
gonococcal infection (A54.83)
Libman-Sacks disease (M32.11)
listerosis (A32.82)
meningococcal infection (A39.51)
rheumatoid arthritis (M05.31)
syphilis (A52.03)
tuberculosis (A18.84)
typhoid fever (A01.02)

I40-   Acute myocarditis
Includes: Subacute myocarditis
Excludes 1:   acute rheumatic myocarditis (I01.2)

I40.0   Infective myocarditis
Septic myocarditis
Use additional code (B95-B97) to identify infectious agent

I40.1   Isolated myocarditis
Fiedler's myocarditis
Giant cell myocarditis
Idiopathic myocarditis

I40.8   Other acute myocarditis

I40.9   Acute myocarditis, unspecified

I41   Myocarditis in diseases classified elsewhere
Code first underlying disease, such as:
Typhus (A75.0-A75.9)
Excludes 1:   myocarditis (in):
Chagas' disease (chronic) (B57.2)
acute (B57.0)
coxsackie (virus) infection (B33.22)
diphtheritic (A36.81)
gonococcal (A54.83)
influenzal (J09.X9, J10.82, J11.82)
meningococcal (A39.52)
mumps (B26.82)
rheumatoid arthritis (M05.31)
sarcoid (D86.85)
syphilis (A52.06)
toxoplasmosis (B58.81)
tuberculous (A18.84)

I42-   Cardiomyopathy
Includes: Myocardiopathy
Code first pre-existing cardiomyopathy complicating pregnancy and
puerperium (O99.4)
Excludes 1:   ischemic cardiomyopathy (I25.5)
peripartum cardiomyopathy (O90.3)
Excludes❷: ventricular hypertrophy (I51.7)

I42.0   Dilated cardiomyopathy
Congestive cardiomyopathy

I42.1   Obstructive hypertrophic cardiomyopathy
Hypertrophic subaortic stenosis (idiopathic)

I42.2   Other hypertrophic cardiomyopathy
Nonobstructive hypertrophic cardiomyopathy

I42.3   Endomyocardial (eosinophilic) disease
Endomyocardial (tropical) fibrosis
Löffler's endocarditis

I42.4   Endocardial fibroelastosis
Congenital cardiomyopathy
Elastomyofibrosis

I
2
5
I
I
4
2

I42.5 **Other restrictive cardiomyopathy**
Constrictive cardiomyopathy NOS

I42.6 **Alcoholic cardiomyopathy**
Code also presence of alcoholism (F10.-)

I42.7 **Cardiomyopathy <u>due to drug and external agent</u>**
Code first poisoning due to drug or toxin, if applicable (T36-T65 with fifth or sixth character 1-4 or 6)
Use additional code for adverse effect, if applicable, to identify drug (T36-T50 with fifth or sixth character 5)

I42.8 **Other cardiomyopathies**

I42.9 **Cardiomyopathy, unspecified**
Cardiomyopathy (primary) (secondary) NOS

I43 **Cardiomyopathy <u>in diseases classified elsewhere</u>**
Code first underlying disease, such as:
Amyloidosis (E85.-)
Glycogen storage disease (E74.0)
Gout (M10.0-)
Thyrotoxicosis (E05.0-E05.9-)
Excludes 1: cardiomyopathy (in):
coxsackie (virus) (B33.24)
diphtheria (A36.81)
sarcoidosis (D86.85)
tuberculosis (A18.84)

I44- **<u>Atrioventricular</u> and left bundle-branch block**

I44.0 **Atrioventricular block, <u>first</u> degree**

I44.1 **Atrioventricular block, <u>second</u> degree**
Atrioventricular block, type I and II
Möbitz block block, type I and II
Second degree block, type I and II
Wenckebach's block

I44.2 **Atrioventricular block, <u>complete</u>**
Complete heart block NOS
Third degree block

I44.3- **Other and unspecified atrioventricular block**
Atrioventricular block NOS

I44.30 **<u>Unspecified</u> atrioventricular block**

I44.39 **<u>Other</u> atrioventricular block**

I44.4 **<u>Left anterior</u> fascicular block**

I44.5 **<u>Left posterior</u> fascicular block**

I44.6- **Other and unspecified fascicular block**

I44.60 **<u>Unspecified</u> fascicular block**
Left bundle-branch hemiblock NOS

I44.69 **<u>Other</u> fascicular block**

I44.7 **Left bundle-branch block, <u>unspecified</u>**

I45- **Other conduction disorders**

I45.0 **<u>Right fascicular</u> block**

I45.1- **Other and unspecified right bundle-branch block**

I45.10 **Unspecified right bundle-branch block**
Right bundle-branch block NOS

I45.19 **Other right bundle-branch block**

I45.2 **Bifascicular block**

I45.3 **Trifascicular block**

I45.4 **Nonspecific intraventricular block**
Bundle-branch block NOS

I45.5 **Other specified heart block**
Sinoatrial block
Sinoauricular block
Excludes 1: heart block NOS (I45.9)

I45.6 **Pre-excitation syndrome**
Accelerated atrioventricular conduction
Accessory atrioventricular conduction
Anomalous atrioventricular excitation
Lown-Ganong-Levine syndrome
Pre-excitation atrioventricular conduction
Wolff-Parkinson-White syndrome

I45.8- **Other specified conduction disorders**

I45.81 **Long QT syndrome**

I45.89 **Other specified conduction disorders**
Atrioventricular [AV] dissociation
Interference dissociation
Isorhythmic dissociation
Nonparoxysmal AV nodal tachycardia

I45.9 **Conduction disorder, unspecified**
Heart block NOS
Stokes-Adams syndrome

I46- **Cardiac arrest**
Excludes 1: cardiogenic shock (R57.0)

I46.2 **Cardiac arrest due to underlying <u>cardiac</u> condition**
Code first underlying cardiac condition

I46.8 **Cardiac arrest due to <u>other</u> underlying condition**
Code first underlying condition

I46.9 **Cardiac arrest, cause <u>unspecified</u>**

I47- **Paroxysmal tachycardia**
Code first tachycardia complicating:
Abortion or ectopic or molar pregnancy (O00-O07, O08.8)
Obstetric surgery and procedures (O75.4)
Excludes 1: sinoauricular tachycardia NOS (R00.0)
sinus [sinusal] tachycardia NOS (R00.0)
tachycardia NOS (R00.0)

I47.0 **Re-entry ventricular arrhythmia**

I47.1 **<u>Supraventricular</u> tachycardia**
Atrial (paroxysmal) tachycardia
Atrioventricular [AV] (paroxysmal) tachycardia
Atrioventricular re-entrant (nodal) tachycardia [AVNRT] [AVRT]
Junctional (paroxysmal) tachycardia
Nodal (paroxysmal) tachycardia

I47.2 **Ventricular tachycardia**

I47.9 **Paroxysmal tachycardia, unspecified**
Bouveret (-Hoffman) syndrome

I48- **<u>Atrial</u> fibrillation and flutter**

I48.0 **<u>Paroxysmal</u> atrial <u>fibrillation</u>**

I48.1 **<u>Persistent</u> atrial <u>fibrillation</u>**

I48.2 **<u>Chronic</u> atrial <u>fibrillation</u>**
Permanent atrial fibrillation

I48.3 **<u>Typical</u> atrial <u>flutter</u>**
Type I atrial flutter

I48.4 **<u>Atypical</u> atrial <u>flutter</u>**
Type II atrial flutter

I48.9- **<u>Unspecified</u> atrial fibrillation and atrial flutter**

I48.91 **Unspecified atrial <u>fibrillation</u>**

I48.92 **Unspecified atrial <u>flutter</u>**

I49- **Other cardiac arrhythmias**
Code first cardiac arrhythmia complicating:
Abortion or ectopic or molar pregnancy (O00-O07, O08.8)
Obstetric surgery and procedures (O75.4)
Excludes 1: bradycardia NOS (R00.1)
neonatal dysrhythmia (P29.1-)
sinoatrial bradycardia (R00.1)
sinus bradycardia (R00.1)
vagal bradycardia (R00.1)

I49.0- **<u>Ventricular</u> fibrillation and flutter**

I49.01 **Ventricular fibrillation**

I49.02 **Ventricular flutter**

I49.1 **Atrial premature depolarization**
Atrial premature beats

I49.2 **Junctional premature depolarization**

I49.3 **Ventricular premature depolarization**

I49.4- **Other and unspecified premature depolarization**

I49.40 **Unspecified premature depolarization**
Premature beats NOS

I49.49 **Other premature depolarization**
Ectopic beats
Extrasystoles
Extrasystolic arrhythmias
Premature contractions

I49.5 **Sick sinus syndrome**
Tachycardia-bradycardia syndrome

I49.8 **Other specified cardiac arrhythmias**
Coronary sinus rhythm disorder
Ectopic rhythm disorder
Nodal rhythm disorder

I49.9 **Cardiac arrhythmia, unspecified**
Arrhythmia (cardiac) NOS

I42 - I60 *(side tab)*

I50- **Heart failure**
    Code first:
      Heart failure complicating abortion or ectopic or molar pregnancy (O00-O07, O08.8)
      Heart failure following surgery (I97.13-)
      Heart failure due to hypertension (I11.0)
      Heart failure due to hypertension with chronic kidney disease (I13.-)
      Obstetric surgery and procedures (O75.4)
      Rheumatic heart failure (I09.81)
    Excludes 1: cardiac arrest (I46.-)
             neonatal cardiac failure (P29.0)

  I50.1 **Left ventricular failure**
      Cardiac asthma
      Edema of lung with heart disease NOS
      Edema of lung with heart failure
      Left heart failure
      Pulmonary edema with heart disease NOS
      Pulmonary edema with heart failure
    Excludes 1: edema of lung without heart disease or heart failure
             (J81.-)
             pulmonary edema without heart disease or failure
             (J81.-)

  I50.2- **Systolic (congestive) heart failure**
    Excludes 1: combined systolic (congestive) and diastolic
             (congestive) heart failure (I50.4-)

    I50.20 **Unspecified** systolic (congestive) heart failure
    I50.21 **Acute** systolic (congestive) heart failure
    I50.22 **Chronic** systolic (congestive) heart failure
    I50.23 **Acute on chronic** systolic (congestive) heart failure

  I50.3- **Diastolic (congestive) heart failure**
    Excludes 1: combined systolic (congestive) and diastolic
             (congestive) heart failure (I50.4-)

    I50.30 **Unspecified** diastolic (congestive) heart failure
    I50.31 **Acute** diastolic (congestive) heart failure
    I50.32 **Chronic** diastolic (congestive) heart failure
    I50.33 **Acute on chronic** diastolic (congestive) heart failure

  I50.4- **Combined** systolic (congestive) and diastolic (congestive) heart failure
    I50.40 **Unspecified** combined systolic (congestive) and diastolic (congestive) heart failure
    I50.41 **Acute** combined systolic (congestive) and diastolic (congestive) heart failure
    I50.42 **Chronic** combined systolic (congestive) and diastolic (congestive) heart failure
    I50.43 **Acute on chronic** combined systolic (congestive) and diastolic (congestive) heart failure

  I50.9 **Heart failure, unspecified**
      Biventricular (heart) failure NOS
      Cardiac, heart or myocardial failure NOS
      Congestive heart disease
      Congestive heart failure NOS
      Right ventricular failure (secondary to left heart failure)
    Excludes 1: fluid overload (E87.70)

I51- **Complications and ill-defined descriptions of heart disease**
    Excludes 1: any condition in I51.4-I51.9 due to hypertension (I11.-)
             any condition in I51.4-I51.9 due to hypertension and chronic
             kidney disease (I13.-)
             heart disease specified as rheumatic (I00-I09)

  I51.0 **Cardiac septal defect, acquired**
      Acquired septal atrial defect (old)
      Acquired septal auricular defect (old)
      Acquired septal ventricular defect (old)
    Excludes 1: cardiac septal defect as current complication following
             acute myocardial infarction (I23.1, I23.2)

  I51.1 **Rupture of chordae tendineae, not elsewhere classified**
    Excludes 1: rupture of chordae tendineae as current complication
             following acute myocardial infarction (I23.4)

  I51.2 **Rupture of papillary muscle, not elsewhere classified**
    Excludes 1: rupture of papillary muscle as current complication
             following acute myocardial infarction (I23.5)

  I51.3 **Intracardiac thrombosis, not elsewhere classified**
      Apical thrombosis (old)
      Atrial thrombosis (old)
      Auricular thrombosis (old)
      Mural thrombosis (old)
      Ventricular thrombosis (old)
    Excludes 1: intracardiac thrombosis as current complication
             following acute myocardial infarction (I23.6)

  I51.4 **Myocarditis, unspecified**
      Chronic (interstitial) myocarditis
      Myocardial fibrosis
      Myocarditis NOS
    Excludes 1: acute or subacute myocarditis (I40.-)

  I51.5 **Myocardial degeneration**
      Fatty degeneration of heart or myocardium
      Myocardial disease
      Senile degeneration of heart or myocardium

  I51.7 **Cardiomegaly**
      Cardiac dilatation
      Cardiac hypertrophy
      Ventricular dilatation

  I51.8- **Other ill-defined heart diseases**
    I51.81 **Takotsubo syndrome**
        Reversible left ventricular dysfunction following sudden emotional stress
        Stress induced cardiomyopathy
        Takotsubo cardiomyopathy
        Transient left ventricular apical ballooning syndrome

    I51.89 **Other ill-defined heart diseases**
        Carditis (acute)(chronic)
        Pancarditis (acute)(chronic)

  I51.9 **Heart disease, unspecified**

I52 **Other heart disorders in diseases classified elsewhere**
    Code first underlying disease, such as:
      Congenital syphilis (A50.5)
      Mucopolysaccharidosis (E76.3)
      Schistosomiasis (B65.0-B65.9)
    Excludes 1: heart disease (in):
             gonococcal infection (A54.83)
             meningococcal infection (A39.50)
             rheumatoid arthritis (M05.31)
             syphilis (A52.06)

Cerebrovascular diseases (I60-I69)

    Use additional code to identify presence of:
      Alcohol abuse and dependence (F10.-)
      Exposure to environmental tobacco smoke (Z77.22)
      History of tobacco use (Z87.891)
      Hypertension (I10-I15)
      Occupational exposure to environmental tobacco smoke (Z57.31)
      Tobacco dependence (F17.-)
      Tobacco use (Z72.0)
    Excludes 1: transient cerebral ischemic attacks and related syndromes
             (G45.-)
             traumatic intracranial hemorrhage (S06.-)

I60- **Nontraumatic subarachnoid hemorrhage**
    Includes: Ruptured cerebral aneurysm
    Excludes 1: sequelae of subarachnoid hemorrhage (I69.0-)
             syphilitic ruptured cerebral aneurysm (A52.05)

  I60.0- **Nontraumatic subarachnoid hemorrhage from carotid siphon and bifurcation**
    I60.00 **Nontraumatic subarachnoid hemorrhage from unspecified carotid siphon and bifurcation**
    I60.01 **Nontraumatic subarachnoid hemorrhage from right carotid siphon and bifurcation**
    I60.02 **Nontraumatic subarachnoid hemorrhage from left carotid siphon and bifurcation**

  I60.1- **Nontraumatic subarachnoid hemorrhage from middle cerebral artery**
    I60.10 **Nontraumatic subarachnoid hemorrhage from unspecified middle cerebral artery**
    I60.11 **Nontraumatic subarachnoid hemorrhage from right middle cerebral artery**
    I60.12 **Nontraumatic subarachnoid hemorrhage from left middle cerebral artery**

  I60.2- **Nontraumatic subarachnoid hemorrhage from anterior communicating artery**
    I60.20 **Nontraumatic subarachnoid hemorrhage from unspecified anterior communicating artery**
    I60.21 **Nontraumatic subarachnoid hemorrhage from right anterior communicating artery**
    I60.22 **Nontraumatic subarachnoid hemorrhage from left anterior communicating artery**

I 4 2 - I 6 0

I60.3- Nontraumatic subarachnoid hemorrhage from posterior communicating artery

  I60.30 Nontraumatic subarachnoid hemorrhage from unspecified posterior communicating artery

  I60.31 Nontraumatic subarachnoid hemorrhage from right posterior communicating artery

  I60.32 Nontraumatic subarachnoid hemorrhage from left posterior communicating artery

I60.4 Nontraumatic subarachnoid hemorrhage from basilar artery

I60.5- Nontraumatic subarachnoid hemorrhage from vertebral artery

  I60.50 Nontraumatic subarachnoid hemorrhage from unspecified vertebral artery

  I60.51 Nontraumatic subarachnoid hemorrhage from right vertebral artery

  I60.52 Nontraumatic subarachnoid hemorrhage from left vertebral artery

I60.6 Nontraumatic subarachnoid hemorrhage from other intracranial arteries

I60.7 Nontraumatic subarachnoid hemorrhage from unspecified intracranial artery
    Ruptured (congenital) berry aneurysm
    Ruptured (congenital) cerebral aneurysm
    Subarachnoid hemorrhage (nontraumatic) from cerebral artery NOS
    Subarachnoid hemorrhage (nontraumatic) from communicating artery NOS
    Excludes 1: berry aneurysm, nonruptured (I67.1)

I60.8 Other nontraumatic subarachnoid hemorrhage
    Meningeal hemorrhage
    Rupture of cerebral arteriovenous malformation

I60.9 Nontraumatic subarachnoid hemorrhage, unspecified

I61- Nontraumatic intracerebral hemorrhage
    Excludes 1: sequelae of intracerebral hemorrhage (I69.1-)

I61.0 Nontraumatic intracerebral hemorrhage in hemisphere, subcortical
    Deep intracerebral hemorrhage (nontraumatic)

I61.1 Nontraumatic intracerebral hemorrhage in hemisphere, cortical
    Cerebral lobe hemorrhage (nontraumatic)
    Superficial intracerebral hemorrhage (nontraumatic)

I61.2 Nontraumatic intracerebral hemorrhage in hemisphere, unspecified

I61.3 Nontraumatic intracerebral hemorrhage in brain stem

I61.4 Nontraumatic intracerebral hemorrhage in cerebellum

I61.5 Nontraumatic intracerebral hemorrhage, intraventricular

I61.6 Nontraumatic intracerebral hemorrhage, multiple localized

I61.8 Other nontraumatic intracerebral hemorrhage

I61.9 Nontraumatic intracerebral hemorrhage, unspecified

I62- Other and unspecified nontraumatic intracranial hemorrhage
    Excludes 1: sequelae of intracranial hemorrhage (I69.2)

I62.0- Nontraumatic subdural hemorrhage

  I62.00 Nontraumatic subdural hemorrhage, unspecified

  I62.01 Nontraumatic acute subdural hemorrhage

  I62.02 Nontraumatic subacute subdural hemorrhage

  I62.03 Nontraumatic chronic subdural hemorrhage

I62.1 Nontraumatic extradural hemorrhage
    Nontraumatic epidural hemorrhage

I62.9 Nontraumatic intracranial hemorrhage, unspecified

I63- Cerebral infarction
    Includes: Occlusion and stenosis of cerebral and precerebral arteries, resulting in cerebral infarction
    Use additional code, if applicable, to identify status post administration of tPA (rtPA) in a different facility within the last 24 hours prior to admission to current facility (Z92.82)
    Excludes 1: sequelae of cerebral infarction (I69.3-)

I63.0- Cerebral infarction due to thrombosis of precerebral arteries

  I63.00 Cerebral infarction due to thrombosis of unspecified precerebral artery

  I63.01- Cerebral infarction due to thrombosis of vertebral artery

    I63.011 Cerebral infarction due to thrombosis of right vertebral artery

    I63.012 Cerebral infarction due to thrombosis of left vertebral artery

    I63.019 Cerebral infarction due to thrombosis of unspecified vertebral artery

  I63.02 Cerebral infarction due to thrombosis of basilar artery

I63.03- Cerebral infarction due to thrombosis of carotid artery

  I63.031 Cerebral infarction due to thrombosis of right carotid artery

  I63.032 Cerebral infarction due to thrombosis of left carotid artery

  I63.039 Cerebral infarction due to thrombosis of unspecified carotid artery

I63.09 Cerebral infarction due to thrombosis of other precerebral artery

I63.1- Cerebral infarction due to embolism of precerebral arteries

  I63.10 Cerebral infarction due to embolism of unspecified precerebral artery

  I63.11- Cerebral infarction due to embolism of vertebral artery

    I63.111 Cerebral infarction due to embolism of right vertebral artery

    I63.112 Cerebral infarction due to embolism of left vertebral artery

    I63.119 Cerebral infarction due to embolism of unspecified vertebral artery

  I63.12 Cerebral infarction due to embolism of basilar artery

  I63.13- Cerebral infarction due to embolism of carotid artery

    I63.131 Cerebral infarction due to embolism of right carotid artery

    I63.132 Cerebral infarction due to embolism of left carotid artery

    I63.139 Cerebral infarction due to embolism of unspecified carotid artery

  I63.19 Cerebral infarction due to embolism of other precerebral artery

I63.2- Cerebral infarction due to unspecified occlusion or stenosis of precerebral arteries

  I63.20 Cerebral infarction due to unspecified occlusion or stenosis of unspecified precerebral arteries

  I63.21- Cerebral infarction due to unspecified occlusion or stenosis of vertebral arteries

    I63.211 Cerebral infarction due to unspecified occlusion or stenosis of right vertebral arteries

    I63.212 Cerebral infarction due to unspecified occlusion or stenosis of left vertebral arteries

    I63.219 Cerebral infarction due to unspecified occlusion or stenosis of unspecified vertebral arteries

  I63.22 Cerebral infarction due to unspecified occlusion or stenosis of basilar arteries

  I63.23- Cerebral infarction due to unspecified occlusion or stenosis of carotid arteries

    I63.231 Cerebral infarction due to unspecified occlusion or stenosis of right carotid arteries

    I63.232 Cerebral infarction due to unspecified occlusion or stenosis of left carotid arteries

    I63.239 Cerebral infarction due to unspecified occlusion or stenosis of unspecified carotid arteries

  I63.29 Cerebral infarction due to unspecified occlusion or stenosis of other precerebral arteries

I63.3- Cerebral infarction due to thrombosis of cerebral arteries

  I63.30 Cerebral infarction due to thrombosis of unspecified cerebral artery

  I63.31- Cerebral infarction due to thrombosis of middle cerebral artery

    I63.311 Cerebral infarction due to thrombosis of right middle cerebral artery

    I63.312 Cerebral infarction due to thrombosis of left middle cerebral artery

    I63.319 Cerebral infarction due to thrombosis of unspecified middle cerebral artery

  I63.32- Cerebral infarction due to thrombosis of anterior cerebral artery

    I63.321 Cerebral infarction due to thrombosis of right anterior cerebral artery

    I63.322 Cerebral infarction due to thrombosis of left anterior cerebral artery

    I63.329 Cerebral infarction due to thrombosis of unspecified anterior cerebral artery

  I63.33- Cerebral infarction due to thrombosis of posterior cerebral artery

    I63.331 Cerebral infarction due to thrombosis of right posterior cerebral artery

    I63.332 Cerebral infarction due to thrombosis of left posterior cerebral artery

    I63.339 Cerebral infarction due to thrombosis of unspecified posterior cerebral artery

I
6
0
-
I
6
7

I63.34- Cerebral infarction due to thrombosis of cerebellar artery
  I63.341 Cerebral infarction due to thrombosis of right cerebellar artery
  I63.342 Cerebral infarction due to thrombosis of left cerebellar artery
  I63.349 Cerebral infarction due to thrombosis of unspecified cerebellar artery
I63.39 Cerebral infarction due to thrombosis of other cerebral artery
I63.4- Cerebral infarction due to embolism of cerebral arteries
  I63.40 Cerebral infarction due to embolism of unspecified cerebral artery
  I63.41- Cerebral infarction due to embolism of middle cerebral artery
    I63.411 Cerebral infarction due to embolism of right middle cerebral artery
    I63.412 Cerebral infarction due to embolism of left middle cerebral artery
    I63.419 Cerebral infarction due to embolism of unspecified middle cerebral artery
  I63.42- Cerebral infarction due to embolism of anterior cerebral artery
    I63.421 Cerebral infarction due to embolism of right anterior cerebral artery
    I63.422 Cerebral infarction due to embolism of left anterior cerebral artery
    I63.429 Cerebral infarction due to embolism of unspecified anterior cerebral artery
  I63.43- Cerebral infarction due to embolism of posterior cerebral artery
    I63.431 Cerebral infarction due to embolism of right posterior cerebral artery
    I63.432 Cerebral infarction due to embolism of left posterior cerebral artery
    I63.439 Cerebral infarction due to embolism of unspecified posterior cerebral artery
  I63.44- Cerebral infarction due to embolism of cerebellar artery
    I63.441 Cerebral infarction due to embolism of right cerebellar artery
    I63.442 Cerebral infarction due to embolism of left cerebellar artery
    I63.449 Cerebral infarction due to embolism of unspecified cerebellar artery
I63.49 Cerebral infarction due to embolism of other cerebral artery
I63.5- Cerebral infarction due to unspecified occlusion or stenosis of cerebral arteries
  I63.50 Cerebral infarction due to unspecified occlusion or stenosis of unspecified cerebral artery
  I63.51- Cerebral infarction due to unspecified occlusion or stenosis of middle cerebral artery
    I63.511 Cerebral infarction due to unspecified occlusion or stenosis of right middle cerebral artery
    I63.512 Cerebral infarction due to unspecified occlusion or stenosis of left middle cerebralartery
    I63.519 Cerebral infarction due to unspecified occlusion or stenosis of unspecified middle cerebral artery
  I63.52- Cerebral infarction due to unspecified occlusion or stenosis of anterior cerebral artery
    I63.521 Cerebral infarction due to unspecified occlusion or stenosis of right anterior cerebral artery
    I63.522 Cerebral infarction due to unspecified occlusion or stenosis of left anterior cerebral artery
    I63.529 Cerebral infarction due to unspecified occlusion or stenosis of unspecified anterior cerebral artery
  I63.53- Cerebral infarction due to unspecified occlusion or stenosis of posterior cerebral artery
    I63.531 Cerebral infarction due to unspecified occlusion or stenosis of right posterior cerebral artery
    I63.532 Cerebral infarction due to unspecified occlusion or stenosis of left posterior cerebral artery
    I63.539 Cerebral infarction due to unspecified occlusion or stenosis of unspecified posterior cerebral artery
  I63.54- Cerebral infarction due to unspecified occlusion or stenosis of cerebellar artery
    I63.541 Cerebral infarction due to unspecified occlusion or stenosis of right cerebellar artery
    I63.542 Cerebral infarction due to unspecified occlusion or stenosis of left cerebellar artery
    I63.549 Cerebral infarction due to unspecified occlusion or stenosis of unspecified cerebellar artery

  I63.59 Cerebral infarction due to unspecified occlusion or stenosis of other cerebral artery
I63.6 Cerebral infarction due to cerebral venous thrombosis, nonpyogenic
I63.8 Other cerebral infarction
I63.9 Cerebral infarction, unspecified
  Stroke NOS
I65- Occlusion and stenosis of precerebral arteries, not resulting in cerebral infarction
  Includes: Embolism of precerebral artery
    Narrowing of precerebral artery
    Obstruction (complete) (partial) of precerebral artery
    Thrombosis of precerebral artery
  Excludes 1: insufficiency, NOS, of precerebral artery (G45.-)
    insufficiency of precerebral arteries causing cerebral infarction (I63.0-I63.2)
I65.0- Occlusion and stenosis of vertebral artery
  I65.01 Occlusion and stenosis of right vertebral artery
  I65.02 Occlusion and stenosis of left vertebral artery
  I65.03 Occlusion and stenosis of bilateral vertebral arteries
  I65.09 Occlusion and stenosis of unspecified vertebral artery
I65.1 Occlusion and stenosis of basilar artery
I65.2- Occlusion and stenosis of carotid artery
  I65.21 Occlusion and stenosis of right carotid artery
  I65.22 Occlusion and stenosis of left carotid artery
  I65.23 Occlusion and stenosis of bilateral carotid arteries
  I65.29 Occlusion and stenosis of unspecified carotid artery
I65.8 Occlusion and stenosis of other precerebral arteries
I65.9 Occlusion and stenosis of unspecified precerebral artery
  Occlusion and stenosis of precerebral artery NOS
I66- Occlusion and stenosis of cerebral arteries, not resulting in cerebral infarction
  Includes: Embolism of cerebral artery
    Narrowing of cerebral artery
    Obstruction (complete) (partial) of cerebral artery
    Thrombosis of cerebral artery
  Excludes 1: occlusion and stenosis of cerebral artery causing cerebral infarction (I63.3-I63.5)
I66.0- Occlusion and stenosis of middle cerebral artery
  I66.01 Occlusion and stenosis of right middle cerebral artery
  I66.02 Occlusion and stenosis of left middle cerebral artery
  I66.03 Occlusion and stenosis of bilateral middle cerebral arteries
  I66.09 Occlusion and stenosis of unspecified middle cerebral artery
I66.1- Occlusion and stenosis of anterior cerebral artery
  I66.11 Occlusion and stenosis of right anterior cerebral artery
  I66.12 Occlusion and stenosis of left anterior cerebral artery
  I66.13 Occlusion and stenosis of bilateral anterior cerebral arteries
  I66.19 Occlusion and stenosis of unspecified anterior cerebral artery
I66.2- Occlusion and stenosis of posterior cerebral artery
  I66.21 Occlusion and stenosis of right posterior cerebral artery
  I66.22 Occlusion and stenosis of left posterior cerebral artery
  I66.23 Occlusion and stenosis of bilateral posterior cerebral arteries
  I66.29 Occlusion and stenosis of unspecified posterior cerebral artery
I66.3 Occlusion and stenosis of cerebellar arteries
I66.8 Occlusion and stenosis of other cerebral arteries
  Occlusion and stenosis of perforating arteries
I66.9 Occlusion and stenosis of unspecified cerebral artery
I67- Other cerebrovascular diseases
  Excludes 1: sequelae of the listed conditions (I69.8)
I67.0 Dissection of cerebral arteries, nonruptured
  Excludes 1: ruptured cerebral arteries (I60.7)
I67.1 Cerebral aneurysm, nonruptured
  Cerebral aneurysm NOS
  Cerebral arteriovenous fistula, acquired
  Internal carotid artery aneurysm, intracranial portion
  Internal carotid artery aneurysm, NOS
  Excludes 1: congenital cerebral aneurysm, nonruptured (Q28.-)
    ruptured cerebral aneurysm (I60.7)
I67.2 Cerebral atherosclerosis
  Atheroma of cerebral and precerebral arteries
I67.3 Progressive vascular leukoencephalopathy
  Binswanger's disease
I67.4 Hypertensive encephalopathy
I67.5 Moyamoya disease

I60 - I67

I67.6   **Nonpyogenic thrombosis of intracranial venous system**
Nonpyogenic thrombosis of cerebral vein
Nonpyogenic thrombosis of intracranial venous sinus
Excludes 1:   nonpyogenic thrombosis of intracranial venous system
causing infarction (I63.6)

I67.7   **Cerebral arteritis, not elsewhere classified**
Granulomatous angiitis of the nervous system
Excludes 1:   allergic granulomatous angiitis (M30.1)

I67.8-   **Other specified cerebrovascular diseases**
I67.81   **Acute cerebrovascular insufficiency**
Acute cerebrovascular insufficiency unspecified as to location
or reversibility

I67.82   **Cerebral ischemia**
Chronic cerebral ischemia

I67.83   **Posterior reversible encephalopathy syndrome**
PRES

I67.84- **Cerebral vasospasm and vasoconstriction**
I67.841   **Reversible cerebrovascular vasoconstriction syndrome**
Call-Fleming syndrome
Code first underlying condition, if applicable, such as
eclampsia (O15.00-O15.9)

I67.848   **Other cerebral vasospasm and vasoconstriction**

I67.89   **Other cerebrovascular disease**

I67.9   **Cerebrovascular disease, unspecified**

I68-   **Cerebrovascular disorders <u>in diseases classified elsewhere</u>**
I68.0   **Cerebral amyloid angiopathy**
Code first underlying amyloidosis (E85.-)

I68.2   **Cerebral arteritis in other diseases classified elsewhere**
Code first underlying disease
Excludes 1:   cerebral arteritis (in):
listerosis (A32.89)
systemic lupus erythematosus (M32.19)
syphilis (A52.04)
tuberculosis (A18.89)

I68.8   **Other cerebrovascular disorders in diseases classified elsewhere**
Code first underlying disease
Excludes 1:   syphilitic cerebral aneurysm (A52.05)

I69-   **<u>Sequelae of cerebrovascular disease</u>**
Note: Category I69 is to be used to indicate conditions in I60-I67 as the
cause of sequelae. The "sequelae" include conditions specified as
such or as residuals which may occur at any time after the onset of
the causal condition.
Excludes 1:   personal history of cerebral infarction without residual deficit
(Z86.73)
personal history of prolonged reversible ischemic neurologic
deficit (PRIND) (Z86.73)
personal history of reversible ischemic neurolcgcial deficit
(RIND) (Z86.73)
sequelae of traumatic intracranial injury (S06.-)
transient ischemic attack (TIA) (G45.9)

I69.0-   **<u>Sequelae of nontraumatic <u>subarachnoid</u> hemorrhage</u>**
I69.00   **<u>Unspecified</u> sequelae of nontraumatic <u>subarachnoid</u>
hemorrhage**

I69.01   **<u>Cognitive</u> deficits following nontraumatic <u>subarachnoid</u>
hemorrhage**

I69.02- **<u>Speech and language</u> deficits following nontraumatic
<u>subarachnoid</u> hemorrhage**
I69.020   **Aphasia following nontraumatic <u>subarachnoid</u>
hemorrhage**
I69.021   **Dysphasia following nontraumatic <u>subarachnoid</u>
hemorrhage**
I69.022   **Dysarthria following nontraumatic <u>subarachnoid</u>
hemorrhage**
I69.023   **Fluency disorder following nontraumatic
<u>subarachnoid</u> hemorrhage**
Stuttering following nontraumatic subarachnoid
hemorrhage
I69.028   **Other speech and language deficits following
nontraumatic <u>subarachnoid</u> hemorrhage**

I69.03- **<u>Monoplegia</u> of <u>upper limb</u> following nontraumatic
<u>subarachnoid</u> hemorrhage**
I69.031   **Monoplegia of upper limb following nontraumatic
<u>subarachnoid</u> hemorrhage affecting <u>right</u> dominant
side**
I69.032   **Monoplegia of upper limb following nontraumatic
<u>subarachnoid</u> hemorrhage affecting <u>left</u> dominant side**
I69.033   **Monoplegia of upper limb following nontraumatic
<u>subarachnoid</u> hemorrhage affecting <u>right</u> <u>non-</u>
dominant side**
I69.034   **Monoplegia of upper limb following nontraumatic
<u>subarachnoid</u> hemorrhage affecting <u>left</u> <u>non</u>-dominant
side**

I69.039   **Monoplegia of upper limb following nontraumatic
<u>subarachnoid</u> hemorrhage affecting <u>unspecified side</u>**

I69.04- **<u>Monoplegia</u> of <u>lower limb</u> following nontraumatic
<u>subarachnoid</u> hemorrhage**
I69.041   **Monoplegia of lower limb following nontraumatic
<u>subarachnoid</u> hemorrhage affecting <u>right</u> dominant
side**
I69.042   **Monoplegia of lower limb following nontraumatic
<u>subarachnoid</u> hemorrhage affecting <u>left</u> dominant side**
I69.043   **Monoplegia of lower limb following nontraumatic
<u>subarachnoid</u> hemorrhage affecting <u>right</u> <u>non</u>-
dominant side**
I69.044   **Monoplegia of lower limb following nontraumatic
<u>subarachnoid</u> hemorrhage affecting <u>left</u> <u>non-dominant</u>
side**
I69.049   **Monoplegia of lower limb following nontraumatic
<u>subarachnoid</u> hemorrhage affecting <u>unspecified side</u>**

I69.05- **<u>Hemiplegia</u> and hemiparesis following nontraumatic
<u>subarachnoid</u> hemorrhage**
I69.051   **Hemiplegia and hemiparesis following nontraumatic
<u>subarachnoid</u> hemorrhage affecting <u>right</u> dominant
side**
I69.052   **Hemiplegia and hemiparesis following nontraumatic
<u>subarachnoid</u> hemorrhage affecting <u>left</u> dominant side**
I69.053   **Hemiplegia and hemiparesis following nontraumatic
<u>subarachnoid</u> hemorrhage affecting <u>right</u> <u>non-</u>
dominant side**
I69.054   **Hemiplegia and hemiparesis following nontraumatic
<u>subarachnoid</u> hemorrhage affecting <u>left</u> <u>non-dominant</u>
side**
I69.059   **Hemiplegia and hemiparesis following nontraumatic
<u>subarachnoid</u> hemorrhage affecting <u>unspecified side</u>**

I69.06- **<u>Other paralytic</u> syndrome following nontraumatic
<u>subarachnoid</u> hemorrhage**
Use additional code to identify type of paralytic syndrome, such
as:
Locked-in state (G83.5)
Quadriplegia (G82.5-)
Excludes 1:   hemiplegia/hemiparesis following nontraumatic
subarachnoid hemorrhage (I69.05-)
monoplegia of lower limb following nontraumatic
subarachnoid hemorrhage (I69.04-)
monoplegia of upper limb following nontraumatic
subarachnoid hemorrhage (I69.03-)
I69.061   **Other paralytic syndrome following nontraumatic
<u>subarachnoid</u> hemorrhage affecting <u>right</u> dominant
side**
I69.062   **Other paralytic syndrome following nontraumatic
<u>subarachnoid</u> hemorrhage affecting <u>left</u> dominant
side**
I69.063   **Other paralytic syndrome following nontraumatic
<u>subarachnoid</u> hemorrhage affecting <u>right</u> <u>non-</u>
dominant side**
I69.064   **Other paralytic syndrome following nontraumatic
<u>subarachnoid</u> hemorrhage affecting <u>left</u> <u>non-dominant</u>
side**
I69.065   **Other paralytic syndrome following nontraumatic
<u>subarachnoid</u> hemorrhage, <u>bilateral</u>**
I69.069   **Other paralytic syndrome following nontraumatic
<u>subarachnoid</u> hemorrhage affecting <u>unspecified side</u>**

I69.09- **<u>Other sequelae</u> of nontraumatic <u>subarachnoid</u> hemorrhage**
I69.090   **Apraxia following nontraumatic <u>subarachnoid</u>
hemorrhage**
I69.091   **Dysphagia following nontraumatic <u>subarachnoid</u>
hemorrhage**
Use additional code to identify the type of dysphagia, if
known (R13.1-)
I69.092   **Facial weakness following nontraumatic <u>subarachnoid</u>
hemorrhage**
Facial droop following nontraumatic subarachnoid
hemorrhage
I69.093   **Ataxia following nontraumatic <u>subarachnoid</u>
hemorrhage**
I69.098   **Other sequelae following nontraumatic <u>subarachnoid</u>
hemorrhage**
Alterations of sensation following nontraumatic
subarachnoid hemorrhage
Disturbance of vision following nontraumatic
subarachnoid hemorrhage
Use additional code to identify the sequelae

I69.1-   **<u>Sequelae of nontraumatic <u>intracerebral</u> hemorrhage</u>**
I69.10   **<u>Unspecified</u> sequelae of nontraumatic <u>intracerebral</u>
hemorrhage**

I
6
7
-
I
6
9

Excludes 1: = NOT CODED HERE! (Do not code both)   **482**   *Excludes ❷:* = Not Included Here

© 2013 Channel Publishing Ltd

I69.11   Cognitive deficits following nontraumatic intracerebral hemorrhage

I69.12-   Speech and language deficits following nontraumatic intracerebral hemorrhage

   I69.120   Aphasia following nontraumatic intracerebral hemorrhage

   I69.121   Dysphasia following nontraumatic intracerebral hemorrhage

   I69.122   Dysarthria following nontraumatic intracerebral hemorrhage

   I69.123   Fluency disorder following nontraumatic intracerebral hemorrhage
      Stuttering following nontraumatic subarachnoid hemorrhage

   I69.128   Other speech and language deficits following nontraumatic intracerebral hemorrhage

I69.13-   Monoplegia of upper limb following nontraumatic intracerebral hemorrhage

   I69.131   Monoplegia of upper limb following nontraumatic intracerebral hemorrhage affecting right dominant side

   I69.132   Monoplegia of upper limb following nontraumatic intracerebral hemorrhage affecting left dominant side

   I69.133   Monoplegia of upper limb following nontraumatic intracerebral hemorrhage affecting right non-dominant side

   I69.134   Monoplegia of upper limb following nontraumatic intracerebral hemorrhage affecting left non-dominant side

   I69.139   Monoplegia of upper limb following nontraumatic intracerebral hemorrhage affecting unspecified side

I69.14-   Monoplegia of lower limb following nontraumatic intracerebral hemorrhage

   I69.141   Monoplegia of lower limb following nontraumatic intracerebral hemorrhage affecting right dominant side

   I69.142   Monoplegia of lower limb following nontraumatic intracerebral hemorrhage affecting left dominant side

   I69.143   Monoplegia of lower limb following nontraumatic intracerebral hemorrhage affecting right non-dominant side

   I69.144   Monoplegia of lower limb following nontraumatic intracerebral hemorrhage affecting left non-dominant side

   I69.149   Monoplegia of lower limb following nontraumatic intracerebral hemorrhage affecting unspecified side

I69.15-   Hemiplegia and hemiparesis following nontraumatic intracerebral hemorrhage

   I69.151   Hemiplegia and hemiparesis following nontraumatic intracerebral hemorrhage affecting right dominant side

   I69.152   Hemiplegia and hemiparesis following nontraumatic intracerebral hemorrhage affecting left dominant side

   I69.153   Hemiplegia and hemiparesis following nontraumatic intracerebral hemorrhage affecting right non-dominant side

   I69.154   Hemiplegia and hemiparesis following nontraumatic intracerebral hemorrhage affecting left non-dominant side

   I69.159   Hemiplegia and hemiparesis following nontraumatic intracerebral hemorrhage affecting unspecified side

I69.16-   Other paralytic syndrome following nontraumatic intracerebral hemorrhage
   Use additional code to identify type of paralytic syndrome, such as:
     Locked-in state (G83.5)
     Quadriplegia (G82.5-)
   Excludes 1:   hemiplegia/hemiparesis following nontraumatic intracerebral hemorrhage (I69.15-)
     monoplegia of lower limb following nontraumatic intracerebral hemorrhage (I69.14-)
     monoplegia of upper limb following nontraumatic intracerebral hemorrhage (I69.13-)

   I69.161   Other paralytic syndrome following nontraumatic intracerebral hemorrhage affecting right dominant side

   I69.162   Other paralytic syndrome following nontraumatic intracerebral hemorrhage affecting left dominant side

   I69.163   Other paralytic syndrome following nontraumatic intracerebral hemorrhage affecting right non-dominant side

   I69.164   Other paralytic syndrome following nontraumatic intracerebral hemorrhage affecting left non-dominant side

   I69.165   Other paralytic syndrome following nontraumatic intracerebral hemorrhage, bilateral

   I69.169   Other paralytic syndrome following nontraumatic intracerebral hemorrhage affecting unspecified side

I69.19-   Other sequelae of nontraumatic intracerebral hemorrhage

   I69.190   Apraxia following nontraumatic intracerebral hemorrhage

   I69.191   Dysphagia following nontraumatic intracerebral hemorrhage
     Use additional code to identify the type of dysphagia, if known (R13.1-)

   I69.192   Facial weakness following nontraumatic intracerebral hemorrhage
     Facial droop following nontraumatic intracerebral hemorrhage

   I69.193   Ataxia following nontraumatic intracerebral hemorrhage

   I69.198   Other sequelae of nontraumatic intracerebral hemorrhage
     Alteration of sensations following nontraumatic intracerebral hemorrhage
     Disturbance of vision following nontraumatic intracerebral hemorrhage
     Use additional code to identify the sequelae

I69.2-   Sequelae of other nontraumatic intracranial hemorrhage

I69.20   Unspecified sequelae of other nontraumatic intracranial hemorrhage

I69.21   Cognitive deficits following other nontraumatic intracranial hemorrhage

I69.22-   Speech and language deficits following other nontraumatic intracranial hemorrhage

   I69.220   Aphasia following other nontraumatic intracranial hemorrhage

   I69.221   Dysphasia following other nontraumatic intracranial hemorrhage

   I69.222   Dysarthria following other nontraumatic intracranial hemorrhage

   I69.223   Fluency disorder following other nontraumatic intracranial hemorrhage
     Stuttering following nontraumatic subarachnoid hemorrhage

   I69.228   Other speech and language deficits following other nontraumatic intracranial hemorrhage

I69.23-   Monoplegia of upper limb following other nontraumatic intracranial hemorrhage

   I69.231   Monoplegia of upper limb following other nontraumatic intracranial hemorrhage affecting right dominant side

   I69.232   Monoplegia of upper limb following other nontraumatic intracranial hemorrhage affecting left dominant side

   I69.233   Monoplegia of upper limb following other nontraumatic intracranial hemorrhage affecting right non-dominant side

   I69.234   Monoplegia of upper limb following other nontraumatic intracranial hemorrhage affecting left non-dominant side

   I69.239   Monoplegia of upper limb following other nontraumatic intracranial hemorrhage affecting unspecified side

I69.24-   Monoplegia of lower limb following other nontraumatic intracranial hemorrhage

   I69.241   Monoplegia of lower limb following other nontraumatic intracranial hemorrhage affecting right dominant side

   I69.242   Monoplegia of lower limb following other nontraumatic intracranial hemorrhage affecting left dominant side

   I69.243   Monoplegia of lower limb following other nontraumatic intracranial hemorrhage affecting right non-dominant side

   I69.244   Monoplegia of lower limb following other nontraumatic intracranial hemorrhage affecting left non-dominant side

   I69.249   Monoplegia of lower limb following other nontraumatic intracranial hemorrhage affecting unspecified side

I67 - I69

I69.25- <u>Hemiplegia</u> and hemiparesis following other nontraumatic <u>intracranial</u> hemorrhage

    I69.251   **Hemiplegia and hemiparesis following other nontraumatic <u>intracranial</u> hemorrhage affecting <u>right</u> dominant side**

    I69.252   **Hemiplegia and hemiparesis following other nontraumatic <u>intracranial</u> hemorrhage affecting <u>left</u> dominant side**

    I69.253   **Hemiplegia and hemiparesis following other nontraumatic <u>intracranial</u> hemorrhage affecting <u>right</u> <u>non</u>-dominant side**

    I69.254   **Hemiplegia and hemiparesis following other nontraumatic <u>intracranial</u> hemorrhage affecting <u>left</u> <u>non</u>-dominant side**

    I69.259   **Hemiplegia and hemiparesis following other nontraumatic <u>intracranial</u> hemorrhage affecting <u>unspecified side</u>**

I69.26- <u>Other paralytic</u> syndrome following other nontraumatic <u>intracranial</u> hemorrhage

    Use additional code to identify type of paralytic syndrome, such as:

       Locked-in state (G83.5)

       Quadriplegia (G82.5-)

    Excludes 1:   *hemiplegia/hemiparesis following other nontraumatic intracranial hemorrhage (I69.25-)*

          monoplegia of lower limb following other nontraumatic intracranial hemorrhage (I69.24-)

          monoplegia of upper limb following other nontraumatic intracranial hemorrhage (I69.23-)

    I69.261   **Other paralytic syndrome following other nontraumatic <u>intracranial</u> hemorrhage affecting <u>right</u> dominant side**

    I69.262   **Other paralytic syndrome following other nontraumatic <u>intracranial</u> hemorrhage affecting <u>left</u> dominant side**

    I69.263   **Other paralytic syndrome following other nontraumatic <u>intracranial</u> hemorrhage affecting <u>right</u> <u>non</u>-dominant side**

    I69.264   **Other paralytic syndrome following other nontraumatic <u>intracranial</u> hemorrhage affecting <u>left</u> <u>non</u>-dominant side**

    I69.265   **Other paralytic syndrome following other nontraumatic <u>intracranial</u> hemorrhage, <u>bilateral</u>**

    I69.269   **Other paralytic syndrome following other nontraumatic <u>intracranial</u> hemorrhage affecting <u>unspecified side</u>**

I69.29- <u>Other sequelae</u> of other nontraumatic <u>intracranial</u> hemorrhage

    I69.290   **Apraxia following other nontraumatic <u>intracranial</u> hemorrhage**

    I69.291   **Dysphagia following other nontraumatic <u>intracranial</u> hemorrhage**

       Use additional code to identify the type of dysphagia, if known (R13.1-)

    I69.292   **Facial weakness following other nontraumatic <u>intracranial</u> hemorrhage**

       Facial droop following other nontraumatic intracranial hemorrhage

    I69.293   **Ataxia following other nontraumatic <u>intracranial</u> hemorrhage**

    I69.298   **Other sequelae of other nontraumatic <u>intracranial</u> hemorrhage**

       Alteration of sensation following other nontraumatic intracranial hemorrhage

       Disturbance of vision following other nontraumatic intracranial hemorrhage

       Use additional code to identify the sequelae

I69.3- <u>Sequelae of cerebral infarction</u>

    Sequelae of stroke NOS

I69.30   <u>Unspecified</u> sequelae of cerebral <u>infarction</u>

I69.31   <u>Cognitive</u> deficits following cerebral <u>infarction</u>

I69.32- <u>Speech and language</u> deficits following cerebral <u>infarction</u>

    I69.320   **Aphasia following cerebral <u>infarction</u>**

    I69.321   **Dysphasia following cerebral <u>infarction</u>**

    I69.322   **Dysarthria following cerebral <u>infarction</u>**

    I69.323   **Fluency disorder following cerebral <u>infarction</u>**

       Stuttering following nontraumatic subarachnoid hemorrhage

    I69.328   **Other speech and language deficits following cerebral infarction**

I69.33- <u>Monoplegia</u> of <u>upper limb</u> following cerebral infarction

    I69.331   **Monoplegia of upper limb following cerebral <u>infarction</u> affecting <u>right</u> dominant side**

    I69.332   **Monoplegia of upper limb following cerebral <u>infarction</u> affecting <u>left</u> dominant side**

    I69.333   **Monoplegia of upper limb following cerebral <u>infarction</u> affecting <u>right</u> <u>non</u>-dominant side**

    I69.334   **Monoplegia of upper limb following cerebral <u>infarction</u> affecting <u>left</u> <u>non</u>-dominant side**

    I69.339   **Monoplegia of upper limb following cerebral <u>infarction</u> affecting <u>unspecified side</u>**

I69.34- <u>Monoplegia</u> of <u>lower limb</u> following cerebral <u>infarction</u>

    I69.341   **Monoplegia of lower limb following cerebral <u>infarction</u> affecting <u>right</u> dominant side**

    I69.342   **Monoplegia of lower limb following cerebral <u>infarction</u> affecting <u>left</u> dominant side**

    I69.343   **Monoplegia of lower limb following cerebral <u>infarction</u> affecting <u>right</u> <u>non</u>-dominant side**

    I69.344   **Monoplegia of lower limb following cerebral <u>infarction</u> affecting <u>left</u> <u>non</u>-dominant side**

    I69.349   **Monoplegia of lower limb following cerebral <u>infarction</u> affecting <u>unspecified side</u>**

I69.35- <u>Hemiplegia</u> and hemiparesis following cerebral <u>infarction</u>

    I69.351   **Hemiplegia and hemiparesis following cerebral <u>infarction</u> affecting <u>right</u> dominant side**

    I69.352   **Hemiplegia and hemiparesis following cerebral <u>infarction</u> affecting <u>left</u> dominant side**

    I69.353   **Hemiplegia and hemiparesis following cerebral <u>infarction</u> affecting <u>right</u> <u>non</u>-dominant side**

    I69.354   **Hemiplegia and hemiparesis following cerebral <u>infarction</u> affecting <u>left</u> <u>non</u>-dominant side**

    I69.359   **Hemiplegia and hemiparesis following cerebral <u>infarction</u> affecting <u>unspecified side</u>**

I69.36- <u>Other paralytic</u> syndrome following cerebral <u>infarction</u>

    Use additional code to identify type of paralytic syndrome, such as:

       Locked-in state (G83.5)

       Quadriplegia (G82.5-)

    Excludes 1:   *hemiplegia/hemiparesis following cerebral infarction (I69.35-)*

          monoplegia of lower limb following cerebral infarction (I69.34-)

          monoplegia of upper limb following cerebral infarction (I69.33-)

    I69.361   **Other paralytic syndrome following cerebral <u>infarction</u> affecting <u>right</u> dominant side**

    I69.362   **Other paralytic syndrome following cerebral <u>infarction</u> affecting <u>left</u> dominant side**

    I69.363   **Other paralytic syndrome following cerebral <u>infarction</u> affecting <u>right</u> <u>non</u>-dominant side**

    I69.364   **Other paralytic syndrome following cerebral <u>infarction</u> affecting <u>left</u> <u>non</u>-dominant side**

    I69.365   **Other paralytic syndrome following cerebral <u>infarction</u>, <u>bilateral</u>**

    I69.369   **Other paralytic syndrome following cerebral <u>infarction</u> affecting <u>unspecified side</u>**

I69.39- <u>Other sequelae</u> of cerebral <u>infarction</u>

    I69.390   **Apraxia following cerebral <u>infarction</u>**

    I69.391   **Dysphagia following cerebral <u>infarction</u>**

       Use additional code to identify the type of dysphagia, if known (R13.1-)

    I69.392   **Facial weakness following cerebral <u>infarction</u>**

       Facial droop following cerebral infarction

    I69.393   **Ataxia following cerebral <u>infarction</u>**

    I69.398   **Other sequelae of cerebral <u>infarction</u>**

       Alteration of sensation following cerebral infarction

       Disturbance of vision following cerebral infarction

       Use additional code to identify the sequelae

I69.8- <u>Sequelae of other cerebrovascular diseases</u>

    Excludes 1:   *sequelae of traumatic intracranial injury (S06.-)*

I69.80   <u>Unspecified</u> sequelae of <u>other</u> cerebrovascular disease

I69.81   <u>Cognitive</u> deficits following <u>other</u> cerebrovascular disease

I69.82- <u>Speech and language</u> deficits following <u>other</u> cerebrovascular disease

    I69.820   **Aphasia following <u>other</u> cerebrovascular disease**

    I69.821   **Dysphasia following <u>other</u> cerebrovascular disease**

    I69.822   **Dysarthria following <u>other</u> cerebrovascular disease**

I69 – I69

I69.823 **Fluency disorder following <u>other</u> cerebrovascular disease**
Stuttering following nontraumatic subarachnoid hemorrhage

I69.828 **Other speech and language deficits following <u>other</u> cerebrovascular disease**

I69.83- <u>Monoplegia</u> of <u>upper limb</u> following <u>other</u> cerebrovascular disease

I69.831 **Monoplegia of upper limb following <u>other</u> cerebrovascular disease affecting <u>right</u> dominant side**

I69.832 **Monoplegia of upper limb following <u>other</u> cerebrovascular disease affecting <u>left</u> dominant side**

I69.833 **Monoplegia of upper limb following <u>other</u> cerebrovascular disease affecting <u>right</u> <u>non</u>-dominant side**

I69.834 **Monoplegia of upper limb following <u>other</u> cerebrovascular disease affecting <u>left</u> <u>non</u>-dominant side**

I69.839 **Monoplegia of upper limb following <u>other</u> cerebrovascular disease affecting <u>unspecified side</u>**

I69.84- <u>Monoplegia</u> of <u>lower limb</u> following <u>other</u> cerebrovascular disease

I69.841 **Monoplegia of lower limb following <u>other</u> cerebrovascular disease affecting <u>right</u> dominant side**

I69.842 **Monoplegia of lower limb following <u>other</u> cerebrovascular disease affecting <u>left</u> dominant side**

I69.843 **Monoplegia of lower limb following <u>other</u> cerebrovascular disease affecting <u>right</u> <u>non</u>-dominant side**

I69.844 **Monoplegia of lower limb following <u>other</u> cerebrovascular disease affecting <u>left</u> <u>non</u>-dominant side**

I69.849 **Monoplegia of lower limb following <u>other</u> cerebrovascular disease affecting <u>unspecified side</u>**

I69.85- <u>Hemiplegia</u> and hemiparesis following <u>other</u> cerebrovascular disease

I69.851 **Hemiplegia and hemiparesis following <u>other</u> cerebrovascular disease affecting <u>right</u> dominant side**

I69.852 **Hemiplegia and hemiparesis following <u>other</u> cerebrovascular disease affecting <u>left</u> dominant side**

I69.853 **Hemiplegia and hemiparesis following <u>other</u> cerebrovascular disease affecting <u>right</u> <u>non</u>-dominant side**

I69.854 **Hemiplegia and hemiparesis following <u>other</u> cerebrovascular disease affecting <u>left</u> <u>non</u>-dominant side**

I69.859 **Hemiplegia and hemiparesis following <u>other</u> cerebrovascular disease affecting <u>unspecified side</u>**

I69.86- <u>Other paralytic</u> syndrome following other cerebrovascular disease
Use additional code to identify type of paralytic syndrome, such as:
Locked-in state (G83.5)
Quadriplegia (G82.5-)
*Excludes 1: hemiplegia/hemiparesis following other cerebrovascular disease (I69.85-)
monoplegia of lower limb following other cerebrovascular disease (I69.84-)
monoplegia of upper limb following other cerebrovascular disease (I69.83-)*

I69.861 **Other paralytic syndrome following <u>other</u> cerebrovascular disease affecting <u>right</u> dominant side**

I69.862 **Other paralytic syndrome following <u>other</u> cerebrovascular disease affecting <u>left</u> dominant side**

I69.863 **Other paralytic syndrome following <u>other</u> cerebrovascular disease affecting <u>right</u> <u>non</u>-dominant side**

I69.864 **Other paralytic syndrome following <u>other</u> cerebrovascular disease affecting <u>left</u> <u>non</u>-dominant side**

I69.865 **Other paralytic syndrome following <u>other</u> cerebrovascular disease, <u>bilateral</u>**

I69.869 **Other paralytic syndrome following <u>other</u> cerebrovascular disease affecting <u>unspecified side</u>**

I69.89- <u>Other sequelae</u> of <u>other</u> cerebrovascular disease

I69.890 **Apraxia following <u>other</u> cerebrovascular disease**

I69.891 **Dysphagia following <u>other</u> cerebrovascular disease**
Use additional code to identify the type of dysphagia, if known (R13.1-)

I69.892 **Facial weakness following <u>other</u> cerebrovascular disease**
Facial droop following other cerebrovascular disease

I69.893 **Ataxia following <u>other</u> cerebrovascular disease**

I69.898 **Other sequelae of <u>other</u> cerebrovascular disease**
Alteration of sensation following other cerebrovascular disease
Disturbance of vision following other cerebrovascular disease
Use additional code to identify the sequelae

I69.9- <u>Sequelae</u> of <u>unspecified</u> cerebrovascular diseases
*Excludes 1: sequelae of stroke (I69.3)
sequelae of traumatic intracranial injury (S06.-)*

I69.90 **<u>Unspecified</u> sequelae of <u>unspecified</u> cerebrovascular disease**

I69.91 **<u>Cognitive</u> deficits following <u>unspecified</u> cerebrovascular disease**

I69.92- <u>Speech and language</u> deficits following <u>unspecified</u> cerebrovascular disease

I69.920 **Aphasia following <u>unspecified</u> cerebrovascular disease**

I69.921 **Dysphasia following <u>unspecified</u> cerebrovascular disease**

I69.922 **Dysarthria following <u>unspecified</u> cerebrovascular disease**

I69.923 **Fluency disorder following <u>unspecified</u> cerebrovascular disease**
Stuttering following nontraumatic subarachnoid hemorrhage

I69.928 **Other speech and language deficits following <u>unspecified</u> cerebrovascular disease**

I69.93- <u>Monoplegia</u> of <u>upper limb</u> following <u>unspecified</u> cerebrovascular disease

I69.931 **Monoplegia of upper limb following <u>unspecified</u> cerebrovascular disease affecting <u>right</u> dominant side**

I69.932 **Monoplegia of upper limb following <u>unspecified</u> cerebrovascular disease affecting <u>left</u> dominant side**

I69.933 **Monoplegia of upper limb following <u>unspecified</u> cerebrovascular disease affecting <u>right</u> <u>non</u>-dominant side**

I69.934 **Monoplegia of upper limb following <u>unspecified</u> cerebrovascular disease affecting <u>left</u> <u>non</u>-dominant side**

I69.939 **Monoplegia of upper limb following <u>unspecified</u> cerebrovascular disease affecting <u>unspecified side</u>**

I69.94- <u>Monoplegia</u> of <u>lower limb</u> following <u>unspecified</u> cerebrovascular disease

I69.941 **Monoplegia of lower limb following <u>unspecified</u> cerebrovascular disease affecting <u>right</u> dominant side**

I69.942 **Monoplegia of lower limb following <u>unspecified</u> cerebrovascular disease affecting <u>left</u> dominant side**

I69.943 **Monoplegia of lower limb following <u>unspecified</u> cerebrovascular disease affecting <u>right</u> <u>non</u>-dominant side**

I69.944 **Monoplegia of lower limb following <u>unspecified</u> cerebrovascular disease affecting <u>left</u> <u>non</u>-dominant side**

I69.949 **Monoplegia of lower limb following <u>unspecified</u> cerebrovascular disease affecting <u>unspecified side</u>**

I69.95- <u>Hemiplegia</u> and hemiparesis following <u>unspecified</u> cerebrovascular disease

I69.951 **Hemiplegia and hemiparesis following <u>unspecified</u> cerebrovascular disease affecting <u>right</u> dominant side**

I69.952 **Hemiplegia and hemiparesis following <u>unspecified</u> cerebrovascular disease affecting <u>left</u> dominant side**

I69.953 **Hemiplegia and hemiparesis following <u>unspecified</u> cerebrovascular disease affecting <u>right</u> <u>non</u>-dominant side**

I69.954 **Hemiplegia and hemiparesis following <u>unspecified</u> cerebrovascular disease affecting <u>left</u> <u>non</u>-dominant side**

I69.959 **Hemiplegia and hemiparesis following <u>unspecified</u> cerebrovascular disease affecting <u>unspecified side</u>**

I69.96- <u>Other paralytic</u> syndrome following <u>unspecified</u> cerebrovascular disease
Use additional code to identify type of paralytic syndrome, such as:
Locked-in state (G83.5)
Quadriplegia (G82.5-)
*Excludes 1: hemiplegia/hemiparesis following unspecified cerebrovascular disease (I69.95-)
monoplegia of lower limb following unspecified cerebrovascular disease (I69.94-)
monoplegia of upper limb following unspecified cerebrovascular disease (I69.93-)*

I69.961 **Other paralytic syndrome following <u>unspecified</u> cerebrovascular disease affecting <u>right</u> dominant side**

I
6
9
-
I
6
9

I69.962   **Other paralytic syndrome following <u>unspecified</u> cerebrovascular disease affecting <u>left</u> dominant side**

I69.963   **Other paralytic syndrome following <u>unspecified</u> cerebrovascular disease affecting <u>right</u> non-dominant side**

I69.964   **Other paralytic syndrome following <u>unspecified</u> cerebrovascular disease affecting <u>left</u> <u>non-</u>dominant side**

I69.965   **Other paralytic syndrome following <u>unspecified</u> cerebrovascular disease, <u>bilateral</u>**

I69.969   **Other paralytic syndrome following <u>unspecified</u> cerebrovascular disease affecting <u>unspecified side</u>**

I69.99- <u>Other sequelae</u> of <u>unspecified</u> cerebrovascular disease

I69.990   **Apraxia following <u>unspecified</u> cerebrovascular disease**

I69.991   **Dysphagia following <u>unspecified</u> cerebrovascular disease**
Use additional code to identify the type of dysphagia, if known (R13.1-)

I69.992   **Facial weakness following <u>unspecified</u> cerebrovascular disease**
Facial droop following unspecified cerebrovascular disease

I69.993   **Ataxia following <u>unspecified</u> cerebrovascular disease**

I69.998   **Other sequelae following <u>unspecified</u> cerebrovascular disease**
Alteration in sensation following unspecified cerebrovascular disease
Disturbance of vision following unspecified cerebrovascular disease
Use additional code to identify the sequelae

Diseases of arteries, arterioles and capillaries (I70-I79)

I70-   <u>Atherosclerosis</u>
Includes: Arteriolosclerosis
Arterial degeneration
Arteriosclerosis
Arteriosclerotic vascular disease
Arteriovascular degeneration
Atheroma
Endarteritis deformans or obliterans
Senile arteritis
Senile endarteritis
Vascular degeneration
Use additional code to identify:
Exposure to environmental tobacco smoke (Z77.22)
History of tobacco use (Z87.891)
Occupational exposure to environmental tobacco smoke (Z57.31)
Tobacco dependence (F17.-)
Tobacco use (Z72.0)
Excludes❷: arteriosclerotic cardiovascular disease (I25.1-)
arteriosclerotic heart disease (I25.1-)
atheroembolism (I75.-)
cerebral atherosclerosis (I67.2)
coronary atherosclerosis (I25.1-)
mesenteric atherosclerosis (K55.1)
precerebral atherosclerosis (I67.2)
primary pulmonary atherosclerosis (I27.0)

I70.0   **Atherosclerosis of aorta**

I70.1   **Atherosclerosis of renal artery**
Goldblatt's kidney
Excludes❷: atherosclerosis of renal arterioles (I12.-)

I70.2-   **Atherosclerosis of <u>native</u> arteries of the extremities**
Mönckeberg's (medial) sclerosis
Use additional code, if applicable, to identify chronic total occlusion of artery of extremity (I70.92)
Excludes❷: atherosclerosis of bypass graft of extremities (I70.30-I70.79)

I70.20- <u>Unspecified</u> atherosclerosis of <u>native</u> arteries of extremities

I70.201   <u>Unspecified</u> atherosclerosis of <u>native</u> arteries of extremities, <u>right</u> leg

I70.202   <u>Unspecified</u> atherosclerosis of <u>native</u> arteries of extremities, <u>left</u> leg

I70.203   <u>Unspecified</u> atherosclerosis of <u>native</u> arteries of extremities, <u>bilateral</u> legs

I70.208   <u>Unspecified</u> atherosclerosis of <u>native</u> arteries of extremities, <u>other extremity</u>

I70.209   <u>Unspecified</u> atherosclerosis of <u>native</u> arteries of extremities, <u>unspecified extremity</u>

I70.21- Atherosclerosis of <u>native</u> arteries of extremities <u>with</u> <u>intermittent claudication</u>

I70.211   **Atherosclerosis of <u>native</u> arteries of extremities <u>with</u> <u>intermittent claudication</u>, <u>right</u> leg**

I70.212   **Atherosclerosis of <u>native</u> arteries of extremities <u>with</u> <u>intermittent claudication</u>, <u>left</u> leg**

I70.213   **Atherosclerosis of <u>native</u> arteries of extremities <u>with</u> <u>intermittent claudication</u>, <u>bilateral</u> legs**

I70.218   **Atherosclerosis of <u>native</u> arteries of extremities <u>with</u> <u>intermittent claudication</u>, <u>other extremity</u>**

I70.219   **Atherosclerosis of <u>native</u> arteries of extremities <u>with</u> <u>intermittent claudication</u>, <u>unspecified extremity</u>**

I70.22- Atherosclerosis of <u>native</u> arteries of extremities <u>with rest pain</u>
Includes: Any condition classifiable to I70.21-

I70.221   **Atherosclerosis of <u>native</u> arteries of extremities <u>with</u> rest pain, <u>right</u> leg**

I70.222   **Atherosclerosis of <u>native</u> arteries of extremities <u>with</u> rest pain, <u>left</u> leg**

I70.223   **Atherosclerosis of <u>native</u> arteries of extremities <u>with</u> rest pain, <u>bilateral</u> legs**

I70.228   **Atherosclerosis of <u>native</u> arteries of extremities <u>with</u> rest pain, <u>other extremity</u>**

I70.229   **Atherosclerosis of native arteries of extremities <u>with</u> rest pain, <u>unspecified extremity</u>**

I70.23- Atherosclerosis of <u>native</u> arteries of <u>right</u> leg <u>with ulceration</u>
Includes: Any condition classifiable to I70.211 and I70.221
Use additional code to identify severity of ulcer (L97.-)

I70.231   **Atherosclerosis of <u>native</u> arteries of <u>right</u> leg <u>with</u> ulceration of <u>thigh</u>**

I70.232   **Atherosclerosis of <u>native</u> arteries of <u>right</u> leg <u>with</u> ulceration of <u>calf</u>**

I70.233   **Atherosclerosis of <u>native</u> arteries of <u>right</u> leg <u>with</u> ulceration of <u>ankle</u>**

I70.234   **Atherosclerosis of <u>native</u> arteries of <u>right</u> leg <u>with</u> ulceration of <u>heel and midfoot</u>**
Atherosclerosis of native arteries of right leg with ulceration of plantar surface of midfoot

I70.235   **Atherosclerosis of <u>native</u> arteries of <u>right</u> leg <u>with</u> ulceration of <u>other part of foot</u>**
Atherosclerosis of native arteries of right leg extremities with ulceration of toe

I70.238   **Atherosclerosis of <u>native</u> arteries of <u>right</u> leg <u>with</u> ulceration of other part of <u>lower right</u> leg**

I70.239   **Atherosclerosis of <u>native</u> arteries of <u>right</u> leg <u>with</u> ulceration of unspecified site**

I70.24- Atherosclerosis of <u>native</u> arteries of <u>left</u> leg <u>with</u> ulceration
Includes: Any condition classifiable to I70.212 and I70.222
Use additional code to identify severity of ulcer (L97.-)

I70.241   **Atherosclerosis of <u>native</u> arteries of <u>left</u> leg <u>with</u> ulceration of <u>thigh</u>**

I70.242   **Atherosclerosis of <u>native</u> arteries of <u>left</u> leg <u>with</u> ulceration of <u>calf</u>**

I70.243   **Atherosclerosis of <u>native</u> arteries of <u>left</u> leg <u>with</u> ulceration of <u>ankle</u>**

I70.244   **Atherosclerosis of <u>native</u> arteries of <u>left</u> leg <u>with</u> ulceration of <u>heel and midfoot</u>**
Atherosclerosis of native arteries of left leg with ulceration of plantar surface of midfoot

I70.245   **Atherosclerosis of <u>native</u> arteries of <u>left</u> leg <u>with</u> ulceration of <u>other part of foot</u>**
Atherosclerosis of native arteries of left leg extremities with ulceration of toe

I70.248   **Atherosclerosis of <u>native</u> arteries of <u>left</u> leg <u>with</u> ulceration of other part of <u>lower left</u> leg**

I70.249   **Atherosclerosis of <u>native</u> arteries of <u>left</u> leg <u>with</u> ulceration of unspecified site**

I70.25   **Atherosclerosis of <u>native</u> arteries of <u>other extremities with</u> ulceration**
Includes: Any condition classifiable to I70.218 and I70.228
Use additional code to identify the severity of the ulcer (L98.49-)

I70.26- Atherosclerosis of <u>native</u> arteries of extremities <u>with</u> gangrene
Includes: Any condition classifiable to I70.21-, I70.22-, I70.23-, I70.24-, and I70.25-
Use additional code to identify the severity of any ulcer (L97.-, L98.49-), if applicable

I70.261   **Atherosclerosis of <u>native</u> arteries of extremities <u>with</u> gangrene, <u>right</u> leg**

I70.262   **Atherosclerosis of <u>native</u> arteries of extremities <u>with</u> gangrene, <u>left</u> leg**

I70.263   **Atherosclerosis of <u>native</u> arteries of extremities <u>with</u> gangrene, <u>bilateral</u> legs**

I70.268   **Atherosclerosis of <u>native</u> arteries of extremities <u>with</u> gangrene, <u>other extremity</u>**

I70.269 Atherosclerosis of <u>native</u> arteries of extremities <u>with gangrene, unspecified extremity</u>

I70.29- <u>Other</u> atherosclerosis of <u>native</u> arteries of extremities

I70.291 <u>Other</u> atherosclerosis of <u>native</u> arteries of extremities, <u>right</u> leg

I70.292 <u>Other</u> atherosclerosis of <u>native</u> arteries of extremities, <u>left</u> leg

I70.293 <u>Other</u> atherosclerosis of <u>native</u> arteries of extremities, <u>bilateral</u> legs

I70.298 <u>Other</u> atherosclerosis of <u>native</u> arteries of extremities, <u>other extremity</u>

I70.299 <u>Other</u> atherosclerosis of <u>native</u> arteries of extremities, <u>unspecified extremity</u>

I70.3- Atherosclerosis of <u>unspecified type of bypass graft(s)</u> of the extremities
Use additional code, if applicable, to identify chronic total occlusion of artery of extremity (I70.92)
Excludes 1: embolism or thrombus of bypass graft(s) of extremities (T82.8-)

I70.30- <u>Unspecified</u> atherosclerosis of <u>unspecified type of bypass graft(s)</u> of the extremities

I70.301 <u>Unspecified</u> atherosclerosis of unspecified type of bypass <u>graft(s)</u> of the extremities, <u>right</u> leg

I70.302 <u>Unspecified</u> atherosclerosis of unspecified type of bypass <u>graft(s)</u> of the extremities, <u>left</u> leg

I70.303 <u>Unspecified</u> atherosclerosis of unspecified type of bypass <u>graft(s)</u> of the extremities, <u>bilateral</u> legs

I70.308 <u>Unspecified</u> atherosclerosis of unspecified type of bypass <u>graft(s)</u> of the extremities, <u>other extremity</u>

I70.309 <u>Unspecified</u> atherosclerosis of unspecified type of bypass <u>graft(s)</u> of the extremities, <u>unspecified extremity</u>

I70.31- Atherosclerosis of <u>unspecified type of bypass graft(s)</u> of the extremities <u>with intermittent claudication</u>

I70.311 Atherosclerosis of unspecified type of bypass <u>graft(s)</u> of the extremities <u>with intermittent claudication, right</u> leg

I70.312 Atherosclerosis of unspecified type of bypass <u>graft(s)</u> of the extremities <u>with intermittent claudication, left</u> leg

I70.313 Atherosclerosis of unspecified type of bypass <u>graft(s)</u> of the extremities <u>with intermittent claudication, bilateral</u> legs

I70.318 Atherosclerosis of unspecified type of bypass graft(s) of the extremities <u>with intermittent claudication, other extremity</u>

I70.319 Atherosclerosis of unspecified type of bypass <u>graft(s)</u> of the extremities <u>with intermittent claudication, unspecified extremity</u>

I70.32- Atherosclerosis of <u>unspecified type of bypass graft(s)</u> of the extremities <u>with rest pain</u>
Includes: Any condition classifiable to I70.31-

I70.321 Atherosclerosis of unspecified type of bypass <u>graft(s)</u> of the extremities <u>with rest pain, right</u> leg

I70.322 Atherosclerosis of unspecified type of bypass <u>graft(s)</u> of the extremities <u>with rest pain, left</u> leg

I70.323 Atherosclerosis of unspecified type of bypass <u>graft(s)</u> of the extremities <u>with rest pain, bilateral</u> legs

I70.328 Atherosclerosis of unspecified type of bypass <u>graft(s)</u> of the extremities <u>with rest pain, other extremity</u>

I70.329 Atherosclerosis of unspecified type of bypass <u>graft(s)</u> of the extremities <u>with rest pain, unspecified extremity</u>

I70.33- Atherosclerosis of <u>unspecified type of bypass graft(s)</u> of the <u>right</u> leg <u>with ulceration</u>
Includes: Any condition classifiable to I70.311 and I70.321
Use additional code to identify severity of ulcer (L97.-)

I70.331 Atherosclerosis of unspecified type of bypass <u>graft(s)</u> of the <u>right</u> leg <u>with ulceration</u> of <u>thigh</u>

I70.332 Atherosclerosis of unspecified type of bypass <u>graft(s)</u> of the <u>right</u> leg <u>with ulceration</u> of <u>calf</u>

I70.333 Atherosclerosis of unspecified type of bypass <u>graft(s)</u> of the <u>right</u> leg <u>with ulceration</u> of <u>ankle</u>

I70.334 Atherosclerosis of unspecified type of bypass <u>graft(s)</u> of the <u>right</u> leg <u>with ulceration</u> of <u>heel and midfoot</u>
Atherosclerosis of unspecified type of bypass graft(s) of right leg with ulceration of plantar surface of midfoot

I70.335 Atherosclerosis of unspecified type of bypass <u>graft(s)</u> of the <u>right</u> leg <u>with ulceration</u> of <u>other part of foot</u>
Atherosclerosis of unspecified type of bypass graft(s) of the right leg with ulceration of toe

I70.338 Atherosclerosis of unspecified type of bypass <u>graft(s)</u> of the <u>right</u> leg <u>with ulceration</u> of <u>other part of lower leg</u>

I70.339 Atherosclerosis of unspecified type of bypass <u>graft(s)</u> of the <u>right</u> leg <u>with ulceration</u> of <u>unspecified site</u>

I70.34- Atherosclerosis of <u>unspecified type of bypass graft(s)</u> of the <u>left</u> leg <u>with ulceration</u>
Includes: Any condition classifiable to I70.312 and I70.322
Use additional code to identify severity of ulcer (L97.-)

I70.341 Atherosclerosis of unspecified type of bypass <u>graft(s)</u> of the <u>left</u> leg <u>with ulceration</u> of <u>thigh</u>

I70.342 Atherosclerosis of unspecified type of bypass <u>graft(s)</u> of the <u>left</u> leg <u>with ulceration</u> of <u>calf</u>

I70.343 Atherosclerosis of unspecified type of bypass <u>graft(s)</u> of the <u>left</u> leg <u>with ulceration</u> of <u>ankle</u>

I70.344 Atherosclerosis of unspecified type of bypass <u>graft(s)</u> of the <u>left</u> leg <u>with ulceration</u> of <u>heel and midfoot</u>
Atherosclerosis of unspecified type of bypass graft(s) of left leg with ulceration of plantar surface of midfoot

I70.345 Atherosclerosis of unspecified type of bypass <u>graft(s)</u> of the <u>left</u> leg <u>with ulceration</u> of <u>other part of foot</u>
Atherosclerosis of unspecified type of bypass graft(s) of the left leg with ulceration of toe

I70.348 Atherosclerosis of unspecified type of bypass <u>graft(s)</u> of the <u>left</u> leg <u>with ulceration</u> of <u>other part of lower leg</u>

I70.349 Atherosclerosis of unspecified type of bypass <u>graft(s)</u> of the <u>left</u> leg <u>with ulceration</u> of <u>unspecified site</u>

I70.35 Atherosclerosis of <u>unspecified type of bypass graft(s)</u> of <u>other extremity with ulceration</u>
Includes: Any condition classifiable to I70.318 and I70.328
Use additional code to identify severity of ulcer (L98.49-)

I70.36- Atherosclerosis of <u>unspecified type of bypass graft(s)</u> of the extremities <u>with gangrene</u>
Includes: Any condition classifiable to I70.31-, I70.32-, I70.33-, I70.34-, I70.35
Use additional code to identify the severity of any ulcer (L97.-, L98.49-), if applicable

I70.361 Atherosclerosis of unspecified type of bypass <u>graft(s)</u> of the extremities <u>with gangrene, right</u> leg

I70.362 Atherosclerosis of unspecified type of bypass <u>graft(s)</u> of the extremities <u>with gangrene, left</u> leg

I70.363 Atherosclerosis of unspecified type of bypass <u>graft(s)</u> of the extremities <u>with gangrene, bilateral</u> legs

I70.368 Atherosclerosis of unspecified type of bypass <u>graft(s)</u> of the extremities <u>with gangrene, other extremity</u>

I70.369 Atherosclerosis of unspecified type of bypass <u>graft(s)</u> of the extremities <u>with gangrene, unspecified extremity</u>

I70.39- <u>Other</u> atherosclerosis of <u>unspecified type of bypass graft(s) of</u> the extremities

I70.391 <u>Other</u> atherosclerosis of unspecified type of bypass <u>graft(s)</u> of the extremities, <u>right</u> leg

I70.392 <u>Other</u> atherosclerosis of unspecified type of bypass <u>graft(s)</u> of the extremities, <u>left</u> leg

I70.393 <u>Other</u> atherosclerosis of unspecified type of bypass <u>graft(s)</u> of the extremities, <u>bilateral</u> legs

I70.398 <u>Other</u> atherosclerosis of unspecified type of bypass <u>graft(s)</u> of the extremities, <u>other extremity</u>

I70.399 <u>Other</u> atherosclerosis of unspecified type of bypass <u>graft(s)</u> of the extremities, <u>unspecified extremity</u>

I70.4- Atherosclerosis of autologous <u>vein</u> bypass graft(s) of the extremities
Use additional code, if applicable, to identify chronic total occlusion of artery of extremity (I70.92)

I70.40- <u>Unspecified</u> atherosclerosis of autologous <u>vein</u> bypass graft(s) of the extremities

I70.401 <u>Unspecified</u> atherosclerosis of autologous <u>vein</u> bypass graft(s) of the extremities, <u>right</u> leg

I70.402 <u>Unspecified</u> atherosclerosis of autologous <u>vein</u> bypass graft(s) of the extremities, <u>left</u> leg

I70.403 <u>Unspecified</u> atherosclerosis of autologous <u>vein</u> bypass graft(s) of the extremities, <u>bilateral</u> legs

I70.408 <u>Unspecified</u> atherosclerosis of autologous <u>vein</u> bypass graft(s) of the extremities, <u>other extremity</u>

I70.409 <u>Unspecified</u> atherosclerosis of autologous <u>vein</u> bypass graft(s) of the extremities, <u>unspecified extremity</u>

I 69 - I 70

I70.41- **Atherosclerosis of autologous <u>vein</u> bypass graft(s) of the extremities <u>with intermittent claudication</u>**

I70.411   **Atherosclerosis of autologous <u>vein</u> bypass graft(s) of the extremities <u>with intermittent claudication</u>, <u>right</u> leg**

I70.412   **Atherosclerosis of autologous <u>vein</u> bypass graft(s) of the extremities <u>with intermittent claudication</u>, <u>left</u> leg**

I70.413   **Atherosclerosis of autologous <u>vein</u> bypass graft(s) of the extremities <u>with intermittent claudication</u>, <u>bilateral</u> legs**

I70.418   **Atherosclerosis of autologous vein bypass graft(s) of the extremities <u>with intermittent claudication</u>, <u>other extremity</u>**

I70.419   **Atherosclerosis of autologous <u>vein</u> bypass graft(s) of the extremities <u>with intermittent claudication</u>, <u>unspecified extremity</u>**

I70.42- **Atherosclerosis of autologous <u>vein</u> bypass graft(s) of the extremities <u>with rest pain</u>**
Includes: Any condition classifiable to I70.41-

I70.421   **Atherosclerosis of autologous vein bypass graft(s) of the extremities <u>with rest pain</u>, <u>right</u> leg**

I70.422   **Atherosclerosis of autologous <u>vein</u> bypass graft(s) of the extremities <u>with rest pain</u>, <u>left</u> leg**

I70.423   **Atherosclerosis of autologous <u>vein</u> bypass graft(s) of the extremities <u>with rest pain</u>, <u>bilateral</u> legs**

I70.428   **Atherosclerosis of autologous <u>vein</u> bypass graft(s) of the extremities <u>with rest pain</u>, <u>other extremity</u>**

I70.429   **Atherosclerosis of autologous <u>vein</u> bypass graft(s) of the extremities <u>with rest pain</u>, <u>unspecified extremity</u>**

I70.43- **Atherosclerosis of autologous vein bypass graft(s) of the <u>right</u> leg <u>with ulceration</u>**
Includes: Any condition classifiable to I70.411 and I70.421
Use additional code to identify severity of ulcer (L97.-)

I70.431   **Atherosclerosis of autologous <u>vein</u> bypass graft(s) of the <u>right</u> leg <u>with ulceration</u> of <u>thigh</u>**

I70.432   **Atherosclerosis of autologous vein bypass graft(s) of the <u>right</u> leg <u>with ulceration</u> of <u>calf</u>**

I70.433   **Atherosclerosis of autologous <u>vein</u> bypass graft(s) of the <u>right</u> leg <u>with ulceration</u> of <u>ankle</u>**

I70.434   **Atherosclerosis of autologous vein bypass graft(s) of the <u>right</u> leg <u>with ulceration</u> of <u>heel and midfoot</u>**
Atherosclerosis of autologous vein bypass graft(s) of right leg with ulceration of plantar surface of midfoot

I70.435   **Atherosclerosis of autologous <u>vein</u> bypass graft(s) of the <u>right</u> leg <u>with ulceration</u> of <u>other part of foot</u>**
Atherosclerosis of autologous vein bypass graft(s) of right leg with ulceration of toe

I70.438   **Atherosclerosis of autologous <u>vein</u> bypass graft(s) of the <u>right</u> leg <u>with ulceration</u> of <u>other part of lower leg</u>**

I70.439   **Atherosclerosis of autologous <u>vein</u> bypass graft(s) of the <u>right</u> leg <u>with ulceration</u> of <u>unspecified site</u>**

I70.44- **Atherosclerosis of autologous <u>vein</u> bypass graft(s) of the <u>left</u> leg <u>with ulceration</u>**
Includes: Any condition classifiable to I70.412 and I70.422
Use additional code to identify severity of ulcer (L97.-)

I70.441   **Atherosclerosis of autologous <u>vein</u> bypass graft(s) of the <u>left</u> leg <u>with ulceration</u> of <u>thigh</u>**

I70.442   **Atherosclerosis of autologous <u>vein</u> bypass graft(s) of the <u>left</u> leg <u>with ulceration</u> of <u>calf</u>**

I70.443   **Atherosclerosis of autologous <u>vein</u> bypass graft(s) of the <u>left</u> leg <u>with ulceration</u> of <u>ankle</u>**

I70.444   **Atherosclerosis of autologous <u>vein</u> bypass graft(s) of the <u>left</u> leg <u>with ulceration</u> of <u>heel and midfoot</u>**
Atherosclerosis of autologous vein bypass graft(s) of left leg with ulceration of plantar surface of midfoot

I70.445   **Atherosclerosis of autologous <u>vein</u> bypass graft(s) of the <u>left</u> leg <u>with ulceration</u> of <u>other part of foot</u>**
Atherosclerosis of autologous vein bypass graft(s) of left leg with ulceration of toe

I70.448   **Atherosclerosis of autologous <u>vein</u> bypass graft(s) of the <u>left</u> leg <u>with ulceration</u> of <u>other part of lower leg</u>**

I70.449   **Atherosclerosis of autologous <u>vein</u> bypass graft(s) of the <u>left</u> leg <u>with ulceration</u> of <u>unspecified site</u>**

I70.45 **Atherosclerosis of autologous <u>vein</u> bypass graft(s) of <u>other extremity</u> <u>with ulceration</u>**
Includes: Any condition classifiable to I70.418, I70.428, and I70.438
Use additional code to identify severity of ulcer (L98.49)

I70.46- **Atherosclerosis of autologous <u>vein</u> bypass graft(s) of the extremities <u>with gangrene</u>**
Includes: Any condition classifiable to I70.41-, I70.42-, and I70.43-, I70.44-, I70.45
Use additional code to identify the severity of any ulcer (L97.-, L98.49-), if applicable

I70.461   **Atherosclerosis of autologous <u>vein</u> bypass graft(s) of the extremities <u>with gangrene</u>, <u>right</u> leg**

I70.462   **Atherosclerosis of autologous <u>vein</u> bypass graft(s) of the extremities <u>with gangrene</u>, <u>left</u> leg**

I70.463   **Atherosclerosis of autologous <u>vein</u> bypass graft(s) of the extremities <u>with gangrene</u>, <u>bilateral</u> legs**

I70.468   **Atherosclerosis of autologous <u>vein</u> bypass graft(s) of the extremities <u>with gangrene</u>, <u>other extremity</u>**

I70.469   **Atherosclerosis of autologous <u>vein</u> bypass graft(s) of the extremities <u>with gangrene</u>, <u>unspecified extremity</u>**

I70.49- **<u>Other</u> atherosclerosis of autologous <u>vein</u> bypass graft(s) of the extremities**

I70.491   **<u>Other</u> atherosclerosis of autologous <u>vein</u> bypass graft(s) of the extremities, <u>right</u> leg**

I70.492   **<u>Other</u> atherosclerosis of autologous <u>vein</u> bypass graft(s) of the extremities, <u>left</u> leg**

I70.493   **<u>Other</u> atherosclerosis of autologous <u>vein</u> bypass graft(s) of the extremities, bilateral legs**

I70.498   **<u>Other</u> atherosclerosis of autologous <u>vein</u> bypass graft(s) of the extremities, other extremity**

I70.499   **<u>Other</u> atherosclerosis of autologous <u>vein</u> bypass graft(s) of the extremities, unspecified extremity**

I70.5- **Atherosclerosis of nonautologous <u>biological</u> bypass graft(s) of the extremities**
Use additional code, if applicable, to identify chronic total occlusion of artery of extremity (I70.92)

I70.50- **<u>Unspecified</u> atherosclerosis of nonautologous <u>biological</u> bypass graft(s) of the extremities**

I70.501   **<u>Unspecified</u> atherosclerosis of nonautologous <u>biological</u> bypass graft(s) of the extremities, <u>right</u> leg**

I70.502   **<u>Unspecified</u> atherosclerosis of nonautologous <u>biological</u> bypass graft(s) of the extremities, <u>left</u> leg**

I70.503   **<u>Unspecified</u> atherosclerosis of nonautologous <u>biological</u> bypass graft(s) of the extremities, <u>bilateral</u> legs**

I70.508   **<u>Unspecified</u> atherosclerosis of nonautologous <u>biological</u> bypass graft(s) of the extremities, <u>other extremity</u>**

I70.509   **<u>Unspecified</u> atherosclerosis of nonautologous <u>biological</u> bypass graft(s) of the extremities, <u>unspecified extremity</u>**

I70.51- **Atherosclerosis of nonautologous <u>biological</u> bypass graft(s) of the extremities <u>with intermittent claudication</u>**

I70.511   **Atherosclerosis of nonautologous <u>biological</u> bypass graft(s) of the extremities <u>with intermittent claudication</u>, <u>right</u> leg**

I70.512   **Atherosclerosis of nonautologous <u>biological</u> bypass graft(s) of the extremities <u>with intermittent claudication</u>, <u>left</u> leg**

I70.513   **Atherosclerosis of nonautologous <u>biological</u> bypass graft(s) of the extremities <u>with intermittent claudication</u>, <u>bilateral</u> legs**

I70.518   **Atherosclerosis of nonautologous <u>biological</u> bypass graft(s) of the extremities <u>with intermittent claudication</u>, <u>other extremity</u>**

I70.519   **Atherosclerosis of nonautologous <u>biological</u> bypass graft(s) of the extremities <u>with intermittent claudication</u>, <u>unspecified extremity</u>**

I70.52- **Atherosclerosis of nonautologous <u>biological</u> bypass graft(s) of the extremities <u>with rest pain</u>**
Includes: Any condition classifiable to I70.51-

I70.521   **Atherosclerosis of nonautologous <u>biological</u> bypass graft(s) of the extremities <u>with rest pain</u>, <u>right</u> leg**

I70.522   **Atherosclerosis of nonautologous <u>biological</u> bypass graft(s) of the extremities <u>with rest pain</u>, <u>left</u> leg**

I70.523   **Atherosclerosis of nonautologous <u>biological</u> bypass graft(s) of the extremities <u>with rest pain</u>, <u>bilateral</u> legs**

I70.528   **Atherosclerosis of nonautologous <u>biological</u> bypass graft(s) of the extremities <u>with rest pain</u>, <u>other extremity</u>**

I70.529   **Atherosclerosis of nonautologous <u>biological</u> bypass graft(s) of the extremities <u>with rest pain</u>, <u>unspecified extremity</u>**

I70
-
I70

I70.53- **Atherosclerosis of nonautologous <u>biological</u> bypass graft(s) of the <u>right</u> leg <u>with ulceration</u>**
Includes: Any condition classifiable to I70.511 and I70.521
Use additional code to identify severity of ulcer (L97.-)

    I70.531 **Atherosclerosis of nonautologous <u>biological</u> bypass graft(s) of the <u>right</u> leg <u>with ulceration</u> of <u>thigh</u>**

    I70.532 **Atherosclerosis of nonautologous <u>biological</u> bypass graft(s) of the <u>right</u> leg <u>with ulceration</u> of <u>calf</u>**

    I70.533 **Atherosclerosis of nonautologous <u>biological</u> bypass graft(s) of the <u>right</u> leg <u>with ulceration</u> of <u>ankle</u>**

    I70.534 **Atherosclerosis of nonautologous <u>biological</u> bypass graft(s) of the <u>right</u> leg <u>with ulceration</u> of <u>heel and midfoot</u>**
        Atherosclerosis of nonautologous biological bypass graft(s) of right leg with ulceration of plantar surface of midfoot

    I70.535 **Atherosclerosis of nonautologous <u>biological</u> bypass graft(s) of the <u>right</u> leg <u>with ulceration</u> of <u>other part of foot</u>**
        Atherosclerosis of nonautologous biological bypass graft(s) of the right leg with ulceration of toe

    I70.538 **Atherosclerosis of nonautologous <u>biological</u> bypass graft(s) of the <u>right</u> leg <u>with ulceration</u> of <u>other part of lower leg</u>**

    I70.539 **Atherosclerosis of nonautologous <u>biological</u> bypass graft(s) of the <u>right</u> leg <u>with ulceration</u> of <u>unspecified site</u>**

I70.54- **Atherosclerosis of nonautologous <u>biological</u> bypass graft(s) of the <u>left</u> leg <u>with ulceration</u>**
Includes: Any condition classifiable to I70.512 and I70.522
Use additional code to identify severity of ulcer (L97.-)

    I70.541 **Atherosclerosis of nonautologous <u>biological</u> bypass graft(s) of the <u>left</u> leg <u>with ulceration</u> of <u>thigh</u>**

    I70.542 **Atherosclerosis of nonautologous <u>biological</u> bypass graft(s) of the <u>left</u> leg <u>with ulceration</u> of <u>calf</u>**

    I70.543 **Atherosclerosis of nonautologous <u>biological</u> bypass graft(s) of the <u>left</u> leg <u>with ulceration</u> of <u>ankle</u>**

    I70.544 **Atherosclerosis of nonautologous <u>biological</u> bypass graft(s) of the <u>left</u> leg <u>with ulceration</u> of <u>heel and midfoot</u>**
        Atherosclerosis of nonautologous biological bypass graft(s) of left leg with ulceration of plantar surface of midfoot

    I70.545 **Atherosclerosis of nonautologous <u>biological</u> bypass graft(s) of the <u>left</u> leg <u>with ulceration</u> of <u>other part of foot</u>**
        Atherosclerosis of nonautologous biological bypass graft(s) of the left leg with ulceration of toe

    I70.548 **Atherosclerosis of nonautologous <u>biological</u> bypass graft(s) of the <u>left</u> leg <u>with ulceration</u> of <u>other part of lower leg</u>**

    I70.549 **Atherosclerosis of nonautologous <u>biological</u> bypass graft(s) of the <u>left</u> leg <u>with ulceration</u> of <u>unspecified site</u>**

I70.55 **Atherosclerosis of nonautologous <u>biological</u> bypass graft(s) of <u>other extremity</u> <u>with ulceration</u>**
Includes: Any condition classifiable to I70.518, I70.528, and I70.538
Use additional code to identify severity of ulcer (L98.49)

I70.56- **Atherosclerosis of nonautologous <u>biological</u> bypass graft(s) of the extremities <u>with gangrene</u>**
Includes: Any condition classifiable to I70.51-, I70.52-, and I70.53-, I70.54-, I70.55
Use additional code to identify the severity of any ulcer (L97.-, L98.49-), if applicable

    I70.561 **Atherosclerosis of nonautologous <u>biological</u> bypass graft(s) of the extremities <u>with gangrene</u>, <u>right</u> leg**

    I70.562 **Atherosclerosis of nonautologous <u>biological</u> bypass graft(s) of the extremities <u>with gangrene</u>, <u>left</u> leg**

    I70.563 **Atherosclerosis of nonautologous <u>biological</u> bypass graft(s) of the extremities <u>with gangrene</u>, <u>bilateral</u> legs**

    I70.568 **Atherosclerosis of nonautologous <u>biological</u> bypass graft(s) of the extremities <u>with gangrene</u>, <u>other extremity</u>**

    I70.569 **Atherosclerosis of nonautologous <u>biological</u> bypass graft(s) of the extremities <u>with gangrene</u>, <u>unspecified extremity</u>**

I70.59- **<u>Other</u> atherosclerosis of nonautologous <u>biological</u> bypass graft(s) of the extremities**

    I70.591 **<u>Other</u> atherosclerosis of nonautologous <u>biological</u> bypass graft(s) of the extremities, <u>right</u> leg**

    I70.592 **<u>Other</u> atherosclerosis of nonautologous <u>biological</u> bypass graft(s) of the extremities, <u>left</u> leg**

    I70.593 **<u>Other</u> atherosclerosis of nonautologous <u>biological</u> bypass graft(s) of the extremities, <u>bilateral</u> legs**

    I70.598 **<u>Other</u> atherosclerosis of nonautologous <u>biological</u> bypass graft(s) of the extremities, <u>other extremity</u>**

    I70.599 **<u>Other</u> atherosclerosis of nonautologous <u>biological</u> bypass graft(s) of the extremities, <u>unspecified extremity</u>**

I70.6- **Atherosclerosis of <u>nonbiological</u> bypass graft(s) of the extremities**
Use additional code, if applicable, to identify chronic total occlusion of artery of extremity (I70.92)

I70.60- **<u>Unspecified</u> atherosclerosis of <u>nonbiological</u> bypass graft(s) of the extremities**

    I70.601 **<u>Unspecified</u> atherosclerosis of <u>nonbiological</u> bypass graft(s) of the extremities, <u>right</u> leg**

    I70.602 **<u>Unspecified</u> atherosclerosis of <u>nonbiological</u> bypass graft(s) of the extremities, <u>left</u> leg**

    I70.603 **<u>Unspecified</u> atherosclerosis of <u>nonbiological</u> bypass graft(s) of the extremities, <u>bilateral</u> legs**

    I70.608 **<u>Unspecified</u> atherosclerosis of <u>nonbiological</u> bypass graft(s) of the extremities, <u>other extremity</u>**

    I70.609 **<u>Unspecified</u> atherosclerosis of <u>nonbiological</u> bypass graft(s) of the extremities, <u>unspecified extremity</u>**

I70.61- **Atherosclerosis of <u>nonbiological</u> bypass graft(s) of the extremities <u>with intermittent claudication</u>**

    I70.611 **Atherosclerosis of <u>nonbiological</u> bypass graft(s) of the extremities <u>with intermittent claudication</u>, <u>right</u> leg**

    I70.612 **Atherosclerosis of <u>nonbiological</u> bypass graft(s) of the extremities <u>with intermittent claudication</u>, <u>left</u> leg**

    I70.613 **Atherosclerosis of <u>nonbiological</u> bypass graft(s) of the extremities <u>with intermittent claudication</u>, <u>bilateral</u> legs**

    I70.618 **Atherosclerosis of <u>nonbiological</u> bypass graft(s) of the extremities <u>with intermittent claudication</u>, <u>other extremity</u>**

    I70.619 **Atherosclerosis of <u>nonbiological</u> bypass graft(s) of the extremities <u>with intermittent claudication</u>, <u>unspecified extremity</u>**

I70.62- **Atherosclerosis of <u>nonbiological</u> bypass graft(s) of the extremities <u>with rest pain</u>**
Includes: Any condition classifiable to I70.61-

    I70.621 **Atherosclerosis of <u>nonbiological</u> bypass graft(s) of the extremities <u>with rest pain</u>, <u>right</u> leg**

    I70.622 **Atherosclerosis of <u>nonbiological</u> bypass graft(s) of the extremities <u>with rest pain</u>, <u>left</u> leg**

    I70.623 **Atherosclerosis of <u>nonbiological</u> bypass graft(s) of the extremities <u>with rest pain</u>, <u>bilateral</u> legs**

    I70.628 **Atherosclerosis of <u>nonbiological</u> bypass graft(s) of the extremities <u>with rest pain</u>, <u>other extremity</u>**

    I70.629 **Atherosclerosis of <u>nonbiological</u> bypass graft(s) of the extremities <u>with rest pain</u>, <u>unspecified extremity</u>**

I70.63- **Atherosclerosis of <u>nonbiological</u> bypass graft(s) of the <u>right</u> leg <u>with ulceration</u>**
Includes: Any condition classifiable to I70.611 and I70.621
Use additional code to identify severity of ulcer (L97.-)

    I70.631 **Atherosclerosis of <u>nonbiological</u> bypass graft(s) of the <u>right</u> leg <u>with ulceration</u> of <u>thigh</u>**

    I70.632 **Atherosclerosis of <u>nonbiological</u> bypass graft(s) of the <u>right</u> leg <u>with ulceration</u> of <u>calf</u>**

    I70.633 **Atherosclerosis of <u>nonbiological</u> bypass graft(s) of the <u>right</u> leg <u>with ulceration</u> of <u>ankle</u>**

    I70.634 **Atherosclerosis of <u>nonbiological</u> bypass graft(s) of the <u>right</u> leg <u>with ulceration</u> of <u>heel and midfoot</u>**
        Atherosclerosis of nonbiological bypass graft(s) of right leg with ulceration of plantar surface of midfoot

    I70.635 **Atherosclerosis of <u>nonbiological</u> bypass graft(s) of the <u>right</u> leg <u>with ulceration</u> of <u>other part of foot</u>**
        Atherosclerosis of nonbiological bypass graft(s) of the right leg with ulceration of toe

    I70.638 **Atherosclerosis of <u>nonbiological</u> bypass graft(s) of the <u>right</u> leg <u>with ulceration</u> of <u>other part of lower leg</u>**

    I70.639 **Atherosclerosis of <u>nonbiological</u> bypass graft(s) of the <u>right</u> leg <u>with ulceration</u> of <u>unspecified site</u>**

I70 - I70

I70.64- Atherosclerosis of <u>nonbiological</u> bypass graft(s) of the <u>left</u> leg <u>with ulceration</u>
Includes: Any condition classifiable to I70.612 and I70.622
Use additional code to identify severity of ulcer (L97.-)

I70.641 Atherosclerosis of <u>nonbiological</u> bypass graft(s) of the <u>left</u> leg <u>with ulceration</u> of <u>thigh</u>

I70.642 Atherosclerosis of <u>nonbiological</u> bypass graft(s) of the <u>left</u> leg <u>with ulceration</u> of <u>calf</u>

I70.643 Atherosclerosis of <u>nonbiological</u> bypass graft(s) of the <u>left</u> leg <u>with ulceration</u> of <u>ankle</u>

I70.644 Atherosclerosis of <u>nonbiological</u> bypass graft(s) of the <u>left</u> leg <u>with ulceration</u> of <u>heel and midfoot</u>
Atherosclerosis of nonbiological bypass graft(s) of left leg with ulceration of plantar surface of midfoot

I70.645 Atherosclerosis of <u>nonbiological</u> bypass graft(s) of the <u>left</u> leg <u>with ulceration</u> of <u>other part of foot</u>
Atherosclerosis of nonbiological bypass graft(s) of the left leg with ulceration of toe

I70.648 Atherosclerosis of <u>nonbiological</u> bypass graft(s) of the <u>left</u> leg <u>with ulceration</u> of <u>other part of lower leg</u>

I70.649 Atherosclerosis of <u>nonbiological</u> bypass graft(s) of the <u>left</u> leg <u>with ulceration</u> of <u>unspecified site</u>

I70.65 Atherosclerosis of <u>nonbiological</u> bypass graft(s) of <u>other extremity</u> <u>with ulceration</u>
Includes: Any condition classifiable to I70.618 and I70.628
Use additional code to identify severity of ulcer (L98.49)

I70.66- Atherosclerosis of <u>nonbiological</u> bypass graft(s) of the extremities <u>with gangrene</u>
Includes: Any condition classifiable to I70.61-, I70.62-, I70.63-, I70.64-, I70.65
Use additional code to identify the severity of any ulcer (L97.-, L98.49-), if applicable

I70.661 Atherosclerosis of <u>nonbiological</u> bypass graft(s) of the extremities <u>with gangrene</u>, <u>right</u> leg

I70.662 Atherosclerosis of <u>nonbiological</u> bypass graft(s) of the extremities <u>with gangrene</u>, <u>left</u> leg

I70.663 Atherosclerosis of <u>nonbiological</u> bypass graft(s) of the extremities <u>with gangrene</u>, <u>bilateral</u> legs

I70.668 Atherosclerosis of <u>nonbiological</u> bypass graft(s) of the extremities <u>with gangrene</u>, other extremity

I70.669 Atherosclerosis of <u>nonbiological</u> bypass graft(s) of the extremities <u>with gangrene</u>, unspecified extremity

I70.69- <u>Other</u> atherosclerosis of <u>nonbiological</u> bypass graft(s) of the extremities

I70.691 <u>Other</u> atherosclerosis of <u>nonbiological</u> bypass graft(s) of the extremities, <u>right</u> leg

I70.692 <u>Other</u> atherosclerosis of <u>nonbiological</u> bypass graft(s) of the extremities, <u>left</u> leg

I70.693 <u>Other</u> atherosclerosis of <u>nonbiological</u> bypass graft(s) of the extremities, <u>bilateral</u> legs

I70.698 <u>Other</u> atherosclerosis of <u>nonbiological</u> bypass graft(s) of the extremities, <u>other extremity</u>

I70.699 <u>Other</u> atherosclerosis of <u>nonbiological</u> bypass graft(s) of the extremities, <u>unspecified extremity</u>

I70.7- Atherosclerosis of <u>other</u> type of bypass graft(s) of the extremities
Use additional code, if applicable, to identify chronic total occlusion of artery of extremity (I70.92)

I70.70- <u>Unspecified</u> atherosclerosis of <u>other</u> type of bypass graft(s) of the extremities

I70.701 <u>Unspecified</u> atherosclerosis of <u>other</u> type of bypass graft(s) of the extremities, <u>right</u> leg

I70.702 <u>Unspecified</u> atherosclerosis of <u>other</u> type of bypass graft(s) of the extremities, <u>left</u> leg

I70.703 <u>Unspecified</u> atherosclerosis of <u>other</u> type of bypass graft(s) of the extremities, <u>bilateral</u> legs

I70.708 <u>Unspecified</u> atherosclerosis of <u>other</u> type of bypass graft(s) of the extremities, <u>other extremity</u>

I70.709 <u>Unspecified</u> atherosclerosis of <u>other</u> type of bypass graft(s) of the extremities, <u>unspecified extremity</u>

I70.71- Atherosclerosis of <u>other</u> type of bypass graft(s) of the extremities <u>with intermittent claudication</u>

I70.711 Atherosclerosis of <u>other</u> type of bypass graft(s) of the extremities <u>with intermittent claudication</u>, <u>right</u> leg

I70.712 Atherosclerosis of <u>other</u> type of bypass graft(s) of the extremities <u>with intermittent claudication</u>, <u>left</u> leg

I70.713 Atherosclerosis of <u>other</u> type of bypass graft(s) of the extremities <u>with intermittent claudication</u>, <u>bilateral</u> legs

I70.718 Atherosclerosis of <u>other</u> type of bypass graft(s) of the extremities <u>with intermittent claudication</u>, <u>other extremity</u>

I70.719 Atherosclerosis of <u>other</u> type of bypass graft(s) of the extremities <u>with intermittent claudication</u>, <u>unspecified extremity</u>

I70.72- Atherosclerosis of <u>other</u> type of bypass graft(s) of the extremities <u>with rest pain</u>
Includes: Any condition classifiable to I70.71-

I70.721 Atherosclerosis of <u>other</u> type of bypass graft(s) of the extremities <u>with rest pain</u>, <u>right</u> leg

I70.722 Atherosclerosis of <u>other</u> type of bypass graft(s) of the extremities <u>with rest pain</u>, <u>left</u> leg

I70.723 Atherosclerosis of <u>other</u> type of bypass graft(s) of the extremities <u>with rest pain</u>, <u>bilateral</u> legs

I70.728 Atherosclerosis of <u>other</u> type of bypass graft(s) of the extremities <u>with rest pain</u>, <u>other extremity</u>

I70.729 Atherosclerosis of <u>other</u> type of bypass graft(s) of the extremities <u>with rest pain</u>, <u>unspecified extremity</u>

I70.73- Atherosclerosis of <u>other</u> type of bypass graft(s) of the <u>right</u> leg <u>with ulceration</u>
Includes: Any condition classifiable to I70.711 and I70.721
Use additional code to identify severity of ulcer (L97.-)

I70.731 Atherosclerosis of <u>other</u> type of bypass graft(s) of the <u>right</u> leg <u>with ulceration</u> of <u>thigh</u>

I70.732 Atherosclerosis of <u>other</u> type of bypass graft(s) of the <u>right</u> leg <u>with ulceration</u> of <u>calf</u>

I70.733 Atherosclerosis of <u>other</u> type of bypass graft(s) of the <u>right</u> leg <u>with ulceration</u> of <u>ankle</u>

I70.734 Atherosclerosis of <u>other</u> type of bypass graft(s) of the <u>right</u> leg <u>with ulceration</u> of <u>heel and midfoot</u>
Atherosclerosis of other type of bypass graft(s) of right leg with ulceration of plantar surface of midfoot

I70.735 Atherosclerosis of <u>other</u> type of bypass graft(s) of the <u>right</u> leg <u>with ulceration</u> of <u>other part of foot</u>
Atherosclerosis of other type of bypass graft(s) of right leg with ulceration of toe

I70.738 Atherosclerosis of <u>other</u> type of bypass graft(s) of the <u>right</u> leg <u>with ulceration</u> of <u>other part of lower leg</u>

I70.739 Atherosclerosis of <u>other</u> type of bypass graft(s) of the <u>right</u> leg <u>with ulceration</u> of <u>unspecified site</u>

I70.74- Atherosclerosis of <u>other</u> type of bypass graft(s) of the <u>left</u> leg <u>with ulceration</u>
Includes: Any condition classifiable to I70.712 and I70.722
Use additional code to identify severity of ulcer (L97.-)

I70.741 Atherosclerosis of <u>other</u> type of bypass graft(s) of the <u>left</u> leg <u>with ulceration</u> of <u>thigh</u>

I70.742 Atherosclerosis of <u>other</u> type of bypass graft(s) of the <u>left</u> leg <u>with ulceration</u> of <u>calf</u>

I70.743 Atherosclerosis of <u>other</u> type of bypass graft(s) of the <u>left</u> leg <u>with ulceration</u> of <u>ankle</u>

I70.744 Atherosclerosis of <u>other</u> type of bypass graft(s) of the <u>left</u> leg <u>with ulceration</u> of <u>heel and midfoot</u>
Atherosclerosis of other type of bypass graft(s) of left leg with ulceration of plantar surface of midfoot

I70.745 Atherosclerosis of <u>other</u> type of bypass graft(s) of the <u>left</u> leg <u>with ulceration</u> of <u>other part of foot</u>
Atherosclerosis of other type of bypass graft(s) of left leg with ulceration of toe

I70.748 Atherosclerosis of <u>other</u> type of bypass graft(s) of the <u>left</u> leg <u>with ulceration</u> of <u>other part of lower leg</u>

I70.749 Atherosclerosis of <u>other</u> type of bypass graft(s) of the <u>left</u> leg <u>with ulceration</u> of <u>unspecified site</u>

I70.75 Atherosclerosis of <u>other</u> type of bypass graft(s) <u>of other extremity</u> <u>with ulceration</u>
Includes: Any condition classifiable to I70.718 and I70.728
Use additional code to identify severity of ulcer (L98.49)

I70.76- Atherosclerosis of <u>other</u> type of bypass graft(s) of the extremities <u>with gangrene</u>
Includes: Any condition classifiable to I70.71-, I70.72-, I70.73-, I70.74-, I70.75
Use additional code to identify the severity of any ulcer (L97.-, L98.49-), if applicable

I70.761 Atherosclerosis of <u>other</u> type of bypass graft(s) of the extremities <u>with gangrene</u>, <u>right</u> leg

I70.762 Atherosclerosis of <u>other</u> type of bypass graft(s) of the extremities <u>with gangrene</u>, <u>left</u> leg

I70.763 Atherosclerosis of <u>other</u> type of bypass graft(s) of the extremities <u>with gangrene</u>, <u>bilateral</u> legs

I70.768 Atherosclerosis of <u>other</u> type of bypass graft(s) of the extremities <u>with gangrene</u>, <u>other extremity</u>

I70.769 Atherosclerosis of <u>other</u> type of bypass graft(s) of the extremities <u>with gangrene</u>, <u>unspecified extremity</u>

I70-I75

I70.79- <u>Other</u> atherosclerosis of <u>other</u> type of bypass graft(s) of the extremities
   I70.791   <u>Other</u> atherosclerosis of <u>other</u> type of bypass graft(s) of the extremities, <u>right</u> leg
   I70.792   <u>Other</u> atherosclerosis of <u>other</u> type of bypass graft(s) of the extremities, <u>left</u> leg
   I70.793   <u>Other</u> atherosclerosis of <u>other</u> type of bypass graft(s) of the extremities, <u>bilateral</u> legs
   I70.798   <u>Other</u> atherosclerosis of <u>other</u> type of bypass graft(s) of the extremities, <u>other extremity</u>
   I70.799   <u>Other</u> atherosclerosis of <u>other</u> type of bypass graft(s) of the extremities, <u>unspecified extremity</u>
I70.8   Atherosclerosis of other arteries
I70.9-   Other and unspecified atherosclerosis
   I70.90   Unspecified atherosclerosis
   I70.91   Generalized atherosclerosis
   I70.92   Chronic total occlusion of artery of the extremities
      Complete occlusion of artery of the extremities
      Total occlusion of artery of the extremities
      Code first atherosclerosis of arteries of the extremities (I70.2-, I70.3-, I70.4-, I70.5-, I70.6-, I70.7-)

I71-   Aortic aneurysm and dissection
   Excludes 1: aortic ectasia (I77.81-)
             syphilitic aortic aneurysm (A52.01)
             traumatic aortic aneurysm (S25.09, S35.09)
   I71.0-   <u>Dissection</u> of aorta
      I71.00   Dissection of unspecified site of aorta
      I71.01   Dissection of <u>thoracic</u> aorta
      I71.02   Dissection of <u>abdominal</u> aorta
      I71.03   Dissection of <u>thoracoabdominal</u> aorta
   I71.1   Thoracic aortic aneurysm, <u>ruptured</u>
   I71.2   Thoracic aortic aneurysm, <u>without</u> rupture
   I71.3   Abdominal aortic aneurysm, <u>ruptured</u>
   I71.4   Abdominal aortic aneurysm, <u>without</u> rupture
   I71.5   Thoracoabdominal aortic aneurysm, <u>ruptured</u>
   I71.6   Thoracoabdominal aortic aneurysm, <u>without</u> rupture
   I71.8   Aortic aneurysm of unspecified site, <u>ruptured</u>
      Rupture of aorta NOS
   I71.9   Aortic aneurysm of unspecified site, <u>without</u> rupture
      Aneurysm of aorta
      Dilatation of aorta
      Hyaline necrosis of aorta

I72-   Other aneurysm
   Includes: Aneurysm (cirsoid) (false) (ruptured)
   Excludes❷: acquired aneurysm (I77.0)
          aneurysm (of) aorta (I71-)
          aneurysm (of) arteriovenous NOS (Q27.3-)
          carotid artery dissection (I77.71)
          cerebral (nonruptured) aneurysm (I67.1)
          coronary aneurysm (I25.4)
          coronary artery dissection (I25.42)
          dissection of artery NEC (I77.79)
          heart aneurysm (I25.3)
          iliac artery dissection (I77.72)
          pulmonary artery aneurysm (I28.1)
          renal artery dissection (I77.73)
          retinal aneurysm (H35.0)
          ruptured cerebral aneurysm (I60.7)
          varicose aneurysm (I77.0)
          vertebral artery dissection (I77.74)
   I72.0   Aneurysm of carotid artery
      Aneurysm of common carotid artery
      Aneurysm of external carotid artery
      Aneurysm of internal carotid artery, extracranial portion
      Excludes 1: aneurysm of internal carotid artery, intracranial portion (I67.1)
               aneurysm of internal carotid artery NOS (I67.1)
   I72.1   Aneurysm of artery of upper extremity
   I72.2   Aneurysm of renal artery
   I72.3   Aneurysm of iliac artery
   I72.4   Aneurysm of artery of lower extremity
   I72.8   Aneurysm of other specified arteries
   I72.9   Aneurysm of unspecified site

I73-   Other peripheral vascular diseases
   Excludes❷: chilblains (T69.1)
          frostbite (T33-T34)
          immersion hand or foot (T69.0-)
          spasm of cerebral artery (G45.9)
   I73.0-   Raynaud's syndrome
      Raynaud's disease
      Raynaud's phenomenon (secondary)
      I73.00   Raynaud's syndrome <u>without</u> gangrene
      I73.01   Raynaud's syndrome <u>with gangrene</u>
   I73.1   Thromboangiitis obliterans [Buerger's disease]
   I73.8-   Other specified peripheral vascular diseases
      Excludes 1: diabetic (peripheral) angiopathy (E08-E13 with .51-.52)
      I73.81   Erythromelalgia
      I73.89   Other specified peripheral vascular diseases
         Acrocyanosis
         Erythrocyanosis
         Simple acroparesthesia [Schultze's type]
         Vasomotor acroparesthesia [Nothnagel's type]
   I73.9   Peripheral vascular disease, unspecified
      Intermittent claudication
      Peripheral angiopathy NOS
      Spasm of artery
      Excludes 1: atherosclerosis of the extremities (I70.2- – I70.7-)

I74-   Arterial <u>embolism and thrombosis</u>
   Includes: Embolic infarction
          Embolic occlusion
          Thrombotic infarction
          Thrombotic occlusion
   Code first embolism and thrombosis complicating abortion or ectopic or molar pregnancy (O00-O07, O08.2)
   Code first embolism and thrombosis complicating pregnancy, childbirth and the puerperium (O88.-)
   Excludes❷: atheroembolism (I75.-)
          basilar embolism and thrombosis (I63.0-I63.2, I65.1)
          carotid embolism and thrombosis (I63.0-I63.2, I65.2)
          cerebral embolism and thrombosis (I63.3-I63.5, I66.-)
          coronary embolism and thrombosis (I21-I25)
          mesenteric embolism and thrombosis (K55.0)
          ophthalmic embolism and thrombosis (H34-)
          precerebral embolism and thrombosis NOS (I63.0-I63.2, I65.9)
          pulmonary embolism and thrombosis (I26-)
          renal embolism and thrombosis (N28.0)
          retinal embolism and thrombosis (H34-)
          septic embolism and thrombosis (I76)
          vertebral embolism and thrombosis (I63.0-I63.2, I65.0)
   I74.0-   Embolism and thrombosis of <u>abdominal</u> aorta
      I74.01   <u>Saddle</u> embolism abdominal aorta
      I74.09   Other arterial embolism and thrombosis of abdominal aorta
         Aortic bifurcation syndrome
         Aortoiliac obstruction
         Leriche's syndrome
   I74.1-   Embolism and thrombosis of other and unspecified parts of aorta
      I74.10   Embolism and thrombosis of unspecified parts of aorta
      I74.11   Embolism and thrombosis of <u>thoracic</u> aorta
      I74.19   Embolism and thrombosis of other parts of aorta
   I74.2   Embolism and thrombosis of arteries of the <u>upper</u> extremities
   I74.3   Embolism and thrombosis of arteries of the <u>lower</u> extremities
   I74.4   Embolism and thrombosis of arteries of extremities, unspecified
      Peripheral arterial embolism NOS
   I74.5   Embolism and thrombosis of <u>iliac</u> artery
   I74.8   Embolism and thrombosis of other arteries
   I74.9   Embolism and thrombosis of unspecified artery

I75-   Atheroembolism
   Includes: Atherothrombotic microembolism
          Cholesterol embolism
   I75.0-   Atheroembolism of <u>extremities</u>
      I75.01-   Atheroembolism of <u>upper</u> extremity
         I75.011   Atheroembolism of <u>right</u> upper extremity
         I75.012   Atheroembolism of <u>left</u> upper extremity
         I75.013   Atheroembolism of <u>bilateral</u> upper extremities
         I75.019   Atheroembolism of <u>unspecified</u> upper extremity
      I75.02-   Atheroembolism of <u>lower</u> extremity
         I75.021   Atheroembolism of <u>right</u> lower extremity
         I75.022   Atheroembolism of <u>left</u> lower extremity
         I75.023   Atheroembolism of <u>bilateral</u> lower extremities
         I75.029   Atheroembolism of <u>unspecified</u> lower extremity

I70 - I75

© 2013 Channel Publishing, Ltd.

I75.8- **Atheroembolism of other sites**
  I75.81 **Atheroembolism of <u>kidney</u>**
    Use additional code for any associated acute kidney failure and chronic kidney disease (N17.-, N18.-)
  I75.89 **Atheroembolism of <u>other site</u>**

I76 **<u>Septic</u> arterial embolism**
  Code first underlying infection, such as:
    Infective endocarditis (I33.0)
    Lung abscess (J85.-)
  Use additional code to identify the site of the embolism (I74.-)
  Excludes❷: septic pulmonary embolism (I26.01, I26.90)

I77- **Other disorders of arteries and arterioles**
  Excludes❷: collagen (vascular) diseases (M30-M36)
    hypersensitivity angiitis (M31.0)
    pulmonary artery (I28.-)
  I77.0 **Arteriovenous fistula, acquired**
    Aneurysmal varix
    Arteriovenous aneurysm, acquired
    Excludes 1: arteriovenous aneurysm NOS (Q27.3-)
      presence of arteriovenous shunt (fistula) for dialysis (Z99.2)
      traumatic — see injury of blood vessel by body region
    Excludes❷: cerebral (I67.1)
      coronary (I25.4)
  I77.1 **Stricture of artery**
    Narrowing of artery
  I77.2 **Rupture of artery**
    Erosion of artery
    Fistula of artery
    Ulcer of artery
    Excludes 1: traumatic rupture of artery — see injury of blood vessel by body region
  I77.3 **Arterial fibromuscular dysplasia**
    Fibromuscular hyperplasia (of) carotid artery
    Fibromuscular hyperplasia (of) renal artery
  I77.4 **Celiac artery compression syndrome**
  I77.5 **Necrosis of artery**
  I77.6 **Arteritis, unspecified**
    Aortitis NOS
    Endarteritis NOS
    Excludes 1: arteritis or endarteritis:
      aortic arch (M31.4)
      cerebral NEC (I67.7)
      coronary (I25.89)
      deformans (I70.-)
      giant cell (M31.5., M31.6)
      obliterans (I70.-)
      senile (I70.-)
  I77.7- **Other arterial dissection**
    Excludes❷: dissection of aorta (I71.0-)
      dissection of coronary artery (I25.42)
    I77.71 **Dissection of carotid artery**
    I77.72 **Dissection of iliac artery**
    I77.73 **Dissection of renal artery**
    I77.74 **Dissection of vertebral artery**
    I77.79 **Dissection of other artery**
  I77.8- **Other specified disorders of arteries and arterioles**
    I77.81- **Aortic ectasia**
      Ectasis aorta
      Excludes 1: aortic aneurysm and dissection (I71.0-)
      I77.810 **Thoracic aortic ectasia**
      I77.811 **Abdominal aortic ectasia**
      I77.812 **Thoracoabdominal aortic ectasia**
      I77.819 **Aortic ectasia, unspecified site**
    I77.89 **Other specified disorders of arteries and arterioles**
  I77.9 **Disorder of arteries and arterioles, unspecified**

I78- **Diseases of capillaries**
  I78.0 **Hereditary hemorrhagic telangiectasia**
    Rendu-Osler-Weber disease
  I78.1 **Nevus, non-neoplastic**
    Araneus nevus
    Senile nevus
    Spider nevus
    Stellar nevus
    Excludes 1: nevus NOS (D22.-)
      vascular NOS (Q82.5)
    Excludes❷: blue nevus (D22.-)
      flammeus nevus (Q82.5)
      hairy nevus (D22.-)
      melanocytic nevus (D22.-)
      pigmented nevus (D22.-)
      portwine nevus (Q82.5)
      sanguineous nevus (Q82.5)
      strawberry nevus (Q82.5)
      verrucous nevus (Q82.5)
  I78.8 **Other diseases of capillaries**
  I78.9 **Disease of capillaries, unspecified**

I79- **Disorders of arteries, arterioles and capillaries <u>in diseases classified elsewhere</u>**
  I79.0 **Aneurysm of aorta in diseases classified elsewhere**
    Code first underlying disease
    Excludes 1: syphilitic aneurysm (A52.01)
  I79.1 **Aortitis in diseases classified elsewhere**
    Code first underlying disease
    Excludes 1: syphilitic aortitis (A52.02)
  I79.8 **Other disorders of arteries, arterioles and capillaries in diseases classified elsewhere**
    Code first underlying disease, such as:
      Amyloidosis (E85.-)
    Excludes 1: diabetic (peripheral) angiopathy (E08-E13 with .51-.52)
      syphilitic endarteritis (A52.09)
      tuberculous endarteritis (A18.89)

Diseases of veins, lymphatic vessels and lymph nodes, not elsewhere classified (I80-I89)

I80- **<u>Phlebitis and thrombophlebitis</u>**
  Includes: Endophlebitis
    Inflammation, vein
    Periphlebitis
    Suppurative phlebitis
  Code first phlebitis and thrombophlebitis complicating abortion, ectopic or molar pregnancy (O00-O07, O08.7)
  Code first phlebitis and thrombophlebitis complicating pregnancy, childbirth and the puerperium (O22-, O87-)
  Excludes 1: venous embolism and thrombosis of lower extremities (I82.4-, I82.5-, I82.81-)
  I80.0- **Phlebitis and thrombophlebitis of <u>superficial</u> vessels of <u>lower</u> extremities**
    Phlebitis and thrombophlebitis of femoropopliteal vein
    I80.00 **Phlebitis and thrombophlebitis of <u>superficial</u> vessels of <u>unspecified</u> lower extremity**
    I80.01 **Phlebitis and thrombophlebitis of <u>superficial</u> vessels of <u>right</u> lower extremity**
    I80.02 **Phlebitis and thrombophlebitis of <u>superficial</u> vessels of <u>left</u> lower extremity**
    I80.03 **Phlebitis and thrombophlebitis of <u>superficial</u> vessels of lower extremities, <u>bilateral</u>**
  I80.1- **Phlebitis and thrombophlebitis of <u>femoral</u> vein**
    I80.10 **Phlebitis and thrombophlebitis of <u>unspecified femoral</u> vein**
    I80.11 **Phlebitis and thrombophlebitis of <u>right femoral</u> vein**
    I80.12 **Phlebitis and thrombophlebitis of <u>left femoral</u> vein**
    I80.13 **Phlebitis and thrombophlebitis of <u>femoral</u> vein, <u>bilateral</u>**
  I80.2- **Phlebitis and thrombophlebitis of other and unspecified deep vessels of lower extremities**
    I80.20- **Phlebitis and thrombophlebitis of <u>unspecified</u> deep vessels of <u>lower</u> extremities**
      I80.201 **Phlebitis and thrombophlebitis of <u>unspecified deep</u> vessels of <u>right</u> lower extremity**
      I80.202 **Phlebitis and thrombophlebitis of <u>unspecified deep</u> vessels of <u>left</u> lower extremity**
      I80.203 **Phlebitis and thrombophlebitis of <u>unspecified deep</u> vessels of lower extremities, <u>bilateral</u>**
      I80.209 **Phlebitis and thrombophlebitis of <u>unspecified deep</u> vessels of <u>unspecified</u> lower extremity**

I75 - I82

I80.21- Phlebitis and thrombophlebitis of <u>iliac</u> vein
  I80.211   Phlebitis and thrombophlebitis of <u>right</u> <u>iliac</u> vein
  I80.212   Phlebitis and thrombophlebitis of <u>left</u> <u>iliac</u> vein
  I80.213   Phlebitis and thrombophlebitis of <u>iliac</u> vein, <u>bilateral</u>
  I80.219   Phlebitis and thrombophlebitis of <u>unspecified</u> <u>iliac</u> vein
I80.22- Phlebitis and thrombophlebitis of <u>popliteal</u> vein
  I80.221   Phlebitis and thrombophlebitis of <u>right</u> <u>popliteal</u> vein
  I80.222   Phlebitis and thrombophlebitis of <u>left</u> <u>popliteal</u> vein
  I80.223   Phlebitis and thrombophlebitis of <u>popliteal</u> vein, <u>bilateral</u>
  I80.229   Phlebitis and thrombophlebitis of <u>unspecified</u> <u>popliteal</u> vein
I80.23- Phlebitis and thrombophlebitis of <u>tibial</u> vein
  I80.231   Phlebitis and thrombophlebitis of <u>right</u> <u>tibial</u> vein
  I80.232   Phlebitis and thrombophlebitis of <u>left</u> <u>tibial</u> vein
  I80.233   Phlebitis and thrombophlebitis of <u>tibial</u> vein, <u>bilateral</u>
  I80.239   Phlebitis and thrombophlebitis of <u>unspecified</u> <u>tibial</u> vein
I80.29- Phlebitis and thrombophlebitis of <u>other deep</u> vessels of <u>lower</u> extremities
  I80.291   Phlebitis and thrombophlebitis of <u>other deep</u> vessels of <u>right</u> <u>lower</u> extremity
  I80.292   Phlebitis and thrombophlebitis of <u>other deep</u> vessels of <u>left</u> <u>lower</u> extremity
  I80.293   Phlebitis and thrombophlebitis of <u>other deep</u> vessels of <u>lower</u> extremity, <u>bilateral</u>
  I80.299   Phlebitis and thrombophlebitis of <u>other deep</u> vessels of <u>unspecified</u> <u>lower</u> extremity
I80.3   Phlebitis and thrombophlebitis of lower extremities, unspecified
I80.8   Phlebitis and thrombophlebitis of other sites
I80.9   Phlebitis and thrombophlebitis of unspecified site

I81   Portal vein thrombosis
    Portal (vein) obstruction
    Excludes❷: hepatic vein thrombosis (I82.0)
             phlebitis of portal vein (K75.1)

I82- Other venous embolism and thrombosis
    Code first venous embolism and thrombosis complicating:
    Abortion, ectopic or molar pregnancy (O00-O07, O08.7)
    Pregnancy, childbirth and the puerperium (O22-, O87-)
    Excludes❷: venous embolism and thrombosis (of):
             cerebral (I63.6, I67.6)
             coronary (I21-I25)
             intracranial and intraspinal, septic or NOS (G08)
             intracranial, nonpyogenic (I67.6)
             intraspinal, nonpyogenic (G95.1)
             mesenteric (K55.0)
             portal (I81)
             pulmonary (I26.-)
  I82.0   Budd-Chiari syndrome
      Hepatic vein thrombosis
  I82.1   Thrombophlebitis migrans
  I82.2- Embolism and thrombosis of vena cava and other thoracic veins
    I82.21- Embolism and thrombosis of <u>superior</u> vena cava
      I82.210   <u>Acute</u> embolism and thrombosis of superior vena cava
          Embolism and thrombosis of superior vena cava NOS
      I82.211   <u>Chronic</u> embolism and thrombosis of superior vena cava
    I82.22- Embolism and thrombosis of <u>inferior</u> vena cava
      I82.220   <u>Acute</u> embolism and thrombosis of inferior vena cava
          Embolism and thrombosis of inferior vena cava NOS
      I82.221   <u>Chronic</u> embolism and thrombosis of inferior vena cava
    I82.29- Embolism and thrombosis of <u>other thoracic</u> veins
        Embolism and thrombosis of brachiocephalic (innominate) vein
      I82.290   <u>Acute</u> embolism and thrombosis of other thoracic veins
      I82.291   <u>Chronic</u> embolism and thrombosis of other thoracic veins
  I82.3   Embolism and thrombosis of renal vein

I82.4- <u>Acute</u> embolism and thrombosis of <u>deep veins</u> of <u>lower extremity</u>
  I82.40- Acute embolism and thrombosis of <u>unspecified</u> <u>deep</u> veins of lower extremity
      Deep vein thrombosis NOS
      DVT NOS
      Excludes 1: acute embolism and thrombosis of unspecified deep veins of distal lower extremity (I82.4Z-)
                   acute embolism and thrombosis of unspecified deep veins of proximal lower extremity (I82.4Y-)
    I82.401   Acute embolism and thrombosis of <u>unspecified</u> <u>deep</u> veins of <u>right</u> lower extremity
    I82.402   Acute embolism and thrombosis of <u>unspecified</u> <u>deep</u> veins of <u>left</u> lower extremity
    I82.403   Acute embolism and thrombosis of <u>unspecified</u> <u>deep</u> veins of lower extremity, <u>bilateral</u>
    I82.409   Acute embolism and thrombosis of <u>unspecified</u> <u>deep</u> veins of <u>unspecified</u> lower extremity
  I82.41- Acute embolism and thrombosis of <u>femoral</u> vein
    I82.411   Acute embolism and thrombosis of <u>right</u> <u>femoral</u> vein
    I82.412   Acute embolism and thrombosis of <u>left</u> <u>femoral</u> vein
    I82.413   Acute embolism and thrombosis of <u>femoral</u> vein, <u>bilateral</u>
    I82.419   Acute embolism and thrombosis of <u>unspecified</u> <u>femoral</u> vein
  I82.42- Acute embolism and thrombosis of <u>iliac</u> vein
    I82.421   Acute embolism and thrombosis of <u>right</u> <u>iliac</u> vein
    I82.422   Acute embolism and thrombosis of <u>left</u> <u>iliac</u> vein
    I82.423   Acute embolism and thrombosis of <u>iliac</u> vein, <u>bilateral</u>
    I82.429   Acute embolism and thrombosis of <u>unspecified</u> <u>iliac</u> vein
  I82.43- Acute embolism and thrombosis of <u>popliteal</u> vein
    I82.431   Acute embolism and thrombosis of <u>right</u> <u>popliteal</u> vein
    I82.432   Acute embolism and thrombosis of <u>left</u> <u>popliteal</u> vein
    I82.433   Acute embolism and thrombosis of <u>popliteal</u> vein, <u>bilateral</u>
    I82.439   Acute embolism and thrombosis of <u>unspecified</u> <u>popliteal</u> vein
  I82.44- Acute embolism and thrombosis of <u>tibial</u> vein
    I82.441   Acute embolism and thrombosis of <u>right</u> <u>tibial</u> vein
    I82.442   Acute embolism and thrombosis of <u>left</u> <u>tibial</u> vein
    I82.443   Acute embolism and thrombosis of <u>tibial</u> vein, <u>bilateral</u>
    I82.449   Acute embolism and thrombosis of <u>unspecified</u> <u>tibial</u> vein
  I82.49- Acute embolism and thrombosis of <u>other specified</u> deep vein of lower extremity
    I82.491   Acute embolism and thrombosis of <u>other specified</u> deep vein of <u>right</u> lower extremity
    I82.492   Acute embolism and thrombosis of <u>other specified</u> deep vein of <u>left</u> lower extremity
    I82.493   Acute embolism and thrombosis of <u>other specified</u> deep vein of lower extremity, <u>bilateral</u>
    I82.499   Acute embolism and thrombosis of <u>other specified</u> deep vein of <u>unspecified</u> lower extremity
  I82.4Y- Acute embolism and thrombosis of <u>unspecified</u> deep veins of <u>proximal</u> lower extremity
      Acute embolism and thrombosis of deep vein of thigh NOS
      Acute embolism and thrombosis of deep vein of upper leg NOS
    I82.4Y1   Acute embolism and thrombosis of <u>unspecified</u> deep veins of <u>right</u> <u>proximal</u> lower extremity
    I82.4Y2   Acute embolism and thrombosis of <u>unspecified</u> deep veins of <u>left</u> <u>proximal</u> lower extremity
    I82.4Y3   Acute embolism and thrombosis of <u>unspecified</u> deep veins of <u>proximal</u> lower extremity, <u>bilateral</u>
    I82.4Y9   Acute embolism and thrombosis of <u>unspecified</u> deep veins of <u>unspecified</u> <u>proximal</u> lower extremity
  I82.4Z- Acute embolism and thrombosis of <u>unspecified</u> deep veins of <u>distal</u> lower extremity
      Acute embolism and thrombosis of deep vein of calf NOS
      Acute embolism and thrombosis of deep vein of lower leg NOS
    I82.4Z1   Acute embolism and thrombosis of <u>unspecified</u> deep veins of <u>right</u> <u>distal</u> lower extremity
    I82.4Z2   Acute embolism and thrombosis of <u>unspecified</u> deep veins of <u>left</u> <u>distal</u> lower extremity
    I82.4Z3   Acute embolism and thrombosis of <u>unspecified</u> deep veins of <u>distal</u> lower extremity, <u>bilateral</u>
    I82.4Z9   Acute embolism and thrombosis of <u>unspecified</u> deep veins of <u>unspecified</u> <u>distal</u> lower extremity

I 7 5 – I 8 2

I82.5- <u>Chronic</u> embolism and thrombosis of deep veins of lower extremity
   Use additional code, if applicable, for associated long-term (current) use of anticoagulants (Z79.01)
   Excludes 1: personal history of venous embolism and thrombosis (Z86.718)

   I82.50- <u>Chronic</u> embolism and thrombosis of <u>unspecified</u> <u>deep</u> veins of lower extremity
      Excludes 1: chronic embolism and thrombosis of unspecified deep veins of distal lower extremity (I82.5Z-) chronic embolism and thrombosis of unspecified deep veins of proximal lower extremity (I82.5Y-)

      I82.501 <u>Chronic</u> embolism and thrombosis of <u>unspecified</u> <u>deep</u> veins of <u>right</u> lower extremity

      I82.502 <u>Chronic</u> embolism and thrombosis of <u>unspecified</u> <u>deep</u> veins of <u>left</u> lower extremity

      I82.503 <u>Chronic</u> embolism and thrombosis of <u>unspecified</u> <u>deep</u> veins of lower extremity, <u>bilateral</u>

      I82.509 <u>Chronic</u> embolism and thrombosis of <u>unspecified</u> <u>deep</u> veins of <u>unspecified</u> lower extremity

   I82.51- <u>Chronic</u> embolism and thrombosis of <u>femoral</u> vein
      I82.511 <u>Chronic</u> embolism and thrombosis of <u>right</u> <u>femoral</u> vein

      I82.512 <u>Chronic</u> embolism and thrombosis of <u>left</u> <u>femoral</u> vein

      I82.513 <u>Chronic</u> embolism and thrombosis of <u>femoral</u> vein, <u>bilateral</u>

      I82.519 <u>Chronic</u> embolism and thrombosis of <u>unspecified</u> <u>femoral</u> vein

   I82.52- <u>Chronic</u> embolism and thrombosis of <u>iliac</u> vein
      I82.521 <u>Chronic</u> embolism and thrombosis of <u>right</u> <u>iliac</u> vein
      I82.522 <u>Chronic</u> embolism and thrombosis of <u>left</u> <u>iliac</u> vein
      I82.523 <u>Chronic</u> embolism and thrombosis of <u>iliac</u> vein, <u>bilateral</u>
      I82.529 <u>Chronic</u> embolism and thrombosis of <u>unspecified</u> <u>iliac</u> vein

   I82.53- <u>Chronic</u> embolism and thrombosis of <u>popliteal</u> vein
      I82.531 <u>Chronic</u> embolism and thrombosis of <u>right</u> <u>popliteal</u> vein
      I82.532 <u>Chronic</u> embolism and thrombosis of <u>left</u> <u>popliteal</u> vein
      I82.533 <u>Chronic</u> embolism and thrombosis of <u>popliteal</u> vein, <u>bilateral</u>
      I82.539 <u>Chronic</u> embolism and thrombosis of <u>unspecified</u> <u>popliteal</u> vein

   I82.54- <u>Chronic</u> embolism and thrombosis of <u>tibial</u> vein
      I82.541 <u>Chronic</u> embolism and thrombosis of <u>right</u> <u>tibial</u> vein
      I82.542 <u>Chronic</u> embolism and thrombosis of <u>left</u> <u>tibial</u> vein
      I82.543 <u>Chronic</u> embolism and thrombosis of <u>tibial</u> vein, <u>bilateral</u>
      I82.549 <u>Chronic</u> embolism and thrombosis of <u>unspecified</u> <u>tibial</u> vein

   I82.59- <u>Chronic</u> embolism and thrombosis of <u>other specified</u> deep vein of lower extremity
      I82.591 <u>Chronic</u> embolism and thrombosis of <u>other specified</u> deep vein of <u>right</u> lower extremity
      I82.592 <u>Chronic</u> embolism and thrombosis of <u>other specified</u> deep vein of <u>left</u> lower extremity
      I82.593 <u>Chronic</u> embolism and thrombosis of <u>other specified</u> deep vein of lower extremity, <u>bilateral</u>
      I82.599 <u>Chronic</u> embolism and thrombosis of <u>other specified</u> deep vein of <u>unspecified</u> lower extremity

   I82.5Y- <u>Chronic</u> embolism and thrombosis of <u>unspecified</u> <u>deep</u> veins of <u>proximal</u> lower extremity
      Chronic embolism and thrombosis of deep veins of thigh NOS
      Chronic embolism and thrombosis of deep veins of upper leg NOS

      I82.5Y1 <u>Chronic</u> embolism and thrombosis of <u>unspecified</u> <u>deep</u> veins of <u>right</u> <u>proximal</u> lower extremity
      I82.5Y2 <u>Chronic</u> embolism and thrombosis of <u>unspecified</u> <u>deep</u> veins of <u>left</u> <u>proximal</u> lower extremity
      I82.5Y3 <u>Chronic</u> embolism and thrombosis of <u>unspecified</u> <u>deep</u> veins of <u>proximal</u> lower extremity, <u>bilateral</u>
      I82.5Y9 <u>Chronic</u> embolism and thrombosis of <u>unspecified</u> <u>deep</u> veins of <u>unspecified</u> <u>proximal</u> lower extremity

   I82.5Z- <u>Chronic</u> embolism and thrombosis of <u>unspecified</u> <u>deep</u> veins of <u>distal</u> lower extremity
      Chronic embolism and thrombosis of deep veins of calf NOS
      Chronic embolism and thrombosis of deep veins of lower leg NOS

      I82.5Z1 <u>Chronic</u> embolism and thrombosis of <u>unspecified</u> <u>deep</u> veins of <u>right</u> <u>distal</u> lower extremity
      I82.5Z2 <u>Chronic</u> embolism and thrombosis of <u>unspecified</u> <u>deep</u> veins of <u>left</u> <u>distal</u> lower extremity
      I82.5Z3 <u>Chronic</u> embolism and thrombosis of <u>unspecified</u> <u>deep</u> veins of <u>distal</u> lower extremity, <u>bilateral</u>
      I82.5Z9 <u>Chronic</u> embolism and thrombosis of <u>unspecified</u> <u>deep</u> veins of unspecified <u>distal</u> lower extremity

I82.6- <u>Acute</u> embolism and thrombosis of <u>veins</u> of <u>upper extremity</u>
   I82.60- <u>Acute</u> embolism and thrombosis of <u>unspecified</u> veins of <u>upper</u> extremity
      I82.601 Acute embolism and thrombosis of <u>unspecified</u> veins of <u>right</u> upper extremity
      I82.602 Acute embolism and thrombosis of <u>unspecified</u> veins of <u>left</u> upper extremity
      I82.603 Acute embolism and thrombosis of <u>unspecified</u> veins of upper extremity, <u>bilateral</u>
      I82.609 Acute embolism and thrombosis of <u>unspecified</u> veins of <u>unspecified</u> upper extremity

   I82.61- Acute embolism and thrombosis of <u>superficial</u> veins of <u>upper</u> extremity
      Acute embolism and thrombosis of antecubital vein
      Acute embolism and thrombosis of basilic vein
      Acute embolism and thrombosis of cephalic vein

      I82.611 Acute embolism and thrombosis of <u>superficial</u> veins of <u>right</u> upper extremity
      I82.612 Acute embolism and thrombosis of <u>superficial</u> veins of <u>left</u> upper extremity
      I82.613 Acute embolism and thrombosis of <u>superficial</u> veins of upper extremity, <u>bilateral</u>
      I82.619 Acute embolism and thrombosis of <u>superficial</u> veins of <u>unspecified</u> upper extremity

   I82.62- Acute embolism and thrombosis of <u>deep</u> veins of <u>upper</u> extremity
      Acute embolism and thrombosis of brachial vein
      Acute embolism and thrombosis of radial vein
      Acute embolism and thrombosis of ulnar vein

      I82.621 Acute embolism and thrombosis of <u>deep</u> veins of <u>right</u> upper extremity
      I82.622 Acute embolism and thrombosis of <u>deep</u> veins of <u>left</u> upper extremity
      I82.623 Acute embolism and thrombosis of <u>deep</u> veins of upper extremity, <u>bilateral</u>
      I82.629 Acute embolism and thrombosis of <u>deep</u> veins of <u>unspecified</u> upper extremity

I82.7- <u>Chronic</u> embolism and thrombosis of veins of <u>upper</u> extremity
   Use additional code, if applicable, for associated long-term (current) use of anticoagulants (Z79.01)
   Excludes 1: personal history of venous embolism and thrombosis (Z86.718)

   I82.70- <u>Chronic</u> embolism and thrombosis of <u>unspecified</u> veins of <u>upper</u> extremity
      I82.701 <u>Chronic</u> embolism and thrombosis of <u>unspecified</u> veins of <u>right</u> upper extremity
      I82.702 <u>Chronic</u> embolism and thrombosis of <u>unspecified</u> veins of <u>left</u> upper extremity
      I82.703 <u>Chronic</u> embolism and thrombosis of <u>unspecified</u> veins of upper extremity, <u>bilateral</u>
      I82.709 <u>Chronic</u> embolism and thrombosis of <u>unspecified</u> veins of <u>unspecified</u> upper extremity

   I82.71- <u>Chronic</u> embolism and thrombosis of <u>superficial</u> veins of <u>upper</u> extremity
      Chronic embolism and thrombosis of antecubital vein
      Chronic embolism and thrombosis of basilic vein
      Chronic embolism and thrombosis of cephalic vein

      I82.711 <u>Chronic</u> embolism and thrombosis of <u>superficial</u> veins of <u>right</u> upper extremity
      I82.712 <u>Chronic</u> embolism and thrombosis of <u>superficial</u> veins of <u>left</u> upper extremity
      I82.713 <u>Chronic</u> embolism and thrombosis of <u>superficial</u> veins of upper extremity, <u>bilateral</u>
      I82.719 <u>Chronic</u> embolism and thrombosis of <u>superficial</u> veins of <u>unspecified</u> upper extremity

I
8
2
|
I
8
3

I82.72- <u>Chronic</u> embolism and thrombosis of <u>deep</u> veins of <u>upper</u> extremity
  Chronic embolism and thrombosis of brachial vein
  Chronic embolism and thrombosis of radial vein
  Chronic embolism and thrombosis of ulnar vein

  I82.721 <u>Chronic</u> embolism and thrombosis of <u>deep</u> veins of <u>right</u> upper extremity
  I82.722 <u>Chronic</u> embolism and thrombosis of <u>deep</u> veins of <u>left</u> upper extremity
  I82.723 <u>Chronic</u> embolism and thrombosis of <u>deep</u> veins of upper extremity, <u>bilateral</u>
  I82.729 <u>Chronic</u> embolism and thrombosis of <u>deep</u> veins of <u>unspecified</u> upper extremity

I82.A- Embolism and thrombosis of axillary vein
  I82.A1- <u>Acute</u> embolism and thrombosis of <u>axillary</u> vein
  I82.A11 Acute embolism and thrombosis of <u>right</u> axillary vein
  I82.A12 Acute embolism and thrombosis of <u>left</u> axillary vein
  I82.A13 Acute embolism and thrombosis of <u>axillary</u> vein, <u>bilateral</u>
  I82.A19 Acute embolism and thrombosis of <u>unspecified</u> axillary vein

  I82.A2- <u>Chronic</u> embolism and thrombosis of <u>axillary</u> vein
  I82.A21 <u>Chronic</u> embolism and thrombosis of <u>right</u> axillary vein
  I82.A22 <u>Chronic</u> embolism and thrombosis of <u>left</u> axillary vein
  I82.A23 <u>Chronic</u> embolism and thrombosis of <u>axillary</u> vein, <u>bilateral</u>
  I82.A29 <u>Chronic</u> embolism and thrombosis of <u>unspecified</u> axillary vein

I82.B- Embolism and thrombosis of <u>subclavian</u> vein
  I82.B1- <u>Acute</u> embolism and thrombosis of <u>subclavian</u> vein
  I82.B11 Acute embolism and thrombosis of <u>right</u> subclavian vein
  I82.B12 Acute embolism and thrombosis of <u>left</u> subclavian vein
  I82.B13 Acute embolism and thrombosis of <u>subclavian</u> vein, <u>bilateral</u>
  I82.B19 Acute embolism and thrombosis of <u>unspecified</u> subclavian vein

  I82.B2- <u>Chronic</u> embolism and thrombosis of <u>subclavian</u> vein
  I82.B21 <u>Chronic</u> embolism and thrombosis of <u>right</u> subclavian vein
  I82.B22 <u>Chronic</u> embolism and thrombosis of <u>left</u> subclavian vein
  I82.B23 <u>Chronic</u> embolism and thrombosis of <u>subclavian</u> vein, <u>bilateral</u>
  I82.B29 <u>Chronic</u> embolism and thrombosis of <u>unspecified</u> subclavian vein

I82.C- Embolism and thrombosis of <u>internal jugular</u> vein
  I82.C1- <u>Acute</u> embolism and thrombosis of <u>internal jugular</u> vein
  I82.C11 Acute embolism and thrombosis of <u>right internal jugular</u> vein
  I82.C12 Acute embolism and thrombosis of <u>left internal jugular</u> vein
  I82.C13 Acute embolism and thrombosis of <u>internal jugular</u> vein, <u>bilateral</u>
  I82.C19 Acute embolism and thrombosis of <u>unspecified internal jugular</u> vein

  I82.C2- <u>Chronic</u> embolism and thrombosis of <u>internal jugular</u> vein
  I82.C21 <u>Chronic</u> embolism and thrombosis of <u>right internal jugular</u> vein
  I82.C22 <u>Chronic</u> embolism and thrombosis of <u>left internal jugular</u> vein
  I82.C23 <u>Chronic</u> embolism and thrombosis of <u>internal jugular</u> vein, <u>bilateral</u>
  I82.C29 <u>Chronic</u> embolism and thrombosis of <u>unspecified internal jugular</u> vein

I82.8- Embolism and thrombosis of <u>other specified</u> veins
  Use additional code, if applicable, for associated long-term (current) use of anticoagulants (Z79.01)

  I82.81- Embolism and thrombosis of <u>superficial</u> veins of <u>lower</u> extremities
    Embolism and thrombosis of saphenous vein (greater) (lesser)
  I82.811 Embolism and thrombosis of <u>superficial</u> veins of <u>right</u> lower extremities
  I82.812 Embolism and thrombosis of <u>superficial</u> veins of <u>left</u> lower extremities
  I82.813 Embolism and thrombosis of <u>superficial</u> veins of lower extremities, <u>bilateral</u>
  I82.819 Embolism and thrombosis of <u>superficial</u> veins of <u>unspecified</u> lower extremities

I82.89- Embolism and thrombosis of <u>other specified veins</u>
  I82.890 <u>Acute</u> embolism and thrombosis of other specified veins
  I82.891 <u>Chronic</u> embolism and thrombosis of other specified veins

I82.9- Embolism and thrombosis of <u>unspecified</u> vein
  I82.90 <u>Acute</u> embolism and thrombosis of unspecified vein
    Embolism of vein NOS
    Thrombosis (vein) NOS
  I82.91 <u>Chronic</u> embolism and thrombosis of unspecified vein

I83- <u>Varicose veins</u> of <u>lower</u> extremities
  Excludes 1: varicose veins complicating pregnancy (O22.0-)
  varicose veins complicating the puerperium (O87.4)

  I83.0- <u>Varicose veins</u> of <u>lower extremities</u> <u>with ulcer</u>
    Use additional code to identify severity of ulcer (L97.-)

  I83.00- Varicose veins of <u>unspecified</u> lower extremity with ulcer
  I83.001 Varicose veins of <u>unspecified</u> lower extremity <u>with</u> ulcer of <u>thigh</u>
  I83.002 Varicose veins of <u>unspecified</u> lower extremity <u>with</u> ulcer of <u>calf</u>
  I83.003 Varicose veins of <u>unspecified</u> lower extremity <u>with</u> ulcer of <u>ankle</u>
  I83.004 Varicose veins of <u>unspecified</u> lower extremity <u>with</u> ulcer of <u>heel and midfoot</u>
    Varicose veins of unspecified lower extremity with ulcer of plantar surface of midfoot
  I83.005 Varicose veins of <u>unspecified</u> lower extremity <u>with</u> ulcer <u>other part of foot</u>
    Varicose veins of unspecified lower extremity with ulcer of toe
  I83.008 Varicose veins of unspecified lower extremity <u>with</u> ulcer <u>other part of lower leg</u>
  I83.009 Varicose veins of <u>unspecified</u> lower extremity <u>with</u> ulcer of <u>unspecified site</u>

  I83.01- Varicose veins of <u>right</u> lower extremity <u>with ulcer</u>
  I83.011 Varicose veins of <u>right</u> lower extremity <u>with ulcer</u> of <u>thigh</u>
  I83.012 Varicose veins of <u>right</u> lower extremity <u>with ulcer</u> of <u>calf</u>
  I83.013 Varicose veins of <u>right</u> lower extremity <u>with ulcer</u> of <u>ankle</u>
  I83.014 Varicose veins of <u>right</u> lower extremity <u>with ulcer</u> of <u>heel and midfoot</u>
    Varicose veins of right lower extremity with ulcer of plantar surface of midfoot
  I83.015 Varicose veins of <u>right</u> lower extremity <u>with ulcer</u> <u>other part of foot</u>
    Varicose veins of right lower extremity with ulcer of toe
  I83.018 Varicose veins of <u>right</u> lower extremity <u>with ulcer</u> <u>other part of lower leg</u>
  I83.019 Varicose veins of <u>right</u> lower extremity <u>with ulcer</u> of <u>unspecified site</u>

  I83.02- Varicose veins of <u>left</u> lower extremity <u>with ulcer</u>
  I83.021 Varicose veins of <u>left</u> lower extremity <u>with ulcer</u> of <u>thigh</u>
  I83.022 Varicose veins of <u>left</u> lower extremity <u>with ulcer</u> of calf
  I83.023 Varicose veins of <u>left</u> lower extremity <u>with ulcer</u> of <u>ankle</u>
  I83.024 Varicose veins of <u>left</u> lower extremity <u>with ulcer</u> of <u>heel and midfoot</u>
    Varicose veins of left lower extremity with ulcer of plantar surface of midfoot
  I83.025 Varicose veins of <u>left</u> lower extremity <u>with ulcer</u> <u>other part of foot</u>
    Varicose veins of left lower extremity with ulcer of toe
  I83.028 Varicose veins of <u>left</u> lower extremity <u>with ulcer</u> <u>other part of lower leg</u>
  I83.029 Varicose veins of <u>left</u> lower extremity <u>with ulcer</u> of <u>unspecified site</u>

I83.1- <u>Varicose veins</u> of <u>lower extremities</u> <u>with inflammation</u>
  Stasis dermatitis
  I83.10 Varicose veins of <u>unspecified</u> lower extremity <u>with inflammation</u>
  I83.11 Varicose veins of <u>right</u> lower extremity <u>with inflammation</u>
  I83.12 Varicose veins of <u>left</u> lower extremity <u>with inflammation</u>

I83.2- <u>Varicose veins</u> of <u>lower extremities with both ulcer and inflammation</u>
  Use additional code to identify severity of ulcer (L97.-)
  I83.20- Varicose veins of <u>unspecified</u> lower extremity <u>with both ulcer and inflammation</u>

I82 - I83

I83.201 Varicose veins of <u>unspecified</u> lower extremity <u>with</u> <u>both ulcer</u> of <u>thigh</u> and <u>inflammation</u>

I83.202 Varicose veins of <u>unspecified</u> lower extremity <u>with</u> <u>both ulcer</u> of <u>calf</u> and <u>inflammation</u>

I83.203 Varicose veins of <u>unspecified</u> lower extremity <u>with</u> <u>both ulcer</u> of <u>ankle</u> and <u>inflammation</u>

I83.204 Varicose veins of <u>unspecified</u> lower extremity <u>with</u> <u>both ulcer</u> of <u>heel and midfoot</u> and <u>inflammation</u>
Varicose veins of unspecified lower extremity with both ulcer of plantar surface of midfoot and inflammation

I83.205 Varicose veins of <u>unspecified</u> lower extremity <u>with</u> <u>both ulcer</u> <u>other part of foot</u> and <u>inflammation</u>
Varicose veins of unspecified lower extremity with both ulcer of toe and inflammation

I83.208 Varicose veins of <u>unspecified</u> lower extremity <u>with</u> <u>both ulcer</u> of <u>other part of lower extremity</u> and <u>inflammation</u>

I83.209 Varicose veins of unspecified lower extremity <u>with</u> <u>both ulcer</u> of <u>unspecified site</u> and <u>inflammation</u>

I83.21- Varicose veins of <u>right</u> lower extremity <u>with both ulcer and inflammation</u>

I83.211 Varicose veins of <u>right</u> lower extremity <u>with both ulcer</u> of <u>thigh</u> and <u>inflammation</u>

I83.212 Varicose veins of <u>right</u> lower extremity <u>with both ulcer</u> of <u>calf</u> and <u>inflammation</u>

I83.213 Varicose veins of <u>right</u> lower extremity <u>with both ulcer</u> of <u>ankle</u> and <u>inflammation</u>

I83.214 Varicose veins of <u>right</u> lower extremity <u>with both ulcer</u> of <u>heel and midfoot</u> and <u>inflammation</u>
Varicose veins of right lower extremity with both ulcer of plantar surface of midfoot and inflammation

I83.215 Varicose veins of <u>right</u> lower extremity <u>with both ulcer</u> <u>other part of foot</u> and <u>inflammation</u>
Varicose veins of right lower extremity with both ulcer of toe and inflammation

I83.218 Varicose veins of <u>right</u> lower extremity <u>with both ulcer</u> of <u>other part of lower extremity</u> and <u>inflammation</u>

I83.219 Varicose veins of <u>right</u> lower extremity <u>with both ulcer</u> of <u>unspecified site</u> and <u>inflammation</u>

I83.22- Varicose veins of <u>left</u> lower extremity <u>with both ulcer and inflammation</u>

I83.221 Varicose veins of <u>left</u> lower extremity <u>with both ulcer</u> of <u>thigh</u> and <u>inflammation</u>

I83.222 Varicose veins of <u>left</u> lower extremity <u>with both ulcer</u> of <u>calf</u> and <u>inflammation</u>

I83.223 Varicose veins of <u>left</u> lower extremity <u>with both ulcer</u> of <u>ankle</u> and <u>inflammation</u>

I83.224 Varicose veins of <u>left</u> lower extremity <u>with both ulcer</u> of <u>heel and midfoot</u> and <u>inflammation</u>
Varicose veins of left lower extremity with both ulcer of plantar surface of midfoot and inflammation

I83.225 Varicose veins of <u>left</u> lower extremity <u>with both ulcer</u> <u>other part of foot</u> and <u>inflammation</u>
Varicose veins of left lower extremity with both ulcer of toe and inflammation

I83.228 Varicose veins of <u>left</u> lower extremity <u>with both ulcer</u> of <u>other part of lower extremity</u> and <u>inflammation</u>

I83.229 Varicose veins of <u>left</u> lower extremity <u>with both ulcer</u> of <u>unspecified site</u> and <u>inflammation</u>

I83.8- Varicose veins <u>of</u> <u>lower extremities with other complications</u>

I83.81- Varicose veins of lower extremities <u>with pain</u>

I83.811 Varicose veins of <u>right</u> lower extremities <u>with pain</u>

I83.812 Varicose veins of <u>left</u> lower extremities <u>with pain</u>

I83.813 Varicose veins of <u>bilateral</u> lower extremities <u>with pain</u>

I83.819 Varicose veins of <u>unspecified</u> lower extremities <u>with pain</u>

I83.89- Varicose veins of lower extremities <u>with other complications</u>
Varicose veins of lower extremities with edema
Varicose veins of lower extremities with swelling

I83.891 Varicose veins of <u>right</u> lower extremities <u>with other complications</u>

I83.892 Varicose veins of <u>left</u> lower extremities <u>with other complications</u>

I83.893 Varicose veins of <u>bilateral</u> lower extremities <u>with other complications</u>

I83.899 Varicose veins of <u>unspecified</u> lower extremities <u>with other complications</u>

I83.9- <u>Asymptomatic</u> varicose veins of lower extremities
Phlebectasia of lower extremities
Varicose veins of lower extremities
Varix of lower extremities

I83.90 Asymptomatic varicose veins of <u>unspecified</u> lower extremity
Varicose veins NOS

I83.91 Asymptomatic varicose veins of <u>right</u> lower extremity

I83.92 Asymptomatic varicose veins of <u>left</u> lower extremity

I83.93 Asymptomatic varicose veins of <u>bilateral</u> lower extremities

I85- Esophageal varices
Use additional code to identify:
Alcohol abuse and dependence (F10.-)

I85.0- Esophageal varices
Idiopathic esophageal varices
Primary esophageal varices

I85.00 Esophageal varices <u>without</u> bleeding
Esophageal varices NOS

I85.01 Esophageal varices <u>with bleeding</u>

I85.1- <u>Secondary</u> esophageal varices
Esophageal varices secondary to alcoholic liver disease
Esophageal varices secondary to cirrhosis of liver
Esophageal varices secondary to schistosomiasis
Esophageal varices secondary to toxic liver disease
Code first underlying disease

I85.10 Secondary esophageal varices <u>without</u> bleeding

I85.11 Secondary esophageal varices <u>with bleeding</u>

I86- Varicose veins of other sites
Excludes 1: varicose veins of unspecified site (I83.9-)
Excludes❷: retinal varices (H35.0-)

I86.0 **Sublingual varices**

I86.1 **Scrotal varices**
Varicocele

I86.2 **Pelvic varices**

I86.3 **Vulval varices**
Excludes 1: vulval varices complicating childbirth and the puerperium (O87.8)
vulval varices complicating pregnancy (O22.1-)

I86.4 **Gastric varices**

I86.8 **Varicose veins of other specified sites**
Varicose ulcer of nasal septum

I87- Other disorders of veins

I87.0- <u>Postthrombotic syndrome</u>
Chronic venous hypertension due to deep vein thrombosis
Postphlebitic syndrome
Excludes 1: chronic venous hypertension without deep vein thrombosis (I87.3-)

I87.00- Postthrombotic syndrome <u>without</u> complications
Asymptomatic Postthrombotic syndrome

I87.001 **Postthrombotic syndrome without complications of <u>right</u> lower extremity**

I87.002 **Postthrombotic syndrome without complications of <u>left</u> lower extremity**

I87.003 **Postthrombotic syndrome without complications of <u>bilateral</u> lower extremity**

I87.009 **Postthrombotic syndrome without complications of <u>unspecified</u> extremity**
Postthrombotic syndrome NOS

I87.01- Postthrombotic syndrome <u>with ulcer</u>
Use additional code to specify site and severity of ulcer (L97.-)

I87.011 **Postthrombotic syndrome <u>with ulcer</u> of <u>right</u> lower extremity**

I87.012 **Postthrombotic syndrome <u>with ulcer</u> of <u>left</u> lower extremity**

I87.013 **Postthrombotic syndrome <u>with ulcer</u> of <u>bilateral</u> lower extremity**

I87.019 **Postthrombotic syndrome <u>with ulcer</u> of <u>unspecified</u> lower extremity**

I87.02- Postthrombotic syndrome <u>with inflammation</u>

I87.021 **Postthrombotic syndrome <u>with inflammation</u> of <u>right</u> lower extremity**

I87.022 **Postthrombotic syndrome <u>with inflammation</u> of <u>left</u> lower extremity**

I87.023 **Postthrombotic syndrome <u>with inflammation</u> of <u>bilateral</u> lower extremity**

I87.029 **Postthrombotic syndrome <u>with inflammation</u> of <u>unspecified</u> lower extremity**

I 8 3 – I 9 6

I87.03-   **Postthrombotic syndrome with ulcer and inflammation**
   Use additional code to specify site and severity of ulcer (L97.-)

I87.031   **Postthrombotic syndrome with ulcer and inflammation of right lower extremity**

I87.032   **Postthrombotic syndrome with ulcer and inflammation of left lower extremity**

I87.033   **Postthrombotic syndrome with ulcer and inflammation of bilateral lower extremity**

I87.039   **Postthrombotic syndrome with ulcer and inflammation of unspecified lower extremity**

I87.09-   **Postthrombotic syndrome with other complications**

I87.091   **Postthrombotic syndrome with other complications of right lower extremity**

I87.092   **Postthrombotic syndrome with other complications of left lower extremity**

I87.093   **Postthrombotic syndrome with other complications of bilateral lower extremity**

I87.099   **Postthrombotic syndrome with other complications of unspecified lower extremity**

I87.1   **Compression of vein**
   Stricture of vein
   Vena cava syndrome (inferior) (superior)
   Excludes❷: compression of pulmonary vein (I28.8)

I87.2   **Venous insufficiency (chronic) (peripheral)**

I87.3-   **Chronic venous hypertension (idiopathic)**
   Stasis edema
   Excludes 1: chronic venous hypertension due to deep vein thrombosis (I87.0-)
   varicose veins of lower extremities (I83.-)

I87.30-   **Chronic venous hypertension (idiopathic) without complications**
   Asymptomatic chronic venous hypertension (idiopathic)

I87.301   **Chronic venous hypertension (idiopathic) without complications of right lower extremity**

I87.302   **Chronic venous hypertension (idiopathic) without complications of left lower extremity**

I87.303   **Chronic venous hypertension (idiopathic) without complications of bilateral lower extremity**

I87.309   **Chronic venous hypertension (idiopathic) without complications of unspecified lower extremity**
   Chronic venous hypertension NOS

I87.31-   **Chronic venous hypertension (idiopathic) with ulcer**
   Use additional code to specify site and severity of ulcer (L97.-)

I87.311   **Chronic venous hypertension (idiopathic) with ulcer of right lower extremity**

I87.312   **Chronic venous hypertension (idiopathic) with ulcer of left lower extremity**

I87.313   **Chronic venous hypertension (idiopathic) with ulcer of bilateral lower extremity**

I87.319   **Chronic venous hypertension (idiopathic) with ulcer of unspecified lower extremity**

I87.32-   **Chronic venous hypertension (idiopathic) with inflammation**

I87.321   **Chronic venous hypertension (idiopathic) with inflammation of right lower extremity**

I87.322   **Chronic venous hypertension (idiopathic) with inflammation of left lower extremity**

I87.323   **Chronic venous hypertension (idiopathic) with inflammation of bilateral lower extremity**

I87.329   **Chronic venous hypertension (idiopathic) with inflammation of unspecified lower extremity**

I87.33-   **Chronic venous hypertension (idiopathic) with ulcer and inflammation**
   Use additional code to specify site and severity of ulcer (L97.-)

I87.331   **Chronic venous hypertension (idiopathic) with ulcer and inflammation of right lower extremity**

I87.332   **Chronic venous hypertension (idiopathic) with ulcer and inflammation of left lower extremity**

I87.333   **Chronic venous hypertension (idiopathic) with ulcer and inflammation of bilateral lower extremity**

I87.339   **Chronic venous hypertension (idiopathic) with ulcer and inflammation of unspecified lower extremity**

I87.39-   **Chronic venous hypertension (idiopathic) with other complications**

I87.391   **Chronic venous hypertension (idiopathic) with other complications of right lower extremity**

I87.392   **Chronic venous hypertension (idiopathic) with other complications of left lower extremity**

I87.393   **Chronic venous hypertension (idiopathic) with other complications of bilateral lower extremity**

I87.399   **Chronic venous hypertension (idiopathic) with other complications of unspecified lower extremity**

I87.8   **Other specified disorders of veins**
   Phlebosclerosis
   Venofibrosis

I87.9   **Disorder of vein, unspecified**

I88-   **Nonspecific lymphadenitis**
   Excludes 1: acute lymphadenitis, except mesenteric (L04.-)
   enlarged lymph nodes NOS (R59.-)
   human immunodeficiency virus [HIV] disease resulting in generalized lymphadenopathy (B20)

I88.0   **Nonspecific mesenteric lymphadenitis**
   Mesenteric lymphadenitis (acute) (chronic)

I88.1   **Chronic lymphadenitis, except mesenteric**
   Adenitis
   Lymphadenitis

I88.8   **Other nonspecific lymphadenitis**

I88.9   **Nonspecific lymphadenitis, unspecified**
   Lymphadenitis NOS

I89-   **Other noninfective disorders of lymphatic vessels and lymph nodes**
   Excludes 1: chylocele, tunica vaginalis (nonfilarial) NOS (N50.8)
   enlarged lymph nodes NOS (R59.-)
   filarial chylocele (B74.-)
   hereditary lymphedema (Q82.0)

I89.0   **Lymphedema, not elsewhere classified**
   Elephantiasis (nonfilarial) NOS
   Lymphangiectasis
   Obliteration, lymphatic vessel
   Praecox lymphedema
   Secondary lymphedema
   Excludes 1: postmastectomy lymphedema (I97.2)

I89.1   **Lymphangitis**
   Chronic lymphangitis
   Lymphangitis NOS
   Subacute lymphangitis
   Excludes 1: acute lymphangitis (L03.-)

I89.8   **Other specified noninfective disorders of lymphatic vessels and lymph nodes**
   Chylocele (nonfilarial)
   Chylous ascites
   Chylous cyst
   Lipomelanotic reticulosis
   Lymph node or vessel fistula
   Lymph node or vessel infarction
   Lymph node or vessel rupture

I89.9   **Noninfective disorder of lymphatic vessels and lymph nodes, unspecified**
   Disease of lymphatic vessels NOS

Other and unspecified disorders of the circulatory system (I95-I99)

I95-   **Hypotension**
   Excludes 1: cardiovascular collapse (R57.9)
   maternal hypotension syndrome (O26.5-)
   nonspecific low blood pressure reading NOS (R03.1)

I95.0   **Idiopathic hypotension**

I95.1   **Orthostatic hypotension**
   Hypotension, postural
   Excludes 1: neurogenic orthostatic hypotension [Shy-Drager] (G90.3)
   orthostatic hypotension due to drugs (I95.2)

I95.2   **Hypotension due to drugs**
   Orthostatic hypotension due to drugs
   Use additional code for adverse effect, if applicable, to identify drug (T36-T50 with fifth or sixth character 5)

I95.3   **Hypotension of hemodialysis**
   Intra-dialytic hypotension

I95.8-   **Other hypotension**

I95.81   **Postprocedural hypotension**

I95.89   **Other hypotension**
   Chronic hypotension

I95.9   **Hypotension, unspecified**

I96   **Gangrene, not elsewhere classified**
   Gangrenous cellulitis
   Excludes 1: gangrene in atherosclerosis of native arteries of the extremities (I70.26)
   gangrene in diabetes mellitus (E08-E13)
   gangrene in hernia (K40.1, K40.4, K41.1, K41.4, K42.1, K43.1-, K44.1, K45.1, K46.1)
   gangrene in other peripheral vascular diseases (I73-)
   gangrene of certain specified sites — see Alphabetical Index
   gas gangrene (A48.0)
   pyoderma gangrenosum (L88)

I83 - I96

I97-   <u>Intraoperative and postprocedural complications</u> and disorders of circulatory system, not elsewhere classified
   Excludes❷: postprocedural shock (T81.1-)
   I97.0   **Postcardiotomy syndrome**
   I97.1-   **Other postprocedural cardiac functional disturbances**
      Excludes❷: acute pulmonary insufficiency following thoracic surgery (J95.1)
         intraoperative cardiac functional disturbances (I97.7-)
      I97.11-   **Postprocedural cardiac insufficiency**
         I97.110   **Postprocedural cardiac insufficiency following cardiac surgery**
         I97.111   **Postprocedural cardiac insufficiency following other surgery**
      I97.12-   **Postprocedural cardiac arrest**
         I97.120   **Postprocedural cardiac arrest following cardiac surgery**
         I97.121   **Postprocedural cardiac arrest following other surgery**
      I97.13-   **Postprocedural heart failure**
         Use additional code to identify the heart failure (I50.-)
         I97.130   **Postprocedural heart failure following cardiac surgery**
         I97.131   **Postprocedural heart failure following other surgery**
      I97.19-   **Other postprocedural cardiac functional disturbances**
         Use additional code, if applicable, to further specify disorder
         I97.190   **Other postprocedural cardiac functional disturbances following cardiac surgery**
         I97.191   **Other postprocedural cardiac functional disturbances following other surgery**
   I97.2   **Postmastectomy lymphedema syndrome**
      Elephantiasis due to mastectomy
      Obliteration of lymphatic vessels
   I97.3   **Postprocedural hypertension**
   I97.4-   <u>Intraoperative hemorrhage and hematoma</u> of a circulatory system organ or structure complicating a procedure
      Excludes 1: intraoperative hemorrhage and hematoma of a circulatory system organ or structure due to accidental puncture and laceration during a procedure (I97.5-)
      Excludes❷: intraoperative cerebrovascular hemorrhage complicating a procedure (G97.3-)
      I97.41-   **Intraoperative hemorrhage and hematoma of a circulatory system organ or structure complicating a circulatory system procedure**
         I97.410   **Intraoperative hemorrhage and hematoma of a circulatory system organ or structure <u>complicating a cardiac catheterization</u>**
         I97.411   **Intraoperative hemorrhage and hematoma of a circulatory system organ or structure <u>complicating a cardiac bypass</u>**
         I97.418   **Intraoperative hemorrhage and hematoma of a circulatory system organ or structure <u>complicating other circulatory system procedure</u>**
      I97.42   **Intraoperative hemorrhage and hematoma of a circulatory system organ or structure <u>complicating other procedure</u>**
   I97.5-   <u>Accidental puncture and laceration</u> of a circulatory system organ or structure during a procedure
      Excludes❷: accidental puncture and laceration of brain during a procedure (G97.4-)
      I97.51   **Accidental puncture and laceration of a circulatory system organ or structure during a <u>circulatory system procedure</u>**
      I97.52   **Accidental puncture and laceration of a circulatory system organ or structure during <u>other procedure</u>**
   I97.6-   <u>Postprocedural hemorrhage and hematoma</u> of a circulatory system organ or structure following a procedure
      Excludes❷: postprocedural cerebrovascular hemorrhage complicating a procedure (G97.5-)
      I97.61-   **Postprocedural hemorrhage and hematoma of a circulatory system organ or structure following a circulatory system procedure**
         I97.610   **Postprocedural hemorrhage and hematoma of a circulatory system organ or <u>structure following a cardiac catheterization</u>**
         I97.611   **Postprocedural hemorrhage and hematoma of a circulatory system organ or <u>structure following cardiac bypass</u>**
         I97.618   **Postprocedural hemorrhage and hematoma of a circulatory system organ or structure <u>following other circulatory system procedure</u>**
      I97.62   **Postprocedural hemorrhage and hematoma of a circulatory system organ or structure <u>following other procedure</u>**

I97.7-   **Intraoperative cardiac functional disturbances**
      Excludes❷: acute pulmonary insufficiency following thoracic surgery (J95.1)
         postprocedural cardiac functional disturbances (I97.1-)
   I97.71-   **Intraoperative cardiac arrest**
      I97.710   **Intraoperative cardiac arrest during <u>cardiac</u> surgery**
      I97.711   **Intraoperative cardiac arrest during <u>other</u> surgery**
   I97.79-   **Other intraoperative cardiac functional disturbances**
      Use additional code, if applicable, to further specify disorder
      I97.790   **Other intraoperative cardiac functional disturbances during <u>cardiac</u> surgery**
      I97.791   **Other intraoperative cardiac functional disturbances during <u>other</u> surgery**
I97.8-   **Other intraoperative and postprocedural complications and disorders of the circulatory system, not elsewhere classified**
      Use additional code, if applicable, to further specify disorder
   I97.81-   **Intraoperative cerebrovascular infarction**
      I97.810   **Intraoperative cerebrovascular infarction during <u>cardiac</u> surgery**
      I97.811   **Intraoperative cerebrovascular infarction during <u>other</u> surgery**
   I97.82-   **Postprocedural cerebrovascular infarction**
      I97.820   **Postprocedural cerebrovascular infarction during <u>cardiac</u> surgery**
      I97.821   **Postprocedural cerebrovascular infarction during <u>other</u> surgery**
   I97.88   **Other intraoperative complications of the circulatory system, <u>not elsewhere classified</u>**
   I97.89   **Other postprocedural complications and disorders of the circulatory system, not elsewhere classified**
I99-   **Other and unspecified disorders of circulatory system**
   I99.8   **Other disorder of circulatory system**
   I99.9   **Unspecified disorder of circulatory system**

I
9
7
-
J
0
3

Excludes 1: = NOT CODED HERE! (Do not code both)   **498**   *Excludes❷: = Not Included Here*

Chapter 10 – Diseases of the respiratory system (J00-J99)

Note: When a respiratory condition is described as occurring in more than one site and is not specifically indexed, it should be classified to the lower anatomic site (e.g. tracheobronchitis to bronchitis in J40).
Use additional code, where applicable, to identify:
  Exposure to environmental tobacco smoke (Z77.22)
  Exposure to tobacco smoke in the perinatal period (P96.81)
  History of tobacco use (Z87.891)
  Occupational exposure to environmental tobacco smoke (Z57.31)
  Tobacco dependence (F17.-)
  Tobacco use (Z72.0)
Excludes❷: certain conditions originating in the perinatal period (P04-P96)
certain infectious and parasitic diseases (A00-B99)
complications of pregnancy, childbirth and the puerperium (O00-O9A)
congenital malformations, deformations and chromosomal abnormalities (Q00-Q99)
endocrine, nutritional and metabolic diseases (E00-E88)
injury, poisoning and certain other consequences of external causes (S00-T88)
neoplasms (C00-D49)
smoke inhalation (T59.81-)
symptoms, signs and abnormal clinical and laboratory findings, not elsewhere classified (R00-R94)
This chapter contains the following blocks:
  J00-J06   Acute upper respiratory infections
  J09-J18   Influenza and pneumonia
  J20-J22   Other acute lower respiratory infections
  J30-J39   Other diseases of upper respiratory tract
  J40-J47   Chronic lower respiratory diseases
  J60-J70   Lung diseases due to external agents
  J80-J84   Other respiratory diseases principally affecting the interstitium
  J85-J86   Suppurative and necrotic conditions of the lower respiratory tract
  J90-J94   Other diseases of the pleura
  J95   Intraoperative and postprocedural complications and disorders of respiratory system, not elsewhere classified
  J96-J99   Other diseases of the respiratory system

Acute upper respiratory infections (J00-J06)

Excludes 1: chronic obstructive pulmonary disease with acute lower respiratory infection (J44.0)
influenza virus with other respiratory manifestations (J09.X2, J10.1, J11.1)

J00   Acute nasopharyngitis [common cold]
  Acute rhinitis
  Coryza (acute)
  Infective nasopharyngitis NOS
  Infective rhinitis
  Nasal catarrh, acute
  Nasopharyngitis NOS
Excludes 1: acute pharyngitis (J02.-)
acute sore throat NOS (J02.9)
pharyngitis NOS (J02.9)
rhinitis NOS (J31.0)
sore throat NOS (J02.9)
Excludes❷: allergic rhinitis (J30.1-J30.9)
chronic pharyngitis (J31.2)
chronic rhinitis (J31.0)
chronic sore throat (J31.2)
nasopharyngitis, chronic (J31.1)
vasomotor rhinitis (J30.0)

J01-   Acute sinusitis
  Includes: Acute abscess of sinus
    Acute empyema of sinus
    Acute infection of sinus
    Acute inflammation of sinus
    Acute suppuration of sinus
  Use additional code (B95-B97) to identify infectious agent
Excludes 1: sinusitis NOS (J32.9)
Excludes❷: chronic sinusitis (J32.0-J32.8)
  J01.0-   Acute maxillary sinusitis
    Acute antritis
    J01.00   Acute maxillary sinusitis, unspecified
    J01.01   Acute recurrent maxillary sinusitis
  J01.1-   Acute frontal sinusitis
    J01.10   Acute frontal sinusitis, unspecified
    J01.11   Acute recurrent frontal sinusitis

J01.2-   Acute ethmoidal sinusitis
  J01.20   Acute ethmoidal sinusitis, unspecified
  J01.21   Acute recurrent ethmoidal sinusitis
J01.3-   Acute sphenoidal sinusitis
  J01.30   Acute sphenoidal sinusitis, unspecified
  J01.31   Acute recurrent sphenoidal sinusitis
J01.4-   Acute pansinusitis
  J01.40   Acute pansinusitis, unspecified
  J01.41   Acute recurrent pansinusitis
J01.8-   Other acute sinusitis
  J01.80   Other acute sinusitis
    Acute sinusitis involving more than one sinus but not pansinusitis
  J01.81   Other acute recurrent sinusitis
    Acute recurrent sinusitis involving more than one sinus but not pansinusitis
J01.9-   Acute sinusitis, unspecified
  J01.90   Acute sinusitis, unspecified
  J01.91   Acute recurrent sinusitis, unspecified
J02-   Acute pharyngitis
  Includes: Acute sore throat
  Excludes 1: acute laryngopharyngitis (J06.0)
  peritonsillar abscess (J36)
  pharyngeal abscess (J39.1)
  retropharyngeal abscess (J39.0)
  Excludes❷: chronic pharyngitis (J31.2)
  J02.0   Streptococcal pharyngitis
    Septic pharyngitis
    Streptococcal sore throat
    Excludes❷: scarlet fever (A38.-)
  J02.8   Acute pharyngitis due to other specified organisms
    Use additional code (B95-B97) to identify infectious agent
    Excludes 1: acute pharyngitis due to coxsackie virus (B08.5)
    acute pharyngitis due to gonococcus (A54.5)
    acute pharyngitis due to herpes [simplex] virus (B00.2)
    acute pharyngitis due to infectious mononucleosis (B27.-)
    enteroviral vesicular pharyngitis (B08.5)
  J02.9   Acute pharyngitis, unspecified
    Gangrenous pharyngitis (acute)
    Infective pharyngitis (acute) NOS
    Pharyngitis (acute) NOS
    Sore throat (acute) NOS
    Suppurative pharyngitis (acute)
    Ulcerative pharyngitis (acute)
J03-   Acute tonsillitis
  Excludes 1: acute sore throat (J02.-)
  hypertrophy of tonsils (J35.1)
  peritonsillar abscess (J36)
  sore throat NOS (J02.9)
  streptococcal sore throat (J02.0)
  Excludes❷: chronic tonsillitis (J35.0)
  J03.0-   Streptococcal tonsillitis
    J03.00   Acute streptococcal tonsillitis, unspecified
    J03.01   Acute recurrent streptococcal tonsillitis
  J03.8-   Acute tonsillitis due to other specified organisms
    Use additional code (B95-B97) to identify infectious agent.
    Excludes 1: diphtheritic tonsillitis (A36.0)
    herpesviral pharyngotonsillitis (B00.2)
    streptococcal tonsillitis (J03.0)
    tuberculous tonsillitis (A15.8)
    Vincent's tonsillitis (A69.1)
    J03.80   Acute tonsillitis due to other specified organisms
    J03.81   Acute recurrent tonsillitis due to other specified organisms
  J03.9-   Acute tonsillitis, unspecified
    Follicular tonsillitis (acute)
    Gangrenous tonsillitis (acute)
    Infective tonsillitis (acute)
    Tonsillitis (acute) NOS
    Ulcerative tonsillitis (acute)
    J03.90   Acute tonsillitis, unspecified
    J03.91   Acute recurrent tonsillitis, unspecified

J97-J03

J04-   Acute laryngitis and tracheitis
Use additional code (B95-B97) to identify infectious agent.
Excludes 1: acute obstructive laryngitis [croup] and epiglottitis (J05.-)
Excludes❷: laryngismus (stridulus) (J38.5)

J04.0   Acute laryngitis
Edematous laryngitis (acute)
Laryngitis (acute) NOS
Subglottic laryngitis (acute)
Suppurative laryngitis (acute)
Ulcerative laryngitis (acute)
Excludes 1: acute obstructive laryngitis (J05.0)
Excludes❷: chronic laryngitis (J37.0)

J04.1-   Acute tracheitis
Acute viral tracheitis
Catarrhal tracheitis (acute)
Tracheitis (acute) NOS
Excludes❷: chronic tracheitis (J42)

J04.10   Acute tracheitis without obstruction
J04.11   Acute tracheitis with obstruction

J04.2   Acute laryngotracheitis
Laryngotracheitis NOS
Tracheitis (acute) with laryngitis (acute)
Excludes 1: acute obstructive laryngotracheitis (J05.0)
Excludes❷: chronic laryngotracheitis (J37.1)

J04.3-   Supraglottitis, unspecified
J04.30   Supraglottitis, unspecified, without obstruction
J04.31   Supraglottitis, unspecified, with obstruction

J05-   Acute obstructive laryngitis [croup] and epiglottitis
Use additional code (B95-B97) to identify infectious agent.

J05.0   Acute obstructive laryngitis [croup]
Obstructive laryngitis (acute) NOS
Obstructive laryngotracheitis NOS

J05.1-   Acute epiglottitis
Excludes❷: epiglottitis, chronic (J37.0)

J05.10   Acute epiglottitis without obstruction
Epiglottitis NOS
J05.11   Acute epiglottitis with obstruction

J06-   Acute upper respiratory infections of multiple and unspecified sites
Excludes 1: acute respiratory infection NOS (J22)
streptococcal pharyngitis (J02.0)

J06.0   Acute laryngopharyngitis

J06.9   Acute upper respiratory infection, unspecified
Upper respiratory disease, acute
Upper respiratory infection NOS

Influenza and pneumonia (J09-J18)

Excludes ❷: allergic or eosinophilic pneumonia (J82)
aspiration pneumonia NOS (J69.0)
congenital pneumonia (P23.9)
lipid pneumonia (J69.1)
meconium pneumonia (P24.01)
neonatal aspiration pneumonia (P24.-)
pneumonia due to solids and liquids (J69.-)
rheumatic pneumonia (I00)
ventilator associated pneumonia (J95.851)

J09-   Influenza due to certain identified influenza viruses
Excludes 1: influenza due to other identified influenza virus (J10-)
influenza due to unidentified influenza virus (J11-)
seasonal influenza due to other identified influenza virus (J10-)
seasonal influenza due to unidentified influenza virus (J11-)

J09.x-   Influenza due to identified novel influenza A virus
Avian influenza
Bird influenza
Influenza A/H5N1
Influenza of other animal origin, not bird or swine
Swine influenza virus (viruses that normally cause infections in pigs)

J09.x1   Influenza due to identified novel influenza A virus with pneumonia
Code also, if applicable, associated:
Lung abscess(J85.1)
Other specified type of pneumonia

J09.x2   Influenza due to identified novel influenza A virus with other respiratory manifestations
Influenza due to identified novel influenza A virus NOS
Influenza due to identified novel influenza A virus with laryngitis
Influenza due to identified novel influenza A virus with pharyngitis
Influenza due to identified novel influenza A virus with upper respiratory symptoms
Use additional code, if applicable, for associated:
Pleural effusion (J91.8)
Sinusitis (J01-)

J09.x3   Influenza due to identified novel influenza A virus with gastrointestinal manifestations
Influenza due to identified novel influenza A virus gastroenteritis
Excludes 1: "intestinal flu" [viral gastroenteritis] (A08-)

J09.x9   Influenza due to identified novel influenza A virus with other manifestations
Influenza due to identified novel influenza A virus with encephalopathy
Influenza due to identified novel influenza A virus with myocarditis
Influenza due to identified novel influenza A virus with otitis media
Use additional code to identify manifestation

J10-   Influenza due to other identified influenza virus
Excludes 1: influenza due to avian influenza virus (J09.X-)
influenza due to swine flu (J09.X-)
influenza due to unidentifed influenza virus (J11-)

J10.0-   Influenza due to other identified influenza virus with pneumonia
Code also associated lung abscess, if applicable (J85.1)

J10.00   Influenza due to other identified influenza virus with unspecified type of pneumonia

J10.01   Influenza due to other identified influenza virus with the same other identified influenza virus pneumonia

J10.08   Influenza due to other identified influenza virus with other specified pneumonia
Code also other specified type of pneumonia

J10.1   Influenza due to other identified influenza virus with other respiratory manifestations
Influenza due to other identified influenza virus NOS
Influenza due to other identified influenza virus with laryngitis
Influenza due to other identified influenza virus with pharyngitis
Influenza due to other identified influenza virus with upper respiratory symptoms
Use additional code for associated pleural effusion, if applicable (J91.8)
Use additional code for associated sinusitis, if applicable (J01.-)

J10.2   Influenza due to other identified influenza virus with gastrointestinal manifestations
Influenza due to other identified influenza virus gastroenteritis
Excludes 1: "intestinal flu" [viral gastroenteritis] (A08.-)

J04 - J17

Excludes 1: = NOT CODED HERE! (Do not code both)

Excludes❷: = Not Included Here

© 2013 Channel Publishing, Ltd.

J10.8-   Influenza due to <u>other</u> identified influenza virus <u>with other manifestations</u>

   J10.81   Influenza due to <u>other</u> identified influenza virus <u>with encephalopathy</u>

   J10.82   Influenza due to <u>other</u> identified influenza virus <u>with myocarditis</u>

   J10.83   Influenza due to <u>other</u> identified influenza virus <u>with otitis media</u>
      Use additional code for any associated perforated tympanic membrane (H72.-)

   J10.89   Influenza due to <u>other</u> identified influenza virus <u>with other manifestations</u>
      Use additional codes to identify the manifestations

J11-   Influenza due to <u>unidentified influenza virus</u>

J11.0-   Influenza due to <u>unidentified</u> influenza virus <u>with pneumonia</u>
      Code also associated lung abscess, if applicable (J85.1)

   J11.00   Influenza due to <u>unidentified</u> influenza virus <u>with unspecified type of pneumonia</u>
      Influenza with pneumonia NOS

   J11.08   Influenza due to <u>unidentified</u> influenza virus <u>with specified pneumonia</u>
      Code also other specified type of pneumonia

J11.1   Influenza due to <u>unidentified</u> influenza virus <u>with other respiratory</u> manifestations
      Influenza NOS
      Influenzal laryngitis NOS
      Influenzal pharyngitis NOS
      Influenza with upper respiratory symptoms NOS
      Use additional code for associated pleural effusion, if applicable (J91.8)
      Use additional code for associated sinusitis, if applicable (J01.-)

J11.2   Influenza due to <u>unidentified</u> influenza virus <u>with gastrointestinal manifestations</u>
      Influenza gastroenteritis NOS
      Excludes 1:   "intestinal flu" [viral gastroenteritis] (A08.-)

J11.8-   Influenza due to <u>unidentified</u> influenza virus <u>with other manifestations</u>

   J11.81   Influenza due to <u>unidentified</u> influenza virus <u>with encephalopathy</u>
      Influenzal encephalopathy NOS

   J11.82   Influenza due to <u>unidentified</u> influenza virus <u>with myocarditis</u>
      Influenzal myocarditis NOS

   J11.83   Influenza due to <u>unidentified</u> influenza virus <u>with otitis media</u>
      Influenzal otitis media NOS
      Use additional code for any associated perforated tympanic membrane (H72.-)

   J11.89   Influenza due to <u>unidentified</u> influenza virus <u>with other manifestations</u>
      Use additional codes to identify the manifestations

J12-   Viral pneumonia, <u>not elsewhere classified</u>
      Includes: Bronchopneumonia due to viruses other than influenza viruses
      Code first associated influenza, if applicable (J09.X1, J10.0-, J11.0-)
      Code also associated abscess, if applicable (J85.1)
      Excludes 1:   aspiration pneumonia due to anesthesia during labor and delivery (O74.0)
         aspiration pneumonia due to anesthesia during pregnancy (O29)
         aspiration pneumonia due to anesthesia during puerperium (O89.0)
         aspiration pneumonia due to solids and liquids (J69.-)
         aspiration pneumonia NOS (J69.0)
         congenital pneumonia (P23.0)
         congenital rubella pneumonitis (P35.0)
         interstitial pneumonia NOS (J84.9)
         lipid pneumonia (J69.1)
         neonatal aspiration pneumonia (P24.-)

J12.0   Adenoviral pneumonia

J12.1   Respiratory syncytial virus pneumonia

J12.2   Parainfluenza virus pneumonia

J12.3   Human metapneumovirus pneumonia

J12.8-   Other viral pneumonia

   J12.81   Pneumonia due to SARS-associated coronavirus
      Severe acute respiratory syndrome NOS

   J12.89   Other viral pneumonia

J12.9   Viral pneumonia, unspecified

J13   Pneumonia due to Streptococcus pneumoniae
      Bronchopneumonia due to S. pneumoniae
      Code first associated influenza, if applicable (J09.X1, J10.0-, J11.0-)
      Code also associated abscess, if applicable (J85.1)
      Excludes 1:   congenital pneumonia due to S. pneumoniae (P23.6)
         lobar pneumonia, unspecified organism (J18.1)
         pneumonia due to other streptococci (J15.3-J15.4)

J14   Pneumonia due to Hemophilus influenzae
      Bronchopneumonia due to H. influenzae
      Code first associated influenza, if applicable (J09.X1, J10.0-, J11.0-)
      Code also associated abscess, if applicable (J85.1)
      Excludes 1:   congenital pneumonia due to H. influenzae (P23.6)

J15-   Bacterial pneumonia, <u>not elsewhere classified</u>
      Includes: Bronchopneumonia due to bacteria other than S. pneumoniae and H. influenzae
      Code first associated influenza, if applicable (J09.X1, J10.0-, J11.0-)
      Code also associated abscess, if applicable (J85.1)
      Excludes 1:   chlamydial pneumonia (J16.0)
         congenital pneumonia (P23.-)
         Legionnaires' disease (A48.1)
         spirochetal pneumonia (A69.8)

J15.0   Pneumonia due to Klebsiella pneumoniae

J15.1   Pneumonia due to Pseudomonas

J15.2-   Pneumonia due to staphylococcus

   J15.20   Pneumonia due to staphylococcus, unspecified

   J15.21-   Pneumonia due to Staphylococcus aureus

      J15.211   Pneumonia due to methicillin susceptible Staphylococcus aureus
         MSSA pneumonia
         Pneumonia due to Staphylococcus aureus NOS

      J15.212   Pneumonia due to methicillin resistant Staphylococcus aureus

   J15.29   Pneumonia due to other staphylococcus

J15.3   Pneumonia due to streptococcus, group B

J15.4   Pneumonia due to other streptococci
      Excludes 1: pneumonia due to streptococcus, group B (J15.3)
         pneumonia due to Streptococcus pneumoniae (J13)

J15.5   Pneumonia due to Escherichia coli

J15.6   Pneumonia due to other aerobic Gram-negative bacteria
      Pneumonia due to Serratia marcescens

J15.7   Pneumonia due to Mycoplasma pneumoniae

J15.8   Pneumonia due to other specified bacteria

J15.9   Unspecified bacterial pneumonia
      Pneumonia due to gram-positive bacteria

J16-   Pneumonia due to other infectious organisms, <u>not elsewhere classified</u>
      Code first associated influenza, if applicable (J09.X1, J10.0-, J11.0-)
      Code also associated abscess, if applicable (J85.1)
      Excludes 1:   congenital pneumonia (P23.-)
         ornithosis (A70)
         pneumocystosis (B59)
         pneumonia NOS (J18.9)

J16.0   Chlamydial pneumonia

J16.8   Pneumonia due to other specified infectious organisms

J17   Pneumonia <u>in diseases classified elsewhere</u>
      Code first underlying disease, such as:
      Q fever (A78)
      Rheumatic fever (I00)
      Schistosomiasis (B65.0-B65.9)
      Excludes 1:   candidial pneumonia (B37.1)
         chlamydial pneumonia (J16.0)
         gonorrheal pneumonia (A54.84)
         histoplasmosis pneumonia (B39.0-B39.2)
         measles pneumonia (B05.2)
         nocardiosis pneumonia (A43.0)
         pneumocystosis (B59)
         pneumonia due to Pneumocystis carinii (B59)
         pneumonia due to Pneumocystis jiroveci (B59)
         pneumonia in actinomycosis (A42.0)
         pneumonia in anthrax (A22.1)
         pneumonia in ascariasis (B77.81)
         pneumonia in aspergillosis (B44.0-B44.1)
         pneumonia in coccidioidomycosis (B38.0-B38.2)
         pneumonia in cytomegalovirus disease (B25.0)
         pneumonia in toxoplasmosis (B58.3)
         rubella pneumonia (B06.81)
         salmonella pneumonia (A02.22)
         spirochetal infection NEC with pneumonia (A69.8)
         tularemia pneumonia (A21.2)
         typhoid fever with pneumonia (A01.03)
         varicella pneumonia (B01.2)
         whooping cough with pneumonia (A37 with fifth-character 1)

J 0 4 - J 1 7

Excludes 1: = NOT CODED HERE! (Do not code both)   *Excludes ❷:* = Not Included Here

J18-   Pneumonia, <u>unspecified organism</u>
Code first associated influenza, if applicable (J09.X1, J10.0-, J11.0-)
Excludes 1: abscess of lung with pneumonia (J85.1)
aspiration pneumonia due to anesthesia during labor and
delivery (O74.0)
aspiration pneumonia due to anesthesia during pregnancy
(O29)
aspiration pneumonia due to anesthesia during puerperium
(O89.0)
aspiration pneumonia due to solids and liquids (J69.-)
aspiration pneumonia NOS (J69.0)
congenital pneumonia (P23.0)
drug-induced interstitial lung disorder (J70.2-J70.4)
interstitial pneumonia NOS (J84.9)
lipid pneumonia (J69.1)
neonatal aspiration pneumonia (P24.-)
pneumonitis due to external agents (J67-J70)
pneumonitis due to fumes and vapors (J68.0)
usual interstitial pneumonia (J84.17)

J18.0   Bronchopneumonia, unspecified organism
Excludes 1: hypostatic bronchopneumonia (J18.2)
lipid pneumonia (J69.1)
Excludes❷: acute bronchiolitis (J21.-)
chronic bronchiolitis (J44.9)

J18.1   Lobar pneumonia, unspecified organism

J18.2   Hypostatic pneumonia, unspecified organism
Hypostatic bronchopneumonia
Passive pneumonia

J18.8   Other pneumonia, unspecified organism

J18.9   Pneumonia, unspecified organism

Other acute lower respiratory infections (J20-J22)

Excludes❷: chronic obstructive pulmonary disease with acute lower
respiratory infection (J44.0)

J20-   Acute bronchitis
Includes: Acute and subacute bronchitis (with) bronchospasm
Acute and subacute bronchitis (with) tracheitis
Acute and subacute bronchitis (with) tracheobronchitis, acute
Acute and subacute fibrinous bronchitis
Acute and subacute membranous bronchitis
Acute and subacute purulent bronchitis
Acute and subacute septic bronchitis
Excludes 1: bronchitis NOS (J40)
tracheobronchitis NOS (J40)
Excludes❷: acute bronchitis with bronchiectasis (J47.0)
acute bronchitis with chronic obstructive asthma (J44.0)
acute bronchitis with chronic obstructive pulmonary disease
(J44.0)
allergic bronchitis NOS (J45.909-)
bronchitis due to chemicals, fumes and vapors (J68.0)
chronic bronchitis NOS (J42)
chronic mucopurulent bronchitis (J41.1)
chronic obstructive bronchitis (J44.-)
chronic obstructive tracheobronchitis (J44.-)
chronic simple bronchitis (J41.0)
chronic tracheobronchitis (J42)

J20.0   Acute bronchitis due to Mycoplasma pneumoniae

J20.1   Acute bronchitis due to Hemophilus influenzae

J20.2   Acute bronchitis due to streptococcus

J20.3   Acute bronchitis due to coxsackievirus

J20.4   Acute bronchitis due to parainfluenza virus

J20.5   Acute bronchitis due to respiratory syncytial virus

J20.6   Acute bronchitis due to rhinovirus

J20.7   Acute bronchitis due to echovirus

J20.8   Acute bronchitis due to other specified organisms

J20.9   Acute bronchitis, unspecified

J21-   Acute bronchiolitis
Includes: Acute bronchiolitis with bronchospasm
Excludes❷: respiratory bronchiolitis interstitial lung disease (J84.115)

J21.0   Acute bronchiolitis due to respiratory syncytial virus

J21.1   Acute bronchiolitis due to human metapneumovirus

J21.8   Acute bronchiolitis due to other specified organisms

J21.9   Acute bronchiolitis, unspecified
Bronchiolitis (acute)
Excludes 1: chronic bronchiolitis (J44-)

J22   Unspecified acute lower respiratory infection
Acute (lower) respiratory (tract) infection NOS
Excludes 1: upper respiratory infection (acute) (J06.9)

Other diseases of upper respiratory tract (J30-J39)

J30-   Vasomotor and allergic rhinitis
Includes: Spasmodic rhinorrhea
Excludes 1: allergic rhinitis with asthma (bronchial) (J45.909)
rhinitis NOS (J31.0)

J30.0   Vasomotor rhinitis

J30.1   Allergic rhinitis due to pollen
Allergy NOS due to pollen
Hay fever
Pollinosis

J30.2   Other seasonal allergic rhinitis

J30.5   Allergic rhinitis due to food

J30.8-   Other allergic rhinitis

J30.81   Allergic rhinitis due to animal (cat) (dog) hair and dander

J30.89   Other allergic rhinitis
Perennial allergic rhinitis

J30.9   Allergic rhinitis, unspecified

J31-   Chronic rhinitis, nasopharyngitis and pharyngitis
Use additional code to identify:
Exposure to environmental tobacco smoke (Z77.22)
Exposure to tobacco smoke in the perinatal period (P96.81)
History of tobacco use (Z87.891)
Occupational exposure to environmental tobacco smoke (Z57.31)
Tobacco dependence (F17.-)
Tobacco use (Z72.0)

J31.0   Chronic rhinitis
Atrophic rhinitis (chronic)
Granulomatous rhinitis (chronic)
Hypertrophic rhinitis (chronic)
Obstructive rhinitis (chronic)
Ozena
Purulent rhinitis (chronic)
Rhinitis (chronic) NOS
Ulcerative rhinitis (chronic)
Excludes 1: allergic rhinitis (J30.1-J30.9)
vasomotor rhinitis (J30.0)

J31.1   Chronic nasopharyngitis
Excludes❷: acute nasopharyngitis (J00)

J31.2   Chronic pharyngitis
Chronic sore throat
Atrophic pharyngitis (chronic)
Granular pharyngitis (chronic)
Hypertrophic pharyngitis (chronic)
Excludes❷: acute pharyngitis (J02.9)

J32-   Chronic sinusitis
Includes: Sinus abscess
Sinus empyema
Sinus infection
Sinus suppuration
Use additional code to identify:
Exposure to environmental tobacco smoke (Z77.22)
Exposure to tobacco smoke in the perinatal period (P96.81)
History of tobacco use (Z87.891)
Infectious agent (B95-B97)
Occupational exposure to environmental tobacco smoke (Z57.31)
Tobacco dependence (F17-)
Tobacco use (Z72.0)
Excludes❷: acute sinusitis (J01-)

J32.0   Chronic maxillary sinusitis
Antritis (chronic)
Maxillary sinusitis NOS

J32.1   Chronic frontal sinusitis
Frontal sinusitis NOS

J32.2   Chronic ethmoidal sinusitis
Ethmoidal sinusitis NOS
Excludes 1: Woakes' ethmoiditis (J33.1)

J32.3   Chronic sphenoidal sinusitis
Sphenoidal sinusitis NOS

J32.4   Chronic pansinusitis
Pansinusitis NOS

J32.8   Other chronic sinusitis
Sinusitis (chronic) involving more than one sinus but not
pansinusitis

J32.9   Chronic sinusitis, unspecified
Sinusitis (chronic) NOS

J
1
8
–
J
3
8

J33-   Nasal polyp
Use additional code to identify:
Exposure to environmental tobacco smoke (Z77.22)
Exposure to tobacco smoke in the perinatal period (P96.81)
History of tobacco use (Z87.891)
Occupational exposure to environmental tobacco smoke (Z57.31)
Tobacco dependence (F17.-)
Tobacco use (Z72.0)
Excludes 1: adenomatous polyps (D14.0)

J33.0   Polyp of nasal cavity
Choanal polyp
Nasopharyngeal polyp

J33.1   Polypoid sinus degeneration
Woakes' syndrome or ethmoiditis

J33.8   Other polyp of sinus
Accessory polyp of sinus
Ethmoidal polyp of sinus
Maxillary polyp of sinus
Sphenoidal polyp of sinus

J33.9   Nasal polyp, unspecified

J34-   Other and unspecified disorders of nose and nasal sinuses
Excludes❷: varicose ulcer of nasal septum (I86.8)

J34.0   Abscess, furuncle and carbuncle of nose
Cellulitis of nose
Necrosis of nose
Ulceration of nose

J34.1   Cyst and mucocele of nose and nasal sinus

J34.2   Deviated nasal septum
Deflection or deviation of septum (nasal) (acquired)
Excludes 1: congenital deviated nasal septum (Q67.4)

J34.3   Hypertrophy of nasal turbinates

J34.8-   Other specified disorders of nose and nasal sinuses

J34.81   Nasal mucositis (ulcerative)
Code also type of associated therapy, such as:
Antineoplastic and immunosuppressive drugs (T45.1x-)
Radiological procedure and radiotherapy (Y84.2)
Excludes❷: gastrointestinal mucositis (ulcerative) (K92.81)
mucositis (ulcerative) of vagina and vulva (N76.81)
oral mucositis (ulcerative) (K12.3-)

J34.89   Other specified disorders of nose and nasal sinuses
Perforation of nasal septum NOS
Rhinolith

J34.9   Unspecified disorder of nose and nasal sinuses

J35-   Chronic diseases of tonsils and adenoids
Use additional code to identify:
Exposure to environmental tobacco smoke (Z77.22)
Exposure to tobacco smoke in the perinatal period (P96.81)
History of tobacco use (Z87.891)
Occupational exposure to environmental tobacco smoke (Z57.31)
Tobacco dependence (F17.-)
Tobacco use (Z72.0)

J35.0-   Chronic tonsillitis and adenoiditis
Excludes❷: acute tonsillitis (J03.-)

J35.01   Chronic tonsillitis

J35.02   Chronic adenoiditis

J35.03   Chronic tonsillitis and adenoiditis

J35.1   Hypertrophy of tonsils
Enlargement of tonsils
Excludes 1: hypertrophy of tonsils with tonsillitis (J35.0-)

J35.2   Hypertrophy of adenoids
Enlargement of adenoids
Excludes 1: hypertrophy of adenoids with adenoiditis (J35.0-)

J35.3   Hypertrophy of tonsils with hypertrophy of adenoids
Excludes 1: hypertrophy of tonsils and adenoids with tonsillitis and
adenoiditis (J35.03)

J35.8   Other chronic diseases of tonsils and adenoids
Adenoid vegetations
Amygdalolith
Calculus, tonsil
Cicatrix of tonsil (and adenoid)
Tonsillar tag
Ulcer of tonsil

J35.9   Chronic disease of tonsils and adenoids, unspecified
Disease (chronic) of tonsils and adenoids NOS

J36   Peritonsillar abscess
Includes: Abscess of tonsil
Peritonsillar cellulitis
Quinsy
Use additional code (B95-B97) to identify infectious agent
Excludes 1: acute tonsillitis (J03.-)
chronic tonsillitis (J35.0)
retropharyngeal abscess (J39.0)
tonsillitis NOS (J03.9-)

J37-   Chronic laryngitis and laryngotracheitis
Use additional code to identify:
Exposure to environmental tobacco smoke (Z77.22)
Exposure to tobacco smoke in the perinatal period (P96.81)
History of tobacco use (Z87.891)
Infectious agent (B95-B97)
Occupational exposure to environmental tobacco smoke (Z57.31)
Tobacco dependence (F17.-)
Tobacco use (Z72.0)

J37.0   Chronic laryngitis
Catarrhal laryngitis
Hypertrophic laryngitis
Sicca laryngitis
Excludes❷: acute laryngitis (J04.0)
obstructive (acute) laryngitis (J05.0)

J37.1   Chronic laryngotracheitis
Laryngitis, chronic, with tracheitis (chronic)
Tracheitis, chronic, with laryngitis
Excludes 1: chronic tracheitis (J42)
Excludes❷: acute laryngotracheitis (J04.2)
acute tracheitis (J04.1)

J38-   Diseases of vocal cords and larynx, not elsewhere classified
Use additional code to identify:
Exposure to environmental tobacco smoke (Z77.22)
Exposure to tobacco smoke in the perinatal period (P96.81)
History of tobacco use (Z87.891)
Occupational exposure to environmental tobacco smoke (Z57.31)
Tobacco dependence (F17.-)
Tobacco use (Z72.0)
Excludes 1: congenital laryngeal stridor (P28.89)
obstructive laryngitis (acute) (J05.0)
postprocedural subglottic stenosis (J95.5)
stridor (R06.1)
ulcerative laryngitis (J04.0)

J38.0-   Paralysis of vocal cords and larynx
Laryngoplegia
Paralysis of glottis

J38.00   Paralysis of vocal cords and larynx, unspecified

J38.01   Paralysis of vocal cords and larynx, unilateral

J38.02   Paralysis of vocal cords and larynx, bilateral

J38.1   Polyp of vocal cord and larynx
Excludes 1: adenomatous polyps (D14.1)

J38.2   Nodules of vocal cords
Chorditis (fibrinous) (nodosa) (tuberosa)
Singer's nodes
Teacher's nodes

J38.3   Other diseases of vocal cords
Abscess of vocal cords
Cellulitis of vocal cords
Granuloma of vocal cords
Leukokeratosis of vocal cords
Leukoplakia of vocal cords

J38.4   Edema of larynx
Edema (of) glottis
Subglottic edema
Supraglottic edema
Excludes 1: acute obstructive laryngitis [croup] (J05.0)
edematous laryngitis (J04.0)

J38.5   Laryngeal spasm
Laryngismus (stridulus)

J38.6   Stenosis of larynx

J38.7   Other diseases of larynx
Abscess of larynx
Cellulitis of larynx
Disease of larynx NOS
Necrosis of larynx
Pachyderma of larynx
Perichondritis of larynx
Ulcer of larynx

J
1
8
–
J
3
8

J39-   Other diseases of upper respiratory tract
Excludes 1:   acute respiratory infection NOS (J22)
acute upper respiratory infection (J06.9)
upper respiratory inflammation due to chemicals, gases, fumes or vapors (J68.2)

J39.0   Retropharyngeal and parapharyngeal abscess
Peripharyngeal abscess
Excludes 1:   peritonsillar abscess (J36)

J39.1   Other abscess of pharynx
Cellulitis of pharynx
Nasopharyngeal abscess

J39.2   Other diseases of pharynx
Cyst of pharynx
Edema of pharynx
Excludes❷: chronic pharyngitis (J31.2)
ulcerative pharyngitis (J02.9)

J39.3   Upper respiratory tract hypersensitivity reaction, site unspecified
Excludes 1:   hypersensitivity reaction of upper respiratory tract, such as:
extrinsic allergic alveolitis (J67.9)
pneumoconiosis (J60-J67.9)

J39.8   Other specified diseases of upper respiratory tract
J39.9   Disease of upper respiratory tract, unspecified

Chronic lower respiratory diseases (J40-J47)

Excludes 1:   bronchitis due to chemicals, gases, fumes and vapors (J68.0)
Excludes❷: cystic fibrosis (E84-)

J40   Bronchitis, not specified as acute or chronic
Bronchitis NOS
Bronchitis with tracheitis NOS
Catarrhal bronchitis
Tracheobronchitis NOS
Use additional code to identify:
Exposure to environmental tobacco smoke (Z77.22)
Exposure to tobacco smoke in the perinatal period (P96.81)
History of tobacco use (Z87.891)
Occupational exposure to environmental tobacco smoke (Z57.31)
Tobacco dependence (F17-)
Tobacco use (Z72.0)
Excludes 1:   acute bronchitis (J20.-)
allergic bronchitis NOS (J45.909-)
asthmatic bronchitis NOS (J45.9-)
bronchitis due to chemicals, gases, fumes and vapors (J68.0)

J41-   Simple and mucopurulent chronic bronchitis
Use additional code to identify:
Exposure to environmental tobacco smoke (Z77.22)
Exposure to tobacco smoke in the perinatal period (P96.81)
History of tobacco use (Z87.891)
Occupational exposure to environmental tobacco smoke (Z57.31)
Tobacco dependence (F17-)
Tobacco use (Z72.0)
Excludes 1:   chronic bronchitis NOS (J42)
chronic obstructive bronchitis (J44-)

J41.0   Simple chronic bronchitis
J41.1   Mucopurulent chronic bronchitis
J41.8   Mixed simple and mucopurulent chronic bronchitis

J42   Unspecified chronic bronchitis
Chronic bronchitis NOS
Chronic tracheitis
Chronic tracheobronchitis
Use additional code to identify:
Exposure to environmental tobacco smoke (Z77.22)
Exposure to tobacco smoke in the perinatal period (P96.81)
History of tobacco use (Z87.891)
Occupational exposure to environmental tobacco smoke (Z57.31)
Tobacco dependence (F17-)
Tobacco use (Z72.0)
Excludes 1:   chronic asthmatic bronchitis (J44-)
chronic bronchitis with airways obstruction (J44-)
chronic emphysematous bronchitis (J44-)
chronic obstructive pulmonary disease NOS (J44.9)
simple and mucopurulent chronic bronchitis (J41-)

J43-   Emphysema
Use additional code to identify:
Exposure to environmental tobacco smoke (Z77.22)
History of tobacco use (Z87.891)
Occupational exposure to environmental tobacco smoke (Z57.31)
Tobacco dependence (F17-)
Tobacco use (Z72.0)
Excludes 1:   compensatory emphysema (J98.3)
emphysema due to inhalation of chemicals, gases, fumes or vapors (J68.4)
emphysema with chronic (obstructive) bronchitis (J44-)
emphysematous (obstructive) bronchitis (J44-)
interstitial emphysema (J98.2)
mediastinal emphysema (J98.2)
neonatal interstitial emphysema (P25.0)
surgical (subcutaneous) emphysema (T81.82)
traumatic subcutaneous emphysema (T79.7)

J43.0   Unilateral pulmonary emphysema [MacLeod's syndrome]
Swyer-James syndrome
Unilateral emphysema
Unilateral hyperlucent lung
Unilateral pulmonary artery functional hypoplasia
Unilateral transparency of lung

J43.1   Panlobular emphysema
Panacinar emphysema

J43.2   Centrilobular emphysema
J43.8   Other emphysema
J43.9   Emphysema, unspecified
Bullous emphysema (lung) (pulmonary)
Emphysema (lung) (pulmonary) NOS
Emphysematous bleb
Vesicular emphysema (lung) (pulmonary)

J44-   Other chronic obstructive pulmonary disease
Includes: Asthma with chronic obstructive pulmonary disease
Chronic asthmatic (obstructive) bronchitis
Chronic bronchitis with airways obstruction
Chronic bronchitis with emphysema
Chronic emphysematous bronchitis
Chronic obstructive asthma
Chronic obstructive bronchitis
Chronic obstructive tracheobronchitis
Use additional code to identify:
Exposure to environmental tobacco smoke (Z77.22)
History of tobacco use (Z87.891)
Occupational exposure to environmental tobacco smoke (Z57.31)
Tobacco dependence (F17-)
Tobacco use (Z72.0)
Code also type of asthma, if applicable (J45.-)
Excludes 1:   bronchiectasis (J47-)
chronic bronchitis NOS (J42)
chronic simple and mucopurulent bronchitis (J41-)
chronic tracheitis (J42)
chronic tracheobronchitis (J42)
emphysema without chronic bronchitis (J43-)
lung diseases due to external agents (J60-J70)

J44.0   Chronic obstructive pulmonary disease with acute lower respiratory infection
Use additional code to identify the infection

J44.1   Chronic obstructive pulmonary disease with (acute) exacerbation
Decompensated COPD
Decompensated COPD with (acute) exacerbation
Excludes❷: chronic obstructive pulmonary disease [COPD] with acute bronchitis (J44.0)

J44.9   Chronic obstructive pulmonary disease, unspecified
Chronic obstructive airway disease NOS
Chronic obstructive lung disease NOS

J45-   Asthma
   Includes: Allergic (predominantly) asthma
             Allergic bronchitis NOS
             Allergic rhinitis with asthma
             Atopic asthma
             Extrinsic allergic asthma
             Hay fever with asthma
             Idiosyncratic asthma
             Intrinsic nonallergic asthma
             Nonallergic asthma
   Use additional code to identify:
       Exposure to environmental tobacco smoke (Z77.22)
       Exposure to tobacco smoke in the perinatal period (P96.81)
       History of tobacco use (Z87.891)
       Occupational exposure to environmental tobacco smoke (Z57.31)
       Tobacco dependence (F17.-)
       Tobacco use (Z72.0)
   Excludes 1:   detergent asthma (J69.8)
             eosinophilic asthma (J82)
             lung diseases due to external agents (J60-J70)
             miner's asthma (J60)
             wheezing NOS (R06.2)
             wood asthma (J67.8)
   Excludes❷: asthma with chronic obstructive pulmonary disease (J44.9)
             chronic asthmatic (obstructive) bronchitis (J44.9)
             chronic obstructive asthma (J44.9)

   J45.2-   Mild intermittent asthma
       J45.20   Mild intermittent asthma, uncomplicated
                Mild intermittent asthma NOS
       J45.21   Mild intermittent asthma with (acute) exacerbation
       J45.22   Mild intermittent asthma with status asthmaticus
   J45.3-   Mild persistent asthma
       J45.30   Mild persistent asthma, uncomplicated
                Mild persistent asthma NOS
       J45.31   Mild persistent asthma with (acute) exacerbation
       J45.32   Mild persistent asthma with status asthmaticus
   J45.4-   Moderate persistent asthma
       J45.40   Moderate persistent asthma, uncomplicated
                Moderate persistent asthma NOS
       J45.41   Moderate persistent asthma with (acute) exacerbation
       J45.42   Moderate persistent asthma with status asthmaticus
   J45.5-   Severe persistent asthma
       J45.50   Severe persistent asthma, uncomplicated
                Severe persistent asthma NOS
       J45.51   Severe persistent asthma with (acute) exacerbation
       J45.52   Severe persistent asthma with status asthmaticus
   J45.9-   Other and unspecified asthma
       J45.90-   Unspecified asthma
                Asthmatic bronchitis NOS
                Childhood asthma NOS
                Late onset asthma
           J45.901   Unspecified asthma with (acute) exacerbation
           J45.902   Unspecified asthma with status asthmaticus
           J45.909   Unspecified asthma, uncomplicated
                    Asthma NOS
       J45.99-   Other asthma
           J45.990   Exercise induced bronchospasm
           J45.991   Cough variant asthma
           J45.998   Other asthma

J47-   Bronchiectasis
   Includes: Bronchiolectasis
   Use additional code to identify:
       Exposure to environmental tobacco smoke (Z77.22)
       Exposure to tobacco smoke in the perinatal period (P96.81)
       History of tobacco use (Z87.891)
       Occupational exposure to environmental tobacco smoke (Z57.31)
       Tobacco dependence (F17.-)
       Tobacco use (Z72.0)
   Excludes 1: congenital bronchiectasis (Q33.4)
             tuberculous bronchiectasis (current disease) (A15.0)
   J47.0   Bronchiectasis with acute lower respiratory infection
            Bronchiectasis with acute bronchitis
   J47.1   Bronchiectasis with (acute) exacerbation
   J47.9   Bronchiectasis, uncomplicated
            Bronchiectasis NOS

Lung diseases due to external agents (J60-J70)

   Excludes❷: asthma (J45-)
             malignant neoplasm of bronchus and lung (C34-)

J60   Coalworker's pneumoconiosis
       Anthracosilicosis
       Anthracosis
       Black lung disease
       Coalworker's lung
   Excludes 1:   coalworker pneumoconiosis with tuberculosis, any type in A15 (J65)

J61   Pneumoconiosis due to asbestos and other mineral fibers
       Asbestosis
   Excludes 1:   pleural plaque with asbestosis (J92.0)
             pneumoconiosis with tuberculosis, any type in A15 (J65)

J62-   Pneumoconiosis due to dust containing silica
   Includes: Silicotic fibrosis (massive) of lung
   Excludes 1:   pneumoconiosis with tuberculosis, any type in A15 (J65)
   J62.0   Pneumoconiosis due to talc dust
   J62.8   Pneumoconiosis due to other dust containing silica
            Silicosis NOS

J63-   Pneumoconiosis due to other inorganic dusts
   Excludes 1:   pneumoconiosis with tuberculosis, any type in A15 (J65)
   J63.0   Aluminosis (of lung)
   J63.1   Bauxite fibrosis (of lung)
   J63.2   Berylliosis
   J63.3   Graphite fibrosis (of lung)
   J63.4   Siderosis
   J63.5   Stannosis
   J63.6   Pneumoconiosis due to other specified inorganic dusts

J64   Unspecified pneumoconiosis
   Excludes 1:   pneumonoconiosis with tuberculosis, any type in A15 (J65)

J65   Pneumoconiosis associated with tuberculosis
       Any condition in J60-J64 with tuberculosis, any type in A15
       Silicotuberculosis

J66-   Airway disease due to specific organic dust
   Excludes❷: allergic alveolitis (J67.-)
             asbestosis (J61)
             bagassosis (J67.1)
             farmer's lung (J67.0)
             hypersensitivity pneumonitis due to organic dust (J67.-)
             reactive airways dysfunction syndrome (J68.3)
   J66.0   Byssinosis
            Airway disease due to cotton dust
   J66.1   Flax-dressers' disease
   J66.2   Cannabinosis
   J66.8   Airway disease due to other specific organic dusts

J67-   Hypersensitivity pneumonitis due to organic dust
   Includes: Allergic alveolitis and pneumonitis due to inhaled organic dust
              and particles of fungal, actinomycetic or other origin
   *Excludes 1:   pneumonitis due to inhalation of chemicals, gases, fumes or
              vapors (J68.0)*
   J67.0   Farmer's lung
            Harvester's lung
            Haymaker's lung
            Moldy hay disease
   J67.1   Bagassosis
            Bagasse disease
            Bagasse pneumonitis
   J67.2   Bird fancier's lung
            Budgerigar fancier's disease or lung
            Pigeon fancier's disease or lung
   J67.3   Suberosis
            Corkhandler's disease or lung
            Corkworker's disease or lung
   J67.4   Maltworker's lung
            Alveolitis due to Aspergillus clavatus
   J67.5   Mushroom-worker's lung
   J67.6   Maple-bark-stripper's lung
            Alveolitis due to Cryptostroma corticale
            Cryptostromosis
   J67.7   Air conditioner and humidifier lung
            Allergic alveolitis due to fungal, thermophilic actinomycetes and
              other organisms growing in ventilation [air conditioning]
              systems

J 3 9 - J 6 7

J67.8 **Hypersensitivity pneumonitis due to other organic dusts**
Cheese-washer's lung
Coffee-worker's lung
Fish-meal worker's lung
Furrier's lung
Sequoiosis

J67.9 **Hypersensitivity pneumonitis due to unspecified organic dust**
Allergic alveolitis (extrinsic) NOS
Hypersensitivity pneumonitis NOS

J68- Respiratory conditions <u>due to inhalation of chemicals, gases, fumes and vapors</u>
Code first (T51-T65) to identify cause
Use additional code to identify associated respiratory conditions, such as:
Acute respiratory failure (J96.0-)

J68.0 **Bronchitis and pneumonitis due to chemicals, gases, fumes and vapors**
Chemical bronchitis (acute)

J68.1 **Pulmonary edema due to chemicals, gases, fumes and vapors**
Chemical pulmonary edema (acute) (chronic)
Excludes 1: pulmonary edema (acute) (chronic) NOS (J81-)

J68.2 **Upper respiratory inflammation due to chemicals, gases, fumes and vapors, not elsewhere classified**

J68.3 **Other acute and subacute respiratory conditions due to chemicals, gases, fumes and vapors**
Reactive airways dysfunction syndrome

J68.4 **Chronic respiratory conditions due to chemicals, gases, fumes and vapors**
Emphysema (diffuse) (chronic) due to inhalation of chemicals, gases, fumes and vapors
Obliterative bronchiolitis (chronic) (subacute) due to inhalation of chemicals, gases, fumes and vapors
Pulmonary fibrosis (chronic) due to inhalation of chemicals, gases, fumes and vapors
Excludes 1: chronic pulmonary edema due to chemicals, gases, fumes and vapors (J68.1)

J68.8 **Other respiratory conditions due to chemicals, gases, fumes and vapors**

J68.9 **Unspecified respiratory condition due to chemicals, gases, fumes and vapors**

J69- Pneumonitis due to solids and liquids
*Excludes 1: neonatal aspiration syndromes (P24-)
postprocedural pneumonitis (J95.4)*

J69.0 **Pneumonitis due to inhalation of food and vomit**
Aspiration pneumonia NOS
Aspiration pneumonia (due to) food (regurgitated)
Aspiration pneumonia (due to) gastric secretions
Aspiration pneumonia (due to) milk
Aspiration pneumonia (due to) vomit
Code also any associated foreign body in respiratory tract (T17-)
*Excludes 1: chemical pneumonitis due to anesthesia (J95.4)
obstetric aspiration pneumonitis (O74.0)*

J69.1 **Pneumonitis due to inhalation of oils and essences**
Exogenous lipoid pneumonia
Lipid pneumonia NOS
Code first (T51-T65) to identify substance
Excludes 1: endogenous lipoid pneumonia (J84.89)

J69.8 **Pneumonitis due to inhalation of other solids and liquids**
Pneumonitis due to aspiration of blood
Pneumonitis due to aspiration of detergent
Code first (T51-T65) to identify substance

J70- Respiratory conditions due to other external agents

J70.0 **Acute pulmonary manifestations due to radiation**
Radiation pneumonitis
Use additional code (W88-W90, X39.0-) to identify the external cause

J70.1 **Chronic and other pulmonary manifestations due to radiation**
Fibrosis of lung following radiation
Use additional code (W88-W90, X39.0-) to identify the external cause

J70.2 **Acute <u>drug-induced</u> interstitial lung disorders**
Use additional code for adverse effect, if applicable, to identify drug (T36-T50 with fifth or sixth character 5)
*Excludes 1: interstitial pneumonia NOS (J84.9)
lymphoid interstitial pneumonia (J84.2)*

J70.3 **Chronic <u>drug-induced</u> interstitial lung disorders**
Use additional code for adverse effect, if applicable, to identify drug (T36-T50 with fifth or sixth character 5)
*Excludes 1: interstitial pneumonia NOS (J84.9)
lymphoid interstitial pneumonia (J84.2)*

J70.4 **<u>Drug-induced</u> interstitial lung disorders, unspecified**
Use additional code for adverse effect, if applicable, to identify drug (T36-T50 with fifth or sixth character 5)
*Excludes 1: interstitial pneumonia NOS (J84.9)
lymphoid interstitial pneumonia (J84.2)*

J70.5 **Respiratory conditions due to smoke inhalation**
Smoke inhalation NOS
Excludes 1: smoke inhalation due to chemicals, gases, fumes and vapors (J68.9)

J70.8 **Respiratory conditions due to other specified external agents**
Code first (T51-T65) to identify the external agent

J70.9 **Respiratory conditions due to unspecified external agent**
Code first (T51-T65) to identify the external agent

Other respiratory diseases principally affecting the interstitium (J80-J84)

J80 **Acute respiratory distress syndrome**
Acute respiratory distress syndrome in adult or child
Adult hyaline membrane disease
Excludes 1: respiratory distress syndrome in newborn (perinatal) (P22.0)

J81- Pulmonary edema
Use additional code to identify:
Exposure to environmental tobacco smoke (Z77.22)
History of tobacco use (Z87.891)
Occupational exposure to environmental tobacco smoke (Z57.31)
Tobacco dependence (F17-)
Tobacco use (Z72.0)
*Excludes 1: chemical (acute) pulmonary edema (J68.1)
hypostatic pneumonia (J18.2)
passive pneumonia (J18.2)
pulmonary edema due to external agents (J60-J70)
pulmonary edema with heart disease NOS (I50.1)
pulmonary edema with heart failure (I50.1)*

J81.0 **<u>Acute</u> pulmonary edema**
Acute edema of lung

J81.1 **<u>Chronic</u> pulmonary edema**
Pulmonary congestion (chronic) (passive)
Pulmonary edema NOS

J82 **Pulmonary eosinophilia, not elsewhere classified**
Allergic pneumonia
Eosinophilic asthma
Eosinophilic pneumonia
Löffler's pneumonia
Tropical (pulmonary) eosinophilia NOS
*Excludes 1: pulmonary eosinophilia due to aspergillosis (B44-)
pulmonary eosinophilia due to drugs (J70.2-J70.4)
pulmonary eosinophilia due to specified parasitic infection (B50-B83)
pulmonary eosinophilia due to systemic connective tissue disorders (M30-M36)
pulmonary infiltrate NOS (R91.8)*

J 6 7 – J 8 6

J84-   Other interstitial pulmonary diseases
  Excludes 1: drug-induced interstitial lung disorders (J70.2-J70.4)
              interstitial emphysema (J98.2)
              lung diseases due to external agents (J60-J70)

  J84.0-   Alveolar and parieto-alveolar conditions
    J84.01   Alveolar proteinosis
    J84.02   Pulmonary alveolar microlithiasis
    J84.03   Idiopathic pulmonary hemosiderosis
            Essential brown induration of lung
            Code first underlying disease, such as:
              Disorders of iron metabolism (E83.1-)
            Excludes 1: acute idiopathic pulmonary hemorrhage in infants
                        [AIPHI] (R04.81)
    J84.09   Other alveolar and parieto-alveolar conditions

  J84.1-   Other interstitial pulmonary diseases with fibrosis
    Excludes 1: pulmonary fibrosis (chronic) due to inhalation of
                chemicals, gases, fumes or vapors (J68.4)
                pulmonary fibrosis (chronic) following radiation
                (J70.1)

    J84.10   Pulmonary fibrosis, unspecified
            Capillary fibrosis of lung
            Cirrhosis of lung (chronic) NOS
            Fibrosis of lung (atrophic) (chronic) (confluent) (massive)
              (perialveolar) (peribronchial) NOS
            Induration of lung (chronic) NOS
            Postinflammatory pulmonary fibrosis

    J84.11-   Idiopathic interstitial pneumonia
      Excludes 1: lymphoid interstitial pneumonia (J84.2)
                  pneumocystis pneumonia (B59)

      J84.111   Idiopathic interstitial pneumonia, not otherwise
                specified

      J84.112   Idiopathic pulmonary fibrosis
              Cryptogenic fibrosing alveolitis
              Idiopathic fibrosing alveolitis

      J84.113   Idiopathic non-specific interstitial pneumonitis
              Excludes 1: non-specific interstitial pneumonia NOS, or
                          due to known underlying cause (J84.89)

      J84.114   Acute interstitial pneumonitis
              Hamman-Rich syndrome
              Excludes 1: pneumocystis pneumonia (B59)

      J84.115   Respiratory bronchiolitis interstitial lung disease
      J84.116   Cryptogenic organizing pneumonia
              Excludes 1: organizing pneumonia NOS, or due to
                          known underlying cause (J84.89)

      J84.117   Desquamative interstitial pneumonia
    J84.17   Other interstitial pulmonary diseases with fibrosis in
              diseases classified elsewhere
            Interstitial pneumonia (nonspecific) (usual) due to collagen
              vascular disease
            Interstitial pneumonia (nonspecific) (usual) in diseases
              classified elsewhere
            Organizing pneumonia due to collagen vascular disease
            Organizing pneumonia in diseases classified elsewhere
            Code first underlying disease, such as:
              Progressive systemic sclerosis (M34.0)
              Rheumatoid arthritis (M05.00-M06.9)
              Systemic lupus erythematosis (M32.0-M32.9)

  J84.2   Lymphoid interstitial pneumonia
          Lymphoid interstitial pneumonitis

  J84.8-   Other specified interstitial pulmonary diseases
    Excludes 1: exogenous lipoid pneumonia (J69.1)
                unspecified lipoid pneumonia (J69.1)

    J84.81   Lymphangioleiomyomatosis
            Lymphangiomyomatosis
    J84.82   Adult pulmonary Langerhans cell histiocytosis
            Adult PLCH
    J84.83   Surfactant mutations of the lung
    J84.84- Other interstitial lung diseases of childhood
      J84.841   Neuroendocrine cell hyperplasia of infancy
      J84.842   Pulmonary interstitial glycogenosis
      J84.843   Alveolar capillary dysplasia with vein misalignment
      J84.848   Other interstitial lung diseases of childhood

    J84.89   Other specified interstitial pulmonary diseases
            Endogenous lipoid pneumonia
            Interstitial pneumonitis
            Non-specific interstitial pneumonitis NOS
            Organizing pneumonia due to known underlying cause
            Organizing pneumonia NOS
            Code first, if applicable:
              Poisoning due to drug or toxin (T51-T65 with fifth or sixth
                character to indicate intent), for toxic pneumonopathy
              Underlying cause of pneumonopathy, if known
            Use additional code, for adverse effect, to identify drug (T36-
              T50 with fifth or sixth character 5), if drug-induced
            Excludes 1: cryptogenic organizing pneumonia (J84.116)
                        idiopathic non-specific interstitial pneumonitis
                        (J84.113)
                        lipoid pneumonia, exogenous or unspecified
                        (J69.1)
                        lymphoid interstitial pneumonia (J84.2)

  J84.9   Interstitial pulmonary disease, unspecified
          Interstitial pneumonia NOS

Suppurative and necrotic conditions of the lower respiratory tract (J85-J86)

J85-   Abscess of lung and mediastinum
        Use additional code (B95-B97) to identify infectious agent

  J85.0   Gangrene and necrosis of lung
  J85.1   Abscess of lung with pneumonia
          Code also the type of pneumonia
  J85.2   Abscess of lung without pneumonia
          Abscess of lung NOS
  J85.3   Abscess of mediastinum

J86-   Pyothorax
        Use additional code (B95-B97) to identify infectious agent
        Excludes 1: abscess of lung (J85.-)
                    pyothorax due to tuberculosis (A15.6)

  J86.0   Pyothorax with fistula
          Any condition classifiable to J86.9 with fistula
          Bronchocutaneous fistula
          Bronchopleural fistula
          Hepatopleural fistula
          Mediastinal fistula
          Pleural fistula
          Thoracic fistula

  J86.9   Pyothorax without fistula
          Abscess of pleura
          Abscess of thorax
          Empyema (chest) (lung) (pleura)
          Fibrinopurulent pleurisy
          Purulent pleurisy
          Pyopneumothorax
          Septic pleurisy
          Seropurulent pleurisy
          Suppurative pleurisy

J 6 7 - J 8 6

Other diseases of the pleura (J90-J94)

J90   Pleural effusion, <u>not elsewhere classified</u>
Encysted pleurisy
Pleural effusion NOS
Pleurisy with effusion (exudative) (serous)
Excludes 1:   chylous (pleural) effusion (J94.0)
malignant pleural effusion (J91.0))
pleurisy NOS (R09.1)
tuberculous pleural effusion (A15.6)

J91-   Pleural effusion <u>in conditions classified elsewhere</u>
Excludes❷: pleural effusion in heart failure (I50.-)
pleural effusion in systemic lupus erythematosus (M32.13)

   J91.0   Malignant pleural effusion
Code first underlying neoplasm

   J91.8   Pleural effusion in other conditions classified elsewhere
Code first underlying disease, such as:
Filariasis (B74.0-B74.9)
Influenza (J09.X2, J10.1, J11.1)

J92-   Pleural plaque
Includes: Pleural thickening

   J92.0   Pleural plaque <u>with presence of asbestos</u>

   J92.9   Pleural plaque <u>without</u> asbestos
Pleural plaque NOS

J93-   Pneumothorax and air leak
Excludes 1:   congenital or perinatal pneumothorax (P25.1)
postprocedural air leak (J95.812)
postprocedural pneumothorax (J95.811)
traumatic pneumothorax (S27.0)
tuberculous (current disease) pneumothorax (A15.-)
pyopneumothorax (J86-)

   J93.0   Spontaneous <u>tension</u> pneumothorax

   J93.1-   Other <u>spontaneous</u> pneumothorax

      J93.11   <u>Primary</u> spontaneous pneumothorax

      J93.12   <u>Secondary</u> spontaneous pneumothorax
Code first underlying condition, such as:
Catamenial pneumothorax due to endometriosis (N80.8)
Cystic fibrosis (E84-)
Eosinophilic pneumonia (J82)
Lymphangioleiomyomatosis (J84.81)
Malignant neoplasm of bronchus amd lung (C34-)
Marfan's syndrome (Q87.4)
Pneumonia due to Pneumocystis carinii (B59)
Secondary malignant neoplasm of lung (C78.0-)
Spontaneous rupture of the esophagus (K22.3)

   J93.8-   Other pneumothorax and air leak

      J93.81   <u>Chronic</u> pneumothorax

      J93.82   Other <u>air leak</u>
Persistent air leak

      J93.83   Other <u>pneumothorax</u>
Acute pneumothorax
Spontaneous pneumothorax NOS

   J93.9   Pneumothorax, unspecified
Pneumothorax NOS

J94-   Other pleural conditions
Excludes 1:   pleurisy NOS (R09.1)
traumatic hemopneumothorax (S27.2)
traumatic hemothorax (S27.1)
tuberculous pleural conditions (current disease) (A15.-)

   J94.0   Chylous effusion
Chyliform effusion

   J94.1   Fibrothorax

   J94.2   Hemothorax
Hemopneumothorax

   J94.8   Other specified pleural conditions
Hydropneumothorax
Hydrothorax

   J94.9   Pleural condition, unspecified

Intraoperative and postprocedural complications and disorders of respiratory system, not elsewhere classified (J95)

J95-   <u>Intraoperative and postprocedural complications</u> and disorders of respiratory system, not elsewhere classified
Excludes❷: aspiration pneumonia (J69.-)
emphysema (subcutaneous) resulting from a procedure (T81.82)
hypostatic pneumonia (J18.2)
pulmonary manifestations due to radiation (J70.0-J70.1)

   J95.0-   Tracheostomy complications

      J95.00   Unspecified tracheostomy complication

      J95.01   Hemorrhage from tracheostomy stoma

      J95.02   Infection of tracheostomy stoma
Use additional code to identify type of infection, such as:
Cellulitis of neck (L03.8)
Sepsis (A40, A41.-)

      J95.03   Malfunction of tracheostomy stoma
Mechanical complication of tracheostomy stoma
Obstruction of tracheostomy airway
Tracheal stenosis due to tracheostomy

      J95.04   Tracheo-esophageal fistula following tracheostomy

      J95.09   Other tracheostomy complication

   J95.1   Acute pulmonary insufficiency following <u>thoracic</u> surgery
Excludes❷: functional disturbances following cardiac surgery (I97.0, I97.1-)

   J95.2   Acute pulmonary insufficiency following <u>non</u>thoracic surgery
Excludes❷: functional disturbances following cardiac surgery (I97.0, I97.1-)

   J95.3   Chronic pulmonary insufficiency following surgery
Excludes❷: functional disturbances following cardiac surgery (I97.0, I97.1-)

   J95.4   Chemical pneumonitis due to anesthesia
Mendelson's syndrome
Postprocedural aspiration pneumonia
Use additional code for adverse effect, if applicable, to identify drug
(T41- with fifth or sixth character 5)
Excludes 1:   aspiration pneumonitis due to anesthesia complicating labor and delivery (O74.0)
aspiration pneumonitis due to anesthesia complicating pregnancy (O29)
aspiration pneumonitis due to anesthesia complicating the puerperium (O89.01)

   J95.5   Postprocedural subglottic stenosis

   J95.6-   <u>Intraoperative hemorrhage and hematoma</u> of a respiratory system organ or structure complicating a procedure
Excludes 1:   intraoperative hemorrhage and hematoma of a respiratory system organ or structure due to accidental puncture and laceration during procedure (J95.7-)

      J95.61   Intraoperative hemorrhage and hematoma of a respiratory system organ or structure complicating a <u>respiratory system procedure</u>

      J95.62   Intraoperative hemorrhage and hematoma of a respiratory system organ or structure complicating <u>other procedure</u>

   J95.7-   Accidental puncture and laceration of a respiratory system organ or structure during a procedure
Excludes❷: postprocedural pneumothorax (J95.811)

      J95.71   Accidental puncture and laceration of a respiratory system organ or structure during a <u>respiratory system procedure</u>

      J95.72   Accidental puncture and laceration of a respiratory system organ or structure during <u>other procedure</u>

Excludes 1: = NOT CODED HERE! (Do not code both)   **508**   *Excludes❷:* = Not Included Here

J95.8-   **Other intraoperative and postprocedural complications and disorders of respiratory system, not elsewhere classified**

   J95.81-   <u>Postprocedural</u> pneumothorax and air leak

      J95.811   Postprocedural <u>pneumothorax</u>

      J95.812   Postprocedural <u>air leak</u>

   J95.82-   <u>Postprocedural respiratory failure</u>

      Excludes 1:   respiratory failure in other conditions (J96-)

      J95.821   <u>Acute</u> postprocedural respiratory failure

         Postprocedural respiratory failure NOS

      J95.822   <u>Acute and chronic</u> postprocedural respiratory failure

   J95.83-   Postprocedural hemorrhage and hematoma of a respiratory system organ or structure following a procedure

      J95.830   Postprocedural hemorrhage and hematoma of a respiratory system organ or structure following a <u>respiratory system procedure</u>

      J95.831   Postprocedural hemorrhage and hematoma of a respiratory system organ or structure following <u>other procedure</u>

   J95.84   Transfusion-related acute lung injury (TRALI)

   J95.85-   Complication of respirator [ventilator]

      J95.850   Mechanical complication of respirator

         Excludes 1:   encounter for respirator [ventilator] dependence during power failure (Z99.12)

      J95.851   Ventilator associated pneumonia

         Ventilator associated pneumonitis

         Use additional code to identify the organism, if known (B95-, B96-, B97-)

         Excludes 1:   ventilator lung in newborn (P27.8)

      J95.859   Other complication of respirator [ventilator]

   J95.88   Other intraoperative complications of respiratory system, not elsewhere classified

   J95.89   Other postprocedural complications and disorders of respiratory system, not elsewhere classified

      Use additional code to identify disorder, such as:

         Aspiration pneumonia (J69.-)

         Bacterial or viral pneumonia (J12-J18)

      Excludes❷: acute pulmonary insufficiency following thoracic surgery (J95.1)

          postprocedural subglottic stenosis (J95.5)

Other diseases of the respiratory system (J96-J99)

J96-   **Respiratory failure, <u>not elsewhere classified</u>**

   Excludes 1:   acute respiratory distress syndrome (J80)

         cardiorespiratory failure (R09.2)

         newborn respiratory distress syndrome (P22.0)

         postprocedural respiratory failure (J95.82-)

         respiratory arrest (R09.2)

         respiratory arrest of newborn (P28.81)

         respiratory failure of newborn (P28.5)

   J96.0-   <u>Acute</u> respiratory failure

      J96.00   Acute respiratory failure, <u>unspecified</u> whether with hypoxia or hypercapnia

      J96.01   Acute respiratory failure <u>with hypoxia</u>

      J96.02   Acute respiratory failure <u>with hypercapnia</u>

   J96.1-   <u>Chronic</u> respiratory failure

      J96.10   Chronic respiratory failure, <u>unspecified</u> whether with hypoxia or hypercapnia

      J96.11   Chronic respiratory failure <u>with hypoxia</u>

      J96.12   Chronic respiratory failure <u>with hypercapnia</u>

   J96.2-   <u>Acute and chronic</u> respiratory failure

      Acute on chronic respiratory failure

      J96.20   Acute and chronic respiratory failure, <u>unspecified</u> whether with hypoxia or hypercapnia

      J96.21   Acute and chronic respiratory failure <u>with hypoxia</u>

      J96.22   Acute and chronic respiratory failure <u>with hypercapnia</u>

   J96.9-   Respiratory failure, <u>unspecified</u>

      J96.90   Respiratory failure, unspecified, <u>unspecified</u> whether with hypoxia or hypercapnia

      J96.91   Respiratory failure, unspecified <u>with hypoxia</u>

      J96.92   Respiratory failure, unspecified <u>with hypercapnia</u>

J98-   **Other respiratory disorders**

   Use additional code to identify:

      Exposure to environmental tobacco smoke (Z77.22)

      Exposure to tobacco smoke in the perinatal period (P96.81)

      History of tobacco use (Z87.891)

      Occupational exposure to environmental tobacco smoke (Z57.31)

      Tobacco dependence (F17.-)

      Tobacco use (Z72.0)

   Excludes 1:   newborn apnea (P28.4)

         newborn sleep apnea (P28.3)

   Excludes❷: apnea NOS (R06.81)

         sleep apnea (G47.3-)

   J98.0-   Diseases of bronchus, <u>not elsewhere classified</u>

      J98.01   Acute bronchospasm

         Excludes 1:   acute bronchiolitis with bronchospasm (J21.-)

           acute bronchitis with bronchospasm (J20.-)

           asthma (J45.-)

           exercise induced bronchospasm (J45.990)

      J98.09   Other diseases of bronchus, not elsewhere classified

         Broncholithiasis

         Calcification of bronchus

         Stenosis of bronchus

         Tracheobronchial collapse

         Tracheobronchial dyskinesia

         Ulcer of bronchus

   J98.1-   Pulmonary collapse

      Excludes 1:   therapeutic collapse of lung status (Z98.3)

      J98.11   Atelectasis

         Excludes 1:   newborn atelectasis

           tuberculous atelectasis (current disease) (A15)

      J98.19   Other pulmonary collapse

   J98.2   Interstitial emphysema

      Mediastinal emphysema

      Excludes 1:   emphysema NOS (J43.9)

         emphysema in newborn (P25.0)

         surgical emphysema (subcutaneous) (T81.82)

         traumatic subcutaneous emphysema (T79.7)

   J98.3   Compensatory emphysema

   J98.4   Other disorders of lung

      Calcification of lung

      Cystic lung disease (acquired)

      Lung disease NOS

      Pulmolithiasis

      Excludes 1:   acute interstitial pneumonitis (J84.114)

         pulmonary insufficiency following surgery (J95.1-J95.2)

J90 - J98

© 2013 Channel Publishing, Ltd.

J98.5   **Diseases of mediastinum, <u>not elsewhere classified</u>**
    Fibrosis of mediastinum
    Hernia of mediastinum
    Retraction of mediastinum
    Mediastinitis
    Excludes❷: abscess of mediastinum (J85.3)

J98.6   **Disorders of diaphragm**
    Diaphragmatitis
    Paralysis of diaphragm
    Relaxation of diaphragm
    Excludes 1: congenital malformation of diaphragm NEC (Q79.1)
    *   congenital diaphragmatic hernia (Q79.0)*
    Excludes❷: diaphragmatic hernia (K44.-)

J98.8   **Other specified respiratory disorders**

J98.9   **Respiratory disorder, unspecified**
    Respiratory disease (chronic) NOS

J99   **Respiratory disorders <u>in diseases classified elsewhere</u>**
    Code first underlying disease, such as:
    Amyloidosis (E85.-)
    Ankylosing spondylitis (M45)
    Congenital syphilis (A50.5)
    Cryoglobulinemia (D89.1)
    Early congenital syphilis (A50.0)
    Schistosomiasis (B65.0-B65.9)
    Excludes 1: respiratory disorders in:
    *   amebiasis (A06.5)*
    *   blastomycosis (B40.0-B40.2)*
    *   candidiasis (B37.1)*
    *   coccidioidomycosis (B38.0-B38.2)*
    *   cystic fibrosis with pulmonary manifestations (E84.0)*
    *   dermatomyositis (M33.01, M33.11)*
    *   histoplasmosis (B39.0-B39.2)*
    *   late syphilis (A52.72, A52.73)*
    *   polymyositis (M33.21)*
    *   sicca syndrome (M35.02)*
    *   systemic lupus erythematosus (M32.13)*
    *   systemic sclerosis (M34.81)*
    *   Wegener's granulomatosis (M31.30-M31.31)*

**J
9
8
–
K
0
3**

Chapter 11 – Diseases of the digestive system (K00-K95)

Excludes❷: *certain conditions originating in the perinatal period*
            (P04-P96)
            certain infectious and parasitic diseases (A00-B99)
            complications of pregnancy, childbirth and the puerperium
            (O00-O9A)
            congenital malformations, deformations and chromosomal
            abnormalities (Q00-Q99)
            endocrine, nutritional and metabolic diseases (E00-E88)
            injury, poisoning and certain other consequences of external
            causes (S00-T88)
            neoplasms (C00-D49)
            symptoms, signs and abnormal clinical and laboratory
            findings, not elsewhere classified (R00-R94)

This chapter contains the following blocks:

K00-K14	Diseases of oral cavity and salivary glands
K20-K31	Diseases of esophagus, stomach and duodenum
K35-K38	Diseases of appendix
K40-K46	Hernia
K50-K52	Noninfective enteritis and colitis
K55-K64	Other diseases of intestines
K65-K68	Diseases of peritoneum and retroperitoneum
K70-K77	Diseases of liver
K80-K87	Disorders of gallbladder, biliary tract and pancreas
K90-K95	Other diseases of the digestive system

Diseases of oral cavity and salivary glands (K00-K14)

K00- Disorders of tooth development and eruption
    Excludes❷: embedded and impacted teeth (K01.-)

K00.0   Anodontia
        Hypodontia
        Oligodontia
        Excludes 1: acquired absence of teeth (K08.1-)

K00.1   Supernumerary teeth
        Distomolar
        Fourth molar
        Mesiodens
        Paramolar
        Supplementary teeth
        Excludes❷: supernumerary roots (K00.2)

K00.2   Abnormalities of size and form of teeth
        Concrescence of teeth
        Fusion of teeth
        Gemination of teeth
        Dens evaginatus
        Dens in dente
        Dens invaginatus
        Enamel pearls
        Macrodontia
        Microdontia
        Peg-shaped [conical] teeth
        Supernumerary roots
        Taurodontism
        Tuberculum paramolare
        Excludes 1:   abnormalities of teeth due to congenital syphilis
                (A50.5)
                tuberculum Carabelli, which is regarded as a normal
                variation and should not be coded

K00.3   Mottled teeth
        Dental fluorosis
        Mottling of enamel
        Nonfluoride enamel opacities
        Excludes❷: deposits [accretions] on teeth (K03.6)

K00.4   Disturbances in tooth formation
        Aplasia and hypoplasia of cementum
        Dilaceration of tooth
        Enamel hypoplasia (neonatal) (postnatal) (prenatal)
        Regional odontodysplasia
        Turner's tooth
        Excludes 1: Hutchinson's teeth and mulberry molars in congenital
                syphilis (A50.5)
        Excludes❷: mottled teeth (K00.3)

**K00.5   Hereditary disturbances in tooth structure, not elsewhere
        classified**
        Amelogenesis imperfecta
        Dentinogenesis imperfecta
        Odontogenesis imperfecta
        Dentinal dysplasia
        Shell teeth

K00.6   Disturbances in tooth eruption
        Dentia praecox
        Natal tooth
        Neonatal tooth
        Premature eruption of tooth
        Premature shedding of primary [deciduous] tooth
        Prenatal teeth
        Retained [persistent] primary tooth
        Excludes❷: embedded and impacted teeth (K01-)

K00.7   Teething syndrome

K00.8   Other disorders of tooth development
        Color changes during tooth formation
        Intrinsic staining of teeth NOS
        Excludes❷: posteruptive color changes (K03.7)

K00.9   Disorder of tooth development, unspecified
        Disorder of odontogenesis NOS

K01- Embedded and impacted teeth
    Excludes 1: abnormal position of fully erupted teeth (M26.3-)

K01.0   Embedded teeth

K01.1   Impacted teeth

K02- Dental caries
    Includes: Dental cavities
            Tooth decay

K02.3   Arrested dental caries
        Arrested coronal and root caries

K02.5- Dental caries on pit and fissure surface
        Dental caries on chewing surface of tooth

    K02.51 Dental caries on pit and fissure surface limited to enamel
            White spot lesions [initial caries] on pit and fissure surface of
                tooth

    **K02.52 Dental caries on pit and fissure surface penetrating into
            dentin**

    K02.53 Dental caries on pit and fissure surface penetrating into pulp

K02.6- Dental caries on smooth surface

    K02.61 Dental caries on smooth surface limited to enamel
            White spot lesions [initial caries] on smooth surface of tooth

    K02.62 Dental caries on smooth surface penetrating into dentin

    K02.63 Dental caries on smooth surface penetrating into pulp

K02.7   Dental root caries

K02.9   Dental caries, unspecified

K03- Other diseases of hard tissues of teeth
    Excludes❷: bruxism (F45.8)
            dental caries (K02.-)
            teeth-grinding NOS (F45.8)

K03.0   Excessive attrition of teeth
        Approximal wear of teeth
        Occlusal wear of teeth

K03.1   Abrasion of teeth
        Dentifrice abrasion of teeth
        Habitual abrasion of teeth
        Occupational abrasion of teeth
        Ritual abrasion of teeth
        Traditional abrasion of teeth
        Wedge defect NOS

K03.2   Erosion of teeth
        Erosion of teeth due to diet
        Erosion of teeth due to drugs and medicaments
        Erosion of teeth due to persistent vomiting
        Erosion of teeth NOS
        Idiopathic erosion of teeth
        Occupational erosion of teeth

K03.3   Pathological resorption of teeth
        Internal granuloma of pulp
        Resorption of teeth (external)

K03.4   Hypercementosis
        Cementation hyperplasia

K03.5   Ankylosis of teeth

K03.6   Deposits [accretions] on teeth
        Betel deposits [accretions] on teeth
        Black deposits [accretions] on teeth
        Extrinsic staining of teeth NOS
        Green deposits [accretions] on teeth
        Materia alba deposits [accretions] on teeth
        Orange deposits [accretions] on teeth
        Staining of teeth NOS
        Subgingival dental calculus
        Supragingival dental calculus
        Tobacco deposits [accretions] on teeth

K03.7   Posteruptive color changes of dental hard tissues
        Excludes❷: deposits [accretions] on teeth (K03.6)

J98 - K03

Excludes 1: = NOT CODED HERE! (Do not code both)

Excludes❷: = Not Included Here

K03.8-   Other specified diseases of hard tissues of teeth

K03.81   Cracked tooth

*Excludes 1:   asymptomatic craze lines in enamel — omit code
broken or fractured tooth due to trauma (S02.5)*

K03.89   Other specified diseases of hard tissues of teeth

K03.9   Disease of hard tissues of teeth, unspecified

K04-   Diseases of pulp and periapical tissues

K04.0   Pulpitis

Acute pulpitis
Chronic (hyperplastic) (ulcerative) pulpitis
Irreversible pulpitis
Reversible pulpitis

K04.1   Necrosis of pulp

Pulpal gangrene

K04.2   Pulp degeneration

Denticles
Pulpal calcifications
Pulpal stones

K04.3   Abnormal hard tissue formation in pulp

Secondary or irregular dentine

K04.4   Acute apical periodontitis of pulpal origin

Acute apical periodontitis NOS

Excludes 1:   acute periodontitis (K05.2-)

K04.5   Chronic apical periodontitis

Apical or periapical granuloma
Apical periodontitis NOS

Excludes 1:   chronic periodontitis (K05.3-)

K04.6   Periapical abscess with sinus

Dental abscess with sinus
Dentoalveolar abscess with sinus

K04.7   Periapical abscess without sinus

Dental abscess without sinus
Dentoalveolar abscess without sinus
Periapical abscess without sinus

K04.8   Radicular cyst

Apical (periodontal) cyst
Periapical cyst
Residual radicular cyst

Excludes ❷: lateral periodontal cyst (K09.0)

K04.9-   Other and unspecified diseases of pulp and periapical tissues

K04.90   Unspecified diseases of pulp and periapical tissues

K04.99   Other diseases of pulp and periapical tissues

K05-   Gingivitis and periodontal diseases

Use additional code to identify:
Alcohol abuse and dependence (F10.-)
Exposure to environmental tobacco smoke (Z77.22)
Exposure to tobacco smoke in the perinatal period (P96.81)
History of tobacco use (Z87.891)
Occupational exposure to environmental tobacco smoke (Z57.31)
Tobacco dependence (F17.-)
Tobacco use (Z72.0)

K05.0-   Acute gingivitis

*Excludes 1:   acute necrotizing ulcerative gingivitis (A69.1)
herpesviral [herpes simplex] gingivostomatitis (B00.2)*

K05.00   Acute gingivitis, <u>plaque</u> induced

Acute gingivitis NOS

K05.01   Acute gingivitis, <u>non</u>-plaque induced

K05.1-   Chronic gingivitis

Desquamative gingivitis (chronic)
Gingivitis (chronic) NOS
Hyperplastic gingivitis (chronic)
Simple marginal gingivitis (chronic)
Ulcerative gingivitis (chronic)

K05.10   Chronic gingivitis, <u>plaque</u> induced

Chronic gingivitis NOS
Gingivitis NOS

K05.11   Chronic gingivitis, <u>non</u>-plaque induced

K05.2-   Aggressive periodontitis

Acute pericoronitis

*Excludes 1:   acute apical periodontitis (K04.4)
periapical abscess (K04.7)
periapical abscess with sinus (K04.6)*

K05.20   Aggressive periodontitis, unspecified

K05.21   Aggressive periodontitis, localized

Periodontal abscess

K05.22   Aggressive periodontitis, generalized

K05.3-   Chronic periodontitis

Chronic pericoronitis
Complex periodontitis
Periodontitis NOS
Simplex periodontitis

Excludes 1:   chronic apical periodontitis (K04.5)

K05.30   Chronic periodontitis, unspecified

K05.31   Chronic periodontitis, localized

K05.32   Chronic periodontitis, generalized

K05.4   Periodontosis

Juvenile periodontosis

K05.5   Other periodontal diseases

Excludes ❷: leukoplakia of gingiva (K13.21)

K05.6   Periodontal disease, unspecified

K06-   Other disorders of gingiva and edentulous alveolar ridge

*Excludes ❷: acute gingivitis (K05.0)
atrophy of edentulous alveolar ridge (K08.2)
chronic gingivitis (K05.1)
gingivitis NOS (K05.1)*

K06.0   Gingival recession

Gingival recession (generalized) (localized) (postinfective)
(postprocedural)

K06.1   Gingival enlargement

Gingival fibromatosis

K06.2   Gingival and edentulous alveolar ridge lesions associated with trauma

Irritative hyperplasia of edentulous ridge [denture hyperplasia]
Use additional code (Chapter 20) to identify external cause or
denture status (Z97.2)

K06.8   Other specified disorders of gingiva and edentulous alveolar ridge

Fibrous epulis
Flabby alveolar ridge
Giant cell epulis
Peripheral giant cell granuloma of gingiva
Pyogenic granuloma of gingiva

Excludes ❷: gingival cyst (K09.0)

K06.9   Disorder of gingiva and edentulous alveolar ridge, unspecified

K08-   Other disorders of teeth and supporting structures

*Excludes ❷: dentofacial anomalies [including malocclusion] (M26.-)
disorders of jaw (M27.-)*

K08.0   Exfoliation of teeth due to systemic causes

Code also underlying systemic condition

K08.1-   <u>Complete loss</u> of teeth

Acquired loss of teeth, complete

*Excludes 1:   congenital absence of teeth (K00.0)
exfoliation of teeth due to systemic causes (K08.0)
partial loss of teeth (K08.4-)*

K08.10-   Complete loss of teeth, <u>unspecified</u> cause

K08.101   Complete loss of teeth, unspecified cause, class I

K08.102   Complete loss of teeth, unspecified cause, class II

K08.103   Complete loss of teeth, unspecified cause, class III

K08.104   Complete loss of teeth, unspecified cause, class IV

K08.109   Complete loss of teeth, unspecified cause, unspecified class

Edentulism NOS

K08.11-   Complete loss of teeth <u>due to trauma</u>

K08.111   Complete loss of teeth due to trauma, class I

K08.112   Complete loss of teeth due to trauma, class II

K08.113   Complete loss of teeth due to trauma, class III

K08.114   Complete loss of teeth due to trauma, class IV

K08.119   Complete loss of teeth due to trauma, unspecified class

K08.12-   Complete loss of teeth <u>due to periodontal diseases</u>

K08.121   Complete loss of teeth due to periodontal diseases, class I

K08.122   Complete loss of teeth due to periodontal diseases, class II

K08.123   Complete loss of teeth due to periodontal diseases, class III

K08.124   Complete loss of teeth due to periodontal diseases, class IV

K08.129   Complete loss of teeth due to periodontal diseases, unspecified class

K08.13-   Complete loss of teeth <u>due to caries</u>

K08.131   Complete loss of teeth due to caries, class I

K08.132   Complete loss of teeth due to caries, class II

K08.133   Complete loss of teeth due to caries, class III

K08.134   Complete loss of teeth due to caries, class IV

K08.139   Complete loss of teeth due to caries, unspecified class

---

Excludes 1: = NOT CODED HERE! (Do not code both)

Excludes ❷: = Not Included Here

K08.19- Complete loss of teeth <u>due to other</u> specified cause

     K08.191   Complete loss of teeth due to other specified cause, class I

     K08.192   Complete loss of teeth due to other specified cause, class II

     K08.193   Complete loss of teeth due to other specified cause, class III

     K08.194   Complete loss of teeth due to other specified cause, class IV

     K08.199   Complete loss of teeth due to other specified cause, unspecified class

K08.2-   Atrophy of edentulous alveolar ridge

     K08.20   Unspecified atrophy of edentulous alveolar ridge
          Atrophy of the mandible NOS
          Atrophy of the maxilla NOS

     K08.21   Minimal atrophy of the mandible
          Minimal atrophy of the edentulous mandible

     K08.22   Moderate atrophy of the mandible
          Moderate atrophy of the edentulous mandible

     K08.23   Severe atrophy of the mandible
          Severe atrophy of the edentulous mandible

     K08.24   Minimal atrophy of maxilla
          Minimal atrophy of the edentulous maxilla

     K08.25   Moderate atrophy of the maxilla
          Moderate atrophy of the edentulous maxilla

     K08.26   Severe atrophy of the maxilla
          Severe atrophy of the edentulous maxilla

K08.3   Retained dental root

K08.4-   <u>Partial loss</u> of teeth
     Acquired loss of teeth, partial
     Excludes 1: complete loss of teeth (K08.1-)
              congenital absence of teeth (K00.0)
     Excludes❷: exfoliation of teeth due to systemic causes (K08.0)

     K08.40- Partial loss of teeth, <u>unspecified</u> cause

       K08.401   Partial loss of teeth, unspecified cause, class I

       K08.402   Partial loss of teeth, unspecified cause, class II

       K08.403   Partial loss of teeth, unspecified cause, class III

       K08.404   Partial loss of teeth, unspecified cause, class IV

       K08.409   Partial loss of teeth, unspecified cause, unspecified class
            Tooth extraction status NOS

     K08.41- Partial loss of teeth <u>due to trauma</u>

       K08.411   Partial loss of teeth due to trauma, class I

       K08.412   Partial loss of teeth due to trauma, class II

       K08.413   Partial loss of teeth due to trauma, class III

       K08.414   Partial loss of teeth due to trauma, class IV

       K08.419   Partial loss of teeth due to trauma, unspecified class

     K08.42- Partial loss of teeth <u>due to periodontal diseases</u>

       K08.421   Partial loss of teeth due to periodontal diseases, class I

       K08.422   Partial loss of teeth due to periodontal diseases, class II

       K08.423   Partial loss of teeth due to periodontal diseases, class III

       K08.424   Partial loss of teeth due to periodontal diseases, class IV

       K08.429   Partial loss of teeth due to periodontal diseases, unspecified class

     K08.43- Partial loss of teeth <u>due to caries</u>

       K08.431   Partial loss of teeth due to caries, class I

       K08.432   Partial loss of teeth due to caries, class II

       K08.433   Partial loss of teeth due to caries, class III

       K08.434   Partial loss of teeth due to caries, class IV

       K08.439   Partial loss of teeth due to caries, unspecified class

     K08.49- Partial loss of teeth <u>due to other</u> specified cause

       K08.491   Partial loss of teeth due to other specified cause, class I

       K08.492   Partial loss of teeth due to other specified cause, class II

       K08.493   Partial loss of teeth due to other specified cause, class III

       K08.494   Partial loss of teeth due to other specified cause, class IV

       K08.499   Partial loss of teeth due to other specified cause, unspecified class

K08.5-   Unsatisfactory restoration of tooth
     Defective bridge, crown, filling
     Defective dental restoration
     Excludes 1: dental restoration status (Z98.811)
     Excludes❷: endosseous dental implant failure (M27.6-)
              unsatisfactory endodontic treatment (M27.5-)

     K08.50   Unsatisfactory restoration of tooth, unspecified
          Defective dental restoration NOS

     K08.51   Open restoration margins of tooth
          Dental restoration failure of marginal integrity
          Open margin on tooth restoration
          Poor gingival margin to tooth restoration

     K08.52   Unrepairable overhanging of dental restorative materials
          Overhanging of tooth restoration

     K08.53- Fractured dental restorative material
       Excludes 1: cracked tooth (K03.81)
              traumatic fracture of tooth (S02.5)

       K08.530   Fractured dental restorative material <u>without</u> loss of material

       K08.531   Fractured dental restorative material <u>with loss of material</u>

       K08.539   Fractured dental restorative material, <u>unspecified</u>

     K08.54   Contour of existing restoration of tooth biologically incompatible with oral health
          Dental restoration failure of periodontal anatomical integrity
          Unacceptable contours of existing restoration of tooth
          Unacceptable morphology of existing restoration of tooth

     K08.55   Allergy to existing dental restorative material
          Use additional code to identify the specific type of allergy

     K08.56   Poor aesthetic of existing restoration of tooth
          Dental restoration aesthetically inadequate or displeasing

     K08.59   Other unsatisfactory restoration of tooth
          Other defective dental restoration

K08.8   Other specified disorders of teeth and supporting structures
     Enlargement of alveolar ridge NOS
     Irregular alveolar process
     Toothache NOS

K08.9   Disorder of teeth and supporting structures, unspecified

K09-   Cysts of oral region, not elsewhere classified
     Includes: Lesions showing histological features both of aneurysmal cyst and of another fibro-osseous lesion
     Excludes❷: cysts of jaw (M27.0-, M27.4-)
              radicular cyst (K04.8)

K09.0   Developmental odontogenic cysts
     Dentigerous cyst
     Eruption cyst
     Follicular cyst
     Gingival cyst
     Lateral periodontal cyst
     Primordial cyst
     Excludes❷: keratocysts (D16.4, D16.5)
              odontogenic keratocystic tumors (D16.4, D16.5)

K09.1   Developmental (nonodontogenic) cysts of oral region
     Cyst (of) incisive canal
     Cyst (of) palatine of papilla
     Globulomaxillary cyst
     Median palatal cyst
     Nasoalveolar cyst
     Nasolabial cyst
     Nasopalatine duct cyst

K09.8   Other cysts of oral region, not elsewhere classified
     Dermoid cyst
     Epidermoid cyst
     Lymphoepithelial cyst
     Epstein's pearl

K09.9   Cyst of oral region, unspecified

K11-   Diseases of salivary glands
     Use additional code to identify:
     Alcohol abuse and dependence (F10.-)
     Exposure to environmental tobacco smoke (Z77.22)
     Exposure to tobacco smoke in the perinatal period (P96.81)
     History of tobacco use (Z87.891)
     Occupational exposure to environmental tobacco smoke (Z57.31)
     Tobacco dependence (F17.-)
     Tobacco use (Z72.0)

K11.0   Atrophy of salivary gland

K11.1   Hypertrophy of salivary gland

K 0 3 - K 1 1

Excludes 1: = NOT CODED HERE! (Do not code both)   **513**   *Excludes❷:* = Not Included Here

K11.2- Sialoadenitis
Parotitis
Excludes 1: epidemic parotitis (B26.-)
mumps (B26.-)
uveoparotid fever [Heerfordt] (D86.89)

K11.20 Sialoadenitis, unspecified
K11.21 Acute sialoadenitis
Excludes 1: acute recurrent sialoadenitis (K11.22)
K11.22 Acute recurrent sialoadenitis
K11.23 Chronic sialoadenitis
K11.3 Abscess of salivary gland
K11.4 Fistula of salivary gland
Excludes 1: congenital fistula of salivary gland (Q38.4)
K11.5 Sialolithiasis
Calculus of salivary gland or duct
Stone of salivary gland or duct
K11.6 Mucocele of salivary gland
Mucous extravasation cyst of salivary gland
Mucous retention cyst of salivary gland
Ranula
K11.7 Disturbances of salivary secretion
Hypoptyalism
Ptyalism
Xerostomia
Excludes❷: dry mouth NOS (R68.2)
K11.8 Other diseases of salivary glands
Benign lymphoepithelial lesion of salivary gland
Mikulicz' disease
Necrotizing sialometaplasia
Sialectasia
Stenosis of salivary duct
Stricture of salivary duct
Excludes 1: sicca syndrome [Sjögren] (M35.0-)
K11.9 Disease of salivary gland, unspecified
Sialoadenopathy NOS

K12- Stomatitis and related lesions
Use additional code to identify:
Alcohol abuse and dependence (F10.-)
Exposure to environmental tobacco smoke (Z77.22)
Exposure to tobacco smoke in the perinatal period (P96.81)
History of tobacco use (Z87.891)
Occupational exposure to environmental tobacco smoke (Z57.31)
Tobacco dependence (F17.-)
Tobacco use (Z72.0)
Excludes 1: cancrum oris (A69.0)
cheilitis (K13.0)
gangrenous stomatitis (A69.0)
herpesviral [herpes simplex] gingivostomatitis (B00.2)
noma (A69.0)
K12.0 Recurrent oral aphthae
Aphthous stomatitis (major) (minor)
Bednar's aphthae
Periadenitis mucosa necrotica recurrens
Recurrent aphthous ulcer
Stomatitis herpetiformis
K12.1 Other forms of stomatitis
Stomatitis NOS
Denture stomatitis
Ulcerative stomatitis
Vesicular stomatitis
Excludes 1: acute necrotizing ulcerative stomatitis (A69.1)
Vincent's stomatitis (A69.1)
K12.2 Cellulitis and abscess of mouth
Cellulitis of mouth (floor)
Submandibular abscess
Excludes❷: abscess of salivary gland (K11.3)
abscess of tongue (K14.0)
periapical abscess (K04.6-K04.7)
periodontal abscess (K05.21)
peritonsillar abscess (J36)
K12.3- Oral mucositis (ulcerative)
Mucositis (oral) (oropharyneal)
Excludes❷: gastrointestinal mucositis (ulcerative) (K92.81)
mucositis (ulcerative) of vagina and vulva (N76.81)
nasal mucositis (ulcerative) (J34.81)

K12.30 Oral mucositis (ulcerative), unspecified
K12.31 Oral mucositis (ulcerative) due to antineoplastic therapy
Use additional code for adverse effect, if applicable, to identify antineoplastic and immunosuppressive drugs (T45.1x5)
Use additional code for other antineoplastic therapy, such as:
Radiological procedure and radiotherapy (Y84.2)

K12.32 Oral mucositis (ulcerative) due to other drugs
Use additional code for adverse effect, if applicable, to identify drug (T36-T50 with fifth or sixth character 5)
K12.33 Oral mucositis (ulcerative) due to radiation
Use additional external cause code (W88-W90, X39.0-) to identify cause
K12.39 Other oral mucositis (ulcerative)
Viral oral mucositis (ulcerative)

K13- Other diseases of lip and oral mucosa
Includes: Epithelial disturbances of tongue
Use additional code to identify:
Alcohol abuse and dependence (F10.-)
Exposure to environmental tobacco smoke (Z77.22)
Exposure to tobacco smoke in the perinatal period (P96.81)
Eistory of tobacco use (Z87.891)
Occupational exposure to environmental tobacco smoke (Z57.31)
Tobacco dependence (F17.-)
Tobacco use (Z72.0)
Excludes❷: certain disorders of gingiva and edentulous alveolar ridge (K05-K06)
cysts of oral region (K09.-)
diseases of tongue (K14.-)
stomatitis and related lesions (K12.-)
K13.0 Diseases of lips
Abscess of lips
Angular cheilitis
Cellulitis of lips
Cheilitis NOS
Cheilodynia
Cheilosis
Exfoliative cheilitis
Fistula of lips
Glandular cheilitis
Hypertrophy of lips
Perlèche NEC
Excludes 1: ariboflavinosis (E53.0)
cheilitis due to radiation-related disorders (L55-L59)
congenital fistula of lips (Q38.0)
congenital hypertrophy of lips (Q18.6)
Perlèche due to candidiasis (B37.83)
Perlèche due to riboflavin deficiency (E53.0)
K13.1 Cheek and lip biting
K13.2- Leukoplakia and other disturbances of oral epithelium, including tongue
Excludes 1: carcinoma in situ of oral epithelium (D00.0-)
hairy leukoplakia (K13.3)
K13.21 Leukoplakia of oral mucosa, including tongue
Leukokeratosis of oral mucosa
Leukoplakia of gingiva, lips, tongue
Excludes 1: hairy leukoplakia (K13.3)
leukokeratosis nicotina palati (K13.24)
K13.22 Minimal keratinized residual ridge mucosa
Minimal keratinization of alveolar ridge mucosa
K13.23 Excessive keratinized residual ridge mucosa
Excessive keratinization of alveolar ridge mucosa
K13.24 Leukokeratosis nicotina palati
Smoker's palate
K13.29 Other disturbances of oral epithelium, including tongue
Erythroplakia of mouth or tongue
Focal epithelial hyperplasia of mouth or tongue
Leukoedema of mouth or tongue
Other oral epithelium disturbances
K13.3 Hairy leukoplakia
K13.4 Granuloma and granuloma-like lesions of oral mucosa
Eosinophilic granuloma
Granuloma pyogenicum
Verrucous xanthoma
K13.5 Oral submucous fibrosis
Submucous fibrosis of tongue
K13.6 Irritative hyperplasia of oral mucosa
Excludes❷: irritative hyperplasia of edentulous ridge [denture hyperplasia] (K06.2)
K13.7- Other and unspecified lesions of oral mucosa
K13.70 Unspecified lesions of oral mucosa
K13.79 Other lesions of oral mucosa
Focal oral mucinosis

K
1
1
-
K
2
5

Excludes 1: = NOT CODED HERE! (Do not code both)

Excludes❷: = Not Included Here

K14- Diseases of tongue
Use additional code to identify:
  Alcohol abuse and dependence (F10.-)
  Exposure to environmental tobacco smoke (Z77.22)
  History of tobacco use (Z87.891)
  Occupational exposure to environmental tobacco smoke (Z57.31)
  Tobacco dependence (F17.-)
  Tobacco use (Z72.0)
Excludes❷: erythroplakia (K13.29)
    focal epithelial hyperplasia (K13.29)
    leukedema of tongue (K13.29)
    leukoplakia of tongue (K13.21)
    hairy leukoplakia (K13.3)
    macroglossia (congenital) (Q38.2)
    submucous fibrosis of tongue (K13.5)

K14.0 Glossitis
  Abscess of tongue
  Ulceration (traumatic) of tongue
  Excludes 1: atrophic glossitis (K14.4)

K14.1 Geographic tongue
  Benign migratory glossitis
  Glossitis areata exfoliativa

K14.2 Median rhomboid glossitis

K14.3 Hypertrophy of tongue papillae
  Black hairy tongue
  Coated tongue
  Hypertrophy of foliate papillae
  Lingua villosa nigra

K14.4 Atrophy of tongue papillae
  Atrophic glossitis

K14.5 Plicated tongue
  Fissured tongue
  Furrowed tongue
  Scrotal tongue
  Excludes 1: fissured tongue, congenital (Q38.3)

K14.6 Glossodynia
  Glossopyrosis
  Painful tongue

K14.8 Other diseases of tongue
  Atrophy of tongue
  Crenated tongue
  Enlargement of tongue
  Glossocele
  Glossoptosis
  Hypertrophy of tongue

K14.9 Disease of tongue, unspecified
  Glossopathy NOS

Diseases of esophagus, stomach and duodenum (K20-K31)

Excludes❷: hiatus hernia (K44.-)

K20- Esophagitis
Use additional code to identify:
  Alcohol abuse and dependence (F10.-)
Excludes 1: erosion of esophagus (K22.1-)
    esophagitis with gastro-esophageal reflux disease (K21.0)
    reflux esophagitis (K21.0)
    ulcerative esophagitis (K22.1-)
Excludes❷: eosinophilic gastritis or gastroenteritis (K52.81)

K20.0 Eosinophilic esophagitis

K20.8 Other esophagitis
  Abscess of esophagus

K20.9 Esophagitis, unspecified
  Esophagitis NOS

K21- Gastro-esophageal reflux disease
Excludes 1: newborn esophageal reflux (P78.83)

K21.0 Gastro-esophageal reflux disease with esophagitis
  Reflux esophagitis

K21.9 Gastro-esophageal reflux disease without esophagitis
  Esophageal reflux NOS

K22- Other diseases of esophagus
Excludes❷: esophageal varices (I85.-)

K22.0 Achalasia of cardia
  Achalasia NOS
  Cardiospasm
  Excludes 1: congenital cardiospasm (Q39.5)

K22.1- Ulcer of esophagus
  Barrett's ulcer
  Erosion of esophagus
  Fungal ulcer of esophagus
  Peptic ulcer of esophagus
  Ulcer of esophagus due to ingestion of chemicals
  Ulcer of esophagus due to ingestion of drugs and medicaments
  Ulcerative esophagitis
Code first poisoning due to drug or toxin, if applicable (T36-T65 with fifth or sixth character 1-4 or 6)
Use additional code for adverse effect, if applicable, to identify drug (T36-T50 with fifth or sixth character 5)
  Excludes 1: Barrett's esophagus (K22.7-)

K22.10 Ulcer of esophagus without bleeding
  Ulcer of esophagus NOS

K22.11 Ulcer of esophagus with bleeding
  Excludes❷: bleeding esophageal varices (I85.01, I85.11)

K22.2 Esophageal obstruction
  Compression of esophagus
  Constriction of esophagus
  Stenosis of esophagus
  Stricture of esophagus
  Excludes 1: congenital stenosis or stricture of esophagus (Q39.3)

K22.3 Perforation of esophagus
  Rupture of esophagus
  Excludes 1: traumatic perforation of (thoracic) esophagus (S27.8-)

K22.4 Dyskinesia of esophagus
  Corkscrew esophagus
  Diffuse esophageal spasm
  Spasm of esophagus
  Excludes 1: cardiospasm (K22.0)

K22.5 Diverticulum of esophagus, acquired
  Esophageal pouch, acquired
  Excludes 1: diverticulum of esophagus (congenital) (Q39.6)

K22.6 Gastro-esophageal laceration-hemorrhage syndrome
  Mallory-Weiss syndrome

K22.7- Barrett's esophagus
  Barrett's disease
  Barrett's syndrome
  Excludes 1: Barrett's ulcer (K22.1)
    malignant neoplasm of esophagus (C15.-)

K22.70 Barrett's esophagus without dysplasia
  Barrett's esophagus NOS

K22.71- Barrett's esophagus with dysplasia
  K22.710 Barrett's esophagus with low grade dysplasia
  K22.711 Barrett's esophagus with high grade dysplasia
  K22.719 Barrett's esophagus with dysplasia, unspecified

K22.8 Other specified diseases of esophagus
  Hemorrhage of esophagus NOS
  Excludes❷: esophageal varices (I85.-)
    Paterson-Kelly syndrome (D50.1)

K22.9 Disease of esophagus, unspecified

K23 Disorders of esophagus in diseases classified elsewhere
Code first underlying disease, such as:
  Congenital syphilis (A50.5)
Excludes 1: late syphilis (A52.79)
    megaesophagus due to Chagas' disease (B57.31)
    tuberculosis (A18.83)

K25- Gastric ulcer
Includes: Erosion (acute) of stomach
    Pylorus ulcer (peptic)
    Stomach ulcer (peptic)
Use additional code to identify:
  Alcohol abuse and dependence (F10.-)
Excludes 1: acute gastritis (K29.0-)
    peptic ulcer NOS (K27.-)

K25.0 Acute gastric ulcer with hemorrhage

K25.1 Acute gastric ulcer with perforation

K25.2 Acute gastric ulcer with both hemorrhage and perforation

K25.3 Acute gastric ulcer without hemorrhage or perforation

K25.4 Chronic or unspecified gastric ulcer with hemorrhage

K25.5 Chronic or unspecified gastric ulcer with perforation

K25.6 Chronic or unspecified gastric ulcer with both hemorrhage and perforation

K25.7 Chronic gastric ulcer without hemorrhage or perforation

K25.9 Gastric ulcer, unspecified as acute or chronic, without hemorrhage or perforation

K
1
1
-
K
2
5

K26- <u>Duodenal</u> ulcer
  Includes: Duodenum ulcer (peptic)
          Erosion (acute) of duodenum
          Postpyloric ulcer (peptic)
  Use additional code to identify:
          Alcohol abuse and dependence (F10.-)
  Excludes 1: peptic ulcer NOS (K27.-)
  K26.0 <u>Acute</u> duodenal ulcer with hemorrhage
  K26.1 <u>Acute</u> duodenal ulcer with perforation
  K26.2 <u>Acute</u> duodenal ulcer with both hemorrhage and perforation
  K26.3 <u>Acute</u> duodenal ulcer without hemorrhage or perforation
  K26.4 Chronic or unspecified duodenal ulcer with hemorrhage
  K26.5 Chronic or unspecified duodenal ulcer with perforation
  K26.6 Chronic or unspecified duodenal ulcer with both hemorrhage and perforation
  K26.7 Chronic duodenal ulcer without hemorrhage or perforation
  K26.9 Duodenal ulcer, <u>unspecified as acute or chronic</u>, without hemorrhage or perforation

K27- <u>Peptic ulcer</u>, site unspecified
  Includes: Gastroduodenal ulcer NOS
          Peptic ulcer NOS
  Use additional code to identify:
          Alcohol abuse and dependence (F10.-)
  Excludes 1: peptic ulcer of newborn (P78.82)
  K27.0 <u>Acute</u> peptic ulcer, site unspecified, with hemorrhage
  K27.1 <u>Acute</u> peptic ulcer, site unspecified, with perforation
  K27.2 <u>Acute</u> peptic ulcer, site unspecified, with both hemorrhage and perforation
  K27.3 <u>Acute</u> peptic ulcer, site unspecified, without hemorrhage or perforation
  K27.4 Chronic or unspecified peptic ulcer, site unspecified, with hemorrhage
  K27.5 Chronic or unspecified peptic ulcer, site unspecified, with perforation
  K27.6 Chronic or unspecified peptic ulcer, site unspecified, with both hemorrhage and perforation
  K27.7 Chronic peptic ulcer, site unspecified, without hemorrhage or perforation
  K27.9 Peptic ulcer, site unspecified, <u>unspecified as acute or chronic</u>, without hemorrhage or perforation

K28- <u>Gastrojejunal</u> ulcer
  Includes: Anastomotic ulcer (peptic) or erosion
          Gastrocolic ulcer (peptic) or erosion
          Gastrointestinal ulcer (peptic) or erosion
          Gastrojejunal ulcer (peptic) or erosion
          Jejunal ulcer (peptic) or erosion
          Marginal ulcer (peptic) or erosion
          Stomal ulcer (peptic) or erosion
  Use additional code to identify:
          Alcohol abuse and dependence (F10.-)
  Excludes 1: primary ulcer of small intestine (K63.3)
  K28.0 <u>Acute</u> gastrojejunal ulcer with hemorrhage
  K28.1 <u>Acute</u> gastrojejunal ulcer with perforation
  K28.2 <u>Acute</u> gastrojejunal ulcer with both hemorrhage and perforation
  K28.3 <u>Acute</u> gastrojejunal ulcer without hemorrhage or perforation
  K28.4 Chronic or unspecified gastrojejunal ulcer with hemorrhage
  K28.5 Chronic or unspecified gastrojejunal ulcer with perforation
  K28.6 Chronic or unspecified gastrojejunal ulcer with both hemorrhage and perforation
  K28.7 Chronic gastrojejunal ulcer without hemorrhage or perforation
  K28.9 Gastrojejunal ulcer, <u>unspecified as acute or chronic</u>, without hemorrhage or perforation

K29- Gastritis and duodenitis
  Excludes 1: eosinophilic gastritis or gastroenteritis (K52.81)
          Zollinger-Ellison syndrome (E16.4)
  K29.0- <u>Acute gastritis</u>
          Use additional code to identify:
              Alcohol abuse and dependence (F10.-)
          Excludes 1: erosion (acute) of stomach (K25.-)
      K29.00 Acute gastritis <u>without</u> bleeding
      K29.01 Acute gastritis <u>with bleeding</u>
  K29.2- <u>Alcoholic</u> gastritis
          Use additional code to identify:
              Alcohol abuse and dependence (F10.-)
      K29.20 Alcoholic gastritis <u>without</u> bleeding
      K29.21 Alcoholic gastritis <u>with bleeding</u>

K29.3- <u>Chronic superficial</u> gastritis
      K29.30 Chronic superficial gastritis <u>without</u> bleeding
      K29.31 Chronic superficial gastritis <u>with bleeding</u>
  K29.4- <u>Chronic atrophic</u> gastritis
          Gastric atrophy
      K29.40 Chronic atrophic gastritis <u>without</u> bleeding
      K29.41 Chronic atrophic gastritis <u>with bleeding</u>
  K29.5- <u>Unspecified chronic</u> gastritis
          Chronic antral gastritis
          Chronic fundal gastritis
      K29.50 Unspecified chronic gastritis <u>without</u> bleeding
      K29.51 Unspecified chronic gastritis <u>with bleeding</u>
  K29.6- <u>Other</u> gastritis
          Giant hypertrophic gastritis
          Granulomatous gastritis
          Ménétrier's disease
      K29.60 Other gastritis <u>without</u> bleeding
      K29.61 Other gastritis <u>with bleeding</u>
  K29.7- Gastritis, <u>unspecified</u>
      K29.70 Gastritis, unspecified, <u>without</u> bleeding
      K29.71 Gastritis, unspecified, <u>with bleeding</u>
  K29.8- <u>Duodenitis</u>
      K29.80 Duodenitis <u>without</u> bleeding
      K29.81 Duodenitis <u>with bleeding</u>
  K29.9- <u>Gastroduodenitis</u>, unspecified
      K29.90 Gastroduodenitis, unspecified, <u>without</u> bleeding
      K29.91 Gastroduodenitis, unspecified, <u>with bleeding</u>

K30 **Functional dyspepsia**
          Indigestion
  Excludes 1: dyspepsia NOS (R10.13)
          heartburn (R12)
          nervous dyspepsia (F45.8)
          neurotic dyspepsia (F45.8)
          psychogenic dyspepsia (F45.8)

K31- **Other diseases of stomach and duodenum**
          Includes: Functional disorders of stomach
  Excludes❷: diabetic gastroparesis (E08.43, E09.43, E10.43, E11.43, E13.43)
          diverticulum of duodenum (K57.00-K57.13)
  K31.0 **Acute dilatation of stomach**
          Acute distention of stomach
  K31.1 **Adult hypertrophic pyloric stenosis**
          Pyloric stenosis NOS
          Excludes 1: congenital or infantile pyloric stenosis (Q40.0)
  K31.2 **Hourglass stricture and stenosis of stomach**
          Excludes 1: congenital hourglass stomach (Q40.2)
              hourglass contraction of stomach (K31.89)
  K31.3 **Pylorospasm, <u>not elsewhere classified</u>**
          Excludes 1: congenital or infantile pylorospasm (Q40.0)
              neurotic pylorospasm (F45.8)
              psychogenic pylorospasm (F45.8)
  K31.4 **Gastric diverticulum**
          Excludes 1: congenital diverticulum of stomach (Q40.2)
  K31.5 **Obstruction of duodenum**
          Constriction of duodenum
          Duodenal ileus (chronic)
          Stenosis of duodenum
          Stricture of duodenum
          Volvulus of duodenum
          Excludes 1: congenital stenosis of duodenum (Q41.0)
  K31.6 **Fistula of stomach and duodenum**
          Gastrocolic fistula
          Gastrojejunocolic fistula
  K31.7 **Polyp of stomach and duodenum**
          Excludes 1: adenomatous polyp of stomach (D13.1)
  K31.8- **Other specified diseases of stomach and duodenum**
      K31.81- **Angiodysplasia of stomach and duodenum**
          K31.811 Angiodysplasia of stomach and duodenum <u>with bleeding</u>
          K31.819 Angiodysplasia of stomach and duodenum <u>without</u> bleeding
                  Angiodysplasia of stomach and duodenum NOS
      K31.82 Dieulafoy lesion (hemorrhagic) of stomach and duodenum
              Excludes❷: Dieulafoy lesion of intestine (K63.81)
      K31.83 Achlorhydria

K
2
6
–
K
4
1

K31.84 Gastroparesis
Gastroparalysis
Code first undrlying disease, if known, such as:
Anorexia nervosa (F50.0-)
Diabetes mellitus (E08.43, E09.43, E10.43, E11.43, E13.43)
Scleroderma (M34-)
K31.89 Other diseases of stomach and duodenum
K31.9 Disease of stomach and duodenum, unspecified

Diseases of appendix (K35-K38)

K35- Acute appendicitis
  K35.2 Acute appendicitis with generalized peritonitis
Appendicitis (acute) with generalized (diffuse) peritonitis
following rupture or perforation of appendix
Perforated appendix NOS
Ruptured appendix NOS
  K35.3 Acute appendicitis with localized peritonitis
Acute appendicitis with or without perforation or rupture NOS
Acute appendicitis with or without perforation or rupture with
localized peritonitis
Acute appendicitis with peritoneal abscess
  K35.8- Other and unspecified acute appendicitis
    K35.80 Unspecified acute appendicitis
Acute appendicitis NOS
Acute appendicitis without (localized) (generalized) peritonitis
    K35.89 Other acute appendicitis
K36 Other appendicitis
Chronic appendicitis
Recurrent appendicitis
K37 Unspecified appendicitis
Excludes 1: unspecified appendicitis with peritonitis (K35.2-K35.3)
K38- Other diseases of appendix
  K38.0 Hyperplasia of appendix
  K38.1 Appendicular concretions
Fecalith of appendix
Stercolith of appendix
  K38.2 Diverticulum of appendix
  K38.3 Fistula of appendix
  K38.8 Other specified diseases of appendix
Intussusception of appendix
  K38.9 Disease of appendix, unspecified

Hernia (K40-K46)

Note: Hernia with both gangrene and obstruction is classified to hernia with
gangrene.
Includes: Acquired hernia
Congenital [except diaphragmatic or hiatus] hernia
Recurrent hernia

K40- Inguinal hernia
Includes: Bubonocele
Direct inguinal hernia
Double inguinal hernia
Indirect inguinal hernia
Inguinal hernia NOS
Oblique inguinal hernia
Scrotal hernia
  K40.0- Bilateral inguinal hernia, with obstruction, without gangrene
Inguinal hernia (bilateral) causing obstruction without gangrene
Incarcerated inguinal hernia (bilateral) without gangrene
Irreducible inguinal hernia (bilateral) without gangrene
Strangulated inguinal hernia (bilateral) without gangrene
    **K40.00 Bilateral inguinal hernia, with obstruction, without
gangrene, not specified as recurrent**
Bilateral inguinal hernia, with obstruction, without gangrene
NOS
    **K40.01 Bilateral inguinal hernia, with obstruction, without
gangrene, recurrent**
  K40.1- Bilateral inguinal hernia, with gangrene
    **K40.10 Bilateral inguinal hernia, with gangrene, not specified as
recurrent**
Bilateral inguinal hernia, with gangrene NOS
    K40.11 Bilateral inguinal hernia, with gangrene, recurrent
  K40.2- Bilateral inguinal hernia, without obstruction or gangrene
    **K40.20 Bilateral inguinal hernia, without obstruction or gangrene,
not specified as recurrent**
Bilateral inguinal hernia NOS
    **K40.21 Bilateral inguinal hernia, without obstruction or gangrene,
recurrent**

K40.3- Unilateral inguinal hernia, with obstruction, without gangrene
Inguinal hernia (unilateral) causing obstruction without gangrene
Incarcerated inguinal hernia (unilateral) without gangrene
Irreducible inguinal hernia (unilateral) without gangrene
Strangulated inguinal hernia (unilateral) without gangrene
  **K40.30 Unilateral inguinal hernia, with obstruction, without
gangrene, not specified as recurrent**
Inguinal hernia, with obstruction NOS
Unilateral inguinal hernia, with obstruction, without gangrene
NOS
  **K40.31 Unilateral inguinal hernia, with obstruction, without
gangrene, recurrent**
K40.4- Unilateral inguinal hernia, with gangrene
  **K40.40 Unilateral inguinal hernia, with gangrene, not specified as
recurrent**
Inguinal hernia with gangrene NOS
Unilateral inguinal hernia with gangrene NOS
  K40.41 Unilateral inguinal hernia, with gangrene, recurrent
K40.9- Unilateral inguinal hernia, without obstruction or gangrene
  **K40.90 Unilateral inguinal hernia, without obstruction or gangrene,
not specified as recurrent**
Inguinal hernia NOS
Unilateral inguinal hernia NOS
  **K40.91 Unilateral inguinal hernia, without obstruction or gangrene,
recurrent**

K41- Femoral hernia
K41.0- Bilateral femoral hernia, with obstruction, without gangrene
Femoral hernia (bilateral) causing obstruction, without gangrene
Incarcerated femoral hernia (bilateral), without gangrene
Irreducible femoral hernia (bilateral), without gangrene
Strangulated femoral hernia (bilateral), without gangrene
  **K41.00 Bilateral femoral hernia, with obstruction, without gangrene,
not specified as recurrent**
Bilateral femoral hernia, with obstruction, without gangrene
NOS
  **K41.01 Bilateral femoral hernia, with obstruction, without gangrene,
recurrent**
K41.1- Bilateral femoral hernia, with gangrene
  **K41.10 Bilateral femoral hernia, with gangrene, not specified as
recurrent**
Bilateral femoral hernia, with gangrene NOS
  K41.11 Bilateral femoral hernia, with gangrene, recurrent
K41.2- Bilateral femoral hernia, without obstruction or gangrene
  **K41.20 Bilateral femoral hernia, without obstruction or gangrene,
not specified as recurrent**
Bilateral femoral hernia NOS
  **K41.21 Bilateral femoral hernia, without obstruction or gangrene,
recurrent**
K41.3- Unilateral femoral hernia, with obstruction, without gangrene
Femoral hernia (unilateral) causing obstruction, without gangrene
Incarcerated femoral hernia (unilateral), without gangrene
Irreducible femoral hernia (unilateral), without gangrene
Strangulated femoral hernia (unilateral), without gangrene
  **K41.30 Unilateral femoral hernia, with obstruction, without
gangrene, not specified as recurrent**
Femoral hernia, with obstruction NOS
Unilateral femoral hernia, with obstruction NOS
  **K41.31 Unilateral femoral hernia, with obstruction, without
gangrene, recurrent**
K41.4- Unilateral femoral hernia, with gangrene
  **K41.40 Unilateral femoral hernia, with gangrene, not specified as
recurrent**
Femoral hernia, with gangrene NOS
Unilateral femoral hernia, with gangrene NOS
  K41.41 Unilateral femoral hernia, with gangrene, recurrent
K41.9- Unilateral femoral hernia, without obstruction or gangrene
  **K41.90 Unilateral femoral hernia, without obstruction or gangrene,
not specified as recurrent**
Femoral hernia NOS
Unilateral femoral hernia NOS
  **K41.91 Unilateral femoral hernia, without obstruction or gangrene,
recurrent**

K
2
6
-
K
4
1

K42- Umbilical hernia
Includes: Paraumbilical hernia
Excludes 1: omphalocele (Q79.2)

K42.0 Umbilical hernia with obstruction, without gangrene
Umbilical hernia causing obstruction, without gangrene
Incarcerated umbilical hernia, without gangrene
Irreducible umbilical hernia, without gangrene
Strangulated umbilical hernia, without gangrene

K42.1 Umbilical hernia with gangrene
Gangrenous umbilical hernia

K42.9 Umbilical hernia without obstruction or gangrene
Umbilical hernia NOS

K43- Ventral hernia

K43.0 Incisional hernia with obstruction, without gangrene
Incarcerated incisional hernia, without gangrene
Incisional hernia causing obstruction, without gangrene
Irreducible incisional hernia, without gangrene
Strangulated incisional hernia, without gangrene

K43.1 Incisional hernia with gangrene
Gangrenous incisional hernia

K43.2 Incisional hernia without obstruction, or gangrene
Incisional hernia NOS

K43.3 Parastomal hernia with obstruction, without gangrene
Incarcerated parastomal hernia, without gangrene
Irreducible parastomal hernia, without gangrene
Parastomal hernia causing obstruction, without gangrene
Strangulated parastomal hernia, without gangrene

K43.4 Parastomal hernia with gangrene
Gangrenous parastomal hernia

K43.5 Parastomal hernia without obstruction, or gangrene
Parastomal hernia NOS

K43.6 Other and unspecified ventral hernia with obstruction, without gangrene
Epigastric hernia, without gangrene
Hypogastric hernia causing obstruction, without gangrene
Incarcerated epigastric hernia, without gangrene
Incarcerated hypogastric hernia, without gangrene
Incarcerated midline hernia, without gangrene
Incarcerated spigelian hernia, without gangrene
Incarcerated subxiphoid hernia, without gangrene
Irreducible epigastric hernia, without gangrene
Irreducible hypogastric hernia, without gangrene
Irreducible midline hernia, without gangrene
Irreducible spigelian hernia, without gangrene
Irreducible subxiphoid hernia, without gangrene
Midline hernia causing obstruction, without gangrene
Spigelian hernia causing obstruction, without gangrene
Strangulated epigastric hernia, without gangrene
Strangulated hypogastric hernia, without gangrene
Strangulated midline hernia, without gangrene
Strangulated spigelian hernia, without gangrene
Strangulated subxiphoid hernia, without gangrene
Subxiphoid hernia causing obstruction, without gangrene

K43.7 Other and unspecified ventral hernia with gangrene
Any condition listed under K43.6 specified as gangenous

K43.9 Ventral hernia without obstruction or gangrene
Epigastric hernia
Ventral hernia NOS

K44- Diaphragmatic hernia
Includes: Hiatus hernia (esophageal) (sliding)
Paraesophageal hernia
*Excludes 1: congenital diaphragmatic hernia (Q79.0)
congenital hiatus hernia (Q40.1)*

K44.0 Diaphragmatic hernia with obstruction, without gangrene
Diaphragmatic hernia causing obstruction
Incarcerated diaphragmatic hernia
Irreducible diaphragmatic hernia
Strangulated diaphragmatic hernia

K44.1 Diaphragmatic hernia with gangrene
Gangrenous diaphragmatic hernia

K44.9 Diaphragmatic hernia without obstruction or gangrene
Diaphragmatic hernia NOS

K45- Other abdominal hernia
Includes: Abdominal hernia, specified site NEC
Lumbar hernia
Obturator hernia
Pudendal hernia
Retroperitoneal hernia
Sciatic hernia

K45.0 Other specified abdominal hernia with obstruction, without gangrene
Other specified abdominal hernia causing obstruction
Other specified incarcerated abdominal hernia
Other specified irreducible abdominal hernia
Other specified strangulated abdominal hernia

K45.1 Other specified abdominal hernia with gangrene
Any condition listed under K45 specified as gangrenous

K45.8 Other specified abdominal hernia without obstruction or gangrene

K46- Unspecified abdominal hernia
Includes: Enterocele
Epiplocele
Hernia NOS
Interstitial hernia
Intestinal hernia
Intra-abdominal hernia
Excludes 1: vaginal enterocele (N81.5)

K46.0 Unspecified abdominal hernia with obstruction, without gangrene
Unspecified abdominal hernia causing obstruction
Unspecified incarcerated abdominal hernia
Unspecified irreducible abdominal hernia
Unspecified strangulated abdominal hernia

K46.1 Unspecified abdominal hernia with gangrene
Any condition listed under K46 specified as gangrenous

K46.9 Unspecified abdominal hernia without obstruction or gangrene
Abdominal hernia NOS

Noninfective enteritis and colitis (K50-K52)

Includes: Noninfective inflammatory bowel disease
*Excludes 1: irritable bowel syndrome (K58.-)
megacolon (K59.3)*

K50- Crohn's disease [regional enteritis]
Includes: Granulomatous enteritis
Use additional code to identify manifestations, such as:
Pyoderma gangrenosum (L88)
Excludes 1: ulcerative colitis (K51.-)

K50.0- Crohn's disease of small intestine
Crohn's disease [regional enteritis] of duodenum
Crohn's disease [regional enteritis] of ileum
Crohn's disease [regional enteritis] of jejunum
Regional ileitis
Terminal ileitis
Excludes 1: Crohn's disease of both small and large intestine (K50.8-)

K50.00 Crohn's disease of small intestine without complications

K50.01- Crohn's disease of small intestine with complications

K50.011 Crohn's disease of small intestine with rectal bleeding

K50.012 Crohn's disease of small intestine with intestinal obstruction

K50.013 Crohn's disease of small intestine with fistula

K50.014 Crohn's disease of small intestine with abscess

K50.018 Crohn's disease of small intestine with other complication

K50.019 Crohn's disease of small intestine with unspecified complications

K50.1- Crohn's disease of large intestine
Crohn's disease [regional enteritis] of colon
Crohn's disease [regional enteritis] of large bowel
Crohn's disease [regional enteritis] of rectum
Granulomatous colitis
Regional colitis
Excludes 1: Crohn's disease of both small and large intestine (K50.8-)

K50.10 Crohn's disease of large intestine without complications

K50.11- Crohn's disease of large intestine with complications

K50.111 Crohn's disease of large intestine with rectal bleeding

K50.112 Crohn's disease of large intestine with intestinal obstruction

K50.113 Crohn's disease of large intestine with fistula

K50.114 Crohn's disease of large intestine with abscess

K50.118 Crohn's disease of large intestine with other complication

K
4
2
-
K
5
2

K50.119   Crohn's disease of large intestine with <u>unspecified</u> complications

K50.8-   Crohn's disease of <u>both small and large intestine</u>

K50.80   Crohn's disease of both small and large intestine <u>without</u> complications

K50.81- Crohn's disease of both small and large intestine <u>with</u> complications

K50.811   Crohn's disease of both small and large intestine with <u>rectal bleeding</u>

K50.812   Crohn's disease of both small and large intestine with <u>intestinal obstruction</u>

K50.813   Crohn's disease of both small and large intestine with <u>fistula</u>

K50.814   Crohn's disease of both small and large intestine with <u>abscess</u>

K50.818   Crohn's disease of both small and large intestine with <u>other</u> complication

K50.819   Crohn's disease of both small and large intestine with <u>unspecified</u> complications

K50.9-   Crohn's disease, <u>unspecified</u>

K50.90   Crohn's disease, unspecified, <u>without</u> complications
Crohn's disease NOS
Regional enteritis NOS

K50.91- Crohn's disease, unspecified, <u>with</u> complications

K50.911   Crohn's disease, unspecified, with <u>rectal bleeding</u>

K50.912   Crohn's disease, unspecified, with <u>intestinal obstruction</u>

K50.913   Crohn's disease, unspecified, with <u>fistula</u>

K50.914   Crohn's disease, unspecified, with <u>abscess</u>

K50.918   Crohn's disease, unspecified, with other complication

K50.919   Crohn's disease, unspecified, with <u>unspecified</u> complications

K51-   <u>Ulcerative colitis</u>
Use additional code to identify manifestations, such as:
Pyoderma gangrenosum (L88)
Excludes 1: Crohn's disease [regional enteritis] (K50.-)

K51.0-   Ulcerative <u>(chronic) pancolitis</u>
Backwash ileitis

K51.00   Ulcerative (chronic) pancolitis <u>without</u> complications
Ulcerative (chronic) pancolitis NOS

K51.01- Ulcerative (chronic) pancolitis <u>with</u> complications

K51.011   Ulcerative (chronic) pancolitis with <u>rectal bleeding</u>

K51.012   Ulcerative (chronic) pancolitis with <u>intestinal obstruction</u>

K51.013   Ulcerative (chronic) pancolitis with <u>fistula</u>

K51.014   Ulcerative (chronic) pancolitis with <u>abscess</u>

K51.018   Ulcerative (chronic) pancolitis with <u>other</u> complication

K51.019   Ulcerative (chronic) pancolitis with <u>unspecified</u> complications

K51.2-   Ulcerative <u>(chronic) proctitis</u>

K51.20   Ulcerative (chronic) proctitis <u>without</u> complications
Ulcerative (chronic) proctitis NOS

K51.21- Ulcerative (chronic) proctitis <u>with</u> complications

K51.211   Ulcerative (chronic) proctitis with <u>rectal bleeding</u>

K51.212   Ulcerative (chronic) proctitis with <u>intestinal obstruction</u>

K51.213   Ulcerative (chronic) proctitis with <u>fistula</u>

K51.214   Ulcerative (chronic) proctitis with <u>abscess</u>

K51.218   Ulcerative (chronic) proctitis with <u>other</u> complication

K51.219   Ulcerative (chronic) proctitis with <u>unspecified</u> complications

K51.3-   Ulcerative <u>(chronic) rectosigmoiditis</u>

K51.30   Ulcerative (chronic) rectosigmoiditis <u>without</u> complications
Ulcerative (chronic) rectosigmoiditis NOS

K51.31- Ulcerative (chronic) rectosigmoiditis <u>with</u> complications

K51.311   Ulcerative (chronic) rectosigmoiditis with <u>rectal bleeding</u>

K51.312   Ulcerative (chronic) rectosigmoiditis with <u>intestinal obstruction</u>

K51.313   Ulcerative (chronic) rectosigmoiditis with <u>fistula</u>

K51.314   Ulcerative (chronic) rectosigmoiditis with <u>abscess</u>

K51.318   Ulcerative (chronic) rectosigmoiditis with <u>other</u> complication

K51.319   Ulcerative (chronic) rectosigmoiditis with <u>unspecified</u> complications

K51.4-   <u>Inflammatory polyps of colon</u>
Excludes 1: adenomatous polyp of colon (D12.6)
polyposis of colon (D12.6)
polyps of colon NOS (K63.5)

K51.40   Inflammatory polyps of colon <u>without</u> complications
Inflammatory polyps of colon NOS

K51.41- Inflammatory polyps of colon <u>with</u> complications

K51.411   Inflammatory polyps of colon with <u>rectal bleeding</u>

K51.412   Inflammatory polyps of colon with <u>intestinal obstruction</u>

K51.413   Inflammatory polyps of colon with <u>fistula</u>

K51.414   Inflammatory polyps of colon with <u>abscess</u>

K51.418   Inflammatory polyps of colon with <u>other</u> complication

K51.419   Inflammatory polyps of colon with <u>unspecified</u> complications

K51.5-   <u>Left sided colitis</u>
Left hemicolitis

K51.50   Left sided colitis <u>without</u> complications
Left sided colitis NOS

K51.51- Left sided colitis <u>with</u> complications

K51.511   Left sided colitis with <u>rectal bleeding</u>

K51.512   Left sided colitis with <u>intestinal obstruction</u>

K51.513   Left sided colitis with <u>fistula</u>

K51.514   Left sided colitis with <u>abscess</u>

K51.518   Left sided colitis with <u>other</u> complication

K51.519   Left sided colitis with <u>unspecified</u> complications

K51.8-   <u>Other ulcerative colitis</u>

K51.80   Other ulcerative colitis <u>without</u> complications

K51.81- Other ulcerative colitis <u>with</u> complications

K51.811   Other ulcerative colitis with <u>rectal bleeding</u>

K51.812   Other ulcerative colitis with <u>intestinal obstruction</u>

K51.813   Other ulcerative colitis with <u>fistula</u>

K51.814   Other ulcerative colitis with <u>abscess</u>

K51.818   Other ulcerative colitis with <u>other</u> complication

K51.819   Other ulcerative colitis with <u>unspecified</u> complications

K51.9-   <u>Ulcerative colitis, unspecified</u>

K51.90   Ulcerative colitis, unspecified, <u>without</u> complications

K51.91- Ulcerative colitis, unspecified, <u>with</u> complications

K51.911   Ulcerative colitis, unspecified with <u>rectal bleeding</u>

K51.912   Ulcerative colitis, unspecified with <u>intestinal obstruction</u>

K51.913   Ulcerative colitis, unspecified with <u>fistula</u>

K51.914   Ulcerative colitis, unspecified with <u>abscess</u>

K51.918   Ulcerative colitis, unspecified with <u>other</u> complication

K51.919   Ulcerative colitis, unspecified with <u>unspecified</u> complications

K52-   Other and unspecified noninfective gastroenteritis and colitis

K52.0   Gastroenteritis and colitis due to radiation

K52.1   Toxic gastroenteritis and colitis
Drug-induced gastroenteritis and colitis
Code first (T51-T65) to identify toxic agent
Use additional code for adverse effect, if applicable, to identify drug (T36-T50 with fifth or sixth character 5)

K52.2   Allergic and dietetic gastroenteritis and colitis
Food hypersensitivity gastroenteritis or colitis
Use additional code to identify type of food allergy (Z91.01-, Z91.02-)

K52.8-   Other specified noninfective gastroenteritis and colitis

K52.81   Eosinophilic gastritis or gastroenteritis
Eosinophilic enteritis
Excludes 1: eosinophilic esophagitis (K20.0)

K52.82   Eosinophilic colitis

K52.89   Other specified noninfective gastroenteritis and colitis
Collagenous colitis
Lymphocytic colitis
Microscopic colitis (collagenous or lymphocytic)

K52.9   Noninfective gastroenteritis and colitis, unspecified
Colitis NOS
Enteritis NOS
Gastroenteritis NOS
Ileitis NOS
Jejunitis NOS
Sigmoiditis NOS
Excludes 1: diarrhea NOS (R19.7)
functional diarrhea (K59.1)
infectious gastroenteritis and colitis NOS (A09)
neonatal diarrhea (noninfective) (P78.3)
psychogenic diarrhea (F45.8)

K 4 2 - K 5 2

Other diseases of intestines (K55-K64)

K55- Vascular disorders of intestine
Excludes 1: necrotizing enterocolitis of newborn (P77.-)

K55.0 Acute vascular disorders of intestine
  Acute fulminant ischemic colitis
  Acute intestinal infarction
  Acute small intestine ischemia
  Infarction of appendices epiploicae
  Mesenteric (artery) (vein) embolism
  Mesenteric (artery) (vein) infarction
  Mesenteric (artery) (vein) thrombosis
  Necrosis of intestine
  Subacute ischemic colitis

K55.1 Chronic vascular disorders of intestine
  Chronic ischemic colitis
  Chronic ischemic enteritis
  Chronic ischemic enterocolitis
  Ischemic stricture of intestine
  Mesenteric atherosclerosis
  Mesenteric vascular insufficiency

K55.2- Angiodysplasia of colon
  K55.20 Angiodysplasia of colon <u>without</u> hemorrhage
  K55.21 Angiodysplasia of colon <u>with hemorrhage</u>

K55.8 Other vascular disorders of intestine

K55.9 Vascular disorder of intestine, unspecified
  Ischemic colitis
  Ischemic enteritis
  Ischemic enterocolitis

K56- Paralytic ileus and intestinal obstruction <u>without</u> hernia
Excludes 1: congenital stricture or stenosis of intestine (Q41-Q42)
* cystic fibrosis with meconium ileus (E84.11)*
* ischemic stricture of intestine (K55.1)*
* meconium ileus NOS (P76.0)*
* neonatal intestinal obstructions classifiable to P76.-*
* obstruction of duodenum (K31.5)*
* postprocedural intestinal obstruction (K91.3)*
* stenosis of anus or rectum (K62.4)*
* intestinal obstruction with hernia (K40-K46)*

K56.0 Paralytic ileus
  Paralysis of bowel
  Paralysis of colon
  Paralysis of intestine
  Excludes 1: gallstone ileus (K56.3)
  * ileus NOS (K56.7)*
  * obstructive ileus NOS (K56.69)*

K56.1 Intussusception
  Intussusception or invagination of bowel
  Intussusception or invagination of colon
  Intussusception or invagination of intestine
  Intussusception or invagination of rectum
  Excludes❷: intussusception of appendix (K38.8)

K56.2 Volvulus
  Strangulation of colon or intestine
  Torsion of colon or intestine
  Twist of colon or intestine
  Excludes❷: volvulus of duodenum (K31.5)

K56.3 Gallstone ileus
  Obstruction of intestine by gallstone

K56.4- Other impaction of intestine
  K56.41 Fecal impaction
    Excludes 1: constipation (K59.0-)
    * incomplete defecation (R15.0)*
  K56.49 Other impaction of intestine

K56.5 Intestinal adhesions [bands] <u>with obstruction</u> (postprocedural) (postinfection)
  Abdominal hernia due to adhesions with obstruction
  Peritoneal adhesions [bands] with intestinal obstruction (postprocedural) (postinfection)

K56.6- Other and unspecified intestinal obstruction
  K56.60 Unspecified intestinal obstruction
    Intestinal obstruction NOS
    Excludes 1: intestinal obstruction due to specified condition-
    * code to condition*
  K56.69 Other intestinal obstruction
    Enterostenosis NOS
    Obstructive ileus NOS
    Occlusion of colon or intestine NOS
    Stenosis of colon or intestine NOS
    Stricture of colon or intestine NOS
    Excludes 1: intestinal obstruction due to specified condition-
    * code to condition*

K56.7 Ileus, unspecified
  Excludes 1: obstructive ileus (K56.69)

K57- <u>Diverticular disease</u> of intestine
Excludes 1: congenital diverticulum of intestine (Q43.8)
* Meckel's diverticulum (Q43.0)*
Excludes❷: diverticulum of appendix (K38.2)

K57.0- Diverticulitis of <u>small</u> intestine <u>with perforation and abscess</u>
  Diverticulitis of small intestine with peritonitis
  Excludes 1: diverticulitis of both small and large intestine with
  * perforation and abscess (K57.4-)*
  K57.00 Diverticulitis of small intestine with perforation and abscess <u>without</u> bleeding
  K57.01 Diverticulitis of small intestine with perforation and abscess <u>with bleeding</u>

K57.1- Diverticular disease of <u>small</u> intestine <u>without perforation or abscess</u>
  Excludes 1: diverticular disease of both small and large intestine
  * without perforation or abscess (K57.5-)*
  K57.10 Divericulo<u>sis</u> of small intestine without perforation or abscess <u>without</u> bleeding
    Diverticular disease of small intestine NOS
  K57.11 Diverticulo<u>sis</u> of small intestine without perforation or abscess <u>with bleeding</u>
  K57.12 <u>Diverticulitis</u> of small intestine without perforation or abscess <u>without</u> bleeding
  K57.13 <u>Diverticulitis</u> of small intestine without perforation or abscess <u>with bleeding</u>

K57.2- Diverticulitis of <u>large</u> intestine <u>with perforation and abscess</u>
  Diverticulitis of colon with peritonitis
  Excludes 1: diverticulitis of both small and large intestine with
  * perforation and abscess (K57.4-)*
  K57.20 Diverticulitis of large intestine with perforation and abscess <u>without</u> bleeding
  K57.21 Diverticulitis of large intestine with perforation and abscess <u>with bleeding</u>

K57.3- Diverticular disease of <u>large</u> intestine <u>without perforation or abscess</u>
  Excludes 1: diverticular disease of both small and large intestine
  * without perforation or abscess (K57.5-)*
  K57.30 Diverticulo<u>sis</u> of large intestine without perforation or abscess <u>without</u> bleeding
    Diverticular disease of colon NOS
  K57.31 Diverticulo<u>sis</u> of large intestine without perforation or abscess <u>with bleeding</u>
  K57.32 <u>Diverticulitis</u> of large intestine without perforation or abscess <u>without</u> bleeding
  K57.33 <u>Diverticulitis</u> of large intestine without perforation or abscess <u>with bleeding</u>

K57.4- Diverticulitis of <u>both small and large</u> intestine <u>with perforation and abscess</u>
  Diverticulitis of both small and large intestine with peritonitis
  K57.40 Diverticulitis of both small and large intestine with perforation and abscess <u>without</u> bleeding
  K57.41 Diverticulitis of both small and large intestine with perforation and abscess <u>with bleeding</u>

K57.5- Diverticular disease of <u>both small and large</u> intestine <u>without perforation or abscess</u>
  K57.50 Diverticulo<u>sis</u> of both small and large intestine without perforation or abscess <u>without</u> bleeding
    Diverticular disease of both small and large intestine NOS
  K57.51 Diverticulo<u>sis</u> of both small and large intestine without perforation or abscess <u>with bleeding</u>
  K57.52 <u>Diverticulitis</u> of both small and large intestine without perforation or abscess <u>without</u> bleeding
  K57.53 <u>Diverticulitis</u> of both small and large intestine without perforation or abscess <u>with bleeding</u>

K57.8- Diverticulitis of intestine, <u>part unspecified</u>, <u>with perforation and abscess</u>
  Diverticulitis of intestine NOS with peritonitis
  K57.80 Diverticulitis of intestine, part unspecified, with perforation and abscess <u>without</u> bleeding
  K57.81 Diverticulitis of intestine, part unspecified, with perforation and abscess <u>with bleeding</u>

K57.9- Diverticular disease of intestine, <u>part unspecified</u>, <u>without perforation or abscess</u>
  K57.90 Diverticulo<u>sis</u> of intestine, part unspecified, without perforation or abscess <u>without</u> bleeding
    Diverticular disease of intestine NOS
  K57.91 Diverticulo<u>sis</u> of intestine, part unspecified, without perforation or abscess <u>with bleeding</u>

K 5 5 - K 6 3

Excludes 1: = NOT CODED HERE! (Do not code both)

Excludes❷: = Not Included Here

K57.92   <u>Diverticulitis</u> of intestine, part unspecified, without perforation or abscess <u>without</u> bleeding

K57.93   <u>Diverticulitis</u> of intestine, part unspecified, without perforation or abscess <u>with bleeding</u>

K58-   **Irritable bowel syndrome**
Includes: Irritable colon
           Spastic colon

K58.0   **Irritable bowel syndrome <u>with diarrhea</u>**

K58.9   **Irritable bowel syndrome <u>without</u> diarrhea**
Irritable bowel syndrome NOS

K59-   **Other functional intestinal disorders**
Excludes 1:   change in bowel habit NOS (R19.4)
*   intestinal malabsorption (K90.-)*
*   psychogenic intestinal disorders (F45.8)*
Excludes❷: functional disorders of stomach (K31.-)

   K59.0-   **Constipation**
Excludes 1:   fecal impaction (K56.41)
*   incomplete defecation (R15.0)*

     K59.00   **Constipation, unspecified**

     K59.01   **Slow transit constipation**

     K59.02   **Outlet dysfunction constipation**

     K59.09   **Other constipation**

   K59.1   **Functional diarrhea**
Excludes 1:   diarrhea NOS (R19.7)
*   irritable bowel syndrome with diarrhea (K58.0)*

   K59.2   **Neurogenic bowel, not elsewhere classified**

   K59.3   **Megacolon, not elsewhere classified**
Dilatation of colon
Toxic megacolon
Code first (T51-T65) to identify toxic agent
Excludes 1:   congenital megacolon (aganglionic) (Q43.1)
*   megacolon (due to) (in) Chagas' disease (B57.32)*
*   megacolon (due to) (in) Clostridium difficile (A04.7)*
*   megacolon (due to) (in) Hirschsprung's disease (Q43.1)*

   K59.4   **Anal spasm**
Proctalgia fugax

   K59.8   **Other specified functional intestinal disorders**
Atony of colon
Pseudo-obstruction (acute) (chronic) of intestine

   K59.9   **Functional intestinal disorder, unspecified**

K60-   **Fissure and fistula of anal and rectal regions**
Excludes 1:   fissure and fistula of anal and rectal regions with abscess or cellulitis (K61.-)
Excludes❷: anal sphincter tear (healed) (nontraumatic) (old) (K62.81)

   K60.0   **Acute anal fissure**

   K60.1   **Chronic anal fissure**

   K60.2   **Anal fissure, unspecified**

   K60.3   **Anal fistula**

   K60.4   **Rectal fistula**
Fistula of rectum to skin
Excludes 1:   rectovaginal fistula (N82.3)
*   vesicorectal fistual (N32.1)*

   K60.5   **Anorectal fistula**

K61-   **Abscess of anal and rectal regions**
Includes: Abscess of anal and rectal regions
           Cellulitis of anal and rectal regions

   K61.0   **Anal abscess**
Perianal abscess
Excludes 1:   intrasphincteric abscess (K61.4)

   K61.1   **Rectal abscess**
Perirectal abscess
Excludes 1:   ischiorectal abscess (K61.3)

   K61.2   **Anorectal abscess**

   K61.3   **Ischiorectal abscess**
Abscess of ischiorectal fossa

   K61.4   **Intrasphincteric abscess**

K62-   **Other diseases of anus and rectum**
Includes: Anal canal
Excludes❷: colostomy and enterostomy malfunction (K94.0-, K94.1-)
*   fecal incontinence (R15.-)*
*   hemorrhoids (K64-)*

   K62.0   **Anal polyp**

   K62.1   **Rectal polyp**
Excludes 1:   adenomatous polyp (D12.8)

   K62.2   **Anal prolapse**
Prolapse of anal canal

   K62.3   **Rectal prolapse**
Prolapse of rectal mucosa

   K62.4   **Stenosis of anus and rectum**
Stricture of anus (sphincter)

   K62.5   **Hemorrhage of anus and rectum**
Excludes 1:   gastrointestinal bleeding NOS (K92.2)
*   melena (K92.1)*
*   neonatal rectal hemorrhage (P54.2)*

   K62.6   **Ulcer of anus and rectum**
Solitary ulcer of anus and rectum
Stercoral ulcer of anus and rectum
Excludes 1:   fissure and fistula of anus and rectum (K60-)
*   ulcerative colitis (K51-)*

   K62.7   **Radiation proctitis**
Use additional code to identify the type of radiation (W90-)

   K62.8-   **Other specified diseases of anus and rectum**
Excludes❷: ulcerative proctitis (K51.2)

     K62.81   **Anal sphincter tear (healed) (nontraumatic) (old)**
Tear of anus, nontraumatic
Use additional code for any associated fecal incontinence (R15.-)
Excludes❷: anal fissure (K60.-)
*   anal sphincter tear (healed) (old) complicating delivery (O34.7-)*
*   traumatic tear of anal sphincter (S31.831)*

     K62.82   **Dysplasia of anus**
Anal intraepithelial neoplasia I and II (AIN I and II) (histologically confirmed)
Dysplasia of anus NOS
Mild and moderate dysplasia of anus (histologically confirmed)
Excludes 1:   abnormal results from anal cytologic examination without histologic confirmation (R85.61-)
*   anal intraepithelial neoplasia III (D01.3)*
*   carcinoma in situ of anus (D01.3)*
*   HGSIL of anus (R85.613)*
*   severe dysplasia of anus (D01.3)*

     K62.89   **Other specified diseases of anus and rectum**
Proctitis NOS
Use additional code for any associated fecal incontinence (R15.-)

   K62.9   **Disease of anus and rectum, unspecified**

K63-   **Other diseases of intestine**

   K63.0   **Abscess of intestine**
Excludes 1:   abscess of intestine with Crohn's disease (K50.014, K50.114, K50.814, K50.914)
*   abscess of intestine with diverticular disease (K57.0, K57.2, K57.4, K57.8)*
*   abscess of intestine with ulcerative colitis (K51.014, K51.214, K51.314, K51.414, K51.514, K51.814, K51.914)*
Excludes❷: abscess of anal and rectal regions (K61-)
*   abscess of appendix (K35.3)*

   K63.1   **Perforation of intestine (nontraumatic)**
Perforation (nontraumatic) of rectum
Excludes 1:   perforation (nontraumatic) of duodenum (K26.-)
*   perforation (nontraumatic) of intestine with diverticular disease (K57.0, K57.2, K57.4, K57.8)*
Excludes❷: perforation (nontraumatic) of appendix (K35.2, K35.3)

   K63.2   **Fistula of intestine**
Excludes 1:   fistula of duodenum (K31.6)
*   fistula of intestine with Crohn's disease (K50.013, K50.113, K50.813, K50.913)*
*   fistula of intestine with ulcerative colitis (K51.013, K51.213, K51.313, K51.413, K51.513, K51.813, K51.913)*
Excludes❷: fistula of anal and rectal regions (K60.-)
*   fistula of appendix (K38.3)*
*   intestinal-genital fistula, female (N82.2-N82.4)*
*   vesicointestinal fistula (N32.1)*

   K63.3   **Ulcer of intestine**
Primary ulcer of small intestine
Excludes 1:   duodenal ulcer (K26-)
*   gastrointestinal ulcer (K28-)*
*   gastrojejunal ulcer (K28-)*
*   jejunal ulcer (K28-)*
*   peptic ulcer, site unspecified (K27-)*
*   ulcer of intestine with perforation (K63.1)*
*   ulcer of anus or rectum (K62.6)*
*   ulcerative colitis (K51-)*

   K63.4   **Enteroptosis**

   K63.5   **Polyp of colon**
Excludes 1:   adenomatous polyp of colon (D12.6)
*   inflammatory polyp of colon (K51.4-)*
*   polyposis of colon (D12.6)*

   K63.8-   **Other specified diseases of intestine**

     K63.81   **Dieulafoy lesion of intestine**
Excludes❷: Dieulafoy lesion of stomach and duodenum (K31.82)

     K63.89   **Other specified diseases of intestine**

   K63.9   **Disease of intestine, unspecified**

K 5 5 - K 6 3

Excludes 1: = NOT CODED HERE! (Do not code both)   *Excludes❷:* = Not Included Here

K64- Hemorrhoids and perianal venous thrombosis
Includes: Piles
*Excludes 1:   hemorrhoids complicating childbirth and the puerperium
(O87.2)
hemorrhoids complicating pregnancy (O22.4)*

K64.0 First degree hemorrhoids
Grade/stage I hemorrhoids
Hemorrhoids (bleeding) without prolapse outside of anal canal

K64.1 Second degree hemorrhoids
Grade/stage II hemorrhoids
Hemorrhoids (bleeding) that prolapse with straining, but retract
spontaneously

K64.2 Third degree hemorrhoids
Grade/stage III hemorrhoids
Hemorrhoids (bleeding) that prolapse with straining and require
manual replacement back inside anal canal

K64.3 Fourth degree hemorrhoids
Grade/stage IV hemorrhoids
Hemorrhoids (bleeding) with prolapsed tissue that cannot be
manually replaced

K64.4 Residual hemorrhoidal skin tags
External hemorrhoids NOS
Skin tags of anus

K64.5 Perianal venous thrombosis
External hemorrhoids with thrombosis
Perianal hematoma
Thrombosed hemorrhoids NOS

K64.8 Other hemorrhoids
Internal hemorrhoids, without mention of degree
Prolapsed hemorrhoids, degree not specified

K64.9 Unspecified hemorrhoids
Hemorrhoids (bleeding) NOS
Hemorrhoids (bleeding) without mention of degree

Diseases of peritoneum and retroperitoneum (K65-K68)

K65- Peritonitis
Use additional code (B95-B97), to identify infectious agent
*Excludes 1:   acute appendicitis with generalized peritonitis (K35.2)
aseptic peritonitis (T81.6)
benign paroxysmal peritonitis (E85.0)
chemical peritonitis (T81.6)
diverticulitis of both small and large intestine with peritonitis
(K57.4-)
diverticulitis of colon with peritonitis (K57.2-)
diverticulitis of intestine, NOS, with peritonitis (K57.8-)
diverticulitis of small intestine with peritonitis (K57.0-)
gonococcal peritonitis (A54.85)
neonatal peritonitis (P78.0-P78.1)
pelvic peritonitis, female (N73.3-N73.5)
periodic familial peritonitis (E85.0)
peritonitis due to talc or other foreign substance (T81.6)
peritonitis in chlamydia (A74.81)
peritonitis in diphtheria (A36.89)
peritonitis in syphilis (late) (A52.74)
peritonitis in tuberculosis (A18.31)
peritonitis with or following abortion or ectopic or molar
pregnancy (O00-O07, O08.0)
peritonitis with or following appendicitis (K35-)
peritonitis with or following diverticular disease of intestine
(K57-)
puerperal peritonitis (O85)
retroperitoneal infections (K68-)*

K65.0 Generalized (acute) peritonitis
Pelvic peritonitis (acute), male
Subphrenic peritonitis (acute)
Suppurative peritonitis (acute)

K65.1 Peritoneal abscess
Abdominopelvic abscess
Abscess (of) omentum
Abscess (of) peritoneum
Mesenteric abscess
Retrocecal abscess
Subdiaphragmatic abscess
Subhepatic abscess
Subphrenic abscess

K65.2 Spontaneous bacterial peritonitis
Excludes 1: bacterial peritonitis NOS (K65.9)

K65.3 Choleperitonitis
Peritonitis due to bile

K65.4 Sclerosing mesenteritis
Fat necrosis of peritoneum
(Idiopathic) sclerosing mesenteric fibrosis
Mesenteric lipodystrophy
Mesenteric panniculitis
Retractile mesenteritis

K65.8 Other peritonitis
Chronic proliferative peritonitis
Peritonitis due to urine

K65.9 Peritonitis, unspecified
Bacterial peritonitis NOS

K66- Other disorders of peritoneum
*Excludes ❷: ascites (R18.-)
peritoneal effusion (chronic) (R18.8)*

K66.0 Peritoneal adhesions (postprocedural) (postinfection)
Adhesions (of) abdominal (wall)
Adhesions (of) diaphragm
Adhesions (of) intestine
Adhesions (of) male pelvis
Adhesions (of) omentum
Adhesions (of) stomach
Adhesive bands
Mesenteric adhesions
*Excludes 1:   female pelvic adhesions [bands] (N73.6)
peritoneal adhesions with intestinal obstruction (K56.5)*

K66.1 Hemoperitoneum
Excludes 1:   traumatic hemoperitoneum (S36.8-)

K66.8 Other specified disorders of peritoneum

K66.9 Disorder of peritoneum, unspecified

K67 Disorders of peritoneum in infectious diseases classified elsewhere
Code first underlying disease, such as :
Congenital syphilis (A50.0)
Helminthiasis (B65.0-B83.9)
*Excludes 1: peritonitis in chlamydia (A74.81)
peritonitis in diphtheria (A36.89)
peritonitis in gonococcal (A54.85)
peritonitis in syphilis (late) (A52.74)
peritonitis in tuberculosis (A18.31)*

K68- Disorders of retroperitoneum

K68.1- Retroperitoneal abscess

K68.11 Postprocedural retroperitoneal abscess

K68.12 Psoas muscle abscess

K68.19 Other retroperitoneal abscess

K68.9 Other disorders of retroperitoneum

Diseases of liver (K70-K77)

Excludes 1: jaundice NOS (R17)
*Excludes ❷: hemochromatosis (E83.11-)
Reye's syndrome (G93.7)
viral hepatitis (B15-B19)
Wilson's disease (E83.0)*

K70- Alcoholic liver disease
Use additional code to identify:
Alcohol abuse and dependence (F10.-)

K70.0 Alcoholic fatty liver

K70.1- Alcoholic hepatitis

K70.10 Alcoholic hepatitis without ascites

K70.11 Alcoholic hepatitis with ascites

K70.2 Alcoholic fibrosis and sclerosis of liver

K70.3- Alcoholic cirrhosis of liver
Alcoholic cirrhosis NOS

K70.30 Alcoholic cirrhosis of liver without ascites

K70.31 Alcoholic cirrhosis of liver with ascites

K70.4- Alcoholic hepatic failure
Acute alcoholic hepatic failure
Alcoholic hepatic failure NOS
Chronic alcoholic hepatic failure
Subacute alcoholic hepatic failure

K70.40 Alcoholic hepatic failure without coma

K70.41 Alcoholic hepatic failure with coma

K70.9 Alcoholic liver disease, unspecified

K
6
4
–
K
7
6

K71-   Toxic liver disease
  Includes: Drug-induced idiosyncratic (unpredictable) liver disease
         Drug-induced toxic (predictable) liver disease
  Code first poisoning due to drug or toxin, if applicable (T36-T65 with fifth
       or sixth character 1-4 or 6)
  Use additional code for adverse effect, if applicable, to identify drug (T36-
       T50 with fifth or sixth character 5)
  Excludes❷: alcoholic liver disease (K70.-)
         Budd-Chiari syndrome (I82.0)
  K71.0   Toxic liver disease with cholestasis
         Cholestasis with hepatocyte injury
         "Pure" cholestasis
  K71.1- Toxic liver disease with hepatic necrosis
         Hepatic failure (acute) (chronic) due to drugs
    K71.10 Toxic liver disease with hepatic necrosis, without coma
    K71.11 Toxic liver disease with hepatic necrosis, with coma
  K71.2   Toxic liver disease with acute hepatitis
  K71.3   Toxic liver disease with chronic persistent hepatitis
  K71.4   Toxic liver disease with chronic lobular hepatitis
  K71.5- Toxic liver disease with chronic active hepatitis
         Toxic liver disease with lupoid hepatitis
    K71.50 Toxic liver disease with chronic active hepatitis without ascites
    K71.51 Toxic liver disease with chronic active hepatitis with ascites
  K71.6   Toxic liver disease with hepatitis, not elsewhere classified
  K71.7   Toxic liver disease with fibrosis and cirrhosis of liver
  K71.8   Toxic liver disease with other disorders of liver
         Toxic liver disease with focal nodular hyperplasia
         Toxic liver disease with hepatic granulomas
         Toxic liver disease with peliosis hepatis
         Toxic liver disease with veno-occlusive disease of liver
  K71.9   Toxic liver disease, unspecified

K72-   Hepatic failure, not elsewhere classified
  Includes: Acute hepatitis NEC, with hepatic failure
         Fulminant hepatitis NEC, with hepatic failure
         Hepatic encephalopathy NOS
         Liver (cell) necrosis with hepatic failure
         Malignant hepatitis NEC, with hepatic failure
         Yellow liver atrophy or dystrophy
  Excludes 1: alcoholic hepatic failure (K70.4)
         hepatic failure with toxic liver disease (K71.1-)
         icterus of newborn (P55-P59)
         postprocedural hepatic failure (K91.82)
         viral hepatitis with hepatic coma (B15-B19)
  Excludes❷: hepatic failure complicating abortion or ectopic or molar
         pregnancy (O00-O07, O08.8)
         hepatic failure complicating pregnancy, childbirth and the
         puerperium (O26.6-)
  K72.0- Acute and subacute hepatic failure
    K72.00 Acute and subacute hepatic failure without coma
    K72.01 Acute and subacute hepatic failure with coma
  K72.1- Chronic hepatic failure
    K72.10 Chronic hepatic failure without coma
    K72.11 Chronic hepatic failure with coma
  K72.9- Hepatic failure, unspecified
    K72.90 Hepatic failure, unspecified without coma
    K72.91 Hepatic failure, unspecified with coma
         Hepatic coma NOS

K73-   Chronic hepatitis, not elsewhere classified
  Excludes 1: alcoholic hepatitis (chronic) (K70.1-)
         drug-induced hepatitis (chronic) (K71.-)
         granulomatous hepatitis (chronic) NEC (K75.3)
         reactive, nonspecific hepatitis (chronic) (K75.2)
         viral hepatitis (chronic) (B15-B19)
  K73.0   Chronic persistent hepatitis, not elsewhere classified
  K73.1   Chronic lobular hepatitis, not elsewhere classified
  K73.2   Chronic active hepatitis, not elsewhere classified
  K73.8   Other chronic hepatitis, not elsewhere classified
  K73.9   Chronic hepatitis, unspecified

K74-   Fibrosis and cirrhosis of liver
  Code also, if applicable, viral hepatitis (acute) (chronic) (B15-B19)
  Excludes 1: alcoholic cirrhosis (of liver) (K70.3)
         alcoholic fibrosis of liver (K70.2)
         cardiac sclerosis of liver (K76.1)
         cirrhosis (of liver) with toxic liver disease (K71.7)
         congenital cirrhosis (of liver) (P78.81)
         pigmentary cirrhosis (of liver) (E83.110)
  K74.0   Hepatic fibrosis
  K74.1   Hepatic sclerosis
  K74.2   Hepatic fibrosis with hepatic sclerosis

K74.3   Primary biliary cirrhosis
         Chronic nonsuppurative destructive cholangitis
K74.4   Secondary biliary cirrhosis
K74.5   Biliary cirrhosis, unspecified
K74.6- Other and unspecified cirrhosis of liver
  K74.60 Unspecified cirrhosis of liver
         Cirrhosis (of liver) NOS
  K74.69 Other cirrhosis of liver
         Cryptogenic cirrhosis (of liver)
         Macronodular cirrhosis (of liver)
         Micronodular cirrhosis (of liver)
         Mixed type cirrhosis (of liver)
         Portal cirrhosis (of liver)
         Postnecrotic cirrhosis (of liver)

K75-   Other inflammatory liver diseases
  Excludes❷: toxic liver disease (K71.-)
  K75.0   Abscess of liver
         Cholangitic hepatic abscess
         Hematogenic hepatic abscess
         Hepatic abscess NOS
         Lymphogenic hepatic abscess
         Pylephlebitic hepatic abscess
         Excludes 1: amebic liver abscess (A06.4)
              cholangitis without liver abscess (K83.0)
              pylephlebitis without liver abscess (K75.1)
  K75.1   Phlebitis of portal vein
         Pylephlebitis
         Excludes 1: pylephlebitic liver abscess (K75.0)
  K75.2   Nonspecific reactive hepatitis
         Excludes 1: acute or subacute hepatitis (K72.0-)
              chronic hepatitis NEC (K73.-)
              viral hepatitis (B15-B19)
  K75.3   Granulomatous hepatitis, not elsewhere classified
         Excludes 1: acute or subacute hepatitis (K72.0-)
              chronic hepatitis NEC (K73.-)
              viral hepatitis (B15-B19)
  K75.4   Autoimmune hepatitis
         Lupoid hepatitis NEC
  K75.8- Other specified inflammatory liver diseases
    K75.81 Nonalcoholic steatohepatitis (NASH)
    K75.89 Other specified inflammatory liver diseases
  K75.9   Inflammatory liver disease, unspecified
         Hepatitis NOS
         Excludes 1: acute or subacute hepatitis (K72.0-)
              chronic hepatitis NEC (K73.-)
              viral hepatitis (B15-B19)

K76-   Other diseases of liver
  Excludes❷: alcoholic liver disease (K70.-)
         amyloid degeneration of liver (E85.-)
         cystic disease of liver (congenital) (Q44.6)
         hepatic vein thrombosis (I82.0)
         hepatomegaly NOS (R16.0)
         pigmentary cirrhosis (of liver) (E83.110)
         portal vein thrombosis (I81)
         toxic liver disease (K71.-)
  K76.0   Fatty (change of) liver, not elsewhere classified
         Nonalcoholic fatty liver disease (NAFLD)
         Excludes 1: nonalcoholic steatohepatitis (NASH) (K75.81)
  K76.1   Chronic passive congestion of liver
         Cardiac cirrhosis
         Cardiac sclerosis
  K76.2   Central hemorrhagic necrosis of liver
         Excludes 1: liver necrosis with hepatic failure (K72-)
  K76.3   Infarction of liver
  K76.4   Peliosis hepatis
         Hepatic angiomatosis
  K76.5   Hepatic veno-occlusive disease
         Excludes 1: Budd-Chiari syndrome (I82.0)
  K76.6   Portal hypertension
         Use additional code for any associated complications, such as:
         Portal hypertensive gastropathy (K31.89)
  K76.7   Hepatorenal syndrome
         Excludes 1: hepatorenal syndrome following labor and delivery
              (O90.4)
              postprocedural hepatorenal syndrome (K91.82)
  K76.8- Other specified diseases of liver
    K76.81 Hepatopulmonary syndrome
         Code first underlying disease, such as:
         Alcoholic cirrhosis of liver (K70.3-)
         Cirrhosis of liver without mention of alcohol (K74.6-)

K
6
4
–
K
7
6

Excludes 1: = NOT CODED HERE! (Do not code both)   **523**   *Excludes❷:* = Not Included Here

K76.89   Other specified diseases of liver
Cyst (simple) of liver
Focal nodular hyperplasia of liver
Hepatoptosis
K76.9   Liver disease, unspecified
K77   Liver disorders <u>in diseases classified elsewhere</u>
Code first underlying disease, such as:
Amyloidosis (E85.-)
Congenital syphilis (A50.0, A50.5)
Congenital toxoplasmosis (P37.1)
Schistosomiasis (B65.0-B65.9)
Excludes 1:   alcoholic hepatitis (K70.1-)
alcoholic liver disease (K70.-)
cytomegaloviral hepatitis (B25.1)
herpesviral [herpes simplex] hepatitis (B00.81)
infectious mononucleosis with liver disease (B27.0-B27.9
with .9)
mumps hepatitis (B26.81)
sarcoidosis with liver disease (D86.89)
secondary syphilis with liver disease (A51.45)
syphilis (late) with liver disease (A52.74)
toxoplasmosis (acquired) hepatitis (B58.1)
tuberculosis with liver disease (A18.83)

Disorders of gallbladder, biliary tract and pancreas
(K80-K87)

K80-   Cholelithiasis
Excludes 1:   retained cholelithiasis following cholecystectomy (K91.86)
K80.0-   Calculus of gallbladder <u>with acute</u> cholecystitis
Any condition listed in K80.2 with acute cholecystitis
K80.00   Calculus of gallbladder with acute cholecystitis <u>without</u> obstruction
K80.01   Calculus of gallbladder with acute cholecystitis <u>with</u> obstruction
K80.1-   Calculus of gallbladder <u>with other</u> cholecystitis
K80.10   Calculus of gallbladder with <u>chronic</u> cholecystitis <u>without</u> obstruction
Cholelithiasis with cholecystitis NOS
K80.11   Calculus of gallbladder with <u>chronic</u> cholecystitis <u>with</u> obstruction
K80.12   Calculus of gallbladder with <u>acute and chronic</u> cholecystitis <u>without</u> obstruction
K80.13   Calculus of gallbladder with <u>acute and chronic</u> cholecystitis <u>with obstruction</u>
K80.18   Calculus of gallbladder with <u>other</u> cholecystitis <u>without</u> obstruction
K80.19   Calculus of gallbladder with <u>other</u> cholecystitis <u>with</u> obstruction
K80.2-   Calculus of gallbladder <u>without</u> cholecystitis
Cholecystolithiasis without cholecystitis
Cholelithiasis (without cholecystitis)
Colic (recurrent) of gallbladder (without cholecystitis)
Gallstone (impacted) of cystic duct (without cholecystitis)
Gallstone (impacted) of gallbladder (without cholecystitis)
K80.20   Calculus of gallbladder without cholecystitis <u>without</u> obstruction
K80.21   Calculus of gallbladder without cholecystitis <u>with</u> obstruction
K80.3-   Calculus of <u>bile duct with cholangitis</u>
Any condition listed in K80.5 with cholangitis
K80.30   Calculus of bile duct with cholangitis, <u>unspecified</u>, <u>without</u> obstruction
K80.31   Calculus of bile duct with cholangitis, <u>unspecified</u>, <u>with</u> obstruction
K80.32   Calculus of bile duct with <u>acute</u> cholangitis <u>without</u> obstruction
K80.33   Calculus of bile duct with <u>acute</u> cholangitis <u>with obstruction</u>
K80.34   Calculus of bile duct with <u>chronic</u> cholangitis <u>without</u> obstruction
K80.35   Calculus of bile duct with <u>chronic</u> cholangitis <u>with</u> obstruction
K80.36   Calculus of bile duct with <u>acute and chronic</u> cholangitis <u>without</u> obstruction
K80.37   Calculus of bile duct with <u>acute and chronic</u> cholangitis <u>with</u> obstruction
K80.4-   Calculus of <u>bile duct with cholecystitis</u>
Any condition listed in K80.5 with cholecystitis (with cholangitis)
K80.40   Calculus of bile duct with cholecystitis, <u>unspecified</u>, <u>without</u> obstruction

K80.41   Calculus of bile duct with cholecystitis, <u>unspecified</u>, <u>with</u> obstruction
K80.42   Calculus of bile duct with <u>acute</u> cholecystitis <u>without</u> obstruction
K80.43   Calculus of bile duct with <u>acute</u> cholecystitis <u>with</u> obstruction
K80.44   Calculus of bile duct with <u>chronic</u> cholecystitis <u>without</u> obstruction
K80.45   Calculus of bile duct with <u>chronic</u> cholecystitis <u>with</u> obstruction
K80.46   Calculus of bile duct with <u>acute and chronic</u> cholecystitis <u>without</u> obstruction
K80.47   Calculus of bile duct with <u>acute and chronic</u> cholecystitis <u>with obstruction</u>
K80.5-   Calculus of <u>bile duct without</u> cholangitis or cholecystitis
Choledocholithiasis (without cholangitis or cholecystitis)
Gallstone (impacted) of bile duct NOS (without cholangitis or cholecystitis)
Gallstone (impacted) of common duct (without cholangitis or cholecystitis)
Gallstone (impacted) of hepatic duct (without cholangitis or cholecystitis)
Hepatic cholelithiasis (without cholangitis or cholecystitis)
Hepatic colic (recurrent) (without cholangitis or cholecystitis)
K80.50   Calculus of bile duct without cholangitis or cholecystitis <u>without</u> obstruction
K80.51   Calculus of bile duct without cholangitis or cholecystitis <u>with</u> obstruction
K80.6-   Calculus of <u>gallbladder and bile duct</u> with cholecystitis
K80.60   Calculus of gallbladder and bile duct with cholecystitis, <u>unspecified</u>, <u>without</u> obstruction
K80.61   Calculus of gallbladder and bile duct with cholecystitis, <u>unspecified</u>, <u>with obstruction</u>
K80.62   Calculus of gallbladder and bile duct with <u>acute</u> cholecystitis <u>without</u> obstruction
K80.63   Calculus of gallbladder and bile duct with <u>acute</u> cholecystitis <u>with obstruction</u>
K80.64   Calculus of gallbladder and bile duct with <u>chronic</u> cholecystitis <u>without</u> obstruction
K80.65   Calculus of gallbladder and bile duct with <u>chronic</u> cholecystitis <u>with obstruction</u>
K80.66   Calculus of gallbladder and bile duct with <u>acute and chronic</u> cholecystitis <u>without</u> obstruction
K80.67   Calculus of gallbladder and bile duct with <u>acute and chronic</u> cholecystitis <u>with</u> obstruction
K80.7-   Calculus of gallbladder and bile duct <u>without</u> cholecystitis
K80.70   Calculus of gallbladder and bile duct without cholecystitis <u>without</u> obstruction
K80.71   Calculus of gallbladder and bile duct without cholecystitis <u>with obstruction</u>
K80.8-   Other cholelithiasis
K80.80   Other cholelithiasis <u>without</u> obstruction
K80.81   Other cholelithiasis <u>with obstruction</u>
K81-   Cholecystitis
Excludes 1:   cholecystitis with cholelithiasis (K80.-)
K81.0   Acute cholecystitis
Abscess of gallbladder
Angiocholecystitis
Emphysematous (acute) cholecystitis
Empyema of gallbladder
Gangrene of gallbladder
Gangrenous cholecystitis
Suppurative cholecystitis
K81.1   Chronic cholecystitis
K81.2   Acute cholecystitis with chronic cholecystitis
K81.9   Cholecystitis, unspecified
K82-   Other diseases of gallbladder
Excludes 1:   nonvisualization of gallbladder (R93.2)
postcholecystectomy syndrome (K91.5)
K82.0   Obstruction of gallbladder
Occlusion of cystic duct or gallbladder without cholelithiasis
Stenosis of cystic duct or gallbladder without cholelithiasis
Stricture of cystic duct or gallbladder without cholelithiasis
Excludes 1:   obstruction of gallbladder with cholelithiasis (K80.-)
K82.1   Hydrops of gallbladder
Mucocele of gallbladder
K82.2   Perforation of gallbladder
Rupture of cystic duct or gallbladder
K82.3   Fistula of gallbladder
Cholecystocolic fistula
Cholecystoduodenal fistula

K82.4   **Cholesterolosis of gallbladder**
　　Strawberry gallbladder
　　Excludes 1:   cholesterolosis of gallbladder with cholecystitis (K81-)
　　　　　　　　cholesterolosis of gallbladder with cholelithiasis (K80-)

K82.8   **Other specified diseases of gallbladder**
　　Adhesions of cystic duct or gallbladder
　　Atrophy of cystic duct or gallbladder
　　Cyst of cystic duct or gallbladder
　　Dyskinesia of cystic duct or gallbladder
　　Hypertrophy of cystic duct or gallbladder
　　Nonfunctioning of cystic duct or gallbladder
　　Ulcer of cystic duct or gallbladder

K82.9   **Disease of gallbladder, unspecified**

K83-   Other diseases of biliary tract
　　Excludes 1:   postcholecystectomy syndrome (K91.5)
　　Excludes❷: conditions involving the gallbladder (K81-K82)
　　　　　　　　conditions involving the cystic duct (K81-K82)

K83.0   **Cholangitis**
　　Ascending cholangitis
　　Cholangitis NOS
　　Primary cholangitis
　　Recurrent cholangitis
　　Sclerosing cholangitis
　　Secondary cholangitis
　　Stenosing cholangitis
　　Suppurative cholangitis
　　Excludes 1:   cholangitic liver abscess (K75.0)
　　　　　　　　cholangitis with choledocholithiasis (K80.3-, K80.4-)
　　　　　　　　chronic nonsuppurative destructive cholangitis (K74.3)

K83.1   **Obstruction of bile duct**
　　Occlusion of bile duct without cholelithiasis
　　Stenosis of bile duct without cholelithiasis
　　Stricture of bile duct without cholelithiasis
　　Excludes 1:   congenital obstruction of bile duct (Q44.3)
　　　　　　　　obstruction of bile duct with cholelithiasis (K80.-)

K83.2   **Perforation of bile duct**
　　Rupture of bile duct

K83.3   **Fistula of bile duct**
　　Choledochoduodenal fistula

K83.4   **Spasm of sphincter of Oddi**

K83.5   **Biliary cyst**

K83.8   **Other specified diseases of biliary tract**
　　Adhesions of biliary tract
　　Atrophy of biliary tract
　　Hypertrophy of biliary tract
　　Ulcer of biliary tract

K83.9   **Disease of biliary tract, unspecified**

K85-   Acute pancreatitis
　　Includes: Abscess of pancreas
　　　　　　　Acute necrosis of pancreas
　　　　　　　Acute (recurrent) pancreatitis
　　　　　　　Gangrene of (gangrenous) pancreas
　　　　　　　Hemorrhagic pancreatitis
　　　　　　　Infective necrosis of pancreas
　　　　　　　Subacute pancreatitis
　　　　　　　Suppurative pancreatitis

K85.0   **Idiopathic acute pancreatitis**

K85.1   **Biliary acute pancreatitis**
　　Gallstone pancreatitis

K85.2   **Alcohol induced acute pancreatitis**
　　Excludes❷: alcohol induced chronic pancreatitis (K86.0)

K85.3   **Drug-induced acute pancreatitis**
　　Use additional code for adverse effect, if applicable, to identify drug
　　　(T36-T50 with fifth or sixth character 5)
　　Use additional code to identify drug abuse and dependence
　　　(F11.-F17.-)

K85.8   **Other acute pancreatitis**

K85.9   **Acute pancreatitis, unspecified**
　　Pancreatitis NOS

K86-   Other diseases of pancreas
　　Excludes❷: fibrocystic disease of pancreas (E84-)
　　　　　　　　islet cell tumor (of pancreas) (D13.7)
　　　　　　　　pancreatic steatorrhea (K90.3)

K86.0   **Alcohol-induced chronic pancreatitis**
　　Use additional code to identify:
　　　Alcohol abuse and dependence (F10-)
　　Excludes❷: alcohol induced acute pancreatitis (K85.2)

K86.1   **Other chronic pancreatitis**
　　Chronic pancreatitis NOS
　　Infectious chronic pancreatitis
　　Recurrent chronic pancreatitis
　　Relapsing chronic pancreatitis

K86.2   **Cyst of pancreas**

K86.3   **Pseudocyst of pancreas**

K86.8   **Other specified diseases of pancreas**
　　Aseptic pancreatic necrosis
　　Atrophy of pancreas
　　Calculus of pancreas
　　Cirrhosis of pancreas
　　Fibrosis of pancreas
　　Pancreatic fat necrosis
　　Pancreatic infantilism
　　Pancreatic necrosis NOS

K86.9   **Disease of pancreas, unspecified**

K87   Disorders of gallbladder, biliary tract and pancreas <u>in diseases classified elsewhere</u>
　　Code first underlying disease
　　Excludes 1:   cytomegaloviral pancreatitis(B25.2)
　　　　　　　　mumps pancreatitis (B26.3)
　　　　　　　　syphilitic gallbladder (A52.74)
　　　　　　　　syphilitic pancreas (A52.74)
　　　　　　　　tuberculosis of gallbladder (A18.83)
　　　　　　　　tuberculosis of pancreas (A18.83)

Other diseases of the digestive system (K90-K95)

K90-   Intestinal malabsorption
　　Excludes 1:   intestinal malabsorption following gastrointestinal surgery
　　　　　　　　(K91.2)

K90.0   **Celiac disease**
　　Gluten-sensitive enteropathy
　　Idiopathic steatorrhea
　　Nontropical sprue
　　Use additional code for associated disorders including:
　　　Dermatitis herpetiformis (L13.0)
　　　Gluten ataxia (G32.81)

K90.1   **Tropical sprue**
　　Sprue NOS
　　Tropical steatorrhea

K90.2   **Blind loop syndrome, not elsewhere classified**
　　Blind loop syndrome NOS
　　Excludes 1:   congenital blind loop syndrome (Q43.8)
　　　　　　　　postsurgical blind loop syndrome (K91.2)

K90.3   **Pancreatic steatorrhea**

K90.4   **Malabsorption due to intolerance, not elsewhere classified**
　　Malabsorption due to intolerance to carbohydrate
　　Malabsorption due to intolerance to fat
　　Malabsorption due to intolerance to protein
　　Malabsorption due to intolerance to starch
　　Excludes❷: gluten-sensitive enteropathy (K90.0)
　　　　　　　　lactose intolerance (E73.-)

K90.8-   Other intestinal malabsorption
　　K90.81   Whipple's disease
　　K90.89   Other intestinal malabsorption

K90.9   **Intestinal malabsorption, unspecified**

K91-   <u>Intraoperative and postprocedural complications</u> and disorders of digestive system, not elsewhere classified
　　Excludes❷: complications of artificial opening of digestive system (K94-)
　　　　　　　　complications of bariatric procedures (K95-)
　　　　　　　　gastrojejunal ulcer (K28-)
　　　　　　　　postprocedural (radiation) retroperitoneal abscess (K68.11)
　　　　　　　　radiation colitis (K52.0)
　　　　　　　　radiation gastroenteritis (K52.0)
　　　　　　　　radiation proctitis (K62.7)

K91.0   **Vomiting following gastrointestinal surgery**

K91.1   **Postgastric surgery syndromes**
　　Dumping syndrome
　　Postgastrectomy syndrome
　　Postvagotomy syndrome

K91.2   **Postsurgical malabsorption, not elsewhere classified**
　　Postsurgical blind loop syndrome
　　Excludes 1:   malabsorption osteomalacia in adults (M83.2)
　　　　　　　　malabsorption osteoporosis, postsurgical (M80.8-,
　　　　　　　　M81.8)

K91.3   **Postprocedural intestinal obstruction**

K91.5   **Postcholecystectomy syndrome**

K 7 6 - K 9 1

© 2013 Channel Publishing, Ltd.

K91.6- <u>Intraoperative hemorrhage and hematoma</u> of a digestive system organ or structure complicating a procedure

    Excludes 1: intraoperative hemorrhage and hematoma of a digestive system organ or structure due to accidental puncture and laceration during a procedure (K91.7-)

    K91.61 Intraoperative hemorrhage and hematoma of a digestive system organ or structure complicating a <u>digestive system procedure</u>

    K91.62 Intraoperative hemorrhage and hematoma of a digestive system organ or structure complicating <u>other procedure</u>

K91.7- <u>Accidental puncture and laceration</u> of a digestive system organ or structure during a procedure

    K91.71 Accidental puncture and laceration of a digestive system organ or structure during a <u>digestive system procedure</u>

    K91.72 Accidental puncture and laceration of a digestive system organ or structure during <u>other procedure</u>

K91.8- Other intraoperative and postprocedural complications and disorders of digestive system

    K91.81 Other intraoperative complications of digestive system

    K91.82 Postprocedural hepatic failure

    K91.83 Postprocedural hepatorenal syndrome

    K91.84- <u>Postprocedural hemorrhage and hematoma</u> of a digestive system organ or structure following a procedure

        K91.840 Postprocedural hemorrhage and hematoma of a digestive system organ or structure following a <u>digestive system procedure</u>

        K91.841 Postprocedural hemorrhage and hematoma of a digestive system organ or structure following <u>other procedure</u>

    K91.85- Complications of intestinal pouch

        K91.850 Pouchitis

            Inflammation of internal ileoanal pouch

        K91.858 Other complications of intestinal pouch

    K91.86 Retained cholelithiasis following cholecystectomy

    K91.89 Other postprocedural complications and disorders of digestive system

        Use additional code, if applicable, to further specify disorder

        Excludes ❷: postprocedural retroperitoneal abscess (K68.11)

K92- Other diseases of digestive system

    Excludes 1: neonatal gastrointestinal hemorrhage (P54.0-P54.3)

    K92.0 Hematemesis

    K92.1 Melena

        Excludes 1: occult blood in feces (R19.5)

    K92.2 Gastrointestinal hemorrhage, unspecified

        Gastric hemorrhage NOS

        Intestinal hemorrhage NOS

        Excludes 1: acute hemorrhagic gastritis (K29.01)

            hemorrhage of anus and rectum (K62.5)

            angiodysplasia of stomach with hemorrhage (K31.811)

            diverticular disease with hemorrhage (K57.-)

            gastritis and duodenitis with hemorrhage (K29.-)

            peptic ulcer with hemorrhage (K25-K28)

    K92.8- Other specified diseases of the digestive system

    K92.81 Gastrointestinal mucositis (ulcerative)

        Code also type of associated therapy, such as:

        Antineoplastic and immunosuppressive drugs (T45.1x-)

        Radiological procedure and radiotherapy (Y84.2)

        Excludes ❷: mucositis (ulcerative) of vagina and vulva (N76.81)

            nasal mucositis (ulcerative) (J34.81)

            oral mucositis (ulcerative) (K12.3-)

    K92.89 Other specified diseases of the digestive system

    K92.9 Disease of digestive system, unspecified

K94- Complications of artificial openings of the digestive system

    K94.0- <u>Colostomy</u> complications

    K94.00 Colostomy complication, unspecified

    K94.01 Colostomy hemorrhage

    K94.02 Colostomy infection

        Use additional code to specify type of infection, such as:

        Cellulitis of abdominal wall (L03.311)

        Sepsis (A40.-, A41.-)

    K94.03 Colostomy malfunction

        Mechanical complication of colostomy

    K94.09 Other complications of colostomy

K94.1- <u>Enterostomy</u> complications

    K94.10 Enterostomy complication, unspecified

    K94.11 Enterostomy hemorrhage

    K94.12 Enterostomy infection

        Use additional code to specify type of infection, such as:

        Cellulitis of abdominal wall (L03.311)

        Sepsis (A40.-, A41.-)

    K94.13 Enterostomy malfunction

        Mechanical complication of enterostomy

    K94.19 Other complications of enterostomy

K94.2- <u>Gastrostomy</u> complications

    K94.20 Gastrostomy complication, unspecified

    K94.21 Gastrostomy hemorrhage

    K94.22 Gastrostomy infection

        Use additional code to specify type of infection, such as:

        Cellulitis of abdominal wall (L03.311)

        Sepsis (A40.-, A41.-)

    K94.23 Gastrostomy malfunction

        Mechanical complication of gastrostomy

    K94.29 Other complications of gastrostomy

K94.3- <u>Esophagostomy</u> complications

    K94.30 Esophagostomy complications, unspecified

    K94.31 Esophagostomy hemorrhage

    K94.32 Esophagostomy infection

        Use additional code to identify the infection

    K94.33 Esophagostomy malfunction

        Mechanical complication of esophagostomy

    K94.39 Other complications of esophagostomy

K95 Complications of bariatric procedures

    K95.0- Complications of gastric band procedure

    K95.01 Infection due to gastric band procedure

        Use additional code to specify type of infection or organism, such as:

        Bacterial and viral infectious agents (B95.-, B96.-)

        Cellulitis of abdominal wall (L03.311)

        Sepsis (A40-, A41-)

    K95.09 Other complications of gastric band procedure

        Use additional code, if applicable, to further specify complication

    K95.8- Complications of other bariatric procedure

        Excludes 1: complications of gastric band surgery (K95.0-)

    K95.81 Infection due to other bariatric procedure

        Use additional code to specify type of infection or organism, such as:

        Bacterial and viral infectious agents (B95.-, B96.-)

        Cellulitis of abdominal wall (L03.311)

        Sepsis (A04.-, A41.-)

    K95.89 Other complications of other bariatric procedure

        Use additional code, if applicable, to further specify complication

K 9 1 - L 0 2

Chapter 12 – Diseases of the skin and subcutaneous tissue (L00-L99)

Excludes❷: certain conditions originating in the perinatal period (P04-P96)
certain infectious and parasitic diseases (A00-B99)
complications of pregnancy, childbirth and the puerperium (O00-O9A)
congenital malformations, deformations, and chromosomal abnormalities (Q00-Q99)
endocrine, nutritional and metabolic diseases (E00-E88)
lipomelanotic reticulosis (I89.8)
neoplasms (C00-D49)
symptoms, signs and abnormal clinical and laboratory findings, not elsewhere classified (R00-R94)
systemic connective tissue disorders (M30-M36)
viral warts (B07-)

This chapter contains the following blocks:
L00-L08   Infections of the skin and subcutaneous tissue
L10-L14   Bullous disorders
L20-L30   Dermatitis and eczema
L40-L45   Papulosquamous disorders
L49-L54   Urticaria and erythema
L55-L59   Radiation-related disorders of the skin and subcutaneous tissue
L60-L75   Disorders of skin appendages
L76   Intraoperative and postprocedural complications of skin and subcutaneous tissue
L80-L99   Other disorders of the skin and subcutaneous tissue

Infections of the skin and subcutaneous tissue (L00-L08)

Use additional code (B95-B97) to identify infectious agent
Excludes❷: hordeolum (H00.0)
infective dermatitis (L30.3)
local infections of skin classified in Chapter 1
lupus panniculitis (L93.2)
panniculitis NOS (M79.3)
panniculitis of neck and back (M54.0-)
Perlèche NOS (K13.0)
Perlèche due to candidiasis (B37.0)
Perlèche due to riboflavin deficiency (E53.0)
pyogenic granuloma (L98.0)
relapsing panniculitis [Weber-Christian] (M35.6)
viral warts (B07.-)
zoster (B02.-)

L00   Staphylococcal scalded skin syndrome
Ritter's disease
Use additional code to identify percentage of skin exfoliation (L49.-)
Excludes 1: bullous impetigo (L01.03)
pemphigus neonatorum (L01.03)
toxic epidermal necrolysis [Lyell] (L51.2)

L01-   Impetigo
Excludes 1: impetigo herpetiformis (L40.1)
L01.0-   Impetigo
Impetigo contagiosa
Impetigo vulgaris
L01.00   Impetigo, unspecified
Impetigo NOS
L01.01   Non-bullous impetigo
L01.02   Bockhart's impetigo
Impetigo follicularis
Perifolliculitis NOS
Superficial pustular perifolliculitis
L01.03   Bullous impetigo
Impetigo neonatorum
Pemphigus neonatorum
L01.09   Other impetigo
Ulcerative impetigo
L01.1   Impetiginization of other dermatoses

L02-   Cutaneous abscess, furuncle and carbuncle
Use additional code to identify organism (B95-B96)
Excludes❷: abscess of anus and rectal regions (K61.-)
abscess of female genital organs (external) (N76.4)
abscess of male genital organs (external) (N48.2, N49.-)
L02.0-   Cutaneous abscess, furuncle and carbuncle of face
Excludes❷: abscess of ear, external (H60.0)
abscess of eyelid (H00.0)
abscess of head [any part, except face] (L02.8)
abscess of lacrimal gland (H04.0)
abscess of lacrimal passages (H04.3)
abscess of mouth (K12.2)
abscess of nose (J34.0)
abscess of orbit (H05.0)
submandibular abscess (K12.2)
L02.01   Cutaneous abscess of face
L02.02   Furuncle of face
Boil of face
Folliculitis of face
L02.03   Carbuncle of face
L02.1-   Cutaneous abscess, furuncle and carbuncle of neck
L02.11   Cutaneous abscess of neck
L02.12   Furuncle of neck
Boil of neck
Folliculitis of neck
L02.13   Carbuncle of neck
L02.2-   Cutaneous abscess, furuncle and carbuncle of trunk
Excludes 1: non-newborn omphalitis (L08.82)
omphalitis of newborn (P38.-)
Excludes❷: abscess of breast (N61)
abscess of buttocks (L02.3)
abscess of female external genital organs (N76.4)
abscess of male external genital organs (N48.2, N49.-)
abscess of hip (L02.4)
L02.21-   Cutaneous abscess of trunk
L02.211   Cutaneous abscess of abdominal wall
L02.212   Cutaneous abscess of back [any part, except buttock]
L02.213   Cutaneous abscess of chest wall
L02.214   Cutaneous abscess of groin
L02.215   Cutaneous abscess of perineum
L02.216   Cutaneous abscess of umbilicus
L02.219   Cutaneous abscess of trunk, unspecified
L02.22-   Furuncle of trunk
Boil of trunk
Folliculitis of trunk
L02.221   Furuncle of abdominal wall
L02.222   Furuncle of back [any part, except buttock]
L02.223   Furuncle of chest wall
L02.224   Furuncle of groin
L02.225   Furuncle of perineum
L02.226   Furuncle of umbilicus
L02.229   Furuncle of trunk, unspecified
L02.23-   Carbuncle of trunk
L02.231   Carbuncle of abdominal wall
L02.232   Carbuncle of back [any part, except buttock]
L02.233   Carbuncle of chest wall
L02.234   Carbuncle of groin
L02.235   Carbuncle of perineum
L02.236   Carbuncle of umbilicus
L02.239   Carbuncle of trunk, unspecified
L02.3-   Cutaneous abscess, furuncle and carbuncle of buttock
Excludes 1: pilonidal cyst with abscess (L05.01)
L02.31   Cutaneous abscess of buttock
Cutaneous abscess of gluteal region
L02.32   Furuncle of buttock
Boil of buttock
Folliculitis of buttock
Furuncle of gluteal region
L02.33   Carbuncle of buttock
Carbuncle of gluteal region

K 9 1 - L 0 2

L02.4- Cutaneous abscess, furuncle and carbuncle of <u>limb</u>
Excludes❷: cutaneous abscess, furuncle and carbuncle of groin
(L02.214, L02.224, L02.234)
cutaneous abscess, furuncle and carbuncle of hand
(L02.5-)
cutaneous abscess, furuncle and carbuncle of foot
(L02.6-)

L02.41- Cutaneous <u>abscess</u> of limb
L02.411   Cutaneous abscess of <u>right</u> <u>axilla</u>
L02.412   Cutaneous abscess of <u>left</u> <u>axilla</u>
L02.413   Cutaneous abscess of <u>right</u> <u>upper</u> limb
L02.414   Cutaneous abscess of <u>left</u> <u>upper</u> limb
L02.415   Cutaneous abscess of <u>right</u> <u>lower</u> limb
L02.416   Cutaneous abscess of <u>left</u> <u>lower</u> limb
L02.419   Cutaneous abscess of limb, <u>unspecified</u>

L02.42- <u>Furuncle</u> of limb
Boil of limb
Folliculitis of limb
L02.421   Furuncle of <u>right</u> <u>axilla</u>
L02.422   Furuncle of <u>left</u> <u>axilla</u>
L02.423   Furuncle of <u>right</u> <u>upper</u> limb
L02.424   Furuncle of <u>left</u> <u>upper</u> limb
L02.425   Furuncle of <u>right</u> <u>lower</u> limb
L02.426   Furuncle of <u>left</u> <u>lower</u> limb
L02.429   Furuncle of limb, <u>unspecified</u>

L02.43- <u>Carbuncle</u> of limb
L02.431   Carbuncle of <u>right</u> <u>axilla</u>
L02.432   Carbuncle of <u>left</u> <u>axilla</u>
L02.433   Carbuncle of <u>right</u> <u>upper</u> limb
L02.434   Carbuncle of <u>left</u> <u>upper</u> limb
L02.435   Carbuncle of <u>right</u> <u>lower</u> limb
L02.436   Carbuncle of <u>left</u> <u>lower</u> limb
L02.439   Carbuncle of limb, <u>unspecified</u>

L02.5- Cutaneous abscess, furuncle and carbuncle of <u>hand</u>
L02.51- Cutaneous <u>abscess</u> of hand
L02.511   Cutaneous abscess of <u>right</u> hand
L02.512   Cutaneous abscess of <u>left</u> hand
L02.519   Cutaneous abscess of <u>unspecified</u> hand

L02.52- <u>Furuncle</u> hand
Boil of hand
Folliculitis of hand
L02.521   Furuncle <u>right</u> hand
L02.522   Furuncle <u>left</u> hand
L02.529   Furuncle <u>unspecified</u> hand

L02.53- <u>Carbuncle</u> of hand
L02.531   Carbuncle of <u>right</u> hand
L02.532   Carbuncle of <u>left</u> hand
L02.539   Carbuncle of <u>unspecified</u> hand

L02.6- Cutaneous abscess, furuncle and carbuncle of <u>foot</u>
L02.61- Cutaneous <u>abscess</u> of foot
L02.611   Cutaneous abscess of <u>right</u> foot
L02.612   Cutaneous abscess of <u>left</u> foot
L02.619   Cutaneous abscess of <u>unspecified</u> foot

L02.62- <u>Furuncle</u> of foot
Boil of foot
Folliculitis of foot
L02.621   Furuncle of <u>right</u> foot
L02.622   Furuncle of <u>left</u> foot
L02.629   Furuncle of <u>unspecified</u> foot

L02.63- <u>Carbuncle</u> of foot
L02.631   Carbuncle of <u>right</u> foot
L02.632   Carbuncle of <u>left</u> foot
L02.639   Carbuncle of <u>unspecified</u> foot

L02.8- Cutaneous abscess, furuncle and carbuncle of <u>other sites</u>
L02.81- Cutaneous <u>abscess</u> of other sites
L02.811   Cutaneous abscess of <u>head</u> [any part, except face]
L02.818   Cutaneous abscess of <u>other</u> sites

L02.82- <u>Furuncle</u> of other sites
Boil of other sites
Folliculitis of other sites
L02.821   Furuncle of <u>head</u> [any part, except face]
L02.828   Furuncle of <u>other</u> sites

L02.83- <u>Carbuncle</u> of other sites
L02.831   Carbuncle of <u>head</u> [any part, except face]
L02.838   Carbuncle of <u>other</u> sites

L02.9- Cutaneous abscess, furuncle and carbuncle, <u>unspecified</u>
L02.91 Cutaneous <u>abscess</u>, unspecified
L02.92 <u>Furuncle</u>, unspecified
Boil NOS
Furunculosis NOS
L02.93 <u>Carbuncle</u>, unspecified

L03- <u>Cellulitis and acute lymphangitis</u>
Excludes❷: cellulitis of anal and rectal region (K61.-)
cellulitis of external auditory canal (H60.1)
cellulitis of eyelid (H00.0)
cellulitis of female external genital organs (N76.4)
cellulitis of lacrimal apparatus (H04.3)
cellulitis of male external genital organs (N48.2, N49.-)
cellulitis of mouth (K12.2)
cellulitis of nose (J34.0)
eosinophilic cellulitis [Wells] (L98.3)
febrile neutrophilic dermatosis [Sweet] (L98.2)
lymphangitis (chronic) (subacute) (I89.1)

L03.0- Cellulitis and acute lymphangitis of finger and toe
Infection of nail
Onychia
Paronychia
Perionychia

L03.01- <u>Cellulitis</u> of finger
Felon
Whitlow
Excludes 1: herpetic whitlow (B00.89)
L03.011   Cellulitis of <u>right</u> finger
L03.012   Cellulitis of <u>left</u> finger
L03.019   Cellulitis of <u>unspecified</u> finger

L03.02- Acute <u>lymphangitis</u> of finger
Hangnail with lymphangitis of finger
L03.021   Acute lymphangitis of <u>right</u> finger
L03.022   Acute lymphangitis of <u>left</u> finger
L03.029   Acute lymphangitis of <u>unspecified</u> finger

L03.03- <u>Cellulitis</u> of toe
L03.031   Cellulitis of <u>right</u> toe
L03.032   Cellulitis of <u>left</u> toe
L03.039   Cellulitis of <u>unspecified</u> toe

L03.04- Acute <u>lymphangitis</u> of toe
Hangnail with lymphangitis of toe
L03.041   Acute lymphangitis of <u>right</u> toe
L03.042   Acute lymphangitis of <u>left</u> toe
L03.049   Acute lymphangitis of <u>unspecified</u> toe

L03.1- Cellulitis and acute lymphangitis of other parts of limb
L03.11- <u>Cellulitis</u> of other parts of <u>limb</u>
Excludes❷: cellulitis of fingers (L03.01-)
cellulitis of toes (L03.03-)
groin (L03.314)
L03.111   Cellulitis of <u>right</u> axilla
L03.112   Cellulitis of <u>left</u> axilla
L03.113   Cellulitis of <u>right</u> <u>upper</u> limb
L03.114   Cellulitis of <u>left</u> <u>upper</u> limb
L03.115   Cellulitis of <u>right</u> <u>lower</u> limb
L03.116   Cellulitis of <u>left</u> <u>lower</u> limb
L03.119   Cellulitis of <u>unspecified</u> part of limb

L03.12- Acute <u>lymphangitis</u> of other parts of <u>limb</u>
Excludes❷: acute lymphangitis of fingers (L03.2-)
acute lymphangitis of toes (L03.04-)
acute lymphangitis of groin (L03.324)
L03.121   Acute lymphangitis of <u>right</u> axilla
L03.122   Acute lymphangitis of <u>left</u> axilla
L03.123   Acute lymphangitis of <u>right</u> <u>upper</u> limb
L03.124   Acute lymphangitis of <u>left</u> <u>upper</u> limb
L03.125   Acute lymphangitis of <u>right</u> <u>lower</u> limb
L03.126   Acute lymphangitis of <u>left</u> <u>lower</u> limb
L03.129   Acute lymphangitis of <u>unspecified</u> part of limb

L03.2- Cellulitis and acute lymphangitis of face and neck
  L03.21- Cellulitis and acute lymphangitis of face
    L03.211   Cellulitis of face
Excludes❷: cellulitis of ear (H60.1-)
cellulitis of eyelid (H00.0-)
cellulitis of head (L03.81-
cellulitis of lacrimal apparatus (H04.3)
cellulitis of lip (K13.0)
cellulitis of mouth (K12.2)
cellulitis of nose (internal) (J34.0)
cellulitis of orbit (H05.0)
cellulitis of scalp (L03.81)
    L03.212   Acute lymphangitis of face
  L03.22- Cellulitis and acute lymphangitis of neck
    L03.221   Cellulitis of neck
    L03.222   Acute lymphangitis of neck
L03.3- Cellulitis and acute lymphangitis of trunk
  L03.31- Cellulitis of trunk
Excludes❷: cellulitis of anal and rectal regions (K61.-)
cellulitis of breast NOS (N61)
cellulitis of female external genital organs (N76.4)
cellulitis of male external genital organs (N48.2, N49.-)
omphalitis of newborn (P38.-)
puerperal cellulitis of breast (O91.2)
    L03.311   Cellulitis of abdominal wall
Excludes❷: cellulitis of umbilicus (L03.316)
cellulitis of groin (L03.314)
    L03.312   Cellulitis of back [any part except buttock]
    L03.313   Cellulitis of chest wall
    L03.314   Cellulitis of groin
    L03.315   Cellulitis of perineum
    L03.316   Cellulitis of umbilicus
    L03.317   Cellulitis of buttock
    L03.319   Cellulitis of trunk, unspecified
  L03.32- Acute lymphangitis of trunk
    L03.321   Acute lymphangitis of abdominal wall
    L03.322   Acute lymphangitis of back [any part except buttock]
    L03.323   Acute lymphangitis of chest wall
    L03.324   Acute lymphangitis of groin
    L03.325   Acute lymphangitis of perineum
    L03.326   Acute lymphangitis of umbilicus
    L03.327   Acute lymphangitis of buttock
    L03.329   Acute lymphangitis of trunk, unspecified
L03.8- Cellulitis and acute lymphangitis of other sites
  L03.81- Cellulitis of other sites
    L03.811   Cellulitis of head [any part, except face]
Cellulitis of scalp
Excludes❷: cellulitis of face (L03.211)
    L03.818   Cellulitis of other sites
  L03.89- Acute lymphangitis of other sites
    L03.891   Acute lymphangitis of head [any part, except face]
    L03.898   Acute lymphangitis of other sites
L03.9- Cellulitis and acute lymphangitis, unspecified
  L03.90   Cellulitis, unspecified
  L03.91   Acute lymphangitis, unspecified
Excludes 1: lymphangitis NOS (I89.1)

L04- Acute lymphadenitis
Includes: Abscess (acute) of lymph nodes, except mesenteric
Acute lymphadenitis, except mesenteric
Excludes 1: chronic or subacute lymphadenitis, except mesenteric (I88.1)
enlarged lymph nodes (R59.-)
human immunodeficiency virus [HIV] disease resulting in generalized lymphadenopathy (B20)
lymphadenitis NOS (I88.9)
nonspecific mesenteric lymphadenitis (I88.0)
  L04.0   Acute lymphadenitis of face, head and neck
  L04.1   Acute lymphadenitis of trunk
  L04.2   Acute lymphadenitis of upper limb
Acute lymphadenitis of axilla
Acute lymphadenitis of shoulder
  L04.3   Acute lymphadenitis of lower limb
Acute lymphadenitis of hip
Excludes❷: acute lymphadenitis of groin (L04.1)
  L04.8   Acute lymphadenitis of other sites
  L04.9   Acute lymphadenitis, unspecified
L05- Pilonidal cyst and sinus
  L05.0- Pilonidal cyst and sinus with abscess
    L05.01   Pilonidal cyst with abscess
Parasacral dimple with abscess
Pilonidal abscess
Pilonidal dimple with abscess
Postanal dimple with abscess
    L05.02   Pilonidal sinus with abscess
Coccygeal fistula with abscess
Coccygeal sinus with abscess
Pilonidal fistula with abscess
  L05.9- Pilonidal cyst and sinus without abscess
    L05.91   Pilonidal cyst without abscess
Parasacral dimple
Pilonidal dimple
Postanal dimple
Pilonidal cyst NOS
    L05.92   Pilonidal sinus without abscess
Coccygeal fistula
Coccygeal sinus without abscess
Pilonidal fistula
L08- Other local infections of skin and subcutaneous tissue
  L08.0   Pyoderma
Dermatitis gangrenosa
Purulent dermatitis
Septic dermatitis
Suppurative dermatitis
Excludes 1: pyoderma gangrenosum (L88)
pyoderma vegetans (L08.81)
  L08.1   Erythrasma
  L08.8- Other specified local infections of the skin and subcutaneous tissue
    L08.81   Pyoderma vegetans
Excludes 1: pyoderma gangrenosum (L88)
pyoderma NOS (L08.0)
    L08.82   Omphalitis not of newborn
Excludes 1: omphalitis of newborn (P38.-)
    L08.89   Other specified local infections of the skin and subcutaneous tissue
  L08.9   Local infection of the skin and subcutaneous tissue, unspecified

L0 2 - L0 8

Bullous disorders (L10-L14)

Excludes 1: *benign familial pemphigus [Hailey-Hailey] (Q82.8)*
staphylococcal scalded skin syndrome (L00)
toxic epidermal necrolysis [Lyell] (L51.2)

L10- Pemphigus
   Excludes 1: *pemphigus neonatorum (L01.03)*
   L10.0 Pemphigus vulgaris
   L10.1 Pemphigus vegetans
   L10.2 Pemphigus foliaceous
   L10.3 Brazilian pemphigus [fogo selvagem]
   L10.4 Pemphigus erythematosus
        Senear-Usher syndrome
   L10.5 Drug-induced pemphigus
        Use additional code for adverse effect, if applicable, to identify drug
        (T36-T50 with fifth or sixth character 5)
   L10.8- Other pemphigus
     L10.81 Paraneoplastic pemphigus
     L10.89 Other pemphigus
   L10.9 Pemphigus, unspecified

L11- Other acantholytic disorders
   L11.0 Acquired keratosis follicularis
        Excludes 1: *keratosis follicularis (congenital) [Darier-White]*
             (Q82.8)
   L11.1 Transient acantholytic dermatosis [Grover]
   L11.8 Other specified acantholytic disorders
   L11.9 Acantholytic disorder, unspecified

L12- Pemphigoid
   Excludes 1: *herpes gestationis (O26.4-)*
            impetigo herpetiformis (L40.1)
   L12.0 Bullous pemphigoid
   L12.1 Cicatricial pemphigoid
        Benign mucous membrane pemphigoid
   L12.2 Chronic bullous disease of childhood
        Juvenile dermatitis herpetiformis
   L12.3- Acquired epidermolysis bullosa
        Excludes 1: *epidermolysis bullosa (congenital) (Q81.-)*
     L12.30 Acquired epidermolysis bullosa, unspecified
     L12.31 Epidermolysis bullosa due to drug
          Use additional code for adverse effect, if applicable, to identify
          drug (T36-T50 with fifth or sixth character 5)
     L12.35 Other acquired epidermolysis bullosa
   L12.8 Other pemphigoid
   L12.9 Pemphigoid, unspecified

L13- Other bullous disorders
   L13.0 Dermatitis herpetiformis
        Duhring's disease
        Hydroa herpetiformis
        Excludes 1: *juvenile dermatitis herpetiformis (L12.2)*
             senile dermatitis herpetiformis (L12.0)
   L13.1 Subcorneal pustular dermatitis
        Sneddon-Wilkinson disease
   L13.8 Other specified bullous disorders
   L13.9 Bullous disorder, unspecified
L14 Bullous disorders <u>in diseases classified elsewhere</u>
        Code first underlying disease

Dermatitis and eczema (L20-L30)

Note: In this block the terms dermatitis and eczema are used synonymously
   and interchangeably.
Excludes ❷: *chronic (childhood) granulomatous disease (D71)*
         dermatitis gangrenosa (L08.0)
         dermatitis herpetiformis (L13.0)
         dry skin dermatitis (L85.3)
         factitial dermatitis (L98.1)
         perioral dermatitis (L71.0)
         radiation-related disorders of the skin and subcutaneous tissue
             (L55-L59)
         stasis dermatitis (I83.1-I83.2)

L20- Atopic dermatitis
   L20.0 Besnier's prurigo
   L20.8- Other atopic dermatitis
        Excludes ❷: *circumscribed neurodermatitis (L28.0)*
     L20.81 Atopic neurodermatitis
          Diffuse neurodermatitis
     L20.82 Flexural eczema
     L20.83 Infantile (acute) (chronic) eczema
     L20.84 Intrinsic (allergic) eczema
     L20.89 Other atopic dermatitis
   L20.9 Atopic dermatitis, unspecified

L21- Seborrheic dermatitis
   Excludes ❷: *infective dermatitis (L30.3)*
            seborrheic keratosis (L82.-)
   L21.0 Seborrhea capitis
        Cradle cap
   L21.1 Seborrheic infantile dermatitis
   L21.8 Other seborrheic dermatitis
   L21.9 Seborrheic dermatitis, unspecified
        Seborrhea NOS

L22 Diaper dermatitis
        Diaper erythema
        Diaper rash
        Psoriasiform diaper rash

L23- <u>Allergic</u> contact dermatitis
   Excludes 1: *allergy NOS (T78.40)*
            contact dermatitis NOS (L25.9)
            dermatitis NOS (L30.9)
   Excludes ❷: *dermatitis due to substances taken internally (L27.-)*
            dermatitis of eyelid (H01.1-)
            diaper dermatitis (L22)
            eczema of external ear (H60.5-)
            irritant contact dermatitis (L24.-)
            perioral dermatitis (L71.0)
            radiation-related disorders of the skin and subcutaneous tissue
                (L55-L59)
   L23.0 Allergic contact dermatitis due to <u>metals</u>
        Allergic contact dermatitis due to chromium
        Allergic contact dermatitis due to nickel
   L23.1 Allergic contact dermatitis due to <u>adhesives</u>
   L23.2 Allergic contact dermatitis due to <u>cosmetics</u>
   L23.3 Allergic contact dermatitis due to <u>drugs in contact with skin</u>
        Use additional code for adverse effect, if applicable, to identify drug
        (T36-T50 with fifth or sixth character 5)
        Excludes ❷: *dermatitis due to ingested drugs and medicaments*
                (L27.0-L27.1)
   L23.4 Allergic contact dermatitis due to <u>dyes</u>
   L23.5 Allergic contact dermatitis due to <u>other chemical products</u>
        Allergic contact dermatitis due to cement
        Allergic contact dermatitis due to insecticide
        Allergic contact dermatitis due to plastic
        Allergic contact dermatitis due to rubber
   L23.6 Allergic contact dermatitis due to <u>food in contact with the skin</u>
        Excludes ❷: *dermatitis due to ingested food (L27.2)*
   L23.7 Allergic contact dermatitis due to <u>plants, except food</u>
        Excludes ❷: *allergy NOS due to pollen (J30.1)*
   L23.8- Allergic contact dermatitis due to other agents
     L23.81 Allergic contact dermatitis due to <u>animal (cat) (dog) dander</u>
          Allergic contact dermatitis due to animal (cat) (dog) hair
     L23.89 Allergic contact dermatitis due to <u>other</u> agents
   L23.9 Allergic contact dermatitis, <u>unspecified</u> cause
        Allergic contact eczema NOS

L 10 - L 30

L24-   Irritant contact dermatitis
  Excludes 1:   *allergy NOS (T78.40)*
         contact dermatitis NOS (L25.9)
         dermatitis NOS (L30.9)
  Excludes❷: *allergic contact dermatitis (L23.-)*
         dermatitis due to substances taken internally (L27.-)
         dermatitis of eyelid (H01.1-)
         diaper dermatitis (L22)
         eczema of external ear (H60.5-)
         perioral dermatitis (L71.0)
         radiation-related disorders of the skin and subcutaneous tissue (L55-L59)

L24.0   Irritant contact dermatitis due to detergents
L24.1   Irritant contact dermatitis due to oils and greases
L24.2   Irritant contact dermatitis due to solvents
         Irritant contact dermatitis due to chlorocompound
         Irritant contact dermatitis due to cyclohexane
         Irritant contact dermatitis due to ester
         Irritant contact dermatitis due to glycol
         Irritant contact dermatitis due to hydrocarbon
         Irritant contact dermatitis due to ketone
L24.3   Irritant contact dermatitis due to cosmetics
L24.4   Irritant contact dermatitis due to drugs in contact with skin
         Use additional code for adverse effect, if applicable, to identify drug
         (T36-T50 with fifth or sixth character 5)
L24.5   Irritant contact dermatitis due to other chemical products
         Irritant contact dermatitis due to cement
         Irritant contact dermatitis due to insecticide
         Irritant contact dermatitis due to plastic
         Irritant contact dermatitis due to rubber
L24.6   Irritant contact dermatitis due to food in contact with skin
         Excludes❷: dermatitis due to ingested food (L27.2)
L24.7   Irritant contact dermatitis due to plants, except food
         Excludes❷: allergy NOS to pollen (J30.1)
L24.8- Irritant contact dermatitis due to other agents
   L24.81   Irritant contact dermatitis due to metals
           Irritant contact dermatitis due to chromium
           Irritant contact dermatitis due to nickel
   L24.89   Irritant contact dermatitis due to other agents
           Irritant contact dermatitis due to dyes
L24.9   Irritant contact dermatitis, unspecified cause
         Irritant contact eczema NOS

L25-   Unspecified contact dermatitis
  Excludes 1:   *allergic contact dermatitis (L23.-)*
         allergy NOS (T78.40)
         dermatitis NOS (L30.9)
         irritant contact dermatitis (L24.-)
  Excludes❷: *dermatitis due to ingested substances (L27.-)*
         dermatitis of eyelid (H01.1-)
         eczema of external ear (H60.5-)
         perioral dermatitis (L71.0)
         radiation-related disorders of the skin and subcutaneous tissue (L55-L59)

L25.0   Unspecified contact dermatitis due to cosmetics
L25.1   Unspecified contact dermatitis due to drugs in contact with skin
         Use additional code for adverse effect, if applicable, to identify drug
         (T36-T50 with fifth or sixth character 5)
         Excludes❷: dermatitis due to ingested drugs and medicaments (L27.0-L27.1)
L25.2   Unspecified contact dermatitis due to dyes
L25.3   Unspecified contact dermatitis due to other chemical products
         Unspecified contact dermatitis due to cement
         Unspecified contact dermatitis due to insecticide
L25.4   Unspecified contact dermatitis due to food in contact with skin
         Excludes❷: dermatitis due to ingested food (L27.2)
L25.5   Unspecified contact dermatitis due to plants, except food
         Excludes 1: nettle rash (L50.9)
         Excludes❷: allergy NOS due to pollen (J30.1)
L25.8   Unspecified contact dermatitis due to other agents
L25.9   Unspecified contact dermatitis, unspecified cause
         Contact dermatitis (occupational) NOS
         Contact eczema (occupational) NOS

L26   Exfoliative dermatitis
       Hebra's pityriasis
       Excludes 1: Ritter's disease (L00)

L27-   Dermatitis due to substances taken internally
  Excludes 1:   *allergy NOS (T78.40)*
  Excludes❷: *adverse food reaction, except dermatitis (T78.0-T78.1)*
         contact dermatitis (L23-L25)
         drug photoallergic response (L56.1)
         drug phototoxic response (L56.0)
         urticaria (L50.-)

L27.0   Generalized skin eruption due to drugs and medicaments taken internally
         Use additional code for adverse effect, if applicable, to identify drug
         (T36-T50 with fifth or sixth character 5)
L27.1   Localized skin eruption due to drugs and medicaments taken internally
         Use additional code for adverse effect, if applicable, to identify drug
         (T36-T50 with fifth or sixth character 5)
L27.2   Dermatitis due to ingested food
         Excludes❷: dermatitis due to food in contact with skin (L23.6, L24.6, L25.4)
L27.8   Dermatitis due to other substances taken internally
L27.9   Dermatitis due to unspecified substance taken internally

L28-   Lichen simplex chronicus and prurigo
L28.0   Lichen simplex chronicus
         Circumscribed neurodermatitis
         Lichen NOS
L28.1   Prurigo nodularis
L28.2   Other prurigo
         Prurigo NOS
         Prurigo Hebra
         Prurigo mitis
         Urticaria papulosa

L29-   Pruritus
  Excludes 1: neurotic excoriation (L98.1)
         psychogenic pruritus (F45.8)
L29.0   Pruritus ani
L29.1   Pruritus scroti
L29.2   Pruritus vulvae
L29.3   Anogenital pruritus, unspecified
L29.8   Other pruritus
L29.9   Pruritus, unspecified
         Itch NOS

L30-   Other and unspecified dermatitis
  Excludes❷: contact dermatitis (L23-L25)
         dry skin dermatitis (L85.3)
         small plaque parapsoriasis (L41.3)
         stasis dermatitis (I83.1-.2)
L30.0   Nummular dermatitis
L30.1   Dyshidrosis [pompholyx]
L30.2   Cutaneous autosensitization
         Candidid [levurid]
         Dermatophytid
         Eczematid
L30.3   Infective dermatitis
         Infectious eczematoid dermatitis
L30.4   Erythema intertrigo
L30.5   Pityriasis alba
L30.8   Other specified dermatitis
L30.9   Dermatitis, unspecified
         Eczema NOS

L
1
0
-
L
3
0

Papulosquamous disorders (L40-L45)

L40- Psoriasis

L40.0 Psoriasis vulgaris
Nummular psoriasis
Plaque psoriasis

L40.1 Generalized pustular psoriasis
Impetigo herpetiformis
Von Zumbusch's disease

L40.2 Acrodermatitis continua

L40.3 Pustulosis palmaris et plantaris

L40.4 Guttate psoriasis

L40.5- Arthropathic psoriasis

L40.50 Arthropathic psoriasis, unspecified

L40.51 Distal interphalangeal psoriatic arthropathy

L40.52 Psoriatic arthritis mutilans

L40.53 Psoriatic spondylitis

L40.54 Psoriatic juvenile arthropathy

L40.59 Other psoriatic arthropathy

L40.8 Other psoriasis
Flexural psoriasis

L40.9 Psoriasis, unspecified

L41- Parapsoriasis
Excludes 1:   poikiloderma vasculare atrophicans (L94.5)

L41.0 Pityriasis lichenoides et varioliformis acuta
Mucha-Habermann disease

L41.1 Pityriasis lichenoides chronica

L41.3 Small plaque parapsoriasis

L41.4 Large plaque parapsoriasis

L41.5 Retiform parapsoriasis

L41.8 Other parapsoriasis

L41.9 Parapsoriasis, unspecified

L42 Pityriasis rosea

L43- Lichen planus
Excludes 1:   lichen planopilaris (L66.1)

L43.0 Hypertrophic lichen planus

L43.1 Bullous lichen planus

L43.2 Lichenoid drug reaction
Use additional code for adverse effect, if applicable, to identify drug (T36-T50 with fifth or sixth character 5)

L43.3 Subacute (active) lichen planus
Lichen planus tropicus

L43.8 Other lichen planus

L43.9 Lichen planus, unspecified

L44- Other papulosquamous disorders

L44.0 Pityriasis rubra pilaris

L44.1 Lichen nitidus

L44.2 Lichen striatus

L44.3 Lichen ruber moniliformis

L44.4 Infantile papular acrodermatitis [Gianotti-Crosti]

L44.8 Other specified papulosquamous disorders

L44.9 Papulosquamous disorder, unspecified

L45 Papulosquamous disorders in diseases classified elsewhere
Code first underlying disease

Urticaria and erythema (L49-L54)

Excludes 1:   Lyme disease (A69.2-)
rosacea (L71.-)

L49- Exfoliation due to erythematous conditions according to extent of body surface involved
Code first erythematous condition causing exfoliation, such as:
Overlap syndrome (L51.3)
Ritter's disease (L00)
(Staphylococcal) scaled skin syndrom (L00)
Stevens-Johnson syndrome (L51.1)
Stevens-Johnson syndrome-toxic epidermal necrolysis
Toxic epidermal necrolysis (L51.2)

L49.0 Exfoliation due to erythematous condition involving less than 10 percent of body surface
Exfoliation due to erythematous condition NOS

L49.1 Exfoliation due to erythematous condition involving 10-19 percent of body surface

L49.2 Exfoliation due to erythematous condition involving 20-29 percent of body surface

L49.3 Exfoliation due to erythematous condition involving 30-39 percent of body surface

L49.4 Exfoliation due to erythematous condition involving 40-49 percent of body surface

L49.5 Exfoliation due to erythematous condition involving 50-59 percent of body surface

L49.6 Exfoliation due to erythematous condition involving 60-69 percent of body surface

L49.7 Exfoliation due to erythematous condition involving 70-79 percent of body surface

L49.8 Exfoliation due to erythematous condition involving 80-89 percent of body surface

L49.9 Exfoliation due to erythematous condition involving 90 or more percent of body surface

L50- Urticaria
Excludes 1:   allergic contact dermatitis (L23-)
angioneurotic edema (T78.3)
giant urticaria (T78.3)
hereditary angio-edema (D84.1)
Quincke's edema (T78.3)
serum urticaria (T80.6-)
solar urticaria (L56.3)
urticaria neonatorum (P83.8)
urticaria papulosa (L28.2)
urticaria pigmentosa (Q82.2)

L50.0 Allergic urticaria

L50.1 Idiopathic urticaria

L50.2 Urticaria due to cold and heat

L50.3 Dermatographic urticaria

L50.4 Vibratory urticaria

L50.5 Cholinergic urticaria

L50.6 Contact urticaria

L50.8 Other urticaria
Chronic urticaria
Recurrent periodic urticaria

L50.9 Urticaria, unspecified

L51- Erythema multiforme
Use additional code for adverse effect, if applicable, to identify drug (T36-T50 with fifth or sixth character 5)
Use additional code to identify associated manifestations, such as:
Arthropathy associated with dermatological disorders (M14.8-)
Conjunctival edema (H11.42)
Conjunctivitis (H10.22-)
Corneal scars and opacities (H17-)
Corneal ulcer (H16.0-)
Edema of eyelid (H02.84)
Inflammation of eyelid (H01.8)
Keratoconjunctivitis sicca (H16.22-)
Mechanical lagophthalmos (H02.22-)
Stomatitis (K12-)
Symblepharon (H11.23-)
Use additional code to identify percentage of skin exfoliation (L49.-)
Excludes 1:   staphylococcal scalded skin syndrome (L00)
Ritter's disease (L00)

L51.0 Nonbullous erythema multiforme

L51.1 Stevens-Johnson syndrome

L51.2 Toxic epidermal necrolysis [Lyell]

L51.3 Stevens-Johnson syndrome-toxic epidermal necrolysis overlap syndrome
SJS-TEN overlap syndrome

L51.8 Other erythema multiforme

L40 - L67

L51.9   **Erythema multiforme, unspecified**
Erythema iris
Erythema multiforme major NOS
Erythema multiforme minor NOS
Herpes iris

L52   **Erythema nodosum**
Excludes 1:   tuberculous erythema nodosum (A18.4)

L53-   **Other erythematous conditions**
*Excludes 1:   erythema ab igne (L59.0)
        erythema due to external agents in contact with skin (L23-
            L25)
        erythema intertrigo (L30.4)*

L53.0   **Toxic erythema**
Code first poisoning due to drug or toxin, if applicable (T36-T65
    with fifth or sixth character 1-4 or 6)
Use additional code for adverse effect, if applicable, to identify drug
    (T36-T50 with fifth or sixth character 5)
Excludes 1:   neonatal erythema toxicum (P83.1)

L53.1   **Erythema annulare centrifugum**
L53.2   **Erythema marginatum**
L53.3   **Other chronic figurate erythema**
L53.8   **Other specified erythematous conditions**
L53.9   **Erythematous condition, unspecified**
Erythema NOS
Erythroderma NOS

L54   **Erythema in diseases classified elsewhere**
Code first underlying disease

Radiation-related disorders of the skin and subcutaneous tissue (L55-L59)

L55-   **Sunburn**
L55.0   **Sunburn of first degree**
L55.1   **Sunburn of second degree**
L55.2   **Sunburn of third degree**
L55.9   **Sunburn, unspecified**

L56-   **Other acute skin changes due to ultraviolet radiation**
Use additional code to identify the source of the ultraviolet radiation (W89,
    X32)

L56.0   **Drug phototoxic response**
Use additional code for adverse effect, if applicable, to identify drug
    (T36-T50 with fifth or sixth character 5)

L56.1   **Drug photoallergic response**
Use additional code for adverse effect, if applicable, to identify drug
    (T36-T50 with fifth or sixth character 5)

L56.2   **Photocontact dermatitis [berloque dermatitis]**
L56.3   **Solar urticaria**
L56.4   **Polymorphous light eruption**
L56.5   **Disseminated superficial actinic porokeratosis (DSAP)**
L56.8   **Other specified acute skin changes due to ultraviolet radiation**
L56.9   **Acute skin change due to ultraviolet radiation, unspecified**

L57-   **Skin changes due to chronic exposure to nonionizing radiation**
Use additional code to identify the source of the ultraviolet radiation (W89,
    X32)

L57.0   **Actinic keratosis**
Keratosis NOS
Senile keratosis
Solar keratosis

L57.1   **Actinic reticuloid**
L57.2   **Cutis rhomboidalis nuchae**
L57.3   **Poikiloderma of Civatte**
L57.4   **Cutis laxa senilis**
Elastosis senilis

L57.5   **Actinic granuloma**
L57.8   **Other skin changes due to chronic exposure to nonionizing radiation**
Farmer's skin
Sailor's skin
Solar dermatitis

L57.9   **Skin changes due to chronic exposure to nonionizing radiation, unspecified**

L58-   **Radiodermatitis**
Use additional code to identify the source of the radiation (W88, W90)

L58.0   **Acute radiodermatitis**
L58.1   **Chronic radiodermatitis**
L58.9   **Radiodermatitis, unspecified**

L59-   **Other disorders of skin and subcutaneous tissue related to radiation**
L59.0   **Erythema ab igne [dermatitis ab igne]**
L59.8   **Other specified disorders of the skin and subcutaneous tissue related to radiation**
L59.9   **Disorder of the skin and subcutaneous tissue related to radiation, unspecified**

Disorders of skin appendages (L60-L75)

Excludes 1:   congenital malformations of integument (Q84.-)

L60-   **Nail disorders**
*Excludes❷: clubbing of nails (R68.3)
        onychia and paronychia (L03.0-)*

L60.0   **Ingrowing nail**
L60.1   **Onycholysis**
L60.2   **Onychogryphosis**
L60.3   **Nail dystrophy**
L60.4   **Beau's lines**
L60.5   **Yellow nail syndrome**
L60.8   **Other nail disorders**
L60.9   **Nail disorder, unspecified**

L62   **Nail disorders in diseases classified elsewhere**
Code first underlying disease, such as:
    Pachydermoperiostosis (M89.4-)

L63-   **Alopecia areata**
L63.0   **Alopecia (capitis) totalis**
L63.1   **Alopecia universalis**
L63.2   **Ophiasis**
L63.8   **Other alopecia areata**
L63.9   **Alopecia areata, unspecified**

L64-   **Androgenic alopecia**
Includes: Male-pattern baldness

L64.0   **Drug-induced androgenic alopecia**
Use additional code for adverse effect, if applicable, to identify drug
    (T36-T50 with fifth or sixth character 5)

L64.8   **Other androgenic alopecia**
L64.9   **Androgenic alopecia, unspecified**

L65-   **Other nonscarring hair loss**
Use additional code for adverse effect, if applicable, to identify drug (T36-
    T50 with fifth or sixth character 5)
Excludes 1:   trichotillomania (F63.3)

L65.0   **Telogen effluvium**
L65.1   **Anagen effluvium**
L65.2   **Alopecia mucinosa**
L65.8   **Other specified nonscarring hair loss**
L65.9   **Nonscarring hair loss, unspecified**
Alopecia NOS

L66-   **Cicatricial alopecia [scarring hair loss]**
L66.0   **Pseudopelade**
L66.1   **Lichen planopilaris**
Follicular lichen planus

L66.2   **Folliculitis decalvans**
L66.3   **Perifolliculitis capitis abscedens**
L66.4   **Folliculitis ulerythematosa reticulata**
L66.8   **Other cicatricial alopecia**
L66.9   **Cicatricial alopecia, unspecified**

L67-   **Hair color and hair shaft abnormalities**
*Excludes 1:   monilethrix (Q84.1)
        pili annulati (Q84.1)
        telogen effluvium (L65.0)*

L67.0   **Trichorrhexis nodosa**
L67.1   **Variations in hair color**
Canities
Greyness, hair (premature)
Heterochromia of hair
Poliosis circumscripta, acquired
Poliosis NOS

L67.8   **Other hair color and hair shaft abnormalities**
Fragilitas crinium

L67.9   **Hair color and hair shaft abnormality, unspecified**

L
4
0
–
L
6
7

Excludes 1: = NOT CODED HERE! (Do not code both)

Excludes❷: = Not Included Here

L68- Hypertrichosis
Includes: Excess hair
Excludes 1:   congenital hypertrichosis (Q84.2)
persistent lanugo (Q84.2)
L68.0 **Hirsutism**
L68.1 **Acquired hypertrichosis lanuginosa**
L68.2 **Localized hypertrichosis**
L68.3 **Polytrichia**
L68.8 **Other hypertrichosis**
L68.9 **Hypertrichosis, unspecified**

L70- Acne
Excludes❷: acne keloid (L73.0)
L70.0 **Acne vulgaris**
L70.1 **Acne conglobata**
L70.2 **Acne varioliformis**
Acne necrotica miliaris
L70.3 **Acne tropica**
L70.4 **Infantile acne**
L70.5 **Acné excoriée des jeunes filles**
Picker's acne
L70.8 **Other acne**
L70.9 **Acne, unspecified**

L71- Rosacea
Use additional code for adverse effect, if applicable, to identify drug (T36-T50 with fifth or sixth character 5)
L71.0 **Perioral dermatitis**
L71.1 **Rhinophyma**
L71.8 **Other rosacea**
L71.9 **Rosacea, unspecified**

L72- Follicular cysts of skin and subcutaneous tissue
L72.0 **Epidermal cyst**
L72.1- **Pilar and trichodermal cyst**
L72.11 **Pilar cyst**
L72.12 **Trichodermal cyst**
Trichilemmal (proliferating) cyst
L72.2 **Steatocystoma multiplex**
L72.3 **Sebaceous cyst**
Excludes❷: pilar cyst (L72.11)
trichilemmal (proliferating) cyst (L72.12)
L72.8 **Other follicular cysts of the skin and subcutaneous tissue**
L72.9 **Follicular cyst of the skin and subcutaneous tissue, unspecified**

L73- Other follicular disorders
L73.0 **Acne keloid**
L73.1 **Pseudofolliculitis barbae**
L73.2 **Hidradenitis suppurativa**
L73.8 **Other specified follicular disorders**
Sycosis barbae
L73.9 **Follicular disorder, unspecified**

L74- Eccrine sweat disorders
Excludes❷: generalized hyperhidrosis (R61)
L74.0 **Miliaria rubra**
L74.1 **Miliaria crystallina**
L74.2 **Miliaria profunda**
Miliaria tropicalis
L74.3 **Miliaria, unspecified**
L74.4 **Anhidrosis**
Hypohidrosis
L74.5- **Focal hyperhidrosis**
L74.51- **Primary focal hyperhidrosis**
L74.510 **Primary focal hyperhidrosis, axilla**
L74.511 **Primary focal hyperhidrosis, face**
L74.512 **Primary focal hyperhidrosis, palms**
L74.513 **Primary focal hyperhidrosis, soles**
L74.519 **Primary focal hyperhidrosis, unspecified**
L74.52 **Secondary focal hyperhidrosis**
Frey's syndrome
L74.8 **Other eccrine sweat disorders**
L74.9 **Eccrine sweat disorder, unspecified**
Sweat gland disorder NOS

L75- Apocrine sweat disorders
Excludes 1: dyshidrosis (L30.1)
hidradenitis suppurativa (L73.2)
L75.0 **Bromhidrosis**
L75.1 **Chromhidrosis**
L75.2 **Apocrine miliaria**
Fox-Fordyce disease
L75.8 **Other apocrine sweat disorders**
L75.9 **Apocrine sweat disorder, unspecified**

Intraoperative and postprocedural complications of skin and subcutaneous tissue (L76)

L76- Intraoperative and postprocedural complications of skin and subcutaneous tissue
L76.0- **Intraoperative hemorrhage and hematoma of skin and subcutaneous tissue complicating a procedure**
Excludes 1: intraoperative hemorrhage and hematoma of skin and subcutaneous tissue due to accidental puncture and laceration during a procedure (L76.1-)
L76.01 **Intraoperative hemorrhage and hematoma of skin and subcutaneous tissue complicating a dermatologic procedure**
L76.02 **Intraoperative hemorrhage and hematoma of skin and subcutaneous tissue complicating other procedure**
L76.1- **Accidental puncture and laceration of skin and subcutaneous tissue during a procedure**
L76.11 **Accidental puncture and laceration of skin and subcutaneous tissue during a dermatologic procedure**
L76.12 **Accidental puncture and laceration of skin and subcutaneous tissue during other procedure**
L76.2- **Postprocedural hemorrhage and hematoma of skin and subcutaneous tissue following a procedure**
L76.21 **Postprocedural hemorrhage and hematoma of skin and subcutaneous tissue following a dermatologic procedure**
L76.22 **Postprocedural hemorrhage and hematoma of skin and subcutaneous tissue following other procedure**
L76.8- **Other intraoperative and postprocedural complications of skin and subcutaneous tissue**
Use additional code, if applicable, to further specify disorder
L76.81 **Other intraoperative complications of skin and subcutaneous tissue**
L76.82 **Other postprocedural complications of skin and subcutaneous tissue**

Other disorders of the skin and subcutaneous tissue (L80-L99)

L80 Vitiligo
Excludes❷: vitiligo of eyelids (H02.73-)
vitiligo of vulva (N90.89)

L81- Other disorders of pigmentation
Excludes 1: birthmark NOS (Q82.5)
Peutz-Jeghers syndrome (Q85.8)
Excludes❷: nevus — see Alphabetical Index
L81.0 **Postinflammatory hyperpigmentation**
L81.1 **Chloasma**
L81.2 **Freckles**
L81.3 **Café au lait spots**
L81.4 **Other melanin hyperpigmentation**
Lentigo
L81.5 **Leukoderma, not elsewhere classified**
L81.6 **Other disorders of diminished melanin formation**
L81.7 **Pigmented purpuric dermatosis**
Angioma serpiginosum
L81.8 **Other specified disorders of pigmentation**
Iron pigmentation
Tattoo pigmentation
L81.9 **Disorder of pigmentation, unspecified**

L82- Seborrheic keratosis
Includes: Dermatosis papulosa nigra
Leser-Trélat disease
Excludes❷: seborrheic dermatitis (L21.-)
L82.0 **Inflamed seborrheic keratosis**
L82.1 **Other seborrheic keratosis**
Seborrheic keratosis NOS

L83 Acanthosis nigricans
Confluent and reticulated papillomatosis

L84 Corns and callosities
Callus
Clavus

L
6
8
I
L
8
9

L85- Other epidermal thickening
Excludes❷: hypertrophic disorders of the skin (L91.-)

L85.0 Acquired ichthyosis
Excludes 1: congenital ichthyosis (Q80.-)

L85.1 Acquired keratosis [keratoderma] palmaris et plantaris
Excludes 1: inherited keratosis palmaris et plantaris (Q82.8)

L85.2 Keratosis punctata (palmaris et plantaris)

L85.3 Xerosis cutis
Dry skin dermatitis

L85.8 Other specified epidermal thickening
Cutaneous horn

L85.9 Epidermal thickening, unspecified

L86 Keratoderma in diseases classified elsewhere
Code first underlying disease, such as:
Reiter's disease (M02.3-)
Excludes 1: gonococcal keratoderma (A54.89)
gonococcal keratosis (A54.89)
keratoderma due to vitamin A deficiency (E50.8)
keratosis due to vitamin A deficiency (E50.8)
xeroderma due to vitamin A deficiency (E50.8)

L87- Transepidermal elimination disorders
Excludes 1: granuloma annulare (perforating) (L92.0)

L87.0 Keratosis follicularis et parafollicularis in cutem penetrans
Kyrle disease
Hyperkeratosis follicularis penetrans

L87.1 Reactive perforating collagenosis

L87.2 Elastosis perforans serpiginosa

L87.8 Other transepidermal elimination disorders

L87.9 Transepidermal elimination disorder, unspecified

L88 Pyoderma gangrenosum
Phagedenic pyoderma
Excludes 1: dermatitis gangrenosa (L08.0)

L89- Pressure ulcer
Includes: Bed sore
Decubitus ulcer
Plaster ulcer
Pressure area
Pressure sore
Code first any associated gangrene (I96)
Excludes❷: decubitus (trophic) ulcer of cervix (uteri) (N86)
diabetic ulcers (E08.621, E08.622, E09.621, E09.622,
E10.621, E10.622, E11.621, E11.622, E13.621, E13.622)
non-pressure chronic ulcer of skin (L97.-)
skin infections (L00-L08)
varicose ulcer (I83.0, I83.2)

L89.0- Pressure ulcer of elbow

L89.00- Pressure ulcer of unspecified elbow

L89.000 Pressure ulcer of unspecified elbow, unstageable

L89.001 Pressure ulcer of unspecified elbow, stage 1
Healing pressure ulcer of unspecified elbow, stage 1
Pressure pre-ulcer skin changes limited to persistent
focal edema, unspecified elbow

L89.002 Pressure ulcer of unspecified elbow, stage 2
Healing pressure ulcer of unspecified elbow, stage 2
Pressure ulcer with abrasion, blister, partial thickness
skin loss involving epidermis and/or dermis,
unspecified elbow

L89.003 Pressure ulcer of unspecified elbow, stage 3
Healing pressure ulcer of unspecified elbow, stage 3
Pressure ulcer with full thickness skin loss involving
damage or necrosis of subcutaneous tissue,
unspecified elbow

L89.004 Pressure ulcer of unspecified elbow, stage 4
Healing pressure ulcer of unspecified elbow, stage 4
Pressure ulcer with necrosis of soft tissues through to
underlying muscle, tendon, or bone, unspecified
elbow

L89.009 Pressure ulcer of unspecified elbow, unspecified stage
Healing pressure ulcer of elbow NOS
Healing pressure ulcer of unspecified elbow,
unspecified stage

L89.01- Pressure ulcer of right elbow

L89.010 Pressure ulcer of right elbow, unstageable

L89.011 Pressure ulcer of right elbow, stage 1
Healing pressure ulcer of right elbow, stage 1
Pressure pre-ulcer skin changes limited to persistent
focal edema, right elbow

L89.012 Pressure ulcer of right elbow, stage 2
Healing pressure ulcer of right elbow, stage 2
Pressure ulcer with abrasion, blister, partial thickness
skin loss involving epidermis and/or dermis, right
elbow

L89.013 Pressure ulcer of right elbow, stage 3
Healing pressure ulcer of right elbow, stage 3
Pressure ulcer with full thickness skin loss involving
damage or necrosis of subcutaneous tissue, right
elbow

L89.014 Pressure ulcer of right elbow, stage 4
Healing pressure ulcer of right elbow, stage 4
Pressure ulcer with necrosis of soft tissues through to
underlying muscle, tendon, or bone, right elbow

L89.019 Pressure ulcer of right elbow, unspecified stage
Healing pressure right of elbow NOS
Healing pressure ulcer of unspecified elbow,
unspecified stage

L89.02- Pressure ulcer of left elbow

L89.020 Pressure ulcer of left elbow, unstageable

L89.021 Pressure ulcer of left elbow, stage 1
Healing pressure ulcer of left elbow, stage 1
Pressure pre-ulcer skin changes limited to persistent
focal edema, left elbow

L89.022 Pressure ulcer of left elbow, stage 2
Healing pressure ulcer of left elbow, stage 2
Pressure ulcer with abrasion, blister, partial thickness
skin loss involving epidermis and/or dermis, left
elbow

L89.023 Pressure ulcer of left elbow, stage 3
Healing pressure ulcer of left elbow, stage 3
Pressure ulcer with full thickness skin loss involving
damage or necrosis of subcutaneous tissue, left
elbow

L89.024 Pressure ulcer of left elbow, stage 4
Healing pressure ulcer of left elbow, stage 4
Pressure ulcer with necrosis of soft tissues through to
underlying muscle, tendon, or bone, left elbow

L89.029 Pressure ulcer of left elbow, unspecified stage
Healing pressure ulcer of left of elbow NOS
Healing pressure ulcer of unspecified elbow,
unspecified stage

L89.1- Pressure ulcer of back

L89.10- Pressure ulcer of unspecified part of back

L89.100 Pressure ulcer of unspecified part of back, unstageable

L89.101 Pressure ulcer of unspecified part of back, stage 1
Healing pressure ulcer of unspecified part of back,
stage 1
Pressure pre-ulcer skin changes limited to persistent
focal edema, unspecified part ofback

L89.102 Pressure ulcer of unspecified part of back, stage 2
Healing pressure ulcer of unspecified part of back,
stage 2
Pressure ulcer with abrasion, blister, partial thickness
skin loss involving epidermis and/or dermis,
unspecified part of back

L89.103 Pressure ulcer of unspecified part of back, stage 3
Healing pressure ulcer of unspecified part of back,
stage 3
Pressure ulcer with full thickness skin loss involving
damage or necrosis of subcutaneous tissue,
unspecified part of back

L89.104 Pressure ulcer of unspecified part of back, stage 4
Healing pressure ulcer of unspecified part of back,
stage 4
Pressure ulcer with necrosis of soft tissues through to
underlying muscle, tendon, or bone, unspecified
part of back

**L89.109 Pressure ulcer of unspecified part of back, unspecified
stage**
Healing pressure ulcer of unspecified part of back NOS
Healing pressure ulcer of unspecified part of back,
unspecified stage

L
6
8
–
L
8
9

L89.11- Pressure ulcer of <u>right upper back</u>
 Pressure ulcer of right shoulder blade

L89.110 Pressure ulcer of <u>right upper back</u>, unstageable

L89.111 Pressure ulcer of <u>right upper back</u>, stage 1
 Healing pressure ulcer of right upper back, stage 1
 Pressure pre-ulcer skin changes limited to persistent focal edema, right upper back

L89.112 Pressure ulcer of <u>right upper back</u>, stage 2
 Healing pressure ulcer of right upper back, stage 2
 Pressure ulcer with abrasion, blister, partial thickness skin loss involving epidermis and/or dermis, right upper back

L89.113 Pressure ulcer of <u>right upper back</u>, stage 3
 Healing pressure ulcer of right upper back, stage 3
 Pressure ulcer with full thickness skin loss involving damage or necrosis of subcutaneous tissue, right upper back

L89.114 Pressure ulcer of <u>right upper back</u>, stage 4
 Healing pressure ulcer of right upper back, stage 4
 Pressure ulcer with necrosis of soft tissues through to underlying muscle, tendon, or bone, right upper back

L89.119 Pressure ulcer of <u>right upper back</u>, unspecified stage
 Healing pressure ulcer of right upper back NOS
 Healing pressure ulcer of right upper back, unspecified stage

L89.12- Pressure ulcer of <u>left upper back</u>
 Pressure ulcer of left shoulder blade

L89.120 Pressure ulcer of <u>left upper back</u>, unstageable

L89.121 Pressure ulcer of <u>left upper back</u>, stage 1
 Healing pressure ulcer of left upper back, stage 1
 Pressure pre-ulcer skin changes limited to persistent focal edema, left upper back

L89.122 Pressure ulcer of <u>left upper back</u>, stage 2
 Healing pressure ulcer of left upper back, stage 2
 Pressure ulcer with abrasion, blister, partial thickness skin loss involving epidermis and/or dermis, left upper back

L89.123 Pressure ulcer of <u>left upper back</u>, stage 3
 Healing pressure ulcer of left upper back, stage 3
 Pressure ulcer with full thickness skin loss involving damage or necrosis of subcutaneous tissue, left upper back

L89.124 Pressure ulcer of <u>left upper back</u>, stage 4
 Healing pressure ulcer of left upper back, stage 4
 Pressure ulcer with necrosis of soft tissues through to underlying muscle, tendon, or bone, left upper back

L89.129 Pressure ulcer of <u>left upper back</u>, unspecified stage
 Healing pressure ulcer of left upper back NOS
 Healing pressure ulcer of left upper back, unspecified stage

L89.13- Pressure ulcer of <u>right lower back</u>

L89.130 Pressure ulcer of <u>right lower back</u>, unstageable

L89.131 Pressure ulcer of <u>right lower back</u>, stage 1
 Healing pressure ulcer of right lower back, stage 1
 Pressure pre-ulcer skin changes limited to persistent focal edema, right lower back

L89.132 Pressure ulcer of <u>right lower back</u>, stage 2
 Healing pressure ulcer of right lower back, stage 2
 Pressure ulcer with abrasion, blister, partial thickness skin loss involving epidermis and/or dermis, right lower back

L89.133 Pressure ulcer of <u>right lower back</u>, stage 3
 Healing pressure ulcer of right lower back, stage 3
 Pressure ulcer with full thickness skin loss involving damage or necrosis of subcutaneous tissue, right lower back

L89.134 Pressure ulcer of <u>right lower back</u>, stage 4
 Healing pressure ulcer of right lower back, stage 4
 Pressure ulcer with necrosis of soft tissues through to underlying muscle, tendon, or bone, right lower back

L89.139 Pressure ulcer of <u>right lower back</u>, unspecified stage
 Healing pressure ulcer of right lower back NOS
 Healing pressure ulcer of right lower back, unspecified stage

L89.14- Pressure ulcer of <u>left lower back</u>

L89.140 Pressure ulcer of <u>left lower back</u>, unstageable

L89.141 Pressure ulcer of <u>left lower back</u>, stage 1
 Healing pressure ulcer of left lower back, stage 1
 Pressure pre-ulcer skin changes limited to persistent focal edema, left lower back

L89.142 Pressure ulcer of <u>left lower back</u>, stage 2
 Healing pressure ulcer of left lower back, stage 2
 Pressure ulcer with abrasion, blister, partial thickness skin loss involving epidermis and/or dermis, left lower back

L89.143 Pressure ulcer of <u>left lower back</u>, stage 3
 Healing pressure ulcer of left lower back, stage 3
 Pressure ulcer with full thickness skin loss involving damage or necrosis of subcutaneous tissue, left lower back

L89.144 Pressure ulcer of <u>left lower back</u>, stage 4
 Healing pressure ulcer of left lower back, stage 4
 Pressure ulcer with necrosis of soft tissues through to underlying muscle, tendon, or bone, left lower back

L89.149 Pressure ulcer of <u>left lower back</u>, unspecified stage
 Healing pressure ulcer of left lower back NOS
 Healing pressure ulcer of left lower back, unspecified stage

L89.15- Pressure ulcer of <u>sacral</u> region
 Pressure ulcer of coccyx
 Pressure ulcer of tailbone

L89.150 Pressure ulcer of <u>sacral</u> region, unstageable

L89.151 Pressure ulcer of <u>sacral</u> region, stage 1
 Healing pressure ulcer of sacral region, stage 1
 Pressure pre-ulcer skin changes limited to persistent focal edema, sacral region

L89.152 Pressure ulcer of <u>sacral</u> region, stage 2
 Healing pressure ulcer of sacral region, stage 2
 Pressure ulcer with abrasion, blister, partial thickness skin loss involving epidermis and/or dermis, sacral region

L89.153 Pressure ulcer of <u>sacral</u> region, stage 3
 Healing pressure ulcer of sacral region, stage 3
 Pressure ulcer with full thickness skin loss involving damage or necrosis of subcutaneous tissue, sacral region

L89.154 Pressure ulcer of <u>sacral</u> region, stage 4
 Healing pressure ulcer of sacral region, stage 4
 Pressure ulcer with necrosis of soft tissues through to underlying muscle, tendon, or bone, sacral region

L89.159 Pressure ulcer of <u>sacral</u> region, unspecified stage
 Healing pressure ulcer of sacral region NOS
 Healing pressure ulcer of sacral region, unspecified stage

L89.2- Pressure ulcer of hip

L89.20- Pressure ulcer of <u>unspecified</u> hip

L89.200 Pressure ulcer of <u>unspecified</u> hip, unstageable

L89.201 Pressure ulcer of <u>unspecified</u> hip, stage 1
 Healing pressure ulcer of unspecified hip back, stage 1
 Pressure pre-ulcer skin changes limited to persistent focal edema, unspecified hip

L89.202 Pressure ulcer of <u>unspecified</u> hip, stage 2
 Healing pressure ulcer of unspecified hip, stage 2
 Pressure ulcer with abrasion, blister, partial thickness skin loss involving epidermis and/or dermis, unspecified hip

L89.203 Pressure ulcer of <u>unspecified</u> hip, stage 3
 Healing pressure ulcer of unspecified hip, stage 3
 Pressure ulcer with full thickness skin loss involving damage or necrosis of subcutaneous tissue, unspecified hip

L89.204 Pressure ulcer of <u>unspecified</u> hip, stage 4
 Healing pressure ulcer of unspecified hip, stage 4
 Pressure ulcer with necrosis of soft tissues through to underlying muscle, tendon, or bone, unspecified hip

L89.209 Pressure ulcer of <u>unspecified</u> hip, unspecified stage
 Healing pressure ulcer of unspecified hip NOS
 Healing pressure ulcer of unspecified hip, unspecified stage

L89.21- Pressure ulcer of <u>right</u> <u>hip</u>
   L89.210   Pressure ulcer of <u>right</u> <u>hip</u>, unstageable
   L89.211   Pressure ulcer of <u>right</u> <u>hip</u>, stage 1
         Healing pressure ulcer of right hip back, stage 1
         Pressure pre-ulcer skin changes limited to persistent focal edema, right hip
   L89.212   Pressure ulcer of <u>right</u> <u>hip</u>, stage 2
         Healing pressure ulcer of right hip, stage 2
         Pressure ulcer with abrasion, blister, partial thickness skin loss involving epidermis and/or dermis, right hip
   L89.213   Pressure ulcer of <u>right</u> <u>hip</u>, stage 3
         Healing pressure ulcer of right hip, stage 3
         Pressure ulcer with full thickness skin loss involving damage or necrosis of subcutaneous tissue, right hip
   L89.214   Pressure ulcer of <u>right</u> <u>hip</u>, stage 4
         Healing pressure ulcer of right hip, stage 4
         Pressure ulcer with necrosis of soft tissues through to underlying muscle, tendon, or bone, right hip
   L89.219   Pressure ulcer of <u>right</u> <u>hip</u>, unspecified stage
         Healing pressure ulcer of right hip NOS
         Healing pressure ulcer of right hip, unspecified stage

L89.22- Pressure ulcer of <u>left</u> <u>hip</u>
   L89.220   Pressure ulcer of <u>left</u> <u>hip</u>, unstageable
   L89.221   Pressure ulcer of <u>left</u> <u>hip</u>, stage 1
         Healing pressure ulcer of left hip back, stage 1
         Pressure pre-ulcer skin changes limited to persistent focal edema, left hip
   L89.222   Pressure ulcer of <u>left</u> <u>hip</u>, stage 2
         Healing pressure ulcer of left hip, stage 2
         Pressure ulcer with abrasion, blister, partial thickness skin loss involving epidermis and/or dermis, left hip
   L89.223   Pressure ulcer of <u>left</u> <u>hip</u>, stage 3
         Healing pressure ulcer of left hip, stage 3
         Pressure ulcer with full thickness skin loss involving damage or necrosis of subcutaneous tissue, left hip
   L89.224   Pressure ulcer of <u>left</u> <u>hip</u>, stage 4
         Healing pressure ulcer of left hip, stage 4
         Pressure ulcer with necrosis of soft tissues through to underlying muscle, tendon, or bone, left hip
   L89.229   Pressure ulcer of <u>left</u> <u>hip</u>, unspecified stage
         Healing pressure ulcer of left hip NOS
         Healing pressure ulcer of left hip, unspecified stage

L89.3- <u>Pressure ulcer of buttock</u>
L89.30- Pressure ulcer of <u>unspecified</u> <u>buttock</u>
   L89.300   Pressure ulcer of <u>unspecified</u> <u>buttock</u>, unstageable
   L89.301   Pressure ulcer of <u>unspecified</u> <u>buttock</u>, stage 1
         Healing pressure ulcer of unspecified buttock, stage 1
         Pressure pre-ulcer skin changes limited to persistent focal edema, unspecified buttock
   L89.302   Pressure ulcer of <u>unspecified</u> <u>buttock</u>, stage 2
         Healing pressure ulcer of unspecified buttock, stage 2
         Pressure ulcer with abrasion, blister, partial thickness skin loss involving epidermis and/or dermis, unspecified buttock
   L89.303   Pressure ulcer of <u>unspecified</u> <u>buttock</u>, stage 3
         Healing pressure ulcer of unspecified buttock, stage 3
         Pressure ulcer with full thickness skin loss involving damage or necrosis of subcutaneous tissue, unspecified buttock
   L89.304   Pressure ulcer of <u>unspecified</u> <u>buttock</u>, stage 4
         Healing pressure ulcer of unspecified buttock, stage 4
         Pressure ulcer with necrosis of soft tissues through to underlying muscle, tendon, or bone, unspecified buttock
   L89.309   Pressure ulcer of <u>unspecified</u> <u>buttock</u>, unspecified stage
         Healing pressure ulcer of unspecified buttock NOS
         Healing pressure ulcer of unspecified buttock, unspecified stage

L89.31- Pressure ulcer of <u>right</u> <u>buttock</u>
   L89.310   Pressure ulcer of <u>right</u> <u>buttock</u>, unstageable
   L89.311   Pressure ulcer of <u>right</u> <u>buttock</u>, stage 1
         Healing pressure ulcer of right buttock, stage 1
         Pressure pre-ulcer skin changes limited to persistent focal edema, right buttock
   L89.312   Pressure ulcer of <u>right</u> <u>buttock</u>, stage 2
         Healing pressure ulcer of right buttock, stage 2
         Pressure ulcer with abrasion, blister, partial thickness skin loss involving epidermis and/or dermis, right buttock

   L89.313   Pressure ulcer of <u>right</u> <u>buttock</u>, stage 3
         Healing pressure ulcer of right buttock, stage 3
         Pressure ulcer with full thickness skin loss involving damage or necrosis of subcutaneous tissue, right buttock
   L89.314   Pressure ulcer of <u>right</u> <u>buttock</u>, stage 4
         Healing pressure ulcer of right buttock, stage 4
         Pressure ulcer with necrosis of soft tissues through to underlying muscle, tendon, or bone, right buttock
   L89.319   Pressure ulcer of <u>right</u> <u>buttock</u>, unspecified stage
         Healing pressure ulcer of right buttock NOS
         Healing pressure ulcer of right buttock, unspecified stage

L89.32- Pressure ulcer of <u>left</u> <u>buttock</u>
   L89.320   Pressure ulcer of <u>left</u> <u>buttock</u>, unstageable
   L89.321   Pressure ulcer of <u>left</u> <u>buttock</u>, stage 1
         Healing pressure ulcer of left buttock, stage 1
         Pressure pre-ulcer skin changes limited to persistent focal edema, left buttock
   L89.322   Pressure ulcer of <u>left</u> <u>buttock</u>, stage 2
         Healing pressure ulcer of left buttock, stage 2
         Pressure ulcer with abrasion, blister, partial thickness skin loss involving epidermis and/or dermis, left buttock
   L89.323   Pressure ulcer of <u>left</u> <u>buttock</u>, stage 3
         Healing pressure ulcer of left buttock, stage 3
         Pressure ulcer with full thickness skin loss involving damage or necrosis of subcutaneous tissue, left buttock
   L89.324   Pressure ulcer of <u>left</u> <u>buttock</u>, stage 4
         Healing pressure ulcer of left buttock, stage 4
         Pressure ulcer with necrosis of soft tissues through to underlying muscle, tendon, or bone, left buttock
   L89.329   Pressure ulcer of <u>left</u> <u>buttock</u>, unspecified stage
         Healing pressure ulcer of left buttock NOS
         Healing pressure ulcer of left buttock, unspecified stage

L89.4- <u>Pressure ulcer</u> of contiguous site of back, buttock and hip
   L89.40   Pressure ulcer of <u>contiguous site of back, buttock and hip,</u> unspecified stage
         Healing pressure ulcer of contiguous site of back, buttock and hip NOS
         Healing pressure ulcer of contiguous site of back, buttock and hip, unspecified stage
   L89.41   Pressure ulcer of <u>contiguous site of back, buttock and hip,</u> stage 1
         Healing pressure ulcer of contiguous site of back, buttock and hip, stage 1
         Pressure pre-ulcer skin changes limited to persistent focal edema, contiguous site of back, buttock and hip
   L89.42   Pressure ulcer of <u>contiguous site of back, buttock and hip,</u> stage 2
         Healing pressure ulcer of contiguous site of back, buttock and hip, stage 2
         Pressure ulcer with abrasion, blister, partial thickness skin loss involving epidermis and/or dermis, contiguous site of back, buttock and hip
   L89.43   Pressure ulcer of <u>contiguous site of back, buttock and hip,</u> stage 3
         Healing pressure ulcer of contiguous site of back, buttock and hip, stage 3
         Pressure ulcer with full thickness skin loss involving damage or necrosis of subcutaneous tissue, contiguous site of back, buttock and hip
   L89.44   Pressure ulcer of <u>contiguous site of back, buttock and hip,</u> stage 4
         Healing pressure ulcer of contiguous site of back, buttock and hip, stage 4
         Pressure ulcer with necrosis of soft tissues through to underlying muscle, tendon, or bone, contiguous site of back, buttock and hip
   L89.45   Pressure ulcer of <u>contiguous site of back, buttock and hip,</u> unstageable

L89

L89 - L89

L89.5- Pressure ulcer of ankle
L89.50- Pressure ulcer of unspecified ankle
- **L89.500** Pressure ulcer of unspecified ankle, unstageable
- **L89.501** Pressure ulcer of unspecified ankle, stage 1
  - Healing pressure ulcer of unspecified ankle, stage 1
  - Pressure pre-ulcer skin changes limited to persistent focal edema, unspecified ankle
- **L89.502** Pressure ulcer of unspecified ankle, stage 2
  - Healing pressure ulcer of unspecified ankle, stage 2
  - Pressure ulcer with abrasion, blister, partial thickness skin loss involving epidermis and/or dermis, unspecified ankle
- **L89.503** Pressure ulcer of unspecified ankle, stage 3
  - Healing pressure ulcer of unspecified ankle, stage 3
  - Pressure ulcer with full thickness skin loss involving damage or necrosis of subcutaneous tissue, unspecified ankle
- **L89.504** Pressure ulcer of unspecified ankle, stage 4
  - Healing pressure ulcer of unspecified ankle, stage 4
  - Pressure ulcer with necrosis of soft tissues through to underlying muscle, tendon, or bone, unspecified ankle
- **L89.509** Pressure ulcer of unspecified ankle, unspecified stage
  - Healing pressure ulcer of unspecified ankle NOS
  - Healing pressure ulcer of unspecified ankle, unspecified stage

L89.51- Pressure ulcer of right ankle
- **L89.510** Pressure ulcer of right ankle, unstageable
- **L89.511** Pressure ulcer of right ankle, stage 1
  - Healing pressure ulcer of right ankle, stage 1
  - Pressure pre-ulcer skin changes limited to persistent focal edema, right ankle
- **L89.512** Pressure ulcer of right ankle, stage 2
  - Healing pressure ulcer of right ankle, stage 2
  - Pressure ulcer with abrasion, blister, partial thickness skin loss involving epidermis and/or dermis, right ankle
- **L89.513** Pressure ulcer of right ankle, stage 3
  - Healing pressure ulcer of right ankle, stage 3
  - Pressure ulcer with full thickness skin loss involving damage or necrosis of subcutaneous tissue, right ankle
- **L89.514** Pressure ulcer of right ankle, stage 4
  - Healing pressure ulcer of right ankle, stage 4
  - Pressure ulcer with necrosis of soft tissues through to underlying muscle, tendon, or bone, right ankle
- **L89.519** Pressure ulcer of right ankle, unspecified stage
  - Healing pressure ulcer of right ankle NOS
  - Healing pressure ulcer of right ankle, unspecified stage

L89.52- Pressure ulcer of left ankle
- **L89.520** Pressure ulcer of left ankle, unstageable
- **L89.521** Pressure ulcer of left ankle, stage 1
  - Healing pressure ulcer of left ankle, stage 1
  - Pressure pre-ulcer skin changes limited to persistnt focal edema, left ankle
- **L89.522** Pressure ulcer of left ankle, stage 2
  - Healing pressure ulcer of left ankle, stage 2
  - Pressure ulcer with abrasion, blister, partial thickness skin loss involving epidermis and/or dermis, left ankle
- **L89.523** Pressure ulcer of left ankle, stage 3
  - Healing pressure ulcer of left ankle, stage 3
  - Pressure ulcer with full thickness skin loss involving damage or necrosis of subcutaneous tissue, left ankle
- **L89.524** Pressure ulcer of left ankle, stage 4
  - Healing pressure ulcer of left ankle, stage 4
  - Pressure ulcer with necrosis of soft tissues through to underlying muscle, tendon, or bone, left ankle
- **L89.529** Pressure ulcer of left ankle, unspecified stage
  - Healing pressure ulcer of left ankle NOS
  - Healing pressure ulcer of left ankle, unspecified stage

L89.6- Pressure ulcer of heel
L89.60- Pressure ulcer of unspecified heel
- **L89.600** Pressure ulcer of unspecified heel, unstageable
- **L89.601** Pressure ulcer of unspecified heel, stage 1
  - Healing pressure ulcer of unspecified heel, stage 1
  - Pressure pre-ulcer skin changes limited to persistent focal edema, unspecified heel
- **L89.602** Pressure ulcer of unspecified heel, stage 2
  - Healing pressure ulcer of unspecified heel, stage 2
  - Pressure ulcer with abrasion, blister, partial thickness skin loss involving epidermis and/or dermis, unspecified heel
- **L89.603** Pressure ulcer of unspecified heel, stage 3
  - Healing pressure ulcer of unspecified heel, stage 3
  - Pressure ulcer with full thickness skin loss involving damage or necrosis of subcutaneous tissue, unspecified heel
- **L89.604** Pressure ulcer of unspecified heel, stage 4
  - Healing pressure ulcer of unspecified heel, stage 4
  - Pressure ulcer with necrosis of soft tissues through to underlying muscle, tendon, or bone, unspecified heel
- **L89.609** Pressure ulcer of unspecified heel, unspecified stage
  - Healing pressure ulcer of unspecified heel NOS
  - Healing pressure ulcer of unspecified heel, unspecified stage

L89.61- Pressure ulcer of right heel
- **L89.610** Pressure ulcer of right heel, unstageable
- **L89.611** Pressure ulcer of right heel, stage 1
  - Healing pressure ulcer of right heel, stage 1
  - Pressure pre-ulcer skin changes limited to persistent focal edema, right heel
- **L89.612** Pressure ulcer of right heel, stage 2
  - Healing pressure ulcer of right heel, stage 2
  - Pressure ulcer with abrasion, blister, partial thickness skin loss involving epidermis and/or dermis, right heel
- **L89.613** Pressure ulcer of right heel, stage 3
  - Healing pressure ulcer of right heel, stage 3
  - Pressure ulcer with full thickness skin loss involving damage or necrosis of subcutaneous tissue, right heel
- **L89.614** Pressure ulcer of right heel, stage 4
  - Healing pressure ulcer of right heel, stage 4
  - Pressure ulcer with necrosis of soft tissues through to underlying muscle, tendon, or bone, right heel
- **L89.619** Pressure ulcer of right heel, unspecified stage
  - Healing pressure ulcer of right heel NOS
  - Healing pressure ulcer of unspecified heel, right stage

L89.62- Pressure ulcer of left heel
- **L89.620** Pressure ulcer of left heel, unstageable
- **L89.621** Pressure ulcer of left heel, stage 1
  - Healing pressure ulcer of left heel, stage 1
  - Pressure pre-ulcer skin changes limited to persistent focal edema, left heel
- **L89.622** Pressure ulcer of left heel, stage 2
  - Healing pressure ulcer of left heel, stage 2
  - Pressure ulcer with abrasion, blister, partial thickness skin loss involving epidermis and/or dermis, left heel
- **L89.623** Pressure ulcer of left heel, stage 3
  - Healing pressure ulcer of left heel, stage 3
  - Pressure ulcer with full thickness skin loss involving damage or necrosis of subcutaneous tissue, left heel
- **L89.624** Pressure ulcer of left heel, stage 4
  - Healing pressure ulcer of left heel, stage 4
  - Pressure ulcer with necrosis of soft tissues through to underlying muscle, tendon, or bone, left heel
- **L89.629** Pressure ulcer of left heel, unspecified stage
  - Healing pressure ulcer of left heel NOS
  - Healing pressure ulcer of left heel, unspecified stage

L89.8- Pressure ulcer of other site
L89.81- Pressure ulcer of head
- Pressure ulcer of face
- **L89.810** Pressure ulcer of head, unstageable
- **L89.811** Pressure ulcer of head, stage 1
  - Healing pressure ulcer of head, stage 1
  - Pressure pre-ulcer skin changes limited to persistent focal edema, head

L89.812   **Pressure ulcer of <u>head</u>, stage 2**
Healing pressure ulcer of head, stage 2
Pressure ulcer with abrasion, blister, partial thickness
skin loss involving epidermis and/or dermis, head

L89.813   **Pressure ulcer of <u>head</u>, stage 3**
Healing pressure ulcer of head, stage 3
Pressure ulcer with full thickness skin loss involving
damage or necrosis of subcutaneous tissue, head

L89.814   **Pressure ulcer of <u>head</u>, stage 4**
Healing pressure ulcer of head, stage 4
Pressure ulcer with necrosis of soft tissues through to
underlying muscle, tendon, or bone, head

L89.819   **Pressure ulcer of <u>head</u>, unspecified stage**
Healing pressure ulcer of head NOS
Healing pressure ulcer of head, unspecified stage

L89.89- **Pressure ulcer of other site**

L89.890   **Pressure ulcer of <u>other</u> site, unstageable**

L89.891   **Pressure ulcer of <u>other</u> site, stage 1**
Healing pressure ulcer of other site, stage 1
Pressure pre-ulcer skin changes limited to persistent
focal edema, other site

L89.892   **Pressure ulcer of <u>other</u> site, stage 2**
Healing pressure ulcer of other site, stage 2
Pressure ulcer with abrasion, blister, partial thickness
skin loss involving epidermis and/or dermis, other
site

L89.893   **Pressure ulcer of <u>other</u> site, stage 3**
Healing pressure ulcer of other site, stage 3
Pressure ulcer with full thickness skin loss involving
damage or necrosis of subcutaneous tissue, other
site

L89.894   **Pressure ulcer of <u>other</u> site, stage 4**
Healing pressure ulcer of other site, stage 4
Pressure ulcer with necrosis of soft tissues through to
underlying muscle, tendon, or bone, other site

L89.899   **Pressure ulcer of <u>other</u> site, unspecified stage**
Healing pressure ulcer of other site NOS
Healing pressure ulcer of other site, unspecified stage

L89.9- **Pressure ulcer of unspecified site**

L89.90   **Pressure ulcer of <u>unspecified site</u>, unspecified stage**
Healing pressure ulcer of unspecified site NOS
Healing pressure ulcer of unspecified site, unspecified stage

L89.91   **Pressure ulcer of <u>unspecified site</u>, stage 1**
Healing pressure ulcer of unspecified site, stage 1
Pressure pre-ulcer skin changes limited to persistent focal
edema, unspecified site

L89.92   **Pressure ulcer of <u>unspecified site</u>, stage 2**
Healing pressure ulcer of unspecified site, stage 2
Pressure ulcer with abrasion, blister, partial thickness skin loss
involving epidermis and/or dermis, unspecified site

L89.93   **Pressure ulcer of <u>unspecified site</u>, stage 3**
Healing pressure ulcer of unspecified site, stage 3
Pressure ulcer with full thickness skin loss involving damage
or necrosis of subcutaneous tissue, unspecified site

L89.94   **Pressure ulcer of <u>unspecified site</u>, stage 4**
Healing pressure ulcer of unspecified site, stage 4
Pressure ulcer with necrosis of soft tissues through to
underlying muscle, tendon, or bone, unspecified site

L89.95   **Pressure ulcer of <u>unspecified site</u>, unstageable**

L90- **Atrophic disorders of skin**

L90.0   **Lichen sclerosus et atrophicus**
*Excludes❷: lichen sclerosus of external female genital organs
(N90.4)
lichen sclerosus of external male genital organs (N48.0)*

L90.1   **Anetoderma of Schweninger-Buzzi**

L90.2   **Anetoderma of Jadassohn-Pellizzari**

L90.3   **Atrophoderma of Pasini and Pierini**

L90.4   **Acrodermatitis chronica atrophicans**

L90.5   **Scar conditions and fibrosis of skin**
Adherent scar (skin)
Cicatrix
Disfigurement of skin due to scar
Fibrosis of skin NOS
Scar NOS
*Excludes❷: hypertrophic scar (L91.0)
keloid scar (L91.0)*

L90.6   **Striae atrophicae**

L90.8   **Other atrophic disorders of skin**

L90.9   **Atrophic disorder of skin, unspecified**

L91- **Hypertrophic disorders of skin**

L91.0   **Hypertrophic scar**
Keloid
Keloid scar
*Excludes❷: acne keloid (L73.0)
scar NOS (L90.5)*

L91.8   **Other hypertrophic disorders of the skin**

L91.9   **Hypertrophic disorder of the skin, unspecified**

L92- **Granulomatous disorders of skin and subcutaneous tissue**
Excludes❷: actinic granuloma (L57.5)

L92.0   **Granuloma annulare**
Perforating granuloma annulare

L92.1   **Necrobiosis lipoidica, not elsewhere classified**
*Excludes 1: necrobiosis lipoidica associated with diabetes mellitus
(E08-E13 with .620)*

L92.2   **Granuloma faciale [eosinophilic granuloma of skin]**

L92.3   **Foreign body granuloma of the skin and subcutaneous tissue**
Use additional code to identify the type of retained foreign body
(Z18.-)

L92.8   **Other granulomatous disorders of the skin and subcutaneous
tissue**

L92.9   **Granulomatous disorder of the skin and subcutaneous tissue,
unspecified**

L93- **Lupus erythematosus**
Use additional code for adverse effect, if applicable, to identify drug (T36-
T50 with fifth or sixth character 5)
*Excludes 1: lupus exedens (A18.4)
lupus vulgaris (A18.4)
scleroderma (M34.-)
systemic lupus erythematosus (M32.-)*

L93.0   **Discoid lupus erythematosus**
Lupus erythematosus NOS

L93.1   **Subacute cutaneous lupus erythematosus**

L93.2   **Other local lupus erythematosus**
Lupus erythematosus profundus
Lupus panniculitis

L94- **Other localized connective tissue disorders**
Excludes 1: systemic connective tissue disorders (M30-M36)

L94.0   **Localized scleroderma [morphea]**
Circumscribed scleroderma

L94.1   **Linear scleroderma**
En coup de sabre lesion

L94.2   **Calcinosis cutis**

L94.3   **Sclerodactyly**

L94.4   **Gottron's papules**

L94.5   **Poikiloderma vasculare atrophicans**

L94.6   **Ainhum**

L94.8   **Other specified localized connective tissue disorders**

L94.9   **Localized connective tissue disorder, unspecified**

L95- **Vasculitis limited to skin, not elsewhere classified**
*Excludes 1: angioma serpiginosum (L81.7)
Henoch(-Schönlein) purpura (D69.0)
hypersensitivity angiitis (M31.0)
lupus panniculitis (L93.2)
panniculitis NOS (M79.3)
panniculitis of neck and back (M54.0-)
polyarteritis nodosa (M30.0)
relapsing panniculitis (M35.6)
rheumatoid vasculitis (M05.2)
serum sickness (T80.6-)
urticaria (L50-)
Wegener's granulomatosis (M31.3-)*

L95.0   **Livedoid vasculitis**
Atrophie blanche (en plaque)

L95.1   **Erythema elevatum diutinum**

L95.8   **Other vasculitis limited to the skin**

L95.9   **Vasculitis limited to the skin, unspecified**

L
8
9
–
L
9
5

L97-　**Non-pressure chronic ulcer** of lower limb, not elsewhere classified
　　Includes:　Chronic ulcer of skin of lower limb NOS
　　　　　　　Non-healing ulcer of skin
　　　　　　　Non-infected sinus of skin
　　　　　　　Trophic ulcer NOS
　　　　　　　Tropical ulcer NOS
　　　　　　　Ulcer of skin of lower limb NOS
　　Code first any associated underlying condition, such as:
　　　Any associated gangrene (I96)
　　　Atherosclerosis of the lower extremities (I70.23-, I70.24-, I70.33-,
　　　　I70.34-, I70.43-, I70.44-, I70.53-, I70.54-, I70.63-, I70.64-, I70.73-,
　　　　I70.74-)
　　　Chronic venous hypertension (I87.31-, I87.33-)
　　　Diabetic ulcers (E08.621, E08.622, E09.621, E09.622, E10.621, E10.622,
　　　　E11.621, E11.622, E13.621, E13.622)
　　　Postphlebitic syndrome (I87.01-, I87.03-)
　　　Postthrombotic syndrome (I87.01-, I87.03-)
　　　Varicose ulcer (I83.0-, I83.2-)
　　Excludes❷:　*pressure ulcer (pressure area) (L89.-)*
　　　　　　　　skin infections (L00-L08)
　　　　　　　　specific infections classified to A00-B99

L97.1-　**Non-pressure chronic ulcer** of thigh

　L97.10-　Non-pressure chronic ulcer of **unspecified thigh**
　　L97.101　Non-pressure chronic ulcer of **unspecified** thigh limited to **breakdown of skin**
　　L97.102　Non-pressure chronic ulcer of **unspecified** thigh **with fat layer exposed**
　　L97.103　Non-pressure chronic ulcer of **unspecified** thigh **with necrosis of muscle**
　　L97.104　Non-pressure chronic ulcer of **unspecified** thigh **with necrosis of bone**
　　L97.109　Non-pressure chronic ulcer of **unspecified** thigh with **unspecified** severity

　L97.11-　Non-pressure chronic ulcer of **right thigh**
　　L97.111　Non-pressure chronic ulcer of **right** thigh limited to **breakdown of skin**
　　L97.112　Non-pressure chronic ulcer of **right** thigh **with fat layer exposed**
　　L97.113　Non-pressure chronic ulcer of **right** thigh **with necrosis of muscle**
　　L97.114　Non-pressure chronic ulcer of **right** thigh **with necrosis of bone**
　　L97.119　Non-pressure chronic ulcer of **right** thigh with **unspecified** severity

　L97.12-　Non-pressure chronic ulcer of **left** thigh
　　L97.121　Non-pressure chronic ulcer of **left** thigh limited to **breakdown of skin**
　　L97.122　Non-pressure chronic ulcer of **left** thigh **with fat layer exposed**
　　L97.123　Non-pressure chronic ulcer of **left** thigh **with necrosis of muscle**
　　L97.124　Non-pressure chronic ulcer of **left** thigh **with necrosis of bone**
　　L97.129　Non-pressure chronic ulcer of **left** thigh with **unspecified** severity

L97.2-　**Non-pressure chronic ulcer** of calf

　L97.20-　Non-pressure chronic ulcer of **unspecified calf**
　　L97.201　Non-pressure chronic ulcer of **unspecified** calf limited to **breakdown of skin**
　　L97.202　Non-pressure chronic ulcer of **unspecified** calf **with fat layer exposed**
　　L97.203　Non-pressure chronic ulcer of **unspecified** calf **with necrosis of muscle**
　　L97.204　Non-pressure chronic ulcer of **unspecified** calf **with necrosis of bone**
　　L97.209　Non-pressure chronic ulcer of **unspecified** calf with **unspecified** severity

　L97.21-　Non-pressure chronic ulcer of **right calf**
　　L97.211　Non-pressure chronic ulcer of **right** calf limited to **breakdown of skin**
　　L97.212　Non-pressure chronic ulcer of **right** calf **with fat layer exposed**
　　L97.213　Non-pressure chronic ulcer of **right** calf **with necrosis of muscle**
　　L97.214　Non-pressure chronic ulcer of **right** calf **with necrosis of bone**
　　L97.219　Non-pressure chronic ulcer of **right** calf with **unspecified** severity

　L97.22-　Non-pressure chronic ulcer of **left calf**
　　L97.221　Non-pressure chronic ulcer of **left** calf limited to **breakdown of skin**
　　L97.222　Non-pressure chronic ulcer of **left** calf **with fat layer exposed**
　　L97.223　Non-pressure chronic ulcer of **left** calf **with necrosis of muscle**
　　L97.224　Non-pressure chronic ulcer of **left** calf **with necrosis of bone**
　　L97.229　Non-pressure chronic ulcer of **left** calf with **unspecified** severity

L97.3-　**Non-pressure chronic ulcer** of ankle

　L97.30-　Non-pressure chronic ulcer of **unspecified ankle**
　　L97.301　Non-pressure chronic ulcer of **unspecified** ankle limited to **breakdown of skin**
　　L97.302　Non-pressure chronic ulcer of **unspecified** ankle **with fat layer exposed**
　　L97.303　Non-pressure chronic ulcer of **unspecified** ankle **with necrosis of muscle**
　　L97.304　Non-pressure chronic ulcer of **unspecified** ankle **with necrosis of bone**
　　L97.309　Non-pressure chronic ulcer of **unspecified** ankle with **unspecified** severity

　L97.31-　Non-pressure chronic ulcer of **right ankle**
　　L97.311　Non-pressure chronic ulcer of **right** ankle limited to **breakdown of skin**
　　L97.312　Non-pressure chronic ulcer of **right** ankle **with fat layer exposed**
　　L97.313　Non-pressure chronic ulcer of **right** ankle **with necrosis of muscle**
　　L97.314　Non-pressure chronic ulcer of **right** ankle **with necrosis of bone**
　　L97.319　Non-pressure chronic ulcer of **right** ankle with **unspecified** severity

　L97.32-　Non-pressure chronic ulcer of **left ankle**
　　L97.321　Non-pressure chronic ulcer of **left** ankle limited to **breakdown of skin**
　　L97.322　Non-pressure chronic ulcer of **left** ankle **with fat layer exposed**
　　L97.323　Non-pressure chronic ulcer of **left** ankle **with necrosis of muscle**
　　L97.324　Non-pressure chronic ulcer of **left** ankle **with necrosis of bone**
　　L97.329　Non-pressure chronic ulcer of **left** ankle with **unspecified** severity

L97.4-　**Non-pressure chronic ulcer** of heel and midfoot
　　　　　Non-pressure chronic ulcer of plantar surface of midfoot

　L97.40-　Non-pressure chronic ulcer of **unspecified heel and midfoot**
　　L97.401　Non-pressure chronic ulcer of **unspecified** heel and midfoot limited to **breakdown of skin**
　　L97.402　Non-pressure chronic ulcer of **unspecified** heel and midfoot **with fat layer exposed**
　　L97.403　Non-pressure chronic ulcer of **unspecified** heel and midfoot **with necrosis of muscle**
　　L97.404　Non-pressure chronic ulcer of **unspecified** heel and midfoot **with necrosis of bone**
　　L97.409　Non-pressure chronic ulcer of unspecified heel and midfoot with **unspecified** severity

　L97.41-　Non-pressure chronic ulcer of **right heel and midfoot**
　　L97.411　Non-pressure chronic ulcer of **right** heel and midfoot limited to **breakdown of skin**
　　L97.412　Non-pressure chronic ulcer of **right** heel and midfoot **with fat layer exposed**
　　L97.413　Non-pressure chronic ulcer of **right** heel and midfoot **with necrosis of muscle**
　　L97.414　Non-pressure chronic ulcer of **right** heel and midfoot **with necrosis of bone**
　　L97.419　Non-pressure chronic ulcer of **right** heel and midfoot with **unspecified** severity

L
9
7
-
L
9
7

L97.42- Non-pressure chronic ulcer of <u>left</u> <u>heel and midfoot</u>

    L97.421 Non-pressure chronic ulcer of <u>left</u> heel and midfoot limited to <u>breakdown of skin</u>

    L97.422 Non-pressure chronic ulcer of <u>left</u> heel and midfoot <u>with fat layer exposed</u>

    L97.423 Non-pressure chronic ulcer of <u>left</u> heel and midfoot <u>with necrosis of muscle</u>

    L97.424 Non-pressure chronic ulcer of <u>left</u> heel and midfoot <u>with necrosis of bone</u>

    L97.429 Non-pressure chronic ulcer of <u>left</u> heel and midfoot with <u>unspecified</u> severity

L97.5- <u>Non-pressure chronic ulcer</u> of <u>other part of foot</u>

    Non-pressure chronic ulcer of toe

L97.50- Non-pressure chronic ulcer of <u>other part of unspecified foot</u>

    L97.501 Non-pressure chronic ulcer of <u>other part of unspecified foot</u> limited to <u>breakdown of skin</u>

    L97.502 Non-pressure chronic ulcer of <u>other part of unspecified foot with fat layer exposed</u>

    L97.503 Non-pressure chronic ulcer of <u>other part of unspecified foot with necrosis of muscle</u>

    L97.504 Non-pressure chronic ulcer of <u>other part of unspecified foot with necrosis of bone</u>

    L97.509 Non-pressure chronic ulcer of <u>other part of unspecified foot</u> with <u>unspecified</u> severity

L97.51- Non-pressure chronic ulcer of <u>other part</u> of <u>right</u> <u>foot</u>

    L97.511 Non-pressure chronic ulcer of <u>other part</u> of <u>right</u> foot limited to <u>breakdown of skin</u>

    L97.512 Non-pressure chronic ulcer of <u>other part</u> of <u>right</u> foot <u>with fat layer exposed</u>

    L97.513 Non-pressure chronic ulcer of <u>other part</u> of <u>right</u> foot <u>with necrosis of muscle</u>

    L97.514 Non-pressure chronic ulcer of <u>other part</u> of <u>right</u> foot <u>with necrosis of bone</u>

    L97.519 Non-pressure chronic ulcer of <u>other part</u> of <u>right</u> foot with <u>unspecified</u> severity

L97.52- Non-pressure chronic ulcer of other part of <u>left</u> <u>foot</u>

    L97.521 Non-pressure chronic ulcer of <u>other part</u> of <u>left</u> foot limited to <u>breakdown of skin</u>

    L97.522 Non-pressure chronic ulcer of <u>other part</u> of <u>left</u> foot <u>with fat layer exposed</u>

    L97.523 Non-pressure chronic ulcer of <u>other part</u> of <u>left</u> foot <u>with necrosis of muscle</u>

    L97.524 Non-pressure chronic ulcer of <u>other part</u> of <u>left</u> foot <u>with necrosis of bone</u>

    L97.529 Non-pressure chronic ulcer of <u>other part</u> of <u>left</u> foot with <u>unspecified</u> severity

L97.8- <u>Non-pressure chronic ulcer</u> of other part of lower leg

L97.80 Non-pressure chronic ulcer of <u>other part of unspecified lower leg</u>

    L97.801 Non-pressure chronic ulcer of other part of unspecified <u>lower leg</u> limited to <u>breakdown of skin</u>

    L97.802 Non-pressure chronic ulcer of other part of unspecified <u>lower leg with fat layer exposed</u>

    L97.803 Non-pressure chronic ulcer of other part of unspecified <u>lower leg with necrosis of muscle</u>

    L97.804 Non-pressure chronic ulcer of other part of unspecified <u>lower leg with necrosis of bone</u>

    L97.809 Non-pressure chronic ulcer of other part of unspecified <u>lower leg</u> with <u>unspecified</u> severity

L97.81- Non-pressure chronic ulcer of <u>other part of right</u> <u>lower leg</u>

    L97.811 Non-pressure chronic ulcer of other part of <u>right</u> lower leg limited to <u>breakdown of skin</u>

    L97.812 Non-pressure chronic ulcer of other part of <u>right</u> lower leg <u>with fat layer exposed</u>

    L97.813 Non-pressure chronic ulcer of other part of <u>right</u> lower leg <u>with necrosis of muscle</u>

    L97.814 Non-pressure chronic ulcer of other part of <u>right</u> lower leg <u>with necrosis of bone</u>

    L97.819 Non-pressure chronic ulcer of other part of <u>right</u> lower leg with <u>unspecified</u> severity

L97.82- Non-pressure chronic ulcer of <u>other part of</u> <u>left</u> lower leg

    L97.821 Non-pressure chronic ulcer of other part of <u>left</u> lower leg limited to <u>breakdown of skin</u>

    L97.822 Non-pressure chronic ulcer of other part of <u>left</u> lower leg <u>with fat layer exposed</u>

    L97.823 Non-pressure chronic ulcer of other part of <u>left</u> lower leg <u>with necrosis of muscle</u>

    L97.824 Non-pressure chronic ulcer of other part of <u>left</u> lower leg <u>with necrosis of bone</u>

    L97.829 Non-pressure chronic ulcer of other part of <u>left</u> lower leg with <u>unspecified</u> severity

L97.9- <u>Non-pressure chronic ulcer</u> of <u>unspecified part of lower leg</u>

L97.90- Non-pressure chronic ulcer of <u>unspecified part of unspecified lower leg</u>

    L97.901 Non-pressure chronic ulcer of unspecified part of <u>unspecified</u> lower leg limited to <u>breakdown of skin</u>

    L97.902 Non-pressure chronic ulcer of unspecified part of <u>unspecified</u> lower leg <u>with fat layer exposed</u>

    L97.903 Non-pressure chronic ulcer of unspecified part of <u>unspecified</u> lower leg <u>with necrosis of muscle</u>

    L97.904 Non-pressure chronic ulcer of unspecified part of <u>unspecified</u> lower leg <u>with necrosis of bone</u>

    L97.909 Non-pressure chronic ulcer of unspecified part of <u>unspecified</u> lower leg with <u>unspecified</u> severity

L97.91- Non-pressure chronic ulcer of <u>unspecified part of right</u> lower leg

    L97.911 Non-pressure chronic ulcer of unspecified part of <u>right</u> lower leg limited to <u>breakdown of skin</u>

    L97.912 Non-pressure chronic ulcer of unspecified part of <u>right</u> lower leg <u>with fat layer exposed</u>

    L97.913 Non-pressure chronic ulcer of unspecified part of <u>right</u> lower leg <u>with necrosis of muscle</u>

    L97.914 Non-pressure chronic ulcer of unspecified part of <u>right</u> lower leg <u>with necrosis of bone</u>

    L97.919 Non-pressure chronic ulcer of unspecified part of <u>right</u> lower leg with <u>unspecified</u> severity

L97.92- Non-pressure chronic ulcer of <u>unspecified part of left</u> lower leg

    L97.921 Non-pressure chronic ulcer of unspecified part of <u>left</u> lower leg limited to <u>breakdown of skin</u>

    L97.922 Non-pressure chronic ulcer of unspecified part of <u>left</u> lower leg <u>with fat layer exposed</u>

    L97.923 Non-pressure chronic ulcer of unspecified part of <u>left</u> lower leg <u>with necrosis of muscle</u>

    L97.924 Non-pressure chronic ulcer of unspecified part of <u>left</u> lower leg <u>with necrosis of bone</u>

    L97.929 Non-pressure chronic ulcer of unspecified part of <u>left</u> lower leg with <u>unspecified</u> severity

L9
7
-
L9
7

Excludes 1: = NOT CODED HERE! (Do not code both)   **541**   *Excludes* ❷ *:* = Not Included Here

L98- Other disorders of skin and subcutaneous tissue, not elsewhere classified

L98.0 Pyogenic granuloma
Excludes❷: pyogenic granuloma of gingiva (K06.8)
pyogenic granuloma of maxillary alveolar ridge (K04.5)
pyogenic granuloma of oral mucosa (K13.4)

L98.1 Factitial dermatitis
Neurotic excoriation

L98.2 Febrile neutrophilic dermatosis [Sweet]

L98.3 Eosinophilic cellulitis [Wells]

L98.4- Non-pressure chronic ulcer of skin, not elsewhere classified
Chronic ulcer of skin NOS
Tropical ulcer NOS
Ulcer of skin NOS
Excludes❷: pressure ulcer (pressure area) (L89.-)
gangrene (I96)
skin infections (L00-L08)
specific infections classified to A00-B99
ulcer of lower limb NEC (L97.-)
varicose ulcer (I83.0-I82.2)

L98.41- Non-pressure chronic ulcer of buttock
L98.411 Non-pressure chronic ulcer of buttock limited to breakdown of skin
L98.412 Non-pressure chronic ulcer of buttock with fat layer exposed
L98.413 Non-pressure chronic ulcer of buttock with necrosis of muscle
L98.414 Non-pressure chronic ulcer of buttock with necrosis of bone
L98.419 Non-pressure chronic ulcer of buttock with unspecified severity

L98.42- Non-pressure chronic ulcer of back
L98.421 Non-pressure chronic ulcer of back limited to breakdown of skin
L98.422 Non-pressure chronic ulcer of back with fat layer exposed
L98.423 Non-pressure chronic ulcer of back with necrosis of muscle
L98.424 Non-pressure chronic ulcer of back with necrosis of bone
L98.429 Non-pressure chronic ulcer of back with unspecified severity

L98.49- Non-pressure chronic ulcer of skin of other sites
Non-pressure chronic ulcer of skin NOS
L98.491 Non-pressure chronic ulcer of skin of other sites limited to breakdown of skin
L98.492 Non-pressure chronic ulcer of skin of other sites with fat layer exposed
L98.493 Non-pressure chronic ulcer of skin of other sites with necrosis of muscle
L98.494 Non-pressure chronic ulcer of skin of other sites with necrosis of bone
L98.499 Non-pressure chronic ulcer of skin of other sites with unspecified severity

L98.5 Mucinosis of the skin
Focal mucinosis
Lichen myxedematosus
Reticular erythematous mucinosis
Excludes 1: focal oral mucinosis (K13.79)
myxedema (E03.9)

L98.6 Other infiltrative disorders of the skin and subcutaneous tissue
Excludes 1: hyalinosis cutis et mucosae (E78.89)

L98.8 Other specified disorders of the skin and subcutaneous tissue

L98.9 Disorder of the skin and subcutaneous tissue, unspecified

L99 Other disorders of skin and subcutaneous tissue in diseases classified elsewhere
Code first underlying disease, such as:
Amyloidosis (E85.-)
Excludes 1: skin disorders in diabetes (E08-E13 with .62)
skin disorders in gonorrhea (A54.89)
skin disorders in syphilis (A51.31, A52.79)

Chapter 13 – Diseases of the musculoskeletal system and connective tissue (M00-M99)

Note: Use an external cause code following the code for the musculoskeletal condition, if applicable, to identify the cause of the musculoskeletal condition

Excludes❷: arthropathic psoriasis (L40.5-)
certain conditions originating in the perinatal period (P04-P96)
certain infectious and parasitic diseases (A00-B99)
compartment syndrome (traumatic) (T79.A-)
complications of pregnancy, childbirth and the puerperium (O00-O9A)
congenital malformations, deformations, and chromosomal abnormalities (Q00-Q99)
endocrine, nutritional and metabolic diseases (E00-E88)
injury, poisoning and certain other consequences of external causes (S00-T88)
neoplasms (C00-D49)
symptoms, signs and abnormal clinical and laboratory findings, not elsewhere classified (R00-R94)

This chapter contains the following blocks:

M00-M02	Infectious arthropathies
M05-M14	Inflammatory polyarthropathies
M15-M19	Osteoarthritis
M20-M25	Other joint disorders
M26-M27	Dentofacial anomalies [including malocclusion] and other disorders of jaw
M30-M36	Systemic connective tissue disorders
M40-M43	Deforming dorsopathies
M45-M49	Spondylopathies
M50-M54	Other dorsopathies
M60-M63	Disorders of muscles
M65-M67	Disorders of synovium and tendon
M70-M79	Other soft tissue disorders
M80-M85	Disorders of bone density and structure
M86-M90	Other osteopathies
M91-M94	Chondropathies
M95	Other disorders of the musculoskeletal system and connective tissue
M96	Intraoperative and postprocedural complications and disorders of musculoskeletal system, not elsewhere classified
M99	Biomechanical lesions, not elsewhere classified

Arthropathies (M00-M25)

Includes: Disorders affecting predominantly peripheral (limb) joints

Infectious arthropathies (M00-M02)

Note: This block comprises arthropathies due to microbiological agents. Distinction is made between the following types of etiological relationship:
  a) direct infection of joint, where organisms invade synovial tissue and microbial antigen is present in the joint;
  b) indirect infection, which may be of two types: a reactive arthropathy, where microbial infection of the body is established but neither organisms nor antigens can be identified in the joint, and a postinfective arthropathy, where microbial antigen is present but recovery of an organism is inconstant and evidence of local multiplication is lacking.

M00- <u>Pyogenic</u> arthritis
  M00.0- <u>Staphylococcal</u> arthritis and polyarthritis
    Use additional code (B95.61-B95.8) to identify bacterial agent
    Excludes❷: infection and inflammatory reaction due to internal joint prosthesis (T84.5-)
  M00.00 Staphylococcal arthritis, <u>unspecified</u> joint
  M00.01- Staphylococcal arthritis, <u>shoulder</u>
    M00.011 Staphylococcal arthritis, <u>right</u> shoulder
    M00.012 Staphylococcal arthritis, <u>left</u> shoulder
    M00.019 Staphylococcal arthritis, <u>unspecified</u> shoulder
  M00.02- Staphylococcal arthritis, <u>elbow</u>
    M00.021 Staphylococcal arthritis, <u>right</u> elbow
    M00.022 Staphylococcal arthritis, <u>left</u> elbow
    M00.029 Staphylococcal arthritis, <u>unspecified</u> elbow
  M00.03- Staphylococcal arthritis, <u>wrist</u>
    Staphylococcal arthritis of carpal bones
    M00.031 Staphylococcal arthritis, <u>right</u> wrist
    M00.032 Staphylococcal arthritis, <u>left</u> wrist
    M00.039 Staphylococcal arthritis, <u>unspecified</u> wrist

M00.04- Staphylococcal arthritis, <u>hand</u>
    Staphylococcal arthritis of metacarpus and phalanges
  M00.041 Staphylococcal arthritis, <u>right</u> hand
  M00.042 Staphylococcal arthritis, <u>left</u> hand
  M00.049 Staphylococcal arthritis, <u>unspecified</u> hand
M00.05- Staphylococcal arthritis, <u>hip</u>
  M00.051 Staphylococcal arthritis, <u>right</u> hip
  M00.052 Staphylococcal arthritis, <u>left</u> hip
  M00.059 Staphylococcal arthritis, <u>unspecified</u> hip
M00.06- Staphylococcal arthritis, <u>knee</u>
  M00.061 Staphylococcal arthritis, <u>right</u> knee
  M00.062 Staphylococcal arthritis, <u>left</u> knee
  M00.069 Staphylococcal arthritis, <u>unspecified</u> knee
M00.07- Staphylococcal arthritis, <u>ankle and foot</u>
    Staphylococcal arthritis, tarsus, metatarsus and phalanges
  M00.071 Staphylococcal arthritis, <u>right</u> ankle and foot
  M00.072 Staphylococcal arthritis, <u>left</u> ankle and foot
  M00.079 Staphylococcal arthritis, <u>unspecified</u> ankle and foot
M00.08 Staphylococcal arthritis, <u>vertebrae</u>
M00.09 Staphylococcal <u>polyarthritis</u>
M00.1- <u>Pneumococcal</u> arthritis and polyarthritis
M00.10 Pneumococcal arthritis, <u>unspecified</u> joint
M00.11- Pneumococcal arthritis, <u>shoulder</u>
  M00.111 Pneumococcal arthritis, <u>right</u> shoulder
  M00.112 Pneumococcal arthritis, <u>left</u> shoulder
  M00.119 Pneumococcal arthritis, <u>unspecified</u> shoulder
M00.12- Pneumococcal arthritis, <u>elbow</u>
  M00.121 Pneumococcal arthritis, <u>right</u> elbow
  M00.122 Pneumococcal arthritis, <u>left</u> elbow
  M00.129 Pneumococcal arthritis, <u>unspecified</u> elbow
M00.13- Pneumococcal arthritis, <u>wrist</u>
    Pneumococcal arthritis of carpal bones
  M00.131 Pneumococcal arthritis, <u>right</u> wrist
  M00.132 Pneumococcal arthritis, <u>left</u> wrist
  M00.139 Pneumococcal arthritis, <u>unspecified</u> wrist
M00.14- Pneumococcal arthritis, <u>hand</u>
    Pneumococcal arthritis of metacarpus and phalanges
  M00.141 Pneumococcal arthritis, <u>right</u> hand
  M00.142 Pneumococcal arthritis, <u>left</u> hand
  M00.149 Pneumococcal arthritis, <u>unspecified</u> hand
M00.15- Pneumococcal arthritis, <u>hip</u>
  M00.151 Pneumococcal arthritis, <u>right</u> hip
  M00.152 Pneumococcal arthritis, <u>left</u> hip
  M00.159 Pneumococcal arthritis, <u>unspecified</u> hip
M00.16- Pneumococcal arthritis, <u>knee</u>
  M00.161 Pneumococcal arthritis, <u>right</u> knee
  M00.162 Pneumococcal arthritis, <u>left</u> knee
  M00.169 Pneumococcal arthritis, <u>unspecified</u> knee
M00.17- Pneumococcal arthritis, <u>ankle and foot</u>
    Pneumococcal arthritis, tarsus, metatarsus and phalanges
  M00.171 Pneumococcal arthritis, <u>right</u> ankle and foot
  M00.172 Pneumococcal arthritis, <u>left</u> ankle and foot
  M00.179 Pneumococcal arthritis, <u>unspecified</u> ankle and foot
M00.18 Pneumococcal arthritis, <u>vertebrae</u>
M00.19 Pneumococcal <u>polyarthritis</u>
M00.2- <u>Other streptococcal</u> arthritis and polyarthritis
    Use additional code (B95.0-B95.2, B95.4-B95.5) to identify bacterial agent
M00.20 Other streptococcal arthritis, <u>unspecified</u> joint
M00.21- Other streptococcal arthritis, <u>shoulder</u>
  M00.211 Other streptococcal arthritis, <u>right</u> shoulder
  M00.212 Other streptococcal arthritis, <u>left</u> shoulder
  M00.219 Other streptococcal arthritis, <u>unspecified</u> shoulder
M00.22- Other streptococcal arthritis, <u>elbow</u>
  M00.221 Other streptococcal arthritis, <u>right</u> elbow
  M00.222 Other streptococcal arthritis, <u>left</u> elbow
  M00.229 Other streptococcal arthritis, <u>unspecified</u> elbow
M00.23- Other streptococcal arthritis, <u>wrist</u>
    Other streptococcal arthritis of carpal bones
  M00.231 Other streptococcal arthritis, <u>right</u> wrist
  M00.232 Other streptococcal arthritis, <u>left</u> wrist
  M00.239 Other streptococcal arthritis, <u>unspecified</u> wrist

M00.24-Other streptococcal arthritis, <u>hand</u>
Other streptococcal arthritis metacarpus and phalanges
    M00.241   Other streptococcal arthritis, <u>right</u> hand
    M00.242   Other streptococcal arthritis, <u>left</u> hand
    M00.249   Other streptococcal arthritis, <u>unspecified</u> hand
M00.25-Other streptococcal arthritis, <u>hip</u>
    M00.251   Other streptococcal arthritis, <u>right</u> hip
    M00.252   Other streptococcal arthritis, <u>left</u> hip
    M00.259   Other streptococcal arthritis, <u>unspecified</u> hip
M00.26-Other streptococcal arthritis, <u>knee</u>
    M00.261   Other streptococcal arthritis, <u>right</u> knee
    M00.262   Other streptococcal arthritis, <u>left</u> knee
    M00.269   Other streptococcal arthritis, <u>unspecified</u> knee
M00.27-Other streptococcal arthritis, <u>ankle and foot</u>
Other streptococcal arthritis, tarsus, metatarsus and phalanges
    M00.271   Other streptococcal arthritis, <u>right</u> ankle and foot
    M00.272   Other streptococcal arthritis, <u>left</u> ankle and foot
    M00.279   Other streptococcal arthritis, <u>unspecified</u> ankle and foot
M00.28 Other streptococcal arthritis, <u>vertebrae</u>
M00.29 Other streptococcal <u>polyarthritis</u>
M00.8- Arthritis and polyarthritis <u>due to other bacteria</u>
Use additional code (B96) to identify bacteria
M00.80 Arthritis due to other bacteria, <u>unspecified</u> joint
M00.81-Arthritis due to other bacteria, <u>shoulder</u>
    M00.811   Arthritis due to other bacteria, <u>right</u> shoulder
    M00.812   Arthritis due to other bacteria, <u>left</u> shoulder
    M00.819   Arthritis due to other bacteria, <u>unspecified</u> shoulder
M00.82-Arthritis due to other bacteria, <u>elbow</u>
    M00.821   Arthritis due to other bacteria, <u>right</u> elbow
    M00.822   Arthritis due to other bacteria, <u>left</u> elbow
    M00.829   Arthritis due to other bacteria, <u>unspecified</u> elbow
M00.83-Arthritis due to other bacteria, <u>wrist</u>
Arthritis due to other bacteria, carpal bones
    M00.831   Arthritis due to other bacteria, <u>right</u> wrist
    M00.832   Arthritis due to other bacteria, <u>left</u> wrist
    M00.839   Arthritis due to other bacteria, <u>unspecified</u> wrist
M00.84-Arthritis due to other bacteria, <u>hand</u>
Arthritis due to other bacteria, metacarpus and phalanges
    M00.841   Arthritis due to other bacteria, <u>right</u> hand
    M00.842   Arthritis due to other bacteria, <u>left</u> hand
    M00.849   Arthritis due to other bacteria, <u>unspecified</u> hand
M00.85-Arthritis due to other bacteria, <u>hip</u>
    M00.851   Arthritis due to other bacteria, <u>right</u> hip
    M00.852   Arthritis due to other bacteria, <u>left</u> hip
    M00.859   Arthritis due to other bacteria, <u>unspecified</u> hip
M00.86-Arthritis due to other bacteria, <u>knee</u>
    M00.861   Arthritis due to other bacteria, <u>right</u> knee
    M00.862   Arthritis due to other bacteria, <u>left</u> knee
    M00.869   Arthritis due to other bacteria, <u>unspecified</u> knee
M00.87-Arthritis due to other bacteria, <u>ankle and foot</u>
Arthritis due to other bacteria, tarsus, metatarsus, and phalanges
    M00.871   Arthritis due to other bacteria, <u>right</u> ankle and foot
    M00.872   Arthritis due to other bacteria, <u>left</u> ankle and foot
    M00.879   Arthritis due to other bacteria, <u>unspecified</u> ankle and foot
M00.88 Arthritis due to other bacteria, <u>vertebrae</u>
M00.89 <u>Polyarthritis</u> due to other bacteria
M00.9   Pyogenic arthritis, <u>unspecified</u>
Infective arthritis NOS

M01- Direct infections of joint <u>in infectious and parasitic diseases classified elsewhere</u>
Code first underlying disease, such as:
    Leprosy [Hansen's disease] (A30.-)
    Mycoses (B35-B49)
    O'nyong-nyong fever (A92.1)
    Paratyphoid fever (A01.1-A01.4)
Excludes 1:   arthropathy in Lyme disease (A69.23)
    gonococcal arthritis (A54.42)
    meningococcal arthritis (A39.83)
    mumps arthritis (B26.85)
    postinfective arthropathy (M02.-)
    postmeningococcal arthritis (A39.84)
    reactive arthritis (M02.3-)
    rubella arthritis (B06.82)
    sarcoidosis arthritis (D86.86)
    typhoid fever arthritis (A01.04)
    tuberculosis arthritis (A18.01-A18.02)
M01.x- Direct infection of joint in infectious and parasitic diseases classified elsewhere
    M01.x0 Direct infection of <u>unspecified</u> joint in infectious and parasitic diseases classified elsewhere
    M01.x1-Direct infection of <u>shoulder</u> joint in infectious and parasitic diseases classified elsewhere
        M01.x11   Direct infection of <u>right</u> shoulder in infectious and parasitic diseases classified elsewhere
        M01.x12   Direct infection of <u>left</u> shoulder in infectious and parasitic diseases classified elsewhere
        M01.x19   Direct infection of <u>unspecified</u> shoulder in infectious and parasitic diseases classified elsewhere
    M01.x2-Direct infection of <u>elbow</u> in infectious and parasitic diseases classified elsewhere
        M01.x21   Direct infection of <u>right</u> elbow in infectious and parasitic diseases classified elsewhere
        M01.x22   Direct infection of <u>left</u> elbow in infectious and parasitic diseases classified elsewhere
        M01.x29   Direct infection of <u>unspecified</u> elbow in infectious and parasitic diseases classified elsewhere
    M01.x3-Direct infection of <u>wrist</u> in infectious and parasitic diseases classified elsewhere
Direct infection of carpal bones in infectious and parasitic diseases classified elsewhere
        M01.x31   Direct infection of <u>right</u> wrist in infectious and parasitic diseases classified elsewhere
        M01.x32   Direct infection of <u>left</u> wrist in infectious and parasitic diseases classified elsewhere
        M01.x39   Direct infection of <u>unspecified</u> wrist in infectious and parasitic diseases classified elsewhere
    M01.x4-Direct infection of <u>hand</u> in infectious and parasitic diseases classified elsewhere
Direct infection of metacarpus and phalanges in infectious and parasitic diseases classified elsewhere
        M01.x41   Direct infection of <u>right</u> hand in infectious and parasitic diseases classified elsewhere
        M01.x42   Direct infection of <u>left</u> hand in infectious and parasitic diseases classified elsewhere
        M01.x49   Direct infection of <u>unspecified</u> hand in infectious and parasitic diseases classified elsewhere
    M01.x5-Direct infection of <u>hip</u> in infectious and parasitic diseases classified elsewhere
        M01.x51   Direct infection of <u>right</u> hip in infectious and parasitic diseases classified elsewhere
        M01.x52   Direct infection of <u>left</u> hip in infectious and parasitic diseases classified elsewhere
        M01.x59   Direct infection of <u>unspecified</u> hip in infectious and parasitic diseases classified elsewhere
    M01.x6-Direct infection of <u>knee</u> in infectious and parasitic diseases classified elsewhere
        M01.x61   Direct infection of <u>right</u> knee in infectious and parasitic diseases classified elsewhere
        M01.x62   Direct infection of <u>left</u> knee in infectious and parasitic diseases classified elsewhere
        M01.x69   Direct infection of <u>unspecified</u> knee in infectious and parasitic diseases classified elsewhere

M00 - M02

M01.x7-Direct infection of <u>ankle and foot</u> **in infectious and parasitic diseases classified elsewhere**
Direct infection of tarsus, metatarsus and phalanges in infectious and parasitic diseases classified elsewhere

    M01.x71   Direct infection of <u>right</u> **ankle and foot in infectious and parasitic diseases classified elsewhere**

    M01.x72   Direct infection of <u>left</u> **ankle and foot in infectious and parasitic diseases classified elsewhere**

    M01.x79   Direct infection of <u>unspecified</u> **ankle and foot in infectious and parasitic diseases classified elsewhere**

M01.x8 Direct infection of <u>vertebrae</u> **in infectious and parasitic diseases classified elsewhere**

M01.x9 Direct infection of <u>multiple joints</u> **in infectious and parasitic diseases classified elsewhere**

M02- <u>Postinfective and reactive arthropathies</u>
Code first underlying disease, such as:
  Congenital syphilis [Clutton's joints] (A50.5)
  Enteritis due to Yersinia enterocolitica (A04.6)
  Infective endocarditis (I33.0)
  Viral hepatitis (B15-B19)
  Excludes 1: Behçet's disease (M35.2)
      direct infections of joint in infectious and parasitic diseases classified elsewhere (M01.-)
      postmeningococcal arthritis (A39.84)
      mumps arthritis (B26.85)
      rubella arthritis (B06.82)
      syphilis arthritis (late) (A52.77)
      rheumatic fever (I00)
      tabetic arthropathy [Charcôt's] (A52.16)

M02.0- Arthropathy <u>following intestinal bypass</u>
M02.00 Arthropathy following intestinal bypass, unspecified site
M02.01-Arthropathy following intestinal bypass, <u>shoulder</u>
  M02.011   Arthropathy following intestinal bypass, <u>right</u> **shoulder**
  M02.012   Arthropathy following intestinal bypass, <u>left</u> **shoulder**
  M02.019   Arthropathy following intestinal bypass, <u>unspecified</u> **shoulder**
M02.02-Arthropathy following intestinal bypass, <u>elbow</u>
  M02.021   Arthropathy following intestinal bypass, <u>right</u> **elbow**
  M02.022   Arthropathy following intestinal bypass, <u>left</u> **elbow**
  M02.029   Arthropathy following intestinal bypass, <u>unspecified</u> **elbow**
M02.03-Arthropathy following intestinal bypass, <u>wrist</u>
Arthropathy following intestinal bypass, carpal bones
  M02.031   Arthropathy following intestinal bypass, <u>right</u> **wrist**
  M02.032   Arthropathy following intestinal bypass, <u>left</u> **wrist**
  M02.039   Arthropathy following intestinal bypass, <u>unspecified</u> **wrist**
M02.04-Arthropathy following intestinal bypass, <u>hand</u>
Arthropathy following intestinal bypass, metacarpals and phalanges
  M02.041   Arthropathy following intestinal bypass, <u>right</u> **hand**
  M02.042   Arthropathy following intestinal bypass, <u>left</u> **hand**
  M02.049   Arthropathy following intestinal bypass, <u>unspecified</u> **hand**
M02.05-Arthropathy following intestinal bypass, <u>hip</u>
  M02.051   Arthropathy following intestinal bypass, <u>right</u> **hip**
  M02.052   Arthropathy following intestinal bypass, <u>left</u> **hip**
  M02.059   Arthropathy following intestinal bypass, <u>unspecified</u> **hip**
M02.06-Arthropathy following intestinal bypass, <u>knee</u>
  M02.061   Arthropathy following intestinal bypass, <u>right</u> **knee**
  M02.062   Arthropathy following intestinal bypass, <u>left</u> **knee**
  M02.069   Arthropathy following intestinal bypass, <u>unspecified</u> **knee**
M02.07-Arthropathy following intestinal bypass, <u>ankle and foot</u>
Arthropathy following intestinal bypass, tarsus, metatarsus and phalanges
  M02.071   Arthropathy following intestinal bypass, <u>right</u> **ankle and foot**
  M02.072   Arthropathy following intestinal bypass, <u>left</u> **ankle and foot**
  M02.079   Arthropathy following intestinal bypass, <u>unspecified</u> **ankle and foot**
M02.08 Arthropathy following intestinal bypass, <u>vertebrae</u>
M02.09 Arthropathy following intestinal bypass, <u>multiple sites</u>

M02.1- <u>Postdysenteric</u> **arthropathy**
M02.10 Postdysenteric arthropathy, <u>unspecified</u> **site**
M02.11-Postdysenteric arthropathy, <u>shoulder</u>
  M02.111   Postdysenteric arthropathy, <u>right</u> **shoulder**
  M02.112   Postdysenteric arthropathy, <u>left</u> **shoulder**
  M02.119   Postdysenteric arthropathy, <u>unspecified</u> **shoulder**
M02.12-Postdysenteric arthropathy, <u>elbow</u>
  M02.121   Postdysenteric arthropathy, <u>right</u> **elbow**
  M02.122   Postdysenteric arthropathy, <u>left</u> **elbow**
  M02.129   Postdysenteric arthropathy, <u>unspecified</u> **elbow**
M02.13-Postdysenteric arthropathy, <u>wrist</u>
Postdysenteric arthropathy, carpal bones
  M02.131   Postdysenteric arthropathy, <u>right</u> **wrist**
  M02.132   Postdysenteric arthropathy, <u>left</u> **wrist**
  M02.139   Postdysenteric arthropathy, <u>unspecified</u> **wrist**
M02.14-Postdysenteric arthropathy, <u>hand</u>
Postdysenteric arthropathy, metacarpus and phalanges
  M02.141   Postdysenteric arthropathy, <u>right</u> **hand**
  M02.142   Postdysenteric arthropathy, <u>left</u> **hand**
  M02.149   Postdysenteric arthropathy, <u>unspecified</u> **hand**
M02.15-Postdysenteric arthropathy, <u>hip</u>
  M02.151   Postdysenteric arthropathy, <u>right</u> **hip**
  M02.152   Postdysenteric arthropathy, <u>left</u> **hip**
  M02.159   Postdysenteric arthropathy, <u>unspecified</u> **hip**
M02.16-Postdysenteric arthropathy, <u>knee</u>
  M02.161   Postdysenteric arthropathy, <u>right</u> **knee**
  M02.162   Postdysenteric arthropathy, <u>left</u> **knee**
  M02.169   Postdysenteric arthropathy, <u>unspecified</u> **knee**
M02.17-Postdysenteric arthropathy, <u>ankle and foot</u>
Postdysenteric arthropathy, tarsus, metatarsus and phalanges
  M02.171   Postdysenteric arthropathy, <u>right</u> **ankle and foot**
  M02.172   Postdysenteric arthropathy, <u>left</u> **ankle and foot**
  M02.179   Postdysenteric arthropathy, <u>unspecified</u> **ankle and foot**
M02.18 Postdysenteric arthropathy, <u>vertebrae</u>
M02.19 Postdysenteric arthropathy, <u>multiple sites</u>
M02.2- <u>Postimmunization</u> **arthropathy**
M02.20 Postimmunization arthropathy, <u>unspecified</u> **site**
M02.21-Postimmunization arthropathy, <u>shoulder</u>
  M02.211   Postimmunization arthropathy, <u>right</u> **shoulder**
  M02.212   Postimmunization arthropathy, <u>left</u> **shoulder**
  M02.219   Postimmunization arthropathy, <u>unspecified</u> **shoulder**
M02.22-Postimmunization arthropathy, <u>elbow</u>
  M02.221   Postimmunization arthropathy, <u>right</u> **elbow**
  M02.222   Postimmunization arthropathy, <u>left</u> **elbow**
  M02.229   Postimmunization arthropathy, <u>unspecified</u> **elbow**
M02.23-Postimmunization arthropathy, <u>wrist</u>
Postimmunization arthropathy, carpal bones
  M02.231   Postimmunization arthropathy, <u>right</u> **wrist**
  M02.232   Postimmunization arthropathy, <u>left</u> **wrist**
  M02.239   Postimmunization arthropathy, <u>unspecified</u> **wrist**
M02.24-Postimmunization arthropathy, <u>hand</u>
Postimmunization arthropathy, metacarpus and phalanges
  M02.241   Postimmunization arthropathy, <u>right</u> **hand**
  M02.242   Postimmunization arthropathy, <u>left</u> **hand**
  M02.249   Postimmunization arthropathy, <u>unspecified</u> **hand**
M02.25-Postimmunization arthropathy, <u>hip</u>
  M02.251   Postimmunization arthropathy, <u>right</u> **hip**
  M02.252   Postimmunization arthropathy, <u>left</u> **hip**
  M02.259   Postimmunization arthropathy, <u>unspecified</u> **hip**
M02.26-Postimmunization arthropathy, <u>knee</u>
  M02.261   Postimmunization arthropathy, <u>right</u> **knee**
  M02.262   Postimmunization arthropathy, <u>left</u> **knee**
  M02.269   Postimmunization arthropathy, <u>unspecified</u> **knee**
M02.27-Postimmunization arthropathy, <u>ankle and foot</u>
Postimmunization arthropathy, tarsus, metatarsus and phalanges
  M02.271   Postimmunization arthropathy, <u>right</u> **ankle and foot**
  M02.272   Postimmunization arthropathy, <u>left</u> **ankle and foot**
  M02.279   Postimmunization arthropathy, <u>unspecified</u> **ankle and foot**
M02.28 Postimmunization arthropathy, <u>vertebrae</u>
M02.29 Postimmunization arthropathy, <u>multiple sites</u>

M 0 0 - M 0 2

© 2013 Channel Publishing, Ltd.

M02.3- Reiter's disease
      Reactive arthritis
  M02.30 Reiter's disease, <u>unspecified</u> site
  M02.31-Reiter's disease, <u>shoulder</u>
    M02.311 Reiter's disease, <u>right</u> shoulder
    M02.312 Reiter's disease, <u>left</u> shoulder
    M02.319 Reiter's disease, <u>unspecified</u> shoulder
  M02.32-Reiter's disease, <u>elbow</u>
    M02.321 Reiter's disease, <u>right</u> elbow
    M02.322 Reiter's disease, <u>left</u> elbow
    M02.329 Reiter's disease, <u>unspecified</u> elbow
  M02.33-Reiter's disease, <u>wrist</u>
      Reiter's disease, carpal bones
    M02.331 Reiter's disease, <u>right</u> wrist
    M02.332 Reiter's disease, <u>left</u> wrist
    M02.339 Reiter's disease, <u>unspecified</u> wrist
  M02.34-Reiter's disease, <u>hand</u>
      Reiter's disease, metacarpus and phalanges
    M02.341 Reiter's disease, <u>right</u> hand
    M02.342 Reiter's disease, <u>left</u> hand
    M02.349 Reiter's disease, <u>unspecified</u> hand
  M02.35-Reiter's disease, <u>hip</u>
    M02.351 Reiter's disease, <u>right</u> hip
    M02.352 Reiter's disease, <u>left</u> hip
    M02.359 Reiter's disease, <u>unspecified</u> hip
  M02.36-Reiter's disease, <u>knee</u>
    M02.361 Reiter's disease, <u>right</u> knee
    M02.362 Reiter's disease, <u>left</u> knee
    M02.369 Reiter's disease, <u>unspecified</u> knee
  M02.37-Reiter's disease, <u>ankle and foot</u>
      Reiter's disease, tarsus, metatarsus and phalanges
    M02.371 Reiter's disease, <u>right</u> ankle and foot
    M02.372 Reiter's disease, <u>left</u> ankle and foot
    M02.379 Reiter's disease, <u>unspecified</u> ankle and foot
  M02.38 Reiter's disease, <u>vertebrae</u>
  M02.39 Reiter's disease, <u>multiple sites</u>
M02.8- <u>Other reactive</u> arthropathies
  M02.80 Other reactive arthropathies, <u>unspecified</u> site
  M02.81-Other reactive arthropathies, <u>shoulder</u>
    M02.811 Other reactive arthropathies, <u>right</u> shoulder
    M02.812 Other reactive arthropathies, <u>left</u> shoulder
    M02.819 Other reactive arthropathies, <u>unspecified</u> shoulder
  M02.82-Other reactive arthropathies, <u>elbow</u>
    M02.821 Other reactive arthropathies, <u>right</u> elbow
    M02.822 Other reactive arthropathies, <u>left</u> elbow
    M02.829 Other reactive arthropathies, <u>unspecified</u> elbow
  M02.83-Other reactive arthropathies, <u>wrist</u>
      Other reactive arthropathies, carpal bones
    M02.831 Other reactive arthropathies, <u>right</u> wrist
    M02.832 Other reactive arthropathies, <u>left</u> wrist
    M02.839 Other reactive arthropathies, <u>unspecified</u> wrist
  M02.84-Other reactive arthropathies, <u>hand</u>
      Other reactive arthropathies, metacarpus and phalanges
    M02.841 Other reactive arthropathies, <u>right</u> hand
    M02.842 Other reactive arthropathies, <u>left</u> hand
    M02.849 Other reactive arthropathies, <u>unspecified</u> hand
  M02.85-Other reactive arthropathies, <u>hip</u>
    M02.851 Other reactive arthropathies, <u>right</u> hip
    M02.852 Other reactive arthropathies, <u>left</u> hip
    M02.859 Other reactive arthropathies, <u>unspecified</u> hip
  M02.86-Other reactive arthropathies, <u>knee</u>
    M02.861 Other reactive arthropathies, <u>right</u> knee
    M02.862 Other reactive arthropathies, <u>left</u> knee
    M02.869 Other reactive arthropathies, <u>unspecified</u> knee
  M02.87-Other reactive arthropathies, <u>ankle and foot</u>
      Other reactive arthropathies, tarsus, metatarsus and phalanges
    M02.871 Other reactive arthropathies, <u>right</u> ankle and foot
    M02.872 Other reactive arthropathies, <u>left</u> ankle and foot
    M02.879 Other reactive arthropathies, <u>unspecified</u> ankle and foot
  M02.88 Other reactive arthropathies, <u>vertebrae</u>
  M02.89 Other reactive arthropathies, <u>multiple sites</u>
M02.9 Reactive arthropathy, <u>unspecified</u>
    Inflammatory polyarthropathies (M05-M14)

Inflammatory polyarthropathies (M05-M14)

M05- Rheumatoid arthritis with rheumatoid factor
  Excludes 1: juvenile rheumatoid arthritis (M08-)
          rheumatic fever (I00)
          rheumatoid arthritis of spine (M45-)
  M05.0- <u>Felty's syndrome</u>
      Rheumatoid arthritis with splenoadenomegaly and leukopenia
    M05.00 Felty's syndrome, <u>unspecified</u> site
    M05.01-Felty's syndrome, <u>shoulder</u>
      M05.011 Felty's syndrome, <u>right</u> shoulder
      M05.012 Felty's syndrome, <u>left</u> shoulder
      M05.019 Felty's syndrome, <u>unspecified</u> shoulder
    M05.02-Felty's syndrome, <u>elbow</u>
      M05.021 Felty's syndrome, <u>right</u> elbow
      M05.022 Felty's syndrome, <u>left</u> elbow
      M05.029 Felty's syndrome, <u>unspecified</u> elbow
    M05.03-Felty's syndrome, <u>wrist</u>
        Felty's syndrome, carpal bones
      M05.031 Felty's syndrome, <u>right</u> wrist
      M05.032 Felty's syndrome, <u>left</u> wrist
      M05.039 Felty's syndrome, <u>unspecified</u> wrist
    M05.04-Felty's syndrome, <u>hand</u>
        Felty's syndrome, metacarpus and phalanges
      M05.041 Felty's syndrome, <u>right</u> hand
      M05.042 Felty's syndrome, <u>left</u> hand
      M05.049 Felty's syndrome, <u>unspecified</u> hand
    M05.05-Felty's syndrome, <u>hip</u>
      M05.051 Felty's syndrome, <u>right</u> hip
      M05.052 Felty's syndrome, <u>left</u> hip
      M05.059 Felty's syndrome, <u>unspecified</u> hip
    M05.06-Felty's syndrome, <u>knee</u>
      M05.061 Felty's syndrome, <u>right</u> knee
      M05.062 Felty's syndrome, <u>left</u> knee
      M05.069 Felty's syndrome, <u>unspecified</u> knee
    M05.07-Felty's syndrome, <u>ankle and foot</u>
        Felty's syndrome, tarsus, metatarsus and phalanges
      M05.071 Felty's syndrome, <u>right</u> ankle and foot
      M05.072 Felty's syndrome, <u>left</u> ankle and foot
      M05.079 Felty's syndrome, <u>unspecified</u> ankle and foot
    M05.09 Felty's syndrome, <u>multiple sites</u>
  M05.1- Rheumatoid <u>lung disease with</u> rheumatoid <u>arthritis</u>
    M05.10 Rheumatoid lung disease with rheumatoid arthritis of <u>unspecified</u> site
    M05.11-Rheumatoid lung disease with rheumatoid arthritis of <u>shoulder</u>
      M05.111 Rheumatoid lung disease with rheumatoid arthritis of <u>right</u> shoulder
      M05.112 Rheumatoid lung disease with rheumatoid arthritis of <u>left</u> shoulder
      M05.119 Rheumatoid lung disease with rheumatoid arthritis of <u>unspecified</u> shoulder
    M05.12-Rheumatoid lung disease with rheumatoid arthritis of <u>elbow</u>
      M05.121 Rheumatoid lung disease with rheumatoid arthritis of <u>right</u> elbow
      M05.122 Rheumatoid lung disease with rheumatoid arthritis of <u>left</u> elbow
      M05.129 Rheumatoid lung disease with rheumatoid arthritis of <u>unspecified</u> elbow
    M05.13-Rheumatoid lung disease with rheumatoid arthritis of <u>wrist</u>
        Rheumatoid lung disease with rheumatoid arthritis, carpal bones
      M05.131 Rheumatoid lung disease with rheumatoid arthritis of <u>right</u> wrist
      M05.132 Rheumatoid lung disease with rheumatoid arthritis of <u>left</u> wrist
      M05.139 Rheumatoid lung disease with rheumatoid arthritis of <u>unspecified</u> wrist
    M05.14-Rheumatoid lung disease with rheumatoid arthritis of <u>hand</u>
        Rheumatoid lung disease with rheumatoid arthritis, metacarpus and phalanges
      M05.141 Rheumatoid lung disease with rheumatoid arthritis of <u>right</u> hand
      M05.142 Rheumatoid lung disease with rheumatoid arthritis of <u>left</u> hand
      M05.149 Rheumatoid lung disease with rheumatoid arthritis of <u>unspecified</u> hand

M02 - M05

M05.15-Rheumatoid lung disease with rheumatoid arthritis of <u>hip</u>

   M05.151 Rheumatoid lung disease with rheumatoid arthritis of <u>right</u> hip

   M05.152 Rheumatoid lung disease with rheumatoid arthritis of <u>left</u> hip

   M05.159 Rheumatoid lung disease with rheumatoid arthritis of <u>unspecified</u> hip

M05.16-Rheumatoid lung disease with rheumatoid arthritis of <u>knee</u>

   M05.161 Rheumatoid lung disease with rheumatoid arthritis of <u>right</u> knee

   M05.162 Rheumatoid lung disease with rheumatoid arthritis of <u>left</u> knee

   M05.169 Rheumatoid lung disease with rheumatoid arthritis of <u>unspecified</u> knee

M05.17-Rheumatoid lung disease with rheumatoid arthritis of <u>ankle and foot</u>
   Rheumatoid lung disease with rheumatoid arthritis, tarsus, metatarsus and phalanges

   M05.171 Rheumatoid lung disease with rheumatoid arthritis of <u>right</u> ankle and foot

   M05.172 Rheumatoid lung disease with rheumatoid arthritis of <u>left</u> ankle and foot

   M05.179 Rheumatoid lung disease with rheumatoid arthritis of <u>unspecified</u> ankle and foot

M05.19 Rheumatoid lung disease with rheumatoid arthritis of <u>multiple sites</u>

M05.2- Rheumatoid <u>vasculitis</u> <u>with</u> rheumatoid <u>arthritis</u>

M05.20 Rheumatoid vasculitis with rheumatoid arthritis of <u>unspecified</u> site

M05.21-Rheumatoid vasculitis with rheumatoid arthritis of <u>shoulder</u>

   M05.211 Rheumatoid vasculitis with rheumatoid arthritis of <u>right</u> shoulder

   M05.212 Rheumatoid vasculitis with rheumatoid arthritis of <u>left</u> shoulder

   M05.219 Rheumatoid vasculitis with rheumatoid arthritis of <u>unspecified</u> shoulder

M05.22-Rheumatoid vasculitis with rheumatoid arthritis of <u>elbow</u>

   M05.221 Rheumatoid vasculitis with rheumatoid arthritis of <u>right</u> elbow

   M05.222 Rheumatoid vasculitis with rheumatoid arthritis of <u>left</u> elbow

   M05.229 Rheumatoid vasculitis with rheumatoid arthritis of <u>unspecified</u> elbow

M05.23-Rheumatoid vasculitis with rheumatoid arthritis of <u>wrist</u>
   Rheumatoid vasculitis with rheumatoid arthritis, carpal bones

   M05.231 Rheumatoid vasculitis with rheumatoid arthritis of <u>right</u> wrist

   M05.232 Rheumatoid vasculitis with rheumatoid arthritis of <u>left</u> wrist

   M05.239 Rheumatoid vasculitis with rheumatoid arthritis of <u>unspecified</u> wrist

M05.24-Rheumatoid vasculitis with rheumatoid arthritis of <u>hand</u>
   Rheumatoid vasculitis with rheumatoid arthritis, metacarpus and phalanges

   M05.241 Rheumatoid vasculitis with rheumatoid arthritis of <u>right</u> hand

   M05.242 Rheumatoid vasculitis with rheumatoid arthritis of <u>left</u> hand

   M05.249 Rheumatoid vasculitis with rheumatoid arthritis of <u>unspecified</u> hand

M05.25-Rheumatoid vasculitis with rheumatoid arthritis of <u>hip</u>

   M05.251 Rheumatoid vasculitis with rheumatoid arthritis of <u>right</u> hip

   M05.252 Rheumatoid vasculitis with rheumatoid arthritis of <u>left</u> hip

   M05.259 Rheumatoid vasculitis with rheumatoid arthritis of <u>unspecified</u> hip

M05.26-Rheumatoid vasculitis with rheumatoid arthritis of <u>knee</u>

   M05.261 Rheumatoid vasculitis with rheumatoid arthritis of <u>right</u> knee

   M05.262 Rheumatoid vasculitis with rheumatoid arthritis of <u>left</u> knee

   M05.269 Rheumatoid vasculitis with rheumatoid arthritis of <u>unspecified</u> knee

M05.27-Rheumatoid vasculitis with rheumatoid arthritis of <u>ankle and foot</u>
   Rheumatoid vasculitis with rheumatoid arthritis, tarsus, metatarsus and phalanges

   M05.271 Rheumatoid vasculitis with rheumatoid arthritis of <u>right</u> ankle and foot

   M05.272 Rheumatoid vasculitis with rheumatoid arthritis of <u>left</u> ankle and foot

   M05.279 Rheumatoid vasculitis with rheumatoid arthritis of <u>unspecified</u> ankle and foot

M05.29 Rheumatoid vasculitis with rheumatoid arthritis of <u>multiple sites</u>

M05.3- Rheumatoid <u>heart</u> disease <u>with</u> rheumatoid <u>arthritis</u>
   Rheumatoid carditis
   Rheumatoid endocarditis
   Rheumatoid myocarditis
   Rheumatoid pericarditis

M05.30 Rheumatoid heart disease with rheumatoid arthritis of <u>unspecified</u> site

M05.31-Rheumatoid heart disease with rheumatoid arthritis of <u>shoulder</u>

   M05.311 Rheumatoid heart disease with rheumatoid arthritis of <u>right</u> shoulder

   M05.312 Rheumatoid heart disease with rheumatoid arthritis of <u>left</u> shoulder

   M05.319 Rheumatoid heart disease with rheumatoid arthritis of <u>unspecified</u> shoulder

M05.32-Rheumatoid heart disease with rheumatoid arthritis of <u>elbow</u>

   M05.321 Rheumatoid heart disease with rheumatoid arthritis of <u>right</u> elbow

   M05.322 Rheumatoid heart disease with rheumatoid arthritis of <u>left</u> elbow

   M05.329 Rheumatoid heart disease with rheumatoid arthritis of <u>unspecified</u> elbow

M05.33-Rheumatoid heart disease with rheumatoid arthritis of <u>wrist</u>
   Rheumatoid heart disease with rheumatoid arthritis, carpal bones

   M05.331 Rheumatoid heart disease with rheumatoid arthritis of <u>right</u> wrist

   M05.332 Rheumatoid heart disease with rheumatoid arthritis of <u>left</u> wrist

   M05.339 Rheumatoid heart disease with rheumatoid arthritis of <u>unspecified</u> wrist

M05.34-Rheumatoid heart disease with rheumatoid arthritis of <u>hand</u>
   Rheumatoid heart disease with rheumatoid arthritis, metacarpus and phalanges

   M05.341 Rheumatoid heart disease with rheumatoid arthritis of <u>right</u> hand

   M05.342 Rheumatoid heart disease with rheumatoid arthritis of <u>left</u> hand

   M05.349 Rheumatoid heart disease with rheumatoid arthritis of <u>unspecified</u> hand

M05.35-Rheumatoid heart disease with rheumatoid arthritis of <u>hip</u>

   M05.351 Rheumatoid heart disease with rheumatoid arthritis of <u>right</u> hip

   M05.352 Rheumatoid heart disease with rheumatoid arthritis of <u>left</u> hip

   M05.359 Rheumatoid heart disease with rheumatoid arthritis of <u>unspecified</u> hip

M05.36-Rheumatoid heart disease with rheumatoid arthritis of <u>knee</u>

   M05.361 Rheumatoid heart disease with rheumatoid arthritis of <u>right</u> knee

   M05.362 Rheumatoid heart disease with rheumatoid arthritis of <u>left</u> knee

   M05.369 Rheumatoid heart disease with rheumatoid arthritis of <u>unspecified</u> knee

M05.37-Rheumatoid heart disease with rheumatoid arthritis of <u>ankle and foot</u>
   Rheumatoid heart disease with rheumatoid arthritis, tarsus, metatarsus and phalanges

   M05.371 Rheumatoid heart disease with rheumatoid arthritis of <u>right</u> ankle and foot

   M05.372 Rheumatoid heart disease with rheumatoid arthritis of <u>left</u> ankle and foot

   M05.379 Rheumatoid heart disease with rheumatoid arthritis of <u>unspecified</u> ankle and foot

M05.39 Rheumatoid heart disease with rheumatoid arthritis of <u>multiple sites</u>

M02 - M05

M05.4- **Rheumatoid <u>myopathy</u> <u>with</u> rheumatoid <u>arthritis</u>**

M05.40 **Rheumatoid myopathy with rheumatoid arthritis of <u>unspecified</u> site**

M05.41-**Rheumatoid myopathy with rheumatoid arthritis of <u>shoulder</u>**

M05.411 **Rheumatoid myopathy with rheumatoid arthritis of <u>right</u> shoulder**

M05.412 **Rheumatoid myopathy with rheumatoid arthritis of <u>left</u> shoulder**

M05.419 **Rheumatoid myopathy with rheumatoid arthritis of <u>unspecified</u> shoulder**

M05.42-**Rheumatoid myopathy with rheumatoid arthritis of <u>elbow</u>**

M05.421 **Rheumatoid myopathy with rheumatoid arthritis of <u>right</u> elbow**

M05.422 **Rheumatoid myopathy with rheumatoid arthritis of <u>left</u> elbow**

M05.429 **Rheumatoid myopathy with rheumatoid arthritis of <u>unspecified</u> elbow**

M05.43-**Rheumatoid myopathy with rheumatoid arthritis of <u>wrist</u>**
   Rheumatoid myopathy with rheumatoid arthritis, carpal bones

M05.431 **Rheumatoid myopathy with rheumatoid arthritis of <u>right</u> wrist**

M05.432 **Rheumatoid myopathy with rheumatoid arthritis of <u>left</u> wrist**

M05.439 **Rheumatoid myopathy with rheumatoid arthritis of <u>unspecified</u> wrist**

M05.44-**Rheumatoid myopathy with rheumatoid arthritis of <u>hand</u>**
   Rheumatoid myopathy with rheumatoid arthritis, metacarpus and phalanges

M05.441 **Rheumatoid myopathy with rheumatoid arthritis of <u>right</u> hand**

M05.442 **Rheumatoid myopathy with rheumatoid arthritis of <u>left</u> hand**

M05.449 **Rheumatoid myopathy with rheumatoid arthritis of <u>unspecified</u> hand**

M05.45-**Rheumatoid myopathy with rheumatoid arthritis of <u>hip</u>**

M05.451 **Rheumatoid myopathy with rheumatoid arthritis of <u>right</u> hip**

M05.452 **Rheumatoid myopathy with rheumatoid arthritis of <u>left</u> hip**

M05.459 **Rheumatoid myopathy with rheumatoid arthritis of <u>unspecified</u> hip**

M05.46-**Rheumatoid myopathy with rheumatoid arthritis of <u>knee</u>**

M05.461 **Rheumatoid myopathy with rheumatoid arthritis of <u>right</u> knee**

M05.462 **Rheumatoid myopathy with rheumatoid arthritis of <u>left</u> knee**

M05.469 **Rheumatoid myopathy with rheumatoid arthritis of <u>unspecified</u> knee**

M05.47-**Rheumatoid myopathy with rheumatoid arthritis of <u>ankle and foot</u>**
   Rheumatoid myopathy with rheumatoid arthritis, tarsus, metatarsus and phalanges

M05.471 **Rheumatoid myopathy with rheumatoid arthritis of <u>right</u> ankle and foot**

M05.472 **Rheumatoid myopathy with rheumatoid arthritis of <u>left</u> ankle and foot**

M05.479 **Rheumatoid myopathy with rheumatoid arthritis of <u>unspecified</u> ankle and foot**

M05.49 **Rheumatoid myopathy with rheumatoid arthritis of <u>multiple</u> sites**

M05.5- **Rheumatoid <u>polyneuropathy</u> <u>with</u> rheumatoid <u>arthritis</u>**

M05.50 **Rheumatoid polyneuropathy with rheumatoid arthritis of <u>unspecified</u> site**

M05.51-**Rheumatoid polyneuropathy with rheumatoid arthritis of <u>shoulder</u>**

M05.511 **Rheumatoid polyneuropathy with rheumatoid arthritis of <u>right</u> shoulder**

M05.512 **Rheumatoid polyneuropathy with rheumatoid arthritis of <u>left</u> shoulder**

M05.519 **Rheumatoid polyneuropathy with rheumatoid arthritis of <u>unspecified</u> shoulder**

M05.52-**Rheumatoid polyneuropathy with rheumatoid arthritis of <u>elbow</u>**

M05.521 **Rheumatoid polyneuropathy with rheumatoid arthritis of <u>right</u> elbow**

M05.522 **Rheumatoid polyneuropathy with rheumatoid arthritis of <u>left</u> elbow**

M05.529 **Rheumatoid polyneuropathy with rheumatoid arthritis of <u>unspecified</u> elbow**

M05.53-**Rheumatoid polyneuropathy with rheumatoid arthritis of <u>wrist</u>**
   Rheumatoid polyneuropathy with rheumatoid arthritis, carpal bones

M05.531 **Rheumatoid polyneuropathy with rheumatoid arthritis of <u>right</u> wrist**

M05.532 **Rheumatoid polyneuropathy with rheumatoid arthritis of <u>left</u> wrist**

M05.539 **Rheumatoid polyneuropathy with rheumatoid arthritis of <u>unspecified</u> wrist**

M05.54-**Rheumatoid polyneuropathy with rheumatoid arthritis of <u>hand</u>**
   Rheumatoid polyneuropathy with rheumatoid arthritis, metacarpus and phalanges

M05.541 **Rheumatoid polyneuropathy with rheumatoid arthritis of <u>right</u> hand**

M05.542 **Rheumatoid polyneuropathy with rheumatoid arthritis of <u>left</u> hand**

M05.549 **Rheumatoid polyneuropathy with rheumatoid arthritis of <u>unspecified</u> hand**

M05.55-**Rheumatoid polyneuropathy with rheumatoid arthritis of <u>hip</u>**

M05.551 **Rheumatoid polyneuropathy with rheumatoid arthritis of <u>right</u> hip**

M05.552 **Rheumatoid polyneuropathy with rheumatoid arthritis of <u>left</u> hip**

M05.559 **Rheumatoid polyneuropathy with rheumatoid arthritis of <u>unspecified</u> hip**

M05.56-**Rheumatoid polyneuropathy with rheumatoid arthritis of <u>knee</u>**

M05.561 **Rheumatoid polyneuropathy with rheumatoid arthritis of <u>right</u> knee**

M05.562 **Rheumatoid polyneuropathy with rheumatoid arthritis of <u>left</u> knee**

M05.569 **Rheumatoid polyneuropathy with rheumatoid arthritis of <u>unspecified</u> knee**

M05.57-**Rheumatoid polyneuropathy with rheumatoid arthritis of <u>ankle and foot</u>**
   Rheumatoid polyneuropathy with rheumatoid arthritis, tarsus, metatarsus and phalanges

M05.571 **Rheumatoid polyneuropathy with rheumatoid arthritis of <u>right</u> ankle and foot**

M05.572 **Rheumatoid polyneuropathy with rheumatoid arthritis of <u>left</u> ankle and foot**

M05.579 **Rheumatoid polyneuropathy with rheumatoid arthritis of <u>unspecified</u> ankle and foot**

M05.59 **Rheumatoid polyneuropathy with rheumatoid arthritis of <u>multiple sites</u>**

M05.6- **Rheumatoid <u>arthritis</u> <u>with</u> involvement of <u>other organs and systems</u>**

M05.60 **Rheumatoid arthritis of <u>unspecified</u> site with involvement of other organs and systems**

M05.61-**Rheumatoid arthritis of <u>shoulder</u> with involvement of other organs and systems**

M05.611 **Rheumatoid arthritis of <u>right</u> shoulder with involvement of other organs and systems**

M05.612 **Rheumatoid arthritis of <u>left</u> shoulder with involvement of other organs and systems**

M05.619 **Rheumatoid arthritis of <u>unspecified</u> shoulder with involvement of other organs and systems**

M05.62-**Rheumatoid arthritis of <u>elbow</u> with involvement of other organs and systems**

M05.621 **Rheumatoid arthritis of <u>right</u> elbow with involvement of other organs and systems**

M05.622 **Rheumatoid arthritis of <u>left</u> elbow with involvement of other organs and systems**

M05.629 **Rheumatoid arthritis of <u>unspecified</u> elbow with involvement of other organs and systems**

M05.63-**Rheumatoid arthritis of <u>wrist</u> with involvement of other organs and systems**
   Rheumatoid arthritis of carpal bones with involvement of other organs and systems

M05.631 **Rheumatoid arthritis of <u>right</u> wrist with involvement of other organs and systems**

M05.632 **Rheumatoid arthritis of <u>left</u> wrist with involvement of other organs and systems**

M05.639 **Rheumatoid arthritis of <u>unspecified</u> wrist with involvement of other organs and systems**

M05
-
M05

M05.64-Rheumatoid arthritis of <u>hand</u> with involvement of other organs and systems
> Rheumatoid arthritis of metacarpus and phalanges with involvement of other organs and systems

- **M05.641** Rheumatoid arthritis of <u>right</u> hand with involvement of other organs and systems
- **M05.642** Rheumatoid arthritis of <u>left</u> hand with involvement of other organs and systems
- **M05.649** Rheumatoid arthritis of <u>unspecified</u> hand with involvement of other organs and systems

M05.65-Rheumatoid arthritis of <u>hip</u> with involvement of other organs and systems

- **M05.651** Rheumatoid arthritis of <u>right</u> hip with involvement of other organs and systems
- **M05.652** Rheumatoid arthritis of <u>left</u> hip with involvement of other organs and systems
- **M05.659** Rheumatoid arthritis of <u>unspecified</u> hip with involvement of other organs and systems

M05.66-Rheumatoid arthritis of <u>knee</u> with involvement of other organs and systems

- **M05.661** Rheumatoid arthritis of <u>right</u> knee with involvement of other organs and systems
- **M05.662** Rheumatoid arthritis of <u>left</u> knee with involvement of other organs and systems
- **M05.669** Rheumatoid arthritis of <u>unspecified</u> knee with involvement of other organs and systems

M05.67-Rheumatoid arthritis of <u>ankle and foot</u> with involvement of other organs and systems
> Rheumatoid arthritis of tarsus, metatarsus and phalanges with involvement of other organs and systems

- **M05.671** Rheumatoid arthritis of <u>right</u> ankle and foot with involvement of other organs and systems
- **M05.672** Rheumatoid arthritis of <u>left</u> ankle and foot with involvement of other organs and systems
- **M05.679** Rheumatoid arthritis of <u>unspecified</u> ankle and foot with involvement of other organs and systems

M05.69 Rheumatoid arthritis of <u>multiple sites</u> with involvement of other organs and systems

M05.7- Rheumatoid <u>arthritis</u> <u>with</u> rheumatoid <u>factor without</u> organ or systems involvement

M05.70 Rheumatoid arthritis with rheumatoid factor of <u>unspecified</u> site without organ or systems involvement

M05.71-Rheumatoid arthritis with rheumatoid factor of <u>shoulder</u> without organ or systems involvement

- **M05.711** Rheumatoid arthritis with rheumatoid factor of <u>right</u> shoulder without organ or systems involvement
- **M05.712** Rheumatoid arthritis with rheumatoid factor of <u>left</u> shoulder without organ or systems involvement
- **M05.719** Rheumatoid arthritis with rheumatoid factor of <u>unspecified</u> shoulder without organ or systems involvement

M05.72-Rheumatoid arthritis with rheumatoid factor of <u>elbow</u> without organ or systems involvement

- **M05.721** Rheumatoid arthritis with rheumatoid factor of <u>right</u> elbow without organ or systems involvement
- **M05.722** Rheumatoid arthritis with rheumatoid factor of <u>left</u> elbow without organ or systems involvement
- **M05.729** Rheumatoid arthritis with rheumatoid factor of <u>unspecified</u> elbow without organ or systems involvement

M05.73-Rheumatoid arthritis with rheumatoid factor of <u>wrist</u> without organ or systems involvement

- **M05.731** Rheumatoid arthritis with rheumatoid factor of <u>right</u> wrist without organ or systems involvement
- **M05.732** Rheumatoid arthritis with rheumatoid factor of <u>left</u> wrist without organ or systems involvement
- **M05.739** Rheumatoid arthritis with rheumatoid factor of <u>unspecified</u> wrist without organ or systems involvement

M05.74-Rheumatoid arthritis with rheumatoid factor of <u>hand</u> without organ or systems involvement

- **M05.741** Rheumatoid arthritis with rheumatoid factor of <u>right</u> hand without organ or systems involvement
- **M05.742** Rheumatoid arthritis with rheumatoid factor of <u>left</u> hand without organ or systems involvement
- **M05.749** Rheumatoid arthritis with rheumatoid factor of <u>unspecified</u> hand without organ or systems involvement

M05.75-Rheumatoid arthritis with rheumatoid factor of <u>hip</u> without organ or systems involvement

- **M05.751** Rheumatoid arthritis with rheumatoid factor of <u>right</u> hip without organ or systems involvement
- **M05.752** Rheumatoid arthritis with rheumatoid factor of <u>left</u> hip without organ or systems involvement
- **M05.759** Rheumatoid arthritis with rheumatoid factor of <u>unspecified</u> hip without organ or systems involvement

M05.76-Rheumatoid arthritis with rheumatoid factor of <u>knee</u> without organ or systems involvement

- **M05.761** Rheumatoid arthritis with rheumatoid factor of <u>right</u> knee without organ or systems involvement
- **M05.762** Rheumatoid arthritis with rheumatoid factor of <u>left</u> knee without organ or systems involvement
- **M05.769** Rheumatoid arthritis with rheumatoid factor of <u>unspecified</u> knee without organ or systems involvement

M05.77-Rheumatoid arthritis with rheumatoid factor of <u>ankle and foot</u> without organ or systems involvement

- **M05.771** Rheumatoid arthritis with rheumatoid factor of <u>right</u> ankle and foot without organ or systems involvement
- **M05.772** Rheumatoid arthritis with rheumatoid factor of <u>left</u> ankle and foot without organ or systems involvement
- **M05.779** Rheumatoid arthritis with rheumatoid factor of <u>unspecified</u> ankle and foot without organ or systems involvement

M05.79 Rheumatoid arthritis with rheumatoid factor of <u>multiple sites</u> without organ or systems involvement

M05.8- Other rheumatoid arthritis <u>with</u> rheumatoid <u>factor</u>

M05.80 Other rheumatoid arthritis with rheumatoid factor of <u>unspecified</u> site

M05.81-Other rheumatoid arthritis with rheumatoid factor of <u>shoulder</u>

- **M05.811** Other rheumatoid arthritis with rheumatoid factor of <u>right</u> shoulder
- **M05.812** Other rheumatoid arthritis with rheumatoid factor of <u>left</u> shoulder
- **M05.819** Other rheumatoid arthritis with rheumatoid factor of <u>unspecified</u> shoulder

M05.82-Other rheumatoid arthritis with rheumatoid factor of <u>elbow</u>

- **M05.821** Other rheumatoid arthritis with rheumatoid factor of <u>right</u> elbow
- **M05.822** Other rheumatoid arthritis with rheumatoid factor of <u>left</u> elbow
- **M05.829** Other rheumatoid arthritis with rheumatoid factor of <u>unspecified</u> elbow

M05.83-Other rheumatoid arthritis with rheumatoid factor of <u>wrist</u>

- **M05.831** Other rheumatoid arthritis with rheumatoid factor of <u>right</u> wrist
- **M05.832** Other rheumatoid arthritis with rheumatoid factor of <u>left</u> wrist
- **M05.839** Other rheumatoid arthritis with rheumatoid factor of <u>unspecified</u> wrist

M05.84-Other rheumatoid arthritis with rheumatoid factor of <u>hand</u>

- **M05.841** Other rheumatoid arthritis with rheumatoid factor of <u>right</u> hand
- **M05.842** Other rheumatoid arthritis with rheumatoid factor of <u>left</u> hand
- **M05.849** Other rheumatoid arthritis with rheumatoid factor of <u>unspecified</u> hand

M05.85-Other rheumatoid arthritis with rheumatoid factor of <u>hip</u>

- **M05.851** Other rheumatoid arthritis with rheumatoid factor of <u>right</u> hip
- **M05.852** Other rheumatoid arthritis with rheumatoid factor of <u>left</u> hip
- **M05.859** Other rheumatoid arthritis with rheumatoid factor of <u>unspecified</u> hip

M05.86-Other rheumatoid arthritis with rheumatoid factor of <u>knee</u>

- **M05.861** Other rheumatoid arthritis with rheumatoid factor of <u>right</u> knee
- **M05.862** Other rheumatoid arthritis with rheumatoid factor of <u>left</u> knee
- **M05.869** Other rheumatoid arthritis with rheumatoid factor of <u>unspecified</u> knee

M 0 5 – M 0 5

Excludes 1: = NOT CODED HERE! (Do not code both)

Excludes ❷: = Not Included Here

M05.87-Other rheumatoid arthritis with rheumatoid factor of <u>ankle</u> <u>and foot</u>
  M05.871   Other rheumatoid arthritis with rheumatoid factor of <u>right</u> ankle and foot
  M05.872   Other rheumatoid arthritis with rheumatoid factor of <u>left</u> ankle and foot
  M05.879   Other rheumatoid arthritis with rheumatoid factor of <u>unspecified</u> ankle and foot
M05.89 Other rheumatoid arthritis with rheumatoid factor of <u>multiple sites</u>
M05.9   Rheumatoid arthritis with rheumatoid factor, <u>unspecified</u>

M06- <u>Other rheumatoid arthritis</u>
M06.0- Rheumatoid <u>arthritis</u> <u>without</u> rheumatoid <u>factor</u>
  M06.00 Rheumatoid arthritis without rheumatoid factor, <u>unspecified</u> site
  M06.01-Rheumatoid arthritis without rheumatoid factor, <u>shoulder</u>
    M06.011   Rheumatoid arthritis without rheumatoid factor, <u>right</u> shoulder
    M06.012   Rheumatoid arthritis without rheumatoid factor, <u>left</u> shoulder
    M06.019   Rheumatoid arthritis without rheumatoid factor, <u>unspecified</u> shoulder
  M06.02-Rheumatoid arthritis without rheumatoid factor, <u>elbow</u>
    M06.021   Rheumatoid arthritis without rheumatoid factor, <u>right</u> elbow
    M06.022   Rheumatoid arthritis without rheumatoid factor, <u>left</u> elbow
    M06.029   Rheumatoid arthritis without rheumatoid factor, <u>unspecified</u> elbow
  M06.03-Rheumatoid arthritis without rheumatoid factor, <u>wrist</u>
    M06.031   Rheumatoid arthritis without rheumatoid factor, <u>right</u> wrist
    M06.032   Rheumatoid arthritis without rheumatoid factor, <u>left</u> wrist
    M06.039   Rheumatoid arthritis without rheumatoid factor, <u>unspecified</u> wrist
  M06.04-Rheumatoid arthritis without rheumatoid factor, <u>hand</u>
    M06.041   Rheumatoid arthritis without rheumatoid factor, <u>right</u> hand
    M06.042   Rheumatoid arthritis without rheumatoid factor, <u>left</u> hand
    M06.049   Rheumatoid arthritis without rheumatoid factor, <u>unspecified</u> hand
  M06.05-Rheumatoid arthritis without rheumatoid factor, <u>hip</u>
    M06.051   Rheumatoid arthritis without rheumatoid factor, <u>right</u> hip
    M06.052   Rheumatoid arthritis without rheumatoid factor, <u>left</u> hip
    M06.059   Rheumatoid arthritis without rheumatoid factor, <u>unspecified</u> hip
  M06.06-Rheumatoid arthritis without rheumatoid factor, <u>knee</u>
    M06.061   Rheumatoid arthritis without rheumatoid factor, <u>right</u> knee
    M06.062   Rheumatoid arthritis without rheumatoid factor, <u>left</u> knee
    M06.069   Rheumatoid arthritis without rheumatoid factor, <u>unspecified</u> knee
  M06.07-Rheumatoid arthritis without rheumatoid factor, <u>ankle and foot</u>
    M06.071   Rheumatoid arthritis without rheumatoid factor, <u>right</u> ankle and foot
    M06.072   Rheumatoid arthritis without rheumatoid factor, <u>left</u> ankle and foot
    M06.079   Rheumatoid arthritis without rheumatoid factor, <u>unspecified</u> ankle and foot
  M06.08 Rheumatoid arthritis without rheumatoid factor, <u>vertebrae</u>
  M06.09 Rheumatoid arthritis without rheumatoid factor, <u>multiple sites</u>
M06.1   Adult-onset Still's disease
  Excludes 1: Still's disease NOS (M08.2-)
M06.2- <u>Rheumatoid bursitis</u>
  M06.20 Rheumatoid bursitis, <u>unspecified</u> site
  M06.21-Rheumatoid bursitis, <u>shoulder</u>
    M06.211   Rheumatoid bursitis, <u>right</u> shoulder
    M06.212   Rheumatoid bursitis, <u>left</u> shoulder
    M06.219   Rheumatoid bursitis, <u>unspecified</u> shoulder

  M06.22-Rheumatoid bursitis, <u>elbow</u>
    M06.221   Rheumatoid bursitis, <u>right</u> elbow
    M06.222   Rheumatoid bursitis, <u>left</u> elbow
    M06.229   Rheumatoid bursitis, <u>unspecified</u> elbow
  M06.23-Rheumatoid bursitis, <u>wrist</u>
    M06.231   Rheumatoid bursitis, <u>right</u> wrist
    M06.232   Rheumatoid bursitis, <u>left</u> wrist
    M06.239   Rheumatoid bursitis, <u>unspecified</u> wrist
  M06.24-Rheumatoid bursitis, <u>hand</u>
    M06.241   Rheumatoid bursitis, <u>right</u> hand
    M06.242   Rheumatoid bursitis, <u>left</u> hand
    M06.249   Rheumatoid bursitis, <u>unspecified</u> hand
  M06.25-Rheumatoid bursitis, <u>hip</u>
    M06.251   Rheumatoid bursitis, <u>right</u> hip
    M06.252   Rheumatoid bursitis, <u>left</u> hip
    M06.259   Rheumatoid bursitis, <u>unspecified</u> hip
  M06.26-Rheumatoid bursitis, <u>knee</u>
    M06.261   Rheumatoid bursitis, <u>right</u> knee
    M06.262   Rheumatoid bursitis, <u>left</u> knee
    M06.269   Rheumatoid bursitis, <u>unspecified</u> knee
  M06.27-Rheumatoid bursitis, <u>ankle and foot</u>
    M06.271   Rheumatoid bursitis, <u>right</u> ankle and foot
    M06.272   Rheumatoid bursitis, <u>left</u> ankle and foot
    M06.279   Rheumatoid bursitis, <u>unspecified</u> ankle and foot
  M06.28 Rheumatoid bursitis, <u>vertebrae</u>
  M06.29 Rheumatoid bursitis, <u>multiple sites</u>
M06.3- <u>Rheumatoid nodule</u>
  M06.30 Rheumatoid nodule, <u>unspecified</u> site
  M06.31-Rheumatoid nodule, <u>shoulder</u>
    M06.311   Rheumatoid nodule, <u>right</u> shoulder
    M06.312   Rheumatoid nodule, <u>left</u> shoulder
    M06.319   Rheumatoid nodule, <u>unspecified</u> shoulder
  M06.32-Rheumatoid nodule, <u>elbow</u>
    M06.321   Rheumatoid nodule, <u>right</u> elbow
    M06.322   Rheumatoid nodule, <u>left</u> elbow
    M06.329   Rheumatoid nodule, <u>unspecified</u> elbow
  M06.33-Rheumatoid nodule, <u>wrist</u>
    M06.331   Rheumatoid nodule, <u>right</u> wrist
    M06.332   Rheumatoid nodule, <u>left</u> wrist
    M06.339   Rheumatoid nodule, <u>unspecified</u> wrist
  M06.34 Rheumatoid nodule, <u>hand</u>
    M06.341   Rheumatoid nodule, <u>right</u> hand
    M06.342   Rheumatoid nodule, <u>left</u> hand
    M06.349   Rheumatoid nodule, <u>unspecified</u> hand
  M06.35-Rheumatoid nodule, <u>hip</u>
    M06.351   Rheumatoid nodule, <u>right</u> hip
    M06.352   Rheumatoid nodule, <u>left</u> hip
    M06.359   Rheumatoid nodule, <u>unspecified</u> hip
  M06.36-Rheumatoid nodule, <u>knee</u>
    M06.361   Rheumatoid nodule, <u>right</u> knee
    M06.362   Rheumatoid nodule, <u>left</u> knee
    M06.369   Rheumatoid nodule, <u>unspecified</u> knee
  M06.37-Rheumatoid nodule, <u>ankle and foot</u>
    M06.371   Rheumatoid nodule, <u>right</u> ankle and foot
    M06.372   Rheumatoid nodule, <u>left</u> ankle and foot
    M06.379   Rheumatoid nodule, <u>unspecified</u> ankle and foot
  M06.38 Rheumatoid nodule, <u>vertebrae</u>
  M06.39 Rheumatoid nodule, <u>multiple sites</u>
M06.4   Inflammatory polyarthropathy
  Excludes 1: polyarthritis NOS (M13.0)
M06.8- <u>Other specified rheumatoid arthritis</u>
  M06.80 Other specified rheumatoid arthritis, <u>unspecified</u> site
  M06.81-Other specified rheumatoid arthritis, <u>shoulder</u>
    M06.811   Other specified rheumatoid arthritis, <u>right</u> shoulder
    M06.812   Other specified rheumatoid arthritis, <u>left</u> shoulder
    M06.819   Other specified rheumatoid arthritis, <u>unspecified</u> shoulder
  M06.82-Other specified rheumatoid arthritis, <u>elbow</u>
    M06.821   Other specified rheumatoid arthritis, <u>right</u> elbow
    M06.822   Other specified rheumatoid arthritis, <u>left</u> elbow
    M06.829   Other specified rheumatoid arthritis, <u>unspecified</u> elbow

M 0 5 - M 0 8

M06.83-Other specified rheumatoid arthritis, <u>wrist</u>
    M06.831 Other specified rheumatoid arthritis, <u>right</u> wrist
    M06.832 Other specified rheumatoid arthritis, <u>left</u> wrist
    M06.839 Other specified rheumatoid arthritis, <u>unspecified</u> wrist
M06.84-Other specified rheumatoid arthritis, <u>hand</u>
    M06.841 Other specified rheumatoid arthritis, <u>right</u> hand
    M06.842 Other specified rheumatoid arthritis, <u>left</u> hand
    M06.849 Other specified rheumatoid arthritis, <u>unspecified</u> hand
M06.85-Other specified rheumatoid arthritis, <u>hip</u>
    M06.851 Other specified rheumatoid arthritis, <u>right</u> hip
    M06.852 Other specified rheumatoid arthritis, <u>left</u> hip
    M06.859 Other specified rheumatoid arthritis, <u>unspecified</u> hip
M06.86-Other specified rheumatoid arthritis, <u>knee</u>
    M06.861 Other specified rheumatoid arthritis, <u>right</u> knee
    M06.862 Other specified rheumatoid arthritis, <u>left</u> knee
    M06.869 Other specified rheumatoid arthritis, <u>unspecified</u> knee
M06.87-Other specified rheumatoid arthritis, <u>ankle and foot</u>
    M06.871 Other specified rheumatoid arthritis, <u>right</u> ankle and foot
    M06.872 Other specified rheumatoid arthritis, <u>left</u> ankle and foot
    M06.879 Other specified rheumatoid arthritis, <u>unspecified</u> ankle and foot
M06.88 Other specified rheumatoid arthritis, <u>vertebrae</u>
M06.89 Other specified rheumatoid arthritis, <u>multiple sites</u>
M06.9 Rheumatoid arthritis, <u>unspecified</u>

M07- Enteropathic arthropathies
  Code also associated enteropathy, such as:
    Regional enteritis [Crohn's disease] (K50.-)
    Ulcerative colitis (K51.-)
  Excludes 1: psoriatic arthropathies (L40.5-)
M07.6- Enteropathic arthropathies
  M07.60 Enteropathic arthropathies, <u>unspecified</u> site
  M07.61-Enteropathic arthropathies, <u>shoulder</u>
    M07.611 Enteropathic arthropathies, <u>right</u> shoulder
    M07.612 Enteropathic arthropathies, <u>left</u> shoulder
    M07.619 Enteropathic arthropathies, <u>unspecified</u> shoulder
  M07.62-Enteropathic arthropathies, <u>elbow</u>
    M07.621 Enteropathic arthropathies, <u>right</u> elbow
    M07.622 Enteropathic arthropathies, <u>left</u> elbow
    M07.629 Enteropathic arthropathies, <u>unspecified</u> elbow
  M07.63-Enteropathic arthropathies, <u>wrist</u>
    M07.631 Enteropathic arthropathies, <u>right</u> wrist
    M07.632 Enteropathic arthropathies, <u>left</u> wrist
    M07.639 Enteropathic arthropathies, <u>unspecified</u> wrist
  M07.64-Enteropathic arthropathies, <u>hand</u>
    M07.641 Enteropathic arthropathies, <u>right</u> hand
    M07.642 Enteropathic arthropathies, <u>left</u> hand
    M07.649 Enteropathic arthropathies, <u>unspecified</u> hand
  M07.65-Enteropathic arthropathies, <u>hip</u>
    M07.651 Enteropathic arthropathies, <u>right</u> hip
    M07.652 Enteropathic arthropathies, <u>left</u> hip
    M07.659 Enteropathic arthropathies, <u>unspecified</u> hip
  M07.66-Enteropathic arthropathies, <u>knee</u>
    M07.661 Enteropathic arthropathies, <u>right</u> knee
    M07.662 Enteropathic arthropathies, <u>left</u> knee
    M07.669 Enteropathic arthropathies, <u>unspecified</u> knee
  M07.67-Enteropathic arthropathies, <u>ankle and foot</u>
    M07.671 Enteropathic arthropathies, <u>right</u> ankle and foot
    M07.672 Enteropathic arthropathies, <u>left</u> ankle and foot
    M07.679 Enteropathic arthropathies, <u>unspecified</u> ankle and foot
  M07.68 Enteropathic arthropathies, <u>vertebrae</u>
  M07.69 Enteropathic arthropathies, <u>multiple sites</u>

M08- <u>Juvenile arthritis</u>
  Code also any associated underlying condition, such as:
    Regional enteritis [Crohn's disease] (K50.-)
    Ulcerative colitis (K51.-)
  Excludes 1: arthropathy in Whipple's disease (M14.8)
          Felty's syndrome (M05.0)
          juvenile dermatomyositis (M33.0-)
          psoriatic juvenile arthropathy (L40.54)
M08.0- <u>Unspecified</u> juvenile rheumatoid arthritis
    Juvenile rheumatoid arthritis with or without rheumatoid factor
  M08.00 Unspecified juvenile rheumatoid arthritis of <u>unspecified</u> site
  M08.01-Unspecified juvenile rheumatoid arthritis, <u>shoulder</u>
    M08.011 Unspecified juvenile rheumatoid arthritis, <u>right</u> shoulder
    M08.012 Unspecified juvenile rheumatoid arthritis, <u>left</u> shoulder
    M08.019 Unspecified juvenile rheumatoid arthritis, <u>unspecified</u> shoulder
  M08.02-Unspecified juvenile rheumatoid arthritis of <u>elbow</u>
    M08.021 Unspecified juvenile rheumatoid arthritis, <u>right</u> elbow
    M08.022 Unspecified juvenile rheumatoid arthritis, <u>left</u> elbow
    M08.029 Unspecified juvenile rheumatoid arthritis, <u>unspecified</u> elbow
  M08.03-Unspecified juvenile rheumatoid arthritis, <u>wrist</u>
    M08.031 Unspecified juvenile rheumatoid arthritis, <u>right</u> wrist
    M08.032 Unspecified juvenile rheumatoid arthritis, <u>left</u> wrist
    M08.039 Unspecified juvenile rheumatoid arthritis, <u>unspecified</u> wrist
  M08.04-Unspecified juvenile rheumatoid arthritis, <u>hand</u>
    M08.041 Unspecified juvenile rheumatoid arthritis, <u>right</u> hand
    M08.042 Unspecified juvenile rheumatoid arthritis, <u>left</u> hand
    M08.049 Unspecified juvenile rheumatoid arthritis, <u>unspecified</u> hand
  M08.05-Unspecified juvenile rheumatoid arthritis, <u>hip</u>
    M08.051 Unspecified juvenile rheumatoid arthritis, <u>right</u> hip
    M08.052 Unspecified juvenile rheumatoid arthritis, <u>left</u> hip
    M08.059 Unspecified juvenile rheumatoid arthritis, <u>unspecified</u> hip
  M08.06-Unspecified juvenile rheumatoid arthritis, <u>knee</u>
    M08.061 Unspecified juvenile rheumatoid arthritis, <u>right</u> knee
    M08.062 Unspecified juvenile rheumatoid arthritis, <u>left</u> knee
    M08.069 Unspecified juvenile rheumatoid arthritis, <u>unspecified</u> knee
  M08.07-Unspecified juvenile rheumatoid arthritis, <u>ankle and foot</u>
    M08.071 Unspecified juvenile rheumatoid arthritis, <u>right</u> ankle and foot
    M08.072 Unspecified juvenile rheumatoid arthritis, <u>left</u> ankle and foot
    M08.079 Unspecified juvenile rheumatoid arthritis, <u>unspecified</u> ankle and foot
  M08.08 Unspecified juvenile rheumatoid arthritis, <u>vertebrae</u>
  M08.09 Unspecified juvenile rheumatoid arthritis, <u>multiple sites</u>
M08.1 Juvenile ankylosing spondylitis
  Excludes 1: ankylosing spondylitis in adults (M45.0-)
M08.2- Juvenile rheumatoid arthritis <u>with systemic onset</u>
    Still's disease NOS
  Excludes 1: adult-onset Still's disease (M06.1-)
  M08.20 Juvenile rheumatoid arthritis with systemic onset, <u>unspecified</u> site
  M08.21-Juvenile rheumatoid arthritis with systemic onset, <u>shoulder</u>
    M08.211 Juvenile rheumatoid arthritis with systemic onset, <u>right</u> shoulder
    M08.212 Juvenile rheumatoid arthritis with systemic onset, <u>left</u> shoulder
    M08.219 Juvenile rheumatoid arthritis with systemic onset, <u>unspecified</u> shoulder
  M08.22-Juvenile rheumatoid arthritis with systemic onset, <u>elbow</u>
    M08.221 Juvenile rheumatoid arthritis with systemic onset, <u>right</u> elbow
    M08.222 Juvenile rheumatoid arthritis with systemic onset, <u>left</u> elbow
    M08.229 Juvenile rheumatoid arthritis with systemic onset, <u>unspecified</u> elbow
  M08.23-Juvenile rheumatoid arthritis with systemic onset, <u>wrist</u>
    M08.231 Juvenile rheumatoid arthritis with systemic onset, <u>right</u> wrist
    M08.232 Juvenile rheumatoid arthritis with systemic onset, <u>left</u> wrist

M05 I M08

M08.239   Juvenile rheumatoid arthritis with systemic onset, <u>unspecified</u> wrist
M08.24-Juvenile rheumatoid arthritis with systemic onset, <u>hand</u>
　　M08.241   Juvenile rheumatoid arthritis with systemic onset, <u>right</u> hand
　　M08.242   Juvenile rheumatoid arthritis with systemic onset, <u>left</u> hand
　　M08.249   Juvenile rheumatoid arthritis with systemic onset, <u>unspecified</u> hand
M08.25-Juvenile rheumatoid arthritis with systemic onset, <u>hip</u>
　　M08.251   Juvenile rheumatoid arthritis with systemic onset, <u>right</u> hip
　　M08.252   Juvenile rheumatoid arthritis with systemic onset, <u>left</u> hip
　　M08.259   Juvenile rheumatoid arthritis with systemic onset, <u>unspecified</u> hip
M08.26-Juvenile rheumatoid arthritis with systemic onset, <u>knee</u>
　　M08.261   Juvenile rheumatoid arthritis with systemic onset, <u>right</u> knee
　　M08.262   Juvenile rheumatoid arthritis with systemic onset, <u>left</u> knee
　　M08.269   Juvenile rheumatoid arthritis with systemic onset, <u>unspecified</u> knee
M08.27-Juvenile rheumatoid arthritis with systemic onset, <u>ankle and foot</u>
　　M08.271   Juvenile rheumatoid arthritis with systemic onset, <u>right</u> ankle and foot
　　M08.272   Juvenile rheumatoid arthritis with systemic onset, <u>left</u> ankle and foot
　　M08.279   Juvenile rheumatoid arthritis with systemic onset, <u>unspecified</u> ankle and foot
M08.28   Juvenile rheumatoid arthritis with systemic onset, <u>vertebrae</u>
M08.29   Juvenile rheumatoid arthritis with systemic onset, <u>multiple sites</u>
M08.3   Juvenile rheumatoid polyarthritis (seronegative)
M08.4-   <u>Pauciarticular</u> juvenile rheumatoid arthritis
M08.40   Pauciarticular juvenile rheumatoid arthritis, <u>unspecified</u> site
M08.41-Pauciarticular juvenile rheumatoid arthritis, <u>shoulder</u>
　　M08.411   Pauciarticular juvenile rheumatoid arthritis, <u>right</u> shoulder
　　M08.412   Pauciarticular juvenile rheumatoid arthritis, <u>left</u> shoulder
　　M08.419   Pauciarticular juvenile rheumatoid arthritis, <u>unspecified</u> shoulder
M08.42-Pauciarticular juvenile rheumatoid arthritis, <u>elbow</u>
　　M08.421   Pauciarticular juvenile rheumatoid arthritis, <u>right</u> elbow
　　M08.422   Pauciarticular juvenile rheumatoid arthritis, <u>left</u> elbow
　　M08.429   Pauciarticular juvenile rheumatoid arthritis, <u>unspecified</u> elbow
M08.43-Pauciarticular juvenile rheumatoid arthritis, <u>wrist</u>
　　M08.431   Pauciarticular juvenile rheumatoid arthritis, <u>right</u> wrist
　　M08.432   Pauciarticular juvenile rheumatoid arthritis, <u>left</u> wrist
　　M08.439   Pauciarticular juvenile rheumatoid arthritis, <u>unspecified</u> wrist
M08.44-Pauciarticular juvenile rheumatoid arthritis, <u>hand</u>
　　M08.441   Pauciarticular juvenile rheumatoid arthritis, <u>right</u> hand
　　M08.442   Pauciarticular juvenile rheumatoid arthritis, <u>left</u> hand
　　M08.449   Pauciarticular juvenile rheumatoid arthritis, <u>unspecified</u> hand
M08.45-Pauciarticular juvenile rheumatoid arthritis, <u>hip</u>
　　M08.451   Pauciarticular juvenile rheumatoid arthritis, <u>right</u> hip
　　M08.452   Pauciarticular juvenile rheumatoid arthritis, <u>left</u> hip
　　M08.459   Pauciarticular juvenile rheumatoid arthritis, <u>unspecified</u> hip
M08.46-Pauciarticular juvenile rheumatoid arthritis, <u>knee</u>
　　M08.461   Pauciarticular juvenile rheumatoid arthritis, <u>right</u> knee
　　M08.462   Pauciarticular juvenile rheumatoid arthritis, <u>left</u> knee
　　M08.469   Pauciarticular juvenile rheumatoid arthritis, <u>unspecified</u> knee

M08.47-Pauciarticular juvenile rheumatoid arthritis, <u>ankle and foot</u>
　　M08.471   Pauciarticular juvenile rheumatoid arthritis, <u>right</u> ankle and foot
　　M08.472   Pauciarticular juvenile rheumatoid arthritis, <u>left</u> ankle and foot
　　M08.479   Pauciarticular juvenile rheumatoid arthritis, <u>unspecified</u> ankle and foot
M08.48   Pauciarticular juvenile rheumatoid arthritis, <u>vertebrae</u>
M08.8-   <u>Other</u> juvenile arthritis
M08.80   Other juvenile arthritis, <u>unspecified</u> site
M08.81-Other juvenile arthritis, <u>shoulder</u>
　　M08.811   Other juvenile arthritis, <u>right</u> shoulder
　　M08.812   Other juvenile arthritis, <u>left</u> shoulder
　　M08.819   Other juvenile arthritis, <u>unspecified</u> shoulder
M08.82-Other juvenile arthritis, <u>elbow</u>
　　M08.821   Other juvenile arthritis, <u>right</u> elbow
　　M08.822   Other juvenile arthritis, <u>left</u> elbow
　　M08.829   Other juvenile arthritis, <u>unspecified</u> elbow
M08.83-Other juvenile arthritis, <u>wrist</u>
　　M08.831   Other juvenile arthritis, <u>right</u> wrist
　　M08.832   Other juvenile arthritis, <u>left</u> wrist
　　M08.839   Other juvenile arthritis, <u>unspecified</u> wrist
M08.84-Other juvenile arthritis, <u>hand</u>
　　M08.841   Other juvenile arthritis, <u>right</u> hand
　　M08.842   Other juvenile arthritis, <u>left</u> hand
　　M08.849   Other juvenile arthritis, <u>unspecified</u> hand
M08.85-Other juvenile arthritis, <u>hip</u>
　　M08.851   Other juvenile arthritis, <u>right</u> hip
　　M08.852   Other juvenile arthritis, <u>left</u> hip
　　M08.859   Other juvenile arthritis, <u>unspecified</u> hip
M08.86-Other juvenile arthritis, <u>knee</u>
　　M08.861   Other juvenile arthritis, <u>right</u> knee
　　M08.862   Other juvenile arthritis, <u>left</u> knee
　　M08.869   Other juvenile arthritis, <u>unspecified</u> knee
M08.87-Other juvenile arthritis, <u>ankle and foot</u>
　　M08.871   Other juvenile arthritis, <u>right</u> ankle and foot
　　M08.872   Other juvenile arthritis, <u>left</u> ankle and foot
　　M08.879   Other juvenile arthritis, <u>unspecified</u> ankle and foot
M08.88   Other juvenile arthritis, <u>other specified site</u>
　　　　Other juvenile arthritis, vertebrae
M08.89   Other juvenile arthritis, <u>multiple sites</u>
M08.9-   Juvenile arthritis, <u>unspecified</u>
　　Excludes 1: juvenile rheumatoid arthritis, unspecified (M08.0-)
M08.90   Juvenile arthritis, unspecified, <u>unspecified</u> site
M08.91-Juvenile arthritis, unspecified, <u>shoulder</u>
　　M08.911   Juvenile arthritis, unspecified, <u>right</u> shoulder
　　M08.912   Juvenile arthritis, unspecified, <u>left</u> shoulder
　　M08.919   Juvenile arthritis, unspecified, <u>unspecified</u> shoulder
M08.92-Juvenile arthritis, unspecified, <u>elbow</u>
　　M08.921   Juvenile arthritis, unspecified, <u>right</u> elbow
　　M08.922   Juvenile arthritis, unspecified, <u>left</u> elbow
　　M08.929   Juvenile arthritis, unspecified, <u>unspecified</u> elbow
M08.93-Juvenile arthritis, unspecified, <u>wrist</u>
　　M08.931   Juvenile arthritis, unspecified, <u>right</u> wrist
　　M08.932   Juvenile arthritis, unspecified, <u>left</u> wrist
　　M08.939   Juvenile arthritis, unspecified, <u>unspecified</u> wrist
M08.94-Juvenile arthritis, unspecified, <u>hand</u>
　　M08.941   Juvenile arthritis, unspecified, <u>right</u> hand
　　M08.942   Juvenile arthritis, unspecified, <u>left</u> hand
　　M08.949   Juvenile arthritis, unspecified, <u>unspecified</u> hand
M08.95-Juvenile arthritis, unspecified, <u>hip</u>
　　M08.951   Juvenile arthritis, unspecified, <u>right</u> hip
　　M08.952   Juvenile arthritis, unspecified, <u>left</u> hip
　　M08.959   Juvenile arthritis, unspecified, <u>unspecified</u> hip
M08.96-Juvenile arthritis, unspecified, <u>knee</u>
　　M08.961   Juvenile arthritis, unspecified, <u>right</u> knee
　　M08.962   Juvenile arthritis, unspecified, <u>left</u> knee
　　M08.969   Juvenile arthritis, unspecified, <u>unspecified</u> knee
M08.97-Juvenile arthritis, unspecified, <u>ankle and foot</u>
　　M08.971   Juvenile arthritis, unspecified, <u>right</u> ankle and foot
　　M08.972   Juvenile arthritis, unspecified, <u>left</u> ankle and foot
　　M08.979   Juvenile arthritis, unspecified, <u>unspecified</u> ankle and foot
M08.98   Juvenile arthritis, unspecified, <u>vertebrae</u>
M08.99   Juvenile arthritis, unspecified, <u>multiple sites</u>

Excludes 1: = NOT CODED HERE! (Do not code both)

Excludes ❷: = Not Included Here

M1A- Chronic gout
  Use additional code to identify:
    Autonomic neuropathy in diseases classified elsewhere (G99.0)
    Calculus of urinary tract in diseases classified elsewhere (N22)
    Cardiomyopathy in diseases classified elsewhere (I43)
    Disorders of external ear in diseases classified elsewhere (H61.1-, H62.8-)
    Disorders of iris and ciliary body in diseases classified elsewhere (H22)
    Glomerular disorders in diseases classified elsewhere (N08)
  Excludes 1:   acute gout (M10.-)
                           gout NOS (M10.-)

The appropriate 7th character is to be added to each code from category M1A:
0   Without tophus (tophi)
1   With tophus (tophi)

M1A.0- Idiopathic chronic gout
    Chronic gouty bursitis
    Primary chronic gout
  M1A.00x- Idiopathic chronic gout, unspecified site
  M1A.01- Idiopathic chronic gout, shoulder
    M1A.011- Idiopathic chronic gout, right shoulder
    M1A.012- Idiopathic chronic gout, left shoulder
    M1A.019- Idiopathic chronic gout, unspecified shoulder
  M1A.02- Idiopathic chronic gout, elbow
    M1A.021- Idiopathic chronic gout, right elbow
    M1A.022- Idiopathic chronic gout, left elbow
    M1A.029- Idiopathic chronic gout, unspecified elbow
  M1A.03- Idiopathic chronic gout, wrist
    M1A.031- Idiopathic chronic gout, right wrist
    M1A.032- Idiopathic chronic gout, left wrist
    M1A.039- Idiopathic chronic gout, unspecified wrist
  M1A.04- Idiopathic chronic gout, hand
    M1A.041- Idiopathic chronic gout, right hand
    M1A.042- Idiopathic chronic gout, left hand
    M1A.049- Idiopathic chronic gout, unspecified hand
  M1A.05- Idiopathic chronic gout, hip
    M1A.051- Idiopathic chronic gout, right hip
    M1A.052- Idiopathic chronic gout, left hip
    M1A.059- Idiopathic chronic gout, unspecified hip
  M1A.06- Idiopathic chronic gout, knee
    M1A.061- Idiopathic chronic gout, right knee
    M1A.062- Idiopathic chronic gout, left knee
    M1A.069- Idiopathic chronic gout, unspecified knee
  M1A.07- Idiopathic chronic gout, ankle and foot
    M1A.071- Idiopathic chronic gout, right ankle and foot
    M1A.072- Idiopathic chronic gout, left ankle and foot
    M1A.079- Idiopathic chronic gout, unspecified ankle and foot
  M1A.08x- Idiopathic chronic gout, vertebrae
  M1A.09x- Idiopathic chronic gout, multiple sites
M1A.1- Lead-induced chronic gout
    Code first toxic effects of lead and its compounds (T56.0-)
  M1A.10x- Lead-induced chronic gout, unspecified site
  M1A.11- Lead-induced chronic gout, shoulder
    M1A.111- Lead-induced chronic gout, right shoulder
    M1A.112- Lead-induced chronic gout, left shoulder
    M1A.119- Lead-induced chronic gout, unspecified shoulder
  M1A.12- Lead-induced chronic gout, elbow
    M1A.121- Lead-induced chronic gout, right elbow
    M1A.122- Lead-induced chronic gout, left elbow
    M1A.129- Lead-induced chronic gout, unspecified elbow
  M1A.13- Lead-induced chronic gout, wrist
    M1A.131- Lead-induced chronic gout, right wrist
    M1A.132- Lead-induced chronic gout, left wrist
    M1A.139- Lead-induced chronic gout, unspecified wrist
  M1A.14- Lead-induced chronic gout, hand
    M1A.141- Lead-induced chronic gout, right hand
    M1A.142- Lead-induced chronic gout, left hand
    M1A.149- Lead-induced chronic gout, unspecified hand
  M1A.15- Lead-induced chronic gout, hip
    M1A.151- Lead-induced chronic gout, right hip
    M1A.152- Lead-induced chronic gout, left hip
    M1A.159- Lead-induced chronic gout, unspecified hip
  M1A.16- Lead-induced chronic gout, knee
    M1A.161- Lead-induced chronic gout, right knee
    M1A.162- Lead-induced chronic gout, left knee
    M1A.169- Lead-induced chronic gout, unspecified knee

  M1A.17- Lead-induced chronic gout, ankle and foot
    M1A.171- Lead-induced chronic gout, right ankle and foot
    M1A.172- Lead-induced chronic gout, left ankle and foot
    M1A.179- Lead-induced chronic gout, unspecified ankle and foot
  M1A.18x- Lead-induced chronic gout, vertebrae
  M1A.19x- Lead-induced chronic gout, multiple sites
M1A.2- Drug-induced chronic gout
    Use additional code for adverse effect, if applicable, to identify drug (T36-T50 with fifth or sixth character 5)
  M1A.20x- Drug-induced chronic gout, unspecified site
  M1A.21- Drug-induced chronic gout, shoulder
    M1A.211- Drug-induced chronic gout, right shoulder
    M1A.212- Drug-induced chronic gout, left shoulder
    M1A.219- Drug-induced chronic gout, unspecified shoulder
  M1A.22- Drug-induced chronic gout, elbow
    M1A.221- Drug-induced chronic gout, right elbow
    M1A.222- Drug-induced chronic gout, left elbow
    M1A.229- Drug-induced chronic gout, unspecified elbow
  M1A.23- Drug-induced chronic gout, wrist
    M1A.231- Drug-induced chronic gout, right wrist
    M1A.232- Drug-induced chronic gout, left wrist
    M1A.239- Drug-induced chronic gout, unspecified wrist
  M1A.24- Drug-induced chronic gout, hand
    M1A.241- Drug-induced chronic gout, right hand
    M1A.242- Drug-induced chronic gout, left hand
    M1A.249- Drug-induced chronic gout, unspecified hand
  M1A.25- Drug-induced chronic gout, hip
    M1A.251- Drug-induced chronic gout, right hip
    M1A.252- Drug-induced chronic gout, left hip
    M1A.259- Drug-induced chronic gout, unspecified hip
  M1A.26- Drug-induced chronic gout, knee
    M1A.261- Drug-induced chronic gout, right knee
    M1A.262- Drug-induced chronic gout, left knee
    M1A.269- Drug-induced chronic gout, unspecified knee
  M1A.27- Drug-induced chronic gout, ankle and foot
    M1A.271- Drug-induced chronic gout, right ankle and foot
    M1A.272- Drug-induced chronic gout, left ankle and foot
    M1A.279- Drug-induced chronic gout, unspecified ankle and foot
  M1A.28x- Drug-induced chronic gout, vertebrae
  M1A.29x- Drug-induced chronic gout, multiple sites
M1A.3- Chronic gout due to renal impairment
    Code first associated renal disease
  M1A.30x- Chronic gout due to renal impairment, unspecified site
  M1A.31- Chronic gout due to renal impairment, shoulder
    M1A.311- Chronic gout due to renal impairment, right shoulder
    M1A.312- Chronic gout due to renal impairment, left shoulder
    M1A.319- Chronic gout due to renal impairment, unspecified shoulder
  M1A.32- Chronic gout due to renal impairment, elbow
    M1A.321- Chronic gout due to renal impairment, right elbow
    M1A.322- Chronic gout due to renal impairment, left elbow
    M1A.329- Chronic gout due to renal impairment, unspecified elbow
  M1A.33- Chronic gout due to renal impairment, wrist
    M1A.331- Chronic gout due to renal impairment, right wrist
    M1A.332- Chronic gout due to renal impairment, left wrist
    M1A.339- Chronic gout due to renal impairment, unspecified wrist
  M1A.34- Chronic gout due to renal impairment, hand
    M1A.341- Chronic gout due to renal impairment, right hand
    M1A.342- Chronic gout due to renal impairment, left hand
    M1A.349- Chronic gout due to renal impairment, unspecified hand
  M1A.35- Chronic gout due to renal impairment, hip
    M1A.351- Chronic gout due to renal impairment, right hip
    M1A.352- Chronic gout due to renal impairment, left hip
    M1A.359- Chronic gout due to renal impairment, unspecified hip
  M1A.36- Chronic gout due to renal impairment, knee
    M1A.361- Chronic gout due to renal impairment, right knee
    M1A.362- Chronic gout due to renal impairment, left knee
    M1A.369- Chronic gout due to renal impairment, unspecified knee

M 0 8 - M 1 A

M1A.37- Chronic gout due to renal impairment, <u>ankle and foot</u>
    M1A.371- Chronic gout due to renal impairment, <u>right</u> ankle and foot
    M1A.372- Chronic gout due to renal impairment, <u>left</u> ankle and foot
    M1A.379- Chronic gout due to renal impairment, <u>unspecified</u> ankle and foot
M1A.38x- Chronic gout due to renal impairment, <u>vertebrae</u>
M1A.39x- Chronic gout due to renal impairment, <u>multiple sites</u>

M1A.4- <u>Other secondary</u> chronic gout
    Code first associated condition
M1A.40x- Other secondary chronic gout, <u>unspecified</u> site
M1A.41- Other secondary chronic gout, <u>shoulder</u>
    M1A.411- Other secondary chronic gout, <u>right</u> shoulder
    M1A.412- Other secondary chronic gout, <u>left</u> shoulder
    M1A.419- Other secondary chronic gout, <u>unspecified</u> shoulder
M1A.42- Other secondary chronic gout, <u>elbow</u>
    M1A.421- Other secondary chronic gout, <u>right</u> elbow
    M1A.422- Other secondary chronic gout, <u>left</u> elbow
    M1A.429- Other secondary chronic gout, <u>unspecified</u> elbow
M1A.43- Other secondary chronic gout, <u>wrist</u>
    M1A.431- Other secondary chronic gout, <u>right</u> wrist
    M1A.432- Other secondary chronic gout, <u>left</u> wrist
    M1A.439- Other secondary chronic gout, <u>unspecified</u> wrist
M1A.44- Other secondary chronic gout, <u>hand</u>
    M1A.441- Other secondary chronic gout, <u>right</u> hand
    M1A.442- Other secondary chronic gout, <u>left</u> hand
    M1A.449- Other secondary chronic gout, <u>unspecified</u> hand
M1A.45- Other secondary chronic gout, <u>hip</u>
    M1A.451- Other secondary chronic gout, <u>right</u> hip
    M1A.452- Other secondary chronic gout, <u>left</u> hip
    M1A.459- Other secondary chronic gout, <u>unspecified</u> hip
M1A.46- Other secondary chronic gout, <u>knee</u>
    M1A.461- Other secondary chronic gout, <u>right</u> knee
    M1A.462- Other secondary chronic gout, <u>left</u> knee
    M1A.469- Other secondary chronic gout, <u>unspecified</u> knee
M1A.47- Other secondary chronic gout, <u>ankle and foot</u>
    M1A.471- Other secondary chronic gout, <u>right</u> ankle and foot
    M1A.472- Other secondary chronic gout, <u>left</u> ankle and foot
    M1A.479- Other secondary chronic gout, <u>unspecified</u> ankle and foot
M1A.48x- Other secondary chronic gout, <u>vertebrae</u>
M1A.49x- Other secondary chronic gout, <u>multiple sites</u>
M1A.9xx- Chronic gout, <u>unspecified</u>

M10- <u>Gout</u>
    <u>Acute</u> gout
    Gout <u>attack</u>
    Gout <u>flare</u>
    Gout <u>NOS</u>
    Podagra
    Use additional code to identify:
    Autonomic neuropathy in diseases classified elsewhere (G99.0)
    Calculus of urinary tract in diseases classified elsewhere (N22)
    Cardiomyopathy in diseases classified elsewhere (I43)
    Disorders of external ear in diseases classified elsewhere (H61.1-, H62.8-)
    Disorders of iris and ciliary body in diseases classified elsewhere (H22)
    Glomerular disorders in diseases classified elsewhere (N08)
    Excludes 1: chronic gout (M1A.-)
M10.0- Idiopathic gout
    Gouty bursitis
    Primary gout
    M10.00 Idiopathic gout, <u>unspecified</u> site
    M10.01-Idiopathic gout, <u>shoulder</u>
        M10.011 Idiopathic gout, <u>right</u> shoulder
        M10.012 Idiopathic gout, <u>left</u> shoulder
        M10.019 Idiopathic gout, <u>unspecified</u> shoulder
    M10.02-Idiopathic gout, <u>elbow</u>
        M10.021 Idiopathic gout, <u>right</u> elbow
        M10.022 Idiopathic gout, <u>left</u> elbow
        M10.029 Idiopathic gout, <u>unspecified</u> elbow
    M10.03-Idiopathic gout, <u>wrist</u>
        M10.031 Idiopathic gout, <u>right</u> wrist
        M10.032 Idiopathic gout, <u>left</u> wrist
        M10.039 Idiopathic gout, <u>unspecified</u> wrist

M10.04-Idiopathic gout, <u>hand</u>
    M10.041 Idiopathic gout, <u>right</u> hand
    M10.042 Idiopathic gout, <u>left</u> hand
    M10.049 Idiopathic gout, <u>unspecified</u> hand
M10.05-Idiopathic gout, <u>hip</u>
    M10.051 Idiopathic gout, <u>right</u> hip
    M10.052 Idiopathic gout, <u>left</u> hip
    M10.059 Idiopathic gout, <u>unspecified</u> hip
M10.06-Idiopathic gout, <u>knee</u>
    M10.061 Idiopathic gout, <u>right</u> knee
    M10.062 Idiopathic gout, <u>left</u> knee
    M10.069 Idiopathic gout, <u>unspecified</u> knee
M10.07-Idiopathic gout, <u>ankle and foot</u>
    M10.071 Idiopathic gout, <u>right</u> ankle and foot
    M10.072 Idiopathic gout, <u>left</u> ankle and foot
    M10.079 Idiopathic gout, <u>unspecified</u> ankle and foot
M10.08 Idiopathic gout, <u>vertebrae</u>
M10.09 Idiopathic gout, <u>multiple sites</u>
M10.1- <u>Lead-induced</u> gout
    Code first toxic effects of lead and its compounds (T56.0-)
    M10.10 Lead-induced gout, <u>unspecified</u> site
    M10.11-Lead-induced gout, <u>shoulder</u>
        M10.111 Lead-induced gout, <u>right</u> shoulder
        M10.112 Lead-induced gout, <u>left</u> shoulder
        M10.119 Lead-induced gout, <u>unspecified</u> shoulder
    M10.12-Lead-induced gout, <u>elbow</u>
        M10.121 Lead-induced gout, <u>right</u> elbow
        M10.122 Lead-induced gout, <u>left</u> elbow
        M10.129 Lead-induced gout, <u>unspecified</u> elbow
    M10.13-Lead-induced gout, <u>wrist</u>
        M10.131 Lead-induced gout, <u>right</u> wrist
        M10.132 Lead-induced gout, <u>left</u> wrist
        M10.139 Lead-induced gout, <u>unspecified</u> wrist
    M10.14-Lead-induced gout, <u>hand</u>
        M10.141 Lead-induced gout, <u>right</u> hand
        M10.142 Lead-induced gout, <u>left</u> hand
        M10.149 Lead-induced gout, <u>unspecified</u> hand
    M10.15-Lead-induced gout, <u>hip</u>
        M10.151 Lead-induced gout, <u>right</u> hip
        M10.152 Lead-induced gout, <u>left</u> hip
        M10.159 Lead-induced gout, <u>unspecified</u> hip
    M10.16-Lead-induced gout, <u>knee</u>
        M10.161 Lead-induced gout, <u>right</u> knee
        M10.162 Lead-induced gout, <u>left</u> knee
        M10.169 Lead-induced gout, <u>unspecified</u> knee
    M10.17-Lead-induced gout, <u>ankle and foot</u>
        M10.171 Lead-induced gout, <u>right</u> ankle and foot
        M10.172 Lead-induced gout, <u>left</u> ankle and foot
        M10.179 Lead-induced gout, <u>unspecified</u> ankle and foot
    M10.18 Lead-induced gout, <u>vertebrae</u>
    M10.19 Lead-induced gout, <u>multiple sites</u>
M10.2- <u>Drug-induced</u> gout
    Use additional code for adverse effect, if applicable, to identify drug (T36-T50 with fifth or sixth character 5)
    M10.20 Drug-induced gout, <u>unspecified</u> site
    M10.21-Drug-induced gout, <u>shoulder</u>
        M10.211 Drug-induced gout, <u>right</u> shoulder
        M10.212 Drug-induced gout, <u>left</u> shoulder
        M10.219 Drug-induced gout, <u>unspecified</u> shoulder
    M10.22-Drug-induced gout, <u>elbow</u>
        M10.221 Drug-induced gout, <u>right</u> elbow
        M10.222 Drug-induced gout, <u>left</u> elbow
        M10.229 Drug-induced gout, <u>unspecified</u> elbow
    M10.23-Drug-induced gout, <u>wrist</u>
        M10.231 Drug-induced gout, <u>right</u> wrist
        M10.232 Drug-induced gout, <u>left</u> wrist
        M10.239 Drug-induced gout, <u>unspecified</u> wrist
    M10.24-Drug-induced gout, <u>hand</u>
        M10.241 Drug-induced gout, <u>right</u> hand
        M10.242 Drug-induced gout, <u>left</u> hand
        M10.249 Drug-induced gout, <u>unspecified</u> hand
    M10.25-Drug-induced gout, <u>hip</u>
        M10.251 Drug-induced gout, <u>right</u> hip
        M10.252 Drug-induced gout, <u>left</u> hip
        M10.259 Drug-induced gout, <u>unspecified</u> hip

M10.26-Drug-induced gout, <u>knee</u>
    M10.261 Drug-induced gout, <u>right</u> knee
    M10.262 Drug-induced gout, <u>left</u> knee
    M10.269 Drug-induced gout, <u>unspecified</u> knee
M10.27-Drug-induced gout, <u>ankle and foot</u>
    M10.271 Drug-induced gout, <u>right</u> ankle and foot
    M10.272 Drug-induced gout, <u>left</u> ankle and foot
    M10.279 Drug-induced gout, <u>unspecified</u> ankle and foot
M10.28 Drug-induced gout, <u>vertebrae</u>
M10.29 Drug-induced gout, <u>multiple sites</u>
M10.3- Gout <u>due to renal impairment</u>
    Code first associated renal disease
M10.30 Gout due to renal impairment, <u>unspecified</u> site
M10.31-Gout due to renal impairment, <u>shoulder</u>
    M10.311 Gout due to renal impairment, <u>right</u> shoulder
    M10.312 Gout due to renal impairment, <u>left</u> shoulder
    M10.319 Gout due to renal impairment, <u>unspecified</u> shoulder
M10.32-Gout due to renal impairment, <u>elbow</u>
    M10.321 Gout due to renal impairment, <u>right</u> elbow
    M10.322 Gout due to renal impairment, <u>left</u> elbow
    M10.329 Gout due to renal impairment, <u>unspecified</u> elbow
M10.33-Gout due to renal impairment, <u>wrist</u>
    M10.331 Gout due to renal impairment, <u>right</u> wrist
    M10.332 Gout due to renal impairment, <u>left</u> wrist
    M10.339 Gout due to renal impairment, <u>unspecified</u> wrist
M10.34-Gout due to renal impairment, <u>hand</u>
    M10.341 Gout due to renal impairment, <u>right</u> hand
    M10.342 Gout due to renal impairment, <u>left</u> hand
    M10.349 Gout due to renal impairment, <u>unspecified</u> hand
M10.35-Gout due to renal impairment, <u>hip</u>
    M10.351 Gout due to renal impairment, <u>right</u> hip
    M10.352 Gout due to renal impairment, <u>left</u> hip
    M10.359 Gout due to renal impairment, <u>unspecified</u> hip
M10.36-Gout due to renal impairment, <u>knee</u>
    M10.361 Gout due to renal impairment, <u>right</u> knee
    M10.362 Gout due to renal impairment, <u>left</u> knee
    M10.369 Gout due to renal impairment, <u>unspecified</u> knee
M10.37-Gout due to renal impairment, <u>ankle and foot</u>
    M10.371 Gout due to renal impairment, <u>right</u> ankle and foot
    M10.372 Gout due to renal impairment, <u>left</u> ankle and foot
    M10.379 Gout due to renal impairment, <u>unspecified</u> ankle and foot
M10.38 Gout due to renal impairment, <u>vertebrae</u>
M10.39 Gout due to renal impairment, <u>multiple sites</u>
M10.4- <u>Other secondary</u> gout
    Code first associated condition
M10.40 Other secondary gout, <u>unspecified</u> site
M10.41-Other secondary gout, <u>shoulder</u>
    M10.411 Other secondary gout, <u>right</u> shoulder
    M10.412 Other secondary gout, <u>left</u> shoulder
    M10.419 Other secondary gout, <u>unspecified</u> shoulder
M10.42-Other secondary gout, <u>elbow</u>
    M10.421 Other secondary gout, <u>right</u> elbow
    M10.422 Other secondary gout, <u>left</u> elbow
    M10.429 Other secondary gout, <u>unspecified</u> elbow
M10.43-Other secondary gout, <u>wrist</u>
    M10.431 Other secondary gout, <u>right</u> wrist
    M10.432 Other secondary gout, <u>left</u> wrist
    M10.439 Other secondary gout, <u>unspecified</u> wrist
M10.44-Other secondary gout, <u>hand</u>
    M10.441 Other secondary gout, <u>right</u> hand
    M10.442 Other secondary gout, <u>left</u> hand
    M10.449 Other secondary gout, <u>unspecified</u> hand
M10.45-Other secondary gout, <u>hip</u>
    M10.451 Other secondary gout, <u>right</u> hip
    M10.452 Other secondary gout, <u>left</u> hip
    M10.459 Other secondary gout, <u>unspecified</u> hip
M10.46-Other secondary gout, <u>knee</u>
    M10.461 Other secondary gout, <u>right</u> knee
    M10.462 Other secondary gout, <u>left</u> knee
    M10.469 Other secondary gout, <u>unspecified</u> knee
M10.47-Other secondary gout, <u>ankle and foot</u>
    M10.471 Other secondary gout, <u>right</u> ankle and foot
    M10.472 Other secondary gout, <u>left</u> ankle and foot
    M10.479 Other secondary gout, <u>unspecified</u> ankle and foot

M10.48 Other secondary gout, <u>vertebrae</u>
M10.49 Other secondary gout, <u>multiple sites</u>
M10.9   Gout, <u>unspecified</u>
    Gout NOS
M11- <u>Other crystal arthropathies</u>
M11.0- <u>Hydroxyapatite deposition</u> disease
    M11.00 Hydroxyapatite deposition disease, <u>unspecified</u> site
    M11.01-Hydroxyapatite deposition disease, <u>shoulder</u>
        M11.011 Hydroxyapatite deposition disease, <u>right</u> shoulder
        M11.012 Hydroxyapatite deposition disease, <u>left</u> shoulder
        M11.019 Hydroxyapatite deposition disease, <u>unspecified</u> shoulder
    M11.02-Hydroxyapatite deposition disease, <u>elbow</u>
        M11.021 Hydroxyapatite deposition disease, <u>right</u> elbow
        M11.022 Hydroxyapatite deposition disease, <u>left</u> elbow
        M11.029 Hydroxyapatite deposition disease, <u>unspecified</u> elbow
    M11.03-Hydroxyapatite deposition disease, <u>wrist</u>
        M11.031 Hydroxyapatite deposition disease, <u>right</u> wrist
        M11.032 Hydroxyapatite deposition disease, <u>left</u> wrist
        M11.039 Hydroxyapatite deposition disease, <u>unspecified</u> wrist
    M11.04-Hydroxyapatite deposition disease, <u>hand</u>
        M11.041 Hydroxyapatite deposition disease, <u>right</u> hand
        M11.042 Hydroxyapatite deposition disease, <u>left</u> hand
        M11.049 Hydroxyapatite deposition disease, <u>unspecified</u> hand
    M11.05-Hydroxyapatite deposition disease, <u>hip</u>
        M11.051 Hydroxyapatite deposition disease, <u>right</u> hip
        M11.052 Hydroxyapatite deposition disease, <u>left</u> hip
        M11.059 Hydroxyapatite deposition disease, <u>unspecified</u> hip
    M11.06-Hydroxyapatite deposition disease, <u>knee</u>
        M11.061 Hydroxyapatite deposition disease, <u>right</u> knee
        M11.062 Hydroxyapatite deposition disease, <u>left</u> knee
        M11.069 Hydroxyapatite deposition disease, <u>unspecified</u> knee
    M11.07-Hydroxyapatite deposition disease, <u>ankle and foot</u>
        M11.071 Hydroxyapatite deposition disease, <u>right</u> ankle and foot
        M11.072 Hydroxyapatite deposition disease, <u>left</u> ankle and foot
        M11.079 Hydroxyapatite deposition disease, <u>unspecified</u> ankle and foot
    M11.08 Hydroxyapatite deposition disease, <u>vertebrae</u>
    M11.09 Hydroxyapatite deposition disease, <u>multiple sites</u>
M11.1- <u>Familial chondrocalcinosis</u>
    M11.10 Familial chondrocalcinosis, <u>unspecified</u> site
    M11.11-Familial chondrocalcinosis, <u>shoulder</u>
        M11.111 Familial chondrocalcinosis, <u>right</u> shoulder
        M11.112 Familial chondrocalcinosis, <u>left</u> shoulder
        M11.119 Familial chondrocalcinosis, <u>unspecified</u> shoulder
    M11.12-Familial chondrocalcinosis, <u>elbow</u>
        M11.121 Familial chondrocalcinosis, <u>right</u> elbow
        M11.122 Familial chondrocalcinosis, <u>left</u> elbow
        M11.129 Familial chondrocalcinosis, <u>unspecified</u> elbow
    M11.13-Familial chondrocalcinosis, <u>wrist</u>
        M11.131 Familial chondrocalcinosis, <u>right</u> wrist
        M11.132 Familial chondrocalcinosis, <u>left</u> wrist
        M11.139 Familial chondrocalcinosis, <u>unspecified</u> wrist
    M11.14-Familial chondrocalcinosis, <u>hand</u>
        M11.141 Familial chondrocalcinosis, <u>right</u> hand
        M11.142 Familial chondrocalcinosis, <u>left</u> hand
        M11.149 Familial chondrocalcinosis, <u>unspecified</u> hand
    M11.15-Familial chondrocalcinosis, <u>hip</u>
        M11.151 Familial chondrocalcinosis, <u>right</u> hip
        M11.152 Familial chondrocalcinosis, <u>left</u> hip
        M11.159 Familial chondrocalcinosis, <u>unspecified</u> hip
    M11.16-Familial chondrocalcinosis, <u>knee</u>
        M11.161 Familial chondrocalcinosis, <u>right</u> knee
        M11.162 Familial chondrocalcinosis, <u>left</u> knee
        M11.169 Familial chondrocalcinosis, <u>unspecified</u> knee
    M11.17-Familial chondrocalcinosis, <u>ankle and foot</u>
        M11.171 Familial chondrocalcinosis, <u>right</u> ankle and foot
        M11.172 Familial chondrocalcinosis, <u>left</u> ankle and foot
        M11.179 Familial chondrocalcinosis, <u>unspecified</u> ankle and foot
    M11.18 Familial chondrocalcinosis, <u>vertebrae</u>
    M11.19 Familial chondrocalcinosis, <u>multiple sites</u>

M
1
A
-
M
1
1

M11.2- Other chondrocalcinosis
    Chondrocalcinosis NOS
  M11.20 Other chondrocalcinosis, unspecified site
  M11.21- Other chondrocalcinosis, shoulder
    M11.211 Other chondrocalcinosis, right shoulder
    M11.212 Other chondrocalcinosis, left shoulder
    M11.219 Other chondrocalcinosis, unspecified shoulder
  M11.22- Other chondrocalcinosis, elbow
    M11.221 Other chondrocalcinosis, right elbow
    M11.222 Other chondrocalcinosis, left elbow
    M11.229 Other chondrocalcinosis, unspecified elbow
  M11.23- Other chondrocalcinosis, wrist
    M11.231 Other chondrocalcinosis, right wrist
    M11.232 Other chondrocalcinosis, left wrist
    M11.239 Other chondrocalcinosis, unspecified wrist
  M11.24- Other chondrocalcinosis, hand
    M11.241 Other chondrocalcinosis, right hand
    M11.242 Other chondrocalcinosis, left hand
    M11.249 Other chondrocalcinosis, unspecified hand
  M11.25- Other chondrocalcinosis, hip
    M11.251 Other chondrocalcinosis, right hip
    M11.252 Other chondrocalcinosis, left hip
    M11.259 Other chondrocalcinosis, unspecified hip
  M11.26- Other chondrocalcinosis, knee
    M11.261 Other chondrocalcinosis, right knee
    M11.262 Other chondrocalcinosis, left knee
    M11.269 Other chondrocalcinosis, unspecified knee
  M11.27- Other chondrocalcinosis, ankle and foot
    M11.271 Other chondrocalcinosis, right ankle and foot
    M11.272 Other chondrocalcinosis, left ankle and foot
    M11.279 Other chondrocalcinosis, unspecified ankle and foot
  M11.28 Other chondrocalcinosis, vertebrae
  M11.29 Other chondrocalcinosis, multiple sites
M11.8- Other specified crystal arthropathies
  M11.80 Other specified crystal arthropathies, unspecified site
  M11.81- Other specified crystal arthropathies, shoulder
    M11.811 Other specified crystal arthropathies, right shoulder
    M11.812 Other specified crystal arthropathies, left shoulder
    M11.819 Other specified crystal arthropathies, unspecified shoulder
  M11.82- Other specified crystal arthropathies, elbow
    M11.821 Other specified crystal arthropathies, right elbow
    M11.822 Other specified crystal arthropathies, left elbow
    M11.829 Other specified crystal arthropathies, unspecified elbow
  M11.83- Other specified crystal arthropathies, wrist
    M11.831 Other specified crystal arthropathies, right wrist
    M11.832 Other specified crystal arthropathies, left wrist
    M11.839 Other specified crystal arthropathies, unspecified wrist
  M11.84- Other specified crystal arthropathies, hand
    M11.841 Other specified crystal arthropathies, right hand
    M11.842 Other specified crystal arthropathies, left hand
    M11.849 Other specified crystal arthropathies, unspecified hand
  M11.85- Other specified crystal arthropathies, hip
    M11.851 Other specified crystal arthropathies, right hip
    M11.852 Other specified crystal arthropathies, left hip
    M11.859 Other specified crystal arthropathies, unspecified hip
  M11.86- Other specified crystal arthropathies, knee
    M11.861 Other specified crystal arthropathies, right knee
    M11.862 Other specified crystal arthropathies, left knee
    M11.869 Other specified crystal arthropathies, unspecified knee
  M11.87- Other specified crystal arthropathies, ankle and foot
    M11.871 Other specified crystal arthropathies, right ankle and foot
    M11.872 Other specified crystal arthropathies, left ankle and foot
    M11.879 Other specified crystal arthropathies, unspecified ankle and foot
  M11.88 Other specified crystal arthropathies, vertebrae
  M11.89 Other specified crystal arthropathies, multiple sites
M11.9 Crystal arthropathy, unspecified

M12- Other and unspecified arthropathy
    Excludes 1: arthrosis (M15-M19)
                 cricoarytenoid arthropathy (J38.7)
  M12.0- Chronic postrheumatic arthropathy [Jaccoud]
    M12.00 Chronic postrheumatic arthropathy [Jaccoud], unspecified site
    M12.01- Chronic postrheumatic arthropathy [Jaccoud], shoulder
      M12.011 Chronic postrheumatic arthropathy [Jaccoud], right shoulder
      M12.012 Chronic postrheumatic arthropathy [Jaccoud], left shoulder
      M12.019 Chronic postrheumatic arthropathy [Jaccoud], unspecified shoulder
    M12.02- Chronic postrheumatic arthropathy [Jaccoud], elbow
      M12.021 Chronic postrheumatic arthropathy [Jaccoud], right elbow
      M12.022 Chronic postrheumatic arthropathy [Jaccoud], left elbow
      M12.029 Chronic postrheumatic arthropathy [Jaccoud], unspecified elbow
    M12.03- Chronic postrheumatic arthropathy [Jaccoud], wrist
      M12.031 Chronic postrheumatic arthropathy [Jaccoud], right wrist
      M12.032 Chronic postrheumatic arthropathy [Jaccoud], left wrist
      M12.039 Chronic postrheumatic arthropathy [Jaccoud], unspecified wrist
    M12.04- Chronic postrheumatic arthropathy [Jaccoud], hand
      M12.041 Chronic postrheumatic arthropathy [Jaccoud], right hand
      M12.042 Chronic postrheumatic arthropathy [Jaccoud], left hand
      M12.049 Chronic postrheumatic arthropathy [Jaccoud], unspecified hand
    M12.05- Chronic postrheumatic arthropathy [Jaccoud], hip
      M12.051 Chronic postrheumatic arthropathy [Jaccoud], right hip
      M12.052 Chronic postrheumatic arthropathy [Jaccoud], left hip
      M12.059 Chronic postrheumatic arthropathy [Jaccoud], unspecified hip
    M12.06- Chronic postrheumatic arthropathy [Jaccoud], knee
      M12.061 Chronic postrheumatic arthropathy [Jaccoud], right knee
      M12.062 Chronic postrheumatic arthropathy [Jaccoud], left knee
      M12.069 Chronic postrheumatic arthropathy [Jaccoud], unspecified knee
    M12.07- Chronic postrheumatic arthropathy [Jaccoud], ankle and foot
      M12.071 Chronic postrheumatic arthropathy [Jaccoud], right ankle and foot
      M12.072 Chronic postrheumatic arthropathy [Jaccoud], left ankle and foot
      M12.079 Chronic postrheumatic arthropathy [Jaccoud], unspecified ankle and foot
    M12.08 Chronic postrheumatic arthropathy [Jaccoud], other specified site
        Chronic postrheumatic arthropathy [Jaccoud], vertebrae
    M12.09 Chronic postrheumatic arthropathy [Jaccoud], multiple sites
  M12.1- Kaschin-Beck disease
      Osteochondroarthrosis deformans endemica
    M12.10 Kaschin-Beck disease, unspecified site
    M12.11- Kaschin-Beck disease, shoulder
      M12.111 Kaschin-Beck disease, right shoulder
      M12.112 Kaschin-Beck disease, left shoulder
      M12.119 Kaschin-Beck disease, unspecified shoulder
    M12.12- Kaschin-Beck disease, elbow
      M12.121 Kaschin-Beck disease, right elbow
      M12.122 Kaschin-Beck disease, left elbow
      M12.129 Kaschin-Beck disease, unspecified elbow
    M12.13- Kaschin-Beck disease, wrist
      M12.131 Kaschin-Beck disease, right wrist
      M12.132 Kaschin-Beck disease, left wrist
      M12.139 Kaschin-Beck disease, unspecified wrist
    M12.14- Kaschin-Beck disease, hand
      M12.141 Kaschin-Beck disease, right hand
      M12.142 Kaschin-Beck disease, left hand
      M12.149 Kaschin-Beck disease, unspecified hand

M
1
1
-
M
1
2

M12.15-Kaschin-Beck disease, <u>hip</u>
  M12.151 Kaschin-Beck disease, <u>right</u> hip
  M12.152 Kaschin-Beck disease, <u>left</u> hip
  M12.159 Kaschin-Beck disease, <u>unspecified</u> hip
M12.16-Kaschin-Beck disease, <u>knee</u>
  M12.161 Kaschin-Beck disease, <u>right</u> knee
  M12.162 Kaschin-Beck disease, <u>left</u> knee
  M12.169 Kaschin-Beck disease, <u>unspecified</u> knee
M12.17-Kaschin-Beck disease, <u>ankle and foot</u>
  M12.171 Kaschin-Beck disease, <u>right</u> ankle and foot
  M12.172 Kaschin-Beck disease, <u>left</u> ankle and foot
  M12.179 Kaschin-Beck disease, <u>unspecified</u> ankle and foot
M12.18 Kaschin-Beck disease, <u>vertebrae</u>
M12.19 Kaschin-Beck disease, <u>multiple sites</u>
M12.2- <u>Villonodular synovitis (pigmented)</u>
M12.20 Villonodular synovitis (pigmented), <u>unspecified</u> site
M12.21-Villonodular synovitis (pigmented), <u>shoulder</u>
  M12.211 Villonodular synovitis (pigmented), <u>right</u> shoulder
  M12.212 Villonodular synovitis (pigmented), <u>left</u> shoulder
  M12.219 Villonodular synovitis (pigmented), <u>unspecified</u> shoulder
M12.22-Villonodular synovitis (pigmented), <u>elbow</u>
  M12.221 Villonodular synovitis (pigmented), <u>right</u> elbow
  M12.222 Villonodular synovitis (pigmented), <u>left</u> elbow
  M12.229 Villonodular synovitis (pigmented), <u>unspecified</u> elbow
M12.23-Villonodular synovitis (pigmented), <u>wrist</u>
  M12.231 Villonodular synovitis (pigmented), <u>right</u> wrist
  M12.232 Villonodular synovitis (pigmented), <u>left</u> wrist
  M12.239 Villonodular synovitis (pigmented), <u>unspecified</u> wrist
M12.24-Villonodular synovitis (pigmented), <u>hand</u>
  M12.241 Villonodular synovitis (pigmented), <u>right</u> hand
  M12.242 Villonodular synovitis (pigmented), <u>left</u> hand
  M12.249 Villonodular synovitis (pigmented), <u>unspecified</u> hand
M12.25-Villonodular synovitis (pigmented), <u>hip</u>
  M12.251 Villonodular synovitis (pigmented), <u>right</u> hip
  M12.252 Villonodular synovitis (pigmented), <u>left</u> hip
  M12.259 Villonodular synovitis (pigmented), <u>unspecified</u> hip
M12.26-Villonodular synovitis (pigmented), <u>knee</u>
  M12.261 Villonodular synovitis (pigmented), <u>right</u> knee
  M12.262 Villonodular synovitis (pigmented), <u>left</u> knee
  M12.269 Villonodular synovitis (pigmented), <u>unspecified</u> knee
M12.27-Villonodular synovitis (pigmented), <u>ankle and foot</u>
  M12.271 Villonodular synovitis (pigmented), <u>right</u> ankle and foot
  M12.272 Villonodular synovitis (pigmented), <u>left</u> ankle and foot
  M12.279 Villonodular synovitis (pigmented), <u>unspecified</u> ankle and foot
M12.28 Villonodular synovitis (pigmented), <u>other specified site</u>
  Villonodular synovitis (pigmented), vertebrae
M12.29 Villonodular synovitis (pigmented), <u>multiple sites</u>
M12.3- <u>Palindromic rheumatism</u>
M12.30 Palindromic rheumatism, <u>unspecified</u> site
M12.31-Palindromic rheumatism, <u>shoulder</u>
  M12.311 Palindromic rheumatism, <u>right</u> shoulder
  M12.312 Palindromic rheumatism, <u>left</u> shoulder
  M12.319 Palindromic rheumatism, <u>unspecified</u> shoulder
M12.32-Palindromic rheumatism, <u>elbow</u>
  M12.321 Palindromic rheumatism, <u>right</u> elbow
  M12.322 Palindromic rheumatism, <u>left</u> elbow
  M12.329 Palindromic rheumatism, <u>unspecified</u> elbow
M12.33-Palindromic rheumatism, <u>wrist</u>
  M12.331 Palindromic rheumatism, <u>right</u> wrist
  M12.332 Palindromic rheumatism, <u>left</u> wrist
  M12.339 Palindromic rheumatism, <u>unspecified</u> wrist
M12.34-Palindromic rheumatism, <u>hand</u>
  M12.341 Palindromic rheumatism, <u>right</u> hand
  M12.342 Palindromic rheumatism, <u>left</u> hand
  M12.349 Palindromic rheumatism, <u>unspecified</u> hand
M12.35-Palindromic rheumatism, <u>hip</u>
  M12.351 Palindromic rheumatism, <u>right</u> hip
  M12.352 Palindromic rheumatism, <u>left</u> hip
  M12.359 Palindromic rheumatism, <u>unspecified</u> hip

M12.36-Palindromic rheumatism, <u>knee</u>
  M12.361 Palindromic rheumatism, <u>right</u> knee
  M12.362 Palindromic rheumatism, <u>left</u> knee
  M12.369 Palindromic rheumatism, <u>unspecified</u> knee
M12.37-Palindromic rheumatism, <u>ankle and foot</u>
  M12.371 Palindromic rheumatism, <u>right</u> ankle and foot
  M12.372 Palindromic rheumatism, <u>left</u> ankle and foot
  M12.379 Palindromic rheumatism, <u>unspecified</u> ankle and foot
M12.38 Palindromic rheumatism, <u>other specified site</u>
  Palindromic rheumatism, vertebrae
M12.39 Palindromic rheumatism, <u>multiple sites</u>
M12.4- <u>Intermittent hydrarthrosis</u>
M12.40 Intermittent hydrarthrosis, <u>unspecified</u> site
M12.41-Intermittent hydrarthrosis, <u>shoulder</u>
  M12.411 Intermittent hydrarthrosis, <u>right</u> shoulder
  M12.412 Intermittent hydrarthrosis, <u>left</u> shoulder
  M12.419 Intermittent hydrarthrosis, <u>unspecified</u> shoulder
M12.42-Intermittent hydrarthrosis, <u>elbow</u>
  M12.421 Intermittent hydrarthrosis, <u>right</u> elbow
  M12.422 Intermittent hydrarthrosis, <u>left</u> elbow
  M12.429 Intermittent hydrarthrosis, <u>unspecified</u> elbow
M12.43-Intermittent hydrarthrosis, <u>wrist</u>
  M12.431 Intermittent hydrarthrosis, <u>right</u> wrist
  M12.432 Intermittent hydrarthrosis, <u>left</u> wrist
  M12.439 Intermittent hydrarthrosis, <u>unspecified</u> wrist
M12.44-Intermittent hydrarthrosis, <u>hand</u>
  M12.441 Intermittent hydrarthrosis, <u>right</u> hand
  M12.442 Intermittent hydrarthrosis, <u>left</u> hand
  M12.449 Intermittent hydrarthrosis, <u>unspecified</u> hand
M12.45-Intermittent hydrarthrosis, <u>hip</u>
  M12.451 Intermittent hydrarthrosis, <u>right</u> hip
  M12.452 Intermittent hydrarthrosis, <u>left</u> hip
  M12.459 Intermittent hydrarthrosis, <u>unspecified</u> hip
M12.46-Intermittent hydrarthrosis, <u>knee</u>
  M12.461 Intermittent hydrarthrosis, <u>right</u> knee
  M12.462 Intermittent hydrarthrosis, <u>left</u> knee
  M12.469 Intermittent hydrarthrosis, <u>unspecified</u> knee
M12.47-Intermittent hydrarthrosis, <u>ankle and foot</u>
  M12.471 Intermittent hydrarthrosis, <u>right</u> ankle and foot
  M12.472 Intermittent hydrarthrosis, <u>left</u> ankle and foot
  M12.479 Intermittent hydrarthrosis, <u>unspecified</u> ankle and foot
M12.48 Intermittent hydrarthrosis, <u>other site</u>
M12.49 Intermittent hydrarthrosis, <u>multiple sites</u>
M12.5- <u>Traumatic arthropathy</u>
  Excludes 1: current injury — see Alphabetic Index
    post-traumatic osteoarthritis of first carpometacarpal joint (M18.2-M18.3)
    post-traumatic osteoarthritis of hip (M16.4-M16.5)
    post-traumatic osteoarthritis of knee (M17.2-M17.3)
    post-traumatic osteoarthritis NOS (M19.1-)
    post-traumatic osteoarthritis of other single joints (M19.1-)
M12.50 Traumatic arthropathy, <u>unspecified</u> site
M12.51-Traumatic arthropathy, <u>shoulder</u>
  M12.511 Traumatic arthropathy, <u>right</u> shoulder
  M12.512 Traumatic arthropathy, <u>left</u> shoulder
  M12.519 Traumatic arthropathy, <u>unspecified</u> shoulder
M12.52-Traumatic arthropathy, <u>elbow</u>
  M12.521 Traumatic arthropathy, <u>right</u> elbow
  M12.522 Traumatic arthropathy, <u>left</u> elbow
  M12.529 Traumatic arthropathy, <u>unspecified</u> elbow
M12.53-Traumatic arthropathy, <u>wrist</u>
  M12.531 Traumatic arthropathy, <u>right</u> wrist
  M12.532 Traumatic arthropathy, <u>left</u> wrist
  M12.539 Traumatic arthropathy, <u>unspecified</u> wrist
M12.54-Traumatic arthropathy, <u>hand</u>
  M12.541 Traumatic arthropathy, <u>right</u> hand
  M12.542 Traumatic arthropathy, <u>left</u> hand
  M12.549 Traumatic arthropathy, <u>unspecified</u> hand
M12.55-Traumatic arthropathy, <u>hip</u>
  M12.551 Traumatic arthropathy, <u>right</u> hip
  M12.552 Traumatic arthropathy, <u>left</u> hip
  M12.559 Traumatic arthropathy, <u>unspecified</u> hip

M 1 1 – M 1 2

M12.56-Traumatic arthropathy, <u>knee</u>
   M12.561 Traumatic arthropathy, <u>right</u> knee
   M12.562 Traumatic arthropathy, <u>left</u> knee
   M12.569 Traumatic arthropathy, <u>unspecified</u> knee
M12.57-Traumatic arthropathy, <u>ankle and foot</u>
   M12.571 Traumatic arthropathy, <u>right</u> ankle and foot
   M12.572 Traumatic arthropathy, <u>left</u> ankle and foot
   M12.579 Traumatic arthropathy, <u>unspecified</u> ankle and foot
M12.58 Traumatic arthropathy, <u>other specified site</u>
    Traumatic arthropathy, vertebrae
M12.59 Traumatic arthropathy, <u>multiple sites</u>
M12.8- <u>Other specific arthropathies</u>, <u>not elsewhere classified</u>
    Transient arthropathy
M12.80 Other specific arthropathies, not elsewhere classified, <u>unspecified</u> site
M12.81-Other specific arthropathies, not elsewhere classified, <u>shoulder</u>
   M12.811 Other specific arthropathies, not elsewhere classified, <u>right</u> shoulder
   M12.812 Other specific arthropathies, not elsewhere classified, <u>left</u> shoulder
   M12.819 Other specific arthropathies, not elsewhere classified, <u>unspecified</u> shoulder
M12.82-Other specific arthropathies, not elsewhere classified, <u>elbow</u>
   M12.821 Other specific arthropathies, not elsewhere classified, <u>right</u> elbow
   M12.822 Other specific arthropathies, not elsewhere classified, <u>left</u> elbow
   M12.829 Other specific arthropathies, not elsewhere classified, <u>unspecified</u> elbow
M12.83-Other specific arthropathies, not elsewhere classified, <u>wrist</u>
   M12.831 Other specific arthropathies, not elsewhere classified, <u>right</u> wrist
   M12.832 Other specific arthropathies, not elsewhere classified, <u>left</u> wrist
   M12.839 Other specific arthropathies, not elsewhere classified, <u>unspecified</u> wrist
M12.84-Other specific arthropathies, not elsewhere classified, <u>hand</u>
   M12.841 Other specific arthropathies, not elsewhere classified, <u>right</u> hand
   M12.842 Other specific arthropathies, not elsewhere classified, <u>left</u> hand
   M12.849 Other specific arthropathies, not elsewhere classified, <u>unspecified</u> hand
M12.85-Other specific arthropathies, not elsewhere classified, <u>hip</u>
   M12.851 Other specific arthropathies, not elsewhere classified, <u>right</u> hip
   M12.852 Other specific arthropathies, not elsewhere classified, <u>left</u> hip
   M12.859 Other specific arthropathies, not elsewhere classified, <u>unspecified</u> hip
M12.86-Other specific arthropathies, not elsewhere classified, <u>knee</u>
   M12.861 Other specific arthropathies, not elsewhere classified, <u>right</u> knee
   M12.862 Other specific arthropathies, not elsewhere classified, <u>left</u> knee
   M12.869 Other specific arthropathies, not elsewhere classified, <u>unspecified</u> knee
M12.87-Other specific arthropathies, not elsewhere classified, <u>ankle and foot</u>
   M12.871 Other specific arthropathies, not elsewhere classified, <u>right</u> ankle and foot
   M12.872 Other specific arthropathies, not elsewhere classified, <u>left</u> ankle and foot
   M12.879 Other specific arthropathies, not elsewhere classified, <u>unspecified</u> ankle and foot
M12.88 Other specific arthropathies, not elsewhere classified, <u>other specified site</u>
    Other specific arthropathies, not elsewhere classified, vertebrae
M12.89 Other specific arthropathies, not elsewhere classified, <u>multiple sites</u>
M12.9 Arthropathy, <u>unspecified</u>

M13- <u>Other arthritis</u>
   Excludes 1: *arthrosis (M15-M19)*
            osteoarthritis (M15-M19)
M13.0 <u>Polyarthritis</u>, <u>unspecified</u>
M13.1- <u>Monoarthritis</u>, <u>not elsewhere classified</u>
  M13.10 Monoarthritis, not elsewhere classified, <u>unspecified</u> site
  M13.11-Monoarthritis, not elsewhere classified, <u>shoulder</u>
    M13.111 Monoarthritis, not elsewhere classified, <u>right</u> shoulder
    M13.112 Monoarthritis, not elsewhere classified, <u>left</u> shoulder
    M13.119 Monoarthritis, not elsewhere classified, <u>unspecified</u> shoulder
  M13.12-Monoarthritis, not elsewhere classified, <u>elbow</u>
    M13.121 Monoarthritis, not elsewhere classified, <u>right</u> elbow
    M13.122 Monoarthritis, not elsewhere classified, <u>left</u> elbow
    M13.129 Monoarthritis, not elsewhere classified, <u>unspecified</u> elbow
  M13.13-Monoarthritis, not elsewhere classified, <u>wrist</u>
    M13.131 Monoarthritis, not elsewhere classified, <u>right</u> wrist
    M13.132 Monoarthritis, not elsewhere classified, <u>left</u> wrist
    M13.139 Monoarthritis, not elsewhere classified, <u>unspecified</u> wrist
  M13.14-Monoarthritis, not elsewhere classified, <u>hand</u>
    M13.141 Monoarthritis, not elsewhere classified, <u>right</u> hand
    M13.142 Monoarthritis, not elsewhere classified, <u>left</u> hand
    M13.149 Monoarthritis, not elsewhere classified, <u>unspecified</u> hand
  M13.15-Monoarthritis, not elsewhere classified, <u>hip</u>
    M13.151 Monoarthritis, not elsewhere classified, <u>right</u> hip
    M13.152 Monoarthritis, not elsewhere classified, <u>left</u> hip
    M13.159 Monoarthritis, not elsewhere classified, <u>unspecified</u> hip
  M13.16-Monoarthritis, not elsewhere classified, <u>knee</u>
    M13.161 Monoarthritis, not elsewhere classified, <u>right</u> knee
    M13.162 Monoarthritis, not elsewhere classified, <u>left</u> knee
    M13.169 Monoarthritis, not elsewhere classified, <u>unspecified</u> knee
  M13.17-Monoarthritis, not elsewhere classified, <u>ankle and foot</u>
    M13.171 Monoarthritis, not elsewhere classified, <u>right</u> ankle and foot
    M13.172 Monoarthritis, not elsewhere classified, <u>left</u> ankle and foot
    M13.179 Monoarthritis, not elsewhere classified, <u>unspecified</u> ankle and foot
M13.8- <u>Other specified arthritis</u>
    Allergic arthritis
   Excludes 1: osteoarthritis (M15-M19)
M13.80 Other specified arthritis, <u>unspecified</u> site
M13.81-Other specified arthritis, <u>shoulder</u>
   M13.811 Other specified arthritis, <u>right</u> shoulder
   M13.812 Other specified arthritis, <u>left</u> shoulder
   M13.819 Other specified arthritis, <u>unspecified</u> shoulder
M13.82-Other specified arthritis, <u>elbow</u>
   M13.821 Other specified arthritis, <u>right</u> elbow
   M13.822 Other specified arthritis, <u>left</u> elbow
   M13.829 Other specified arthritis, <u>unspecified</u> elbow
M13.83-Other specified arthritis, <u>wrist</u>
   M13.831 Other specified arthritis, <u>right</u> wrist
   M13.832 Other specified arthritis, <u>left</u> wrist
   M13.839 Other specified arthritis, <u>unspecified</u> wrist
M13.84-Other specified arthritis, <u>hand</u>
   M13.841 Other specified arthritis, <u>right</u> hand
   M13.842 Other specified arthritis, <u>left</u> hand
   M13.849 Other specified arthritis, <u>unspecified</u> hand
M13.85-Other specified arthritis, <u>hip</u>
   M13.851 Other specified arthritis, <u>right</u> hip
   M13.852 Other specified arthritis, <u>left</u> hip
   M13.859 Other specified arthritis, <u>unspecified</u> hip
M13.86-Other specified arthritis, <u>knee</u>
   M13.861 Other specified arthritis, <u>right</u> knee
   M13.862 Other specified arthritis, <u>left</u> knee
   M13.869 Other specified arthritis, <u>unspecified</u> knee
M13.87-Other specified arthritis, <u>ankle and foot</u>
   M13.871 Other specified arthritis, <u>right</u> ankle and foot
   M13.872 Other specified arthritis, <u>left</u> ankle and foot
   M13.879 Other specified arthritis, <u>unspecified</u> ankle and foot

M12 - M16

M13.88 Other specified arthritis, <u>other site</u>

M13.89 Other specified arthritis, <u>multiple sites</u>

M14- Arthropathies <u>in other diseases classified elsewhere</u>

  Excludes 1: arthropathy in:
      diabetes mellitus (E08-E13 with .61-)
      hematological disorders (M36.2-M36.3)
      hypersensitivity reactions (M36.4)
      neoplastic disease (M36.1)
      neurosyphillis (A52.16)
      sarcoidosis (D86.86)
      enteropathic arthropathies (M07.-)
      juvenile psoriatic arthropathy (L40.54)
      lipoid dermatoarthritis (E78.81)

M14.6- <u>Charcôt's joint</u>
  Neuropathic arthropathy
  Excludes 1: Charcôt's joint in diabetes mellitus (E08-E13 with .610)
      Charcôt's joint in tabes dorsalis (A52.16)

M14.60 Charcôt's joint, <u>unspecified</u> site

M14.61- Charcôt's joint, <u>shoulder</u>

  M14.611 Charcôt's joint, <u>right</u> shoulder

  M14.612 Charcôt's joint, <u>left</u> shoulder

  M14.619 Charcôt's joint, <u>unspecified</u> shoulder

M14.62- Charcôt's joint, <u>elbow</u>

  M14.621 Charcôt's joint, <u>right</u> elbow

  M14.622 Charcôt's joint, <u>left</u> elbow

  M14.629 Charcôt's joint, <u>unspecified</u> elbow

M14.63- Charcôt's joint, <u>wrist</u>

  M14.631 Charcôt's joint, <u>right</u> wrist

  M14.632 Charcôt's joint, <u>left</u> wrist

  M14.639 Charcôt's joint, <u>unspecified</u> wrist

M14.64- Charcôt's joint, <u>hand</u>

  M14.641 Charcôt's joint, <u>right</u> hand

  M14.642 Charcôt's joint, <u>left</u> hand

  M14.649 Charcôt's joint, <u>unspecified</u> hand

M14.65- Charcôt's joint, <u>hip</u>

  M14.651 Charcôt's joint, <u>right</u> hip

  M14.652 Charcôt's joint, <u>left</u> hip

  M14.659 Charcôt's joint, <u>unspecified</u> hip

M14.66- Charcôt's joint, <u>knee</u>

  M14.661 Charcôt's joint, <u>right</u> knee

  M14.662 Charcôt's joint, <u>left</u> knee

  M14.669 Charcôt's joint, <u>unspecified</u> knee

M14.67- Charcôt's joint, <u>ankle and foot</u>

  M14.671 Charcôt's joint, <u>right</u> ankle and foot

  M14.672 Charcôt's joint, <u>left</u> ankle and foot

  M14.679 Charcôt's joint, <u>unspecified</u> ankle and foot

M14.68 Charcôt's joint, <u>vertebrae</u>

M14.69 Charcôt's joint, <u>multiple sites</u>

M14.8- Arthropathies <u>in other specified diseases classified elsewhere</u>
  Code first underlying disease, such as:
    Amyloidosis (E85.-)
    Erythema multiforme (L51-)
    Erythema nodosum (L52)
    Hemochromatosis (E83.11-)
    Hyperparathyroidism (E21-)
    Hypothyroidism (E00-E03)
    Sickle-cell disorders (D57-)
    Thyrotoxicosis [hyperthyroidism] (E05-)
    Whipple's disease (K90.81)

M14.80 Arthropathies in other specified diseases classified elsewhere, <u>unspecified</u> site

M14.81- Arthropathies in other specified diseases classified elsewhere, <u>shoulder</u>

  M14.811 Arthropathies in other specified diseases classified elsewhere, <u>right</u> shoulder

  M14.812 Arthropathies in other specified diseases classified elsewhere, <u>left</u> shoulder

  M14.819 Arthropathies in other specified diseases classified elsewhere, <u>unspecified</u> shoulder

M14.82- Arthropathies in other specified diseases classified elsewhere, <u>elbow</u>

  M14.821 Arthropathies in other specified diseases classified elsewhere, <u>right</u> elbow

  M14.822 Arthropathies in other specified diseases classified elsewhere, <u>left</u> elbow

  M14.829 Arthropathies in other specified diseases classified elsewhere, <u>unspecified</u> elbow

M14.83- Arthropathies in other specified diseases classified elsewhere, <u>wrist</u>

  M14.831 Arthropathies in other specified diseases classified elsewhere, <u>right</u> wrist

  M14.832 Arthropathies in other specified diseases classified elsewhere, <u>left</u> wrist

  M14.839 Arthropathies in other specified diseases classified elsewhere, <u>unspecified</u> wrist

M14.84- Arthropathies in other specified diseases classified elsewhere, <u>hand</u>

  M14.841 Arthropathies in other specified diseases classified elsewhere, <u>right</u> hand

  M14.842 Arthropathies in other specified diseases classified elsewhere, <u>left</u> hand

  M14.849 Arthropathies in other specified diseases classified elsewhere, <u>unspecified</u> hand

M14.85- Arthropathies in other specified diseases classified elsewhere, <u>hip</u>

  M14.851 Arthropathies in other specified diseases classified elsewhere, <u>right</u> hip

  M14.852 Arthropathies in other specified diseases classified elsewhere, <u>left</u> hip

  M14.859 Arthropathies in other specified diseases classified elsewhere, <u>unspecified</u> hip

M14.86- Arthropathies in other specified diseases classified elsewhere, <u>knee</u>

  M14.861 Arthropathies in other specified diseases classified elsewhere, <u>right</u> knee

  M14.862 Arthropathies in other specified diseases classified elsewhere, <u>left</u> knee

  M14.869 Arthropathies in other specified diseases classified elsewhere, <u>unspecified</u> knee

M14.87- Arthropathies in other specified diseases classified elsewhere, <u>ankle and foot</u>

  M14.871 Arthropathies in other specified diseases classified elsewhere, <u>right</u> ankle and foot

  M14.872 Arthropathies in other specified diseases classified elsewhere, <u>left</u> ankle and foot

  M14.879 Arthropathies in other specified diseases classified elsewhere, <u>unspecified</u> ankle and foot

M14.88 Arthropathies in other specified diseases classified elsewhere, <u>vertebrae</u>

M14.89 Arthropathies in other specified diseases classified elsewhere, <u>multiple sites</u>

Osteoarthritis (M15-M19)

Excludes❷: osteoarthritis of spine (M47.-)

M15- <u>Polyosteoarthritis</u>
  Includes: arthritis of multiple sites
  Excludes 1: bilateral involvement of single joint (M16-M19)

M15.0 Primary generalized (osteo)arthritis

M15.1 Heberden's nodes (with arthropathy)
  Interphalangeal distal osteoarthritis

M15.2 Bouchard's nodes (with arthropathy)
  Juxtaphalangeal distal osteoarthritis

M15.3 Secondary multiple arthritis
  Post-traumatic polyosteoarthritis

M15.4 Erosive (osteo)arthritis

M15.8 Other polyosteoarthritis

M15.9 Polyosteoarthritis, <u>unspecified</u>
  Generalized osteoarthritis NOS

M16- Osteoarthritis <u>of hip</u>

M16.0 <u>Bilateral primary</u> osteoarthritis of hip

M16.1- <u>Unilateral primary</u> osteoarthritis of hip
  Primary osteoarthritis of hip NOS

  M16.10 Unilateral primary osteoarthritis, <u>unspecified</u> hip

  M16.11 Unilateral primary osteoarthritis, <u>right</u> hip

  M16.12 Unilateral primary osteoarthritis, <u>left</u> hip

M16.2 <u>Bilateral</u> osteoarthritis <u>resulting from hip dysplasia</u>

M16.3- <u>Unilateral</u> osteoarthritis <u>resulting from hip dysplasia</u>
  Dysplastic osteoarthritis of hip NOS

  M16.30 Unilateral osteoarthritis resulting from hip dysplasia, <u>unspecified</u> hip

  M16.31 Unilateral osteoarthritis resulting from hip dysplasia, <u>right</u> hip

  M16.32 Unilateral osteoarthritis resulting from hip dysplasia, <u>left</u> hip

M16.4 <u>Bilateral post-traumatic</u> osteoarthritis of hip

M12-M16

M16.5- **Unilateral** **post-traumatic** osteoarthritis of hip
    Post-traumatic osteoarthritis of hip NOS
  M16.50 Unilateral post-traumatic osteoarthritis, **unspecified** hip
  M16.51 Unilateral post-traumatic osteoarthritis, **right** hip
  M16.52 Unilateral post-traumatic osteoarthritis, **left** hip
M16.6 **Other** **bilateral** secondary osteoarthritis of hip
M16.7 **Other** **unilateral** secondary osteoarthritis of hip
    Secondary osteoarthritis of hip NOS
M16.9 Osteoarthritis of hip, **unspecified**

M17- **Osteoarthritis** of **knee**
M17.0 **Bilateral** **primary** osteoarthritis of knee
M17.1- **Unilateral** **primary** osteoarthritis of knee
    Primary osteoarthritis of knee NOS
  M17.10 Unilateral primary osteoarthritis, **unspecified** knee
  M17.11 Unilateral primary osteoarthritis, **right** knee
  M17.12 Unilateral primary osteoarthritis, **left** knee
M17.2 **Bilateral** **post-traumatic** osteoarthritis of knee
M17.3- **Unilateral** **post-traumatic** osteoarthritis of knee
    Post-traumatic osteoarthritis of knee NOS
  M17.30 Unilateral post-traumatic osteoarthritis, **unspecified** knee
  M17.31 Unilateral post-traumatic osteoarthritis, **right** knee
  M17.32 Unilateral post-traumatic osteoarthritis, **left** knee
M17.4 **Other** **bilateral** secondary osteoarthritis of knee
M17.5 **Other** **unilateral** secondary osteoarthritis of knee
    Secondary osteoarthritis of knee NOS
M17.9 Osteoarthritis of knee, **unspecified**

M18- **Osteoarthritis** of **first carpometacarpal** joint
M18.0 **Bilateral** **primary** osteoarthritis of first carpometacarpal joints
M18.1- **Unilateral** **primary** osteoarthritis of first carpometacarpal joint
    Primary osteoarthritis of first carpometacarpal joint NOS
  M18.10 Unilateral primary osteoarthritis of first carpometacarpal joint, **unspecified** hand
  M18.11 Unilateral primary osteoarthritis of first carpometacarpal joint, **right** hand
  M18.12 Unilateral primary osteoarthritis of first carpometacarpal joint, **left** hand
M18.2 **Bilateral** **post-traumatic** osteoarthritis of first carpometacarpal joints
M18.3- **Unilateral** **post-traumatic** osteoarthritis of first carpometacarpal joint
    Post-traumatic osteoarthritis of first carpometacarpal joint NOS
  M18.30 Unilateral post-traumatic osteoarthritis of first carpometacarpal joint, **unspecified** hand
  M18.31 Unilateral post-traumatic osteoarthritis of first carpometacarpal joint, **right** hand
  M18.32 Unilateral post-traumatic osteoarthritis of first carpometacarpal joint, **left** hand
M18.4 **Other** **bilateral** secondary osteoarthritis of first carpometacarpal joints
M18.5- **Other** **unilateral** secondary osteoarthritis of first carpometacarpal joint
    Secondary osteoarthritis of first carpometacarpal joint NOS
  M18.50 Other unilateral secondary osteoarthritis of first carpometacarpal joint, **unspecified** hand
  M18.51 Other unilateral secondary osteoarthritis of first carpometacarpal joint, **right** hand
  M18.52 Other unilateral secondary osteoarthritis of first carpometacarpal joint, **left** hand
M18.9 Osteoarthritis of first carpometacarpal joint, **unspecified**

M19 **Other and unspecified** osteoarthritis
    Excludes 1: polyarthritis (M15.-)
    Excludes❷: arthrosis of spine (M47.-)
              hallux rigidus (M20.2)
              osteoarthritis of spine (M47.-)
M19.0- **Primary** osteoarthritis of other joints
  M19.01-Primary osteoarthritis, **shoulder**
    M19.011 Primary osteoarthritis, **right** shoulder
    M19.012 Primary osteoarthritis, **left** shoulder
    M19.019 Primary osteoarthritis, **unspecified** shoulder
  M19.02-Primary osteoarthritis, **elbow**
    M19.021 Primary osteoarthritis, **right** elbow
    M19.022 Primary osteoarthritis, **left** elbow
    M19.029 Primary osteoarthritis, **unspecified** elbow
  M19.03-Primary osteoarthritis, **wrist**
    M19.031 Primary osteoarthritis, **right** wrist
    M19.032 Primary osteoarthritis, **left** wrist
    M19.039 Primary osteoarthritis, **unspecified** wrist

M19.04-Primary osteoarthritis, **hand**
    Excludes❷: primary osteoarthritis of first carpometacarpal joint (M18.0-, M18.1-)
    M19.041 Primary osteoarthritis, **right** hand
    M19.042 Primary osteoarthritis, **left** hand
    M19.049 Primary osteoarthritis, **unspecified** hand
  M19.07-Primary osteoarthritis **ankle and foot**
    M19.071 Primary osteoarthritis, **right** ankle and foot
    M19.072 Primary osteoarthritis, **left** ankle and foot
    M19.079 Primary osteoarthritis, **unspecified** ankle and foot
M19.1- **Post-traumatic** osteoarthritis of other joints
  M19.11-Post-traumatic osteoarthritis, **shoulder**
    M19.111 Post-traumatic osteoarthritis, **right** shoulder
    M19.112 Post-traumatic osteoarthritis, **left** shoulder
    M19.119 Post-traumatic osteoarthritis, **unspecified** shoulder
  M19.12-Post-traumatic osteoarthritis, **elbow**
    M19.121 Post-traumatic osteoarthritis, **right** elbow
    M19.122 Post-traumatic osteoarthritis, **left** elbow
    M19.129 Post-traumatic osteoarthritis, **unspecified** elbow
  M19.13-Post-traumatic osteoarthritis, **wrist**
    M19.131 Post-traumatic osteoarthritis, **right** wrist
    M19.132 Post-traumatic osteoarthritis, **left** wrist
    M19.139 Post-traumatic osteoarthritis, **unspecified** wrist
  M19.14-Post-traumatic osteoarthritis, **hand**
    Excludes❷: post-traumatic osteoarthritis of first carpometacarpal joint (M18.2-, M18.3-)
    M19.141 Post-traumatic osteoarthritis, **right** hand
    M19.142 Post-traumatic osteoarthritis, **left** hand
    M19.149 Post-traumatic osteoarthritis, **unspecified** hand
  M19.17-Post-traumatic osteoarthritis, **ankle and foot**
    M19.171 Post-traumatic osteoarthritis, **right** ankle and foot
    M19.172 Post-traumatic osteoarthritis, **left** ankle and foot
    M19.179 Post-traumatic osteoarthritis, **unspecified** ankle and foot
M19.2- **Secondary** osteoarthritis of other joints
  M19.21-Secondary osteoarthritis, **shoulder**
    M19.211 Secondary osteoarthritis, **right** shoulder
    M19.212 Secondary osteoarthritis, **left** shoulder
    M19.219 Secondary osteoarthritis, **unspecified** shoulder
  M19.22-Secondary osteoarthritis, **elbow**
    M19.221 Secondary osteoarthritis, **right** elbow
    M19.222 Secondary osteoarthritis, **left** elbow
    M19.229 Secondary osteoarthritis, **unspecified** elbow
  M19.23-Secondary osteoarthritis, **wrist**
    M19.231 Secondary osteoarthritis, **right** wrist
    M19.232 Secondary osteoarthritis, **left** wrist
    M19.239 Secondary osteoarthritis, **unspecified** wrist
  M19.24-Secondary osteoarthritis, **hand**
    M19.241 Secondary osteoarthritis, **right** hand
    M19.242 Secondary osteoarthritis, **left** hand
    M19.249 Secondary osteoarthritis, **unspecified** hand
  M19.27-Secondary osteoarthritis, **ankle and foot**
    M19.271 Secondary osteoarthritis, **right** ankle and foot
    M19.272 Secondary osteoarthritis, **left** ankle and foot
    M19.279 Secondary osteoarthritis, **unspecified** ankle and foot
M19.9- **Osteoarthritis, unspecified site**
  M19.90 **Unspecified** osteoarthritis, unspecified site
    Arthrosis NOS
    Arthritis NOS
    Osteoarthritis NOS
  M19.91 **Primary** osteoarthritis, unspecified site
    Primary osteoarthritis NOS
  M19.92 **Post-traumatic** osteoarthritis, unspecified site
    Post-traumatic osteoarthritis NOS
  M19.93 **Secondary** osteoarthritis, unspecified site
    Secondary osteoarthritis NOS

M 1 6 - M 2 1 *(side tab)*

Other joint disorders (M20-M25)

Excludes❷: joints of the spine (M40-M54)

M20- Acquired deformities of fingers and toes
    Excludes 1: acquired absence of fingers and toes (Z89.-)
    congenital absence of fingers and toes (Q71.3-, Q72.3-)
    congenital deformities and malformations of fingers and toes
    (Q66.-, Q68-Q70, Q74.-)

  M20.0- Deformity of finger(s)
    Excludes 1: clubbing of fingers (R68.3)
    palmar fascial fibromatosis [Dupuytren] (M72.0)
    trigger finger (M65.3)

    M20.00- Unspecified deformity of finger(s)
      M20.001 Unspecified deformity of right finger(s)
      M20.002 Unspecified deformity of left finger(s)
      M20.009 Unspecified deformity of unspecified finger(s)

    M20.01- Mallet finger
      M20.011 Mallet finger of right finger(s)
      M20.012 Mallet finger of left finger(s)
      M20.019 Mallet finger of unspecified finger(s)

    M20.02- Boutonnière deformity
      M20.021 Boutonnière deformity of right finger(s)
      M20.022 Boutonnière deformity of left finger(s)
      M20.029 Boutonnière deformity of unspecified finger(s)

    M20.03- Swan-neck deformity
      M20.031 Swan-neck deformity of right finger(s)
      M20.032 Swan-neck deformity of left finger(s)
      M20.039 Swan-neck deformity of unspecified finger(s)

    M20.09- Other deformity of finger(s)
      M20.091 Other deformity of right finger(s)
      M20.092 Other deformity of left finger(s)
      M20.099 Other deformity of finger(s), unspecified finger(s)

  M20.1- Hallux valgus (acquired)
    Bunion
    M20.10 Hallux valgus (acquired), unspecified foot
    M20.11 Hallux valgus (acquired), right foot
    M20.12 Hallux valgus (acquired), left foot

  M20.2- Hallux rigidus
    M20.20 Hallux rigidus, unspecified foot
    M20.21 Hallux rigidus, right foot
    M20.22 Hallux rigidus, left foot

  M20.3- Hallux varus (acquired)
    M20.30 Hallux varus (acquired), unspecified foot
    M20.31 Hallux varus (acquired), right foot
    M20.32 Hallux varus (acquired), left foot

  M20.4- Other hammer toe(s) (acquired)
    M20.40 Other hammer toe(s) (acquired), unspecified foot
    M20.41 Other hammer toe(s) (acquired), right foot
    M20.42 Other hammer toe(s) (acquired), left foot

  M20.5- Other deformities of toe(s) (acquired)
    M20.5x- Other deformities of toe(s) (acquired)
      M20.5x1 Other deformities of toe(s) (acquired), right foot
      M20.5x2 Other deformities of toe(s) (acquired), left foot
      M20.5x9 Other deformities of toe(s) (acquired), unspecified foot

  M20.6- Acquired deformities of toe(s), unspecified
    M20.60 Acquired deformities of toe(s), unspecified, unspecified foot
    M20.61 Acquired deformities of toe(s), unspecified, right foot
    M20.62 Acquired deformities of toe(s), unspecified, left foot

M21- Other acquired deformities of limbs
    Excludes 1: acquired absence of limb (Z89.-)
    congenital absence of limbs (Q71-Q73)
    congenital deformities and malformations of limbs (Q65-Q66,
    Q68-Q74)
    Excludes❷: acquired deformities of fingers or toes (M20.-)
    coxa plana (M91.2)

  M21.0- Valgus deformity, not elsewhere classified
    Excludes 1: metatarsus valgus (Q66.6)
    talipes calcaneovalgus (Q66.4)
    M21.00 Valgus deformity, not elsewhere classified, unspecified site
    M21.02- Valgus deformity, not elsewhere classified, elbow
      Cubitus valgus
      M21.021 Valgus deformity, not elsewhere classified, right elbow
      M21.022 Valgus deformity, not elsewhere classified, left elbow
      M21.029 Valgus deformity, not elsewhere classified, unspecified elbow

    M21.05- Valgus deformity, not elsewhere classified, hip
      M21.051 Valgus deformity, not elsewhere classified, right hip
      M21.052 Valgus deformity, not elsewhere classified, left hip
      M21.059 Valgus deformity, not elsewhere classified, unspecified hip

    M21.06- Valgus deformity, not elsewhere classified, knee
      Genu valgum
      Knock knee
      M21.061 Valgus deformity, not elsewhere classified, right knee
      M21.062 Valgus deformity, not elsewhere classified, left knee
      M21.069 Valgus deformity, not elsewhere classified, unspecified knee

    M21.07- Valgus deformity, not elsewhere classified, ankle
      M21.071 Valgus deformity, not elsewhere classified, right ankle
      M21.072 Valgus deformity, not elsewhere classified, left ankle
      M21.079 Valgus deformity, not elsewhere classified, unspecified ankle

  M21.1- Varus deformity, not elsewhere classified
    Excludes 1: metatarsus varus (Q66.2)
    tibia vara (M92.5)
    M21.10 Varus deformity, not elsewhere classified, unspecified site
    M21.12- Varus deformity, not elsewhere classified, elbow
      Cubitus varus, elbow
      M21.121 Varus deformity, not elsewhere classified, right elbow
      M21.122 Varus deformity, not elsewhere classified, left elbow
      M21.129 Varus deformity, not elsewhere classified, unspecified elbow

    M21.15- Varus deformity, not elsewhere classified, hip
      M21.151 Varus deformity, not elsewhere classified, right hip
      M21.152 Varus deformity, not elsewhere classified, left hip
      M21.159 Varus deformity, not elsewhere classified, unspecified hip

    M21.16- Varus deformity, not elsewhere classified, knee
      Bow leg
      Genu varum
      M21.161 Varus deformity, not elsewhere classified, right knee
      M21.162 Varus deformity, not elsewhere classified, left knee
      M21.169 Varus deformity, not elsewhere classified, unspecified knee

    M21.17- Varus deformity, not elsewhere classified, ankle
      M21.171 Varus deformity, not elsewhere classified, right ankle
      M21.172 Varus deformity, not elsewhere classified, left ankle
      M21.179 Varus deformity, not elsewhere classified, unspecified ankle

  M21.2- Flexion deformity
    M21.20 Flexion deformity, unspecified site
    M21.21- Flexion deformity, shoulder
      M21.211 Flexion deformity, right shoulder
      M21.212 Flexion deformity, left shoulder
      M21.219 Flexion deformity, unspecified shoulder
    M21.22- Flexion deformity, elbow
      M21.221 Flexion deformity, right elbow
      M21.222 Flexion deformity, left elbow
      M21.229 Flexion deformity, unspecified elbow
    M21.23- Flexion deformity, wrist
      M21.231 Flexion deformity, right wrist
      M21.232 Flexion deformity, left wrist
      M21.239 Flexion deformity, unspecified wrist
    M21.24- Flexion deformity, finger joints
      M21.241 Flexion deformity, right finger joints
      M21.242 Flexion deformity, left finger joints
      M21.249 Flexion deformity, unspecified finger joints
    M21.25- Flexion deformity, hip
      M21.251 Flexion deformity, right hip
      M21.252 Flexion deformity, left hip
      M21.259 Flexion deformity, unspecified hip
    M21.26- Flexion deformity, knee
      M21.261 Flexion deformity, right knee
      M21.262 Flexion deformity, left knee
      M21.269 Flexion deformity, unspecified knee
    M21.27- Flexion deformity, ankle and toes
      M21.271 Flexion deformity, right ankle and toes
      M21.272 Flexion deformity, left ankle and toes
      M21.279 Flexion deformity, unspecified ankle and toes

M 16 - M 21

M21.3- Wrist or foot drop (acquired)
  M21.33-Wrist drop (acquired)
    M21.331 Wrist drop, right wrist
    M21.332 Wrist drop, left wrist
    M21.339 Wrist drop, unspecified wrist
  M21.37-Foot drop (acquired)
    M21.371 Foot drop, right foot
    M21.372 Foot drop, left foot
    M21.379 Foot drop, unspecified foot
M21.4- Flat foot [pes planus] (acquired)
    Excludes 1: congenital pes planus (Q66.5-)
  M21.40 Flat foot [pes planus] (acquired), unspecified foot
  M21.41 Flat foot [pes planus] (acquired), right foot
  M21.42 Flat foot [pes planus] (acquired), left foot
M21.5- Acquired clawhand, clubhand, clawfoot and clubfoot
    Excludes 1: clubfoot, not specified as acquired (Q66.89)
  M21.51-Acquired clawhand
    M21.511 Acquired clawhand, right hand
    M21.512 Acquired clawhand, left hand
    M21.519 Acquired clawhand, unspecified hand
  M21.52-Acquired clubhand
    M21.521 Acquired clubhand, right hand
    M21.522 Acquired clubhand, left hand
    M21.529 Acquired clubhand, unspecified hand
  M21.53-Acquired clawfoot
    M21.531 Acquired clawfoot, right foot
    M21.532 Acquired clawfoot, left foot
    M21.539 Acquired clawfoot, unspecified foot
  M21.54-Acquired clubfoot
    M21.541 Acquired clubfoot, right foot
    M21.542 Acquired clubfoot, left foot
    M21.549 Acquired clubfoot, unspecified foot
M21.6- Other acquired deformities of foot
    Excludes❷: deformities of toe (acquired) (M20.1-M20.6)
  M21.6x-Other acquired deformities of foot
    M21.6x1 Other acquired deformities of right foot
    M21.6x2 Other acquired deformities of left foot
    M21.6x9 Other acquired deformities of unspecified foot
M21.7- Unequal limb length (acquired)
    Note: The site used should correspond to the shorter limb
  M21.70 Unequal limb length (acquired), unspecified site
  M21.72-Unequal limb length (acquired), humerus
    M21.721 Unequal limb length (acquired), right humerus
    M21.722 Unequal limb length (acquired), left humerus
    M21.729 Unequal limb length (acquired), unspecified humerus
  M21.73-Unequal limb length (acquired), ulna and radius
    M21.731 Unequal limb length (acquired), right ulna
    M21.732 Unequal limb length (acquired), left ulna
    M21.733 Unequal limb length (acquired), right radius
    M21.734 Unequal limb length (acquired), left radius
    M21.739 Unequal limb length (acquired), unspecified ulna and radius
  M21.75-Unequal limb length (acquired), femur
    M21.751 Unequal limb length (acquired), right femur
    M21.752 Unequal limb length (acquired), left femur
    M21.759 Unequal limb length (acquired), unspecified femur
  M21.76-Unequal limb length (acquired), tibia and fibula
    M21.761 Unequal limb length (acquired), right tibia
    M21.762 Unequal limb length (acquired), left tibia
    M21.763 Unequal limb length (acquired), right fibula
    M21.764 Unequal limb length (acquired), left fibula
    M21.769 Unequal limb length (acquired), unspecified tibia and fibula
M21.8- Other specified acquired deformities of limbs
    Excludes❷: coxa plana (M91.2)
  M21.80 Other specified acquired deformities of unspecified limb
  M21.82-Other specified acquired deformities of upper arm
    M21.821 Other specified acquired deformities of right upper arm
    M21.822 Other specified acquired deformities of left upper arm
    M21.829 Other specified acquired deformities of unspecified upper arm

M21.83-Other specified acquired deformities of forearm
    M21.831 Other specified acquired deformities of right forearm
    M21.832 Other specified acquired deformities of left forearm
    M21.839 Other specified acquired deformities of unspecified forearm
M21.85-Other specified acquired deformities of thigh
    M21.851 Other specified acquired deformities of right thigh
    M21.852 Other specified acquired deformities of left thigh
    M21.859 Other specified acquired deformities of unspecified thigh
M21.86-Other specified acquired deformities of lower leg
    M21.861 Other specified acquired deformities of right lower leg
    M21.862 Other specified acquired deformities of left lower leg
    M21.869 Other specified acquired deformities of unspecified lower leg
M21.9- Unspecified acquired deformity of limb and hand
  M21.90 Unspecified acquired deformity of unspecified limb
  M21.92-Unspecified acquired deformity of upper arm
    M21.921 Unspecified acquired deformity of right upper arm
    M21.922 Unspecified acquired deformity of left upper arm
    M21.929 Unspecified acquired deformity of unspecified upper arm
  M21.93-Unspecified acquired deformity of forearm
    M21.931 Unspecified acquired deformity of right forearm
    M21.932 Unspecified acquired deformity of left forearm
    M21.939 Unspecified acquired deformity of unspecified forearm
  M21.94-Unspecified acquired deformity of hand
    M21.941 Unspecified acquired deformity of hand, right hand
    M21.942 Unspecified acquired deformity of hand, left hand
    M21.949 Unspecified acquired deformity of hand, unspecified hand
  M21.95-Unspecified acquired deformity of thigh
    M21.951 Unspecified acquired deformity of right thigh
    M21.952 Unspecified acquired deformity of left thigh
    M21.959 Unspecified acquired deformity of unspecified thigh
  M21.96-Unspecified acquired deformity of lower leg
    M21.961 Unspecified acquired deformity of right lower leg
    M21.962 Unspecified acquired deformity of left lower leg
    M21.969 Unspecified acquired deformity of unspecified lower leg
M22- Disorder of patella
    Excludes 1: traumatic dislocation of patella (S83.0-)
  M22.0- Recurrent dislocation of patella
    M22.00 Recurrent dislocation of patella, unspecified knee
    M22.01 Recurrent dislocation of patella, right knee
    M22.02 Recurrent dislocation of patella, left knee
  M22.1- Recurrent subluxation of patella
      Incomplete dislocation of patella
    M22.10 Recurrent subluxation of patella, unspecified knee
    M22.11 Recurrent subluxation of patella, right knee
    M22.12 Recurrent subluxation of patella, left knee
  M22.2- Patellofemoral disorders
    M22.2x-Patellofemoral disorders
      M22.2x1 Patellofemoral disorders, right knee
      M22.2x2 Patellofemoral disorders, left knee
      M22.2x9 Patellofemoral disorders, unspecified knee
  M22.3- Other derangements of patella
    M22.3x-Other derangements of patella
      M22.3x1 Other derangements of patella, right knee
      M22.3x2 Other derangements of patella, left knee
      M22.3x9 Other derangements of patella, unspecified knee
  M22.4- Chondromalacia patellae
    M22.40 Chondromalacia patellae, unspecified knee
    M22.41 Chondromalacia patellae, right knee
    M22.42 Chondromalacia patellae, left knee
  M22.8- Other disorders of patella
    M22.8x-Other disorders of patella
      M22.8x1 Other disorders of patella, right knee
      M22.8x2 Other disorders of patella, left knee
      M22.8x9 Other disorders of patella, unspecified knee
  M22.9- Unspecified disorder of patella
    M22.90 Unspecified disorder of patella, unspecified knee
    M22.91 Unspecified disorder of patella, right knee
    M22.92 Unspecified disorder of patella, left knee

M 2 1 - M 2 3

M23- **Internal derangement** of **knee**
   Excludes 1:   ankylosis (M24.66)
                 current injury — see injury of knee and lower leg (S80-S89)
                 deformity of knee (M21.-)
                 osteochondritis dissecans (M93.2)
                 recurrent dislocation or subluxation of joints (M24.4)
                 recurrent dislocation or subluxation of patella (M22.0-M22.1)

M23.0- **Cystic meniscus**
   M23.00-Cystic meniscus, **unspecified meniscus**
         Cystic meniscus, unspecified lateral meniscus
         Cystic meniscus, unspecified medial meniscus
     M23.000 **Cystic meniscus, unspecified lateral meniscus, right** knee
     M23.001 **Cystic meniscus, unspecified lateral meniscus, left** knee
     M23.002 **Cystic meniscus, unspecified lateral meniscus, unspecified** knee
     M23.003 **Cystic meniscus, unspecified medial meniscus, right** knee
     M23.004 **Cystic meniscus, unspecified medial meniscus, left** knee
     M23.005 **Cystic meniscus, unspecified medial meniscus, unspecified** knee
     M23.006 **Cystic meniscus, unspecified meniscus, right** knee
     M23.007 **Cystic meniscus, unspecified meniscus, left** knee
     M23.009 **Cystic meniscus, unspecified meniscus, unspecified** knee
   M23.01-Cystic meniscus, **anterior horn** of **medial** meniscus
     M23.011 **Cystic meniscus, anterior horn of medial meniscus, right** knee
     M23.012 **Cystic meniscus, anterior horn of medial meniscus, left** knee
     M23.019 **Cystic meniscus, anterior horn of medial meniscus, unspecified** knee
   M23.02-Cystic meniscus, **posterior horn** of **medial** meniscus
     M23.021 **Cystic meniscus, posterior horn of medial meniscus, right** knee
     M23.022 **Cystic meniscus, posterior horn of medial meniscus, left** knee
     M23.029 **Cystic meniscus, posterior horn of medial meniscus, unspecified** knee
   M23.03-Cystic meniscus, **other medial meniscus**
     M23.031 **Cystic meniscus, other medial meniscus, right** knee
     M23.032 **Cystic meniscus, other medial meniscus, left** knee
     M23.039 **Cystic meniscus, other medial meniscus, unspecified** knee
   M23.04-Cystic meniscus, **anterior horn** of **lateral** meniscus
     M23.041 **Cystic meniscus, anterior horn of lateral meniscus, right** knee
     M23.042 **Cystic meniscus, anterior horn of lateral meniscus, left** knee
     M23.049 **Cystic meniscus, anterior horn of lateral meniscus, unspecified** knee
   M23.05-Cystic meniscus, **posterior horn** of **lateral** meniscus
     M23.051 **Cystic meniscus, posterior horn of lateral meniscus, right** knee
     M23.052 **Cystic meniscus, posterior horn of lateral meniscus, left** knee
     M23.059 **Cystic meniscus, posterior horn of lateral meniscus, unspecified** knee
   M23.06-Cystic meniscus, **other lateral** meniscus
     M23.061 **Cystic meniscus, other lateral meniscus, right** knee
     M23.062 **Cystic meniscus, other lateral meniscus, left** knee
     M23.069 **Cystic meniscus, other lateral meniscus, unspecified** knee
M23.2- **Derangement of meniscus** **due to old tear or injury**
        Old bucket-handle tear
   M23.20-Derangement of **unspecified** meniscus due to old tear or injury
        Derangement of unspecified lateral meniscus due to old tear or injury
        Derangement of unspecified medial meniscus due to old tear or injury
     M23.200 **Derangement of unspecified lateral meniscus due to old tear or injury, right** knee
     M23.201 **Derangement of unspecified lateral meniscus due to old tear or injury, left** knee
     M23.202 **Derangement of unspecified lateral meniscus due to old tear or injury, unspecified** knee

     M23.203 **Derangement of unspecified medial meniscus due to old tear or injury, right** knee
     M23.204 **Derangement of unspecified medial meniscus due to old tear or injury, left** knee
     M23.205 **Derangement of unspecified medial meniscus due to old tear or injury, unspecified** knee
     M23.206 **Derangement of unspecified meniscus due to old tear or injury, right** knee
     M23.207 **Derangement of unspecified meniscus due to old tear or injury, left** knee
     M23.209 **Derangement of unspecified meniscus due to old tear or injury, unspecified** knee
   M23.21-Derangement of **anterior horn** of medial meniscus due to old tear or injury
     M23.211 **Derangement of anterior horn of medial meniscus due to old tear or injury, right** knee
     M23.212 **Derangement of anterior horn of medial meniscus due to old tear or injury, left** knee
     M23.219 **Derangement of anterior horn of medial meniscus due to old tear or injury, unspecified** knee
   M23.22-Derangement of **posterior horn** of **medial** meniscus due to old tear or injury
     M23.221 **Derangement of posterior horn of medial meniscus due to old tear or injury, right** knee
     M23.222 **Derangement of posterior horn of medial meniscus due to old tear or injury, left** knee
     M23.229 **Derangement of posterior horn of medial meniscus due to old tear or injury, unspecified** knee
   M23.23-Derangement of other medial meniscus due to old tear or injury
     M23.231 **Derangement of other medial meniscus due to old tear or injury, right** knee
     M23.232 **Derangement of other medial meniscus due to old tear or injury, left** knee
     M23.239 **Derangement of other medial meniscus due to old tear or injury, unspecified** knee
   M23.24-Derangement of **anterior horn** of **lateral** meniscus due to old tear or injury
     M23.241 **Derangement of anterior horn of lateral meniscus due to old tear or injury, right** knee
     M23.242 **Derangement of anterior horn of lateral meniscus due to old tear or injury, left** knee
     M23.249 **Derangement of anterior horn of lateral meniscus due to old tear or injury, unspecified** knee
   M23.25-Derangement of **posterior horn** of **lateral** meniscus due to old tear or injury
     M23.251 **Derangement of posterior horn of lateral meniscus due to old tear or injury, right** knee
     M23.252 **Derangement of posterior horn of lateral meniscus due to old tear or injury, left** knee
     M23.259 **Derangement of posterior horn of lateral meniscus due to old tear or injury, unspecified** knee
   M23.26-Derangement of **other lateral** meniscus due to old tear or injury
     M23.261 **Derangement of other lateral meniscus due to old tear or injury, right** knee
     M23.262 **Derangement of other lateral meniscus due to old tear or injury, left** knee
     M23.269 **Derangement of other lateral meniscus due to old tear or injury, unspecified** knee
M23.3- **Other meniscus derangements**
        Degenerate meniscus
        Detached meniscus
        Retained meniscus
   M23.30-Other meniscus derangements, **unspecified** meniscus
        Other meniscus derangements, unspecified lateral meniscus
        Other meniscus derangements, unspecified medial meniscus
     M23.300 **Other meniscus derangements, unspecified lateral meniscus, right** knee
     M23.301 **Other meniscus derangements, unspecified lateral meniscus, left** knee
     M23.302 **Other meniscus derangements, unspecified lateral meniscus, unspecified** knee
     M23.303 **Other meniscus derangements, unspecified medial meniscus, right** knee
     M23.304 **Other meniscus derangements, unspecified medial meniscus, left** knee
     M23.305 **Other meniscus derangements, unspecified medial meniscus, unspecified** knee
     M23.306 **Other meniscus derangements, unspecified meniscus, right** knee

M23.307   Other meniscus derangements, <u>unspecified</u> meniscus, <u>left</u> knee

M23.309   Other meniscus derangements, <u>unspecified</u> meniscus, <u>unspecified</u> knee

M23.31-Other meniscus derangements, <u>anterior horn</u> of <u>medial</u> meniscus

M23.311   Other meniscus derangements, anterior horn of medial meniscus, <u>right</u> knee

M23.312   Other meniscus derangements, anterior horn of medial meniscus, <u>left</u> knee

M23.319   Other meniscus derangements, anterior horn of medial meniscus, <u>unspecified</u> knee

M23.32-Other meniscus derangements, <u>posterior horn</u> of <u>medial</u> meniscus

M23.321   Other meniscus derangements, posterior horn of medial meniscus, <u>right</u> knee

M23.322   Other meniscus derangements, posterior horn of medial meniscus, <u>left</u> knee

M23.329   Other meniscus derangements, posterior horn of medial meniscus, <u>unspecified</u> knee

M23.33-Other meniscus derangements, <u>other medial</u> meniscus

M23.331   Other meniscus derangements, other medial meniscus, <u>right</u> knee

M23.332   Other meniscus derangements, other medial meniscus, <u>left</u> knee

M23.339   Other meniscus derangements, other medial meniscus, <u>unspecified</u> knee

M23.34-Other meniscus derangements, <u>anterior horn</u> of <u>lateral</u> meniscus

M23.341   Other meniscus derangements, anterior horn of lateral meniscus, <u>right</u> knee

M23.342   Other meniscus derangements, anterior horn of lateral meniscus, <u>left</u> knee

M23.349   Other meniscus derangements, anterior horn of lateral meniscus, <u>unspecified</u> knee

M23.35-Other meniscus derangements, posterior horn of <u>lateral</u> meniscus

M23.351   Other meniscus derangements, posterior horn of lateral meniscus, <u>right</u> knee

M23.352   Other meniscus derangements, posterior horn of lateral meniscus, <u>left</u> knee

M23.359   Other meniscus derangements, posterior horn of lateral meniscus, <u>unspecified</u> knee

M23.36-Other meniscus derangements, <u>other lateral</u> meniscus

M23.361   Other meniscus derangements, other lateral meniscus, <u>right</u> knee

M23.362   Other meniscus derangements, other lateral meniscus, <u>left</u> knee

M23.369   Other meniscus derangements, other lateral meniscus, <u>unspecified</u> knee

M23.4- <u>Loose body</u> in <u>knee</u>

M23.40 Loose body in knee, <u>unspecified</u> knee

M23.41 Loose body in knee, <u>right</u> knee

M23.42 Loose body in knee, <u>left</u> knee

M23.5- <u>Chronic instability</u> of <u>knee</u>

M23.50 Chronic instability of knee, <u>unspecified</u> knee

M23.51 Chronic instability of knee, <u>right</u> knee

M23.52 Chronic instability of knee, <u>left</u> knee

M23.6- <u>Other spontaneous disruption of ligament(s) of knee</u>

M23.60-Other spontaneous disruption of <u>unspecified</u> <u>ligament</u> of knee

M23.601   Other spontaneous disruption of <u>unspecified</u> ligament of <u>right</u> knee

M23.602   Other spontaneous disruption of <u>unspecified</u> ligament of <u>left</u> knee

M23.609   Other spontaneous disruption of <u>unspecified</u> ligament of <u>unspecified</u> knee

M23.61-Other spontaneous disruption of <u>anterior cruciate ligament</u> of knee

M23.611   Other spontaneous disruption of anterior cruciate ligament of <u>right</u> knee

M23.612   Other spontaneous disruption of anterior cruciate ligament of <u>left</u> knee

M23.619   Other spontaneous disruption of anterior cruciate ligament of <u>unspecified</u> knee

M23.62-Other spontaneous disruption of <u>posterior cruciate ligament</u> of knee

M23.621   Other spontaneous disruption of posterior cruciate ligament of <u>right</u> knee

M23.622   Other spontaneous disruption of posterior cruciate ligament of <u>left</u> knee

M23.629   Other spontaneous disruption of posterior cruciate ligament of <u>unspecified</u> knee

M23.63-Other spontaneous disruption of <u>medial collateral ligament</u> of knee

M23.631   Other spontaneous disruption of medial collateral ligament of <u>right</u> knee

M23.632   Other spontaneous disruption of medial collateral ligament of <u>left</u> knee

M23.639   Other spontaneous disruption of medial collateral ligament of <u>unspecified</u> knee

M23.64-Other spontaneous disruption of <u>lateral collateral ligament</u> of knee

M23.641   Other spontaneous disruption of lateral collateral ligament of <u>right</u> knee

M23.642   Other spontaneous disruption of lateral collateral ligament of <u>left</u> knee

M23.649   Other spontaneous disruption of lateral collateral ligament of <u>unspecified</u> knee

M23.67-Other spontaneous disruption of <u>capsular ligament</u> of knee

M23.671   Other spontaneous disruption of capsular ligament of <u>right</u> knee

M23.672   Other spontaneous disruption of capsular ligament of <u>left</u> knee

M23.679   Other spontaneous disruption of capsular ligament of <u>unspecified</u> knee

M23.8- Other internal derangements of knee
        Laxity of ligament of knee
        Snapping knee

M23.8x-<u>Other internal derangements</u> of knee

M23.8x1 Other internal derangements of <u>right</u> knee

M23.8x2 Other internal derangements of <u>left</u> knee

M23.8x9 Other internal derangements of <u>unspecified</u> knee

M23.9- <u>Unspecified</u> internal derangement of knee

M23.90 Unspecified internal derangement of <u>unspecified</u> knee

M23.91 Unspecified internal derangement of <u>right</u> knee

M23.92 Unspecified internal derangement of <u>left</u> knee

M24- Other specific joint derangements
      Excludes 1:   current injury — see injury of joint by body region
      Excludes❷: ganglion (M67.4)
                    snapping knee (M23.8-)
                    temporomandibular joint disorders (M26.6-)

M24.0- <u>Loose body in joint</u>
        Excludes❷: loose body in knee (M23.4)

M24.00 Loose body in <u>unspecified</u> joint

M24.01-Loose body in <u>shoulder</u>

M24.011   Loose body in <u>right</u> shoulder

M24.012   Loose body in <u>left</u> shoulder

M24.019   Loose body in <u>unspecified</u> shoulder

M24.02-Loose body in <u>elbow</u>

M24.021   Loose body in <u>right</u> elbow

M24.022   Loose body in <u>left</u> elbow

M24.029   Loose body in <u>unspecified</u> elbow

M24.03-Loose body in <u>wrist</u>

M24.031   Loose body in <u>right</u> wrist

M24.032   Loose body in <u>left</u> wrist

M24.039   Loose body in <u>unspecified</u> wrist

M24.04-Loose body in <u>finger</u> joints

M24.041   Loose body in <u>right</u> finger joint(s)

M24.042   Loose body in <u>left</u> finger joint(s)

M24.049   Loose body in <u>unspecified</u> finger joint(s)

M24.05-Loose body in <u>hip</u>

M24.051   Loose body in <u>right</u> hip

M24.052   Loose body in <u>left</u> hip

M24.059   Loose body in <u>unspecified</u> hip

M24.07-Loose body in <u>ankle and toe</u> joints

M24.071   Loose body in <u>right</u> ankle

M24.072   Loose body in <u>left</u> ankle

M24.073   Loose body in <u>unspecified</u> ankle

M24.074   Loose body in <u>right</u> toe joint(s)

M24.075   Loose body in <u>left</u> toe joint(s)

M24.076   Loose body in <u>unspecified</u> toe joints

M
2
3
–
M
2
4

M24.08 Loose body, <u>other site</u>
M24.1- <u>Other articular cartilage disorders</u>
> *Excludes❷:* *chondrocalcinosis (M11.1, M11.2-)*
> *internal derangement of knee (M23.-)*
> *metastatic calcification (E83.5)*
> *ochronosis (E70.2)*

M24.10 Other articular cartilage disorders, <u>unspecified</u> site
M24.11- Other articular cartilage disorders, <u>shoulder</u>
   M24.111   Other articular cartilage disorders, <u>right</u> shoulder
   M24.112   Other articular cartilage disorders, <u>left</u> shoulder
   M24.119   Other articular cartilage disorders, <u>unspecified</u> shoulder
M24.12- Other articular cartilage disorders, <u>elbow</u>
   M24.121   Other articular cartilage disorders, <u>right</u> elbow
   M24.122   Other articular cartilage disorders, <u>left</u> elbow
   M24.129   Other articular cartilage disorders, <u>unspecified</u> elbow
M24.13- Other articular cartilage disorders, <u>wrist</u>
   M24.131   Other articular cartilage disorders, <u>right</u> wrist
   M24.132   Other articular cartilage disorders, <u>left</u> wrist
   M24.139   Other articular cartilage disorders, <u>unspecified</u> wrist
M24.14- Other articular cartilage disorders, <u>hand</u>
   M24.141   Other articular cartilage disorders, <u>right</u> hand
   M24.142   Other articular cartilage disorders, <u>left</u> hand
   M24.149   Other articular cartilage disorders, <u>unspecified</u> hand
M24.15- Other articular cartilage disorders, <u>hip</u>
   M24.151   Other articular cartilage disorders, <u>right</u> hip
   M24.152   Other articular cartilage disorders, <u>left</u> hip
   M24.159   Other articular cartilage disorders, <u>unspecified</u> hip
M24.17- Other articular cartilage disorders, <u>ankle and foot</u>
   M24.171   Other articular cartilage disorders, <u>right</u> ankle
   M24.172   Other articular cartilage disorders, <u>left</u> ankle
   M24.173   Other articular cartilage disorders, <u>unspecified</u> ankle
   M24.174   Other articular cartilage disorders, <u>right</u> foot
   M24.175   Other articular cartilage disorders, <u>left</u> foot
   M24.176   Other articular cartilage disorders, <u>unspecified</u> foot
M24.2- <u>Disorder of ligament</u>
> Instability secondary to old ligament injury
> Ligamentous laxity NOS
> *Excludes 1: familial ligamentous laxity (M35.7)*
> *Excludes❷: internal derangement of knee (M23.5-M23.89)*

M24.20 Disorder of ligament, <u>unspecified</u> site
M24.21- Disorder of ligament, <u>shoulder</u>
   M24.211   Disorder of ligament, <u>right</u> shoulder
   M24.212   Disorder of ligament, <u>left</u> shoulder
   M24.219   Disorder of ligament, <u>unspecified</u> shoulder
M24.22- Disorder of ligament, <u>elbow</u>
   M24.221   Disorder of ligament, <u>right</u> elbow
   M24.222   Disorder of ligament, <u>left</u> elbow
   M24.229   Disorder of ligament, <u>unspecified</u> elbow
M24.23- Disorder of ligament, <u>wrist</u>
   M24.231   Disorder of ligament, <u>right</u> wrist
   M24.232   Disorder of ligament, <u>left</u> wrist
   M24.239   Disorder of ligament, <u>unspecified</u> wrist
M24.24- Disorder of ligament, <u>hand</u>
   M24.241   Disorder of ligament, <u>right</u> hand
   M24.242   Disorder of ligament, <u>left</u> hand
   M24.249   Disorder of ligament, <u>unspecified</u> hand
M24.25- Disorder of ligament, <u>hip</u>
   M24.251   Disorder of ligament, <u>right</u> hip
   M24.252   Disorder of ligament, <u>left</u> hip
   M24.259   Disorder of ligament, <u>unspecified</u> hip
M24.27- Disorder of ligament, <u>ankle and foot</u>
   M24.271   Disorder of ligament, <u>right</u> ankle
   M24.272   Disorder of ligament, <u>left</u> ankle
   M24.273   Disorder of ligament, <u>unspecified</u> ankle
   M24.274   Disorder of ligament, <u>right</u> foot
   M24.275   Disorder of ligament, <u>left</u> foot
   M24.276   Disorder of ligament, <u>unspecified</u> foot
M24.28 Disorder of ligament, <u>vertebrae</u>

M24.3- <u>Pathological dislocation of joint, not elsewhere classified</u>
> *Excludes 1: congenital dislocation or displacement of joint — see*
> *congenital malformations and deformations of the*
> *musculoskeletal system (Q65-Q79)*
> *current injury — see injury of joints and ligaments by*
> *body region*
> *recurrent dislocation of joint (M24.4-)*

M24.30 Pathological dislocation of <u>unspecified</u> joint, not elsewhere classified
M24.31- Pathological dislocation of <u>shoulder</u>, not elsewhere classified
   M24.311   Pathological dislocation of <u>right</u> shoulder, not elsewhere classified
   M24.312   Pathological dislocation of <u>left</u> shoulder, not elsewhere classified
   M24.319   Pathological dislocation of <u>unspecified</u> shoulder, not elsewhere classified
M24.32- Pathological dislocation of <u>elbow</u>, not elsewhere classified
   M24.321   Pathological dislocation of <u>right</u> elbow, not elsewhere classified
   M24.322   Pathological dislocation of <u>left</u> elbow, not elsewhere classified
   M24.329   Pathological dislocation of <u>unspecified</u> elbow, not elsewhere classified
M24.33- Pathological dislocation of <u>wrist</u>, not elsewhere classified
   M24.331   Pathological dislocation of <u>right</u> wrist, not elsewhere classified
   M24.332   Pathological dislocation of <u>left</u> wrist, not elsewhere classified
   M24.339   Pathological dislocation of <u>unspecified</u> wrist, not elsewhere classified
M24.34- Pathological dislocation of <u>hand</u>, not elsewhere classified
   M24.341   Pathological dislocation of <u>right</u> hand, not elsewhere classified
   M24.342   Pathological dislocation of <u>left</u> hand, not elsewhere classified
   M24.349   Pathological dislocation of <u>unspecified</u> hand, not elsewhere classified
M24.35- Pathological dislocation of <u>hip</u>, not elsewhere classified
   M24.351   Pathological dislocation of <u>right</u> hip, not elsewhere classified
   M24.352   Pathological dislocation of <u>left</u> hip, not elsewhere classified
   M24.359   Pathological dislocation of <u>unspecified</u> hip, not elsewhere classified
M24.36- Pathological dislocation of <u>knee</u>, not elsewhere classified
   M24.361   Pathological dislocation of <u>right</u> knee, not elsewhere classified
   M24.362   Pathological dislocation of <u>left</u> knee, not elsewhere classified
   M24.369   Pathological dislocation of <u>unspecified</u> knee, not elsewhere classified
M24.37- Pathological dislocation of <u>ankle and foot</u>, not elsewhere classified
   M24.371   Pathological dislocation of <u>right</u> ankle, not elsewhere classified
   M24.372   Pathological dislocation of <u>left</u> ankle, not elsewhere classified
   M24.373   Pathological dislocation of <u>unspecified</u> ankle, not elsewhere classified
   M24.374   Pathological dislocation of <u>right</u> foot, not elsewhere classified
   M24.375   Pathological dislocation of <u>left</u> foot, not elsewhere classified
   M24.376   Pathological dislocation of <u>unspecified</u> foot, not elsewhere classified
M24.4- <u>Recurrent</u> <u>dislocation</u> of joint
> Recurrent subluxation of joint
> *Excludes❷: recurrent dislocation of patella (M22.0-M22.1)*
> *recurrent vertebral dislocation (M43.3-, M43.4,*
> *M43.5-)*

M24.40 Recurrent dislocation, <u>unspecified</u> joint
M24.41- Recurrent dislocation, <u>shoulder</u>
   M24.411   Recurrent dislocation, <u>right</u> shoulder
   M24.412   Recurrent dislocation, <u>left</u> shoulder
   M24.419   Recurrent dislocation, <u>unspecified</u> shoulder
M24.42- Recurrent dislocation, <u>elbow</u>
   M24.421   Recurrent dislocation, <u>right</u> elbow
   M24.422   Recurrent dislocation, <u>left</u> elbow
   M24.429   Recurrent dislocation, <u>unspecified</u> elbow

M
2
3
|
M
2
4

Excludes 1: = NOT CODED HERE! (Do not code both)

Excludes❷: = Not Included Here

M24.43-Recurrent dislocation, <u>wrist</u>
   M24.431   Recurrent dislocation, <u>right</u> wrist
   M24.432   Recurrent dislocation, <u>left</u> wrist
   M24.439   Recurrent dislocation, <u>unspecified</u> wrist
M24.44-Recurrent dislocation, <u>hand and finger(s)</u>
   M24.441   Recurrent dislocation, <u>right</u> hand
   M24.442   Recurrent dislocation, <u>left</u> hand
   M24.443   Recurrent dislocation, <u>unspecified</u> hand
   M24.444   Recurrent dislocation, <u>right</u> finger
   M24.445   Recurrent dislocation, <u>left</u> finger
   M24.446   Recurrent dislocation, <u>unspecified</u> finger
M24.45-Recurrent dislocation, <u>hip</u>
   M24.451   Recurrent dislocation, <u>right</u> hip
   M24.452   Recurrent dislocation, <u>left</u> hip
   M24.459   Recurrent dislocation, <u>unspecified</u> hip
M24.46-Recurrent dislocation, <u>knee</u>
   M24.461   Recurrent dislocation, <u>right</u> knee
   M24.462   Recurrent dislocation, <u>left</u> knee
   M24.469   Recurrent dislocation, <u>unspecified</u> knee
M24.47-Recurrent dislocation, <u>ankle, foot and toes</u>
   M24.471   Recurrent dislocation, <u>right</u> ankle
   M24.472   Recurrent dislocation, <u>left</u> ankle
   M24.473   Recurrent dislocation, <u>unspecified</u> ankle
   M24.474   Recurrent dislocation, <u>right</u> foot
   M24.475   Recurrent dislocation, <u>left</u> foot
   M24.476   Recurrent dislocation, <u>unspecified</u> foot
   M24.477   Recurrent dislocation, <u>right</u> toe(s)
   M24.478   Recurrent dislocation, <u>left</u> toe(s)
   M24.479   Recurrent dislocation, <u>unspecified</u> toe(s)
M24.5- <u>Contracture</u> of joint
   Excludes 1: *contracture of muscle without contracture of joint*
       (M62.4-)
       contracture of tendon (sheath) without contracture of
       joint (M62.4-)
       Dupuytren's contracture (M72.0)
   Excludes❷: *acquired deformities of limbs (M20-M21)*
M24.50 Contracture, <u>unspecified</u> joint
M24.51-Contracture, <u>shoulder</u>
   M24.511   Contracture, <u>right</u> shoulder
   M24.512   Contracture, <u>left</u> shoulder
   M24.519   Contracture, <u>unspecified</u> shoulder
M24.52-Contracture, <u>elbow</u>
   M24.521   Contracture, <u>right</u> elbow
   M24.522   Contracture, <u>left</u> elbow
   M24.529   Contracture, <u>unspecified</u> elbow
M24.53-Contracture, <u>wrist</u>
   M24.531   Contracture, <u>right</u> wrist
   M24.532   Contracture, <u>left</u> wrist
   M24.539   Contracture, <u>unspecified</u> wrist
M24.54-Contracture, <u>hand</u>
   M24.541   Contracture, <u>right</u> hand
   M24.542   Contracture, <u>left</u> hand
   M24.549   Contracture, <u>unspecified</u> hand
M24.55-Contracture, <u>hip</u>
   M24.551   Contracture, <u>right</u> hip
   M24.552   Contracture, <u>left</u> hip
   M24.559   Contracture, <u>unspecified</u> hip
M24.56-Contracture, <u>knee</u>
   M24.561   Contracture, <u>right</u> knee
   M24.562   Contracture, <u>left</u> knee
   M24.569   Contracture, <u>unspecified</u> knee
M24.57-Contracture, <u>ankle and foot</u>
   M24.571   Contracture, <u>right</u> ankle
   M24.572   Contracture, <u>left</u> ankle
   M24.573   Contracture, <u>unspecified</u> ankle
   M24.574   Contracture, <u>right</u> foot
   M24.575   Contracture, <u>left</u> foot
   M24.576   Contracture, <u>unspecified</u> foot
M24.6- <u>Ankylosis</u> of joint
   Excludes 1: *stiffness of joint without ankylosis (M25.6-)*
   Excludes❷: *spine (M43.2-)*
M24.60 Ankylosis, <u>unspecified</u> joint

M24.61-Ankylosis, <u>shoulder</u>
   M24.611   Ankylosis, <u>right</u> shoulder
   M24.612   Ankylosis, <u>left</u> shoulder
   M24.619   Ankylosis, <u>unspecified</u> shoulder
M24.62-Ankylosis, <u>elbow</u>
   M24.621   Ankylosis, <u>right</u> elbow
   M24.622   Ankylosis, <u>left</u> elbow
   M24.629   Ankylosis, <u>unspecified</u> elbow
M24.63-Ankylosis, <u>wrist</u>
   M24.631   Ankylosis, <u>right</u> wrist
   M24.632   Ankylosis, <u>left</u> wrist
   M24.639   Ankylosis, <u>unspecified</u> wrist
M24.64-Ankylosis, <u>hand</u>
   M24.641   Ankylosis, <u>right</u> hand
   M24.642   Ankylosis, <u>left</u> hand
   M24.649   Ankylosis, <u>unspecified</u> hand
M24.65-Ankylosis, <u>hip</u>
   M24.651   Ankylosis, <u>right</u> hip
   M24.652   Ankylosis, <u>left</u> hip
   M24.659   Ankylosis, <u>unspecified</u> hip
M24.66-Ankylosis, <u>knee</u>
   M24.661   Ankylosis, <u>right</u> knee
   M24.662   Ankylosis, <u>left</u> knee
   M24.669   Ankylosis, <u>unspecified</u> knee
M24.67-Ankylosis, <u>ankle and foot</u>
   M24.671   Ankylosis, <u>right</u> ankle
   M24.672   Ankylosis, <u>left</u> ankle
   M24.673   Ankylosis, <u>unspecified</u> ankle
   M24.674   Ankylosis, <u>right</u> foot
   M24.675   Ankylosis, <u>left</u> foot
   M24.676   Ankylosis, <u>unspecified</u> foot
M24.7   Protrusio acetabuli
M24.8- <u>Other specific</u> joint derangements, <u>not elsewhere classified</u>
   Excludes❷: *iliotibial band syndrome (M76.3)*
M24.80 Other specific joint derangements of <u>unspecified</u> joint, not
    elsewhere classified
M24.81-Other specific joint derangements of <u>shoulder</u>, not elsewhere
    classified
   M24.811   Other specific joint derangements of <u>right</u> shoulder,
         not elsewhere classified
   M24.812   Other specific joint derangements of <u>left</u> shoulder, not
         elsewhere classified
   M24.819   Other specific joint derangements of <u>unspecified</u>
         shoulder, not elsewhere classified
M24.82-Other specific joint derangements of <u>elbow</u>, not elsewhere
    classified
   M24.821   Other specific joint derangements of <u>right</u> elbow, not
         elsewhere classified
   M24.822   Other specific joint derangements of <u>left</u> elbow, not
         elsewhere classified
   M24.829   Other specific joint derangements of <u>unspecified</u>
         elbow, not elsewhere classified
M24.83-Other specific joint derangements of wrist, not elsewhere
    classified
   M24.831   Other specific joint derangements of <u>right</u> wrist, not
         elsewhere classified
   M24.832   Other specific joint derangements of <u>left</u> wrist, not
         elsewhere classified
   M24.839   Other specific joint derangements of <u>unspecified</u> wrist,
         not elsewhere classified
M24.84-Other specific joint derangements of <u>hand</u>, not elsewhere
    classified
   M24.841   Other specific joint derangements of <u>right</u> hand, not
         elsewhere classified
   M24.842   Other specific joint derangements of <u>left</u> hand, not
         elsewhere classified
   M24.849   Other specific joint derangements of <u>unspecified</u> hand,
         not elsewhere classified
M24.85-Other specific joint derangements of <u>hip</u>, not elsewhere
    classified
     Irritable hip
   M24.851   Other specific joint derangements of <u>right</u> hip, not
         elsewhere classified
   M24.852   Other specific joint derangements of <u>left</u> hip, not
         elsewhere classified
   M24.859   Other specific joint derangements of <u>unspecified</u> hip,
         not elsewhere classified

M
2
4
-
M
2
5

M24.87-Other specific joint derangements of <u>ankle and foot</u>, not elsewhere classified

  M24.871   Other specific joint derangements of <u>right</u> ankle, not elsewhere classified

  M24.872   Other specific joint derangements of <u>left</u> ankle, not elsewhere classified

  M24.873   Other specific joint derangements of <u>unspecified</u> ankle, not elsewhere classified

  M24.874   Other specific joint derangements of <u>right</u> foot, not elsewhere classified

  M24.875   Other specific joint derangements <u>left</u> foot, not elsewhere classified

  M24.876   Other specific joint derangements of <u>unspecified</u> foot, not elsewhere classified

M24.9   Joint derangement, <u>unspecified</u>

M25-   <u>Other joint disorder</u>, <u>not elsewhere classified</u>

Excludes❷: abnormality of gait and mobility (R26.-)
acquired deformities of limb (M20-M21)
calcification of bursa (M71.4-)
calcification of shoulder (joint) (M75.3)
calcification of tendon (M65.2-)
difficulty in walking (R26.2)
temporomandibular joint disorder (M26.6-)

M25.0-   <u>Hemarthrosis</u>

Excludes 1:   current injury — see injury of joint by body region
hemophilic arthropathy (M36.2)

M25.00 Hemarthrosis, <u>unspecified</u> joint

M25.01-Hemarthrosis, <u>shoulder</u>

  M25.011   Hemarthrosis, <u>right</u> shoulder
  M25.012   Hemarthrosis, <u>left</u> shoulder
  M25.019   Hemarthrosis, <u>unspecified</u> shoulder

M25.02-Hemarthrosis, <u>elbow</u>

  M25.021   Hemarthrosis, <u>right</u> elbow
  M25.022   Hemarthrosis, <u>left</u> elbow
  M25.029   Hemarthrosis, <u>unspecified</u> elbow

M25.03-Hemarthrosis, <u>wrist</u>

  M25.031   Hemarthrosis, <u>right</u> wrist
  M25.032   Hemarthrosis, <u>left</u> wrist
  M25.039   Hemarthrosis, <u>unspecified</u> wrist

M25.04-Hemarthrosis, <u>hand</u>

  M25.041   Hemarthrosis, <u>right</u> hand
  M25.042   Hemarthrosis, <u>left</u> hand
  M25.049   Hemarthrosis, <u>unspecified</u> hand

M25.05-Hemarthrosis, <u>hip</u>

  M25.051   Hemarthrosis, <u>right</u> hip
  M25.052   Hemarthrosis, <u>left</u> hip
  M25.059   Hemarthrosis, <u>unspecified</u> hip

M25.06-Hemarthrosis, <u>knee</u>

  M25.061   Hemarthrosis, <u>right</u> knee
  M25.062   Hemarthrosis, <u>left</u> knee
  M25.069   Hemarthrosis, <u>unspecified</u> knee

M25.07-Hemarthrosis, <u>ankle and foot</u>

  M25.071   Hemarthrosis, <u>right</u> ankle
  M25.072   Hemarthrosis, <u>left</u> ankle
  M25.073   Hemarthrosis, <u>unspecified</u> ankle
  M25.074   Hemarthrosis, <u>right</u> foot
  M25.075   Hemarthrosis, <u>left</u> foot
  M25.076   Hemarthrosis, <u>unspecified</u> foot

M25.08 Hemarthrosis, <u>other specified site</u>

  Hemarthrosis, vertebrae

M25.1-   Fistula of joint

M25.10 Fistula, <u>unspecified</u> joint

M25.11-Fistula, <u>shoulder</u>

  M25.111   Fistula, <u>right</u> shoulder
  M25.112   Fistula, <u>left</u> shoulder
  M25.119   Fistula, <u>unspecified</u> shoulder

M25.12-Fistula, <u>elbow</u>

  M25.121   Fistula, <u>right</u> elbow
  M25.122   Fistula, <u>left</u> elbow
  M25.129   Fistula, <u>unspecified</u> elbow

M25.13-Fistula, wrist

  M25.131   Fistula, <u>right</u> wrist
  M25.132   Fistula, <u>left</u> wrist
  M25.139   Fistula, <u>unspecified</u> wrist

M25.14-Fistula, <u>hand</u>

  M25.141   Fistula, <u>right</u> hand
  M25.142   Fistula, <u>left</u> hand

  M25.149   Fistula, <u>unspecified</u> hand

M25.15-Fistula, <u>hip</u>

  M25.151   Fistula, <u>right</u> hip
  M25.152   Fistula, <u>left</u> hip
  M25.159   Fistula, <u>unspecified</u> hip

M25.16-Fistula, <u>knee</u>

  M25.161   Fistula, <u>right</u> knee
  M25.162   Fistula, <u>left</u> knee
  M25.169   Fistula, <u>unspecified</u> knee

M25.17-Fistula, <u>ankle and foot</u>

  M25.171   Fistula, <u>right</u> ankle
  M25.172   Fistula, <u>left</u> ankle
  M25.173   Fistula, <u>unspecified</u> ankle
  M25.174   Fistula, <u>right</u> foot
  M25.175   Fistula, <u>left</u> foot
  M25.176   Fistula, <u>unspecified</u> foot

M25.18 Fistula, <u>other specified site</u>

  Fistula, vertebrae

M25.2-   <u>Flail joint</u>

M25.20 Flail joint, <u>unspecified</u> joint

M25.21-Flail joint, <u>shoulder</u>

  M25.211   Flail joint, <u>right</u> shoulder
  M25.212   Flail joint, <u>left</u> shoulder
  M25.219   Flail joint, <u>unspecified</u> shoulder

M25.22-Flail joint, <u>elbow</u>

  M25.221   Flail joint, <u>right</u> elbow
  M25.222   Flail joint, <u>left</u> elbow
  M25.229   Flail joint, <u>unspecified</u> elbow

M25.23-Flail joint, <u>wrist</u>

  M25.231   Flail joint, <u>right</u> wrist
  M25.232   Flail joint, <u>left</u> wrist
  M25.239   Flail joint, <u>unspecified</u> wrist

M25.24-Flail joint, <u>hand</u>

  M25.241   Flail joint, <u>right</u> hand
  M25.242   Flail joint, <u>left</u> hand
  M25.249   Flail joint, <u>unspecified</u> hand

M25.25-Flail joint, <u>hip</u>

  M25.251   Flail joint, <u>right</u> hip
  M25.252   Flail joint, <u>left</u> hip
  M25.259   Flail joint, <u>unspecified</u> hip

M25.26-Flail joint, <u>knee</u>

  M25.261   Flail joint, <u>right</u> knee
  M25.262   Flail joint, <u>left</u> knee
  M25.269   Flail joint, <u>unspecified</u> knee

M25.27-Flail joint, <u>ankle and foot</u>

  M25.271   Flail joint, <u>right</u> ankle and foot
  M25.272   Flail joint, <u>left</u> ankle and foot
  M25.279   Flail joint, <u>unspecified</u> ankle and foot

M25.28 Flail joint, <u>other site</u>

M25.3-   <u>Other instability</u> of joint

Excludes 1:   instability of joint secondary to old ligament injury (M24.2-)
instability of joint secondary to removal of joint prosthesis (M96.8-)
Excludes❷: spinal instabilities (M53.2-)

M25.30 Other instability, <u>unspecified</u> joint

M25.31-Other instability, <u>shoulder</u>

  M25.311   Other instability, <u>right</u> shoulder
  M25.312   Other instability, <u>left</u> shoulder
  M25.319   Other instability, <u>unspecified</u> shoulder

M25.32-Other instability, <u>elbow</u>

  M25.321   Other instability, <u>right</u> elbow
  M25.322   Other instability, <u>left</u> elbow
  M25.329   Other instability, <u>unspecified</u> elbow

M25.33-Other instability, <u>wrist</u>

  M25.331   Other instability, <u>right</u> wrist
  M25.332   Other instability, <u>left</u> wrist
  M25.339   Other instability, <u>unspecified</u> wrist

M25.34-Other instability, <u>hand</u>

  M25.341   Other instability, <u>right</u> hand
  M25.342   Other instability, <u>left</u> hand
  M25.349   Other instability, <u>unspecified</u> hand

M25.35-Other instability, <u>hip</u>

  M25.351   Other instability, <u>right</u> hip
  M25.352   Other instability, <u>left</u> hip
  M25.359   Other instability, <u>unspecified</u> hip

M 2 4 - M 2 5

M25.36-Other instability, <u>knee</u>
  M25.361 Other instability, <u>right</u> knee
  M25.362 Other instability, <u>left</u> knee
  M25.369 Other instability, <u>unspecified</u> knee
M25.37-Other instability, <u>ankle and foot</u>
  M25.371 Other instability, <u>right</u> ankle
  M25.372 Other instability, <u>left</u> ankle
  M25.373 Other instability, <u>unspecified</u> ankle
  M25.374 Other instability, <u>right</u> foot
  M25.375 Other instability, <u>left</u> foot
  M25.376 Other instability, <u>unspecified</u> foot
M25.4- <u>Effusion</u> of joint
  Excludes 1: *hydrarthrosis in yaws (A66.6)*
          intermittent hydrarthrosis (M12.4-)
          other infective (teno)synovitis (M65.1-)
M25.40 Effusion, <u>unspecified</u> joint
M25.41-Effusion, <u>shoulder</u>
  M25.411 Effusion, <u>right</u> shoulder
  M25.412 Effusion, <u>left</u> shoulder
  M25.419 Effusion, <u>unspecified</u> shoulder
M25.42-Effusion, <u>elbow</u>
  M25.421 Effusion, <u>right</u> elbow
  M25.422 Effusion, <u>left</u> elbow
  M25.429 Effusion, <u>unspecified</u> elbow
M25.43-Effusion, <u>wrist</u>
  M25.431 Effusion, <u>right</u> wrist
  M25.432 Effusion, <u>left</u> wrist
  M25.439 Effusion, <u>unspecified</u> wrist
M25.44-Effusion, <u>hand</u>
  M25.441 Effusion, <u>right</u> hand
  M25.442 Effusion, <u>left</u> hand
  M25.449 Effusion, <u>unspecified</u> hand
M25.45-Effusion, <u>hip</u>
  M25.451 Effusion, <u>right</u> hip
  M25.452 Effusion, <u>left</u> hip
  M25.459 Effusion, <u>unspecified</u> hip
M25.46-Effusion, <u>knee</u>
  M25.461 Effusion, <u>right</u> knee
  M25.462 Effusion, <u>left</u> knee
  M25.469 Effusion, <u>unspecified</u> knee
M25.47-Effusion, <u>ankle and foot</u>
  M25.471 Effusion, <u>right</u> ankle
  M25.472 Effusion, <u>left</u> ankle
  M25.473 Effusion, <u>unspecified</u> ankle
  M25.474 Effusion, <u>right</u> foot
  M25.475 Effusion, <u>left</u> foot
  M25.476 Effusion, <u>unspecified</u> foot
M25.48 Effusion, <u>other site</u>
M25.5- <u>Pain in</u> joint
  Excludes ❷: *pain in hand (M79.64-)*
          pain in fingers (M79.64-)
          pain in foot (M79.67-)
          pain in limb (M79.6-)
          pain in toes (M79.67-)
M25.50 Pain in <u>unspecified</u> joint
M25.51-Pain in <u>shoulder</u>
  M25.511 Pain in <u>right</u> shoulder
  M25.512 Pain in <u>left</u> shoulder
  M25.519 Pain in <u>unspecified</u> shoulder
M25.52-Pain in <u>elbow</u>
  M25.521 Pain in <u>right</u> elbow
  M25.522 Pain in <u>left</u> elbow
  M25.529 Pain in <u>unspecified</u> elbow
M25.53-Pain in <u>wrist</u>
  M25.531 Pain in <u>right</u> wrist
  M25.532 Pain in <u>left</u> wrist
  M25.539 Pain in <u>unspecified</u> wrist
M25.55-Pain in hip
  M25.551 Pain in <u>right</u> hip
  M25.552 Pain in <u>left</u> hip
  M25.559 Pain in <u>unspecified</u> hip
M25.56-Pain in <u>knee</u>
  M25.561 Pain in <u>right</u> knee
  M25.562 Pain in <u>left</u> knee
  M25.569 Pain in <u>unspecified</u> knee

M25.57-Pain in <u>ankle and joints of foot</u>
  M25.571 Pain in <u>right</u> ankle and joints of right foot
  M25.572 Pain in <u>left</u> ankle and joints of left foot
  M25.579 Pain in <u>unspecified</u> ankle and joints of unspecified foot
M25.6- <u>Stiffness</u> of joint, <u>not elsewhere classified</u>
  Excludes 1: *ankylosis of joint (M24.6-)*
          contracture of joint (M24.5-)
M25.60 Stiffness of <u>unspecified</u> joint, not elsewhere classified
M25.61-Stiffness of <u>shoulder</u>, not elsewhere classified
  M25.611 Stiffness of <u>right</u> shoulder, not elsewhere classified
  M25.612 Stiffness of <u>left</u> shoulder, not elsewhere classified
  M25.619 Stiffness of <u>unspecified</u> shoulder, not elsewhere classified
M25.62-Stiffness of <u>elbow</u>, not elsewhere classified
  M25.621 Stiffness of <u>right</u> elbow, not elsewhere classified
  M25.622 Stiffness of <u>left</u> elbow, not elsewhere classified
  M25.629 Stiffness of <u>unspecified</u> elbow, not elsewhere classified
M25.63-Stiffness of <u>wrist</u>, not elsewhere classified
  M25.631 Stiffness of <u>right</u> wrist, not elsewhere classified
  M25.632 Stiffness of <u>left</u> wrist, not elsewhere classified
  M25.639 Stiffness of <u>unspecified</u> wrist, not elsewhere classified
M25.64-Stiffness of <u>hand</u>, not elsewhere classified
  M25.641 Stiffness of <u>right</u> hand, not elsewhere classified
  M25.642 Stiffness of <u>left</u> hand, not elsewhere classified
  M25.649 Stiffness of <u>unspecified</u> hand, not elsewhere classified
M25.65-Stiffness of <u>hip</u>, not elsewhere classified
  M25.651 Stiffness of <u>right</u> hip, not elsewhere classified
  M25.652 Stiffness of <u>left</u> hip, not elsewhere classified
  M25.659 Stiffness of <u>unspecified</u> hip, not elsewhere classified
M25.66-Stiffness of <u>knee</u>, not elsewhere classified
  M25.661 Stiffness of <u>right</u> knee, not elsewhere classified
  M25.662 Stiffness of <u>left</u> knee, not elsewhere classified
  M25.669 Stiffness of <u>unspecified</u> knee, not elsewhere classified
M25.67-Stiffness of <u>ankle and foot</u>, not elsewhere classified
  M25.671 Stiffness of <u>right</u> ankle, not elsewhere classified
  M25.672 Stiffness of <u>left</u> ankle, not elsewhere classified
  M25.673 Stiffness of <u>unspecified</u> ankle, not elsewhere classified
  M25.674 Stiffness of <u>right</u> foot, not elsewhere classified
  M25.675 Stiffness of <u>left</u> foot, not elsewhere classified
  M25.676 Stiffness of <u>unspecified</u> foot, not elsewhere classified
M25.7- <u>Osteophyte</u>
M25.70 Osteophyte, <u>unspecified</u> joint
M25.71-Osteophyte, <u>shoulder</u>
  M25.711 Osteophyte, <u>right</u> shoulder
  M25.712 Osteophyte, <u>left</u> shoulder
  M25.719 Osteophyte, <u>unspecified</u> shoulder
M25.72-Osteophyte, <u>elbow</u>
  M25.721 Osteophyte, <u>right</u> elbow
  M25.722 Osteophyte, <u>left</u> elbow
  M25.729 Osteophyte, <u>unspecified</u> elbow
M25.73-Osteophyte, <u>wrist</u>
  M25.731 Osteophyte, <u>right</u> wrist
  M25.732 Osteophyte, <u>left</u> wrist
  M25.739 Osteophyte, <u>unspecified</u> wrist
M25.74-Osteophyte, <u>hand</u>
  M25.741 Osteophyte, <u>right</u> hand
  M25.742 Osteophyte, <u>left</u> hand
  M25.749 Osteophyte, <u>unspecified</u> hand
M25.75-Osteophyte, <u>hip</u>
  M25.751 Osteophyte, <u>right</u> hip
  M25.752 Osteophyte, <u>left</u> hip
  M25.759 Osteophyte, <u>unspecified</u> hip
M25.76-Osteophyte, <u>knee</u>
  M25.761 Osteophyte, <u>right</u> knee
  M25.762 Osteophyte, <u>left</u> knee
  M25.769 Osteophyte, <u>unspecified</u> knee
M25.77-Osteophyte, <u>ankle and foot</u>
  M25.771 Osteophyte, <u>right</u> ankle
  M25.772 Osteophyte, <u>left</u> ankle
  M25.773 Osteophyte, <u>unspecified</u> ankle
  M25.774 Osteophyte, <u>right</u> foot
  M25.775 Osteophyte, <u>left</u> foot
  M25.776 Osteophyte, <u>unspecified</u> foot
M25.78 Osteophyte, <u>vertebrae</u>

M25 - M26

Excludes 1: = NOT CODED HERE! (Do not code both)

Excludes ❷: = Not Included Here

M25.8- Other specified joint disorders
    M25.80 Other specified joint disorders, unspecified joint
    M25.81-Other specified joint disorders, shoulder
        M25.811 Other specified joint disorders, right shoulder
        M25.812 Other specified joint disorders, left shoulder
        M25.819 Other specified joint disorders, unspecified shoulder
    M25.82-Other specified joint disorders, elbow
        M25.821 Other specified joint disorders, right elbow
        M25.822 Other specified joint disorders, left elbow
        M25.829 Other specified joint disorders, unspecified elbow
    M25.83-Other specified joint disorders, wrist
        M25.831 Other specified joint disorders, right wrist
        M25.832 Other specified joint disorders, left wrist
        M25.839 Other specified joint disorders, unspecified wrist
    M25.84-Other specified joint disorders, hand
        M25.841 Other specified joint disorders, right hand
        M25.842 Other specified joint disorders, left hand
        M25.849 Other specified joint disorders, unspecified hand
    M25.85-Other specified joint disorders, hip
        M25.851 Other specified joint disorders, right hip
        M25.852 Other specified joint disorders, left hip
        M25.859 Other specified joint disorders, unspecified hip
    M25.86-Other specified joint disorders, knee
        M25.861 Other specified joint disorders, right knee
        M25.862 Other specified joint disorders, left knee
        M25.869 Other specified joint disorders, unspecified knee
    M25.87-Other specified joint disorders, ankle and foot
        M25.871 Other specified joint disorders, right ankle and foot
        M25.872 Other specified joint disorders, left ankle and foot
        M25.879 Other specified joint disorders, unspecified ankle and foot
M25.9 Joint disorder, unspecified

Dentofacial anomalies [including malocclusion] and other disorders of jaw (M26-M27)

Excludes 1: *hemifacial atrophy or hypertrophy (Q67.4)*
             unilateral condylar hyperplasia or hypoplasia (M27.8)

M26- Dentofacial anomalies [including malocclusion]
M26.0- Major anomalies of jaw size
    Excludes 1: *acromegaly (E22.0)*
             Robin's syndrome (Q87.0)
    M26.00 Unspecified anomaly of jaw size
    M26.01 Maxillary hyperplasia
    M26.02 Maxillary hypoplasia
    M26.03 Mandibular hyperplasia
    M26.04 Mandibular hypoplasia
    M26.05 Macrogenia
    M26.06 Microgenia
    M26.07 Excessive tuberosity of jaw
        Entire maxillary tuberosity
    M26.09 Other specified anomalies of jaw size
M26.1- Anomalies of jaw-cranial base relationship
    M26.10 Unspecified anomaly of jaw-cranial base relationship
    M26.11 Maxillary asymmetry
    M26.12 Other jaw asymmetry
    M26.19 Other specified anomalies of jaw-cranial base relationship
M26.2- Anomalies of dental arch relationship
    M26.20 Unspecified anomaly of dental arch relationship
    M26.21-Malocclusion, Angle's class
        M26.211 Malocclusion, Angle's class I
            Neutro-occlusion
        M26.212 Malocclusion, Angle's class II
            Disto-occlusion Division I
            Disto-occlusion Division II
        M26.213 Malocclusion, Angle's class III
            Mesio-occlusion
        M26.219 Malocclusion, Angle's class, unspecified
    M26.22-Open occlusal relationship
        M26.220 Open anterior occlusal relationship
            Anterior openbite
        M26.221 Open posterior occlusal relationship
            Posterior openbite
    M26.23 Excessive horizontal overlap
        Excessive horizontal overjet

    M26.24 Reverse articulation
        Crossbite (anterior) (posterior)
    M26.25 Anomalies of interarch distance
    M26.29 Other anomalies of dental arch relationship
        Midline deviation of dental arch
        Overbite (excessive) deep
        Overbite (excessive) horizontal
        Overbite (excessive) vertical
        Posterior lingual occlusion of mandibular teeth
M26.3- Anomalies of tooth position of fully erupted tooth or teeth
    Excludes❷: embedded and impacted teeth (K01.-)
    M26.30 Unspecified anomaly of tooth position of fully erupted tooth or teeth
        Abnormal spacing of fully erupted tooth or teeth NOS
        Displacement of fully erupted tooth or teeth NOS
        Transposition of fully erupted tooth or teeth NOS
    M26.31 Crowding of fully erupted teeth
    M26.32 Excessive spacing of fully erupted teeth
        Diastema of fully erupted tooth or teeth NOS
    M26.33 Horizontal displacement of fully erupted tooth or teeth
        Tipped tooth or teeth
        Tipping of fully erupted tooth
    M26.34 Vertical displacement of fully erupted tooth or teeth
        Extruded tooth
        Infraeruption of tooth or teeth
        Supraeruption of tooth or teeth
    M26.35 Rotation of fully erupted tooth or teeth
    M26.36 Insufficient interocclusal distance of fully erupted teeth (ridge)
        Lack of adequate intermaxillary vertical dimension of fully erupted teeth
    M26.37 Excessive interocclusal distance of fully erupted teeth
        Excessive intermaxillary vertical dimension of fully erupted teeth
        Loss of occlusal vertical dimension of fully erupted teeth
    M26.39 Other anomalies of tooth position of fully erupted tooth or teeth
M26.4 Malocclusion, unspecified
M26.5- Dentofacial functional abnormalities
    Excludes 1: *bruxism (F45.8)*
             teeth-grinding NOS (F45.8)
    M26.50 Dentofacial functional abnormalities, unspecified
    M26.51 Abnormal jaw closure
    M26.52 Limited mandibular range of motion
    M26.53 Deviation in opening and closing of the mandible
    M26.54 Insufficient anterior guidance
        Insufficient anterior occlusal guidance
    M26.55 Centric occlusion maximum intercuspation discrepancy
        Excludes 1: centric occlusion NOS (M26.59)
    M26.56 Non-working side interference
        Balancing side interference
    M26.57 Lack of posterior occlusal support
    M26.59 Other dentofacial functional abnormalities
        Centric occlusion (of teeth) NOS
        Malocclusion due to abnormal swallowing
        Malocclusion due to mouth breathing
        Malocclusion due to tongue, lip or finger habits
M26.6- Temporomandibular joint disorders
    Excludes❷: current temporomandibular joint dislocation (S03.0)
             current temporomandibular joint sprain (S03.4)
    M26.60 Temporomandibular joint disorder, unspecified
    M26.61 Adhesions and ankylosis of temporomandibular joint
    M26.62 Arthralgia of temporomandibular joint
    M26.63 Articular disc disorder of temporomandibular joint
    M26.69 Other specified disorders of temporomandibular joint
M26.7- Dental alveolar anomalies
    M26.70 Unspecified alveolar anomaly
    M26.71 Alveolar maxillary hyperplasia
    M26.72 Alveolar mandibular hyperplasia
    M26.73 Alveolar maxillary hypoplasia
    M26.74 Alveolar mandibular hypoplasia
    M26.79 Other specified alveolar anomalies
M26.8- Other dentofacial anomalies
    M26.81 Anterior soft tissue impingement
        Anterior soft tissue impingement on teeth
    M26.82 Posterior soft tissue impingement
        Posterior soft tissue impingement on teeth
    M26.89 Other dentofacial anomalies
M26.9 Dentofacial anomaly, unspecified

M
2
5
I
M
2
6

© 2013 Channel Publishing, Ltd.

Excludes 1: = NOT CODED HERE! (Do not code both)

Excludes❷: = Not Included Here

M27- Other diseases of jaws

M27.0   Developmental disorders of jaws
Latent bone cyst of jaw
Stafne's cyst
Torus mandibularis
Torus palatinus

M27.1   Giant cell granuloma, central
Giant cell granuloma NOS
Excludes 1: peripheral giant cell granuloma (K06.8)

M27.2   Inflammatory conditions of jaws
Osteitis of jaw(s)
Osteomyelitis (neonatal) jaw(s)
Osteoradionecrosis jaw(s)
Periostitis jaw(s)
Sequestrum of jaw bone
Use additional code (W88-W90, X39.0) to identify radiation, if
radiation-induced
Excludes❷: osteonecrosis of jaw due to drug (M87.180)

M27.3   Alveolitis of jaws
Alveolar osteitis
Dry socket

M27.4-   Other and unspecified cysts of jaw
Excludes 1: cysts of oral region (K09.-)
latent bone cyst of jaw (M27.0)
Stafne's cyst (M27.0)

M27.40   Unspecified cyst of jaw
Cyst of jaw NOS

M27.49   Other cysts of jaw
Aneurysmal cyst of jaw
Hemorrhagic cyst of jaw
Traumatic cyst of jaw

**M27.5-   Periradicular pathology associated with previous endodontic
treatment**

M27.51   Perforation of root canal space due to endodontic treatment

M27.52   Endodontic overfill

M27.53   Endodontic underfill

**M27.59   Other periradicular pathology associated with previous
endodontic treatment**

M27.6-   Endosseous dental implant failure

M27.61   Osseointegration failure of dental implant
Hemorrhagic complications of dental implant placement
Iatrogenic osseointegration failure of dental implant
Osseointegration failure of dental implant due to
complications of systemic disease
Osseointegration failure of dental implant due to poor bone
quality
Pre-integration failure of dental implant NOS
Pre-osseointegration failure of dental implant

M27.62   Post-osseointegration biological failure of dental implant
Failure of dental implant due to lack of attached gingiva
Failure of dental implant due to occlusal trauma (caused by
poor prosthetic design)
Failure of dental implant due to parafunctional habits
Failure of dental implant due to periodontal infection (peri-
implantitis)
Failure of dental implant due to poor oral hygiene
Iatrogenic post-osseointegration failure of dental implant
Post-osseointegration failure of dental implant due to
complications of systemic disease

M27.63   Post-osseointegration mechanical failure of dental implant
Failure of dental prosthesis causing loss of dental implant
Fracture of dental implant
Excludes❷: cracked tooth (K03.81)
*fractured dental restorative material with loss of
material (K08.531)*
*fractured dental restorative material without loss
of material (K08.530)*
fractured tooth (S02.5)

M27.69   Other endosseous dental implant failure
Dental implant failure NOS

M27.8   Other specified diseases of jaws
Cherubism
Exostosis
Fibrous dysplasia
Unilateral condylar hyperplasia
Unilateral condylar hypoplasia
Excludes 1: jaw pain (R68.84)

M27.9   Disease of jaws, unspecified

Systemic connective tissue disorders (M30-M36)

Includes: Autoimmune disease NOS
Collagen (vascular) disease NOS
Systemic autoimmune disease
Systemic collagen (vascular) disease
*Excludes 1: autoimmune disease, single organ or single cell-type — code
to relevant condition category*

M30- Polyarteritis nodosa and related conditions
Excludes 1: microscopic polyarteritis (M31.7)

M30.0   Polyarteritis nodosa

M30.1   Polyarteritis with lung involvement [Churg-Strauss]
Allergic granulomatous angiitis

M30.2   Juvenile polyarteritis

M30.3   Mucocutaneous lymph node syndrome [Kawasaki]

M30.8   Other conditions related to polyarteritis nodosa
Polyangiitis overlap syndrome

M31- Other necrotizing vasculopathies

M31.0   Hypersensitivity angiitis
Goodpasture's syndrome

M31.1   Thrombotic microangiopathy
Thrombotic thrombocytopenic purpura

M31.2   Lethal midline granuloma

M31.3-   Wegener's granulomatosis
Necrotizing respiratory granulomatosis

M31.30   Wegener's granulomatosis without renal involvement
Wegener's granulomatosis NOS

M31.31   Wegener's granulomatosis with renal involvement

M31.4   Aortic arch syndrome [Takayasu]

M31.5   Giant cell arteritis with polymyalgia rheumatica

M31.6   Other giant cell arteritis

M31.7   Microscopic polyangiitis
Microscopic polyarteritis
Excludes 1: polyarteritis nodosa (M30.0)

M31.8   Other specified necrotizing vasculopathies
Hypocomplementemic vasculitis
Septic vasculitis

M31.9   Necrotizing vasculopathy, unspecified

M32- Systemic lupus erythematosus (SLE)
Excludes 1: lupus erythematosus (discoid) (NOS) (L93.0)

M32.0   Drug-induced systemic lupus erythematosus
Use additional code for adverse effect, if applicable, to identify drug
(T36-T50 with fifth or sixth character 5)

M32.1-   Systemic lupus erythematosus with organ or system involvement

**M32.10   Systemic lupus erythematosus, organ or system involvement
unspecified**

M32.11   Endocarditis in systemic lupus erythematosus
Libman-Sacks disease

M32.12   Pericarditis in systemic lupus erythematosus
Lupus pericarditis

M32.13   Lung involvement in systemic lupus erythematosus
Pleural effusion due to systemic lupus erythematosus

M32.14   Glomerular disease in systemic lupus erythematosus
Lupus renal disease NOS

**M32.15   Tubulo-interstitial nephropathy in systemic lupus
erythematosus**

**M32.19   Other organ or system involvement in systemic lupus
erythematosus**

M32.8   Other forms of systemic lupus erythematosus

M32.9   Systemic lupus erythematosus, unspecified
SLE NOS
Systemic lupus erythematosus NOS
Systemic lupus erythematosus without organ involvement

M33- Dermatopolymyositis

M33.0-   Juvenile dermatopolymyositis

**M33.00   Juvenile dermatopolymyositis, organ involvement
unspecified**

M33.01   Juvenile dermatopolymyositis with respiratory involvement

M33.02   Juvenile dermatopolymyositis with myopathy

M33.09   Juvenile dermatopolymyositis with other organ involvement

M33.1-   Other dermatopolymyositis

M33.10   Other dermatopolymyositis, organ involvement unspecified

M33.11   Other dermatopolymyositis with respiratory involvement

M33.12   Other dermatopolymyositis with myopathy

M33.19   Other dermatopolymyositis with other organ involvement

M33.2-   Polymyositis

M33.20   Polymyositis, organ involvement unspecified

M33.21   Polymyositis with respiratory involvement

M
2
7
-
M
4
1

M33.22 Polymyositis <u>with myopathy</u>

M33.29 Polymyositis <u>with other organ involvement</u>

M33.9- Dermatopolymyositis, <u>unspecified</u>

   M33.90 Dermatopolymyositis, unspecified, organ involvement unspecified

   M33.91 Dermatopolymyositis, unspecified <u>with respiratory involvement</u>

   M33.92 Dermatopolymyositis, unspecified <u>with myopathy</u>

   M33.99 Dermatopolymyositis, unspecified <u>with other organ involvement</u>

M34- Systemic sclerosis [scleroderma]
   Excludes 1: circumscribed scleroderma (L94.0)
             neonatal scleroderma (P83.8)

   M34.0 Progressive systemic sclerosis

   M34.1 CR(E)ST syndrome
      Combination of calcinosis, Raynaud's phenomenon, esophageal dysfunction, sclerodactyly, telangiectasia

   M34.2 Systemic sclerosis induced by drug and chemical
      Code first poisoning due to drug or toxin, if applicable (T36-T65 with fifth or sixth character 1-4 or 6)
      Use additional code for adverse effect, if applicable, to identify drug (T36-T50 with fifth or sixth character 5)

   M34.8- Other forms of systemic sclerosis

   M34.81 Systemic sclerosis <u>with lung involvement</u>

   M34.82 Systemic sclerosis <u>with myopathy</u>

   M34.83 Systemic sclerosis <u>with polyneuropathy</u>

   M34.89 Other systemic sclerosis

   M34.9 Systemic sclerosis, unspecified

M35- Other systemic involvement of connective tissue
   Excludes 1: reactive perforating collagenosis (L87.1)

   M35.0- <u>Sicca syndrome</u> **[Sjögren]**

   M35.00 Sicca syndrome, <u>unspecified</u>

   M35.01 Sicca syndrome <u>with keratoconjunctivitis</u>

   M35.02 Sicca syndrome <u>with lung involvement</u>

   M35.03 Sicca syndrome <u>with myopathy</u>

   M35.04 Sicca syndrome <u>with tubulo-interstitial nephropathy</u>
      Renal tubular acidosis in sicca syndrome

   M35.09 Sicca syndrome <u>with other organ involvement</u>

   M35.1 Other overlap syndromes
      Mixed connective tissue disease
      Excludes 1: polyangiitis overlap syndrome (M30.8)

   M35.2 Behçet's disease

   M35.3 Polymyalgia rheumatica
      Excludes 1: polymyalgia rheumatica with giant cell arteritis (M31.5)

   M35.4 Diffuse (eosinophilic) fasciitis

   M35.5 Multifocal fibrosclerosis

   M35.6 Relapsing panniculitis [Weber-Christian]
      Excludes 1: lupus panniculitis (L93.2)
             panniculitis NOS (M79.3-)

   M35.7 Hypermobility syndrome
      Familial ligamentous laxity
      Excludes 1: Ehlers-Danlos syndrome (Q79.6)
             ligamentous laxity, NOS (M24.2-)

   M35.8 Other specified systemic involvement of connective tissue

   M35.9 Systemic involvement of connective tissue, unspecified
      Autoimmune disease (systemic) NOS
      Collagen (vascular) disease NOS

M36- Systemic disorders of connective tissue in diseases classified elsewhere
   Excludes❷: arthropathies in diseases classified elsewhere (M14.-)

   M36.0 Dermato(poly)myositis in neoplastic disease
      Code first underlying neoplasm (C00-D49)

   M36.1 Arthropathy in neoplastic disease
      Code first underlying neoplasm, such as:
        Leukemia (C91-C95)
        Malignant histiocytosis (C96.A)
        Multiple myeloma (C90.0)

   M36.2 Hemophilic arthropathy
      Hemarthrosis in hemophilic arthropathy
      Code first underlying disease, such as:
        Factor VIII deficiency (D66)
          With vascular defect (D68.0)
        Factor IX deficiency (D67)
        Hemophilia (classical) (D66)
        Hemophilia B (D67)
        Hemophilia C (D68.1)

   M36.3 Arthropathy in other blood disorders

   M36.4 Arthropathy in hypersensitivity reactions classified elsewhere
      Code first underlying disease, such as:
        Henoch (-Schönlein) purpura (D69.0)
        Serum sickness (T80.6-)

   M36.8 Systemic disorders of connective tissue <u>in other diseases classified elsewhere</u>
      Code first underlying disease, such as:
        Alkaptonuria (E70.2)
        Hypogammaglobulinemia (D80.-)
        Ochronosis (E70.2)

Dorsopathies (M40-M54)

Deforming dorsopathies (M40-M43)

M40- Kyphosis and lordosis
   Excludes 1: congenital kyphosis and lordosis (Q76.4)
             kyphoscoliosis (M41.-)
             postprocedural kyphosis and lordosis (M96.-)

   M40.0- Postural kyphosis
      Excludes 1: osteochondrosis of spine (M42.-)

   M40.00 Postural kyphosis, site <u>unspecified</u>

   M40.03 Postural kyphosis, <u>cervicothoracic</u> **region**

   M40.04 Postural kyphosis, <u>thoracic</u> **region**

   M40.05 Postural kyphosis, <u>thoracolumbar</u> **region**

   M40.1- Other secondary kyphosis

   M40.10 Other secondary kyphosis, site <u>unspecified</u>

   M40.12 Other secondary kyphosis, <u>cervical</u> **region**

   M40.13 Other secondary kyphosis, <u>cervicothoracic</u> **region**

   M40.14 Other secondary kyphosis, <u>thoracic</u> **region**

   M40.15 Other secondary kyphosis, <u>thoracolumbar</u> **region**

   M40.2- Other and unspecified kyphosis

   M40.20- <u>Unspecified</u> **kyphosis**

      M40.202 Unspecified kyphosis, cervical region

      M40.203 Unspecified kyphosis, <u>cervicothoracic</u> **region**

      M40.204 Unspecified kyphosis, <u>thoracic</u> **region**

      M40.205 Unspecified kyphosis, <u>thoracolumbar</u> **region**

      M40.209 Unspecified kyphosis, <u>site unspecified</u>

   M40.29- <u>Other</u> **kyphosis**

      M40.292 Other kyphosis, <u>cervical</u> **region**

      M40.293 Other kyphosis, <u>cervicothoracic</u> **region**

      M40.294 Other kyphosis, <u>thoracic</u> **region**

      M40.295 Other kyphosis, <u>thoracolumbar</u> **region**

      M40.299 Other kyphosis, site <u>unspecified</u>

   M40.3- Flatback syndrome

   M40.30 Flatback syndrome, <u>site unspecified</u>

   M40.35 Flatback syndrome, <u>thoracolumbar</u> **region**

   M40.36 Flatback syndrome, <u>lumbar</u> **region**

   M40.37 Flatback syndrome, <u>lumbosacral</u> **region**

   M40.4- Postural lordosis
      Acquired lordosis

   M40.40 Postural lordosis, <u>site unspecified</u>

   M40.45 Postural lordosis, <u>thoracolumbar</u> **region**

   M40.46 Postural lordosis, <u>lumbar</u> **region**

   M40.47 Postural lordosis, <u>lumbosacral</u> **region**

   M40.5- Lordosis, <u>unspecified</u>

   M40.50 Lordosis, unspecified, site <u>unspecified</u>

   M40.55 Lordosis, unspecified, <u>thoracolumbar</u> **region**

   M40.56 Lordosis, unspecified, <u>lumbar</u> **region**

   M40.57 Lordosis, unspecified, <u>lumbosacral</u> **region**

M41- Scoliosis
   Includes: kyphoscoliosis
   Excludes 1: congenital scoliosis NOS (Q67.5)
             congenital scoliosis due to bony malformation (Q76.3)
             postural congenital scoliosis (Q67.5)
             kyphoscoliotic heart disease (I27.1)
             postprocedural scoliosis (M96.-)

   M41.0- <u>Infantile idiopathic</u> **scoliosis**

   M41.00 Infantile idiopathic scoliosis, <u>site unspecified</u>

   M41.02 Infantile idiopathic scoliosis, <u>cervical</u> **region**

   M41.03 Infantile idiopathic scoliosis, <u>cervicothoracic</u> **region**

   M41.04 Infantile idiopathic scoliosis, <u>thoracic</u> **region**

   M41.05 Infantile idiopathic scoliosis, <u>thoracolumbar</u> **region**

   M41.06 Infantile idiopathic scoliosis, <u>lumbar</u> **region**

   M41.07 Infantile idiopathic scoliosis, <u>lumbosacral</u> **region**

   M41.08 Infantile idiopathic scoliosis, <u>sacral and sacrococcygeal</u> **region**

M 2 7 I M 4 1

M41.1- Juvenile and adolescent idiopathic scoliosis
  M41.11- <u>Juvenile idiopathic</u> scoliosis
    M41.112 Juvenile idiopathic scoliosis, <u>cervical</u> region
    M41.113 Juvenile idiopathic scoliosis, <u>cervicothoracic</u> region
    M41.114 Juvenile idiopathic scoliosis, <u>thoracic</u> region
    M41.115 Juvenile idiopathic scoliosis, <u>thoracolumbar</u> region
    M41.116 Juvenile idiopathic scoliosis, <u>lumbar</u> region
    M41.117 Juvenile idiopathic scoliosis, <u>lumbosacral</u> region
    M41.119 Juvenile idiopathic scoliosis, <u>site unspecified</u>
  M41.12-<u>Adolescent</u> scoliosis
    M41.122 Adolescent idiopathic scoliosis, <u>cervical</u> region
    M41.123 Adolescent idiopathic scoliosis, <u>cervicothoracic</u> region
    M41.124 Adolescent idiopathic scoliosis, <u>thoracic</u> region
    M41.125 Adolescent idiopathic scoliosis, <u>thoracolumbar</u> region
    M41.126 Adolescent idiopathic scoliosis, <u>lumbar</u> region
    M41.127 Adolescent idiopathic scoliosis, <u>lumbosacral</u> region
    M41.129 Adolescent idiopathic scoliosis, <u>site unspecified</u>
M41.2- <u>Other idiopathic</u> scoliosis
  M41.20 Other idiopathic scoliosis, <u>site unspecified</u>
  M41.22 Other idiopathic scoliosis, <u>cervical</u> region
  M41.23 Other idiopathic scoliosis, <u>cervicothoracic</u> region
  M41.24 Other idiopathic scoliosis, <u>thoracic</u> region
  M41.25 Other idiopathic scoliosis, <u>thoracolumbar</u> region
  M41.26 Other idiopathic scoliosis, <u>lumbar</u> region
  M41.27 Other idiopathic scoliosis, <u>lumbosacral</u> region
M41.3- <u>Thoracogenic</u> scoliosis
  M41.30 Thoracogenic scoliosis, <u>site unspecified</u>
  M41.34 Thoracogenic scoliosis, <u>thoracic</u> region
  M41.35 Thoracogenic scoliosis, <u>thoracolumbar</u> region
M41.4- <u>Neuromuscular</u> scoliosis
    Scoliosis secondary to cerebral palsy, Friedreich's ataxia, poliomyelitis and other neuromuscular disorders
    Code also underlying condition
  M41.40 Neuromuscular scoliosis, <u>site unspecified</u>
  M41.41 Neuromuscular scoliosis, <u>occipito-atlanto-axial</u> region
  M41.42 Neuromuscular scoliosis, <u>cervical</u> region
  M41.43 Neuromuscular scoliosis, <u>cervicothoracic</u> region
  M41.44 Neuromuscular scoliosis, <u>thoracic</u> region
  M41.45 Neuromuscular scoliosis, <u>thoracolumbar</u> region
  M41.46 Neuromuscular scoliosis, <u>lumbar</u> region
  M41.47 Neuromuscular scoliosis, <u>lumbosacral</u> region
M41.5- <u>Other secondary</u> scoliosis
  M41.50 Other secondary scoliosis, <u>site unspecified</u>
  M41.52 Other secondary scoliosis, <u>cervical</u> region
  M41.53 Other secondary scoliosis, <u>cervicothoracic</u> region
  M41.54 Other secondary scoliosis, <u>thoracic</u> region
  M41.55 Other secondary scoliosis, <u>thoracolumbar</u> region
  M41.56 Other secondary scoliosis, <u>lumbar</u> region
  M41.57 Other secondary scoliosis, <u>lumbosacral</u> region
M41.8- <u>Other forms</u> of scoliosis
  M41.80 Other forms of scoliosis, <u>site unspecified</u>
  M41.82 Other forms of scoliosis, <u>cervical</u> region
  M41.83 Other forms of scoliosis, <u>cervicothoracic</u> region
  M41.84 Other forms of scoliosis, <u>thoracic</u> region
  M41.85 Other forms of scoliosis, <u>thoracolumbar</u> region
  M41.86 Other forms of scoliosis, <u>lumbar</u> region
  M41.87 Other forms of scoliosis, <u>lumbosacral</u> region
M41.9 Scoliosis, unspecified

M42- Spinal osteochondrosis
M42.0- <u>Juvenile</u> osteochondrosis of spine
    Calvé's disease
    Scheuermann's disease
    Excludes 1: postural kyphosis (M40.0)
  M42.00 Juvenile osteochondrosis of spine, <u>site unspecified</u>
  M42.01 Juvenile osteochondrosis of spine, <u>occipito-atlanto-axial</u> region
  M42.02 Juvenile osteochondrosis of spine, <u>cervical</u> region
  M42.03 Juvenile osteochondrosis of spine, <u>cervicothoracic</u> region
  M42.04 Juvenile osteochondrosis of spine, <u>thoracic</u> region
  M42.05 Juvenile osteochondrosis of spine, <u>thoracolumbar</u> region
  M42.06 Juvenile osteochondrosis of spine, <u>lumbar</u> region
  M42.07 Juvenile osteochondrosis of spine, <u>lumbosacral</u> region
  M42.08 Juvenile osteochondrosis of spine, <u>sacral and sacrococcygeal</u> region
  M42.09 Juvenile osteochondrosis of spine, <u>multiple sites</u> in spine

M42.1- <u>Adult</u> osteochondrosis of spine
  M42.10 Adult osteochondrosis of spine, <u>site unspecified</u>
  M42.11 Adult osteochondrosis of spine, <u>occipito-atlanto-axial</u> region
  M42.12 Adult osteochondrosis of spine, <u>cervical</u> region
  M42.13 Adult osteochondrosis of spine, <u>cervicothoracic</u> region
  M42.14 Adult osteochondrosis of spine, <u>thoracic</u> region
  M42.15 Adult osteochondrosis of spine, <u>thoracolumbar</u> region
  M42.16 Adult osteochondrosis of spine, <u>lumbar</u> region
  M42.17 Adult osteochondrosis of spine, <u>lumbosacral</u> region
  M42.18 Adult osteochondrosis of spine, <u>sacral and sacrococcygeal</u> region
  M42.19 Adult osteochondrosis of spine, <u>multiple sites</u> in spine
M42.9 Spinal osteochondrosis, unspecified

M43- Other deforming dorsopathies
  Excludes 1: congenital spondylolysis and spondylolisthesis (Q76.2)
          hemivertebra (Q76.3-Q76.4)
          Klippel-Feil syndrome (Q76.1)
          lumbarization and sacralization (Q76.4)
          platyspondylisis (Q76.4)
          spina bifida occulta (Q76.0)
          spinal curvature in osteoporosis (M80.-)
          spinal curvature in Paget's disease of bone [osteitis deformans] (M88.-)
M43.0- <u>Spondylolysis</u>
  Excludes 1: congenital spondylolysis (Q76.2)
          spondylolisthesis (M43.1)
  M43.00 Spondylolysis, <u>site unspecified</u>
  M43.01 Spondylolysis, <u>occipito-atlanto-axial</u> region
  M43.02 Spondylolysis, <u>cervical</u> region
  M43.03 Spondylolysis, <u>cervicothoracic</u> region
  M43.04 Spondylolysis, <u>thoracic</u> region
  M43.05 Spondylolysis, <u>thoracolumbar</u> region
  M43.06 Spondylolysis, <u>lumbar</u> region
  M43.07 Spondylolysis, <u>lumbosacral</u> region
  M43.08 Spondylolysis, <u>sacral and sacrococcygeal</u> region
  M43.09 Spondylolysis, <u>multiple sites</u> in spine
M43.1- <u>Spondylolisthesis</u>
  Excludes 1: acute traumatic of lumbosacral region (S33.1)
          acute traumatic of sites other than lumbosacral — code to Fracture, vertebra, by region
          congenital spondylolisthesis (Q76.2)
  M43.10 Spondylolisthesis, <u>site unspecified</u>
  M43.11 Spondylolisthesis, <u>occipito-atlanto-axial</u> region
  M43.12 Spondylolisthesis, <u>cervical</u> region
  M43.13 Spondylolisthesis, <u>cervicothoracic</u> region
  M43.14 Spondylolisthesis, <u>thoracic</u> region
  M43.15 Spondylolisthesis, <u>thoracolumbar</u> region
  M43.16 Spondylolisthesis, <u>lumbar</u> region
  M43.17 Spondylolisthesis, <u>lumbosacral</u> region
  M43.18 Spondylolisthesis, <u>sacral and sacrococcygeal</u> region
  M43.19 Spondylolisthesis, <u>multiple sites</u> in spine
M43.2- <u>Fusion of spine</u>
    Ankylosis of spinal joint
  Excludes 1: ankylosing spondylitis (M45.0-)
          congenital fusion of spine (Q76.4)
  Excludes❷: arthrodesis status (Z98.1)
          pseudoarthrosis after fusion or arthrodesis (M96.0)
  M43.20 Fusion of spine, <u>site unspecified</u>
  M43.21 Fusion of spine, <u>occipito-atlanto-axial</u> region
  M43.22 Fusion of spine, <u>cervical</u> region
  M43.23 Fusion of spine, <u>cervicothoracic</u> region
  M43.24 Fusion of spine, <u>thoracic</u> region
  M43.25 Fusion of spine, <u>thoracolumbar</u> region
  M43.26 Fusion of spine, <u>lumbar</u> region
  M43.27 Fusion of spine, <u>lumbosacral</u> region
  M43.28 Fusion of spine, <u>sacral and sacrococcygeal</u> region
M43.3 Recurrent atlantoaxial dislocation with myelopathy
M43.4 Other recurrent atlantoaxial dislocation
M43.5- Other recurrent vertebral dislocation
  Excludes 1: biomechanical lesions NEC (M99.-)
  M43.5x-<u>Other recurrent vertebral dislocation</u>
    M43.5x2 Other recurrent vertebral dislocation, <u>cervical</u> region
    M43.5x3 Other recurrent vertebral dislocation, <u>cervicothoracic</u> region
    M43.5x4 Other recurrent vertebral dislocation, <u>thoracic</u> region
    M43.5x5 Other recurrent vertebral dislocation, <u>thoracolumbar</u> region
    M43.5x6 Other recurrent vertebral dislocation, <u>lumbar</u> region

M41 - M46

M43.5x7 Other recurrent vertebral dislocation, <u>lumbosacral</u> region

M43.5x8 Other recurrent vertebral dislocation, <u>sacral and sacrococcygeal</u> region

M43.5x9 Other recurrent vertebral dislocation, <u>site unspecified</u>

M43.6 Torticollis
Excludes 1: *congenital (sternomastoid) torticollis (Q68.0)*
current injury — see Injury, of spine, by body region
ocular torticollis (R29.891)
psychogenic torticollis (F45.8)
spasmodic torticollis (G24.3)
torticollis due to birth injury (P15.2)

M43.8- Other specified deforming dorsopathies
Excludes❷: kyphosis and lordosis (M40.-)
scoliosis (M41.-)

M43.8x-<u>Other specified deforming dorsopathies</u>

M43.8x1 Other specified deforming dorsopathies, <u>occipito-atlanto-axial</u> region

M43.8x2 Other specified deforming dorsopathies, <u>cervical</u> region

M43.8x3 Other specified deforming dorsopathies, <u>cervicothoracic</u> region

M43.8x4 Other specified deforming dorsopathies, <u>thoracic</u> region

M43.8x5 Other specified deforming dorsopathies, <u>thoracolumbar</u> region

M43.8x6 Other specified deforming dorsopathies, <u>lumbar</u> region

M43.8x7 Other specified deforming dorsopathies, <u>lumbosacral</u> region

M43.8x8 Other specified deforming dorsopathies, <u>sacral and sacrococcygeal</u> region

M43.8x9 Other specified deforming dorsopathies, <u>site unspecified</u>

M43.9 Deforming dorsopathy, unspecified
Curvature of spine NOS

Spondylopathies (M45-M49)

M45- <u>Ankylosing spondylitis</u>
Rheumatoid arthritis of spine
Excludes 1: arthropathy in Reiter's disease (M02.3-)
juvenile (ankylosing) spondylitis (M08.1)
Excludes❷: Behçet's disease (M35.2)

M45.0 Ankylosing spondylitis of <u>multiple sites</u> in spine
M45.1 Ankylosing spondylitis of <u>occipito-atlanto-axial</u> region
M45.2 Ankylosing spondylitis of <u>cervical</u> region
M45.3 Ankylosing spondylitis of <u>cervicothoracic</u> region
M45.4 Ankylosing spondylitis of <u>thoracic</u> region
M45.5 Ankylosing spondylitis of <u>thoracolumbar</u> region
M45.6 Ankylosing spondylitis of <u>lumbar</u> region
M45.7 Ankylosing spondylitis of <u>lumbosacral</u> region
M45.8 Ankylosing spondylitis <u>sacral and sacrococcygeal</u> region
M45.9 Ankylosing spondylitis of <u>unspecified</u> sites in spine

M46- Other inflammatory spondylopathies
M46.0- <u>Spinal enthesopathy</u>
Disorder of ligamentous or muscular attachments of spine
M46.00 Spinal enthesopathy, <u>site unspecified</u>
M46.01 Spinal enthesopathy, <u>occipito-atlanto-axial</u> region
M46.02 Spinal enthesopathy, <u>cervical</u> region
M46.03 Spinal enthesopathy, <u>cervicothoracic</u> region
M46.04 Spinal enthesopathy, <u>thoracic</u> region
M46.05 Spinal enthesopathy, <u>thoracolumbar</u> region
M46.06 Spinal enthesopathy, <u>lumbar</u> region
M46.07 Spinal enthesopathy, <u>lumbosacral</u> region
M46.08 Spinal enthesopathy, <u>sacral and sacrococcygeal</u> region
M46.09 Spinal enthesopathy, <u>multiple sites</u> in spine
M46.1 Sacroiliitis, not elsewhere classified
M46.2- <u>Osteomyelitis</u> of vertebra
M46.20 Osteomyelitis of vertebra, <u>site unspecified</u>
M46.21 Osteomyelitis of vertebra, <u>occipito-atlanto-axial</u> region
M46.22 Osteomyelitis of vertebra, <u>cervical</u> region
M46.23 Osteomyelitis of vertebra, <u>cervicothoracic</u> region
M46.24 Osteomyelitis of vertebra, <u>thoracic</u> region
M46.25 Osteomyelitis of vertebra, <u>thoracolumbar</u> region
M46.26 Osteomyelitis of vertebra, <u>lumbar</u> region
M46.27 Osteomyelitis of vertebra, <u>lumbosacral</u> region
M46.28 Osteomyelitis of vertebra, <u>sacral and sacrococcygeal</u> region

M46.3- <u>Infection of intervertebral disc (pyogenic)</u>
Use additional code (B95-B97) to identify infectious agent
M46.30 Infection of intervertebral disc (pyogenic), <u>site unspecified</u>
M46.31 Infection of intervertebral disc (pyogenic), <u>occipito-atlanto-axial</u> region
M46.32 Infection of intervertebral disc (pyogenic), <u>cervical</u> region
M46.33 Infection of intervertebral disc (pyogenic), <u>cervicothoracic</u> region
M46.34 Infection of intervertebral disc (pyogenic), <u>thoracic</u> region
M46.35 Infection of intervertebral disc (pyogenic), <u>thoracolumbar</u> region
M46.36 Infection of intervertebral disc (pyogenic), <u>lumbar</u> region
M46.37 Infection of intervertebral disc (pyogenic), <u>lumbosacral</u> region
M46.38 Infection of intervertebral disc (pyogenic), <u>sacral and sacrococcygeal</u> region
M46.39 Infection of intervertebral disc (pyogenic), <u>multiple sites</u> in spine

M46.4- <u>Discitis, unspecified</u>
M46.40 Discitis, unspecified, <u>site unspecified</u>
M46.41 Discitis, unspecified, <u>occipito-atlanto-axial</u> region
M46.42 Discitis, unspecified, <u>cervical</u> region
M46.43 Discitis, unspecified, <u>cervicothoracic</u> region
M46.44 Discitis, unspecified, <u>thoracic</u> region
M46.45 Discitis, unspecified, <u>thoracolumbar</u> region
M46.46 Discitis, unspecified, <u>lumbar</u> region
M46.47 Discitis, unspecified, <u>lumbosacral</u> region
M46.48 Discitis, unspecified, <u>sacral and sacrococcygeal</u> region
M46.49 Discitis, unspecified, <u>multiple sites</u> in spine

M46.5- <u>Other infective</u> spondylopathies
M46.50 Other infective spondylopathies, <u>site unspecified</u>
M46.51 Other infective spondylopathies, <u>occipito-atlanto-axial</u> region
M46.52 Other infective spondylopathies, <u>cervical</u> region
M46.53 Other infective spondylopathies, <u>cervicothoracic</u> region
M46.54 Other infective spondylopathies, <u>thoracic</u> region
M46.55 Other infective spondylopathies, <u>thoracolumbar</u> region
M46.56 Other infective spondylopathies, <u>lumbar</u> region
M46.57 Other infective spondylopathies, <u>lumbosacral</u> region
M46.58 Other infective spondylopathies, <u>sacral and sacrococcygeal</u> region
M46.59 Other infective spondylopathies, <u>multiple sites</u> in spine

M46.8- <u>Other specified inflammatory</u> spondylopathies
M46.80 Other specified inflammatory spondylopathies, <u>site unspecified</u>
M46.81 Other specified inflammatory spondylopathies, <u>occipito-atlanto-axial</u> region
M46.82 Other specified inflammatory spondylopathies, <u>cervical</u> region
M46.83 Other specified inflammatory spondylopathies, <u>cervicothoracic</u> region
M46.84 Other specified inflammatory spondylopathies, <u>thoracic</u> region
M46.85 Other specified inflammatory spondylopathies, <u>thoracolumbar</u> region
M46.86 Other specified inflammatory spondylopathies, <u>lumbar</u> region
M46.87 Other specified inflammatory spondylopathies, <u>lumbosacral</u> region
M46.88 Other specified inflammatory spondylopathies, <u>sacral and sacrococcygeal</u> region
M46.89 Other specified inflammatory spondylopathies, <u>multiple sites</u> in spine

M46.9- <u>Unspecified</u> inflammatory spondylopathy
M46.90 Unspecified inflammatory spondylopathy, <u>site unspecified</u>
M46.91 Unspecified inflammatory spondylopathy, <u>occipito-atlanto-axial</u> region
M46.92 Unspecified inflammatory spondylopathy, <u>cervical</u> region
M46.93 Unspecified inflammatory spondylopathy, <u>cervicothoracic</u> region
M46.94 Unspecified inflammatory spondylopathy, <u>thoracic</u> region
M46.95 Unspecified inflammatory spondylopathy, <u>thoracolumbar</u> region
M46.96 Unspecified inflammatory spondylopathy, <u>lumbar</u> region
M46.97 Unspecified inflammatory spondylopathy, <u>lumbosacral</u> region
M46.98 Unspecified inflammatory spondylopathy, <u>sacral and sacrococcygeal</u> region

M41 - M46

Excludes 1: = NOT CODED HERE! (Do not code both)   **573**   *Excludes❷:* = Not Included Here

M46.99 Unspecified inflammatory spondylopathy, <u>multiple sites</u> in spine

M47- <u>Spondylosis</u>
Includes: Arthrosis or osteoarthritis of spine
         Degeneration of facet joints

M47.0- Anterior spinal and vertebral artery compression syndromes

M47.01-<u>Anterior spinal artery compression syndromes</u>

M47.011 Anterior spinal artery compression syndromes, <u>occipito-atlanto-axial</u> region

M47.012 Anterior spinal artery compression syndromes, <u>cervical</u> region

M47.013 Anterior spinal artery compression syndromes, <u>cervicothoracic</u> region

M47.014 Anterior spinal artery compression syndromes, <u>thoracic</u> region

M47.015 Anterior spinal artery compression syndromes, <u>thoracolumbar</u> region

M47.016 Anterior spinal artery compression syndromes, <u>lumbar</u> region

M47.019 Anterior spinal artery compression syndromes, <u>site unspecified</u>

M47.02-<u>Vertebral artery compression syndromes</u>

M47.021 Vertebral artery compression syndromes, <u>occipito-atlanto-axial</u> region

M47.022 Vertebral artery compression syndromes, <u>cervical</u> region

M47.029 Vertebral artery compression syndromes, <u>site unspecified</u>

M47.1- <u>Other</u> spondylosis <u>with myelopathy</u>
Spondylogenic compression of spinal cord
Excludes 1: vertebral subluxation (M43.3-M43.59)

M47.10 Other spondylosis with myelopathy, <u>site unspecified</u>

M47.11 Other spondylosis with myelopathy, <u>occipito-atlanto-axial</u> region

M47.12 Other spondylosis with myelopathy, <u>cervical</u> region

M47.13 Other spondylosis with myelopathy, <u>cervicothoracic</u> region

M47.14 Other spondylosis with myelopathy, <u>thoracic</u> region

M47.15 Other spondylosis with myelopathy, <u>thoracolumbar</u> region

M47.16 Other spondylosis with myelopathy, <u>lumbar</u> region

M47.2- <u>Other</u> spondylosis <u>with radiculopathy</u>

M47.20 Other spondylosis with radiculopathy, <u>site unspecified</u>

M47.21 Other spondylosis with radiculopathy, <u>occipito-atlanto-axial</u> region

M47.22 Other spondylosis with radiculopathy, <u>cervical</u> region

M47.23 Other spondylosis with radiculopathy, <u>cervicothoracic</u> region

M47.24 Other spondylosis with radiculopathy, <u>thoracic</u> region

M47.25 Other spondylosis with radiculopathy, <u>thoracolumbar</u> region

M47.26 Other spondylosis with radiculopathy, <u>lumbar</u> region

M47.27 Other spondylosis with radiculopathy, <u>lumbosacral</u> region

M47.28 Other spondylosis with radiculopathy, <u>sacral and sacrococcygeal</u> region

M47.8- <u>Other</u> spondylosis

M47.81-Spondylosis <u>without</u> myelopathy or radiculopathy

M47.811 Spondylosis without myelopathy or radiculopathy, <u>occipito-atlanto-axial</u> region

M47.812 Spondylosis without myelopathy or radiculopathy, <u>cervical</u> region

M47.813 Spondylosis without myelopathy or radiculopathy, <u>cervicothoracic</u> region

M47.814 Spondylosis without myelopathy or radiculopathy, <u>thoracic</u> region

M47.815 Spondylosis without myelopathy or radiculopathy, <u>thoracolumbar</u> region

M47.816 Spondylosis without myelopathy or radiculopathy, <u>lumbar</u> region

M47.817 Spondylosis without myelopathy or radiculopathy, <u>lumbosacral</u> region

M47.818 Spondylosis without myelopathy or radiculopathy, <u>sacral and sacrococcygeal</u> region

M47.819 Spondylosis without myelopathy or radiculopathy, <u>site unspecified</u>

M47.89-Other spondylosis

M47.891 Other spondylosis, <u>occipito-atlanto-axial</u> region

M47.892 Other spondylosis, <u>cervical</u> region

M47.893 Other spondylosis, <u>cervicothoracic</u> region

M47.894 Other spondylosis, <u>thoracic</u> region

M47.895 Other spondylosis, <u>thoracolumbar</u> region

M47.896 Other spondylosis, <u>lumbar</u> region

M47.897 Other spondylosis, <u>lumbosacral</u> region

M47.898 Other spondylosis, <u>sacral and sacrococcygeal</u> region

M47.899 Other spondylosis, <u>site unspecified</u>

M47.9 Spondylosis, unspecified

M48- Other spondylopathies

M48.0- <u>Spinal stenosis</u>
Caudal stenosis

M48.00 Spinal stenosis, <u>site unspecified</u>

M48.01 Spinal stenosis, <u>occipito-atlanto-axial</u> region

M48.02 Spinal stenosis, <u>cervical</u> region

M48.03 Spinal stenosis, <u>cervicothoracic</u> region

M48.04 Spinal stenosis, <u>thoracic</u> region

M48.05 Spinal stenosis, <u>thoracolumbar</u> region

M48.06 Spinal stenosis, <u>lumbar</u> region

M48.07 Spinal stenosis, <u>lumbosacral</u> region

M48.08 Spinal stenosis, <u>sacral and sacrococcygeal</u> region

M48.1- <u>Ankylosing hyperostosis [Forestier]</u>
Diffuse idiopathic skeletal hyperostosis [DISH]

M48.10 Ankylosing hyperostosis [Forestier], <u>site unspecified</u>

M48.11 Ankylosing hyperostosis [Forestier], <u>occipito-atlanto-axial</u> region

M48.12 Ankylosing hyperostosis [Forestier], <u>cervical</u> region

M48.13 Ankylosing hyperostosis [Forestier], <u>cervicothoracic</u> region

M48.14 Ankylosing hyperostosis [Forestier], <u>thoracic</u> region

M48.15 Ankylosing hyperostosis [Forestier], <u>thoracolumbar</u> region

M48.16 Ankylosing hyperostosis [Forestier], <u>lumbar</u> region

M48.17 Ankylosing hyperostosis [Forestier], <u>lumbosacral</u> region

M48.18 Ankylosing hyperostosis [Forestier], <u>sacral and sacrococcygeal</u> region

M48.19 Ankylosing hyperostosis [Forestier], <u>multiple sites</u> in spine

M48.2- <u>Kissing spine</u>

M48.20 Kissing spine, <u>site unspecified</u>

M48.21 Kissing spine, <u>occipito-atlanto-axial</u> region

M48.22 Kissing spine, <u>cervical</u> region

M48.23 Kissing spine, <u>cervicothoracic</u> region

M48.24 Kissing spine, <u>thoracic</u> region

M48.25 Kissing spine, <u>thoracolumbar</u> region

M48.26 Kissing spine, <u>lumbar</u> region

M48.27 Kissing spine, <u>lumbosacral</u> region

M48.3- <u>Traumatic spondylopathy</u>

M48.30 Traumatic spondylopathy, <u>site unspecified</u>

M48.31 Traumatic spondylopathy, <u>occipito-atlanto-axial</u> region

M48.32 Traumatic spondylopathy, <u>cervical</u> region

M48.33 Traumatic spondylopathy, <u>cervicothoracic</u> region

M48.34 Traumatic spondylopathy, <u>thoracic</u> region

M48.35 Traumatic spondylopathy, <u>thoracolumbar</u> region

M48.36 Traumatic spondylopathy, <u>lumbar</u> region

M48.37 Traumatic spondylopathy, <u>lumbosacral</u> region

M48.38 Traumatic spondylopathy, <u>sacral and sacrococcygeal</u> region

M48.4- <u>Fatigue fracture</u> of vertebra
Stress fracture of vertebra
Excludes 1: pathological fracture NOS (M84.4-)
*   pathological fracture of vertebra due to neoplasm (M84.58)*
*   pathological fracture of vertebra due to other diagnosis (M84.68)*
*   pathological fracture of vertebra due to osteoporosis (M80-)*
*   traumatic fracture of vertebrae (S12.0-S12.3-, S22.0-, S32.0-)*

The appropriate 7th character is to be added to each code from subcategory M48.4:
A   Initial encounter for fracture
D   Subsequent encounter for fracture with routine healing
G   Subsequent encounter for fracture with delayed healing
S   Sequela of fracture

M48.40x- Fatigue fracture of vertebra, <u>site unspecified</u>

M48.41x- Fatigue fracture of vertebra, <u>occipito-atlanto-axial</u> region

M48.42x- Fatigue fracture of vertebra, <u>cervical</u> region

M48.43x- Fatigue fracture of vertebra, <u>cervicothoracic</u> region

M48.44x- Fatigue fracture of vertebra, <u>thoracic</u> region

M48.45x- Fatigue fracture of vertebra, <u>thoracolumbar</u> region

M48.46x- Fatigue fracture of vertebra, <u>lumbar</u> region

M48.47x- Fatigue fracture of vertebra, <u>lumbosacral</u> region

M48.48x- Fatigue fracture of vertebra, <u>sacral and sacrococcygeal</u> region

M46 - M50

© 2013 Channel Publishing Ltd

M48.5- Collapsed vertebra, not elsewhere classified
Collapsed vertebra NOS
Wedging of vertebra NOS
Excludes 1: current injury — see Injury of spine, by body region
fatigue fracture of vertebra (M48.4)
pathological fracture of vertebra due to neoplasm (M84.58)
pathological fracture of vertebra due to other diagnosis (M84.68)
pathological fracture of vertebra due to osteoporosis (M80.-)
pathological fracture NOS (M84.4-)
stress fracture of vertebra (M48.4-)
traumatic fracture of vertebra (S12.-, S22.-, S32.-)

The appropriate 7th character is to be added to each code from subcategory M48.5:
A   Initial encounter for fracture
D   Subsequent encounter for fracture with routine healing
G   Subsequent encounter for fracture with delayed healing
S   Sequela of fracture

M48.50x- Collapsed vertebra, not elsewhere classified, site unspecified
M48.51x- Collapsed vertebra, not elsewhere classified, occipito-atlanto-axial region
M48.52x- Collapsed vertebra, not elsewhere classified, cervical region
M48.53x- Collapsed vertebra, not elsewhere classified, cervicothoracic region
M48.54x- Collapsed vertebra, not elsewhere classified, thoracic region
M48.55x- Collapsed vertebra, not elsewhere classified, thoracolumbar region
M48.56x- Collapsed vertebra, not elsewhere classified, lumbar region
M48.57x- Collapsed vertebra, not elsewhere classified, lumbosacral region
M48.58x- Collapsed vertebra, not elsewhere classified, sacral and sacrococcygeal region

M48.8- Other specified spondylopathies
Ossification of posterior longitudinal ligament
M48.8x-Other specified spondylopathies
M48.8x1 Other specified spondylopathies, occipito-atlanto-axial region
M48.8x2 Other specified spondylopathies, cervical region
M48.8x3 Other specified spondylopathies, cervicothoracic region
M48.8x4 Other specified spondylopathies, thoracic region
M48.8x5 Other specified spondylopathies, thoracolumbar region
M48.8x6 Other specified spondylopathies, lumbar region
M48.8x7 Other specified spondylopathies, lumbosacral region
M48.8x8 Other specified spondylopathies, sacral and sacrococcygeal region
M48.8x9 Other specified spondylopathies, site unspecified
M48.9 Spondylopathy, unspecified

M49- Spondylopathies in diseases classified elsewhere
Includes: Curvature of spine in diseases classified elsewhere
Deformity of spine in diseases classified elsewhere
Kyphosis in diseases classified elsewhere
Scoliosis in diseases classified elsewhere
Spondylopathy in diseases classified elsewhere
Code first underlying disease, such as:
Brucellosis (A23.-)
Charcot-Marie-Tooth disease (G60.0)
Enterobacterial infections (A01-A04)
Osteitis fibrosa cystica (E21.0)
Excludes 1: curvature of spine in tuberculosis [Pott's] (A18.01)
enteropathic arthropathies (M07.-)
gonococcal spondylitis (A54.41)
neuropathic spondylopathy in syringomyelia (G95.0)
neuropathic spondylopathy in tabes dorsalis (A52.11)
neuropathic [tabes dorsalis] spondylitis (A52.11)
nonsyphilitic neuropathic spondylopathy NEC (G98.0)
spondylitis in syphilis (acquired) (A52.77)
tuberculosis spondylitis (A18.01)
typhoid fever spondylitis (A01.05)
M49.8- Spondylopathy in diseases classified elsewhere
M49.80 Spondylopathy in diseases classified elsewhere, site unspecified
M49.81 Spondylopathy in diseases classified elsewhere, occipito-atlanto-axial region
M49.82 Spondylopathy in diseases classified elsewhere, cervical region
M49.83 Spondylopathy in diseases classified elsewhere, cervicothoracic region
M49.84 Spondylopathy in diseases classified elsewhere, thoracic region
M49.85 Spondylopathy in diseases classified elsewhere, thoracolumbar region
M49.86 Spondylopathy in diseases classified elsewhere, lumbar region
M49.87 Spondylopathy in diseases classified elsewhere, lumbosacral region
M49.88 Spondylopathy in diseases classified elsewhere, sacral and sacrococcygeal region
M49.89 Spondylopathy in diseases classified elsewhere, multiple sites in spine

Other dorsopathies (M50-M54)

Excludes 1: current injury — see injury of spine by body region
discitis NOS (M46.4-)

M50- Cervical disc disorders
Note: Code to the most superior level of disorder
Includes: Cervicothoracic disc disorders with cervicalgia
Cervicothoracic disc disorders
M50.0- Cervical disc disorder with myelopathy
M50.00 Cervical disc disorder with myelopathy, unspecified cervical region
M50.01 Cervical disc disorder with myelopathy, high cervical region
C2-C3 disc disorder with myelopathy
C3-C4 disc disorder with myelopathy
M50.02 Cervical disc disorder with myelopathy, mid-cervical region
C4-C5 disc disorder with myelopathy
C5-C6 disc disorder with myelopathy
C6-C7 disc disorder with myelopathy
M50.03 Cervical disc disorder with myelopathy, cervicothoracic region
C7-T1 disc disorder with myelopathy
M50.1- Cervical disc disorder with radiculopathy
Excludes❷: brachial radiculitis NOS (M54.13)
M50.10 Cervical disc disorder with radiculopathy, unspecified cervical region
M50.11 Cervical disc disorder with radiculopathy, high cervical region
C2-C3 disc disorder with radiculopathy
C3 radiculopathy due to disc disorder
C3-C4 disc disorder with radiculopathy
C4 radiculopathy due to disc disorder
M50.12 Cervical disc disorder with radiculopathy, mid-cervical region
C4-C5 disc disorder with radiculopathy
C5 radiculopathy due to disc disorder
C5-C6 disc disorder with radiculopathy
C6 radiculopathy due to disc disorder
C6-C7 disc disorder with radiculopathy
C7 radiculopathy due to disc disorder
M50.13 Cervical disc disorder with radiculopathy, cervicothoracic region
C7-T1 disc disorder with radiculopathy
C8 radiculopathy due to disc disorder
M50.2- Other cervical disc displacement
M50.20 Other cervical disc displacement, unspecified cervical region
M50.21 Other cervical disc displacement, high cervical region
Other C2-C3 cervical disc displacement
Other C3-C4 cervical disc displacement
M50.22 Other cervical disc displacement, mid-cervical region
Other C4-C5 cervical disc displacement
Other C5-C6 cervical disc displacement
Other C6-C7 cervical disc displacement
M50.23 Other cervical disc displacement, cervicothoracic region
Other C7-T1 cervical disc displacement
M50.3- Other cervical disc degeneration
M50.30 Other cervical disc degeneration, unspecified cervical region
M50.31 Other cervical disc degeneration, high cervical region
Other C2-C3 cervical disc degeneration
Other C3-C4 cervical disc degeneration
M50.32 Other cervical disc degeneration, mid-cervical region
Other C4-C5 cervical disc degeneration
Other C5-C6 cervical disc degeneration
Other C6-C7 cervical disc degeneration
M50.33 Other cervical disc degeneration, cervicothoracic region
Other C7-T1 cervical disc degeneration

M46 I M50

M50.8- <u>Other cervical disc disorders</u>

M50.80 Other cervical disc disorders, <u>unspecified</u> <u>cervical</u> region

M50.81 Other cervical disc disorders, <u>high cervical</u> region
   Other C2-C3 cervical disc disorders
   Other C3-C4 cervical disc disorders

M50.82 Other cervical disc disorders, <u>mid-cervical</u> region
   Other C4-C5 cervical disc disorders
   Other C5-C6 cervical disc disorders
   Other C6-C7 cervical disc disorders

M50.83 Other cervical disc disorders, <u>cervicothoracic</u> region
   Other C7-T1 cervical disc disorders

M50.9- Cervical disc disorder, <u>unspecified</u>

M50.90 Cervical disc disorder, unspecified, <u>unspecified</u> <u>cervical</u> region

M50.91 Cervical disc disorder, unspecified, <u>high cervical</u> region
   C2-C3 cervical disc disorder, unspecified
   C3-C4 cervical disc disorder, unspecified

M50.92 Cervical disc disorder, unspecified, <u>mid-cervical</u> region
   C4-C5 cervical disc disorder, unspecified
   C5-C6 cervical disc disorder, unspecified
   C6-C7 cervical disc disorder, unspecified

M50.93 Cervical disc disorder, unspecified, <u>cervicothoracic</u> region
   C7-T1 cervical disc disorder, unspecified

M51- <u>Thoracic, thoracolumbar, and lumbosacral intervertebral disc</u> <u>disorders</u>
   Excludes❷: cervical and cervicothoracic disc disorders (M50.-)
      sacral and sacrococcygeal disorders (M53.3)

M51.0- Thoracic, thoracolumbar and lumbosacral intervertebral disc disorders <u>with myelopathy</u>

M51.04 Intervertebral disc disorders with myelopathy, <u>thoracic</u> region

M51.05 Intervertebral disc disorders with myelopathy, <u>thoracolumbar</u> region

M51.06 Intervertebral disc disorders with myelopathy, <u>lumbar</u> region

M51.1- Thoracic, thoracolumbar and lumbosacral intervertebral disc disorders <u>with radiculopathy</u>
   Sciatica due to intervertebral disc disorder
   Excludes 1: lumbar radiculitis NOS (M54.16)
      sciatica NOS (M54.3)

M51.14 Intervertebral disc disorders with radiculopathy, <u>thoracic</u> region

M51.15 Intervertebral disc disorders with radiculopathy, <u>thoracolumbar</u> region

M51.16 Intervertebral disc disorders with radiculopathy, <u>lumbar</u> region

M51.17 Intervertebral disc disorders with radiculopathy, <u>lumbosacral</u> region

M51.2- <u>Other</u> thoracic, thoracolumbar and lumbosacral intervertebral disc <u>displacement</u>
   Lumbago due to displacement of intervertebral disc

M51.24 Other intervertebral disc displacement, <u>thoracic</u> region

M51.25 Other intervertebral disc displacement, <u>thoracolumbar</u> region

M51.26 Other intervertebral disc displacement, <u>lumbar</u> region

M51.27 Other intervertebral disc displacement, <u>lumbosacral</u> region

M51.3- <u>Other</u> thoracic, thoracolumbar and lumbosacral intervertebral disc <u>degeneration</u>

M51.34 Other intervertebral disc degeneration, <u>thoracic</u> region

M51.35 Other intervertebral disc degeneration, <u>thoracolumbar</u> region

M51.36 Other intervertebral disc degeneration, <u>lumbar</u> region

M51.37 Other intervertebral disc degeneration, <u>lumbosacral</u> region

M51.4- <u>Schmorl's nodes</u>

M51.44 Schmorl's nodes, <u>thoracic</u> region

M51.45 Schmorl's nodes, <u>thoracolumbar</u> region

M51.46 Schmorl's nodes, <u>lumbar</u> region

M51.47 Schmorl's nodes, <u>lumbosacral</u> region

M51.8- <u>Other</u> thoracic, thoracolumbar and lumbosacral intervertebral disc <u>disorders</u>

M51.84 Other intervertebral disc disorders, <u>thoracic</u> region

M51.85 Other intervertebral disc disorders, <u>thoracolumbar</u> region

M51.86 Other intervertebral disc disorders, <u>lumbar</u> region

M51.87 Other intervertebral disc disorders, <u>lumbosacral</u> region

M51.9 <u>Unspecified</u> thoracic, thoracolumbar and lumbosacral intervertebral disc disorder

M53- <u>Other</u> and <u>unspecified</u> dorsopathies, <u>not elsewhere classified</u>

M53.0 Cervicocranial syndrome
   Posterior cervical sympathetic syndrome

M53.1 Cervicobrachial syndrome
   Excludes❷: cervical disc disorder (M50.-)
      thoracic outlet syndrome (G54.0)

M53.2- Spinal instabilities

M53.2x-<u>Spinal instabilities</u>

M53.2x1 Spinal instabilities, <u>occipito-atlanto-axial</u> region

M53.2x2 Spinal instabilities, <u>cervical</u> region

M53.2x3 Spinal instabilities, <u>cervicothoracic</u> region

M53.2x4 Spinal instabilities, <u>thoracic</u> region

M53.2x5 Spinal instabilities, <u>thoracolumbar</u> region

M53.2x6 Spinal instabilities, <u>lumbar</u> region

M53.2x7 Spinal instabilities, <u>lumbosacral</u> region

M53.2x8 Spinal instabilities, <u>sacral and sacrococcygeal</u> region

M53.2x9 Spinal instabilities, <u>site unspecified</u>

M53.3 Sacrococcygeal disorders, not elsewhere classified
   Coccygodynia

M53.8- <u>Other specified dorsopathies</u>

M53.80 Other specified dorsopathies, <u>site unspecified</u>

M53.81 Other specified dorsopathies, <u>occipito-atlanto-axial</u> region

M53.82 Other specified dorsopathies, <u>cervical</u> region

M53.83 Other specified dorsopathies, <u>cervicothoracic</u> region

M53.84 Other specified dorsopathies, <u>thoracic</u> region

M53.85 Other specified dorsopathies, <u>thoracolumbar</u> region

M53.86 Other specified dorsopathies, <u>lumbar</u> region

M53.87 Other specified dorsopathies, <u>lumbosacral</u> region

M53.88 Other specified dorsopathies, <u>sacral and sacrococcygeal</u> region

M53.9 Dorsopathy, <u>unspecified</u>

M54- <u>Dorsalgia</u>
   Excludes 1: psychogenic dorsalgia (F45.41)

M54.0- <u>Panniculitis affecting regions of neck and back</u>
   Excludes 1: lupus panniculitis (L93.2)
      panniculitis NOS (M79.3)
      relapsing [Weber-Christian] panniculitis (M35.6)

M54.00 Panniculitis affecting regions of neck and back, <u>site unspecified</u>

M54.01 Panniculitis affecting regions of neck and back, <u>occipito-atlanto-axial</u> region

M54.02 Panniculitis affecting regions of neck and back, <u>cervical</u> region

M54.03 Panniculitis affecting regions of neck and back, <u>cervicothoracic</u> region

M54.04 Panniculitis affecting regions of neck and back, <u>thoracic</u> region

M54.05 Panniculitis affecting regions of neck and back, <u>thoracolumbar</u> region

M54.06 Panniculitis affecting regions of neck and back, <u>lumbar</u> region

M54.07 Panniculitis affecting regions of neck and back, <u>lumbosacral</u> region

M54.08 Panniculitis affecting regions of neck and back, <u>sacral and sacrococcygeal</u> region

M54.09 Panniculitis affecting regions, neck and back, <u>multiple sites</u> in spine

M54.1- <u>Radiculopathy</u>
   Brachial neuritis or radiculitis NOS
   Lumbar neuritis or radiculitis NOS
   Lumbosacral neuritis or radiculitis NOS
   Thoracic neuritis or radiculitis NOS
   Radiculitis NOS
   Excludes 1: neuralgia and neuritis NOS (M79.2)
      radiculopathy with cervical disc disorder (M50.1)
      radiculopathy with lumbar and other intervertebral disc
         disorder (M51.1-)
      radiculopathy with spondylosis (M47.2-)

M54.10 Radiculopathy, <u>site unspecified</u>

M54.11 Radiculopathy, <u>occipito-atlanto-axial</u> region

M54.12 Radiculopathy, <u>cervical</u> region

M54.13 Radiculopathy, <u>cervicothoracic</u> region

M54.14 Radiculopathy, <u>thoracic</u> region

M54.15 Radiculopathy, <u>thoracolumbar</u> region

M54.16 Radiculopathy, <u>lumbar</u> region

M54.17 Radiculopathy, <u>lumbosacral</u> region

M54.18 Radiculopathy, <u>sacral and sacrococcygeal</u> region

M50 - M60 *(side tab)*

© 2013 Channel Publishing Ltd

M54.2　Cervicalgia
　　Excludes 1:　cervicalgia due to intervertebral cervical disc disorder
　　　　　　　　　(M50.-)

M54.3-　Sciatica
　　Excludes 1:　lesion of sciatic nerve (G57.0)
　　　　　　　　　sciatica due to intervertebral disc disorder (M51.1-)
　　　　　　　　　sciatica with lumbago (M54.4-)

　　M54.30　Sciatica, unspecified side
　　M54.31　Sciatica, right side
　　M54.32　Sciatica, left side

M54.4-　Lumbago with sciatica
　　Excludes 1:　lumbago with sciatica due to intervertebral disc
　　　　　　　　　disorder (M51.1-)

　　M54.40　Lumbago with sciatica, unspecified side
　　M54.41　Lumbago with sciatica, right side
　　M54.42　Lumbago with sciatica, left side

M54.5　Low back pain
　　　Loin pain
　　　Lumbago NOS
　　Excludes 1:　low back strain (S39.012)
　　　　　　　　　lumbago due to intervertebral disc displacement
　　　　　　　　　(M51.2-)
　　　　　　　　　lumbago with sciatica (M54.4-)

M54.6　Pain in thoracic spine
　　Excludes 1:　pain in thoracic spine due to intervertebral disc
　　　　　　　　　disorder (M51.-)

M54.8-　Other dorsalgia
　　Excludes 1:　dorsalgia in thoracic region (M54.6)
　　　　　　　　　low back pain (M54.5)

　　M54.81　Occipital neuralgia
　　M54.89　Other dorsalgia

M54.9　Dorsalgia, unspecified
　　　Backache NOS
　　　Back pain NOS

Soft tissue disorders (M60-M79)

Disorders of muscles (M60-M63)

Excludes 1:　dermatopolymyositis (M33-)
　　　　　　　muscular dystrophies and myopathies (G71-G72)
　　　　　　　myopathy in amyloidosis (E85.-)
　　　　　　　myopathy in polyarteritis nodosa (M30.0)
　　　　　　　myopathy in rheumatoid arthritis (M05.32)
　　　　　　　myopathy in scleroderma (M34.-)
　　　　　　　myopathy in Sjögren's syndrome (M35.03)
　　　　　　　myopathy in systemic lupus erythematosus (M32.-)

M60-　Myositis
　　Excludes ❷:　inclusion body myositis [IBM] (G72.41)

M60.0-　Infective myositis
　　　Tropical pyomyositis
　　　Use additional code (B95-B97) to identify infectious agent

　　M60.00-Infective myositis, unspecified site
　　　M60.000　Infective myositis, unspecified right arm
　　　　　　Infective myositis, right upper limb NOS
　　　M60.001　Infective myositis, unspecified left arm
　　　　　　Infective myositis, left upper limb NOS
　　　M60.002　Infective myositis, unspecified arm
　　　　　　Infective myositis, upper limb NOS
　　　M60.003　Infective myositis, unspecified right leg
　　　　　　Infective myositis, right lower limb NOS
　　　M60.004　Infective myositis, unspecified left leg
　　　　　　Infective myositis, left lower limb NOS
　　　M60.005　Infective myositis, unspecified leg
　　　　　　Infective myositis, lower limb NOS
　　　M60.009　Infective myositis, unspecified site

　　M60.01-Infective myositis, shoulder
　　　M60.011　Infective myositis, right shoulder
　　　M60.012　Infective myositis, left shoulder
　　　M60.019　Infective myositis, unspecified shoulder

　　M60.02-Infective myositis, upper arm
　　　M60.021　Infective myositis, right upper arm
　　　M60.022　Infective myositis, left upper arm
　　　M60.029　Infective myositis, unspecified upper arm

　　M60.03-Infective myositis, forearm
　　　M60.031　Infective myositis, right forearm
　　　M60.032　Infective myositis, left forearm
　　　M60.039　Infective myositis, unspecified forearm

M60.04-Infective myositis, hand and fingers
　　M60.041　Infective myositis, right hand
　　M60.042　Infective myositis, left hand
　　M60.043　Infective myositis, unspecified hand
　　M60.044　Infective myositis, right finger(s)
　　M60.045　Infective myositis, left finger(s)
　　M60.046　Infective myositis, unspecified finger(s)

M60.05-Infective myositis, thigh
　　M60.051　Infective myositis, right thigh
　　M60.052　Infective myositis, left thigh
　　M60.059　Infective myositis, unspecified thigh

M60.06-Infective myositis, lower leg
　　M60.061　Infective myositis, right lower leg
　　M60.062　Infective myositis, left lower leg
　　M60.069　Infective myositis, unspecified lower leg

M60.07-Infective myositis, ankle, foot and toes
　　M60.070　Infective myositis, right ankle
　　M60.071　Infective myositis, left ankle
　　M60.072　Infective myositis, unspecified ankle
　　M60.073　Infective myositis, right foot
　　M60.074　Infective myositis, left foot
　　M60.075　Infective myositis, unspecified foot
　　M60.076　Infective myositis, right toe(s)
　　M60.077　Infective myositis, left toe(s)
　　M60.078　Infective myositis, unspecified toe(s)

M60.08　Infective myositis, other site
M60.09　Infective myositis, multiple sites

M60.1-　Interstitial myositis
M60.10　Interstitial myositis of unspecified site

M60.11-Interstitial myositis, shoulder
　　M60.111　Interstitial myositis, right shoulder
　　M60.112　Interstitial myositis, left shoulder
　　M60.119　Interstitial myositis, unspecified shoulder

M60.12-Interstitial myositis, upper arm
　　M60.121　Interstitial myositis, right upper arm
　　M60.122　Interstitial myositis, left upper arm
　　M60.129　Interstitial myositis, unspecified upper arm

M60.13-Interstitial myositis, forearm
　　M60.131　Interstitial myositis, right forearm
　　M60.132　Interstitial myositis, left forearm
　　M60.139　Interstitial myositis, unspecified forearm

M60.14-Interstitial myositis, hand
　　M60.141　Interstitial myositis, right hand
　　M60.142　Interstitial myositis, left hand
　　M60.149　Interstitial myositis, unspecified hand

M60.15-Interstitial myositis, thigh
　　M60.151　Interstitial myositis, right thigh
　　M60.152　Interstitial myositis, left thigh
　　M60.159　Interstitial myositis, unspecified thigh

M60.16-Interstitial myositis, lower leg
　　M60.161　Interstitial myositis, right lower leg
　　M60.162　Interstitial myositis, left lower leg
　　M60.169　Interstitial myositis, unspecified lower leg

M60.17-Interstitial myositis, ankle and foot
　　M60.171　Interstitial myositis, right ankle and foot
　　M60.172　Interstitial myositis, left ankle and foot
　　M60.179　Interstitial myositis, unspecified ankle and foot

M60.18　Interstitial myositis, other site
M60.19　Interstitial myositis, multiple sites

M60.2-　Foreign body granuloma of soft tissue, not elsewhere classified
　　　Use additional code to identify the type of retained foreign body
　　　　(Z18.-)
　　Excludes 1:　foreign body granuloma of skin and subcutaneous
　　　　　　　　　tissue (L92.3)

M60.20　Foreign body granuloma of soft tissue, not elsewhere classified, unspecified site
M60.21-Foreign body granuloma of soft tissue, not elsewhere classified, shoulder
　　M60.211　Foreign body granuloma of soft tissue, not elsewhere classified, right shoulder
　　M60.212　Foreign body granuloma of soft tissue, not elsewhere classified, left shoulder
　　M60.219　Foreign body granuloma of soft tissue, not elsewhere classified, unspecified shoulder

---

Excludes 1: = NOT CODED HERE! (Do not code both)　　　**577**　　　*Excludes ❷: = Not Included Here*

M60.22-Foreign body granuloma of soft tissue, not elsewhere classified, <u>upper arm</u>
- M60.221 Foreign body granuloma of soft tissue, not elsewhere classified, <u>right</u> upper arm
- M60.222 Foreign body granuloma of soft tissue, not elsewhere classified, <u>left</u> upper arm
- M60.229 Foreign body granuloma of soft tissue, not elsewhere classified, <u>unspecified</u> upper arm

M60.23-Foreign body granuloma of soft tissue, not elsewhere classified, <u>forearm</u>
- M60.231 Foreign body granuloma of soft tissue, not elsewhere classified, <u>right</u> forearm
- M60.232 Foreign body granuloma of soft tissue, not elsewhere classified, <u>left</u> forearm
- M60.239 Foreign body granuloma of soft tissue, not elsewhere classified, <u>unspecified</u> forearm

M60.24-Foreign body granuloma of soft tissue, not elsewhere classified, <u>hand</u>
- M60.241 Foreign body granuloma of soft tissue, not elsewhere classified, <u>right</u> hand
- M60.242 Foreign body granuloma of soft tissue, not elsewhere classified, <u>left</u> hand
- M60.249 Foreign body granuloma of soft tissue, not elsewhere classified, <u>unspecified</u> hand

M60.25-Foreign body granuloma of soft tissue, not elsewhere classified, <u>thigh</u>
- M60.251 Foreign body granuloma of soft tissue, not elsewhere classified, <u>right</u> thigh
- M60.252 Foreign body granuloma of soft tissue, not elsewhere classified, <u>left</u> thigh
- M60.259 Foreign body granuloma of soft tissue, not elsewhere classified, <u>unspecified</u> thigh

M60.26-Foreign body granuloma of soft tissue, not elsewhere classified, <u>lower leg</u>
- M60.261 Foreign body granuloma of soft tissue, not elsewhere classified, <u>right</u> lower leg
- M60.262 Foreign body granuloma of soft tissue, not elsewhere classified, <u>left</u> lower leg
- M60.269 Foreign body granuloma of soft tissue, not elsewhere classified, <u>unspecified</u> lower leg

M60.27-Foreign body granuloma of soft tissue, not elsewhere classified, <u>ankle and foot</u>
- M60.271 Foreign body granuloma of soft tissue, not elsewhere classified, <u>right</u> ankle and foot
- M60.272 Foreign body granuloma of soft tissue, not elsewhere classified, <u>left</u> ankle and foot
- M60.279 Foreign body granuloma of soft tissue, not elsewhere classified, <u>unspecified</u> ankle and foot

M60.28 Foreign body granuloma of soft tissue, not elsewhere classified, <u>other</u> <u>site</u>

M60.8- <u>Other myositis</u>
- M60.80 Other myositis, <u>unspecified site</u>
- M60.81-Other myositis <u>shoulder</u>
  - M60.811 Other myositis, <u>right</u> shoulder
  - M60.812 Other myositis, <u>left</u> shoulder
  - M60.819 Other myositis, <u>unspecified</u> shoulder
- M60.82-Other myositis, <u>upper arm</u>
  - M60.821 Other myositis, <u>right</u> upper arm
  - M60.822 Other myositis, <u>left</u> upper arm
  - M60.829 Other myositis, <u>unspecified</u> upper arm
- M60.83-Other myositis, <u>forearm</u>
  - M60.831 Other myositis, <u>right</u> forearm
  - M60.832 Other myositis, <u>left</u> forearm
  - M60.839 Other myositis, <u>unspecified</u> forearm
- M60.84-Other myositis, <u>hand</u>
  - M60.841 Other myositis, <u>right</u> hand
  - M60.842 Other myositis, <u>left</u> hand
  - M60.849 Other myositis, <u>unspecified</u> hand
- M60.85-Other myositis, <u>thigh</u>
  - M60.851 Other myositis, <u>right</u> thigh
  - M60.852 Other myositis, <u>left</u> thigh
  - M60.859 Other myositis, <u>unspecified</u> thigh
- M60.86-Other myositis, <u>lower leg</u>
  - M60.861 Other myositis, <u>right</u> lower leg
  - M60.862 Other myositis, <u>left</u> lower leg
  - M60.869 Other myositis, <u>unspecified</u> lower leg

M60.87-Other myositis, <u>ankle and foot</u>
- M60.871 Other myositis, <u>right</u> ankle and foot
- M60.872 Other myositis, <u>left</u> ankle and foot
- M60.879 Other myositis, <u>unspecified</u> ankle and foot
M60.88 Other myositis, <u>other site</u>
M60.89 Other myositis, <u>multiple sites</u>
M60.9 Myositis, <u>unspecified</u>

M61- <u>Calcification and ossification of muscle</u>
M61.0- Myositis ossificans <u>traumatica</u>
- M61.00 Myositis ossificans traumatica, <u>unspecified site</u>
- M61.01-Myositis ossificans traumatica, <u>shoulder</u>
  - M61.011 Myositis ossificans traumatica, <u>right</u> shoulder
  - M61.012 Myositis ossificans traumatica, <u>left</u> shoulder
  - M61.019 Myositis ossificans traumatica, <u>unspecified</u> shoulder
- M61.02-Myositis ossificans traumatica, <u>upper arm</u>
  - M61.021 Myositis ossificans traumatica, <u>right</u> upper arm
  - M61.022 Myositis ossificans traumatica, <u>left</u> upper arm
  - M61.029 Myositis ossificans traumatica, <u>unspecified</u> upper arm
- M61.03-Myositis ossificans traumatica, <u>forearm</u>
  - M61.031 Myositis ossificans traumatica, <u>right</u> forearm
  - M61.032 Myositis ossificans traumatica, <u>left</u> forearm
  - M61.039 Myositis ossificans traumatica, <u>unspecified</u> forearm
- M61.04-Myositis ossificans traumatica, <u>hand</u>
  - M61.041 Myositis ossificans traumatica, <u>right</u> hand
  - M61.042 Myositis ossificans traumatica, <u>left</u> hand
  - M61.049 Myositis ossificans traumatica, <u>unspecified</u> hand
- M61.05-Myositis ossificans traumatica, <u>thigh</u>
  - M61.051 Myositis ossificans traumatica, <u>right</u> thigh
  - M61.052 Myositis ossificans traumatica, <u>left</u> thigh
  - M61.059 Myositis ossificans traumatica, <u>unspecified</u> thigh
- M61.06-Myositis ossificans traumatica, <u>lower leg</u>
  - M61.061 Myositis ossificans traumatica, <u>right</u> lower leg
  - M61.062 Myositis ossificans traumatica, <u>left</u> lower leg
  - M61.069 Myositis ossificans traumatica, <u>unspecified</u> lower leg
- M61.07-Myositis ossificans traumatica, <u>ankle and foot</u>
  - M61.071 Myositis ossificans traumatica, <u>right</u> ankle and foot
  - M61.072 Myositis ossificans traumatica, <u>left</u> ankle and foot
  - M61.079 Myositis ossificans traumatica, <u>unspecified</u> ankle and foot
- M61.08 Myositis ossificans traumatica, <u>other site</u>
- M61.09 Myositis ossificans traumatica, <u>multiple sites</u>
M61.1- Myositis ossificans <u>progressiva</u>
  Fibrodysplasia ossificans progressiva
- M61.10 Myositis ossificans progressiva, <u>unspecified site</u>
- M61.11-Myositis ossificans progressiva, <u>shoulder</u>
  - M61.111 Myositis ossificans progressiva, <u>right</u> shoulder
  - M61.112 Myositis ossificans progressiva, <u>left</u> shoulder
  - M61.119 Myositis ossificans progressiva, <u>unspecified</u> shoulder
- M61.12-Myositis ossificans progressiva, <u>upper arm</u>
  - M61.121 Myositis ossificans progressiva, <u>right</u> upper arm
  - M61.122 Myositis ossificans progressiva, <u>left</u> upper arm
  - M61.129 Myositis ossificans progressiva, <u>unspecified</u> arm
- M61.13-Myositis ossificans progressiva, <u>forearm</u>
  - M61.131 Myositis ossificans progressiva, <u>right</u> forearm
  - M61.132 Myositis ossificans progressiva, <u>left</u> forearm
  - M61.139 Myositis ossificans progressiva, <u>unspecified</u> forearm
- M61.14-Myositis ossificans progressiva, <u>hand and finger(s)</u>
  - M61.141 Myositis ossificans progressiva, <u>right</u> hand
  - M61.142 Myositis ossificans progressiva, <u>left</u> hand
  - M61.143 Myositis ossificans progressiva, <u>unspecified</u> hand
  - M61.144 Myositis ossificans progressiva, <u>right</u> finger(s)
  - M61.145 Myositis ossificans progressiva, <u>left</u> finger(s)
  - M61.146 Myositis ossificans progressiva, <u>unspecified</u> finger(s)
- M61.15-Myositis ossificans progressiva, <u>thigh</u>
  - M61.151 Myositis ossificans progressiva, <u>right</u> thigh
  - M61.152 Myositis ossificans progressiva, <u>left</u> thigh
  - M61.159 Myositis ossificans progressiva, <u>unspecified</u> thigh
- M61.16-Myositis ossificans progressiva, <u>lower leg</u>
  - M61.161 Myositis ossificans progressiva, <u>right</u> lower leg
  - M61.162 Myositis ossificans progressiva, <u>left</u> lower leg
  - M61.169 Myositis ossificans progressiva, <u>unspecified</u> lower leg
- M61.17-Myositis ossificans progressiva, <u>ankle, foot and toe(s)</u>
  - M61.171 Myositis ossificans progressiva, <u>right</u> ankle
  - M61.172 Myositis ossificans progressiva, <u>left</u> ankle

M60
|
M61

© 2013 Channel Publishing, Ltd.

M61.173   Myositis ossificans progressiva, <u>unspecified</u> ankle
M61.174   Myositis ossificans progressiva, <u>right</u> foot
M61.175   Myositis ossificans progressiva, <u>left</u> foot
M61.176   Myositis ossificans progressiva, <u>unspecified</u> foot
M61.177   Myositis ossificans progressiva, <u>right</u> toe(s)
M61.178   Myositis ossificans progressiva, <u>left</u> toe(s)
M61.179   Myositis ossificans progressiva, <u>unspecified</u> toe(s)
M61.18   Myositis ossificans progressiva, <u>other site</u>
M61.19   Myositis ossificans progressiva, <u>multiple sites</u>
M61.2-   <u>Paralytic calcification and ossification of muscle</u>
    Myositis ossificans associated with quadriplegia or paraplegia
M61.20   Paralytic calcification and ossification of muscle, <u>unspecified site</u>
M61.21-Paralytic calcification and ossification of muscle, <u>shoulder</u>
M61.211   Paralytic calcification and ossification of muscle, <u>right</u> shoulder
M61.212   Paralytic calcification and ossification of muscle, <u>left</u> shoulder
M61.219   Paralytic calcification and ossification of muscle, <u>unspecified</u> shoulder
M61.22-Paralytic calcification and ossification of muscle, <u>upper arm</u>
M61.221   Paralytic calcification and ossification of muscle, <u>right</u> upper arm
M61.222   Paralytic calcification and ossification of muscle, <u>left</u> upper arm
M61.229   Paralytic calcification and ossification of muscle, <u>unspecified</u> upper arm
M61.23-Paralytic calcification and ossification of muscle, <u>forearm</u>
M61.231   Paralytic calcification and ossification of muscle, <u>right</u> forearm
M61.232   Paralytic calcification and ossification of muscle, <u>left</u> forearm
M61.239   Paralytic calcification and ossification of muscle, <u>unspecified</u> forearm
M61.24-Paralytic calcification and ossification of muscle, <u>hand</u>
M61.241   Paralytic calcification and ossification of muscle, <u>right</u> hand
M61.242   Paralytic calcification and ossification of muscle, <u>left</u> hand
M61.249   Paralytic calcification and ossification of muscle, <u>unspecified</u> hand
M61.25-Paralytic calcification and ossification of muscle, <u>thigh</u>
M61.251   Paralytic calcification and ossification of muscle, <u>right</u> thigh
M61.252   Paralytic calcification and ossification of muscle, <u>left</u> thigh
M61.259   Paralytic calcification and ossification of muscle, <u>unspecified</u> thigh
M61.26-Paralytic calcification and ossification of muscle, <u>lower leg</u>
M61.261   Paralytic calcification and ossification of muscle, <u>right</u> lower leg
M61.262   Paralytic calcification and ossification of muscle, <u>left</u> lower leg
M61.269   Paralytic calcification and ossification of muscle, <u>unspecified</u> lower leg
M61.27-Paralytic calcification and ossification of muscle, <u>ankle and foot</u>
M61.271   Paralytic calcification and ossification of muscle, <u>right</u> ankle and foot
M61.272   Paralytic calcification and ossification of muscle, <u>left</u> ankle and foot
M61.279   Paralytic calcification and ossification of muscle, <u>unspecified</u> ankle and foot
M61.28   Paralytic calcification and ossification of muscle, <u>other site</u>
M61.29   Paralytic calcification and ossification of muscle, <u>multiple sites</u>
M61.3-   <u>Calcification and ossification of muscles associated with burns</u>
    Myositis ossificans associated with burns
M61.30   Calcification and ossification of muscles associated with burns, <u>unspecified site</u>
M61.31-Calcification and ossification of muscles associated with burns, <u>shoulder</u>
M61.311   Calcification and ossification of muscles associated with burns, <u>right</u> shoulder
M61.312   Calcification and ossification of muscles associated with burns, <u>left</u> shoulder
M61.319   Calcification and ossification of muscles associated with burns, <u>unspecified</u> shoulder

M61.32-Calcification and ossification of muscles associated with burns, <u>upper arm</u>
M61.321   Calcification and ossification of muscles associated with burns, <u>right</u> upper arm
M61.322   Calcification and ossification of muscles associated with burns, <u>left</u> upper arm
M61.329   Calcification and ossification of muscles associated with burns, <u>unspecified</u> upper arm
M61.33-Calcification and ossification of muscles associated with burns, <u>forearm</u>
M61.331   Calcification and ossification of muscles associated with burns, <u>right</u> forearm
M61.332   Calcification and ossification of muscles associated with burns, <u>left</u> forearm
M61.339   Calcification and ossification of muscles associated with burns, <u>unspecified</u> forearm
M61.34-Calcification and ossification of muscles associated with burns, <u>hand</u>
M61.341   Calcification and ossification of muscles associated with burns, <u>right</u> hand
M61.342   Calcification and ossification of muscles associated with burns, <u>left</u> hand
M61.349   Calcification and ossification of muscles associated with burns, <u>unspecified</u> hand
M61.35-Calcification and ossification of muscles associated with burns, <u>thigh</u>
M61.351   Calcification and ossification of muscles associated with burns, <u>right</u> thigh
M61.352   Calcification and ossification of muscles associated with burns, <u>left</u> thigh
M61.359   Calcification and ossification of muscles associated with burns, <u>unspecified</u> thigh
M61.36-Calcification and ossification of muscles associated with burns, <u>lower leg</u>
M61.361   Calcification and ossification of muscles associated with burns, <u>right</u> lower leg
M61.362   Calcification and ossification of muscles associated with burns, <u>left</u> lower leg
M61.369   Calcification and ossification of muscles associated with burns, <u>unspecified</u> lower leg
M61.37-Calcification and ossification of muscles associated with burns, <u>ankle and foot</u>
M61.371   Calcification and ossification of muscles associated with burns, <u>right</u> ankle and foot
M61.372   Calcification and ossification of muscles associated with burns, <u>left</u> ankle and foot
M61.379   Calcification and ossification of muscles associated with burns, <u>unspecified</u> ankle and foot
M61.38   Calcification and ossification of muscles associated with burns, <u>other site</u>
M61.39   Calcification and ossification of muscles associated with burns, <u>multiple sites</u>
M61.4-   <u>Other calcification</u> of muscle
    Excludes 1: calcific tendinitis NOS (M65.2-)
              calcific tendinitis of shoulder (M75.3)
M61.40   Other calcification of muscle, <u>unspecified site</u>
M61.41-Other calcification of muscle, <u>shoulder</u>
M61.411   Other calcification of muscle, <u>right</u> shoulder
M61.412   Other calcification of muscle, <u>left</u> shoulder
M61.419   Other calcification of muscle, <u>unspecified</u> shoulder
M61.42-Other calcification of muscle, <u>upper arm</u>
M61.421   Other calcification of muscle, <u>right</u> upper arm
M61.422   Other calcification of muscle, <u>left</u> upper arm
M61.429   Other calcification of muscle, <u>unspecified</u> upper arm
M61.43-Other calcification of muscle, <u>forearm</u>
M61.431   Other calcification of muscle, <u>right</u> forearm
M61.432   Other calcification of muscle, <u>left</u> forearm
M61.439   Other calcification of muscle, <u>unspecified</u> forearm
M61.44-Other calcification of muscle, <u>hand</u>
M61.441   Other calcification of muscle, <u>right</u> hand
M61.442   Other calcification of muscle, <u>left</u> hand
M61.449   Other calcification of muscle, <u>unspecified</u> hand
M61.45-Other calcification of muscle, <u>thigh</u>
M61.451   Other calcification of muscle, <u>right</u> thigh
M61.452   Other calcification of muscle, <u>left</u> thigh
M61.459   Other calcification of muscle, <u>unspecified</u> thigh

M 6 0 – M 6 1

M61.46-Other calcification of muscle, <u>lower leg</u>
    M61.461 Other calcification of muscle, <u>right</u> lower leg
    M61.462 Other calcification of muscle, <u>left</u> lower leg
    M61.469 Other calcification of muscle, <u>unspecified</u> lower leg
M61.47-Other calcification of muscle, ankle and foot
    M61.471 Other calcification of muscle, <u>right</u> ankle and foot
    M61.472 Other calcification of muscle, <u>left</u> ankle and foot
    M61.479 Other calcification of muscle, <u>unspecified</u> ankle and foot
M61.48 Other calcification of muscle, other site
M61.49 Other calcification of muscle, <u>multiple sites</u>
M61.5- <u>Other ossification</u> of muscle
M61.50 Other ossification of muscle, <u>unspecified site</u>
M61.51-Other ossification of muscle, <u>shoulder</u>
    M61.511 Other ossification of muscle, <u>right</u> shoulder
    M61.512 Other ossification of muscle, <u>left</u> shoulder
    M61.519 Other ossification of muscle, <u>unspecified</u> shoulder
M61.52-Other ossification of muscle, <u>upper arm</u>
    M61.521 Other ossification of muscle, <u>right</u> upper arm
    M61.522 Other ossification of muscle, <u>left</u> upper arm
    M61.529 Other ossification of muscle, <u>unspecified</u> upper arm
M61.53-Other ossification of muscle, <u>forearm</u>
    M61.531 Other ossification of muscle, <u>right</u> forearm
    M61.532 Other ossification of muscle, <u>left</u> forearm
    M61.539 Other ossification of muscle, <u>unspecified</u> forearm
M61.54-Other ossification of muscle, <u>hand</u>
    M61.541 Other ossification of muscle, <u>right</u> hand
    M61.542 Other ossification of muscle, <u>left</u> hand
    M61.549 Other ossification of muscle, <u>unspecified</u> hand
M61.55-Other ossification of muscle, <u>thigh</u>
    M61.551 Other ossification of muscle, <u>right</u> thigh
    M61.552 Other ossification of muscle, <u>left</u> thigh
    M61.559 Other ossification of muscle, <u>unspecified</u> thigh
M61.56-Other ossification of muscle, <u>lower leg</u>
    M61.561 Other ossification of muscle, <u>right</u> lower leg
    M61.562 Other ossification of muscle, <u>left</u> lower leg
    M61.569 Other ossification of muscle, <u>unspecified</u> lower leg
M61.57-Other ossification of muscle, <u>ankle and foot</u>
    M61.571 Other ossification of muscle, <u>right</u> ankle and foot
    M61.572 Other ossification of muscle, <u>left</u> ankle and foot
    M61.579 Other ossification of muscle, <u>unspecified</u> ankle and foot
M61.58 Other ossification of muscle, <u>other site</u>
M61.59 Other ossification of muscle, <u>multiple sites</u>
M61.9 Calcification and ossification of muscle, <u>unspecified</u>

M62- Other disorders of muscle
   Excludes 1: alcoholic myopathy (G72.1)
               cramp and spasm (R25.2)
               drug-induced myopathy (G72.0)
               myalgia (M79.1)
               stiff-man syndrome (G25.82)
   Excludes❷: nontraumatic hematoma of muscle (M79.81)
M62.0- <u>Separation of muscle (nontraumatic)</u>
    Diastasis of muscle
   Excludes 1: diastasis recti complicating pregnancy, labor and delivery (O71.8)
               traumatic separation of muscle — see strain of muscle by body region
M62.00 Separation of muscle (nontraumatic), <u>unspecified site</u>
M62.01-Separation of muscle (nontraumatic), <u>shoulder</u>
    M62.011 Separation of muscle (nontraumatic), <u>right</u> shoulder
    M62.012 Separation of muscle (nontraumatic), <u>left</u> shoulder
    M62.019 Separation of muscle (nontraumatic), <u>unspecified</u> shoulder
M62.02-Separation of muscle (nontraumatic), <u>upper arm</u>
    M62.021 Separation of muscle (nontraumatic), <u>right</u> upper arm
    M62.022 Separation of muscle (nontraumatic), <u>left</u> upper arm
    M62.029 Separation of muscle (nontraumatic), <u>unspecified</u> upper arm
M62.03-Separation of muscle (nontraumatic), <u>forearm</u>
    M62.031 Separation of muscle (nontraumatic), <u>right</u> forearm
    M62.032 Separation of muscle (nontraumatic), <u>left</u> forearm
    M62.039 Separation of muscle (nontraumatic), <u>unspecified</u> forearm

M62.04-Separation of muscle (nontraumatic), <u>hand</u>
    M62.041 Separation of muscle (nontraumatic), <u>right</u> hand
    M62.042 Separation of muscle (nontraumatic), <u>left</u> hand
    M62.049 Separation of muscle (nontraumatic), <u>unspecified</u> hand
M62.05-Separation of muscle (nontraumatic), <u>thigh</u>
    M62.051 Separation of muscle (nontraumatic), <u>right</u> thigh
    M62.052 Separation of muscle (nontraumatic), <u>left</u> thigh
    M62.059 Separation of muscle (nontraumatic), <u>unspecified</u> thigh
M62.06-Separation of muscle (nontraumatic), <u>lower leg</u>
    M62.061 Separation of muscle (nontraumatic), <u>right</u> lower leg
    M62.062 Separation of muscle (nontraumatic), <u>left</u> lower leg
    M62.069 Separation of muscle (nontraumatic), <u>unspecified</u> lower leg
M62.07-Separation of muscle (nontraumatic), <u>ankle and foot</u>
    M62.071 Separation of muscle (nontraumatic), <u>right</u> ankle and foot
    M62.072 Separation of muscle (nontraumatic), <u>left</u> ankle and foot
    M62.079 Separation of muscle (nontraumatic), <u>unspecified</u> ankle and foot
M62.08 Separation of muscle (nontraumatic), <u>other site</u>
M62.1- <u>Other rupture</u> of muscle (nontraumatic)
   Excludes 1: traumatic rupture of muscle — see strain of muscle by body region
   Excludes❷: rupture of tendon (M66.-)
M62.10 Other rupture of muscle (nontraumatic), <u>unspecified site</u>
M62.11-Other rupture of muscle (nontraumatic), <u>shoulder</u>
    M62.111 Other rupture of muscle (nontraumatic), <u>right</u> shoulder
    M62.112 Other rupture of muscle (nontraumatic), <u>left</u> shoulder
    M62.119 Other rupture of muscle (nontraumatic), <u>unspecified</u> shoulder
M62.12-Other rupture of muscle (nontraumatic), <u>upper arm</u>
    M62.121 Other rupture of muscle (nontraumatic), <u>right</u> upper arm
    M62.122 Other rupture of muscle (nontraumatic), <u>left</u> upper arm
    M62.129 Other rupture of muscle (nontraumatic), <u>unspecified</u> upper arm
M62.13-Other rupture of muscle (nontraumatic), <u>forearm</u>
    M62.131 Other rupture of muscle (nontraumatic), <u>right</u> forearm
    M62.132 Other rupture of muscle (nontraumatic), <u>left</u> forearm
    M62.139 Other rupture of muscle (nontraumatic), <u>unspecified</u> forearm
M62.14-Other rupture of muscle (nontraumatic), <u>hand</u>
    M62.141 Other rupture of muscle (nontraumatic), <u>right</u> hand
    M62.142 Other rupture of muscle (nontraumatic), <u>left</u> hand
    M62.149 Other rupture of muscle (nontraumatic), <u>unspecified</u> hand
M62.15-Other rupture of muscle (nontraumatic), <u>thigh</u>
    M62.151 Other rupture of muscle (nontraumatic), <u>right</u> thigh
    M62.152 Other rupture of muscle (nontraumatic), <u>left</u> thigh
    M62.159 Other rupture of muscle (nontraumatic), <u>unspecified</u> thigh
M62.16-Other rupture of muscle (nontraumatic), <u>lower leg</u>
    M62.161 Other rupture of muscle (nontraumatic), <u>right</u> lower leg
    M62.162 Other rupture of muscle (nontraumatic), <u>left</u> lower leg
    M62.169 Other rupture of muscle (nontraumatic), <u>unspecified</u> lower leg
M62.17-Other rupture of muscle (nontraumatic), <u>ankle and foot</u>
    M62.171 Other rupture of muscle (nontraumatic), <u>right</u> ankle and foot
    M62.172 Other rupture of muscle (nontraumatic), <u>left</u> ankle and foot
    M62.179 Other rupture of muscle (nontraumatic), <u>unspecified</u> ankle and foot
M62.18 Other rupture of muscle (nontraumatic), <u>other site</u>

M61 – M62

M62.2- <u>Nontraumatic ischemic infarction</u> of muscle
   Excludes 1:   compartment syndrome (traumatic) (T79.A-)
   nontraumatic compartment syndrome (M79.A-)
   traumatic ischemia of muscle (T79.6)
   rhabdomyolysis (M62.82)
   Volkmann's ischemic contracture (T79.6)

M62.20 Nontraumatic ischemic infarction of muscle, <u>unspecified</u> <u>site</u>
M62.21-Nontraumatic ischemic infarction of muscle, <u>shoulder</u>
   M62.211   Nontraumatic ischemic infarction of muscle, <u>right</u> shoulder
   M62.212   Nontraumatic ischemic infarction of muscle, <u>left</u> shoulder
   M62.219   Nontraumatic ischemic infarction of muscle, <u>unspecified</u> shoulder
M62.22-Nontraumatic ischemic infarction of muscle, <u>upper arm</u>
   M62.221   Nontraumatic ischemic infarction of muscle, <u>right</u> upper arm
   M62.222   Nontraumatic ischemic infarction of muscle, <u>left</u> upper arm
   M62.229   Nontraumatic ischemic infarction of muscle, <u>unspecified</u> upper arm
M62.23-Nontraumatic ischemic infarction of muscle, <u>forearm</u>
   M62.231   Nontraumatic ischemic infarction of muscle, <u>right</u> forearm
   M62.232   Nontraumatic ischemic infarction of muscle, <u>left</u> forearm
   M62.239   Nontraumatic ischemic infarction of muscle, <u>unspecified</u> forearm
M62.24-Nontraumatic ischemic infarction of muscle, <u>hand</u>
   M62.241   Nontraumatic ischemic infarction of muscle, <u>right</u> hand
   M62.242   Nontraumatic ischemic infarction of muscle, <u>left</u> hand
   M62.249   Nontraumatic ischemic infarction of muscle, <u>unspecified</u> hand
M62.25-Nontraumatic ischemic infarction of muscle, <u>thigh</u>
   M62.251   Nontraumatic ischemic infarction of muscle, <u>right</u> thigh
   M62.252   Nontraumatic ischemic infarction of muscle, <u>left</u> thigh
   M62.259   Nontraumatic ischemic infarction of muscle, <u>unspecified</u> thigh
M62.26-Nontraumatic ischemic infarction of muscle, <u>lower leg</u>
   M62.261   Nontraumatic ischemic infarction of muscle, <u>right</u> lower leg
   M62.262   Nontraumatic ischemic infarction of muscle, <u>left</u> lower leg
   M62.269   Nontraumatic ischemic infarction of muscle, <u>unspecified</u> lower leg
M62.27-Nontraumatic ischemic infarction of muscle, <u>ankle and foot</u>
   M62.271   Nontraumatic ischemic infarction of muscle, <u>right</u> ankle and foot
   M62.272   Nontraumatic ischemic infarction of muscle, <u>left</u> ankle and foot
   M62.279   Nontraumatic ischemic infarction of muscle, <u>unspecified</u> ankle and foot
M62.28 Nontraumatic ischemic infarction of muscle, <u>other site</u>
M62.3 Immobility syndrome (paraplegic)
M62.4- <u>Contracture</u> of muscle
   Contracture of tendon (sheath)
   Excludes 1:   contracture of joint (M24.5-)
M62.40 Contracture of muscle, <u>unspecified</u> site
M62.41-Contracture of muscle, <u>shoulder</u>
   M62.411   Contracture of muscle, <u>right</u> shoulder
   M62.412   Contracture of muscle, <u>left</u> shoulder
   M62.419   Contracture of muscle, <u>unspecified</u> shoulder
M62.42-Contracture of muscle, <u>upper arm</u>
   M62.421   Contracture of muscle, <u>right</u> upper arm
   M62.422   Contracture of muscle, <u>left</u> upper arm
   M62.429   Contracture of muscle, <u>unspecified</u> upper arm
M62.43-Contracture of muscle, <u>forearm</u>
   M62.431   Contracture of muscle, <u>right</u> forearm
   M62.432   Contracture of muscle, <u>left</u> forearm
   M62.439   Contracture of muscle, <u>unspecified</u> forearm
M62.44-Contracture of muscle, <u>hand</u>
   M62.441   Contracture of muscle, <u>right</u> hand
   M62.442   Contracture of muscle, <u>left</u> hand
   M62.449   Contracture of muscle, <u>unspecified</u> hand

M62.45-Contracture of muscle, <u>thigh</u>
   M62.451   Contracture of muscle, <u>right</u> thigh
   M62.452   Contracture of muscle, <u>left</u> thigh
   M62.459   Contracture of muscle, <u>unspecified</u> thigh
M62.46-Contracture of muscle, <u>lower leg</u>
   M62.461   Contracture of muscle, <u>right</u> lower leg
   M62.462   Contracture of muscle, <u>left</u> lower leg
   M62.469   Contracture of muscle, <u>unspecified</u> lower leg
M62.47-Contracture of muscle, <u>ankle and foot</u>
   M62.471   Contracture of muscle, <u>right</u> ankle and foot
   M62.472   Contracture of muscle, <u>left</u> ankle and foot
   M62.479   Contracture of muscle, <u>unspecified</u> ankle and foot
M62.48 Contracture of muscle, <u>other site</u>
M62.49 Contracture of muscle, <u>multiple sites</u>
M62.5- <u>Muscle wasting and atrophy, not elsewhere classified</u>
   Disuse atrophy NEC
   Excludes 1:   neuralgic amyotrophy (G54.5)
   progressive muscular atrophy (G12.29)
   Excludes ❷: pelvic muscle wasting (N81.84)
M62.50 Muscle wasting and atrophy, not elsewhere classified, <u>unspecified site</u>
M62.51-Muscle wasting and atrophy, not elsewhere classified, <u>shoulder</u>
   M62.511   Muscle wasting and atrophy, not elsewhere classified, <u>right</u> shoulder
   M62.512   Muscle wasting and atrophy, not elsewhere classified, <u>left</u> shoulder
   M62.519   Muscle wasting and atrophy, not elsewhere classified, <u>unspecified</u> shoulder
M62.52-Muscle wasting and atrophy, not elsewhere classified, <u>upper arm</u>
   M62.521   Muscle wasting and atrophy, not elsewhere classified, <u>right</u> upper arm
   M62.522   Muscle wasting and atrophy, not elsewhere classified, <u>left</u> upper arm
   M62.529   Muscle wasting and atrophy, not elsewhere classified, <u>unspecified</u> upper arm
M62.53-Muscle wasting and atrophy, not elsewhere classified, <u>forearm</u>
   M62.531   Muscle wasting and atrophy, not elsewhere classified, <u>right</u> forearm
   M62.532   Muscle wasting and atrophy, not elsewhere classified, <u>left</u> forearm
   M62.539   Muscle wasting and atrophy, not elsewhere classified, <u>unspecified</u> forearm
M62.54-Muscle wasting and atrophy, not elsewhere classified, <u>hand</u>
   M62.541   Muscle wasting and atrophy, not elsewhere classified, <u>right</u> hand
   M62.542   Muscle wasting and atrophy, not elsewhere classified, <u>left</u> hand
   M62.549   Muscle wasting and atrophy, not elsewhere classified, <u>unspecified</u> hand
M62.55-Muscle wasting and atrophy, not elsewhere classified, <u>thigh</u>
   M62.551   Muscle wasting and atrophy, not elsewhere classified, <u>right</u> thigh
   M62.552   Muscle wasting and atrophy, not elsewhere classified, <u>left</u> thigh
   M62.559   Muscle wasting and atrophy, not elsewhere classified, <u>unspecified</u> thigh
M62.56-Muscle wasting and atrophy, not elsewhere classified, <u>lower leg</u>
   M62.561   Muscle wasting and atrophy, not elsewhere classified, <u>right</u> lower leg
   M62.562   Muscle wasting and atrophy, not elsewhere classified, <u>left</u> lower leg
   M62.569   Muscle wasting and atrophy, not elsewhere classified, <u>unspecified</u> lower leg
M62.57-Muscle wasting and atrophy, not elsewhere classified, <u>ankle and foot</u>
   M62.571   Muscle wasting and atrophy, not elsewhere classified, <u>right</u> ankle and foot
   M62.572   Muscle wasting and atrophy, not elsewhere classified, <u>left</u> ankle and foot
   M62.579   Muscle wasting and atrophy, not elsewhere classified, <u>unspecified</u> ankle and foot
M62.58 Muscle wasting and atrophy, not elsewhere classified, <u>other site</u>
M62.59 Muscle wasting and atrophy, not elsewhere classified, <u>multiple sites</u>

M 6 1 I M 6 2

M62.8- Other specified disorders of muscle
  Excludes❷: nontraumatic hematoma of muscle (M79.81)
  M62.81 Muscle weakness (generalized)
  M62.82 Rhabdomyolysis
    Excludes 1: traumatic rhabdomyolysis (T79.6)
  M62.83-Muscle spasm
    M62.830 Muscle spasm of back
    M62.831 Muscle spasm of calf
      Charley-horse
    M62.838 Other muscle spasm
  M62.89 Other specified disorders of muscle
    Muscle (sheath) hernia
  M62.9 Disorder of muscle, unspecified
M63- Disorders of muscle <u>in diseases classified elsewhere</u>
  Code first underlying disease, such as:
    Leprosy (A30.-)
    Neoplasm (C49.-, C79.89, D21.-, D48.1)
    Schistosomiasis (B65.-)
    Trichinellosis (B75)
  Excludes 1: myopathy in cysticercosis (B69.81)
    myopathy in endocrine diseases (G73.7)
    myopathy in metabolic diseases (G73.7)
    myopathy in sarcoidosis (D86.87)
    myopathy in secondary syphilis (A51.49)
    myopathy in syphilis (late) (A52.78)
    myopathy in toxoplasmosis (B58.82)
    myopathy in tuberculosis (A18.09)
  M63.8- Disorders of muscle in diseases classified elsewhere
    M63.80 Disorders of muscle in diseases classified elsewhere, <u>unspecified site</u>
    M63.81-Disorders of muscle in diseases classified elsewhere, <u>shoulder</u>
      M63.811 Disorders of muscle in diseases classified elsewhere, <u>right</u> shoulder
      M63.812 Disorders of muscle in diseases classified elsewhere, <u>left</u> shoulder
      M63.819 Disorders of muscle in diseases classified elsewhere, <u>unspecified</u> shoulder
    M63.82-Disorders of muscle in diseases classified elsewhere, <u>upper arm</u>
      M63.821 Disorders of muscle in diseases classified elsewhere, <u>right</u> upper arm
      M63.822 Disorders of muscle in diseases classified elsewhere, <u>left</u> upper arm
      M63.829 Disorders of muscle in diseases classified elsewhere, <u>unspecified</u> upper arm
    M63.83-Disorders of muscle in diseases classified elsewhere, <u>forearm</u>
      M63.831 Disorders of muscle in diseases classified elsewhere, <u>right</u> forearm
      M63.832 Disorders of muscle in diseases classified elsewhere, <u>left</u> forearm
      M63.839 Disorders of muscle in diseases classified elsewhere, <u>unspecified</u> forearm
    M63.84-Disorders of muscle in diseases classified elsewhere, <u>hand</u>
      M63.841 Disorders of muscle in diseases classified elsewhere, <u>right</u> hand
      M63.842 Disorders of muscle in diseases classified elsewhere, <u>left</u> hand
      M63.849 Disorders of muscle in diseases classified elsewhere, <u>unspecified</u> hand
    M63.85-Disorders of muscle in diseases classified elsewhere, <u>thigh</u>
      M63.851 Disorders of muscle in diseases classified elsewhere, <u>right</u> thigh
      M63.852 Disorders of muscle in diseases classified elsewhere, <u>left</u> thigh
      M63.859 Disorders of muscle in diseases classified elsewhere, <u>unspecified</u> thigh
    M63.86-Disorders of muscle in diseases classified elsewhere, <u>lower leg</u>
      M63.861 Disorders of muscle in diseases classified elsewhere, <u>right</u> lower leg
      M63.862 Disorders of muscle in diseases classified elsewhere, <u>left</u> lower leg
      M63.869 Disorders of muscle in diseases classified elsewhere, <u>unspecified</u> lower leg

M63.87-Disorders of muscle in diseases classified elsewhere, <u>ankle and foot</u>
  M63.871 Disorders of muscle in diseases classified elsewhere, <u>right</u> ankle and foot
  M63.872 Disorders of muscle in diseases classified elsewhere, <u>left</u> ankle and foot
  M63.879 Disorders of muscle in diseases classified elsewhere, <u>unspecified</u> ankle and foot
M63.88 Disorders of muscle in diseases classified elsewhere, <u>other site</u>
M63.89 Disorders of muscle in diseases classified elsewhere, <u>multiple sites</u>

Disorders of synovium and tendon (M65-M67)

M65- <u>Synovitis and tenosynovitis</u>
  Excludes 1: chronic crepitant synovitis of hand and wrist (M70.0-)
    current injury — see injury of ligament or tendon by body region
    soft tissue disorders related to use, overuse and pressure (M70.-)
  M65.0- <u>Abscess of tendon sheath</u>
    Use additional code (B95-B96) to identify bacterial agent.
    M65.00 Abscess of tendon sheath, <u>unspecified site</u>
    M65.01-Abscess of tendon sheath, <u>shoulder</u>
      M65.011 Abscess of tendon sheath, <u>right</u> shoulder
      M65.012 Abscess of tendon sheath, <u>left</u> shoulder
      M65.019 Abscess of tendon sheath, <u>unspecified</u> shoulder
    M65.02-Abscess of tendon sheath, <u>upper arm</u>
      M65.021 Abscess of tendon sheath, <u>right</u> upper arm
      M65.022 Abscess of tendon sheath, <u>left</u> upper arm
      M65.029 Abscess of tendon sheath, <u>unspecified</u> upper arm
    M65.03-Abscess of tendon sheath, <u>forearm</u>
      M65.031 Abscess of tendon sheath, <u>right</u> forearm
      M65.032 Abscess of tendon sheath, <u>left</u> forearm
      M65.039 Abscess of tendon sheath, <u>unspecified</u> forearm
    M65.04-Abscess of tendon sheath, <u>hand</u>
      M65.041 Abscess of tendon sheath, <u>right</u> hand
      M65.042 Abscess of tendon sheath, <u>left</u> hand
      M65.049 Abscess of tendon sheath, <u>unspecified</u> hand
    M65.05-Abscess of tendon sheath, thigh
      M65.051 Abscess of tendon sheath, <u>right</u> thigh
      M65.052 Abscess of tendon sheath, <u>left</u> thigh
      M65.059 Abscess of tendon sheath, <u>unspecified</u> thigh
    M65.06-Abscess of tendon sheath, <u>lower leg</u>
      M65.061 Abscess of tendon sheath, <u>right</u> lower leg
      M65.062 Abscess of tendon sheath, <u>left</u> lower leg
      M65.069 Abscess of tendon sheath, <u>unspecified</u> lower leg
    M65.07-Abscess of tendon sheath, <u>ankle and foot</u>
      M65.071 Abscess of tendon sheath, <u>right</u> ankle and foot
      M65.072 Abscess of tendon sheath, <u>left</u> ankle and foot
      M65.079 Abscess of tendon sheath, <u>unspecified</u> ankle and foot
    M65.08 Abscess of tendon sheath, <u>other site</u>
  M65.1- <u>Other infective (teno)synovitis</u>
    M65.10 Other infective (teno)synovitis, <u>unspecified site</u>
    M65.11- Other infective (teno)synovitis, <u>shoulder</u>
      M65.111 Other infective (teno)synovitis, <u>right</u> shoulder
      M65.112 Other infective (teno)synovitis, <u>left</u> shoulder
      M65.119 Other infective (teno)synovitis, <u>unspecified</u> shoulder
    M65.12-Other infective (teno)synovitis, <u>elbow</u>
      M65.121 Other infective (teno)synovitis, <u>right</u> elbow
      M65.122 Other infective (teno)synovitis, <u>left</u> elbow
      M65.129 Other infective (teno)synovitis, <u>unspecified</u> elbow
    M65.13-Other infective (teno)synovitis, <u>wrist</u>
      M65.131 Other infective (teno)synovitis, <u>right</u> wrist
      M65.132 Other infective (teno)synovitis, <u>left</u> wrist
      M65.139 Other infective (teno)synovitis, <u>unspecified</u> wrist
    M65.14-Other infective (teno)synovitis, <u>hand</u>
      M65.141 Other infective (teno)synovitis, <u>right</u> hand
      M65.142 Other infective (teno)synovitis, <u>left</u> hand
      M65.149 Other infective (teno)synovitis, <u>unspecified</u> hand
    M65.15-Other infective (teno)synovitis, <u>hip</u>
      M65.151 Other infective (teno)synovitis, <u>right</u> hip
      M65.152 Other infective (teno)synovitis, <u>left</u> hip
      M65.159 Other infective (teno)synovitis, <u>unspecified</u> hip

M65.16-Other infective (teno)synovitis, <u>knee</u>
   M65.161 Other infective (teno)synovitis, <u>right</u> knee
   M65.162 Other infective (teno)synovitis, <u>left</u> knee
   M65.169 Other infective (teno)synovitis, <u>unspecified</u> knee
M65.17-Other infective (teno)synovitis, <u>ankle and foot</u>
   M65.171 Other infective (teno)synovitis, <u>right</u> ankle and foot
   M65.172 Other infective (teno)synovitis, <u>left</u> ankle and foot
   M65.179 Other infective (teno)synovitis, <u>unspecified</u> ankle and foot
M65.18 Other infective (teno)synovitis, <u>other site</u>
M65.19 Other infective (teno)synovitis, <u>multiple sites</u>
M65.2- <u>Calcific tendinitis</u>
   Excludes 1: tendinitis as classified in M75-M77
            calcified tendinitis of shoulder (M75.3)
M65.20 Calcific tendinitis, <u>unspecified</u> site
M65.22-Calcific tendinitis, <u>upper arm</u>
   M65.221 Calcific tendinitis, <u>right</u> upper arm
   M65.222 Calcific tendinitis, <u>left</u> upper arm
   M65.229 Calcific tendinitis, <u>unspecified</u> upper arm
M65.23-Calcific tendinitis, <u>forearm</u>
   M65.231 Calcific tendinitis, <u>right</u> forearm
   M65.232 Calcific tendinitis, <u>left</u> forearm
   M65.239 Calcific tendinitis, <u>unspecified</u> forearm
M65.24-Calcific tendinitis, <u>hand</u>
   M65.241 Calcific tendinitis, <u>right</u> hand
   M65.242 Calcific tendinitis, <u>left</u> hand
   M65.249 Calcific tendinitis, <u>unspecified</u> hand
M65.25-Calcific tendinitis, <u>thigh</u>
   M65.251 Calcific tendinitis, <u>right</u> thigh
   M65.252 Calcific tendinitis, <u>left</u> thigh
   M65.259 Calcific tendinitis, <u>unspecified</u> thigh
M65.26-Calcific tendinitis, <u>lower leg</u>
   M65.261 Calcific tendinitis, <u>right</u> lower leg
   M65.262 Calcific tendinitis, <u>left</u> lower leg
   M65.269 Calcific tendinitis, <u>unspecified</u> lower leg
M65.27-Calcific tendinitis, <u>ankle and foot</u>
   M65.271 Calcific tendinitis, <u>right</u> ankle and foot
   M65.272 Calcific tendinitis, <u>left</u> ankle and foot
   M65.279 Calcific tendinitis, <u>unspecified</u> ankle and foot
M65.28 Calcific tendinitis, <u>other site</u>
M65.29 Calcific tendinitis, <u>multiple sites</u>
M65.3- <u>Trigger finger</u>
   Nodular tendinous disease
M65.30 Trigger finger, <u>unspecified</u> finger
M65.31-Trigger <u>thumb</u>
   M65.311 Trigger thumb, <u>right</u> thumb
   M65.312 Trigger thumb, <u>left</u> thumb
   M65.319 Trigger thumb, <u>unspecified</u> thumb
M65.32-Trigger finger, <u>index</u> finger
   M65.321 Trigger finger, <u>right</u> index finger
   M65.322 Trigger finger, <u>left</u> index finger
   M65.329 Trigger finger, <u>unspecified</u> index finger
M65.33-Trigger finger, <u>middle</u> finger
   M65.331 Trigger finger, <u>right</u> middle finger
   M65.332 Trigger finger, <u>left</u> middle finger
   M65.339 Trigger finger, <u>unspecified</u> middle finger
M65.34-Trigger finger, <u>ring</u> finger
   M65.341 Trigger finger, <u>right</u> ring finger
   M65.342 Trigger finger, <u>left</u> ring finger
   M65.349 Trigger finger, <u>unspecified</u> ring finger
M65.35-Trigger finger, <u>little</u> finger
   M65.351 Trigger finger, <u>right</u> little finger
   M65.352 Trigger finger, <u>left</u> little finger
   M65.359 Trigger finger, <u>unspecified</u> little finger
M65.4 Radial styloid tenosynovitis [de Quervain]
M65.8- <u>Other synovitis and tenosynovitis</u>
M65.80 Other synovitis and tenosynovitis, <u>unspecified</u> site
M65.81-Other synovitis and tenosynovitis, <u>shoulder</u>
   M65.811 Other synovitis and tenosynovitis, <u>right</u> shoulder
   M65.812 Other synovitis and tenosynovitis, <u>left</u> shoulder
   M65.819 Other synovitis and tenosynovitis, <u>unspecified</u> shoulder

M65.82-Other synovitis and tenosynovitis, <u>upper arm</u>
   M65.821 Other synovitis and tenosynovitis, <u>right</u> upper arm
   M65.822 Other synovitis and tenosynovitis, <u>left</u> upper arm
   M65.829 Other synovitis and tenosynovitis, <u>unspecified</u> upper arm
M65.83-Other synovitis and tenosynovitis, <u>forearm</u>
   M65.831 Other synovitis and tenosynovitis, <u>right</u> forearm
   M65.832 Other synovitis and tenosynovitis, <u>left</u> forearm
   M65.839 Other synovitis and tenosynovitis, <u>unspecified</u> forearm
M65.84-Other synovitis and tenosynovitis, <u>hand</u>
   M65.841 Other synovitis and tenosynovitis, <u>right</u> hand
   M65.842 Other synovitis and tenosynovitis, <u>left</u> hand
   M65.849 Other synovitis and tenosynovitis, <u>unspecified</u> hand
M65.85-Other synovitis and tenosynovitis, <u>thigh</u>
   M65.851 Other synovitis and tenosynovitis, <u>right</u> thigh
   M65.852 Other synovitis and tenosynovitis, <u>left</u> thigh
   M65.859 Other synovitis and tenosynovitis, <u>unspecified</u> thigh
M65.86-Other synovitis and tenosynovitis, <u>lower leg</u>
   M65.861 Other synovitis and tenosynovitis, <u>right</u> lower leg
   M65.862 Other synovitis and tenosynovitis, <u>left</u> lower leg
   M65.869 Other synovitis and tenosynovitis, <u>unspecified</u> lower leg
M65.87-Other synovitis and tenosynovitis, <u>ankle and foot</u>
   M65.871 Other synovitis and tenosynovitis, <u>right</u> ankle and foot
   M65.872 Other synovitis and tenosynovitis, <u>left</u> ankle and foot
   M65.879 Other synovitis and tenosynovitis, <u>unspecified</u> ankle and foot
M65.88 Other synovitis and tenosynovitis, <u>other site</u>
M65.89 Other synovitis and tenosynovitis, multiple sites
M65.9 Synovitis and tenosynovitis, <u>unspecified</u>
M66- <u>Spontaneous rupture of synovium and tendon</u>
   Includes: Rupture that occurs when a normal force is applied to tissues
             that are inferred to have less than normal strength
   Excludes❷: rotator cuff syndrome (M75.1-)
               rupture where an abnormal force is applied to normal
               tissue — see injury of tendon by body region
M66.0 Rupture of popliteal cyst
M66.1- Rupture of <u>synovium</u>
   Rupture of synovial cyst
   Excludes❷: rupture of popliteal cyst (M66.0)
M66.10 Rupture of synovium, <u>unspecified</u> joint
M66.11-Rupture of synovium, <u>shoulder</u>
   M66.111 Rupture of synovium, <u>right</u> shoulder
   M66.112 Rupture of synovium, <u>left</u> shoulder
   M66.119 Rupture of synovium, <u>unspecified</u> shoulder
M66.12-Rupture of synovium, <u>elbow</u>
   M66.121 Rupture of synovium, <u>right</u> elbow
   M66.122 Rupture of synovium, <u>left</u> elbow
   M66.129 Rupture of synovium, <u>unspecified</u> elbow
M66.13-Rupture of synovium, <u>wrist</u>
   M66.131 Rupture of synovium, <u>right</u> wrist
   M66.132 Rupture of synovium, <u>left</u> wrist
   M66.139 Rupture of synovium, <u>unspecified</u> wrist
M66.14-Rupture of synovium, <u>hand and fingers</u>
   M66.141 Rupture of synovium, <u>right</u> hand
   M66.142 Rupture of synovium, <u>left</u> hand
   M66.143 Rupture of synovium, <u>unspecified</u> hand
   M66.144 Rupture of synovium, <u>right</u> finger(s)
   M66.145 Rupture of synovium, <u>left</u> finger(s)
   M66.146 Rupture of synovium, <u>unspecified</u> finger(s)
M66.15-Rupture of synovium, <u>hip</u>
   M66.151 Rupture of synovium, <u>right</u> hip
   M66.152 Rupture of synovium, <u>left</u> hip
   M66.159 Rupture of synovium, <u>unspecified</u> hip
M66.17-Rupture of synovium, <u>ankle, foot and toes</u>
   M66.171 Rupture of synovium, <u>right</u> ankle
   M66.172 Rupture of synovium, <u>left</u> ankle
   M66.173 Rupture of synovium, <u>unspecified</u> ankle
   M66.174 Rupture of synovium, <u>right</u> foot
   M66.175 Rupture of synovium, <u>left</u> foot
   M66.176 Rupture of synovium, <u>unspecified</u> foot
   M66.177 Rupture of synovium, <u>right</u> toe(s)
   M66.178 Rupture of synovium, <u>left</u> toe(s)
   M66.179 Rupture of synovium, <u>unspecified</u> toe(s)
M66.18 Rupture of synovium, <u>other site</u>

M62
–
M66

M66.2- Spontaneous rupture of <u>extensor</u> tendons
  M66.20 Spontaneous rupture of extensor tendons, <u>unspecified</u> <u>site</u>
  M66.21-Spontaneous rupture of extensor tendons, <u>shoulder</u>
    M66.211 Spontaneous rupture of extensor tendons, <u>right</u> shoulder
    M66.212 Spontaneous rupture of extensor tendons, <u>left</u> shoulder
    M66.219 Spontaneous rupture of extensor tendons, <u>unspecified</u> shoulder
  M66.22-Spontaneous rupture of extensor tendons, <u>upper arm</u>
    M66.221 Spontaneous rupture of extensor tendons, <u>right</u> upper arm
    M66.222 Spontaneous rupture of extensor tendons, <u>left</u> upper arm
    M66.229 Spontaneous rupture of extensor tendons, <u>unspecified</u> upper arm
  M66.23-Spontaneous rupture of extensor tendons, <u>forearm</u>
    M66.231 Spontaneous rupture of extensor tendons, <u>right</u> forearm
    M66.232 Spontaneous rupture of extensor tendons, <u>left</u> forearm
    M66.239 Spontaneous rupture of extensor tendons, <u>unspecified</u> forearm
  M66.24-Spontaneous rupture of extensor tendons, <u>hand</u>
    M66.241 Spontaneous rupture of extensor tendons, <u>right</u> hand
    M66.242 Spontaneous rupture of extensor tendons, <u>left</u> hand
    M66.249 Spontaneous rupture of extensor tendons, <u>unspecified</u> hand
  M66.25-Spontaneous rupture of extensor tendons, <u>thigh</u>
    M66.251 Spontaneous rupture of extensor tendons, <u>right</u> thigh
    M66.252 Spontaneous rupture of extensor tendons, <u>left</u> thigh
    M66.259 Spontaneous rupture of extensor tendons, <u>unspecified</u> thigh
  M66.26-Spontaneous rupture of extensor tendons, <u>lower leg</u>
    M66.261 Spontaneous rupture of extensor tendons, <u>right</u> lower leg
    M66.262 Spontaneous rupture of extensor tendons, <u>left</u> lower leg
    M66.269 Spontaneous rupture of extensor tendons, <u>unspecified</u> lower leg
  M66.27-Spontaneous rupture of extensor tendons, <u>ankle and foot</u>
    M66.271 Spontaneous rupture of extensor tendons, <u>right</u> ankle and foot
    M66.272 Spontaneous rupture of extensor tendons, <u>left</u> ankle and foot
    M66.279 Spontaneous rupture of extensor tendons, <u>unspecified</u> ankle and foot
  M66.28 Spontaneous rupture of extensor tendons, <u>other site</u>
  M66.29 Spontaneous rupture of extensor tendons, <u>multiple sites</u>
M66.3- Spontaneous rupture of <u>flexor</u> tendons
  M66.30 Spontaneous rupture of flexor tendons, <u>unspecified</u> <u>site</u>
  M66.31-Spontaneous rupture of flexor tendons, <u>shoulder</u>
    M66.311 Spontaneous rupture of flexor tendons, <u>right</u> shoulder
    M66.312 Spontaneous rupture of flexor tendons, <u>left</u> shoulder
    M66.319 Spontaneous rupture of flexor tendons, <u>unspecified</u> shoulder
  M66.32-Spontaneous rupture of flexor tendons, <u>upper arm</u>
    M66.321 Spontaneous rupture of flexor tendons, <u>right</u> upper arm
    M66.322 Spontaneous rupture of flexor tendons, <u>left</u> upper arm
    M66.329 Spontaneous rupture of flexor tendons, <u>unspecified</u> upper arm
  M66.33-Spontaneous rupture of flexor tendons, <u>forearm</u>
    M66.331 Spontaneous rupture of flexor tendons, <u>right</u> forearm
    M66.332 Spontaneous rupture of flexor tendons, <u>left</u> forearm
    M66.339 Spontaneous rupture of flexor tendons, <u>unspecified</u> forearm
  M66.34-Spontaneous rupture of flexor tendons, <u>hand</u>
    M66.341 Spontaneous rupture of flexor tendons, <u>right</u> hand
    M66.342 Spontaneous rupture of flexor tendons, <u>left</u> hand
    M66.349 Spontaneous rupture of flexor tendons, <u>unspecified</u> hand
  M66.35-Spontaneous rupture of flexor tendons, <u>thigh</u>
    M66.351 Spontaneous rupture of flexor tendons, <u>right</u> thigh
    M66.352 Spontaneous rupture of flexor tendons, <u>left</u> thigh
    M66.359 Spontaneous rupture of flexor tendons, <u>unspecified</u> thigh

M66.36-Spontaneous rupture of flexor tendons, <u>lower leg</u>
  M66.361 Spontaneous rupture of flexor tendons, <u>right</u> lower leg
  M66.362 Spontaneous rupture of flexor tendons, <u>left</u> lower leg
  M66.369 Spontaneous rupture of flexor tendons, <u>unspecified</u> lower leg
M66.37-Spontaneous rupture of flexor tendons, <u>ankle and foot</u>
  M66.371 Spontaneous rupture of flexor tendons, <u>right</u> ankle and foot
  M66.372 Spontaneous rupture of flexor tendons, <u>left</u> ankle and foot
  M66.379 Spontaneous rupture of flexor tendons, <u>unspecified</u> ankle and foot
M66.38 Spontaneous rupture of flexor tendons, <u>other site</u>
M66.39 Spontaneous rupture of flexor tendons, <u>multiple sites</u>
M66.8- Spontaneous rupture of <u>other</u> tendons
  M66.80 Spontaneous rupture of other tendons, <u>unspecified</u> <u>site</u>
  M66.81-Spontaneous rupture of other tendons, <u>shoulder</u>
    M66.811 Spontaneous rupture of other tendons, <u>right</u> shoulder
    M66.812 Spontaneous rupture of other tendons, <u>left</u> shoulder
    M66.819 Spontaneous rupture of other tendons, <u>unspecified</u> shoulder
  M66.82-Spontaneous rupture of other tendons, <u>upper arm</u>
    M66.821 Spontaneous rupture of other tendons, <u>right</u> upper arm
    M66.822 Spontaneous rupture of other tendons, <u>left</u> upper arm
    M66.829 Spontaneous rupture of other tendons, <u>unspecified</u> upper arm
  M66.83-Spontaneous rupture of other tendons, <u>forearm</u>
    M66.831 Spontaneous rupture of other tendons, <u>right</u> forearm
    M66.832 Spontaneous rupture of other tendons, <u>left</u> forearm
    M66.839 Spontaneous rupture of other tendons, <u>unspecified</u> forearm
  M66.84-Spontaneous rupture of other tendons, <u>hand</u>
    M66.841 Spontaneous rupture of other tendons, <u>right</u> hand
    M66.842 Spontaneous rupture of other tendons, <u>left</u> hand
    M66.849 Spontaneous rupture of other tendons, <u>unspecified</u> hand
  M66.85-Spontaneous rupture of other tendons, <u>thigh</u>
    M66.851 Spontaneous rupture of other tendons, <u>right</u> thigh
    M66.852 Spontaneous rupture of other tendons, <u>left</u> thigh
    M66.859 Spontaneous rupture of other tendons, <u>unspecified</u> thigh
  M66.86-Spontaneous rupture of other tendons, <u>lower leg</u>
    M66.861 Spontaneous rupture of other tendons, <u>right</u> lower leg
    M66.862 Spontaneous rupture of other tendons, <u>left</u> lower leg
    M66.869 Spontaneous rupture of other tendons, <u>unspecified</u> lower leg
  M66.87-Spontaneous rupture of other tendons, <u>ankle and foot</u>
    M66.871 Spontaneous rupture of other tendons, <u>right</u> ankle and foot
    M66.872 Spontaneous rupture of other tendons, <u>left</u> ankle and foot
    M66.879 Spontaneous rupture of other tendons, <u>unspecified</u> ankle and foot
  M66.88 Spontaneous rupture of other tendons, <u>other</u>
  M66.89 Spontaneous rupture of other tendons, <u>multiple sites</u>
M66.9 Spontaneous rupture of <u>unspecified</u> tendon
    Rupture at musculotendinous junction, nontraumatic

M67- <u>Other disorders</u> of synovium and tendon
  Excludes 1: palmar fascial fibromatosis [Dupuytren] (M72.0)
        tendinitis NOS (M77.9-)
        xanthomatosis localized to tendons (E78.2)
  M67.0- <u>Short Achilles tendon (acquired)</u>
    M67.00 Short Achilles tendon (acquired), <u>unspecified</u> ankle
    M67.01 Short Achilles tendon (acquired), <u>right</u> ankle
    M67.02 Short Achilles tendon (acquired), <u>left</u> ankle
  M67.2- <u>Synovial hypertrophy</u>, <u>not elsewhere classified</u>
    Excludes 1: villonodular synovitis (pigmented) (M12.2-)
    M67.20 Synovial hypertrophy, not elsewhere classified, <u>unspecified site</u>
    M67.21-Synovial hypertrophy, not elsewhere classified, <u>shoulder</u>
      M67.211 Synovial hypertrophy, not elsewhere classified, <u>right</u> shoulder
      M67.212 Synovial hypertrophy, not elsewhere classified, <u>left</u> shoulder
      M67.219 Synovial hypertrophy, not elsewhere classified, <u>unspecified</u> shoulder

M 6 6 I M 6 7

M67.22-Synovial hypertrophy, not elsewhere classified, <u>upper arm</u>
   M67.221 Synovial hypertrophy, not elsewhere classified, <u>right</u> upper arm
   M67.222 Synovial hypertrophy, not elsewhere classified, <u>left</u> upper arm
   M67.229 Synovial hypertrophy, not elsewhere classified, <u>unspecified</u> upper arm
M67.23-Synovial hypertrophy, not elsewhere classified, <u>forearm</u>
   M67.231 Synovial hypertrophy, not elsewhere classified, <u>right</u> forearm
   M67.232 Synovial hypertrophy, not elsewhere classified, <u>left</u> forearm
   M67.239 Synovial hypertrophy, not elsewhere classified, <u>unspecified</u> forearm
M67.24-Synovial hypertrophy, not elsewhere classified, <u>hand</u>
   M67.241 Synovial hypertrophy, not elsewhere classified, <u>right</u> hand
   M67.242 Synovial hypertrophy, not elsewhere classified, <u>left</u> hand
   M67.249 Synovial hypertrophy, not elsewhere classified, <u>unspecified</u> hand
M67.25-Synovial hypertrophy, not elsewhere classified, <u>thigh</u>
   M67.251 Synovial hypertrophy, not elsewhere classified, <u>right</u> thigh
   M67.252 Synovial hypertrophy, not elsewhere classified, <u>left</u> thigh
   M67.259 Synovial hypertrophy, not elsewhere classified, <u>unspecified</u> thigh
M67.26-Synovial hypertrophy, not elsewhere classified, <u>lower leg</u>
   M67.261 Synovial hypertrophy, not elsewhere classified, <u>right</u> lower leg
   M67.262 Synovial hypertrophy, not elsewhere classified, <u>left</u> lower leg
   M67.269 Synovial hypertrophy, not elsewhere classified, <u>unspecified</u> lower leg
M67.27-Synovial hypertrophy, not elsewhere classified, <u>ankle and foot</u>
   M67.271 Synovial hypertrophy, not elsewhere classified, <u>right</u> ankle and foot
   M67.272 Synovial hypertrophy, not elsewhere classified, <u>left</u> ankle and foot
   M67.279 Synovial hypertrophy, not elsewhere classified, <u>unspecified</u> ankle and foot
M67.28 Synovial hypertrophy, not elsewhere classified, <u>other site</u>
M67.29 Synovial hypertrophy, not elsewhere classified, <u>multiple sites</u>
M67.3- <u>Transient</u> synovitis
     Toxic synovitis
     Excludes 1: palindromic rheumatism (M12.3-)
M67.30 Transient synovitis, <u>unspecified site</u>
M67.31-Transient synovitis, <u>shoulder</u>
   M67.311 Transient synovitis, <u>right</u> shoulder
   M67.312 Transient synovitis, <u>left</u> shoulder
   M67.319 Transient synovitis, <u>unspecified</u> shoulder
M67.32-Transient synovitis, <u>elbow</u>
   M67.321 Transient synovitis, <u>right</u> elbow
   M67.322 Transient synovitis, <u>left</u> elbow
   M67.329 Transient synovitis, <u>unspecified</u> elbow
M67.33-Transient synovitis, <u>wrist</u>
   M67.331 Transient synovitis, <u>right</u> wrist
   M67.332 Transient synovitis, <u>left</u> wrist
   M67.339 Transient synovitis, <u>unspecified</u> wrist
M67.34-Transient synovitis, <u>hand</u>
   M67.341 Transient synovitis, <u>right</u> hand
   M67.342 Transient synovitis, <u>left</u> hand
   M67.349 Transient synovitis, <u>unspecified</u> hand
M67.35-Transient synovitis, <u>hip</u>
   M67.351 Transient synovitis, <u>right</u> hip
   M67.352 Transient synovitis, <u>left</u> hip
   M67.359 Transient synovitis, <u>unspecified</u> hip
M67.36-Transient synovitis, <u>knee</u>
   M67.361 Transient synovitis, <u>right</u> knee
   M67.362 Transient synovitis, <u>left</u> knee
   M67.369 Transient synovitis, <u>unspecified</u> knee

M67.37-Transient synovitis, <u>ankle and foot</u>
   M67.371 Transient synovitis, <u>right</u> ankle and foot
   M67.372 Transient synovitis, <u>left</u> ankle and foot
   M67.379 Transient synovitis, <u>unspecified</u> ankle and foot
M67.38 Transient synovitis, <u>other site</u>
M67.39 Transient synovitis, <u>multiple sites</u>
M67.4- <u>Ganglion</u>
     Ganglion of joint or tendon (sheath)
     Excludes 1: ganglion in yaws (A66.6)
     Excludes ❷: cyst of bursa (M71.2-M71.3)
                  cyst of synovium (M71.2-M71.3)
M67.40 Ganglion, <u>unspecified site</u>
M67.41-Ganglion, <u>shoulder</u>
   M67.411 Ganglion, <u>right</u> shoulder
   M67.412 Ganglion, <u>left</u> shoulder
   M67.419 Ganglion, <u>unspecified</u> shoulder
M67.42-Ganglion, <u>elbow</u>
   M67.421 Ganglion, <u>right</u> elbow
   M67.422 Ganglion, <u>left</u> elbow
   M67.429 Ganglion, <u>unspecified</u> elbow
M67.43-Ganglion, <u>wrist</u>
   M67.431 Ganglion, <u>right</u> wrist
   M67.432 Ganglion, <u>left</u> wrist
   M67.439 Ganglion, <u>unspecified</u> wrist
M67.44-Ganglion, <u>hand</u>
   M67.441 Ganglion, <u>right</u> hand
   M67.442 Ganglion, <u>left</u> hand
   M67.449 Ganglion, <u>unspecified</u> hand
M67.45-Ganglion, <u>hip</u>
   M67.451 Ganglion, <u>right</u> hip
   M67.452 Ganglion, <u>left</u> hip
   M67.459 Ganglion, <u>unspecified</u> hip
M67.46-Ganglion, <u>knee</u>
   M67.461 Ganglion, <u>right</u> knee
   M67.462 Ganglion, <u>left</u> knee
   M67.469 Ganglion, <u>unspecified</u> knee
M67.47-Ganglion, <u>ankle and foot</u>
   M67.471 Ganglion, <u>right</u> ankle and foot
   M67.472 Ganglion, <u>left</u> ankle and foot
   M67.479 Ganglion, <u>unspecified</u> ankle and foot
M67.48 Ganglion, <u>other site</u>
M67.49 Ganglion, <u>multiple sites</u>
M67.5- <u>Plica syndrome</u>
     Plica knee
M67.50 Plica syndrome, <u>unspecified</u> knee
M67.51 Plica syndrome, <u>right</u> knee
M67.52 Plica syndrome, <u>left</u> knee
M67.8- <u>Other specified</u> disorders of synovium and tendon
M67.80 Other specified disorders of synovium and tendon, <u>unspecified site</u>
M67.81-Other specified disorders of synovium and tendon, <u>shoulder</u>
   M67.811 Other specified disorders of synovium, <u>right</u> shoulder
   M67.812 Other specified disorders of synovium, <u>left</u> shoulder
   M67.813 Other specified disorders of tendon, <u>right</u> shoulder
   M67.814 Other specified disorders of tendon, <u>left</u> shoulder
   M67.819 Other specified disorders of synovium and tendon, <u>unspecified</u> shoulder
M67.82-Other specified disorders of synovium and tendon, <u>elbow</u>
   M67.821 Other specified disorders of synovium, <u>right</u> elbow
   M67.822 Other specified disorders of synovium, <u>left</u> elbow
   M67.823 Other specified disorders of tendon, <u>right</u> elbow
   M67.824 Other specified disorders of tendon, <u>left</u> elbow
   M67.829 Other specified disorders of synovium and tendon, <u>unspecified</u> elbow
M67.83-Other specified disorders of synovium and tendon, <u>wrist</u>
   M67.831 Other specified disorders of synovium, <u>right</u> wrist
   M67.832 Other specified disorders of synovium, <u>left</u> wrist
   M67.833 Other specified disorders of tendon, <u>right</u> wrist
   M67.834 Other specified disorders of tendon, <u>left</u> wrist
   M67.839 Other specified disorders of synovium and tendon, <u>unspecified</u> forearm

M 6 6 I M 6 7

M67.84-Other specified disorders of synovium and tendon, <u>hand</u>
> M67.841 Other specified disorders of synovium, <u>right</u> hand
> M67.842 Other specified disorders of synovium, <u>left</u> hand
> M67.843 Other specified disorders of tendon, <u>right</u> hand
> M67.844 Other specified disorders of tendon, <u>left</u> hand
> M67.849 Other specified disorders of synovium and tendon, <u>unspecified</u> hand

M67.85-Other specified disorders of synovium and tendon, <u>hip</u>
> M67.851 Other specified disorders of synovium, <u>right</u> hip
> M67.852 Other specified disorders of synovium, <u>left</u> hip
> M67.853 Other specified disorders of tendon, <u>right</u> hip
> M67.854 Other specified disorders of tendon, <u>left</u> hip
> M67.859 Other specified disorders of synovium and tendon, <u>unspecified</u> hip

M67.86-Other specified disorders of synovium and tendon, <u>knee</u>
> M67.861 Other specified disorders of synovium, <u>right</u> knee
> M67.862 Other specified disorders of synovium, <u>left</u> knee
> M67.863 Other specified disorders of tendon, <u>right</u> knee
> M67.864 Other specified disorders of tendon, <u>left</u> knee
> M67.869 Other specified disorders of synovium and tendon, <u>unspecified</u> knee

M67.87-Other specified disorders of synovium and tendon, <u>ankle and foot</u>
> M67.871 Other specified disorders of synovium, <u>right</u> ankle and foot
> M67.872 Other specified disorders of synovium, <u>left</u> ankle and foot
> M67.873 Other specified disorders of tendon, <u>right</u> ankle and foot
> M67.874 Other specified disorders of tendon, <u>left</u> ankle and foot
> M67.879 Other specified disorders of synovium and tendon, <u>unspecified</u> ankle and foot

M67.88 Other specified disorders of synovium and tendon, <u>other site</u>
M67.89 Other specified disorders of synovium and tendon, <u>multiple sites</u>

M67.9- Unspecified disorder of synovium and tendon
> M67.90 Unspecified disorder of synovium and tendon, <u>unspecified site</u>

M67.91-Unspecified disorder of synovium and tendon, <u>shoulder</u>
> M67.911 Unspecified disorder of synovium and tendon, <u>right</u> shoulder
> M67.912 Unspecified disorder of synovium and tendon, <u>left</u> shoulder
> M67.919 Unspecified disorder of synovium and tendon, <u>unspecified</u> shoulder

M67.92-Unspecified disorder of synovium and tendon, <u>upper arm</u>
> M67.921 Unspecified disorder of synovium and tendon, <u>right</u> upper arm
> M67.922 Unspecified disorder of synovium and tendon, <u>left</u> upper arm
> M67.929 Unspecified disorder of synovium and tendon, <u>unspecified</u> upper arm

M67.93-Unspecified disorder of synovium and tendon, <u>forearm</u>
> M67.931 Unspecified disorder of synovium and tendon, <u>right</u> forearm
> M67.932 Unspecified disorder of synovium and tendon, <u>left</u> forearm
> M67.939 Unspecified disorder of synovium and tendon, <u>unspecified</u> forearm

M67.94-Unspecified disorder of synovium and tendon, <u>hand</u>
> M67.941 Unspecified disorder of synovium and tendon, <u>right</u> hand
> M67.942 Unspecified disorder of synovium and tendon, <u>left</u> hand
> M67.949 Unspecified disorder of synovium and tendon, <u>unspecified</u> hand

M67.95-Unspecified disorder of synovium and tendon, <u>thigh</u>
> M67.951 Unspecified disorder of synovium and tendon, <u>right</u> thigh
> M67.952 Unspecified disorder of synovium and tendon, <u>left</u> thigh
> M67.959 Unspecified disorder of synovium and tendon, <u>unspecified</u> thigh

M67.96-Unspecified disorder of synovium and tendon, <u>lower leg</u>
> M67.961 Unspecified disorder of synovium and tendon, <u>right</u> lower leg
> M67.962 Unspecified disorder of synovium and tendon, <u>left</u> lower leg
> M67.969 Unspecified disorder of synovium and tendon, <u>unspecified</u> lower leg

M67.97-Unspecified disorder of synovium and tendon, <u>ankle and foot</u>
> M67.971 Unspecified disorder of synovium and tendon, <u>right</u> ankle and foot
> M67.972 Unspecified disorder of synovium and tendon, <u>left</u> ankle and foot
> M67.979 Unspecified disorder of synovium and tendon, <u>unspecified</u> ankle and foot

M67.98 Unspecified disorder of synovium and tendon, <u>other site</u>
M67.99 Unspecified disorder of synovium and tendon, <u>multiple sites</u>

Other soft tissue disorders (M70-M79)

M70- <u>Soft tissue disorders related to use, overuse and pressure</u>
Includes: soft tissue disorders of occupational origin
Use additional external cause code to identify activity causing disorder (Y93.-)
Excludes 1: bursitis NOS (M71.9-)
Excludes ❷: bursitis of shoulder (M75.5)
enthesopathies (M76-M77)
pressure ulcer (pressure area) (L89.-)

M70.0- <u>Crepitant synovitis</u> (acute) (chronic) of hand and wrist
> M70.03-Crepitant synovitis (acute) (chronic), <u>wrist</u>
> > M70.031 Crepitant synovitis (acute) (chronic), <u>right</u> wrist
> > M70.032 Crepitant synovitis (acute) (chronic), <u>left</u> wrist
> > M70.039 Crepitant synovitis (acute) (chronic), <u>unspecified</u> wrist

> M70.04-Crepitant synovitis (acute) (chronic), <u>hand</u>
> > M70.041 Crepitant synovitis (acute) (chronic), <u>right</u> hand
> > M70.042 Crepitant synovitis (acute) (chronic), <u>left</u> hand
> > M70.049 Crepitant synovitis (acute) (chronic), <u>unspecified</u> hand

M70.1- <u>Bursitis</u> of hand
> M70.10 Bursitis, <u>unspecified</u> hand
> M70.11 Bursitis, <u>right</u> hand
> M70.12 Bursitis, <u>left</u> hand

M70.2- <u>Olecranon</u> bursitis
> M70.20 Olecranon bursitis, <u>unspecified</u> elbow
> M70.21 Olecranon bursitis, <u>right</u> elbow
> M70.22 Olecranon bursitis, <u>left</u> elbow

M70.3- <u>Other</u> bursitis of <u>elbow</u>
> M70.30 Other bursitis of elbow, <u>unspecified</u> elbow
> M70.31 Other bursitis of elbow, <u>right</u> elbow
> M70.32 Other bursitis of elbow, <u>left</u> elbow

M70.4- <u>Prepatellar</u> bursitis
> M70.40 Prepatellar bursitis, <u>unspecified</u> knee
> M70.41 Prepatellar bursitis, <u>right</u> knee
> M70.42 Prepatellar bursitis, <u>left</u> knee

M70.5- <u>Other</u> bursitis of <u>knee</u>
> M70.50 Other bursitis of knee, <u>unspecified</u> knee
> M70.51 Other bursitis of knee, <u>right</u> knee
> M70.52 Other bursitis of knee, <u>left</u> knee

M70.6- <u>Trochanteric</u> bursitis
> Trochanteric tendinitis
> M70.60 Trochanteric bursitis, <u>unspecified</u> hip
> M70.61 Trochanteric bursitis, <u>right</u> hip
> M70.62 Trochanteric bursitis, <u>left</u> hip

M70.7- <u>Other</u> bursitis of <u>hip</u>
> Ischial bursitis
> M70.70 Other bursitis of hip, <u>unspecified</u> hip
> M70.71 Other bursitis of hip, <u>right</u> hip
> M70.72 Other bursitis of hip, <u>left</u> hip

M70.8- <u>Other soft tissue disorders</u> related to use, overuse and pressure
> M70.80 Other soft tissue disorders related to use, overuse and pressure of <u>unspecified</u> site
> M70.81-Other soft tissue disorders related to use, overuse and pressure of <u>shoulder</u>
> > M70.811 Other soft tissue disorders related to use, overuse and pressure, <u>right</u> shoulder
> > M70.812 Other soft tissue disorders related to use, overuse and pressure, <u>left</u> shoulder
> > M70.819 Other soft tissue disorders related to use, overuse and pressure, <u>unspecified</u> shoulder

M 6 7
I
M 7 1

M70.82-Other soft tissue disorders related to use, overuse and pressure of <u>upper arm</u>
M70.821 Other soft tissue disorders related to use, overuse and pressure, <u>right</u> upper arm
M70.822 Other soft tissue disorders related to use, overuse and pressure, <u>left</u> upper arm
M70.829 Other soft tissue disorders related to use, overuse and pressure, <u>unspecified</u> upper arms

M70.83-Other soft tissue disorders related to use, overuse and pressure of <u>forearm</u>
M70.831 Other soft tissue disorders related to use, overuse and pressure, <u>right</u> forearm
M70.832 Other soft tissue disorders related to use, overuse and pressure, <u>left</u> forearm
M70.839 Other soft tissue disorders related to use, overuse and pressure, <u>unspecified</u> forearm

M70.84-Other soft tissue disorders related to use, overuse and pressure of <u>hand</u>
M70.841 Other soft tissue disorders related to use, overuse and pressure, <u>right</u> hand
M70.842 Other soft tissue disorders related to use, overuse and pressure, <u>left</u> hand
M70.849 Other soft tissue disorders related to use, overuse and pressure, <u>unspecified</u> hand

M70.85-Other soft tissue disorders related to use, overuse and pressure of <u>thigh</u>
M70.851 Other soft tissue disorders related to use, overuse and pressure, <u>right</u> thigh
M70.852 Other soft tissue disorders related to use, overuse and pressure, <u>left</u> thigh
M70.859 Other soft tissue disorders related to use, overuse and pressure, <u>unspecified</u> thigh

M70.86 Other soft tissue disorders related to use, overuse and pressure <u>lower leg</u>
M70.861 Other soft tissue disorders related to use, overuse and pressure, <u>right</u> lower leg
M70.862 Other soft tissue disorders related to use, overuse and pressure, <u>left</u> lower leg
M70.869 Other soft tissue disorders related to use, overuse and pressure, <u>unspecified</u> leg

M70.87-Other soft tissue disorders related to use, overuse and pressure of <u>ankle and foot</u>
M70.871 Other soft tissue disorders related to use, overuse and pressure, <u>right</u> ankle and foot
M70.872 Other soft tissue disorders related to use, overuse and pressure, <u>left</u> ankle and foot
M70.879 Other soft tissue disorders related to use, overuse and pressure, <u>unspecified</u> ankle and foot

M70.88 Other soft tissue disorders related to use, overuse and pressure <u>other site</u>
M70.89 Other soft tissue disorders related to use, overuse and pressure <u>multiple sites</u>

M70.9- <u>Unspecified</u> soft tissue disorder related to use, overuse and pressure
M70.90 Unspecified soft tissue disorder related to use, overuse and pressure of <u>unspecified site</u>
M70.91-Unspecified soft tissue disorder related to use, overuse and pressure of <u>shoulder</u>
M70.911 Unspecified soft tissue disorder related to use, overuse and pressure, <u>right</u> shoulder
M70.912 Unspecified soft tissue disorder related to use, overuse and pressure, <u>left</u> shoulder
M70.919 Unspecified soft tissue disorder related to use, overuse and pressure, <u>unspecified</u> shoulder

M70.92-Unspecified soft tissue disorder related to use, overuse and pressure of <u>upper arm</u>
M70.921 Unspecified soft tissue disorder related to use, overuse and pressure, <u>right</u> upperarm
M70.922 Unspecified soft tissue disorder related to use, overuse and pressure, <u>left</u> upperarm
M70.929 Unspecified soft tissue disorder related to use, overuse and pressure, <u>unspecified</u> upper arm

M70.93-Unspecified soft tissue disorder related to use, overuse and pressure of <u>forearm</u>
M70.931 Unspecified soft tissue disorder related to use, overuse and pressure, <u>right</u> forearm
M70.932 Unspecified soft tissue disorder related to use, overuse and pressure, <u>left</u> forearm
M70.939 Unspecified soft tissue disorder related to use, overuse and pressure, <u>unspecified</u> forearm

M70.94-Unspecified soft tissue disorder related to use, overuse and pressure of <u>hand</u>
M70.941 Unspecified soft tissue disorder related to use, overuse and pressure, <u>right</u> hand
M70.942 Unspecified soft tissue disorder related to use, overuse and pressure, <u>left</u> hand
M70.949 Unspecified soft tissue disorder related to use, overuse and pressure, <u>unspecified</u> hand

M70.95-Unspecified soft tissue disorder related to use, overuse and pressure of <u>thigh</u>
M70.951 Unspecified soft tissue disorder related to use, overuse and pressure, <u>right</u> thigh
M70.952 Unspecified soft tissue disorder related to use, overuse and pressure, <u>left</u> thigh
M70.959 Unspecified soft tissue disorder related to use, overuse and pressure, <u>unspecified</u> thigh

M70.96-Unspecified soft tissue disorder related to use, overuse and pressure <u>lower leg</u>
M70.961 Unspecified soft tissue disorder related to use, overuse and pressure, <u>right</u> lower leg
M70.962 Unspecified soft tissue disorder related to use, overuse and pressure, <u>left</u> lower leg
M70.969 Unspecified soft tissue disorder related to use, overuse and pressure, <u>unspecified</u> lower leg

M70.97-Unspecified soft tissue disorder related to use, overuse and pressure of <u>ankle and foot</u>
M70.971 Unspecified soft tissue disorder related to use, overuse and pressure, <u>right</u> ankle and foot
M70.972 Unspecified soft tissue disorder related to use, overuse and pressure, <u>left</u> ankle and foot
M70.979 Unspecified soft tissue disorder related to use, overuse and pressure, <u>unspecified</u> ankle and foot

M70.98 Unspecified soft tissue disorder related to use, overuse and pressure <u>other</u>
M70.99 Unspecified soft tissue disorder related to use, overuse and pressure <u>multiple sites</u>

M71- Other bursopathies
Excludes 1: bunion (M20.1)
    bursitis related to use, overuse or pressure (M70.-)
    enthesopathies (M76-M77)

M71.0- <u>Abscess of bursa</u>
Use additional code (B95.-, B96.-) to identify causative organism
M71.00 Abscess of bursa, <u>unspecified site</u>
M71.01-Abscess of bursa, <u>shoulder</u>
M71.011 Abscess of bursa, <u>right</u> shoulder
M71.012 Abscess of bursa, <u>left</u> shoulder
M71.019 Abscess of bursa, <u>unspecified</u> shoulder
M71.02-Abscess of bursa, <u>elbow</u>
M71.021 Abscess of bursa, <u>right</u> elbow
M71.022 Abscess of bursa, <u>left</u> elbow
M71.029 Abscess of bursa, <u>unspecified</u> elbow
M71.03-Abscess of bursa, <u>wrist</u>
M71.031 Abscess of bursa, <u>right</u> wrist
M71.032 Abscess of bursa, <u>left</u> wrist
M71.039 Abscess of bursa, <u>unspecified</u> wrist
M71.04-Abscess of bursa, <u>hand</u>
M71.041 Abscess of bursa, <u>right</u> hand
M71.042 Abscess of bursa, <u>left</u> hand
M71.049 Abscess of bursa, <u>unspecified</u> hand
M71.05-Abscess of bursa, <u>hip</u>
M71.051 Abscess of bursa, <u>right</u> hip
M71.052 Abscess of bursa, <u>left</u> hip
M71.059 Abscess of bursa, <u>unspecified</u> hip
M71.06-Abscess of bursa, <u>knee</u>
M71.061 Abscess of bursa, <u>right</u> knee
M71.062 Abscess of bursa, <u>left</u> knee
M71.069 Abscess of bursa, <u>unspecified</u> knee
M71.07-Abscess of bursa, <u>ankle and foot</u>
M71.071 Abscess of bursa, <u>right</u> ankle and foot
M71.072 Abscess of bursa, <u>left</u> ankle and foot
M71.079 Abscess of bursa, <u>unspecified</u> ankle and foot
M71.08 Abscess of bursa, other site
M71.09 Abscess of bursa, <u>multiple sites</u>

M 6 7 - M 7 1

© 2013 Channel Publishing, Ltd.

M71.1- **Other infective** bursitis
    Use additional code (B95.-, B96.-) to identify causative organism
  M71.10 Other infective bursitis, <u>unspecified</u> <u>site</u>
  M71.11- Other infective bursitis, <u>shoulder</u>
    M71.111   Other infective bursitis, <u>right</u> shoulder
    M71.112   Other infective bursitis, <u>left</u> shoulder
    M71.119   Other infective bursitis, <u>unspecified</u> shoulder
  M71.12- Other infective bursitis, <u>elbow</u>
    M71.121   Other infective bursitis, <u>right</u> elbow
    M71.122   Other infective bursitis, <u>left</u> elbow
    M71.129   Other infective bursitis, <u>unspecified</u> elbow
  M71.13- Other infective bursitis, <u>wrist</u>
    M71.131   Other infective bursitis, <u>right</u> wrist
    M71.132   Other infective bursitis, <u>left</u> wrist
    M71.139   Other infective bursitis, <u>unspecified</u> wrist
  M71.14- Other infective bursitis, <u>hand</u>
    M71.141   Other infective bursitis, <u>right</u> hand
    M71.142   Other infective bursitis, <u>left</u> hand
    M71.149   Other infective bursitis, <u>unspecified</u> hand
  M71.15- Other infective bursitis, <u>hip</u>
    M71.151   Other infective bursitis, <u>right</u> hip
    M71.152   Other infective bursitis, <u>left</u> hip
    M71.159   Other infective bursitis, <u>unspecified</u> hip
  M71.16- Other infective bursitis, <u>knee</u>
    M71.161   Other infective bursitis, <u>right</u> knee
    M71.162   Other infective bursitis, <u>left</u> knee
    M71.169   Other infective bursitis, <u>unspecified</u> knee
  M71.17- Other infective bursitis, <u>ankle and foot</u>
    M71.171   Other infective bursitis, <u>right</u> ankle and foot
    M71.172   Other infective bursitis, <u>left</u> ankle and foot
    M71.179   Other infective bursitis, <u>unspecified</u> ankle and foot
  M71.18 Other infective bursitis, other site
  M71.19 Other infective bursitis, <u>multiple sites</u>
M71.2- **Synovial cyst of popliteal space [Baker]**
    Excludes 1: synovial cyst of popliteal space with rupture (M66.0)
  M71.20 Synovial cyst of popliteal space [Baker], <u>unspecified</u> knee
  M71.21 Synovial cyst of popliteal space [Baker], <u>right</u> knee
  M71.22 Synovial cyst of popliteal space [Baker], <u>left</u> knee
M71.3- **Other bursal cyst**
    Synovial cyst NOS
    Excludes 1: synovial cyst with rupture (M66.1-)
  M71.30 Other bursal cyst, <u>unspecified</u> <u>site</u>
  M71.31- Other bursal cyst, <u>shoulder</u>
    M71.311   Other bursal cyst, <u>right</u> shoulder
    M71.312   Other bursal cyst, <u>left</u> shoulder
    M71.319   Other bursal cyst, <u>unspecified</u> shoulder
  M71.32- Other bursal cyst, <u>elbow</u>
    M71.321   Other bursal cyst, <u>right</u> elbow
    M71.322   Other bursal cyst, <u>left</u> elbow
    M71.329   Other bursal cyst, <u>unspecified</u> elbow
  M71.33- Other bursal cyst, <u>wrist</u>
    M71.331   Other bursal cyst, <u>right</u> wrist
    M71.332   Other bursal cyst, <u>left</u> wrist
    M71.339   Other bursal cyst, <u>unspecified</u> wrist
  M71.34- Other bursal cyst, <u>hand</u>
    M71.341   Other bursal cyst, <u>right</u> hand
    M71.342   Other bursal cyst, <u>left</u> hand
    M71.349   Other bursal cyst, <u>unspecified</u> hand
  M71.35- Other bursal cyst, <u>hip</u>
    M71.351   Other bursal cyst, <u>right</u> hip
    M71.352   Other bursal cyst, <u>left</u> hip
    M71.359   Other bursal cyst, <u>unspecified</u> hip
  M71.37- Other bursal cyst, <u>ankle and foot</u>
    M71.371   Other bursal cyst, <u>right</u> ankle and foot
    M71.372   Other bursal cyst, <u>left</u> ankle and foot
    M71.379   Other bursal cyst, <u>unspecified</u> ankle and foot
  M71.38 Other bursal cyst, <u>other site</u>
  M71.39 Other bursal cyst, <u>multiple sites</u>
M71.4- **Calcium deposit** in bursa
    Excludes❷: calcium deposit in bursa of shoulder (M75.3)
  M71.40 Calcium deposit in bursa, <u>unspecified</u> <u>site</u>
  M71.42- Calcium deposit in bursa, <u>elbow</u>
    M71.421   Calcium deposit in bursa, <u>right</u> elbow
    M71.422   Calcium deposit in bursa, <u>left</u> elbow
    M71.429   Calcium deposit in bursa, <u>unspecified</u> elbow

M71.43- Calcium deposit in bursa, wrist
    M71.431   Calcium deposit in bursa, <u>right</u> wrist
    M71.432   Calcium deposit in bursa, <u>left</u> wrist
    M71.439   Calcium deposit in bursa, <u>unspecified</u> wrist
  M71.44- Calcium deposit in bursa, hand
    M71.441   Calcium deposit in bursa, <u>right</u> hand
    M71.442   Calcium deposit in bursa, <u>left</u> hand
    M71.449   Calcium deposit in bursa, <u>unspecified</u> hand
  M71.45- Calcium deposit in bursa, <u>hip</u>
    M71.451   Calcium deposit in bursa, <u>right</u> hip
    M71.452   Calcium deposit in bursa, <u>left</u> hip
    M71.459   Calcium deposit in bursa, <u>unspecified</u> hip
  M71.46- Calcium deposit in bursa, <u>knee</u>
    M71.461   Calcium deposit in bursa, <u>right</u> knee
    M71.462   Calcium deposit in bursa, <u>left</u> knee
    M71.469   Calcium deposit in bursa, <u>unspecified</u> knee
  M71.47- Calcium deposit in bursa, <u>ankle and foot</u>
    M71.471   Calcium deposit in bursa, <u>right</u> ankle and foot
    M71.472   Calcium deposit in bursa, <u>left</u> ankle and foot
    M71.479   Calcium deposit in bursa, <u>unspecified</u> ankle and foot
  M71.48 Calcium deposit in bursa, <u>other site</u>
  M71.49 Calcium deposit in bursa, <u>multiple sites</u>
M71.5- **Other** bursitis, <u>not elsewhere classified</u>
    Excludes 1: bursitis NOS (M71.9-)
    Excludes❷: bursitis of shoulder (M75.5)
        bursitis of tibial collateral [Pellegrini-Stieda] (M76.4)
  M71.50 Other bursitis, not elsewhere classified, <u>unspecified site</u>
  M71.52- Other bursitis, not elsewhere classified, <u>elbow</u>
    M71.521   Other bursitis, not elsewhere classified, <u>right</u> elbow
    M71.522   Other bursitis, not elsewhere classified, <u>left</u> elbow
    M71.529   Other bursitis, not elsewhere classified, <u>unspecified</u> elbow
  M71.53- Other bursitis, not elsewhere classified, <u>wrist</u>
    M71.531   Other bursitis, not elsewhere classified, <u>right</u> wrist
    M71.532   Other bursitis, not elsewhere classified, <u>left</u> wrist
    M71.539   Other bursitis, not elsewhere classified, <u>unspecified</u> wrist
  M71.54- Other bursitis, not elsewhere classified, <u>hand</u>
    M71.541   Other bursitis, not elsewhere classified, <u>right</u> hand
    M71.542   Other bursitis, not elsewhere classified, <u>left</u> hand
    M71.549   Other bursitis, not elsewhere classified, <u>unspecified</u> hand
  M71.55- Other bursitis, not elsewhere classified, <u>hip</u>
    M71.551   Other bursitis, not elsewhere classified, <u>right</u> hip
    M71.552   Other bursitis, not elsewhere classified, <u>left</u> hip
    M71.559   Other bursitis, not elsewhere classified, <u>unspecified</u> hip
  M71.56- Other bursitis, not elsewhere classified, <u>knee</u>
    M71.561   Other bursitis, not elsewhere classified, <u>right</u> knee
    M71.562   Other bursitis, not elsewhere classified, <u>left</u> knee
    M71.569   Other bursitis, not elsewhere classified, <u>unspecified</u> knee
  M71.57- Other bursitis, not elsewhere classified, <u>ankle and foot</u>
    M71.571   Other bursitis, not elsewhere classified, <u>right</u> ankle and foot
    M71.572   Other bursitis, not elsewhere classified, <u>left</u> ankle and foot
    M71.579   Other bursitis, not elsewhere classified, <u>unspecified</u> ankle and foot
  M71.58 Other bursitis, not elsewhere classified, <u>other site</u>
M71.8- **Other specified bursopathies**
  M71.80 Other specified bursopathies, <u>unspecified site</u>
  M71.81- Other specified bursopathies, <u>shoulder</u>
    M71.811   Other specified bursopathies, <u>right</u> shoulder
    M71.812   Other specified bursopathies, <u>left</u> shoulder
    M71.819   Other specified bursopathies, <u>unspecified</u> shoulder
  M71.82- Other specified bursopathies, <u>elbow</u>
    M71.821   Other specified bursopathies, <u>right</u> elbow
    M71.822   Other specified bursopathies, <u>left</u> elbow
    M71.829   Other specified bursopathies, <u>unspecified</u> elbow
  M71.83- Other specified bursopathies, <u>wrist</u>
    M71.831   Other specified bursopathies, <u>right</u> wrist
    M71.832   Other specified bursopathies, <u>left</u> wrist
    M71.839   Other specified bursopathies, <u>unspecified</u> wrist

M71 - M76

M71.84-Other specified bursopathies, <u>hand</u>

    M71.841 Other specified bursopathies, <u>right</u> hand

    M71.842 Other specified bursopathies, <u>left</u> hand

    M71.849 Other specified bursopathies, <u>unspecified</u> hand

M71.85-Other specified bursopathies, <u>hip</u>

    M71.851 Other specified bursopathies, <u>right</u> hip

    M71.852 Other specified bursopathies, <u>left</u> hip

    M71.859 Other specified bursopathies, <u>unspecified</u> hip

M71.86-Other specified bursopathies, <u>knee</u>

    M71.861 Other specified bursopathies, <u>right</u> knee

    M71.862 Other specified bursopathies, <u>left</u> knee

    M71.869 Other specified bursopathies, <u>unspecified</u> knee

M71.87-Other specified bursopathies, <u>ankle and foot</u>

    M71.871 Other specified bursopathies, <u>right</u> ankle and foot

    M71.872 Other specified bursopathies, <u>left</u> ankle and foot

    M71.879 Other specified bursopathies, <u>unspecified</u> ankle and foot

  M71.88 Other specified bursopathies, <u>other site</u>

  M71.89 Other specified bursopathies, <u>multiple sites</u>

M71.9   **Bursopathy, <u>unspecified</u>**

    Bursitis NOS

M72- Fibroblastic disorders

    Excludes❷: retroperitoneal fibromatosis (D48.3)

M72.0   **Palmar fascial fibromatosis [Dupuytren]**

M72.1   **Knuckle pads**

M72.2   **Plantar fascial fibromatosis**

    Plantar fasciitis

M72.4   **Pseudosarcomatous fibromatosis**

    Nodular fasciitis

M72.6   **Necrotizing fasciitis**

    Use additional code (B95.-, B96.-) to identify causative organism

M72.8   **Other fibroblastic disorders**

    Abscess of fascia

    Fasciitis NEC

    Other infective fasciitis

    Use additional code to (B95.-, B96.-) identify causative organism

    Excludes 1: diffuse (eosinophilic) fasciitis (M35.4)

        necrotizing fasciitis (M72.6)

        nodular fasciitis (M72.4)

        perirenal fasciitis NOS (N13.5)

        perirenal fasciitis with infection (N13.6)

        plantar fasciitis (M72.2)

M72.9   **Fibroblastic disorder, unspecified**

    Fasciitis NOS

    Fibromatosis NOS

M75- <u>Shoulder lesions</u>

    Excludes❷: shoulder-hand syndrome (M89.0-)

M75.0- <u>Adhesive capsulitis</u> of shoulder

    Frozen shoulder

    Periarthritis of shoulder

  M75.00 Adhesive capsulitis of <u>unspecified</u> shoulder

  M75.01 Adhesive capsulitis of <u>right</u> shoulder

  M75.02 Adhesive capsulitis of <u>left</u> shoulder

M75.1- <u>Rotator cuff tear or rupture</u>, <u>not specified as traumatic</u>

    Rotator cuff syndrome

    Supraspinatus tear or rupture, not specified as traumatic

    Excludes 1: tear of rotator cuff, traumatic (S46.01-)

  M75.10-<u>Unspecified</u> rotator cuff tear or rupture, not specified as traumatic

    M75.100 Unspecified rotator cuff tear or rupture of <u>unspecified</u> shoulder, not specified as traumatic

    M75.101 Unspecified rotator cuff tear or rupture of <u>right</u> shoulder, not specified as traumatic

    M75.102 Unspecified rotator cuff tear or rupture of <u>left</u> shoulder, not specified as traumatic

  M75.11-<u>Incomplete</u> rotator cuff tear or rupture, not specified as traumatic

    M75.110 Incomplete rotator cuff tear or rupture of <u>unspecified</u> shoulder, not specified as traumatic

    M75.111 Incomplete rotator cuff tear or rupture of <u>right</u> shoulder, not specified as traumatic

    M75.112 Incomplete rotator cuff tear or rupture of <u>left</u> shoulder, not specified as traumatic

  M75.12-<u>Complete</u> rotator cuff tear or rupture, not specified as traumatic

    M75.120 Complete rotator cuff tear or rupture of <u>unspecified</u> shoulder, not specified as traumatic

    M75.121 Complete rotator cuff tear or rupture of <u>right</u> shoulder, not specified as traumatic

    M75.122 Complete rotator cuff tear or rupture of <u>left</u> shoulder, not specified as traumatic

M75.2- <u>Bicipital</u> tendinitis

  M75.20 Bicipital tendinitis, <u>unspecified</u> shoulder

  M75.21 Bicipital tendinitis, <u>right</u> shoulder

  M75.22 Bicipital tendinitis, <u>left</u> shoulder

M75.3- <u>Calcific</u> tendinitis of shoulder

    Calcified bursa of shoulder

  M75.30 Calcific tendinitis of <u>unspecified</u> shoulder

  M75.31 Calcific tendinitis of <u>right</u> shoulder

  M75.32 Calcific tendinitis of <u>left</u> shoulder

M75.4- <u>Impingement syndrome</u> of shoulder

  M75.40 Impingement syndrome of <u>unspecified</u> shoulder

  M75.41 Impingement syndrome of <u>right</u> shoulder

  M75.42 Impingement syndrome of <u>left</u> shoulder

M75.5- <u>Bursitis</u> of shoulder

  M75.50 Bursitis of <u>unspecified</u> shoulder

  M75.51 Bursitis of <u>right</u> shoulder

  M75.52 Bursitis of <u>left</u> shoulder

M75.8- <u>Other</u> shoulder lesions

  M75.80 Other shoulder lesions, <u>unspecified</u> shoulder

  M75.81 Other shoulder lesions, <u>right</u> shoulder

  M75.82 Other shoulder lesions, <u>left</u> shoulder

M75.9- <u>Shoulder lesion, unspecified</u>

  M75.90 Shoulder lesion, unspecified, <u>unspecified</u> shoulder

  M75.91 Shoulder lesion, unspecified, <u>right</u> shoulder

  M75.92 Shoulder lesion, unspecified, <u>left</u> shoulder

M76- Enthesopathies, lower limb, excluding foot

    Excludes❷: bursitis due to use, overuse and pressure (M70-)

            enthesopathies of ankle and foot (M77.5-)

M76.0- <u>Gluteal</u> tendinitis

  M76.00 Gluteal tendinitis, <u>unspecified</u> hip

  M76.01 Gluteal tendinitis, <u>right</u> hip

  M76.02 Gluteal tendinitis, <u>left</u> hip

M76.1- <u>Psoas</u> tendinitis

  M76.10 Psoas tendinitis, <u>unspecified</u> hip

  M76.11 Psoas tendinitis, <u>right</u> hip

  M76.12 Psoas tendinitis, <u>left</u> hip

M76.2- <u>Iliac crest spur</u>

  M76.20 Iliac crest spur, <u>unspecified</u> hip

  M76.21 Iliac crest spur, <u>right</u> hip

  M76.22 Iliac crest spur, <u>left</u> hip

M76.3- <u>Iliotibial band syndrome</u>

  M76.30 Iliotibial band syndrome, <u>unspecified</u> leg

  M76.31 Iliotibial band syndrome, <u>right</u> leg

  M76.32 Iliotibial band syndrome, <u>left</u> leg

M76.4- <u>Tibial collateral bursitis [Pellegrini-Stieda]</u>

  M76.40 Tibial collateral bursitis [Pellegrini-Stieda], <u>unspecified</u> leg

  M76.41 Tibial collateral bursitis [Pellegrini-Stieda], <u>right</u> leg

  M76.42 Tibial collateral bursitis [Pellegrini-Stieda], <u>left</u> leg

M76.5- <u>Patellar</u> tendinitis

  M76.50 Patellar tendinitis, <u>unspecified</u> knee

  M76.51 Patellar tendinitis, <u>right</u> knee

  M76.52 Patellar tendinitis, <u>left</u> knee

M76.6- <u>Achilles</u> tendinitis

    Achilles bursitis

  M76.60 Achilles tendinitis, <u>unspecified</u> leg

  M76.61 Achilles tendinitis, <u>right</u> leg

  M76.62 Achilles tendinitis, <u>left</u> leg

M76.7- <u>Peroneal</u> tendinitis

  M76.70 Peroneal tendinitis, <u>unspecified</u> leg

  M76.71 Peroneal tendinitis, <u>right</u> leg

  M76.72 Peroneal tendinitis, <u>left</u> leg

M76.8- <u>Other specified</u> enthesopathies of lower limb, excluding foot

  M76.81-<u>Anterior tibial syndrome</u>

    M76.811 Anterior tibial syndrome, <u>right</u> leg

    M76.812 Anterior tibial syndrome, <u>left</u> leg

    M76.819 Anterior tibial syndrome, <u>unspecified</u> leg

  M76.82-<u>Posterior tibial tendinitis</u>

    M76.821 Posterior tibial tendinitis, <u>right</u> leg

    M76.822 Posterior tibial tendinitis, <u>left</u> leg

    M76.829 Posterior tibial tendinitis, <u>unspecified</u> leg

M 7 1 - M 7 6

Excludes 1: = NOT CODED HERE! (Do not code both)

Excludes❷: = Not Included Here

M76.89-Other specified enthesopathies of <u>lower limb</u>, excluding foot

    M76.891   Other specified enthesopathies of <u>right</u> lower limb, excluding foot

    M76.892   Other specified enthesopathies of <u>left</u> lower limb, excluding foot

    M76.899   Other specified enthesopathies of <u>unspecified</u> lower limb, excluding foot

M76.9   Unspecified enthesopathy, lower limb, excluding foot

M77- Other enthesopathies
   Excludes 1: bursitis NOS (M71.9-)
   Excludes ❷: bursitis due to use, overuse and pressure (M70.-)
          osteophyte (M25.7)
          spinal enthesopathy (M46.0-)

M77.0- <u>Medial</u> epicondylitis
   M77.00 Medial epicondylitis, <u>unspecified</u> elbow
   M77.01 Medial epicondylitis, <u>right</u> elbow
   M77.02 Medial epicondylitis, <u>left</u> elbow

M77.1- <u>Lateral</u> epicondylitis
    Tennis elbow
   M77.10 Lateral epicondylitis, <u>unspecified</u> elbow
   M77.11 Lateral epicondylitis, <u>right</u> elbow
   M77.12 Lateral epicondylitis, <u>left</u> elbow

M77.2- <u>Periarthritis</u> of <u>wrist</u>
   M77.20 Periarthritis, <u>unspecified</u> wrist
   M77.21 Periarthritis, <u>right</u> wrist
   M77.22 Periarthritis, <u>left</u> wrist

M77.3- <u>Calcaneal spur</u>
   M77.30 Calcaneal spur, <u>unspecified</u> foot
   M77.31 Calcaneal spur, <u>right</u> foot
   M77.32 Calcaneal spur, <u>left</u> foot

M77.4- <u>Metatarsalgia</u>
   Excludes 1: Morton's metatarsalgia (G57.6)
   M77.40 Metatarsalgia, <u>unspecified</u> foot
   M77.41 Metatarsalgia, <u>right</u> foot
   M77.42 Metatarsalgia, <u>left</u> foot

M77.5- <u>Other</u> enthesopathy of foot
   M77.50 Other enthesopathy of <u>unspecified</u> foot
   M77.51 Other enthesopathy of <u>right</u> foot
   M77.52 Other enthesopathy of <u>left</u> foot

M77.8   Other enthesopathies, not elsewhere classified
M77.9   Enthesopathy, unspecified
    Bone spur NOS
    Capsulitis NOS
    Periarthritis NOS
    Tendinitis NOS

M79- Other and unspecified soft tissue disorders, <u>not elsewhere classified</u>
   Excludes 1: psychogenic rheumatism (F45.8)
          soft tissue pain, psychogenic (F45.41)

M79.0 Rheumatism, unspecified
   Excludes 1: fibromyalgia (M79.7)
          palindromic rheumatism (M12.3-)

M79.1 Myalgia
    Myofascial pain syndrome
   Excludes 1: fibromyalgia (M79.7)
          myositis (M60.-)

M79.2 Neuralgia and neuritis, unspecified
   Excludes 1: brachial radiculitis NOS (M54.1)
          lumbosacral radiculitis NOS (M54.1)
          mononeuropathies (G56-G58)
          radiculitis NOS (M54.1)
          sciatica (M54.3-M54.4)

M79.3 Panniculitis, unspecified
   Excludes 1: lupus panniculitis (L93.2)
          neck and back panniculitis (M54.0-)
          relapsing [Weber-Christian] panniculitis (M35.6)

M79.4 Hypertrophy of (infrapatellar) fat pad
M79.5 Residual foreign body in soft tissue
   Excludes 1: foreign body granuloma of skin and subcutaneous tissue (L92.3)
          foreign body granuloma of soft tissue (M60.2-)

M79.6- Pain in limb, hand, foot, fingers and toes
   Excludes ❷: pain in joint (M25.5-)
   M79.60-Pain in limb, <u>unspecified</u>
    M79.601   Pain in <u>right</u> arm
         Pain in right upper limb NOS
    M79.602   Pain in <u>left</u> arm
         Pain in left upper limb NOS
    M79.603   Pain in arm, <u>unspecified</u>
         Pain in upper limb NOS

    M79.604   Pain in <u>right</u> leg
         Pain in right lower limb NOS
    M79.605   Pain in <u>left</u> leg
         Pain in left lower limb NOS
    M79.606   Pain in leg, <u>unspecified</u>
         Pain in lower limb NOS
    M79.609   Pain in <u>unspecified</u> limb
         Pain in limb NOS

   M79.62-Pain in <u>upper arm</u>
         Pain in axillary region
    M79.621   Pain in <u>right</u> upper arm
    M79.622   Pain in <u>left</u> upper arm
    M79.629   Pain in <u>unspecified</u> upper arm

   M79.63-Pain in <u>forearm</u>
    M79.631   Pain in <u>right</u> forearm
    M79.632   Pain in <u>left</u> forearm
    M79.639   Pain in <u>unspecified</u> forearm

   M79.64-Pain in <u>hand and fingers</u>
    M79.641   Pain in <u>right</u> hand
    M79.642   Pain in <u>left</u> hand
    M79.643   Pain in <u>unspecified</u> hand
    M79.644   Pain in <u>right</u> finger(s)
    M79.645   Pain in <u>left</u> finger(s)
    M79.646   Pain in <u>unspecified</u> finger(s)

   M79.65-Pain in <u>thigh</u>
    M79.651   Pain in <u>right</u> thigh
    M79.652   Pain in <u>left</u> thigh
    M79.659   Pain in <u>unspecified</u> thigh

   M79.66-Pain in <u>lower leg</u>
    M79.661   Pain in <u>right</u> lower leg
    M79.662   Pain in <u>left</u> lower leg
    M79.669   Pain in <u>unspecified</u> lower leg

   M79.67-Pain in <u>foot and toes</u>
    M79.671   Pain in <u>right</u> foot
    M79.672   Pain in <u>left</u> foot
    M79.673   Pain in <u>unspecified</u> foot
    M79.674   Pain in <u>right</u> toe(s)
    M79.675   Pain in <u>left</u> toe(s)
    M79.676   Pain in <u>unspecified</u> toe(s)

M79.7 Fibromyalgia
    Fibromyositis
    Fibrositis
    Myofibrositis

M79.A- <u>Nontraumatic compartment syndrome</u>
   Code first, if applicable, associated postprocedural complication
   Excludes 1: compartment syndrome NOS (T79.A-)
          fibromyalgia (M79.7)
          nontraumatic ischemic infarction of muscle (M62.2-)
          traumatic compartment syndrome (T79.A-)

   M79.A1- Nontraumatic compartment syndrome of <u>upper extremity</u>
       Nontraumatic compartment syndrome of shoulder, arm, forearm, wrist, hand, and fingers
    M79.A11   Nontraumatic compartment syndrome of <u>right</u> upper extremity
    M79.A12   Nontraumatic compartment syndrome of <u>left</u> upper extremity
    M79.A19   Nontraumatic compartment syndrome of <u>unspecified</u> upper extremity

   M79.A2- Nontraumatic compartment syndrome of <u>lower extremity</u>
       Nontraumatic compartment syndrome of hip, buttock, thigh, leg, foot, and toes
    M79.A21   Nontraumatic compartment syndrome of <u>right</u> lower extremity
    M79.A22   Nontraumatic compartment syndrome of <u>left</u> lower extremity
    M79.A29   Nontraumatic compartment syndrome of <u>unspecified</u> lower extremity

   M79.A3   Nontraumatic compartment syndrome of <u>abdomen</u>
   M79.A9   Nontraumatic compartment syndrome of <u>other sites</u>

M79.8- Other specified soft tissue disorders
   M79.81 Nontraumatic hematoma of soft tissue
        Nontraumatic hematoma of muscle
        Nontraumatic seroma of muscle and soft tissue
   M79.89 Other specified soft tissue disorders
        Polyalgia

M79.9 Soft tissue disorder, unspecified

Excludes 1: = NOT CODED HERE! (Do not code both)   **590**   *Excludes ❷: = Not Included Here*

Osteopathies and chondropathies (M80-M94)

Disorders of bone density and structure (M80-M85)

M80- <u>Osteoporosis</u> <u>with current pathological fracture</u>
Includes: Osteoporosis with current fragility fracture
Use additional code to identify major osseous defect, if applicable (M89.7-)
Excludes 1: collapsed vertebra NOS (M48.5)
pathological fracture NOS (M84.4)
wedging of vertebra NOS (M48.5)
Excludes ❷: personal history of (healed) osteoporosis fracture (Z87.310)

The appropriate 7th character is to be added to each code from category M80:
A   Initial encounter for fracture
D   Subsequent encounter for fracture with routine healing
G   Subsequent encounter for fracture with delayed healing
K   Subsequent encounter for fracture with nonunion
P   Subsequent encounter for fracture with malunion
S   Sequela

M80.0- <u>Age-related</u> osteoporosis <u>with current pathological fracture</u>
Involutional osteoporosis with current pathological fracture
Osteoporosis NOS with current pathological fracture
Postmenopausal osteoporosis with current pathological fracture
Senile osteoporosis with current pathological fracture

M80.00x- Age-related osteoporosis with current pathological fracture, <u>unspecified</u> site

M80.01- Age-related osteoporosis with current pathological fracture, <u>shoulder</u>

M80.011- Age-related osteoporosis with current pathological fracture, <u>right</u> shoulder

M80.012- Age-related osteoporosis with current pathological fracture, <u>left</u> shoulder

M80.019- Age-related osteoporosis with current pathological fracture, <u>unspecified</u> shoulder

M80.02- Age-related osteoporosis with current pathological fracture, <u>humerus</u>

M80.021- Age-related osteoporosis with current pathological fracture, <u>right</u> humerus

M80.022- Age-related osteoporosis with current pathological fracture, <u>left</u> humerus

M80.029- Age-related osteoporosis with current pathological fracture, <u>unspecified</u> humerus

M80.03- Age-related osteoporosis with current pathological fracture, <u>forearm</u>
Age-related osteoporosis with current pathological fracture of wrist

M80.031- Age-related osteoporosis with current pathological fracture, <u>right</u> forearm

M80.032- Age-related osteoporosis with current pathological fracture, <u>left</u> forearm

M80.039- Age-related osteoporosis with current pathological fracture, <u>unspecified</u> forearm

M80.04- Age-related osteoporosis with current pathological fracture, <u>hand</u>

M80.041- Age-related osteoporosis with current pathological fracture, <u>right</u> hand

M80.042- Age-related osteoporosis with current pathological fracture, <u>left</u> hand

M80.049- Age-related osteoporosis with current pathological fracture, <u>unspecified</u> hand

M80.05- Age-related osteoporosis with current pathological fracture, <u>femur</u>
Age-related osteoporosis with current pathological fracture of hip

M80.051- Age-related osteoporosis with current pathological fracture, <u>right</u> femur

M80.052- Age-related osteoporosis with current pathological fracture, <u>left</u> femur

M80.059- Age-related osteoporosis with current pathological fracture, <u>unspecified</u> femur

M80.06- Age-related osteoporosis with current pathological fracture, <u>lower leg</u>

M80.061- Age-related osteoporosis with current pathological fracture, <u>right</u> lower leg

M80.062- Age-related osteoporosis with current pathological fracture, <u>left</u> lower leg

M80.069- Age-related osteoporosis with current pathological fracture, <u>unspecified</u> lower leg

M80.07- Age-related osteoporosis with current pathological fracture, <u>ankle and foot</u>

M80.071- Age-related osteoporosis with current pathological fracture, <u>right</u> ankle and foot

M80.072- Age-related osteoporosis with current pathological fracture, <u>left</u> ankle and foot

M80.079- Age-related osteoporosis with current pathological fracture, <u>unspecified</u> ankle and foot

M80.08x- Age-related osteoporosis with current pathological fracture, <u>vertebra(e)</u>

M80.8- <u>Other</u> osteoporosis <u>with current pathological fracture</u>
Drug-induced osteoporosis with current pathological fracture
Idiopathic osteoporosis with current pathological fracture
Osteoporosis of disuse with current pathological fracture
Postoophorectomy osteoporosis with current pathological fracture
Postsurgical malabsorption osteoporosis with current pathological fracture
Post-traumatic osteoporosis with current pathological fracture
Use additional code for adverse effect, if applicable, to identify drug (T36-T50 with fifth or sixth character 5)

M80.80x- Other osteoporosis with current pathological fracture, <u>unspecified</u> site

M80.81- Other osteoporosis with pathological fracture, <u>shoulder</u>

M80.811- Other osteoporosis with current pathological fracture, <u>right</u> shoulder

M80.812- Other osteoporosis with current pathological fracture, <u>left</u> shoulder

M80.819- Other osteoporosis with current pathological fracture, <u>unspecified</u> shoulder

M80.82- Other osteoporosis with current pathological fracture, <u>humerus</u>

M80.821- Other osteoporosis with current pathological fracture, <u>right</u> humerus

M80.822- Other osteoporosis with current pathological fracture, <u>left</u> humerus

M80.829- Other osteoporosis with current pathological fracture, <u>unspecified</u> humerus

M80.83- Other osteoporosis with current pathological fracture, <u>forearm</u>
Other osteoporosis with current pathological fracture of wrist

M80.831- Other osteoporosis with current pathological fracture, <u>right</u> forearm

M80.832- Other osteoporosis with current pathological fracture, <u>left</u> forearm

M80.839- Other osteoporosis with current pathological fracture, <u>unspecified</u> forearm

M80.84- Other osteoporosis with current pathological fracture, <u>hand</u>

M80.841- Other osteoporosis with current pathological fracture, <u>right</u> hand

M80.842- Other osteoporosis with current pathological fracture, <u>left</u> hand

M80.849- Other osteoporosis with current pathological fracture, <u>unspecified</u> hand

M80.85- Other osteoporosis with current pathological fracture, <u>femur</u>
Other osteoporosis with current pathological fracture of hip

M80.851- Other osteoporosis with current pathological fracture, <u>right</u> femur

M80.852- Other osteoporosis with current pathological fracture, <u>left</u> femur

M80.859- Other osteoporosis with current pathological fracture, <u>unspecified</u> femur

M80.86- Other osteoporosis with current pathological fracture, <u>lower leg</u>

M80.861- Other osteoporosis with current pathological fracture, <u>right</u> lower leg

M80.862- Other osteoporosis with current pathological fracture, <u>left</u> lower leg

M80.869- Other osteoporosis with current pathological fracture, <u>unspecified</u> lower leg

M
7
6
I
M
8
0

Excludes 1: = NOT CODED HERE! (Do not code both)

Excludes ❷: = Not Included Here

M80.87-   Other osteoporosis with current pathological fracture, <u>ankle and foot</u>

   M80.871-   Other osteoporosis with current pathological fracture, <u>right</u> ankle and foot

   M80.872-   Other osteoporosis with current pathological fracture, <u>left</u> ankle and foot

   M80.879-   Other osteoporosis with current pathological fracture, <u>unspecified</u> ankle and foot

M80.88x-   Other osteoporosis with current pathological fracture, vertebra(e)

M81-   Osteoporosis <u>without</u> current pathological fracture
Use additional code to identify:
Major osseous defect, if applicable (M89.7-)
Personal history of (healed) osteoporosis fracture, if applicable (Z87.310)
Excludes 1:   osteoporosis with current pathological fracture (M80.-)
Sudeck's atrophy (M89.0)

M81.0   <u>Age-related</u> **osteoporosis without current pathological fracture**
Involutional osteoporosis without current pathological fracture
Osteoporosis NOS
Postmenopausal osteoporosis without current pathological fracture
Senile osteoporosis without current pathological fracture

M81.6   <u>Localized</u> **osteoporosis [Lequesne]**
Excludes 1:   Sudeck's atrophy (M89.0)

M81.8   <u>Other</u> **osteoporosis without current pathological fracture**
Drug-induced osteoporosis without current pathological fracture
Idiopathic osteoporosis without current pathological fracture
Osteoporosis of disuse without current pathological fracture
Postoophorectomy osteoporosis without current pathological fracture
Postsurgical malabsorption osteoporosis without current pathological fracture
Post-traumatic osteoporosis without current pathological fracture
Use additional code for adverse effect, if applicable, to identify drug (T36-T50 with fifth or sixth character 5)

M83-   <u>Adult osteomalacia</u>
Excludes 1:   infantile and juvenile osteomalacia (E55.0)
renal osteodystrophy (N25.0)
rickets (active) (E55.0)
rickets (active) sequelae (E64.3)
vitamin D-resistant osteomalacia (E83.3)
vitamin D-resistant rickets (active) (E83.3)

M83.0   Puerperal osteomalacia

M83.1   Senile osteomalacia

M83.2   Adult osteomalacia due to malabsorption
Postsurgical malabsorption osteomalacia in adults

M83.3   Adult osteomalacia due to malnutrition

M83.4   Aluminum bone disease

M83.5   Other drug-induced osteomalacia in adults
Use additional code for adverse effect, if applicable, to identify drug (T36-T50 with fifth or sixth character 5)

M83.8   Other adult osteomalacia

M83.9   Adult osteomalacia, unspecified

M84-   Disorder of continuity of bone
Excludes❷: traumatic fracture of bone-see fracture, by site

M84.3-   <u>Stress fracture</u>
Fatigue fracture
March fracture
Stress fracture NOS
Stress reaction
Use additional external cause code(s) to identify the cause of the stress fracture
Excludes 1:   pathological fracture NOS (M84.4.-)
pathological fracture due to osteoporosis (M80.-)
traumatic fracture (S12.-, S22.-, S32.-, S42.-, S52.-, S62.-, S72.-, S82.-, S92.-)
Excludes❷: personal history of (healed) stress (fatigue) fracture (Z87.312)
stress fracture of vertebra (M48.4-)

The appropriate 7th character is to be added to each code from subcategory M84.3:
A   Initial encounter for fracture
D   Subsequent encounter for fracture with routine healing
G   Subsequent encounter for fracture with delayed healing
K   Subsequent encounter for fracture with nonunion
P   Subsequent encounter for fracture with malunion
S   Sequela

M84.30x-   Stress fracture, <u>unspecified</u> <u>site</u>

M84.31-   Stress fracture, <u>shoulder</u>

   M84.311-   Stress fracture, <u>right</u> shoulder

   M84.312-   Stress fracture, <u>left</u> shoulder

   M84.319-   Stress fracture, <u>unspecified</u> shoulder

M84.32-   Stress fracture, <u>humerus</u>

   M84.321-   Stress fracture, <u>right</u> humerus

   M84.322-   Stress fracture, <u>left</u> humerus

   M84.329-   Stress fracture, <u>unspecified</u> humerus

M84.33-   Stress fracture, <u>ulna and radius</u>

   M84.331-   Stress fracture, <u>right</u> ulna

   M84.332-   Stress fracture, <u>left</u> ulna

   M84.333-   Stress fracture, <u>right</u> radius

   M84.334-   Stress fracture, <u>left</u> radius

   M84.339-   Stress fracture, <u>unspecified</u> ulna and radius

M84.34-   Stress fracture, <u>hand and fingers</u>

   M84.341-   Stress fracture, <u>right</u> hand

   M84.342-   Stress fracture, <u>left</u> hand

   M84.343-   Stress fracture, <u>unspecified</u> hand

   M84.344-   Stress fracture, <u>right</u> finger(s)

   M84.345-   Stress fracture, <u>left</u> finger(s)

   M84.346-   Stress fracture, <u>unspecified</u> finger(s)

M84.35-   Stress fracture, <u>pelvis and femur</u>
Stress fracture, hip

   M84.350-   Stress fracture, pelvis

   M84.351-   Stress fracture, <u>right</u> femur

   M84.352-   Stress fracture, <u>left</u> femur

   M84.353-   Stress fracture, <u>unspecified</u> femur

   M84.359-   Stress fracture, hip, <u>unspecified</u>

M84.36-   Stress fracture, <u>tibia and fibula</u>

   M84.361-   Stress fracture, <u>right</u> tibia

   M84.362-   Stress fracture, <u>left</u> tibia

   M84.363-   Stress fracture, <u>right</u> fibula

   M84.364-   Stress fracture, <u>left</u> fibula

   M84.369-   Stress fracture, <u>unspecified</u> tibia and fibula

M84.37-   Stress fracture, <u>ankle, foot and toes</u>

   M84.371-   Stress fracture, <u>right</u> ankle

   M84.372-   Stress fracture, <u>left</u> ankle

   M84.373-   Stress fracture, <u>unspecified</u> ankle

   M84.374-   Stress fracture, <u>right</u> foot

   M84.375-   Stress fracture, <u>left</u> foot

   M84.376-   Stress fracture, <u>unspecified</u> foot

   M84.377-   Stress fracture, <u>right</u> toe(s)

   M84.378-   Stress fracture, <u>left</u> toe(s)

   M84.379-   Stress fracture, <u>unspecified</u> toe(s)

M84.38x-   Stress fracture, <u>other site</u>
Excludes❷: stress fracture of vertebra (M48.4-)

M84.4-   Pathological fracture, <u>not elsewhere classified</u>
Chronic fracture
Pathological fracture NOS
Excludes 1:   collapsed vertebra NEC (M48.5)
pathological fracture in neoplastic disease (M84.5-)
pathological fracture in osteoporosis (M80.-)
pathological fracture in other disease (M84.6-)
stress fracture (M84.3-)
traumatic fracture (S12.-, S22.-, S32.-, S42.-, S52.-, S62.-, S72.-, S82.-, S92.-)
Excludes❷: personal history of (healed) pathological fracture (Z87.311)

The appropriate 7th character is to be added to each code from subcategory M84.4:
A   Initial encounter for fracture
D   Subsequent encounter for fracture with routine healing
G   Subsequent encounter for fracture with delayed healing
K   Subsequent encounter for fracture with nonunion
P   Subsequent encounter for fracture with malunion
S   Sequela

M84.40x-   Pathological fracture, <u>unspecified</u> <u>site</u>

M84.41-   Pathological fracture, <u>shoulder</u>

   M84.411-   Pathological fracture, <u>right</u> shoulder

   M84.412-   Pathological fracture, <u>left</u> shoulder

   M84.419-   Pathological fracture, <u>unspecified</u> shoulder

M84.42-   Pathological fracture, <u>humerus</u>

   M84.421-   Pathological fracture, <u>right</u> humerus

   M84.422-   Pathological fracture, <u>left</u> humerus

   M84.429-   Pathological fracture, <u>unspecified</u> humerus

M84.43-   Pathological fracture, <u>ulna and radius</u>

   M84.431-   Pathological fracture, <u>right</u> ulna

   M84.432-   Pathological fracture, <u>left</u> ulna

   M84.433-   Pathological fracture, <u>right</u> radius

   M84.434-   Pathological fracture, <u>left</u> radius

   M84.439-   Pathological fracture, <u>unspecified</u> ulna and radius

M
8
0
–
M
8
4

M84.44-   Pathological fracture, <u>hand and fingers</u>
   M84.441- Pathological fracture, <u>right</u> hand
   M84.442- Pathological fracture, <u>left</u> hand
   M84.443- Pathological fracture, <u>unspecified</u> hand
   M84.444- Pathological fracture, <u>right</u> finger(s)
   M84.445- Pathological fracture, <u>left</u> finger(s)
   M84.446- Pathological fracture, <u>unspecified</u> finger(s)
M84.45-   Pathological fracture, <u>femur and pelvis</u>
   M84.451- Pathological fracture, <u>right</u> femur
   M84.452- Pathological fracture, <u>left</u> femur
   M84.453- Pathological fracture, <u>unspecified</u> femur
   M84.454- Pathological fracture, pelvis
   M84.459- Pathological fracture, hip, <u>unspecified</u>
M84.46-   Pathological fracture, <u>tibia and fibula</u>
   M84.461- Pathological fracture, <u>right</u> tibia
   M84.462- Pathological fracture, <u>left</u> tibia
   M84.463- Pathological fracture, <u>right</u> fibula
   M84.464- Pathological fracture, <u>left</u> fibula
   M84.469- Pathological fracture, <u>unspecified</u> tibia and fibula
M84.47-   Pathological fracture, <u>ankle, foot and toes</u>
   M84.471- Pathological fracture, <u>right</u> ankle
   M84.472- Pathological fracture, <u>left</u> ankle
   M84.473- Pathological fracture, <u>unspecified</u> ankle
   M84.474- Pathological fracture, <u>right</u> foot
   M84.475- Pathological fracture, <u>left</u> foot
   M84.476- Pathological fracture, <u>unspecified</u> foot
   M84.477- Pathological fracture, <u>right</u> toe(s)
   M84.478- Pathological fracture, <u>left</u> toe(s)
   M84.479- Pathological fracture, <u>unspecified</u> toe(s)
M84.48x- Pathological fracture, <u>other site</u>
M84.5-   Pathological fracture <u>in neoplastic disease</u>
Code also underlying neoplasm
The appropriate 7th character is to be added to each code from subcategory M84.5:
  A   Initial encounter for fracture
  D   Subsequent encounter for fracture with routine healing
  G   Subsequent encounter for fracture with delayed healing
  K   Subsequent encounter for fracture with nonunion
  P   Subsequent encounter for fracture with malunion
  S   Sequela
M84.50x- Pathological fracture in neoplastic disease, <u>unspecified</u> <u>site</u>
M84.51- Pathological fracture in neoplastic disease, <u>shoulder</u>
   M84.511- Pathological fracture in neoplastic disease, <u>right</u> shoulder
   M84.512- Pathological fracture in neoplastic disease, <u>left</u> shoulder
   M84.519- Pathological fracture in neoplastic disease, <u>unspecified</u> shoulder
M84.52- Pathological fracture in neoplastic disease, <u>humerus</u>
   M84.521- Pathological fracture in neoplastic disease, <u>right</u> humerus
   M84.522- Pathological fracture in neoplastic disease, <u>left</u> humerus
   M84.529- Pathological fracture in neoplastic disease, <u>unspecified</u> humerus
M84.53- Pathological fracture in neoplastic disease, <u>ulna and radius</u>
   M84.531- Pathological fracture in neoplastic disease, <u>right</u> ulna
   M84.532- Pathological fracture in neoplastic disease, <u>left</u> ulna
   M84.533- Pathological fracture in neoplastic disease, <u>right</u> radius
   M84.534- Pathological fracture in neoplastic disease, <u>left</u> radius
   M84.539- Pathological fracture in neoplastic disease, <u>unspecified</u> ulna and radius
M84.54- Pathological fracture in neoplastic disease, <u>hand</u>
   M84.541- Pathological fracture in neoplastic disease, <u>right</u> hand
   M84.542- Pathological fracture in neoplastic disease, <u>left</u> hand
   M84.549- Pathological fracture in neoplastic disease, <u>unspecified</u> hand
M84.55- Pathological fracture in neoplastic disease, <u>pelvis and femur</u>
   M84.550- Pathological fracture in neoplastic disease, pelvis
   M84.551- Pathological fracture in neoplastic disease, <u>right</u> femur
   M84.552- Pathological fracture in neoplastic disease, <u>left</u> femur
   M84.553- Pathological fracture in neoplastic disease, <u>unspecified</u> femur
   M84.559- Pathological fracture in neoplastic disease, hip, <u>unspecified</u>

M84.56- Pathological fracture in neoplastic disease, <u>tibia and fibula</u>
   M84.561- Pathological fracture in neoplastic disease, <u>right</u> tibia
   M84.562- Pathological fracture in neoplastic disease, <u>left</u> tibia
   M84.563- Pathological fracture in neoplastic disease, <u>right</u> fibula
   M84.564- Pathological fracture in neoplastic disease, <u>left</u> fibula
   M84.569- Pathological fracture in neoplastic disease, <u>unspecified</u> tibia and fibula
M84.57- Pathological fracture in neoplastic disease, <u>ankle and foot</u>
   M84.571- Pathological fracture in neoplastic disease, <u>right</u> ankle
   M84.572- Pathological fracture in neoplastic disease, <u>left</u> ankle
   M84.573- Pathological fracture in neoplastic disease, <u>unspecified</u> ankle
   M84.574- Pathological fracture in neoplastic disease, <u>right</u> foot
   M84.575- Pathological fracture in neoplastic disease, <u>left</u> foot
   M84.576- Pathological fracture in neoplastic disease, <u>unspecified</u> foot
M84.58x- Pathological fracture in neoplastic disease, <u>other specified site</u>
   Pathological fracture in neoplastic disease, vertebrae
M84.6- Pathological fracture <u>in other disease</u>
Code also underlying condition
Excludes 1: pathological fracture in osteoporosis (M80.-)
The appropriate 7th character is to be added to each code from subcategory M84.6:
  A   Initial encounter for fracture
  D   Subsequent encounter for fracture with routine healing
  G   Subsequent encounter for fracture with delayed healing
  K   Subsequent encounter for fracture with nonunion
  P   Subsequent encounter for fracture with malunion
  S   Sequela
M84.60x- Pathological fracture in other disease, <u>unspecified site</u>
M84.61- Pathological fracture in other disease, <u>shoulder</u>
   M84.611- Pathological fracture in other disease, <u>right</u> shoulder
   M84.612- Pathological fracture in other disease, <u>left</u> shoulder
   M84.619- Pathological fracture in other disease, <u>unspecified</u> shoulder
M84.62- Pathological fracture in other disease, <u>humerus</u>
   M84.621- Pathological fracture in other disease, <u>right</u> humerus
   M84.622- Pathological fracture in other disease, <u>left</u> humerus
   M84.629- Pathological fracture in other disease, <u>unspecified</u> humerus
M84.63- Pathological fracture in other disease, <u>ulna and radius</u>
   M84.631- Pathological fracture in other disease, <u>right</u> ulna
   M84.632- Pathological fracture in other disease, <u>left</u> ulna
   M84.633- Pathological fracture in other disease, <u>right</u> radius
   M84.634- Pathological fracture in other disease, <u>left</u> radius
   M84.639- Pathological fracture in other disease, <u>unspecified</u> ulna and radius
M84.64- Pathological fracture in other disease, <u>hand</u>
   M84.641- Pathological fracture in other disease, <u>right</u> hand
   M84.642- Pathological fracture in other disease, <u>left</u> hand
   M84.649- Pathological fracture in other disease, <u>unspecified</u> hand
M84.65- Pathological fracture in other disease, <u>pelvis and femur</u>
   M84.650- Pathological fracture in other disease, pelvis
   M84.651- Pathological fracture in other disease, <u>right</u> femur
   M84.652- Pathological fracture in other disease, <u>left</u> femur
   M84.653- Pathological fracture in other disease, <u>unspecified</u> femur
   M84.659- Pathological fracture in other disease, hip, <u>unspecified</u>
M84.66- Pathological fracture in other disease, <u>tibia and fibula</u>
   M84.661- Pathological fracture in other disease, <u>right</u> tibia
   M84.662- Pathological fracture in other disease, <u>left</u> tibia
   M84.663- Pathological fracture in other disease, <u>right</u> fibula
   M84.664- Pathological fracture in other disease, <u>left</u> fibula
   M84.669- Pathological fracture in other disease, <u>unspecified</u> tibia and fibula
M84.67   Pathological fracture in other disease, ankle and foot
   M84.671- Pathological fracture in other disease, <u>right</u> ankle
   M84.672- Pathological fracture in other disease, <u>left</u> ankle
   M84.673- Pathological fracture in other disease, <u>unspecified</u> ankle
   M84.674- Pathological fracture in other disease, <u>right</u> foot
   M84.675- Pathological fracture in other disease, <u>left</u> foot
   M84.676- Pathological fracture in other disease, <u>unspecified</u> foot
M84.68x- Pathological fracture in other disease, <u>other site</u>

M80 - M84

M84.8- Other disorders of continuity of bone
  M84.80 Other disorders of continuity of bone, unspecified site
  M84.81- Other disorders of continuity of bone, shoulder
    M84.811 Other disorders of continuity of bone, right shoulder
    M84.812 Other disorders of continuity of bone, left shoulder
    M84.819 Other disorders of continuity of bone, unspecified shoulder
  M84.82- Other disorders of continuity of bone, humerus
    M84.821 Other disorders of continuity of bone, right humerus
    M84.822 Other disorders of continuity of bone, left humerus
    M84.829 Other disorders of continuity of bone, unspecified humerus
  M84.83- Other disorders of continuity of bone, ulna and radius
    M84.831 Other disorders of continuity of bone, right ulna
    M84.832 Other disorders of continuity of bone, left ulna
    M84.833 Other disorders of continuity of bone, right radius
    M84.834 Other disorders of continuity of bone, left radius
    M84.839 Other disorders of continuity of bone, unspecified ulna and radius
  M84.84- Other disorders of continuity of bone, hand
    M84.841 Other disorders of continuity of bone, right hand
    M84.842 Other disorders of continuity of bone, left hand
    M84.849 Other disorders of continuity of bone, unspecified hand
  M84.85- Other disorders of continuity of bone, pelvic region and thigh
    M84.851 Other disorders of continuity of bone, right pelvic region and thigh
    M84.852 Other disorders of continuity of bone, left pelvic region and thigh
    M84.859 Other disorders of continuity of bone, unspecified pelvic region and thigh
  M84.86- Other disorders of continuity of bone, tibia and fibula
    M84.861 Other disorders of continuity of bone, right tibia
    M84.862 Other disorders of continuity of bone, left tibia
    M84.863 Other disorders of continuity of bone, right fibula
    M84.864 Other disorders of continuity of bone, left fibula
    M84.869 Other disorders of continuity of bone, unspecified tibia and fibula
  M84.87- Other disorders of continuity of bone, ankle and foot
    M84.871 Other disorders of continuity of bone, right ankle and foot
    M84.872 Other disorders of continuity of bone, left ankle and foot
    M84.879 Other disorders of continuity of bone, unspecified ankle and foot
  M84.88 Other disorders of continuity of bone, other site
M84.9 Disorder of continuity of bone, unspecified

M85- Other disorders of bone density and structure
  Excludes 1: *osteogenesis imperfecta (Q78.0)*
    osteopetrosis (Q78.2)
    osteopoikilosis (Q78.8)
    polyostotic fibrous dysplasia (Q78.1)
  M85.0- Fibrous dysplasia (monostotic)
    Excludes❷: *fibrous dysplasia of jaw (M27.8)*
  M85.00 Fibrous dysplasia (monostotic), unspecified site
  M85.01- Fibrous dysplasia (monostotic), shoulder
    M85.011 Fibrous dysplasia (monostotic), right shoulder
    M85.012 Fibrous dysplasia (monostotic), left shoulder
    M85.019 Fibrous dysplasia (monostotic), unspecified shoulder
  M85.02- Fibrous dysplasia (monostotic), upper arm
    M85.021 Fibrous dysplasia (monostotic), right upper arm
    M85.022 Fibrous dysplasia (monostotic), left upper arm
    M85.029 Fibrous dysplasia (monostotic), unspecified upper arm
  M85.03- Fibrous dysplasia (monostotic), forearm
    M85.031 Fibrous dysplasia (monostotic), right forearm
    M85.032 Fibrous dysplasia (monostotic), left forearm
    M85.039 Fibrous dysplasia (monostotic), unspecified forearm
  M85.04- Fibrous dysplasia (monostotic), hand
    M85.041 Fibrous dysplasia (monostotic), right hand
    M85.042 Fibrous dysplasia (monostotic), left hand
    M85.049 Fibrous dysplasia (monostotic), unspecified hand
  M85.05- Fibrous dysplasia (monostotic), thigh
    M85.051 Fibrous dysplasia (monostotic), right thigh
    M85.052 Fibrous dysplasia (monostotic), left thigh
    M85.059 Fibrous dysplasia (monostotic), unspecified thigh

  M85.06- Fibrous dysplasia (monostotic), lower leg
    M85.061 Fibrous dysplasia (monostotic), right lower leg
    M85.062 Fibrous dysplasia (monostotic), left lower leg
    M85.069 Fibrous dysplasia (monostotic), unspecified lower leg
  M85.07 Fibrous dysplasia (monostotic), ankle and foot
    M85.071 Fibrous dysplasia (monostotic), right ankle and foot
    M85.072 Fibrous dysplasia (monostotic), left ankle and foot
    M85.079 Fibrous dysplasia (monostotic), unspecified ankle and foot
  M85.08 Fibrous dysplasia (monostotic), other site
  M85.09 Fibrous dysplasia (monostotic), multiple sites
M85.1- Skeletal fluorosis
  M85.10 Skeletal fluorosis, unspecified site
  M85.11- Skeletal fluorosis, shoulder
    M85.111 Skeletal fluorosis, right shoulder
    M85.112 Skeletal fluorosis, left shoulder
    M85.119 Skeletal fluorosis, unspecified shoulder
  M85.12- Skeletal fluorosis, upper arm
    M85.121 Skeletal fluorosis, right upper arm
    M85.122 Skeletal fluorosis, left upper arm
    M85.129 Skeletal fluorosis, unspecified upper arm
  M85.13- Skeletal fluorosis, forearm
    M85.131 Skeletal fluorosis, right forearm
    M85.132 Skeletal fluorosis, left forearm
    M85.139 Skeletal fluorosis, unspecified forearm
  M85.14- Skeletal fluorosis, hand
    M85.141 Skeletal fluorosis, right hand
    M85.142 Skeletal fluorosis, left hand
    M85.149 Skeletal fluorosis, unspecified hand
  M85.15- Skeletal fluorosis, thigh
    M85.151 Skeletal fluorosis, right thigh
    M85.152 Skeletal fluorosis, left thigh
    M85.159 Skeletal fluorosis, unspecified thigh
  M85.16- Skeletal fluorosis, lower leg
    M85.161 Skeletal fluorosis, right lower leg
    M85.162 Skeletal fluorosis, left lower leg
    M85.169 Skeletal fluorosis, unspecified lower leg
  M85.17- Skeletal fluorosis, ankle and foot
    M85.171 Skeletal fluorosis, right ankle and foot
    M85.172 Skeletal fluorosis, left ankle and foot
    M85.179 Skeletal fluorosis, unspecified ankle and foot
  M85.18 Skeletal fluorosis, other site
  M85.19 Skeletal fluorosis, multiple sites
M85.2 Hyperostosis of skull
M85.3- Osteitis condensans
  M85.30 Osteitis condensans, unspecified site
  M85.31- Osteitis condensans, shoulder
    M85.311 Osteitis condensans, right shoulder
    M85.312 Osteitis condensans, left shoulder
    M85.319 Osteitis condensans, unspecified shoulder
  M85.32- Osteitis condensans, upper arm
    M85.321 Osteitis condensans, right upper arm
    M85.322 Osteitis condensans, left upper arm
    M85.329 Osteitis condensans, unspecified upper arm
  M85.33- Osteitis condensans, forearm
    M85.331 Osteitis condensans, right forearm
    M85.332 Osteitis condensans, left forearm
    M85.339 Osteitis condensans, unspecified forearm
  M85.34- Osteitis condensans, hand
    M85.341 Osteitis condensans, right hand
    M85.342 Osteitis condensans, left hand
    M85.349 Osteitis condensans, unspecified hand
  M85.35- Osteitis condensans, thigh
    M85.351 Osteitis condensans, right thigh
    M85.352 Osteitis condensans, left thigh
    M85.359 Osteitis condensans, unspecified thigh
  M85.36- Osteitis condensans, lower leg
    M85.361 Osteitis condensans, right lower leg
    M85.362 Osteitis condensans, left lower leg
    M85.369 Osteitis condensans, unspecified lower leg

M84 - M85

M85.37-Osteitis condensans, <u>ankle and foot</u>
  M85.371 Osteitis condensans, <u>right</u> ankle and foot
  M85.372 Osteitis condensans, <u>left</u> ankle and foot
  M85.379 Osteitis condensans, <u>unspecified</u> ankle and foot
M85.38 Osteitis condensans, <u>other site</u>
M85.39 Osteitis condensans, <u>multiple sites</u>

M85.4- <u>Solitary bone cyst</u>
  Excludes❷: solitary cyst of jaw (M27.4)
M85.40 Solitary bone cyst, <u>unspecified site</u>
M85.41-Solitary bone cyst, <u>shoulder</u>
  M85.411 Solitary bone cyst, <u>right</u> shoulder
  M85.412 Solitary bone cyst, <u>left</u> shoulder
  M85.419 Solitary bone cyst, <u>unspecified</u> shoulder
M85.42-Solitary bone cyst, <u>humerus</u>
  M85.421 Solitary bone cyst, <u>right</u> humerus
  M85.422 Solitary bone cyst, <u>left</u> humerus
  M85.429 Solitary bone cyst, <u>unspecified</u> humerus
M85.43-Solitary bone cyst, <u>ulna and radius</u>
  M85.431 Solitary bone cyst, <u>right</u> ulna and radius
  M85.432 Solitary bone cyst, <u>left</u> ulna and radius
  M85.439 Solitary bone cyst, <u>unspecified</u> ulna and radius
M85.44-Solitary bone cyst, <u>hand</u>
  M85.441 Solitary bone cyst, <u>right</u> hand
  M85.442 Solitary bone cyst, <u>left</u> hand
  M85.449 Solitary bone cyst, <u>unspecified</u> hand
M85.45-Solitary bone cyst, <u>pelvis</u>
  M85.451 Solitary bone cyst, <u>right</u> pelvis
  M85.452 Solitary bone cyst, <u>left</u> pelvis
  M85.459 Solitary bone cyst, <u>unspecified</u> pelvis
M85.46-Solitary bone cyst, <u>tibia and fibula</u>
  M85.461 Solitary bone cyst, <u>right</u> tibia and fibula
  M85.462 Solitary bone cyst, <u>left</u> tibia and fibula
  M85.469 Solitary bone cyst, <u>unspecified</u> tibia and fibula
M85.47-Solitary bone cyst, <u>ankle and foot</u>
  M85.471 Solitary bone cyst, <u>right</u> ankle and foot
  M85.472 Solitary bone cyst, <u>left</u> ankle and foot
  M85.479 Solitary bone cyst, <u>unspecified</u> ankle and foot
M85.48 Solitary bone cyst, <u>other site</u>

M85.5- <u>Aneurysmal bone cyst</u>
  Excludes❷: aneurysmal cyst of jaw (M27.4)
M85.50 Aneurysmal bone cyst, <u>unspecified site</u>
M85.51-Aneurysmal bone cyst, <u>shoulder</u>
  M85.511 Aneurysmal bone cyst, <u>right</u> shoulder
  M85.512 Aneurysmal bone cyst, <u>left</u> shoulder
  M85.519 Aneurysmal bone cyst, <u>unspecified</u> shoulder
M85.52-Aneurysmal bone cyst, <u>upper arm</u>
  M85.521 Aneurysmal bone cyst, <u>right</u> upper arm
  M85.522 Aneurysmal bone cyst, <u>left</u> upper arm
  M85.529 Aneurysmal bone cyst, <u>unspecified</u> upper arm
M85.53-Aneurysmal bone cyst, <u>forearm</u>
  M85.531 Aneurysmal bone cyst, <u>right</u> forearm
  M85.532 Aneurysmal bone cyst, <u>left</u> forearm
  M85.539 Aneurysmal bone cyst, <u>unspecified</u> forearm
M85.54-Aneurysmal bone cyst, <u>hand</u>
  M85.541 Aneurysmal bone cyst, <u>right</u> hand
  M85.542 Aneurysmal bone cyst, <u>left</u> hand
  M85.549 Aneurysmal bone cyst, <u>unspecified</u> hand
M85.55-Aneurysmal bone cyst, <u>thigh</u>
  M85.551 Aneurysmal bone cyst, <u>right</u> thigh
  M85.552 Aneurysmal bone cyst, <u>left</u> thigh
  M85.559 Aneurysmal bone cyst, <u>unspecified</u> thigh
M85.56-Aneurysmal bone cyst, <u>lower leg</u>
  M85.561 Aneurysmal bone cyst, <u>right</u> lower leg
  M85.562 Aneurysmal bone cyst, <u>left</u> lower leg
  M85.569 Aneurysmal bone cyst, <u>unspecified</u> lower leg
M85.57-Aneurysmal bone cyst, <u>ankle and foot</u>
  M85.571 Aneurysmal bone cyst, <u>right</u> ankle and foot
  M85.572 Aneurysmal bone cyst, <u>left</u> ankle and foot
  M85.579 Aneurysmal bone cyst, <u>unspecified</u> ankle and foot
M85.58 Aneurysmal bone cyst, <u>other site</u>
M85.59 Aneurysmal bone cyst, <u>multiple sites</u>

M85.6- <u>Other cyst</u> of bone
  Excludes 1: cyst of jaw NEC (M27.4)
          osteitis fibrosa cystica generalisata [von
            Recklinghausen's disease of bone] (E21.0)
M85.60 Other cyst of bone, <u>unspecified</u> site
M85.61-Other cyst of bone, <u>shoulder</u>
  M85.611 Other cyst of bone, <u>right</u> shoulder
  M85.612 Other cyst of bone, <u>left</u> shoulder
  M85.619 Other cyst of bone, <u>unspecified</u> shoulder
M85.62-Other cyst of bone, <u>upper arm</u>
  M85.621 Other cyst of bone, <u>right</u> upper arm
  M85.622 Other cyst of bone, <u>left</u> upper arm
  M85.629 Other cyst of bone, <u>unspecified</u> upper arm
M85.63-Other cyst of bone, <u>forearm</u>
  M85.631 Other cyst of bone, <u>right</u> forearm
  M85.632 Other cyst of bone, <u>left</u> forearm
  M85.639 Other cyst of bone, <u>unspecified</u> forearm
M85.64-Other cyst of bone, <u>hand</u>
  M85.641 Other cyst of bone, <u>right</u> hand
  M85.642 Other cyst of bone, <u>left</u> hand
  M85.649 Other cyst of bone, <u>unspecified</u> hand
M85.65-Other cyst of bone, <u>thigh</u>
  M85.651 Other cyst of bone, <u>right</u> thigh
  M85.652 Other cyst of bone, <u>left</u> thigh
  M85.659 Other cyst of bone, <u>unspecified</u> thigh
M85.66-Other cyst of bone, <u>lower leg</u>
  M85.661 Other cyst of bone, <u>right</u> lower leg
  M85.662 Other cyst of bone, <u>left</u> lower leg
  M85.669 Other cyst of bone, <u>unspecified</u> lower leg
M85.67-Other cyst of bone, <u>ankle and foot</u>
  M85.671 Other cyst of bone, <u>right</u> ankle and foot
  M85.672 Other cyst of bone, <u>left</u> ankle and foot
  M85.679 Other cyst of bone, <u>unspecified</u> ankle and foot
M85.68 Other cyst of bone, <u>other site</u>
M85.69 Other cyst of bone, <u>multiple sites</u>

M85.8- <u>Other specified</u> disorders of bone density and structure
  Hyperostosis of bones, except skull
  Osteosclerosis, acquired
  Excludes 1: diffuse idiopathic skeletal hyperostosis [DISH] (M48.1)
            osteosclerosis congenita (Q77.4)
            osteosclerosis fragilitas (generalista) (Q78.2)
            osteosclerosis myelofibrosis (D75.81)
M85.80 Other specified disorders of bone density and structure, <u>unspecified</u> site
M85.81-Other specified disorders of bone density and structure, <u>shoulder</u>
  M85.811 Other specified disorders of bone density and structure, <u>right</u> shoulder
  M85.812 Other specified disorders of bone density and structure, <u>left</u> shoulder
  M85.819 Other specified disorders of bone density and structure, <u>unspecified</u> shoulder
M85.82-Other specified disorders of bone density and structure, <u>upper arm</u>
  M85.821 Other specified disorders of bone density and structure, <u>right</u> upper arm
  M85.822 Other specified disorders of bone density and structure, <u>left</u> upper arm
  M85.829 Other specified disorders of bone density and structure, <u>unspecified</u> upper arm
M85.83-Other specified disorders of bone density and structure, <u>forearm</u>
  M85.831 Other specified disorders of bone density and structure, <u>right</u> forearm
  M85.832 Other specified disorders of bone density and structure, <u>left</u> forearm
  M85.839 Other specified disorders of bone density and structure, <u>unspecified</u> forearm
M85.84-Other specified disorders of bone density and structure, <u>hand</u>
  M85.841 Other specified disorders of bone density and structure, <u>right</u> hand
  M85.842 Other specified disorders of bone density and structure, <u>left</u> hand
  M85.849 Other specified disorders of bone density and structure, <u>unspecified</u> hand

M
8
4
I
M
8
5

M85.85-Other specified disorders of bone density and structure, <u>thigh</u>
>   M85.851   Other specified disorders of bone density and structure, <u>right</u> thigh
>   M85.852   Other specified disorders of bone density and structure, <u>left</u> thigh
>   M85.859   Other specified disorders of bone density and structure, <u>unspecified</u> thigh

M85.86-Other specified disorders of bone density and structure, <u>lower leg</u>
>   M85.861   Other specified disorders of bone density and structure, <u>right</u> lower leg
>   M85.862   Other specified disorders of bone density and structure, <u>left</u> lower leg
>   M85.869   Other specified disorders of bone density and structure, <u>unspecified</u> lower leg

M85.87-Other specified disorders of bone density and structure, <u>ankle and foot</u>
>   M85.871   Other specified disorders of bone density and structure, <u>right</u> ankle and foot
>   M85.872   Other specified disorders of bone density and structure, <u>left</u> ankle and foot
>   M85.879   Other specified disorders of bone density and structure, <u>unspecified</u> ankle and foot

M85.88   Other specified disorders of bone density and structure, <u>other site</u>

M85.89   Other specified disorders of bone density and structure, <u>multiple sites</u>

M85.9   Disorder of bone density and structure, <u>unspecified</u>

Other osteopathies (M86-M90)

Excludes 1: postprocedural osteopathies (M96.-)

M86-   <u>Osteomyelitis</u>
Use additional code (B95-B97) to identify infectious agent
Use additional code to identify major osseous defect, if applicable (M89.7-)
Excludes 1: osteomyelitis due to:
>   *echinococcus (B67.2)*
>   *gonococcus (A54.43)*
>   *salmonella (A02.24)*

Excludes❷: ostemyelitis of:
>   *orbit (H05.0-)*
>   *petrous bone (H70.2-)*
>   *vertebra (M46.2-)*

M86.0-   <u>Acute hematogenous</u> osteomyelitis
M86.00   Acute hematogenous osteomyelitis, <u>unspecified</u> site
M86.01-Acute hematogenous osteomyelitis, <u>shoulder</u>
>   M86.011   Acute hematogenous osteomyelitis, <u>right</u> shoulder
>   M86.012   Acute hematogenous osteomyelitis, <u>left</u> shoulder
>   M86.019   Acute hematogenous osteomyelitis, <u>unspecified</u> shoulder

M86.02-Acute hematogenous osteomyelitis, <u>humerus</u>
>   M86.021   Acute hematogenous osteomyelitis, <u>right</u> humerus
>   M86.022   Acute hematogenous osteomyelitis, <u>left</u> humerus
>   M86.029   Acute hematogenous osteomyelitis, <u>unspecified</u> humerus

M86.03-Acute hematogenous osteomyelitis, <u>radius and ulna</u>
>   M86.031   Acute hematogenous osteomyelitis, <u>right</u> radius and ulna
>   M86.032   Acute hematogenous osteomyelitis, <u>left</u> radius and ulna
>   M86.039   Acute hematogenous osteomyelitis, <u>unspecified</u> radius and ulna

M86.04-Acute hematogenous osteomyelitis, <u>hand</u>
>   M86.041   Acute hematogenous osteomyelitis, <u>right</u> hand
>   M86.042   Acute hematogenous osteomyelitis, <u>left</u> hand
>   M86.049   Acute hematogenous osteomyelitis, <u>unspecified</u> hand

M86.05-Acute hematogenous osteomyelitis, <u>femur</u>
>   M86.051   Acute hematogenous osteomyelitis, <u>right</u> femur
>   M86.052   Acute hematogenous osteomyelitis, <u>left</u> femur
>   M86.059   Acute hematogenous osteomyelitis, <u>unspecified</u> femur

M86.06-Acute hematogenous osteomyelitis, <u>tibia and fibula</u>
>   M86.061   Acute hematogenous osteomyelitis, <u>right</u> tibia and fibula
>   M86.062   Acute hematogenous osteomyelitis, <u>left</u> tibia and fibula
>   M86.069   Acute hematogenous osteomyelitis, <u>unspecified</u> tibia and fibula

M86.07-Acute hematogenous osteomyelitis, <u>ankle and foot</u>
>   M86.071   Acute hematogenous osteomyelitis, <u>right</u> ankle and foot
>   M86.072   Acute hematogenous osteomyelitis, <u>left</u> ankle and foot
>   M86.079   Acute hematogenous osteomyelitis, <u>unspecified</u> ankle and foot

M86.08   Acute hematogenous osteomyelitis, <u>other sites</u>
M86.09   Acute hematogenous osteomyelitis, <u>multiple sites</u>

M86.1-   <u>Other acute</u> osteomyelitis
M86.10   Other acute osteomyelitis, <u>unspecified</u> site
M86.11-Other acute osteomyelitis, <u>shoulder</u>
>   M86.111   Other acute osteomyelitis, <u>right</u> shoulder
>   M86.112   Other acute osteomyelitis, <u>left</u> shoulder
>   M86.119   Other acute osteomyelitis, <u>unspecified</u> shoulder

M86.12-Other acute osteomyelitis, <u>humerus</u>
>   M86.121   Other acute osteomyelitis, <u>right</u> humerus
>   M86.122   Other acute osteomyelitis, <u>left</u> humerus
>   M86.129   Other acute osteomyelitis, <u>unspecified</u> humerus

M86.13-Other acute osteomyelitis, <u>radius and ulna</u>
>   M86.131   Other acute osteomyelitis, <u>right</u> radius and ulna
>   M86.132   Other acute osteomyelitis, <u>left</u> radius and ulna
>   M86.139   Other acute osteomyelitis, <u>unspecified</u> radius and ulna

M86.14-Other acute osteomyelitis, <u>hand</u>
>   M86.141   Other acute osteomyelitis, <u>right</u> hand
>   M86.142   Other acute osteomyelitis, <u>left</u> hand
>   M86.149   Other acute osteomyelitis, <u>unspecified</u> hand

M86.15-Other acute osteomyelitis, <u>femur</u>
>   M86.151   Other acute osteomyelitis, <u>right</u> femur
>   M86.152   Other acute osteomyelitis, <u>left</u> femur
>   M86.159   Other acute osteomyelitis, <u>unspecified</u> femur

M86.16-Other acute osteomyelitis, <u>tibia and fibula</u>
>   M86.161   Other acute osteomyelitis, <u>right</u> tibia and fibula
>   M86.162   Other acute osteomyelitis, <u>left</u> tibia and fibula
>   M86.169   Other acute osteomyelitis, <u>unspecified</u> tibia and fibula

M86.17-Other acute osteomyelitis, <u>ankle and foot</u>
>   M86.171   Other acute osteomyelitis, <u>right</u> ankle and foot
>   M86.172   Other acute osteomyelitis, <u>left</u> ankle and foot
>   M86.179   Other acute osteomyelitis, <u>unspecified</u> ankle and foot

M86.18   Other acute osteomyelitis, <u>other site</u>
M86.19   Other acute osteomyelitis, <u>multiple sites</u>

M86.2-   <u>Subacute</u> osteomyelitis
M86.20   Subacute osteomyelitis, <u>unspecified</u> site
M86.21-Subacute osteomyelitis, <u>shoulder</u>
>   M86.211   Subacute osteomyelitis, <u>right</u> shoulder
>   M86.212   Subacute osteomyelitis, <u>left</u> shoulder
>   M86.219   Subacute osteomyelitis, <u>unspecified</u> shoulder

M86.22-Subacute osteomyelitis, <u>humerus</u>
>   M86.221   Subacute osteomyelitis, <u>right</u> humerus
>   M86.222   Subacute osteomyelitis, <u>left</u> humerus
>   M86.229   Subacute osteomyelitis, <u>unspecified</u> humerus

M86.23-Subacute osteomyelitis, <u>radius and ulna</u>
>   M86.231   Subacute osteomyelitis, <u>right</u> radius and ulna
>   M86.232   Subacute osteomyelitis, <u>left</u> radius and ulna
>   M86.239   Subacute osteomyelitis, <u>unspecified</u> radius and ulna

M86.24-Subacute osteomyelitis, <u>hand</u>
>   M86.241   Subacute osteomyelitis, <u>right</u> hand
>   M86.242   Subacute osteomyelitis, <u>left</u> hand
>   M86.249   Subacute osteomyelitis, <u>unspecified</u> hand

M86.25-Subacute osteomyelitis, <u>femur</u>
>   M86.251   Subacute osteomyelitis, <u>right</u> femur
>   M86.252   Subacute osteomyelitis, <u>left</u> femur
>   M86.259   Subacute osteomyelitis, <u>unspecified</u> femur

M86.26-Subacute osteomyelitis, <u>tibia and fibula</u>
>   M86.261   Subacute osteomyelitis, <u>right</u> tibia and fibula
>   M86.262   Subacute osteomyelitis, <u>left</u> tibia and fibula
>   M86.269   Subacute osteomyelitis, <u>unspecified</u> tibia and fibula

M86.27-Subacute osteomyelitis, <u>ankle and foot</u>
>   M86.271   Subacute osteomyelitis, <u>right</u> ankle and foot
>   M86.272   Subacute osteomyelitis, <u>left</u> ankle and foot
>   M86.279   Subacute osteomyelitis, <u>unspecified</u> ankle and foot

M86.28   Subacute osteomyelitis, <u>other site</u>
M86.29   Subacute osteomyelitis, <u>multiple sites</u>

M85
-
M86

M86.3- Chronic multifocal osteomyelitis
   M86.30 Chronic multifocal osteomyelitis, unspecified site
   M86.31-Chronic multifocal osteomyelitis, shoulder
      M86.311   Chronic multifocal osteomyelitis, right shoulder
      M86.312   Chronic multifocal osteomyelitis, left shoulder
      M86.319   Chronic multifocal osteomyelitis, unspecified shoulder
   M86.32-Chronic multifocal osteomyelitis, humerus
      M86.321   Chronic multifocal osteomyelitis, right humerus
      M86.322   Chronic multifocal osteomyelitis, left humerus
      M86.329   Chronic multifocal osteomyelitis, unspecified humerus
   M86.33-Chronic multifocal osteomyelitis, radius and ulna
      M86.331   Chronic multifocal osteomyelitis, right radius and ulna
      M86.332   Chronic multifocal osteomyelitis, left radius and ulna
      M86.339   Chronic multifocal osteomyelitis, unspecified radius and ulna
   M86.34-Chronic multifocal osteomyelitis, hand
      M86.341   Chronic multifocal osteomyelitis, right hand
      M86.342   Chronic multifocal osteomyelitis, left hand
      M86.349   Chronic multifocal osteomyelitis, unspecified hand
   M86.35-Chronic multifocal osteomyelitis, femur
      M86.351   Chronic multifocal osteomyelitis, right femur
      M86.352   Chronic multifocal osteomyelitis, left femur
      M86.359   Chronic multifocal osteomyelitis, unspecified femur
   M86.36-Chronic multifocal osteomyelitis, tibia and fibula
      M86.361   Chronic multifocal osteomyelitis, right tibia and fibula
      M86.362   Chronic multifocal osteomyelitis, left tibia and fibula
      M86.369   Chronic multifocal osteomyelitis, unspecified tibia and fibula
   M86.37-Chronic multifocal osteomyelitis, ankle and foot
      M86.371   Chronic multifocal osteomyelitis, right ankle and foot
      M86.372   Chronic multifocal osteomyelitis, left ankle and foot
      M86.379   Chronic multifocal osteomyelitis, unspecified ankle and foot
   M86.38 Chronic multifocal osteomyelitis, other site
   M86.39 Chronic multifocal osteomyelitis, multiple sites
M86.4- Chronic osteomyelitis with draining sinus
   M86.40 Chronic osteomyelitis with draining sinus, unspecified site
   M86.41-Chronic osteomyelitis with draining sinus, shoulder
      M86.411   Chronic osteomyelitis with draining sinus, right shoulder
      M86.412   Chronic osteomyelitis with draining sinus, left shoulder
      M86.419   Chronic osteomyelitis with draining sinus, unspecified shoulder
   M86.42-Chronic osteomyelitis with draining sinus, humerus
      M86.421   Chronic osteomyelitis with draining sinus, right humerus
      M86.422   Chronic osteomyelitis with draining sinus, left humerus
      M86.429   Chronic osteomyelitis with draining sinus, unspecified humerus
   M86.43-Chronic osteomyelitis with draining sinus, radius and ulna
      M86.431   Chronic osteomyelitis with draining sinus, right radius and ulna
      M86.432   Chronic osteomyelitis with draining sinus, left radius and ulna
      M86.439   Chronic osteomyelitis with draining sinus, unspecified radius and ulna
   M86.44-Chronic osteomyelitis with draining sinus, hand
      M86.441   Chronic osteomyelitis with draining sinus, right hand
      M86.442   Chronic osteomyelitis with draining sinus, left hand
      M86.449   Chronic osteomyelitis with draining sinus, unspecified hand
   M86.45-Chronic osteomyelitis with draining sinus, femur
      M86.451   Chronic osteomyelitis with draining sinus, right femur
      M86.452   Chronic osteomyelitis with draining sinus, left femur
      M86.459   Chronic osteomyelitis with draining sinus, unspecified femur
   M86.46-Chronic osteomyelitis with draining sinus, tibia and fibula
      M86.461   Chronic osteomyelitis with draining sinus, right tibia and fibula
      M86.462   Chronic osteomyelitis with draining sinus, left tibia and fibula
      M86.469   Chronic osteomyelitis with draining sinus, unspecified tibia and fibula

M86.47-Chronic osteomyelitis with draining sinus, ankle and foot
      M86.471   Chronic osteomyelitis with draining sinus, right ankle and foot
      M86.472   Chronic osteomyelitis with draining sinus, left ankle and foot
      M86.479   Chronic osteomyelitis with draining sinus, unspecified ankle and foot
   M86.48 Chronic osteomyelitis with draining sinus, other site
   M86.49 Chronic osteomyelitis with draining sinus, multiple sites
M86.5- Other chronic hematogenous osteomyelitis
   M86.50 Other chronic hematogenous osteomyelitis, unspecified site
   M86.51-Other chronic hematogenous osteomyelitis, shoulder
      M86.511   Other chronic hematogenous osteomyelitis, right shoulder
      M86.512   Other chronic hematogenous osteomyelitis, left shoulder
      M86.519   Other chronic hematogenous osteomyelitis, unspecified shoulder
   M86.52-Other chronic hematogenous osteomyelitis, humerus
      M86.521   Other chronic hematogenous osteomyelitis, right humerus
      M86.522   Other chronic hematogenous osteomyelitis, left humerus
      M86.529   Other chronic hematogenous osteomyelitis, unspecified humerus
   M86.53-Other chronic hematogenous osteomyelitis, radius and ulna
      M86.531   Other chronic hematogenous osteomyelitis, right radius and ulna
      M86.532   Other chronic hematogenous osteomyelitis, left radius and ulna
      M86.539   Other chronic hematogenous osteomyelitis, unspecified radius and ulna
   M86.54-Other chronic hematogenous osteomyelitis, hand
      M86.541   Other chronic hematogenous osteomyelitis, right hand
      M86.542   Other chronic hematogenous osteomyelitis, left hand
      M86.549   Other chronic hematogenous osteomyelitis, unspecified hand
   M86.55-Other chronic hematogenous osteomyelitis, femur
      M86.551   Other chronic hematogenous osteomyelitis, right femur
      M86.552   Other chronic hematogenous osteomyelitis, left femur
      M86.559   Other chronic hematogenous osteomyelitis, unspecified femur
   M86.56-Other chronic hematogenous osteomyelitis, tibia and fibula
      M86.561   Other chronic hematogenous osteomyelitis, right tibia and fibula
      M86.562   Other chronic hematogenous osteomyelitis, left tibia and fibula
      M86.569   Other chronic hematogenous osteomyelitis, unspecified tibia and fibula
   M86.57-Other chronic hematogenous osteomyelitis, ankle and foot
      M86.571   Other chronic hematogenous osteomyelitis, right ankle and foot
      M86.572   Other chronic hematogenous osteomyelitis, left ankle and foot
      M86.579   Other chronic hematogenous osteomyelitis, unspecified ankle and foot
   M86.58 Other chronic hematogenous osteomyelitis, other site
   M86.59 Other chronic hematogenous osteomyelitis, multiple sites
M86.6- Other chronic osteomyelitis
   M86.60 Other chronic osteomyelitis, unspecified site
   M86.61-Other chronic osteomyelitis, shoulder
      M86.611   Other chronic osteomyelitis, right shoulder
      M86.612   Other chronic osteomyelitis, left shoulder
      M86.619   Other chronic osteomyelitis, unspecified shoulder
   M86.62-Other chronic osteomyelitis, humerus
      M86.621   Other chronic osteomyelitis, right humerus
      M86.622   Other chronic osteomyelitis, left humerus
      M86.629   Other chronic osteomyelitis, unspecified humerus
   M86.63-Other chronic osteomyelitis, radius and ulna
      M86.631   Other chronic osteomyelitis, right radius and ulna
      M86.632   Other chronic osteomyelitis, left radius and ulna
      M86.639   Other chronic osteomyelitis, unspecified radius and ulna

M8 5 I M8 6

Excludes 1: = NOT CODED HERE! (Do not code both)

Excludes❷: = Not Included Here

M86.64-Other chronic osteomyelitis, <u>hand</u>
    M86.641 Other chronic osteomyelitis, <u>right</u> hand
    M86.642 Other chronic osteomyelitis, <u>left</u> hand
    M86.649 Other chronic osteomyelitis, <u>unspecified</u> hand
M86.65-Other chronic osteomyelitis, <u>thigh</u>
    M86.651 Other chronic osteomyelitis, <u>right</u> thigh
    M86.652 Other chronic osteomyelitis, <u>left</u> thigh
    M86.659 Other chronic osteomyelitis, <u>unspecified</u> thigh
M86.66-Other chronic osteomyelitis, <u>tibia and fibula</u>
    M86.661 Other chronic osteomyelitis, <u>right</u> tibia and fibula
    M86.662 Other chronic osteomyelitis, <u>left</u> tibia and fibula
    M86.669 Other chronic osteomyelitis, <u>unspecified</u> tibia and fibula
M86.67-Other chronic osteomyelitis, <u>ankle and foot</u>
    M86.671 Other chronic osteomyelitis, <u>right</u> ankle and foot
    M86.672 Other chronic osteomyelitis, <u>left</u> ankle and foot
    M86.679 Other chronic osteomyelitis, <u>unspecified</u> ankle and foot
M86.68 Other chronic osteomyelitis, <u>other site</u>
M86.69 Other chronic osteomyelitis, <u>multiple sites</u>
M86.8- Other osteomyelitis
    Brodie's abscess
 M86.8x-<u>Other</u> osteomyelitis
    M86.8x0 Other osteomyelitis, multiple sites
    M86.8x1 Other osteomyelitis, shoulder
    M86.8x2 Other osteomyelitis, upper arm
    M86.8x3 Other osteomyelitis, forearm
    M86.8x4 Other osteomyelitis, hand
    M86.8x5 Other osteomyelitis, thigh
    M86.8x6 Other osteomyelitis, lower leg
    M86.8x7 Other osteomyelitis, ankle and foot
    M86.8x8 Other osteomyelitis, other site
    M86.8x9 Other osteomyelitis, unspecified sites
M86.9 Osteomyelitis, <u>unspecified</u>
    Infection of bone NOS
    Periostitis without osteomyelitis

M87- Osteonecrosis
    Includes: avascular necrosis of bone
    Use additional code to identify major osseous defect, if applicable (M89.7-)
    Excludes 1: juvenile osteonecrosis (M91-M92)
    *   osteochondropathies (M90-M93)*
 M87.0- <u>Idiopathic aseptic necrosis of bone</u>
  M87.00 Idiopathic aseptic necrosis of <u>unspecified</u> <u>bone</u>
  M87.01-Idiopathic aseptic necrosis of <u>shoulder</u>
      Idiopathic aseptic necrosis of clavicle and scapula
    M87.011 Idiopathic aseptic necrosis of <u>right</u> shoulder
    M87.012 Idiopathic aseptic necrosis of <u>left</u> shoulder
    M87.019 Idiopathic aseptic necrosis of <u>unspecified</u> shoulder
  M87.02-Idiopathic aseptic necrosis of <u>humerus</u>
    M87.021 Idiopathic aseptic necrosis of <u>right</u> humerus
    M87.022 Idiopathic aseptic necrosis of <u>left</u> humerus
    M87.029 Idiopathic aseptic necrosis of <u>unspecified</u> humerus
  M87.03-Idiopathic aseptic necrosis of <u>radius, ulna and carpus</u>
    M87.031 Idiopathic aseptic necrosis of <u>right</u> radius
    M87.032 Idiopathic aseptic necrosis of <u>left</u> radius
    M87.033 Idiopathic aseptic necrosis of <u>unspecified</u> radius
    M87.034 Idiopathic aseptic necrosis of <u>right</u> ulna
    M87.035 Idiopathic aseptic necrosis of <u>left</u> ulna
    M87.036 Idiopathic aseptic necrosis of <u>unspecified</u> ulna
    M87.037 Idiopathic aseptic necrosis of <u>right</u> carpus
    M87.038 Idiopathic aseptic necrosis of <u>left</u> carpus
    M87.039 Idiopathic aseptic necrosis of <u>unspecified</u> carpus
  M87.04-Idiopathic aseptic necrosis of <u>hand and fingers</u>
      Idiopathic aseptic necrosis of metacarpals and phalanges of hands
    M87.041 Idiopathic aseptic necrosis of <u>right</u> hand
    M87.042 Idiopathic aseptic necrosis of <u>left</u> hand
    M87.043 Idiopathic aseptic necrosis of <u>unspecified</u> hand
    M87.044 Idiopathic aseptic necrosis of <u>right</u> finger(s)
    M87.045 Idiopathic aseptic necrosis of <u>left</u> finger(s)
    M87.046 Idiopathic aseptic necrosis of <u>unspecified</u> finger(s)
  M87.05-Idiopathic aseptic necrosis of <u>pelvis and femur</u>
    M87.050 Idiopathic aseptic necrosis of pelvis
    M87.051 Idiopathic aseptic necrosis of <u>right</u> femur
    M87.052 Idiopathic aseptic necrosis of <u>left</u> femur

    M87.059 Idiopathic aseptic necrosis of <u>unspecified</u> femur
      Idiopathic aseptic necrosis of hip NOS
  M87.06-Idiopathic aseptic necrosis of <u>tibia and fibula</u>
    M87.061 Idiopathic aseptic necrosis of <u>right</u> tibia
    M87.062 Idiopathic aseptic necrosis of <u>left</u> tibia
    M87.063 Idiopathic aseptic necrosis of <u>unspecified</u> tibia
    M87.064 Idiopathic aseptic necrosis of <u>right</u> fibula
    M87.065 Idiopathic aseptic necrosis of <u>left</u> fibula
    M87.066 Idiopathic aseptic necrosis of <u>unspecified</u> fibula
  M87.07-Idiopathic aseptic necrosis of <u>ankle, foot and toes</u>
      Idiopathic aseptic necrosis of metatarsus, tarsus, and phalanges of toes
    M87.071 Idiopathic aseptic necrosis of <u>right</u> ankle
    M87.072 Idiopathic aseptic necrosis of <u>left</u> ankle
    M87.073 Idiopathic aseptic necrosis of <u>unspecified</u> ankle
    M87.074 Idiopathic aseptic necrosis of <u>right</u> foot
    M87.075 Idiopathic aseptic necrosis of <u>left</u> foot
    M87.076 Idiopathic aseptic necrosis of <u>unspecified</u> foot
    M87.077 Idiopathic aseptic necrosis of <u>right</u> toe(s)
    M87.078 Idiopathic aseptic necrosis of <u>left</u> toe(s)
    M87.079 Idiopathic aseptic necrosis of <u>unspecified</u> toe(s)
  M87.08 Idiopathic aseptic necrosis of bone, <u>other site</u>
  M87.09 Idiopathic aseptic necrosis of bone, <u>multiple sites</u>
 M87.1- Osteonecrosis <u>due to drugs</u>
    Use additional code for adverse effect, if applicable, to identify drug (T36-T50 with fifth or sixth character 5)
  M87.10 Osteonecrosis due to drugs, <u>unspecified</u> <u>bone</u>
  M87.11-Osteonecrosis due to drugs, <u>shoulder</u>
    M87.111 Osteonecrosis due to drugs, <u>right</u> shoulder
    M87.112 Osteonecrosis due to drugs, <u>left</u> shoulder
    M87.119 Osteonecrosis due to drugs, <u>unspecified</u> shoulder
  M87.12-Osteonecrosis due to drugs, <u>humerus</u>
    M87.121 Osteonecrosis due to drugs, <u>right</u> humerus
    M87.122 Osteonecrosis due to drugs, <u>left</u> humerus
    M87.129 Osteonecrosis due to drugs, <u>unspecified</u> humerus
  M87.13-Osteonecrosis due to drugs of <u>radius, ulna and carpus</u>
    M87.131 Osteonecrosis due to drugs of <u>right</u> radius
    M87.132 Osteonecrosis due to drugs of <u>left</u> radius
    M87.133 Osteonecrosis due to drugs of <u>unspecified</u> radius
    M87.134 Osteonecrosis due to drugs of <u>right</u> ulna
    M87.135 Osteonecrosis due to drugs of <u>left</u> ulna
    M87.136 Osteonecrosis due to drugs of <u>unspecified</u> ulna
    M87.137 Osteonecrosis due to drugs of <u>right</u> carpus
    M87.138 Osteonecrosis due to drugs of <u>left</u> carpus
    M87.139 Osteonecrosis due to drugs of <u>unspecified</u> carpus
  M87.14-Osteonecrosis due to drugs, <u>hand and fingers</u>
    M87.141 Osteonecrosis due to drugs, <u>right</u> hand
    M87.142 Osteonecrosis due to drugs, <u>left</u> hand
    M87.143 Osteonecrosis due to drugs, <u>unspecified</u> hand
    M87.144 Osteonecrosis due to drugs, <u>right</u> finger(s)
    M87.145 Osteonecrosis due to drugs, <u>left</u> finger(s)
    M87.146 Osteonecrosis due to drugs, <u>unspecified</u> finger(s)
  M87.15-Osteonecrosis due to drugs, <u>pelvis and femur</u>
    M87.150 Osteonecrosis due to drugs, pelvis
    M87.151 Osteonecrosis due to drugs, <u>right</u> femur
    M87.152 Osteonecrosis due to drugs, <u>left</u> femur
    M87.159 Osteonecrosis due to drugs, <u>unspecified</u> femur
  M87.16-Osteonecrosis due to drugs, <u>tibia and fibula</u>
    M87.161 Osteonecrosis due to drugs, <u>right</u> tibia
    M87.162 Osteonecrosis due to drugs, <u>left</u> tibia
    M87.163 Osteonecrosis due to drugs, <u>unspecified</u> tibia
    M87.164 Osteonecrosis due to drugs, <u>right</u> fibula
    M87.165 Osteonecrosis due to drugs, <u>left</u> fibula
    M87.166 Osteonecrosis due to drugs, <u>unspecified</u> fibula
  M87.17-Osteonecrosis due to drugs, <u>ankle, foot and toes</u>
    M87.171 Osteonecrosis due to drugs, <u>right</u> ankle
    M87.172 Osteonecrosis due to drugs, <u>left</u> ankle
    M87.173 Osteonecrosis due to drugs, <u>unspecified</u> ankle
    M87.174 Osteonecrosis due to drugs, <u>right</u> foot
    M87.175 Osteonecrosis due to drugs, <u>left</u> foot
    M87.176 Osteonecrosis due to drugs, <u>unspecified</u> foot
    M87.177 Osteonecrosis due to drugs, <u>right</u> toe(s)
    M87.178 Osteonecrosis due to drugs, <u>left</u> toe(s)
    M87.179 Osteonecrosis due to drugs, <u>unspecified</u> toe(s)

M
8
6
I
M
8
7

M87.18-Osteonecrosis due to drugs, <u>other site</u>
   M87.180 Osteonecrosis due to drugs, <u>jaw</u>
   M87.188 Osteonecrosis due to drugs, <u>other site</u>
M87.19 Osteonecrosis due to drugs, <u>multiple sites</u>
M87.2- Osteonecrosis <u>due to previous trauma</u>
M87.20 Osteonecrosis due to previous trauma, <u>unspecified</u> <u>bone</u>
M87.21-Osteonecrosis due to previous trauma, <u>shoulder</u>
   M87.211 Osteonecrosis due to previous trauma, <u>right</u> shoulder
   M87.212 Osteonecrosis due to previous trauma, <u>left</u> shoulder
   M87.219 Osteonecrosis due to previous trauma, <u>unspecified</u> shoulder
M87.22-Osteonecrosis due to previous trauma, <u>humerus</u>
   M87.221 Osteonecrosis due to previous trauma, <u>right</u> humerus
   M87.222 Osteonecrosis due to previous trauma, <u>left</u> humerus
   M87.229 Osteonecrosis due to previous trauma, <u>unspecified</u> humerus
M87.23-Osteonecrosis due to previous trauma of <u>radius, ulna and carpus</u>
   M87.231 Osteonecrosis due to previous trauma of <u>right</u> radius
   M87.232 Osteonecrosis due to previous trauma of <u>left</u> radius
   M87.233 Osteonecrosis due to previous trauma of <u>unspecified</u> radius
   M87.234 Osteonecrosis due to previous trauma of <u>right</u> ulna
   M87.235 Osteonecrosis due to previous trauma of <u>left</u> ulna
   M87.236 Osteonecrosis due to previous trauma of <u>unspecified</u> ulna
   M87.237 Osteonecrosis due to previous trauma of <u>right</u> carpus
   M87.238 Osteonecrosis due to previous trauma of <u>left</u> carpus
   M87.239 Osteonecrosis due to previous trauma of <u>unspecified</u> carpus
M87.24-Osteonecrosis due to previous trauma, <u>hand and fingers</u>
   M87.241 Osteonecrosis due to previous trauma, <u>right</u> hand
   M87.242 Osteonecrosis due to previous trauma, <u>left</u> hand
   M87.243 Osteonecrosis due to previous trauma, <u>unspecified</u> hand
   M87.244 Osteonecrosis due to previous trauma, <u>right</u> finger(s)
   M87.245 Osteonecrosis due to previous trauma, <u>left</u> finger(s)
   M87.246 Osteonecrosis due to previous trauma, <u>unspecified</u> finger(s)
M87.25-Osteonecrosis due to previous trauma, <u>pelvis and femur</u>
   M87.250 Osteonecrosis due to previous trauma, pelvis
   M87.251 Osteonecrosis due to previous trauma, <u>right</u> femur
   M87.252 Osteonecrosis due to previous trauma, <u>left</u> femur
   M87.256 Osteonecrosis due to previous trauma, <u>unspecified</u> femur
M87.26-Osteonecrosis due to previous trauma, <u>tibia and fibula</u>
   M87.261 Osteonecrosis due to previous trauma, <u>right</u> tibia
   M87.262 Osteonecrosis due to previous trauma, <u>left</u> tibia
   M87.263 Osteonecrosis due to previous trauma, <u>unspecified</u> tibia
   M87.264 Osteonecrosis due to previous trauma, <u>right</u> fibula
   M87.265 Osteonecrosis due to previous trauma, <u>left</u> fibula
   M87.266 Osteonecrosis due to previous trauma, <u>unspecified</u> fibula
M87.27-Osteonecrosis due to previous trauma, <u>ankle, foot and toes</u>
   M87.271 Osteonecrosis due to previous trauma, <u>right</u> ankle
   M87.272 Osteonecrosis due to previous trauma, <u>left</u> ankle
   M87.273 Osteonecrosis due to previous trauma, <u>unspecified</u> ankle
   M87.274 Osteonecrosis due to previous trauma, <u>right</u> foot
   M87.275 Osteonecrosis due to previous trauma, <u>left</u> foot
   M87.276 Osteonecrosis due to previous trauma, <u>unspecified</u> foot
   M87.277 Osteonecrosis due to previous trauma, <u>right</u> toe(s)
   M87.278 Osteonecrosis due to previous trauma, <u>left</u> toe(s)
   M87.279 Osteonecrosis due to previous trauma, <u>unspecified</u> toe(s)
M87.28 Osteonecrosis due to previous trauma, <u>other site</u>
M87.29 Osteonecrosis due to previous trauma, <u>multiple sites</u>
M87.3- <u>Other secondary</u> osteonecrosis
M87.30 Other secondary osteonecrosis, <u>unspecified bone</u>
M87.31-Other secondary osteonecrosis, <u>shoulder</u>
   M87.311 Other secondary osteonecrosis, <u>right</u> shoulder
   M87.312 Other secondary osteonecrosis, <u>left</u> shoulder
   M87.319 Other secondary osteonecrosis, <u>unspecified</u> shoulder

M87.32-Other secondary osteonecrosis, <u>humerus</u>
   M87.321 Other secondary osteonecrosis, <u>right</u> humerus
   M87.322 Other secondary osteonecrosis, <u>left</u> humerus
   M87.329 Other secondary osteonecrosis, <u>unspecified</u> humerus
M87.33-Other secondary osteonecrosis of <u>radius, ulna and carpus</u>
   M87.331 Other secondary osteonecrosis of <u>right</u> radius
   M87.332 Other secondary osteonecrosis of <u>left</u> radius
   M87.333 Other secondary osteonecrosis of <u>unspecified</u> radius
   M87.334 Other secondary osteonecrosis of <u>right</u> ulna
   M87.335 Other secondary osteonecrosis of <u>left</u> ulna
   M87.336 Other secondary osteonecrosis of <u>unspecified</u> ulna
   M87.337 Other secondary osteonecrosis of <u>right</u> carpus
   M87.338 Other secondary osteonecrosis of <u>left</u> carpus
   M87.339 Other secondary osteonecrosis of <u>unspecified</u> carpus
M87.34-Other secondary osteonecrosis, <u>hand and fingers</u>
   M87.341 Other secondary osteonecrosis, <u>right</u> hand
   M87.342 Other secondary osteonecrosis, <u>left</u> hand
   M87.343 Other secondary osteonecrosis, <u>unspecified</u> hand
   M87.344 Other secondary osteonecrosis, <u>right</u> finger(s)
   M87.345 Other secondary osteonecrosis, <u>left</u> finger(s)
   M87.346 Other secondary osteonecrosis, <u>unspecified</u> finger(s)
M87.35-Other secondary osteonecrosis, <u>pelvis and femur</u>
   M87.350 Other secondary osteonecrosis, pelvis
   M87.351 Other secondary osteonecrosis, <u>right</u> femur
   M87.352 Other secondary osteonecrosis, <u>left</u> femur
   M87.353 Other secondary osteonecrosis, <u>unspecified</u> femur
M87.36-Other secondary osteonecrosis, <u>tibia and fibula</u>
   M87.361 Other secondary osteonecrosis, <u>right</u> tibia
   M87.362 Other secondary osteonecrosis, <u>left</u> tibia
   M87.363 Other secondary osteonecrosis, <u>unspecified</u> tibia
   M87.364 Other secondary osteonecrosis, <u>right</u> fibula
   M87.365 Other secondary osteonecrosis, <u>left</u> fibula
   M87.366 Other secondary osteonecrosis, <u>unspecified</u> fibula
M87.37-Other secondary osteonecrosis, <u>ankle and foot</u>
   M87.371 Other secondary osteonecrosis, <u>right</u> ankle
   M87.372 Other secondary osteonecrosis, <u>left</u> ankle
   M87.373 Other secondary osteonecrosis, <u>unspecified</u> ankle
   M87.374 Other secondary osteonecrosis, <u>right</u> foot
   M87.375 Other secondary osteonecrosis, <u>left</u> foot
   M87.376 Other secondary osteonecrosis, <u>unspecified</u> foot
   M87.377 Other secondary osteonecrosis, <u>right</u> toe(s)
   M87.378 Other secondary osteonecrosis, <u>left</u> toe(s)
   M87.379 Other secondary osteonecrosis, <u>unspecified</u> toe(s)
M87.38 Other secondary osteonecrosis, <u>other site</u>
M87.39 Other secondary osteonecrosis, <u>multiple sites</u>
M87.8- <u>Other</u> osteonecrosis
M87.80 Other osteonecrosis, <u>unspecified bone</u>
M87.81-Other osteonecrosis, <u>shoulder</u>
   M87.811 Other osteonecrosis, <u>right</u> shoulder
   M87.812 Other osteonecrosis, <u>left</u> shoulder
   M87.819 Other osteonecrosis, <u>unspecified</u> shoulder
M87.82-Other osteonecrosis, <u>humerus</u>
   M87.821 Other osteonecrosis, <u>right</u> humerus
   M87.822 Other osteonecrosis, <u>left</u> humerus
   M87.829 Other osteonecrosis, <u>unspecified</u> humerus
M87.83-Other osteonecrosis of <u>radius, ulna and carpus</u>
   M87.831 Other osteonecrosis of <u>right</u> radius
   M87.832 Other osteonecrosis of <u>left</u> radius
   M87.833 Other osteonecrosis of <u>unspecified</u> radius
   M87.834 Other osteonecrosis of <u>right</u> ulna
   M87.835 Other osteonecrosis of <u>left</u> ulna
   M87.836 Other osteonecrosis of <u>unspecified</u> ulna
   M87.837 Other osteonecrosis of <u>right</u> carpus
   M87.838 Other osteonecrosis of <u>left</u> carpus
   M87.839 Other osteonecrosis of <u>unspecified</u> carpus
M87.84-Other osteonecrosis, <u>hand and fingers</u>
   M87.841 Other osteonecrosis, <u>right</u> hand
   M87.842 Other osteonecrosis, <u>left</u> hand
   M87.843 Other osteonecrosis, <u>unspecified</u> hand
   M87.844 Other osteonecrosis, <u>right</u> finger(s)
   M87.845 Other osteonecrosis, <u>left</u> finger(s)
   M87.849 Other osteonecrosis, <u>unspecified</u> finger(s)

M86
|
M87

Excludes 1: = NOT CODED HERE! (Do not code both)   **599**   *Excludes* ❷: = Not Included Here

M87.85-Other osteonecrosis, <u>pelvis and femur</u>
   M87.850 Other osteonecrosis, pelvis
   M87.851 Other osteonecrosis, <u>right</u> femur
   M87.852 Other osteonecrosis, <u>left</u> femur
   M87.859 Other osteonecrosis, <u>unspecified</u> femur
M87.86-Other osteonecrosis, <u>tibia and fibula</u>
   M87.861 Other osteonecrosis, <u>right</u> tibia
   M87.862 Other osteonecrosis, <u>left</u> tibia
   M87.863 Other osteonecrosis, <u>unspecified</u> tibia
   M87.864 Other osteonecrosis, <u>right</u> fibula
   M87.865 Other osteonecrosis, <u>left</u> fibula
   M87.869 Other osteonecrosis, <u>unspecified</u> fibula
M87.87-Other osteonecrosis, <u>ankle, foot and toes</u>
   M87.871 Other osteonecrosis, <u>right</u> ankle
   M87.872 Other osteonecrosis, <u>left</u> ankle
   M87.873 Other osteonecrosis, <u>unspecified</u> ankle
   M87.874 Other osteonecrosis, <u>right</u> foot
   M87.875 Other osteonecrosis, <u>left</u> foot
   M87.876 Other osteonecrosis, <u>unspecified</u> foot
   M87.877 Other osteonecrosis, <u>right</u> toe(s)
   M87.878 Other osteonecrosis, <u>left</u> toe(s)
   M87.879 Other osteonecrosis, <u>unspecified</u> toe(s)
M87.88 Other osteonecrosis, <u>other site</u>
M87.89 Other osteonecrosis, <u>multiple sites</u>
M87.9 Osteonecrosis, <u>unspecified</u>
   Necrosis of bone NOS

M88- <u>Osteitis deformans [Paget's disease of bone]</u>
   Excludes 1: osteitis deformans in neoplastic disease (M90.6)
M88.0 Osteitis deformans of <u>skull</u>
M88.1 Osteitis deformans of <u>vertebrae</u>
M88.8- Osteitis deformans of <u>other bones</u>
  M88.81-Osteitis deformans of <u>shoulder</u>
   M88.811 Osteitis deformans of <u>right</u> shoulder
   M88.812 Osteitis deformans of <u>left</u> shoulder
   M88.819 Osteitis deformans of <u>unspecified</u> shoulder
  M88.82-Osteitis deformans of <u>upper arm</u>
   M88.821 Osteitis deformans of <u>right</u> upper arm
   M88.822 Osteitis deformans of <u>left</u> upper arm
   M88.829 Osteitis deformans of <u>unspecified</u> upper arm
  M88.83-Osteitis deformans of <u>forearm</u>
   M88.831 Osteitis deformans of <u>right</u> forearm
   M88.832 Osteitis deformans of <u>left</u> forearm
   M88.839 Osteitis deformans of <u>unspecified</u> forearm
  M88.84-Osteitis deformans of <u>hand</u>
   M88.841 Osteitis deformans of <u>right</u> hand
   M88.842 Osteitis deformans of <u>left</u> hand
   M88.849 Osteitis deformans of <u>unspecified</u> hand
  M88.85-Osteitis deformans of <u>thigh</u>
   M88.851 Osteitis deformans of <u>right</u> thigh
   M88.852 Osteitis deformans of <u>left</u> thigh
   M88.859 Osteitis deformans of <u>unspecified</u> thigh
  M88.86-Osteitis deformans of <u>lower leg</u>
   M88.861 Osteitis deformans of <u>right</u> lower leg
   M88.862 Osteitis deformans of <u>left</u> lower leg
   M88.869 Osteitis deformans of <u>unspecified</u> lower leg
  M88.87-Osteitis deformans of <u>ankle and foot</u>
   M88.871 Osteitis deformans of <u>right</u> ankle and foot
   M88.872 Osteitis deformans of <u>left</u> ankle and foot
   M88.879 Osteitis deformans of <u>unspecified</u> ankle and foot
  M88.88 Osteitis deformans of <u>other bones</u>
   Excludes❷: osteitis deformans of skull (M88.0)
           osteitis deformans of vertebrae (M88.1)
  M88.89 Osteitis deformans of <u>multiple sites</u>
M88.9 Osteitis deformans of <u>unspecified</u> bone

M89- Other disorders of bone
  M89.0- <u>Algoneurodystrophy</u>
     Shoulder-hand syndrome
     Sudeck's atrophy
     Excludes 1: causalgia, lower limb (G57.7-)
             causalgia, upper limb (G56.4-)
             complex regional pain syndrome II, lower limb
               (G57.7-)
             complex regional pain syndrome II, upper limb
               (G56.4-)
             reflex sympathetic dystrophy (G90.5-)
  M89.00 Algoneurodystrophy, <u>unspecified site</u>
  M89.01-Algoneurodystrophy, <u>shoulder</u>
   M89.011 Algoneurodystrophy, <u>right</u> shoulder
   M89.012 Algoneurodystrophy, <u>left</u> shoulder
   M89.019 Algoneurodystrophy, <u>unspecified</u> shoulder
  M89.02-Algoneurodystrophy, <u>upper arm</u>
   M89.021 Algoneurodystrophy, <u>right</u> upper arm
   M89.022 Algoneurodystrophy, <u>left</u> upper arm
   M89.029 Algoneurodystrophy, <u>unspecified</u> upper arm
  M89.03-Algoneurodystrophy, <u>forearm</u>
   M89.031 Algoneurodystrophy, <u>right</u> forearm
   M89.032 Algoneurodystrophy, <u>left</u> forearm
   M89.039 Algoneurodystrophy, <u>unspecified</u> forearm
  M89.04-Algoneurodystrophy, <u>hand</u>
   M89.041 Algoneurodystrophy, <u>right</u> hand
   M89.042 Algoneurodystrophy, <u>left</u> hand
   M89.049 Algoneurodystrophy, <u>unspecified</u> hand
  M89.05-Algoneurodystrophy, <u>thigh</u>
   M89.051 Algoneurodystrophy, <u>right</u> thigh
   M89.052 Algoneurodystrophy, <u>left</u> thigh
   M89.059 Algoneurodystrophy, <u>unspecified</u> thigh
  M89.06-Algoneurodystrophy, <u>lower leg</u>
   M89.061 Algoneurodystrophy, <u>right</u> lower leg
   M89.062 Algoneurodystrophy, <u>left</u> lower leg
   M89.069 Algoneurodystrophy, <u>unspecified</u> lower leg
  M89.07-Algoneurodystrophy, <u>ankle and foot</u>
   M89.071 Algoneurodystrophy, <u>right</u> ankle and foot
   M89.072 Algoneurodystrophy, <u>left</u> ankle and foot
   M89.079 Algoneurodystrophy, <u>unspecified</u> ankle and foot
  M89.08 Algoneurodystrophy, <u>other site</u>
  M89.09 Algoneurodystrophy, <u>multiple sites</u>
  M89.1- <u>Physeal arrest</u>
     Arrest of growth plate
     Epiphyseal arrest
     Growth plate arrest
  M89.12-Physeal arrest, <u>humerus</u>
   M89.121 <u>Complete</u> physeal arrest, <u>right</u> proximal humerus
   M89.122 <u>Complete</u> physeal arrest, <u>left</u> proximal humerus
   M89.123 Partial physeal arrest, <u>right</u> proximal humerus
   M89.124 Partial physeal arrest, <u>left</u> proximal humerus
   M89.125 <u>Complete</u> physeal arrest, <u>right</u> distal humerus
   M89.126 <u>Complete</u> physeal arrest, <u>left</u> distal humerus
   M89.127 Partial physeal arrest, <u>right</u> distal humerus
   M89.128 Partial physeal arrest, <u>left</u> distal humerus
   M89.129 Physeal arrest, humerus, <u>unspecified</u>
  M89.13-Physeal arrest, <u>forearm</u>
   M89.131 <u>Complete</u> physeal arrest, <u>right</u> distal radius
   M89.132 <u>Complete</u> physeal arrest, <u>left</u> distal radius
   M89.133 Partial physeal arrest, <u>right</u> distal radius
   M89.134 Partial physeal arrest, <u>left</u> distal radius
   M89.138 Other physeal arrest of forearm
   M89.139 Physeal arrest, forearm, <u>unspecified</u>
  M89.15-Physeal arrest, <u>femur</u>
   M89.151 <u>Complete</u> physeal arrest, <u>right</u> proximal femur
   M89.152 <u>Complete</u> physeal arrest, <u>left</u> proximal femur
   M89.153 Partial physeal arrest, <u>right</u> proximal femur
   M89.154 Partial physeal arrest, <u>left</u> proximal femur
   M89.155 <u>Complete</u> physeal arrest, <u>right</u> distal femur
   M89.156 <u>Complete</u> physeal arrest, <u>left</u> distal femur
   M89.157 Partial physeal arrest, <u>right</u> distal femur
   M89.158 Partial physeal arrest, <u>left</u> distal femur
   M89.159 Physeal arrest, femur, <u>unspecified</u>

M 8 7 – M 8 9

M89.16-Physeal arrest, <u>lower leg</u>
- M89.160 <u>Complete</u> physeal arrest, <u>right</u> proximal tibia
- M89.161 <u>Complete</u> physeal arrest, <u>left</u> proximal tibia
- M89.162 Partial physeal arrest, <u>right</u> proximal tibia
- M89.163 Partial physeal arrest, <u>left</u> proximal tibia
- M89.164 <u>Complete</u> physeal arrest, <u>right</u> distal tibia
- M89.165 <u>Complete</u> physeal arrest, <u>left</u> distal tibia
- M89.166 Partial physeal arrest, <u>right</u> distal tibia
- M89.167 Partial physeal arrest, <u>left</u> distal tibia
- M89.168 Other physeal arrest of lower leg
- M89.169 Physeal arrest, lower leg, <u>unspecified</u>

M89.18 Physeal arrest, other site

M89.2- <u>Other disorders of bone development and growth</u>
- M89.20 Other disorders of bone development and growth, <u>unspecified site</u>
- M89.21-Other disorders of bone development and growth, <u>shoulder</u>
  - M89.211 Other disorders of bone development and growth, <u>right</u> shoulder
  - M89.212 Other disorders of bone development and growth, <u>left</u> shoulder
  - M89.219 Other disorders of bone development and growth, <u>unspecified</u> shoulder
- M89.22-Other disorders of bone development and growth, <u>humerus</u>
  - M89.221 Other disorders of bone development and growth, <u>right</u> humerus
  - M89.222 Other disorders of bone development and growth, <u>left</u> humerus
  - M89.229 Other disorders of bone development and growth, <u>unspecified</u> humerus
- M89.23-Other disorders of bone development and growth, <u>ulna and radius</u>
  - M89.231 Other disorders of bone development and growth, <u>right</u> ulna
  - M89.232 Other disorders of bone development and growth, <u>left</u> ulna
  - M89.233 Other disorders of bone development and growth, <u>right</u> radius
  - M89.234 Other disorders of bone development and growth, <u>left</u> radius
  - M89.239 Other disorders of bone development and growth, <u>unspecified</u> ulna and radius
- M89.24-Other disorders of bone development and growth, <u>hand</u>
  - M89.241 Other disorders of bone development and growth, <u>right</u> hand
  - M89.242 Other disorders of bone development and growth, <u>left</u> hand
  - M89.249 Other disorders of bone development and growth, <u>unspecified</u> hand
- M89.25-Other disorders of bone development and growth, <u>femur</u>
  - M89.251 Other disorders of bone development and growth, <u>right</u> femur
  - M89.252 Other disorders of bone development and growth, <u>left</u> femur
  - M89.259 Other disorders of bone development and growth, <u>unspecified</u> femur
- M89.26-Other disorders of bone development and growth, <u>tibia and fibula</u>
  - M89.261 Other disorders of bone development and growth, <u>right</u> tibia
  - M89.262 Other disorders of bone development and growth, <u>left</u> tibia
  - M89.263 Other disorders of bone development and growth, <u>right</u> fibula
  - M89.264 Other disorders of bone development and growth, <u>left</u> fibula
  - M89.269 Other disorders of bone development and growth, <u>unspecified</u> lower leg
- M89.27-Other disorders of bone development and growth, <u>ankle and foot</u>
  - M89.271 Other disorders of bone development and growth, <u>right</u> ankle and foot
  - M89.272 Other disorders of bone development and growth, <u>left</u> ankle and foot
  - M89.279 Other disorders of bone development and growth, <u>unspecified</u> ankle and foot
- M89.28 Other disorders of bone development and growth, <u>other site</u>
- M89.29 Other disorders of bone development and growth, <u>multiple sites</u>

M89.3- <u>Hypertrophy</u> of bone
- M89.30 Hypertrophy of bone, <u>unspecified site</u>
- M89.31-Hypertrophy of bone, <u>shoulder</u>
  - M89.311 Hypertrophy of bone, <u>right</u> shoulder
  - M89.312 Hypertrophy of bone, <u>left</u> shoulder
  - M89.319 Hypertrophy of bone, <u>unspecified</u> shoulder
- M89.32-Hypertrophy of bone, <u>humerus</u>
  - M89.321 Hypertrophy of bone, <u>right</u> humerus
  - M89.322 Hypertrophy of bone, <u>left</u> humerus
  - M89.329 Hypertrophy of bone, <u>unspecified</u> humerus
- M89.33-Hypertrophy of bone, <u>ulna and radius</u>
  - M89.331 Hypertrophy of bone, <u>right</u> ulna
  - M89.332 Hypertrophy of bone, <u>left</u> ulna
  - M89.333 Hypertrophy of bone, <u>right</u> radius
  - M89.334 Hypertrophy of bone, <u>left</u> radius
  - M89.339 Hypertrophy of bone, <u>unspecified</u> ulna and radius
- M89.34-Hypertrophy of bone, <u>hand</u>
  - M89.341 Hypertrophy of bone, <u>right</u> hand
  - M89.342 Hypertrophy of bone, <u>left</u> hand
  - M89.349 Hypertrophy of bone, <u>unspecified</u> hand
- M89.35-Hypertrophy of bone, <u>femur</u>
  - M89.351 Hypertrophy of bone, <u>right</u> femur
  - M89.352 Hypertrophy of bone, <u>left</u> femur
  - M89.359 Hypertrophy of bone, <u>unspecified</u> femur
- M89.36-Hypertrophy of bone, <u>tibia and fibula</u>
  - M89.361 Hypertrophy of bone, <u>right</u> tibia
  - M89.362 Hypertrophy of bone, <u>left</u> tibia
  - M89.363 Hypertrophy of bone, <u>right</u> fibula
  - M89.364 Hypertrophy of bone, <u>left</u> fibula
  - M89.369 Hypertrophy of bone, <u>unspecified</u> tibia and fibula
- M89.37-Hypertrophy of bone, <u>ankle and foot</u>
  - M89.371 Hypertrophy of bone, <u>right</u> ankle and foot
  - M89.372 Hypertrophy of bone, <u>left</u> ankle and foot
  - M89.379 Hypertrophy of bone, <u>unspecified</u> ankle and foot
- M89.38 Hypertrophy of bone, <u>other site</u>
- M89.39 Hypertrophy of bone, <u>multiple sites</u>

M89.4- <u>Other hypertrophic</u> osteoarthropathy
  Marie-Bamberger disease
  Pachydermoperiostosis
- M89.40 Other hypertrophic osteoarthropathy, <u>unspecified site</u>
- M89.41-Other hypertrophic osteoarthropathy, <u>shoulder</u>
  - M89.411 Other hypertrophic osteoarthropathy, <u>right</u> shoulder
  - M89.412 Other hypertrophic osteoarthropathy, <u>left</u> shoulder
  - M89.419 Other hypertrophic osteoarthropathy, <u>unspecified</u> shoulder
- M89.42-Other hypertrophic osteoarthropathy, <u>upper arm</u>
  - M89.421 Other hypertrophic osteoarthropathy, <u>right</u> upper arm
  - M89.422 Other hypertrophic osteoarthropathy, <u>left</u> upper arm
  - M89.429 Other hypertrophic osteoarthropathy, <u>unspecified</u> upper arm
- M89.43-Other hypertrophic osteoarthropathy, <u>forearm</u>
  - M89.431 Other hypertrophic osteoarthropathy, <u>right</u> forearm
  - M89.432 Other hypertrophic osteoarthropathy, <u>left</u> forearm
  - M89.439 Other hypertrophic osteoarthropathy, <u>unspecified</u> forearm
- M89.44-Other hypertrophic osteoarthropathy, <u>hand</u>
  - M89.441 Other hypertrophic osteoarthropathy, <u>right</u> hand
  - M89.442 Other hypertrophic osteoarthropathy, <u>left</u> hand
  - M89.449 Other hypertrophic osteoarthropathy, <u>unspecified</u> hand
- M89.45-Other hypertrophic osteoarthropathy, <u>thigh</u>
  - M89.451 Other hypertrophic osteoarthropathy, <u>right</u> thigh
  - M89.452 Other hypertrophic osteoarthropathy, <u>left</u> thigh
  - M89.459 Other hypertrophic osteoarthropathy, <u>unspecified</u> thigh
- M89.46-Other hypertrophic osteoarthropathy, <u>lower leg</u>
  - M89.461 Other hypertrophic osteoarthropathy, <u>right</u> lower leg
  - M89.462 Other hypertrophic osteoarthropathy, <u>left</u> lower leg
  - M89.469 Other hypertrophic osteoarthropathy, <u>unspecified</u> lower leg

M87 - M89

Excludes 1: = NOT CODED HERE! (Do not code both)   *Excludes ❷:* = Not Included Here

M89.47-Other hypertrophic osteoarthropathy, <u>ankle and foot</u>
> **M89.471** Other hypertrophic osteoarthropathy, <u>right</u> ankle and foot
> **M89.472** Other hypertrophic osteoarthropathy, <u>left</u> ankle and foot
> **M89.479** Other hypertrophic osteoarthropathy, <u>unspecified</u> ankle and foot

M89.48 Other hypertrophic osteoarthropathy, <u>other site</u>
M89.49 Other hypertrophic osteoarthropathy, <u>multiple sites</u>
M89.5- <u>Osteolysis</u>
> Use additional code to identify major osseous defect, if applicable (M89.7-)
> *Excludes❷: periprosthetic osteolysis of internal prosthetic joint (T84.05-)*

M89.50 Osteolysis, <u>unspecified site</u>
M89.51-Osteolysis, <u>shoulder</u>
> **M89.511** Osteolysis, <u>right</u> shoulder
> **M89.512** Osteolysis, <u>left</u> shoulder
> **M89.519** Osteolysis, <u>unspecified</u> shoulder

M89.52-Osteolysis, <u>upper arm</u>
> **M89.521** Osteolysis, <u>right</u> upper arm
> **M89.522** Osteolysis, <u>left</u> upper arm
> **M89.529** Osteolysis, <u>unspecified</u> upper arm

M89.53-Osteolysis, <u>forearm</u>
> **M89.531** Osteolysis, <u>right</u> forearm
> **M89.532** Osteolysis, <u>left</u> forearm
> **M89.539** Osteolysis, <u>unspecified</u> forearm

M89.54-Osteolysis, <u>hand</u>
> **M89.541** Osteolysis, <u>right</u> hand
> **M89.542** Osteolysis, <u>left</u> hand
> **M89.549** Osteolysis, <u>unspecified</u> hand

M89.55-Osteolysis, <u>thigh</u>
> **M89.551** Osteolysis, <u>right</u> thigh
> **M89.552** Osteolysis, <u>left</u> thigh
> **M89.559** Osteolysis, <u>unspecified</u> thigh

M89.56-Osteolysis, <u>lower leg</u>
> **M89.561** Osteolysis, <u>right</u> lower leg
> **M89.562** Osteolysis, <u>left</u> lower leg
> **M89.569** Osteolysis, <u>unspecified</u> lower leg

M89.57-Osteolysis, <u>ankle and foot</u>
> **M89.571** Osteolysis, <u>right</u> ankle and foot
> **M89.572** Osteolysis, <u>left</u> ankle and foot
> **M89.579** Osteolysis, <u>unspecified</u> ankle and foot

M89.58 Osteolysis, <u>other site</u>
M89.59 Osteolysis, <u>multiple sites</u>
M89.6- <u>Osteopathy after poliomyelitis</u>
> Use additional code (B91) to identify previous poliomyelitis
> *Excludes 1: postpolio syndrome (G14)*

M89.60 Osteopathy after poliomyelitis, <u>unspecified site</u>
M89.61-Osteopathy after poliomyelitis, <u>shoulder</u>
> **M89.611** Osteopathy after poliomyelitis, <u>right</u> shoulder
> **M89.612** Osteopathy after poliomyelitis, <u>left</u> shoulder
> **M89.619** Osteopathy after poliomyelitis, <u>unspecified</u> shoulder

M89.62-Osteopathy after poliomyelitis, <u>upper arm</u>
> **M89.621** Osteopathy after poliomyelitis, <u>right</u> upper arm
> **M89.622** Osteopathy after poliomyelitis, <u>left</u> upper arm
> **M89.629** Osteopathy after poliomyelitis, <u>unspecified</u> upper arm

M89.63-Osteopathy after poliomyelitis, <u>forearm</u>
> **M89.631** Osteopathy after poliomyelitis, <u>right</u> forearm
> **M89.632** Osteopathy after poliomyelitis, <u>left</u> forearm
> **M89.639** Osteopathy after poliomyelitis, <u>unspecified</u> forearm

M89.64-Osteopathy after poliomyelitis, <u>hand</u>
> **M89.641** Osteopathy after poliomyelitis, <u>right</u> hand
> **M89.642** Osteopathy after poliomyelitis, <u>left</u> hand
> **M89.649** Osteopathy after poliomyelitis, <u>unspecified</u> hand

M89.65-Osteopathy after poliomyelitis, <u>thigh</u>
> **M89.651** Osteopathy after poliomyelitis, <u>right</u> thigh
> **M89.652** Osteopathy after poliomyelitis, <u>left</u> thigh
> **M89.659** Osteopathy after poliomyelitis, <u>unspecified</u> thigh

M89.66-Osteopathy after poliomyelitis, <u>lower leg</u>
> **M89.661** Osteopathy after poliomyelitis, <u>right</u> lower leg
> **M89.662** Osteopathy after poliomyelitis, <u>left</u> lower leg
> **M89.669** Osteopathy after poliomyelitis, <u>unspecified</u> lower leg

M89.67-Osteopathy after poliomyelitis, <u>ankle and foot</u>
> **M89.671** Osteopathy after poliomyelitis, <u>right</u> ankle and foot
> **M89.672** Osteopathy after poliomyelitis, <u>left</u> ankle and foot
> **M89.679** Osteopathy after poliomyelitis, <u>unspecified</u> ankle and foot

M89.68 Osteopathy after poliomyelitis, <u>other site</u>
M89.69 Osteopathy after poliomyelitis, <u>multiple sites</u>
M89.7- <u>Major osseous defect</u>
> Code first underlying disease, if known, such as:
>   Aseptic necrosis of bone (M87.-)
>   Malignant neoplasm of bone (C40.-)
>   Osteolysis (M89.5)
>   Osteomyelitis (M86.-)
>   Osteonecrosis (M87.-)
>   Osteoporosis (M80.-, M81.-)
>   Periprosthetic osteolysis (T84.05-)

M89.70 Major osseous defect, <u>unspecified site</u>
M89.71-Major osseous defect, <u>shoulder region</u>
> Major osseous defect clavicle or scapula
> **M89.711** Major osseous defect, <u>right</u> shoulder region
> **M89.712** Major osseous defect, <u>left</u> shoulder region
> **M89.719** Major osseous defect, <u>unspecified</u> shoulder region

M89.72-Major osseous defect, <u>humerus</u>
> **M89.721** Major osseous defect, <u>right</u> humerus
> **M89.722** Major osseous defect, <u>left</u> humerus
> **M89.729** Major osseous defect, <u>unspecified</u> humerus

M89.73-Major osseous defect, <u>forearm</u>
> Major osseous defect of radius and ulna
> **M89.731** Major osseous defect, <u>right</u> forearm
> **M89.732** Major osseous defect, <u>left</u> forearm
> **M89.739** Major osseous defect, <u>unspecified</u> forearm

M89.74-Major osseous defect, <u>hand</u>
> Major osseous defect of carpus, fingers, metacarpus
> **M89.741** Major osseous defect, <u>right</u> hand
> **M89.742** Major osseous defect, <u>left</u> hand
> **M89.749** Major osseous defect, <u>unspecified</u> hand

M89.75-Major osseous defect, <u>pelvic region and thigh</u>
> Major osseous defect of femur and pelvis
> **M89.751** Major osseous defect, <u>right</u> pelvic region and thigh
> **M89.752** Major osseous defect, <u>left</u> pelvic region and thigh
> **M89.759** Major osseous defect, <u>unspecified</u> pelvic region and thigh

M89.76-Major osseous defect, <u>lower leg</u>
> Major osseous defect of fibula and tibia
> **M89.761** Major osseous defect, <u>right</u> lower leg
> **M89.762** Major osseous defect, <u>left</u> lower leg
> **M89.769** Major osseous defect, <u>unspecified</u> lower leg

M89.77-Major osseous defect, <u>ankle and foot</u>
> Major osseous defect of metatarsus, tarsus, toes
> **M89.771** Major osseous defect, <u>right</u> ankle and foot
> **M89.772** Major osseous defect, <u>left</u> ankle and foot
> **M89.779** Major osseous defect, <u>unspecified</u> ankle and foot

M89.78 Major osseous defect, <u>other site</u>
M89.79 Major osseous defect, <u>multiple sites</u>
M89.8- <u>Other specified</u> disorders of bone
> Infantile cortical hyperostoses
> Post-traumatic subperiosteal ossification

M89.8x-Other specified disorders of bone
> **M89.8x0** Other specified disorders of bone, multiple sites
> **M89.8x1** Other specified disorders of bone, shoulder
> **M89.8x2** Other specified disorders of bone, upper arm
> **M89.8x3** Other specified disorders of bone, forearm
> **M89.8x4** Other specified disorders of bone, hand
> **M89.8x5** Other specified disorders of bone, thigh
> **M89.8x6** Other specified disorders of bone, lower leg
> **M89.8x7** Other specified disorders of bone, ankle and foot
> **M89.8x8** Other specified disorders of bone, other site
> **M89.8x9** Other specified disorders of bone, unspecified site

M89.9 Disorder of bone, <u>unspecified</u>

M89 - M90

M90- **Osteopathies** in diseases classified elsewhere
    Excludes 1: osteochondritis, osteomyelitis, and osteopathy (in):
        cryptococcosis (B45.3)
        diabetes mellitus (E08-E13 with .61-)
        gonococcal (A54.43)
        neurogenic syphilis (A52.11)
        renal osteodystrophy (N25.0)
        salmonellosis (A02.24)
        secondary syphilis (A51.46)
        syphilis (late) (A52.77)

M90.5- **Osteonecrosis** in diseases classified elsewhere
    Code first underlying disease, such as:
      Caisson disease (T70.3)
      Hemoglobinopathy (D50-D64)

  M90.50 Osteonecrosis in diseases classified elsewhere, <u>unspecified site</u>

  M90.51-Osteonecrosis in diseases classified elsewhere, <u>shoulder</u>
    M90.511 Osteonecrosis in diseases classified elsewhere, <u>right</u> shoulder
    M90.512 Osteonecrosis in diseases classified elsewhere, <u>left</u> shoulder
    M90.519 Osteonecrosis in diseases classified elsewhere, <u>unspecified</u> shoulder

  M90.52-Osteonecrosis in diseases classified elsewhere, <u>upper arm</u>
    M90.521 Osteonecrosis in diseases classified elsewhere, <u>right</u> upper arm
    M90.522 Osteonecrosis in diseases classified elsewhere, <u>left</u> upper arm
    M90.529 Osteonecrosis in diseases classified elsewhere, <u>unspecified</u> upper arm

  M90.53-Osteonecrosis in diseases classified elsewhere, <u>forearm</u>
    M90.531 Osteonecrosis in diseases classified elsewhere, <u>right</u> forearm
    M90.532 Osteonecrosis in diseases classified elsewhere, <u>left</u> forearm
    M90.539 Osteonecrosis in diseases classified elsewhere, <u>unspecified</u> forearm

  M90.54-Osteonecrosis in diseases classified elsewhere, <u>hand</u>
    M90.541 Osteonecrosis in diseases classified elsewhere, <u>right</u> hand
    M90.542 Osteonecrosis in diseases classified elsewhere, <u>left</u> hand
    M90.549 Osteonecrosis in diseases classified elsewhere, <u>unspecified</u> hand

  M90.55-Osteonecrosis in diseases classified elsewhere, <u>thigh</u>
    M90.551 Osteonecrosis in diseases classified elsewhere, <u>right</u> thigh
    M90.552 Osteonecrosis in diseases classified elsewhere, <u>left</u> thigh
    M90.559 Osteonecrosis in diseases classified elsewhere, <u>unspecified</u> thigh

  M90.56-Osteonecrosis in diseases classified elsewhere, <u>lower leg</u>
    M90.561 Osteonecrosis in diseases classified elsewhere, <u>right</u> lower leg
    M90.562 Osteonecrosis in diseases classified elsewhere, <u>left</u> lower leg
    M90.569 Osteonecrosis in diseases classified elsewhere, <u>unspecified</u> lower leg

  M90.57-Osteonecrosis in diseases classified elsewhere, <u>ankle and foot</u>
    M90.571 Osteonecrosis in diseases classified elsewhere, <u>right</u> ankle and foot
    M90.572 Osteonecrosis in diseases classified elsewhere, <u>left</u> ankle and foot
    M90.579 Osteonecrosis in diseases classified elsewhere, <u>unspecified</u> ankle and foot

  M90.58 Osteonecrosis in diseases classified elsewhere, <u>other site</u>
  M90.59 Osteonecrosis in diseases classified elsewhere, <u>multiple sites</u>

M90.6- **Osteitis deformans** in neoplastic diseases
    Osteitis deformans in malignant neoplasm of bone
    Code first the neoplasm (C40.-, C41.-)
    Excludes 1: osteitis deformans [Paget's disease of bone] (M88.-)

  M90.60 Osteitis deformans in neoplastic diseases, <u>unspecified site</u>
  M90.61-Osteitis deformans in neoplastic diseases, <u>shoulder</u>
    M90.611 Osteitis deformans in neoplastic diseases, <u>right</u> shoulder
    M90.612 Osteitis deformans in neoplastic diseases, <u>left</u> shoulder
    M90.619 Osteitis deformans in neoplastic diseases, <u>unspecified</u> shoulder

  M90.62-Osteitis deformans in neoplastic diseases, <u>upper arm</u>
    M90.621 Osteitis deformans in neoplastic diseases, <u>right</u> upper arm
    M90.622 Osteitis deformans in neoplastic diseases, <u>left</u> upper arm
    M90.629 Osteitis deformans in neoplastic diseases, <u>unspecified</u> upper arm

  M90.63-Osteitis deformans in neoplastic diseases, <u>forearm</u>
    M90.631 Osteitis deformans in neoplastic diseases, <u>right</u> forearm
    M90.632 Osteitis deformans in neoplastic diseases, <u>left</u> forearm
    M90.639 Osteitis deformans in neoplastic diseases, <u>unspecified</u> forearm

  M90.64-Osteitis deformans in neoplastic diseases, <u>hand</u>
    M90.641 Osteitis deformans in neoplastic diseases, <u>right</u> hand
    M90.642 Osteitis deformans in neoplastic diseases, <u>left</u> hand
    M90.649 Osteitis deformans in neoplastic diseases, <u>unspecified</u> hand

  M90.65-Osteitis deformans in neoplastic diseases, <u>thigh</u>
    M90.651 Osteitis deformans in neoplastic diseases, <u>right</u> thigh
    M90.652 Osteitis deformans in neoplastic diseases, <u>left</u> thigh
    M90.659 Osteitis deformans in neoplastic diseases, <u>unspecified</u> thigh

  M90.66-Osteitis deformans in neoplastic diseases, <u>lower leg</u>
    M90.661 Osteitis deformans in neoplastic diseases, <u>right</u> lower leg
    M90.662 Osteitis deformans in neoplastic diseases, <u>left</u> lower leg
    M90.669 Osteitis deformans in neoplastic diseases, <u>unspecified</u> lower leg

  M90.67-Osteitis deformans in neoplastic diseases, <u>ankle and foot</u>
    M90.671 Osteitis deformans in neoplastic diseases, <u>right</u> ankle and foot
    M90.672 Osteitis deformans in neoplastic diseases, <u>left</u> ankle and foot
    M90.679 Osteitis deformans in neoplastic diseases, <u>unspecified</u> ankle and foot

  M90.68 Osteitis deformans in neoplastic diseases, <u>other site</u>
  M90.69 Osteitis deformans in neoplastic diseases, <u>multiple sites</u>

M90.8- **Osteopathy** in diseases classified elsewhere
    Code first underlying disease, such as:
      Rickets (E55.0)
      Vitamin-D-resistant rickets (E83.3)

  M90.80 Osteopathy in diseases classified elsewhere, <u>unspecified site</u>
  M90.81-Osteopathy in diseases classified elsewhere, <u>shoulder</u>
    M90.811 Osteopathy in diseases classified elsewhere, <u>right</u> shoulder
    M90.812 Osteopathy in diseases classified elsewhere, <u>left</u> shoulder
    M90.819 Osteopathy in diseases classified elsewhere, <u>unspecified</u> shoulder

  M90.82-Osteopathy in diseases classified elsewhere, <u>upper arm</u>
    M90.821 Osteopathy in diseases classified elsewhere, <u>right</u> upper arm
    M90.822 Osteopathy in diseases classified elsewhere, <u>left</u> upper arm
    M90.829 Osteopathy in diseases classified elsewhere, <u>unspecified</u> upper arm

  M90.83-Osteopathy in diseases classified elsewhere, <u>forearm</u>
    M90.831 Osteopathy in diseases classified elsewhere, <u>right</u> forearm
    M90.832 Osteopathy in diseases classified elsewhere, <u>left</u> forearm
    M90.839 Osteopathy in diseases classified elsewhere, <u>unspecified</u> forearm

  M90.84-Osteopathy in diseases classified elsewhere, <u>hand</u>
    M90.841 Osteopathy in diseases classified elsewhere, <u>right</u> hand
    M90.842 Osteopathy in diseases classified elsewhere, <u>left</u> hand
    M90.849 Osteopathy in diseases classified elsewhere, <u>unspecified</u> hand

  M90.85-Osteopathy in diseases classified elsewhere, <u>thigh</u>
    M90.851 Osteopathy in diseases classified elsewhere, <u>right</u> thigh
    M90.852 Osteopathy in diseases classified elsewhere, <u>left</u> thigh
    M90.859 Osteopathy in diseases classified elsewhere, <u>unspecified</u> thigh

M89 - M90

© 2013 Channel Publishing, Ltd.

M90.86-Osteopathy in diseases classified elsewhere, <u>lower leg</u>
   M90.861 Osteopathy in diseases classified elsewhere, <u>right</u> lower leg
   M90.862 Osteopathy in diseases classified elsewhere, <u>left</u> lower leg
   M90.869 Osteopathy in diseases classified elsewhere, <u>unspecified</u> lower leg
M90.87-Osteopathy in diseases classified elsewhere, <u>ankle and foot</u>
   M90.871 Osteopathy in diseases classified elsewhere, <u>right</u> ankle and foot
   M90.872 Osteopathy in diseases classified elsewhere, <u>left</u> ankle and foot
   M90.879 Osteopathy in diseases classified elsewhere, <u>unspecified</u> ankle and foot
M90.88 Osteopathy in diseases classified elsewhere, <u>other site</u>
M90.89 Osteopathy in diseases classified elsewhere, <u>multiple sites</u>

Chondropathies (M91-M94)

Excludes 1: postprocedural chondropathies (M96.-)

M91- <u>Juvenile osteochondrosis of hip and pelvis</u>
  Excludes 1: slipped upper femoral epiphysis (nontraumatic) (M93.0)
M91.0 Juvenile osteochondrosis of <u>pelvis</u>
   Osteochondrosis (juvenile) of acetabulum
   Osteochondrosis (juvenile) of iliac crest [Buchanan]
   Osteochondrosis (juvenile) of ischiopubic synchondrosis [van Neck]
   Osteochondrosis (juvenile) of symphysis pubis [Pierson]
M91.1- Juvenile osteochondrosis of <u>head of femur [Legg-Calvé-Perthes]</u>
   M91.10 Juvenile osteochondrosis of head of femur [Legg-Calvé-Perthes], <u>unspecified</u> leg
   M91.11 Juvenile osteochondrosis of head of femur [Legg-Calvé-Perthes], <u>right</u> leg
   M91.12 Juvenile osteochondrosis of head of femur [Legg-Calvé-Perthes], <u>left</u> leg
M91.2- <u>Coxa plana</u>
   Hip deformity due to previous juvenile osteochondrosis
   M91.20 Coxa plana, <u>unspecified</u> hip
   M91.21 Coxa plana, <u>right</u> hip
   M91.22 Coxa plana, <u>left</u> hip
M91.3- <u>Pseudocoxalgia</u>
   M91.30 Pseudocoxalgia, <u>unspecified</u> hip
   M91.31 Pseudocoxalgia, <u>right</u> hip
   M91.32 Pseudocoxalgia, <u>left</u> hip
M91.4- <u>Coxa magna</u>
   M91.40 Coxa magna, <u>unspecified</u> hip
   M91.41 Coxa magna, <u>right</u> hip
   M91.42 Coxa magna, <u>left</u> hip
M91.8- <u>Other</u> juvenile osteochondrosis of hip and pelvis
   Juvenile osteochondrosis after reduction of congenital dislocation of hip
   M91.80 Other juvenile osteochondrosis of hip and pelvis, <u>unspecified</u> leg
   M91.81 Other juvenile osteochondrosis of hip and pelvis, <u>right</u> leg
   M91.82 Other juvenile osteochondrosis of hip and pelvis, <u>left</u> leg
M91.9- Juvenile osteochondrosis of hip and pelvis, <u>unspecified</u>
   M91.90 Juvenile osteochondrosis of hip and pelvis, unspecified, <u>unspecified</u> leg
   M91.91 Juvenile osteochondrosis of hip and pelvis, unspecified, <u>right</u> leg
   M91.92 Juvenile osteochondrosis of hip and pelvis, unspecified, <u>left</u> leg

M92- <u>Other</u> juvenile osteochondrosis
M92.0- Juvenile osteochondrosis of <u>humerus</u>
   Osteochondrosis (juvenile) of capitulum of humerus [Panner]
   Osteochondrosis (juvenile) of head of humerus [Haas]
   M92.00 Juvenile osteochondrosis of humerus, <u>unspecified</u> arm
   M92.01 Juvenile osteochondrosis of humerus, <u>right</u> arm
   M92.02 Juvenile osteochondrosis of humerus, <u>left</u> arm
M92.1- Juvenile osteochondrosis of <u>radius and ulna</u>
   Osteochondrosis (juvenile) of lower ulna [Burns]
   Osteochondrosis (juvenile) of radial head [Brailsford]
   M92.10 Juvenile osteochondrosis of radius and ulna, <u>unspecified</u> arm
   M92.11 Juvenile osteochondrosis of radius and ulna, <u>right</u> arm
   M92.12 Juvenile osteochondrosis of radius and ulna, <u>left</u> arm
M92.2- Juvenile osteochondrosis, <u>hand</u>
   M92.20-Unspecified juvenile osteochondrosis, hand
     M92.201 Unspecified juvenile osteochondrosis, <u>right</u> hand
     M92.202 Unspecified juvenile osteochondrosis, <u>left</u> hand
     M92.209 Unspecified juvenile osteochondrosis, <u>unspecified</u> hand
   M92.21-Osteochondrosis (juvenile) of <u>carpal lunate [Kienböck]</u>
     M92.211 Osteochondrosis (juvenile) of carpal lunate [Kienböck], <u>right</u> hand
     M92.212 Osteochondrosis (juvenile) of carpal lunate [Kienböck], <u>left</u> hand
     M92.219 Osteochondrosis (juvenile) of carpal lunate [Kienböck], <u>unspecified</u> hand
   M92.22-Osteochondrosis (juvenile) of <u>metacarpal heads [Mauclaire]</u>
     M92.221 Osteochondrosis (juvenile) of metacarpal heads [Mauclaire], <u>right</u> hand
     M92.222 Osteochondrosis (juvenile) of metacarpal heads [Mauclaire], <u>left</u> hand
     M92.229 Osteochondrosis (juvenile) of metacarpal heads [Mauclaire], <u>unspecified</u> hand
   M92.29-<u>Other</u> juvenile osteochondrosis, <u>hand</u>
     M92.291 Other juvenile osteochondrosis, <u>right</u> hand
     M92.292 Other juvenile osteochondrosis, <u>left</u> hand
     M92.299 Other juvenile osteochondrosis, <u>unspecified</u> hand
M92.3- <u>Other</u> juvenile osteochondrosis, <u>upper limb</u>
   M92.30 Other juvenile osteochondrosis, <u>unspecified</u> upper limb
   M92.31 Other juvenile osteochondrosis, <u>right</u> upper limb
   M92.32 Other juvenile osteochondrosis, <u>left</u> upper limb
M92.4- Juvenile osteochondrosis of <u>patella</u>
   Osteochondrosis (juvenile) of primary patellar center [Köhler]
   Osteochondrosis (juvenile) of secondary patellar centre [Sinding Larsen]
   M92.40 Juvenile osteochondrosis of patella, <u>unspecified</u> knee
   M92.41 Juvenile osteochondrosis of patella, <u>right</u> knee
   M92.42 Juvenile osteochondrosis of patella, <u>left</u> knee
M92.5- Juvenile osteochondrosis of <u>tibia and fibula</u>
   Osteochondrosis (juvenile) of proximal tibia [Blount]
   Osteochondrosis (juvenile) of tibial tubercle [Osgood-Schlatter]
   Tibia vara
   M92.50 Juvenile osteochondrosis of tibia and fibula, <u>unspecified</u> leg
   M92.51 Juvenile osteochondrosis of tibia and fibula, <u>right</u> leg
   M92.52 Juvenile osteochondrosis of tibia and fibula, <u>left</u> leg
M92.6- Juvenile osteochondrosis of <u>tarsus</u>
   Osteochondrosis (juvenile) of calcaneum [Sever]
   Osteochondrosis (juvenile) of os tibiale externum [Haglund]
   Osteochondrosis (juvenile) of talus [Diaz]
   Osteochondrosis (juvenile) of tarsal navicular [Köhler]
   M92.60 Juvenile osteochondrosis of tarsus, <u>unspecified</u> ankle
   M92.61 Juvenile osteochondrosis of tarsus, <u>right</u> ankle
   M92.62 Juvenile osteochondrosis of tarsus, <u>left</u> ankle
M92.7- Juvenile osteochondrosis of <u>metatarsus</u>
   Osteochondrosis (juvenile) of fifth metatarsus [Iselin]
   Osteochondrosis (juvenile) of second metatarsus [Freiberg]
   M92.70 Juvenile osteochondrosis of metatarsus, <u>unspecified</u> foot
   M92.71 Juvenile osteochondrosis of metatarsus, <u>right</u> foot
   M92.72 Juvenile osteochondrosis of metatarsus, <u>left</u> foot
M92.8 <u>Other specified</u> juvenile osteochondrosis
   Calcaneal apophysitis
M92.9 Juvenile osteochondrosis, <u>unspecified</u>
   Juvenile apophysitis NOS
   Juvenile epiphysitis NOS
   Juvenile osteochondritis NOS
   Juvenile osteochondrosis NOS

M90 - M93

M93- Other osteochondropathies
  Excludes❷: osteochondrosis of spine (M42.-)
  M93.0- Slipped upper femoral epiphysis (nontraumatic)
    Use additional code for associated chondrolysis (M94.3)
    M93.00-Unspecified slipped upper femoral epiphysis (nontraumatic)
      M93.001 Unspecified slipped upper femoral epiphysis (nontraumatic), **right** hip
      M93.002 Unspecified slipped upper femoral epiphysis (nontraumatic), **left** hip
      M93.003 Unspecified slipped upper femoral epiphysis (nontraumatic), **unspecified** hip
    M93.01-Acute slipped upper femoral epiphysis (nontraumatic)
      M93.011 Acute slipped upper femoral epiphysis (nontraumatic), **right** hip
      M93.012 Acute slipped upper femoral epiphysis (nontraumatic), **left** hip
      M93.013 Acute slipped upper femoral epiphysis (nontraumatic), **unspecified** hip
    M93.02-Chronic slipped upper femoral epiphysis (nontraumatic)
      M93.021 Chronic slipped upper femoral epiphysis (nontraumatic), **right** hip
      M93.022 Chronic slipped upper femoral epiphysis (nontraumatic), **left** hip
      M93.023 Chronic slipped upper femoral epiphysis (nontraumatic), **unspecified** hip
    M93.03-Acute on chronic slipped upper femoral epiphysis (nontraumatic)
      M93.031 Acute on chronic slipped upper femoral epiphysis (nontraumatic), **right** hip
      M93.032 Acute on chronic slipped upper femoral epiphysis (nontraumatic), **left** hip
      M93.033 Acute on chronic slipped upper femoral epiphysis (nontraumatic), **unspecified** hip
  M93.1 Kienböck's disease of adults
    Adult osteochondrosis of carpal lunates
  M93.2- Osteochondritis dissecans
    M93.20 Osteochondritis dissecans of **unspecified site**
    M93.21-Osteochondritis dissecans of shoulder
      M93.211 Osteochondritis dissecans, **right** shoulder
      M93.212 Osteochondritis dissecans, **left** shoulder
      M93.219 Osteochondritis dissecans, **unspecified** shoulder
    M93.22-Osteochondritis dissecans of elbow
      M93.221 Osteochondritis dissecans, **right** elbow
      M93.222 Osteochondritis dissecans, **left** elbow
      M93.229 Osteochondritis dissecans, **unspecified** elbow
    M93.23-Osteochondritis dissecans of wrist
      M93.231 Osteochondritis dissecans, **right** wrist
      M93.232 Osteochondritis dissecans, **left** wrist
      M93.239 Osteochondritis dissecans, **unspecified** wrist
    M93.24-Osteochondritis dissecans of joints of hand
      M93.241 Osteochondritis dissecans, joints of **right** hand
      M93.242 Osteochondritis dissecans, joints of **left** hand
      M93.249 Osteochondritis dissecans, joints of **unspecified** hand
    M93.25-Osteochondritis dissecans of hip
      M93.251 Osteochondritis dissecans, **right** hip
      M93.252 Osteochondritis dissecans, **left** hip
      M93.259 Osteochondritis dissecans, **unspecified** hip
    M93.26-Osteochondritis dissecans knee
      M93.261 Osteochondritis dissecans, **right** knee
      M93.262 Osteochondritis dissecans, **left** knee
      M93.269 Osteochondritis dissecans, **unspecified** knee
    M93.27-Osteochondritis dissecans of ankle and joints of foot
      M93.271 Osteochondritis dissecans, **right** ankle and joints of **right** foot
      M93.272 Osteochondritis dissecans, **left** ankle and joints of **left** foot
      M93.279 Osteochondritis dissecans, **unspecified** ankle and joints of foot
    M93.28 Osteochondritis dissecans **other site**
    M93.29 Osteochondritis dissecans **multiple sites**
  M93.8- Other specified osteochondropathies
    M93.80 Other specified osteochondropathies of **unspecified site**
    M93.81-Other specified osteochondropathies of shoulder
      M93.811 Other specified osteochondropathies, **right** shoulder
      M93.812 Other specified osteochondropathies, **left** shoulder
      M93.819 Other specified osteochondropathies, **unspecified** shoulder

    M93.82-Other specified osteochondropathies of upper arm
      M93.821 Other specified osteochondropathies, **right** upper arm
      M93.822 Other specified osteochondropathies, **left** upper arm
      M93.829 Other specified osteochondropathies, **unspecified** upper arm
    M93.83-Other specified osteochondropathies of forearm
      M93.831 Other specified osteochondropathies, **right** forearm
      M93.832 Other specified osteochondropathies, **left** forearm
      M93.839 Other specified osteochondropathies, **unspecified** forearm
    M93.84-Other specified osteochondropathies of hand
      M93.841 Other specified osteochondropathies, **right** hand
      M93.842 Other specified osteochondropathies, **left** hand
      M93.849 Other specified osteochondropathies, **unspecified** hand
    M93.85-Other specified osteochondropathies of thigh
      M93.851 Other specified osteochondropathies, **right** thigh
      M93.852 Other specified osteochondropathies, **left** thigh
      M93.859 Other specified osteochondropathies, **unspecified** thigh
    M93.86-Other specified osteochondropathies lower leg
      M93.861 Other specified osteochondropathies, **right** lower leg
      M93.862 Other specified osteochondropathies, **left** lower leg
      M93.869 Other specified osteochondropathies, **unspecified** lower leg
    M93.87-Other specified osteochondropathies of ankle and foot
      M93.871 Other specified osteochondropathies, **right** ankle and foot
      M93.872 Other specified osteochondropathies, **left** ankle and foot
      M93.879 Other specified osteochondropathies, **unspecified** ankle and foot
    M93.88 Other specified osteochondropathies **other**
    M93.89 Other specified osteochondropathies **multiple sites**
  M93.9- Osteochondropathy, unspecified
    Apophysitis NOS
    Epiphysitis NOS
    Osteochondritis NOS
    Osteochondrosis NOS
    M93.90 Osteochondropathy, unspecified of **unspecified site**
    M93.91-Osteochondropathy, unspecified of shoulder
      M93.911 Osteochondropathy, unspecified, **right** shoulder
      M93.912 Osteochondropathy, unspecified, **left** shoulder
      M93.919 Osteochondropathy, unspecified, **unspecified** shoulder
    M93.92-Osteochondropathy, unspecified of upper arm
      M93.921 Osteochondropathy, unspecified, **right** upper arm
      M93.922 Osteochondropathy, unspecified, **left** upper arm
      M93.929 Osteochondropathy, unspecified, **unspecified** upper arm
    M93.93-Osteochondropathy, unspecified of forearm
      M93.931 Osteochondropathy, unspecified, **right** forearm
      M93.932 Osteochondropathy, unspecified, **left** forearm
      M93.939 Osteochondropathy, unspecified, **unspecified** forearm
    M93.94-Osteochondropathy, unspecified of hand
      M93.941 Osteochondropathy, unspecified, **right** hand
      M93.942 Osteochondropathy, unspecified, **left** hand
      M93.949 Osteochondropathy, unspecified, **unspecified** hand
    M93.95-Osteochondropathy, unspecified of thigh
      M93.951 Osteochondropathy, unspecified, **right** thigh
      M93.952 Osteochondropathy, unspecified, **left** thigh
      M93.959 Osteochondropathy, unspecified, **unspecified** thigh
    M93.96-Osteochondropathy, unspecified lower leg
      M93.961 Osteochondropathy, unspecified, **right** lower leg
      M93.962 Osteochondropathy, unspecified, **left** lower leg
      M93.969 Osteochondropathy, unspecified, **unspecified** lower leg
    M93.97-Osteochondropathy, unspecified of ankle and foot
      M93.971 Osteochondropathy, unspecified, **right** ankle and foot
      M93.972 Osteochondropathy, unspecified, **left** ankle and foot
      M93.979 Osteochondropathy, unspecified, **unspecified** ankle and foot
    M93.98 Osteochondropathy, unspecified **other**
    M93.99 Osteochondropathy, unspecified **multiple sites**

M90 - M93

M94- Other disorders of cartilage

M94.0 Chondrocostal junction syndrome [Tietze]
Costochondritis

M94.1 Relapsing polychondritis

M94.2- Chondromalacia
Excludes 1: chondromalacia patellae (M22.4)

M94.20 Chondromalacia, unspecified site

M94.21-Chondromalacia, shoulder
    M94.211 Chondromalacia, right shoulder
    M94.212 Chondromalacia, left shoulder
    M94.219 Chondromalacia, unspecified shoulder

M94.22-Chondromalacia, elbow
    M94.221 Chondromalacia, right elbow
    M94.222 Chondromalacia, left elbow
    M94.229 Chondromalacia, unspecified elbow

M94.23-Chondromalacia, wrist
    M94.231 Chondromalacia, right wrist
    M94.232 Chondromalacia, left wrist
    M94.239 Chondromalacia, unspecified wrist

M94.24-Chondromalacia, joints of hand
    M94.241 Chondromalacia, joints of right hand
    M94.242 Chondromalacia, joints of left hand
    M94.249 Chondromalacia, joints of unspecified hand

M94.25-Chondromalacia, hip
    M94.251 Chondromalacia, right hip
    M94.252 Chondromalacia, left hip
    M94.259 Chondromalacia, unspecified hip

M94.26-Chondromalacia, knee
    M94.261 Chondromalacia, right knee
    M94.262 Chondromalacia, left knee
    M94.269 Chondromalacia, unspecified knee

M94.27-Chondromalacia, ankle and joints of foot
    M94.271 Chondromalacia, right ankle and joints of right foot
    M94.272 Chondromalacia, left ankle and joints of left foot
    M94.279 Chondromalacia, unspecified ankle and joints of foot

M94.28 Chondromalacia, other site

M94.29 Chondromalacia, multiple sites

M94.3- Chondrolysis
Code first any associated slipped upper femoral epiphysis (nontraumatic) (M93.0-)

M94.35-Chondrolysis, hip
    M94.351 Chondrolysis, right hip
    M94.352 Chondrolysis, left hip
    M94.359 Chondrolysis, unspecified hip

M94.8- Other specified disorders of cartilage

M94.8x-Other specified disorders of cartilage
    M94.8x0 Other specified disorders of cartilage, multiple sites
    M94.8x1 Other specified disorders of cartilage, shoulder
    M94.8x2 Other specified disorders of cartilage, upper arm
    M94.8x3 Other specified disorders of cartilage, forearm
    M94.8x4 Other specified disorders of cartilage, hand
    M94.8x5 Other specified disorders of cartilage, thigh
    M94.8x6 Other specified disorders of cartilage, lower leg
    M94.8x7 Other specified disorders of cartilage, ankle and foot
    M94.8x8 Other specified disorders of cartilage, other site
    M94.8x9 Other specified disorders of cartilage, unspecified sites

M94.9 Disorder of cartilage, unspecified

Other disorders of the musculoskeletal system and connective tissue (M95)

M95- Other acquired deformities of musculoskeletal system and connective tissue
Excludes❷: acquired absence of limbs and organs (Z89-Z90)
acquired deformities of limbs (M20-M21)
congenital malformations and deformations of the musculoskeletal system (Q65-Q79)
deforming dorsopathies (M40-M43)
dentofacial anomalies [including malocclusion] (M26.-)
postprocedural musculoskeletal disorders (M96.-)

M95.0 Acquired deformity of nose
Excludes❷: deviated nasal septum (J34.2)

M95.1- Cauliflower ear
Excludes❷: other acquired deformities of ear (H61.1)

M95.10 Cauliflower ear, unspecified ear
M95.11 Cauliflower ear, right ear
M95.12 Cauliflower ear, left ear

M95.2 Other acquired deformity of head
M95.3 Acquired deformity of neck
M95.4 Acquired deformity of chest and rib
M95.5 Acquired deformity of pelvis
Excludes 1: maternal care for known or suspected disproportion (O33.-)

M95.8 Other specified acquired deformities of musculoskeletal system
M95.9 Acquired deformity of musculoskeletal system, unspecified

M
9
4
–
M
9
9

Intraoperative and postprocedural complications and disorders of musculoskeletal system, not elsewhere classified (M96)

M96- Intraoperative and postprocedural complications and disorders of musculoskeletal system, not elsewhere classified
> Excludes❷: *arthropathy following intestinal bypass (M02.0-)*
> *complications of internal orthopedic prosthetic devices, implants and grafts (T84.-)*
> *disorders associated with osteoporosis (M80)*
> *presence of functional implants and other devices (Z96-Z97)*

M96.0 Pseudarthrosis after fusion or arthrodesis

M96.1 Postlaminectomy syndrome, not elsewhere classified

M96.2 Postradiation kyphosis

M96.3 Postlaminectomy kyphosis

M96.4 Postsurgical lordosis

M96.5 Postradiation scoliosis

M96.6- Fracture of bone following insertion of orthopedic implant, joint prosthesis, or bone plate
> Intraoperative fracture of bone during insertion of orthopedic implant, joint prosthesis, or bone plate
> Excludes❷: *complication of internal orthopedic devices, implants or grafts (T84.-)*

M96.62- Fracture of humerus following insertion of orthopedic implant, joint prosthesis, or bone plate

> **M96.621 Fracture of humerus following insertion of orthopedic implant, joint prosthesis, or bone plate, right arm**

> **M96.622 Fracture of humerus following insertion of orthopedic implant, joint prosthesis, or bone plate, left arm**

> **M96.629 Fracture of humerus following insertion of orthopedic implant, joint prosthesis, or bone plate, unspecified arm**

M96.63- Fracture of radius or ulna following insertion of orthopedic implant, joint prosthesis, or bone plate

> **M96.631 Fracture of radius or ulna following insertion of orthopedic implant, joint prosthesis, or bone plate, right arm**

> **M96.632 Fracture of radius or ulna following insertion of orthopedic implant, joint prosthesis, or bone plate, left arm**

> **M96.639 Fracture of radius or ulna following insertion of orthopedic implant, joint prosthesis, or bone plate, unspecified arm**

M96.65 Fracture of pelvis following insertion of orthopedic implant, joint prosthesis, or bone plate

M96.66- Fracture of femur following insertion of orthopedic implant, joint prosthesis, or bone plate

> **M96.661 Fracture of femur following insertion of orthopedic implant, joint prosthesis, or bone plate, right leg**

> **M96.662 Fracture of femur following insertion of orthopedic implant, joint prosthesis, or bone plate, left leg**

> **M96.669 Fracture of femur following insertion of orthopedic implant, joint prosthesis, or bone plate, unspecified leg**

M96.67- Fracture of tibia or fibula following insertion of orthopedic implant, joint prosthesis, or bone plate

> **M96.671 Fracture of tibia or fibula following insertion of orthopedic implant, joint prosthesis, or bone plate, right leg**

> **M96.672 Fracture of tibia or fibula following insertion of orthopedic implant, joint prosthesis, or bone plate, left leg**

> **M96.679 Fracture of tibia or fibula following insertion of orthopedic implant, joint prosthesis, or bone plate, unspecified leg**

M96.69 Fracture of other bone following insertion of orthopedic implant, joint prosthesis, or bone plate

M96.8- Other intraoperative and postprocedural complications and disorders of musculoskeletal system, not elsewhere classified

M96.81- Intraoperative hemorrhage and hematoma of a musculoskeletal structure complicating a procedure
> Excludes 1: *intraoperative hemorrhage and hematoma of a musculoskeletal structure due to accidental puncture and laceration during a procedure (M96.82-)*

> **M96.810 Intraoperative hemorrhage and hematoma of a musculoskeletal structure complicating a musculoskeletal system procedure**

> **M96.811 Intraoperative hemorrhage and hematoma of a musculoskeletal structure complicating other procedure**

M96.82- Accidental puncture and laceration of a musculoskeletal structure during a procedure

> **M96.820 Accidental puncture and laceration of a musculoskeletal structure during a musculoskeletal system procedure**

> **M96.821 Accidental puncture and laceration of a musculoskeletal structure during other procedure**

M96.83- Postprocedural hemorrhage and hematoma of a musculoskeletal structure following a procedure

> **M96.830 Postprocedural hemorrhage and hematoma of a musculoskeletal structure following a musculoskeletal system procedure**

> **M96.831 Postprocedural hemorrhage and hematoma of a musculoskeletal structure following other procedure**

M96.89 Other intraoperative and postprocedural complications and disorders of the musculoskeletal system
> Instability of joint secondary to removal of joint prosthesis
> Use additional code, if applicable, to further specify disorder

Biomechanical lesions, not elsewhere classified (M99)

M99- Biomechanical lesions, not elsewhere classified
> Note: This category should not be used if the condition can be classified elsewhere.

M99.0- Segmental and somatic dysfunction

> **M99.00 Segmental and somatic dysfunction of head region**

> **M99.01 Segmental and somatic dysfunction of cervical region**

> **M99.02 Segmental and somatic dysfunction of thoracic region**

> **M99.03 Segmental and somatic dysfunction of lumbar region**

> **M99.04 Segmental and somatic dysfunction of sacral region**

> **M99.05 Segmental and somatic dysfunction of pelvic region**

> **M99.06 Segmental and somatic dysfunction of lower extremity**

> **M99.07 Segmental and somatic dysfunction of upper extremity**

> **M99.08 Segmental and somatic dysfunction of rib cage**

> **M99.09 Segmental and somatic dysfunction of abdomen and other regions**

M99.1- Subluxation complex (vertebral)

> **M99.10 Subluxation complex (vertebral) of head region**

> **M99.11 Subluxation complex (vertebral) of cervical region**

> **M99.12 Subluxation complex (vertebral) of thoracic region**

> **M99.13 Subluxation complex (vertebral) of lumbar region**

> **M99.14 Subluxation complex (vertebral) of sacral region**

> **M99.15 Subluxation complex (vertebral) of pelvic region**

> **M99.16 Subluxation complex (vertebral) of lower extremity**

> **M99.17 Subluxation complex (vertebral) of upper extremity**

> **M99.18 Subluxation complex (vertebral) of rib cage**

> **M99.19 Subluxation complex (vertebral) of abdomen and other regions**

M99.2- Subluxation stenosis of neural canal

> **M99.20 Subluxation stenosis of neural canal of head region**

> **M99.21 Subluxation stenosis of neural canal of cervical region**

> **M99.22 Subluxation stenosis of neural canal of thoracic region**

> **M99.23 Subluxation stenosis of neural canal of lumbar region**

> **M99.24 Subluxation stenosis of neural canal of sacral region**

> **M99.25 Subluxation stenosis of neural canal of pelvic region**

> **M99.26 Subluxation stenosis of neural canal of lower extremity**

> **M99.27 Subluxation stenosis of neural canal of upper extremity**

> **M99.28 Subluxation stenosis of neural canal of rib cage**

> **M99.29 Subluxation stenosis of neural canal of abdomen and other regions**

M99.3- Osseous stenosis of neural canal

> **M99.30 Osseous stenosis of neural canal of head region**

> **M99.31 Osseous stenosis of neural canal of cervical region**

> **M99.32 Osseous stenosis of neural canal of thoracic region**

> **M99.33 Osseous stenosis of neural canal of lumbar region**

> **M99.34 Osseous stenosis of neural canal of sacral region**

> **M99.35 Osseous stenosis of neural canal of pelvic region**

> **M99.36 Osseous stenosis of neural canal of lower extremity**

> **M99.37 Osseous stenosis of neural canal of upper extremity**

> **M99.38 Osseous stenosis of neural canal of rib cage**

> **M99.39 Osseous stenosis of neural canal of abdomen and other regions**

M 9 4 - M 9 9

M99.4- <u>Connective tissue stenosis</u> of neural canal

   M99.40 Connective tissue stenosis of neural canal of head region
   M99.41 Connective tissue stenosis of neural canal of cervical region
   M99.42 Connective tissue stenosis of neural canal of thoracic region
   M99.43 Connective tissue stenosis of neural canal of lumbar region
   M99.44 Connective tissue stenosis of neural canal of sacral region
   M99.45 Connective tissue stenosis of neural canal of pelvic region
   M99.46 Connective tissue stenosis of neural canal of lower extremity
   M99.47 Connective tissue stenosis of neural canal of upper extremity
   M99.48 Connective tissue stenosis of neural canal of rib cage
   M99.49 Connective tissue stenosis of neural canal of abdomen and other regions

M99.5- <u>Intervertebral disc stenosis</u> of neural canal

   M99.50 Intervertebral disc stenosis of neural canal of head region
   M99.51 Intervertebral disc stenosis of neural canal of cervical region
   M99.52 Intervertebral disc stenosis of neural canal of thoracic region
   M99.53 Intervertebral disc stenosis of neural canal of lumbar region
   M99.54 Intervertebral disc stenosis of neural canal of sacral region
   M99.55 Intervertebral disc stenosis of neural canal of pelvic region
   M99.56 Intervertebral disc stenosis of neural canal of lower extremity
   M99.57 Intervertebral disc stenosis of neural canal of upper extremity
   M99.58 Intervertebral disc stenosis of neural canal of rib cage
   M99.59 Intervertebral disc stenosis of neural canal of abdomen and other regions

M99.6- <u>Osseous and subluxation stenosis</u> of intervertebral foramina

   M99.60 Osseous and subluxation stenosis of intervertebral foramina of head region
   M99.61 Osseous and subluxation stenosis of intervertebral foramina of cervical region
   M99.62 Osseous and subluxation stenosis of intervertebral foramina of thoracic region
   M99.63 Osseous and subluxation stenosis of intervertebral foramina of lumbar region
   M99.64 Osseous and subluxation stenosis of intervertebral foramina of sacral region
   M99.65 Osseous and subluxation stenosis of intervertebral foramina of pelvic region
   M99.66 Osseous and subluxation stenosis of intervertebral foramina of lower extremity
   M99.67 Osseous and subluxation stenosis of intervertebral foramina of upper extremity
   M99.68 Osseous and subluxation stenosis of intervertebral foramina of rib cage
   M99.69 Osseous and subluxation stenosis of intervertebral foramina of abdomen and other regions

M99.7- <u>Connective tissue and disc stenosis</u> of intervertebral foramina

   M99.70 Connective tissue and disc stenosis of intervertebral foramina of head region
   M99.71 Connective tissue and disc stenosis of intervertebral foramina of cervical region
   M99.72 Connective tissue and disc stenosis of intervertebral foramina of thoracic region
   M99.73 Connective tissue and disc stenosis of intervertebral foramina of lumbar region
   M99.74 Connective tissue and disc stenosis of intervertebral foramina of sacral region
   M99.75 Connective tissue and disc stenosis of intervertebral foramina of pelvic region
   M99.76 Connective tissue and disc stenosis of intervertebral foramina of lower extremity
   M99.77 Connective tissue and disc stenosis of intervertebral foramina of upper extremity
   M99.78 Connective tissue and disc stenosis of intervertebral foramina of rib cage
   M99.79 Connective tissue and disc stenosis of intervertebral foramina of abdomen and other regions

M99.8- <u>Other</u> biomechanical lesions

   M99.80 Other biomechanical lesions of head region
   M99.81 Other biomechanical lesions of cervical region
   M99.82 Other biomechanical lesions of thoracic region
   M99.83 Other biomechanical lesions of lumbar region
   M99.84 Other biomechanical lesions of sacral region
   M99.85 Other biomechanical lesions of pelvic region
   M99.86 Other biomechanical lesions of lower extremity
   M99.87 Other biomechanical lesions of upper extremity
   M99.88 Other biomechanical lesions of rib cage
   M99.89 Other biomechanical lesions of abdomen and other regions

M99.9 Biomechanical lesion, <u>unspecified</u>

M99 : N03

Chapter 14 – Diseases of the genitourinary system (N00-N99)

Excludes❷: *certain conditions originating in the perinatal period (P04-P96)*
certain infectious and parasitic diseases (A00-B99)
complications of pregnancy, childbirth and the puerperium (O00-O9A)
congenital malformations, deformations and chromosomal abnormalities (Q00-Q99)
endocrine, nutritional and metabolic diseases (E00-E88)
injury, poisoning and certain other consequences of external causes (S00-T88)
neoplasms (C00-D49)
symptoms, signs and abnormal clinical and laboratory findings, not elsewhere classified (R00-R94)

This chapter contains the following blocks:
N00-N08   Glomerular diseases
N10-N16   Renal tubulo-interstitial diseases
N17-N19   Acute kidney failure and chronic kidney disease
N20-N23   Urolithiasis
N25-N29   Other disorders of kidney and ureter
N30-N39   Other diseases of the urinary system
N40-N53   Diseases of male genital organs
N60-N65   Disorders of breast
N70-N77   Inflammatory diseases of female pelvic organs
N80-N98   Noninflammatory disorders of female genital tract
N99   Intraoperative and postprocedural complications and disorders of genitourinary system, not elsewhere classified

Glomerular diseases (N00-N08)

Excludes 1: *hypertensive chronic kidney disease (I12.-)*
Code also any associated kidney failure (N17-N19).

N00-   Acute nephritic syndrome
Includes: Acute glomerular disease
Acute glomerulonephritis
Acute nephritis
Excludes 1: *acute tubulo-interstitial nephritis (N10)*
nephritic syndrome NOS (N05.-)

N00.0   Acute nephritic syndrome with minor glomerular abnormality
Acute nephritic syndrome with minimal change lesion

N00.1   Acute nephritic syndrome with focal and segmental glomerular lesions
Acute nephritic syndrome with focal and segmental hyalinosis
Acute nephritic syndrome with focal and segmental sclerosis
Acute nephritic syndrome with focal glomerulonephritis

N00.2   Acute nephritic syndrome with diffuse membranous glomerulonephritis

N00.3   Acute nephritic syndrome with diffuse mesangial proliferative glomerulonephritis

N00.4   Acute nephritic syndrome with diffuse endocapillary proliferative glomerulonephritis

N00.5   Acute nephritic syndrome with diffuse mesangiocapillary glomerulonephritis
Acute nephritic syndrome with membranoproliferative glomerulonephritis, types 1 and 3, or NOS

N00.6   Acute nephritic syndrome with dense deposit disease
Acute nephritic syndrome with membranoproliferative glomerulonephritis, type 2

N00.7   Acute nephritic syndrome with diffuse crescentic glomerulonephritis
Acute nephritic syndrome with extracapillary glomerulonephritis

N00.8   Acute nephritic syndrome with other morphologic changes
Acute nephritic syndrome with proliferative glomerulonephritis NOS

N00.9   Acute nephritic syndrome with unspecified morphologic changes

N01-   Rapidly progressive nephritic syndrome
Includes: Rapidly progressive glomerular disease
Rapidly progressive glomerulonephritis
Rapidly progressive nephritis
Excludes 1: *nephritic syndrome NOS (N05.-)*

N01.0   Rapidly progressive nephritic syndrome with minor glomerular abnormality
Rapidly progressive nephritic syndrome with minimal change lesion

N01.1   Rapidly progressive nephritic syndrome with focal and segmental glomerular lesions
Rapidly progressive nephritic syndrome with focal and segmental hyalinosis
Rapidly progressive nephritic syndrome with focal and segmental sclerosis
Rapidly progressive nephritic syndrome with focal glomerulonephritis

N01.2   Rapidly progressive nephritic syndrome with diffuse membranous glomerulonephritis

N01.3   Rapidly progressive nephritic syndrome with diffuse mesangial proliferative glomerulonephritis

N01.4   Rapidly progressive nephritic syndrome with diffuse endocapillary proliferative glomerulonephritis

N01.5   Rapidly progressive nephritic syndrome with diffuse mesangiocapillary glomerulonephritis
Rapidly progressive nephritic syndrome with membranoproliferative glomerulonephritis, types 1 and 3, or NOS

N01.6   Rapidly progressive nephritic syndrome with dense deposit disease
Rapidly progressive nephritic syndrome with membranoproliferative glomerulonephritis, type 2

N01.7   Rapidly progressive nephritic syndrome with diffuse crescentic glomerulonephritis
Rapidly progressive nephritic syndrome with extracapillary glomerulonephritis

N01.8   Rapidly progressive nephritic syndrome with other morphologic changes
Rapidly progressive nephritic syndrome with proliferative glomerulonephritis NOS

N01.9   Rapidly progressive nephritic syndrome with unspecified morphologic changes

N02-   Recurrent and persistent hematuria
Excludes 1: *acute cystitis with hematuria (N30.01)*
hematuria NOS (R31.9)
hematuria not associated with specified morphologic lesions (R31.-)

N02.0   Recurrent and persistent hematuria with minor glomerular abnormality
Recurrent and persistent hematuria with minimal change lesion

N02.1   Recurrent and persistent hematuria with focal and segmental glomerular lesions
Recurrent and persistent hematuria with focal and segmental hyalinosis
Recurrent and persistent hematuria with focal and segmental sclerosis
Recurrent and persistent hematuria with focal glomerulonephritis

N02.2   Recurrent and persistent hematuria with diffuse membranous glomerulonephritis

N02.3   Recurrent and persistent hematuria with diffuse mesangial proliferative glomerulonephritis

N02.4   Recurrent and persistent hematuria with diffuse endocapillary proliferative glomerulonephritis

N02.5   Recurrent and persistent hematuria with diffuse mesangiocapillary glomerulonephritis
Recurrent and persistent hematuria with membranoproliferative glomerulonephritis, types 1 and 3, or NOS

N02.6   Recurrent and persistent hematuria with dense deposit disease
Recurrent and persistent hematuria with membranoproliferative glomerulonephritis, type 2

N02.7   Recurrent and persistent hematuria with diffuse crescentic glomerulonephritis
Recurrent and persistent hematuria with extracapillary glomerulonephritis

N02.8   Recurrent and persistent hematuria with other morphologic changes
Recurrent and persistent hematuria with proliferative glomerulonephritis NOS

N02.9   Recurrent and persistent hematuria with unspecified morphologic changes

N03-   Chronic nephritic syndrome
Includes: Chronic glomerular disease
Chronic glomerulonephritis
Chronic nephritis
Excludes 1: *chronic tubulo-interstitial nephritis (N11.-)*
diffuse sclerosing glomerulonephritis (N05.8-)
nephritic syndrome NOS (N05.-)

N03.0   Chronic nephritic syndrome with minor glomerular abnormality
Chronic nephritic syndrome with minimal change lesion

N03.1   Chronic nephritic syndrome with focal and segmental glomerular lesions
Chronic nephritic syndrome with focal and segmental hyalinosis
Chronic nephritic syndrome with focal and segmental sclerosis
Chronic nephritic syndrome with focal glomerulonephritis

N03.2   Chronic nephritic syndrome with diffuse membranous glomerulonephritis

N03.3   Chronic nephritic syndrome with diffuse mesangial proliferative glomerulonephritis

M99 - N03

N03.4   **Chronic nephritic syndrome <u>with</u> diffuse endocapillary proliferative glomerulonephritis**

N03.5   **Chronic nephritic syndrome <u>with</u> diffuse mesangiocapillary glomerulonephritis**
      Chronic nephritic syndrome with membranoproliferative glomerulonephritis, types 1 and 3, or NOS

N03.6   **Chronic nephritic syndrome <u>with</u> dense deposit disease**
      Chronic nephritic syndrome with membranoproliferative glomerulonephritis, type 2

N03.7   **Chronic nephritic syndrome <u>with</u> diffuse crescentic glomerulonephritis**
      Chronic nephritic syndrome with extracapillary glomerulonephritis

N03.8   **Chronic nephritic syndrome <u>with</u> other morphologic changes**
      Chronic nephritic syndrome with proliferative glomerulonephritis NOS

N03.9   **Chronic nephritic syndrome <u>with</u> unspecified morphologic changes**

N04-   <u>**Nephrotic**</u> **syndrome**
      Includes: Congenital nephrotic syndrome
            Lipoid nephrosis

N04.0   **Nephrotic syndrome <u>with</u> minor glomerular abnormality**
      Nephrotic syndrome with minimal change lesion

N04.1   **Nephrotic syndrome <u>with</u> focal and segmental glomerular lesions**
      Nephrotic syndrome with focal and segmental hyalinosis
      Nephrotic syndrome with focal and segmental sclerosis
      Nephrotic syndrome with focal glomerulonephritis

N04.2   **Nephrotic syndrome <u>with</u> diffuse membranous glomerulonephritis**

N04.3   **Nephrotic syndrome <u>with</u> diffuse mesangial proliferative glomerulonephritis**

N04.4   **Nephrotic syndrome <u>with</u> diffuse endocapillary proliferative glomerulonephritis**

N04.5   **Nephrotic syndrome <u>with</u> diffuse mesangiocapillary glomerulonephritis**
      Nephrotic syndrome with membranoproliferative glomerulonephritis, types 1 and 3, or NOS

N04.6   **Nephrotic syndrome <u>with</u> dense deposit disease**
      Nephrotic syndrome with membranoproliferative glomerulonephritis, type 2

N04.7   **Nephrotic syndrome <u>with</u> diffuse crescentic glomerulonephritis**
      Nephrotic syndrome with extracapillary glomerulonephritis

N04.8   **Nephrotic syndrome <u>with</u> other morphologic changes**
      Nephrotic syndrome with proliferative glomerulonephritis NOS

N04.9   **Nephrotic syndrome <u>with</u> unspecified morphologic changes**

N05-   <u>**Unspecified**</u> **nephritic syndrome**
      Includes: Glomerular disease NOS
            Glomerulonephritis NOS
            Nephritis NOS
            Nephropathy NOS and renal disease NOS with morphological lesion specified in .0-.8
      Excludes 1:   *nephropathy NOS with no stated morphological lesion (N28.9)*
            renal disease NOS with no stated morphological lesion (N28.9)
            tubulo-interstitial nephritis NOS (N12)

N05.0   **Unspecified nephritic syndrome <u>with</u> minor glomerular abnormality**
      Unspecified nephritic syndrome with minimal change lesion

N05.1   **Unspecified nephritic syndrome <u>with</u> focal and segmental glomerular lesions**
      Unspecified nephritic syndrome with focal and segmental hyalinosis
      Unspecified nephritic syndrome with focal and segmental sclerosis
      Unspecified nephritic syndrome with focal glomerulonephritis

N05.2   **Unspecified nephritic syndrome <u>with</u> diffuse membranous glomerulonephritis**

N05.3   **Unspecified nephritic syndrome <u>with</u> diffuse mesangial proliferative glomerulonephritis**

N05.4   **Unspecified nephritic syndrome <u>with</u> diffuse endocapillary proliferative glomerulonephritis**

N05.5   **Unspecified nephritic syndrome <u>with</u> diffuse mesangiocapillary glomerulonephritis**
      Unspecified nephritic syndrome with membranoproliferative glomerulonephritis, types 1 and 3, or NOS

N05.6   **Unspecified nephritic syndrome <u>with</u> dense deposit disease**
      Unspecified nephritic syndrome with membranoproliferative glomerulonephritis, type 2

N05.7   **Unspecified nephritic syndrome <u>with</u> diffuse crescentic glomerulonephritis**
      Unspecified nephritic syndrome with extracapillary glomerulonephritis

N05.8   **Unspecified nephritic syndrome <u>with</u> other morphologic changes**
      Unspecified nephritic syndrome with proliferative glomerulonephritis NOS

N05.9   **Unspecified nephritic syndrome <u>with</u> unspecified morphologic changes**

N06-   <u>**Isolated proteinuria with specified morphological lesion**</u>
      Excludes 1:   proteinuria not associated with specific morphologic lesions (R80.0)

N06.0   **Isolated proteinuria <u>with</u> minor glomerular abnormality**
      Isolated proteinuria with minimal change lesion

N06.1   **Isolated proteinuria <u>with</u> focal and segmental glomerular lesions**
      Isolated proteinuria with focal and segmental hyalinosis
      Isolated proteinuria with focal and segmental sclerosis
      Isolated proteinuria with focal glomerulonephritis

N06.2   **Isolated proteinuria <u>with</u> diffuse membranous glomerulonephritis**

N06.3   **Isolated proteinuria <u>with</u> diffuse mesangial proliferative glomerulonephritis**

N06.4   **Isolated proteinuria <u>with</u> diffuse endocapillary proliferative glomerulonephritis**

N06.5   **Isolated proteinuria <u>with</u> diffuse mesangiocapillary glomerulonephritis**
      Isolated proteinuria with membranoproliferative glomerulonephritis, types 1 and 3, or NOS

N06.6   **Isolated proteinuria <u>with</u> dense deposit disease**
      Isolated proteinuria with membranoproliferative glomerulonephritis, type 2

N06.7   **Isolated proteinuria <u>with</u> diffuse crescentic glomerulonephritis**
      Isolated proteinuria with extracapillary glomerulonephritis

N06.8   **Isolated proteinuria <u>with</u> other morphologic lesion**
      Isolated proteinuria with proliferative glomerulonephritis NOS

N06.9   **Isolated proteinuria <u>with</u> unspecified morphologic lesion**

N07-   <u>**Hereditary nephropathy, not elsewhere classified**</u>
      Excludes❷: Alport's syndrome (Q87.81-)
            hereditary amyloid nephropathy (E85.-)
            nail patella syndrome (Q87.2)
            non-neuropathic heredofamilial amyloidosis (E85.-)

N07.0   **Hereditary nephropathy, not elsewhere classified <u>with</u> minor glomerular abnormality**
      Hereditary nephropathy, not elsewhere classified with minimal change lesion

N07.1   **Hereditary nephropathy, not elsewhere classified <u>with</u> focal and segmental glomerular lesions**
      Hereditary nephropathy, not elsewhere classified with focal and segmental hyalinosis
      Hereditary nephropathy, not elsewhere classified with focal and segmental sclerosis
      Hereditary nephropathy, not elsewhere classified with focal glomerulonephritis

N07.2   **Hereditary nephropathy, not elsewhere classified <u>with</u> diffuse membranous glomerulonephritis**

N07.3   **Hereditary nephropathy, not elsewhere classified <u>with</u> diffuse mesangial proliferative glomerulonephritis**

N07.4   **Hereditary nephropathy, not elsewhere classified <u>with</u> diffuse endocapillary proliferative glomerulonephritis**

N07.5   **Hereditary nephropathy, not elsewhere classified <u>with</u> diffuse mesangiocapillary glomerulonephritis**
      Hereditary nephropathy, not elsewhere classified with membranoproliferative glomerulonephritis, types 1 and 3, or NOS

N07.6   **Hereditary nephropathy, not elsewhere classified <u>with</u> dense deposit disease**
      Hereditary nephropathy, not elsewhere classified with membranoproliferative glomerulonephritis, type 2

N07.7   **Hereditary nephropathy, not elsewhere classified <u>with</u> diffuse crescentic glomerulonephritis**
      Hereditary nephropathy, not elsewhere classified with extracapillary glomerulonephritis

N07.8   **Hereditary nephropathy, not elsewhere classified <u>with</u> other morphologic lesions**
      Hereditary nephropathy, not elsewhere classified with proliferative glomerulonephritis NOS

N07.9   **Hereditary nephropathy, not elsewhere classified <u>with</u> unspecified morphologic lesions**

N
0
3
I
N
1
5

Excludes 1: = NOT CODED HERE! (Do not code both)

Excludes❷: = Not Included Here

N08   Glomerular disorders in diseases classified elsewhere
Glomerulonephritis
Nephritis
Nephropathy
Code first underlying disease, such as:
Amyloidosis (E85.-)
Congenital syphilis (A50.5)
Cryoglobulinemia (D89.1)
Disseminated intravascular coagulation (D65)
Gout (M1A.-, M10.-)
Microscopic polyangiitis (M31.7)
Multiple myeloma (C90.0-)
Sepsis (A40.0-A41.9)
Sickle-cell disease (D57.0-D57.8)
Excludes 1:   glomerulonephritis, nephritis and nephropathy (in):
antiglomerular basement membrane disease (M31.0)
diabetes (E08-E13 with .21)
gonococcal (A54.21)
Goodpasture's syndrome (M31.0)
hemolytic-uremic syndrome (D59.3)
lupus (M32.14)
mumps (B26.83)
syphilis (A52.75)
systemic lupus erythematosus (M32.14)
Wegener's granulomatosis (M31.31)
pyelonephritis in diseases classified elsewhere (N16)
renal tubulo-interstitial disorders classified elsewhere (N16)

Renal tubulo-interstitial diseases (N10-N16)

Includes: Pyelonephritis
Excludes 1:   pyeloureteritis cystica (N28.85)

N10   Acute tubulo-interstitial nephritis
Acute infectious interstitial nephritis
Acute pyelitis
Acute pyelonephritis
Hemoglobin nephrosis
Myoglobin nephrosis
Use additional code (B95-B97), to identify infectious agent.

N11-   Chronic tubulo-interstitial nephritis
Includes: Chronic infectious interstitial nephritis
Chronic pyelitis
Chronic pyelonephritis
Use additional code (B95-B97), to identify infectious agent.

N11.0   Nonobstructive reflux-associated chronic pyelonephritis
Pyelonephritis (chronic) associated with (vesicoureteral) reflux
Excludes 1:   vesicoureteral reflux NOS (N13.70)

N11.1   Chronic obstructive pyelonephritis
Pyelonephritis (chronic) associated with anomaly of pelviureteric junction
Pyelonephritis (chronic) associated with anomaly of pyeloureteric junction
Pyelonephritis (chronic) associated with crossing of vessel
Pyelonephritis (chronic) associated with kinking of ureter
Pyelonephritis (chronic) associated with obstruction of ureter
Pyelonephritis (chronic) associated with stricture of pelviureteric junction
Pyelonephritis (chronic) associated with stricture of ureter
Excludes 1:   calculous pyelonephritis (N20.9)
obstructive uropathy (N13.-)

N11.8   Other chronic tubulo-interstitial nephritis
Nonobstructive chronic pyelonephritis NOS

N11.9   Chronic tubulo-interstitial nephritis, unspecified
Chronic interstitial nephritis NOS
Chronic pyelitis NOS
Chronic pyelonephritis NOS

N12   Tubulo-interstitial nephritis, not specified as acute or chronic
Interstitial nephritis NOS
Pyelitis NOS
Pyelonephritis NOS
Excludes 1:   calculous pyelonephritis (N20.9)

N13-   Obstructive and reflux uropathy
Excludes❷: calculus of kidney and ureter without hydronephrosis (N20.-)
congenital obstructive defects of renal pelvis and ureter (Q62.0-Q62.3)
hydronephrosis with ureteropelvic junction obstruction (Q62.1)
obstructive pyelonephritis (N11.1)

N13.1   Hydronephrosis with ureteral stricture, not elsewhere classified
Excludes 1:   hydronephrosis with ureteral stricture with infection (N13.6)

N13.2   Hydronephrosis with renal and ureteral calculous obstruction
Excludes 1:   hydronephrosis with renal and ureteral calculous obstruction with infection (N13.6)

N13.3-   Other and unspecified hydronephrosis
Excludes 1:   hydronephrosis with infection (N13.6)
N13.30   Unspecified hydronephrosis
N13.39   Other hydronephrosis

N13.4   Hydroureter
Excludes 1:   congenital hydroureter (Q62.3-)
hydroureter with infection (N13.6)
vesicoureteral-reflux with hydroureter (N13.73-)

N13.5   Crossing vessel and stricture of ureter without hydronephrosis
Kinking and stricture of ureter without hydronephrosis
Excludes 1:   crossing vessel and stricture of ureter without hydronephrosis with infection (N13.6)

N13.6   Pyonephrosis
Conditions in N13.1-N13.5 with infection
Obstructive uropathy with infection
Use additional code (B95-B97), to identify infectious agent

N13.7-   Vesicoureteral-reflux
Excludes 1:   reflux-associated pyelonephritis (N11.0)

N13.70   Vesicoureteral-reflux, unspecified
Vesicoureteral-reflux NOS

N13.71   Vesicoureteral-reflux without reflux nephropathy

N13.72- Vesicoureteral-reflux with reflux nephropathy without hydroureter

N13.721   Vesicoureteral-reflux with reflux nephropathy without hydroureter, unilateral

N13.722   Vesicoureteral-reflux with reflux nephropathy without hydroureter, bilateral

N13.729   Vesicoureteral-reflux with reflux nephropathy without hydroureter, unspecified

N13.73- Vesicoureteral-reflux with reflux nephropathy with hydroureter

N13.731   Vesicoureteral-reflux with reflux nephropathy with hydroureter, unilateral

N13.732   Vesicoureteral-reflux with reflux nephropathy with hydroureter, bilateral

N13.739   Vesicoureteral-reflux with reflux nephropathy with hydroureter, unspecified

N13.8   Other obstructive and reflux uropathy
Urinary tract obstruction due to specified cause
Code first, if applicable, any causal condition, such as:
Enlarged prostate (N40.1)

N13.9   Obstructive and reflux uropathy, unspecified
Urinary tract obstruction NOS

N14-   Drug- and heavy-metal-induced tubulo-interstitial and tubular conditions
Code first poisoning due to drug or toxin, if applicable (T36-T65 with fifth or sixth character 1-4 or 6)
Use additional code for adverse effect, if applicable, to identify drug (T36-T50 with fifth or sixth character 5)

N14.0   Analgesic nephropathy
N14.1   Nephropathy induced by other drugs, medicaments and biological substances
N14.2   Nephropathy induced by unspecified drug, medicament or biological substance
N14.3   Nephropathy induced by heavy metals
N14.4   Toxic nephropathy, not elsewhere classified

N15-   Other renal tubulo-interstitial diseases
N15.0   Balkan nephropathy
Balkan endemic nephropathy
N15.1   Renal and perinephric abscess
N15.8   Other specified renal tubulo-interstitial diseases
N15.9   Renal tubulo-interstitial disease, unspecified
Infection of kidney NOS
Excludes 1:   urinary tract infection NOS (N39.0)

N 0 3 - N 1 5

N16 **Renal tubulo-interstitial disorders <u>in diseases classified elsewhere</u>**
 Pyelonephritis
 Tubulo-interstitial nephritis
 Code first underlying disease, such as:
  Brucellosis (A23.0-A23.9)
  Cryoglobulinemia (D89.1)
  Glycogen storage disease (E74.0)
  Leukemia (C91-C95)
  Lymphoma (C81.0-C85.9, C96.0-C96.9)
  Multiple myeloma (C90.0-)
  Sepsis (A40.0-A41.9)
  Wilson's disease (E83.0)
 Excludes 1: diphtheritic pyelonephritis and tubulo-interstitial nephritis (A36.84)
   pyelonephritis and tubulo-interstitial nephritis in candidiasis (B37.49)
   pyelonephritis and tubulo-interstitial nephritis in cystinosis (E72.0)
   pyelonephritis and tubulo-interstitial nephritis in salmonella infection (A02.25)
   pyelonephritis and tubulo-interstitial nephritis in sarcoidosis (D86.84)
   pyelonephritis and tubulo-interstitial nephritis in sicca syndrome [Sjogren's] (M35.04)
   pyelonephritis and tubulo-interstitial nephritis in systemic lupus erythematosus (M32.15)
   pyelonephritis and tubulo-interstitial nephritis in toxoplasmosis (B58.83)
   renal tubular degeneration in diabetes (E08-E13 with .29)
   syphilitic pyelonephritis and tubulo-interstitial nephritis (A52.75)

Acute kidney failure and chronic kidney disease (N17-N19)

 Excludes❷: congenital renal failure (P96.0)
   drug- and heavy-metal-induced tubulo-interstitial and tubular conditions (N14.-)
   extrarenal uremia (R39.2)
   hemolytic-uremic syndrome (D59.3)
   hepatorenal syndrome (K76.7)
   postpartum hepatorenal syndrome (O90.4)
   posttraumatic renal failure (T79.5)
   prerenal uremia (R39.2)
   renal failure complicating abortion or ectopic or molar pregnancy (O00-O07, O08.4)
   renal failure following labor and delivery (O90.4)
   renal failure postprocedural (N99.0)

N17- **<u>Acute</u> kidney failure**
 Code also associated underlying condition
 Excludes 1: posttraumatic renal failure (T79.5)
 N17.0 **Acute kidney failure <u>with tubular necrosis</u>**
   Acute tubular necrosis
   Renal tubular necrosis
   Tubular necrosis NOS
 N17.1 **Acute kidney failure <u>with acute cortical necrosis</u>**
   Acute cortical necrosis
   Cortical necrosis NOS
   Renal cortical necrosis
 N17.2 **Acute kidney failure <u>with medullary necrosis</u>**
   Medullary [papillary] necrosis NOS
   Acute medullary [papillary] necrosis
   Renal medullary [papillary] necrosis
 N17.8 **<u>Other</u> acute kidney failure**
 N17.9 **Acute kidney failure, <u>unspecified</u>**
   Acute kidney injury (nontraumatic)
   Excludes❷: traumatic kidney injury (S37.0-)

N18- **<u>Chronic</u> kidney disease (CKD)**
 Code first any associated:
  Diabetic chronic kidney disease (E08.22, E09.22, E10.22, E11.22, E13.22)
  Hypertensive chronic kidney disease (I12.-, I13.-)
 Use additional code to identify kidney transplant status, if applicable, (Z94.0)
 N18.1 **Chronic kidney disease, stage 1**
 N18.2 **Chronic kidney disease, stage 2 (mild)**
 N18.3 **Chronic kidney disease, stage 3 (moderate)**
 N18.4 **Chronic kidney disease, stage 4 (severe)**
 N18.5 **Chronic kidney disease, stage 5**
   Excludes 1: chronic kidney disease, stage 5 requiring chronic dialysis (N18.6)
 N18.6 **<u>End stage renal disease</u>**
   Chronic kidney disease requiring chronic dialysis
   Use additional code to identify dialysis status (Z99.2)

N18.9 **Chronic kidney disease, <u>unspecified</u>**
   Chronic renal disease
   Chronic renal failure NOS
   Chronic renal insufficiency
   Chronic uremia
N19 **<u>Unspecified</u> kidney failure**
   Uremia NOS
   Excludes 1: acute kidney failure (N17.-)
    chronic kidney disease (N18.-)
    chronic uremia (N18.9)
    extrarenal uremia (R39.2)
    prerenal uremia (R39.2)
    renal insufficiency (acute) (N28.9)
    uremia of newborn (P96.0)

Urolithiasis (N20-N23)

N20- **Calculus of kidney and ureter**
   Calculous pyelonephritis
   Excludes 1: nephrocalcinosis (E83.5)
    that with hydronephrosis (N13.2)
 N20.0 **Calculus of kidney**
   Nephrolithiasis NOS
   Renal calculus
   Renal stone
   Staghorn calculus
   Stone in kidney
 N20.1 **Calculus of ureter**
   Ureteric stone
 N20.2 **Calculus of kidney with calculus of ureter**
 N20.9 **Urinary calculus, unspecified**
N21- **Calculus of lower urinary tract**
   Includes: Calculus of lower urinary tract with cystitis and urethritis
 N21.0 **Calculus in bladder**
   Calculus in diverticulum of bladder
   Urinary bladder stone
   Excludes❷: staghorn calculus (N20.0)
 N21.1 **Calculus in urethra**
   Excludes❷: calculus of prostate (N42.0)
 N21.8 **Other lower urinary tract calculus**
 N21.9 **Calculus of lower urinary tract, unspecified**
   Excludes 1: calculus of urinary tract NOS (N20.9)
N22 **Calculus of urinary tract <u>in diseases classified elsewhere</u>**
   Code first underlying disease, such as:
    Gout (M1A.-, M10.-)
    Schistosomiasis (B65.0-B65.9)
N23 **Unspecified renal colic**

Other disorders of kidney and ureter (N25-N29)

   Excludes❷: disorders of kidney and ureter with urolithiasis (N20-N23)
N25- **Disorders resulting from impaired renal tubular function**
   Excludes 1: metabolic disorders classifiable to E70-E88
 N25.0 **Renal osteodystrophy**
   Azotemic osteodystrophy
   Phosphate-losing tubular disorders
   Renal rickets
   Renal short stature
 N25.1 **Nephrogenic diabetes insipidus**
   Excludes 1: diabetes insipidus NOS (E23.2)
 N25.8- **Other disorders resulting from impaired renal tubular function**
  N25.81 **Secondary hyperparathyroidism of renal origin**
    Excludes 1: secondary hyperparathyroidism, non-renal (E21.1)
  N25.89 **Other disorders resulting from impaired renal tubular function**
    Hypokalemic nephropathy
    Lightwood-Albright syndrome
    Renal tubular acidosis NOS
 N25.9 **Disorder resulting from impaired renal tubular function, unspecified**
N26- **Unspecified contracted kidney**
   Excludes 1: contracted kidney due to hypertension (I12.-)
    diffuse sclerosing glomerulonephritis (N05.8.-)
    hypertensive nephrosclerosis (arteriolar) (arteriosclerotic) (I12.-)
    small kidney of unknown cause (N27.-)
 N26.1 **Atrophy of kidney (terminal)**
 N26.2 **Page kidney**
 N26.9 **Renal sclerosis, unspecified**

N
1
6
-
N
3
4

N27- Small kidney of unknown cause
   Includes: oligonephronia

N27.0   Small kidney, <u>unilateral</u>

N27.1   Small kidney, <u>bilateral</u>

N27.9   Small kidney, <u>unspecified</u>

N28- Other disorders of kidney and ureter, not elsewhere classified

N28.0   Ischemia and infarction of kidney
   Renal artery embolism
   Renal artery obstruction
   Renal artery occlusion
   Renal artery thrombosis
   Renal infarct
   Excludes 1: atherosclerosis of renal artery (extrarenal part) (I70.1)
             congenital stenosis of renal artery (Q27.1)
             Goldblatt's kidney (I70.1)

N28.1   Cyst of kidney, acquired
   Cyst (multiple) (solitary) of kidney, acquired
   Excludes 1: cystic kidney disease (congenital) (Q61.-)

N28.8- Other specified disorders of kidney and ureter
   Excludes 1: hydroureter (N13.4)
             ureteric stricture with hydronephrosis (N13.1)
             ureteric stricture without hydronephrosis (N13.5)

N28.81 Hypertrophy of kidney

N28.82 Megaloureter

N28.83 Nephroptosis

N28.84 Pyelitis cystica

N28.85 Pyeloureteritis cystica

N28.86 Ureteritis cystica

N28.89 Other specified disorders of kidney and ureter

N28.9   Disorder of kidney and ureter, unspecified
   Nephropathy NOS
   Renal disease (acute) NOS
   Renal insufficiency (acute)
   Excludes 1: chronic renal insufficiency (N18.9)
             unspecified nephritic syndrome (N05.-)

N29 Other disorders of kidney and ureter <u>in diseases classified elsewhere</u>
   Code first underlying disease, such as:
   Amyloidosis (E85.-)
   Nephrocalcinosis (E83.5)
   Schistosomiasis (B65.0-B65.9)
   Excludes 1: disorders of kidney and ureter in:
             cystinosis (E72.0)
             gonorrhea (A54.21)
             syphilis (A52.75)
             tuberculosis (A18.11)

Other diseases of the urinary system (N30-N39)

   Excludes 1: urinary infection (complicating):
             abortion or ectopic or molar pregnancy (O00-O07, O08.8)
             pregnancy, childbirth and the puerperium (O23.-, O75.3,
             O86.2-)

N30- <u>Cystitis</u>
   Use additional code to identify infectious agent (B95-B97)
   Excludes 1: prostatocystitis (N41.3)

N30.0- <u>Acute</u> cystitis
   Excludes 1: irradiation cystitis (N30.4-)
             trigonitis (N30.3-)

N30.00 Acute cystitis <u>without</u> hematuria

N30.01 Acute cystitis <u>with</u> hematuria

N30.1- <u>Interstitial</u> cystitis (chronic)

N30.10 Interstitial cystitis (chronic) <u>without</u> hematuria

N30.11 Interstitial cystitis (chronic) <u>with</u> hematuria

N30.2- Other chronic cystitis

N30.20 Other chronic cystitis <u>without</u> hematuria

N30.21 Other chronic cystitis <u>with</u> hematuria

N30.3- <u>Trigonitis</u>
   Urethrotrigonitis

N30.30 Trigonitis <u>without</u> hematuria

N30.31 Trigonitis <u>with</u> hematuria

N30.4- <u>Irradiation</u> cystitis

N30.40 Irradiation cystitis <u>without</u> hematuria

N30.41 Irradiation cystitis <u>with</u> hematuria

N30.8- <u>Other</u> cystitis
   Abscess of bladder

N30.80 Other cystitis <u>without</u> hematuria

N30.81 Other cystitis <u>with</u> hematuria

N30.9- Cystitis, <u>unspecified</u>

N30.90 Cystitis, unspecified <u>without</u> hematuria

N30.91 Cystitis, unspecified <u>with</u> hematuria

N31- Neuromuscular dysfunction of bladder, <u>not elsewhere classified</u>
   Use additional code to identify any associated urinary incontinence (N39.3-N39.4-)
   Excludes 1: cord bladder NOS (G95.89)
             neurogenic bladder due to cauda equina syndrome (G83.4)
             neuromuscular dysfunction due to spinal cord lesion (G95.89)

N31.0   Uninhibited neuropathic bladder, not elsewhere classified

N31.1   Reflex neuropathic bladder, not elsewhere classified

N31.2   Flaccid neuropathic bladder, not elsewhere classified
   Atonic (motor) (sensory) neuropathic bladder
   Autonomous neuropathic bladder
   Nonreflex neuropathic bladder

N31.8   Other neuromuscular dysfunction of bladder

N31.9   Neuromuscular dysfunction of bladder, unspecified
   Neurogenic bladder dysfunction NOS

N32- Other disorders of bladder
   Excludes❷: calculus of bladder (N21.0)
             cystocele (N81.1-)
             hernia or prolapse of bladder, female (N81.1-)

N32.0   Bladder-neck obstruction
   Bladder-neck stenosis (acquired)
   Excludes 1: congenital bladder-neck obstruction (Q64.3-)

N32.1   Vesicointestinal fistula
   Vesicorectal fistula

N32.2   Vesical fistula, not elsewhere classified
   Excludes 1: fistula between bladder and female genital tract
             (N82.0-N82.1)

N32.3   Diverticulum of bladder
   Excludes 1: congenital diverticulum of bladder (Q64.6)
             diverticulitis of bladder (N30.8-)

N32.8- Other specified disorders of bladder

N32.81 Overactive bladder
   Detrusor muscle hyperactivity
   Excludes 1: frequent urination due to specified bladder
             condition — code to condition

N32.89 Other specified disorders of bladder
   Bladder hemorrhage
   Bladder hypertrophy
   Calcified bladder
   Contracted bladder

N32.9   Bladder disorder, unspecified

N33 Bladder disorders <u>in diseases classified elsewhere</u>
   Code first underlying disease, such as:
   Schistosomiasis (B65.0-B65.9)
   Excludes 1: bladder disorder in syphilis (A52.76)
             bladder disorder in tuberculosis (A18.12)
             candidal cystitis (B37.41)
             chlamydial cystitis (A56.01)
             cystitis in gonorrhea (A54.01)
             cystitis in neurogenic bladder (N31.-)
             diphtheritic cystitis (A36.85)
             syphilitic cystitis (A52.76)
             trichomonal cystitis (A59.03)

N34- Urethritis and urethral syndrome
   Use additional code (B95-B97), to identify infectious agent
   Excludes❷: Reiter's disease (M02.3-)
             urethritis in diseases with a predominantly sexual mode of
             transmission (A50-A64)
             urethrotrigonitis (N30.3-)

N34.0   Urethral abscess
   Abscess (of) Cowper's gland
   Abscess (of) Littré's gland
   Abscess (of) urethral (gland)
   Periurethral abscess
   Excludes 1: urethral caruncle (N36.2)

N34.1   Nonspecific urethritis
   Nongonococcal urethritis
   Nonvenereal urethritis

N34.2   Other urethritis
   Meatitis, urethral
   Postmenopausal urethritis
   Ulcer of urethra (meatus)
   Urethritis NOS

N34.3   Urethral syndrome, unspecified

N
1
6
I
N
3
4

Excludes 1: = NOT CODED HERE! (Do not code both)

Excludes❷: = Not Included Here

N35- Urethral stricture
Excludes 1: congenital urethral stricture (Q64.3-)
postprocedural urethral stricture (N99.1-)

N35.0- Post-traumatic urethral stricture
Urethral stricture due to injury
Excludes 1: postprocedural urethral stricture (N99.1-)

N35.01- Post-traumatic urethral stricture, male
N35.010 Post-traumatic urethral stricture, male, meatal
N35.011 Post-traumatic bulbous urethral stricture
N35.012 Post-traumatic membranous urethral stricture
N35.013 Post-traumatic anterior urethral stricture
N35.014 Post-traumatic urethral stricture, male, unspecified

N35.02- Post-traumatic urethral stricture, female
N35.021 Urethral stricture due to childbirth
N35.028 Other post-traumatic urethral stricture, female

N35.1- Postinfective urethral stricture, not elsewhere classified
Excludes 1: urethral stricture associated with schistosomiasis (B65.-, N29)
gonococcal urethral stricture (A54.01)
syphilitic urethral stricture (A52.76)

N35.11- Postinfective urethral stricture, not elsewhere classified, male
N35.111 Postinfective urethral stricture, not elsewhere classified, male, meatal
N35.112 Postinfective bulbous urethral stricture, not elsewhere classified
N35.113 Postinfective membranous urethral stricture, not elsewhere classified
N35.114 Postinfective anterior urethral stricture, not elsewhere classified
N35.119 Postinfective urethral stricture, not elsewhere classified, male, unspecified

N35.12 Postinfective urethral stricture, not elsewhere classified, female

N35.8 Other urethral stricture
Excludes 1: postprocedural urethral stricture (N99.1-)

N35.9 Urethral stricture, unspecified

N36- Other disorders of urethra
N36.0 Urethral fistula
Urethroperineal fistula
Urethrorectal fistula
Urinary fistula NOS
Excludes 1: urethroscrotal fistula (N50.8)
urethrovaginal fistula (N82.1)
urethrovesicovaginal fistula (N82.1)

N36.1 Urethral diverticulum
N36.2 Urethral caruncle
N36.4- Urethral functional and muscular disorders
Use additional code to identify associated urinary stress incontinence (N39.3)
N36.41 Hypermobility of urethra
N36.42 Intrinsic sphincter deficiency (ISD)
N36.43 Combined hypermobility of urethra and intrinsic sphincter deficiency
N36.44 Muscular disorders of urethra
Bladder sphincter dyssynergy
N36.5 Urethral false passage
N36.8 Other specified disorders of urethra
N36.9 Urethral disorder, unspecified

N37 Urethral disorders in diseases classified elsewhere
Code first underlying disease
Excludes 1: urethritis (in):
candidal infection (B37.41)
chlamydial (A56.01)
gonorrhea (A54.01)
syphilis (A52.76)
trichomonal infection (A59.03)
tuberculosis (A18.13)

N39- Other disorders of urinary system
Excludes❷: hematuria NOS (R31.-)
recurrent or persistent hematuria (N02.-)
recurrent or persistent hematuria with specified morphological lesion (N02.-)
proteinuria NOS (R80.-)

N39.0 Urinary tract infection, site not specified
Use additional code (B95-B97), to identify infectious agent.
Excludes 1: candidiasis of urinary tract (B37.4-)
neonatal urinary tract infection (P39.3)
urinary tract infection of specified site, such as:
cystitis (N30.-)
urethritis (N34.-)

N39.3 Stress incontinence (female) (male)
Code also any associated overactive bladder (N32.81)
Excludes 1: mixed incontinence (N39.46)

N39.4- Other specified urinary incontinence
Code also any associated overactive bladder (N32.81)
Excludes 1: enuresis NOS (R32)
functional urinary incontinence (R39.81)
urinary incontinence associated with cognitive impairment (R39.81)
urinary incontinence NOS (R32)
urinary incontinence of nonorganic origin (F98.0)

N39.41 Urge incontinence
Excludes 1: mixed incontinence (N39.46)
N39.42 Incontinence without sensory awareness
N39.43 Post-void dribbling
N39.44 Nocturnal enuresis
N39.45 Continuous leakage
N39.46 Mixed incontinence
Urge and stress incontinence
N39.49- Other specified urinary incontinence
N39.490 Overflow incontinence
N39.498 Other specified urinary incontinence
Reflex incontinence
Total incontinence

N39.8 Other specified disorders of urinary system
N39.9 Disorder of urinary system, unspecified

Diseases of male genital organs (N40-N53)

N40- Enlarged prostate
Includes: Adenofibromatous hypertrophy of prostate
Benign hypertrophy of the prostate
Benign prostatic hyperplasia
Benign prostatic hypertrophy
BPH
Nodular prostate
Polyp of prostate
Excludes 1: benign neoplasms of prostate (adenoma, benign) (fibroadenoma) (fibroma) (myoma) (D29.1)
Excludes❷: malignant neoplasm of prostate (C61)

N40.0 Enlarged prostate without lower urinary tract symptoms
Enlarged prostate NOS
Enlarged prostate without LUTS

N40.1 Enlarged prostate with lower urinary tract symptoms
Enlarged prostate with LUTS
Use additional code for associated symptoms, when specified:
Incomplete bladder emptying (R39.14)
Nocturia (R35.1)
Straining on urination (R39.16)
Urinary frequency (R35.0)
Urinary hesitancy (R39.11)
Urinary incontinence (N39.4-)
Urinary obstruction (N13.8)
Urinary retention (R33.8)
Urinary urgency (R39.15)
Weak urinary stream (R39.12)

N40.2 Nodular prostate without lower urinary tract symptoms
Nodular prostate without LUTS

N40.3 Nodular prostate with lower urinary tract symptoms
Use additional code for associated symptoms, when specified:
Incomplete bladder emptying (R39.14)
Nocturia (R35.1)
Straining on urination (R39.16)
Urinary frequency (R35.0)
Urinary hesitancy (R39.11)
Urinary incontinence (N39.4-)
Urinary obstruction (N13.8)
Urinary retention (R33.8)
Urinary urgency (R39.15)
Weak urinary stream (R39.12)

N
3
5
-
N
4
8

N41-   Inflammatory diseases of prostate
Use additional code (B95-B97), to identify infectious agent

N41.0   Acute prostatitis

N41.1   Chronic prostatitis

N41.2   Abscess of prostate

N41.3   Prostatocystitis

N41.4   Granulomatous prostatitis

N41.8   Other inflammatory diseases of prostate

N41.9   Inflammatory disease of prostate, unspecified
Prostatitis NOS

N42-   Other and unspecified disorders of prostate

N42.0   Calculus of prostate
Prostatic stone

N42.1   Congestion and hemorrhage of prostate
Excludes 1:   enlarged prostate (N40.-)
              hematuria (R31.-)
              hyperplasia of prostate (N40.-)
              inflammatory diseases of prostate (N41.-)

N42.3   Dysplasia of prostate
Prostatic intraepithelial neoplasia I (PIN I)
Prostatic intraepithelial neoplasia II (PIN II)
Excludes 1:   prostatic intraepithelial neoplasia III (PIN III) (D07.5)

N42.8-   Other specified disorders of prostate

N42.81   Prostatodynia syndrome
Painful prostate syndrome

N42.82   Prostatosis syndrome

N42.83   Cyst of prostate

N42.89   Other specified disorders of prostate

N42.9   Disorder of prostate, unspecified

N43-   Hydrocele and spermatocele
Includes: Hydrocele of spermatic cord, testis or tunica vaginalis
Excludes 1:   congenital hydrocele (P83.5)

N43.0   Encysted hydrocele

N43.1   Infected hydrocele
Use additional code (B95-B97), to identify infectious agent

N43.2   Other hydrocele

N43.3   Hydrocele, unspecified

N43.4-   Spermatocele of epididymis
Spermatic cyst

N43.40   Spermatocele of epididymis, unspecified

N43.41   Spermatocele of epididymis, single

N43.42   Spermatocele of epididymis, multiple

N44-   Noninflammatory disorders of testis

N44.0-   Torsion of testis

N44.00   Torsion of testis, unspecified

N44.01   Extravaginal torsion of spermatic cord

N44.02   Intravaginal torsion of spermatic cord
Torsion of spermatic cord NOS

N44.03   Torsion of appendix testis

N44.04   Torsion of appendix epididymis

N44.1   Cyst of tunica albuginea testis

N44.2   Benign cyst of testis

N44.8   Other noninflammatory disorders of the testis

N45-   Orchitis and epididymitis
Use additional code (B95-B97), to identify infectious agent.

N45.1   Epididymitis

N45.2   Orchitis

N45.3   Epididymo-orchitis

N45.4   Abscess of epididymis or testis

N46-   Male infertility
Excludes 1:   vasectomy status (Z98.52)

N46.0-   Azoospermia
Absolute male infertility
Male infertility due to germinal (cell) aplasia
Male infertility due to spermatogenic arrest (complete)

N46.01   Organic azoospermia
Azoospermia NOS

N46.02-   Azoospermia due to extratesticular causes
Code also associated cause

N46.021   Azoospermia due to drug therapy

N46.022   Azoospermia due to infection

N46.023   Azoospermia due to obstruction of efferent ducts

N46.024   Azoospermia due to radiation

N46.025   Azoospermia due to systemic disease

N46.029   Azoospermia due to other extratesticular causes

N46.1-   Oligospermia
Male infertility due to germinal cell desquamation
Male infertility due to hypospermatogenesis
Male infertility due to incomplete spermatogenic arrest

N46.11   Organic oligospermia
Oligospermia NOS

N46.12-   Oligospermia due to extratesticular causes
Code also associated cause

N46.121   Oligospermia due to drug therapy

N46.122   Oligospermia due to infection

N46.123   Oligospermia due to obstruction of efferent ducts

N46.124   Oligospermia due to radiation

N46.125   Oligospermia due to systemic disease

N46.129   Oligospermia due to other extratesticular causes

N46.8   Other male infertility

N46.9   Male infertility, unspecified

N47-   Disorders of prepuce

N47.0   Adherent prepuce, newborn

N47.1   Phimosis

N47.2   Paraphimosis

N47.3   Deficient foreskin

N47.4   Benign cyst of prepuce

N47.5   Adhesions of prepuce and glans penis

N47.6   Balanoposthitis
Use additional code (B95-B97), to identify infectious agent
Excludes 1:   balanitis (N48.1)

N47.7   Other inflammatory diseases of prepuce
Use additional code (B95-B97), to identify infectious agent

N47.8   Other disorders of prepuce

N48-   Other disorders of penis

N48.0   Leukoplakia of penis
Balanitis xerotica obliterans
Kraurosis of penis
Lichen sclerosus of external male genital organs
Excludes 1:   carcinoma in situ of penis (D07.4)

N48.1   Balanitis
Use additional code (B95-B97), to identify infectious agent
Excludes 1:   amebic balanitis (A06.8)
              balanitis xerotica obliterans (N48.0)
              candidal balanitis (B37.42)
              gonococcal balanitis (A54.23)
              herpesviral [herpes simplex] balanitis (A60.01)

N48.2-   Other inflammatory disorders of penis
Use additional code (B95-B97), to identify infectious agent.
Excludes 1:   balanitis (N48.1)
              balanitis xerotica obliterans (N48.0)
              balanoposthitis (N47.6)

N48.21   Abscess of corpus cavernosum and penis

N48.22   Cellulitis of corpus cavernosum and penis

N48.29   Other inflammatory disorders of penis

N48.3-   Priapism
Painful erection
Code first underlying cause

N48.30   Priapism, unspecified

N48.31   Priapism due to trauma

N48.32   Priapism due to disease classified elsewhere

N48.33   Priapism, drug-induced

N48.39   Other priapism

N48.5   Ulcer of penis

N48.6   Induration penis plastica
Peyronie's disease
Plastic induration of penis

N48.8-   Other specified disorders of penis

N48.81   Thrombosis of superficial vein of penis

N48.82   Acquired torsion of penis
Acquired torsion of penis NOS
Excludes 1:   congenital torsion of penis (Q55.63)

N48.83   Acquired buried penis
Excludes 1:   congenital hidden penis (Q55.64)

N48.89   Other specified disorders of penis

N48.9   Disorder of penis, unspecified

N35 - N48

Excludes 1: = NOT CODED HERE! (Do not code both)

Excludes❷: = Not Included Here

N49- Inflammatory disorders of male genital organs, <u>not elsewhere classified</u>
Use additional code (B95-B97), to identify infectious agent
Excludes 1: inflammation of penis (N48.1, N48.2-)
orchitis and epididymitis (N45.-)

N49.0   Inflammatory disorders of seminal vesicle
Vesiculitis NOS

N49.1   Inflammatory disorders of spermatic cord, tunica vaginalis and vas deferens
Vasitis

N49.2   Inflammatory disorders of scrotum

N49.3   Fournier gangrene

N49.8   Inflammatory disorders of other specified male genital organs
Inflammation of multiple sites in male genital organs

N49.9   Inflammatory disorder of unspecified male genital organ
Abscess of unspecified male genital organ
Boil of unspecified male genital organ
Carbuncle of unspecified male genital organ
Cellulitis of unspecified male genital organ

N50- Other and unspecified disorders of male genital organs
Excludes❷: torsion of testis (N44.0-)

N50.0   Atrophy of testis

N50.1   Vascular disorders of male genital organs
Hematocele, NOS, of male genital organs
Hemorrhage of male genital organs
Thrombosis of male genital organs

N50.3   Cyst of epididymis

N50.8   Other specified disorders of male genital organs
Atrophy of scrotum, seminal vesicle, spermatic cord, tunica vaginalis and vas deferens
Chylocele, tunica vaginalis (nonfilarial) NOS
Edema of scrotum, seminal vesicle, spermatic cord, testis, tunica vaginalis and vas deferens
Hypertrophy of scrotum, seminal vesicle, spermatic cord, testis, tunica vaginalis and vas deferens
Stricture of spermatic cord, tunica vaginalis, and vas deferens
Ulcer of scrotum, seminal vesicle, spermatic cord, testis, tunica vaginalis and vas deferens
Urethroscrotal fistula

N50.9   Disorder of male genital organs, unspecified

N51   Disorders of male genital organs <u>in diseases classified elsewhere</u>
Code first underlying disease, such as:
Filariasis (B74.0-B74.9)
Excludes 1: amebic balanitis (A06.8)
candidal balanitis (B37.42)
gonococcal balanitis (A54.23)
gonococcal prostatitis (A54.22)
herpesviral [herpes simplex] balanitis (A60.01)
trichomonal prostatitis (A59.02)
tuberculous prostatitis (A18.14)

N52- <u>Male erectile dysfunction</u>
Excludes 1: psychogenic impotence (F52.21)

N52.0- <u>Vasculogenic</u> erectile dysfunction
N52.01   Erectile dysfunction due to arterial insufficiency
N52.02   Corporo-venous occlusive erectile dysfunction
N52.03   Combined arterial insufficiency and corporo-venous occlusive erectile dysfunction

N52.1   Erectile dysfunction <u>due to diseases classified elsewhere</u>
Code first underlying disease

N52.2   Drug-induced erectile dysfunction

N52.3- Post-surgical erectile dysfunction
N52.31   Erectile dysfunction following radical prostatectomy
N52.32   Erectile dysfunction following radical cystectomy
N52.33   Erectile dysfunction following urethral surgery
N52.34   Erectile dysfunction following simple prostatectomy
N52.39   Other post-surgical erectile dysfunction

N52.8   <u>Other</u> male erectile dysfunction

N52.9   Male erectile dysfunction, <u>unspecified</u>
Impotence NOS

N53- Other male sexual dysfunction
Excludes 1: psychogenic sexual dysfunction (F52.-)

N53.1- Ejaculatory dysfunction
Excludes 1: premature ejaculation (F52.4)
N53.11   Retarded ejaculation
N53.12   Painful ejaculation
N53.13   Anejaculatory orgasm
N53.14   Retrograde ejaculation
N53.19   Other ejaculatory dysfunction
Ejaculatory dysfunction NOS

N53.8   Other male sexual dysfunction

N53.9   Unspecified male sexual dysfunction

Disorders of breast (N60-N65)

Excludes 1: disorders of breast associated with childbirth (O91-O92)

N60- Benign mammary dysplasia
Includes: Fibrocystic mastopathy

N60.0- <u>Solitary cyst</u> of breast
Cyst of breast
N60.01   Solitary cyst of <u>right</u> breast
N60.02   Solitary cyst of <u>left</u> breast
N60.09   Solitary cyst of <u>unspecified</u> breast

N60.1- <u>Diffuse cystic mastopathy</u>
Cystic breast
Fibrocystic disease of breast
Excludes 1: diffuse cystic mastopathy with epithelial proliferation (N60.3-)
N60.11   Diffuse cystic mastopathy of <u>right</u> breast
N60.12   Diffuse cystic mastopathy of <u>left</u> breast
N60.19   Diffuse cystic mastopathy of <u>unspecified</u> breast

N60.2- <u>Fibroadenosis</u> of breast
Adenofibrosis of breast
Excludes❷: fibroadenoma of breast (D24.-)
N60.21   Fibroadenosis of <u>right</u> breast
N60.22   Fibroadenosis of <u>left</u> breast
N60.29   Fibroadenosis of <u>unspecified</u> breast

N60.3- <u>Fibrosclerosis</u> of breast
Cystic mastopathy with epithelial proliferation
N60.31   Fibrosclerosis of <u>right</u> breast
N60.32   Fibrosclerosis of <u>left</u> breast
N60.39   Fibrosclerosis of unspecified breast

N60.4- <u>Mammary duct ectasia</u>
N60.41   Mammary duct ectasia of <u>right</u> breast
N60.42   Mammary duct ectasia of <u>left</u> breast
N60.49   Mammary duct ectasia of <u>unspecified</u> breast

N60.8- <u>Other</u> benign mammary dysplasias
N60.81   Other benign mammary dysplasias of <u>right</u> breast
N60.82   Other benign mammary dysplasias of <u>left</u> breast
N60.89   Other benign mammary dysplasias of <u>unspecified</u> breast

N60.9- <u>Unspecified</u> benign mammary dysplasia
N60.91   Unspecified benign mammary dysplasia of <u>right</u> breast
N60.92   Unspecified benign mammary dysplasia of <u>left</u> breast
N60.99   Unspecified benign mammary dysplasia of unspecified breast

N61   Inflammatory disorders of breast
Abscess (acute) (chronic) (nonpuerperal) of areola
Abscess (acute) (chronic) (nonpuerperal) of breast
Carbuncle of breast
Infective mastitis (acute) (subacute) (nonpuerperal)
Mastitis (acute) (subacute) (nonpuerperal) NOS
Excludes 1: inflammatory carcinoma of breast (C50.9)
inflammatory disorder of breast associated with childbirth (O91.-)
neonatal infective mastitis (P39.0)
thrombophlebitis of breast [Mondor's disease] (I80.8)

N62   Hypertrophy of breast
Gynecomastia
Hypertrophy of breast NOS
Massive pubertal hypertrophy of breast
Excludes 1: breast engorgement of newborn (P83.4)
disproportion of reconstructed breast (N65.1)

N63   Unspecified lump in breast
Nodule(s) NOS in breast

N64- Other disorders of breast
Excludes❷: mechanical complication of breast prosthesis and implant (T85.4-)
N64.0   Fissure and fistula of nipple
N64.1   Fat necrosis of breast
Fat necrosis (segmental) of breast
Code first breast necrosis due to breast graft (T85.89)
N64.2   Atrophy of breast
N64.3   Galactorrhea not associated with childbirth
N64.4   Mastodynia

N64.5-   Other signs and symptoms in breast
Excludes❷: abnormal findings on diagnostic imaging of breast (R92.-)

N64.51 Induration of breast
N64.52 Nipple discharge
Excludes 1: abnormal findings in nipple discharge (R89.-)
N64.53 Retraction of nipple
N64.59 Other signs and symptoms in breast
N64.8-   Other specified disorders of breast
N64.81 Ptosis of breast
Excludes 1: ptosis of native breast in relation to reconstructed breast (N65.1)
N64.82 Hypoplasia of breast
Micromastia
Excludes 1: congenital absence of breast (Q83.0)
hypoplasia of native breast in relation to reconstructed breast (N65.1)
N64.89 Other specified disorders of breast
Galactocele
Subinvolution of breast (postlactational)
N64.9   Disorder of breast, unspecified
N65- Deformity and disproportion of reconstructed breast
N65.0   Deformity of reconstructed breast
Contour irregularity in reconstructed breast
Excess tissue in reconstructed breast
Misshapen reconstructed breast
N65.1   Disproportion of reconstructed breast
Breast asymmetry between native breast and reconstructed breast
Disproportion between native breast and reconstructed breast

Inflammatory diseases of female pelvic organs (N70-N77)

Excludes 1: inflammatory diseases of female pelvic organs complicating:
abortion or ectopic or molar pregnancy (O00-O07, O08.0)
pregnancy, childbirth and the puerperium (O23.-, O75.3, O85, O86.-)

N70-   Salpingitis and oophoritis
Includes: Abscess (of) fallopian tube
Abscess (of) ovary
Pyosalpinx
Salpingo-oophoritis
Tubo-ovarian abscess
Tubo-ovarian inflammatory disease
Use additional code (B95-B97), to identify infectious agent
Excludes 1: gonococcal infection (A54.24)
tuberculous infection (A18.17)

N70.0-   Acute salpingitis and oophoritis
N70.01 Acute salpingitis
N70.02 Acute oophoritis
N70.03 Acute salpingitis and oophoritis
N70.1-   Chronic salpingitis and oophoritis
Hydrosalpinx
N70.11 Chronic salpingitis
N70.12 Chronic oophoritis
N70.13 Chronic salpingitis and oophoritis
N70.9-   Salpingitis and oophoritis, unspecified
N70.91 Salpingitis, unspecified
N70.92 Oophoritis, unspecified
N70.93 Salpingitis and oophoritis, unspecified
N71-   Inflammatory disease of uterus, except cervix
Includes: Endo (myo) metritis
Metritis
Myometritis
Pyometra
Uterine abscess
Use additional code (B95-B97), to identify infectious agent
Excludes 1: hyperplastic endometritis (N85.0-)
infection of uterus following delivery (O85, O86.-)
N71.0   Acute inflammatory disease of uterus
N71.1   Chronic inflammatory disease of uterus
N71.9   Inflammatory disease of uterus, unspecified

N72   Inflammatory disease of cervix uteri
Includes: Cervicitis (with or without erosion or ectropion)
Endocervicitis (with or without erosion or ectropion)
Exocervicitis (with or without erosion or ectropion)
Use additional code (B95-B97), to identify infectious agent
Excludes 1: erosion and ectropion of cervix without cervicitis (N86)

N73-   Other female pelvic inflammatory diseases
Use additional code (B95-B97), to identify infectious agent
N73.0   Acute parametritis and pelvic cellulitis
Abscess of broad ligament
Abscess of parametrium
Pelvic cellulitis, female
N73.1   Chronic parametritis and pelvic cellulitis
Any condition in N73.0 specified as chronic
Excludes 1: tuberculous parametritis and pelvic cellultis (A18.17)
N73.2   Unspecified parametritis and pelvic cellulitis
Any condition in N73.0 unspecified whether acute or chronic
N73.3   Female acute pelvic peritonitis
N73.4   Female chronic pelvic peritonitis
Excludes 1: tuberculous pelvic (female) peritonitis (A18.17)
N73.5   Female pelvic peritonitis, unspecified
N73.6   Female pelvic peritoneal adhesions (postinfective)
Excludes❷: postprocedural pelvic peritoneal adhesions (N99.4)
N73.8   Other specified female pelvic inflammatory diseases
N73.9   Female pelvic inflammatory disease, unspecified
Female pelvic infection or inflammation NOS
N74   Female pelvic inflammatory disorders in diseases classified elsewhere
Code first underlying disease
Excludes 1: chlamydial cervicitis (A56.02)
chlamydial pelvic inflammatory disease (A56.11)
gonococcal cervicitis (A54.03)
gonococcal pelvic inflammatory disease (A54.24)
herpesviral [herpes simplex] cervicitis (A60.03)
herpesviral [herpes simplex] pelvic inflammatory disease (A60.09)
syphilitic cervicitis (A52.76)
syphilitic pelvic inflammatory disease (A52.76)
trichomonal cervicitis (A59.09)
tuberculous cervicitis (A18.16)
tuberculous pelvic inflammatory disease (A18.17)
N75- Diseases of Bartholin's gland
N75.0   Cyst of Bartholin's gland
N75.1   Abscess of Bartholin's gland
N75.8   Other diseases of Bartholin's gland
Bartholinitis
N75.9   Disease of Bartholin's gland, unspecified
N76- Other inflammation of vagina and vulva
Use additional code (B95-B97), to identify infectious agent
Excludes❷: senile (atrophic) vaginitis (N95.2)
vulvar vestibulitis (N94.810)
N76.0   Acute vaginitis
Acute vulvovaginitis
Vaginitis NOS
Vulvovaginitis NOS
N76.1   Subacute and chronic vaginitis
Chronic vulvovaginitis
Subacute vulvovaginitis
N76.2   Acute vulvitis
Vulvitis NOS
N76.3   Subacute and chronic vulvitis
N76.4   Abscess of vulva
Furuncle of vulva
N76.5   Ulceration of vagina
N76.6   Ulceration of vulva
N76.8-   Other specified inflammation of vagina and vulva
N76.81 Mucositis (ulcerative) of vagina and vulva
Code also type of associated therapy, such as:
Antineoplastic and immunosuppressive drugs (T45.1x-)
Radiological procedure and radiotherapy (Y84.2)
Excludes❷: gastrointestinal mucositis (ulcerative) (K92.81)
nasal mucositis (ulcerative) (J34.81)
oral mucositis (ulcerative) (K12.3-)
N76.89 Other specified inflammation of vagina and vulva

Excludes 1: = NOT CODED HERE! (Do not code both)   **617**   *Excludes❷:* = Not Included Here

N77- Vulvovaginal ulceration and inflammation <u>in diseases classified elsewhere</u>

N77.0 Ulceration of vulva in diseases classified elsewhere
Code first underlying disease, such as:
Behçet's disease (M35.2)
Excludes 1: ulceration of vulva in gonococcal infection (A54.02)
ulceration of vulva in herpesviral [herpes simplex]
infection (A60.04)
ulceration of vulva in syphilis (A51.0)
ulceration of vulva in tuberculosis (A18.18)

N77.1 Vaginitis, vulvitis and vulvovaginitis in diseases classified elsewhere
Code first underlying disease, such as:
Pinworm (B80)
Excludes 1: candidal vulvovaginitis (B37.3)
chlamydial vulvovaginitis (A56.02)
gonococcal vulvovaginitis (A54.02)
herpesviral [herpes simplex] vulvovaginitis (A60.04)
trichomonal vulvovaginitis (A59.01)
tuberculous vulvovaginitis (A18.18)
vulvovaginitis in early syphilis (A51.0)
vulvovaginitis in late syphilis (A52.76)

Noninflammatory disorders of female genital tract (N80-N98)

N80- Endometriosis

N80.0 Endometriosis of uterus
Adenomyosis
Excludes 1: stromal endometriosis (D39.0)

N80.1 Endometriosis of ovary

N80.2 Endometriosis of fallopian tube

N80.3 Endometriosis of pelvic peritoneum

N80.4 Endometriosis of rectovaginal septum and vagina

N80.5 Endometriosis of intestine

N80.6 Endometriosis in cutaneous scar

N80.8 Other endometriosis

N80.9 Endometriosis, unspecified

N81- <u>Female genital prolapse</u>
Excludes 1: genital prolapse complicating pregnancy, labor or delivery
(O34.5-)
prolapse and hernia of ovary and fallopian tube (N83.4)
prolapse of vaginal vault after hysterectomy (N99.3)

N81.0 Urethrocele
Excludes 1: urethrocele with cystocele (N81.1-)
urethrocele with prolapse of uterus (N81.2-N81.4)

N81.1- Cystocele
Cystocele with urethrocele
Cystourethrocele
Excludes 1: cystocele with prolapse of uterus (N81.2-N81.4)

N81.10 Cystocele, unspecified
Prolapse of (anterior) vaginal wall NOS

N81.11 Cystocele, midline

N81.12 Cystocele, lateral
Paravaginal cystocele

N81.2 Incomplete uterovaginal prolapse
First degree uterine prolapse
Prolapse of cervix NOS
Second degree uterine prolapse
Excludes 1: cervical stump prolaspe (N81.85)

N81.3 Complete uterovaginal prolapse
Procidentia (uteri) NOS
Third degree uterine prolapse

N81.4 Uterovaginal prolapse, unspecified
Prolapse of uterus NOS

N81.5 Vaginal enterocele
Excludes 1: enterocele with prolapse of uterus (N81.2-N81.4)

N81.6 Rectocele
Prolapse of posterior vaginal wall
Use additional code for any associated fecal incontinence, if
applicable (R15.-)
Excludes❷: perineocele (N81.81)
rectal prolapse (K62.3)
rectocele with prolapse of uterus (N81.2-N81.4)

N81.8- Other female genital prolapse

N81.81 Perineocele

N81.82 Incompetence or weakening of pubocervical tissue

N81.83 Incompetence or weakening of rectovaginal tissue

N81.84 Pelvic muscle wasting
Disuse atrophy of pelvic muscles and anal sphincter

N81.85 Cervical stump prolapse

N81.89 Other female genital prolapse
Deficient perineum
Old laceration of muscles of pelvic floor

N81.9 Female genital prolapse, unspecified

N82- Fistulae involving female genital tract
Excludes 1: vesicointestinal fistulae (N32.1)

N82.0 Vesicovaginal fistula

N82.1 Other female urinary-genital tract fistulae
Cervicovesical fistula
Ureterovaginal fistula
Urethrovaginal fistula
Uteroureteric fistula
Uterovesical fistula

N82.2 Fistula of vagina to small intestine

N82.3 Fistula of vagina to large intestine
Rectovaginal fistula

N82.4 Other female intestinal-genital tract fistulae
Intestinouterine fistula

N82.5 Female genital tract-skin fistulae
Uterus to abdominal wall fistula
Vaginoperineal fistula

N82.8 Other female genital tract fistulae

N82.9 Female genital tract fistula, unspecified

N83- Noninflammatory disorders of ovary, fallopian tube and broad ligament
Excludes❷: hydrosalpinx (N70.1-)

N83.0 Follicular cyst of ovary
Cyst of graafian follicle
Hemorrhagic follicular cyst (of ovary)

N83.1 Corpus luteum cyst
Hemorrhagic corpus luteum cyst

N83.2- Other and unspecified ovarian cysts
Excludes 1: developmental ovarian cyst (Q50.1)
neoplastic ovarian cyst (D27.-)
polycystic ovarian syndrome (E28.2)
Stein-Leventhal syndrome (E28.2)

N83.20 Unspecified ovarian cysts

N83.29 Other ovarian cysts
Retention cyst of ovary
Simple cyst of ovary

N83.3- Acquired atrophy of ovary and fallopian tube

N83.31 Acquired atrophy of ovary

N83.32 Acquired atrophy of fallopian tube

N83.33 Acquired atrophy of ovary and fallopian tube

N83.4 Prolapse and hernia of ovary and fallopian tube

N83.5- Torsion of ovary, ovarian pedicle and fallopian tube
Torsion of accessory tube

N83.51 Torsion of ovary and ovarian pedicle

N83.52 Torsion of fallopian tube
Torsion of hydatid of Morgagni

N83.53 Torsion of ovary, ovarian pedicle and fallopian tube

N83.6 Hematosalpinx
Excludes 1: hematosalpinx (with) (in):
hematocolpos (N89.7)
hematometra (N85.7)
tubal pregnancy (O00.1)

N83.7 Hematoma of broad ligament

N83.8 Other noninflammatory disorders of ovary, fallopian tube and broad ligament
Broad ligament laceration syndrome [Allen-Masters]

N83.9 Noninflammatory disorder of ovary, fallopian tube and broad ligament, unspecified

N84- Polyp of female genital tract
Excludes 1: adenomatous polyp (D28.-)
placental polyp (O90.89)

N84.0 Polyp of corpus uteri
Polyp of endometrium
Polyp of uterus NOS
Excludes 1: polypoid endometrial hyperplasia (N85.0-)

N84.1 Polyp of cervix uteri
Mucous polyp of cervix

N84.2 Polyp of vagina

N84.3 Polyp of vulva
Polyp of labia

N84.8 Polyp of other parts of female genital tract

N84.9 Polyp of female genital tract, unspecified

N85- Other noninflammatory disorders of uterus, except cervix
Excludes 1: endometriosis (N80.-)
inflammatory diseases of uterus (N71.-)
noninflammatory disorders of cervix, except malposition
(N86-N88)
polyp of corpus uteri (N84.0)
uterine prolapse (N81.-)

N85.0- Endometrial hyperplasia

N85.00 Endometrial hyperplasia, unspecified
Hyperplasia (adenomatous) (cystic) (glandular) of
endometrium
Hyperplastic endometritis

N85.01 Benign endometrial hyperplasia
Endometrial hyperplasia (complex) (simple) without atypia

N85.02 Endometrial intraepithelial neoplasia [EIN]
Endometrial hyperplasia with atypia
Excludes 1: malignant neoplasm of endometrium (with
endometrial intraepithelial neoplasia [EIN])
(C54.1)

N85.2 Hypertrophy of uterus
Bulky or enlarged uterus
Excludes 1: puerperal hypertrophy of uterus (O90.89)

N85.3 Subinvolution of uterus
Excludes 1: puerperal subinvolution of uterus (O90.89)

N85.4 Malposition of uterus
Anteversion of uterus
Retroflexion of uterus
Retroversion of uterus
Excludes 1: malposition of uterus complicating pregnancy, labor or
delivery (O34.5-, O65.5)

N85.5 Inversion of uterus
Excludes 1: current obstetric trauma (O71.2)
postpartum inversion of uterus (O71.2)

N85.6 Intrauterine synechiae

N85.7 Hematometra
Hematosalpinx with hematometra
Excludes 1: hematometra with hematocolpos (N89.7)

N85.8 Other specified noninflammatory disorders of uterus
Atrophy of uterus, acquired
Fibrosis of uterus NOS

N85.9 Noninflammatory disorder of uterus, unspecified
Disorder of uterus NOS

N86 Erosion and ectropion of cervix uteri
Decubitus (trophic) ulcer of cervix
Eversion of cervix
Excludes 1: erosion and ectropion of cervix with cervicitis (N72)

N87- <u>Dysplasia of cervix uteri</u>
Excludes 1: abnormal results from cervical cytological examination without
histologic confirmation (R87.61-)
carcinoma in situ of cervix uteri (D06.-)
cervical intraepithelial neoplasia III [CIN III] (D06.-)
HGSIL of cervix (R87.613)
severe dysplasia of cervix uteri (D06.-)

N87.0 <u>Mild</u> cervical dysplasia
Cervical intraepithelial neoplasia I [CIN I]

N87.1 <u>Moderate</u> cervical dysplasia
Cervical intraepithelial neoplasia II [CIN II]

N87.9 Dysplasia of cervix uteri, <u>unspecified</u>
Anaplasia of cervix
Cervical atypism
Cervical dysplasia NOS

N88- Other noninflammatory disorders of cervix uteri
Excludes ❷: inflammatory disease of cervix (N72)
polyp of cervix (N84.1)

N88.0 Leukoplakia of cervix uteri

N88.1 Old laceration of cervix uteri
Adhesions of cervix
Excludes 1: current obstetric trauma (O71.3)

N88.2 Stricture and stenosis of cervix uteri
Excludes 1: stricture and stenosis of cervix uteri complicating labor
(O65.5)

N88.3 Incompetence of cervix uteri
Investigation and management of (suspected) cervical
incompetence in a nonpregnant woman
Excludes 1: cervical incompetence complicating pregnancy
(O34.3-)

N88.4 Hypertrophic elongation of cervix uteri

N88.8 Other specified noninflammatory disorders of cervix uteri
Excludes 1: current obstetric trauma (O71.3)

N88.9 Noninflammatory disorder of cervix uteri, unspecified

N89- Other noninflammatory disorders of vagina
Excludes 1: abnormal results from vaginal cytologic examination without
histologic confirmation (R87.62-)
carcinoma in situ of vagina (D07.2)
HGSIL of vagina (R87.623)
inflammation of vagina (N76.-)
senile (atrophic) vaginitis (N95.2)
severe dysplasia of vagina (D07.2)
trichomonal leukorrhea (A59.00)
vaginal intraepithelial neoplasia [VAIN], grade III (D07.2)

N89.0 <u>Mild</u> <u>vaginal</u> dysplasia
Vaginal intraepithelial neoplasia [VAIN], grade I

N89.1 <u>Moderate</u> <u>vaginal</u> dysplasia
Vaginal intraepithelial neoplasia [VAIN], grade II

N89.3 Dysplasia of <u>vagina, unspecified</u>

N89.4 Leukoplakia of vagina

N89.5 Stricture and atresia of vagina
Vaginal adhesions
Vaginal stenosis
Excludes 1: congenital atresia or stricture (Q52.4)
postprocedural adhesions of vagina (N99.2)

N89.6 Tight hymenal ring
Rigid hymen
Tight introitus
Excludes 1: imperforate hymen (Q52.3)

N89.7 Hematocolpos
Hematocolpos with hematometra or hematosalpinx

N89.8 Other specified noninflammatory disorders of vagina
Leukorrhea NOS
Old vaginal laceration
Pessary ulcer of vagina
Excludes 1: current obstetric trauma (O70.-, O71.4, O71.7-O71.8)
old laceration involving muscles of pelvic floor (N81.8)

N89.9 Noninflammatory disorder of vagina, unspecified

N90- Other noninflammatory disorders of vulva and perineum
Excludes 1: anogenital (venereal) warts (A63.0)
carcinoma in situ of vulva (D07.1)
condyloma acuminatum (A63.0)
current obstetric trauma (O70.-, O71.7-O71.8)
inflammation of vulva (N76.-)
severe dysplasia of vulva (D07.1)
vulvar intraepithelial neoplasm III [VIN III] (D07.1)

N90.0 <u>Mild</u> <u>vulvar</u> dysplasia
Vulvar intrepithelial neoplasia [VIN], grade I

N90.1 <u>Moderate</u> <u>vulvar</u> dysplasia
Vulvar intraepithelial neoplasia [VIN], grade II

N90.3 Dysplasia of <u>vulva, unspecified</u>

N90.4 Leukoplakia of vulva
Dystrophy of vulva
Kraurosis of vulva
Lichen sclerosus of external female genital organs

N90.5 Atrophy of vulva
Stenosis of vulva

N90.6 Hypertrophy of vulva
Hypertrophy of labia

N90.7 Vulvar cyst

Excludes 1: = NOT CODED HERE! (Do not code both)

Excludes ❷: = Not Included Here

N90.8-   **Other specified noninflammatory disorders of vulva and perineum**

N90.81- Female genital mutilation status
Female genital cutting status

N90.810   **Female genital mutilation status, unspecified**
Female genital cutting status, unspecified
Female genital mutilation status NOS

N90.811   **Female genital mutilation Type I status**
Clitorectomy status
Female genital cutting Type I status

N90.812   **Female genital mutilation Type II status**
Clitorectomy with excision of labia minora status
Female genital cutting Type II status

N90.813   **Female genital mutilation Type III status**
Female genital cutting Type III status
Infibulation status

N90.818   **Other female genital mutilation status**
Female genital cutting Type IV status
Female genital mutilation Type IV status
Other female genital cutting status

N90.89   **Other specified noninflammatory disorders of vulva and perineum**
Adhesions of vulva
Hypertrophy of clitoris

N90.9   **Noninflammatory disorder of vulva and perineum, unspecified**

N91-   Absent, scanty and rare menstruation
Excludes 1: ovarian dysfunction (E28.-)

N91.0   **Primary amenorrhea**

N91.1   **Secondary amenorrhea**

N91.2   **Amenorrhea, unspecified**

N91.3   **Primary oligomenorrhea**

N91.4   **Secondary oligomenorrhea**

N91.5   **Oligomenorrhea, unspecified**
Hypomenorrhea NOS

N92-   Excessive, frequent and irregular menstruation
Excludes 1: postmenopausal bleeding (N95.0)
precocious puberty (menstruation) (E30.1)

N92.0   **Excessive and frequent menstruation with regular cycle**
Heavy periods NOS
Menorrhagia NOS
Polymenorrhea

N92.1   **Excessive and frequent menstruation with irregular cycle**
Irregular intermenstrual bleeding
Irregular, shortened intervals between menstrual bleeding
Menometrorrhagia
Metrorrhagia

N92.2   **Excessive menstruation at puberty**
Excessive bleeding associated with onset of menstrual periods
Pubertal menorrhagia
Puberty bleeding

N92.3   **Ovulation bleeding**
Regular intermenstrual bleeding

N92.4   **Excessive bleeding in the premenopausal period**
Climacteric menorrhagia or metrorrhagia
Menopausal menorrhagia or metrorrhagia
Preclimacteric menorrhagia or metrorrhagia
Premenopausal menorrhagia or metrorrhagia

N92.5   **Other specified irregular menstruation**

N92.6   **Irregular menstruation, unspecified**
Irregular bleeding NOS
Irregular periods NOS
Excludes 1: irregular menstruation with:
lengthened intervals or scanty bleeding (N91.3-N91.5)
shortened intervals or excessive bleeding (N92.1)

N93-   Other abnormal uterine and vaginal bleeding
Excludes 1: neonatal vaginal hemorrhage (P54.6)
precocious puberty (menstruation) (E30.1)
pseudomenses (P54.6)

N93.0   **Postcoital and contact bleeding**

N93.8   **Other specified abnormal uterine and vaginal bleeding**
Dysfunctional or functional uterine or vaginal bleeding NOS

N93.9   **Abnormal uterine and vaginal bleeding, unspecified**

N94-   Pain and other conditions associated with female genital organs and menstrual cycle

N94.0   **Mittelschmerz**

N94.1   **Dyspareunia**
Excludes 1: psychogenic dyspareunia (F52.6)

N94.2   **Vaginismus**
Excludes 1: psychogenic vaginismus (F52.5)

N94.3   **Premenstrual tension syndrome**
Premenstrual dysphoric disorder
Code also associated menstrual migraine (G43.82-, G43.83-)

N94.4   **Primary dysmenorrhea**

N94.5   **Secondary dysmenorrhea**

N94.6   **Dysmenorrhea, unspecified**
Excludes 1: psychogenic dysmenorrhea (F45.8)

N94.8-   Other specified conditions associated with female genital organs and menstrual cycle

N94.81- Vulvodynia

N94.810   **Vulvar vestibulitis**

N94.818   **Other vulvodynia**

N94.819   **Vulvodynia, unspecified**
Vulvodynia NOS

N94.89   **Other specified conditions associated with female genital organs and menstrual cycle**

N94.9   **Unspecified condition associated with female genital organs and menstrual cycle**

N95-   Menopausal and other perimenopausal disorders
Menopausal and other perimenopausal disorders due to naturally occurring (age-related) menopause and perimenopause
Excludes 1: excessive bleeding in the premenopausal period (N92.4)
menopausal and perimenopausal disorders due to artificial or premature menopause (E89.4-, E28.31-)
premature menopause (E28.31-)
Excludes❷: postmenopausal osteoporosis (M81.0-)
postmenopausal osteoporosis with current pathological fracture (M80.0-)
postmenopausal urethritis (N34.2)

N95.0   **Postmenopausal bleeding**

N95.1   **Menopausal and female climacteric states**
Symptoms such as flushing, sleeplessness, headache, lack of concentration, associated with natural (age-related) menopause
Use additional code for associated symptoms
Excludes 1: asymptomatic menopausal state (Z78.0)
symptoms associated with artificial menopause (E89.41)
symptoms associated with premature menopause (E28.310)

N95.2   **Postmenopausal atrophic vaginitis**
Senile (atrophic) vaginitis

N95.8   **Other specified menopausal and perimenopausal disorders**

N95.9   **Unspecified menopausal and perimenopausal disorder**

N96   Recurrent pregnancy loss
Investigation or care in a nonpregnant woman with history of recurrent pregnancy loss
Excludes 1: recurrent pregacy loss with current pregnancy (O26.2-)

N97-   Female infertility
Includes: Inability to achieve a pregnancy
Sterility, female NOS
Excludes 1: female infertility associated with:
hypopituitarism (E23.0)
Stein-Leventhal syndrome (E28.2)
Excludes❷: incompetence of cervix uteri (N88.3)

N97.0   **Female infertility associated with anovulation**

N97.1   **Female infertility of tubal origin**
Female infertility associated with congenital anomaly of tube
Female infertility due to tubal block
Female infertility due to tubal occlusion
Female infertility due to tubal stenosis

N97.2   **Female infertility of uterine origin**
Female infertility associated with congenital anomaly of uterus
Female infertility due to nonimplantation of ovum

N97.8   **Female infertility of other origin**

N97.9   **Female infertility, unspecified**

N98- Complications associated with artificial fertilization

N98.0 Infection associated with artificial insemination

N98.1 Hyperstimulation of ovaries
Hyperstimulation of ovaries NOS
Hyperstimulation of ovaries associated with induced ovulation

N98.2 Complications of attempted introduction of fertilized ovum following in vitro fertilization

N98.3 Complications of attempted introduction of embryo in embryo transfer

N98.8 Other complications associated with artificial fertilization

N98.9 Complication associated with artificial fertilization, unspecified

Intraoperative and postprocedural complications and disorders of genitourinary system, not elsewhere classified (N99)

N99- Intraoperative and postprocedural complications and disorders of genitourinary system, not elsewhere classified
Excludes❷: irradiation cystitis (N30.4-)
postoophorectomy osteoporosis with current pathological fracture (M80.8-)
postoophorectomy osteoporosis without current pathological fracture (M81.8)

N99.0 **Postprocedural (acute) (chronic) kidney failure**
Use additional code to type of kidney disease

N99.1- Postprocedural urethral stricture
Postcatheterization urethral stricture

   N99.11- Postprocedural urethral stricture, male

      N99.110 Postprocedural urethral stricture, male, meatal

      N99.111 Postprocedural bulbous urethral stricture

      N99.112 Postprocedural membranous urethral stricture

      N99.113 Postprocedural anterior urethral stricture

      N99.114 Postprocedural urethral stricture, male, unspecified

   N99.12 Postprocedural urethral stricture, female

N99.2 Postprocedural adhesions of vagina

N99.3 Prolapse of vaginal vault after hysterectomy

N99.4 Postprocedural pelvic peritoneal adhesions
Excludes❷: pelvic peritoneal adhesions NOS (N73.6)
postinfective pelvic peritoneal adhesions (N73.6)

N99.5- Complications of stoma of urinary tract
Excludes❷: mechanical complication of urinary (indwelling) catheter (T83.0-)

   N99.51- Complication of cystostomy

      N99.510 **Cystostomy hemorrhage**

      N99.511 **Cystostomy infection**

      N99.512 **Cystostomy malfunction**

      N99.518 **Other cystostomy complication**

   N99.52- Complication of other external stoma of urinary tract

      N99.520 **Hemorrhage of other external stoma of urinary tract**

      N99.521 **Infection of other external stoma of urinary tract**

      N99.522 **Malfunction of other external stoma of urinary tract**

      N99.528 **Other complication of other external stoma of urinary tract**

   N99.53- Complication of other stoma of urinary tract

      N99.530 **Hemorrhage of other stoma of urinary tract**

      N99.531 **Infection of other stoma of urinary tract**

      N99.532 **Malfunction of other stoma of urinary tract**

      N99.538 **Other complication of other stoma of urinary tract**

N99.6- Intraoperative hemorrhage and hematoma of a genitourinary system organ or structure complicating a procedure
Excludes 1: intraoperative hemorrhage and hematoma of a genitourinary system organ or structure due to accidental puncture or laceration during a procedure (N99.7-)

   N99.61 Intraoperative hemorrhage and hematoma of a genitourinary system organ or structure complicating a genitourinary system procedure

   N99.62 Intraoperative hemorrhage and hematoma of a genitourinary system organ or structure complicating other procedure

N99.7- Accidental puncture and laceration of a genitourinary system organ or structure during a procedure

   N99.71 Accidental puncture and laceration of a genitourinary system organ or structure during a genitourinary system procedure

   N99.72 Accidental puncture and laceration of a genitourinary system organ or structure during other procedure

N99.8- Other intraoperative and postprocedural complications and disorders of genitourinary system

   N99.81 Other intraoperative complications of genitourinary system

   N99.82- Postprocedural hemorrhage and hematoma of a genitourinary system organ or structure following a procedure

      N99.820 Postprocedural hemorrhage and hematoma of a genitourinary system organ or structure following a genitourinary system procedure

      N99.821 Postprocedural hemorrhage and hematoma of a genitourinary system organ or structure following other procedure

   N99.83 Residual ovary syndrome

   N99.89 Other postprocedural complications and disorders of genitourinary system

N90 – N99

Excludes 1: = NOT CODED HERE! (Do not code both)

Excludes❷: = Not Included Here

This page is intentionally blank.

N
9
9
–
O
0
3

Chapter 15 – Pregnancy, childbirth and the puerperium (O00-O9A)

Note: CODES FROM THIS CHAPTER ARE FOR USE ONLY ON MATERNAL RECORDS, NEVER ON NEWBORN RECORDS.
Codes from this chapter are for use for conditions related to or aggravated by the pregnancy, childbirth, or by the puerperium (maternal causes or obstetric causes)

Use additional code from category Z3A, Weeks of gestation, to identify the specific week of the pregnancy

Trimesters are counted from the first day of the last menstrual period. They are defined as follows:
1st trimester- less than 14 weeks 0 days
2nd trimester- 14 weeks 0 days to less than 28 weeks 0 days
3rd trimester- 28 weeks 0 days until delivery

Excludes 1: supervision of normal pregnancy (Z34.-)
Excludes❷: mental and behavioral disorders associated with the puerperium (F53)
obstetrical tetanus (A34)
postpartum necrosis of pituitary gland (E23.0)
puerperal osteomalacia (M83.0)

This chapter contains the following blocks:

O00-O08	Pregnancy with abortive outcome
O09	Supervision of high risk pregnancy
O10-O16	Edema, proteinuria and hypertensive disorders in pregnancy, childbirth and the puerperium
O20-O29	Other maternal disorders predominantly related to pregnancy
O30-O48	Maternal care related to the fetus and amniotic cavity and possible delivery problems
O60-O77	Complications of labor and delivery
O80-O82	Encounter for delivery
O85-O92	Complications predominantly related to the puerperium
O94-O9A	Other obstetric conditions, not elsewhere classified

Pregnancy with abortive outcome (O00-O08)

Excludes 1: continuing pregnancy in multiple gestation after abortion of one fetus or more (O31.1-, O31.3-)

O00- Ectopic pregnancy
Includes: Ruptured ectopic pregnancy
Use additional code from category O08 to identify any associated complication

O00.0 Abdominal pregnancy
Excludes 1: maternal care for viable fetus in abdominal pregnancy (O36.7-)

O00.1 Tubal pregnancy
Fallopian pregnancy
Rupture of (fallopian) tube due to pregnancy
Tubal abortion

O00.2 Ovarian pregnancy

O00.8 Other ectopic pregnancy
Cervical pregnancy
Cornual pregnancy
Intraligamentous pregnancy
Mural pregnancy

O00.9 Ectopic pregnancy, unspecified

O01- Hydatidiform mole
Use additional code from category O08 to identify any associated complication
Excludes 1: chorioadenoma (destruens) (D39.2)
malignant hydatidiform mole (D39.2)

O01.0 Classical hydatidiform mole
Complete hydatidiform mole

O01.1 Incomplete and partial hydatidiform mole

O01.9 Hydatidiform mole, unspecified
Trophoblastic disease NOS
Vesicular mole NOS

O02- Other abnormal products of conception
Use additional code from category O08 to identify any associated complication
Excludes 1: papyraceous fetus (O31.0-)

O02.0 Blighted ovum and nonhydatidiform mole
Carneous mole
Fleshy mole
Intrauterine mole NOS
Molar pregnancy NEC
Pathological ovum

O02.1 Missed abortion
Early fetal death, before completion of 20 weeks of gestation, with retention of dead fetus
Excludes 1: failed induced abortion (O07-)
fetal death (intrauterine) (late) (O36.4)
missed abortion with blighted ovum (O02.0)
missed abortion with hydatidiform mole (O01-)
missed abortion with nonhydatidiform (O02.0)
missed abortion with other abnormal products of conception (O02.8-)
missed delivery (O36.4)
stillbirth (P95)

O02.8- Other specified abnormal products of conception
Excludes 1: abnormal products of conception with blighted ovum (O02.0)
abnormal products of conception with hydatidiform mole (O01.-)
abnormal products of conception with nonhydatidiform mole (O02.0)

O02.81 Inappropriate change in quantitative human chorionic gonadotropin (hCG) in early pregnancy
Biochemical pregnancy
Chemical pregnancy
Inappropriate level of quantitative human chorionic gonadotropin (hCG) for gestational age in early pregnancy

O02.89 Other specified abnormal products of conception

O02.9 Abnormal product of conception, unspecified

O03- Spontaneous abortion
Note: Incomplete abortion includes retained products of conception following spontaneous abortion
Includes: Miscarriage

O03.0 Genital tract and pelvic infection following incomplete spontaneous abortion
Endometritis following incomplete spontaneous abortion
Oophoritis following incomplete spontaneous abortion
Parametritis following incomplete spontaneous abortion
Pelvic peritonitis following incomplete spontaneous abortion
Salpingitis following incomplete spontaneous abortion
Salpingo-oophoritis following incomplete spontaneous abortion
Excludes 1: sepsis following incomplete spontaneous abortion (O03.37)
urinary tract infection following incomplete spontaneous abortion (O03.38)

O03.1 Delayed or excessive hemorrhage following incomplete spontaneous abortion
Afibrinogenemia following incomplete spontaneous abortion
Defibrination syndrome following incomplete spontaneous abortion
Hemolysis following incomplete spontaneous abortion
Intravascular coagulation following incomplete spontaneous abortion

O03.2 Embolism following incomplete spontaneous abortion
Air embolism following incomplete spontaneous abortion
Amniotic fluid embolism following incomplete spontaneous abortion
Blood-clot embolism following incomplete spontaneous abortion
Embolism NOS following incomplete spontaneous abortion
Fat embolism following incomplete spontaneous abortion
Pulmonary embolism following incomplete spontaneous abortion
Pyemic embolism following incomplete spontaneous abortion
Septic or septicopyemic embolism following incomplete spontaneous abortion
Soap embolism following incomplete spontaneous abortion

O03.3- Other and unspecified complications following incomplete spontaneous abortion

O03.30 Unspecified complication following incomplete spontaneous abortion

O03.31 Shock following incomplete spontaneous abortion
Circulatory collapse following incomplete spontaneous abortion
Shock (postprocedural) following incomplete spontaneous abortion
Excludes 1: shock due to infection following incomplete spontaneous abortion (O03.37)

O03.32 Renal failure following incomplete spontaneous abortion
Kidney failure (acute) following incomplete spontaneous abortion
Oliguria following incomplete spontaneous abortion
Renal shutdown following incomplete spontaneous abortion
Renal tubular necrosis following incomplete spontaneous abortion
Uremia following incomplete spontaneous abortion

O03.33 Metabolic disorder following incomplete spontaneous abortion

O03 - O03 O03

O03.34 **Damage to pelvic organs following incomplete spontaneous abortion**
  Laceration, perforation, tear or chemical damage of bladder following incomplete spontaneous abortion
  Laceration, perforation, tear or chemical damage of bowel following incomplete spontaneous abortion
  Laceration, perforation, tear or chemical damage of broad ligament following incomplete spontaneous abortion
  Laceration, perforation, tear or chemical damage of cervix following incomplete spontaneous abortion
  Laceration, perforation, tear or chemical damage of periurethral tissue following incomplete spontaneous abortion
  Laceration, perforation, tear or chemical damage of uterus following incomplete spontaneous abortion
  Laceration, perforation, tear or chemical damage of vagina following incomplete spontaneous abortion

O03.35 **Other venous complications following incomplete spontaneous abortion**

O03.36 **Cardiac arrest following incomplete spontaneous abortion**

O03.37 **Sepsis following incomplete spontaneous abortion**
  Use additional code to identify infectious agent (B95-B97)
  Use additional code to identify severe sepsis, if applicable (R65.2-)
  Excludes 1: septic or septicopyemic embolism following incomplete spontaneous abortion (O03.2)

O03.38 **Urinary tract infection following incomplete spontaneous abortion**
  Cystitis following incomplete spontaneous abortion

O03.39 **Incomplete spontaneous abortion with other complications**

O03.4 **Incomplete spontaneous abortion without complication**

O03.5 **Genital tract and pelvic infection following complete or unspecified spontaneous abortion**
  Endometritis following complete or unspecified spontaneous abortion
  Oophoritis following complete or unspecified spontaneous abortion
  Parametritis following complete or unspecified spontaneous abortion
  Pelvic peritonitis following complete or unspecified spontaneous abortion
  Salpingitis following complete or unspecified spontaneous abortion
  Salpingo-oophoritis following complete or unspecified spontaneous abortion
  Excludes 1: sepsis following complete or unspecified spontaneous abortion (O03.87)
    urinary tract infection following complete or unspecified spontaneous abortion (O03.88)

O03.6 **Delayed or excessive hemorrhage following complete or unspecified spontaneous abortion**
  Afibrinogenemia following complete or unspecified spontaneous abortion
  Defibrination syndrome following complete or unspecified spontaneous abortion
  Hemolysis following complete or unspecified spontaneous abortion
  Intravascular coagulation following complete or unspecified spontaneous abortion

O03.7 **Embolism following complete or unspecified spontaneous abortion**
  Air embolism following complete or unspecified spontaneous abortion
  Amniotic fluid embolism following complete or unspecified spontaneous abortion
  Blood-clot embolism following complete or unspecified spontaneous abortion
  Embolism NOS following complete or unspecified spontaneous abortion
  Fat embolism following complete or unspecified spontaneous abortion
  Pulmonary embolism following complete or unspecified spontaneous abortion
  Pyemic embolism following complete or unspecified spontaneous abortion
  Septic or septicopyemic embolism following complete or unspecified spontaneous abortion
  Soap embolism following complete or unspecified spontaneous abortion

O03.8- **Other and unspecified complications following complete or unspecified spontaneous abortion**

O03.80 **Unspecified complication following complete or unspecified spontaneous abortion**

O03.81 **Shock following complete or unspecified spontaneous abortion**
  Circulatory collapse following complete or unspecified spontaneous abortion
  Shock (postprocedural) following complete or unspecified spontaneous abortion
  Excludes 1: shock due to infection following complete or unspecified spontaneous abortion (O03.87)

O03.82 **Renal failure following complete or unspecified spontaneous abortion**
  Kidney failure (acute) following complete or unspecified spontaneous abortion
  Oliguria following complete or unspecified spontaneous abortion
  Renal shutdown following complete or unspecified spontaneous abortion
  Renal tubular necrosis following complete or unspecified spontaneous abortion
  Uremia following complete or unspecified spontaneous abortion

O03.83 **Metabolic disorder following complete or unspecified spontaneous abortion**

O03.84 **Damage to pelvic organs following complete or unspecified spontaneous abortion**
  Laceration, perforation, tear or chemical damage of bladder following complete or unspecified spontaneous abortion
  Laceration, perforation, tear or chemical damage of bowel following complete or unspecified spontaneous abortion
  Laceration, perforation, tear or chemical damage of broad ligament following complete or unspecified spontaneous abortion
  Laceration, perforation, tear or chemical damage of cervix following complete or unspecified spontaneous abortion
  Laceration, perforation, tear or chemical damage of periurethral tissue following complete or unspecified spontaneous abortion
  Laceration, perforation, tear or chemical damage of uterus following complete or unspecified spontaneous abortion
  Laceration, perforation, tear or chemical damage of vagina following complete or unspecified spontaneous abortion

O03.85 **Other venous complications following complete or unspecified spontaneous abortion**

O03.86 **Cardiac arrest following complete or unspecified spontaneous abortion**

O03.87 **Sepsis following complete or unspecified spontaneous abortion**
  Use additional code to identify infectious agent (B95-B97)
  Use additional code to identify severe sepsis, if applicable (R65.2-)
  Excludes 1: septic or septicopyemic embolism following complete or unspecified spontaneousabortion (O03.7)

O03.88 **Urinary tract infection following complete or unspecified spontaneous abortion**
  Cystitis following complete or unspecified spontaneous abortion

O03.89 **Complete or unspecified spontaneous abortion with other complications**

O03.9 **Complete or unspecified spontaneous abortion without complication**
  Miscarriage NOS
  Spontaneous abortion NOS

O04- Complications following (induced) termination of pregnancy
  Includes: Complications following (induced) termination of pregnancy
  Excludes 1: encounter for elective termination of pregnancy, uncomplicated (Z33.2)
    failed attempted termination of pregnancy (O07.-)

O04.5 **Genital tract and pelvic infection following (induced) termination of pregnancy**
  Endometritis following (induced) termination of pregnancy
  Oophoritis following (induced) termination of pregnancy
  Parametritis following (induced) termination of pregnancy
  Pelvic peritonitis following (induced) termination of pregnancy
  Salpingitis following (induced) termination of pregnancy
  Salpingo-oophoritis following (induced) termination of pregnancy
  Excludes 1: sepsis following (induced) termination of pregnancy (O04.87)
    urinary tract infection following (induced) termination of pregnancy (O04.88)

O 0 3 - O 0 7

Excludes 1: = NOT CODED HERE! (Do not code both)

Excludes❷: = Not Included Here

O04.6   **Delayed or excessive hemorrhage following** (induced) **termination** of pregnancy
    Afibrinogenemia following (induced) termination of pregnancy
    Defibrination syndrome following (induced) termination of pregnancy
    Hemolysis following (induced) termination of pregnancy
    Intravascular coagulation following (induced) termination of pregnancy

O04.7   **Embolism following** (induced) **termination** of pregnancy
    Air embolism following (induced) termination of pregnancy
    Amniotic fluid embolism following (induced) termination of pregnancy
    Blood-clot embolism following (induced) termination of pregnancy
    Embolism NOS following (induced) termination of pregnancy
    Fat embolism following (induced) termination of pregnancy
    Pulmonary embolism following (induced) termination of pregnancy
    Pyemic embolism following (induced) termination of pregnancy
    Septic or septicopyemic embolism following (induced) termination of pregnancy
    Soap embolism following (induced) termination of pregnancy

O04.8-   **(Induced) termination** of pregnancy **with other** and unspecified complications

  O04.80 **(Induced) termination** of pregnancy **with unspecified complications**

  O04.81 **Shock following** (induced) **termination** of pregnancy
    Circulatory collapse following (induced) termination of pregnancy
    Shock (postprocedural) following (induced) termination of pregnancy
    Excludes 1:   shock due to infection following (induced) termination of pregnancy (O04.87)

  O04.82 **Renal failure following** (induced) **termination** of pregnancy
    Kidney failure (acute) following (induced) termination of pregnancy
    Oliguria following (induced) termination of pregnancy
    Renal shutdown following (induced) termination of pregnancy
    Renal tubular necrosis following (induced) termination of pregnancy
    Uremia following (induced) termination of pregnancy

  O04.83 **Metabolic disorder following** (induced) **termination** of pregnancy

  O04.84 **Damage to pelvic organs following** (induced) **termination** of pregnancy
    Laceration, perforation, tear or chemical damage of bladder following (induced) termination of pregnancy
    Laceration, perforation, tear or chemical damage of bowel following (induced) termination of pregnancy
    Laceration, perforation, tear or chemical damage of broad ligament following (induced) termination of pregnancy
    Laceration, perforation, tear or chemical damage of cervix following (induced) termination of pregnancy
    Laceration, perforation, tear or chemical damage of periurethral tissue following (induced) termination of pregnancy
    Laceration, perforation, tear or chemical damage of uterus following (induced) termination of pregnancy
    Laceration, perforation, tear or chemical damage of vagina following (induced) termination of pregnancy

  O04.85 **Other venous complications following** (induced) **termination** of pregnancy

  O04.86 **Cardiac arrest following** (induced) **termination** of pregnancy

  O04.87 **Sepsis following** (induced) **termination** of pregnancy
    Use additional code to identify infectious agent (B95-B97)
    Use additional code to identify severe sepsis, if applicable (R65.2-)
    Excludes 1:   septic or septicopyemic embolism following (induced) termination of pregnancy (O04.7)

  O04.88 **Urinary tract infection following** (induced) **termination** of pregnancy
    Cystitis following (induced) termination of pregnancy

  O04.89 **(Induced) termination** of pregnancy **with other complications**

O07-   **Failed attempted termination of pregnancy**
    Includes: Failure of attempted induction of termination of pregnancy
    Incomplete elective abortion
    Excludes 1:   incomplete spontaneous abortion (O03.0-)

O07.0   **Genital tract and pelvic infection following** failed **attempted termination of pregnancy**
    Endometritis following failed attempted termination of pregnancy
    Oophoritis following failed attempted termination of pregnancy
    Parametritis following failed attempted termination of pregnancy
    Pelvic peritonitis following failed attempted termination of pregnancy
    Salpingitis following failed attempted termination of pregnancy
    Salpingo-oophoritis following failed attempted termination of pregnancy
    Excludes 1:   sepsis following failed attempted termination of pregnancy (O07.37)
        urinary tract infection following failed attempted termination of pregnancy (O07.38)

O07.1   **Delayed or excessive hemorrhage following** failed **attempted termination of pregnancy**
    Afibrinogenemia following failed attempted termination of pregnancy
    Defibrination syndrome following failed attempted termination of pregnancy
    Hemolysis following failed attempted termination of pregnancy
    Intravascular coagulation following failed attempted termination of pregnancy

O07.2   **Embolism following** failed **attempted termination of pregnancy**
    Air embolism following failed attempted termination of pregnancy
    Amniotic fluid embolism following failed attempted termination of pregnancy
    Blood-clot embolism following failed attempted termination of pregnancy
    Embolism NOS following failed attempted termination of pregnancy
    Fat embolism following failed attempted termination of pregnancy
    Pulmonary embolism following failed attempted termination of pregnancy
    Pyemic embolism following failed attempted termination of pregnancy
    Septic or septicopyemic embolism following failed attempted termination of pregnancy
    Soap embolism following failed attempted termination of pregnancy

O07.3-   **Failed attempted termination of pregnancy with other** and unspecified complications

  O07.30 **Failed attempted termination of pregnancy with unspecified complications**

  O07.31 **Shock following** failed **attempted termination of pregnancy**
    Circulatory collapse following failed attempted termination of pregnancy
    Shock (postprocedural) following failed attempted termination of pregnancy
    Excludes 1:   shock due to infection following failed attempted termination of pregnancy (O07.37)

  O07.32 **Renal failure following** failed **attempted termination of pregnancy**
    Kidney failure (acute) following failed attempted termination of pregnancy
    Oliguria following failed attempted termination of pregnancy
    Renal shutdown following failed attempted termination of pregnancy
    Renal tubular necrosis following failed attempted termination of pregnancy
    Uremia following failed attempted termination of pregnancy

  O07.33 **Metabolic disorder following** failed **attempted termination of pregnancy**

  O07.34 **Damage to pelvic organs following** failed **attempted termination of pregnancy**
    Laceration, perforation, tear or chemical damage of bladder following failed attempted termination of pregnancy
    Laceration, perforation, tear or chemical damage of bowel following failed attempted termination of pregnancy
    Laceration, perforation, tear or chemical damage of broad ligament following failed attempted termination of pregnancy
    Laceration, perforation, tear or chemical damage of cervix following failed attempted termination of pregnancy
    Laceration, perforation, tear or chemical damage of periurethral tissue following failed attempted termination of pregnancy
    Laceration, perforation, tear or chemical damage of uterus following failed attempted termination of pregnancy
    Laceration, perforation, tear or chemical damage of vagina following failed attempted termination of pregnancy

O03 - O07

Excludes 1: = NOT CODED HERE! (Do not code both)

Excludes ❷: = Not Included Here

O07.35 Other venous complications following failed attempted termination of pregnancy

O07.36 Cardiac arrest following failed attempted termination of pregnancy

O07.37 Sepsis following failed attempted termination of pregnancy
Use additional code (B95-B97), to identify infectious agent
Use additional code (R65.2-) to identify severe sepsis, if applicable
Excludes 1: septic or septicopyemic embolism following failed attempted termination of pregnancy (O07.2)

O07.38 Urinary tract infection following failed attempted termination of pregnancy
Cystitis following failed attempted termination of pregnancy

O07.39 Failed attempted termination of pregnancy with other complications

O07.4 Failed attempted termination of pregnancy without complication

O08- Complications following ectopic and molar pregnancy
This category is for use with categories O00-O02 to identify any associated complications

O08.0 Genital tract and pelvic infection following ectopic and molar pregnancy
Endometritis following ectopic and molar pregnancy
Oophoritis following ectopic and molar pregnancy
Parametritis following ectopic and molar pregnancy
Pelvic peritonitis following ectopic and molar pregnancy
Salpingitis following ectopic and molar pregnancy
Salpingo-oophoritis following ectopic and molar pregnancy
Excludes 1: sepsis following ectopic and molar pregnancy (O08.82)
urinary tract infection (O08.83)

O08.1 Delayed or excessive hemorrhage following ectopic and molar pregnancy
Afibrinogenemia following ectopic and molar pregnancy
Defibrination syndrome following ectopic and molar pregnancy
Hemolysis following ectopic and molar pregnancy
Intravascular coagulation following ectopic and molar pregnancy
Excludes 1: delayed or excessive hemorrhage due to incomplete abortion (O03.1)

O08.2 Embolism following ectopic and molar pregnancy
Air embolism following ectopic and molar pregnancy
Amniotic fluid embolism following ectopic and molar pregnancy
Blood-clot embolism following ectopic and molar pregnancy
Embolism NOS following ectopic and molar pregnancy
Fat embolism following ectopic and molar pregnancy
Pulmonary embolism following ectopic and molar pregnancy
Pyemic embolism following ectopic and molar pregnancy
Septic or septicopyemic embolism following ectopic and molar pregnancy
Soap embolism following ectopic and molar pregnancy

O08.3 Shock following ectopic and molar pregnancy
Circulatory collapse following ectopic and molar pregnancy
Shock (postprocedural) following ectopic and molar pregnancy
Excludes 1: shock due to infection following ectopic and molar pregnancy (O08.82)

O08.4 Renal failure following ectopic and molar pregnancy
Kidney failure (acute) following ectopic and molar pregnancy
Oliguria following ectopic and molar pregnancy
Renal shutdown following ectopic and molar pregnancy
Renal tubular necrosis following ectopic and molar pregnancy
Uremia following ectopic and molar pregnancy

O08.5 Metabolic disorders following an ectopic and molar pregnancy

O08.6 Damage to pelvic organs and tissues following an ectopic and molar pregnancy
Laceration, perforation, tear or chemical damage of bladder following an ectopic and molar pregnancy
Laceration, perforation, tear or chemical damage of bowel following an ectopic and molar pregnancy
Laceration, perforation, tear or chemical damage of broad ligament following an ectopic and molar pregnancy
Laceration, perforation, tear or chemical damage of cervix following an ectopic and molar pregnancy
Laceration, perforation, tear or chemical damage of periurethral tissue following an ectopic and molar pregnancy
Laceration, perforation, tear or chemical damage of uterus following an ectopic and molar pregnancy
Laceration, perforation, tear or chemical damage of vagina following an ectopic and molar pregnancy

O08.7 Other venous complications following an ectopic and molar pregnancy

O08.8- Other complications following an ectopic and molar pregnancy

O08.81 Cardiac arrest following an ectopic and molar pregnancy

O08.82 Sepsis following ectopic and molar pregnancy
Use additional code (B95-B97), to identify infectious agent
Use additional code (R65.2-) to identify severe sepsis, if applicable
Excludes 1: septic or septicopyemic embolism following ectopic and molar pregnancy (O08.2)

O08.83 Urinary tract infection following an ectopic and molar pregnancy
Cystitis following an ectopic and molar pregnancy

O08.89 Other complications following an ectopic and molar pregnancy

O08.9 Unspecified complication following an ectopic and molar pregnancy

Supervision of high risk pregnancy (O09)

O09- Supervision of high risk pregnancy

O09.0- Supervision of pregnancy with history of infertility

O09.00 Supervision of pregnancy with history of infertility, unspecified trimester

O09.01 Supervision of pregnancy with history of infertility, first trimester

O09.02 Supervision of pregnancy with history of infertility, second trimester

O09.03 Supervision of pregnancy with history of infertility, third trimester

O09.1- Supervision of pregnancy with history of ectopic or molar pregnancy

O09.10 Supervision of pregnancy with history of ectopic or molar pregnancy, unspecified trimester

O09.11 Supervision of pregnancy with history of ectopic or molar pregnancy, first trimester

O09.12 Supervision of pregnancy with history of ectopic or molar pregnancy, second trimester

O09.13 Supervision of pregnancy with history of ectopic or molar pregnancy, third trimester

O09.2- Supervision of pregnancy with other poor reproductive or obstetric history
Excludes ❷: pregnancy care for patient with history of recurrent pregnancy loss (O26.2-)

O09.21- Supervision of pregnancy with history of pre-term labor

O09.211 Supervision of pregnancy with history of pre-term labor, first trimester

O09.212 Supervision of pregnancy with history of pre-term labor, second trimester

O09.213 Supervision of pregnancy with history of pre-term labor, third trimester

O09.219 Supervision of pregnancy with history of pre-term labor, unspecified trimester

O09.29- Supervision of pregnancy with other poor reproductive or obstetric history
Supervision of pregnancy with history of neonatal death
Supervision of pregnancy with history of stillbirth

O09.291 Supervision of pregnancy with other poor reproductive or obstetric history, first trimester

O09.292 Supervision of pregnancy with other poor reproductive or obstetric history, second trimester

O09.293 Supervision of pregnancy with other poor reproductive or obstetric history, third trimester

O09.299 Supervision of pregnancy with other poor reproductive or obstetric history, unspecified trimester

O09.3- Supervision of pregnancy with insufficient antenatal care
Supervision of concealed pregnancy
Supervision of hidden pregnancy

O09.30 Supervision of pregnancy with insufficient antenatal care, unspecified trimester

O09.31 Supervision of pregnancy with insufficient antenatal care, first trimester

O09.32 Supervision of pregnancy with insufficient antenatal care, second trimester

O09.33 Supervision of pregnancy with insufficient antenatal care, third trimester

O09.4- Supervision of pregnancy with grand multiparity

O09.40 Supervision of pregnancy with grand multiparity, unspecified trimester

O09.41 Supervision of pregnancy with grand multiparity, first trimester

O07 - O10

O09.42 Supervision of pregnancy with grand multiparity, <u>second</u> trimester

O09.43 Supervision of pregnancy with grand multiparity, <u>third</u> trimester

O09.5- Supervision of elderly primigravida and multigravida
Pregnancy for a female 35 years and older at expected date of delivery

O09.51- <u>Supervision of elderly primigravida</u>

   O09.511 Supervision of elderly primigravida, <u>first</u> trimester

   O09.512 Supervision of elderly primigravida, <u>second</u> trimester

   O09.513 Supervision of elderly primigravida, <u>third</u> trimester

   O09.519 Supervision of elderly primigravida, <u>unspecified</u> trimester

O09.52- <u>Supervision of elderly multigravida</u>

   O09.521 Supervision of elderly multigravida, <u>first</u> trimester

   O09.522 Supervision of elderly multigravida, <u>second</u> trimester

   O09.523 Supervision of elderly multigravida, <u>third</u> trimester

   O09.529 Supervision of elderly multigravida, <u>unspecified</u> trimester

O09.6- Supervision of young primigravida and multigravida
Supervision of pregnancy for a female less than 16 years old at expected date of delivery

O09.61- <u>Supervision of young primigravida</u>

   O09.611 Supervision of young primigravida, <u>first</u> trimester

   O09.612 Supervision of young primigravida, <u>second</u> trimester

   O09.613 Supervision of young primigravida, <u>third</u> trimester

   O09.619 Supervision of young primigravida, <u>unspecified</u> trimester

O09.62- <u>Supervision of young multigravida</u>

   O09.621 Supervision of young multigravida, <u>first</u> trimester

   O09.622 Supervision of young multigravida, <u>second</u> trimester

   O09.623 Supervision of young multigravida, <u>third</u> trimester

   O09.629 Supervision of young multigravida, <u>unspecified</u> trimester

O09.7- <u>Supervision of high risk pregnancy due to social problems</u>

   O09.70 Supervision of high risk pregnancy due to social problems, <u>unspecified</u> trimester

   O09.71 Supervision of high risk pregnancy due to social problems, <u>first</u> trimester

   O09.72 Supervision of high risk pregnancy due to social problems, <u>second</u> trimester

   O09.73 Supervision of high risk pregnancy due to social problems, <u>third</u> trimester

O09.8- Supervision of other high risk pregnancies

O09.81- Supervision of pregnancy <u>resulting from assisted reproductive technology</u>
Supervision of pregnancy resulting from in-vitro fertilization

   O09.811 Supervision of pregnancy resulting from assisted reproductive technology, <u>first</u> trimester

   O09.812 Supervision of pregnancy resulting from assisted reproductive technology, <u>second</u> trimester

   O09.813 Supervision of pregnancy resulting from assisted reproductive technology, <u>third</u> trimester

   O09.819 Supervision of pregnancy resulting from assisted reproductive technology, <u>unspecified</u> trimester

O09.82- Supervision of pregnancy <u>with history of in utero procedure during previous pregnancy</u>

   O09.821 Supervision of pregnancy with history of in utero procedure during previous pregnancy, <u>first</u> trimester

   O09.822 Supervision of pregnancy with history of in utero procedure during previous pregnancy, <u>second</u> trimester

   O09.823 Supervision of pregnancy with history of in utero procedure during previous pregnancy, <u>third</u> trimester

   O09.829 Supervision of pregnancy with history of in utero procedure during previous pregnancy, <u>unspecified</u> trimester

   Excludes 1: supervision of pregnancy affected by in utero procedure during current pregnancy (O35.7)

O09.89- Supervision of other high risk pregnancies

   O09.891 Supervision of other high risk pregnancies, <u>first</u> trimester

   O09.892 Supervision of other high risk pregnancies, <u>second</u> trimester

   O09.893 Supervision of other high risk pregnancies, <u>third</u> trimester

   O09.899 Supervision of other high risk pregnancies, <u>unspecified</u> trimester

O09.9- Supervision of high risk pregnancy, <u>unspecified</u>

   O09.90 Supervision of high risk pregnancy, unspecified, <u>unspecified</u> trimester

   O09.91 Supervision of high risk pregnancy, unspecified, <u>first</u> trimester

   O09.92 Supervision of high risk pregnancy, unspecified, <u>second</u> trimester

   O09.93 Supervision of high risk pregnancy, unspecified, <u>third</u> trimester

Edema, proteinuria and hypertensive disorders in pregnancy, childbirth and the puerperium (O10-O16)

O10- <u>Pre-existing hypertension</u> complicating pregnancy, childbirth and the puerperium
Includes: Pre-existing hypertension with pre-existing proteinuria complicating pregnancy, childbirth and the puerperium
Excludes ❷: pre-existing hypertension with superimposed pre-eclampsia complicating pregnancy, childbirth and the puerperium (O11.-)

O10.0- Pre-existing <u>essential</u> hypertension complicating pregnancy, childbirth and the puerperium
Any condition in I10 specified as a reason for obstetric care during pregnancy, childbirth or the puerperium

O10.01- Pre-existing essential hypertension <u>complicating pregnancy</u>,

   O10.011 Pre-existing essential hypertension complicating pregnancy, <u>first</u> trimester

   O10.012 Pre-existing essential hypertension complicating pregnancy, <u>second</u> trimester

   O10.013 Pre-existing essential hypertension complicating pregnancy, <u>third</u> trimester

   O10.019 Pre-existing essential hypertension complicating pregnancy, <u>unspecified</u> trimester

O10.02 Pre-existing essential hypertension <u>complicating childbirth</u>

O10.03 Pre-existing essential hypertension <u>complicating the puerperium</u>

O10.1- Pre-existing <u>hypertensive heart disease</u> complicating pregnancy, childbirth and the puerperium
Any condition in I11 specified as a reason for obstetric care during pregnancy, childbirth or the puerperium
Use additional code from I11 to identify the type of hypertensive heart disease

O10.11- Pre-existing hypertensive heart disease <u>complicating pregnancy</u>

   O10.111 Pre-existing hypertensive heart disease complicating pregnancy, <u>first</u> trimester

   O10.112 Pre-existing hypertensive heart disease complicating pregnancy, <u>second</u> trimester

   O10.113 Pre-existing hypertensive heart disease complicating pregnancy, <u>third</u> trimester

   O10.119 Pre-existing hypertensive heart disease complicating pregnancy, <u>unspecified</u> trimester

O10.12 Pre-existing hypertensive heart disease <u>complicating childbirth</u>

O10.13 Pre-existing hypertensive heart disease <u>complicating the puerperium</u>

O10.2- Pre-existing <u>hypertensive chronic kidney disease</u> complicating pregnancy, childbirth and the puerperium
Any condition in I12 specified as a reason for obstetric care during pregnancy, childbirth or the puerperium
Use additional code from I12 to identify the type of hypertensive chronic kidney disease

O10.21- Pre-existing hypertensive chronic kidney disease complicating pregnancy

   O10.211 Pre-existing hypertensive chronic kidney disease complicating pregnancy, <u>first</u> trimester

   O10.212 Pre-existing hypertensive chronic kidney disease complicating pregnancy, <u>second</u> trimester

   O10.213 Pre-existing hypertensive chronic kidney disease complicating pregnancy, <u>third</u> trimester

   O10.219 Pre-existing hypertensive chronic kidney disease complicating pregnancy, <u>unspecified</u> trimester

O10.22 Pre-existing hypertensive chronic kidney disease <u>complicating childbirth</u>

O10.23 Pre-existing hypertensive chronic kidney disease <u>complicating the puerperium</u>

O 0 7 - O 1 0

O10.3- Pre-existing <u>hypertensive heart and chronic kidney disease</u> complicating pregnancy, childbirth and the puerperium
> Any condition in I13 specified as a reason for obstetric care during pregnancy, childbirth or the puerperium
> Use additional code from I13 to identify the type of hypertensive heart and chronic kidney disease

O10.31- Pre-existing hypertensive heart and chronic kidney disease <u>complicating pregnancy</u>

    O10.311 Pre-existing hypertensive heart and chronic kidney disease complicating pregnancy, <u>first</u> trimester

    O10.312 Pre-existing hypertensive heart and chronic kidney disease complicating pregnancy, <u>second</u> trimester

    O10.313 Pre-existing hypertensive heart and chronic kidney disease complicating pregnancy, <u>third</u> trimester

    O10.319 Pre-existing hypertensive heart and chronic kidney disease complicating pregnancy, <u>unspecified</u> trimester

O10.32 Pre-existing hypertensive heart and chronic kidney disease <u>complicating childbirth</u>

O10.33 Pre-existing hypertensive heart and chronic kidney disease <u>complicating the puerperium</u>

O10.4- Pre-existing <u>secondary</u> hypertension complicating pregnancy, childbirth and the puerperium
> Any condition in I15 specified as a reason for obstetric care during pregnancy, childbirth or the puerperium
> Use additional code from I15 to identify the type of secondary hypertension

O10.41- Pre-existing secondary hypertension <u>complicating pregnancy</u>

    O10.411 Pre-existing secondary hypertension complicating pregnancy, <u>first</u> trimester

    O10.412 Pre-existing secondary hypertension complicating pregnancy, <u>second</u> trimester

    O10.413 Pre-existing secondary hypertension complicating pregnancy, <u>third</u> trimester

    O10.419 Pre-existing secondary hypertension complicating pregnancy, <u>unspecified</u> trimester

O10.42 Pre-existing secondary hypertension <u>complicating childbirth</u>

O10.43 Pre-existing secondary hypertension <u>complicating the puerperium</u>

O10.9- <u>Unspecified</u> pre-existing <u>hypertension</u> complicating pregnancy, childbirth and the puerperium

O10.91- Unspecified pre-existing hypertension <u>complicating pregnancy</u>

    O10.911 Unspecified pre-existing hypertension complicating pregnancy, <u>first</u> trimester

    O10.912 Unspecified pre-existing hypertension complicating pregnancy, <u>second</u> trimester

    O10.913 Unspecified pre-existing hypertension complicating pregnancy, <u>third</u> trimester

    O10.919 Unspecified pre-existing hypertension complicating pregnancy, <u>unspecified</u> trimester

O10.92 Unspecified pre-existing hypertension <u>complicating childbirth</u>

O10.93 Unspecified pre-existing hypertension <u>complicating the puerperium</u>

O11- Pre-existing hypertension <u>with pre-eclampsia</u>
> Includes: Conditions in O10 complicated by pre-eclampsia
>   Pre-eclampsia superimposed pre-existing hypertension
> Use additional code from O10 to identify the type of hypertension

O11.1 Pre-existing hypertension with pre-eclampsia, <u>first</u> trimester

O11.2 Pre-existing hypertension with pre-eclampsia, <u>second</u> trimester

O11.3 Pre-existing hypertension with pre-eclampsia, <u>third</u> trimester

O11.9 Pre-existing hypertension with pre-eclampsia, <u>unspecified</u> trimester

O12- Gestational [pregnancy-induced] edema and proteinuria <u>without hypertension</u>

O12.0- <u>Gestational edema</u>

    O12.00 Gestational edema, <u>unspecified</u> trimester

    O12.01 Gestational edema, <u>first</u> trimester

    O12.02 Gestational edema, <u>second</u> trimester

    O12.03 Gestational edema, <u>third</u> trimester

O12.1- <u>Gestational proteinuria</u>

    O12.10 Gestational proteinuria, <u>unspecified</u> trimester

    O12.11 Gestational proteinuria, <u>first</u> trimester

    O12.12 Gestational proteinuria, <u>second</u> trimester

    O12.13 Gestational proteinuria, <u>third</u> trimester

O12.2- <u>Gestational edema with proteinuria</u>

    O12.20 Gestational edema with proteinuria, <u>unspecified</u> trimester

    O12.21 Gestational edema with proteinuria, <u>first</u> trimester

    O12.22 Gestational edema with proteinuria, <u>second</u> trimester

    O12.23 Gestational edema with proteinuria, <u>third</u> trimester

O13- Gestational [pregnancy-induced] hypertension <u>without significant proteinuria</u>
> Includes: Gestational hypertension NOS

O13.1 Gestational [pregnancy-induced] hypertension without significant proteinuria, <u>first</u> trimester

O13.2 Gestational [pregnancy-induced] hypertension without significant proteinuria, <u>second</u> trimester

O13.3 Gestational [pregnancy-induced] hypertension without significant proteinuria, <u>third</u> trimester

O13.9 Gestational [pregnancy-induced] hypertension without significant proteinuria, <u>unspecified</u> trimester

O14- <u>Pre-eclampsia</u>
> *Excludes 1: pre-existing hypertension with pre-eclampsia (O11)*

O14.0- <u>Mild to moderate</u> pre-eclampsia

    O14.00 Mild to moderate pre-eclampsia, <u>unspecified</u> trimester

    O14.02 Mild to moderate pre-eclampsia, <u>second</u> trimester

    O14.03 Mild to moderate pre-eclampsia, <u>third</u> trimester

O14.1- <u>Severe</u> pre-eclampsia
> *Excludes 1: HELLP syndrome (O14.2-)*

    O14.10 Severe pre-eclampsia, <u>unspecified</u> trimester

    O14.12 Severe pre-eclampsia, <u>second</u> trimester

    O14.13 Severe pre-eclampsia, <u>third</u> trimester

O14.2- <u>HELLP syndrome</u>
> Severe pre-eclampsia with hemolysis, elevated liver enzymes and low platelet count (HELLP)

    O14.20 HELLP syndrome (HELLP), <u>unspecified</u> trimester

    O14.22 HELLP syndrome (HELLP), <u>second</u> trimester

    O14.23 HELLP syndrome (HELLP), <u>third</u> trimester

O14.9- <u>Unspecified</u> pre-eclampsia

    O14.90 Unspecified pre-eclampsia, <u>unspecified</u> trimester

    O14.92 Unspecified pre-eclampsia, <u>second</u> trimester

    O14.93 Unspecified pre-eclampsia, <u>third</u> trimester

O15- <u>Eclampsia</u>
> Includes: Convulsions following conditions in O10-O14 and O16

O15.0- Eclampsia <u>in pregnancy</u>

    O15.00 Eclampsia in pregnancy, unspecified trimester

    O15.02 Eclampsia in pregnancy, <u>second</u> trimester

    O15.03 Eclampsia in pregnancy, <u>third</u> trimester

O15.1 Eclampsia <u>in labor</u>

O15.2 Eclampsia <u>in the puerperium</u>

O15.9 Eclampsia, <u>unspecified</u> as to time period
> Eclampsia NOS

O16- <u>Unspecified</u> maternal hypertension

O16.1 Unspecified maternal hypertension, <u>first</u> trimester

O16.2 Unspecified maternal hypertension, <u>second</u> trimester

O16.3 Unspecified maternal hypertension, <u>third</u> trimester

O16.9 Unspecified maternal hypertension, <u>unspecified</u> trimester

Other maternal disorders predominantly related to pregnancy (O20-O29)

> *Excludes❷: maternal care related to the fetus and amniotic cavity and possible delivery problems (O30-O48)*
> *   maternal diseases classifiable elsewhere but complicating pregnancy, labor and delivery, and the puerperium (O98-O99)*

O20- Hemorrhage in early pregnancy
> Includes: Hemorrhage before completion of 20 weeks gestation
> *Excludes 1: pregnancy with abortive outcome (O00-O08)*

O20.0 Threatened abortion
> Hemorrhage specified as due to threatened abortion

O20.8 Other hemorrhage in early pregnancy

O20.9 Hemorrhage in early pregnancy, unspecified

O21- Excessive vomiting in pregnancy

O21.0 Mild hyperemesis gravidarum
> Hyperemesis gravidarum, mild or unspecified, starting before the end of the 20th week of gestation

O21.1 Hyperemesis gravidarum <u>with metabolic disturbance</u>
> Hyperemesis gravidarum, starting before the end of the 20th week of gestation, with metabolic disturbance such as carbohydrate depletion
> Hyperemesis gravidarum, starting before the end of the 20th week of gestation, with metabolic disturbance such as dehydration
> Hyperemesis gravidarum, starting before the end of the 20th week of gestation, with metabolic disturbance such as electrolyte imbalance

O 10 - 023 *(side tab)*

O21.2   **Late vomiting of pregnancy**
Excessive vomiting starting after 20 completed weeks of gestation

O21.8   **Other vomiting complicating pregnancy**
Vomiting due to diseases classified elsewhere, complicating pregnancy
Use additional code, to identify cause.

O21.9   **Vomiting of pregnancy, unspecified**

O22-   Venous complications and hemorrhoids in pregnancy
Excludes 1: venous complications of:
abortion NOS (O03.9)
ectopic or molar pregnancy (O08.7)
failed attempted abortion (O07.35)
induced abortion (O04.85)
spontaneous abortion (O03.89)
Excludes❷: obstetric pulmonary embolism (O88-)
venous complications and hemorrhoids of childbirth and the puerperium   (O87-)

O22.0- Varicose veins of lower extremity in pregnancy
Varicose veins NOS in pregnancy

O22.00 Varicose veins of lower extremity in pregnancy, unspecified trimester

O22.01 Varicose veins of lower extremity in pregnancy, first trimester

O22.02 Varicose veins of lower extremity in pregnancy, second trimester

O22.03 Varicose veins of lower extremity in pregnancy, third trimester

O22.1- Genital varices in pregnancy
Perineal varices in pregnancy
Vaginal varices in pregnancy
Vulval varices in pregnancy

O22.10 Genital varices in pregnancy, unspecified trimester

O22.11 Genital varices in pregnancy, first trimester

O22.12 Genital varices in pregnancy, second trimester

O22.13 Genital varices in pregnancy, third trimester

O22.2- Superficial thrombophlebitis in pregnancy
Phlebitis in pregnancy NOS
Thrombophlebitis of legs in pregnancy
Thrombosis in pregnancy NOS
Use additional code to identify the superficial thrombophlebitis (I80.0-)

O22.20 Superficial thrombophlebitis in pregnancy, unspecified trimester

O22.21 Superficial thrombophlebitis in pregnancy, first trimester

O22.22 Superficial thrombophlebitis in pregnancy, second trimester

O22.23 Superficial thrombophlebitis in pregnancy, third trimester

O22.3- Deep phlebothrombosis in pregnancy
Deep vein thrombosis, antepartum
Use additional code to identify the deep vein thrombosis (I82.4-, I82.5-, I82.62-. I82.72-)
Use additional code, if applicable, for associated long-term (current) use of anticoagulants (Z79.01)

O22.30 Deep phlebothrombosis in pregnancy, unspecified trimester

O22.31 Deep phlebothrombosis in pregnancy, first trimester

O22.32 Deep phlebothrombosis in pregnancy, second trimester

O22.33 Deep phlebothrombosis in pregnancy, third trimester

O22.4- Hemorrhoids in pregnancy

O22.40 Hemorrhoids in pregnancy, unspecified trimester

O22.41 Hemorrhoids in pregnancy, first trimester

O22.42 Hemorrhoids in pregnancy, second trimester

O22.43 Hemorrhoids in pregnancy, third trimester

O22.5- Cerebral venous thrombosis in pregnancy
Cerebrovenous sinus thrombosis in pregnancy

O22.50 Cerebral venous thrombosis in pregnancy, unspecified trimester

O22.51 Cerebral venous thrombosis in pregnancy, first trimester

O22.52 Cerebral venous thrombosis in pregnancy, second trimester

O22.53 Cerebral venous thrombosis in pregnancy, third trimester

O22.8- Other venous complications in pregnancy

O22.8x- Other venous complications in pregnancy

O22.8x1   Other venous complications in pregnancy, first trimester

O22.8x2   Other venous complications in pregnancy, second trimester

O22.8x3   Other venous complications in pregnancy, third trimester

O22.8x9   Other venous complications in pregnancy, unspecified trimester

O22.9- Venous complication in pregnancy, unspecified
Gestational phlebitis NOS
Gestational phlebopathy NOS
Gestational thrombosis NOS

O22.90 Venous complication in pregnancy, unspecified, unspecified trimester

O22.91 Venous complication in pregnancy, unspecified, first trimester

O22.92 Venous complication in pregnancy, unspecified, second trimester

O22.93 Venous complication in pregnancy, unspecified, third trimester

O23-   Infections of genitourinary tract in pregnancy
Use additional code to identify organism (B95-, B96-)
Excludes❷: gonococcal infections complicating pregnancy, childbirth and the puerperium (O98.2)
infections with a predominantly sexual mode of transmission NOS complicating pregnancy, childbirth and the puerperium (O98.3)
syphilis complicating pregnancy, childbirth and the puerperium (O98.1)
tuberculosis of genitourinary system complicating pregnancy, childbirth and the puerperium (O98.0)
venereal disease NOS complicating pregnancy, childbirth and the puerperium (O98.3)

O23.0- Infections of kidney in pregnancy
Pyelonephritis in pregnancy

O23.00 Infections of kidney in pregnancy, unspecified trimester

O23.01 Infections of kidney in pregnancy, first trimester

O23.02 Infections of kidney in pregnancy, second trimester

O23.03 Infections of kidney in pregnancy, third trimester

O23.1- Infections of bladder in pregnancy

O23.10 Infections of bladder in pregnancy, unspecified trimester

O23.11 Infections of bladder in pregnancy, first trimester

O23.12 Infections of bladder in pregnancy, second trimester

O23.13 Infections of bladder in pregnancy, third trimester

O23.2- Infections of urethra in pregnancy

O23.20 Infections of urethra in pregnancy, unspecified trimester

O23.21 Infections of urethra in pregnancy, first trimester

O23.22 Infections of urethra in pregnancy, second trimester

O23.23 Infections of urethra in pregnancy, third trimester

O23.3- Infections of other parts of urinary tract in pregnancy

O23.30 Infections of other parts of urinary tract in pregnancy, unspecified trimester

O23.31 Infections of other parts of urinary tract in pregnancy, first trimester

O23.32 Infections of other parts of urinary tract in pregnancy, second trimester

O23.33 Infections of other parts of urinary tract in pregnancy, third trimester

O23.4- Unspecified infection of urinary tract in pregnancy

O23.40 Unspecified infection of urinary tract in pregnancy, unspecified trimester

O23.41 Unspecified infection of urinary tract in pregnancy, first trimester

O23.42 Unspecified infection of urinary tract in pregnancy, second trimester

O23.43 Unspecified infection of urinary tract in pregnancy, third trimester

O23.5- Infections of the genital tract in pregnancy

O23.51- Infection of cervix in pregnancy

O23.511   Infections of cervix in pregnancy, first trimester

O23.512   Infections of cervix in pregnancy, second trimester

O23.513   Infections of cervix in pregnancy, third trimester

O23.519   Infections of cervix in pregnancy, unspecified trimester

O23.52- Salpingo-oophoritis in pregnancy
Oophoritis in pregnancy
Salpingitis in pregnancy

O23.521   Salpingo-oophoritis in pregnancy, first trimester

O23.522   Salpingo-oophoritis in pregnancy, second trimester

O23.523   Salpingo-oophoritis in pregnancy, third trimester

O23.529   Salpingo-oophoritis in pregnancy, unspecified trimester

O23.59- Infection of other part of genital tract in pregnancy

O23.591   Infection of other part of genital tract in pregnancy, first trimester

O23.592   Infection of other part of genital tract in pregnancy, second trimester

O
1
0
-
O
2
3

Excludes 1: = NOT CODED HERE! (Do not code both)   **629**   *Excludes❷:* = Not Included Here

O23.593 Infection of other part of genital tract in pregnancy, <u>third</u> trimester

O23.599 Infection of other part of genital tract in pregnancy, <u>unspecified</u> trimester

O23.9- <u>Unspecified</u> genitourinary tract infection in pregnancy
Genitourinary tract infection in pregnancy NOS

O23.90 Unspecified genitourinary tract infection in pregnancy, <u>unspecified</u> trimester

O23.91 Unspecified genitourinary tract infection in pregnancy, <u>first</u> trimester

O23.92 Unspecified genitourinary tract infection in pregnancy, <u>second</u> trimester

O23.93 Unspecified genitourinary tract infection in pregnancy, <u>third</u> trimester

O24- <u>Diabetes mellitus</u> in pregnancy, childbirth, and the puerperium

O24.0- <u>Pre-existing diabetes mellitus</u>, <u>type 1</u>, in pregnancy, childbirth and the puerperium
Juvenile onset diabetes mellitus, in pregnancy, childbirth and the puerperium
Ketosis-prone diabetes mellitus in pregnancy, childbirth and the puerperium
Use additional code from category E10 to further identify any manifestations

O24.01- Pre-existing diabetes mellitus, type 1, <u>in pregnancy</u>

O24.011 Pre-existing diabetes mellitus, type 1, in pregnancy, <u>first</u> trimester

O24.012 Pre-existing diabetes mellitus, type 1, in pregnancy, <u>second</u> trimester

O24.013 Pre-existing diabetes mellitus, type 1, in pregnancy, <u>third</u> trimester

O24.019 Pre-existing diabetes mellitus, type 1, in pregnancy, <u>unspecified</u> trimester

O24.02 Pre-existing diabetes mellitus, type 1, <u>in childbirth</u>

O24.03 Pre-existing diabetes mellitus, type 1, <u>in the puerperium</u>

O24.1- Pre-existing diabetes mellitus, <u>type 2</u>, in pregnancy, childbirth and the puerperium
Insulin-resistant diabetes mellitus in pregnancy, childbirth and the puerperium
Use additional code (for):
From category E11 to further identify any manifestations
Long-term (current) use of insulin (Z79.4)

O24.11- Pre-existing diabetes mellitus, <u>type 2</u>, <u>in pregnancy</u>

O24.111 Pre-existing diabetes mellitus, type 2, in pregnancy, <u>first</u> trimester

O24.112 Pre-existing diabetes mellitus, type 2, in pregnancy, <u>second</u> trimester

O24.113 Pre-existing diabetes mellitus, type 2, in pregnancy, <u>third</u> trimester

O24.119 Pre-existing diabetes mellitus, type 2, in pregnancy, <u>unspecified</u> trimester

O24.12 Pre-existing diabetes mellitus, <u>type 2</u>, <u>in childbirth</u>

O24.13 Pre-existing diabetes mellitus, <u>type 2</u>, <u>in the puerperium</u>

O24.3- <u>Unspecified</u> pre-existing diabetes mellitus in pregnancy, childbirth and the puerperium
Use additional code (for):
From category E11 to further identify any manifestation
Long-term (current) use of insulin (Z79.4)

O24.31- <u>Unspecified</u> pre-existing diabetes mellitus in pregnancy

O24.311 Unspecified pre-existing diabetes mellitus in pregnancy, <u>first</u> trimester

O24.312 Unspecified pre-existing diabetes mellitus in pregnancy, <u>second</u> trimester

O24.313 Unspecified pre-existing diabetes mellitus in pregnancy, <u>third</u> trimester

O24.319 Unspecified pre-existing diabetes mellitus in pregnancy, <u>unspecified</u> trimester

O24.32 <u>Unspecified</u> pre-existing diabetes mellitus <u>in childbirth</u>

O24.33 <u>Unspecified</u> pre-existing diabetes mellitus <u>in the puerperium</u>

O24.4- <u>Gestational</u> diabetes mellitus
Diabetes mellitus arising in pregnancy
Gestational diabetes mellitus NOS

O24.41- Gestational diabetes mellitus <u>in pregnancy</u>

O24.410 Gestational diabetes mellitus in pregnancy, <u>diet controlled</u>

O24.414 Gestational diabetes mellitus in pregnancy, <u>insulin controlled</u>

O24.419 Gestational diabetes mellitus in pregnancy, <u>unspecified control</u>

O24.42- Gestational diabetes mellitus <u>in childbirth</u>

O24.420 Gestational diabetes mellitus in childbirth, <u>diet controlled</u>

O24.424 Gestational diabetes mellitus in childbirth, <u>insulin controlled</u>

O24.429 Gestational diabetes mellitus in childbirth, <u>unspecified control</u>

O24.43- Gestational diabetes mellitus <u>in the puerperium</u>

O24.430 Gestational diabetes mellitus in the puerperium, <u>diet controlled</u>

O24.434 Gestational diabetes mellitus in the puerperium, <u>insulin controlled</u>

O24.439 Gestational diabetes mellitus in the puerperium, <u>unspecified control</u>

O24.8- <u>Other pre-existing diabetes mellitus</u> in pregnancy, childbirth, and the puerperium
Use additional code (for):
From categories E08, E09 and E13 to further identify any manifestation
Long-term (current) use of insulin (Z79.4)

O24.81- Other pre-existing diabetes mellitus <u>in pregnancy</u>

O24.811 Other pre-existing diabetes mellitus in pregnancy, <u>first</u> trimester

O24.812 Other pre-existing diabetes mellitus in pregnancy, <u>second</u> trimester

O24.813 Other pre-existing diabetes mellitus in pregnancy, <u>third</u> trimester

O24.819 Other pre-existing diabetes mellitus in pregnancy, <u>unspecified</u> trimester

O24.82 Other pre-existing diabetes mellitus <u>in childbirth</u>

O24.83 Other pre-existing diabetes mellitus <u>in the puerperium</u>

O24.9- <u>Unspecified</u> diabetes mellitus in pregnancy, childbirth and the puerperium
Use additional code for long-term (current) use of insulin (Z79.4)

O24.91- Unspecified diabetes mellitus <u>in pregnancy</u>

O24.911 Unspecified diabetes mellitus in pregnancy, <u>first</u> trimester

O24.912 Unspecified diabetes mellitus in pregnancy, <u>second</u> trimester

O24.913 Unspecified diabetes mellitus in pregnancy, <u>third</u> trimester

O24.919 Unspecified diabetes mellitus in pregnancy, <u>unspecified</u> trimester

O24.92 Unspecified diabetes mellitus <u>in childbirth</u>

O24.93 Unspecified diabetes mellitus <u>in the puerperium</u>

O25- <u>Malnutrition</u> in pregnancy, childbirth and the puerperium

O25.1- Malnutrition in pregnancy

O25.10 Malnutrition in pregnancy, <u>unspecified</u> trimester

O25.11 Malnutrition in pregnancy, <u>first</u> trimester

O25.12 Malnutrition in pregnancy, <u>second</u> trimester

O25.13 Malnutrition in pregnancy, <u>third</u> trimester

O25.2 Malnutrition <u>in childbirth</u>

O25.3 Malnutrition <u>in the puerperium</u>

O26- <u>Maternal care for other conditions predominantly related to pregnancy</u>

O26.0- <u>Excessive weight gain</u> in pregnancy
Excludes❷: gestational edema (O12.0, O12.2)

O26.00 Excessive weight gain in pregnancy, <u>unspecified</u> trimester

O26.01 Excessive weight gain in pregnancy, <u>first</u> trimester

O26.02 Excessive weight gain in pregnancy, <u>second</u> trimester

O26.03 Excessive weight gain in pregnancy, <u>third</u> trimester

O26.1- <u>Low weight gain</u> in pregnancy

O26.10 Low weight gain in pregnancy, <u>unspecified</u> trimester

O26.11 Low weight gain in pregnancy, <u>first</u> trimester

O26.12 Low weight gain in pregnancy, <u>second</u> trimester

O26.13 Low weight gain in pregnancy, <u>third</u> trimester

O26.2- Pregnancy care for patient <u>with recurrent pregnancy loss</u>

O26.20 Pregnancy care for patient with recurrent pregnancy loss, <u>unspecified</u> trimester

O26.21 Pregnancy care for patient with recurrent pregnancy loss, <u>first</u> trimester

O26.22 Pregnancy care for patient with recurrent pregnancy loss, <u>second</u> trimester

O26.23 Pregnancy care for patient with recurrent pregnancy loss, <u>third</u> trimester

O 2 3 - O 2 9

O26.3- Retained intrauterine contraceptive device in pregnancy
  O26.30 Retained intrauterine contraceptive device in pregnancy, unspecified trimester
  O26.31 Retained intrauterine contraceptive device in pregnancy, first trimester
  O26.32 Retained intrauterine contraceptive device in pregnancy, second trimester
  O26.33 Retained intrauterine contraceptive device in pregnancy, third trimester
O26.4- Herpes gestationis
  O26.40 Herpes gestationis, unspecified trimester
  O26.41 Herpes gestationis, first trimester
  O26.42 Herpes gestationis, second trimester
  O26.43 Herpes gestationis, third trimester
O26.5- Maternal hypotension syndrome
    Supine hypotensive syndrome
  O26.50 Maternal hypotension syndrome, unspecified trimester
  O26.51 Maternal hypotension syndrome, first trimester
  O26.52 Maternal hypotension syndrome, second trimester
  O26.53 Maternal hypotension syndrome, third trimester
O26.6- Liver and biliary tract disorders in pregnancy, childbirth and the puerperium
    Use additional code to identify the specific disorder
    Excludes❷: hepatorenal syndrome following labor and delivery (O90.4)
  O26.61- Liver and biliary tract disorders in pregnancy
    O26.611 Liver and biliary tract disorders in pregnancy, first trimester
    O26.612 Liver and biliary tract disorders in pregnancy, second trimester
    O26.613 Liver and biliary tract disorders in pregnancy, third trimester
    O26.619 Liver and biliary tract disorders in pregnancy, unspecified trimester
  O26.62 Liver and biliary tract disorders in childbirth
  O26.63 Liver and biliary tract disorders in the puerperium
O26.7- Subluxation of symphysis (pubis) in pregnancy, childbirth and the puerperium
    Excludes 1: traumatic separation of symphysis (pubis) during childbirth (O71.6)
  O26.71- Subluxation of symphysis (pubis) in pregnancy
    O26.711 Subluxation of symphysis (pubis) in pregnancy, first trimester
    O26.712 Subluxation of symphysis (pubis) in pregnancy, second trimester
    O26.713 Subluxation of symphysis (pubis) in pregnancy, third trimester
    O26.719 Subluxation of symphysis (pubis) in pregnancy, unspecified trimester
  O26.72 Subluxation of symphysis (pubis) in childbirth
  O26.73 Subluxation of symphysis (pubis) in the puerperium
O26.8- Other specified pregnancy related conditions
  O26.81- Pregnancy related exhaustion and fatigue
    O26.811 Pregnancy related exhaustion and fatigue, first trimester
    O26.812 Pregnancy related exhaustion and fatigue, second trimester
    O26.813 Pregnancy related exhaustion and fatigue, third trimester
    O26.819 Pregnancy related exhaustion and fatigue, unspecified trimester
  O26.82- Pregnancy related peripheral neuritis
    O26.821 Pregnancy related peripheral neuritis, first trimester
    O26.822 Pregnancy related peripheral neuritis, second trimester
    O26.823 Pregnancy related peripheral neuritis, third trimester
    O26.829 Pregnancy related peripheral neuritis, unspecified trimester
  O26.83- Pregnancy related renal disease
      Use additional code to identify the specific disorder
    O26.831 Pregnancy related renal disease, first trimester
    O26.832 Pregnancy related renal disease, second trimester
    O26.833 Pregnancy related renal disease, third trimester
    O26.839 Pregnancy related renal disease, unspecified trimester

O26.84- Uterine size-date discrepancy complicating pregnancy
    Excludes 1: encounter for suspected problem with fetal growth ruled out (Z03.74)
  O26.841 Uterine size-date discrepancy, first trimester
  O26.842 Uterine size-date discrepancy, second trimester
  O26.843 Uterine size-date discrepancy, third trimester
  O26.849 Uterine size-date discrepancy, unspecified trimester
O26.85- Spotting complicating pregnancy
  O26.851 Spotting complicating pregnancy, first trimester
  O26.852 Spotting complicating pregnancy, second trimester
  O26.853 Spotting complicating pregnancy, third trimester
  O26.859 Spotting complicating pregnancy, unspecified trimester
O26.86 Pruritic urticarial papules and plaques of pregnancy (PUPPP)
    Polymorphic eruption of pregnancy
O26.87- Cervical shortening
    Excludes 1: encounter for suspected cervical shortening ruled out (Z03.75)
  O26.872 Cervical shortening, second trimester
  O26.873 Cervical shortening, third trimester
  O26.879 Cervical shortening, unspecified trimester
O26.89- Other specified pregnancy related conditions
  O26.891 Other specified pregnancy related conditions, first trimester
  O26.892 Other specified pregnancy related conditions, second trimester
  O26.893 Other specified pregnancy related conditions, third trimester
  O26.899 Other specified pregnancy related conditions, unspecified trimester
O26.9- Pregnancy related conditions, unspecified
  O26.90 Pregnancy related conditions, unspecified, unspecified trimester
  O26.91 Pregnancy related conditions, unspecified, first trimester
  O26.92 Pregnancy related conditions, unspecified, second trimester
  V26.93 Pregnancy related conditions, unspecified, third trimester
O28- Abnormal findings on antenatal screening of mother
    Excludes 1: diagnostic findings classified elsewhere — see Alphabetical Index
  O28.0 Abnormal hematological finding on antenatal screening of mother
  O28.1 Abnormal biochemical finding on antenatal screening of mother
  O28.2 Abnormal cytological finding on antenatal screening of mother
  O28.3 Abnormal ultrasonic finding on antenatal screening of mother
  O28.4 Abnormal radiological finding on antenatal screening of mother
  O28.5 Abnormal chromosomal and genetic finding on antenatal screening of mother
  O28.8 Other abnormal findings on antenatal screening of mother
  O28.9 Unspecified abnormal findings on antenatal screening of mother
O29- Complications of anesthesia during pregnancy
    Includes: Maternal complications arising from the administration of a general, regional or local anesthetic, analgesic or other sedation during pregnancy
    Use additional code, if necessary, to identify the complication
    Excludes❷: complications of anesthesia during labor and delivery (O74.-)
    complicatios of anesthesia during the puerperium (O89.-)
  O29.0- Pulmonary complications of anesthesia during pregnancy
    O29.01- Aspiration pneumonitis due to anesthesia during pregnancy
        Inhalation of stomach contents or secretions NOS due to anesthesia during pregnancy
        Mendelson's syndrome due to anesthesia during pregnancy
      O29.011 Aspiration pneumonitis due to anesthesia during pregnancy, first trimester
      O29.012 Aspiration pneumonitis due to anesthesia during pregnancy, second trimester
      O29.013 Aspiration pneumonitis due to anesthesia during pregnancy, third trimester
      O29.019 Aspiration pneumonitis due to anesthesia during pregnancy, unspecified trimester
    O29.02- Pressure collapse of lung due to anesthesia during pregnancy
      O29.021 Pressure collapse of lung due to anesthesia during pregnancy, first trimester
      O29.022 Pressure collapse of lung due to anesthesia during pregnancy, second trimester
      O29.023 Pressure collapse of lung due to anesthesia during pregnancy, third trimester
      O29.029 Pressure collapse of lung due to anesthesia during pregnancy, unspecified trimester

O 2 3 I O 2 9

Excludes 1: = NOT CODED HERE! (Do not code both)   **631**   *Excludes❷: = Not Included Here*

O29.09- <u>Other pulmonary</u> complications of anesthesia during pregnancy
    O29.091 Other pulmonary complications of anesthesia during pregnancy, <u>first</u> trimester
    O29.092 Other pulmonary complications of anesthesia during pregnancy, <u>second</u> trimester
    O29.093 Other pulmonary complications of anesthesia during pregnancy, <u>third</u> trimester
    O29.099 Other pulmonary complications of anesthesia during pregnancy, <u>unspecified</u> trimester

O29.1- <u>Cardiac complications</u> of anesthesia during pregnancy
  O29.11- <u>Cardiac arrest</u> due to anesthesia during pregnancy
    O29.111 Cardiac arrest due to anesthesia during pregnancy, <u>first</u> trimester
    O29.112 Cardiac arrest due to anesthesia during pregnancy, <u>second</u> trimester
    O29.113 Cardiac arrest due to anesthesia during pregnancy, <u>third</u> trimester
    O29.119 Cardiac arrest due to anesthesia during pregnancy, <u>unspecified</u> trimester

  O29.12- <u>Cardiac failure</u> due to anesthesia during pregnancy
    O29.121 Cardiac failure due to anesthesia during pregnancy, <u>first</u> trimester
    O29.122 Cardiac failure due to anesthesia during pregnancy, <u>second</u> trimester
    O29.123 Cardiac failure due to anesthesia during pregnancy, <u>third</u> trimester
    O29.129 Cardiac failure due to anesthesia during pregnancy, <u>unspecified</u> trimester

  O29.19- <u>Other cardiac complications</u> of anesthesia during pregnancy
    O29.191 Other cardiac complications of anesthesia during pregnancy, <u>first</u> trimester
    O29.192 Other cardiac complications of anesthesia during pregnancy, <u>second</u> trimester
    O29.193 Other cardiac complications of anesthesia during pregnancy, <u>third</u> trimester
    O29.199 Other cardiac complications of anesthesia during pregnancy, <u>unspecified</u> trimester

O29.2- <u>Central nervous system complications</u> of anesthesia during pregnancy
  O29.21- <u>Cerebral anoxia</u> due to anesthesia during pregnancy
    O29.211 Cerebral anoxia due to anesthesia during pregnancy, <u>first</u> trimester
    O29.212 Cerebral anoxia due to anesthesia during pregnancy, <u>second</u> trimester
    O29.213 Cerebral anoxia due to anesthesia during pregnancy, <u>third</u> trimester
    O29.219 Cerebral anoxia due to anesthesia during pregnancy, <u>unspecified</u> trimester

  O29.29- <u>Other central nervous system complications</u> of anesthesia during pregnancy
    O29.291 Other central nervous system complications of anesthesia during pregnancy, <u>first</u> trimester
    O29.292 Other central nervous system complications of anesthesia during pregnancy, <u>second</u> trimester
    O29.293 Other central nervous system complications of anesthesia during pregnancy, <u>third</u> trimester
    O29.299 Other central nervous system complications of anesthesia during pregnancy, <u>unspecified</u> trimester

O29.3- <u>Toxic reaction to local anesthesia</u> during pregnancy
  O29.3x- Toxic reaction to local anesthesia during pregnancy
    O29.3x1 Toxic reaction to local anesthesia during pregnancy, <u>first</u> trimester
    O29.3x2 Toxic reaction to local anesthesia during pregnancy, <u>second</u> trimester
    O29.3x3 Toxic reaction to local anesthesia during pregnancy, <u>third</u> trimester
    O29.3x9 Toxic reaction to local anesthesia during pregnancy, <u>unspecified</u> trimester

O29.4- <u>Spinal and epidural anesthesia induced headache</u> during pregnancy
    O29.40 Spinal and epidural anesthesia induced headache during pregnancy, <u>unspecified</u> trimester
    O29.41 Spinal and epidural anesthesia induced headache during pregnancy, <u>first</u> trimester
    O29.42 Spinal and epidural anesthesia induced headache during pregnancy, <u>second</u> trimester
    O29.43 Spinal and epidural anesthesia induced headache during pregnancy, <u>third</u> trimester

O29.5- <u>Other complications of spinal and epidural anesthesia</u> during pregnancy
  O29.5x- Other complications of spinal and epidural anesthesia during pregnancy
    O29.5x1 Other complications of spinal and epidural anesthesia during pregnancy, <u>first</u> trimester
    O29.5x2 Other complications of spinal and epidural anesthesia during pregnancy, <u>second</u> trimester
    O29.5x3 Other complications of spinal and epidural anesthesia during pregnancy, <u>third</u> trimester
    O29.5x9 Other complications of spinal and epidural anesthesia during pregnancy, <u>unspecified</u> trimester

O29.6- <u>Failed or difficult intubation for anesthesia</u> during pregnancy
    O29.60 Failed or difficult intubation for anesthesia during pregnancy, <u>unspecified</u> trimester
    O29.61 Failed or difficult intubation for anesthesia during pregnancy, <u>first</u> trimester
    O29.62 Failed or difficult intubation for anesthesia during pregnancy, <u>second</u> trimester
    O29.63 Failed or difficult intubation for anesthesia during pregnancy, <u>third</u> trimester

O29.8- <u>Other complications of anesthesia</u> during pregnancy
  O29.8x- Other complications of anesthesia during pregnancy
    O29.8x1 Other complications of anesthesia during pregnancy, <u>first</u> trimester
    O29.8x2 Other complications of anesthesia during pregnancy, <u>second</u> trimester
    O29.8x3 Other complications of anesthesia during pregnancy, <u>third</u> trimester
    O29.8x9 Other complications of anesthesia during pregnancy, <u>unspecified</u> trimester

O29.9- <u>Unspecified</u> complication of anesthesia during pregnancy
    O29.90 Unspecified complication of anesthesia during pregnancy, <u>unspecified</u> trimester
    O29.91 Unspecified complication of anesthesia during pregnancy, <u>first</u> trimester
    O29.92 Unspecified complication of anesthesia during pregnancy, <u>second</u> trimester
    O29.93 Unspecified complication of anesthesia during pregnancy, <u>third</u> trimester

Maternal care related to the fetus and amniotic cavity and possible delivery problems (O30-O48)

O30- <u>Multiple gestation</u>
  Code also any complications specific to multiple gestation
  O30.0- <u>Twin pregnancy</u>
    O30.00- Twin pregnancy, <u>unspecified number</u> of placenta and <u>unspecified number</u> of amniotic sacs
      O30.001 Twin pregnancy, unspecified number of placenta and unspecified number of amniotic sacs, <u>first</u> trimester
      O30.002 Twin pregnancy, unspecified number of placenta and unspecified number of amniotic sacs, <u>second</u> trimester
      O30.003 Twin pregnancy, unspecified number of placenta and unspecified number of amniotic sacs, <u>third</u> trimester
      O30.009 Twin pregnancy, unspecified number of placenta and unspecified number of amniotic sacs, <u>unspecified</u> trimester

    O30.01- Twin pregnancy, <u>monochorionic/monoamniotic</u>
      Twin pregnancy, one placenta, one amniotic sac
      Excludes 1: conjoined twins (O30.02-)
      O30.011 Twin pregnancy, monochorionic/monoamniotic, <u>first</u> trimester
      O30.012 Twin pregnancy, monochorionic/monoamniotic, <u>second</u> trimester
      O30.013 Twin pregnancy, monochorionic/monoamniotic, <u>third</u> trimester
      O30.019 Twin pregnancy, monochorionic/monoamniotic, <u>unspecified</u> trimester

    O30.02- <u>Conjoined twin</u> pregnancy
      O30.021 Conjoined twin pregnancy, <u>first</u> trimester
      O30.022 Conjoined twin pregnancy, <u>second</u> trimester
      O30.023 Conjoined twin pregnancy, <u>third</u> trimester
      O30.029 Conjoined twin pregnancy, <u>unspecified</u> trimester

O29 - O30 (side tab)

O30.03- Twin pregnancy, <u>monochorionic/diamniotic</u>
　　Twin pregnancy, one placenta, two amniotic sacs

O30.031 Twin pregnancy, monochorionic/diamniotic, <u>first</u> trimester

O30.032 Twin pregnancy, monochorionic/diamniotic, <u>second</u> trimester

O30.033 Twin pregnancy, monochorionic/diamniotic, <u>third</u> trimester

O30.039 Twin pregnancy, monochorionic/diamniotic, <u>unspecified</u> trimester

O30.04- Twin pregnancy, <u>dichorionic/diamniotic</u>
　　Twin pregnancy, two placentae, two amniotic sacs

O30.041 Twin pregnancy, dichorionic/diamniotic, <u>first</u> trimester

O30.042 Twin pregnancy, dichorionic/diamniotic, <u>second</u> trimester

O30.043 Twin pregnancy, dichorionic/diamniotic, <u>third</u> trimester

O30.049 Twin pregnancy, dichorionic/diamniotic, <u>unspecified</u> trimester

O30.09- Twin pregnancy, <u>unable to determine number</u> of placenta and number of amniotic sacs

O30.091 Twin pregnancy, unable to determine number of placenta and number of amniotic sacs, <u>first</u> trimester

O30.092 Twin pregnancy, unable to determine number of placenta and number of amniotic sacs, <u>second</u> trimester

O30.093 Twin pregnancy, unable to determine number of placenta and number of amniotic sacs, <u>third</u> trimester

O30.099 Twin pregnancy, unable to determine number of placenta and number of amniotic sacs, <u>unspecified</u> trimester

O30.1- <u>Triplet</u> pregnancy

O30.10- Triplet pregnancy, <u>unspecified number</u> of placenta and <u>unspecified number</u> of amniotic sacs

O30.101 Triplet pregnancy, unspecified number of placenta and unspecified number of amniotic sacs, <u>first</u> trimester

O30.102 Triplet pregnancy, unspecified number of placenta and unspecified number of amniotic sacs, <u>second</u> trimester

O30.103 Triplet pregnancy, unspecified number of placenta and unspecified number of amniotic sacs, <u>third</u> trimester

O30.109 Triplet pregnancy, unspecified number of placenta and unspecified number of amniotic sacs, <u>unspecified</u> trimester

O30.11- Triplet pregnancy <u>with two or more monochorionic</u> fetuses

O30.111 Triplet pregnancy with two or more monochorionic fetuses, <u>first</u> trimester

O30.112 Triplet pregnancy with two or more monochorionic fetuses, <u>second</u> trimester

O30.113 Triplet pregnancy with two or more monochorionic fetuses, <u>third</u> trimester

O30.119 Triplet pregnancy with two or more monochorionic fetuses, <u>unspecified</u> trimester

O30.12- Triplet pregnancy <u>with two or more monoamniotic</u> fetuses

O30.121 Triplet pregnancy with two or more monoamniotic fetuses, <u>first</u> trimester

O30.122 Triplet pregnancy with two or more monoamniotic fetuses, <u>second</u> trimester

O30.123 Triplet pregnancy with two or more monoamniotic fetuses, <u>third</u> trimester

O30.129 Triplet pregnancy with two or more monoamniotic fetuses, <u>unspecified</u> trimester

O30.19- Triplet pregnancy, <u>unable to determine number</u> of placenta and number of amniotic sacs

O30.191 Triplet pregnancy, unable to determine number of placenta and number of amniotic sacs, <u>first</u> trimester

O30.192 Triplet pregnancy, unable to determine number of placenta and number of amniotic sacs, <u>second</u> trimester

O30.193 Triplet pregnancy, unable to determine number of placenta and number of amniotic sacs, <u>third</u> trimester

O30.199 Triplet pregnancy, unable to determine number of placenta and number of amniotic sacs, <u>unspecified</u> trimester

O30.2- <u>Quadruplet</u> pregnancy

O30.20- Quadruplet pregnancy, <u>unspecified number</u> of placenta and <u>unspecified number</u> of amnioticsacs

O30.201 Quadruplet pregnancy, unspecified number of placenta and unspecified number of amniotic sacs, <u>first</u> trimester

O30.202 Quadruplet pregnancy, unspecified number of placenta and unspecified number of amniotic sacs, <u>second</u> trimester

O30.203 Quadruplet pregnancy, unspecified number of placenta and unspecified number of amniotic sacs, <u>third</u> trimester

O30.209 Quadruplet pregnancy, unspecified number of placenta and unspecified number of amniotic sacs, <u>unspecified</u> trimester

O30.21- Quadruplet pregnancy <u>with two or more monochorionic</u> fetuses

O30.211 Quadruplet pregnancy with two or more monochorionic fetuses, <u>first</u> trimester

O30.212 Quadruplet pregnancy with two or more monochorionic fetuses, <u>second</u> trimester

O30.213 Quadruplet pregnancy with two or more monochorionic fetuses, <u>third</u> trimester

O30.219 Quadruplet pregnancy with two or more monochorionic fetuses, <u>unspecified</u> trimester

O30.22- Quadruplet pregnancy <u>with two or more monoamniotic</u> fetuses

O30.221 Quadruplet pregnancy with two or more monoamniotic fetuses, <u>first</u> trimester

O30.222 Quadruplet pregnancy with two or more monoamniotic fetuses, <u>second</u> trimester

O30.223 Quadruplet pregnancy with two or more monoamniotic fetuses, <u>third</u> trimester

O30.229 Quadruplet pregnancy with two or more monoamniotic fetuses, <u>unspecified</u> trimester

O30.29- Quadruplet pregnancy, <u>unable to determine number</u> of placenta and number of amniotic sacs

O30.291 Quadruplet pregnancy, unable to determine number of placenta and number of amniotic sacs, <u>first</u> trimester

O30.292 Quadruplet pregnancy, unable to determine number of placenta and number of amniotic sacs, <u>second</u> trimester

O30.293 Quadruplet pregnancy, unable to determine number of placenta and number of amniotic sacs, <u>third</u> trimester

O30.299 Quadruplet pregnancy, unable to determine number of placenta and number of amniotic sacs, <u>unspecified</u> trimester

O30.8- <u>Other specified</u> multiple gestation
　　Multiple gestation pregnancy greater then quadruplets

O30.80- Other specified multiple gestation, <u>unspecified number</u> of placenta and <u>unspecified number</u> of amniotic sacs

O30.801 Other specified multiple gestation, unspecified number of placenta and unspecified number of amniotic sacs, <u>first</u> trimester

O30.802 Other specified multiple gestation, unspecified number of placenta and unspecified number of amniotic sacs, <u>second</u> trimester

O30.803 Other specified multiple gestation, unspecified number of placenta and unspecified number of amniotic sacs, <u>third</u> trimester

O30.809 Other specified multiple gestation, unspecified number of placenta and unspecified number of amniotic sacs, <u>unspecified</u> trimester

O30.81- Other specified multiple gestation <u>with two or more monochorionic</u> fetuses

O30.811 Other specified multiple gestation with two or more monochorionic fetuses, <u>first</u> trimester

O30.812 Other specified multiple gestation with two or more monochorionic fetuses, <u>second</u> trimester

O30.813 Other specified multiple gestation with two or more monochorionic fetuses, <u>third</u> trimester

O30.819 Other specified multiple gestation with two or more monochorionic fetuses, <u>unspecified</u> trimester

O30.82- Other specified multiple gestation <u>with two or more monoamniotic</u> fetuses

O30.821 Other specified multiple gestation with two or more monoamniotic fetuses, <u>first</u> trimester

O30.822 Other specified multiple gestation with two or more monoamniotic fetuses, <u>second</u> trimester

O29 - O30

Excludes 1: = NOT CODED HERE! (Do not code both)

Excludes ❷: = Not Included Here

O30.823 Other specified multiple gestation with two or more monoamniotic fetuses, <u>third</u> trimester

O30.829 Other specified multiple gestation with two or more monoamniotic fetuses, <u>unspecified</u> trimester

O30.89- Other specified multiple gestation, <u>unable to determine number</u> of placenta and number of amniotic sacs

O30.891 Other specified multiple gestation, unable to determine number of placenta and number of amniotic sacs, <u>first</u> trimester

O30.892 Other specified multiple gestation, unable to determine number of placenta and number of amniotic sacs, <u>second</u> trimester

O30.893 Other specified multiple gestation, unable to determine number of placenta and number of amniotic sacs, <u>third</u> trimester

O30.899 Other specified multiple gestation, unable to determine number of placenta and number of amniotic sacs, <u>unspecified</u> trimester

O30.9- Multiple gestation, <u>unspecified</u>
Multiple pregnancy NOS

O30.90 Multiple gestation, unspecified, <u>unspecified</u> trimester

O30.91 Multiple gestation, unspecified, <u>first</u> trimester

O30.92 Multiple gestation, unspecified, <u>second</u> trimester

O30.93 Multiple gestation, unspecified, <u>third</u> trimester

O31- <u>Complications specific to multiple gestation</u>
Excludes❷: delayed delivery of second twin, triplet, etc. (O63.2)
malpresentation of one fetus or more (O32.9)
placental transfusion syndromes (O43.0-)

One of the following 7th characters is to be assigned to each code under category O31. 7th character 0 is for single gestations and multiple gestations where the fetus is unspecified. 7th characters 1 through 9 are for cases of multiple gestations to identify the fetus for which the code applies. The appropriate code from category O30, Multiple gestation, must also be assigned when assigning a code from category O31 that has a 7th character of 1 through 9.
- **0** Not applicable or unspecified
- **1** Fetus 1
- **2** Fetus 2
- **3** Fetus 3
- **4** Fetus 4
- **5** Fetus 5
- **9** Other fetus

O31.0- <u>Papyraceous fetus</u>
Fetus compressus

O31.00x- Papyraceous fetus, <u>unspecified</u> trimester

O31.01x- Papyraceous fetus, <u>first</u> trimester

O31.02x- Papyraceous fetus, <u>second</u> trimester

O31.03x- Papyraceous fetus, <u>third</u> trimester

O31.1- <u>Continuing pregnancy after spontaneous abortion</u> of one fetus or more

O31.10x- Continuing pregnancy after spontaneous abortion of one fetus or more, <u>unspecified</u> trimester

O31.11x- Continuing pregnancy after spontaneous abortion of one fetus or more, <u>first</u> trimester

O31.12x- Continuing pregnancy after spontaneous abortion of one fetus or more, <u>second</u> trimester

O31.13x- Continuing pregnancy after spontaneous abortion of one fetus or more, <u>third</u> trimester

O31.2- <u>Continuing pregnancy after intrauterine death</u> of one fetus or more

O31.20x- Continuing pregnancy after intrauterine death of one fetus or more, <u>unspecified</u> trimester

O31.21x- Continuing pregnancy after intrauterine death of one fetus or more, <u>first</u> trimester

O31.22x- Continuing pregnancy after intrauterine death of one fetus or more, <u>second</u> trimester

O31.23x- Continuing pregnancy after intrauterine death of one fetus or more, <u>third</u> trimester

O31.3- <u>Continuing pregnancy after elective fetal reduction</u> of one fetus or more
Continuing pregnancy after selective termination of one fetus or more

O31.30x- Continuing pregnancy after elective fetal reduction of one fetus or more, <u>unspecified</u> trimester

O31.31x- Continuing pregnancy after elective fetal reduction of one fetus or more, <u>first</u> trimester

O31.32x- Continuing pregnancy after elective fetal reduction of one fetus or more, <u>second</u> trimester

O31.33x- Continuing pregnancy after elective fetal reduction of one fetus or more, <u>third</u> trimester

O31.8- Other complications specific to multiple gestation

O31.8x- <u>Other complications specific to multiple gestation</u>

O31.8x1- Other complications specific to multiple gestation, <u>first</u> trimester

O31.8x2- Other complications specific to multiple gestation, <u>second</u> trimester

O31.8x3- Other complications specific to multiple gestation, <u>third</u> trimester

O31.8x9- Other complications specific to multiple gestation, <u>unspecified</u> trimester

O32- <u>Maternal care for malpresentation of fetus</u>
Includes: The listed conditions as a reason for observation, hospitalization or other obstetric care of the mother, or for cesarean delivery before onset of labor
Excludes 1: malpresentation of fetus with obstructed labor (O64.-)

One of the following 7th characters is to be assigned to each code under category O32. 7th character 0 is for single gestations and multiple gestations where the fetus is unspecified. 7th characters 1 through 9 are for cases of multiple gestations to identify the fetus for which the code applies. The appropriate code from category O30, Multiple gestation, must also be assigned when assigning a code from category O32 that has a 7th character of 1 through 9.
- **0** Not applicable or unspecified
- **1** Fetus 1
- **2** Fetus 2
- **3** Fetus 3
- **4** Fetus 4
- **5** Fetus 5
- **9** Other fetus

O32.0xx- Maternal care for <u>unstable lie</u>

O32.1xx- Maternal care for <u>breech presentation</u>
Maternal care for buttocks presentation
Maternal care for complete breech
Maternal care for frank breech
Excludes 1: footling presentation (O32.8)
incomplete breech (O32.8)

O32.2xx- Maternal care for <u>transverse and oblique lie</u>
Maternal care for oblique presentation
Maternal care for transverse presentation

O32.3xx- Maternal care for <u>face, brow and chin presentation</u>

O32.4xx- Maternal care for <u>high head at term</u>
Maternal care for failure of head to enter pelvic brim

O32.6xx- Maternal care for <u>compound presentation</u>

O32.8xx- Maternal care for <u>other</u> malpresentation of fetus
Maternal care for footling presentation
Maternal care for incomplete breech

O32.9xx- Maternal care for malpresentation of fetus, <u>unspecified</u>

O33- Maternal care <u>for disproportion</u>
Includes: The listed conditions as a reason for observation, hospitalization or other obstetric care of the mother, or for cesarean delivery before onset of labor
Excludes 1: disproportion with obstructed labor (O65-O66)

O33.0 Maternal care for disproportion due to <u>deformity of maternal pelvic bones</u>
Maternal care for disproportion due to pelvic deformity causing disproportion NOS

O33.1 Maternal care for disproportion due to <u>generally contracted pelvis</u>
Maternal care for disproportion due to contracted pelvis NOS causing disproportion

O33.2 Maternal care for disproportion due to <u>inlet contraction of pelvis</u>
Maternal care for disproportion due to inlet contraction (pelvis) causing disproportion

O33.3xx- Maternal care for disproportion due to <u>outlet contraction of pelvis</u>
Maternal care for disproportion due to mid-cavity contraction (pelvis)
Maternal care for disproportion due to outlet contraction (pelvis)

One of the following 7th characters is to be assigned to code O33.3. 7th character 0 is for single gestations and multiple gestations where the fetus is unspecified. 7th characters 1 through 9 are for cases of multiple gestations to identify the fetus for which the code applies. The appropriate code from category O30, Multiple gestation, must also be assigned when assigning code O33.3 with a 7th character of 1 through 9.
- **0** Not applicable or unspecified
- **1** Fetus 1
- **2** Fetus 2
- **3** Fetus 3
- **4** Fetus 4
- **5** Fetus 5
- **9** Other fetus

O 3 0 - O 3 4

O33.4xx- Maternal care for disproportion of <u>mixed maternal and fetal origin</u>

One of the following 7th characters is to be assigned to code O33.4. 7th character 0 is for single gestations and multiple gestations where the fetus is unspecified. 7th characters 1 through 9 are for cases of multiple gestations to identify the fetus for which the code applies. The appropriate code from category O30, Multiple gestation, must also be assigned when assigning code O33.4 with a 7th character of 1 through 9.

   0   Not applicable or unspecified
   1   Fetus 1
   2   Fetus 2
   3   Fetus 3
   4   Fetus 4
   5   Fetus 5
   9   Other fetus

O33.5xx- Maternal care for disproportion due to <u>unusually large fetus</u>

Maternal care for disproportion due to disproportion of fetal origin with normally formed fetus
Maternal care for disproportion due to fetal disproportion NOS

One of the following 7th characters is to be assigned to code O33.5. 7th character 0 is for single gestations and multiple gestations where the fetus is unspecified. 7th characters 1 through 9 are for cases of multiple gestations to identify the fetus for which the code applies. The appropriate code from category O30, Multiple gestation, must also be assigned when assigning code O33.5 with a 7th character of 1 through 9.

   0   Not applicable or unspecified
   1   Fetus 1
   2   Fetus 2
   3   Fetus 3
   4   Fetus 4
   5   Fetus 5
   9   Other fetus

O33.6xx- Maternal care for disproportion due to <u>hydrocephalic fetus</u>

One of the following 7th characters is to be assigned to code O33.6. 7th character 0 is for single gestations and multiple gestations where the fetus is unspecified. 7th characters 1 through 9 are for cases of multiple gestations to identify the fetus for which the code applies. The appropriate code from category O30, Multiple gestation, must also be assigned when assigning code O33.6 with a 7th character of 1 through 9.

   0   Not applicable or unspecified
   1   Fetus 1
   2   Fetus 2
   3   Fetus 3
   4   Fetus 4
   5   Fetus 5
   9   Other fetus

O33.7 Maternal care for disproportion due to other <u>fetal deformities</u>

Maternal care for disproportion due to fetal ascites
Maternal care for disproportion due to fetal hydrops
Maternal care for disproportion due to fetal meningomyelocele
Maternal care for disproportion due to fetal sacral teratoma
Maternal care for disproportion due to fetal tumor
Excludes 1: obstructed labor due to other fetal deformities (O66.3)

O33.8 Maternal care for disproportion of <u>other</u> origin

O33.9 Maternal care for disproportion, <u>unspecified</u>

Maternal care for disproportion due to cephalopelvic disproportion NOS
Maternal care for disproportion due to fetopelvic disproportion NOS

O34- Maternal care for <u>abnormality of pelvic organs</u>

Includes: The listed conditions as a reason for hospitalization or other obstetric care of the mother, or for cesarean delivery before onset of labor
Code first any associated obstructed labor (O65.5)
Use additional code for specific condition

O34.0- Maternal care for <u>congenital malformation of uterus</u>

O34.00 Maternal care for unspecified congenital malformation of uterus, <u>unspecified</u> trimester

O34.01 Maternal care for unspecified congenital malformation of uterus, <u>first</u> trimester

O34.02 Maternal care for unspecified congenital malformation of uterus, <u>second</u> trimester

O34.03 Maternal care for unspecified congenital malformation of uterus, <u>third</u> trimester

O34.1- Maternal care for <u>benign tumor of corpus uteri</u>

Excludes❷: maternal care for benign tumor of cervix (O34.4-)
maternal care for malignant neoplasm of uterus (O9A.1-)

O34.10 Maternal care for benign tumor of corpus uteri, <u>unspecified</u> trimester

O34.11 Maternal care for benign tumor of corpus uteri, <u>first</u> trimester

O34.12 Maternal care for benign tumor of corpus uteri, <u>second</u> trimester

O34.13 Maternal care for benign tumor of corpus uteri, <u>third</u> trimester

O34.2- Maternal care due to uterine scar from previous surgery

O34.21 Maternal care for <u>scar from previous cesarean delivery</u>

O34.29 Maternal care due to <u>uterine scar from other previous surgery</u>

O34.3- Maternal care for <u>cervical incompetence</u>

Maternal care for cerclage with or without cervical incompetence
Maternal care for Shirodkar suture with or without cervical incompetence

O34.30 Maternal care for cervical incompetence, <u>unspecified</u> trimester

O34.31 Maternal care for cervical incompetence, <u>first</u> trimester

O34.32 Maternal care for cervical incompetence, <u>second</u> trimester

O34.33 Maternal care for cervical incompetence, <u>third</u> trimester

O34.4- Maternal care for other abnormalities of cervix

O34.40 Maternal care for other abnormalities of cervix, <u>unspecified</u> trimester

O34.41 Maternal care for other abnormalities of cervix, <u>first</u> trimester

O34.42 Maternal care for other abnormalities of cervix, <u>second</u> trimester

O34.43 Maternal care for other abnormalities of cervix, <u>third</u> trimester

O34.5- Maternal care for other abnormalities of gravid uterus

O34.51- Maternal care for <u>incarceration of gravid uterus</u>

O34.511 Maternal care for incarceration of gravid uterus, <u>first</u> trimester

O34.512 Maternal care for incarceration of gravid uterus, <u>second</u> trimester

O34.513 Maternal care for incarceration of gravid uterus, <u>third</u> trimester

O34.519 Maternal care for incarceration of gravid uterus, <u>unspecified</u> trimester

O34.52- Maternal care for <u>prolapse of gravid uterus</u>

O34.521 Maternal care for prolapse of gravid uterus, <u>first</u> trimester

O34.522 Maternal care for prolapse of gravid uterus, <u>second</u> trimester

O34.523 Maternal care for prolapse of gravid uterus, <u>third</u> trimester

O34.529 Maternal care for prolapse of gravid uterus, <u>unspecified</u> trimester

O34.53- Maternal care for retroversion of <u>gravid uterus</u>

O34.531 Maternal care for retroversion of gravid uterus, <u>first</u> trimester

O34.532 Maternal care for retroversion of gravid uterus, <u>second</u> trimester

O34.533 Maternal care for retroversion of gravid uterus, <u>third</u> trimester

O34.539 Maternal care for retroversion of gravid uterus, <u>unspecified</u> trimester

O34.59- Maternal care for <u>other</u> abnormalities of gravid uterus

O34.591 Maternal care for other abnormalities of gravid uterus, <u>first</u> trimester

O34.592 Maternal care for other abnormalities of gravid uterus, <u>second</u> trimester

O34.593 Maternal care for other abnormalities of gravid uterus, <u>third</u> trimester

O34.599 Maternal care for other abnormalities of gravid uterus, <u>unspecified</u> trimester

O34.6- Maternal care for <u>abnormality of vagina</u>

Excludes❷: maternal care for vaginal varices in pregnancy (O22.1-)

O34.60 Maternal care for abnormality of vagina, <u>unspecified</u> trimester

O34.61 Maternal care for abnormality of vagina, <u>first</u> trimester

O34.62 Maternal care for abnormality of vagina, <u>second</u> trimester

O34.63 Maternal care for abnormality of vagina, <u>third</u> trimester

O30 - O34

O34.7- Maternal care for <u>abnormality of vulva and perineum</u>
Excludes❷: maternal care for perineal and vulval varices in pregnancy (O22.1-)
O34.70 Maternal care for abnormality of vulva and perineum, <u>unspecified</u> trimester
O34.71 Maternal care for abnormality of vulva and perineum, <u>first</u> trimester
O34.72 Maternal care for abnormality of vulva and perineum, <u>second</u> trimester
O34.73 Maternal care for abnormality of vulva and perineum, <u>third</u> trimester
O34.8- Maternal care for <u>other</u> abnormalities of <u>pelvic organs</u>
O34.80 Maternal care for other abnormalities of pelvic organs, <u>unspecified</u> trimester
O34.81 Maternal care for other abnormalities of pelvic organs, <u>first</u> trimester
O34.82 Maternal care for other abnormalities of pelvic organs, <u>second</u> trimester
O34.83 Maternal care for other abnormalities of pelvic organs, <u>third</u> trimester
O34.9- Maternal care for abnormality of pelvic organ, <u>unspecified</u>
O34.90 Maternal care for abnormality of pelvic organ, unspecified, <u>unspecified</u> trimester
O34.91 Maternal care for abnormality of pelvic organ, unspecified, <u>first</u> trimester
O34.92 Maternal care for abnormality of pelvic organ, unspecified, <u>second</u> trimester
O34.93 Maternal care for abnormality of pelvic organ, unspecified, <u>third</u> trimester

O35- Maternal care for <u>known or suspected fetal abnormality and damage</u>
Includes: The listed conditions in the fetus as a reason for hospitalization or other obstetric care to the mother, or for termination of pregnancy
Code also any associated maternal condition
Excludes 1: encounter for suspected maternal and fetal conditions ruled out (Z03.7-)
One of the following 7th characters is to be assigned to each code under category O35. 7th character 0 is for single gestations and multiple gestations where the fetus is unspecified. 7th characters 1 through 9 are for cases of multiple gestations to identify the fetus for which the code applies. The appropriate code from category O30, Multiple gestation, must also be assigned when assigning a code from category O35 that has a 7th character of 1 through 9.
0 Not applicable or unspecified
1 Fetus 1
2 Fetus 2
3 Fetus 3
4 Fetus 4
5 Fetus 5
9 Other fetus
O35.0xx- Maternal care for (suspected) <u>central nervous system malformation in fetus</u>
Maternal care for fetal anencephaly
Maternal care for fetal hydrocephalus
Maternal care for fetal spina bifida
Excludes❷: chromosomal abnormality in fetus (O35.1)
O35.1xx- Maternal care for (suspected) <u>chromosomal abnormality in fetus</u>
O35.2xx- Maternal care for (suspected) <u>hereditary disease in fetus</u>
Excludes❷: chromosomal abnormality in fetus (O35.1)
O35.3xx- Maternal care for (suspected) <u>damage to fetus from viral disease in mother</u>
Maternal care for damage to fetus from maternal cytomegalovirus infection
Maternal care for damage to fetus from maternal rubella
O35.4xx- Maternal care for (suspected) damage to fetus <u>from alcohol</u>
O35.5xx- Maternal care for (suspected) damage to fetus <u>by drugs</u>
Maternal care for damage to fetus from drug addiction
O35.6xx- Maternal care for (suspected) damage to fetus <u>by radiation</u>
O35.7xx- Maternal care for (suspected) damage to fetus <u>by other medical procedures</u>
Maternal care for damage to fetus by amniocentesis
Maternal care for damage to fetus by biopsy procedures
Maternal care for damage to fetus by hematological investigation
Maternal care for damage to fetus by intrauterine contraceptive device
Maternal care for damage to fetus by intrauterine surgery
O35.8xx- Maternal care for <u>other</u> (suspected) fetal abnormality and damage
Maternal care for damage to fetus from maternal listeriosis
Maternal care for damage to fetus from maternal toxoplasmosis

O35.9xx- Maternal care for (suspected) fetal abnormality and damage, <u>unspecified</u>
O36- Maternal care <u>for other fetal problems</u>
Includes: The listed conditions in the fetus as a reason for hospitalization or other obstetric care of the mother, or for termination of pregnancy
Excludes 1: encounter for suspected maternal and fetal conditions ruled out (Z03.7-)
placental transfusion syndromes (O43.0-)
Excludes❷: labor and delivery complicated by fetal stress (O77.-)
One of the following 7th characters is to be assigned to each code under category O36. 7th character 0 is for single gestations and multiple gestations where the fetus is unspecified. 7th characters 1 through 9 are for cases of multiple gestations to identify the fetus for which the code applies. The appropriate code from category O30, Multiple gestation, must also be assigned when assigning a code from category O36 that has a 7th character of 1 through 9.
0 Not applicable or unspecified
1 Fetus 1
2 Fetus 2
3 Fetus 3
4 Fetus 4
5 Fetus 5
9 Other fetus
O36.0- Maternal care for rhesus isoimmunization
Maternal care for Rh incompatibility (with hydrops fetalis)
O36.01- Maternal care for <u>anti-D [Rh] antibodies</u>
O36.011- Maternal care for anti-D [Rh] antibodies, <u>first</u> trimester
O36.012- Maternal care for anti-D [Rh] antibodies, <u>second</u> trimester
O36.013- Maternal care for anti-D [Rh] antibodies, <u>third</u> trimester
O36.019- Maternal care for anti-D [Rh] antibodies, <u>unspecified</u> trimester
O36.09- Maternal care for other <u>rhesus isoimmunization</u>
O36.091- Maternal care for other rhesus isoimmunization, <u>first</u> trimester
O36.092- Maternal care for other rhesus isoimmunization, <u>second</u> trimester
O36.093- Maternal care for other rhesus isoimmunization, <u>third</u> trimester
O36.099- Maternal care for other rhesus <u>isoimmunization, unspecified</u> trimester
O36.1- Maternal care for other isoimmunization
Maternal care for ABO isoimmunization
O36.11- Maternal care for <u>Anti-A sensitization</u>
Maternal care for isoimmunization NOS (with hydrops fetalis)
O36.111- Maternal care for Anti-A sensitization, <u>first</u> trimester
O36.112- Maternal care for Anti-A sensitization, <u>second</u> trimester
O36.113- Maternal care for Anti-A sensitization, <u>third</u> trimester
O36.119- Maternal care for Anti-A sensitization, <u>unspecified</u> trimester
O36.19- Maternal care for <u>other isoimmunization</u>
Maternal care for Anti-B sensitization
O36.191- Maternal care for other isoimmunization, <u>first</u> trimester
O36.192- Maternal care for other isoimmunization, <u>second</u> trimester
O36.193- Maternal care for other isoimmunization, <u>third</u> trimester
O36.199- Maternal care for other isoimmunization, <u>unspecified</u> trimester
O36.2- Maternal care for <u>hydrops fetalis</u>
Maternal care for hydrops fetalis NOS
Maternal care for hydrops fetalis not associated with isoimmunization
Excludes 1: hydrops fetalis associated with ABO isoimmunization (O36.1-)
hydrops fetalis associated with rhesus isoimmunization (O36.0-)
O36.20x- Maternal care for hydrops fetalis, <u>unspecified</u> trimester
O36.21x- Maternal care for hydrops fetalis, <u>first</u> trimester
O36.22x- Maternal care for hydrops fetalis, <u>second</u> trimester
O36.23x- Maternal care for hydrops fetalis, <u>third</u> trimester

O 3 4 - O 4 1

O36.4xx- Maternal care for intrauterine death
Maternal care for intrauterine fetal death NOS
Maternal care for intrauterine fetal death after completion of 20 weeks of gestation
Maternal care for late fetal death
Maternal care for missed delivery
Excludes 1: missed abortion (O02.1)
stillbirth (P95)

O36.5- Maternal care for known or suspected <u>poor fetal growth</u>
O36.51- Maternal care for known or suspected <u>placental insufficiency</u>
O36.511- Maternal care for known or suspected placental insufficiency, <u>first</u> trimester
O36.512- Maternal care for known or suspected placental insufficiency, <u>second</u> trimester
O36.513- Maternal care for known or suspected placental insufficiency, <u>third</u> trimester
O36.519- Maternal care for known or suspected placental insufficiency, <u>unspecified</u> trimester
O36.59- Maternal care for <u>other</u> known or suspected poor fetal growth
Maternal care for known or suspected light-for-dates NOS
Maternal care for known or suspected small-for-dates NOS
O36.591- Maternal care for other known or suspected poor fetal growth, <u>first</u> trimester
O36.592- Maternal care for other known or suspected poor fetal growth, <u>second</u> trimester
O36.593- Maternal care for other known or suspected poor fetal growth, <u>third</u> trimester
O36.599- Maternal care for other known or suspected poor fetal growth, <u>unspecified</u> trimester

O36.6- Maternal care for <u>excessive fetal growth</u>
Maternal care for known or suspected large-for-dates
O36.60x- Maternal care for excessive fetal growth, <u>unspecified</u> trimester
O36.61x- Maternal care for excessive fetal growth, <u>first</u> trimester
O36.62x- Maternal care for excessive fetal growth, <u>second</u> trimester
O36.63x- Maternal care for excessive fetal growth, <u>third</u> trimester

O36.7- Maternal care for <u>viable fetus in abdominal</u> pregnancy
O36.70x- Maternal care for viable fetus in abdominal pregnancy, <u>unspecified</u> trimester
O36.71x- Maternal care for viable fetus in abdominal pregnancy, <u>first</u> trimester
O36.72x- Maternal care for viable fetus in abdominal pregnancy, <u>second</u> trimester
O36.73x- Maternal care for viable fetus in abdominal pregnancy, <u>third</u> trimester

O36.8- Maternal care for other specified fetal problems
O36.80 Pregnancy with <u>inconclusive fetal viability</u>
Encounter to determine fetal viability of pregnancy
O36.81- <u>Decreased fetal movements</u>
O36.812- Decreased fetal movements, <u>second</u> trimester
O36.813- Decreased fetal movements, <u>third</u> trimester
O36.819- Decreased fetal movements, <u>unspecified</u> trimester
O36.82- <u>Fetal anemia and thrombocytopenia</u>
O36.821- Fetal anemia and thrombocytopenia, <u>first</u> trimester
O36.822- Fetal anemia and thrombocytopenia, <u>second</u> trimester
O36.823- Fetal anemia and thrombocytopenia, <u>third</u> trimester
O36.829- Fetal anemia and thrombocytopenia, <u>unspecified</u> trimester
O36.89- Maternal care for <u>other specified</u> fetal problems
O36.891- Maternal care for other specified fetal problems, <u>first</u> trimester
O36.892- Maternal care for other specified fetal problems, <u>second</u> trimester
O36.893- Maternal care for other specified fetal problems, <u>third</u> trimester
O36.899- Maternal care for other specified fetal problems, <u>unspecified</u> trimester

O36.9- Maternal care for fetal problem, <u>unspecified</u>
O36.90x- Maternal care for fetal problem, unspecified, <u>unspecified</u> trimester
O36.91x- Maternal care for fetal problem, unspecified, <u>first</u> trimester
O36.92x- Maternal care for fetal problem, unspecified, <u>second</u> trimester
O36.93x- Maternal care for fetal problem, unspecified, <u>third</u> trimester

O40- <u>Polyhydramnios</u>
Includes: Hydramnios
Excludes 1: encounter for suspected maternal and fetal conditions ruled out (Z03.7-)
One of the following 7th characters is to be assigned to each code under category O40. 7th character 0 is for single gestations and multiple gestations where the fetus is unspecified. 7th characters 1 through 9 are for cases of multiple gestations to identify the fetus for which the code applies. The appropriate code from category O30, Multiple gestation, must also be assigned when assigning a code from category O40 that has a 7th character of 1 through 9.
0 Not applicable or unspecified
1 Fetus 1
2 Fetus 2
3 Fetus 3
4 Fetus 4
5 Fetus 5
9 Other fetus
O40.1xx- Polyhydramnios, <u>first</u> trimester
O40.2xx- Polyhydramnios, <u>second</u> trimester
O40.3xx- Polyhydramnios, <u>third</u> trimester
O40.9xx- Polyhydramnios, <u>unspecified</u> trimester

O41- Other disorders of amniotic fluid and membranes
Excludes 1: encounter for suspected maternal and fetal conditions ruled out (Z03.7-)
One of the following 7th characters is to be assigned to each code under category O41. 7th character 0 is for single gestations and multiple gestations where the fetus is unspecified. 7th characters 1 through 9 are for cases of multiple gestations to identify the fetus for which the code applies. The appropriate code from category O30, Multiple gestation, must also be assigned when assigning a code from category O41 that has a 7th character of 1 through 9.
0 Not applicable or unspecified
1 Fetus 1
2 Fetus 2
3 Fetus 3
4 Fetus 4
5 Fetus 5
9 Other fetus
O41.0- <u>Oligohydramnios</u>
Oligohydramnios without rupture of membranes
O41.00x- Oligohydramnios, <u>unspecified</u> trimester
O41.01x- Oligohydramnios, <u>first</u> trimester
O41.02x- Oligohydramnios, <u>second</u> trimester
O41.03x- Oligohydramnios, <u>third</u> trimester
O41.1- Infection of amniotic sac and membranes
O41.10- <u>Infection of amniotic sac and membranes, unspecified</u>
O41.101- Infection of amniotic sac and membranes, unspecified, <u>first</u> trimester
O41.102- Infection of amniotic sac and membranes, unspecified, <u>second</u> trimester
O41.103- Infection of amniotic sac and membranes, unspecified, <u>third</u> trimester
O41.109- Infection of amniotic sac and membranes, unspecified, <u>unspecified</u> trimester
O41.12- <u>Chorioamnionitis</u>
O41.121- Chorioamnionitis, <u>first</u> trimester
O41.122- Chorioamnionitis, <u>second</u> trimester
O41.123- Chorioamnionitis, <u>third</u> trimester
O41.129- Chorioamnionitis, <u>unspecified</u> trimester
O41.14- <u>Placentitis</u>
O41.141- Placentitis, <u>first</u> trimester
O41.142- Placentitis, <u>second</u> trimester
O41.143- Placentitis, <u>third</u> trimester
O41.149- Placentitis, <u>unspecified</u> trimester
O41.8- Other specified disorders of amniotic fluid and membranes
O41.8x- <u>Other specified</u> disorders of amniotic fluid and membranes
O41.8x1- Other specified disorders of amniotic fluid and membranes, <u>first</u> trimester
O41.8x2- Other specified disorders of amniotic fluid and membranes, <u>second</u> trimester
O41.8x3- Other specified disorders of amniotic fluid and membranes, <u>third</u> trimester
O41.8x9- Other specified disorders of amniotic fluid and membranes, <u>unspecified</u> trimester
O41.9- Disorder of amniotic fluid and membranes, <u>unspecified</u>
O41.90x- Disorder of amniotic fluid and membranes, unspecified, <u>unspecified</u> trimester
O41.91x- Disorder of amniotic fluid and membranes, unspecified, <u>first</u> trimester

O34 - O41

O41.92x- Disorder of amniotic fluid and membranes, unspecified, <u>second</u> trimester

O41.93x- Disorder of amniotic fluid and membranes, unspecified, <u>third</u> trimester

O42- <u>Premature rupture of membranes</u>

O42.0- Premature rupture of membranes, <u>onset of labor within 24 hours of rupture</u>

O42.00 Premature rupture of membranes, onset of labor within 24 hours of rupture, <u>unspecified</u> weeks of gestation

O42.01- <u>Preterm</u> premature rupture of membranes, onset of labor within 24 hours of rupture
Premature rupture of membranes before 37 completed weeks of gestation

O42.011 Preterm premature rupture of membranes, onset of labor within 24 hours of rupture, <u>first</u> trimester

O42.012 Preterm premature rupture of membranes, onset of labor within 24 hours of rupture, <u>second</u> trimester

O42.013 Preterm premature rupture of membranes, onset of labor within 24 hours of rupture, <u>third</u> trimester

O42.019 Preterm premature rupture of membranes, onset of labor within 24 hours of rupture, <u>unspecified</u> trimester

O42.02 <u>Full-term</u> premature rupture of membranes, onset of labor within 24 hours of rupture
Premature rupture of membranes after 37 completed weeks of gestation

O42.1- Premature rupture of membranes, onset of labor <u>more than 24</u> hours following rupture

O42.10 Premature rupture of membranes, onset of labor more than 24 hours following rupture, unspecified weeks of gestation

O42.11- Preterm premature rupture of membranes, onset of labor more than 24 hours following rupture
Premature rupture of membranes before 37 completed weeks of gestation

O42.111 Preterm premature rupture of membranes, onset of labor more than 24 hours following rupture, <u>first</u> trimester

O42.112 Preterm premature rupture of membranes, onset of labor more than 24 hours following rupture, <u>second</u> trimester

O42.113 Preterm premature rupture of membranes, onset of labor more than 24 hours following rupture, <u>third</u> trimester

O42.119 Preterm premature rupture of membranes, onset of labor more than 24 hours following rupture, <u>unspecified</u> trimester

O42.12 <u>Full-term</u> premature rupture of membranes, onset of labor more than 24 hours following rupture
Premature rupture of membranes after 37 completed weeks of gestation

O42.9- Premature rupture of membranes, <u>unspecified as to length of time</u> between rupture and onset of labor

O42.90 Premature rupture of membranes, unspecified as to length of time between rupture and onset of labor, unspecified weeks of gestation

O42.91- <u>Preterm</u> premature rupture of membranes, unspecified as to length of time between rupture and onset of labor
Premature rupture of membranes before 37 completed weeks of gestation

O42.911 Preterm premature rupture of membranes, unspecified as to length of time between rupture and onset of labor, <u>first</u> trimester

O42.912 Preterm premature rupture of membranes, unspecified as to length of time between rupture and onset of labor, <u>second</u> trimester

O42.913 Preterm premature rupture of membranes, unspecified as to length of time between rupture and onset of labor, <u>third</u> trimester

O42.919 Preterm premature rupture of membranes, unspecified as to length of time between rupture and onset of labor, <u>unspecified</u> trimester

O42.92 <u>Full-term</u> premature rupture of membranes, unspecified as to length of time between rupture and onset of labor
Premature rupture of membranes after 37 completed weeks of gestation

O43- Placental disorders
Excludes❷: maternal care for poor fetal growth due to placental insufficiency (O36.5-)
placenta previa (O44.-)
placental polyp (O90.89)
placentitis (O41.14-)
premature separation of placenta [abruptio placentae] (O45.-)

O43.0- <u>Placental transfusion syndromes</u>

O43.01- <u>Fetomaternal</u> placental transfusion syndrome
Maternofetal placental transfusion syndrome

O43.011 Fetomaternal placental transfusion syndrome, <u>first</u> trimester

O43.012 Fetomaternal placental transfusion syndrome, <u>second</u> trimester

O43.013 Fetomaternal placental transfusion syndrome, <u>third</u> trimester

O43.019 Fetomaternal placental transfusion syndrome, <u>unspecified</u> trimester

O43.02- <u>Fetus-to-fetus</u> placental transfusion syndrome

O43.021 Fetus-to-fetus placental transfusion syndrome, <u>first</u> trimester

O43.022 Fetus-to-fetus placental transfusion syndrome, <u>second</u> trimester

O43.023 Fetus-to-fetus placental transfusion syndrome, <u>third</u> trimester

O43.029 Fetus-to-fetus placental transfusion syndrome, <u>unspecified</u> trimester

O43.1- Malformation of placenta

O43.10- <u>Malformation</u> of placenta, <u>unspecified</u>
Abnormal placenta NOS

O43.101 Malformation of placenta, unspecified, <u>first</u> trimester

O43.102 Malformation of placenta, unspecified, <u>second</u> trimester

O43.103 Malformation of placenta, unspecified, <u>third</u> trimester

O43.109 Malformation of placenta, unspecified, <u>unspecified</u> trimester

O43.11- <u>Circumvallate</u> placenta

O43.111 Circumvallate placenta, <u>first</u> trimester

O43.112 Circumvallate placenta, <u>second</u> trimester

O43.113 Circumvallate placenta, <u>third</u> trimester

O43.119 Circumvallate placenta, <u>unspecified</u> trimester

O43.12- <u>Velamentous</u> insertion of umbilical cord

O43.121 Velamentous insertion of umbilical cord, <u>first</u> trimester

O43.122 Velamentous insertion of umbilical cord, <u>second</u> trimester

O43.123 Velamentous insertion of umbilical cord, <u>third</u> trimester

O43.129 Velamentous insertion of umbilical cord, <u>unspecified</u> trimester

O43.19- <u>Other</u> malformation of placenta

O43.191 Other malformation of placenta, <u>first</u> trimester

O43.192 Other malformation of placenta, <u>second</u> trimester

O43.193 Other malformation of placenta, <u>third</u> trimester

O43.199 Other malformation of placenta, <u>unspecified</u> trimester

O43.2- Morbidly adherent placenta
Code also associated third stage postpartum hemorrhage, if applicable (O72.0)
Excludes 1: retained placenta (O73.-)

O43.21- Placenta <u>accreta</u>

O43.211 Placenta accreta, <u>first</u> trimester

O43.212 Placenta accreta, <u>second</u> trimester

O43.213 Placenta accreta, <u>third</u> trimester

O43.219 Placenta accreta, <u>unspecified</u> trimester

O43.22- Placenta <u>increta</u>

O43.221 Placenta increta, <u>first</u> trimester

O43.222 Placenta increta, <u>second</u> trimester

O43.223 Placenta increta, <u>third</u> trimester

O43.229 Placenta increta, <u>unspecified</u> trimester

O43.23- Placenta <u>percreta</u>

O43.231 Placenta percreta, <u>first</u> trimester

O43.232 Placenta percreta, <u>second</u> trimester

O43.233 Placenta percreta, <u>third</u> trimester

O43.239 Placenta percreta, <u>unspecified</u> trimester

O 4 1 - O 4 6

© 2013 Channel Publishing Ltd

O43.8- Other placental disorders
  O43.81- Placental <u>infarction</u>
    O43.811   Placental infarction, <u>first</u> trimester
    O43.812   Placental infarction, <u>second</u> trimester
    O43.813   Placental infarction, <u>third</u> trimester
    O43.819   Placental infarction, <u>unspecified</u> trimester
  O43.89- <u>Other</u> placental disorders
    Placental dysfunction
    O43.891   Other placental disorders, <u>first</u> trimester
    O43.892   Other placental disorders, <u>second</u> trimester
    O43.893   Other placental disorders, <u>third</u> trimester
    O43.899   Other placental disorders, <u>unspecified</u> trimester
  O43.9- <u>Unspecified</u> placental disorder
    O43.90 Unspecified placental disorder, <u>unspecified</u> trimester
    O43.91 Unspecified placental disorder, <u>first</u> trimester
    O43.92 Unspecified placental disorder, <u>second</u> trimester
    O43.93 Unspecified placental disorder, <u>third</u> trimester

O44- <u>Placenta previa</u>
  O44.0- Placenta previa <u>specified as without hemorrhage</u>
    Low implantation of placenta specified as without hemorrhage
    O44.00 Placenta previa specified as without hemorrhage, <u>unspecified</u> trimester
    O44.01 Placenta previa specified as without hemorrhage, <u>first</u> trimester
    O44.02 Placenta previa specified as without hemorrhage, <u>second</u> trimester
    O44.03 Placenta previa specified as without hemorrhage, <u>third</u> trimester
  O44.1- Placenta previa <u>with hemorrhage</u>
    Low implantation of placenta, NOS or with hemorrhage
    Marginal placenta previa, NOS or with hemorrhage
    Partial placenta previa, NOS or with hemorrhage
    Total placenta previa, NOS or with hemorrhage
    Excludes 1: labor and delivery complicated by hemorrhage from vasa previa (O69.4)
    O44.10 Placenta previa with hemorrhage, <u>unspecified</u> trimester
    O44.11 Placenta previa with hemorrhage, <u>first</u> trimester
    O44.12 Placenta previa with hemorrhage, <u>second</u> trimester
    O44.13 Placenta previa with hemorrhage, <u>third</u> trimester

O45- <u>Premature separation of placenta [abruptio placentae]</u>
  O45.0- Premature separation of placenta <u>with coagulation defect</u>
    O45.00- Premature separation of placenta with coagulation defect, <u>unspecified</u>
      O45.001   Premature separation of placenta with coagulation defect, unspecified, <u>first</u> trimester
      O45.002   Premature separation of placenta with coagulation defect, unspecified, <u>second</u> trimester
      O45.003   Premature separation of placenta with coagulation defect, unspecified, <u>third</u> trimester
      O45.009   Premature separation of placenta with coagulation defect, unspecified, <u>unspecified</u> trimester
    O45.01- Premature separation of placenta <u>with afibrinogenemia</u>
      Premature separation of placenta with hypofibrinogenemia
      O45.011   Premature separation of placenta with afibrinogenemia, <u>first</u> trimester
      O45.012   Premature separation of placenta with afibrinogenemia, <u>second</u> trimester
      O45.013   Premature separation of placenta with afibrinogenemia, <u>third</u> trimester
      O45.019   Premature separation of placenta with afibrinogenemia, <u>unspecified</u> trimester
    O45.02- Premature separation of placenta <u>with disseminated intravascular coagulation</u>
      O45.021   Premature separation of placenta with disseminated intravascular coagulation, <u>first</u> trimester
      O45.022   Premature separation of placenta with disseminated intravascular coagulation, <u>second</u> trimester
      O45.023   Premature separation of placenta with disseminated intravascular coagulation, <u>third</u> trimester
      O45.029   Premature separation of placenta with disseminated intravascular coagulation, <u>unspecified</u> trimester
    O45.09- Premature separation of placenta <u>with other coagulation defect</u>
      O45.091   Premature separation of placenta with other coagulation defect, <u>first</u> trimester
      O45.092   Premature separation of placenta with other coagulation defect, <u>second</u> trimester

O45.093   Premature separation of placenta with other coagulation defect, <u>third</u> trimester
O45.099   Premature separation of placenta with other coagulation defect, <u>unspecified</u> trimester
  O45.8- Other premature separation of placenta
    O45.8x- <u>Other</u> premature separation of placenta
      O45.8x1   Other premature separation of placenta, <u>first</u> trimester
      O45.8x2   Other premature separation of placenta, <u>second</u> trimester
      O45.8x3   Other premature separation of placenta, <u>third</u> trimester
      O45.8x9   Other premature separation of placenta, <u>unspecified</u> trimester
  O45.9- Premature separation of placenta, <u>unspecified</u>
    Abruptio placentae NOS
    O45.90 Premature separation of placenta, unspecified, <u>unspecified</u> trimester
    O45.91 Premature separation of placenta, unspecified, <u>first</u> trimester
    O45.92 Premature separation of placenta, unspecified, <u>second</u> trimester
    O45.93 Premature separation of placenta, unspecified, <u>third</u> trimester

O46- <u>Antepartum hemorrhage</u>, <u>not elsewhere classified</u>
  Excludes 1: hemorrhage in early pregnancy (O20.-)
        intrapartum hemorrhage NEC (O67.-)
        placenta previa (O44.-)
        premature separation of placenta [abruptio placentae] (O45.-)
  O46.0- Antepartum hemorrhage with coagulation defect
    O46.00- Antepartum hemorrhage <u>with coagulation defect, unspecified</u>
      O46.001   Antepartum hemorrhage with coagulation defect, unspecified, <u>first</u> trimester
      O46.002   Antepartum hemorrhage with coagulation defect, unspecified, <u>second</u> trimester
      O46.003   Antepartum hemorrhage with coagulation defect, unspecified, <u>third</u> trimester
      O46.009   Antepartum hemorrhage with coagulation defect, unspecified, <u>unspecified</u> trimester
    O46.01- Antepartum hemorrhage <u>with afibrinogenemia</u>
      Antepartum hemorrhage with hypofibrinogenemia
      O46.011   Antepartum hemorrhage with afibrinogenemia, <u>first</u> trimester
      O46.012   Antepartum hemorrhage with afibrinogenemia, <u>second</u> trimester
      O46.013   Antepartum hemorrhage with afibrinogenemia, <u>third</u> trimester
      O46.019   Antepartum hemorrhage with afibrinogenemia, <u>unspecified</u> trimester
    O46.02- Antepartum hemorrhage <u>with disseminated intravascular coagulation</u>
      O46.021   Antepartum hemorrhage with disseminated intravascular coagulation, <u>first</u> trimester
      O46.022   Antepartum hemorrhage with disseminated intravascular coagulation, <u>second</u> trimester
      O46.023   Antepartum hemorrhage with disseminated intravascular coagulation, <u>third</u> trimester
      O46.029   Antepartum hemorrhage with disseminated intravascular coagulation, <u>unspecified</u> trimester
    O46.09- Antepartum hemorrhage <u>with other coagulation defect</u>
      O46.091   Antepartum hemorrhage with other coagulation defect, <u>first</u> trimester
      O46.092   Antepartum hemorrhage with other coagulation defect, <u>second</u> trimester
      O46.093   Antepartum hemorrhage with other coagulation defect, <u>third</u> trimester
      O46.099   Antepartum hemorrhage with other coagulation defect, <u>unspecified</u> trimester
  O46.8- Other antepartum hemorrhage
    O46.8x- <u>Other antepartum hemorrhage</u>
      O46.8x1   Other antepartum hemorrhage, <u>first</u> trimester
      O46.8x2   Other antepartum hemorrhage, <u>second</u> trimester
      O46.8x3   Other antepartum hemorrhage, <u>third</u> trimester
      O46.8x9   Other antepartum hemorrhage, unspecified trimester
  O46.9- Antepartum hemorrhage, <u>unspecified</u>
    O46.90 Antepartum hemorrhage, unspecified, <u>unspecified</u> trimester
    O46.91 Antepartum hemorrhage, unspecified, <u>first</u> trimester
    O46.92 Antepartum hemorrhage, unspecified, <u>second</u> trimester
    O46.93 Antepartum hemorrhage, unspecified, <u>third</u> trimester

O 4 1 - O 4 6

Excludes 1: = NOT CODED HERE! (Do not code both)   **639**   *Excludes ❷:* = Not Included Here

O47- False labor
  Includes: Braxton Hicks contractions
              Threatened labor
  Excludes 1: preterm labor (O60.-)
  O47.0- False labor before 37 completed weeks of gestation
    O47.00 False labor before 37 completed weeks of gestation, unspecified trimester
    O47.02 False labor before 37 completed weeks of gestation, second trimester
    O47.03 False labor before 37 completed weeks of gestation, third trimester
  O47.1 False labor at or after 37 completed weeks of gestation
  O47.9 False labor, unspecified
O48- Late pregnancy
  O48.0 Post-term pregnancy
      Pregnancy over 40 completed weeks to 42 completed weeks gestation
  O48.1 Prolonged pregnancy
      Pregnancy which has advanced beyond 42 completed weeks gestation

Complications of labor and delivery (O60-O77)

O60- Preterm labor
  Includes: Onset (spontaneous) of labor before 37 completed weeks of gestation
  Excludes 1: false labor (O47.0-)
            threatened labor NOS (O47.0-)
  O60.0- Preterm labor without delivery
    O60.00 Preterm labor without delivery, unspecified trimester
    O60.02 Preterm labor without delivery, second trimester
    O60.03 Preterm labor without delivery, third trimester
  O60.1- Preterm labor with preterm delivery
      One of the following 7th characters is to be assigned to each code under subcategory O60.1. 7th character 0 is for single gestations and multiple gestations where the fetus is unspecified. 7th characters 1 through 9 are for cases of multiple gestations to identify the fetus for which the code applies. The appropriate code from category O30, Multiple gestation, must also be assigned when assigning a code from subcategory O60.1 that has a 7th character of 1 through 9.
      0 Not applicable or unspecified
      1 Fetus 1
      2 Fetus 2
      3 Fetus 3
      4 Fetus 4
      5 Fetus 5
      9 Other fetus
    O60.10x- Preterm labor with preterm delivery, unspecified trimester
        Preterm labor with delivery NOS
    O60.12x- Preterm labor second trimester with preterm delivery second trimester
    O60.13x- Preterm labor second trimester with preterm delivery third trimester
    O60.14x- Preterm labor third trimester with preterm delivery third trimester
  O60.2- Term delivery with preterm labor
      One of the following 7th characters is to be assigned to each code under subcategory O60.2. 7th character 0 is for single gestations and multiple gestations where the fetus is unspecified. 7th characters 1 through 9 are for cases of multiple gestations to identify the fetus for which the code applies. The appropriate code from category O30, Multiple gestation, must also be assigned when assigning a code from subcategory O60.2 that has a 7th character of 1 through 9.
      0 Not applicable or unspecified
      1 Fetus 1
      2 Fetus 2
      3 Fetus 3
      4 Fetus 4
      5 Fetus 5
      9 Other fetus
    O60.20x- Term delivery with preterm labor, unspecified trimester
    O60.22x- Term delivery with preterm labor, second trimester
    O60.23x- Term delivery with preterm labor, third trimester

O61- Failed induction of labor
  O61.0 Failed medical induction of labor
      Failed induction (of labor) by oxytocin
      Failed induction (of labor) by prostaglandins
  O61.1- Failed instrumental induction of labor
      Failed mechanical induction (of labor)
      Failed surgical induction (of labor)
  O61.8 Other failed induction of labor
  O61.9 Failed induction of labor, unspecified
O62- Abnormalities of forces of labor
  O62.0 Primary inadequate contractions
      Failure of cervical dilatation
      Primary hypotonic uterine dysfunction
      Uterine inertia during latent phase of labor
  O62.1 Secondary uterine inertia
      Arrested active phase of labor
      Secondary hypotonic uterine dysfunction
  O62.2 Other uterine inertia
      Atony of uterus without hemorrhage
      Atony of uterus NOS
      Desultory labor
      Hypotonic uterine dysfunction NOS
      Irregular labor
      Poor contractions
      Slow slope active phase of labor
      Uterine inertia NOS
      Excludes 1: atony of uterus with hemorrhage (postpartum) (O72.1)
                postpartum atony of uterus without hemorrhage (O75.89)
  O62.3 Precipitate labor
  O62.4 Hypertonic, incoordinate, and prolonged uterine contractions
      Cervical spasm
      Contraction ring dystocia
      Dyscoordinate labor
      Hour-glass contraction of uterus
      Hypertonic uterine dysfunction
      Incoordinate uterine action
      Tetanic contractions
      Uterine dystocia NOS
      Uterine spasm
      Excludes 1: dystocia (fetal) (maternal) NOS (O66.9)
  O62.8 Other abnormalities of forces of labor
  O62.9 Abnormality of forces of labor, unspecified
O63- Long labor
  O63.0 Prolonged first stage (of labor)
  O63.1 Prolonged second stage (of labor)
  O63.2 Delayed delivery of second twin, triplet, etc.
  O63.9 Long labor, unspecified
      Prolonged labor NOS
O64- Obstructed labor due to malposition and malpresentation of fetus
      One of the following 7th characters is to be assigned to each code under category O64. 7th character 0 is for single gestations and multiple gestations where the fetus is unspecified. 7th characters 1 through 9 are for cases of multiple gestations to identify the fetus for which the code applies. The appropriate code from category O30, Multiple gestation, must also be assigned when assigning a code from category O64 that has a 7th character of 1 through 9.
      0 Not applicable or unspecified
      1 Fetus 1
      2 Fetus 2
      3 Fetus 3
      4 Fetus 4
      5 Fetus 5
      9 Other fetus
  O64.0xx- Obstructed labor due to incomplete rotation of fetal head
      Deep transverse arrest
      Obstructed labor due to persistent occipitoiliac (position)
      Obstructed labor due to persistent occipitoposterior (position)
      Obstructed labor due to persistent occipitosacral (position)
      Obstructed labor due to persistent occipitotransverse (position)
  O64.1xx- Obstructed labor due to breech presentation
      Obstructed labor due to buttocks presentation
      Obstructed labor due to complete breech presentation
      Obstructed labor due to frank breech presentation
  O64.2xx- Obstructed labor due to face presentation
      Obstructed labor due to chin presentation
  O64.3xx- Obstructed labor due to brow presentation
  O64.4xx- Obstructed labor due to shoulder presentation
      Prolapsed arm
      Excludes 1: impacted shoulders (O66.0)
                shoulder dystocia (O66.0)

O64.5xx- Obstructed labor <u>due to compound presentation</u>

O64.8xx- Obstructed labor <u>due to other</u> malposition and malpresentation
Obstructed labor due to footling presentation
Obstructed labor due to incomplete breech presentation

O64.9xx- Obstructed labor due to malposition and malpresentation, <u>unspecified</u>

O65- Obstructed labor <u>due to maternal pelvic abnormality</u>

O65.0 Obstructed labor due to deformed pelvis

O65.1 Obstructed labor due to generally contracted pelvis

O65.2 Obstructed labor due to pelvic inlet contraction

O65.3 Obstructed labor due to pelvic outlet and mid-cavity contraction

O65.4 Obstructed labor due to fetopelvic disproportion, unspecified
Excludes 1: dystocia due to abnormality of fetus (O66.2-O66.3)

O65.5 Obstructed labor due to abnormality of maternal pelvic organs
Obstructed labor due to conditions listed in O34.-
Use additional code to identify abnormality of pelvic organs O34.-

O65.8 Obstructed labor due to other maternal pelvic abnormalities

O65.9 Obstructed labor due to maternal pelvic abnormality, unspecified

O66- <u>Other</u> obstructed labor

O66.0 Obstructed labor <u>due to shoulder dystocia</u>
Impacted shoulders

O66.1 Obstructed labor <u>due to locked twins</u>

O66.2 Obstructed labor <u>due to unusually large fetus</u>

O66.3 Obstructed labor <u>due to other abnormalities of fetus</u>
Dystocia due to fetal ascites
Dystocia due to fetal hydrops
Dystocia due to fetal meningomyelocele
Dystocia due to fetal sacral teratoma
Dystocia due to fetal tumor
Dystocia due to hydrocephalic fetus
Use additional code to identify cause of obstruction

O66.4- <u>Failed trial of labor</u>

O66.40 Failed trial of labor, unspecified

O66.41 Failed attempted vaginal birth after previous cesarean delivery
Code first rupture of uterus, if applicable (O71.0-, O71.1)

O66.5 Attempted application of vacuum extractor and forceps
Attempted application of vacuum or forceps, with subsequent delivery by forceps or cesarean delivery

O66.6 Obstructed labor due to other multiple fetuses

O66.8 Other specified obstructed labor
Use additional code to identify cause of obstruction

O66.9 Obstructed labor, <u>unspecified</u>
Dystocia NOS
Fetal dystocia NOS
Maternal dystocia NOS

O67- Labor and delivery <u>complicated by intrapartum hemorrhage</u>, not <u>elsewhere classified</u>
Excludes 1: antepartum hemorrhage NEC (O46.-)
placenta previa (O44.-)
premature separation of placenta [abruptio placentae] (O45.-)
Excludes ❷: postpartum hemorrhage (O72.-)

O67.0 Intrapartum hemorrhage <u>with coagulation defect</u>
Intrapartum hemorrhage (excessive) associated with afibrinogenemia
Intrapartum hemorrhage (excessive) associated with disseminated intravascular coagulation
Intrapartum hemorrhage (excessive) associated with hyperfibrinolysis
Intrapartum hemorrhage (excessive) associated with hypofibrinogenemia

O67.8 Other intrapartum hemorrhage
Excessive intrapartum hemorrhage

O67.9 Intrapartum hemorrhage, <u>unspecified</u>

O68 Labor and delivery complicated by abnormality of fetal acid-base balance
Fetal acidemia complicating labor and delivery
Fetal acidosis complicating labor and delivery
Fetal alkalosis complicating labor and delivery
Fetal metabolic acidemia complicating labor and delivery
Excludes 1: fetal stress NOS (O77.9)
labor and delivery complicated by electrocardiographic evidence of fetal stress (O77.8)
labor and delivery complicated by ultrasonic evidence of fetal stress (O77.8)
Excludes ❷: abnormality in fetal heart rate or rhythm (O76)
labor and delivery complicated by meconium in amniotic fluid (O77.0)

O69- Labor and delivery <u>complicated by umbilical cord complications</u>
One of the following 7th characters is to be assigned to each code under category O69. 7th character 0 is for single gestations and multiple gestations where the fetus is unspecified. 7th characters 1 through 9 are for cases of multiple gestations to identify the fetus for which the code applies. The appropriate code from category O30, Multiple gestation, must also be assigned when assigning a code from category O69 that has a 7th character of 1 through 9.
0   Not applicable or unspecified
1   Fetus 1
2   Fetus 2
3   Fetus 3
4   Fetus 4
5   Fetus 5
9   Other fetus

O69.0xx- Labor and delivery complicated by <u>prolapse of cord</u>

O69.1xx- Labor and delivery complicated by <u>cord around neck</u>, <u>with compression</u>
Excludes 1: labor and delivery complicated by cord around neck, without compression (O69.81)

O69.2xx- Labor and delivery complicated by <u>other cord entanglement</u>, <u>with compression</u>
Labor and delivery complicated by compression of cord NOS
Labor and delivery complicated by entanglement of cords of twins in monoamniotic sac
Labor and delivery complicated by knot in cord
Excludes 1: labor and delivery complicated by other cord entanglement, without compression (O69.82)

O69.3xx- Labor and delivery complicated by <u>short cord</u>

O69.4xx- Labor and delivery complicated by <u>vasa previa</u>
Labor and delivery complicated by hemorrhage from vasa previa

O69.5xx- Labor and delivery complicated by <u>vascular lesion of cord</u>
Labor and delivery complicated by cord bruising
Labor and delivery complicated by cord hematoma
Labor and delivery complicated by thrombosis of umbilical vessels

O69.8- Labor and delivery complicated by <u>other cord</u> complications

O69.81x- Labor and delivery complicated by cord around neck, <u>without</u> compression

O69.82x- Labor and delivery complicated by other cord entanglement, <u>without</u> compression

O69.89x- Labor and delivery complicated by <u>other</u> cord complications

O69.9xx- Labor and delivery complicated by cord complication, <u>unspecified</u>

O70- <u>Perineal laceration during delivery</u>
Includes: Episiotomy extended by laceration
Excludes 1: obstetric high vaginal laceration alone (O71.4)

O70.0 First degree perineal laceration during delivery
Perineal laceration, rupture or tear involving fourchette during delivery
Perineal laceration, rupture or tear involving labia during delivery
Perineal laceration, rupture or tear involving skin during delivery
Perineal laceration, rupture or tear involving vagina during delivery
Perineal laceration, rupture or tear involving vulva during delivery
Slight perineal laceration, rupture or tear during delivery

O70.1 Second degree perineal laceration during delivery
Perineal laceration, rupture or tear during delivery as in O70.0, also involving pelvic floor
Perineal laceration, rupture or tear during delivery as in O70.0, also involving perineal muscles
Perineal laceration, rupture or tear during delivery as in O70.0, also involving vaginal muscles
Excludes 1: perineal laceration involving anal sphincter (O70.2)

O70.2 Third degree perineal laceration during delivery
Perineal laceration, rupture or tear during delivery as in O70.1, also involving anal sphincter
Perineal laceration, rupture or tear during delivery as in O70.1, also involving rectovaginal septum
Perineal laceration, rupture or tear during delivery as in O70.1, also involving sphincter NOS
Excludes 1: anal sphincter tear during delivery without third degree perineal laceration (O70.4)
perineal laceration involving anal or rectal mucosa (O70.3)

O70.3 Fourth degree perineal laceration during delivery
Perineal laceration, rupture or tear during delivery as in O70.2, also involving anal mucosa
Perineal laceration, rupture or tear during delivery as in O70.2, also involving rectal mucosa

O47 - O70

O70.4   Anal sphincter tear complicating delivery, <u>not associated with third degree laceration</u>
    Excludes 1:   anal sphincter tear with third degree perineal laceration (O70.2)

O70.9   Perineal laceration during delivery, unspecified

O71-   **Other obstetric trauma**
    Includes: obstetric damage from instruments

O71.0-   <u>Rupture of uterus (spontaneous) before onset of labor</u>
    Excludes 1:   disruption of (current) cesarean delivery wound (O90.0)
        laceration of uterus, NEC (O71.81)

    O71.00   Rupture of uterus before onset of labor, <u>unspecified</u> trimester

    O71.02   Rupture of uterus before onset of labor, <u>second</u> trimester

    O71.03   Rupture of uterus before onset of labor, <u>third</u> trimester

O71.1   Rupture of uterus <u>during labor</u>
    Rupture of uterus not stated as occurring before onset of labor
    Excludes 1:   disruption of cesarean delivery wound (O90.0)
        laceration of uterus, NEC (O71.81)

O71.2   Postpartum inversion of uterus

O71.3   Obstetric laceration of cervix
    Annular detachment of cervix

O71.4   Obstetric high vaginal laceration alone
    Laceration of vaginal wall without perineal laceration
    Excludes 1:   obstetric high vaginal laceration with perineal laceration (O70.-)

O71.5   Other obstetric injury to pelvic organs
    Obstetric injury to bladder
    Obstetric injury to urethra
    Excludes❷: obstetric periurethral trauma (O71.82)

O71.6   Obstetric damage to pelvic joints and ligaments
    Obstetric avulsion of inner symphyseal cartilage
    Obstetric damage to coccyx
    Obstetric traumatic separation of symphysis (pubis)

O71.7   Obstetric hematoma of pelvis
    Obstetric hematoma of perineum
    Obstetric hematoma of vagina
    Obstetric hematoma of vulva

O71.8-   Other specified obstetric trauma

    O71.81   Laceration of uterus, not elsewhere classified

    O71.82   Other specified trauma to perineum and vulva
        Obstetric periurethral trauma

    O71.89   Other specified obstetric trauma

O71.9   Obstetric trauma, unspecified

O72-   <u>Postpartum hemorrhage</u>
    Includes: Hemorrhage after delivery of fetus or infant

O72.0   Third-stage hemorrhage
    Hemorrhage associated with retained, trapped or adherent placenta
    Retained placenta NOS
    Code also type of adherent placenta (O43.2-)

O72.1   Other immediate postpartum hemorrhage
    Hemorrhage following delivery of placenta
    Postpartum hemorrhage (atonic) NOS
    Uterine atony with hemorrhage
    Excludes 1:   uterine atony NOS (O62.2)
        uterine atony without hemorrhage (O62.2)
        postpartum atony of uterus without hemorrhage (O75.89)

O72.2   Delayed and secondary postpartum hemorrhage
    Hemorrhage associated with retained portions of placenta or membranes after the first 24 hours following delivery of placenta
    Retained products of conception NOS, following delivery

O72.3   Postpartum coagulation defects
    Postpartum afibrinogenemia
    Postpartum fibrinolysis

O73-   <u>Retained placenta and membranes, without</u> hemorrhage
    Excludes 1:   placenta accreta (O43.21-)
        placenta increta (O43.22-)
        placenta percreta (O43.23-)

O73.0   Retained placenta without hemorrhage
    Adherent placenta, without hemorrhage
    Trapped placenta without hemorrhage

O73.1   Retained portions of placenta and membranes, without hemorrhage
    Retained products of conception following delivery, without hemorrhage

O74-   <u>Complications of anesthesia during labor and delivery</u>
    Includes: Maternal complications arising from the administration of a general, regional or local anesthetic, analgesic or other sedation during labor and delivery
    Use additional code, if applicable, to identify specific complication

O74.0   <u>Aspiration pneumonitis</u> due to anesthesia during labor and delivery
    Inhalation of stomach contents or secretions NOS due to anesthesia during labor and delivery
    Mendelson's syndrome due to anesthesia during labor and delivery

O74.1   Other pulmonary complications of anesthesia during labor and delivery

O74.2   <u>Cardiac complications</u> of anesthesia during labor and delivery

O74.3   <u>Central nervous system</u> complications of anesthesia during labor and delivery

O74.4   Toxic reaction to local anesthesia during labor and delivery

O74.5   <u>Spinal and epidural anesthesia-induced headache</u> during labor and delivery

O74.6   <u>Other complications of spinal and epidural anesthesia</u> during labor and delivery

O74.7   <u>Failed or difficult intubation for anesthesia</u> during labor and delivery

O74.8   <u>Other</u> complications of anesthesia during labor and delivery

O74.9   Complication of anesthesia during labor and delivery, <u>unspecified</u>

O75-   Other complications of labor and delivery, <u>not elsewhere classified</u>
    Excludes❷: puerperal (postpartum) infection (O86.-)
        puerperal (postpartum) sepsis (O85)

O75.0   Maternal distress during labor and delivery

O75.1   Shock during or following labor and delivery
    Obstetric shock following labor and delivery

O75.2   Pyrexia during labor, not elsewhere classified

O75.3   Other infection during labor
    Sepsis during labor
    Use additional code (B95-B97), to identify infectious agent

O75.4   Other complications of obstetric surgery and procedures
    Cardiac arrest following obstetric surgery or procedures
    Cardiac failure following obstetric surgery or procedures
    Cerebral anoxia following obstetric surgery or procedures
    Pulmonary edema following obstetric surgery or procedures
    Use additional code to identify specific complication
    Excludes❷: complications of anesthesia during labor and delivery (O74.-)
        disruption of obstetrical (surgical) wound (O90.0-O90.1)
        hematoma of obstetrical (surgical) wound (O90.2)
        infection of obstetrical (surgical) wound (O86.0)

O75.5   Delayed delivery after artificial rupture of membranes

O75.8-   Other specified complications of labor and delivery

    O75.81   Maternal exhaustion complicating labor and delivery

    O75.82   Onset (spontaneous) of labor after 37 completed weeks of gestation but before 39 completed weeks of gestation, with delivery by (planned) cesarean section
        Delivery by (planned) cesarean section occurring after 37 completed weeks of gestation but before 39 completed weeks gestation due to (spontaneous) onset of labor
        Code first to specify reason for planned cesarean section, such as:
        Cephalopelvic disproportion (normally formed fetus) (O33.9)
        Previous cesarean delivery (O34.21)

    O75.89   Other specified complications of labor and delivery

O75.9   Complication of labor and delivery, unspecified

O76   <u>Abnormality in fetal heart rate</u> and rhythm complicating labor and delivery
    Depressed fetal heart rate tones complicating labor and delivery
    Fetal bradycardia complicating labor and delivery
    Fetal heart rate decelerations complicating labor and delivery
    Fetal heart rate irregularity complicating labor and delivery
    Fetal heart rate abnormal variability complicating labor and delivery
    Fetal tachycardia complicating labor and delivery
    Non-reassuring fetal heart rate or rhythm complicating labor and delivery
    Excludes 1:   fetal stress NOS (O77.9)
        labor and delivery complicated by electrocardiographic evidence of fetal stress (O77.8)
        labor and delivery complicated by ultrasonic evidence of fetal stress (O77.8)
    Excludes❷: fetal metabolic acidemia (O68)
        other fetal stress (O77.0-O77.1)

O70
-
O88

© 2013 Channel Publishing Ltd

O77- Other fetal stress complicating labor and delivery

O77.0 Labor and delivery complicated by meconium in amniotic fluid

O77.1 Fetal stress in labor or delivery due to drug administration

O77.8 Labor and delivery complicated by other evidence of fetal stress
Labor and delivery complicated by electrocardiographic evidence of fetal stress
Labor and delivery complicated by ultrasonic evidence of fetal stress
Excludes 1: abnormality of fetal acid-base balance (O68)
abnormality in fetal heart rate or rhythm (O76)
fetal metabolic acidemia (O68)

O77.9 Labor and delivery complicated by fetal stress, unspecified
Excludes 1: abnormality of fetal acid-base balance (O68)
abnormality in fetal heart rate or rhythm (O76)
fetal metabolic acidemia (O68)

Encounter for delivery (O80-O82)

O80 Encounter for full-term uncomplicated delivery
Delivery requiring minimal or no assistance, with or without episiotomy, without fetal manipulation [e.g., rotation version] or instrumentation [forceps] of a spontaneous, cephalic, vaginal, full-term, single, live-born infant. This code is for use as a single diagnosis code and is not to be used with any other code from chapter 15.
Use additional code to indicate outcome of delivery (Z37.0)

O82 Encounter for cesarean delivery without indication
Use additional code to indicate outcome of delivery (Z37.0)

Complications predominantly related to the puerperium (O85-O92)

Excludes❷: mental and behavioral disorders associated with the puerperium (F53)
obstetrical tetanus (A34)
puerperal osteomalacia (M83.0)

O85 Puerperal sepsis
Postpartum sepsis
Puerperal peritonitis
Puerperal pyemia
Use additional code (B95-B97), to identify infectious agent
Use additional code (R65.2-) to identify severe sepsis, if applicable
Excludes 1: fever of unknown origin following delivery (O86.4)
genital tract infection following delivery (O86.1-)
obstetric pyemic and septic embolism (O88.3-)
puerperal septic thrombophlebitis (O86.81)
urinary tract infection following delivery (O86.2-)
Excludes❷: sepsis during labor (O75.3)

O86- Other puerperal infections
Use additional code (B95-B97), to identify infectious agent
Excludes❷: infection during labor (O75.3)
obstetrical tetanus (A34)

O86.0 Infection of obstetric surgical wound
Infected cesarean delivery wound following delivery
Infected perineal repair following delivery

O86.1- Other infection of genital tract following delivery
O86.11 Cervicitis following delivery
O86.12 Endometritis following delivery
O86.13 Vaginitis following delivery
O86.19 Other infection of genital tract following delivery

O86.2- Urinary tract infection following delivery
O86.20 Urinary tract infection following delivery, unspecified
Puerperal urinary tract infection NOS
O86.21 Infection of kidney following delivery
O86.22 Infection of bladder following delivery
Infection of urethra following delivery
O86.29 Other urinary tract infection following delivery

O86.4 Pyrexia of unknown origin following delivery
Puerperal infection NOS following delivery
Puerperal pyrexia NOS following delivery
Excludes❷: pyrexia during labor (O75.2)

O86.8- Other specified puerperal infections
O86.81 Puerperal septic thrombophlebitis
O86.89 Other specified puerperal infections

O87- Venous complications and hemorrhoids in the puerperium
Includes: Venous complications in labor, delivery and the puerperium
Excludes❷: obstetric embolism (O88-)
puerperal septic thrombophlebitis (O86.81)
venous complications in pregnancy (O22-)

O87.0 Superficial thrombophlebitis in the puerperium
Puerperal phlebitis NOS
Puerperal thrombosis NOS

O87.1 Deep phlebothrombosis in the puerperium
Deep vein thrombosis, postpartum
Pelvic thrombophlebitis, postpartum
Use additional code to identify the deep vein thrombosis (I82.4-, I82.5-, I82.62-. I82.72-)
Use additional code, if applicable, for associated long-term (current) use of anticoagulants (Z79.01)

O87.2 Hemorrhoids in the puerperium

O87.3 Cerebral venous thrombosis in the puerperium
Cerebrovenous sinus thrombosis in the puerperium

O87.4 Varicose veins of lower extremity in the puerperium

O87.8 Other venous complications in the puerperium
Genital varices in the puerperium

O87.9 Venous complication in the puerperium, unspecified
Puerperal phlebopathy NOS

O88- Obstetric embolism
Excludes 1: embolism complicating abortion NOS (O03.2)
embolism complicating ectopic or molar pregnancy (O08.2)
embolism complicating failed attempted abortion (O07.2)
embolism complicating induced abortion (O04.7)
embolism complicating spontaneous abortion (O03.2, O03.7)

O88.0- Obstetric air embolism
O88.01- Obstetric air embolism in pregnancy
O88.011 Air embolism in pregnancy, first trimester
O88.012 Air embolism in pregnancy, second trimester
O88.013 Air embolism in pregnancy, third trimester
O88.019 Air embolism in pregnancy, unspecified trimester
O88.02 Air embolism in childbirth
O88.03 Air embolism in the puerperium

O88.1- Amniotic fluid embolism
Anaphylactoid syndrome in pregnancy
O88.11- Amniotic fluid embolism in pregnancy
O88.111 Amniotic fluid embolism in pregnancy, first trimester
O88.112 Amniotic fluid embolism in pregnancy, second trimester
O88.113 Amniotic fluid embolism in pregnancy, third trimester
O88.119 Amniotic fluid embolism in pregnancy, unspecified trimester
O88.12 Amniotic fluid embolism in childbirth
O88.13 Amniotic fluid embolism in the puerperium

O88.2- Obstetric thromboembolism
O88.21- Thromboembolism in pregnancy
Obstetric (pulmonary) embolism NOS
O88.211 Thromboembolism in pregnancy, first trimester
O88.212 Thromboembolism in pregnancy, second trimester
O88.213 Thromboembolism in pregnancy, third trimester
O88.219 Thromboembolism in pregnancy, unspecified trimester
O88.22 Thromboembolism in childbirth
O88.23 Thromboembolism in the puerperium
Puerperal (pulmonary) embolism NOS

O88.3- Obstetric pyemic and septic embolism
O88.31- Pyemic and septic embolism in pregnancy
O88.311 Pyemic and septic embolism in pregnancy, first trimester
O88.312 Pyemic and septic embolism in pregnancy, second trimester
O88.313 Pyemic and septic embolism in pregnancy, third trimester
O88.319 Pyemic and septic embolism in pregnancy, unspecified trimester
O88.32 Pyemic and septic embolism in childbirth
O88.33 Pyemic and septic embolism in the puerperium

O88.8- Other obstetric embolism
Obstetric fat embolism
O88.81- Other embolism in pregnancy
O88.811 Other embolism in pregnancy, first trimester
O88.812 Other embolism in pregnancy, second trimester
O88.813 Other embolism in pregnancy, third trimester
O88.819 Other embolism in pregnancy, unspecified trimester

O
7
0
|
O
8
8

O88.82 Other embolism <u>in childbirth</u>

O88.83 Other embolism <u>in the puerperium</u>

O89- <u>Complications of anesthesia</u> <u>during the puerperium</u>

Includes: Maternal complications arising from the administration of a general, regional or local anesthetic, analgesic or other sedation during the puerperium

Use additional code, if applicable, to identify specific complication

O89.0- <u>Pulmonary complications</u> of anesthesia during the puerperium

O89.01 Aspiration pneumonitis due to anesthesia during the puerperium

Inhalation of stomach contents or secretions NOS due to anesthesia during the puerperium

Mendelson's syndrome due to anesthesia during the puerperium

O89.09 Other pulmonary complications of anesthesia during the puerperium

O89.1 <u>Cardiac</u> **complications of anesthesia during the puerperium**

O89.2 <u>Central nervous system</u> **complications of anesthesia during the puerperium**

O89.3 <u>Toxic reaction</u> **to local anesthesia during the puerperium**

O89.4 <u>Spinal and epidural anesthesia-induced headache</u> **during the puerperium**

O89.5 <u>Other complications of spinal and epidural anesthesia</u> **during the puerperium**

O89.6 <u>Failed or difficult intubation</u> **for anesthesia during the puerperium**

O89.8 <u>Other</u> **complications of anesthesia during the puerperium**

O89.9 Complication of anesthesia during the puerperium, <u>unspecified</u>

O90- Complications of the puerperium, <u>not elsewhere classified</u>

O90.0 Disruption of cesarean delivery wound

Dehiscence of cesarean delivery wound

Excludes 1:   rupture of uterus (spontaneous) before onset of labor (O71.0-)
rupture of uterus during labor (O71.1)

O90.1 Disruption of perineal obstetric wound

Disruption of wound of episiotomy

Disruption of wound of perineal laceration

Secondary perineal tear

O90.2 Hematoma of obstetric wound

O90.3 Peripartum cardiomyopathy

Conditions in I42.- arising during pregnancy and the puerperium

Excludes 1:   pre-existing heart disease complicating pregnancy and the puerperium (O99.4-)

O90.4 Postpartum acute kidney failure

Hepatorenal syndrome following labor and delivery

O90.5 Postpartum thyroiditis

O90.6 Postpartum mood disturbance

Postpartum blues

Postpartum dysphoria

Postpartum sadness

Excludes 1:   postpartum depression (F53)
puerperal psychosis (F53)

O90.8- Other complications of the puerperium, <u>not elsewhere classified</u>

O90.81 Anemia of the puerperium

Postpartum anemia NOS

Excludes 1:   pre-existing anemia complicating the puerperium (O99.03)

O90.89 Other complications of the puerperium, not elsewhere classified

Placental polyp

O90.9 Complication of the puerperium, unspecified

O91- Infections of breast associated with pregnancy, the puerperium and lactation

Use additional code to identify infection

O91.0- <u>Infection of nipple</u> **associated with pregnancy, the puerperium and lactation**

O91.01- Infection of nipple <u>associated with pregnancy</u>

Gestational abscess of nipple

O91.011 Infection of nipple associated with pregnancy, <u>first</u> **trimester**

O91.012 Infection of nipple associated with pregnancy, <u>second</u> **trimester**

O91.013 Infection of nipple associated with pregnancy, <u>third</u> **trimester**

O91.019 Infection of nipple associated with pregnancy, <u>unspecified</u> **trimester**

O91.02 Infection of nipple <u>associated with the puerperium</u>

Puerperal abscess of nipple

O91.03 Infection of nipple <u>associated with lactation</u>

Abscess of nipple associated with lactation

O91.1- <u>Abscess of breast</u> **associated with pregnancy, the puerperium and lactation**

O91.11- Abscess of breast <u>associated with pregnancy</u>

Gestational mammary abscess

Gestational purulent mastitis

Gestational subareolar abscess

O91.111 Abscess of breast associated with pregnancy, <u>first</u> **trimester**

O91.112 Abscess of breast associated with pregnancy, <u>second</u> **trimester**

O91.113 Abscess of breast associated with pregnancy, <u>third</u> **trimester**

O91.119 Abscess of breast associated with pregnancy, <u>unspecified</u> **trimester**

O91.12 Abscess of breast <u>associated with the puerperium</u>

Puerperal mammary abscess

Puerperal purulent mastitis

Puerperal subareolar abscess

O91.13 Abscess of breast <u>associated with lactation</u>

Mammary abscess associated with lactation

Purulent mastitis associated with lactation

Subareolar abscess associated with lactation

O91.2- <u>Nonpurulent mastitis</u> **associated with pregnancy, the puerperium and lactation**

O91.21- Nonpurulent mastitis <u>associated with pregnancy</u>

Gestational interstitial mastitis

Gestational lymphangitis of breast

Gestational mastitis NOS

Gestational parenchymatous mastitis

O91.211 Nonpurulent mastitis associated with pregnancy, <u>first</u> **trimester**

O91.212 Nonpurulent mastitis associated with pregnancy, <u>second</u> **trimester**

O91.213 Nonpurulent mastitis associated with pregnancy, <u>third</u> **trimester**

O91.219 Nonpurulent mastitis associated with pregnancy, <u>unspecified</u> **trimester**

O91.22 Nonpurulent mastitis <u>associated with the puerperium</u>

Puerperal interstitial mastitis

Puerperal lymphangitis of breast

Puerperal mastitis NOS

Puerperal parenchymatous mastitis

O91.23 Nonpurulent mastitis <u>associated with lactation</u>

Interstitial mastitis associated with lactation

Lymphangitis of breast associated with lactation

Mastitis NOS associated with lactation

Parenchymatous mastitis associated with lactation

O92- <u>Other disorders of breast</u> **and disorders of lactation associated with pregnancy and the puerperium**

O92.0- <u>Retracted nipple</u> **associated with pregnancy, the puerperium, and lactation**

O92.01- Retracted nipple <u>associated with pregnancy</u>

O92.011 Retracted nipple associated with pregnancy, <u>first</u> **trimester**

O92.012 Retracted nipple associated with pregnancy, <u>second</u> **trimester**

O92.013 Retracted nipple associated with pregnancy, <u>third</u> **trimester**

O92.019 Retracted nipple associated with pregnancy, <u>unspecified</u> **trimester**

O92.02 Retracted nipple associated <u>with the puerperium</u>

O92.03 Retracted nipple associated <u>with lactation</u>

O92.1- <u>Cracked nipple</u> **associated with pregnancy, the puerperium, and lactation**

Fissure of nipple, gestational or puerperal

O92.11- Cracked nipple <u>associated with pregnancy</u>

O92.111 Cracked nipple associated with pregnancy, <u>first</u> **trimester**

O92.112 Cracked nipple associated with pregnancy, <u>second</u> **trimester**

O92.113 Cracked nipple associated with pregnancy, <u>third</u> **trimester**

O92.119 Cracked nipple associated with pregnancy, unspecified trimester

O92.12 Cracked nipple <u>associated with the puerperium</u>

O92.13 Cracked nipple <u>associated with lactation</u>

O88
|
O98

O92.2- Other and unspecified disorders of breast associated with pregnancy and the puerperium

  O92.20 Unspecified disorder of breast associated with pregnancy and the puerperium

  O92.29 Other disorders of breast associated with pregnancy and the puerperium

O92.3 Agalactia
  Primary agalactia
  Excludes 1: elective agalactia (O92.5)
        secondary agalactia (O92.5)
        therapeutic agalactia (O92.5)

O92.4 Hypogalactia

O92.5 Suppressed lactation
  Elective agalactia
  Secondary agalactia
  Therapeutic agalactia
  Excludes 1: primary agalactia (O92.3)

O92.6 Galactorrhea

O92.7- Other and unspecified disorders of lactation

  O92.70 Unspecified disorders of lactation

  O92.79 Other disorders of lactation
      Puerperal galactocele

Other obstetric conditions, not elsewhere classified (O94-O9A)

O94 Sequelae of complication of pregnancy, childbirth, and the puerperium
  Note: This category is to be used to indicate conditions in O00-O77-, O85-O94 and O98-O9A- as the cause of late effects. The sequelae include conditions specified as such, or as late effects, which may occur at any time after the puerperium.
  Code first condition resulting from (sequela) of complication of pregnancy, childbirth, and the puerperium

O98 Maternal infectious and parasitic diseases classifiable elsewhere but complicating pregnancy, childbirth and the puerperium
  Includes: The listed conditions when complicating the pregnant state, when aggravated by the pregnancy, or as a reason for obstetric care
  Use additional code (Chapter 1), to identify specific infectious or parasitic disease
  Excludes❷: herpes gestationis (O26.4-)
      infectious carrier state (O99.82-, O99.83-)
      obstetrical tetanus (A34)
      puerperal infection (O86.-)
      puerperal sepsis (O85)
      when the reason for maternal care is that the disease is known or suspected to have affected the fetus (O35-O36)

O98.0- Tuberculosis complicating pregnancy, childbirth and the puerperium
  Conditions in A15-A19

  O98.01- Tuberculosis complicating pregnancy

    O98.011 Tuberculosis complicating pregnancy, first trimester

    O98.012 Tuberculosis complicating pregnancy, second trimester

    O98.013 Tuberculosis complicating pregnancy, third trimester

    O98.019 Tuberculosis complicating pregnancy, unspecified trimester

  O98.02 Tuberculosis complicating childbirth

  O98.03 Tuberculosis complicating the puerperium

O98.1- Syphilis complicating pregnancy, childbirth and the puerperium
  Conditions in A50-A53

  O98.11- Syphilis complicating pregnancy

    O98.111 Syphilis complicating pregnancy, first trimester

    O98.112 Syphilis complicating pregnancy, second trimester

    O98.113 Syphilis complicating pregnancy, third trimester

    O98.119 Syphilis complicating pregnancy, unspecified trimester

  O98.12 Syphilis complicating childbirth

  O98.13 Syphilis complicating the puerperium

O98.2- Gonorrhea complicating pregnancy, childbirth and the puerperium
  Conditions in A54.-

  O98.21- Gonorrhea complicating pregnancy

    O98.211 Gonorrhea complicating pregnancy, first trimester

    O98.212 Gonorrhea complicating pregnancy, second trimester

    O98.213 Gonorrhea complicating pregnancy, third trimester

    O98.219 Gonorrhea complicating pregnancy, unspecified trimester

  O98.22 Gonorrhea complicating childbirth

  O98.23 Gonorrhea complicating the puerperium

O98.3- Other infections with a predominantly sexual mode of transmission complicating pregnancy, childbirth and the puerperium
  Conditions in A55-A64

  O98.31- Other infections with a predominantly sexual mode of transmission complicating pregnancy

    O98.311 Other infections with a predominantly sexual mode of transmission complicating pregnancy, first trimester

    O98.312 Other infections with a predominantly sexual mode of transmission complicating pregnancy, second trimester

    O98.313 Other infections with a predominantly sexual mode of transmission complicating pregnancy, third trimester

    O98.319 Other infections with a predominantly sexual mode of transmission complicating pregnancy, unspecified trimester

  O98.32 Other infections with a predominantly sexual mode of transmission complicating childbirth

  O98.33 Other infections with a predominantly sexual mode of transmission complicating the puerperium

O98.4- Viral hepatitis complicating pregnancy, childbirth and the puerperium
  Conditions in B15-B19

  O98.41- Viral hepatitis complicating pregnancy

    O98.411 Viral hepatitis complicating pregnancy, first trimester

    O98.412 Viral hepatitis complicating pregnancy, second trimester

    O98.413 Viral hepatitis complicating pregnancy, third trimester

    O98.419 Viral hepatitis complicating pregnancy, unspecified trimester

  O98.42 Viral hepatitis complicating childbirth

  O98.43 Viral hepatitis complicating the puerperium

O98.5- Other viral diseases complicating pregnancy, childbirth and the puerperium
  Conditions in A80-B09, B25-B34, R87.81-, R87.82-
  Excludes 1: human immunodeficiency virus [HIV] disease complicating pregnancy, childbirth and the puerperium (O98.7-)

  O98.51- Other viral diseases complicating pregnancy

    O98.511 Other viral diseases complicating pregnancy, first trimester

    O98.512 Other viral diseases complicating pregnancy, second trimester

    O98.513 Other viral diseases complicating pregnancy, third trimester

    O98.519 Other viral diseases complicating pregnancy, unspecified trimester

  O98.52 Other viral diseases complicating childbirth

  O98.53 Other viral diseases complicating the puerperium

O98.6- Protozoal diseases complicating pregnancy, childbirth and the puerperium
  Conditions in B50-B64

  O98.61- Protozoal diseases complicating pregnancy

    O98.611 Protozoal diseases complicating pregnancy, first trimester

    O98.612 Protozoal diseases complicating pregnancy, second trimester

    O98.613 Protozoal diseases complicating pregnancy, third trimester

    O98.619 Protozoal diseases complicating pregnancy, unspecified trimester

  O98.62 Protozoal diseases complicating childbirth

  O98.63 Protozoal diseases complicating the puerperium

O98.7- Human immunodeficiency virus [HIV] disease complicating pregnancy, childbirth and the puerperium
  Use additional code to identify the type of HIV disease:
    Acquired immune deficiency syndrome (AIDS) (B20)
    Asymptomatic HIV status (Z21)
    HIV positive NOS (Z21)
    Symptomatic HIV disease (B20)

  O98.71- Human immunodeficiency virus [HIV] disease complicating pregnancy

    O98.711 Human immunodeficiency virus [HIV] disease complicating pregnancy, first trimester

    O98.712 Human immunodeficiency virus [HIV] disease complicating pregnancy, second trimester

    O98.713 Human immunodeficiency virus [HIV] disease complicating pregnancy, third trimester

    O98.719 Human immunodeficiency virus [HIV] disease complicating pregnancy, unspecified trimester

O88 - O98

O98.72 Human immunodeficiency virus [HIV] disease complicating <u>childbirth</u>

O98.73 Human immunodeficiency virus [HIV] disease complicating <u>the puerperium</u>

O98.8- <u>Other</u> maternal infectious and parasitic diseases complicating pregnancy, childbirth and the puerperium

O98.81- Other maternal infectious and parasitic diseases complicating <u>pregnancy</u>

O98.811 Other maternal infectious and parasitic diseases complicating pregnancy, <u>first</u> trimester

O98.812 Other maternal infectious and parasitic diseases complicating pregnancy, <u>second</u> trimester

O98.813 Other maternal infectious and parasitic diseases complicating pregnancy, <u>third</u> trimester

O98.819 Other maternal infectious and parasitic diseases complicating pregnancy, <u>unspecified</u> trimester

O98.82 Other maternal infectious and parasitic diseases complicating <u>childbirth</u>

O98.83 Other maternal infectious and parasitic diseases complicating <u>the puerperium</u>

O98.9- <u>Unspecified</u> maternal infectious and parasitic disease complicating pregnancy, childbirth and the puerperium

O98.91- Unspecified maternal infectious and parasitic disease complicating <u>pregnancy</u>

O98.911 Unspecified maternal infectious and parasitic disease complicating pregnancy, <u>first</u> trimester

O98.912 Unspecified maternal infectious and parasitic disease complicating pregnancy, <u>second</u> trimester

O98.913 Unspecified maternal infectious and parasitic disease complicating pregnancy, <u>third</u> trimester

O98.919 Unspecified maternal infectious and parasitic disease complicating pregnancy, <u>unspecified</u> trimester

O98.92 Unspecified maternal infectious and parasitic disease complicating <u>childbirth</u>

O98.93 Unspecified maternal infectious and parasitic disease complicating <u>the puerperium</u>

O99- <u>Other maternal diseases classifiable elsewhere</u> but complicating pregnancy, childbirth and the puerperium
Includes: Conditions which complicate the pregnant state, are aggravated by the pregnancy or are a main reason for obstetric care
Use additional code to identify specific condition
Excludes❷: when the reason for maternal care is that the condition is known or suspected to have affected the fetus (O35-O36)

O99.0- <u>Anemia</u> complicating pregnancy, childbirth and the puerperium
Conditions in D50-D64
Excludes 1: anemia arising in the puerperium (O90.81)
postpartum anemia NOS (O90.81)

O99.01- Anemia complicating <u>pregnancy</u>

O99.011 Anemia complicating pregnancy, <u>first</u> trimester

O99.012 Anemia complicating pregnancy, <u>second</u> trimester

O99.013 Anemia complicating pregnancy, <u>third</u> trimester

O99.019 Anemia complicating pregnancy, <u>unspecified</u> trimester

O99.02 Anemia complicating <u>childbirth</u>

O99.03 Anemia complicating <u>the puerperium</u>
Excludes 1: postpartum anemia not pre-existing prior to delivery (O90.81)

O99.1- <u>Other diseases of the blood and blood-forming organs and certain disorders involving the immune mechanism</u> complicating pregnancy, childbirth and the puerperium
Conditions in D65-D89
Excludes❷: hemorrhage with coagulation defects (O45.-, O46.0-, O67.0, O72.3)

O99.11- Other diseases of the blood and blood-forming organs and certain disorders involving the immune mechanism complicating <u>pregnancy</u>

O99.111 Other diseases of the blood and blood-forming organs and certain disorders involving the immune mechanism complicating pregnancy, <u>first</u> trimester

O99.112 Other diseases of the blood and blood-forming organs and certain disorders involving the immune mechanism complicating pregnancy, <u>second</u> trimester

O99.113 Other diseases of the blood and blood-forming organs and certain disorders involving the immune mechanism complicating pregnancy, <u>third</u> trimester

O99.119 Other diseases of the blood and blood-forming organs and certain disorders involving the immune mechanism complicating pregnancy, <u>unspecified</u> trimester

O99.12 Other diseases of the blood and blood-forming organs and certain disorders involving the immune mechanism complicating <u>childbirth</u>

O99.13 Other diseases of the blood and blood-forming organs and certain disorders involving the immune mechanism complicating <u>the puerperium</u>

O99.2- <u>Endocrine, nutritional and metabolic diseases</u> complicating pregnancy, childbirth and the puerperium
Conditions in E00-E88
Excludes❷: diabetes mellitus (O24.-)
malnutrition (O25.-)
postpartum thyroiditis (O90.5)

O99.21- <u>Obesity</u> complicating pregnancy, childbirth, and the puerperium
Use additional code to identify the type of obesity (E66.-)

O99.210 Obesity complicating <u>pregnancy, unspecified</u> trimester

O99.211 Obesity complicating <u>pregnancy, first</u> trimester

O99.212 Obesity complicating <u>pregnancy, second</u> trimester

O99.213 Obesity complicating <u>pregnancy, third</u> trimester

O99.214 Obesity complicating <u>childbirth</u>

O99.215 Obesity complicating <u>the puerperium</u>

O99.28- <u>Other</u> endocrine, nutritional and metabolic diseases complicating pregnancy, childbirth and the puerperium

O99.280 Endocrine, nutritional and metabolic diseases complicating <u>pregnancy, unspecified</u> trimester

O99.281 Endocrine, nutritional and metabolic diseases complicating <u>pregnancy, first</u> trimester

O99.282 Endocrine, nutritional and metabolic diseases complicating <u>pregnancy, second</u> trimester

O99.283 Endocrine, nutritional and metabolic diseases complicating <u>pregnancy, third</u> trimester

O99.284 Endocrine, nutritional and metabolic diseases complicating <u>childbirth</u>

O99.285 Endocrine, nutritional and metabolic diseases complicating <u>the puerperium</u>

O99.3- <u>Mental disorders and diseases of the nervous system</u> complicating pregnancy, childbirth and the puerperium

O99.31- <u>Alcohol use</u> complicating pregnancy, childbirth, and the puerperium
Use additional code(s) from F10 to identify manifestations of the alcohol use

O99.310 Alcohol use complicating <u>pregnancy, unspecified</u> trimester

O99.311 Alcohol use complicating <u>pregnancy, first</u> trimester

O99.312 Alcohol use complicating <u>pregnancy, second</u> trimester

O99.313 Alcohol use complicating <u>pregnancy, third</u> trimester

O99.314 Alcohol use complicating <u>childbirth</u>

O99.315 Alcohol use complicating <u>the puerperium</u>

O99.32- <u>Drug use</u> complicating pregnancy, childbirth, and the puerperium
Use additional code(s) from F11-F16 and F18-F19 to identify manifestations of the drug use

O99.320 Drug use complicating <u>pregnancy, unspecified</u> trimester

O99.321 Drug use complicating <u>pregnancy, first</u> trimester

O99.322 Drug use complicating <u>pregnancy, second</u> trimester

O99.323 Drug use complicating <u>pregnancy, third</u> trimester

O99.324 Drug use complicating <u>childbirth</u>

O99.325 Drug use complicating <u>the puerperium</u>

O99.33- <u>Smoking</u> (tobacco) complicating pregnancy, childbirth, and the puerperium
Use additional code from F17 to identify type of tobacco

O99.330 Smoking (tobacco) complicating <u>pregnancy, unspecified</u> trimester

O99.331 Smoking (tobacco) complicating <u>pregnancy, first</u> trimester

O99.332 Smoking (tobacco) complicating <u>pregnancy, second</u> trimester

O99.333 Smoking (tobacco) complicating <u>pregnancy, third</u> trimester

O99.334 Smoking (tobacco) complicating <u>childbirth</u>

O99.335 Smoking (tobacco) complicating <u>the puerperium</u>

O99.34- <u>Other mental disorders</u> complicating pregnancy, childbirth, and the puerperium
Conditions in F01-F09 and F20-F99
Excludes❷: postpartum mood disturbance (O90.6)
postnatal psychosis (F53)
puerperal psychosis (F53)

O99.340 Other mental disorders complicating <u>pregnancy, unspecified</u> trimester

O99.341 Other mental disorders complicating <u>pregnancy, first</u> trimester

O99.342 Other mental disorders complicating <u>pregnancy, second</u> trimester

O99.343 Other mental disorders complicating <u>pregnancy, third</u> trimester

O99.344 Other mental disorders complicating <u>childbirth</u>

O99.345 Other mental disorders complicating <u>the puerperium</u>

O99.35- <u>Diseases of the nervous system</u> complicating pregnancy, childbirth, and the puerperium
Conditions in G00-G99
Excludes❷: pregnancy related peripheral neuritis (O26.8-)

O99.350 Diseases of the nervous system complicating <u>pregnancy, unspecified</u> trimester

O99.351 Diseases of the nervous system complicating <u>pregnancy, first</u> trimester

O99.352 Diseases of the nervous system complicating <u>pregnancy, second</u> trimester

O99.353 Diseases of the nervous system complicating <u>pregnancy, third</u> trimester

O99.354 Diseases of the nervous system complicating <u>childbirth</u>

O99.355 Diseases of the nervous system complicating <u>the puerperium</u>

O99.4- <u>Diseases of the circulatory system</u> complicating pregnancy, childbirth and the puerperium
Conditions in I00-I99
Excludes 1: peripartum cardiomyopathy (O90.3)
Excludes❷: hypertensive disorders (O10-O16)
obstetric embolism (O88.-)
venous complications and cerebrovenous sinus thrombosis in labor, childbirth and the puerperium (O87-)
venous complications and cerebrovenous sinus thrombosis in pregnancy (O22-)

O99.41- Diseases of the circulatory system complicating <u>pregnancy</u>

O99.411 Diseases of the circulatory system complicating pregnancy, <u>first</u> trimester

O99.412 Diseases of the circulatory system complicating pregnancy, <u>second</u> trimester

O99.413 Diseases of the circulatory system complicating pregnancy, <u>third</u> trimester

O99.419 Diseases of the circulatory system complicating pregnancy, <u>unspecified</u> trimester

O99.42 Diseases of the circulatory system complicating <u>childbirth</u>

O99.43 Diseases of the circulatory system complicating <u>the puerperium</u>

O99.5- <u>Diseases of the respiratory system</u> complicating pregnancy, childbirth and the puerperium
Conditions in J00-J99

O99.51- Diseases of the respiratory system complicating <u>pregnancy</u>

O99.511 Diseases of the respiratory system complicating pregnancy, <u>first</u> trimester

O99.512 Diseases of the respiratory system complicating pregnancy, <u>second</u> trimester

O99.513 Diseases of the respiratory system complicating pregnancy, <u>third</u> trimester

O99.519 Diseases of the respiratory system complicating pregnancy, <u>unspecified</u> trimester

O99.52 Diseases of the respiratory system complicating <u>childbirth</u>

O99.53 Diseases of the respiratory system complicating <u>the puerperium</u>

O99.6- <u>Diseases of the digestive system</u> complicating pregnancy, childbirth and the puerperium
Conditions in K00-K93
Excludes❷: liver and biliary tract disorders in pregnancy, childbirth and the puerperium (O26.6-)

O99.61- Diseases of the digestive system complicating <u>pregnancy</u>

O99.611 Diseases of the digestive system complicating pregnancy, <u>first</u> trimester

O99.612 Diseases of the digestive system complicating pregnancy, <u>second</u> trimester

O99.613 Diseases of the digestive system complicating pregnancy, <u>third</u> trimester

O99.619 Diseases of the digestive system complicating pregnancy, <u>unspecified</u> trimester

O99.62 Diseases of the digestive system complicating <u>childbirth</u>

O99.63 Diseases of the digestive system complicating <u>the puerperium</u>

O99.7- <u>Diseases of the skin and subcutaneous tissue</u> complicating pregnancy, childbirth and the puerperium
Conditions in L00-L99
Excludes❷: herpes gestationis (O26.4)
pruritic urticarial papules and plaques of pregnancy (PUPPP) (O26.86)

O99.71- Diseases of the skin and subcutaneous tissue complicating <u>pregnancy</u>

O99.711 Diseases of the skin and subcutaneous tissue complicating pregnancy, <u>first</u> trimester

O99.712 Diseases of the skin and subcutaneous tissue complicating pregnancy, <u>second</u> trimester

O99.713 Diseases of the skin and subcutaneous tissue complicating pregnancy, <u>third</u> trimester

O99.719 Diseases of the skin and subcutaneous tissue complicating pregnancy, <u>unspecified</u> trimester

O99.72 Diseases of the skin and subcutaneous tissue complicating <u>childbirth</u>

O99.73 Diseases of the skin and subcutaneous tissue complicating <u>the puerperium</u>

O99.8- <u>Other specified diseases and conditions</u> complicating pregnancy, childbirth and the puerperium
Conditions in D00-D48, H00-H95, M00-N99, and Q00-Q99
Use additional code to identify condition
Excludes❷: genitourinary infections in pregnancy (O23-)
infection of genitourinary tract following delivery (O86.1-O86.3)
malignant neoplasm complicating pregnancy, childbirth and the puerperium (O9A.1-)
maternal care for known or suspected abnormality of maternal pelvic organs (O34-)
postpartum acute kidney failure (O90.4)
traumatic injuries in pregnancy (O9A.2-)

O99.81- <u>Abnormal glucose</u> complicating pregnancy, childbirth and the puerperium
Excludes 1: gestational diabetes (O24.4-)

O99.810 Abnormal glucose complicating <u>pregnancy</u>

O99.814 Abnormal glucose complicating <u>childbirth</u>

O99.815 Abnormal glucose complicating <u>the puerperium</u>

O99.82- <u>Streptococcus B carrier state</u> complicating pregnancy, childbirth and the puerperium

O99.820 Streptococcus B carrier state complicating <u>pregnancy</u>

O99.824 Streptococcus B carrier state complicating <u>childbirth</u>

O99.825 Streptococcus B carrier state complicating <u>the puerperium</u>

O99.83- <u>Other infection carrier state</u> complicating pregnancy, childbirth and the puerperium
Use additional code to identify the carrier state (Z22.-)

O99.830 Other infection carrier state complicating <u>pregnancy</u>

O99.834 Other infection carrier state complicating <u>childbirth</u>

O99.835 Other infection carrier state complicating <u>the puerperium</u>

O99.84- <u>Bariatric surgery status</u> complicating pregnancy, childbirth and the puerperium
Gastric banding status complicating pregnancy, childbirth and the puerperium
Gastric bypass status for obesity complicating pregnancy, childbirth and the puerperium
Obesity surgery status complicating pregnancy, childbirth and the puerperium

O99.840 Bariatric surgery status complicating <u>pregnancy, unspecified</u> trimester

O99.841 Bariatric surgery status complicating <u>pregnancy, first</u> trimester

O99.842 Bariatric surgery status complicating <u>pregnancy, second</u> trimester

O99.843 Bariatric surgery status complicating <u>pregnancy, third</u> trimester

O99.844 Bariatric surgery status complicating <u>childbirth</u>

O99.845 Bariatric surgery status complicating <u>the puerperium</u>

O99.89 <u>Other specified</u> diseases and conditions complicating pregnancy, childbirth and the puerperium

O
9
8
I
O
9
9

Excludes 1: = NOT CODED HERE! (Do not code both)

Excludes❷: = Not Included Here

O9A- **Maternal malignant neoplasms, traumatic injuries and abuse classifiable elsewhere but complicating pregnancy, childbirth and the puerperium**

O9A.1- <u>Malignant neoplasm</u> complicating pregnancy, childbirth and the puerperium
> Conditions in C00-C96
> Use additional code to identify neoplasm
> *Excludes❷: maternal care for benign tumor of corpus uteri (O34.1-)*
> *maternal care for benign tumor of cervix (O34.4-)*

O9A.11-Malignant neoplasm complicating <u>pregnancy</u>

O9A.111 Malignant neoplasm complicating pregnancy, <u>first</u> trimester

O9A.112 Malignant neoplasm complicating pregnancy, <u>second</u> trimester

O9A.113 Malignant neoplasm complicating pregnancy, <u>third</u> trimester

O9A.119 Malignant neoplasm complicating pregnancy, <u>unspecified</u> trimester

O9A.12 Malignant neoplasm complicating <u>childbirth</u>

O9A.13 Malignant neoplasm complicating <u>the puerperium</u>

O9A.2- <u>Injury, poisoning and certain other consequences of external causes</u> complicating pregnancy, childbirth and the puerperium
> Conditions in S00-T88, except T74 and T76
> Use additional code(s) to identify the injury or poisoning
> *Excludes❷: physical, sexual and psychological abuse complicating pregnancy, childbirth and the puerperium (O9A.3-, O9A.4-, O9A.5-)*

O9A.21- Injury, poisoning and certain other consequences of external causes complicating <u>pregnancy</u>

O9A.211 Injury, poisoning and certain other consequences of external causes complicating pregnancy, <u>first</u> trimester

O9A.212 Injury, poisoning and certain other consequences of external causes complicating pregnancy, <u>second</u> trimester

O9A.213 Injury, poisoning and certain other consequences of external causes complicating pregnancy, <u>third</u> trimester

O9A.219 Injury, poisoning and certain other consequences of external causes complicating pregnancy, <u>unspecified</u> trimester

O9A.22 Injury, poisoning and certain other consequences of external causes complicating <u>childbirth</u>

O9A.23 Injury, poisoning and certain other consequences of external causes complicating <u>the puerperium</u>

O9A.3- <u>Physical abuse</u> complicating pregnancy, childbirth and the puerperium
> Conditions in T74.11 or T76.11
> Use additional code (if applicable):
> To identify any associated current injury due to physical abuse
> To identify the perpetrator of abuse (Y07.-)
> *Excludes❷: sexual abuse complicating pregnancy, childbirth and the puerperium (O9A.4-)*

O9A.31- Physical abuse complicating <u>pregnancy</u>

O9A.311 Physical abuse complicating pregnancy, <u>first</u> trimester

O9A.312 Physical abuse complicating pregnancy, <u>second</u> trimester

O9A.313 Physical abuse complicating pregnancy, <u>third</u> trimester

O9A.319 Physical abuse complicating pregnancy, <u>unspecified</u> trimester

O9A.32 Physical abuse complicating <u>childbirth</u>

O9A.33 Physical abuse complicating <u>the puerperium</u>

O9A.4- <u>Sexual abuse</u> complicating pregnancy, childbirth and the puerperium
> Conditions in T74.21 or T76.21
> Use additional code (if applicable):
> To identify any associated current injury due to sexual abuse
> To identify the perpetrator of abuse (Y07.-)

O9A.41- Sexual abuse complicating <u>pregnancy</u>

O9A.411 Sexual abuse complicating pregnancy, <u>first</u> trimester

O9A.412 Sexual abuse complicating pregnancy, <u>second</u> trimester

O9A.413 Sexual abuse complicating pregnancy, <u>third</u> trimester

O9A.419 Sexual abuse complicating pregnancy, <u>unspecified</u> trimester

O9A.42 Sexual abuse complicating <u>childbirth</u>

O9A.43 Sexual abuse complicating <u>the puerperium</u>

O9A.5- <u>Psychological abuse</u> complicating pregnancy, childbirth and the puerperium
> Conditions in T74.31 or T76.31
> Use additional code to identify the perpetrator of abuse (Y07.-)

O9A.51- Psychological abuse complicating <u>pregnancy</u>

O9A.511 Psychological abuse complicating pregnancy, <u>first</u> trimester

O9A.512 Psychological abuse complicating pregnancy, <u>second</u> trimester

O9A.513 Psychological abuse complicating pregnancy, <u>third</u> trimester

O9A.519 Psychological abuse complicating pregnancy, <u>unspecified</u> trimester

O9A.52 Psychological abuse complicating <u>childbirth</u>

O9A.53 Psychological abuse complicating <u>the puerperium</u>

O
9
A
I
P
0
2

Excludes 1: = NOT CODED HERE! (Do not code both)

Excludes❷: = Not Included Here

Chapter 16 – Certain conditions originating in the perinatal period (P00-P96)

Note: Codes from this chapter are for use on newborn records only, never on maternal records

Includes: Conditions that have their origin in the fetal or perinatal period (before birth through the first 28 days after birth) even if morbidity occurs later

Excludes❷: congenital malformations, deformations and chromosomal abnormalities (Q00-Q99)
endocrine, nutritional and metabolic diseases (E00-E88)
injury, poisoning and certain other consequences of external causes (S00-T88)
neoplasms (C00-D49)
tetanus neonatorum (A33)

This chapter contains the following blocks:

P00-P04 Newborn affected by maternal factors and by complications of pregnancy, labor, and delivery
P05-P08 Disorders of newborn related to length of gestation and fetal growth
P09 Abnormal findings on neonatal screening
P10-P15 Birth trauma
P19-P29 Respiratory and cardiovascular disorders specific to the perinatal period
P35-P39 Infections specific to the perinatal period
P50-P61 Hemorrhagic and hematological disorders of newborn
P70-P74 Transitory endocrine and metabolic disorders specific to newborn
P76-P78 Digestive system disorders of newborn
P80-P83 Conditions involving the integument and temperature regulation of newborn
P84 Other problems with newborn
P90-P96 Other disorders originating in the perinatal period

Newborn affected by maternal factors and by complications of pregnancy, labor, and delivery (P00-P04)

Note: These codes are for use when the listed maternal conditions are specified as the cause of confirmed morbidity or potential morbidity which have their origin in the perinatal period (before birth through the first 28 days after birth). Codes from these categories are also for use for newborns who are suspected of having an abnormal condition resulting from exposure from the mother or the birth process, but without signs or symptoms, and, which after examination and observation, is found not to exist. These codes may be used even if treatment is begun for a suspected condition that is ruled out.

P00- **Newborn (suspected to be) affected by <u>maternal conditions</u> that may be <u>unrelated</u> to present pregnancy**
Code first any current condition in newborn
Excludes❷: newborn (suspected to be) affected by maternal complications of pregnancy (P01.-)
newborn affected by maternal endocrine and metabolic disorders (P70-P74)
newborn affected by noxious substances transmitted via placenta or breast milk (P04.-)

P00.0 **Newborn (suspected to be) affected by maternal hypertensive disorders**
Newborn (suspected to be) affected by maternal conditions classifiable to O10-O11, O13-O16

P00.1 **Newborn (suspected to be) affected by maternal renal and urinary tract diseases**
Newborn (suspected to be) affected by maternal conditions classifiable to N00-N39

P00.2 **Newborn (suspected to be) affected by maternal infectious and parasitic diseases**
Newborn (suspected to be) affected by maternal infectious disease classifiable to A00-B99, J09 and J10
Excludes 1: infections specific to the perinatal period (P35-P39)
maternal genital tract or other localized infections (P00.8)

P00.3 **Newborn (suspected to be) affected by other maternal circulatory and respiratory diseases**
Newborn (suspected to be) affected by maternal conditions classifiable to I00-I99, J00-J99, Q20-Q34 and not included in P00.0, P00.2

P00.4 **Newborn (suspected to be) affected by maternal nutritional disorders**
Newborn (suspected to be) affected by maternal disorders classifiable to E40-E64
Maternal malnutrition NOS

P00.5 **Newborn (suspected to be) affected by maternal injury**
Newborn (suspected to be) affected by maternal conditions classifiable to O9A.2-

P00.6 **Newborn (suspected to be) affected by surgical procedure on mother**
Newborn (suspected to be) affected by amniocentesis
Excludes 1: cesarean delivery for present delivery (P03.4)
damage to placenta from amniocentesis, cesarean delivery or surgical induction (P02.1)
previous surgery to uterus or pelvic organs (P03.89)
Excludes❷: newborn affected by complication of (fetal) intrauterine procedure (P96.5)

P00.7 **Newborn (suspected to be) affected by other medical procedures on mother, not elsewhere classified**
Newborn (suspected to be) affected by radiation to mother
Excludes 1: damage to placenta from amniocentesis, cesarean delivery or surgical induction (P02.1)
newborn affected by other complications of labor and delivery (P03.-)

P00.8- **Newborn (suspected to be) affected by other maternal conditions**

P00.81 **Newborn (suspected to be) affected by periodontal disease in mother**

P00.89 **Newborn (suspected to be) affected by other maternal conditions**
Newborn (suspected to be) affected by conditions classifiable to T80-T88
Newborn (suspected to be) affected by maternal genital tract or other localized infections
Newborn (suspected to be) affected by maternal systemic lupus erythematosus

P00.9 **Newborn (suspected to be) affected by unspecified maternal condition**

P01- **Newborn (suspected to be) affected by <u>maternal complications</u> of pregnancy**
Code first any current condition in newborn

P01.0 **Newborn (suspected to be) affected by incompetent cervix**

P01.1 **Newborn (suspected to be) affected by premature rupture of membranes**

P01.2 **Newborn (suspected to be) affected by oligohydramnios**
Excludes 1: oligohydramnios due to premature rupture of membranes (P01.1)

P01.3 **Newborn (suspected to be) affected by polyhydramnios**
Newborn (suspected to be) affected by hydramnios

P01.4 **Newborn (suspected to be) affected by ectopic pregnancy**
Newborn (suspected to be) affected by abdominal pregnancy

P01.5 **Newborn (suspected to be) affected by multiple pregnancy**
Newborn (suspected to be) affected by triplet (pregnancy)
Newborn (suspected to be) affected by twin (pregnancy)

P01.6 **Newborn (suspected to be) affected by maternal death**

P01.7 **Newborn (suspected to be) affected by malpresentation before labor**
Newborn (suspected to be) affected by breech presentation before labor
Newborn (suspected to be) affected by external version before labor
Newborn (suspected to be) affected by face presentation before labor
Newborn (suspected to be) affected by transverse lie before labor
Newborn (suspected to be) affected by unstable lie before labor

P01.8 **Newborn (suspected to be) affected by other maternal complications of pregnancy**

P01.9 **Newborn (suspected to be) affected by maternal complication of pregnancy, unspecified**

P02- **Newborn (suspected to be) affected by <u>complications</u> of placenta, cord and membranes**
Code first any current condition in newborn

P02.0 **Newborn (suspected to be) affected by placenta previa**

P02.1 **Newborn (suspected to be) affected by other forms of placental separation and hemorrhage**
Newborn (suspected to be) affected by abruptio placenta
Newborn (suspected to be) affected by accidental hemorrhage
Newborn (suspected to be) affected by antepartum hemorrhage
Newborn (suspected to be) affected by damage to placenta from amniocentesis, cesarean delivery or surgical induction
Newborn (suspected to be) affected by maternal blood loss
Newborn (suspected to be) affected by premature separation of placenta

P02.2- **Newborn (suspected to be) affected by other and unspecified morphological and functional abnormalities of placenta**

P02.20 **Newborn (suspected to be) affected by unspecified morphological and functional abnormalities of placenta**

P02.29 **Newborn (suspected to be) affected by other morphological and functional abnormalities of placenta**
Newborn (suspected to be) affected by placental dysfunction
Newborn (suspected to be) affected by placental infarction
Newborn (suspected to be) affected by placental insufficiency

O9A - P02

© 2013 Channel Publishing, Ltd.

P02.3 Newborn (suspected to be) affected by placental transfusion syndromes
Newborn (suspected to be) affected by placental and cord abnormalities resulting in twin-to-twin or other transplacental transfusion

P02.4 Newborn (suspected to be) affected by prolapsed cord

P02.5 Newborn (suspected to be) affected by other compression of umbilical cord
Newborn (suspected to be) affected by umbilical cord (tightly) around neck
Newborn (suspected to be) affected by entanglement of umbilical cord
Newborn (suspected to be) affected by knot in umbilical cord

P02.6- Newborn (suspected to be) affected by other and unspecified conditions of umbilical cord

P02.60 Newborn (suspected to be) affected by unspecified conditions of umbilical cord

P02.69 Newborn (suspected to be) affected by other conditions of umbilical cord
Newborn (suspected to be) affected by short umbilical cord
Newborn (suspected to be) affected by vasa previa
Excludes 1: newborn affected by single umbilical artery (Q27.0)

P02.7 Newborn (suspected to be) affected by chorioamnionitis
Newborn (suspected to be) affected by amnionitis
Newborn (suspected to be) affected by membranitis
Newborn (suspected to be) affected by placentitis

P02.8 Newborn (suspected to be) affected by other abnormalities of membranes

P02.9 Newborn (suspected to be) affected by abnormality of membranes, unspecified

P03- Newborn (suspected to be) affected by other complications of labor and delivery
Code first any current condition in newborn

P03.0 Newborn (suspected to be) affected by breech delivery and extraction

P03.1 Newborn (suspected to be) affected by other malpresentation, malposition and disproportion during labor and delivery
Newborn (suspected to be) affected by contracted pelvis
Newborn (suspected to be) affected by conditions classifiable to O64-O66
Newborn (suspected to be) affected by persistent occipitoposterior
Newborn (suspected to be) affected by transverse lie

P03.2 Newborn (suspected to be) affected by forceps delivery

P03.3 Newborn (suspected to be) affected by delivery by vacuum extractor [ventouse]

P03.4 Newborn (suspected to be) affected by cesarean delivery

P03.5 Newborn (suspected to be) affected by precipitate delivery
Newborn (suspected to be) affected by rapid second stage

P03.6 Newborn (suspected to be) affected by abnormal uterine contractions
Newborn (suspected to be) affected by conditions classifiable to O62.-, except O62.3
Newborn (suspected to be) affected by hypertonic labor
Newborn (suspected to be) affected by uterine inertia

P03.8- Newborn (suspected to be) affected by other specified complications of labor and delivery

P03.81- Newborn (suspected to be) affected by abnormality in fetal (intrauterine) heart rate or rhythm
Excludes 1: neonatal cardiac dysrhythmia (P29.1-)

P03.810 Newborn (suspected to be) affected by abnormality in fetal (intrauterine) heart rate or rhythm before the onset of labor

P03.811 Newborn (suspected to be) affected by abnormality in fetal (intrauterine) heart rate or rhythm during labor

P03.819 Newborn (suspected to be) affected by abnormality in fetal (intrauterine) heart rate or rhythm, unspecified as to time of onset

P03.82 Meconium passage during delivery
Excludes 1: meconium aspiration (P24.00, P24.01)
meconium staining (P96.83)

P03.89 Newborn (suspected to be) affected by other specified complications of labor and delivery
Newborn (suspected to be) affected by abnormality of maternal soft tissues
Newborn (suspected to be) affected by conditions classifiable to O60-O75 and by procedures used in labor and delivery not included in P02.- and P03.0-P03.6
Newborn (suspected to be) affected by induction of labor

P03.9 Newborn (suspected to be) affected by complication of labor and delivery, unspecified

P04- Newborn (suspected to be) affected by noxious substances transmitted via placenta or breast milk
Includes: Nonteratogenic effects of substances transmitted via placenta
Excludes❷: congenital malformations (Q00-Q99)
neonatal jaundice from excessive hemolysis due to drugs or toxins transmitted from mother (P58.4)
newborn in contact with and (suspected) exposures hazardous to health not transmitted via placenta or breast milk (Z77.-)

P04.0 Newborn (suspected to be) affected by maternal anesthesia and analgesia in pregnancy, labor and delivery
Newborn (suspected to be) affected by reactions and intoxications from maternal opiates and tranquilizers administered during labor and delivery

P04.1 Newborn (suspected to be) affected by other maternal medication
Newborn (suspected to be) affected by cancer chemotherapy
Newborn (suspected to be) affected by cytotoxic drugs
Excludes 1: dysmorphism due to warfarin (Q86.2)
fetal hydantoin syndrome (Q86.1)
maternal use of drugs of addiction (P04.4-)

P04.2 Newborn (suspected to be) affected by maternal use of tobacco
Newborn (suspected to be) affected by exposure in utero to tobacco smoke
Excludes❷: newborn exposure to environmental tobacco smoke (P96.81)

P04.3 Newborn (suspected to be) affected by maternal use of alcohol
Excludes 1: fetal alcohol syndrome (Q86.0)

P04.4- Newborn (suspected to be) affected by maternal use of drugs of addiction

P04.41 Newborn (suspected to be) affected by maternal use of cocaine
"Crack baby"

P04.49 Newborn (suspected to be) affected by maternal use of other drugs of addiction
Excludes❷: newborn (suspected to be) affected by maternal anesthesia and analgesia (P04.0)
withdrawal symptoms from maternal use of drugs of addiction (P96.1)

P04.5 Newborn (suspected to be) affected by maternal use of nutritional chemical substances

P04.6 Newborn (suspected to be) affected by maternal exposure to environmental chemical substances

P04.8 Newborn (suspected to be) affected by other maternal noxious substances

P04.9 Newborn (suspected to be) affected by maternal noxious substance, unspecified

Disorders of newborn related to length of gestation and fetal growth (P05-P08)

P05- Disorders of newborn related to slow fetal growth and fetal malnutrition

P05.0- Newborn light for gestational age
Newborn light-for-dates

P05.00 Newborn light for gestational age, unspecified weight
P05.01 Newborn light for gestational age, less than 500 grams
P05.02 Newborn light for gestational age, 500-749 grams
P05.03 Newborn light for gestational age, 750-999 grams
P05.04 Newborn light for gestational age, 1000-1249 grams
P05.05 Newborn light for gestational age, 1250-1499 grams
P05.06 Newborn light for gestational age, 1500-1749 grams
P05.07 Newborn light for gestational age, 1750-1999 grams
P05.08 Newborn light for gestational age, 2000-2499 grams

P05.1- Newborn small for gestational age
Newborn small-and-light-for-dates
Newborn small-for-dates

P05.10 Newborn small for gestational age, unspecified weight
P05.11 Newborn small for gestational age, less than 500 grams
P05.12 Newborn small for gestational age, 500-749 grams
P05.13 Newborn small for gestational age, 750-999 grams
P05.14 Newborn small for gestational age, 1000-1249 grams
P05.15 Newborn small for gestational age, 1250-1499 grams
P05.16 Newborn small for gestational age, 1500-1749 grams
P05.17 Newborn small for gestational age, 1750-1999 grams
P05.18 Newborn small for gestational age, 2000-2499 grams

P05.2 **Newborn affected by fetal (intrauterine) malnutrition <u>not light or</u> <u>small for gestational age</u>**
Infant, not light or small for gestational age, showing signs of fetal malnutrition, such as dry, peeling skin and loss of subcutaneous tissue
Excludes 1: *newborn affected by fetal malnutrition with light for gestational age (P05.0-)*
newborn affected by fetal malnutrition with small for gestational age (P05.1-)

P05.9 **Newborn affected by slow intrauterine growth, unspecified**
Newborn affected by fetal growth retardation NOS

P07- **Disorders of newborn related to short gestation and low birth weight, not elsewhere classified**
Note: When both birth weight and gestational age of the newborn are available, both should be coded with birth weight sequenced before gestational age
Includes: The listed conditions, without further specification, as the cause of morbidity or additional care, in newborn
Excludes 1: *low birth weight due to slow fetal growth and fetal malnutrition (P05.-)*

P07.0- **<u>Extremely low birth weight</u> newborn**
Newborn birth weight 999 g. or less

P07.00 **Extremely low birth weight newborn, unspecified weight**
P07.01 **Extremely low birth weight newborn, less than 500 grams**
P07.02 **Extremely low birth weight newborn, 500-749 grams**
P07.03 **Extremely low birth weight newborn, 750-999 grams**

P07.1- **<u>Other low birth weight</u> newborn**
Newborn birth weight 1000-2499 g.

P07.10 **Other low birth weight newborn, unspecified weight**
P07.14 **Other low birth weight newborn, 1000-1249 grams**
P07.15 **Other low birth weight newborn, 1250-1499 grams**
P07.16 **Other low birth weight newborn, 1500-1749 grams**
P07.17 **Other low birth weight newborn, 1750-1999 grams**
P07.18 **Other low birth weight newborn, 2000-2499 grams**

P07.2- **<u>Extreme immaturity</u> of newborn**
Less than 28 completed weeks (less than 196 completed days) of gestation

P07.20 **Extreme immaturity of newborn, unspecified weeks of gestation**
Gestational age less than 28 completed weeks NOS

P07.21 **Extreme immaturity of newborn, gestational age less than 23 completed weeks**
Extreme immaturity of newborn, gestational age less than 23 weeks, 0 days

P07.22 **Extreme immaturity of newborn, gestational age 23 completed weeks**
Extreme immaturity of newborn, gestational age 23 weeks, 0 days through 23 weeks, 6 days

P07.23 **Extreme immaturity of newborn, gestational age 24 completed weeks**
Extreme immaturity of newborn, gestational age 24 weeks, 0 days through 24 weeks, 6 days

P07.24 **Extreme immaturity of newborn, gestational age 25 completed weeks**
Extreme immaturity of newborn, gestational age 25 weeks, 0 days through 25 weeks, 6 days

P07.25 **Extreme immaturity of newborn, gestational age 26 completed weeks**
Extreme immaturity of newborn, gestational age 26 weeks, 0 days through 26 weeks, 6 days

P07.26 **Extreme immaturity of newborn, gestational age 27 completed weeks**
Extreme immaturity of newborn, gestational age 27 weeks, 0 days through 27 weeks, 6 days

P07.3- **<u>Preterm</u> [premature] newborn [other]**
28 completed weeks or more but less than 37 completed weeks (196 completed days but less than 259 completed days) of gestation.
Prematurity NOS

P07.30 **Preterm newborn, unspecified weeks of gestation**
P07.31 **Preterm newborn, gestational age 28 completed weeks**
Preterm newborn, gestational age 28 weeks, 0 days through 28 weeks, 6 days

P07.32 **Preterm newborn, gestational age 29 completed weeks**
Preterm newborn, gestational age 29 weeks, 0 days through 29 weeks, 6 days

P07.33 **Preterm newborn, gestational age 30 completed weeks**
Preterm newborn, gestational age 30 weeks, 0 days through 30 weeks, 6 days

P07.34 **Preterm newborn, gestational age 31 completed weeks**
Preterm newborn, gestational age 31 weeks, 0 days through 31 weeks, 6 days

P07.35 **Preterm newborn, gestational age 32 completed weeks**
Preterm newborn, gestational age 32 weeks, 0 days through 32 weeks, 6 days

P07.36 **Preterm newborn, gestational age 33 completed weeks**
Preterm newborn, gestational age 33 weeks, 0 days through 33 weeks, 6 days

P07.37 **Preterm newborn, gestational age 34 completed weeks**
Preterm newborn, gestational age 34 weeks, 0 days through 34 weeks, 6 days

P07.38 **Preterm newborn, gestational age 35 completed weeks**
Preterm newborn, gestational age 35 weeks, 0 days through 35 weeks, 6 days

P07.39 **Preterm newborn, gestational age 36 completed weeks**
Preterm newborn, gestational age 36 weeks, 0 days through 36 weeks, 6 days

P08- **Disorders of newborn related to <u>long gestation and high birth weight</u>**
Note: When both birth weight and gestational age of the newborn are available, priority of assignment should be given to birth weight
Includes: The listed conditions, without further specification, as causes of morbidity or additional care, in newborn

P08.0 **Exceptionally large newborn baby**
Usually implies a birth weight of 4500 g. or more
Excludes 1: *syndrome of infant of diabetic mother (P70.1)*
syndrome of infant of mother with gestational diabetes (P70.0)

P08.1 **Other heavy for gestational age newborn**
Other newborn heavy- or large-for-dates regardless of period of gestation
Usually implies a birth weight of 4000 g. to 4499 g.
Excludes 1: *newborn with a birth weight of 4500 or more (P08.0)*
syndrome of infant of diabetic mother (P70.1)
syndrome of infant of mother with gestational diabetes (P70.0).

P08.2- **Late newborn, not heavy for gestational age**

P08.21 **Post-term newborn**
Newborn with gestation period over 40 completed weeks to 42 completed weeks

P08.22 **Prolonged gestation of newborn**
Newborn with gestation period over 42 completed weeks (294 days or more), not heavy- or large-for-dates
Postmaturity NOS

Abnormal findings on neonatal screening (P09)

P09 **Abnormal findings on neonatal screening**
Use additional code to identify signs, symptoms and conditions associated with the screening
Excludes ❷: *nonspecific serologic evidence of human immunodeficiency virus [HIV] (R75)*

P 0 2 – P 0 9

Birth trauma (P10-P15)

P10- <u>Intracranial laceration and hemorrhage due to birth injury</u>
Excludes 1: intracranial hemorrhage of newborn NOS (P52.9)
intracranial hemorrhage of newborn due to anoxia or hypoxia (P52.-)
nontraumatic intracranial hemorrhage of newborn (P52.-)

P10.0 **Subdural hemorrhage due to birth injury**
Subdural hematoma (localized) due to birth injury
Excludes 1: subdural hemorrhage accompanying tentorial tear (P10.4)

P10.1 **Cerebral hemorrhage due to birth injury**
P10.2 **Intraventricular hemorrhage due to birth injury**
P10.3 **Subarachnoid hemorrhage due to birth injury**
P10.4 **Tentorial tear due to birth injury**
P10.8 **Other intracranial lacerations and hemorrhages due to birth injury**
P10.9 **Unspecified intracranial laceration and hemorrhage due to birth injury**

P11- <u>Other</u> birth injuries to <u>central nervous system</u>
P11.0 **Cerebral edema due to birth injury**
P11.1 **Other specified brain damage due to birth injury**
P11.2 **Unspecified brain damage due to birth injury**
P11.3 **Birth injury to facial nerve**
Facial palsy due to birth injury
P11.4 **Birth injury to other cranial nerves**
P11.5 **Birth injury to spine and spinal cord**
Fracture of spine due to birth injury
P11.9 **Birth injury to central nervous system, unspecified**

P12- Birth injury to <u>scalp</u>
P12.0 **Cephalhematoma due to birth injury**
P12.1 **Chignon (from vacuum extraction) due to birth injury**
P12.2 **Epicranial subaponeurotic hemorrhage due to birth injury**
Subgaleal hemorrhage
P12.3 **Bruising of scalp due to birth injury**
P12.4 **Injury of scalp of newborn due to monitoring equipment**
Sampling incision of scalp of newborn
Scalp clip (electrode) injury of newborn
P12.8- **Other birth injuries to scalp**
  P12.81 **Caput succedaneum**
  P12.89 **Other birth injuries to scalp**
P12.9 **Birth injury to scalp, unspecified**

P13- Birth injury to <u>skeleton</u>
Excludes❷: birth injury to spine (P11.5)
P13.0 **Fracture of skull due to birth injury**
P13.1 **Other birth injuries to skull**
Excludes 1: cephalhematoma (P12.0)
P13.2 **Birth injury to femur**
P13.3 **Birth injury to other long bones**
P13.4 **Fracture of clavicle due to birth injury**
P13.8 **Birth injuries to other parts of skeleton**
P13.9 **Birth injury to skeleton, unspecified**

P14- Birth injury to <u>peripheral nervous system</u>
P14.0 **Erb's paralysis due to birth injury**
P14.1 **Klumpke's paralysis due to birth injury**
P14.2 **Phrenic nerve paralysis due to birth injury**
P14.3 **Other brachial plexus birth injuries**
P14.8 **Birth injuries to other parts of peripheral nervous system**
P14.9 **Birth injury to peripheral nervous system, unspecified**

P15- <u>Other birth injuries</u>
P15.0 **Birth injury to liver**
Rupture of liver due to birth injury
P15.1 **Birth injury to spleen**
Rupture of spleen due to birth injury
P15.2 **Sternomastoid injury due to birth injury**
P15.3 **Birth injury to eye**
Subconjunctival hemorrhage due to birth injury
Traumatic glaucoma due to birth injury
P15.4 **Birth injury to face**
Facial congestion due to birth injury
P15.5 **Birth injury to external genitalia**
P15.6 **Subcutaneous fat necrosis due to birth injury**
P15.8 **Other specified birth injuries**
P15.9 **Birth injury, unspecified**

Respiratory and cardiovascular disorders specific to the perinatal period (P19-P29)

P19- Metabolic acidemia in newborn
Includes: Metabolic acidemia in newborn
P19.0 **Metabolic acidemia in newborn first noted before onset of labor**
P19.1 **Metabolic acidemia in newborn first noted during labor**
P19.2 **Metabolic acidemia noted at birth**
P19.9 **Metabolic acidemia, unspecified**

P22- <u>Respiratory distress of newborn</u>
Excludes 1: respiratory arrest of newborn (P28.81)
respiratory failure of newborn NOS (P28.5)
P22.0 **Respiratory distress syndrome of newborn**
Cardiorespiratory distress syndrome of newborn
Hyaline membrane disease
Idiopathic respiratory distress syndrome [IRDS or RDS] of newborn
Pulmonary hypoperfusion syndrome
Respiratory distress syndrome, type I
P22.1 **Transient tachypnea of newborn**
Idiopathic tachypnea of newborn
Respiratory distress syndrome, type II
Wet lung syndrome
P22.8 **Other respiratory distress of newborn**
P22.9 **Respiratory distress of newborn, unspecified**

P23- <u>Congenital pneumonia</u>
Includes: Infective pneumonia acquired in utero or during birth
Excludes 1: neonatal pneumonia resulting from aspiration (P24.-)
P23.0 **Congenital pneumonia due to viral agent**
Use additional code (B97) to identify organism
Excludes 1: congenital rubella pneumonitis (P35.0)
P23.1 **Congenital pneumonia due to Chlamydia**
P23.2 **Congenital pneumonia due to staphylococcus**
P23.3 **Congenital pneumonia due to streptococcus, group B**
P23.4 **Congenital pneumonia due to Escherichia coli**
P23.5 **Congenital pneumonia due to Pseudomonas**
P23.6 **Congenital pneumonia due to other bacterial agents**
Congenital pneumonia due to Hemophilus influenzae
Congenital pneumonia due to Klebsiella pneumoniae
Congenital pneumonia due to Mycoplasma
Congenital pneumonia due to Streptococcus, except group B
Use additional code (B95-B96) to identify organism
P23.8 **Congenital pneumonia due to other organisms**
P23.9 **Congenital pneumonia, unspecified**

P24- <u>Neonatal aspiration</u>
Includes: Aspiration in utero and during delivery
P24.0- <u>Meconium</u> aspiration
Excludes 1: meconium passage (without aspiration) during delivery (P03.82)
meconium staining (P96.83)
  P24.00 **Meconium aspiration <u>without</u> respiratory symptoms**
Meconium aspiration NOS
  P24.01 **Meconium aspiration <u>with respiratory symptoms</u>**
Meconium aspiration pneumonia
Meconium aspiration pneumonitis
Meconium aspiration syndrome NOS
Use additional code to identify any secondary pulmonary hypertension, if applicable (I27.2)
P24.1- Neonatal aspiration of (clear) <u>amniotic fluid</u> and mucus
Neonatal aspiration of liquor (amnii)
  P24.10 **Neonatal aspiration of (clear) amniotic fluid and mucus <u>without</u> respiratory symptoms**
Neonatal aspiration of amniotic fluid and mucus NOS
  P24.11 **Neonatal aspiration of (clear) amniotic fluid and mucus <u>with respiratory symptoms</u>**
Neonatal aspiration of amniotic fluid and mucus with pneumonia
Neonatal aspiration of amniotic fluid and mucus with pneumonitis
Use additional code to identify any secondary pulmonary hypertension, if applicable (I27.2)
P24.2- Neonatal aspiration of <u>blood</u>
  P24.20 **Neonatal aspiration of blood <u>without</u> respiratory symptoms**
Neonatal aspiration of blood NOS
  P24.21 **Neonatal aspiration of blood <u>with respiratory symptoms</u>**
Neonatal aspiration of blood with pneumonia
Neonatal aspiration of blood with pneumonitis
Use additional code to identify any secondary pulmonary hypertension, if applicable (I27.2)

P
1
0
-
P
3
6

P24.3- Neonatal aspiration of <u>milk and regurgitated food</u>
    Neonatal aspiration of stomach contents
  P24.30 Neonatal aspiration of milk and regurgitated food <u>without respiratory symptoms</u>
    Neonatal aspiration of milk and regurgitated food NOS
  P24.31 Neonatal aspiration of milk and regurgitated food <u>with respiratory symptoms</u>
    Neonatal aspiration of milk and regurgitated food with pneumonia
    Neonatal aspiration of milk and regurgitated food with pneumonitis
    Use additional code to identify any secondary pulmonary hypertension, if applicable (I27.2)

P24.8- <u>Other</u> neonatal aspiration
  P24.80 Other neonatal aspiration <u>without</u> respiratory symptoms
    Neonatal aspiration NEC
  P24.81 Other neonatal aspiration <u>with respiratory symptoms</u>
    Neonatal aspiration pneumonia NEC
    Neonatal aspiration with pneumonitis NEC
    Neonatal aspiration with pneumonia NOS
    Neonatal aspiration with pneumonitis NOS
    Use additional code to identify any secondary pulmonary hypertension, if applicable (I27.2)

P24.9 Neonatal aspiration, <u>unspecified</u>

P25- <u>Interstitial emphysema</u> and related conditions originating in the perinatal period
  P25.0 Interstitial emphysema originating in the perinatal period
  P25.1 Pneumothorax originating in the perinatal period
  P25.2 Pneumomediastinum originating in the perinatal period
  P25.3 Pneumopericardium originating in the perinatal period
  P25.8 Other conditions related to interstitial emphysema originating in the perinatal period

P26- <u>Pulmonary hemorrhage</u> originating in the perinatal period
  Excludes 1: acute idiopathic hemorrhage in infants over 28 days old (R04.81)
  P26.0 Tracheobronchial hemorrhage originating in the perinatal period
  P26.1 Massive pulmonary hemorrhage originating in the perinatal period
  P26.8 Other pulmonary hemorrhages originating in the perinatal period
  P26.9 Unspecified pulmonary hemorrhage originating in the perinatal period

P27- <u>Chronic respiratory disease</u> originating in the perinatal period
  Excludes 1: respiratory distress of newborn (P22.0-P22.9)
  P27.0 Wilson-Mikity syndrome
    Pulmonary dysmaturity
  P27.1 Bronchopulmonary dysplasia originating in the perinatal period
  P27.8 Other chronic respiratory diseases originating in the perinatal period
    Congenital pulmonary fibrosis
    Ventilator lung in newborn
  P27.9 Unspecified chronic respiratory disease originating in the perinatal period

P28- <u>Other respiratory conditions</u> originating in the perinatal period
  Excludes 1: congenital malformations of the respiratory system (Q30-Q34)
  P28.0 Primary atelectasis of newborn
    Primary failure to expand terminal respiratory units
    Pulmonary hypoplasia associated with short gestation
    Pulmonary immaturity NOS
  P28.1- Other and unspecified atelectasis of newborn
    P28.10 Unspecified atelectasis of newborn
      Atelectasis of newborn NOS
    P28.11 Resorption atelectasis without respiratory distress syndrome
      Excludes 1: resorption atelectasis with respiratory distress syndrome (P22.0)
    P28.19 Other atelectasis of newborn
      Partial atelectasis of newborn
      Secondary atelectasis of newborn
  P28.2 Cyanotic attacks of newborn
    Excludes 1: apnea of newborn (P28.3-P28.4)
  P28.3 Primary sleep apnea of newborn
    Central sleep apnea of newborn
    Obstructive sleep apnea of newborn
    Sleep apnea of newborn NOS
  P28.4 Other apnea of newborn
    Apnea of prematurity
    Obstructive apnea of newborn
    Excludes 1: obstructive sleep apnea of newborn (P28.3)

P28.5 Respiratory failure of newborn
  Excludes 1: respiratory arrest of newborn (P28.81)
    respiratory distress of newborn (P22.0-)
P28.8- Other specified respiratory conditions of newborn
  P28.81 Respiratory arrest of newborn
  P28.89 Other specified respiratory conditions of newborn
    Congenital laryngeal stridor
    Sniffles in newborn
    Snuffles in newborn
    Excludes 1: early congenital syphilitic rhinitis (A50.05)
P28.9 Respiratory condition of newborn, unspecified
    Respiratory depression in newborn

P29- <u>Cardiovascular disorders</u> originating in the perinatal period
  Excludes 1: congenital malformations of the circulatory system (Q20-Q28)
  P29.0 Neonatal cardiac failure
  P29.1- Neonatal cardiac dysrhythmia
    P29.11 Neonatal tachycardia
    P29.12 Neonatal bradycardia
  P29.2 Neonatal hypertension
  P29.3 Persistent fetal circulation
    Delayed closure of ductus arteriosus
    (Persistent) pulmonary hypertension of newborn
  P29.4 Transient myocardial ischemia in newborn
  P29.8- Other cardiovascular disorders originating in the perinatal period
    P29.81 Cardiac arrest of newborn
    P29.89 Other cardiovascular disorders originating in the perinatal period
  P29.9 Cardiovascular disorder originating in the perinatal period, unspecified

Infections specific to the perinatal period (P35-P39)

Infections acquired in utero, during birth via the umbilicus, or during the first 28 days after birth
Excludes❷: asymptomatic human immunodeficiency virus [HIV] infection status (Z21)
  congenital gonococcal infection (A54.-)
  congenital pneumonia (P23.-)
  congenital syphilis (A50.-)
  human immunodeficiency virus [HIV] disease (B20)
  infant botulism (A48.51)
  infectious diseases not specific to the perinatal period (A00-B99, J09, J10.-)
  intestinal infectious disease (A00-A09)
  laboratory evidence of human immunodeficiency virus [HIV] (R75)
  tetanus neonatorum (A33)

P35- <u>Congenital viral diseases</u>
  Includes: Infections acquired in utero or during birth
  P35.0 Congenital rubella syndrome
    Congenital rubella pneumonitis
  P35.1 Congenital cytomegalovirus infection
  P35.2 Congenital herpesviral [herpes simplex] infection
  P35.3 Congenital viral hepatitis
  P35.8 Other congenital viral diseases
    Congenital varicella [chickenpox]
  P35.9 Congenital viral disease, unspecified

P36- <u>Bacterial sepsis</u> of newborn
  Includes: Congenital sepsis
  Use additional code(s), if applicable, to identify severe sepsis (R65.2-) and associated acute organ dysfunction(s)
  P36.0 Sepsis of newborn due to streptococcus, group B
  P36.1- Sepsis of newborn due to other and unspecified streptococci
    P36.10 Sepsis of newborn due to unspecified streptococci
    P36.19 Sepsis of newborn due to other streptococci
  P36.2 Sepsis of newborn due to Staphylococcus aureus
  P36.3- Sepsis of newborn due to other and unspecified staphylococci
    P36.30 Sepsis of newborn due to unspecified staphylococci
    P36.39 Sepsis of newborn due to other staphylococci
  P36.4 Sepsis of newborn due to Escherichia coli
  P36.5 Sepsis of newborn due to anaerobes
  P36.8 Other bacterial sepsis of newborn
    Use additional code from category B96 to identify organism
  P36.9 Bacterial sepsis of newborn, unspecified

P10 - P36

P37- Other congenital infectious and parasitic diseases
  Excludes❷: congenital syphilis (A50.-)
    infectious neonatal diarrhea (A00-A09)
    necrotizing enterocolitis in newborn (P77.-)
    noninfectious neonatal diarrhea (P78.3)
    ophthalmia neonatorum due to gonococcus (A54.31)
    tetanus neonatorum (A33)
  P37.0 Congenital tuberculosis
  P37.1 Congenital toxoplasmosis
    Hydrocephalus due to congenital toxoplasmosis
  P37.2 Neonatal (disseminated) listeriosis
  P37.3 Congenital falciparum malaria
  P37.4 Other congenital malaria
  P37.5 Neonatal candidiasis
  P37.8 Other specified congenital infectious and parasitic diseases
  P37.9 Congenital infectious or parasitic disease, unspecified

P38- Omphalitis of newborn
  Excludes 1: omphalitis not of newborn (L08.82)
    tetanus omphalitis (A33)
    umbilical hemorrhage of newborn (P51.-)
  P38.1 Omphalitis with mild hemorrhage
  P38.9 Omphalitis without hemorrhage
    Omphalitis of newborn NOS

P39- Other infections specific to the perinatal period
  Use additional code to identify organism or specific infection
  P39.0 Neonatal infective mastitis
    Excludes 1: breast engorgement of newborn (P83.4)
      noninfective mastitis of newborn (P83.4)
  P39.1 Neonatal conjunctivitis and dacryocystitis
    Neonatal chlamydial conjunctivitis
    Ophthalmia neonatorum NOS
    Excludes 1: gonococcal conjunctivitis (A54.31)
  P39.2 Intra-amniotic infection affecting newborn, not elsewhere classified
  P39.3 Neonatal urinary tract infection
  P39.4 Neonatal skin infection
    Neonatal pyoderma
    Excludes 1: pemphigus neonatorum (L00)
      staphylococcal scalded skin syndrome (L00)
  P39.8 Other specified infections specific to the perinatal period
  P39.9 Infection specific to the perinatal period, unspecified

Hemorrhagic and hematological disorders of newborn (P50-P61)

Excludes 1: congenital stenosis and stricture of bile ducts (Q44.3)
  Crigler-Najjar syndrome (E80.5)
  Dubin-Johnson syndrome (E80.6)
  Gilbert syndrome (E80.4)
  hereditary hemolytic anemias (D55-D58)

P50- Newborn affected by intrauterine (fetal) blood loss
  Excludes 1: congenital anemia from intrauterine (fetal) blood loss (P61.3)
  P50.0 Newborn affected by intrauterine (fetal) blood loss from vasa previa
  P50.1 Newborn affected by intrauterine (fetal) blood loss from ruptured cord
  P50.2 Newborn affected by intrauterine (fetal) blood loss from placenta
  P50.3 Newborn affected by hemorrhage into co-twin
  P50.4 Newborn affected by hemorrhage into maternal circulation
  P50.5 Newborn affected by intrauterine (fetal) blood loss from cut end of co-twin's cord
  P50.8 Newborn affected by other intrauterine (fetal) blood loss
  P50.9 Newborn affected by intrauterine (fetal) blood loss, unspecified
    Newborn affected by fetal hemorrhage NOS

P51- Umbilical hemorrhage of newborn
  Excludes 1: omphalitis with mild hemorrhage (P38.1)
    umbilical hemorrhage from cut end of co-twins cord (P50.5)
  P51.0 Massive umbilical hemorrhage of newborn
  P51.8 Other umbilical hemorrhages of newborn
    Slipped umbilical ligature NOS
  P51.9 Umbilical hemorrhage of newborn, unspecified

P52- Intracranial nontraumatic hemorrhage of newborn
  Includes: Intracranial hemorrhage due to anoxia or hypoxia
  Excludes 1: intracranial hemorrhage due to birth injury (P10.-)
    intracranial hemorrhage due to other injury (S06.-)
  P52.0 Intraventricular (nontraumatic) hemorrhage, grade 1, of newborn
    Subependymal hemorrhage (without intraventricular extension)
    Bleeding into germinal matrix
  P52.1 Intraventricular (nontraumatic) hemorrhage, grade 2, of newborn
    Subependymal hemorrhage with intraventricular extension
    Bleeding into ventricle
  P52.2- Intraventricular (nontraumatic) hemorrhage, grade 3 and grade 4, of newborn
    P52.21 Intraventricular (nontraumatic) hemorrhage, grade 3, of newborn
      Subependymal hemorrhage with intraventricular extension with enlargement of ventricle
    P52.22 Intraventricular (nontraumatic) hemorrhage, grade 4, of newborn
      Bleeding into cerebral cortex
      Subependymal hemorrhage with intracerebral extension
  P52.3 Unspecified intraventricular (nontraumatic) hemorrhage of newborn
  P52.4 Intracerebral (nontraumatic) hemorrhage of newborn
  P52.5 Subarachnoid (nontraumatic) hemorrhage of newborn
  P52.6 Cerebellar (nontraumatic) and posterior fossa hemorrhage of newborn
  P52.8 Other intracranial (nontraumatic) hemorrhages of newborn
  P52.9 Intracranial (nontraumatic) hemorrhage of newborn, unspecified

P53 Hemorrhagic disease of newborn
  Vitamin K deficiency of newborn

P54- Other neonatal hemorrhages
  Excludes 1: newborn affected by (intrauterine) blood loss (P50.-)
    pulmonary hemorrhage originating in the perinatal period (P26.-)
  P54.0 Neonatal hematemesis
    Excludes 1: neonatal hematemesis due to swallowed maternal blood (P78.2)
  P54.1 Neonatal melena
    Excludes 1: neonatal melena due to swallowed maternal blood (P78.2)
  P54.2 Neonatal rectal hemorrhage
  P54.3 Other neonatal gastrointestinal hemorrhage
  P54.4 Neonatal adrenal hemorrhage
  P54.5 Neonatal cutaneous hemorrhage
    Neonatal bruising
    Neonatal ecchymoses
    Neonatal petechiae
    Neonatal superficial hematoma
    Excludes❷: bruising of scalp due to birth injury (P12.3)
      cephalhematoma due to birth injury (P12.0)
  P54.6 Neonatal vaginal hemorrhage
    Neonatal pseudomenses
  P54.8 Other specified neonatal hemorrhages
  P54.9 Neonatal hemorrhage, unspecified

P55- Hemolytic disease of newborn
  P55.0 Rh isoimmunization of newborn
  P55.1 ABO isoimmunization of newborn
  P55.8 Other hemolytic diseases of newborn
  P55.9 Hemolytic disease of newborn, unspecified

P56- Hydrops fetalis due to hemolytic disease
  Excludes 1: hydrops fetalis NOS (P83.2)
  P56.0 Hydrops fetalis due to isoimmunization
  P56.9- Hydrops fetalis due to other and unspecified hemolytic disease
    P56.90 Hydrops fetalis due to unspecified hemolytic disease
    P56.99 Hydrops fetalis due to other hemolytic disease

P57- Kernicterus
  P57.0 Kernicterus due to isoimmunization
  P57.8 Other specified kernicterus
    Excludes 1: Crigler-Najjar syndrome (E80.5)
  P57.9 Kernicterus, unspecified

P58- Neonatal jaundice due to other excessive hemolysis
  Excludes 1: jaundice due to isoimmunization (P55-P57)
  P58.0 Neonatal jaundice due to bruising
  P58.1 Neonatal jaundice due to bleeding
  P58.2 Neonatal jaundice due to infection
  P58.3 Neonatal jaundice due to polycythemia

Excludes 1: = NOT CODED HERE! (Do not code both)   **654**   *Excludes❷: = Not Included Here*

P
3
7
-
P
7
8

P58.4- **Neonatal jaundice due to drugs or toxins transmitted from mother or given to newborn**
Code first poisoning due to drug or toxin, if applicable (T36-T65 with fifth or sixth character 1-4 or 6)
Use additional code for adverse effect, if applicable, to identify drug (T36-T50 with fifth or sixth character 5)

    P58.41 **Neonatal jaundice due to drugs or toxins transmitted from mother**

    P58.42 **Neonatal jaundice due to drugs or toxins given to newborn**

P58.5 **Neonatal jaundice due to swallowed maternal blood**

P58.8 **Neonatal jaundice due to other specified excessive hemolysis**

P58.9 **Neonatal jaundice due to excessive hemolysis, unspecified**

P59- **Neonatal jaundice from other and unspecified causes**
Excludes 1: *jaundice due to inborn errors of metabolism (E70-E88)*
              kernicterus (P57.-)

P59.0 **Neonatal jaundice associated with preterm delivery**
Hyperbilirubinemia of prematurity
Jaundice due to delayed conjugation associated with preterm delivery

P59.1 **Inspissated bile syndrome**

P59.2- **Neonatal jaundice from other and unspecified hepatocellular damage**
Excludes 1: *congenital viral hepatitis (P35.3)*

    P59.20 **Neonatal jaundice from unspecified hepatocellular damage**

    P59.29 **Neonatal jaundice from other hepatocellular damage**
Neonatal giant cell hepatitis
Neonatal (idiopathic) hepatitis

P59.3 **Neonatal jaundice from breast milk inhibitor**

P59.8 **Neonatal jaundice from other specified causes**

P59.9 **Neonatal jaundice, unspecified**
Neonatal physiological jaundice (intense) (prolonged) NOS

P60 **Disseminated intravascular coagulation of newborn**
Defibrination syndrome of newborn

P61- **Other perinatal hematological disorders**
Excludes 1: *transient hypogammaglobulinemia of infancy (D80.7)*

P61.0 **Transient neonatal thrombocytopenia**
Neonatal thrombocytopenia due to exchange transfusion
Neonatal thrombocytopenia due to idiopathic maternal thrombocytopenia
Neonatal thrombocytopenia due to isoimmunization

P61.1 **Polycythemia neonatorum**

P61.2 **Anemia of prematurity**

P61.3 **Congenital anemia from fetal blood loss**

P61.4 **Other congenital anemias, not elsewhere classified**
Congenital anemia NOS

P61.5 **Transient neonatal neutropenia**
Excludes 1: *congenital neutropenia (nontransient) (D70.0)*

P61.6 **Other transient neonatal disorders of coagulation**

P61.8 **Other specified perinatal hematological disorders**

P61.9 **Perinatal hematological disorder, unspecified**

Transitory endocrine and metabolic disorders specific to newborn (P70-P74)

Includes: Transitory endocrine and metabolic disturbances caused by the infant's response to maternal endocrine and metabolic factors, or its adjustment to extrauterine environment

P70- **Transitory disorders of carbohydrate metabolism specific to newborn**

P70.0 **Syndrome of infant of mother with gestational diabetes**
Newborn (with hypoglycemia) affected by maternal gestational diabetes
Excludes 1: *newborn (with hypoglycemia) affected by maternal (pre-existing) diabetes mellitus (P70.1)*
            syndrome of infant of a diabetic mother (P70.1)

P70.1 **Syndrome of infant of a diabetic mother**
Newborn (with hypoglycemia) affected by maternal (pre-existing) diabetes mellitus
Excludes 1: *newborn (with hypoglycemia) affected by maternal gestational diabetes (P70.0)*
            syndrome of infant of mother with gestational diabetes (P70.0)

P70.2 **Neonatal diabetes mellitus**

P70.3 **Iatrogenic neonatal hypoglycemia**

P70.4 **Other neonatal hypoglycemia**
Transitory neonatal hypoglycemia

P70.8 **Other transitory disorders of carbohydrate metabolism of newborn**

P70.9 **Transitory disorder of carbohydrate metabolism of newborn, unspecified**

P71- **Transitory neonatal disorders of calcium and magnesium metabolism**

P71.0 **Cow's milk hypocalcemia in newborn**

P71.1 **Other neonatal hypocalcemia**
Excludes 1: *neonatal hypoparathyroidism (P71.4)*

P71.2 **Neonatal hypomagnesemia**

P71.3 **Neonatal tetany without calcium or magnesium deficiency**
Neonatal tetany NOS

P71.4 **Transitory neonatal hypoparathyroidism**

P71.8 **Other transitory neonatal disorders of calcium and magnesium metabolism**

P71.9 **Transitory neonatal disorder of calcium and magnesium metabolism, unspecified**

P72- **Other transitory neonatal endocrine disorders**
Excludes 1: *congenital hypothyroidism with or without goiter (E03.0-E03.1)*
            dyshormogenetic goiter (E07.1)
            Pendred's syndrome (E07.1)

P72.0 **Neonatal goiter, not elsewhere classified**
Transitory congenital goiter with normal functioning

P72.1 **Transitory neonatal hyperthyroidism**
Neonatal thyrotoxicosis

P72.2 **Other transitory neonatal disorders of thyroid function, not elsewhere classified**
Transitory neonatal hypothyroidism

P72.8 **Other specified transitory neonatal endocrine disorders**

P72.9 **Transitory neonatal endocrine disorder, unspecified**

P74- **Other transitory neonatal electrolyte and metabolic disturbances**

P74.0 **Late metabolic acidosis of newborn**
Excludes 1: *(fetal) metabolic acidosis of newborn (P19)*

P74.1 **Dehydration of newborn**

P74.2 **Disturbances of sodium balance of newborn**

P74.3 **Disturbances of potassium balance of newborn**

P74.4 **Other transitory electrolyte disturbances of newborn**

P74.5 **Transitory tyrosinemia of newborn**

P74.6 **Transitory hyperammonemia of newborn**

P74.8 **Other transitory neonatal metabolic disturbances of newborn**
Amino-acid metabolic disorders described as transitory

P74.9 **Transitory metabolic disturbance of newborn, unspecified**

Digestive system disorders of newborn (P76-P78)

P76- **Other intestinal obstruction of newborn**

P76.0 **Meconium plug syndrome**
Meconium ileus NOS
Excludes 1: *meconium ileus in cystic fibrosis (E84.11)*

P76.1 **Transitory ileus of newborn**
Excludes 1: *Hirschsprung's disease (Q43.1)*

P76.2 **Intestinal obstruction due to inspissated milk**

P76.8 **Other specified intestinal obstruction of newborn**
Excludes 1: *intestinal obstruction classifiable to K56.-*

P76.9 **Intestinal obstruction of newborn, unspecified**

P77- **Necrotizing enterocolitis of newborn**

P77.1 **Stage 1 necrotizing enterocolitis in newborn**
Necrotizing enterocolitis without pneumatosis, without perforation

P77.2 **Stage 2 necrotizing enterocolitis in newborn**
Necrotizing enterocolitis with pneumatosis, without perforation

P77.3 **Stage 3 necrotizing enterocolitis in newborn**
Necrotizing enterocolitis with perforation
Necrotizing enterocolitis with pneumatosis and perforation

P77.9 **Necrotizing enterocolitis in newborn, unspecified**
Necrotizing enterocolitis in newborn, NOS

P78- **Other perinatal digestive system disorders**
Excludes 1: *cystic fibrosis (E84.0-E84.9)*
            neonatal gastrointestinal hemorrhages (P54.0-P54.3)

P78.0 **Perinatal intestinal perforation**
Meconium peritonitis

P78.1 **Other neonatal peritonitis**
Neonatal peritonitis NOS

P78.2 **Neonatal hematemesis and melena due to swallowed maternal blood**

P78.3 **Noninfective neonatal diarrhea**
Neonatal diarrhea NOS

P78.8- **Other specified perinatal digestive system disorders**

    P78.81 **Congenital cirrhosis (of liver)**

    P78.82 **Peptic ulcer of newborn**

    P78.83 **Newborn esophageal reflux**
Neonatal esophageal reflux

    P78.89 **Other specified perinatal digestive system disorders**

P78.9 **Perinatal digestive system disorder, unspecified**

P37 - P78

Excludes 1: = NOT CODED HERE! (Do not code both)

Excludes❷: = Not Included Here

Conditions involving the integument and temperature regulation of newborn (P80-P83)

P80- Hypothermia of newborn

P80.0 Cold injury syndrome
Severe and usually chronic hypothermia associated with a pink flushed appearance, edema and neurological and biochemical abnormalities
Excludes 1: mild hypothermia of newborn (P80.8)

P80.8 Other hypothermia of newborn
Mild hypothermia of newborn

P80.9 Hypothermia of newborn, unspecified

P81- Other disturbances of temperature regulation of newborn

P81.0 Environmental hyperthermia of newborn

P81.8 Other specified disturbances of temperature regulation of newborn

P81.9 Disturbance of temperature regulation of newborn, unspecified
Fever of newborn NOS

P83- Other conditions of integument specific to newborn
Excludes 1: congenital malformations of skin and integument (Q80-Q84)
hydrops fetalis due to hemolytic disease (P56.-)
neonatal skin infection (P39.4)
staphylococcal scalded skin syndrome (L00)
Excludes❷: cradle cap (L21.0)
diaper [napkin] dermatitis (L22)

P83.0 Sclerema neonatorum

P83.1 Neonatal erythema toxicum

P83.2 Hydrops fetalis not due to hemolytic disease
Hydrops fetalis NOS

P83.3- Other and unspecified edema specific to newborn

P83.30 Unspecified edema specific to newborn

P83.39 Other edema specific to newborn

P83.4 Breast engorgement of newborn
Noninfective mastitis of newborn

P83.5 Congenital hydrocele

P83.6 Umbilical polyp of newborn

P83.8 Other specified conditions of integument specific to newborn
Bronze baby syndrome
Neonatal scleroderma
Urticaria neonatorum

P83.9 Condition of the integument specific to newborn, unspecified

Other problems with newborn (P84)

P84 Other problems with newborn
Acidemia of newborn
Acidosis of newborn
Anoxia of newborn NOS
Asphyxia of newborn NOS
Hypercapnia of newborn
Hypoxemia of newborn
Hypoxia of newborn NOS
Mixed metabolic and respiratory acidosis of newborn
Excludes 1: intracranial hemorrhage due to anoxia or hypoxia (P52.-)
hypoxic ischemic encephalopathy [HIE] (P91.6-)
late metabolic acidosis of newborn (P74.0)

Other disorders originating in the perinatal period (P90-P96)

P90 Convulsions of newborn
Excludes 1: benign myoclonic epilepsy in infancy (G40.3-)
benign neonatal convulsions (familial) (G40.3-)

P91- Other disturbances of cerebral status of newborn

P91.0 Neonatal cerebral ischemia

P91.1 Acquired periventricular cysts of newborn

P91.2 Neonatal cerebral leukomalacia
Periventricular leukomalacia

P91.3 Neonatal cerebral irritability

P91.4 Neonatal cerebral depression

P91.5 Neonatal coma

P91.6- Hypoxic ischemic encephalopathy [HIE]

P91.60 Hypoxic ischemic encephalopathy [HIE], unspecified

P91.61 Mild hypoxic ischemic encephalopathy [HIE]

P91.62 Moderate hypoxic ischemic encephalopathy [HIE]

P91.63 Severe hypoxic ischemic encephalopathy [HIE]

P91.8 Other specified disturbances of cerebral status of newborn

P91.9 Disturbance of cerebral status of newborn, unspecified

P92- Feeding problems of newborn
Excludes 1: feeding problems in child over 28 days old (R63.3)

P92.0- Vomiting of newborn
Excludes 1: vomiting of child over 28 days old (R11.-)

P92.01 Bilious vomiting of newborn
Excludes 1: bilious vomiting in child over 28 days old (R11.14)

P92.09 Other vomiting of newborn
Excludes 1: regurgitation of food in newborn (P92.1)

P92.1 Regurgitation and rumination of newborn

P92.2 Slow feeding of newborn

P92.3 Underfeeding of newborn

P92.4 Overfeeding of newborn

P92.5 Neonatal difficulty in feeding at breast

P92.6 Failure to thrive in newborn
Excludes 1: failure to thrive in child over 28 days old (R62.51)

P92.8 Other feeding problems of newborn

P92.9 Feeding problem of newborn, unspecified

P93- Reactions and intoxications due to drugs administered to newborn
Includes: Reactions and intoxications due to drugs administered to fetus affecting newborn
Excludes 1: jaundice due to drugs or toxins transmitted from mother or given to newborn (P58.4-)
reactions and intoxications from maternal opiates, tranquilizers and other medication (P04.0-P04.1, P04.4)
withdrawal symptoms from maternal use of drugs of addiction (P96.1)
withdrawal symptoms from therapeutic use of drugs in newborn (P96.2)

P93.0 Grey baby syndrome
Grey syndrome from chloramphenicol administration in newborn

P93.8 Other reactions and intoxications due to drugs administered to newborn
Use additional code for adverse effect, if applicable, to identify drug (T36-T50 with fifth or sixth character 5)

P94- Disorders of muscle tone of newborn

P94.0 Transient neonatal myasthenia gravis
Excludes 1: myasthenia gravis (G70.0)

P94.1 Congenital hypertonia

P94.2 Congenital hypotonia
Floppy baby syndrome, unspecified

P94.8 Other disorders of muscle tone of newborn

P94.9 Disorder of muscle tone of newborn, unspecified

P95 Stillbirth
Deadborn fetus NOS
Fetal death of unspecified cause
Stillbirth NOS
Excludes 1: maternal care for intrauterine death (O36.4)
missed abortion (O02.1)
outcome of delivery, stillbirth (Z37.1, Z37.3, Z37.4, Z37.7)

P96- Other conditions originating in the perinatal period

P96.0 Congenital renal failure
Uremia of newborn

P96.1 Neonatal withdrawal symptoms from maternal use of drugs of addiction
Drug withdrawal syndrome in infant of dependent mother
Neonatal abstinence syndrome
Excludes 1: reactions and intoxications from maternal opiates and tranquilizers administered during labor and delivery (P04.0)

P96.2 Withdrawal symptoms from therapeutic use of drugs in newborn

P96.3 Wide cranial sutures of newborn
Neonatal craniotabes

P96.5 Complication to newborn due to (fetal) intrauterine procedure
Excludes❷: newborn (suspected to be) affected by amniocentesis (P00.6)

P96.8- Other specified conditions originating in the perinatal period

P96.81 Exposure to (parental) (environmental) tobacco smoke in the perinatal period
Excludes❷: newborn affected by in utero exposure to tobacco (P04.2)
exposure to environmental tobacco smoke after the perinatal period (Z77.22)

P96.82 Delayed separation of umbilical cord

P96.83 Meconium staining
Excludes 1: meconium aspiration (P24.00, P24.01)
meconium passage during delivery (P03.82)

P96.89 Other specified conditions originating in the perinatal period
Use additional code to specify condition

P96.9 Condition originating in the perinatal period, unspecified
Congenital debility NOS

P
8
0
–
Q
0
7

Chapter 17 – Congenital malformations, deformations and chromosomal abnormalities (Q00-Q99)

Note: Codes from this chapter are not for use on maternal or fetal records
Excludes❷: inborn errors of metabolism (E70-E88)
This chapter contains the following blocks:

Q00-Q07 Congenital malformations of the nervous system
Q10-Q18 Congenital malformations of eye, ear, face and neck
Q20-Q28 Congenital malformations of the circulatory system
Q30-Q34 Congenital malformations of the respiratory system
Q35-Q37 Cleft lip and cleft palate
Q38-Q45 Other congenital malformations of the digestive system
Q50-Q56 Congenital malformations of genital organs
Q60-Q64 Congenital malformations of the urinary system
Q65-Q79 Congenital malformations and deformations of the musculoskeletal system
Q80-Q89 Other congenital malformations
Q90-Q99 Chromosomal abnormalities, not elsewhere classified

Congenital malformations of the nervous system (Q00-Q07)

Q00- Anencephaly and similar malformations

Q00.0 Anencephaly
Acephaly
Acrania
Amyelencephaly
Hemianencephaly
Hemicephaly

Q00.1 Craniorachischisis

Q00.2 Iniencephaly

Q01- Encephalocele
Includes: Arnold-Chiari syndrome, type III
Encephalocystocele
Encephalomyelocele
Hydroencephalocele
Hydromeningocele, cranial
Meningocele, cerebral
Meningoencephalocele
Excludes 1: Meckel-Gruber syndrome (Q61.9)

Q01.0 Frontal encephalocele

Q01.1 Nasofrontal encephalocele

Q01.2 Occipital encephalocele

Q01.8 Encephalocele of other sites

Q01.9 Encephalocele, unspecified

Q02 Microcephaly
Includes: Hydromicrocephaly
Micrencephalon
Excludes 1: Meckel-Gruber syndrome (Q61.9)

Q03- Congenital hydrocephalus
Includes: Hydrocephalus in newborn
Excludes 1: Arnold-Chiari syndrome, type II (Q07.0-)
acquired hydrocephalus (G91.-)
hydrocephalus due to congenital toxoplasmosis (P37.1)
hydrocephalus with spina bifida (Q05.0-Q05.4)

Q03.0 Malformations of aqueduct of Sylvius
Anomaly of aqueduct of Sylvius
Obstruction of aqueduct of Sylvius, congenital
Stenosis of aqueduct of Sylvius

Q03.1 Atresia of foramina of Magendie and Luschka
Dandy-Walker syndrome

Q03.8 Other congenital hydrocephalus

Q03.9 Congenital hydrocephalus, unspecified

Q04- Other congenital malformations of brain
Excludes 1: cyclopia (Q87.0)
macrocephaly (Q75.3)

Q04.0 Congenital malformations of corpus callosum
Agenesis of corpus callosum

Q04.1 Arhinencephaly

Q04.2 Holoprosencephaly

Q04.3 Other reduction deformities of brain
Absence of part of brain
Agenesis of part of brain
Agyria
Aplasia of part of brain
Hydranencephaly
Hypoplasia of part of brain
Lissencephaly
Microgyria
Pachygyria
Excludes 1: congenital malformations of corpus callosum (Q04.0)

Q04.4 Septo-optic dysplasia of brain
Q04.5 Megalencephaly
Q04.6 Congenital cerebral cysts
Porencephaly
Schizencephaly
Excludes 1: acquired porencephalic cyst (G93.0)

Q04.8 Other specified congenital malformations of brain
Arnold-Chiari syndrome, type IV
Macrogyria

Q04.9 Congenital malformation of brain, unspecified
Congenital anomaly NOS of brain
Congenital deformity NOS of brain
Congenital disease or lesion NOS of brain
Multiple anomalies NOS of brain, congenital

Q05- Spina bifida
Includes: Hydromeningocele (spinal)
Meningocele (spinal)
Meningomyelocele
Myelocele
Myelomeningocele
Rachischisis
Spina bifida (aperta) (cystica)
Syringomyelocele
Use additional code for any associated paraplegia (paraparesis) (G82.2-)
Excludes 1: Arnold-Chiari syndrome, type II (Q07.0-)
spina bifida occulta (Q76.0)

Q05.0 Cervical spina bifida with hydrocephalus
Q05.1 Thoracic spina bifida with hydrocephalus
Dorsal spina bifida with hydrocephalus
Thoracolumbar spina bifida with hydrocephalus
Q05.2 Lumbar spina bifida with hydrocephalus
Lumbosacral spina bifida with hydrocephalus
Q05.3 Sacral spina bifida with hydrocephalus
Q05.4 Unspecified spina bifida with hydrocephalus
Q05.5 Cervical spina bifida without hydrocephalus
Q05.6 Thoracic spina bifida without hydrocephalus
Dorsal spina bifida NOS
Thoracolumbar spina bifida NOS
Q05.7 Lumbar spina bifida without hydrocephalus
Lumbosacral spina bifida NOS
Q05.8 Sacral spina bifida without hydrocephalus
Q05.9 Spina bifida, unspecified

Q06- Other congenital malformations of spinal cord
Q06.0 Amyelia
Q06.1 Hypoplasia and dysplasia of spinal cord
Atelomyelia
Myelatelia
Myelodysplasia of spinal cord
Q06.2 Diastematomyelia
Q06.3 Other congenital cauda equina malformations
Q06.4 Hydromyelia
Hydrorachis
Q06.8 Other specified congenital malformations of spinal cord
Q06.9 Congenital malformation of spinal cord, unspecified
Congenital anomaly NOS of spinal cord
Congenital deformity NOS of spinal cord
Congenital disease or lesion NOS of spinal cord

Q07- Other congenital malformations of nervous system
Excludes❷: congenital central alveolar hypoventilation syndrome (G47.35)
familial dysautonomia [Riley-Day] (G90.1)
neurofibromatosis (nonmalignant) (Q85.0-)
Q07.0- Arnold-Chiari syndrome
Arnold-Chiari syndrome, type II
Excludes 1: Arnold-Chiari syndrome, type III (Q01.-)
Arnold-Chiari syndrome, type IV (Q04.8)
Q07.00 Arnold-Chiari syndrome without spina bifida or hydrocephalus
Q07.01 Arnold-Chiari syndrome with spina bifida
Q07.02 Arnold-Chiari syndrome with hydrocephalus
Q07.03 Arnold-Chiari syndrome with spina bifida and hydrocephalus
Q07.8 Other specified congenital malformations of nervous system
Agenesis of nerve
Displacement of brachial plexus
Jaw-winking syndrome
Marcus Gunn's syndrome
Q07.9 Congenital malformation of nervous system, unspecified
Congenital anomaly NOS of nervous system
Congenital deformity NOS of nervous system
Congenital disease or lesion NOS of nervous system

P80-Q07

© 2013 Channel Publishing, Ltd.

Congenital malformations of eye, ear, face and neck
(Q10-Q18)

Excludes❷: cleft lip and cleft palate (Q35-Q37)
congenital malformation of cervical spine (Q05.0, Q05.5,
Q67.5, Q76.0-Q76.4)
congenital malformation of larynx (Q31.-)
congenital malformation of lip NEC (Q38.0)
congenital malformation of nose (Q30.-)
congenital malformation of parathyroid gland (Q89.2)
congenital malformation of thyroid gland (Q89.2)

Q10- **Congenital malformations of eyelid, lacrimal apparatus and orbit**
Excludes 1: cryptophthalmos NOS (Q11.2)
cryptophthalmos syndrome (Q87.0)

Q10.0 **Congenital ptosis**
Q10.1 **Congenital ectropion**
Q10.2 **Congenital entropion**
Q10.3 **Other congenital malformations of eyelid**
Ablepharon
Blepharophimosis, congenital
Coloboma of eyelid
Congenital absence or agenesis of cilia
Congenital absence or agenesis of eyelid
Congenital accessory eyelid
Congenital accessory eye muscle
Congenital malformation of eyelid NOS
Q10.4 **Absence and agenesis of lacrimal apparatus**
Congenital absence of punctum lacrimale
Q10.5 **Congenital stenosis and stricture of lacrimal duct**
Q10.6 **Other congenital malformations of lacrimal apparatus**
Congenital malformation of lacrimal apparatus NOS
Q10.7 **Congenital malformation of orbit**

Q11- **Anophthalmos, microphthalmos and macrophthalmos**
Q11.0 **Cystic eyeball**
Q11.1 **Other anophthalmos**
Anophthalmos NOS
Agenesis of eye
Aplasia of eye
Q11.2 **Microphthalmos**
Cryptophthalmos NOS
Dysplasia of eye
Hypoplasia of eye
Rudimentary eye
Excludes 1: cryptophthalmos syndrome (Q87.0)
Q11.3 **Macrophthalmos**
Excludes 1: macrophthalmos in congenital glaucoma (Q15.0)

Q12- **Congenital lens malformations**
Q12.0 **Congenital cataract**
Q12.1 **Congenital displaced lens**
Q12.2 **Coloboma of lens**
Q12.3 **Congenital aphakia**
Q12.4 **Spherophakia**
Q12.8 **Other congenital lens malformations**
Microphakia
Q12.9 **Congenital lens malformation, unspecified**

Q13- **Congenital malformations of anterior segment of eye**
Q13.0 **Coloboma of iris**
Coloboma NOS
Q13.1 **Absence of iris**
Aniridia
Use additional code for associated glaucoma (H42)
Q13.2 **Other congenital malformations of iris**
Anisocoria, congenital
Atresia of pupil
Congenital malformation of iris NOS
Corectopia
Q13.3 **Congenital corneal opacity**
Q13.4 **Other congenital corneal malformations**
Congenital malformation of cornea NOS
Microcornea
Peter's anomaly
Q13.5 **Blue sclera**
Q13.8- **Other congenital malformations of anterior segment of eye**
Q13.81 **Rieger's anomaly**
Use additional code for associated glaucoma (H42)
Q13.89 **Other congenital malformations of anterior segment of eye**
Q13.9 **Congenital malformation of anterior segment of eye, unspecified**

Q14- **Congenital malformations of posterior segment of eye**
Excludes❷: optic nerve hypoplasia (H47.03-)
Q14.0 **Congenital malformation of vitreous humor**
Congenital vitreous opacity
Q14.1 **Congenital malformation of retina**
Congenital retinal aneurysm
Q14.2 **Congenital malformation of optic disc**
Coloboma of optic disc
Q14.3 **Congenital malformation of choroid**
Q14.8 **Other congenital malformations of posterior segment of eye**
Coloboma of the fundus
Q14.9 **Congenital malformation of posterior segment of eye, unspecified**

Q15- **Other congenital malformations of eye**
Excludes 1: congenital nystagmus (H55.01)
ocular albinism (E70.31-)
optic nerve hypoplasia (H47.03-)
retinitis pigmentosa (H35.52)
Q15.0 **Congenital glaucoma**
Axenfeld's anomaly
Buphthalmos
Glaucoma of childhood
Glaucoma of newborn
Hydrophthalmos
Keratoglobus, congenital, with glaucoma
Macrocornea with glaucoma
Macrophthalmos in congenital glaucoma
Megalocornea with glaucoma
Q15.8 **Other specified congenital malformations of eye**
Q15.9 **Congenital malformation of eye, unspecified**
Congenital anomaly of eye
Congenital deformity of eye

Q16- **Congenital malformations of ear causing impairment of hearing**
Excludes 1: congenital deafness (H90.-)
Q16.0 **Congenital absence of (ear) auricle**
Q16.1 **Congenital absence, atresia and stricture of auditory canal (external)**
Congenital atresia or stricture of osseous meatus
Q16.2 **Absence of eustachian tube**
Q16.3 **Congenital malformation of ear ossicles**
Congenital fusion of ear ossicles
Q16.4 **Other congenital malformations of middle ear**
Congenital malformation of middle ear NOS
Q16.5 **Congenital malformation of inner ear**
Congenital anomaly of membranous labyrinth
Congenital anomaly of organ of Corti
Q16.9 **Congenital malformation of ear causing impairment of hearing, unspecified**
Congenital absence of ear NOS

Q17- **Other congenital malformations of ear**
Excludes 1: congenital malformations of ear with impairment of hearing (Q16.0-Q16.9)
preauricular sinus (Q18.1)
Q17.0 **Accessory auricle**
Accessory tragus
Polyotia
Preauricular appendage or tag
Supernumerary ear
Supernumerary lobule
Q17.1 **Macrotia**
Q17.2 **Microtia**
Q17.3 **Other misshapen ear**
Pointed ear
Q17.4 **Misplaced ear**
Low-set ears
Excludes 1: cervical auricle (Q18.2)
Q17.5 **Prominent ear**
Bat ear
Q17.8 **Other specified congenital malformations of ear**
Congenital absence of lobe of ear
Q17.9 **Congenital malformation of ear, unspecified**
Congenital anomaly of ear NOS

Q10-Q25

Q18- **Other congenital malformations of face and neck**
  Excludes 1:   *cleft lip and cleft palate (Q35-Q37)*
       conditions classified to Q67.0-Q67.4
       congenital malformations of skull and face bones (Q75.-)
       cyclopia (Q87.0)
       dentofacial anomalies [including malocclusion] (M26.-)
       malformation syndromes affecting facial appearance (Q87.0)
       persistent thyroglossal duct (Q89.2)

   Q18.0   **Sinus, fistula and cyst of branchial cleft**
      Branchial vestige

   Q18.1   **Preauricular sinus and cyst**
      Fistula of auricle, congenital
      Cervicoaural fistula

   Q18.2   **Other branchial cleft malformations**
      Branchial cleft malformation NOS
      Cervical auricle
      Otocephaly

   Q18.3   **Webbing of neck**
      Pterygium colli

   Q18.4   **Macrostomia**

   Q18.5   **Microstomia**

   Q18.6   **Macrocheilia**
      Hypertrophy of lip, congenital

   Q18.7   **Microcheilia**

   Q18.8   **Other specified congenital malformations of face and neck**
      Medial cyst of face and neck
      Medial fistula of face and neck
      Medial sinus of face and neck

   Q18.9   **Congenital malformation of face and neck, unspecified**
      Congenital anomaly NOS of face and neck

Congenital malformations of the circulatory system (Q20-Q28)

Q20- **Congenital malformations of cardiac chambers and connections**
  Excludes 1:   *dextrocardia with situs inversus (Q89.3)*
       mirror-image atrial arrangement with situs inversus (Q89.3)

   Q20.0   **Common arterial trunk**
      Persistent truncus arteriosus
      Excludes 1:   *aortic septal defect (Q21.4)*

   Q20.1   **Double outlet right ventricle**
      Taussig-Bing syndrome

   Q20.2   **Double outlet left ventricle**

   Q20.3   **Discordant ventriculoarterial connection**
      Dextrotransposition of aorta
      Transposition of great vessels (complete)

   Q20.4   **Double inlet ventricle**
      Common ventricle
      Cor triloculare biatriatum
      Single ventricle

   Q20.5   **Discordant atrioventricular connection**
      Corrected transposition
      Levotransposition
      Ventricular inversion

   Q20.6   **Isomerism of atrial appendages**
      Isomerism of atrial appendages with asplenia or polysplenia

   Q20.8   **Other congenital malformations of cardiac chambers and connections**
      Cor binoculare

   Q20.9   **Congenital malformation of cardiac chambers and connections, unspecified**

Q21- **Congenital malformations of cardiac septa**
  Excludes 1:   *acquired cardiac septal defect (I51.0)*

   Q21.0   **Ventricular septal defect**
      Roger's disease

   Q21.1   **Atrial septal defect**
      Coronary sinus defect
      Patent or persistent foramen ovale
      Patent or persistent ostium secundum defect (type II)
      Patent or persistent sinus venosus defect

   Q21.2   **Atrioventricular septal defect**
      Common atrioventricular canal
      Endocardial cushion defect
      Ostium primum atrial septal defect (type I)

   Q21.3   **Tetralogy of Fallot**
      Ventricular septal defect with pulmonary stenosis or atresia, dextroposition of aorta and hypertrophy of right ventricle

   Q21.4   **Aortopulmonary septal defect**
      Aortic septal defect
      Aortopulmonary window

   Q21.8   **Other congenital malformations of cardiac septa**
      Eisenmenger's defect
      Pentalogy of Fallot
      Excludes 1:   *Eisenmenger's complex (I27.8)*
          Eisenmenger's syndrome (I27.8)

   Q21.9   **Congenital malformation of cardiac septum, unspecified**
      Septal (heart) defect NOS

Q22- **Congenital malformations of pulmonary and tricuspid valves**

   Q22.0   **Pulmonary valve atresia**

   Q22.1   **Congenital pulmonary valve stenosis**

   Q22.2   **Congenital pulmonary valve insufficiency**
      Congenital pulmonary valve regurgitation

   Q22.3   **Other congenital malformations of pulmonary valve**
      Congenital malformation of pulmonary valve NOS
      Supernumerary cusps of pulmonary valve

   Q22.4   **Congenital tricuspid stenosis**
      Congenital tricuspid atresia

   Q22.5   **Ebstein's anomaly**

   Q22.6   **Hypoplastic right heart syndrome**

   Q22.8   **Other congenital malformations of tricuspid valve**

   Q22.9   **Congenital malformation of tricuspid valve, unspecified**

Q23- **Congenital malformations of aortic and mitral valves**

   Q23.0   **Congenital stenosis of aortic valve**
      Congenital aortic atresia
      Congenital aortic stenosis NOS
      Excludes 1:   *congenital stenosis of aortic valve in hypoplastic left heart syndrome (Q23.4)*
          congenital subaortic stenosis (Q24.4)
          supravalvular aortic stenosis (congenital) (Q25.3)

   Q23.1   **Congenital insufficiency of aortic valve**
      Bicuspid aortic valve
      Congenital aortic insufficiency

   Q23.2   **Congenital mitral stenosis**
      Congenital mitral atresia

   Q23.3   **Congenital mitral insufficiency**

   Q23.4   **Hypoplastic left heart syndrome**

   Q23.8   **Other congenital malformations of aortic and mitral valves**

   Q23.9   **Congenital malformation of aortic and mitral valves, unspecified**

Q24- **Other congenital malformations of heart**
  Excludes 1:   *endocardial fibroelastosis (I42.4)*

   Q24.0   **Dextrocardia**
      Excludes 1:   *dextrocardia with situs inversus (Q89.3)*
          isomerism of atrial appendages (with asplenia or polysplenia) (Q20.6)
          mirror-image atrial arrangement with situs inversus (Q89.3)

   Q24.1   **Levocardia**

   Q24.2   **Cor triatriatum**

   Q24.3   **Pulmonary infundibular stenosis**
      Subvalvular pulmonic stenosis

   Q24.4   **Congenital subaortic stenosis**

   Q24.5   **Malformation of coronary vessels**
      Congenital coronary (artery) aneurysm

   Q24.6   **Congenital heart block**

   Q24.8   **Other specified congenital malformations of heart**
      Congenital diverticulum of left ventricle
      Congenital malformation of myocardium
      Congenital malformation of pericardium
      Malposition of heart
      Uhl's disease

   Q24.9   **Congenital malformation of heart, unspecified**
      Congenital anomaly of heart
      Congenital disease of heart

Q25- **Congenital malformations of great arteries**

   Q25.0   **Patent ductus arteriosus**
      Patent ductus Botallo
      Persistent ductus arteriosus

   Q25.1   **Coarctation of aorta**
      Coarctation of aorta (preductal) (postductal)

   Q25.2   **Atresia of aorta**

   Q25.3   **Supravalvular aortic stenosis**
      Excludes 1:   *congenital aortic stenosis NOS (Q23.0)*
          congenital stenosis of aortic valve (Q23.0)

Q 10 - Q 25

Excludes 1: = NOT CODED HERE! (Do not code both)   **659**   *Excludes ❷: = Not Included Here*

Q25.4 Other congenital malformations of aorta
Absence of aorta
Aneurysm of sinus of Valsalva (ruptured)
Aplasia of aorta
Congenital aneurysm of aorta
Congenital malformations of aorta
Congenital dilatation of aorta
Double aortic arch [vascular ring of aorta]
Hypoplasia of aorta
Persistent convolutions of aortic arch
Persistent right aortic arch
Excludes 1: hypoplasia of aorta in hypoplastic left heart syndrome (Q23.4)

Q25.5 Atresia of pulmonary artery

Q25.6 Stenosis of pulmonary artery
Supravalvular pulmonary stenosis

Q25.7- Other congenital malformations of pulmonary artery

Q25.71 Coarctation of pulmonary artery

Q25.72 Congenital pulmonary arteriovenous malformation
Congenital pulmonary arteriovenous aneurysm

Q25.79 Other congenital malformations of pulmonary artery
Aberrant pulmonary artery
Agenesis of pulmonary artery
Congenital aneurysm of pulmonary artery
Congenital anomaly of pulmonary artery
Hypoplasia of pulmonary artery

Q25.8 Other congenital malformations of other great arteries

Q25.9 Congenital malformation of great arteries, unspecified

Q26- Congenital malformations of great veins

Q26.0 Congenital stenosis of vena cava
Congenital stenosis of vena cava (inferior) (superior)

Q26.1 Persistent left superior vena cava

Q26.2 Total anomalous pulmonary venous connection
Total anomalous pulmonary venous return [TAPVR], subdiaphragmatic
Total anomalous pulmonary venous return [TAPVR], supradiaphragmatic

Q26.3 Partial anomalous pulmonary venous connection
Partial anomalous pulmonary venous return

Q26.4 Anomalous pulmonary venous connection, unspecified

Q26.5 Anomalous portal venous connection

Q26.6 Portal vein-hepatic artery fistula

Q26.8 Other congenital malformations of great veins
Absence of vena cava (inferior) (superior)
Azygos continuation of inferior vena cava
Persistent left posterior cardinal vein
Scimitar syndrome

Q26.9 Congenital malformation of great vein, unspecified
Congenital anomaly of vena cava (inferior) (superior) NOS

Q27- Other congenital malformations of peripheral vascular system
*Excludes❷: anomalies of cerebral and precerebral vessels (Q28.0-Q28.3)
anomalies of coronary vessels (Q24.5)
anomalies of pulmonary artery (Q25.5-Q25.7)
congenital retinal aneurysm (Q14.1)
hemangioma and lymphangioma (D18.-)*

Q27.0 Congenital absence and hypoplasia of umbilical artery
Single umbilical artery

Q27.1 Congenital renal artery stenosis

Q27.2 Other congenital malformations of renal artery
Congenital malformation of renal artery NOS
Multiple renal arteries

Q27.3- Arteriovenous malformation (peripheral)
Arteriovenous aneurysm
Excludes 1: acquired arteriovenous aneurysm (I77.0)
*Excludes❷: arteriovenous malformation of cerebral vessels (Q28.2)
arteriovenous malformation of precerebral vessels (Q28.0)*

Q27.30 Arteriovenous malformation, site unspecified

Q27.31 Arteriovenous malformation of vessel of upper limb

Q27.32 Arteriovenous malformation of vessel of lower limb

Q27.33 Arteriovenous malformation of digestive system vessel

Q27.34 Arteriovenous malformation of renal vessel

Q27.39 Arteriovenous malformation, other site

Q27.4 Congenital phlebectasia

Q27.8 Other specified congenital malformations of peripheral vascular system
Absence of peripheral vascular system
Atresia of peripheral vascular system
Congenital aneurysm (peripheral)
Congenital stricture, artery
Congenital varix
Excludes 1: arteriovenous malformation (Q27.3-)

Q27.9 Congenital malformation of peripheral vascular system, unspecified
Anomaly of artery or vein NOS

Q28- Other congenital malformations of circulatory system
*Excludes 1: congenital aneurysm NOS (Q27.8)
congenital coronary aneurysm (Q24.5)
ruptured cerebral arteriovenous malformation (I60.8)
ruptured malformation of precerebral vessels (I72.0)*
*Excludes❷: congenital peripheral aneurysm (Q27.8)
congenital pulmonary aneurysm (Q25.79)
congenital retinal aneurysm (Q14.1)*

Q28.0 Arteriovenous malformation of precerebral vessels
Congenital arteriovenous precerebral aneurysm (nonruptured)

Q28.1 Other malformations of precerebral vessels
Congenital malformation of precerebral vessels NOS
Congenital precerebral aneurysm (nonruptured)

Q28.2 Arteriovenous malformation of cerebral vessels
Arteriovenous malformation of brain NOS
Congenital arteriovenous cerebral aneurysm (nonruptured)

Q28.3 Other malformations of cerebral vessels
Congenital cerebral aneurysm (nonruptured)
Congenital malformation of cerebral vessels NOS
Developmental venous anomaly

Q28.8 Other specified congenital malformations of circulatory system
Congenital aneurysm, specified site NEC
Spinal vessel anomaly

Q28.9 Congenital malformation of circulatory system, unspecified

Congenital malformations of the respiratory system (Q30-Q34)

Q30- Congenital malformations of nose
Excludes 1: congenital deviation of nasal septum (Q67.4)

Q30.0 Choanal atresia
Atresia of nares (anterior) (posterior)
Congenital stenosis of nares (anterior) (posterior)

Q30.1 Agenesis and underdevelopment of nose
Congenital absent of nose

Q30.2 Fissured, notched and cleft nose

Q30.3 Congenital perforated nasal septum

Q30.8 Other congenital malformations of nose
Accessory nose
Congenital anomaly of nasal sinus wall

Q30.9 Congenital malformation of nose, unspecified

Q31- Congenital malformations of larynx
Excludes 1: congenital laryngeal stridor NOS (P28.89)

Q31.0 Web of larynx
Glottic web of larynx
Subglottic web of larynx
Web of larynx NOS

Q31.1 Congenital subglottic stenosis

Q31.2 Laryngeal hypoplasia

Q31.3 Laryngocele

Q31.5 Congenital laryngomalacia

Q31.8 Other congenital malformations of larynx
Absence of larynx
Agenesis of larynx
Atresia of larynx
Congenital cleft thyroid cartilage
Congenital fissure of epiglottis
Congenital stenosis of larynx NEC
Posterior cleft of cricoid cartilage

Q31.9 Congenital malformation of larynx, unspecified

Q32- Congenital malformations of trachea and bronchus
Excludes 1: congenital bronchiectasis (Q33.4)

Q32.0 Congenital tracheomalacia

Q32.1 Other congenital malformations of trachea
Atresia of trachea
Congenital anomaly of tracheal cartilage
Congenital dilatation of trachea
Congenital malformation of trachea
Congenital stenosis of trachea
Congenital tracheocele

Q 2 5 - Q 4 0

Q32.2   **Congenital bronchomalacia**

Q32.3   **Congenital stenosis of bronchus**

Q32.4   **Other congenital malformations of bronchus**
Absence of bronchus
Agenesis of bronchus
Atresia of bronchus
Congenital diverticulum of bronchus
Congenital malformation of bronchus NOS

Q33-   **Congenital malformations of lung**

Q33.0   **Congenital cystic lung**
Congenital cystic lung disease
Congenital honeycomb lung
Congenital polycystic lung disease
Excludes 1: cystic fibrosis (E84.0)
cystic lung disease, acquired or unspecified (J98.4)

Q33.1   **Accessory lobe of lung**
Azygos lobe (fissured), lung

Q33.2   **Sequestration of lung**

Q33.3   **Agenesis of lung**
Congenital absence of lung (lobe)

Q33.4   **Congenital bronchiectasis**

Q33.5   **Ectopic tissue in lung**

Q33.6   **Congenital hypoplasia and dysplasia of lung**
Excludes 1: pulmonary hypoplasia associated with short gestation
(P28.0)

Q33.8   **Other congenital malformations of lung**

Q33.9   **Congenital malformation of lung, unspecified**

Q34-   **Other congenital malformations of respiratory system**
Excludes❷: congenital central alveolar hypoventilation syndrome
(G47.35)

Q34.0   **Anomaly of pleura**

Q34.1   **Congenital cyst of mediastinum**

Q34.8   **Other specified congenital malformations of respiratory system**
Atresia of nasopharynx

Q34.9   **Congenital malformation of respiratory system, unspecified**
Congenital absence of respiratory system
Congenital anomaly of respiratory system NOS

Cleft lip and cleft palate (Q35-Q37)

Use additional code to identify associated malformation of the nose (Q30.2)
Excludes 1: Robin's syndrome (Q87.0)

Q35-   **Cleft palate**
Includes: Fissure of palate
Palatoschisis
Excludes 1: cleft palate with cleft lip (Q37-)

Q35.1   **Cleft hard palate**

Q35.3   **Cleft soft palate**

Q35.5   **Cleft hard palate with cleft soft palate**

Q35.7   **Cleft uvula**

Q35.9   **Cleft palate, unspecified**
Cleft palate NOS

Q36-   **Cleft lip**
Includes: Cheiloschisis
Congenital fissure of lip
Harelip
Labium leporinum
Excludes 1: cleft lip with cleft palate (Q37-)

Q36.0   **Cleft lip, bilateral**

Q36.1   **Cleft lip, median**

Q36.9   **Cleft lip, unilateral**
Cleft lip NOS

Q37-   **Cleft palate with cleft lip**
Includes: Cheilopalatoschisis

Q37.0   **Cleft hard palate with bilateral cleft lip**

Q37.1   **Cleft hard palate with unilateral cleft lip**
Cleft hard palate with cleft lip NOS

Q37.2   **Cleft soft palate with bilateral cleft lip**

Q37.3   **Cleft soft palate with unilateral cleft lip**
Cleft soft palate with cleft lip NOS

Q37.4   **Cleft hard and soft palate with bilateral cleft lip**

Q37.5   **Cleft hard and soft palate with unilateral cleft lip**
Cleft hard and soft palate with cleft lip NOS

Q37.8   **Unspecified cleft palate with bilateral cleft lip**

Q37.9   **Unspecified cleft palate with unilateral cleft lip**
Cleft palate with cleft lip NOS

Other congenital malformations of the digestive system (Q38-Q45)

Q38-   **Other congenital malformations of tongue, mouth and pharynx**
Excludes 1: dentofacial anomalies (M26.-)
macrostomia (Q18.4)
microstomia (Q18.5)

Q38.0   **Congenital malformations of lips, not elsewhere classified**
Congenital fistula of lip
Congenital malformation of lip NOS
Van der Woude's syndrome
Excludes 1: cleft lip (Q36.-)
cleft lip with cleft palate (Q37.-)
macrocheilia (Q18.6)
microcheilia (Q18.7)

Q38.1   **Ankyloglossia**
Tongue tie

Q38.2   **Macroglossia**
Congenital hypertrophy of tongue

Q38.3   **Other congenital malformations of tongue**
Aglossia
Bifid tongue
Congenital adhesion of tongue
Congenital fissure of tongue
Congenital malformation of tongue NOS
Double tongue
Hypoglossia
Hypoplasia of tongue
Microglossia

Q38.4   **Congenital malformations of salivary glands and ducts**
Atresia of salivary glands and ducts
Congenital absence of salivary glands and ducts
Congenital accessory salivary glands and ducts
Congenital fistula of salivary gland

Q38.5   **Congenital malformations of palate, not elsewhere classified**
Congenital absence of uvula
Congenital malformation of palate NOS
Congenital high arched palate
Excludes 1: cleft palate (Q35.-)
cleft palate with cleft lip (Q37.-)

Q38.6   **Other congenital malformations of mouth**
Congenital malformation of mouth NOS

Q38.7   **Congenital pharyngeal pouch**
Congenital diverticulum of pharynx
Excludes 1: pharyngeal pouch syndrome (D82.1)

Q38.8   **Other congenital malformations of pharynx**
Congenital malformation of pharynx NOS
Imperforate pharynx

Q39-   **Congenital malformations of esophagus**

Q39.0   **Atresia of esophagus without fistula**
Atresia of esophagus NOS

Q39.1   **Atresia of esophagus with tracheo-esophageal fistula**
Atresia of esophagus with broncho-esophageal fistula

Q39.2   **Congenital tracheo-esophageal fistula without atresia**
Congenital tracheo-esophageal fistula NOS

Q39.3   **Congenital stenosis and stricture of esophagus**

Q39.4   **Esophageal web**

Q39.5   **Congenital dilatation of esophagus**
Congenital cardiospasm

Q39.6   **Congenital diverticulum of esophagus**
Congenital esophageal pouch

Q39.8   **Other congenital malformations of esophagus**
Congenital absence of esophagus
Congenital displacement of esophagus
Congenital duplication of esophagus

Q39.9   **Congenital malformation of esophagus, unspecified**

Q40-   **Other congenital malformations of upper alimentary tract**

Q40.0   **Congenital hypertrophic pyloric stenosis**
Congenital or infantile constriction
Congenital or infantile hypertrophy
Congenital or infantile spasm
Congenital or infantile stenosis
Congenital or infantile stricture

Q40.1   **Congenital hiatus hernia**
Congenital displacement of cardia through esophageal hiatus
Excludes 1: congenital diaphragmatic hernia (Q79.0)

Q25-Q40

Excludes 1: = NOT CODED HERE! (Do not code both)   **661**   *Excludes❷: = Not Included Here*

Q40.2   **Other specified congenital malformations of stomach**
Congenital displacement of stomach
Congenital diverticulum of stomach
Congenital hourglass stomach
Congenital duplication of stomach
Megalogastria
Microgastria

Q40.3   **Congenital malformation of stomach, unspecified**

Q40.8   **Other specified congenital malformations of upper alimentary tract**

Q40.9   **Congenital malformation of upper alimentary tract, unspecified**
Congenital anomaly of upper alimentary tract
Congenital deformity of upper alimentary tract

Q41-   Congenital absence, atresia and stenosis of small intestine
Includes: Congenital obstruction, occlusion or stricture of small intestine or intestine NOS
Excludes 1:   cystic fibrosis with intestinal manifestation (E84.11)
meconium ileus NOS (without cystic fibrosis) (P76.0)

Q41.0   **Congenital absence, atresia and stenosis of duodenum**

Q41.1   **Congenital absence, atresia and stenosis of jejunum**
Apple peel syndrome
Imperforate jejunum

Q41.2   **Congenital absence, atresia and stenosis of ileum**

Q41.8   **Congenital absence, atresia and stenosis of other specified parts of small intestine**

Q41.9   **Congenital absence, atresia and stenosis of small intestine, part unspecified**
Congenital absence, atresia and stenosis of intestine NOS

Q42-   Congenital absence, atresia and stenosis of large intestine
Includes: Congenital obstruction, occlusion and stricture of large intestine

Q42.0   **Congenital absence, atresia and stenosis of rectum with fistula**

Q42.1   **Congenital absence, atresia and stenosis of rectum without fistula**
Imperforate rectum

Q42.2   **Congenital absence, atresia and stenosis of anus with fistula**

Q42.3   **Congenital absence, atresia and stenosis of anus without fistula**
Imperforate anus

Q42.8   **Congenital absence, atresia and stenosis of other parts of large intestine**

Q42.9   **Congenital absence, atresia and stenosis of large intestine, part unspecified**

Q43-   Other congenital malformations of intestine

Q43.0   **Meckel's diverticulum (displaced) (hypertrophic)**
Persistent omphalomesenteric duct
Persistent vitelline duct

Q43.1   **Hirschsprung's disease**
Aganglionosis
Congenital (aganglionic) megacolon

Q43.2   **Other congenital functional disorders of colon**
Congenital dilatation of colon

Q43.3   **Congenital malformations of intestinal fixation**
Congenital omental, anomalous adhesions [bands]
Congenital peritoneal adhesions [bands]
Incomplete rotation of cecum and colon
Insufficient rotation of cecum and colon
Jackson's membrane
Malrotation of colon
Rotation failure of cecum and colon
Universal mesentery

Q43.4   **Duplication of intestine**

Q43.5   **Ectopic anus**

Q43.6   **Congenital fistula of rectum and anus**
Excludes 1:   congenital fistula of anus with absence, atresia and stenosis (Q42.2)
congenital fistula of rectum with absence, atresia and stenosis (Q42.0)
congenital rectovaginal fistula (Q52.2)
congenital urethrorectal fistula (Q64.73)
pilonidal fistula or sinus (L05.-)

Q43.7   **Persistent cloaca**
Cloaca NOS

Q43.8   **Other specified congenital malformations of intestine**
Congenital blind loop syndrome
Congenital diverticulitis, colon
Congenital diverticulum, intestine
Dolichocolon
Megaloappendix
Megaloduodenum
Microcolon
Transposition of appendix
Transposition of colon
Transposition of intestine

Q43.9   **Congenital malformation of intestine, unspecified**

Q44-   Congenital malformations of gallbladder, bile ducts and liver

Q44.0   **Agenesis, aplasia and hypoplasia of gallbladder**
Congenital absence of gallbladder

Q44.1   **Other congenital malformations of gallbladder**
Congenital malformation of gallbladder NOS
Intrahepatic gallbladder

Q44.2   **Atresia of bile ducts**

Q44.3   **Congenital stenosis and stricture of bile ducts**

Q44.4   **Choledochal cyst**

Q44.5   **Other congenital malformations of bile ducts**
Accessory hepatic duct
Biliary duct duplication
Congenital malformation of bile duct NOS
Cystic duct duplication

Q44.6   **Cystic disease of liver**
Fibrocystic disease of liver

Q44.7   **Other congenital malformations of liver**
Accessory liver
Alagille's syndrome
Congenital absence of liver
Congenital hepatomegaly
Congenital malformation of liver NOS

Q45-   Other congenital malformations of digestive system
Excludes ❷: congenital diaphragmatic hernia (Q79.0)
congenital hiatus hernia (Q40.1)

Q45.0   **Agenesis, aplasia and hypoplasia of pancreas**
Congenital absence of pancreas

Q45.1   **Annular pancreas**

Q45.2   **Congenital pancreatic cyst**

Q45.3   **Other congenital malformations of pancreas and pancreatic duct**
Accessory pancreas
Congenital malformation of pancreas or pancreatic duct NOS
Excludes 1:   congenital diabetes mellitus (E10.-)
cystic fibrosis (E84.0-E84.9)
fibrocystic disease of pancreas (E84.-)
neonatal diabetes mellitus (P70.2)

Q45.8   **Other specified congenital malformations of digestive system**
Absence (complete) (partial) of alimentary tract NOS
Duplication of digestive system
Malposition, congenital of digestive system

Q45.9   **Congenital malformation of digestive system, unspecified**
Congenital anomaly of digestive system
Congenital deformity of digestive system

Congenital malformations of genital organs (Q50-Q56)

Excludes 1:   androgen insensitivity syndrome (E34.5-)
syndromes associated with anomalies in the number and form of chromosomes (Q90-Q99)

Q50-   Congenital malformations of ovaries, fallopian tubes and broad ligaments

Q50.0-   Congenital absence of ovary
Excludes 1:   Turner's syndrome (Q96.-)

Q50.01   Congenital absence of ovary, unilateral

Q50.02   Congenital absence of ovary, bilateral

Q50.1   **Developmental ovarian cyst**

Q50.2   **Congenital torsion of ovary**

Q50.3-   Other congenital malformations of ovary

Q50.31   Accessory ovary

Q50.32   Ovarian streak
46, XX with streak gonads

Q50.39   Other congenital malformation of ovary
Congenital malformation of ovary NOS

Q50.4   **Embryonic cyst of fallopian tube**
Fimbrial cyst

Q50.5   **Embryonic cyst of broad ligament**
Epoophoron cyst
Parovarian cyst

Q50.6   **Other congenital malformations of fallopian tube and broad ligament**
Absence of fallopian tube and broad ligament
Accessory fallopian tube and broad ligament
Atresia of fallopian tube and broad ligament
Congenital malformation of fallopian tube or broad ligament NOS

Q 40 – Q 56

Q51- Congenital malformations of uterus and cervix

Q51.0 **Agenesis and aplasia of uterus**
Congenital absence of uterus

Q51.1- **Doubling of uterus with doubling of cervix and vagina**

Q51.10 **Doubling of uterus with doubling of cervix and vagina without obstruction**
Doubling of uterus with doubling of cervix and vagina NOS

Q51.11 **Doubling of uterus with doubling of cervix and vagina with obstruction**

Q51.2 **Other doubling of uterus**
Doubling of uterus NOS
Septate uterus, complete or partial

Q51.3 **Bicornate uterus**
Bicornate uterus, complete or partial

Q51.4 **Unicornate uterus**
Unicornate uterus with or without a separate uterine horn
Uterus with only one functioning horn

Q51.5 **Agenesis and aplasia of cervix**
Congenital absence of cervix

Q51.6 **Embryonic cyst of cervix**

Q51.7 **Congenital fistulae between uterus and digestive and urinary tracts**

Q51.8- **Other congenital malformations of uterus and cervix**

Q51.81- **Other congenital malformations of uterus**

Q51.810 **Arcuate uterus**
Arcuatus uterus

Q51.811 **Hypoplasia of uterus**

Q51.818 **Other congenital malformations of uterus**
Müllerian anomaly of uterus NEC

Q51.82- **Other congenital malformations of cervix**

Q51.820 **Cervical duplication**

Q51.821 **Hypoplasia of cervix**

Q51.828 **Other congenital malformations of cervix**

Q51.9 **Congenital malformation of uterus and cervix, unspecified**

Q52- Other congenital malformations of female genitalia

Q52.0 **Congenital absence of vagina**
Vaginal agenesis, total or partial

Q52.1- **Doubling of vagina**
Excludes 1: doubling of vagina with doubling of uterus and cervix (Q51.1-)

Q52.10 **Doubling of vagina, unspecified**
Septate vagina NOS

Q52.11 **Transverse vaginal septum**

Q52.12 **Longitudinal vaginal septum**
Longitudinal vaginal septum with or without obstruction

Q52.2 **Congenital rectovaginal fistula**
Excludes 1: cloaca (Q43.7)

Q52.3 **Imperforate hymen**

Q52.4 **Other congenital malformations of vagina**
Canal of Nuck cyst, congenital
Congenital malformation of vagina NOS
Embryonic vaginal cyst
Gartner's duct cyst

Q52.5 **Fusion of labia**

Q52.6 **Congenital malformation of clitoris**

Q52.7- **Other and unspecified congenital malformations of vulva**

Q52.70 **Unspecified congenital malformations of vulva**
Congenital malformation of vulva NOS

Q52.71 **Congenital absence of vulva**

Q52.79 **Other congenital malformations of vulva**
Congenital cyst of vulva

Q52.8 **Other specified congenital malformations of female genitalia**

Q52.9 **Congenital malformation of female genitalia, unspecified**

Q53- Undescended and ectopic testicle

Q53.0- **Ectopic testis**

Q53.00 **Ectopic testis, unspecified**

Q53.01 **Ectopic testis, unilateral**

Q53.02 **Ectopic testes, bilateral**

Q53.1- **Undescended testicle, unilateral**

Q53.10 **Unspecified undescended testicle, unilateral**

Q53.11 **Abdominal testis, unilateral**

Q53.12 **Ectopic perineal testis, unilateral**

Q53.2- **Undescended testicle, bilateral**

Q53.20 **Undescended testicle, unspecified, bilateral**

Q53.21 **Abdominal testis, bilateral**

Q53.22 **Ectopic perineal testis, bilateral**

Q53.9 **Undescended testicle, unspecified**
Cryptorchism NOS

Q54- Hypospadias
Excludes 1: epispadias (Q64.0)

Q54.0 **Hypospadias, balanic**
Hypospadias, coronal
Hypospadias, glandular

Q54.1 **Hypospadias, penile**

Q54.2 **Hypospadias, penoscrotal**

Q54.3 **Hypospadias, perineal**

Q54.4 **Congenital chordee**
Chordee without hypospadias

Q54.8 **Other hypospadias**
Hypospadias with intersex state

Q54.9 **Hypospadias, unspecified**

Q55- Other congenital malformations of male genital organs
Excludes 1: congenital hydrocele (P83.5)
hypospadias (Q54.-)

Q55.0 **Absence and aplasia of testis**
Monorchism

Q55.1 **Hypoplasia of testis and scrotum**
Fusion of testes

Q55.2- **Other and unspecified congenital malformations of testis and scrotum**

Q55.20 **Unspecified congenital malformations of testis and scrotum**
Congenital malformation of testis or scrotum NOS

Q55.21 **Polyorchism**

Q55.22 **Retractile testis**

Q55.23 **Scrotal transposition**

Q55.29 **Other congenital malformations of testis and scrotum**

Q55.3 **Atresia of vas deferens**
Code first any associated cystic fibrosis (E84.-)

Q55.4 **Other congenital malformations of vas deferens, epididymis, seminal vesicles and prostate**
Absence or aplasia of prostate
Absence or aplasia of spermatic cord
Congenital malformation of vas deferens, epididymis, seminal vesicles or prostate NOS

Q55.5 **Congenital absence and aplasia of penis**

Q55.6- **Other congenital malformations of penis**

Q55.61 **Curvature of penis (lateral)**

Q55.62 **Hypoplasia of penis**
Micropenis

Q55.63 **Congenital torsion of penis**
Excludes 1: acquired torsion of penis (N48.82)

Q55.64 **Hidden penis**
Buried penis
Concealed penis
Excludes 1: acquired buried penis (N48.83)

Q55.69 **Other congenital malformation of penis**
Congenital malformation of penis NOS

Q55.7 **Congenital vasocutaneous fistula**

Q55.8 **Other specified congenital malformations of male genital organs**

Q55.9 **Congenital malformation of male genital organ, unspecified**
Congenital anomaly of male genital organ
Congenital deformity of male genital organ

Q56- Indeterminate sex and pseudohermaphroditism
Excludes 1: 46,XX true hermaphrodite (Q99.1)
androgen insensitivity syndrome (E34.5-)
chimera 46,XX/46,XY true hermaphrodite (Q99.0)
female pseudohermaphroditism with adrenocortical disorder (E25.-)
pseudohermaphroditism with specified chromosomal anomaly (Q96-Q99)
pure gonadal dysgenesis (Q99.1)

Q56.0 **Hermaphroditism, not elsewhere classified**
Ovotestis

Q56.1 **Male pseudohermaphroditism, not elsewhere classified**
46, XY with streak gonads
Male pseudohermaphroditism NOS

Q56.2 **Female pseudohermaphroditism, not elsewhere classified**
Female pseudohermaphroditism NOS

Q56.3 **Pseudohermaphroditism, unspecified**

Q56.4 **Indeterminate sex, unspecified**
Ambiguous genitalia

Q40 - Q56

Congenital malformations of the urinary system (Q60-Q64)

Q60- Renal agenesis and other reduction defects of kidney
Includes: Congenital absence of kidney
Congenital atrophy of kidney
Infantile atrophy of kidney
Q60.0   Renal <u>agenesis</u>, <u>unilateral</u>
Q60.1   Renal <u>agenesis</u>, <u>bilateral</u>
Q60.2   Renal <u>agenesis</u>, <u>unspecified</u>
Q60.3   Renal hypoplasia, <u>unilateral</u>
Q60.4   Renal hypoplasia, <u>bilateral</u>
Q60.5   Renal hypoplasia, <u>unspecified</u>
Q60.6   Potter's syndrome

Q61- Cystic kidney disease
Excludes 1:   acquired cyst of kidney (N28.1)
Potter's syndrome (Q60.6)
Q61.0- Congenital renal cyst
Q61.00   Congenital renal cyst, unspecified
Cyst of kidney NOS (congenital)
Q61.01   Congenital single renal cyst
Q61.02   Congenital multiple renal cysts
Q61.1- Polycystic kidney, infantile type
Polycystic kidney, autosomal recessive
Q61.11   Cystic dilatation of collecting ducts
Q61.19   Other polycystic kidney, infantile type
Q61.2   Polycystic kidney, adult type
Polycystic kidney, autosomal dominant
Q61.3   Polycystic kidney, unspecified
Q61.4   Renal dysplasia
Multicystic dysplastic kidney
Multicystic kidney (development)
Multicystic kidney disease
Multicystic renal dysplasia
Excludes 1:   polycystic kidney disease (Q61.11-Q61.3)
Q61.5   Medullary cystic kidney
Nephronopthisis
Sponge kidney NOS
Q61.8   Other cystic kidney diseases
Fibrocystic kidney
Fibrocystic renal degeneration or disease
Q61.9   Cystic kidney disease, unspecified
Meckel-Gruber syndrome

Q62- Congenital obstructive defects of renal pelvis and congenital malformations of ureter
Q62.0   Congenital hydronephrosis
Q62.1- Congenital occlusion of ureter
Atresia and stenosis of ureter
Q62.10   Congenital occlusion of ureter, unspecified
Q62.11   Congenital occlusion of ureteropelvic junction
Q62.12   Congenital occlusion of ureterovesical orifice
Q62.2   Congenital megaureter
Congenital dilatation of ureter
Q62.3- Other obstructive defects of renal pelvis and ureter
Q62.31   Congenital ureterocele, orthotopic
Q62.32   Cecoureterocele
Ectopic ureterocele
Q62.39   Other obstructive defects of renal pelvis and ureter
Ureteropelvic junction obstruction NOS
Q62.4   Agenesis of ureter
Congenital absence ureter
Q62.5   Duplication of ureter
Accessory ureter
Double ureter
Q62.6- Malposition of ureter
Q62.60   Malposition of ureter, unspecified
Q62.61   Deviation of ureter
Q62.62   Displacement of ureter
Q62.63   Anomalous implantation of ureter
Ectopia of ureter
Ectopic ureter
Q62.69   Other malposition of ureter
Q62.7   Congenital vesico-uretero-renal reflux
Q62.8   Other congenital malformations of ureter
Anomaly of ureter NOS

Q63- Other congenital malformations of kidney
Excludes 1:   congenital nephrotic syndrome (N04.-)
Q63.0   Accessory kidney
Q63.1   Lobulated, fused and horseshoe kidney
Q63.2   Ectopic kidney
Congenital displaced kidney
Malrotation of kidney
Q63.3   Hyperplastic and giant kidney
Compensatory hypertrophy of kidney
Q63.8   Other specified congenital malformations of kidney
Congenital renal calculi
Q63.9   Congenital malformation of kidney, unspecified

Q64- Other congenital malformations of urinary system
Q64.0   Epispadias
Excludes 1:   hypospadias (Q54.-)
Q64.1- Exstrophy of urinary bladder
Q64.10   Exstrophy of urinary bladder, unspecified
Ectopia vesicae
Q64.11   Supravesical fissure of urinary bladder
Q64.12   Cloacal extrophy of urinary bladder
Q64.19   Other exstrophy of urinary bladder
Extroversion of bladder
Q64.2   Congenital posterior urethral valves
Q64.3- Other atresia and stenosis of urethra and bladder neck
Q64.31   Congenital bladder neck obstruction
Congenital obstruction of vesicourethral orifice
Q64.32   Congenital stricture of urethra
Q64.33   Congenital stricture of urinary meatus
Q64.39   Other atresia and stenosis of urethra and bladder neck
Atresia and stenosis of urethra and bladder neck NOS
Q64.4   Malformation of urachus
Cyst of urachus
Patent urachus
Prolapse of urachus
Q64.5   Congenital absence of bladder and urethra
Q64.6   Congenital diverticulum of bladder
Q64.7- Other and unspecified congenital malformations of bladder and urethra
Excludes 1:   congenital prolapse of bladder (mucosa) (Q79.4)
Q64.70   Unspecified congenital malformation of bladder and urethra
Malformation of bladder or urethra NOS
Q64.71   Congenital prolapse of urethra
Q64.72   Congenital prolapse of urinary meatus
Q64.73   Congenital urethrorectal fistula
Q64.74   Double urethra
Q64.75   Double urinary meatus
Q64.79   Other congenital malformations of bladder and urethra
Q64.8   Other specified congenital malformations of urinary system
Q64.9   Congenital malformation of urinary system, unspecified
Congenital anomaly NOS of urinary system
Congenital deformity NOS of urinary system

Congenital malformations and deformations of the musculoskeletal system (Q65-Q79)

Q65- <u>Congenital deformities of hip</u>
Excludes 1:   clicking hip (R29.4)
Q65.0- Congenital dislocation of hip, <u>unilateral</u>
Q65.00   Congenital dislocation of <u>unspecified</u> hip, unilateral
Q65.01   Congenital dislocation of <u>right</u> hip, unilateral
Q65.02   Congenital dislocation of <u>left</u> hip, unilateral
Q65.1   Congenital dislocation of hip, <u>bilateral</u>
Q65.2   Congenital dislocation of hip, <u>unspecified</u>
Q65.3- Congenital <u>partial</u> dislocation of hip, <u>unilateral</u>
Q65.30   Congenital partial dislocation of <u>unspecified</u> hip, unilateral
Q65.31   Congenital partial dislocation of <u>right</u> hip, unilateral
Q65.32   Congenital partial dislocation of <u>left</u> hip, unilateral
Q65.4   Congenital <u>partial</u> dislocation of hip, <u>bilateral</u>
Q65.5   Congenital <u>partial</u> dislocation of hip, <u>unspecified</u>
Q65.6   Congenital unstable hip
Congenital dislocatable hip

Q60 - Q71

Q65.8- Other congenital deformities of hip
    Q65.81 Congenital coxa valga
    Q65.82 Congenital coxa vara
    Q65.89 Other specified congenital deformities of hip
        Anteversion of femoral neck
        Congenital acetabular dysplasia
Q65.9 Congenital deformity of hip, unspecified

Q66- Congenital deformities of feet
    Excludes 1: reduction defects of feet (Q72.-)
                valgus deformities (acquired) (M21.0-)
                varus deformities (acquired) (M21.1-)

Q66.0 Congenital talipes equinovarus
Q66.1 Congenital talipes calcaneovarus
Q66.2 Congenital metatarsus (primus) varus
Q66.3 Other congenital varus deformities of feet
    Hallux varus, congenital
Q66.4 Congenital talipes calcaneovalgus
Q66.5- Congenital pes planus
    Congenital flat foot
    Congenital rigid flat foot
    Congenital spastic (everted) flat foot
    Excludes 1: pes planus, acquired (M21.4)
    Q66.50 Congenital pes planus, unspecified foot
    Q66.51 Congenital pes planus, <u>right</u> foot
    Q66.52 Congenital pes planus, <u>left</u> foot
Q66.6 Other congenital valgus deformities of feet
    Congenital metatarsus valgus
Q66.7 Congenital pes cavus
Q66.8- Other congenital deformities of feet
    Q66.80 Congenital vertical talus deformity, unspecified foot
    Q66.81 Congenital vertical talus deformity, <u>right</u> foot
    Q66.82 Congenital vertical talus deformity, <u>left</u> foot
    Q66.89 Other congenital deformities of feet
        Congenital asymmetric talipes
        Congenital clubfoot NOS
        Congenital talipes NOS
        Congenital tarsal coalition
        Hammer toe, congenital
Q66.9 Congenital deformity of feet, unspecified

Q67- Congenital musculoskeletal deformities of head, face, spine and chest
    Excludes 1: congenital malformation syndromes classified to Q87.-
                Potter's syndrome (Q60.6)
Q67.0 Congenital facial asymmetry
Q67.1 Congenital compression facies
Q67.2 Dolichocephaly
Q67.3 Plagiocephaly
Q67.4 Other congenital deformities of skull, face and jaw
    Congenital depressions in skull
    Congenital hemifacial atrophy or hypertrophy
    Deviation of nasal septum, congenital
    Squashed or bent nose, congenital
    Excludes 1: dentofacial anomalies [including malocclusion] (M26.-)
                syphilitic saddle nose (A50.5)
Q67.5 Congenital deformity of spine
    Congenital postural scoliosis
    Congenital scoliosis NOS
    Excludes 1: infantile idiopathic scoliosis (M41.0)
                scoliosis due to congenital bony malformation (Q76.3)
Q67.6 Pectus excavatum
    Congenital funnel chest
Q67.7 Pectus carinatum
    Congenital pigeon chest
Q67.8 Other congenital deformities of chest
    Congenital deformity of chest wall NOS

Q68- Other congenital musculoskeletal deformities
    Excludes 1: reduction defects of limb(s) (Q71-Q73)
    Excludes ❷: congenital myotonic chondrodystrophy (G71.13)
Q68.0 Congenital deformity of sternocleidomastoid muscle
    Congenital contracture of sternocleidomastoid (muscle)
    Congenital (sternomastoid) torticollis
    Sternomastoid tumor (congenital)
Q68.1 Congenital deformity of finger(s) and hand
    Congenital clubfinger
    Spade-like hand (congenital)
Q68.2 Congenital deformity of knee
    Congenital dislocation of knee
    Congenital genu recurvatum
Q68.3 Congenital bowing of femur
    Excludes 1: anteversion of femur (neck) (Q65.89)

Q68.4 Congenital bowing of tibia and fibula
Q68.5 Congenital bowing of long bones of leg, unspecified
Q68.6 Discoid meniscus
Q68.8 Other specified congenital musculoskeletal deformities
    Congenital deformity of clavicle
    Congenital deformity of elbow
    Congenital deformity of forearm
    Congenital deformity of scapula
    Congenital deformity of wrist
    Congenital dislocation of elbow
    Congenital dislocation of shoulder
    Congenital dislocation of wrist

Q69- Polydactyly
Q69.0 Accessory finger(s)
Q69.1 Accessory thumb(s)
Q69.2 Accessory toe(s)
    Accessory hallux
Q69.9 Polydactyly, unspecified
    Supernumerary digit(s) NOS

Q70- Syndactyly
Q70.0- <u>Fused fingers</u>
    Complex syndactyly of fingers with synostosis
    Q70.00 Fused fingers, <u>unspecified</u> hand
    Q70.01 Fused fingers, <u>right</u> hand
    Q70.02 Fused fingers, <u>left</u> hand
    Q70.03 Fused fingers, <u>bilateral</u>
Q70.1- <u>Webbed fingers</u>
    Simple syndactyly of fingers without synostosis
    Q70.10 Webbed fingers, <u>unspecified</u> hand
    Q70.11 Webbed fingers, <u>right</u> hand
    Q70.12 Webbed fingers, <u>left</u> hand
    Q70.13 Webbed fingers, <u>bilateral</u>
Q70.2- <u>Fused toes</u>
    Complex syndactyly of toes with synostosis
    Q70.20 Fused toes, <u>unspecified</u> foot
    Q70.21 Fused toes, <u>right</u> foot
    Q70.22 Fused toes, <u>left</u> foot
    Q70.23 Fused toes, <u>bilateral</u>
Q70.3- <u>Webbed toes</u>
    Simple syndactyly of toes without synostosis
    Q70.30 Webbed toes, <u>unspecified</u> foot
    Q70.31 Webbed toes, <u>right</u> foot
    Q70.32 Webbed toes, <u>left</u> foot
    Q70.33 Webbed toes, <u>bilateral</u>
Q70.4 Polysyndactyly, unspecified
    Excludes 1: specified syndactyly of hand and feet — code to
                specified conditions (Q70.0-Q70.3-)
Q70.9 Syndactyly, unspecified
    Symphalangy NOS

Q71- Reduction defects of upper limb
Q71.0- Congenital <u>complete absence</u> of <u>upper</u> limb
    Q71.00 Congenital complete absence of <u>unspecified</u> upper limb
    Q71.01 Congenital complete absence of <u>right</u> upper limb
    Q71.02 Congenital complete absence of <u>left</u> upper limb
    Q71.03 Congenital complete absence of upper limb, <u>bilateral</u>
Q71.1- Congenital <u>absence of upper arm and forearm with hand present</u>
    Q71.10 Congenital absence of <u>unspecified</u> upper arm and forearm with hand present
    Q71.11 Congenital absence of <u>right</u> upper arm and forearm with hand present
    Q71.12 Congenital absence of <u>left</u> upper arm and forearm with hand present
    Q71.13 Congenital absence of upper arm and forearm with hand present, <u>bilateral</u>
Q71.2- Congenital <u>absence of both forearm and hand</u>
    Q71.20 Congenital absence of both forearm and hand, <u>unspecified</u> upper limb
    Q71.21 Congenital absence of both forearm and hand, <u>right</u> upper limb
    Q71.22 Congenital absence of both forearm and hand, <u>left</u> upper limb
    Q71.23 Congenital absence of both forearm and hand, <u>bilateral</u>
Q71.3- Congenital <u>absence of hand and finger</u>
    Q71.30 Congenital absence of <u>unspecified</u> hand and finger
    Q71.31 Congenital absence of <u>right</u> hand and finger
    Q71.32 Congenital absence of <u>left</u> hand and finger
    Q71.33 Congenital absence of hand and finger, <u>bilateral</u>

Q 60 - Q 71

Q71.4- Longitudinal reduction defect of radius
   Clubhand (congenital)
   Radial clubhand
 Q71.40 Longitudinal reduction defect of unspecified radius
 Q71.41 Longitudinal reduction defect of right radius
 Q71.42 Longitudinal reduction defect of left radius
 Q71.43 Longitudinal reduction defect of radius, bilateral
Q71.5- Longitudinal reduction defect of ulna
 Q71.50 Longitudinal reduction defect of unspecified ulna
 Q71.51 Longitudinal reduction defect of right ulna
 Q71.52 Longitudinal reduction defect of left ulna
 Q71.53 Longitudinal reduction defect of ulna, bilateral
Q71.6- Lobster-claw hand
 Q71.60 Lobster-claw hand, unspecified hand
 Q71.61 Lobster-claw right hand
 Q71.62 Lobster-claw left hand
 Q71.63 Lobster-claw hand, bilateral
Q71.8- Other reduction defects of upper limb
 Q71.81- Congenital shortening of upper limb
  Q71.811 Congenital shortening of right upper limb
  Q71.812 Congenital shortening of left upper limb
  Q71.813 Congenital shortening of upper limb, bilateral
  Q71.819 Congenital shortening of unspecified upper limb
 Q71.89- Other reduction defects of upper limb
  Q71.891 Other reduction defects of right upper limb
  Q71.892 Other reduction defects of left upper limb
  Q71.893 Other reduction defects of upper limb, bilateral
  Q71.899 Other reduction defects of unspecified upper limb
Q71.9- Unspecified reduction defect of upper limb
 Q71.90 Unspecified reduction defect of unspecified upper limb
 Q71.91 Unspecified reduction defect of right upper limb
 Q71.92 Unspecified reduction defect of left upper limb
 Q71.93 Unspecified reduction defect of upper limb, bilateral

Q72- Reduction defects of lower limb
Q72.0- Congenital complete absence of lower limb
 Q72.00 Congenital complete absence of unspecified lower limb
 Q72.01 Congenital complete absence of right lower limb
 Q72.02 Congenital complete absence of left lower limb
 Q72.03 Congenital complete absence of lower limb, bilateral
Q72.1- Congenital absence of thigh and lower leg with foot present
 Q72.10 Congenital absence of unspecified thigh and lower leg with foot present
 Q72.11 Congenital absence of right thigh and lower leg with foot present
 Q72.12 Congenital absence of left thigh and lower leg with foot present
 Q72.13 Congenital absence of thigh and lower leg with foot present, bilateral
Q72.2- Congenital absence of both lower leg and foot
 Q72.20 Congenital absence of both lower leg and foot, unspecified lower limb
 Q72.21 Congenital absence of both lower leg and foot, right lower limb
 Q72.22 Congenital absence of both lower leg and foot, left lower limb
 Q72.23 Congenital absence of both lower leg and foot, bilateral
Q72.3- Congenital absence of foot and toe(s)
 Q72.30 Congenital absence of unspecified foot and toe(s)
 Q72.31 Congenital absence of right foot and toe(s)
 Q72.32 Congenital absence of left foot and toe(s)
 Q72.33 Congenital absence of foot and toe(s), bilateral
Q72.4- Longitudinal reduction defect of femur
   Proximal femoral focal deficiency
 Q72.40 Longitudinal reduction defect of unspecified femur
 Q72.41 Longitudinal reduction defect of right femur
 Q72.42 Longitudinal reduction defect of left femur
 Q72.43 Longitudinal reduction defect of femur, bilateral
Q72.5- Longitudinal reduction defect of tibia
 Q72.50 Longitudinal reduction defect of unspecified tibia
 Q72.51 Longitudinal reduction defect of right tibia
 Q72.52 Longitudinal reduction defect of left tibia
 Q72.53 Longitudinal reduction defect of tibia, bilateral

Q72.6- Longitudinal reduction defect of fibula
 Q72.60 Longitudinal reduction defect of unspecified fibula
 Q72.61 Longitudinal reduction defect of right fibula
 Q72.62 Longitudinal reduction defect of left fibula
 Q72.63 Longitudinal reduction defect of fibula, bilateral
Q72.7- Split foot
 Q72.70 Split foot, unspecified lower limb
 Q72.71 Split foot, right lower limb
 Q72.72 Split foot, left lower limb
 Q72.73 Split foot, bilateral
Q72.8- Other reduction defects of lower limb
 Q72.81- Congenital shortening of lower limb
  Q72.811 Congenital shortening of right lower limb
  Q72.812 Congenital shortening of left lower limb
  Q72.813 Congenital shortening of lower limb, bilateral
  Q72.819 Congenital shortening of unspecified lower limb
 Q72.89- Other reduction defects of lower limb
  Q72.891 Other reduction defects of right lower limb
  Q72.892 Other reduction defects of left lower limb
  Q72.893 Other reduction defects of lower limb, bilateral
  Q72.899 Other reduction defects of unspecified lower limb
Q72.9- Unspecified reduction defect of lower limb
 Q72.90 Unspecified reduction defect of unspecified lower limb
 Q72.91 Unspecified reduction defect of right lower limb
 Q72.92 Unspecified reduction defect of left lower limb
 Q72.93 Unspecified reduction defect of lower limb, bilateral

Q73- Reduction defects of unspecified limb
Q73.0 Congenital absence of unspecified limb(s)
   Amelia NOS
Q73.1 Phocomelia, unspecified limb(s)
   Phocomelia NOS
Q73.8 Other reduction defects of unspecified limb(s)
   Longitudinal reduction deformity of unspecified limb(s)
   Ectromelia of limb NOS
   Hemimelia of limb NOS
   Reduction defect of limb NOS

Q74- Other congenital malformations of limb(s)
 Excludes 1: *polydactyly (Q69.-)*
     reduction defect of limb (Q71-Q73)
     syndactyly (Q70.-)
Q74.0 Other congenital malformations of upper limb(s), including shoulder girdle
   Accessory carpal bones
   Cleidocranial dysostosis
   Congenital pseudarthrosis of clavicle
   Macrodactylia (fingers)
   Madelung's deformity
   Radioulnar synostosis
   Sprengel's deformity
   Triphalangeal thumb
Q74.1 Congenital malformation of knee
   Congenital absence of patella
   Congenital dislocation of patella
   Congenital genu valgum
   Congenital genu varum
   Rudimentary patella
  Excludes 1: *congenital dislocation of knee (Q68.2)*
      congenital genu recurvatum (Q68.2)
      nail patella syndrome (Q87.2)
Q74.2 Other congenital malformations of lower limb(s), including pelvic girdle
   Congenital fusion of sacroiliac joint
   Congenital malformation of ankle joint
   Congenital malformation of sacroiliac joint
  Excludes 1: *anteversion of femur (neck) (Q65.89)*
Q74.3 Arthrogryposis multiplex congenita
Q74.8 Other specified congenital malformations of limb(s)
Q74.9 Unspecified congenital malformation of limb(s)
   Congenital anomaly of limb(s) NOS

Q 7 1 - Q 7 9

Q75-   **Other congenital malformations of skull and face bones**
    Excludes 1: *congenital malformation of face NOS (Q18-)*
              congenital malformation syndromes classified to Q87-
              dentofacial anomalies [including malocclusion] (M26-)
              musculoskeletal deformities of head and face (Q67.0-Q67.4)
              skull defects associated with congenital anomalies of brain
                  such as:
                  anencephaly (Q00.0)
                  encephalocele (Q01-)
                  hydrocephalus (Q03-)
                  microcephaly (Q02)

Q75.0   **Craniosynostosis**
    Acrocephaly
    Imperfect fusion of skull
    Oxycephaly
    Trigonocephaly

Q75.1   **Craniofacial dysostosis**
    Crouzon's disease

Q75.2   **Hypertelorism**

Q75.3   **Macrocephaly**

Q75.4   **Mandibulofacial dysostosis**
    Franceschetti syndrome
    Treacher Collins syndrome

Q75.5   **Oculomandibular dysostosis**

Q75.8   **Other specified congenital malformations of skull and face bones**
    Absence of skull bone, congenital
    Congenital deformity of forehead
    Platybasia

Q75.9   **Congenital malformation of skull and face bones, unspecified**
    Congenital anomaly of face bones NOS
    Congenital anomaly of skull NOS

Q76-   **Congenital malformations of spine and bony thorax**
    Excludes 1: *congenital musculoskeletal deformities of spine and chest*
              (Q67.5-Q67.8)

Q76.0   **Spina bifida occulta**
    Excludes 1: *meningocele (spinal) (Q05.-)*
              spina bifida (aperta) (cystica) (Q05.-)

Q76.1   **Klippel-Feil syndrome**
    Cervical fusion syndrome

Q76.2   **Congenital spondylolisthesis**
    Congenital spondylolysis
    Excludes 1: *spondylolisthesis (acquired) (M43.1-)*
              spondylolysis (acquired) (M43.0-)

Q76.3   **Congenital scoliosis due to congenital bony malformation**
    Hemivertebra fusion or failure of segmentation with scoliosis

Q76.4-   **Other congenital malformations of spine, not associated with scoliosis**

    Q76.41-   **Congenital kyphosis**

        Q76.411   **Congenital kyphosis, occipito-atlanto-axial region**
        Q76.412   **Congenital kyphosis, cervical region**
        Q76.413   **Congenital kyphosis, cervicothoracic region**
        Q76.414   **Congenital kyphosis, thoracic region**
        Q76.415   **Congenital kyphosis, thoracolumbar region**
        Q76.419   **Congenital kyphosis, unspecified region**

    Q76.42-   **Congenital lordosis**

        Q76.425   **Congenital lordosis, thoracolumbar region**
        Q76.426   **Congenital lordosis, lumbar region**
        Q76.427   **Congenital lordosis, lumbosacral region**
        Q76.428   **Congenital lordosis, sacral and sacrococcygeal region**
        Q76.429   **Congenital lordosis, unspecified region**

    Q76.49   **Other congenital malformations of spine, not associated with scoliosis**
        Congenital absence of vertebra NOS
        Congenital fusion of spine NOS
        Congenital malformation of lumbosacral (joint) (region) NOS
        Congenital malformation of spine NOS
        Hemivertebra NOS
        Malformation of spine NOS
        Platyspondylisis NOS
        Supernumerary vertebra NOS

Q76.5   **Cervical rib**
    Supernumerary rib in cervical region

Q76.6   **Other congenital malformations of ribs**
    Accessory rib
    Congenital absence of rib
    Congenital fusion of ribs
    Congenital malformation of ribs NOS
    Excludes 1: *short rib syndrome (Q77.2)*

Q76.7   **Congenital malformation of sternum**
    Congenital absence of sternum
    Sternum bifidum

Q76.8   **Other congenital malformations of bony thorax**

Q76.9   **Congenital malformation of bony thorax, unspecified**

Q77-   **Osteochondrodysplasia with defects of growth of tubular bones and spine**
    Excludes 1: *mucopolysaccharidosis (E76.0-E76.3)*
    Excludes❷: *congenital myotonic chondrodystrophy (G71.13)*

Q77.0   **Achondrogenesis**
    Hypochondrogenesis

Q77.1   **Thanatophoric short stature**

Q77.2   **Short rib syndrome**
    Asphyxiating thoracic dysplasia [Jeune]

Q77.3   **Chondrodysplasia punctata**
    Excludes 1: *Rhizomelic chondrodysplasia punctata (E71.43)*

Q77.4   **Achondroplasia**
    Hypochondroplasia
    Osteosclerosis congenita

Q77.5   **Diastrophic dysplasia**

Q77.6   **Chondroectodermal dysplasia**
    Ellis-van Creveld syndrome

Q77.7   **Spondyloepiphyseal dysplasia**

Q77.8   **Other osteochondrodysplasia with defects of growth of tubular bones and spine**

Q77.9   **Osteochondrodysplasia with defects of growth of tubular bones and spine, unspecified**

Q78-   **Other osteochondrodysplasias**
    Excludes❷: *congenital myotonic chondrodystrophy (G71.13)*

Q78.0   **Osteogenesis imperfecta**
    Fragilitas ossium
    Osteopsathyrosis

Q78.1   **Polyostotic fibrous dysplasia**
    Albright(-McCune)(-Sternberg) syndrome

Q78.2   **Osteopetrosis**
    Albers-Schönberg syndrome
    Osteosclerosis NOS

Q78.3   **Progressive diaphyseal dysplasia**
    Camurati-Engelmann syndrome

Q78.4   **Enchondromatosis**
    Maffucci's syndrome
    Ollier's disease

Q78.5   **Metaphyseal dysplasia**
    Pyle's syndrome

Q78.6   **Multiple congenital exostoses**
    Diaphyseal aclasis

Q78.8   **Other specified osteochondrodysplasias**
    Osteopoikilosis

Q78.9   **Osteochondrodysplasia, unspecified**
    Chondrodystrophy NOS
    Osteodystrophy NOS

Q79-   **Congenital malformations of musculoskeletal system, not elsewhere classified**
    Excludes❷: *congenital (sternomastoid) torticollis (Q68.0)*

Q79.0   **Congenital diaphragmatic hernia**
    Excludes 1: *congenital hiatus hernia (Q40.1)*

Q79.1   **Other congenital malformations of diaphragm**
    Absence of diaphragm
    Congenital malformation of diaphragm NOS
    Eventration of diaphragm

Q79.2   **Exomphalos**
    Omphalocele
    Excludes 1: *umbilical hernia (K42.-)*

Q79.3   **Gastroschisis**

Q79.4   **Prune belly syndrome**
    Congenital prolapse of bladder mucosa
    Eagle-Barrett syndrome

Q79.5-   **Other congenital malformations of abdominal wall**
    Excludes 1: *umbilical hernia (K42.-)*

    Q79.51   **Congenital hernia of bladder**

    Q79.59   **Other congenital malformations of abdominal wall**

Q79.6   **Ehlers-Danlos syndrome**

Q79.8   **Other congenital malformations of musculoskeletal system**
    Absence of muscle
    Absence of tendon
    Accessory muscle
    Amyotrophia congenita
    Congenital constricting bands
    Congenital shortening of tendon
    Poland syndrome

Q71 - Q79

Q79.9   Congenital malformation of musculoskeletal system, unspecified
Congenital anomaly of musculoskeletal system NOS
Congenital deformity of musculoskeletal system NOS

Other congenital malformations (Q80-Q89)

Q80- Congenital ichthyosis
Excludes 1:   Refsum's disease (G60.1)

Q80.0   Ichthyosis vulgaris

Q80.1   X-linked ichthyosis

Q80.2   Lamellar ichthyosis
Collodion baby

Q80.3   Congenital bullous ichthyosiform erythroderma

Q80.4   Harlequin fetus

Q80.8   Other congenital ichthyosis

Q80.9   Congenital ichthyosis, unspecified

Q81- Epidermolysis bullosa

Q81.0   Epidermolysis bullosa simplex
Excludes 1:   Cockayne's syndrome (Q87.1)

Q81.1   Epidermolysis bullosa letalis
Herlitz' syndrome

Q81.2   Epidermolysis bullosa dystrophica

Q81.8   Other epidermolysis bullosa

Q81.9   Epidermolysis bullosa, unspecified

Q82- Other congenital malformations of skin
Excludes 1:   acrodermatitis enteropathica (E83.2)
congenital erythropoietic porphyria (E80.0)
pilonidal cyst or sinus (L05.-)
Sturge-Weber (-Dimitri) syndrome (Q85.8)

Q82.0   Hereditary lymphedema

Q82.1   Xeroderma pigmentosum

Q82.2   Mastocytosis
Urticaria pigmentosa
Excludes 1:   malignant mastocytosis (C96.2)

Q82.3   Incontinentia pigmenti

Q82.4   Ectodermal dysplasia (anhidrotic)
Excludes 1:   Ellis-van Creveld syndrome (Q77.6)

Q82.5   Congenital non-neoplastic nevus
Birthmark NOS
Flammeus nevus
Portwine nevus
Sanguineous nevus
Strawberry nevus
Vascular nevus NOS
Verrucous nevus
Excludes❷: café au lait spots (L81.3)
lentigo (L81.4)
nevus NOS (D22.-)
araneus nevus (I78.1)
melanocytic nevus (D22.-)
pigmented nevus (D22.-)
spider nevus (I78.1)
stellar nevus (I78.1)

Q82.8   Other specified congenital malformations of skin
Abnormal palmar creases
Accessory skin tags
Benign familial pemphigus [Hailey-Hailey]
Congenital poikiloderma
Cutis laxa (hyperelastica)
Dermatoglyphic anomalies
Inherited keratosis palmaris et plantaris
Keratosis follicularis [Darier-White]
Excludes 1:   Ehlers-Danlos syndrome (Q79.6)

Q82.9   Congenital malformation of skin, unspecified

Q83- Congenital malformations of breast
Excludes❷: absence of pectoral muscle (Q79.8)
hypoplasia of breast (N64.82)
micromastia (N64.82)

Q83.0   Congenital absence of breast with absent nipple

Q83.1   Accessory breast
Supernumerary breast

Q83.2   Absent nipple

Q83.3   Accessory nipple
Supernumerary nipple

Q83.8   Other congenital malformations of breast

Q83.9   Congenital malformation of breast, unspecified

Q84- Other congenital malformations of integument

Q84.0   Congenital alopecia
Congenital atrichosis

Q84.1   Congenital morphological disturbances of hair, not elsewhere classified
Beaded hair
Monilethrix
Pili annulati
Excludes 1:   Menkes' kinky hair syndrome (E83.0)

Q84.2   Other congenital malformations of hair
Congenital hypertrichosis
Congenital malformation of hair NOS
Persistent lanugo

Q84.3   Anonychia
Excludes 1:   nail patella syndrome (Q87.2)

Q84.4   Congenital leukonychia

Q84.5   Enlarged and hypertrophic nails
Congenital onychauxis
Pachyonychia

Q84.6   Other congenital malformations of nails
Congenital clubnail
Congenital koilonychia
Congenital malformation of nail NOS

Q84.8   Other specified congenital malformations of integument
Aplasia cutis congenita

Q84.9   Congenital malformation of integument, unspecified
Congenital anomaly of integument NOS
Congenital deformity of integument NOS

Q85- Phakomatoses, not elsewhere classified
Excludes 1:   ataxia telangiectasia [Louis-Bar] (G11.3)
familial dysautonomia [Riley-Day] (G90.1)

Q85.0- Neurofibromatosis (nonmalignant)

Q85.00 Neurofibromatosis, unspecified

Q85.01 Neurofibromatosis, type 1
Von Recklinghausen disease

Q85.02 Neurofibromatosis, type 2
Acoustic neurofibromatosis

Q85.03 Schwannomatosis

Q85.09 Other neurofibromatosis

Q85.1   Tuberous sclerosis
Bourneville's disease
Epiloia

Q85.8   Other phakomatoses, not elsewhere classified
Peutz-Jeghers Syndrome
Sturge-Weber(-Dimitri) syndrome
von Hippel-Lindau syndrome
Excludes 1:   Meckel-Gruber syndrome (Q61.9)

Q85.9   Phakomatosis, unspecified
Hamartosis NOS

Q86- Congenital malformation syndromes due to known exogenous causes, not elsewhere classified
Excludes❷: iodine-deficiency-related hypothyroidism (E00-E02)
nonteratogenic effects of substances transmitted via placenta or breast milk (P04.-)

Q86.0   Fetal alcohol syndrome (dysmorphic)

Q86.1   Fetal hydantoin syndrome
Meadow's syndrome

Q86.2   Dysmorphism due to warfarin

Q86.8   Other congenital malformation syndromes due to known exogenous causes

Q87- Other specified congenital malformation syndromes affecting multiple systems
Use additional code(s) to identify all associated manifestations

Q87.0   Congenital malformation syndromes predominantly affecting facial appearance
Acrocephalopolysyndactyly
Acrocephalosyndactyly [Apert]
Cryptophthalmos syndrome
Cyclopia
Goldenhar syndrome
Moebius syndrome
Oro-facial-digital syndrome
Robin syndrome
Whistling face

Q
7
9
-
Q
9
3

© 2013 Channel Publishing, Ltd.

Q87.1   Congenital malformation syndromes predominantly associated with short stature
Aarskog syndrome
Cockayne syndrome
De Lange syndrome
Dubowitz syndrome
Noonan syndrome
Prader-Willi syndrome
Robinow-Silverman-Smith syndrome
Russell-Silver syndrome
Seckel syndrome
*Excludes 1:   Ellis-van Creveld syndrome (Q77.6)
Smith-Lemli-Opitz syndrome (E78.72)*

Q87.2   Congenital malformation syndromes predominantly involving limbs
Holt-Oram syndrome
Klippel-Trenaunay-Weber syndrome
Nail patella syndrome
Rubinstein-Taybi syndrome
Sirenomelia syndrome
Thrombocytopenia with absent radius [TAR] syndrome
VATER syndrome

Q87.3   Congenital malformation syndromes involving early overgrowth
Beckwith-Wiedemann syndrome
Sotos syndrome
Weaver syndrome

Q87.4- Marfan's syndrome

Q87.40   Marfan's syndrome, unspecified

Q87.41- Marfan's syndrome with cardiovascular manifestations

Q87.410   Marfan's syndrome with aortic dilation

Q87.418   Marfan's syndrome with other cardiovascular manifestations

Q87.42   Marfan's syndrome with ocular manifestations

Q87.43   Marfan's syndrome with skeletal manifestation

Q87.5   Other congenital malformation syndromes with other skeletal changes

Q87.8- Other specified congenital malformation syndromes, not elsewhere classified
Excludes 1: Zellweger syndrome (E71.510)

Q87.81   Alport syndrome
Use additional code to identify stage of chronic kidney disease (N18.1-N18.6)

Q87.89   Other specified congenital malformation syndromes, not elsewhere classified
Laurence-Moon (-Bardet)-Biedl syndrome

Q89- Other congenital malformations, not elsewhere classified

Q89.0- Congenital absence and malformations of spleen
Excludes 1:   isomerism of atrial appendages (with asplenia or polysplenia) (Q20.6)

Q89.01   Asplenia (congenital)

Q89.09   Congenital malformations of spleen
Congenital splenomegaly

Q89.1   Congenital malformations of adrenal gland
*Excludes 1: adrenogenital disorders (E25.-)
congenital adrenal hyperplasia (E25.0)*

Q89.2   Congenital malformations of other endocrine glands
Congenital malformation of parathyroid or thyroid gland
Persistent thyroglossal duct
Thyroglossal cyst
*Excludes 1: congenital goiter (E03.0)
congenital hypothyroidism (E03.1)*

Q89.3   Situs inversus
Dextrocardia with situs inversus
Mirror-image atrial arrangement with situs inversus
Situs inversus or transversus abdominalis
Situs inversus or transversus thoracis
Transposition of abdominal viscera
Transposition of thoracic viscera
Excludes 1: dextrocardia NOS (Q24.0)

Q89.4   Conjoined twins
Craniopagus
Dicephaly
Pygopagus
Thoracopagus

Q89.7   Multiple congenital malformations, not elsewhere classified
Multiple congenital anomalies NOS
Multiple congenital deformities NOS
Excludes 1: congenital malformation syndromes affecting multiple systems (Q87.-)

Q89.8   Other specified congenital malformations
Use additional code(s) to identify all associated manifestations

Q89.9   Congenital malformation, unspecified
Congenital anomaly NOS
Congenital deformity NOS

Chromosomal abnormalities, not elsewhere classified (Q90-Q99)

Excludes ❷: mitochondrial metabolic disorders (E88.4-)

Q90- Down syndrome
Use additional code(s) to identify any associated physical conditions and degree of intellectual disabilities (F70-F79)

Q90.0   Trisomy 21, nonmosaicism (meiotic nondisjunction)

Q90.1   Trisomy 21, mosaicism (mitotic nondisjunction)

Q90.2   Trisomy 21, translocation

Q90.9   Down syndrome, unspecified
Trisomy 21 NOS

Q91- Trisomy 18 and Trisomy 13

Q91.0   Trisomy 18, nonmosaicism (meiotic nondisjunction)

Q91.1   Trisomy 18, mosaicism (mitotic nondisjunction)

Q91.2   Trisomy 18, translocation

Q91.3   Trisomy 18, unspecified

Q91.4   Trisomy 13, nonmosaicism (meiotic nondisjunction)

Q91.5   Trisomy 13, mosaicism (mitotic nondisjunction)

Q91.6   Trisomy 13, translocation

Q91.7   Trisomy 13, unspecified

Q92- Other trisomies and partial trisomies of the autosomes, not elsewhere classified
Includes: Unbalanced translocations and insertions
Excludes 1: trisomies of chromosomes 13, 18, 21 (Q90-Q91)

Q92.0   Whole chromosome trisomy, nonmosaicism (meiotic nondisjunction)

Q92.1   Whole chromosome trisomy, mosaicism (mitotic nondisjunction)

Q92.2   Partial trisomy
Less than whole arm duplicated
Whole arm or more duplicated
Excludes 1: partial trisomy due to unbalanced translocation (Q92.5)

Q92.5   Duplications with other complex rearrangements
Partial trisomy due to unbalanced translocations
Code also any associated deletions due to unbalanced translocations, inversions and insertions (Q93.7)

Q92.6- Marker chromosomes
Trisomies due to dicentrics
Trisomies due to extra rings
Trisomies due to isochromosomes
Individual with marker heterochromatin

Q92.61   Marker chromosomes in normal individual

Q92.62   Marker chromosomes in abnormal individual

Q92.7   Triploidy and polyploidy

Q92.8   Other specified trisomies and partial trisomies of autosomes
Duplications identified by fluorescence in situ hybridization (FISH)
Duplications identified by in situ hybridization (ISH)
Duplications seen only at prometaphase

Q92.9   Trisomy and partial trisomy of autosomes, unspecified

Q93- Monosomies and deletions from the autosomes, not elsewhere classified

Q93.0   Whole chromosome monosomy, nonmosaicism (meiotic nondisjunction)

Q93.1   Whole chromosome monosomy, mosaicism (mitotic nondisjunction)

Q93.2   Chromosome replaced with ring, dicentric or isochromosome

Q93.3   Deletion of short arm of chromosome 4
Wolff-Hirschorn syndrome

Q93.4   Deletion of short arm of chromosome 5
Cri-du-chat syndrome

Q93.5   Other deletions of part of a chromosome
Angelman syndrome

Q93.7   Deletions with other complex rearrangements
Deletions due to unbalanced translocations, inversions and insertions
Code also any associated duplications due to unbalanced translocations, inversions and insertions (Q92.5)

Q79 - Q93

Excludes 1: = NOT CODED HERE! (Do not code both)   **669**   *Excludes ❷:* = Not Included Here

Q93.8- Other deletions from the autosomes
> **Q93.81 Velo-cardio-facial syndrome**
>> Deletion 22q11.2
> **Q93.88 Other microdeletions**
>> Miller-Dieker syndrome
>> Smith-Magenis syndrome
> **Q93.89 Other deletions from the autosomes**
>> Deletions identified by fluorescence in situ hybridization (FISH)
>> Deletions identified by in situ hybridization (ISH)
>> Deletions seen only at prometaphase
Q93.9 Deletion from autosomes, unspecified

Q95- Balanced rearrangements and structural markers, not elsewhere classified
> Includes: Robertsonian and balanced reciprocal translocations and insertions
Q95.0 Balanced translocation and insertion in normal individual
Q95.1 Chromosome inversion in normal individual
Q95.2 Balanced autosomal rearrangement in abnormal individual
Q95.3 Balanced sex/autosomal rearrangement in abnormal individual
Q95.5 Individual with autosomal fragile site
Q95.8 Other balanced rearrangements and structural markers
Q95.9 Balanced rearrangement and structural marker, unspecified

Q96- Turner's syndrome
> *Excludes 1:   Noonan syndrome (Q87.1)*
Q96.0 Karyotype 45, X
Q96.1 Karyotype 46, X iso (Xq)
> Karyotype 46, isochromosome Xq
Q96.2 Karyotype 46, X with abnormal sex chromosome, except iso (Xq)
> Karyotype 46, X with abnormal sex chromosome, except isochromosome Xq
Q96.3 Mosaicism, 45, X/46, XX or XY
Q96.4 Mosaicism, 45, X/other cell line(s) with abnormal sex chromosome
Q96.8 Other variants of Turner's syndrome
Q96.9 Turner's syndrome, unspecified

Q97- Other sex chromosome abnormalities, female phenotype, not elsewhere classified
> *Excludes 1:   Turner's syndrome (Q96.-)*
Q97.0 Karyotype 47, XXX
Q97.1 Female with more than three X chromosomes
Q97.2 Mosaicism, lines with various numbers of X chromosomes
Q97.3 Female with 46, XY karyotype
Q97.8 Other specified sex chromosome abnormalities, female phenotype
Q97.9 Sex chromosome abnormality, female phenotype, unspecified

Q98- Other sex chromosome abnormalities, male phenotype, not elsewhere classified
Q98.0 Klinefelter syndrome karyotype 47, XXY
Q98.1 Klinefelter syndrome, male with more than two X chromosomes
Q98.3 Other male with 46, XX karyotype
Q98.4 Klinefelter syndrome, unspecified
Q98.5 Karyotype 47, XYY
Q98.6 Male with structurally abnormal sex chromosome
Q98.7 Male with sex chromosome mosaicism
Q98.8 Other specified sex chromosome abnormalities, male phenotype
Q98.9 Sex chromosome abnormality, male phenotype, unspecified

Q99- Other chromosome abnormalities, not elsewhere classified
Q99.0 Chimera 46, XX/46, XY
> Chimera 46, XX/46, XY true hermaphrodite
Q99.1 46, XX true hermaphrodite
> 46, XX with streak gonads
> 46, XY with streak gonads
> Pure gonadal dysgenesis
Q99.2 Fragile X chromosome
> Fragile X syndrome
Q99.8 Other specified chromosome abnormalities
Q99.9 Chromosomal abnormality, unspecified

Q 9 3 | R 0 6

Chapter 18 – Symptoms, signs and abnormal clinical and laboratory findings, not elsewhere classified (R00-R99)

Note: This chapter includes symptoms, signs, abnormal results of clinical or other investigative procedures, and ill-defined conditions regarding which no diagnosis classifiable elsewhere is recorded. Signs and symptoms that point rather definitely to a given diagnosis have been assigned to a category in other chapters of the classification. In general, categories in this chapter include the less well-defined conditions and symptoms that, without the necessary study of the case to establish a final diagnosis, point perhaps equally to two or more diseases or to two or more systems of the body. Practically all categories in the chapter could be designated "not otherwise specified", "unknown etiology" or "transient". The Alphabetical Index should be consulted to determine which symptoms and signs are to be allocated here and which to other chapters. The residual subcategories, numbered .8, are generally provided for other relevant symptoms that cannot be allocated elsewhere in the classification.

The conditions and signs or symptoms included in categories R00-R94 consist of:
- (a) cases for which no more specific diagnosis can be made even after all the facts bearing on the case have been investigated;
- (b) signs or symptoms existing at the time of initial encounter that proved to be transient and whose causes could not be determined;
- (c) provisional diagnosis in a patient who failed to return for further investigation or care;
- (d) cases referred elsewhere for investigation or treatment before the diagnosis was made;
- (e) cases in which a more precise diagnosis was not available for any other reason;
- (f) certain symptoms, for which supplementary information is provided, that represent important problems in medical care in their own right.

Excludes❷: abnormal findings on antenatal screening of mother (O28-)
certain conditions originating in the perinatal period (P04-P96)
signs and symptoms classified in the body system chapters
signs and symptoms of breast (N63, N64.5)

This chapter contains the following blocks:
R00-R09	Symptoms and signs involving the circulatory and respiratory systems
R10-R19	Symptoms and signs involving the digestive system and abdomen
R20-R23	Symptoms and signs involving the skin and subcutaneous tissue
R25-R29	Symptoms and signs involving the nervous and musculoskeletal systems
R30-R39	Symptoms and signs involving the genitourinary system
R40-R46	Symptoms and signs involving cognition, perception, emotional state and behavior
R47-R49	Symptoms and signs involving speech and voice
R50-R69	General symptoms and signs
R70-R79	Abnormal findings on examination of blood, without diagnosis
R80-R82	Abnormal findings on examination of urine, without diagnosis
R83-R89	Abnormal findings on examination of other body fluids, substances and tissues, without diagnosis
R90-R94	Abnormal findings on diagnostic imaging and in function studies, without diagnosis
R97	Abnormal tumor markers
R99	Ill-defined and unknown cause of mortality

Symptoms and signs involving the circulatory and respiratory systems (R00-R09)

R00- Abnormalities of heart beat
Excludes 1: abnormalities originating in the perinatal period (P29.1-)
specified arrhythmias (I47-I49)

R00.0 Tachycardia, unspecified
Rapid heart beat
Sinoauricular tachycardia NOS
Sinus [sinusal] tachycardia NOS
Excludes 1: neonatal tachycardia (P29.11)
paroxysmal tachycardia (I47.-)

R00.1 Bradycardia, unspecified
Sinoatrial bradycardia
Sinus bradycardia
Slow heart beat
Vagal bradycardia
Use additional code for adverse effect, if applicable, to identify drug (T36-T50 with fifth or sixth character 5)
Excludes 1: neonatal bradycardia (P29.12)

R00.2 Palpitations
Awareness of heart beat
R00.8 Other abnormalities of heart beat
R00.9 Unspecified abnormalities of heart beat

R01- Cardiac murmurs and other cardiac sounds
Excludes 1: cardiac murmurs and sounds originating in the perinatal period (P29.8)

R01.0 Benign and innocent cardiac murmurs
Functional cardiac murmur
R01.1 Cardiac murmur, unspecified
Cardiac bruit NOS
Heart murmur NOS
R01.2 Other cardiac sounds
Cardiac dullness, increased or decreased
Precordial friction

R03- Abnormal blood-pressure reading, without diagnosis
R03.0 Elevated blood-pressure reading, without diagnosis of hypertension
Note: This category is to be used to record an episode of elevated blood pressure in a patient in whom no formal diagnosis of hypertension has been made, or as an isolated incidental finding.
R03.1 Nonspecific low blood-pressure reading
Excludes 1: hypotension (I95-)
maternal hypotension syndrome (O26.5-)
neurogenic orthostatic hypotension (G90.3)

R04- Hemorrhage from respiratory passages
R04.0 Epistaxis
Hemorrhage from nose
Nosebleed
R04.1 Hemorrhage from throat
Excludes❷: hemoptysis (R04.2)
R04.2 Hemoptysis
Blood-stained sputum
Cough with hemorrhage
R04.8- Hemorrhage from other sites in respiratory passages
R04.81 Acute idiopathic pulmonary hemorrhage in infants
AIPHI
Acute idiopathic hemorrhage in infants over 28 days old
Excludes 1: perinatal pulmonary hemorrhage (P26.-)
von Willebrand's disease (D68.0)
R04.89 Hemorrhage from other sites in respiratory passages
Pulmonary hemorrhage NOS
R04.9 Hemorrhage from respiratory passages, unspecified

R05 Cough
Excludes 1: cough with hemorrhage (R04.2)
smoker's cough (J41.0)

R06- Abnormalities of breathing
Excludes 1: acute respiratory distress syndrome (J80)
respiratory arrest (R09.2)
respiratory arrest of newborn (P28.81)
respiratory distress syndrome of newborn (P22.-)
respiratory failure (J96.-)
respiratory failure of newborn (P28.5)

R06.0- Dyspnea
Excludes 1: tachypnea NOS (R06.82)
transient tachypnea of newborn (P22.1)
R06.00 Dyspnea, unspecified
R06.01 Orthopnea
R06.02 Shortness of breath
R06.09 Other forms of dyspnea
R06.1 Stridor
Excludes 1: congenital laryngeal stridor (P28.89)
laryngismus (stridulus) (J38.5)
R06.2 Wheezing
Excludes 1: Asthma (J45-)
R06.3 Periodic breathing
Cheyne-Stokes breathing
R06.4 Hyperventilation
Excludes 1: psychogenic hyperventilation (F45.8)
R06.5 Mouth breathing
Excludes❷: dry mouth NOS (R68.2)
R06.6 Hiccough
Excludes 1: psychogenic hiccough (F45.8)
R06.7 Sneezing
R06.8- Other abnormalities of breathing
R06.81 Apnea, not elsewhere classified
Apnea NOS
Excludes 1: apnea (of) newborn (P28.4)
sleep apnea (G47.3-)
sleep apnea of newborn (primary) (P28.3)

Q93 – R06

© 2013 Channel Publishing, Ltd.

R06.82 Tachypnea, not elsewhere classified
Tachypnea NOS
Excludes 1: transitory tachypnea of newborn (P22.1)

R06.83 Snoring

R06.89 Other abnormalities of breathing
Breath-holding (spells)
Sighing

R06.9 Unspecified abnormalities of breathing

R07- Pain in throat and chest
Excludes 1: epidemic myalgia (B33.0)
Excludes❷: jaw pain R68.84
pain in breast (N64.4)

R07.0 Pain in throat
Excludes 1: chronic sore throat (J31.2)
sore throat (acute) NOS (J02.9)
Excludes❷: dysphagia (R13.1-)
pain in neck (M54.2)

R07.1 Chest pain on breathing
Painful respiration

R07.2 Precordial pain

R07.8- Other chest pain

R07.81 Pleurodynia
Pleurodynia NOS
Excludes 1: epidemic pleurodynia (B33.0)

R07.82 Intercostal pain

R07.89 Other chest pain
Anterior chest-wall pain NOS

R07.9 Chest pain, unspecified

R09- Other symptoms and signs involving the circulatory and respiratory system
Excludes 1: acute respiratory distress syndrome (J80)
respiratory arrest of newborn (P28.81)
respiratory distress syndrome of newborn (P22.0)
respiratory failure (J96.-)
respiratory failure of newborn (P28.5)

R09.0- Asphyxia and hypoxemia
Excludes 1: asphyxia due to carbon monoxide (T58.-)
asphyxia due to foreign body in respiratory tract (T17.-)
birth (intrauterine) asphyxia (P84)
hypercapnia (R06.4)
hyperventilation (R06.4)
traumatic asphyxia (T71.-)

R09.01 Asphyxia

R09.02 Hypoxemia

R09.1 Pleurisy
Excludes 1: pleurisy with effusion (J90)

R09.2 Respiratory arrest
Cardiorespiratory failure
Excludes 1: cardiac arrest (I46.-)
respiratory arrest of newborn (P28.81)
respiratory distress of newborn (P22.0)
respiratory failure (J96.-)
respiratory failure of newborn (P28.5)
respiratory insufficiency (R06.89)
respiratory insufficiency of newborn (P28.5)

R09.3 Abnormal sputum
Abnormal amount of sputum
Abnormal color of sputum
Abnormal odor of sputum
Excessive sputum
Excludes 1: blood-stained sputum (R04.2)

R09.8- Other specified symptoms and signs involving the circulatory and respiratory systems

R09.81 Nasal congestion

R09.82 Postnasal drip

R09.89 Other specified symptoms and signs involving the circulatory and respiratory systems
Bruit (arterial)
Abnormal chest percussion
Feeling of foreign body in throat
Friction sounds in chest
Chest tympany
Choking sensation
Rales
Weak pulse
Excludes❷: foreign body in throat (T17.2-)
wheezing (R06.2)

Symptoms and signs involving the digestive system and abdomen (R10-R19)

Excludes 1: congenital or infantile pylorospasm (Q40.0)
gastrointestinal hemorrhage (K92.0-K92.2)
intestinal obstruction (K56.-)
newborn gastrointestinal hemorrhage (P54.0-P54.3)
newborn intestinal obstruction (P76.-)
pylorospasm (K31.3)
signs and symptoms involving the urinary system (R30-R39)
symptoms referable to female genital organs (N94.-)
symptoms referable to male genital organs male (N48-N50)

R10- Abdominal and pelvic pain
Excludes 1: renal colic (N23)
Excludes❷: dorsalgia (M54.-)
flatulence and related conditions (R14.-)

R10.0 Acute abdomen
Severe abdominal pain (generalized) (with abdominal rigidity)
Excludes 1: abdominal rigidity NOS (R19.3)
generalized abdominal pain NOS (R10.84)
localized abdominal pain (R10.1-R10.3-)

R10.1- Pain localized to upper abdomen

R10.10 Upper abdominal pain, unspecified

R10.11 Right upper quadrant pain

R10.12 Left upper quadrant pain

R10.13 Epigastric pain
Dyspepsia
Excludes 1: functional dyspepsia (K30)

R10.2 Pelvic and perineal pain
Excludes 1: vulvodynia (N94.81)

R10.3- Pain localized to other parts of lower abdomen

R10.30 Lower abdominal pain, unspecified

R10.31 Right lower quadrant pain

R10.32 Left lower quadrant pain

R10.33 Periumbilical pain

R10.8- Other abdominal pain

R10.81- Abdominal tenderness
Abdominal tenderness NOS

R10.811 Right upper quadrant abdominal tenderness

R10.812 Left upper quadrant abdominal tenderness

R10.813 Right lower quadrant abdominal tenderness

R10.814 Left lower quadrant abdominal tenderness

R10.815 Periumbilic abdominal tenderness

R10.816 Epigastric abdominal tenderness

R10.817 Generalized abdominal tenderness

R10.819 Abdominal tenderness, unspecified site

R10.82- Rebound abdominal tenderness

R10.821 Right upper quadrant rebound abdominal tenderness

R10.822 Left upper quadrant rebound abdominal tenderness

R10.823 Right lower quadrant rebound abdominal tenderness

R10.824 Left lower quadrant rebound abdominal tenderness

R10.825 Periumbilic rebound abdominal tenderness

R10.826 Epigastric rebound abdominal tenderness

R10.827 Generalized rebound abdominal tenderness

R10.829 Rebound abdominal tenderness, unspecified site

R10.83 Colic
Colic NOS
Infantile colic
Excludes 1: colic in adult and child over 12 months old (R10.84)

R10.84 Generalized abdominal pain
Excludes 1: generalized abdominal pain associated with acute abdomen (R10.0)

R10.9 Unspecified abdominal pain

R11- Nausea and vomiting
Excludes 1: cyclical vomiting associated with migraine (G43.A-)
excessive vomiting in pregnancy (O21-)
hematemesis (K92.0)
neonatal hematemesis (P54.0)
newborn vomiting (P92.0-)
psychogenic vomiting (F50.8)
vomiting associated with bulimia nervosa (F50.2)
vomiting following gastrointestinal surgery (K91.0)

R11.0 Nausea
Nausea NOS
Nausea without vomiting

Excludes 1: = NOT CODED HERE! (Do not code both)

Excludes❷: = Not Included Here

R11.1-   **Vomiting**
    R11.10   Vomiting, unspecified
        Vomiting NOS
    R11.11   Vomiting without nausea
    R11.12   Projectile vomiting
    R11.13   Vomiting of fecal matter
    R11.14   Bilious vomiting
        Bilious emesis
R11.2   **Nausea with vomiting, unspecified**
    Persistent nausea with vomiting NOS

R12   **Heartburn**
    Excludes 1: dyspepsia NOS (R10.13)
               functional dyspepsia (K30)

R13-   **Aphagia and dysphagia**
  R13.0   Aphagia
    Inability to swallow
    Excludes 1: psychogenic aphagia (F50.9)
  R13.1-   Dysphagia
    Code first, if applicable, dysphagia following cerebrovascular disease
        (I69. with final characters -91)
    Excludes 1: psychogenic dysphagia (F45.8)
    R13.10   Dysphagia, unspecified
        Difficulty in swallowing NOS
    R13.11   Dysphagia, oral phase
    R13.12   Dysphagia, oropharyngeal phase
    R13.13   Dysphagia, pharyngeal phase
    R13.14   Dysphagia, pharyngoesophageal phase
    R13.19   Other dysphagia
        Cervical dysphagia
        Neurogenic dysphagia

R14-   **Flatulence and related conditions**
    Excludes 1: psychogenic aerophagy (F45.8)
  R14.0   Abdominal distension (gaseous)
    Bloating
    Tympanites (abdominal) (intestinal)
  R14.1   Gas pain
  R14.2   Eructation
  R14.3   Flatulence

R15-   **Fecal incontinence**
    Includes: Encopresis NOS
    Excludes 1: fecal incontinence of nonorganic origin (F98.1)
  R15.0   Incomplete defecation
    Excludes 1: constipation (K59.0-)
            fecal impaction (K56.41)
  R15.1   Fecal smearing
    Fecal soiling
  R15.2   Fecal urgency
  R15.9   Full incontinence of feces
    Fecal incontinence NOS

R16-   **Hepatomegaly and splenomegaly, <u>not elsewhere classified</u>**
  R16.0   Hepatomegaly, not elsewhere classified
    Hepatomegaly NOS
  R16.1   Splenomegaly, not elsewhere classified
    Splenomegaly NOS
  R16.2   Hepatomegaly with splenomegaly, not elsewhere classified
    Hepatosplenomegaly NOS

R17   **Unspecified jaundice**
    Excludes 1: neonatal jaundice (P55, P57-P59)

R18-   **Ascites**
    Includes: Fluid in peritoneal cavity
    Excludes 1: ascites in alcoholic cirrhosis (K70.31)
            ascites in alcoholic hepatitis (K70.11)
            ascites in toxic liver disease with chronic active hepatitis
                (K71.51)
  R18.0   Malignant ascites
    Code first malignancy, such as:
      Malignant neoplasm of ovary (C56.-)
      Secondary malignant neoplasm of retroperitoneum and peritoneum
        (C78.6)
  R18.8   Other ascites
    Ascites NOS
    Peritoneal effusion (chronic)

R19-   **Other symptoms and signs involving the digestive system and abdomen**
    Excludes 1: acute abdomen (R10.0)
  R19.0-   Intra-abdominal and pelvic swelling, mass and lump
    Excludes 1: abdominal distension (gaseous) (R14.-)
            ascites (R18.-)
    R19.00   Intra-abdominal and pelvic swelling, mass and lump, <u>unspecified</u> site
    R19.01   <u>Right</u> <u>upper</u> quadrant abdominal swelling, mass and lump
    R19.02   <u>Left</u> <u>upper</u> quadrant abdominal swelling, mass and lump
    R19.03   <u>Right</u> <u>lower</u> quadrant abdominal swelling, mass and lump
    R19.04   <u>Left</u> <u>lower</u> quadrant abdominal swelling, mass and lump
    R19.05   Periumbilic swelling, mass or lump
        Diffuse or generalized umbilical swelling or mass
    R19.06   Epigastric swelling, mass or lump
    R19.07   Generalized intra-abdominal and pelvic swelling, mass and lump
        Diffuse or generalized intra-abdominal swelling or mass NOS
        Diffuse or generalized pelvic swelling or mass NOS
    R19.09   Other intra-abdominal and pelvic swelling, mass and lump
  R19.1-   Abnormal bowel sounds
    R19.11   Absent bowel sounds
    R19.12   Hyperactive bowel sounds
    R19.15   Other abnormal bowel sounds
        Abnormal bowel sounds NOS
  R19.2   Visible peristalsis
    Hyperperistalsis
  R19.3-   <u>Abdominal rigidity</u>
    Excludes 1: abdominal rigidity with severe abdominal pain (R10.0)
    R19.30   Abdominal rigidity, unspecified site
    R19.31   <u>Right</u> <u>upper</u> quadrant abdominal rigidity
    R19.32   <u>Left</u> <u>upper</u> quadrant abdominal rigidity
    R19.33   <u>Right</u> <u>lower</u> quadrant abdominal rigidity
    R19.34   <u>Left</u> <u>lower</u> quadrant abdominal rigidity
    R19.35   Periumbilic abdominal rigidity
    R19.36   Epigastric abdominal rigidity
    R19.37   Generalized abdominal rigidity
  R19.4   Change in bowel habit
    Excludes 1: constipation (K59.0-)
            functional diarrhea (K59.1)
  R19.5   Other fecal abnormalities
    Abnormal stool color
    Bulky stools
    Mucus in stools
    Occult blood in feces
    Occult blood in stools
    Excludes 1: melena (K92.1)
            neonatal melena (P54.1)
  R19.6   Halitosis
  R19.7   Diarrhea, unspecified
    Diarrhea NOS
    Excludes 1: functional diarrhea (K59.1)
            neonatal diarrhea (P78.3)
            psychogenic diarrhea (F45.8)
  R19.8   Other specified symptoms and signs involving the digestive system and abdomen

Symptoms and signs involving the skin and subcutaneous tissue (R20-R23)

Excludes ❷: symptoms relating to breast (N64.4-N64.5)

R20-   **Disturbances of skin sensation**
    Excludes 1: dissociative anesthesia and sensory loss (F44.6)
            psychogenic disturbances (F45.8)
  R20.0   Anesthesia of skin
  R20.1   Hypoesthesia of skin
  R20.2   Paresthesia of skin
    Formication
    Pins and needles
    Tingling skin
    Excludes 1: acroparesthesia (I73.8)
  R20.3   Hyperesthesia
  R20.8   Other disturbances of skin sensation
  R20.9   Unspecified disturbances of skin sensation

R21   **Rash and other nonspecific skin eruption**
    Includes: Rash NOS
    Excludes 1: specified type of rash — code to condition
            vesicular eruption (R23.8)

R 0 6 ı R 2 1

R22- <u>Localized swelling, mass and lump</u> of skin and subcutaneous tissue
Includes: Subcutaneous nodules (localized) (superficial)
Excludes 1: abnormal findings on diagnostic imaging (R90-R93)
edema (R60-)
enlarged lymph nodes (R59-)
localized adiposity (E65)
swelling of joint (M25.4-)

R22.0   Localized swelling, mass and lump, <u>head</u>
R22.1   Localized swelling, mass and lump, <u>neck</u>
R22.2   Localized swelling, mass and lump, <u>trunk</u>
Excludes 1:   intra-abdominal or pelvic mass and lump (R19.0-)
intra-abdominal or pelvic swelling (R19.0-)
Excludes❷: breast mass and lump (N63)

R22.3-   Localized swelling, mass and lump, <u>upper limb</u>
R22.30   Localized swelling, mass and lump, <u>unspecified</u> upper limb
R22.31   Localized swelling, mass and lump, <u>right</u> upper limb
R22.32   Localized swelling, mass and lump, <u>left</u> upper limb
R22.33   Localized swelling, mass and lump, upper limb, <u>bilateral</u>

R22.4-   Localized swelling, mass and lump, <u>lower limb</u>
R22.40   Localized swelling, mass and lump, <u>unspecified</u> lower limb
R22.41   Localized swelling, mass and lump, <u>right</u> lower limb
R22.42   Localized swelling, mass and lump, <u>left</u> lower limb
R22.43   Localized swelling, mass and lump, lower limb, <u>bilateral</u>

R22.9   Localized swelling, mass and lump, <u>unspecified</u>

R23-   Other skin changes
R23.0   Cyanosis
Excludes 1:   acrocyanosis (I73.8)
cyanotic attacks of newborn (P28.2)

R23.1   Pallor
Clammy skin

R23.2   Flushing
Excessive blushing
Code first, if applicable, menopausal and female climacteric states
(N95.1)

R23.3   Spontaneous ecchymoses
Petechiae
Excludes 1:   ecchymoses of newborn (P54.5)
purpura (D69.-)

R23.4   Changes in skin texture
Desquamation of skin
Induration of skin
Scaling of skin
Excludes 1: epidermal thickening NOS (L85.9)

R23.8   Other skin changes
R23.9   Unspecified skin changes

Symptoms and signs involving the nervous and musculoskeletal systems (R25-R29)

R25-   Abnormal involuntary movements
Excludes 1:   specific movement disorders (G20-G26)
stereotyped movement disorders (F98.4)
tic disorders (F95.-)

R25.0   Abnormal head movements
R25.1   Tremor, unspecified
Excludes 1:   chorea NOS (G25.5)
essential tremor (G25.0)
hysterical tremor (F44.4)
intention tremor (G25.2)

R25.2   Cramp and spasm
Excludes❷: carpopedal spasm (R29.0)
charley-horse (M62.831)
infantile spasms (G40.4-)
muscle spasm of back (M62.830)
muscle spasm of calf (M62.831)

R25.3   Fasciculation
Twitching NOS

R25.8   Other abnormal involuntary movements
R25.9   Unspecified abnormal involuntary movements

R26-   Abnormalities of gait and mobility
Excludes 1:   ataxia NOS (R27.0)
hereditary ataxia (G11.-)
locomotor (syphilitic) ataxia (A52.11)
immobility syndrome (paraplegic) (M62.3)

R26.0   Ataxic gait
Staggering gait

R26.1   Paralytic gait
Spastic gait

R26.2   Difficulty in walking, <u>not elsewhere classified</u>
Excludes 1: falling (R29.6)
unsteadiness on feet (R26.81)

R26.8-   Other abnormalities of gait and mobility
R26.81   Unsteadiness on feet
R26.89   Other abnormalities of gait and mobility
R26.9   Unspecified abnormalities of gait and mobility

R27-   Other lack of coordination
Excludes 1: ataxic gait (R26.0)
hereditary ataxia (G11.-)
vertigo NOS (R42)

R27.0   Ataxia, unspecified
*Excludes 1: ataxia following cerebrovascular disease (I69. with
final characters -93)*

R27.8   Other lack of coordination
R27.9   Unspecified lack of coordination

R29-   Other symptoms and signs involving the nervous and musculoskeletal
systems
R29.0   Tetany
Carpopedal spasm
Excludes 1:   hysterical tetany (F44.5)
neonatal tetany (P71.3)
parathyroid tetany (E20.9)
post-thyroidectomy tetany (E89.2)

R29.1   Meningismus
R29.2   Abnormal reflex
Excludes❷: abnormal pupillary reflex (H57.0)
hyperactive gag reflex (J39.2)
vasovagal reaction or syncope (R55)

R29.3   Abnormal posture
R29.4   Clicking hip
Excludes 1: congenital deformities of hip (Q65.-)

R29.5   Transient paralysis
Code first any associated spinal cord injury (S14.0, S14.1-, S24.0,
S24.1-, S34.0-, S34.1-)
Excludes 1:   transient ischemic attack (G45.9)

R29.6   Repeated falls
Falling
Tendency to fall
Excludes❷: at risk for falling (Z91.81)
history of falling (Z91.81)

R29.8-   Other symptoms and signs involving the nervous and
musculoskeletal systems
R29.81-   Other symptoms and signs involving the nervous system
R29.810   Facial weakness
Facial droop
Excludes 1:   Bell's palsy (G51.0)
*facial weakness following cerebrovascular
disease (I69. with final characters-92)*

R29.818   Other symptoms and signs involving the nervous
system
R29.89-   Other symptoms and signs involving the musculoskeletal
system
Excludes❷: pain in limb (M79.6-)
R29.890   Loss of height
Excludes 1:   osteoporosis (M80-M81)
R29.891   Ocular torticollis
Excludes 1:   congenital (sternomastoid) torticollis Q68.0
psychogenic torticollis (F45.8)
spasmodic torticollis (G24.3)
torticollis due to birth injury (P15.8)
torticollis NOS M43.6
R29.898   Other symptoms and signs involving the
musculoskeletal system

R29.9-   Unspecified symptoms and signs involving the nervous and
musculoskeletal systems
R29.90   Unspecified symptoms and signs involving the nervous
system
R29.91   Unspecified symptoms and signs involving the
musculoskeletal system

Symptoms and signs involving the genitourinary system (R30-R39)

R30-   Pain associated with micturition
Excludes 1: psychogenic pain associated with micturition (F45.8)
R30.0   Dysuria
Strangury
R30.1   Vesical tenesmus
R30.9   Painful micturition, unspecified
Painful urination NOS

Excludes 1: = NOT CODED HERE! (Do not code both)

Excludes❷ = Not Included Here

**R
2
2
-
R
4
0**

R31-   Hematuria
  Excludes 1:   hematuria included with underlying conditions, such as:
      acute cystitis with hematuria (N30.01)
      recurrent and persistent hematuria in glomerular diseases
         (N02.-)
  R31.0   Gross hematuria
  R31.1   Benign essential microscopic hematuria
  R31.2   Other microscopic hematuria
  R31.9   Hematuria, unspecified
R32   Unspecified urinary incontinence
      Enuresis NOS
  Excludes 1:   functional urinary incontinence (R39.81)
      nonorganic enuresis (F98.0)
      stress incontinence and other specified urinary incontinence
         (N39.3-N39.4-)
      urinary incontinence associated with cognitive impairment
         (R39.81)
R33-   Retention of urine
  Excludes 1:   psychogenic retention of urine (F45.8)
  R33.0   Drug-induced retention of urine
      Use additional code for adverse effect, if applicable, to identify drug
         (T36-T50 with fifth or sixth character 5)
  R33.8   Other retention of urine
      Code first, if applicable, any causal condition, such as:
         Enlarged prostate (N40.1)
  R33.9   Retention of urine, unspecified
R34   Anuria and oliguria
  Excludes 1:   anuria and oliguria complicating abortion or ectopic or molar
      pregnancy (O00-O07, O08.4)
      anuria and oliguria complicating pregnancy (O26.83-)
      anuria and oliguria complicating the puerperium (O90.4)
R35-   Polyuria
      Code first, if applicable, any causal condition, such as:
         Enlarged prostate (N40.1)
  Excludes 1:   psychogenic polyuria (F45.8)
  R35.0   Frequency of micturition
  R35.1   Nocturia
  R35.8   Other polyuria
      Polyuria NOS
R36-   Urethral discharge
  R36.0   Urethral discharge without blood
  R36.1   Hematospermia
  R36.9   Urethral discharge, unspecified
      Penile discharge NOS
      Urethrorrhea
R37   Sexual dysfunction, unspecified
**R39-   Other and unspecified symptoms and signs involving the genitourinary
    system**
  R39.0   Extravasation of urine
  R39.1-   Other difficulties with micturition
      Code first, if applicable, any causal condition, such as:
         Enlarged prostate (N40.1)
    R39.11   Hesitancy of micturition
    R39.12   Poor urinary stream
        Weak urinary steam
    R39.13   Splitting of urinary stream
    R39.14   Feeling of incomplete bladder emptying
    R39.15   Urgency of urination
        Excludes 1:   urge incontinence (N39.41, N39.46)
    R39.16   Straining to void
    R39.19   Other difficulties with micturition
  R39.2   Extrarenal uremia
      Prerenal uremia
      Excludes 1:   uremia NOS (N19)
  R39.8-   Other symptoms and signs involving the genitourinary system
    R39.81   Functional urinary incontinence
        Urinary incontinence due to cognitive impairment, or severe
           physical disability or immobility
        Excludes 1:   stress incontinence and other specified urinary
           incontinence (N39.3-N39.4-)
           urinary incontinence NOS (R32)
    **R39.89   Other symptoms and signs involving the genitourinary
        system**
  **R39.9   Unspecified symptoms and signs involving the genitourinary
      system**

Symptoms and signs involving cognition, perception, emotional state and behavior (R40-R46)

*Excludes 1:   symptoms and signs constituting part of a pattern of mental
      disorder (F01-F99)*

R40-   Somnolence, stupor and coma
  Excludes 1:   neonatal coma (P91.5)
      somnolence, stupor and coma in diabetes (E08-E13)
      somnolence, stupor and coma in hepatic failure (K72-)
      somnolence, stupor and coma in hypoglycemia (nondiabetic) (E15)
  R40.0   Somnolence
      Drowsiness
      Excludes 1:   coma (R40.2-)
  R40.1   Stupor
      Catatonic stupor
      Semicoma
      Excludes 1:   catatonic schizophrenia (F20.2)
         coma (R40.2-)
         depressive stupor (F31-F33)
         dissociative stupor (F44.2)
         manic stupor (F30.2)
  R40.2-   Coma
      Code first any associated:
         Fracture of skull (S02.-)
         Intracranial injury (S06.-)
      Note: One code from subcategories R40.21-R40.23 is required to
         complete the coma scale
    R40.20   Unspecified coma
        Coma NOS
        Unconsciousness NOS
    R40.21-   Coma scale, eyes open
        **The following appropriate 7th character is to be added to
           subcategory R40.21-:**
        0 - Unspecified time
        1 - In the field [EMT or ambulance]
        2 - At arrival to emergency department
        3 - At hospital admission
        4 - 24 hours or more after hospital admission
      R40.211-   Coma scale, eyes open, never
      R40.212-   Coma scale, eyes open, to pain
      R40.213-   Coma scale, eyes open, to sound
      R40.214-   Coma scale, eyes open, spontaneous
    R40.22-   Coma scale, best verbal response
        **The following appropriate 7th character is to be added to
           subcategory R40.22-:**
        0 - Unspecified time
        1 - In the field [EMT or ambulance]
        2 - At arrival to emergency department
        3 - At hospital admission
        4 - 24 hours or more after hospital admission
      R40.221-   Coma scale, best verbal response, none
      **R40.222-   Coma scale, best verbal response, incomprehensible
          words**
      R40.223-   Coma scale, best verbal response, inappropriate words
      **R40.224-   Coma scale, best verbal response, confused
          conversation**
      R40.225-   Coma scale, best verbal response, oriented
    R40.23-   Coma scale, best motor response
        **The following appropriate 7th character is to be added to
           subcategory R40.23-:**
        0 - Unspecified time
        1 - In the field [EMT or ambulance]
        2 - At arrival to emergency department
        3 - At hospital admission
        4 - 24 hours or more after hospital admission
      R40.231-   Coma scale, best motor response, none
      R40.232-   Coma scale, best motor response, extension
      R40.233-   Coma scale, best motor response, abnormal
      R40.234-   Coma scale, best motor response, flexion withdrawal
      R40.235-   Coma scale, best motor response, localizes pain
      R40.236-   Coma scale, best motor response, obeys commands
    R40.24-   Glasgow coma scale, total score
        Use codes R40.21- through R40.23- only when the individual
           score(s) are documented
      R40.241   Glasgow coma scale score 13-15
      R40.242   Glasgow coma scale score 9-12
      R40.243   Glasgow coma scale score 3-8
      **R40.244   Other coma, without documented Glasgow coma scale
          score, or with partial score reported**
  R40.3   Persistent vegetative state
  R40.4   Transient alteration of awareness

R
2
2
|
R
4
0

R41- **Other symptoms and signs involving cognitive functions and awareness**
  Excludes 1:   dissociative [conversion] disorders (F44-)
  mild cognitive impairment, so stated (G31.84)

R41.0 **Disorientation, unspecified**
  Confusion NOS
  Delirium NOS

R41.1 **Anterograde amnesia**

R41.2 **Retrograde amnesia**

R41.3 **Other amnesia**
  Amnesia NOS
  Memory loss NOS
  Excludes 1:   amnestic disorder due to known physiologic condition (F04)
  amnestic syndrome due to psychoactive substance use (F10-F19 with 5th character .6)
  mild memory disturbance due to known physiological condition (F06.8)
  transient global amnesia (G45.4)

R41.4 **Neurologic neglect syndrome**
  Asomatognosia
  Hemi-akinesia
  Hemi-inattention
  Hemispatial neglect
  Left-sided neglect
  Sensory neglect
  Visuospatial neglect
  Excludes 1:   visuospatial deficit (R41.842)

R41.8- **Other symptoms and signs involving cognitive functions and awareness**
  R41.81 **Age-related cognitive decline**
    Senility NOS
  R41.82 **Altered mental status, unspecified**
    Change in mental status NOS
    Excludes 1:   altered level of consciousness (R40.-)
    altered mental status due to known condition — code to condition
    delirium NOS (R41.0)
  R41.83 **Borderline intellectual functioning**
    IQ level 71 to 84
    Excludes 1:   intellectual disabilities (F70-F79)
  R41.84- **Other specified cognitive deficit**
    R41.840 **Attention and concentration deficit**
      Excludes 1:   attention-deficit hyperactivity disorders (F90.-)
    R41.841 **Cognitive communication deficit**
    R41.842 **Visuospatial deficit**
    R41.843 **Psychomotor deficit**
    R41.844 **Frontal lobe and executive function deficit**
  R41.89 **Other symptoms and signs involving cognitive functions and awareness**
    Anosognosia

R41.9 **Unspecified symptoms and signs involving cognitive functions and awareness**

R42 **Dizziness and giddiness**
  Light-headedness
  Vertigo NOS
  Excludes 1:   vertiginous syndromes (H81.-)
  vertigo from infrasound (T75.23)

R43- **Disturbances of smell and taste**
  R43.0 **Anosmia**
  R43.1 **Parosmia**
  R43.2 **Parageusia**
  R43.8 **Other disturbances of smell and taste**
    Mixed disturbance of smell and taste
  R43.9 **Unspecified disturbances of smell and taste**

R44- **Other symptoms and signs involving general sensations and perceptions**
  Excludes 1:   alcoholic hallucinations (F1.5)
  hallucinations in drug psychosis (F11-F19 with .5)
  hallucinations in mood disorders with psychotic symptoms (F30.2, F31.5, F32.3, F33.3)
  hallucinations in schizophrenia, schizotypal and delusional disorders (F20-F29)
  Excludes❷: disturbances of skin sensation (R20.-)
  R44.0 **Auditory hallucinations**
  R44.1 **Visual hallucinations**
  R44.2 **Other hallucinations**
  R44.3 **Hallucinations, unspecified**
  R44.8 **Other symptoms and signs involving general sensations and perceptions**
  R44.9 **Unspecified symptoms and signs involving general sensations and perceptions**

R45- **Symptoms and signs involving emotional state**
  R45.0 **Nervousness**
    Nervous tension
  R45.1 **Restlessness and agitation**
  R45.2 **Unhappiness**
  R45.3 **Demoralization and apathy**
    Excludes 1:   anhedonia (R45.84)
  R45.4 **Irritability and anger**
  R45.5 **Hostility**
  R45.6 **Violent behavior**
  R45.7 **State of emotional shock and stress, unspecified**
  R45.8- **Other symptoms and signs involving emotional state**
    R45.81 **Low self-esteem**
    R45.82 **Worries**
    R45.83 **Excessive crying of child, adolescent or adult**
      Excludes 1:   excessive crying of infant (baby) R68.11
    R45.84 **Anhedonia**
    R45.85- **Homicidal and suicidal ideations**
      Excludes 1:   suicide attempt (T14.91)
      R45.850 **Homicidal ideations**
      R45.851 **Suicidal ideations**
    R45.86 **Emotional lability**
    R45.87 **Impulsiveness**
    R45.89 **Other symptoms and signs involving emotional state**

R46- **Symptoms and signs involving appearance and behavior**
  Excludes 1:   appearance and behavior in schizophrenia, schizotypal and delusional disorders (F20-F29)
  mental and behavioral disorders (F01-F99)
  R46.0 **Very low level of personal hygiene**
  R46.1 **Bizarre personal appearance**
  R46.2 **Strange and inexplicable behavior**
  R46.3 **Overactivity**
  R46.4 **Slowness and poor responsiveness**
    Excludes 1:   stupor (R40.1)
  R46.5 **Suspiciousness and marked evasiveness**
  R46.6 **Undue concern and preoccupation with stressful events**
  R46.7 **Verbosity and circumstantial detail obscuring reason for contact**
  R46.8- **Other symptoms and signs involving appearance and behavior**
    R46.81 **Obsessive-compulsive behavior**
      Excludes 1:   obsessive-compulsive disorder (F42)
    R46.89 **Other symptoms and signs involving appearance and behavior**

Symptoms and signs involving speech and voice (R47-R49)

R47- **Speech disturbances, not elsewhere classified**
  Excludes 1:   autism (F84.0)
  cluttering (F80.81)
  specific developmental disorders of speech and language (F80.-)
  stuttering (F80.81)
  R47.0- **Dysphasia and aphasia**
    R47.01 **Aphasia**
      Excludes 1:   aphasia following cerebrovascular disease (I69. with final characters -20)
      progressive isolated aphasia (G31.01)
    R47.02 **Dysphasia**
      Excludes 1:   dysphasia following cerebrovascular disease (I69. with final characters -21)
  R47.1 **Dysarthria and anarthria**
    Excludes 1:   dysarthria following cerebrovascular disease (I69. with final characters -22)
  R47.8- **Other speech disturbances**
    Excludes 1:   dysarthria following cerebrovascular disease (I69. with final characters -28)
    R47.81 **Slurred speech**
    R47.82 **Fluency disorder in conditions classified elsewhere**
      Stuttering in conditions classified elsewhere
      Code first underlying disease or condition, such as:
        Parkinson's disease (G20)
      Excludes 1:   adult onset fluency disorder (F98.5)
      childhood onset fluency disorder (F80.81)
      fluency disorder (stuttering) following cerebrovascular disease (I69. with final characters-23)
    R47.89 **Other speech disturbances**
  R47.9 **Unspecified speech disturbances**

R48- Dyslexia and other symbolic dysfunctions, not elsewhere classified
   Excludes 1: specific developmental disorders of scholastic skills (F81-)
   R48.0   Dyslexia and alexia
   R48.1   Agnosia
            Astereognosia (astereognosis)
            Autotopagnosia
            Excludes 1: visual object agnosia (R48.3)
   R48.2   Apraxia
            *Excludes 1: apraxia following cerebrovascular disease (I69. with
                        final characters -90)*
   R48.3   Visual agnosia
            Prosopagnosia
            Simultanagnosia (asimultagnosia)
   R48.8   Other symbolic dysfunctions
            Acalculia
            Agraphia
   R48.9   Unspecified symbolic dysfunctions

R49- Voice and resonance disorders
   Excludes 1: psychogenic voice and resonance disorders (F44.4)
   R49.0   Dysphonia
            Hoarseness
   R49.1   Aphonia
            Loss of voice
   R49.2-   Hypernasality and hyponasality
      R49.21   Hypernasality
      R49.22   Hyponasality
   R49.8   Other voice and resonance disorders
   R49.9   Unspecified voice and resonance disorder
            Change in voice NOS
            Resonance disorder NOS

General symptoms and signs (R50-R69)

R50- Fever of other and unknown origin
   Excludes 1: chills without fever (R68.83)
               febrile convulsions (R56.0-)
               fever of unknown origin during labor (O75.2)
               fever of unknown origin in newborn (P81.9)
               hypothermia due to illness (R68.0)
               malignant hyperthermia due to anesthesia (T88.3)
               puerperal pyrexia NOS (O86.4)
   R50.2   Drug-induced fever
            Use additional code for adverse effect, if applicable, to identify drug
               (T36-T50 with fifth or sixth character 5)
            Excludes 1: postvaccination (postimmunization) fever (R50.83)
   R50.8-   Other specified fever
      R50.81   Fever presenting with conditions classified elsewhere
               Code first underlying condition when associated fever is present,
                  such as with:
               Leukemia (C91-C95)
               Neutropenia (D70-)
               Sickle-cell disease (D57-)
      R50.82   Postprocedural fever
               Excludes 1: postprocedural infection (T81.4)
                           posttransfusion fever (R50.84)
                           postvaccination (postimmunization) fever (R50.83)
      R50.83   Postvaccination fever
               Postimmunization fever
      R50.84   Febrile nonhemolytic transfusion reaction
               FNHTR
               Posttransfusion fever
   R50.9   Fever, unspecified
            Fever NOS
            Fever of unknown origin [FUO]
            Fever with chills
            Fever with rigors
            Hyperpyrexia NOS
            Persistent fever
            Pyrexia NOS

R51   Headache
      Facial pain NOS
      Excludes 1: atypical face pain (G50.1)
                  migraine and other headache syndromes (G43-G44)
                  trigeminal neuralgia (G50.0)

R52   Pain, unspecified
      Acute pain NOS
      Generalized pain NOS
      Pain NOS
      Excludes 1: acute and chronic pain, not elsewhere classified (G89-)
                  *localized pain, unspecified type — code to pain by site, such
                     as:*
                     abdomen pain (R10-)
                     back pain (M54.9)
                     breast pain (N64.4)
                     chest pain (R07.1-R07.9)
                     ear pain (H92.0-)
                     eye pain (H57.1)
                     headache (R51)
                     joint pain (M25.5-)
                     limb pain (M79.6-)
                     lumbar region pain (M54.5)
                     pelvic and perineal pain (R10.2)
                     shoulder pain (M25.51-)
                     spine pain (M54-)
                     throat pain (R07.0)
                     tongue pain (K14.6)
                     tooth pain (K08.8)
                  *pain disorders exclusively related to psychological factors
                     (F45.41)*
                  renal colic (N23)

R53- Malaise and fatigue
   R53.0   Neoplastic (malignant) related fatigue
            Code first associated neoplasm
   R53.1   Weakness
            Asthenia NOS
            Excludes 1: age-related weakness (R54)
                        muscle weakness (M62.8-)
                        senile asthenia (R54)
   R53.2   Functional quadriplegia
            Complete immobility due to severe physical disability or frailty
            Excludes 1: frailty NOS (R54)
                        hysterical paralysis (F44.4)
                        immobility syndrome (M62.3)
                        neurologic quadriplegia (G82.5-)
                        quadriplegia (G82.50)
   R53.8-   Other malaise and fatigue
            Excludes 1: combat exhaustion and fatigue (F43.0)
                        congenital debility (P96.9)
                        exhaustion and fatigue due to depressive episode (F32.-)
                        *exhaustion and fatigue due to excessive exertion
                           (T73.3)*
                        exhaustion and fatigue due to exposure (T73.2)
                        exhaustion and fatigue due to heat (T67.-)
                        exhaustion and fatigue due to pregnancy (O26.8-)
                        *exhaustion and fatigue due to recurrent depressive
                           episode (F33)*
                        exhaustion and fatigue due to senile debility (R54)
      R53.81   Other malaise
               Chronic debility
               Debility NOS
               General physical deterioration
               Malaise NOS
               Nervous debility
               Excludes 1: age-related physical debility (R54)
      R53.82   Chronic fatigue, unspecified
               Chronic fatigue syndrome NOS
               Excludes 1: postviral fatigue syndrome (G93.3)
      R53.83   Other fatigue
               Fatigue NOS
               Lack of energy
               Lethargy
               Tiredness

R54   Age-related physical debility
      Frailty
      Old age
      Senescence
      Senile asthenia
      Senile debility
      Excludes 1: age-related cognitive decline (R41.81)
                  senile psychosis (F03)
                  senility NOS (R41.81)

R
4
1
-
R
5
4

Excludes 1: = NOT CODED HERE! (Do not code both)   **677**   *Excludes ❷: = Not Included Here*

R55   Syncope and collapse
Blackout
Fainting
Vasovagal attack
Excludes 1:   cardiogenic shock (R57.0)
carotid sinus syncope (G90.01)
heat syncope (T67.1)
neurocirculatory asthenia (F45.8)
neurogenic orthostatic hypotension (G90.3)
orthostatic hypotension (I95.1)
postprocedural shock (T81.1-)
psychogenic syncope (F48.8)
shock NOS (R57.9)
shock complicating or following abortion or ectopic or molar
pregnancy (O00-O07, O08.3)
shock complicating or following labor and delivery (O75.1)
Stokes-Adams attack (I45.9)
unconsciousness NOS (R40.2-)

R56- Convulsions, not elsewhere classified
Excludes 1:   dissociative convulsions and seizures (F44.5)
epileptic convulsions and seizures (G40.-)
newborn convulsions and seizures (P90)

  R56.0- Febrile convulsions
   R56.00 Simple febrile convulsions
Febrile convulsion NOS
Febrile seizure NOS
   R56.01 Complex febrile convulsions
Atypical febrile seizure
Complex febrile seizure
Complicated febrile seizure
Excludes 1: status epilepticus (G40.901)
  R56.1   Post traumatic seizures
Excludes 1: post traumatic epilepsy (G40.-)
  R56.9   Unspecified convulsions
Convulsion disorder
Fit NOS
Recurrent convulsions
Seizure(s) (convulsive) NOS

R57- Shock, not elsewhere classified
Excludes 1:   anaphylactic reaction or shock due to adverse food reaction
(T78.0-)
anaphylactic shock due to adverse effect of correct drug or
medicament properly administered (T88.6)
anaphylactic shock due to serum (T80.5-)
anaphylactic shock NOS (T78.2)
anesthetic shock (T88.3)
electric shock (T75.4)
obstetric shock (O75.1)
postprocedural shock (T81.1-)
psychic shock (F43.0)
septic shock (R65.21)
shock complicating or following ectopic or molar pregnancy
(O00-O07, O08.3)
shock due to lightning (T75.01)
traumatic shock (T79.4)
toxic shock syndrome (A48.3)

  R57.0   Cardiogenic shock
  R57.1   Hypovolemic shock
  R57.8   Other shock
  R57.9   Shock, unspecified
Failure of peripheral circulation NOS

R58   Hemorrhage, not elsewhere classified
Hemorrhage NOS
Excludes 1:   hemorrhage included with underlying conditions, such as:
acute duodenal ulcer with hemorrhage (K26.0)
acute gastritis with bleeding (K29.01)
ulcerative enterocolitis with rectal bleeding (K51.01)

R59- Enlarged lymph nodes
Includes: swollen glands
Excludes 1:   lymphadenitis NOS (I88.9)
acute lymphadenitis (L04.-)
chronic lymphadenitis (I88.1)
mesenteric (acute) (chronic) lymphadenitis (I88.0)

  R59.0   Localized enlarged lymph nodes
  R59.1   Generalized enlarged lymph nodes
Lymphadenopathy NOS
  R59.9   Enlarged lymph nodes, unspecified

R60- Edema, not elsewhere classified
Excludes 1:   angioneurotic edema (T78.3)
ascites (R18-)
cerebral edema (G93.6)
cerebral edema due to birth injury (P11.0)
edema of larynx (J38.4)
edema of nasopharynx (J39.2)
edema of pharynx (J39.2)
gestational edema (O12.0-)
hereditary edema (Q82.0)
hydrops fetalis NOS (P83.2)
hydrothorax (J94.8)
newborn edema (P83.3)
nutritional edema (E40-E46)
pulmonary edema (J81-)

  R60.0   Localized edema
  R60.1   Generalized edema
  R60.9   Edema, unspecified
Fluid retention NOS

R61   Generalized hyperhidrosis
Excessive sweating
Night sweats
Secondary hyperhidrosis
Code first, if applicable, menopausal and female climacteric states (N95.1)
Excludes 1:   focal (primary) (secondary) hyperhidrosis (L74.5-)
Frey's syndrome (L74.52)
localized (primary) (secondary) hyperhidrosis (L74.5-)

R62- Lack of expected normal physiological development in childhood and
adults
Excludes 1:   delayed puberty (E30.0)
gonadal dysgenesis (Q99.1)
hypopituitarism (E23.0)

  R62.0   Delayed milestone in childhood
Delayed attainment of expected physiological developmental stage
Late talker
Late walker
  R62.5- Other and unspecified lack of expected normal physiological
development in childhood
Excludes 1:   HIV disease resulting in failure to thrive (B20)
physical retardation due to malnutrition (E45)
   R62.50 Unspecified lack of expected normal physiological
development in childhood
Infantilism NOS
   R62.51 Failure to thrive (child)
Failure to gain weight
Excludes 1: failure to thrive in child under 28 days old (P92.6)
   R62.52 Short stature (child)
Lack of growth
Physical retardation
Short stature NOS
Excludes 1: short stature due to endocrine disorder (E34.3)
   R62.59 Other lack of expected normal physiological development in
childhood
  R62.7   Adult failure to thrive

R63- Symptoms and signs concerning food and fluid intake
Excludes 1:   bulimia NOS (F50.2)
eating disorders of nonorganic origin (F50.-)
malnutrition (E40-E46)

  R63.0   Anorexia
Loss of appetite
Excludes 1: anorexia nervosa (F50.0-)
loss of appetite of nonorganic origin (F50.8)
  R63.1   Polydipsia
Excessive thirst
  R63.2   Polyphagia
Excessive eating
Hyperalimentation NOS
  R63.3   Feeding difficulties
Feeding problem (elderly) (infant) NOS
Excludes 1: feeding problems of newborn (P92.-)
infant feeding disorder of nonorganic origin (F98.2-)
  R63.4   Abnormal weight loss
  R63.5   Abnormal weight gain
Excludes 1: excessive weight gain in pregnancy (O26.0-)
obesity (E66.-)
  R63.6   Underweight
Use additional code to identify body mass index (BMI), if known
(Z68.-)
Excludes 1: abnormal weight loss (R63.4)
anorexia nervosa (F50.0-)
malnutrition (E40-E46)
  R63.8   Other symptoms and signs concerning food and fluid intake

R64   Cachexia
Wasting syndrome
Code first underlying condition, if known
Excludes 1:   abnormal weight loss (R63.4)
nutritional marasmus (E41)

R65-   Symptoms and signs specifically associated with systemic inflammation and infection

R65.1-   Systemic inflammatory response syndrome (SIRS) of non-infectious origin
Code first underlying condition, such as:
Heatstroke (T67.0)
Injury and trauma (S00-T88)
Excludes 1:   sepsis — code to infection
severe sepsis (R65.2)

R65.10   Systemic inflammatory response syndrome (SIRS) of non-infectious origin without acute organ dysfunction
Systemic inflammatory response syndrome (SIRS) NOS

R65.11   Systemic inflammatory response syndrome (SIRS) of non-infectious origin with acute organ dysfunction
Use additional code to identify specific acute organ dysfunction, such as:
Acute kidney failure (N17.-)
Acute respiratory failure (J96.0-)
Critical illness myopathy (G72.81)
Critical illness polyneuropathy (G62.81)
Disseminated intravascular coagulopathy [DIC] (D65)
Encephalopathy (metabolic) (septic) (G93.41)
Hepatic failure (K72.0-)

R65.2-   Severe sepsis
Infection with associated acute organ dysfunction
Sepsis with acute organ dysfunction
Sepsis with multiple organ dysfunction
Systemic inflammatory response syndrome due to infectious process with acute organ dysfunction
Code first underlying infection, such as:
Infection following a procedure (T81.4)
Infections following infusion, transfusion and therapeutic injection (T80.2-)
Puerperal sepsis (O85)
Sepsis following complete or unspecified spontaneous abortion (O03.87)
Sepsis following ectopic and molar pregnancy (O08.82)
Sepsis following incomplete spontaneous abortion (O03.37)
Sepsis following (induced) termination of pregnancy (O04.87)
Sepsis NOS (A41.9)
Use additional code to identify specific acute organ dysfunction, such as:
Acute kidney failure (N17.-)
Acute respiratory failure (J96.0-)
Critical illness myopathy (G72.81)
Critical illness polyneuropathy (G62.81)
Disseminated intravascular coagulopathy [DIC] (D65)
Encephalopathy (metabolic) (septic) (G93.41)
Hepatic failure (K72.0-)

R65.20   Severe sepsis without septic shock
Severe sepsis NOS

R65.21   Severe sepsis with septic shock

R68-   Other general symptoms and signs

R68.0   Hypothermia, not associated with low environmental temperature
Excludes 1:   hypothermia NOS (accidental) (T68)
hypothermia due to anesthesia (T88.51)
hypothermia due to low environmental temperature (T68)
newborn hypothermia (P80.-)

R68.1-   Nonspecific symptoms peculiar to infancy
Excludes 1:   colic, infantile (R10.83)
neonatal cerebral irritability (P91.3)
teething syndrome (K00.7)

R68.11   Excessive crying of infant (baby)
Excludes 1:   excessive crying of child, adolescent, or adult (R45.83)

R68.12   Fussy infant (baby)
Irritable infant

R68.13   Apparent life threatening event in infant (ALTE)
Apparent life threatening event in newborn
Code first confirmed diagnosis, if known
Use additional code(s) for associated signs and symptoms if no confirmed diagnosis established, or if signs and symptoms are not associated routinely with confirmed diagnosis, or provide additional information for cause of ALTE

R68.19   Other nonspecific symptoms peculiar to infancy

R68.2   Dry mouth, unspecified
Excludes 1:   dry mouth due to dehydration (E86.0)
dry mouth due to sicca syndrome [Sjögren] (M35.0-)
salivary gland hyposecretion (K11.7)

R68.3   Clubbing of fingers
Clubbing of nails
Excludes 1:   congenital clubfinger (Q68.1)

R68.8-   Other general symptoms and signs

R68.81   Early satiety

R68.82   Decreased libido
Decreased sexual desire

R68.83   Chills (without fever)
Chills NOS
Excludes 1:   chills with fever (R50.9)

R68.84   Jaw pain
Mandibular pain
Maxilla pain
Excludes 1:   temporomandibular joint arthralgia (M26.62)

R68.89   Other general symptoms and signs

R69   Illness, unspecified
Unknown and unspecified cases of morbidity

Abnormal findings on examination of blood, without diagnosis (R70-R79)

Excludes 1:   abnormalities (of) (on):
abnormal findings on antenatal screening of mother (O28.-)
coagulation hemorrhagic disorders (D65-D68)
lipids (E78.-)
platelets and thrombocytes (D69.-)
white blood cells classified elsewhere (D70-D72)
diagnostic abnormal findings classified elsewhere — see Alphabetical Index
hemorrhagic and hematological disorders of newborn (P50-P61)

R70-   Elevated erythrocyte sedimentation rate and abnormality of plasma viscosity

R70.0   Elevated erythrocyte sedimentation rate

R70.1   Abnormal plasma viscosity

R71-   Abnormality of red blood cells
Excludes 1:   anemias (D50-D64)
anemia of premature infant (P61.2)
benign (familial) polycythemia (D75.0)
congenital anemias (P61.2-P61.4)
newborn anemia due to isoimmunization (P55.-)
polycythemia neonatorum (P61.1)
polycythemia NOS (D75.1)
polycythemia vera (D45)
secondary polycythemia (D75.1)

R71.0   Precipitous drop in hematocrit
Drop (precipitous) in hemoglobin
Drop in hematocrit

R71.8   Other abnormality of red blood cells
Abnormal red-cell morphology NOS
Abnormal red-cell volume NOS
Anisocytosis
Poikilocytosis

R73-   Elevated blood glucose level
Excludes 1:   diabetes mellitus (E08-E13)
diabetes mellitus in pregnancy, childbirth and the puerperium (O24.-)
neonatal disorders (P70.0-P70.2)
postsurgical hypoinsulinemia (E89.1)

R73.0-   Abnormal glucose
Excludes 1:   abnormal glucose in pregnancy (O99.81-)
diabetes mellitus (E08-E13)
dysmetabolic syndrome X (E88.81)
gestational diabetes (O24.4-)
glycosuria (R81)
hypoglycemia (E16.2)

R73.01   Impaired fasting glucose
Elevated fasting glucose

R73.02   Impaired glucose tolerance (oral)
Elevated glucose tolerance

R73.09   Other abnormal glucose
Abnormal glucose NOS
Abnormal non-fasting glucose tolerance
Latent diabetes
Prediabetes

R73.9   Hyperglycemia, unspecified

R
5
5
–
R
7
3

Excludes 1: = NOT CODED HERE! (Do not code both)   **679**   *Excludes ❷: = Not Included Here*

R74- Abnormal serum enzyme levels

R74.0 Nonspecific elevation of levels of transaminase and lactic acid dehydrogenase [LDH]

R74.8 Abnormal levels of other serum enzymes
Abnormal level of acid phosphatase
Abnormal level of alkaline phosphatase
Abnormal level of amylase
Abnormal level of lipase [triacylglycerol lipase]

R74.9 Abnormal serum enzyme level, unspecified

R75 Inconclusive laboratory evidence of human immunodeficiency virus [HIV]
Nonconclusive HIV-test finding in infants
Excludes 1: asymptomatic human immunodeficiency virus [HIV] infection status (Z21)
human immunodeficiency virus [HIV] disease (B20)

R76- Other abnormal immunological findings in serum

R76.0 Raised antibody titer
Excludes 1: isoimmunization in pregnancy (O36.0-O36.1)
isoimmunization affecting newborn (P55-)

R76.1- Nonspecific reaction to test for tuberculosis

R76.11 Nonspecific reaction to tuberculin skin test without active tuberculosis
Abnormal result of Mantoux test
PPD positive
Tuberculin (skin test) positive
Tuberculin (skin test) reactor
Excludes 1: nonspecific reaction to cell mediated immunity measurement of gamma interferon antigen response without active tuberculosis (R76.12)

R76.12 Nonspecific reaction to cell mediated immunity measurement of gamma interferon antigen response without active tuberculosis
Nonspecific reaction to QuantiFERON-TB test (QFT) without active tuberculosis
Excludes 1: nonspecific reaction to tuberculin skin test without active tuberculosis (R76.11)
positive tuberculin skin test (R76.11)

R76.8 Other specified abnormal immunological findings in serum
Raised level of immunoglobulins NOS

R76.9 Abnormal immunological finding in serum, unspecified

R77- Other abnormalities of plasma proteins
Excludes 1: disorders of plasma-protein metabolism (E88.0)

R77.0 Abnormality of albumin

R77.1 Abnormality of globulin
Hyperglobulinemia NOS

R77.2 Abnormality of alphafetoprotein

R77.8 Other specified abnormalities of plasma proteins

R77.9 Abnormality of plasma protein, unspecified

R78- Findings of drugs and other substances, not normally found in blood
Use additional code to identify the any retained foreign body, if applicable (Z18.-)
Excludes 1: mental or behavioral disorders due to psychoactive substance use (F10-F19)

R78.0 Finding of alcohol in blood
Use additional external cause code (Y90.-), for detail regarding alcohol level

R78.1 Finding of opiate drug in blood

R78.2 Finding of cocaine in blood

R78.3 Finding of hallucinogen in blood

R78.4 Finding of other drugs of addictive potential in blood

R78.5 Finding of other psychotropic drug in blood

R78.6 Finding of steroid agent in blood

R78.7- Finding of abnormal level of heavy metals in blood

R78.71 Abnormal lead level in blood
Excludes 1: lead poisoning (T56.0-)

R78.79 Finding of abnormal level of heavy metals in blood

R78.8- Finding of other specified substances, not normally found in blood

R78.81 Bacteremia
Excludes 1: sepsis-code to specified infection (A00-B99)

R78.89 Finding of other specified substances, not normally found in blood
Finding of abnormal level of lithium in blood

R78.9 Finding of unspecified substance, not normally found in blood

R79- Other abnormal findings of blood chemistry
Use additional code to identify any retained foreign body, if applicable (Z18-)
Excludes 1: abnormality of fluid, electrolyte or acid-base balance (E86-E87)
asymptomatic hyperuricemia (E79.0)
hyperglycemia NOS (R73.9)
hypoglycemia NOS (E16.2)
neonatal hypoglycemia (P70.3-P70.4)
specific findings indicating disorder of amino-acid metabolism (E70-E72)
specific findings indicating disorder of carbohydrate metabolism (E73-E74)
specific findings indicating disorder of lipid metabolism (E75.-)

R79.0 Abnormal level of blood mineral
Abnormal blood level of cobalt
Abnormal blood level of copper
Abnormal blood level of iron
Abnormal blood level of magnesium
Abnormal blood level of mineral NEC
Abnormal blood level of zinc
Excludes 1: abnormal level of lithium (R78.89)
disorders of mineral metabolism (E83.-)
neonatal hypomagnesemia (P71.2)
nutritional mineral deficiency (E58-E61)

R79.1 Abnormal coagulation profile
Abnormal or prolonged bleeding time
Abnormal or prolonged coagulation time
Abnormal or prolonged partial thromboplastin time [PTT]
Abnormal or prolonged prothrombin time [PT]
Excludes 1: coagulation defects (D68.-)

R79.8- Other specified abnormal findings of blood chemistry

R79.81 Abnormal blood-gas level

R79.82 Elevated C-reactive protein (CRP)

R79.89 Other specified abnormal findings of blood chemistry

R79.9 Abnormal finding of blood chemistry, unspecified

Abnormal findings on examination of urine, without diagnosis (R80-R82)

Excludes 1: abnormal findings on antenatal screening of mother (O28.-)
diagnostic abnormal findings classified elsewhere — see Alphabetical Index
specific findings indicating disorder of amino-acid metabolism (E70-E72)
specific findings indicating disorder of carbohydrate metabolism (E73-E74)

R80- Proteinuria
Excludes 1: gestational proteinuria (O12.1-)

R80.0 Isolated proteinuria
Idiopathic proteinuria
Excludes 1: isolated proteinuria with specific morphological lesion (N06.-)

R80.1 Persistent proteinuria, unspecified

R80.2 Orthostatic proteinuria, unspecified
Postural proteinuria

R80.3 Bence Jones proteinuria

R80.8 Other proteinuria

R80.9 Proteinuria, unspecified
Albuminuria NOS

R81 Glycosuria
Excludes 1: renal glycosuria (E74.8)

R82- Other and unspecified abnormal findings in urine
Includes: Chromoabnormalities in urine
Use additional code to identify any retained foreign body, if applicable (Z18.-)
Excludes❷: hematuria (R31.-)

R82.0 Chyluria
Excludes 1: filarial chyluria (B74.-)

R82.1 Myoglobinuria

R82.2 Biliuria

R82.3 Hemoglobinuria
Excludes 1: hemoglobinuria due to hemolysis from external causes NEC (D59.6)
hemoglobinuria due to paroxysmal nocturnal [Marchiafava-Micheli] (D59.5)

R82.4 Acetonuria
Ketonuria

R82.5 Elevated urine levels of drugs, medicaments and biological substances
Elevated urine levels of catecholamines
Elevated urine levels of indoleacetic acid
Elevated urine levels of 17-ketosteroids
Elevated urine levels of steroids

R 7 4 - R 8 5

R82.6   Abnormal urine levels of substances chiefly nonmedicinal as to source
Abnormal urine level of heavy metals

R82.7   Abnormal findings on microbiological examination of urine
Positive culture findings of urine
Excludes 1: colonization status (Z22.-)

R82.8   Abnormal findings on cytological and histological examination of urine

R82.9-   Other and unspecified abnormal findings in urine

   R82.90   Unspecified abnormal findings in urine

   R82.91   Other chromoabnormalities of urine
Chromoconversion (dipstick)
Idiopathic dipstick converts positive for blood with no cellular forms in sediment
Excludes 1: hemoglobinuria (R82.3)
myoglobinuria (R82.1)

   R82.99   Other abnormal findings in urine
Cells and casts in urine
Crystalluria
Melanuria

Abnormal findings on examination of other body fluids, substances and tissues, without diagnosis (R83-R89)

Excludes 1: abnormal findings on antenatal screening of mother (O28.-)
diagnostic abnormal findings classified elsewhere — see Alphabetical Index
Excludes❷: abnormal findings on examination of blood, without diagnosis (R70-R79)
abnormal findings on examination of urine, without diagnosis (R80-R82)
abnormal tumor markers (R97.-)

R83-   Abnormal findings in cerebrospinal fluid

R83.0   Abnormal level of enzymes in cerebrospinal fluid

R83.1   Abnormal level of hormones in cerebrospinal fluid

R83.2   Abnormal level of other drugs, medicaments and biological substances in cerebrospinal fluid

R83.3   Abnormal level of substances chiefly nonmedicinal as to source in cerebrospinal fluid

R83.4   Abnormal immunological findings in cerebrospinal fluid

R83.5   Abnormal microbiological findings in cerebrospinal fluid
Positive culture findings in cerebrospinal fluid
Excludes 1: colonization status (Z22.-)

R83.6   Abnormal cytological findings in cerebrospinal fluid

R83.8   Other abnormal findings in cerebrospinal fluid
Abnormal chromosomal findings in cerebrospinal fluid

R83.9   Unspecified abnormal finding in cerebrospinal fluid

R84-   Abnormal findings in specimens from respiratory organs and thorax
Includes: Abnormal findings in bronchial washings
Abnormal findings in nasal secretions
Abnormal findings in pleural fluid
Abnormal findings in sputum
Abnormal findings in throat scrapings
Excludes 1: blood-stained sputum (R04.2)

R84.0   Abnormal level of enzymes in specimens from respiratory organs and thorax

R84.1   Abnormal level of hormones in specimens from respiratory organs and thorax

R84.2   Abnormal level of other drugs, medicaments and biological substances in specimens from respiratory organs and thorax

R84.3   Abnormal level of substances chiefly nonmedicinal as to source in specimens from respiratory organs and thorax

R84.4   Abnormal immunological findings in specimens from respiratory organs and thorax

R84.5   Abnormal microbiological findings in specimens from respiratory organs and thorax
Positive culture findings in specimens from respiratory organs and thorax
Excludes 1: colonization status (Z22.-)

R84.6   Abnormal cytological findings in specimens from respiratory organs and thorax

R84.7   Abnormal histological findings in specimens from respiratory organs and thorax

R84.8   Other abnormal findings in specimens from respiratory organs and thorax
Abnormal chromosomal findings in specimens from respiratory organs and thorax

R84.9   Unspecified abnormal finding in specimens from respiratory organs and thorax

R85-   Abnormal findings in specimens from digestive organs and abdominal cavity
Includes: Abnormal findings in peritoneal fluid
Abnormal findings in saliva
Excludes 1: cloudy peritoneal dialysis effluent (R88.0)
fecal abnormalities (R19.5)

R85.0   Abnormal level of enzymes in specimens from digestive organs and abdominal cavity

R85.1   Abnormal level of hormones in specimens from digestive organs and abdominal cavity

R85.2   Abnormal level of other drugs, medicaments and biological substances in specimens from digestive organs and abdominal cavity

R85.3   Abnormal level of substances chiefly nonmedicinal as to source in specimens from digestive organs and abdominal cavity

R85.4   Abnormal immunological findings in specimens from digestive organs and abdominal cavity

R85.5   Abnormal microbiological findings in specimens from digestive organs and abdominal cavity
Positive culture findings in specimens from digestive organs and abdominal cavity
Excludes 1: colonization status (Z22.-)

R85.6-   Abnormal cytological findings in specimens from digestive organs and abdominal cavity

   R85.61- Abnormal cytologic smear of anus
Excludes 1: abnormal cytological findings in specimens from other digestive organs and abdominal cavity (R85.69)
anal intraepithelial neoplasia I [AIN I] (K62.82)
anal intraepithelial neoplasia II [AIN II] (K62.82)
anal intraepithelial neoplasia III [AIN III] (D01.3)
carcinoma in situ of anus (histologically confirmed) (D01.3)
dysplasia (mild) (moderate) of anus (histologically confirmed) (K62.82)
severe dysplasia of anus (histologically confirmed) (D01.3)
Excludes❷: anal high risk human papillomavirus (HPV) DNA test positive (R85.81)
anal low risk human papillomavirus (HPV) DNA test positive (R85.82)

     R85.610   Atypical squamous cells of undetermined significance on cytologic smear of anus (ASC-US)

     R85.611   Atypical squamous cells cannot exclude high grade squamous intraepithelial lesion on cytologic smear of anus (ASC-H)

     R85.612   Low grade squamous intraepithelial lesion on cytologic smear of anus (LGSIL)

     R85.613   High grade squamous intraepithelial lesion on cytologic smear of anus (HGSIL)

     R85.614   Cytologic evidence of malignancy on smear of anus

     R85.615   Unsatisfactory cytologic smear of anus
Inadequate sample of cytologic smear of anus

     R85.616   Satisfactory anal smear but lacking transformation zone

     R85.618   Other abnormal cytological findings on specimens from anus

     R85.619   Unspecified abnormal cytological findings in specimens from anus
Abnormal anal cytology NOS
Atypical glandular cells of anus NOS

   R85.69   Abnormal cytological findings in specimens from other digestive organs and abdominal cavity

R85.7   Abnormal histological findings in specimens from digestive organs and abdominal cavity

R85.8-   Other abnormal findings in specimens from digestive organs and abdominal cavity

   R85.81   Anal high risk human papillomavirus (HPV) DNA test positive
Excludes 1: anogenital warts due to human papillomavirus (HPV) (A63.0)
condyloma acuminatum (A63.0)

   R85.82   Anal low risk human papillomavirus (HPV) DNA test positive
Use additional code for associated human papillomavirus (B97.7)

   R85.89   Other abnormal findings in specimens from digestive organs and abdominal cavity
Abnormal chromosomal findings in specimens from digestive organs and abdominal cavity

R85.9   Unspecified abnormal finding in specimens from digestive organs and abdominal cavity

R
7
4
-
R
8
5

R86-   Abnormal findings in specimens from <u>male</u> genital organs
  Includes: Abnormal findings in prostatic secretions
           Abnormal findings in semen, seminal fluid
           Abnormal spermatozoa
  Excludes 1:   azoospermia (N46.0-)
              oligospermia (N46.1-)

R86.0   Abnormal level of enzymes in specimens from male genital
         organs
R86.1   Abnormal level of hormones in specimens from male genital
         organs
R86.2   Abnormal level of other drugs, medicaments and biological
         substances in specimens from male genital organs
R86.3   Abnormal level of substances chiefly nonmedicinal as to source in
         specimens from male genital organs
R86.4   Abnormal immunological findings in specimens from male
         genital organs
R86.5   Abnormal microbiological findings in specimens from male
         genital organs
             Positive culture findings in specimens from male genital organs
         Excludes 1:   colonization status (Z22.-)
R86.6   Abnormal cytological findings in specimens from male genital
         organs
R86.7   Abnormal histological findings in specimens from male genital
         organs
R86.8   Other abnormal findings in specimens from male genital organs
             Abnormal chromosomal findings in specimens from male genital
             organs
R86.9   Unspecified abnormal finding in specimens from male genital
         organs

R87-   Abnormal findings in specimens from <u>female</u> genital organs
  Includes: Abnormal findings in secretion and smears from cervix uteri
           Abnormal findings in secretion and smears from vagina
           Abnormal findings in secretion and smears from vulva

R87.0   Abnormal level of enzymes in specimens from female genital
         organs
R87.1   Abnormal level of hormones in specimens from female genital
         organs
R87.2   Abnormal level of other drugs, medicaments and biological
         substances in specimens from female genital organs
R87.3   Abnormal level of substances chiefly nonmedicinal as to source in
         specimens from female genital organs
R87.4   Abnormal immunological findings in specimens from female
         genital organs
R87.5   Abnormal microbiological findings in specimens from female
         genital organs
             Positive culture findings in specimens from female genital organs
         Excludes 1:   colonization status (Z22.-)
R87.6-   Abnormal cytological findings in specimens from <u>female</u> genital
         organs

  R87.61-   <u>Abnormal cytological findings in specimens from cervix uteri</u>
         Excludes 1:   abnormal cytological findings in specimens from
                    other female genital organs (R87.69)
                    abnormal cytological findings in specimens from
                    vagina (R87.62-)
                    carcinoma in situ of cervix uteri (histologically
                    confirmed) (D06.-)
                    cervical intraepithelial neoplasia I [CIN I] (N87.0)
                    cervical intraepithelial neoplasia II [CIN II]
                    (N87.1)
                    cervical intraepithelial neoplasia III [CIN III]
                    (D06.-)
                    dysplasia (mild) (moderate) of cervix uteri
                    (histologically confirmed) (N87.-)
                    severe dysplasia of cervix uteri (histologically
                    confirmed) (D06.-)
         Excludes❷: cervical high risk human papillomavirus (HPV)
                    DNA test positive (R87.810)
                    cervical low risk human papillomavirus (HPV)
                    DNA test positive (R87.820)

  R87.610   <u>Atypical squamous cells</u> of <u>undetermined</u> significance
            on cytologic smear of cervix (ASC-US)
  R87.611   <u>Atypical squamous cells</u> <u>cannot exclude high grade</u>
            <u>squamous intraepithelial lesion</u> on cytologic smear of
            cervix (ASC-H)
  R87.612   <u>Low grade squamous intraepithelial</u> lesion on
            cytologic smear of cervix (LGSIL)
  R87.613   <u>High grade squamous intraepithelial</u> lesion on
            cytologic smear of cervix (HGSIL)
  R87.614   <u>Cytologic evidence of malignancy</u> on smear of cervix
  R87.615   <u>Unsatisfactory</u> cytologic smear of cervix
               Inadequate sample of cytologic smear of cervix

R87.616   <u>Satisfactory</u> cervical smear <u>but lacking transformation</u>
          <u>zone</u>
R87.618   <u>Other</u> abnormal cytological findings on specimens
          from cervix uteri
R87.619   <u>Unspecified</u> abnormal cytological findings in
          specimens from cervix uteri
             Abnormal cervical cytology NOS
             Abnormal Papanicolaou smear of cervix NOS
             Abnormal thin preparation smear of cervix NOS
             Atypical endocervical cells of cervix NOS
             Atypical endometrial cells of cervix NOS
             Atypical glandular cells of cervix NOS

R87.62-   <u>Abnormal cytological findings in specimens from vagina</u>
          Use additional code to identify acquired absence of uterus and
          cervix, if applicable (Z90.71-)
         Excludes 1:   abnormal cytological findings in specimens from
                    cervix uteri (R87.61-)
                    abnormal cytological findings in specimens from
                    other female genital organs (R87.69)
                    carcinoma in situ of vagina (histologically
                    confirmed) (D07.2)
                    dysplasia (mild) (moderate) of vagina
                    (histologically confirmed) (N89.-)
                    severe dysplasia of vagina (histologically
                    confirmed) (D07.2)
                    vaginal intraepithelial neoplasia I [VAIN I]
                    (N89.0)
                    vaginal intraepithelial neoplasia II [VAIN II]
                    (N89.1)
                    vaginal intraepithelial neoplasia III [VAIN III]
                    (D07.2)
         Excludes❷: vaginal high risk human papillomavirus (HPV)
                    DNA test positive (R87.811)
                    vaginal low risk human papillomavirus (HPV)
                    DNA test positive (R87.821)

  R87.620   <u>Atypical squamous cells</u> of <u>undetermined</u> significance
            on cytologic smear of vagina (ASC-US)
  R87.621   <u>Atypical squamous cells</u> <u>cannot exclude high grade</u>
            <u>squamous intraepithelial lesion</u> on cytologic smear of
            vagina (ASC-H)
  R87.622   <u>Low grade squamous intraepithelial</u> lesion on
            cytologic smear of vagina (LGSIL)
  R87.623   <u>High grade squamous intraepithelial</u> lesion on
            cytologic smear of vagina (HGSIL)
  R87.624   <u>Cytologic evidence of malignancy</u> on smear of vagina
  R87.625   <u>Unsatisfactory</u> cytologic smear of vagina
               Inadequate sample of cytologic smear of vagina
  R87.628   <u>Other</u> abnormal cytological findings on specimens
            from vagina
  R87.629   <u>Unspecified</u> abnormal cytological findings in
            specimens from vagina
               Abnormal Papanicolaou smear of vagina NOS
               Abnormal thin preparation smear of vagina NOS
               Abnormal vaginal cytology NOS
               Atypical endocervical cells of vagina NOS
               Atypical endometrial cells of vagina NOS
               Atypical glandular cells of vagina NOS

R87.69   Abnormal cytological findings in specimens from other
         female genital organs
             Abnormal cytological findings in specimens from female
             genital organs NOS
         Excludes 1:   dysplasia of vulva (histologically confirmed)
                    (N90.0-N90.3)

R87.7   Abnormal histological findings in specimens from female genital
         organs
         Excludes 1:   carcinoma in situ (histologically confirmed) of female
                    genital organs (D06-D07.3)
                    cervical intraepithelial neoplasia I [CIN I] (N87.0)
                    cervical intraepithelial neoplasia II [CIN II] (N87.1)
                    cervical intraepithelial neoplasia III [CIN III] (D06.-)
                    dysplasia (mild) (moderate) of cervix uteri
                    (histologically confirmed) (N87.-)
                    dysplasia (mild) (moderate) of vagina (histologically
                    confirmed) (N89.-)
                    severe dysplasia of cervix uteri (histologically
                    confirmed) (D06.-)
                    severe dysplasia of vagina (histologically confirmed)
                    (D07.2)
                    vaginal intraepithelial neoplasia I [VAIN I] (N89.0)
                    vaginal intraepithelial neoplasia II [VAIN II] (N89.1)
                    vaginal intraepithelial neoplasia III [VAIN III] (D07.2)

R
8
6
I
R
9
3

Excludes 1: = NOT CODED HERE! (Do not code both)   *Excludes❷:* = Not Included Here

R87.8- **Other abnormal findings in specimens from female genital organs**

R87.81- **High risk human papillomavirus (HPV) DNA test positive from female genital organs**
Excludes 1: anogenital warts due to human papillomavirus (HPV) (A63.0)
condyloma acuminatum (A63.0)

R87.810 Cervical <u>high risk</u> human papillomavirus (HPV) DNA test positive

R87.811 Vaginal <u>high risk</u> human papillomavirus (HPV) DNA test positive

R87.82- **Low risk human papillomavirus (HPV) DNA test positive from female genital organs**
Use additional code for associated human papillomavirus (B97.7)

R87.820 Cervical <u>low risk</u> human papillomavirus (HPV) DNA test positive

R87.821 Vaginal <u>low risk</u> human papillomavirus (HPV) DNA test positive

R87.89 **Other abnormal findings in specimens from female genital organs**
Abnormal chromosomal findings in specimens from female genital organs

R87.9 **Unspecified abnormal finding in specimens from female genital organs**

R88- **Abnormal findings in other body fluids and substances**

R88.0 **Cloudy (hemodialysis) (peritoneal) dialysis effluent**

R88.8 **Abnormal findings in other body fluids and substances**

R89- **Abnormal findings in specimens from other organs, systems and tissues**
Includes: Abnormal findings in nipple discharge
Abnormal findings in synovial fluid
Abnormal findings in wound secretions

R89.0 **Abnormal level of enzymes in specimens from other organs, systems and tissues**

R89.1 **Abnormal level of hormones in specimens from other organs, systems and tissues**

R89.2 **Abnormal level of other drugs, medicaments and biological substances in specimens from other organs, systems and tissues**

R89.3 **Abnormal level of substances chiefly nonmedicinal as to source in specimens from other organs, systems and tissues**

R89.4 **Abnormal immunological findings in specimens from other organs, systems and tissues**

R89.5 **Abnormal microbiological findings in specimens from other organs, systems and tissues**
Positive culture findings in specimens from other organs, systems and tissues
Excludes 1: colonization status (Z22.-)

R89.6 **Abnormal cytological findings in specimens from other organs, systems and tissues**

R89.7 **Abnormal histological findings in specimens from other organs, systems and tissues**

R89.8 **Other abnormal findings in specimens from other organs, systems and tissues**
Abnormal chromosomal findings in specimens from other organs, systems and tissues

R89.9 **Unspecified abnormal finding in specimens from other organs, systems and tissues**

Abnormal findings on diagnostic imaging and in function studies, without diagnosis (R90-R94)

Includes: Nonspecific abnormal findings on diagnostic imaging by computerized axial tomography [CAT scan]
Nonspecific abnormal findings on diagnostic imaging by magnetic resonance imaging [MRI][NMR]
Nonspecific abnormal findings on diagnostic imaging by positron emission tomography [PET scan]
Nonspecific abnormal findings on diagnostic imaging by thermography
Nonspecific abnormal findings on diagnostic imaging by ultrasound [echogram]
Nonspecific abnormal findings on diagnostic imaging by X-ray examination
Excludes 1: abnormal findings on antenatal screening of mother (O28.-)
diagnostic abnormal findings classified elsewhere — see Alphabetical Index

R90- **Abnormal findings on diagnostic imaging of central nervous system**

R90.0 **Intracranial space-occupying lesion found on diagnostic imaging of central nervous system**

R90.8- **Other abnormal findings on diagnostic imaging of central nervous system**

R90.81 **Abnormal echoencephalogram**

R90.82 **White matter disease, unspecified**

R90.89 **Other abnormal findings on diagnostic imaging of central nervous system**
Other cerebrovascular abnormality found on diagnostic imaging of central nervous system

R91- **Abnormal findings on diagnostic imaging of lung**

R91.1 **Solitary pulmonary nodule**
Coin lesion lung
Solitary pulmonary nodule, subsegmental branch of the bronchial tree

R91.8 **Other nonspecific abnormal finding of lung field**
Lung mass NOS found on diagnostic imaging of lung
Pulmonary infiltrate NOS
Shadow, lung

R92- **Abnormal and inconclusive findings on diagnostic imaging of breast**

R92.0 **Mammographic microcalcification found on diagnostic imaging of breast**
Excludes ❷: mammographic calcification (calculus) found on diagnostic imaging of breast (R92.1)

R92.1 **Mammographic calcification found on diagnostic imaging of breast**
Mammographic calculus found on diagnostic imaging of breast

R92.2 **Inconclusive mammogram**
Dense breasts NOS
Inconclusive mammogram NEC
Inconclusive mammography due to dense breasts
Inconclusive mammography NEC

R92.8 **Other abnormal and inconclusive findings on diagnostic imaging of breast**

R93- **Abnormal findings on diagnostic imaging of other body structures**

R93.0 **Abnormal findings on diagnostic imaging of skull and head, not elsewhere classified**
Excludes 1: intracranial space-occupying lesion found on diagnostic imaging (R90.0)

R93.1 **Abnormal findings on diagnostic imaging of heart and coronary circulation**
Abnormal echocardiogram NOS
Abnormal heart shadow

R93.2 **Abnormal findings on diagnostic imaging of liver and biliary tract**
Nonvisualization of gallbladder

R93.3 **Abnormal findings on diagnostic imaging of other parts of digestive tract**

R93.4 **Abnormal findings on diagnostic imaging of urinary organs**
Filling defect of bladder found on diagnostic imaging
Filling defect of kidney found on diagnostic imaging
Filling defect of ureter found on diagnostic imaging
Excludes 1: hypertrophy of kidney (N28.81)

R93.5 **Abnormal findings on diagnostic imaging of other abdominal regions, including retroperitoneum**

R93.6 **Abnormal findings on diagnostic imaging of limbs**
Excludes ❷: abnormal finding in skin and subcutaneous tissue (R93.8)

R93.7 **Abnormal findings on diagnostic imaging of other parts of musculoskeletal system**
Excludes ❷: abnormal findings on diagnostic imaging of skull (R93.0)

R
8
6
–
R
9
3

R93.8 **Abnormal findings on diagnostic imaging of other specified body structures**
   Abnormal finding by radioisotope localization of placenta
   Abnormal radiological finding in skin and subcutaneous tissue
   Mediastinal shift

R93.9 **Diagnostic imaging inconclusive due to excess body fat of patient**

R94- **Abnormal results of function studies**
   Includes: Abnormal results of radionuclide [radioisotope] uptake studies
      Abnormal results of scintigraphy

R94.0- **Abnormal results of function studies of central nervous system**

   R94.01 **Abnormal electroencephalogram [EEG]**

   R94.02 **Abnormal brain scan**

   R94.09 **Abnormal results of other function studies of central nervous system**

R94.1- **Abnormal results of function studies of peripheral nervous system and special senses**

   R94.11- **Abnormal results of function studies of eye**

      R94.110 **Abnormal electro-oculogram [EOG]**

      R94.111 **Abnormal electroretinogram [ERG]**
         Abnormal retinal function study

      R94.112 **Abnormal visually evoked potential [VEP]**

      R94.113 **Abnormal oculomotor study**

      R94.118 **Abnormal results of other function studies of eye**

   R94.12- **Abnormal results of function studies of ear and other special senses**

      R94.120 **Abnormal auditory function study**

      R94.121 **Abnormal vestibular function study**

      R94.128 **Abnormal results of other function studies of ear and other special senses**

   R94.13- **Abnormal results of function studies of peripheral nervous system**

      R94.130 **Abnormal response to nerve stimulation, unspecified**

      R94.131 **Abnormal electromyogram [EMG]**
         Excludes 1: electromyogram of eye (R94.113)

      R94.138 **Abnormal results of other function studies of peripheral nervous system**

R94.2 **Abnormal results of pulmonary function studies**
   Reduced ventilatory capacity
   Reduced vital capacity

R94.3- **Abnormal results of cardiovascular function studies**

   R94.30 **Abnormal result of cardiovascular function study, unspecified**

   R94.31 **Abnormal electrocardiogram [ECG] [EKG]**
      Excludes 1: long QT syndrome (I45.81)

   R94.39 **Abnormal result of other cardiovascular function study**
      Abnormal electrophysiological intracardiac studies
      Abnormal phonocardiogram
      Abnormal vectorcardiogram

R94.4 **Abnormal results of kidney function studies**
   Abnormal renal function test

R94.5 **Abnormal results of liver function studies**

R94.6 **Abnormal results of thyroid function studies**

R94.7 **Abnormal results of other endocrine function studies**
   Excludes❷: abnormal glucose (R73.0-)

R94.8 **Abnormal results of function studies of other organs and systems**
   Abnormal basal metabolic rate [BMR]
   Abnormal bladder function test
   Abnormal splenic function test

Abnormal tumor markers (R97)

R97- **Abnormal tumor markers**
   Elevated tumor associated antigens [TAA]
   Elevated tumor specific antigens [TSA]

R97.0 **Elevated carcinoembryonic antigen [CEA]**

R97.1 **Elevated cancer antigen 125 [CA 125]**

R97.2 **Elevated prostate specific antigen [PSA]**

R97.8 **Other abnormal tumor markers**

Ill-defined and unknown cause of mortality (R99)

R99 **Ill-defined and unknown cause of mortality**
   Death (unexplained) NOS
   Unspecified cause of mortality

© 2013 Channel Publishing, Ltd.

Chapter 19 – Injury, poisoning and certain other consequences of external causes (S00-T88)

Use additional code to identify any retained foreign body, if applicable (Z18-)
Excludes 1: birth trauma (P10-P15)
obstetric trauma (O70-O71)
This chapter contains the following blocks:

S00-S09	Injuries to the head
S10-S19	Injuries to the neck
S20-S29	Injuries to the thorax
S30-S39	Injuries to the abdomen, lower back, lumbar spine, pelvis and external genitals
S40-S49	Injuries to the shoulder and upper arm
S50-S59	Injuries to the elbow and forearm
S60-S69	Injuries to the wrist, hand and fingers
S70-S79	Injuries to the hip and thigh
S80-S89	Injuries to the knee and lower leg
S90-S99	Injuries to the ankle and foot
T07	Injuries involving multiple body regions
T14	Injury of unspecified body region
T15-T19	Effects of foreign body entering through natural orifice
T20-T25	Burns and corrosions of external body surface, specified by site
T26-T28	Burns and corrosions confined to eye and internal organs
T30-T32	Burns and corrosions of multiple and unspecified body regions
T33-T34	Frostbite
T36-T50	Poisoning by, adverse effects of and underdosing of drugs, medicaments and biological substances
T51-T65	Toxic effects of substances chiefly nonmedicinal as to source
T66-T78	Other and unspecified effects of external causes
T79	Certain early complications of trauma
T80-T88	Complications of surgical and medical care, not elsewhere classified

Note: Use secondary code(s) from Chapter 20, External causes of morbidity, to indicate cause of injury. Codes within the T section that include the external cause do not require an additional external cause code

The chapter uses the S-section for coding different types of injuries related to single body regions and the T-section to cover injuries to unspecified body regions as well as poisoning and certain other consequences of external causes.

Injuries to the head (S00-S09)

Includes: Injuries of ear
Injuries of eye
Injuries of face [any part]
Injuries of gum
Injuries of jaw
Injuries of oral cavity
Injuries of palate
Injuries of periocular area
Injuries of scalp
Injuries of temporomandibular joint area
Injuries of tongue
Injuries of tooth
Code also for any associated infection
Excludes❷: burns and corrosions (T20-T32)
effects of foreign body in ear (T16)
effects of foreign body in larynx (T17.3)
effects of foreign body in mouth NOS (T18.0)
effects of foreign body in nose (T17.0-T17.1)
effects of foreign body in pharynx (T17.2)
effects of foreign body on external eye (T15.-)
frostbite (T33-T34)
insect bite or sting, venomous (T63.4)

S00- Superficial injury of head
Excludes 1: diffuse cerebral contusion (S06.2-)
focal cerebral contusion (S06.3-)
injury of eye and orbit (S05.-)
open wound of head (S01.-)

The appropriate 7th character is to be added to each code from category S00:
A Initial encounter
D Subsequent encounter
S Sequela

S00.0- Superficial injury of scalp
S00.00x- Unspecified superficial injury of scalp
S00.01x- Abrasion of scalp
S00.02x- Blister (nonthermal) of scalp

S00.03x- Contusion of scalp
Bruise of scalp
Hematoma of scalp
S00.04x- External constriction of part of scalp
S00.05x- Superficial foreign body of scalp
Splinter in the scalp
S00.06x- Insect bite (nonvenomous) of scalp
S00.07x- Other superficial bite of scalp
Excludes 1: open bite of scalp (S01.05)

S00.1- Contusion of eyelid and periocular area
Black eye
Excludes❷: contusion of eyeball and orbital tissues (S05.1)
S00.10x- Contusion of unspecified eyelid and periocular area
S00.11x- Contusion of right eyelid and periocular area
S00.12x- Contusion of left eyelid and periocular area

S00.2- Other and unspecified superficial injuries of eyelid and periocular area
Excludes❷: superficial injury of conjunctiva and cornea (S05.0-)
S00.20- Unspecified superficial injury of eyelid and periocular area
S00.201- Unspecified superficial injury of right eyelid and periocular area
S00.202- Unspecified superficial injury of left eyelid and periocular area
S00.209- Unspecified superficial injury of unspecified eyelid and periocular area
S00.21- Abrasion of eyelid and periocular area
S00.211- Abrasion of right eyelid and periocular area
S00.212- Abrasion of left eyelid and periocular area
S00.219- Abrasion of unspecified eyelid and periocular area
S00.22- Blister (nonthermal) of eyelid and periocular area
S00.221- Blister (nonthermal) of right eyelid and periocular area
S00.222- Blister (nonthermal) of left eyelid and periocular area
S00.229- Blister (nonthermal) of unspecified eyelid and periocular area
S00.24- External constriction of eyelid and periocular area
S00.241- External constriction of right eyelid and periocular area
S00.242- External constriction of left eyelid and periocular area
S00.249- External constriction of unspecified eyelid and periocular area
S00.25- Superficial foreign body of eyelid and periocular area
Splinter of eyelid and periocular area
Excludes❷: retained foreign body in eyelid (H02.81-)
S00.251- Superficial foreign body of right eyelid and periocular area
S00.252- Superficial foreign body of left eyelid and periocular area
S00.259- Superficial foreign body of unspecified eyelid and periocular area
S00.26- Insect bite (nonvenomous) of eyelid and periocular area
S00.261- Insect bite (nonvenomous) of right eyelid and periocular area
S00.262- Insect bite (nonvenomous) of left eyelid and periocular area
S00.269- Insect bite (nonvenomous) of unspecified eyelid and periocular area
S00.27- Other superficial bite of eyelid and periocular area
Excludes 1: open bite of eyelid and periocular area (S01.15)
S00.271- Other superficial bite of right eyelid and periocular area
S00.272- Other superficial bite of left eyelid and periocular area
S00.279- Other superficial bite of unspecified eyelid and periocular area
S00.3- Superficial injury of nose
S00.30x- Unspecified superficial injury of nose
S00.31x- Abrasion of nose
S00.32x- Blister (nonthermal) of nose
S00.33x- Contusion of nose
Bruise of nose
Hematoma of nose
S00.34x- External constriction of nose
S00.35x- Superficial foreign body of nose
Splinter in the nose
S00.36x- Insect bite (nonvenomous) of nose
S00.37x- Other superficial bite of nose
Excludes 1: open bite of nose (S01.25)

R93 I S00

Excludes 1: = NOT CODED HERE! (Do not code both) *Excludes❷ = Not Included Here*

S00.4-   Superficial injury of ear
  S00.40-   Unspecified superficial injury of ear
    S00.401- Unspecified superficial injury of right ear
    S00.402- Unspecified superficial injury of left ear
    S00.409- Unspecified superficial injury of unspecified ear
  S00.41-   Abrasion of ear
    S00.411- Abrasion of right ear
    S00.412- Abrasion of left ear
    S00.419- Abrasion of unspecified ear
  S00.42-   Blister (nonthermal) of ear
    S00.421- Blister (nonthermal) of right ear
    S00.422- Blister (nonthermal) of left ear
    S00.429- Blister (nonthermal) of unspecified ear
  S00.43-   Contusion of ear
    Bruise of ear
    Hematoma of ear
    S00.431- Contusion of right ear
    S00.432- Contusion of left ear
    S00.439- Contusion of unspecified ear
  S00.44-   External constriction of ear
    S00.441- External constriction of right ear
    S00.442- External constriction of left ear
    S00.449- External constriction of unspecified ear
  S00.45-   Superficial foreign body of ear
    Splinter in the ear
    S00.451- Superficial foreign body of right ear
    S00.452- Superficial foreign body of left ear
    S00.459- Superficial foreign body of unspecified ear
  S00.46-   Insect bite (nonvenomous) of ear
    S00.461- Insect bite (nonvenomous) of right ear
    S00.462- Insect bite (nonvenomous) of left ear
    S00.469- Insect bite (nonvenomous) of unspecified ear
  S00.47-   Other superficial bite of ear
    Excludes 1: open bite of ear (S01.35)
    S00.471- Other superficial bite of right ear
    S00.472- Other superficial bite of left ear
    S00.479- Other superficial bite of unspecified ear
S00.5-   Superficial injury of lip and oral cavity
  S00.50-   Unspecified superficial injury of lip and oral cavity
    S00.501- Unspecified superficial injury of lip
    S00.502- Unspecified superficial injury of oral cavity
  S00.51-   Abrasion of lip and oral cavity
    S00.511- Abrasion of lip
    S00.512- Abrasion of oral cavity
  S00.52-   Blister (nonthermal) of lip and oral cavity
    S00.521- Blister (nonthermal) of lip
    S00.522- Blister (nonthermal) of oral cavity
  S00.53-   Contusion of lip and oral cavity
    S00.531- Contusion of lip
      Bruise of lip
      Hematoma of oral cavity
    S00.532- Contusion of oral cavity
      Bruise of lip
      Hematoma of oral cavity
  S00.54-   External constriction of lip and oral cavity
    S00.541- External constriction of lip
    S00.542- External constriction of oral cavity
  S00.55-   Superficial foreign body of lip and oral cavity
    S00.551- Superficial foreign body of lip
      Splinter of lip and oral cavity
    S00.552- Superficial foreign body of oral cavity
      Splinter of lip and oral cavity
  S00.56-   Insect bite (nonvenomous) of lip and oral cavity
    S00.561- Insect bite (nonvenomous) of lip
    S00.562- Insect bite (nonvenomous) of oral cavity
  S00.57-   Other superficial bite of lip and oral cavity
    S00.571- Other superficial bite of lip
      Excludes 1: open bite of lip (S01.551)
    S00.572- Other superficial bite of oral cavity
      Excludes 1: open bite of oral cavity (S01.552)
S00.8-   Superficial injury of other parts of head
  S00.80x- Unspecified superficial injury of other part of head
  S00.81x- Abrasion of other part of head
  S00.82x- Blister (nonthermal) of other part of head

S00.83x-   Contusion of other part of head
  Bruise of other part of head
  Hematoma of other part of head
S00.84x-   External constriction of other part of head
S00.85x-   Superficial foreign body of other part of head
  Splinter in other part of head
S00.86x-   Insect bite (nonvenomous) of other part of head
S00.87x-   Other superficial bite of other part of head
  Excludes 1: open bite of other part of head (S01.85)
S00.9-   Superficial injury of unspecified part of head
  S00.90x- Unspecified superficial injury of unspecified part of head
  S00.91x- Abrasion of unspecified part of head
  S00.92x- Blister (nonthermal) of unspecified part of head
  S00.93x- Contusion of unspecified part of head
    Bruise of head
    Hematoma of head
  S00.94x- External constriction of unspecified part of head
  S00.95x- Superficial foreign body of unspecified part of head
    Splinter of head
  S00.96x- Insect bite (nonvenomous) of unspecified part of head
  S00.97x- Other superficial bite of unspecified part of head
    Excludes 1: open bite of head (S01.95)

S01- Open wound of head
Code also any associated:
  Injury of cranial nerve (S04.-)
  Injury of muscle and tendon of head (S09.1-)
  Intracranial injury (S06.-)
  Wound infection
Excludes 1: open skull fracture (S02.- with 7th character B)
Excludes❷: injury of eye and orbit (S05.-)
    traumatic amputation of part of head (S08.-)

The appropriate 7th character is to be added to each code from category S01:
  A   Initial encounter
  D   Subsequent encounter
  S   Sequela

S01.0-   Open wound of scalp
    Excludes 1: avulsion of scalp (S08.0)
  S01.00x- Unspecified open wound of scalp
  S01.01x- Laceration without foreign body of scalp
  S01.02x- Laceration with foreign body of scalp
  S01.03x- Puncture wound without foreign body of scalp
  S01.04x- Puncture wound with foreign body of scalp
  S01.05x- Open bite of scalp
    Bite of scalp NOS
    Excludes 1: superficial bite of scalp (S00.06, S00.07-)
S01.1-   Open wound of eyelid and periocular area
    Open wound of eyelid and periocular area with or without involvement of lacrimal passages
  S01.10-   Unspecified open wound of eyelid and periocular area
    S01.101- Unspecified open wound of right eyelid and periocular area
    S01.102- Unspecified open wound of left eyelid and periocular area
    S01.109- Unspecified open wound of unspecified eyelid and periocular area
  S01.11-   Laceration without foreign body of eyelid and periocular area
    S01.111- Laceration without foreign body of right eyelid and periocular area
    S01.112- Laceration without foreign body of left eyelid and periocular area
    S01.119- Laceration without foreign body of unspecified eyelid and periocular area
  S01.12-   Laceration with foreign body of eyelid and periocular area
    S01.121- Laceration with foreign body of right eyelid and periocular area
    S01.122- Laceration with foreign body of left eyelid and periocular area
    S01.129- Laceration with foreign body of unspecified eyelid and periocular area
  S01.13-   Puncture wound without foreign body of eyelid and periocular area
    S01.131- Puncture wound without foreign body of right eyelid and periocular area
    S01.132- Puncture wound without foreign body of left eyelid and periocular area
    S01.139- Puncture wound without foreign body of unspecified eyelid and periocular area

S00 - S01

© 2013 Channel Publishing, Ltd.

S01.14- <u>Puncture</u> wound <u>with foreign body</u> of eyelid and periocular area

  S01.141- Puncture wound <u>with foreign body</u> of <u>right</u> eyelid and periocular area

  S01.142- Puncture wound <u>with foreign body</u> of <u>left</u> eyelid and periocular area

  S01.149- Puncture wound <u>with foreign body</u> of <u>unspecified</u> eyelid and periocular area

S01.15- <u>Open bite</u> of eyelid and periocular area
    Bite of eyelid and periocular area NOS
    Excludes 1: superficial bite of eyelid and periocular area (S00.26, S00.27)

  S01.151- Open bite of <u>right</u> eyelid and periocular area

  S01.152- Open bite of <u>left</u> eyelid and periocular area

  S01.159- Open bite of <u>unspecified</u> eyelid and periocular area

S01.2- Open wound of <u>nose</u>

  S01.20x- Unspecified open wound of nose

  S01.21x- Laceration <u>without</u> foreign body of nose

  S01.22x- Laceration <u>with foreign body</u> of nose

  S01.23x- Puncture wound <u>without</u> foreign body of nose

  S01.24x- Puncture wound <u>with foreign body</u> of nose

  S01.25x- Open bite of nose
    Bite of nose NOS
    Excludes 1: superficial bite of nose (S00.36, S00.37)

S01.3- Open wound of <u>ear</u>

  S01.30- <u>Unspecified</u> open wound of ear

    S01.301- Unspecified open wound of <u>right</u> ear

    S01.302- Unspecified open wound of <u>left</u> ear

    S01.309- Unspecified open wound of <u>unspecified</u> ear

  S01.31- <u>Laceration</u> <u>without</u> foreign body of ear

    S01.311- Laceration <u>without</u> foreign body of <u>right</u> ear

    S01.312- Laceration <u>without</u> foreign body of <u>left</u> ear

    S01.319- Laceration <u>without</u> foreign body of <u>unspecified</u> ear

  S01.32- <u>Laceration</u> <u>with foreign body</u> of ear

    S01.321- Laceration <u>with foreign body</u> of <u>right</u> ear

    S01.322- Laceration <u>with foreign body</u> of <u>left</u> ear

    S01.329- Laceration <u>with foreign body</u> of <u>unspecified</u> ear

  S01.33- <u>Puncture</u> wound <u>without</u> foreign body of ear

    S01.331- Puncture wound <u>without</u> foreign body of <u>right</u> ear

    S01.332- Puncture wound <u>without</u> foreign body of <u>left</u> ear

    S01.339- Puncture wound <u>without</u> foreign body of <u>unspecified</u> ear

  S01.34- <u>Puncture</u> wound <u>with foreign body</u> of ear

    S01.341- Puncture wound <u>with foreign body</u> of <u>right</u> ear

    S01.342- Puncture wound <u>with foreign body</u> of <u>left</u> ear

    S01.349- Puncture wound <u>with foreign body</u> of <u>unspecified</u> ear

  S01.35- <u>Open bite</u> of ear
    Bite of ear NOS
    Excludes 1: superficial bite of ear (S00.46, S00.47)

    S01.351- Open bite of <u>right</u> ear

    S01.352- Open bite of <u>left</u> ear

    S01.359- Open bite of <u>unspecified</u> ear

S01.4- Open wound of <u>cheek and temporomandibular area</u>

  S01.40- <u>Unspecified</u> open wound of cheek and temporomandibular area

    S01.401- Unspecified open wound of <u>right</u> cheek and temporomandibular area

    S01.402- Unspecified open wound of <u>left</u> cheek and temporomandibular area

    S01.409- Unspecified open wound of <u>unspecified</u> cheek and temporomandibular area

  S01.41- <u>Laceration</u> <u>without</u> foreign body of cheek and temporomandibular area

    S01.411- Laceration <u>without</u> foreign body of <u>right</u> cheek and temporomandibular area

    S01.412- Laceration <u>without</u> foreign body of <u>left</u> cheek and temporomandibular area

    S01.419- Laceration <u>without</u> foreign body of <u>unspecified</u> cheek and temporomandibular area

  S01.42- <u>Laceration</u> <u>with foreign body</u> of cheek and temporomandibular area

    S01.421- Laceration <u>with foreign body</u> of <u>right</u> cheek and temporomandibular area

    S01.422- Laceration <u>with foreign body</u> of <u>left</u> cheek and temporomandibular area

    S01.429- Laceration <u>with foreign body</u> of <u>unspecified</u> cheek and temporomandibular area

S01.43- <u>Puncture</u> wound <u>without</u> foreign body of cheek and temporomandibular area

  S01.431- Puncture wound <u>without</u> foreign body of <u>right</u> cheek and temporomandibular area

  S01.432- Puncture wound <u>without</u> foreign body of <u>left</u> cheek and temporomandibular area

  S01.439- Puncture wound <u>without</u> foreign body of <u>unspecified</u> cheek andtemporomandibular area

S01.44- <u>Puncture</u> wound <u>with foreign body</u> of cheek and temporomandibular area

  S01.441- Puncture wound <u>with foreign body</u> of <u>right</u> cheek and temporomandibular area

  S01.442- Puncture wound <u>with foreign body</u> of <u>left</u> cheek and temporomandibular area

  S01.449- Puncture wound <u>with foreign body</u> of <u>unspecified</u> cheek and temporomandibular area

S01.45- <u>Open bite</u> of cheek and temporomandibular area
    Bite of cheek and temporomandibular area NOS
    Excludes ❷: superficial bite of cheek and temporomandibular area (S00.86, S00.87)

  S01.451- Open bite of <u>right</u> cheek and temporomandibular area

  S01.452- Open bite of <u>left</u> cheek and temporomandibular area

  S01.459- Open bite of <u>unspecified</u> cheek and temporomandibular area

S01.5- Open wound of <u>lip and oral cavity</u>
  Excludes ❷: tooth dislocation (S03.2)
        tooth fracture (S02.5)

  S01.50- <u>Unspecified</u> open wound of lip and oral cavity

    S01.501- Unspecified open wound of <u>lip</u>

    S01.502- Unspecified open wound of <u>oral cavity</u>

  S01.51- <u>Laceration</u> of lip and oral cavity <u>without</u> foreign body

    S01.511- Laceration <u>without</u> foreign body of <u>lip</u>

    S01.512- Laceration <u>without</u> foreign body of <u>oral cavity</u>

  S01.52- <u>Laceration</u> of lip and oral cavity <u>with foreign body</u>

    S01.521- Laceration <u>with foreign body</u> of <u>lip</u>

    S01.522- Laceration <u>with foreign body</u> of <u>oral cavity</u>

  S01.53- <u>Puncture</u> wound of lip and oral cavity <u>without</u> foreign body

    S01.531- Puncture wound <u>without</u> foreign body of <u>lip</u>

    S01.532- Puncture wound <u>without</u> foreign body of <u>oral cavity</u>

  S01.54- <u>Puncture</u> wound of lip and oral cavity <u>with foreign body</u>

    S01.541- Puncture wound <u>with foreign body</u> of <u>lip</u>

    S01.542- Puncture wound <u>with foreign body</u> of <u>oral cavity</u>

  S01.55- <u>Open bite</u> of lip and oral cavity

    S01.551- Open bite of <u>lip</u>
      Bite of lip NOS
      Excludes 1: superficial bite of lip (S00.571)

    S01.552- Open bite of <u>oral cavity</u>
      Bite of oral cavity NOS
      Excludes 1: superficial bite of oral cavity (S00.572)

S01.8- Open wound of <u>other parts of head</u>

  S01.80x- Unspecified open wound of other part of head

  S01.81x- Laceration <u>without</u> foreign body of other part of head

  S01.82x- Laceration <u>with foreign body</u> of other part of head

  S01.83x- Puncture wound <u>without</u> foreign body of other part of head

  S01.84x- Puncture wound <u>with foreign body</u> of other part of head

  S01.85x- Open bite of other part of head
    Bite of other part of head NOS
    Excludes 1: superficial bite of other part of head (S00.85)

S01.9- Open wound of <u>unspecified part of head</u>

  S01.90x- Unspecified open wound of unspecified part of head

  S01.91x- Laceration <u>without</u> foreign body of unspecified part of head

  S01.92x- Laceration <u>with foreign body</u> of unspecified part of head

  S01.93x- Puncture wound <u>without</u> foreign body of unspecified part of head

  S01.94x- Puncture wound <u>with foreign body</u> of unspecified part of head

  S01.95x- Open bite of unspecified part of head
    Bite of head NOS
    Excludes 1: superficial bite of head NOS (S00.97)

S00 - S01

Excludes 1: = NOT CODED HERE! (Do not code both)

Excludes ❷: = Not Included Here

S02- Fracture of skull and facial bones
Note: A fracture not indicated as open or closed should be coded to closed
Code also any associated intracranial injury (S06.-)
The appropriate 7th character is to be added to each code from category S02:
A   Initial encounter for closed fracture
B   Initial encounter for open fracture
D   Subsequent encounter for fracture with routine healing
G   Subsequent encounter for fracture with delayed healing
K   Subsequent encounter for fracture with nonunion
S   Sequela

S02.0xx-   Fracture of vault of skull
   Fracture of frontal bone
   Fracture of parietal bone
S02.1-   Fracture of base of skull
   Excludes 1: orbit NOS (S02.8)
   Excludes❷: orbital floor (S02.3-)
S02.10x-   Unspecified fracture of base of skull
S02.11-   Fracture of occiput
S02.110-   Type I occipital condyle fracture
S02.111-   Type II occipital condyle fracture
S02.112-   Type III occipital condyle fracture
S02.113-   Unspecified occipital condyle fracture
S02.118-   Other fracture of occiput
S02.119-   Unspecified fracture of occiput
S02.19x-   Other fracture of base of skull
   Fracture of anterior fossa of base of skull
   Fracture of ethmoid sinus
   Fracture of frontal sinus
   Fracture of middle fossa of base of skull
   Fracture of orbital roof
   Fracture of posterior fossa of base of skull
   Fracture of sphenoid
   Fracture of temporal bone
S02.2xx-   Fracture of nasal bones
S02.3xx-   Fracture of orbital floor
   Excludes 1: orbit NOS (S02.8)
   Excludes❷: orbital roof (S02.1-)
S02.4-   Fracture of malar, maxillary and zygoma bones
   Fracture of superior maxilla
   Fracture of upper jaw (bone)
   Fracture of zygomatic process of temporal bone
S02.40-   Fracture of malar, maxillary and zygoma bones, unspecified
S02.400-   Malar fracture unspecified
S02.401-   Maxillary fracture, unspecified
S02.402-   Zygomatic fracture, unspecified
S02.41-   LeFort fracture
S02.411-   LeFort I fracture
S02.412-   LeFort II fracture
S02.413-   LeFort III fracture
S02.42x-   Fracture of alveolus of maxilla
S02.5xx-   Fracture of tooth (traumatic)
   Broken tooth
   Excludes 1: cracked tooth (nontraumatic) (K03.81)
S02.6-   Fracture of mandible
   Fracture of lower jaw (bone)
S02.60-   Fracture of mandible, unspecified
S02.600-   Fracture of unspecified part of body of mandible
S02.609-   Fracture of mandible, unspecified
S02.61x-   Fracture of condylar process of mandible
S02.62x-   Fracture of subcondylar process of mandible
S02.63x-   Fracture of coronoid process of mandible
S02.64x-   Fracture of ramus of mandible
S02.65x-   Fracture of angle of mandible
S02.66x-   Fracture of symphysis of mandible
S02.67x-   Fracture of alveolus of mandible
S02.69x-   Fracture of mandible of other specified site
S02.8xx-   Fractures of other specified skull and facial bones
   Fracture of orbit NOS
   Fracture of palate
   Excludes 1: fracture of orbital floor (S02.3-)
              fracture of orbital roof (S02.1-)
S02.9-   Fracture of unspecified skull and facial bones
S02.91x-   Unspecified fracture of skull
S02.92x-   Unspecified fracture of facial bones

S03- Dislocation and sprain of joints and ligaments of head
Includes: Avulsion of joint (capsule) or ligament of head
   Laceration of cartilage, joint (capsule) or ligament of head
   Sprain of cartilage, joint (capsule) or ligament of head
   Traumatic hemarthrosis of joint or ligament of head
   Traumatic rupture of joint or ligament of head
   Traumatic subluxation of joint or ligament of head
   Traumatic tear of joint or ligament of head
Code also any associated open wound
   Excludes❷: Strain of muscle or tendon of head (S09.1)
The appropriate 7th character is to be added to each code from category S03:
A   Initial encounter
D   Subsequent encounter
S   Sequela

S03.0xx-   Dislocation of jaw
   Dislocation of jaw (cartilage) (meniscus)
   Dislocation of mandible
   Dislocation of temporomandibular (joint)
S03.1xx-   Dislocation of septal cartilage of nose
S03.2xx-   Dislocation of tooth
S03.4xx-   Sprain of jaw
   Sprain of temporomandibular (joint) (ligament)
S03.8xx-   Sprain of joints and ligaments of other parts of head
S03.9xx-   Sprain of joints and ligaments of unspecified parts of head

S04- Injury of cranial nerve
The selection of side should be based on the side of the body being affected
Code first any associated intracranial injury (S06.-)
Code also any associated:
   Open wound of head (S01.-)
   Skull fracture (S02.-)
The appropriate 7th character is to be added to each code from category S04:
A   Initial encounter
D   Subsequent encounter
S   Sequela

S04.0-   Injury of optic nerve and pathways
   Use additional code to identify any visual field defect or blindness (H53.4-, H54)
S04.01-   Injury of optic nerve
   Injury of 2nd cranial nerve
S04.011-   Injury of optic nerve, right eye
S04.012-   Injury of optic nerve, left eye
S04.019-   Injury of optic nerve, unspecified eye
   Injury of optic nerve NOS
S04.02x-   Injury of optic chiasm
S04.03-   Injury of optic tract and pathways
   Injury of optic radiation
S04.031-   Injury of optic tract and pathways, right eye
S04.032-   Injury of optic tract and pathways, left eye
S04.039-   Injury of optic tract and pathways, unspecified eye
   Injury of optic tract and pathways NOS
S04.04-   Injury of visual cortex
S04.041-   Injury of visual cortex, right eye
S04.042-   Injury of visual cortex, left eye
S04.049-   Injury of visual cortex, unspecified eye
   Injury of visual cortex NOS
S04.1-   Injury of oculomotor nerve
   Injury of 3rd cranial nerve
S04.10x-   Injury of oculomotor nerve, unspecified side
S04.11x-   Injury of oculomotor nerve, right side
S04.12x-   Injury of oculomotor nerve, left side
S04.2-   Injury of trochlear nerve
   Injury of 4th cranial nerve
S04.20x-   Injury of trochlear nerve, unspecified side
S04.21x-   Injury of trochlear nerve, right side
S04.22x-   Injury of trochlear nerve, left side
S04.3-   Injury of trigeminal nerve
   Injury of 5th cranial nerve
S04.30x-   Injury of trigeminal nerve, unspecified side
S04.31x-   Injury of trigeminal nerve, right side
S04.32x-   Injury of trigeminal nerve, left side
S04.4-   Injury of abducent nerve
   Injury of 6th cranial nerve
S04.40x-   Injury of abducent nerve, unspecified side
S04.41x-   Injury of abducent nerve, right side
S04.42x-   Injury of abducent nerve, left side

S02 - S06

S04.5- Injury of facial nerve
Injury of 7th cranial nerve
  S04.50x- Injury of facial nerve, unspecified side
  S04.51x- Injury of facial nerve, right side
  S04.52x- Injury of facial nerve, left side
S04.6- Injury of acoustic nerve
Injury of auditory nerve
Injury of 8th cranial nerve
  S04.60x- Injury of acoustic nerve, unspecified side
  S04.61x- Injury of acoustic nerve, right side
  S04.62x- Injury of acoustic nerve, left side
S04.7- Injury of accessory nerve
Injury of 11th cranial nerve
  S04.70x- Injury of accessory nerve, unspecified side
  S04.71x- Injury of accessory nerve, right side
  S04.72x- Injury of accessory nerve, left side
S04.8- Injury of other cranial nerves
  S04.81- Injury of olfactory [1st] nerve
    S04.811- Injury of olfactory [1st] nerve, right side
    S04.812- Injury of olfactory [1st] nerve, left side
    S04.819- Injury of olfactory [1st] nerve, unspecified side
  S04.89- Injury of other cranial nerves
Injury of vagus [10th] nerve
    S04.891- Injury of other cranial nerves, right side
    S04.892- Injury of other cranial nerves, left side
    S04.899- Injury of other cranial nerves, unspecified side
S04.9xx- Injury of unspecified cranial nerve

S05- Injury of eye and orbit
Includes: Open wound of eye and orbit
Excludes❷: 2nd cranial [optic] nerve injury (S04.0-)
  3rd cranial [oculomotor] nerve injury (S04.1-)
  open wound of eyelid and periocular area (S01.1-)
  orbital bone fracture (S02.1-, S02.3-, S02.8-)
  superficial injury of eyelid (S00.1-S00.2)

The appropriate 7th character is to be added to each code from category S05:
  A   Initial encounter
  D   Subsequent encounter
  S   Sequela

S05.0- Injury of conjunctiva and corneal abrasion without foreign body
Excludes 1: foreign body in conjunctival sac (T15.1)
  foreign body in cornea (T15.0)
  S05.00x- Injury of conjunctiva and corneal abrasion without foreign body, unspecified eye
  S05.01x- Injury of conjunctiva and corneal abrasion without foreign body, right eye
  S05.02x- Injury of conjunctiva and corneal abrasion without foreign body, left eye
S05.1- Contusion of eyeball and orbital tissues
Traumatic hyphema
Excludes❷: black eye NOS (S00.1)
  contusion of eyelid and periocular area (S00.1)
  S05.10x- Contusion of eyeball and orbital tissues, unspecified eye
  S05.11x- Contusion of eyeball and orbital tissues, right eye
  S05.12x- Contusion of eyeball and orbital tissues, left eye
S05.2- Ocular laceration and rupture with prolapse or loss of intraocular tissue
  S05.20x- Ocular laceration and rupture with prolapse or loss of intraocular tissue, unspecified eye
  S05.21x- Ocular laceration and rupture with prolapse or loss of intraocular tissue, right eye
  S05.22x- Ocular laceration and rupture with prolapse or loss of intraocular tissue, left eye
S05.3- Ocular laceration without prolapse or loss of intraocular tissue
Laceration of eye NOS
  S05.30x- Ocular laceration without prolapse or loss of intraocular tissue, unspecified eye
  S05.31x- Ocular laceration without prolapse or loss of intraocular tissue, right eye
  S05.32x- Ocular laceration without prolapse or loss of intraocular tissue, left eye
S05.4- Penetrating wound of orbit with or without foreign body
Excludes❷: retained (old) foreign body following penetrating wound in orbit (H05.5-)
  S05.40x- Penetrating wound of orbit with or without foreign body, unspecified eye
  S05.41x- Penetrating wound of orbit with or without foreign body, right eye
  S05.42x- Penetrating wound of orbit with or without foreign body, left eye

S05.5- Penetrating wound with foreign body of eyeball
Excludes❷: retained (old) intraocular foreign body (H44.6-, H44.7)
  S05.50x- Penetrating wound with foreign body of unspecified eyeball
  S05.51x- Penetrating wound with foreign body of right eyeball
  S05.52x- Penetrating wound with foreign body of left eyeball
S05.6- Penetrating wound without foreign body of eyeball
Ocular penetration NOS
  S05.60x- Penetrating wound without foreign body of unspecified eyeball
  S05.61x- Penetrating wound without foreign body of right eyeball
  S05.62x- Penetrating wound without foreign body of left eyeball
S05.7- Avulsion of eye
Traumatic enucleation
  S05.70x- Avulsion of unspecified eye
  S05.71x- Avulsion of right eye
  S05.72x- Avulsion of left eye
S05.8- Other injuries of eye and orbit
Lacrimal duct injury
  S05.8x- Other injuries of eye and orbit
    S05.8x1- Other injuries of right eye and orbit
    S05.8x2- Other injuries of left eye and orbit
    S05.8x9- Other injuries of unspecified eye and orbit
S05.9- Unspecified injury of eye and orbit
Injury of eye NOS
  S05.90x- Unspecified injury of unspecified eye and orbit
  S05.91x- Unspecified injury of right eye and orbit
  S05.92x- Unspecified injury of left eye and orbit

S06- Intracranial injury
Includes: Traumatic brain injury
Code also any associated:
  Open wound of head (S01.-)
  Skull fracture (S02.-)
Excludes 1: head injury NOS (S09.90)

The appropriate 7th character is to be added to each code from category S06:
  A   Initial encounter
  D   Subsequent encounter
  S   Sequela

S06.0- Concussion
Commotio cerebri
Excludes 1: concussion with other intracranial injuries classified in category S06- code to specified intracranial injury
  S06.0x- Concussion
    S06.0x0- Concussion without loss of consciousness
    S06.0x1- Concussion with loss of consciousness of 30 minutes or less
    S06.0x2- Concussion with loss of consciousness of 31 minutes to 59 minutes
    S06.0x3- Concussion with loss of consciousness of 1 hour to 5 hours 59 minutes
    S06.0x4- Concussion with loss of consciousness of 6 hours to 24 hours
    S06.0x5- Concussion with loss of consciousness greater than 24 hours with return to pre-existing conscious level
    S06.0x6- Concussion with loss of consciousness greater than 24 hours without return to pre-existing conscious level with patient surviving
    S06.0x7- Concussion with loss of consciousness of any duration with death due to brain injury prior to regaining consciousness
    S06.0x8- Concussion with loss of consciousness of any duration with death due to other cause prior to regaining consciousness
    S06.0x9- Concussion with loss of consciousness of unspecified duration
Concussion NOS
S06.1- Traumatic cerebral edema
Diffuse traumatic cerebral edema
Focal traumatic cerebral edema
  S06.1x- Traumatic cerebral edema
    S06.1x0- Traumatic cerebral edema without loss of consciousness
    S06.1x1- Traumatic cerebral edema with loss of consciousness of 30 minutes or less
    S06.1x2- Traumatic cerebral edema with loss of consciousness of 31 minutes to 59 minutes
    S06.1x3- Traumatic cerebral edema with loss of consciousness of 1 hour to 5 hours 59 minutes

S02 - S06

S06.1x4-   Traumatic cerebral edema <u>with</u> loss of consciousness of <u>6 hours to 24 hours</u>

S06.1x5-   Traumatic cerebral edema <u>with</u> loss of consciousness <u>greater than 24</u> hours <u>with return</u> to pre-existing conscious level

S06.1x6-   Traumatic cerebral edema <u>with</u> loss of consciousness <u>greater than 24</u> hours <u>without</u> return to pre-existing conscious level <u>with patient surviving</u>

S06.1x7-   Traumatic cerebral edema <u>with</u> loss of consciousness of <u>any duration with death</u> due to <u>brain injury</u> prior to regaining consciousness

S06.1x8-   Traumatic cerebral edema <u>with</u> loss of consciousness of <u>any duration with death</u> due to <u>other cause</u> prior to regaining consciousness

S06.1x9-   Traumatic cerebral edema with loss of consciousness of <u>unspecified</u> duration
   Traumatic cerebral edema NOS

S06.2-   **Diffuse traumatic brain injury**
  Diffuse axonal brain injury
  Excludes 1: traumatic diffuse cerebral edema (S06.1x-)

S06.2x-   **Diffuse traumatic brain injury**

S06.2x0-   **Diffuse traumatic brain injury <u>without</u> loss of consciousness**

S06.2x1-   **Diffuse traumatic brain injury <u>with</u> loss of consciousness of <u>30 minutes or less</u>**

S06.2x2-   **Diffuse traumatic brain injury <u>with</u> loss of consciousness of <u>31 minutes to 59 minutes</u>**

S06.2x3-   **Diffuse traumatic brain injury <u>with</u> loss of consciousness of <u>1 hour to 5 hours 59 minutes</u>**

S06.2x4-   **Diffuse traumatic brain injury <u>with</u> loss of consciousness of <u>6 hours to 24 hours</u>**

S06.2x5-   **Diffuse traumatic brain injury <u>with</u> loss of consciousness <u>greater than 24</u> hours <u>with return</u> to pre-existing conscious levels**

S06.2x6-   **Diffuse traumatic brain injury <u>with</u> loss of consciousness <u>greater than 24</u> hours <u>without return</u> to pre-existing conscious level <u>with patient surviving</u>**

S06.2x7-   **Diffuse traumatic brain injury <u>with</u> loss of consciousness of <u>any duration with death</u> due to <u>brain injury</u> prior to regaining consciousness**

S06.2x8-   **Diffuse traumatic brain injury <u>with</u> loss of consciousness of <u>any duration with death</u> due to <u>other cause</u> prior to regaining consciousness**

S06.2x9-   **Diffuse traumatic brain injury <u>with</u> loss of consciousness of <u>unspecified</u> duration**
   Diffuse traumatic brain injury NOS

S06.3-   <u>Focal traumatic brain injury</u>
  Excludes 1: any condition classifiable to S06.4-S06.6
    focal cerebral edema (S06.1)

S06.30-   <u>Unspecified</u> focal traumatic brain injury

S06.300-   Unspecified focal traumatic brain injury <u>without</u> loss of consciousness

S06.301-   Unspecified focal traumatic brain injury <u>with</u> loss of consciousness of <u>30 minutes or less</u>

S06.302-   Unspecified focal traumatic brain injury <u>with</u> loss of consciousness of <u>31 minutes to 59 minutes</u>

S06.303-   Unspecified focal traumatic brain injury <u>with</u> loss of consciousness of <u>1 hour to 5 hours 59 minutes</u>

S06.304-   Unspecified focal traumatic brain injury <u>with</u> loss of consciousness of <u>6 hours to 24 hours</u>

S06.305-   Unspecified focal traumatic brain injury <u>with</u> loss of consciousness <u>greater than 24</u> hours <u>with return</u> to pre-existing conscious level

S06.306-   Unspecified focal traumatic brain injury <u>with</u> loss of consciousness <u>greater than 24</u> hours <u>without return</u> to pre-existing conscious level <u>with patient surviving</u>

S06.307-   Unspecified focal traumatic brain injury <u>with</u> loss of consciousness of <u>any duration with death</u> due to <u>brain injury</u> prior to regaining consciousness

S06.308-   Unspecified focal traumatic brain injury <u>with</u> loss of consciousness of <u>any duration with death</u> due to <u>other cause</u> prior to regaining consciousness

S06.309-   Unspecified focal traumatic brain injury <u>with</u> loss of consciousness of <u>unspecified</u> duration
   Unspecified focal traumatic brain injury NOS

S06.31-   <u>Contusion and laceration</u> of <u>right</u> cerebrum

S06.310-   Contusion and laceration of <u>right</u> cerebrum <u>without</u> loss of consciousness

S06.311-   Contusion and laceration of <u>right</u> cerebrum <u>with</u> loss of consciousness of <u>30 minutes or less</u>

S06.312-   Contusion and laceration of <u>right</u> cerebrum <u>with</u> loss of consciousness of <u>31 minutes to 59 minutes</u>

S06.313-   Contusion and laceration of <u>right</u> cerebrum <u>with</u> loss of consciousness of <u>1 hour to 5 hours 59 minutes</u>

S06.314-   Contusion and laceration of <u>right</u> cerebrum <u>with</u> loss of consciousness of <u>6 hours to 24 hours</u>

S06.315-   Contusion and laceration of <u>right</u> cerebrum <u>with</u> loss of consciousness <u>greater than 24</u> hours <u>with return</u> to pre-existing conscious level

S06.316-   Contusion and laceration of <u>right</u> cerebrum <u>with</u> loss of consciousness <u>greater than 24</u> hours <u>without return</u> to pre-existing conscious level <u>with patient surviving</u>

S06.317-   Contusion and laceration of <u>right</u> cerebrum <u>with</u> loss of consciousness of <u>any duration with death</u> due to <u>brain injury</u> prior to regaining consciousness

S06.318-   Contusion and laceration of <u>right</u> cerebrum <u>with</u> loss of consciousness of <u>any duration with death</u> due to <u>other cause</u> prior to regaining consciousness

S06.319-   Contusion and laceration of <u>right</u> cerebrum <u>with</u> loss of consciousness of <u>unspecified</u> duration
   Contusion and laceration of right cerebrum NOS

S06.32-   <u>Contusion and laceration</u> of <u>left</u> cerebrum

S06.320-   Contusion and laceration of <u>left</u> cerebrum <u>without</u> loss of consciousness

S06.321-   Contusion and laceration of <u>left</u> cerebrum <u>with</u> loss of consciousness of <u>30 minutes or less</u>

S06.322-   Contusion and laceration of <u>left</u> cerebrum <u>with</u> loss of consciousness of <u>31 minutes to 59 minutes</u>

S06.323-   Contusion and laceration of <u>left</u> cerebrum <u>with</u> loss of consciousness of <u>1 hour to 5 hours 59 minutes</u>

S06.324-   Contusion and laceration of <u>left</u> cerebrum <u>with</u> loss of consciousness of <u>6 hours to 24 hours</u>

S06.325-   Contusion and laceration of <u>left</u> cerebrum <u>with</u> loss of consciousness <u>greater than 24</u> hours <u>with return</u> to pre-existing conscious level

S06.326-   Contusion and laceration of <u>left</u> cerebrum <u>with</u> loss of consciousness <u>greater than 24</u> hours <u>without return</u> to pre-existing conscious level <u>with patient surviving</u>

S06.327-   Contusion and laceration of <u>left</u> cerebrum <u>with</u> loss of consciousness of <u>any duration with death</u> due to <u>brain injury</u> prior to regaining consciousness

S06.328-   Contusion and laceration of <u>left</u> cerebrum <u>with</u> loss of consciousness of <u>any duration with death</u> due to <u>other cause</u> prior to regaining consciousness

S06.329-   Contusion and laceration of <u>left</u> cerebrum <u>with</u> loss of consciousness of <u>unspecified</u> duration
   Contusion and laceration of left cerebrum NOS

S06.33-   <u>Contusion and laceration</u> of cerebrum, <u>unspecified</u>

S06.330-   Contusion and laceration of cerebrum, <u>unspecified</u>, <u>without</u> loss of consciousness

S06.331-   Contusion and laceration of cerebrum, <u>unspecified</u>, <u>with</u> loss of consciousness of <u>30 minutes or less</u>

S06.332-   Contusion and laceration of cerebrum, <u>unspecified</u>, <u>with</u> loss of consciousness of <u>31 minutes to 59 minutes</u>

S06.333-   Contusion and laceration of cerebrum, <u>unspecified</u>, <u>with</u> loss of consciousness of <u>1 hour to 5 hours 59 minutes</u>

S06.334-   Contusion and laceration of cerebrum, <u>unspecified</u>, <u>with</u> loss of consciousness of <u>6 hours to 24 hours</u>

S06.335-   Contusion and laceration of cerebrum, <u>unspecified</u>, <u>with</u> loss of consciousness <u>greater than 24</u> hours <u>with return</u> to pre-existing conscious level

S06.336-   Contusion and laceration of cerebrum, <u>unspecified</u>, <u>with</u> loss of consciousness <u>greater than 24</u> hours <u>without return</u> to pre-existing conscious level <u>with patient surviving</u>

S06.337-   Contusion and laceration of cerebrum, <u>unspecified</u>, <u>with</u> loss of consciousness of <u>any duration with death</u> due to <u>brain injury</u> prior to regaining consciousness

S06.338-   Contusion and laceration of cerebrum, <u>unspecified</u>, <u>with</u> loss of consciousness of <u>any duration with death</u> due to <u>other cause</u> prior to regaining consciousness

S06.339-   Contusion and laceration of cerebrum, <u>unspecified</u>, <u>with</u> loss of consciousness of <u>unspecified</u> duration
   Contusion and laceration of cerebrum NOS

S06 - S06

S06.34- <u>Traumatic hemorrhage</u> of <u>right</u> cerebrum
Traumatic intracerebral hemorrhage and hematoma of right cerebrum

S06.340- Traumatic hemorrhage of <u>right</u> cerebrum <u>without</u> loss of consciousness

S06.341- Traumatic hemorrhage of <u>right</u> cerebrum <u>with</u> loss of consciousness of <u>30 minutes or less</u>

S06.342- Traumatic hemorrhage of <u>right</u> cerebrum <u>with</u> loss of consciousness of <u>31 minutes to 59 minutes</u>

S06.343- Traumatic hemorrhage of <u>right</u> cerebrum <u>with</u> loss of consciousness of <u>1 hours to 5 hours 59 minutes</u>

S06.344- Traumatic hemorrhage of <u>right</u> cerebrum <u>with</u> loss of consciousness of <u>6 hours to 24 hours</u>

S06.345- Traumatic hemorrhage of <u>right</u> cerebrum <u>with</u> loss of consciousness greater than 24 hours <u>with return</u> to pre-existing conscious level

S06.346- Traumatic hemorrhage of <u>right</u> cerebrum <u>with</u> loss of consciousness <u>greater than 24</u> hours <u>without</u> return to pre-existing conscious level <u>with patient surviving</u>

S06.347- Traumatic hemorrhage of <u>right</u> cerebrum <u>with</u> loss of consciousness of <u>any duration with death</u> due to <u>brain injury</u> prior to regaining consciousness

S06.348- Traumatic hemorrhage of <u>right</u> cerebrum <u>with</u> loss of consciousness of <u>any duration with death</u> due to <u>other cause</u> prior to regaining consciousness

S06.349- Traumatic hemorrhage of <u>right</u> cerebrum <u>with</u> loss of consciousness of <u>unspecified</u> duration
Traumatic hemorrhage of right cerebrum NOS

S06.35- <u>Traumatic hemorrhage</u> of <u>left</u> cerebrum
Traumatic intracerebral hemorrhage and hematoma of left cerebrum

S06.350- Traumatic hemorrhage of <u>left</u> cerebrum <u>without</u> loss of consciousness

S06.351- Traumatic hemorrhage of <u>left</u> cerebrum <u>with</u> loss of consciousness of <u>30 minutes or less</u>

S06.352- Traumatic hemorrhage of <u>left</u> cerebrum <u>with</u> loss of consciousness of <u>31 minutes to 59 minutes</u>

S06.353- Traumatic hemorrhage of <u>left</u> cerebrum <u>with</u> loss of consciousness of <u>1 hours to 5 hours 59 minutes</u>

S06.354- Traumatic hemorrhage of <u>left</u> cerebrum <u>with</u> loss of consciousness of <u>6 hours to 24 hours</u>

S06.355- Traumatic hemorrhage of <u>left</u> cerebrum <u>with</u> loss of consciousness <u>greater than 24</u> hours <u>with return</u> to pre-existing conscious level

S06.356- Traumatic hemorrhage of <u>left</u> cerebrum <u>with</u> loss of consciousness greater than 24 hours <u>without</u> return to pre-existing conscious level <u>with patient surviving</u>

S06.357- Traumatic hemorrhage of <u>left</u> cerebrum <u>with</u> loss of consciousness of <u>any duration with death</u> due to <u>brain injury</u> prior to regaining consciousness

S06.358- Traumatic hemorrhage of <u>left</u> cerebrum <u>with</u> loss of consciousness of <u>any duration with death</u> due to <u>other cause</u> prior to regaining consciousness

S06.359- Traumatic hemorrhage of <u>left</u> cerebrum <u>with</u> loss of consciousness of <u>unspecified</u> duration
Traumatic hemorrhage of left cerebrum NOS

S06.36- <u>Traumatic hemorrhage</u> of cerebrum, <u>unspecified</u>
Traumatic intracerebral hemorrhage and hematoma, unspecified

S06.360- Traumatic hemorrhage of cerebrum, <u>unspecified</u>, <u>without</u> loss of consciousness

S06.361- Traumatic hemorrhage of cerebrum, <u>unspecified</u>, <u>with</u> loss of consciousness of <u>30 minutes or less</u>

S06.362- Traumatic hemorrhage of cerebrum, <u>unspecified</u>, <u>with</u> loss of consciousness of <u>31 minutes to 59 minutes</u>

S06.363- Traumatic hemorrhage of cerebrum, <u>unspecified</u>, <u>with</u> loss of consciousness of <u>1 hours to 5 hours 59 minutes</u>

S06.364- Traumatic hemorrhage of cerebrum, <u>unspecified</u>, <u>with</u> loss of consciousness of <u>6 hours to 24 hours</u>

S06.365- Traumatic hemorrhage of cerebrum, <u>unspecified</u>, <u>with</u> loss of consciousness <u>greater than 24</u> hours <u>with return</u> to pre-existing conscious level

S06.366- Traumatic hemorrhage of cerebrum, <u>unspecified</u>, <u>with</u> loss of consciousness <u>greater than 24</u> hours <u>without</u> <u>return</u> to pre-existing conscious level <u>with patient surviving</u>

S06.367- Traumatic hemorrhage of cerebrum, <u>unspecified</u>, <u>with</u> loss of consciousness of <u>any duration with death</u> due to <u>brain injury</u> prior to regaining consciousness

S06.368- Traumatic hemorrhage of cerebrum, <u>unspecified</u>, <u>with</u> loss of consciousness of <u>any duration with death</u> due to <u>other cause</u> prior to regaining consciousness

S06.369- Traumatic hemorrhage of cerebrum, <u>unspecified</u>, <u>with</u> loss of consciousness of <u>unspecified</u> duration
Traumatic hemorrhage of cerebrum NOS

S06.37- <u>Contusion, laceration, and hemorrhage</u> of <u>cerebellum</u>

S06.370- Contusion, laceration, and hemorrhage of cerebellum <u>without</u> loss of consciousness

S06.371- Contusion, laceration, and hemorrhage of cerebellum <u>with</u> loss of consciousness of <u>30 minutes or less</u>

S06.372- Contusion, laceration, and hemorrhage of cerebellum <u>with</u> loss of consciousness of <u>31 minutes to 59 minutes</u>

S06.373- Contusion, laceration, and hemorrhage of cerebellum <u>with</u> loss of consciousness of <u>1 hour to 5 hours 59 minutes</u>

S06.374- Contusion, laceration, and hemorrhage of cerebellum <u>with</u> loss of consciousness of <u>6 hours to 24 hours</u>

S06.375- Contusion, laceration, and hemorrhage of cerebellum <u>with</u> loss of consciousness <u>greater than 24</u> hours <u>with return</u> to pre-existing conscious level

S06.376- Contusion, laceration, and hemorrhage of cerebellum <u>with</u> loss of consciousness <u>greater than 24</u> hours <u>without return</u> to pre-existing conscious level <u>with patient surviving</u>

S06.377- Contusion, laceration, and hemorrhage of cerebellum <u>with</u> loss of consciousness of <u>any duration with death</u> due to <u>brain injury</u> prior to regaining consciousness

S06.378- Contusion, laceration, and hemorrhage of cerebellum <u>with</u> loss of consciousness of <u>any duration with death</u> due to <u>other cause</u> prior to regaining consciousness

S06.379- Contusion, laceration, and hemorrhage of cerebellum <u>with</u> loss of consciousness of <u>unspecified</u> duration
Contusion, laceration, and hemorrhage of cerebellum NOS

S06.38- <u>Contusion, laceration, and hemorrhage</u> of <u>brainstem</u>

S06.380- Contusion, laceration, and hemorrhage of brainstem <u>without</u> loss of consciousness

S06.381- Contusion, laceration, and hemorrhage of brainstem <u>with</u> loss of consciousness of <u>30 minutes or less</u>

S06.382- Contusion, laceration, and hemorrhage of brainstem <u>with</u> loss of consciousness of <u>31 minutes to 59 minutes</u>

S06.383- Contusion, laceration, and hemorrhage of brainstem <u>with</u> loss of consciousness of <u>1 hour to 5 hours 59 minutes</u>

S06.384- Contusion, laceration, and hemorrhage of brainstem <u>with</u> loss of consciousness of <u>6 hours to 24 hours</u>

S06.385- Contusion, laceration, and hemorrhage of brainstem <u>with</u> loss of consciousness <u>greater than 24</u> hours <u>with return</u> to pre-existing conscious level

S06.386- Contusion, laceration, and hemorrhage of brainstem <u>with</u> loss of consciousness <u>greater than 24</u> hours <u>without return</u> to pre-existing conscious level <u>with patient surviving</u>

S06.387- Contusion, laceration, and hemorrhage of brainstem <u>with</u> loss of consciousness of <u>any duration with death</u> due to <u>brain injury</u> prior to regaining consciousness

S06.388- Contusion, laceration, and hemorrhage of brainstem <u>with</u> loss of consciousness of <u>any duration with death</u> due to <u>other cause</u> prior to regaining consciousness

S06.389- Contusion, laceration, and hemorrhage of brainstem <u>with</u> loss of consciousness of <u>unspecified</u> duration
Contusion, laceration, and hemorrhage of brainstem NOS

S06.4- **Epidural hemorrhage**
Extradural hemorrhage NOS
Extradural hemorrhage (traumatic)

S06.4x- <u>Epidural hemorrhage</u>

S06.4x0- Epidural hemorrhage <u>without</u> loss of consciousness

S06.4x1- Epidural hemorrhage <u>with</u> loss of consciousness of <u>30 minutes or less</u>

S06.4x2- Epidural hemorrhage <u>with</u> loss of consciousness of <u>31 minutes to 59 minutes</u>

S06.4x3- Epidural hemorrhage <u>with</u> loss of consciousness of <u>1 hour to 5 hours 59 minutes</u>

S06.4x4- Epidural hemorrhage <u>with</u> loss of consciousness of <u>6 hours to 24 hours</u>

S06.4x5- Epidural hemorrhage <u>with</u> loss of consciousness greater than 24 hours <u>with return</u> to pre-existing conscious level

S06.4x6- Epidural hemorrhage <u>with</u> loss of consciousness greater than 24 hours <u>without return</u> to pre-existing conscious level <u>with patient surviving</u>

S 0 6
6
I
S 0 6
6

S06.4x7- Epidural hemorrhage <u>with</u> loss of consciousness of <u>any duration with death</u> due to <u>brain injury</u> prior to regaining consciousness

S06.4x8- Epidural hemorrhage <u>with</u> loss of consciousness of <u>any duration with death</u> due to <u>other causes</u> prior to regaining consciousness

S06.4x9- Epidural hemorrhage <u>with</u> loss of consciousness of <u>unspecified</u> duration
　　Epidural hemorrhage NOS

S06.5- Traumatic subdural hemorrhage
S06.5x- <u>Traumatic subdural hemorrhage</u>

S06.5x0- Traumatic subdural hemorrhage <u>without</u> loss of consciousness

S06.5x1- Traumatic subdural hemorrhage <u>with</u> loss of consciousness of <u>30 minutes or less</u>

S06.5x2- Traumatic subdural hemorrhage <u>with</u> loss of consciousness of <u>31 minutes to 59 minutes</u>

S06.5x3- Traumatic subdural hemorrhage <u>with</u> loss of consciousness of <u>1 hour to 5 hours 59 minutes</u>

S06.5x4- Traumatic subdural hemorrhage <u>with</u> loss of consciousness of <u>6 hours to 24 hours</u>

S06.5x5- Traumatic subdural hemorrhage <u>with</u> loss of consciousness <u>greater than 24</u> hours <u>with return</u> to pre-existing conscious level

S06.5x6- Traumatic subdural hemorrhage <u>with</u> loss of consciousness <u>greater than 24</u> hours <u>without return</u> to pre-existing conscious level <u>with patient surviving</u>

S06.5x7- Traumatic subdural hemorrhage <u>with</u> loss of <u>any duration with death</u> due to <u>brain injury</u> before regaining consciousness

S06.5x8- Traumatic subdural hemorrhage <u>with</u> loss of consciousness of <u>any duration with death</u> due to <u>other cause</u> before regaining consciousness

S06.5x9- Traumatic subdural hemorrhage <u>with</u> loss of consciousness of <u>unspecified</u> duration
　　Traumatic subdural hemorrhage NOS

S06.6- Traumatic subarachnoid hemorrhage
S06.6x- <u>Traumatic subarachnoid hemorrhage</u>

S06.6x0- Traumatic subarachnoid hemorrhage <u>without</u> loss of consciousness

S06.6x1- Traumatic subarachnoid hemorrhage <u>with</u> loss of consciousness of <u>30 minutes or less</u>

S06.6x2- Traumatic subarachnoid hemorrhage <u>with</u> loss of consciousness of <u>31 minutes to 59 minutes</u>

S06.6x3- Traumatic subarachnoid hemorrhage <u>with</u> loss of consciousness of <u>1 hour to 5 hours 59 minutes</u>

S06.6x4- Traumatic subarachnoid hemorrhage <u>with</u> loss of consciousness of <u>6 hours to 24 hours</u>

S06.6x5- Traumatic subarachnoid hemorrhage <u>with</u> loss of consciousness <u>greater than 24</u> hours <u>with return</u> to pre-existing conscious level

S06.6x6- Traumatic subarachnoid hemorrhage <u>with</u> loss of consciousness <u>greater than 24</u> hours <u>without return</u> to pre-existing conscious level <u>with patient surviving</u>

S06.6x7- Traumatic subarachnoid hemorrhage <u>with</u> loss of consciousness of <u>any duration with death</u> due to <u>brain injury</u> prior to regaining consciousness

S06.6x8- Traumatic subarachnoid hemorrhage <u>with</u> loss of consciousness of <u>any duration with death</u> due to <u>other cause</u> prior to regaining consciousness

S06.6x9- Traumatic subarachnoid hemorrhage <u>with</u> loss of consciousness of <u>unspecified</u> duration
　　Traumatic subarachnoid hemorrhage NOS

S06.8- Other specified intracranial injuries
S06.81- Injury of <u>right internal carotid artery, intracranial portion, not elsewhere classified</u>

S06.810- Injury of <u>right</u> internal carotid artery, intracranial portion, not elsewhere classified <u>without</u> loss of consciousness

S06.811- Injury of <u>right</u> internal carotid artery, intracranial portion, not elsewhere classified <u>with</u> loss of consciousness of <u>30 minutes or less</u>

S06.812- Injury of <u>right</u> internal carotid artery, intracranial portion, not elsewhere classified <u>with</u> loss of consciousness of <u>31 minutes to 59 minutes</u>

S06.813- Injury of <u>right</u> internal carotid artery, intracranial portion, not elsewhere classified <u>with</u> loss of consciousness of <u>1 hour to 5 hours 59 minutes</u>

S06.814- Injury of <u>right</u> internal carotid artery, intracranial portion, not elsewhere classified <u>with</u> loss of consciousness of <u>6 hours to 24 hours</u>

S06.815- Injury of <u>right</u> internal carotid artery, intracranial portion, not elsewhere classified <u>with</u> loss of consciousness <u>greater than 24</u> hours <u>with return</u> to pre-existing conscious level

S06.816- Injury of <u>right</u> internal carotid artery, intracranial portion, not elsewhere classified <u>with</u> loss of consciousness <u>greater than 24</u> hours <u>without return</u> to pre-existing conscious level <u>with patient surviving</u>

S06.817- Injury of <u>right</u> internal carotid artery, intracranial portion, not elsewhere classified <u>with</u> loss of consciousness of <u>any duration with death</u> due to <u>brain injury</u> prior to regaining consciousness

S06.818- Injury of <u>right</u> internal carotid artery, intracranial portion, not elsewhere classified <u>with</u> loss of consciousness of <u>any duration with death</u> due to <u>other cause</u> prior to regaining consciousness

S06.819- Injury of <u>right</u> internal carotid artery, intracranial portion, not elsewhere classified <u>with</u> loss of consciousness of <u>unspecified</u> duration
　　Injury of right internal carotid artery, intracranial portion, not elsewhere classified NOS

S06.82- Injury of <u>left internal carotid artery, intracranial portion, not elsewhere classified</u>

S06.820- Injury of <u>left</u> internal carotid artery, intracranial portion, not elsewhere classified <u>without</u> loss of consciousness

S06.821- Injury of <u>left</u> internal carotid artery, intracranial portion, not elsewhere classified <u>with</u> loss of consciousness of <u>30 minutes or less</u>

S06.822- Injury of <u>left</u> internal carotid artery, intracranial portion, not elsewhere classified <u>with</u> loss of consciousness of <u>31 minutes to 59 minutes</u>

S06.823- Injury of <u>left</u> internal carotid artery, intracranial portion, not elsewhere classified <u>with</u> loss of consciousness of <u>1 hour to 5 hours 59 minutes</u>

S06.824- Injury of <u>left</u> internal carotid artery, intracranial portion, not elsewhere classified <u>with</u> loss of consciousness of <u>6 hours to 24 hours</u>

S06.825- Injury of <u>left</u> internal carotid artery, intracranial portion, not elsewhere classified <u>with</u> loss of consciousness <u>greater than 24</u> hours <u>with return</u> to pre-existing conscious level

S06.826- Injury of <u>left</u> internal carotid artery, intracranial portion, not elsewhere classified <u>with</u> loss of consciousness <u>greater than 24</u> hours <u>without return</u> to pre-existing conscious level <u>with patient surviving</u>

S06.827- Injury of <u>left</u> internal carotid artery, intracranial portion, not elsewhere classified <u>with</u> loss of consciousness of <u>any duration with death</u> due to <u>brain injury</u> prior to regaining consciousness

S06.828- Injury of <u>left</u> internal carotid artery, intracranial portion, not elsewhere classified <u>with</u> loss of consciousness of <u>any duration with death</u> due to <u>other cause</u> prior to regaining consciousness

S06.829- Injury of <u>left</u> internal carotid artery, intracranial portion, not elsewhere classified <u>with</u> loss of consciousness of <u>unspecified</u> duration
　　Injury of left internal carotid artery, intracranial portion, not elsewhere classified NOS

S06.89- <u>Other specified intracranial injury</u>

S06.890- Other specified intracranial injury <u>without</u> loss of consciousness

S06.891- Other specified intracranial injury <u>with</u> loss of consciousness of <u>30 minutes or less</u>

S06.892- Other specified intracranial injury <u>with</u> loss of consciousness of <u>31 minutes to 59 minutes</u>

S06.893- Other specified intracranial injury <u>with</u> loss of consciousness of <u>1 hour to 5 hours 59 minutes</u>

S06.894- Other specified intracranial injury <u>with</u> loss of consciousness of <u>6 hours to 24 hours</u>

S06.895- Other specified intracranial injury <u>with</u> loss of consciousness <u>greater than 24</u> hours <u>with return</u> to pre-existing conscious level

S06.896- Other specified intracranial injury <u>with</u> loss of consciousness <u>greater than 24</u> hours <u>without return</u> to pre-existing conscious level <u>with patient surviving</u>

S06.897- Other specified intracranial injury <u>with</u> loss of consciousness of <u>any duration with death</u> due to <u>brain injury</u> prior to regaining consciousness

S06.898- Other specified intracranial injury <u>with</u> loss of consciousness of <u>any duration with death</u> due to <u>other cause</u> prior to regaining consciousness

S06.899- Other specified intracranial injury **with** loss of consciousness of **unspecified** duration

S06.9- Unspecified intracranial injury
Brain injury NOS
Head injury NOS with loss of consciousness
Excludes 1: head injury NOS (S09.90)

S06.9x- Unspecified intracranial injury

S06.9x0- Unspecified intracranial injury **without** loss of consciousness

S06.9x1- Unspecified intracranial injury **with** loss of consciousness of **30 minutes or less**

S06.9x2- Unspecified intracranial injury **with** loss of consciousness of **31 minutes to 59 minutes**

S06.9x3- Unspecified intracranial injury **with** loss of consciousness of **1 hour to 5 hours 59 minutes**

S06.9x4- Unspecified intracranial injury **with** loss of consciousness of **6 hours to 24 hours**

S06.9x5- Unspecified intracranial injury **with** loss of consciousness **greater than 24** hours **with return** to pre-existing conscious level

S06.9x6- Unspecified intracranial injury **with** loss of consciousness **greater than 24** hours **without return** to pre-existing conscious level **with patient surviving**

S06.9x7- Unspecified intracranial injury **with** loss of consciousness of **any duration with death** due to **brain injury** prior to regaining consciousness

S06.9x8- Unspecified intracranial injury **with** loss of consciousness of **any duration with death** due to **other cause** prior to regaining consciousness

S06.9x9- Unspecified intracranial injury **with** loss of consciousness of **unspecified** duration

S07- Crushing injury of head
Use additional code for all associated injuries, such as:
Intracranial injuries (S06.-)
Skull fractures (S02.-)

The appropriate 7th character is to be added to each code from category S07:
A **Initial** encounter
D **Subsequent** encounter
S **Sequela**

S07.0xx- Crushing injury of face
S07.1xx- Crushing injury of skull
S07.8xx- Crushing injury of other parts of head
S07.9xx- Crushing injury of head, part **unspecified**

S08- Avulsion and traumatic amputation of **part of head**
Note: An amputation not identified as partial or complete should be coded to complete

The appropriate 7th character is to be added to each code from category S08:
A **Initial** encounter
D **Subsequent** encounter
S **Sequela**

S08.0xx- Avulsion of scalp
S08.1- Traumatic amputation of **ear**
S08.11- **Complete** traumatic amputation of ear
S08.111- Complete traumatic amputation of **right** ear
S08.112- Complete traumatic amputation of **left** ear
S08.119- Complete traumatic amputation of **unspecified** ear
S08.12- **Partial** traumatic amputation of ear
S08.121- Partial traumatic amputation of **right** ear
S08.122- Partial traumatic amputation of **left** ear
S08.129- Partial traumatic amputation of **unspecified** ear
S08.8- Traumatic amputation of other parts of head
S08.81- Traumatic amputation of **nose**
S08.811- Complete traumatic amputation of nose
S08.812- Partial traumatic amputation of nose
S08.89x- Traumatic amputation of other parts of head

S09- Other and unspecified injuries of head

The appropriate 7th character is to be added to each code from category S09:
A **Initial** encounter
D **Subsequent** encounter
S **Sequela**

S09.0xx- Injury of blood vessels of head, **not elsewhere classified**
Excludes 1: injury of cerebral blood vessels (S06.-)
injury of precerebral blood vessels (S15.-)

S09.1- Injury of muscle and tendon of head
Code also any associated open wound (S01.-)
Excludes ❷: sprain to joints and ligament of head (S03.9)

S09.10x- Unspecified injury of muscle and tendon of head
Injury of muscle and tendon of head NOS
S09.11x- Strain of muscle and tendon of head
S09.12x- Laceration of muscle and tendon of head
S09.19x- Other specified injury of muscle and tendon of head

S09.2- Traumatic rupture of ear drum
Excludes 1: traumatic rupture of ear drum due to blast injury (S09.31-)
S09.20x- Traumatic rupture of **unspecified** ear drum
S09.21x- Traumatic rupture of **right** ear drum
S09.22x- Traumatic rupture of **left** ear drum

S09.3- Other specified and unspecified injury of **middle and inner ear**
Excludes 1: injury to ear NOS (S09.91-)
Excludes ❷: injury to external ear (S00.4-, S01.3-, S08.1-)
S09.30- **Unspecified** injury of middle and inner ear
S09.301- Unspecified injury of **right** middle and inner ear
S09.302- Unspecified injury of **left** middle and inner ear
S09.309- Unspecified injury of **unspecified** middle and inner ear
S09.31- **Primary blast** injury of ear
Blast injury of ear NOS
S09.311- Primary blast injury of **right** ear
S09.312- Primary blast injury of **left** ear
S09.313- Primary blast injury of ear, **bilateral**
S09.319- Primary blast injury of **unspecified** ear
S09.39- **Other specified** injury of middle and inner ear
Secondary blast injury to ear
S09.391- Other specified injury of **right** middle and inner ear
S09.392- Other specified injury of **left** middle and inner ear
S09.399- Other specified injury of **unspecified** middle and inner ear

S09.8xx- **Other** specified injuries of head
S09.9- **Unspecified** injury of face and head
S09.90x- Unspecified injury of **head**
Head injury NOS
Excludes 1: brain injury NOS (S06.9-)
head injury NOS with loss of consciousness (S06.9-)
intracranial injury NOS (S06.9-)
S09.91x- Unspecified injury of **ear**
Injury of ear NOS
S09.92x- Unspecified injury of **nose**
Injury of nose NOS
S09.93x- Unspecified injury of **face**
Injury of face NOS

Injuries to the neck (S10-S19)

Includes: Injuries of nape
Injuries of supraclavicular region
Injuries of throat
Excludes ❷: burns and corrosions (T20-T32)
effects of foreign body in esophagus (T18.1)
effects of foreign body in larynx (T17.3)
effects of foreign body in pharynx (T17.2)
effects of foreign body in trachea (T17.4)
frostbite (T33-T34)
insect bite or sting, venomous (T63.4)

S10- Superficial injury of neck
The appropriate 7th character is to be added to each code from category S10:
A **Initial** encounter
D **Subsequent** encounter
S **Sequela**
S10.0xx- Contusion of throat
Contusion of cervical esophagus
Contusion of larynx
Contusion of pharynx
Contusion of trachea
S10.1- Other and unspecified superficial injuries of throat
S10.10x- Unspecified superficial injuries of throat
S10.11x- Abrasion of throat
S10.12x- Blister (nonthermal) of throat
S10.14x- External constriction of part of throat
S10.15x- Superficial foreign body of throat
Splinter in the throat
S10.16x- Insect bite (nonvenomous) of throat

S06 - S10

S10.17x-   Other superficial bite of throat
            Excludes 1: open bite of throat (S11.85)
S10.8-   Superficial injury of <u>other specified parts</u> of neck
    S10.80x-   Unspecified superficial injury of other specified part of neck
    S10.81x-   Abrasion of other specified part of neck
    S10.82x-   Blister (nonthermal) of other specified part of neck
    S10.83x-   Contusion of other specified part of neck
    S10.84x-   External constriction of other specified part of neck
    S10.85x-   Superficial foreign body of other specified part of neck
                Splinter in other specified part of neck
    S10.86x-   Insect bite of other specified part of neck
    S10.87x-   Other superficial bite of other specified part of neck
                *Excludes 1: open bite of other specified parts of neck
                              (S11.85)*
S10.9-   Superficial injury of <u>unspecified</u> part of neck
    S10.90x-   Unspecified superficial injury of unspecified part of neck
    S10.91x-   Abrasion of unspecified part of neck
    S10.92x-   Blister (nonthermal) of unspecified part of neck
    S10.93x-   Contusion of unspecified part of neck
    S10.94x-   External constriction of unspecified part of neck
    S10.95x-   Superficial foreign body of unspecified part of neck
    S10.96x-   Insect bite of unspecified part of neck
    S10.97x-   Other superficial bite of unspecified part of neck

S11-   <u>Open wound</u> of <u>neck</u>
        Code also any associated:
          Spinal cord injury (S14.0, S14.1-)
          Wound infection
        Excludes❷: open fracture of vertebra (S12.- with 7th character B)
        **The appropriate 7th character is to be added to each code from
          category S11:**
        A   <u>Initial</u> encounter
        D   <u>Subsequent</u> encounter
        S   <u>Sequela</u>
    S11.0-   Open wound of larynx and trachea
        S11.01-   Open wound of <u>larynx</u>
                    Excludes❷: open wound of vocal cord (S11.03)
            S11.011-   Laceration <u>without</u> foreign body of larynx
            S11.012-   Laceration <u>with foreign body</u> of larynx
            S11.013-   <u>Puncture</u> wound <u>without</u> foreign body of larynx
            S11.014-   <u>Puncture</u> wound <u>with foreign body</u> of larynx
            S11.015-   Open bite of larynx
                        Bite of larynx NOS
            S11.019-   Unspecified open wound of larynx
        S11.02-   Open wound of <u>trachea</u>
                    Open wound of cervical trachea
                    Open wound of trachea NOS
                    Excludes❷: open wound of thoracic trachea (S27.5-)
            S11.021-   Laceration <u>without</u> foreign body of trachea
            S11.022-   Laceration <u>with foreign body</u> of trachea
            S11.023-   <u>Puncture</u> wound <u>without</u> foreign body of trachea
            S11.024-   <u>Puncture</u> wound <u>with foreign body</u> of trachea
            S11.025-   Open bite of trachea
                        Bite of trachea NOS
            S11.029-   Unspecified open wound of trachea
        S11.03-   Open wound of <u>vocal cord</u>
            S11.031-   Laceration <u>without</u> foreign body of vocal cord
            S11.032-   Laceration <u>with foreign body</u> of vocal cord
            S11.033-   <u>Puncture</u> wound <u>without</u> foreign body of vocal cord
            S11.034-   <u>Puncture</u> wound <u>with foreign body</u> of vocal cord
            S11.035-   Open bite of vocal cord
                        Bite of vocal cord NOS
            S11.039-   Unspecified open wound of vocal cord
    S11.1-   Open wound of <u>thyroid gland</u>
        S11.10x-   Unspecified open wound of thyroid gland
        S11.11x-   Laceration <u>without</u> foreign body of thyroid gland
        S11.12x-   <u>Laceration</u> <u>with foreign body</u> of thyroid gland
        S11.13x-   <u>Puncture</u> wound <u>without</u> foreign body of thyroid gland
        S11.14x-   <u>Puncture</u> wound <u>with foreign body</u> of thyroid gland
        S11.15x-   Open bite of thyroid gland
                    Bite of thyroid gland NOS
    S11.2-   Open wound of <u>pharynx and cervical esophagus</u>
                Excludes 1: open wound of esophagus NOS (S27.8-)
        S11.20x-   Unspecified open wound of pharynx and cervical
                    esophagus
        S11.21x-   <u>Laceration</u> <u>without</u> foreign body of pharynx and cervical
                    esophagus

S11.22x-   <u>Laceration</u> <u>with foreign body</u> of pharynx and cervical
            esophagus
S11.23x-   <u>Puncture</u> wound <u>without</u> foreign body of pharynx and
            cervical esophagus
S11.24x-   <u>Puncture</u> wound <u>with foreign body</u> of pharynx and
            cervical esophagus
S11.25x-   Open bite of pharynx and cervical esophagus
            Bite of pharynx and cervical esophagus NOS
S11.8-   Open wound of <u>other specified parts</u> of neck
    S11.80x-   Unspecified open wound of other specified part of neck
    S11.81x-   <u>Laceration</u> <u>without</u> foreign body of other specified part of
                neck
    S11.82x-   <u>Laceration</u> <u>with foreign body</u> of other specified part of
                neck
    S11.83x-   <u>Puncture</u> wound <u>without</u> foreign body of other specified
                part of neck
    S11.84x-   <u>Puncture</u> wound <u>with foreign body</u> of other specified part
                of neck
    S11.85x-   Open bite of other specified part of neck
                Bite of other specified part of neck NOS
                *Excludes 1: superficial bite of other specified part of neck
                              (S10.87)*
    S11.89x-   Other open wound of other specified part of neck
S11.9-   Open wound of <u>unspecified</u> part of neck
    S11.90x-   Unspecified open wound of unspecified part of neck
    S11.91x-   <u>Laceration</u> <u>without</u> foreign body of unspecified part of
                neck
    S11.92x-   <u>Laceration</u> <u>with foreign body</u> of unspecified part of neck
    S11.93x-   <u>Puncture</u> wound <u>without</u> foreign body of unspecified part
                of neck
    S11.94x-   <u>Puncture</u> wound <u>with foreign body</u> of unspecified part of
                neck
    S11.95x-   Open bite of unspecified part of neck
                Bite of neck NOS
                Excludes 1: superficial bite of neck (S10.97)

S12-   <u>Fracture</u> of <u>cervical vertebra</u> and other parts of neck
        Note: A fracture not indicated as nondisplaced or displaced should be
                classified to displaced
        Note: A fracture not indicated as open or closed should be coded to closed
        Includes: Fracture of cervical neural arch
                    Fracture of cervical spine
                    Fracture of cervical spinous process
                    Fracture of cervical transverse process
                    Fracture of cervical vertebral arch
                    Fracture of neck
        Code first any associated cervical spinal cord injury (S14.0, S14.1-)
        **The appropriate 7th character is to be added to all codes from
          subcategories S12.0-S12.6:**
        A   <u>Initial</u> encounter for <u>closed</u> fracture
        B   <u>Initial</u> encounter for <u>open</u> fracture
        D   <u>Subsequent</u> encounter for fracture <u>with routine healing</u>
        G   <u>Subsequent</u> encounter for fracture <u>with delayed healing</u>
        K   <u>Subsequent</u> encounter for fracture <u>with nonunion</u>
        S   <u>Sequela</u>
    S12.0-   Fracture of <u>first</u> cervical vertebra
                Atlas
        S12.00-   <u>Unspecified fracture</u> of first cervical vertebra
            S12.000-   Unspecified <u>displaced</u> fracture of first cervical
                        vertebra
            S12.001-   Unspecified <u>nondisplaced</u> fracture of first cervical
                        vertebra
        S12.01x-   <u>Stable burst</u> fracture of first cervical vertebra
        S12.02x-   <u>Unstable burst</u> fracture of first cervical vertebra
        S12.03-   <u>Posterior arch</u> fracture of first cervical vertebra
            S12.030-   <u>Displaced</u> posterior arch fracture of first cervical
                        vertebra
            S12.031-   <u>Nondisplaced</u> posterior arch fracture of first cervical
                        vertebra
        S12.04-   <u>Lateral mass</u> fracture of first cervical vertebra
            S12.040-   <u>Displaced</u> lateral mass fracture of first cervical
                        vertebra
            S12.041-   <u>Nondisplaced</u> lateral mass fracture of first cervical
                        vertebra
        S12.09-   <u>Other</u> fracture of first cervical vertebra
            S12.090-   Other <u>displaced</u> fracture of first cervical vertebra
            S12.091-   Other <u>nondisplaced</u> fracture of first cervical vertebra

**S10
-
S12**

S12.1-   Fracture of <u>second</u> cervical vertebra
     Axis
  S12.10- <u>Unspecified</u> <u>fracture</u> of second cervical vertebra
    S12.100- Unspecified <u>displaced</u> fracture of second cervical vertebra
    S12.101- Unspecified <u>nondisplaced</u> fracture of second cervical vertebra
  S12.11- Type II dens fracture
    S12.110- <u>Anterior</u> <u>displaced</u> Type II dens fracture
    S12.111- <u>Posterior</u> <u>displaced</u> Type II dens fracture
    S12.112- <u>Nondisplaced</u> Type II dens fracture
  S12.12- <u>Other dens</u> fracture
    S12.120- Other <u>displaced</u> dens fracture
    S12.121- Other <u>nondisplaced</u> dens fracture
  S12.13- <u>Unspecified</u> <u>traumatic spondylolisthesis</u> of second cervical vertebra
    S12.130- Unspecified traumatic <u>displaced</u> spondylolisthesis of second cervical vertebra
    S12.131- Unspecified traumatic <u>nondisplaced</u> spondylolisthesis of second cervical vertebra
  S12.14x- <u>Type III traumatic spondylolisthesis</u> of second cervical vertebra
  S12.15- <u>Other traumatic spondylolisthesis</u> of second cervical vertebra
    S12.150- Other traumatic <u>displaced</u> spondylolisthesis of second cervical vertebra
    S12.151- Other traumatic <u>nondisplaced</u> spondylolisthesis of second cervical vertebra
  S12.19- <u>Other fracture</u> of second cervical vertebra
    S12.190- Other <u>displaced</u> fracture of second cervical vertebra
    S12.191- Other <u>nondisplaced</u> fracture of second cervical vertebra
S12.2-   Fracture of <u>third</u> cervical vertebra
  S12.20- <u>Unspecified</u> <u>fracture</u> of third cervical vertebra
    S12.200- Unspecified <u>displaced</u> fracture of third cervical vertebra
    S12.201- Unspecified <u>nondisplaced</u> fracture of third cervical vertebra
  S12.23- <u>Unspecified</u> <u>traumatic spondylolisthesis</u> of third cervical vertebra
    S12.230- Unspecified traumatic <u>displaced</u> spondylolisthesis of third cervical vertebra
    S12.231- Unspecified traumatic <u>nondisplaced</u> spondylolisthesis of third cervical vertebra
  S12.24x- <u>Type III traumatic spondylolisthesis</u> of third cervical vertebra
  S12.25- <u>Other traumatic spondylolisthesis</u> of third cervical vertebra
    S12.250- Other traumatic <u>displaced</u> spondylolisthesis of third cervical vertebra
    S12.251- Other traumatic <u>nondisplaced</u> spondylolisthesis of third cervical vertebra
  S12.29- <u>Other fracture</u> of third cervical vertebra
    S12.290- Other <u>displaced</u> fracture of third cervical vertebra
    S12.291- Other <u>nondisplaced</u> fracture of third cervical vertebra
S12.3-   <u>Fracture</u> of <u>fourth</u> cervical vertebra
  S12.30- <u>Unspecified</u> <u>fracture</u> of fourth cervical vertebra
    S12.300- Unspecified <u>displaced</u> fracture of fourth cervical vertebra
    S12.301- Unspecified <u>nondisplaced</u> fracture of fourth cervical vertebra
  S12.33- <u>Unspecified</u> <u>traumatic spondylolisthesis</u> of fourth cervical vertebra
    S12.330- Unspecified traumatic <u>displaced</u> spondylolisthesis of fourth cervical vertebra
    S12.331- Unspecified traumatic <u>nondisplaced</u> spondylolisthesis of fourth cervical vertebra
  S12.34x- <u>Type III traumatic spondylolisthesis</u> of fourth cervical vertebra
  S12.35- <u>Other traumatic spondylolisthesis</u> of fourth cervical vertebra
    S12.350- Other traumatic <u>displaced</u> spondylolisthesis of fourth cervical vertebra
    S12.351- Other traumatic <u>nondisplaced</u> spondylolisthesis of fourth cervical vertebra
  S12.39- <u>Other fracture</u> of fourth cervical vertebra
    S12.390- Other <u>displaced</u> fracture of fourth cervical vertebra
    S12.391- Other <u>nondisplaced</u> fracture of fourth cervical vertebra

S12.4-   <u>Fracture</u> of <u>fifth</u> cervical vertebra
  S12.40- <u>Unspecified</u> <u>fracture</u> of fifth cervical vertebra
    S12.400- Unspecified <u>displaced</u> fracture of fifth cervical vertebra
    S12.401- Unspecified <u>nondisplaced</u> fracture of fifth cervical vertebra
  S12.43- <u>Unspecified</u> <u>traumatic spondylolisthesis</u> of fifth cervical vertebra
    S12.430- Unspecified traumatic <u>displaced</u> spondylolisthesis of fifth cervical vertebra
    S12.431- Unspecified traumatic <u>nondisplaced</u> spondylolisthesis of fifth cervical vertebra
  S12.44x- <u>Type III traumatic spondylolisthesis</u> of fifth cervical vertebra
  S12.45- <u>Other traumatic spondylolisthesis</u> of fifth cervical vertebra
    S12.450- Other traumatic <u>displaced</u> spondylolisthesis of fifth cervical vertebra
    S12.451- Other traumatic <u>nondisplaced</u> spondylolisthesis of fifth cervical vertebra
  S12.49- <u>Other fracture</u> of fifth cervical vertebra
    S12.490- Other <u>displaced</u> fracture of fifth cervical vertebra
    S12.491- Other <u>nondisplaced</u> fracture of fifth cervical vertebra
S12.5-   <u>Fracture</u> of <u>sixth</u> cervical vertebra
  S12.50- <u>Unspecified</u> <u>fracture</u> of sixth cervical vertebra
    S12.500- Unspecified <u>displaced</u> fracture of sixth cervical vertebra
    S12.501- Unspecified <u>nondisplaced</u> fracture of sixth cervical vertebra
  S12.53- <u>Unspecified</u> <u>traumatic spondylolisthesis</u> of sixth cervical vertebra
    S12.530- Unspecified traumatic <u>displaced</u> spondylolisthesis of sixth cervical vertebra
    S12.531- Unspecified traumatic <u>nondisplaced</u> spondylolisthesis of sixth cervical vertebra
  S12.54x- <u>Type III traumatic spondylolisthesis</u> of sixth cervical vertebra
  S12.55- <u>Other traumatic spondylolisthesis</u> of sixth cervical vertebra
    S12.550- Other traumatic <u>displaced</u> spondylolisthesis of sixth cervical vertebra
    S12.551- Other traumatic <u>nondisplaced</u> spondylolisthesis of sixth cervical vertebra
  S12.59- <u>Other fracture</u> of sixth cervical vertebra
    S12.590- Other <u>displaced</u> fracture of sixth cervical vertebra
    S12.591- Other <u>nondisplaced</u> fracture of sixth cervical vertebra
S12.6-   <u>Fracture</u> of <u>seventh</u> cervical vertebra
  S12.60- <u>Unspecified</u> <u>fracture</u> of seventh cervical vertebra
    S12.600- Unspecified <u>displaced</u> fracture of seventh cervical vertebra
    S12.601- Unspecified <u>nondisplaced</u> fracture of seventh cervical vertebra
  S12.63- <u>Unspecified</u> <u>traumatic spondylolisthesis</u> of seventh cervical vertebra
    S12.630- Unspecified traumatic <u>displaced</u> spondylolisthesis of seventh cervical vertebra
    S12.631- Unspecified traumatic <u>nondisplaced</u> spondylolisthesis of seventh cervical vertebra
  S12.64x- <u>Type III traumatic spondylolisthesis</u> of seventh cervical vertebra
  S12.65- <u>Other traumatic spondylolisthesis</u> of seventh cervical vertebra
    S12.650- Other traumatic <u>displaced</u> spondylolisthesis of seventh cervical vertebra
    S12.651- Other traumatic <u>nondisplaced</u> spondylolisthesis of seventh cervical vertebra
  S12.69- <u>Other fracture</u> of seventh cervical vertebra
    S12.690- Other <u>displaced</u> fracture of seventh cervical vertebra
    S12.691- Other <u>nondisplaced</u> fracture of seventh cervical vertebra

S1 0 - S1 2

Excludes 1: = NOT CODED HERE! (Do not code both)

Excludes ❷: = Not Included Here

S12.8xx- **Fracture** of **other parts of neck**
    Hyoid bone
    Larynx
    Thyroid cartilage
    Trachea
    The appropriate 7th character is to be added to code S12.8:
    A **Initial** encounter
    D **Subsequent** encounter
    S **Sequela**

S12.9xx- **Fracture** of **neck, unspecified**
    Fracture of neck NOS
    Fracture of cervical spine NOS
    Fracture of cervical vertebra NOS
    The appropriate 7th character is to be added to code S12.9:
    A **Initial** encounter
    D **Subsequent** encounter
    S **Sequela**

S13- **Dislocation and sprain** of joints and ligaments at **neck** level
    Includes: Avulsion of joint or ligament at neck level
      Laceration of cartilage, joint or ligament at neck level
      Sprain of cartilage, joint or ligament at neck level
      Traumatic hemarthrosis of joint or ligament at neck level
      Traumatic rupture of joint or ligament at neck level
      Traumatic subluxation of joint or ligament at neck level
      Traumatic tear of joint or ligament at neck level
    Code also any associated open wound
    Excludes❷: strain of muscle or tendon at neck level (S16.1)
    The appropriate 7th character is to be added to each code from category S13:
    A **Initial** encounter
    D **Subsequent** encounter
    S **Sequela**

S13.0xx- **Traumatic rupture** of **cervical intervertebral disc**
    Excludes 1: rupture or displacement (nontraumatic) of cervical intervertebral disc NOS (M50.-)

S13.1- **Subluxation and dislocation** of **cervical vertebrae**
    Code also any associated:
      Open wound of neck (S11.-)
      Spinal cord injury (S14.1-)
    Excludes❷: fracture of cervical vertebrae (S12.0-S12.3-)
  S13.10- Subluxation and dislocation of **unspecified** cervical vertebrae
    S13.100- **Subluxation** of unspecified cervical vertebrae
    S13.101- **Dislocation** of unspecified cervical vertebrae
  S13.11- Subluxation and dislocation of **C0/C1** cervical vertebrae
    Subluxation and dislocation of atlantooccipital joint
    Subluxation and dislocation of atloidooccipital joint
    Subluxation and dislocation of occipitoatloid joint
    S13.110- **Subluxation** of C0/C1 cervical vertebrae
    S13.111- **Dislocation** of C0/C1 cervical vertebrae
  S13.12- Subluxation and dislocation of **C1/C2** cervical vertebrae
    Subluxation and dislocation of atlantoaxial joint
    S13.120- **Subluxation** of C1/C2 cervical vertebrae
    S13.121- **Dislocation** of C1/C2 cervical vertebrae
  S13.13- Subluxation and dislocation of **C2/C3** cervical vertebrae
    S13.130- **Subluxation** of C2/C3 cervical vertebrae
    S13.131- **Dislocation** of C2/C3 cervical vertebrae
  S13.14- Subluxation and dislocation of **C3/C4** cervical vertebrae
    S13.140- **Subluxation** of C3/C4 cervical vertebrae
    S13.141- **Dislocation** of C3/C4 cervical vertebrae
  S13.15- Subluxation and dislocation of **C4/C5** cervical vertebrae
    S13.150- **Subluxation** of C4/C5 cervical vertebrae
    S13.151- **Dislocation** of C4/C5 cervical vertebrae
  S13.16- Subluxation and dislocation of **C5/C6** cervical vertebrae
    S13.160- **Subluxation** of C5/C6 cervical vertebrae
    S13.161- **Dislocation** of C5/C6 cervical vertebrae
  S13.17- Subluxation and dislocation of **C6/C7** cervical vertebrae
    S13.170- **Subluxation** of C6/C7 cervical vertebrae
    S13.171- **Dislocation** of C6/C7 cervical vertebrae
  S13.18- Subluxation and dislocation of **C7/T1** cervical vertebrae
    S13.180- **Subluxation** of C7/T1 cervical vertebrae
    S13.181- **Dislocation** of C7/T1 cervical vertebrae
S13.2- Dislocation of other and **unspecified** parts of neck
  S13.20x- Dislocation of **unspecified** parts of neck
  S13.29x- Dislocation of **other** parts of neck
S13.4xx- **Sprain of ligaments** of cervical spine
    Sprain of anterior longitudinal (ligament), cervical
    Sprain of atlanto-axial (joints)
    Sprain of atlanto-occipital (joints)
    Whiplash injury of cervical spine

S13.5xx- **Sprain of thyroid region**
    Sprain of cricoarytenoid (joint) (ligament)
    Sprain of cricothyroid (joint) (ligament)
    Sprain of thyroid cartilage
S13.8xx- **Sprain of joints and ligaments of other parts of neck**
S13.9xx- **Sprain of joints and ligaments of unspecified parts of neck**

S14- **Injury of nerves and spinal cord** at **neck** level
    Note: Code to highest level of cervical cord injury
    Code also any associated:
      Fracture of cervical vertebra (S12.0--S12.6.-)
      Open wound of neck (S11.-)
      Transient paralysis (R29.5)
    The appropriate 7th character is to be added to each code from category S14:
    A **Initial** encounter
    D **Subsequent** encounter
    S **Sequela**

S14.0xx- **Concussion and edema** of cervical spinal cord
S14.1- Other and unspecified injuries of cervical spinal cord
  S14.10- **Unspecified injury** of cervical spinal cord
    S14.101- Unspecified injury at **C1** level of cervical spinal cord
    S14.102- Unspecified injury at **C2** level of cervical spinal cord
    S14.103- Unspecified injury at **C3** level of cervical spinal cord
    S14.104- Unspecified injury at **C4** level of cervical spinal cord
    S14.105- Unspecified injury at **C5** level of cervical spinal cord
    S14.106- Unspecified injury at **C6** level of cervical spinal cord
    S14.107- Unspecified injury at **C7** level of cervical spinal cord
    S14.108- Unspecified injury at **C8** level of cervical spinal cord
    S14.109- Unspecified injury at **unspecified** level of cervical spinal cord
      Injury of cervical spinal cord NOS
  S14.11- **Complete lesion** of cervical spinal cord
    S14.111- **Complete lesion at C1** level of cervical spinal cord
    S14.112- **Complete lesion at C2** level of cervical spinal cord
    S14.113- **Complete lesion at C3** level of cervical spinal cord
    S14.114- **Complete lesion at C4** level of cervical spinal cord
    S14.115- **Complete lesion at C5** level of cervical spinal cord
    S14.116- **Complete lesion at C6** level of cervical spinal cord
    S14.117- **Complete lesion at C7** level of cervical spinal cord
    S14.118- **Complete lesion at C8** level of cervical spinal cord
    S14.119- **Complete lesion at unspecified** level of cervical spinal cord
  S14.12- **Central cord syndrome** of cervical spinal cord
    S14.121- **Central cord syndrome at C1** level of cervical spinal cord
    S14.122- **Central cord syndrome at C2** level of cervical spinal cord
    S14.123- **Central cord syndrome at C3** level of cervical spinal cord
    S14.124- **Central cord syndrome at C4** level of cervical spinal cord
    S14.125- **Central cord syndrome at C5** level of cervical spinal cord
    S14.126- **Central cord syndrome at C6** level of cervical spinal cord
    S14.127- **Central cord syndrome at C7** level of cervical spinal cord
    S14.128- **Central cord syndrome at C8** level of cervical spinal cord
    S14.129- **Central cord syndrome at unspecified** level of cervical spinal cord
  S14.13- **Anterior cord syndrome** of cervical spinal cord
    S14.131- **Anterior cord syndrome at C1** level of cervical spinal cord
    S14.132- **Anterior cord syndrome at C2** level of cervical spinal cord
    S14.133- **Anterior cord syndrome at C3** level of cervical spinal cord
    S14.134- **Anterior cord syndrome at C4** level of cervical spinal cord
    S14.135- **Anterior cord syndrome at C5** level of cervical spinal cord
    S14.136- **Anterior cord syndrome at C6** level of cervical spinal cord
    S14.137- **Anterior cord syndrome at C7** level of cervical spinal cord
    S14.138- **Anterior cord syndrome at C8** level of cervical spinal cord

S12 - S15

S14.139-   Anterior cord syndrome at <u>unspecified</u> level of cervical spinal cord
S14.14-   <u>Brown-Séquard syndrome</u> of cervical spinal cord
   S14.141-   Brown-Séquard syndrome at <u>C1</u> level of cervical spinal cord
   S14.142-   Brown-Séquard syndrome at <u>C2</u> level of cervical spinal cord
   S14.143-   Brown-Séquard syndrome at <u>C3</u> level of cervical spinal cord
   S14.144-   Brown-Séquard syndrome at <u>C4</u> level of cervical spinal cord
   S14.145-   Brown-Séquard syndrome at <u>C5</u> level of cervical spinal cord
   S14.146-   Brown-Séquard syndrome at <u>C6</u> level of cervical spinal cord
   S14.147-   Brown-Séquard syndrome at <u>C7</u> level of cervical spinal cord
   S14.148-   Brown-Séquard syndrome at <u>C8</u> level of cervical spinal cord
   S14.149-   Brown-Séquard syndrome at <u>unspecified</u> level of cervical spinal cord
S14.15-   <u>Other incomplete lesions</u> of cervical spinal cord
   Incomplete lesion of cervical spinal cord NOS
   Posterior cord syndrome of cervical spinal cord
   S14.151-   Other incomplete lesion at <u>C1</u> level of cervical spinal cord
   S14.152-   Other incomplete lesion at <u>C2</u> level of cervical spinal cord
   S14.153-   Other incomplete lesion at <u>C3</u> level of cervical spinal cord
   S14.154-   Other incomplete lesion at <u>C4</u> level of cervical spinal cord
   S14.155-   Other incomplete lesion at <u>C5</u> level of cervical spinal cord
   S14.156-   Other incomplete lesion at <u>C6</u> level of cervical spinal cord
   S14.157-   Other incomplete lesion at <u>C7</u> level of cervical spinal cord
   S14.158-   Other incomplete lesion at <u>C8</u> level of cervical spinal cord
   S14.159-   Other incomplete lesion at <u>unspecified</u> level of cervical spinal cord
S14.2xx-   Injury of nerve root of cervical spine
S14.3xx-   Injury of brachial plexus
S14.4xx-   Injury of peripheral nerves of neck
S14.5xx-   Injury of cervical sympathetic nerves
S14.8xx-   Injury of <u>other</u> specified nerves of neck
S14.9xx-   Injury of <u>unspecified</u> nerves of neck
S15-   <u>Injury of blood vessels</u> at <u>neck</u> level
   Code also any associated open wound (S11.-)

The appropriate 7th character is to be added to each code from category S15:
  A   <u>Initial</u> encounter
  D   <u>Subsequent</u> encounter
  S   <u>Sequela</u>

S15.0-   Injury of <u>carotid artery</u> of neck
   Injury of carotid artery (common) (external) (internal, extracranial portion)
   Injury of carotid artery NOS
   Excludes 1:   injury of internal carotid artery, intracranial portion (S06.8)
   S15.00-   <u>Unspecified</u> injury of carotid artery
     S15.001-   Unspecified injury of <u>right</u> carotid artery
     S15.002-   Unspecified injury of <u>left</u> carotid artery
     S15.009-   Unspecified injury of <u>unspecified</u> carotid artery
   S15.01-   <u>Minor laceration</u> of carotid artery
     Incomplete transection of carotid artery
     Laceration of carotid artery NOS
     Superficial laceration of carotid artery
     S15.011-   Minor laceration of <u>right</u> carotid artery
     S15.012-   Minor laceration of <u>left</u> carotid artery
     S15.019-   Minor laceration of <u>unspecified</u> carotid artery
   S15.02-   <u>Major laceration</u> of carotid artery
     Complete transection of carotid artery
     Traumatic rupture of carotid artery
     S15.021-   Major laceration of <u>right</u> carotid artery
     S15.022-   Major laceration of <u>left</u> carotid artery
     S15.029-   Major laceration of <u>unspecified</u> carotid artery

   S15.09-   <u>Other specified</u> injury of carotid artery
     S15.091-   Other specified injury of <u>right</u> carotid artery
     S15.092-   Other specified injury of <u>left</u> carotid artery
     S15.099-   Other specified injury of <u>unspecified</u> carotid artery
S15.1-   Injury of <u>vertebral artery</u>
   S15.10-   <u>Unspecified</u> injury of vertebral artery
     S15.101-   Unspecified injury of <u>right</u> vertebral artery
     S15.102-   Unspecified injury of <u>left</u> vertebral artery
     S15.109-   Unspecified injury of <u>unspecified</u> vertebral artery
   S15.11-   <u>Minor laceration</u> of vertebral artery
     Incomplete transection of vertebral artery
     Laceration of vertebral artery NOS
     Superficial laceration of vertebral artery
     S15.111-   Minor laceration of <u>right</u> vertebral artery
     S15.112-   Minor laceration of <u>left</u> vertebral artery
     S15.119-   Minor laceration of <u>unspecified</u> vertebral artery
   S15.12-   <u>Major laceration</u> of vertebral artery
     Complete transection of vertebral artery
     Traumatic rupture of vertebral artery
     S15.121-   Major laceration of <u>right</u> vertebral artery
     S15.122-   Major laceration of <u>left</u> vertebral artery
     S15.129-   Major laceration of <u>unspecified</u> vertebral artery
   S15.19-   <u>Other specified</u> injury of vertebral artery
     S15.191-   Other specified injury of <u>right</u> vertebral artery
     S15.192-   Other specified injury of <u>left</u> vertebral artery
     S15.199-   Other specified injury of <u>unspecified</u> vertebral artery
S15.2-   Injury of <u>external jugular vein</u>
   S15.20-   <u>Unspecified</u> injury of external jugular vein
     S15.201-   Unspecified injury of <u>right</u> external jugular vein
     S15.202-   Unspecified injury of <u>left</u> external jugular vein
     S15.209-   Unspecified injury of <u>unspecified</u> external jugular vein
   S15.21-   <u>Minor laceration</u> of external jugular vein
     Incomplete transection of external jugular vein
     Laceration of external jugular vein NOS
     Superficial laceration of external jugular vein
     S15.211-   Minor laceration of <u>right</u> external jugular vein
     S15.212-   Minor laceration of <u>left</u> external jugular vein
     S15.219-   Minor laceration of <u>unspecified</u> external jugular vein
   S15.22-   <u>Major laceration</u> of external jugular vein
     Complete transection of external jugular vein
     Traumatic rupture of external jugular vein
     S15.221-   Major laceration of <u>right</u> external jugular vein
     S15.222-   Major laceration of <u>left</u> external jugular vein
     S15.229-   Major laceration of <u>unspecified</u> external jugular vein
   S15.29-   <u>Other specified</u> injury of external jugular vein
     S15.291-   Other specified injury of <u>right</u> external jugular vein
     S15.292-   Other specified injury of <u>left</u> external jugular vein
     S15.299-   Other specified injury of <u>unspecified</u> external jugular vein
S15.3-   Injury of <u>internal jugular vein</u>
   S15.30-   <u>Unspecified</u> injury of internal jugular vein
     S15.301-   Unspecified injury of <u>right</u> internal jugular vein
     S15.302-   Unspecified injury of <u>left</u> internal jugular vein
     S15.309-   Unspecified injury of <u>unspecified</u> internal jugular vein
   S15.31-   <u>Minor laceration</u> of internal jugular vein
     Incomplete transection of internal jugular vein
     Laceration of internal jugular vein NOS
     Superficial laceration of internal jugular vein
     S15.311-   Minor laceration of <u>right</u> internal jugular vein
     S15.312-   Minor laceration of <u>left</u> internal jugular vein
     S15.319-   Minor laceration of <u>unspecified</u> internal jugular vein
   S15.32-   <u>Major laceration</u> of internal jugular vein
     Complete transection of internal jugular vein
     Traumatic rupture of internal jugular vein
     S15.321-   Major laceration of <u>right</u> internal jugular vein
     S15.322-   Major laceration of <u>left</u> internal jugular vein
     S15.329-   Major laceration of <u>unspecified</u> internal jugular vein
   S15.39-   <u>Other specified</u> injury of internal jugular vein
     S15.391-   Other specified injury of <u>right</u> internal jugular vein
     S15.392-   Other specified injury of <u>left</u> internal jugular vein
     S15.399-   Other specified injury of <u>unspecified</u> internal jugular vein
S15.8xx-   Injury of <u>other</u> specified blood vessels at neck level
S15.9xx-   Injury of <u>unspecified</u> blood vessel at neck level

S 1 2 – S 1 5

S16- <u>Injury of muscle, fascia and tendon</u> at <u>neck</u> level
Code also any associated open wound (S11.-)
Excludes❷: sprain of joint or ligament at neck level (S13.9)

The appropriate 7th character is to be added to each code from category S16:
A <u>Initial</u> encounter
D <u>Subsequent</u> encounter
S <u>Sequela</u>

S16.1xx- <u>Strain</u> of muscle, fascia and tendon at neck level
S16.2xx- <u>Laceration</u> of muscle, fascia and tendon at neck level
S16.8xx- <u>Other</u> specified injury of muscle, fascia and tendon at neck level
S16.9xx- <u>Unspecified</u> injury of muscle, fascia and tendon at neck level

S17- <u>Crushing</u> injury of neck
Use additional code for all associated injuries, such as:
Injury of blood vessels (S15.-)
Open wound of neck (S11.-)
Spinal cord injury (S14.0, S14.1-)
Vertebral fracture (S12.0--S12.3-)

The appropriate 7th character is to be added to each code from category S17:
A <u>Initial</u> encounter
D <u>Subsequent</u> encounter
S <u>Sequela</u>

S17.0xx- Crushing injury of <u>larynx and trachea</u>
S17.8xx- Crushing injury of <u>other</u> specified parts of neck
S17.9xx- Crushing injury of neck, part <u>unspecified</u>

S19- Other specified and unspecified injuries of neck

The appropriate 7th character is to be added to each code from category S19:
A <u>Initial</u> encounter
D <u>Subsequent</u> encounter
S <u>Sequela</u>

S19.8- <u>Other specified</u> injuries of neck
S19.80x- Other specified injuries of <u>unspecified</u> part of neck
S19.81x- Other specified injuries of <u>larynx</u>
S19.82x- Other specified injuries of <u>cervical trachea</u>
Excludes❷: other specified injury of thoracic trachea (S27.5-)
S19.83x- Other specified injuries of <u>vocal cord</u>
S19.84x- Other specified injuries of <u>thyroid gland</u>
S19.85x- Other specified injuries of <u>pharynx and cervical esophagus</u>
S19.89x- Other specified injuries of <u>other specified</u> part of neck
S19.9xx- <u>Unspecified</u> injury of neck

Injuries to the thorax (S20-S29)

Includes: Injuries of breast
Injuries of chest (wall)
Injuries of interscapular area
Excludes❷: burns and corrosions (T20-T32)
effects of foreign body in bronchus (T17.5)
effects of foreign body in esophagus (T18.1)
effects of foreign body in lung (T17.8)
effects of foreign body in trachea (T17.4)
frostbite (T33-T34)
injuries of axilla
injuries of clavicle
injuries of scapular region
injuries of shoulder
insect bite or sting, venomous (T63.4)

S20- <u>Superficial injury</u> of thorax

The appropriate 7th character is to be added to each code from category S20:
A <u>Initial</u> encounter
D <u>Subsequent</u> encounter
S <u>Sequela</u>

S20.0- <u>Contusion</u> of <u>breast</u>
S20.00x- Contusion of breast, <u>unspecified</u> breast
S20.01x- Contusion of <u>right</u> breast
S20.02x- Contusion of <u>left</u> breast
S20.1- Other and unspecified superficial injuries of <u>breast</u>
S20.10- <u>Unspecified</u> superficial injuries of breast
S20.101- Unspecified superficial injuries of breast, <u>right</u> breast
S20.102- Unspecified superficial injuries of breast, <u>left</u> breast
S20.109- Unspecified superficial injuries of breast, <u>unspecified</u> breast
S20.11- <u>Abrasion</u> of breast
S20.111- Abrasion of breast, <u>right</u> breast
S20.112- Abrasion of breast, <u>left</u> breast
S20.119- Abrasion of breast, <u>unspecified</u> breast

S20.12- <u>Blister</u> (nonthermal) of breast
S20.121- Blister (nonthermal) of breast, <u>right</u> breast
S20.122- Blister (nonthermal) of breast, <u>left</u> breast
S20.129- Blister (nonthermal) of breast, <u>unspecified</u> breast
S20.14- <u>External constriction</u> of part of breast
S20.141- External constriction of part of breast, <u>right</u> breast
S20.142- External constriction of part of breast, <u>left</u> breast
S20.149- External constriction of part of breast, <u>unspecified</u> breast
S20.15- <u>Superficial foreign body</u> of breast
Splinter in the breast
S20.151- Superficial foreign body of breast, <u>right</u> breast
S20.152- Superficial foreign body of breast, <u>left</u> breast
S20.159- Superficial foreign body of breast, <u>unspecified</u> breast
S20.16- <u>Insect bite (nonvenomous)</u> of breast
S20.161- Insect bite (nonvenomous) of breast, <u>right</u> breast
S20.162- Insect bite (nonvenomous) of breast, <u>left</u> breast
S20.169- Insect bite (nonvenomous) of breast, <u>unspecified</u> breast
S20.17- <u>Other superficial bite</u> of breast
Excludes 1: open bite of breast (S21.05-)
S20.171- Other superficial bite of breast, <u>right</u> breast
S20.172- Other superficial bite of breast, <u>left</u> breast
S20.179- Other superficial bite of breast, <u>unspecified</u> breast
S20.2- <u>Contusion</u> of <u>thorax</u>
S20.20x- Contusion of thorax, <u>unspecified</u>
S20.21- Contusion of <u>front wall</u> of thorax
S20.211- Contusion of <u>right</u> front wall of thorax
S20.212- Contusion of <u>left</u> front wall of thorax
S20.219- Contusion of <u>unspecified</u> front wall of thorax
S20.22- Contusion of <u>back wall</u> of thorax
S20.221- Contusion of <u>right</u> back wall of thorax
S20.222- Contusion of <u>left</u> back wall of thorax
S20.229- Contusion of <u>unspecified</u> back wall of thorax
S20.3- Other and unspecified superficial injuries of <u>front wall</u> of thorax
S20.30- <u>Unspecified</u> superficial injuries of <u>front wall</u> of thorax
S20.301- Unspecified superficial injuries of <u>right</u> front wall of thorax
S20.302- Unspecified superficial injuries of <u>left</u> front wall of thorax
S20.309- Unspecified superficial injuries of <u>unspecified</u> front wall of thorax
S20.31- <u>Abrasion</u> of <u>front wall</u> of thorax
S20.311- Abrasion of <u>right</u> front wall of thorax
S20.312- Abrasion of <u>left</u> front wall of thorax
S20.319- Abrasion of <u>unspecified</u> front wall of thorax
S20.32- <u>Blister</u> (nonthermal) of <u>front wall</u> of thorax
S20.321- Blister (nonthermal) of <u>right</u> front wall of thorax
S20.322- Blister (nonthermal) of <u>left</u> front wall of thorax
S20.329- Blister (nonthermal) of <u>unspecified</u> front wall of thorax
S20.34- <u>External constriction</u> of <u>front wall</u> of thorax
S20.341- External constriction of <u>right</u> front wall of thorax
S20.342- External constriction of <u>left</u> front wall of thorax
S20.349- External constriction of <u>unspecified</u> front wall of thorax
S20.35- <u>Superficial foreign body</u> of <u>front wall</u> of thorax
Splinter in front wall of thorax
S20.351- Superficial foreign body of <u>right</u> front wall of thorax
S20.352- Superficial foreign body of <u>left</u> front wall of thorax
S20.359- Superficial foreign body of <u>unspecified</u> front wall of thorax
S20.36- <u>Insect bite (nonvenomous)</u> of <u>front wall</u> of thorax
S20.361- Insect bite (nonvenomous) of <u>right</u> front wall of thorax
S20.362- Insect bite (nonvenomous) of <u>left</u> front wall of thorax
S20.369- Insect bite (nonvenomous) of <u>unspecified</u> front wall of thorax
S20.37- <u>Other superficial bite</u> of <u>front wall</u> of thorax
Excludes 1: open bite of front wall of thorax (S21.14)
S20.371- Other superficial bite of <u>right</u> front wall of thorax
S20.372- Other superficial bite of <u>left</u> front wall of thorax
S20.379- Other superficial bite of <u>unspecified</u> front wall of thorax

Excludes 1: = NOT CODED HERE! (Do not code both)   **698**   *Excludes❷: = Not Included Here*

S20.4- Other and unspecified superficial injuries of back wall of <u>thorax</u>
   S20.40- <u>Unspecified</u> superficial injuries of <u>back wall</u> of thorax
      S20.401- Unspecified superficial injuries of <u>right</u> back wall of thorax
      S20.402- Unspecified superficial injuries of <u>left</u> back wall of thorax
      S20.409- Unspecified superficial injuries of <u>unspecified</u> back wall of thorax
   S20.41- <u>Abrasion</u> of <u>back wall</u> of thorax
      S20.411- Abrasion of <u>right</u> back wall of thorax
      S20.412- Abrasion of <u>left</u> back wall of thorax
      S20.419- Abrasion of <u>unspecified</u> back wall of thorax
   S20.42- <u>Blister</u> (nonthermal) of <u>back wall</u> of thorax
      S20.421- Blister (nonthermal) of <u>right</u> back wall of thorax
      S20.422- Blister (nonthermal) of <u>left</u> back wall of thorax
      S20.429- Blister (nonthermal) of <u>unspecified</u> back wall of thorax
   S20.44- <u>External constriction</u> of <u>back wall</u> of thorax
      S20.441- External constriction of <u>right</u> back wall of thorax
      S20.442- External constriction of <u>left</u> back wall of thorax
      S20.449- External constriction of <u>unspecified</u> back wall of thorax
   S20.45- <u>Superficial foreign body</u> of back wall of thorax
      Splinter of back wall of thorax
      S20.451- Superficial foreign body of <u>right</u> back wall of thorax
      S20.452- Superficial foreign body of <u>left</u> back wall of thorax
      S20.459- Superficial foreign body of <u>unspecified</u> back wall of thorax
   S20.46- <u>Insect bite (nonvenomous)</u> of <u>back wall</u> of thorax
      S20.461- Insect bite (nonvenomous) of <u>right</u> back wall of thorax
      S20.462- Insect bite (nonvenomous) of <u>left</u> back wall of thorax
      S20.469- Insect bite (nonvenomous) of <u>unspecified</u> back wall of thorax
   S20.47- <u>Other superficial bite</u> of <u>back wall</u> of thorax
      Excludes 1: open bite of back wall of thorax (S21.24)
      S20.471- Other superficial bite of <u>right</u> back wall of thorax
      S20.472- Other superficial bite of <u>left</u> back wall of thorax
      S20.479- Other superficial bite of <u>unspecified</u> back wall of thorax
S20.9- Superficial injury of <u>unspecified</u> parts of thorax
   Excludes 1: contusion of thorax NOS (S20.20)
   S20.90x- <u>Unspecified</u> superficial injury of <u>unspecified</u> parts of thorax
      Superficial injury of thoracic wall NOS
   S20.91x- Abrasion of <u>unspecified</u> parts of thorax
   S20.92x- Blister (nonthermal) of <u>unspecified</u> parts of thorax
   S20.94x- External constriction of <u>unspecified</u> parts of thorax
   S20.95x- Superficial foreign body of <u>unspecified</u> parts of thorax
      Splinter in thorax NOS
   S20.96x- Insect bite (nonvenomous) of <u>unspecified</u> parts of thorax
   S20.97x- Other superficial bite of <u>unspecified</u> parts of thorax
      Excludes 1: open bite of thorax NOS (S21.95)

S21- <u>Open wound</u> of thorax
   Code also any associated injury, such as :
   Injury of heart (S26.-)
   Injury of intrathoracic organs (S27.-)
   Rib fracture (S22.3-, S22.4-)
   Spinal cord injury (S24.0-, S24.1-)
   Traumatic hemothorax (S27.1)
   Traumatic hemopneumothorax (S27.3)
   Traumatic pneumothorax (S27.0)
   Wound infection
   Excludes 1: traumatic amputation (partial) of thorax (S28.1)
   The appropriate 7th character is to be added to each code from category S21:
    A <u>Initial</u> encounter
    D <u>Subsequent</u> encounter
    S <u>Sequela</u>
S21.0- Open wound of <u>breast</u>
   S21.00- <u>Unspecified</u> open wound of breast
      S21.001- Unspecified open wound of <u>right</u> breast
      S21.002- Unspecified open wound of <u>left</u> breast
      S21.009- Unspecified open wound of <u>unspecified</u> breast
   S21.01- <u>Laceration</u> <u>without</u> foreign body of breast
      S21.011- Laceration <u>without</u> foreign body of <u>right</u> breast
      S21.012- Laceration <u>without</u> foreign body of <u>left</u> breast
      S21.019- Laceration <u>without</u> foreign body of <u>unspecified</u> breast

S21.02- <u>Laceration</u> <u>with foreign body</u> of breast
      S21.021- Laceration <u>with foreign body</u> of <u>right</u> breast
      S21.022- Laceration <u>with foreign body</u> of <u>left</u> breast
      S21.029- Laceration <u>with foreign body</u> of <u>unspecified</u> breast
S21.03- <u>Puncture</u> wound <u>without</u> foreign body of breast
      S21.031- Puncture wound <u>without</u> foreign body of <u>right</u> breast
      S21.032- Puncture wound <u>without</u> foreign body of <u>left</u> breast
      S21.039- Puncture wound <u>without</u> foreign body of <u>unspecified</u> breast
S21.04- <u>Puncture</u> wound <u>with foreign body</u> of breast
      S21.041- Puncture wound <u>with foreign body</u> of <u>right</u> breast
      S21.042- Puncture wound <u>with foreign body</u> of <u>left</u> breast
      S21.049- Puncture wound <u>with foreign body</u> of <u>unspecified</u> breast
S21.05- <u>Open bite</u> of breast
      Bite of breast NOS
      Excludes 1: superficial bite of breast (S20.17)
      S21.051- Open bite of <u>right</u> breast
      S21.052- Open bite of <u>left</u> breast
      S21.059- Open bite of <u>unspecified</u> breast
S21.1- <u>Open wound</u> of <u>front wall</u> of <u>thorax</u> <u>without</u> penetration into thoracic cavity
   Open wound of chest without penetration into thoracic cavity
   S21.10- <u>Unspecified</u> open wound of <u>front wall</u> of thorax <u>without</u> penetration into thoracic cavity
      S21.101- Unspecified open wound of <u>right</u> front wall of thorax <u>without</u> penetration into thoracic cavity
      S21.102- Unspecified open wound of <u>left</u> front wall of thorax <u>without</u> penetration into thoracic cavity
      S21.109- Unspecified open wound of <u>unspecified</u> front wall of thorax <u>without</u> penetration into thoracic cavity
   S21.11- <u>Laceration</u> <u>without</u> foreign body of front wall of thorax <u>without</u> penetration into thoracic cavity
      S21.111- Laceration <u>without</u> foreign body of <u>right</u> front wall of thorax <u>without</u> penetration into thoracic cavity
      S21.112- Laceration <u>without</u> foreign body of <u>left</u> front wall of thorax <u>without</u> penetration into thoracic cavity
      S21.119- Laceration <u>without</u> foreign body of <u>unspecified</u> front wall of thorax <u>without</u> penetration into thoracic cavity
   S21.12- Laceration <u>with foreign body</u> of front wall of thorax <u>without</u> penetration into thoracic cavity
      S21.121- Laceration <u>with foreign body</u> of <u>right</u> front wall of thorax <u>without</u> penetration into thoracic cavity
      S21.122- Laceration <u>with foreign body</u> of <u>left</u> front wall of thorax <u>without</u> penetration into thoracic cavity
      S21.129- Laceration <u>with foreign body</u> of <u>unspecified</u> front wall of thorax <u>without</u> penetration into thoracic cavity
   S21.13- <u>Puncture</u> wound <u>without</u> foreign body of front wall of thorax <u>without</u> penetration into thoracic cavity
      S21.131- Puncture wound <u>without</u> foreign body of <u>right</u> front wall of thorax <u>without</u> penetration into thoracic cavity
      S21.132- Puncture wound <u>without</u> foreign body of <u>left</u> front wall of thorax <u>without</u> penetration into thoracic cavity
      S21.139- Puncture wound <u>without</u> foreign body of <u>unspecified</u> front wall of thorax <u>without</u> penetration into thoracic cavity
   S21.14- <u>Puncture</u> wound <u>with foreign body</u> of front wall of thorax <u>without</u> penetration into thoracic cavity
      S21.141- Puncture wound <u>with foreign body</u> of <u>right</u> front wall of thorax <u>without</u> penetration into thoracic cavity
      S21.142- Puncture wound <u>with foreign body</u> of <u>left</u> front wall of thorax <u>without</u> penetration into thoracic cavity
      S21.149- Puncture wound <u>with foreign body</u> of <u>unspecified</u> front wall of thorax <u>without</u> penetration into thoracic cavity
   S21.15- <u>Open bite</u> of front wall of thorax <u>without</u> penetration into thoracic cavity
      Bite of front wall of thorax NOS
      Excludes 1: superficial bite of front wall of thorax (S20.37)
      S21.151- Open bite of <u>right</u> front wall of thorax <u>without</u> penetration into thoracic cavity
      S21.152- Open bite of <u>left</u> front wall of thorax <u>without</u> penetration into thoracic cavity
      S21.159- Open bite of <u>unspecified</u> front wall of thorax <u>without</u> penetration into thoracic cavity

S 1 6 I S 2 1

S21.2-   Open wound of back wall of thorax without penetration into thoracic cavity

   S21.20-   Unspecified open wound of back wall of thorax without penetration into thoracic cavity

      S21.201-   Unspecified open wound of right back wall of thorax without penetration into thoracic cavity

      S21.202-   Unspecified open wound of left back wall of thorax without penetration into thoracic cavity

      S21.209-   Unspecified open wound of unspecified back wall of thorax without penetration into thoracic cavity

   S21.21-   Laceration without foreign body of back wall of thorax without penetration into thoracic cavity

      S21.211-   Laceration without foreign body of right back wall of thorax without penetration into thoracic cavity

      S21.212-   Laceration without foreign body of left back wall of thorax without penetration into thoracic cavity

      S21.219-   Laceration without foreign body of unspecified back wall of thorax without penetration into thoracic cavity

   S21.22-   Laceration with foreign body of back wall of thorax without penetration into thoracic cavity

      S21.221-   Laceration with foreign body of right back wall of thorax without penetration into thoracic cavity

      S21.222-   Laceration with foreign body of left back wall of thorax without penetration into thoracic cavity

      S21.229-   Laceration with foreign body of unspecified back wall of thorax without penetration into thoracic cavity

   S21.23-   Puncture wound without foreign body of back wall of thorax without penetration into thoracic cavity

      S21.231-   Puncture wound without foreign body of right back wall of thorax without penetration into thoracic cavity

      S21.232-   Puncture wound without foreign body of left back wall of thorax without penetration into thoracic cavity

      S21.239-   Puncture wound without foreign body of unspecified back wall of thorax without penetration into thoracic cavity

   S21.24-   Puncture wound with foreign body of back wall of thorax without penetration into thoracic cavity

      S21.241-   Puncture wound with foreign body of right back wall of thorax without penetration into thoracic cavity

      S21.242-   Puncture wound with foreign body of left back wall of thorax without penetration into thoracic cavity

      S21.249-   Puncture wound with foreign body of unspecified back wall of thorax without penetration into thoracic cavity

   S21.25-   Open bite of back wall of thorax without penetration into thoracic cavity
      Bite of back wall of thorax NOS
      Excludes 1: superficial bite of back wall of thorax (S20.47)

      S21.251-   Open bite of right back wall of thorax without penetration into thoracic cavity

      S21.252-   Open bite of left back wall of thorax without penetration into thoracic cavity

      S21.259-   Open bite of unspecified back wall of thorax without penetration into thoracic cavity

S21.3-   Open wound of front wall of thorax with penetration into thoracic cavity
      Open wound of chest with penetration into thoracic cavity

   S21.30-   Unspecified open wound of front wall of thorax with penetration into thoracic cavity

      S21.301-   Unspecified open wound of right front wall of thorax with penetration into thoracic cavity

      S21.302-   Unspecified open wound of left front wall of thorax with penetration into thoracic cavity

      S21.309-   Unspecified open wound of unspecified front wall of thorax with penetration into thoracic cavity

   S21.31-   Laceration without foreign body of front wall of thorax with penetration into thoracic cavity

      S21.311-   Laceration without foreign body of right front wall of thorax with penetration into thoracic cavity

      S21.312-   Laceration without foreign body of left front wall of thorax with penetration into thoracic cavity

      S21.319-   Laceration without foreign body of unspecified front wall of thorax with penetration into thoracic cavity

   S21.32-   Laceration with foreign body of front wall of thorax with penetration into thoracic cavity

      S21.321-   Laceration with foreign body of right front wall of thorax with penetration into thoracic cavity

      S21.322-   Laceration with foreign body of left front wall of thorax with penetration into thoracic cavity

      S21.329-   Laceration with foreign body of unspecified front wall of thorax with penetration into thoracic cavity

S21.33-   Puncture wound without foreign body of front wall of thorax with penetration into thoracic cavity

   S21.331-   Puncture wound without foreign body of right front wall of thorax with penetration into thoracic cavity

   S21.332-   Puncture wound without foreign body of left front wall of thorax with penetration into thoracic cavity

   S21.339-   Puncture wound without foreign body of unspecified front wall of thorax with penetration into thoracic cavity

S21.34-   Puncture wound with foreign body of front wall of thorax with penetration into thoracic cavity

   S21.341-   Puncture wound with foreign body of right front wall of thorax with penetration into thoracic cavity

   S21.342-   Puncture wound with foreign body of left front wall of thorax with penetration into thoracic cavity

   S21.349-   Puncture wound with foreign body of unspecified front wall of thorax with penetration into thoracic cavity

S21.35-   Open bite of front wall of thorax with penetration into thoracic cavity
      Excludes 1: superficial bite of front wall of thorax (S20.37)

   S21.351-   Open bite of right front wall of thorax with penetration into thoracic cavity

   S21.352-   Open bite of left front wall of thorax with penetration into thoracic cavity

   S21.359-   Open bite of unspecified front wall of thorax with penetration into thoracic cavity

S21.4-   Open wound of back wall of thorax with penetration into thoracic cavity

   S21.40-   Unspecified open wound of back wall of thorax with penetration into thoracic cavity

      S21.401-   Unspecified open wound of right back wall of thorax with penetration into thoracic cavity

      S21.402-   Unspecified open wound of left back wall of thorax with penetration into thoracic cavity

      S21.409-   Unspecified open wound of unspecified back wall of thorax with penetration into thoracic cavity

   S21.41-   Laceration without foreign body of back wall of thorax with penetration into thoracic cavity

      S21.411-   Laceration without foreign body of right back wall of thorax with penetration into thoracic cavity

      S21.412-   Laceration without foreign body of left back wall of thorax with penetration into thoracic cavity

      S21.419-   Laceration without foreign body of unspecified back wall of thorax with penetration into thoracic cavity

   S21.42-   Laceration with foreign body of back wall of thorax with penetration into thoracic cavity

      S21.421-   Laceration with foreign body of right back wall of thorax with penetration into thoracic cavity

      S21.422-   Laceration with foreign body of left back wall of thorax with penetration into thoracic cavity

      S21.429-   Laceration with foreign body of unspecified back wall of thorax with penetration into thoracic cavity

   S21.43-   Puncture wound without foreign body of back wall of thorax with penetration into thoracic cavity

      S21.431-   Puncture wound without foreign body of right back wall of thorax with penetration into thoracic cavity

      S21.432-   Puncture wound without foreign body of left back wall of thorax with penetration into thoracic cavity

      S21.439-   Puncture wound without foreign body of unspecified back wall of thorax with penetration into thoracic cavity

   S21.44-   Puncture wound with foreign body of back wall of thorax with penetration into thoracic cavity

      S21.441-   Puncture wound with foreign body of right back wall of thorax with penetration into thoracic cavity

      S21.442-   Puncture wound with foreign body of left back wall of thorax with penetration into thoracic cavity

      S21.449-   Puncture wound with foreign body of unspecified back wall of thorax with penetration into thoracic cavity

   S21.45-   Open bite of back wall of thorax with penetration into thoracic cavity
      Bite of back wall of thorax NOS
      Excludes 1: superficial bite of back wall of thorax (S20.47)

      S21.451-   Open bite of right back wall of thorax with penetration into thoracic cavity

      S21.452-   Open bite of left back wall of thorax with penetration into thoracic cavity

      S21.459-   Open bite of unspecified back wall of thorax with penetration into thoracic cavity

S21-S23

S21.9- Open wound of unspecified part of thorax
    Open wound of thoracic wall NOS
  S21.90x- Unspecified open wound of unspecified part of thorax
  S21.91x- Laceration without foreign body of unspecified part of thorax
  S21.92x- Laceration with foreign body of unspecified part of thorax
  S21.93x- Puncture wound without foreign body of unspecified part of thorax
  S21.94x- Puncture wound with foreign body of unspecified part of thorax
  S21.95x- Open bite of unspecified part of thorax
    Excludes 1: superficial bite of thorax (S20.97)

S22- Fracture of rib(s), sternum and thoracic spine
Note: A fracture not indicated as nondisplaced or displaced should be classified to displaced
Note: A fracture not indicated as open or closed should be coded to closed
Includes: Fracture of thoracic neural arch
   Fracture of thoracic spinous process
   Fracture of thoracic transverse process
   Fracture of thoracic vertebra
   Fracture of thoracic vertebral arch
Code first any associated:
  Injury of intrathoracic organ (S27.-)
  Spinal cord injury (S24.0-, S24.1-)
Excludes 1: transection of thorax (S28.1)
Excludes❷: fracture of clavicle (S42.0-)
    fracture of scapula (S42.1-)

The appropriate 7th character is to be added to each code from category S22:
  A Initial encounter for closed fracture
  B Initial encounter for open fracture
  D Subsequent encounter for fracture with routine healing
  G Subsequent encounter for fracture with delayed healing
  K Subsequent encounter for fracture with nonunion
  S Sequela

S22.0- Fracture of thoracic vertebra
  S22.00- Fracture of unspecified thoracic vertebra
   S22.000- Wedge compression fracture of unspecified thoracic vertebra
   S22.001- Stable burst fracture of unspecified thoracic vertebra
   S22.002- Unstable burst fracture of unspecified thoracic vertebra
   S22.008- Other fracture of unspecified thoracic vertebra
   S22.009- Unspecified fracture of unspecified thoracic vertebra
  S22.01- Fracture of first thoracic vertebra
   S22.010- Wedge compression fracture of first thoracic vertebra
   S22.011- Stable burst fracture of first thoracic vertebra
   S22.012- Unstable burst fracture of first thoracic vertebra
   S22.018- Other fracture of first thoracic vertebra
   S22.019- Unspecified fracture of first thoracic vertebra
  S22.02- Fracture of second thoracic vertebra
   S22.020- Wedge compression fracture of second thoracic vertebra
   S22.021- Stable burst fracture of second thoracic vertebra
   S22.022- Unstable burst fracture of second thoracic vertebra
   S22.028- Other fracture of second thoracic vertebra
   S22.029- Unspecified fracture of second thoracic vertebra
  S22.03- Fracture of third thoracic vertebra
   S22.030- Wedge compression fracture of third thoracic vertebra
   S22.031- Stable burst fracture of third thoracic vertebra
   S22.032- Unstable burst fracture of third thoracic vertebra
   S22.038- Other fracture of third thoracic vertebra
   S22.039- Unspecified fracture of third thoracic vertebra
  S22.04- Fracture of fourth thoracic vertebra
   S22.040- Wedge compression fracture of fourth thoracic vertebra
   S22.041- Stable burst fracture of fourth thoracic vertebra
   S22.042- Unstable burst fracture of fourth thoracic vertebra
   S22.048- Other fracture of fourth thoracic vertebra
   S22.049- Unspecified fracture of fourth thoracic vertebra
  S22.05- Fracture of T5-T6 vertebra
   S22.050- Wedge compression fracture of T5-T6 vertebra
   S22.051- Stable burst fracture of T5-T6 vertebra
   S22.052- Unstable burst fracture of T5-T6 vertebra
   S22.058- Other fracture of T5-T6 vertebra
   S22.059- Unspecified fracture of T5-T6 vertebra

  S22.06- Fracture of T7-T8 vertebra
   S22.060- Wedge compression fracture of T7-T8 vertebra
   S22.061- Stable burst fracture of T7-T8 vertebra
   S22.062- Unstable burst fracture of T7-T8 vertebra
   S22.068- Other fracture of T7-T8 thoracic vertebra
   S22.069- Unspecified fracture of T7-T8 vertebra
  S22.07- Fracture of T9-T10 vertebra
   S22.070- Wedge compression fracture of T9-T10 vertebra
   S22.071- Stable burst fracture of T9-T10 vertebra
   S22.072- Unstable burst fracture of T9-T10 vertebra
   S22.078- Other fracture of T9-T10 vertebra
   S22.079- Unspecified fracture of T9-T10 vertebra
  S22.08- Fracture of T11-T12 vertebra
   S22.080- Wedge compression fracture of T11-T12 vertebra
   S22.081- Stable burst fracture of T11-T12 vertebra
   S22.082- Unstable burst fracture of T11-T12 vertebra
   S22.088- Other fracture of T11-T12 vertebra
   S22.089- Unspecified fracture of T11-T12 vertebra
  S22.2- Fracture of sternum
   S22.20x- Unspecified fracture of sternum
   S22.21x- Fracture of manubrium
   S22.22x- Fracture of body of sternum
   S22.23x- Sternal manubrial dissociation
   S22.24x- Fracture of xiphoid process
  S22.3- Fracture of one rib
   S22.31x- Fracture of one rib, right side
   S22.32x- Fracture of one rib, left side
   S22.39x- Fracture of one rib, unspecified side
  S22.4- Multiple fractures of ribs
    Fractures of two or more ribs
    Excludes 1: flail chest (S22.5-)
   S22.41x- Multiple fractures of ribs, right side
   S22.42x- Multiple fractures of ribs, left side
   S22.43x- Multiple fractures of ribs, bilateral
   S22.49x- Multiple fractures of ribs, unspecified side
  S22.5xx- Flail chest
  S22.9xx- Fracture of bony thorax, part unspecified

S23- Dislocation and sprain of joints and ligaments of thorax
Includes: Avulsion of joint or ligament of thorax
   Laceration of cartilage, joint or ligament of thorax
   Sprain of cartilage, joint or ligament of thorax
   Traumatic hemarthrosis of joint or ligament of thorax
   Traumatic rupture of joint or ligament of thorax
   Traumatic subluxation of joint or ligament of thorax
   Traumatic tear of joint or ligament of thorax
Code also any associated open wound
Excludes❷: dislocation, sprain of sternoclavicular joint (S43.2, S43.6)
    strain of muscle or tendon of thorax (S29.01-)

The appropriate 7th character is to be added to each code from category S23:
  A Initial encounter
  D Subsequent encounter
  S Sequela

S23.0xx- Traumatic rupture of thoracic intervertebral disc
    Excludes 1: rupture or displacement (nontraumatic) of thoracic intervertebral disc NOS (M51.- with fifth character 4)
S23.1- Subluxation and dislocation of thoracic vertebra
  Code also any associated:
   Open wound of thorax (S21.-)
   Spinal cord injury (S24.0-, S24.1-)
  Excludes❷: fracture of thoracic vertebrae (S22.0-)
  S23.10- Subluxation and dislocation of unspecified thoracic vertebra
   S23.100- Subluxation of unspecified thoracic vertebra
   S23.101- Dislocation of unspecified thoracic vertebra
  S23.11- Subluxation and dislocation of T1/T2 thoracic vertebra
   S23.110- Subluxation of T1/T2 thoracic vertebra
   S23.111- Dislocation of T1/T2 thoracic vertebra
  S23.12- Subluxation and dislocation of T2/T3-T3/T4 thoracic vertebra
   S23.120- Subluxation of T2/T3 thoracic vertebra
   S23.121- Dislocation of T2/T3 thoracic vertebra
   S23.122- Subluxation of T3/T4 thoracic vertebra
   S23.123- Dislocation of T3/T4 thoracic vertebra

S21 - S23

S23.13- Subluxation and dislocation of T4/T5-T5/T6 thoracic vertebra
    S23.130- Subluxation of T4/T5 thoracic vertebra
    S23.131- Dislocation of T4/T5 thoracic vertebra
    S23.132- Subluxation of T5/T6 thoracic vertebra
    S23.133- Dislocation of T5/T6 thoracic vertebra
S23.14- Subluxation and dislocation of T6/T7-T7/T8 thoracic vertebra
    S23.140- Subluxation of T6/T7 thoracic vertebra
    S23.141- Dislocation of T6/T7 thoracic vertebra
    S23.142- Subluxation of T7/T8 thoracic vertebra
    S23.143- Dislocation of T7/T8 thoracic vertebra
S23.15- Subluxation and dislocation of T8/T9-T9/T10 thoracic vertebra
    S23.150- Subluxation of T8/T9 thoracic vertebra
    S23.151- Dislocation of T8/T9 thoracic vertebra
    S23.152- Subluxation of T9/T10 thoracic vertebra
    S23.153- Dislocation of T9/T10 thoracic vertebra
S23.16- Subluxation and dislocation of T10/T11-T11/T12 thoracic vertebra
    S23.160- Subluxation of T10/T11 thoracic vertebra
    S23.161- Dislocation of T10/T11 thoracic vertebra
    S23.162- Subluxation of T11/T12 thoracic vertebra
    S23.163- Dislocation of T11/T12 thoracic vertebra
S23.17- Subluxation and dislocation of T12/L1 thoracic vertebra
    S23.170- Subluxation of T12/L1 thoracic vertebra
    S23.171- Dislocation of T12/L1 thoracic vertebra
S23.2- Dislocation of other and unspecified parts of thorax
    S23.20x- Dislocation of unspecified part of thorax
    S23.29x- Dislocation of other parts of thorax
S23.3xx- Sprain of ligaments of thoracic spine
S23.4- Sprain of ribs and sternum
    S23.41x- Sprain of ribs
    S23.42- Sprain of sternum
        S23.420- Sprain of sternoclavicular (joint) (ligament)
        S23.421- Sprain of chondrosternal joint
        S23.428- Other sprain of sternum
        S23.429- Unspecified sprain of sternum
S23.8xx- Sprain of other specified parts of thorax
S23.9xx- Sprain of unspecified parts of thorax

S24- Injury of nerves and spinal cord at thorax level
  Note: Code to highest level of thoracic spinal cord injury
    Injuries to the spinal cord (S24.0 and S24.1) refer to the cord level and not bone level injury, and can affect nerve roots at and below the level given.
  Code also any associated:
    Fracture of thoracic vertebra (S22.0-)
    Open wound of thorax (S21.-)
    Transient paralysis (R29.5)
  Excludes❷: injury of brachial plexus (S14.3)

The appropriate 7th character is to be added to each code from category S24:
  A Initial encounter
  D Subsequent encounter
  S Sequela

S24.0xx- Concussion and edema of thoracic spinal cord
S24.1- Other and unspecified injuries of thoracic spinal cord
    S24.10- Unspecified injury of thoracic spinal cord
        S24.101- Unspecified injury at T1 level of thoracic spinal cord
        S24.102- Unspecified injury at T2-T6 level of thoracic spinal cord
        S24.103- Unspecified injury at T7-T10 level of thoracic spinal cord
        S24.104- Unspecified injury at T11-T12 level of thoracic spinal cord
        S24.109- Unspecified injury at unspecified level of thoracic spinal cord
          Injury of thoracic spinal cord NOS
    S24.11- Complete lesion of thoracic spinal cord
        S24.111- Complete lesion at T1 level of thoracic spinal cord
        S24.112- Complete lesion at T2-T6 level of thoracic spinal cord
        S24.113- Complete lesion at T7-T10 level of thoracic spinal cord
        S24.114- Complete lesion at T11-T12 level of thoracic spinal cord
        S24.119- Complete lesion at unspecified level of thoracic spinal cord

S24.13- Anterior cord syndrome of thoracic spinal cord
    S24.131- Anterior cord syndrome at T1 level of thoracic spinal cord
    S24.132- Anterior cord syndrome at T2-T6 level of thoracic spinal cord
    S24.133- Anterior cord syndrome at T7-T10 level of thoracic spinal cord
    S24.134- Anterior cord syndrome at T11-T12 level of thoracic spinal cord
    S24.139- Anterior cord syndrome at unspecified level of thoracic spinal cord
S24.14- Brown-Séquard syndrome of thoracic spinal cord
    S24.141- Brown-Séquard syndrome at T1 level of thoracic spinal cord
    S24.142- Brown-Séquard syndrome at T2-T6 level of thoracic spinal cord
    S24.143- Brown-Séquard syndrome at T7-T10 level of thoracic spinal cord
    S24.144- Brown-Séquard syndrome at T11-T12 level of thoracic spinal cord
    S24.149- Brown-Séquard syndrome at unspecified level of thoracic spinal cord
S24.15- Other incomplete lesions of thoracic spinal cord
    Incomplete lesion of thoracic spinal cord NOS
    Posterior cord syndrome of thoracic spinal cord
    S24.151- Other incomplete lesion at T1 level of thoracic spinal cord
    S24.152- Other incomplete lesion at T2-T6 level of thoracic spinal cord
    S24.153- Other incomplete lesion at T7-T10 level of thoracic spinal cord
    S24.154- Other incomplete lesion at T11-T12 level of thoracic spinal cord
    S24.159- Other incomplete lesion at unspecified level of thoracic spinal cord
S24.2xx- Injury of nerve root of thoracic spine
S24.3xx- Injury of peripheral nerves of thorax
S24.4xx- Injury of thoracic sympathetic nervous system
    Injury of cardiac plexus
    Injury of esophageal plexus
    Injury of pulmonary plexus
    Injury of stellate ganglion
    Injury of thoracic sympathetic ganglion
S24.8xx- Injury of other specified nerves of thorax
S24.9xx- Injury of unspecified nerve of thorax

S25- Injury of blood vessels of thorax
  Code also any associated open wound (S21.-)

The appropriate 7th character is to be added to each code from category S25:
  A Initial encounter
  D Subsequent encounter
  S Sequela

S25.0- Injury of thoracic aorta
    Injury of aorta NOS
    S25.00x- Unspecified injury of thoracic aorta
    S25.01x- Minor laceration of thoracic aorta
        Incomplete transection of thoracic aorta
        Laceration of thoracic aorta NOS
        Superficial laceration of thoracic aorta
    S25.02x- Major laceration of thoracic aorta
        Complete transection of thoracic aorta
        Traumatic rupture of thoracic aorta
    S25.09x- Other specified injury of thoracic aorta
S25.1- Injury of innominate or subclavian artery
    S25.10- Unspecified injury of innominate or subclavian artery
        S25.101- Unspecified injury of right innominate or subclavian artery
        S25.102- Unspecified injury of left innominate or subclavian artery
        S25.109- Unspecified injury of unspecified innominate or subclavian artery
    S25.11- Minor laceration of innominate or subclavian artery
        Incomplete transection of innominate or subclavian artery
        Laceration of innominate or subclavian artery NOS
        Superficial laceration of innominate or subclavian artery
        S25.111- Minor laceration of right innominate or subclavian artery
        S25.112- Minor laceration of left innominate or subclavian artery
        S25.119- Minor laceration of unspecified innominate or subclavian artery

S23 - S26

S25.12- <u>Major laceration</u> of <u>innominate or subclavian artery</u>
Complete transection of innominate or subclavian artery
Traumatic rupture of innominate or subclavian artery

S25.121- Major laceration of <u>right</u> innominate or subclavian <u>artery</u>

S25.122- Major laceration of <u>left</u> innominate or subclavian <u>artery</u>

S25.129- Major laceration of <u>unspecified</u> innominate or subclavian <u>artery</u>

S25.19- <u>Other specified injury</u> of <u>innominate or subclavian artery</u>

S25.191- Other specified injury of <u>right</u> innominate or subclavian <u>artery</u>

S25.192- Other specified injury of <u>left</u> innominate or subclavian <u>artery</u>

S25.199- Other specified injury of <u>unspecified</u> innominate or subclavian <u>artery</u>

S25.2- Injury of <u>superior vena cava</u>
Injury of vena cava NOS

S25.20x- <u>Unspecified</u> injury of <u>superior vena cava</u>

S25.21x- <u>Minor laceration</u> of <u>superior vena cava</u>
Incomplete transection of superior vena cava
Laceration of superior vena cava NOS
Superficial laceration of superior vena cava

S25.22x- <u>Major laceration</u> of <u>superior vena cava</u>
Complete transection of superior vena cava
Traumatic rupture of superior vena cava

S25.29x- <u>Other</u> specified injury of superior vena cava

S25.3- Injury of <u>innominate or subclavian vein</u>

S25.30- <u>Unspecified</u> injury of <u>innominate or subclavian vein</u>

S25.301- Unspecified injury of <u>right</u> innominate or subclavian <u>vein</u>

S25.302- Unspecified injury of <u>left</u> innominate or subclavian <u>vein</u>

S25.309- Unspecified injury of <u>unspecified</u> innominate or subclavian <u>vein</u>

S25.31- <u>Minor laceration</u> of <u>innominate or subclavian vein</u>
Incomplete transection of innominate or subclavian vein
Laceration of innominate or subclavian vein NOS
Superficial laceration of innominate or subclavian vein

S25.311- Minor laceration of <u>right</u> innominate or subclavian <u>vein</u>

S25.312- Minor laceration of <u>left</u> innominate or subclavian <u>vein</u>

S25.319- Minor laceration of <u>unspecified</u> innominate or subclavian <u>vein</u>

S25.32- <u>Major laceration</u> of <u>innominate or subclavian vein</u>
Complete transection of innominate or subclavian vein
Traumatic rupture of innominate or subclavian vein

S25.321- Major laceration of <u>right</u> innominate or subclavian <u>vein</u>

S25.322- Major laceration of <u>left</u> innominate or subclavian <u>vein</u>

S25.329- Major laceration of <u>unspecified</u> innominate or subclavian <u>vein</u>

S25.39- <u>Other</u> specified injury of <u>innominate or subclavian vein</u>

S25.391- Other specified injury of <u>right</u> innominate or subclavian <u>vein</u>

S25.392- Other specified injury of <u>left</u> innominate or subclavian <u>vein</u>

S25.399- Other specified injury of <u>unspecified</u> innominate or subclavian <u>vein</u>

S25.4- Injury of <u>pulmonary blood vessels</u>

S25.40- <u>Unspecified</u> injury of <u>pulmonary blood vessels</u>

S25.401- Unspecified injury of <u>right</u> pulmonary blood vessels

S25.402- Unspecified injury of <u>left</u> pulmonary blood vessels

S25.409- Unspecified injury of <u>unspecified</u> pulmonary blood vessels

S25.41- <u>Minor laceration</u> of <u>pulmonary blood vessels</u>
Incomplete transection of pulmonary blood vessels
Laceration of pulmonary blood vessels NOS
Superficial laceration of pulmonary blood vessels

S25.411- Minor laceration of <u>right</u> pulmonary blood vessels

S25.412- Minor laceration of <u>left</u> pulmonary blood vessels

S25.419- Minor laceration of <u>unspecified</u> pulmonary blood vessels

S25.42- <u>Major laceration</u> of <u>pulmonary blood vessels</u>
Complete transection of pulmonary blood vessels
Traumatic rupture of pulmonary blood vessels

S25.421- Major laceration of <u>right</u> pulmonary blood vessels

S25.422- Major laceration of <u>left</u> pulmonary blood vessels

S25.429- Major laceration of <u>unspecified</u> pulmonary blood vessels

S25.49- <u>Other specified injury</u> of <u>pulmonary blood vessels</u>

S25.491- Other specified injury of <u>right</u> pulmonary blood vessels

S25.492- Other specified injury of <u>left</u> pulmonary blood vessels

S25.499- Other specified injury of <u>unspecified</u> pulmonary blood vessels

S25.5- Injury of <u>intercostal blood vessels</u>

S25.50- <u>Unspecified</u> injury of <u>intercostal blood vessels</u>

S25.501- Unspecified injury of intercostal blood vessels, <u>right</u> side

S25.502- Unspecified injury of intercostal blood vessels, <u>left</u> side

S25.509- Unspecified injury of intercostal blood vessels, <u>unspecified</u> side

S25.51- <u>Laceration</u> of <u>intercostal blood vessels</u>

S25.511- Laceration of intercostal blood vessels, <u>right</u> side

S25.512- Laceration of intercostal blood vessels, <u>left</u> side

S25.519- Laceration of intercostal blood vessels, <u>unspecified</u> side

S25.59- <u>Other</u> specified injury of <u>intercostal blood vessels</u>

S25.591- Other specified injury of intercostal blood vessels, <u>right</u> side

S25.592- Other specified injury of intercostal blood vessels, <u>left</u> side

S25.599- Other specified injury of intercostal blood vessels, <u>unspecified</u> side

S25.8- Injury of <u>other blood vessels of thorax</u>
Injury of azygos vein
Injury of mammary artery or vein

S25.80- <u>Unspecified</u> injury of <u>other blood vessels of thorax</u>

S25.801- Unspecified injury of other blood vessels of thorax, <u>right</u> side

S25.802- Unspecified injury of other blood vessels of thorax, <u>left</u> side

S25.809- Unspecified injury of other blood vessels of thorax, <u>unspecified</u> side

S25.81- <u>Laceration</u> of <u>other blood vessels of thorax</u>

S25.811- Laceration of other blood vessels of thorax, <u>right</u> side

S25.812- Laceration of other blood vessels of thorax, <u>left</u> side

S25.819- Laceration of other blood vessels of thorax, <u>unspecified</u> side

S25.89- <u>Other</u> specified injury of <u>other blood vessels of thorax</u>

S25.891- Other specified injury of other blood vessels of thorax, <u>right</u> side

S25.892- Other specified injury of other blood vessels of thorax, <u>left</u> side

S25.899- Other specified injury of other blood vessels of thorax, <u>unspecified</u> side

S25.9- Injury of <u>unspecified</u> <u>blood vessel of thorax</u>

S25.90x- <u>Unspecified</u> injury of <u>unspecified</u> <u>blood vessel of thorax</u>

S25.91x- <u>Laceration</u> of <u>unspecified</u> <u>blood vessel of thorax</u>

S25.99x- <u>Other</u> specified injury of <u>unspecified</u> <u>blood vessel of thorax</u>

S26- Injury of <u>heart</u>
Code also any associated:
Open wound of thorax (S21.-)
Traumatic hemopneumothorax (S27.2)
Traumatic hemothorax (S27.1)
Traumatic pneumothorax (S27.0)

The appropriate 7th character is to be added to each code from category S26:
A   <u>Initial</u> encounter
D   <u>Subsequent</u> encounter
S   <u>Sequela</u>

S26.0- Injury of <u>heart with hemopericardium</u>

S26.00x- <u>Unspecified</u> injury of heart with hemopericardium

S26.01x- <u>Contusion</u> of heart with hemopericardium

S26.02- <u>Laceration</u> of heart <u>with hemopericardium</u>

S26.020- <u>Mild</u> laceration of heart <u>with hemopericardium</u>
Laceration of heart without penetration of heart chamber

S26.021- <u>Moderate</u> laceration of heart <u>with hemopericardium</u>
Laceration of heart with penetration of heart chamber

S26.022- <u>Major</u> laceration of heart <u>with hemopericardium</u>
Laceration of heart with penetration of multiple heart chambers

S26.09x- <u>Other</u> injury of heart <u>with hemopericardium</u>

S 2 3 – S 2 6

S26.1- Injury of <u>heart</u> <u>without</u> hemopericardium
  S26.10x- <u>Unspecified</u> injury of heart <u>without</u> hemopericardium
  S26.11x- <u>Contusion</u> of heart <u>without</u> hemopericardium
  S26.12x- <u>Laceration</u> of heart <u>without</u> hemopericardium
  S26.19x- <u>Other</u> injury of heart <u>without</u> hemopericardium
S26.9- Injury of heart, <u>unspecified with or without</u> hemopericardium
  S26.90x- <u>Unspecified</u> injury of heart, <u>unspecified with or without</u> hemopericardium
  S26.91x- <u>Contusion</u> of heart, <u>unspecified with or without</u> hemopericardium
  S26.92x- <u>Laceration</u> of heart, <u>unspecified with or without</u> hemopericardium
    Laceration of heart NOS
  S26.99x- <u>Other</u> injury of heart, <u>unspecified with or without</u> hemopericardium

S27- Injury of <u>other and unspecified</u> <u>intrathoracic organs</u>
  Code also any associated open wound of thorax (S21.-)
  Excludes❷: injury of cervical esophagus (S10-S19)
       injury of trachea (cervical) (S10-S19)

The appropriate 7th character is to be added to each code from category S27:
  A <u>Initial</u> encounter
  D <u>Subsequent</u> encounter
  S <u>Sequela</u>

S27.0xx- Traumatic <u>pneumothorax</u>
  Excludes 1: spontaneous pneumothorax (J93.-)
S27.1xx- Traumatic <u>hemothorax</u>
S27.2xx- Traumatic <u>hemopneumothorax</u>
S27.3- Other and unspecified injuries of <u>lung</u>
  S27.30- <u>Unspecified</u> injury of lung
    S27.301- Unspecified injury of lung, <u>unilateral</u>
    S27.302- Unspecified injury of lung, <u>bilateral</u>
    S27.309- Unspecified injury of lung, <u>unspecified</u>
  S27.31- <u>Primary blast</u> injury of lung
    Blast injury of lung NOS
    S27.311- Primary blast injury of lung, <u>unilateral</u>
    S27.312- Primary blast injury of lung, <u>bilateral</u>
    S27.319- Primary blast injury of lung, <u>unspecified</u>
  S27.32- <u>Contusion</u> of lung
    S27.321- Contusion of lung, <u>unilateral</u>
    S27.322- Contusion of lung, <u>bilateral</u>
    S27.329- Contusion of lung, <u>unspecified</u>
  S27.33- <u>Laceration</u> of lung
    S27.331- Laceration of lung, <u>unilateral</u>
    S27.332- Laceration of lung, <u>bilateral</u>
    S27.339- Laceration of lung, <u>unspecified</u>
  S27.39- <u>Other</u> injuries of lung
    Secondary blast injury of lung
    S27.391- Other injuries of lung, <u>unilateral</u>
    S27.392- Other injuries of lung, <u>bilateral</u>
    S27.399- Other injuries of lung, <u>unspecified</u>
S27.4- Injury of <u>bronchus</u>
  S27.40- <u>Unspecified</u> injury of bronchus
    S27.401- Unspecified injury of bronchus, <u>unilateral</u>
    S27.402- Unspecified injury of bronchus, <u>bilateral</u>
    S27.409- Unspecified injury of bronchus, <u>unspecified</u>
  S27.41- <u>Primary blast</u> injury of bronchus
    Blast injury of bronchus NOS
    S27.411- Primary blast injury of bronchus, <u>unilateral</u>
    S27.412- Primary blast injury of bronchus, <u>bilateral</u>
    S27.419- Primary blast injury of bronchus, <u>unspecified</u>
  S27.42- <u>Contusion</u> of bronchus
    S27.421- Contusion of bronchus, <u>unilateral</u>
    S27.422- Contusion of bronchus, <u>bilateral</u>
    S27.429- Contusion of bronchus, <u>unspecified</u>
  S27.43- <u>Laceration</u> of bronchus
    S27.431- Laceration of bronchus, <u>unilateral</u>
    S27.432- Laceration of bronchus, <u>bilateral</u>
    S27.439- Laceration of bronchus, <u>unspecified</u>
  S27.49- <u>Other</u> injury of bronchus
    Secondary blast injury of bronchus
    S27.491- Other injury of bronchus, <u>unilateral</u>
    S27.492- Other injury of bronchus, <u>bilateral</u>
    S27.499- Other injury of bronchus, <u>unspecified</u>

S27.5- Injury of <u>thoracic trachea</u>
  S27.50x- <u>Unspecified</u> injury of thoracic trachea
  S27.51x- <u>Primary blast</u> injury of thoracic trachea
    Blast injury of thoracic trachea NOS
  S27.52x- <u>Contusion</u> of thoracic trachea
  S27.53x- <u>Laceration</u> of thoracic trachea
  S27.59x- <u>Other</u> injury of thoracic trachea
    Secondary blast injury of thoracic trachea
S27.6- Injury of <u>pleura</u>
  S27.60x- <u>Unspecified</u> injury of pleura
  S27.63x- <u>Laceration</u> of pleura
  S27.69x- <u>Other</u> injury of pleura
S27.8- Injury of <u>other specified</u> intrathoracic organs
  S27.80- Injury of <u>diaphragm</u>
    S27.802- <u>Contusion</u> of diaphragm
    S27.803- <u>Laceration</u> of diaphragm
    S27.808- <u>Other</u> injury of diaphragm
    S27.809- <u>Unspecified</u> injury of diaphragm
  S27.81- Injury of <u>esophagus (thoracic part)</u>
    S27.812- <u>Contusion</u> of esophagus (thoracic part)
    S27.813- <u>Laceration</u> of esophagus (thoracic part)
    S27.818- <u>Other</u> injury of esophagus (thoracic part)
    S27.819- <u>Unspecified</u> injury of esophagus (thoracic part)
  S27.89- Injury of <u>other specified</u> intrathoracic organs
    Injury of lymphatic thoracic duct
    Injury of thymus gland
    S27.892- <u>Contusion</u> of other specified intrathoracic organs
    S27.893- <u>Laceration</u> of other specified intrathoracic organs
    S27.898- <u>Other</u> injury of other specified intrathoracic organs
    S27.899- <u>Unspecified</u> injury of other specified intrathoracic organs
S27.9xx- Injury of <u>unspecified</u> intrathoracic organ

S28- Crushing injury of <u>thorax</u>, and traumatic amputation of part of thorax
The appropriate 7th character is to be added to each code from category S28:
  A <u>Initial</u> encounter
  D <u>Subsequent</u> encounter
  S <u>Sequela</u>
S28.0xx- <u>Crushed</u> chest
  Use additional code for all associated injuries
  Excludes 1: flail chest (S22.5)
S28.1xx- <u>Traumatic amputation</u> (partial) of <u>part of thorax</u>, <u>except</u> breast
S28.2- <u>Traumatic amputation</u> of <u>breast</u>
  S28.21- <u>Complete</u> traumatic amputation of breast
    Traumatic amputation of breast NOS
    S28.211- Complete traumatic amputation of <u>right</u> breast
    S28.212- Complete traumatic amputation of <u>left</u> breast
    S28.219- Complete traumatic amputation of <u>unspecified</u> breast
  S28.22- <u>Partial</u> traumatic amputation of <u>breast</u>
    S28.221- Partial traumatic amputation of <u>right</u> breast
    S28.222- Partial traumatic amputation of <u>left</u> breast
    S28.229- Partial traumatic amputation of <u>unspecified</u> breast

S29- Other and <u>unspecified</u> injuries of thorax
  Code also any associated open wound (S21.-)
The appropriate 7th character is to be added to each code from category S29:
  A <u>Initial</u> encounter
  D <u>Subsequent</u> encounter
  S <u>Sequela</u>
S29.0- Injury of <u>muscle and tendon</u> at <u>thorax</u> level
  S29.00- <u>Unspecified</u> injury of muscle and tendon of thorax
    S29.001- Unspecified injury of muscle and tendon of <u>front wall</u> of thorax
    S29.002- Unspecified injury of muscle and tendon of <u>back wall</u> of thorax
    S29.009- Unspecified injury of muscle and tendon of <u>unspecified</u> wall of thorax
  S29.01- <u>Strain</u> of muscle and tendon of thorax
    S29.011- Strain of muscle and tendon of <u>front wall</u> of thorax
    S29.012- Strain of muscle and tendon of <u>back wall</u> of thorax
    S29.019- Strain of muscle and tendon of <u>unspecified</u> wall of thorax

S29.02-   <u>Laceration</u> of muscle and tendon of thorax
 S29.021- Laceration of muscle and tendon of <u>front wall</u> of thorax
 S29.022- Laceration of muscle and tendon of <u>back wall</u> of thorax
 S29.029- Laceration of muscle and tendon of <u>unspecified</u> wall of thorax
S29.09-   <u>Other</u> injury of muscle and tendon of thorax
 S29.091- Other injury of muscle and tendon of <u>front wall</u> of thorax
 S29.092- Other injury of muscle and tendon of <u>back wall</u> of thorax
 S29.099- Other injury of muscle and tendon of <u>unspecified</u> wall of thorax
S29.8xx-   <u>Other</u> specified injuries of thorax
S29.9xx-   <u>Unspecified</u> injury of thorax

Injuries to the abdomen, lower back, lumbar spine, pelvis and external genitals (S30-S39)

Includes: Injuries to the abdominal wall
   Injuries to the anus
   Injuries to the buttock
   Injuries to the external genitalia
   Injuries to the flank
   Injuries to the groin
Excludes❷: burns and corrosions (T20-T32)
   effects of foreign body in anus and rectum (T18.5)
   effects of foreign body in genitourinary tract (T19.-)
   effects of foreign body in stomach, small intestine and colon (T18.2-T18.4)
   frostbite (T33-T34)
   insect bite or sting, venomous (T63.4)

S30-   <u>Superficial injury</u> of <u>abdomen, lower back, pelvis and external genitals</u>
Excludes❷: superficial injury of hip (S70.-)
The appropriate 7th character is to be added to each code from category S30:
 A <u>Initial</u> encounter
 D <u>Subsequent</u> encounter
 S <u>Sequela</u>
S30.0xx-   <u>Contusion</u> of <u>lower back and pelvis</u>
  Contusion of buttock
S30.1xx-   <u>Contusion</u> of <u>abdominal wall</u>
  Contusion of flank
  Contusion of groin
S30.2-   <u>Contusion</u> of <u>external genital organs</u>
 S30.20- Contusion of <u>unspecified</u> external genital organ
  S30.201- Contusion of unspecified external genital organ, <u>male</u>
  S30.202- Contusion of unspecified external genital organ, <u>female</u>
 S30.21x- Contusion of penis
 S30.22x- Contusion of scrotum and testes
 S30.23x- Contusion of vagina and vulva
S30.3xx-   Contusion of anus
S30.8-   <u>Other</u> superficial injuries of abdomen, lower back, pelvis and external genitals
 S30.81- <u>Abrasion</u> of abdomen, lower back, pelvis and external genitals
  S30.810- Abrasion of lower back and pelvis
  S30.811- Abrasion of abdominal wall
  S30.812- Abrasion of penis
  S30.813- Abrasion of scrotum and testes
  S30.814- Abrasion of vagina and vulva
  S30.815- Abrasion of <u>unspecified</u> external genital organs, <u>male</u>
  S30.816- Abrasion of <u>unspecified</u> external genital organs, <u>female</u>
  S30.817- Abrasion of anus
 S30.82- <u>Blister</u> (nonthermal) of abdomen, lower back, pelvis and external genitals
  S30.820- Blister (nonthermal) of lower back and pelvis
  S30.821- Blister (nonthermal) of abdominal wall
  S30.822- Blister (nonthermal) of penis
  S30.823- Blister (nonthermal) of scrotum and testes
  S30.824- Blister (nonthermal) of vagina and vulva
  S30.825- Blister (nonthermal) of <u>unspecified</u> external genital organs, <u>male</u>
  S30.826- Blister (nonthermal) of <u>unspecified</u> external genital organs, <u>female</u>
  S30.827- Blister (nonthermal) of anus

S30.84-   <u>External constriction</u> of abdomen, lower back, pelvis and external genitals
 S30.840- External constriction of lower back and pelvis
 S30.841- External constriction of abdominal wall
 S30.842- External constriction of penis
   Hair tourniquet syndrome of penis
   Use additional cause code to identify the constricting item (W49.0-)
 S30.843- External constriction of scrotum and testes
 S30.844- External constriction of vagina and vulva
 S30.845- External constriction of <u>unspecified</u> external genital organs, <u>male</u>
 S30.846- External constriction of <u>unspecified</u> external genital organs, <u>female</u>
S30.85-   <u>Superficial foreign body</u> of abdomen, lower back, pelvis and external genitals
  Splinter in the abdomen, lower back, pelvis and external genitals
 S30.850- Superficial foreign body of lower back and pelvis
 S30.851- Superficial foreign body of abdominal wall
 S30.852- Superficial foreign body of penis
 S30.853- Superficial foreign body of scrotum and testes
 S30.854- Superficial foreign body of vagina and vulva
 S30.855- Superficial foreign body of <u>unspecified</u> external genital organs, <u>male</u>
 S30.856- Superficial foreign body of <u>unspecified</u> external genital organs, <u>female</u>
 S30.857- Superficial foreign body of anus
S30.86-   <u>Insect bite (nonvenomous)</u> of abdomen, lower back, pelvis and external genitals
 S30.860- Insect bite (nonvenomous) of lower back and pelvis
 S30.861- Insect bite (nonvenomous) of abdominal wall
 S30.862- Insect bite (nonvenomous) of penis
 S30.863- Insect bite (nonvenomous) of scrotum and testes
 S30.864- Insect bite (nonvenomous) of vagina and vulva
 S30.865- Insect bite (nonvenomous) of <u>unspecified</u> external genital organs, <u>male</u>
 S30.866- Insect bite (nonvenomous) of <u>unspecified</u> external genital organs, <u>female</u>
 S30.867- Insect bite (nonvenomous) of anus
S30.87-   <u>Other superficial bite</u> of abdomen, lower back, pelvis and external genitals
 Excludes 1: open bite of abdomen, lower back, pelvis and external genitals (S31.05, S31.15, S31.25, S31.35, S31.45, S31.55)
 S30.870- Other superficial bite of lower back and pelvis
 S30.871- Other superficial bite of abdominal wall
 S30.872- Other superficial bite of penis
 S30.873- Other superficial bite of scrotum and testes
 S30.874- Other superficial bite of vagina and vulva
 S30.875- Other superficial bite of <u>unspecified</u> external genital organs, <u>male</u>
 S30.876- Other superficial bite of <u>unspecified</u> external genital organs, <u>female</u>
 S30.877- Other superficial bite of anus
S30.9-   <u>Unspecified superficial injury</u> of abdomen, lower back, pelvis and external genitals
 S30.91x- Unspecified superficial injury of lower back and pelvis
 S30.92x- Unspecified superficial injury of abdominal wall
 S30.93x- Unspecified superficial injury of penis
 S30.94x- Unspecified superficial injury of scrotum and testes
 S30.95x- Unspecified superficial injury of vagina and vulva
 S30.96x- Unspecified superficial injury of <u>unspecified</u> external genital organs, <u>male</u>
 S30.97x- Unspecified superficial injury of <u>unspecified</u> external genital organs, <u>female</u>
 S30.98x- Unspecified superficial injury of anus

S 2 6 - S 3 0

Excludes 1: = NOT CODED HERE! (Do not code both)   **705**   *Excludes❷:* = Not Included Here

S31- Open wound of abdomen, lower back, pelvis and external genitals
Code also any associated:
Spinal cord injury (S24.0, S24.1-, S34.0-, S34.1-)
Wound infection
Excludes 1: traumatic amputation of part of abdomen, lower back and pelvis (S38.2-, S38.3)
Excludes❷: open wound of hip (S71.00-S71.02)
open fracture of pelvis (S32.1--S32.9 with 7th character B)

The appropriate 7th character is to be added to each code from
category S31:
A Initial encounter
D Subsequent encounter
S Sequela

S31.0- Open wound of lower back and pelvis
S31.00- Unspecified open wound of lower back and pelvis
S31.000- Unspecified open wound of lower back and pelvis without penetration into retroperitoneum
Unspecified open wound of lower back and pelvis NOS
S31.001- Unspecified open wound of lower back and pelvis with penetration into retroperitoneum
S31.01- Laceration without foreign body of lower back and pelvis
S31.010- Laceration without foreign body of lower back and pelvis without penetration into retroperitoneum
Laceration without foreign body of lower back and pelvis NOS
S31.011- Laceration without foreign body of lower back and pelvis with penetration into retroperitoneum
S31.02- Laceration with foreign body of lower back and pelvis
S31.020- Laceration with foreign body of lower back and pelvis without penetration into retroperitoneum
Laceration with foreign body of lower back and pelvis NOS
S31.021- Laceration with foreign body of lower back and pelvis with penetration into retroperitoneum
S31.03- Puncture wound without foreign body of lower back and pelvis
S31.030- Puncture wound without foreign body of lower back and pelvis without penetration into retroperitoneum
Puncture wound without foreign body of lower back and pelvis NOS
S31.031- Puncture wound without foreign body of lower back and pelvis with penetration into retroperitoneum
S31.04- Puncture wound with foreign body of lower back and pelvis
S31.040- Puncture wound with foreign body of lower back and pelvis without penetration into retroperitoneum
Puncture wound with foreign body of lower back and pelvis NOS
S31.041- Puncture wound with foreign body of lower back and pelvis with penetration into retroperitoneum
S31.05- Open bite of lower back and pelvis
Bite of lower back and pelvis NOS
Excludes 1: superficial bite of lower back and pelvis (S30.860, S30.870)
S31.050- Open bite of lower back and pelvis without penetration into retroperitoneum
Open bite of lower back and pelvis NOS
S31.051- Open bite of lower back and pelvis with penetration into retroperitoneum
S31.1- Open wound of abdominal wall without penetration into peritoneal cavity
Open wound of abdominal wall NOS
Excludes❷: open wound of abdominal wall with penetration into peritoneal cavity (S31.6-)
S31.10- Unspecified open wound of abdominal wall without penetration into peritoneal cavity
S31.100- Unspecified open wound of abdominal wall, right upper quadrant without penetration into peritoneal cavity
S31.101- Unspecified open wound of abdominal wall, left upper quadrant without penetration into peritoneal cavity
S31.102- Unspecified open wound of abdominal wall, epigastric region without penetration into peritoneal cavity
S31.103- Unspecified open wound of abdominal wall, right lower quadrant without penetration into peritoneal cavity
S31.104- Unspecified open wound of abdominal wall, left lower quadrant without penetration into peritoneal cavity
S31.105- Unspecified open wound of abdominal wall, periumbilic region without penetration into peritoneal cavity

S31.109- Unspecified open wound of abdominal wall, unspecified quadrant without penetration into peritoneal cavity
Unspecified open wound of abdominal wall NOS
S31.11- Laceration without foreign body of abdominal wall without penetration into peritoneal cavity
S31.110- Laceration without foreign body of abdominal wall, right upper quadrant without penetration into peritoneal cavity
S31.111- Laceration without foreign body of abdominal wall, left upper quadrant without penetration into peritoneal cavity
S31.112- Laceration without foreign body of abdominal wall, epigastric region without penetration into peritoneal cavity
S31.113- Laceration without foreign body of abdominal wall, right lower quadrant without penetration into peritoneal cavity
S31.114- Laceration without foreign body of abdominal wall, left lower quadrant without penetration into peritoneal cavity
S31.115- Laceration without foreign body of abdominal wall, periumbilic region without penetration into peritoneal cavity
S31.119- Laceration without foreign body of abdominal wall, unspecified quadrant without penetration into peritoneal cavity
S31.12- Laceration with foreign body of abdominal wall without penetration into peritoneal cavity
S31.120- Laceration of abdominal wall with foreign body, right upper quadrant without penetration into peritoneal cavity
S31.121- Laceration of abdominal wall with foreign body, left upper quadrant without penetration into peritoneal cavity
S31.122- Laceration of abdominal wall with foreign body, epigastric region without penetration into peritoneal cavity
S31.123- Laceration of abdominal wall with foreign body, right lower quadrant without penetration into peritoneal cavity
S31.124- Laceration of abdominal wall with foreign body, left lower quadrant without penetration into peritoneal cavity
S31.125- Laceration of abdominal wall with foreign body, periumbilic region without penetration into peritoneal cavity
S31.129- Laceration of abdominal wall with foreign body, unspecified quadrant without penetration into peritoneal cavity
S31.13- Puncture wound of abdominal wall without foreign body without penetration into peritoneal cavity
S31.130- Puncture wound of abdominal wall without foreign body, right upper quadrant without penetration into peritoneal cavity
S31.131- Puncture wound of abdominal wall without foreign body, left upper quadrant without penetration into peritoneal cavity
S31.132- Puncture wound of abdominal wall without foreign body, epigastric region without penetration into peritoneal cavity
S31.133- Puncture wound of abdominal wall without foreign body, right lower quadrant without penetration into peritoneal cavity
S31.134- Puncture wound of abdominal wall without foreign body, left lower quadrant without penetration into peritoneal cavity
S31.135- Puncture wound of abdominal wall without foreign body, periumbilic region without penetration into peritoneal cavity
S31.139- Puncture wound of abdominal wall without foreign body, unspecified quadrant without penetration into peritoneal cavity
S31.14- Puncture wound of abdominal wall with foreign body without penetration into peritoneal cavity
S31.140- Puncture wound of abdominal wall with foreign body, right upper quadrant without penetration into peritoneal cavity
S31.141- Puncture wound of abdominal wall with foreign body, left upper quadrant without penetration into peritoneal cavity

© 2013 Channel Publishing, Ltd.

S31.142- Puncture wound of abdominal wall <u>with foreign body</u>, <u>epigastric region</u> <u>without</u> penetration into peritoneal cavity

S31.143- Puncture wound of abdominal wall <u>with foreign body</u>, <u>right</u> <u>lower</u> quadrant <u>without</u> penetration into peritoneal cavity

S31.144- Puncture wound of abdominal wall <u>with foreign body</u>, <u>left</u> <u>lower</u> quadrant <u>without</u> penetration into peritoneal cavity

S31.145- Puncture wound of abdominal wall <u>with foreign body</u>, <u>periumbilic region</u> <u>without</u> penetration into peritoneal cavity

S31.149- Puncture wound of abdominal wall <u>with foreign body</u>, <u>unspecified</u> <u>quadrant</u> <u>without</u> penetration into peritoneal cavity

S31.15- <u>Open bite</u> of abdominal wall <u>without</u> penetration into peritoneal cavity
   Bite of abdominal wall NOS
   Excludes 1: superficial bite of abdominal wall (S30.871)

S31.150- Open bite of abdominal wall, <u>right</u> <u>upper</u> quadrant <u>without</u> penetration into peritoneal cavity

S31.151- Open bite of abdominal wall, <u>left</u> <u>upper</u> quadrant <u>without</u> penetration into peritoneal cavity

S31.152- Open bite of abdominal wall, <u>epigastric region</u> <u>without</u> penetration into peritoneal cavity

S31.153- Open bite of abdominal wall, <u>right</u> <u>lower</u> quadrant <u>without</u> penetration into peritoneal cavity

S31.154- Open bite of abdominal wall, <u>left</u> <u>lower</u> quadrant <u>without</u> penetration into peritoneal cavity

S31.155- Open bite of abdominal wall, <u>periumbilic region</u> <u>without</u> penetration into peritoneal cavity

S31.159- Open bite of abdominal wall, <u>unspecified</u> <u>quadrant</u> <u>without</u> penetration into peritoneal cavity

S31.2- Open wound of <u>penis</u>

S31.20x- Unspecified open wound of penis

S31.21x- Laceration <u>without</u> foreign body of penis

S31.22x- Laceration <u>with foreign body</u> of penis

S31.23x- Puncture wound <u>without</u> foreign body of penis

S31.24x- Puncture wound <u>with foreign body</u> of penis

S31.25x- Open bite of penis
   Bite of penis NOS
   Excludes 1: superficial bite of penis (S30.862, S30.872)

S31.3- Open wound of <u>scrotum and testes</u>

S31.30x- Unspecified open wound of scrotum and testes

S31.31x- Laceration <u>without</u> foreign body of scrotum and testes

S31.32x- Laceration <u>with foreign body</u> of scrotum and testes

S31.33x- Puncture wound <u>without</u> foreign body of scrotum and testes

S31.34x- Puncture wound <u>with foreign body</u> of scrotum and testes

S31.35x- Open bite of scrotum and testes
   Bite of scrotum and testes NOS
   Excludes 1: superficial bite of scrotum and testes (S30.863, S30.873)

S31.4- Open wound of <u>vagina and vulva</u>
   Excludes 1: injury to vagina and vulva during delivery (O70.-, O71.4)

S31.40x- Unspecified open wound of vagina and vulva

S31.41x- Laceration <u>without</u> foreign body of vagina and vulva

S31.42x- Laceration <u>with foreign body</u> of vagina and vulva

S31.43x- Puncture wound <u>without</u> foreign body of vagina and vulva

S31.44x- Puncture wound <u>with foreign body</u> of vagina and vulva

S31.45x- Open bite of vagina and vulva
   Bite of vagina and vulva NOS
   Excludes 1: superficial bite of vagina and vulva (S30.864, S30.874)

S31.5- Open wound of <u>unspecified external genital organs</u>
   Excludes 1: traumatic amputation of external genital organs (S38.21, S38.22)

S31.50- <u>Unspecified</u> open wound of <u>unspecified</u> external genital organs

S31.501- Unspecified open wound of <u>unspecified</u> external genital organs, <u>male</u>

S31.502- Unspecified open wound of <u>unspecified</u> external genital organs, <u>female</u>

S31.51- <u>Laceration</u> <u>without</u> foreign body of <u>unspecified</u> external genital organs

S31.511- Laceration <u>without</u> foreign body of <u>unspecified</u> external genital organs, <u>male</u>

S31.512- Laceration <u>without</u> foreign body of <u>unspecified</u> external genital organs, <u>female</u>

S31.52- Laceration <u>with foreign body</u> of <u>unspecified</u> external genital organs

S31.521- Laceration <u>with foreign body</u> of <u>unspecified</u> external genital organs, <u>male</u>

S31.522- Laceration <u>with foreign body</u> of <u>unspecified</u> external genital organs, <u>female</u>

S31.53- <u>Puncture</u> wound <u>without</u> foreign body of <u>unspecified</u> external genital organs

S31.531- Puncture wound <u>without</u> foreign body of <u>unspecified</u> external genital organs, <u>male</u>

S31.532- Puncture wound <u>without</u> foreign body of <u>unspecified</u> external genital organs, <u>female</u>

S31.54- <u>Puncture</u> wound <u>with foreign body</u> of <u>unspecified</u> external genital organs

S31.541- Puncture wound <u>with foreign body</u> of <u>unspecified</u> external genital organs, <u>male</u>

S31.542- Puncture wound <u>with foreign body</u> of <u>unspecified</u> external genital organs, <u>female</u>

S31.55- <u>Open bite</u> of <u>unspecified external genital organs</u>
   Bite of unspecified external genital organs NOS
   Excludes 1: superficial bite of unspecified external genital organs (S30.865, S30.866, S30.875, S30.876)

S31.551- Open bite of <u>unspecified</u> external genital organs, <u>male</u>

S31.552- Open bite of <u>unspecified</u> external genital organs, <u>female</u>

S31.6- <u>Open wound</u> of <u>abdominal wall</u> <u>with penetration</u> into peritoneal cavity

S31.60- <u>Unspecified</u> open wound of <u>abdominal wall</u> <u>with penetration</u> into peritoneal cavity

S31.600- Unspecified open wound of abdominal wall, <u>right</u> <u>upper</u> quadrant <u>with penetration</u> into peritoneal cavity

S31.601- Unspecified open wound of abdominal wall, <u>left</u> <u>upper</u> quadrant <u>with penetration</u> into peritoneal cavity

S31.602- Unspecified open wound of abdominal wall, <u>epigastric region</u> <u>with penetration</u> into peritoneal cavity

S31.603- Unspecified open wound of abdominal wall, <u>right</u> <u>lower</u> quadrant <u>with penetration</u> into peritoneal cavity

S31.604- Unspecified open wound of abdominal wall, <u>left</u> <u>lower</u> quadrant <u>with penetration</u> into peritoneal cavity

S31.605- Unspecified open wound of abdominal wall, <u>periumbilic region</u> <u>with penetration</u> into peritoneal cavity

S31.609- Unspecified open wound of abdominal wall, <u>unspecified</u> <u>quadrant</u> <u>with penetration</u> into peritoneal cavity

S31.61- <u>Laceration</u> <u>without</u> foreign body of abdominal wall <u>with penetration</u> into peritoneal cavity

S31.610- Laceration <u>without</u> foreign body of abdominal wall, <u>right</u> <u>upper</u> quadrant <u>with penetration</u> into peritoneal cavity

S31.611- Laceration <u>without</u> foreign body of abdominal wall, <u>left</u> <u>upper</u> quadrant <u>with penetration</u> into peritoneal cavity

S31.612- Laceration <u>without</u> foreign body of abdominal wall, <u>epigastric region</u> <u>with penetration</u> into peritoneal cavity

S31.613- Laceration <u>without</u> foreign body of abdominal wall, <u>right</u> <u>lower</u> quadrant <u>with penetration</u> into peritoneal cavity

S31.614- Laceration <u>without</u> foreign body of abdominal wall, <u>left</u> <u>lower</u> quadrant <u>with penetration</u> into peritoneal cavity

S31.615- Laceration <u>without</u> foreign body of abdominal wall, <u>periumbilic region</u> <u>with penetration</u> into peritoneal cavity

S31.619- Laceration <u>without</u> foreign body of abdominal wall, <u>unspecified</u> <u>quadrant</u> <u>with penetration</u> into peritoneal cavity

S31.62- <u>Laceration</u> <u>with foreign body</u> of abdominal wall <u>with penetration</u> into peritoneal cavity

S31.620- Laceration <u>with foreign body</u> of abdominal wall, <u>right</u> <u>upper</u> quadrant <u>with penetration</u> into peritoneal cavity

S31.621- Laceration <u>with foreign body</u> of abdominal wall, <u>left</u> <u>upper</u> quadrant <u>with penetration</u> into peritoneal cavity

S31.622- Laceration <u>with foreign body</u> of abdominal wall, <u>epigastric region</u> <u>with penetration</u> into peritoneal cavity

S
3
1
–
S
3
1

S31.623- Laceration <u>with foreign body</u> of abdominal wall, <u>right lower</u> quadrant <u>with penetration</u> into peritoneal cavity

S31.624- Laceration <u>with foreign body</u> of abdominal wall, <u>left lower</u> quadrant <u>with penetration</u> into peritoneal cavity

S31.625- Laceration <u>with foreign body</u> of abdominal wall, <u>periumbilic region</u> <u>with penetration</u> into peritoneal cavity

S31.629- Laceration <u>with foreign body</u> of abdominal wall, <u>unspecified quadrant</u> <u>with penetration</u> into peritoneal cavity

S31.63- <u>Puncture</u> wound <u>without</u> foreign body of abdominal wall <u>with penetration</u> into peritoneal cavity

S31.630- Puncture wound <u>without</u> foreign body of abdominal wall, <u>right upper</u> quadrant <u>with penetration</u> into peritoneal cavity

S31.631- Puncture wound <u>without</u> foreign body of abdominal wall, <u>left upper</u> quadrant <u>with penetration</u> into peritoneal cavity

S31.632- Puncture wound <u>without</u> foreign body of abdominal wall, <u>epigastric region</u> <u>with penetration</u> into peritoneal cavity

S31.633- Puncture wound <u>without</u> foreign body of abdominal wall, <u>right lower</u> quadrant <u>with penetration</u> into peritoneal cavity

S31.634- Puncture wound <u>without</u> foreign body of abdominal wall, <u>left lower</u> quadrant <u>with penetration</u> into peritoneal cavity

S31.635- Puncture wound <u>without</u> foreign body of abdominal wall, <u>periumbilic region</u> <u>with penetration</u> into peritoneal cavity

S31.639- Puncture wound <u>without</u> foreign body of abdominal wall, <u>unspecified quadrant</u> <u>with penetration</u> into peritoneal cavity

S31.64- <u>Puncture</u> wound <u>with foreign body</u> of abdominal wall <u>with penetration</u> into peritoneal cavity

S31.640- Puncture wound <u>with foreign body</u> of abdominal wall, <u>right upper</u> quadrant <u>with penetration</u> into peritoneal cavity

S31.641- Puncture wound <u>with foreign body</u> of abdominal wall, <u>left upper</u> quadrant <u>with penetration</u> into peritoneal cavity

S31.642- Puncture wound <u>with foreign body</u> of abdominal wall, <u>epigastric region</u> <u>with penetration</u> into peritoneal cavity

S31.643- Puncture wound <u>with foreign body</u> of abdominal wall, <u>right lower</u> quadrant <u>with penetration</u> into peritoneal cavity

S31.644- Puncture wound <u>with foreign body</u> of abdominal wall, <u>left lower</u> quadrant <u>with penetration</u> into peritoneal cavity

S31.645- Puncture wound <u>with foreign body</u> of abdominal wall, <u>periumbilic region</u> <u>with penetration</u> into peritoneal cavity

S31.649- Puncture wound <u>with foreign body</u> of abdominal wall, <u>unspecified quadrant</u> <u>with penetration</u> into peritoneal cavity

S31.65- <u>Open bite</u> of abdominal wall <u>with penetration</u> into peritoneal cavity
    Excludes 1: superficial bite of abdominal wall (S30.861, S30.871)

S31.650- Open bite of abdominal wall, <u>right upper</u> quadrant <u>with penetration</u> into peritoneal cavity

S31.651- Open bite of abdominal wall, <u>left upper</u> quadrant <u>with penetration</u> into peritoneal cavity

S31.652- Open bite of abdominal wall, <u>epigastric region</u> <u>with penetration</u> into peritoneal cavity

S31.653- Open bite of abdominal wall, <u>right lower</u> quadrant <u>with penetration</u> into peritoneal cavity

S31.654- Open bite of abdominal wall, <u>left lower</u> quadrant <u>with penetration</u> into peritoneal cavity

S31.655- Open bite of abdominal wall, <u>periumbilic region</u> <u>with penetration</u> into peritoneal cavity

S31.659- Open bite of abdominal wall, <u>unspecified quadrant</u> <u>with penetration</u> into peritoneal cavity

S31.8- <u>Open wound</u> of <u>other parts of abdomen, lower back and pelvis</u>

S31.80- Open wound of <u>unspecified</u> buttock

S31.801- <u>Laceration without</u> foreign body of <u>unspecified</u> buttock

S31.802- <u>Laceration with foreign body</u> of <u>unspecified</u> buttock

S31.803- <u>Puncture</u> wound <u>without</u> foreign body of <u>unspecified</u> buttock

S31.804- <u>Puncture</u> wound <u>with foreign body</u> of <u>unspecified</u> buttock

S31.805- <u>Open bite</u> of <u>unspecified</u> buttock
    Bite of buttock NOS
    Excludes 1: superficial bite of buttock (S30.870)

S31.809- <u>Unspecified</u> open wound of <u>unspecified</u> buttock

S31.81- Open wound of <u>right</u> <u>buttock</u>

S31.811- <u>Laceration without</u> foreign body of <u>right</u> buttock

S31.812- <u>Laceration with foreign body</u> of <u>right</u> buttock

S31.813- <u>Puncture</u> wound <u>without</u> foreign body of <u>right</u> buttock

S31.814- <u>Puncture</u> wound <u>with foreign body</u> of <u>right</u> buttock

S31.815- <u>Open bite</u> of <u>right</u> buttock
    Bite of right buttock NOS
    Excludes 1: superficial bite of buttock (S30.870)

S31.819- <u>Unspecified</u> open wound of <u>right</u> buttock

S31.82- Open wound of <u>left</u> <u>buttock</u>

S31.821- <u>Laceration without</u> foreign body of <u>left</u> buttock

S31.822- <u>Laceration with foreign body</u> of <u>left</u> buttock

S31.823- <u>Puncture</u> wound <u>without</u> foreign body of <u>left</u> buttock

S31.824- <u>Puncture</u> wound <u>with foreign body</u> of <u>left</u> buttock

S31.825- <u>Open bite</u> of <u>left</u> buttock
    Bite of left buttock NOS
    Excludes 1: superficial bite of buttock (S30.870)

S31.829- <u>Unspecified</u> open wound of <u>left</u> buttock

S31.83- Open wound of <u>anus</u>

S31.831- <u>Laceration without</u> foreign body of anus

S31.832- <u>Laceration with foreign body</u> of anus

S31.833- <u>Puncture</u> wound <u>without</u> foreign body of anus

S31.834- <u>Puncture</u> wound <u>with foreign body</u> of anus

S31.835- <u>Open bite</u> of anus
    Bite of anus NOS
    Excludes 1: superficial bite of anus (S30.877)

S31.839- <u>Unspecified</u> open wound of anus

S32- <u>Fracture</u> of <u>lumbar</u> spine and pelvis
  Note: A fracture not indicated as displaced or nondisplaced should be coded to displaced
  Note: A fracture not indicated as opened or closed should be coded to closed
  Includes: Fracture of lumbosacral neural arch
          Fracture of lumbosacral spinous process
          Fracture of lumbosacral transverse process
          Fracture of lumbosacral vertebra
          Fracture of lumbosacral vertebral arch
  Code first any associated spinal cord and spinal nerve injury (S34.-)
  Excludes 1: transection of abdomen (S38.3)
  Excludes❷: fracture of hip NOS (S72.0-)

The appropriate 7th character is to be added to each code from category S32:
A   <u>Initial</u> encounter for <u>closed</u> fracture
B   <u>Initial</u> encounter for <u>open</u> fracture
D   <u>Subsequent</u> encounter for fracture <u>with routine healing</u>
G   <u>Subsequent</u> encounter for fracture <u>with delayed healing</u>
K   <u>Subsequent</u> encounter for fracture <u>with nonunion</u>
S   <u>Sequela</u>

S32.0- <u>Fracture</u> of <u>lumbar</u> <u>vertebra</u>
    Fracture of lumbar spine NOS

S32.00- Fracture of <u>unspecified</u> <u>lumbar</u> vertebra

S32.000- <u>Wedge</u> compression fracture of <u>unspecified</u> lumbar vertebra

S32.001- <u>Stable burst</u> fracture of <u>unspecified</u> lumbar vertebra

S32.002- <u>Unstable burst</u> fracture of <u>unspecified</u> lumbar vertebra

S32.008- <u>Other</u> fracture of <u>unspecified</u> lumbar vertebra

S32.009- <u>Unspecified</u> fracture of <u>unspecified</u> lumbar vertebra

S32.01- Fracture of <u>first</u> lumbar vertebra

S32.010- <u>Wedge</u> compression fracture of first lumbar vertebra

S32.011- <u>Stable burst</u> fracture of first lumbar vertebra

S32.012- <u>Unstable burst</u> fracture of first lumbar vertebra

S32.018- <u>Other</u> fracture of first lumbar vertebra

S32.019- <u>Unspecified</u> fracture of first lumbar vertebra

S32.02- Fracture of <u>second</u> lumbar vertebra

S32.020- <u>Wedge</u> compression fracture of second lumbar vertebra

S32.021- <u>Stable burst</u> fracture of second lumbar vertebra

S32.022- <u>Unstable burst</u> fracture of second lumbar vertebra

S32.028- <u>Other</u> fracture of second lumbar vertebra

S32.029- <u>Unspecified</u> fracture of second lumbar vertebra

S
3
1
-
S
3
2

S32.03- Fracture of _third_ lumbar vertebra
  S32.030- _Wedge_ compression fracture of third lumbar vertebra
  S32.031- _Stable burst_ fracture of third lumbar vertebra
  S32.032- _Unstable burst_ fracture of third lumbar vertebra
  S32.038- _Other_ fracture of third lumbar vertebra
  S32.039- _Unspecified_ fracture of third lumbar vertebra
S32.04- Fracture of _fourth_ lumbar vertebra
  S32.040- _Wedge_ compression fracture of fourth lumbar vertebra
  S32.041- _Stable burst_ fracture of fourth lumbar vertebra
  S32.042- _Unstable burst_ fracture of fourth lumbar vertebra
  S32.048- _Other_ fracture of fourth lumbar vertebra
  S32.049- _Unspecified_ fracture of fourth lumbar vertebra
S32.05- Fracture of _fifth_ lumbar vertebra
  S32.050- _Wedge_ compression fracture of fifth lumbar vertebra
  S32.051- _Stable burst_ fracture of fifth lumbar vertebra
  S32.052- _Unstable burst_ fracture of fifth lumbar vertebra
  S32.058- _Other_ fracture of fifth lumbar vertebra
  S32.059- _Unspecified_ fracture of fifth lumbar vertebra
S32.1- Fracture of _sacrum_
  Note: For vertical fractures, code to most medial fracture extension
  Note: Use two codes if both a vertical and transverse fracture are present
  Code also any associated fracture of pelvic ring (S32.8-)
  S32.10x- _Unspecified_ fracture of sacrum
  S32.11- _Zone I_ fracture of sacrum
    Vertical sacral ala fracture of sacrum
    S32.110- _Nondisplaced_ Zone I fracture of sacrum
    S32.111- _Minimally displaced_ Zone I fracture of sacrum
    S32.112- _Severely displaced_ Zone I fracture of sacrum
    S32.119- _Unspecified_ Zone I fracture of sacrum
  S32.12- _Zone II_ fracture of sacrum
    Vertical foraminal region fracture of sacrum
    S32.120- _Nondisplaced_ Zone II fracture of sacrum
    S32.121- _Minimally displaced_ Zone II fracture of sacrum
    S32.122- _Severely displaced_ Zone II fracture of sacrum
    S32.129- _Unspecified_ Zone II fracture of sacrum
  S32.13- _Zone III_ fracture of sacrum
    Vertical fracture into spinal canal region of sacrum
    S32.130- _Nondisplaced_ Zone III fracture of sacrum
    S32.131- _Minimally displaced_ Zone III fracture of sacrum
    S32.132- _Severely displaced_ Zone III fracture of sacrum
    S32.139- _Unspecified_ Zone III fracture of sacrum
  S32.14x- Type 1 fracture of sacrum
    Transverse flexion fracture of sacrum without displacement
  S32.15x- Type 2 fracture of sacrum
    Transverse flexion fracture of sacrum with posterior displacement
  S32.16x- Type 3 fracture of sacrum
    Transverse extension fracture of sacrum with anterior displacement
  S32.17x- Type 4 fracture of sacrum
    Transverse segmental comminution of upper sacrum
  S32.19x- _Other_ fracture of sacrum
S32.2xx- Fracture of coccyx
S32.3- Fracture of _ilium_
  Excludes 1: fracture of ilium with associated disruption of pelvic ring (S32.8-)
  S32.30- _Unspecified_ fracture of ilium
    S32.301- Unspecified fracture of _right_ ilium
    S32.302- Unspecified fracture of _left_ ilium
    S32.309- Unspecified fracture of _unspecified_ ilium
  S32.31- _Avulsion_ fracture of ilium
    S32.311- _Displaced_ avulsion fracture of _right_ ilium
    S32.312- _Displaced_ avulsion fracture of _left_ ilium
    S32.313- _Displaced_ avulsion fracture of _unspecified_ ilium
    S32.314- _Nondisplaced_ avulsion fracture of _right_ ilium
    S32.315- _Nondisplaced_ avulsion fracture of _left_ ilium
    S32.316- _Nondisplaced_ avulsion fracture of _unspecified_ ilium
  S32.39- _Other_ fracture of ilium
    S32.391- Other fracture of _right_ ilium
    S32.392- Other fracture of _left_ ilium
    S32.399- Other fracture of _unspecified_ ilium

S32.4- Fracture of _acetabulum_
  Code also any associated fracture of pelvic ring (S32.8-)
  S32.40- _Unspecified_ fracture of acetabulum
    S32.401- Unspecified fracture of _right_ acetabulum
    S32.402- Unspecified fracture of _left_ acetabulum
    S32.409- Unspecified fracture of _unspecified_ acetabulum
  S32.41- Fracture of _anterior wall_ of acetabulum
    S32.411- _Displaced_ fracture of anterior wall of _right_ acetabulum
    S32.412- _Displaced_ fracture of anterior wall of _left_ acetabulum
    S32.413- _Displaced_ fracture of anterior wall of _unspecified_ acetabulum
    S32.414- _Nondisplaced_ fracture of anterior wall of _right_ acetabulum
    S32.415- _Nondisplaced_ fracture of anterior wall of _left_ acetabulum
    S32.416- _Nondisplaced_ fracture of anterior wall of _unspecified_ acetabulum
  S32.42- Fracture of _posterior wall_ of acetabulum
    S32.421- _Displaced_ fracture of posterior wall of _right_ acetabulum
    S32.422- _Displaced_ fracture of posterior wall of _left_ acetabulum
    S32.423- _Displaced_ fracture of posterior wall of _unspecified_ acetabulum
    S32.424- _Nondisplaced_ fracture of posterior wall of _right_ acetabulum
    S32.425- _Nondisplaced_ fracture of posterior wall of _left_ acetabulum
    S32.426- _Nondisplaced_ fracture of posterior wall of _unspecified_ acetabulum
  S32.43- Fracture of _anterior column [iliopubic]_ of acetabulum
    S32.431- _Displaced_ fracture of anterior column [iliopubic] of _right_ acetabulum
    S32.432- _Displaced_ fracture of anterior column [iliopubic] of _left_ acetabulum
    S32.433- _Displaced_ fracture of anterior column [iliopubic] of _unspecified_ acetabulum
    S32.434- _Nondisplaced_ fracture of anterior column [iliopubic] of _right_ acetabulum
    S32.435- _Nondisplaced_ fracture of anterior column [iliopubic] of _left_ acetabulum
    S32.436- _Nondisplaced_ fracture of anterior column [iliopubic] of _unspecified_ acetabulum
  S32.44- Fracture of _posterior column [ilioischial]_ of acetabulum
    S32.441- _Displaced_ fracture of posterior column [ilioischial] of _right_ acetabulum
    S32.442- _Displaced_ fracture of posterior column [ilioischial] of _left_ acetabulum
    S32.443- _Displaced_ fracture of posterior column [ilioischial] of _unspecified_ acetabulum
    S32.444- _Nondisplaced_ fracture of posterior column [ilioischial] of _right_ acetabulum
    S32.445- _Nondisplaced_ fracture of posterior column [ilioischial] of _left_ acetabulum
    S32.446- _Nondisplaced_ fracture of posterior column [ilioischial] of _unspecified_ acetabulum
  S32.45- _Transverse_ fracture of acetabulum
    S32.451- _Displaced_ transverse fracture of _right_ acetabulum
    S32.452- _Displaced_ transverse fracture of _left_ acetabulum
    S32.453- _Displaced_ transverse fracture of _unspecified_ acetabulum
    S32.454- _Nondisplaced_ transverse fracture of _right_ acetabulum
    S32.455- _Nondisplaced_ transverse fracture of _left_ acetabulum
    S32.456- _Nondisplaced_ transverse fracture of _unspecified_ acetabulum
  S32.46- _Associated transverse-posterior_ fracture of acetabulum
    S32.461- _Displaced_ associated transverse-posterior fracture of _right_ acetabulum
    S32.462- _Displaced_ associated transverse-posterior fracture of _left_ acetabulum
    S32.463- _Displaced_ associated transverse-posterior fracture of _unspecified_ acetabulum
    S32.464- _Nondisplaced_ associated transverse-posterior fracture of _right_ acetabulum
    S32.465- _Nondisplaced_ associated transverse-posterior fracture of _left_ acetabulum
    S32.466- _Nondisplaced_ associated transverse-posterior fracture of _unspecified_ acetabulum

S 3 1 - S 3 2

Excludes 1: = NOT CODED HERE! (Do not code both)

Excludes ❷: = Not Included Here

S32.47-   Fracture of <u>medial wall</u> of acetabulum
    S32.471-   <u>Displaced</u> fracture of medial wall of <u>right</u> acetabulum
    S32.472-   <u>Displaced</u> fracture of medial wall of <u>left</u> acetabulum
    S32.473-   <u>Displaced</u> fracture of medial wall of <u>unspecified</u> acetabulum
    S32.474-   <u>Nondisplaced</u> fracture of medial wall of <u>right</u> acetabulum
    S32.475-   <u>Nondisplaced</u> fracture of medial wall of <u>left</u> acetabulum
    S32.476-   <u>Nondisplaced</u> fracture of medial wall of <u>unspecified</u> acetabulum
S32.48-   <u>Dome</u> fracture of acetabulum
    S32.481-   <u>Displaced</u> dome fracture of <u>right</u> acetabulum
    S32.482-   <u>Displaced</u> dome fracture of <u>left</u> acetabulum
    S32.483-   <u>Displaced</u> dome fracture of <u>unspecified</u> acetabulum
    S32.484-   <u>Nondisplaced</u> dome fracture of <u>right</u> acetabulum
    S32.485-   <u>Nondisplaced</u> dome fracture of <u>left</u> acetabulum
    S32.486-   <u>Nondisplaced</u> dome fracture of <u>unspecified</u> acetabulum
S32.49-   <u>Other specified</u> fracture of acetabulum
    S32.491-   Other specified fracture of <u>right</u> acetabulum
    S32.492-   Other specified fracture of <u>left</u> acetabulum
    S32.499-   Other specified fracture of <u>unspecified</u> acetabulum
S32.5-   Fracture of <u>pubis</u>
    Excludes 1: fracture of pubis with associated disruption of pelvic ring (S32.8-)
S32.50-   <u>Unspecified</u> fracture of pubis
    S32.501-   Unspecified fracture of <u>right</u> pubis
    S32.502-   Unspecified fracture of <u>left</u> pubis
    S32.509-   Unspecified fracture of <u>unspecified</u> pubis
S32.51-   Fracture of <u>superior rim</u> of pubis
    S32.511-   Fracture of superior rim of <u>right</u> pubis
    S32.512-   Fracture of superior rim of <u>left</u> pubis
    S32.519-   Fracture of superior rim of <u>unspecified</u> pubis
S32.59-   <u>Other specified</u> fracture of pubis
    S32.591-   Other specified fracture of <u>right</u> pubis
    S32.592-   Other specified fracture of <u>left</u> pubis
    S32.599-   Other specified fracture of <u>unspecified</u> pubis
S32.6-   Fracture of <u>ischium</u>
    Excludes 1: fracture of ischium with associated disruption of pelvic ring (S32.8-)
S32.60-   <u>Unspecified</u> fracture of ischium
    S32.601-   Unspecified fracture of <u>right</u> ischium
    S32.602-   Unspecified fracture of <u>left</u> ischium
    S32.609-   Unspecified fracture of <u>unspecified</u> ischium
S32.61-   <u>Avulsion</u> fracture of ischium
    S32.611-   <u>Displaced</u> avulsion fracture of <u>right</u> ischium
    S32.612-   <u>Displaced</u> avulsion fracture of <u>left</u> ischium
    S32.613-   <u>Displaced</u> avulsion fracture of <u>unspecified</u> ischium
    S32.614-   <u>Nondisplaced</u> avulsion fracture of <u>right</u> ischium
    S32.615-   <u>Nondisplaced</u> avulsion fracture of <u>left</u> ischium
    S32.616-   <u>Nondisplaced</u> avulsion fracture of <u>unspecified</u> ischium
S32.69-   <u>Other specified</u> fracture of ischium
    S32.691-   Other specified fracture of <u>right</u> ischium
    S32.692-   Other specified fracture of <u>left</u> ischium
    S32.699-   Other specified fracture of <u>unspecified</u> ischium
S32.8-   Fracture of <u>other parts of pelvis</u>
    Code also any associated:
      Fracture of acetabulum (S32.4-)
      Sacral fracture (S32.1-)
S32.81-   <u>Multiple</u> fractures of pelvis <u>with disruption of pelvic ring</u>
    Multiple pelvic fractures with disruption of pelvic circle
    S32.810-   Multiple fractures of pelvis with <u>stable</u> disruption of pelvic ring
    S32.811-   Multiple fractures of pelvis with <u>unstable</u> disruption of pelvic ring
S32.82x-   <u>Multiple</u> fractures of pelvis <u>without</u> disruption of pelvic ring
    Multiple pelvic fractures without disruption of pelvic circle
S32.89x-   Fracture of <u>other</u> parts of pelvis
S32.9xx-   Fracture of <u>unspecified</u> parts of lumbosacral spine and pelvis
    Fracture of lumbosacral spine NOS
    Fracture of pelvis NOS

S33   <u>Dislocation and sprain</u> of joints and ligaments of lumbar spine and pelvis
    Includes: Avulsion of joint or ligament of lumbar spine and pelvis
      Laceration of cartilage, joint or ligament of lumbar spine and pelvis
      Sprain of cartilage, joint or ligament of lumbar spine and pelvis
      Traumatic hemarthrosis of joint or ligament of lumbar spine and pelvis
      Traumatic rupture of joint or ligament of lumbar spine and pelvis
      Traumatic subluxation of joint or ligament of lumbar spine and pelvis
      Traumatic tear of joint or ligament of lumbar spine and pelvis
    Code also any associated open wound
    Excludes 1: nontraumatic rupture or displacement of lumbar intervertebral disc NOS (M51.-)
      obstetric damage to pelvic joints and ligaments (O71.6)
    Excludes❷: dislocation and sprain of joints and ligaments of hip (S73.-)
      strain of muscle of lower back and pelvis (S39.01-)

> **The appropriate 7th character is to be added to each code from category S33:**
>   **A**   <u>Initial</u> encounter
>   **D**   <u>Subsequent</u> encounter
>   **S**   <u>Sequela</u>

S33.0xx-   <u>Traumatic rupture</u> of <u>lumbar</u> intervertebral disc
    Excludes 1: rupture or displacement (nontraumatic) of lumbar intervertebral disc NOS (M51.- with fifth character 6)
S33.1-   <u>Subluxation and dislocation of lumbar vertebra</u>
    Code also any associated:
      Open wound of abdomen, lower back and pelvis (S31)
      Spinal cord injury (S24.0, S24.1-, S34.0-, S34.1-)
    Excludes❷: fracture of lumbar vertebrae (S32.0-)
    S33.10-   Subluxation and dislocation of <u>unspecified</u> <u>lumbar</u> vertebra
      S33.100-   <u>Subluxation</u> of <u>unspecified</u> <u>lumbar</u> vertebra
      S33.101-   <u>Dislocation</u> of <u>unspecified</u> <u>lumbar</u> vertebra
    S33.11-   Subluxation and dislocation of <u>L1/L2</u> lumbar vertebra
      S33.110-   <u>Subluxation</u> of <u>L1/L2</u> lumbar vertebra
      S33.111-   <u>Dislocation</u> of <u>L1/L2</u> lumbar vertebra
    S33.12-   Subluxation and dislocation of <u>L2/L3</u> lumbar vertebra
      S33.120-   <u>Subluxation</u> of <u>L2/L3</u> lumbar vertebra
      S33.121-   <u>Dislocation</u> of <u>L2/L3</u> lumbar vertebra
    S33.13-   Subluxation and dislocation of <u>L3/L4</u> lumbar vertebra
      S33.130-   <u>Subluxation</u> of <u>L3/L4</u> lumbar vertebra
      S33.131-   <u>Dislocation</u> of <u>L3/L4</u> lumbar vertebra
    S33.14-   Subluxation and dislocation of <u>L4/L5</u> lumbar vertebra
      S33.140-   <u>Subluxation</u> of <u>L4/L5</u> lumbar vertebra
      S33.141-   <u>Dislocation</u> of <u>L4/L5</u> lumbar vertebra
S33.2xx-   Dislocation of <u>sacroiliac and sacrococcygeal joint</u>
S33.3-   Dislocation of <u>other and unspecified</u> parts of lumbar spine and pelvis
    S33.30x-   Dislocation of <u>unspecified</u> parts of lumbar spine and pelvis
    S33.39x-   Dislocation of <u>other</u> parts of lumbar spine and pelvis
S33.4xx-   <u>Traumatic rupture</u> of <u>symphysis pubis</u>
S33.5xx-   <u>Sprain</u> of <u>ligaments of lumbar spine</u>
S33.6xx-   <u>Sprain</u> of <u>sacroiliac joint</u>
S33.8xx-   <u>Sprain</u> of <u>other</u> parts of lumbar spine and pelvis
S33.9xx-   <u>Sprain</u> of <u>unspecified</u> parts of lumbar spine and pelvis

S34-   Injury of <u>lumbar and sacral spinal cord and nerves</u> at <u>abdomen, lower back and pelvis</u> level
    Note: Code to highest level of lumbar cord injury
      Injuries to the spinal cord (S34.0 and S34.1) refer to the cord level and not bone level injury, and can affect nerve roots at and below the level given.
    Code also any associated:
      Fracture of vertebra (S22.0-, S32.0-)
      Open wound of abdomen, lower back and pelvis (S31.-)
      Transient paralysis (R29.5)

> **The appropriate 7th character is to be added to each code from category S34:**
>   **A**   <u>Initial</u> encounter
>   **D**   <u>Subsequent</u> encounter
>   **S**   <u>Sequela</u>

S34.0-   <u>Concussion and edema</u> of <u>lumbar and sacral spinal cord</u>
    S34.01x-   Concussion and edema of <u>lumbar</u> spinal cord
    S34.02x-   Concussion and edema of <u>sacral</u> spinal cord
      Concussion and edema of conus medullaris
S34.1-   <u>Other and unspecified</u> injury of <u>lumbar and sacral spinal cord</u>
    S34.10-   <u>Unspecified</u> injury to lumbar spinal cord
      S34.101-   Unspecified injury to <u>L1</u> level of lumbar spinal cord
      S34.102-   Unspecified injury to <u>L2</u> level of lumbar spinal cord
      S34.103-   Unspecified injury to <u>L3</u> level of lumbar spinal cord

S34.104-   Unspecified injury to <u>L4</u> level of lumbar spinal cord

S34.105-   Unspecified injury to <u>L5</u> level of lumbar spinal cord

S34.109-   Unspecified injury to <u>unspecified</u> level of lumbar spinal cord

S34.11-   <u>Complete</u> lesion of lumbar spinal cord

     S34.111-   Complete lesion of <u>L1</u> level of lumbar spinal cord

     S34.112-   Complete lesion of <u>L2</u> level of lumbar spinal cord

     S34.113-   Complete lesion of <u>L3</u> level of lumbar spinal cord

     S34.114-   Complete lesion of <u>L4</u> level of lumbar spinal cord

     S34.115-   Complete lesion of <u>L5</u> level of lumbar spinal cord

     S34.119-   Complete lesion of <u>unspecified</u> level of lumbar spinal cord

S34.12-   <u>Incomplete</u> lesion of lumbar spinal cord

     S34.121-   Incomplete lesion of <u>L1</u> level of lumbar spinal cord

     S34.122-   Incomplete lesion of <u>L2</u> level of lumbar spinal cord

     S34.123-   Incomplete lesion of <u>L3</u> level of lumbar spinal cord

     S34.124-   Incomplete lesion of <u>L4</u> level of lumbar spinal cord

     S34.125-   Incomplete lesion of <u>L5</u> level of lumbar spinal cord

     S34.129-   Incomplete lesion of <u>unspecified</u> level of lumbar spinal cord

S34.13-   <u>Other and unspecified</u> injury to <u>sacral spinal cord</u>
       Other injury to conus medullaris

     S34.131-   <u>Complete</u> lesion of sacral spinal cord
             Complete lesion of conus medullaris

     S34.132-   <u>Incomplete</u> lesion of sacral spinal cord
             Incomplete lesion of conus medullaris

     S34.139-   <u>Unspecified</u> injury to sacral spinal cord
             Unspecified injury of conus medullaris

S34.2-   Injury of <u>nerve root of lumbar and sacral spine</u>

     S34.21x-   Injury of nerve root of <u>lumbar</u> spine

     S34.22x-   Injury of nerve root of <u>sacral</u> spine

S34.3xx-   Injury of cauda equina

S34.4xx-   Injury of lumbosacral plexus

S34.5xx-   Injury of lumbar, sacral and pelvic sympathetic nerves
       Injury of celiac ganglion or plexus
       Injury of hypogastric plexus
       Injury of mesenteric plexus (inferior) (superior)
       Injury of splanchnic nerve

S34.6xx-   Injury of peripheral nerve(s) at abdomen, lower back and pelvis level

S34.8xx-   Injury of <u>other</u> nerves at abdomen, lower back and pelvis level

S34.9xx-   Injury of <u>unspecified</u> nerves at abdomen, lower back and pelvis level

S35-   <u>Injury of blood vessels</u> at <u>abdomen, lower back and pelvis level</u>
     Code also any associated open wound (S31.-)
     The appropriate 7th character is to be added to each code from category S35:
     A   <u>**Initial** encounter</u>
     D   <u>**Subsequent** encounter</u>
     S   <u>**Sequela**</u>

S35.0-   Injury of <u>abdominal aorta</u>
      Excludes 1: injury of aorta NOS (S25.0)

     S35.00x-   <u>Unspecified</u> injury of abdominal aorta

     S35.01x-   <u>Minor laceration</u> of abdominal aorta
             Incomplete transection of abdominal aorta
             Laceration of abdominal aorta NOS
             Superficial laceration of abdominal aorta

     S35.02x-   <u>Major laceration</u> of abdominal aorta
             Complete transection of abdominal aorta
             Traumatic rupture of abdominal aorta

     S35.09x-   <u>Other</u> injury of abdominal aorta

S35.1-   Injury of <u>inferior vena cava</u>
       Injury of hepatic vein
      Excludes 1: injury of vena cava NOS (S25.2)

     S35.10x-   <u>Unspecified</u> injury of inferior vena cava

     S35.11x-   <u>Minor laceration</u> of inferior vena cava
             Incomplete transection of inferior vena cava
             Laceration of inferior vena cava NOS
             Superficial laceration of inferior vena cava

     S35.12x-   <u>Major laceration</u> of inferior vena cava
             Complete transection of inferior vena cava
             Traumatic rupture of inferior vena cava

     S35.19x-   <u>Other</u> injury of inferior vena cava

S35.2-   Injury of <u>celiac or mesenteric</u> artery <u>and branches</u>

S35.21-   Injury of <u>celiac artery</u>

     S35.211-   <u>Minor laceration</u> of celiac <u>artery</u>
             Incomplete transection of celiac artery
             Laceration of celiac artery NOS
             Superficial laceration of celiac artery

     S35.212-   <u>Major laceration</u> of celiac <u>artery</u>
             Complete transection of celiac artery
             Traumatic rupture of celiac artery

     S35.218-   <u>Other</u> injury of celiac <u>artery</u>

     S35.219-   <u>Unspecified</u> injury of celiac <u>artery</u>

S35.22-   Injury of <u>superior mesenteric artery</u>

     S35.221-   <u>Minor laceration</u> of superior mesenteric <u>artery</u>
             Incomplete transection of superior mesenteric artery
             Laceration of superior mesenteric artery NOS
             Superficial laceration of superior mesenteric artery

     S35.222-   <u>Major laceration</u> of superior mesenteric artery
             Complete transection of superior mesenteric artery
             Traumatic rupture of superior mesenteric artery

     S35.228-   <u>Other</u> injury of superior mesenteric <u>artery</u>

     S35.229-   <u>Unspecified</u> injury of superior mesenteric <u>artery</u>

S35.23-   Injury of inferior mesenteric <u>artery</u>

     S35.231-   <u>Minor laceration</u> of inferior mesenteric <u>artery</u>
             Incomplete transection of inferior mesenteric artery
             Laceration of inferior mesenteric artery NOS
             Superficial laceration of inferior mesenteric artery

     S35.232-   <u>Major laceration</u> of inferior mesenteric <u>artery</u>
             Complete transection of inferior mesenteric artery
             Traumatic rupture of inferior mesenteric artery

     S35.238-   <u>Other</u> injury of inferior mesenteric <u>artery</u>

     S35.239-   <u>Unspecified</u> injury of inferior mesenteric <u>artery</u>

S35.29-   Injury of <u>branches of celiac and mesenteric artery</u>
       Injury of gastric artery
       Injury of gastroduodenal artery
       Injury of hepatic artery
       Injury of splenic artery

     S35.291-   <u>Minor laceration</u> of <u>branches</u> of celiac and mesenteric <u>artery</u>
             Incomplete transection of branches of celiac and mesenteric artery
             Laceration of branches of celiac and mesenteric artery NOS
             Superficial laceration of branches of celiac and mesenteric artery

     S35.292-   <u>Major laceration</u> of <u>branches</u> of celiac and mesenteric <u>artery</u>
             Complete transection of branches of celiac and mesenteric artery
             Traumatic rupture of branches of celiac and mesenteric artery

     S35.298-   <u>Other</u> injury of <u>branches</u> of celiac and mesenteric <u>artery</u>

     S35.299-   <u>Unspecified</u> injury of <u>branches</u> of celiac and mesenteric <u>artery</u>

S35.3-   Injury of <u>portal or splenic vein</u> and <u>branches</u>

S35.31-   Injury of <u>portal vein</u>

     S35.311-   <u>Laceration</u> of portal <u>vein</u>

     S35.318-   <u>Other</u> specified injury of portal <u>vein</u>

     S35.319-   <u>Unspecified</u> injury of portal <u>vein</u>

S35.32-   Injury of <u>splenic vein</u>

     S35.321-   Laceration of splenic <u>vein</u>

     S35.328-   Other specified injury of splenic <u>vein</u>

     S35.329-   Unspecified injury of splenic <u>vein</u>

S35.33-   Injury of <u>superior mesenteric vein</u>

     S35.331-   <u>Laceration</u> of superior mesenteric <u>vein</u>

     S35.338-   <u>Other</u> specified injury of superior mesenteric <u>vein</u>

     S35.339-   <u>Unspecified</u> injury of superior mesenteric <u>vein</u>

S35.34-   Injury of <u>inferior mesenteric vein</u>

     S35.341-   <u>Laceration</u> of inferior mesenteric <u>vein</u>

     S35.348-   <u>Other</u> specified injury of inferior mesenteric <u>vein</u>

     S35.349-   <u>Unspecified</u> injury of inferior mesenteric <u>vein</u>

S35.4-   Injury of <u>renal blood vessels</u>

S35.40-   <u>Unspecified</u> injury of renal blood vessel

     S35.401-   Unspecified injury of <u>right</u> renal <u>artery</u>

     S35.402-   Unspecified injury of <u>left</u> renal <u>artery</u>

     S35.403-   Unspecified injury of <u>unspecified</u> renal <u>artery</u>

     S35.404-   Unspecified injury of <u>right</u> renal <u>vein</u>

     S35.405-   Unspecified injury of <u>left</u> renal <u>vein</u>

     S35.406-   Unspecified injury of <u>unspecified</u> renal <u>vein</u>

S
3
2
–
S
3
5

S35.41- Laceration of renal blood vessel
   S35.411- Laceration of right renal artery
   S35.412- Laceration of left renal artery
   S35.413- Laceration of unspecified renal artery
   S35.414- Laceration of right renal vein
   S35.415- Laceration of left renal vein
   S35.416- Laceration of unspecified renal vein
S35.49- Other specified injury of renal blood vessel
   S35.491- Other specified injury of right renal artery
   S35.492- Other specified injury of left renal artery
   S35.493- Other specified injury of unspecified renal artery
   S35.494- Other specified injury of right renal vein
   S35.495- Other specified injury of left renal vein
   S35.496- Other specified injury of unspecified renal vein
S35.5- Injury of iliac blood vessels
  S35.50x- Injury of unspecified iliac blood vessel(s)
  S35.51- Injury of iliac artery or vein
    Injury of hypogastric artery or vein
   S35.511- Injury of right iliac artery
   S35.512- Injury of left iliac artery
   S35.513- Injury of unspecified iliac artery
   S35.514- Injury of right iliac vein
   S35.515- Injury of left iliac vein
   S35.516- Injury of unspecified iliac vein
  S35.53- Injury of uterine artery or vein
   S35.531- Injury of right uterine artery
   S35.532- Injury of left uterine artery
   S35.533- Injury of unspecified uterine artery
   S35.534- Injury of right uterine vein
   S35.535- Injury of left uterine vein
   S35.536- Injury of unspecified uterine vein
  S35.59x- Injury of other iliac blood vessels
S35.8- Injury of other blood vessels at abdomen, lower back and pelvis level
   Injury of ovarian artery or vein
  S35.8x- Injury of other blood vessels at abdomen, lower back and pelvis level
   S35.8x1- Laceration of other blood vessels at abdomen, lower back and pelvis level
   S35.8x8- Other specified injury of other blood vessels at abdomen, lower back and pelvis level
   S35.8x9- Unspecified injury of other blood vessels at abdomen, lower back and pelvis level
S35.9- Injury of unspecified blood vessel at abdomen, lower back and pelvis level
  S35.90x- Unspecified injury of unspecified blood vessel at abdomen, lower back and pelvis level
  S35.91x- Laceration of unspecified blood vessel at abdomen, lower back and pelvis level
  S35.99x- Other specified injury of unspecified blood vessel at abdomen, lower back and pelvis level

S36- Injury of intra-abdominal organs
  Code also any associated open wound (S31.-)
  The appropriate 7th character is to be added to each code from category S36:
   A **Initial** encounter
   D **Subsequent** encounter
   S **Sequela**
S36.0- Injury of spleen
  S36.00x- Unspecified injury of spleen
  S36.02- Contusion of spleen
   S36.020- Minor contusion of spleen
     Contusion of spleen less than 2 cm
   S36.021- Major contusion of spleen
     Contusion of spleen greater than 2 cm
   S36.029- Unspecified contusion of spleen
  S36.03- Laceration of spleen
   S36.030- Superficial (capsular) laceration of spleen
     Laceration of spleen less than 1 cm
     Minor laceration of spleen
   S36.031- Moderate laceration of spleen
     Laceration of spleen 1 to 3 cm
   S36.032- Major laceration of spleen
     Avulsion of spleen
     Laceration of spleen greater than 3 cm
     Massive laceration of spleen
     Multiple moderate lacerations of spleen
     Stellate laceration of spleen

   S36.039- Unspecified laceration of spleen
  S36.09x- Other injury of spleen
S36.1- Injury of liver and gallbladder and bile duct
  S36.11- Injury of liver
   S36.112- Contusion of liver
   S36.113- Laceration of liver, unspecified degree
   S36.114- Minor laceration of liver
     Laceration involving capsule only, or, without significant involvement of hepatic parenchyma [i.e., less than 1 cm deep]
   S36.115- Moderate laceration of liver
     Laceration involving parenchyma but without major disruption of parenchyma [i.e., less than 10 cm long and less than 3 cm deep]
   S36.116- Major laceration of liver
     Laceration with significant disruption of hepatic parenchyma [i.e., greater than 10 cm long and 3 cm deep]
     Multiple moderate lacerations, with or without hematoma
     Stellate laceration of liver
   S36.118- Other injury of liver
   S36.119- Unspecified injury of liver
  S36.12- Injury of gallbladder
   S36.122- Contusion of gallbladder
   S36.123- Laceration of gallbladder
   S36.128- Other injury of gallbladder
   S36.129- Unspecified injury of gallbladder
  S36.13x- Injury of bile duct
S36.2- Injury of pancreas
  S36.20- Unspecified injury of pancreas
   S36.200- Unspecified injury of head of pancreas
   S36.201- Unspecified injury of body of pancreas
   S36.202- Unspecified injury of tail of pancreas
   S36.209- Unspecified injury of unspecified part of pancreas
  S36.22- Contusion of pancreas
   S36.220- Contusion of head of pancreas
   S36.221- Contusion of body of pancreas
   S36.222- Contusion of tail of pancreas
   S36.229- Contusion of unspecified part of pancreas
  S36.23- Laceration of pancreas, unspecified degree
   S36.230- Laceration of head of pancreas, unspecified degree
   S36.231- Laceration of body of pancreas, unspecified degree
   S36.232- Laceration of tail of pancreas, unspecified degree
   S36.239- Laceration of unspecified part of pancreas, unspecified degree
  S36.24- Minor laceration of pancreas
   S36.240- Minor laceration of head of pancreas
   S36.241- Minor laceration of body of pancreas
   S36.242- Minor laceration of tail of pancreas
   S36.249- Minor laceration of unspecified part of pancreas
  S36.25- Moderate laceration of pancreas
   S36.250- Moderate laceration of head of pancreas
   S36.251- Moderate laceration of body of pancreas
   S36.252- Moderate laceration of tail of pancreas
   S36.259- Moderate laceration of unspecified part of pancreas
  S36.26- Major laceration of pancreas
   S36.260- Major laceration of head of pancreas
   S36.261- Major laceration of body of pancreas
   S36.262- Major laceration of tail of pancreas
   S36.269- Major laceration of unspecified part of pancreas
  S36.29- Other injury of pancreas
   S36.290- Other injury of head of pancreas
   S36.291- Other injury of body of pancreas
   S36.292- Other injury of tail of pancreas
   S36.299- Other injury of unspecified part of pancreas
S36.3- Injury of stomach
  S36.30x- Unspecified injury of stomach
  S36.32x- Contusion of stomach
  S36.33x- Laceration of stomach
  S36.39x- Other injury of stomach

S36.4-　Injury of <u>small intestine</u>
　S36.40-　<u>Unspecified</u> injury of small intestine
　　S36.400-　Unspecified injury of <u>duodenum</u>
　　S36.408-　Unspecified injury of <u>other</u> part of small intestine
　　S36.409-　Unspecified injury of <u>unspecified</u> part of small intestine
　S36.41-　<u>Primary blast</u> injury of small intestine
　　　Blast injury of small intestine NOS
　　S36.410-　Primary blast injury of <u>duodenum</u>
　　S36.418-　Primary blast injury of <u>other</u> part of small intestine
　　S36.419-　Primary blast injury of <u>unspecified</u> part of small intestine
　S36.42-　<u>Contusion</u> of small intestine
　　S36.420-　Contusion of <u>duodenum</u>
　　S36.428-　Contusion of <u>other</u> part of small intestine
　　S36.429-　Contusion of <u>unspecified</u> part of small intestine
　S36.43-　<u>Laceration</u> of small intestine
　　S36.430-　Laceration of <u>duodenum</u>
　　S36.438-　Laceration of <u>other</u> part of small intestine
　　S36.439-　Laceration of <u>unspecified</u> part of small intestine
　S36.49-　<u>Other</u> injury of small intestine
　　S36.490-　Other injury of <u>duodenum</u>
　　S36.498-　Other injury of <u>other</u> part of small intestine
　　S36.499-　Other injury of <u>unspecified</u> part of small intestine
S36.5-　Injury of <u>colon</u>
　　Excludes❷: injury of rectum (S36.6-)
　S36.50-　<u>Unspecified</u> injury of colon
　　S36.500-　Unspecified injury of <u>ascending</u> [<u>right</u>] colon
　　S36.501-　Unspecified injury of <u>transverse</u> colon
　　S36.502-　Unspecified injury of <u>descending</u> [<u>left</u>] colon
　　S36.503-　Unspecified injury of <u>sigmoid</u> colon
　　S36.508-　Unspecified injury of <u>other</u> part of colon
　　S36.509-　Unspecified injury of <u>unspecified</u> part of colon
　S36.51-　<u>Primary blast</u> injury of colon
　　　Blast injury of colon NOS
　　S36.510-　Primary blast injury of <u>ascending</u> [<u>right</u>] colon
　　S36.511-　Primary blast injury of <u>transverse</u> colon
　　S36.512-　Primary blast injury of <u>descending</u> [<u>left</u>] colon
　　S36.513-　Primary blast injury of <u>sigmoid</u> colon
　　S36.518-　Primary blast injury of <u>other</u> part of colon
　　S36.519-　Primary blast injury of <u>unspecified</u> part of colon
　S36.52-　<u>Contusion</u> of colon
　　S36.520-　Contusion of <u>ascending</u> [<u>right</u>] colon
　　S36.521-　Contusion of <u>transverse</u> colon
　　S36.522-　Contusion of <u>descending</u> [<u>left</u>] colon
　　S36.523-　Contusion of <u>sigmoid</u> colon
　　S36.528-　Contusion of <u>other</u> part of colon
　　S36.529-　Contusion of <u>unspecified</u> part of colon
　S36.53-　<u>Laceration</u> of colon
　　S36.530-　Laceration of <u>ascending</u> [<u>right</u>] colon
　　S36.531-　Laceration of <u>transverse</u> colon
　　S36.532-　Laceration of <u>descending</u> [<u>left</u>] colon
　　S36.533-　Laceration of <u>sigmoid</u> colon
　　S36.538-　Laceration of <u>other</u> part of colon
　　S36.539-　Laceration of <u>unspecified</u> part of colon
　S36.59-　<u>Other</u> injury of colon
　　　Secondary blast injury of colon
　　S36.590-　Other injury of <u>ascending</u> [<u>right</u>] colon
　　S36.591-　Other injury of <u>transverse</u> colon
　　S36.592-　Other injury of <u>descending</u> [<u>left</u>] colon
　　S36.593-　Other injury of <u>sigmoid</u> colon
　　S36.598-　Other injury of <u>other</u> part of colon
　　S36.599-　Other injury of <u>unspecified</u> part of colon
S36.6-　Injury of <u>rectum</u>
　S36.60x-　<u>Unspecified</u> injury of rectum
　S36.61x-　<u>Primary blast</u> injury of rectum
　　　Blast injury of rectum NOS
　S36.62x-　<u>Contusion</u> of rectum
　S36.63x-　<u>Laceration</u> of rectum
　S36.69x-　<u>Other</u> injury of rectum
　　　Secondary blast injury of rectum

S36.8-　Injury of <u>other intra-abdominal organs</u>
　S36.81x-　Injury of <u>peritoneum</u>
　S36.89-　Injury of <u>other intra-abdominal organs</u>
　　　Injury of retroperitoneum
　　S36.892-　<u>Contusion</u> of other intra-abdominal organs
　　S36.893-　<u>Laceration</u> of other intra-abdominal organs
　　S36.898-　<u>Other</u> injury of other intra-abdominal organs
　　S36.899-　<u>Unspecified</u> injury of other intra-abdominal organs
S36.9-　Injury of <u>unspecified</u> intra-abdominal organ
　S36.90x-　<u>Unspecified</u> injury of unspecified intra-abdominal organ
　S36.92x-　<u>Contusion</u> of unspecified intra-abdominal organ
　S36.93x-　<u>Laceration</u> of unspecified intra-abdominal organ
　S36.99x-　<u>Other</u> injury of unspecified intra-abdominal organ

S37-　Injury of <u>urinary and pelvic organs</u>
　　Code also any associated open wound (S31.-)
　　Excludes 1: obstetric trauma to pelvic organs (O71.-)
　　Excludes❷: injury of peritoneum (S36.81)
　　　　　　injury of retroperitoneum (S36.89-)
　　The appropriate 7th character is to be added to each code from category S37:
　　A　<u>Initial</u> encounter
　　D　<u>Subsequent</u> encounter
　　S　<u>Sequela</u>
S37.0-　Injury of <u>kidney</u>
　　Excludes❷: acute kidney injury (nontraumatic) (N17.9)
　S37.00-　<u>Unspecified</u> injury of kidney
　　S37.001-　Unspecified injury of <u>right</u> kidney
　　S37.002-　Unspecified injury of <u>left</u> kidney
　　S37.009-　Unspecified injury of <u>unspecified</u> kidney
　S37.01-　<u>Minor contusion</u> of kidney
　　　Contusion of kidney less than 2 cm
　　　Contusion of kidney NOS
　　S37.011-　Minor contusion of <u>right</u> kidney
　　S37.012-　Minor contusion of <u>left</u> kidney
　　S37.019-　Minor contusion of <u>unspecified</u> kidney
　S37.02-　<u>Major contusion</u> of kidney
　　　Contusion of kidney greater than 2 cm
　　S37.021-　Major contusion of <u>right</u> kidney
　　S37.022-　Major contusion of <u>left</u> kidney
　　S37.029-　Major contusion of <u>unspecified</u> kidney
　S37.03-　<u>Laceration</u> of kidney, <u>unspecified</u> degree
　　S37.031-　Laceration of <u>right</u> kidney, unspecified degree
　　S37.032-　Laceration of <u>left</u> kidney, unspecified degree
　　S37.039-　Laceration of <u>unspecified</u> kidney, unspecified degree
　S37.04-　<u>Minor laceration</u> of kidney
　　　Laceration of kidney less than 1 cm
　　S37.041-　Minor laceration of <u>right</u> kidney
　　S37.042-　Minor laceration of <u>left</u> kidney
　　S37.049-　Minor laceration of <u>unspecified</u> kidney
　S37.05-　<u>Moderate laceration</u> of kidney
　　　Laceration of kidney 1 to 3 cm
　　S37.051-　Moderate laceration of <u>right</u> kidney
　　S37.052-　Moderate laceration of <u>left</u> kidney
　　S37.059-　Moderate laceration of <u>unspecified</u> kidney
　S37.06-　<u>Major laceration</u> of kidney
　　　Avulsion of kidney
　　　Laceration of kidney greater than 3 cm
　　　Massive laceration of kidney
　　　Multiple moderate lacerations of kidney
　　　Stellate laceration of kidney
　　S37.061-　Major laceration of <u>right</u> kidney
　　S37.062-　Major laceration of <u>left</u> kidney
　　S37.069-　Major laceration of <u>unspecified</u> kidney
　S37.09-　<u>Other</u> injury of kidney
　　S37.091-　Other injury of <u>right</u> kidney
　　S37.092-　Other injury of <u>left</u> kidney
　　S37.099-　Other injury of <u>unspecified</u> kidney
　S37.1-　Injury of <u>ureter</u>
　　S37.10x-　<u>Unspecified</u> injury of ureter
　　S37.12x-　<u>Contusion</u> of ureter
　　S37.13x-　<u>Laceration</u> of ureter
　　S37.19x-　Other injury of ureter
　S37.2-　Injury of <u>bladder</u>
　　S37.20x-　<u>Unspecified</u> injury of bladder
　　S37.22x-　<u>Contusion</u> of bladder
　　S37.23x-　<u>Laceration</u> of bladder
　　S37.29x-　<u>Other</u> injury of bladder

S
3
5
–
S
3
7

S37.3- Injury of <u>urethra</u>
  S37.30x- <u>Unspecified</u> injury of urethra
  S37.32x- <u>Contusion</u> of urethra
  S37.33x- <u>Laceration</u> of urethra
  S37.39x- <u>Other</u> injury of urethra
S37.4- Injury of <u>ovary</u>
  S37.40- <u>Unspecified</u> injury of ovary
    S37.401- Unspecified injury of ovary, <u>unilateral</u>
    S37.402- Unspecified injury of ovary, <u>bilateral</u>
    S37.409- Unspecified injury of ovary, <u>unspecified</u>
  S37.42- <u>Contusion</u> of ovary
    S37.421- Contusion of ovary, <u>unilateral</u>
    S37.422- Contusion of ovary, <u>bilateral</u>
    S37.429- Contusion of ovary, <u>unspecified</u>
  S37.43- <u>Laceration</u> of ovary
    S37.431- Laceration of ovary, <u>unilateral</u>
    S37.432- Laceration of ovary, <u>bilateral</u>
    S37.439- Laceration of ovary, <u>unspecified</u>
  S37.49- <u>Other</u> injury of ovary
    S37.491- Other injury of ovary, <u>unilateral</u>
    S37.492- Other injury of ovary, <u>bilateral</u>
    S37.499- Other injury of ovary, <u>unspecified</u>
S37.5- Injury of <u>fallopian tube</u>
  S37.50- <u>Unspecified</u> injury of fallopian tube
    S37.501- Unspecified injury of fallopian tube, <u>unilateral</u>
    S37.502- Unspecified injury of fallopian tube, <u>bilateral</u>
    S37.509- Unspecified injury of fallopian tube, <u>unspecified</u>
  S37.51- <u>Primary blast</u> injury of fallopian tube
    Blast injury of fallopian tube NOS
    S37.511- Primary blast injury of fallopian tube, <u>unilateral</u>
    S37.512- Primary blast injury of fallopian tube, <u>bilateral</u>
    S37.519- Primary blast injury of fallopian tube, <u>unspecified</u>
  S37.52- <u>Contusion</u> of fallopian tube
    S37.521- Contusion of fallopian tube, <u>unilateral</u>
    S37.522- Contusion of fallopian tube, <u>bilateral</u>
    S37.529- Contusion of fallopian tube, <u>unspecified</u>
  S37.53- <u>Laceration</u> of fallopian tube
    S37.531- Laceration of fallopian tube, <u>unilateral</u>
    S37.532- Laceration of fallopian tube, <u>bilateral</u>
    S37.539- Laceration of fallopian tube, <u>unspecified</u>
  S37.59- <u>Other</u> injury of fallopian tube
    Secondary blast injury of fallopian tube
    S37.591- Other injury of fallopian tube, <u>unilateral</u>
    S37.592- Other injury of fallopian tube, <u>bilateral</u>
    S37.599- Other injury of fallopian tube, <u>unspecified</u>
S37.6- Injury of <u>uterus</u>
  Excludes 1: injury to gravid uterus (O9A.2-)
        injury to uterus during delivery (O71.-)
  S37.60x- <u>Unspecified</u> injury of uterus
  S37.62x- <u>Contusion</u> of uterus
  S37.63x- <u>Laceration</u> of uterus
  S37.69x- <u>Other</u> injury of uterus
S37.8- Injury of <u>other urinary and pelvic organs</u>
  S37.81- Injury of <u>adrenal gland</u>
    S37.812- <u>Contusion</u> of adrenal gland
    S37.813- <u>Laceration</u> of adrenal gland
    S37.818- <u>Other</u> injury of adrenal gland
    S37.819- <u>Unspecified</u> injury of adrenal gland
  S37.82- Injury of <u>prostate</u>
    S37.822- <u>Contusion</u> of prostate
    S37.823- <u>Laceration</u> of prostate
    S37.828- <u>Other</u> injury of prostate
    S37.829- <u>Unspecified</u> injury of prostate
  S37.89- Injury of other urinary and pelvic organ
    S37.892- <u>Contusion</u> of other urinary and pelvic organ
    S37.893- <u>Laceration</u> of other urinary and pelvic organ
    S37.898- <u>Other</u> injury of other urinary and pelvic organ
    S37.899- <u>Unspecified</u> injury of other urinary and pelvic organ
S37.9- Injury of <u>unspecified urinary and pelvic organ</u>
  S37.90x- <u>Unspecified</u> injury of unspecified urinary and pelvic organ
  S37.92x- <u>Contusion</u> of unspecified urinary and pelvic organ
  S37.93x- <u>Laceration</u> of unspecified urinary and pelvic organ
  S37.99x- <u>Other</u> injury of unspecified urinary and pelvic organ

S38- <u>Crushing injury</u> and <u>traumatic amputation</u> of <u>abdomen, lower back, pelvis and external genitals</u>
  Note: An amputation not identified as partial or complete should be coded to complete
  The appropriate 7th character is to be added to each code from category S38:
    A <u>Initial</u> encounter
    D <u>Subsequent</u> encounter
    S <u>Sequela</u>
S38.0- <u>Crushing</u> injury of <u>external genital organs</u>
  Use additional code for any associated injuries
  S38.00- Crushing injury of <u>unspecified</u> external genital organs
    S38.001- Crushing injury of <u>unspecified</u> external genital organs, <u>male</u>
    S38.002- Crushing injury of <u>unspecified</u> external genital organs, <u>female</u>
  S38.01x- Crushing injury of <u>penis</u>
  S38.02x- Crushing injury of <u>scrotum and testis</u>
  S38.03x- Crushing injury of <u>vulva</u>
S38.1xx- Crushing injury of <u>abdomen, lower back, and pelvis</u>
  Use additional code for all associated injuries, such as:
    Fracture of thoracic or lumbar spine and pelvis (S22.0-, S32.-)
    Injury to intra-abdominal organs (S36.-)
    Injury to urinary and pelvic organs (S37.-)
    Open wound of abdominal wall (S31.-)
    Spinal cord injury (S34.0, S34.1-)
    Excludes❷: crushing injury of external genital organs (S38.0-)
S38.2- <u>Traumatic amputation</u> of <u>external genital organs</u>
  S38.21- Traumatic amputation of <u>female external genital organs</u>
    Traumatic amputation of clitoris
    Traumatic amputation of labium (majus) (minus)
    Traumatic amputation of vulva
    S38.211- <u>Complete</u> traumatic amputation of female external genital organs
    S38.212- <u>Partial</u> traumatic amputation of female external genital organs
  S38.22- Traumatic amputation of <u>penis</u>
    S38.221- <u>Complete</u> traumatic amputation of penis
    S38.222- <u>Partial</u> traumatic amputation of penis
  S38.23- Traumatic amputation of <u>scrotum and testis</u>
    S38.231- <u>Complete</u> traumatic amputation of scrotum and testis
    S38.232- <u>Partial</u> traumatic amputation of scrotum and testis
S38.3xx- Transection (partial) of <u>abdomen</u>
S39- <u>Other and unspecified</u> injuries of <u>abdomen, lower back, pelvis and external genitals</u>
  Code also any associated open wound (S31.-)
  Excludes❷: sprain of joints and ligaments of lumbar spine and pelvis (S33.-)
  The appropriate 7th character is to be added to each code from category S39:
    A <u>Initial</u> encounter
    D <u>Subsequent</u> encounter
    S <u>Sequela</u>
S39.0- Injury of <u>muscle, fascia and tendon</u> of <u>abdomen, lower back and pelvis</u>
  S39.00- <u>Unspecified</u> injury of muscle, fascia and tendon of abdomen, lower back and pelvis
    S39.001- Unspecified injury of muscle, fascia and tendon of <u>abdomen</u>
    S39.002- Unspecified injury of muscle, fascia and tendon of <u>lower back</u>
    S39.003- Unspecified injury of muscle, fascia and tendon of <u>pelvis</u>
  S39.01- <u>Strain</u> of muscle, fascia and tendon of abdomen, lower back and pelvis
    S39.011- Strain of muscle, fascia and tendon of <u>abdomen</u>
    S39.012- Strain of muscle, fascia and tendon of <u>lower back</u>
    S39.013- Strain of muscle, fascia and tendon of <u>pelvis</u>
  S39.02- <u>Laceration</u> of muscle, fascia and tendon of abdomen, lower back and pelvis
    S39.021- Laceration of muscle, fascia and tendon of <u>abdomen</u>
    S39.022- Laceration of muscle, fascia and tendon of <u>lower back</u>
    S39.023- Laceration of muscle, fascia and tendon of <u>pelvis</u>
  S39.09- <u>Other injury</u> of muscle, fascia and tendon of abdomen, lower back and pelvis
    S39.091- Other injury of muscle, fascia and tendon of <u>abdomen</u>
    S39.092- Other injury of muscle, fascia and tendon of <u>lower back</u>
    S39.093- Other injury of muscle, fascia and tendon of <u>pelvis</u>

S37 - S41

Excludes 1: = NOT CODED HERE! (Do not code both)

Excludes❷: = Not Included Here

S39.8- <u>Other specified</u> injuries of abdomen, lower back, pelvis and external genitals
  S39.81x- Other specified injuries of <u>abdomen</u>
  S39.82x- Other specified injuries of <u>lower back</u>
  S39.83x- Other specified injuries of <u>pelvis</u>
  S39.84- Other specified injuries of <u>external genitals</u>
    S39.840- <u>Fracture</u> of <u>corpus cavernosum penis</u>
    S39.848- <u>Other</u> specified injuries of external genitals
S39.9- <u>Unspecified</u> injury of abdomen, lower back, pelvis and external genitals
  S39.91x- Unspecified injury of <u>abdomen</u>
  S39.92x- Unspecified injury of <u>lower back</u>
  S39.93x- Unspecified injury of <u>pelvis</u>
  S39.94x- Unspecified injury of <u>external genitals</u>

Injuries to the shoulder and upper arm (S40-S49)

Includes: Injuries of axilla
           Injuries of scapular region
Excludes❷: burns and corrosions (T20-T32)
           frostbite (T33-T34)
           injuries of elbow (S50-S59)
           insect bite or sting, venomous (T63.4)

S40- Superficial injury of <u>shoulder and upper arm</u>
  The appropriate 7th character is to be added to each code from category S40:
    A <u>Initial</u> encounter
    D <u>Subsequent</u> encounter
    S <u>Sequela</u>
  S40.0- <u>Contusion</u> of shoulder and upper arm
    S40.01- <u>Contusion</u> of <u>shoulder</u>
      S40.011- Contusion of <u>right</u> shoulder
      S40.012- Contusion of <u>left</u> shoulder
      S40.019- Contusion of <u>unspecified</u> shoulder
    S40.02- Contusion of <u>upper arm</u>
      S40.021- Contusion of <u>right</u> upper arm
      S40.022- Contusion of <u>left</u> upper arm
      S40.029- Contusion of <u>unspecified</u> upper arm
  S40.2- Other superficial injuries of shoulder
    S40.21- <u>Abrasion</u> of <u>shoulder</u>
      S40.211- Abrasion of <u>right</u> shoulder
      S40.212- Abrasion of <u>left</u> shoulder
      S40.219- Abrasion of <u>unspecified</u> shoulder
    S40.22- <u>Blister</u> (nonthermal) of <u>shoulder</u>
      S40.221- Blister (nonthermal) of <u>right</u> shoulder
      S40.222- Blister (nonthermal) of <u>left</u> shoulder
      S40.229- Blister (nonthermal) of <u>unspecified</u> shoulder
    S40.24- <u>External constriction</u> of <u>shoulder</u>
      S40.241- External constriction of <u>right</u> shoulder
      S40.242- External constriction of <u>left</u> shoulder
      S40.249- External constriction of <u>unspecified</u> shoulder
    S40.25- <u>Superficial foreign body</u> of <u>shoulder</u>
      Splinter in the shoulder
      S40.251- Superficial foreign body of <u>right</u> shoulder
      S40.252- Superficial foreign body of <u>left</u> shoulder
      S40.259- Superficial foreign body of <u>unspecified</u> shoulder
    S40.26- <u>Insect bite (nonvenomous)</u> of <u>shoulder</u>
      S40.261- Insect bite (nonvenomous) of <u>right</u> shoulder
      S40.262- Insect bite (nonvenomous) of <u>left</u> shoulder
      S40.269- Insect bite (nonvenomous) of <u>unspecified</u> shoulder
    S40.27- <u>Other superficial bite</u> of <u>shoulder</u>
      Excludes 1: open bite of shoulder (S41.05)
      S40.271- Other superficial bite of <u>right</u> shoulder
      S40.272- Other superficial bite of <u>left</u> shoulder
      S40.279- Other superficial bite of <u>unspecified</u> shoulder
  S40.8- Other superficial injuries of <u>upper arm</u>
    S40.81- <u>Abrasion</u> of <u>upper arm</u>
      S40.811- Abrasion of <u>right</u> upper arm
      S40.812- Abrasion of <u>left</u> upper arm
      S40.819- Abrasion of <u>unspecified</u> upper arm
    S40.82- <u>Blister</u> (nonthermal) of <u>upper arm</u>
      S40.821- Blister (nonthermal) of <u>right</u> upper arm
      S40.822- Blister (nonthermal) of <u>left</u> upper arm
      S40.829- Blister (nonthermal) of <u>unspecified</u> upper arm

    S40.84- <u>External constriction</u> of <u>upper arm</u>
      S40.841- External constriction of <u>right</u> upper arm
      S40.842- External constriction of <u>left</u> upper arm
      S40.849- External constriction of <u>unspecified</u> upper arm
    S40.85- <u>Superficial foreign body</u> of <u>upper arm</u>
      Splinter in the upper arm
      S40.851- Superficial foreign body of <u>right</u> upper arm
      S40.852- Superficial foreign body of <u>left</u> upper arm
      S40.859- Superficial foreign body of <u>unspecified</u> upper arm
    S40.86- <u>Insect bite (nonvenomous)</u> of <u>upper arm</u>
      S40.861- Insect bite (nonvenomous) of <u>right</u> upper arm
      S40.862- Insect bite (nonvenomous) of <u>left</u> upper arm
      S40.869- Insect bite (nonvenomous) of <u>unspecified</u> upper arm
    S40.87- <u>Other superficial bite</u> of <u>upper arm</u>
      Excludes 1: open bite of upper arm (S41.14)
      Excludes❷: other superficial bite of shoulder (S40.27-)
      S40.871- Other superficial bite of <u>right</u> upper arm
      S40.872- Other superficial bite of <u>left</u> upper arm
      S40.879- Other superficial bite of <u>unspecified</u> upper arm
  S40.9- Unspecified superficial injury of shoulder and upper arm
    S40.91- <u>Unspecified superficial injury</u> of <u>shoulder</u>
      S40.911- Unspecified superficial injury of <u>right</u> shoulder
      S40.912- Unspecified superficial injury of <u>left</u> shoulder
      S40.919- Unspecified superficial injury of <u>unspecified</u> shoulder
    S40.92- <u>Unspecified superficial injury</u> of <u>upper arm</u>
      S40.921- Unspecified superficial injury of <u>right</u> upper arm
      S40.922- Unspecified superficial injury of <u>left</u> upper arm
      S40.929- Unspecified superficial injury of <u>unspecified</u> upper arm

S41- Open wound of <u>shoulder and upper arm</u>
  Code also any associated wound infection
  Excludes 1: traumatic amputation of shoulder and upper arm (S48.-)
  Excludes❷: open fracture of shoulder and upper arm (S42.- with 7th character B or C)
  The appropriate 7th character is to be added to each code from category S41:
    A <u>Initial</u> encounter
    D <u>Subsequent</u> encounter
    S <u>Sequela</u>
  S41.0- <u>Open wound</u> of <u>shoulder</u>
    S41.00- <u>Unspecified</u> open wound of <u>shoulder</u>
      S41.001- Unspecified open wound of <u>right</u> shoulder
      S41.002- Unspecified open wound of <u>left</u> shoulder
      S41.009- Unspecified open wound of <u>unspecified</u> shoulder
    S41.01- <u>Laceration</u> <u>without</u> foreign body of <u>shoulder</u>
      S41.011- Laceration <u>without</u> foreign body of <u>right</u> shoulder
      S41.012- Laceration <u>without</u> foreign body of <u>left</u> shoulder
      S41.019- Laceration <u>without</u> foreign body of <u>unspecified</u> shoulder
    S41.02- <u>Laceration</u> <u>with foreign body</u> of <u>shoulder</u>
      S41.021- Laceration <u>with foreign body</u> of <u>right</u> shoulder
      S41.022- Laceration <u>with foreign body</u> of <u>left</u> shoulder
      S41.029- Laceration <u>with foreign body</u> of <u>unspecified</u> shoulder
    S41.03- <u>Puncture</u> wound <u>without</u> foreign body of <u>shoulder</u>
      S41.031- Puncture wound <u>without</u> foreign body of <u>right</u> shoulder
      S41.032- Puncture wound <u>without</u> foreign body of <u>left</u> shoulder
      S41.039- Puncture wound <u>without</u> foreign body of <u>unspecified</u> shoulder
    S41.04- <u>Puncture</u> wound <u>with foreign body</u> of shoulder
      S41.041- Puncture wound <u>with foreign body</u> of <u>right</u> shoulder
      S41.042- Puncture wound <u>with foreign body</u> of <u>left</u> shoulder
      S41.049- Puncture wound <u>with foreign body</u> of <u>unspecified</u> shoulder
    S41.05- Open bite of <u>shoulder</u>
      Bite of shoulder NOS
      Excludes 1: superficial bite of shoulder (S40.27)
      S41.051- Open bite of <u>right</u> shoulder
      S41.052- Open bite of <u>left</u> shoulder
      S41.059- Open bite of <u>unspecified</u> shoulder

© 2013 Channel Publishing, Ltd.

S 3 7 - S 4 1

S41.1- Open wound of upper arm
  S41.10- Unspecified open wound of upper arm
    S41.101- Unspecified open wound of right upper arm
    S41.102- Unspecified open wound of left upper arm
    S41.109- Unspecified open wound of unspecified upper arm
  S41.11- Laceration without foreign body of upper arm
    S41.111- Laceration without foreign body of right upper arm
    S41.112- Laceration without foreign body of left upper arm
    S41.119- Laceration without foreign body of unspecified upper arm
  S41.12- Laceration with foreign body of upper arm
    S41.121- Laceration with foreign body of right upper arm
    S41.122- Laceration with foreign body of left upper arm
    S41.129- Laceration with foreign body of unspecified upper arm
  S41.13- Puncture wound without foreign body of upper arm
    S41.131- Puncture wound without foreign body of right upper arm
    S41.132- Puncture wound without foreign body of left upper arm
    S41.139- Puncture wound without foreign body of unspecified upper arm
  S41.14- Puncture wound with foreign body of upper arm
    S41.141- Puncture wound with foreign body of right upper arm
    S41.142- Puncture wound with foreign body of left upper arm
    S41.149- Puncture wound with foreign body of unspecified upper arm
  S41.15- Open bite of upper arm
    Bite of upper arm NOS
    Excludes 1: superficial bite of upper arm (S40.87)
    S41.151- Open bite of right upper arm
    S41.152- Open bite of left upper arm
    S41.159- Open bite of unspecified upper arm

S42- Fracture of shoulder and upper arm
  Note: A fracture not indicated as displaced or nondisplaced should be coded to displaced
  Note: A fracture not indicated as open or closed should be coded to closed
  Excludes 1: traumatic amputation of shoulder and upper arm (S48.-)
  The appropriate 7th character is to be added to all codes from category S42:
  A Initial encounter for closed fracture
  B Initial encounter for open fracture
  D Subsequent encounter for fracture with routine healing
  G Subsequent encounter for fracture with delayed healing
  K Subsequent encounter for fracture with nonunion
  P Subsequent encounter for fracture with malunion
  S Sequela
  S42.0- Fracture of clavicle
    S42.00- Fracture of unspecified part of clavicle
      S42.001- Fracture of unspecified part of right clavicle
      S42.002- Fracture of unspecified part of left clavicle
      S42.009- Fracture of unspecified part of unspecified clavicle
    S42.01- Fracture of sternal end of clavicle
      S42.011- Anterior displaced fracture of sternal end of right clavicle
      S42.012- Anterior displaced fracture of sternal end of left clavicle
      S42.013- Anterior displaced fracture of sternal end of unspecified clavicle
        Displaced fracture of sternal end of clavicle NOS
      S42.014- Posterior displaced fracture of sternal end of right clavicle
      S42.015- Posterior displaced fracture of sternal end of left clavicle
      S42.016- Posterior displaced fracture of sternal end of unspecified clavicle
      S42.017- Nondisplaced fracture of sternal end of right clavicle
      S42.018- Nondisplaced fracture of sternal end of left clavicle
      S42.019- Nondisplaced fracture of sternal end of unspecified clavicle
    S42.02- Fracture of shaft of clavicle
      S42.021- Displaced fracture of shaft of right clavicle
      S42.022- Displaced fracture of shaft of left clavicle
      S42.023- Displaced fracture of shaft of unspecified clavicle
      S42.024- Nondisplaced fracture of shaft of right clavicle
      S42.025- Nondisplaced fracture of shaft of left clavicle
      S42.026- Nondisplaced fracture of shaft of unspecified clavicle

S42.03- Fracture of lateral end of clavicle
    Fracture of acromial end of clavicle
  S42.031- Displaced fracture of lateral end of right clavicle
  S42.032- Displaced fracture of lateral end of left clavicle
  S42.033- Displaced fracture of lateral end of unspecified clavicle
  S42.034- Nondisplaced fracture of lateral end of right clavicle
  S42.035- Nondisplaced fracture of lateral end of left clavicle
  S42.036- Nondisplaced fracture of lateral end of unspecified clavicle

S42.1- Fracture of scapula
  S42.10- Fracture of unspecified part of scapula
    S42.101- Fracture of unspecified part of scapula, right shoulder
    S42.102- Fracture of unspecified part of scapula, left shoulder
    S42.109- Fracture of unspecified part of scapula, unspecified shoulder
  S42.11- Fracture of body of scapula
    S42.111- Displaced fracture of body of scapula, right shoulder
    S42.112- Displaced fracture of body of scapula, left shoulder
    S42.113- Displaced fracture of body of scapula, unspecified shoulder
    S42.114- Nondisplaced fracture of body of scapula, right shoulder
    S42.115- Nondisplaced fracture of body of scapula, left shoulder
    S42.116- Nondisplaced fracture of body of scapula, unspecified shoulder
  S42.12- Fracture of acromial process
    S42.121- Displaced fracture of acromial process, right shoulder
    S42.122- Displaced fracture of acromial process, left shoulder
    S42.123- Displaced fracture of acromial process, unspecified shoulder
    S42.124- Nondisplaced fracture of acromial process, right shoulder
    S42.125- Nondisplaced fracture of acromial process, left shoulder
    S42.126- Nondisplaced fracture of acromial process, unspecified shoulder
  S42.13- Fracture of coracoid process
    S42.131- Displaced fracture of coracoid process, right shoulder
    S42.132- Displaced fracture of coracoid process, left shoulder
    S42.133- Displaced fracture of coracoid process, unspecified shoulder
    S42.134- Nondisplaced fracture of coracoid process, right shoulder
    S42.135- Nondisplaced fracture of coracoid process, left shoulder
    S42.136- Nondisplaced fracture of coracoid process, unspecified shoulder
  S42.14- Fracture of glenoid cavity of scapula
    S42.141- Displaced fracture of glenoid cavity of scapula, right shoulder
    S42.142- Displaced fracture of glenoid cavity of scapula, left shoulder
    S42.143- Displaced fracture of glenoid cavity of scapula, unspecified shoulder
    S42.144- Nondisplaced fracture of glenoid cavity of scapula, right shoulder
    S42.145- Nondisplaced fracture of glenoid cavity of scapula, left shoulder
    S42.146- Nondisplaced fracture of glenoid cavity of scapula, unspecified shoulder
  S42.15- Fracture of neck of scapula
    S42.151- Displaced fracture of neck of scapula, right shoulder
    S42.152- Displaced fracture of neck of scapula, left shoulder
    S42.153- Displaced fracture of neck of scapula, unspecified shoulder
    S42.154- Nondisplaced fracture of neck of scapula, right shoulder
    S42.155- Nondisplaced fracture of neck of scapula, left shoulder
    S42.156- Nondisplaced fracture of neck of scapula, unspecified shoulder
  S42.19- Fracture of other part of scapula
    S42.191- Fracture of other part of scapula, right shoulder
    S42.192- Fracture of other part of scapula, left shoulder
    S42.199- Fracture of other part of scapula, unspecified shoulder

S42.2-   Fracture of upper end of humerus
Fracture of proximal end of humerus
Excludes❷: *fracture of shaft of humerus (S42.3-)*
physeal fracture of upper end of humerus (S49.0-)

S42.20-   Unspecified fracture of upper end of humerus
S42.201-   Unspecified fracture of upper end of right humerus
S42.202-   Unspecified fracture of upper end of left humerus
S42.209-   Unspecified fracture of upper end of unspecified humerus

S42.21-   Unspecified fracture of surgical neck of humerus
Fracture of neck of humerus NOS
S42.211-   Unspecified displaced fracture of surgical neck of right humerus
S42.212-   Unspecified displaced fracture of surgical neck of left humerus
S42.213-   Unspecified displaced fracture of surgical neck of unspecified humerus
S42.214-   Unspecified nondisplaced fracture of surgical neck of right humerus
S42.215-   Unspecified nondisplaced fracture of surgical neck of left humerus
S42.216-   Unspecified nondisplaced fracture of surgical neck of unspecified humerus

S42.22-   2-part fracture of surgical neck of humerus
S42.221-   2-part displaced fracture of surgical neck of right humerus
S42.222-   2-part displaced fracture of surgical neck of left humerus
S42.223-   2-part displaced fracture of surgical neck of unspecified humerus
S42.224-   2-part nondisplaced fracture of surgical neck of right humerus
S42.225-   2-part nondisplaced fracture of surgical neck of left humerus
S42.226-   2-part nondisplaced fracture of surgical neck of unspecified humerus

S42.23-   3-part fracture of surgical neck of humerus
S42.231-   3-part fracture of surgical neck of right humerus
S42.232-   3-part fracture of surgical neck of left humerus
S42.239-   3-part fracture of surgical neck of unspecified humerus

S42.24-   4-part fracture of surgical neck of humerus
S42.241-   4-part fracture of surgical neck of right humerus
S42.242-   4-part fracture of surgical neck of left humerus
S42.249-   4-part fracture of surgical neck of unspecified humerus

S42.25-   Fracture of greater tuberosity of humerus
S42.251-   Displaced fracture of greater tuberosity of right humerus
S42.252-   Displaced fracture of greater tuberosity of left humerus
S42.253-   Displaced fracture of greater tuberosity of unspecified humerus
S42.254-   Nondisplaced fracture of greater tuberosity of right humerus
S42.255-   Nondisplaced fracture of greater tuberosity of left humerus
S42.256-   Nondisplaced fracture of greater tuberosity of unspecified humerus

S42.26-   Fracture of lesser tuberosity of humerus
S42.261-   Displaced fracture of lesser tuberosity of right humerus
S42.262-   Displaced fracture of lesser tuberosity of left humerus
S42.263-   Displaced fracture of lesser tuberosity of unspecified humerus
S42.264-   Nondisplaced fracture of lesser tuberosity of right humerus
S42.265-   Nondisplaced fracture of lesser tuberosity of left humerus
S42.266-   Nondisplaced fracture of lesser tuberosity of unspecified humerus

S42.27-   Torus fracture of upper end of humerus
The appropriate 7th character is to be added to all codes in subcategory S42.27:
A   Initial encounter for closed fracture
D   Subsequent encounter for fracture with routine healing
G   Subsequent encounter for fracture with delayed healing
K   Subsequent encounter for fracture with nonunion
P   Subsequent encounter for fracture with malunion
S   Sequela
S42.271-   Torus fracture of upper end of right humerus
S42.272-   Torus fracture of upper end of left humerus
S42.279-   Torus fracture of upper end of unspecified humerus

S42.29-   Other fracture of upper end of humerus
Fracture of anatomical neck of humerus
Fracture of articular head of humerus
S42.291-   Other displaced fracture of upper end of right humerus
S42.292-   Other displaced fracture of upper end of left humerus
S42.293-   Other displaced fracture of upper end of unspecified humerus
S42.294-   Other nondisplaced fracture of upper end of right humerus
S42.295-   Other nondisplaced fracture of upper end of left humerus
S42.296-   Other nondisplaced fracture of upper end of unspecified humerus

S42.3-   Fracture of shaft of humerus
Fracture of humerus NOS
Fracture of upper arm NOS
Excludes❷: *physeal fractures of upper end of humerus (S49.0-)*
physeal fractures of lower end of humerus (S49.1-)

S42.30-   Unspecified fracture of shaft of humerus
S42.301-   Unspecified fracture of shaft of humerus, right arm
S42.302-   Unspecified fracture of shaft of humerus, left arm
S42.309-   Unspecified fracture of shaft of humerus, unspecified arm

S42.31-   Greenstick fracture of shaft of humerus
The appropriate 7th character is to be added to all codes in subcategory S42.31:
A   Initial encounter for closed fracture
D   Subsequent encounter for fracture with routine healing
G   Subsequent encounter for fracture with delayed healing
K   Subsequent encounter for fracture with nonunion
P   Subsequent encounter for fracture with malunion
S   Sequela
S42.311-   Greenstick fracture of shaft of humerus, right arm
S42.312-   Greenstick fracture of shaft of humerus, left arm
S42.319-   Greenstick fracture of shaft of humerus, unspecified arm

S42.32-   Transverse fracture of shaft of humerus
S42.321-   Displaced transverse fracture of shaft of humerus, right arm
S42.322-   Displaced transverse fracture of shaft of humerus, left arm
S42.323-   Displaced transverse fracture of shaft of humerus, unspecified arm
S42.324-   Nondisplaced transverse fracture of shaft of humerus, right arm
S42.325-   Nondisplaced transverse fracture of shaft of humerus, left arm
S42.326-   Nondisplaced transverse fracture of shaft of humerus, unspecified arm

S42.33-   Oblique fracture of shaft of humerus
S42.331-   Displaced oblique fracture of shaft of humerus, right arm
S42.332-   Displaced oblique fracture of shaft of humerus, left arm
S42.333-   Displaced oblique fracture of shaft of humerus, unspecified arm
S42.334-   Nondisplaced oblique fracture of shaft of humerus, right arm
S42.335-   Nondisplaced oblique fracture of shaft of humerus, left arm
S42.336-   Nondisplaced oblique fracture of shaft of humerus, unspecified arm

S 4 1 – S 4 2

S42.34- <u>Spiral</u> fracture of <u>shaft</u> of <u>humerus</u>
- S42.341- <u>Displaced</u> spiral fracture of shaft of humerus, <u>right</u> arm
- S42.342- <u>Displaced</u> spiral fracture of shaft of humerus, <u>left</u> arm
- S42.343- <u>Displaced</u> spiral fracture of shaft of humerus, <u>unspecified</u> arm
- S42.344- <u>Nondisplaced</u> spiral fracture of shaft of humerus, <u>right</u> arm
- S42.345- <u>Nondisplaced</u> spiral fracture of shaft of humerus, <u>left</u> arm
- S42.346- <u>Nondisplaced</u> spiral fracture of shaft of humerus, <u>unspecified</u> arm

S42.35- <u>Comminuted</u> fracture of <u>shaft</u> of <u>humerus</u>
- S42.351- <u>Displaced</u> comminuted fracture of shaft of humerus, <u>right</u> arm
- S42.352- <u>Displaced</u> comminuted fracture of shaft of humerus, <u>left</u> arm
- S42.353- <u>Displaced</u> comminuted fracture of shaft of humerus, <u>unspecified</u> arm
- S42.354- <u>Nondisplaced</u> comminuted fracture of shaft of humerus, <u>right</u> arm
- S42.355- <u>Nondisplaced</u> comminuted fracture of shaft of humerus, <u>left</u> arm
- S42.356- <u>Nondisplaced</u> comminuted fracture of shaft of humerus, <u>unspecified</u> arm

S42.36- <u>Segmental</u> fracture of <u>shaft</u> of <u>humerus</u>
- S42.361- <u>Displaced</u> segmental fracture of shaft of humerus, <u>right</u> arm
- S42.362- <u>Displaced</u> segmental fracture of shaft of humerus, <u>left</u> arm
- S42.363- <u>Displaced</u> segmental fracture of shaft of humerus, <u>unspecified</u> arm
- S42.364- <u>Nondisplaced</u> segmental fracture of shaft of humerus, <u>right</u> arm
- S42.365- <u>Nondisplaced</u> segmental fracture of shaft of humerus, <u>left</u> arm
- S42.366- <u>Nondisplaced</u> segmental fracture of shaft of humerus, <u>unspecified</u> arm

S42.39- <u>Other</u> fracture of <u>shaft</u> of <u>humerus</u>
- S42.391- Other fracture of shaft of <u>right</u> humerus
- S42.392- Other fracture of shaft of <u>left</u> humerus
- S42.399- Other fracture of shaft of <u>unspecified</u> humerus

S42.4- Fracture of <u>lower end</u> of <u>humerus</u>
Fracture of distal end of humerus
Excludes❷: fracture of shaft of humerus (S42.3-)
physeal fracture of lower end of humerus (S49.1-)

S42.40- <u>Unspecified</u> fracture of <u>lower end</u> of <u>humerus</u>
Fracture of elbow NOS
- S42.401- Unspecified fracture of lower end of <u>right</u> humerus
- S42.402- Unspecified fracture of lower end of <u>left</u> humerus
- S42.409- Unspecified fracture of lower end of <u>unspecified</u> humerus

S42.41- Simple supracondylar fracture <u>without</u> intercondylar fracture of humerus
- S42.411- <u>Displaced</u> simple supracondylar fracture <u>without</u> intercondylar fracture of <u>right</u> humerus
- S42.412- <u>Displaced</u> simple supracondylar fracture <u>without</u> intercondylar fracture of <u>left</u> humerus
- S42.413- <u>Displaced</u> simple supracondylar fracture <u>without</u> intercondylar fracture of <u>unspecified</u> humerus
- S42.414- <u>Nondisplaced</u> simple supracondylar fracture <u>without</u> intercondylar fracture of <u>right</u> humerus
- S42.415- <u>Nondisplaced</u> simple supracondylar fracture <u>without</u> intercondylar fracture of <u>left</u> humerus
- S42.416- <u>Nondisplaced</u> simple supracondylar fracture <u>without</u> intercondylar fracture of <u>unspecified</u> humerus

S42.42- <u>Comminuted supracondylar</u> fracture <u>without</u> intercondylar fracture of humerus
- S42.421- <u>Displaced</u> comminuted supracondylar fracture <u>without</u> intercondylar fracture of <u>right</u> humerus
- S42.422- <u>Displaced</u> comminuted supracondylar fracture <u>without</u> intercondylar fracture of <u>left</u> humerus
- S42.423- <u>Displaced</u> comminuted supracondylar fracture <u>without</u> intercondylar fracture of <u>unspecified</u> humerus
- S42.424- <u>Nondisplaced</u> comminuted supracondylar fracture <u>without</u> intercondylar fracture of <u>right</u> humerus
- S42.425- <u>Nondisplaced</u> comminuted supracondylar fracture <u>without</u> intercondylar fracture of <u>left</u> humerus
- S42.426- <u>Nondisplaced</u> comminuted supracondylar fracture <u>without</u> intercondylar fracture of <u>unspecified</u> humerus

S42.43- Fracture (avulsion) of <u>lateral epicondyle</u> of <u>humerus</u>
- S42.431- <u>Displaced</u> fracture (avulsion) of lateral epicondyle of <u>right</u> humerus
- S42.432- <u>Displaced</u> fracture (avulsion) of lateral epicondyle of <u>left</u> humerus
- S42.433- <u>Displaced</u> fracture (avulsion) of lateral epicondyle of <u>unspecified</u> humerus
- S42.434- <u>Nondisplaced</u> fracture (avulsion) of lateral epicondyle of <u>right</u> humerus
- S42.435- <u>Nondisplaced</u> fracture (avulsion) of lateral epicondyle of <u>left</u> humerus
- S42.436- <u>Nondisplaced</u> fracture (avulsion) of lateral epicondyle of <u>unspecified</u> humerus

S42.44- Fracture (avulsion) of <u>medial epicondyle</u> of humerus
- S42.441- <u>Displaced</u> fracture (avulsion) of medial epicondyle of <u>right</u> humerus
- S42.442- <u>Displaced</u> fracture (avulsion) of medial epicondyle of <u>left</u> humerus
- S42.443- <u>Displaced</u> fracture (avulsion) of medial epicondyle of <u>unspecified</u> humerus
- S42.444- <u>Nondisplaced</u> fracture (avulsion) of medial epicondyle of <u>right</u> humerus
- S42.445- <u>Nondisplaced</u> fracture (avulsion) of medial epicondyle of <u>left</u> humerus
- S42.446- <u>Nondisplaced</u> fracture (avulsion) of medial epicondyle of <u>unspecified</u> humerus
- S42.447- <u>Incarcerated</u> fracture (avulsion) of medial epicondyle of <u>right</u> humerus
- S42.448- <u>Incarcerated</u> fracture (avulsion) of medial epicondyle of <u>left</u> humerus
- S42.449- <u>Incarcerated</u> fracture (avulsion) of medial epicondyle of <u>unspecified</u> humerus

S42.45- Fracture of <u>lateral condyle</u> of <u>humerus</u>
Fracture of capitellum of humerus
- S42.451- <u>Displaced</u> fracture of lateral condyle of <u>right</u> humerus
- S42.452- <u>Displaced</u> fracture of lateral condyle of <u>left</u> humerus
- S42.453- <u>Displaced</u> fracture of lateral condyle of <u>unspecified</u> humerus
- S42.454- <u>Nondisplaced</u> fracture of lateral condyle of <u>right</u> humerus
- S42.455- <u>Nondisplaced</u> fracture of lateral condyle of <u>left</u> humerus
- S42.456- <u>Nondisplaced</u> fracture of lateral condyle of <u>unspecified</u> humerus

S42.46- Fracture of <u>medial condyle</u> of <u>humerus</u>
Trochlea fracture of humerus
- S42.461- <u>Displaced</u> fracture of medial condyle of <u>right</u> humerus
- S42.462- <u>Displaced</u> fracture of medial condyle of <u>left</u> humerus
- S42.463- <u>Displaced</u> fracture of medial condyle of <u>unspecified</u> humerus
- S42.464- <u>Nondisplaced</u> fracture of medial condyle of <u>right</u> humerus
- S42.465- <u>Nondisplaced</u> fracture of medial condyle of <u>left</u> humerus
- S42.466- <u>Nondisplaced</u> fracture of medial condyle of <u>unspecified</u> humerus

S42.47- <u>Transcondylar</u> fracture of <u>humerus</u>
- S42.471- <u>Displaced</u> transcondylar fracture of <u>right</u> humerus
- S42.472- <u>Displaced</u> transcondylar fracture of <u>left</u> humerus
- S42.473- <u>Displaced</u> transcondylar fracture of <u>unspecified</u> humerus
- S42.474- <u>Nondisplaced</u> transcondylar fracture of <u>right</u> humerus
- S42.475- <u>Nondisplaced</u> transcondylar fracture of <u>left</u> humerus
- S42.476- <u>Nondisplaced</u> transcondylar fracture of <u>unspecified</u> humerus

S42.48- <u>Torus</u> fracture of <u>lower end</u> of <u>humerus</u>

The appropriate 7th character is to be added to all codes in subcategory S42.48:
- A   <u>Initial</u> encounter for <u>closed</u> fracture
- D   <u>Subsequent</u> encounter for fracture <u>with routine healing</u>
- G   <u>Subsequent</u> encounter for fracture <u>with delayed healing</u>
- K   <u>Subsequent</u> encounter for fracture <u>with nonunion</u>
- P   <u>Subsequent</u> encounter for fracture <u>with malunion</u>
- S   Sequela

- S42.481- Torus fracture of lower end of <u>right</u> humerus
- S42.482- Torus fracture of lower end of <u>left</u> humerus
- S42.489- Torus fracture of lower end of <u>unspecified</u> humerus

S
4
2
–
S
4
3

S42.49- Other fracture of lower end of humerus
- **S42.491-** Other displaced fracture of lower end of right humerus
- **S42.492-** Other displaced fracture of lower end of left humerus
- **S42.493-** Other displaced fracture of lower end of unspecified humerus
- **S42.494-** Other nondisplaced fracture of lower end of right humerus
- **S42.495-** Other nondisplaced fracture of lower end of left humerus
- **S42.496-** Other nondisplaced fracture of lower end of unspecified humerus

S42.9- Fracture of shoulder girdle, part unspecified
Fracture of shoulder NOS
- **S42.90x-** Fracture of unspecified shoulder girdle, part unspecified
- **S42.91x-** Fracture of right shoulder girdle, part unspecified
- **S42.92x-** Fracture of left shoulder girdle, part unspecified

S43- Dislocation and sprain of joints and ligaments of shoulder girdle
Includes: Avulsion of joint or ligament of shoulder girdle
Laceration of cartilage, joint or ligament of shoulder girdle
Sprain of cartilage, joint or ligament of shoulder girdle
Traumatic hemarthrosis of joint or ligament of shoulder girdle
Traumatic rupture of joint or ligament of shoulder girdle
Traumatic subluxation of joint or ligament of shoulder girdle
Traumatic tear of joint or ligament of shoulder girdle
Code also any associated open wound
Excludes❷: strain of muscle, fascia and tendon of shoulder and upper arm (S46.-)

The appropriate 7th character is to be added to each code from category S43:
A Initial encounter
D Subsequent encounter
S Sequela

S43.0- Subluxation and dislocation of shoulder joint
Dislocation of glenohumeral joint
Subluxation of glenohumeral joint
- **S43.00-** Unspecified subluxation and dislocation of shoulder joint
Dislocation of humerus NOS
Subluxation of humerus NOS
  - **S43.001-** Unspecified subluxation of right shoulder joint
  - **S43.002-** Unspecified subluxation of left shoulder joint
  - **S43.003-** Unspecified subluxation of unspecified shoulder joint
  - **S43.004-** Unspecified dislocation of right shoulder joint
  - **S43.005-** Unspecified dislocation of left shoulder joint
  - **S43.006-** Unspecified dislocation of unspecified shoulder joint
- **S43.01-** Anterior subluxation and dislocation of humerus
  - **S43.011-** Anterior subluxation of right humerus
  - **S43.012-** Anterior subluxation of left humerus
  - **S43.013-** Anterior subluxation of unspecified humerus
  - **S43.014-** Anterior dislocation of right humerus
  - **S43.015-** Anterior dislocation of left humerus
  - **S43.016-** Anterior dislocation of unspecified humerus
- **S43.02-** Posterior subluxation and dislocation of humerus
  - **S43.021-** Posterior subluxation of right humerus
  - **S43.022-** Posterior subluxation of left humerus
  - **S43.023-** Posterior subluxation of unspecified humerus
  - **S43.024-** Posterior dislocation of right humerus
  - **S43.025-** Posterior dislocation of left humerus
  - **S43.026-** Posterior dislocation of unspecified humerus
- **S43.03-** Inferior subluxation and dislocation of humerus
  - **S43.031-** Inferior subluxation of right humerus
  - **S43.032-** Inferior subluxation of left humerus
  - **S43.033-** Inferior subluxation of unspecified humerus
  - **S43.034-** Inferior dislocation of right humerus
  - **S43.035-** Inferior dislocation of left humerus
  - **S43.036-** Inferior dislocation of unspecified humerus
- **S43.08-** Other subluxation and dislocation of shoulder joint
  - **S43.081-** Other subluxation of right shoulder joint
  - **S43.082-** Other subluxation of left shoulder joint
  - **S43.083-** Other subluxation of unspecified shoulder joint
  - **S43.084-** Other dislocation of right shoulder joint
  - **S43.085-** Other dislocation of left shoulder joint
  - **S43.086-** Other dislocation of unspecified shoulder joint

S43.1- Subluxation and dislocation of acromioclavicular joint
- **S43.10-** Unspecified dislocation of acromioclavicular joint
  - **S43.101-** Unspecified dislocation of right acromioclavicular joint
  - **S43.102-** Unspecified dislocation of left acromioclavicular joint
  - **S43.109-** Unspecified dislocation of unspecified acromioclavicular joint
- **S43.11-** Subluxation of acromioclavicular joint
  - **S43.111-** Subluxation of right acromioclavicular joint
  - **S43.112-** Subluxation of left acromioclavicular joint
  - **S43.119-** Subluxation of unspecified acromioclavicular joint
- **S43.12-** Dislocation of acromioclavicular joint, 100%-200% displacement
  - **S43.121-** Dislocation of right acromioclavicular joint, 100%-200% displacement
  - **S43.122-** Dislocation of left acromioclavicular joint, 100%-200% displacement
  - **S43.129-** Dislocation of unspecified acromioclavicular joint, 100%-200% displacement
- **S43.13-** Dislocation of acromioclavicular joint, greater than 200% displacement
  - **S43.131-** Dislocation of right acromioclavicular joint, greater than 200% displacement
  - **S43.132-** Dislocation of left acromioclavicular joint, greater than 200% displacement
  - **S43.139-** Dislocation of unspecified acromioclavicular joint, greater than 200% displacement
- **S43.14-** Inferior dislocation of acromioclavicular joint
  - **S43.141-** Inferior dislocation of right acromioclavicular joint
  - **S43.142-** Inferior dislocation of left acromioclavicular joint
  - **S43.149-** Inferior dislocation of unspecified acromioclavicular joint
- **S43.15-** Posterior dislocation of acromioclavicular joint
  - **S43.151-** Posterior dislocation of right acromioclavicular joint
  - **S43.152-** Posterior dislocation of left acromioclavicular joint
  - **S43.159-** Posterior dislocation of unspecified acromioclavicular joint

S43.2- Subluxation and dislocation of sternoclavicular joint
- **S43.20-** Unspecified subluxation and dislocation of sternoclavicular joint
  - **S43.201-** Unspecified subluxation of right sternoclavicular joint
  - **S43.202-** Unspecified subluxation of left sternoclavicular joint
  - **S43.203-** Unspecified subluxation of unspecified sternoclavicular joint
  - **S43.204-** Unspecified dislocation of right sternoclavicular joint
  - **S43.205-** Unspecified dislocation of left sternoclavicular joint
  - **S43.206-** Unspecified dislocation of unspecified sternoclavicular joint
- **S43.21-** Anterior subluxation and dislocation of sternoclavicular joint
  - **S43.211-** Anterior subluxation of right sternoclavicular joint
  - **S43.212-** Anterior subluxation of left sternoclavicular joint
  - **S43.213-** Anterior subluxation of unspecified sternoclavicular joint
  - **S43.214-** Anterior dislocation of right sternoclavicular joint
  - **S43.215-** Anterior dislocation of left sternoclavicular joint
  - **S43.216-** Anterior dislocation of unspecified sternoclavicular joint
- **S43.22-** Posterior subluxation and dislocation of sternoclavicular joint
  - **S43.221-** Posterior subluxation of right sternoclavicular joint
  - **S43.222-** Posterior subluxation of left sternoclavicular joint
  - **S43.223-** Posterior subluxation of unspecified sternoclavicular joint
  - **S43.224-** Posterior dislocation of right sternoclavicular joint
  - **S43.225-** Posterior dislocation of left sternoclavicular joint
  - **S43.226-** Posterior dislocation of unspecified sternoclavicular joint

S42 - S43

S43.3-   Subluxation and dislocation of other and unspecified parts of shoulder girdle

S43.30-   Subluxation and dislocation of unspecified parts of shoulder girdle
   Dislocation of shoulder girdle NOS
   Subluxation of shoulder girdle NOS

S43.301-   Subluxation of unspecified parts of right shoulder girdle
S43.302-   Subluxation of unspecified parts of left shoulder girdle
S43.303-   Subluxation of unspecified parts of unspecified shoulder girdle
S43.304-   Dislocation of unspecified parts of right shoulder girdle
S43.305-   Dislocation of unspecified parts of left shoulder girdle
S43.306-   Dislocation of unspecified parts of unspecified shoulder girdle

S43.31-   Subluxation and dislocation of scapula
S43.311-   Subluxation of right scapula
S43.312-   Subluxation of left scapula
S43.313-   Subluxation of unspecified scapula
S43.314-   Dislocation of right scapula
S43.315-   Dislocation of left scapula
S43.316-   Dislocation of unspecified scapula

S43.39-   Subluxation and dislocation of other parts of shoulder girdle
S43.391-   Subluxation of other parts of right shoulder girdle
S43.392-   Subluxation of other parts of left shoulder girdle
S43.393-   Subluxation of other parts of unspecified shoulder girdle
S43.394-   Dislocation of other parts of right shoulder girdle
S43.395-   Dislocation of other parts of left shoulder girdle
S43.396-   Dislocation of other parts of unspecified shoulder girdle

S43.4-   Sprain of shoulder joint
S43.40-   Unspecified sprain of shoulder joint
S43.401-   Unspecified sprain of right shoulder joint
S43.402-   Unspecified sprain of left shoulder joint
S43.409-   Unspecified sprain of unspecified shoulder joint

S43.41-   Sprain of coracohumeral (ligament)
S43.411-   Sprain of right coracohumeral (ligament)
S43.412-   Sprain of left coracohumeral (ligament)
S43.419-   Sprain of unspecified coracohumeral (ligament)

S43.42-   Sprain of rotator cuff capsule
   Excludes 1:   rotator cuff syndrome (complete) (incomplete), not specified as traumatic (M75.1-)
   Excludes❷: injury of tendon of rotator cuff (S46.0-)
S43.421-   Sprain of right rotator cuff capsule
S43.422-   Sprain of left rotator cuff capsule
S43.429-   Sprain of unspecified rotator cuff capsule

S43.43-   Superior glenoid labrum lesion
   SLAP lesion
S43.431-   Superior glenoid labrum lesion of right shoulder
S43.432-   Superior glenoid labrum lesion of left shoulder
S43.439-   Superior glenoid labrum lesion of unspecified shoulder

S43.49-   Other sprain of shoulder joint
S43.491-   Other sprain of right shoulder joint
S43.492-   Other sprain of left shoulder joint
S43.499-   Other sprain of unspecified shoulder joint

S43.5-   Sprain of acromioclavicular joint
   Sprain of acromioclavicular ligament
S43.50x-   Sprain of unspecified acromioclavicular joint
S43.51x-   Sprain of right acromioclavicular joint
S43.52x-   Sprain of left acromioclavicular joint

S43.6-   Sprain of sternoclavicular joint
S43.60x-   Sprain of unspecified sternoclavicular joint
S43.61x-   Sprain of right sternoclavicular joint
S43.62x-   Sprain of left sternoclavicular joint

S43.8-   Sprain of other specified parts of shoulder girdle
S43.80x-   Sprain of other specified parts of unspecified shoulder girdle
S43.81x-   Sprain of other specified parts of right shoulder girdle
S43.82x-   Sprain of other specified parts of left shoulder girdle

S43.9-   Sprain of unspecified parts of shoulder girdle
S43.90x-   Sprain of unspecified parts of unspecified shoulder girdle
   Sprain of shoulder girdle NOS
S43.91x-   Sprain of unspecified parts of right shoulder girdle
S43.92x-   Sprain of unspecified parts of left shoulder girdle

S44-   Injury of nerves at shoulder and upper arm level
   Code also any associated open wound (S41.-)
   Excludes❷: injury of brachial plexus (S14.3-)
   The appropriate 7th character is to be added to each code from category S44:
   A   Initial encounter
   D   Subsequent encounter
   S   Sequela

S44.0-   Injury of ulnar nerve at upper arm level
   Excludes 1:   ulnar nerve NOS (S54.0)
S44.00x-   Injury of ulnar nerve at upper arm level, unspecified arm
S44.01x-   Injury of ulnar nerve at upper arm level, right arm
S44.02x-   Injury of ulnar nerve at upper arm level, left arm

S44.1-   Injury of median nerve at upper arm level
   Excludes 1:   median nerve NOS (S54.1)
S44.10x-   Injury of median nerve at upper arm level, unspecified arm
S44.11x-   Injury of median nerve at upper arm level, right arm
S44.12x-   Injury of median nerve at upper arm level, left arm

S44.2-   Injury of radial nerve at upper arm level
   Excludes 1:   radial nerve NOS (S54.2)
S44.20x-   Injury of radial nerve at upper arm level, unspecified arm
S44.21x-   Injury of radial nerve at upper arm level, right arm
S44.22x-   Injury of radial nerve at upper arm level, left arm

S44.3-   Injury of axillary nerve
S44.30x-   Injury of axillary nerve, unspecified arm
S44.31x-   Injury of axillary nerve, right arm
S44.32x-   Injury of axillary nerve, left arm

S44.4-   Injury of musculocutaneous nerve
S44.40x-   Injury of musculocutaneous nerve, unspecified arm
S44.41x-   Injury of musculocutaneous nerve, right arm
S44.42x-   Injury of musculocutaneous nerve, left arm

S44.5-   Injury of cutaneous sensory nerve at shoulder and upper arm level
S44.50x-   Injury of cutaneous sensory nerve at shoulder and upper arm level, unspecified arm
S44.51x-   Injury of cutaneous sensory nerve at shoulder and upper arm level, right arm
S44.52x-   Injury of cutaneous sensory nerve at shoulder and upper arm level, left arm

S44.8-   Injury of other nerves at shoulder and upper arm level
S44.8x-   Injury of other nerves at shoulder and upper arm level
S44.8x1-   Injury of other nerves at shoulder and upper arm level, right arm
S44.8x2-   Injury of other nerves at shoulder and upper arm level, left arm
S44.8x9-   Injury of other nerves at shoulder and upper arm level, unspecified arm

S44.9-   Injury of unspecified nerve at shoulder and upper arm level
S44.90x-   Injury of unspecified nerve at shoulder and upper arm level, unspecified arm
S44.91x-   Injury of unspecified nerve at shoulder and upper arm level, right arm
S44.92x-   Injury of unspecified nerve at shoulder and upper arm level, left arm

S45-   Injury of blood vessels at shoulder and upper arm level
   Code also any associated open wound (S41.-)
   Excludes❷: injury of subclavian artery (S25.1)
             injury of subclavian vein (S25.3)
   The appropriate 7th character is to be added to each code from category S45:
   A   Initial encounter
   D   Subsequent encounter
   S   Sequela

S45.0-   Injury of axillary artery
S45.00-   Unspecified injury of axillary artery
S45.001-   Unspecified injury of axillary artery, right side
S45.002-   Unspecified injury of axillary artery, left side
S45.009-   Unspecified injury of axillary artery, unspecified side

S45.01-   Laceration of axillary artery
S45.011-   Laceration of axillary artery, right side
S45.012-   Laceration of axillary artery, left side
S45.019-   Laceration of axillary artery, unspecified side

S45.09-   Other specified injury of axillary artery
S45.091-   Other specified injury of axillary artery, right side
S45.092-   Other specified injury of axillary artery, left side
S45.099-   Other specified injury of axillary artery, unspecified side

S
4
3
|
S
4
6

Excludes 1: = NOT CODED HERE! (Do not code both)   **720**   *Excludes❷:* = Not Included Here

S45.1-   Injury of <u>brachial artery</u>
- S45.10-   <u>Unspecified</u> injury of <u>brachial artery</u>
  - S45.101-   Unspecified injury of brachial artery, <u>right</u> side
  - S45.102-   Unspecified injury of brachial artery, <u>left</u> side
  - S45.109-   Unspecified injury of brachial artery, <u>unspecified</u> side
- S45.11-   <u>Laceration</u> of <u>brachial artery</u>
  - S45.111-   Laceration of brachial artery, <u>right</u> side
  - S45.112-   Laceration of brachial artery, <u>left</u> side
  - S45.119-   Laceration of brachial artery, <u>unspecified</u> side
- S45.19-   <u>Other</u> specified injury of <u>brachial artery</u>
  - S45.191-   Other specified injury of brachial artery, <u>right</u> side
  - S45.192-   Other specified injury of brachial artery, <u>left</u> side
  - S45.199-   Other specified injury of brachial artery, <u>unspecified</u> side

S45.2-   Injury of <u>axillary or brachial vein</u>
- S45.20-   <u>Unspecified</u> injury of <u>axillary or brachial vein</u>
  - S45.201-   Unspecified injury of axillary or brachial vein, <u>right</u> side
  - S45.202-   Unspecified injury of axillary or brachial vein, <u>left</u> side
  - S45.209-   Unspecified injury of axillary or brachial vein, <u>unspecified</u> side
- S45.21-   <u>Laceration</u> of <u>axillary or brachial vein</u>
  - S45.211-   Laceration of axillary or brachial vein, <u>right</u> side
  - S45.212-   Laceration of axillary or brachial vein, <u>left</u> side
  - S45.219-   Laceration of axillary or brachial vein, <u>unspecified</u> side
- S45.29-   <u>Other</u> specified injury of <u>axillary or brachial vein</u>
  - S45.291-   Other specified injury of axillary or brachial vein, <u>right</u> side
  - S45.292-   Other specified injury of axillary or brachial vein, <u>left</u> side
  - S45.299-   Other specified injury of axillary or brachial vein, <u>unspecified</u> side

S45.3-   Injury of <u>superficial vein at shoulder and upper arm level</u>
- S45.30-   <u>Unspecified</u> injury of <u>superficial vein at shoulder and upper arm level</u>
  - S45.301-   Unspecified injury of superficial vein at shoulder and upper arm level, <u>right</u> arm
  - S45.302-   Unspecified injury of superficial vein at shoulder and upper arm level, <u>left</u> arm
  - S45.309-   Unspecified injury of superficial vein at shoulder and upper arm level, <u>unspecified</u> arm
- S45.31-   <u>Laceration</u> of <u>superficial vein at shoulder and upper arm level</u>
  - S45.311-   Laceration of superficial vein at shoulder and upper arm level, <u>right</u> arm
  - S45.312-   Laceration of superficial vein at shoulder and upper arm level, <u>left</u> arm
  - S45.319-   Laceration of superficial vein at shoulder and upper arm level, <u>unspecified</u> arm
- S45.39-   <u>Other specified</u> injury of <u>superficial vein at shoulder and upper arm level</u>
  - S45.391-   Other specified injury of superficial vein at shoulder and upper arm level, <u>right</u> arm
  - S45.392-   Other specified injury of superficial vein at shoulder and upper arm level, <u>left</u> arm
  - S45.399-   Other specified injury of superficial vein at shoulder and upper arm level, <u>unspecified</u> arm

S45.8-   Injury of <u>other specified blood vessels</u> at shoulder and upper arm level
- S45.80-   <u>Unspecified</u> injury of <u>other specified blood vessels at shoulder and upper arm level</u>
  - S45.801-   Unspecified injury of other specified blood vessels at shoulder and upper arm level, <u>right</u> arm
  - S45.802-   Unspecified injury of other specified blood vessels at shoulder and upper arm level, <u>left</u> arm
  - S45.809-   Unspecified injury of other specified blood vessels at shoulder and upper arm level, <u>unspecified</u> arm
- S45.81-   <u>Laceration</u> of <u>other specified blood vessels at shoulder and upper arm level</u>
  - S45.811-   Laceration of other specified blood vessels at shoulder and upper arm level, <u>right</u> arm
  - S45.812-   Laceration of other specified blood vessels at shoulder and upper arm level, <u>left</u> arm
  - S45.819-   Laceration of other specified blood vessels at shoulder and upper arm level, <u>unspecified</u> arm

S45.89-   <u>Other specified injury</u> of <u>other specified blood vessels</u> at <u>shoulder and upper arm level</u>
  - S45.891-   Other specified injury of other specified blood vessels at shoulder and upper arm level, <u>right</u> arm
  - S45.892-   Other specified injury of other specified blood vessels at shoulder and upper arm level, <u>left</u> arm
  - S45.899-   Other specified injury of other specified blood vessels at shoulder and upper arm level, <u>unspecified</u> arm

S45.9-   Injury of <u>unspecified blood vessel at shoulder and upper arm level</u>
- S45.90-   <u>Unspecified</u> injury of <u>unspecified blood vessel at shoulder and upper arm level</u>
  - S45.901-   Unspecified injury of unspecified blood vessel at shoulder and upper arm level, <u>right</u> arm
  - S45.902-   Unspecified injury of unspecified blood vessel at shoulder and upper arm level, <u>left</u> arm
  - S45.909-   Unspecified injury of unspecified blood vessel at shoulder and upper arm level, <u>unspecified</u> arm
- S45.91-   <u>Laceration</u> of <u>unspecified blood vessel at shoulder and upper arm level</u>
  - S45.911-   Laceration of unspecified blood vessel at shoulder and upper arm level, <u>right</u> arm
  - S45.912-   Laceration of unspecified blood vessel at shoulder and upper arm level, <u>left</u> arm
  - S45.919-   Laceration of unspecified blood vessel at shoulder and upper arm level, <u>unspecified</u> arm
- S45.99-   <u>Other specified injury</u> of <u>unspecified blood vessel at shoulder and upper arm level</u>
  - S45.991-   Other specified injury of unspecified blood vessel at shoulder and upper arm level, <u>right</u> arm
  - S45.992-   Other specified injury of unspecified blood vessel at shoulder and upper arm level, <u>left</u> arm
  - S45.999-   Other specified injury of unspecified blood vessel at shoulder and upper arm level, <u>unspecified</u> arm

S46-   Injury of <u>muscle, fascia and tendon at shoulder and upper arm level</u>
Code also any associated open wound (S41.-)
Excludes ❷: injury of muscle, fascia and tendon at elbow (S56.-)
sprain of joints and ligaments of shoulder girdle (S43.9)

The appropriate 7th character is to be added to each code from category S46:
- A   <u>Initial</u> encounter
- D   <u>Subsequent</u> encounter
- S   <u>Sequela</u>

S46.0-   Injury of <u>muscle(s) and tendon(s)</u> of the <u>rotator cuff of shoulder</u>
- S46.00-   <u>Unspecified</u> injury of <u>muscle(s) and tendon(s)</u> of the <u>rotator cuff of shoulder</u>
  - S46.001-   Unspecified injury of muscle(s) and tendon(s) of the rotator cuff of <u>right</u> shoulder
  - S46.002-   Unspecified injury of muscle(s) and tendon(s) of the rotator cuff of <u>left</u> shoulder
  - S46.009-   Unspecified injury of muscle(s) and tendon(s) of the rotator cuff of <u>unspecified</u> shoulder
- S46.01-   <u>Strain</u> of <u>muscle(s) and tendon(s)</u> of the <u>rotator cuff of shoulder</u>
  - S46.011-   Strain of muscle(s) and tendon(s) of the rotator cuff of <u>right</u> shoulder
  - S46.012-   Strain of muscle(s) and tendon(s) of the rotator cuff of <u>left</u> shoulder
  - S46.019-   Strain of muscle(s) and tendon(s) of the rotator cuff of <u>unspecified</u> shoulder
- S46.02-   <u>Laceration</u> of <u>muscle(s) and tendon(s)</u> of the <u>rotator cuff of shoulder</u>
  - S46.021-   Laceration of muscle(s) and tendon(s) of the rotator cuff of <u>right</u> shoulder
  - S46.022-   Laceration of muscle(s) and tendon(s) of the rotator cuff of <u>left</u> shoulder
  - S46.029-   Laceration of muscle(s) and tendon(s) of the rotator cuff of <u>unspecified</u> shoulder
- S46.09-   <u>Other injury</u> of <u>muscle(s) and tendon(s)</u> of the <u>rotator cuff of shoulder</u>
  - S46.091-   Other injury of muscle(s) and tendon(s) of the rotator cuff of <u>right</u> shoulder
  - S46.092-   Other injury of muscle(s) and tendon(s) of the rotator cuff of <u>left</u> shoulder
  - S46.099-   Other injury of muscle(s) and tendon(s) of the rotator cuff of <u>unspecified</u> shoulder

S43 - S46

S46.1- Injury of <u>muscle, fascia and tendon</u> of <u>long head of biceps</u>
  S46.10- <u>Unspecified</u> injury of <u>muscle, fascia and tendon</u> of <u>long head of biceps</u>
    S46.101- Unspecified injury of muscle, fascia and tendon of long head of biceps, <u>right</u> arm
    S46.102- Unspecified injury of muscle, fascia and tendon of long head of biceps, <u>left</u> arm
    S46.109- Unspecified injury of muscle, fascia and tendon of long head of biceps, <u>unspecified</u> arm
  S46.11- <u>Strain</u> of <u>muscle, fascia and tendon</u> of <u>long head of biceps</u>
    S46.111- Strain of muscle, fascia and tendon of long head of biceps, <u>right</u> arm
    S46.112- Strain of muscle, fascia and tendon of long head of biceps, <u>left</u> arm
    S46.119- Strain of muscle, fascia and tendon of long head of biceps, <u>unspecified</u> arm
  S46.12- <u>Laceration</u> of <u>muscle, fascia and tendon</u> of <u>long head of biceps</u>
    S46.121- Laceration of muscle, fascia and tendon of long head of biceps, <u>right</u> arm
    S46.122- Laceration of muscle, fascia and tendon of long head of biceps, <u>left</u> arm
    S46.129- Laceration of muscle, fascia and tendon of long head of biceps, <u>unspecified</u> arm
  S46.19- <u>Other</u> injury of <u>muscle, fascia and tendon</u> of <u>long head of biceps</u>
    S46.191- Other injury of muscle, fascia and tendon of long head of biceps, <u>right</u> arm
    S46.192- Other injury of muscle, fascia and tendon of long head of biceps, <u>left</u> arm
    S46.199- Other injury of muscle, fascia and tendon of long head of biceps, <u>unspecified</u> arm
S46.2- Injury of <u>muscle, fascia and tendon</u> of <u>other parts of biceps</u>
  S46.20- <u>Unspecified</u> injury of <u>muscle, fascia and tendon</u> of <u>other parts of biceps</u>
    S46.201- Unspecified injury of muscle, fascia and tendon of other parts of biceps, <u>right</u> arm
    S46.202- Unspecified injury of muscle, fascia and tendon of other parts of biceps, <u>left</u> arm
    S46.209- Unspecified injury of muscle, fascia and tendon of other parts of biceps, <u>unspecified</u> arm
  S46.21- <u>Strain</u> of <u>muscle, fascia and tendon</u> of <u>other parts of biceps</u>
    S46.211- Strain of muscle, fascia and tendon of other parts of biceps, <u>right</u> arm
    S46.212- Strain of muscle, fascia and tendon of other parts of biceps, <u>left</u> arm
    S46.219- Strain of muscle, fascia and tendon of other parts of biceps, <u>unspecified</u> arm
  S46.22- <u>Laceration</u> of <u>muscle, fascia and tendon</u> of <u>other parts of biceps</u>
    S46.221- Laceration of muscle, fascia and tendon of other parts of biceps, <u>right</u> arm
    S46.222- Laceration of muscle, fascia and tendon of other parts of biceps, <u>left</u> arm
    S46.229- Laceration of muscle, fascia and tendon of other parts of biceps, <u>unspecified</u> arm
  S46.29- <u>Other</u> injury of <u>muscle, fascia and tendon</u> of <u>other parts of biceps</u>
    S46.291- Other injury of muscle, fascia and tendon of other parts of biceps, <u>right</u> arm
    S46.292- Other injury of muscle, fascia and tendon of other parts of biceps, <u>left</u> arm
    S46.299- Other injury of muscle, fascia and tendon of other parts of biceps, <u>unspecified</u> arm
S46.3- Injury of <u>muscle, fascia and tendon</u> of <u>triceps</u>
  S46.30- <u>Unspecified</u> injury of <u>muscle, fascia and tendon</u> of <u>triceps</u>
    S46.301- Unspecified injury of muscle, fascia and tendon of triceps, <u>right</u> arm
    S46.302- Unspecified injury of muscle, fascia and tendon of triceps, <u>left</u> arm
    S46.309- Unspecified injury of muscle, fascia and tendon of triceps, <u>unspecified</u> arm
  S46.31- <u>Strain</u> of <u>muscle, fascia and tendon</u> of <u>triceps</u>
    S46.311- Strain of muscle, fascia and tendon of triceps, <u>right</u> arm
    S46.312- Strain of muscle, fascia and tendon of triceps, <u>left</u> arm
    S46.319- Strain of muscle, fascia and tendon of triceps, <u>unspecified</u> arm

S46.32- <u>Laceration</u> of <u>muscle, fascia and tendon</u> of <u>triceps</u>
    S46.321- Laceration of muscle, fascia and tendon of triceps, <u>right</u> arm
    S46.322- Laceration of muscle, fascia and tendon of triceps, <u>left</u> arm
    S46.329- Laceration of muscle, fascia and tendon of triceps, <u>unspecified</u> arm
  S46.39- <u>Other injury</u> of muscle, fascia and tendon of <u>triceps</u>
    S46.391- Other injury of muscle, fascia and tendon of triceps, <u>right</u> arm
    S46.392- Other injury of muscle, fascia and tendon of triceps, <u>left</u> arm
    S46.399- Other injury of muscle, fascia and tendon of triceps, <u>unspecified</u> arm
S46.8- <u>Injury</u> of <u>other muscles, fascia and tendons</u> at <u>shoulder and upper arm level</u>
  S46.80- <u>Unspecified</u> injury of <u>other muscles, fascia and tendons</u> at <u>shoulder and upper arm level</u>
    S46.801- Unspecified injury of other muscles, fascia and tendons at shoulder and upper arm level, <u>right</u> arm
    S46.802- Unspecified injury of other muscles, fascia and tendons at shoulder and upper arm level, <u>left</u> arm
    S46.809- Unspecified injury of other muscles, fascia and tendons at shoulder and upper arm level, <u>unspecified</u> arm
  S46.81- <u>Strain</u> of <u>other muscles, fascia and tendons</u> at <u>shoulder and upper arm level</u>
    S46.811- Strain of other muscles, fascia and tendons at shoulder and upper arm level, <u>right</u> arm
    S46.812- Strain of other muscles, fascia and tendons at shoulder and upper arm level, <u>left</u> arm
    S46.819- Strain of other muscles, fascia and tendons at shoulder and upper arm level, <u>unspecified</u> arm
  S46.82- <u>Laceration</u> of <u>other muscles, fascia and tendons</u> at <u>shoulder and upper arm level</u>
    S46.821- Laceration of other muscles, fascia and tendons at shoulder and upper arm level, <u>right</u> arm
    S46.822- Laceration of other muscles, fascia and tendons at shoulder and upper arm level, <u>left</u> arm
    S46.829- Laceration of other muscles, fascia and tendons at shoulder and upper arm level, <u>unspecified</u> arm
  S46.89- <u>Other injury</u> of <u>other muscles, fascia and tendons</u> at <u>shoulder and upper arm level</u>
    S46.891- Other injury of other muscles, fascia and tendons at shoulder and upper arm level, <u>right</u> arm
    S46.892- Other injury of other muscles, fascia and tendons at shoulder and upper arm level, <u>left</u> arm
    S46.899- Other injury of other muscles, fascia and tendons at shoulder and upper arm level, <u>unspecified</u> arm
S46.9- Injury of <u>unspecified</u> <u>muscle, fascia and tendon</u> at <u>shoulder and upper arm level</u>
  S46.90- <u>Unspecified</u> injury of <u>unspecified</u> <u>muscle, fascia and tendon</u> at <u>shoulder and upper arm level</u>
    S46.901- Unspecified injury of unspecified muscle, fascia and tendon at shoulder and upper arm level, <u>right</u> arm
    S46.902- Unspecified injury of unspecified muscle, fascia and tendon at shoulder and upper arm level, <u>left</u> arm
    S46.909- Unspecified injury of <u>unspecified</u> muscle, fascia and tendon at shoulder and upper arm level, <u>unspecified</u> arm
  S46.91- <u>Strain</u> of <u>unspecified</u> <u>muscle, fascia and tendon</u> at <u>shoulder and upper arm level</u>
    S46.911- Strain of unspecified muscle, fascia and tendon at shoulder and upper arm level, <u>right</u> arm
    S46.912- Strain of unspecified muscle, fascia and tendon at shoulder and upper arm level, <u>left</u> arm
    S46.919- Strain of unspecified muscle, fascia and tendon at shoulder and upper arm level, <u>unspecified</u> arm
  S46.92- <u>Laceration</u> of <u>unspecified</u> <u>muscle, fascia and tendon</u> at <u>shoulder and upper arm level</u>
    S46.921- Laceration of unspecified muscle, fascia and tendon at shoulder and upper arm level, <u>right</u> arm
    S46.922- Laceration of unspecified muscle, fascia and tendon at shoulder and upper arm level, <u>left</u> arm
    S46.929- Laceration of unspecified muscle, fascia and tendon at shoulder and upper arm level, <u>unspecified</u> arm

S46 - S49

S46.99- Other injury of unspecified muscle, fascia and tendon at shoulder and upper arm level

    S46.991- Other injury of unspecified muscle, fascia and tendon at shoulder and upper arm level, right arm

    S46.992- Other injury of unspecified muscle, fascia and tendon at shoulder and upper arm level, left arm

    S46.999- Other injury of unspecified muscle, fascia and tendon at shoulder and upper arm level, unspecified arm

S47- Crushing injury of shoulder and upper arm
    Use additional code for all associated injuries
    Excludes❷: crushing injury of elbow (S57.0-)

    The appropriate 7th character is to be added to each code from category S47:
    A Initial encounter
    D Subsequent encounter
    S Sequela

S47.1xx- Crushing injury of right shoulder and upper arm

S47.2xx- Crushing injury of left shoulder and upper arm

S47.9xx- Crushing injury of shoulder and upper arm, unspecified arm

S48- Traumatic amputation of shoulder and upper arm
    Note: An amputation not identified as partial or complete should be coded to complete
    Excludes 1: traumatic amputation at elbow level (S58.0)

    The appropriate 7th character is to be added to each code from category S48:
    A Initial encounter
    D Subsequent encounter
    S Sequela

S48.0- Traumatic amputation at shoulder joint
    S48.01- Complete traumatic amputation at shoulder joint
        S48.011- Complete traumatic amputation at right shoulder joint
        S48.012- Complete traumatic amputation at left shoulder joint
        S48.019- Complete traumatic amputation at unspecified shoulder joint
    S48.02- Partial traumatic amputation at shoulder joint
        S48.021- Partial traumatic amputation at right shoulder joint
        S48.022- Partial traumatic amputation at left shoulder joint
        S48.029- Partial traumatic amputation at unspecified shoulder joint

S48.1- Traumatic amputation at level between shoulder and elbow
    S48.11- Complete traumatic amputation at level between shoulder and elbow
        S48.111- Complete traumatic amputation at level between right shoulder and elbow
        S48.112- Complete traumatic amputation at level between left shoulder and elbow
        S48.119- Complete traumatic amputation at level between unspecified shoulder and elbow
    S48.12- Partial traumatic amputation at level between shoulder and elbow
        S48.121- Partial traumatic amputation at level between right shoulder and elbow
        S48.122- Partial traumatic amputation at level between left shoulder and elbow
        S48.129- Partial traumatic amputation at level between unspecified shoulder and elbow

S48.9- Traumatic amputation of shoulder and upper arm, level unspecified
    S48.91- Complete traumatic amputation of shoulder and upper arm, level unspecified
        S48.911- Complete traumatic amputation of right shoulder and upper arm, level unspecified
        S48.912- Complete traumatic amputation of left shoulder and upper arm, level unspecified
        S48.919- Complete traumatic amputation of unspecified shoulder and upper arm, level unspecified
    S48.92- Partial traumatic amputation of shoulder and upper arm, level unspecified
        S48.921- Partial traumatic amputation of right shoulder and upper arm, level unspecified
        S48.922- Partial traumatic amputation of left shoulder and upper arm, level unspecified
        S48.929- Partial traumatic amputation of unspecified shoulder and upper arm, level unspecified

S49- Other and unspecified injuries of shoulder and upper arm
    The appropriate 7th character is to be added to each code from subcategories S49.0 and S49.1:
    A Initial encounter for closed fracture
    D Subsequent encounter for fracture with routine healing
    G Subsequent encounter for fracture with delayed healing
    K Subsequent encounter for fracture with nonunion
    P Subsequent encounter for fracture with malunion
    S Sequela

S49.0- Physeal fracture of upper end of humerus
    S49.00- Unspecified physeal fracture of upper end of humerus
        S49.001- Unspecified physeal fracture of upper end of humerus, right arm
        S49.002- Unspecified physeal fracture of upper end of humerus, left arm
        S49.009- Unspecified physeal fracture of upper end of humerus, unspecified arm
    S49.01- Salter-Harris Type I physeal fracture of upper end of humerus
        S49.011- Salter-Harris Type I physeal fracture of upper end of humerus, right arm
        S49.012- Salter-Harris Type I physeal fracture of upper end of humerus, left arm
        S49.019- Salter-Harris Type I physeal fracture of upper end of humerus, unspecified arm
    S49.02- Salter-Harris Type II physeal fracture of upper end of humerus
        S49.021- Salter-Harris Type II physeal fracture of upper end of humerus, right arm
        S49.022- Salter-Harris Type II physeal fracture of upper end of humerus, left arm
        S49.029- Salter-Harris Type II physeal fracture of upper end of humerus, unspecified arm
    S49.03- Salter-Harris Type III physeal fracture of upper end of humerus
        S49.031- Salter Harris Type III physeal fracture of upper end of humerus, right arm
        S49.032- Salter-Harris Type III physeal fracture of upper end of humerus, left arm
        S49.039- Salter Harris Type III physeal fracture of upper end of humerus, unspecified arm
    S49.04- Salter-Harris Type IV physeal fracture of upper end of humerus
        S49.041- Salter-Harris Type IV physeal fracture of upper end of humerus, right arm
        S49.042- Salter-Harris Type IV physeal fracture of upper end of humerus, left arm
        S49.049- Salter-Harris Type IV physeal fracture of upper end of humerus, unspecified arm
    S49.09- Other physeal fracture of upper end of humerus
        S49.091- Other physeal fracture of upper end of humerus, right arm
        S49.092- Other physeal fracture of upper end of humerus, left arm
        S49.099- Other physeal fracture of upper end of humerus, unspecified arm

S49.1- Physeal fracture of lower end of humerus
    S49.10- Unspecified physeal fracture of lower end of humerus
        S49.101- Unspecified physeal fracture of lower end of humerus, right arm
        S49.102- Unspecified physeal fracture of lower end of humerus, left arm
        S49.109- Unspecified physeal fracture of lower end of humerus, unspecified arm
    S49.11- Salter-Harris Type I physeal fracture of lower end of humerus
        S49.111- Salter-Harris Type I physeal fracture of lower end of humerus, right arm
        S49.112- Salter-Harris Type I physeal fracture of lower end of humerus, left arm
        S49.119- Salter-Harris Type I physeal fracture of lower end of humerus, unspecified arm
    S49.12- Salter-Harris Type II physeal fracture of lower end of humerus
        S49.121- Salter-Harris Type II physeal fracture of lower end of humerus, right arm
        S49.122- Salter-Harris Type II physeal fracture of lower end of humerus, left arm
        S49.129- Salter-Harris Type II physeal fracture of lower end of humerus, unspecified arm

S46 - S49

S49.13- Salter Harris Type III physeal fracture of lower end of humerus
    S49.131- Salter Harris Type III physeal fracture of lower end of humerus, right arm
    S49.132- Salter Harris Type III physeal fracture of lower end of humerus, left arm
    S49.139- Salter Harris Type III physeal fracture of lower end of humerus, unspecified arm

S49.14- Salter-Harris Type IV physeal fracture of lower end of humerus
    S49.141- Salter-Harris Type IV physeal fracture of lower end of humerus, right arm
    S49.142- Salter-Harris Type IV physeal fracture of lower end of humerus, left arm
    S49.149- Salter-Harris Type IV physeal fracture of lower end of humerus, unspecified arm

S49.19- Other physeal fracture of lower end of humerus
    S49.191- Other physeal fracture of lower end of humerus, right arm
    S49.192- Other physeal fracture of lower end of humerus, left arm
    S49.199- Other physeal fracture of lower end of humerus, unspecified arm

S49.8- Other specified injuries of shoulder and upper arm
> The appropriate 7th character is to be added to each code in subcategory S49.8:
> A Initial encounter
> D Subsequent encounter
> S Sequela

S49.80x- Other specified injuries of shoulder and upper arm, unspecified arm
S49.81x- Other specified injuries of right shoulder and upper arm
S49.82x- Other specified injuries of left shoulder and upper arm

S49.9- Unspecified injury of shoulder and upper arm
> The appropriate 7th character is to be added to each code in subcategory S49.9:
> A Initial encounter
> D Subsequent encounter
> S Sequela

S49.90x- Unspecified injury of shoulder and upper arm, unspecified arm
S49.91x- Unspecified injury of right shoulder and upper arm
S49.92x- Unspecified injury of left shoulder and upper arm

Injuries to the elbow and forearm (S50-S59)

Excludes❷: burns and corrosions (T20-T32)
     frostbite (T33-T34)
     injuries of wrist and hand (S60-S69)
     insect bite or sting, venomous (T63.4)

S50- Superficial injury of elbow and forearm
Excludes❷: superficial injury of wrist and hand (S60.-)
> The appropriate 7th character is to be added to each code from category S50:
> A Initial encounter
> D Subsequent encounter
> S Sequela

S50.0- Contusion of elbow
    S50.00x- Contusion of unspecified elbow
    S50.01x- Contusion of right elbow
    S50.02x- Contusion of left elbow

S50.1- Contusion of forearm
    S50.10x- Contusion of unspecified forearm
    S50.11x- Contusion of right forearm
    S50.12x- Contusion of left forearm

S50.3- Other superficial injuries of elbow
  S50.31- Abrasion of elbow
    S50.311- Abrasion of right elbow
    S50.312- Abrasion of left elbow
    S50.319- Abrasion of unspecified elbow
  S50.32- Blister (nonthermal) of elbow
    S50.321- Blister (nonthermal) of right elbow
    S50.322- Blister (nonthermal) of left elbow
    S50.329- Blister (nonthermal) of unspecified elbow
  S50.34- External constriction of elbow
    S50.341- External constriction of right elbow
    S50.342- External constriction of left elbow
    S50.349- External constriction of unspecified elbow

  S50.35- Superficial foreign body of elbow
     Splinter in the elbow
    S50.351- Superficial foreign body of right elbow
    S50.352- Superficial foreign body of left elbow
    S50.359- Superficial foreign body of unspecified elbow
  S50.36- Insect bite (nonvenomous) of elbow
    S50.361- Insect bite (nonvenomous) of right elbow
    S50.362- Insect bite (nonvenomous) of left elbow
    S50.369- Insect bite (nonvenomous) of unspecified elbow
  S50.37- Other superficial bite of elbow
     Excludes 1: open bite of elbow (S51.04)
    S50.371- Other superficial bite of right elbow
    S50.372- Other superficial bite of left elbow
    S50.379- Other superficial bite of unspecified elbow

S50.8- Other superficial injuries of forearm
  S50.81- Abrasion of forearm
    S50.811- Abrasion of right forearm
    S50.812- Abrasion of left forearm
    S50.819- Abrasion of unspecified forearm
  S50.82- Blister (nonthermal) of forearm
    S50.821- Blister (nonthermal) of right forearm
    S50.822- Blister (nonthermal) of left forearm
    S50.829- Blister (nonthermal) of unspecified forearm
  S50.84- External constriction of forearm
    S50.841- External constriction of right forearm
    S50.842- External constriction of left forearm
    S50.849- External constriction of unspecified forearm
  S50.85- Superficial foreign body of forearm
     Splinter in the forearm
    S50.851- Superficial foreign body of right forearm
    S50.852- Superficial foreign body of left forearm
    S50.859- Superficial foreign body of unspecified forearm
  S50.86- Insect bite (nonvenomous) of forearm
    S50.861- Insect bite (nonvenomous) of right forearm
    S50.862- Insect bite (nonvenomous) of left forearm
    S50.869- Insect bite (nonvenomous) of unspecified forearm
  S50.87- Other superficial bite of forearm
     Excludes 1: open bite of forearm (S51.84)
    S50.871- Other superficial bite of right forearm
    S50.872- Other superficial bite of left forearm
    S50.879- Other superficial bite of unspecified forearm

S50.9- Unspecified superficial injury of elbow and forearm
  S50.90- Unspecified superficial injury of elbow
    S50.901- Unspecified superficial injury of right elbow
    S50.902- Unspecified superficial injury of left elbow
    S50.909- Unspecified superficial injury of unspecified elbow
  S50.91- Unspecified superficial injury of forearm
    S50.911- Unspecified superficial injury of right forearm
    S50.912- Unspecified superficial injury of left forearm
    S50.919- Unspecified superficial injury of unspecified forearm

S51- Open wound of elbow and forearm
Code also any associated wound infection
Excludes 1: open fracture of elbow and forearm (S52.- with open fracture 7th character)
     traumatic amputation of elbow and forearm (S58.-)
Excludes❷: open wound of wrist and hand (S61.-)
> The appropriate 7th character is to be added to each code from category S51:
> A Initial encounter
> D Subsequent encounter
> S Sequela

S51.0- Open wound of elbow
  S51.00- Unspecified open wound of elbow
    S51.001- Unspecified open wound of right elbow
    S51.002- Unspecified open wound of left elbow
    S51.009- Unspecified open wound of unspecified elbow
     Open wound of elbow NOS
  S51.01- Laceration without foreign body of elbow
    S51.011- Laceration without foreign body of right elbow
    S51.012- Laceration without foreign body of left elbow
    S51.019- Laceration without foreign body of unspecified elbow
  S51.02- Laceration with foreign body of elbow
    S51.021- Laceration with foreign body of right elbow
    S51.022- Laceration with foreign body of left elbow
    S51.029- Laceration with foreign body of unspecified elbow

S49 - S52

S51.03- <u>Puncture</u> wound <u>without</u> foreign body of <u>elbow</u>
  S51.031- Puncture wound <u>without</u> foreign body of <u>right</u> elbow
  S51.032- Puncture wound <u>without</u> foreign body of <u>left</u> elbow
  S51.039- Puncture wound <u>without</u> foreign body of <u>unspecified</u> elbow
S51.04- <u>Puncture</u> wound <u>with foreign body</u> of <u>elbow</u>
  S51.041- Puncture wound <u>with foreign body</u> of <u>right</u> elbow
  S51.042- Puncture wound <u>with foreign body</u> of <u>left</u> elbow
  S51.049- Puncture wound <u>with foreign body</u> of <u>unspecified</u> elbow
S51.05- <u>Open bite</u> of <u>elbow</u>
  Bite of elbow NOS
  Excludes 1: superficial bite of elbow (S50.36, S50.37)
  S51.051- Open bite, <u>right</u> elbow
  S51.052- Open bite, <u>left</u> elbow
  S51.059- Open bite, <u>unspecified</u> elbow
S51.8- <u>Open wound</u> of <u>forearm</u>
  Excludes❷: open wound of elbow (S51.0-)
  S51.80- <u>Unspecified</u> open wound of <u>forearm</u>
    S51.801- Unspecified open wound of <u>right</u> forearm
    S51.802- Unspecified open wound of <u>left</u> forearm
    S51.809- Unspecified open wound of <u>unspecified</u> forearm
      Open wound of forearm NOS
  S51.81- <u>Laceration</u> <u>without</u> foreign body of <u>forearm</u>
    S51.811- Laceration <u>without</u> foreign body of <u>right</u> forearm
    S51.812- Laceration <u>without</u> foreign body of <u>left</u> forearm
    S51.819- Laceration <u>without</u> foreign body of <u>unspecified</u> forearm
  S51.82- <u>Laceration</u> <u>with foreign body</u> of <u>forearm</u>
    S51.821- Laceration <u>with foreign body</u> of <u>right</u> forearm
    S51.822- Laceration <u>with foreign body</u> of <u>left</u> forearm
    S51.829- Laceration <u>with foreign body</u> of <u>unspecified</u> forearm
  S51.83- <u>Puncture</u> wound <u>without</u> foreign body of <u>forearm</u>
    S51.831- Puncture wound <u>without</u> foreign body of <u>right</u> forearm
    S51.832- Puncture wound <u>without</u> foreign body of <u>left</u> forearm
    S51.839- Puncture wound <u>without</u> foreign body of <u>unspecified</u> forearm
  S51.84- <u>Puncture</u> wound <u>with foreign body</u> of <u>forearm</u>
    S51.841- Puncture wound <u>with foreign body</u> of <u>right</u> forearm
    S51.842- Puncture wound <u>with foreign body</u> of <u>left</u> forearm
    S51.849- Puncture wound <u>with foreign body</u> of <u>unspecified</u> forearm
  S51.85- <u>Open bite</u> of <u>forearm</u>
    Bite of forearm NOS
    Excludes 1: superficial bite of forearm (S50.86, S50.87)
    S51.851- Open bite of <u>right</u> forearm
    S51.852- Open bite of <u>left</u> forearm
    S51.859- Open bite of <u>unspecified</u> forearm

S52- <u>Fracture</u> of <u>forearm</u>
  Note: A fracture not indicated as displaced or nondisplaced should be coded to displaced
  Note: A fracture not indicated as open or closed should be coded to closed
  Note: The open fracture designations are based on the Gustilo open fracture classification
  Excludes 1: traumatic amputation of forearm (S58.-)
  Excludes❷: fracture at wrist and hand level (S62.-)
  The appropriate 7th character is to be added to all codes from category S52:
    A <u>Initial</u> encounter for <u>closed</u> fracture
    B <u>Initial</u> encounter for <u>open</u> fracture <u>type I or II</u>
      <u>Initial</u> encounter for <u>open</u> fracture <u>NOS</u>
    C <u>Initial</u> encounter for <u>open</u> fracture <u>type IIIA, IIIB, or IIIC</u>
    D <u>Subsequent</u> encounter for <u>closed</u> fracture <u>with routine healing</u>
    E <u>Subsequent</u> encounter for <u>open</u> fracture <u>type I or II</u> <u>with routine healing</u>
    F <u>Subsequent</u> encounter for <u>open</u> fracture <u>type IIIA, IIIB, or IIIC</u> <u>with routine healing</u>
    G <u>Subsequent</u> encounter for <u>closed</u> fracture <u>with delayed healing</u>
    H <u>Subsequent</u> encounter for <u>open</u> fracture <u>type I or II</u> <u>with delayed healing</u>
    J <u>Subsequent</u> encounter for <u>open</u> fracture <u>type IIIA, IIIB, or IIIC</u> <u>with delayed healing</u>
    K <u>Subsequent</u> encounter for <u>closed</u> fracture <u>with nonunion</u>
    M <u>Subsequent</u> encounter for <u>open</u> fracture <u>type I or II</u> <u>with nonunion</u>
    N <u>Subsequent</u> encounter for <u>open</u> fracture <u>type IIIA, IIIB, or IIIC</u> <u>with nonunion</u>
    P <u>Subsequent</u> encounter for <u>closed</u> fracture <u>with malunion</u>
    Q <u>Subsequent</u> encounter for <u>open</u> fracture <u>type I or II</u> <u>with malunion</u>
    R <u>Subsequent</u> encounter for <u>open</u> fracture <u>type IIIA, IIIB, or IIIC</u> <u>with malunion</u>
    S <u>Sequela</u>
  S52.0- <u>Fracture</u> of <u>upper end</u> of <u>ulna</u>
    Fracture of proximal end of ulna
    Excludes❷: fracture of elbow NOS (S42.40-)
    fractures of shaft of ulna (S52.2-)
    S52.00- <u>Unspecified</u> fracture of <u>upper end</u> of <u>ulna</u>
      S52.001- Unspecified fracture of upper end of <u>right</u> ulna
      S52.002- Unspecified fracture of upper end of <u>left</u> ulna
      S52.009- Unspecified fracture of upper end of <u>unspecified</u> ulna
    S52.01- <u>Torus</u> fracture of <u>upper end</u> of <u>ulna</u>
      The appropriate 7th character is to be added to all codes in subcategory S52.01:
        A <u>Initial</u> encounter for <u>closed</u> fracture
        D <u>Subsequent</u> encounter for fracture <u>with routine healing</u>
        G <u>Subsequent</u> encounter for fracture <u>with delayed healing</u>
        K <u>Subsequent</u> encounter for fracture <u>with nonunion</u>
        P <u>Subsequent</u> encounter for fracture <u>with malunion</u>
        S <u>Sequela</u>
      S52.011- Torus fracture of upper end of <u>right</u> ulna
      S52.012- Torus fracture of upper end of <u>left</u> ulna
      S52.019- Torus fracture of upper end of <u>unspecified</u> ulna
    S52.02- Fracture of <u>olecranon process</u> <u>without</u> intraarticular extension of <u>ulna</u>
      S52.021- <u>Displaced</u> fracture of olecranon process <u>without</u> intraarticular extension of <u>right</u> ulna
      S52.022- <u>Displaced</u> fracture of olecranon process <u>without</u> intraarticular extension of <u>left</u> ulna
      S52.023- <u>Displaced</u> fracture of olecranon process <u>without</u> intraarticular extension of <u>unspecified</u> ulna
      S52.024- <u>Nondisplaced</u> fracture of olecranon process <u>without</u> intraarticular extension of <u>right</u> ulna
      S52.025- <u>Nondisplaced</u> fracture of olecranon process <u>without</u> intraarticular extension of <u>left</u> ulna
      S52.026- <u>Nondisplaced</u> fracture of olecranon process <u>without</u> intraarticular extension of <u>unspecified</u> ulna
    S52.03- Fracture of <u>olecranon process</u> <u>with intraarticular extension</u> of <u>ulna</u>
      S52.031- <u>Displaced</u> fracture of olecranon process with intraarticular extension of <u>right</u> ulna
      S52.032- <u>Displaced</u> fracture of olecranon process with intraarticular extension of <u>left</u> ulna
      S52.033- <u>Displaced</u> fracture of olecranon process with intraarticular extension of <u>unspecified</u> ulna
      S52.034- <u>Nondisplaced</u> fracture of olecranon process with intraarticular extension of <u>right</u> ulna

S49 – S52

S52.035-   <u>Nondisplaced</u> fracture of olecranon process with intraarticular extension of <u>left</u> ulna

S52.036-   <u>Nondisplaced</u> fracture of olecranon process with intraarticular extension of <u>unspecified</u> ulna

S52.04-   Fracture of <u>coronoid process</u> of <u>ulna</u>

S52.041-   <u>Displaced</u> fracture of coronoid process of <u>right</u> ulna

S52.042-   <u>Displaced</u> fracture of coronoid process of <u>left</u> ulna

S52.043-   <u>Displaced</u> fracture of coronoid process of <u>unspecified</u> ulna

S52.044-   <u>Nondisplaced</u> fracture of coronoid process of <u>right</u> ulna

S52.045-   <u>Nondisplaced</u> fracture of coronoid process of <u>left</u> ulna

S52.046-   <u>Nondisplaced</u> fracture of coronoid process of <u>unspecified</u> ulna

S52.09-   <u>Other</u> fracture of <u>upper end</u> of <u>ulna</u>

S52.091-   Other fracture of upper end of <u>right</u> ulna

S52.092-   Other fracture of upper end of <u>left</u> ulna

S52.099-   Other fracture of upper end of <u>unspecified</u> ulna

S52.1-   Fracture of <u>upper end</u> of <u>radius</u>
Fracture of proximal end of radius
Excludes❷: physeal fractures of upper end of radius (S59.2-)
fracture of shaft of radius (S52.3-)

S52.10-   <u>Unspecified</u> fracture of <u>upper end</u> of <u>radius</u>

S52.101-   Unspecified fracture of upper end of <u>right</u> radius

S52.102-   Unspecified fracture of upper end of <u>left</u> radius

S52.109-   Unspecified fracture of upper end of <u>unspecified</u> radius

S52.11-   <u>Torus</u> fracture of <u>upper end</u> of <u>radius</u>

The appropriate 7th character is to be added to all codes in subcategory S52.11:
A   <u>Initial</u> encounter for <u>closed</u> fracture
D   <u>Subsequent</u> encounter for fracture <u>with routine healing</u>
G   <u>Subsequent</u> encounter for fracture <u>with delayed healing</u>
K   <u>Subsequent</u> encounter for fracture <u>with nonunion</u>
P   <u>Subsequent</u> encounter for fracture <u>with malunion</u>
S   <u>Sequela</u>

S52.111-   Torus fracture of upper end of <u>right</u> radius

S52.112-   Torus fracture of upper end of <u>left</u> radius

S52.119-   Torus fracture of upper end of <u>unspecified</u> radius

S52.12-   Fracture of <u>head</u> of <u>radius</u>

S52.121-   <u>Displaced</u> fracture of head of <u>right</u> radius

S52.122-   <u>Displaced</u> fracture of head of <u>left</u> radius

S52.123-   <u>Displaced</u> fracture of head of <u>unspecified</u> radius

S52.124-   <u>Nondisplaced</u> fracture of head of <u>right</u> radius

S52.125-   <u>Nondisplaced</u> fracture of head of <u>left</u> radius

S52.126-   <u>Nondisplaced</u> fracture of head of <u>unspecified</u> radius

S52.13-   Fracture of <u>neck</u> of <u>radius</u>

S52.131-   <u>Displaced</u> fracture of neck of <u>right</u> radius

S52.132-   <u>Displaced</u> fracture of neck of <u>left</u> radius

S52.133-   <u>Displaced</u> fracture of neck of <u>unspecified</u> radius

S52.134-   <u>Nondisplaced</u> fracture of neck of <u>right</u> radius

S52.135-   <u>Nondisplaced</u> fracture of neck of <u>left</u> radius

S52.136-   <u>Nondisplaced</u> fracture of neck of <u>unspecified</u> radius

S52.18-   <u>Other</u> fracture of <u>upper end</u> of <u>radius</u>

S52.181-   Other fracture of upper end of <u>right</u> radius

S52.182-   Other fracture of upper end of <u>left</u> radius

S52.189-   Other fracture of upper end of <u>unspecified</u> radius

S52.2-   Fracture of <u>shaft</u> of <u>ulna</u>

S52.20-   <u>Unspecified</u> fracture of <u>shaft</u> of <u>ulna</u>
Fracture of ulna NOS

S52.201-   Unspecified fracture of shaft of <u>right</u> ulna

S52.202-   Unspecified fracture of shaft of <u>left</u> ulna

S52.209-   Unspecified fracture of shaft of <u>unspecified</u> ulna

S52.21-   <u>Greenstick</u> fracture of <u>shaft</u> of <u>ulna</u>

The appropriate 7th character is to be added to all codes in subcategory S52.21:
A   <u>Initial</u> encounter for <u>closed</u> fracture
D   <u>Subsequent</u> encounter for fracture <u>with routine healing</u>
G   <u>Subsequent</u> encounter for fracture <u>with delayed healing</u>
K   <u>Subsequent</u> encounter for fracture <u>with nonunion</u>
P   <u>Subsequent</u> encounter for fracture <u>with malunion</u>
S   <u>Sequela</u>

S52.211-   Greenstick fracture of shaft of <u>right</u> ulna

S52.212-   Greenstick fracture of shaft of <u>left</u> ulna

S52.219-   Greenstick fracture of shaft of <u>unspecified</u> ulna

S52.22-   <u>Transverse</u> fracture of <u>shaft</u> of <u>ulna</u>

S52.221-   <u>Displaced</u> transverse fracture of shaft of <u>right</u> ulna

S52.222-   <u>Displaced</u> transverse fracture of shaft of <u>left</u> ulna

S52.223-   <u>Displaced</u> transverse fracture of shaft of <u>unspecified</u> ulna

S52.224-   <u>Nondisplaced</u> transverse fracture of shaft of <u>right</u> ulna

S52.225-   <u>Nondisplaced</u> transverse fracture of shaft of <u>left</u> ulna

S52.226-   <u>Nondisplaced</u> transverse fracture of shaft of <u>unspecified</u> ulna

S52.23-   <u>Oblique</u> fracture of <u>shaft</u> of <u>ulna</u>

S52.231-   <u>Displaced</u> oblique fracture of shaft of <u>right</u> ulna

S52.232-   <u>Displaced</u> oblique fracture of shaft of <u>left</u> ulna

S52.233-   <u>Displaced</u> oblique fracture of shaft of <u>unspecified</u> ulna

S52.234-   <u>Nondisplaced</u> oblique fracture of shaft of <u>right</u> ulna

S52.235-   <u>Nondisplaced</u> oblique fracture of shaft of <u>left</u> ulna

S52.236-   <u>Nondisplaced</u> oblique fracture of shaft of <u>unspecified</u> ulna

S52.24-   <u>Spiral</u> fracture of <u>shaft</u> of <u>ulna</u>

S52.241-   <u>Displaced</u> spiral fracture of shaft of ulna, <u>right</u> arm

S52.242-   <u>Displaced</u> spiral fracture of shaft of ulna, <u>left</u> arm

S52.243-   <u>Displaced</u> spiral fracture of shaft of ulna, <u>unspecified</u> arm

S52.244-   <u>Nondisplaced</u> spiral fracture of shaft of ulna, <u>right</u> arm

S52.245-   <u>Nondisplaced</u> spiral fracture of shaft of ulna, <u>left</u> arm

S52.246-   <u>Nondisplaced</u> spiral fracture of shaft of ulna, <u>unspecified</u> arm

S52.25-   <u>Comminuted</u> fracture of <u>shaft</u> of <u>ulna</u>

S52.251-   <u>Displaced</u> comminuted fracture of shaft of ulna, <u>right</u> arm

S52.252-   <u>Displaced</u> comminuted fracture of shaft of ulna, <u>left</u> arm

S52.253-   <u>Displaced</u> comminuted fracture of shaft of ulna, <u>unspecified</u> arm

S52.254-   <u>Nondisplaced</u> comminuted fracture of shaft of ulna, <u>right</u> arm

S52.255-   <u>Nondisplaced</u> comminuted fracture of shaft of ulna, <u>left</u> arm

S52.256-   <u>Nondisplaced</u> comminuted fracture of shaft of ulna, <u>unspecified</u> arm

S52.26-   <u>Segmental</u> fracture of <u>shaft</u> of <u>ulna</u>

S52.261-   <u>Displaced</u> segmental fracture of shaft of ulna, <u>right</u> arm

S52.262-   <u>Displaced</u> segmental fracture of shaft of ulna, <u>left</u> arm

S52.263-   <u>Displaced</u> segmental fracture of shaft of ulna, <u>unspecified</u> arm

S52.264-   <u>Nondisplaced</u> segmental fracture of shaft of ulna, <u>right</u> arm

S52.265-   <u>Nondisplaced</u> segmental fracture of shaft of ulna, <u>left</u> arm

S52.266-   <u>Nondisplaced</u> segmental fracture of shaft of ulna, <u>unspecified</u> arm

S52.27-   <u>Monteggia's</u> fracture of <u>ulna</u>
Fracture of upper shaft of ulna with dislocation of radial head

S52.271-   Monteggia's fracture of <u>right</u> ulna

S52.272-   Monteggia's fracture of <u>left</u> ulna

S52.279-   Monteggia's fracture of <u>unspecified</u> ulna

S52.28-   <u>Bent bone</u> of <u>ulna</u>

S52.281-   Bent bone of <u>right</u> ulna

S52.282-   Bent bone of <u>left</u> ulna

S52.283-   Bent bone of <u>unspecified</u> ulna

S52.29-   <u>Other</u> fracture of <u>shaft</u> of <u>ulna</u>

S52.291-   Other fracture of shaft of <u>right</u> ulna

S52.292-   Other fracture of shaft of <u>left</u> ulna

S52.299-   Other fracture of shaft of <u>unspecified</u> ulna

S52.3-   Fracture of <u>shaft</u> of <u>radius</u>

S52.30-   <u>Unspecified</u> fracture of <u>shaft</u> of <u>radius</u>

S52.301-   Unspecified fracture of shaft of <u>right</u> radius

S52.302-   Unspecified fracture of shaft of <u>left</u> radius

S52.309-   Unspecified fracture of shaft of <u>unspecified</u> radius

S 5 2 – S 5 2

S52.31- Greenstick fracture of <u>shaft</u> of <u>radius</u>

The appropriate 7th character is to be added to all codes in subcategory S52.31:
- A   <u>Initial</u> encounter for <u>closed</u> fracture
- D   <u>Subsequent</u> encounter for fracture <u>with routine healing</u>
- G   <u>Subsequent</u> encounter for fracture <u>with delayed healing</u>
- K   <u>Subsequent</u> encounter for fracture <u>with nonunion</u>
- P   <u>Subsequent</u> encounter for fracture <u>with malunion</u>
- S   <u>Sequela</u>

- S52.311- Greenstick fracture of shaft of radius, <u>right</u> arm
- S52.312- Greenstick fracture of shaft of radius, <u>left</u> arm
- S52.319- Greenstick fracture of shaft of radius, <u>unspecified</u> arm

S52.32- <u>Transverse</u> fracture of <u>shaft</u> of <u>radius</u>
- S52.321- <u>Displaced</u> transverse fracture of shaft of <u>right</u> radius
- S52.322- <u>Displaced</u> transverse fracture of shaft of <u>left</u> radius
- S52.323- <u>Displaced</u> transverse fracture of shaft of <u>unspecified</u> radius
- S52.324- <u>Nondisplaced</u> transverse fracture of shaft of <u>right</u> radius
- S52.325- <u>Nondisplaced</u> transverse fracture of shaft of <u>left</u> radius
- S52.326- <u>Nondisplaced</u> transverse fracture of shaft of <u>unspecified</u> radius

S52.33- <u>Oblique</u> fracture of <u>shaft</u> of <u>radius</u>
- S52.331- <u>Displaced</u> oblique fracture of shaft of <u>right</u> radius
- S52.332- <u>Displaced</u> oblique fracture of shaft of <u>left</u> radius
- S52.333- <u>Displaced</u> oblique fracture of shaft of <u>unspecified</u> radius
- S52.334- <u>Nondisplaced</u> oblique fracture of shaft of <u>right</u> radius
- S52.335- <u>Nondisplaced</u> oblique fracture of shaft of <u>left</u> radius
- S52.336- <u>Nondisplaced</u> oblique fracture of shaft of <u>unspecified</u> radius

S52.34- <u>Spiral</u> fracture of <u>shaft</u> of <u>radius</u>
- S52.341- <u>Displaced</u> spiral fracture of shaft of radius, <u>right</u> arm
- S52.342- <u>Displaced</u> spiral fracture of shaft of radius, <u>left</u> arm
- S52.343- <u>Displaced</u> spiral fracture of shaft of radius, <u>unspecified</u> arm
- S52.344- <u>Nondisplaced</u> spiral fracture of shaft of radius, <u>right</u> arm
- S52.345- <u>Nondisplaced</u> spiral fracture of shaft of radius, <u>left</u> arm
- S52.346- <u>Nondisplaced</u> spiral fracture of shaft of radius, <u>unspecified</u> arm

S52.35- <u>Comminuted</u> fracture of <u>shaft</u> of <u>radius</u>
- S52.351- <u>Displaced</u> comminuted fracture of shaft of radius, <u>right</u> arm
- S52.352- <u>Displaced</u> comminuted fracture of shaft of radius, <u>left</u> arm
- S52.353- <u>Displaced</u> comminuted fracture of shaft of radius, <u>unspecified</u> arm
- S52.354- <u>Nondisplaced</u> comminuted fracture of shaft of radius, <u>right</u> arm
- S52.355- <u>Nondisplaced</u> comminuted fracture of shaft of radius, <u>left</u> arm
- S52.356- <u>Nondisplaced</u> comminuted fracture of shaft of radius, <u>unspecified</u> arm

S52.36- <u>Segmental</u> fracture of <u>shaft</u> of <u>radius</u>
- S52.361- <u>Displaced</u> segmental fracture of shaft of radius, <u>right</u> arm
- S52.362- <u>Displaced</u> segmental fracture of shaft of radius, <u>left</u> arm
- S52.363- <u>Displaced</u> segmental fracture of shaft of radius, <u>unspecified</u> arm
- S52.364- <u>Nondisplaced</u> segmental fracture of shaft of radius, <u>right</u> arm
- S52.365- <u>Nondisplaced</u> segmental fracture of shaft of radius, <u>left</u> arm
- S52.366- <u>Nondisplaced</u> segmental fracture of shaft of radius, <u>unspecified</u> arm

S52.37- <u>Galeazzi's</u> fracture
    Fracture of lower shaft of radius with radioulnar joint dislocation
- S52.371- Galeazzi's fracture of <u>right</u> radius
- S52.372- Galeazzi's fracture of <u>left</u> radius
- S52.379- Galeazzi's fracture of <u>unspecified</u> radius

S52.38- <u>Bent bone</u> of <u>radius</u>
- S52.381- Bent bone of <u>right</u> radius
- S52.382- Bent bone of <u>left</u> radius
- S52.389- Bent bone of <u>unspecified</u> radius

S52.39- <u>Other</u> fracture of <u>shaft</u> of <u>radius</u>
- S52.391- Other fracture of shaft of radius, <u>right</u> arm
- S52.392- Other fracture of shaft of radius, <u>left</u> arm
- S52.399- Other fracture of shaft of radius, <u>unspecified</u> arm

S52.5- Fracture of <u>lower end</u> of <u>radius</u>
    Fracture of distal end of radius
    Excludes❷: physeal fractures of lower end of radius (S59.2-)

S52.50- <u>Unspecified</u> fracture of the <u>lower end</u> of <u>radius</u>
- S52.501- Unspecified fracture of the lower end of <u>right</u> radius
- S52.502- Unspecified fracture of the lower end of <u>left</u> radius
- S52.509- Unspecified fracture of the lower end of <u>unspecified</u> radius

S52.51- <u>Fracture</u> of <u>radial styloid process</u>
- S52.511- <u>Displaced</u> fracture of <u>right</u> radial styloid process
- S52.512- <u>Displaced</u> fracture of <u>left</u> radial styloid process
- S52.513- <u>Displaced</u> fracture of <u>unspecified</u> radial styloid process
- S52.514- <u>Nondisplaced</u> fracture of <u>right</u> radial styloid process
- S52.515- <u>Nondisplaced</u> fracture of <u>left</u> radial styloid process
- S52.516- <u>Nondisplaced</u> fracture of <u>unspecified</u> radial styloid process

S52.52- <u>Torus</u> fracture of <u>lower end</u> of <u>radius</u>

The appropriate 7th character is to be added to all codes in subcategory S52.52:
- A   <u>Initial</u> encounter for <u>closed</u> fracture
- D   <u>Subsequent</u> encounter for fracture <u>with routine healing</u>
- G   <u>Subsequent</u> encounter for fracture <u>with delayed healing</u>
- K   <u>Subsequent</u> encounter for fracture <u>with nonunion</u>
- P   <u>Subsequent</u> encounter for fracture <u>with malunion</u>
- S   <u>Sequela</u>

- S52.521- Torus fracture of lower end of <u>right</u> radius
- S52.522- Torus fracture of lower end of <u>left</u> radius
- S52.529- Torus fracture of lower end of <u>unspecified</u> radius

S52.53- <u>Colles'</u> fracture
- S52.531- Colles' fracture of <u>right</u> radius
- S52.532- Colles' fracture of <u>left</u> radius
- S52.539- Colles' fracture of <u>unspecified</u> radius

S52.54- <u>Smith's</u> fracture
- S52.541- Smith's fracture of <u>right</u> radius
- S52.542- Smith's fracture of <u>left</u> radius
- S52.549- Smith's fracture of <u>unspecified</u> radius

S52.55- <u>Other</u> <u>extraarticular</u> fracture of <u>lower end</u> of <u>radius</u>
- S52.551- Other extraarticular fracture of lower end of <u>right</u> radius
- S52.552- Other extraarticular fracture of lower end of <u>left</u> radius
- S52.559- Other extraarticular fracture of lower end of <u>unspecified</u> radius

S52.56- <u>Barton's</u> fracture
- S52.561- Barton's fracture of <u>right</u> radius
- S52.562- Barton's fracture of <u>left</u> radius
- S52.569- Barton's fracture of <u>unspecified</u> radius

S52.57- <u>Other</u> <u>intraarticular</u> fracture of <u>lower end</u> of <u>radius</u>
- S52.571- Other intraarticular fracture of lower end of <u>right</u> radius
- S52.572- Other intraarticular fracture of lower end of <u>left</u> radius
- S52.579- Other intraarticular fracture of lower end of <u>unspecified</u> radius

S52.59- <u>Other</u> fractures of <u>lower end</u> of <u>radius</u>
- S52.591- Other fractures of lower end of <u>right</u> radius
- S52.592- Other fractures of lower end of <u>left</u> radius
- S52.599- Other fractures of lower end of <u>unspecified</u> radius

S52.6- Fracture of <u>lower end</u> of <u>ulna</u>

S52.60- <u>Unspecified</u> fracture of <u>lower end</u> of <u>ulna</u>
- S52.601- Unspecified fracture of lower end of <u>right</u> ulna
- S52.602- Unspecified fracture of lower end of <u>left</u> ulna
- S52.609- Unspecified fracture of lower end of <u>unspecified</u> ulna

S52 – S52

S52.61- Fracture of <u>ulna styloid process</u>
    S52.611- <u>Displaced</u> fracture of <u>right</u> ulna styloid process
    S52.612- <u>Displaced</u> fracture of <u>left</u> ulna styloid process
    S52.613- <u>Displaced</u> fracture of <u>unspecified</u> ulna styloid process
    S52.614- <u>Nondisplaced</u> fracture of <u>right</u> ulna styloid process
    S52.615- <u>Nondisplaced</u> fracture of <u>left</u> ulna styloid process
    S52.616- <u>Nondisplaced</u> fracture of <u>unspecified</u> ulna styloid process
S52.62- <u>Torus</u> fracture of <u>lower end</u> of <u>ulna</u>

> **The appropriate 7th character is to be added to all codes in subcategory S52.62:**
> **A**   <u>Initial</u> encounter for <u>closed</u> fracture
> **D**   <u>Subsequent</u> encounter for fracture <u>with routine healing</u>
> **G**   <u>Subsequent</u> encounter for fracture <u>with delayed healing</u>
> **K**   <u>Subsequent</u> encounter for fracture <u>with nonunion</u>
> **P**   <u>Subsequent</u> encounter for fracture <u>with malunion</u>
> **S**   <u>Sequela</u>

    S52.621- Torus fracture of lower end of <u>right</u> ulna
    S52.622- Torus fracture of lower end of <u>left</u> ulna
    S52.629- Torus fracture of lower end of <u>unspecified</u> ulna
S52.69- <u>Other</u> fracture of <u>lower end</u> of <u>ulna</u>
    S52.691- Other fracture of lower end of <u>right</u> ulna
    S52.692- Other fracture of lower end of <u>left</u> ulna
    S52.699- Other fracture of lower end of <u>unspecified</u> ulna
S52.9- <u>Unspecified</u> fracture of <u>forearm</u>
    S52.90x- Unspecified fracture of <u>unspecified</u> forearm
    S52.91x- Unspecified fracture of <u>right</u> forearm
    S52.92x- Unspecified fracture of <u>left</u> forearm

S53- <u>Dislocation and sprain</u> of joints and ligaments of <u>elbow</u>
  Includes: Avulsion of joint or ligament of elbow
              Laceration of cartilage, joint or ligament of elbow
              Sprain of cartilage, joint or ligament of elbow
              Traumatic hemarthrosis of joint or ligament of elbow
              Traumatic rupture of joint or ligament of elbow
              Traumatic subluxation of joint or ligament of elbow
              Traumatic tear of joint or ligament of elbow
  Code also any associated open wound
  Excludes❷: strain of muscle, fascia and tendon at forearm level (S56.-)

> **The appropriate 7th character is to be added to each code from category S53:**
> **A**   <u>Initial</u> encounter
> **D**   <u>Subsequent</u> encounter
> **S**   <u>Sequela</u>

S53.0- <u>Subluxation and dislocation</u> of <u>radial head</u>
     Dislocation of radiohumeral joint
     Subluxation of radiohumeral joint
     Excludes 1: Monteggia's fracture-dislocation (S52.27-)
    S53.00- <u>Unspecified</u> subluxation and dislocation of <u>radial head</u>
      S53.001- Unspecified <u>subluxation</u> of <u>right</u> radial head
      S53.002- Unspecified <u>subluxation</u> of <u>left</u> radial head
      S53.003- Unspecified <u>subluxation</u> of <u>unspecified</u> radial head
      S53.004- Unspecified <u>dislocation</u> of <u>right</u> radial head
      S53.005- Unspecified <u>dislocation</u> of <u>left</u> radial head
      S53.006- Unspecified <u>dislocation</u> of <u>unspecified</u> radial head
    S53.01- <u>Anterior</u> subluxation and dislocation of <u>radial head</u>
       Anteriomedial subluxation and dislocation of radial head
      S53.011- Anterior <u>subluxation</u> of <u>right</u> radial head
      S53.012- Anterior <u>subluxation</u> of <u>left</u> radial head
      S53.013- Anterior <u>subluxation</u> of <u>unspecified</u> radial head
      S53.014- Anterior <u>dislocation</u> of <u>right</u> radial head
      S53.015- Anterior <u>dislocation</u> of <u>left</u> radial head
      S53.016- Anterior <u>dislocation</u> of <u>unspecified</u> radial head
    S53.02- <u>Posterior</u> subluxation and dislocation of <u>radial head</u>
       Posteriolateral subluxation and dislocation of radial head
      S53.021- Posterior <u>subluxation</u> of <u>right</u> radial head
      S53.022- Posterior <u>subluxation</u> of <u>left</u> radial head
      S53.023- Posterior <u>subluxation</u> of <u>unspecified</u> radial head
      S53.024- Posterior <u>dislocation</u> of <u>right</u> radial head
      S53.025- Posterior <u>dislocation</u> of <u>left</u> radial head
      S53.026- Posterior <u>dislocation</u> of <u>unspecified</u> radial head
    S53.03- <u>Nursemaid's</u> elbow
      S53.031- Nursemaid's elbow, <u>right</u> elbow
      S53.032- Nursemaid's elbow, <u>left</u> elbow
      S53.033- Nursemaid's elbow, <u>unspecified</u> elbow

S53.09- <u>Other</u> subluxation and dislocation of <u>radial head</u>
    S53.091- Other <u>subluxation</u> of <u>right</u> radial head
    S53.092- Other <u>subluxation</u> of <u>left</u> radial head
    S53.093- Other <u>subluxation</u> of <u>unspecified</u> radial head
    S53.094- Other <u>dislocation</u> of <u>right</u> radial head
    S53.095- Other <u>dislocation</u> of <u>left</u> radial head
    S53.096- Other <u>dislocation</u> of <u>unspecified</u> radial head
S53.1- <u>Subluxation and dislocation</u> of <u>ulnohumeral joint</u>
   Subluxation and dislocation of elbow NOS
   Excludes 1: dislocation of radial head alone (S53.0-)
    S53.10- <u>Unspecified</u> subluxation and dislocation of <u>ulnohumeral joint</u>
      S53.101- Unspecified <u>subluxation</u> of <u>right</u> ulnohumeral joint
      S53.102- Unspecified <u>subluxation</u> of <u>left</u> ulnohumeral joint
      S53.103- Unspecified <u>subluxation</u> of <u>unspecified</u> ulnohumeral joint
      S53.104- Unspecified <u>dislocation</u> of <u>right</u> ulnohumeral joint
      S53.105- Unspecified <u>dislocation</u> of <u>left</u> ulnohumeral joint
      S53.106- Unspecified <u>dislocation</u> of <u>unspecified</u> ulnohumeral joint
    S53.11- <u>Anterior</u> subluxation and dislocation of <u>ulnohumeral joint</u>
      S53.111- Anterior <u>subluxation</u> of <u>right</u> ulnohumeral joint
      S53.112- Anterior <u>subluxation</u> of <u>left</u> ulnohumeral joint
      S53.113- Anterior <u>subluxation</u> of <u>unspecified</u> ulnohumeral joint
      S53.114- Anterior <u>dislocation</u> of <u>right</u> ulnohumeral joint
      S53.115- Anterior <u>dislocation</u> of <u>left</u> ulnohumeral joint
      S53.116- Anterior <u>dislocation</u> of <u>unspecified</u> ulnohumeral joint
    S53.12- <u>Posterior</u> subluxation and dislocation of <u>ulnohumeral joint</u>
      S53.121- Posterior <u>subluxation</u> of <u>right</u> ulnohumeral joint
      S53.122- Posterior <u>subluxation</u> of <u>left</u> ulnohumeral joint
      S53.123- Posterior <u>subluxation</u> of <u>unspecified</u> ulnohumeral joint
      S53.124- Posterior <u>dislocation</u> of <u>right</u> ulnohumeral joint
      S53.125- Posterior <u>dislocation</u> of <u>left</u> ulnohumeral joint
      S53.126- Posterior <u>dislocation</u> of <u>unspecified</u> ulnohumeral joint
    S53.13- <u>Medial</u> subluxation and dislocation of <u>ulnohumeral joint</u>
      S53.131- Medial <u>subluxation</u> of <u>right</u> ulnohumeral joint
      S53.132- Medial <u>subluxation</u> of <u>left</u> ulnohumeral joint
      S53.133- Medial <u>subluxation</u> of <u>unspecified</u> ulnohumeral joint
      S53.134- Medial <u>dislocation</u> of <u>right</u> ulnohumeral joint
      S53.135- Medial <u>dislocation</u> of <u>left</u> ulnohumeral joint
      S53.136- Medial <u>dislocation</u> of <u>unspecified</u> ulnohumeral joint
    S53.14- <u>Lateral</u> subluxation and dislocation of <u>ulnohumeral joint</u>
      S53.141- Lateral <u>subluxation</u> of <u>right</u> ulnohumeral joint
      S53.142- Lateral <u>subluxation</u> of <u>left</u> ulnohumeral joint
      S53.143- Lateral <u>subluxation</u> of <u>unspecified</u> ulnohumeral joint
      S53.144- Lateral <u>dislocation</u> of <u>right</u> ulnohumeral joint
      S53.145- Lateral <u>dislocation</u> of <u>left</u> ulnohumeral joint
      S53.146- Lateral <u>dislocation</u> of <u>unspecified</u> ulnohumeral joint
    S53.19- <u>Other</u> subluxation and dislocation of <u>ulnohumeral joint</u>
      S53.191- Other <u>subluxation</u> of <u>right</u> ulnohumeral joint
      S53.192- Other <u>subluxation</u> of <u>left</u> ulnohumeral joint
      S53.193- Other <u>subluxation</u> of <u>unspecified</u> ulnohumeral joint
      S53.194- Other <u>dislocation</u> of <u>right</u> ulnohumeral joint
      S53.195- Other <u>dislocation</u> of <u>left</u> ulnohumeral joint
      S53.196- Other <u>dislocation</u> of <u>unspecified</u> ulnohumeral joint
S53.2- <u>Traumatic rupture</u> of <u>radial collateral ligament</u>
   Excludes 1: sprain of radial collateral ligament NOS (S53.43-)
    S53.20x- Traumatic rupture of <u>unspecified</u> radial collateral ligament
    S53.21x- Traumatic rupture of <u>right</u> radial collateral ligament
    S53.22x- Traumatic rupture of <u>left</u> radial collateral ligament
S53.3- <u>Traumatic rupture</u> of <u>ulnar collateral ligament</u>
   Excludes 1: sprain of ulnar collateral ligament (S53.44-)
    S53.30x- Traumatic rupture of <u>unspecified</u> ulnar collateral ligament
    S53.31x- Traumatic rupture of <u>right</u> ulnar collateral ligament
    S53.32x- Traumatic rupture of <u>left</u> ulnar collateral ligament
S53.4- <u>Sprain</u> of <u>elbow</u>
   Excludes❷: traumatic rupture of radial collateral ligament (S53.2-)
              traumatic rupture of ulnar collateral ligament (S53.3-)
    S53.40- <u>Unspecified</u> sprain of <u>elbow</u>
      S53.401- Unspecified sprain of <u>right</u> elbow
      S53.402- Unspecified sprain of <u>left</u> elbow
      S53.409- Unspecified sprain of <u>unspecified</u> elbow
         Sprain of elbow NOS

S52 - S55

S53.41- Radiohumeral (joint) sprain
- **S53.411-** Radiohumeral (joint) sprain of right elbow
- **S53.412-** Radiohumeral (joint) sprain of left elbow
- **S53.419-** Radiohumeral (joint) sprain of unspecified elbow

S53.42- Ulnohumeral (joint) sprain
- **S53.421-** Ulnohumeral (joint) sprain of right elbow
- **S53.422-** Ulnohumeral (joint) sprain of left elbow
- **S53.429-** Ulnohumeral (joint) sprain of unspecified elbow

S53.43- Radial collateral ligament sprain
- **S53.431-** Radial collateral ligament sprain of right elbow
- **S53.432-** Radial collateral ligament sprain of left elbow
- **S53.439-** Radial collateral ligament sprain of unspecified elbow

S53.44- Ulnar collateral ligament sprain
- **S53.441-** Ulnar collateral ligament sprain of right elbow
- **S53.442-** Ulnar collateral ligament sprain of left elbow
- **S53.449-** Ulnar collateral ligament sprain of unspecified elbow

S53.49- Other sprain of elbow
- **S53.491-** Other sprain of right elbow
- **S53.492-** Other sprain of left elbow
- **S53.499-** Other sprain of unspecified elbow

S54- Injury of nerves at forearm level
Code also any associated open wound (S51.-)
Excludes❷: injury of nerves at wrist and hand level (S64.-)
The appropriate 7th character is to be added to each code from category S54:
- **A**   Initial encounter
- **D**   Subsequent encounter
- **S**   Sequela

S54.0- Injury of ulnar nerve at forearm level
Injury of ulnar nerve NOS
- **S54.00x-** Injury of ulnar nerve at forearm level, unspecified arm
- **S54.01x-** Injury of ulnar nerve at forearm level, right arm
- **S54.02x-** Injury of ulnar nerve at forearm level, left arm

S54.1- Injury of median nerve at forearm level
Injury of median nerve NOS
- **S54.10x-** Injury of median nerve at forearm level, unspecified arm
- **S54.11x-** Injury of median nerve at forearm level, right arm
- **S54.12x-** Injury of median nerve at forearm level, left arm

S54.2- Injury of radial nerve at forearm level
Injury of radial nerve NOS
- **S54.20x-** Injury of radial nerve at forearm level, unspecified arm
- **S54.21x-** Injury of radial nerve at forearm level, right arm
- **S54.22x-** Injury of radial nerve at forearm level, left arm

S54.3- Injury of cutaneous sensory nerve at forearm level
- **S54.30x-** Injury of cutaneous sensory nerve at forearm level, unspecified arm
- **S54.31x-** Injury of cutaneous sensory nerve at forearm level, right arm
- **S54.32x-** Injury of cutaneous sensory nerve at forearm level, left arm

S54.8- Injury of other nerves at forearm level
- **S54.8x-** Unspecified injury of other nerves at forearm level
  - **S54.8x1-** Unspecified injury of other nerves at forearm level, right arm
  - **S54.8x2-** Unspecified injury of other nerves at forearm level, left arm
  - **S54.8x9-** Unspecified injury of other nerves at forearm level, unspecified arm

S54.9- Injury of unspecified nerve at forearm level
- **S54.90x-** Injury of unspecified nerve at forearm level, unspecified arm
- **S54.91x-** Injury of unspecified nerve at forearm level, right arm
- **S54.92x-** Injury of unspecified nerve at forearm level, left arm

S55- Injury of blood vessels at forearm level
Code also any associated open wound (S51.-)
Excludes❷: injury of blood vessels at wrist and hand level (S65.-)
          injury of brachial vessels (S45.1-S45.2)
The appropriate 7th character is to be added to each code from category S55:
- **A**   Initial encounter
- **D**   Subsequent encounter
- **S**   Sequela

S55.0- Injury of ulnar artery at forearm level
- **S55.00-** Unspecified injury of ulnar artery at forearm level
  - **S55.001-** Unspecified injury of ulnar artery at forearm level, right arm
  - **S55.002-** Unspecified injury of ulnar artery at forearm level, left arm
  - **S55.009-** Unspecified injury of ulnar artery at forearm level, unspecified arm
- **S55.01-** Laceration of ulnar artery at forearm level
  - **S55.011-** Laceration of ulnar artery at forearm level, right arm
  - **S55.012-** Laceration of ulnar artery at forearm level, left arm
  - **S55.019-** Laceration of ulnar artery at forearm level, unspecified arm
- **S55.09-** Other specified injury of ulnar artery at forearm level
  - **S55.091-** Other specified injury of ulnar artery at forearm level, right arm
  - **S55.092-** Other specified injury of ulnar artery at forearm level, left arm
  - **S55.099-** Other specified injury of ulnar artery at forearm level, unspecified arm

S55.1- Injury of radial artery at forearm level
- **S55.10-** Unspecified injury of radial artery at forearm level
  - **S55.101-** Unspecified injury of radial artery at forearm level, right arm
  - **S55.102-** Unspecified injury of radial artery at forearm level, left arm
  - **S55.109-** Unspecified injury of radial artery at forearm level, unspecified arm
- **S55.11-** Laceration of radial artery at forearm level
  - **S55.111-** Laceration of radial artery at forearm level, right arm
  - **S55.112-** Laceration of radial artery at forearm level, left arm
  - **S55.119-** Laceration of radial artery at forearm level, unspecified arm
- **S55.19-** Other specified injury of radial artery at forearm level
  - **S55.191-** Other specified injury of radial artery at forearm level, right arm
  - **S55.192-** Other specified injury of radial artery at forearm level, left arm
  - **S55.199-** Other specified injury of radial artery at forearm level, unspecified arm

S55.2- Injury of vein at forearm level
- **S55.20-** Unspecified injury of vein at forearm level
  - **S55.201-** Unspecified injury of vein at forearm level, right arm
  - **S55.202-** Unspecified injury of vein at forearm level, left arm
  - **S55.209-** Unspecified injury of vein at forearm level, unspecified arm
- **S55.21-** Laceration of vein at forearm level
  - **S55.211-** Laceration of vein at forearm level, right arm
  - **S55.212-** Laceration of vein at forearm level, left arm
  - **S55.219-** Laceration of vein at forearm level, unspecified arm
- **S55.29-** Other specified injury of vein at forearm level
  - **S55.291-** Other specified injury of vein at forearm level, right arm
  - **S55.292-** Other specified injury of vein at forearm level, left arm
  - **S55.299-** Other specified injury of vein at forearm level, unspecified arm

S55.8- Injury of other blood vessels at forearm level
- **S55.80-** Unspecified injury of other blood vessels at forearm level
  - **S55.801-** Unspecified injury of other blood vessels at forearm level, right arm
  - **S55.802-** Unspecified injury of other blood vessels at forearm level, left arm
  - **S55.809-** Unspecified injury of other blood vessels at forearm level, unspecified arm

S 5 2 – S 5 5

© 2013 Channel Publishing, Ltd.

S55.81-   Laceration of other blood vessels at forearm level

  S55.811-   Laceration of other blood vessels at forearm level, right arm

  S55.812-   Laceration of other blood vessels at forearm level, left arm

  S55.819-   Laceration of other blood vessels at forearm level, unspecified arm

S55.89-   Other specified injury of other blood vessels at forearm level

  S55.891-   Other specified injury of other blood vessels at forearm level, right arm

  S55.892-   Other specified injury of other blood vessels at forearm level, left arm

  S55.899-   Other specified injury of other blood vessels at forearm level, unspecified arm

S55.9-   Injury of unspecified blood vessel at forearm level

  S55.90-   Unspecified injury of unspecified blood vessel at forearm level

    S55.901-   Unspecified injury of unspecified blood vessel at forearm level, right arm

    S55.902-   Unspecified injury of unspecified blood vessel at forearm level, left arm

    S55.909-   Unspecified injury of unspecified blood vessel at forearm level, unspecified arm

  S55.91-   Laceration of unspecified blood vessel at forearm level

    S55.911-   Laceration of unspecified blood vessel at forearm level, right arm

    S55.912-   Laceration of unspecified blood vessel at forearm level, left arm

    S55.919-   Laceration of unspecified blood vessel at forearm level, unspecified arm

  S55.99-   Other specified injury of unspecified blood vessel at forearm level

    S55.991-   Other specified injury of unspecified blood vessel at forearm level, right arm

    S55.992-   Other specified injury of unspecified blood vessel at forearm level, left arm

    S55.999-   Other specified injury of unspecified blood vessel at forearm level, unspecified arm

S56-   Injury of muscle, fascia and tendon at forearm level

Code also any associated open wound (S51.-)

Excludes❷: injury of muscle, fascia and tendon at or below wrist (S66.-)
sprain of joints and ligaments of elbow (S53.4-)

The appropriate 7th character is to be added to each code from category S56:
A   Initial encounter
D   Subsequent encounter
S   Sequela

S56.0-   Injury of flexor muscle, fascia and tendon of thumb at forearm level

  S56.00-   Unspecified injury of flexor muscle, fascia and tendon of thumb at forearm level

    S56.001-   Unspecified injury of flexor muscle, fascia and tendon of right thumb at forearm level

    S56.002-   Unspecified injury of flexor muscle, fascia and tendon of left thumb at forearm level

    S56.009-   Unspecified injury of flexor muscle, fascia and tendon of unspecified thumb at forearm level

  S56.01-   Strain of flexor muscle, fascia and tendon of thumb at forearm level

    S56.011-   Strain of flexor muscle, fascia and tendon of right thumb at forearm level

    S56.012-   Strain of flexor muscle, fascia and tendon of left thumb at forearm level

    S56.019-   Strain of flexor muscle, fascia and tendon of unspecified thumb at forearm level

  S56.02-   Laceration of flexor muscle, fascia and tendon of thumb at forearm level

    S56.021-   Laceration of flexor muscle, fascia and tendon of right thumb at forearm level

    S56.022-   Laceration of flexor muscle, fascia and tendon of left thumb at forearm level

    S56.029-   Laceration of flexor muscle, fascia and tendon of unspecified thumb at forearm level

  S56.09-   Other injury of flexor muscle, fascia and tendon of thumb at forearm level

    S56.091-   Other injury of flexor muscle, fascia and tendon of right thumb at forearm level

    S56.092-   Other injury of flexor muscle, fascia and tendon of left thumb at forearm level

    S56.099-   Other injury of flexor muscle, fascia and tendon of unspecified thumb at forearm level

S56.1-   Injury of flexor muscle, fascia and tendon of other and unspecified finger at forearm level

  S56.10-   Unspecified injury of flexor muscle, fascia and tendon of other and unspecified finger at forearm level

    S56.101-   Unspecified injury of flexor muscle, fascia and tendon of right index finger at forearm level

    S56.102-   Unspecified injury of flexor muscle, fascia and tendon of left index finger at forearm level

    S56.103-   Unspecified injury of flexor muscle, fascia and tendon of right middle finger at forearm level

    S56.104-   Unspecified injury of flexor muscle, fascia and tendon of left middle finger at forearm level

    S56.105-   Unspecified injury of flexor muscle, fascia and tendon of right ring finger at forearm level

    S56.106-   Unspecified injury of flexor muscle, fascia and tendon of left ring finger at forearm level

    S56.107-   Unspecified injury of flexor muscle, fascia and tendon of right little finger at forearm level

    S56.108-   Unspecified injury of flexor muscle, fascia and tendon of left little finger at forearm level

    S56.109-   Unspecified injury of flexor muscle, fascia and tendon of unspecified finger at forearm level

  S56.11-   Strain of flexor muscle, fascia and tendon of other and unspecified finger at forearm level

    S56.111-   Strain of flexor muscle, fascia and tendon of right index finger at forearm level

    S56.112-   Strain of flexor muscle, fascia and tendon of left index finger at forearm level

    S56.113-   Strain of flexor muscle, fascia and tendon of right middle finger at forearm level

    S56.114-   Strain of flexor muscle, fascia and tendon of left middle finger at forearm level

    S56.115-   Strain of flexor muscle, fascia and tendon of right ring finger at forearm level

    S56.116-   Strain of flexor muscle, fascia and tendon of left ring finger at forearm level

    S56.117-   Strain of flexor muscle, fascia and tendon of right little finger at forearm level

    S56.118-   Strain of flexor muscle, fascia and tendon of left little finger at forearm level

    S56.119-   Strain of flexor muscle, fascia and tendon of finger of unspecified finger at forearm level

  S56.12-   Laceration of flexor muscle, fascia and tendon of other and unspecified finger at forearm level

    S56.121-   Laceration of flexor muscle, fascia and tendon of right index finger at forearm level

    S56.122-   Laceration of flexor muscle, fascia and tendon of left index finger at forearm level

    S56.123-   Laceration of flexor muscle, fascia and tendon of right middle finger at forearm level

    S56.124-   Laceration of flexor muscle, fascia and tendon of left middle finger at forearm level

    S56.125-   Laceration of flexor muscle, fascia and tendon of right ring finger at forearm level

    S56.126-   Laceration of flexor muscle, fascia and tendon of left ring finger at forearm level

    S56.127-   Laceration of flexor muscle, fascia and tendon of right little finger at forearm level

    S56.128-   Laceration of flexor muscle, fascia and tendon of left little finger at forearm level

    S56.129-   Laceration of flexor muscle, fascia and tendon of unspecified finger at forearm level

  S56.19-   Other injury of flexor muscle, fascia and tendon of other and unspecified finger at forearm level

    S56.191-   Other injury of flexor muscle, fascia and tendon of right index finger at forearm level

    S56.192-   Other injury of flexor muscle, fascia and tendon of left index finger at forearm level

    S56.193-   Other injury of flexor muscle, fascia and tendon of right middle finger at forearm level

    S56.194-   Other injury of flexor muscle, fascia and tendon of left middle finger at forearm level

    S56.195-   Other injury of flexor muscle, fascia and tendon of right ring finger at forearm level

    S56.196-   Other injury of flexor muscle, fascia and tendon of left ring finger at forearm level

    S56.197-   Other injury of flexor muscle, fascia and tendon of right little finger at forearm level

S56.198-   Other injury of flexor muscle, fascia and tendon of <u>left</u> <u>little</u> finger at forearm level

S56.199-   Other injury of flexor muscle, fascia and tendon of <u>unspecified</u> <u>finger</u> at forearm level

S56.2-   <u>Injury</u> of <u>other flexor</u> muscle, fascia and tendon at <u>forearm level</u>

  S56.20-   <u>Unspecified</u> injury of <u>other flexor</u> muscle, fascia and tendon at <u>forearm level</u>

    S56.201-   Unspecified injury of other flexor muscle, fascia and tendon at forearm level, <u>right</u> arm

    S56.202-   Unspecified injury of other flexor muscle, fascia and tendon at forearm level, <u>left</u> arm

    S56.209-   Unspecified injury of other flexor muscle, fascia and tendon at forearm level, <u>unspecified</u> arm

  S56.21-   <u>Strain</u> of <u>other flexor</u> muscle, fascia and tendon at <u>forearm level</u>

    S56.211-   Strain of other flexor muscle, fascia and tendon at forearm level, <u>right</u> arm

    S56.212-   Strain of other flexor muscle, fascia and tendon at forearm level, <u>left</u> arm

    S56.219-   Strain of other flexor muscle, fascia and tendon at forearm level, <u>unspecified</u> arm

  S56.22-   <u>Laceration</u> of <u>other flexor</u> muscle, fascia and tendon at <u>forearm level</u>

    S56.221-   Laceration of other flexor muscle, fascia and tendon at forearm level, <u>right</u> arm

    S56.222-   Laceration of other flexor muscle, fascia and tendon at forearm level, <u>left</u> arm

    S56.229-   Laceration of other flexor muscle, fascia and tendon at forearm level, <u>unspecified</u> arm

  S56.29-   <u>Other injury</u> of <u>other flexor</u> muscle, fascia and tendon at <u>forearm level</u>

    S56.291-   Other injury of other flexor muscle, fascia and tendon at forearm level, <u>right</u> arm

    S56.292-   Other injury of other flexor muscle, fascia and tendon at forearm level, <u>left</u> arm

    S56.299-   Other injury of other flexor muscle, fascia and tendon at forearm level, <u>unspecified</u> arm

S56.3-   <u>Injury</u> of <u>extensor or abductor</u> muscles, fascia and tendons of <u>thumb</u> at <u>forearm level</u>

  S56.30-   <u>Unspecified</u> injury of <u>extensor or abductor</u> muscles, fascia and tendons of <u>thumb</u> at <u>forearm level</u>

    S56.301-   Unspecified injury of extensor or abductor muscles, fascia and tendons of <u>right</u> thumb at forearm level

    S56.302-   Unspecified injury of extensor or abductor muscles, fascia and tendons of <u>left</u> thumb at forearm level

    S56.309-   Unspecified injury of extensor or abductor muscles, fascia and tendons of <u>unspecified</u> thumb at forearm level

  S56.31-   <u>Strain</u> of <u>extensor or abductor muscles</u>, fascia and tendons of <u>thumb</u> at <u>forearm level</u>

    S56.311-   Strain of extensor or abductor muscles, fascia and tendons of <u>right</u> thumb at forearm level

    S56.312-   Strain of extensor or abductor muscles, fascia and tendons of <u>left</u> thumb at forearm level

    S56.319-   Strain of extensor or abductor muscles, fascia and tendons of <u>unspecified</u> thumb at forearm level

  S56.32-   <u>Laceration</u> of <u>extensor or abductor</u> muscles, fascia and tendons of <u>thumb</u> at <u>forearm level</u>

    S56.321-   Laceration of extensor or abductor muscles, fascia and tendons of <u>right</u> thumb at forearm level

    S56.322-   Laceration of extensor or abductor muscles, fascia and tendons of <u>left</u> thumb at forearm level

    S56.329-   Laceration of extensor or abductor muscles, fascia and tendons of <u>unspecified</u> thumb at forearm level

  S56.39-   <u>Other injury</u> of <u>extensor or abductor</u> muscles, fascia and tendons of <u>thumb</u> at <u>forearm level</u>

    S56.391-   Other injury of extensor or abductor muscles, fascia and tendons of <u>right</u> thumb at forearm level

    S56.392-   Other injury of extensor or abductor muscles, fascia and tendons of <u>left</u> thumb at forearm level

    S56.399-   Other injury of extensor or abductor muscles, fascia and tendons of <u>unspecified</u> thumb at forearm level

S56.4-   <u>Injury</u> of <u>extensor</u> muscle, fascia and tendon of other and unspecified <u>finger</u> at <u>forearm level</u>

  S56.40-   <u>Unspecified</u> injury of <u>extensor</u> muscle, fascia and tendon of other and unspecified <u>finger</u> at <u>forearm level</u>

    S56.401-   Unspecified injury of extensor muscle, fascia and tendon of <u>right</u> <u>index</u> finger at forearm level

    S56.402-   Unspecified injury of extensor muscle, fascia and tendon of <u>left</u> <u>index</u> finger at forearm level

    S56.403-   Unspecified injury of extensor muscle, fascia and tendon of <u>right</u> <u>middle</u> finger at forearm level

    S56.404-   Unspecified injury of extensor muscle, fascia and tendon of <u>left</u> <u>middle</u> finger at forearm level

    S56.405-   Unspecified injury of extensor muscle, fascia and tendon of <u>right</u> <u>ring</u> finger at forearm level

    S56.406-   Unspecified injury of extensor muscle, fascia and tendon of <u>left</u> <u>ring</u> finger at forearm level

    S56.407-   Unspecified injury of extensor muscle, fascia and tendon of <u>right</u> <u>little</u> finger at forearm level

    S56.408-   Unspecified injury of extensor muscle, fascia and tendon of <u>left</u> <u>little</u> finger at forearm level

    S56.409-   Unspecified injury of extensor muscle, fascia and tendon of <u>unspecified</u> <u>finger</u> atforearm level

  S56.41-   <u>Strain</u> of <u>extensor</u> muscle, fascia and tendon of other and unspecified <u>finger</u> at <u>forearm level</u>

    S56.411-   Strain of extensor muscle, fascia and tendon of <u>right</u> <u>index</u> finger at forearm level

    S56.412-   Strain of extensor muscle, fascia and tendon of <u>left</u> <u>index</u> finger at forearm level

    S56.413-   Strain of extensor muscle, fascia and tendon of <u>right</u> <u>middle</u> finger at forearm level

    S56.414-   Strain of extensor muscle, fascia and tendon of <u>left</u> <u>middle</u> finger at forearm level

    S56.415-   Strain of extensor muscle, fascia and tendon of <u>right</u> <u>ring</u> finger at forearm level

    S56.416-   Strain of extensor muscle, fascia and tendon of <u>left</u> <u>ring</u> finger at forearm level

    S56.417-   Strain of extensor muscle, fascia and tendon of <u>right</u> <u>little</u> finger at forearm level

    S56.418-   Strain of extensor muscle, fascia and tendon of <u>left</u> <u>little</u> finger at forearm level

    S56.419-   Strain of extensor muscle, fascia and tendon of finger, <u>unspecified</u> <u>finger</u> at forearm level

  S56.42-   <u>Laceration</u> of <u>extensor</u> muscle, fascia and tendon of other and unspecified <u>finger</u> at forearm level

    S56.421-   Laceration of extensor muscle, fascia and tendon of <u>right</u> <u>index</u> finger at forearm level

    S56.422-   Laceration of extensor muscle, fascia and tendon of <u>left</u> <u>index</u> finger at forearm level

    S56.423-   Laceration of extensor muscle, fascia and tendon of <u>right</u> <u>middle</u> finger at forearm level

    S56.424-   Laceration of extensor muscle, fascia and tendon of <u>left</u> <u>middle</u> finger at forearm level

    S56.425-   Laceration of extensor muscle, fascia and tendon of <u>right</u> <u>ring</u> finger at forearm level

    S56.426-   Laceration of extensor muscle, fascia and tendon of <u>left</u> <u>ring</u> finger at forearm level

    S56.427-   Laceration of extensor muscle, fascia and tendon of <u>right</u> <u>little</u> finger at forearm level

    S56.428-   Laceration of extensor muscle, fascia and tendon of <u>left</u> <u>little</u> finger at forearm level

    S56.429-   Laceration of extensor muscle, fascia and tendon of <u>unspecified</u> <u>finger</u> at forearm level

  S56.49-   <u>Other injury</u> of <u>extensor</u> muscle, fascia and tendon of other and unspecified <u>finger</u> at <u>forearm level</u>

    S56.491-   Other injury of extensor muscle, fascia and tendon of <u>right</u> <u>index</u> finger at forearm level

    S56.492-   Other injury of extensor muscle, fascia and tendon of <u>left</u> <u>index</u> finger at forearm level

    S56.493-   Other injury of extensor muscle, fascia and tendon of <u>right</u> <u>middle</u> finger at forearm level

    S56.494-   Other injury of extensor muscle, fascia and tendon of <u>left</u> <u>middle</u> finger at forearm level

    S56.495-   Other injury of extensor muscle, fascia and tendon of <u>right</u> <u>ring</u> finger at forearm level

    S56.496-   Other injury of extensor muscle, fascia and tendon of <u>left</u> <u>ring</u> finger at forearm level

    S56.497-   Other injury of extensor muscle, fascia and tendon of <u>right</u> <u>little</u> finger at forearm level

    S56.498-   Other injury of extensor muscle, fascia and tendon of <u>left</u> <u>little</u> finger at forearm level

    S56.499-   Other injury of extensor muscle, fascia and tendon of <u>unspecified</u> <u>finger</u> at forearm level

S 5 5 – S 5 6

S56.5- Injury of other extensor muscle, fascia and tendon at forearm level

S56.50- Unspecified injury of other extensor muscle, fascia and tendon at forearm level

S56.501- Unspecified injury of other extensor muscle, fascia and tendon at forearm level, right arm

S56.502- Unspecified injury of other extensor muscle, fascia and tendon at forearm level, left arm

S56.509- Unspecified injury of other extensor muscle, fascia and tendon at forearm level, unspecified arm

S56.51- Strain of other extensor muscle, fascia and tendon at forearm level

S56.511- Strain of other extensor muscle, fascia and tendon at forearm level, right arm

S56.512- Strain of other extensor muscle, fascia and tendon at forearm level, left arm

S56.519- Strain of other extensor muscle, fascia and tendon at forearm level, unspecified arm

S56.52- Laceration of other extensor muscle, fascia and tendon at forearm level

S56.521- Laceration of other extensor muscle, fascia and tendon at forearm level, right arm

S56.522- Laceration of other extensor muscle, fascia and tendon at forearm level, left arm

S56.529- Laceration of other extensor muscle, fascia and tendon at forearm level, unspecified arm

S56.59- Other injury of other extensor muscle, fascia and tendon at forearm level

S56.591- Other injury of other extensor muscle, fascia and tendon at forearm level, right arm

S56.592- Other injury of other extensor muscle, fascia and tendon at forearm level, left arm

S56.599- Other injury of other extensor muscle, fascia and tendon at forearm level, unspecified arm

S56.8- Injury of other muscles, fascia and tendons at forearm level

S56.80- Unspecified injury of other muscles, fascia and tendons at forearm level

S56.801- Unspecified injury of other muscles, fascia and tendons at forearm level, right arm

S56.802- Unspecified injury of other muscles, fascia and tendons at forearm level, left arm

S56.809- Unspecified injury of other muscles, fascia and tendons at forearm level, unspecified arm

S56.81- Strain of other muscles, fascia and tendons at forearm level

S56.811- Strain of other muscles, fascia and tendons at forearm level, right arm

S56.812- Strain of other muscles, fascia and tendons at forearm level, left arm

S56.819- Strain of other muscles, fascia and tendons at forearm level, unspecified arm

S56.82- Laceration of other muscles, fascia and tendons at forearm level

S56.821- Laceration of other muscles, fascia and tendons at forearm level, right arm

S56.822- Laceration of other muscles, fascia and tendons at forearm level, left arm

S56.829- Laceration of other muscles, fascia and tendons at forearm level, unspecified arm

S56.89- Other injury of other muscles, fascia and tendons at forearm level

S56.891- Other injury of other muscles, fascia and tendons at forearm level, right arm

S56.892- Other injury of other muscles, fascia and tendons at forearm level, left arm

S56.899- Other injury of other muscles, fascia and tendons at forearm level, unspecified arm

S56.9- Injury of unspecified muscles, fascia and tendons at forearm level

S56.90- Unspecified injury of unspecified muscles, fascia and tendons at forearm level

S56.901- Unspecified injury of unspecified muscles, fascia and tendons at forearm level, right arm

S56.902- Unspecified injury of unspecified muscles, fascia and tendons at forearm level, left arm

S56.909- Unspecified injury of unspecified muscles, fascia and tendons at forearm level, unspecified arm

S56.91- Strain of unspecified muscles, fascia and tendons at forearm level

S56.911- Strain of unspecified muscles, fascia and tendons at forearm level, right arm

S56.912- Strain of unspecified muscles, fascia and tendons at forearm level, left arm

S56.919- Strain of unspecified muscles, fascia and tendons at forearm level, unspecified arm

S56.92- Laceration of unspecified muscles, fascia and tendons at forearm level

S56.921- Laceration of unspecified muscles, fascia and tendons at forearm level, right arm

S56.922- Laceration of unspecified muscles, fascia and tendons at forearm level, left arm

S56.929- Laceration of unspecified muscles, fascia and tendons at forearm level, unspecified arm

S56.99- Other injury of unspecified muscles, fascia and tendons at forearm level

S56.991- Other injury of unspecified muscles, fascia and tendons at forearm level, right arm

S56.992- Other injury of unspecified muscles, fascia and tendons at forearm level, left arm

S56.999- Other injury of unspecified muscles, fascia and tendons at forearm level, unspecified arm

S57- Crushing injury of elbow and forearm
Use additional code(s) for all associated injuries
Excludes❷: crushing injury of wrist and hand (S67.-)

The appropriate 7th character is to be added to each code from category S57:
A Initial encounter
D Subsequent encounter
S Sequela

S57.0- Crushing injury of elbow

S57.00x- Crushing injury of unspecified elbow

S57.01x- Crushing injury of right elbow

S57.02x- Crushing injury of left elbow

S57.8- Crushing injury of forearm

S57.80x- Crushing injury of unspecified forearm

S57.81x- Crushing injury of right forearm

S57.82x- Crushing injury of left forearm

S58- Traumatic amputation of elbow and forearm
Note: An amputation not identified as partial or complete should be coded to complete
Excludes 1: traumatic amputation of wrist and hand (S68.-)

The appropriate 7th character is to be added to each code from category S58:
A Initial encounter
D Subsequent encounter
S Sequela

S58.0- Traumatic amputation at elbow level

S58.01- Complete traumatic amputation at elbow level

S58.011- Complete traumatic amputation at elbow level, right arm

S58.012- Complete traumatic amputation at elbow level, left arm

S58.019- Complete traumatic amputation at elbow level, unspecified arm

S58.02- Partial traumatic amputation at elbow level

S58.021- Partial traumatic amputation at elbow level, right arm

S58.022- Partial traumatic amputation at elbow level, left arm

S58.029- Partial traumatic amputation at elbow level, unspecified arm

S58.1- Traumatic amputation at level between elbow and wrist

S58.11- Complete traumatic amputation at level between elbow and wrist

S58.111- Complete traumatic amputation at level between elbow and wrist, right arm

S58.112- Complete traumatic amputation at level between elbow and wrist, left arm

S58.119- Complete traumatic amputation at level between elbow and wrist, unspecified arm

S58.12- Partial traumatic amputation at level between elbow and wrist

S58.121- Partial traumatic amputation at level between elbow and wrist, right arm

S58.122- Partial traumatic amputation at level between elbow and wrist, left arm

S58.129- Partial traumatic amputation at level between elbow and wrist, unspecified arm

S
5
6
I
S
5
9

S58.9- Traumatic amputation of forearm, level unspecified
  Excludes 1: traumatic amputation of wrist (S68.-)

  S58.91- Complete traumatic amputation of forearm, level unspecified

  S58.911- Complete traumatic amputation of right forearm, level unspecified

  S58.912- Complete traumatic amputation of left forearm, level unspecified

  S58.919- Complete traumatic amputation of unspecified forearm, level unspecified

  S58.92- Partial traumatic amputation of forearm, level unspecified

  S58.921- Partial traumatic amputation of right forearm, level unspecified

  S58.922- Partial traumatic amputation of left forearm, level unspecified

  S58.929- Partial traumatic amputation of unspecified forearm, level unspecified

S59- Other and unspecified injuries of elbow and forearm
  Excludes ❷: other and unspecified injuries of wrist and hand (S69.-)

  The appropriate 7th character is to be added to each code from subcategories S59.0, S59.1, and S59.2:
  A   Initial encounter for closed fracture
  D   Subsequent encounter for fracture with routine healing
  G   Subsequent encounter for fracture with delayed healing
  K   Subsequent encounter for fracture with nonunion
  P   Subsequent encounter for fracture with malunion
  S   Sequela

  S59.0- Physeal fracture of lower end of ulna

  S59.00- Unspecified physeal fracture of lower end of ulna

  S59.001- Unspecified physeal fracture of lower end of ulna, right arm

  S59.002- Unspecified physeal fracture of lower end of ulna, left arm

  S59.009- Unspecified physeal fracture of lower end of ulna, unspecified arm

  S59.01- Salter-Harris Type I physeal fracture of lower end of ulna

  S59.011- Salter-Harris Type I physeal fracture of lower end of ulna, right arm

  S59.012- Salter-Harris Type I physeal fracture of lower end of ulna, left arm

  S59.019- Salter-Harris Type I physeal fracture of lower end of ulna, unspecified arm

  S59.02- Salter-Harris Type II physeal fracture of lower end of ulna

  S59.021- Salter-Harris Type II physeal fracture of lower end of ulna, right arm

  S59.022- Salter-Harris Type II physeal fracture of lower end of ulna, left arm

  S59.029- Salter-Harris Type II physeal fracture of lower end of ulna, unspecified arm

  S59.03- Salter-Harris Type III physeal fracture of lower end of ulna

  S59.031- Salter-Harris Type III physeal fracture of lower end of ulna, right arm

  S59.032- Salter-Harris Type III physeal fracture of lower end of ulna, left arm

  S59.039- Salter-Harris Type III physeal fracture of lower end of ulna, unspecified arm

  S59.04- Salter-Harris Type IV physeal fracture of lower end of ulna

  S59.041- Salter-Harris Type IV physeal fracture of lower end of ulna, right arm

  S59.042- Salter-Harris Type IV physeal fracture of lower end of ulna, left arm

  S59.049- Salter-Harris Type IV physeal fracture of lower end of ulna, unspecified arm

  S59.09- Other physeal fracture of lower end of ulna

  S59.091- Other physeal fracture of lower end of ulna, right arm

  S59.092- Other physeal fracture of lower end of ulna, left arm

  S59.099- Other physeal fracture of lower end of ulna, unspecified arm

  S59.1- Physeal fracture of upper end of radius

  S59.10- Unspecified physeal fracture of upper end of radius

  S59.101- Unspecified physeal fracture of upper end of radius, right arm

  S59.102- Unspecified physeal fracture of upper end of radius, left arm

  S59.109- Unspecified physeal fracture of upper end of radius, unspecified arm

  S59.11- Salter-Harris Type I physeal fracture of upper end of radius

  S59.111- Salter-Harris Type I physeal fracture of upper end of radius, right arm

  S59.112- Salter-Harris Type I physeal fracture of upper end of radius, left arm

  S59.119- Salter-Harris Type I physeal fracture of upper end of radius, unspecified arm

  S59.12- Salter-Harris Type II physeal fracture of upper end of radius

  S59.121- Salter-Harris Type II physeal fracture of upper end of radius, right arm

  S59.122- Salter-Harris Type II physeal fracture of upper end of radius, left arm

  S59.129- Salter-Harris Type II physeal fracture of upper end of radius, unspecified arm

  S59.13- Salter-Harris Type III physeal fracture of upper end of radius

  S59.131- Salter-Harris Type III physeal fracture of upper end of radius, right arm

  S59.132- Salter-Harris Type III physeal fracture of upper end of radius, left arm

  S59.139- Salter-Harris Type III physeal fracture of upper end of radius, unspecified arm

  S59.14- Salter-Harris Type IV physeal fracture of upper end of radius

  S59.141- Salter-Harris Type IV physeal fracture of upper end of radius, right arm

  S59.142- Salter-Harris Type IV physeal fracture of upper end of radius, left arm

  S59.149- Salter-Harris Type IV physeal fracture of upper end of radius, unspecified arm

  S59.19- Other physeal fracture of upper end of radius

  S59.191- Other physeal fracture of upper end of radius, right arm

  S59.192- Other physeal fracture of upper end of radius, left arm

  S59.199- Other physeal fracture of upper end of radius, unspecified arm

S59.2- Physeal fracture of lower end of radius

  S59.20- Unspecified physeal fracture of lower end of radius

  S59.201- Unspecified physeal fracture of lower end of radius, right arm

  S59.202- Unspecified physeal fracture of lower end of radius, left arm

  S59.209- Unspecified physeal fracture of lower end of radius, unspecified arm

  S59.21- Salter-Harris Type I physeal fracture of lower end of radius

  S59.211- Salter-Harris Type I physeal fracture of lower end of radius, right arm

  S59.212- Salter-Harris Type I physeal fracture of lower end of radius, left arm

  S59.219- Salter-Harris Type I physeal fracture of lower end of radius, unspecified arm

  S59.22- Salter-Harris Type II physeal fracture of lower end of radius

  S59.221- Salter-Harris Type II physeal fracture of lower end of radius, right arm

  S59.222- Salter-Harris Type II physeal fracture of lower end of radius, left arm

  S59.229- Salter-Harris Type II physeal fracture of lower end of radius, unspecified arm

  S59.23- Salter-Harris Type III physeal fracture of lower end of radius

  S59.231- Salter-Harris Type III physeal fracture of lower end of radius, right arm

  S59.232- Salter-Harris Type III physeal fracture of lower end of radius, left arm

  S59.239- Salter-Harris Type III physeal fracture of lower end of radius, unspecified arm

  S59.24- Salter-Harris Type IV physeal fracture of lower end of radius

  S59.241- Salter-Harris Type IV physeal fracture of lower end of radius, right arm

  S59.242- Salter-Harris Type IV physeal fracture of lower end of radius, left arm

  S59.249- Salter-Harris Type IV physeal fracture of lower end of radius, unspecified arm

  S59.29- Other physeal fracture of lower end of radius

  S59.291- Other physeal fracture of lower end of radius, right arm

  S59.292- Other physeal fracture of lower end of radius, left arm

  S59.299- Other physeal fracture of lower end of radius, unspecified arm

S 5 6 ı S 5 9

S59.8-   <u>Other specified injuries</u> of <u>elbow and forearm</u>
          The appropriate 7th character is to be added to each code in
              subcategory S59.8:
          A   <u>Initial</u> encounter
          D   <u>Subsequent</u> encounter
          S   <u>Sequela</u>
     S59.80-   <u>Other specified injuries</u> of <u>elbow</u>
         S59.801-   Other specified injuries of <u>right</u> elbow
         S59.802-   Other specified injuries of <u>left</u> elbow
         S59.809-   Other specified injuries of <u>unspecified</u> elbow
     S59.81-   <u>Other specified injuries</u> of <u>forearm</u>
         S59.811-   Other specified injuries <u>right</u> forearm
         S59.812-   Other specified injuries <u>left</u> forearm
         S59.819-   Other specified injuries <u>unspecified</u> forearm
S59.9-   <u>Unspecified injury</u> of <u>elbow and forearm</u>
          The appropriate 7th character is to be added to each code in
              subcategory S59.9:
          A   <u>Initial</u> encounter
          D   <u>Subsequent</u> encounter
          S   <u>Sequela</u>
     S59.90-   <u>Unspecified injury</u> of <u>elbow</u>
         S59.901-   Unspecified injury of <u>right</u> elbow
         S59.902-   Unspecified injury of <u>left</u> elbow
         S59.909-   Unspecified injury of <u>unspecified</u> elbow
     S59.91-   <u>Unspecified injury</u> of <u>forearm</u>
         S59.911-   Unspecified injury of <u>right</u> forearm
         S59.912-   Unspecified injury of <u>left</u> forearm
         S59.919-   Unspecified injury of <u>unspecified</u> forearm

Injuries to the wrist, hand and fingers (S60-S69)

Excludes❷: burns and corrosions (T20-T32)
            frostbite (T33-T34)
            insect bite or sting, venomous (T63.4)

S60-   <u>Superficial injury</u> of <u>wrist, hand and fingers</u>
        The appropriate 7th character is to be added to each code from
            category S60:
        A   <u>Initial</u> encounter
        D   <u>Subsequent</u> encounter
        S   <u>Sequela</u>
   S60.0-   <u>Contusion</u> of <u>finger without</u> damage to nail
            Excludes 1: contusion involving nail (matrix) (S60.1)
       S60.00x-   <u>Contusion</u> of <u>unspecified</u> finger <u>without</u> damage to nail
                   Contusion of finger(s) NOS
       S60.01-   <u>Contusion</u> of <u>thumb without</u> damage to nail
           S60.011-   Contusion of <u>right</u> thumb without damage to nail
           S60.012-   Contusion of <u>left</u> thumb without damage to nail
           S60.019-   Contusion of <u>unspecified</u> thumb without damage to
                       nail
       S60.02-   <u>Contusion</u> of <u>index</u> finger <u>without</u> damage to nail
           S60.021-   Contusion of <u>right</u> index finger without damage to nail
           S60.022-   Contusion of <u>left</u> index finger without damage to nail
           S60.029-   Contusion of <u>unspecified</u> index finger without damage
                       to nail
       S60.03-   <u>Contusion</u> of <u>middle</u> finger <u>without</u> damage to nail
           S60.031-   Contusion of <u>right</u> middle finger without damage to
                       nail
           S60.032-   Contusion of <u>left</u> middle finger without damage to nail
           S60.039-   Contusion of <u>unspecified</u> middle finger without
                       damage to nail
       S60.04-   <u>Contusion</u> of <u>ring</u> finger <u>without</u> damage to nail
           S60.041-   Contusion of <u>right</u> ring finger without damage to nail
           S60.042-   Contusion of <u>left</u> ring finger without damage to nail
           S60.049-   Contusion of <u>unspecified</u> ring finger without damage
                       to nail
       S60.05-   <u>Contusion</u> of <u>little</u> finger <u>without</u> damage to nail
           S60.051-   Contusion of <u>right</u> little finger without damage to nail
           S60.052-   Contusion of <u>left</u> little finger without damage to nail
           S60.059-   Contusion of <u>unspecified</u> little finger without damage
                       to nail

S60.1-   <u>Contusion</u> of <u>finger with</u> damage to nail
     S60.10x-   Contusion of <u>unspecified</u> finger <u>with damage to nail</u>
     S60.11-   <u>Contusion</u> of <u>thumb with</u> damage to nail
         S60.111-   Contusion of <u>right</u> thumb with damage to nail
         S60.112-   Contusion of <u>left</u> thumb with damage to nail
         S60.119-   Contusion of <u>unspecified</u> thumb with damage to nail
     S60.12-   <u>Contusion</u> of <u>index</u> finger <u>with</u> damage to nail
         S60.121-   Contusion of <u>right</u> index finger with damage to nail
         S60.122-   Contusion of <u>left</u> index finger with damage to nail
         S60.129-   Contusion of <u>unspecified</u> index finger with damage to
                     nail
     S60.13-   <u>Contusion</u> of <u>middle</u> finger <u>with</u> damage to nail
         S60.131-   Contusion of <u>right</u> middle finger with damage to nail
         S60.132-   Contusion of <u>left</u> middle finger with damage to nail
         S60.139-   Contusion of <u>unspecified</u> middle finger with damage to
                     nail
     S60.14-   <u>Contusion</u> of <u>ring</u> finger <u>with</u> damage to nail
         S60.141-   Contusion of <u>right</u> ring finger with damage to nail
         S60.142-   Contusion of <u>left</u> ring finger with damage to nail
         S60.149-   Contusion of <u>unspecified</u> ring finger with damage to
                     nail
     S60.15-   <u>Contusion</u> of <u>little</u> finger <u>with</u> damage to nail
         S60.151-   Contusion of <u>right</u> little finger with damage to nail
         S60.152-   Contusion of <u>left</u> little finger with damage to nail
         S60.159-   Contusion of <u>unspecified</u> little finger with damage to
                     nail
S60.2-   <u>Contusion</u> of <u>wrist and hand</u>
          Excludes❷: contusion of fingers (S60.0-, S60.1-)
     S60.21-   <u>Contusion</u> of <u>wrist</u>
         S60.211-   Contusion of <u>right</u> wrist
         S60.212-   Contusion of <u>left</u> wrist
         S60.219-   Contusion of <u>unspecified</u> wrist
     S60.22-   <u>Contusion</u> of <u>hand</u>
         S60.221-   Contusion of <u>right</u> hand
         S60.222-   Contusion of <u>left</u> hand
         S60.229-   Contusion of <u>unspecified</u> hand
S60.3-   <u>Other superficial injuries</u> of <u>thumb</u>
     S60.31-   <u>Abrasion</u> of <u>thumb</u>
         S60.311-   Abrasion of <u>right</u> thumb
         S60.312-   Abrasion of <u>left</u> thumb
         S60.319-   Abrasion of <u>unspecified</u> thumb
     S60.32-   <u>Blister</u> (nonthermal) of <u>thumb</u>
         S60.321-   Blister (nonthermal) of <u>right</u> thumb
         S60.322-   Blister (nonthermal) of <u>left</u> thumb
         S60.329-   Blister (nonthermal) of <u>unspecified</u> thumb
     S60.34-   <u>External constriction</u> of <u>thumb</u>
                Hair tourniquet syndrome of thumb
                Use additional cause code to identify the constricting item
                     (W49.0-)
         S60.341-   External constriction of <u>right</u> thumb
         S60.342-   External constriction of <u>left</u> thumb
         S60.349-   External constriction of <u>unspecified</u> thumb
     S60.35-   <u>Superficial foreign body</u> of <u>thumb</u>
                Splinter in the thumb
         S60.351-   Superficial foreign body of <u>right</u> thumb
         S60.352-   Superficial foreign body of <u>left</u> thumb
         S60.359-   Superficial foreign body of <u>unspecified</u> thumb
     S60.36-   <u>Insect bite</u> (nonvenomous) of <u>thumb</u>
         S60.361-   Insect bite (nonvenomous) of <u>right</u> thumb
         S60.362-   Insect bite (nonvenomous) of <u>left</u> thumb
         S60.369-   Insect bite (nonvenomous) of <u>unspecified</u> thumb
     S60.37-   <u>Other superficial bite</u> of <u>thumb</u>
                Excludes 1: open bite of thumb (S61.05-, S61.15-)
         S60.371-   Other superficial bite of <u>right</u> thumb
         S60.372-   Other superficial bite of <u>left</u> thumb
         S60.379-   Other superficial bite of <u>unspecified</u> thumb
     S60.39-   <u>Other superficial injuries</u> of <u>thumb</u>
         S60.391-   Other superficial injuries of <u>right</u> thumb
         S60.392-   Other superficial injuries of <u>left</u> thumb
         S60.399-   Other superficial injuries of <u>unspecified</u> thumb

S 5 9 - S 6 0

S60.4- <u>Other superficial injuries</u> of <u>other fingers</u>
  S60.41- <u>Abrasion</u> of <u>fingers</u>
    S60.410- Abrasion of <u>right index</u> finger
    S60.411- Abrasion of <u>left index</u> finger
    S60.412- Abrasion of <u>right middle</u> finger
    S60.413- Abrasion of <u>left middle</u> finger
    S60.414- Abrasion of <u>right ring</u> finger
    S60.415- Abrasion of <u>left ring</u> finger
    S60.416- Abrasion of <u>right little</u> finger
    S60.417- Abrasion of <u>left little</u> finger
    S60.418- Abrasion of <u>other</u> finger
      Abrasion of specified finger with unspecified laterality
    S60.419- Abrasion of <u>unspecified</u> finger
  S60.42- <u>Blister (nonthermal)</u> of <u>fingers</u>
    S60.420- Blister (nonthermal) of <u>right index</u> finger
    S60.421- Blister (nonthermal) of <u>left index</u> finger
    S60.422- Blister (nonthermal) of <u>right middle</u> finger
    S60.423- Blister (nonthermal) of <u>left middle</u> finger
    S60.424- Blister (nonthermal) of <u>right ring</u> finger
    S60.425- Blister (nonthermal) of <u>left ring</u> finger
    S60.426- Blister (nonthermal) of <u>right little</u> finger
    S60.427- Blister (nonthermal) of <u>left little</u> finger
    S60.428- Blister (nonthermal) of <u>other</u> finger
      Blister (nonthermal) of specified finger with unspecified laterality
    S60.429- Blister (nonthermal) of <u>unspecified</u> finger
  S60.44- <u>External constriction</u> of <u>fingers</u>
    Hair tourniquet syndrome of finger
    Use additional cause code to identify the constricting item (W49.0-)
    S60.440- External constriction of <u>right index</u> finger
    S60.441- External constriction of <u>left index</u> finger
    S60.442- External constriction of <u>right middle</u> finger
    S60.443- External constriction of <u>left middle</u> finger
    S60.444- External constriction of <u>right ring</u> finger
    S60.445- External constriction of <u>left ring</u> finger
    S60.446- External constriction of <u>right little</u> finger
    S60.447- External constriction of <u>left little</u> finger
    S60.448- External constriction of <u>other</u> finger
      External constriction of specified finger with unspecified laterality
    S60.449- External constriction of <u>unspecified</u> finger
  S60.45- <u>Superficial foreign body</u> of <u>fingers</u>
    Splinter in the finger(s)
    S60.450- Superficial foreign body of <u>right index</u> finger
    S60.451- Superficial foreign body of <u>left index</u> finger
    S60.452- Superficial foreign body of <u>right middle</u> finger
    S60.453- Superficial foreign body of <u>left middle</u> finger
    S60.454- Superficial foreign body of <u>right ring</u> finger
    S60.455- Superficial foreign body of <u>left ring</u> finger
    S60.456- Superficial foreign body of <u>right little</u> finger
    S60.457- Superficial foreign body of <u>left little</u> finger
    S60.458- Superficial foreign body of <u>other</u> finger
      Superficial foreign body of specified finger with unspecified laterality
    S60.459- Superficial foreign body of <u>unspecified</u> finger
  S60.46- <u>Insect bite (nonvenomous)</u> of <u>fingers</u>
    S60.460- Insect bite (nonvenomous) of <u>right index</u> finger
    S60.461- Insect bite (nonvenomous) of <u>left index</u> finger
    S60.462- Insect bite (nonvenomous) of <u>right middle</u> finger
    S60.463- Insect bite (nonvenomous) of <u>left middle</u> finger
    S60.464- Insect bite (nonvenomous) of <u>right ring</u> finger
    S60.465- Insect bite (nonvenomous) of <u>left ring</u> finger
    S60.466- Insect bite (nonvenomous) of <u>right little</u> finger
    S60.467- Insect bite (nonvenomous) of <u>left little</u> finger
    S60.468- Insect bite (nonvenomous) of <u>other</u> finger
      Insect bite (nonvenomous) of specified finger with unspecified laterality
    S60.469- Insect bite (nonvenomous) of <u>unspecified</u> finger
  S60.47- <u>Other superficial bite</u> of <u>fingers</u>
    Excludes 1: open bite of fingers (S61.25-, S61.35-)
    S60.470- Other superficial bite of <u>right index</u> finger
    S60.471- Other superficial bite of <u>left index</u> finger
    S60.472- Other superficial bite of <u>right middle</u> finger
    S60.473- Other superficial bite of <u>left middle</u> finger
    S60.474- Other superficial bite of <u>right ring</u> finger
    S60.475- Other superficial bite of <u>left ring</u> finger
    S60.476- Other superficial bite of <u>right little</u> finger
    S60.477- Other superficial bite of <u>left little</u> finger
    S60.478- Other superficial bite of <u>other</u> finger
      Other superficial bite of specified finger with unspecified laterality
    S60.479- Other superficial bite of <u>unspecified</u> finger
S60.5- <u>Other superficial injuries</u> of <u>hand</u>
  Excludes❷: superficial injuries of fingers (S60.3-, S60.4-)
  S60.51- <u>Abrasion</u> of <u>hand</u>
    S60.511- Abrasion of <u>right</u> hand
    S60.512- Abrasion of <u>left</u> hand
    S60.519- Abrasion of <u>unspecified</u> hand
  S60.52- <u>Blister (nonthermal)</u> of <u>hand</u>
    S60.521- Blister (nonthermal) of <u>right</u> hand
    S60.522- Blister (nonthermal) of <u>left</u> hand
    S60.529- Blister (nonthermal) of <u>unspecified</u> hand
  S60.54- <u>External constriction</u> of <u>hand</u>
    S60.541- External constriction of <u>right</u> hand
    S60.542- External constriction of <u>left</u> hand
    S60.549- External constriction of <u>unspecified</u> hand
  S60.55- <u>Superficial foreign body</u> of <u>hand</u>
    Splinter in the hand
    S60.551- Superficial foreign body of <u>right</u> hand
    S60.552- Superficial foreign body of <u>left</u> hand
    S60.559- Superficial foreign body of <u>unspecified</u> hand
  S60.56- <u>Insect bite (nonvenomous)</u> of <u>hand</u>
    S60.561- Insect bite (nonvenomous) of <u>right</u> hand
    S60.562- Insect bite (nonvenomous) of <u>left</u> hand
    S60.569- Insect bite (nonvenomous) of <u>unspecified</u> hand
  S60.57- <u>Other superficial bite</u> of <u>hand</u>
    Excludes 1: open bite of hand (S61.45-)
    S60.571- Other superficial bite of hand of <u>right</u> hand
    S60.572- Other superficial bite of hand of <u>left</u> hand
    S60.579- Other superficial bite of hand of <u>unspecified</u> hand
S60.8- <u>Other superficial injuries</u> of <u>wrist</u>
  S60.81- <u>Abrasion</u> of <u>wrist</u>
    S60.811- Abrasion of <u>right</u> wrist
    S60.812- Abrasion of <u>left</u> wrist
    S60.819- Abrasion of <u>unspecified</u> wrist
  S60.82- <u>Blister (nonthermal)</u> of <u>wrist</u>
    S60.821- Blister (nonthermal) of <u>right</u> wrist
    S60.822- Blister (nonthermal) of <u>left</u> wrist
    S60.829- Blister (nonthermal) of <u>unspecified</u> wrist
  S60.84- <u>External constriction</u> of <u>wrist</u>
    S60.841- External constriction of <u>right</u> wrist
    S60.842- External constriction of <u>left</u> wrist
    S60.849- External constriction of <u>unspecified</u> wrist
  S60.85- <u>Superficial foreign body</u> of <u>wrist</u>
    Splinter in the wrist
    S60.851- Superficial foreign body of <u>right</u> wrist
    S60.852- Superficial foreign body of <u>left</u> wrist
    S60.859- Superficial foreign body of <u>unspecified</u> wrist
  S60.86- <u>Insect bite (nonvenomous)</u> of <u>wrist</u>
    S60.861- Insect bite (nonvenomous) of <u>right</u> wrist
    S60.862- Insect bite (nonvenomous) of <u>left</u> wrist
    S60.869- Insect bite (nonvenomous) of <u>unspecified</u> wrist
  S60.87- <u>Other superficial bite</u> of <u>wrist</u>
    Excludes 1: open bite of wrist (S61.55)
    S60.871- Other superficial bite of <u>right</u> wrist
    S60.872- Other superficial bite of <u>left</u> wrist
    S60.879- Other superficial bite of <u>unspecified</u> wrist
S60.9- <u>Unspecified superficial injury</u> of wrist, hand and fingers
  S60.91- <u>Unspecified superficial injury</u> of <u>wrist</u>
    S60.911- Unspecified superficial injury of <u>right</u> wrist
    S60.912- Unspecified superficial injury of <u>left</u> wrist
    S60.919- Unspecified superficial injury of <u>unspecified</u> wrist
  S60.92- <u>Unspecified superficial injury</u> of <u>hand</u>
    S60.921- Unspecified superficial injury of <u>right</u> hand
    S60.922- Unspecified superficial injury of <u>left</u> hand
    S60.929- Unspecified superficial injury of <u>unspecified</u> hand
  S60.93- <u>Unspecified superficial injury</u> of <u>thumb</u>
    S60.931- Unspecified superficial injury of <u>right</u> thumb
    S60.932- Unspecified superficial injury of <u>left</u> thumb
    S60.939- Unspecified superficial injury of <u>unspecified</u> thumb

S59 - S60

S60.94- Unspecified superficial injury of other fingers
    S60.940- Unspecified superficial injury of right index finger
    S60.941- Unspecified superficial injury of left index finger
    S60.942- Unspecified superficial injury of right middle finger
    S60.943- Unspecified superficial injury of left middle finger
    S60.944- Unspecified superficial injury of right ring finger
    S60.945- Unspecified superficial injury of left ring finger
    S60.946- Unspecified superficial injury of right little finger
    S60.947- Unspecified superficial injury of left little finger
    S60.948- Unspecified superficial injury of other finger
        Unspecified superficial injury of specified finger with unspecified laterality
    S60.949- Unspecified superficial injury of unspecified finger

S61- **Open wound of wrist, hand and fingers**
    Code also any associated wound infection
    Excludes 1: open fracture of wrist, hand and finger (S62.- with 7th character B)
    traumatic amputation of wrist and hand (S68.-)

    The appropriate 7th character is to be added to each code from category S61:
    A   Initial encounter
    D   Subsequent encounter
    S   Sequela

S61.0- Open wound of thumb without damage to nail
    Excludes 1: open wound of thumb with damage to nail (S61.1-)
    S61.00- Unspecified open wound of thumb without damage to nail
        S61.001- Unspecified open wound of right thumb without damage to nail
        S61.002- Unspecified open wound of left thumb without damage to nail
        S61.009- Unspecified open wound of unspecified thumb without damage to nail
    S61.01- Laceration without foreign body of thumb without damage to nail
        S61.011- Laceration without foreign body of right thumb without damage to nail
        S61.012- Laceration without foreign body of left thumb without damage to nail
        S61.019- Laceration without foreign body of unspecified thumb without damage to nail
    S61.02- Laceration with foreign body of thumb without damage to nail
        S61.021- Laceration with foreign body of right thumb without damage to nail
        S61.022- Laceration with foreign body of left thumb without damage to nail
        S61.029- Laceration with foreign body of unspecified thumb without damage to nail
    S61.03- Puncture wound without foreign body of thumb without damage to nail
        S61.031- Puncture wound without foreign body of right thumb without damage to nail
        S61.032- Puncture wound without foreign body of left thumb without damage to nail
        S61.039- Puncture wound without foreign body of unspecified thumb without damage to nail
    S61.04- Puncture wound with foreign body of thumb without damage to nail
        S61.041- Puncture wound with foreign body of right thumb without damage to nail
        S61.042- Puncture wound with foreign body of left thumb without damage to nail
        S61.049- Puncture wound with foreign body of unspecified thumb without damage to nail
    S61.05- Open bite of thumb without damage to nail
        Bite of thumb NOS
        Excludes 1: superficial bite of thumb (S60.36-, S60.37-)
        S61.051- Open bite of right thumb without damage to nail
        S61.052- Open bite of left thumb without damage to nail
        S61.059- Open bite of unspecified thumb without damage to nail

S61.1- Open wound of thumb with damage to nail
    S61.10- Unspecified open wound of thumb with damage to nail
        S61.101- Unspecified open wound of right thumb with damage to nail
        S61.102- Unspecified open wound of left thumb with damage to nail
        S61.109- Unspecified open wound of unspecified thumb with damage to nail

S61.11- Laceration without foreign body of thumb with damage to nail
    S61.111- Laceration without foreign body of right thumb with damage to nail
    S61.112- Laceration without foreign body of left thumb with damage to nail
    S61.119- Laceration without foreign body of unspecified thumb with damage to nail
S61.12- Laceration with foreign body of thumb with damage to nail
    S61.121- Laceration with foreign body of right thumb with damage to nail
    S61.122- Laceration with foreign body of left thumb with damage to nail
    S61.129- Laceration with foreign body of unspecified thumb with damage to nail
S61.13- Puncture wound without foreign body of thumb with damage to nail
    S61.131- Puncture wound without foreign body of right thumb with damage to nail
    S61.132- Puncture wound without foreign body of left thumb with damage to nail
    S61.139- Puncture wound without foreign body of unspecified thumb with damage to nail
S61.14- Puncture wound with foreign body of thumb with damage to nail
    S61.141- Puncture wound with foreign body of right thumb with damage to nail
    S61.142- Puncture wound with foreign body of left thumb with damage to nail
    S61.149- Puncture wound with foreign body of unspecified thumb with damage to nail
S61.15- Open bite of thumb with damage to nail
    Bite of thumb with damage to nail NOS
    Excludes 1: superficial bite of thumb (S60.36-, S60.37-)
    S61.151- Open bite of right thumb with damage to nail
    S61.152- Open bite of left thumb with damage to nail
    S61.159- Open bite of unspecified thumb with damage to nail

S61.2- Open wound of other finger without damage to nail
    Excludes 1: open wound of finger involving nail (matrix) (S61.3-)
    Excludes❷: open wound of thumb without damage to nail (S61.0-)
    S61.20- Unspecified open wound of other finger without damage to nail
        S61.200- Unspecified open wound of right index finger without damage to nail
        S61.201- Unspecified open wound of left index finger without damage to nail
        S61.202- Unspecified open wound of right middle finger without damage to nail
        S61.203- Unspecified open wound of left middle finger without damage to nail
        S61.204- Unspecified open wound of right ring finger without damage to nail
        S61.205- Unspecified open wound of left ring finger without damage to nail
        S61.206- Unspecified open wound of right little finger without damage to nail
        S61.207- Unspecified open wound of left little finger without damage to nail
        S61.208- Unspecified open wound of other finger without damage to nail
            Unspecified open wound of specified finger with unspecified laterality without damage to nail
        S61.209- Unspecified open wound of unspecified finger without damage to nail
    S61.21- Laceration without foreign body of finger without damage to nail
        S61.210- Laceration without foreign body of right index finger without damage to nail
        S61.211- Laceration without foreign body of left index finger without damage to nail
        S61.212- Laceration without foreign body of right middle finger without damage to nail
        S61.213- Laceration without foreign body of left middle finger without damage to nail
        S61.214- Laceration without foreign body of right ring finger without damage to nail
        S61.215- Laceration without foreign body of left ring finger without damage to nail
        S61.216- Laceration without foreign body of right little finger without damage to nail

S61.217-   Laceration <u>without</u> foreign body of <u>left</u> <u>little</u> finger <u>without</u> damage to nail

S61.218-   Laceration <u>without</u> foreign body of <u>other</u> finger <u>without</u> damage to nail
> Laceration without foreign body of specified finger with unspecified laterality without damage to nail

S61.219-   Laceration <u>without</u> foreign body of <u>unspecified</u> finger <u>without</u> damage to nail

S61.22-   <u>Laceration with foreign body</u> of <u>finger</u> <u>without</u> damage to nail

S61.220-   Laceration <u>with foreign body</u> of <u>right</u> <u>index</u> finger <u>without</u> damage to nail

S61.221-   Laceration <u>with foreign body</u> of <u>left</u> <u>index</u> finger <u>without</u> damage to nail

S61.222-   Laceration <u>with foreign body</u> of <u>right</u> <u>middle</u> finger <u>without</u> damage to nail

S61.223-   Laceration <u>with foreign body</u> of <u>left</u> <u>middle</u> finger <u>without</u> damage to nail

S61.224-   Laceration <u>with foreign body</u> of <u>right</u> <u>ring</u> finger <u>without</u> damage to nail

S61.225-   Laceration <u>with foreign body</u> of <u>left</u> <u>ring</u> finger <u>without</u> damage to nail

S61.226-   Laceration <u>with foreign body</u> of <u>right</u> <u>little</u> finger <u>without</u> damage to nail

S61.227-   Laceration <u>with foreign body</u> of <u>left</u> <u>little</u> finger <u>without</u> damage to nail

S61.228-   Laceration <u>with foreign body</u> of <u>other</u> finger <u>without</u> damage to nail
> Laceration with foreign body of specified finger with unspecified laterality without damage to nail

S61.229-   Laceration <u>with foreign body</u> of <u>unspecified</u> finger <u>without</u> damage to nail

S61.23-   <u>Puncture</u> wound <u>without</u> foreign body of finger <u>without</u> damage to nail

S61.230-   Puncture wound <u>without</u> foreign body of <u>right</u> <u>index</u> finger <u>without</u> damage to nail

S61.231-   Puncture wound <u>without</u> foreign body of <u>left</u> <u>index</u> finger <u>without</u> damage to nail

S61.232-   Puncture wound <u>without</u> foreign body of <u>right</u> <u>middle</u> finger <u>without</u> damage to nail

S61.233-   Puncture wound <u>without</u> foreign body of <u>left</u> <u>middle</u> finger <u>without</u> damage to nail

S61.234-   Puncture wound <u>without</u> foreign body of <u>right</u> <u>ring</u> finger <u>without</u> damage to nail

S61.235-   Puncture wound <u>without</u> foreign body of <u>left</u> <u>ring</u> finger <u>without</u> damage to nail

S61.236-   Puncture wound <u>without</u> foreign body of <u>right</u> <u>little</u> finger <u>without</u> damage to nail

S61.237-   Puncture wound <u>without</u> foreign body of <u>left</u> <u>little</u> finger <u>without</u> damage to nail

S61.238-   Puncture wound <u>without</u> foreign body of other <u>finger</u> <u>without</u> damage to nail
> Puncture wound without foreign body of specified finger with unspecified laterality without damage to nail

S61.239-   Puncture wound <u>without</u> foreign body of <u>unspecified</u> finger <u>without</u> damage to nail

S61.24-   <u>Puncture</u> wound <u>with foreign body</u> of finger <u>without</u> damage to nail

S61.240-   Puncture wound <u>with foreign body</u> of <u>right</u> <u>index</u> finger <u>without</u> damage to nail

S61.241-   Puncture wound <u>with foreign body</u> of <u>left</u> <u>index</u> finger <u>without</u> damage to nail

S61.242-   Puncture wound <u>with foreign body</u> of <u>right</u> <u>middle</u> finger <u>without</u> damage to nail

S61.243-   Puncture wound <u>with foreign body</u> of <u>left</u> <u>middle</u> finger <u>without</u> damage to nail

S61.244-   Puncture wound <u>with foreign body</u> of <u>right</u> <u>ring</u> finger <u>without</u> damage to nail

S61.245-   Puncture wound <u>with foreign body</u> of <u>left</u> <u>ring</u> finger <u>without</u> damage to nail

S61.246-   Puncture wound <u>with foreign body</u> of <u>right</u> <u>little</u> finger <u>without</u> damage to nail

S61.247-   Puncture wound <u>with foreign body</u> of <u>left</u> <u>little</u> finger <u>without</u> damage to nail

S61.248-   Puncture wound <u>with foreign body</u> of <u>other</u> finger <u>without</u> damage to nail
> Puncture wound with foreign body of specified finger with unspecified laterality without damage to nail

S61.249-   Puncture wound <u>with foreign body</u> of <u>unspecified</u> finger <u>without</u> damage to nail

S61.25-   <u>Open bite</u> of finger <u>without</u> damage to nail
> Bite of finger without damage to nail NOS
> *Excludes 1:   superficial bite of finger (S60.46-, S60.47-)*

S61.250-   Open bite of <u>right</u> <u>index</u> finger <u>without</u> damage to nail

S61.251-   Open bite of <u>left</u> <u>index</u> finger <u>without</u> damage to nail

S61.252-   Open bite of <u>right</u> <u>middle</u> finger <u>without</u> damage to nail

S61.253-   Open bite of <u>left</u> <u>middle</u> finger <u>without</u> damage to nail

S61.254-   Open bite of <u>right</u> <u>ring</u> finger <u>without</u> damage to nail

S61.255-   Open bite of <u>left</u> <u>ring</u> finger <u>without</u> damage to nail

S61.256-   Open bite of <u>right</u> <u>little</u> finger <u>without</u> damage to nail

S61.257-   Open bite of <u>left</u> <u>little</u> finger <u>without</u> damage to nail

S61.258-   Open bite of other <u>finger</u> <u>without</u> damage to nail
> Open bite of specified finger with unspecified laterality without damage to nail

S61.259-   Open bite of <u>unspecified</u> finger <u>without</u> damage to nail

S61.3-   <u>Open wound of</u> other finger <u>with damage to nail</u>

S61.30-   <u>Unspecified open wound</u> of finger <u>with damage to nail</u>

S61.300-   Unspecified open wound of <u>right</u> <u>index</u> finger <u>with</u> <u>damage to nail</u>

S61.301-   Unspecified open wound of <u>left</u> <u>index</u> finger <u>with</u> <u>damage to nail</u>

S61.302-   Unspecified open wound of <u>right</u> <u>middle</u> finger <u>with</u> <u>damage to nail</u>

S61.303-   Unspecified open wound of <u>left</u> <u>middle</u> finger <u>with</u> <u>damage to nail</u>

S61.304-   Unspecified open wound of <u>right</u> <u>ring</u> finger <u>with</u> <u>damage to nail</u>

S61.305-   Unspecified open wound of <u>left</u> <u>ring</u> finger <u>with</u> <u>damage to nail</u>

S61.306-   Unspecified open wound of <u>right</u> <u>little</u> finger <u>with</u> <u>damage to nail</u>

S61.307-   Unspecified open wound of <u>left</u> <u>little</u> finger <u>with</u> <u>damage to nail</u>

S61.308-   Unspecified open wound of <u>other</u> finger <u>with damage to nail</u>
> Unspecified open wound of specified finger with unspecified laterality with damage to nail

S61.309-   Unspecified open wound of <u>unspecified</u> finger <u>with</u> <u>damage to nail</u>

S61.31-   <u>Laceration</u> <u>without</u> foreign body of <u>finger</u> <u>with damage to</u> nail

S61.310-   Laceration <u>without</u> foreign body of <u>right</u> <u>index</u> finger <u>with damage to nail</u>

S61.311-   Laceration <u>without</u> foreign body of <u>left</u> <u>index</u> finger <u>with damage to nail</u>

S61.312-   Laceration <u>without</u> foreign body of <u>right</u> <u>middle</u> finger <u>with damage to nail</u>

S61.313-   Laceration <u>without</u> foreign body of <u>left</u> <u>middle</u> finger <u>with damage to nail</u>

S61.314-   Laceration <u>without</u> foreign body of <u>right</u> <u>ring</u> finger <u>with damage to nail</u>

S61.315-   Laceration <u>without</u> foreign body of <u>left</u> <u>ring</u> finger <u>with damage to nail</u>

S61.316-   Laceration <u>without</u> foreign body of <u>right</u> <u>little</u> finger <u>with damage to nail</u>

S61.317-   Laceration <u>without</u> foreign body of <u>left</u> <u>little</u> finger <u>with damage to nail</u>

S61.318-   Laceration <u>without</u> foreign body of <u>other</u> finger <u>with</u> <u>damage to nail</u>
> Laceration without foreign body of specified finger with unspecified laterality with damage to nail

S61.319-   Laceration <u>without</u> foreign body of <u>unspecified</u> finger <u>with</u> damage to nail

S61.32-   <u>Laceration with foreign body</u> of <u>finger</u> <u>with damage to nail</u>

S61.320-   Laceration <u>with foreign body</u> of <u>right</u> <u>index</u> finger <u>with damage to nail</u>

S61.321-   Laceration <u>with foreign body</u> of <u>left</u> <u>index</u> finger <u>with</u> <u>damage to nail</u>

S61.322-   Laceration <u>with foreign body</u> of <u>right</u> <u>middle</u> finger <u>with damage to nail</u>

S61.323-   Laceration <u>with foreign body</u> of <u>left</u> <u>middle</u> finger <u>with</u> <u>damage to nail</u>

S61.324-   Laceration <u>with foreign body</u> of <u>right</u> <u>ring</u> finger <u>with</u> <u>damage to nail</u>

S61.325-   Laceration <u>with foreign body</u> of <u>left</u> <u>ring</u> finger <u>with</u> <u>damage to nail</u>

S61.326-   Laceration <u>with foreign body</u> of <u>right</u> <u>little</u> finger <u>with</u> <u>damage to nail</u>

S 6 0 – S 6 1

S61.327- Laceration <u>with foreign body</u> of <u>left</u> <u>little</u> finger <u>with damage to nail</u>

S61.328- Laceration <u>with foreign body</u> of <u>other</u> finger <u>with damage to nail</u>
Laceration with foreign body of specified finger with unspecified laterality with damage to nail

S61.329- Laceration <u>with foreign body</u> of <u>unspecified</u> finger <u>with damage to nail</u>

S61.33- <u>Puncture</u> wound <u>without</u> foreign body of <u>finger</u> <u>with damage to nail</u>

S61.330- Puncture wound <u>without</u> foreign body of <u>right</u> <u>index</u> finger <u>with damage to nail</u>

S61.331- Puncture wound <u>without</u> foreign body of <u>left</u> <u>index</u> finger <u>with damage to nail</u>

S61.332- Puncture wound <u>without</u> foreign body of <u>right</u> <u>middle</u> finger <u>with damage to nail</u>

S61.333- Puncture wound <u>without</u> foreign body of <u>left</u> <u>middle</u> finger <u>with damage to nail</u>

S61.334- Puncture wound <u>without</u> foreign body of <u>right</u> <u>ring</u> finger <u>with damage to nail</u>

S61.335- Puncture wound <u>without</u> foreign body of <u>left</u> <u>ring</u> finger <u>with damage to nail</u>

S61.336- Puncture wound <u>without</u> foreign body of <u>right</u> <u>little</u> finger <u>with damage to nail</u>

S61.337- Puncture wound <u>without</u> foreign body of <u>left</u> <u>little</u> finger <u>with damage to nail</u>

S61.338- Puncture wound <u>without</u> foreign body of <u>other</u> finger <u>with damage to nail</u>
Puncture wound without foreign body of specified finger with unspecified laterality with damage to nail

S61.339- Puncture wound <u>without</u> foreign body of <u>unspecified</u> finger <u>with damage to nail</u>

S61.34- <u>Puncture</u> wound <u>with foreign body</u> of <u>finger</u> <u>with damage to nail</u>

S61.340- Puncture wound <u>with foreign body</u> of <u>right</u> <u>index</u> finger <u>with damage to nail</u>

S61.341- Puncture wound <u>with foreign body</u> of <u>left</u> <u>index</u> finger <u>with damage to nail</u>

S61.342- Puncture wound <u>with foreign body</u> of <u>right</u> <u>middle</u> finger <u>with damage to nail</u>

S61.343- Puncture wound <u>with foreign body</u> of <u>left</u> <u>middle</u> finger <u>with damage to nail</u>

S61.344- Puncture wound <u>with foreign body</u> of <u>right</u> <u>ring</u> finger <u>with damage to nail</u>

S61.345- Puncture wound <u>with foreign body</u> of <u>left</u> <u>ring</u> finger <u>with damage to nail</u>

S61.346- Puncture wound <u>with foreign body</u> of <u>right</u> <u>little</u> finger <u>with damage to nail</u>

S61.347- Puncture wound <u>with foreign body</u> of <u>left</u> <u>little</u> finger <u>with damage to nail</u>

S61.348- Puncture wound <u>with foreign body</u> of <u>other</u> finger <u>with damage to nail</u>
Puncture wound with foreign body of specified finger with unspecified laterality with damage to nail

S61.349- Puncture wound <u>with foreign body</u> of <u>unspecified</u> finger <u>with damage to nail</u>

S61.35- <u>Open bite</u> of <u>finger</u> <u>with damage to nail</u>
Bite of finger with damage to nail NOS
Excludes 1: superficial bite of finger (S60.46-, S60.47-)

S61.350- Open bite of <u>right</u> <u>index</u> finger <u>with damage to nail</u>
S61.351- Open bite of <u>left</u> <u>index</u> finger <u>with damage to nail</u>
S61.352- Open bite of <u>right</u> <u>middle</u> finger <u>with damage to nail</u>
S61.353- Open bite of <u>left</u> <u>middle</u> finger <u>with damage to nail</u>
S61.354- Open bite of <u>right</u> <u>ring</u> finger <u>with damage to nail</u>
S61.355- Open bite of <u>left</u> <u>ring</u> finger <u>with damage to nail</u>
S61.356- Open bite of <u>right</u> <u>little</u> finger <u>with damage to nail</u>
S61.357- Open bite of <u>left</u> <u>little</u> finger <u>with damage to nail</u>
S61.358- Open bite of <u>other</u> finger <u>with damage to nail</u>
Open bite of specified finger with unspecified laterality with damage to nail

S61.359- Open bite of <u>unspecified</u> finger <u>with damage to nail</u>

S61.4- <u>Open wound</u> of <u>hand</u>

S61.40- <u>Unspecified open wound</u> of <u>hand</u>
S61.401- Unspecified open wound of <u>right</u> hand
S61.402- Unspecified open wound of <u>left</u> hand
S61.409- Unspecified open wound of <u>unspecified</u> hand

S61.41- <u>Laceration</u> <u>without</u> foreign body of <u>hand</u>
S61.411- Laceration <u>without</u> foreign body of <u>right</u> hand
S61.412- Laceration <u>without</u> foreign body of <u>left</u> hand
S61.419- Laceration <u>without</u> foreign body of <u>unspecified</u> hand

S61.42- <u>Laceration</u> <u>with foreign body</u> of <u>hand</u>
S61.421- Laceration <u>with foreign body</u> of <u>right</u> hand
S61.422- Laceration <u>with foreign body</u> of <u>left</u> hand
S61.429- Laceration <u>with foreign body</u> of <u>unspecified</u> hand

S61.43- <u>Puncture</u> wound <u>without</u> foreign body of <u>hand</u>
S61.431- Puncture wound <u>without</u> foreign body of <u>right</u> hand
S61.432- Puncture wound <u>without</u> foreign body of <u>left</u> hand
S61.439- Puncture wound <u>without</u> foreign body of <u>unspecified</u> hand

S61.44- <u>Puncture</u> wound <u>with foreign body</u> of <u>hand</u>
S61.441- Puncture wound <u>with foreign body</u> of <u>right</u> hand
S61.442- Puncture wound <u>with foreign body</u> of <u>left</u> hand
S61.449- Puncture wound <u>with foreign body</u> of <u>unspecified</u> hand

S61.45- <u>Open bite</u> of <u>hand</u>
Bite of hand NOS
Excludes 1: superficial bite of hand (S60.56-, S60.57-)

S61.451- Open bite of <u>right</u> hand
S61.452- Open bite of <u>left</u> hand
S61.459- Open bite of <u>unspecified</u> hand

S61.5- <u>Open wound</u> of <u>wrist</u>

S61.50- <u>Unspecified open wound</u> of <u>wrist</u>
S61.501- Unspecified open wound of <u>right</u> wrist
S61.502- Unspecified open wound of <u>left</u> wrist
S61.509- Unspecified open wound of <u>unspecified</u> wrist

S61.51- <u>Laceration</u> <u>without</u> foreign body of <u>wrist</u>
S61.511- Laceration <u>without</u> foreign body of <u>right</u> wrist
S61.512- Laceration <u>without</u> foreign body of <u>left</u> wrist
S61.519- Laceration <u>without</u> foreign body of <u>unspecified</u> wrist

S61.52- <u>Laceration</u> <u>with foreign body</u> of <u>wrist</u>
S61.521- Laceration <u>with foreign body</u> of <u>right</u> wrist
S61.522- Laceration <u>with foreign body</u> of <u>left</u> wrist
S61.529- Laceration <u>with foreign body</u> of <u>unspecified</u> wrist

S61.53- <u>Puncture</u> wound <u>without</u> foreign body of <u>wrist</u>
S61.531- Puncture wound <u>without</u> foreign body of <u>right</u> wrist
S61.532- Puncture wound <u>without</u> foreign body of <u>left</u> wrist
S61.539- Puncture wound <u>without</u> foreign body of <u>unspecified</u> wrist

S61.54- <u>Puncture</u> wound <u>with foreign body</u> of <u>wrist</u>
S61.541- Puncture wound <u>with foreign body</u> of <u>right</u> wrist
S61.542- Puncture wound <u>with foreign body</u> of <u>left</u> wrist
S61.549- Puncture wound <u>with foreign body</u> of <u>unspecified</u> wrist

S61.55- <u>Open bite</u> of <u>wrist</u>
Bite of wrist NOS
Excludes 1: superficial bite of wrist (S60.86-, S60.87-)

S61.551- Open bite of <u>right</u> wrist
S61.552- Open bite of <u>left</u> wrist
S61.559- Open bite of <u>unspecified</u> wrist

S62- <u>Fracture</u> at <u>wrist and hand level</u>
Note: A fracture not indicated as displaced or nondisplaced should be coded to displaced
Note: A fracture not indicated as open or closed should be coded to closed
Excludes 1: traumatic amputation of wrist and hand (S68.-)
Excludes ❷: fracture of distal parts of ulna and radius (S52.-)

The appropriate 7th character is to be added to each code from category S62:
A <u>Initial</u> encounter for <u>closed</u> fracture
B <u>Initial</u> encounter for <u>open</u> fracture
D <u>Subsequent</u> encounter for fracture <u>with routine healing</u>
G <u>Subsequent</u> encounter for fracture <u>with delayed healing</u>
K <u>Subsequent</u> encounter for fracture <u>with nonunion</u>
P <u>Subsequent</u> encounter for fracture <u>with malunion</u>
S <u>Sequela</u>

S62.0- <u>Fracture</u> of <u>navicular [scaphoid] bone</u> of <u>wrist</u>

S62.00- <u>Unspecified</u> fracture of <u>navicular [scaphoid] bone</u> of <u>wrist</u>
S62.001- Unspecified fracture of navicular [scaphoid] bone of <u>right</u> wrist
S62.002- Unspecified fracture of navicular [scaphoid] bone of <u>left</u> wrist
S62.009- Unspecified fracture of navicular [scaphoid] bone of <u>unspecified</u> wrist

S 6 1 – S 6 2

Excludes 1: = NOT CODED HERE! (Do not code both)

Excludes ❷: = Not Included Here

S62.01- Fracture of <u>distal pole</u> of <u>navicular [scaphoid]</u> bone of <u>wrist</u>
Fracture of volar tuberosity of navicular [scaphoid] bone of wrist

S62.011- <u>Displaced</u> fracture of distal pole of navicular [scaphoid] bone of <u>right</u> wrist

S62.012- <u>Displaced</u> fracture of distal pole of navicular [scaphoid] bone of <u>left</u> wrist

S62.013- <u>Displaced</u> fracture of distal pole of navicular [scaphoid] bone of <u>unspecified</u> wrist

S62.014- <u>Nondisplaced</u> fracture of distal pole of navicular [scaphoid] bone of <u>right</u> wrist

S62.015- <u>Nondisplaced</u> fracture of distal pole of navicular [scaphoid] bone of <u>left</u> wrist

S62.016- <u>Nondisplaced</u> fracture of distal pole of navicular [scaphoid] bone of <u>unspecified</u> wrist

S62.02- Fracture of <u>middle third</u> of <u>navicular [scaphoid]</u> bone of <u>wrist</u>

S62.021- <u>Displaced</u> fracture of middle third of navicular [scaphoid] bone of <u>right</u> wrist

S62.022- <u>Displaced</u> fracture of middle third of navicular [scaphoid] bone of <u>left</u> wrist

S62.023- <u>Displaced</u> fracture of middle third of navicular [scaphoid] bone of <u>unspecified</u> wrist

S62.024- <u>Nondisplaced</u> fracture of middle third of navicular [scaphoid] bone of <u>right</u> wrist

S62.025- <u>Nondisplaced</u> fracture of middle third of navicular [scaphoid] bone of <u>left</u> wrist

S62.026- <u>Nondisplaced</u> fracture of middle third of navicular [scaphoid] bone of <u>unspecified</u> wrist

S62.03- Fracture of <u>proximal third</u> of <u>navicular [scaphoid]</u> bone of <u>wrist</u>

S62.031- <u>Displaced</u> fracture of proximal third of navicular [scaphoid] bone of <u>right</u> wrist

S62.032- <u>Displaced</u> fracture of proximal third of navicular [scaphoid] bone of <u>left</u> wrist

S62.033- <u>Displaced</u> fracture of proximal third of navicular [scaphoid] bone of <u>unspecified</u> wrist

S62.034- <u>Nondisplaced</u> fracture of proximal third of navicular [scaphoid] bone of <u>right</u> wrist

S62.035- <u>Nondisplaced</u> fracture of proximal third of navicular [scaphoid] bone of <u>left</u> wrist

S62.036- <u>Nondisplaced</u> fracture of proximal third of navicular [scaphoid] bone of <u>unspecified</u> wrist

S62.1- Fracture of <u>other and unspecified</u> <u>carpal bone(s)</u>
Excludes❷: fracture of scaphoid of wrist (S62.0-)

S62.10- Fracture of <u>unspecified</u> <u>carpal</u> bone
Fracture of wrist NOS

S62.101- Fracture of <u>unspecified</u> carpal bone, <u>right</u> wrist

S62.102- Fracture of <u>unspecified</u> carpal bone, <u>left</u> wrist

S62.109- Fracture of <u>unspecified</u> carpal bone, <u>unspecified</u> wrist

S62.11- Fracture of <u>triquetrum [cuneiform]</u> bone of <u>wrist</u>

S62.111- <u>Displaced</u> fracture of triquetrum [cuneiform] bone, <u>right</u> wrist

S62.112- <u>Displaced</u> fracture of triquetrum [cuneiform] bone, <u>left</u> wrist

S62.113- <u>Displaced</u> fracture of triquetrum [cuneiform] bone, <u>unspecified</u> wrist

S62.114- <u>Nondisplaced</u> fracture of triquetrum [cuneiform] bone, <u>right</u> wrist

S62.115- <u>Nondisplaced</u> fracture of triquetrum [cuneiform] bone, <u>left</u> wrist

S62.116- <u>Nondisplaced</u> fracture of triquetrum [cuneiform] bone, <u>unspecified</u> wrist

S62.12- Fracture of <u>lunate [semilunar]</u>

S62.121- <u>Displaced</u> fracture of lunate [semilunar], <u>right</u> wrist

S62.122- <u>Displaced</u> fracture of lunate [semilunar], <u>left</u> wrist

S62.123- <u>Displaced</u> fracture of lunate [semilunar], <u>unspecified</u> wrist

S62.124- <u>Nondisplaced</u> fracture of lunate [semilunar], <u>right</u> wrist

S62.125- <u>Nondisplaced</u> fracture of lunate [semilunar], <u>left</u> wrist

S62.126- <u>Nondisplaced</u> fracture of lunate [semilunar], <u>unspecified</u> wrist

S62.13- Fracture of <u>capitate [os magnum]</u> bone

S62.131- <u>Displaced</u> fracture of capitate [os magnum] bone, <u>right</u> wrist

S62.132- <u>Displaced</u> fracture of capitate [os magnum] bone, <u>left</u> wrist

S62.133- <u>Displaced</u> fracture of capitate [os magnum] bone, <u>unspecified</u> wrist

S62.134- <u>Nondisplaced</u> fracture of capitate [os magnum] bone, <u>right</u> wrist

S62.135- <u>Nondisplaced</u> fracture of capitate [os magnum] bone, <u>left</u> wrist

S62.136- <u>Nondisplaced</u> fracture of capitate [os magnum] bone, <u>unspecified</u> wrist

S62.14- Fracture of <u>body of hamate [unciform]</u> bone
Fracture of hamate [unciform] bone NOS

S62.141- <u>Displaced</u> fracture of body of hamate [unciform] bone, <u>right</u> wrist

S62.142- <u>Displaced</u> fracture of body of hamate [unciform] bone, <u>left</u> wrist

S62.143- <u>Displaced</u> fracture of body of hamate [unciform] bone, <u>unspecified</u> wrist

S62.144- <u>Nondisplaced</u> fracture of body of hamate [unciform] bone, <u>right</u> wrist

S62.145- <u>Nondisplaced</u> fracture of body of hamate [unciform] bone, <u>left</u> wrist

S62.146- <u>Nondisplaced</u> fracture of body of hamate [unciform] bone, <u>unspecified</u> wrist

S62.15- Fracture of <u>hook process</u> of <u>hamate [unciform]</u> bone
Fracture of unciform process of hamate [unciform] bone

S62.151- <u>Displaced</u> fracture of hook process of hamate [unciform] bone, <u>right</u> wrist

S62.152- <u>Displaced</u> fracture of hook process of hamate [unciform] bone, <u>left</u> wrist

S62.153- <u>Displaced</u> fracture of hook process of hamate [unciform] bone, <u>unspecified</u> wrist

S62.154- <u>Nondisplaced</u> fracture of hook process of hamate [unciform] bone, <u>right</u> wrist

S62.155- <u>Nondisplaced</u> fracture of hook process of hamate [unciform] bone, <u>left</u> wrist

S62.156- <u>Nondisplaced</u> fracture of hook process of hamate [unciform] bone, <u>unspecified</u> wrist

S62.16- Fracture of <u>pisiform</u>

S62.161- <u>Displaced</u> fracture of pisiform, <u>right</u> wrist

S62.162- <u>Displaced</u> fracture of pisiform, <u>left</u> wrist

S62.163- <u>Displaced</u> fracture of pisiform, <u>unspecified</u> wrist

S62.164- <u>Nondisplaced</u> fracture of pisiform, <u>right</u> wrist

S62.165- <u>Nondisplaced</u> fracture of pisiform, <u>left</u> wrist

S62.166- <u>Nondisplaced</u> fracture of pisiform, <u>unspecified</u> wrist

S62.17- Fracture of <u>trapezium [larger multangular]</u>

S62.171- <u>Displaced</u> fracture of trapezium [larger multangular], <u>right</u> wrist

S62.172- <u>Displaced</u> fracture of trapezium [larger multangular], <u>left</u> wrist

S62.173- <u>Displaced</u> fracture of trapezium [larger multangular], <u>unspecified</u> wrist

S62.174- <u>Nondisplaced</u> fracture of trapezium [larger multangular], <u>right</u> wrist

S62.175- <u>Nondisplaced</u> fracture of trapezium [larger multangular], <u>left</u> wrist

S62.176- <u>Nondisplaced</u> fracture of trapezium [larger multangular], <u>unspecified</u> wrist

S62.18- Fracture of <u>trapezoid [smaller multangular]</u>

S62.181- <u>Displaced</u> fracture of trapezoid [smaller multangular], <u>right</u> wrist

S62.182- <u>Displaced</u> fracture of trapezoid [smaller multangular], <u>left</u> wrist

S62.183- <u>Displaced</u> fracture of trapezoid [smaller multangular], <u>unspecified</u> wrist

S62.184- <u>Nondisplaced</u> fracture of trapezoid [smaller multangular], <u>right</u> wrist

S62.185- <u>Nondisplaced</u> fracture of trapezoid [smaller multangular], <u>left</u> wrist

S62.186- <u>Nondisplaced</u> fracture of trapezoid [smaller multangular], <u>unspecified</u> wrist

S62.2- Fracture of <u>first metacarpal</u> bone

S62.20- <u>Unspecified</u> fracture of <u>first metacarpal</u> bone

S62.201- Unspecified fracture of first metacarpal bone, <u>right</u> hand

S62.202- Unspecified fracture of first metacarpal bone, <u>left</u> hand

S62.209- Unspecified fracture of first metacarpal bone, <u>unspecified</u> hand

S62.21- <u>Bennett's fracture</u>

S62.211- Bennett's fracture, <u>right</u> hand
S62.212- Bennett's fracture, <u>left</u> hand
S62.213- Bennett's fracture, <u>unspecified</u> hand

S 6 1 - S 6 2

S62.22- Rolando's fracture
- S62.221- <u>Displaced</u> Rolando's fracture, <u>right</u> hand
- S62.222- <u>Displaced</u> Rolando's fracture, <u>left</u> hand
- S62.223- <u>Displaced</u> Rolando's fracture, <u>unspecified</u> hand
- S62.224- <u>Nondisplaced</u> Rolando's fracture, <u>right</u> hand
- S62.225- <u>Nondisplaced</u> Rolando's fracture, <u>left</u> hand
- S62.226- <u>Nondisplaced</u> Rolando's fracture, <u>unspecified</u> hand

S62.23- <u>Other</u> fracture of <u>base</u> of <u>first</u> <u>metacarpal</u> bone
- S62.231- Other <u>displaced</u> fracture of base of first metacarpal bone, <u>right</u> hand
- S62.232- Other <u>displaced</u> fracture of base of first metacarpal bone, <u>left</u> hand
- S62.233- Other <u>displaced</u> fracture of base of first metacarpal bone, <u>unspecified</u> hand
- S62.234- Other <u>nondisplaced</u> fracture of base of first metacarpal bone, <u>right</u> hand
- S62.235- Other <u>nondisplaced</u> fracture of base of first metacarpal bone, <u>left</u> hand
- S62.236- Other <u>nondisplaced</u> fracture of base of first metacarpal bone, <u>unspecified</u> hand

S62.24- Fracture of <u>shaft</u> of <u>first</u> <u>metacarpal</u> bone
- S62.241- <u>Displaced</u> fracture of shaft of first metacarpal bone, <u>right</u> hand
- S62.242- <u>Displaced</u> fracture of shaft of first metacarpal bone, <u>left</u> hand
- S62.243- <u>Displaced</u> fracture of shaft of first metacarpal bone, <u>unspecified</u> hand
- S62.244- <u>Nondisplaced</u> fracture of shaft of first metacarpal bone, <u>right</u> hand
- S62.245- <u>Nondisplaced</u> fracture of shaft of first metacarpal bone, <u>left</u> hand
- S62.246- <u>Nondisplaced</u> fracture of shaft of first metacarpal bone, <u>unspecified</u> hand

S62.25- Fracture of <u>neck</u> of <u>first</u> <u>metacarpal</u> bone
- S62.251- <u>Displaced</u> fracture of neck of first metacarpal bone, <u>right</u> hand
- S62.252- <u>Displaced</u> fracture of neck of first metacarpal bone, <u>left</u> hand
- S62.253- <u>Displaced</u> fracture of neck of first metacarpal bone, <u>unspecified</u> hand
- S62.254- <u>Nondisplaced</u> fracture of neck of first metacarpal bone, <u>right</u> hand
- S62.255- <u>Nondisplaced</u> fracture of neck of first metacarpal bone, <u>left</u> hand
- S62.256- <u>Nondisplaced</u> fracture of neck of first metacarpal bone, <u>unspecified</u> hand

S62.29- <u>Other</u> fracture of <u>first</u> <u>metacarpal</u> bone
- S62.291- Other fracture of first metacarpal bone, <u>right</u> hand
- S62.292- Other fracture of first metacarpal bone, <u>left</u> hand
- S62.299- Other fracture of first metacarpal bone, <u>unspecified</u> hand

S62.3- Fracture of <u>other and unspecified</u> <u>metacarpal</u> bone
Excludes❷: fracture of first metacarpal bone (S62.2-)

S62.30- <u>Unspecified</u> fracture of <u>other</u> <u>metacarpal</u> bone
- S62.300- Unspecified fracture of <u>second</u> metacarpal bone, <u>right</u> hand
- S62.301- Unspecified fracture of <u>second</u> metacarpal bone, <u>left</u> hand
- S62.302- Unspecified fracture of <u>third</u> metacarpal bone, <u>right</u> hand
- S62.303- Unspecified fracture of <u>third</u> metacarpal bone, <u>left</u> hand
- S62.304- Unspecified fracture of <u>fourth</u> metacarpal bone, <u>right</u> hand
- S62.305- Unspecified fracture of <u>fourth</u> metacarpal bone, <u>left</u> hand
- S62.306- Unspecified fracture of <u>fifth</u> metacarpal bone, <u>right</u> hand
- S62.307- Unspecified fracture of <u>fifth</u> metacarpal bone, <u>left</u> hand
- S62.308- Unspecified fracture of <u>other</u> metacarpal bone
  Unspecified fracture of specified metacarpal bone with unspecified laterality
- S62.309- Unspecified fracture of <u>unspecified</u> metacarpal bone

S62.31- <u>Displaced</u> fracture of <u>base</u> of <u>other</u> <u>metacarpal</u> bone
- S62.310- <u>Displaced</u> fracture of <u>base</u> of <u>second</u> metacarpal bone, <u>right</u> hand
- S62.311- <u>Displaced</u> fracture of <u>base</u> of <u>second</u> metacarpal bone. <u>left</u> hand
- S62.312- <u>Displaced</u> fracture of <u>base</u> of <u>third</u> metacarpal bone, <u>right</u> hand
- S62.313- <u>Displaced</u> fracture of <u>base</u> of <u>third</u> metacarpal bone, <u>left</u> hand
- S62.314- <u>Displaced</u> fracture of <u>base</u> of <u>fourth</u> metacarpal bone, <u>right</u> hand
- S62.315- <u>Displaced</u> fracture of <u>base</u> of <u>fourth</u> metacarpal bone, <u>left</u> hand
- S62.316- <u>Displaced</u> fracture of <u>base</u> of <u>fifth</u> metacarpal bone, <u>right</u> hand
- S62.317- <u>Displaced</u> fracture of <u>base</u> of <u>fifth</u> metacarpal bone. <u>left</u> hand
- S62.318- <u>Displaced</u> fracture of <u>base</u> of <u>other</u> metacarpal bone
  Displaced fracture of base of specified metacarpal bone with unspecified laterality
- S62.319- <u>Displaced</u> fracture of <u>base</u> of <u>unspecified</u> metacarpal bone

S62.32- <u>Displaced</u> fracture of <u>shaft</u> of <u>other</u> <u>metacarpal</u> bone
- S62.320- <u>Displaced</u> fracture of <u>shaft</u> of <u>second</u> metacarpal bone, <u>right</u> hand
- S62.321- <u>Displaced</u> fracture of <u>shaft</u> of <u>second</u> metacarpal bone, <u>left</u> hand
- S62.322- <u>Displaced</u> fracture of <u>shaft</u> of <u>third</u> metacarpal bone, <u>right</u> hand
- S62.323- <u>Displaced</u> fracture of <u>shaft</u> of <u>third</u> metacarpal bone, <u>left</u> hand
- S62.324- <u>Displaced</u> fracture of <u>shaft</u> of <u>fourth</u> metacarpal bone, <u>right</u> hand
- S62.325- <u>Displaced</u> fracture of <u>shaft</u> of <u>fourth</u> metacarpal bone, <u>left</u> hand
- S62.326- <u>Displaced</u> fracture of <u>shaft</u> of <u>fifth</u> metacarpal bone, <u>right</u> hand
- S62.327- <u>Displaced</u> fracture of <u>shaft</u> of <u>fifth</u> metacarpal bone, <u>left</u> hand
- S62.328- <u>Displaced</u> fracture of <u>shaft</u> of <u>other</u> metacarpal bone
  Displaced fracture of shaft of specified metacarpal bone with unspecified laterality
- S62.329- <u>Displaced</u> fracture of <u>shaft</u> of <u>unspecified</u> metacarpal bone

S62.33- <u>Displaced</u> fracture of <u>neck</u> of <u>other</u> <u>metacarpal</u> bone
- S62.330- <u>Displaced</u> fracture of <u>neck</u> of <u>second</u> metacarpal bone, <u>right</u> hand
- S62.331- <u>Displaced</u> fracture of <u>neck</u> of <u>second</u> metacarpal bone, <u>left</u> hand
- S62.332- <u>Displaced</u> fracture of <u>neck</u> of <u>third</u> metacarpal bone, <u>right</u> hand
- S62.333- <u>Displaced</u> fracture of <u>neck</u> of <u>third</u> metacarpal bone, <u>left</u> hand
- S62.334- <u>Displaced</u> fracture of <u>neck</u> of <u>fourth</u> metacarpal bone, <u>right</u> hand
- S62.335- <u>Displaced</u> fracture of <u>neck</u> of <u>fourth</u> metacarpal bone, <u>left</u> hand
- S62.336- <u>Displaced</u> fracture of <u>neck</u> of <u>fifth</u> metacarpal bone, <u>right</u> hand
- S62.337- <u>Displaced</u> fracture of <u>neck</u> of <u>fifth</u> metacarpal bone, <u>left</u> hand
- S62.338- <u>Displaced</u> fracture of <u>neck</u> of <u>other</u> metacarpal bone
  Displaced fracture of neck of specified metacarpal bone with unspecified laterality
- S62.339- <u>Displaced</u> fracture of <u>neck</u> of <u>unspecified</u> metacarpal bone

S62.34- <u>Nondisplaced</u> fracture of <u>base</u> of <u>other</u> <u>metacarpal</u> bone
- S62.340- <u>Nondisplaced</u> fracture of <u>base</u> of <u>second</u> metacarpal bone, <u>right</u> hand
- S62.341- <u>Nondisplaced</u> fracture of <u>base</u> of <u>second</u> metacarpal bone. <u>left</u> hand
- S62.342- <u>Nondisplaced</u> fracture of <u>base</u> of <u>third</u> metacarpal bone, <u>right</u> hand
- S62.343- <u>Nondisplaced</u> fracture of <u>base</u> of <u>third</u> metacarpal bone, <u>left</u> hand
- S62.344- <u>Nondisplaced</u> fracture of <u>base</u> of <u>fourth</u> metacarpal bone, <u>right</u> hand
- S62.345- <u>Nondisplaced</u> fracture of <u>base</u> of <u>fourth</u> metacarpal bone, <u>left</u> hand

S
6
2
I
S
6
2

© 2013 Channel Publishing Ltd

S62.346-   Nondisplaced fracture of base of fifth metacarpal bone, right hand

S62.347-   Nondisplaced fracture of base of fifth metacarpal bone. left hand

S62.348-   Nondisplaced fracture of base of other metacarpal bone
            Nondisplaced fracture of base of specified metacarpal bone with unspecified laterality

S62.349-   Nondisplaced fracture of base of unspecified metacarpal bone

S62.35- Nondisplaced fracture of shaft of other metacarpal bone

S62.350-   Nondisplaced fracture of shaft of second metacarpal bone, right hand

S62.351-   Nondisplaced fracture of shaft of second metacarpal bone, left hand

S62.352-   Nondisplaced fracture of shaft of third metacarpal bone, right hand

S62.353-   Nondisplaced fracture of shaft of third metacarpal bone, left hand

S62.354-   Nondisplaced fracture of shaft of fourth metacarpal bone, right hand

S62.355-   Nondisplaced fracture of shaft of fourth metacarpal bone, left hand

S62.356-   Nondisplaced fracture of shaft of fifth metacarpal bone, right hand

S62.357-   Nondisplaced fracture of shaft of fifth metacarpal bone, left hand

S62.358-   Nondisplaced fracture of shaft of other metacarpal bone
            Nondisplaced fracture of shaft of specified metacarpal bone with unspecified laterality

S62.359-   Nondisplaced fracture of shaft of unspecified metacarpal bone

S62.36- Nondisplaced fracture of neck of other metacarpal bone

S62.360-   Nondisplaced fracture of neck of second metacarpal bone, right hand

S62.361-   Nondisplaced fracture of neck of second metacarpal bone, left hand

S62.362-   Nondisplaced fracture of neck of third metacarpal bone, right hand

S62.363-   Nondisplaced fracture of neck of third metacarpal bone, left hand

S62.364-   Nondisplaced fracture of neck of fourth metacarpal bone, right hand

S62.365-   Nondisplaced fracture of neck of fourth metacarpal bone, left hand

S62.366-   Nondisplaced fracture of neck of fifth metacarpal bone, right hand

S62.367-   Nondisplaced fracture of neck of fifth metacarpal bone, left hand

S62.368-   Nondisplaced fracture of neck of other metacarpal bone
            Nondisplaced fracture of neck of specified metacarpal bone with unspecified laterality

S62.369-   Nondisplaced fracture of neck of unspecified metacarpal bone

S62.39- Other fracture of other metacarpal bone

S62.390-   Other fracture of second metacarpal bone, right hand

S62.391-   Other fracture of second metacarpal bone, left hand

S62.392-   Other fracture of third metacarpal bone, right hand

S62.393-   Other fracture of third metacarpal bone, left hand

S62.394-   Other fracture of fourth metacarpal bone, right hand

S62.395-   Other fracture of fourth metacarpal bone, left hand

S62.396-   Other fracture of fifth metacarpal bone, right hand

S62.397-   Other fracture of fifth metacarpal bone, left hand

S62.398-   Other fracture of other metacarpal bone
            Other fracture of specified metacarpal bone with unspecified laterality

S62.399-   Other fracture of unspecified metacarpal bone

S62.5-   Fracture of thumb

S62.50- Fracture of unspecified phalanx of thumb

S62.501-   Fracture of unspecified phalanx of right thumb

S62.502-   Fracture of unspecified phalanx of left thumb

S62.509-   Fracture of unspecified phalanx of unspecified thumb

S62.51- Fracture of proximal phalanx of thumb

S62.511-   Displaced fracture of proximal phalanx of right thumb

S62.512-   Displaced fracture of proximal phalanx of left thumb

S62.513-   Displaced fracture of proximal phalanx of unspecified thumb

S62.514-   Nondisplaced fracture of proximal phalanx of right thumb

S62.515-   Nondisplaced fracture of proximal phalanx of left thumb

S62.516-   Nondisplaced fracture of proximal phalanx of unspecified thumb

S62.52- Fracture of distal phalanx of thumb

S62.521-   Displaced fracture of distal phalanx of right thumb

S62.522-   Displaced fracture of distal phalanx of left thumb

S62.523-   Displaced fracture of distal phalanx of unspecified thumb

S62.524-   Nondisplaced fracture of distal phalanx of right thumb

S62.525-   Nondisplaced fracture of distal phalanx of left thumb

S62.526-   Nondisplaced fracture of distal phalanx of unspecified thumb

S62.6-   Fracture of other and unspecified finger(s)
         Excludes ❷: fracture of thumb (S62.5-)

S62.60- Fracture of unspecified phalanx of finger

S62.600-   Fracture of unspecified phalanx of right index finger

S62.601-   Fracture of unspecified phalanx of left index finger

S62.602-   Fracture of unspecified phalanx of right middle finger

S62.603-   Fracture of unspecified phalanx of left middle finger

S62.604-   Fracture of unspecified phalanx of right ring finger

S62.605-   Fracture of unspecified phalanx of left ring finger

S62.606-   Fracture of unspecified phalanx of right little finger

S62.607-   Fracture of unspecified phalanx of left little finger

S62.608-   Fracture of unspecified phalanx of other finger
            Fracture of unspecified phalanx of specified finger with unspecified laterality

S62.609-   Fracture of unspecified phalanx of unspecified finger

S62.61- Displaced fracture of proximal phalanx of finger

S62.610-   Displaced fracture of proximal phalanx of right index finger

S62.611-   Displaced fracture of proximal phalanx of left index finger

S62.612-   Displaced fracture of proximal phalanx of right middle finger

S62.613-   Displaced fracture of proximal phalanx of left middle finger

S62.614-   Displaced fracture of proximal phalanx of right ring finger

S62.615-   Displaced fracture of proximal phalanx of left ring finger

S62.616-   Displaced fracture of proximal phalanx of right little finger

S62.617-   Displaced fracture of proximal phalanx of left little finger

S62.618-   Displaced fracture of proximal phalanx of other finger
            Displaced fracture of proximal phalanx of specified finger with unspecified laterality

S62.619-   Displaced fracture of proximal phalanx of unspecified finger

S62.62- Displaced fracture of medial phalanx of finger

S62.620-   Displaced fracture of medial phalanx of right index finger

S62.621-   Displaced fracture of medial phalanx of left index finger

S62.622-   Displaced fracture of medial phalanx of right middle finger

S62.623-   Displaced fracture of medial phalanx of left middle finger

S62.624-   Displaced fracture of medial phalanx of right ring finger

S62.625-   Displaced fracture of medial phalanx of left ring finger

S62.626-   Displaced fracture of medial phalanx of right little finger

S62.627-   Displaced fracture of medial phalanx of left little finger

S62.628-   Displaced fracture of medial phalanx of other finger
            Displaced fracture of medial phalanx of specified finger with unspecified laterality

S62.629-   Displaced fracture of medial phalanx of unspecified finger

S62 - S62

S62.63- Displaced fracture of distal phalanx of finger

S62.630- Displaced fracture of distal phalanx of right index finger

S62.631- Displaced fracture of distal phalanx of left index finger

S62.632- Displaced fracture of distal phalanx of right middle finger

S62.633- Displaced fracture of distal phalanx of left middle finger

S62.634- Displaced fracture of distal phalanx of right ring finger

S62.635- Displaced fracture of distal phalanx of left ring finger

S62.636- Displaced fracture of distal phalanx of right little finger

S62.637- Displaced fracture of distal phalanx of left little finger

S62.638- Displaced fracture of distal phalanx of other finger
Displaced fracture of distal phalanx of specified finger with unspecified laterality

S62.639- Displaced fracture of distal phalanx of unspecified finger

S62.64- Nondisplaced fracture of proximal phalanx of finger

S62.640- Nondisplaced fracture of proximal phalanx of right index finger

S62.641- Nondisplaced fracture of proximal phalanx of left index finger

S62.642- Nondisplaced fracture of proximal phalanx of right middle finger

S62.643- Nondisplaced fracture of proximal phalanx of left middle finger

S62.644- Nondisplaced fracture of proximal phalanx of right ring finger

S62.645- Nondisplaced fracture of proximal phalanx of left ring finger

S62.646- Nondisplaced fracture of proximal phalanx of right little finger

S62.647- Nondisplaced fracture of proximal phalanx of left little finger

S62.648- Nondisplaced fracture of proximal phalanx of other finger
Nondisplaced fracture of proximal phalanx of specified finger with unspecified laterality

S62.649- Nondisplaced fracture of proximal phalanx of unspecified finger

S62.65- Nondisplaced fracture of medial phalanx of finger

S62.650- Nondisplaced fracture of medial phalanx of right index finger

S62.651- Nondisplaced fracture of medial phalanx of left index finger

S62.652- Nondisplaced fracture of medial phalanx of right middle finger

S62.653- Nondisplaced fracture of medial phalanx of left middle finger

S62.654- Nondisplaced fracture of medial phalanx of right ring finger

S62.655- Nondisplaced fracture of medial phalanx of left ring finger

S62.656- Nondisplaced fracture of medial phalanx of right little finger

S62.657- Nondisplaced fracture of medial phalanx of left little finger

S62.658- Nondisplaced fracture of medial phalanx of other finger
Nondisplaced fracture of medial phalanx of specified finger with unspecified laterality

S62.659- Nondisplaced fracture of medial phalanx of unspecified finger

S62.66- Nondisplaced fracture of distal phalanx of finger

S62.660- Nondisplaced fracture of distal phalanx of right index finger

S62.661- Nondisplaced fracture of distal phalanx of left index finger

S62.662- Nondisplaced fracture of distal phalanx of right middle finger

S62.663- Nondisplaced fracture of distal phalanx of left middle finger

S62.664- Nondisplaced fracture of distal phalanx of right ring finger

S62.665- Nondisplaced fracture of distal phalanx of left ring finger

S62.666- Nondisplaced fracture of distal phalanx of right little finger

S62.667- Nondisplaced fracture of distal phalanx of left little finger

S62.668- Nondisplaced fracture of distal phalanx of other finger
Nondisplaced fracture of distal phalanx of specified finger with unspecified laterality

S62.669- Nondisplaced fracture of distal phalanx of unspecified finger

S62.9- Unspecified fracture of wrist and hand

S62.90x- Unspecified fracture of unspecified wrist and hand

S62.91x- Unspecified fracture of right wrist and hand

S62.92x- Unspecified fracture of left wrist and hand

S63- Dislocation and sprain of joints and ligaments at wrist and hand level
Includes: Avulsion of joint or ligament at wrist and hand level
Laceration of cartilage, joint or ligament at wrist and hand level
Sprain of cartilage, joint or ligament at wrist and hand level
Traumatic hemarthrosis of joint or ligament at wrist and hand level
Traumatic rupture of joint or ligament at wrist and hand level
Traumatic subluxation of joint or ligament at wrist and hand level
Traumatic tear of joint or ligament at wrist and hand level
Code also any associated open wound
Excludes❷: strain of muscle, fascia and tendon of wrist and hand (S66.-)

The appropriate 7th character is to be added to each code from category S63:
A Initial encounter
D Subsequent encounter
S Sequela

S63.0- Subluxation and dislocation of wrist and hand joints

S63.00- Unspecified subluxation and dislocation of wrist and hand
Dislocation of carpal bone NOS
Dislocation of distal end of radius NOS
Subluxation of carpal bone NOS
Subluxation of distal end of radius NOS

S63.001- Unspecified subluxation of right wrist and hand

S63.002- Unspecified subluxation of left wrist and hand

S63.003- Unspecified subluxation of unspecified wrist and hand

S63.004- Unspecified dislocation of right wrist and hand

S63.005- Unspecified dislocation of left wrist and hand

S63.006- Unspecified dislocation of unspecified wrist and hand

S63.01- Subluxation and dislocation of distal radioulnar joint

S63.011- Subluxation of distal radioulnar joint of right wrist

S63.012- Subluxation of distal radioulnar joint of left wrist

S63.013- Subluxation of distal radioulnar joint of unspecified wrist

S63.014- Dislocation of distal radioulnar joint of right wrist

S63.015- Dislocation of distal radioulnar joint of left wrist

S63.016- Dislocation of distal radioulnar joint of unspecified wrist

S63.02- Subluxation and dislocation of radiocarpal joint

S63.021- Subluxation of radiocarpal joint of right wrist

S63.022- Subluxation of radiocarpal joint of left wrist

S63.023- Subluxation of radiocarpal joint of unspecified wrist

S63.024- Dislocation of radiocarpal joint of right wrist

S63.025- Dislocation of radiocarpal joint of left wrist

S63.026- Dislocation of radiocarpal joint of unspecified wrist

S63.03- Subluxation and dislocation of midcarpal joint

S63.031- Subluxation of midcarpal joint of right wrist

S63.032- Subluxation of midcarpal joint of left wrist

S63.033- Subluxation of midcarpal joint of unspecified wrist

S63.034- Dislocation of midcarpal joint of right wrist

S63.035- Dislocation of midcarpal joint of left wrist

S63.036- Dislocation of midcarpal joint of unspecified wrist

S63.04- Subluxation and dislocation of carpometacarpal joint of thumb
Excludes❷: interphalangeal subluxation and dislocation of thumb (S63.1-)

S63.041- Subluxation of carpometacarpal joint of right thumb

S63.042- Subluxation of carpometacarpal joint of left thumb

S63.043- Subluxation of carpometacarpal joint of unspecified thumb

S63.044- Dislocation of carpometacarpal joint of right thumb

S63.045- Dislocation of carpometacarpal joint of left thumb

S63.046- Dislocation of carpometacarpal joint of unspecified thumb

S 6 2 - S 6 3

S63.05- Subluxation and dislocation of <u>other carpometacarpal joint</u>
  Excludes❷: subluxation and dislocation of carpometacarpal joint of thumb (S63.04-)
  S63.051- <u>Subluxation</u> of other carpometacarpal joint of <u>right</u> hand
  S63.052- <u>Subluxation</u> of other carpometacarpal joint of <u>left</u> hand
  S63.053- <u>Subluxation</u> of other carpometacarpal joint of <u>unspecified</u> hand
  S63.054- <u>Dislocation</u> of other carpometacarpal joint of <u>right</u> hand
  S63.055- <u>Dislocation</u> of other carpometacarpal joint of <u>left</u> hand
  S63.056- <u>Dislocation</u> of other carpometacarpal joint of <u>unspecified</u> hand

S63.06- Subluxation and dislocation of <u>metacarpal (bone), proximal end</u>
  S63.061- <u>Subluxation</u> of metacarpal (bone), proximal end of <u>right</u> hand
  S63.062- <u>Subluxation</u> of metacarpal (bone), proximal end of <u>left</u> hand
  S63.063- <u>Subluxation</u> of metacarpal (bone), proximal end of <u>unspecified</u> hand
  S63.064- <u>Dislocation</u> of metacarpal (bone), proximal end of <u>right</u> hand
  S63.065- <u>Dislocation</u> of metacarpal (bone), proximal end of <u>left</u> hand
  S63.066- <u>Dislocation</u> of metacarpal (bone), proximal end of <u>unspecified</u> hand

S63.07- Subluxation and dislocation of <u>distal end of ulna</u>
  S63.071- <u>Subluxation</u> of distal end of <u>right</u> ulna
  S63.072- <u>Subluxation</u> of distal end of <u>left</u> ulna
  S63.073- <u>Subluxation</u> of distal end of <u>unspecified</u> ulna
  S63.074- <u>Dislocation</u> of distal end of <u>right</u> ulna
  S63.075- <u>Dislocation</u> of distal end of <u>left</u> ulna
  S63.076- <u>Dislocation</u> of distal end of <u>unspecified</u> ulna

S63.09- <u>Other</u> subluxation and dislocation of <u>wrist and hand</u>
  S63.091- Other <u>subluxation</u> of <u>right</u> wrist and hand
  S63.092- Other <u>subluxation</u> of <u>left</u> wrist and hand
  S63.093- Other <u>subluxation</u> of <u>unspecified</u> wrist and hand
  S63.094- Other <u>dislocation</u> of <u>right</u> wrist and hand
  S63.095- Other <u>dislocation</u> of <u>left</u> wrist and hand
  S63.096- Other <u>dislocation</u> of <u>unspecified</u> wrist and hand

S63.1- Subluxation and dislocation of <u>thumb</u>
  S63.10- <u>Unspecified</u> subluxation and dislocation of <u>thumb</u>
    S63.101- Unspecified <u>subluxation</u> of <u>right</u> thumb
    S63.102- Unspecified <u>subluxation</u> of <u>left</u> thumb
    S63.103- Unspecified <u>subluxation</u> of <u>unspecified</u> thumb
    S63.104- Unspecified <u>dislocation</u> of <u>right</u> thumb
    S63.105- Unspecified <u>dislocation</u> of <u>left</u> thumb
    S63.106- Unspecified <u>dislocation</u> of <u>unspecified</u> thumb

  S63.11- Subluxation and dislocation of <u>metacarpophalangeal joint</u> of <u>thumb</u>
    S63.111- <u>Subluxation</u> of metacarpophalangeal joint of <u>right</u> thumb
    S63.112- <u>Subluxation</u> of metacarpophalangeal joint of <u>left</u> thumb
    S63.113- <u>Subluxation</u> of metacarpophalangeal joint of <u>unspecified</u> thumb
    S63.114- <u>Dislocation</u> of metacarpophalangeal joint of <u>right</u> thumb
    S63.115- <u>Dislocation</u> of metacarpophalangeal joint of <u>left</u> thumb
    S63.116- <u>Dislocation</u> of metacarpophalangeal joint of <u>unspecified</u> thumb

  S63.12- Subluxation and dislocation of <u>unspecified interphalangeal joint</u> of <u>thumb</u>
    S63.121- <u>Subluxation</u> of unspecified interphalangeal joint of <u>right</u> thumb
    S63.122- <u>Subluxation</u> of unspecified interphalangeal joint of <u>left</u> thumb
    S63.123- <u>Subluxation</u> of unspecified interphalangeal joint of <u>unspecified</u> thumb
    S63.124- <u>Dislocation</u> of unspecified interphalangeal joint of <u>right</u> thumb
    S63.125- <u>Dislocation</u> of unspecified interphalangeal joint of <u>left</u> thumb
    S63.126- <u>Dislocation</u> of unspecified interphalangeal joint of <u>unspecified</u> thumb

S63.13- Subluxation and dislocation of <u>proximal interphalangeal joint</u> of <u>thumb</u>
  S63.131- <u>Subluxation</u> of proximal interphalangeal joint of <u>right</u> thumb
  S63.132- <u>Subluxation</u> of proximal interphalangeal joint of <u>left</u> thumb
  S63.133- <u>Subluxation</u> of proximal interphalangeal joint of <u>unspecified</u> thumb
  S63.134- <u>Dislocation</u> of proximal interphalangeal joint of <u>right</u> thumb
  S63.135- <u>Dislocation</u> of proximal interphalangeal joint of <u>left</u> thumb
  S63.136- <u>Dislocation</u> of proximal interphalangeal joint of <u>unspecified</u> thumb

S63.14- Subluxation and dislocation of <u>distal interphalangeal joint</u> of <u>thumb</u>
  S63.141- <u>Subluxation</u> of distal interphalangeal joint of <u>right</u> thumb
  S63.142- <u>Subluxation</u> of distal interphalangeal joint of <u>left</u> thumb
  S63.143- <u>Subluxation</u> of distal interphalangeal joint of <u>unspecified</u> thumb
  S63.144- <u>Dislocation</u> of distal interphalangeal joint of <u>right</u> thumb
  S63.145- <u>Dislocation</u> of distal interphalangeal joint of <u>left</u> thumb
  S63.146- <u>Dislocation</u> of distal interphalangeal joint of <u>unspecified</u> thumb

S63.2- Subluxation and dislocation of <u>other finger(s)</u>
  Excludes❷: subluxation and dislocation of thumb (S63.1-)
  S63.20- <u>Unspecified subluxation</u> of other <u>finger</u>
    S63.200- Unspecified subluxation of <u>right</u> <u>index</u> finger
    S63.201- Unspecified subluxation of <u>left</u> <u>index</u> finger
    S63.202- Unspecified subluxation of <u>right</u> <u>middle</u> finger
    S63.203- Unspecified subluxation of <u>left</u> <u>middle</u> finger
    S63.204- Unspecified subluxation of <u>right</u> <u>ring</u> finger
    S63.205- Unspecified subluxation of <u>left</u> <u>ring</u> finger
    S63.206- Unspecified subluxation of <u>right</u> <u>little</u> finger
    S63.207- Unspecified subluxation of <u>left</u> <u>little</u> finger
    S63.208- Unspecified subluxation of <u>other</u> finger
      Unspecified subluxation of specified finger with unspecified laterality
    S63.209- Unspecified subluxation of <u>unspecified</u> finger

  S63.21- <u>Subluxation</u> of <u>metacarpophalangeal joint</u> of <u>finger</u>
    S63.210- Subluxation of metacarpophalangeal joint of <u>right</u> <u>index</u> finger
    S63.211- Subluxation of metacarpophalangeal joint of <u>left index</u> finger
    S63.212- Subluxation of metacarpophalangeal joint of <u>right</u> <u>middle</u> finger
    S63.213- Subluxation of metacarpophalangeal joint of <u>left</u> <u>middle</u> finger
    S63.214- Subluxation of metacarpophalangeal joint of <u>right</u> <u>ring</u> finger
    S63.215- Subluxation of metacarpophalangeal joint of <u>left ring</u> finger
    S63.216- Subluxation of metacarpophalangeal joint of <u>right</u> <u>little</u> finger
    S63.217- Subluxation of metacarpophalangeal joint of <u>left little</u> finger
    S63.218- Subluxation of metacarpophalangeal joint of <u>other</u> finger
      Subluxation of metacarpophalangeal joint of specified finger with unspecified laterality
    S63.219- Subluxation of metacarpophalangeal joint of <u>unspecified</u> finger

  S63.22- <u>Subluxation</u> of <u>unspecified interphalangeal joint</u> of <u>finger</u>
    S63.220- Subluxation of unspecified interphalangeal joint of <u>right</u> <u>index</u> finger
    S63.221- Subluxation of unspecified interphalangeal joint of <u>left</u> <u>index</u> finger
    S63.222- Subluxation of unspecified interphalangeal joint of <u>right</u> <u>middle</u> finger
    S63.223- Subluxation of unspecified interphalangeal joint of <u>left</u> <u>middle</u> finger
    S63.224- Subluxation of unspecified interphalangeal joint of <u>right</u> <u>ring</u> finger
    S63.225- Subluxation of unspecified interphalangeal joint of <u>left</u> <u>ring</u> finger

S 6 2 - S 6 3

S63.226- Subluxation of unspecified interphalangeal joint of <u>right</u> <u>little</u> finger

S63.227- Subluxation of unspecified interphalangeal joint of <u>left</u> <u>little</u> finger

S63.228- Subluxation of unspecified interphalangeal joint of <u>other</u> finger
    Subluxation of unspecified interphalangeal joint of specified finger with unspecified laterality

S63.229- Subluxation of unspecified interphalangeal joint of <u>unspecified</u> finger

S63.23- <u>Subluxation</u> of <u>proximal interphalangeal joint</u> of <u>finger</u>

S63.230- Subluxation of proximal interphalangeal joint of <u>right</u> <u>index</u> finger

S63.231- Subluxation of proximal interphalangeal joint of <u>left</u> <u>index</u> finger

S63.232- Subluxation of proximal interphalangeal joint of <u>right</u> <u>middle</u> finger

S63.233- Subluxation of proximal interphalangeal joint of <u>left</u> <u>middle</u> finger

S63.234- Subluxation of proximal interphalangeal joint of <u>right</u> ring finger

S63.235- Subluxation of proximal interphalangeal joint of <u>left</u> ring finger

S63.236- Subluxation of proximal interphalangeal joint of <u>right</u> <u>little</u> finger

S63.237- Subluxation of proximal interphalangeal joint of <u>left</u> <u>little</u> finger

S63.238- Subluxation of proximal interphalangeal joint of <u>other</u> finger
    Subluxation of proximal interphalangeal joint of specified finger with unspecified laterality

S63.239- Subluxation of proximal interphalangeal joint of <u>unspecified</u> finger

S63.24- <u>Subluxation</u> of <u>distal interphalangeal joint</u> of <u>finger</u>

S63.240- Subluxation of distal interphalangeal joint of <u>right</u> <u>index</u> finger

S63.241- Subluxation of distal interphalangeal joint of <u>left</u> <u>index</u> finger

S63.242- Subluxation of distal interphalangeal joint of <u>right</u> <u>middle</u> finger

S63.243- Subluxation of distal interphalangeal joint of <u>left</u> <u>middle</u> finger

S63.244- Subluxation of distal interphalangeal joint of <u>right</u> ring finger

S63.245- Subluxation of distal interphalangeal joint of <u>left</u> ring finger

S63.246- Subluxation of distal interphalangeal joint of <u>right</u> <u>little</u> finger

S63.247- Subluxation of distal interphalangeal joint of <u>left</u> <u>little</u> finger

S63.248- Subluxation of distal interphalangeal joint of <u>other</u> finger
    Subluxation of distal interphalangeal joint of specified finger with unspecified laterality

S63.249- Subluxation of distal interphalangeal joint of <u>unspecified</u> finger

S63.25- <u>Unspecified</u> <u>dislocation</u> of <u>other</u> <u>finger</u>

S63.250- Unspecified dislocation of <u>right</u> <u>index</u> finger
S63.251- Unspecified dislocation of <u>left</u> <u>index</u> finger
S63.252- Unspecified dislocation of <u>right</u> <u>middle</u> finger
S63.253- Unspecified dislocation of <u>left</u> <u>middle</u> finger
S63.254- Unspecified dislocation of <u>right</u> ring finger
S63.255- Unspecified dislocation of <u>left</u> ring finger
S63.256- Unspecified dislocation of <u>right</u> <u>little</u> finger
S63.257- Unspecified dislocation of <u>left</u> <u>little</u> finger
S63.258- Unspecified dislocation of <u>other</u> finger
    Unspecified dislocation of specified finger with unspecified laterality
S63.259- Unspecified dislocation of <u>unspecified</u> finger
    Unspecified dislocation of specified finger with unspecified laterality

S63.26- <u>Dislocation</u> of <u>metacarpophalangeal joint</u> of <u>finger</u>

S63.260- Dislocation of metacarpophalangeal joint of <u>right</u> <u>index</u> finger

S63.261- Dislocation of metacarpophalangeal joint of <u>left</u> <u>index</u> finger

S63.262- Dislocation of metacarpophalangeal joint of <u>right</u> <u>middle</u> finger

S63.263- Dislocation of metacarpophalangeal joint of <u>left</u> <u>middle</u> finger

S63.264- Dislocation of metacarpophalangeal joint of <u>right</u> ring finger

S63.265- Dislocation of metacarpophalangeal joint of <u>left</u> ring finger

S63.266- Dislocation of metacarpophalangeal joint of <u>right</u> <u>little</u> finger

S63.267- Dislocation of metacarpophalangeal joint of <u>left</u> <u>little</u> finger

S63.268- Dislocation of metacarpophalangeal joint of <u>other</u> finger
    Dislocation of metacarpophalangeal joint of specified finger with unspecified laterality

S63.269- Dislocation of metacarpophalangeal joint of <u>unspecified</u> finger

S63.27- <u>Dislocation</u> of <u>unspecified interphalangeal joint</u> of <u>finger</u>

S63.270- Dislocation of unspecified interphalangeal joint of <u>right</u> <u>index</u> finger

S63.271- Dislocation of unspecified interphalangeal joint of <u>left</u> <u>index</u> finger

S63.272- Dislocation of unspecified interphalangeal joint of <u>right</u> <u>middle</u> finger

S63.273- Dislocation of unspecified interphalangeal joint of <u>left</u> <u>middle</u> finger

S63.274- Dislocation of unspecified interphalangeal joint of <u>right</u> ring finger

S63.275- Dislocation of unspecified interphalangeal joint of <u>left</u> ring finger

S63.276- Dislocation of unspecified interphalangeal joint of <u>right</u> <u>little</u> finger

S63.277- Dislocation of unspecified interphalangeal joint of <u>left</u> <u>little</u> finger

S63.278- Dislocation of unspecified interphalangeal joint of <u>other</u> finger
    Dislocation of unspecified interphalangeal joint of specified finger with unspecified laterality

S63.279- Dislocation of unspecified interphalangeal joint of <u>unspecified</u> finger
    Dislocation of unspecified interphalangeal joint of specified finger without specified laterality

S63.28- <u>Dislocation</u> of <u>proximal interphalangeal joint</u> of <u>finger</u>

S63.280- Dislocation of proximal interphalangeal joint of <u>right</u> <u>index</u> finger

S63.281- Dislocation of proximal interphalangeal joint of <u>left</u> <u>index</u> finger

S63.282- Dislocation of proximal interphalangeal joint of <u>right</u> <u>middle</u> finger

S63.283- Dislocation of proximal interphalangeal joint of <u>left</u> <u>middle</u> finger

S63.284- Dislocation of proximal interphalangeal joint of <u>right</u> ring finger

S63.285- Dislocation of proximal interphalangeal joint of <u>left</u> ring finger

S63.286- Dislocation of proximal interphalangeal joint of <u>right</u> <u>little</u> finger

S63.287- Dislocation of proximal interphalangeal joint of <u>left</u> <u>little</u> finger

S63.288- Dislocation of proximal interphalangeal joint of <u>other</u> finger
    Dislocation of proximal interphalangeal joint of specified finger with unspecified laterality

S63.289- Dislocation of proximal interphalangeal joint of <u>unspecified</u> finger

S63.29- <u>Dislocation</u> of <u>distal interphalangeal joint</u> of <u>finger</u>

S63.290- Dislocation of distal interphalangeal joint of <u>right</u> <u>index</u> finger

S63.291- Dislocation of distal interphalangeal joint of <u>left</u> <u>index</u> finger

S63.292- Dislocation of distal interphalangeal joint of <u>right</u> <u>middle</u> finger

S63.293- Dislocation of distal interphalangeal joint of <u>left</u> <u>middle</u> finger

S63.294- Dislocation of distal interphalangeal joint of <u>right</u> ring finger

S63.295- Dislocation of distal interphalangeal joint of <u>left</u> ring finger

S63.296- Dislocation of distal interphalangeal joint of <u>right</u> <u>little</u> finger

S63.297- Dislocation of distal interphalangeal joint of <u>left</u> <u>little</u> finger

S63 - S63

S63.298-   Dislocation of distal interphalangeal joint of <u>other</u> finger
> Dislocation of distal interphalangeal joint of specified finger with unspecified laterality

S63.299-   Dislocation of distal interphalangeal joint of <u>unspecified</u> finger

S63.3-   <u>Traumatic rupture</u> of <u>ligament</u> of <u>wrist</u>

S63.30-   <u>Traumatic rupture</u> of <u>unspecified ligament</u> of <u>wrist</u>

S63.301-   Traumatic rupture of unspecified ligament of <u>right</u> wrist

S63.302-   Traumatic rupture of unspecified ligament of <u>left</u> wrist

S63.309-   Traumatic rupture of unspecified ligament of <u>unspecified</u> wrist

S63.31-   <u>Traumatic rupture</u> of <u>collateral</u> ligament of <u>wrist</u>

S63.311-   Traumatic rupture of collateral ligament of <u>right</u> wrist

S63.312-   Traumatic rupture of collateral ligament of <u>left</u> wrist

S63.319-   Traumatic rupture of collateral ligament of <u>unspecified</u> wrist

S63.32-   <u>Traumatic rupture</u> of <u>radiocarpal</u> ligament

S63.321-   Traumatic rupture of <u>right</u> radiocarpal ligament

S63.322-   Traumatic rupture of <u>left</u> radiocarpal ligament

S63.329-   Traumatic rupture of <u>unspecified</u> radiocarpal ligament

S63.33-   <u>Traumatic rupture</u> of <u>ulnocarpal (palmar)</u> ligament

S63.331-   Traumatic rupture of <u>right</u> ulnocarpal (palmar) ligament

S63.332-   Traumatic rupture of <u>left</u> ulnocarpal (palmar) ligament

S63.339-   Traumatic rupture of <u>unspecified</u> ulnocarpal (palmar) ligament

S63.39-   <u>Traumatic rupture</u> of <u>other ligament</u> of <u>wrist</u>

S63.391-   Traumatic rupture of other ligament of <u>right</u> wrist

S63.392-   Traumatic rupture of other ligament of <u>left</u> wrist

S63.399-   Traumatic rupture of other ligament of <u>unspecified</u> wrist

S63.4-   <u>Traumatic rupture</u> of <u>ligament</u> of <u>finger</u> at <u>metacarpophalangeal and interphalangeal joint(s)</u>

S63.40-   <u>Traumatic rupture</u> of <u>unspecified ligament</u> of <u>finger</u> at <u>metacarpophalangeal and interphalangeal joint</u>

S63.400-   Traumatic rupture of unspecified ligament of <u>right index</u> finger at metacarpophalangeal and interphalangeal joint

S63.401-   Traumatic rupture of unspecified ligament of <u>left index</u> finger at metacarpophalangeal and interphalangeal joint

S63.402-   Traumatic rupture of unspecified ligament of <u>right middle</u> finger at metacarpophalangeal and interphalangeal joint

S63.403-   Traumatic rupture of unspecified ligament of <u>left middle</u> finger at metacarpophalangeal and interphalangeal joint

S63.404-   Traumatic rupture of unspecified ligament of <u>right ring</u> finger at metacarpophalangeal and interphalangeal joint

S63.405-   Traumatic rupture of unspecified ligament of <u>left ring</u> finger at metacarpophalangeal and interphalangeal joint

S63.406-   Traumatic rupture of unspecified ligament of <u>right little</u> finger at metacarpophalangeal and interphalangeal joint

S63.407-   Traumatic rupture of unspecified ligament of <u>left little</u> finger at metacarpophalangeal and interphalangeal joint

S63.408-   Traumatic rupture of unspecified ligament of <u>other</u> finger at metacarpophalangeal and interphalangeal joint
> Traumatic rupture of unspecified ligament of specified finger with unspecified laterality at metacarpophalangeal and interphalangeal joint

S63.409-   Traumatic rupture of unspecified ligament of <u>unspecified</u> finger at metacarpophalangeal and interphalangeal joint

S63.41-   <u>Traumatic rupture</u> of <u>collateral</u> ligament of <u>finger</u> at <u>metacarpophalangeal and interphalangeal joint</u>

S63.410-   Traumatic rupture of collateral ligament of <u>right index</u> finger at metacarpophalangeal and interphalangeal joint

S63.411-   Traumatic rupture of collateral ligament of <u>left index</u> finger at metacarpophalangeal and interphalangeal joint

S63.412-   Traumatic rupture of collateral ligament of <u>right middle</u> finger at metacarpophalangeal and interphalangeal joint

S63.413-   Traumatic rupture of collateral ligament of <u>left middle</u> finger at metacarpophalangeal and interphalangeal joint

S63.414-   Traumatic rupture of collateral ligament of <u>right ring</u> finger at metacarpophalangeal and interphalangeal joint

S63.415-   Traumatic rupture of collateral ligament of <u>left ring</u> finger at metacarpophalangeal and interphalangeal joint

S63.416-   Traumatic rupture of collateral ligament of <u>right little</u> finger at metacarpophalangeal and interphalangeal joint

S63.417-   Traumatic rupture of collateral ligament of <u>left little</u> finger at metacarpophalangeal and interphalangeal joint

S63.418-   Traumatic rupture of collateral ligament of <u>other</u> finger at metacarpophalangeal and interphalangeal joint
> Traumatic rupture of collateral ligament of specified finger with unspecified laterality at metacarpophalangeal and interphalangeal joint

S63.419-   Traumatic rupture of collateral ligament of <u>unspecified</u> finger at metacarpophalangeal and interphalangeal joint

S63.42-   <u>Traumatic rupture</u> of <u>palmar ligament</u> of <u>finger</u> at <u>metacarpophalangeal and interphalangeal joint</u>

S63.420-   Traumatic rupture of palmar ligament of <u>right index</u> finger at metacarpophalangeal and interphalangeal joint

S63.421-   Traumatic rupture of palmar ligament of <u>left index</u> finger at metacarpophalangeal and interphalangeal joint

S63.422-   Traumatic rupture of palmar ligament of <u>right middle</u> finger at metacarpophalangeal and interphalangeal joint

S63.423-   Traumatic rupture of palmar ligament of <u>left middle</u> finger at metacarpophalangeal and interphalangeal joint

S63.424-   Traumatic rupture of palmar ligament of <u>right ring</u> finger at metacarpophalangeal and interphalangeal joint

S63.425-   Traumatic rupture of palmar ligament of <u>left ring</u> finger at metacarpophalangeal and interphalangeal joint

S63.426-   Traumatic rupture of palmar ligament of <u>right little</u> finger at metacarpophalangeal and interphalangeal joint

S63.427-   Traumatic rupture of palmar ligament of <u>left little</u> finger at metacarpophalangeal and interphalangeal joint

S63.428-   Traumatic rupture of palmar ligament of <u>other</u> finger at metacarpophalangeal and interphalangeal joint
> Traumatic rupture of palmar ligament of specified finger with unspecified laterality at metacarpophalangeal and interphalangeal joint

S63.429-   Traumatic rupture of palmar ligament of <u>unspecified</u> finger at metacarpophalangeal and interphalangeal joint

S63.43-   <u>Traumatic rupture</u> of <u>volar plate</u> of <u>finger</u> at <u>metacarpophalangeal and interphalangeal joint</u>

S63.430-   Traumatic rupture of volar plate of <u>right index</u> finger at metacarpophalangeal and interphalangeal joint

S63.431-   Traumatic rupture of volar plate of <u>left index</u> finger at metacarpophalangeal and interphalangeal joint

S63.432-   Traumatic rupture of volar plate of <u>right middle</u> finger at metacarpophalangeal and interphalangeal joint

S63.433-   Traumatic rupture of volar plate of <u>left middle</u> finger at metacarpophalangeal and interphalangeal joint

S63.434-   Traumatic rupture of volar plate of <u>right ring</u> finger at metacarpophalangeal and interphalangeal joint

S63.435-   Traumatic rupture of volar plate of <u>left ring</u> finger at metacarpophalangeal and interphalangeal joint

S63.436-   Traumatic rupture of volar plate of <u>right little</u> finger at metacarpophalangeal and interphalangeal joint

S63.437-   Traumatic rupture of volar plate of <u>left little</u> finger at metacarpophalangeal and interphalangeal joint

S63 - S63

S63.438- Traumatic rupture of volar plate of <u>other</u> finger at
metacarpophalangeal and interphalangeal joint
  Traumatic rupture of volar plate of specified finger with
  unspecified laterality at metacarpophalangeal and
  interphalangeal joint
S63.439- Traumatic rupture of volar plate of <u>unspecified</u> finger
at metacarpophalangeal and interphalangeal joint
S63.49- <u>Traumatic rupture</u> of <u>other ligament</u> of <u>finger</u> at
<u>metacarpophalangeal and interphalangeal joint</u>
  S63.490- Traumatic rupture of other ligament of <u>right index</u>
  finger at metacarpophalangeal and interphalangeal
  joint
  S63.491- Traumatic rupture of other ligament of <u>left index</u>
  finger at metacarpophalangeal and interphalangeal
  joint
  S63.492- Traumatic rupture of other ligament of <u>right middle</u>
  finger at metacarpophalangeal and interphalangeal
  joint
  S63.493- Traumatic rupture of other ligament of <u>left middle</u>
  finger at metacarpophalangeal and interphalangeal
  joint
  S63.494- Traumatic rupture of other ligament of <u>right ring</u>
  finger at metacarpophalangeal and interphalangeal
  joint
  S63.495- Traumatic rupture of other ligament of <u>left ring</u> finger
  at metacarpophalangeal and interphalangeal joint
  S63.496- Traumatic rupture of other ligament of <u>right little</u>
  finger at metacarpophalangeal and interphalangeal
  joint
  S63.497- Traumatic rupture of other ligament of <u>left little</u> finger
  at metacarpophalangeal and interphalangeal joint
  S63.498- Traumatic rupture of other ligament of <u>other</u> finger at
  metacarpophalangeal and interphalangeal joint
    Traumatic rupture of ligament of specified finger with
    unspecified laterality at metacarpophalangeal and
    interphalangeal joint
  S63.499- Traumatic rupture of other ligament of <u>unspecified</u>
  finger at metacarpophalangeal and interphalangeal
  joint
S63.5- <u>Other and unspecified</u> <u>sprain</u> of <u>wrist</u>
  S63.50- <u>Unspecified</u> sprain of <u>wrist</u>
    S63.501- Unspecified sprain of <u>right</u> wrist
    S63.502- Unspecified sprain of <u>left</u> wrist
    S63.509- Unspecified sprain of <u>unspecified</u> wrist
  S63.51- <u>Sprain</u> of <u>carpal (joint)</u>
    S63.511- Sprain of carpal joint of <u>right</u> wrist
    S63.512- Sprain of carpal joint of <u>left</u> wrist
    S63.519- Sprain of carpal joint of <u>unspecified</u> wrist
  S63.52- <u>Sprain</u> of <u>radiocarpal joint</u>
    *Excludes 1: traumatic rupture of radiocarpal ligament
                  (S63.32-)*
    S63.521- Sprain of radiocarpal joint of <u>right</u> wrist
    S63.522- Sprain of radiocarpal joint of <u>left</u> wrist
    S63.529- Sprain of radiocarpal joint of <u>unspecified</u> wrist
  S63.59- <u>Other specified sprain</u> of <u>wrist</u>
    S63.591- Other specified sprain of <u>right</u> wrist
    S63.592- Other specified sprain of <u>left</u> wrist
    S63.599- Other specified sprain of <u>unspecified</u> wrist
S63.6- <u>Other and unspecified</u> <u>sprain</u> of <u>finger(s)</u>
    *Excludes 1: traumatic rupture of ligament of finger at
                  metacarpophalangeal and interphalangeal joint(s)
                  (S63.4-)*
  S63.60- <u>Unspecified</u> <u>sprain</u> of <u>thumb</u>
    S63.601- Unspecified sprain of <u>right</u> thumb
    S63.602- Unspecified sprain of <u>left</u> thumb
    S63.609- Unspecified sprain of <u>unspecified</u> thumb
  S63.61- <u>Unspecified</u> <u>sprain</u> of other and <u>unspecified</u> <u>finger(s)</u>
    S63.610- Unspecified sprain of <u>right index</u> finger
    S63.611- Unspecified sprain of <u>left index</u> finger
    S63.612- Unspecified sprain of <u>right middle</u> finger
    S63.613- Unspecified sprain of <u>left middle</u> finger
    S63.614- Unspecified sprain of <u>right ring</u> finger
    S63.615- Unspecified sprain of <u>left ring</u> finger
    S63.616- Unspecified sprain of <u>right little</u> finger
    S63.617- Unspecified sprain of <u>left little</u> finger
    S63.618- Unspecified sprain of other <u>finger</u>
      Unspecified sprain of specified finger with unspecified
      laterality
    S63.619- Unspecified sprain of <u>unspecified</u> finger

S63.62- <u>Sprain</u> of <u>interphalangeal joint</u> of <u>thumb</u>
    S63.621- Sprain of interphalangeal joint of <u>right</u> thumb
    S63.622- Sprain of interphalangeal joint of <u>left</u> thumb
    S63.629- Sprain of interphalangeal joint of <u>unspecified</u> thumb
  S63.63- <u>Sprain</u> of <u>interphalangeal joint</u> of <u>other and unspecified</u>
<u>finger(s)</u>
    S63.630- Sprain of interphalangeal joint of <u>right index</u> finger
    S63.631- Sprain of interphalangeal joint of <u>left index</u> finger
    S63.632- Sprain of interphalangeal joint of <u>right middle</u> finger
    S63.633- Sprain of interphalangeal joint of <u>left middle</u> finger
    S63.634- Sprain of interphalangeal joint of <u>right ring</u> finger
    S63.635- Sprain of interphalangeal joint of <u>left ring</u> finger
    S63.636- Sprain of interphalangeal joint of <u>right little</u> finger
    S63.637- Sprain of interphalangeal joint of <u>left little</u> finger
    S63.638- Sprain of interphalangeal joint of <u>other</u> finger
    S63.639- Sprain of interphalangeal joint of <u>unspecified</u> finger
  S63.64- <u>Sprain</u> of <u>metacarpophalangeal joint</u> of <u>thumb</u>
    S63.641- Sprain of metacarpophalangeal joint of <u>right</u> thumb
    S63.642- Sprain of metacarpophalangeal joint of <u>left</u> thumb
    S63.649- Sprain of metacarpophalangeal joint of <u>unspecified</u>
    thumb
  S63.65- <u>Sprain</u> of <u>metacarpophalangeal joint</u> of <u>other and</u>
<u>unspecified finger(s)</u>
    S63.650- Sprain of metacarpophalangeal joint of <u>right index</u>
    finger
    S63.651- Sprain of metacarpophalangeal joint of <u>left index</u>
    finger
    S63.652- Sprain of metacarpophalangeal joint of <u>right middle</u>
    finger
    S63.653- Sprain of metacarpophalangeal joint of <u>left middle</u>
    finger
    S63.654- Sprain of metacarpophalangeal joint of <u>right ring</u>
    finger
    S63.655- Sprain of metacarpophalangeal joint of <u>left ring</u> finger
    S63.656- Sprain of metacarpophalangeal joint of <u>right little</u>
    finger
    S63.657- Sprain of metacarpophalangeal joint of <u>left little</u>
    finger
    S63.658- Sprain of metacarpophalangeal joint of <u>other</u> finger
      Sprain of metacarpophalangeal joint of specified finger
      with unspecified laterality
    S63.659- Sprain of metacarpophalangeal joint of <u>unspecified</u>
    finger
  S63.68- <u>Other sprain</u> of <u>thumb</u>
    S63.681- Other sprain of <u>right</u> thumb
    S63.682- Other sprain of <u>left</u> thumb
    S63.689- Other sprain of <u>unspecified</u> thumb
  S63.69- <u>Other sprain</u> of <u>other and unspecified</u> <u>finger(s)</u>
    S63.690- Other sprain of <u>right index</u> finger
    S63.691- Other sprain of <u>left index</u> finger
    S63.692- Other sprain of <u>right middle</u> finger
    S63.693- Other sprain of <u>left middle</u> finger
    S63.694- Other sprain of <u>right ring</u> finger
    S63.695- Other sprain of <u>left ring</u> finger
    S63.696- Other sprain of <u>right little</u> finger
    S63.697- Other sprain of <u>left little</u> finger
    S63.698- Other sprain of <u>other</u> finger
      Other sprain of specified finger with unspecified
      laterality
    S63.699- Other sprain of <u>unspecified</u> finger
S63.8- <u>Sprain</u> of other part of <u>wrist and hand</u>
  S63.8x- <u>Sprain</u> of <u>other part</u> of <u>wrist and hand</u>
    S63.8x1- Sprain of other part of <u>right</u> wrist and hand
    S63.8x2- Sprain of other part of <u>left</u> wrist and hand
    S63.8x9- Sprain of other part of <u>unspecified</u> wrist and hand
S63.9- <u>Sprain</u> of <u>unspecified part</u> of <u>wrist and hand</u>
  S63.90x- Sprain of unspecified part of <u>unspecified</u> wrist and hand
  S63.91x- Sprain of unspecified part of <u>right</u> wrist and hand
  S63.92x- Sprain of unspecified part of <u>left</u> wrist and hand

S64- Injury of nerves at wrist and hand level
Code also any associated open wound (S61.-)
The appropriate 7th character is to be added to each code from
   category S64:
   A Initial encounter
   D Subsequent encounter
   S Sequela

S64.0- Injury of ulnar nerve at wrist and hand level
   S64.00x- Injury of ulnar nerve at wrist and hand level of unspecified arm
   S64.01x- Injury of ulnar nerve at wrist and hand level of right arm
   S64.02x- Injury of ulnar nerve at wrist and hand level of left arm
S64.1- Injury of median nerve at wrist and hand level
   S64.10x- Injury of median nerve at wrist and hand level of unspecified arm
   S64.11x- Injury of median nerve at wrist and hand level of right arm
   S64.12x- Injury of median nerve at wrist and hand level of left arm
S64.2- Injury of radial nerve at wrist and hand level
   S64.20x- Injury of radial nerve at wrist and hand level of unspecified arm
   S64.21x- Injury of radial nerve at wrist and hand level of right arm
   S64.22x- Injury of radial nerve at wrist and hand level of left arm
S64.3- Injury of digital nerve of thumb
   S64.30x- Injury of digital nerve of unspecified thumb
   S64.31x- Injury of digital nerve of right thumb
   S64.32x- Injury of digital nerve of left thumb
S64.4- Injury of digital nerve of other and unspecified finger
   S64.40x- Injury of digital nerve of unspecified finger
   S64.49- Injury of digital nerve of other finger
      S64.490- Injury of digital nerve of right index finger
      S64.491- Injury of digital nerve of left index finger
      S64.492- Injury of digital nerve of right middle finger
      S64.493- Injury of digital nerve of left middle finger
      S64.494- Injury of digital nerve of right ring finger
      S64.495- Injury of digital nerve of left ring finger
      S64.496- Injury of digital nerve of right little finger
      S64.497- Injury of digital nerve of left little finger
      S64.498- Injury of digital nerve of other finger
         Injury of digital nerve of specified finger with unspecified laterality
S64.8- Injury of other nerves at wrist and hand level
   S64.8x- Injury of other nerves at wrist and hand level
      S64.8x1- Injury of other nerves at wrist and hand level of right arm
      S64.8x2- Injury of other nerves at wrist and hand level of left arm
      S64.8x9- Injury of other nerves at wrist and hand level of unspecified arm
S64.9- Injury of unspecified nerve at wrist and hand level
   S64.90x- Injury of unspecified nerve at wrist and hand level of unspecified arm
   S64.91x- Injury of unspecified nerve at wrist and hand level of right arm
   S64.92x- Injury of unspecified nerve at wrist and hand level of left arm

S65- Injury of blood vessels at wrist and hand level
Code also any associated open wound (S61.-)
The appropriate 7th character is to be added to each code from
   category S65:
   A Initial encounter
   D Subsequent encounter
   S Sequela

S65.0- Injury of ulnar artery at wrist and hand level
   S65.00- Unspecified injury of ulnar artery at wrist and hand level
      S65.001- Unspecified injury of ulnar artery at wrist and hand level of right arm
      S65.002- Unspecified injury of ulnar artery at wrist and hand level of left arm
      S65.009- Unspecified injury of ulnar artery at wrist and hand level of unspecified arm
   S65.01- Laceration of ulnar artery at wrist and hand level
      S65.011- Laceration of ulnar artery at wrist and hand level of right arm
      S65.012- Laceration of ulnar artery at wrist and hand level of left arm
      S65.019- Laceration of ulnar artery at wrist and hand level of unspecified arm

   S65.09- Other specified injury of ulnar artery at wrist and hand level
      S65.091- Other specified injury of ulnar artery at wrist and hand level of right arm
      S65.092- Other specified injury of ulnar artery at wrist and hand level of left arm
      S65.099- Other specified injury of ulnar artery at wrist and hand level of unspecified arm
S65.1- Injury of radial artery at wrist and hand level
   S65.10- Unspecified injury of radial artery at wrist and hand level
      S65.101- Unspecified injury of radial artery at wrist and hand level of right arm
      S65.102- Unspecified injury of radial artery at wrist and hand level of left arm
      S65.109- Unspecified injury of radial artery at wrist and hand level of unspecified arm
   S65.11- Laceration of radial artery at wrist and hand level
      S65.111- Laceration of radial artery at wrist and hand level of right arm
      S65.112- Laceration of radial artery at wrist and hand level of left arm
      S65.119- Laceration of radial artery at wrist and hand level of unspecified arm
   S65.19- Other specified injury of radial artery at wrist and hand level
      S65.191- Other specified injury of radial artery at wrist and hand level of right arm
      S65.192- Other specified injury of radial artery at wrist and hand level of left arm
      S65.199- Other specified injury of radial artery at wrist and hand level of unspecified arm
S65.2- Injury of superficial palmar arch
   S65.20- Unspecified injury of superficial palmar arch
      S65.201- Unspecified injury of superficial palmar arch of right hand
      S65.202- Unspecified injury of superficial palmar arch of left hand
      S65.209- Unspecified injury of superficial palmar arch of unspecified hand
   S65.21- Laceration of superficial palmar arch
      S65.211- Laceration of superficial palmar arch of right hand
      S65.212- Laceration of superficial palmar arch of left hand
      S65.219- Laceration of superficial palmar arch of unspecified hand
   S65.29- Other specified injury of superficial palmar arch
      S65.291- Other specified injury of superficial palmar arch of right hand
      S65.292- Other specified injury of superficial palmar arch of left hand
      S65.299- Other specified injury of superficial palmar arch of unspecified hand
S65.3- Injury of deep palmar arch
   S65.30- Unspecified injury of deep palmar arch
      S65.301- Unspecified injury of deep palmar arch of right hand
      S65.302- Unspecified injury of deep palmar arch of left hand
      S65.309- Unspecified injury of deep palmar arch of unspecified hand
   S65.31- Laceration of deep palmar arch
      S65.311- Laceration of deep palmar arch of right hand
      S65.312- Laceration of deep palmar arch of left hand
      S65.319- Laceration of deep palmar arch of unspecified hand
   S65.39- Other specified injury of deep palmar arch
      S65.391- Other specified injury of deep palmar arch of right hand
      S65.392- Other specified injury of deep palmar arch of left hand
      S65.399- Other specified injury of deep palmar arch of unspecified hand
S65.4- Injury of blood vessel of thumb
   S65.40- Unspecified injury of blood vessel of thumb
      S65.401- Unspecified injury of blood vessel of right thumb
      S65.402- Unspecified injury of blood vessel of left thumb
      S65.409- Unspecified injury of blood vessel of unspecified thumb
   S65.41- Laceration of blood vessel of thumb
      S65.411- Laceration of blood vessel of right thumb
      S65.412- Laceration of blood vessel of left thumb
      S65.419- Laceration of blood vessel of unspecified thumb

S 6 3 - S 6 5

Excludes 1: = NOT CODED HERE! (Do not code both)   **747**   *Excludes ❷:* = Not Included Here

S65.49- <u>Other specified injury</u> of <u>blood vessel</u> of <u>thumb</u>
  S65.491- Other specified injury of blood vessel of <u>right</u> thumb
  S65.492- Other specified injury of blood vessel of <u>left</u> thumb
  S65.499- Other specified injury of blood vessel of <u>unspecified</u> thumb
S65.5- <u>Injury of blood vessel</u> of <u>other and unspecified</u> <u>finger</u>
  S65.50- <u>Unspecified</u> injury of <u>blood vessel</u> of <u>other and unspecified</u> <u>finger</u>
    S65.500- Unspecified injury of blood vessel of <u>right index</u> finger
    S65.501- Unspecified injury of blood vessel of <u>left index</u> finger
    S65.502- Unspecified injury of blood vessel of <u>right middle</u> finger
    S65.503- Unspecified injury of blood vessel of <u>left middle</u> finger
    S65.504- Unspecified injury of blood vessel of <u>right ring</u> finger
    S65.505- Unspecified injury of blood vessel of <u>left ring</u> finger
    S65.506- Unspecified injury of blood vessel of <u>right little</u> finger
    S65.507- Unspecified injury of blood vessel of <u>left little</u> finger
    S65.508- Unspecified injury of blood vessel of <u>other</u> finger
      Unspecified injury of blood vessel of specified finger with unspecified laterality
    S65.509- Unspecified injury of blood vessel of <u>unspecified</u> finger
  S65.51- <u>Laceration</u> of <u>blood vessel</u> of <u>other and unspecified finger</u>
    S65.510- Laceration of blood vessel of <u>right index</u> finger
    S65.511- Laceration of blood vessel of <u>left index</u> finger
    S65.512- Laceration of blood vessel of <u>right middle</u> finger
    S65.513- Laceration of blood vessel of <u>left middle</u> finger
    S65.514- Laceration of blood vessel of <u>right ring</u> finger
    S65.515- Laceration of blood vessel of <u>left ring</u> finger
    S65.516- Laceration of blood vessel of <u>right little</u> finger
    S65.517- Laceration of blood vessel of <u>left little</u> finger
    S65.518- Laceration of blood vessel of <u>other</u> finger
      Laceration of blood vessel of specified finger with unspecified laterality
    S65.519- Laceration of blood vessel of <u>unspecified</u> finger
  S65.59- <u>Other specified injury</u> of <u>blood vessel</u> of <u>other and unspecified finger</u>
    S65.590- Other specified injury of blood vessel of <u>right index</u> finger
    S65.591- Other specified injury of blood vessel of <u>left index</u> finger
    S65.592- Other specified injury of blood vessel of <u>right middle</u> finger
    S65.593- Other specified injury of blood vessel of <u>left middle</u> finger
    S65.594- Other specified injury of blood vessel of <u>right ring</u> finger
    S65.595- Other specified injury of blood vessel of <u>left ring</u> finger
    S65.596- Other specified injury of blood vessel of <u>right little</u> finger
    S65.597- Other specified injury of blood vessel of <u>left little</u> finger
    S65.598- Other specified injury of blood vessel of <u>other</u> finger
      Other specified injury of blood vessel of specified finger with unspecified laterality
    S65.599- Other specified injury of blood vessel of <u>unspecified</u> finger
S65.8- Injury of <u>other blood vessels</u> at <u>wrist and hand level</u>
  S65.80- <u>Unspecified</u> injury of <u>other blood vessels</u> at <u>wrist and hand level</u>
    S65.801- Unspecified injury of other blood vessels at wrist and hand level of <u>right</u> arm
    S65.802- Unspecified injury of other blood vessels at wrist and hand level of <u>left</u> arm
    S65.809- Unspecified injury of other blood vessels at wrist and hand level of <u>unspecified</u> arm
  S65.81- <u>Laceration</u> of <u>other blood vessels</u> at <u>wrist and hand level</u>
    S65.811- Laceration of other blood vessels at wrist and hand level of <u>right</u> arm
    S65.812- Laceration of other blood vessels at wrist and hand level of <u>left</u> arm
    S65.819- Laceration of other blood vessels at wrist and hand level of <u>unspecified</u> arm
  S65.89- <u>Other specified injury</u> of <u>other blood vessels</u> at <u>wrist and hand level</u>
    S65.891- Other specified injury of other blood vessels at wrist and hand level of <u>right</u> arm
    S65.892- Other specified injury of other blood vessels at wrist and hand level of <u>left</u> arm

  S65.899- Other specified injury of other blood vessels at wrist and hand level of <u>unspecified</u> arm
S65.9- Injury of <u>unspecified blood vessel</u> at <u>wrist and hand level</u>
  S65.90- <u>Unspecified</u> injury of unspecified blood vessel at wrist and hand level
    S65.901- Unspecified injury of unspecified blood vessel at wrist and hand level of <u>right</u> arm
    S65.902- Unspecified injury of unspecified blood vessel at wrist and hand level of <u>left</u> arm
    S65.909- Unspecified injury of unspecified blood vessel at wrist and hand level of <u>unspecified</u> arm
  S65.91- <u>Laceration</u> of <u>unspecified blood vessel</u> at <u>wrist and hand level</u>
    S65.911- Laceration of unspecified blood vessel at wrist and hand level of <u>right</u> arm
    S65.912- Laceration of unspecified blood vessel at wrist and hand level of <u>left</u> arm
    S65.919- Laceration of unspecified blood vessel at wrist and hand level of <u>unspecified</u> arm
  S65.99- <u>Other specified injury</u> of <u>unspecified blood vessel</u> at <u>wrist and hand level</u>
    S65.991- Other specified injury of unspecified blood vessel at wrist and hand of <u>right</u> arm
    S65.992- Other specified injury of unspecified blood vessel at wrist and hand of <u>left</u> arm
    S65.999- Other specified injury of unspecified blood vessel at wrist and hand of <u>unspecified</u> arm

S66- <u>Injury of muscle, fascia and tendon at wrist and hand level</u>
  Code also any associated open wound (S61.-)
  Excludes❷: sprain of joints and ligaments of wrist and hand (S63.-)
  The appropriate 7th character is to be added to each code from category S66:
  A <u>Initial</u> encounter
  D <u>Subsequent</u> encounter
  S <u>Sequela</u>
S66.0- Injury of <u>long flexor muscle, fascia and tendon</u> of <u>thumb</u> at <u>wrist and hand level</u>
  S66.00- <u>Unspecified</u> injury of <u>long flexor</u> muscle, fascia and tendon of <u>thumb</u> at <u>wrist and hand level</u>
    S66.001- Unspecified injury of long flexor muscle, fascia and tendon of <u>right</u> thumb at wrist and hand level
    S66.002- Unspecified injury of long flexor muscle, fascia and tendon of <u>left</u> thumb at wrist and hand level
    S66.009- Unspecified injury of long flexor muscle, fascia and tendon of <u>unspecified</u> thumb at wrist and hand level
  S66.01- <u>Strain</u> of <u>long flexor</u> muscle, fascia and tendon of <u>thumb</u> at <u>wrist and hand level</u>
    S66.011- Strain of long flexor muscle, fascia and tendon of <u>right</u> thumb at wrist and hand level
    S66.012- Strain of long flexor muscle, fascia and tendon of <u>left</u> thumb at wrist and hand level
    S66.019- Strain of long flexor muscle, fascia and tendon of <u>unspecified</u> thumb at wrist and hand level
  S66.02- <u>Laceration</u> of <u>long flexor</u> muscle, fascia and tendon of <u>thumb</u> at <u>wrist and hand level</u>
    S66.021- Laceration of long flexor muscle, fascia and tendon of <u>right</u> thumb at wrist and hand level
    S66.022- Laceration of long flexor muscle, fascia and tendon of <u>left</u> thumb at wrist and hand level
    S66.029- Laceration of long flexor muscle, fascia and tendon of <u>unspecified</u> thumb at wrist and hand level
  S66.09- <u>Other specified injury</u> of <u>long flexor</u> muscle, fascia and tendon of <u>thumb</u> at <u>wrist and hand level</u>
    S66.091- Other specified injury of long flexor muscle, fascia and tendon of <u>right</u> thumb at wrist and hand level
    S66.092- Other specified injury of long flexor muscle, fascia and tendon of <u>left</u> thumb at wrist and hand level
    S66.099- Other specified injury of long flexor muscle, fascia and tendon of <u>unspecified</u> thumb at wrist and hand level
S66.1- <u>Injury of flexor muscle, fascia and tendon</u> of <u>other and unspecified finger</u> at <u>wrist and hand level</u>
  Excludes❷: Injury of long flexor muscle, fascia and tendon of thumb at wrist and hand level (S66.0-)
  S66.10- <u>Unspecified</u> injury of <u>flexor muscle, fascia and tendon</u> of <u>other and unspecified finger</u> at <u>wrist and hand level</u>
    S66.100- Unspecified injury of flexor muscle, fascia and tendon of <u>right index</u> finger at wrist and hand level
    S66.101- Unspecified injury of flexor muscle, fascia and tendon of <u>left index</u> finger at wrist and hand level
    S66.102- Unspecified injury of flexor muscle, fascia and tendon of <u>right middle</u> finger at wrist and hand level

S 65 – S 66

© 2013 Channel Publishing, Ltd.

S66.103-   Unspecified injury of flexor muscle, fascia and tendon of left middle finger at wrist and hand level

S66.104-   Unspecified injury of flexor muscle, fascia and tendon of right ring finger at wrist and hand level

S66.105-   Unspecified injury of flexor muscle, fascia and tendon of left ring finger at wrist and hand level

S66.106-   Unspecified injury of flexor muscle, fascia and tendon of right little finger at wristand hand level

S66.107-   Unspecified injury of flexor muscle, fascia and tendon of left little finger at wristand hand level

S66.108-   Unspecified injury of flexor muscle, fascia and tendon of other finger at wrist and hand level
           Unspecified injury of flexor muscle, fascia and tendon of specified finger with unspecified laterality at wrist and hand level

S66.109-   Unspecified injury of flexor muscle, fascia and tendon of unspecified finger at wrist and hand level

S66.11-   Strain of flexor muscle, fascia and tendon of other and unspecified finger at wrist and hand level

S66.110-   Strain of flexor muscle, fascia and tendon of right index finger at wrist and hand level

S66.111-   Strain of flexor muscle, fascia and tendon of left index finger at wrist and hand level

S66.112-   Strain of flexor muscle, fascia and tendon of right middle finger at wrist and hand level

S66.113-   Strain of flexor muscle, fascia and tendon of left middle finger at wrist and hand level

S66.114-   Strain of flexor muscle, fascia and tendon of right ring finger at wrist and hand level

S66.115-   Strain of flexor muscle, fascia and tendon of left ring finger at wrist and hand level

S66.116-   Strain of flexor muscle, fascia and tendon of right little finger at wrist and hand level

S66.117-   Strain of flexor muscle, fascia and tendon of left little finger at wrist and hand level

S66.118-   Strain of flexor muscle, fascia and tendon of other finger at wrist and hand level
           Strain of flexor muscle, fascia and tendon of specified finger with unspecified laterality at wrist and hand level

S66.119-   Strain of flexor muscle, fascia and tendon of unspecified finger at wrist and hand level

S66.12-   Laceration of flexor muscle, fascia and tendon of other and unspecified finger at wrist and hand level

S66.120-   Laceration of flexor muscle, fascia and tendon of right index finger at wrist and hand level

S66.121-   Laceration of flexor muscle, fascia and tendon of left index finger at wrist and hand level

S66.122-   Laceration of flexor muscle, fascia and tendon of right middle finger at wrist and hand level

S66.123-   Laceration of flexor muscle, fascia and tendon of left middle finger at wrist and hand level

S66.124-   Laceration of flexor muscle, fascia and tendon of right ring finger at wrist and hand level

S66.125-   Laceration of flexor muscle, fascia and tendon of left ring finger at wrist and hand level

S66.126-   Laceration of flexor muscle, fascia and tendon of right little finger at wrist and hand level

S66.127-   Laceration of flexor muscle, fascia and tendon of left little finger at wrist and hand level

S66.128-   Laceration of flexor muscle, fascia and tendon of other finger at wrist and hand level
           Laceration of flexor muscle, fascia and tendon of specified finger with unspecified laterality at wrist and hand level

S66.129-   Laceration of flexor muscle, fascia and tendon of unspecified finger at wrist and hand level

S66.19-   Other injury of flexor muscle, fascia and tendon of other and unspecified finger at wrist and hand level

S66.190-   Other injury of flexor muscle, fascia and tendon of right index finger at wrist and hand level

S66.191-   Other injury of flexor muscle, fascia and tendon of left index finger at wrist and hand level

S66.192-   Other injury of flexor muscle, fascia and tendon of right middle finger at wrist and hand level

S66.193-   Other injury of flexor muscle, fascia and tendon of left middle finger at wrist and hand level

S66.194-   Other injury of flexor muscle, fascia and tendon of right ring finger at wrist and hand level

S66.195-   Other injury of flexor muscle, fascia and tendon of left ring finger at wrist and hand level

S66.196-   Other injury of flexor muscle, fascia and tendon of right little finger at wrist and hand level

S66.197-   Other injury of flexor muscle, fascia and tendon of left little finger at wrist and hand level

S66.198-   Other injury of flexor muscle, fascia and tendon of other finger at wrist and hand level
           Other injury of flexor muscle, fascia and tendon of specified finger with unspecified laterality at wrist and hand level

S66.199-   Other injury of flexor muscle, fascia and tendon of unspecified finger at wrist and hand level

S66.2-   Injury of extensor muscle, fascia and tendon of thumb at wrist and hand level

S66.20-   Unspecified injury of extensor muscle, fascia and tendon of thumb at wrist and hand level

S66.201-   Unspecified injury of extensor muscle, fascia and tendon of right thumb at wrist and hand level

S66.202-   Unspecified injury of extensor muscle, fascia and tendon of left thumb at wrist and hand level

S66.209-   Unspecified injury of extensor muscle, fascia and tendon of unspecified thumb at wrist and hand level

S66.21-   Strain of extensor muscle, fascia and tendon of thumb at wrist and hand level

S66.211-   Strain of extensor muscle, fascia and tendon of right thumb at wrist and hand level

S66.212-   Strain of extensor muscle, fascia and tendon of left thumb at wrist and hand level

S66.219-   Strain of extensor muscle, fascia and tendon of unspecified thumb at wrist and hand level

S66.22-   Laceration of extensor muscle, fascia and tendon of thumb at wrist and hand level

S66.221-   Laceration of extensor muscle, fascia and tendon of right thumb at wrist and hand level

S66.222-   Laceration of extensor muscle, fascia and tendon of left thumb at wrist and hand level

S66.229-   Laceration of extensor muscle, fascia and tendon of unspecified thumb at wrist and hand level

S66.29-   Other specified injury of extensor muscle, fascia and tendon of thumb at wrist and hand level

S66.291-   Other specified injury of extensor muscle, fascia and tendon of right thumb at wrist and hand level

S66.292-   Other specified injury of extensor muscle, fascia and tendon of left thumb at wrist and hand level

S66.299-   Other specified injury of extensor muscle, fascia and tendon of unspecified thumb at wrist and hand level

S66.3-   Injury of extensor muscle, fascia and tendon of other and unspecified finger at wrist and hand level
           Excludes❷: Injury of extensor muscle, fascia and tendon of thumb at wrist and hand level (S66.2-)

S66.30-   Unspecified injury of extensor muscle, fascia and tendon of other and unspecified finger at wrist and hand level

S66.300-   Unspecified injury of extensor muscle, fascia and tendon of right index finger at wrist and hand level

S66.301-   Unspecified injury of extensor muscle, fascia and tendon of left index finger at wrist and hand level

S66.302-   Unspecified injury of extensor muscle, fascia and tendon of right middle finger at wrist and hand level

S66.303-   Unspecified injury of extensor muscle, fascia and tendon of left middle finger at wrist and hand level

S66.304-   Unspecified injury of extensor muscle, fascia and tendon of right ring finger at wrist and hand level

S66.305-   Unspecified injury of extensor muscle, fascia and tendon of left ring finger at wrist and hand level

S66.306-   Unspecified injury of extensor muscle, fascia and tendon of right little finger at wrist and hand level

S66.307-   Unspecified injury of extensor muscle, fascia and tendon of left little finger at wrist and hand level

S66.308-   Unspecified injury of extensor muscle, fascia and tendon of other finger at wrist and hand level
           Unspecified injury of extensor muscle, fascia and tendon of specified finger with unspecified laterality at wrist and hand level

S66.309-   Unspecified injury of extensor muscle, fascia and tendon of unspecified finger at wrist and hand level

S
6
5
I
S
6
6

S66.31- <u>Strain</u> of <u>extensor</u> muscle, fascia and tendon of <u>other and unspecified finger</u> at <u>wrist and hand level</u>

 S66.310- Strain of extensor muscle, fascia and tendon of <u>right index</u> finger at wrist and hand level

 S66.311- Strain of extensor muscle, fascia and tendon of <u>left index</u> finger at wrist and hand level

 S66.312- Strain of extensor muscle, fascia and tendon of <u>right middle</u> finger at wrist and hand level

 S66.313- Strain of extensor muscle, fascia and tendon of <u>left middle</u> finger at wrist and hand level

 S66.314- Strain of extensor muscle, fascia and tendon of <u>right ring</u> finger at wrist and hand level

 S66.315- Strain of extensor muscle, fascia and tendon of <u>left ring</u> finger at wrist and hand level

 S66.316- Strain of extensor muscle, fascia and tendon of <u>right little</u> finger at wrist and hand level

 S66.317- Strain of extensor muscle, fascia and tendon of <u>left little</u> finger at wrist and hand level

 S66.318- Strain of extensor muscle, fascia and tendon of <u>other</u> finger at wrist and hand level
  Strain of extensor muscle, fascia and tendon of specified finger with unspecified laterality at wrist and hand level

 S66.319- Strain of extensor muscle, fascia and tendon of <u>unspecified</u> finger at wrist and hand level

S66.32- <u>Laceration</u> of <u>extensor</u> muscle, fascia and tendon of <u>other and unspecified finger</u> at <u>wrist and hand level</u>

 S66.320- Laceration of extensor muscle, fascia and tendon of <u>right index</u> finger at wrist and hand level

 S66.321- Laceration of extensor muscle, fascia and tendon of <u>left index</u> finger at wrist and hand level

 S66.322- Laceration of extensor muscle, fascia and tendon of <u>right</u> middle finger at wrist and hand level

 S66.323- Laceration of extensor muscle, fascia and tendon of <u>left middle</u> finger at wrist and hand level

 S66.324- Laceration of extensor muscle, fascia and tendon of <u>right ring</u> finger at wrist and hand level

 S66.325- Laceration of extensor muscle, fascia and tendon of <u>left ring</u> finger at wrist and hand level

 S66.326- Laceration of extensor muscle, fascia and tendon of <u>right little</u> finger at wrist and hand level

 S66.327- Laceration of extensor muscle, fascia and tendon of <u>left little</u> finger at wrist and hand level

 S66.328- Laceration of extensor muscle, fascia and tendon of <u>other</u> finger at wrist and hand level
  Laceration of extensor muscle, fascia and tendon of specified finger with unspecified laterality at wrist and hand level

 S66.329- Laceration of extensor muscle, fascia and tendon of <u>unspecified</u> finger at wrist and hand level

S66.39- <u>Other injury</u> of <u>extensor</u> muscle, fascia and tendon of <u>other and unspecified finger</u> at <u>wrist and hand level</u>

 S66.390- Other injury of extensor muscle, fascia and tendon of <u>right index</u> finger at wrist and hand level

 S66.391- Other injury of extensor muscle, fascia and tendon of <u>left index</u> finger at wrist and hand level

 S66.392- Other injury of extensor muscle, fascia and tendon of <u>right middle</u> finger at wrist and hand level

 S66.393- Other injury of extensor muscle, fascia and tendon of <u>left middle</u> finger at wrist and hand level

 S66.394- Other injury of extensor muscle, fascia and tendon of <u>right ring</u> finger at wrist and hand level

 S66.395- Other injury of extensor muscle, fascia and tendon of <u>left ring</u> finger at wrist and hand level

 S66.396- Other injury of extensor muscle, fascia and tendon of <u>right little</u> finger at wrist and hand level

 S66.397- Other injury of extensor muscle, fascia and tendon of <u>left little</u> finger at wrist and hand level

 S66.398- Other injury of extensor muscle, fascia and tendon of <u>other</u> finger at wrist and hand level
  Other injury of extensor muscle, fascia and tendon of specified finger with unspecified laterality at wrist and hand level

 S66.399- Other injury of extensor muscle, fascia and tendon of <u>unspecified</u> finger at wrist and hand level

S66.4- <u>Injury</u> of <u>intrinsic</u> muscle, fascia and tendon of <u>thumb</u> at wrist and hand level

 S66.40- <u>Unspecified</u> injury of <u>intrinsic</u> muscle, fascia and tendon of <u>thumb</u> at <u>wrist and hand level</u>

  S66.401- Unspecified injury of intrinsic muscle, fascia and tendon of <u>right</u> thumb at wrist and hand level

  S66.402- Unspecified injury of intrinsic muscle, fascia and tendon of <u>left</u> thumb at wrist and hand level

  S66.409- Unspecified injury of intrinsic muscle, fascia and tendon of <u>unspecified</u> thumb at wrist and hand level

 S66.41- <u>Strain</u> of <u>intrinsic</u> muscle, fascia and tendon of <u>thumb</u> at <u>wrist and hand level</u>

  S66.411- Strain of intrinsic muscle, fascia and tendon of <u>right</u> thumb at wrist and hand level

  S66.412- Strain of intrinsic muscle, fascia and tendon of <u>left</u> thumb at wrist and hand level

  S66.419- Strain of intrinsic muscle, fascia and tendon of <u>unspecified</u> thumb at wrist and hand level

 S66.42- <u>Laceration</u> of <u>intrinsic</u> muscle, fascia and tendon of <u>thumb</u> at <u>wrist and hand level</u>

  S66.421- Laceration of intrinsic muscle, fascia and tendon of <u>right</u> thumb at wrist and hand level

  S66.422- Laceration of intrinsic muscle, fascia and tendon of <u>left</u> thumb at wrist and hand level

  S66.429- Laceration of intrinsic muscle, fascia and tendon of <u>unspecified</u> thumb at wrist and hand level

 S66.49- <u>Other specified injury</u> of <u>intrinsic</u> muscle, fascia and tendon of <u>thumb</u> at <u>wrist and hand level</u>

  S66.491- Other specified injury of intrinsic muscle, fascia and tendon of <u>right</u> thumb at wrist and hand level

  S66.492- Other specified injury of intrinsic muscle, fascia and tendon of <u>left</u> thumb at wrist and hand level

  S66.499- Other specified injury of intrinsic muscle, fascia and tendon of <u>unspecified</u> thumb at wrist and hand level

S66.5- <u>Injury</u> of <u>intrinsic</u> muscle, fascia and tendon of <u>other and unspecified finger</u> at <u>wrist and hand level</u>
 Excludes ❷: injury of intrinsic muscle, fascia and tendon of thumb at wrist and hand level (S66.4-)

 S66.50- <u>Unspecified</u> injury of <u>intrinsic</u> muscle, fascia and tendon of <u>other and unspecified finger</u> at <u>wrist and hand level</u>

  S66.500- Unspecified injury of intrinsic muscle, fascia and tendon of <u>right index</u> finger at wrist and hand level

  S66.501- Unspecified injury of intrinsic muscle, fascia and tendon of <u>left index</u> finger at wrist and hand level

  S66.502- Unspecified injury of intrinsic muscle, fascia and tendon of <u>right middle</u> finger at wrist and hand level

  S66.503- Unspecified injury of intrinsic muscle, fascia and tendon of <u>left middle</u> finger at wrist and hand level

  S66.504- Unspecified injury of intrinsic muscle, fascia and tendon of <u>right ring</u> finger at wrist and hand level

  S66.505- Unspecified injury of intrinsic muscle, fascia and tendon of <u>left ring</u> finger at wrist and hand level

  S66.506- Unspecified injury of intrinsic muscle, fascia and tendon of <u>right little</u> finger at wrist and hand level

  S66.507- Unspecified injury of intrinsic muscle, fascia and tendon of <u>left little</u> finger at wrist and hand level

  S66.508- Unspecified injury of intrinsic muscle, fascia and tendon of <u>other</u> finger at wrist and hand level
   Unspecified injury of intrinsic muscle, fascia and tendon of specified finger with unspecified laterality at wrist and hand level

  S66.509- Unspecified injury of intrinsic muscle, fascia and tendon of <u>unspecified</u> finger at wrist and hand level

 S66.51- <u>Strain</u> of <u>intrinsic</u> muscle, fascia and tendon of <u>other and unspecified finger</u> at <u>wrist and hand level</u>

  S66.510- Strain of intrinsic muscle, fascia and tendon of <u>right index</u> finger at wrist and hand level

  S66.511- Strain of intrinsic muscle, fascia and tendon of <u>left index</u> finger at wrist and hand level

  S66.512- Strain of intrinsic muscle, fascia and tendon of <u>right middle</u> finger at wrist and hand level

  S66.513- Strain of intrinsic muscle, fascia and tendon of <u>left middle</u> finger at wrist and hand level

  S66.514- Strain of intrinsic muscle, fascia and tendon of <u>right ring</u> finger at wrist and hand level

  S66.515- Strain of intrinsic muscle, fascia and tendon of <u>left ring</u> finger at wrist and hand level

  S66.516- Strain of intrinsic muscle, fascia and tendon of <u>right little</u> finger at wrist and hand level

S 6 6 - S 6 7

S66.517- Strain of intrinsic muscle, fascia and tendon of <u>left little</u> finger at wrist and hand level

S66.518- Strain of intrinsic muscle, fascia and tendon of <u>other</u> finger at wrist and hand level
      Strain of intrinsic muscle, fascia and tendon of specified finger with unspecified laterality at wrist and hand level

S66.519- Strain of intrinsic muscle, fascia and tendon of <u>unspecified</u> finger at wrist and hand level

S66.52- <u>Laceration</u> of <u>intrinsic</u> muscle, fascia and tendon of <u>other and unspecified finger</u> at <u>wrist and hand level</u>

  S66.520- Laceration of intrinsic muscle, fascia and tendon of <u>right index</u> finger at wrist and hand level

  S66.521- Laceration of intrinsic muscle, fascia and tendon of <u>left index</u> finger at wrist and hand level

  S66.522- Laceration of intrinsic muscle, fascia and tendon of <u>right middle</u> finger at wrist and hand level

  S66.523- Laceration of intrinsic muscle, fascia and tendon of <u>left middle</u> finger at wrist and hand level

  S66.524- Laceration of intrinsic muscle, fascia and tendon of <u>right ring</u> finger at wrist and hand level

  S66.525- Laceration of intrinsic muscle, fascia and tendon of <u>left ring</u> finger at wrist and hand level

  S66.526- Laceration of intrinsic muscle, fascia and tendon of <u>right little</u> finger at wrist and hand level

  S66.527- Laceration of intrinsic muscle, fascia and tendon of <u>left</u> little finger at wrist and hand level

  S66.528- Laceration of intrinsic muscle, fascia and tendon of <u>other</u> finger at wrist and hand level
      Laceration of intrinsic muscle, fascia and tendon of specified finger with unspecified laterality at wrist and hand level

  S66.529- Laceration of intrinsic muscle, fascia and tendon of <u>unspecified</u> finger at wrist and hand level

S66.59- <u>Other injury</u> of <u>intrinsic</u> muscle, fascia and tendon of <u>other and unspecified finger</u> at <u>wrist and hand level</u>

  S66.590- Other injury of intrinsic muscle, fascia and tendon of <u>right index</u> finger at wrist andhand level

  S66.591- Other injury of intrinsic muscle, fascia and tendon of <u>left index</u> finger at wrist and hand level

  S66.592- Other injury of intrinsic muscle, fascia and tendon of <u>right middle</u> finger at wrist and hand level

  S66.593- Other injury of intrinsic muscle, fascia and tendon of <u>left middle</u> finger at wrist and hand level

  S66.594- Other injury of intrinsic muscle, fascia and tendon of <u>right ring</u> finger at wrist and hand level

  S66.595- Other injury of intrinsic muscle, fascia and tendon of <u>left ring</u> finger at wrist and hand level

  S66.596- Other injury of intrinsic muscle, fascia and tendon of <u>right little</u> finger at wrist and hand level

  S66.597- Other injury of intrinsic muscle, fascia and tendon of <u>left little</u> finger at wrist and hand level

  S66.598- Other injury of intrinsic muscle, fascia and tendon of <u>other</u> finger at wrist and hand level
      Other injury of intrinsic muscle, fascia and tendon of specified finger with unspecified laterality at wrist and hand level

  S66.599- Other injury of intrinsic muscle, fascia and tendon of <u>unspecified</u> finger at wrist and hand level

S66.8- <u>Injury</u> of <u>other specified</u> muscles, fascia and tendons at <u>wrist and hand level</u>

  S66.80- <u>Unspecified</u> injury of <u>other specified</u> muscles, fascia and tendons at <u>wrist and hand level</u>

  S66.801- Unspecified injury of other specified muscles, fascia and tendons at wrist and hand level, <u>right</u> hand

  S66.802- Unspecified injury of other specified muscles, fascia and tendons at wrist and hand level, <u>left</u> hand

  S66.809- Unspecified injury of other specified muscles, fascia and tendons at wrist and hand level, <u>unspecified</u> hand

  S66.81- <u>Strain</u> of <u>other specified</u> muscles, fascia and tendons at <u>wrist and hand level</u>

  S66.811- Strain of other specified muscles, fascia and tendons at wrist and hand level, <u>right</u> hand

  S66.812- Strain of other specified muscles, fascia and tendons at wrist and hand level, <u>left</u> hand

  S66.819- Strain of other specified muscles, fascia and tendons at wrist and hand level, <u>unspecified</u> hand

S66.82- <u>Laceration</u> of <u>other specified</u> muscles, fascia and tendons at <u>wrist and hand level</u>

  S66.821- Laceration of other specified muscles, fascia and tendons at wrist and hand level, <u>right</u> hand

  S66.822- Laceration of other specified muscles, fascia and tendons at wrist and hand level, <u>left</u> hand

  S66.829- Laceration of other specified muscles, fascia and tendons at wrist and hand level, <u>unspecified</u> hand

S66.89- <u>Other injury</u> of <u>other specified</u> muscles, fascia and tendons at <u>wrist and hand level</u>

  S66.891- Other injury of other specified muscles, fascia and tendons at wrist and hand level, <u>right</u> hand

  S66.892- Other injury of other specified muscles, fascia and tendons at wrist and hand level, <u>left</u> hand

  S66.899- Other injury of other specified muscles, fascia and tendons at wrist and hand level, <u>unspecified</u> hand

S66.9- Injury of <u>unspecified</u> muscle, fascia and tendon at <u>wrist and hand level</u>

  S66.90- <u>Unspecified</u> injury of <u>unspecified</u> muscle, fascia and tendon at <u>wrist and hand level</u>

  S66.901- Unspecified injury of unspecified muscle, fascia and tendon at wrist and hand level, <u>right</u> hand

  S66.902- Unspecified injury of unspecified muscle, fascia and tendon at wrist and hand level, <u>left</u> hand

  S66.909- Unspecified injury of unspecified muscle, fascia and tendon at wrist and hand level, <u>unspecified</u> hand

  S66.91- <u>Strain</u> of <u>unspecified</u> muscle, fascia and tendon at <u>wrist and hand level</u>

  S66.911- Strain of unspecified muscle, fascia and tendon at wrist and hand level, <u>right</u> hand

  S66.912- Strain of unspecified muscle, fascia and tendon at wrist and hand level, <u>left</u> hand

  S66.919- Strain of unspecified muscle, fascia and tendon at wrist and hand level, <u>unspecified</u> hand

  S66.92- <u>Laceration</u> of <u>unspecified</u> muscle, fascia and tendon at <u>wrist and hand level</u>

  S66.921- Laceration of unspecified muscle, fascia and tendon at wrist and hand level, <u>right</u> hand

  S66.922- Laceration of unspecified muscle, fascia and tendon at wrist and hand level, <u>left</u> hand

  S66.929- Laceration of unspecified muscle, fascia and tendon at wrist and hand level, <u>unspecified</u> hand

  S66.99- <u>Other injury</u> of <u>unspecified</u> muscle, fascia and tendon at <u>wrist and hand level</u>

  S66.991- Other injury of unspecified muscle, fascia and tendon at wrist and hand level, <u>right</u> hand

  S66.992- Other injury of unspecified muscle, fascia and tendon at wrist and hand level, <u>left</u> hand

  S66.999- Other injury of unspecified muscle, fascia and tendon at wrist and hand level, <u>unspecified</u> hand

S67- <u>Crushing injury</u> of <u>wrist, hand and fingers</u>
Use additional code for all associated injuries, such as:
  Fracture of wrist and hand (S62.-)
  Open wound of wrist and hand (S61.-)
The appropriate 7th character is to be added to each code from category S67:
A <u>Initial</u> encounter
D <u>Subsequent</u> encounter
S <u>Sequela</u>

S67.0- <u>Crushing</u> injury of <u>thumb</u>
  S67.00x- Crushing injury of <u>unspecified</u> thumb
  S67.01x- Crushing injury of <u>right</u> thumb
  S67.02x- Crushing injury of <u>left</u> thumb

S67.1- <u>Crushing</u> injury of <u>other and unspecified finger(s)</u>
  Excludes❷: crushing injury of thumb (S67.0-)
  S67.10x- Crushing injury of <u>unspecified</u> finger(s)
  S67.19- Crushing injury of <u>other</u> finger(s)
    S67.190- Crushing injury of <u>right index</u> finger
    S67.191- Crushing injury of <u>left index</u> finger
    S67.192- Crushing injury of <u>right middle</u> finger
    S67.193- Crushing injury of <u>left middle</u> finger
    S67.194- Crushing injury of <u>right ring</u> finger
    S67.195- Crushing injury of <u>left ring</u> finger
    S67.196- Crushing injury of <u>right little</u> finger
    S67.197- Crushing injury of <u>left little</u> finger
    S67.198- Crushing injury of <u>other</u> finger
      Crushing injury of specified finger with unspecified laterality

Excludes 1: = NOT CODED HERE! (Do not code both)   *Excludes❷:* = Not Included Here

S66 - S67

S67.2- <u>Crushing</u> injury of <u>hand</u>
Excludes❷: *crushing injury of fingers (S67.1-)*
crushing injury of thumb (S67.0-)

S67.20x- Crushing injury of <u>unspecified</u> hand

S67.21x- Crushing injury of <u>right</u> hand

S67.22x- Crushing injury of <u>left</u> hand

S67.3- <u>Crushing</u> injury of <u>wrist</u>

S67.30x- Crushing injury of <u>unspecified</u> wrist

S67.31x- Crushing injury of <u>right</u> wrist

S67.32x- Crushing injury of <u>left</u> wrist

S67.4- <u>Crushing</u> injury of <u>wrist and hand</u>
Excludes 1: *crushing injury of hand alone (S67.2-)*
crushing injury of wrist alone (S67.3-)
Excludes❷: *crushing injury of fingers (S67.1-)*
crushing injury of thumb (S67.0-)

S67.40x- Crushing injury of <u>unspecified</u> wrist and hand

S67.41x- Crushing injury of <u>right</u> wrist and hand

S67.42x- Crushing injury of <u>left</u> wrist and hand

S67.9- <u>Crushing</u> injury of <u>unspecified part(s)</u> of <u>wrist, hand and fingers</u>

S67.90x- Crushing injury of unspecified part(s) of <u>unspecified</u> wrist, hand and fingers

S67.91x- Crushing injury of unspecified part(s) of <u>right</u> wrist, hand and fingers

S67.92x- Crushing injury of unspecified part(s) of <u>left</u> wrist, hand and fingers

S68- <u>Traumatic amputation</u> of <u>wrist, hand and fingers</u>
Note: An amputation not identified as partial or complete should be coded to complete

The appropriate 7th character is to be added to each code from category S68:
A   <u>Initial</u> encounter
D   <u>Subsequent</u> encounter
S   <u>Sequela</u>

S68.0- Traumatic <u>metacarpophalangeal</u> <u>amputation</u> of <u>thumb</u>
Traumatic amputation of thumb NOS

S68.01- <u>Complete</u> traumatic <u>metacarpophalangeal</u> <u>amputation</u> of <u>thumb</u>

S68.011- Complete traumatic metacarpophalangeal amputation of <u>right</u> thumb

S68.012- Complete traumatic metacarpophalangeal amputation of <u>left</u> thumb

S68.019- Complete traumatic metacarpophalangeal amputation of <u>unspecified</u> thumb

S68.02- <u>Partial</u> traumatic <u>metacarpophalangeal</u> <u>amputation</u> of <u>thumb</u>

S68.021- Partial traumatic metacarpophalangeal amputation of <u>right</u> thumb

S68.022- Partial traumatic metacarpophalangeal amputation of <u>left</u> thumb

S68.029- Partial traumatic metacarpophalangeal amputation of <u>unspecified</u> thumb

S68.1- <u>Traumatic</u> <u>metacarpophalangeal</u> <u>amputation</u> of <u>other and unspecified</u> <u>finger</u>
Traumatic amputation of finger NOS
Excludes❷: *traumatic metacarpophalangeal amputation of thumb (S68.0-)*

S68.11- <u>Complete</u> traumatic <u>metacarpophalangeal</u> amputation of <u>other and unspecified</u> <u>finger</u>

S68.110- Complete traumatic metacarpophalangeal amputation of <u>right</u> <u>index</u> finger

S68.111- Complete traumatic metacarpophalangeal amputation of <u>left</u> <u>index</u> finger

S68.112- Complete traumatic metacarpophalangeal amputation of <u>right</u> <u>middle</u> finger

S68.113- Complete traumatic metacarpophalangeal amputation of <u>left</u> <u>middle</u> finger

S68.114- Complete traumatic metacarpophalangeal amputation of <u>right</u> <u>ring</u> finger

S68.115- Complete traumatic metacarpophalangeal amputation of <u>left</u> <u>ring</u> finger

S68.116- Complete traumatic metacarpophalangeal amputation of <u>right</u> <u>little</u> finger

S68.117- Complete traumatic metacarpophalangeal amputation of <u>left</u> <u>little</u> finger

S68.118- Complete traumatic metacarpophalangeal amputation of <u>other</u> finger
Complete traumatic metacarpophalangeal amputation of specified finger with unspecified laterality

S68.119- Complete traumatic metacarpophalangeal amputation of <u>unspecified</u> finger

S68.12- <u>Partial</u> traumatic <u>metacarpophalangeal</u> <u>amputation</u> of <u>other and unspecified</u> <u>finger</u>

S68.120- Partial traumatic metacarpophalangeal amputation of <u>right</u> <u>index</u> finger

S68.121- Partial traumatic metacarpophalangeal amputation of <u>left</u> <u>index</u> finger

S68.122- Partial traumatic metacarpophalangeal amputation of <u>right</u> <u>middle</u> finger

S68.123- Partial traumatic metacarpophalangeal amputation of <u>left</u> <u>middle</u> finger

S68.124- Partial traumatic metacarpophalangeal amputation of <u>right</u> <u>ring</u> finger

S68.125- Partial traumatic metacarpophalangeal amputation of <u>left</u> <u>ring</u> finger

S68.126- Partial traumatic metacarpophalangeal amputation of <u>right</u> <u>little</u> finger

S68.127- Partial traumatic metacarpophalangeal amputation of <u>left</u> <u>little</u> finger

S68.128- Partial traumatic metacarpophalangeal amputation of <u>other</u> finger
Partial traumatic metacarpophalangeal amputation of specified finger with unspecified laterality

S68.129- Partial traumatic metacarpophalangeal amputation of <u>unspecified</u> finger

S68.4- Traumatic <u>amputation</u> of <u>hand</u> at <u>wrist level</u>
Traumatic amputation of hand NOS
Traumatic amputation of wrist

S68.41- <u>Complete</u> traumatic <u>amputation</u> of <u>hand</u> at <u>wrist level</u>

S68.411- Complete traumatic amputation of <u>right</u> hand at wrist level

S68.412- Complete traumatic amputation of <u>left</u> hand at wrist level

S68.419- Complete traumatic amputation of <u>unspecified</u> hand at wrist level

S68.42- <u>Partial</u> traumatic <u>amputation</u> of <u>hand</u> at <u>wrist level</u>

S68.421- Partial traumatic amputation of <u>right</u> hand at wrist level

S68.422- Partial traumatic amputation of <u>left</u> hand at wrist level

S68.429- Partial traumatic amputation of <u>unspecified</u> hand at wrist level

S68.5- Traumatic <u>transphalangeal</u> <u>amputation</u> of <u>thumb</u>
Traumatic interphalangeal joint amputation of thumb

S68.51- <u>Complete</u> traumatic <u>transphalangeal</u> <u>amputation</u> of <u>thumb</u>

S68.511- Complete traumatic transphalangeal amputation of <u>right</u> thumb

S68.512- Complete traumatic transphalangeal amputation of <u>left</u> thumb

S68.519- Complete traumatic transphalangeal amputation of <u>unspecified</u> thumb

S68.52- <u>Partial</u> traumatic <u>transphalangeal</u> <u>amputation</u> of <u>thumb</u>

S68.521- Partial traumatic transphalangeal amputation of <u>right</u> thumb

S68.522- Partial traumatic transphalangeal amputation of <u>left</u> thumb

S68.529- Partial traumatic transphalangeal amputation of <u>unspecified</u> thumb

S68.6- Traumatic <u>transphalangeal</u> <u>amputation</u> of <u>other and unspecified</u> <u>finger</u>

S68.61- <u>Complete</u> traumatic <u>transphalangeal</u> <u>amputation</u> of <u>other and unspecified</u> <u>finger(s)</u>

S68.610- Complete traumatic transphalangeal amputation of <u>right</u> <u>index</u> finger

S68.611- Complete traumatic transphalangeal amputation of <u>left</u> <u>index</u> finger

S68.612- Complete traumatic transphalangeal amputation of <u>right</u> <u>middle</u> finger

S68.613- Complete traumatic transphalangeal amputation of <u>left</u> <u>middle</u> finger

S68.614- Complete traumatic transphalangeal amputation of <u>right</u> <u>ring</u> finger

S68.615- Complete traumatic transphalangeal amputation of <u>left</u> <u>ring</u> finger

S68.616- Complete traumatic transphalangeal amputation of <u>right</u> <u>little</u> finger

S68.617- Complete traumatic transphalangeal amputation of <u>left</u> <u>little</u> finger

S67 – S70

S68.618-   Complete traumatic transphalangeal amputation of <u>other</u> finger
    Complete traumatic transphalangeal amputation of specified finger with unspecified laterality
S68.619-   Complete traumatic transphalangeal amputation of <u>unspecified</u> finger
S68.62-   <u>Partial</u> traumatic <u>transphalangeal amputation</u> of <u>other and unspecified finger</u>
S68.620-   Partial traumatic transphalangeal amputation of <u>right index</u> finger
S68.621-   Partial traumatic transphalangeal amputation of <u>left index</u> finger
S68.622-   Partial traumatic transphalangeal amputation of <u>right middle</u> finger
S68.623-   Partial traumatic transphalangeal amputation of <u>left middle</u> finger
S68.624-   Partial traumatic transphalangeal amputation of <u>right ring</u> finger
S68.625-   Partial traumatic transphalangeal amputation of <u>left ring</u> finger
S68.626-   Partial traumatic transphalangeal amputation of <u>right little</u> finger
S68.627-   Partial traumatic transphalangeal amputation of <u>left little</u> finger
S68.628-   Partial traumatic transphalangeal amputation of <u>other</u> finger
    Partial traumatic transphalangeal amputation of specified finger with unspecified laterality
S68.629-   Partial traumatic transphalangeal amputation of <u>unspecified</u> finger
S68.7-   <u>Traumatic transmetacarpal amputation</u> of <u>hand</u>
S68.71-   <u>Complete</u> traumatic <u>transmetacarpal amputation</u> of <u>hand</u>
S68.711-   Complete traumatic transmetacarpal amputation of <u>right</u> hand
S68.712-   Complete traumatic transmetacarpal amputation of <u>left</u> hand
S68.719-   Complete traumatic transmetacarpal amputation of <u>unspecified</u> hand
S68.72-   <u>Partial</u> traumatic <u>transmetacarpal amputation</u> of <u>hand</u>
S68.721-   Partial traumatic transmetacarpal amputation of <u>right</u> hand
S68.722-   Partial traumatic transmetacarpal amputation of <u>left</u> hand
S68.729-   Partial traumatic transmetacarpal amputation of <u>unspecified</u> hand
S69-   <u>Other and unspecified injuries</u> of <u>wrist, hand and finger(s)</u>
The appropriate 7th character is to be added to each code from category S69:
   A   <u>Initial</u> encounter
   D   <u>Subsequent</u> encounter
   S   <u>Sequela</u>
S69.8-   <u>Other specified injuries</u> of <u>wrist, hand and finger(s)</u>
S69.80x-   Other specified injuries of <u>unspecified</u> wrist, hand and finger(s)
S69.81x-   Other specified injuries of <u>right</u> wrist, hand and finger(s)
S69.82x-   Other specified injuries of <u>left</u> wrist, hand and finger(s)
S69.9-   <u>Unspecified injury</u> of <u>wrist, hand and finger(s)</u>
S69.90x-   Unspecified injury of <u>unspecified</u> wrist, hand and finger(s)
S69.91x-   Unspecified injury of <u>right</u> wrist, hand and finger(s)
S69.92x-   Unspecified injury of <u>left</u> wrist, hand and finger(s)

Injuries to the hip and thigh (S70-S79)

Excludes❷: burns and corrosions (T20-T32)
    frostbite (T33-T34)
    snake bite (T63.0-)
    venomous insect bite or sting (T63.4-)

S70-   <u>Superficial injury</u> of <u>hip and thigh</u>
The appropriate 7th character is to be added to each code from category S70:
   A   <u>Initial</u> encounter
   D   <u>Subsequent</u> encounter
   S   <u>Sequela</u>
S70.0-   <u>Contusion</u> of <u>hip</u>
S70.00x-   Contusion of <u>unspecified</u> hip
S70.01x-   Contusion of <u>right</u> hip
S70.02x-   Contusion of <u>left</u> hip

S70.1-   <u>Contusion</u> of <u>thigh</u>
S70.10x-   Contusion of <u>unspecified</u> thigh
S70.11x-   Contusion of <u>right</u> thigh
S70.12x-   Contusion of <u>left</u> thigh
S70.2-   <u>Other superficial injuries</u> of <u>hip</u>
S70.21-   <u>Abrasion</u> of <u>hip</u>
S70.211-   Abrasion, <u>right</u> hip
S70.212-   Abrasion, <u>left</u> hip
S70.219-   Abrasion, <u>unspecified</u> hip
S70.22-   <u>Blister</u> (nonthermal) of <u>hip</u>
S70.221-   Blister (nonthermal), <u>right</u> hip
S70.222-   Blister (nonthermal), <u>left</u> hip
S70.229-   Blister (nonthermal), <u>unspecified</u> hip
S70.24-   <u>External constriction</u> of <u>hip</u>
S70.241-   External constriction, <u>right</u> hip
S70.242-   External constriction, <u>left</u> hip
S70.249-   External constriction, <u>unspecified</u> hip
S70.25-   <u>Superficial foreign body</u> of <u>hip</u>
    Splinter in the hip
S70.251-   Superficial foreign body, <u>right</u> hip
S70.252-   Superficial foreign body, <u>left</u> hip
S70.259-   Superficial foreign body, <u>unspecified</u> hip
S70.26-   <u>Insect bite (nonvenomous)</u> of <u>hip</u>
S70.261-   Insect bite (nonvenomous), <u>right</u> hip
S70.262-   Insect bite (nonvenomous), <u>left</u> hip
S70.269-   Insect bite (nonvenomous), <u>unspecified</u> hip
S70.27-   <u>Other superficial bite</u> of <u>hip</u>
    Excludes 1:   open bite of hip (S71.05-)
S70.271-   Other superficial bite of hip, <u>right</u> hip
S70.272-   Other superficial bite of hip, <u>left</u> hip
S70.279-   Other superficial bite of hip, <u>unspecified</u> hip
S70.3-   <u>Other superficial injuries</u> of <u>thigh</u>
S70.31-   <u>Abrasion</u> of <u>thigh</u>
S70.311-   Abrasion, <u>right</u> thigh
S70.312-   Abrasion, <u>left</u> thigh
S70.319-   Abrasion, <u>unspecified</u> thigh
S70.32-   <u>Blister</u> (nonthermal) of <u>thigh</u>
S70.321-   Blister (nonthermal), <u>right</u> thigh
S70.322-   Blister (nonthermal), <u>left</u> thigh
S70.329-   Blister (nonthermal), <u>unspecified</u> thigh
S70.34-   <u>External constriction</u> of <u>thigh</u>
S70.341-   External constriction, <u>right</u> thigh
S70.342-   External constriction, <u>left</u> thigh
S70.349-   External constriction, <u>unspecified</u> thigh
S70.35-   <u>Superficial foreign body</u> of <u>thigh</u>
    Splinter in the thigh
S70.351-   Superficial foreign body, <u>right</u> thigh
S70.352-   Superficial foreign body, <u>left</u> thigh
S70.359-   Superficial foreign body, <u>unspecified</u> thigh
S70.36-   <u>Insect bite (nonvenomous)</u> of <u>thigh</u>
S70.361-   Insect bite (nonvenomous), <u>right</u> thigh
S70.362-   Insect bite (nonvenomous), <u>left</u> thigh
S70.369-   Insect bite (nonvenomous), <u>unspecified</u> thigh
S70.37-   <u>Other superficial bite</u> of <u>thigh</u>
    Excludes 1:   open bite of thigh (S71.15)
S70.371-   Other superficial bite of <u>right</u> thigh
S70.372-   Other superficial bite of <u>left</u> thigh
S70.379-   Other superficial bite of <u>unspecified</u> thigh
S70.9-   <u>Unspecified superficial injury</u> of <u>hip and thigh</u>
S70.91-   <u>Unspecified</u> superficial injury of <u>hip</u>
S70.911-   Unspecified superficial injury of <u>right</u> hip
S70.912-   Unspecified superficial injury of <u>left</u> hip
S70.919-   Unspecified superficial injury of <u>unspecified</u> hip
S70.92-   <u>Unspecified</u> superficial injury of <u>thigh</u>
S70.921-   Unspecified superficial injury of <u>right</u> thigh
S70.922-   Unspecified superficial injury of <u>left</u> thigh
S70.929-   Unspecified superficial injury of <u>unspecified</u> thigh

S 6 7 I S 7 0

Excludes 1: = NOT CODED HERE! (Do not code both)   **753**   *Excludes❷: = Not Included Here*

S71-　Open wound of hip and thigh
　　Code also any associated wound infection
　　Excludes 1:　*open fracture of hip and thigh (S72.-)*
　　　　　　　　traumatic amputation of hip and thigh (S78.-)
　　Excludes❷:　*bite of venomous animal (T63.-)*
　　　　　　　　open wound of ankle, foot and toes (S91.-)
　　　　　　　　open wound of knee and lower leg (S81.-)

The appropriate 7th character is to be added to each code from category S71:
　　A　**Initial** encounter
　　D　**Subsequent** encounter
　　S　**Sequela**

S71.0-　Open wound of hip
　S71.00-　Unspecified open wound of hip
　　S71.001-　Unspecified open wound, right hip
　　S71.002-　Unspecified open wound, left hip
　　S71.009-　Unspecified open wound, unspecified hip
　S71.01-　Laceration without foreign body of hip
　　S71.011-　Laceration without foreign body, right hip
　　S71.012-　Laceration without foreign body, left hip
　　S71.019-　Laceration without foreign body, unspecified hip
　S71.02-　Laceration with foreign body of hip
　　S71.021-　Laceration with foreign body, right hip
　　S71.022-　Laceration with foreign body, left hip
　　S71.029-　Laceration with foreign body, unspecified hip
　S71.03-　Puncture wound without foreign body of hip
　　S71.031-　Puncture wound without foreign body, right hip
　　S71.032-　Puncture wound without foreign body, left hip
　　S71.039-　Puncture wound without foreign body, unspecified hip
　S71.04-　Puncture wound with foreign body of hip
　　S71.041-　Puncture wound with foreign body, right hip
　　S71.042-　Puncture wound with foreign body, left hip
　　S71.049-　Puncture wound with foreign body, unspecified hip
　S71.05-　Open bite of hip
　　　Bite of hip NOS
　　　Excludes 1:　*superficial bite of hip (S70.26, S70.27)*
　　S71.051-　Open bite, right hip
　　S71.052-　Open bite, left hip
　　S71.059-　Open bite, unspecified hip

S71.1-　Open wound of thigh
　S71.10-　Unspecified open wound of thigh
　　S71.101-　Unspecified open wound, right thigh
　　S71.102-　Unspecified open wound, left thigh
　　S71.109-　Unspecified open wound, unspecified thigh
　S71.11-　Laceration without foreign body of thigh
　　S71.111-　Laceration without foreign body, right thigh
　　S71.112-　Laceration without foreign body, left thigh
　　S71.119-　Laceration without foreign body, unspecified thigh
　S71.12-　Laceration with foreign body of thigh
　　S71.121-　Laceration with foreign body, right thigh
　　S71.122-　Laceration with foreign body, left thigh
　　S71.129-　Laceration with foreign body, unspecified thigh
　S71.13-　Puncture wound without foreign body of thigh
　　S71.131-　Puncture wound without foreign body, right thigh
　　S71.132-　Puncture wound without foreign body, left thigh
　　S71.139-　Puncture wound without foreign body, unspecified thigh
　S71.14-　Puncture wound with foreign body of thigh
　　S71.141-　Puncture wound with foreign body, right thigh
　　S71.142-　Puncture wound with foreign body, left thigh
　　S71.149-　Puncture wound with foreign body, unspecified thigh
　S71.15-　Open bite of thigh
　　　Bite of thigh NOS
　　　Excludes 1:　*superficial bite of thigh (S70.37-)*
　　S71.151-　Open bite, right thigh
　　S71.152-　Open bite, left thigh
　　S71.159-　Open bite, unspecified thigh

S72-　Fracture of femur
　　Note: A fracture not indicated as displaced or nondisplaced should be coded to displaced
　　Note: A fracture not indicated as open or closed should be coded to closed
　　Note: The open fracture designations are based on the Gustilo open fracture classification
　　Excludes 1:　*traumatic amputation of hip and thigh (S78.-)*
　　Excludes❷:　*fracture of lower leg and ankle (S82.-)*
　　　　　　　　fracture of foot (S92.-)
　　　　　　　　periprosthetic fracture of prosthetic implant of hip (T84.040, T84.041)

The appropriate 7th character is to be added to all codes from category S72:
　　A　**Initial** encounter for **closed** fracture
　　B　**Initial** encounter for **open** fracture **type I or II**
　　　　Initial encounter for open fracture NOS
　　C　**Initial** encounter for **open** fracture **type IIIA, IIIB, or IIIC**
　　D　**Subsequent** encounter for **closed** fracture **with routine healing**
　　E　**Subsequent** encounter for **open** fracture **type I or II with routine healing**
　　F　**Subsequent** encounter for **open** fracture **type IIIA, IIIB, or IIIC with routine healing**
　　G　**Subsequent** encounter for **closed** fracture **with delayed healing**
　　H　**Subsequent** encounter for **open** fracture **type I or II with delayed healing**
　　J　**Subsequent** encounter for **open** fracture **type IIIA, IIIB, or IIIC with delayed healing**
　　K　**Subsequent** encounter for **closed** fracture **with nonunion**
　　M　**Subsequent** encounter for **open** fracture **type I or II with nonunion**
　　N　**Subsequent** encounter for **open** fracture **type IIIA, IIIB, or IIIC with nonunion**
　　P　**Subsequent** encounter for **closed** fracture **with malunion**
　　Q　**Subsequent** encounter for **open** fracture **type I or II with malunion**
　　R　**Subsequent** encounter for **open** fracture **type IIIA, IIIB, or IIIC with malunion**
　　S　**Sequela**

S72.0-　Fracture of head and neck of femur
　　　Excludes❷:　*physeal fracture of upper end of femur (S79.0-)*
　S72.00-　Fracture of unspecified part of neck of femur
　　　Fracture of hip NOS
　　　Fracture of neck of femur NOS
　　S72.001-　Fracture of unspecified part of neck of right femur
　　S72.002-　Fracture of unspecified part of neck of left femur
　　S72.009-　Fracture of unspecified part of neck of unspecified femur
　S72.01-　Unspecified intracapsular fracture of femur
　　　Subcapital fracture of femur
　　S72.011-　Unspecified intracapsular fracture of right femur
　　S72.012-　Unspecified intracapsular fracture of left femur
　　S72.019-　Unspecified intracapsular fracture of unspecified femur
　S72.02-　Fracture of epiphysis (separation) (upper) of femur
　　　Transepiphyseal fracture of femur
　　　Excludes 1:　*capital femoral epiphyseal fracture (pediatric) of femur (S79.01-)*
　　　　　　　　Salter-Harris Type I physeal fracture of upper end of femur (S79.01-)
　　S72.021-　Displaced fracture of epiphysis (separation) (upper) of right femur
　　S72.022-　Displaced fracture of epiphysis (separation) (upper) of left femur
　　S72.023-　Displaced fracture of epiphysis (separation) (upper) of unspecified femur
　　S72.024-　Nondisplaced fracture of epiphysis (separation) (upper) of right femur
　　S72.025-　Nondisplaced fracture of epiphysis (separation) (upper) of left femur
　　S72.026-　Nondisplaced fracture of epiphysis (separation) (upper) of unspecified femur
　S72.03-　Midcervical fracture of femur
　　　Transcervical fracture of femur NOS
　　S72.031-　Displaced midcervical fracture of right femur
　　S72.032-　Displaced midcervical fracture of left femur
　　S72.033-　Displaced midcervical fracture of unspecified femur
　　S72.034-　Nondisplaced midcervical fracture of right femur
　　S72.035-　Nondisplaced midcervical fracture of left femur
　　S72.036-　Nondisplaced midcervical fracture of unspecified femur

S
7
1
-
S
7
2

S72.04- Fracture of <u>base of neck</u> of femur
    Cervicotrochanteric fracture of femur
  S72.041- <u>Displaced</u> fracture of base of neck of <u>right</u> femur
  S72.042- <u>Displaced</u> fracture of base of neck of <u>left</u> femur
  S72.043- <u>Displaced</u> fracture of base of neck of <u>unspecified</u> femur
  S72.044- <u>Nondisplaced</u> fracture of base of neck of <u>right</u> femur
  S72.045- <u>Nondisplaced</u> fracture of base of neck of <u>left</u> femur
  S72.046- <u>Nondisplaced</u> fracture of base of neck of <u>unspecified</u> femur

S72.05- <u>Unspecified</u> fracture of <u>head</u> of femur
    Fracture of head of femur NOS
  S72.051- Unspecified fracture of head of <u>right</u> femur
  S72.052- Unspecified fracture of head of <u>left</u> femur
  S72.059- Unspecified fracture of head of <u>unspecified</u> femur

S72.06- <u>Articular</u> fracture of <u>head</u> of femur
  S72.061- <u>Displaced</u> articular fracture of head of <u>right</u> femur
  S72.062- <u>Displaced</u> articular fracture of head of <u>left</u> femur
  S72.063- <u>Displaced</u> articular fracture of head of <u>unspecified</u> femur
  S72.064- <u>Nondisplaced</u> articular fracture of head of <u>right</u> femur
  S72.065- <u>Nondisplaced</u> articular fracture of head of <u>left</u> femur
  S72.066- <u>Nondisplaced</u> articular fracture of head of <u>unspecified</u> femur

S72.09- <u>Other fracture</u> of <u>head and neck</u> of femur
  S72.091- Other fracture of head and neck of <u>right</u> femur
  S72.092- Other fracture of head and neck of <u>left</u> femur
  S72.099- Other fracture of head and neck of <u>unspecified</u> femur

S72.1- <u>Pertrochanteric fracture</u>
  S72.10- <u>Unspecified</u> trochanteric fracture of femur
    Fracture of trochanter NOS
    S72.101- Unspecified trochanteric fracture of <u>right</u> femur
    S72.102- Unspecified trochanteric fracture of <u>left</u> femur
    S72.109- Unspecified trochanteric fracture of <u>unspecified</u> femur

  S72.11- Fracture of <u>greater trochanter</u> of femur
    S72.111- <u>Displaced</u> fracture of greater trochanter of <u>right</u> femur
    S72.112- <u>Displaced</u> fracture of greater trochanter of <u>left</u> femur
    S72.113- <u>Displaced</u> fracture of greater trochanter of <u>unspecified</u> femur
    S72.114- <u>Nondisplaced</u> fracture of greater trochanter of <u>right</u> femur
    S72.115- <u>Nondisplaced</u> fracture of greater trochanter of <u>left</u> femur
    S72.116- <u>Nondisplaced</u> fracture of greater trochanter of <u>unspecified</u> femur

  S72.12- Fracture of <u>lesser trochanter</u> of femur
    S72.121- <u>Displaced</u> fracture of lesser trochanter of <u>right</u> femur
    S72.122- <u>Displaced</u> fracture of lesser trochanter of <u>left</u> femur
    S72.123- <u>Displaced</u> fracture of lesser trochanter of <u>unspecified</u> femur
    S72.124- <u>Nondisplaced</u> fracture of lesser trochanter of <u>right</u> femur
    S72.125- <u>Nondisplaced</u> fracture of lesser trochanter of <u>left</u> femur
    S72.126- <u>Nondisplaced</u> fracture of lesser trochanter of <u>unspecified</u> femur

  S72.13- <u>Apophyseal</u> fracture of femur
    Excludes 1: chronic (nontraumatic) slipped upper femoral epiphysis (M93.0-)
    S72.131- <u>Displaced</u> apophyseal fracture of <u>right</u> femur
    S72.132- <u>Displaced</u> apophyseal fracture of <u>left</u> femur
    S72.133- <u>Displaced</u> apophyseal fracture of <u>unspecified</u> femur
    S72.134- <u>Nondisplaced</u> apophyseal fracture of <u>right</u> femur
    S72.135- <u>Nondisplaced</u> apophyseal fracture of <u>left</u> femur
    S72.136- <u>Nondisplaced</u> apophyseal fracture of <u>unspecified</u> femur

  S72.14- <u>Intertrochanteric</u> fracture of femur
    S72.141- <u>Displaced</u> intertrochanteric fracture of <u>right</u> femur
    S72.142- <u>Displaced</u> intertrochanteric fracture of <u>left</u> femur
    S72.143- <u>Displaced</u> intertrochanteric fracture of <u>unspecified</u> femur
    S72.144- <u>Nondisplaced</u> intertrochanteric fracture of <u>right</u> femur
    S72.145- <u>Nondisplaced</u> intertrochanteric fracture of <u>left</u> femur
    S72.146- <u>Nondisplaced</u> intertrochanteric fracture of <u>unspecified</u> femur

S72.2- <u>Subtrochanteric</u> fracture of femur
  S72.21x- <u>Displaced</u> subtrochanteric fracture of <u>right</u> femur
  S72.22x- <u>Displaced</u> subtrochanteric fracture of <u>left</u> femur
  S72.23x- <u>Displaced</u> subtrochanteric fracture of <u>unspecified</u> femur
  S72.24x- <u>Nondisplaced</u> subtrochanteric fracture of <u>right</u> femur
  S72.25x- <u>Nondisplaced</u> subtrochanteric fracture of <u>left</u> femur
  S72.26x- <u>Nondisplaced</u> subtrochanteric fracture of <u>unspecified</u> femur

S72.3- Fracture of <u>shaft</u> of femur
  S72.30- <u>Unspecified</u> fracture of <u>shaft</u> of femur
    S72.301- Unspecified fracture of shaft of <u>right</u> femur
    S72.302- Unspecified fracture of shaft of <u>left</u> femur
    S72.309- Unspecified fracture of shaft of <u>unspecified</u> femur

  S72.32- <u>Transverse</u> fracture of <u>shaft</u> of femur
    S72.321- <u>Displaced</u> transverse fracture of shaft of <u>right</u> femur
    S72.322- <u>Displaced</u> transverse fracture of shaft of <u>left</u> femur
    S72.323- <u>Displaced</u> transverse fracture of shaft of <u>unspecified</u> femur
    S72.324- <u>Nondisplaced</u> transverse fracture of shaft of <u>right</u> femur
    S72.325- <u>Nondisplaced</u> transverse fracture of shaft of <u>left</u> femur
    S72.326- <u>Nondisplaced</u> transverse fracture of shaft of <u>unspecified</u> femur

  S72.33- <u>Oblique</u> fracture of <u>shaft</u> of femur
    S72.331- <u>Displaced</u> oblique fracture of shaft of <u>right</u> femur
    S72.332- <u>Displaced</u> oblique fracture of shaft of <u>left</u> femur
    S72.333- <u>Displaced</u> oblique fracture of shaft of <u>unspecified</u> femur
    S72.334- <u>Nondisplaced</u> oblique fracture of shaft of <u>right</u> femur
    S72.335- <u>Nondisplaced</u> oblique fracture of shaft of <u>left</u> femur
    S72.336- <u>Nondisplaced</u> oblique fracture of shaft of <u>unspecified</u> femur

  S72.34- <u>Spiral</u> fracture of <u>shaft</u> of femur
    S72.341- <u>Displaced</u> spiral fracture of shaft of <u>right</u> femur
    S72.342- <u>Displaced</u> spiral fracture of shaft of <u>left</u> femur
    S72.343- <u>Displaced</u> spiral fracture of shaft of <u>unspecified</u> femur
    S72.344- <u>Nondisplaced</u> spiral fracture of shaft of <u>right</u> femur
    S72.345- <u>Nondisplaced</u> spiral fracture of shaft of <u>left</u> femur
    S72.346- <u>Nondisplaced</u> spiral fracture of shaft of <u>unspecified</u> femur

  S72.35- <u>Comminuted</u> fracture of <u>shaft</u> of femur
    S72.351- <u>Displaced</u> comminuted fracture of shaft of <u>right</u> femur
    S72.352- <u>Displaced</u> comminuted fracture of shaft of <u>left</u> femur
    S72.353- <u>Displaced</u> comminuted fracture of shaft of <u>unspecified</u> femur
    S72.354- <u>Nondisplaced</u> comminuted fracture of shaft of <u>right</u> femur
    S72.355- <u>Nondisplaced</u> comminuted fracture of shaft of <u>left</u> femur
    S72.356- <u>Nondisplaced</u> comminuted fracture of shaft of <u>unspecified</u> femur

  S72.36- <u>Segmental</u> fracture of <u>shaft</u> of femur
    S72.361- <u>Displaced</u> segmental fracture of shaft of <u>right</u> femur
    S72.362- <u>Displaced</u> segmental fracture of shaft of <u>left</u> femur
    S72.363- <u>Displaced</u> segmental fracture of shaft of <u>unspecified</u> femur
    S72.364- <u>Nondisplaced</u> segmental fracture of shaft of <u>right</u> femur
    S72.365- <u>Nondisplaced</u> segmental fracture of shaft of <u>left</u> femur
    S72.366- <u>Nondisplaced</u> segmental fracture of shaft of <u>unspecified</u> femur

  S72.39- <u>Other fracture</u> of <u>shaft</u> of femur
    S72.391- Other fracture of shaft of <u>right</u> femur
    S72.392- Other fracture of shaft of <u>left</u> femur
    S72.399- Other fracture of shaft of <u>unspecified</u> femur

S71 - S72

S72.4- Fracture of <u>lower end</u> of femur
Fracture of distal end of femur
Excludes❷: fracture of shaft of femur (S72.3-)
physeal fracture of lower end of femur (S79.1-)

S72.40- <u>Unspecified</u> fracture of <u>lower end</u> of femur

S72.401- Unspecified fracture of lower end of <u>right</u> femur

S72.402- Unspecified fracture of lower end of <u>left</u> femur

S72.409- Unspecified fracture of lower end of <u>unspecified</u> femur

S72.41- <u>Unspecified condyle</u> fracture of <u>lower end</u> of femur
Condyle fracture of femur NOS

S72.411- <u>Displaced</u> unspecified condyle fracture of lower end of <u>right</u> femur

S72.412- <u>Displaced</u> unspecified condyle fracture of lower end of <u>left</u> femur

S72.413- <u>Displaced</u> unspecified condyle fracture of lower end of <u>unspecified</u> femur

S72.414- <u>Nondisplaced</u> unspecified condyle fracture of lower end of <u>right</u> femur

S72.415- <u>Nondisplaced</u> unspecified condyle fracture of lower end of <u>left</u> femur

S72.416- <u>Nondisplaced</u> unspecified condyle fracture of lower end of <u>unspecified</u> femur

S72.42- Fracture of <u>lateral condyle</u> of femur

S72.421- <u>Displaced</u> fracture of lateral condyle of <u>right</u> femur

S72.422- <u>Displaced</u> fracture of lateral condyle of <u>left</u> femur

S72.423- <u>Displaced</u> fracture of lateral condyle of <u>unspecified</u> femur

S72.424- <u>Nondisplaced</u> fracture of lateral condyle of <u>right</u> femur

S72.425- <u>Nondisplaced</u> fracture of lateral condyle of <u>left</u> femur

S72.426- <u>Nondisplaced</u> fracture of lateral condyle of <u>unspecified</u> femur

S72.43- Fracture of <u>medial condyle</u> of femur

S72.431- <u>Displaced</u> fracture of medial condyle of <u>right</u> femur

S72.432- <u>Displaced</u> fracture of medial condyle of <u>left</u> femur

S72.433- <u>Displaced</u> fracture of medial condyle of <u>unspecified</u> femur

S72.434- <u>Nondisplaced</u> fracture of medial condyle of <u>right</u> femur

S72.435- <u>Nondisplaced</u> fracture of medial condyle of <u>left</u> femur

S72.436- <u>Nondisplaced</u> fracture of medial condyle of <u>unspecified</u> femur

S72.44- Fracture of <u>lower epiphysis</u> (separation) of femur
Excludes 1: Salter-Harris Type I physeal fracture of lower end of femur (S79.11-)

S72.441- <u>Displaced</u> fracture of lower epiphysis (separation) of <u>right</u> femur

S72.442- <u>Displaced</u> fracture of lower epiphysis (separation) of <u>left</u> femur

S72.443- <u>Displaced</u> fracture of lower epiphysis (separation) of <u>unspecified</u> femur

S72.444- <u>Nondisplaced</u> fracture of lower epiphysis (separation) of <u>right</u> femur

S72.445- <u>Nondisplaced</u> fracture of lower epiphysis (separation) of <u>left</u> femur

S72.446- <u>Nondisplaced</u> fracture of lower epiphysis (separation) of <u>unspecified</u> femur

S72.45- <u>Supracondylar</u> fracture <u>without</u> intracondylar extension of lower end of femur
Supracondylar fracture of lower end of femur NOS
Excludes 1: supracondylar fracture with intracondylar extension of lower end of femur (S72.46-)

S72.451- <u>Displaced</u> supracondylar fracture <u>without</u> intracondylar extension of lower end of <u>right</u> femur

S72.452- <u>Displaced</u> supracondylar fracture <u>without</u> intracondylar extension of lower end of <u>left</u> femur

S72.453- <u>Displaced</u> supracondylar fracture <u>without</u> intracondylar extension of lower end of <u>unspecified</u> femur

S72.454- <u>Nondisplaced</u> supracondylar fracture <u>without</u> intracondylar extension of lower end of <u>right</u> femur

S72.455- <u>Nondisplaced</u> supracondylar fracture <u>without</u> intracondylar extension of lower end of <u>left</u> femur

S72.456- <u>Nondisplaced</u> supracondylar fracture <u>without</u> intracondylar extension of lower end of <u>unspecified</u> femur

S72.46- <u>Supracondylar</u> fracture <u>with intracondylar extension</u> of lower end of femur
Excludes 1: supracondylar fracture without intracondylar extension of lower end of femur (S72.45-)

S72.461- <u>Displaced</u> supracondylar fracture <u>with intracondylar extension</u> of lower end of <u>right</u> femur

S72.462- <u>Displaced</u> supracondylar fracture <u>with intracondylar extension</u> of lower end of <u>left</u> femur

S72.463- <u>Displaced</u> supracondylar fracture <u>with intracondylar extension</u> of lower end of <u>unspecified</u> femur

S72.464- <u>Nondisplaced</u> supracondylar fracture <u>with intracondylar extension</u> of lower end of <u>right</u> femur

S72.465- <u>Nondisplaced</u> supracondylar fracture <u>with intracondylar extension</u> of lower end of <u>left</u> femur

S72.466- <u>Nondisplaced</u> supracondylar fracture <u>with intracondylar extension</u> of lower end of <u>unspecified</u> femur

S72.47- <u>Torus</u> fracture of <u>lower end</u> of femur
The appropriate 7th character is to be added to all codes in subcategory S72.47:
  A <u>Initial</u> encounter for <u>closed</u> fracture
  D <u>Subsequent</u> encounter for fracture <u>with routine healing</u>
  G <u>Subsequent</u> encounter for fracture <u>with delayed healing</u>
  K <u>Subsequent</u> encounter for fracture <u>with nonunion</u>
  P <u>Subsequent</u> encounter for fracture <u>with malunion</u>
  S <u>Sequela</u>

S72.471- Torus fracture of lower end of <u>right</u> femur

S72.472- Torus fracture of lower end of <u>left</u> femur

S72.479- Torus fracture of lower end of <u>unspecified</u> femur

S72.49- <u>Other fracture</u> of <u>lower end</u> of femur

S72.491- Other fracture of lower end of <u>right</u> femur

S72.492- Other fracture of lower end of <u>left</u> femur

S72.499- Other fracture of lower end of <u>unspecified</u> femur

S72.8- Other fracture of femur

S72.8x- <u>Other fracture</u> of femur

S72.8x1- Other fracture of <u>right</u> femur

S72.8x2- Other fracture of <u>left</u> femur

S72.8x9- Other fracture of <u>unspecified</u> femur

S72.9- <u>Unspecified</u> fracture of femur
Fracture of thigh NOS
Fracture of upper leg NOS
Excludes 1: fracture of hip NOS (S72.00-, S72.01-)

S72.90x- Unspecified fracture of <u>unspecified</u> femur

S72.91x- Unspecified fracture of <u>right</u> femur

S72.92x- Unspecified fracture of <u>left</u> femur

S73- <u>Dislocation and sprain</u> of joint and ligaments of <u>hip</u>
Includes: Avulsion of joint or ligament of hip
Laceration of cartilage, joint or ligament of hip
Sprain of cartilage, joint or ligament of hip
Traumatic hemarthrosis of joint or ligament of hip
Traumatic rupture of joint or ligament of hip
Traumatic subluxation of joint or ligament of hip
Traumatic tear of joint or ligament of hip
Code also any associated open wound
Excludes❷: strain of muscle, fascia and tendon of hip and thigh (S76.-)
The appropriate 7th character is to be added to each code from category S73:
  A <u>Initial</u> encounter
  D <u>Subsequent</u> encounter
  S <u>Sequela</u>

S73.0- <u>Subluxation and dislocation</u> of hip
Excludes 2: dislocation and subluxation of hip prosthesis (T84.020, T84.021)

S73.00- <u>Unspecified</u> subluxation and dislocation of hip
Dislocation of hip NOS
Subluxation of hip NOS

S73.001- Unspecified <u>subluxation</u> of <u>right</u> hip

S73.002- Unspecified <u>subluxation</u> of <u>left</u> hip

S73.003- Unspecified <u>subluxation</u> of <u>unspecified</u> hip

S73.004- Unspecified <u>dislocation</u> of <u>right</u> hip

S73.005- Unspecified <u>dislocation</u> of <u>left</u> hip

S73.006- Unspecified <u>dislocation</u> of <u>unspecified</u> hip

S73.01- <u>Posterior</u> subluxation and dislocation of hip

S73.011- Posterior <u>subluxation</u> of <u>right</u> hip

S73.012- Posterior <u>subluxation</u> of <u>left</u> hip

S73.013- Posterior <u>subluxation</u> of <u>unspecified</u> hip

S73.014- Posterior <u>dislocation</u> of <u>right</u> hip

S73.015- Posterior <u>dislocation</u> of <u>left</u> hip

Excludes❷: = Not Included Here

S73.016- Posterior <u>dislocation</u> of <u>unspecified</u> hip
S73.02- Obturator subluxation and dislocation of hip
    S73.021- Obturator <u>subluxation</u> of <u>right</u> hip
    S73.022- Obturator <u>subluxation</u> of <u>left</u> hip
    S73.023- Obturator <u>subluxation</u> of <u>unspecified</u> hip
    S73.024- Obturator <u>dislocation</u> of <u>right</u> hip
    S73.025- Obturator <u>dislocation</u> of <u>left</u> hip
    S73.026- Obturator <u>dislocation</u> of <u>unspecified</u> hip
S73.03- <u>Other anterior</u> dislocation of hip
    S73.031- Other anterior <u>subluxation</u> of <u>right</u> hip
    S73.032- Other anterior <u>subluxation</u> of <u>left</u> hip
    S73.033- Other anterior <u>subluxation</u> of <u>unspecified</u> hip
    S73.034- Other anterior <u>dislocation</u> of <u>right</u> hip
    S73.035- Other anterior <u>dislocation</u> of <u>left</u> hip
    S73.036- Other anterior <u>dislocation</u> of <u>unspecified</u> hip
S73.04- <u>Central</u> dislocation of hip
    S73.041- Central <u>subluxation</u> of <u>right</u> hip
    S73.042- Central <u>subluxation</u> of <u>left</u> hip
    S73.043- Central <u>subluxation</u> of <u>unspecified</u> hip
    S73.044- Central <u>dislocation</u> of <u>right</u> hip
    S73.045- Central <u>dislocation</u> of <u>left</u> hip
    S73.046- Central <u>dislocation</u> of <u>unspecified</u> hip
S73.1- <u>Sprain</u> of <u>hip</u>
  S73.10- <u>Unspecified sprain</u> of hip
    S73.101- Unspecified sprain of <u>right</u> hip
    S73.102- Unspecified sprain of <u>left</u> hip
    S73.109- Unspecified sprain of <u>unspecified</u> hip
  S73.11- <u>Iliofemoral ligament sprain</u> of hip
    S73.111- Iliofemoral ligament sprain of <u>right</u> hip
    S73.112- Iliofemoral ligament sprain of <u>left</u> hip
    S73.119- Iliofemoral ligament sprain of <u>unspecified</u> hip
  S73.12- <u>Ischiocapsular (ligament) sprain</u> of hip
    S73.121- Ischiocapsular ligament sprain of <u>right</u> hip
    S73.122- Ischiocapsular ligament sprain of <u>left</u> hip
    S73.129- Ischiocapsular ligament sprain of <u>unspecified</u> hip
  S73.19- <u>Other sprain</u> of hip
    S73.191- Other sprain of <u>right</u> hip
    S73.192- Other sprain of <u>left</u> hip
    S73.199- Other sprain of <u>unspecified</u> hip

S74- <u>Injury of nerves</u> at <u>hip and thigh level</u>
Code also any associated open wound (S71.-)
Excludes❷: injury of nerves at ankle and foot level (S94.-)
    injury of nerves at lower leg level (S84.-)

The appropriate 7th character is to be added to each code from
  category S74:
  A <u>Initial</u> encounter
  D <u>Subsequent</u> encounter
  S <u>Sequela</u>

S74.0- Injury of <u>sciatic</u> nerve at <u>hip and thigh level</u>
  S74.00x- Injury of sciatic nerve at hip and thigh level, <u>unspecified</u> leg
  S74.01x- Injury of sciatic nerve at hip and thigh level, <u>right</u> leg
  S74.02x- Injury of sciatic nerve at hip and thigh level, <u>left</u> leg
S74.1- Injury of <u>femoral</u> nerve at <u>hip and thigh level</u>
  S74.10x- Injury of femoral nerve at hip and thigh level, <u>unspecified</u> leg
  S74.11x- Injury of femoral nerve at hip and thigh level, <u>right</u> leg
  S74.12x- Injury of femoral nerve at hip and thigh level, <u>left</u> leg
S74.2- Injury of <u>cutaneous sensory</u> nerve at <u>hip and thigh level</u>
  S74.20x- Injury of cutaneous sensory nerve at hip and thigh level, <u>unspecified</u> leg
  S74.21x- Injury of cutaneous sensory nerve at hip and high level, <u>right</u> leg
  S74.22x- Injury of cutaneous sensory nerve at hip and thigh level, <u>left</u> leg
S74.8- Injury of <u>other nerves</u> at <u>hip and thigh level</u>
  S74.8x- Injury of <u>other nerves</u> at <u>hip and thigh level</u>
    S74.8x1- Injury of other nerves at hip and thigh level, <u>right</u> leg
    S74.8x2- Injury of other nerves at hip and thigh level, <u>left</u> leg
    S74.8x9- Injury of other nerves at hip and thigh level, <u>unspecified</u> leg
S74.9- Injury of <u>unspecified</u> nerve at <u>hip and thigh level</u>
  S74.90x- Injury of unspecified nerve at hip and thigh level, <u>unspecified</u> leg
  S74.91x- Injury of unspecified nerve at hip and thigh level, <u>right</u> leg
  S74.92x- Injury of unspecified nerve at hip and thigh level, <u>left</u> leg

S75- <u>Injury of blood vessels</u> at <u>hip and thigh level</u>
Code also any associated open wound (S71.-)
Excludes❷: injury of blood vessels at lower leg level (S85.-)
    injury of popliteal artery (S85.0)

The appropriate 7th character is to be added to each code from
  category S75:
  A <u>Initial</u> encounter
  D <u>Subsequent</u> encounter
  S <u>Sequela</u>

S75.0- Injury of <u>femoral artery</u>
  S75.00- <u>Unspecified</u> injury of <u>femoral artery</u>
    S75.001- Unspecified injury of femoral artery, <u>right</u> leg
    S75.002- Unspecified injury of femoral artery, <u>left</u> leg
    S75.009- Unspecified injury of femoral artery, <u>unspecified</u> leg
  S75.01- <u>Minor laceration</u> of <u>femoral artery</u>
    Incomplete transection of femoral artery
    Laceration of femoral artery NOS
    Superficial laceration of femoral artery
    S75.011- Minor laceration of femoral artery, <u>right</u> leg
    S75.012- Minor laceration of femoral artery, <u>left</u> leg
    S75.019- Minor laceration of femoral artery, <u>unspecified</u> leg
  S75.02- <u>Major laceration</u> of <u>femoral artery</u>
    Complete transection of femoral artery
    Traumatic rupture of femoral artery
    S75.021- Major laceration of femoral artery, <u>right</u> leg
    S75.022- Major laceration of femoral artery, <u>left</u> leg
    S75.029- Major laceration of femoral artery, <u>unspecified</u> leg
  S75.09- <u>Other specified injury</u> of <u>femoral artery</u>
    S75.091- Other specified injury of femoral artery, <u>right</u> leg
    S75.092- Other specified injury of femoral artery, <u>left</u> leg
    S75.099- Other specified injury of femoral artery, <u>unspecified</u> leg
S75.1- Injury of <u>femoral vein</u> at <u>hip and thigh level</u>
  S75.10- <u>Unspecified</u> injury of <u>femoral vein</u> at <u>hip and thigh level</u>
    S75.101- Unspecified injury of femoral vein at hip and thigh level, <u>right</u> leg
    S75.102- Unspecified injury of femoral vein at hip and thigh level, <u>left</u> leg
    S75.109- Unspecified injury of femoral vein at hip and thigh level, <u>unspecified</u> leg
  S75.11- <u>Minor laceration</u> of <u>femoral vein</u> at <u>hip and thigh level</u>
    Incomplete transection of femoral vein at hip and thigh level
    Laceration of femoral vein at hip and thigh level NOS
    Superficial laceration of femoral vein at hip and thigh level
    S75.111- Minor laceration of femoral vein at hip and thigh level, <u>right</u> leg
    S75.112- Minor laceration of femoral vein at hip and thigh level, <u>left</u> leg
    S75.119- Minor laceration of femoral vein at hip and thigh level, <u>unspecified</u> leg
  S75.12- <u>Major laceration</u> of <u>femoral vein</u> at <u>hip and thigh level</u>
    Complete transection of femoral vein at hip and thigh level
    Traumatic rupture of femoral vein at hip and thigh level
    S75.121- Major laceration of femoral vein at hip and thigh level, <u>right</u> leg
    S75.122- Major laceration of femoral vein at hip and thigh level, <u>left</u> leg
    S75.129- Major laceration of femoral vein at hip and thigh level, <u>unspecified</u> leg
  S75.19- <u>Other specified injury</u> of <u>femoral vein</u> at <u>hip and thigh level</u>
    S75.191- Other specified injury of femoral vein at hip and thigh level, <u>right</u> leg
    S75.192- Other specified injury of femoral vein at hip and thigh level, <u>left</u> leg
    S75.199- Other specified injury of femoral vein at hip and thigh level, <u>unspecified</u> leg
S75.2- Injury of <u>greater saphenous</u> vein at <u>hip and thigh level</u>
  Excludes 1: greater saphenous vein NOS (S85.3)
  S75.20- <u>Unspecified</u> injury of <u>greater saphenous vein</u> at <u>hip and thigh level</u>
    S75.201- Unspecified injury of greater saphenous vein at hip and thigh level, <u>right</u> leg
    S75.202- Unspecified injury of greater saphenous vein at hip and thigh level, <u>left</u> leg
    S75.209- Unspecified injury of greater saphenous vein at hip and thigh level, <u>unspecified</u> leg

S72 - S75

Excludes 1: = NOT CODED HERE! (Do not code both)

Excludes❷: = Not Included Here

S75.21- Minor laceration of greater saphenous vein at hip and thigh level

    Incomplete transection of greater saphenous vein at hip and thigh level

    Laceration of greater saphenous vein at hip and thigh level NOS

    Superficial laceration of greater saphenous vein at hip and thigh level

    S75.211- Minor laceration of greater saphenous vein at hip and thigh level, right leg

    S75.212- Minor laceration of greater saphenous vein at hip and thigh level, left leg

    S75.219- Minor laceration of greater saphenous vein at hip and thigh level, unspecified leg

S75.22- Major laceration of greater saphenous vein at hip and thigh level

    Complete transection of greater saphenous vein at hip and thigh level

    Traumatic rupture of greater saphenous vein at hip and thigh level

    S75.221- Major laceration of greater saphenous vein at hip and thigh level, right leg

    S75.222- Major laceration of greater saphenous vein at hip and thigh level, left leg

    S75.229- Major laceration of greater saphenous vein at hip and thigh level, unspecified leg

S75.29- Other specified injury of greater saphenous vein at hip and thigh level

    S75.291- Other specified injury of greater saphenous vein at hip and thigh level, right leg

    S75.292- Other specified injury of greater saphenous vein at hip and thigh level, left leg

    S75.299- Other specified injury of greater saphenous vein at hip and thigh level, unspecified leg

S75.8- Injury of other blood vessels at hip and thigh level

S75.80- Unspecified injury of other blood vessels at hip and thigh level

    S75.801- Unspecified injury of other blood vessels at hip and thigh level, right leg

    S75.802- Unspecified injury of other blood vessels at hip and thigh level, left leg

    S75.809- Unspecified injury of other blood vessels at hip and thigh level, unspecified leg

S75.81- Laceration of other blood vessels at hip and thigh level

    S75.811- Laceration of other blood vessels at hip and thigh level, right leg

    S75.812- Laceration of other blood vessels at hip and thigh level, left leg

    S75.819- Laceration of other blood vessels at hip and thigh level, unspecified leg

S75.89- Other specified injury of other blood vessels at hip and thigh level

    S75.891- Other specified injury of other blood vessels at hip and thigh level, right leg

    S75.892- Other specified injury of other blood vessels at hip and thigh level, left leg

    S75.899- Other specified injury of other blood vessels at hip and thigh level, unspecified leg

S75.9- Injury of unspecified blood vessel at hip and thigh level

S75.90- Unspecified injury of unspecified blood vessel at hip and thigh level

    S75.901- Unspecified injury of unspecified blood vessel at hip and thigh level, right leg

    S75.902- Unspecified injury of unspecified blood vessel at hip and thigh level, left leg

    S75.909- Unspecified injury of unspecified blood vessel at hip and thigh level, unspecified leg

S75.91- Laceration of unspecified blood vessel at hip and thigh level

    S75.911- Laceration of unspecified blood vessel at hip and thigh level, right leg

    S75.912- Laceration of unspecified blood vessel at hip and thigh level, left leg

    S75.919- Laceration of unspecified blood vessel at hip and thigh level, unspecified leg

S75.99- Other specified injury of unspecified blood vessel at hip and thigh level

    S75.991- Other specified injury of unspecified blood vessel at hip and thigh level, right leg

    S75.992- Other specified injury of unspecified blood vessel at hip and thigh level, left leg

    S75.999- Other specified injury of unspecified blood vessel at hip and thigh level, unspecified leg

S76- Injury of muscle, fascia and tendon at hip and thigh level

Code also any associated open wound (S71.-)

Excludes❷: injury of muscle, fascia and tendon at lower leg level (S86)

sprain of joint and ligament of hip (S73.1)

The appropriate 7th character is to be added to each code from category S76:

A Initial encounter

D Subsequent encounter

S Sequela

S76.0- Injury of muscle, fascia and tendon of hip

S76.00- Unspecified injury of muscle, fascia and tendon of hip

    S76.001- Unspecified injury of muscle, fascia and tendon of right hip

    S76.002- Unspecified injury of muscle, fascia and tendon of left hip

    S76.009- Unspecified injury of muscle, fascia and tendon of unspecified hip

S76.01- Strain of muscle, fascia and tendon of hip

    S76.011- Strain of muscle, fascia and tendon of right hip

    S76.012- Strain of muscle, fascia and tendon of left hip

    S76.019- Strain of muscle, fascia and tendon of unspecified hip

S76.02- Laceration of muscle, fascia and tendon of hip

    S76.021- Laceration of muscle, fascia and tendon of right hip

    S76.022- Laceration of muscle, fascia and tendon of left hip

    S76.029- Laceration of muscle, fascia and tendon of unspecified hip

S76.09- Other specified injury of muscle, fascia and tendon of hip

    S76.091- Other specified injury of muscle, fascia and tendon of right hip

    S76.092- Other specified injury of muscle, fascia and tendon of left hip

    S76.099- Other specified injury of muscle, fascia and tendon of unspecified hip

S76.1- Injury of quadriceps muscle, fascia and tendon

    Injury of patellar ligament (tendon)

S76.10- Unspecified injury of quadriceps muscle, fascia and tendon

    S76.101- Unspecified injury of right quadriceps muscle, fascia and tendon

    S76.102- Unspecified injury of left quadriceps muscle, fascia and tendon

    S76.109- Unspecified injury of unspecified quadriceps muscle, fascia and tendon

S76.11- Strain of quadriceps muscle, fascia and tendon

    S76.111- Strain of right quadriceps muscle, fascia and tendon

    S76.112- Strain of left quadriceps muscle, fascia and tendon

    S76.119- Strain of unspecified quadriceps muscle, fascia and tendon

S76.12- Laceration of quadriceps muscle, fascia and tendon

    S76.121- Laceration of right quadriceps muscle, fascia and tendon

    S76.122- Laceration of left quadriceps muscle, fascia and tendon

    S76.129- Laceration of unspecified quadriceps muscle, fascia and tendon

S76.19- Other specified injury of quadriceps muscle, fascia and tendon

    S76.191- Other specified injury of right quadriceps muscle, fascia and tendon

    S76.192- Other specified injury of left quadriceps muscle, fascia and tendon

    S76.199- Other specified injury of unspecified quadriceps muscle, fascia and tendon

S76.2- Injury of adductor muscle, fascia and tendon of thigh

S76.20- Unspecified injury of adductor muscle, fascia and tendon of thigh

    S76.201- Unspecified injury of adductor muscle, fascia and tendon of right thigh

    S76.202- Unspecified injury of adductor muscle, fascia and tendon of left thigh

    S76.209- Unspecified injury of adductor muscle, fascia and tendon of unspecified thigh

S75 - S77

S76.21- Strain of adductor muscle, fascia and tendon of thigh
    S76.211- Strain of adductor muscle, fascia and tendon of right thigh
    S76.212- Strain of adductor muscle, fascia and tendon of left thigh
    S76.219- Strain of adductor muscle, fascia and tendon of unspecified thigh
S76.22- Laceration of adductor muscle, fascia and tendon of thigh
    S76.221- Laceration of adductor muscle, fascia and tendon of right thigh
    S76.222- Laceration of adductor muscle, fascia and tendon of left thigh
    S76.229- Laceration of adductor muscle, fascia and tendon of unspecified thigh
S76.29- Other injury of adductor muscle, fascia and tendon of thigh
    S76.291- Other injury of adductor muscle, fascia and tendon of right thigh
    S76.292- Other injury of adductor muscle, fascia and tendon of left thigh
    S76.299- Other injury of adductor muscle, fascia and tendon of unspecified thigh
S76.3- Injury of muscle, fascia and tendon of the posterior muscle group at thigh level
    S76.30- Unspecified injury of muscle, fascia and tendon of the posterior muscle group at thigh level
        S76.301- Unspecified injury of muscle, fascia and tendon of the posterior muscle group at thigh level, right thigh
        S76.302- Unspecified injury of muscle, fascia and tendon of the posterior muscle group at thigh level, left thigh
        S76.309- Unspecified injury of muscle, fascia and tendon of the posterior muscle group at thigh level, unspecified thigh
    S76.31- Strain of muscle, fascia and tendon of the posterior muscle group at thigh level
        S76.311- Strain of muscle, fascia and tendon of the posterior muscle group at thigh level, right thigh
        S76.312- Strain of muscle, fascia and tendon of the posterior muscle group at thigh level, left thigh
        S76.319- Strain of muscle, fascia and tendon of the posterior muscle group at thigh level, unspecified thigh
    S76.32- Laceration of muscle, fascia and tendon of the posterior muscle group at thigh level
        S76.321- Laceration of muscle, fascia and tendon of the posterior muscle group at thigh level, right thigh
        S76.322- Laceration of muscle, fascia and tendon of the posterior muscle group at thigh level, left thigh
        S76.329- Laceration of muscle, fascia and tendon of the posterior muscle group at thigh level, unspecified thigh
    S76.39- Other specified injury of muscle, fascia and tendon of the posterior muscle group at thigh level
        S76.391- Other specified injury of muscle, fascia and tendon of the posterior muscle group at thigh level, right thigh
        S76.392- Other specified injury of muscle, fascia and tendon of the posterior muscle group at thigh level, left thigh
        S76.399- Other specified injury of muscle, fascia and tendon of the posterior muscle group at thigh level, unspecified thigh
S76.8- Injury of other specified muscles, fascia and tendons at thigh level
    S76.80- Unspecified injury of other specified muscles, fascia and tendons at thigh level
        S76.801- Unspecified injury of other specified muscles, fascia and tendons at thigh level, right thigh
        S76.802- Unspecified injury of other specified muscles, fascia and tendons at thigh level, left thigh
        S76.809- Unspecified injury of other specified muscles, fascia and tendons at thigh level, unspecified thigh
    S76.81- Strain of other specified muscles, fascia and tendons at thigh level
        S76.811- Strain of other specified muscles, fascia and tendons at thigh level, right thigh
        S76.812- Strain of other specified muscles, fascia and tendons at thigh level, left thigh
        S76.819- Strain of other specified muscles, fascia and tendons at thigh level, unspecified thigh

S76.82- Laceration of other specified muscles, fascia and tendons at thigh level
    S76.821- Laceration of other specified muscles, fascia and tendons at thigh level, right thigh
    S76.822- Laceration of other specified muscles, fascia and tendons at thigh level, left thigh
    S76.829- Laceration of other specified muscles, fascia and tendons at thigh level, unspecified thigh
S76.89- Other injury of other specified muscles, fascia and tendons at thigh level
    S76.891- Other injury of other specified muscles, fascia and tendons at thigh level, right thigh
    S76.892- Other injury of other specified muscles, fascia and tendons at thigh level, left thigh
    S76.899- Other injury of other specified muscles, fascia and tendons at thigh level, unspecified thigh
S76.9- Injury of unspecified muscles, fascia and tendons at thigh level
    S76.90- Unspecified injury of unspecified muscles, fascia and tendons at thigh level
        S76.901- Unspecified injury of unspecified muscles, fascia and tendons at thigh level, right thigh
        S76.902- Unspecified injury of unspecified muscles, fascia and tendons at thigh level, left thigh
        S76.909- Unspecified injury of unspecified muscles, fascia and tendons at thigh level, unspecified thigh
    S76.91- Strain of unspecified muscles, fascia and tendons at thigh level
        S76.911- Strain of unspecified muscles, fascia and tendons at thigh level, right thigh
        S76.912- Strain of unspecified muscles, fascia and tendons at thigh level, left thigh
        S76.919- Strain of unspecified muscles, fascia and tendons at thigh level, unspecified thigh
    S76.92- Laceration of unspecified muscles, fascia and tendons at thigh level
        S76.921- Laceration of unspecified muscles, fascia and tendons at thigh level, right thigh
        S76.922- Laceration of unspecified muscles, fascia and tendons at thigh level, left thigh
        S76.929- Laceration of unspecified muscles, fascia and tendons at thigh level, unspecified thigh
    S76.99- Other specified injury of unspecified muscles, fascia and tendons at thigh level
        S76.991- Other specified injury of unspecified muscles, fascia and tendons at thigh level, right thigh
        S76.992- Other specified injury of unspecified muscles, fascia and tendons at thigh level, left thigh
        S76.999- Other specified injury of unspecified muscles, fascia and tendons at thigh level, unspecified thigh

S77- Crushing injury of hip and thigh
Use additional code(s) for all associated injuries
Excludes❷: crushing injury of ankle and foot (S97.-)
crushing injury of lower leg (S87.-)
The appropriate 7th character is to be added to each code from category S77:
  A Initial encounter
  D Subsequent encounter
  S Sequela
S77.0- Crushing injury of hip
    S77.00x- Crushing injury of unspecified hip
    S77.01x- Crushing injury of right hip
    S77.02x- Crushing injury of left hip
S77.1- Crushing injury of thigh
    S77.10x- Crushing injury of unspecified thigh
    S77.11x- Crushing injury of right thigh
    S77.12x- Crushing injury of left thigh
S77.2- Crushing injury of hip with thigh
    S77.20x- Crushing injury of unspecified hip with thigh
    S77.21x- Crushing injury of right hip with thigh
    S77.22x- Crushing injury of left hip with thigh

S75 - S77

S78-   <u>Traumatic amputation</u> of <u>hip</u> and <u>thigh</u>
     Note: An amputation not identified as partial or complete should be coded
       to complete
     Excludes 1: traumatic amputation of knee (S88.0-)

     The appropriate 7th character is to be added to each code from
       category S78:
       A   <u>Initial</u> encounter
       D   <u>Subsequent</u> encounter
       S   <u>Sequela</u>

   S78.0-   Traumatic <u>amputation</u> at <u>hip joint</u>
     S78.01-   <u>Complete</u> traumatic <u>amputation</u> at <u>hip joint</u>
       S78.011-   Complete traumatic amputation at <u>right</u> hip joint
       S78.012-   Complete traumatic amputation at <u>left</u> hip joint
       S78.019-   Complete traumatic amputation at <u>unspecified</u> hip
          joint
     S78.02-   <u>Partial</u> traumatic <u>amputation</u> at <u>hip joint</u>
       S78.021-   Partial traumatic amputation at <u>right</u> hip joint
       S78.022-   Partial traumatic amputation at <u>left</u> hip joint
       S78.029-   Partial traumatic amputation at <u>unspecified</u> hip joint
   S78.1-   Traumatic <u>amputation</u> at <u>level between hip and knee</u>
     Excludes 1: traumatic amputation of knee (S88.0-)
     S78.11-   <u>Complete</u> traumatic amputation at <u>level between hip and</u>
       <u>knee</u>
       S78.111-   Complete traumatic amputation at level between <u>right</u>
          hip and knee
       S78.112-   Complete traumatic amputation at level between <u>left</u>
          hip and knee
       S78.119-   Complete traumatic amputation at level between
          <u>unspecified</u> hip and knee
     S78.12-   <u>Partial</u> traumatic amputation at <u>level between hip and knee</u>
       S78.121-   Partial traumatic amputation at level between <u>right</u>
          hip and knee
       S78.122-   Partial traumatic amputation at level between <u>left</u> hip
          and knee
       S78.129-   Partial traumatic amputation at level between
          <u>unspecified</u> hip and knee
   S78.9-   Traumatic <u>amputation</u> of <u>hip and thigh</u>, <u>level unspecified</u>
     S78.91-   <u>Complete</u> traumatic <u>amputation</u> of <u>hip and thigh</u>, <u>level</u>
       <u>unspecified</u>
       S78.911-   Complete traumatic amputation of <u>right</u> hip and
          thigh, level unspecified
       S78.912-   Complete traumatic amputation of <u>left</u> hip and thigh,
          level unspecified
       S78.919-   Complete traumatic amputation of <u>unspecified</u> hip
          and thigh, level unspecified
     S78.92-   <u>Partial</u> traumatic <u>amputation</u> of <u>hip and thigh</u>, <u>level</u>
       <u>unspecified</u>
       S78.921-   Partial traumatic amputation of <u>right</u> hip and thigh,
          level unspecified
       S78.922-   Partial traumatic amputation of <u>left</u> hip and thigh,
          level unspecified
       S78.929-   Partial traumatic amputation of <u>unspecified</u> hip and
          thigh, level unspecified

S79-   <u>Other and unspecified injuries</u> of <u>hip</u> and <u>thigh</u>
     Note: A fracture not indicated as open or closed should be coded to closed
     The appropriate 7th character is to be added to each code from
       subcategories S79.0 and S79.1:
       A   <u>Initial</u> encounter for closed fracture
       D   <u>Subsequent</u> encounter for fracture with routine healing
       G   <u>Subsequent</u> encounter for fracture with delayed healing
       K   <u>Subsequent</u> encounter for fracture with nonunion
       P   <u>Subsequent</u> encounter for fracture with malunion
       S   <u>Sequela</u>
   S79.0-   <u>Physeal</u> <u>fracture</u> of <u>upper end</u> of <u>femur</u>
     Excludes 1: apophyseal fracture of upper end of femur (S72.13-)
             nontraumatic slipped upper femoral epiphysis (M93.0-)
     S79.00-   <u>Unspecified</u> <u>physeal</u> fracture of <u>upper end</u> of <u>femur</u>
       S79.001-   Unspecified physeal fracture of upper end of <u>right</u>
          femur
       S79.002-   Unspecified physeal fracture of upper end of <u>left</u>
          femur
       S79.009-   Unspecified physeal fracture of upper end of
          <u>unspecified</u> femur

     S79.01-   <u>Salter-Harris Type I</u> physeal fracture of <u>upper end</u> of <u>femur</u>
       Acute on chronic slipped capital femoral epiphysis (traumatic)
       Acute slipped capital femoral epiphysis (traumatic)
       Capital femoral epiphyseal fracture
       Excludes 1: chronic slipped upper femoral epiphysis
             (nontraumatic) (M93.02-)
       S79.011-   Salter-Harris Type I physeal fracture of upper end of
          <u>right</u> femur
       S79.012-   Salter-Harris Type I physeal fracture of upper end of
          <u>left</u> femur
       S79.019-   Salter-Harris Type I physeal fracture of upper end of
          <u>unspecified</u> femur
     S79.09-   <u>Other physeal</u> fracture of <u>upper end</u> of <u>femur</u>
       S79.091-   Other physeal fracture of upper end of <u>right</u> femur
       S79.092-   Other physeal fracture of upper end of <u>left</u> femur
       S79.099-   Other physeal fracture of upper end of <u>unspecified</u>
          femur
   S79.1-   <u>Physeal</u> <u>fracture</u> of <u>lower end</u> of <u>femur</u>
     S79.10-   <u>Unspecified</u> <u>physeal</u> fracture of <u>lower end</u> of <u>femur</u>
       S79.101-   Unspecified physeal fracture of lower end of <u>right</u>
          femur
       S79.102-   Unspecified physeal fracture of lower end of <u>left</u> femur
       S79.109-   Unspecified physeal fracture of lower end of
          <u>unspecified</u> femur
     S79.11-   <u>Salter-Harris Type I</u> physeal fracture of <u>lower end</u> of <u>femur</u>
       S79.111-   Salter-Harris Type I physeal fracture of lower end of
          <u>right</u> femur
       S79.112-   Salter-Harris Type I physeal fracture of lower end of
          <u>left</u> femur
       S79.119-   Salter-Harris Type I physeal fracture of lower end of
          <u>unspecified</u> femur
     S79.12-   <u>Salter-Harris Type II</u> physeal fracture of <u>lower end</u> of <u>femur</u>
       S79.121-   Salter-Harris Type II physeal fracture of lower end of
          <u>right</u> femur
       S79.122-   Salter-Harris Type II physeal fracture of lower end of
          <u>left</u> femur
       S79.129-   Salter-Harris Type II physeal fracture of lower end of
          <u>unspecified</u> femur
     S79.13-   <u>Salter-Harris Type III</u> physeal fracture of <u>lower end</u> of <u>femur</u>
       S79.131-   Salter-Harris Type III physeal fracture of lower end of
          <u>right</u> femur
       S79.132-   Salter-Harris Type III physeal fracture of lower end of
          <u>left</u> femur
       S79.139-   Salter-Harris Type III physeal fracture of lower end of
          <u>unspecified</u> femur
     S79.14-   <u>Salter-Harris Type IV</u> physeal fracture of <u>lower end</u> of <u>femur</u>
       S79.141-   Salter-Harris Type IV physeal fracture of lower end of
          <u>right</u> femur
       S79.142-   Salter-Harris Type IV physeal fracture of lower end of
          <u>left</u> femur
       S79.149-   Salter-Harris Type IV physeal fracture of lower end of
          <u>unspecified</u> femur
     S79.19-   <u>Other physeal</u> fracture of <u>lower end</u> of <u>femur</u>
       S79.191-   Other physeal fracture of lower end of <u>right</u> femur
       S79.192-   Other physeal fracture of lower end of <u>left</u> femur
       S79.199-   Other physeal fracture of lower end of <u>unspecified</u>
          femur
   S79.8-   <u>Other specified injuries</u> of <u>hip</u> and <u>thigh</u>
     The appropriate 7th character is to be added to each code in
       subcategory S79.8:
       A   <u>Initial</u> encounter
       D   <u>Subsequent</u> encounter
       S   <u>Sequela</u>
     S79.81-   <u>Other specified injuries</u> of <u>hip</u>
       S79.811-   Other specified injuries of <u>right</u> hip
       S79.812-   Other specified injuries of <u>left</u> hip
       S79.819-   Other specified injuries of <u>unspecified</u> hip
     S79.82-   <u>Other specified injuries</u> of <u>thigh</u>
       S79.821-   Other specified injuries of <u>right</u> thigh
       S79.822-   Other specified injuries of <u>left</u> thigh
       S79.829-   Other specified injuries of <u>unspecified</u> thigh

S78 - S81

S79.9-   Unspecified injury of hip and thigh
The appropriate 7th character is to be added to each code in subcategory S79.9:
  A   Initial encounter
  D   Subsequent encounter
  S   Sequela
S79.91- Unspecified injury of hip
  S79.911- Unspecified injury of right hip
  S79.912- Unspecified injury of left hip
  S79.919- Unspecified injury of unspecified hip
S79.92- Unspecified injury of thigh
  S79.921- Unspecified injury of right thigh
  S79.922- Unspecified injury of left thigh
  S79.929- Unspecified injury of unspecified thigh

Injuries to the knee and lower leg (S80-S89)

Excludes❷: burns and corrosions (T20-T32)
          frostbite (T33-T34)
          injuries of ankle and foot, except fracture of ankle and
              malleolus (S90-S99)
          insect bite or sting, venomous (T63.4)

S80-   Superficial injury of knee and lower leg
Excludes❷: superficial injury of ankle and foot (S90.-)
The appropriate 7th character is to be added to each code from category S80:
  A   Initial encounter
  D   Subsequent encounter
  S   Sequela
S80.0- Contusion of knee
  S80.00x- Contusion of unspecified knee
  S80.01x- Contusion of right knee
  S80.02x- Contusion of left knee
S80.1- Contusion of lower leg
  S80.10x- Contusion of unspecified lower leg
  S80.11x- Contusion of right lower leg
  S80.12x- Contusion of left lower leg
S80.2- Other superficial injuries of knee
  S80.21- Abrasion of knee
    S80.211- Abrasion, right knee
    S80.212- Abrasion, left knee
    S80.219- Abrasion, unspecified knee
  S80.22- Blister (nonthermal) of knee
    S80.221- Blister (nonthermal), right knee
    S80.222- Blister (nonthermal), left knee
    S80.229- Blister (nonthermal), unspecified knee
  S80.24- External constriction of knee
    S80.241- External constriction, right knee
    S80.242- External constriction, left knee
    S80.249- External constriction, unspecified knee
  S80.25- Superficial foreign body of knee
      Splinter in the knee
    S80.251- Superficial foreign body, right knee
    S80.252- Superficial foreign body, left knee
    S80.259- Superficial foreign body, unspecified knee
  S80.26- Insect bite (nonvenomous) of knee
    S80.261- Insect bite (nonvenomous), right knee
    S80.262- Insect bite (nonvenomous), left knee
    S80.269- Insect bite (nonvenomous), unspecified knee
  S80.27- Other superficial bite of knee
      Excludes 1: open bite of knee (S81.05-)
    S80.271- Other superficial bite of right knee
    S80.272- Other superficial bite of left knee
    S80.279- Other superficial bite of unspecified knee
S80.8- Other superficial injuries of lower leg
  S80.81- Abrasion of lower leg
    S80.811- Abrasion, right lower leg
    S80.812- Abrasion, left lower leg
    S80.819- Abrasion, unspecified lower leg
  S80.82- Blister (nonthermal) of lower leg
    S80.821- Blister (nonthermal), right lower leg
    S80.822- Blister (nonthermal), left lower leg
    S80.829- Blister (nonthermal), unspecified lower leg
  S80.84- External constriction of lower leg
    S80.841- External constriction, right lower leg
    S80.842- External constriction, left lower leg
    S80.849- External constriction, unspecified lower leg

  S80.85- Superficial foreign body of lower leg
      Splinter in the lower leg
    S80.851- Superficial foreign body, right lower leg
    S80.852- Superficial foreign body, left lower leg
    S80.859- Superficial foreign body, unspecified lower leg
  S80.86- Insect bite (nonvenomous) of lower leg
    S80.861- Insect bite (nonvenomous), right lower leg
    S80.862- Insect bite (nonvenomous), left lower leg
    S80.869- Insect bite (nonvenomous), unspecified lower leg
  S80.87- Other superficial bite of lower leg
      Excludes 1: open bite of lower leg (S81.85-)
    S80.871- Other superficial bite, right lower leg
    S80.872- Other superficial bite, left lower leg
    S80.879- Other superficial bite, unspecified lower leg
S80.9- Unspecified superficial injury of knee and lower leg
  S80.91- Unspecified superficial injury of knee
    S80.911- Unspecified superficial injury of right knee
    S80.912- Unspecified superficial injury of left knee
    S80.919- Unspecified superficial injury of unspecified knee
  S80.92- Unspecified superficial injury of lower leg
    S80.921- Unspecified superficial injury of right lower leg
    S80.922- Unspecified superficial injury of left lower leg
    S80.929- Unspecified superficial injury of unspecified lower leg
S81-   Open wound of knee and lower leg
Code also any associated wound infection
Excludes 1: open fracture of knee and lower leg (S82.-)
          traumatic amputation of lower leg (S88.-)
Excludes❷: open wound of ankle and foot (S91.-)
The appropriate 7th character is to be added to each code from category S81:
  A   Initial encounter
  D   Subsequent encounter
  S   Sequela
S81.0- Open wound of knee
  S81.00- Unspecified open wound of knee
    S81.001- Unspecified open wound, right knee
    S81.002- Unspecified open wound, left knee
    S81.009- Unspecified open wound, unspecified knee
  S81.01- Laceration without foreign body of knee
    S81.011- Laceration without foreign body, right knee
    S81.012- Laceration without foreign body, left knee
    S81.019- Laceration without foreign body, unspecified knee
  S81.02- Laceration with foreign body of knee
    S81.021- Laceration with foreign body, right knee
    S81.022- Laceration with foreign body, left knee
    S81.029- Laceration with foreign body, unspecified knee
  S81.03- Puncture wound without foreign body of knee
    S81.031- Puncture wound without foreign body, right knee
    S81.032- Puncture wound without foreign body, left knee
    S81.039- Puncture wound without foreign body, unspecified knee
  S81.04- Puncture wound with foreign body of knee
    S81.041- Puncture wound with foreign body, right knee
    S81.042- Puncture wound with foreign body, left knee
    S81.049- Puncture wound with foreign body, unspecified knee
  S81.05- Open bite of knee
      Bite of knee NOS
      Excludes 1: superficial bite of knee (S80.27-)
    S81.051- Open bite, right knee
    S81.052- Open bite, left knee
    S81.059- Open bite, unspecified knee
S81.8- Open wound of lower leg
  S81.80- Unspecified open wound of lower leg
    S81.801- Unspecified open wound, right lower leg
    S81.802- Unspecified open wound, left lower leg
    S81.809- Unspecified open wound, unspecified lower leg
  S81.81- Laceration without foreign body of lower leg
    S81.811- Laceration without foreign body, right lower leg
    S81.812- Laceration without foreign body, left lower leg
    S81.819- Laceration without foreign body, unspecified lower leg
  S81.82- Laceration with foreign body of lower leg
    S81.821- Laceration with foreign body, right lower leg
    S81.822- Laceration with foreign body, left lower leg
    S81.829- Laceration with foreign body, unspecified lower leg

S
7
8
–
S
8
1

S81.83- <u>Puncture</u> wound <u>without</u> foreign body of lower leg
  S81.831- Puncture wound <u>without</u> foreign body, <u>right</u> lower leg
  S81.832- Puncture wound <u>without</u> foreign body, <u>left</u> lower leg
  S81.839- Puncture wound <u>without</u> foreign body, <u>unspecified</u> lower leg
S81.84- <u>Puncture</u> wound <u>with foreign body</u> of lower leg
  S81.841- Puncture wound <u>with foreign body</u>, <u>right</u> lower leg
  S81.842- Puncture wound <u>with foreign body</u>, <u>left</u> lower leg
  S81.849- Puncture wound <u>with foreign body</u>, <u>unspecified</u> lower leg
S81.85- <u>Open bite</u> of lower leg
    Bite of lower leg NOS
    Excludes 1: superficial bite of lower leg (S80.86-, S80.87-)
  S81.851- Open bite, <u>right</u> lower leg
  S81.852- Open bite, <u>left</u> lower leg
  S81.859- Open bite, <u>unspecified</u> lower leg
S82- <u>Fracture</u> of <u>lower leg, including ankle</u>
    Note: A fracture not indicated as displaced or nondisplaced should be coded to displaced
    Note: A fracture not indicated as open or closed should be coded to closed
    Note: The open fracture designations are based on the Gustilo open fracture classification
    Includes: Fracture of malleolus
    Excludes 1: traumatic amputation of lower leg (S88.-)
    Excludes ❷: fracture of foot, except ankle (S92.-)
    *   periprosthetic fracture of prosthetic implant of knee (T84.042, T84.043)*

The appropriate 7th character is to be added to all codes from category S82:
  A <u>Initial</u> encounter for <u>closed</u> fracture
  B <u>Initial</u> encounter for <u>open fracture type I or II</u>
    <u>Initial</u> encounter for open fracture NOS
  C <u>Initial</u> encounter for <u>open fracture type IIIA, IIIB, or IIIC</u>
  D <u>Subsequent</u> encounter for <u>closed</u> fracture <u>with routine healing</u>
  E <u>Subsequent</u> encounter for <u>open fracture type I or II with routine healing</u>
  F <u>Subsequent</u> encounter for <u>open fracture type IIIA, IIIB, or IIIC with routine healing</u>
  G <u>Subsequent</u> encounter for <u>closed</u> fracture <u>with delayed healing</u>
  H <u>Subsequent</u> encounter for <u>open fracture type I or II with delayed healing</u>
  J <u>Subsequent</u> encounter for <u>open fracture type IIIA, IIIB, or IIIC with delayed healing</u>
  K <u>Subsequent</u> encounter for <u>closed</u> fracture <u>with nonunion</u>
  M <u>Subsequent</u> encounter for <u>open fracture type I or II with nonunion</u>
  N <u>Subsequent</u> encounter for <u>open fracture type IIIA, IIIB, or IIIC with nonunion</u>
  P <u>Subsequent</u> encounter for <u>closed</u> fracture <u>with malunion</u>
  Q <u>Subsequent</u> encounter for <u>open fracture type I or II with malunion</u>
  R <u>Subsequent</u> encounter for <u>open fracture type IIIA, IIIB, or IIIC with malunion</u>
  S <u>Sequela</u>

S82.0- <u>Fracture</u> of <u>patella</u>
    Knee cap
  S82.00- <u>Unspecified</u> fracture of <u>patella</u>
    S82.001- Unspecified fracture of <u>right</u> patella
    S82.002- Unspecified fracture of <u>left</u> patella
    S82.009- Unspecified fracture of <u>unspecified</u> patella
  S82.01- <u>Osteochondral</u> fracture of <u>patella</u>
    S82.011- <u>Displaced</u> osteochondral fracture of <u>right</u> patella
    S82.012- <u>Displaced</u> osteochondral fracture of <u>left</u> patella
    S82.013- <u>Displaced</u> osteochondral fracture of <u>unspecified</u> patella
    S82.014- <u>Nondisplaced</u> osteochondral fracture of <u>right</u> patella
    S82.015- <u>Nondisplaced</u> osteochondral fracture of <u>left</u> patella
    S82.016- <u>Nondisplaced</u> osteochondral fracture of <u>unspecified</u> patella
  S82.02- <u>Longitudinal</u> fracture of <u>patella</u>
    S82.021- <u>Displaced</u> longitudinal fracture of <u>right</u> patella
    S82.022- <u>Displaced</u> longitudinal fracture of <u>left</u> patella
    S82.023- <u>Displaced</u> longitudinal fracture of <u>unspecified</u> patella
    S82.024- <u>Nondisplaced</u> longitudinal fracture of <u>right</u> patella
    S82.025- <u>Nondisplaced</u> longitudinal fracture of <u>left</u> patella
    S82.026- <u>Nondisplaced</u> longitudinal fracture of <u>unspecified</u> patella

S82.03- <u>Transverse</u> fracture of <u>patella</u>
  S82.031- <u>Displaced</u> transverse fracture of <u>right</u> patella
  S82.032- <u>Displaced</u> transverse fracture of <u>left</u> patella
  S82.033- <u>Displaced</u> transverse fracture of <u>unspecified</u> patella
  S82.034- <u>Nondisplaced</u> transverse fracture of <u>right</u> patella
  S82.035- <u>Nondisplaced</u> transverse fracture of <u>left</u> patella
  S82.036- <u>Nondisplaced</u> transverse fracture of <u>unspecified</u> patella
S82.04- <u>Comminuted</u> fracture of <u>patella</u>
  S82.041- <u>Displaced</u> comminuted fracture of <u>right</u> patella
  S82.042- <u>Displaced</u> comminuted fracture of <u>left</u> patella
  S82.043- <u>Displaced</u> comminuted fracture of <u>unspecified</u> patella
  S82.044- <u>Nondisplaced</u> comminuted fracture of <u>right</u> patella
  S82.045- <u>Nondisplaced</u> comminuted fracture of <u>left</u> patella
  S82.046- <u>Nondisplaced</u> comminuted fracture of <u>unspecified</u> patella
S82.09- <u>Other fracture</u> of <u>patella</u>
  S82.091- Other fracture of <u>right</u> patella
  S82.092- Other fracture of <u>left</u> patella
  S82.099- Other fracture of <u>unspecified</u> patella
S82.1- <u>Fracture</u> of <u>upper end</u> of <u>tibia</u>
    Fracture of proximal end of tibia
    Excludes ❷: fracture of shaft of tibia (S82.2-)
    *   physeal fracture of upper end of tibia (S89.0-)*
  S82.10- <u>Unspecified</u> fracture of <u>upper end</u> of <u>tibia</u>
    S82.101- Unspecified fracture of upper end of <u>right</u> tibia
    S82.102- Unspecified fracture of upper end of <u>left</u> tibia
    S82.109- Unspecified fracture of upper end of <u>unspecified</u> tibia
  S82.11- Fracture of <u>tibial spine</u>
    S82.111- <u>Displaced</u> fracture of <u>right</u> tibial spine
    S82.112- <u>Displaced</u> fracture of <u>left</u> tibial spine
    S82.113- <u>Displaced</u> fracture of <u>unspecified</u> tibial spine
    S82.114- <u>Nondisplaced</u> fracture of <u>right</u> tibial spine
    S82.115- <u>Nondisplaced</u> fracture of <u>left</u> tibial spine
    S82.116- <u>Nondisplaced</u> fracture of <u>unspecified</u> tibial spine
  S82.12- Fracture of <u>lateral condyle</u> of <u>tibia</u>
    S82.121- <u>Displaced</u> fracture of lateral condyle of <u>right</u> tibia
    S82.122- <u>Displaced</u> fracture of lateral condyle of <u>left</u> tibia
    S82.123- <u>Displaced</u> fracture of lateral condyle of <u>unspecified</u> tibia
    S82.124- <u>Nondisplaced</u> fracture of lateral condyle of <u>right</u> tibia
    S82.125- <u>Nondisplaced</u> fracture of lateral condyle of <u>left</u> tibia
    S82.126- <u>Nondisplaced</u> fracture of lateral condyle of <u>unspecified</u> tibia
  S82.13- Fracture of <u>medial condyle</u> of <u>tibia</u>
    S82.131- <u>Displaced</u> fracture of medial condyle of <u>right</u> tibia
    S82.132- <u>Displaced</u> fracture of medial condyle of <u>left</u> tibia
    S82.133- <u>Displaced</u> fracture of medial condyle of <u>unspecified</u> tibia
    S82.134- <u>Nondisplaced</u> fracture of medial condyle of <u>right</u> tibia
    S82.135- <u>Nondisplaced</u> fracture of medial condyle of <u>left</u> tibia
    S82.136- <u>Nondisplaced</u> fracture of medial condyle of <u>unspecified</u> tibia
  S82.14- <u>Bicondylar</u> fracture of <u>tibia</u>
    Fracture of tibial plateau NOS
    S82.141- <u>Displaced</u> bicondylar fracture of <u>right</u> tibia
    S82.142- <u>Displaced</u> bicondylar fracture of <u>left</u> tibia
    S82.143- <u>Displaced</u> bicondylar fracture of <u>unspecified</u> tibia
    S82.144- <u>Nondisplaced</u> bicondylar fracture of <u>right</u> tibia
    S82.145- <u>Nondisplaced</u> bicondylar fracture of <u>left</u> tibia
    S82.146- <u>Nondisplaced</u> bicondylar fracture of <u>unspecified</u> tibia
  S82.15- Fracture of <u>tibial tuberosity</u>
    S82.151- <u>Displaced</u> fracture of <u>right</u> tibial tuberosity
    S82.152- <u>Displaced</u> fracture of <u>left</u> tibial tuberosity
    S82.153- <u>Displaced</u> fracture of <u>unspecified</u> tibial tuberosity
    S82.154- <u>Nondisplaced</u> fracture of <u>right</u> tibial tuberosity
    S82.155- <u>Nondisplaced</u> fracture of <u>left</u> tibial tuberosity
    S82.156- <u>Nondisplaced</u> fracture of <u>unspecified</u> tibial tuberosity

S82.16- Torus fracture of upper end of tibia
The appropriate 7th character is to be added to all codes in subcategory S82.16:
  A Initial encounter for closed fracture
  D Subsequent encounter for fracture with routine healing
  G Subsequent encounter for fracture with delayed healing
  K Subsequent encounter for fracture with nonunion
  P Subsequent encounter for fracture with malunion
  S Sequela

  S82.161- Torus fracture of upper end of right tibia
  S82.162- Torus fracture of upper end of left tibia
  S82.169- Torus fracture of upper end of unspecified tibia

S82.19- Other fracture of upper end of tibia
  S82.191- Other fracture of upper end of right tibia
  S82.192- Other fracture of upper end of left tibia
  S82.199- Other fracture of upper end of unspecified tibia

S82.2- Fracture of shaft of tibia
S82.20- Unspecified fracture of shaft of tibia
    Fracture of tibia NOS
  S82.201- Unspecified fracture of shaft of right tibia
  S82.202- Unspecified fracture of shaft of left tibia
  S82.209- Unspecified fracture of shaft of unspecified tibia

S82.22- Transverse fracture of shaft of tibia
  S82.221- Displaced transverse fracture of shaft of right tibia
  S82.222- Displaced transverse fracture of shaft of left tibia
  S82.223- Displaced transverse fracture of shaft of unspecified tibia
  S82.224- Nondisplaced transverse fracture of shaft of right tibia
  S82.225- Nondisplaced transverse fracture of shaft of left tibia
  S82.226- Nondisplaced transverse fracture of shaft of unspecified tibia

S82.23- Oblique fracture of shaft of tibia
  S82.231- Displaced oblique fracture of shaft of right tibia
  S82.232- Displaced oblique fracture of shaft of left tibia
  S82.233- Displaced oblique fracture of shaft of unspecified tibia
  S82.234- Nondisplaced oblique fracture of shaft of right tibia
  S82.235- Nondisplaced oblique fracture of shaft of left tibia
  S82.236- Nondisplaced oblique fracture of shaft of unspecified tibia

S82.24- Spiral fracture of shaft of tibia
    Toddler fracture
  S82.241- Displaced spiral fracture of shaft of right tibia
  S82.242- Displaced spiral fracture of shaft of left tibia
  S82.243- Displaced spiral fracture of shaft of unspecified tibia
  S82.244- Nondisplaced spiral fracture of shaft of right tibia
  S82.245- Nondisplaced spiral fracture of shaft of left tibia
  S82.246- Nondisplaced spiral fracture of shaft of unspecified tibia

S82.25- Comminuted fracture of shaft of tibia
  S82.251- Displaced comminuted fracture of shaft of right tibia
  S82.252- Displaced comminuted fracture of shaft of left tibia
  S82.253- Displaced comminuted fracture of shaft of unspecified tibia
  S82.254- Nondisplaced comminuted fracture of shaft of right tibia
  S82.255- Nondisplaced comminuted fracture of shaft of left tibia
  S82.256- Nondisplaced comminuted fracture of shaft of unspecified tibia

S82.26- Segmental fracture of shaft of tibia
  S82.261- Displaced segmental fracture of shaft of right tibia
  S82.262- Displaced segmental fracture of shaft of left tibia
  S82.263- Displaced segmental fracture of shaft of unspecified tibia
  S82.264- Nondisplaced segmental fracture of shaft of right tibia
  S82.265- Nondisplaced segmental fracture of shaft of left tibia
  S82.266- Nondisplaced segmental fracture of shaft of unspecified tibia

S82.29- Other fracture of shaft of tibia
  S82.291- Other fracture of shaft of right tibia
  S82.292- Other fracture of shaft of left tibia
  S82.299- Other fracture of shaft of unspecified tibia

S82.3- Fracture of lower end of tibia
  Excludes 1: bimalleolar fracture of lower leg (S82.84-)
    fracture of medial malleolus alone (S82.5-)
    Maisonneuve's fracture (S82.86-)
    pilon fracture of distal tibia (S82.87-)
    trimalleolar fractures of lower leg (S82.85-)

S82.30- Unspecified fracture of lower end of tibia
  S82.301- Unspecified fracture of lower end of right tibia
  S82.302- Unspecified fracture of lower end of left tibia
  S82.309- Unspecified fracture of lower end of unspecified tibia

S82.31- Torus fracture of lower end of tibia
The appropriate 7th character is to be added to all codes in subcategory S82.31:
  A Initial encounter for closed fracture
  D Subsequent encounter for fracture with routine healing
  G Subsequent encounter for fracture with delayed healing
  K Subsequent encounter for fracture with nonunion
  P Subsequent encounter for fracture with malunion
  S Sequela

  S82.311- Torus fracture of lower end of right tibia
  S82.312- Torus fracture of lower end of left tibia
  S82.319- Torus fracture of lower end of unspecified tibia

S82.39- Other fracture of lower end of tibia
  S82.391- Other fracture of lower end of right tibia
  S82.392- Other fracture of lower end of left tibia
  S82.399- Other fracture of lower end of unspecified tibia

S82.4- Fracture of shaft of fibula
  Excludes ❷: fracture of lateral malleolus alone (S82.6-)

S82.40- Unspecified fracture of shaft of fibula
  S82.401- Unspecified fracture of shaft of right fibula
  S82.402- Unspecified fracture of shaft of left fibula
  S82.409- Unspecified fracture of shaft of unspecified fibula

S82.42- Transverse fracture of shaft of fibula
  S82.421- Displaced transverse fracture of shaft of right fibula
  S82.422- Displaced transverse fracture of shaft of left fibula
  S82.423- Displaced transverse fracture of shaft of unspecified fibula
  S82.424- Nondisplaced transverse fracture of shaft of right fibula
  S82.425- Nondisplaced transverse fracture of shaft of left fibula
  S82.426- Nondisplaced transverse fracture of shaft of unspecified fibula

S82.43- Oblique fracture of shaft of fibula
  S82.431- Displaced oblique fracture of shaft of right fibula
  S82.432- Displaced oblique fracture of shaft of left fibula
  S82.433- Displaced oblique fracture of shaft of unspecified fibula
  S82.434- Nondisplaced oblique fracture of shaft of right fibula
  S82.435- Nondisplaced oblique fracture of shaft of left fibula
  S82.436- Nondisplaced oblique fracture of shaft of unspecified fibula

S82.44- Spiral fracture of shaft of fibula
  S82.441- Displaced spiral fracture of shaft of right fibula
  S82.442- Displaced spiral fracture of shaft of left fibula
  S82.443- Displaced spiral fracture of shaft of unspecified fibula
  S82.444- Nondisplaced spiral fracture of shaft of right fibula
  S82.445- Nondisplaced spiral fracture of shaft of left fibula
  S82.446- Nondisplaced spiral fracture of shaft of unspecified fibula

S82.45- Comminuted fracture of shaft of fibula
  S82.451- Displaced comminuted fracture of shaft of right fibula
  S82.452- Displaced comminuted fracture of shaft of left fibula
  S82.453- Displaced comminuted fracture of shaft of unspecified fibula
  S82.454- Nondisplaced comminuted fracture of shaft of right fibula
  S82.455- Nondisplaced comminuted fracture of shaft of left fibula
  S82.456- Nondisplaced comminuted fracture of shaft of unspecified fibula

S 8 1 – S 8 2

S82.46- <u>Segmental</u> fracture of <u>shaft</u> of <u>fibula</u>
  S82.461- <u>Displaced</u> segmental fracture of shaft of <u>right</u> fibula
  S82.462- <u>Displaced</u> segmental fracture of shaft of <u>left</u> fibula
  S82.463- <u>Displaced</u> segmental fracture of shaft of <u>unspecified</u> fibula
  S82.464- <u>Nondisplaced</u> segmental fracture of shaft of <u>right</u> fibula
  S82.465- <u>Nondisplaced</u> segmental fracture of shaft of <u>left</u> fibula
  S82.466- <u>Nondisplaced</u> segmental fracture of shaft of <u>unspecified</u> fibula
S82.49- <u>Other fracture</u> of <u>shaft</u> of <u>fibula</u>
  S82.491- Other fracture of shaft of <u>right</u> fibula
  S82.492- Other fracture of shaft of <u>left</u> fibula
  S82.499- Other fracture of shaft of <u>unspecified</u> fibula
S82.5- Fracture of <u>medial malleolus</u>
  Excludes 1: pilon fracture of distal tibia (S82.87-)
  Salter-Harris type III of lower end of tibia (S89.13-)
  Salter-Harris type IV of lower end of tibia (S89.14-)
  S82.51x- <u>Displaced</u> fracture of medial malleolus of <u>right</u> <u>tibia</u>
  S82.52x- <u>Displaced</u> fracture of medial malleolus of <u>left</u> <u>tibia</u>
  S82.53x- <u>Displaced</u> fracture of medial malleolus of <u>unspecified</u> <u>tibia</u>
  S82.54x- <u>Nondisplaced</u> fracture of medial malleolus of <u>right</u> <u>tibia</u>
  S82.55x- <u>Nondisplaced</u> fracture of medial malleolus of <u>left</u> <u>tibia</u>
  S82.56x- <u>Nondisplaced</u> fracture of medial malleolus of <u>unspecified</u> <u>tibia</u>
S82.6- Fracture of <u>lateral malleolus</u>
  Excludes 1: pilon fracture of distal tibia (S82.87-)
  S82.61x- <u>Displaced</u> fracture of lateral malleolus of <u>right</u> <u>fibula</u>
  S82.62x- <u>Displaced</u> fracture of lateral malleolus of <u>left</u> <u>fibula</u>
  S82.63x- <u>Displaced</u> fracture of lateral malleolus of <u>unspecified</u> <u>fibula</u>
  S82.64x- <u>Nondisplaced</u> fracture of lateral malleolus of <u>right</u> <u>fibula</u>
  S82.65x- <u>Nondisplaced</u> fracture of lateral malleolus of <u>left</u> <u>fibula</u>
  S82.66x- <u>Nondisplaced</u> fracture of lateral malleolus of <u>unspecified</u> <u>fibula</u>
S82.8- <u>Other fractures</u> of <u>lower leg</u>
  S82.81- <u>Torus</u> fracture of <u>upper end</u> of <u>fibula</u>
  The appropriate 7th character is to be added to all codes in subcategory S82.81:
    A <u>Initial</u> encounter for <u>closed</u> fracture
    D <u>Subsequent</u> encounter for fracture <u>with routine healing</u>
    G <u>Subsequent</u> encounter for fracture <u>with delayed healing</u>
    K <u>Subsequent</u> encounter for fracture <u>with nonunion</u>
    P <u>Subsequent</u> encounter for fracture <u>with malunion</u>
    S <u>Sequela</u>
  S82.811- Torus fracture of upper end of <u>right</u> fibula
  S82.812- Torus fracture of upper end of <u>left</u> fibula
  S82.819- Torus fracture of upper end of <u>unspecified</u> fibula
  S82.82- <u>Torus</u> fracture of <u>lower end</u> of <u>fibula</u>
  The appropriate 7th character is to be added to all codes in subcategory S82.82:
    A <u>Initial</u> encounter for <u>closed</u> fracture
    D <u>Subsequent</u> encounter for fracture <u>with routine healing</u>
    G <u>Subsequent</u> encounter for fracture <u>with delayed healing</u>
    K <u>Subsequent</u> encounter for fracture <u>with nonunion</u>
    P <u>Subsequent</u> encounter for fracture <u>with malunion</u>
    S <u>Sequela</u>
  S82.821- Torus fracture of lower end of <u>right</u> fibula
  S82.822- Torus fracture of lower end of <u>left</u> fibula
  S82.829- Torus fracture of lower end of <u>unspecified</u> fibula
  S82.83- <u>Other fracture</u> of <u>upper and lower end</u> of <u>fibula</u>
  S82.831- Other fracture of upper and lower end of <u>right</u> fibula
  S82.832- Other fracture of upper and lower end of <u>left</u> fibula
  S82.839- Other fracture of upper and lower end of <u>unspecified</u> fibula
  S82.84- <u>Bimalleolar</u> fracture of <u>lower leg</u>
  S82.841- <u>Displaced</u> bimalleolar fracture of <u>right</u> lower leg
  S82.842- <u>Displaced</u> bimalleolar fracture of <u>left</u> lower leg
  S82.843- <u>Displaced</u> bimalleolar fracture of <u>unspecified</u> lower leg
  S82.844- <u>Nondisplaced</u> bimalleolar fracture of <u>right</u> lower leg
  S82.845- <u>Nondisplaced</u> bimalleolar fracture of <u>left</u> lower leg
  S82.846- <u>Nondisplaced</u> bimalleolar fracture of <u>unspecified</u> lower leg

S82.85- <u>Trimalleolar</u> fracture of <u>lower leg</u>
  S82.851- <u>Displaced</u> trimalleolar fracture of <u>right</u> lower leg
  S82.852- <u>Displaced</u> trimalleolar fracture of <u>left</u> lower leg
  S82.853- <u>Displaced</u> trimalleolar fracture of <u>unspecified</u> lower leg
  S82.854- <u>Nondisplaced</u> trimalleolar fracture of <u>right</u> lower leg
  S82.855- <u>Nondisplaced</u> trimalleolar fracture of <u>left</u> lower leg
  S82.856- <u>Nondisplaced</u> trimalleolar fracture of <u>unspecified</u> lower leg
S82.86- <u>Maisonneuve's</u> fracture
  S82.861- <u>Displaced</u> Maisonneuve's fracture of <u>right</u> leg
  S82.862- <u>Displaced</u> Maisonneuve's fracture of <u>left</u> leg
  S82.863- <u>Displaced</u> Maisonneuve's fracture of <u>unspecified</u> leg
  S82.864- <u>Nondisplaced</u> Maisonneuve's fracture of <u>right</u> leg
  S82.865- <u>Nondisplaced</u> Maisonneuve's fracture of <u>left</u> leg
  S82.866- <u>Nondisplaced</u> Maisonneuve's fracture of <u>unspecified</u> leg
S82.87- <u>Pilon</u> fracture of <u>tibia</u>
  S82.871- <u>Displaced</u> pilon fracture of <u>right</u> tibia
  S82.872- <u>Displaced</u> pilon fracture of <u>left</u> tibia
  S82.873- <u>Displaced</u> pilon fracture of <u>unspecified</u> tibia
  S82.874- <u>Nondisplaced</u> pilon fracture of <u>right</u> tibia
  S82.875- <u>Nondisplaced</u> pilon fracture of <u>left</u> tibia
  S82.876- <u>Nondisplaced</u> pilon fracture of <u>unspecified</u> tibia
S82.89- <u>Other</u> fractures of <u>lower leg</u>
  Fracture of ankle NOS
  S82.891- Other fracture of <u>right</u> lower leg
  S82.892- Other fracture of <u>left</u> lower leg
  S82.899- Other fracture of <u>unspecified</u> lower leg
S82.9- <u>Unspecified</u> fracture of <u>lower leg</u>
  S82.90x- Unspecified fracture of <u>unspecified</u> lower leg
  S82.91x- Unspecified fracture of <u>right</u> lower leg
  S82.92x- Unspecified fracture of <u>left</u> lower leg
S83- <u>Dislocation and sprain</u> of joints and ligaments of <u>knee</u>
  Includes: Avulsion of joint or ligament of knee
    Laceration of cartilage, joint or ligament of knee
    Sprain of cartilage, joint or ligament of knee
    Traumatic hemarthrosis of joint or ligament of knee
    Traumatic rupture of joint or ligament of knee
    Traumatic subluxation of joint or ligament of knee
    Traumatic tear of joint or ligament of knee
  Code also any associated open wound
  Excludes 1: derangement of patella (M22.0-M22.3)
    injury of patellar ligament (tendon) (S76.1-)
    internal derangement of knee (M23.-)
    old dislocation of knee (M24.36)
    pathological dislocation of knee (M24.36)
    recurrent dislocation of knee (M22.0)
  Excludes ❷: strain of muscle, fascia and tendon of lower leg (S86.-)
  The appropriate 7th character is to be added to each code from category S83:
    A <u>Initial</u> encounter
    D <u>Subsequent</u> encounter
    S <u>Sequela</u>
S83.0- <u>Subluxation and dislocation</u> of <u>patella</u>
  S83.00- <u>Unspecified</u> subluxation and dislocation of <u>patella</u>
  S83.001- Unspecified <u>subluxation</u> of <u>right</u> patella
  S83.002- Unspecified <u>subluxation</u> of <u>left</u> patella
  S83.003- Unspecified <u>subluxation</u> of <u>unspecified</u> patella
  S83.004- Unspecified <u>dislocation</u> of <u>right</u> patella
  S83.005- Unspecified <u>dislocation</u> of <u>left</u> patella
  S83.006- Unspecified <u>dislocation</u> of <u>unspecified</u> patella
  S83.01- <u>Lateral</u> subluxation and dislocation of <u>patella</u>
  S83.011- Lateral <u>subluxation</u> of <u>right</u> patella
  S83.012- Lateral <u>subluxation</u> of <u>left</u> patella
  S83.013- Lateral <u>subluxation</u> of <u>unspecified</u> patella
  S83.014- Lateral <u>dislocation</u> of <u>right</u> patella
  S83.015- Lateral <u>dislocation</u> of <u>left</u> patella
  S83.016- Lateral <u>dislocation</u> of <u>unspecified</u> patella
  S83.09- <u>Other</u> subluxation and dislocation of <u>patella</u>
  S83.091- Other <u>subluxation</u> of <u>right</u> patella
  S83.092- Other <u>subluxation</u> of <u>left</u> patella
  S83.093- Other <u>subluxation</u> of <u>unspecified</u> patella
  S83.094- Other <u>dislocation</u> of <u>right</u> patella
  S83.095- Other <u>dislocation</u> of <u>left</u> patella
  S83.096- Other <u>dislocation</u> of <u>unspecified</u> patella

S 8 2 - S 8 3

S83.1-   Subluxation and dislocation of knee
     Excludes ❷: instability of knee prosthesis (T84.022, T84.023)
     S83.10-   Unspecified subluxation and dislocation of knee
         S83.101-   Unspecified subluxation of right knee
         S83.102-   Unspecified subluxation of left knee
         S83.103-   Unspecified subluxation of unspecified knee
         S83.104-   Unspecified dislocation of right knee
         S83.105-   Unspecified dislocation of left knee
         S83.106-   Unspecified dislocation of unspecified knee
     S83.11-   Anterior subluxation and dislocation of proximal end of tibia
         Posterior subluxation and dislocation of distal end of femur
         S83.111-   Anterior subluxation of proximal end of tibia, right knee
         S83.112-   Anterior subluxation of proximal end of tibia, left knee
         S83.113-   Anterior subluxation of proximal end of tibia, unspecified knee
         S83.114-   Anterior dislocation of proximal end of tibia, right knee
         S83.115-   Anterior dislocation of proximal end of tibia, left knee
         S83.116-   Anterior dislocation of proximal end of tibia, unspecified knee
     S83.12-   Posterior subluxation and dislocation of proximal end of tibia
         Anterior dislocation of distal end of femur
         S83.121-   Posterior subluxation of proximal end of tibia, right knee
         S83.122-   Posterior subluxation of proximal end of tibia, left knee
         S83.123-   Posterior subluxation of proximal end of tibia, unspecified knee
         S83.124-   Posterior dislocation of proximal end of tibia, right knee
         S83.125-   Posterior dislocation of proximal end of tibia, left knee
         S83.126-   Posterior dislocation of proximal end of tibia, unspecified knee
     S83.13-   Medial subluxation and dislocation of proximal end of tibia
         S83.131-   Medial subluxation of proximal end of tibia, right knee
         S83.132-   Medial subluxation of proximal end of tibia, left knee
         S83.133-   Medial subluxation of proximal end of tibia, unspecified knee
         S83.134-   Medial dislocation of proximal end of tibia, right knee
         S83.135-   Medial dislocation of proximal end of tibia, left knee
         S83.136-   Medial dislocation of proximal end of tibia, unspecified knee
     S83.14-   Lateral subluxation and dislocation of proximal end of tibia
         S83.141-   Lateral subluxation of proximal end of tibia, right knee
         S83.142-   Lateral subluxation of proximal end of tibia, left knee
         S83.143-   Lateral subluxation of proximal end of tibia, unspecified knee
         S83.144-   Lateral dislocation of proximal end of tibia, right knee
         S83.145-   Lateral dislocation of proximal end of tibia, left knee
         S83.146-   Lateral dislocation of proximal end of tibia, unspecified knee
     S83.19-   Other subluxation and dislocation of knee
         S83.191-   Other subluxation of right knee
         S83.192-   Other subluxation of left knee
         S83.193-   Other subluxation of unspecified knee
         S83.194-   Other dislocation of right knee
         S83.195-   Other dislocation of left knee
         S83.196-   Other dislocation of unspecified knee
S83.2-   Tear of meniscus, current injury
     Excludes 1:   old bucket-handle tear (M23.2)
     S83.20-   Tear of unspecified meniscus, current injury
         Tear of meniscus of knee NOS
         S83.200-   Bucket-handle tear of unspecified meniscus, current injury, right knee
         S83.201-   Bucket-handle tear of unspecified meniscus, current injury, left knee
         S83.202-   Bucket-handle tear of unspecified meniscus, current injury, unspecified knee
         S83.203-   Other tear of unspecified meniscus, current injury, right knee

S83.204-   Other tear of unspecified meniscus, current injury, left knee
S83.205-   Other tear of unspecified meniscus, current injury, unspecified knee
S83.206-   Unspecified tear of unspecified meniscus, current injury, right knee
S83.207-   Unspecified tear of unspecified meniscus, current injury, left knee
S83.209-   Unspecified tear of unspecified meniscus, current injury, unspecified knee
     S83.21-   Bucket-handle tear of medial meniscus, current injury
         S83.211-   Bucket-handle tear of medial meniscus, current injury, right knee
         S83.212-   Bucket-handle tear of medial meniscus, current injury, left knee
         S83.219-   Bucket-handle tear of medial meniscus, current injury, unspecified knee
     S83.22-   Peripheral tear of medial meniscus, current injury
         S83.221-   Peripheral tear of medial meniscus, current injury, right knee
         S83.222-   Peripheral tear of medial meniscus, current injury, left knee
         S83.229-   Peripheral tear of medial meniscus, current injury, unspecified knee
     S83.23-   Complex tear of medial meniscus, current injury
         S83.231-   Complex tear of medial meniscus, current injury, right knee
         S83.232-   Complex tear of medial meniscus, current injury, left knee
         S83.239-   Complex tear of medial meniscus, current injury, unspecified knee
     S83.24-   Other tear of medial meniscus, current injury
         S83.241-   Other tear of medial meniscus, current injury, right knee
         S83.242-   Other tear of medial meniscus, current injury, left knee
         S83.249-   Other tear of medial meniscus, current injury, unspecified knee
     S83.25-   Bucket-handle tear of lateral meniscus, current injury
         S83.251-   Bucket-handle tear of lateral meniscus, current injury, right knee
         S83.252-   Bucket-handle tear of lateral meniscus, current injury, left knee
         S83.259-   Bucket-handle tear of lateral meniscus, current injury, unspecified knee
     S83.26-   Peripheral tear of lateral meniscus, current injury
         S83.261-   Peripheral tear of lateral meniscus, current injury, right knee
         S83.262-   Peripheral tear of lateral meniscus, current injury, left knee
         S83.269-   Peripheral tear of lateral meniscus, current injury, unspecified knee
     S83.27-   Complex tear of lateral meniscus, current injury
         S83.271-   Complex tear of lateral meniscus, current injury, right knee
         S83.272-   Complex tear of lateral meniscus, current injury, left knee
         S83.279-   Complex tear of lateral meniscus, current injury, unspecified knee
     S83.28-   Other tear of lateral meniscus, current injury
         S83.281-   Other tear of lateral meniscus, current injury, right knee
         S83.282-   Other tear of lateral meniscus, current injury, left knee
         S83.289-   Other tear of lateral meniscus, current injury, unspecified knee
S83.3-   Tear of articular cartilage of knee, current
     S83.30x-   Tear of articular cartilage of unspecified knee, current
     S83.31x-   Tear of articular cartilage of right knee, current
     S83.32x-   Tear of articular cartilage of left knee, current
S83.4-   Sprain of collateral ligament of knee
     S83.40-   Sprain of unspecified collateral ligament of knee
         S83.401-   Sprain of unspecified collateral ligament of right knee
         S83.402-   Sprain of unspecified collateral ligament of left knee
         S83.409-   Sprain of unspecified collateral ligament of unspecified knee

S 8 2 - S 8 3

S83.41- Sprain of medial collateral ligament of knee
    Sprain of tibial collateral ligament
    S83.411- Sprain of medial collateral ligament of right knee
    S83.412- Sprain of medial collateral ligament of left knee
    S83.419- Sprain of medial collateral ligament of unspecified knee
S83.42- Sprain of lateral collateral ligament of knee
    Sprain of fibular collateral ligament
    S83.421- Sprain of lateral collateral ligament of right knee
    S83.422- Sprain of lateral collateral ligament of left knee
    S83.429- Sprain of lateral collateral ligament of unspecified knee
S83.5- Sprain of cruciate ligament of knee
    S83.50- Sprain of unspecified cruciate ligament of knee
        S83.501- Sprain of unspecified cruciate ligament of right knee
        S83.502- Sprain of unspecified cruciate ligament of left knee
        S83.509- Sprain of unspecified cruciate ligament of unspecified knee
    S83.51- Sprain of anterior cruciate ligament of knee
        S83.511- Sprain of anterior cruciate ligament of right knee
        S83.512- Sprain of anterior cruciate ligament of left knee
        S83.519- Sprain of anterior cruciate ligament of unspecified knee
    S83.52- Sprain of posterior cruciate ligament of knee
        S83.521- Sprain of posterior cruciate ligament of right knee
        S83.522- Sprain of posterior cruciate ligament of left knee
        S83.529- Sprain of posterior cruciate ligament of unspecified knee
S83.6- Sprain of the superior tibiofibular joint and ligament
    S83.60x- Sprain of the superior tibiofibular joint and ligament, unspecified knee
    S83.61x- Sprain of the superior tibiofibular joint and ligament, right knee
    S83.62x- Sprain of the superior tibiofibular joint and ligament, left knee
S83.8- Sprain of other specified parts of knee
    S83.8x- Sprain of other specified parts of knee
        S83.8x1- Sprain of other specified parts of right knee
        S83.8x2- Sprain of other specified parts of left knee
        S83.8x9- Sprain of other specified parts of unspecified knee
S83.9- Sprain of unspecified site of knee
    S83.90x- Sprain of unspecified site of unspecified knee
    S83.91x- Sprain of unspecified site of right knee
    S83.92x- Sprain of unspecified site of left knee

S84- Injury of nerves at lower leg level
    Code also any associated open wound (S81-)
    Excludes❷: injury of nerves at ankle and foot level (S94-)
    The appropriate 7th character is to be added to each code from category S84:
    A   Initial encounter
    D   Subsequent encounter
    S   Sequela
S84.0- Injury of tibial nerve at lower leg level
    S84.00x- Injury of tibial nerve at lower leg level, unspecified leg
    S84.01x- Injury of tibial nerve at lower leg level, right leg
    S84.02x- Injury of tibial nerve at lower leg level, left leg
S84.1- Injury of peroneal nerve at lower leg level
    S84.10x- Injury of peroneal nerve at lower leg level, unspecified leg
    S84.11x- Injury of peroneal nerve at lower leg level, right leg
    S84.12x- Injury of peroneal nerve at lower leg level, left leg
S84.2- Injury of cutaneous sensory nerve at lower leg level
    S84.20x- Injury of cutaneous sensory nerve at lower leg level, unspecified leg
    S84.21x- Injury of cutaneous sensory nerve at lower leg level, right leg
    S84.22x- Injury of cutaneous sensory nerve at lower leg level, left leg
S84.8- Injury of other nerves at lower leg level
    S84.80- Injury of other nerves at lower leg level
        S84.801- Injury of other nerves at lower leg level, right leg
        S84.802- Injury of other nerves at lower leg level, left leg
        S84.809- Injury of other nerves at lower leg level, unspecified leg

S84.9- Injury of unspecified nerve at lower leg level
    S84.90x- Injury of unspecified nerve at lower leg level, unspecified leg
    S84.91x- Injury of unspecified nerve at lower leg level, right leg
    S84.92x- Injury of unspecified nerve at lower leg level, left leg
S85- Injury of blood vessels at lower leg level
    Code also any associated open wound (S81.-)
    Excludes❷: injury of blood vessels at ankle and foot level (S95.-)
    The appropriate 7th character is to be added to each code from category S85:
    A   Initial encounter
    D   Subsequent encounter
    S   Sequela
S85.0- Injury of popliteal artery
    S85.00- Unspecified injury of popliteal artery
        S85.001- Unspecified injury of popliteal artery, right leg
        S85.002- Unspecified injury of popliteal artery, left leg
        S85.009- Unspecified injury of popliteal artery, unspecified leg
    S85.01- Laceration of popliteal artery
        S85.011- Laceration of popliteal artery, right leg
        S85.012- Laceration of popliteal artery, left leg
        S85.019- Laceration of popliteal artery, unspecified leg
    S85.09- Other specified injury of popliteal artery
        S85.091- Other specified injury of popliteal artery, right leg
        S85.092- Other specified injury of popliteal artery, left leg
        S85.099- Other specified injury of popliteal artery, unspecified leg
S85.1- Injury of tibial artery
    S85.10- Unspecified injury of unspecified tibial artery
        Injury of tibial artery NOS
        S85.101- Unspecified injury of unspecified tibial artery, right leg
        S85.102- Unspecified injury of unspecified tibial artery, left leg
        S85.109- Unspecified injury of unspecified tibial artery, unspecified leg
    S85.11- Laceration of unspecified tibial artery
        S85.111- Laceration of unspecified tibial artery, right leg
        S85.112- Laceration of unspecified tibial artery, left leg
        S85.119- Laceration of unspecified tibial artery, unspecified leg
    S85.12- Other specified injury of unspecified tibial artery
        S85.121- Other specified injury of unspecified tibial artery, right leg
        S85.122- Other specified injury of unspecified tibial artery, left leg
        S85.129- Other specified injury of unspecified tibial artery, unspecified leg
    S85.13- Unspecified injury of anterior tibial artery
        S85.131- Unspecified injury of anterior tibial artery, right leg
        S85.132- Unspecified injury of anterior tibial artery, left leg
        S85.139- Unspecified injury of anterior tibial artery, unspecified leg
    S85.14- Laceration of anterior tibial artery
        S85.141- Laceration of anterior tibial artery, right leg
        S85.142- Laceration of anterior tibial artery, left leg
        S85.149- Laceration of anterior tibial artery, unspecified leg
    S85.15- Other specified injury of anterior tibial artery
        S85.151- Other specified injury of anterior tibial artery, right leg
        S85.152- Other specified injury of anterior tibial artery, left leg
        S85.159- Other specified injury of anterior tibial artery, unspecified leg
    S85.16- Unspecified injury of posterior tibial artery
        S85.161- Unspecified injury of posterior tibial artery, right leg
        S85.162- Unspecified injury of posterior tibial artery, left leg
        S85.169- Unspecified injury of posterior tibial artery, unspecified leg
    S85.17- Laceration of posterior tibial artery
        S85.171- Laceration of posterior tibial artery, right leg
        S85.172- Laceration of posterior tibial artery, left leg
        S85.179 Laceration of posterior tibial artery, unspecified leg
    S85.18- Other specified injury of posterior tibial artery
        S85.181- Other specified injury of posterior tibial artery, right leg
        S85.182- Other specified injury of posterior tibial artery, left leg
        S85.189 Other specified injury of posterior tibial artery, unspecified leg

S 8 3 - S 8 6

S85.2- Injury of peroneal artery
    S85.20- Unspecified injury of peroneal artery
        S85.201- Unspecified injury of peroneal artery, right leg
        S85.202- Unspecified injury of peroneal artery, left leg
        S85.209 Unspecified injury of peroneal artery, unspecified leg
    S85.21- Laceration of peroneal artery
        S85.211- Laceration of peroneal artery, right leg
        S85.212- Laceration of peroneal artery, left leg
        S85.219- Laceration of peroneal artery, unspecified leg
    S85.29- Other specified injury of peroneal artery
        S85.291- Other specified injury of peroneal artery, right leg
        S85.292- Other specified injury of peroneal artery, left leg
        S85.299- Other specified injury of peroneal artery, unspecified leg
S85.3- Injury of greater saphenous vein at lower leg level
    Injury of greater saphenous vein NOS
    Injury of saphenous vein NOS
    S85.30- Unspecified injury of greater saphenous vein at lower leg level
        S85.301- Unspecified injury of greater saphenous vein at lower leg level, right leg
        S85.302- Unspecified injury of greater saphenous vein at lower leg level, left leg
        S85.309- Unspecified injury of greater saphenous vein at lower leg level, unspecified leg
    S85.31- Laceration of greater saphenous vein at lower leg level
        S85.311- Laceration of greater saphenous vein at lower leg level, right leg
        S85.312- Laceration of greater saphenous vein at lower leg level, left leg
        S85.319- Laceration of greater saphenous vein at lower leg level, unspecified leg
    S85.39- Other specified injury of greater saphenous vein at lower leg level
        S85.391- Other specified injury of greater saphenous vein at lower leg level, right leg
        S85.392- Other specified injury of greater saphenous vein at lower leg level, left leg
        S85.399- Other specified injury of greater saphenous vein at lower leg level, unspecified leg
S85.4- Injury of lesser saphenous vein at lower leg level
    S85.40- Unspecified injury of lesser saphenous vein at lower leg level
        S85.401- Unspecified injury of lesser saphenous vein at lower leg level, right leg
        S85.402- Unspecified injury of lesser saphenous vein at lower leg level, left leg
        S85.409- Unspecified injury of lesser saphenous vein at lower leg level, unspecified leg
    S85.41- Laceration of lesser saphenous vein at lower leg level
        S85.411- Laceration of lesser saphenous vein at lower leg level, right leg
        S85.412- Laceration of lesser saphenous vein at lower leg level, left leg
        S85.419- Laceration of lesser saphenous vein at lower leg level, unspecified leg
    S85.49- Other specified injury of lesser saphenous vein at lower leg level
        S85.491- Other specified injury of lesser saphenous vein at lower leg level, right leg
        S85.492- Other specified injury of lesser saphenous vein at lower leg level, left leg
        S85.499- Other specified injury of lesser saphenous vein at lower leg level, unspecified leg
S85.5- Injury of popliteal vein
    S85.50- Unspecified injury of popliteal vein
        S85.501- Unspecified injury of popliteal vein, right leg
        S85.502- Unspecified injury of popliteal vein, left leg
        S85.509- Unspecified injury of popliteal vein, unspecified leg
    S85.51- Laceration of popliteal vein
        S85.511- Laceration of popliteal vein, right leg
        S85.512- Laceration of popliteal vein, left leg
        S85.519- Laceration of popliteal vein, unspecified leg
    S85.59- Other specified injury of popliteal vein
        S85.591- Other specified injury of popliteal vein, right leg
        S85.592- Other specified injury of popliteal vein, left leg
        S85.599- Other specified injury of popliteal vein, unspecified leg

S85.8- Injury of other blood vessels at lower leg level
    S85.80- Unspecified injury of other blood vessels at lower leg level
        S85.801- Unspecified injury of other blood vessels at lower leg level, right leg
        S85.802- Unspecified injury of other blood vessels at lower leg level, left leg
        S85.809- Unspecified injury of other blood vessels at lower leg level, unspecified leg
    S85.81- Laceration of other blood vessels at lower leg level
        S85.811- Laceration of other blood vessels at lower leg level, right leg
        S85.812- Laceration of other blood vessels at lower leg level, left leg
        S85.819- Laceration of other blood vessels at lower leg level, unspecified leg
    S85.89- Other specified injury of other blood vessels at lower leg level
        S85.891- Other specified injury of other blood vessels at lower leg level, right leg
        S85.892- Other specified injury of other blood vessels at lower leg level, left leg
        S85.899- Other specified injury of other blood vessels at lower leg level, unspecified leg
S85.9- Injury of unspecified blood vessel at lower leg level
    S85.90- Unspecified injury of unspecified blood vessel at lower leg level
        S85.901- Unspecified injury of unspecified blood vessel at lower leg level, right leg
        S85.902- Unspecified injury of unspecified blood vessel at lower leg level, left leg
        S85.909- Unspecified injury of unspecified blood vessel at lower leg level, unspecified leg
    S85.91- Laceration of unspecified blood vessel at lower leg level
        S85.911- Laceration of unspecified blood vessel at lower leg level, right leg
        S85.912- Laceration of unspecified blood vessel at lower leg level, left leg
        S85.919- Laceration of unspecified blood vessel at lower leg level, unspecified leg
    S85.99- Other specified injury of unspecified blood vessel at lower leg level
        S85.991- Other specified injury of unspecified blood vessel at lower leg level, right leg
        S85.992- Other specified injury of unspecified blood vessel at lower leg level, left leg
        S85.999- Other specified injury of unspecified blood vessel at lower leg level, unspecified leg

S86- Injury of muscle, fascia and tendon at lower leg level
    Code also any associated open wound (S81.-)
    Excludes❷: injury of muscle, fascia and tendon at ankle (S96.-)
        injury of patellar ligament (tendon) (S76.1-)
        sprain of joints and ligaments of knee (S83.-)
    The appropriate 7th character is to be added to each code from category S86:
    A **Initial** encounter
    D **Subsequent** encounter
    S **Sequela**
S86.0- Injury of Achilles tendon
    S86.00- Unspecified injury of Achilles tendon
        S86.001- Unspecified injury of right Achilles tendon
        S86.002- Unspecified injury of left Achilles tendon
        S86.009- Unspecified injury of unspecified Achilles tendon
    S86.01- Strain of Achilles tendon
        S86.011- Strain of right Achilles tendon
        S86.012- Strain of left Achilles tendon
        S86.019- Strain of unspecified Achilles tendon
    S86.02- Laceration of Achilles tendon
        S86.021- Laceration of right Achilles tendon
        S86.022- Laceration of left Achilles tendon
        S86.029- Laceration of unspecified Achilles tendon
    S86.09- Other specified injury of Achilles tendon
        S86.091- Other specified injury of right Achilles tendon
        S86.092- Other specified injury of left Achilles tendon
        S86.099- Other specified injury of unspecified Achilles tendon

S83 – S86

S86.1-   Injury of other muscle(s) and tendon(s) of posterior muscle group at lower leg level

 S86.10-   Unspecified injury of other muscle(s) and tendon(s) of posterior muscle group at lower leg level

  S86.101-   Unspecified injury of other muscle(s) and tendon(s) of posterior muscle group at lower leg level, right leg

  S86.102-   Unspecified injury of other muscle(s) and tendon(s) of posterior muscle group at lower leg level, left leg

  S86.109-   Unspecified injury of other muscle(s) and tendon(s) of posterior muscle group at lower leg level, unspecified leg

 S86.11-   Strain of other muscle(s) and tendon(s) of posterior muscle group at lower leg level

  S86.111-   Strain of other muscle(s) and tendon(s) of posterior muscle group at lower leg level, right leg

  S86.112-   Strain of other muscle(s) and tendon(s) of posterior muscle group at lower leg level, left leg

  S86.119-   Strain of other muscle(s) and tendon(s) of posterior muscle group at lower leg level, unspecified leg

 S86.12-   Laceration of other muscle(s) and tendon(s) of posterior muscle group at lower leg level

  S86.121-   Laceration of other muscle(s) and tendon(s) of posterior muscle group at lower leg level, right leg

  S86.122-   Laceration of other muscle(s) and tendon(s) of posterior muscle group at lower leg level, left leg

  S86.129-   Laceration of other muscle(s) and tendon(s) of posterior muscle group at lower leg level, unspecified leg

 S86.19-   Other injury of other muscle(s) and tendon(s) of posterior muscle group at lower leg level

  S86.191-   Other injury of other muscle(s) and tendon(s) of posterior muscle group at lower leg level, right leg

  S86.192-   Other injury of other muscle(s) and tendon(s) of posterior muscle group at lower leg level, left leg

  S86.199-   Other injury of other muscle(s) and tendon(s) of posterior muscle group at lower leg level, unspecified leg

S86.2-   Injury of muscle(s) and tendon(s) of anterior muscle group at lower leg level

 S86.20-   Unspecified injury of muscle(s) and tendon(s) of anterior muscle group at lower leg level

  S86.201-   Unspecified injury of muscle(s) and tendon(s) of anterior muscle group at lower leg level, right leg

  S86.202-   Unspecified injury of muscle(s) and tendon(s) of anterior muscle group at lower leg level, left leg

  S86.209-   Unspecified injury of muscle(s) and tendon(s) of anterior muscle group at lower leg level, unspecified leg

 S86.21-   Strain of muscle(s) and tendon(s) of anterior muscle group at lower leg level

  S86.211-   Strain of muscle(s) and tendon(s) of anterior muscle group at lower leg level, right leg

  S86.212-   Strain of muscle(s) and tendon(s) of anterior muscle group at lower leg level, left leg

  S86.219-   Strain of muscle(s) and tendon(s) of anterior muscle group at lower leg level, unspecified leg

 S86.22-   Laceration of muscle(s) and tendon(s) of anterior muscle group at lower leg level

  S86.221-   Laceration of muscle(s) and tendon(s) of anterior muscle group at lower leg level, right leg

  S86.222-   Laceration of muscle(s) and tendon(s) of anterior muscle group at lower leg level, left leg

  S86.229-   Laceration of muscle(s) and tendon(s) of anterior muscle group at lower leg level, unspecified leg

 S86.29-   Other injury of muscle(s) and tendon(s) of anterior muscle group at lower leg level

  S86.291-   Other injury of muscle(s) and tendon(s) of anterior muscle group at lower leg level, right leg

  S86.292-   Other injury of muscle(s) and tendon(s) of anterior muscle group at lower leg level, left leg

  S86.299-   Other injury of muscle(s) and tendon(s) of anterior muscle group at lower leg level, unspecified leg

S86.3-   Injury of muscle(s) and tendon(s) of peroneal muscle group at lower leg level

 S86.30-   Unspecified injury of muscle(s) and tendon(s) of peroneal muscle group at lower leg level

  S86.301-   Unspecified injury of muscle(s) and tendon(s) of peroneal muscle group at lower leg level, right leg

  S86.302-   Unspecified injury of muscle(s) and tendon(s) of peroneal muscle group at lower leg level, left leg

  S86.309-   Unspecified injury of muscle(s) and tendon(s) of peroneal muscle group at lower leg level, unspecified leg

 S86.31-   Strain of muscle(s) and tendon(s) of peroneal muscle group at lower leg level

  S86.311-   Strain of muscle(s) and tendon(s) of peroneal muscle group at lower leg level, right leg

  S86.312-   Strain of muscle(s) and tendon(s) of peroneal muscle group at lower leg level, left leg

  S86.319-   Strain of muscle(s) and tendon(s) of peroneal muscle group at lower leg level, unspecified leg

 S86.32-   Laceration of muscle(s) and tendon(s) of peroneal muscle group at lower leg level

  S86.321-   Laceration of muscle(s) and tendon(s) of peroneal muscle group at lower leg level, right leg

  S86.322-   Laceration of muscle(s) and tendon(s) of peroneal muscle group at lower leg level, left leg

  S86.329-   Laceration of muscle(s) and tendon(s) of peroneal muscle group at lower leg level, unspecified leg

 S86.39-   Other injury of muscle(s) and tendon(s) of peroneal muscle group at lower leg level

  S86.391-   Other injury of muscle(s) and tendon(s) of peroneal muscle group at lower leg level, right leg

  S86.392-   Other injury of muscle(s) and tendon(s) of peroneal muscle group at lower leg level, left leg

  S86.399-   Other injury of muscle(s) and tendon(s) of peroneal muscle group at lower leg level, unspecified leg

S86.8-   Injury of other muscles and tendons at lower leg level

 S86.80-   Unspecified injury of other muscles and tendons at lower leg level

  S86.801-   Unspecified injury of other muscle(s) and tendon(s) at lower leg level, right leg

  S86.802-   Unspecified injury of other muscle(s) and tendon(s) at lower leg level, left leg

  S86.809-   Unspecified injury of other muscle(s) and tendon(s) at lower leg level, unspecified leg

 S86.81-   Strain of other muscles and tendons at lower leg level

  S86.811-   Strain of other muscle(s) and tendon(s) at lower leg level, right leg

  S86.812-   Strain of other muscle(s) and tendon(s) at lower leg level, left leg

  S86.819-   Strain of other muscle(s) and tendon(s) at lower leg level, unspecified leg

 S86.82-   Laceration of other muscles and tendons at lower leg level

  S86.821-   Laceration of other muscle(s) and tendon(s) at lower leg level, right leg

  S86.822-   Laceration of other muscle(s) and tendon(s) at lower leg level, left leg

  S86.829-   Laceration of other muscle(s) and tendon(s) at lower leg level, unspecified leg

 S86.89-   Other injury of other muscles and tendons at lower leg level

  S86.891-   Other injury of other muscle(s) and tendon(s) at lower leg level, right leg

  S86.892-   Other injury of other muscle(s) and tendon(s) at lower leg level, left leg

  S86.899-   Other injury of other muscle(s) and tendon(s) at lower leg level, unspecified leg

S86.9-   Injury of unspecified muscle and tendon at lower leg level

 S86.90-   Unspecified injury of unspecified muscle and tendon at lower leg level

  S86.901-   Unspecified injury of unspecified muscle(s) and tendon(s) at lower leg level, right leg

  S86.902-   Unspecified injury of unspecified muscle(s) and tendon(s) at lower leg level, left leg

  S86.909-   Unspecified injury of unspecified muscle(s) and tendon(s) at lower leg level, unspecified leg

 S86.91-   Strain of unspecified muscle and tendon at lower leg level

  S86.911-   Strain of unspecified muscle(s) and tendon(s) at lower leg level, right leg

  S86.912-   Strain of unspecified muscle(s) and tendon(s) at lower leg level, left leg

S86
-
S89

S86.919- Strain of unspecified muscle(s) and tendon(s) at lower leg level, unspecified leg
S86.92- Laceration of unspecified muscle and tendon at lower leg level
    S86.921- Laceration of unspecified muscle(s) and tendon(s) at lower leg level, right leg
    S86.922- Laceration of unspecified muscle(s) and tendon(s) at lower leg level, left leg
    S86.929- Laceration of unspecified muscle(s) and tendon(s) at lower leg level, unspecified leg
S86.99- Other injury of unspecified muscle and tendon at lower leg level
    S86.991- Other injury of unspecified muscle(s) and tendon(s) at lower leg level, right leg
    S86.992- Other injury of unspecified muscle(s) and tendon(s) at lower leg level, left leg
    S86.999- Other injury of unspecified muscle(s) and tendon(s) at lower leg level, unspecified leg

S87- Crushing injury of lower leg
Use additional code(s) for all associated injuries
Excludes❷: crushing injury of ankle and foot (S97.-)
The appropriate 7th character is to be added to each code from category S87:
  A Initial encounter
  D Subsequent encounter
  S Sequela
S87.0- Crushing injury of knee
    S87.00x- Crushing injury of unspecified knee
    S87.01x- Crushing injury of right knee
    S87.02x- Crushing injury of left knee
S87.8- Crushing injury of lower leg
    S87.80x- Crushing injury of unspecified lower leg
    S87.81x- Crushing injury of right lower leg
    S87.82x- Crushing injury of left lower leg

S88- Traumatic amputation of lower leg
Note: An amputation not identified as partial or complete should be coded to complete
Excludes 1: traumatic amputation of ankle and foot (S98.-)
The appropriate 7th character is to be added to each code from category S88:
  A Initial encounter
  D Subsequent encounter
  S Sequela
S88.0- Traumatic amputation at knee level
  S88.01- Complete traumatic amputation at knee level
    S88.011- Complete traumatic amputation at knee level, right lower leg
    S88.012- Complete traumatic amputation at knee level, left lower leg
    S88.019- Complete traumatic amputation at knee level, unspecified lower leg
  S88.02- Partial traumatic amputation at knee level
    S88.021- Partial traumatic amputation at knee level, right lower leg
    S88.022- Partial traumatic amputation at knee level, left lower leg
    S88.029- Partial traumatic amputation at knee level, unspecified lower leg
S88.1- Traumatic amputation at level between knee and ankle
  S88.11- Complete traumatic amputation at level between knee and ankle
    S88.111- Complete traumatic amputation at level between knee and ankle, right lower leg
    S88.112- Complete traumatic amputation at level between knee and ankle, left lower leg
    S88.119- Complete traumatic amputation at level between knee and ankle, unspecified lower leg
  S88.12- Partial traumatic amputation at level between knee and ankle
    S88.121- Partial traumatic amputation at level between knee and ankle, right lower leg
    S88.122- Partial traumatic amputation at level between knee and ankle, left lower leg
    S88.129- Partial traumatic amputation at level between knee and ankle, unspecified lower leg

S88.9- Traumatic amputation of lower leg, level unspecified
  S88.91- Complete traumatic amputation of lower leg, level unspecified
    S88.911- Complete traumatic amputation of right lower leg, level unspecified
    S88.912- Complete traumatic amputation of left lower leg, level unspecified
    S88.919- Complete traumatic amputation of unspecified lower leg, level unspecified
  S88.92- Partial traumatic amputation of lower leg, level unspecified
    S88.921- Partial traumatic amputation of right lower leg, level unspecified
    S88.922- Partial traumatic amputation of left lower leg, level unspecified
    S88.929- Partial traumatic amputation of unspecified lower leg, level unspecified

S89- Other and unspecified injuries of lower leg
Note: A fracture not indicated as open or closed should be coded to closed
Excludes❷: other and unspecified injuries of ankle and foot (S99.-)
The appropriate 7th character is to be added to each code from subcategories S89.0, S89.1, S89.2, and S89.3:
  A Initial encounter for closed fracture
  D Subsequent encounter for fracture with routine healing
  G Subsequent encounter for fracture with delayed healing
  K Subsequent encounter for fracture with nonunion
  P Subsequent encounter for fracture with malunion
  S Sequela
S89.0- Physeal fracture of upper end of tibia
  S89.00- Unspecified physeal fracture of upper end of tibia
    S89.001- Unspecified physeal fracture of upper end of right tibia
    S89.002- Unspecified physeal fracture of upper end of left tibia
    S89.009- Unspecified physeal fracture of upper end of unspecified tibia
  S89.01- Salter-Harris Type I physeal fracture of upper end of tibia
    S89.011- Salter-Harris Type I physeal fracture of upper end of right tibia
    S89.012- Salter-Harris Type I physeal fracture of upper end of left tibia
    S89.019- Salter-Harris Type I physeal fracture of upper end of unspecified tibia
  S89.02- Salter-Harris Type II physeal fracture of upper end of tibia
    S89.021- Salter-Harris Type II physeal fracture of upper end of right tibia
    S89.022- Salter-Harris Type II physeal fracture of upper end of left tibia
    S89.029- Salter-Harris Type II physeal fracture of upper end of unspecified tibia
  S89.03- Salter-Harris Type III physeal fracture of upper end of tibia
    S89.031- Salter-Harris Type III physeal fracture of upper end of right tibia
    S89.032- Salter-Harris Type III physeal fracture of upper end of left tibia
    S89.039- Salter-Harris Type III physeal fracture of upper end of unspecified tibia
  S89.04- Salter-Harris Type IV physeal fracture of upper end of tibia
    S89.041- Salter-Harris Type IV physeal fracture of upper end of right tibia
    S89.042- Salter-Harris Type IV physeal fracture of upper end of left tibia
    S89.049- Salter-Harris Type IV physeal fracture of upper end of unspecified tibia
  S89.09- Other physeal fracture of upper end of tibia
    S89.091- Other physeal fracture of upper end of right tibia
    S89.092- Other physeal fracture of upper end of left tibia
    S89.099- Other physeal fracture of upper end of unspecified tibia

S86 - S89

S89.1- __Physeal__ fracture of __lower end__ of __tibia__
  S89.10- __Unspecified physeal__ fracture of __lower end__ of __tibia__
    S89.101- Unspecified physeal fracture of lower end of __right__ tibia
    S89.102- Unspecified physeal fracture of lower end of __left__ tibia
    S89.109- Unspecified physeal fracture of lower end of __unspecified__ tibia
  S89.11- __Salter-Harris Type I__ physeal fracture of __lower end__ of __tibia__
    S89.111- Salter-Harris Type I physeal fracture of lower end of __right__ tibia
    S89.112- Salter-Harris Type I physeal fracture of lower end of __left__ tibia
    S89.119- Salter-Harris Type I physeal fracture of lower end of __unspecified__ tibia
  S89.12- __Salter-Harris Type II__ physeal fracture of __lower end__ of __tibia__
    S89.121- Salter-Harris Type II physeal fracture of lower end of __right__ tibia
    S89.122- Salter-Harris Type II physeal fracture of lower end of __left__ tibia
    S89.129- Salter-Harris Type II physeal fracture of lower end of __unspecified__ tibia
  S89.13- __Salter-Harris Type III__ physeal fracture of __lower end__ of __tibia__
    Excludes 1: fracture of medial malleolus (adult) (S82.5-)
    S89.131- Salter-Harris Type III physeal fracture of lower end of __right__ tibia
    S89.132- Salter-Harris Type III physeal fracture of lower end of __left__ tibia
    S89.139- Salter-Harris Type III physeal fracture of lower end of __unspecified__ tibia
  S89.14- __Salter-Harris Type IV__ physeal fracture of __lower end__ of __tibia__
    Excludes 1: fracture of medial malleolus (adult) (S82.5-)
    S89.141- Salter-Harris Type IV physeal fracture of lower end of __right__ tibia
    S89.142- Salter-Harris Type IV physeal fracture of lower end of __left__ tibia
    S89.149- Salter-Harris Type IV physeal fracture of lower end of __unspecified__ tibia
  S89.19- __Other physeal__ fracture of __lower end__ of __tibia__
    S89.191- Other physeal fracture of lower end of __right__ tibia
    S89.192- Other physeal fracture of lower end of __left__ tibia
    S89.199- Other physeal fracture of lower end of __unspecified__ tibia
S89.2- __Physeal fracture__ of __upper end__ of __fibula__
  S89.20- __Unspecified physeal__ fracture of __upper end__ of __fibula__
    S89.201- Unspecified physeal fracture of upper end of __right__ fibula
    S89.202- Unspecified physeal fracture of upper end of __left__ fibula
    S89.209- Unspecified physeal fracture of upper end of __unspecified__ fibula
  S89.21- __Salter-Harris Type I__ physeal fracture of __upper end__ of __fibula__
    S89.211- Salter-Harris Type I physeal fracture of upper end of __right__ fibula
    S89.212- Salter-Harris Type I physeal fracture of upper end of __left__ fibula
    S89.219- Salter-Harris Type I physeal fracture of upper end of __unspecified__ fibula
  S89.22- __Salter-Harris Type II__ physeal fracture of __upper end__ of __fibula__
    S89.221- Salter-Harris Type II physeal fracture of upper end of __right__ fibula
    S89.222- Salter-Harris Type II physeal fracture of upper end of __left__ fibula
    S89.229- Salter-Harris Type II physeal fracture of upper end of __unspecified__ fibula
  S89.29- __Other physeal__ fracture of __upper end__ of __fibula__
    S89.291- Other physeal fracture of upper end of __right__ fibula
    S89.292- Other physeal fracture of upper end of __left__ fibula
    S89.299- Other physeal fracture of upper end of __unspecified__ fibula
S89.3- __Physeal__ fracture of __lower end__ of __fibula__
  S89.30- Unspecified physeal fracture of lower end of fibula
    S89.301- Unspecified physeal fracture of lower end of __right__ fibula
    S89.302- Unspecified physeal fracture of lower end of __left__ fibula
    S89.309- Unspecified physeal fracture of lower end of __unspecified__ fibula

S89.31- __Salter-Harris Type I__ physeal fracture of __lower end__ of __fibula__
    S89.311- Salter-Harris Type I physeal fracture of lower end of __right__ fibula
    S89.312- Salter-Harris Type I physeal fracture of lower end of __left__ fibula
    S89.319- Salter-Harris Type I physeal fracture of lower end of __unspecified__ fibula
  S89.32- __Salter-Harris Type II__ physeal fracture of __lower end__ of __fibula__
    S89.321- Salter-Harris Type II physeal fracture of lower end of __right__ fibula
    S89.322- Salter-Harris Type II physeal fracture of lower end of __left__ fibula
    S89.329- Salter-Harris Type II physeal fracture of lower end of __unspecified__ fibula
  S89.39- __Other physeal__ fracture of __lower end__ of __fibula__
    S89.391- Other physeal fracture of lower end of __right__ fibula
    S89.392- Other physeal fracture of lower end of __left__ fibula
    S89.399- Other physeal fracture of lower end of __unspecified__ fibula
S89.8- __Other specified injuries__ of __lower leg__
  The appropriate 7th character is to be added to each code in subcategory S89.8:
    A __Initial__ encounter
    D __Subsequent__ encounter
    S __Sequela__
  S89.80x- Other specified injuries of __unspecified__ lower leg
  S89.81x- Other specified injuries of __right__ lower leg
  S89.82x- Other specified injuries of __left__ lower leg
S89.9- __Unspecified injury__ of __lower leg__
  The appropriate 7th character is to be added to each code in subcategory S89.9:
    A __Initial__ encounter
    D __Subsequent__ encounter
    S __Sequela__
  S89.90x- Unspecified injury of __unspecified__ lower leg
  S89.91x- Unspecified injury of __right__ lower leg
  S89.92x- Unspecified injury of __left__ lower leg

Injuries to the ankle and foot (S90-S99)

Excludes ❷: burns and corrosions (T20-T32)
   fracture of ankle and malleolus (S82.-)
   frostbite (T33-T34)
   insect bite or sting, venomous (T63.4)

S90- __Superficial injury__ of __ankle, foot and toes__
  The appropriate 7th character is to be added to each code from category S90:
    A __Initial__ encounter
    D __Subsequent__ encounter
    S __Sequela__
S90.0- __Contusion__ of __ankle__
  S90.00x- Contusion of __unspecified__ ankle
  S90.01x- Contusion of __right__ ankle
  S90.02x- Contusion of __left__ ankle
S90.1- __Contusion__ of __toe without__ damage to nail
  S90.11- __Contusion__ of __great toe without__ damage to nail
    S90.111- Contusion of __right__ great toe __without__ damage to nail
    S90.112- Contusion of __left__ great toe __without__ damage to nail
    S90.119- Contusion of __unspecified__ great toe __without__ damage to nail
  S90.12- __Contusion__ of __lesser toe without__ damage to nail
    S90.121- Contusion of __right__ lesser toe(s) __without__ damage to nail
    S90.122- Contusion of __left__ lesser toe(s) __without__ damage to nail
    S90.129- Contusion of __unspecified__ lesser toe(s) __without__ damage to nail
      Contusion of toe NOS
S90.2- __Contusion__ of __toe with__ damage to nail
  S90.21- Contusion of __great toe with__ damage to nail
    S90.211- Contusion of __right__ great toe with damage to nail
    S90.212- Contusion of __left__ great toe with damage to nail
    S90.219- Contusion of __unspecified__ great toe with damage to nail
  S90.22- __Contusion__ of __lesser toe with__ damage to nail
    S90.221- Contusion of __right__ lesser toe(s) with damage to nail
    S90.222- Contusion of __left__ lesser toe(s) with damage to nail
    S90.229- Contusion of __unspecified__ lesser toe(s) with damage to nail

S89 - S91

S90.3- **Contusion** of foot
Excludes❷: contusion of toes (S90.1-, S90.2-)
S90.30x- Contusion of unspecified foot
Contusion of foot NOS
S90.31x- Contusion of right foot
S90.32x- Contusion of left foot
S90.4- **Other superficial injuries** of toe
S90.41- **Abrasion** of toe
S90.411- Abrasion, right great toe
S90.412- Abrasion, left great toe
S90.413- Abrasion, unspecified great toe
S90.414- Abrasion, right lesser toe(s)
S90.415- Abrasion, left lesser toe(s)
S90.416- Abrasion, unspecified lesser toe(s)
S90.42- **Blister** (nonthermal) of toe
S90.421- Blister (nonthermal), right great toe
S90.422- Blister (nonthermal), left great toe
S90.423- Blister (nonthermal), unspecified great toe
S90.424- Blister (nonthermal), right lesser toe(s)
S90.425- Blister (nonthermal), left lesser toe(s)
S90.426- Blister (nonthermal), unspecified lesser toe(s)
S90.44- **External constriction** of toe
Hair tourniquet syndrome of toe
S90.441- External constriction, right great toe
S90.442- External constriction, left great toe
S90.443- External constriction, unspecified great toe
S90.444- External constriction, right lesser toe(s)
S90.445- External constriction, left lesser toe(s)
S90.446- External constriction, unspecified lesser toe(s)
S90.45- **Superficial foreign body** of toe
Splinter in the toe
S90.451- Superficial foreign body, right great toe
S90.452- Superficial foreign body, left great toe
S90.453- Superficial foreign body, unspecified great toe
S90.454- Superficial foreign body, right lesser toe(s)
S90.455- Superficial foreign body, left lesser toe(s)
S90.456- Superficial foreign body, unspecified lesser toe(s)
S90.46- **Insect bite** (nonvenomous) of toe
S90.461- Insect bite (nonvenomous), right great toe
S90.462- Insect bite (nonvenomous), left great toe
S90.463- Insect bite (nonvenomous), unspecified great toe
S90.464- Insect bite (nonvenomous), right lesser toe(s)
S90.465- Insect bite (nonvenomous), left lesser toe(s)
S90.466- Insect bite (nonvenomous), unspecified lesser toe(s)
S90.47- **Other superficial bite** of toe
Excludes 1: open bite of toe (S91.15-, S91.25-)
S90.471- Other superficial bite of right great toe
S90.472- Other superficial bite of left great toe
S90.473- Other superficial bite of unspecified great toe
S90.474- Other superficial bite of right lesser toe(s)
S90.475- Other superficial bite of left lesser toe(s)
S90.476- Other superficial bite of unspecified lesser toe(s)
S90.5- **Other superficial injuries** of ankle
S90.51- **Abrasion** of ankle
S90.511- Abrasion, right ankle
S90.512- Abrasion, left ankle
S90.519- Abrasion, unspecified ankle
S90.52- **Blister** (nonthermal) of ankle
S90.521- Blister (nonthermal), right ankle
S90.522- Blister (nonthermal), left ankle
S90.529- Blister (nonthermal), unspecified ankle
S90.54- **External constriction** of ankle
S90.541- External constriction, right ankle
S90.542- External constriction, left ankle
S90.549- External constriction, unspecified ankle
S90.55- **Superficial foreign body** of ankle
Splinter in the ankle
S90.551- Superficial foreign body, right ankle
S90.552- Superficial foreign body, left ankle
S90.559- Superficial foreign body, unspecified ankle
S90.56- **Insect bite** (nonvenomous) of ankle
S90.561- Insect bite (nonvenomous), right ankle
S90.562- Insect bite (nonvenomous), left ankle
S90.569- Insect bite (nonvenomous), unspecified ankle

S90.57- **Other superficial bite** of ankle
Excludes 1: open bite of ankle (S91.05-)
S90.571- Other superficial bite of ankle, right ankle
S90.572- Other superficial bite of ankle, left ankle
S90.579- Other superficial bite of ankle, unspecified ankle
S90.8- **Other superficial injuries** of foot
S90.81- **Abrasion** of foot
S90.811- Abrasion, right foot
S90.812- Abrasion, left foot
S90.819- Abrasion, unspecified foot
S90.82- **Blister** (nonthermal) of foot
S90.821- Blister (nonthermal), right foot
S90.822- Blister (nonthermal), left foot
S90.829- Blister (nonthermal), unspecified foot
S90.84- **External constriction** of foot
S90.841- External constriction, right foot
S90.842- External constriction, left foot
S90.849- External constriction, unspecified foot
S90.85- **Superficial foreign body** of foot
Splinter in the foot
S90.851- Superficial foreign body, right foot
S90.852- Superficial foreign body, left foot
S90.859- Superficial foreign body, unspecified foot
S90.86- **Insect bite** (nonvenomous) of foot
S90.861- Insect bite (nonvenomous), right foot
S90.862- Insect bite (nonvenomous), left foot
S90.869- Insect bite (nonvenomous), unspecified foot
S90.87- **Other superficial bite** of foot
Excludes 1: open bite of foot (S91.35-)
S90.871- Other superficial bite of right foot
S90.872- Other superficial bite of left foot
S90.879- Other superficial bite of unspecified foot
S90.9- **Unspecified superficial injury** of ankle, foot and toe
S90.91- **Unspecified** superficial injury of ankle
S90.911- Unspecified superficial injury of right ankle
S90.912- Unspecified superficial injury of left ankle
S90.919- Unspecified superficial injury of unspecified ankle
S90.92- **Unspecified** superficial injury of foot
S90.921- Unspecified superficial injury of right foot
S90.922- Unspecified superficial injury of left foot
S90.929- Unspecified superficial injury of unspecified foot
S90.93- **Unspecified** superficial injury of toes
S90.931- Unspecified superficial injury of right great toe
S90.932- Unspecified superficial injury of left great toe
S90.933- Unspecified superficial injury of unspecified great toe
S90.934- Unspecified superficial injury of right lesser toe(s)
S90.935- Unspecified superficial injury of left lesser toe(s)
S90.936- Unspecified superficial injury of unspecified lesser toe(s)
S91- **Open wound** of ankle, foot and toes
Code also any associated wound infection
Excludes 1: open fracture of ankle, foot and toes (S92.-with 7th character B)
traumatic amputation of ankle and foot (S98.-)
The appropriate 7th character is to be added to each code from category S91:
A Initial encounter
D Subsequent encounter
S Sequela
S91.0- **Open wound** of ankle
S91.00- **Unspecified** open wound of ankle
S91.001- Unspecified open wound, right ankle
S91.002- Unspecified open wound, left ankle
S91.009- Unspecified open wound, unspecified ankle
S91.01- **Laceration** without foreign body of ankle
S91.011- Laceration without foreign body, right ankle
S91.012- Laceration without foreign body, left ankle
S91.019- Laceration without foreign body, unspecified ankle
S91.02- **Laceration** with foreign body of ankle
S91.021- Laceration with foreign body, right ankle
S91.022- Laceration with foreign body, left ankle
S91.029- Laceration with foreign body, unspecified ankle

S89 - S91

S91.03- Puncture wound without foreign body of ankle
  S91.031- Puncture wound without foreign body, right ankle
  S91.032- Puncture wound without foreign body, left ankle
  S91.039- Puncture wound without foreign body, unspecified ankle
S91.04- Puncture wound with foreign body of ankle
  S91.041- Puncture wound with foreign body, right ankle
  S91.042- Puncture wound with foreign body, left ankle
  S91.049- Puncture wound with foreign body, unspecified ankle
S91.05- Open bite of ankle
  Excludes 1: superficial bite of ankle (S90.56-, S90.57-)
  S91.051- Open bite, right ankle
  S91.052- Open bite, left ankle
  S91.059- Open bite, unspecified ankle
S91.1- Open wound of toe without damage to nail
  S91.10- Unspecified open wound of toe without damage to nail
    S91.101- Unspecified open wound of right great toe without damage to nail
    S91.102- Unspecified open wound of left great toe without damage to nail
    S91.103- Unspecified open wound of unspecified great toe without damage to nail
    S91.104- Unspecified open wound of right lesser toe(s) without damage to nail
    S91.105- Unspecified open wound of left lesser toe(s) without damage to nail
    S91.106- Unspecified open wound of unspecified lesser toe(s) without damage to nail
    S91.109- Unspecified open wound of unspecified toe(s) without damage to nail
  S91.11- Laceration without foreign body of toe without damage to nail
    S91.111- Laceration without foreign body of right great toe without damage to nail
    S91.112- Laceration without foreign body of left great toe without damage to nail
    S91.113- Laceration without foreign body of unspecified great toe without damage to nail
    S91.114- Laceration without foreign body of right lesser toe(s) without damage to nail
    S91.115- Laceration without foreign body of left lesser toe(s) without damage to nail
    S91.116- Laceration without foreign body of unspecified lesser toe(s) without damage to nail
    S91.119- Laceration without foreign body of unspecified toe without damage to nail
  S91.12- Laceration with foreign body of toe without damage to nail
    S91.121- Laceration with foreign body of right great toe without damage to nail
    S91.122- Laceration with foreign body of left great toe without damage to nail
    S91.123- Laceration with foreign body of unspecified great toe without damage to nail
    S91.124- Laceration with foreign body of right lesser toe(s) without damage to nail
    S91.125- Laceration with foreign body of left lesser toe(s) without damage to nail
    S91.126- Laceration with foreign body of unspecified lesser toe(s) without damage to nail
    S91.129- Laceration with foreign body of unspecified toe(s) without damage to nail
  S91.13- Puncture wound without foreign body of toe without damage to nail
    S91.131- Puncture wound without foreign body of right great toe without damage to nail
    S91.132- Puncture wound without foreign body of left great toe without damage to nail
    S91.133- Puncture wound without foreign body of unspecified great toe without damage to nail
    S91.134- Puncture wound without foreign body of right lesser toe(s) without damage to nail
    S91.135- Puncture wound without foreign body of left lesser toe(s) without damage to nail
    S91.136- Puncture wound without foreign body of unspecified lesser toe(s) without damage to nail
    S91.139- Puncture wound without foreign body of unspecified toe(s) without damage to nail

S91.14- Puncture wound with foreign body of toe without damage to nail
  S91.141- Puncture wound with foreign body of right great toe without damage to nail
  S91.142- Puncture wound with foreign body of left great toe without damage to nail
  S91.143- Puncture wound with foreign body of unspecified great toe without damage to nail
  S91.144- Puncture wound with foreign body of right lesser toe(s) without damage to nail
  S91.145- Puncture wound with foreign body of left lesser toe(s) without damage to nail
  S91.146- Puncture wound with foreign body of unspecified lesser toe(s) without damage to nail
  S91.149- Puncture wound with foreign body of unspecified toe(s) without damage to nail
S91.15- Open bite of toe without damage to nail
  Bite of toe NOS
  Excludes 1: superficial bite of toe (S90.46-, S90.47-)
  S91.151- Open bite of right great toe without damage to nail
  S91.152- Open bite of left great toe without damage to nail
  S91.153- Open bite of unspecified great toe without damage to nail
  S91.154- Open bite of right lesser toe(s) without damage to nail
  S91.155- Open bite of left lesser toe(s) without damage to nail
  S91.156- Open bite of unspecified lesser toe(s) without damage to nail
  S91.159- Open bite of unspecified toe(s) without damage to nail
S91.2- Open wound of toe with damage to nail
  S91.20- Unspecified open wound of toe with damage to nail
    S91.201- Unspecified open wound of right great toe with damage to nail
    S91.202- Unspecified open wound of left great toe with damage to nail
    S91.203- Unspecified open wound of unspecified great toe with damage to nail
    S91.204- Unspecified open wound of right lesser toe(s) with damage to nail
    S91.205- Unspecified open wound of left lesser toe(s) with damage to nail
    S91.206- Unspecified open wound of unspecified lesser toe(s) with damage to nail
    S91.209- Unspecified open wound of unspecified toe(s) with damage to nail
  S91.21- Laceration without foreign body of toe with damage to nail
    S91.211- Laceration without foreign body of right great toe with damage to nail
    S91.212- Laceration without foreign body of left great toe with damage to nail
    S91.213- Laceration without foreign body of unspecified great toe with damage to nail
    S91.214- Laceration without foreign body of right lesser toe(s) with damage to nail
    S91.215- Laceration without foreign body of left lesser toe(s) with damage to nail
    S91.216- Laceration without foreign body of unspecified lesser toe(s) with damage to nail
    S91.219- Laceration without foreign body of unspecified toe(s) with damage to nail
  S91.22- Laceration with foreign body of toe with damage to nail
    S91.221- Laceration with foreign body of right great toe with damage to nail
    S91.222- Laceration with foreign body of left great toe with damage to nail
    S91.223- Laceration with foreign body of unspecified great toe with damage to nail
    S91.224- Laceration with foreign body of right lesser toe(s) with damage to nail
    S91.225- Laceration with foreign body of left lesser toe(s) with damage to nail
    S91.226- Laceration with foreign body of unspecified lesser toe(s) with damage to nail
    S91.229- Laceration with foreign body of unspecified toe(s) with damage to nail

S91.23- Puncture wound without foreign body of toe with damage to nail

    S91.231- Puncture wound without foreign body of right great toe with damage to nail

    S91.232- Puncture wound without foreign body of left great toe with damage to nail

    S91.233- Puncture wound without foreign body of unspecified great toe with damage to nail

    S91.234- Puncture wound without foreign body of right lesser toe(s) with damage to nail

    S91.235- Puncture wound without foreign body of left lesser toe(s) with damage to nail

    S91.236- Puncture wound without foreign body of unspecified lesser toe(s) with damage to nail

    S91.239- Puncture wound without foreign body of unspecified toe(s) with damage to nail

S91.24- Puncture wound with foreign body of toe with damage to nail

    S91.241- Puncture wound with foreign body of right great toe with damage to nail

    S91.242- Puncture wound with foreign body of left great toe with damage to nail

    S91.243- Puncture wound with foreign body of unspecified great toe with damage to nail

    S91.244- Puncture wound with foreign body of right lesser toe(s) with damage to nail

    S91.245- Puncture wound with foreign body of left lesser toe(s) with damage to nail

    S91.246- Puncture wound with foreign body of unspecified lesser toe(s) with damage to nail

    S91.249- Puncture wound with foreign body of unspecified toe(s) with damage to nail

S91.25- Open bite of toe with damage to nail
    Bite of toe with damage to nail NOS
    Excludes 1: superficial bite of toe (S90.46-, S90.47-)

    S91.251- Open bite of right great toe with damage to nail
    S91.252- Open bite of left great toe with damage to nail
    S91.253- Open bite of unspecified great toe with damage to nail
    S91.254- Open bite of right lesser toe(s) with damage to nail
    S91.255- Open bite of left lesser toe(s) with damage to nail
    S91.256- Open bite of unspecified lesser toe(s) with damage to nail
    S91.259- Open bite of unspecified toe(s) with damage to nail

S91.3- Open wound of foot
  S91.30- Unspecified open wound of foot
    S91.301- Unspecified open wound, right foot
    S91.302- Unspecified open wound, left foot
    S91.309- Unspecified open wound, unspecified foot
  S91.31- Laceration without foreign body of foot
    S91.311- Laceration without foreign body, right foot
    S91.312- Laceration without foreign body, left foot
    S91.319- Laceration without foreign body, unspecified foot
  S91.32- Laceration with foreign body of foot
    S91.321- Laceration with foreign body, right foot
    S91.322- Laceration with foreign body, left foot
    S91.329- Laceration with foreign body, unspecified foot
  S91.33- Puncture wound without foreign body of foot
    S91.331- Puncture wound without foreign body, right foot
    S91.332- Puncture wound without foreign body, left foot
    S91.339- Puncture wound without foreign body, unspecified foot
  S91.34- Puncture wound with foreign body of foot
    S91.341- Puncture wound with foreign body, right foot
    S91.342- Puncture wound with foreign body, left foot
    S91.349- Puncture wound with foreign body, unspecified foot
  S91.35- Open bite of foot
    Excludes 1: superficial bite of foot (S90.86-, S90.87-)
    S91.351- Open bite, right foot
    S91.352- Open bite, left foot
    S91.359- Open bite, unspecified foot

S92- Fracture of foot and toe, except ankle
  Note: A fracture not indicated as displaced or nondisplaced should be coded to displaced
  Note: A fracture not indicated as open or closed should be coded to closed
  Excludes 1: traumatic amputation of ankle and foot (S98.-)
  Excludes ❷: fracture of ankle (S82.-)
            fracture of malleolus (S82.-)

The appropriate 7th character is to be added to each code from category S92:
A   Initial encounter for closed fracture
B   Initial encounter for open fracture
D   Subsequent encounter for fracture with routine healing
G   Subsequent encounter for fracture with delayed healing
K   Subsequent encounter for fracture with nonunion
P   Subsequent encounter for fracture with malunion
S   Sequela

S92.0- Fracture of calcaneus
  Heel bone
  Os calcis
  S92.00- Unspecified fracture of calcaneus
    S92.001- Unspecified fracture of right calcaneus
    S92.002- Unspecified fracture of left calcaneus
    S92.009- Unspecified fracture of unspecified calcaneus
  S92.01- Fracture of body of calcaneus
    S92.011- Displaced fracture of body of right calcaneus
    S92.012- Displaced fracture of body of left calcaneus
    S92.013- Displaced fracture of body of unspecified calcaneus
    S92.014- Nondisplaced fracture of body of right calcaneus
    S92.015- Nondisplaced fracture of body of left calcaneus
    S92.016- Nondisplaced fracture of body of unspecified calcaneus
  S92.02- Fracture of anterior process of calcaneus
    S92.021- Displaced fracture of anterior process of right calcaneus
    S92.022- Displaced fracture of anterior process of left calcaneus
    S92.023- Displaced fracture of anterior process of unspecified calcaneus
    S92.024- Nondisplaced fracture of anterior process of right calcaneus
    S92.025- Nondisplaced fracture of anterior process of left calcaneus
    S92.026- Nondisplaced fracture of anterior process of unspecified calcaneus
  S92.03- Avulsion fracture of tuberosity of calcaneus
    S92.031- Displaced avulsion fracture of tuberosity of right calcaneus
    S92.032- Displaced avulsion fracture of tuberosity of left calcaneus
    S92.033- Displaced avulsion fracture of tuberosity of unspecified calcaneus
    S92.034- Nondisplaced avulsion fracture of tuberosity of right calcaneus
    S92.035- Nondisplaced avulsion fracture of tuberosity of left calcaneus
    S92.036- Nondisplaced avulsion fracture of tuberosity of unspecified calcaneus
  S92.04- Other fracture of tuberosity of calcaneus
    S92.041- Displaced other fracture of tuberosity of right calcaneus
    S92.042- Displaced other fracture of tuberosity of left calcaneus
    S92.043- Displaced other fracture of tuberosity of unspecified calcaneus
    S92.044- Nondisplaced other fracture of tuberosity of right calcaneus
    S92.045- Nondisplaced other fracture of tuberosity of left calcaneus
    S92.046- Nondisplaced other fracture of tuberosity of unspecified calcaneus
  S92.05- Other extraarticular fracture of calcaneus
    S92.051- Displaced other extraarticular fracture of right calcaneus
    S92.052- Displaced other extraarticular fracture of left calcaneus
    S92.053- Displaced other extraarticular fracture of unspecified calcaneus
    S92.054- Nondisplaced other extraarticular fracture of right calcaneus

S91
-
S92

S92.055- <u>Nondisplaced</u> other extraarticular fracture of <u>left</u> calcaneus

S92.056- <u>Nondisplaced</u> other extraarticular fracture of <u>unspecified</u> calcaneus

S92.06- <u>Intraarticular</u> fracture of <u>calcaneus</u>

S92.061- <u>Displaced</u> intraarticular fracture of <u>right</u> calcaneus

S92.062- <u>Displaced</u> intraarticular fracture of <u>left</u> calcaneus

S92.063- <u>Displaced</u> intraarticular fracture of <u>unspecified</u> calcaneus

S92.064- <u>Nondisplaced</u> intraarticular fracture of <u>right</u> calcaneus

S92.065- <u>Nondisplaced</u> intraarticular fracture of <u>left</u> calcaneus

S92.066- <u>Nondisplaced</u> intraarticular fracture of <u>unspecified</u> calcaneus

S92.1- <u>Fracture</u> of <u>talus</u>
   Astragalus

S92.10- <u>Unspecified</u> fracture of <u>talus</u>

S92.101- Unspecified fracture of <u>right</u> talus

S92.102- Unspecified fracture of <u>left</u> talus

S92.109- Unspecified fracture of <u>unspecified</u> talus

S92.11- Fracture of <u>neck</u> of <u>talus</u>

S92.111- <u>Displaced</u> fracture of neck of <u>right</u> talus

S92.112- <u>Displaced</u> fracture of neck of <u>left</u> talus

S92.113- <u>Displaced</u> fracture of neck of <u>unspecified</u> talus

S92.114- <u>Nondisplaced</u> fracture of neck of <u>right</u> talus

S92.115- <u>Nondisplaced</u> fracture of neck of <u>left</u> talus

S92.116- <u>Nondisplaced</u> fracture of neck of <u>unspecified</u> talus

S92.12- Fracture of <u>body</u> of <u>talus</u>

S92.121- <u>Displaced</u> fracture of body of <u>right</u> talus

S92.122- <u>Displaced</u> fracture of body of <u>left</u> talus

S92.123- <u>Displaced</u> fracture of body of <u>unspecified</u> talus

S92.124- <u>Nondisplaced</u> fracture of body of <u>right</u> talus

S92.125- <u>Nondisplaced</u> fracture of body of <u>left</u> talus

S92.126- <u>Nondisplaced</u> fracture of body of <u>unspecified</u> talus

S92.13- Fracture of <u>posterior process</u> of <u>talus</u>

S92.131- <u>Displaced</u> fracture of posterior process of <u>right</u> talus

S92.132- <u>Displaced</u> fracture of posterior process of <u>left</u> talus

S92.133- <u>Displaced</u> fracture of posterior process of <u>unspecified</u> talus

S92.134- <u>Nondisplaced</u> fracture of posterior process of <u>right</u> talus

S92.135- <u>Nondisplaced</u> fracture of posterior process of <u>left</u> talus

S92.136- <u>Nondisplaced</u> fracture of posterior process of <u>unspecified</u> talus

S92.14- <u>Dome</u> fracture of <u>talus</u>
   Excludes 1: osteochondritis dissecans (M93.2)

S92.141- <u>Displaced</u> dome fracture of <u>right</u> talus

S92.142- <u>Displaced</u> dome fracture of <u>left</u> talus

S92.143- <u>Displaced</u> dome fracture of <u>unspecified</u> talus

S92.144- <u>Nondisplaced</u> dome fracture of <u>right</u> talus

S92.145- <u>Nondisplaced</u> dome fracture of <u>left</u> talus

S92.146- <u>Nondisplaced</u> dome fracture of <u>unspecified</u> talus

S92.15- <u>Avulsion</u> fracture (chip fracture) of <u>talus</u>

S92.151- <u>Displaced</u> avulsion fracture (chip fracture) of <u>right</u> talus

S92.152- <u>Displaced</u> avulsion fracture (chip fracture) of <u>left</u> talus

S92.153- <u>Displaced</u> avulsion fracture (chip fracture) of <u>unspecified</u> talus

S92.154- <u>Nondisplaced</u> avulsion fracture (chip fracture) of <u>right</u> talus

S92.155- <u>Nondisplaced</u> avulsion fracture (chip fracture) of <u>left</u> talus

S92.156- <u>Nondisplaced</u> avulsion fracture (chip fracture) of <u>unspecified</u> talus

S92.19- <u>Other fracture</u> of <u>talus</u>

S92.191- Other fracture of <u>right</u> talus

S92.192- Other fracture of <u>left</u> talus

S92.199- Other fracture of <u>unspecified</u> talus

S92.2- Fracture of <u>other and unspecified</u> <u>tarsal</u> bone(s)

S92.20- Fracture of <u>unspecified</u> tarsal bone(s)

S92.201- Fracture of <u>unspecified</u> tarsal bone(s) of <u>right</u> foot

S92.202- Fracture of <u>unspecified</u> tarsal bone(s) of <u>left</u> foot

S92.209- Fracture of <u>unspecified</u> tarsal bone(s) of <u>unspecified</u> foot

S92.21- Fracture of <u>cuboid</u> bone

S92.211- <u>Displaced</u> fracture of cuboid bone of <u>right</u> foot

S92.212- <u>Displaced</u> fracture of cuboid bone of <u>left</u> foot

S92.213- <u>Displaced</u> fracture of cuboid bone of <u>unspecified</u> foot

S92.214- <u>Nondisplaced</u> fracture of cuboid bone of <u>right</u> foot

S92.215- <u>Nondisplaced</u> fracture of cuboid bone of <u>left</u> foot

S92.216- <u>Nondisplaced</u> fracture of cuboid bone of <u>unspecified</u> foot

S92.22- Fracture of <u>lateral cuneiform</u>

S92.221- <u>Displaced</u> fracture of lateral cuneiform of <u>right</u> foot

S92.222- <u>Displaced</u> fracture of lateral cuneiform of <u>left</u> foot

S92.223- <u>Displaced</u> fracture of lateral cuneiform of <u>unspecified</u> foot

S92.224- <u>Nondisplaced</u> fracture of lateral cuneiform of <u>right</u> foot

S92.225- <u>Nondisplaced</u> fracture of lateral cuneiform of <u>left</u> foot

S92.226- <u>Nondisplaced</u> fracture of lateral cuneiform of <u>unspecified</u> foot

S92.23- Fracture of <u>intermediate cuneiform</u>

S92.231- <u>Displaced</u> fracture of intermediate cuneiform of <u>right</u> foot

S92.232- <u>Displaced</u> fracture of intermediate cuneiform of <u>left</u> foot

S92.233- <u>Displaced</u> fracture of intermediate cuneiform of <u>unspecified</u> foot

S92.234- <u>Nondisplaced</u> fracture of intermediate cuneiform of <u>right</u> foot

S92.235- <u>Nondisplaced</u> fracture of intermediate cuneiform of <u>left</u> foot

S92.236- <u>Nondisplaced</u> fracture of intermediate cuneiform of <u>unspecified</u> foot

S92.24- Fracture of <u>medial cuneiform</u>

S92.241- <u>Displaced</u> fracture of medial cuneiform of <u>right</u> foot

S92.242- <u>Displaced</u> fracture of medial cuneiform of <u>left</u> foot

S92.243- <u>Displaced</u> fracture of medial cuneiform of <u>unspecified</u> foot

S92.244- <u>Nondisplaced</u> fracture of medial cuneiform of <u>right</u> foot

S92.245- <u>Nondisplaced</u> fracture of medial cuneiform of <u>left</u> foot

S92.246- <u>Nondisplaced</u> fracture of medial cuneiform of <u>unspecified</u> foot

S92.25- Fracture of <u>navicular [scaphoid]</u> of <u>foot</u>

S92.251- <u>Displaced</u> fracture of navicular [scaphoid] of <u>right</u> foot

S92.252- <u>Displaced</u> fracture of navicular [scaphoid] of <u>left</u> foot

S92.253- <u>Displaced</u> fracture of navicular [scaphoid] of <u>unspecified</u> foot

S92.254- <u>Nondisplaced</u> fracture of navicular [scaphoid] of <u>right</u> foot

S92.255- <u>Nondisplaced</u> fracture of navicular [scaphoid] of <u>left</u> foot

S92.256- <u>Nondisplaced</u> fracture of navicular [scaphoid] of <u>unspecified</u> foot

S92.3- <u>Fracture</u> of <u>metatarsal</u> bone(s)

S92.30- Fracture of <u>unspecified</u> <u>metatarsal</u> bone(s)

S92.301- Fracture of <u>unspecified</u> metatarsal bone(s), <u>right</u> foot

S92.302- Fracture of <u>unspecified</u> metatarsal bone(s), <u>left</u> foot

S92.309- Fracture of <u>unspecified</u> metatarsal bone(s), <u>unspecified</u> foot

S92.31- Fracture of first metatarsal bone

S92.311- <u>Displaced</u> fracture of first metatarsal bone, <u>right</u> foot

S92.312- <u>Displaced</u> fracture of first metatarsal bone, <u>left</u> foot

S92.313- <u>Displaced</u> fracture of first metatarsal bone, <u>unspecified</u> foot

S92.314- <u>Nondisplaced</u> fracture of first metatarsal bone, <u>right</u> foot

S92.315- <u>Nondisplaced</u> fracture of first metatarsal bone, <u>left</u> foot

S92.316- <u>Nondisplaced</u> fracture of first metatarsal bone, <u>unspecified</u> foot

S92.32- Fracture of <u>second</u> metatarsal bone
    S92.321- <u>Displaced</u> fracture of second metatarsal bone, <u>right</u> foot
    S92.322- <u>Displaced</u> fracture of second metatarsal bone, <u>left</u> foot
    S92.323- <u>Displaced</u> fracture of second metatarsal bone, <u>unspecified</u> foot
    S92.324- <u>Nondisplaced</u> fracture of second metatarsal bone, <u>right</u> foot
    S92.325- <u>Nondisplaced</u> fracture of second metatarsal bone, <u>left</u> foot
    S92.326- <u>Nondisplaced</u> fracture of second metatarsal bone, <u>unspecified</u> foot
S92.33- Fracture of <u>third</u> metatarsal bone
    S92.331- <u>Displaced</u> fracture of third metatarsal bone, <u>right</u> foot
    S92.332- <u>Displaced</u> fracture of third metatarsal bone, <u>left</u> foot
    S92.333- <u>Displaced</u> fracture of third metatarsal bone, <u>unspecified</u> foot
    S92.334- <u>Nondisplaced</u> fracture of third metatarsal bone, <u>right</u> foot
    S92.335- <u>Nondisplaced</u> fracture of third metatarsal bone, <u>left</u> foot
    S92.336- <u>Nondisplaced</u> fracture of third metatarsal bone, <u>unspecified</u> foot
S92.34- Fracture of <u>fourth</u> metatarsal bone
    S92.341- <u>Displaced</u> fracture of fourth metatarsal bone, <u>right</u> foot
    S92.342- <u>Displaced</u> fracture of fourth metatarsal bone, <u>left</u> foot
    S92.343- <u>Displaced</u> fracture of fourth metatarsal bone, <u>unspecified</u> foot
    S92.344- <u>Nondisplaced</u> fracture of fourth metatarsal bone, <u>right</u> foot
    S92.345- <u>Nondisplaced</u> fracture of fourth metatarsal bone, <u>left</u> foot
    S92.346- <u>Nondisplaced</u> fracture of fourth metatarsal bone, <u>unspecified</u> foot
S92.35- Fracture of <u>fifth</u> metatarsal bone
    S92.351- <u>Displaced</u> fracture of fifth metatarsal bone, <u>right</u> foot
    S92.352- <u>Displaced</u> fracture of fifth metatarsal bone, <u>left</u> foot
    S92.353- <u>Displaced</u> fracture of fifth metatarsal bone, <u>unspecified</u> foot
    S92.354- <u>Nondisplaced</u> fracture of fifth metatarsal bone, <u>right</u> foot
    S92.355- <u>Nondisplaced</u> fracture of fifth metatarsal bone, <u>left</u> foot
    S92.356- <u>Nondisplaced</u> fracture of fifth metatarsal bone, <u>unspecified</u> foot
S92.4- <u>Fracture</u> of <u>great toe</u>
    S92.40- <u>Unspecified</u> fracture of <u>great</u> <u>toe</u>
        S92.401- <u>Displaced</u> unspecified fracture of <u>right</u> great toe
        S92.402- <u>Displaced</u> unspecified fracture of <u>left</u> great toe
        S92.403- <u>Displaced</u> unspecified fracture of <u>unspecified</u> great toe
        S92.404- <u>Nondisplaced</u> unspecified fracture of <u>right</u> great toe
        S92.405- <u>Nondisplaced</u> unspecified fracture of <u>left</u> great toe
        S92.406- <u>Nondisplaced</u> unspecified fracture of <u>unspecified</u> great toe
    S92.41- Fracture of <u>proximal phalanx</u> of <u>great</u> <u>toe</u>
        S92.411- <u>Displaced</u> fracture of proximal phalanx of <u>right</u> great toe
        S92.412- <u>Displaced</u> fracture of proximal phalanx of <u>left</u> great toe
        S92.413- <u>Displaced</u> fracture of proximal phalanx of <u>unspecified</u> great toe
        S92.414- <u>Nondisplaced</u> fracture of proximal phalanx of <u>right</u> great toe
        S92.415- <u>Nondisplaced</u> fracture of proximal phalanx of <u>left</u> great toe
        S92.416- <u>Nondisplaced</u> fracture of proximal phalanx of <u>unspecified</u> great toe
    S92.42- Fracture of <u>distal phalanx</u> of <u>great</u> <u>toe</u>
        S92.421- <u>Displaced</u> fracture of distal phalanx of <u>right</u> great toe
        S92.422- <u>Displaced</u> fracture of distal phalanx of <u>left</u> great toe
        S92.423- <u>Displaced</u> fracture of distal phalanx of <u>unspecified</u> great toe
        S92.424- <u>Nondisplaced</u> fracture of distal phalanx of <u>right</u> great toe
        S92.425- <u>Nondisplaced</u> fracture of distal phalanx of <u>left</u> great toe
        S92.426- <u>Nondisplaced</u> fracture of distal phalanx of <u>unspecified</u> great toe

S92.49- <u>Other fracture</u> of <u>great toe</u>
    S92.491- Other fracture of <u>right</u> great toe
    S92.492- Other fracture of <u>left</u> great toe
    S92.499- Other fracture of <u>unspecified</u> great toe
S92.5- <u>Fracture</u> of <u>lesser toe(s)</u>
    S92.50- <u>Unspecified</u> fracture of <u>lesser toe(s)</u>
        S92.501- <u>Displaced</u> unspecified fracture of <u>right</u> lesser toe(s)
        S92.502- <u>Displaced</u> unspecified fracture of <u>left</u> lesser toe(s)
        S92.503- <u>Displaced</u> unspecified fracture of <u>unspecified</u> lesser toe(s)
        S92.504- <u>Nondisplaced</u> unspecified fracture of <u>right</u> lesser toe(s)
        S92.505- <u>Nondisplaced</u> unspecified fracture of <u>left</u> lesser toe(s)
        S92.506- <u>Nondisplaced</u> unspecified fracture of <u>unspecified</u> lesser toe(s)
    S92.51- Fracture of <u>proximal phalanx</u> of <u>lesser toe(s)</u>
        S92.511- <u>Displaced</u> fracture of proximal phalanx of <u>right</u> lesser toe(s)
        S92.512- <u>Displaced</u> fracture of proximal phalanx of <u>left</u> lesser toe(s)
        S92.513- <u>Displaced</u> fracture of proximal phalanx of <u>unspecified</u> lesser toe(s)
        S92.514- <u>Nondisplaced</u> fracture of proximal phalanx of <u>right</u> lesser toe(s)
        S92.515- <u>Nondisplaced</u> fracture of proximal phalanx of <u>left</u> lesser toe(s)
        S92.516- <u>Nondisplaced</u> fracture of proximal phalanx of <u>unspecified</u> lesser toe(s)
    S92.52- Fracture of <u>medial phalanx</u> of <u>lesser toe(s)</u>
        S92.521- <u>Displaced</u> fracture of medial phalanx of <u>right</u> lesser toe(s)
        S92.522- <u>Displaced</u> fracture of medial phalanx of <u>left</u> lesser toe(s)
        S92.523- <u>Displaced</u> fracture of medial phalanx of <u>unspecified</u> lesser toe(s)
        S92.524- <u>Nondisplaced</u> fracture of medial phalanx of <u>right</u> lesser toe(s)
        S92.525- <u>Nondisplaced</u> fracture of medial phalanx of <u>left</u> lesser toe(s)
        S92.526- <u>Nondisplaced</u> fracture of medial phalanx of <u>unspecified</u> lesser toe(s)
    S92.53- Fracture of <u>distal phalanx</u> of <u>lesser toe(s)</u>
        S92.531- <u>Displaced</u> fracture of distal phalanx of <u>right</u> lesser toe(s)
        S92.532- <u>Displaced</u> fracture of distal phalanx of <u>left</u> lesser toe(s)
        S92.533- <u>Displaced</u> fracture of distal phalanx of <u>unspecified</u> lesser toe(s)
        S92.534- <u>Nondisplaced</u> fracture of distal phalanx of <u>right</u> lesser toe(s)
        S92.535- <u>Nondisplaced</u> fracture of distal phalanx of <u>left</u> lesser toe(s)
        S92.536- <u>Nondisplaced</u> fracture of distal phalanx of <u>unspecified</u> lesser toe(s)
    S92.59- <u>Other fracture</u> of <u>lesser toe(s)</u>
        S92.591- Other fracture of <u>right</u> lesser toe(s)
        S92.592- Other fracture of <u>left</u> lesser toe(s)
        S92.599- Other fracture of <u>unspecified</u> lesser toe(s)
S92.9- Unspecified fracture of foot and toe
    S92.90- <u>Unspecified</u> fracture of <u>foot</u>
        S92.901- Unspecified fracture of <u>right</u> foot
        S92.902- Unspecified fracture of <u>left</u> foot
        S92.909- Unspecified fracture of <u>unspecified</u> foot
    S92.91- <u>Unspecified</u> fracture of <u>toe</u>
        S92.911- Unspecified fracture of <u>right</u> toe(s)
        S92.912- Unspecified fracture of <u>left</u> toe(s)
        S92.919- Unspecified fracture of <u>unspecified</u> toe(s)

S92 – S92

Excludes 1: = NOT CODED HERE! (Do not code both)   **775**   *Excludes* ❷*:* = Not Included Here

S93-   <u>Dislocation and sprain</u> of joints and ligaments at <u>ankle, foot and toe level</u>
Includes: Avulsion of joint or ligament of ankle, foot and toe
           Laceration of cartilage, joint or ligament of ankle, foot and toe
           Sprain of cartilage, joint or ligament of ankle, foot and toe
           Traumatic hemarthrosis of joint or ligament of ankle, foot and toe
           Traumatic rupture of joint or ligament of ankle, foot and toe
           Traumatic subluxation of joint or ligament of ankle, foot and toe
           Traumatic tear of joint or ligament of ankle, foot and toe
Code also any associated open wound
Excludes❷: strain of muscle and tendon of ankle and foot (S96.-)

The appropriate 7th character is to be added to each code from category S93:
A   <u>Initial</u> encounter
D   <u>Subsequent</u> encounter
S   <u>Sequela</u>

S93.0-   Subluxation and dislocation of <u>ankle joint</u>
        Subluxation and dislocation of astragalus
        Subluxation and dislocation of fibula, lower end
        Subluxation and dislocation of talus
        Subluxation and dislocation of tibia, lower end
    S93.01x-   <u>Subluxation</u> of <u>right</u> ankle joint
    S93.02x-   <u>Subluxation</u> of <u>left</u> ankle joint
    S93.03x-   <u>Subluxation</u> of <u>unspecified</u> ankle joint
    S93.04x-   <u>Dislocation</u> of <u>right</u> ankle joint
    S93.05x-   <u>Dislocation</u> of <u>left</u> ankle joint
    S93.06x-   <u>Dislocation</u> of <u>unspecified</u> ankle joint
S93.1-   Subluxation and dislocation of toe
    S93.10-   <u>Unspecified</u> subluxation and dislocation of <u>toe</u>
           Dislocation of toe NOS
           Subluxation of toe NOS
       S93.101-   Unspecified <u>subluxation</u> of <u>right</u> toe(s)
       S93.102-   Unspecified <u>subluxation</u> of <u>left</u> toe(s)
       S93.103-   Unspecified <u>subluxation</u> of <u>unspecified</u> toe(s)
       S93.104-   Unspecified <u>dislocation</u> of <u>right</u> toe(s)
       S93.105-   Unspecified <u>dislocation</u> of <u>left</u> toe(s)
       S93.106-   Unspecified <u>dislocation</u> of <u>unspecified</u> toe(s)
    S93.11-   <u>Dislocation</u> of <u>interphalangeal joint</u>
       S93.111-   Dislocation of interphalangeal joint of <u>right</u> <u>great</u> toe
       S93.112-   Dislocation of interphalangeal joint of <u>left</u> <u>great</u> toe
       S93.113-   Dislocation of interphalangeal joint of <u>unspecified</u> <u>great</u> toe
       S93.114-   Dislocation of interphalangeal joint of <u>right</u> <u>lesser</u> toe(s)
       S93.115-   Dislocation of interphalangeal joint of <u>left</u> <u>lesser</u> toe(s)
       S93.116-   Dislocation of interphalangeal joint of <u>unspecified</u> <u>lesser</u> toe(s)
       S93.119-   Dislocation of interphalangeal joint of <u>unspecified</u> toe(s)
    S93.12-   <u>Dislocation</u> of <u>metatarsophalangeal joint</u>
       S93.121-   Dislocation of metatarsophalangeal joint of <u>right</u> <u>great</u> toe
       S93.122-   Dislocation of metatarsophalangeal joint of <u>left</u> <u>great</u> toe
       S93.123-   Dislocation of metatarsophalangeal joint of <u>unspecified</u> <u>great</u> toe
       S93.124-   Dislocation of metatarsophalangeal joint of <u>right</u> <u>lesser</u> toe(s)
       S93.125-   Dislocation of metatarsophalangeal joint of <u>left</u> <u>lesser</u> toe(s)
       S93.126-   Dislocation of metatarsophalangeal joint of <u>unspecified</u> lesser toe(s)
       S93.129-   Dislocation of metatarsophalangeal joint of <u>unspecified</u> toe(s)
    S93.13-   <u>Subluxation</u> of <u>interphalangeal joint</u>
       S93.131-   Subluxation of interphalangeal joint of <u>right</u> <u>great</u> toe
       S93.132-   Subluxation of interphalangeal joint of <u>left</u> <u>great</u> toe
       S93.133-   Subluxation of interphalangeal joint of <u>unspecified</u> <u>great</u> toe
       S93.134-   Subluxation of interphalangeal joint of <u>right</u> <u>lesser</u> toe(s)
       S93.135-   Subluxation of interphalangeal joint of <u>left</u> <u>lesser</u> toe(s)
       S93.136-   Subluxation of interphalangeal joint of <u>unspecified</u> <u>lesser</u> toe(s)
       S93.139-   Subluxation of interphalangeal joint of <u>unspecified</u> toe(s)

S93.14-   <u>Subluxation</u> of <u>metatarsophalangeal joint</u>
    S93.141-   Subluxation of metatarsophalangeal joint of <u>right</u> <u>great</u> toe
    S93.142-   Subluxation of metatarsophalangeal joint of <u>left</u> <u>great</u> toe
    S93.143-   Subluxation of metatarsophalangeal joint of <u>unspecified</u> <u>great</u> toe
    S93.144-   Subluxation of metatarsophalangeal joint of <u>right</u> <u>lesser</u> toe(s)
    S93.145-   Subluxation of metatarsophalangeal joint of <u>left</u> <u>lesser</u> toe(s)
    S93.146-   Subluxation of metatarsophalangeal joint of <u>unspecified</u> <u>lesser</u> toe(s)
    S93.149-   Subluxation of metatarsophalangeal joint of <u>unspecified</u> toe(s)
S93.3-   Subluxation and dislocation of <u>foot</u>
    Excludes❷: dislocation of toe (S93.1-)
    S93.30-   <u>Unspecified</u> subluxation and dislocation of <u>foot</u>
           Dislocation of foot NOS
           Subluxation of foot NOS
       S93.301-   Unspecified <u>subluxation</u> of <u>right</u> foot
       S93.302-   Unspecified <u>subluxation</u> of <u>left</u> foot
       S93.303-   Unspecified <u>subluxation</u> of <u>unspecified</u> foot
       S93.304-   Unspecified <u>dislocation</u> of <u>right</u> foot
       S93.305-   Unspecified <u>dislocation</u> of <u>left</u> foot
       S93.306-   Unspecified <u>dislocation</u> of <u>unspecified</u> foot
    S93.31-   Subluxation and dislocation of <u>tarsal joint</u>
       S93.311-   <u>Subluxation</u> of tarsal joint of <u>right</u> foot
       S93.312-   <u>Subluxation</u> of tarsal joint of <u>left</u> foot
       S93.313-   <u>Subluxation</u> of tarsal joint of <u>unspecified</u> foot
       S93.314-   <u>Dislocation</u> of tarsal joint of <u>right</u> foot
       S93.315-   <u>Dislocation</u> of tarsal joint of <u>left</u> foot
       S93.316-   <u>Dislocation</u> of tarsal joint of <u>unspecified</u> foot
    S93.32-   Subluxation and dislocation of <u>tarsometatarsal joint</u>
       S93.321-   <u>Subluxation</u> of tarsometatarsal joint of <u>right</u> foot
       S93.322-   <u>Subluxation</u> of tarsometatarsal joint of <u>left</u> foot
       S93.323-   <u>Subluxation</u> of tarsometatarsal joint of <u>unspecified</u> foot
       S93.324-   <u>Dislocation</u> of tarsometatarsal joint of <u>right</u> foot
       S93.325-   <u>Dislocation</u> of tarsometatarsal joint of <u>left</u> foot
       S93.326-   <u>Dislocation</u> of tarsometatarsal joint of <u>unspecified</u> foot
    S93.33-   <u>Other</u> subluxation and dislocation of <u>foot</u>
       S93.331-   Other <u>subluxation</u> of <u>right</u> foot
       S93.332-   Other <u>subluxation</u> of <u>left</u> foot
       S93.333-   Other <u>subluxation</u> of <u>unspecified</u> foot
       S93.334-   Other <u>dislocation</u> of <u>right</u> foot
       S93.335-   Other <u>dislocation</u> of <u>left</u> foot
       S93.336-   Other <u>dislocation</u> of <u>unspecified</u> foot
S93.4-   <u>Sprain</u> of <u>ankle</u>
    Excludes❷: injury of Achilles tendon (S86.0-)
    S93.40-   <u>Sprain</u> of <u>unspecified</u> ligament of <u>ankle</u>
           Sprain of ankle NOS
           Sprained ankle NOS
       S93.401-   Sprain of unspecified ligament of <u>right</u> ankle
       S93.402-   Sprain of unspecified ligament of <u>left</u> ankle
       S93.409-   Sprain of unspecified ligament of <u>unspecified</u> ankle
    S93.41-   <u>Sprain</u> of <u>calcaneofibular</u> ligament
       S93.411-   Sprain of calcaneofibular ligament of <u>right</u> ankle
       S93.412-   Sprain of calcaneofibular ligament of <u>left</u> ankle
       S93.419-   Sprain of calcaneofibular ligament of <u>unspecified</u> ankle
    S93.42-   <u>Sprain</u> of <u>deltoid</u> ligament
       S93.421-   Sprain of deltoid ligament of <u>right</u> ankle
       S93.422-   Sprain of deltoid ligament of <u>left</u> ankle
       S93.429-   Sprain of deltoid ligament of <u>unspecified</u> ankle
    S93.43-   <u>Sprain</u> of <u>tibiofibular</u> ligament
       S93.431-   Sprain of tibiofibular ligament of <u>right</u> ankle
       S93.432-   Sprain of tibiofibular ligament of <u>left</u> ankle
       S93.439-   Sprain of tibiofibular ligament of <u>unspecified</u> ankle
    S93.49-   <u>Sprain</u> of <u>other ligament</u> of <u>ankle</u>
           Sprain of internal collateral ligament
           Sprain of talofibular ligament
       S93.491-   Sprain of other ligament of <u>right</u> ankle
       S93.492-   Sprain of other ligament of <u>left</u> ankle
       S93.499-   Sprain of other ligament of <u>unspecified</u> ankle

S93 - S95

S93.5-   Sprain of toe
   S93.50-   Unspecified sprain of toe
      S93.501-   Unspecified sprain of right great toe
      S93.502-   Unspecified sprain of left great toe
      S93.503-   Unspecified sprain of unspecified great toe
      S93.504-   Unspecified sprain of right lesser toe(s)
      S93.505-   Unspecified sprain of left lesser toe(s)
      S93.506-   Unspecified sprain of unspecified lesser toe(s)
      S93.509-   Unspecified sprain of unspecified toe(s)
   S93.51-   Sprain of interphalangeal joint of toe
      S93.511-   Sprain of interphalangeal joint of right great toe
      S93.512-   Sprain of interphalangeal joint of left great toe
      S93.513-   Sprain of interphalangeal joint of unspecified great toe
      S93.514-   Sprain of interphalangeal joint of right lesser toe(s)
      S93.515-   Sprain of interphalangeal joint of left lesser toe(s)
      S93.516-   Sprain of interphalangeal joint of unspecified lesser toe(s)
      S93.519-   Sprain of interphalangeal joint of unspecified toe(s)
   S93.52-   Sprain of metatarsophalangeal joint of toe
      S93.521-   Sprain of metatarsophalangeal joint of right great toe
      S93.522-   Sprain of metatarsophalangeal joint of left great toe
      S93.523-   Sprain of metatarsophalangeal joint of unspecified great toe
      S93.524-   Sprain of metatarsophalangeal joint of right lesser toe(s)
      S93.525-   Sprain of metatarsophalangeal joint of left lesser toe(s)
      S93.526-   Sprain of metatarsophalangeal joint of unspecified lesser toe(s)
      S93.529-   Sprain of metatarsophalangeal joint of unspecified toe(s)
S93.6-   Sprain of foot
   Excludes❷: sprain of metatarsophalangeal joint of toe (S93.52-)
              sprain of toe (S93.5-)
   S93.60-   Unspecified sprain of foot
      S93.601-   Unspecified sprain of right foot
      S93.602-   Unspecified sprain of left foot
      S93.609-   Unspecified sprain of unspecified foot
   S93.61-   Sprain of tarsal ligament of foot
      S93.611-   Sprain of tarsal ligament of right foot
      S93.612-   Sprain of tarsal ligament of left foot
      S93.619-   Sprain of tarsal ligament of unspecified foot
   S93.62-   Sprain of tarsometatarsal ligament of foot
      S93.621-   Sprain of tarsometatarsal ligament of right foot
      S93.622-   Sprain of tarsometatarsal ligament of left foot
      S93.629-   Sprain of tarsometatarsal ligament of unspecified foot
   S93.69-   Other sprain of foot
      S93.691-   Other sprain of right foot
      S93.692-   Other sprain of left foot
      S93.699-   Other sprain of unspecified foot

S94-   Injury of nerves at ankle and foot level
   Code also any associated open wound (S91.-)
   The appropriate 7th character is to be added to each code from category S94:
   A   Initial encounter
   D   Subsequent encounter
   S   Sequela
   S94.0-   Injury of lateral plantar nerve
      S94.00x-   Injury of lateral plantar nerve, unspecified leg
      S94.01x-   Injury of lateral plantar nerve, right leg
      S94.02x-   Injury of lateral plantar nerve, left leg
   S94.1-   Injury of medial plantar nerve
      S94.10x-   Injury of medial plantar nerve, unspecified leg
      S94.11x-   Injury of medial plantar nerve, right leg
      S94.12x-   Injury of medial plantar nerve, left leg
   S94.2-   Injury of deep peroneal nerve at ankle and foot level
      Injury of terminal, lateral branch of deep peroneal nerve
      S94.20x-   Injury of deep peroneal nerve at ankle and foot level, unspecified leg
      S94.21x-   Injury of deep peroneal nerve at ankle and foot level, right leg
      S94.22x-   Injury of deep peroneal nerve at ankle and foot level, left leg

S94.3-   Injury of cutaneous sensory nerve at ankle and foot level
      S94.30x-   Injury of cutaneous sensory nerve at ankle and foot level, unspecified leg
      S94.31x-   Injury of cutaneous sensory nerve at ankle and foot level, right leg
      S94.32x-   Injury of cutaneous sensory nerve at ankle and foot level, left leg
S94.8-   Injury of other nerves at ankle and foot level
   S94.8x-   Injury of other nerves at ankle and foot level
      S94.8x1-   Injury of other nerves at ankle and foot level, right leg
      S94.8x2-   Injury of other nerves at ankle and foot level, left leg
      S94.8x9-   Injury of other nerves at ankle and foot level, unspecified leg
S94.9-   Injury of unspecified nerve at ankle and foot level
      S94.90x-   Injury of unspecified nerve at ankle and foot level, unspecified leg
      S94.91x-   Injury of unspecified nerve at ankle and foot level, right leg
      S94.92x-   Injury of unspecified nerve at ankle and foot level, left leg

S95-   Injury of blood vessels at ankle and foot level
   Code also any associated open wound (S91.-)
   Excludes❷: injury of posterior tibial artery and vein (S85.1-, S85.8-)
   The appropriate 7th character is to be added to each code from category S95:
   A   Initial encounter
   D   Subsequent encounter
   S   Sequela
   S95.0-   Injury of dorsal artery of foot
      S95.00-   Unspecified injury of dorsal artery of foot
         S95.001-   Unspecified injury of dorsal artery of right foot
         S95.002-   Unspecified injury of dorsal artery of left foot
         S95.009-   Unspecified injury of dorsal artery of unspecified foot
      S95.01-   Laceration of dorsal artery of foot
         S95.011-   Laceration of dorsal artery of right foot
         S95.012-   Laceration of dorsal artery of left foot
         S95.019-   Laceration of dorsal artery of unspecified foot
      S95.09-   Other specified injury of dorsal artery of foot
         S95.091-   Other specified injury of dorsal artery of right foot
         S95.092-   Other specified injury of dorsal artery of left foot
         S95.099-   Other specified injury of dorsal artery of unspecified foot
   S95.1-   Injury of plantar artery of foot
      S95.10-   Unspecified injury of plantar artery of foot
         S95.101-   Unspecified injury of plantar artery of right foot
         S95.102-   Unspecified injury of plantar artery of left foot
         S95.109-   Unspecified injury of plantar artery of unspecified foot
      S95.11-   Laceration of plantar artery of foot
         S95.111-   Laceration of plantar artery of right foot
         S95.112-   Laceration of plantar artery of left foot
         S95.119-   Laceration of plantar artery of unspecified foot
      S95.19-   Other specified injury of plantar artery of foot
         S95.191-   Other specified injury of plantar artery of right foot
         S95.192-   Other specified injury of plantar artery of left foot
         S95.199-   Other specified injury of plantar artery of unspecified foot
   S95.2-   Injury of dorsal vein of foot
      S95.20-   Unspecified injury of dorsal vein of foot
         S95.201-   Unspecified injury of dorsal vein of right foot
         S95.202-   Unspecified injury of dorsal vein of left foot
         S95.209-   Unspecified injury of dorsal vein of unspecified foot
      S95.21-   Laceration of dorsal vein of foot
         S95.211-   Laceration of dorsal vein of right foot
         S95.212-   Laceration of dorsal vein of left foot
         S95.219-   Laceration of dorsal vein of unspecified foot
      S95.29-   Other specified injury of dorsal vein of foot
         S95.291-   Other specified injury of dorsal vein of right foot
         S95.292-   Other specified injury of dorsal vein of left foot
         S95.299-   Other specified injury of dorsal vein of unspecified foot

S93 - S95

S95.8- **Injury** of other blood vessels at ankle and foot level
S95.80- **Unspecified** injury of other blood vessels at ankle and foot level
S95.801- Unspecified injury of other blood vessels at ankle and foot level, right leg
S95.802- Unspecified injury of other blood vessels at ankle and foot level, left leg
S95.809- Unspecified injury of other blood vessels at ankle and foot level, unspecified leg
S95.81- **Laceration** of other blood vessels at ankle and foot level
S95.811- Laceration of other blood vessels at ankle and foot level, right leg
S95.812- Laceration of other blood vessels at ankle and foot level, left leg
S95.819- Laceration of other blood vessels at ankle and foot level, unspecified leg
S95.89- **Other specified injury** of other blood vessels at ankle and foot level
S95.891- Other specified injury of other blood vessels at ankle and foot level, right leg
S95.892- Other specified injury of other blood vessels at ankle and foot level, left leg
S95.899- Other specified injury of other blood vessels at ankle and foot level, unspecified leg
S95.9- Injury of unspecified blood vessel at ankle and foot level
S95.90- **Unspecified** injury of unspecified blood vessel at ankle and foot level
S95.901- Unspecified injury of unspecified blood vessel at ankle and foot level, right leg
S95.902- Unspecified injury of unspecified blood vessel at ankle and foot level, left leg
S95.909- Unspecified injury of unspecified blood vessel at ankle and foot level, unspecified leg
S95.91- **Laceration** of unspecified blood vessel at ankle and foot level
S95.911- Laceration of unspecified blood vessel at ankle and foot level, right leg
S95.912- Laceration of unspecified blood vessel at ankle and foot level, left leg
S95.919- Laceration of unspecified blood vessel at ankle and foot level, unspecified leg
S95.99- **Other specified injury** of unspecified blood vessel at ankle and foot level
S95.991- Other specified injury of unspecified blood vessel at ankle and foot level, right leg
S95.992- Other specified injury of unspecified blood vessel at ankle and foot level, left leg
S95.999- Other specified injury of unspecified blood vessel at ankle and foot level, unspecified leg

S96- **Injury** of muscle and tendon at ankle and foot level
Code also any associated open wound (S91.-)
Excludes ❷: injury of Achilles tendon (S86.0-)
sprain of joints and ligaments of ankle and foot (S93.-)

The appropriate 7th character is to be added to each code from category S96:
A **Initial** encounter
D **Subsequent** encounter
S **Sequela**

S96.0- **Injury** of muscle and tendon of long flexor muscle of toe at ankle and foot level
S96.00- **Unspecified** injury of muscle and tendon of long flexor muscle of toe at ankle and foot level
S96.001- Unspecified injury of muscle and tendon of long flexor muscle of toe at ankle and foot level, right foot
S96.002- Unspecified injury of muscle and tendon of long flexor muscle of toe at ankle and foot level, left foot
S96.009- Unspecified injury of muscle and tendon of long flexor muscle of toe at ankle and foot level, unspecified foot
S96.01- **Strain** of muscle and tendon of long flexor muscle of toe at ankle and foot level
S96.011- Strain of muscle and tendon of long flexor muscle of toe at ankle and foot level, right foot
S96.012- Strain of muscle and tendon of long flexor muscle of toe at ankle and foot level, left foot
S96.019- Strain of muscle and tendon of long flexor muscle of toe at ankle and foot level, unspecified foot

S96.02- **Laceration** of muscle and tendon of long flexor muscle of toe at ankle and foot level
S96.021- Laceration of muscle and tendon of long flexor muscle of toe at ankle and foot level, right foot
S96.022- Laceration of muscle and tendon of long flexor muscle of toe at ankle and foot level, left foot
S96.029- Laceration of muscle and tendon of long flexor muscle of toe at ankle and foot level, unspecified foot
S96.09- **Other injury** of muscle and tendon of long flexor muscle of toe at ankle and foot level
S96.091- Other injury of muscle and tendon of long flexor muscle of toe at ankle and foot level, right foot
S96.092- Other injury of muscle and tendon of long flexor muscle of toe at ankle and foot level, left foot
S96.099- Other injury of muscle and tendon of long flexor muscle of toe at ankle and foot level, unspecified foot
S96.1- **Injury** of muscle and tendon of long extensor muscle of toe at ankle and foot level
S96.10- **Unspecified** injury of muscle and tendon of long extensor muscle of toe at ankle and foot level
S96.101- Unspecified injury of muscle and tendon of long extensor muscle of toe at ankle and foot level, right foot
S96.102- Unspecified injury of muscle and tendon of long extensor muscle of toe at ankle and foot level, left foot
S96.109- Unspecified injury of muscle and tendon of long extensor muscle of toe at ankle and foot level, unspecified foot
S96.11- **Strain** of muscle and tendon of long extensor muscle of toe at ankle and foot level
S96.111- Strain of muscle and tendon of long extensor muscle of toe at ankle and foot level, right foot
S96.112- Strain of muscle and tendon of long extensor muscle of toe at ankle and foot level, left foot
S96.119- Strain of muscle and tendon of long extensor muscle of toe at ankle and foot level, unspecified foot
S96.12- **Laceration** of muscle and tendon of long extensor muscle of toe at ankle and foot level
S96.121- Laceration of muscle and tendon of long extensor muscle of toe at ankle and foot level, right foot
S96.122- Laceration of muscle and tendon of long extensor muscle of toe at ankle and foot level, left foot
S96.129- Laceration of muscle and tendon of long extensor muscle of toe at ankle and foot level, unspecified foot
S96.19- **Other specified injury** of muscle and tendon of long extensor muscle of toe at ankle and foot level
S96.191- Other specified injury of muscle and tendon of long extensor muscle of toe at ankle and foot level, right foot
S96.192- Other specified injury of muscle and tendon of long extensor muscle of toe at ankle and foot level, left foot
S96.199- Other specified injury of muscle and tendon of long extensor muscle of toe at ankle and foot level, unspecified foot
S96.2- **Injury** of intrinsic muscle and tendon at ankle and foot level
S96.20- **Unspecified** injury of intrinsic muscle and tendon at ankle and foot level
S96.201- Unspecified injury of intrinsic muscle and tendon at ankle and foot level, right foot
S96.202- Unspecified injury of intrinsic muscle and tendon at ankle and foot level, left foot
S96.209- Unspecified injury of intrinsic muscle and tendon at ankle and foot level, unspecified foot
S96.21- **Strain** of intrinsic muscle and tendon at ankle and foot level
S96.211- Strain of intrinsic muscle and tendon at ankle and foot level, right foot
S96.212- Strain of intrinsic muscle and tendon at ankle and foot level, left foot
S96.219- Strain of intrinsic muscle and tendon at ankle and foot level, unspecified foot
S96.22- **Laceration** of intrinsic muscle and tendon at ankle and foot level
S96.221- Laceration of intrinsic muscle and tendon at ankle and foot level, right foot
S96.222- Laceration of intrinsic muscle and tendon at ankle and foot level, left foot
S96.229- Laceration of intrinsic muscle and tendon at ankle and foot level, unspecified foot

S95 - S98

© 2013 Channel Publishing, Ltd.

S96.29- Other specified injury of intrinsic muscle and tendon at ankle and foot level

    S96.291- Other specified injury of intrinsic muscle and tendon at ankle and foot level, right foot

    S96.292- Other specified injury of intrinsic muscle and tendon at ankle and foot level, left foot

    S96.299- Other specified injury of intrinsic muscle and tendon at ankle and foot level, unspecified foot

S96.8- Injury of other specified muscles and tendons at ankle and foot level

   S96.80- Unspecified injury of other specified muscles and tendons at ankle and foot level

    S96.801- Unspecified injury of other specified muscles and tendons at ankle and foot level, right foot

    S96.802- Unspecified injury of other specified muscles and tendons at ankle and foot level, left foot

    S96.809- Unspecified injury of other specified muscles and tendons at ankle and foot level, unspecified foot

   S96.81- Strain of other specified muscles and tendons at ankle and foot level

    S96.811- Strain of other specified muscles and tendons at ankle and foot level, right foot

    S96.812- Strain of other specified muscles and tendons at ankle and foot level, left foot

    S96.819- Strain of other specified muscles and tendons at ankle and foot level, unspecified foot

   S96.82- Laceration of other specified muscles and tendons at ankle and foot level

    S96.821- Laceration of other specified muscles and tendons at ankle and foot level, right foot

    S96.822- Laceration of other specified muscles and tendons at ankle and foot level, left foot

    S96.829- Laceration of other specified muscles and tendons at ankle and foot level, unspecified foot

   S96.89- Other specified injury of other specified muscles and tendons at ankle and foot level

    S96.891- Other specified injury of other specified muscles and tendons at ankle and foot level, right foot

    S96.892- Other specified injury of other specified muscles and tendons at ankle and foot level, left foot

    S96.899- Other specified injury of other specified muscles and tendons at ankle and foot level, unspecified foot

S96.9- Injury of unspecified muscle and tendon at ankle and foot level

   S96.90- Unspecified injury of unspecified muscle and tendon at ankle and foot level

    S96.901- Unspecified injury of unspecified muscle and tendon at ankle and foot level, right foot

    S96.902- Unspecified injury of unspecified muscle and tendon at ankle and foot level, left foot

    S96.909- Unspecified injury of unspecified muscle and tendon at ankle and foot level, unspecified foot

   S96.91- Strain of unspecified muscle and tendon at ankle and foot level

    S96.911- Strain of unspecified muscle and tendon at ankle and foot level, right foot

    S96.912- Strain of unspecified muscle and tendon at ankle and foot level, left foot

    S96.919- Strain of unspecified muscle and tendon at ankle and foot level, unspecified foot

   S96.92- Laceration of unspecified muscle and tendon at ankle and foot level

    S96.921- Laceration of unspecified muscle and tendon at ankle and foot level, right foot

    S96.922- Laceration of unspecified muscle and tendon at ankle and foot level, left foot

    S96.929- Laceration of unspecified muscle and tendon at ankle and foot level, unspecified foot

   S96.99- Other specified injury of unspecified muscle and tendon at ankle and foot level

    S96.991- Other specified injury of unspecified muscle and tendon at ankle and foot level, right foot

    S96.992- Other specified injury of unspecified muscle and tendon at ankle and foot level, left foot

    S96.999- Other specified injury of unspecified muscle and tendon at ankle and foot level, unspecified foot

S97- Crushing injury of ankle and foot

Use additional code(s) for all associated injuries

The appropriate 7th character is to be added to each code from category S97:

  A Initial encounter
  D Subsequent encounter
  S Sequela

S97.0- Crushing injury of ankle

   S97.00x- Crushing injury of unspecified ankle

   S97.01x- Crushing injury of right ankle

   S97.02x- Crushing injury of left ankle

S97.1- Crushing injury of toe

   S97.10- Crushing injury of unspecified toe(s)

    S97.101- Crushing injury of unspecified right toe(s)

    S97.102- Crushing injury of unspecified left toe(s)

    S97.109- Crushing injury of unspecified toe(s)
      Crushing injury of toe NOS

   S97.11- Crushing injury of great toe

    S97.111- Crushing injury of right great toe

    S97.112- Crushing injury of left great toe

    S97.119- Crushing injury of unspecified great toe

   S97.12- Crushing injury of lesser toe(s)

    S97.121- Crushing injury of right lesser toe(s)

    S97.122- Crushing injury of left lesser toe(s)

    S97.129- Crushing injury of unspecified lesser toe(s)

S97.8- Crushing injury of foot

   S97.80x- Crushing injury of unspecified foot
      Crushing injury of foot NOS

   S97.81x- Crushing injury of right foot

   S97.82x- Crushing injury of left foot

S98- Traumatic amputation of ankle and foot

Note: An amputation not identified as partial or complete should be coded to complete

The appropriate 7th character is to be added to each code from category S98:

  A Initial encounter
  D Subsequent encounter
  S Sequela

S98.0- Traumatic amputation of foot at ankle level

   S98.01- Complete traumatic amputation of foot at ankle level

    S98.011- Complete traumatic amputation of right foot at ankle level

    S98.012- Complete traumatic amputation of left foot at ankle level

    S98.019- Complete traumatic amputation of unspecified foot at ankle level

   S98.02- Partial traumatic amputation of foot at ankle level

    S98.021- Partial traumatic amputation of right foot at ankle level

    S98.022- Partial traumatic amputation of left foot at ankle level

    S98.029- Partial traumatic amputation of unspecified foot at ankle level

S98.1- Traumatic amputation of one toe

   S98.11- Complete traumatic amputation of great toe

    S98.111- Complete traumatic amputation of right great toe

    S98.112- Complete traumatic amputation of left great toe

    S98.119- Complete traumatic amputation of unspecified great toe

   S98.12- Partial traumatic amputation of great toe

    S98.121- Partial traumatic amputation of right great toe

    S98.122- Partial traumatic amputation of left great toe

    S98.129- Partial traumatic amputation of unspecified great toe

   S98.13- Complete traumatic amputation of one lesser toe
      Traumatic amputation of toe NOS

    S98.131- Complete traumatic amputation of one right lesser toe

    S98.132- Complete traumatic amputation of one left lesser toe

    S98.139- Complete traumatic amputation of one unspecified lesser toe

   S98.14- Partial traumatic amputation of one lesser toe

    S98.141- Partial traumatic amputation of one right lesser toe

    S98.142- Partial traumatic amputation of one left lesser toe

    S98.149- Partial traumatic amputation of one unspecified lesser toe

S95 – S98

Excludes 1: = NOT CODED HERE! (Do not code both)   *Excludes ❷:* = Not Included Here

S98.2- Traumatic amputation of two or more lesser toes

  S98.21- Complete traumatic amputation of two or more lesser toes

    S98.211- Complete traumatic amputation of two or more right lesser toes

    S98.212- Complete traumatic amputation of two or more left lesser toes

    S98.219- Complete traumatic amputation of two or more unspecified lesser toes

  S98.22- Partial traumatic amputation of two or more lesser toes

    S98.221- Partial traumatic amputation of two or more right lesser toes

    S98.222- Partial traumatic amputation of two or more left lesser toes

    S98.229- Partial traumatic amputation of two or more unspecified lesser toes

S98.3- Traumatic amputation of midfoot

  S98.31- Complete traumatic amputation of midfoot

    S98.311- Complete traumatic amputation of right midfoot

    S98.312- Complete traumatic amputation of left midfoot

    S98.319- Complete traumatic amputation of unspecified midfoot

  S98.32- Partial traumatic amputation of midfoot

    S98.321- Partial traumatic amputation of right midfoot

    S98.322- Partial traumatic amputation of left midfoot

    S98.329- Partial traumatic amputation of unspecified midfoot

S98.9- Traumatic amputation of foot, level unspecified

  S98.91- Complete traumatic amputation of foot, level unspecified

    S98.911- Complete traumatic amputation of right foot, level unspecified

    S98.912- Complete traumatic amputation of left foot, level unspecified

    S98.919- Complete traumatic amputation of unspecified foot, level unspecified

  S98.92- Partial traumatic amputation of foot, level unspecified

    S98.921- Partial traumatic amputation of right foot, level unspecified

    S98.922- Partial traumatic amputation of left foot, level unspecified

    S98.929- Partial traumatic amputation of unspecified foot, level unspecified

S99- Other and unspecified injuries of ankle and foot

> The appropriate 7th character is to be added to each code from category S99:
> **A** Initial encounter
> **D** Subsequent encounter
> **S** Sequela

S99.8- Other specified injuries of ankle and foot

  S99.81- Other specified injuries of ankle

    S99.811- Other specified injuries of right ankle

    S99.812- Other specified injuries of left ankle

    S99.819- Other specified injuries of unspecified ankle

  S99.82- Other specified injuries of foot

    S99.821- Other specified injuries of right foot

    S99.822- Other specified injuries of left foot

    S99.829- Other specified injuries of unspecified foot

S99.9- Unspecified injury of ankle and foot

  S99.91- Unspecified injury of ankle

    S99.911- Unspecified injury of right ankle

    S99.912- Unspecified injury of left ankle

    S99.919- Unspecified injury of unspecified ankle

  S99.92- Unspecified injury of foot

    S99.921- Unspecified injury of right foot

    S99.922- Unspecified injury of left foot

    S99.929- Unspecified injury of unspecified foot

S98 - T17

Injury, poisoning and certain other consequences of external causes (T07-T88)

Injuries involving multiple body regions (T07)

Excludes 1: burns and corrosions (T20-T32)
           frostbite (T33-T34)
           insect bite or sting, venomous (T63.4)
           sunburn (L55-)

T07   Unspecified multiple injuries
    Excludes 1: injury NOS (T14-)

Injury of unspecified body region (T14)

T14-   Injury of unspecified body region
    Excludes 1: multiple unspecified injuries (T07)
    T14.8   <u>Other injury</u> of <u>unspecified</u> body region
            Abrasion NOS
            Contusion NOS
            Crush injury NOS
            Fracture NOS
            Skin injury NOS
            Vascular injury NOS
    T14.9-   Unspecified injury
        T14.90   <u>Injury, unspecified</u>
                Injury NOS
        T14.91   Suicide attempt
                Attempted suicide NOS

Effects of foreign body entering through natural orifice (T15-T19)

Excludes❷: foreign body accidentally left in operation wound (T81.5-)
          foreign body in penetrating wound — see open wound by body region
          residual foreign body in soft tissue (M79.5)
          splinter, without open wound — see superficial injury by body region

T15-   <u>Foreign body</u> on <u>external eye</u>
    Excludes❷: foreign body in penetrating wound of orbit and eye ball (S05.4-, S05.5-)
              open wound of eyelid and periocular area (S01.1-)
              retained foreign body in eyelid (H02.8-)
              retained (old) foreign body in penetrating wound of orbit and eye ball (H05.5-, H44.6-, H44.7-)
              superficial foreign body of eyelid and periocular area (S00.25-)

The appropriate 7th character is to be added to each code from category T15:
    A   <u>Initial</u> encounter
    D   <u>Subsequent</u> encounter
    S   <u>Sequela</u>

    T15.0-   Foreign body in <u>cornea</u>
        T15.00x-   Foreign body in cornea, <u>unspecified</u> eye
        T15.01x-   Foreign body in cornea, <u>right</u> eye
        T15.02x-   Foreign body in cornea, <u>left</u> eye
    T15.1-   Foreign body in <u>conjunctival sac</u>
        T15.10x-   Foreign body in conjunctival sac, <u>unspecified</u> eye
        T15.11x-   Foreign body in conjunctival sac, <u>right</u> eye
        T15.12x-   Foreign body in conjunctival sac, <u>left</u> eye
    T15.8-   Foreign body <u>in other and multiple parts of external eye</u>
            Foreign body in lacrimal punctum
        T15.80x-   Foreign body in other and multiple parts of external eye, <u>unspecified</u> eye
        T15.81x-   Foreign body in other and multiple parts of external eye, <u>right</u> eye
        T15.82x-   Foreign body in other and multiple parts of external eye, <u>left</u> eye
    T15.9-   Foreign body on <u>external eye, part unspecified</u>
        T15.90x-   Foreign body on external eye, part unspecified, <u>unspecified</u> eye
        T15.91x-   Foreign body on external eye, part unspecified, <u>right</u> eye
        T15.92x-   Foreign body on external eye, part unspecified, <u>left</u> eye

T16-   <u>Foreign body</u> in <u>ear</u>
    Includes: Foreign body in auditory canal
    The appropriate 7th character is to be added to each code from category T16:
        A   <u>Initial</u> encounter
        D   <u>Subsequent</u> encounter
        S   <u>Sequela</u>
    T16.1xx-   Foreign body in <u>right</u> ear
    T16.2xx-   Foreign body in <u>left</u> ear
    T16.9xx-   Foreign body in ear, <u>unspecified</u> ear

T17-   <u>Foreign body</u> in <u>respiratory tract</u>
    The appropriate 7th character is to be added to each code from category T17:
        A   <u>Initial</u> encounter
        D   <u>Subsequent</u> encounter
        S   <u>Sequela</u>
    T17.0xx-   Foreign body in nasal sinus
    T17.1xx-   Foreign body in nostril
            Foreign body in nose NOS
    T17.2-   Foreign body in <u>pharynx</u>
            Foreign body in nasopharynx
            Foreign body in throat NOS
        T17.20-   <u>Unspecified</u> foreign body in pharynx
            T17.200-   Unspecified foreign body in pharynx <u>causing asphyxiation</u>
            T17.208-   Unspecified foreign body in pharynx <u>causing other injury</u>
        T17.21-   <u>Gastric contents</u> in pharynx
                Aspiration of gastric contents into pharynx
                Vomitus in pharynx
            T17.210-   Gastric contents in pharynx <u>causing asphyxiation</u>
            T17.218-   Gastric contents in pharynx <u>causing other injury</u>
        T17.22-   <u>Food</u> in pharynx
                Bones in pharynx
                Seeds in pharynx
            T17.220-   Food in pharynx <u>causing asphyxiation</u>
            T17.228-   Food in pharynx <u>causing other injury</u>
        T17.29-   <u>Other foreign object</u> in pharynx
            T17.290-   Other foreign object in pharynx <u>causing asphyxiation</u>
            T17.298-   Other foreign object in pharynx <u>causing other injury</u>
    T17.3-   Foreign body in <u>larynx</u>
        T17.30-   <u>Unspecified</u> foreign body in larynx
            T17.300-   Unspecified foreign body in larynx <u>causing asphyxiation</u>
            T17.308-   Unspecified foreign body in larynx <u>causing other injury</u>
        T17.31-   Gastric contents in <u>larynx</u>
                Aspiration of gastric contents into larynx
                Vomitus in larynx
            T17.310-   Gastric contents in larynx <u>causing asphyxiation</u>
            T17.318-   Gastric contents in larynx <u>causing other injury</u>
        T17.32-   Food in <u>larynx</u>
                Bones in larynx
                Seeds in larynx
            T17.320-   Food in larynx <u>causing asphyxiation</u>
            T17.328-   Food in larynx <u>causing other injury</u>
        T17.39-   <u>Other foreign object</u> in larynx
            T17.390-   Other foreign object in larynx <u>causing asphyxiation</u>
            T17.398-   Other foreign object in larynx <u>causing other injury</u>
    T17.4-   Foreign body in <u>trachea</u>
        T17.40-   <u>Unspecified</u> foreign body in trachea
            T17.400-   Unspecified foreign body in trachea <u>causing asphyxiation</u>
            T17.408-   Unspecified foreign body in trachea <u>causing other injury</u>
        T17.41-   Gastric contents in <u>trachea</u>
                Aspiration of gastric contents into trachea
                Vomitus in trachea
            T17.410-   Gastric contents in trachea <u>causing asphyxiation</u>
            T17.418-   Gastric contents in trachea <u>causing other injury</u>
        T17.42-   Food in <u>trachea</u>
                Bones in trachea
                Seeds in trachea
            T17.420-   Food in trachea <u>causing asphyxiation</u>
            T17.428-   Food in trachea <u>causing other injury</u>
        T17.49-   <u>Other foreign object</u> in trachea
            T17.490-   Other foreign object in trachea <u>causing asphyxiation</u>
            T17.498-   Other foreign object in trachea <u>causing other injury</u>

S 9 8 – T 1 7

Excludes 1: = NOT CODED HERE! (Do not code both)   *Excludes❷:* = Not Included Here

T17.5- Foreign body in <u>bronchus</u>
  T17.50- <u>Unspecified</u> foreign body in <u>bronchus</u>
    T17.500- Unspecified foreign body in bronchus <u>causing asphyxiation</u>
    T17.508- Unspecified foreign body in bronchus <u>causing other injury</u>
  T17.51- <u>Gastric contents</u> in <u>bronchus</u>
        Aspiration of gastric contents into bronchus
        Vomitus in bronchus
    T17.510- Gastric contents in bronchus <u>causing asphyxiation</u>
    T17.518- Gastric contents in bronchus <u>causing other injury</u>
  T17.52- <u>Food</u> in <u>bronchus</u>
        Bones in bronchus
        Seeds in bronchus
    T17.520- Food in bronchus <u>causing asphyxiation</u>
    T17.528- Food in bronchus <u>causing other injury</u>
  T17.59- <u>Other foreign object</u> in <u>bronchus</u>
    T17.590- Other foreign object in bronchus <u>causing asphyxiation</u>
    T17.598- Other foreign object in bronchus <u>causing other injury</u>
T17.8- Foreign body <u>in other parts of respiratory tract</u>
      Foreign body in bronchioles
      Foreign body in lung
  T17.80- <u>Unspecified</u> foreign body <u>in other parts of respiratory tract</u>
    T17.800- Unspecified foreign body in other parts of respiratory tract <u>causing asphyxiation</u>
    T17.808- Unspecified foreign body in other parts of respiratory tract <u>causing other injury</u>
  T17.81- <u>Gastric contents</u> <u>in other parts of respiratory tract</u>
        Aspiration of gastric contents into other parts of respiratory tract
        Vomitus in other parts of respiratory tract
    T17.810- Gastric contents in other parts of respiratory tract <u>causing asphyxiation</u>
    T17.818- Gastric contents in other parts of respiratory tract <u>causing other injury</u>
  T17.82- <u>Food</u> <u>in other parts of respiratory tract</u>
        Bones in other parts of respiratory tract
        Seeds in other parts of respiratory tract
    T17.820- Food in other parts of respiratory tract <u>causing asphyxiation</u>
    T17.828- Food in other parts of respiratory tract <u>causing other injury</u>
  T17.89- <u>Other foreign object</u> <u>in other parts of respiratory tract</u>
    T17.890- Other foreign object in other parts of respiratory tract <u>causing asphyxiation</u>
    T17.898- Other foreign object in other parts of respiratory tract <u>causing other injury</u>
T17.9- Foreign body <u>in respiratory tract</u>, <u>part unspecified</u>
  T17.90- <u>Unspecified</u> foreign body in respiratory tract, part unspecified
    T17.900- Unspecified foreign body in respiratory tract, part unspecified <u>causing asphyxiation</u>
    T17.908- Unspecified foreign body in respiratory tract, part unspecified <u>causing other injury</u>
  T17.91- <u>Gastric contents</u> in respiratory tract, <u>part unspecified</u>
        Aspiration of gastric contents into respiratory tract, part unspecified
        Vomitus in trachea respiratory tract, part unspecified
    T17.910- Gastric contents in respiratory tract, part unspecified <u>causing asphyxiation</u>
    T17.918- Gastric contents in respiratory tract, part unspecified <u>causing other injury</u>
  T17.92- <u>Food</u> <u>in respiratory tract</u>, <u>part unspecified</u>
        Bones in respiratory tract, part unspecified
        Seeds in respiratory tract, part unspecified
    T17.920- Food in respiratory tract, part unspecified <u>causing asphyxiation</u>
    T17.928- Food in respiratory tract, part unspecified <u>causing other injury</u>
  T17.99- <u>Other foreign object</u> <u>in respiratory tract</u>, <u>part unspecified</u>
    T17.990- Other foreign object in respiratory tract, part unspecified in <u>causing asphyxiation</u>
    T17.998- Other foreign object in respiratory tract, part unspecified <u>causing other injury</u>

T18- <u>Foreign body</u> <u>in alimentary tract</u>
      Excludes❷: foreign body in pharynx (T17.2-)
      The appropriate 7th character is to be added to each code from category T18:
      A <u>Initial</u> encounter
      D <u>Subsequent</u> encounter
      S <u>Sequela</u>
T18.0xx- Foreign body in <u>mouth</u>
T18.1- Foreign body in <u>esophagus</u>
      Excludes❷: foreign body in respiratory tract (T17.-)
  T18.10- <u>Unspecified</u> foreign body in <u>esophagus</u>
    T18.100- Unspecified foreign body in esophagus <u>causing compression of trachea</u>
          Unspecified foreign body in esophagus causing obstruction of respiration
    T18.108- Unspecified foreign body in esophagus <u>causing other injury</u>
  T18.11- <u>Gastric contents</u> in <u>esophagus</u>
        Vomitus in esophagus
    T18.110- Gastric contents in esophagus <u>causing compression of trachea</u>
          Gastric contents in esophagus causing obstruction of respiration
    T18.118- Gastric contents in esophagus <u>causing other injury</u>
  T18.12- <u>Food</u> in <u>esophagus</u>
        Bones in esophagus
        Seeds in esophagus
    T18.120- Food in esophagus <u>causing compression of trachea</u>
          Food in esophagus causing obstruction of respiration
    T18.128- Food in esophagus <u>causing other injury</u>
  T18.19- <u>Other foreign object</u> in <u>esophagus</u>
    T18.190- Other foreign object in esophagus <u>causing compression of trachea</u>
          Other foreign body in esophagus causing obstruction of respiration
    T18.198- Other foreign object in esophagus <u>causing other injury</u>
T18.2xx- Foreign body in stomach
T18.3xx- Foreign body in small intestine
T18.4xx- Foreign body in colon
T18.5xx- Foreign body in anus and rectum
          Foreign body in rectosigmoid (junction)
T18.8xx- Foreign body in other parts of alimentary tract
T18.9xx- Foreign body of alimentary tract, part unspecified
          Foreign body in digestive system NOS
          Swallowed foreign body NOS

T19- <u>Foreign body</u> <u>in genitourinary tract</u>
      Excludes❷: complications due to implanted mesh (T83.7-)
          mechanical complications of contraceptive device (intrauterine) (vaginal) (T83.3-)
          presence of contraceptive device (intrauterine) (vaginal) (Z97.5)
      The appropriate 7th character is to be added to each code from category T19:
      A <u>Initial</u> encounter
      D <u>Subsequent</u> encounter
      S <u>Sequela</u>
T19.0xx- Foreign body in urethra
T19.1xx- Foreign body in bladder
T19.2xx- Foreign body in vulva and vagina
T19.3xx- Foreign body in uterus
T19.4xx- Foreign body in penis
T19.8xx- Foreign body in other parts of genitourinary tract
T19.9xx- Foreign body in genitourinary tract, part unspecified

T 1 7 - T 2 0

Excludes 1: = NOT CODED HERE! (Do not code both)   **782**   *Excludes❷: = Not Included Here*

Burns and corrosions (T20-T32)

Includes: Burns (thermal) from electrical heating appliances
Burns (thermal) from electricity
Burns (thermal) from flame
Burns (thermal) from friction
Burns (thermal) from hot air and hot gases
Burns (thermal) from hot objects
Burns (thermal) from lightning
Burns (thermal) from radiation
Chemical burn [corrosion] (external) (internal)
Scalds

*Excludes❷: erythema [dermatitis] ab igne (L59.0)
radiation-related disorders of the skin and subcutaneous tissue
(L55-L59)
sunburn (L55.-)*

Burns and corrosions of external body surface, specified by site (T20-T25)

Includes: Burns and corrosions of first degree [erythema]
Burns and corrosions of second degree [blisters][epidermal loss]
Burns and corrosions of third degree [deep necrosis of
underlying tissue] [full- thickness skin loss]
Use additional code from category T31 or T32 to identify extent of body
surface involved

T20- <u>Burn and corrosion</u> of <u>head, face, and neck</u>
*Excludes❷: burn and corrosion of ear drum (T28.41, T28.91)
burn and corrosion of eye and adnexa (T26.-)
burn and corrosion of mouth and pharynx (T28.0)*

**The appropriate 7th character is to be added to each code from
category T20:**
A <u>Initial</u> encounter
D <u>Subsequent</u> encounter
S <u>Sequela</u>

T20.0- Burn of <u>unspecified degree</u> of head, face, and neck
Use additional external cause code to identify the source, place and
intent of the burn (X00-X19, X75-X77, X96-X98, Y92)

T20.00x- Burn of <u>unspecified degree</u> of <u>head, face, and neck,
unspecified</u> site

T20.01- Burn of <u>unspecified degree</u> of <u>ear</u> [any part, except ear
drum]
Excludes❷: burn of ear drum (T28.41-)

T20.011- Burn of <u>unspecified degree</u> of <u>right</u> ear [any part,
except ear drum]

T20.012- Burn of <u>unspecified degree</u> of <u>left</u> ear [any part, except
ear drum]

T20.019- Burn of <u>unspecified degree</u> of <u>unspecified</u> ear [any
part, except ear drum]

T20.02x- Burn of <u>unspecified degree</u> of lip(s)
T20.03x- Burn of <u>unspecified degree</u> of chin
T20.04x- Burn of <u>unspecified degree</u> of nose (septum)
T20.05x- Burn of <u>unspecified degree</u> of scalp [any part]
T20.06x- Burn of <u>unspecified degree</u> of forehead and cheek
T20.07x- Burn of <u>unspecified degree</u> of neck
T20.09x- Burn of <u>unspecified degree</u> of multiple sites of head, face,
and neck

T20.1- Burn of <u>first</u> degree of <u>head, face, and neck</u>
Use additional external cause code to identify the source, place and
intent of the burn (X00-X19, X75-X77, X96-X98, Y92)

T20.10x- Burn of <u>first</u> degree of head, face, and neck, <u>unspecified</u>
site

T20.11- Burn of <u>first</u> degree of <u>ear</u> [any part, except ear drum]
Excludes❷: burn of ear drum (T28.41-)

T20.111- Burn of <u>first</u> degree of <u>right</u> ear [any part, except ear
drum]

T20.112- Burn of <u>first</u> degree of <u>left</u> ear [any part, except ear
drum]

T20.119- Burn of <u>first</u> degree of <u>unspecified</u> ear [any part,
except ear drum]

T20.12x- Burn of <u>first</u> degree of lip(s)
T20.13x- Burn of <u>first</u> degree of chin
T20.14x- Burn of <u>first</u> degree of nose (septum)
T20.15x- Burn of <u>first</u> degree of scalp [any part]
T20.16x- Burn of <u>first</u> degree of forehead and cheek
T20.17x- Burn of <u>first</u> degree of neck
T20.19x- Burn of <u>first</u> degree of multiple sites of head, face, and
neck

T20.2- Burn of <u>second</u> degree of head, face, and neck
Use additional external cause code to identify the source, place and
intent of the burn (X00-X19, X75-X77, X96-X98, Y92)

T20.20x- Burn of <u>second</u> degree of head, face, and neck, <u>unspecified</u>
site

T20.21- Burn of <u>second</u> degree of <u>ear</u> [any part, except ear drum]
Excludes❷: burn of ear drum (T28.41-)

T20.211- Burn of <u>second</u> degree of <u>right</u> ear [any part, except
ear drum]

T20.212- Burn of <u>second</u> degree of <u>left</u> ear [any part, except ear
drum]

T20.219- Burn of <u>second</u> degree of <u>unspecified</u> ear [any part,
except ear drum]

T20.22x- Burn of <u>second</u> degree of lip(s)
T20.23x- Burn of <u>second</u> degree of chin
T20.24x- Burn of <u>second</u> degree of nose (septum)
T20.25x- Burn of <u>second</u> degree of scalp [any part]
T20.26x- Burn of <u>second</u> degree of forehead and cheek
T20.27x- Burn of <u>second</u> degree of neck
T20.29x- Burn of <u>second</u> degree of multiple sites of head, face, and
neck

T20.3- Burn of <u>third</u> degree of <u>head, face, and neck</u>
Use additional external cause code to identify the source, place and
intent of the burn (X00-X19, X75-X77, X96-X98, Y92)

T20.30x- Burn of <u>third</u> degree of <u>head, face, and neck, unspecified</u>
site

T20.31- Burn of <u>third</u> degree of <u>ear</u> [any part, except ear drum]
Excludes❷: burn of ear drum (T28.41-)

T20.311- Burn of <u>third</u> degree of <u>right</u> ear [any part, except ear
drum]

T20.312- Burn of <u>third</u> degree of <u>left</u> ear [any part, except ear
drum]

T20.319- Burn of <u>third</u> degree of <u>unspecified</u> ear [any part,
except ear drum]

T20.32x- Burn of <u>third</u> degree of lip(s)
T20.33x- Burn of <u>third</u> degree of chin
T20.34x- Burn of <u>third</u> degree of nose (septum)
T20.35x- Burn of <u>third</u> degree of scalp [any part]
T20.36x- Burn of <u>third</u> degree of forehead and cheek
T20.37x- Burn of <u>third</u> degree of neck
T20.39x- Burn of <u>third</u> degree of multiple sites of head, face, and
neck

T20.4- <u>Corrosion</u> of <u>unspecified degree</u> of <u>head, face, and neck</u>
Code first (T51-T65) to identify chemical and intent
Use additional external cause code to identify place (Y92)

T20.40x- <u>Corrosion</u> of <u>unspecified degree</u> of <u>head, face, and neck,
unspecified</u> site

T20.41- <u>Corrosion</u> of <u>unspecified degree</u> of <u>ear</u> [any part, except
ear drum]
Excludes❷: corrosion of ear drum (T28.91-)

T20.411- Corrosion of unspecified degree of <u>right</u> ear [any part,
except ear drum]

T20.412- Corrosion of unspecified degree of <u>left</u> ear [any part,
except ear drum]

T20.419- Corrosion of unspecified degree of <u>unspecified</u> ear
[any part, except ear drum]

T
1
7
-
T
2
0

T20.42x- Corrosion of unspecified degree of lip(s)

T20.43x- Corrosion of unspecified degree of chin

T20.44x- Corrosion of unspecified degree of nose (septum)

T20.45x- Corrosion of unspecified degree of scalp [any part]

T20.46x- Corrosion of unspecified degree of forehead and cheek

T20.47x- Corrosion of unspecified degree of neck

T20.49x- Corrosion of unspecified degree of multiple sites of head, face, and neck

T20.5- Corrosion of first degree of head, face, and neck
Code first (T51-T65) to identify chemical and intent
Use additional external cause code to identify place (Y92)

T20.50x- Corrosion of first degree of head, face, and neck, unspecified site

T20.51- Corrosion of first degree of ear [any part, except ear drum]
Excludes❷: corrosion of ear drum (T28.91-)

T20.511- Corrosion of first degree of right ear [any part, except ear drum]

T20.512- Corrosion of first degree of left ear [any part, except ear drum]

T20.519- Corrosion of first degree of unspecified ear [any part, except ear drum]

T20.52x- Corrosion of first degree of lip(s)

T20.53x- Corrosion of first degree of chin

T20.54x- Corrosion of first degree of nose (septum)

T20.55x- Corrosion of first degree of scalp [any part]

T20.56x- Corrosion of first degree of forehead and cheek

T20.57x- Corrosion of first degree of neck

T20.59x- Corrosion of first degree of multiple sites of head, face, and neck

T20.6- Corrosion of second degree of head, face, and neck
Code first (T51-T65) to identify chemical and intent
Use additional external cause code to identify place (Y92)

T20.60x- Corrosion of second degree of head, face, and neck, unspecified site

T20.61- Corrosion of second degree of ear [any part, except ear drum]
Excludes❷: corrosion of ear drum (T28.91-)

T20.611- Corrosion of second degree of right ear [any part, except ear drum]

T20.612- Corrosion of second degree of left ear [any part, except ear drum]

T20.619- Corrosion of second degree of unspecified ear [any part, except ear drum]

T20.62x- Corrosion of second degree of lip(s)

T20.63x- Corrosion of second degree of chin

T20.64x- Corrosion of second degree of nose (septum)

T20.65x- Corrosion of second degree of scalp [any part]

T20.66x- Corrosion of second degree of forehead and cheek

T20.67x- Corrosion of second degree of neck

T20.69x- Corrosion of second degree of multiple sites of head, face, and neck

T20.7- Corrosion of third degree of head, face, and neck
Code first (T51-T65) to identify chemical and intent
Use additional external cause code to identify place (Y92)

T20.70x- Corrosion of third degree of head, face, and neck, unspecified site

T20.71- Corrosion of third degree of ear [any part, except ear drum]
Excludes❷: corrosion of ear drum (T28.91-)

T20.711- Corrosion of third degree of right ear [any part, except ear drum]

T20.712- Corrosion of third degree of left ear [any part, except ear drum]

T20.719- Corrosion of third degree of unspecified ear [any part, except ear drum]

T20.72x- Corrosion of third degree of lip(s)

T20.73x- Corrosion of third degree of chin

T20.74x- Corrosion of third degree of nose (septum)

T20.75x- Corrosion of third degree of scalp [any part]

T20.76x- Corrosion of third degree of forehead and cheek

T20.77x- Corrosion of third degree of neck

T20.79x- Corrosion of third degree of multiple sites of head, face, and neck

T21- Burn and corrosion of trunk
Includes: Burns and corrosion of hip region
Excludes❷: burns and corrosion of axilla (T22.- with fifth character 4)
burns and corrosion of scapular region (T22.- with fifth character 6)
burns and corrosion of shoulder (T22. with fifth character 5)

The appropriate 7th character is to be added to each code from category T21:
A Initial encounter
D Subsequent encounter
S Sequela

T21.0- Burn of unspecified degree of trunk
Use additional external cause code to identify the source, place and intent of the burn (X00-X19, X75-X77, X96-X98, Y92)

T21.00x- Burn of unspecified degree of trunk, unspecified site

T21.01x- Burn of unspecified degree of chest wall
Burn of of unspecified degree of breast

T21.02x- Burn of unspecified degree of abdominal wall
Burn of unspecified degree of flank
Burn of unspecified degree of groin

T21.03x- Burn of unspecified degree of upper back
Burn of unspecified degree of interscapular region

T21.04x- Burn of unspecified degree of lower back

T21.05x- Burn of unspecified degree of buttock
Burn of unspecified degree of anus

T21.06x- Burn of unspecified degree of male genital region
Burn of unspecified degree of penis
Burn of unspecified degree of scrotum
Burn of unspecified degree of testis

T21.07x- Burn of unspecified degree of female genital region
Burn of unspecified degree of labium (majus) (minus)
Burn of unspecified degree of perineum
Burn of unspecified degree of vulva
Excludes❷: burn of vagina (T28.3)

T21.09x- Burn of unspecified degree of other site of trunk

T21.1- Burn of first degree of trunk
Use additional external cause code to identify the source, place and intent of the burn (X00-X19, X75-X77, X96-X98, Y92)

T21.10x- Burn of first degree of trunk, unspecified site

T21.11x- Burn of first degree of chest wall
Burn of first degree of breast

T21.12x- Burn of first degree of abdominal wall
Burn of first degree of flank
Burn of first degree of groin

T21.13x- Burn of first degree of upper back
Burn of first degree of interscapular region

T21.14x- Burn of first degree of lower back

T21.15x- Burn of first degree of buttock
Burn of first degree of anus

T21.16x- Burn of first degree of male genital region
Burn of first degree of penis
Burn of first degree of scrotum
Burn of first degree of testis

T21.17x- Burn of first degree of female genital region
Burn of first degree of labium (majus) (minus)
Burn of first degree of perineum
Burn of first degree of vulva
Excludes❷: burn of vagina (T28.3)

T21.19x- Burn of first degree of other site of trunk

T21.2- Burn of second degree of trunk
Use additional external cause code to identify the source, place and intent of the burn (X00-X19, X75-X77, X96-X98, Y92)

T21.20x- Burn of second degree of trunk, unspecified site

T21.21x- Burn of second degree of chest wall
Burn of second degree of breast

T21.22x- Burn of second degree of abdominal wall
Burn of second degree of flank
Burn of second degree of groin

T21.23x- Burn of second degree of upper back
Burn of second degree of interscapular region

T21.24x- Burn of second degree of lower back

T21.25x- Burn of second degree of buttock
Burn of second degree of anus

T21.26x- Burn of second degree of male genital region
Burn of second degree of penis
Burn of second degree of scrotum
Burn of second degree of testis

T
2
0
-
T
2
2

T21.27x- Burn of <u>second</u> degree of <u>female genital region</u>
    Burn of second degree of labium (majus) (minus)
    Burn of second degree of perineum
    Burn of second degree of vulva
    Excludes❷: burn of vagina (T28.3)

T21.29x- Burn of <u>second</u> degree of <u>other</u> site of trunk

T21.3- Burn of <u>third</u> degree of <u>trunk</u>
    Use additional external cause code to identify the source, place and
    intent of the burn (X00-X19, X75-X77, X96-X98, Y92)

T21.30x- Burn of <u>third</u> degree of trunk, <u>unspecified</u> site

T21.31x- Burn of <u>third</u> degree of <u>chest wall</u>
    Burn of third degree of breast

T21.32x- Burn of <u>third</u> degree of <u>abdominal wall</u>
    Burn of third degree of flank
    Burn of third degree of groin

T21.33x- Burn of <u>third</u> degree of <u>upper back</u>
    Burn of third degree of interscapular region

T21.34x- Burn of <u>third</u> degree of <u>lower back</u>

T21.35x- Burn of <u>third</u> degree of <u>buttock</u>
    Burn of third degree of anus

T21.36x- Burn of <u>third</u> degree of <u>male genital region</u>
    Burn of third degree of penis
    Burn of third degree of scrotum
    Burn of third degree of testis

T21.37x- Burn of <u>third</u> degree of <u>female genital region</u>
    Burn of third degree of labium (majus) (minus)
    Burn of third degree of perineum
    Burn of third degree of vulva
    Excludes❷: burn of vagina (T28.3)

T21.39x- Burn of <u>third</u> degree of <u>other</u> site of trunk

T21.4- Corrosion of <u>unspecified degree</u> of <u>trunk</u>
    Code first (T51-T65) to identify chemical and intent
    Use additional external cause code to identify place (Y92)

T21.40x- Corrosion of <u>unspecified degree</u> of trunk, <u>unspecified</u> site

T21.41x- Corrosion of <u>unspecified degree</u> of <u>chest wall</u>
    Corrosion of unspecified degree of breast

T21.42x- Corrosion of <u>unspecified degree</u> of <u>abdominal wall</u>
    Corrosion of unspecified degree of flank
    Corrosion of unspecified degree of groin

T21.43x- Corrosion of <u>unspecified degree</u> of <u>upper back</u>
    Corrosion of unspecified degree of interscapular region

T21.44x- Corrosion of <u>unspecified degree</u> of <u>lower back</u>

T21.45x- Corrosion of <u>unspecified degree</u> of <u>buttock</u>
    Corrosion of unspecified degree of anus

T21.46x- Corrosion of <u>unspecified degree</u> of <u>male genital region</u>
    Corrosion of unspecified degree of penis
    Corrosion of unspecified degree of scrotum
    Corrosion of unspecified degree of testis

T21.47x- Corrosion of <u>unspecified degree</u> of <u>female genital region</u>
    Corrosion of unspecified degree of labium (majus) (minus)
    Corrosion of unspecified degree of perineum
    Corrosion of unspecified degree of vulva
    Excludes❷: corrosion of vagina (T28.8)

T21.49x- Corrosion of <u>unspecified degree</u> of <u>other</u> site of trunk

T21.5- Corrosion of <u>first</u> degree of <u>trunk</u>
    Code first (T51-T65) to identify chemical and intent
    Use additional external cause code to identify place (Y92)

T21.50x- Corrosion of <u>first</u> degree of trunk, <u>unspecified</u> site

T21.51x- Corrosion of <u>first</u> degree of <u>chest wall</u>
    Corrosion of first degree of breast

T21.52x- Corrosion of <u>first</u> degree of <u>abdominal wall</u>
    Corrosion of first degree of flank
    Corrosion of first degree of groin

T21.53x- Corrosion of <u>first</u> degree of <u>upper back</u>
    Corrosion of first degree of interscapular region

T21.54x- Corrosion of <u>first</u> degree of <u>lower back</u>

T21.55x- Corrosion of <u>first</u> degree of <u>buttock</u>
    Corrosion of first degree of anus

T21.56x- Corrosion of <u>first</u> degree of <u>male genital region</u>
    Corrosion of first degree of penis
    Corrosion of first degree of scrotum
    Corrosion of first degree of testis

T21.57x- Corrosion of <u>first</u> degree of <u>female genital region</u>
    Corrosion of first degree of labium (majus) (minus)
    Corrosion of first degree of perineum
    Corrosion of first degree of vulva
    Excludes❷: corrosion of vagina (T28.8)

T21.59x- Corrosion of <u>first</u> degree of <u>other</u> site of trunk

T21.6- Corrosion of <u>second</u> degree of <u>trunk</u>
    Code first (T51-T65) to identify chemical and intent
    Use additional external cause code to identify place (Y92)

T21.60x- Corrosion of <u>second</u> degree of trunk, <u>unspecified</u> site

T21.61x- Corrosion of <u>second</u> degree of <u>chest wall</u>
    Corrosion of second degree of breast

T21.62x- Corrosion of <u>second</u> degree of <u>abdominal wall</u>
    Corrosion of second degree of flank
    Corrosion of second degree of groin

T21.63x- Corrosion of <u>second</u> degree of <u>upper back</u>
    Corrosion of second degree of interscapular region

T21.64x- Corrosion of <u>second</u> degree of <u>lower back</u>

T21.65x- Corrosion of <u>second</u> degree of <u>buttock</u>
    Corrosion of second degree of anus

T21.66x- Corrosion of <u>second</u> degree of <u>male genital region</u>
    Corrosion of second degree of penis
    Corrosion of second degree of scrotum
    Corrosion of second degree of testis

T21.67x- Corrosion of <u>second</u> degree of <u>female genital region</u>
    Corrosion of second degree of labium (majus) (minus)
    Corrosion of second degree of perineum
    Corrosion of second degree of vulva
    Excludes❷: corrosion of vagina (T28.8)

T21.69x- Corrosion of <u>second</u> degree of <u>other</u> site of trunk

T21.7- Corrosion of <u>third</u> degree of <u>trunk</u>
    Code first (T51-T65) to identify chemical and intent
    Use additional external cause code to identify place (Y92)

T21.70x- Corrosion of <u>third</u> degree of trunk, <u>unspecified</u> site

T21.71x- Corrosion of <u>third</u> degree of <u>chest wall</u>
    Corrosion of third degree of breast

T21.72x- Corrosion of <u>third</u> degree of <u>abdominal wall</u>
    Corrosion of third degree of flank
    Corrosion of third degree of groin

T21.73x- Corrosion of <u>third</u> degree of <u>upper back</u>
    Corrosion of third degree of interscapular region

T21.74x- Corrosion of <u>third</u> degree of <u>lower back</u>

T21.75x- Corrosion of <u>third</u> degree of <u>buttock</u>
    Corrosion of third degree of anus

T21.76x- Corrosion of <u>third</u> degree of <u>male genital region</u>
    Corrosion of third degree of penis
    Corrosion of third degree of scrotum
    Corrosion of third degree of testis

T21.77x- Corrosion of <u>third</u> degree of <u>female genital region</u>
    Corrosion of third degree of labium (majus) (minus)
    Corrosion of third degree of perineum
    Corrosion of third degree of vulva
    Excludes❷: corrosion of vagina (T28.8)

T21.79x- Corrosion of <u>third</u> degree of <u>other</u> site of trunk

T22- Burn and corrosion of <u>shoulder and upper limb</u>, except wrist and hand
    Excludes❷: burn and corrosion of interscapular region (T21.-)
    burn and corrosion of wrist and hand (T23.-)

The appropriate 7th character is to be added to each code from
category T22:
A <u>Initial</u> encounter
D <u>Subsequent</u> encounter
S <u>Sequela</u>

T22.0- Burn of <u>unspecified degree</u> of <u>shoulder and upper limb</u>, except
wrist and hand
    Use additional external cause code to identify the source, place and
    intent of the burn (X00-X19, X75-X77, X96-X98, Y92)

T22.00x- Burn of <u>unspecified degree</u> of <u>shoulder and upper limb</u>,
except wrist and hand, <u>unspecified</u> site

T22.01- Burn of <u>unspecified degree</u> of <u>forearm</u>
    T22.011- Burn of unspecified degree of <u>right</u> forearm
    T22.012- Burn of unspecified degree of <u>left</u> forearm
    T22.019- Burn of unspecified degree of <u>unspecified</u> forearm

T22.02- Burn of <u>unspecified degree</u> of <u>elbow</u>
    T22.021- Burn of unspecified degree of <u>right</u> elbow
    T22.022- Burn of unspecified degree of <u>left</u> elbow
    T22.029- Burn of unspecified degree of <u>unspecified</u> elbow

T22.03- Burn of <u>unspecified degree</u> of <u>upper arm</u>
    T22.031- Burn of unspecified degree of <u>right</u> upper arm
    T22.032- Burn of unspecified degree of <u>left</u> upper arm
    T22.039- Burn of unspecified degree of <u>unspecified</u> upper arm

T22.04- Burn of <u>unspecified degree</u> of <u>axilla</u>
    T22.041- Burn of unspecified degree of <u>right</u> axilla
    T22.042- Burn of unspecified degree of <u>left</u> axilla
    T22.049- Burn of unspecified degree of <u>unspecified</u> axilla

T
2
0
–
T
2
2

Excludes 1: = NOT CODED HERE! (Do not code both)

Excludes❷: = Not Included Here

T22.05- Burn of <u>unspecified degree</u> of <u>shoulder</u>
  T22.051- Burn of unspecified degree of <u>right</u> shoulder
  T22.052- Burn of unspecified degree of <u>left</u> shoulder
  T22.059- Burn of unspecified degree of <u>unspecified</u> shoulder
T22.06- Burn of <u>unspecified degree</u> of <u>scapular region</u>
  T22.061- Burn of unspecified degree of <u>right</u> scapular region
  T22.062- Burn of unspecified degree of <u>left</u> scapular region
  T22.069- Burn of unspecified degree of <u>unspecified</u> scapular region
T22.09- Burn of <u>unspecified degree</u> of <u>multiple</u> sites of shoulder and upper limb, except wrist and hand
  T22.091- Burn of unspecified degree of multiple sites of <u>right</u> shoulder and upper limb, except wrist and hand
  T22.092- Burn of unspecified degree of multiple sites of <u>left</u> shoulder and upper limb, except wrist and hand
  T22.099- Burn of unspecified degree of multiple sites of <u>unspecified</u> shoulder and upper limb, except wrist and hand

T22.1- Burn of <u>first</u> degree of <u>shoulder and upper limb</u>, <u>except wrist and hand</u>
  Use additional external cause code to identify the source, place and intent of the burn (X00-X19, X75-X77, X96-X98, Y92)
  T22.10x- Burn of <u>first</u> degree of <u>shoulder and upper limb</u>, except wrist and hand, <u>unspecified</u> site
T22.11- Burn of <u>first</u> degree of <u>forearm</u>
  T22.111- Burn of first degree of <u>right</u> forearm
  T22.112- Burn of first degree of <u>left</u> forearm
  T22.119- Burn of first degree of <u>unspecified</u> forearm
T22.12- Burn of <u>first</u> degree of <u>elbow</u>
  T22.121- Burn of first degree of <u>right</u> elbow
  T22.122- Burn of first degree of <u>left</u> elbow
  T22.129- Burn of first degree of <u>unspecified</u> elbow
T22.13- Burn of <u>first</u> degree of <u>upper arm</u>
  T22.131- Burn of first degree of <u>right</u> upper arm
  T22.132- Burn of first degree of <u>left</u> upper arm
  T22.139- Burn of first degree of <u>unspecified</u> upper arm
T22.14- Burn of <u>first</u> degree of <u>axilla</u>
  T22.141- Burn of first degree of <u>right</u> axilla
  T22.142- Burn of first degree of <u>left</u> axilla
  T22.149- Burn of first degree of <u>unspecified</u> axilla
T22.15- Burn of <u>first</u> degree of <u>shoulder</u>
  T22.151- Burn of first degree of <u>right</u> shoulder
  T22.152- Burn of first degree of <u>left</u> shoulder
  T22.159- Burn of first degree of <u>unspecified</u> shoulder
T22.16- Burn of <u>first</u> degree of <u>scapular region</u>
  T22.161- Burn of first degree of <u>right</u> scapular region
  T22.162- Burn of first degree of <u>left</u> scapular region
  T22.169- Burn of first degree of <u>unspecified</u> scapular region
T22.19- Burn of <u>first</u> degree of <u>multiple</u> sites of shoulder and upper limb, except wrist and hand
  T22.191- Burn of first degree of multiple sites of <u>right</u> shoulder and upper limb, except wrist and hand
  T22.192- Burn of first degree of multiple sites of <u>left</u> shoulder and upper limb, except wrist and hand
  T22.199- Burn of first degree of multiple sites of <u>unspecified</u> shoulder and upper limb, except wrist and hand

T22.2- Burn of <u>second</u> degree of <u>shoulder and upper limb</u>, <u>except wrist and hand</u>
  Use additional external cause code to identify the source, place and intent of the burn (X00-X19, X75-X77, X96-X98, Y92)
  T22.20x- Burn of <u>second</u> degree of <u>shoulder and upper limb</u>, except wrist and hand, <u>unspecified</u> site
T22.21- Burn of <u>second</u> degree of <u>forearm</u>
  T22.211- Burn of second degree of <u>right</u> forearm
  T22.212- Burn of second degree of <u>left</u> forearm
  T22.219- Burn of second degree of <u>unspecified</u> forearm
T22.22- Burn of <u>second</u> degree of <u>elbow</u>
  T22.221- Burn of second degree of <u>right</u> elbow
  T22.222- Burn of second degree of <u>left</u> elbow
  T22.229- Burn of second degree of <u>unspecified</u> elbow
T22.23- Burn of <u>second</u> degree of <u>upper arm</u>
  T22.231- Burn of second degree of <u>right</u> upper arm
  T22.232- Burn of second degree of <u>left</u> upper arm
  T22.239- Burn of second degree of <u>unspecified</u> upper arm

T22.24- Burn of <u>second</u> degree of <u>axilla</u>
  T22.241- Burn of second degree of <u>right</u> axilla
  T22.242- Burn of second degree of <u>left</u> axilla
  T22.249- Burn of second degree of <u>unspecified</u> axilla
T22.25- Burn of <u>second</u> degree of <u>shoulder</u>
  T22.251- Burn of second degree of <u>right</u> shoulder
  T22.252- Burn of second degree of <u>left</u> shoulder
  T22.259- Burn of second degree of <u>unspecified</u> shoulder
T22.26- Burn of <u>second</u> degree of <u>scapular region</u>
  T22.261- Burn of second degree of <u>right</u> scapular region
  T22.262- Burn of second degree of <u>left</u> scapular region
  T22.269- Burn of second degree of <u>unspecified</u> scapular region
T22.29- Burn of <u>second</u> degree of <u>multiple</u> sites of shoulder and upper limb, except wrist and hand
  T22.291- Burn of second degree of multiple sites of <u>right</u> shoulder and upper limb, except wrist and hand
  T22.292- Burn of second degree of multiple sites of <u>left</u> shoulder and upper limb, except wrist and hand
  T22.299- Burn of second degree of multiple sites of <u>unspecified</u> shoulder and upper limb, except wrist and hand

T22.3- Burn of <u>third</u> degree of <u>shoulder and upper limb</u>, <u>except wrist and hand</u>
  Use additional external cause code to identify the source, place and intent of the burn (X00-X19, X75-X77, X96-X98, Y92)
  T22.30x- Burn of <u>third</u> degree of shoulder and upper limb, except wrist and hand, <u>unspecified</u> site
T22.31- Burn of <u>third</u> degree of <u>forearm</u>
  T22.311- Burn of third degree of <u>right</u> forearm
  T22.312- Burn of third degree of <u>left</u> forearm
  T22.319- Burn of third degree of <u>unspecified</u> forearm
T22.32- Burn of <u>third</u> degree of <u>elbow</u>
  T22.321- Burn of third degree of <u>right</u> elbow
  T22.322- Burn of third degree of <u>left</u> elbow
  T22.329- Burn of third degree of <u>unspecified</u> elbow
T22.33- Burn of <u>third</u> degree of <u>upper arm</u>
  T22.331- Burn of third degree of <u>right</u> upper arm
  T22.332- Burn of third degree of <u>left</u> upper arm
  T22.339- Burn of third degree of <u>unspecified</u> upper arm
T22.34- Burn of <u>third</u> degree of <u>axilla</u>
  T22.341- Burn of third degree of <u>right</u> axilla
  T22.342- Burn of third degree of left axilla
  T22.349- Burn of third degree of <u>unspecified</u> axilla
T22.35- Burn of <u>third</u> degree of <u>shoulder</u>
  T22.351- Burn of third degree of <u>right</u> shoulder
  T22.352- Burn of third degree of <u>left</u> shoulder
  T22.359- Burn of third degree of <u>unspecified</u> shoulder
T22.36- Burn of <u>third</u> degree of <u>scapular region</u>
  T22.361- Burn of third degree of <u>right</u> scapular region
  T22.362- Burn of third degree of <u>left</u> scapular region
  T22.369- Burn of third degree of <u>unspecified</u> scapular region
T22.39- Burn of <u>third</u> degree of <u>multiple</u> sites of shoulder and upper limb, except wrist and hand
  T22.391- Burn of third degree of multiple sites of <u>right</u> shoulder and upper limb, except wrist and hand
  T22.392- Burn of third degree of multiple sites of <u>left</u> shoulder and upper limb, except wrist and hand
  T22.399- Burn of third degree of multiple sites of <u>unspecified</u> shoulder and upper limb, except wrist and hand

T22.4- <u>Corrosion</u> of <u>unspecified degree</u> of <u>shoulder and upper limb, except wrist and hand</u>
  Code first (T51-T65) to identify chemical and intent
  Use additional external cause code to identify place (Y92)
  T22.40x- <u>Corrosion</u> of <u>unspecified degree</u> of <u>shoulder and upper limb, except wrist and hand, unspecified</u> site
T22.41- <u>Corrosion</u> of <u>unspecified degree</u> of <u>forearm</u>
  T22.411- Corrosion of unspecified degree of <u>right</u> forearm
  T22.412- Corrosion of unspecified degree of <u>left</u> forearm
  T22.419- Corrosion of unspecified degree of <u>unspecified</u> forearm
T22.42- <u>Corrosion</u> of <u>unspecified degree</u> of <u>elbow</u>
  T22.421- Corrosion of unspecified degree of <u>right</u> elbow
  T22.422- Corrosion of unspecified degree of <u>left</u> elbow
  T22.429- Corrosion of unspecified degree of <u>unspecified</u> elbow
T22.43- <u>Corrosion</u> of <u>unspecified degree</u> of <u>upper arm</u>
  T22.431- Corrosion of unspecified degree of <u>right</u> upper arm
  T22.432- Corrosion of unspecified degree of <u>left</u> upper arm

---

Excludes 1: = NOT CODED HERE! (Do not code both)   **786**   *Excludes ❷:* = Not Included Here

T 2 2 - T 2 2

T22.439- Corrosion of unspecified degree of <u>unspecified</u> upper arm

T22.44- <u>Corrosion</u> of <u>unspecified degree</u> of <u>axilla</u>

    T22.441- Corrosion of unspecified degree of <u>right</u> axilla

    T22.442- Corrosion of unspecified degree of <u>left</u> axilla

    T22.449- Corrosion of unspecified degree of <u>unspecified</u> axilla

T22.45- <u>Corrosion</u> of <u>unspecified degree</u> of <u>shoulder</u>

    T22.451- Corrosion of unspecified degree of <u>right</u> shoulder

    T22.452- Corrosion of unspecified degree of <u>left</u> shoulder

    T22.459- Corrosion of unspecified degree of <u>unspecified</u> shoulder

T22.46- <u>Corrosion</u> of <u>unspecified degree</u> of <u>scapular region</u>

    T22.461- Corrosion of unspecified degree of <u>right</u> scapular region

    T22.462- Corrosion of unspecified degree of <u>left</u> scapular region

    T22.469- Corrosion of unspecified degree of <u>unspecified</u> scapular region

T22.49- <u>Corrosion</u> of <u>unspecified degree</u> of <u>multiple</u> sites of shoulder and upper limb, except wrist and hand

    T22.491- Corrosion of unspecified degree of multiple sites of <u>right</u> shoulder and upper limb, except wrist and hand

    T22.492- Corrosion of unspecified degree of multiple sites of <u>left</u> shoulder and upper limb, except wrist and hand

    T22.499- Corrosion of unspecified degree of multiple sites of <u>unspecified</u> shoulder and upper limb, except wrist and hand

T22.5- <u>Corrosion</u> of <u>first</u> degree of <u>shoulder and upper limb, except wrist and hand</u>

    Code first (T51-T65) to identify chemical and intent

    Use additional external cause code to identify place (Y92)

    T22.50x- <u>Corrosion</u> of <u>first</u> degree of <u>shoulder and upper limb</u>, except wrist and hand <u>unspecified</u> site

T22.51- <u>Corrosion</u> of <u>first</u> degree of <u>forearm</u>

    T22.511- Corrosion of first degree of <u>right</u> forearm

    T22.512- Corrosion of first degree of <u>left</u> forearm

    T22.519- Corrosion of first degree of <u>unspecified</u> forearm

T22.52- <u>Corrosion</u> of <u>first</u> degree of <u>elbow</u>

    T22.521- Corrosion of first degree of <u>right</u> elbow

    T22.522- Corrosion of first degree of <u>left</u> elbow

    T22.529- Corrosion of first degree of <u>unspecified</u> elbow

T22.53- <u>Corrosion</u> of <u>first</u> degree of <u>upper arm</u>

    T22.531- Corrosion of first degree of <u>right</u> upper arm

    T22.532- Corrosion of first degree of <u>left</u> upper arm

    T22.539- Corrosion of first degree of <u>unspecified</u> upper arm

T22.54- <u>Corrosion</u> of <u>first</u> degree of <u>axilla</u>

    T22.541- Corrosion of first degree of <u>right</u> axilla

    T22.542- Corrosion of first degree of <u>left</u> axilla

    T22.549- Corrosion of first degree of <u>unspecified</u> axilla

T22.55- <u>Corrosion</u> of <u>first</u> degree of <u>shoulder</u>

    T22.551- Corrosion of first degree of <u>right</u> shoulder

    T22.552- Corrosion of first degree of <u>left</u> shoulder

    T22.559- Corrosion of first degree of <u>unspecified</u> shoulder

T22.56- <u>Corrosion</u> of <u>first</u> degree of <u>scapular region</u>

    T22.561- Corrosion of first degree of <u>right</u> scapular region

    T22.562- Corrosion of first degree of <u>left</u> scapular region

    T22.569- Corrosion of first degree of <u>unspecified</u> scapular region

T22.59- <u>Corrosion</u> of <u>first</u> degree of <u>multiple</u> sites of shoulder and upper limb, except wrist and hand

    T22.591- Corrosion of first degree of multiple sites of <u>right</u> shoulder and upper limb, except wrist and hand

    T22.592- Corrosion of first degree of multiple sites of <u>left</u> shoulder and upper limb, except wrist and hand

    T22.599- Corrosion of first degree of multiple sites of <u>unspecified</u> shoulder and upper limb, except wrist and hand

T22.6- <u>Corrosion</u> of <u>second</u> degree of <u>shoulder and upper limb, except wrist and hand</u>

    Code first (T51-T65) to identify chemical and intent

    Use additional external cause code to identify place (Y92)

    T22.60x- <u>Corrosion</u> of <u>second</u> degree of shoulder and upper limb, except wrist and hand, <u>unspecified</u> site

T22.61- <u>Corrosion</u> of <u>second</u> degree of <u>forearm</u>

    T22.611- Corrosion of second degree of <u>right</u> forearm

    T22.612- Corrosion of second degree of <u>left</u> forearm

    T22.619- Corrosion of second degree of <u>unspecified</u> forearm

T22.62- <u>Corrosion</u> of <u>second</u> degree of <u>elbow</u>

    T22.621- Corrosion of second degree of <u>right</u> elbow

    T22.622- Corrosion of second degree of <u>left</u> elbow

    T22.629- Corrosion of second degree of <u>unspecified</u> elbow

T22.63- <u>Corrosion</u> of <u>second</u> degree of <u>upper arm</u>

    T22.631- Corrosion of second degree of <u>right</u> upper arm

    T22.632- Corrosion of second degree of <u>left</u> upper arm

    T22.639- Corrosion of second degree of <u>unspecified</u> upper arm

T22.64- <u>Corrosion</u> of <u>second</u> degree of <u>axilla</u>

    T22.641- Corrosion of second degree of <u>right</u> axilla

    T22.642- Corrosion of second degree of <u>left</u> axilla

    T22.649- Corrosion of second degree of <u>unspecified</u> axilla

T22.65- <u>Corrosion</u> of <u>second</u> degree of <u>shoulder</u>

    T22.651- Corrosion of second degree of <u>right</u> shoulder

    T22.652- Corrosion of second degree of <u>left</u> shoulder

    T22.659- Corrosion of second degree of <u>unspecified</u> shoulder

T22.66- <u>Corrosion</u> of <u>second</u> degree of <u>scapular region</u>

    T22.661- Corrosion of second degree of <u>right</u> scapular region

    T22.662- Corrosion of second degree of <u>left</u> scapular region

    T22.669- Corrosion of second degree of <u>unspecified</u> scapular region

T22.69- <u>Corrosion</u> of <u>second</u> degree of <u>multiple</u> sites of shoulder and upper limb, except wrist and hand

    T22.691- Corrosion of second degree of multiple sites of <u>right</u> shoulder and upper limb, except wrist and hand

    T22.692- Corrosion of second degree of multiple sites of <u>left</u> shoulder and upper limb, except wrist and hand

    T22.699- Corrosion of second degree of multiple sites of <u>unspecified</u> shoulder and upper limb, except wrist and hand

T22.7- <u>Corrosion</u> of <u>third</u> degree of <u>shoulder and upper limb</u>, except wrist and hand

    Code first (T51-T65) to identify chemical and intent

    Use additional external cause code to identify place (Y92)

    T22.70x- <u>Corrosion</u> of <u>third</u> degree of shoulder and upper limb, except wrist and hand, <u>unspecified</u> site

T22.71- <u>Corrosion</u> of <u>third</u> degree of <u>forearm</u>

    T22.711- Corrosion of third degree of <u>right</u> forearm

    T22.712- Corrosion of third degree of <u>left</u> forearm

    T22.719- Corrosion of third degree of <u>unspecified</u> forearm

T22.72- <u>Corrosion</u> of <u>third</u> degree of <u>elbow</u>

    T22.721- Corrosion of third degree of <u>right</u> elbow

    T22.722- Corrosion of third degree of <u>left</u> elbow

    T22.729- Corrosion of third degree of <u>unspecified</u> elbow

T22.73- <u>Corrosion</u> of <u>third</u> degree of <u>upper arm</u>

    T22.731- Corrosion of third degree of <u>right</u> upper arm

    T22.732- Corrosion of third degree of <u>left</u> upper arm

    T22.739- Corrosion of third degree of <u>unspecified</u> upper arm

T22.74- <u>Corrosion</u> of <u>third</u> degree of <u>axilla</u>

    T22.741- Corrosion of third degree of <u>right</u> axilla

    T22.742- Corrosion of third degree of <u>left</u> axilla

    T22.749- Corrosion of third degree of <u>unspecified</u> axilla

T22.75- <u>Corrosion</u> of <u>third</u> degree of <u>shoulder</u>

    T22.751- Corrosion of third degree of <u>right</u> shoulder

    T22.752- Corrosion of third degree of <u>left</u> shoulder

    T22.759- Corrosion of third degree of <u>unspecified</u> shoulder

T22.76- <u>Corrosion</u> of <u>third</u> degree of <u>scapular region</u>

    T22.761- Corrosion of third degree of <u>right</u> scapular region

    T22.762- Corrosion of third degree of <u>left</u> scapular region

    T22.769- Corrosion of third degree of <u>unspecified</u> scapular region

T22.79- <u>Corrosion</u> of <u>third</u> degree of <u>multiple</u> sites of shoulder and upper limb, except wrist and hand

    T22.791- Corrosion of third degree of multiple sites of <u>right</u> shoulder and upper limb, except wrist and hand

    T22.792- Corrosion of third degree of multiple sites of <u>left</u> shoulder and upper limb, except wrist and hand

    T22.799- Corrosion of third degree of multiple sites of <u>unspecified</u> shoulder and upper limb, except wrist and hand

T22 - T22

© 2013 Channel Publishing, Ltd.

T23-   Burn and corrosion of wrist and hand
       The appropriate 7th character is to be added to each code from
       category T23:
       A   Initial encounter
       D   Subsequent encounter
       S   Sequela

T23.0- Burn of unspecified degree of wrist and hand
        Use additional external cause code to identify the source, place and
        intent of the burn (X00-X19, X75-X77, X96-X98, Y92)

T23.00- Burn of unspecified degree of hand, unspecified site
   T23.001- Burn of unspecified degree of right hand, unspecified
             site
   T23.002- Burn of unspecified degree of left hand, unspecified
             site
   T23.009- Burn of unspecified degree of unspecified hand,
             unspecified site

T23.01- Burn of unspecified degree of thumb (nail)
   T23.011- Burn of unspecified degree of right thumb (nail)
   T23.012- Burn of unspecified degree of left thumb (nail)
   T23.019- Burn of unspecified degree of unspecified thumb (nail)

T23.02- Burn of unspecified degree of single finger (nail) except
         thumb
   T23.021- Burn of unspecified degree of single right finger (nail)
             except thumb
   T23.022- Burn of unspecified degree of single left finger (nail)
             except thumb
   T23.029- Burn of unspecified degree of unspecified single finger
             (nail) except thumb

T23.03- Burn of unspecified degree of multiple fingers (nail), not
         including thumb
   T23.031- Burn of unspecified degree of multiple right fingers
             (nail), not including thumb
   T23.032- Burn of unspecified degree of multiple left fingers
             (nail), not including thumb
   T23.039- Burn of unspecified degree of unspecified multiple
             fingers (nail), not including thumb

T23.04- Burn of unspecified degree of multiple fingers (nail),
         including thumb
   T23.041- Burn of unspecified degree of multiple right fingers
             (nail), including thumb
   T23.042- Burn of unspecified degree of multiple left fingers
             (nail), including thumb
   T23.049- Burn of unspecified degree of unspecified multiple
             fingers (nail), including thumb

T23.05- Burn of unspecified degree of palm
   T23.051- Burn of unspecified degree of right palm
   T23.052- Burn of unspecified degree of left palm
   T23.059- Burn of unspecified degree of unspecified palm

T23.06- Burn of unspecified degree of back of hand
   T23.061- Burn of unspecified degree of back of right hand
   T23.062- Burn of unspecified degree of back of left hand
   T23.069- Burn of unspecified degree of back of unspecified
             hand

T23.07- Burn of unspecified degree of wrist
   T23.071- Burn of unspecified degree of right wrist
   T23.072- Burn of unspecified degree of left wrist
   T23.079- Burn of unspecified degree of unspecified wrist

T23.09- Burn of unspecified degree of multiple sites of wrist and
         hand
   T23.091- Burn of unspecified degree of multiple sites of right
             wrist and hand
   T23.092- Burn of unspecified degree of multiple sites of left
             wrist and hand
   T23.099- Burn of unspecified degree of multiple sites of
             unspecified wrist and hand

T23.1- Burn of first degree of wrist and hand
        Use additional external cause code to identify the source, place and
        intent of the burn (X00-X19, X75-X77, X96-X98, Y92)

T23.10- Burn of first degree of hand, unspecified site
   T23.101- Burn of first degree of right hand, unspecified site
   T23.102- Burn of first degree of left hand, unspecified site
   T23.109- Burn of first degree of unspecified hand, unspecified
             site

T23.11- Burn of first degree of thumb (nail)
   T23.111- Burn of first degree of right thumb (nail)
   T23.112- Burn of first degree of left thumb (nail)
   T23.119- Burn of first degree of unspecified thumb (nail)

T23.12- Burn of first degree of single finger (nail) except thumb
   T23.121- Burn of first degree of single right finger (nail) except
             thumb
   T23.122- Burn of first degree of single left finger (nail) except
             thumb
   T23.129- Burn of first degree of unspecified single finger (nail)
             except thumb

T23.13- Burn of first degree of multiple fingers (nail), not including
         thumb
   T23.131- Burn of first degree of multiple right fingers (nail), not
             including thumb
   T23.132- Burn of first degree of multiple left fingers (nail), not
             including thumb
   T23.139- Burn of first degree of unspecified multiple fingers
             (nail), not including thumb

T23.14- Burn of first degree of multiple fingers (nail), including
         thumb
   T23.141- Burn of first degree of multiple right fingers (nail),
             including thumb
   T23.142- Burn of first degree of multiple left fingers (nail),
             including thumb
   T23.149- Burn of first degree of unspecified multiple fingers
             (nail), including thumb

T23.15- Burn of first degree of palm
   T23.151- Burn of first degree of right palm
   T23.152- Burn of first degree of left palm
   T23.159- Burn of first degree of unspecified palm

T23.16- Burn of first degree of back of hand
   T23.161- Burn of first degree of back of right hand
   T23.162- Burn of first degree of back of left hand
   T23.169- Burn of first degree of back of unspecified hand

T23.17- Burn of first degree of wrist
   T23.171- Burn of first degree of right wrist
   T23.172- Burn of first degree of left wrist
   T23.179- Burn of first degree of unspecified wrist

T23.19- Burn of first degree of multiple sites of wrist and hand
   T23.191- Burn of first degree of multiple sites of right wrist and
             hand
   T23.192- Burn of first degree of multiple sites of left wrist and
             hand
   T23.199- Burn of first degree of multiple sites of unspecified
             wrist and hand

T23.2- Burn of second degree of wrist and hand
        Use additional external cause code to identify the source, place and
        intent of the burn (X00-X19, X75-X77, X96-X98, Y92)

T23.20- Burn of second degree of hand, unspecified site
   T23.201- Burn of second degree of right hand, unspecified site
   T23.202- Burn of second degree of left hand, unspecified site
   T23.209- Burn of second degree of unspecified hand,
             unspecified site

T23.21- Burn of second degree of thumb (nail)
   T23.211- Burn of second degree of right thumb (nail)
   T23.212- Burn of second degree of left thumb (nail)
   T23.219- Burn of second degree of unspecified thumb (nail)

T23.22- Burn of second degree of single finger (nail) except thumb
   T23.221- Burn of second degree of single right finger (nail)
             except thumb
   T23.222- Burn of second degree of single left finger (nail) except
             thumb
   T23.229- Burn of second degree of unspecified single finger
             (nail) except thumb

T23.23- Burn of second degree of multiple fingers (nail), not
         including thumb
   T23.231- Burn of second degree of multiple right fingers (nail),
             not including thumb
   T23.232- Burn of second degree of multiple left fingers (nail),
             not including thumb
   T23.239- Burn of second degree of unspecified multiple fingers
             (nail), not including thumb

T23.24- Burn of second degree of multiple fingers (nail), including
         thumb
   T23.241- Burn of second degree of multiple right fingers (nail),
             including thumb
   T23.242- Burn of second degree of multiple left fingers (nail),
             including thumb
   T23.249- Burn of second degree of unspecified multiple fingers
             (nail), including thumb

T 2 3 - T 2 3

T23.25- Burn of second degree of palm
   T23.251- Burn of second degree of right palm
   T23.252- Burn of second degree of left palm
   T23.259- Burn of second degree of unspecified palm
T23.26- Burn of second degree of back of hand
   T23.261- Burn of second degree of back of right hand
   T23.262- Burn of second degree of back of left hand
   T23.269- Burn of second degree of back of unspecified hand
T23.27- Burn of second degree of wrist
   T23.271- Burn of second degree of right wrist
   T23.272- Burn of second degree of left wrist
   T23.279- Burn of second degree of unspecified wrist
T23.29- Burn of second degree of multiple sites of wrist and hand
   T23.291- Burn of second degree of multiple sites of right wrist and hand
   T23.292- Burn of second degree of multiple sites of left wrist and hand
   T23.299- Burn of second degree of multiple sites of unspecified wrist and hand

T23.3- Burn of third degree of wrist and hand
   Use additional external cause code to identify the source, place and intent of the burn (X00-X19, X75-X77, X96-X98, Y92)
T23.30- Burn of third degree of hand, unspecified site
   T23.301- Burn of third degree of right hand, unspecified site
   T23.302- Burn of third degree of left hand, unspecified site
   T23.309- Burn of third degree of unspecified hand, unspecified site
T23.31- Burn of third degree of thumb (nail)
   T23.311- Burn of third degree of right thumb (nail)
   T23.312- Burn of third degree of left thumb (nail)
   T23.319- Burn of third degree of unspecified thumb (nail)
T23.32- Burn of third degree of single finger (nail) except thumb
   T23.321- Burn of third degree of single right finger (nail) except thumb
   T23.322- Burn of third degree of single left finger (nail) except thumb
   T23.329- Burn of third degree of unspecified single finger (nail) except thumb
T23.33- Burn of third degree of multiple fingers (nail), not including thumb
   T23.331- Burn of third degree of multiple right fingers (nail), not including thumb
   T23.332- Burn of third degree of multiple left fingers (nail), not including thumb
   T23.339- Burn of third degree of unspecified multiple fingers (nail), not including thumb
T23.34- Burn of third degree of multiple fingers (nail), including thumb
   T23.341- Burn of third degree of multiple right fingers (nail), including thumb
   T23.342- Burn of third degree of multiple left fingers (nail), including thumb
   T23.349- Burn of third degree of unspecified multiple fingers (nail), including thumb
T23.35- Burn of third degree of palm
   T23.351- Burn of third degree of right palm
   T23.352- Burn of third degree of left palm
   T23.359- Burn of third degree of unspecified palm
T23.36- Burn of third degree of back of hand
   T23.361- Burn of third degree of back of right hand
   T23.362- Burn of third degree of back of left hand
   T23.369- Burn of third degree of back of unspecified hand
T23.37- Burn of third degree of wrist
   T23.371- Burn of third degree of right wrist
   T23.372- Burn of third degree of left wrist
   T23.379- Burn of third degree of unspecified wrist
T23.39- Burn of third degree of multiple sites of wrist and hand
   T23.391- Burn of third degree of multiple sites of right wrist and hand
   T23.392- Burn of third degree of multiple sites of left wrist and hand
   T23.399- Burn of third degree of multiple sites of unspecified wrist and hand

T23.4- Corrosion of unspecified degree of wrist and hand
   Code first (T51-T65) to identify chemical and intent
   Use additional external cause code to identify place (Y92)
T23.40- Corrosion of unspecified degree of hand, unspecified site
   T23.401- Corrosion of unspecified degree of right hand, unspecified site
   T23.402- Corrosion of unspecified degree of left hand, unspecified site
   T23.409- Corrosion of unspecified degree of unspecified hand, unspecified site
T23.41- Corrosion of unspecified degree of thumb (nail)
   T23.411- Corrosion of unspecified degree of right thumb (nail)
   T23.412- Corrosion of unspecified degree of left thumb (nail)
   T23.419- Corrosion of unspecified degree of unspecified thumb (nail)
T23.42- Corrosion of unspecified degree of single finger (nail) except thumb
   T23.421- Corrosion of unspecified degree of single right finger (nail) except thumb
   T23.422- Corrosion of unspecified degree of single left finger (nail) except thumb
   T23.429- Corrosion of unspecified degree of unspecified single finger (nail) except thumb
T23.43- Corrosion of unspecified degree of multiple fingers (nail), not including thumb
   T23.431- Corrosion of unspecified degree of multiple right fingers (nail), not including thumb
   T23.432- Corrosion of unspecified degree of multiple left fingers (nail), not including thumb
   T23.439- Corrosion of unspecified degree of unspecified multiple fingers (nail), not including thumb
T23.44- Corrosion of unspecified degree of multiple fingers (nail), including thumb
   T23.441- Corrosion of unspecified degree of multiple right fingers (nail), including thumb
   T23.442- Corrosion of unspecified degree of multiple left fingers (nail), including thumb
   T23.449- Corrosion of unspecified degree of unspecified multiple fingers (nail), including thumb
T23.45- Corrosion of unspecified degree of palm
   T23.451- Corrosion of unspecified degree of right palm
   T23.452- Corrosion of unspecified degree of left palm
   T23.459- Corrosion of unspecified degree of unspecified palm
T23.46- Corrosion of unspecified degree of back of hand
   T23.461- Corrosion of unspecified degree of back of right hand
   T23.462- Corrosion of unspecified degree of back of left hand
   T23.469- Corrosion of unspecified degree of back of unspecified hand
T23.47- Corrosion of unspecified degree of wrist
   T23.471- Corrosion of unspecified degree of right wrist
   T23.472- Corrosion of unspecified degree of left wrist
   T23.479- Corrosion of unspecified degree of unspecified wrist
T23.49- Corrosion of unspecified degree of multiple sites of wrist and hand
   T23.491- Corrosion of unspecified degree of multiple sites of right wrist and hand
   T23.492- Corrosion of unspecified degree of multiple sites of left wrist and hand
   T23.499- Corrosion of unspecified degree of multiple sites of unspecified wrist and hand
T23.5- Corrosion of first degree of wrist and hand
   Code first (T51-T65) to identify chemical and intent
   Use additional external cause code to identify place (Y92)
T23.50- Corrosion of first degree of hand, unspecified site
   T23.501- Corrosion of first degree of right hand, unspecified site
   T23.502- Corrosion of first degree of left hand, unspecified site
   T23.509- Corrosion of first degree of unspecified hand, unspecified site
T23.51- Corrosion of first degree of thumb (nail)
   T23.511- Corrosion of first degree of right thumb (nail)
   T23.512- Corrosion of first degree of left thumb (nail)
   T23.519- Corrosion of first degree of unspecified thumb (nail)
T23.52- Corrosion of first degree of single finger (nail) except thumb
   T23.521- Corrosion of first degree of single right finger (nail) except thumb
   T23.522- Corrosion of first degree of single left finger (nail) except thumb
   T23.529- Corrosion of first degree of unspecified single finger (nail) except thumb

T23 - T23

Excludes 1: = NOT CODED HERE! (Do not code both)   Excludes ❷ = Not Included Here

T23.53- Corrosion of first degree of multiple fingers (nail), not including thumb
  - T23.531- Corrosion of first degree of multiple right fingers (nail), not including thumb
  - T23.532- Corrosion of first degree of multiple left fingers (nail), not including thumb
  - T23.539- Corrosion of first degree of unspecified multiple fingers (nail), not including thumb

T23.54- Corrosion of first degree of multiple fingers (nail), including thumb
  - T23.541- Corrosion of first degree of multiple right fingers (nail), including thumb
  - T23.542- Corrosion of first degree of multiple left fingers (nail), including thumb
  - T23.549- Corrosion of first degree of unspecified multiple fingers (nail), including thumb

T23.55- Corrosion of first degree of palm
  - T23.551- Corrosion of first degree of right palm
  - T23.552- Corrosion of first degree of left palm
  - T23.559- Corrosion of first degree of unspecified palm

T23.56- Corrosion of first degree of back of hand
  - T23.561- Corrosion of first degree of back of right hand
  - T23.562- Corrosion of first degree of back of left hand
  - T23.569- Corrosion of first degree of back of unspecified hand

T23.57- Corrosion of first degree of wrist
  - T23.571- Corrosion of first degree of right wrist
  - T23.572- Corrosion of first degree of left wrist
  - T23.579- Corrosion of first degree of unspecified wrist

T23.59- Corrosion of first degree of multiple sites of wrist and hand
  - T23.591- Corrosion of first degree of multiple sites of right wrist and hand
  - T23.592- Corrosion of first degree of multiple sites of left wrist and hand
  - T23.599- Corrosion of first degree of multiple sites of unspecified wrist and hand

T23.6- Corrosion of second degree of wrist and hand
  Code first (T51-T65) to identify chemical and intent
  Use additional external cause code to identify place (Y92)

T23.60- Corrosion of second degree of hand, unspecified site
  - T23.601- Corrosion of second degree of right hand, unspecified site
  - T23.602- Corrosion of second degree of left hand, unspecified site
  - T23.609- Corrosion of second degree of unspecified hand, unspecified site

T23.61- Corrosion of second degree of thumb (nail)
  - T23.611- Corrosion of second degree of right thumb (nail)
  - T23.612- Corrosion of second degree of left thumb (nail)
  - T23.619- Corrosion of second degree of unspecified thumb (nail)

T23.62- Corrosion of second degree of single finger (nail) except thumb
  - T23.621- Corrosion of second degree of single right finger (nail) except thumb
  - T23.622- Corrosion of second degree of single left finger (nail) except thumb
  - T23.629- Corrosion of second degree of unspecified single finger (nail) except thumb

T23.63- Corrosion of second degree of multiple fingers (nail), not including thumb
  - T23.631- Corrosion of second degree of multiple right fingers (nail), not including thumb
  - T23.632- Corrosion of second degree of multiple left fingers (nail), not including thumb
  - T23.639- Corrosion of second degree of unspecified multiple fingers (nail), not including thumb

T23.64- Corrosion of second degree of multiple fingers (nail), including thumb
  - T23.641- Corrosion of second degree of multiple right fingers (nail), including thumb
  - T23.642- Corrosion of second degree of multiple left fingers (nail), including thumb
  - T23.649- Corrosion of second degree of unspecified multiple fingers (nail), including thumb

T23.65- Corrosion of second degree of palm
  - T23.651- Corrosion of second degree of right palm
  - T23.652- Corrosion of second degree of left palm
  - T23.659- Corrosion of second degree of unspecified palm

T23.66- Corrosion of second degree of back of hand
  - T23.661- Corrosion of second degree back of right hand
  - T23.662- Corrosion of second degree back of left hand
  - T23.669- Corrosion of second degree back of unspecified hand

T23.67- Corrosion of second degree of wrist
  - T23.671- Corrosion of second degree of right wrist
  - T23.672- Corrosion of second degree of left wrist
  - T23.679- Corrosion of second degree of unspecified wrist

T23.69- Corrosion of second degree of multiple sites of wrist and hand
  - T23.691- Corrosion of second degree of multiple sites of right wrist and hand
  - T23.692- Corrosion of second degree of multiple sites of left wrist and hand
  - T23.699- Corrosion of second degree of multiple sites of unspecified wrist and hand

T23.7- Corrosion of third degree of wrist and hand
  Code first (T51-T65) to identify chemical and intent
  Use additional external cause code to identify place (Y92)

T23.70- Corrosion of third degree of hand, unspecified site
  - T23.701- Corrosion of third degree of right hand, unspecified site
  - T23.702- Corrosion of third degree of left hand, unspecified site
  - T23.709- Corrosion of third degree of unspecified hand, unspecified site

T23.71- Corrosion of third degree of thumb (nail)
  - T23.711- Corrosion of third degree of right thumb (nail)
  - T23.712- Corrosion of third degree of left thumb (nail)
  - T23.719- Corrosion of third degree of unspecified thumb (nail)

T23.72- Corrosion of third degree of single finger (nail) except thumb
  - T23.721- Corrosion of third degree of single right finger (nail) except thumb
  - T23.722- Corrosion of third degree of single left finger (nail) except thumb
  - T23.729- Corrosion of third degree of unspecified single finger (nail) except thumb

T23.73- Corrosion of third degree of multiple fingers (nail), not including thumb
  - T23.731- Corrosion of third degree of multiple right fingers (nail), not including thumb
  - T23.732- Corrosion of third degree of multiple left fingers (nail), not including thumb
  - T23.739- Corrosion of third degree of unspecified multiple fingers (nail), not including thumb

T23.74- Corrosion of third degree of multiple fingers (nail), including thumb
  - T23.741- Corrosion of third degree of multiple right fingers (nail), including thumb
  - T23.742- Corrosion of third degree of multiple left fingers (nail), including thumb
  - T23.749- Corrosion of third degree of unspecified multiple fingers (nail), including thumb

T23.75- Corrosion of third degree of palm
  - T23.751- Corrosion of third degree of right palm
  - T23.752- Corrosion of third degree of left palm
  - T23.759- Corrosion of third degree of unspecified palm

T23.76- Corrosion of third degree of back of hand
  - T23.761- Corrosion of third degree of back of right hand
  - T23.762- Corrosion of third degree of back of left hand
  - T23.769- Corrosion of third degree back of unspecified hand

T23.77- Corrosion of third degree of wrist
  - T23.771- Corrosion of third degree of right wrist
  - T23.772- Corrosion of third degree of left wrist
  - T23.779- Corrosion of third degree of unspecified wrist

T23.79- Corrosion of third degree of multiple sites of wrist and hand
  - T23.791- Corrosion of third degree of multiple sites of right wrist and hand
  - T23.792- Corrosion of third degree of multiple sites of left wrist and hand
  - T23.799- Corrosion of third degree of multiple sites of unspecified wrist and hand

T
2
3
-
T
2
4

Excludes 1: = NOT CODED HERE! (Do not code both)   **790**   *Excludes ❷:* = Not Included Here

T24-   Burn and corrosion of lower limb, except ankle and foot
    Excludes❷: burn and corrosion of ankle and foot (T25.-)
    burn and corrosion of hip region (T21.-)

The appropriate 7th character is to be added to each code from category T24:
    A   Initial encounter
    D   Subsequent encounter
    S   Sequela

T24.0- Burn of unspecified degree of lower limb, except ankle and foot
    Use additional external cause code to identify the source, place and intent of the burn (X00-X19, X75-X77, X96-X98, Y92)

  T24.00- Burn of unspecified degree of unspecified site of lower limb, except ankle and foot
    T24.001- Burn of unspecified degree of unspecified site of right lower limb, except ankle and foot
    T24.002- Burn of unspecified degree of unspecified site of left lower limb, except ankle and foot
    T24.009- Burn of unspecified degree of unspecified site of unspecified lower limb, except ankle and foot

  T24.01- Burn of unspecified degree of thigh
    T24.011- Burn of unspecified degree of right thigh
    T24.012- Burn of unspecified degree of left thigh
    T24.019- Burn of unspecified degree of unspecified thigh

  T24.02- Burn of unspecified degree of knee
    T24.021- Burn of unspecified degree of right knee
    T24.022- Burn of unspecified degree of left knee
    T24.029- Burn of unspecified degree of unspecified knee

  T24.03- Burn of unspecified degree of lower leg
    T24.031- Burn of unspecified degree of right lower leg
    T24.032- Burn of unspecified degree of left lower leg
    T24.039- Burn of unspecified degree of unspecified lower leg

  T24.09- Burn of unspecified degree of multiple sites of lower limb, except ankle and foot
    T24.091- Burn of unspecified degree of multiple sites of right lower limb, except ankle and foot
    T24.092- Burn of unspecified degree of multiple sites of left lower limb, except ankle and foot
    T24.099- Burn of unspecified degree of multiple sites of unspecified lower limb, except ankle and foot

T24.1- Burn of first degree of lower limb, except ankle and foot
    Use additional external cause code to identify the source, place and intent of the burn (X00-X19, X75-X77, X96-X98, Y92)

  T24.10- Burn of first degree of unspecified site of lower limb, except ankle and foot
    T24.101- Burn of first degree of unspecified site of right lower limb, except ankle and foot
    T24.102- Burn of first degree of unspecified site of left lower limb, except ankle and foot
    T24.109- Burn of first degree of unspecified site of unspecified lower limb, except ankle and foot

  T24.11- Burn of first degree of thigh
    T24.111- Burn of first degree of right thigh
    T24.112- Burn of first degree of left thigh
    T24.119- Burn of first degree of unspecified thigh

  T24.12- Burn of first degree of knee
    T24.121- Burn of first degree of right knee
    T24.122- Burn of first degree of left knee
    T24.129- Burn of first degree of unspecified knee

  T24.13- Burn of first degree of lower leg
    T24.131- Burn of first degree of right lower leg
    T24.132- Burn of first degree of left lower leg
    T24.139- Burn of first degree of unspecified lower leg

  T24.19- Burn of first degree of multiple sites of lower limb, except ankle and foot
    T24.191- Burn of first degree of multiple sites of right lower limb, except ankle and foot
    T24.192- Burn of first degree of multiple sites of left lower limb, except ankle and foot
    T24.199- Burn of first degree of multiple sites of unspecified lower limb, except ankle and foot

T24.2- Burn of second degree of lower limb, except ankle and foot
    Use additional external cause code to identify the source, place and intent of the burn (X00-X19, X75-X77, X96-X98, Y92)

  T24.20- Burn of second degree of unspecified site of lower limb, except ankle and foot
    T24.201- Burn of second degree of unspecified site of right lower limb, except ankle and foot
    T24.202- Burn of second degree of unspecified site of left lower limb, except ankle and foot
    T24.209- Burn of second degree of unspecified site of unspecified lower limb, except ankle and foot

  T24.21- Burn of second degree of thigh
    T24.211- Burn of second degree of right thigh
    T24.212- Burn of second degree of left thigh
    T24.219- Burn of second degree of unspecified thigh

  T24.22- Burn of second degree of knee
    T24.221- Burn of second degree of right knee
    T24.222- Burn of second degree of left knee
    T24.229- Burn of second degree of unspecified knee

  T24.23- Burn of second degree of lower leg
    T24.231- Burn of second degree of right lower leg
    T24.232- Burn of second degree of left lower leg
    T24.239- Burn of second degree of unspecified lower leg

  T24.29- Burn of second degree of multiple sites of lower limb, except ankle and foot
    T24.291- Burn of second degree of multiple sites of right lower limb, except ankle and foot
    T24.292- Burn of second degree of multiple sites of left lower limb, except ankle and foot
    T24.299- Burn of second degree of multiple sites of unspecified lower limb, except ankle and foot

T24.3- Burn of third degree of lower limb, except ankle and foot
    Use additional external cause code to identify the source, place and intent of the burn (X00-X19, X75-X77, X96-X98, Y92)

  T24.30- Burn of third degree of unspecified site of lower limb, except ankle and foot
    T24.301- Burn of third degree of unspecified site of right lower limb, except ankle and foot
    T24.302- Burn of third degree of unspecified site of left lower limb, except ankle and foot
    T24.309- Burn of third degree of unspecified site of unspecified lower limb, except ankle and foot

  T24.31- Burn of third degree of thigh
    T24.311- Burn of third degree of right thigh
    T24.312- Burn of third degree of left thigh
    T24.319- Burn of third degree of unspecified thigh

  T24.32- Burn of third degree of knee
    T24.321- Burn of third degree of right knee
    T24.322- Burn of third degree of left knee
    T24.329- Burn of third degree of unspecified knee

  T24.33- Burn of third degree of lower leg
    T24.331- Burn of third degree of right lower leg
    T24.332- Burn of third degree of left lower leg
    T24.339- Burn of third degree of unspecified lower leg

  T24.39- Burn of third degree of multiple sites of lower limb, except ankle and foot
    T24.391- Burn of third degree of multiple sites of right lower limb, except ankle and foot
    T24.392- Burn of third degree of multiple sites of left lower limb, except ankle and foot
    T24.399- Burn of third degree of multiple sites of unspecified lower limb, except ankle and foot

T24.4- Corrosion of unspecified degree of lower limb, except ankle and foot
    Code first (T51-T65) to identify chemical and intent
    Use additional external cause code to identify place (Y92)

  T24.40- Corrosion of unspecified degree of unspecified site of lower limb, except ankle and foot
    T24.401- Corrosion of unspecified degree of unspecified site of right lower limb, except ankle and foot
    T24.402- Corrosion of unspecified degree of unspecified site of left lower limb, except ankle and foot
    T24.409- Corrosion of unspecified degree of unspecified site of unspecified lower limb, except ankle and foot

  T24.41- Corrosion of unspecified degree of thigh
    T24.411- Corrosion of unspecified degree of right thigh
    T24.412- Corrosion of unspecified degree of left thigh
    T24.419- Corrosion of unspecified degree of unspecified thigh

T23 – T24

T24.42- Corrosion of unspecified degree of knee
　　T24.421- Corrosion of unspecified degree of right knee
　　T24.422- Corrosion of unspecified degree of left knee
　　T24.429- Corrosion of unspecified degree of unspecified knee
T24.43- Corrosion of unspecified degree of lower leg
　　T24.431- Corrosion of unspecified degree of right lower leg
　　T24.432- Corrosion of unspecified degree of left lower leg
　　T24.439- Corrosion of unspecified degree of unspecified lower leg
T24.49- Corrosion of unspecified degree of multiple sites of lower limb, except ankle and foot
　　T24.491- Corrosion of unspecified degree of multiple sites of right lower limb, except ankle and foot
　　T24.492- Corrosion of unspecified degree of multiple sites of left lower limb, except ankle and foot
　　T24.499- Corrosion of unspecified degree of multiple sites of unspecified lower limb, except ankle and foot
T24.5- Corrosion of first degree of lower limb, except ankle and foot
　　Code first (T51-T65) to identify chemical and intent
　　Use additional external cause code to identify place (Y92)
　　T24.50- Corrosion of first degree of unspecified site of lower limb, except ankle and foot
　　　　T24.501- Corrosion of first degree of unspecified site of right lower limb, except ankle and foot
　　　　T24.502- Corrosion of first degree of unspecified site of left lower limb, except ankle and foot
　　　　T24.509- Corrosion of first degree of unspecified site of unspecified lower limb, except ankle and foot
　　T24.51- Corrosion of first degree of thigh
　　　　T24.511- Corrosion of first degree of right thigh
　　　　T24.512- Corrosion of first degree of left thigh
　　　　T24.519- Corrosion of first degree of unspecified thigh
　　T24.52- Corrosion of first degree of knee
　　　　T24.521- Corrosion of first degree of right knee
　　　　T24.522- Corrosion of first degree of left knee
　　　　T24.529- Corrosion of first degree of unspecified knee
　　T24.53- Corrosion of first degree of lower leg
　　　　T24.531- Corrosion of first degree of right lower leg
　　　　T24.532- Corrosion of first degree of left lower leg
　　　　T24.539- Corrosion of first degree of unspecified lower leg
　　T24.59- Corrosion of first degree of multiple sites of lower limb, except ankle and foot
　　　　T24.591- Corrosion of first degree of multiple sites of right lower limb, except ankle and foot
　　　　T24.592- Corrosion of first degree of multiple sites of left lower limb, except ankle and foot
　　　　T24.599- Corrosion of first degree of multiple sites of unspecified lower limb, except ankle and foot
T24.6- Corrosion of second degree of lower limb, except ankle and foot
　　Code first (T51-T65) to identify chemical and intent
　　Use additional external cause code to identify place (Y92)
　　T24.60- Corrosion of second degree of unspecified site of lower limb, except ankle and foot
　　　　T24.601- Corrosion of second degree of unspecified site of right lower limb, except ankle and foot
　　　　T24.602- Corrosion of second degree of unspecified site of left lower limb, except ankle and foot
　　　　T24.609- Corrosion of second degree of unspecified site of unspecified lower limb, except ankle and foot
　　T24.61- Corrosion of second degree of thigh
　　　　T24.611- Corrosion of second degree of right thigh
　　　　T24.612- Corrosion of second degree of left thigh
　　　　T24.619- Corrosion of second degree of unspecified thigh
　　T24.62- Corrosion of second degree of knee
　　　　T24.621- Corrosion of second degree of right knee
　　　　T24.622- Corrosion of second degree of left knee
　　　　T24.629- Corrosion of second degree of unspecified knee
　　T24.63- Corrosion of second degree of lower leg
　　　　T24.631- Corrosion of second degree of right lower leg
　　　　T24.632- Corrosion of second degree of left lower leg
　　　　T24.639- Corrosion of second degree of unspecified lower leg
　　T24.69- Corrosion of second degree of multiple sites of lower limb, except ankle and foot
　　　　T24.691- Corrosion of second degree of multiple sites of right lower limb, except ankle and foot
　　　　T24.692- Corrosion of second degree of multiple sites of left lower limb, except ankle and foot

T24.699- Corrosion of second degree of multiple sites of unspecified lower limb, except ankle and foot
T24.7- Corrosion of third degree of lower limb, except ankle and foot
　　Code first (T51-T65) to identify chemical and intent
　　Use additional external cause code to identify place (Y92)
　　T24.70- Corrosion of third degree of unspecified site of lower limb, except ankle and foot
　　　　T24.701- Corrosion of third degree of unspecified site of right lower limb, except ankle and foot
　　　　T24.702- Corrosion of third degree of unspecified site of left lower limb, except ankle and foot
　　　　T24.709- Corrosion of third degree of unspecified site of unspecified lower limb, except ankle and foot
　　T24.71- Corrosion of third degree of thigh
　　　　T24.711- Corrosion of third degree of right thigh
　　　　T24.712- Corrosion of third degree of left thigh
　　　　T24.719- Corrosion of third degree of unspecified thigh
　　T24.72- Corrosion of third degree of knee
　　　　T24.721- Corrosion of third degree of right knee
　　　　T24.722- Corrosion of third degree of left knee
　　　　T24.729- Corrosion of third degree of unspecified knee
　　T24.73- Corrosion of third degree of lower leg
　　　　T24.731- Corrosion of third degree of right lower leg
　　　　T24.732- Corrosion of third degree of left lower leg
　　　　T24.739- Corrosion of third degree of unspecified lower leg
　　T24.79- Corrosion of third degree of multiple sites of lower limb, except ankle and foot
　　　　T24.791- Corrosion of third degree of multiple sites of right lower limb, except ankle and foot
　　　　T24.792- Corrosion of third degree of multiple sites of left lower limb, except ankle and foot
　　　　T24.799- Corrosion of third degree of multiple sites of unspecified lower limb, except ankle and foot

T25- Burn and corrosion of ankle and foot
　　The appropriate 7th character is to be added to each code from category T25:
　　A　Initial encounter
　　D　Subsequent encounter
　　S　Sequela
T25.0- Burn of unspecified degree of ankle and foot
　　Use additional external cause code to identify the source, place and intent of the burn (X00-X19, X75-X77, X96-X98, Y92)
　　T25.01- Burn of unspecified degree of ankle
　　　　T25.011- Burn of unspecified degree of right ankle
　　　　T25.012- Burn of unspecified degree of left ankle
　　　　T25.019- Burn of unspecified degree of unspecified ankle
　　T25.02- Burn of unspecified degree of foot
　　　　Excludes❷: burn of unspecified degree of toe(s) (nail) (T25.03-)
　　　　T25.021- Burn of unspecified degree of right foot
　　　　T25.022- Burn of unspecified degree of left foot
　　　　T25.029- Burn of unspecified degree of unspecified foot
　　T25.03- Burn of unspecified degree of toe(s) (nail)
　　　　T25.031- Burn of unspecified degree of right toe(s) (nail)
　　　　T25.032- Burn of unspecified degree of left toe(s) (nail)
　　　　T25.039- Burn of unspecified degree of unspecified toe(s) (nail)
　　T25.09- Burn of unspecified degree of multiple sites of ankle and foot
　　　　T25.091- Burn of unspecified degree of multiple sites of right ankle and foot
　　　　T25.092- Burn of unspecified degree of multiple sites of left ankle and foot
　　　　T25.099- Burn of unspecified degree of multiple sites of unspecified ankle and foot
T25.1- Burn of first degree of ankle and foot
　　Use additional external cause code to identify the source, place and intent of the burn (X00-X19, X75-X77, X96-X98, Y92)
　　T25.11- Burn of first degree of ankle
　　　　T25.111- Burn of first degree of right ankle
　　　　T25.112- Burn of first degree of left ankle
　　　　T25.119- Burn of first degree of unspecified ankle
　　T25.12- Burn of first degree of foot
　　　　Excludes❷: burn of first degree of toe(s) (nail) (T25.13-)
　　　　T25.121- Burn of first degree of right foot
　　　　T25.122- Burn of first degree of left foot
　　　　T25.129- Burn of first degree of unspecified foot

T 2 4 - T 2 5

T25.13- Burn of <u>first</u> degree of <u>toe(s)</u> (nail)
    T25.131- Burn of first degree of <u>right</u> toe(s) (nail)
    T25.132- Burn of first degree of <u>left</u> toe(s) (nail)
    T25.139- Burn of first degree of <u>unspecified</u> toe(s) (nail)
T25.19- Burn of <u>first</u> degree of <u>multiple</u> sites of <u>ankle and foot</u>
    T25.191- Burn of first degree of multiple sites of <u>right</u> ankle and foot
    T25.192- Burn of first degree of multiple sites of <u>left</u> ankle and foot
    T25.199- Burn of first degree of multiple sites of <u>unspecified</u> ankle and foot

T25.2- Burn of <u>second</u> degree of <u>ankle and foot</u>
    Use additional external cause code to identify the source, place and intent of the burn (X00-X19, X75-X77, X96-X98, Y92)
  T25.21- Burn of <u>second</u> degree of <u>ankle</u>
    T25.211- Burn of second degree of <u>right</u> ankle
    T25.212- Burn of second degree of <u>left</u> ankle
    T25.219- Burn of second degree of <u>unspecified</u> ankle
  T25.22- Burn of <u>second</u> degree of <u>foot</u>
    Excludes❷: burn of second degree of toe(s) (nail) (T25.23-)
    T25.221- Burn of second degree of <u>right</u> foot
    T25.222- Burn of second degree of <u>left</u> foot
    T25.229- Burn of second degree of <u>unspecified</u> foot
  T25.23- Burn of <u>second</u> degree of <u>toe(s)</u> (nail)
    T25.231- Burn of second degree of <u>right</u> toe(s) (nail)
    T25.232- Burn of second degree of <u>left</u> toe(s) (nail)
    T25.239- Burn of second degree of <u>unspecified</u> toe(s) (nail)
  T25.29- Burn of <u>second</u> degree of <u>multiple</u> sites of <u>ankle and foot</u>
    T25.291- Burn of second degree of multiple sites of <u>right</u> ankle and foot
    T25.292- Burn of second degree of multiple sites of <u>left</u> ankle and foot
    T25.299- Burn of second degree of multiple sites of <u>unspecified</u> ankle and foot

T25.3- Burn of <u>third</u> degree of <u>ankle and foot</u>
    Use additional external cause code to identify the source, place and intent of the burn (X00-X19, X75-X77, X96-X98, Y92)
  T25.31- Burn of <u>third</u> degree of <u>ankle</u>
    T25.311- Burn of third degree of <u>right</u> ankle
    T25.312- Burn of third degree of <u>left</u> ankle
    T25.319- Burn of third degree of <u>unspecified</u> ankle
  T25.32- Burn of <u>third</u> degree of <u>foot</u>
    Excludes❷: burn of third degree of toe(s) (nail) (T25.33-)
    T25.321- Burn of third degree of <u>right</u> foot
    T25.322- Burn of third degree of <u>left</u> foot
    T25.329- Burn of third degree of <u>unspecified</u> foot
  T25.33- Burn of <u>third</u> degree of <u>toe(s)</u> (nail)
    T25.331- Burn of third degree of <u>right</u> toe(s) (nail)
    T25.332- Burn of third degree of <u>left</u> toe(s) (nail)
    T25.339- Burn of third degree of <u>unspecified</u> toe(s) (nail)
  T25.39- Burn of <u>third</u> degree of <u>multiple</u> sites of <u>ankle and foot</u>
    T25.391- Burn of third degree of multiple sites of <u>right</u> ankle and foot
    T25.392- Burn of third degree of multiple sites of <u>left</u> ankle and foot
    T25.399- Burn of third degree of multiple sites of <u>unspecified</u> ankle and foot

T25.4- <u>Corrosion</u> of <u>unspecified degree</u> of <u>ankle and foot</u>
    Code first (T51-T65) to identify chemical and intent
    Use additional external cause code to identify place (Y92)
  T25.41- <u>Corrosion</u> of <u>unspecified degree</u> of <u>ankle</u>
    T25.411- Corrosion of unspecified degree of <u>right</u> ankle
    T25.412- Corrosion of unspecified degree of <u>left</u> ankle
    T25.419- Corrosion of unspecified degree of <u>unspecified</u> ankle
  T25.42- <u>Corrosion</u> of <u>unspecified degree</u> of <u>foot</u>
    Excludes❷: corrosion of unspecified degree of toe(s) (nail) (T25.43-)
    T25.421- Corrosion of unspecified degree of <u>right</u> foot
    T25.422- Corrosion of unspecified degree of <u>left</u> foot
    T25.429- Corrosion of unspecified degree of <u>unspecified</u> foot
  T25.43- <u>Corrosion</u> of <u>unspecified degree</u> of <u>toe(s)</u> (nail)
    T25.431- Corrosion of unspecified degree of <u>right</u> toe(s) (nail)
    T25.432- Corrosion of unspecified degree of <u>left</u> toe(s) (nail)
    T25.439- Corrosion of unspecified degree of <u>unspecified</u> toe(s) (nail)

T25.49- <u>Corrosion</u> of <u>unspecified degree</u> of <u>multiple</u> sites of <u>ankle and foot</u>
    T25.491- Corrosion of unspecified degree of multiple sites of <u>right</u> ankle and foot
    T25.492- Corrosion of unspecified degree of multiple sites of <u>left</u> ankle and foot
    T25.499- Corrosion of unspecified degree of multiple sites of <u>unspecified</u> ankle and foot

T25.5- <u>Corrosion</u> of <u>first</u> degree of <u>ankle and foot</u>
    Code first (T51-T65) to identify chemical and intent
    Use additional external cause code to identify place (Y92)
  T25.51- <u>Corrosion</u> of <u>first</u> degree of <u>ankle</u>
    T25.511- Corrosion of first degree of <u>right</u> ankle
    T25.512- Corrosion of first degree of <u>left</u> ankle
    T25.519- Corrosion of first degree of <u>unspecified</u> ankle
  T25.52- <u>Corrosion</u> of <u>first</u> degree of <u>foot</u>
    Excludes❷: corrosion of first degree of toe(s) (nail) (T25.53-)
    T25.521- Corrosion of first degree of <u>right</u> foot
    T25.522- Corrosion of first degree of <u>left</u> foot
    T25.529- Corrosion of first degree of <u>unspecified</u> foot
  T25.53- <u>Corrosion</u> of <u>first</u> degree of <u>toe(s)</u> (nail)
    T25.531- Corrosion of first degree of <u>right</u> toe(s) (nail)
    T25.532- Corrosion of first degree of <u>left</u> toe(s) (nail)
    T25.539- Corrosion of first degree of <u>unspecified</u> toe(s) (nail)
  T25.59- <u>Corrosion</u> of <u>first</u> degree of <u>multiple</u> sites of <u>ankle and foot</u>
    T25.591- Corrosion of first degree of multiple sites of <u>right</u> ankle and foot
    T25.592- Corrosion of first degree of multiple sites of <u>left</u> ankle and foot
    T25.599- Corrosion of first degree of multiple sites of <u>unspecified</u> ankle and foot

T25.6- <u>Corrosion</u> of <u>second</u> degree of <u>ankle and foot</u>
    Code first (T51-T65) to identify chemical and intent
    Use additional external cause code to identify place (Y92)
  T25.61- <u>Corrosion</u> of <u>second</u> degree of <u>ankle</u>
    T25.611- Corrosion of second degree of <u>right</u> ankle
    T25.612- Corrosion of second degree of <u>left</u> ankle
    T25.619- Corrosion of second degree of <u>unspecified</u> ankle
  T25.62- <u>Corrosion</u> of <u>second</u> degree of <u>foot</u>
    Excludes❷: corrosion of second degree of toe(s) (nail) (T25.63-)
    T25.621- Corrosion of second degree of <u>right</u> foot
    T25.622- Corrosion of second degree of <u>left</u> foot
    T25.629- Corrosion of second degree of <u>unspecified</u> foot
  T25.63- <u>Corrosion</u> of <u>second</u> degree of <u>toe(s)</u> (nail)
    T25.631- Corrosion of second degree of <u>right</u> toe(s) (nail)
    T25.632- Corrosion of second degree of <u>left</u> toe(s) (nail)
    T25.639- Corrosion of second degree of <u>unspecified</u> toe(s) (nail)
  T25.69 <u>Corrosion</u> of <u>second</u> degree of <u>multiple</u> sites of <u>ankle and foot</u>
    T25.691- Corrosion of second degree of <u>right</u> ankle and foot
    T25.692- Corrosion of second degree of <u>left</u> ankle and foot
    T25.699- Corrosion of second degree of <u>unspecified</u> ankle and foot

T25.7- <u>Corrosion</u> of <u>third</u> degree of <u>ankle and foot</u>
    Code first (T51-T65) to identify chemical and intent
    Use additional external cause code to identify place (Y92)
  T25.71- <u>Corrosion</u> of <u>third</u> degree of <u>ankle</u>
    T25.711- Corrosion of third degree of <u>right</u> ankle
    T25.712- Corrosion of third degree of <u>left</u> ankle
    T25.719- Corrosion of third degree of <u>unspecified</u> ankle
  T25.72- <u>Corrosion</u> of <u>third</u> degree of <u>foot</u>
    Excludes❷: corrosion of third degree of toe(s) (nail) (T25.73-)
    T25.721- Corrosion of third degree of <u>right</u> foot
    T25.722- Corrosion of third degree of <u>left</u> foot
    T25.729- Corrosion of third degree of <u>unspecified</u> foot
  T25.73- <u>Corrosion</u> of <u>third</u> degree of <u>toe(s)</u> (nail)
    T25.731- Corrosion of third degree of <u>right</u> toe(s) (nail)
    T25.732- Corrosion of third degree of <u>left</u> toe(s) (nail)
    T25.739- Corrosion of third degree of <u>unspecified</u> toe(s) (nail)
  T25.79- <u>Corrosion</u> of <u>third</u> degree of <u>multiple</u> sites of <u>ankle and foot</u>
    T25.791- Corrosion of third degree of multiple sites of <u>right</u> ankle and foot
    T25.792- Corrosion of third degree of multiple sites of <u>left</u> ankle and foot
    T25.799- Corrosion of third degree of multiple sites of <u>unspecified</u> ankle and foot

T24 - T25

Excludes 1: = NOT CODED HERE! (Do not code both)

Excludes❷: = Not Included Here

Burns and corrosions confined to eye and internal organs (T26-T28)

T26- Burn and corrosion confined to eye and adnexa

> **The appropriate 7th character is to be added to each code from category T26:**
> A   **Initial** encounter
> D   **Subsequent** encounter
> S   **Sequela**

T26.0- Burn of eyelid and periocular area
Use additional external cause code to identify the source, place and intent of the burn (X00-X19, X75-X77, X96-X98, Y92)

  T26.00x- Burn of unspecified eyelid and periocular area
  T26.01x- Burn of right eyelid and periocular area
  T26.02x- Burn of left eyelid and periocular area

T26.1- Burn of cornea and conjunctival sac
Use additional external cause code to identify the source, place and intent of the burn (X00-X19, X75-X77, X96-X98, Y92)

  T26.10x- Burn of cornea and conjunctival sac, unspecified eye
  T26.11x- Burn of cornea and conjunctival sac, right eye
  T26.12x- Burn of cornea and conjunctival sac, left eye

T26.2- Burn with resulting rupture and destruction of eyeball
Use additional external cause code to identify the source, place and intent of the burn (X00-X19, X75-X77, X96-X98, Y92)

  T26.20x- Burn with resulting rupture and destruction of unspecified eyeball
  T26.21x- Burn with resulting rupture and destruction of right eyeball
  T26.22x- Burn with resulting rupture and destruction of left eyeball

T26.3- Burns of other specified parts of eye and adnexa
Use additional external cause code to identify the source, place and intent of the burn (X00-X19, X75-X77, X96-X98, Y92)

  T26.30x- Burns of other specified parts of unspecified eye and adnexa
  T26.31x- Burns of other specified parts of right eye and adnexa
  T26.32x- Burns of other specified parts of left eye and adnexa

T26.4- Burn of eye and adnexa, part unspecified
Use additional external cause code to identify the source, place and intent of the burn (X00-X19, X75-X77, X96-X98, Y92)

  T26.40x- Burn of unspecified eye and adnexa, part unspecified
  T26.41x- Burn of right eye and adnexa, part unspecified
  T26.42x- Burn of left eye and adnexa, part unspecified

T26.5- Corrosion of eyelid and periocular area
Code first (T51-T65) to identify chemical and intent
Use additional external cause code to identify place (Y92)

  T26.50x- Corrosion of unspecified eyelid and periocular area
  T26.51x- Corrosion of right eyelid and periocular area
  T26.52x- Corrosion of left eyelid and periocular area

T26.6- Corrosion of cornea and conjunctival sac
Code first (T51-T65) to identify chemical and intent
Use additional external cause code to identify place (Y92)

  T26.60x- Corrosion of cornea and conjunctival sac, unspecified eye
  T26.61x- Corrosion of cornea and conjunctival sac, right eye
  T26.62x- Corrosion of cornea and conjunctival sac, left eye

T26.7- Corrosion with resulting rupture and destruction of eyeball
Code first (T51-T65) to identify chemical and intent
Use additional external cause code to identify place (Y92)

  T26.70x- Corrosion with resulting rupture and destruction of unspecified eyeball
  T26.71x- Corrosion with resulting rupture and destruction of right eyeball
  T26.72x- Corrosion with resulting rupture and destruction of left eyeball

T26.8- Corrosions of other specified parts of eye and adnexa
Code first (T51-T65) to identify chemical and intent
Use additional external cause code to identify place (Y92)

  T26.80x- Corrosions of other specified parts of unspecified eye and adnexa
  T26.81x- Corrosions of other specified parts of right eye and adnexa
  T26.82x- Corrosions of other specified parts of left eye and adnexa

T26.9- Corrosion of eye and adnexa, part unspecified
Code first (T51-T65) to identify chemical and intent
Use additional external cause code to identify place (Y92)

  T26.90x- Corrosion of unspecified eye and adnexa, part unspecified
  T26.91x- Corrosion of right eye and adnexa, part unspecified
  T26.92x- Corrosion of left eye and adnexa, part unspecified

T27- Burn and corrosion of respiratory tract
Use additional external cause code to identify the source and intent of the burn (X00-X19, X75-X77, X96-X98)
Use additional external cause code to identify place (Y92)

> **The appropriate 7th character is to be added to each code from category T27:**
> A   **Initial** encounter
> D   **Subsequent** encounter
> S   **Sequela**

T27.0xx- Burn of larynx and trachea
T27.1xx- Burn involving larynx and trachea with lung
T27.2xx- Burn of other parts of respiratory tract
  Burn of thoracic cavity
T27.3xx- Burn of respiratory tract, part unspecified
  Code first (T51-T65) to identify chemical and intent for codes T27.4-T27.7
T27.4xx- Corrosion of larynx and trachea
T27.5xx- Corrosion involving larynx and trachea with lung
T27.6xx- Corrosion of other parts of respiratory tract
T27.7xx- Corrosion of respiratory tract, part unspecified

T28- Burn and corrosion of other internal organs
Use additional external cause code to identify the source and intent of the burn (X00-X19, X75-X77, X96-X98)
Use additional external cause code to identify place (Y92)

> **The appropriate 7th character is to be added to each code from category T28:**
> A   **Initial** encounter
> D   **Subsequent** encounter
> S   **Sequela**

T28.0xx- Burn of mouth and pharynx
T28.1xx- Burn of esophagus
T28.2xx- Burn of other parts of alimentary tract
T28.3xx- Burn of internal genitourinary organs
T28.4xx- Burns of other and unspecified internal organs
  T28.40x- Burn of unspecified internal organ
  T28.41- Burn of ear drum
    T28.411- Burn of right ear drum
    T28.412- Burn of left ear drum
    T28.419- Burn of unspecified ear drum
  T28.49x- Burn of other internal organ
    Code first (T51-T65) to identify chemical and intent for T28.5-T28.9-

T28.5xx- Corrosion of mouth and pharynx
T28.6xx- Corrosion of esophagus
T28.7xx- Corrosion of other parts of alimentary tract
T28.8xx- Corrosion of internal genitourinary organs
T28.9xx- Corrosions of other and unspecified internal organs
  T28.90x- Corrosions of unspecified internal organs
  T28.91- Corrosions of ear drum
    T28.911- Corrosions of right ear drum
    T28.912- Corrosions of left ear drum
    T28.919- Corrosions of unspecified ear drum
  T28.99x- Corrosions of other internal organs

Burns and corrosions of multiple and unspecified body regions (T30-T32)

T30- Burn and corrosion, body region unspecified
  T30.0 Burn of unspecified body region, unspecified degree
    Note: This code is not for inpatient use. Code to specified site and degree of burns
    Burn NOS
    Multiple burns NOS

  T30.4 Corrosion of unspecified body region, unspecified degree
    Note: This code is not for inpatient use. Code to specified site and degree of corrosion
    Corrosion NOS
    Multiple corrosion NOS

T31- Burns classified according to extent of body surface involved
  Note: This category is to be used as the primary code only when the site of the burn is unspecified. It should be used as a supplementary code with categories T20-T25 when the site is specified.

  T31.0 Burns involving less than 10% of body surface
  T31.1- Burns involving 10-19% of body surface
    T31.10 Burns involving 10-19% of body surface with 0% to 9% third degree burns
      Burns involving 10-19% of body surface NOS

T 2 6 - T 3 2

T31.11   **Burns involving 10-19% of body surface <u>with 10-19% third</u> <u>degree</u> burns**

T31.2-   Burns involving <u>20-29% of body surface</u>

     T31.20   **Burns involving 20-29% of body surface <u>with 0% to 9%</u> <u>third</u> degree burns**
         Burns involving 20-29% of body surface NOS

     T31.21   **Burns involving 20-29% of body surface <u>with 10-19% third</u> degree burns**

     T31.22   **Burns involving 20-29% of body surface <u>with 20-29% third</u> degree burns**

T31.3-   Burns involving <u>30-39% of body surface</u>

     T31.30   **Burns involving 30-39% of body surface <u>with 0% to 9%</u> <u>third</u> degree burns**
         Burns involving 30-39% of body surface NOS

     T31.31   **Burns involving 30-39% of body surface <u>with 10-19% third</u> degree burns**

     T31.32   **Burns involving 30-39% of body surface <u>with 20-29% third</u> degree burns**

     T31.33   **Burns involving 30-39% of body surface <u>with 30-39% third</u> degree burns**

T31.4-   Burns involving <u>40-49% of body surface</u>

     T31.40   **Burns involving 40-49% of body surface <u>with 0% to 9%</u> <u>third</u> degree burns**
         Burns involving 40-49% of body surface NOS

     T31.41   **Burns involving 40-49% of body surface <u>with 10-19% third</u> degree burns**

     T31.42   **Burns involving 40-49% of body surface <u>with 20-29% third</u> degree burns**

     T31.43   **Burns involving 40-49% of body surface <u>with 30-39% third</u> degree burns**

     T31.44   **Burns involving 40-49% of body surface <u>with 40-49% third</u> degree burns**

T31.5-   Burns involving <u>50-59% of body surface</u>

     T31.50   **Burns involving 50-59% of body surface <u>with 0% to 9%</u> <u>third</u> degree burns**
         Burns involving 50-59% of body surface NOS

     T31.51   **Burns involving 50-59% of body surface <u>with 10-19% third</u> degree burns**

     T31.52   **Burns involving 50-59% of body surface <u>with 20-29% third</u> degree burns**

     T31.53   **Burns involving 50-59% of body surface <u>with 30-39% third</u> degree burns**

     T31.54   **Burns involving 50-59% of body surface <u>with 40-49% third</u> degree burns**

     T31.55   **Burns involving 50-59% of body surface <u>with 50-59% third</u> degree burns**

T31.6-   Burns involving <u>60-69% of body surface</u>

     T31.60   **Burns involving 60-69% of body surface <u>with 0% to 9%</u> <u>third</u> degree burns**
         Burns involving 60-69% of body surface NOS

     T31.61   **Burns involving 60-69% of body surface <u>with 10-19% third</u> degree burns**

     T31.62   **Burns involving 60-69% of body surface <u>with 20-29% third</u> degree burns**

     T31.63   **Burns involving 60-69% of body surface <u>with 30-39% third</u> degree burns**

     T31.64   **Burns involving 60-69% of body surface <u>with 40-49% third</u> degree burns**

     T31.65   **Burns involving 60-69% of body surface <u>with 50-59% third</u> degree burns**

     T31.66   **Burns involving 60-69% of body surface <u>with 60-69% third</u> degree burns**

T31.7-   Burns involving <u>70-79% of body surface</u>

     T31.70   **Burns involving 70-79% of body surface <u>with 0% to 9%</u> <u>third</u> degree burns**
         Burns involving 70-79% of body surface NOS

     T31.71   **Burns involving 70-79% of body surface <u>with 10-19% third</u> degree burns**

     T31.72   **Burns involving 70-79% of body surface <u>with 20-29% third</u> degree burns**

     T31.73   **Burns involving 70-79% of body surface <u>with 30-39% third</u> degree burns**

     T31.74   **Burns involving 70-79% of body surface <u>with 40-49% third</u> degree burns**

     T31.75   **Burns involving 70-79% of body surface <u>with 50-59% third</u> degree burns**

     T31.76   **Burns involving 70-79% of body surface <u>with 60-69% third</u> degree burns**

     T31.77   **Burns involving 70-79% of body surface <u>with 70-79% third</u> degree burns**

T31.8-   Burns involving <u>80-89% of body surface</u>

     T31.80   **Burns involving 80-89% of body surface <u>with 0% to 9%</u> <u>third</u> degree burns**
         Burns involving 80-89% of body surface NOS

     T31.81   **Burns involving 80-89% of body surface <u>with 10-19% third</u> degree burns**

     T31.82   **Burns involving 80-89% of body surface <u>with 20-29% third</u> degree burns**

     T31.83   **Burns involving 80-89% of body surface <u>with 30-39% third</u> degree burns**

     T31.84   **Burns involving 80-89% of body surface <u>with 40-49% third</u> degree burns**

     T31.85   **Burns involving 80-89% of body surface <u>with 50-59% third</u> degree burns**

     T31.86   **Burns involving 80-89% of body surface <u>with 60-69% third</u> degree burns**

     T31.87   **Burns involving 80-89% of body surface <u>with 70-79% third</u> degree burns**

     T31.88   **Burns involving 80-89% of body surface <u>with 80-89% third</u> degree burns**

T31.9-   Burns involving <u>90% or more of body surface</u>

     T31.90   **Burns involving 90% or more of body surface <u>with 0% to</u> <u>9% third</u> degree burns**
         Burns involving 90% or more of body surface NOS

     T31.91   **Burns involving 90% or more of body surface <u>with 10-19%</u> <u>third</u> degree burns**

     T31.92   **Burns involving 90% or more of body surface <u>with 20-29%</u> <u>third</u> degree burns**

     T31.93   **Burns involving 90% or more of body surface <u>with 30-39%</u> <u>third</u> degree burns**

     T31.94   **Burns involving 90% or more of body surface <u>with 40-49%</u> <u>third</u> degree burns**

     T31.95   **Burns involving 90% or more of body surface <u>with 50-59%</u> <u>third</u> degree burns**

     T31.96   **Burns involving 90% or more of body surface <u>with 60-69%</u> <u>third</u> degree burns**

     T31.97   **Burns involving 90% or more of body surface <u>with 70-79%</u> <u>third</u> degree burns**

     T31.98   **Burns involving 90% or more of body surface <u>with 80-89%</u> <u>third</u> degree burns**

     T31.99   **Burns involving 90% or more of body surface <u>with 90% or</u> <u>more third</u> degree burns**

T32-   <u>Corrosions classified according to extent of body surface involved</u>
     Note: This category is to be used as the primary code only when the site of the corrosion is unspecified. It may be used as a supplementary code with categories T20-T25 when the site is specified.

T32.0   <u>Corrosions</u> involving <u>less than 10% of body surface</u>

T32.1-   <u>Corrosions</u> involving <u>10-19% of body surface</u>

     T32.10   **Corrosions involving 10-19% of body surface <u>with 0% to 9%</u> <u>third</u> degree corrosion**
         Corrosions involving 10-19% of body surface NOS

     T32.11   **Corrosions involving 10-19% of body surface <u>with 10-19%</u> <u>third</u> degree corrosion**

T32.2-   <u>Corrosions</u> involving <u>20-29% of body surface</u>

     T32.20   **Corrosions involving 20-29% of body surface <u>with 0% to 9%</u> <u>third</u> degree corrosion**

     T32.21   **Corrosions involving 20-29% of body surface <u>with 10-19%</u> <u>third</u> degree corrosion**

     T32.22   **Corrosions involving 20-29% of body surface <u>with 20-29%</u> <u>third</u> degree corrosion**

T32.3-   <u>Corrosions</u> involving <u>30-39% of body surface</u>

     T32.30   **Corrosions involving 30-39% of body surface <u>with 0% to 9%</u> <u>third</u> degree corrosion**

     T32.31   **Corrosions involving 30-39% of body surface <u>with 10-19%</u> <u>third</u> degree corrosion**

     T32.32   **Corrosions involving 30-39% of body surface <u>with 20-29%</u> <u>third</u> degree corrosion**

     T32.33   **Corrosions involving 30-39% of body surface <u>with 30-39%</u> <u>third</u> degree corrosion**

T32.4-   <u>Corrosions</u> involving <u>40-49% of body surface</u>

     T32.40   **Corrosions involving 40-49% of body surface <u>with 0% to 9%</u> <u>third</u> degree corrosion**

     T32.41   **Corrosions involving 40-49% of body surface <u>with 10-19%</u> <u>third</u> degree corrosion**

     T32.42   **Corrosions involving 40-49% of body surface <u>with 20-29%</u> <u>third</u> degree corrosion**

     T32.43   **Corrosions involving 40-49% of body surface <u>with 30-39%</u> <u>third</u> degree corrosion**

T26 - T32

Excludes 1: = NOT CODED HERE! (Do not code both)   **795**   *Excludes ❷:* = Not Included Here

T32.44 Corrosions involving 40-49% of body surface <u>with 40-49% third</u> degree corrosion

T32.5- <u>Corrosions</u> involving <u>50-59% of body surface</u>

  T32.50 Corrosions involving 50-59% of body surface <u>with 0% to 9% third</u> degree corrosion

  T32.51 Corrosions involving 50-59% of body surface <u>with 10-19% third</u> degree corrosion

  T32.52 Corrosions involving 50-59% of body surface <u>with 20-29% third</u> degree corrosion

  T32.53 Corrosions involving 50-59% of body surface <u>with 30-39% third</u> degree corrosion

  T32.54 Corrosions involving 50-59% of body surface <u>with 40-49% third</u> degree corrosion

  T32.55 Corrosions involving 50-59% of body surface <u>with 50-59% third</u> degree corrosion

T32.6- <u>Corrosions</u> involving <u>60-69% of body surface</u>

  T32.60 Corrosions involving 60-69% of body surface <u>with 0% to 9% third</u> degree corrosion

  T32.61 Corrosions involving 60-69% of body surface <u>with 10-19% third</u> degree corrosion

  T32.62 Corrosions involving 60-69% of body surface <u>with 20-29% third</u> degree corrosion

  T32.63 Corrosions involving 60-69% of body surface <u>with 30-39% third</u> degree corrosion

  T32.64 Corrosions involving 60-69% of body surface <u>with 40-49% third</u> degree corrosion

  T32.65 Corrosions involving 60-69% of body surface <u>with 50-59% third</u> degree corrosion

  T32.66 Corrosions involving 60-69% of body surface <u>with 60-69% third</u> degree corrosion

T32.7- <u>Corrosions</u> involving <u>70-79% of body surface</u>

  T32.70 Corrosions involving 70-79% of body surface <u>with 0% to 9% third</u> degree corrosion

  T32.71 Corrosions involving 70-79% of body surface <u>with 10-19% third</u> degree corrosion

  T32.72 Corrosions involving 70-79% of body surface <u>with 20-29% third</u> degree corrosion

  T32.73 Corrosions involving 70-79% of body surface <u>with 30-39% third</u> degree corrosion

  T32.74 Corrosions involving 70-79% of body surface <u>with 40-49% third</u> degree corrosion

  T32.75 Corrosions involving 70-79% of body surface <u>with 50-59% third</u> degree corrosion

  T32.76 Corrosions involving 70-79% of body surface <u>with 60-69% third</u> degree corrosion

  T32.77 Corrosions involving 70-79% of body surface <u>with 70-79% third</u> degree corrosion

T32.8- <u>Corrosions</u> involving <u>80-89% of body surface</u>

  T32.80 Corrosions involving 80-89% of body surface <u>with 0% to 9% third</u> degree corrosion

  T32.81 Corrosions involving 80-89% of body surface <u>with 10-19% third</u> degree corrosion

  T32.82 Corrosions involving 80-89% of body surface <u>with 20-29% third</u> degree corrosion

  T32.83 Corrosions involving 80-89% of body surface <u>with 30-39% third</u> degree corrosion

  T32.84 Corrosions involving 80-89% of body surface <u>with 40-49% third</u> degree corrosion

  T32.85 Corrosions involving 80-89% of body surface <u>with 50-59% third</u> degree corrosion

  T32.86 Corrosions involving 80-89% of body surface <u>with 60-69% third</u> degree corrosion

  T32.87 Corrosions involving 80-89% of body surface <u>with 70-79% third</u> degree corrosion

  T32.88 Corrosions involving 80-89% of body surface <u>with 80-89% third</u> degree corrosion

T32.9- <u>Corrosions</u> involving <u>90% or more of body surface</u>

  T32.90 Corrosions involving 90% or more of body surface <u>with 0% to 9% third</u> degree corrosion

  T32.91 Corrosions involving 90% or more of body surface <u>with 10-19% third</u> degree corrosion

  T32.92 Corrosions involving 90% or more of body surface <u>with 20-29% third</u> degree corrosion

  T32.93 Corrosions involving 90% or more of body surface <u>with 30-39% third</u> degree corrosion

  T32.94 Corrosions involving 90% or more of body surface <u>with 40-49% third</u> degree corrosion

  T32.95 Corrosions involving 90% or more of body surface <u>with 50-59% third</u> degree corrosion

  T32.96 Corrosions involving 90% or more of body surface <u>with 60-69% third</u> degree corrosion

  T32.97 Corrosions involving 90% or more of body surface <u>with 70-79% third</u> degree corrosion

  T32.98 Corrosions involving 90% or more of body surface <u>with 80-89% third</u> degree corrosion

  T32.99 Corrosions involving 90% or more of body surface <u>with 90% or more third</u> degree corrosion

Frostbite (T33-T34)

Excludes❷: hypothermia and other effects of reduced temperature (T68, T69.-)

T33- <u>Superficial frostbite</u>

Includes: Frostbite with partial thickness skin loss

The appropriate 7th character is to be added to each code from category T33:
  A   <u>Initial</u> encounter
  D   <u>Subsequent</u> encounter
  S   <u>Sequela</u>

T33.0- Superficial frostbite of head

  T33.01- Superficial frostbite of <u>ear</u>

    T33.011- Superficial frostbite of <u>right</u> ear

    T33.012- Superficial frostbite of <u>left</u> ear

    T33.019- Superficial frostbite of <u>unspecified</u> ear

  T33.02x- Superficial frostbite of nose

  T33.09x- Superficial frostbite of other part of head

T33.1xx- Superficial frostbite of neck

T33.2xx- Superficial frostbite of thorax

T33.3xx- Superficial frostbite of abdominal wall, lower back and pelvis

T33.4- Superficial frostbite of <u>arm</u>

  Excludes❷: superficial frostbite of wrist and hand (T33.5-)

  T33.40x- Superficial frostbite of <u>unspecified</u> arm

  T33.41x- Superficial frostbite of <u>right</u> arm

  T33.42x- Superficial frostbite of <u>left</u> arm

T33.5- Superficial frostbite of wrist, hand, and fingers

  T33.51- Superficial frostbite of <u>wrist</u>

    T33.511- Superficial frostbite of <u>right</u> wrist

    T33.512- Superficial frostbite of <u>left</u> wrist

    T33.519- Superficial frostbite of <u>unspecified</u> wrist

  T33.52- Superficial frostbite of <u>hand</u>

    Excludes❷: superficial frostbite of fingers (T33.53-)

    T33.521- Superficial frostbite of <u>right</u> hand

    T33.522- Superficial frostbite of <u>left</u> hand

    T33.529- Superficial frostbite of <u>unspecified</u> hand

  T33.53- Superficial frostbite of <u>finger(s)</u>

    T33.531- Superficial frostbite of <u>right</u> finger(s)

    T33.532- Superficial frostbite of <u>left</u> finger(s)

    T33.539- Superficial frostbite of <u>unspecified</u> finger(s)

T33.6- Superficial frostbite of <u>hip and thigh</u>

  T33.60x- Superficial frostbite of <u>unspecified</u> hip and thigh

  T33.61x- Superficial frostbite of <u>right</u> hip and thigh

  T33.62x- Superficial frostbite of <u>left</u> hip and thigh

T33.7- Superficial frostbite of <u>knee and lower leg</u>

  Excludes❷: superficial frostbite of ankle and foot (T33.8-)

  T33.70x- Superficial frostbite of <u>unspecified</u> knee and lower leg

  T33.71x- Superficial frostbite of <u>right</u> knee and lower leg

  T33.72x- Superficial frostbite of <u>left</u> knee and lower leg

T33.8- Superficial frostbite of ankle, foot, and toe(s)

  T33.81- Superficial frostbite of <u>ankle</u>

    T33.811- Superficial frostbite of <u>right</u> ankle

    T33.812- Superficial frostbite of <u>left</u> ankle

    T33.819- Superficial frostbite of <u>unspecified</u> ankle

  T33.82- Superficial frostbite of <u>foot</u>

    T33.821- Superficial frostbite of <u>right</u> foot

    T33.822- Superficial frostbite of <u>left</u> foot

    T33.829- Superficial frostbite of <u>unspecified</u> foot

  T33.83- Superficial frostbite of <u>toe(s)</u>

    T33.831- Superficial frostbite of <u>right</u> toe(s)

    T33.832- Superficial frostbite of <u>left</u> toe(s)

    T33.839- Superficial frostbite of <u>unspecified</u> toe(s)

T33.9- Superficial frostbite of other and unspecified sites

  T33.90x- Superficial frostbite of <u>unspecified</u> sites

    Superficial frostbite NOS

  T33.99x- Superficial frostbite of <u>other</u> sites

    Superficial frostbite of leg NOS

    Superficial frostbite of trunk NOS

Excludes 1: = NOT CODED HERE! (Do not code both)

Excludes❷: = Not Included Here

T34-   Frostbite with tissue necrosis

> The appropriate 7th character is to be added to each code from category T34:
> A   Initial encounter
> D   Subsequent encounter
> S   Sequela

T34.0-   Frostbite with tissue necrosis of head

T34.01-   Frostbite with tissue necrosis of ear

T34.011-   Frostbite with tissue necrosis of right ear

T34.012-   Frostbite with tissue necrosis of left ear

T34.019-   Frostbite with tissue necrosis of unspecified ear

T34.02x-   Frostbite with tissue necrosis of nose

T34.09x-   Frostbite with tissue necrosis of other part of head

T34.1xx-   Frostbite with tissue necrosis of neck

T34.2xx-   Frostbite with tissue necrosis of thorax

T34.3xx-   Frostbite with tissue necrosis of abdominal wall, lower back and pelvis

T34.4-   Frostbite with tissue necrosis of arm
Excludes❷: frostbite with tissue necrosis of wrist and hand (T34.5-)

T34.40x-   Frostbite with tissue necrosis of unspecified arm

T34.41x-   Frostbite with tissue necrosis of right arm

T34.42x-   Frostbite with tissue necrosis of left arm

T34.5-   Frostbite with tissue necrosis of wrist, hand, and finger(s)

T34.51-   Frostbite with tissue necrosis of wrist

T34.511-   Frostbite with tissue necrosis of right wrist

T34.512-   Frostbite with tissue necrosis of left wrist

T34.519-   Frostbite with tissue necrosis of unspecified wrist

T34.52-   Frostbite with tissue necrosis of hand
Excludes❷: frostbite with tissue necrosis of finger(s) (T34.53-)

T34.521-   Frostbite with tissue necrosis of right hand

T34.522-   Frostbite with tissue necrosis of left hand

T34.529-   Frostbite with tissue necrosis of unspecified hand

T34.53-   Frostbite with tissue necrosis of finger(s)

T34.531-   Frostbite with tissue necrosis of right finger(s)

T34.532-   Frostbite with tissue necrosis of left finger(s)

T34.539-   Frostbite with tissue necrosis of unspecified finger(s)

T34.6-   Frostbite with tissue necrosis of hip and thigh

T34.60x-   Frostbite with tissue necrosis of unspecified hip and thigh

T34.61x-   Frostbite with tissue necrosis of right hip and thigh

T34.62x-   Frostbite with tissue necrosis of left hip and thigh

T34.7-   Frostbite with tissue necrosis of knee and lower leg
Excludes❷: frostbite with tissue necrosis of ankle and foot (T34.8-)

T34.70x-   Frostbite with tissue necrosis of unspecified knee and lower leg

T34.71x-   Frostbite with tissue necrosis of right knee and lower leg

T34.72x-   Frostbite with tissue necrosis of left knee and lower leg

T34.8-   Frostbite with tissue necrosis of ankle, foot, and toe(s)

T34.81-   Frostbite with tissue necrosis of ankle

T34.811-   Frostbite with tissue necrosis of right ankle

T34.812-   Frostbite with tissue necrosis of left ankle

T34.819-   Frostbite with tissue necrosis of unspecified ankle

T34.82-   Frostbite with tissue necrosis of foot

T34.821-   Frostbite with tissue necrosis of right foot

T34.822-   Frostbite with tissue necrosis of left foot

T34.829-   Frostbite with tissue necrosis of unspecified foot

T34.83-   Frostbite with tissue necrosis of toe(s)

T34.831-   Frostbite with tissue necrosis of right toe(s)

T34.832-   Frostbite with tissue necrosis of left toe(s)

T34.839-   Frostbite with tissue necrosis of unspecified toe(s)

T34.9-   Frostbite with tissue necrosis of other and unspecified sites

T34.90x-   Frostbite with tissue necrosis of unspecified sites
Frostbite with tissue necrosis NOS

T34.99x-   Frostbite with tissue necrosis of other sites
Frostbite with tissue necrosis of leg NOS
Frostbite with tissue necrosis of trunk NOS

Poisoning by, adverse effects of and underdosing of drugs, medicaments and biological substances (T36-T50)

Includes: Adverse effect of correct substance properly administered
Poisoning by overdose of substance
Poisoning by wrong substance given or taken in error
Underdosing by (inadvertently) (deliberately) taking less substance than prescribed or instructed

Code first, for adverse effects, the nature of the adverse effect, such as:
Adverse effect NOS (T88.7)
Aspirin gastritis (K29-)
Blood disorders (D56-D76)
Contact dermatitis (L23-L25)
Dermatitis due to substances taken internally (L27-)
Nephropathy (N14.0-N14.2)

Note: The drug giving rise to the adverse effect should be identified by use of codes from categories T36-T50 with fifth or sixth character 5.

Use additional code(s) to specify:
Manifestations of poisoning
Underdosing of medication regime (Z91.12-, Z91.13-)
Underdosing or failure in dosage during medical and surgical care (Y63.6, Y63.8-Y63.9)

Excludes 1: toxic reaction to local anesthesia in pregnancy (O29.3-)
Excludes❷: abuse and dependence of psychoactive substances (F10-F19)
abuse of non-dependence-producing substances (F55-)
drug reaction and poisoning affecting newborn (P00-P96)
pathological drug intoxication (inebriation) (F10-F19)

T36-   Poisoning by, adverse effect of and underdosing of systemic antibiotics
Excludes 1: antineoplastic antibiotics (T45.1-)
locally applied antibiotic NEC (T49.0)
topically used antibiotic for ear, nose and throat (T49.6)
topically used antibiotic for eye (T49.5)

> The appropriate 7th character is to be added to each code from category T36:
> A   Initial encounter
> D   Subsequent encounter
> S   Sequela

T36.0-   Poisoning by, adverse effect of and underdosing of penicillins

T36.0x-   Poisoning by, adverse effect of and underdosing of penicillins

T36.0x1-   Poisoning by penicillins, accidental (unintentional)
Poisoning by penicillins NOS

T36.0x2-   Poisoning by penicillins, intentional self-harm

T36.0x3-   Poisoning by penicillins, assault

T36.0x4-   Poisoning by penicillins, undetermined

T36.0x5-   Adverse effect of penicillins

T36.0x6-   Underdosing of penicillins

T36.1-   Poisoning by, adverse effect of and underdosing of cephalosporins and other beta-lactam antibiotics

T36.1x-   Poisoning by, adverse effect of and underdosing of cephalosporins and other beta-lactam antibiotics

T36.1x1-   Poisoning by cephalosporins and other beta-lactam antibiotics, accidental (unintentional)
Poisoning by cephalosporins and other beta-lactam antibiotics NOS

T36.1x2-   Poisoning by cephalosporins and other beta-lactam antibiotics, intentional self-harm

T36.1x3-   Poisoning by cephalosporins and other beta-lactam antibiotics, assault

T36.1x4-   Poisoning by cephalosporins and other beta-lactam antibiotics, undetermined

T36.1x5-   Adverse effect of cephalosporins and other beta-lactam antibiotics

T36.1x6-   Underdosing of cephalosporins and other beta-lactam antibiotics

T36.2-   Poisoning by, adverse effect of and underdosing of chloramphenicol group

T36.2x-   Poisoning by, adverse effect of and underdosing of chloramphenicol group

T36.2x1-   Poisoning by chloramphenicol group, accidental (unintentional)
Poisoning by chloramphenicol group NOS

T36.2x2-   Poisoning by chloramphenicol group, intentional self-harm

T36.2x3-   Poisoning by chloramphenicol group, assault

T36.2x4-   Poisoning by chloramphenicol group, undetermined

T36.2x5-   Adverse effect of chloramphenicol group

T36.2x6-   Underdosing of chloramphenicol group

T32 - T36

Excludes 1: = NOT CODED HERE! (Do not code both)   *Excludes❷ = Not Included Here*

T36.3- Poisoning by, adverse effect of and underdosing of macrolides
- **T36.3x-** Poisoning by, adverse effect of and underdosing of <u>macrolides</u>
  - **T36.3x1-** Poisoning by macrolides, <u>accidental</u> (unintentional)
    Poisoning by macrolides NOS
  - **T36.3x2-** Poisoning by macrolides, <u>intentional</u> self-harm
  - **T36.3x3-** Poisoning by macrolides, <u>assault</u>
  - **T36.3x4-** Poisoning by macrolides, <u>undetermined</u>
  - **T36.3x5-** <u>Adverse effect</u> of macrolides
  - **T36.3x6-** <u>Underdosing</u> of macrolides

T36.4- Poisoning by, adverse effect of and underdosing of tetracyclines
- **T36.4x-** Poisoning by, adverse effect of and underdosing of <u>tetracyclines</u>
  - **T36.4x1-** Poisoning by tetracyclines, <u>accidental</u> (unintentional)
    Poisoning by tetracyclines NOS
  - **T36.4x2-** Poisoning by tetracyclines, <u>intentional</u> self-harm
  - **T36.4x3-** Poisoning by tetracyclines, <u>assault</u>
  - **T36.4x4-** Poisoning by tetracyclines, <u>undetermined</u>
  - **T36.4x5-** <u>Adverse effect</u> of tetracyclines
  - **T36.4x6-** <u>Underdosing</u> of tetracyclines

T36.5- Poisoning by, adverse effect of and underdosing of aminoglycosides
  Poisoning by, adverse effect of and underdosing of streptomycin
- **T36.5x-** Poisoning by, adverse effect of and underdosing of <u>aminoglycosides</u>
  - **T36.5x1-** Poisoning by aminoglycosides, <u>accidental</u> (unintentional)
    Poisoning by aminoglycosides NOS
  - **T36.5x2-** Poisoning by aminoglycosides, <u>intentional</u> self-harm
  - **T36.5x3-** Poisoning by aminoglycosides, <u>assault</u>
  - **T36.5x4-** Poisoning by aminoglycosides, <u>undetermined</u>
  - **T36.5x5-** <u>Adverse effect</u> of aminoglycosides
  - **T36.5x6-** <u>Underdosing</u> of aminoglycosides

T36.6- Poisoning by, adverse effect of and underdosing of rifampicins
- **T36.6x-** Poisoning by, adverse effect of and underdosing of <u>rifampicins</u>
  - **T36.6x1-** Poisoning by rifampicins, <u>accidental</u> (unintentional)
    Poisoning by rifampicins NOS
  - **T36.6x2-** Poisoning by rifampicins, <u>intentional</u> self-harm
  - **T36.6x3-** Poisoning by rifampicins, <u>assault</u>
  - **T36.6x4-** Poisoning by rifampicins, <u>undetermined</u>
  - **T36.6x5-** <u>Adverse effect</u> of rifampicins
  - **T36.6x6-** <u>Underdosing</u> of rifampicins

T36.7- Poisoning by, adverse effect of and underdosing of antifungal antibiotics, systemically used
- **T36.7x-** Poisoning by, adverse effect of and underdosing of <u>antifungal antibiotics, systemically used</u>
  - **T36.7x1-** Poisoning by antifungal antibiotics, systemically used, <u>accidental</u> (unintentional)
    Poisoning by antifungal antibiotics, systemically used NOS
  - **T36.7x2-** Poisoning by antifungal antibiotics, systemically used, <u>intentional</u> self-harm
  - **T36.7x3-** Poisoning by antifungal antibiotics, systemically used, <u>assault</u>
  - **T36.7x4-** Poisoning by antifungal antibiotics, systemically used, <u>undetermined</u>
  - **T36.7x5-** <u>Adverse effect</u> of antifungal antibiotics, systemically used
  - **T36.7x6-** <u>Underdosing</u> of antifungal antibiotics, systemically used

T36.8- Poisoning by, adverse effect of and underdosing of other systemic antibiotics
- **T36.8x-** Poisoning by, adverse effect of and underdosing of <u>other systemic antibiotics</u>
  - **T36.8x1-** Poisoning by other systemic antibiotics, <u>accidental</u> (unintentional)
    Poisoning by other systemic antibiotics NOS
  - **T36.8x2-** Poisoning by other systemic antibiotics, <u>intentional</u> self-harm
  - **T36.8x3-** Poisoning by other systemic antibiotics, <u>assault</u>
  - **T36.8x4-** Poisoning by other systemic antibiotics, <u>undetermined</u>
  - **T36.8x5-** <u>Adverse effect</u> of other systemic antibiotics
  - **T36.8x6-** <u>Underdosing</u> of other systemic antibiotics

T36.9- Poisoning by, adverse effect of and underdosing of <u>unspecified systemic antibiotic</u>
- **T36.91x-** Poisoning by unspecified systemic antibiotic, <u>accidental</u> (unintentional)
    Poisoning by systemic antibiotic NOS
- **T36.92x-** Poisoning by unspecified systemic antibiotic, <u>intentional</u> self-harm
- **T36.93x-** Poisoning by unspecified systemic antibiotic, <u>assault</u>
- **T36.94x-** Poisoning by unspecified systemic antibiotic, <u>undetermined</u>
- **T36.95x-** <u>Adverse effect</u> of unspecified systemic antibiotic
- **T36.96x-** <u>Underdosing</u> of unspecified systemic antibiotic

T37- Poisoning by, adverse effect of and underdosing of <u>other systemic anti-infectives and antiparasitics</u>
  Excludes 1: *anti-infectives topically used for ear, nose and throat (T49.6-)*
    anti-infectives topically used for eye (T49.5-)
    locally applied anti-infectives NEC (T49.0-)

  The appropriate 7th character is to be added to each code from category T37:
  A <u>Initial</u> encounter
  D <u>Subsequent</u> encounter
  S <u>Sequela</u>

T37.0- Poisoning by, adverse effect of and underdosing of sulfonamides
- **T37.0x-** Poisoning by, adverse effect of and underdosing of <u>sulfonamides</u>
  - **T37.0x1-** Poisoning by sulfonamides, <u>accidental</u> (unintentional)
    Poisoning by sulfonamides NOS
  - **T37.0x2-** Poisoning by sulfonamides, <u>intentional</u> self-harm
  - **T37.0x3-** Poisoning by sulfonamides, <u>assault</u>
  - **T37.0x4-** Poisoning by sulfonamides, <u>undetermined</u>
  - **T37.0x5-** <u>Adverse effect</u> of sulfonamides
  - **T37.0x6-** <u>Underdosing</u> of sulfonamides

T37.1- Poisoning by, adverse effect of and underdosing of antimycobacterial drugs
  Excludes 1: *rifampicins (T36.6-)*
    streptomycin (T36.5-)
- **T37.1x-** Poisoning by, adverse effect of and underdosing of <u>antimycobacterial drugs</u>
  - **T37.1x1-** Poisoning by antimycobacterial drugs, <u>accidental</u> (unintentional)
    Poisoning by antimycobacterial drugs NOS
  - **T37.1x2-** Poisoning by antimycobacterial drugs, <u>intentional</u> self-harm
  - **T37.1x3-** Poisoning by antimycobacterial drugs, <u>assault</u>
  - **T37.1x4-** Poisoning by antimycobacterial drugs, <u>undetermined</u>
  - **T37.1x5-** <u>Adverse effect</u> of antimycobacterial drugs
  - **T37.1x6-** <u>Underdosing</u> of antimycobacterial drugs

T37.2- Poisoning by, adverse effect of and underdosing of antimalarials and drugs acting on other blood protozoa
  Excludes 1: *hydroxyquinoline derivatives (T37.8-)*
- **T37.2x-** Poisoning by, adverse effect of and underdosing of <u>antimalarials and drugs acting on other blood protozoa</u>
  - **T37.2x1-** Poisoning by antimalarials and drugs acting on other blood protozoa, <u>accidental</u> (unintentional)
    Poisoning by antimalarials and drugs acting on other blood protozoa NOS
  - **T37.2x2-** Poisoning by antimalarials and drugs acting on other blood protozoa, <u>intentional</u> self-harm
  - **T37.2x3-** Poisoning by antimalarials and drugs acting on other blood protozoa, <u>assault</u>
  - **T37.2x4-** Poisoning by antimalarials and drugs acting on other blood protozoa, <u>undetermined</u>
  - **T37.2x5-** <u>Adverse effect</u> of antimalarials and drugs acting on other blood protozoa
  - **T37.2x6-** <u>Underdosing</u> of antimalarials and drugs acting on other blood protozoa

T37.3- Poisoning by, adverse effect of and underdosing of other antiprotozoal drugs
- **T37.3x-** Poisoning by, adverse effect of and underdosing of <u>other antiprotozoal drugs</u>
  - **T37.3x1-** Poisoning by other antiprotozoal drugs, <u>accidental</u> (unintentional)
    Poisoning by other antiprotozoal drugs NOS
  - **T37.3x2-** Poisoning by other antiprotozoal drugs, <u>intentional</u> self-harm
  - **T37.3x3-** Poisoning by other antiprotozoal drugs, <u>assault</u>
  - **T37.3x4-** Poisoning by other antiprotozoal drugs, <u>undetermined</u>
  - **T37.3x5-** <u>Adverse effect</u> of other antiprotozoal drugs
  - **T37.3x6-** <u>Underdosing</u> of other antiprotozoal drugs

T 3 6 - T 3 8

T37.4- Poisoning by, adverse effect of and underdosing of anthelminthics

    T37.4x- Poisoning by, adverse effect of and underdosing of <u>anthelminthics</u>

        T37.4x1- Poisoning by anthelminthics, <u>accidental</u> (unintentional)
            Poisoning by anthelminthics NOS

        T37.4x2- Poisoning by anthelminthics, <u>intentional</u> self-harm

        T37.4x3- Poisoning by anthelminthics, <u>assault</u>

        T37.4x4- Poisoning by anthelminthics, <u>undetermined</u>

        T37.4x5- <u>Adverse effect</u> of anthelminthics

        T37.4x6- <u>Underdosing</u> of anthelminthics

T37.5- Poisoning by, adverse effect of and underdosing of antiviral drugs
    Excludes 1: amantadine (T42.8-)
           cytarabine (T45.1-)

    T37.5x- Poisoning by, adverse effect of and underdosing of <u>antiviral drugs</u>

        T37.5x1- Poisoning by antiviral drugs, <u>accidental</u> (unintentional)
            Poisoning by antiviral drugs NOS

        T37.5x2- Poisoning by antiviral drugs, <u>intentional</u> self-harm

        T37.5x3- Poisoning by antiviral drugs, <u>assault</u>

        T37.5x4- Poisoning by antiviral drugs, <u>undetermined</u>

        T37.5x5- <u>Adverse effect</u> of antiviral drugs

        T37.5x6- <u>Underdosing</u> of antiviral drugs

T37.8- Poisoning by, adverse effect of and underdosing of other specified systemic anti-infectives and antiparasitics
    Poisoning by, adverse effect of and underdosing of hydroxyquinoline derivatives
    Excludes 1: antimalarial drugs (T37.2-)

    T37.8x- Poisoning by, adverse effect of and underdosing of <u>other specified systemic anti-infectives and antiparasitics</u>

        T37.8x1- Poisoning by other specified systemic anti-infectives and antiparasitics, <u>accidental</u> (unintentional)
            Poisoning by other specified systemic anti-infectives and antiparasitics NOS

        T37.8x2- Poisoning by other specified systemic anti-infectives and antiparasitics, <u>intentional</u> self-harm

        T37.8x3- Poisoning by other specified systemic anti-infectives and antiparasitics, <u>assault</u>

        T37.8x4- Poisoning by other specified systemic anti-infectives and antiparasitics, <u>undetermined</u>

        T37.8x5- <u>Adverse effect</u> of other specified systemic anti-infectives and antiparasitics

        T37.8x6- <u>Underdosing</u> of other specified systemic anti-infectives and antiparasitics

T37.9- Poisoning by, adverse effect of and underdosing of <u>unspecified systemic anti-infective and antiparasitics</u>

    T37.91x- Poisoning by unspecified systemic anti-infective and antiparasitics, <u>accidental</u> (unintentional)
        Poisoning by, adverse effect of and underdosing of systemic anti-infective and antiparasitics NOS

    T37.92x- Poisoning by unspecified systemic anti-infective and antiparasitics, <u>intentional</u> self-harm

    T37.93x- Poisoning by unspecified systemic anti-infective and antiparasitics, <u>assault</u>

    T37.94x- Poisoning by unspecified systemic anti-infective and antiparasitics, <u>undetermined</u>

    T37.95x- <u>Adverse effect</u> of unspecified systemic anti-infective and antiparasitic

    T37.96x- <u>Underdosing</u> of unspecified systemic anti-infectives and antiparasitics

T38- Poisoning by, adverse effect of and underdosing of <u>hormones and their synthetic substitutes and antagonists, not elsewhere classified</u>
    Excludes 1: mineralocorticoids and their antagonists (T50.0-)
           oxytocic hormones (T48.0-)
           parathyroid hormones and derivatives (T50.9-)

The appropriate 7th character is to be added to each code from category T38:
  A   <u>Initial</u> encounter
  D   <u>Subsequent</u> encounter
  S   <u>Sequela</u>

T38.0- Poisoning by, adverse effect of and underdosing of glucocorticoids and synthetic analogues
    Excludes 1: glucocorticoids, topically used (T49.-)

    T38.0x- Poisoning by, adverse effect of and underdosing of <u>glucocorticoids and synthetic analogues</u>

        T38.0x1- Poisoning by glucocorticoids and synthetic analogues, <u>accidental</u> (unintentional)
            Poisoning by glucocorticoids and synthetic analogues NOS

        T38.0x2- Poisoning by glucocorticoids and synthetic analogues, <u>intentional</u> self-harm

        T38.0x3- Poisoning by glucocorticoids and synthetic analogues, <u>assault</u>

        T38.0x4- Poisoning by glucocorticoids and synthetic analogues, <u>undetermined</u>

        T38.0x5- <u>Adverse effect</u> of glucocorticoids and synthetic analogues

        T38.0x6- <u>Underdosing</u> of glucocorticoids and synthetic analogues

T38.1- Poisoning by, adverse effect of and underdosing of thyroid hormones and substitutes

    T38.1x- Poisoning by, adverse effect of and underdosing of <u>thyroid hormones and substitutes</u>

        T38.1x1- Poisoning by thyroid hormones and substitutes, <u>accidental</u> (unintentional)
            Poisoning by thyroid hormones and substitutes NOS

        T38.1x2- Poisoning by thyroid hormones and substitutes, <u>intentional</u> self-harm

        T38.1x3- Poisoning by thyroid hormones and substitutes, <u>assault</u>

        T38.1x4- Poisoning by thyroid hormones and substitutes, <u>undetermined</u>

        T38.1x5- <u>Adverse effect</u> of thyroid hormones and substitutes

        T38.1x6- <u>Underdosing</u> of thyroid hormones and substitutes

T38.2- Poisoning by, adverse effect of and underdosing of antithyroid drugs

    T38.2x- Poisoning by, adverse effect of and underdosing of <u>antithyroid drugs</u>

        T38.2x1- Poisoning by antithyroid drugs, <u>accidental</u> (unintentional)
            Poisoning by antithyroid drugs NOS

        T38.2x2- Poisoning by antithyroid drugs, <u>intentional</u> self-harm

        T38.2x3- Poisoning by antithyroid drugs, <u>assault</u>

        T38.2x4- Poisoning by antithyroid drugs, <u>undetermined</u>

        T38.2x5- <u>Adverse effect</u> of antithyroid drugs

        T38.2x6- <u>Underdosing</u> of antithyroid drugs

T38.3- Poisoning by, adverse effect of and underdosing of insulin and oral hypoglycemic [antidiabetic] drugs

    T38.3x- Poisoning by, adverse effect of and underdosing of <u>insulin and oral hypoglycemic [antidiabetic] drugs</u>

        T38.3x1- Poisoning by insulin and oral hypoglycemic [antidiabetic] drugs, <u>accidental</u> (unintentional)
            Poisoning by insulin and oral hypoglycemic [antidiabetic] drugs NOS

        T38.3x2- Poisoning by insulin and oral hypoglycemic [antidiabetic] drugs, <u>intentional</u> self-harm

        T38.3x3- Poisoning by insulin and oral hypoglycemic [antidiabetic] drugs, <u>assault</u>

        T38.3x4- Poisoning by insulin and oral hypoglycemic [antidiabetic] drugs, <u>undetermined</u>

        T38.3x5- <u>Adverse effect</u> of insulin and oral hypoglycemic [antidiabetic] drugs

        T38.3x6- <u>Underdosing</u> of insulin and oral hypoglycemic [antidiabetic] drugs

T 3 6 - T 3 8

T38.4- **Poisoning by, adverse effect of and underdosing of oral contraceptives**
Poisoning by, adverse effect of and underdosing of multiple- and single-ingredient oral contraceptive preparations

T38.4x- Poisoning by, adverse effect of and underdosing of <u>oral contraceptives</u>

T38.4x1- Poisoning by oral contraceptives, <u>accidental (unintentional)</u>
Poisoning by oral contraceptives NOS

T38.4x2- Poisoning by oral contraceptives, <u>intentional</u> self-harm

T38.4x3- Poisoning by oral contraceptives, <u>assault</u>

T38.4x4- Poisoning by oral contraceptives, <u>undetermined</u>

T38.4x5- <u>Adverse effect</u> of oral contraceptives

T38.4x6- <u>Underdosing</u> of oral contraceptives

T38.5- **Poisoning by, adverse effect of and underdosing of other estrogens and progestogens**
Poisoning by, adverse effect of and underdosing of estrogens and progestogens mixtures and substitutes

T38.5x- Poisoning by, adverse effect of and underdosing of <u>other estrogens and progestogens</u>

T38.5x1- Poisoning by other estrogens and progestogens, <u>accidental (unintentional)</u>
Poisoning by other estrogens and progestogens NOS

T38.5x2- Poisoning by other estrogens and progestogens, <u>intentional</u> self-harm

T38.5x3- Poisoning by other estrogens and progestogens, <u>assault</u>

T38.5x4- Poisoning by other estrogens and progestogens, <u>undetermined</u>

T38.5x5- <u>Adverse effect</u> of other estrogens and progestogens

T38.5x6- <u>Underdosing</u> of other estrogens and progestogens

T38.6- **Poisoning by, adverse effect of and underdosing of antigonadotrophins, antiestrogens, antiandrogens, not elsewhere classified**
Poisoning by, adverse effect of and underdosing of tamoxifen

T38.6x- Poisoning by, adverse effect of and underdosing of <u>antigonadotrophins, antiestrogens, antiandrogens, not elsewhere classified</u>

T38.6x1- Poisoning by antigonadotrophins, antiestrogens, antiandrogens, not elsewhere classified, <u>accidental (unintentional)</u>
Poisoning by antigonadotrophins, antiestrogens, antiandrogens, not elsewhere classified NOS

T38.6x2- Poisoning by antigonadotrophins, antiestrogens, antiandrogens, not elsewhere classified, <u>intentional</u> self-harm

T38.6x3- Poisoning by antigonadotrophins, antiestrogens, antiandrogens, not elsewhere classified, <u>assault</u>

T38.6x4- Poisoning by antigonadotrophins, antiestrogens, antiandrogens, not elsewhere classified, <u>undetermined</u>

T38.6x5- <u>Adverse effect</u> of antigonadotrophins, antiestrogens, antiandrogens, not elsewhere classified

T38.6x6- <u>Underdosing</u> of antigonadotrophins, antiestrogens, antiandrogens, not elsewhere classified

T38.7- **Poisoning by, adverse effect of and underdosing of androgens and anabolic congeners**

T38.7x- Poisoning by, adverse effect of and underdosing of <u>androgens and anabolic congeners</u>

T38.7x1- Poisoning by androgens and anabolic congeners, <u>accidental (unintentional)</u>
Poisoning by androgens and anabolic congeners NOS

T38.7x2- Poisoning by androgens and anabolic congeners, <u>intentional</u> self-harm

T38.7x3- Poisoning by androgens and anabolic congeners, <u>assault</u>

T38.7x4- Poisoning by androgens and anabolic congeners, <u>undetermined</u>

T38.7x5- <u>Adverse effect</u> of androgens and anabolic congeners

T38.7x6- <u>Underdosing</u> of androgens and anabolic congeners

T38.8- **Poisoning by, adverse effect of and underdosing of other and unspecified hormones and synthetic substitutes**

T38.80- Poisoning by, adverse effect of and underdosing of <u>unspecified hormones and synthetic substitutes</u>

T38.801- Poisoning by unspecified hormones and synthetic substitutes, <u>accidental (unintentional)</u>
Poisoning by unspecified hormones and synthetic substitutes NOS

T38.802- Poisoning by unspecified hormones and synthetic substitutes, <u>intentional</u> self-harm

T38.803- Poisoning by unspecified hormones and synthetic substitutes, <u>assault</u>

T38.804- Poisoning by unspecified hormones and synthetic substitutes, <u>undetermined</u>

T38.805- <u>Adverse effect</u> of unspecified hormones and synthetic substitutes

T38.806- <u>Underdosing</u> of unspecified hormones and synthetic substitutes

T38.81- Poisoning by, adverse effect of and underdosing of <u>anterior pituitary [adenohypophyseal] hormones</u>

T38.811- Poisoning by anterior pituitary [adenohypophyseal] hormones, <u>accidental (unintentional)</u>
Poisoning by anterior pituitary [adenohypophyseal] hormones NOS

T38.812- Poisoning by anterior pituitary [adenohypophyseal] hormones, <u>intentional</u> self-harm

T38.813- Poisoning by anterior pituitary [adenohypophyseal] hormones, <u>assault</u>

T38.814- Poisoning by anterior pituitary [adenohypophyseal] hormones, <u>undetermined</u>

T38.815- <u>Adverse effect</u> of anterior pituitary [adenohypophyseal] hormones

T38.816- <u>Underdosing</u> of anterior pituitary [adenohypophyseal] hormones

T38.89- Poisoning by, adverse effect of and underdosing of <u>other hormones and synthetic substitutes</u>

T38.891- Poisoning by other hormones and synthetic substitutes, <u>accidental (unintentional)</u>
Poisoning by other hormones and synthetic substitutes NOS

T38.892- Poisoning by other hormones and synthetic substitutes, <u>intentional</u> self-harm

T38.893- Poisoning by other hormones and synthetic substitutes, <u>assault</u>

T38.894- Poisoning by other hormones and synthetic substitutes, <u>undetermined</u>

T38.895- <u>Adverse effect</u> of other hormones and synthetic substitutes

T38.896- <u>Underdosing</u> of other hormones and synthetic substitutes

T38.9- **Poisoning by, adverse effect of and underdosing of other and unspecified hormone antagonists**

T38.90- Poisoning by, adverse effect of and underdosing of <u>unspecified hormone antagonists</u>

T38.901- Poisoning by unspecified hormone antagonists, <u>accidental (unintentional)</u>
Poisoning by unspecified hormone antagonists NOS

T38.902- Poisoning by unspecified hormone antagonists, <u>intentional</u> self-harm

T38.903- Poisoning by unspecified hormone antagonists, <u>assault</u>

T38.904- Poisoning by unspecified hormone antagonists, <u>undetermined</u>

T38.905- <u>Adverse effect</u> of unspecified hormone antagonists

T38.906- <u>Underdosing</u> of unspecified hormone antagonists

T38.99- Poisoning by, adverse effect of and underdosing of <u>other hormone antagonists</u>

T38.991- Poisoning by other hormone antagonists, <u>accidental (unintentional)</u>
Poisoning by other hormone antagonists NOS

T38.992- Poisoning by other hormone antagonists, <u>intentional</u> self-harm

T38.993- Poisoning by other hormone antagonists, <u>assault</u>

T38.994- Poisoning by other hormone antagonists, <u>undetermined</u>

T38.995- <u>Adverse effect</u> of other hormone antagonists

T38.996- <u>Underdosing</u> of other hormone antagonists

T39- **Poisoning by, adverse effect of and underdosing of <u>nonopioid analgesics, antipyretics and antirheumatics</u>**

The appropriate 7th character is to be added to each code from category T39:
A   <u>Initial</u> encounter
D   <u>Subsequent</u> encounter
S   <u>Sequela</u>

T39.0- Poisoning by, adverse effect of and underdosing of <u>salicylates</u>

T39.01- Poisoning by, adverse effect of and underdosing of <u>aspirin</u>
Poisoning by, adverse effect of and underdosing of acetylsalicylic acid

T39.011- Poisoning by aspirin, <u>accidental</u> (unintentional)

T39.012- Poisoning by aspirin, <u>intentional</u> self-harm

T39.013- Poisoning by aspirin, <u>assault</u>

T39.014- Poisoning by aspirin, <u>undetermined</u>

T39.015- <u>Adverse effect</u> of aspirin

T
3
8
-
T
4
0

Excludes 1: = NOT CODED HERE! (Do not code both)

Excludes ❷: = Not Included Here

T39.016- <u>Underdosing</u> of aspirin

T39.09- Poisoning by, adverse effect of and underdosing of <u>other salicylates</u>

    T39.091- Poisoning by salicylates, <u>accidental</u> (unintentional)
        Poisoning by salicylates NOS

    T39.092- Poisoning by salicylates, <u>intentional</u> self-harm

    T39.093- Poisoning by salicylates, <u>assault</u>

    T39.094- Poisoning by salicylates, <u>undetermined</u>

    T39.095- <u>Adverse effect</u> of salicylates

    T39.096- <u>Underdosing</u> of salicylates

T39.1- Poisoning by, adverse effect of and underdosing of <u>4-Aminophenol derivatives</u>

    T39.1x- Poisoning by, adverse effect of and underdosing of 4-Aminophenol derivatives

    T39.1x1- Poisoning by 4-Aminophenol derivatives, <u>accidental</u> (unintentional)
        Poisoning by 4-Aminophenol derivatives NOS

    T39.1x2- Poisoning by 4-Aminophenol derivatives, <u>intentional</u> self-harm

    T39.1x3- Poisoning by 4-Aminophenol derivatives, <u>assault</u>

    T39.1x4- Poisoning by 4-Aminophenol derivatives, <u>undetermined</u>

    T39.1x5- <u>Adverse effect</u> of 4-Aminophenol derivatives

    T39.1x6- <u>Underdosing</u> of 4-Aminophenol derivatives

T39.2- Poisoning by, adverse effect of and underdosing of pyrazolone derivatives

    T39.2x- Poisoning by, adverse effect of and underdosing of <u>pyrazolone derivatives</u>

    T39.2x1- Poisoning by pyrazolone derivatives, <u>accidental</u> (unintentional)
        Poisoning by pyrazolone derivatives NOS

    T39.2x2- Poisoning by pyrazolone derivatives, <u>intentional</u> self-harm

    T39.2x3- Poisoning by pyrazolone derivatives, <u>assault</u>

    T39.2x4- Poisoning by pyrazolone derivatives, <u>undetermined</u>

    T39.2x5- <u>Adverse effect</u> of pyrazolone derivatives

    T39.2x6- <u>Underdosing</u> of pyrazolone derivatives

T39.3- Poisoning by, adverse effect of and underdosing of <u>other nonsteroidal anti-inflammatory drugs [NSAID]</u>

    T39.31- Poisoning by, adverse effect of and underdosing of <u>propionic acid derivatives</u>
        Poisoning by, adverse effect of and underdosing of fenoprofen
        Poisoning by, adverse effect of and underdosing of flurbiprofen
        Poisoning by, adverse effect of and underdosing of ibuprofen
        Poisoning by, adverse effect of and underdosing of ketoprofen
        Poisoning by, adverse effect of and underdosing of naproxen
        Poisoning by, adverse effect of and underdosing of oxaprozin

    T39.311- Poisoning by propionic acid derivatives, <u>accidental</u> (unintentional)

    T39.312- Poisoning by propionic acid derivatives, <u>intentional</u> self-harm

    T39.313- Poisoning by propionic acid derivatives, <u>assault</u>

    T39.314- Poisoning by propionic acid derivatives, <u>undetermined</u>

    T39.315- <u>Adverse effect</u> of propionic acid derivatives

    T39.316- <u>Underdosing</u> of propionic acid derivatives

    T39.39- Poisoning by, adverse effect of and underdosing of <u>other nonsteroidal anti-inflammatory drugs [NSAID]</u>

    T39.391- Poisoning by other nonsteroidal anti-inflammatory drugs [NSAID], <u>accidental</u> (unintentional)
        Poisoning by other nonsteroidal anti-inflammatory drugs NOS

    T39.392- Poisoning by other nonsteroidal anti-inflammatory drugs [NSAID], <u>intentional</u> self-harm

    T39.393- Poisoning by other nonsteroidal anti-inflammatory drugs [NSAID], <u>assault</u>

    T39.394- Poisoning by other nonsteroidal anti-inflammatory drugs [NSAID], <u>undetermined</u>

    T39.395- <u>Adverse effect</u> of other nonsteroidal anti-inflammatory drugs [NSAID]

    T39.396- <u>Underdosing</u> of other nonsteroidal anti-inflammatory drugs [NSAID]

T39.4- Poisoning by, adverse effect of and underdosing of antirheumatics, not elsewhere classified
    Excludes 1: poisoning by, adverse effect of and underdosing of glucocorticoids (T38.0-)
        poisoning by, adverse effect of and underdosing of salicylates (T39.0-)

    T39.4x- Poisoning by, adverse effect of and underdosing of <u>antirheumatics, not elsewhere classified</u>

    T39.4x1- Poisoning by antirheumatics, not elsewhere classified, <u>accidental</u> (unintentional)
        Poisoning by antirheumatics, not elsewhere classified NOS

    T39.4x2- Poisoning by antirheumatics, not elsewhere classified, <u>intentional</u> self-harm

    T39.4x3- Poisoning by antirheumatics, not elsewhere classified, <u>assault</u>

    T39.4x4- Poisoning by antirheumatics, not elsewhere classified, <u>undetermined</u>

    T39.4x5- <u>Adverse effect</u> of antirheumatics, not elsewhere classified

    T39.4x6- <u>Underdosing</u> of antirheumatics, not elsewhere classified

T39.8- Poisoning by, adverse effect of and underdosing of other nonopioid analgesics and antipyretics, not elsewhere classified

    T39.8x- Poisoning by, adverse effect of and underdosing of <u>other nonopioid analgesics and antipyretics, not elsewhere classified</u>

    T39.8x1- Poisoning by other nonopioid analgesics and antipyretics, not elsewhere classified, <u>accidental</u> (unintentional)
        Poisoning by other nonopioid analgesics and antipyretics, not elsewhere classified NOS

    T39.8x2- Poisoning by other nonopioid analgesics and antipyretics, not elsewhere classified, <u>intentional</u> self-harm

    T39.8x3- Poisoning by other nonopioid analgesics and antipyretics, not elsewhere classified, <u>assault</u>

    T39.8x4- Poisoning by other nonopioid analgesics and antipyretics, not elsewhere classified, <u>undetermined</u>

    T39.8x5- <u>Adverse effect</u> of other nonopioid analgesics and antipyretics, not elsewhere classified

    T39.8x6- <u>Underdosing</u> of other nonopioid analgesics and antipyretics, not elsewhere classified

T39.9- Poisoning by, adverse effect of and underdosing of <u>unspecified nonopioid analgesic, antipyretic and antirheumatic</u>

    T39.91x- Poisoning by unspecified nonopioid analgesic, antipyretic and antirheumatic, <u>accidental</u> (unintentional)
        Poisoning by nonopioid analgesic, antipyretic and antirheumatic NOS

    T39.92x- Poisoning by unspecified nonopioid analgesic, antipyretic and antirheumatic, <u>intentional</u> self-harm

    T39.93x- Poisoning by unspecified nonopioid analgesic, antipyretic and antirheumatic, <u>assault</u>

    T39.94x- Poisoning by unspecified nonopioid analgesic, antipyretic and antirheumatic, <u>undetermined</u>

    T39.95x- <u>Adverse effect</u> of unspecified nonopioid analgesic, antipyretic and antirheumatic

    T39.96x- <u>Underdosing</u> of unspecified nonopioid analgesic, antipyretic and antirheumatic

T40- Poisoning by, adverse effect of and underdosing of <u>narcotics and psychodysleptics [hallucinogens]</u>
    Excludes❷: drug dependence and related mental and behavioral disorders due to psychoactive substance use (F10.-F19.-)

    The appropriate 7th character is to be added to each code from category T40:
    A <u>Initial</u> encounter
    D <u>Subsequent</u> encounter
    S <u>Sequela</u>

T40.0- Poisoning by, adverse effect of and underdosing of opium

    T40.0x- Poisoning by, adverse effect of and underdosing of <u>opium</u>

    T40.0x1- Poisoning by opium, <u>accidental</u> (unintentional)
        Poisoning by opium NOS

    T40.0x2- Poisoning by opium, <u>intentional</u> self-harm

    T40.0x3- Poisoning by opium, <u>assault</u>

    T40.0x4- Poisoning by opium, <u>undetermined</u>

    T40.0x5- <u>Adverse effect</u> of opium

    T40.0x6- <u>Underdosing</u> of opium

T38 – T40

T40.1-   Poisoning by and adverse effect of heroin
   T40.1x- Poisoning by and adverse effect of <u>heroin</u>
      T40.1x1- Poisoning by heroin, <u>accidental</u> (unintentional)
         Poisoning by heroin NOS
      T40.1x2- Poisoning by heroin, <u>intentional</u> self-harm
      T40.1x3- Poisoning by heroin, <u>assault</u>
      T40.1x4- Poisoning by heroin, <u>undetermined</u>
T40.2-   Poisoning by, adverse effect of and underdosing of other opioids
   T40.2x- Poisoning by, adverse effect of and underdosing of <u>other opioids</u>
      T40.2x1- Poisoning by other opioids, <u>accidental</u> (unintentional)
         Poisoning by other opioids NOS
      T40.2x2- Poisoning by other opioids, <u>intentional</u> self-harm
      T40.2x3- Poisoning by other opioids, <u>assault</u>
      T40.2x4- Poisoning by other opioids, <u>undetermined</u>
      T40.2x5- <u>Adverse effect</u> of other opioids
      T40.2x6- <u>Underdosing</u> of other opioids
T40.3-   Poisoning by, adverse effect of and underdosing of methadone
   T40.3x- Poisoning by, adverse effect of and underdosing of <u>methadone</u>
      T40.3x1- Poisoning by methadone, <u>accidental</u> (unintentional)
         Poisoning by methadone NOS
      T40.3x2- Poisoning by methadone, <u>intentional</u> self-harm
      T40.3x3- Poisoning by methadone, <u>assault</u>
      T40.3x4- Poisoning by methadone, <u>undetermined</u>
      T40.3x5- <u>Adverse effect</u> of methadone
      T40.3x6- <u>Underdosing</u> of methadone
T40.4-   Poisoning by, adverse effect of and underdosing of other synthetic narcotics
   T40.4x- Poisoning by, adverse effect of and underdosing of <u>other synthetic narcotics</u>
      T40.4x1- Poisoning by other synthetic narcotics, <u>accidental</u> (unintentional)
         Poisoning by other synthetic narcotics NOS
      T40.4x2- Poisoning by other synthetic narcotics, <u>intentional</u> self-harm
      T40.4x3- Poisoning by other synthetic narcotics, <u>assault</u>
      T40.4x4- Poisoning by other synthetic narcotics, <u>undetermined</u>
      T40.4x5- <u>Adverse effect</u> of other synthetic narcotics
      T40.4x6- <u>Underdosing</u> of other synthetic narcotics
T40.5-   Poisoning by, adverse effect of and underdosing of cocaine
   T40.5x- Poisoning by, adverse effect of and underdosing of <u>cocaine</u>
      T40.5x1- Poisoning by cocaine, <u>accidental</u> (unintentional)
         Poisoning by cocaine NOS
      T40.5x2- Poisoning by cocaine, <u>intentional</u> self-harm
      T40.5x3- Poisoning by cocaine, <u>assault</u>
      T40.5x4- Poisoning by cocaine, <u>undetermined</u>
      T40.5x5- <u>Adverse effect</u> of cocaine
      T40.5x6- <u>Underdosing</u> of cocaine
T40.6-   Poisoning by, adverse effect of and underdosing of other and unspecified narcotics
   T40.60- Poisoning by, adverse effect of and underdosing of <u>unspecified</u> narcotics
      T40.601- Poisoning by unspecified narcotics, <u>accidental</u> (unintentional)
         Poisoning by narcotics NOS
      T40.602- Poisoning by unspecified narcotics, <u>intentional</u> self-harm
      T40.603- Poisoning by unspecified narcotics, <u>assault</u>
      T40.604- Poisoning by unspecified narcotics, <u>undetermined</u>
      T40.605- <u>Adverse effect</u> of unspecified narcotics
      T40.606- <u>Underdosing</u> of unspecified narcotics
   T40.69- Poisoning by, adverse effect of and underdosing of <u>other</u> narcotics
      T40.691- Poisoning by other narcotics, <u>accidental</u> (unintentional)
         Poisoning by other narcotics NOS
      T40.692- Poisoning by other narcotics, <u>intentional</u> self-harm
      T40.693- Poisoning by other narcotics, <u>assault</u>
      T40.694- Poisoning by other narcotics, <u>undetermined</u>
      T40.695- <u>Adverse effect</u> of other narcotics
      T40.696- <u>Underdosing</u> of other narcotics

T40.7-   Poisoning by, adverse effect of and underdosing of cannabis (derivatives)
   T40.7x- Poisoning by, adverse effect of and underdosing of <u>cannabis (derivatives)</u>
      T40.7x1- Poisoning by cannabis (derivatives), <u>accidental</u> (unintentional)
         Poisoning by cannabis NOS
      T40.7x2- Poisoning by cannabis (derivatives), <u>intentional</u> self-harm
      T40.7x3- Poisoning by cannabis (derivatives), <u>assault</u>
      T40.7x4- Poisoning by cannabis (derivatives), <u>undetermined</u>
      T40.7x5- <u>Adverse effect</u> of cannabis (derivatives)
      T40.7x6- <u>Underdosing</u> of cannabis (derivatives)
T40.8-   Poisoning by and adverse effect of lysergide [LSD]
   T40.8x- Poisoning by and adverse effect of lysergide [LSD]
      T40.8x1- Poisoning by lysergide [LSD], <u>accidental</u> (unintentional)
         Poisoning by lysergide [LSD] NOS
      T40.8x2- Poisoning by lysergide [LSD], <u>intentional</u> self-harm
      T40.8x3- Poisoning by lysergide [LSD], <u>assault</u>
      T40.8x4- Poisoning by lysergide [LSD], <u>undetermined</u>
T40.9-   Poisoning by, adverse effect of and underdosing of other and unspecified psychodysleptics [hallucinogens]
   T40.90- Poisoning by, adverse effect of and underdosing of <u>unspecified psychodysleptics [hallucinogens]</u>
      T40.901- Poisoning by unspecified psychodysleptics [hallucinogens], <u>accidental</u> (unintentional)
      T40.902- Poisoning by unspecified psychodysleptics [hallucinogens], <u>intentional</u> self-harm
      T40.903- Poisoning by unspecified psychodysleptics [hallucinogens], <u>assault</u>
      T40.904- Poisoning by unspecified psychodysleptics [hallucinogens], <u>undetermined</u>
      T40.905- <u>Adverse effect</u> of unspecified psychodysleptics [hallucinogens]
      T40.906- <u>Underdosing</u> of unspecified psychodysleptics
   T40.99- Poisoning by, adverse effect of and underdosing of <u>other psychodysleptics [hallucinogens]</u>
      T40.991- Poisoning by other psychodysleptics [hallucinogens], <u>accidental</u> (unintentional)
         Poisoning by other psychodysleptics [hallucinogens] NOS
      T40.992- Poisoning by other psychodysleptics [hallucinogens], <u>intentional</u> self-harm
      T40.993- Poisoning by other psychodysleptics [hallucinogens], <u>assault</u>
      T40.994- Poisoning by other psychodysleptics [hallucinogens], <u>undetermined</u>
      T40.995- <u>Adverse effect</u> of other psychodysleptics [hallucinogens]
      T40.996- <u>Underdosing</u> of other psychodysleptics
T41-   Poisoning by, adverse effect of and underdosing of <u>anesthetics and therapeutic gases</u>
   Excludes 1: *benzodiazepines (T42.4-)*
              cocaine (T40.5-)
              complications of anesthesia during pregnancy (O29.-)
              complications of anesthesia during labor and delivery (O74.-)
              complications of anesthesia during the puerperium (O89.-)
              opioids (T40.0-T40.2-)

The appropriate 7th character is to be added to each code from category T41:
  A <u>Initial</u> encounter
  D <u>Subsequent</u> encounter
  S <u>Sequela</u>

T41.0-   Poisoning by, adverse effect of and underdosing of inhaled anesthetics
   Excludes 1: *oxygen (T41.5-)*
   T41.0x- Poisoning by, adverse effect of and underdosing of <u>inhaled anesthetics</u>
      T41.0x1- Poisoning by inhaled anesthetics, <u>accidental</u> (unintentional)
         Poisoning by inhaled anesthetics NOS
      T41.0x2- Poisoning by inhaled anesthetics, <u>intentional</u> self-harm
      T41.0x3- Poisoning by inhaled anesthetics, <u>assault</u>
      T41.0x4- Poisoning by inhaled anesthetics, <u>undetermined</u>
      T41.0x5- <u>Adverse effect</u> of inhaled anesthetics
      T41.0x6- <u>Underdosing</u> of inhaled anesthetics

T40 – T42

T41.1- Poisoning by, adverse effect of and underdosing of intravenous anesthetics
> Poisoning by, adverse effect of and underdosing of thiobarbiturates

T41.1x- Poisoning by, adverse effect of and underdosing of <u>intravenous anesthetics</u>

T41.1x1- Poisoning by intravenous anesthetics, <u>accidental</u> (unintentional)
> Poisoning by intravenous anesthetics NOS

T41.1x2- Poisoning by intravenous anesthetics, <u>intentional</u> self-harm

T41.1x3- Poisoning by intravenous anesthetics, <u>assault</u>

T41.1x4- Poisoning by intravenous anesthetics, <u>undetermined</u>

T41.1x5- <u>Adverse effect</u> of intravenous anesthetics

T41.1x6- <u>Underdosing</u> of intravenous anesthetics

T41.2- Poisoning by, adverse effect of and underdosing of other and unspecified general anesthetics

T41.20- Poisoning by, adverse effect of and underdosing of <u>unspecified general anesthetics</u>

T41.201- Poisoning by unspecified general anesthetics, <u>accidental</u> (unintentional)
> Poisoning by general anesthetics NOS

T41.202- Poisoning by unspecified general anesthetics, <u>intentional</u> self-harm

T41.203- Poisoning by unspecified general anesthetics, <u>assault</u>

T41.204- Poisoning by unspecified general anesthetics, <u>undetermined</u>

T41.205- <u>Adverse effect</u> of unspecified general anesthetics

T41.206- <u>Underdosing</u> of unspecified general anesthetics

T41.29- Poisoning by, adverse effect of and underdosing of <u>other general anesthetics</u>

T41.291- Poisoning by other general anesthetics, <u>accidental</u> (unintentional)
> Poisoning by other general anesthetics NOS

T41.292- Poisoning by other general anesthetics, <u>intentional</u> self-harm

T41.293- Poisoning by other general anesthetics, <u>assault</u>

T41.294- Poisoning by other general anesthetics, <u>undetermined</u>

T41.295- <u>Adverse effect</u> of other general anesthetics

T41.296- <u>Underdosing</u> of other general anesthetics

T41.3- Poisoning by, adverse effect of and underdosing of local anesthetics

T41.3x- Poisoning by, adverse effect of and underdosing of <u>local anesthetics</u>
> Cocaine (topical)
> *Excludes❷: poisoning by cocaine used as a central nervous system stimulant (T40.5x1-T40.5x4)*

T41.3x1- Poisoning by local anesthetics, <u>accidental</u> (unintentional)
> Poisoning by local anesthetics NOS

T41.3x2- Poisoning by local anesthetics, <u>intentional</u> self-harm

T41.3x3- Poisoning by local anesthetics, <u>assault</u>

T41.3x4- Poisoning by local anesthetics, <u>undetermined</u>

T41.3x5- <u>Adverse effect</u> of local anesthetics

T41.3x6- <u>Underdosing</u> of local anesthetics

T41.4- Poisoning by, adverse effect of and underdosing of <u>unspecified anesthetic</u>

T41.41x- Poisoning by unspecified anesthetic, <u>accidental</u> (unintentional)
> Poisoning by anesthetic NOS

T41.42x- Poisoning by unspecified anesthetic, <u>intentional</u> self-harm

T41.43x- Poisoning by unspecified anesthetic, <u>assault</u>

T41.44x- Poisoning by unspecified anesthetic, <u>undetermined</u>

T41.45x- <u>Adverse effect</u> of unspecified anesthetic

T41.46x- <u>Underdosing</u> of unspecified anesthetics

T41.5- Poisoning by, adverse effect of and underdosing of therapeutic gases

T41.5x- Poisoning by, adverse effect of and underdosing of <u>therapeutic gases</u>

T41.5x1- Poisoning by therapeutic gases, <u>accidental</u> (unintentional)
> Poisoning by therapeutic gases NOS

T41.5x2- Poisoning by therapeutic gases, <u>intentional</u> self-harm

T41.5x3- Poisoning by therapeutic gases, <u>assault</u>

T41.5x4- Poisoning by therapeutic gases, <u>undetermined</u>

T41.5x5- <u>Adverse effect</u> of therapeutic gases

T41.5x6- <u>Underdosing</u> of therapeutic gases

T42- Poisoning by, adverse effect of and underdosing of <u>antiepileptic, sedative-hypnotic and antiparkinsonism drugs</u>
> *Excludes❷: drug dependence and related mental and behavioral disorders due to psychoactive substance use (F10.-F19.-)*

> The appropriate 7th character is to be added to each code from category T42:
> **A** <u>Initial</u> encounter
> **D** <u>Subsequent</u> encounter
> **S** <u>Sequela</u>

T42.0- Poisoning by, adverse effect of and underdosing of hydantoin derivatives

T42.0x- Poisoning by, adverse effect of and underdosing of <u>hydantoin derivatives</u>

T42.0x1- Poisoning by hydantoin derivatives, <u>accidental</u> (unintentional)
> Poisoning by hydantoin derivatives NOS

T42.0x2- Poisoning by hydantoin derivatives, <u>intentional</u> self-harm

T42.0x3- Poisoning by hydantoin derivatives, <u>assault</u>

T42.0x4- Poisoning by hydantoin derivatives, <u>undetermined</u>

T42.0x5- <u>Adverse effect</u> of hydantoin derivatives

T42.0x6- <u>Underdosing</u> of hydantoin derivatives

T42.1- Poisoning by, adverse effect of and underdosing of iminostilbenes
> Poisoning by, adverse effect of and underdosing of carbamazepine

T42.1x- Poisoning by, adverse effect of and underdosing of <u>iminostilbenes</u>

T42.1x1- Poisoning by iminostilbenes, <u>accidental</u> (unintentional)
> Poisoning by iminostilbenes NOS

T42.1x2- Poisoning by iminostilbenes, <u>intentional</u> self-harm

T42.1x3- Poisoning by iminostilbenes, <u>assault</u>

T42.1x4- Poisoning by iminostilbenes, <u>undetermined</u>

T42.1x5- <u>Adverse effect</u> of iminostilbenes

T42.1x6- <u>Underdosing</u> of iminostilbenes

T42.2- Poisoning by, adverse effect of and underdosing of succinimides and oxazolidinediones

T42.2x- Poisoning by, adverse effect of and underdosing of <u>succinimides and oxazolidinediones</u>

T42.2x1- Poisoning by succinimides and oxazolidinediones, <u>accidental</u> (unintentional)
> Poisoning by succinimides and oxazolidinediones NOS

T42.2x2- Poisoning by succinimides and oxazolidinediones, <u>intentional</u> self-harm

T42.2x3- Poisoning by succinimides and oxazolidinediones, <u>assault</u>

T42.2x4- Poisoning by succinimides and oxazolidinediones, <u>undetermined</u>

T42.2x5- <u>Adverse effect</u> of succinimides and oxazolidinediones

T42.2x6- <u>Underdosing</u> of succinimides and oxazolidinediones

T42.3- Poisoning by, adverse effect of and underdosing of barbiturates
> *Excludes 1: poisoning by, adverse effect of and underdosing of thiobarbiturates (T41.1-)*

T42.3x- Poisoning by, adverse effect of and underdosing of <u>barbiturates</u>

T42.3x1- Poisoning by barbiturates, <u>accidental</u> (unintentional)
> Poisoning by barbiturates NOS

T42.3x2- Poisoning by barbiturates, <u>intentional</u> self-harm

T42.3x3- Poisoning by barbiturates, <u>assault</u>

T42.3x4- Poisoning by barbiturates, <u>undetermined</u>

T42.3x5- <u>Adverse effect</u> of barbiturates

T42.3x6- <u>Underdosing</u> of barbiturates

T42.4- Poisoning by, adverse effect of and underdosing of benzodiazepines

T42.4x- Poisoning by, adverse effect of and underdosing of <u>benzodiazepines</u>

T42.4x1- Poisoning by benzodiazepines, <u>accidental</u> (unintentional)
> Poisoning by benzodiazepines NOS

T42.4x2- Poisoning by benzodiazepines, <u>intentional</u> self-harm

T42.4x3- Poisoning by benzodiazepines, <u>assault</u>

T42.4x4- Poisoning by benzodiazepines, <u>undetermined</u>

T42.4x5- <u>Adverse effect</u> of benzodiazepines

T42.4x6- <u>Underdosing</u> of benzodiazepines

T40 – T42

T42.5- **Poisoning by, adverse effect of and underdosing of mixed antiepileptics**

  T42.5x- **Poisoning by, adverse effect of and underdosing of** <u>antiepileptics</u>

   T42.5x1- **Poisoning by mixed antiepileptics, <u>accidental</u> (unintentional)**
     Poisoning by mixed antiepileptics NOS

   T42.5x2- **Poisoning by mixed antiepileptics, <u>intentional</u> self-harm**

   T42.5x3- **Poisoning by mixed antiepileptics, <u>assault</u>**

   T42.5x4- **Poisoning by mixed antiepileptics, <u>undetermined</u>**

   T42.5x5- **<u>Adverse effect</u> of mixed antiepileptics**

   T42.5x6- **<u>Underdosing</u> of mixed antiepileptics**

T42.6- **Poisoning by, adverse effect of and underdosing of other antiepileptic and sedative-hypnotic drugs**
     Poisoning by, adverse effect of and underdosing of methaqualone
     Poisoning by, adverse effect of and underdosing of valproic acid
     Excludes 1: poisoning by, adverse effect of and underdosing of carbamazepine (T42.1-)

  T42.6x- **Poisoning by, adverse effect of and underdosing of <u>other antiepileptic and sedative-hypnotic drugs</u>**

   T42.6x1- **Poisoning by other antiepileptic and sedative-hypnotic drugs, <u>accidental</u> (unintentional)**
     Poisoning by other antiepileptic and sedative-hypnotic drugs NOS

   T42.6x2- **Poisoning by other antiepileptic and sedative-hypnotic drugs, <u>intentional</u> self-harm**

   T42.6x3- **Poisoning by other antiepileptic and sedative-hypnotic drugs, <u>assault</u>**

   T42.6x4- **Poisoning by other antiepileptic and sedative-hypnotic drugs, <u>undetermined</u>**

   T42.6x5- **<u>Adverse effect</u> of other antiepileptic and sedative-hypnotic drugs**

   T42.6x6- **<u>Underdosing</u> of other antiepileptic and sedative-hypnotic drugs**

T42.7- **Poisoning by, adverse effect of and underdosing of <u>unspecified antiepileptic and sedative-hypnotic drugs</u>**

  T42.71x- **Poisoning by unspecified antiepileptic and sedative-hypnotic drugs, <u>accidental</u> (unintentional)**
     Poisoning by antiepileptic and sedative-hypnotic drugs NOS

  T42.72x- **Poisoning by unspecified antiepileptic and sedative-hypnotic drugs, <u>intentional</u> self-harm**

  T42.73x- **Poisoning by unspecified antiepileptic and sedative-hypnotic drugs, <u>assault</u>**

  T42.74x- **Poisoning by unspecified antiepileptic and sedative-hypnotic drugs, <u>undetermined</u>**

  T42.75x- **<u>Adverse effect</u> of unspecified antiepileptic and sedative-hypnotic drugs**

  T42.76x- **<u>Underdosing</u> of unspecified antiepileptic and sedative-hypnotic drugs**

T42.8- **Poisoning by, adverse effect of and underdosing of antiparkinsonism drugs and other central muscle-tone depressants**
     Poisoning by, adverse effect of and underdosing of amantadine

  T42.8x- **Poisoning by, adverse effect of and underdosing of <u>antiparkinsonism drugs and other central muscle-tone depressants</u>**

   T42.8x1- **Poisoning by antiparkinsonism drugs and other central muscle-tone depressants, <u>accidental</u> (unintentional)**
     Poisoning by antiparkinsonism drugs and other central muscle-tone depressants NOS

   T42.8x2- **Poisoning by antiparkinsonism drugs and other central muscle-tone depressants, <u>intentional</u> self-harm**

   T42.8x3- **Poisoning by antiparkinsonism drugs and other central muscle-tone depressants, <u>assault</u>**

   T42.8x4- **Poisoning by antiparkinsonism drugs and other central muscle-tone depressants, <u>undetermined</u>**

   T42.8x5- **<u>Adverse effect</u> of antiparkinsonism drugs and other central muscle-tone depressants**

   T42.8x6- **<u>Underdosing</u> of antiparkinsonism drugs and other central muscle-tone depressants**

T43- **Poisoning by, adverse effect of and underdosing of <u>psychotropic drugs, not elsewhere classified</u>**
     Excludes 1: appetite depressants (T50.5-)
       barbiturates (T42.3-)
       benzodiazepines (T42.4-)
       methaqualone (T42.6-)
       psychodysleptics [hallucinogens] (T40.7-T40.9-)
     Excludes ❷: drug dependence and related mental and behavioral disorders due to psychoactive substance use (F10.--F19.-)

The appropriate 7th character is to be added to each code from category T43:
  A **<u>Initial</u> encounter**
  D **<u>Subsequent</u> encounter**
  S **<u>Sequela</u>**

T43.0- **Poisoning by, adverse effect of and underdosing of tricyclic and tetracyclic antidepressants**

  T43.01- **Poisoning by, adverse effect of and underdosing of <u>tricyclic antidepressants</u>**

   T43.011- **Poisoning by tricyclic antidepressants, <u>accidental</u> (unintentional)**
     Poisoning by tricyclic antidepressants NOS

   T43.012- **Poisoning by tricyclic antidepressants, <u>intentional</u> self-harm**

   T43.013- **Poisoning by tricyclic antidepressants, <u>assault</u>**

   T43.014- **Poisoning by tricyclic antidepressants, <u>undetermined</u>**

   T43.015- **<u>Adverse effect</u> of tricyclic antidepressants**

   T43.016- **<u>Underdosing</u> of tricyclic antidepressants**

  T43.02- **Poisoning by, adverse effect of and underdosing of <u>tetracyclic antidepressants</u>**

   T43.021- **Poisoning by tetracyclic antidepressants, <u>accidental</u> (unintentional)**
     Poisoning by tetracyclic antidepressants NOS

   T43.022- **Poisoning by tetracyclic antidepressants, <u>intentional</u> self-harm**

   T43.023- **Poisoning by tetracyclic antidepressants, <u>assault</u>**

   T43.024- **Poisoning by tetracyclic antidepressants, <u>undetermined</u>**

   T43.025- **<u>Adverse effect</u> of tetracyclic antidepressants**

   T43.026- **<u>Underdosing</u> of tetracyclic antidepressants**

T43.1- **Poisoning by, adverse effect of and underdosing of monoamine-oxidase-inhibitor antidepressants**

  T43.1x- **Poisoning by, adverse effect of and underdosing of <u>monoamine-oxidase-inhibitor antidepressants</u>**

   T43.1x1- **Poisoning by monoamine-oxidase-inhibitor antidepressants, <u>accidental</u> (unintentional)**
     Poisoning by monoamine-oxidase-inhibitor antidepressants NOS

   T43.1x2- **Poisoning by monoamine-oxidase-inhibitor antidepressants, <u>intentional</u> self-harm**

   T43.1x3- **Poisoning by monoamine-oxidase-inhibitor antidepressants, <u>assault</u>**

   T43.1x4- **Poisoning by monoamine-oxidase-inhibitor antidepressants, <u>undetermined</u>**

   T43.1x5- **<u>Adverse effect</u> of monoamine-oxidase-inhibitor antidepressants**

   T43.1x6- **<u>Underdosing</u> of monoamine-oxidase-inhibitor antidepressants**

T43.2- **Poisoning by, adverse effect of and underdosing of other and unspecified antidepressants**

  T43.20- **Poisoning by, adverse effect of and underdosing of <u>unspecified antidepressants</u>**

   T43.201- **Poisoning by unspecified antidepressants, <u>accidental</u> (unintentional)**
     Poisoning by antidepressants NOS

   T43.202- **Poisoning by unspecified antidepressants, <u>intentional</u> self-harm**

   T43.203- **Poisoning by unspecified antidepressants, <u>assault</u>**

   T43.204- **Poisoning by unspecified antidepressants, <u>undetermined</u>**

   T43.205- **<u>Adverse effect</u> of unspecified antidepressants**

   T43.206- **<u>Underdosing</u> of unspecified antidepressants**

  T43.21- **Poisoning by, adverse effect of and underdosing of <u>selective serotonin and norepinephrinere uptake inhibitors</u>**
     Poisoning by, adverse effect of and underdosing of SSNRI antidepressants

   T43.211- **Poisoning by selective serotonin and norepinephrine reuptake inhibitors, <u>accidental</u> (unintentional)**

   T43.212- **Poisoning by selective serotonin and norepinephrine reuptake inhibitors, <u>intentional</u> self-harm**

   T43.213- **Poisoning by selective serotonin and norepinephrine reuptake inhibitors, <u>assault</u>**

T
4
2
I
T
4
3

T43.214- Poisoning by selective serotonin and norepinephrine reuptake inhibitors, <u>undetermined</u>

T43.215- <u>Adverse effect</u> of selective serotonin and norepinephrine reuptake inhibitors

T43.216- <u>Underdosing</u> of selective serotonin and norepinephrine reuptake inhibitors

T43.22- Poisoning by, adverse effect of and underdosing of <u>selective serotonin reuptake inhibitors</u>
  Poisoning by, adverse effect of and underdosing of SSRI antidepressants

T43.221- Poisoning by selective serotonin reuptake inhibitors, <u>accidental</u> (unintentional)

T43.222- Poisoning by selective serotonin reuptake inhibitors, <u>intentional</u> self-harm

T43.223- Poisoning by selective serotonin reuptake inhibitors, <u>assault</u>

T43.224- Poisoning by selective serotonin reuptake inhibitors, <u>undetermined</u>

T43.225- <u>Adverse effect</u> of selective serotonin reuptake inhibitors

T43.226- <u>Underdosing</u> of selective serotonin reuptake inhibitors

T43.29- Poisoning by, adverse effect of and underdosing of <u>other antidepressants</u>

T43.291- Poisoning by other antidepressants, <u>accidental</u> (unintentional)
  Poisoning by other antidepressants NOS

T43.292- Poisoning by other antidepressants, <u>intentional</u> self-harm

T43.293- Poisoning by other antidepressants, <u>assault</u>

T43.294- Poisoning by other antidepressants, <u>undetermined</u>

T43.295- <u>Adverse effect</u> of other antidepressants

T43.296- <u>Underdosing</u> of other antidepressants

T43.3- Poisoning by, adverse effect of and underdosing of phenothiazine antipsychotics and neuroleptics

T43.3x- Poisoning by, adverse effect of and underdosing of <u>phenothiazine antipsychotics and neuroleptics</u>

T43.3x1- Poisoning by phenothiazine antipsychotics and neuroleptics, <u>accidental</u> (unintentional)
  Poisoning by phenothiazine antipsychotics and neuroleptics NOS

T43.3x2- Poisoning by phenothiazine antipsychotics and neuroleptics, <u>intentional</u> self-harm

T43.3x3- Poisoning by phenothiazine antipsychotics and neuroleptics, <u>assault</u>

T43.3x4- Poisoning by phenothiazine antipsychotics and neuroleptics, <u>undetermined</u>

T43.3x5- <u>Adverse effect</u> of phenothiazine antipsychotics and neuroleptics

T43.3x6- <u>Underdosing</u> of phenothiazine antipsychotics and neuroleptics

T43.4- Poisoning by, adverse effect of and underdosing of butyrophenone and thiothixene neuroleptics

T43.4x- Poisoning by, adverse effect of and underdosing of <u>butyrophenone and thiothixene neuroleptics</u>

T43.4x1- Poisoning by butyrophenone and thiothixene neuroleptics, <u>accidental</u> (unintentional)
  Poisoning by butyrophenone and thiothixene neuroleptics NOS

T43.4x2- Poisoning by butyrophenone and thiothixene neuroleptics, <u>intentional</u> self-harm

T43.4x3- Poisoning by butyrophenone and thiothixene neuroleptics, <u>assault</u>

T43.4x4- Poisoning by butyrophenone and thiothixene neuroleptics, <u>undetermined</u>

T43.4x5- <u>Adverse effect</u> of butyrophenone and thiothixene neuroleptics

T43.4x6- <u>Underdosing</u> of butyrophenone and thiothixene neuroleptics

T43.5- Poisoning by, adverse effect of and underdosing of other and unspecified antipsychotics and neuroleptics
  Excludes 1: poisoning by, adverse effect of and underdosing of rauwolfia (T46.5-)

T43.50- Poisoning by, adverse effect of and underdosing of <u>unspecified antipsychotics and neuroleptics</u>

T43.501- Poisoning by unspecified antipsychotics and neuroleptics, <u>accidental</u> (unintentional)
  Poisoning by antipsychotics and neuroleptics NOS

T43.502- Poisoning by unspecified antipsychotics and neuroleptics, <u>intentional</u> self-harm

T43.503- Poisoning by unspecified antipsychotics and neuroleptics, <u>assault</u>

T43.504- Poisoning by unspecified antipsychotics and neuroleptics, <u>undetermined</u>

T43.505- <u>Adverse effect</u> of unspecified antipsychotics and neuroleptics

T43.506- <u>Underdosing</u> of unspecified antipsychotics and neuroleptics

T43.59- Poisoning by, adverse effect of and underdosing of <u>other antipsychotics and neuroleptics</u>

T43.591- Poisoning by other antipsychotics and neuroleptics, <u>accidental</u> (unintentional)
  Poisoning by other antipsychotics and neuroleptics NOS

T43.592- Poisoning by other antipsychotics and neuroleptics, <u>intentional</u> self-harm

T43.593- Poisoning by other antipsychotics and neuroleptics, <u>assault</u>

T43.594- Poisoning by other antipsychotics and neuroleptics, <u>undetermined</u>

T43.595- <u>Adverse effect</u> of other antipsychotics and neuroleptics

T43.596- <u>Underdosing</u> of other antipsychotics and neuroleptics

T43.6- Poisoning by, adverse effect of and underdosing of <u>psychostimulants</u>
  Excludes 1: poisoning by, adverse effect of and underdosing of cocaine (T40.5-)

T43.60- Poisoning by, adverse effect of and underdosing of <u>unspecified psychostimulant</u>

T43.601- Poisoning by unspecified psychostimulants, <u>accidental</u> (unintentional)
  Poisoning by psychostimulants NOS

T43.602- Poisoning by unspecified psychostimulants, <u>intentional</u> self-harm

T43.603- Poisoning by unspecified psychostimulants, <u>assault</u>

T43.604- Poisoning by unspecified psychostimulants, <u>undetermined</u>

T43.605- <u>Adverse effect</u> of unspecified psychostimulants

T43.606- <u>Underdosing</u> of unspecified psychostimulants

T43.61- Poisoning by, adverse effect of and underdosing of <u>caffeine</u>

T43.611- Poisoning by caffeine, <u>accidental</u> (unintentional)
  Poisoning by caffeine NOS

T43.612- Poisoning by caffeine, <u>intentional</u> self-harm

T43.613- Poisoning by caffeine, <u>assault</u>

T43.614- Poisoning by caffeine, <u>undetermined</u>

T43.615- <u>Adverse effect</u> of caffeine

T43.616- <u>Underdosing</u> of caffeine

T43.62- Poisoning by, adverse effect of and underdosing of <u>amphetamines</u>
  Poisoning by, adverse effect of and underdosing of methamphetamines

T43.621- Poisoning by amphetamines, <u>accidental</u> (unintentional)
  Poisoning by amphetamines NOS

T43.622- Poisoning by amphetamines, <u>intentional</u> self-harm

T43.623- Poisoning by amphetamines, <u>assault</u>

T43.624- Poisoning by amphetamines, <u>undetermined</u>

T43.625- <u>Adverse effect</u> of amphetamines

T43.626- <u>Underdosing</u> of amphetamines

T43.63- Poisoning by, adverse effect of and underdosing of <u>methylphenidate</u>

T43.631- Poisoning by methylphenidate, <u>accidental</u> (unintentional)
  Poisoning by methylphenidate NOS

T43.632- Poisoning by methylphenidate, <u>intentional</u> self-harm

T43.633- Poisoning by methylphenidate, <u>assault</u>

T43.634- Poisoning by methylphenidate, <u>undetermined</u>

T43.635- <u>Adverse effect</u> of methylphenidate

T43.636- <u>Underdosing</u> of methylphenidate

T43.69- Poisoning by, adverse effect of and underdosing of <u>other psychostimulants</u>

T43.691- Poisoning by other psychostimulants, <u>accidental</u> (unintentional)
  Poisoning by other psychostimulants NOS

T43.692- Poisoning by other psychostimulants, <u>intentional</u> self-harm

T43.693- Poisoning by other psychostimulants, <u>assault</u>

T43.694- Poisoning by other psychostimulants, <u>undetermined</u>

T43.695- <u>Adverse effect</u> of other psychostimulants

T43.696- <u>Underdosing</u> of other psychostimulants

T
4
2
-
T
4
3

T43.8- Poisoning by, adverse effect of and underdosing of other psychotropic drugs

    T43.8x- Poisoning by, adverse effect of and underdosing of <u>other psychotropic drugs</u>

        T43.8x1- Poisoning by other psychotropic drugs, <u>accidental</u> (unintentional)
            Poisoning by other psychotropic drugs NOS

        T43.8x2- Poisoning by other psychotropic drugs, <u>intentional</u> self-harm

        T43.8x3- Poisoning by other psychotropic drugs, <u>assault</u>

        T43.8x4- Poisoning by other psychotropic drugs, <u>undetermined</u>

        T43.8x5- <u>Adverse effect</u> of other psychotropic drugs

        T43.8x6- <u>Underdosing</u> of other psychotropic drugs

T43.9- Poisoning by, adverse effect of and underdosing of <u>unspecified psychotropic drug</u>

    T43.91x- Poisoning by unspecified psychotropic drug, <u>accidental</u> (unintentional)
        Poisoning by psychotropic drug NOS

    T43.92x- Poisoning by unspecified psychotropic drug, <u>intentional</u> self-harm

    T43.93x- Poisoning by unspecified psychotropic drug, <u>assault</u>

    T43.94x- Poisoning by unspecified psychotropic drug, <u>undetermined</u>

    T43.95x- <u>Adverse effect</u> of unspecified psychotropic drug

    T43.96x- <u>Underdosing</u> of unspecified psychotropic drug

T44- Poisoning by, adverse effect of and underdosing of <u>drugs primarily affecting the autonomic nervous system</u>

> **The appropriate 7th character is to be added to each code from category T44:**
> **A** <u>Initial</u> encounter
> **D** <u>Subsequent</u> encounter
> **S** <u>Sequela</u>

T44.0- Poisoning by, adverse effect of and underdosing of anticholinesterase agents

    T44.0x- Poisoning by, adverse effect of and underdosing of <u>anticholinesterase agents</u>

        T44.0x1- Poisoning by anticholinesterase agents, <u>accidental</u> (unintentional)
            Poisoning by anticholinesterase agents NOS

        T44.0x2- Poisoning by anticholinesterase agents, <u>intentional</u> self-harm

        T44.0x3- Poisoning by anticholinesterase agents, <u>assault</u>

        T44.0x4- Poisoning by anticholinesterase agents, <u>undetermined</u>

        T44.0x5- <u>Adverse effect</u> of anticholinesterase agents

        T44.0x6- <u>Underdosing</u> of anticholinesterase agents

T44.1- Poisoning by, adverse effect of and underdosing of other parasympathomimetics [cholinergics]

    T44.1x- Poisoning by, adverse effect of and underdosing of <u>other parasympathomimetics [cholinergics]</u>

        T44.1x1- Poisoning by other parasympathomimetics [cholinergics], <u>accidental</u> (unintentional)
            Poisoning by other parasympathomimetics [cholinergics] NOS

        T44.1x2- Poisoning by other parasympathomimetics [cholinergics], <u>intentional</u> self-harm

        T44.1x3- Poisoning by other parasympathomimetics [cholinergics], <u>assault</u>

        T44.1x4- Poisoning by other parasympathomimetics [cholinergics], <u>undetermined</u>

        T44.1x5- <u>Adverse effect</u> of other parasympathomimetics [cholinergics]

        T44.1x6- <u>Underdosing</u> of other parasympathomimetics

T44.2- Poisoning by, adverse effect of and underdosing of ganglionic blocking drugs

    T44.2x- Poisoning by, adverse effect of and underdosing of <u>ganglionic blocking drugs</u>

        T44.2x1- Poisoning by ganglionic blocking drugs, <u>accidental</u> (unintentional)
            Poisoning by ganglionic blocking drugs NOS

        T44.2x2- Poisoning by ganglionic blocking drugs, <u>intentional</u> self-harm

        T44.2x3- Poisoning by ganglionic blocking drugs, <u>assault</u>

        T44.2x4- Poisoning by ganglionic blocking drugs, <u>undetermined</u>

        T44.2x5- <u>Adverse effect</u> of ganglionic blocking drugs

        T44.2x6- <u>Underdosing</u> of ganglionic blocking drugs

T44.3- Poisoning by, adverse effect of and underdosing of other parasympatholytics [anticholinergics and antimuscarinics] and spasmolytics
    Poisoning by, adverse effect of and underdosing of papaverine

    T44.3x- Poisoning by, adverse effect of and underdosing of <u>other parasympatholytics [anticholinergics and antimuscarinics] and spasmolytics</u>

        T44.3x1- Poisoning by other parasympatholytics [anticholinergics and antimuscarinics] and spasmolytics, <u>accidental</u> (unintentional)
            Poisoning by other parasympatholytics [anticholinergics and antimuscarinics] and spasmolytics NOS

        T44.3x2- Poisoning by other parasympatholytics [anticholinergics and antimuscarinics] and spasmolytics, <u>intentional</u> self-harm

        T44.3x3- Poisoning by other parasympatholytics [anticholinergics and antimuscarinics] and spasmolytics, <u>assault</u>

        T44.3x4- Poisoning by other parasympatholytics [anticholinergics and antimuscarinics] and spasmolytics, <u>undetermined</u>

        T44.3x5- <u>Adverse effect</u> of other parasympatholytics [anticholinergics and antimuscarinics] and spasmolytics

        T44.3x6- <u>Underdosing</u> of other parasympatholytics [anticholinergics and antimuscarinics] and spasmolytics

T44.4- Poisoning by, adverse effect of and underdosing of predominantly alpha-adrenoreceptor agonists
    Poisoning by, adverse effect of and underdosing of metaraminol

    T44.4x- Poisoning by, adverse effect of and underdosing of <u>predominantly alpha-adrenoreceptor agonists</u>

        T44.4x1- Poisoning by predominantly alpha-adrenoreceptor agonists, <u>accidental</u> (unintentional)
            Poisoning by predominantly alpha-adrenoreceptor agonists NOS

        T44.4x2- Poisoning by predominantly alpha-adrenoreceptor agonists, <u>intentional</u> self-harm

        T44.4x3- Poisoning by predominantly alpha-adrenoreceptor agonists, <u>assault</u>

        T44.4x4- Poisoning by predominantly alpha-adrenoreceptor agonists, <u>undetermined</u>

        T44.4x5- <u>Adverse effect</u> of predominantly alpha-adrenoreceptor agonists

        T44.4x6- <u>Underdosing</u> of predominantly alpha-adrenoreceptor agonists

T44.5- Poisoning by, adverse effect of and underdosing of predominantly beta-adrenoreceptor agonists
    Excludes 1: poisoning by, adverse effect of and underdosing of beta-adrenoreceptor agonists used in asthmatherapy (T48.6-)

    T44.5x- Poisoning by, adverse effect of and underdosing of <u>predominantly beta-adrenoreceptor agonists</u>

        T44.5x1- Poisoning by predominantly beta-adrenoreceptor agonists, <u>accidental</u> (unintentional)
            Poisoning by predominantly beta-adrenoreceptor agonists NOS

        T44.5x2- Poisoning by predominantly beta-adrenoreceptor agonists, <u>intentional</u> self-harm

        T44.5x3- Poisoning by predominantly beta-adrenoreceptor agonists, <u>assault</u>

        T44.5x4- Poisoning by predominantly beta-adrenoreceptor agonists, <u>undetermined</u>

        T44.5x5- <u>Adverse effect</u> of predominantly beta-adrenoreceptor agonists

        T44.5x6- <u>Underdosing</u> of predominantly beta-adrenoreceptor agonists

T44.6- Poisoning by, adverse effect of and underdosing of alpha-adrenoreceptor antagonists
    Excludes 1: poisoning by, adverse effect of and underdosing of ergot alkaloids (T48.0)

    T44.6x- Poisoning by, adverse effect of and underdosing of <u>alpha-adrenoreceptor antagonists</u>

        T44.6x1- Poisoning by alpha-adrenoreceptor antagonists, <u>accidental</u> (unintentional)
            Poisoning by alpha-adrenoreceptor antagonists NOS

        T44.6x2- Poisoning by alpha-adrenoreceptor antagonists, <u>intentional</u> self-harm

        T44.6x3- Poisoning by alpha-adrenoreceptor antagonists, <u>assault</u>

T43 - T45

T44.6x4- Poisoning by alpha-adrenoreceptor antagonists, **undetermined**

T44.6x5- **Adverse effect** of alpha-adrenoreceptor antagonists

T44.6x6- **Underdosing** of alpha-adrenoreceptor antagonists

T44.7- Poisoning by, adverse effect of and underdosing of beta-adrenoreceptor antagonists

T44.7x- Poisoning by, adverse effect of and underdosing of **beta-adrenoreceptor antagonists**

T44.7x1- Poisoning by beta-adrenoreceptor antagonists, **accidental** (unintentional)
Poisoning by beta-adrenoreceptor antagonists NOS

T44.7x2- Poisoning by beta-adrenoreceptor antagonists, **intentional** self-harm

T44.7x3- Poisoning by beta-adrenoreceptor antagonists, **assault**

T44.7x4- Poisoning by beta-adrenoreceptor antagonists, **undetermined**

T44.7x5- **Adverse effect** of beta-adrenoreceptor antagonists

T44.7x6- **Underdosing** of beta-adrenoreceptor antagonists

T44.8- Poisoning by, adverse effect of and underdosing of centrally-acting and adrenergic-neuron-blocking agents
Excludes 1: poisoning by, adverse effect of and underdosing of clonidine (T46.5)
poisoning by, adverse effect of and underdosing of guanethidine (T46.5)

T44.8x- Poisoning by, adverse effect of and underdosing of **centrally-acting and adrenergic-neuron-blocking agents**

T44.8x1- Poisoning by centrally-acting and adrenergic-neuron-blocking agents, **accidental** (unintentional)
Poisoning by centrally-acting and adrenergic-neuron-blocking agents NOS

T44.8x2- Poisoning by centrally-acting and adrenergic-neuron-blocking agents, **intentional** self-harm

T44.8x3- Poisoning by centrally-acting and adrenergic-neuron-blocking agents, **assault**

T44.8x4- Poisoning by centrally-acting and adrenergic-neuron-blocking agents, **undetermined**

T44.8x5- **Adverse effect** of centrally-acting and adrenergic-neuron-blocking agents

T44.8x6- **Underdosing** of centrally-acting and adrenergic-neuron-blocking agents

T44.9- Poisoning by, adverse effect of and underdosing of other and unspecified drugs primarily affecting the autonomic nervous system
Poisoning by, adverse effect of and underdosing of drug stimulating both alpha and beta-adrenoreceptors

T44.90- Poisoning by, adverse effect of and underdosing of **unspecified drugs primarily affecting the autonomic nervous system**

T44.901- Poisoning by unspecified drugs primarily affecting the autonomic nervous system, **accidental** (unintentional)
Poisoning by unspecified drugs primarily affecting the autonomic nervous system NOS

T44.902- Poisoning by unspecified drugs primarily affecting the autonomic nervous system, **intentional** self-harm

T44.903- Poisoning by unspecified drugs primarily affecting the autonomic nervous system, **assault**

T44.904- Poisoning by unspecified drugs primarily affecting the autonomic nervous system, **undetermined**

T44.905- **Adverse effect** of unspecified drugs primarily affecting the autonomic nervous system

T44.906- **Underdosing** of unspecified drugs primarily affecting the autonomic nervous system

T44.99- Poisoning by, adverse effect of and underdosing of **other drugs primarily affecting the autonomic nervous system**

T44.991- Poisoning by other drug primarily affecting the autonomic nervous system, **accidental** (unintentional)
Poisoning by other drugs primarily affecting the autonomic nervous system NOS

T44.992- Poisoning by other drug primarily affecting the autonomic nervous system, **intentional** self-harm

T44.993- Poisoning by other drug primarily affecting the autonomic nervous system, **assault**

T44.994- Poisoning by other drug primarily affecting the autonomic nervous system, **undetermined**

T44.995- **Adverse effect** of other drug primarily affecting the autonomic nervous system

T44.996- **Underdosing** of other drug primarily affecting the autonomic nervous system

T45- Poisoning by, adverse effect of and underdosing of **primarily systemic and hematological agents**, **not elsewhere classified**
The appropriate 7th character is to be added to each code from category T45:
A **Initial** encounter
D **Subsequent** encounter
S **Sequela**

T45.0- Poisoning by, adverse effect of and underdosing of antiallergic and antiemetic drugs
Excludes 1: poisoning by, adverse effect of and underdosing of phenothiazine-based neuroleptics (T43.3)

T45.0x- Poisoning by, adverse effect of and underdosing of **antiallergic and antiemetic drugs**

T45.0x1- Poisoning by antiallergic and antiemetic drugs, **accidental** (unintentional)
Poisoning by antiallergic and antiemetic drugs NOS

T45.0x2- Poisoning by antiallergic and antiemetic drugs, **intentional** self-harm

T45.0x3- Poisoning by antiallergic and antiemetic drugs, **assault**

T45.0x4- Poisoning by antiallergic and antiemetic drugs, **undetermined**

T45.0x5- **Adverse effect** of antiallergic and antiemetic drugs

T45.0x6- **Underdosing** of antiallergic and antiemetic drugs

T45.1- Poisoning by, adverse effect of and underdosing of antineoplastic and immunosuppressive drugs
Excludes 1: poisoning by, adverse effect of and underdosing of tamoxifen (T38.6)

T45.1x- Poisoning by, adverse effect of and underdosing of **antineoplastic and immunosuppressive drugs**

T45.1x1- Poisoning by antineoplastic and immunosuppressive drugs, **accidental** (unintentional)
Poisoning by antineoplastic and immunosuppressive drugs NOS

T45.1x2- Poisoning by antineoplastic and immunosuppressive drugs, **intentional** self-harm

T45.1x3- Poisoning by antineoplastic and immunosuppressive drugs, **assault**

T45.1x4- Poisoning by antineoplastic and immunosuppressive drugs, **undetermined**

T45.1x5- **Adverse effect** of antineoplastic and immunosuppressive drugs

T45.1x6- **Underdosing** of antineoplastic and immunosuppressive drugs

T45.2- Poisoning by, adverse effect of and underdosing of vitamins
Excludes ❷: poisoning by, adverse effect of and underdosing of nicotinic acid (derivatives) (T46.7)
poisoning by, adverse effect of and underdosing of iron (T45.4)
poisoning by, adverse effect of and underdosing of vitamin K (T45.7)

T45.2x- Poisoning by, adverse effect of and underdosing of **vitamins**

T45.2x1- Poisoning by vitamins, **accidental** (unintentional)
Poisoning by vitamins NOS

T45.2x2- Poisoning by vitamins, **intentional** self-harm

T45.2x3- Poisoning by vitamins, **assault**

T45.2x4- Poisoning by vitamins, **undetermined**

T45.2x5- **Adverse effect** of vitamins

T45.2x6- **Underdosing** of vitamins
Excludes 1: vitamin deficiencies (E50-E56)

T45.3- Poisoning by, adverse effect of and underdosing of enzymes

T45.3x- Poisoning by, adverse effect of and underdosing of **enzymes**

T45.3x1- Poisoning by enzymes, **accidental** (unintentional)
Poisoning by enzymes NOS

T45.3x2- Poisoning by enzymes, **intentional** self-harm

T45.3x3- Poisoning by enzymes, **assault**

T45.3x4- Poisoning by enzymes, **undetermined**

T45.3x5- **Adverse effect** of enzymes

T45.3x6- **Underdosing** of enzymes

T43 - T45

T45.4- Poisoning by, adverse effect of and underdosing of iron and its compounds

    T45.4x- Poisoning by, adverse effect of and underdosing of <u>iron and its compounds</u>

        T45.4x1- Poisoning by iron and its compounds, <u>accidental</u> (unintentional)
            Poisoning by iron and its compounds NOS

        T45.4x2- Poisoning by iron and its compounds, <u>intentional</u> self-harm

        T45.4x3- Poisoning by iron and its compounds, <u>assault</u>

        T45.4x4- Poisoning by iron and its compounds, <u>undetermined</u>

        T45.4x5- <u>Adverse effect</u> of iron and its compounds

        T45.4x6- <u>Underdosing</u> of iron and its compounds
           Excludes 1: iron deficiency (E61.1)

T45.5- Poisoning by, adverse effect of and underdosing of anticoagulants and antithrombotic drugs

    T45.51- Poisoning by, adverse effect of and underdosing of <u>anticoagulants</u>

        T45.511- Poisoning by anticoagulants, <u>accidental</u> (unintentional)
            Poisoning by anticoagulants NOS

        T45.512- Poisoning by anticoagulants, <u>intentional</u> self-harm

        T45.513- Poisoning by anticoagulants, <u>assault</u>

        T45.514- Poisoning by anticoagulants, <u>undetermined</u>

        T45.515- <u>Adverse effect</u> of anticoagulants

        T45.516- <u>Underdosing</u> of anticoagulants

    T45.52- Poisoning by, adverse effect of and underdosing of <u>antithrombotic drugs</u>
        Poisoning by, adverse effect of and underdosing of antiplatelet drugs
        Excludes❷: poisoning by, adverse effect of and underdosing of aspirin (T39.01-)
                poisoning by, adverse effect of and underdosing of acetylsalicylic acid (T39.01-)

        T45.521- Poisoning by antithrombotic drugs, <u>accidental</u> (unintentional)
            Poisoning by antithrombotic drug NOS

        T45.522- Poisoning by antithrombotic drugs, <u>intentional</u> self-harm

        T45.523- Poisoning by antithrombotic drugs, <u>assault</u>

        T45.524- Poisoning by antithrombotic drugs, <u>undetermined</u>

        T45.525- <u>Adverse effect</u> of antithrombotic drugs

        T45.526- <u>Underdosing</u> of antithrombotic drugs

T45.6- Poisoning by, adverse effect of and underdosing of fibrinolysis-affecting drugs

    T45.60- Poisoning by, adverse effect of and underdosing of <u>unspecified fibrinolysis-affecting drugs</u>

        T45.601- Poisoning by unspecified fibrinolysis-affecting drugs, <u>accidental</u> (unintentional)
            Poisoning by fibrinolysis-affecting drug NOS

        T45.602- Poisoning by unspecified fibrinolysis-affecting drugs, <u>intentional</u> self-harm

        T45.603- Poisoning by unspecified fibrinolysis-affecting drugs, <u>assault</u>

        T45.604- Poisoning by unspecified fibrinolysis-affecting drugs, <u>undetermined</u>

        T45.605- <u>Adverse effect</u> of unspecified fibrinolysis-affecting drugs

        T45.606- <u>Underdosing</u> of unspecified fibrinolysis-affecting drugs

    T45.61- Poisoning by, adverse effect of and underdosing of <u>thrombolytic drugs</u>

        T45.611- Poisoning by thrombolytic drug, <u>accidental</u> (unintentional)
            Poisoning by thrombolytic drug NOS

        T45.612- Poisoning by thrombolytic drug, <u>intentional</u> self-harm

        T45.613- Poisoning by thrombolytic drug, <u>assault</u>

        T45.614- Poisoning by thrombolytic drug, <u>undetermined</u>

        T45.615- <u>Adverse effect</u> of thrombolytic drugs

        T45.616- <u>Underdosing</u> of thrombolytic drugs

    T45.62- Poisoning by, adverse effect of and underdosing of <u>hemostatic drugs</u>

        T45.621- Poisoning by hemostatic drug, <u>accidental</u> (unintentional)
            Poisoning by hemostatic drug NOS

        T45.622- Poisoning by hemostatic drug, <u>intentional</u> self-harm

        T45.623- Poisoning by hemostatic drug, <u>assault</u>

        T45.624- Poisoning by hemostatic drug, <u>undetermined</u>

        T45.625- <u>Adverse effect</u> of hemostatic drug

        T45.626- <u>Underdosing</u> of hemostatic drugs

    T45.69- Poisoning by, adverse effect of and underdosing of <u>other fibrinolysis-affecting drugs</u>

        T45.691- Poisoning by other fibrinolysis-affecting drugs, <u>accidental</u> (unintentional)
            Poisoning by other fibrinolysis-affecting drug NOS

        T45.692- Poisoning by other fibrinolysis-affecting drugs, <u>intentional</u> self-harm

        T45.693- Poisoning by other fibrinolysis-affecting drugs, <u>assault</u>

        T45.694- Poisoning by other fibrinolysis-affecting drugs, <u>undetermined</u>

        T45.695- <u>Adverse effect</u> of other fibrinolysis-affecting drugs

        T45.696- <u>Underdosing</u> of other fibrinolysis-affecting drugs

T45.7- Poisoning by, adverse effect of and underdosing of anticoagulant antagonists, vitamin K and other coagulants

    T45.7x- Poisoning by, adverse effect of and underdosing of <u>anticoagulant antagonists, vitamin K and other coagulants</u>

        T45.7x1- Poisoning by anticoagulant antagonists, vitamin K and other coagulants, <u>accidental</u> (unintentional)
            Poisoning by anticoagulant antagonists, vitamin K and other coagulants NOS

        T45.7x2- Poisoning by anticoagulant antagonists, vitamin K and other coagulants, <u>intentional</u> self-harm

        T45.7x3- Poisoning by anticoagulant antagonists, vitamin K and other coagulants, <u>assault</u>

        T45.7x4- Poisoning by anticoagulant antagonists, vitamin K and other coagulants, <u>undetermined</u>

        T45.7x5- <u>Adverse effect</u> of anticoagulant antagonists, vitamin K and other coagulants

        T45.7x6- <u>Underdosing</u> of anticoagulant antagonist, vitamin K and other coagulants
            Excludes 1: vitamin K deficiency (E56.1)

T45.8- Poisoning by, adverse effect of and underdosing of other primarily systemic and hematological agents
    Poisoning by, adverse effect of and underdosing of liver preparations and other antianemic agents
    Poisoning by, adverse effect of and underdosing of natural blood and blood products
    Poisoning by, adverse effect of and underdosing of plasma substitute
    Excludes❷: poisoning by, adverse effect of and underdosing of immunoglobulin (T50.Z1)
                poisoning by, adverse effect of and underdosing of iron (T45.4)
                transfusion reactions (T80-)

    T45.8x- Poisoning by, adverse effect of and underdosing of <u>other primarily systemic and hematological agents</u>

        T45.8x1- Poisoning by other primarily systemic and hematological agents, <u>accidental</u> (unintentional)
            Poisoning by other primarily systemic and hematological agents NOS

        T45.8x2- Poisoning by other primarily systemic and hematological agents, <u>intentional</u> self-harm

        T45.8x3- Poisoning by other primarily systemic and hematological agents, <u>assault</u>

        T45.8x4- Poisoning by other primarily systemic and hematological agents, <u>undetermined</u>

        T45.8x5- <u>Adverse effect</u> of other primarily systemic and hematological agents

        T45.8x6- <u>Underdosing</u> of other primarily systemic and hematological agents

T45.9- Poisoning by, adverse effect of and underdosing of <u>unspecified primarily systemic and hematological agent</u>

    T45.91x- Poisoning by unspecified primarily systemic and hematological agent, <u>accidental</u> (unintentional)
        Poisoning by primarily systemic and hematological agent NOS

    T45.92x- Poisoning by unspecified primarily systemic and hematological agent, <u>intentional</u> self-harm

    T45.93x- Poisoning by unspecified primarily systemic and hematological agent, <u>assault</u>

    T45.94x- Poisoning by unspecified primarily systemic and hematological agent, <u>undetermined</u>

    T45.95x- <u>Adverse effect</u> of unspecified primarily systemic and hematological agent

    T45.96x- <u>Underdosing</u> of unspecified primarily systemic and hematological agent

T45 - T46

T46- Poisoning by, adverse effect of and underdosing of agents <u>primarily affecting the cardiovascular system</u>
   Excludes 1: *poisoning by, adverse effect of and underdosing of metaraminol (T44.4)*

   The appropriate 7th character is to be added to each code from category T46:
   A   <u>Initial</u> encounter
   D   <u>Subsequent</u> encounter
   S   <u>Sequela</u>

T46.0- Poisoning by, adverse effect of and underdosing of cardiac-stimulant glycosides and drugs of similar action
   T46.0x- Poisoning by, adverse effect of and underdosing of <u>cardiac-stimulant glycosides and drugs of similar action</u>
      T46.0x1- Poisoning by cardiac-stimulant glycosides and drugs of similar action, <u>accidental</u> (unintentional)
            Poisoning by cardiac-stimulant glycosides and drugs of similar action NOS
      T46.0x2- Poisoning by cardiac-stimulant glycosides and drugs of similar action, <u>intentional</u> self-harm
      T46.0x3- Poisoning by cardiac-stimulant glycosides and drugs of similar action, <u>assault</u>
      T46.0x4- Poisoning by cardiac-stimulant glycosides and drugs of similar action, <u>undetermined</u>
      T46.0x5- <u>Adverse effect</u> of cardiac-stimulant glycosides and drugs of similar action
      T46.0x6- <u>Underdosing</u> of cardiac-stimulant glycosides and drugs of similar action

T46.1- Poisoning by, adverse effect of and underdosing of calcium-channel blockers
   T46.1x- Poisoning by, adverse effect of and underdosing of <u>calcium-channel blockers</u>
      T46.1x1- Poisoning by calcium-channel blockers, <u>accidental</u> (unintentional)
            Poisoning by calcium-channel blockers NOS
      T46.1x2- Poisoning by calcium-channel blockers, <u>intentional</u> self-harm
      T46.1x3- Poisoning by calcium-channel blockers, <u>assault</u>
      T46.1x4- Poisoning by calcium-channel blockers, <u>undetermined</u>
      T46.1x5- <u>Adverse effect</u> of calcium-channel blockers
      T46.1x6- <u>Underdosing</u> of calcium-channel blockers

T46.2- Poisoning by, adverse effect of and underdosing of other antidysrhythmic drugs, not elsewhere classified
   Excludes 1: *poisoning by, adverse effect of and underdosing of beta-adrenoreceptor antagonists (T44.7-)*
   T46.2x- Poisoning by, adverse effect of and underdosing of <u>other antidysrhythmic drugs</u>
      T46.2x1- Poisoning by other antidysrhythmic drugs, <u>accidental</u> (unintentional)
            Poisoning by other antidysrhythmic drugs NOS
      T46.2x2- Poisoning by other antidysrhythmic drugs, <u>intentional</u> self-harm
      T46.2x3- Poisoning by other antidysrhythmic drugs, <u>assault</u>
      T46.2x4- Poisoning by other antidysrhythmic drugs, <u>undetermined</u>
      T46.2x5- <u>Adverse effect</u> of other antidysrhythmic drugs
      T46.2x6- <u>Underdosing</u> of other antidysrhythmic drugs

T46.3- Poisoning by, adverse effect of and underdosing of coronary vasodilators
         Poisoning by, adverse effect of and underdosing of dipyridamole
   Excludes 1: *poisoning by, adverse effect of and underdosing of calcium-channel blockers (T46.1)*
   T46.3x- Poisoning by, adverse effect of and underdosing of <u>coronary vasodilators</u>
      T46.3x1- Poisoning by coronary vasodilators, <u>accidental</u> (unintentional)
            Poisoning by coronary vasodilators NOS
      T46.3x2- Poisoning by coronary vasodilators, <u>intentional</u> self-harm
      T46.3x3- Poisoning by coronary vasodilators, <u>assault</u>
      T46.3x4- Poisoning by coronary vasodilators, <u>undetermined</u>
      T46.3x5- <u>Adverse effect</u> of coronary vasodilators
      T46.3x6- <u>Underdosing</u> of coronary vasodilators

T46.4- Poisoning by, adverse effect of and underdosing of angiotensin-converting-enzyme inhibitors
   T46.4x- Poisoning by, adverse effect of and underdosing of <u>angiotensin-converting-enzyme inhibitors</u>
      T46.4x1- Poisoning by angiotensin-converting-enzyme inhibitors, <u>accidental</u> (unintentional)
            Poisoning by angiotensin-converting-enzyme inhibitors NOS
      T46.4x2- Poisoning by angiotensin-converting-enzyme inhibitors, <u>intentional</u> self-harm
      T46.4x3- Poisoning by angiotensin-converting-enzyme inhibitors, <u>assault</u>
      T46.4x4- Poisoning by angiotensin-converting-enzyme inhibitors, <u>undetermined</u>
      T46.4x5- <u>Adverse effect</u> of angiotensin-converting-enzyme inhibitors
      T46.4x6- <u>Underdosing</u> of angiotensin-converting-enzyme inhibitors

T46.5- Poisoning by, adverse effect of and underdosing of other antihypertensive drugs
   Excludes ❷: *poisoning by, adverse effect of and underdosing of beta-adrenoreceptor antagonists (T44.7)*
         poisoning by, adverse effect of and underdosing of calcium-channel blockers (T46.1)
         poisoning by, adverse effect of and underdosing of diuretics (T50.0-T50.2)
   T46.5x- Poisoning by, adverse effect of and underdosing of <u>other antihypertensive drugs</u>
      T46.5x1- Poisoning by other antihypertensive drugs, <u>accidental</u> (unintentional)
            Poisoning by other antihypertensive drugs NOS
      T46.5x2- Poisoning by other antihypertensive drugs, <u>intentional</u> self-harm
      T46.5x3- Poisoning by other antihypertensive drugs, <u>assault</u>
      T46.5x4- Poisoning by other antihypertensive drugs, <u>undetermined</u>
      T46.5x5- <u>Adverse effect</u> of other antihypertensive drugs
      T46.5x6- <u>Underdosing</u> of other antihypertensive drugs

T46.6- Poisoning by, adverse effect of and underdosing of antihyperlipidemic and antiarteriosclerotic drugs
   T46.6x- Poisoning by, adverse effect of and underdosing of <u>antihyperlipidemic and antiarteriosclerotic drugs</u>
      T46.6x1- Poisoning by antihyperlipidemic and antiarteriosclerotic drugs, <u>accidental</u> (unintentional)
            Poisoning by antihyperlipidemic and antiarteriosclerotic drugs NOS
      T46.6x2- Poisoning by antihyperlipidemic and antiarteriosclerotic drugs, <u>intentional</u> self-harm
      T46.6x3- Poisoning by antihyperlipidemic and antiarteriosclerotic drugs, <u>assault</u>
      T46.6x4- Poisoning by antihyperlipidemic and antiarteriosclerotic drugs, <u>undetermined</u>
      T46.6x5- <u>Adverse effect</u> of antihyperlipidemic and antiarteriosclerotic drugs
      T46.6x6- <u>Underdosing</u> of antihyperlipidemic and antiarteriosclerotic drugs

T46.7- Poisoning by, adverse effect of and underdosing of peripheral vasodilators
         Poisoning by, adverse effect of and underdosing of nicotinic acid (derivatives)
   Excludes 1: *poisoning by, adverse effect of and underdosing of papaverine (T44.3)*
   T46.7x- Poisoning by, adverse effect of and underdosing of <u>peripheral vasodilators</u>
      T46.7x1- Poisoning by peripheral vasodilators, <u>accidental</u> (unintentional)
            Poisoning by peripheral vasodilators NOS
      T46.7x2- Poisoning by peripheral vasodilators, <u>intentional</u> self-harm
      T46.7x3- Poisoning by peripheral vasodilators, <u>assault</u>
      T46.7x4- Poisoning by peripheral vasodilators, <u>undetermined</u>
      T46.7x5- <u>Adverse effect</u> of peripheral vasodilators
      T46.7x6- <u>Underdosing</u> of peripheral vasodilators

T45 - T46

T46.8-   Poisoning by, adverse effect of and underdosing of antivaricose drugs, including sclerosing agents

　　T46.8x- Poisoning by, adverse effect of and underdosing of <u>antivaricose drugs, including sclerosing agents</u>

　　　　T46.8x1- Poisoning by antivaricose drugs, including sclerosing agents, <u>accidental</u> (unintentional)
　　　　　　Poisoning by antivaricose drugs, including sclerosing agents NOS

　　　　T46.8x2- Poisoning by antivaricose drugs, including sclerosing agents, <u>intentional</u> self-harm

　　　　T46.8x3- Poisoning by antivaricose drugs, including sclerosing agents, <u>assault</u>

　　　　T46.8x4- Poisoning by antivaricose drugs, including sclerosing agents, <u>undetermined</u>

　　　　T46.8x5- <u>Adverse effect</u> of antivaricose drugs, including sclerosing agents

　　　　T46.8x6- <u>Underdosing</u> of antivaricose drugs, including sclerosing agents

T46.9-   Poisoning by, adverse effect of and underdosing of other and unspecified agents primarily affecting the cardiovascular system

　　T46.90- Poisoning by, adverse effect of and underdosing of <u>unspecified agents primarily affecting the cardiovascular system</u>

　　　　T46.901- Poisoning by unspecified agents primarily affecting the cardiovascular system, <u>accidental</u> (unintentional)

　　　　T46.902- Poisoning by unspecified agents primarily affecting the cardiovascular system, <u>intentional</u> self-harm

　　　　T46.903- Poisoning by unspecified agents primarily affecting the cardiovascular system, <u>assault</u>

　　　　T46.904- Poisoning by unspecified agents primarily affecting the cardiovascular system, <u>undetermined</u>

　　　　T46.905- <u>Adverse effect</u> of unspecified agents primarily affecting the cardiovascular system

　　　　T46.906- <u>Underdosing</u> of unspecified agents primarily affecting the cardiovascular system

　　T46.99- Poisoning by, adverse effect of and underdosing of <u>other agents primarily affecting the cardiovascular system</u>

　　　　T46.991- Poisoning by other agents primarily affecting the cardiovascular system, <u>accidental</u> (unintentional)

　　　　T46.992- Poisoning by other agents primarily affecting the cardiovascular system, <u>intentional</u> self-harm

　　　　T46.993- Poisoning by other agents primarily affecting the cardiovascular system, <u>assault</u>

　　　　T46.994- Poisoning by other agents primarily affecting the cardiovascular system, <u>undetermined</u>

　　　　T46.995- <u>Adverse effect</u> of other agents primarily affecting the cardiovascular system

　　　　T46.996- <u>Underdosing</u> of other agents primarily affecting the cardiovascular system

T47-   Poisoning by, adverse effect of and underdosing of <u>agents primarily affecting the gastrointestinal system</u>

The appropriate 7th character is to be added to each code from category T47:
　A   <u>Initial</u> encounter
　D   <u>Subsequent</u> encounter
　S   <u>Sequela</u>

T47.0-   Poisoning by, adverse effect of and underdosing of histamine H2-receptor blockers

　　T47.0x- Poisoning by, adverse effect of and underdosing of <u>histamine H2-receptor blockers</u>

　　　　T47.0x1- Poisoning by histamine H2-receptor blockers, <u>accidental</u> (unintentional)
　　　　　　Poisoning by histamine H2-receptor blockers NOS

　　　　T47.0x2- Poisoning by histamine H2-receptor blockers, <u>intentional</u> self-harm

　　　　T47.0x3- Poisoning by histamine H2-receptor blockers, <u>assault</u>

　　　　T47.0x4- Poisoning by histamine H2-receptor blockers, <u>undetermined</u>

　　　　T47.0x5- <u>Adverse effect</u> of histamine H2-receptor blockers

　　　　T47.0x6- <u>Underdosing</u> of histamine H2-receptor blockers

T47.1-   Poisoning by, adverse effect of and underdosing of other antacids and anti-gastric-secretion drugs

　　T47.1x- Poisoning by, adverse effect of and underdosing of <u>other antacids and anti-gastric-secretion drugs</u>

　　　　T47.1x1- Poisoning by other antacids and anti-gastric-secretion drugs, <u>accidental</u> (unintentional)
　　　　　　Poisoning by other antacids and anti-gastric-secretion drugs NOS

　　　　T47.1x2- Poisoning by other antacids and anti-gastric-secretion drugs, <u>intentional</u> self-harm

　　　　T47.1x3- Poisoning by other antacids and anti-gastric-secretion drugs, <u>assault</u>

　　　　T47.1x4- Poisoning by other antacids and anti-gastric-secretion drugs, <u>undetermined</u>

　　　　T47.1x5- <u>Adverse effect</u> of other antacids and anti-gastric-secretion drugs

　　　　T47.1x6- <u>Underdosing</u> of other antacids and anti-gastric-secretion drugs

T47.2-   Poisoning by, adverse effect of and underdosing of stimulant laxatives

　　T47.2x- Poisoning by, adverse effect of and underdosing of <u>stimulant laxatives</u>

　　　　T47.2x1- Poisoning by stimulant laxatives, <u>accidental</u> (unintentional)
　　　　　　Poisoning by stimulant laxatives NOS

　　　　T47.2x2- Poisoning by stimulant laxatives, <u>intentional</u> self-harm

　　　　T47.2x3- Poisoning by stimulant laxatives, <u>assault</u>

　　　　T47.2x4- Poisoning by stimulant laxatives, <u>undetermined</u>

　　　　T47.2x5- <u>Adverse effect</u> of stimulant laxatives

　　　　T47.2x6- <u>Underdosing</u> of stimulant laxatives

T47.3-   Poisoning by, adverse effect of and underdosing of saline and osmotic laxatives

　　T47.3x- Poisoning by and adverse effect of <u>saline and osmotic laxatives</u>

　　　　T47.3x1- Poisoning by saline and osmotic laxatives, <u>accidental</u> (unintentional)
　　　　　　Poisoning by saline and osmotic laxatives NOS

　　　　T47.3x2- Poisoning by saline and osmotic laxatives, <u>intentional</u> self-harm

　　　　T47.3x3- Poisoning by saline and osmotic laxatives, <u>assault</u>

　　　　T47.3x4- Poisoning by saline and osmotic laxatives, <u>undetermined</u>

　　　　T47.3x5- <u>Adverse effect</u> of saline and osmotic laxatives

　　　　T47.3x6   <u>Underdosing</u> of saline and osmotic laxatives

T47.4-   Poisoning by, adverse effect of and underdosing of other laxatives

　　T47.4x- Poisoning by, adverse effect of and underdosing of <u>other laxatives</u>

　　　　T47.4x1- Poisoning by other laxatives, <u>accidental</u> (unintentional)
　　　　　　Poisoning by other laxatives NOS

　　　　T47.4x2- Poisoning by other laxatives, <u>intentional</u> self-harm

　　　　T47.4x3- Poisoning by other laxatives, <u>assault</u>

　　　　T47.4x4- Poisoning by other laxatives, <u>undetermined</u>

　　　　T47.4x5- <u>Adverse effect</u> of other laxatives

　　　　T47.4x6- <u>Underdosing</u> of other laxatives

T47.5-   Poisoning by, adverse effect of and underdosing of digestants

　　T47.5x- Poisoning by, adverse effect of and underdosing of <u>digestants</u>

　　　　T47.5x1- Poisoning by digestants, <u>accidental</u> (unintentional)
　　　　　　Poisoning by digestants NOS

　　　　T47.5x2- Poisoning by digestants, <u>intentional</u> self-harm

　　　　T47.5x3- Poisoning by digestants, <u>assault</u>

　　　　T47.5x4- Poisoning by digestants, <u>undetermined</u>

　　　　T47.5x5- <u>Adverse effect</u> of digestants

　　　　T47.5x6- <u>Underdosing</u> of digestants

T47.6-   Poisoning by, adverse effect of and underdosing of antidiarrheal drugs

　　Excludes❷: poisoning by, adverse effect of and underdosing of systemic antibiotics and other anti-infectives (T36-T37)

　　T47.6x- Poisoning by, adverse effect of and underdosing of <u>antidiarrheal drugs</u>

　　　　T47.6x1- Poisoning by antidiarrheal drugs, <u>accidental</u> (unintentional)
　　　　　　Poisoning by antidiarrheal drugs NOS

　　　　T47.6x2- Poisoning by antidiarrheal drugs, <u>intentional</u> self-harm

　　　　T47.6x3- Poisoning by antidiarrheal drugs, <u>assault</u>

　　　　T47.6x4- Poisoning by antidiarrheal drugs, <u>undetermined</u>

　　　　T47.6x5- <u>Adverse effect</u> of antidiarrheal drugs

　　　　T47.6x6- <u>Underdosing</u> of antidiarrheal drugs

T 4 6 – T 4 8

T47.7-   Poisoning by, adverse effect of and underdosing of emetics
   T47.7x- Poisoning by, adverse effect of and underdosing of <u>emetics</u>
      T47.7x1- Poisoning by emetics, <u>accidental</u> (unintentional)
               Poisoning by emetics NOS
      T47.7x2- Poisoning by emetics, <u>intentional</u> self-harm
      T47.7x3- Poisoning by emetics, <u>assault</u>
      T47.7x4- Poisoning by emetics, <u>undetermined</u>
      T47.7x5- <u>Adverse effect</u> of emetics
      T47.7x6- <u>Underdosing</u> of emetics
T47.8-   Poisoning by, adverse effect of and underdosing of other agents
         primarily affecting gastrointestinal system
   T47.8x- Poisoning by, adverse effect of and underdosing of <u>other
            agents primarily affecting gastrointestinal system</u>
      T47.8x1- Poisoning by other agents primarily affecting
               gastrointestinal system, <u>accidental</u> (unintentional)
               Poisoning by other agents primarily affecting
                  gastrointestinal system NOS
      T47.8x2- Poisoning by other agents primarily affecting
               gastrointestinal system, <u>intentional</u> self-harm
      T47.8x3- Poisoning by other agents primarily affecting
               gastrointestinal system, <u>assault</u>
      T47.8x4- Poisoning by other agents primarily affecting
               gastrointestinal system, <u>undetermined</u>
      T47.8x5- <u>Adverse effect</u> of other agents primarily affecting
               gastrointestinal system
      T47.8x6- <u>Underdosing</u> of other agents primarily affecting
               gastrointestinal system
T47.9-   Poisoning by, adverse effect of and underdosing of <u>unspecified
         agents primarily affecting the gastrointestinal system</u>
   T47.91x- Poisoning by unspecified agents primarily affecting the
            gastrointestinal system, <u>accidental</u> (unintentional)
            Poisoning by agents primarily affecting the gastrointestinal
               system NOS
   T47.92x- Poisoning by unspecified agents primarily affecting the
            gastrointestinal system, <u>intentional</u> self-harm
   T47.93x- Poisoning by unspecified agents primarily affecting the
            gastrointestinal system, <u>assault</u>
   T47.94x- Poisoning by unspecified agents primarily affecting the
            gastrointestinal system, <u>undetermined</u>
   T47.95x- <u>Adverse effect</u> of unspecified agents primarily affecting the
            gastrointestinal system
   T47.96x- <u>Underdosing</u> of unspecified agents primarily affecting the
            gastrointestinal system
T48-   Poisoning by, adverse effect of and underdosing of <u>agents primarily
       acting on smooth and skeletal muscles and the respiratory system</u>
       The appropriate 7th character is to be added to each code from
          category T48:
       A   <u>Initial</u> encounter
       D   <u>Subsequent</u> encounter
       S   <u>Sequela</u>
T48.0-   Poisoning by, adverse effect of and underdosing of oxytocic drugs
         *Excludes 1: poisoning by, adverse effect of and underdosing of
                  estrogens, progestogens and antagonists (T38.4-
                  T38.6)*
   T48.0x- Poisoning by, adverse effect of and underdosing of <u>oxytocic
            drugs</u>
      T48.0x1- Poisoning by oxytocic drugs, <u>accidental</u> (unintentional)
               Poisoning by oxytocic drugs NOS
      T48.0x2- Poisoning by oxytocic drugs, <u>intentional</u> self-harm
      T48.0x3- Poisoning by oxytocic drugs, <u>assault</u>
      T48.0x4- Poisoning by oxytocic drugs, <u>undetermined</u>
      T48.0x5- <u>Adverse effect</u> of oxytocic drugs
      T48.0x6- <u>Underdosing</u> of oxytocic drugs
T48.1-   Poisoning by, adverse effect of and underdosing of skeletal
         muscle relaxants [neuromuscular blocking agents]
   T48.1x- Poisoning by, adverse effect of and underdosing of <u>skeletal
            muscle relaxants [neuromuscular blocking agents]</u>
      T48.1x1- Poisoning by skeletal muscle relaxants [neuromuscular
               blocking agents], <u>accidental</u> (unintentional)
               Poisoning by skeletal muscle relaxants [neuromuscular
                  blocking agents] NOS
      T48.1x2- Poisoning by skeletal muscle relaxants [neuromuscular
               blocking agents], <u>intentional</u> self-harm
      T48.1x3- Poisoning by skeletal muscle relaxants [neuromuscular
               blocking agents], <u>assault</u>
      T48.1x4- Poisoning by skeletal muscle relaxants [neuromuscular
               blocking agents], <u>undetermined</u>
      T48.1x5- <u>Adverse effect</u> of skeletal muscle relaxants
               [neuromuscular blocking agents]

      T48.1x6- <u>Underdosing</u> of skeletal muscle relaxants
               [neuromuscular blocking agents]
T48.2-   Poisoning by, adverse effect of and underdosing of other and
         unspecified drugs acting on muscles
   T48.20- Poisoning by, adverse effect of and underdosing of
            <u>unspecified drugs acting on muscles</u>
      T48.201- Poisoning by unspecified drugs acting on muscles,
               <u>accidental</u> (unintentional)
               Poisoning by unspecified drugs acting on muscles NOS
      T48.202- Poisoning by unspecified drugs acting on muscles,
               <u>intentional</u> self-harm
      T48.203- Poisoning by unspecified drugs acting on muscles,
               <u>assault</u>
      T48.204- Poisoning by unspecified drugs acting on muscles,
               <u>undetermined</u>
      T48.205- <u>Adverse effect</u> of unspecified drugs acting on muscles
      T48.206- <u>Underdosing</u> of unspecified drugs acting on muscles
   T48.29- Poisoning by, adverse effect of and underdosing of <u>other
            drugs acting on muscles</u>
      T48.291- Poisoning by other drugs acting on muscles, <u>accidental</u>
               (unintentional)
               Poisoning by other drugs acting on muscles NOS
      T48.292- Poisoning by other drugs acting on muscles,
               <u>intentional</u> self-harm
      T48.293- Poisoning by other drugs acting on muscles, <u>assault</u>
      T48.294- Poisoning by other drugs acting on muscles,
               <u>undetermined</u>
      T48.295- <u>Adverse effect</u> of other drugs acting on muscles
      T48.296- <u>Underdosing</u> of other drugs acting on muscles
T48.3-   Poisoning by, adverse effect of and underdosing of antitussives
   T48.3x- Poisoning by, adverse effect of and underdosing of
            <u>antitussives</u>
      T48.3x1- Poisoning by antitussives, <u>accidental</u> (unintentional)
               Poisoning by antitussives NOS
      T48.3x2- Poisoning by antitussives, <u>intentional</u> self-harm
      T48.3x3- Poisoning by antitussives, <u>assault</u>
      T48.3x4- Poisoning by antitussives, <u>undetermined</u>
      T48.3x5- <u>Adverse effect</u> of antitussives
      T48.3x6- <u>Underdosing</u> of antitussives
T48.4-   Poisoning by, adverse effect of and underdosing of expectorants
   T48.4x- Poisoning by, adverse effect of and underdosing of
            <u>expectorants</u>
      T48.4x1- Poisoning by expectorants, <u>accidental</u> (unintentional)
               Poisoning by expectorants NOS
      T48.4x2- Poisoning by expectorants, <u>intentional</u> self-harm
      T48.4x3- Poisoning by expectorants, <u>assault</u>
      T48.4x4- Poisoning by expectorants, <u>undetermined</u>
      T48.4x5- <u>Adverse effect</u> of expectorants
      T48.4x6- <u>Underdosing</u> of expectorants
T48.5-   Poisoning by, adverse effect of and underdosing of other anti-
         common-cold drugs
         Poisoning by, adverse effect of and underdosing of decongestants
         *Excludes❷: poisoning by, adverse effect of and underdosing of
                  antipyretics, NEC (T39.9-)
                  poisoning by, adverse effect of and underdosing of non-
                  steroidal antiinflammatory drugs (T39.3-)
                  poisoning by, adverse effect of and underdosing of
                  salicylates (T39.0-)*
   T48.5x- Poisoning by, adverse effect of and underdosing of <u>other
            anti-common-cold drugs</u>
      T48.5x1- Poisoning by other anti-common-cold drugs,
               <u>accidental</u> (unintentional)
               Poisoning by other anti-common-cold drugs NOS
      T48.5x2- Poisoning by other anti-common-cold drugs,
               <u>intentional</u> self-harm
      T48.5x3- Poisoning by other anti-common-cold drugs, <u>assault</u>
      T48.5x4- Poisoning by other anti-common-cold drugs,
               <u>undetermined</u>
      T48.5x5- <u>Adverse effect</u> of other anti-common-cold drugs
      T48.5x6- <u>Underdosing</u> of other anti-common-cold drugs

T46 - T48

T48.6-   Poisoning by, adverse effect of and underdosing of antiasthmatics, not elsewhere classified
Poisoning by, adverse effect of and underdosing of beta-adrenoreceptor agonists used in asthma therapy
Excludes 1:   poisoning by, adverse effect of and underdosing of beta-adrenoreceptor agonists not used in asthma therapy (T44.5)
poisoning by, adverse effect of and underdosing of anterior pituitary [adenohypophyseal] hormones (T38.8)

T48.6x- Poisoning by, adverse effect of and underdosing of antiasthmatics

T48.6x1-   Poisoning by antiasthmatics, accidental (unintentional)
Poisoning by antiasthmatics NOS

T48.6x2-   Poisoning by antiasthmatics, intentional self-harm

T48.6x3-   Poisoning by antiasthmatics, assault

T48.6x4-   Poisoning by antiasthmatics, undetermined

T48.6x5-   Adverse effect of antiasthmatics

T48.6x6-   Underdosing of antiasthmatics

T48.9-   Poisoning by, adverse effect of and underdosing of other and unspecified agents primarily acting on the respiratory system

T48.90- Poisoning by, adverse effect of and underdosing of unspecified agents primarily acting on the respiratory system

T48.901-   Poisoning by unspecified agents primarily acting on the respiratory system, accidental (unintentional)

T48.902-   Poisoning by unspecified agents primarily acting on the respiratory system, intentional self-harm

T48.903-   Poisoning by unspecified agents primarily acting on the respiratory system, assault

T48.904-   Poisoning by unspecified agents primarily acting on the respiratory system, undetermined

T48.905-   Adverse effect of unspecified agents primarily acting on the respiratory system

T48.906-   Underdosing of unspecified agents primarily acting on the respiratory system

T48.99- Poisoning by, adverse effect of and underdosing of other agents primarily acting on the respiratory system

T48.991-   Poisoning by other agents primarily acting on the respiratory system, accidental (unintentional)

T48.992-   Poisoning by other agents primarily acting on the respiratory system, intentional self-harm

T48.993-   Poisoning by other agents primarily acting on the respiratory system, assault

T48.994-   Poisoning by other agents primarily acting on the respiratory system, undetermined

T48.995-   Adverse effect of other agents primarily acting on the respiratory system

T48.996-   Underdosing of other agents primarily acting on the respiratory system

T49- Poisoning by, adverse effect of and underdosing of topical agents primarily affecting skin and mucous membrane and by ophthalmological, otorhinorlaryngological and dental drugs
Includes: Poisoning by, adverse effect of and underdosing of glucocorticoids, topically used

The appropriate 7th character is to be added to each code from category T49:
A   Initial encounter
D   Subsequent encounter
S   Sequela

T49.0-   Poisoning by, adverse effect of and underdosing of local antifungal, anti-infective and anti-inflammatory drugs

T49.0x- Poisoning by, adverse effect of and underdosing of local antifungal, anti-infective and anti-inflammatory drugs

T49.0x1-   Poisoning by local antifungal, anti-infective and anti-inflammatory drugs, accidental (unintentional)
Poisoning by local antifungal, anti-infective and anti-inflammatory drugs NOS

T49.0x2-   Poisoning by local antifungal, anti-infective and anti-inflammatory drugs, intentional self-harm

T49.0x3-   Poisoning by local antifungal, anti-infective and anti-inflammatory drugs, assault

T49.0x4-   Poisoning by local antifungal, anti-infective and anti-inflammatory drugs, undetermined

T49.0x5-   Adverse effect of local antifungal, anti-infective and anti-inflammatory drugs

T49.0x6-   Underdosing of local antifungal, anti-infective and anti-inflammatory drugs

T49.1-   Poisoning by, adverse effect of and underdosing of antipruritics

T49.1x- Poisoning by, adverse effect of and underdosing of antipruritics

T49.1x1-   Poisoning by antipruritics, accidental (unintentional)
Poisoning by antipruritics NOS

T49.1x2-   Poisoning by antipruritics, intentional self-harm

T49.1x3-   Poisoning by antipruritics, assault

T49.1x4-   Poisoning by antipruritics, undetermined

T49.1x5-   Adverse effect of antipruritics

T49.1x6-   Underdosing of antipruritics

T49.2-   Poisoning by, adverse effect of and underdosing of local astringents and local detergents

T49.2x- Poisoning by, adverse effect of and underdosing of local astringents and local detergents

T49.2x1-   Poisoning by local astringents and local detergents, accidental (unintentional)
Poisoning by local astringents and local detergents NOS

T49.2x2-   Poisoning by local astringents and local detergents, intentional self-harm

T49.2x3-   Poisoning by local astringents and local detergents, assault

T49.2x4-   Poisoning by local astringents and local detergents, undetermined

T49.2x5-   Adverse effect of local astringents and local detergents

T49.2x6-   Underdosing of local astringents and local detergents

T49.3-   Poisoning by, adverse effect of and underdosing of emollients, demulcents and protectants

T49.3x- Poisoning by, adverse effect of and underdosing of emollients, demulcents and protectants

T49.3x1-   Poisoning by emollients, demulcents and protectants, accidental (unintentional)
Poisoning by emollients, demulcents and protectants NOS

T49.3x2-   Poisoning by emollients, demulcents and protectants, intentional self-harm

T49.3x3-   Poisoning by emollients, demulcents and protectants, assault

T49.3x4-   Poisoning by emollients, demulcents and protectants, undetermined

T49.3x5-   Adverse effect of emollients, demulcents and protectants

T49.3x6-   Underdosing of emollients, demulcents and protectants

T49.4-   Poisoning by, adverse effect of and underdosing of keratolytics, keratoplastics, and other hair treatment drugs and preparations

T49.4x- Poisoning by, adverse effect of and underdosing of keratolytics, keratoplastics, and other hair treatment drugs and preparations

T49.4x1-   Poisoning by keratolytics, keratoplastics, and other hair treatment drugs and preparations, accidental (unintentional)
Poisoning by keratolytics, keratoplastics, and other hair treatment drugs and preparations NOS

T49.4x2-   Poisoning by keratolytics, keratoplastics, and other hair treatment drugs and preparations, intentional self-harm

T49.4x3-   Poisoning by keratolytics, keratoplastics, and other hair treatment drugs and preparations, assault

T49.4x4-   Poisoning by keratolytics, keratoplastics, and other hair treatment drugs and preparations, undetermined

T49.4x5-   Adverse effect of keratolytics, keratoplastics, and other hair treatment drugs and preparations

T49.4x6-   Underdosing of keratolytics, keratoplastics, and other hair treatment drugs and preparations

T49.5-   Poisoning by, adverse effect of and underdosing of ophthalmological drugs and preparations

T49.5x- Poisoning by, adverse effect of and underdosing of ophthalmological drugs and preparations

T49.5x1-   Poisoning by ophthalmological drugs and preparations, accidental (unintentional)
Poisoning by ophthalmological drugs and preparations NOS

T49.5x2-   Poisoning by ophthalmological drugs and preparations, intentional self-harm

T49.5x3-   Poisoning by ophthalmological drugs and preparations, assault

T49.5x4-   Poisoning by ophthalmological drugs and preparations, undetermined

T48 - T50

T49.5x5-   Adverse effect of ophthalmological drugs and preparations

T49.5x6-   Underdosing of ophthalmological drugs and preparations

T49.6-   Poisoning by, adverse effect of and underdosing of otorhinolaryngological drugs and preparations

T49.6x-   Poisoning by, adverse effect of and underdosing of otorhinolaryngological drugs and preparations

T49.6x1-   Poisoning by otorhinolaryngological drugs and preparations, accidental (unintentional)
Poisoning by otorhinolaryngological drugs and preparations NOS

T49.6x2-   Poisoning by otorhinolaryngological drugs and preparations, intentional self-harm

T49.6x3-   Poisoning by otorhinolaryngological drugs and preparations, assault

T49.6x4-   Poisoning by otorhinolaryngological drugs and preparations, undetermined

T49.6x5-   Adverse effect of otorhinolaryngological drugs and preparations

T49.6x6-   Underdosing of otorhinolaryngological drugs and preparations

T49.7-   Poisoning by, adverse effect of and underdosing of dental drugs, topically applied

T49.7x-   Poisoning by, adverse effect of and underdosing of dental drugs, topically applied

T49.7x1-   Poisoning by dental drugs, topically applied, accidental (unintentional)
Poisoning by dental drugs, topically applied NOS

T49.7x2-   Poisoning by dental drugs, topically applied, intentional self-harm

T49.7x3-   Poisoning by dental drugs, topically applied, assault

T49.7x4-   Poisoning by dental drugs, topically applied, undetermined

T49.7x5-   Adverse effect of dental drugs, topically applied

T49.7x6-   Underdosing of dental drugs, topically applied

T49.8-   Poisoning by, adverse effect of and underdosing of other topical agents
Poisoning by, adverse effect of and underdosing of spermicides

T49.8x-   Poisoning by, adverse effect of and underdosing of other topical agents

T49.8x1-   Poisoning by other topical agents, accidental (unintentional)
Poisoning by other topical agents NOS

T49.8x2-   Poisoning by other topical agents, intentional self-harm

T49.8x3-   Poisoning by other topical agents, assault

T49.8x4-   Poisoning by other topical agents, undetermined

T49.8x5-   Adverse effect of other topical agents

T49.8x6-   Underdosing of other topical agents

T49.9-   Poisoning by, adverse effect of and underdosing of unspecified topical agent

T49.91x-   Poisoning by unspecified topical agent, accidental (unintentional)

T49.92x-   Poisoning by unspecified topical agent, intentional self-harm

T49.93x-   Poisoning by unspecified topical agent, assault

T49.94x-   Poisoning by unspecified topical agent, undetermined

T49.95x-   Adverse effect of unspecified topical agent

T49.96x-   Underdosing of unspecified topical agent

T50-   Poisoning by, adverse effect of and underdosing of diuretics and other and unspecified drugs, medicaments and biological substances

The appropriate 7th character is to be added to each code from category T50:
A   Initial encounter
D   Subsequent encounter
S   Sequela

T50.0-   Poisoning by, adverse effect of and underdosing of mineralocorticoids and their antagonists

T50.0x-   Poisoning by, adverse effect of and underdosing of mineralocorticoids and their antagonists

T50.0x1-   Poisoning by mineralocorticoids and their antagonists, accidental (unintentional)
Poisoning by mineralocorticoids and their antagonists NOS

T50.0x2-   Poisoning by mineralocorticoids and their antagonists, intentional self-harm

T50.0x3-   Poisoning by mineralocorticoids and their antagonists, assault

T50.0x4-   Poisoning by mineralocorticoids and their antagonists, undetermined

T50.0x5-   Adverse effect of mineralocorticoids and their antagonists

T50.0x6-   Underdosing of mineralocorticoids and their antagonists

T50.1-   Poisoning by, adverse effect of and underdosing of loop [high-ceiling] diuretics

T50.1x-   Poisoning by, adverse effect of and underdosing of loop [high-ceiling] diuretics

T50.1x1-   Poisoning by loop [high-ceiling] diuretics, accidental (unintentional)
Poisoning by loop [high-ceiling] diuretics NOS

T50.1x2-   Poisoning by loop [high-ceiling] diuretics, intentional self-harm

T50.1x3-   Poisoning by loop [high-ceiling] diuretics, assault

T50.1x4-   Poisoning by loop [high-ceiling] diuretics, undetermined

T50.1x5-   Adverse effect of loop [high-ceiling] diuretics

T50.1x6-   Underdosing of loop [high-ceiling] diuretics

T50.2-   Poisoning by, adverse effect of and underdosing of carbonic-anhydrase inhibitors, benzothiadiazides and other diuretics
Poisoning by, adverse effect of and underdosing of acetazolamide

T50.2x-   Poisoning by, adverse effect of and underdosing of carbonic-anhydrase inhibitors, benzothiadiazides and other diuretics

T50.2x1-   Poisoning by carbonic-anhydrase inhibitors, benzothiadiazides and other diuretics, accidental (unintentional)
Poisoning by carbonic-anhydrase inhibitors, benzothiadiazides and other diuretics NOS

T50.2x2-   Poisoning by carbonic-anhydrase inhibitors, benzothiadiazides and other diuretics, intentional self-harm

T50.2x3-   Poisoning by carbonic-anhydrase inhibitors, benzothiadiazides and other diuretics, assault

T50.2x4-   Poisoning by carbonic-anhydrase inhibitors, benzothiadiazides and other diuretics, undetermined

T50.2x5-   Adverse effect of carbonic-anhydrase inhibitors, benzothiadiazides and other diuretics

T50.2x6-   Underdosing of carbonic-anhydrase inhibitors, benzothiadiazides and other diuretics

T50.3-   Poisoning by, adverse effect of and underdosing of electrolytic, caloric and water-balance agents
Poisoning by, adverse effect of and underdosing of oral rehydration salts

T50.3x-   Poisoning by, adverse effect of and underdosing of electrolytic, caloric and water-balance agents

T50.3x1-   Poisoning by electrolytic, caloric and water-balance agents, accidental (unintentional)
Poisoning by electrolytic, caloric and water-balance agents NOS

T50.3x2-   Poisoning by electrolytic, caloric and water-balance agents, intentional self-harm

T50.3x3-   Poisoning by electrolytic, caloric and water-balance agents, assault

T50.3x4-   Poisoning by electrolytic, caloric and water-balance agents, undetermined

T50.3x5-   Adverse effect of electrolytic, caloric and water-balance agents

T50.3x6-   Underdosing of electrolytic, caloric and water-balance agents

T50.4-   Poisoning by, adverse effect of and underdosing of drugs affecting uric acid metabolism

T50.4x-   Poisoning by, adverse effect of and underdosing of drugs affecting uric acid metabolism

T50.4x1-   Poisoning by drugs affecting uric acid metabolism, accidental (unintentional)
Poisoning by drugs affecting uric acid metabolism NOS

T50.4x2-   Poisoning by drugs affecting uric acid metabolism, intentional self-harm

T50.4x3-   Poisoning by drugs affecting uric acid metabolism, assault

T50.4x4-   Poisoning by drugs affecting uric acid metabolism, undetermined

T50.4x5-   Adverse effect of drugs affecting uric acid metabolism

T50.4x6-   Underdosing of drugs affecting uric acid metabolism

T48 - T50

T50.5-   Poisoning by, adverse effect of and underdosing of appetite depressants

   T50.5x-   Poisoning by, adverse effect of and underdosing of <u>appetite depressants</u>

      T50.5x1-   Poisoning by appetite depressants, <u>accidental</u> (unintentional)
         Poisoning by appetite depressants NOS

      T50.5x2-   Poisoning by appetite depressants, <u>intentional</u> self-harm

      T50.5x3-   Poisoning by appetite depressants, <u>assault</u>

      T50.5x4-   Poisoning by appetite depressants, <u>undetermined</u>

      T50.5x5-   <u>Adverse effect</u> of appetite depressants

      T50.5x6-   <u>Underdosing</u> of appetite depressants

T50.6-   Poisoning by, adverse effect of and underdosing of antidotes and chelating agents
   Poisoning by, adverse effect of and underdosing of alcohol deterrents

   T50.6x-   Poisoning by, adverse effect of and underdosing of <u>antidotes and chelating agents</u>

      T50.6x1-   Poisoning by antidotes and chelating agents, <u>accidental</u> (unintentional)
         Poisoning by antidotes and chelating agents NOS

      T50.6x2-   Poisoning by antidotes and chelating agents, <u>intentional</u> self-harm

      T50.6x3-   Poisoning by antidotes and chelating agents, <u>assault</u>

      T50.6x4-   Poisoning by antidotes and chelating agents, <u>undetermined</u>

      T50.6x5-   <u>Adverse effect</u> of antidotes and chelating agents

      T50.6x6-   <u>Underdosing</u> of antidotes and chelating agents

T50.7-   Poisoning by, adverse effect of and underdosing of analeptics and opioid receptor antagonists

   T50.7x-   Poisoning by, adverse effect of and underdosing of <u>analeptics and opioid receptor antagonists</u>

      T50.7x1-   Poisoning by analeptics and opioid receptor antagonists, <u>accidental</u> (unintentional)
         Poisoning by analeptics and opioid receptor antagonists NOS

      T50.7x2-   Poisoning by analeptics and opioid receptor antagonists, <u>intentional</u> self-harm

      T50.7x3-   Poisoning by analeptics and opioid receptor antagonists, <u>assault</u>

      T50.7x4-   Poisoning by analeptics and opioid receptor antagonists, <u>undetermined</u>

      T50.7x5-   <u>Adverse effect</u> of analeptics and opioid receptor antagonists

      T50.7x6-   <u>Underdosing</u> of analeptics and opioid receptor antagonists

T50.8-   Poisoning by, adverse effect of and underdosing of diagnostic agents

   T50.8x-   Poisoning by, adverse effect of and underdosing of <u>diagnostic agents</u>

      T50.8x1-   Poisoning by diagnostic agents, <u>accidental</u> (unintentional)
         Poisoning by diagnostic agents NOS

      T50.8x2-   Poisoning by diagnostic agents, <u>intentional</u> self-harm

      T50.8x3-   Poisoning by diagnostic agents, <u>assault</u>

      T50.8x4-   Poisoning by diagnostic agents, <u>undetermined</u>

      T50.8x5-   <u>Adverse effect</u> of diagnostic agents

      T50.8x6-   <u>Underdosing</u> of diagnostic agents

T50.A-   Poisoning by, adverse effect of and underdosing of bacterial vaccines

   T50.A1- Poisoning by, adverse effect of and underdosing of <u>pertussis vaccine, including combinations with a pertussis component</u>

      T50.A11- Poisoning by pertussis vaccine, including combinations with a pertussis component, <u>accidental</u> (unintentional)

      T50.A12- Poisoning by pertussis vaccine, including combinations with a pertussis component, <u>intentional</u> self-harm

      T50.A13- Poisoning by pertussis vaccine, including combinations with a pertussis component, <u>assault</u>

      T50.A14- Poisoning by pertussis vaccine, including combinations with a pertussis component, <u>undetermined</u>

      T50.A15- <u>Adverse effect</u> of pertussis vaccine, including combinations with a pertussis component

      T50.A16- <u>Underdosing</u> of pertussis vaccine, including combinations with a pertussis component

---

T50.A2- Poisoning by, adverse effect of and underdosing of <u>mixed bacterial vaccines without a pertussis component</u>

      T50.A21- Poisoning by mixed bacterial vaccines without a pertussis component, <u>accidental</u> (unintentional)

      T50.A22- Poisoning by mixed bacterial vaccines without a pertussis component, <u>intentional</u> self-harm

      T50.A23- Poisoning by mixed bacterial vaccines without a pertussis component, <u>assault</u>

      T50.A24- Poisoning by mixed bacterial vaccines without a pertussis component, <u>undetermined</u>

      T50.A25- <u>Adverse effect</u> of mixed bacterial vaccines without a pertussis component

      T50.A26- <u>Underdosing</u> of mixed bacterial vaccines without a pertussis component

T50.A9- Poisoning by, adverse effect of and underdosing of <u>other bacterial vaccines</u>

      T50.A91- Poisoning by other bacterial vaccines, <u>accidental</u> (unintentional)

      T50.A92- Poisoning by other bacterial vaccines, <u>intentional</u> self-harm

      T50.A93- Poisoning by other bacterial vaccines, <u>assault</u>

      T50.A94- Poisoning by other bacterial vaccines, <u>undetermined</u>

      T50.A95- <u>Adverse effect</u> of other bacterial vaccines

      T50.A96- <u>Underdosing</u> of other bacterial vaccines

T50.B-   Poisoning by, adverse effect of and underdosing of viral vaccines

   T50.B1- Poisoning by, adverse effect of and underdosing of <u>smallpox vaccines</u>

      T50.B11- Poisoning by smallpox vaccines, <u>accidental</u> (unintentional)

      T50.B12- Poisoning by smallpox vaccines, <u>intentional</u> self-harm

      T50.B13- Poisoning by smallpox vaccines, <u>assault</u>

      T50.B14- Poisoning by smallpox vaccines, <u>undetermined</u>

      T50.B15- <u>Adverse effect</u> of smallpox vaccines

      T50.B16- <u>Underdosing</u> of smallpox vaccines

T50.B9- Poisoning by, adverse effect of and underdosing of <u>other viral vaccines</u>

      T50.B91- Poisoning by other viral vaccines, <u>accidental</u> (unintentional)

      T50.B92- Poisoning by other viral vaccines, <u>intentional</u> self-harm

      T50.B93- Poisoning by other viral vaccines, <u>assault</u>

      T50.B94- Poisoning by other viral vaccines, <u>undetermined</u>

      T50.B95- <u>Adverse effect</u> of other viral vaccines

      T50.B96- <u>Underdosing</u> of other viral vaccines

T50.Z-   Poisoning by, adverse effect of and underdosing of other vaccines and biological substances

   T50.Z1- Poisoning by, adverse effect of and underdosing of <u>immunoglobulin</u>

      T50.Z11- Poisoning by immunoglobulin, <u>accidental</u> (unintentional)

      T50.Z12- Poisoning by immunoglobulin, <u>intentional</u> self-harm

      T50.Z13- Poisoning by immunoglobulin, <u>assault</u>

      T50.Z14- Poisoning by immunoglobulin, <u>undetermined</u>

      T50.Z15- <u>Adverse effect</u> of immunoglobulin

      T50.Z16- <u>Underdosing</u> of immunoglobulin

T50.Z9- Poisoning by, adverse effect of and underdosing of <u>other vaccines and biological substances</u>

      T50.Z91- Poisoning by other vaccines and biological substances, <u>accidental</u> (unintentional)

      T50.Z92- Poisoning by other vaccines and biological substances, <u>intentional</u> self-harm

      T50.Z93- Poisoning by other vaccines and biological substances, <u>assault</u>

      T50.Z94- Poisoning by other vaccines and biological substances, <u>undetermined</u>

      T50.Z95- <u>Adverse effect</u> of other vaccines and biological substances

      T50.Z96- <u>Underdosing</u> of other vaccines and biological substances

T50 - T52

Excludes 1: = NOT CODED HERE! (Do not code both)

Excludes ❷: = Not Included Here

T50.9-	Poisoning by, adverse effect of and underdosing of other and unspecified drugs, medicaments and biological substances

T50.90- Poisoning by, adverse effect of and underdosing of <u>unspecified drugs, medicaments and biological substances</u>

T50.901-	Poisoning by unspecified drugs, medicaments and biological substances, <u>accidental</u> (unintentional)

T50.902-	Poisoning by unspecified drugs, medicaments and biological substances, <u>intentional</u> self-harm

T50.903-	Poisoning by unspecified drugs, medicaments and biological substances, <u>assault</u>

T50.904-	Poisoning by unspecified drugs, medicaments and biological substances, <u>undetermined</u>

T50.905-	<u>Adverse effect</u> of unspecified drugs, medicaments and biological substances

T50.906-	<u>Underdosing</u> of unspecified drugs, medicaments and biological substances

T50.99- Poisoning by, adverse effect of and underdosing of <u>other drugs, medicaments and biological substances</u>

T50.991-	Poisoning by other drugs, medicaments and biological substances, <u>accidental</u> (unintentional)

T50.992-	Poisoning by other drugs, medicaments and biological substances, <u>intentional</u> self-harm

T50.993-	Poisoning by other drugs, medicaments and biological substances, <u>assault</u>

T50.994-	Poisoning by other drugs, medicaments and biological substances, <u>undetermined</u>

T50.995-	<u>Adverse effect</u> of other drugs, medicaments and biological substances

T50.996-	<u>Underdosing</u> of other drugs, medicaments and biological substances

Toxic effects of substances chiefly nonmedicinal as to source (T51-T65)

Note:	When no intent is indicated code to accidental. Undetermined intent is only for use when there is specific documentation in the record that the intent of the toxic effect cannot be determined.

Use additional code(s):
For all associated manifestations of toxic effect, such as: respiratory conditions due to external agents (J60-J70)
Personal history of foreign body fully removed (Z87.821)
To identify any retained foreign body, if applicable (Z18.-)
Excludes 1: contact with and (suspected) exposure to toxic substances (Z77.-)

T51-	Toxic effect of <u>alcohol</u>

The appropriate 7th character is to be added to each code from category T51:
A	<u>Initial</u> encounter
D	<u>Subsequent</u> encounter
S	<u>Sequela</u>

T51.0-	Toxic effect of ethanol
Toxic effect of ethyl alcohol
Excludes❷: acute alcohol intoxication or "hangover" effects (F10.129, F10.229, F10.929)
drunkenness (F10.129, F10.229, F10.929)
pathological alcohol intoxication (F10.129, F10.229, F10.929)

T51.0x- Toxic effect of <u>ethanol</u>
T51.0x1-	Toxic effect of ethanol, <u>accidental</u> (unintentional)
Toxic effect of ethanol NOS
T51.0x2-	Toxic effect of ethanol, <u>intentional</u> self-harm
T51.0x3-	Toxic effect of ethanol, <u>assault</u>
T51.0x4-	Toxic effect of ethanol, <u>undetermined</u>

T51.1-	Toxic effect of methanol
Toxic effect of methyl alcohol
T51.1x- Toxic effect of <u>methanol</u>
T51.1x1-	Toxic effect of methanol, <u>accidental</u> (unintentional)
Toxic effect of methanol NOS
T51.1x2-	Toxic effect of methanol, <u>intentional</u> self-harm
T51.1x3-	Toxic effect of methanol, <u>assault</u>
T51.1x4-	Toxic effect of methanol, <u>undetermined</u>

T51.2-	Toxic effect of 2-Propanol
Toxic effect of isopropyl alcohol
T51.2x- Toxic effect of <u>2-Propanol</u>
T51.2x1-	Toxic effect of 2-Propanol, <u>accidental</u> (unintentional)
Toxic effect of 2-Propanol NOS
T51.2x2-	Toxic effect of 2-Propanol, <u>intentional</u> self-harm
T51.2x3-	Toxic effect of 2-Propanol, <u>assault</u>
T51.2x4-	Toxic effect of 2-Propanol, <u>undetermined</u>

T51.3-	Toxic effect of fusel oil
Toxic effect of amyl alcohol
Toxic effect of butyl [1-butanol] alcohol
Toxic effect of propyl [1-propanol] alcohol
T51.3x- Toxic effect of <u>fusel oil</u>
T51.3x1-	Toxic effect of fusel oil, <u>accidental</u> (unintentional)
Toxic effect of fusel oil NOS
T51.3x2-	Toxic effect of fusel oil, <u>intentional</u> self-harm
T51.3x3-	Toxic effect of fusel oil, <u>assault</u>
T51.3x4-	Toxic effect of fusel oil, <u>undetermined</u>

T51.8-	Toxic effect of other alcohols
T51.8x- Toxic effect of <u>other alcohols</u>
T51.8x1-	Toxic effect of other alcohols, <u>accidental</u> (unintentional)
Toxic effect of other alcohols NOS
T51.8x2-	Toxic effect of other alcohols, <u>intentional</u> self-harm
T51.8x3-	Toxic effect of other alcohols, <u>assault</u>
T51.8x4-	Toxic effect of other alcohols, <u>undetermined</u>

T51.9-	Toxic effect of <u>unspecified alcohol</u>
T51.91x-	Toxic effect of unspecified alcohol, <u>accidental</u> (unintentional)
T51.92x-	Toxic effect of unspecified alcohol, <u>intentional</u> self-harm
T51.93x-	Toxic effect of unspecified alcohol, <u>assault</u>
T51.94x-	Toxic effect of unspecified alcohol, <u>undetermined</u>

T52-	Toxic effect of <u>organic solvents</u>
Excludes 1: halogen derivatives of aliphatic and aromatic hydrocarbons (T53.-)

The appropriate 7th character is to be added to each code from category T52:
A	<u>Initial</u> encounter
D	<u>Subsequent</u> encounter
S	<u>Sequela</u>

T52.0-	Toxic effects of petroleum products
Toxic effects of gasoline [petrol]
Toxic effects of kerosene [paraffin oil]
Toxic effects of paraffin wax
Toxic effects of ether petroleum
Toxic effects of naphtha petroleum
Toxic effects of spirit petroleum
T52.0x- Toxic effects of <u>petroleum products</u>
T52.0x1-	Toxic effect of petroleum products, <u>accidental</u> (unintentional)
Toxic effects of petroleum products NOS
T52.0x2-	Toxic effect of petroleum products, <u>intentional</u> self-harm
T52.0x3-	Toxic effect of petroleum products, <u>assault</u>
T52.0x4-	Toxic effect of petroleum products, <u>undetermined</u>

T52.1-	Toxic effects of benzene
Excludes 1: homologues of benzene (T52.2)
nitroderivatives and aminoderivatives of benzene and its homologues (T65.3)
T52.1x- Toxic effects of <u>benzene</u>
T52.1x1-	Toxic effect of benzene, <u>accidental</u> (unintentional)
Toxic effects of benzene NOS
T52.1x2-	Toxic effect of benzene, <u>intentional</u> self-harm
T52.1x3-	Toxic effect of benzene, <u>assault</u>
T52.1x4-	Toxic effect of benzene, <u>undetermined</u>

T52.2-	Toxic effects of homologues of benzene
Toxic effects of toluene [methylbenzene]
Toxic effects of xylene [dimethylbenzene]
T52.2x- Toxic effects of <u>homologues of benzene</u>
T52.2x1-	Toxic effect of homologues of benzene, <u>accidental</u> (unintentional)
Toxic effects of homologues of benzene NOS
T52.2x2-	Toxic effect of homologues of benzene, <u>intentional</u> self-harm
T52.2x3-	Toxic effect of homologues of benzene, <u>assault</u>
T52.2x4-	Toxic effect of homologues of benzene, <u>undetermined</u>

T52.3-	Toxic effects of glycols
T52.3x- Toxic effects of <u>glycols</u>
T52.3x1-	Toxic effect of glycols, <u>accidental</u> (unintentional)
Toxic effects of glycols NOS
T52.3x2-	Toxic effect of glycols, <u>intentional</u> self-harm
T52.3x3-	Toxic effect of glycols, <u>assault</u>
T52.3x4-	Toxic effect of glycols, <u>undetermined</u>

T52.4- Toxic effects of ketones
    T52.4x- Toxic effects of <u>ketones</u>
       T52.4x1- Toxic effect of ketones, <u>accidental</u> (unintentional)
          Toxic effects of ketones NOS
       T52.4x2- Toxic effect of ketones, <u>intentional</u> self-harm
       T52.4x3- Toxic effect of ketones, <u>assault</u>
       T52.4x4- Toxic effect of ketones, <u>undetermined</u>
T52.8- Toxic effects of other organic solvents
    T52.8x- Toxic effects of <u>other organic solvents</u>
       T52.8x1- Toxic effect of other organic solvents, <u>accidental</u> (unintentional)
          Toxic effects of other organic solvents NOS
       T52.8x2- Toxic effect of other organic solvents, <u>intentional</u> self-harm
       T52.8x3- Toxic effect of other organic solvents, <u>assault</u>
       T52.8x4- Toxic effect of other organic solvents, <u>undetermined</u>
T52.9- Toxic effects of <u>unspecified organic solvent</u>
    T52.91x- Toxic effect of unspecified organic solvent, <u>accidental</u> (unintentional)
    T52.92x- Toxic effect of unspecified organic solvent, <u>intentional</u> self-harm
    T52.93x- Toxic effect of unspecified organic solvent, <u>assault</u>
    T52.94x- Toxic effect of unspecified organic solvent, <u>undetermined</u>
T53-   Toxic effect of <u>halogen derivatives of aliphatic and aromatic hydrocarbons</u>

The appropriate 7th character is to be added to each code from category T53:
  A <u>Initial</u> encounter
  D <u>Subsequent</u> encounter
  S <u>Sequela</u>

T53.0- Toxic effects of carbon tetrachloride
    Toxic effects of tetrachloromethane
    T53.0x- Toxic effects of <u>carbon tetrachloride</u>
       T53.0x1- Toxic effect of carbon tetrachloride, <u>accidental</u> (unintentional)
          Toxic effects of carbon tetrachloride NOS
       T53.0x2- Toxic effect of carbon tetrachloride, <u>intentional</u> self-harm
       T53.0x3- Toxic effect of carbon tetrachloride, <u>assault</u>
       T53.0x4- Toxic effect of carbon tetrachloride, <u>undetermined</u>
T53.1- Toxic effects of chloroform
    Toxic effects of trichloromethane
    T53.1x- Toxic effects of <u>chloroform</u>
       T53.1x1- Toxic effect of chloroform, <u>accidental</u> (unintentional)
          Toxic effects of chloroform NOS
       T53.1x2- Toxic effect of chloroform, <u>intentional</u> self-harm
       T53.1x3- Toxic effect of chloroform, <u>assault</u>
       T53.1x4- Toxic effect of chloroform, <u>undetermined</u>
T53.2- Toxic effects of trichloroethylene
    Toxic effects of trichloroethene
    T53.2x- Toxic effects of <u>trichloroethylene</u>
       T53.2x1- Toxic effect of trichloroethylene, <u>accidental</u> (unintentional)
          Toxic effects of trichloroethylene NOS
       T53.2x2- Toxic effect of trichloroethylene, <u>intentional</u> self-harm
       T53.2x3- Toxic effect of trichloroethylene, <u>assault</u>
       T53.2x4- Toxic effect of trichloroethylene, <u>undetermined</u>
T53.3- Toxic effects of tetrachloroethylene
    Toxic effects of perchloroethylene
    Toxic effect of tetrachloroethene
    T53.3x- Toxic effects of <u>tetrachloroethylene</u>
       T53.3x1- Toxic effect of tetrachloroethylene, <u>accidental</u> (unintentional)
          Toxic effects of tetrachloroethylene NOS
       T53.3x2- Toxic effect of tetrachloroethylene, <u>intentional</u> self-harm
       T53.3x3- Toxic effect of tetrachloroethylene, <u>assault</u>
       T53.3x4- Toxic effect of tetrachloroethylene, <u>undetermined</u>
T53.4- Toxic effects of dichloromethane
    Toxic effects of methylene chloride
    T53.4x- Toxic effects of <u>dichloromethane</u>
       T53.4x1- Toxic effect of dichloromethane, <u>accidental</u> (unintentional)
          Toxic effects of dichloromethane NOS
       T53.4x2- Toxic effect of dichloromethane, <u>intentional</u> self-harm
       T53.4x3- Toxic effect of dichloromethane, <u>assault</u>
       T53.4x4- Toxic effect of dichloromethane, <u>undetermined</u>

T53.5- Toxic effects of chlorofluorocarbons
    T53.5x- Toxic effects of <u>chlorofluorocarbons</u>
       T53.5x1- Toxic effect of chlorofluorocarbons, <u>accidental</u> (unintentional)
          Toxic effects of chlorofluorocarbons NOS
       T53.5x2- Toxic effect of chlorofluorocarbons, <u>intentional</u> self-harm
       T53.5x3- Toxic effect of chlorofluorocarbons, <u>assault</u>
       T53.5x4- Toxic effect of chlorofluorocarbons, <u>undetermined</u>
T53.6- Toxic effects of other halogen derivatives of aliphatic hydrocarbons
    T53.6x- Toxic effects of <u>other halogen derivatives of aliphatic hydrocarbons</u>
       T53.6x1- Toxic effect of other halogen derivatives of aliphatic hydrocarbons, <u>accidental</u> (unintentional)
          Toxic effects of other halogen derivatives of aliphatic hydrocarbons NOS
       T53.6x2- Toxic effect of other halogen derivatives of aliphatic hydrocarbons, <u>intentional</u> self-harm
       T53.6x3- Toxic effect of other halogen derivatives of aliphatic hydrocarbons, <u>assault</u>
       T53.6x4- Toxic effect of other halogen derivatives of aliphatic hydrocarbons, <u>undetermined</u>
T53.7- Toxic effects of other halogen derivatives of aromatic hydrocarbons
    T53.7x- Toxic effects of <u>other halogen derivatives of aromatic hydrocarbons</u>
       T53.7x1- Toxic effect of other halogen derivatives of aromatic hydrocarbons, <u>accidental</u> (unintentional)
          Toxic effects of other halogen derivatives of aromatic hydrocarbons NOS
       T53.7x2- Toxic effect of other halogen derivatives of aromatic hydrocarbons, <u>intentional</u> self-harm
       T53.7x3- Toxic effect of other halogen derivatives of aromatic hydrocarbons, <u>assault</u>
       T53.7x4- Toxic effect of other halogen derivatives of aromatic hydrocarbons, <u>undetermined</u>
T53.9- Toxic effects of <u>unspecified halogen derivatives of aliphatic and aromatic hydrocarbons</u>
    T53.91x- Toxic effect of unspecified halogen derivatives of aliphatic and aromatic hydrocarbons, <u>accidental</u> (unintentional)
    T53.92x- Toxic effect of unspecified halogen derivatives of aliphatic and aromatic hydrocarbons, <u>intentional</u> self-harm
    T53.93x- Toxic effect of unspecified halogen derivatives of aliphatic and aromatic hydrocarbons, <u>assault</u>
    T53.94x- Toxic effect of unspecified halogen derivatives of aliphatic and aromatic hydrocarbons, <u>undetermined</u>

T54-   Toxic effect of <u>corrosive substances</u>

The appropriate 7th character is to be added to each code from category T54:
  A <u>Initial</u> encounter
  D <u>Subsequent</u> encounter
  S <u>Sequela</u>

T54.0- Toxic effects of phenol and phenol homologues
    T54.0x- Toxic effects of <u>phenol and phenol homologues</u>
       T54.0x1- Toxic effect of phenol and phenol homologues, <u>accidental</u> (unintentional)
          Toxic effects of phenol and phenol homologues NOS
       T54.0x2- Toxic effect of phenol and phenol homologues, <u>intentional</u> self-harm
       T54.0x3- Toxic effect of phenol and phenol homologues, <u>assault</u>
       T54.0x4- Toxic effect of phenol and phenol homologues, <u>undetermined</u>
T54.1- Toxic effects of other corrosive organic compounds
    T54.1x- Toxic effects of <u>other corrosive organic compounds</u>
       T54.1x1- Toxic effect of other corrosive organic compounds, <u>accidental</u> (unintentional)
          Toxic effects of other corrosive organic compounds NOS
       T54.1x2- Toxic effect of other corrosive organic compounds, <u>intentional</u> self-harm
       T54.1x3- Toxic effect of other corrosive organic compounds, <u>assault</u>
       T54.1x4- Toxic effect of other corrosive organic compounds, <u>undetermined</u>

T52 - T56

T54.2- Toxic effects of corrosive acids and acid-like substances
    Toxic effects of hydrochloric acid
    Toxic effects of sulfuric acid

  T54.2x- Toxic effects of <u>corrosive acids and acid-like substances</u>

    T54.2x1- Toxic effect of corrosive acids and acid-like substances, <u>accidental</u> (unintentional)
      Toxic effects of corrosive acids and acid-like substances NOS

    T54.2x2- Toxic effect of corrosive acids and acid-like substances, <u>intentional</u> self-harm

    T54.2x3- Toxic effect of corrosive acids and acid-like substances, <u>assault</u>

    T54.2x4- Toxic effect of corrosive acids and acid-like substances, <u>undetermined</u>

T54.3- Toxic effects of corrosive alkalis and alkali-like substances
    Toxic effects of potassium hydroxide
    Toxic effects of sodium hydroxide

  T54.3x- Toxic effects of <u>corrosive alkalis and alkali-like substances</u>

    T54.3x1- Toxic effect of corrosive alkalis and alkali-like substances, <u>accidental</u> (unintentional)
      Toxic effects of corrosive alkalis and alkali-like substances NOS

    T54.3x2- Toxic effect of corrosive alkalis and alkali-like substances, <u>intentional</u> self-harm

    T54.3x3- Toxic effect of corrosive alkalis and alkali-like substances, <u>assault</u>

    T54.3x4- Toxic effect of corrosive alkalis and alkali-like substances, <u>undetermined</u>

T54.9- Toxic effects of <u>unspecified corrosive substance</u>

  T54.91x- Toxic effect of unspecified corrosive substance, <u>accidental</u> (unintentional)

  T54.92x- Toxic effect of unspecified corrosive substance, <u>intentional</u> self-harm

  T54.93x- Toxic effect of unspecified corrosive substance, <u>assault</u>

  T54.94x- Toxic effect of unspecified corrosive substance, <u>undetermined</u>

T55- Toxic effect of <u>soaps and detergents</u>

The appropriate 7th character is to be added to each code from category T55:
  A   <u>Initial</u> encounter
  D   <u>Subsequent</u> encounter
  S   <u>Sequela</u>

T55.0- Toxic effect of soaps

  T55.0x- Toxic effect of <u>soaps</u>

    T55.0x1- Toxic effect of soaps, <u>accidental</u> (unintentional)
      Toxic effect of soaps NOS

    T55.0x2- Toxic effect of soaps, <u>intentional</u> self-harm

    T55.0x3- Toxic effect of soaps, <u>assault</u>

    T55.0x4- Toxic effect of soaps, <u>undetermined</u>

T55.1- Toxic effect of detergents

  T55.1x- Toxic effect of <u>detergents</u>

    T55.1x1- Toxic effect of detergents, <u>accidental</u> (unintentional)
      Toxic effect of detergents NOS

    T55.1x2- Toxic effect of detergents, <u>intentional</u> self-harm

    T55.1x3- Toxic effect of detergents, <u>assault</u>

    T55.1x4- Toxic effect of detergents, <u>undetermined</u>

T56- Toxic effect of <u>metals</u>
  Includes: Toxic effects of fumes and vapors of metals
      Toxic effects of metals from all sources, except medicinal substances
  Use additional code to identify any retained metal foreign body, if applicable (Z18.0-, T18.1-)
  Excludes 1:   arsenic and its compounds (T57.0)
      manganese and its compounds (T57.2)

The appropriate 7th character is to be added to each code from category T56:
  A   <u>Initial</u> encounter
  D   <u>Subsequent</u> encounter
  S   <u>Sequela</u>

T56.0- Toxic effects of lead and its compounds

  T56.0x- Toxic effects of <u>lead and its compounds</u>

    T56.0x1- Toxic effect of lead and its compounds, <u>accidental</u> (unintentional)
      Toxic effects of lead and its compounds NOS

    T56.0x2- Toxic effect of lead and its compounds, <u>intentional</u> self-harm

    T56.0x3- Toxic effect of lead and its compounds, <u>assault</u>

    T56.0x4- Toxic effect of lead and its compounds, <u>undetermined</u>

T56.1- Toxic effects of mercury and its compounds

  T56.1x- Toxic effects of <u>mercury and its compounds</u>

    T56.1x1- Toxic effect of mercury and its compounds, <u>accidental</u> (unintentional)
      Toxic effects of mercury and its compounds NOS

    T56.1x2- Toxic effect of mercury and its compounds, <u>intentional</u> self-harm

    T56.1x3- Toxic effect of mercury and its compounds, <u>assault</u>

    T56.1x4- Toxic effect of mercury and its compounds, <u>undetermined</u>

T56.2- Toxic effects of chromium and its compounds

  T56.2x- Toxic effects of <u>chromium and its compounds</u>

    T56.2x1- Toxic effect of chromium and its compounds, <u>accidental</u> (unintentional)
      Toxic effects of chromium and its compounds NOS

    T56.2x2- Toxic effect of chromium and its compounds, <u>intentional</u> self-harm

    T56.2x3- Toxic effect of chromium and its compounds, <u>assault</u>

    T56.2x4- Toxic effect of chromium and its compounds, <u>undetermined</u>

T56.3- Toxic effects of cadmium and its compounds

  T56.3x- Toxic effects of <u>cadmium and its compounds</u>

    T56.3x1- Toxic effect of cadmium and its compounds, <u>accidental</u> (unintentional)
      Toxic effects of cadmium and its compounds NOS

    T56.3x2- Toxic effect of cadmium and its compounds, <u>intentional</u> self-harm

    T56.3x3- Toxic effect of cadmium and its compounds, <u>assault</u>

    T56.3x4- Toxic effect of cadmium and its compounds, <u>undetermined</u>

T56.4- Toxic effects of copper and its compounds

  T56.4x- Toxic effects of <u>copper and its compounds</u>

    T56.4x1- Toxic effect of copper and its compounds, <u>accidental</u> (unintentional)
      Toxic effects of copper and its compounds NOS

    T56.4x2- Toxic effect of copper and its compounds, <u>intentional</u> self-harm

    T56.4x3- Toxic effect of copper and its compounds, <u>assault</u>

    T56.4x4- Toxic effect of copper and its compounds, <u>undetermined</u>

T56.5- Toxic effects of zinc and its compounds

  T56.5x- Toxic effects of <u>zinc and its compounds</u>

    T56.5x1- Toxic effect of zinc and its compounds, <u>accidental</u> (unintentional)
      Toxic effects of zinc and its compounds NOS

    T56.5x2- Toxic effect of zinc and its compounds, <u>intentional</u> self-harm

    T56.5x3- Toxic effect of zinc and its compounds, <u>assault</u>

    T56.5x4- Toxic effect of zinc and its compounds, <u>undetermined</u>

T56.6- Toxic effects of tin and its compounds

  T56.6x- Toxic effects of <u>tin and its compounds</u>

    T56.6x1- Toxic effect of tin and its compounds, <u>accidental</u> (unintentional)
      Toxic effects of tin and its compounds NOS

    T56.6x2- Toxic effect of tin and its compounds, <u>intentional</u> self-harm

    T56.6x3- Toxic effect of tin and its compounds, <u>assault</u>

    T56.6x4- Toxic effect of tin and its compounds, <u>undetermined</u>

T56.7- Toxic effects of beryllium and its compounds

  T56.7x- Toxic effects of <u>beryllium and its compounds</u>

    T56.7x1- Toxic effect of beryllium and its compounds, <u>accidental</u> (unintentional)
      Toxic effects of beryllium and its compounds NOS

    T56.7x2- Toxic effect of beryllium and its compounds, <u>intentional</u> self-harm

    T56.7x3- Toxic effect of beryllium and its compounds, <u>assault</u>

    T56.7x4- Toxic effect of beryllium and its compounds, <u>undetermined</u>

T56.8- Toxic effects of other metals

  T56.81- Toxic effect of <u>thallium</u>

    T56.811- Toxic effect of thallium, <u>accidental</u> (unintentional)
      Toxic effect of thallium NOS

    T56.812- Toxic effect of thallium, <u>intentional</u> self-harm

    T56.813- Toxic effect of thallium, <u>assault</u>

    T56.814- Toxic effect of thallium, <u>undetermined</u>

T52 - T56

Excludes 1: = NOT CODED HERE! (Do not code both)   **817**   *Excludes ❷:* = Not Included Here

T56.89- Toxic effects of other metals
- **T56.891-** Toxic effect of other metals, accidental (unintentional)
  - Toxic effects of other metals NOS
- **T56.892-** Toxic effect of other metals, intentional self-harm
- **T56.893-** Toxic effect of other metals, assault
- **T56.894-** Toxic effect of other metals, undetermined

T56.9- Toxic effects of unspecified metal
- **T56.91x-** Toxic effect of unspecified metal, accidental (unintentional)
- **T56.92x-** Toxic effect of unspecified metal, intentional self-harm
- **T56.93x-** Toxic effect of unspecified metal, assault
- **T56.94x-** Toxic effect of unspecified metal, undetermined

T57- Toxic effect of other inorganic substances

The appropriate 7th character is to be added to each code from category T57:
- **A** Initial encounter
- **D** Subsequent encounter
- **S** Sequela

T57.0- Toxic effect of arsenic and its compounds
- **T57.0x-** Toxic effect of arsenic and its compounds
  - **T57.0x1-** Toxic effect of arsenic and its compounds, accidental (unintentional)
    - Toxic effect of arsenic and its compounds NOS
  - **T57.0x2-** Toxic effect of arsenic and its compounds, intentional self-harm
  - **T57.0x3-** Toxic effect of arsenic and its compounds, assault
  - **T57.0x4-** Toxic effect of arsenic and its compounds, undetermined

T57.1- Toxic effect of phosphorus and its compounds
Excludes 1: organophosphate insecticides (T60.0)
- **T57.1x-** Toxic effect of phosphorus and its compounds
  - **T57.1x1-** Toxic effect of phosphorus and its compounds, accidental (unintentional)
    - Toxic effect of phosphorus and its compounds NOS
  - **T57.1x2-** Toxic effect of phosphorus and its compounds, intentional self-harm
  - **T57.1x3-** Toxic effect of phosphorus and its compounds, assault
  - **T57.1x4-** Toxic effect of phosphorus and its compounds, undetermined

T57.2- Toxic effect of manganese and its compounds
- **T57.2x-** Toxic effect of manganese and its compounds
  - **T57.2x1-** Toxic effect of manganese and its compounds, accidental (unintentional)
    - Toxic effect of manganese and its compounds NOS
  - **T57.2x2-** Toxic effect of manganese and its compounds, intentional self-harm
  - **T57.2x3-** Toxic effect of manganese and its compounds, assault
  - **T57.2x4-** Toxic effect of manganese and its compounds, undetermined

T57.3- Toxic effect of hydrogen cyanide
- **T57.3x-** Toxic effect of hydrogen cyanide
  - **T57.3x1-** Toxic effect of hydrogen cyanide, accidental (unintentional)
    - Toxic effect of hydrogen cyanide NOS
  - **T57.3x2-** Toxic effect of hydrogen cyanide, intentional self-harm
  - **T57.3x3-** Toxic effect of hydrogen cyanide, assault
  - **T57.3x4-** Toxic effect of hydrogen cyanide, undetermined

T57.8- Toxic effect of other specified inorganic substances
- **T57.8x-** Toxic effect of other specified inorganic substances
  - **T57.8x1-** Toxic effect of other specified inorganic substances, accidental (unintentional)
    - Toxic effect of other specified inorganic substances NOS
  - **T57.8x2-** Toxic effect of other specified inorganic substances, intentional self-harm
  - **T57.8x3-** Toxic effect of other specified inorganic substances, assault
  - **T57.8x4-** Toxic effect of other specified inorganic substances, undetermined

T57.9- Toxic effect of unspecified inorganic substance
- **T57.91x-** Toxic effect of unspecified inorganic substance, accidental (unintentional)
- **T57.92x-** Toxic effect of unspecified inorganic substance, intentional self-harm
- **T57.93x-** Toxic effect of unspecified inorganic substance, assault
- **T57.94x-** Toxic effect of unspecified inorganic substance, undetermined

T58- Toxic effect of carbon monoxide
Includes: Asphyxiation from carbon monoxide
Toxic effect of carbon monoxide from all sources

The appropriate 7th character is to be added to each code from category T58:
- **A** Initial encounter
- **D** Subsequent encounter
- **S** Sequela

T58.0- Toxic effect of carbon monoxide from motor vehicle exhaust
Toxic effect of exhaust gas from gas engine
Toxic effect of exhaust gas from motor pump
- **T58.01x-** Toxic effect of carbon monoxide from motor vehicle exhaust, accidental (unintentional)
- **T58.02x-** Toxic effect of carbon monoxide from motor vehicle exhaust, intentional self-harm
- **T58.03x-** Toxic effect of carbon monoxide from motor vehicle exhaust, assault
- **T58.04x-** Toxic effect of carbon monoxide from motor vehicle exhaust, undetermined

T58.1- Toxic effect of carbon monoxide from utility gas
Toxic effect of acetylene
Toxic effect of gas NOS used for lighting, heating, cooking
Toxic effect of water gas
- **T58.11x-** Toxic effect of carbon monoxide from utility gas, accidental (unintentional)
- **T58.12x-** Toxic effect of carbon monoxide from utility gas, intentional self-harm
- **T58.13x-** Toxic effect of carbon monoxide from utility gas, assault
- **T58.14x-** Toxic effect of carbon monoxide from utility gas, undetermined

T58.2- Toxic effect of carbon monoxide from incomplete combustion of other domestic fuels
Toxic effect of carbon monoxide from incomplete combustion of coal, coke, kerosene, wood
- **T58.2x-** Toxic effect of carbon monoxide from incomplete combustion of other domestic fuels
  - **T58.2x1-** Toxic effect of carbon monoxide from incomplete combustion of other domestic fuels, accidental (unintentional)
  - **T58.2x2-** Toxic effect of carbon monoxide from incomplete combustion of other domestic fuels, intentional self-harm
  - **T58.2x3-** Toxic effect of carbon monoxide from incomplete combustion of other domestic fuels, assault
  - **T58.2x4-** Toxic effect of carbon monoxide from incomplete combustion of other domestic fuels, undetermined

T58.8- Toxic effect of carbon monoxide from other source
Toxic effect of carbon monoxide from blast furnace gas
Toxic effect of carbon monoxide from fuels in industrial use
Toxic effect of carbon monoxide from kiln vapor
- **T58.8x-** Toxic effect of carbon monoxide from other source
  - **T58.8x1-** Toxic effect of carbon monoxide from other source, accidental (unintentional)
  - **T58.8x2-** Toxic effect of carbon monoxide from other source, intentional self-harm
  - **T58.8x3-** Toxic effect of carbon monoxide from other source, assault
  - **T58.8x4-** Toxic effect of carbon monoxide from other source, undetermined

T58.9- Toxic effect of carbon monoxide from unspecified source
- **T58.91x-** Toxic effect of carbon monoxide from unspecified source, accidental (unintentional)
- **T58.92x-** Toxic effect of carbon monoxide from unspecified source, intentional self-harm
- **T58.93x-** Toxic effect of carbon monoxide from unspecified source, assault
- **T58.94x-** Toxic effect of carbon monoxide from unspecified source, undetermined

T
5
6
-
T
6
0

T59-   Toxic effect of <u>other gases, fumes and vapors</u>
   Includes: Aerosol propellants
   Excludes 1: chlorofluorocarbons (T53.5)

The appropriate 7th character is to be added to each code from category T59:
   A   <u>Initial</u> encounter
   D   <u>Subsequent</u> encounter
   S   <u>Sequela</u>

  T59.0-   Toxic effect of nitrogen oxides
    T59.0x- Toxic effect of <u>nitrogen oxides</u>
      T59.0x1- Toxic effect of nitrogen oxides, <u>accidental</u> (unintentional)
          Toxic effect of nitrogen oxides NOS
      T59.0x2- Toxic effect of nitrogen oxides, <u>intentional</u> self-harm
      T59.0x3- Toxic effect of nitrogen oxides, <u>assault</u>
      T59.0x4- Toxic effect of nitrogen oxides, <u>undetermined</u>

  T59.1-   Toxic effect of sulfur dioxide
    T59.1x- Toxic effect of <u>sulfur dioxide</u>
      T59.1x1- Toxic effect of sulfur dioxide, <u>accidental</u> (unintentional)
          Toxic effect of sulfur dioxide NOS
      T59.1x2- Toxic effect of sulfur dioxide, <u>intentional</u> self-harm
      T59.1x3- Toxic effect of sulfur dioxide, <u>assault</u>
      T59.1x4- Toxic effect of sulfur dioxide, <u>undetermined</u>

  T59.2-   Toxic effect of formaldehyde
    T59.2x- Toxic effect of <u>formaldehyde</u>
      T59.2x1- Toxic effect of formaldehyde, <u>accidental</u> (unintentional)
          Toxic effect of formaldehyde NOS
      T59.2x2- Toxic effect of formaldehyde, <u>intentional</u> self-harm
      T59.2x3- Toxic effect of formaldehyde, <u>assault</u>
      T59.2x4- Toxic effect of formaldehyde, <u>undetermined</u>

  T59.3-   Toxic effect of lacrimogenic gas
      Toxic effect of tear gas
    T59.3x- Toxic effect of <u>lacrimogenic gas</u>
      T59.3x1- Toxic effect of lacrimogenic gas, <u>accidental</u> (unintentional)
          Toxic effect of lacrimogenic gas NOS
      T59.3x2- Toxic effect of lacrimogenic gas, <u>intentional</u> self-harm
      T59.3x3- Toxic effect of lacrimogenic gas, <u>assault</u>
      T59.3x4- Toxic effect of lacrimogenic gas, <u>undetermined</u>

  T59.4-   Toxic effect of chlorine gas
    T59.4x- Toxic effect of <u>chlorine gas</u>
      T59.4x1- Toxic effect of chlorine gas, <u>accidental</u> (unintentional)
          Toxic effect of chlorine gas NOS
      T59.4x2- Toxic effect of chlorine gas, <u>intentional</u> self-harm
      T59.4x3- Toxic effect of chlorine gas, <u>assault</u>
      T59.4x4- Toxic effect of chlorine gas, <u>undetermined</u>

  T59.5-   Toxic effect of fluorine gas and hydrogen fluoride
    T59.5x- Toxic effect of <u>fluorine gas and hydrogen fluoride</u>
      T59.5x1- Toxic effect of fluorine gas and hydrogen fluoride, <u>accidental</u> (unintentional)
          Toxic effect of fluorine gas and hydrogen fluoride NOS
      T59.5x2- Toxic effect of fluorine gas and hydrogen fluoride, <u>intentional</u> self-harm
      T59.5x3- Toxic effect of fluorine gas and hydrogen fluoride, <u>assault</u>
      T59.5x4- Toxic effect of fluorine gas and hydrogen fluoride, <u>undetermined</u>

  T59.6-   Toxic effect of hydrogen sulfide
    T59.6x- Toxic effect of <u>hydrogen sulfide</u>
      T59.6x1- Toxic effect of hydrogen sulfide, <u>accidental</u> (unintentional)
          Toxic effect of hydrogen sulfide NOS
      T59.6x2- Toxic effect of hydrogen sulfide, <u>intentional</u> self-harm
      T59.6x3- Toxic effect of hydrogen sulfide, <u>assault</u>
      T59.6x4- Toxic effect of hydrogen sulfide, <u>undetermined</u>

  T59.7-   Toxic effect of carbon dioxide
    T59.7x- Toxic effect of <u>carbon dioxide</u>
      T59.7x1- Toxic effect of carbon dioxide, <u>accidental</u> (unintentional)
          Toxic effect of carbon dioxide NOS
      T59.7x2- Toxic effect of carbon dioxide, <u>intentional</u> self-harm
      T59.7x3- Toxic effect of carbon dioxide, <u>assault</u>
      T59.7x4- Toxic effect of carbon dioxide, <u>undetermined</u>

  T59.8-   Toxic effect of other specified gases, fumes and vapors
    T59.81- Toxic effect of <u>smoke</u>
      Smoke inhalation
      Excludes❷: toxic effect of cigarette (tobacco) smoke (T65.22-)
      T59.811- Toxic effect of smoke, <u>accidental</u> (unintentional)
          Toxic effect of smoke NOS
      T59.812- Toxic effect of smoke, <u>intentional</u> self-harm
      T59.813- Toxic effect of smoke, <u>assault</u>
      T59.814- Toxic effect of smoke, <u>undetermined</u>
    T59.89- Toxic effect of <u>other specified gases, fumes and vapors</u>
      T59.891- Toxic effect of other specified gases, fumes and vapors, <u>accidental</u> (unintentional)
      T59.892- Toxic effect of other specified gases, fumes and vapors, <u>intentional</u> self-harm
      T59.893- Toxic effect of other specified gases, fumes and vapors, <u>assault</u>
      T59.894- Toxic effect of other specified gases, fumes and vapors, <u>undetermined</u>

  T59.9-   Toxic effect of <u>unspecified gases, fumes and vapors</u>
    T59.91x- Toxic effect of unspecified gases, fumes and vapors, <u>accidental</u> (unintentional)
    T59.92x- Toxic effect of unspecified gases, fumes and vapors, <u>intentional</u> self-harm
    T59.93x- Toxic effect of unspecified gases, fumes and vapors, <u>assault</u>
    T59.94x- Toxic effect of unspecified gases, fumes and vapors, <u>undetermined</u>

T60-   Toxic effect of <u>pesticides</u>
   Includes: Toxic effect of wood preservatives

The appropriate 7th character is to be added to each code from category T60:
   A   <u>Initial</u> encounter
   D   <u>Subsequent</u> encounter
   S   <u>Sequela</u>

  T60.0-   Toxic effect of organophosphate and carbamate insecticides
    T60.0x- Toxic effect of <u>organophosphate and carbamate insecticides</u>
      T60.0x1- Toxic effect of organophosphate and carbamate insecticides, <u>accidental</u> (unintentional)
          Toxic effect of organophosphate and carbamate insecticides NOS
      T60.0x2- Toxic effect of organophosphate and carbamate insecticides, <u>intentional</u> self-harm
      T60.0x3- Toxic effect of organophosphate and carbamate insecticides, <u>assault</u>
      T60.0x4- Toxic effect of organophosphate and carbamate insecticides, <u>undetermined</u>

  T60.1-   Toxic effect of halogenated insecticides
    Excludes 1: chlorinated hydrocarbon (T53.-)
    T60.1x- Toxic effect of <u>halogenated insecticides</u>
      T60.1x1- Toxic effect of halogenated insecticides, <u>accidental</u> (unintentional)
          Toxic effect of halogenated insecticides NOS
      T60.1x2- Toxic effect of halogenated insecticides, <u>intentional</u> self-harm
      T60.1x3- Toxic effect of halogenated insecticides, <u>assault</u>
      T60.1x4- Toxic effect of halogenated insecticides, <u>undetermined</u>

  T60.2-   Toxic effect of other insecticides
    T60.2x- Toxic effect of <u>other insecticides</u>
      T60.2x1- Toxic effect of other insecticides, <u>accidental</u> (unintentional)
          Toxic effect of other insecticides NOS
      T60.2x2- Toxic effect of other insecticides, <u>intentional</u> self-harm
      T60.2x3- Toxic effect of other insecticides, <u>assault</u>
      T60.2x4- Toxic effect of other insecticides, <u>undetermined</u>

  T60.3-   Toxic effect of herbicides and fungicides
    T60.3x- Toxic effect of <u>herbicides and fungicides</u>
      T60.3x1- Toxic effect of herbicides and fungicides, <u>accidental</u> (unintentional)
          Toxic effect of herbicides and fungicides NOS
      T60.3x2- Toxic effect of herbicides and fungicides, <u>intentional</u> self-harm
      T60.3x3- Toxic effect of herbicides and fungicides, <u>assault</u>
      T60.3x4- Toxic effect of herbicides and fungicides, <u>undetermined</u>

T56 - T60

T60.4- Toxic effect of rodenticides
Excludes 1: strychnine and its salts (T65.1)
thallium (T56.81-)

T60.4x- Toxic effect of <u>rodenticides</u>

T60.4x1- Toxic effect of rodenticides, <u>accidental</u> (unintentional)
Toxic effect of rodenticides NOS

T60.4x2- Toxic effect of rodenticides, <u>intentional</u> self-harm

T60.4x3- Toxic effect of rodenticides, <u>assault</u>

T60.4x4- Toxic effect of rodenticides, <u>undetermined</u>

T60.8- Toxic effect of other pesticides

T60.8x- Toxic effect of <u>other pesticides</u>

T60.8x1- Toxic effect of other pesticides, <u>accidental</u> (unintentional)
Toxic effect of other pesticides NOS

T60.8x2- Toxic effect of other pesticides, <u>intentional</u> self-harm

T60.8x3- Toxic effect of other pesticides, <u>assault</u>

T60.8x4- Toxic effect of other pesticides, <u>undetermined</u>

T60.9- Toxic effect of <u>unspecified pesticide</u>

T60.91x- Toxic effect of unspecified pesticide, <u>accidental</u> (unintentional)

T60.92x- Toxic effect of unspecified pesticide, <u>intentional</u> self-harm

T60.93x- Toxic effect of unspecified pesticide, <u>assault</u>

T60.94x- Toxic effect of unspecified pesticide, <u>undetermined</u>

T61- Toxic effect of <u>noxious substances eaten as seafood</u>
Excludes 1: allergic reaction to food, such as:
anaphylactic reaction or shock due to adverse food reaction (T78.0-)
bacterial foodborne intoxications (A05.-)
dermatitis (L23.6, L25.4, L27.2)
gastroenteritis (noninfective) (K52.2)
toxic effect of aflatoxin and other mycotoxins (T64)
toxic effect of cyanides (T65.0-)
toxic effect of harmful algae bloom (T65.82-)
toxic effect of hydrogen cyanide (T57.3-)
toxic effect of mercury (T56.1-)
toxic effect of red tide (T65.82-)

The appropriate 7th character is to be added to each code from category T61:
A <u>Initial</u> encounter
D <u>Subsequent</u> encounter
S <u>Sequela</u>

T61.0- <u>Ciguatera fish</u> poisoning

T61.01x- Ciguatera fish poisoning, <u>accidental</u> (unintentional)

T61.02x- Ciguatera fish poisoning, <u>intentional</u> self-harm

T61.03x- Ciguatera fish poisoning, <u>assault</u>

T61.04x- Ciguatera fish poisoning, <u>undetermined</u>

T61.1- <u>Scombroid fish</u> poisoning
Histamine-like syndrome

T61.11x- Scombroid fish poisoning, <u>accidental</u> (unintentional)

T61.12x- Scombroid fish poisoning, <u>intentional</u> self-harm

T61.13x- Scombroid fish poisoning, <u>assault</u>

T61.14x- Scombroid fish poisoning, <u>undetermined</u>

T61.7- Other fish and shellfish poisoning

T61.77- <u>Other fish</u> poisoning

T61.771- Other fish poisoning, <u>accidental</u> (unintentional)

T61.772- Other fish poisoning, <u>intentional</u> self-harm

T61.773- Other fish poisoning, <u>assault</u>

T61.774- Other fish poisoning, <u>undetermined</u>

T61.78- <u>Other shellfish</u> poisoning

T61.781- Other shellfish poisoning, <u>accidental</u> (unintentional)

T61.782- Other shellfish poisoning, <u>intentional</u> self-harm

T61.783- Other shellfish poisoning, <u>assault</u>

T61.784- Other shellfish poisoning, <u>undetermined</u>

T61.8- Toxic effect of other seafood

T61.8x- Toxic effect of <u>other seafood</u>

T61.8x1- Toxic effect of other seafood, <u>accidental</u> (unintentional)

T61.8x2- Toxic effect of other seafood, <u>intentional</u> self-harm

T61.8x3- Toxic effect of other seafood, <u>assault</u>

T61.8x4- Toxic effect of other seafood, <u>undetermined</u>

T61.9- Toxic effect of <u>unspecified seafood</u>

T61.91x- Toxic effect of unspecified seafood, <u>accidental</u> (unintentional)

T61.92x- Toxic effect of unspecified seafood, <u>intentional</u> self-harm

T61.93x- Toxic effect of unspecified seafood, <u>assault</u>

T61.94x- Toxic effect of unspecified seafood, <u>undetermined</u>

T62- Toxic effect of <u>other noxious substances eaten as food</u>
Excludes 1: allergic reaction to food, such as:
anaphylactic shock (reaction) due to adverse food reaction (T78.0-)
bacterial food borne intoxications (A05.-)
dermatitis (L23.6, L25.4, L27.2)
gastroenteritis (noninfective) (K52.2)
toxic effect of aflatoxin and other mycotoxins (T64)
toxic effect of cyanides (T65.0-)
toxic effect of hydrogen cyanide (T57.3-)
toxic effect of mercury (T56.1-)

The appropriate 7th character is to be added to each code from category T62:
A <u>Initial</u> encounter
D <u>Subsequent</u> encounter
S <u>Sequela</u>

T62.0- Toxic effect of ingested mushrooms

T62.0x- Toxic effect of <u>ingested mushrooms</u>

T62.0x1- Toxic effect of ingested mushrooms, <u>accidental</u> (unintentional)
Toxic effect of ingested mushrooms NOS

T62.0x2- Toxic effect of ingested mushrooms, <u>intentional</u> self-harm

T62.0x3- Toxic effect of ingested mushrooms, <u>assault</u>

T62.0x4- Toxic effect of ingested mushrooms, <u>undetermined</u>

T62.1- Toxic effect of ingested berries

T62.1x- Toxic effect of <u>ingested berries</u>

T62.1x1- Toxic effect of ingested berries, <u>accidental</u> (unintentional)
Toxic effect of ingested berries NOS

T62.1x2- Toxic effect of ingested berries, <u>intentional</u> self-harm

T62.1x3- Toxic effect of ingested berries, <u>assault</u>

T62.1x4- Toxic effect of ingested berries, <u>undetermined</u>

T62.2- Toxic effect of other ingested (parts of) plant(s)

T62.2x- Toxic effect of <u>other ingested (parts of) plant(s)</u>

T62.2x1- Toxic effect of other ingested (parts of) plant(s), <u>accidental</u> (unintentional)
Toxic effect of other ingested (parts of) plant(s) NOS

T62.2x2- Toxic effect of other ingested (parts of) plant(s), <u>intentional</u> self-harm

T62.2x3- Toxic effect of other ingested (parts of) plant(s), <u>assault</u>

T62.2x4- Toxic effect of other ingested (parts of) plant(s), <u>undetermined</u>

T62.8- Toxic effect of other specified noxious substances eaten as food

T62.8x- Toxic effect of <u>other specified noxious substances eaten as food</u>

T62.8x1- Toxic effect of other specified noxious substances eaten as food, <u>accidental</u> (unintentional)
Toxic effect of other specified noxious substances eaten as food NOS

T62.8x2- Toxic effect of other specified noxious substances eaten as food, <u>intentional</u> self-harm

T62.8x3- Toxic effect of other specified noxious substances eaten as food, <u>assault</u>

T62.8x4- Toxic effect of other specified noxious substances eaten as food, <u>undetermined</u>

T62.9- Toxic effect of <u>unspecified noxious substance eaten as food</u>

T62.91x- Toxic effect of unspecified noxious substance eaten as food, <u>accidental</u> (unintentional)
Toxic effect of unspecified noxious substance eaten as food NOS

T62.92x- Toxic effect of unspecified noxious substance eaten as food, <u>intentional</u> self-harm

T62.93x- Toxic effect of unspecified noxious substance eaten as food, <u>assault</u>

T62.94x- Toxic effect of unspecified noxious substance eaten as food, <u>undetermined</u>

T60 - T63

© 2013 Channel Publishing, Ltd.

T63-   Toxic effect of <u>contact with venomous animals and plants</u>
    Includes: Bite or touch of venomous animal
                Pricked or stuck by thorn or leaf
    Excludes❷: ingestion of toxic animal or plant (T61.-, T62.-)
    The appropriate 7th character is to be added to each code from category T63:
    A   <u>Initial</u> encounter
    D   <u>Subsequent</u> encounter
    S   <u>Sequela</u>

T63.0-   Toxic effect of snake venom
    T63.00-   Toxic effect of <u>unspecified snake venom</u>
        T63.001-   Toxic effect of unspecified snake venom, <u>accidental</u> (unintentional)
                Toxic effect of unspecified snake venom NOS
        T63.002-   Toxic effect of unspecified snake venom, <u>intentional</u> self-harm
        T63.003-   Toxic effect of unspecified snake venom, <u>assault</u>
        T63.004-   Toxic effect of unspecified snake venom, <u>undetermined</u>
    T63.01-   Toxic effect of <u>rattlesnake venom</u>
        T63.011-   Toxic effect of rattlesnake venom, <u>accidental</u> (unintentional)
                Toxic effect of rattlesnake venom NOS
        T63.012-   Toxic effect of rattlesnake venom, <u>intentional</u> self-harm
        T63.013-   Toxic effect of rattlesnake venom, <u>assault</u>
        T63.014-   Toxic effect of rattlesnake venom, <u>undetermined</u>
    T63.02-   Toxic effect of <u>coral snake venom</u>
        T63.021-   Toxic effect of coral snake venom, <u>accidental</u> (unintentional)
                Toxic effect of coral snake venom NOS
        T63.022-   Toxic effect of coral snake venom, <u>intentional</u> self-harm
        T63.023-   Toxic effect of coral snake venom, <u>assault</u>
        T63.024-   Toxic effect of coral snake venom, <u>undetermined</u>
    T63.03-   Toxic effect of <u>taipan venom</u>
        T63.031-   Toxic effect of taipan venom, <u>accidental</u> (unintentional)
                Toxic effect of taipan venom NOS
        T63.032-   Toxic effect of taipan venom, <u>intentional</u> self-harm
        T63.033-   Toxic effect of taipan venom, <u>assault</u>
        T63.034-   Toxic effect of taipan venom, <u>undetermined</u>
    T63.04-   Toxic effect of <u>cobra venom</u>
        T63.041-   Toxic effect of cobra venom, <u>accidental</u> (unintentional)
                Toxic effect of cobra venom NOS
        T63.042-   Toxic effect of cobra venom, <u>intentional</u> self-harm
        T63.043-   Toxic effect of cobra venom, <u>assault</u>
        T63.044-   Toxic effect of cobra venom, <u>undetermined</u>
    T63.06-   Toxic effect of venom of <u>other North and South American snake</u>
        T63.061-   Toxic effect of venom of other North and South American snake, <u>accidental</u> (unintentional)
                Toxic effect of venom of other North and South American snake NOS
        T63.062-   Toxic effect of venom of other North and South American snake, <u>intentional</u> self-harm
        T63.063-   Toxic effect of venom of other North and South American snake, <u>assault</u>
        T63.064-   Toxic effect of venom of other North and South American snake, <u>undetermined</u>
    T63.07-   Toxic effect of venom of <u>other Australian snake</u>
        T63.071-   Toxic effect of venom of other Australian snake, <u>accidental</u> (unintentional)
                Toxic effect of venom of other Australian snake NOS
        T63.072-   Toxic effect of venom of other Australian snake, <u>intentional</u> self-harm
        T63.073-   Toxic effect of venom of other Australian snake, <u>assault</u>
        T63.074-   Toxic effect of venom of other Australian snake, <u>undetermined</u>
    T63.08-   Toxic effect of venom of <u>other African and Asian snake</u>
        T63.081-   Toxic effect of venom of other African and Asian snake, <u>accidental</u> (unintentional)
                Toxic effect of venom of other African and Asian snake NOS
        T63.082-   Toxic effect of venom of other African and Asian snake, <u>intentional</u> self-harm
        T63.083-   Toxic effect of venom of other African and Asian snake, <u>assault</u>
        T63.084-   Toxic effect of venom of other African and Asian snake, <u>undetermined</u>

T63.09-   Toxic effect of <u>venom of other snake</u>
        T63.091-   Toxic effect of venom of other snake, <u>accidental</u> (unintentional)
                Toxic effect of venom of other snake NOS
        T63.092-   Toxic effect of venom of other snake, <u>intentional</u> self-harm
        T63.093-   Toxic effect of venom of other snake, <u>assault</u>
        T63.094-   Toxic effect of venom of other snake, <u>undetermined</u>
T63.1-   Toxic effect of <u>venom of other reptiles</u>
    T63.11-   Toxic effect of <u>venom of gila monster</u>
        T63.111-   Toxic effect of venom of gila monster, <u>accidental</u> (unintentional)
                Toxic effect of venom of gila monster NOS
        T63.112-   Toxic effect of venom of gila monster, <u>intentional</u> self-harm
        T63.113-   Toxic effect of venom of gila monster, <u>assault</u>
        T63.114-   Toxic effect of venom of gila monster, <u>undetermined</u>
    T63.12-   Toxic effect of <u>venom of other venomous lizard</u>
        T63.121-   Toxic effect of venom of other venomous lizard, <u>accidental</u> (unintentional)
                Toxic effect of venom of other venomous lizard NOS
        T63.122-   Toxic effect of venom of other venomous lizard, <u>intentional</u> self-harm
        T63.123-   Toxic effect of venom of other venomous lizard, <u>assault</u>
        T63.124-   Toxic effect of venom of other venomous lizard, <u>undetermined</u>
    T63.19-   Toxic effect of <u>venom of other reptiles</u>
        T63.191-   Toxic effect of venom of other reptiles, <u>accidental</u> (unintentional)
                Toxic effect of venom of other reptiles NOS
        T63.192-   Toxic effect of venom of other reptiles, <u>intentional</u> self-harm
        T63.193-   Toxic effect of venom of other reptiles, <u>assault</u>
        T63.194-   Toxic effect of venom of other reptiles, <u>undetermined</u>
T63.2-   Toxic effect of venom of scorpion
    T63.2x-   Toxic effect of <u>venom of scorpion</u>
        T63.2x1-   Toxic effect of venom of scorpion, <u>accidental</u> (unintentional)
                Toxic effect of venom of scorpion NOS
        T63.2x2-   Toxic effect of venom of scorpion, <u>intentional</u> self-harm
        T63.2x3-   Toxic effect of venom of scorpion, <u>assault</u>
        T63.2x4-   Toxic effect of venom of scorpion, <u>undetermined</u>
T63.3-   Toxic effect of venom of spider
    T63.30-   Toxic effect of <u>unspecified spider venom</u>
        T63.301-   Toxic effect of unspecified spider venom, <u>accidental</u> (unintentional)
        T63.302-   Toxic effect of unspecified spider venom, <u>intentional</u> self-harm
        T63.303-   Toxic effect of unspecified spider venom, <u>assault</u>
        T63.304-   Toxic effect of unspecified spider venom, <u>undetermined</u>
    T63.31-   Toxic effect of <u>venom of black widow spider</u>
        T63.311-   Toxic effect of venom of black widow spider, <u>accidental</u> (unintentional)
        T63.312-   Toxic effect of venom of black widow spider, <u>intentional</u> self-harm
        T63.313-   Toxic effect of venom of black widow spider, <u>assault</u>
        T63.314-   Toxic effect of venom of black widow spider, <u>undetermined</u>
    T63.32-   Toxic effect of <u>venom of tarantula</u>
        T63.321-   Toxic effect of venom of tarantula, <u>accidental</u> (unintentional)
        T63.322-   Toxic effect of venom of tarantula, <u>intentional</u> self-harm
        T63.323-   Toxic effect of venom of tarantula, <u>assault</u>
        T63.324-   Toxic effect of venom of tarantula, <u>undetermined</u>
    T63.33-   Toxic effect of <u>venom of brown recluse spider</u>
        T63.331-   Toxic effect of venom of brown recluse spider, <u>accidental</u> (unintentional)
        T63.332-   Toxic effect of venom of brown recluse spider, <u>intentional</u> self-harm
        T63.333-   Toxic effect of venom of brown recluse spider, <u>assault</u>
        T63.334-   Toxic effect of venom of brown recluse spider, <u>undetermined</u>

T
6
0
|
T
6
3

Excludes 1: = NOT CODED HERE! (Do not code both)   **821**   *Excludes❷:* = Not Included Here

T63.39- Toxic effect of <u>venom of other spider</u>
    T63.391- Toxic effect of venom of other spider, <u>accidental</u> (unintentional)
    T63.392- Toxic effect of venom of other spider, <u>intentional</u> self-harm
    T63.393- Toxic effect of venom of other spider, <u>assault</u>
    T63.394- Toxic effect of venom of other spider, <u>undetermined</u>

T63.4- Toxic effect of venom of other arthropods
  T63.41- Toxic effect of <u>venom of centipedes and venomous millipedes</u>
    T63.411- Toxic effect of venom of centipedes and venomous millipedes, <u>accidental</u> (unintentional)
    T63.412- Toxic effect of venom of centipedes and venomous millipedes, <u>intentional</u> self-harm
    T63.413- Toxic effect of venom of centipedes and venomous millipedes, <u>assault</u>
    T63.414- Toxic effect of venom of centipedes and venomous millipedes, <u>undetermined</u>

  T63.42- Toxic effect of <u>venom of ants</u>
    T63.421- Toxic effect of venom of ants, <u>accidental</u> (unintentional)
    T63.422- Toxic effect of venom of ants, <u>intentional</u> self-harm
    T63.423- Toxic effect of venom of ants, <u>assault</u>
    T63.424- Toxic effect of venom of ants, <u>undetermined</u>

  T63.43- Toxic effect of <u>venom of caterpillars</u>
    T63.431- Toxic effect of venom of caterpillars, <u>accidental</u> (unintentional)
    T63.432- Toxic effect of venom of caterpillars, <u>intentional</u> self-harm
    T63.433- Toxic effect of venom of caterpillars, <u>assault</u>
    T63.434- Toxic effect of venom of caterpillars, <u>undetermined</u>

  T63.44- Toxic effect of <u>venom of bees</u>
    T63.441- Toxic effect of venom of bees, <u>accidental</u> (unintentional)
    T63.442- Toxic effect of venom of bees, <u>intentional</u> self-harm
    T63.443- Toxic effect of venom of bees, <u>assault</u>
    T63.444- Toxic effect of venom of bees, <u>undetermined</u>

  T63.45- Toxic effect of <u>venom of hornets</u>
    T63.451- Toxic effect of venom of hornets, <u>accidental</u> (unintentional)
    T63.452- Toxic effect of venom of hornets, <u>intentional</u> self-harm
    T63.453- Toxic effect of venom of hornets, <u>assault</u>
    T63.454- Toxic effect of venom of hornets, <u>undetermined</u>

  T63.46- Toxic effect of <u>venom of wasps</u>
    Toxic effect of yellow jacket
    T63.461- Toxic effect of venom of wasps, <u>accidental</u> (unintentional)
    T63.462- Toxic effect of venom of wasps, <u>intentional</u> self-harm
    T63.463- Toxic effect of venom of wasps, <u>assault</u>
    T63.464- Toxic effect of venom of wasps, <u>undetermined</u>

  T63.48- Toxic effect of <u>venom of other arthropod</u>
    T63.481- Toxic effect of venom of other arthropod, <u>accidental</u> (unintentional)
    T63.482- Toxic effect of venom of other arthropod, <u>intentional</u> self-harm
    T63.483- Toxic effect of venom of other arthropod, <u>assault</u>
    T63.484- Toxic effect of venom of other arthropod, <u>undetermined</u>

T63.5- Toxic effect of <u>contact with venomous fish</u>
  Excludes❷: poisoning by ingestion of fish (T61.-)
  T63.51- Toxic effect of <u>contact with stingray</u>
    T63.511- Toxic effect of contact with stingray, <u>accidental</u> (unintentional)
    T63.512- Toxic effect of contact with stingray, <u>intentional</u> self-harm
    T63.513- Toxic effect of contact with stingray, <u>assault</u>
    T63.514- Toxic effect of contact with stingray, <u>undetermined</u>

  T63.59- Toxic effect of <u>contact with other venomous fish</u>
    T63.591- Toxic effect of contact with other venomous fish, <u>accidental</u> (unintentional)
    T63.592- Toxic effect of contact with other venomous fish, <u>intentional</u> self-harm
    T63.593- Toxic effect of contact with other venomous fish, <u>assault</u>
    T63.594- Toxic effect of contact with other venomous fish, <u>undetermined</u>

T63.6- Toxic effect of <u>contact with other venomous marine animals</u>
  Excludes 1: sea-snake venom (T63.09)
  Excludes❷: poisoning by ingestion of shellfish (T61.78-)
  T63.61- Toxic effect of <u>contact with Portugese Man-o-war</u>
    Toxic effect of contact with bluebottle
    T63.611- Toxic effect of contact with Portugese Man-o-war, <u>accidental</u> (unintentional)
    T63.612- Toxic effect of contact with Portugese Man-o-war, <u>intentional</u> self-harm
    T63.613- Toxic effect of contact with Portugese Man-o-war, <u>assault</u>
    T63.614- Toxic effect of contact with Portugese Man-o-war, <u>undetermined</u>

  T63.62- Toxic effect of <u>contact with other jellyfish</u>
    T63.621- Toxic effect of contact with other jellyfish, <u>accidental</u> (unintentional)
    T63.622- Toxic effect of contact with other jellyfish, <u>intentional</u> self-harm
    T63.623- Toxic effect of contact with other jellyfish, <u>assault</u>
    T63.624- Toxic effect of contact with other jellyfish, <u>undetermined</u>

  T63.63- Toxic effect of <u>contact with sea anemone</u>
    T63.631- Toxic effect of contact with sea anemone, <u>accidental</u> (unintentional)
    T63.632- Toxic effect of contact with sea anemone, <u>intentional</u> self-harm
    T63.633- Toxic effect of contact with sea anemone, <u>assault</u>
    T63.634- Toxic effect of contact with sea anemone, <u>undetermined</u>

  T63.69- Toxic effect of <u>contact with other venomous marine animals</u>
    T63.691- Toxic effect of contact with other venomous marine animals, <u>accidental</u> (unintentional)
    T63.692- Toxic effect of contact with other venomous marine animals, <u>intentional</u> self-harm
    T63.693- Toxic effect of contact with other venomous marine animals, <u>assault</u>
    T63.694- Toxic effect of contact with other venomous marine animals, <u>undetermined</u>

T63.7- Toxic effect of contact with venomous plant
  T63.71- Toxic effect of <u>contact with venomous marine plant</u>
    T63.711- Toxic effect of contact with venomous marine plant, <u>accidental</u> (unintentional)
    T63.712- Toxic effect of contact with venomous marine plant, <u>intentional</u> self-harm
    T63.713- Toxic effect of contact with venomous marine plant, <u>assault</u>
    T63.714- Toxic effect of contact with venomous marine plant, <u>undetermined</u>

  T63.79- Toxic effect of <u>contact with other venomous plant</u>
    T63.791- Toxic effect of contact with other venomous plant, <u>accidental</u> (unintentional)
    T63.792- Toxic effect of contact with other venomous plant, <u>intentional</u> self-harm
    T63.793- Toxic effect of contact with other venomous plant, <u>assault</u>
    T63.794- Toxic effect of contact with other venomous plant, <u>undetermined</u>

T63.8- Toxic effect of contact with other venomous animals
  T63.81- Toxic effect of <u>contact with venomous frog</u>
    Excludes 1: contact with nonvenomous frog (W62.0)
    T63.811- Toxic effect of contact with venomous frog, <u>accidental</u> (unintentional)
    T63.812- Toxic effect of contact with venomous frog, <u>intentional</u> self-harm
    T63.813- Toxic effect of contact with venomous frog, <u>assault</u>
    T63.814- Toxic effect of contact with venomous frog, <u>undetermined</u>

  T63.82- Toxic effect of contact <u>with venomous toad</u>
    Excludes 1: contact with nonvenomous toad (W62.1)
    T63.821- Toxic effect of contact with venomous toad, <u>accidental</u> (unintentional)
    T63.822- Toxic effect of contact with venomous toad, <u>intentional</u> self-harm
    T63.823- Toxic effect of contact with venomous toad, <u>assault</u>
    T63.824- Toxic effect of contact with venomous toad, <u>undetermined</u>

T 6 3 ı T 6 5

T63.83- Toxic effect of contact with other venomous amphibian
Excludes 1: contact with nonvenomous amphibian (W62.9)
- **T63.831- Toxic effect of contact with other venomous amphibian, accidental (unintentional)**
- **T63.832- Toxic effect of contact with other venomous amphibian, intentional self-harm**
- **T63.833- Toxic effect of contact with other venomous amphibian, assault**
- **T63.834- Toxic effect of contact with other venomous amphibian, undetermined**

T63.89- Toxic effect of contact with other venomous animals
- **T63.891- Toxic effect of contact with other venomous animals, accidental (unintentional)**
- **T63.892- Toxic effect of contact with other venomous animals, intentional self-harm**
- **T63.893- Toxic effect of contact with other venomous animals, assault**
- **T63.894- Toxic effect of contact with other venomous animals, undetermined**

T63.9- Toxic effect of contact with unspecified venomous animal
- **T63.91x- Toxic effect of contact with unspecified venomous animal, accidental (unintentional)**
- **T63.92x- Toxic effect of contact with unspecified venomous animal, intentional self-harm**
- **T63.93x- Toxic effect of contact with unspecified venomous animal, assault**
- **T63.94x- Toxic effect of contact with unspecified venomous animal, undetermined**

T64- Toxic effect of aflatoxin and other mycotoxin food contaminants
The appropriate 7th character is to be added to each code from category T64:
- A Initial encounter
- D Subsequent encounter
- S Sequela

T64.0- Toxic effect of aflatoxin
- **T64.01x- Toxic effect of aflatoxin, accidental (unintentional)**
- **T64.02x- Toxic effect of aflatoxin, intentional self-harm**
- **T64.03x- Toxic effect of aflatoxin, assault**
- **T64.04x- Toxic effect of aflatoxin, undetermined**

T64.8- Toxic effect of other mycotoxin food contaminants
- **T64.81x- Toxic effect of other mycotoxin food contaminants, accidental (unintentional)**
- **T64.82x- Toxic effect of other mycotoxin food contaminants, intentional self-harm**
- **T64.83x- Toxic effect of other mycotoxin food contaminants, assault**
- **T64.84x- Toxic effect of other mycotoxin food contaminants, undetermined**

T65- Toxic effect of other and unspecified substances
The appropriate 7th character is to be added to each code from category T65:
- A Initial encounter
- D Subsequent encounter
- S Sequela

T65.0- Toxic effect of cyanides
Excludes 1: hydrogen cyanide (T57.3-)
T65.0x- Toxic effect of cyanides
- **T65.0x1- Toxic effect of cyanides, accidental (unintentional)**
  Toxic effect of cyanides NOS
- **T65.0x2- Toxic effect of cyanides, intentional self-harm**
- **T65.0x3- Toxic effect of cyanides, assault**
- **T65.0x4- Toxic effect of cyanides, undetermined**

T65.1- Toxic effect of strychnine and its salts
T65.1x- Toxic effect of strychnine and its salts
- **T65.1x1- Toxic effect of strychnine and its salts, accidental (unintentional)**
  Toxic effect of strychnine and its salts NOS
- **T65.1x2- Toxic effect of strychnine and its salts, intentional self-harm**
- **T65.1x3- Toxic effect of strychnine and its salts, assault**
- **T65.1x4- Toxic effect of strychnine and its salts, undetermined**

T65.2- Toxic effect of tobacco and nicotine
Excludes ❷: nicotine dependence (F17.-)
T65.21- Toxic effect of chewing tobacco
- **T65.211- Toxic effect of chewing tobacco, accidental (unintentional)**
  Toxic effect of chewing tobacco NOS
- **T65.212- Toxic effect of chewing tobacco, intentional self-harm**
- **T65.213- Toxic effect of chewing tobacco, assault**
- **T65.214- Toxic effect of chewing tobacco, undetermined**

T65.22- Toxic effect of tobacco cigarettes
Toxic effect of tobacco smoke
Use additional code for exposure to second hand tobacco smoke (Z57.31, Z77.22)
- **T65.221- Toxic effect of tobacco cigarettes, accidental (unintentional)**
  Toxic effect of tobacco cigarettes NOS
- **T65.222- Toxic effect of tobacco cigarettes, intentional self-harm**
- **T65.223- Toxic effect of tobacco cigarettes, assault**
- **T65.224- Toxic effect of tobacco cigarettes, undetermined**

T65.29- Toxic effect of other tobacco and nicotine
- **T65.291- Toxic effect of other tobacco and nicotine, accidental (unintentional)**
  Toxic effect of other tobacco and nicotine NOS
- **T65.292- Toxic effect of other tobacco and nicotine, intentional self-harm**
- **T65.293- Toxic effect of other tobacco and nicotine, assault**
- **T65.294- Toxic effect of other tobacco and nicotine, undetermined**

T65.3- Toxic effect of nitroderivatives and aminoderivatives of benzene and its homologues
Toxic effect of anilin [benzenamine]
Toxic effect of nitrobenzene
Toxic effect of trinitrotoluene
T65.3x- Toxic effect of nitroderivatives and aminoderivatives of benzene and its homologues
- **T65.3x1- Toxic effect of nitroderivatives and aminoderivatives of benzene and its homologues, accidental (unintentional)**
  Toxic effect of nitroderivatives and aminoderivatives of benzene and its homologues NOS
- **T65.3x2- Toxic effect of nitroderivatives and aminoderivatives of benzene and its homologues, intentional self-harm**
- **T65.3x3- Toxic effect of nitroderivatives and aminoderivatives of benzene and its homologues, assault**
- **T65.3x4- Toxic effect of nitroderivatives and aminoderivatives of benzene and its homologues, undetermined**

T65.4- Toxic effect of carbon disulfide
T65.4x- Toxic effect of carbon disulfide
- **T65.4x1- Toxic effect of carbon disulfide, accidental (unintentional)**
  Toxic effect of carbon disulfide NOS
- **T65.4x2- Toxic effect of carbon disulfide, intentional self-harm**
- **T65.4x3- Toxic effect of carbon disulfide, assault**
- **T65.4x4- Toxic effect of carbon disulfide, undetermined**

T65.5- Toxic effect of nitroglycerin and other nitric acids and esters
Toxic effect of 1,2,3-Propanetriol trinitrate
T65.5x- Toxic effect of nitroglycerin and other nitric acids and esters
- **T65.5x1- Toxic effect of nitroglycerin and other nitric acids and esters, accidental (unintentional)**
  Toxic effect of nitroglycerin and other nitric acids and esters NOS
- **T65.5x2- Toxic effect of nitroglycerin and other nitric acids and esters, intentional self-harm**
- **T65.5x3- Toxic effect of nitroglycerin and other nitric acids and esters, assault**
- **T65.5x4- Toxic effect of nitroglycerin and other nitric acids and esters, undetermined**

T65.6- Toxic effect of paints and dyes, not elsewhere classified
T65.6x- Toxic effect of paints and dyes, not elsewhere classified
- **T65.6x1- Toxic effect of paints and dyes, not elsewhere classified, accidental (unintentional)**
  Toxic effect of paints and dyes NOS
- **T65.6x2- Toxic effect of paints and dyes, not elsewhere classified, intentional self-harm**
- **T65.6x3- Toxic effect of paints and dyes, not elsewhere classified, assault**
- **T65.6x4- Toxic effect of paints and dyes, not elsewhere classified, undetermined**

T65.8- Toxic effect of other specified substances
T65.81- Toxic effect of latex
- **T65.811- Toxic effect of latex, accidental (unintentional)**
  Toxic effect of latex NOS
- **T65.812- Toxic effect of latex, intentional self-harm**
- **T65.813- Toxic effect of latex, assault**
- **T65.814- Toxic effect of latex, undetermined**

T 6 3 - T 6 5

T65.82- Toxic effect of <u>harmful algae and algae toxins</u>
    Toxic effect of (harmful) algae bloom NOS
    Toxic effect of blue-green algae bloom
    Toxic effect of brown tide
    Toxic effect of cyanobacteria bloom
    Toxic effect of Florida red tide
    Toxic effect of pfiesteria piscicida
    Toxic effect of red tide

    T65.821- Toxic effect of harmful algae and algae toxins, <u>accidental</u> **(unintentional)**
        Toxic effect of harmful algae and algae toxins NOS

    T65.822- Toxic effect of harmful algae and algae toxins, <u>intentional</u> **self-harm**

    T65.823- Toxic effect of harmful algae and algae toxins, <u>assault</u>

    T65.824- Toxic effect of harmful algae and algae toxins, <u>undetermined</u>

T65.83- Toxic effect of <u>fiberglass</u>

    T65.831- Toxic effect of fiberglass, <u>accidental</u> **(unintentional)**
        Toxic effect of fiberglass NOS

    T65.832- Toxic effect of fiberglass, <u>intentional</u> **self-harm**

    T65.833- Toxic effect of fiberglass, <u>assault</u>

    T65.834- Toxic effect of fiberglass, <u>undetermined</u>

T65.89- Toxic effect of <u>other specified substances</u>

    T65.891- Toxic effect of other specified substances, <u>accidental</u> **(unintentional)**
        Toxic effect of other specified substances NOS

    T65.892- Toxic effect of other specified substances, <u>intentional</u> **self-harm**

    T65.893- Toxic effect of other specified substances, <u>assault</u>

    T65.894- Toxic effect of other specified substances, <u>undetermined</u>

T65.9- Toxic effect of <u>unspecified substance</u>

    T65.91x- Toxic effect of unspecified substance, <u>accidental</u> **(unintentional)**
        Poisoning NOS

    T65.92x- Toxic effect of unspecified substance, <u>intentional</u> **self-harm**

    T65.93x- Toxic effect of unspecified substance, <u>assault</u>

    T65.94x- Toxic effect of unspecified substance, <u>undetermined</u>

Other and unspecified effects of external causes (T66-T78)

T66xxx- Radiation sickness, <u>unspecified</u>
  Excludes 1: radiation gastroenteritis and colitis (K52.0)
       radiation pneumonitis (J70.0)
       radiation related disorders of the skin and
         subcutaneous tissue (L55-L59)
       specified adverse effects of radiation, such as:
         burns (T20-T31)
         leukemia (C91-C95)
         sunburn (L55.-)

  The appropriate 7th character is to be added to code T66:
    A <u>Initial</u> **encounter**
    D <u>Subsequent</u> **encounter**
    S <u>Sequela</u>

T67- Effects of heat and light
  Excludes 1: erythema [dermatitis] ab igne (L59.0)
       malignant hyperpyrexia due to anesthesia (T88.3)
       radiation-related disorders of the skin and subcutaneous tissue
         (L55-L59)
  Excludes❷: burns (T20-T31)
       sunburn (L55.-)
       sweat disorder due to heat (L74-L75)

  The appropriate 7th character is to be added to each code from category T67:
    A <u>Initial</u> **encounter**
    D <u>Subsequent</u> **encounter**
    S <u>Sequela</u>

  T67.0xx- Heatstroke and sunstroke
    Heat apoplexy
    Heat pyrexia
    Siriasis
    Thermoplegia
    Use additional code(s) to identify any associated complications of
      heatstroke, such as:
    Coma and stupor (R40.-)
    Systemic inflammatory response syndrome (R65.1-)

  T67.1xx- Heat syncope
    Heat collapse

  T67.2xx- Heat cramp

  T67.3xx- Heat exhaustion, anhydrotic
    Heat prostration due to water depletion
    Excludes 1: heat exhaustion due to salt depletion (T67.4)

  T67.4xx- Heat exhaustion due to salt depletion
    Heat prostration due to salt (and water) depletion

  T67.5xx- Heat exhaustion, <u>unspecified</u>
    Heat prostration NOS

  T67.6xx- Heat fatigue, transient

  T67.7xx- Heat edema

  T67.8xx- Other effects of heat and light

  T67.9xx- Effect of heat and light, <u>unspecified</u>

T68xxx- Hypothermia
    Accidental hypothermia
    Hypothermia NOS
    Use additional code to identify source of exposure:
      Exposure to excessive cold of man-made origin (W93)
      Exposure to excessive cold of natural origin (X31)
  Excludes 1: hypothermia following anesthesia (T88.51)
       hypothermia not associated with low environmental
         temperature (R68.0)
       hypothermia of newborn (P80.-)
  Excludes❷: frostbite (T33-T34)

  The appropriate 7th character is to be added to code T68:
    A <u>Initial</u> **encounter**
    D <u>Subsequent</u> **encounter**
    S <u>Sequela</u>

T69- Other effects of reduced temperature
    Use additional code to identify source of exposure:
      Exposure to excessive cold of man-made origin (W93)
      Exposure to excessive cold of natural origin (X31)
  Excludes❷: frostbite (T33-T34)

  The appropriate 7th character is to be added to each code from category T69:
    A <u>Initial</u> **encounter**
    D <u>Subsequent</u> **encounter**
    S <u>Sequela</u>

  T69.0- Immersion hand and foot

    T69.01- Immersion <u>hand</u>

      T69.011- Immersion hand, <u>right</u> **hand**

      T69.012- Immersion hand, <u>left</u> **hand**

      T69.019- Immersion hand, <u>unspecified</u> **hand**

    T69.02- Immersion <u>foot</u>
      Trench foot

      T69.021- Immersion foot, <u>right</u> **foot**

      T69.022- Immersion foot, <u>left</u> **foot**

      T69.029- Immersion foot, <u>unspecified</u> **foot**

  T69.1xx- Chilblains

  T69.8xx- Other specified effects of reduced temperature

  T69.9xx- Effect of reduced temperature, unspecified

T70- Effects of air pressure and water pressure
  The appropriate 7th character is to be added to each code from category T70:
    A <u>Initial</u> **encounter**
    D <u>Subsequent</u> **encounter**
    S <u>Sequela</u>

  T70.0xx- Otitic barotrauma
    Aero-otitis media
    Effects of change in ambient atmospheric pressure or water
      pressure on ears

  T70.1xx- Sinus barotrauma
    Aerosinusitis
    Effects of change in ambient atmospheric pressure on sinuses

  T70.2- Other and <u>unspecified</u> **effects of high altitude**
    Excludes❷: polycythemia due to high altitude (D75.1)

    T70.20x- Unspecified effects of high altitude

    T70.29x- Other effects of high altitude
      Alpine sickness
      Anoxia due to high altitude
      Barotrauma NOS
      Hypobaropathy
      Mountain sickness

  T70.3xx- Caisson disease [decompression sickness]
    Compressed-air disease
    Diver's palsy or paralysis

  T70.4xx- Effects of high-pressure fluids
    Hydraulic jet injection (industrial)
    Pneumatic jet injection (industrial)
    Traumatic jet injection (industrial)

  T70.8xx- Other effects of air pressure and water pressure

  T70.9xx- Effect of air pressure and water pressure, unspecified

---

Excludes 1: = NOT CODED HERE! (Do not code both)   **824**   *Excludes❷:* = Not Included Here

T71- Asphyxiation
Mechanical suffocation
Traumatic suffocation
Excludes 1:   *acute respiratory distress (syndrome) (J80)*
anoxia due to high altitude (T70.2)
asphyxia NOS (R09.01)
asphyxia from carbon monoxide (T58-)
asphyxia from inhalation of food or foreign body (T17-)
asphyxia from other gases, fumes and vapors (T59-)
respiratory distress (syndrome) in newborn (P22-)

The appropriate 7th character is to be added to each code from category T71:
  A   Initial encounter
  D   Subsequent encounter
  S   Sequela

T71.1- Asphyxiation due to mechanical threat to breathing
Suffocation due to mechanical threat to breathing

T71.11- Asphyxiation due to smothering under pillow

T71.111- Asphyxiation due to smothering under pillow, accidental
Asphyxiation due to smothering under pillow NOS

T71.112- Asphyxiation due to smothering under pillow, intentional self-harm

T71.113- Asphyxiation due to smothering under pillow, assault

T71.114- Asphyxiation due to smothering under pillow, undetermined

T71.12- Asphyxiation due to plastic bag

T71.121- Asphyxiation due to plastic bag, accidental
Asphyxiation due to plastic bag NOS

T71.122- Asphyxiation due to plastic bag, intentional self-harm

T71.123- Asphyxiation due to plastic bag, assault

T71.124- Asphyxiation due to plastic bag, undetermined

T71.13- Asphyxiation due to being trapped in bed linens

T71.131- Asphyxiation due to being trapped in bed linens, accidental
Asphyxiation due to being trapped in bed linens NOS

T71.132- Asphyxiation due to being trapped in bed linens, intentional self-harm

T71.133- Asphyxiation due to being trapped in bed linens, assault

T71.134- Asphyxiation due to being trapped in bed linens, undetermined

T71.14- Asphyxiation due to smothering under another person's body (in bed)

T71.141- Asphyxiation due to smothering under another person's body (in bed), accidental
Asphyxiation due to smothering under another person's body (in bed) NOS

T71.143- Asphyxiation due to smothering under another person's body (in bed), assault

T71.144- Asphyxiation due to smothering under another person's body (in bed), undetermined

T71.15- Asphyxiation due to smothering in furniture

T71.151- Asphyxiation due to smothering in furniture, accidental
Asphyxiation due to smothering in furniture NOS

T71.152- Asphyxiation due to smothering in furniture, intentional self-harm

T71.153- Asphyxiation due to smothering in furniture, assault

T71.154- Asphyxiation due to smothering in furniture, undetermined

T71.16- Asphyxiation due to hanging
Hanging by window shade cord
Use additional code for any associated injuries, such as:
Crushing injury of neck (S17.-)
Fracture of cervical vertebrae (S12.0-S12.2-)
Open wound of neck (S11.-)

T71.161- Asphyxiation due to hanging, accidental
Asphyxiation due to hanging NOS
Hanging NOS

T71.162- Asphyxiation due to hanging, intentional self-harm

T71.163- Asphyxiation due to hanging, assault

T71.164- Asphyxiation due to hanging, undetermined

T71.19- Asphyxiation due to mechanical threat to breathing due to other causes

T71.191- Asphyxiation due to mechanical threat to breathing due to other causes, accidental
Asphyxiation due to other causes NOS

T71.192- Asphyxiation due to mechanical threat to breathing due to other causes, intentional self-harm

T71.193- Asphyxiation due to mechanical threat to breathing due to other causes, assault

T71.194- Asphyxiation due to mechanical threat to breathing due to other causes, undetermined

T71.2- Asphyxiation due to systemic oxygen deficiency due to low oxygen content in ambient air
Suffocation due to systemic oxygen deficiency due to low oxygen content in ambient air

T71.20x- Asphyxiation due to systemic oxygen deficiency due to low oxygen content in ambient air due to unspecified cause

T71.21x- Asphyxiation due to cave-in or falling earth
Use additional code for any associated cataclysm (X34-X38)

T71.22- Asphyxiation due to being trapped in a car trunk

T71.221- Asphyxiation due to being trapped in a car trunk, accidental

T71.222- Asphyxiation due to being trapped in a car trunk, intentional self-harm

T71.223- Asphyxiation due to being trapped in a car trunk, assault

T71.224- Asphyxiation due to being trapped in a car trunk, undetermined

T71.23- Asphyxiation due to being trapped in a (discarded) refrigerator

T71.231- Asphyxiation due to being trapped in a (discarded) refrigerator, accidental

T71.232- Asphyxiation due to being trapped in a (discarded) refrigerator, intentional self-harm

T71.233- Asphyxiation due to being trapped in a (discarded) refrigerator, assault

T71.234- Asphyxiation due to being trapped in a (discarded) refrigerator, undetermined

T71.29x- Asphyxiation due to being trapped in other low oxygen environment

T71.9xx- Asphyxiation due to unspecified cause
Suffocation (by strangulation) due to unspecified cause
Suffocation NOS
Systemic oxygen deficiency due to low oxygen content in ambient air due to unspecified cause
Systemic oxygen deficiency due to mechanical threat to breathing due to unspecified cause
Traumatic asphyxia NOS

T73- Effects of other deprivation
The appropriate 7th character is to be added to each code from category T73:
  A   Initial encounter
  D   Subsequent encounter
  S   Sequela

T73.0xx- Starvation
Deprivation of food

T73.1xx- Deprivation of water

T73.2xx- Exhaustion due to exposure

T73.3xx- Exhaustion due to excessive exertion
Exhaustion due to overexertion

T73.8xx- Other effects of deprivation

T73.9xx- Effect of deprivation, unspecified

T74- Adult and child abuse, neglect and other maltreatment, confirmed
Use additional code, if applicable, to identify any associated current injury
Use additional external cause code to identify perpetrator, if known (Y07-)
Excludes 1:   *abuse and maltreatment in pregnancy (O9A.3-, O9A.4-, O9A.5-)*
adult and child maltreatment, suspected (T76-)

The appropriate 7th character is to be added to each code from category T74:
  A   Initial encounter
  D   Subsequent encounter
  S   Sequela

T74.0- Neglect or abandonment, confirmed

T74.01x- Adult neglect or abandonment, confirmed

T74.02x- Child neglect or abandonment, confirmed

T74.1- Physical abuse, confirmed
Excludes❷: sexual abuse (T74.2-)

T74.11x- Adult physical abuse, confirmed

T74.12x- Child physical abuse, confirmed
Excludes❷: shaken infant syndrome (T74.4)

T74.2- Sexual abuse, confirmed
Rape, confirmed
Sexual assault, confirmed

T74.21x- Adult sexual abuse, confirmed

T74.22x- Child sexual abuse, confirmed

T
6
5
-
T
7
4

T74.3- __Psychological abuse, confirmed__

   T74.31x- __Adult__ psychological abuse, __confirmed__

   T74.32x- __Child__ psychological abuse, __confirmed__

T74.4xx- Shaken infant syndrome

T74.9- __Unspecified maltreatment, confirmed__

   T74.91x- Unspecified __adult__ maltreatment, __confirmed__

   T74.92x- Unspecified __child__ maltreatment, __confirmed__

T75- Other and unspecified effects of other external causes

  Excludes 1: adverse effects NEC (T78.-)

  Excludes❷: burns (electric) (T20-T31)

  The appropriate 7th character is to be added to each code from category T75:

  A __Initial__ encounter

  D __Subsequent__ encounter

  S __Sequela__

T75.0- Effects of lightning

   Struck by lightning

  T75.00x- __Unspecified effects of lightning__

   Struck by lightning NOS

  T75.01x- __Shock due to being struck by lightning__

  T75.09x- __Other effects of lightning__

   Use additional code for other effects of lightning

T75.1xx- Unspecified effects of drowning and nonfatal submersion

   Immersion

   Excludes 1: specified effects of drowning — code to effects

T75.2- Effects of vibration

  T75.20x- __Unspecified effects of vibration__

  T75.21x- __Pneumatic hammer syndrome__

  T75.22x- __Traumatic vasospastic syndrome__

  T75.23x- __Vertigo from infrasound__

   Excludes 1: vertigo NOS (R42)

  T75.29- Other effects of vibration

T75.3xx- Motion sickness

   Airsickness

   Seasickness

   Travel sickness

   Use additional external cause code to identify vehicle or type of motion (Y92.81-, Y93.5-)

T75.4xx- Electrocution

   Shock from electric current

   Shock from electroshock gun (taser)

T75.8- Other specified effects of external causes

  T75.81x- __Effects of abnormal gravitation [G] forces__

  T75.82x- __Effects of weightlessness__

  T75.89x- __Other specified effects of external causes__

T76- Adult and child abuse, neglect and other maltreatment, __suspected__

  Use additional code, if applicable, to identify any associated current injury

  Excludes 1: adult and child maltreatment, confirmed (T74.-)

   suspected abuse and maltreatment in pregnancy (O9A.3-, O9A.4-, O9A.5-)

   suspected adult physical abuse, ruled out (Z04.71)

   suspected adult sexual abuse, ruled out (Z04.41)

   suspected child physical abuse, ruled out (Z04.72)

   suspected child sexual abuse, ruled out (Z04.42)

  The appropriate 7th character is to be added to each code from category T76:

  A __Initial__ encounter

  D __Subsequent__ encounter

  S __Sequela__

T76.0- __Neglect or abandonment, suspected__

  T76.01x- __Adult__ neglect or abandonment, suspected

  T76.02x- __Child__ neglect or abandonment, suspected

T76.1- __Physical abuse, suspected__

  T76.11x- __Adult__ physical abuse, suspected

  T76.12x- __Child__ physical abuse, suspected

T76.2- __Sexual abuse, suspected__

   Rape, suspected

   Sexual abuse, suspected

   Excludes 1: alleged abuse, ruled out (Z04.7)

  T76.21x- __Adult__ sexual abuse, suspected

  T76.22x- __Child__ sexual abuse, suspected

T76.3- __Psychological abuse, suspected__

  T76.31x- __Adult__ psychological abuse, suspected

  T76.32x- __Child__ psychological abuse, suspected

T76.9- __Unspecified maltreatment, suspected__

  T76.91x- Unspecified __adult__ maltreatment, suspected

  T76.92x- Unspecified __child__ maltreatment, suspected

T78- Adverse effects, __not elsewhere classified__

  Excludes❷: complications of surgical and medical care NEC (T80-T88)

  The appropriate 7th character is to be added to each code from category T78:

  A __Initial__ encounter

  D __Subsequent__ encounter

  S __Sequela__

T78.0- __Anaphylactic reaction due to food__

   Anaphylactic reaction due to adverse food reaction

   Anaphylactic shock or reaction due to nonpoisonous foods

   Anaphylactoid reaction due to food

  T78.00x- **Anaphylactic reaction due to unspecified food**

  T78.01x- **Anaphylactic reaction due to peanuts**

  T78.02x- **Anaphylactic reaction due to shellfish (crustaceans)**

  T78.03x- **Anaphylactic reaction due to other fish**

  T78.04x- **Anaphylactic reaction due to fruits and vegetables**

  T78.05x- **Anaphylactic reaction due to tree nuts and seeds**

   Excludes 1: anaphylactic reaction due to peanuts (T78.01)

  T78.06x- **Anaphylactic reaction due to food additives**

  T78.07x- **Anaphylactic reaction due to milk and dairy products**

  T78.08x- **Anaphylactic reaction due to eggs**

  T78.09x- **Anaphylactic reaction due to other food products**

T78.1xx- Other adverse food reactions, __not elsewhere classified__

   Use additional code to identify the type of reaction

   Excludes 1: anaphylactic reaction or shock due to adverse food reaction (T78.0-)

    anaphylactic reaction due to food (T78.0-)

    bacterial food borne intoxications (A05-)

   Excludes❷: allergic and dietetic gastroenteritis and colitis (K52.2)

    allergic rhinitis due to food (J30.5)

    dermatitis due to food in contact with skin (L23.6, L24.6, L25.4)

    dermatitis due to ingested food (L27.2)

T78.2xx- Anaphylactic shock, __unspecified__

   Allergic shock

   Anaphylactic reaction

   Anaphylaxis

   Excludes 1: anaphylactic reaction or shock due to adverse effect of correct medicinal substance properly administered (T88.6)

    anaphylactic reaction or shock due to adverse food reaction (T78.0-)

    anaphylactic reaction or shock due to serum (T80.5)

T78.3xx- Angioneurotic edema

   Allergic angioedema

   Giant urticaria

   Quincke's edema

   Excludes 1: serum urticaria (T80.6-)

    urticaria (L50-)

T78.4- Other and unspecified allergy

   Excludes 1: specified types of allergic reaction such as:

    allergic diarrhea (K52.2)

    allergic gastroenteritis and colitis (K52.2)

    dermatitis (L23-L25, L27.-)

    hay fever (J30.1)

  T78.40x- **Allergy, unspecified**

   Allergic reaction NOS

   Hypersensitivity NOS

  T78.41x- **Arthus phenomenon**

   Arthus reaction

  T78.49x- **Other allergy**

T78.8xx- Other adverse effects, not elsewhere classified

Excludes 1: = NOT CODED HERE! (Do not code both)

Excludes❷: = Not Included Here

Certain early complications of trauma (T79)

T79- Certain early complications of trauma, <u>not elsewhere classified</u>
  Excludes❷: *acute respiratory distress syndrome (J80)*
        complications occurring during or following medical
            procedures (T80-T88)
        complications of surgical and medical care NEC (T80-T88)
        newborn respiratory distress syndrome (P22.0)

  The appropriate 7th character is to be added to each code from
    category T79:
    A <u>**Initial**</u> **encounter**
    D <u>**Subsequent**</u> **encounter**
    S <u>**Sequela**</u>

T79.0xx- **Air embolism (traumatic)**
  Excludes 1: *air embolism complicating abortion or ectopic or*
        molar pregnancy (O00-O07, O08.2)
      air embolism complicating pregnancy, childbirth and
        the puerperium (O88.0)
      air embolism following infusion, transfusion, and
        therapeutic injection (T80.0)
      air embolism following procedure NEC (T81.7-)

T79.1xx- **Fat embolism (traumatic)**
  Excludes 1: *fat embolism complicating:*
        abortion or ectopic or molar pregnancy (O00-O07,
          O08.2)
        pregnancy, childbirth and the puerperium (O88.8)

T79.2xx- **Traumatic secondary and recurrent hemorrhage and seroma**

T79.4xx- **Traumatic shock**
    Shock (immediate) (delayed) following injury
  Excludes 1: *anaphylactic shock due to adverse food reaction*
        (T78.0-)
      anaphylactic shock due to correct medicinal
        substance properly administered (T88.6)
      anaphylactic shock due to serum (T80.5-)
      anaphylactic shock NOS (T78.2)
      anesthetic shock (T88.2)
      electric shock (T75.4)
      nontraumatic shock NEC (R57-)
      obstetric shock (O75.1)
      postprocedural shock (T81.1-)
      septic shock (R65.21)
      shock complicating abortion or ectopic or molar
        pregnancy (O00-O07, O08.3)
      shock due to lightning (T75.01)
      shock NOS (R57.9)

T79.5xx- **Traumatic anuria**
    Crush syndrome
    Renal failure following crushing

T79.6xx- **Traumatic ischemia of muscle**
    Traumatic rhabdomyolysis
    Volkmann's ischemic contracture
  Excludes❷: *anterior tibial syndrome (M76.8)*
      compartment syndrome (traumatic) (T79.A-)
      nontraumatic ischemia of muscle (M62.2-)

T79.7xx- **Traumatic subcutaneous emphysema**
  Excludes 1: *emphysema NOS (J43)*
      emphysema (subcutaneous) resulting from a
        procedure (T81.82)

T79.A- **Traumatic compartment syndrome**
  Excludes 1: *fibromyalgia (M79.7)*
      nontraumatic compartment syndrome (M79.A-)
      traumatic ischemic infarction of muscle (T79.6)

  T79.A0- **Compartment syndrome, <u>unspecified</u>**
      Compartment syndrome NOS

  T79.A1- **Traumatic compartment syndrome of <u>upper extremity</u>**
      Traumatic compartment syndrome of shoulder, arm, forearm,
        wrist, hand, and fingers

    T79.A11- **Traumatic compartment syndrome of <u>right</u> upper extremity**

    T79.A12- **Traumatic compartment syndrome of <u>left</u> upper extremity**

    T79.A19- **Traumatic compartment syndrome of <u>unspecified</u> upper extremity**

  T79.A2- **Traumatic compartment syndrome of <u>lower extremity</u>**
      Traumatic compartment syndrome of hip, buttock, thigh, leg,
        foot, and toes

    T79.A21- **Traumatic compartment syndrome of <u>right</u> lower extremity**

    T79.A22- **Traumatic compartment syndrome of <u>left</u> lower extremity**

    T79.A29- **Traumatic compartment syndrome of <u>unspecified</u> lower extremity**

T79.A3x- Traumatic compartment syndrome of <u>abdomen</u>
T79.A9x- Traumatic compartment syndrome of <u>other</u> sites
T79.8xx- Other early complications of trauma
T79.9xx- Unspecified early complication of trauma

Complications of surgical and medical care, not elsewhere classified (T80-T88)

Use additional code for adverse effect, if applicable, to identify drug (T36-T50 with fifth or sixth character 5)
Use additional code(s) to identify the specified condition resulting from the complication
Use additional code to identify devices involved and details of circumstances (Y62-Y82)
  Excludes❷: *any encounters with medical care for postprocedural*
        conditions in which no complications are present, such
        as:
      artificial opening status (Z93-)
      closure of external stoma (Z43-)
      fitting and adjustment of external prosthetic device (Z44-)
    burns and corrosions from local applications and irradiation
        (T20-T32)
    complications of surgical procedures during pregnancy,
        childbirth and the puerperium (O00-O9A)
    mechanical complication of respirator [ventilator] (J95.850)
    poisoning and toxic effects of drugs and chemicals (T36-T65
        with fifth or sixth characters 1-4 or 6)
    postprocedural fever (R50.82)
    specified complications classified elsewhere, such as:
      cerebrospinal fluid leak from spinal puncture (G97.0)
      colostomy malfunction (K94.0-)
      disorders of fluid and electrolyte imbalance (E86-E87)
      functional disturbances following cardiac surgery (I97.0-
        I97.1)
      intraoperative and postprocedural complications of
        specified body systems (D78-, E36-, E89-, G97.3-,
        G97.4, H59.3-, H59-, H95.2-, H95.3, I97.4-, I97.5,
        J95.6-, J95.7, K91.6-, L76-, M96-, N99-)
      ostomy complications (J95.0-, K94.-, N99.5-)
      postgastric surgery syndromes (K91.1)
      postlaminectomy syndrome NEC (M96.1)
      postmastectomy lymphedema syndrome (I97.2)
      postsurgical blind-loop syndrome (K91.2)
      ventilator associated pneumonia (J95.851)

T80- **Complications following <u>infusion, transfusion and therapeutic injection</u>**
  Includes: complications following perfusion
  Excludes❷: *bone marrow transplant rejection (T86.01)*
      febrile nonhemolytic transfusion reaction (R50.84)
      fluid overload due to transfusion (E87.71)
      posttransfusion purpura (D69.51)
      transfusion associated circulatory overload (TACO) (E87.71)
      transfusion (red blood cell) associated hemochromatosis
        (E83.111)
      transfusion related acute lung injury (TRALI) (J95.84)

  The appropriate 7th character is to be added to each code from
    category T80:
    A <u>**Initial**</u> **encounter**
    D <u>**Subsequent**</u> **encounter**
    S <u>**Sequela**</u>

T80.0xx- <u>**Air embolism**</u> **following infusion, transfusion and therapeutic injection**

T80.1xx- <u>**Vascular complications**</u> **following infusion, transfusion and therapeutic injection**
    Use additional code to identify the vascular complication
  Excludes❷: *extravasation of vesicant agent (T80.81-)*
      infiltration of vesicant agent (T80.81-)
      postprocedural vascular complications (T81.7-)
      vascular complications specified as due to prosthetic
        devices, implants and grafts (T82.8-, T83.8,
        T84.8-, T85.8)

T
7
4
–
T
8
0

T80.2- <u>Infections</u> following infusion, transfusion and therapeutic injection

Use additional code to identify the specific infection, such as:
Sepsis (A41.9)

Use additional code (R65.2-) to identify severe sepsis, if applicable

Excludes❷: infections specified as due to prosthetic devices, implants and grafts (T82.6-T82.7, T83.5-T83.6, T84.5-T84.7, T85.7)
postprocedural infections (T81.4)

T80.21- Infection <u>due to central venous catheter</u>

T80.211- <u>Bloodstream</u> infection due to central venous catheter

Catheter-related bloodstream infection (CRBSI) NOS

Central line-associated bloodstream infection (CLABSI)

Bloodstream infection due to Hickman catheter

Bloodstream infection due to peripherally inserted central catheter (PICC)

Bloodstream infection due to portacath (port-a-cath)

Bloodstream infection due to triple lumen catheter

Bloodstream infection due to umbilical venous catheter

T80.212- <u>Local</u> infection due to central venous catheter

Exit or insertion site infection

Local infection due to Hickman catheter

Local infection due to peripherally inserted central catheter (PICC)

Local infection due to portacath (port-a-cath)

Local infection due to triple lumen catheter

Local infection due to umbilical venous catheter

Port or reservoir infection

Tunnel infection

T80.218- <u>Other</u> infection due to central venous catheter

Other central line-associated infection

Other infection due to Hickman catheter

Other infection due to peripherally inserted central catheter (PICC)

Other infection due to portacath (port-a-cath)

Other infection due to triple lumen catheter

Other infection due to umbilical venous catheter

T80.219- <u>Unspecified</u> infection due to central venous catheter

Central line-associated infection NOS

Unspecified infection due to Hickman catheter

Unspecified infection due to peripherally inserted central catheter (PICC)

Unspecified infection due to portacath (port-a-cath)

Unspecified infection due to triple lumen catheter

Unspecified infection due to umbilical venous catheter

T80.22x- <u>Acute infection</u> following transfusion, infusion, or injection of <u>blood and blood products</u>

T80.29x- Infection following <u>other infusion, transfusion and therapeutic injection</u>

T80.3- <u>ABO incompatibility reaction</u> due to transfusion of blood or blood products

Excludes 1: minor blood group antigens reactions (Duffy) (E) (K(ell)) (Kidd) (Lewis) (M) (N) (P) (S) (T80.A)

T80.30- ABO incompatibility reaction due to transfusion of blood or blood products, <u>unspecified</u>

ABO incompatibility blood transfusion NOS

Reaction to ABO incompatibility from transfusion NOS

T80.31- ABO incompatibility <u>with hemolytic transfusion reaction</u>

T80.310- ABO incompatibility with <u>acute</u> hemolytic transfusion reaction

ABO incompatibility with hemolytic transfusion reaction less than 24 hours after transfusion

Acute hemolytic transfusion reaction (AHTR) due to ABO incompatibility

T80.311- ABO incompatibility with <u>delayed</u> hemolytic transfusion reaction

ABO incompatibility with hemolytic transfusion reaction 24 hours or more after transfusion

Delayed hemolytic transfusion reaction (DHTR) due to ABO incompatibility

T80.319- ABO incompatibility with hemolytic transfusion reaction, <u>unspecified</u>

ABO incompatibility with hemolytic transfusion reaction at unspecified time after transfusion

Hemolytic transfusion reaction (HTR) due to ABO incompatibility NOS

T80.39x- <u>Other</u> ABO incompatibility reaction due to transfusion of blood or blood products

Delayed serologic transfusion reaction (DSTR) from ABO incompatibility

Other ABO incompatible blood transfusion

Other reaction to ABO incompatible blood transfusion

T80.4- <u>Rh incompatibility reaction</u> due to transfusion of blood or blood products

Reaction due to incompatibility of Rh antigens (C) (c) (D) (E) (e)

T80.40x- Rh incompatibility reaction due to transfusion of blood or blood products, <u>unspecified</u>

Reaction due to Rh factor in transfusion NOS

Rh incompatible blood transfusion NOS

T80.41- Rh incompatibility <u>with hemolytic transfusion reaction</u>

T80.410- Rh incompatibility with <u>acute</u> hemolytic transfusion reaction

Acute hemolytic transfusion reaction (AHTR) due to Rh incompatibility

Rh incompatibility with hemolytic transfusion reaction less than 24 hours after transfusion

T80.411- Rh incompatibility with <u>delayed</u> hemolytic transfusion reaction

Delayed hemolytic transfusion reaction (DHTR) due to Rh incompatibility

Rh incompatibility with hemolytic transfusion reaction 24 hours or more after transfusion

T80.419- Rh incompatibility with hemolytic transfusion reaction, <u>unspecified</u>

Rh incompatibility with hemolytic transfusion reaction at unspecified time after transfusion

Hemolytic transfusion reaction (HTR) due to Rh incompatibility NOS

T80.49x- <u>Other</u> Rh incompatibility reaction due to transfusion of blood or blood products

Delayed serologic transfusion reaction (DSTR) from Rh incompatibility

Other reaction to Rh incompatible blood transfusion

T80.A- <u>Non-ABO incompatibility reaction</u> due to transfusion of blood or blood products

Reaction due to incompatibility of minor antigens (Duffy) (Kell) (Kidd) (Lewis) (M) (N) (P) (S)

T80.A0x- Non-ABO incompatibility reaction due to transfusion of blood or blood products, <u>unspecified</u>

Non-ABO antigen incompatibility reaction from transfusion NOS

T80.A1- Non-ABO incompatibility <u>with hemolytic transfusion reaction</u>

T80.A10- Non-ABO incompatibility with <u>acute</u> hemolytic transfusion reaction

Acute hemolytic transfusion reaction (AHTR) due to non-ABO incompatibility

Non-ABO incompatibility with hemolytic transfusion reaction less than 24 hours after transfusion

T80.A11- Non-ABO incompatibility with <u>delayed</u> hemolytic transfusion reaction

Delayed hemolytic transfusion reaction (DHTR) due to non-ABO incompatibility

Non-ABO incompatibility with hemolytic transfusion reaction 24 or more hours after transfusion

T80.A19- Non-ABO incompatibility with hemolytic transfusion reaction, <u>unspecified</u>

Hemolytic transfusion reaction (HTR) due to non-ABO incompatibility NOS

Non-ABO incompatibility with hemolytic transfusion reaction at unspecified time after transfusion

T80.A9x- <u>Other</u> non-ABO incompatibility reaction due to transfusion of blood or blood products

Delayed serologic transfusion reaction (DSTR) from non-ABO incompatibility

Other reaction to non-ABO incompatible blood transfusion

T80.5- Anaphylactic reaction due to serum

Allergic shock due to serum

Anaphylactic shock due to serum

Anaphylactoid reaction due to serum

Anaphylaxis due to serum

Excludes 1: ABO incompatibility reaction due to transfusion of blood or blood products (T80.3-)
allergic reaction or shock NOS (T78.2)
anaphylactic reaction or shock NOS (T78.2)
anaphylactic reaction or shock due to adverse effect of correct medicinal substance properly administered (T88.6)
other serum reaction (T80.6-)

T80.51x- Anaphylactic reaction due to administration of blood and blood products

T80.52x- Anaphylactic reaction due to vaccination

T80.59x- Anaphylactic reaction due to other serum

T
8
0
-
T
8
1

T80.6- **Other serum reactions**
　　Intoxication by serum
　　Protein sickness
　　Serum rash
　　Serum sickness
　　Serum urticaria
　　Excludes❷: serum hepatitis (B16-)

　T80.61x- Other serum reaction due to administration of blood and blood products

　T80.62x- Other serum reaction due to vaccination

　T80.69x- Other serum reaction due to other serum

T80.8- **Other complications following infusion, transfusion and therapeutic injection**

　T80.81- Extravasation of vesicant agent
　　Infiltration of vesicant agent

　　T80.810- Extravasation of vesicant antineoplastic chemotherapy
　　　Infiltration of vesicant antineoplastic chemotherapy

　　T80.818- Extravasation of other vesicant agent
　　　Infiltration of other vesicant agent

　T80.89x- Other complications following infusion, transfusion and therapeutic injection
　　Delayed serologic transfusion reaction (DSTR), unspecified incompatibility
　　Use additional code to identify graft-versus-host reaction, if applicable, (D89.81-)

T80.9- **Unspecified complication following infusion, transfusion and therapeutic injection**

　T80.90x- Unspecified complication following infusion and therapeutic injection

　T80.91- Hemolytic transfusion reaction, unspecified incompatibility
　　Excludes 1: ABO incompatibility with hemolytic transfusion reaction (T80.31-)
　　　Non-ABO incompatibility with hemolytic transfusion reaction (T80.A1-)
　　　Rh incompatibility with hemolytic transfusion reaction (T80.41-)

　　T80.910- Acute hemolytic transfusion reaction, unspecified incompatibility

　　T80.911- Delayed hemolytic transfusion reaction, unspecified incompatibility

　　T80.919- Hemolytic transfusion reaction, unspecified incompatibility, unspecified as acute ordelayed
　　　Hemolytic transfusion reaction NOS

　T80.92x- Unspecified transfusion reaction
　　Transfusion reaction NOS

T81- **Complications of procedures, not elsewhere classified**
　Use additional code for adverse effect, if applicable, to identify drug (T36-T50 with fifth or sixth character 5)
　Excludes❷: complications following immunization (T88.0-T88.1)
　　complications following infusion, transfusion and therapeutic injection (T80-)
　　complications of transplanted organs and tissue (T86-)
　　specified complications classified elsewhere, such as:
　　　complication of prosthetic devices, implants and grafts (T82-T85)
　　　dermatitis due to drugs and medicaments (L23.3, L24.4, L25.1, L27.0-L27.1)
　　　endosseous dental implant failure (M27.6-)
　　　floppy iris syndrome (IFIS) (intraoperative) H21.81
　　　intraoperative and postprocedural complications of specific body system (D78.-, E36.-, E89.-, G97.3-, G97.4, H59.3-, H59.-, H95.2-, H95.3, I97.4-, I97.5, J95, K91.-, L76.-, M96.-, N99.-)
　　　ostomy complications (J95.0-, K94.-, N99.5-)
　　　plateau iris syndrome (post-iridectomy) (postprocedural) H21.82
　　　poisoning and toxic effects of drugs and chemicals (T36-T65 with fifth or sixth character 1-4 or 6)

The appropriate 7th character is to be added to each code from category T81:
A   Initial encounter
D   Subsequent encounter
S   Sequela

T81.1- Postprocedural shock
　Shock during or resulting from a procedure, not elsewhere classified
　Excludes 1: anaphylactic shock NOS (T78.2)
　　anaphylactic shock due to correct substance properly administered (T88.6)
　　anaphylactic shock due to serum (T80.5-)
　　anesthetic shock (T88.2)
　　electric shock (T75.4)
　　obstetric shock (O75.1)
　　septic shock (R65.21)
　　shock following abortion or ectopic or molar pregnancy (O00-O07, O08.3)
　　traumatic shock (T79.4)

　T81.10x- Postprocedural shock, unspecified
　　Collapse NOS during or resulting from a procedure, not elsewhere classified
　　Postprocedural failure of peripheral circulation
　　Postprocedural shock NOS

　T81.11x- Postprocedural cardiogenic shock

　T81.12x- Postprocedural septic shock
　　Postprocedural endotoxic shock during or resulting from a procedure, not elsewhere classified
　　Postprocedural gram-negative shock during or resulting from a procedure, not elsewhere classified
　　Code first underlying infection
　　Use additional code, to identify any associated acute organ dysfunction, if applicable

　T81.19x- Other postprocedural shock
　　Postprocedural hypovolemic shock

T81.3- Disruption of wound, not elsewhere classified
　Disruption of any suture materials or other closure methods
　Excludes 1: breakdown (mechanical) of permanent sutures (T85.612)
　　displacement of permanent sutures (T85.622)
　　disruption of cesarean delivery wound (O90.0)
　　disruption of perineal obstetric wound (O90.1)
　　mechanical complication of permanent sutures NEC (T85.692)

　T81.30x- Disruption of wound, unspecified
　　Disruption of wound NOS

　T81.31x- Disruption of external operation (surgical) wound, not elsewhere classified
　　Dehiscence of operation wound NOS
　　Disruption of operation wound NOS
　　Disruption or dehiscence of closure of cornea
　　Disruption or dehiscence of closure of mucosa
　　Disruption or dehiscence of closure of skin and subcutaneous tissue
　　Full-thickness skin disruption or dehiscence
　　Superficial disruption or dehiscence of operation wound
　　Excludes 1: dehiscence of amputation stump (T87.81)

T80 - T81

Excludes 1: = NOT CODED HERE! (Do not code both)   **829**   *Excludes❷: = Not Included Here*

T81.32x- Disruption of <u>internal</u> operation (surgical) wound, not elsewhere classified
Deep disruption or dehiscence of operation wound NOS
Disruption or dehiscence of closure of internal organ or other internal tissue
Disruption or dehiscence of closure of muscle or muscle flap
Disruption or dehiscence of closure of ribs or rib cage
Disruption or dehiscence of closure of skull or craniotomy
Disruption or dehiscence of closure of sternum or sternotomy
Disruption or dehiscence of closure of tendon or ligament
Disruption or dehiscence of closure of superficial or muscular fascia

T81.33x- Disruption of <u>traumatic</u> injury wound repair
Disruption or dehiscence of closure of traumatic laceration (external) (internal)

T81.4xx- Infection following a procedure
Intra-abdominal abscess following a procedure
Postprocedural infection, not elsewhere classified
Sepsis following a procedure
Stitch abscess following a procedure
Subphrenic abscess following a procedure
Wound abscess following a procedure
Use additional code to identify infection
Use additional code (R65.2-) to identify severe sepsis, if applicable
Excludes 1:   obstetric surgical wound infection (O86.0)
postprocedural fever NOS (R50.82)
postprocedural retroperitoneal abscess (K68.11)
Excludes❷: bleb associated endophthalmitis (H59.4-)
infection due to infusion, transfusion and therapeutic injection (T80.2-)
infection due to prosthetic devices, implants and grafts (T82.6-T82.7, T83.5-T83.6, T84.5-T84.7, T85.7)

T81.5-   Complications of foreign body accidentally left in body following procedure
T81.50- <u>Unspecified complication</u> of <u>foreign body accidentally left in body following procedure</u>
T81.500-   Unspecified complication of foreign body accidentally left in body following <u>surgical operation</u>
T81.501-   Unspecified complication of foreign body accidentally left in body following <u>infusion or transfusion</u>
T81.502-   Unspecified complication of foreign body accidentally left in body following <u>kidney dialysis</u>
T81.503-   Unspecified complication of foreign body accidentally left in body following <u>injection or immunization</u>
T81.504-   Unspecified complication of foreign body accidentally left in body following <u>endoscopic examination</u>
T81.505-   Unspecified complication of foreign body accidentally left in body following <u>heart catheterization</u>
T81.506-   Unspecified complication of foreign body accidentally left in body following <u>aspiration, puncture or other catheterization</u>
T81.507-   Unspecified complication of foreign body accidentally left in body following <u>removal of catheter or packing</u>
T81.508-   Unspecified complication of foreign body accidentally left in body following <u>other procedure</u>
T81.509-   Unspecified complication of foreign body accidentally left in body following <u>unspecified procedure</u>
T81.51- <u>Adhesions</u> due to <u>foreign body accidentally left in body following procedure</u>
T81.510-   Adhesions due to foreign body accidentally left in body following <u>surgical operation</u>
T81.511-   Adhesions due to foreign body accidentally left in body following <u>infusion or transfusion</u>
T81.512-   Adhesions due to foreign body accidentally left in body following <u>kidney dialysis</u>
T81.513-   Adhesions due to foreign body accidentally left in body following <u>injection or immunization</u>
T81.514-   Adhesions due to foreign body accidentally left in body following <u>endoscopic examination</u>
T81.515-   Adhesions due to foreign body accidentally left in body following <u>heart catheterization</u>
T81.516-   Adhesions due to foreign body accidentally left in body following <u>aspiration, puncture or other catheterization</u>
T81.517-   Adhesions due to foreign body accidentally left in body following <u>removal of catheter or packing</u>
T81.518-   Adhesions due to foreign body accidentally left in body following <u>other procedure</u>
T81.519-   Adhesions due to foreign body accidentally left in body following <u>unspecified procedure</u>

T81.52- <u>Obstruction</u> due to <u>foreign body accidentally left in body following procedure</u>
T81.520-   Obstruction due to foreign body accidentally left in body following <u>surgical operation</u>
T81.521-   Obstruction due to foreign body accidentally left in body following <u>infusion or transfusion</u>
T81.522-   Obstruction due to foreign body accidentally <u>left</u> in body following <u>kidney dialysis</u>
T81.523-   Obstruction due to foreign body accidentally left in body following <u>injection or immunization</u>
T81.524-   Obstruction due to foreign body accidentally <u>left</u> in body following <u>endoscopic examination</u>
T81.525-   Obstruction due to foreign body accidentally left in body following <u>heart catheterization</u>
T81.526-   Obstruction due to foreign body accidentally left in body following <u>aspiration, puncture or other catheterization</u>
T81.527-   Obstruction due to foreign body accidentally left in body following <u>removal of catheter or packing</u>
T81.528-   Obstruction due to foreign body accidentally left in body following <u>other procedure</u>
T81.529-   Obstruction due to foreign body accidentally left in body following <u>unspecified procedure</u>

T81.53- <u>Perforation</u> due to <u>foreign body accidentally left in body following procedure</u>
T81.530-   Perforation due to foreign body accidentally left in body following <u>surgical operation</u>
T81.531-   Perforation due to foreign body accidentally left in body following <u>infusion or transfusion</u>
T81.532-   Perforation due to foreign body accidentally left in body following <u>kidney dialysis</u>
T81.533-   Perforation due to foreign body accidentally left in body following <u>injection or immunization</u>
T81.534-   Perforation due to foreign body accidentally <u>left</u> in body following <u>endoscopic examination</u>
T81.535-   Perforation due to foreign body accidentally left in body following <u>heart catheterization</u>
T81.536-   Perforation due to foreign body accidentally <u>left</u> in body following <u>aspiration, puncture or other catheterization</u>
T81.537-   Perforation due to foreign body accidentally left in body following <u>removal of catheter or packing</u>
T81.538-   Perforation due to foreign body accidentally left in body following <u>other procedure</u>
T81.539-   Perforation due to foreign body accidentally left in body following <u>unspecified procedure</u>

T81.59- <u>Other complications</u> of <u>foreign body accidentally left in body following procedure</u>
Excludes❷: obstruction or perforation due to prosthetic devices and implants intentionally left in body (T82.0-T82.5, T83.0-T83.4, T83.7, T84.0-T84.4, T85.0-T85.6)
T81.590-   Other complications of foreign body accidentally left in body following <u>surgical operation</u>
T81.591-   Other complications of foreign body accidentally left in body following <u>infusion or transfusion</u>
T81.592-   Other complications of foreign body accidentally left in body following <u>kidneydialysis</u>
T81.593-   Other complications of foreign body accidentally left in body following <u>injection or immunization</u>
T81.594-   Other complications of foreign body accidentally left in body following <u>endoscopic examination</u>
T81.595-   Other complications of foreign body accidentally left in body following <u>heart catheterization</u>
T81.596-   Other complications of foreign body accidentally left in body following <u>aspiration, puncture or other catheterization</u>
T81.597-   Other complications of foreign body accidentally left in body following <u>removal of catheter or packing</u>
T81.598-   Other complications of foreign body accidentally left in body following <u>other procedure</u>
T81.599-   Other complications of foreign body accidentally left in body following <u>unspecified procedure</u>

T81.6-   <u>Acute reaction</u> to <u>foreign substance accidentally left during a procedure</u>
Excludes❷: complications of foreign body accidentally left in body cavity or operation wound following procedure (T81.5-)
T81.60x- <u>Unspecified</u> acute reaction to foreign substance accidentally left during a procedure

Excludes 1: = NOT CODED HERE! (Do not code both)   **830**   *Excludes❷:* = Not Included Here

T81.61x- **Aseptic peritonitis** due to foreign substance accidentally left during a procedure
   Chemical peritonitis

T81.69x- **Other acute reaction** to foreign substance accidentally left during a procedure

T81.7- **Vascular complications following a procedure, not elsewhere classified**
   Air embolism following procedure NEC
   Phlebitis or thrombophlebitis resulting from a procedure
   Excludes 1: embolism complicating abortion or ectopic or molar pregnancy (O00-O07, O08.2)
   embolism complicating pregnancy, childbirth and the puerperium (O88.-)
   traumatic embolism (T79.0)
   Excludes❷: embolism due to prosthetic devices, implants and grafts (T82.8-, T83.8, T84.8-, T85.8)
   embolism following infusion, transfusion and therapeutic injection (T80.0)

T81.71- Complication of **artery** following a procedure, not elsewhere classified

   T81.710- Complication of **mesenteric** artery following a procedure, not elsewhere classified

   T81.711- Complication of **renal** artery following a procedure, not elsewhere classified

   T81.718- Complication of **other artery** following a procedure, not elsewhere classified

   T81.719- Complication of **unspecified artery** following a procedure, not elsewhere classified

T81.72x- Complication of **vein** following a procedure, not elsewhere classified

T81.8- **Other complications of procedures, not elsewhere classified**
   Excludes❷: hypothermia following anesthesia (T88.51)
   malignant hyperpyrexia due to anesthesia (T88.3)

T81.81x- **Complication of inhalation therapy**

T81.82x- **Emphysema (subcutaneous) resulting from a procedure**

T81.83x- **Persistent postprocedural fistula**

T81.89x- **Other complications of procedures, not elsewhere classified**
   Use additional code to specify complication, such as:
   Postprocedural delirium (F05)

T81.9xx- **Unspecified complication of procedure**

T82- **Complications of cardiac and vascular prosthetic devices, implants and grafts**
   Excludes❷: failure and rejection of transplanted organs and tissue (T86.-)
   The appropriate 7th character is to be added to each code from category T82:
   A **Initial** encounter
   D **Subsequent** encounter
   S **Sequela**

T82.0- **Mechanical** complication of **heart valve prosthesis**
   Mechanical complication of artificial heart valve
   Excludes 1: mechanical complication of biological heart valve graft (T82.22-)

T82.01x- **Breakdown (mechanical) of heart valve prosthesis**

T82.02x- **Displacement of heart valve prosthesis**
   Malposition of heart valve prosthesis

T82.03x- **Leakage of heart valve prosthesis**

T82.09x- **Other mechanical complication of heart valve prosthesis**
   Obstruction (mechanical) of heart valve prosthesis
   Perforation of heart valve prosthesis
   Protrusion of heart valve prosthesis

T82.1- **Mechanical** complication of **cardiac electronic device**

T82.11- Breakdown (mechanical) of cardiac electronic device

   T82.110- **Breakdown (mechanical) of cardiac electrode**

   T82.111- **Breakdown (mechanical) of cardiac pulse generator (battery)**

   T82.118- **Breakdown (mechanical) of other cardiac electronic device**

   T82.119- **Breakdown (mechanical) of unspecified cardiac electronic device**

T82.12- **Displacement** of **cardiac electronic device**
   Malposition of cardiac electronic device

   T82.120- **Displacement of cardiac electrode**

   T82.121- **Displacement of cardiac pulse generator (battery)**

   T82.128- **Displacement of other cardiac electronic device**

   T82.129- **Displacement of unspecified cardiac electronic device**

T82.19- **Other mechanical** complication of **cardiac electronic device**
   Leakage of cardiac electronic device
   Obstruction of cardiac electronic device
   Perforation of cardiac electronic device
   Protrusion of cardiac electronic device

   T82.190- **Other mechanical complication of cardiac electrode**

   T82.191- **Other mechanical complication of cardiac pulse generator (battery)**

   T82.198- **Other mechanical complication of other cardiac electronic device**

   T82.199- **Other mechanical complication of unspecified cardiac device**

T82.2- **Mechanical complication of coronary artery bypass graft and biological heart valve graft**
   Excludes 1: mechanical complication of artificial heart valve prosthesis (T82.0-)

T82.21- **Mechanical** complication of **coronary artery bypass graft**

   T82.211- **Breakdown (mechanical) of coronary artery bypass graft**

   T82.212- **Displacement of coronary artery bypass graft**
   Malposition of coronary artery bypass graft

   T82.213- **Leakage of coronary artery bypass graft**

   T82.218- **Other mechanical complication of coronary artery bypass graft**
   Obstruction, mechanical of coronary artery bypass graft
   Perforation of coronary artery bypass graft
   Protrusion of coronary artery bypass graft

T82.22- **Mechanical** complication of **biological heart valve graft**

   T82.221- **Breakdown (mechanical) of biological heart valve graft**

   T82.222- **Displacement of biological heart valve graft**
   Malposition of biological heart valve graft

   T82.223- **Leakage of biological heart valve graft**

   T82.228- **Other mechanical complication of biological heart valve graft**
   Obstruction of biological heart valve graft
   Perforation of biological heart valve graft
   Protrusion of biological heart valve graft

T82.3- **Mechanical** complication of **other vascular grafts**

T82.31- **Breakdown** (mechanical) of other vascular grafts

   T82.310- **Breakdown (mechanical) of aortic (bifurcation) graft (replacement)**

   T82.311- **Breakdown (mechanical) of carotid arterial graft (bypass)**

   T82.312- **Breakdown (mechanical) of femoral arterial graft (bypass)**

   T82.318- **Breakdown (mechanical) of other vascular grafts**

   T82.319- **Breakdown (mechanical) of unspecified vascular grafts**

T82.32- **Displacement** of other vascular grafts
   Malposition of other vascular grafts

   T82.320- **Displacement of aortic (bifurcation) graft (replacement)**

   T82.321- **Displacement of carotid arterial graft (bypass)**

   T82.322- **Displacement of femoral arterial graft (bypass)**

   T82.328- **Displacement of other vascular grafts**

   T82.329- **Displacement of unspecified vascular grafts**

T82.33- **Leakage** of other vascular grafts

   T82.330- **Leakage of aortic (bifurcation) graft (replacement)**

   T82.331- **Leakage of carotid arterial graft (bypass)**

   T82.332- **Leakage of femoral arterial graft (bypass)**

   T82.338- **Leakage of other vascular grafts**

   T82.339- **Leakage of unspecified vascular graft**

T82.39- **Other mechanical** complication of other vascular grafts
   Obstruction (mechanical) of other vascular grafts
   Perforation of other vascular grafts
   Protrusion of other vascular grafts

   T82.390- **Other mechanical complication of aortic (bifurcation) graft (replacement)**

   T82.391- **Other mechanical complication of carotid arterial graft (bypass)**

   T82.392- **Other mechanical complication of femoral arterial graft (bypass)**

   T82.398- **Other mechanical complication of other vascular grafts**

   T82.399- **Other mechanical complication of unspecified vascular grafts**

T82.4- **Mechanical** complication of **vascular dialysis catheter**
   Mechanical complication of hemodialysis catheter
   Excludes 1: mechanical complication of intraperitoneal dialysis catheter (T85.62)

T82.41x- **Breakdown (mechanical) of vascular dialysis catheter**

T82.42x- **Displacement of vascular dialysis catheter**
   Malposition of vascular dialysis catheter

T82.43x- **Leakage of vascular dialysis catheter**

T82.49x- Other complication of vascular dialysis catheter
Obstruction (mechanical) of vascular dialysis catheter
Perforation of vascular dialysis catheter
Protrusion of vascular dialysis catheter

T82.5- Mechanical complication of other cardiac and vascular devices and implants
Excludes❷: mechanical complication of epidural and subdural infusion catheter (T85.61)

T82.51- Breakdown (mechanical) of other cardiac and vascular devices and implants

T82.510- Breakdown (mechanical) of surgically created arteriovenous fistula

T82.511- Breakdown (mechanical) of surgically created arteriovenous shunt

T82.512- Breakdown (mechanical) of artificial heart

T82.513- Breakdown (mechanical) of balloon (counterpulsation) device

T82.514- Breakdown (mechanical) of infusion catheter

T82.515- Breakdown (mechanical) of umbrella device

T82.518- Breakdown (mechanical) of other cardiac and vascular devices and implants

T82.519- Breakdown (mechanical) of unspecified cardiac and vascular devices and implants

T82.52- Displacement of other cardiac and vascular devices and implants
Malposition of other cardiac and vascular devices and implants

T82.520- Displacement of surgically created arteriovenous fistula

T82.521- Displacement of surgically created arteriovenous shunt

T82.522- Displacement of artificial heart

T82.523- Displacement of balloon (counterpulsation) device

T82.524- Displacement of infusion catheter

T82.525- Displacement of umbrella device

T82.528- Displacement of other cardiac and vascular devices and implants

T82.529- Displacement of unspecified cardiac and vascular devices and implants

T82.53- Leakage of other cardiac and vascular devices and implants

T82.530- Leakage of surgically created arteriovenous fistula

T82.531- Leakage of surgically created arteriovenous shunt

T82.532- Leakage of artificial heart

T82.533- Leakage of balloon (counterpulsation) device

T82.534- Leakage of infusion catheter

T82.535- Leakage of umbrella device

T82.538- Leakage of other cardiac and vascular devices and implants

T82.539- Leakage of unspecified cardiac and vascular devices and implants

T82.59- Other mechanical complication of other cardiac and vascular devices and implants
Obstruction (mechanical) of other cardiac and vascular devices and implants
Perforation of other cardiac and vascular devices and implants
Protrusion of other cardiac and vascular devices and implants

T82.590- Other mechanical complication of surgically created arteriovenous fistula

T82.591- Other mechanical complication of surgically created arteriovenous shunt

T82.592- Other mechanical complication of artificial heart

T82.593- Other mechanical complication of balloon (counterpulsation) device

T82.594- Other mechanical complication of infusion catheter

T82.595- Other mechanical complication of umbrella device

T82.598- Other mechanical complication of other cardiac and vascular devices and implants

T82.599- Other mechanical complication of unspecified cardiac and vascular devices and implants

T82.6xx- Infection and inflammatory reaction due to cardiac valve prosthesis
Use additional code to identify infection

T82.7xx- Infection and inflammatory reaction due to other cardiac and vascular devices, implants and grafts
Use additional code to identify infection

T82.8- Other specified complications of cardiac and vascular prosthetic devices, implants and grafts

T82.81- Embolism of cardiac and vascular prosthetic devices, implants and grafts

T82.817- Embolism of cardiac prosthetic devices, implants and grafts

T82.818- Embolism of vascular prosthetic devices, implants and grafts

T82.82- Fibrosis of cardiac and vascular prosthetic devices, implants and grafts

T82.827- Fibrosis of cardiac prosthetic devices, implants and grafts

T82.828- Fibrosis of vascular prosthetic devices, implants and grafts

T82.83- Hemorrhage of cardiac and vascular prosthetic devices, implants and grafts

T82.837- Hemorrhage of cardiac prosthetic devices, implants and grafts

T82.838- Hemorrhage of vascular prosthetic devices, implants and grafts

T82.84- Pain from cardiac and vascular prosthetic devices, implants and grafts

T82.847- Pain from cardiac prosthetic devices, implants and grafts

T82.848- Pain from vascular prosthetic devices, implants and grafts

T82.85- Stenosis of cardiac and vascular prosthetic devices, implants and grafts

T82.857- Stenosis of cardiac prosthetic devices, implants and grafts

T82.858- Stenosis of vascular prosthetic devices, implants and grafts

T82.86- Thrombosis of cardiac and vascular prosthetic devices, implants and grafts

T82.867- Thrombosis of cardiac prosthetic devices, implants and grafts

T82.868- Thrombosis of vascular prosthetic devices, implants and grafts

T82.89- Other specified complication of cardiac and vascular prosthetic devices, implants and grafts

T82.897- Other specified complication of cardiac prosthetic devices, implants and grafts

T82.898- Other specified complication of vascular prosthetic devices, implants and grafts

T82.9xx- Unspecified complication of cardiac and vascular prosthetic device, implant and graft

T83- Complications of genitourinary prosthetic devices, implants and grafts
Excludes❷: failure and rejection of transplanted organs and tissue (T86.-)
The appropriate 7th character is to be added to each code from category T83:
A Initial encounter
D Subsequent encounter
S Sequela

T83.0- Mechanical complication of urinary (indwelling) catheter
Excludes❷: complications of stoma of urinary tract (N99.5-)

T83.01- Breakdown (mechanical) of urinary (indwelling) catheter

T83.010- Breakdown (mechanical) of cystostomy catheter

T83.018- Breakdown (mechanical) of other indwelling urethral catheter

T83.02- Displacement of urinary (indwelling) catheter
Malposition of urinary (indwelling) catheter

T83.020- Displacement of cystostomy catheter

T83.028- Displacement of other indwelling urethral catheter

T83.03- Leakage of urinary (indwelling) catheter

T83.030- Leakage of cystostomy catheter

T83.038- Leakage of other indwelling urethral catheter

T83.09- Other mechanical complication of urinary (indwelling) catheter
Obstruction (mechanical) of urinary (indwelling) catheter
Perforation of urinary (indwelling) catheter
Protrusion of urinary (indwelling) catheter

T83.090- Other mechanical complication of cystostomy catheter

T83.098- Other mechanical complication of other indwelling urethral catheter

T83.1- Mechanical complication of other urinary devices and implants

T83.11- Breakdown (mechanical) of other urinary devices and implants

T83.110- Breakdown (mechanical) of urinary electronic stimulator device

T83.111- Breakdown (mechanical) of urinary sphincter implant

T83.112- Breakdown (mechanical) of urinary stent

T83.118- Breakdown (mechanical) of other urinary devices and implants

T83.12- Displacement of other urinary devices and implants
Malposition of other urinary devices and implants

T83.120- Displacement of urinary electronic stimulator device

T
8
2
-
T
8
4

Excludes 1: = NOT CODED HERE! (Do not code both)

Excludes❷: = Not Included Here

T83.121- Displacement of urinary sphincter implant
T83.122- Displacement of urinary stent
T83.128- Displacement of other urinary devices and implants
T83.19- Other mechanical complication of other urinary devices and implants
 Leakage of other urinary devices and implants
 Obstruction (mechanical) of other urinary devices and implants
 Perforation of other urinary devices and implants
 Protrusion of other urinary devices and implants
 T83.190- Other mechanical complication of urinary electronic stimulator device
 T83.191- Other mechanical complication of urinary sphincter implant
 T83.192- Other mechanical complication of urinary stent
 T83.198- Other mechanical complication of other urinary devices and implants
T83.2- Mechanical complication of graft of urinary organ
T83.21x- Breakdown (mechanical) of graft of urinary organ
T83.22x- Displacement of graft of urinary organ
 Malposition of graft of urinary organ
T83.23x- Leakage of graft of urinary organ
T83.29x- Other mechanical complication of graft of urinary organ
 Obstruction (mechanical) of graft of urinary organ
 Perforation of graft of urinary organ
 Protrusion of graft of urinary organ
T83.3- Mechanical complication of intrauterine contraceptive device
T83.31x- Breakdown (mechanical) of intrauterine contraceptive device
T83.32x- Displacement of intrauterine contraceptive device
 Malposition of intrauterine contraceptive device
T83.39x- Other mechanical complication of intrauterine contraceptive device
 Leakage of intrauterine contraceptive device
 Obstruction (mechanical) of intrauterine contraceptive device
 Perforation of intrauterine contraceptive device
 Protrusion of intrauterine contraceptive device
T83.4- Mechanical complication of other prosthetic devices, implants and grafts of genital tract
T83.41- Breakdown (mechanical) of other prosthetic devices, implants and grafts of genital tract
 T83.410- Breakdown (mechanical) of penile (implanted) prosthesis
 T83.418- Breakdown (mechanical) of other prosthetic devices, implants and grafts of genital tract
T83.42- Displacement of other prosthetic devices and grafts of genital tract
 Malposition of other prosthetic devices, implants and grafts of genital tract
 T83.420- Displacement of penile (implanted) prosthesis
 T83.428- Displacement of other prosthetic devices, implants and grafts of genital tract
T83.49- Other mechanical complication of other prosthetic devices, implants and grafts of genital tract
 Leakage of other prosthetic devices and grafts of genital tract
 Obstruction, mechanical of other prosthetic devices, implants and grafts of genital tract
 Perforation of other prosthetic devices, implants and grafts of genital tract
 Protrusion of other prosthetic devices, implants and grafts of genital tract
 T83.490- Other mechanical complication of penile (implanted) prosthesis
 T83.498- Other mechanical complication of other prosthetic devices, implants and grafts of genital tract
T83.5- Infection and inflammatory reaction due to prosthetic device, implant and graft in urinary system
 Use additional code to identify infection
T83.51x- Infection and inflammatory reaction due to indwelling urinary catheter
 Excludes❷: complications of stoma of urinary tract (N99.5-)
T83.59x- Infection and inflammatory reaction due to prosthetic device, implant and graft in urinary system

T83.6xx- Infection and inflammatory reaction due to prosthetic device, implant and graft in genital tract
 Use additional code to identify infection
T83.7- Complications due to implanted mesh and other prosthetic materials
T83.71- Erosion of implanted mesh and other prosthetic materials to surrounding organ or tissue
 T83.711- Erosion of implanted vaginal mesh and other prosthetic materials to surrounding organ or tissue
  Erosion of implanted vaginal mesh and other prosthetic materials into the pelvic floor muscles
 T83.718- Erosion of other implanted mesh and other prosthetic materials to surrounding organ or tissue
T83.72- Exposure of implanted mesh and other prosthetic materials into surrounding organ or tissue
 T83.721- Exposure of implanted vaginal mesh and other prosthetic materials into vagina
  Exposure of implanted vaginal mesh and other prosthetic materials through vaginal wall
 T83.728- Exposure of other implanted mesh and other prosthetic materials to surrounding organ or tissue
T83.8- Other specified complications of genitourinary prosthetic devices, implants and grafts
 T83.81x- Embolism of genitourinary prosthetic devices, implants and grafts
 T83.82x- Fibrosis of genitourinary prosthetic devices, implants and grafts
 T83.83x- Hemorrhage of genitourinary prosthetic devices, implants and grafts
 T83.84x- Pain from genitourinary prosthetic devices, implants and grafts
 T83.85x- Stenosis of genitourinary prosthetic devices, implants and grafts
 T83.86x- Thrombosis of genitourinary prosthetic devices, implants and grafts
 T83.89x- Other specified complication of genitourinary prosthetic devices, implants and grafts
T83.9xx- Unspecified complication of genitourinary prosthetic device, implant and graft

T84- Complications of internal orthopedic prosthetic devices, implants and grafts
 Excludes❷: failure and rejection of transplanted organs and tissues (T86.-)
  fracture of bone following insertion of orthopedic implant, joint prosthesis or bone plate (M96.6)

The appropriate 7th character is to be added to each code from category T84:
A Initial encounter
D Subsequent encounter
S Sequela

T84.0- Mechanical complication of internal joint prosthesis
T84.01- Broken internal joint prosthesis
 Breakage (fracture) of prosthetic joint
 Broken prosthetic joint implant
 Excludes 1: periprosthetic joint implant fracture (T84.04)
 T84.010- Broken internal right hip prosthesis
 T84.011- Broken internal left hip prosthesis
 T84.012- Broken internal right knee prosthesis
 T84.013- Broken internal left knee prosthesis
 T84.018- Broken internal joint prosthesis, other site
  Use additional code to identify the joint (Z96.6-)
 T84.019- Broken internal joint prosthesis, unspecified site
T84.02- Dislocation of internal joint prosthesis
 Instability of internal joint prosthesis
 Subluxation of internal joint prosthesis
 T84.020- Dislocation of internal right hip prosthesis
 T84.021- Dislocation of internal left hip prosthesis
 T84.022- Instability of internal right knee prosthesis
 T84.023- Instability of internal left knee prosthesis
 T84.028- Dislocation of other internal joint prosthesis
  Use additional code to identify the joint (Z96.6-)
 T84.029- Dislocation of unspecified internal joint prosthesis
T84.03- Mechanical loosening of internal prosthetic joint
 Aseptic loosening of prosthetic joint
 T84.030- Mechanical loosening of internal right hip prosthetic joint
 T84.031- Mechanical loosening of internal left hip prosthetic joint
 T84.032- Mechanical loosening of internal right knee prosthetic joint
 T84.033- Mechanical loosening of internal left knee prosthetic joint

T
8
2
|
T
8
4

T84.038- Mechanical loosening of <u>other</u> internal prosthetic joint
Use additional code to identify the joint (Z96.6-)

T84.039- Mechanical loosening of <u>unspecified</u> internal prosthetic joint

T84.04- <u>Periprosthetic fracture</u> around internal prosthetic joint
Excludes❷: breakage (fracture) of prosthetic joint (T84.01)

T84.040- Periprosthetic fracture around internal prosthetic <u>right hip</u> joint

T84.041- Periprosthetic fracture around internal prosthetic <u>left hip</u> joint

T84.042- Periprosthetic fracture around internal prosthetic <u>right knee</u> joint

T84.043- Periprosthetic fracture around internal prosthetic <u>left knee</u> joint

T84.048- Periprosthetic fracture around <u>other</u> internal prosthetic joint
Use additional code to identify the joint (Z96.6-)

T84.049- Periprosthetic fracture around <u>unspecified</u> internal prosthetic joint

T84.05- <u>Periprosthetic osteolysis</u> of internal prosthetic joint
Use additional code to identify major osseous defect, if applicable (M89.7-)

T84.050- Periprosthetic osteolysis of internal prosthetic <u>right hip</u> joint

T84.051- Periprosthetic osteolysis of internal prosthetic <u>left hip</u> joint

T84.052- Periprosthetic osteolysis of internal prosthetic <u>right knee</u> joint

T84.053- Periprosthetic osteolysis of internal prosthetic <u>left knee</u> joint

T84.058- Periprosthetic osteolysis of <u>other</u> internal prosthetic joint
Use additional code to identify the joint (Z96.6-)

T84.059- Periprosthetic osteolysis of <u>unspecified</u> internal prosthetic joint

T84.06- <u>Wear of articular bearing surface</u> of internal prosthetic joint

T84.060- Wear of articular bearing surface of internal prosthetic <u>right hip</u> joint

T84.061- Wear of articular bearing surface of internal prosthetic <u>left hip</u> joint

T84.062- Wear of articular bearing surface of internal prosthetic <u>right knee</u> joint

T84.063- Wear of articular bearing surface of internal prosthetic <u>left knee</u> joint

T84.068- Wear of articular bearing surface of <u>other</u> internal prosthetic joint
Use additional code to identify the joint (Z96.6-)

T84.069- Wear of articular bearing surface of <u>unspecified</u> internal prosthetic joint

T84.09- <u>Other mechanical complication</u> of internal joint prosthesis
Prosthetic joint implant failure NOS

T84.090- Other mechanical complication of internal <u>right hip</u> prosthesis

T84.091- Other mechanical complication of internal <u>left hip</u> prosthesis

T84.092- Other mechanical complication of internal <u>right knee</u> prosthesis

T84.093- Other mechanical complication of internal <u>left knee</u> prosthesis

T84.098- Other mechanical complication of <u>other</u> internal joint prosthesis
Use additional code to identify the joint (Z96.6-)

T84.099- Other mechanical complication of <u>unspecified</u> internal joint prosthesis

T84.1- <u>Mechanical complication of internal fixation device of bones of limb</u>
Excludes❷: mechanical complication of internal fixation device of bones of feet (T84.2-)
mechanical complication of internal fixation device of bones of fingers (T84.2-)
mechanical complication of internal fixation device of bones of hands (T84.2-)
mechanical complication of internal fixation device of bones of toes (T84.2-)

T84.11- <u>Breakdown</u> (mechanical) of internal fixation device of bones of limb

T84.110- Breakdown (mechanical) of internal fixation device of <u>right humerus</u>

T84.111- Breakdown (mechanical) of internal fixation device of <u>left humerus</u>

T84.112- Breakdown (mechanical) of internal fixation device of bone of <u>right forearm</u>

T84.113- Breakdown (mechanical) of internal fixation device of bone of <u>left forearm</u>

T84.114- Breakdown (mechanical) of internal fixation device of <u>right femur</u>

T84.115- Breakdown (mechanical) of internal fixation device of <u>left femur</u>

T84.116- Breakdown (mechanical) of internal fixation device of bone of <u>right lower leg</u>

T84.117- Breakdown (mechanical) of internal fixation device of bone of <u>left lower leg</u>

T84.119- Breakdown (mechanical) of internal fixation device of <u>unspecified</u> bone of limb

T84.12- <u>Displacement</u> of internal fixation device of bones of limb
Malposition of internal fixation device of bones of limb

T84.120- Displacement of internal fixation device of <u>right humerus</u>

T84.121- Displacement of internal fixation device of <u>left humerus</u>

T84.122- Displacement of internal fixation device of bone of <u>right forearm</u>

T84.123- Displacement of internal fixation device of bone of <u>left forearm</u>

T84.124- Displacement of internal fixation device of <u>right femur</u>

T84.125- Displacement of internal fixation device of <u>left femur</u>

T84.126- Displacement of internal fixation device of bone of <u>right lower leg</u>

T84.127- Displacement of internal fixation device of bone of <u>left lower leg</u>

T84.129- Displacement of internal fixation device of <u>unspecified</u> bone of limb

T84.19- <u>Other mechanical complication</u> of internal fixation device of bones of limb
Obstruction (mechanical) of internal fixation device of bones of limb
Perforation of internal fixation device of bones of limb
Protrusion of internal fixation device of bones of limb

T84.190- Other mechanical complication of internal fixation device of <u>right humerus</u>

T84.191- Other mechanical complication of internal fixation device of <u>left humerus</u>

T84.192- Other mechanical complication of internal fixation device of bone of <u>right forearm</u>

T84.193- Other mechanical complication of internal fixation device of bone of <u>left forearm</u>

T84.194- Other mechanical complication of internal fixation device of <u>right femur</u>

T84.195- Other mechanical complication of internal fixation device of <u>left femur</u>

T84.196- Other mechanical complication of internal fixation device of bone of <u>right lower leg</u>

T84.197- Other mechanical complication of internal fixation device of bone of <u>left lower leg</u>

T84.199- Other mechanical complication of internal fixation device of <u>unspecified</u> bone of limb

T84.2- <u>Mechanical complication of internal fixation device of other bones</u>

T84.21- <u>Breakdown</u> (mechanical) of internal fixation device of other bones

T84.210- Breakdown (mechanical) of internal fixation device of bones of <u>hand and fingers</u>

T84.213- Breakdown (mechanical) of internal fixation device of bones of <u>foot and toes</u>

T84.216- Breakdown (mechanical) of internal fixation device of <u>vertebrae</u>

T84.218- Breakdown (mechanical) of internal fixation device of <u>other bones</u>

T84.22- <u>Displacement</u> of internal fixation device of other bones
Malposition of internal fixation device of other bones

T84.220- Displacement of internal fixation device of bones of <u>hand and fingers</u>

T84.223- Displacement of internal fixation device of bones of <u>foot and toes</u>

T84.226- Displacement of internal fixation device of <u>vertebrae</u>

T84.228- Displacement of internal fixation device of <u>other bones</u>

T
8
4
-
T
8
5

T84.29- **Other mechanical complication** of internal fixation device of **other bones**
    Obstruction (mechanical) of internal fixation device of other bones
    Perforation of internal fixation device of other bones
    Protrusion of internal fixation device of other bones
   T84.290- **Other mechanical complication of internal fixation device of bones of hand and fingers**
   T84.293- **Other mechanical complication of internal fixation device of bones of foot and toes**
   T84.296- **Other mechanical complication of internal fixation device of vertebrae**
   T84.298- **Other mechanical complication of internal fixation device of other bones**

T84.3- **Mechanical complication** of **other bone devices, implants and grafts**
    Excludes❷: *other complications of bone graft (T86.83-)*
   T84.31- **Breakdown** (mechanical) of other bone devices, implants and grafts
    T84.310- **Breakdown (mechanical) of electronic bone stimulator**
    T84.318- **Breakdown (mechanical) of other bone devices, implants and grafts**
   T84.32- **Displacement** of other bone devices, implants and grafts
    Malposition of other bone devices, implants and grafts
    T84.320- **Displacement of electronic bone stimulator**
    T84.328- **Displacement of other bone devices, implants and grafts**
   T84.39- **Other mechanical complication** of other bone devices, implants and grafts
    Obstruction (mechanical) of other bone devices, implants and grafts
    Perforation of other bone devices, implants and grafts
    Protrusion of other bone devices, implants and grafts
    T84.390- **Other mechanical complication of electronic bone stimulator**
    T84.398- **Other mechanical complication of other bone devices, implants and grafts**

T84.4- **Mechanical complication of other internal orthopedic devices, implants and grafts**
   T84.41- **Breakdown** (mechanical) of other internal orthopedic devices, implants and grafts
    T84.410- **Breakdown (mechanical) of muscle and tendon graft**
    T84.418- **Breakdown (mechanical) of other internal orthopedic devices, implants and grafts**
   T84.42- **Displacement** of other internal orthopedic devices, implants and grafts
    Malposition of other internal orthopedic devices, implants and grafts
    T84.420- **Displacement of muscle and tendon graft**
    T84.428- **Displacement of other internal orthopedic devices, implants and grafts**
   T84.49- **Other mechanical complication** of other internal orthopedic devices, implants and grafts
    Mechanical complication of other internal orthopedic devices, implants and grafts NOS
    Obstruction (mechanical) of other internal orthopedic devices, implants and grafts
    Perforation of other internal orthopedic devices, implants and grafts
    Protrusion of other internal orthopedic devices, implants and grafts
    T84.490- **Other mechanical complication of muscle and tendon graft**
    T84.498- **Other mechanical complication of other internal orthopedic devices, implants and grafts**

T84.5- **Infection and inflammatory reaction** due to **internal joint prosthesis**
    Use additional code to identify infection
   T84.50x- **Infection and inflammatory reaction due to unspecified internal joint prosthesis**
   T84.51x- **Infection and inflammatory reaction due to internal right hip prosthesis**
   T84.52x- **Infection and inflammatory reaction due to internal left hip prosthesis**
   T84.53x- **Infection and inflammatory reaction due to internal right knee prosthesis**
   T84.54x- **Infection and inflammatory reaction due to internal left knee prosthesis**
   T84.59x- **Infection and inflammatory reaction due to other internal joint prosthesis**

T84.6- **Infection and inflammatory reaction** due to **internal fixation device**
    Use additional code to identify infection
   T84.60x- **Infection and inflammatory reaction due to internal fixation device of unspecified site**
   T84.61- Infection and inflammatory reaction due to internal fixation device of **arm**
    T84.610- **Infection and inflammatory reaction due to internal fixation device of right humerus**
    T84.611- **Infection and inflammatory reaction due to internal fixation device of left humerus**
    T84.612- **Infection and inflammatory reaction due to internal fixation device of right radius**
    T84.613- **Infection and inflammatory reaction due to internal fixation device of left radius**
    T84.614- **Infection and inflammatory reaction due to internal fixation device of right ulna**
    T84.615- **Infection and inflammatory reaction due to internal fixation device of left ulna**
    T84.619- **Infection and inflammatory reaction due to internal fixation device of unspecified bone of arm**
   T84.62- Infection and inflammatory reaction due to internal fixation device of **leg**
    T84.620- **Infection and inflammatory reaction due to internal fixation device of right femur**
    T84.621- **Infection and inflammatory reaction due to internal fixation device of left femur**
    T84.622- **Infection and inflammatory reaction due to internal fixation device of right tibia**
    T84.623- **Infection and inflammatory reaction due to internal fixation device of left tibia**
    T84.624- **Infection and inflammatory reaction due to internal fixation device of right fibula**
    T84.625- **Infection and inflammatory reaction due to internal fixation device of left fibula**
    T84.629- **Infection and inflammatory reaction due to internal fixation device of unspecified bone of leg**
   T84.63x- **Infection and inflammatory reaction due to internal fixation device of spine**
   T84.69x- **Infection and inflammatory reaction due to internal fixation device of other site**

T84.7xx- **Infection and inflammatory reaction** due to **other internal orthopedic prosthetic devices, implants and grafts**
    Use additional code to identify infection

T84.8- **Other specified complications** of **internal orthopedic prosthetic devices, implants and grafts**
   T84.81x- **Embolism** due to internal orthopedic prosthetic devices, implants and grafts
   T84.82x- **Fibrosis** due to internal orthopedic prosthetic devices, implants and grafts
   T84.83x- **Hemorrhage** due to internal orthopedic prosthetic devices, implants and grafts
   T84.84x- **Pain** due to internal orthopedic prosthetic devices, implants and grafts
   T84.85x- **Stenosis** due to internal orthopedic prosthetic devices, implants and grafts
   T84.86x- **Thrombosis** due to internal orthopedic prosthetic devices, implants and grafts
   T84.89x- **Other specified complication** of internal orthopedic prosthetic devices, implants and grafts

T84.9xx- **Unspecified** complication of internal orthopedic prosthetic device, implant and graft

T85- **Complications of other internal prosthetic devices, implants and grafts**
    Excludes❷: *failure and rejection of transplanted organs and tissue (T86-)*
    The appropriate 7th character is to be added to each code from category T85:
    A **Initial** encounter
    D **Subsequent** encounter
    S **Sequela**

T85.0- **Mechanical complication of ventricular intracranial (communicating) shunt**
   T85.01x- **Breakdown** (mechanical) of ventricular intracranial (communicating) shunt
   T85.02x- **Displacement** of ventricular intracranial (communicating) shunt
    Malposition of ventricular intracranial (communicating) shunt
   T85.03x- **Leakage** of ventricular intracranial (communicating) shunt

T 8 4 - T 8 5

Excludes 1: = NOT CODED HERE! (Do not code both)

Excludes❷: = Not Included Here

T85.09x- <u>Other mechanical</u> complication of ventricular intracranial (communicating) shunt
> Obstruction (mechanical) of ventricular intracranial (communicating) shunt
> Perforation of ventricular intracranial (communicating) shunt
> Protrusion of ventricular intracranial (communicating) shunt

T85.1- <u>Mechanical</u> complication of <u>implanted electronic stimulator of nervous system</u>

T85.11- <u>Breakdown</u> (mechanical) of implanted electronic stimulator of nervous system

T85.110- **Breakdown (mechanical) of implanted electronic neurostimulator (electrode) of <u>brain</u>**

T85.111- **Breakdown (mechanical) of implanted electronic neurostimulator (electrode) of <u>peripheral nerve</u>**

T85.112- **Breakdown (mechanical) of implanted electronic neurostimulator (electrode) of <u>spinal cord</u>**

T85.118- **Breakdown (mechanical) of <u>other</u> implanted electronic stimulator of nervous system**

T85.12- <u>Displacement</u> of implanted electronic stimulator of nervous system
> Malposition of implanted electronic stimulator of nervous system

T85.120- **Displacement of implanted electronic neurostimulator (electrode) of <u>brain</u>**

T85.121- **Displacement of implanted electronic neurostimulator (electrode) of <u>peripheral nerve</u>**

T85.122- **Displacement of implanted electronic neurostimulator (electrode) of <u>spinal cord</u>**

T85.128- **Displacement of <u>other</u> implanted electronic stimulator of nervous system**

T85.19- <u>Other mechanical</u> complication of implanted electronic stimulator of nervous system
> Leakage of implanted electronic stimulator of nervous system
> Obstruction (mechanical) of implanted electronic stimulator of nervous system
> Perforation of implanted electronic stimulator of nervous system
> Protrusion of implanted electronic stimulator of nervous system

T85.190- **Other mechanical complication of implanted electronic neurostimulator (electrode) of <u>brain</u>**

T85.191- **Other mechanical complication of implanted electronic neurostimulator (electrode) of <u>peripheral nerve</u>**

T85.192- **Other mechanical complication of implanted electronic neurostimulator (electrode) of <u>spinal cord</u>**

T85.199- **Other mechanical complication of <u>other</u> implanted electronic stimulator of nervous system**

T85.2- <u>Mechanical</u> complication of <u>intraocular lens</u>

T85.21x- <u>Breakdown</u> (mechanical) of intraocular lens

T85.22x- <u>Displacement</u> of intraocular lens
> Malposition of intraocular lens

T85.29x- <u>Other mechanical</u> complication of intraocular lens
> Obstruction (mechanical) of intraocular lens
> Perforation of intraocular lens
> Protrusion of intraocular lens

T85.3- <u>Mechanical</u> complication of <u>other ocular prosthetic devices, implants and grafts</u>
Excludes❷: other complications of corneal graft (T86.84-)

T85.31- <u>Breakdown</u> (mechanical) of other ocular prosthetic devices, implants and grafts

T85.310- **Breakdown (mechanical) of prosthetic orbit of <u>right</u> eye**

T85.311- **Breakdown (mechanical) of prosthetic orbit of <u>left</u> eye**

T85.318- **Breakdown (mechanical) of <u>other</u> ocular prosthetic devices, implants and grafts**

T85.32- <u>Displacement</u> of other ocular prosthetic devices, implants and grafts
> Malposition of other ocular prosthetic devices, implants and grafts

T85.320- **Displacement of prosthetic orbit of <u>right</u> eye**

T85.321- **Displacement of prosthetic orbit of <u>left</u> eye**

T85.328- **Displacement of <u>other</u> ocular prosthetic devices, implants and grafts**

T85.39- <u>Other mechanical</u> complication of other ocular prosthetic devices, implants and grafts
> Obstruction (mechanical) of other ocular prosthetic devices, implants and grafts
> Perforation of other ocular prosthetic devices, implants and grafts
> Protrusion of other ocular prosthetic devices, implants and grafts

T85.390- **Other mechanical complication of prosthetic orbit of <u>right</u> eye**

T85.391- **Other mechanical complication of prosthetic orbit of <u>left</u> eye**

T85.398- **Other mechanical complication of <u>other</u> ocular prosthetic devices, implants and grafts**

T85.4- <u>Mechanical</u> complication of <u>breast prosthesis and implant</u>

T85.41x- <u>Breakdown</u> (mechanical) of breast prosthesis and implant

T85.42x- <u>Displacement</u> of breast prosthesis and implant
> Malposition of breast prosthesis and implant

T85.43x- <u>Leakage</u> of breast prosthesis and implant

T85.44x- <u>Capsular contracture</u> of breast implant

T85.49x- <u>Other mechanicalm</u> complication of breast prosthesis and implant
> Obstruction (mechanical) of breast prosthesis and implant
> Perforation of breast prosthesis and implant
> Protrusion of breast prosthesis and implant

T85.5- <u>Mechanical</u> complication of <u>gastrointestinal prosthetic devices, implants and grafts</u>

T85.51- <u>Breakdown</u> (mechanical) of gastrointestinal prosthetic devices, implants and grafts

T85.510- **Breakdown (mechanical) of <u>bile duct prosthesis</u>**

T85.511- **Breakdown (mechanical) of <u>esophageal anti-reflux device</u>**

T85.518- **Breakdown (mechanical) of <u>other</u> gastrointestinal prosthetic devices, implants and grafts**

T85.52- <u>Displacement</u> of gastrointestinal prosthetic devices, implants and grafts
> Malposition of gastrointestinal prosthetic devices, implants and grafts

T85.520- **Displacement of <u>bile duct prosthesis</u>**

T85.521- **Displacement of <u>esophageal anti-reflux device</u>**

T85.528- **Displacement of <u>other</u> gastrointestinal prosthetic devices, implants and grafts**

T85.59- <u>Other mechanical</u> complication of gastrointestinal prosthetic devices, implants and
> Obstruction, mechanical of gastrointestinal prosthetic devices, implants and grafts
> Perforation of gastrointestinal prosthetic devices, implants and grafts
> Protrusion of gastrointestinal prosthetic devices, implants and grafts

T85.590- **Other mechanical complication of <u>bile duct prosthesis</u>**

T85.591- **Other mechanical complication of <u>esophageal anti-reflux device</u>**

T85.598- **Other mechanical complication of <u>other</u> gastrointestinal prosthetic devices, implants and grafts**

T85.6- <u>Mechanical</u> complication of <u>other specified internal and external prosthetic devices, implants and grafts</u>

T85.61- <u>Breakdown</u> (mechanical) of other specified internal prosthetic devices, implants and grafts

T85.610- **Breakdown (mechanical) of <u>epidural and subdural infusion catheter</u>**

T85.611- **Breakdown (mechanical) of <u>intraperitoneal dialysis catheter</u>**
Excludes 1: mechanical complication of vascular dialysis catheter (T82.4-)

T85.612- **Breakdown (mechanical) of <u>permanent sutures</u>**
Excludes 1: mechanical complication of permanent (wire) suture used in bone repair (T84.1-T84.2)

T85.613- **Breakdown (mechanical) of <u>artificial skin graft and decellularized allodermis</u>**
> Failure of artificial skin graft and decellularized allodermis
> Non-adherence of artificial skin graft and decellularized allodermis
> Poor incorporation of artificial skin graft and decellularized allodermis
> Shearing of artificial skin graft and decellularized allodermis

T85.614- **Breakdown (mechanical) of <u>insulin pump</u>**

T85.618- **Breakdown (mechanical) of <u>other</u> specified internal prosthetic devices, implants and grafts**

T 8 5 - T 8 6

© 2013 Channel Publishing, Ltd.

T85.62-   <u>Displacement</u> of other specified internal prosthetic devices, implants and grafts
> Malposition of other specified internal prosthetic devices, implants and grafts

T85.620-   Displacement of <u>epidural and subdural infusion catheter</u>

T85.621-   Displacement of <u>intraperitoneal dialysis catheter</u>
> *Excludes 1: mechanical complication of vascular dialysis catheter (T82.4-)*

T85.622-   Displacement of <u>permanent sutures</u>
> *Excludes 1: mechanical complication of permanent (wire) suture used in bone repair (T84.1-T84.2)*

T85.623-   Displacement of <u>artificial skin graft and decellularized allodermis</u>
> Dislodgement of artificial skin graft and decellularized allodermis
> Displacement of artificial skin graft and decellularized allodermis

T85.624-   Displacement of <u>insulin pump</u>

T85.628-   Displacement of <u>other</u> specified internal prosthetic devices, implants and grafts

T85.63-   <u>Leakage</u> of other specified internal prosthetic devices, implants and grafts

T85.630-   Leakage of <u>epidural and subdural infusion catheter</u>

T85.631-   Leakage of <u>intraperitoneal dialysis catheter</u>
> *Excludes 1: mechanical complication of vascular dialysis catheter (T82.4)*

T85.633-   Leakage of <u>insulin pump</u>

T85.638-   Leakage of <u>other</u> specified internal prosthetic devices, implants and grafts

T85.69-   <u>Other mechanical</u> complication of other specified internal prosthetic devices, implants and grafts
> Obstruction, mechanical of other specified internal prosthetic devices, implants and grafts
> Perforation of other specified internal prosthetic devices, implants and grafts
> Protrusion of other specified internal prosthetic devices, implants and grafts

T85.690-   Other mechanical complication of <u>epidural and subdural infusion catheter</u>

T85.691-   Other mechanical complication of <u>intraperitoneal dialysis catheter</u>
> *Excludes 1: mechanical complication of vascular dialysis catheter (T82.4)*

T85.692-   Other mechanical complication of <u>permanent sutures</u>
> *Excludes 1: mechanical complication of permanent (wire) suture used in bone repair (T84.1-T84.2)*

T85.693-   Other mechanical complication of <u>artificial skin graft and decellularized allodermis</u>

T85.694-   Other mechanical complication of <u>insulin pump</u>

T85.698-   Other mechanical complication of <u>other</u> specified internal prosthetic devices, implants and grafts
> Mechanical complication of nonabsorbable surgical material NOS

T85.7-   <u>Infection and inflammatory reaction</u> due to <u>other</u> internal prosthetic devices, implants and grafts
> Use additional code to identify infection

T85.71x-   Infection and inflammatory reaction due to <u>peritoneal dialysis catheter</u>

T85.72x-   Infection and inflammatory reaction due to <u>insulin pump</u>

T85.79x-   Infection and inflammatory reaction due to <u>other</u> internal prosthetic devices, implants and grafts

T85.8-   <u>Other specified complications</u> of internal prosthetic devices, implants and grafts, not elsewhere classified

T85.81x-   <u>Embolism</u> due to internal prosthetic devices, implants and grafts, not elsewhere classified

T85.82x-   <u>Fibrosis</u> due to internal prosthetic devices, implants and grafts, not elsewhere classified

T85.83x-   <u>Hemorrhage</u> due to internal prosthetic devices, implants and grafts, not elsewhere classified

T85.84x-   <u>Pain</u> due to internal prosthetic devices, implants and grafts, not elsewhere classified

T85.85x-   <u>Stenosis</u> due to internal prosthetic devices, implants and grafts, not elsewhere classified

T85.86x-   <u>Thrombosis</u> due to internal prosthetic devices, implants and grafts, not elsewhere classified

T85.89x-   <u>Other specified complication</u> of internal prosthetic devices, implants and grafts, not elsewhere classified

T85.9xx-   <u>Unspecified</u> complication of internal prosthetic device, implant and graft
> Complication of internal prosthetic device, implant and graft NOS

T86-   <u>Complications of transplanted organs and tissue</u>
> Use additional code to identify other transplant complications, such as:
> Graft-versus-host disease (D89.81-)
> Malignancy associated with organ transplant (C80.2)
> Post-transplant lymphoproliferative disorders (PTLD) (D47.Z1)

T86.0-   Complications of <u>bone marrow transplant</u>

T86.00   <u>Unspecified</u> complication of bone marrow transplant

T86.01   Bone marrow transplant <u>rejection</u>

T86.02   Bone marrow transplant <u>failure</u>

T86.03   Bone marrow transplant <u>infection</u>

T86.09   <u>Other</u> complications of bone marrow transplant

T86.1-   Complications of <u>kidney transplant</u>

T86.10   <u>Unspecified</u> complication of kidney transplant

T86.11   Kidney transplant <u>rejection</u>

T86.12   Kidney transplant <u>failure</u>

T86.13   Kidney transplant <u>infection</u>
> Use additional code to specify infection

T86.19   <u>Other</u> complication of kidney transplant

T86.2-   Complications of <u>heart transplant</u>
> *Excludes 1: complication of:*
> *artificial heart device (T82.5)*
> *heart-lung transplant (T86.3)*

T86.20   <u>Unspecified</u> complication of heart transplant

T86.21   Heart transplant <u>rejection</u>

T86.22   Heart transplant <u>failure</u>

T86.23   Heart transplant <u>infection</u>
> Use additional code to specify infection

T86.29-   <u>Other</u> complications of heart transplant

T86.290   <u>Cardiac allograft vasculopathy</u>
> *Excludes 1: atherosclerosis of coronary arteries (I25.75-, I25.76-, I25.81-)*

T86.298   <u>Other</u> complications of heart transplant

T86.3-   Complications of <u>heart-lung transplant</u>

T86.30   <u>Unspecified</u> complication of heart-lung transplant

T86.31   Heart-lung transplant <u>rejection</u>

T86.32   Heart-lung transplant <u>failure</u>

T86.33   Heart-lung transplant <u>infection</u>
> Use additional code to specify infection

T86.39   <u>Other</u> complications of heart-lung transplant

T86.4-   Complications of <u>liver transplant</u>

T86.40   <u>Unspecified</u> complication of liver transplant

T86.41   Liver transplant <u>rejection</u>

T86.42   Liver transplant <u>failure</u>

T86.43   Liver transplant <u>infection</u>
> Use additional code to identify infection, such as:
> Cytomegalovirus (CMV) infection (B25.-)

T86.49   <u>Other</u> complications of liver transplant

T86.5   Complications of <u>stem cell transplant</u>
> Complications from stem cells from peripheral blood
> Complications from stem cells from umbilical cord

T86.8-   Complications of other transplanted organs and tissues

T86.81-   Complications of <u>lung transplant</u>
> *Excludes 1: complication of heart-lung transplant (T86.3-)*

T86.810   Lung transplant <u>rejection</u>

T86.811   Lung transplant <u>failure</u>

T86.812   Lung transplant <u>infection</u>
> Use additional code to specify infection

T86.818   <u>Other</u> complications of lung transplant

T86.819   <u>Unspecified</u> complication of lung transplant

T86.82-   Complications of <u>skin graft (allograft) (autograft)</u>
> *Excludes❷: complication of artificial skin graft (T85.693)*

T86.820   Skin graft (allograft) <u>rejection</u>

T86.821   Skin graft (allograft) (autograft) <u>failure</u>

T86.822   Skin graft (allograft) (autograft) <u>infection</u>
> Use additional code to specify infection

T86.828   <u>Other</u> complications of skin graft (allograft) (autograft)

T86.829   <u>Unspecified</u> complication of skin graft (allograft) (autograft)

T86.83-   Complications of <u>bone graft</u>
> *Excludes❷: mechanical complications of bone graft (T84.3-)*

T86.830   Bone graft <u>rejection</u>

T86.831   Bone graft <u>failure</u>

Excludes 1: = NOT CODED HERE! (Do not code both)   **837**   *Excludes❷:* = Not Included Here

T
8
5
–
T
8
6

T86.832 **Bone graft** <u>infection</u>
Use additional code to specify infection

T86.838 <u>Other</u> complications of bone graft

T86.839 <u>Unspecified</u> complication of bone graft

T86.84- Complications of <u>corneal transplant</u>
Excludes❷: mechanical complications of corneal graft (T85.3-)

T86.840 Corneal transplant <u>rejection</u>

T86.841 Corneal transplant <u>failure</u>

T86.842 Corneal transplant <u>infection</u>
Use additional code to specify infection

T86.848 <u>Other</u> complications of corneal transplant

T86.849 <u>Unspecified</u> complication of corneal transplant

T86.85- Complication of <u>intestine transplant</u>

T86.850 Intestine transplant <u>rejection</u>

T86.851 Intestine transplant <u>failure</u>

T86.852 Intestine transplant <u>infection</u>
Use additional code to specify infection

T86.858 <u>Other</u> complications of intestine transplant

T86.859 <u>Unspecified</u> complication of intestine transplant

T86.89- Complications of <u>other transplanted tissue</u>
Transplant failure or rejection of pancreas

T86.890 Other transplanted tissue <u>rejection</u>

T86.891 Other transplanted tissue <u>failure</u>

T86.892 Other transplanted tissue <u>infection</u>
Use additional code to specify infection

T86.898 <u>Other</u> complications of other transplanted tissue

T86.899 <u>Unspecified</u> complication of other transplanted tissue

T86.9- Complication of <u>unspecified transplanted organ and tissue</u>

T86.90 <u>Unspecified</u> complication of unspecified transplanted organ and tissue

T86.91 Unspecified transplanted organ and tissue <u>rejection</u>

T86.92 Unspecified transplanted organ and tissue <u>failure</u>

T86.93 Unspecified transplanted organ and tissue <u>infection</u>
Use additional code to specify infection

T86.99 <u>Other</u> complications of unspecified transplanted organ and tissue

T87- <u>Complications peculiar to reattachment and amputation</u>

T87.0- Complications of reattached (part of) upper extremity

T87.0x- <u>Complications</u> of <u>reattached (part of)</u> upper extremity

T87.0x1 Complications of reattached (part of) <u>right</u> upper extremity

T87.0x2 Complications of reattached (part of) <u>left</u> extremity

T87.0x9 Complications of reattached (part of) <u>unspecified</u> upper extremity

T87.1- Complications of reattached (part of) <u>lower extremity</u>

T87.1x- <u>Complications</u> of <u>reattached (part of)</u> lower extremity

T87.1x1 Complications of reattached (part of) <u>right</u> lower extremity

T87.1x2 Complications of reattached (part of) <u>left</u> lower extremity

T87.1x9 Complications of reattached (part of) <u>unspecified</u> lower extremity

T87.2 Complications of <u>other reattached body part</u>

T87.3- <u>Neuroma</u> of <u>amputation stump</u>

T87.30 Neuroma of amputation stump, <u>unspecified</u> extremity

T87.31 Neuroma of amputation stump, <u>right</u> <u>upper</u> extremity

T87.32 Neuroma of amputation stump, <u>left</u> <u>upper</u> extremity

T87.33 Neuroma of amputation stump, <u>right</u> <u>lower</u> extremity

T87.34 Neuroma of amputation stump, <u>left</u> <u>lower</u> extremity

T87.4- <u>Infection</u> of <u>amputation stump</u>

T87.40 Infection of amputation stump, <u>unspecified</u> extremity

T87.41 Infection of amputation stump, <u>right</u> <u>upper</u> extremity

T87.42 Infection of amputation stump, <u>left</u> <u>upper</u> extremity

T87.43 Infection of amputation stump, <u>right</u> <u>lower</u> extremity

T87.44 Infection of amputation stump, <u>left</u> <u>lower</u> extremity

T87.5- <u>Necrosis</u> of <u>amputation stump</u>

T87.50 Necrosis of amputation stump, <u>unspecified</u> extremity

T87.51 Necrosis of amputation stump, <u>right</u> <u>upper</u> extremity

T87.52 Necrosis of amputation stump, <u>left</u> <u>upper</u> extremity

T87.53 Necrosis of amputation stump, <u>right</u> <u>lower</u> extremity

T87.54 Necrosis of amputation stump, <u>left</u> <u>lower</u> extremity

T87.8- Other complications of amputation stump

T87.81 <u>Dehiscence</u> of amputation stump

T87.89 <u>Other</u> complications of amputation stump
Amputation stump contracture
Amputation stump contracture of next proximal joint
Amputation stump edema
Amputation stump flexion
Amputation stump hematoma
Excludes❷: phantom limb syndrome (G54.6-G54.7)

T87.9 <u>Unspecified</u> complications of amputation stump

T88- Other complications of surgical and medical care, <u>not elsewhere classified</u>
Excludes❷: complication following infusion, transfusion and therapeutic injection (T80.-)
complication following procedure NEC (T81.-)
complications of anesthesia in labor and delivery (O74.-)
complications of anesthesia in pregnancy (O29.-)
complications of anesthesia in puerperium (O89.-)
complications of devices, implants and grafts (T82-T85)
complications of obstetric surgery and procedure (O75.4)
dermatitis due to drugs and medicaments (L23.3, L24.4, L25.1, L27.0-L27.1)
poisoning and toxic effects of drugs and chemicals (T36-T65 with fifth or sixth character 1-4 or 6)
specified complications classified elsewhere

The appropriate 7th character is to be added to each code from category T88:
A   <u>Initial</u> encounter
D   <u>Subsequent</u> encounter
S   <u>Sequela</u>

T88.0xx- **Infection following immunization**
Sepsis following immunization

T88.1xx- **Other complications following immunization, <u>not elsewhere classified</u>**
Generalized vaccinia
Rash following immunization
Excludes 1: vaccinia not from vaccine (B08.011)
Excludes❷: anaphylactic shock due to serum (T80.5-)
other serum reactions (T80.6-)
postimmunization arthropathy (M02.2)
postimmunization encephalitis (G04.02)
postimmunization fever (R50.83)

T88.2xx- **Shock due to anesthesia**
Use additional code for adverse effect, if applicable, to identify drug (T41- with fifth or sixth character 5)
Excludes 1: complications of anesthesia (in):
labor and delivery (O74-)
pregnancy (O29-)
puerperium (O89-)
postprocedural shock NOS (T81.1-)

T88.3xx- **Malignant hyperthermia due to anesthesia**
Use additional code for adverse effect, if applicable, to identify drug (T41- with fifth or sixth character 5)

T88.4xx- **Failed or difficult intubation**

T88.5- **Other complications of anesthesia**
Use additional code for adverse effect, if applicable, to identify drug (T41- with fifth or sixth character 5)

T88.51x- **Hypothermia following anesthesia**

T88.52x- **Failed moderate sedation during procedure**
Failed conscious sedation during procedure
Excludes❷: personal history of failed moderate sedation (Z92.83)

T88.59x- **Other complications of anesthesia**

T88.6xx- **Anaphylactic reaction due to adverse effect of correct drug or medicament properly administered**
Anaphylactic shock due to adverse effect of correct drug or medicament properly administered
Anaphylactoid reaction NOS
Use additional code for adverse effect, if applicable, to identify drug (T36-T50 with fifth or sixth character 5)
Excludes 1: anaphylactic reaction due to serum (T80.5)

T88.7xx- **Unspecified adverse effect of drug or medicament**
Drug hypersensitivity NOS
Drug reaction NOS
Use additional code for adverse effect, if applicable, to identify drug (T36-T50 with fifth or sixth character 5)
Excludes 1: specified adverse effects of drugs and medicaments (A00-R94 and T80-T88.6, T88.8)

T88.8xx- **Other specified complications of surgical and medical care, not elsewhere classified**
Use additional code to identify the complication

T88.9xx- **Complication of surgical and medical care, unspecified**

T86 - V00

Chapter 20 – External causes of morbidity (V00-Y99)

Note: This chapter permits the classification of environmental events and circumstances as the cause of injury, and other adverse effects. Where a code from this section is applicable, it is intended that it shall be used secondary to a code from another chapter of the Classification indicating the nature of the condition. Most often, the condition will be classifiable to Chapter 19, Injury, poisoning and certain other consequences of external causes (S00-T88). Other conditions that may be stated to be due to external causes are classified in Chapters I to XVIII. For these conditions, codes from Chapter 20 should be used to provide additional information as to the cause of the condition.

This chapter contains the following blocks:

V00-X58	Accidents
V00-V99	Transport accidents
V00-V09	Pedestrian injured in transport accident
V10-V19	Pedal cycle rider injured in transport accident
V20-V29	Motorcycle rider injured in transport accident
V30-V39	Occupant of three-wheeled motor vehicle injured in transport accident
V40-V49	Car occupant injured in transport accident
V50-V59	Occupant of pick-up truck or van injured in transport accident
V60-V69	Occupant of heavy transport vehicle injured in transport accident
V70-V79	Bus occupant injured in transport accident
V80-V89	Other land transport accidents
V90-V94	Water transport accidents
V95-V97	Air and space transport accidents
V98-V99	Other and unspecified transport accidents
W00-W19	Slipping, tripping, stumbling and falls
W20-W49	Exposure to inanimate mechanical forces
W50-W64	Exposure to animate mechanical forces
W65-W74	Accidental non-transport drowning and submersion
W85-W99	Exposure to electric current, radiation and extreme ambient air temperature and pressure
X00-X08	Exposure to smoke, fire and flames
X10-X19	Contact with heat and hot substances
X30-X39	Exposure to forces of nature
X52-X58	Accidental exposure to other specified factors
X71-X83	Intentional self-harm
X92-Y09	Assault
Y21-Y33	Event of undetermined intent
Y35-Y38	Legal intervention, operations of war, military operations, and terrorism
Y62-Y69	Misadventures to patients during surgical and medical care
Y70-Y82	Medical devices associated with adverse incidents in diagnostic and therapeutic use
Y83-Y84	Surgical and other medical procedures as the cause of abnormal reaction of the patient, or of later complication, without mention of misadventure at the time of the procedure
Y90-Y99	Supplementary factors related to causes of morbidity classified elsewhere

Accidents (V00-X58)

Transport accidents (V00-V99)

Note: This section is structured in 12 groups. Those relating to land transport accidents (V01-V89) reflect the victim's mode of transport and are subdivided to identify the victim's "counterpart" or the type of event. The vehicle of which the injured person is an occupant is identified in the first two characters since it is seen as the most important factor to identify for prevention purposes. A transport accident is one in which the vehicle involved must be moving or running or in use for transport purposes at the time of the accident.

Use additional code to identify:
Airbag injury (W22.1)
Type of street or road (Y92.4-)
Use of cellular telephone and other electronic equipment at the time of the transport accident (Y93.C-)

Excludes 1:   agricultural vehicles in stationary use or maintenance (W31-)
  assault by crashing of motor vehicle (Y03-)
  automobile or motor cycle in stationary use or maintenance — code to type of accident
  crashing of motor vehicle, undetermined intent (Y32)
  intentional self-harm by crashing of motor vehicle (X82)

Excludes❷: transport accidents due to cataclysm (X34-X38)

Definitions of transport vehicles:

(a) A **transport accident** is any accident involving a device designed primarily for, or used at the time primarily for, conveying persons or goods from one place to another.

(b) A **public highway [trafficway] or street** is the entire width between property lines (or other boundary lines) of land open to the public as a matter of right or custom for purposes of moving persons or property from one place to another. A roadway is that part of the public highway designed, improved and customarily used for vehicular traffic.

(c) A **traffic accident** is any vehicle accident occurring on the public highway [i.e. originating on, terminating on, or involving a vehicle partially on the highway]. A vehicle accident is assumed to have occurred on the public highway unless another place is specified, except in the case of accidents involving only off-road motor vehicles, which are classified as nontraffic accidents unless the contrary is stated.

(d) A **nontraffic accident** is any vehicle accident that occurs entirely in any place other than a public highway.

(e) A **pedestrian** is any person involved in an accident who was not at the time of the accident riding in or on a motor vehicle, railway train, streetcar or animal-drawn or other vehicle, or on a pedal cycle or animal. This includes, a person changing a tire or working on a parked car. It also includes the use of a pedestrian conveyance such as a baby carriage, ice-skates, roller skates, a skateboard, nonmotorized or motorized wheelchair, motorized mobility scooter, or nonmotorized scooter.

(f) A **driver** is an occupant of a transport vehicle who is operating or intending to operate it.

(g) A **passenger** is any occupant of a transport vehicle other than the driver, except a person traveling on the outside of the vehicle.

(h) A **person on the outside of a vehicle** is any person being transported by a vehicle but not occupying the space normally reserved for the driver or passengers, or the space intended for the transport of property. This includes the body, bumper, fender, roof, running board or step of a vehicle.

(i) A **pedal cycle** is any land transport vehicle operated solely by nonmotorized pedals including a bicycle or tricycle.

(j) A **pedal cyclist** is any person riding a pedal cycle or in a sidecar or trailer attached to a pedal cycle.

(k) A **motorcycle** is a two-wheeled motor vehicle with one or two riding saddles and sometimes with a third wheel for the support of a sidecar. The sidecar is considered part of the motorcycle.

(l) A **motorcycle rider** is any person riding a motorcycle or in a sidecar or trailer attached to the motorcycle.

(m) A **three-wheeled motor vehicle** is a motorized tricycle designed primarily for on-road use. This includes a motor-driven tricycle, a motorized rickshaw, or a three-wheeled motor car.

(n) A **car [automobile]** is a four-wheeled motor vehicle designed primarily for carrying up to 7 persons. A trailer being towed by the car is considered part of the car.

(o) A **pick-up truck or van** is a four or six-wheeled motor vehicle designed for carrying passengers as well as property or cargo weighing less than the local limit for classification as a heavy goods vehicle, and not requiring a special driver's license. This includes a minivan and a sport-utility vehicle (SUV).

(p) A **heavy transport vehicle** is a motor vehicle designed primarily for carrying property, meeting local criteria for classification as a heavy goods vehicle in terms of weight and requiring a special driver's license.

(q) A **bus (coach)** is a motor vehicle designed or adapted primarily for carrying more than 10 passengers, and requiring a special driver's license.

(r) A **railway train or railway vehicle** is any device, with or without freight or passenger cars coupled to it, designed for traffic on a railway track. This includes subterranean (subways) or elevated trains.

(s) A **streetcar**, is a device designed and used primarily for transporting passengers within a municipality, running on rails, usually subject to normal traffic control signals, and operated principally on a right-of-way that forms part of the roadway. This includes a tram or trolley that runs on rails. A trailer being towed by a streetcar is considered part of the streetcar.

(t) A **special vehicle mainly used on industrial premises** is a motor vehicle designed primarily for use within the buildings and premises of industrial or commercial establishments. This includes battery-powered trucks, forklifts, coal-cars in a coal mine, logging cars and trucks used in mines or quarries.

(u) A **special vehicle mainly used in agriculture** is a motor vehicle designed specifically for use in farming and agriculture (horticulture), to work the land, tend and harvest crops and transport materials on the farm. This includes harvesters, farm machinery and tractor and trailers.

(v) A **special construction vehicle** is a motor vehicle designed specifically for use on construction and demolition sites. This includes bulldozers, diggers, earth levellers, dump trucks, backhoes, front-end loaders, pavers, and mechanical shovels.

(w) A **special all-terrain vehicle** is a motor vehicle of special design to enable it to negotiate over rough or soft terrain, snow or sand. This includes snow mobiles, all-terrain vehicles (ATV), and dune buggies. It does not include passenger vehicle designated as Sport Utility Vehicles (SUV).

T86-I-V00

(x) A **watercraft** is any device designed for transporting passengers or goods on water. This includes motor or sail boats, ships, and hovercraft.

(y) An **aircraft** is any device for transporting passengers or goods in the air. This includes hot-air balloons, gliders, helicopters and airplanes.

(z) A **military vehicle** is any motorized vehicle operating on a public roadway owned by the military and being operated by a member of the military.

Pedestrian injured in transport accident (V00-V09)

Includes: Person changing tire on transport vehicle
            Person examining engine of vehicle broken down in (on side of) road
*Excludes 1:   fall due to non-transport collision with other person (W03)
            pedestrian on foot falling (slipping) on ice and snow (W00-)
            struck or bumped by another person (W51)*

V00-   Pedestrian conveyance accident
Use additional place of occurrence and activity external cause codes, if known (Y92-, Y93-)
*Excludes 1:   collision with another person without fall (W51)
            fall due to person on foot colliding with another person on foot (W03)
            fall from non-moving wheelchair, nonmotorized scooter and motorized mobility scooter without collision (W05-)
            pedestrian (conveyance) collision with other land transport vehicle (V01-V09)
            pedestrian on foot falling (slipping) on ice and snow (W00-)*

The appropriate 7th character is to be added to each code from category V00:
   A   Initial encounter
   D   Subsequent encounter
   S   Sequela

V00.0-   Pedestrian on foot injured in collision with pedestrian conveyance
   V00.01x-   Pedestrian on foot injured in collision with roller-skater
   V00.02x-   Pedestrian on foot injured in collision with skateboarder
   V00.09x-   Pedestrian on foot injured in collision with other pedestrian conveyance
V00.1-   Rolling-type pedestrian conveyance accident
      *Excludes 1:   accident with babystroller (V00.82-)
               accident with wheelchair (powered) (V00.81-)
               accident with motorized mobility scooter (V00.83-)*
   V00.11-   In-line roller-skate accident
      V00.111-   Fall from in-line roller-skates
      V00.112-   In-line roller-skater colliding with stationary object
      V00.118-   Other in-line roller-skate accident
         Excludes 1:   roller-skater collision with other land transport vehicle (V01-V09 with 5th character 1)
   V00.12-   Non-in- line roller-skate accident
      V00.121-   Fall from non-in-line roller-skates
      V00.122-   Non-in-line roller-skater colliding with stationary object
      V00.128-   Other non-in-line roller-skating accident
         Excludes 1:   roller-skater collision with other land transport vehicle (V01-V09 with 5th character 1)
   V00.13-   Skateboard accident
      V00.131-   Fall from skateboard
      V00.132-   Skateboarder colliding with stationary object
      V00.138-   Other skateboard accident
         Excludes 1:   skateboarder collision with other land transport vehicle (V01-V09 with 5th character 2)
   V00.14-   Scooter (nonmotorized) accident
         Excludes 1:   motorscooter accident (V20-V29)
      V00.141-   Fall from scooter (nonmotorized)
      V00.142-   Scooter (nonmotorized) colliding with stationary object
      V00.148-   Other scooter (nonmotorized) accident
         Excludes 1:   scooter (nonmotorized) collision with other land transport vehicle (V01-V09 with fifth character 9)
   V00.15-   Heelies accident
         Rolling shoe
         Wheeled shoe
         Wheelies accident
      V00.151-   Fall from heelies
      V00.152-   Heelies colliding with stationary object
      V00.158-   Other heelies accident

V00.18-   Accident on other rolling-type pedestrian conveyance
   V00.181-   Fall from other rolling-type pedestrian conveyance
   V00.182-   Pedestrian on other rolling-type pedestrian conveyance colliding with stationary object
   V00.188-   Other accident on other rolling-type pedestrian conveyance
V00.2-   Gliding-type pedestrian conveyance accident
   V00.21-   Ice-skates accident
      V00.211-   Fall from ice-skates
      V00.212-   Ice-skater colliding with stationary object
      V00.218-   Other ice-skates accident
         Excludes 1:   ice-skater collision with other land transport vehicle (V01-V09 with 5th digit 9)
   V00.22-   Sled accident
      V00.221-   Fall from sled
      V00.222-   Sledder colliding with stationary object
      V00.228-   Other sled accident
         Excludes 1:   sled collision with other land transport vehicle (V01-V09 with 5th digit 9)
   V00.28-   Other gliding-type pedestrian conveyance accident
      V00.281-   Fall from other gliding-type pedestrian conveyance
      V00.282-   Pedestrian on other gliding-type pedestrian conveyance colliding with stationary object
      V00.288-   Other accident on other gliding-type pedestrian conveyance
         Excludes 1:   gliding-type pedestrian conveyance collision with other land transport vehicle (V01-V09 with 5th digit 9)
V00.3-   Flat-bottomed pedestrian conveyance accident
   V00.31-   Snowboard accident
      V00.311-   Fall from snowboard
      V00.312-   Snowboarder colliding with stationary object
      V00.318-   Other snowboard accident
         Excludes 1:   snowboarder collision with other land transport vehicle (V01-V09 with 5th digit 9)
   V00.32-   Snow-ski accident
      V00.321-   Fall from snow-skis
      V00.322-   Snow-skier colliding with stationary object
      V00.328-   Other snow-ski accident
         Excludes 1:   snow-skier collision with other land transport vehicle (V01-V09 with 5th digit 9)
   V00.38-   Other flat-bottomed pedestrian conveyance accident
      V00.381-   Fall from other flat-bottomed pedestrian conveyance
      V00.382-   Pedestrian on other flat-bottomed pedestrian conveyance colliding with stationary object
      V00.388-   Other accident on other flat-bottomed pedestrian conveyance
V00.8-   Accident on other pedestrian conveyance
   V00.81-   Accident with wheelchair (powered)
      V00.811-   Fall from moving wheelchair (powered)
         Excludes 1:   fall from non-moving wheelchair (W05.0)
      V00.812-   Wheelchair (powered) colliding with stationary object
      V00.818-   Other accident with wheelchair (powered)
   V00.82-   Accident with babystroller
      V00.821-   Fall from babystroller
      V00.822-   Babystroller colliding with stationary object
      V00.828-   Other accident with babystroller
   V00.83-   Accident with motorized mobility scooter
      V00.831-   Fall from motorized mobility scooter
         Excludes 1:   fall from non-moving motorized mobility scooter (W05.2)
      V00.832-   Motorized mobility scooter colliding with stationary object
      V00.838-   Other accident with motorized mobility scooter
   V00.89-   Accident on other pedestrian conveyance
      V00.891-   Fall from other pedestrian conveyance
      V00.892-   Pedestrian on other pedestrian conveyance colliding with stationary object
      V00.898-   Other accident on other pedestrian conveyance
         Excludes 1:   other pedestrian (conveyance) collision with other land transport vehicle (V01-V09 with 5th digit 9)

V00 - V02

V01- **Pedestrian injured in collision** with **pedal cycle**
The appropriate 7th character is to be added to each code from category V01:
A   **Initial** encounter
D   **Subsequent** encounter
S   **Sequela**

V01.0- **Pedestrian injured in collision** with **pedal cycle** in **nontraffic** accident

V01.00x- **Pedestrian on foot injured in collision with pedal cycle in nontraffic accident**
Pedestrian NOS injured in collision with pedal cycle in nontraffic accident

V01.01x- **Pedestrian on roller-skates injured in collision with pedal cycle in nontraffic accident**

V01.02x- **Pedestrian on skateboard injured in collision with pedal cycle in nontraffic accident**

V01.09x- **Pedestrian with other conveyance injured in collision with pedal cycle in nontraffic accident**
Pedestrian with babystroller injured in collision with pedal cycle in nontraffic accident
Pedestrian on ice-skates injured in collision with pedal cycle in nontraffic accident
Pedestrian on nonmotorized scooter injured in collision with pedal cycle in nontraffic accident
Pedestrian on sled injured in collision with pedal cycle in nontraffic accident
Pedestrian on snowboard injured in collision with pedal cycle in nontraffic accident
Pedestrian on snow-skis injured in collision with pedal cycle in nontraffic accident
Pedestrian in wheelchair (powered) injured in collision with pedal cycle in nontraffic accident
Pedestrian in motorized mobility scooter injured in collision with pedal cycle in nontraffic accident

V01.1- **Pedestrian injured in collision** with **pedal cycle** in **traffic** accident

V01.10x- **Pedestrian on foot injured in collision with pedal cycle in traffic accident**
Pedestrian NOS injured in collision with pedal cycle in traffic accident

V01.11x- **Pedestrian on roller-skates injured in collision with pedal cycle in traffic accident**

V01.12x- **Pedestrian on skateboard injured in collision with pedal cycle in traffic accident**

V01.19x- **Pedestrian with other conveyance injured in collision with pedal cycle in traffic accident**
Pedestrian with babystroller injured in collision with pedal cycle in traffic accident
Pedestrian on ice-skates injured in collision with pedal cycle in traffic accident
Pedestrian on nonmotorized scooter injured in collision with pedal cycle in traffic accident
Pedestrian on sled injured in collision with pedal cycle in traffic accident
Pedestrian on snowboard injured in collision with pedal cycle in traffic accident
Pedestrian on snow-skis injured in collision with pedal cycle in traffic accident
Pedestrian in wheelchair (powered) injured in collision with pedal cycle in traffic accident
Pedestrian in motorized mobility scooter injured in collision with pedal cycle in traffic accident

V01.9- **Pedestrian injured in collision** with **pedal cycle, unspecified** whether traffic or nontraffic accident

V01.90x- **Pedestrian on foot injured in collision with pedal cycle, unspecified whether traffic or nontraffic accident**
Pedestrian NOS injured in collision with pedal cycle, unspecified whether traffic or nontraffic accident

V01.91x- **Pedestrian on roller-skates injured in collision with pedal cycle, unspecified whether traffic or nontraffic accident**

V01.92x- **Pedestrian on skateboard injured in collision with pedal cycle, unspecified whether traffic or nontraffic accident**

V01.99x- **Pedestrian with other conveyance injured in collision with pedal cycle, unspecified whether traffic or nontraffic accident**
Pedestrian with babystroller injured in collision with pedal cycle, unspecified whether traffic or nontraffic accident
Pedestrian on ice-skates injured in collision with pedal cycle unspecified, whether traffic or nontraffic accident
Pedestrian on nonmotorized scooter injured in collision with pedal cycle, unspecified whether traffic or nontraffic accident
Pedestrian on sled injured in collision with pedal cycle unspecified, whether traffic or nontraffic accident
Pedestrian on snowboard injured in collision with pedal cycle, unspecified whether traffic or nontraffic accident
Pedestrian on snow-skis injured in collision with pedal cycle, unspecified whether traffic or nontraffic accident
Pedestrian in wheelchair (powered) injured in collision with pedal cycle, unspecified whether traffic or nontraffic accident
Pedestrian in motorized mobility scooter injured in collision with pedal cycle, unspecified whether traffic or nontraffic accident

V02- **Pedestrian injured in collision** with **two- or three-wheeled motor vehicle**
The appropriate 7th character is to be added to each code from category V02:
A   **Initial** encounter
D   **Subsequent** encounter
S   **Sequela**

V02.0- **Pedestrian injured in collision** with **two- or three-wheeled motor vehicle** in **nontraffic** accident

V02.00x- **Pedestrian on foot injured in collision with two- or three-wheeled motor vehicle in nontraffic accident**
Pedestrian NOS injured in collision with two- or three-wheeled motor vehicle in nontraffic accident

V02.01x- **Pedestrian on roller-skates injured in collision with two- or three-wheeled motor vehicle in nontraffic accident**

V02.02x- **Pedestrian on skateboard injured in collision with two- or three-wheeled motor vehicle in nontraffic accident**

V02.09x- **Pedestrian with other conveyance injured in collision with two- or three-wheeled motorvehicle in nontraffic accident**
Pedestrian with babystroller injured in collision with two- or three-wheeled motor vehicle in nontraffic accident
Pedestrian on ice-skates injured in collision with two- or three-wheeled motor vehicle in nontraffic accident
Pedestrian on nonmotorized scooter injured in collision with two- or three-wheeled motor vehicle in nontraffic accident
Pedestrian on sled injured in collision with two- or three-wheeled motor vehicle in nontraffic accident
Pedestrian on snowboard injured in collision with two- or three-wheeled motor vehicle in nontraffic accident
Pedestrian on snow-skis injured in collision with two- or three-wheeled motor vehicle in nontraffic accident
Pedestrian in wheelchair (powered) injured in collision with two- or three-wheeled motor vehicle in nontraffic accident
Pedestrian in motorized mobility scooter injured in collision with two- or three-wheeled motor vehicle in nontraffic accident

V02.1- **Pedestrian injured in collision** with **two- or three-wheeled motor vehicle** in **traffic** accident

V02.10x- **Pedestrian on foot injured in collision with two- or three-wheeled motor vehicle in traffic accident**
Pedestrian NOS injured in collision with two- or three-wheeled motor vehicle in traffic accident

V02.11x- **Pedestrian on roller-skates injured in collision with two- or three-wheeled motor vehicle intraffic accident**

V02.12x- **Pedestrian on skateboard injured in collision with two- or three-wheeled motor vehicle intraffic accident**

V
0
0
–
V
0
2

V02.19x- **Pedestrian with other conveyance injured in collision with two- or three-wheeled motorvehicle in traffic accident**
Pedestrian with babystroller injured in collision with two- or three-wheeled motor vehicle in traffic accident
Pedestrian on ice-skates injured in collision with two- or three-wheeled motor vehicle in traffic accident
Pedestrian on nonmotorized scooter injured in collision with two- or three-wheeled motor vehicle in traffic accident
Pedestrian on sled injured in collision with two- or three-wheeled motor vehicle in traffic accident
Pedestrian on snowboard injured in collision with two- or three-wheeled motor vehicle in traffic accident
Pedestrian on snow-skis injured in collision with two- or three-wheeled motor vehicle in traffic accident
Pedestrian in wheelchair (powered) injured in collision with two- or three-wheeled motor vehicle in traffic accident
Pedestrian in motorized mobility scooter injured in collision with two- or three-wheeled motor vehicle in traffic accident

V02.9- **Pedestrian injured in collision with two- or three-wheeled motor vehicle, unspecified whether traffic or nontraffic accident**
V02.90x- **Pedestrian on foot injured in collision with two- or three-wheeled motor vehicle, unspecified whether traffic or nontraffic accident**
Pedestrian NOS injured in collision with two- or three-wheeled motor vehicle, unspecified whether traffic or nontraffic accident

V02.91x- **Pedestrian on roller-skates injured in collision with two- or three-wheeled motor vehicle, unspecified whether traffic or nontraffic accident**

V02.92x- **Pedestrian on skateboard injured in collision with two- or three-wheeled motor vehicle, unspecified whether traffic or nontraffic accident**

V02.99x- **Pedestrian with other conveyance injured in collision with two- or three-wheeled motor vehicle, unspecified whether traffic or nontraffic accident**
Pedestrian with babystroller injured in collision with two- or three-wheeled motor vehicle, unspecified whether traffic or nontraffic accident
Pedestrian on ice-skates injured in collision with two- or three-wheeled motor vehicle, unspecified whether traffic or nontraffic accident
Pedestrian on nonmotorized scooter injured in collision with two- or three-wheeled motor vehicle, unspecified whether traffic or nontraffic accident
Pedestrian on sled injured in collision with two- or three-wheeled motor vehicle, unspecified whether traffic or nontraffic accident
Pedestrian on snowboard injured in collision with two- or three-wheeled motor vehicle, unspecified whether traffic or nontraffic accident
Pedestrian on snow-skis injured in collision with two- or three-wheeled motor vehicle, unspecified whether traffic or nontraffic accident
Pedestrian in wheelchair (powered) injured in collision with two- or three-wheeled motor vehicle, unspecified whether traffic or nontraffic accident
Pedestrian in motorized mobility scooter injured in collision with two- or three-wheeled motor vehicle, unspecified whether traffic or nontraffic accident

V03- **Pedestrian injured in collision with car, pick-up truck or van**
The appropriate 7th character is to be added to each code from category V03:
A   Initial encounter
D   Subsequent encounter
S   Sequela

V03.0- **Pedestrian injured in collision with car, pick-up truck or van in nontraffic accident**
V03.00x- **Pedestrian on foot injured in collision with car, pick-up truck or van in nontraffic accident**
Pedestrian NOS injured in collision with car, pick-up truck or van in nontraffic accident

V03.01x- **Pedestrian on roller-skates injured in collision with car, pick-up truck or van in nontraffic accident**

V03.02x- **Pedestrian on skateboard injured in collision with car, pick-up truck or van in nontraffic accident**

V03.09x- **Pedestrian with other conveyance injured in collision with car, pick-up truck or van in nontraffic accident**
Pedestrian with babystroller injured in collision with car, pick-up truck or van in nontraffic accident
Pedestrian on ice-skates injured in collision with car, pick-up truck or van in nontraffic accident
Pedestrian on nonmotorized scooter injured in collision with car, pick-up truck or van in nontraffic accident
Pedestrian on sled injured in collision with car, pick-up truck or van in nontraffic accident
Pedestrian on snowboard injured in collision with car, pick-up truck or van in nontraffic accident
Pedestrian on snow-skis injured in collision with car, pick-up truck or van in nontraffic accident
Pedestrian in wheelchair (powered) injured in collision with car, pick-up truck or van in nontraffic accident
Pedestrian in motorized mobility scooter injured in collision with car, pick-up truck or van in nontraffic accident

V03.1- **Pedestrian injured in collision with car, pick-up truck or van in traffic accident**
V03.10x- **Pedestrian on foot injured in collision with car, pick-up truck or van in traffic accident**
Pedestrian NOS injured in collision with car, pick-up truck or van in traffic accident

V03.11x- **Pedestrian on roller-skates injured in collision with car, pick-up truck or van in traffic accident**

V03.12x- **Pedestrian on skateboard injured in collision with car, pick-up truck or van in traffic accident**

V03.19x- **Pedestrian with other conveyance injured in collision with car, pick-up truck or van in traffic accident**
Pedestrian with babystroller injured in collision with car, pick-up truck or van in traffic accident
Pedestrian on ice-skates injured in collision with car, pick-up truck or van in traffic accident
Pedestrian on nonmotorized scooter injured in collision with car, pick-up truck or van in traffic accident
Pedestrian on sled injured in collision with car, pick-up truck or van in traffic accident
Pedestrian on snowboard injured in collision with car, pick-up truck or van in traffic accident
Pedestrian on snow-skis injured in collision with car, pick-up truck or van in traffic accident
Pedestrian in wheelchair (powered) injured in collision with car, pick-up truck or van in traffic accident
Pedestrian in motorized mobility scooter injured in collision with car, pick-up truck or van in traffic accident

V03.9- **Pedestrian injured in collision with car, pick-up truck or van, unspecified whether traffic or nontraffic accident**
V03.90x- **Pedestrian on foot injured in collision with car, pick-up truck or van, unspecified whether traffic or nontraffic accident**
Pedestrian NOS injured in collision with car, pick-up truck or van, unspecified whether traffic or nontraffic accident

V03.91x- **Pedestrian on roller-skates injured in collision with car, pick-up truck or van, unspecified whether traffic or nontraffic accident**

V03.92x- **Pedestrian on skateboard injured in collision with car, pick-up truck or van, unspecified whether traffic or nontraffic accident**

V03.99x- **Pedestrian with other conveyance injured in collision with car, pick-up truck or van, unspecified whether traffic or nontraffic accident**
Pedestrian with babystroller injured in collision with car, pick-up truck or van, unspecified whether traffic or nontraffic accident
Pedestrian on ice-skates injured in collision with car, pick-up truck or van, unspecified whether traffic or nontraffic accident
Pedestrian on nonmotorized scooter injured in collision with car, pick-up truck or van, unspecified whether traffic or nontraffic accident
Pedestrian on sled injured in collision with car, pick-up truck or van in nontraffic accident
Pedestrian on snowboard injured in collision with car, pick-up truck or van, unspecified whether traffic or nontraffic accident
Pedestrian on snow-skis injured in collision with car, pick-up truck or van, unspecified whether traffic or nontraffic accident
Pedestrian in wheelchair (powered) injured in collision with car, pick-up truck or van, unspecified whether traffic or nontraffic accident
Pedestrian in motorized mobility scooter injured in collision with car, pick-up truck or van, unspecified whether traffic or nontraffic accident

**V
0
2
-
V
0
5**

© 2013 Channel Publishing, Ltd.

V04-   **Pedestrian injured in collision** with <u>heavy transport vehicle or bus</u>
  Excludes 1:   pedestrian injured in collision with military vehicle (V09.01, V09.21)

The appropriate 7th character is to be added to each code from category V04:
  A   <u>Initial</u> encounter
  D   <u>Subsequent</u> encounter
  S   <u>Sequela</u>

V04.0-   **Pedestrian injured in collision** with <u>heavy transport vehicle or bus</u> in <u>nontraffic</u> accident

  V04.00x-   **Pedestrian on foot injured in collision with heavy transport vehicle or bus in nontraffic accident**
       Pedestrian NOS injured in collision with heavy transport vehicle or bus in nontraffic accident

  V04.01x-   **Pedestrian on roller-skates injured in collision with heavy transport vehicle or bus in nontraffic accident**

  V04.02x-   **Pedestrian on skateboard injured in collision with heavy transport vehicle or bus in nontraffic accident**

  V04.09x-   **Pedestrian with other conveyance injured in collision with heavy transport vehicle or bus in nontraffic accident**
       Pedestrian with babystroller injured in collision with heavy transport vehicle or bus in nontraffic accident
       Pedestrian on ice-skates injured in collision with heavy transport vehicle or bus in nontraffic accident
       Pedestrian on nonmotorized scooter injured in collision with heavy transport vehicle or bus in nontraffic accident
       Pedestrian on sled injured in collision with heavy transport vehicle or bus in nontraffic accident
       Pedestrian on snowboard injured in collision with heavy transport vehicle or bus in nontraffic accident
       Pedestrian on snow-skis injured in collision with heavy transport vehicle or bus in nontraffic accident
       Pedestrian in wheelchair (powered) injured in collision with heavy transport vehicle or bus in nontraffic accident
       Pedestrian in motorized mobility scooter injured in collision with heavy transport vehicle or bus in nontraffic accident

V04.1-   **Pedestrian injured in collision** with <u>heavy transport vehicle or bus</u> in <u>traffic</u> accident

  V04.10x-   **Pedestrian on foot injured in collision with heavy transport vehicle or bus in traffic accident**
       Pedestrian NOS injured in collision with heavy transport vehicle or bus in traffic accident

  V04.11x-   **Pedestrian on roller-skates injured in collision with heavy transport vehicle or bus in traffic accident**

  V04.12x-   **Pedestrian on skateboard injured in collision with heavy transport vehicle or bus in traffic accident**

  V04.19x-   **Pedestrian with other conveyance injured in collision with heavy transport vehicle or bus in traffic accident**
       Pedestrian with babystroller injured in collision with heavy transport vehicle or bus in traffic accident
       Pedestrian on ice-skates injured in collision with heavy transport vehicle or bus in traffic accident
       Pedestrian on nonmotorized scooter injured in collision with heavy transport vehicle or bus in traffic accident
       Pedestrian on sled injured in collision with heavy transport vehicle or bus in traffic accident
       Pedestrian on snowboard injured in collision with heavy transport vehicle or bus in traffic accident
       Pedestrian on snow-skis injured in collision with heavy transport vehicle or bus in traffic accident
       Pedestrian in wheelchair (powered) injured in collision with heavy transport vehicle or bus in traffic accident
       Pedestrian in motorized mobility scooter injured in collision with heavy transport vehicle or bus in traffic accident

V04.9-   **Pedestrian injured in collision** with <u>heavy transport vehicle or bus</u>, <u>unspecified</u> whether traffic or nontraffic accident

  V04.90x-   **Pedestrian on foot injured in collision with heavy transport vehicle or bus, unspecified whether traffic or nontraffic accident**
       Pedestrian NOS injured in collision with heavy transport vehicle or bus, unspecified whether traffic or nontraffic accident

  V04.91x-   **Pedestrian on roller-skates injured in collision with heavy transport vehicle or bus, unspecified whether traffic or nontraffic accident**

  V04.92x-   **Pedestrian on skateboard injured in collision with heavy transport vehicle or bus, unspecified whether traffic or nontraffic accident**

  V04.99x-   **Pedestrian with other conveyance injured in collision with heavy transport vehicle or bus, unspecified whether traffic or nontraffic accident**
       Pedestrian with babystroller injured in collision with heavy transport vehicle or bus, unspecified whether traffic or nontraffic accident
       Pedestrian on ice-skates injured in collision with heavy transport vehicle or bus, unspecified whether traffic or nontraffic accident
       Pedestrian on nonmotorized scooter injured in collision with heavy transport vehicle or bus, unspecified whether traffic or nontraffic accident
       Pedestrian on sled injured in collision with heavy transport vehicle or bus, unspecified whether traffic or nontraffic accident
       Pedestrian on snowboard injured in collision with heavy transport vehicle or bus, unspecified whether traffic or nontraffic accident
       Pedestrian on snow-skis injured in collision with heavy transport vehicle or bus, unspecified whether traffic or nontraffic accident
       Pedestrian in wheelchair (powered) injured in collision with heavy transport vehicle or bus, unspecified whether traffic or nontraffic accident
       Pedestrian in motorized mobility scooter injured in collision with heavy transport vehicle or bus, unspecified whether traffic or nontraffic accident

V05-   **Pedestrian injured in collision** with <u>railway train or railway vehicle</u>
The appropriate 7th character is to be added to each code from category V05:
  A   <u>Initial</u> encounter
  D   <u>Subsequent</u> encounter
  S   <u>Sequela</u>

V05.0-   **Pedestrian injured in collision** with <u>railway train or railway vehicle</u> in <u>nontraffic</u> accident

  V05.00x-   **Pedestrian on foot injured in collision with railway train or railway vehicle in nontraffic accident**
       Pedestrian NOS injured in collision with railway train or railway vehicle in nontraffic accident

  V05.01x-   **Pedestrian on roller-skates injured in collision with railway train or railway vehicle in nontraffic accident**

  V05.02x-   **Pedestrian on skateboard injured in collision with railway train or railway vehicle in nontraffic accident**

  V05.09x-   **Pedestrian with other conveyance injured in collision with railway train or railway vehicle in nontraffic accident**
       Pedestrian with babystroller injured in collision with railway train or railway vehicle in nontraffic accident
       Pedestrian on ice-skates injured in collision with railway train or railway vehicle in nontraffic accident
       Pedestrian on nonmotorized scooter injured in collision with railway train or railway vehicle in nontraffic accident
       Pedestrian on sled injured in collision with railway train or railway vehicle in nontraffic accident
       Pedestrian on snowboard injured in collision with railway train or railway vehicle in nontraffic accident
       Pedestrian on snow-skis injured in collision with railway train or railway vehicle in nontraffic accident
       Pedestrian in wheelchair (powered) injured in collision with railway train or railway vehicle in nontraffic accident
       Pedestrian in motorized mobility scooter injured in collision with railway train or railway vehicle in nontraffic accident

V05.1-   **Pedestrian injured in collision** with <u>railway train or railway vehicle</u> in <u>traffic</u> accident

  V05.10x-   **Pedestrian on foot injured in collision with railway train or railway vehicle in traffic accident**
       Pedestrian NOS injured in collision with railway train or railway vehicle in traffic accident

  V05.11x-   **Pedestrian on roller-skates injured in collision with railway train or railway vehicle in traffic accident**

  V05.12x-   **Pedestrian on skateboard injured in collision with railway train or railway vehicle in traffic accident**

V
0
2
–
V
0
5

V05.19x- Pedestrian with other conveyance injured in collision with railway train or railway vehicle in traffic accident
> Pedestrian with babystroller injured in collision with railway train or railway vehicle in traffic accident
> Pedestrian on ice-skates injured in collision with railway train or railway vehicle in traffic accident
> Pedestrian on nonmotorized scooter injured in collision with railway train or railway vehicle in traffic accident
> Pedestrian on sled injured in collision with railway train or railway vehicle in traffic accident
> Pedestrian on snowboard injured in collision with railway train or railway vehicle in traffic accident
> Pedestrian on snow-skis injured in collision with railway train or railway vehicle in traffic accident
> Pedestrian in wheelchair (powered) injured in collision with railway train or railway vehicle in traffic accident
> Pedestrian in motorized mobility scooter injured in collision with railway train or railway vehicle in traffic accident

V05.9- Pedestrian injured in collision with railway train or railway vehicle, unspecified whether traffic or nontraffic accident

V05.90x- Pedestrian on foot injured in collision with railway train or railway vehicle, unspecified whether traffic or nontraffic accident
> Pedestrian NOS injured in collision with railway train or railway vehicle, unspecified whether traffic or nontraffic accident

V05.91x- Pedestrian on roller-skates injured in collision with railway train or railway vehicle, unspecified whether traffic or nontraffic accident

V05.92x- Pedestrian on skateboard injured in collision with railway train or railway vehicle, unspecified whether traffic or nontraffic accident

V05.99x- Pedestrian with other conveyance injured in collision with railway train or railway vehicle, unspecified whether traffic or nontraffic accident
> Pedestrian with babystroller injured in collision with railway train or railway vehicle, unspecified whether traffic or nontraffic
> Pedestrian on ice-skates injured in collision with railway train or railway vehicle, unspecified whether traffic or nontraffic
> Pedestrian on nonmotorized scooter injured in collision with railway train or railway vehicle, unspecified whether traffic or nontraffic
> Pedestrian on sled injured in collision with railway train or railway vehicle, unspecified whether traffic or nontraffic
> Pedestrian on snowboard injured in collision with railway train or railway vehicle, unspecified whether traffic or nontraffic
> Pedestrian on snow-skis injured in collision with railway train or railway vehicle, unspecified whether traffic or nontraffic
> Pedestrian in wheelchair (powered) injured in collision with railway train or railway vehicle, unspecified whether traffic or nontraffic
> Pedestrian in motorized mobility scooter injured in collision with railway train or railway vehicle, unspecified whether traffic or nontraffic

V06- Pedestrian injured in collision with other nonmotor vehicle
> Includes: Collision with animal-drawn vehicle, animal being ridden, nonpowered streetcar
> *Excludes 1:* pedestrian injured in collision with pedestrian conveyance (V00.0-)

> **The appropriate 7th character is to be added to each code from category V06:**
> **A** Initial encounter
> **D** Subsequent encounter
> **S** Sequela

V06.0- Pedestrian injured in collision with other nonmotor vehicle in nontraffic accident

V06.00x- Pedestrian on foot injured in collision with other nonmotor vehicle in nontraffic accident
> Pedestrian NOS injured in collision with other nonmotor vehicle in nontraffic accident

V06.01x- Pedestrian on roller-skates injured in collision with other nonmotor vehicle in nontraffic accident

V06.02x- Pedestrian on skateboard injured in collision with other nonmotor vehicle in nontraffic accident

V06.09x- Pedestrian with other conveyance injured in collision with other nonmotor vehicle in nontraffic accident
> Pedestrian with babystroller injured in collision with other nonmotor vehicle in nontraffic accident
> Pedestrian on ice-skates injured in collision with other nonmotor vehicle in nontraffic accident
> Pedestrian on nonmotorized scooter injured in collision with other nonmotor vehicle in nontraffic accident
> Pedestrian on sled injured in collision with other nonmotor vehicle in nontraffic accident
> Pedestrian on snowboard injured in collision with other nonmotor vehicle in nontraffic accident
> Pedestrian on snow-skis injured in collision with other nonmotor vehicle in nontraffic accident
> Pedestrian in wheelchair (powered) injured in collision with other nonmotor vehicle in nontraffic accident
> Pedestrian in motorized mobility scooter injured in collision with other nonmotor vehicle in nontraffic accident

V06.1- Pedestrian injured in collision with other nonmotor vehicle in traffic accident

V06.10x- Pedestrian on foot injured in collision with other nonmotor vehicle in traffic accident
> Pedestrian NOS injured in collision with other nonmotor vehicle in traffic accident

V06.11x- Pedestrian on roller-skates injured in collision with other nonmotor vehicle in traffic accident

V06.12x- Pedestrian on skateboard injured in collision with other nonmotor vehicle in traffic accident

V06.19x- Pedestrian with other conveyance injured in collision with other nonmotor vehicle in traffic accident
> Pedestrian with babystroller injured in collision with other nonmotor vehicle in nontraffic accident
> Pedestrian on ice-skates injured in collision with other nonmotor vehicle in traffic accident
> Pedestrian on nonmotorized scooter injured in collision with other nonmotor vehicle in traffic accident
> Pedestrian on sled injured in collision with other nonmotor vehicle in traffic accident
> Pedestrian on snowboard injured in collision with other nonmotor vehicle in traffic accident
> Pedestrian on snow-skis injured in collision with other nonmotor vehicle in traffic accident
> Pedestrian in wheelchair (powered) injured in collision with other nonmotor vehicle in traffic accident
> Pedestrian in motorized mobility scooter injured in collision with other nonmotor vehicle in traffic accident

V06.9- Pedestrian injured in collision with other nonmotor vehicle, unspecified whether traffic or nontraffic accident

V06.90x- Pedestrian on foot injured in collision with other nonmotor vehicle, unspecified whether traffic or nontraffic accident
> Pedestrian NOS injured in collision with other nonmotor vehicle, unspecified whether traffic or nontraffic accident

V06.91x- Pedestrian on roller-skates injured in collision with other nonmotor vehicle, unspecified whether traffic or nontraffic accident

V06.92x- Pedestrian on skateboard injured in collision with other nonmotor vehicle, unspecified whether traffic or nontraffic accident

V06.99x- Pedestrian with other conveyance injured in collision with other nonmotor vehicle, unspecified whether traffic or nontraffic accident
> Pedestrian with babystroller injured in collision with other nonmotor vehicle, unspecified whether traffic or nontraffic accident
> Pedestrian on ice-skates injured in collision with other nonmotor vehicle, unspecified whether traffic or nontraffic accident
> Pedestrian on nonmotorized scooter injured in collision with other nonmotor vehicle, unspecified whether traffic or nontraffic accident
> Pedestrian on sled injured in collision with other nonmotor vehicle, unspecified whether traffic or nontraffic accident
> Pedestrian on snowboard injured in collision with other nonmotor vehicle, unspecified whether traffic or nontraffic accident
> Pedestrian on snow-skis injured in collision with other nonmotor vehicle, unspecified whether traffic or nontraffic accident
> Pedestrian in wheelchair (powered) injured in collision with other nonmotor vehicle, unspecified whether traffic or nontraffic accident
> Pedestrian in motorized mobility scooter injured in collision with other nonmotor vehicle, unspecified whether traffic or nontraffic accident

V05 - V15

V09- Pedestrian injured in other and unspecified transport accidents
The appropriate 7th character is to be added to each code from category V09:
A Initial encounter
D Subsequent encounter
S Sequela
  V09.0- Pedestrian injured in nontraffic accident involving other and unspecified motor vehicles
    V09.00x- Pedestrian injured in nontraffic accident involving unspecified motor vehicles
    V09.01x- Pedestrian injured in nontraffic accident involving military vehicle
    V09.09x- Pedestrian injured in nontraffic accident involving other motor vehicles
        Pedestrian injured in nontraffic accident by special vehicle
  V09.1xx- Pedestrian injured in unspecified nontraffic accident
  V09.2- Pedestrian injured in traffic accident involving other and unspecified motor vehicles
    V09.20x- Pedestrian injured in traffic accident involving unspecified motor vehicles
    V09.21x- Pedestrian injured in traffic accident involving military vehicle
    V09.29x- Pedestrian injured in traffic accident involving other motor vehicles
  V09.3xx- Pedestrian injured in unspecified traffic accident
  V09.9xx- Pedestrian injured in unspecified transport accident

Pedal cycle rider injured in transport accident (V10-V19)

Includes: Any non-motorized vehicle, excluding an animal-drawn vehicle, or a sidecar or trailer attached to the pedal cycle
Excludes❷: rupture of pedal cycle tire (W37.0)

V10- Pedal cycle rider injured in collision with pedestrian or animal
Excludes 1: pedal cycle rider collision with animal-drawn vehicle or animal being ridden (V16.-)
The appropriate 7th character is to be added to each code from category V10:
A Initial encounter
D Subsequent encounter
S Sequela
  V10.0xx- Pedal cycle driver injured in collision with pedestrian or animal in nontraffic accident
  V10.1xx- Pedal cycle passenger injured in collision with pedestrian or animal in nontraffic accident
  V10.2xx- Unspecified pedal cyclist injured in collision with pedestrian or animal in nontraffic accident
  V10.3xx- Person boarding or alighting a pedal cycle injured in collision with pedestrian or animal
  V10.4xx- Pedal cycle driver injured in collision with pedestrian or animal in traffic accident
  V10.5xx- Pedal cycle passenger injured in collision with pedestrian or animal in traffic accident
  V10.9xx- Unspecified pedal cyclist injured in collision with pedestrian or animal in traffic accident

V11- Pedal cycle rider injured in collision with other pedal cycle
The appropriate 7th character is to be added to each code from category V11:
A Initial encounter
D Subsequent encounter
S Sequela
  V11.0xx- Pedal cycle driver injured in collision with other pedal cycle in nontraffic accident
  V11.1xx- Pedal cycle passenger injured in collision with other pedal cycle in nontraffic accident
  V11.2xx- Unspecified pedal cyclist injured in collision with other pedal cycle in nontraffic accident
  V11.3xx- Person boarding or alighting a pedal cycle injured in collision with other pedal cycle
  V11.4xx- Pedal cycle driver injured in collision with other pedal cycle in traffic accident
  V11.5xx- Pedal cycle passenger injured in collision with other pedal cycle in traffic accident
  V11.9xx- Unspecified pedal cyclist injured in collision with other pedal cycle in traffic accident

V12- Pedal cycle rider injured in collision with two- or three-wheeled motor vehicle
The appropriate 7th character is to be added to each code from category V12:
A Initial encounter
D Subsequent encounter
S Sequela
  V12.0xx- Pedal cycle driver injured in collision with two- or three-wheeled motor vehicle in nontraffic accident
  V12.1xx- Pedal cycle passenger injured in collision with two- or three-wheeled motor vehicle in nontraffic accident
  V12.2xx- Unspecified pedal cyclist injured in collision with two- or three-wheeled motor vehicle in nontraffic accident
  V12.3xx- Person boarding or alighting a pedal cycle injured in collision with two- or three-wheeled motor vehicle
  V12.4xx- Pedal cycle driver injured in collision with two- or three-wheeled motor vehicle in traffic accident
  V12.5xx- Pedal cycle passenger injured in collision with two- or three-wheeled motor vehicle in traffic accident
  V12.9xx- Unspecified pedal cyclist injured in collision with two- or three-wheeled motor vehicle in traffic accident

V13- Pedal cycle rider injured in collision with car, pick-up truck or van
The appropriate 7th character is to be added to each code from category V13:
A Initial encounter
D Subsequent encounter
S Sequela
  V13.0xx- Pedal cycle driver injured in collision with car, pick-up truck or van in nontraffic accident
  V13.1xx- Pedal cycle passenger injured in collision with car, pick-up truck or van in nontraffic accident
  V13.2xx- Unspecified pedal cyclist injured in collision with car, pick-up truck or van in nontraffic accident
  V13.3xx- Person boarding or alighting a pedal cycle injured in collision with car, pick-up truck or van
  V13.4xx- Pedal cycle driver injured in collision with car, pick-up truck or van in traffic accident
  V13.5xx- Pedal cycle passenger injured in collision with car, pick-up truck or van in traffic accident
  V13.9xx- Unspecified pedal cyclist injured in collision with car, pick-up truck or van in traffic accident

V14- Pedal cycle rider injured in collision with heavy transport vehicle or bus
Excludes 1: pedal cycle rider injured in collision with military vehicle (V19.81)
The appropriate 7th character is to be added to each code from category V14:
A Initial encounter
D Subsequent encounter
S Sequela
  V14.0xx- Pedal cycle driver injured in collision with heavy transport vehicle or bus in nontraffic accident
  V14.1xx- Pedal cycle passenger injured in collision with heavy transport vehicle or bus in nontraffic accident
  V14.2xx- Unspecified pedal cyclist injured in collision with heavy transport vehicle or bus in nontraffic accident
  V14.3xx- Person boarding or alighting a pedal cycle injured in collision with heavy transport vehicle or bus
  V14.4xx- Pedal cycle driver injured in collision with heavy transport vehicle or bus in traffic accident
  V14.5xx- Pedal cycle passenger injured in collision with heavy transport vehicle or bus in traffic accident
  V14.9xx- Unspecified pedal cyclist injured in collision with heavy transport vehicle or bus in traffic accident

V15- Pedal cycle rider injured in collision with railway train or railway vehicle
The appropriate 7th character is to be added to each code from category V15:
A Initial encounter
D Subsequent encounter
S Sequela
  V15.0xx- Pedal cycle driver injured in collision with railway train or railway vehicle in nontraffic accident
  V15.1xx- Pedal cycle passenger injured in collision with railway train or railway vehicle in nontraffic accident
  V15.2xx- Unspecified pedal cyclist injured in collision with railway train or railway vehicle in nontraffic accident
  V15.3xx- Person boarding or alighting a pedal cycle injured in collision with railway train or railway vehicle
  V15.4xx- Pedal cycle driver injured in collision with railway train or railway vehicle in traffic accident

V
0
5
-
V
1
5

Excludes 1: = NOT CODED HERE! (Do not code both)   *Excludes❷: = Not Included Here*

V15.5xx- Pedal cycle passenger injured in collision with railway train or railway vehicle in traffic accident

V15.9xx- Unspecified pedal cyclist injured in collision with railway train or railway vehicle in traffic accident

V16- <u>Pedal cycle rider injured in collision</u> with <u>other nonmotor vehicle</u>
Includes: Collision with animal-drawn vehicle, animal being ridden, streetcar

The appropriate 7th character is to be added to each code from category V16:
 A <u>Initial</u> encounter
 D <u>Subsequent</u> encounter
 S <u>Sequela</u>

V16.0xx- Pedal cycle driver injured in collision with other nonmotor vehicle in nontraffic accident

V16.1xx- Pedal cycle passenger injured in collision with other nonmotor vehicle in nontraffic accident

V16.2xx- Unspecified pedal cyclist injured in collision with other nonmotor vehicle in nontraffic accident

V16.3xx- Person boarding or alighting a pedal cycle injured in collision with other nonmotor vehicle in nontraffic accident

V16.4xx- Pedal cycle driver injured in collision with other nonmotor vehicle in traffic accident

V16.5xx- Pedal cycle passenger injured in collision with other nonmotor vehicle in traffic accident

V16.9xx- Unspecified pedal cyclist injured in collision with other nonmotor vehicle in traffic accident

V17- <u>Pedal cycle rider injured in collision</u> with <u>fixed or stationary object</u>

The appropriate 7th character is to be added to each code from category V17:
 A <u>Initial</u> encounter
 D <u>Subsequent</u> encounter
 S <u>Sequela</u>

V17.0xx- Pedal cycle driver injured in collision with fixed or stationary object in nontraffic accident

V17.1xx- Pedal cycle passenger injured in collision with fixed or stationary object in nontraffic accident

V17.2xx- Unspecified pedal cyclist injured in collision with fixed or stationary object in nontraffic accident

V17.3xx- Person boarding or alighting a pedal cycle injured in collision with fixed or stationary object

V17.4xx- Pedal cycle driver injured in collision with fixed or stationary object in traffic accident

V17.5xx- Pedal cycle passenger injured in collision with fixed or stationary object in traffic accident

V17.9xx- Unspecified pedal cyclist injured in collision with fixed or stationary object in traffic accident

V18- <u>Pedal cycle rider injured</u> in <u>noncollision</u> transport accident
Includes: Fall or thrown from pedal cycle (without antecedent collision)
Overturning pedal cycle NOS
Overturning pedal cycle without collision

The appropriate 7th character is to be added to each code from category V18:
 A <u>Initial</u> encounter
 D <u>Subsequent</u> encounter
 S <u>Sequela</u>

V18.0xx- Pedal cycle driver injured in noncollision transport accident in nontraffic accident

V18.1xx- Pedal cycle passenger injured in noncollision transport accident in nontraffic accident

V18.2xx- Unspecified pedal cyclist injured in noncollision transport accident in nontraffic accident

V18.3xx- Person boarding or alighting a pedal cycle injured in noncollision transport accident

V18.4xx- Pedal cycle driver injured in noncollision transport accident in traffic accident

V18.5xx- Pedal cycle passenger injured in noncollision transport accident in traffic accident

V18.9xx- Unspecified pedal cyclist injured in noncollision transport accident in traffic accident

V19- <u>Pedal cycle rider injured</u> in <u>other and unspecified</u> transport accidents

The appropriate 7th character is to be added to each code from category V19:
 A <u>Initial</u> encounter
 D <u>Subsequent</u> encounter
 S <u>Sequela</u>

V19.0- Pedal cycle driver injured in collision with other and unspecified motor vehicles in nontraffic accident

V19.00x- Pedal cycle driver injured in collision with unspecified motor vehicles in nontraffic accident

V19.09x- Pedal cycle driver injured in collision with other motor vehicles in nontraffic accident

V19.1- Pedal cycle passenger injured in collision with other and unspecified motor vehicles in nontraffic accident

V19.10x- Pedal cycle passenger injured in collision with unspecified motor vehicles in nontraffic accident

V19.19x- Pedal cycle passenger injured in collision with other motor vehicles in nontraffic accident

V19.2- Unspecified pedal cyclist injured in collision with other and unspecified motor vehicles in nontraffic accident

V19.20x- Unspecified pedal cyclist injured in collision with unspecified motor vehicles in nontraffic accident
Pedal cycle collision NOS, nontraffic

V19.29x- Unspecified pedal cyclist injured in collision with other motor vehicles in nontraffic accident

V19.3xx- Pedal cyclist (driver) (passenger) injured in unspecified nontraffic accident
Pedal cycle accident NOS, nontraffic
Pedal cyclist injured in nontraffic accident NOS

V19.4- Pedal cycle driver injured in collision with other and unspecified motor vehicles in traffic accident

V19.40x- Pedal cycle driver injured in collision with unspecified motor vehicles in traffic accident

V19.49x- Pedal cycle driver injured in collision with other motor vehicles in traffic accident

V19.5- Pedal cycle passenger injured in collision with other and unspecified motor vehicles in traffic accident

V19.50x- Pedal cycle passenger injured in collision with unspecified motor vehicles in traffic accident

V19.59x- Pedal cycle passenger injured in collision with other motor vehicles in traffic accident

V19.6- Unspecified pedal cyclist injured in collision with other and unspecified motor vehicles in traffic accident

V19.60x- Unspecified pedal cyclist injured in collision with unspecified motor vehicles in traffic accident
Pedal cycle collision NOS (traffic)

V19.69x- Unspecified pedal cyclist injured in collision with other motor vehicles in traffic accident

V19.8- Pedal cyclist (driver) (passenger) injured in other specified transport accidents

V19.81x- Pedal cyclist (driver) (passenger) injured in transport accident with military vehicle

V19.88x- Pedal cyclist (driver) (passenger) injured in other specified transport accidents

V19.9xx- Pedal cyclist (driver) (passenger) injured in unspecified traffic accident
Pedal cycle accident NOS

Motorcycle rider injured in transport accident (V20-V29)

Includes: Moped
Motorcycle with sidecar
Motorized bicycle
Motor scooter
Excludes 1: three-wheeled motor vehicle (V30-V39)

V20- <u>Motorcycle rider injured in collision</u> with <u>pedestrian or animal</u>
Excludes 1: motorcycle rider collision with animal-drawn vehicle or animal being ridden (V26.-)

The appropriate 7th character is to be added to each code from category V20:
 A <u>Initial</u> encounter
 D <u>Subsequent</u> encounter
 S <u>Sequela</u>

V20.0xx- Motorcycle driver injured in collision with pedestrian or animal in nontraffic accident

V20.1xx- Motorcycle passenger injured in collision with pedestrian or animal in nontraffic accident

V20.2xx- Unspecified motorcycle rider injured in collision with pedestrian or animal in nontraffic accident

V20.3xx- Person boarding or alighting a motorcycle injured in collision with pedestrian or animal

V20.4xx- Motorcycle driver injured in collision with pedestrian or animal in traffic accident

V20.5xx- Motorcycle passenger injured in collision with pedestrian or animal in traffic accident

V20.9xx- Unspecified motorcycle rider injured in collision with pedestrian or animal in traffic accident

V
1
5
I
V
2
8

V21- Motorcycle rider injured in collision with pedal cycle

The appropriate 7th character is to be added to each code from category V21:
- **A** Initial encounter
- **D** Subsequent encounter
- **S** Sequela

V21.0xx- Motorcycle driver injured in collision with pedal cycle in nontraffic accident

V21.1xx- Motorcycle passenger injured in collision with pedal cycle in nontraffic accident

V21.2xx- Unspecified motorcycle rider injured in collision with pedal cycle in nontraffic accident

V21.3xx- Person boarding or alighting a motorcycle injured in collision with pedal cycle

V21.4xx- Motorcycle driver injured in collision with pedal cycle in traffic accident

V21.5xx- Motorcycle passenger injured in collision with pedal cycle in traffic accident

V21.9xx- Unspecified motorcycle rider injured in collision with pedal cycle in traffic accident

V22- Motorcycle rider injured in collision with two- or three-wheeled motor vehicle

The appropriate 7th character is to be added to each code from category V22:
- **A** Initial encounter
- **D** Subsequent encounter
- **S** Sequela

V22.0xx- Motorcycle driver injured in collision with two- or three-wheeled motor vehicle in nontraffic accident

V22.1xx- Motorcycle passenger injured in collision with two- or three-wheeled motor vehicle in nontraffic accident

V22.2xx- Unspecified motorcycle rider injured in collision with two- or three-wheeled motor vehicle in nontraffic accident

V22.3xx- Person boarding or alighting a motorcycle injured in collision with two- or three-wheeled motor vehicle

V22.4xx- Motorcycle driver injured in collision with two- or three-wheeled motor vehicle in traffic accident

V22.5xx- Motorcycle passenger injured in collision with two- or three-wheeled motor vehicle in traffic accident

V22.9xx- Unspecified motorcycle rider injured in collision with two- or three-wheeled motor vehicle in traffic accident

V23- Motorcycle rider injured in collision with car, pick-up truck or van

The appropriate 7th character is to be added to each code from category V23:
- **A** Initial encounter
- **D** Subsequent encounter
- **S** Sequela

V23.0xx- Motorcycle driver injured in collision with car, pick-up truck or van in nontraffic accident

V23.1xx- Motorcycle passenger injured in collision with car, pick-up truck or van in nontraffic accident

V23.2xx- Unspecified motorcycle rider injured in collision with car, pick-up truck or van in nontraffic accident

V23.3xx- Person boarding or alighting a motorcycle injured in collision with car, pick-up truck or van

V23.4xx- Motorcycle driver injured in collision with car, pick-up truck or van in traffic accident

V23.5xx- Motorcycle passenger injured in collision with car, pick-up truck or van in traffic accident

V23.9xx- Unspecified motorcycle rider injured in collision with car, pick-up truck or van in traffic accident

V24- Motorcycle rider injured in collision with heavy transport vehicle or bus

Excludes 1: motorcycle rider injured in collision with military vehicle (V29.81)

The appropriate 7th character is to be added to each code from category V24:
- **A** Initial encounter
- **D** Subsequent encounter
- **S** Sequela

V24.0xx- Motorcycle driver injured in collision with heavy transport vehicle or bus in nontraffic accident

V24.1xx- Motorcycle passenger injured in collision with heavy transport vehicle or bus in nontraffic accident

V24.2xx- Unspecified motorcycle rider injured in collision with heavy transport vehicle or bus in nontraffic accident

V24.3xx- Person boarding or alighting a motorcycle injured in collision with heavy transport vehicle or bus

V24.4xx- Motorcycle driver injured in collision with heavy transport vehicle or bus in traffic accident

V24.5xx- Motorcycle passenger injured in collision with heavy transport vehicle or bus in traffic accident

V24.9xx- Unspecified motorcycle rider injured in collision with heavy transport vehicle or bus in traffic accident

V25- Motorcycle rider injured in collision with railway train or railway vehicle

The appropriate 7th character is to be added to each code from category V25:
- **A** Initial encounter
- **D** Subsequent encounter
- **S** Sequela

V25.0xx- Motorcycle driver injured in collision with railway train or railway vehicle in nontraffic accident

V25.1xx- Motorcycle passenger injured in collision with railway train or railway vehicle in nontraffic accident

V25.2xx- Unspecified motorcycle rider injured in collision with railway train or railway vehicle in nontraffic accident

V25.3xx- Person boarding or alighting a motorcycle injured in collision with railway train or railway vehicle

V25.4xx- Motorcycle driver injured in collision with railway train or railway vehicle in traffic accident

V25.5xx- Motorcycle passenger injured in collision with railway train or railway vehicle in traffic accident

V25.9xx- Unspecified motorcycle rider injured in collision with railway train or railway vehicle in traffic accident

V26- Motorcycle rider injured in collision with other nonmotor vehicle

Includes: Collision with animal-drawn vehicle, animal being ridden, streetcar

The appropriate 7th character is to be added to each code from category V26:
- **A** Initial encounter
- **D** Subsequent encounter
- **S** Sequela

V26.0xx- Motorcycle driver injured in collision with other nonmotor vehicle in nontraffic accident

V26.1xx- Motorcycle passenger injured in collision with other nonmotor vehicle in nontraffic accident

V26.2xx- Unspecified motorcycle rider injured in collision with other nonmotor vehicle in nontraffic accident

V26.3xx- Person boarding or alighting a motorcycle injured in collision with other nonmotor vehicle

V26.4xx- Motorcycle driver injured in collision with other nonmotor vehicle in traffic accident

V26.5xx- Motorcycle passenger injured in collision with other nonmotor vehicle in traffic accident

V26.9xx- Unspecified motorcycle rider injured in collision with other nonmotor vehicle in traffic accident

V27- Motorcycle rider injured in collision with fixed or stationary object

The appropriate 7th character is to be added to each code from category V27:
- **A** Initial encounter
- **D** Subsequent encounter
- **S** Sequela

V27.0xx- Motorcycle driver injured in collision with fixed or stationary object in nontraffic accident

V27.1xx- Motorcycle passenger injured in collision with fixed or stationary object in nontraffic accident

V27.2xx- Unspecified motorcycle rider injured in collision with fixed or stationary object in nontraffic accident

V27.3xx- Person boarding or alighting a motorcycle injured in collision with fixed or stationary object

V27.4xx- Motorcycle driver injured in collision with fixed or stationary object in traffic accident

V27.5xx- Motorcycle passenger injured in collision with fixed or stationary object in traffic accident

V27.9xx- Unspecified motorcycle rider injured in collision with fixed or stationary object in traffic accident

V28- Motorcycle rider injured in noncollision transport accident

Includes: Fall or thrown from motorcycle (without antecedent collision)
Overturning motorcycle NOS
Overturning motorcycle without collision

The appropriate 7th character is to be added to each code from category V28:
- **A** Initial encounter
- **D** Subsequent encounter
- **S** Sequela

V28.0xx- Motorcycle driver injured in noncollision transport accident in nontraffic accident

V28.1xx- Motorcycle passenger injured in noncollision transport accident in nontraffic accident

V
1
5
-
V
2
8

© 2013 Channel Publishing, Ltd.

V28.2xx- Unspecified motorcycle rider injured in noncollision transport accident in nontraffic accident

V28.3xx- Person boarding or alighting a motorcycle injured in noncollision transport accident

V28.4xx- Motorcycle driver injured in noncollision transport accident in traffic accident

V28.5xx- Motorcycle passenger injured in noncollision transport accident in traffic accident

V28.9xx- Unspecified motorcycle rider injured in noncollision transport accident in traffic accident

V29- Motorcycle rider injured in other and unspecified transport accidents

The appropriate 7th character is to be added to each code from category V29:
A   Initial encounter
D   Subsequent encounter
S   Sequela

V29.0- Motorcycle driver injured in collision with other and unspecified motor vehicles in nontraffic accident

   V29.00x- Motorcycle driver injured in collision with unspecified motor vehicles in nontraffic accident

   V29.09x- Motorcycle driver injured in collision with other motor vehicles in nontraffic accident

V29.1- Motorcycle passenger injured in collision with other and unspecified motor vehicles in nontraffic accident

   V29.10x- Motorcycle passenger injured in collision with unspecified motor vehicles in nontraffic accident

   V29.19x- Motorcycle passenger injured in collision with other motor vehicles in nontraffic accident

V29.2- Unspecified motorcycle rider injured in collision with other and unspecified motor vehicles in nontraffic accident

   V29.20x- Unspecified motorcycle rider injured in collision with unspecified motor vehicles in nontraffic accident
     Motorcycle collision NOS, nontraffic

   V29.29x- Unspecified motorcycle rider injured in collision with other motor vehicles in nontraffic accident

V29.3xx- Motorcycle rider (driver) (passenger) injured in unspecified nontraffic accident
     Motorcycle accident NOS, nontraffic
     Motorcycle rider injured in nontraffic accident NOS

V29.4- Motorcycle driver injured in collision with other and unspecified motor vehicles in traffic accident

   V29.40x- Motorcycle driver injured in collision with unspecified motor vehicles in traffic accident

   V29.49x- Motorcycle driver injured in collision with other motor vehicles in traffic accident

V29.5- Motorcycle passenger injured in collision with other and unspecified motor vehicles in traffic accident

   V29.50x- Motorcycle passenger injured in collision with unspecified motor vehicles in traffic accident

   V29.59x- Motorcycle passenger injured in collision with other motor vehicles in traffic accident

V29.6- Unspecified motorcycle rider injured in collision with other and unspecified motor vehicles in traffic accident

   V29.60x- Unspecified motorcycle rider injured in collision with unspecified motor vehicles in traffic accident
     Motorcycle collision NOS (traffic)

   V29.69x- Unspecified motorcycle rider injured in collision with other motor vehicles in traffic accident

V29.8- Motorcycle rider (driver) (passenger) injured in other specified transport accidents

   V29.81x- Motorcycle rider (driver) (passenger) injured in transport accident with military vehicle

   V29.88x- Motorcycle rider (driver) (passenger) injured in other specified transport accidents

V29.9xx- Motorcycle rider (driver) (passenger) injured in unspecified traffic accident
     Motorcycle accident NOS

Occupant of three-wheeled motor vehicle injured in transport accident (V30-V39)

Includes: Motorized tricycle
          Motorized rickshaw
          Three-wheeled motor car
Excludes 1:   *all-terrain vehicles (V86.-)*
           motorcycle with sidecar (V20-V29)
           vehicle designed primarily for off-road use (V86.-)

V30- Occupant of three-wheeled motor vehicle injured in collision with pedestrian or animal
Excludes 1:   *three-wheeled motor vehicle collision with animal-drawn vehicle or animal being ridden (V36.-)*

The appropriate 7th character is to be added to each code from category V30:
A   Initial encounter
D   Subsequent encounter
S   Sequela

V30.0xx- Driver of three-wheeled motor vehicle injured in collision with pedestrian or animal in nontraffic accident

V30.1xx- Passenger in three-wheeled motor vehicle injured in collision with pedestrian or animal in nontraffic accident

V30.2xx- Person on outside of three-wheeled motor vehicle injured in collision with pedestrian or animal in nontraffic accident

V30.3xx- Unspecified occupant of three-wheeled motor vehicle injured in collision with pedestrian or animal in nontraffic accident

V30.4xx- Person boarding or alighting a three-wheeled motor vehicle injured in collision with pedestrian or animal

V30.5xx- Driver of three-wheeled motor vehicle injured in collision with pedestrian or animal in traffic accident

V30.6xx- Passenger in three-wheeled motor vehicle injured in collision with pedestrian or animal in traffic accident

V30.7xx- Person on outside of three-wheeled motor vehicle injured in collision with pedestrian or animal in traffic accident

V30.9xx- Unspecified occupant of three-wheeled motor vehicle injured in collision with pedestrian or animal in traffic accident

V31- Occupant of three-wheeled motor vehicle injured in collision with pedal cycle

The appropriate 7th character is to be added to each code from category V31:
A   Initial encounter
D   Subsequent encounter
S   Sequela

V31.0xx- Driver of three-wheeled motor vehicle injured in collision with pedal cycle in nontraffic accident

V31.1xx- Passenger in three-wheeled motor vehicle injured in collision with pedal cycle in nontraffic accident

V31.2xx- Person on outside of three-wheeled motor vehicle injured in collision with pedal cycle in nontraffic accident

V31.3xx- Unspecified occupant of three-wheeled motor vehicle injured in collision with pedal cycle in nontraffic accident

V31.4xx- Person boarding or alighting a three-wheeled motor vehicle injured in collision with pedal cycle

V31.5xx- Driver of three-wheeled motor vehicle injured in collision with pedal cycle in traffic accident

V31.6xx- Passenger in three-wheeled motor vehicle injured in collision with pedal cycle in traffic accident

V31.7xx- Person on outside of three-wheeled motor vehicle injured in collision with pedal cycle in traffic accident

V31.9xx- Unspecified occupant of three-wheeled motor vehicle injured in collision with pedal cycle in traffic accident

V32- Occupant of three-wheeled motor vehicle injured in collision with two- or three-wheeled motor vehicle

The appropriate 7th character is to be added to each code from category V32:
A   Initial encounter
D   Subsequent encounter
S   Sequela

V32.0xx- Driver of three-wheeled motor vehicle injured in collision with two- or three-wheeled motor vehicle in nontraffic accident

V32.1xx- Passenger in three-wheeled motor vehicle injured in collision with two- or three-wheeled motor vehicle in nontraffic accident

V32.2xx- Person on outside of three-wheeled motor vehicle injured in collision with two- or three-wheeled motor vehicle in nontraffic accident

V32.3xx- Unspecified occupant of three-wheeled motor vehicle injured in collision with two- or three-wheeled motor vehicle in nontraffic accident

V32.4xx- Person boarding or alighting a three-wheeled motor vehicle injured in collision with two- or three-wheeled motor vehicle

V 2 8 - V 3 8

V32.5xx- Driver of three-wheeled motor vehicle injured in collision with two- or three-wheeled motor vehicle in traffic accident

V32.6xx- Passenger in three-wheeled motor vehicle injured in collision with two- or three-wheeled motor vehicle in traffic accident

V32.7xx- Person on outside of three-wheeled motor vehicle injured in collision with two- or three-wheeled motor vehicle in traffic accident

V32.9xx- Unspecified occupant of three-wheeled motor vehicle injured in collision with two- or three-wheeled motor vehicle in traffic accident

V33- Occupant of three-wheeled motor vehicle injured in collision with car, pick-up truck or van

The appropriate 7th character is to be added to each code from category V33:
A   Initial encounter
D   Subsequent encounter
S   Sequela

V33.0xx- Driver of three-wheeled motor vehicle injured in collision with car, pick-up truck or van in nontraffic accident

V33.1xx- Passenger in three-wheeled motor vehicle injured in collision with car, pick-up truck or van in nontraffic accident

V33.2xx- Person on outside of three-wheeled motor vehicle injured in collision with car, pick-up truck or van in nontraffic accident

V33.3xx- Unspecified occupant of three-wheeled motor vehicle injured in collision with car, pick-up truck or van in nontraffic accident

V33.4xx- Person boarding or alighting a three-wheeled motor vehicle injured in collision with car, pick-up truck or van

V33.5xx- Driver of three-wheeled motor vehicle injured in collision with car, pick-up truck or van in traffic accident

V33.6xx- Passenger in three-wheeled motor vehicle injured in collision with car, pick-up truck or van in traffic accident

V33.7xx- Person on outside of three-wheeled motor vehicle injured in collision with car, pick-up truck or van in traffic accident

V33.9xx- Unspecified occupant of three-wheeled motor vehicle injured in collision with car, pick-up truck or van in traffic accident

V34- Occupant of three-wheeled motor vehicle injured in collision with heavy transport vehicle or bus
Excludes 1: occupant of three-wheeled motor vehicle injured in collision with military vehicle (V39.81)

The appropriate 7th character is to be added to each code from category V34:
A   Initial encounter
D   Subsequent encounter
S   Sequela

V34.0xx- Driver of three-wheeled motor vehicle injured in collision with heavy transport vehicle or bus in nontraffic accident

V34.1xx- Passenger in three-wheeled motor vehicle injured in collision with heavy transport vehicle or bus in nontraffic accident

V34.2xx- Person on outside of three-wheeled motor vehicle injured in collision with heavy transport vehicle or bus in nontraffic accident

V34.3xx- Unspecified occupant of three-wheeled motor vehicle injured in collision with heavy transport vehicle or bus in nontraffic accident

V34.4xx- Person boarding or alighting a three-wheeled motor vehicle injured in collision with heavy transport vehicle or bus

V34.5xx- Driver of three-wheeled motor vehicle injured in collision with heavy transport vehicle or bus in traffic accident

V34.6xx- Passenger in three-wheeled motor vehicle injured in collision with heavy transport vehicle or bus in traffic accident

V34.7xx- Person on outside of three-wheeled motor vehicle injured in collision with heavy transport vehicle or bus in traffic accident

V34.9xx- Unspecified occupant of three-wheeled motor vehicle injured in collision with heavy transport vehicle or bus in traffic accident

V35- Occupant of three-wheeled motor vehicle injured in collision with railway train or railway vehicle

The appropriate 7th character is to be added to each code from category V35:
A   Initial encounter
D   Subsequent encounter
S   Sequela

V35.0xx- Driver of three-wheeled motor vehicle injured in collision with railway train or railway vehicle in nontraffic accident

V35.1xx- Passenger in three-wheeled motor vehicle injured in collision with railway train or railway vehicle in nontraffic accident

V35.2xx- Person on outside of three-wheeled motor vehicle injured in collision with railway train or railway vehicle in nontraffic accident

V35.3xx- Unspecified occupant of three-wheeled motor vehicle injured in collision with railway train or railway vehicle in nontraffic accident

V35.4xx- Person boarding or alighting a three-wheeled motor vehicle injured in collision with railway train or railway vehicle

V35.5xx- Driver of three-wheeled motor vehicle injured in collision with railway train or railway vehicle in traffic accident

V35.6xx- Passenger in three-wheeled motor vehicle injured in collision with railway train or railway vehicle in traffic accident

V35.7xx- Person on outside of three-wheeled motor vehicle injured in collision with railway train or railway vehicle in traffic accident

V35.9xx- Unspecified occupant of three-wheeled motor vehicle injured in collision with railway train or railway vehicle in traffic accident

V36- Occupant of three-wheeled motor vehicle injured in collision with other nonmotor vehicle
Includes: Collision with animal-drawn vehicle, animal being ridden, streetcar

The appropriate 7th character is to be added to each code from category V36:
A   Initial encounter
D   Subsequent encounter
S   Sequela

V36.0xx- Driver of three-wheeled motor vehicle injured in collision with other nonmotor vehicle in nontraffic accident

V36.1xx- Passenger in three-wheeled motor vehicle injured in collision with other nonmotor vehicle in nontraffic accident

V36.2xx- Person on outside of three-wheeled motor vehicle injured in collision with other nonmotor vehicle in nontraffic accident

V36.3xx- Unspecified occupant of three-wheeled motor vehicle injured in collision with other nonmotor vehicle in nontraffic accident

V36.4xx- Person boarding or alighting a three-wheeled motor vehicle injured in collision with other nonmotor vehicle

V36.5xx- Driver of three-wheeled motor vehicle injured in collision with other nonmotor vehicle in traffic accident

V36.6xx- Passenger in three-wheeled motor vehicle injured in collision with other nonmotor vehicle in traffic accident

V36.7xx- Person on outside of three-wheeled motor vehicle injured in collision with other nonmotor vehicle in traffic accident

V36.9xx- Unspecified occupant of three-wheeled motor vehicle injured in collision with other nonmotor vehicle in traffic accident

V37- Occupant of three-wheeled motor vehicle injured in collision with fixed or stationary object

The appropriate 7th character is to be added to each code from category V37:
A   Initial encounter
D   Subsequent encounter
S   Sequela

V37.0xx- Driver of three-wheeled motor vehicle injured in collision with fixed or stationary object in nontraffic accident

V37.1xx- Passenger in three-wheeled motor vehicle injured in collision with fixed or stationary object in nontraffic accident

V37.2xx- Person on outside of three-wheeled motor vehicle injured in collision with fixed or stationary object in nontraffic accident

V37.3xx- Unspecified occupant of three-wheeled motor vehicle injured in collision with fixed or stationary object in nontraffic accident

V37.4xx- Person boarding or alighting a three-wheeled motor vehicle injured in collision with fixed or stationary object

V37.5xx- Driver of three-wheeled motor vehicle injured in collision with fixed or stationary object in traffic accident

V37.6xx- Passenger in three-wheeled motor vehicle injured in collision with fixed or stationary object in traffic accident

V37.7xx- Person on outside of three-wheeled motor vehicle injured in collision with fixed or stationary object in traffic accident

V37.9xx- Unspecified occupant of three-wheeled motor vehicle injured in collision with fixed or stationary object in traffic accident

V38- Occupant of three-wheeled motor vehicle injured in noncollision transport accident
Includes: Fall or thrown from three-wheeled motor vehicle
Overturning of three-wheeled motor vehicle NOS
Overturning of three-wheeled motor vehicle without collision

The appropriate 7th character is to be added to each code from category V38:
A   Initial encounter
D   Subsequent encounter
S   Sequela

V38.0xx- Driver of three-wheeled motor vehicle injured in noncollision transport accident in nontraffic accident

V38.1xx- Passenger in three-wheeled motor vehicle injured in noncollision transport accident in nontraffic accident

V38.2xx- Person on outside of three-wheeled motor vehicle injured in noncollision transport accident in nontraffic accident

V38.3xx- Unspecified occupant of three-wheeled motor vehicle injured in noncollision transport accident in nontraffic accident

V28 – V38

V38.4xx- Person boarding or alighting a three-wheeled motor vehicle injured in noncollision transport accident

V38.5xx- Driver of three-wheeled motor vehicle injured in noncollision transport accident in traffic accident

V38.6xx- Passenger in three-wheeled motor vehicle injured in noncollision transport accident in traffic accident

V38.7xx- Person on outside of three-wheeled motor vehicle injured in noncollision transport accident in traffic accident

V38.9xx- Unspecified occupant of three-wheeled motor vehicle injured in noncollision transport accident in traffic accident

V39- Occupant of three-wheeled motor vehicle injured in other and unspecified transport accidents

The appropriate 7th character is to be added to each code from category V39:
A Initial encounter
D Subsequent encounter
S Sequela

V39.0- Driver of three-wheeled motor vehicle injured in collision with other and unspecified motor vehicles in nontraffic accident

V39.00x- Driver of three-wheeled motor vehicle injured in collision with unspecified motor vehicles in nontraffic accident

V39.09x- Driver of three-wheeled motor vehicle injured in collision with other motor vehicles in nontraffic accident

V39.1- Passenger in three-wheeled motor vehicle injured in collision with other and unspecified motor vehicles in nontraffic accident

V39.10x- Passenger in three-wheeled motor vehicle injured in collision with unspecified motor vehicles in nontraffic accident

V39.19x- Passenger in three-wheeled motor vehicle injured in collision with other motor vehicles in nontraffic accident

V39.2- Unspecified occupant of three-wheeled motor vehicle injured in collision with other and unspecified motor vehicles in nontraffic accident

V39.20x- Unspecified occupant of three-wheeled motor vehicle injured in collision with unspecified motor vehicles in nontraffic accident
　　Collision NOS involving three-wheeled motor vehicle, nontraffic

V39.29x- Unspecified occupant of three-wheeled motor vehicle injured in collision with other motor vehicles in nontraffic accident

V39.3xx- Occupant (driver) (passenger) of three-wheeled motor vehicle injured in unspecified nontraffic accident
　　Accident NOS involving three-wheeled motor vehicle, nontraffic
　　Occupant of three-wheeled motor vehicle injured in nontraffic accident NOS

V39.4- Driver of three-wheeled motor vehicle injured in collision with other and unspecified motor vehicles in traffic accident

V39.40x- Driver of three-wheeled motor vehicle injured in collision with unspecified motor vehicles in traffic accident

V39.49x- Driver of three-wheeled motor vehicle injured in collision with other motor vehicles in traffic accident

V39.5- Passenger in three-wheeled motor vehicle injured in collision with other and unspecified motor vehicles in traffic accident

V39.50x- Passenger in three-wheeled motor vehicle injured in collision with unspecified motor vehicles in traffic accident

V39.59x- Passenger in three-wheeled motor vehicle injured in collision with other motor vehicles in traffic accident

V39.6- Unspecified occupant of three-wheeled motor vehicle injured in collision with other and unspecified motor vehicles in traffic accident

V39.60x- Unspecified occupant of three-wheeled motor vehicle injured in collision with unspecified motor vehicles in traffic accident
　　Collision NOS involving three-wheeled motor vehicle (traffic)

V39.69x- Unspecified occupant of three-wheeled motor vehicle injured in collision with other motor vehicles in traffic accident

V39.8- Occupant (driver) (passenger) of three-wheeled motor vehicle injured in other specified transport accidents

V39.81x- Occupant (driver) (passenger) of three-wheeled motor vehicle injured in transport accident with military vehicle

V39.89x- Occupant (driver) (passenger) of three-wheeled motor vehicle injured in other specified transport accidents

V39.9xx- Occupant (driver) (passenger) of three-wheeled motor vehicle injured in unspecified traffic accident
　　Accident NOS involving three-wheeled motor vehicle

Car occupant injured in transport accident (V40-V49)

Includes: A four-wheeled motor vehicle designed primarily for carrying passengers
Automobile (pulling a trailer or camper)
Excludes 1: *bus (V50-V59)*
minibus (V50-V59)
minivan (V50-V59)
motorcoach (V70-V79)
pick-up truck (V50-V59)
sport utility vehicle (SUV) (V50-V59)

V40- Car occupant injured in collision with pedestrian or animal
Excludes 1: *car collision with animal-drawn vehicle or animal being ridden (V46.-)*

The appropriate 7th character is to be added to each code from category V40:
A Initial encounter
D Subsequent encounter
S Sequela

V40.0xx- Car driver injured in collision with pedestrian or animal in nontraffic accident

V40.1xx- Car passenger injured in collision with pedestrian or animal in nontraffic accident

V40.2xx- Person on outside of car injured in collision with pedestrian or animal in nontraffic accident

V40.3xx- Unspecified car occupant injured in collision with pedestrian or animal in nontraffic accident

V40.4xx- Person boarding or alighting a car injured in collision with pedestrian or animal

V40.5xx- Car driver injured in collision with pedestrian or animal in traffic accident

V40.6xx- Car passenger injured in collision with pedestrian or animal in traffic accident

V40.7xx- Person on outside of car injured in collision with pedestrian or animal in traffic accident

V40.9xx- Unspecified car occupant injured in collision with pedestrian or animal in traffic accident

V41- Car occupant injured in collision with pedal cycle
The appropriate 7th character is to be added to each code from category V41:
A Initial encounter
D Subsequent encounter
S Sequela

V41.0xx- Car driver injured in collision with pedal cycle in nontraffic accident

V41.1xx- Car passenger injured in collision with pedal cycle in nontraffic accident

V41.2xx- Person on outside of car injured in collision with pedal cycle in nontraffic accident

V41.3xx- Unspecified car occupant injured in collision with pedal cycle in nontraffic accident

V41.4xx- Person boarding or alighting a car injured in collision with pedal cycle

V41.5xx- Car driver injured in collision with pedal cycle in traffic accident

V41.6xx- Car passenger injured in collision with pedal cycle in traffic accident

V41.7xx- Person on outside of car injured in collision with pedal cycle in traffic accident

V41.9xx- Unspecified car occupant injured in collision with pedal cycle in traffic accident

V42- Car occupant injured in collision with two- or three-wheeled motor vehicle
The appropriate 7th character is to be added to each code from category V42:
A Initial encounter
D Subsequent encounter
S Sequela

V42.0xx- Car driver injured in collision with two- or three-wheeled motor vehicle in nontraffic accident

V42.1xx- Car passenger injured in collision with two- or three-wheeled motor vehicle in nontraffic accident

V42.2xx- Person on outside of car injured in collision with two- or three-wheeled motor vehicle in nontraffic accident

V42.3xx- Unspecified car occupant injured in collision with two- or three-wheeled motor vehicle in nontraffic accident

V42.4xx- Person boarding or alighting a car injured in collision with two- or three-wheeled motor vehicle

V42.5xx- Car driver injured in collision with two- or three-wheeled motor vehicle in traffic accident

V42.6xx- Car passenger injured in collision with two- or three-wheeled motor vehicle in traffic accident

V42.7xx- Person on outside of car injured in collision with two- or three-wheeled motor vehicle in traffic accident

V42.9xx- Unspecified car occupant injured in collision with two- or three-wheeled motor vehicle in traffic accident

V43- Car occupant injured in collision with car, pick-up truck or van
The appropriate 7th character is to be added to each code from category V43:
A Initial encounter
D Subsequent encounter
S Sequela

V43.0- Car driver injured in collision with car, pick-up truck or van in nontraffic accident

V43.01x- Car driver injured in collision with sport utility vehicle in nontraffic accident

V43.02x- Car driver injured in collision with other type car in nontraffic accident

V43.03x- Car driver injured in collision with pick-up truck in nontraffic accident

V43.04x- Car driver injured in collision with van in nontraffic accident

V43.1- Car passenger injured in collision with car, pick-up truck or van in nontraffic accident

V43.11x- Car passenger injured in collision with sport utility vehicle in nontraffic accident

V43.12x- Car passenger injured in collision with other type car in nontraffic accident

V43.13x- Car passenger injured in collision with pick-up in nontraffic accident

V43.14x- Car passenger injured in collision with van in nontraffic accident

V43.2- Person on outside of car injured in collision with car, pick-up truck or van in nontraffic accident

V43.21x- Person on outside of car injured in collision with sport utility vehicle in nontraffic accident

V43.22x- Person on outside of car injured in collision with other type car in nontraffic accident

V43.23x- Person on outside of car injured in collision with pick-up truck in nontraffic accident

V43.24x- Person on outside of car injured in collision with van in nontraffic accident

V43.3- Unspecified car occupant injured in collision with car, pick-up truck or van in nontraffic accident

V43.31x- Unspecified car occupant injured in collision with sport utility vehicle in nontraffic accident

V43.32x- Unspecified car occupant injured in collision with other type car in nontraffic accident

V43.33x- Unspecified car occupant injured in collision with pick-up truck in nontraffic accident

V43.34x- Unspecified car occupant injured in collision with van in nontraffic accident

V43.4- Person boarding or alighting a car injured in collision with car, pick-up truck or van

V43.41x- Person boarding or alighting a car injured in collision with sport utility vehicle

V43.42x- Person boarding or alighting a car injured in collision with other type car

V43.43x- Person boarding or alighting a car injured in collision with pick-up truck

V43.44x- Person boarding or alighting a car injured in collision with van

V43.5- Car driver injured in collision with car, pick-up truck or van in traffic accident

V43.51x- Car driver injured in collision with sport utility vehicle in traffic accident

V43.52x- Car driver injured in collision with other type car in traffic accident

V43.53x- Car driver injured in collision with pick-up truck in traffic accident

V43.54x- Car driver injured in collision with van in traffic accident

V43.6- Car passenger injured in collision with car, pick-up truck or van in traffic accident

V43.61x- Car passenger injured in collision with sport utility vehicle in traffic accident

V43.62x- Car passenger injured in collision with other type car in traffic accident

V43.63x- Car passenger injured in collision with pick-up truck in traffic accident

V43.64x- Car passenger injured in collision with van in traffic accident

V43.7- Person on outside of car injured in collision with car, pick-up truck or van in traffic accident

V43.71x- Person on outside of car injured in collision with sport utility vehicle in traffic accident

V43.72x- Person on outside of car injured in collision with other type car in traffic accident

V43.73x- Person on outside of car injured in collision with pick-up truck in traffic accident

V43.74x- Person on outside of car injured in collision with van in traffic accident

V43.9- Unspecified car occupant injured in collision with car, pick-up truck or van in traffic accident

V43.91x- Unspecified car occupant injured in collision with sport utility vehicle in traffic accident

V43.92x- Unspecified car occupant injured in collision with other type car in traffic accident

V43.93x- Unspecified car occupant injured in collision with pick-up truck in traffic accident

V43.94x- Unspecified car occupant injured in collision with van in traffic accident

V44- Car occupant injured in collision with heavy transport vehicle or bus
Excludes 1: car occupant injured in collision with military vehicle (V49.81)
The appropriate 7th character is to be added to each code from category V44:
A Initial encounter
D Subsequent encounter
S Sequela

V44.0xx- Car driver injured in collision with heavy transport vehicle or bus in nontraffic accident

V44.1xx- Car passenger injured in collision with heavy transport vehicle or bus in nontraffic accident

V44.2xx- Person on outside of car injured in collision with heavy transport vehicle or bus in nontraffic accident

V44.3xx- Unspecified car occupant injured in collision with heavy transport vehicle or bus in nontraffic accident

V44.4xx- Person boarding or alighting a car injured in collision with heavy transport vehicle or bus

V44.5xx- Car driver injured in collision with heavy transport vehicle or bus in traffic accident

V44.6xx- Car passenger injured in collision with heavy transport vehicle or bus in traffic accident

V44.7xx- Person on outside of car injured in collision with heavy transport vehicle or bus in traffic accident

V44.9xx- Unspecified car occupant injured in collision with heavy transport vehicle or bus in traffic accident

V45- Car occupant injured in collision with railway train or railway vehicle
The appropriate 7th character is to be added to each code from category V45:
A Initial encounter
D Subsequent encounter
S Sequela

V45.0xx- Car driver injured in collision with railway train or railway vehicle in nontraffic accident

V45.1xx- Car passenger injured in collision with railway train or railway vehicle in nontraffic accident

V45.2xx- Person on outside of car injured in collision with railway train or railway vehicle in nontraffic accident

V45.3xx- Unspecified car occupant injured in collision with railway train or railway vehicle in nontraffic accident

V45.4xx- Person boarding or alighting a car injured in collision with railway train or railway vehicle

V45.5xx- Car driver injured in collision with railway train or railway vehicle in traffic accident

V45.6xx- Car passenger injured in collision with railway train or railway vehicle in traffic accident

V45.7xx- Person on outside of car injured in collision with railway train or railway vehicle in traffic accident

V45.9xx- Unspecified car occupant injured in collision with railway train or railway vehicle in traffic accident

V46- Car occupant injured in collision with other nonmotor vehicle
Includes: Collision with animal-drawn vehicle, animal being ridden, streetcar
The appropriate 7th character is to be added to each code from category V46:
A Initial encounter
D Subsequent encounter
S Sequela

V46.0xx- Car driver injured in collision with other nonmotor vehicle in nontraffic accident

V
3
8
|
V
4
6

V46.1xx-   Car passenger injured in collision with other nonmotor vehicle in nontraffic accident

V46.2xx-   Person on outside of car injured in collision with other nonmotor vehicle in nontraffic accident

V46.3xx-   Unspecified car occupant injured in collision with other nonmotor vehicle in nontraffic accident

V46.4xx-   Person boarding or alighting a car injured in collision with other nonmotor vehicle

V46.5xx-   Car driver injured in collision with other nonmotor vehicle in traffic accident

V46.6xx-   Car passenger injured in collision with other nonmotor vehicle in traffic accident

V46.7xx-   Person on outside of car injured in collision with other nonmotor vehicle in traffic accident

V46.9xx-   Unspecified car occupant injured in collision with other nonmotor vehicle in traffic accident

V47-   Car occupant injured in collision with fixed or stationary object

The appropriate 7th character is to be added to each code from category V47:
A   Initial encounter
D   Subsequent encounter
S   Sequela

V47.0-   Car driver injured in collision with fixed or stationary object in nontraffic accident

V47.01x-   Driver of sport utility vehicle injured in collision with fixed or stationary object in nontraffic accident

V47.02x-   Driver of other type car injured in collision with fixed or stationary object in nontraffic accident

V47.1-   Car passenger injured in collision with fixed or stationary object in nontraffic accident

V47.11x-   Passenger of sport utility vehicle injured in collision with fixed or stationary object in nontraffic accident

V47.12x-   Passenger of other type car injured in collision with fixed or stationary object in nontraffic accident

V47.2xx-   Person on outside of car injured in collision with fixed or stationary object in nontraffic accident

V47.3-   Unspecified car occupant injured in collision with fixed or stationary object in nontraffic accident

V47.31x-   Unspecified occupant of sport utility vehicle injured in collision with fixed or stationary object in nontraffic accident

V47.32x-   Unspecified occupant of other type car injured in collision with fixed or stationary object in nontraffic accident

V47.4-   Person boarding or alighting a car injured in collision with fixed or stationary object

V47.5-   Car driver injured in collision with fixed or stationary object in traffic accident

V47.51x-   Driver of sport utility vehicle injured in collision with fixed or stationary object in traffic accident

V47.52x-   Driver of other type car injured in collision with fixed or stationary object in traffic accident

V47.6-   Car passenger injured in collision with fixed or stationary object in traffic accident

V47.61x-   Passenger of sport utility vehicle injured in collision with fixed or stationary object in traffic accident

V47.62x-   Passenger of other type car injured in collision with fixed or stationary object in traffic accident

V47.7xx-   Person on outside of car injured in collision with fixed or stationary object in traffic accident

V47.9-   Unspecified car occupant injured in collision with fixed or stationary object in traffic accident

V47.91x-   Unspecified occupant of sport utility vehicle injured in collision with fixed or stationary object in traffic accident

V47.92x-   Unspecified occupant of other type car injured in collision with fixed or stationary object in traffic accident

V48-   Car occupant injured in noncollision transport accident
Includes: Overturning car NOS
            Overturning car without collision

The appropriate 7th character is to be added to each code from category V48:
A   Initial encounter
D   Subsequent encounter
S   Sequela

V48.0xx-   Car driver injured in noncollision transport accident in nontraffic accident

V48.1xx-   Car passenger injured in noncollision transport accident in nontraffic accident

V48.2xx-   Person on outside of car injured in noncollision transport accident in nontraffic accident

V48.3xx-   Unspecified car occupant injured in noncollision transport accident in nontraffic accident

V48.4xx-   Person boarding or alighting a car injured in noncollision transport accident

V48.5xx-   Car driver injured in noncollision transport accident in traffic accident

V48.6xx-   Car passenger injured in noncollision transport accident in traffic accident

V48.7xx-   Person on outside of car injured in noncollision transport accident in traffic accident

V48.9xx-   Unspecified car occupant injured in noncollision transport accident in traffic accident

V49-   Car occupant injured in other and unspecified transport accidents

The appropriate 7th character is to be added to each code from category V49:
A   Initial encounter
D   Subsequent encounter
S   Sequela

V49.0-   Driver injured in collision with other and unspecified motor vehicles in nontraffic accident

V49.00x-   Driver injured in collision with unspecified motor vehicles in nontraffic accident

V49.09x-   Driver injured in collision with other motor vehicles in nontraffic accident

V49.1-   Passenger injured in collision with other and unspecified motor vehicles in nontraffic accident

V49.10x-   Passenger injured in collision with unspecified motor vehicles in nontraffic accident

V49.19x-   Passenger injured in collision with other motor vehicles in nontraffic accident

V49.2-   Unspecified car occupant injured in collision with other and unspecified motor vehicles in nontraffic accident

V49.20x-   Unspecified car occupant injured in collision with unspecified motor vehicles in nontraffic accident
            Car collision NOS, nontraffic

V49.29x-   Unspecified car occupant injured in collision with other motor vehicles in nontraffic accident

V49.3xx-   Car occupant (driver) (passenger) injured in unspecified nontraffic accident
            Car accident NOS, nontraffic
            Car occupant injured in nontraffic accident NOS

V49.4-   Driver injured in collision with other and unspecified motor vehicles in traffic accident

V49.40x-   Driver injured in collision with unspecified motor vehicles in traffic accident

V49.49x-   Driver injured in collision with other motor vehicles in traffic accident

V49.5-   Passenger injured in collision with other and unspecified motor vehicles in traffic accident

V49.50x-   Passenger injured in collision with unspecified motor vehicles in traffic accident

V49.59x-   Passenger injured in collision with other motor vehicles in traffic accident

V49.6-   Unspecified car occupant injured in collision with other and unspecified motor vehicles in traffic accident

V49.60x-   Unspecified car occupant injured in collision with unspecified motor vehicles in traffic accident
            Car collision NOS (traffic)

V49.69x-   Unspecified car occupant injured in collision with other motor vehicles in traffic accident

V49.8-   Car occupant (driver) (passenger) injured in other specified transport accidents

V49.81x-   Car occupant (driver) (passenger) injured in transport accident with military vehicle

V49.88x-   Car occupant (driver) (passenger) injured in other specified transport accidents

V49.9xx-   Car occupant (driver) (passenger) injured in unspecified traffic accident
            Car accident NOS

V
4
6
I
V
5
5

Occupant of pick-up truck or van injured in transport accident (V50-V59)

Includes: A four or six wheel motor vehicle designed primarily for carrying passengers and property but weighing less than the local limit for classification as a heavy goods vehicle
        Minibus
        Minivan
        Sport utility vehicle (SUV)
        Truck
        Van

Excludes 1: heavy transport vehicle (V60-V69)

V50- **Occupant of pick-up truck or van injured in collision** with **pedestrian or animal**
    Excludes 1: pick-up truck or van collision with animal-drawn vehicle or animal being ridden (V56.-)

The appropriate 7th character is to be added to each code from category V50:
    A **Initial** encounter
    D **Subsequent** encounter
    S **Sequela**

V50.0xx- Driver of pick-up truck or van injured in collision with pedestrian or animal in nontraffic accident

V50.1xx- Passenger in pick-up truck or van injured in collision with pedestrian or animal in nontraffic accident

V50.2xx- Person on outside of pick-up truck or van injured in collision with pedestrian or animal in nontraffic accident

V50.3xx- Unspecified occupant of pick-up truck or van injured in collision with pedestrian or animal in nontraffic accident

V50.4xx- Person boarding or alighting a pick-up truck or van injured in collision with pedestrian or animal

V50.5xx- Driver of pick-up truck or van injured in collision with pedestrian or animal in traffic accident

V50.6xx- Passenger in pick-up truck or van injured in collision with pedestrian or animal in traffic accident

V50.7xx- Person on outside of pick-up truck or van injured in collision with pedestrian or animal in traffic accident

V50.9xx- Unspecified occupant of pick-up truck or van injured in collision with pedestrian or animal in traffic accident

V51- **Occupant of pick-up truck or van injured in collision** with **pedal cycle**
The appropriate 7th character is to be added to each code from category V51:
    A **Initial** encounter
    D **Subsequent** encounter
    S **Sequela**

V51.0xx- Driver of pick-up truck or van injured in collision with pedal cycle in nontraffic accident

V51.1xx- Passenger in pick-up truck or van injured in collision with pedal cycle in nontraffic accident

V51.2xx- Person on outside of pick-up truck or van injured in collision with pedal cycle in nontraffic accident

V51.3xx- Unspecified occupant of pick-up truck or van injured in collision with pedal cycle in nontraffic accident

V51.4xx- Person boarding or alighting a pick-up truck or van injured in collision with pedal cycle

V51.5xx- Driver of pick-up truck or van injured in collision with pedal cycle in traffic accident

V51.6xx- Passenger in pick-up truck or van injured in collision with pedal cycle in traffic accident

V51.7xx- Person on outside of pick-up truck or van injured in collision with pedal cycle in traffic accident

V51.9xx- Unspecified occupant of pick-up truck or van injured in collision with pedal cycle in traffic accident

V52- **Occupant of pick-up truck or van injured in collision** with **two- or three-wheeled motor vehicle**
The appropriate 7th character is to be added to each code from category V52:
    A **Initial** encounter
    D **Subsequent** encounter
    S **Sequela**

V52.0xx- Driver of pick-up truck or van injured in collision with two- or three-wheeled motor vehicle in nontraffic accident

V52.1xx- Passenger in pick-up truck or van injured in collision with two- or three-wheeled motor vehicle in nontraffic accident

V52.2xx- Person on outside of pick-up truck or van injured in collision with two- or three-wheeled motor vehicle in nontraffic accident

V52.3xx- Unspecified occupant of pick-up truck or van injured in collision with two- or three-wheeled motor vehicle in nontraffic accident

V52.4xx- Person boarding or alighting a pick-up truck or van injured in collision with two- or three-wheeled motor vehicle

V52.5xx- Driver of pick-up truck or van injured in collision with two- or three-wheeled motor vehicle in traffic accident

V52.6xx- Passenger in pick-up truck or van injured in collision with two- or three-wheeled motor vehicle in traffic accident

V52.7xx- Person on outside of pick-up truck or van injured in collision with two- or three-wheeled motor vehicle in traffic accident

V52.9xx- Unspecified occupant of pick-up truck or van injured in collision with two- or three-wheeled motor vehicle in traffic accident

V53- **Occupant of pick-up truck or van injured in collision** with **car, pick-up truck or van**
The appropriate 7th character is to be added to each code from category V53:
    A **Initial** encounter
    D **Subsequent** encounter
    S **Sequela**

V53.0xx- Driver of pick-up truck or van injured in collision with car, pick-up truck or van in nontraffic accident

V53.1xx- Passenger in pick-up truck or van injured in collision with car, pick-up truck or van in nontraffic accident

V53.2xx- Person on outside of pick-up truck or van injured in collision with car, pick-up truck or van in nontraffic accident

V53.3xx- Unspecified occupant of pick-up truck or van injured in collision with car, pick-up truck or van in nontraffic accident

V53.4xx- Person boarding or alighting a pick-up truck or van injured in collision with car, pick-up truck or van

V53.5xx- Driver of pick-up truck or van injured in collision with car, pick-up truck or van in traffic accident

V53.6xx- Passenger in pick-up truck or van injured in collision with car, pick-up truck or van in traffic accident

V53.7xx- Person on outside of pick-up truck or van injured in collision with car, pick-up truck or van in traffic accident

V53.9xx- Unspecified occupant of pick-up truck or van injured in collision with car, pick-up truck or van in traffic accident

V54- **Occupant of pick-up truck or van injured in collision** with **heavy transport vehicle or bus**
    Excludes 1: occupant of pick-up truck or van injured in collision with military vehicle (V59.81)

The appropriate 7th character is to be added to each code from category V54:
    A **Initial** encounter
    D **Subsequent** encounter
    S **Sequela**

V54.0xx- Driver of pick-up truck or van injured in collision with heavy transport vehicle or bus in nontraffic accident

V54.1xx- Passenger in pick-up truck or van injured in collision with heavy transport vehicle or bus in nontraffic accident

V54.2xx- Person on outside of pick-up truck or van injured in collision with heavy transport vehicle or bus in nontraffic accident

V54.3xx- Unspecified occupant of pick-up truck or van injured in collision with heavy transport vehicle or bus in nontraffic accident

V54.4xx- Person boarding or alighting a pick-up truck or van injured in collision with heavy transport vehicle or bus

V54.5xx- Driver of pick-up truck or van injured in collision with heavy transport vehicle or bus in traffic accident

V54.6xx- Passenger in pick-up truck or van injured in collision with heavy transport vehicle or bus in traffic accident

V54.7xx- Person on outside of pick-up truck or van injured in collision with heavy transport vehicle or bus in traffic accident

V54.9xx- Unspecified occupant of pick-up truck or van injured in collision with heavy transport vehicle or bus in traffic accident

V55- **Occupant of pick-up truck or van injured in collision** with **railway train or railway vehicle**
The appropriate 7th character is to be added to each code from category V55:
    A **Initial** encounter
    D **Subsequent** encounter
    S **Sequela**

V55.0xx- Driver of pick-up truck or van injured in collision with railway train or railway vehicle in nontraffic accident

V55.1xx- Passenger in pick-up truck or van injured in collision with railway train or railway vehicle in nontraffic accident

V55.2xx- Person on outside of pick-up truck or van injured in collision with railway train or railway vehicle in nontraffic accident

V55.3xx- Unspecified occupant of pick-up truck or van injured in collision with railway train or railway vehicle in nontraffic accident

V55.4xx- Person boarding or alighting a pick-up truck or van injured in collision with railway train or railway vehicle

V
4
6
I
V
5
5

V55.5xx- Driver of pick-up truck or van injured in collision with railway train or railway vehicle in traffic accident

V55.6xx- Passenger in pick-up truck or van injured in collision with railway train or railway vehicle in traffic accident

V55.7xx- Person on outside of pick-up truck or van injured in collision with railway train or railway vehicle in traffic accident

V55.9xx- Unspecified occupant of pick-up truck or van injured in collision with railway train or railway vehicle in traffic accident

V56- Occupant of pick-up truck or van injured in collision with other nonmotor vehicle
    Includes: Collision with animal-drawn vehicle, animal being ridden, streetcar
    The appropriate 7th character is to be added to each code from category V56:
    A   Initial encounter
    D   Subsequent encounter
    S   Sequela

V56.0xx- Driver of pick-up truck or van injured in collision with other nonmotor vehicle in nontraffic accident

V56.1xx- Passenger in pick-up truck or van injured in collision with other nonmotor vehicle in nontraffic accident

V56.2xx- Person on outside of pick-up truck or van injured in collision with other nonmotor vehicle in nontraffic accident

V56.3xx- Unspecified occupant of pick-up truck or van injured in collision with other nonmotor vehicle in nontraffic accident

V56.4xx- Person boarding or alighting a pick-up truck or van injured in collision with other nonmotor vehicle

V56.5xx- Driver of pick-up truck or van injured in collision with other nonmotor vehicle in traffic accident

V56.6xx- Passenger in pick-up truck or van injured in collision with other nonmotor vehicle in traffic accident

V56.7xx- Person on outside of pick-up truck or van injured in collision with other nonmotor vehicle in traffic accident

V56.9xx- Unspecified occupant of pick-up truck or van injured in collision with other nonmotor vehicle in traffic accident

V57- Occupant of pick-up truck or van injured in collision with fixed or stationary object
    The appropriate 7th character is to be added to each code from category V57:
    A   Initial encounter
    D   Subsequent encounter
    S   Sequela

V57.0xx- Driver of pick-up truck or van injured in collision with fixed or stationary object in nontraffic accident

V57.1xx- Passenger in pick-up truck or van injured in collision with fixed or stationary object in nontraffic accident

V57.2xx- Person on outside of pick-up truck or van injured in collision with fixed or stationary object in nontraffic accident

V57.3xx- Unspecified occupant of pick-up truck or van injured in collision with fixed or stationary object in nontraffic accident

V57.4xx- Person boarding or alighting a pick-up truck or van injured in collision with fixed or stationary object

V57.5xx- Driver of pick-up truck or van injured in collision with fixed or stationary object in traffic accident

V57.6xx- Passenger in pick-up truck or van injured in collision with fixed or stationary object in traffic accident

V57.7xx- Person on outside of pick-up truck or van injured in collision with fixed or stationary object in traffic accident

V57.9xx- Unspecified occupant of pick-up truck or van injured in collision with fixed or stationary object in traffic accident

V58- Occupant of pick-up truck or van injured in noncollision transport accident
    Includes: Overturning pick-up truck or van NOS
                Overturning pick-up truck or van without collision
    The appropriate 7th character is to be added to each code from category V58:
    A   Initial encounter
    D   Subsequent encounter
    S   Sequela

V58.0xx- Driver of pick-up truck or van injured in noncollision transport accident in nontraffic accident

V58.1xx- Passenger in pick-up truck or van injured in noncollision transport accident in nontraffic accident

V58.2xx- Person on outside of pick-up truck or van injured in noncollision transport accident in nontraffic accident

V58.3xx- Unspecified occupant of pick-up truck or van injured in noncollision transport accident in nontraffic accident

V58.4xx- Person boarding or alighting a pick-up truck or van injured in noncollision transport accident

V58.5xx- Driver of pick-up truck or van injured in noncollision transport accident in traffic accident

V58.6xx- Passenger in pick-up truck or van injured in noncollision transport accident in traffic accident

V58.7xx- Person on outside of pick-up truck or van injured in noncollision transport accident in traffic accident

V58.9xx- Unspecified occupant of pick-up truck or van injured in noncollision transport accident in traffic accident

V59- Occupant of pick-up truck or van injured in other and unspecified transport accidents
    The appropriate 7th character is to be added to each code from category V59:
    A   Initial encounter
    D   Subsequent encounter
    S   Sequela

V59.0- Driver of pick-up truck or van injured in collision with other and unspecified motor vehicles in nontraffic accident

V59.00x- Driver of pick-up truck or van injured in collision with unspecified motor vehicles in nontraffic accident

V59.09x- Driver of pick-up truck or van injured in collision with other motor vehicles in nontraffic accident

V59.1- Passenger in pick-up truck or van injured in collision with other and unspecified motor vehicles in nontraffic accident

V59.10x- Passenger in pick-up truck or van injured in collision with unspecified motor vehicles in nontraffic accident

V59.19x- Passenger in pick-up truck or van injured in collision with other motor vehicles in nontraffic accident

V59.2- Unspecified occupant of pick-up truck or van injured in collision with other and unspecified motor vehicles in nontraffic accident

V59.20x- Unspecified occupant of pick-up truck or van injured in collision with unspecified motor vehicles in nontraffic accident
    Collision NOS involving pick-up truck or van, nontraffic

V59.29x- Unspecified occupant of pick-up truck or van injured in collision with other motor vehicles in nontraffic accident

V59.3xx- Occupant (driver) (passenger) of pick-up truck or van injured in unspecified nontraffic accident
    Accident NOS involving pick-up truck or van, nontraffic
    Occupant of pick-up truck or van injured in nontraffic accident NOS

V59.4- Driver of pick-up truck or van injured in collision with other and unspecified motor vehicles in traffic accident

V59.40x- Driver of pick-up truck or van injured in collision with unspecified motor vehicles in traffic accident

V59.49x- Driver of pick-up truck or van injured in collision with other motor vehicles in traffic accident

V59.5- Passenger in pick-up truck or van injured in collision with other and unspecified motor vehicles in traffic accident

V59.50x- Passenger in pick-up truck or van injured in collision with unspecified motor vehicles in traffic accident

V59.59x- Passenger in pick-up truck or van injured in collision with other motor vehicles in traffic accident

V59.6- Unspecified occupant of pick-up truck or van injured in collision with other and unspecified motor vehicles in traffic accident

V59.60x- Unspecified occupant of pick-up truck or van injured in collision with unspecified motor vehicles in traffic accident
    Collision NOS involving pick-up truck or van (traffic)

V59.69x- Unspecified occupant of pick-up truck or van injured in collision with other motor vehicles in traffic accident

V59.8- Occupant (driver) (passenger) of pick-up truck or van injured in other specified transport accidents

V59.81x- Occupant (driver) (passenger) of pick-up truck or van injured in transport accident with military vehicle

V59.88x- Occupant (driver) (passenger) of pick-up truck or van injured in other specified transport accidents

V59.9xx- Occupant (driver) (passenger) of pick-up truck or van injured in unspecified traffic accident
    Accident NOS involving pick-up truck or van

Excludes 1: = NOT CODED HERE! (Do not code both)   Excludes ❷: = Not Included Here

Occupant of heavy transport vehicle injured in transport accident (V60-V69)

Includes: 18 wheeler
            Armored car
            Panel truck
Excludes 1:   bus
            motorcoach

V60-   Occupant of heavy transport vehicle injured in collision with pedestrian or animal
Excludes 1:   heavy transport vehicle collision with animal-drawn vehicle or animal being ridden (V66.-)

The appropriate 7th character is to be added to each code from category V60:
  A   Initial encounter
  D   Subsequent encounter
  S   Sequela

V60.0xx-   Driver of heavy transport vehicle injured in collision with pedestrian or animal in nontraffic accident

V60.1xx-   Passenger in heavy transport vehicle injured in collision with pedestrian or animal in nontraffic accident

V60.2xx-   Person on outside of heavy transport vehicle injured in collision with pedestrian or animal in nontraffic accident

V60.3xx-   Unspecified occupant of heavy transport vehicle injured in collision with pedestrian or animal in nontraffic accident

V60.4xx-   Person boarding or alighting a heavy transport vehicle injured in collision with pedestrian or animal

V60.5xx-   Driver of heavy transport vehicle injured in collision with pedestrian or animal in traffic accident

V60.6xx-   Passenger in heavy transport vehicle injured in collision with pedestrian or animal in traffic accident

V60.7xx-   Person on outside of heavy transport vehicle injured in collision with pedestrian or animal in traffic accident

V60.9xx-   Unspecified occupant of heavy transport vehicle injured in collision with pedestrian or animal in traffic accident

V61-   Occupant of heavy transport vehicle injured in collision with pedal cycle

The appropriate 7th character is to be added to each code from category V61:
  A   Initial encounter
  D   Subsequent encounter
  S   Sequela

V61.0xx-   Driver of heavy transport vehicle injured in collision with pedal cycle in nontraffic accident

V61.1xx-   Passenger in heavy transport vehicle injured in collision with pedal cycle in nontraffic accident

V61.2xx-   Person on outside of heavy transport vehicle injured in collision with pedal cycle in nontraffic accident

V61.3xx-   Unspecified occupant of heavy transport vehicle injured in collision with pedal cycle in nontraffic accident

V61.4xx-   Person boarding or alighting a heavy transport vehicle injured in collision with pedal cycle while boarding or alighting

V61.5xx-   Driver of heavy transport vehicle injured in collision with pedal cycle in traffic accident

V61.6xx-   Passenger in heavy transport vehicle injured in collision with pedal cycle in traffic accident

V61.7xx-   Person on outside of heavy transport vehicle injured in collision with pedal cycle in traffic accident

V61.9xx-   Unspecified occupant of heavy transport vehicle injured in collision with pedal cycle in traffic accident

V62-   Occupant of heavy transport vehicle injured in collision with two- or three-wheeled motor vehicle

The appropriate 7th character is to be added to each code from category V62:
  A   Initial encounter
  D   Subsequent encounter
  S   Sequela

V62.0xx-   Driver of heavy transport vehicle injured in collision with two- or three-wheeled motor vehicle in nontraffic accident

V62.1xx-   Passenger in heavy transport vehicle injured in collision with two- or three-wheeled motor vehicle in nontraffic accident

V62.2xx-   Person on outside of heavy transport vehicle injured in collision with two- or three-wheeled motor vehicle in nontraffic accident

V62.3xx-   Unspecified occupant of heavy transport vehicle injured in collision with two- or three-wheeled motor vehicle in nontraffic accident

V62.4xx-   Person boarding or alighting a heavy transport vehicle injured in collision with two- or three-wheeled motor vehicle

V62.5xx-   Driver of heavy transport vehicle injured in collision with two- or three-wheeled motor vehicle in traffic accident

V62.6xx-   Passenger in heavy transport vehicle injured in collision with two- or three-wheeled motor vehicle in traffic accident

V62.7xx-   Person on outside of heavy transport vehicle injured in collision with two- or three-wheeled motor vehicle in traffic accident

V62.9xx-   Unspecified occupant of heavy transport vehicle injured in collision with two- or three-wheeled motor vehicle in traffic accident

V63-   Occupant of heavy transport vehicle injured in collision with car, pick-up truck or van

The appropriate 7th character is to be added to each code from category V63:
  A   Initial encounter
  D   Subsequent encounter
  S   Sequela

V63.0xx-   Driver of heavy transport vehicle injured in collision with car, pick-up truck or van in nontraffic accident

V63.1xx-   Passenger in heavy transport vehicle injured in collision with car, pick-up truck or van in nontraffic accident

V63.2xx-   Person on outside of heavy transport vehicle injured in collision with car, pick-up truck or van in nontraffic accident

V63.3xx-   Unspecified occupant of heavy transport vehicle injured in collision with car, pick-up truck or van in nontraffic accident

V63.4xx-   Person boarding or alighting a heavy transport vehicle injured in collision with car, pick-up truck or van

V63.5xx-   Driver of heavy transport vehicle injured in collision with car, pick-up truck or van in traffic accident

V63.6xx-   Passenger in heavy transport vehicle injured in collision with car, pick-up truck or van in traffic accident

V63.7xx-   Person on outside of heavy transport vehicle injured in collision with car, pick-up truck or van in traffic accident

V63.9xx-   Unspecified occupant of heavy transport vehicle injured in collision with car, pick-up truck or van in traffic accident

V64-   Occupant of heavy transport vehicle injured in collision with heavy transport vehicle or bus
Excludes 1:   occupant of heavy transport vehicle injured in collision with military vehicle (V69.81)

The appropriate 7th character is to be added to each code from category V64:
  A   Initial encounter
  D   Subsequent encounter
  S   Sequela

V64.0xx-   Driver of heavy transport vehicle injured in collision with heavy transport vehicle or bus in nontraffic accident

V64.1xx-   Passenger in heavy transport vehicle injured in collision with heavy transport vehicle or bus in nontraffic accident

V64.2xx-   Person on outside of heavy transport vehicle injured in collision with heavy transport vehicle or bus in nontraffic accident

V64.3xx-   Unspecified occupant of heavy transport vehicle injured in collision with heavy transport vehicle or bus in nontraffic accident

V64.4xx-   Person boarding or alighting a heavy transport vehicle injured in collision with heavy transport vehicle or bus while boarding or alighting

V64.5xx-   Driver of heavy transport vehicle injured in collision with heavy transport vehicle or bus in traffic accident

V64.6xx-   Passenger in heavy transport vehicle injured in collision with heavy transport vehicle or bus in traffic accident

V64.7xx-   Person on outside of heavy transport vehicle injured in collision with heavy transport vehicle or bus in traffic accident

V64.9xx-   Unspecified occupant of heavy transport vehicle injured in collision with heavy transport vehicle or bus in traffic accident

V65-   Occupant of heavy transport vehicle injured in collision with railway train or railway vehicle

The appropriate 7th character is to be added to each code from category V65:
  A   Initial encounter
  D   Subsequent encounter
  S   Sequela

V65.0xx-   Driver of heavy transport vehicle injured in collision with railway train or railway vehicle in nontraffic accident

V65.1xx-   Passenger in heavy transport vehicle injured in collision with railway train or railway vehicle in nontraffic accident

V65.2xx-   Person on outside of heavy transport vehicle injured in collision with railway train or railway vehicle in nontraffic accident

V65.3xx-   Unspecified occupant of heavy transport vehicle injured in collision with railway train or railway vehicle in nontraffic accident

V65.4xx-   Person boarding or alighting a heavy transport vehicle injured in collision with railway train or railway vehicle

V 5 5 - V 6 5

V65.5xx- Driver of heavy transport vehicle injured in collision with railway train or railway vehicle in traffic accident

V65.6xx- Passenger in heavy transport vehicle injured in collision with railway train or railway vehicle in traffic accident

V65.7xx- Person on outside of heavy transport vehicle injured in collision with railway train or railway vehicle in traffic accident

V65.9xx- Unspecified occupant of heavy transport vehicle injured in collision with railway train or railway vehicle in traffic accident

V66- Occupant of heavy transport vehicle injured in collision with other nonmotor vehicle

Includes: Collision with animal-drawn vehicle, animal being ridden, streetcar

The appropriate 7th character is to be added to each code from category V66:
   A   Initial encounter
   D   Subsequent encounter
   S   Sequela

V66.0xx- Driver of heavy transport vehicle injured in collision with other nonmotor vehicle in nontraffic accident

V66.1xx- Passenger in heavy transport vehicle injured in collision with other nonmotor vehicle in nontraffic accident

V66.2xx- Person on outside of heavy transport vehicle injured in collision with other nonmotor vehicle in nontraffic accident

V66.3xx- Unspecified occupant of heavy transport vehicle injured in collision with other nonmotor vehicle in nontraffic accident

V66.4xx- Person boarding or alighting a heavy transport vehicle injured in collision with other nonmotor vehicle

V66.5xx- Driver of heavy transport vehicle injured in collision with other nonmotor vehicle in traffic accident

V66.6xx- Passenger in heavy transport vehicle injured in collision with other nonmotor vehicle in traffic accident

V66.7xx- Person on outside of heavy transport vehicle injured in collision with other nonmotor vehicle in traffic accident

V66.9xx- Unspecified occupant of heavy transport vehicle injured in collision with other nonmotor vehicle in traffic accident

V67- Occupant of heavy transport vehicle injured in collision with fixed or stationary object

The appropriate 7th character is to be added to each code from category V67:
   A   Initial encounter
   D   Subsequent encounter
   S   Sequela

V67.0xx- Driver of heavy transport vehicle injured in collision with fixed or stationary object in nontraffic accident

V67.1xx- Passenger in heavy transport vehicle injured in collision with fixed or stationary object in nontraffic accident

V67.2xx- Person on outside of heavy transport vehicle injured in collision with fixed or stationary object in nontraffic accident

V67.3xx- Unspecified occupant of heavy transport vehicle injured in collision with fixed or stationary object in nontraffic accident

V67.4xx- Person boarding or alighting a heavy transport vehicle injured in collision with fixed or stationary object

V67.5xx- Driver of heavy transport vehicle injured in collision with fixed or stationary object in traffic accident

V67.6xx- Passenger in heavy transport vehicle injured in collision with fixed or stationary object in traffic accident

V67.7xx- Person on outside of heavy transport vehicle injured in collision with fixed or stationary object in traffic accident

V67.9xx- Unspecified occupant of heavy transport vehicle injured in collision with fixed or stationary object in traffic accident

V68- Occupant of heavy transport vehicle injured in noncollision transport accident

Includes: Overturning heavy transport vehicle NOS
            Overturning heavy transport vehicle without collision

The appropriate 7th character is to be added to each code from category V68:
   A   Initial encounter
   D   Subsequent encounter
   S   Sequela

V68.0xx- Driver of heavy transport vehicle injured in noncollision transport accident in nontraffic accident

V68.1xx- Passenger in heavy transport vehicle injured in noncollision transport accident in nontraffic accident

V68.2xx- Person on outside of heavy transport vehicle injured in noncollision transport accident in nontraffic accident

V68.3xx- Unspecified occupant of heavy transport vehicle injured in noncollision transport accident in nontraffic accident

V68.4xx- Person boarding or alighting a heavy transport vehicle injured in noncollision transport accident

V68.5xx- Driver of heavy transport vehicle injured in noncollision transport accident in traffic accident

V68.6xx- Passenger in heavy transport vehicle injured in noncollision transport accident in traffic accident

V68.7xx- Person on outside of heavy transport vehicle injured in noncollision transport accident in traffic accident

V68.9xx- Unspecified occupant of heavy transport vehicle injured in noncollision transport accident in traffic accident

V69- Occupant of heavy transport vehicle injured in other and unspecified transport accidents

The appropriate 7th character is to be added to each code from category V69:
   A   Initial encounter
   D   Subsequent encounter
   S   Sequela

V69.0- Driver of heavy transport vehicle injured in collision with other and unspecified motor vehicles in nontraffic accident

V69.00x- Driver of heavy transport vehicle injured in collision with unspecified motor vehicles in nontraffic accident

V69.09x- Driver of heavy transport vehicle injured in collision with other motor vehicles in nontraffic accident

V69.1- Passenger in heavy transport vehicle injured in collision with other and unspecified motor vehicles in nontraffic accident

V69.10x- Passenger in heavy transport vehicle injured in collision with unspecified motor vehicles in nontraffic accident

V69.19x- Passenger in heavy transport vehicle injured in collision with other motor vehicles in nontraffic accident

V69.2- Unspecified occupant of heavy transport vehicle injured in collision with other and unspecified motor vehicles in nontraffic accident

V69.20x- Unspecified occupant of heavy transport vehicle injured in collision with unspecified motor vehicles in nontraffic accident
         Collision NOS involving heavy transport vehicle, nontraffic

V69.29x- Unspecified occupant of heavy transport vehicle injured in collision with other motor vehicles in nontraffic accident

V69.3xx- Occupant (driver) (passenger) of heavy transport vehicle injured in unspecified nontraffic accident
         Accident NOS involving heavy transport vehicle, nontraffic
         Occupant of heavy transport vehicle injured in nontraffic accident NOS

V69.4- Driver of heavy transport vehicle injured in collision with other and unspecified motor vehicles intraffic accident

V69.40x- Driver of heavy transport vehicle injured in collision with unspecified motor vehicles in traffic accident

V69.49x- Driver of heavy transport vehicle injured in collision with other motor vehicles in traffic accident

V69.5- Passenger in heavy transport vehicle injured in collision with other and unspecified motor vehicles in traffic accident

V69.50x- Passenger in heavy transport vehicle injured in collision with unspecified motor vehicles in traffic accident

V69.59x- Passenger in heavy transport vehicle injured in collision with other motor vehicles in traffic accident

V69.6- Unspecified occupant of heavy transport vehicle injured in collision with other and unspecified motor vehicles in traffic accident

V69.60x- Unspecified occupant of heavy transport vehicle injured in collision with unspecified motor vehicles in traffic accident
         Collision NOS involving heavy transport vehicle (traffic)

V69.69x- Unspecified occupant of heavy transport vehicle injured in collision with other motor vehicles in traffic accident

V69.8- Occupant (driver) (passenger) of heavy transport vehicle injured in other specified transport accidents

V69.81x- Occupant (driver) (passenger) of heavy transport vehicle injured in transport accidents with military vehicle

V69.88x- Occupant (driver) (passenger) of heavy transport vehicle injured in other specified transport accidents

V69.9xx- Occupant (driver) (passenger) of heavy transport vehicle injured in unspecified traffic accident
         Accident NOS involving heavy transport vehicle

Bus occupant injured in transport accident (V70-V79)

Includes: Motorcoach
Excludes 1: *minibus (V50-V59)*

V70- Bus occupant injured in collision with pedestrian or animal
    Excludes 1: *bus collision with animal-drawn vehicle or animal being ridden (V76.-)*

The appropriate 7th character is to be added to each code from category V70:
A   Initial encounter
D   Subsequent encounter
S   Sequela

V70.0xx- Driver of bus injured in collision with pedestrian or animal in nontraffic accident
V70.1xx- Passenger on bus injured in collision with pedestrian or animal in nontraffic accident
V70.2xx- Person on outside of bus injured in collision with pedestrian or animal in nontraffic accident
V70.3xx- Unspecified occupant of bus injured in collision with pedestrian or animal in nontraffic accident
V70.4xx- Person boarding or alighting from bus injured in collision with pedestrian or animal
V70.5xx- Driver of bus injured in collision with pedestrian or animal in traffic accident
V70.6xx- Passenger on bus injured in collision with pedestrian or animal in traffic accident
V70.7xx- Person on outside of bus injured in collision with pedestrian or animal in traffic accident
V70.9xx- Unspecified occupant of bus injured in collision with pedestrian or animal in traffic accident

V71- Bus occupant injured in collision with pedal cycle
The appropriate 7th character is to be added to each code from category V71:
A   Initial encounter
D   Subsequent encounter
S   Sequela

V71.0xx- Driver of bus injured in collision with pedal cycle in nontraffic accident
V71.1xx- Passenger on bus injured in collision with pedal cycle in nontraffic accident
V71.2xx- Person on outside of bus injured in collision with pedal cycle in nontraffic accident
V71.3xx- Unspecified occupant of bus injured in collision with pedal cycle in nontraffic accident
V71.4xx- Person boarding or alighting from bus injured in collision with pedal cycle
V71.5xx- Driver of bus injured in collision with pedal cycle in traffic accident
V71.6xx- Passenger on bus injured in collision with pedal cycle in traffic accident
V71.7xx- Person on outside of bus injured in collision with pedal cycle in traffic accident
V71.9xx- Unspecified occupant of bus injured in collision with pedal cycle in traffic accident

V72- Bus occupant injured in collision with two- or three-wheeled motor vehicle
The appropriate 7th character is to be added to each code from category V72:
A   Initial encounter
D   Subsequent encounter
S   Sequela

V72.0xx- Driver of bus injured in collision with two- or three-wheeled motor vehicle in nontraffic accident
V72.1xx- Passenger on bus injured in collision with two- or three-wheeled motor vehicle in nontraffic accident
V72.2xx- Person on outside of bus injured in collision with two- or three-wheeled motor vehicle in nontraffic accident
V72.3xx- Unspecified occupant of bus injured in collision with two- or three-wheeled motor vehicle in nontraffic accident
V72.4xx- Person boarding or alighting from bus injured in collision with two- or three-wheeled motor vehicle
V72.5xx- Driver of bus injured in collision with two- or three-wheeled motor vehicle in traffic accident
V72.6xx- Passenger on bus injured in collision with two- or three-wheeled motor vehicle in traffic accident
V72.7xx- Person on outside of bus injured in collision with two- or three-wheeled motor vehicle in traffic accident
V72.9xx- Unspecified occupant of bus injured in collision with two- or three-wheeled motor vehicle in traffic accident

V73- Bus occupant injured in collision with car, pick-up truck or van
The appropriate 7th character is to be added to each code from category V73:
A   Initial encounter
D   Subsequent encounter
S   Sequela

V73.0xx- Driver of bus injured in collision with car, pick-up truck or van in nontraffic accident
V73.1xx- Passenger on bus injured in collision with car, pick-up truck or van in nontraffic accident
V73.2xx- Person on outside of bus injured in collision with car, pick-up truck or van in nontraffic accident
V73.3xx- Unspecified occupant of bus injured in collision with car, pick-up truck or van in nontraffic accident
V73.4xx- Person boarding or alighting from bus injured in collision with car, pick-up truck or van
V73.5xx- Driver of bus injured in collision with car, pick-up truck or van in traffic accident
V73.6xx- Passenger on bus injured in collision with car, pick-up truck or van in traffic accident
V73.7xx- Person on outside of bus injured in collision with car, pick-up truck or van in traffic accident
V73.9xx- Unspecified occupant of bus injured in collision with car, pick-up truck or van in traffic accident

V74- Bus occupant injured in collision with heavy transport vehicle or bus
    Excludes 1: *bus occupant injured in collision with military vehicle (V79.81)*

The appropriate 7th character is to be added to each code from category V74:
A   Initial encounter
D   Subsequent encounter
S   Sequela

V74.0xx- Driver of bus injured in collision with heavy transport vehicle or bus in nontraffic accident
V74.1xx- Passenger on bus injured in collision with heavy transport vehicle or bus in nontraffic accident
V74.2xx- Person on outside of bus injured in collision with heavy transport vehicle or bus in nontraffic accident
V74.3xx- Unspecified occupant of bus injured in collision with heavy transport vehicle or bus in nontraffic accident
V74.4xx- Person boarding or alighting from bus injured in collision with heavy transport vehicle or bus
V74.5xx- Driver of bus injured in collision with heavy transport vehicle or bus in traffic accident
V74.6xx- Passenger on bus injured in collision with heavy transport vehicle or bus in traffic accident
V74.7xx- Person on outside of bus injured in collision with heavy transport vehicle or bus in traffic accident
V74.9xx- Unspecified occupant of bus injured in collision with heavy transport vehicle or bus in traffic accident

V75- Bus occupant injured in collision with railway train or railway vehicle
The appropriate 7th character is to be added to each code from category V75:
A   Initial encounter
D   Subsequent encounter
S   Sequela

V75.0xx- Driver of bus injured in collision with railway train or railway vehicle in nontraffic accident
V75.1xx- Passenger on bus injured in collision with railway train or railway vehicle in nontraffic accident
V75.2xx- Person on outside of bus injured in collision with railway train or railway vehicle in nontraffic accident
V75.3xx- Unspecified occupant of bus injured in collision with railway train or railway vehicle in nontraffic accident
V75.4xx- Person boarding or alighting from bus injured in collision with railway train or railway vehicle
V75.5xx- Driver of bus injured in collision with railway train or railway vehicle in traffic accident
V75.6xx- Passenger on bus injured in collision with railway train or railway vehicle in traffic accident
V75.7xx- Person on outside of bus injured in collision with railway train or railway vehicle in traffic accident
V75.9xx- Unspecified occupant of bus injured in collision with railway train or railway vehicle in traffic accident

V 6 5 – V 7 5

V76-   <u>Bus occupant injured in collision</u> with <u>other nonmotor vehicle</u>

    Includes: Collision with animal-drawn vehicle, animal being ridden, streetcar

The appropriate 7th character is to be added to each code from category V76:
- A   <u>Initial</u> encounter
- D   <u>Subsequent</u> encounter
- S   <u>Sequela</u>

V76.0xx-   Driver of bus injured in collision with other nonmotor vehicle in nontraffic accident

V76.1xx-   Passenger on bus injured in collision with other nonmotor vehicle in nontraffic accident

V76.2xx-   Person on outside of bus injured in collision with other nonmotor vehicle in nontraffic accident

V76.3xx-   Unspecified occupant of bus injured in collision with other nonmotor vehicle in nontraffic accident

V76.4xx-   Person boarding or alighting from bus injured in collision with other nonmotor vehicle

V76.5xx-   Driver of bus injured in collision with other nonmotor vehicle in traffic accident

V76.6xx-   Passenger on bus injured in collision with other nonmotor vehicle in traffic accident

V76.7xx-   Person on outside of bus injured in collision with other nonmotor vehicle in traffic accident

V76.9xx-   Unspecified occupant of bus injured in collision with other nonmotor vehicle in traffic accident

V77-   <u>Bus occupant injured in collision</u> with <u>fixed or stationary object</u>

The appropriate 7th character is to be added to each code from category V77:
- A   <u>Initial</u> encounter
- D   <u>Subsequent</u> encounter
- S   <u>Sequela</u>

V77.0xx-   Driver of bus injured in collision with fixed or stationary object in nontraffic accident

V77.1xx-   Passenger on bus injured in collision with fixed or stationary object in nontraffic accident

V77.2xx-   Person on outside of bus injured in collision with fixed or stationary object in nontraffic accident

V77.3xx-   Unspecified occupant of bus injured in collision with fixed or stationary object in nontraffic accident

V77.4xx-   Person boarding or alighting from bus injured in collision with fixed or stationary object

V77.5xx-   Driver of bus injured in collision with fixed or stationary object in traffic accident

V77.6xx-   Passenger on bus injured in collision with fixed or stationary object in traffic accident

V77.7xx-   Person on outside of bus injured in collision with fixed or stationary object in traffic accident

V77.9xx-   Unspecified occupant of bus injured in collision with fixed or stationary object in traffic accident

V78-   <u>Bus occupant injured</u> in <u>noncollision</u> transport accident

    Includes: Overturning bus NOS

           Overturning bus without collision

The appropriate 7th character is to be added to each code from category V78:
- A   <u>Initial</u> encounter
- D   <u>Subsequent</u> encounter
- S   <u>Sequela</u>

V78.0xx-   Driver of bus injured in noncollision transport accident in nontraffic accident

V78.1xx-   Passenger on bus injured in noncollision transport accident in nontraffic accident

V78.2xx-   Person on outside of bus injured in noncollision transport accident in nontraffic accident

V78.3xx-   Unspecified occupant of bus injured in noncollision transport accident in nontraffic accident

V78.4xx-   Person boarding or alighting from bus injured in noncollision transport accident

V78.5xx-   Driver of bus injured in noncollision transport accident in traffic accident

V78.6xx-   Passenger on bus injured in noncollision transport accident in traffic accident

V78.7xx-   Person on outside of bus injured in noncollision transport accident in traffic accident

V78.9xx-   Unspecified occupant of bus injured in noncollision transport accident in traffic accident

V79-   <u>Bus occupant injured</u> in <u>other and unspecified transport accidents</u>

The appropriate 7th character is to be added to each code from category V79:
- A   <u>Initial</u> encounter
- D   <u>Subsequent</u> encounter
- S   <u>Sequela</u>

V79.0-   Driver of bus injured in collision with other and unspecified motor vehicles in nontraffic accident

V79.00x-   Driver of bus injured in collision with unspecified motor vehicles in nontraffic accident

V79.09x-   Driver of bus injured in collision with other motor vehicles in nontraffic accident

V79.1-   Passenger on bus injured in collision with other and unspecified motor vehicles in nontraffic accident

V79.10x-   Passenger on bus injured in collision with unspecified motor vehicles in nontraffic accident

V79.19x-   Passenger on bus injured in collision with other motor vehicles in nontraffic accident

V79.2-   Unspecified bus occupant injured in collision with other and unspecified motor vehicles in nontraffic accident

V79.20x-   Unspecified bus occupant injured in collision with unspecified motor vehicles in nontraffic accident

      Bus collision NOS, nontraffic

V79.29x-   Unspecified bus occupant injured in collision with other motor vehicles in nontraffic accident

V79.3xx-   Bus occupant (driver) (passenger) injured in unspecified nontraffic accident

      Bus accident NOS, nontraffic

      Bus occupant injured in nontraffic accident NOS

V79.4-   Driver of bus injured in collision with other and unspecified motor vehicles in traffic accident

V79.40x-   Driver of bus injured in collision with unspecified motor vehicles in traffic accident

V79.49x-   Driver of bus injured in collision with other motor vehicles in traffic accident

V79.5-   Passenger on bus injured in collision with other and unspecified motor vehicles in traffic accident

V79.50x-   Passenger on bus injured in collision with unspecified motor vehicles in traffic accident

V79.59x-   Passenger on bus injured in collision with other motor vehicles in traffic accident

V79.6-   Unspecified bus occupant injured in collision with other and unspecified motor vehicles in traffic accident

V79.60x-   Unspecified bus occupant injured in collision with unspecified motor vehicles in traffic accident

      Bus collision NOS (traffic)

V79.69x-   Unspecified bus occupant injured in collision with other motor vehicles in traffic accident

V79.8-   Bus occupant (driver) (passenger) injured in other specified transport accidents

V79.81x-   Bus occupant (driver) (passenger) injured in transport accidents with military vehicle

V79.88x-   Bus occupant (driver) (passenger) injured in other specified transport accidents

V79.9xx-   Bus occupant (driver) (passenger) injured in unspecified traffic accident

      Bus accident NOS

Other land transport accidents (V80-V89)

V80-   <u>Animal-rider or occupant of animal-drawn vehicle injured in transport accident</u>

The appropriate 7th character is to be added to each code from category V80:
- A   <u>Initial</u> encounter
- D   <u>Subsequent</u> encounter
- S   <u>Sequela</u>

V80.0-   Animal-rider or occupant of animal drawn vehicle injured <u>by fall from or being thrown from animal or animal-drawn vehicle in noncollision accident</u>

V80.01-   Animal-rider injured by fall from or being thrown from animal in noncollision accident

V80.010-   Animal-rider injured by fall from or being thrown from horse in noncollision accident

V80.018-   Animal-rider injured by fall from or being thrown from other animal in noncollision accident

V80.02x-   Occupant of animal-drawn vehicle injured by fall from or being thrown from animal-drawn vehicle in noncollision accident

      Overturning animal-drawn vehicle NOS

      Overturning animal-drawn vehicle without collision

V80.1- Animal-rider or occupant of animal-drawn vehicle injured in collision with pedestrian or animal
  Excludes 1: animal-rider or animal-drawn vehicle collision with animal-drawn vehicle or animal being ridden (V80.7)
  V80.11x- Animal-rider injured in collision with pedestrian or animal
  V80.12x- Occupant of animal-drawn vehicle injured in collision with pedestrian or animal
V80.2- Animal-rider or occupant of animal-drawn vehicle injured in collision with pedal cycle
  V80.21x- Animal-rider injured in collision with pedal cycle
  V80.22x- Occupant of animal-drawn vehicle injured in collision with pedal cycle
V80.3- Animal-rider or occupant of animal-drawn vehicle injured in collision with two- or three-wheeled motor vehicle
  V80.31x- Animal-rider injured in collision with two- or three-wheeled motor vehicle
  V80.32x- Occupant of animal-drawn vehicle injured in collision with two- or three-wheeled motor vehicle
V80.4- Animal-rider or occupant of animal-drawn vehicle injured in collision with car, pick-up truck, van, heavy transport vehicle or bus
  Excludes 1: animal-rider injured in collision with military vehicle (V80.910)
  occupant of animal-drawn vehicle injured in collision with military vehicle (V80.920)
  V80.41x- Animal-rider injured in collision with car, pick-up truck, van, heavy transport vehicle or bus
  V80.42x- Occupant of animal-drawn vehicle injured in collision with car, pick-up truck, van, heavy transport vehicle or bus
V80.5- Animal-rider or occupant of animal-drawn vehicle injured in collision with other specified motor vehicle
  V80.51x- Animal-rider injured in collision with other specified motor vehicle
  V80.52x- Occupant of animal-drawn vehicle injured in collision with other specified motor vehicle
V80.6- Animal-rider or occupant of animal-drawn vehicle injured in collision with railway train or railway vehicle
  V80.61x- Animal-rider injured in collision with railway train or railway vehicle
  V80.62x- Occupant of animal-drawn vehicle injured in collision with railway train or railway vehicle
V80.7- Animal-rider or occupant of animal-drawn vehicle injured in collision with other nonmotor vehicles
  V80.71- Animal-rider or occupant of animal-drawn vehicle injured in collision with animal being ridden
    V80.710- Animal-rider injured in collision with other animal being ridden
    V80.711- Occupant of animal-drawn vehicle injured in collision with animal being ridden
  V80.72- Animal-rider or occupant of animal-drawn vehicle injured in collision with other animal-drawn vehicle
    V80.720- Animal-rider injured in collision with animal-drawn vehicle
    V80.721- Occupant of animal-drawn vehicle injured in collision with other animal-drawn vehicle
  V80.73- Animal-rider or occupant of animal-drawn vehicle injured in collision with streetcar
    V80.730- Animal-rider injured in collision with streetcar
    V80.731- Occupant of animal-drawn vehicle injured in collision with streetcar
  V80.79- Animal-rider or occupant of animal-drawn vehicle injured in collision with other nonmotor vehicles
    V80.790- Animal-rider injured in collision with other nonmotor vehicles
    V80.791- Occupant of animal-drawn vehicle injured in collision with other nonmotor vehicles
V80.8- Animal-rider or occupant of animal-drawn vehicle injured in collision with fixed or stationary object
  V80.81x- Animal-rider injured in collision with fixed or stationary object
  V80.82x- Occupant of animal-drawn vehicle injured in collision with fixed or stationary object

V80.9- Animal-rider or occupant of animal-drawn vehicle injured in other and unspecified transport accidents
  V80.91- Animal-rider injured in other and unspecified transport accidents
    V80.910- Animal-rider injured in transport accident with military vehicle
    V80.918- Animal-rider injured in other transport accident
    V80.919- Animal-rider injured in unspecified transport accident
      Animal rider accident NOS
  V80.92- Occupant of animal-drawn vehicle injured in other and unspecified transport accidents
    V80.920- Occupant of animal-drawn vehicle injured in transport accident with military vehicle
    V80.928- Occupant of animal-drawn vehicle injured in other transport accident
    V80.929- Occupant of animal-drawn vehicle injured in unspecified transport accident
      Animal-drawn vehicle accident NOS
V81- Occupant of railway train or railway vehicle injured in transport accident
  Includes: Derailment of railway train or railway vehicle
    Person on outside of train
  Excludes 1: streetcar (V82.-)
  The appropriate 7th character is to be added to each code from category V81:
    A Initial encounter
    D Subsequent encounter
    S Sequela
  V81.0xx- Occupant of railway train or railway vehicle injured in collision with motor vehicle in nontraffic accident
    Excludes 1: Occupant of railway train or railway vehicle injured due to collision with military vehicle (V81.83)
  V81.1xx- Occupant of railway train or railway vehicle injured in collision with motor vehicle in traffic accident
    Excludes 1: Occupant of railway train or railway vehicle injured due to collision with military vehicle (V81.83)
  V81.2xx- Occupant of railway train or railway vehicle injured in collision with or hit by rolling stock
  V81.3xx- Occupant of railway train or railway vehicle injured in collision with other object
    Railway collision NOS
  V81.4xx- Person injured while boarding or alighting from railway train or railway vehicle
  V81.5xx- Occupant of railway train or railway vehicle injured by fall in railway train or railway vehicle
  V81.6xx- Occupant of railway train or railway vehicle injured by fall from railway train or railway vehicle
  V81.7xx- Occupant of railway train or railway vehicle injured in derailment without antecedent collision
  V81.8- Occupant of railway train or railway vehicle injured in other specified railway accidents
    V81.81x- Occupant of railway train or railway vehicle injured due to explosion or fire on train
    V81.82x- Occupant of railway train or railway vehicle injured due to object falling onto train
      Occupant of railway train or railway vehicle injured due to falling earth onto train
      Occupant of railway train or railway vehicle injured due to falling rocks onto train
      Occupant of railway train or railway vehicle injured due to falling snow onto train
      Occupant of railway train or railway vehicle injured due to falling trees onto train
    V81.83x- Occupant of railway train or railway vehicle injured due to collision with military vehicle
    V81.89x- Occupant of railway train or railway vehicle injured due to other specified railway accident
  V81.9xx- Occupant of railway train or railway vehicle injured in unspecified railway accident
    Railway accident NOS

V76 - V81

V82- __Occupant of powered streetcar injured__ in __transport accident__
Includes: Interurban electric car
            Person on outside of streetcar
            Tram (car)
            Trolley (car)
Excludes 1: bus (V70-V79)
            motorcoach (V70-V79)
            nonpowered streetcar (V76.-)
            train (V81.-)

The appropriate 7th character is to be added to each code from
  category V82:
  A __Initial__ encounter
  D __Subsequent__ encounter
  S __Sequela__

V82.0xx- Occupant of streetcar injured in collision with motor vehicle in nontraffic accident

V82.1xx- Occupant of streetcar injured in collision with motor vehicle in traffic accident

V82.2xx- Occupant of streetcar injured in collision with or hit by rolling stock

V82.3xx- Occupant of streetcar injured in collision with other object
Excludes 1: collision with animal-drawn vehicle or animal being ridden (V82.8)

V82.4xx- Person injured while boarding or alighting from streetcar

V82.5xx- Occupant of streetcar injured by fall in streetcar
Excludes 1: fall in streetcar:
            while boarding or alighting (V82.4)
            with antecedent collision (V82.0-V82.3)

V82.6xx- Occupant of streetcar injured by fall from streetcar
Excludes 1: fall from streetcar:
            while boarding or alighting (V82.4)
            with antecedent collision (V82.0-V82.3)

V82.7xx- Occupant of streetcar injured in derailment without antecedent collision
Excludes 1: occupant of streetcar injured in derailment with antecedent collision (V82.0-V82.3)

V82.8xx- Occupant of streetcar injured in other specified transport accidents
            Streetcar collision with military vehicle
            Streetcar collision with train or nonmotor vehicles

V82.9xx- Occupant of streetcar injured in unspecified traffic accident
            Streetcar accident NOS

V83- __Occupant of special vehicle mainly used on industrial premises injured__ in __transport accident__
Includes: Battery-powered airport passenger vehicle
            Battery-powered truck (baggage) (mail)
            Voal-car in mine
            Forklift (truck)
            Logging car
            Self-propelled industrial truck
            Station baggage truck (powered)
            Tram, truck, or tub (powered) in mine or quarry
Excludes 1: special construction vehicles (V85.-)
            special industrial vehicle in stationary use or maintenance (W31.-)

The appropriate 7th character is to be added to each code from
  category V83:
  A __Initial__ encounter
  D __Subsequent__ encounter
  S __Sequela__

V83.0xx- Driver of special industrial vehicle injured in traffic accident

V83.1xx- Passenger of special industrial vehicle injured in traffic accident

V83.2xx- Person on outside of special industrial vehicle injured in traffic accident

V83.3xx- Unspecified occupant of special industrial vehicle injured in traffic accident

V83.4xx- Person injured while boarding or alighting from special industrial vehicle

V83.5xx- Driver of special industrial vehicle injured in nontraffic accident

V83.6xx- Passenger of special industrial vehicle injured in nontraffic accident

V83.7xx- Person on outside of special industrial vehicle injured in nontraffic accident

V83.9xx- Unspecified occupant of special industrial vehicle injured in nontraffic accident
            Special-industrial-vehicle accident NOS

V84- __Occupant of special vehicle mainly used in agriculture injured__ in __transport accident__
Includes: Self-propelled farm machinery
            Tractor (and trailer)
Excludes 1: animal-powered farm machinery accident (W30.8-)
            contact with combine harvester (W30.0)
            special agricultural vehicle in stationary use or maintenance (W30.-)

The appropriate 7th character is to be added to each code from
  category V84:
  A __Initial__ encounter
  D __Subsequent__ encounter
  S __Sequela__

V84.0xx- Driver of special agricultural vehicle injured in traffic accident

V84.1xx- Passenger of special agricultural vehicle injured in traffic accident

V84.2xx- Person on outside of special agricultural vehicle injured in traffic accident

V84.3xx- Unspecified occupant of special agricultural vehicle injured in traffic accident

V84.4xx- Person injured while boarding or alighting from special agricultural vehicle

V84.5xx- Driver of special agricultural vehicle injured in nontraffic accident

V84.6xx- Passenger of special agricultural vehicle injured in nontraffic accident

V84.7xx- Person on outside of special agricultural vehicle injured in nontraffic accident

V84.9xx- Unspecified occupant of special agricultural vehicle injured in nontraffic accident
            Special-agricultural vehicle accident NOS

V85- __Occupant of special construction vehicle injured__ in __transport accident__
Includes: Bulldozer
            Digger
            Dump truck
            Earth-leveller
            Mechanical shovel
            Road-roller
Excludes 1: special industrial vehicle (V83.-)
            special construction vehicle in stationary use or maintenance (W31.-)

The appropriate 7th character is to be added to each code from
  category V85:
  A __Initial__ encounter
  D __Subsequent__ encounter
  S __Sequela__

V85.0xx- Driver of special construction vehicle injured in traffic accident

V85.1xx- Passenger of special construction vehicle injured in traffic accident

V85.2xx- Person on outside of special construction vehicle injured in traffic accident

V85.3xx- Unspecified occupant of special construction vehicle injured in traffic accident

V85.4xx- Person injured while boarding or alighting from special construction vehicle

V85.5xx- Driver of special construction vehicle injured in nontraffic accident

V85.6xx- Passenger of special construction vehicle injured in nontraffic accident

V85.7xx- Person on outside of special construction vehicle injured in nontraffic accident

V85.9xx- Unspecified occupant of special construction vehicle injured in nontraffic accident
            Special-construction-vehicle accident NOS

V86- __Occupant of special all-terrain or other off-road motor vehicle, injured__ in __transport accident__
Excludes 1: special all-terrain vehicle in stationary use or maintenance (W31.-)
            sport-utility vehicle (V50-V59)
            three-wheeled motor vehicle designed for on-road use (V30-V39)

The appropriate 7th character is to be added to each code from
  category V86:
  A __Initial__ encounter
  D __Subsequent__ encounter
  S __Sequela__

V86.0- Driver of special all-terrain or other off-road motor vehicle injured in traffic accident

V86.01x- Driver of ambulance or fire engine injured in traffic accident

V86.02x- Driver of snowmobile injured in traffic accident

V86.03x- Driver of dune buggy injured in traffic accident

V 8 2 - V 8 7

V86.04x- Driver of military vehicle injured in traffic accident
V86.09x- Driver of other special all-terrain or other off-road motor
          vehicle injured in traffic accident
              Driver of dirt bike injured in traffic accident
              Driver of go cart injured in traffic accident
              Driver of golf cart injured in traffic accident
V86.1- Passenger of special all-terrain or other off-road motor vehicle
        injured in traffic accident
V86.11x- Passenger of ambulance or fire engine injured in traffic
          accident
V86.12x- Passenger of snowmobile injured in traffic accident
V86.13x- Passenger of dune buggy injured in traffic accident
V86.14x- Passenger of military vehicle injured in traffic accident
V86.19x- Passenger of other special all-terrain or other off-road
          motor vehicle injured in traffic accident
              Passenger of dirt bike injured in traffic accident
              Passenger of go cart injured in traffic accident
              Passenger of golf cart injured in traffic accident
V86.2- Person on outside of special all-terrain or other off-road motor
        vehicle injured in traffic accident
V86.21x- Person on outside of ambulance or fire engine injured in
          traffic accident
V86.22x- Person on outside of snowmobile injured in traffic accident
V86.23x- Person on outside of dune buggy injured in traffic accident
V86.24x- Person on outside of military vehicle injured in traffic
          accident
V86.29x- Person on outside of other special all-terrain or other off-
          road motor vehicle injured in traffic accident
              Person on outside of dirt bike injured in traffic accident
              Person on outside of go cart injured in traffic accident
              Person on outside of golf cart injured in traffic accident
V86.3- Unspecified occupant of special all-terrain or other off-road
        motor vehicle injured in traffic accident
V86.31x- Unspecified occupant of ambulance or fire engine injured
          in traffic accident
V86.32x- Unspecified occupant of snowmobile injured in traffic
          accident
V86.33x- Unspecified occupant of dune buggy injured in traffic
          accident
V86.34x- Unspecified occupant of military vehicle injured in traffic
          accident
V86.39x- Unspecified occupant of other special all-terrain or other
          off-road motor vehicle injured in traffic accident
              Unspecified occupant of dirt bike injured in traffic accident
              Unspecified occupant of go cart injured in traffic accident
              Unspecified occupant of golf cart injured in traffic accident
V86.4- Person injured while boarding or alighting from special all-
        terrain or other off-road motor vehicle
V86.41x- Person injured while boarding or alighting from
          ambulance or fire engine
V86.42x- Person injured while boarding or alighting from
          snowmobile
V86.43x- Person injured while boarding or alighting from dune
          buggy
V86.44x- Person injured while boarding or alighting from military
          vehicle
V86.49x- Person injured while boarding or alighting from other
          special all-terrain or other off-road motor vehicle
              Person injured while boarding or alighting from dirt bike
              Person injured while boarding or alighting from go cart
              Person injured while boarding or alighting from golf cart
V86.5- Driver of special all-terrain or other off-road motor vehicle
        injured in nontraffic accident
V86.51x- Driver of ambulance or fire engine injured in nontraffic
          accident
V86.52x- Driver of snowmobile injured in nontraffic accident
V86.53x- Driver of dune buggy injured in nontraffic accident
V86.54x- Driver of military vehicle injured in nontraffic accident
V86.59x- Driver of other special all-terrain or other off-road motor
          vehicle injured in nontraffic accident
              Driver of dirt bike injured in nontraffic accident
              Driver of go cart injured in nontraffic accident
              Driver of golf cart injured in nontraffic accident

V86.6- Passenger of special all-terrain or other off-road motor vehicle
        injured in nontraffic accident
V86.61x- Passenger of ambulance or fire engine injured in
          nontraffic accident
V86.62x- Passenger of snowmobile injured in nontraffic accident
V86.63x- Passenger of dune buggy injured in nontraffic accident
V86.64x- Passenger of military vehicle injured in nontraffic accident
V86.69x- Passenger of other special all-terrain or other off-road
          motor vehicle injured in nontraffic accident
              Passenger of dirt bike injured in nontraffic accident
              Passenger of go cart injured in nontraffic accident
              Passenger of golf cart injured in nontraffic accident
V86.7- Person on outside of special all-terrain or other off-road motor
        vehicle injured in nontraffic accident
V86.71x- Person on outside of ambulance or fire engine injured in
          nontraffic accident
V86.72x- Person on outside of snowmobile injured in nontraffic
          accident
V86.73x- Person on outside of dune buggy injured in nontraffic
          accident
V86.74x- Person on outside of military vehicle injured in nontraffic
          accident
V86.79x- Person on outside of other special all-terrain or other off-
          road motor vehicles injured in nontraffic accident
              Person on outside of dirt bike injured in nontraffic accident
              Person on outside of go cart injured in nontraffic accident
              Person on outside of golf cart injured in nontraffic accident
V86.9- Unspecified occupant of special all-terrain or other off-road
        motor vehicle injured in nontraffic accident
V86.91x- Unspecified occupant of ambulance or fire engine injured
          in nontraffic accident
V86.92x- Unspecified occupant of snowmobile injured in nontraffic
          accident
V86.93x- Unspecified occupant of dune buggy injured in nontraffic
          accident
V86.94x- Unspecified occupant of military vehicle injured in
          nontraffic accident
V86.99x- Unspecified occupant of other special all-terrain or other
          off-road motor vehicle injured in nontraffic accident
              All-terrain motor-vehicle accident NOS
              Off-road motor-vehicle accident NOS
              Other motor-vehicle accident NOS
              Unspecified occupant of dirt bike injured in nontraffic
                accident
              Unspecified occupant of go cart injured in nontraffic
                accident
              Unspecified occupant of golf cart injured in nontraffic
                accident
V87- Traffic accident of specified type but victim's mode of transport
      unknown
      Excludes 1: *collision involving:*
                   pedal cycle (V10-V19)
                   pedestrian (V01-V09)
      The appropriate 7th character is to be added to each code from
        category V87:
        A   Initial encounter
        D   Subsequent encounter
        S   Sequela
V87.0xx- Person injured in collision between car and two- or three-
          wheeled powered vehicle (traffic)
V87.1xx- Person injured in collision between other motor vehicle and
          two- or three-wheeled motor vehicle (traffic)
V87.2xx- Person injured in collision between car and pick-up truck or
          van (traffic)
V87.3xx- Person injured in collision between car and bus (traffic)
V87.4xx- Person injured in collision between car and heavy transport
          vehicle (traffic)
V87.5xx- Person injured in collision between heavy transport vehicle
          and bus (traffic)
V87.6xx- Person injured in collision between railway train or railway
          vehicle and car (traffic)
V87.7xx- Person injured in collision between other specified motor
          vehicles (traffic)
V87.8xx- Person injured in other specified noncollision transport
          accidents involving motor vehicle (traffic)
V87.9xx- Person injured in other specified (collision) (noncollision)
          transport accidents involving nonmotor vehicle (traffic)

V
8
2
–
V
8
7

V88- Nontraffic accident of specified type but victim's mode of transport unknown

Excludes 1:   collision involving:
   pedal cycle (V10-V19)
   pedestrian (V01-V09)

The appropriate 7th character is to be added to each code from category V88:
   A Initial encounter
   D Subsequent encounter
   S Sequela

V88.0xx- Person injured in collision between car and two- or three-wheeled motor vehicle, nontraffic

V88.1xx- Person injured in collision between other motor vehicle and two- or three-wheeled motor vehicle, nontraffic

V88.2xx- Person injured in collision between car and pick-up truck or van, nontraffic

V88.3xx- Person injured in collision between car and bus, nontraffic

V88.4xx- Person injured in collision between car and heavy transport vehicle, nontraffic

V88.5xx- Person injured in collision between heavy transport vehicle and bus, nontraffic

V88.6xx- Person injured in collision between railway train or railway vehicle and car, nontraffic

V88.7xx- Person injured in collision between other specified motor vehicle, nontraffic

V88.8xx- Person injured in other specified noncollision transport accidents involving motor vehicle, nontraffic

V88.9xx- Person injured in other specified (collision)(noncollision) transport accidents involving nonmotor vehicle, nontraffic

V89- Motor- or nonmotor-vehicle accident, type of vehicle unspecified

The appropriate 7th character is to be added to each code from category V89:
   A Initial encounter
   D Subsequent encounter
   S Sequela

V89.0xx- Person injured in unspecified motor-vehicle accident, nontraffic
   Motor-vehicle accident NOS, nontraffic

V89.1xx- Person injured in unspecified nonmotor-vehicle accident, nontraffic
   Nonmotor-vehicle accident NOS (nontraffic)

V89.2xx- Person injured in unspecified motor-vehicle accident, traffic
   Motor-vehicle accident [MVA] NOS
   Road (traffic) accident [RTA] NOS

V89.3xx- Person injured in unspecified nonmotor-vehicle accident, traffic
   Nonmotor-vehicle traffic accident NOS

V89.9xx- Person injured in unspecified vehicle accident
   Collision NOS

Water transport accidents (V90-V94)

V90- Drowning and submersion due to accident to watercraft

Excludes 1:   civilian water transport accident involving military watercraft (V94.81-)
   fall into water not from watercraft (W16.-)
   military watercraft accident in military or war operations (Y36.0-, Y37.0-)
   water-transport-related drowning or submersion without accident to watercraft (V92.-)

The appropriate 7th character is to be added to each code from category V90:
   A Initial encounter
   D Subsequent encounter
   S Sequela

V90.0- Drowning and submersion due to watercraft overturning

V90.00x- Drowning and submersion due to merchant ship overturning

V90.01x- Drowning and submersion due to passenger ship overturning
   Drowning and submersion due to Ferry-boat overturning
   Drowning and submersion due to Liner overturning

V90.02x- Drowning and submersion due to fishing boat overturning

V90.03x- Drowning and submersion due to other powered watercraft overturning
   Drowning and submersion due to Hovercraft (on open water) overturning
   Drowning and submersion due to Jet ski overturning

V90.04x- Drowning and submersion due to sailboat overturning

V90.05x- Drowning and submersion due to canoe or kayak overturning

V90.06x- Drowning and submersion due to (nonpowered) inflatable craft overturning

V90.08x- Drowning and submersion due to other unpowered watercraft overturning
   Drowning and submersion due to windsurfer overturning

V90.09x- Drowning and submersion due to unspecified watercraft overturning
   Drowning and submersion due to boat NOS overturning
   Drowning and submersion due to ship NOS overturning
   Drowning and submersion due to watercraft NOS overturning

V90.1- Drowning and submersion due to watercraft sinking

V90.10x- Drowning and submersion due to merchant ship sinking

V90.11x- Drowning and submersion due to passenger ship sinking
   Drowning and submersion due to Ferry-boat sinking
   Drowning and submersion due to Liner sinking

V90.12x- Drowning and submersion due to fishing boat sinking

V90.13x- Drowning and submersion due to other powered watercraft sinking
   Drowning and submersion due to Hovercraft (on open water) sinking
   Drowning and submersion due to Jet ski sinking

V90.14x- Drowning and submersion due to sailboat sinking

V90.15x- Drowning and submersion due to canoe or kayak sinking

V90.16x- Drowning and submersion due to (nonpowered) inflatable craft sinking

V90.18x- Drowning and submersion due to other unpowered watercraft sinking

V90.19x- Drowning and submersion due to unspecified watercraft sinking
   Drowning and submersion due to boat NOS sinking
   Drowning and submersion due to ship NOS sinking
   Drowning and submersion due to watercraft NOS sinking

V90.2- Drowning and submersion due to falling or jumping from burning watercraft

V90.20x- Drowning and submersion due to falling or jumping from burning merchant ship

V90.21x- Drowning and submersion due to falling or jumping from burning passenger ship
   Drowning and submersion due to falling or jumping from burning Ferry-boat
   Drowning and submersion due to falling or jumping from burning Liner

V90.22x- Drowning and submersion due to falling or jumping from burning fishing boat

V90.23x- Drowning and submersion due to falling or jumping from other burning powered watercraft
   Drowning and submersion due to falling and jumping from burning Hovercraft (on open water)
   Drowning and submersion due to falling and jumping from burning Jet ski

V90.24x- Drowning and submersion due to falling or jumping from burning sailboat

V90.25x- Drowning and submersion due to falling or jumping from burning canoe or kayak

V90.26x- Drowning and submersion due to falling or jumping from burning (nonpowered) inflatable craft

V90.27x- Drowning and submersion due to falling or jumping from burning water-skis

V90.28x- Drowning and submersion due to falling or jumping from other burning unpowered watercraft
   Drowning and submersion due to falling and jumping from burning surf-board
   Drowning and submersion due to falling and jumping from burning windsurfer

V90.29x- Drowning and submersion due to falling or jumping from unspecified burning watercraft
   Drowning and submersion due to falling or jumping from burning boat NOS
   Drowning and submersion due to falling or jumping from burning ship NOS
   Drowning and submersion due to falling or jumping from burning watercraft NOS

V 8 8 - V 9 1

V90.3- **Drowning and submersion** <u>due to falling or jumping from crushed watercraft</u>

V90.30x- Drowning and submersion due to falling or jumping from crushed merchant ship

V90.31x- Drowning and submersion due to falling or jumping from crushed passenger ship
> Drowning and submersion due to falling and jumping from crushed Ferry boat
> Drowning and submersion due to falling and jumping from crushed Liner

V90.32x- Drowning and submersion due to falling or jumping from crushed fishing boat

V90.33x- Drowning and submersion due to falling or jumping from other crushed powered watercraft
> Drowning and submersion due to falling and jumping from crushed Hovercraft
> Drowning and submersion due to falling and jumping from crushed Jet ski

V90.34x- Drowning and submersion due to falling or jumping from crushed sailboat

V90.35x- Drowning and submersion due to falling or jumping from crushed canoe or kayak

V90.36x- Drowning and submersion due to falling or jumping from crushed (nonpowered) inflatable craft

V90.37x- Drowning and submersion due to falling or jumping from crushed water-skis

V90.38x- Drowning and submersion due to falling or jumping from other crushed unpowered watercraft
> Drowning and submersion due to falling and jumping from crushed surf-board
> Drowning and submersion due to falling and jumping from crushed windsurfer

V90.39x- Drowning and submersion due to falling or jumping from crushed unspecified watercraft
> Drowning and submersion due to falling and jumping from crushed boat NOS
> Drowning and submersion due to falling and jumping from crushed ship NOS
> Drowning and submersion due to falling and jumping from crushed watercraft NOS

V90.8- **Drowning and submersion** <u>due to other accident to watercraft</u>

V90.80x- Drowning and submersion due to other accident to merchant ship

V90.81x- Drowning and submersion due to other accident to passenger ship
> Drowning and submersion due to other accident to Ferry-boat
> Drowning and submersion due to other accident to Liner

V90.82x- Drowning and submersion due to other accident to fishing boat

V90.83x- Drowning and submersion due to other accident to other powered watercraft
> Drowning and submersion due to other accident to Hovercraft (on open water)
> Drowning and submersion due to other accident to Jet ski

V90.84x- Drowning and submersion due to other accident to sailboat

V90.85x- Drowning and submersion due to other accident to canoe or kayak

V90.86x- Drowning and submersion due to other accident to (nonpowered) inflatable craft

V90.87x- Drowning and submersion due to other accident to water-skis

V90.88x- Drowning and submersion due to other accident to other unpowered watercraft
> Drowning and submersion due to other accident to surf-board
> Drowning and submersion due to other accident to windsurfer

V90.89x- Drowning and submersion due to other accident to unspecified watercraft
> Drowning and submersion due to other accident to boat NOS
> Drowning and submersion due to other accident to ship NOS
> Drowning and submersion due to other accident to watercraft NOS

V91- <u>Other injury due to accident to watercraft</u>

Includes: Any injury except drowning and submersion as a result of an accident to watercraft

Excludes 1:   civilian water transport accident involving military watercraft (V94.81-)
military watercraft accident in military or war operations (Y36, Y37.-)

Excludes ❷: drowning and submersion due to accident to watercraft (V90.-)

The appropriate 7th character is to be added to each code from category V91:
A <u>Initial</u> encounter
D <u>Subsequent</u> encounter
S <u>Sequela</u>

V91.0- <u>Burn</u> due to watercraft on fire
> *Excludes 1: burn from localized fire or explosion on board ship without accident to watercraft (V93.-)*

V91.00x- Burn due to merchant ship on fire

V91.01x- Burn due to passenger ship on fire
> Burn due to Ferry-boat on fire
> Burn due to Liner on fire

V91.02x- Burn due to fishing boat on fire

V91.03x- Burn due to other powered watercraft on fire
> Burn due to Hovercraft (on open water) on fire
> Burn due to Jet ski on fire

V91.04x- Burn due to sailboat on fire

V91.05x- Burn due to canoe or kayak on fire

V91.06x- Burn due to (nonpowered) inflatable craft on fire

V91.07x- Burn due to water-skis on fire

V91.08x- Burn due to other unpowered watercraft on fire

V91.09x- Burn due to unspecified watercraft on fire
> Burn due to boat NOS on fire
> Burn due to ship NOS on fire
> Burn due to watercraft NOS on fire

V91.1- <u>Crushed</u> between watercraft and other watercraft or other object due to collision
> Crushed by lifeboat after abandoning ship in a collision
> NOTE: Select the specified type of watercraft that the victim was on at the time of the collision

V91.10x- Crushed between merchant ship and other watercraft or other object due to collision

V91.11x- Crushed between passenger ship and other watercraft or other object due to collision
> Crushed between Ferry-boat and other watercraft or other object due to collision
> Crushed between Liner and other watercraft or other object due to collision

V91.12x- Crushed between fishing boat and other watercraft or other object due to collision

V91.13x- Crushed between other powered watercraft and other watercraft or other object due to collision
> Crushed between Hovercraft (on open water) and other watercraft or other object due to collision
> Crushed between Jet ski and other watercraft or other object due to collision

V91.14x- Crushed between sailboat and other watercraft or other object due to collision

V91.15x- Crushed between canoe or kayak and other watercraft or other object due to collision

V91.16x- Crushed between (nonpowered) inflatable craft and other watercraft or other object due to collision

V91.18x- Crushed between other unpowered watercraft and other watercraft or other object due to collision
> Crushed between surfboard and other watercraft or other object due to collision
> Crushed between windsurfer and other watercraft or other object due to collision

V91.19x- Crushed between unspecified watercraft and other watercraft or other object due to collision
> Crushed between boat NOS and other watercraft or other object due to collision
> Crushed between ship NOS and other watercraft or other object due to collision
> Crushed between watercraft NOS and other watercraft or other object due to collision

V 8 8 – V 9 1

V91.2- **Fall** due to collision between watercraft and other watercraft or other object

Fall while remaining on watercraft after collision

Note: Select the specified type of watercraft that the victim was on at the time of the collision

Excludes 1: crushed between watercraft and other watercraft and other object due to collision (V91.1-)
drowning and submersion due to falling from crushed watercraft (V90.3-)

V91.20x- Fall due to collision between merchant ship and other watercraft or other object

V91.21x- Fall due to collision between passenger ship and other watercraft or other object

Fall due to collision between Ferry-boat and other watercraft or other object

Fall due to collision between Liner and other watercraft or other object

V91.22x- Fall due to collision between fishing boat and other watercraft or other object

V91.23x- Fall due to collision between other powered watercraft and other watercraft or other object

Fall due to collision between Hovercraft (on open water) and other watercraft or other object

Fall due to collision between Jet ski and other watercraft or other object

V91.24x- Fall due to collision between sailboat and other watercraft or other object

V91.25x- Fall due to collision between canoe or kayak and other watercraft or other object

V91.26x- Fall due to collision between (nonpowered) inflatable craft and other watercraft or other object

V91.29x- Fall due to collision between unspecified watercraft and other watercraft or other object

Fall due to collision between boat NOS and other watercraft or other object

Fall due to collision between ship NOS and other watercraft or other object

Fall due to collision between watercraft NOS and other watercraft or other object

V91.3- **Hit or struck by falling object** due to accident to watercraft

Hit or struck by falling object (part of damaged watercraft or other object) after falling or jumping from damaged watercraft

Excludes❷: drowning or submersion due to fall or jumping from damaged watercraft (V90.2-, V90.3-)

V91.30x- Hit or struck by falling object due to accident to merchant ship

V91.31x- Hit or struck by falling object due to accident to passenger ship

Hit or struck by falling object due to accident to Ferry-boat

Hit or struck by falling object due to accident to Liner

V91.32x- Hit or struck by falling object due to accident to fishing boat

V91.33x- Hit or struck by falling object due to accident to other powered watercraft

Hit or struck by falling object due to accident to Hovercraft (on open water)

Hit or struck by falling object due to accident to Jet ski

V91.34x- Hit or struck by falling object due to accident to sailboat

V91.35x- Hit or struck by falling object due to accident to canoe or kayak

V91.36x- Hit or struck by falling object due to accident to (nonpowered) inflatable craft

V91.37x- Hit or struck by falling object due to accident to water-skis

Hit by water-skis after jumping off of waterskis

V91.38x- Hit or struck by falling object due to accident to other unpowered watercraft

Hit or struck by surf-board after falling off damaged surf-board

Hit or struck by object after falling off damaged windsurfer

V91.39x- Hit or struck by falling object due to accident to unspecified watercraft

Hit or struck by falling object due to accident to boat NOS

Hit or struck by falling object due to accident to ship NOS

Hit or struck by falling object due to accident to watercraft NOS

V91.8- **Other injury** due to other accident to watercraft

V91.80x- Other injury due to other accident to merchant ship

V91.81x- Other injury due to other accident to passenger ship

Other injury due to other accident to Ferry-boat

Other injury due to other accident to Liner

V91.82x- Other injury due to other accident to fishing boat

V91.83x- Other injury due to other accident to other powered watercraft

Other injury due to other accident to Hovercraft (on open water)

Other injury due to other accident to Jet ski

V91.84x- Other injury due to other accident to sailboat

V91.85x- Other injury due to other accident to canoe or kayak

V91.86x- Other injury due to other accident to (nonpowered) inflatable craft

V91.87x- Other injury due to other accident to water-skis

V91.88x- Other injury due to other accident to other unpowered watercraft

Other injury due to other accident to surf-board

Other injury due to other accident to windsurfer

V91.89x- Other injury due to other accident to unspecified watercraft

Other injury due to other accident to boat NOS

Other injury due to other accident to ship NOS

Other injury due to other accident to watercraft NOS

V92- **Drowning and submersion due to accident on board watercraft, without accident to watercraft**

Excludes 1: civilian water transport accident involving military watercraft (V94.81-)
drowning or submersion due to accident to watercraft (V90-V91)
drowning or submersion of diver who voluntarily jumps from boat not involved in an accident (W16.711, W16.721)
fall into water without watercraft (W16.-)
military watercraft accident in military or war operations (Y36, Y37)

> The appropriate 7th character is to be added to each code from category V92:
> **A** **Initial** encounter
> **D** **Subsequent** encounter
> **S** **Sequela**

V92.0- **Drowning and submersion due to fall off watercraft**

Drowning and submersion due to fall from gangplank of watercraft

Drowning and submersion due to fall overboard watercraft

Excludes❷: hitting head on object or bottom of body of water due to fall from watercraft (V94.0-)

V92.00x- Drowning and submersion due to fall off merchant ship

V92.01x- Drowning and submersion due to fall off passenger ship

Drowning and submersion due to fall off Ferry-boat

Drowning and submersion due to fall off Liner

V92.02x- Drowning and submersion due to fall off fishing boat

V92.03x- Drowning and submersion due to fall off other powered watercraft

Drowning and submersion due to fall off Hovercraft (on open water)

Drowning and submersion due to fall off Jet ski

V92.04x- Drowning and submersion due to fall off sailboat

V92.05x- Drowning and submersion due to fall off canoe or kayak

V92.06x- Drowning and submersion due to fall off (nonpowered) inflatable craft

V92.07x- Drowning and submersion due to fall off water-skis

Excludes 1: drowning and submersion due to falling off burning water-skis (V90.27)
drowning and submersion due to falling off crushed water-skis (V90.37)
hit by boat while water-skiing NOS (V94.-)

V92.08x- Drowning and submersion due to fall off other unpowered watercraft

Drowning and submersion due to fall off surf-board

Drowning and submersion due to fall off windsurfer

Excludes 1: drowning and submersion due to fall off burning unpowered watercraft (V90.28)
drowning and submersion due to fall off crushed unpowered watercraft (V90.38)
drowning and submersion due to fall off damaged unpowered watercraft (V90.88)
drowning and submersion due to rider of nonpowered watercraft being hit by other watercraft (V94.2-)
other injury due to rider of nonpowered watercraft being hit by other watercraft (V94.2-)

V92.09x- Drowning and submersion due to fall off unspecified watercraft

Drowning and submersion due to fall off boat NOS

Drowning and submersion due to fall off ship

Drowning and submersion due to fall off watercraft NOS

V92.1- Drowning and submersion <u>due to being thrown overboard by motion of watercraft</u>
> *Excludes 1:* *drowning and submersion due to fall off surf-board (V92.08)*
> *drowning and submersion due to fall off water-skis (V92.07)*
> *drowning and submersion due to fall off windsurfer (V92.08)*

V92.10x- Drowning and submersion due to being thrown overboard by motion of merchant ship

V92.11x- Drowning and submersion due to being thrown overboard by motion of passenger ship
> Drowning and submersion due to being thrown overboard by motion of Ferry-boat
> Drowning and submersion due to being thrown overboard by motion of Liner

V92.12x- Drowning and submersion due to being thrown overboard by motion of fishing boat

V92.13x- Drowning and submersion due to being thrown overboard by motion of other powered watercraft
> Drowning and submersion due to being thrown overboard by motion of Hovercraft

V92.14x- Drowning and submersion due to being thrown overboard by motion of sailboat

V92.15x- Drowning and submersion due to being thrown overboard by motion of canoe or kayak

V92.16x- Drowning and submersion due to being thrown overboard by motion of (nonpowered) inflatable craft

V92.19x- Drowning and submersion due to being thrown overboard by motion of unspecified watercraft
> Drowning and submersion due to being thrown overboard by motion of boat NOS
> Drowning and submersion due to being thrown overboard by motion of ship NOS
> Drowning and submersion due to being thrown overboard by motion of watercraft NOS

V92.2- Drowning and submersion <u>due to being washed overboard from watercraft</u>
> Code first any associated cataclysm (X37.0-)

V92.20x- Drowning and submersion due to being washed overboard from merchant ship

V92.21x- Drowning and submersion due to being washed overboard from passenger ship
> Drowning and submersion due to being washed overboard from Ferry-boat
> Drowning and submersion due to being washed overboard from Liner

V92.22x- Drowning and submersion due to being washed overboard from fishing boat

V92.23x- Drowning and submersion due to being washed overboard from other powered watercraft
> Drowning and submersion due to being washed overboard from Hovercraft (on open water)
> Drowning and submersion due to being washed overboard from Jet ski

V92.24x- Drowning and submersion due to being washed overboard from sailboat

V92.25x- Drowning and submersion due to being washed overboard from canoe or kayak

V92.26x- Drowning and submersion due to being washed overboard from (nonpowered) inflatable craft

V92.27x- Drowning and submersion due to being washed overboard from water-skis
> *Excludes 1:* *drowning and submersion due to fall off water-skis (V92.07)*

V92.28x- Drowning and submersion due to being washed overboard from other unpowered watercraft
> Drowning and submersion due to being washed overboard from surf-board
> Drowning and submersion due to being washed overboard from windsurfer

V92.29x- Drowning and submersion due to being washed overboard from unspecified watercraft
> Drowning and submersion due to being washed overboard from boat NOS
> Drowning and submersion due to being washed overboard from ship NOS
> Drowning and submersion due to being washed overboard from watercraft NOS

V93- Other injury due to accident on board watercraft, <u>without accident to watercraft</u>
> *Excludes 1:* *civilian water transport accident involving military watercraft (V94.81-)*
> *other injury due to accident to watercraft (V91.-)*
> *military watercraft accident in military or war operations (Y36, Y37.-)*
> *Excludes ❷:* *drowning and submersion due to accident on board watercraft, without accident to watercraft (V92.-)*

> The appropriate 7th character is to be added to each code from category V93:
> **A** <u>Initial</u> encounter
> **D** <u>Subsequent</u> encounter
> **S** <u>Sequela</u>

V93.0- <u>Burn</u> due to localized fire on board watercraft
> *Excludes 1:* *burn due to watercraft on fire (V91.0-)*

V93.00x- Burn due to localized fire on board merchant vessel

V93.01x- Burn due to localized fire on board passenger vessel
> Burn due to localized fire on board Ferry-boat
> Burn due to localized fire on board Liner

V93.02x- Burn due to localized fire on board fishing boat

V93.03x- Burn due to localized fire on board other powered watercraft
> Burn due to localized fire on board Hovercraft
> Burn due to localized fire on board Jet ski

V93.04x- Burn due to localized fire on board sailboat

V93.09x- Burn due to localized fire on board unspecified watercraft
> Burn due to localized fire on board boat NOS
> Burn due to localized fire on board ship NOS
> Burn due to localized fire on board watercraft NOS

V93.1- <u>Other burn</u> on board watercraft
> Burn due to source other than fire on board watercraft
> *Excludes 1:* *burn due to watercraft on fire (V91.0-)*

V93.10x- Other burn on board merchant vessel

V93.11x- Other burn on board passenger vessel
> Other burn on board Ferry-boat
> Other burn on board Liner

V93.12x- Other burn on board fishing boat

V93.13x- Other burn on board other powered watercraft
> Other burn on board Hovercraft
> Other burn on board Jet ski

V93.14x- Other burn on board sailboat

V93.19x- Other burn on board unspecified watercraft
> Other burn on board boat NOS
> Other burn on board ship NOS
> Other burn on board watercraft NOS

V93.2- <u>Heat exposure</u> on board watercraft
> *Excludes 1:* *exposure to man-made heat not aboard watercraft (W92)*
> *exposure to natural heat while on board watercraft (X30)*
> *exposure to sunlight while on board watercraft (X32)*
> *Excludes ❷:* *burn due to fire on board watercraft (V93.0-)*

V93.20x- Heat exposure on board merchant ship

V93.21x- Heat exposure on board passenger ship
> Heat exposure on board Ferry-boat
> Heat exposure on board Liner

V93.22x- Heat exposure on board fishing boat

V93.23x- Heat exposure on board other powered watercraft
> Heat exposure on board hovercraft

V93.24x- Heat exposure on board sailboat

V93.29x- Heat exposure on board unspecified watercraft
> Heat exposure on board boat NOS
> Heat exposure on board ship NOS
> Heat exposure on board watercraft NOS

V93.3- <u>Fall</u> on board watercraft
> *Excludes 1:* *fall due to collision of watercraft (V91.2-)*

V93.30x- Fall on board merchant ship

V93.31x- Fall on board passenger ship
> Fall on board Ferry-boat
> Fall on board Liner

V93.32x- Fall on board fishing boat

V93.33x- Fall on board other powered watercraft
> Fall on board Hovercraft (on open water)
> Fall on board Jet ski

V93.34x- Fall on board sailboat

V93.35x- Fall on board canoe or kayak

V93.36x- Fall on board (nonpowered) inflatable craft

V93.38x- Fall on board other unpowered watercraft

V93.39x- Fall on board unspecified watercraft
> Fall on board boat NOS
> Fall on board ship NOS
> Fall on board watercraft NOS

V 9 1 – V 9 3

Excludes 1: = NOT CODED HERE! (Do not code both)

Excludes ❷: = Not Included Here

V93.4-   Struck by falling object on board watercraft
   Hit by falling object on board watercraft
   Excludes 1:   struck by falling object due to accident to watercraft (V91.3)

V93.40x-   Struck by falling object on merchant ship

V93.41x-   Struck by falling object on passenger ship
   Struck by falling object on Ferry-boat
   Struck by falling object on Liner

V93.42x-   Struck by falling object on fishing boat

V93.43x-   Struck by falling object on other powered watercraft
   Struck by falling object on Hovercraft

V93.44x-   Struck by falling object on sailboat

V93.48x-   Struck by falling object on other unpowered watercraft

V93.49x-   Struck by falling object on unspecified watercraft

V93.5-   Explosion on board watercraft
   Boiler explosion on steamship
   Excludes❷: fire on board watercraft (V93.0-)

V93.50x-   Explosion on board merchant ship

V93.51x-   Explosion on board passenger ship
   Explosion on board Ferry-boat
   Explosion on board Liner

V93.52x-   Explosion on board fishing boat

V93.53x-   Explosion on board other powered watercraft
   Explosion on board Hovercraft
   Explosion on board Jet ski

V93.54x-   Explosion on board sailboat

V93.59x-   Explosion on board unspecified watercraft
   Explosion on board boat NOS
   Explosion on board ship NOS
   Explosion on board watercraft NOS

V93.6-   Machinery accident on board watercraft
   Excludes 1:   machinery explosion on board watercraft (V93.4-)
   machinery fire on board watercraft (V93.0-)

V93.60x-   Machinery accident on board merchant ship

V93.61x-   Machinery accident on board passenger ship
   Machinery accident on board Ferry-boat
   Machinery accident on board Liner

V93.62x-   Machinery accident on board fishing boat

V93.63x-   Machinery accident on board other powered watercraft
   Machinery accident on board Hovercraft

V93.64x-   Machinery accident on board sailboat

V93.69x-   Machinery accident on board unspecified watercraft
   Machinery accident on board boat NOS
   Machinery accident on board ship NOS
   Machinery accident on board watercraft NOS

V93.8-   Other injury due to other accident on board watercraft
   Accidental poisoning by gases or fumes on watercraft

V93.80x-   Other injury due to other accident on board merchant ship

V93.81x-   Other injury due to other accident on board passenger ship
   Other injury due to other accident on board Ferry-boat
   Other injury due to other accident on board Liner

V93.82x-   Other injury due to other accident on board fishing boat

V93.83x-   Other injury due to other accident on board other powered watercraft
   Other injury due to other accident on board Hovercraft
   Other injury due to other accident on board Jet ski

V93.84x-   Other injury due to other accident on board sailboat

V93.85x-   Other injury due to other accident on board canoe or kayak

V93.86x-   Other injury due to other accident on board (nonpowered) inflatable craft

V93.87x-   Other injury due to other accident on board water-skis
   Hit or struck by object while waterskiing

V93.88x-   Other injury due to other accident on board other unpowered watercraft
   Hit or struck by object while surfing
   Hit or struck by object while on board windsurfer

V93.89x-   Other injury due to other accident on board unspecified watercraft
   Other injury due to other accident on board boat NOS
   Other injury due to other accident on board ship NOS
   Other injury due to other accident on board watercraft NOS

V94-   Other and unspecified water transport accidents
   Excludes 1:   military watercraft accidents in military or war operations (Y36, Y37)
   The appropriate 7th character is to be added to each code from category V94:
   A   Initial encounter
   D   Subsequent encounter
   S   Sequela

V94.0xx-   Hitting object or bottom of body of water due to fall from watercraft
   Excludes❷: drowning and submersion due to fall from watercraft (V92.0-)

V94.1-   Bather struck by watercraft
   Swimmer hit by watercraft

V94.11x-   Bather struck by powered watercraft

V94.12x-   Bather struck by nonpowered watercraft

V94.2-   Rider of nonpowered watercraft struck by other watercraft

V94.21x-   Rider of nonpowered watercraft struck by other nonpowered watercraft
   Canoer hit by other nonpowered watercraft
   Surfer hit by other nonpowered watercraft
   Windsurfer hit by other nonpowered watercraft

V94.22x-   Rider of nonpowered watercraft struck by powered watercraft
   Canoer hit by motorboat
   Surfer hit by motorboat
   Windsurfer hit by motorboat

V94.3-   Injury to rider of (inflatable) watercraft being pulled behind other watercraft

V94.31x-   Injury to rider of (inflatable) recreational watercraft being pulled behind other watercraft
   Injury to rider of inner-tube pulled behind motor boat

V94.32x-   Injury to rider of non-recreational watercraft being pulled behind other watercraft
   Injury to occupant of dingy being pulled behind boat or ship
   Injury to occupant of life-raft being pulled behind boat or ship

V94.4xx-   Injury to barefoot water-skier
   Injury to person being pulled behind boat or ship

V94.8-   Other water transport accident

V94.81-   Water transport accident involving military watercraft

V94.810-   Civilian watercraft involved in water transport accident with military watercraft
   Passenger on civilian watercraft injured due to accident with military watercraft

V94.811-   Civilian in water injured by military watercraft

V94.818-   Other water transport accident involving military watercraft

V94.89x-   Other water transport accident

V94.9xx-   Unspecified water transport accident
   Water transport accident NOS

Air and space transport accidents (V95-V97)

Excludes 1:   military aircraft accidents in military or war operations (Y36, Y37)

V95-   Accident to powered aircraft causing injury to occupant
   The appropriate 7th character is to be added to each code from category V95:
   A   Initial encounter
   D   Subsequent encounter
   S   Sequela

V95.0-   Helicopter accident injuring occupant

V95.00x-   Unspecified helicopter accident injuring occupant

V95.01x-   Helicopter crash injuring occupant

V95.02x-   Forced landing of helicopter injuring occupant

V95.03x-   Helicopter collision injuring occupant
   Helicopter collision with any object, fixed, movable or moving

V95.04x-   Helicopter fire injuring occupant

V95.05x-   Helicopter explosion injuring occupant

V95.09x-   Other helicopter accident injuring occupant

V95.1-   Ultralight, microlight or powered-glider accident injuring occupant

V95.10x-   Unspecified ultralight, microlight or powered-glider accident injuring occupant

V95.11x-   Ultralight, microlight or powered-glider crash injuring occupant

V95.12x-   Forced landing of ultralight, microlight or powered-glider injuring occupant

V
9
3
–
V
9
9

V95.13x- Ultralight, microlight or powered-glider collision injuring occupant
  Ultralight, microlight or powered-glider collision with any object, fixed, movable or moving

V95.14x- Ultralight, microlight or powered-glider fire injuring occupant

V95.15x- Ultralight, microlight or powered-glider explosion injuring occupant

V95.19x- Other ultralight, microlight or powered-glider accident injuring occupant

V95.2- Other private fixed-wing aircraft accident injuring occupant

V95.20x- Unspecified accident to other private fixed-wing aircraft, injuring occupant

V95.21x- Other private fixed-wing aircraft crash injuring occupant

V95.22x- Forced landing of other private fixed-wing aircraft injuring occupant

V95.23x- Other private fixed-wing aircraft collision injuring occupant
  Other private fixed-wing aircraft collision with any object, fixed, movable or moving

V95.24x- Other private fixed-wing aircraft fire injuring occupant

V95.25x- Other private fixed-wing aircraft explosion injuring occupant

V95.29x- Other accident to other private fixed-wing aircraft injuring occupant

V95.3- Commercial fixed-wing aircraft accident injuring occupant

V95.30x- Unspecified accident to commercial fixed-wing aircraft injuring occupant

V95.31x- Commercial fixed-wing aircraft crash injuring occupant

V95.32x- Forced landing of commercial fixed-wing aircraft injuring occupant

V95.33x- Commercial fixed-wing aircraft collision injuring occupant
  Commercial fixed-wing aircraft collision with any object, fixed, movable or moving

V95.34x- Commercial fixed-wing aircraft fire injuring occupant

V95.35x- Commercial fixed-wing aircraft explosion injuring occupant

V95.39x- Other accident to commercial fixed-wing aircraft injuring occupant

V95.4- Spacecraft accident injuring occupant

V95.40x- Unspecified spacecraft accident injuring occupant

V95.41x- Spacecraft crash injuring occupant

V95.42x- Forced landing of spacecraft injuring occupant

V95.43x- Spacecraft collision injuring occupant
  Spacecraft collision with any object, fixed, moveable or moving

V95.44x- Spacecraft fire injuring occupant

V95.45x- Spacecraft explosion injuring occupant

V95.49x- Other spacecraft accident injuring occupant

V95.8xx- Other powered aircraft accidents injuring occupant

V95.9xx- Unspecified aircraft accident injuring occupant
  Aircraft accident NOS
  Air transport accident NOS

V96- Accident to nonpowered aircraft causing injury to occupant

> The appropriate 7th character is to be added to each code from category V96:
> **A** Initial encounter
> **D** Subsequent encounter
> **S** Sequela

V96.0- Balloon accident injuring occupant

V96.00x- Unspecified balloon accident injuring occupant

V96.01x- Balloon crash injuring occupant

V96.02x- Forced landing of balloon injuring occupant

V96.03x- Balloon collision injuring occupant
  Balloon collision with any object, fixed, moveable or moving

V96.04x- Balloon fire injuring occupant

V96.05x- Balloon explosion injuring occupant

V96.09x- Other balloon accident injuring occupant

V96.1- Hang-glider accident injuring occupant

V96.10x- Unspecified hang-glider accident injuring occupant

V96.11x- Hang-glider crash injuring occupant

V96.12x- Forced landing of hang-glider injuring occupant

V96.13x- Hang-glider collision injuring occupant
  Hang-glider collision with any object, fixed, moveable or moving

V96.14x- Hang-glider fire injuring occupant

V96.15x- Hang-glider explosion injuring occupant

V96.19x- Other hang-glider accident injuring occupant

V96.2- Glider (nonpowered) accident injuring occupant

V96.20x- Unspecified glider (nonpowered) accident injuring occupant

V96.21x- Glider (nonpowered) crash injuring occupant

V96.22x- Forced landing of glider (nonpowered) injuring occupant

V96.23x- Glider (nonpowered) collision injuring occupant
  Glider (nonpowered) collision with any object, fixed, moveable or moving

V96.24x- Glider (nonpowered) fire injuring occupant

V96.25x- Glider (nonpowered) explosion injuring occupant

V96.29x- Other glider (nonpowered) accident injuring occupant

V96.8xx- Other nonpowered-aircraft accidents injuring occupant
  Kite carrying a person accident injuring occupant

V96.9xx- Unspecified nonpowered-aircraft accident injuring occupant
  Nonpowered-aircraft accident NOS

V97- Other specified air transport accidents

> The appropriate 7th character is to be added to each code from category V97:
> **A** Initial encounter
> **D** Subsequent encounter
> **S** Sequela

V97.0xx- Occupant of aircraft injured in other specified air transport accidents
  Fall in, on or from aircraft in air transport accident
  Excludes 1: accident while boarding or alighting aircraft (V97.1)

V97.1xx- Person injured while boarding or alighting from aircraft

V97.2- Parachutist accident

V97.21x- Parachutist entangled in object
  Parachutist landing in tree

V97.22x- Parachutist injured on landing

V97.29x- Other parachutist accident

V97.3- Person on ground injured in air transport accident

V97.31x- Hit by object falling from aircraft
  Hit by crashing aircraft
  Injured by aircraft hitting house
  Injured by aircraft hitting car

V97.32x- Injured by rotating propeller

V97.33x- Sucked into jet engine

V97.39x- Other injury to person on ground due to air transport accident

V97.8- Other air transport accidents, not elsewhere classified
  Excludes 1: aircraft accident NOS (V95.9)
    exposure to changes in air pressure during ascent or descent (W94.-)

V97.81- Air transport accident involving military aircraft

V97.810- Civilian aircraft involved in air transport accident with military aircraft
  Passenger in civilian aircraft injured due to accident with military aircraft

V97.811- Civilian injured by military aircraft

V97.818- Other air transport accident involving military aircraft

V97.89x- Other air transport accidents, not elsewhere classified
  Injury from machinery on aircraft

Other and unspecified transport accidents (V98-V99)

Excludes 1: vehicle accident, type of vehicle unspecified (V89.-)

V98- Other specified transport accidents

> The appropriate 7th character is to be added to each code from category V98:
> **A** Initial encounter
> **D** Subsequent encounter
> **S** Sequela

V98.0xx- Accident to, on or involving cable-car, not on rails
  Caught or dragged by cable-car, not on rails
  Fall or jump from cable-car, not on rails
  Object thrown from or in cable-car, not on rails

V98.1xx- Accident to, on or involving land-yacht

V98.2xx- Accident to, on or involving ice yacht

V98.3xx- Accident to, on or involving ski lift
  Accident to, on or involving ski chair-lift
  Accident to, on or involving ski-lift with gondola

V98.8xx- Other specified transport accidents

V99.xxx- Unspecified transport accident

> The appropriate 7th character is to be added to code V99
> **A** Initial encounter
> **D** Subsequent encounter
> **S** Sequela

V93 – V99

Other external causes of accidental injury (W00-X58)

Slipping, tripping, stumbling and falls (W00-W19)

Excludes 1: *assault involving a fall (Y01-Y02)*
fall from animal (V80.-)
fall (in) (from) machinery (in operation) (W28-W31)
fall (in) (from) transport vehicle (V01-V99)
intentional self-harm involving a fall (X80-X81)
Excludes ❷: *at risk for fall (history of fall) Z91.81*
fall (in) (from) burning building (X00.-)
fall into fire (X00-X04, X08-X09)

W00- Fall due to ice and snow
Includes: Pedestrian on foot falling (slipping) on ice and snow
Excludes 1: *fall on (from) ice and snow involving pedestrian conveyance (V00.-)*
fall from stairs and steps not due to ice and snow (W10.-)

The appropriate 7th character is to be added to each code from category W00:
  A   Initial encounter
  D   Subsequent encounter
  S   Sequela

W00.0xx- Fall on same level due to ice and snow
W00.1xx- Fall from stairs and steps due to ice and snow
W00.2xx- Other fall from one level to another due to ice and snow
W00.9xx- Unspecified fall due to ice and snow

W01- Fall on same level from slipping, tripping and stumbling
Includes: Fall on moving sidewalk
Excludes 1: *fall due to bumping (striking) against object (W18.0-)*
fall in shower or bathtub (W18.2-)
fall on same level NOS (W18.30)
fall on same level from slipping, tripping and stumbling due to ice or snow (W00.0)
fall off or from toilet (W18.1-)
slipping, tripping and stumbling NOS (W18.40)
slipping, tripping and stumbling without falling (W18.4-)

The appropriate 7th character is to be added to each code from category W01:
  A   Initial encounter
  D   Subsequent encounter
  S   Sequela

W01.0xx- Fall on same level from slipping, tripping and stumbling without subsequent striking against object
  Falling over animal
W01.1- Fall on same level from slipping, tripping and stumbling with subsequent striking against object
  W01.10x- Fall on same level from slipping, tripping and stumbling with subsequent striking against unspecified object
  W01.11-   Fall on same level from slipping, tripping and stumbling with subsequent striking against sharp object
    W01.110- Fall on same level from slipping, tripping and stumbling with subsequent striking against sharp glass
    W01.111- Fall on same level from slipping, tripping and stumbling with subsequent striking against power tool or machine
    W01.118- Fall on same level from slipping, tripping and stumbling with subsequent striking against other sharp object
    W01.119- Fall on same level from slipping, tripping and stumbling with subsequent striking against unspecified sharp object
  W01.19- Fall on same level from slipping, tripping and stumbling with subsequent striking against other object
    W01.190- Fall on same level from slipping, tripping and stumbling with subsequent striking against furniture
    W01.198- Fall on same level from slipping, tripping and stumbling with subsequent striking against other object

W03.xxx- Other fall on same level due to collision with another person
Fall due to non-transport collision with other person
Excludes 1: *collision with another person without fall (W51)*
crushed or pushed by a crowd or human stampede (W52)
fall involving pedestrian conveyance (V00-V09)
fall due to ice or snow (W00)
fall on same level NOS (W18.30)

The appropriate 7th character is to be added to code W03:
  A   Initial encounter
  D   Subsequent encounter
  S   Sequela

W04.xxx- Fall while being carried or supported by other persons
Accidentally dropped while being carried
The appropriate 7th character is to be added to code W04:
  A   Initial encounter
  D   Subsequent encounter
  S   Sequela

W05- Fall from non-moving wheelchair, nonmotorized scooter and motorized mobility scooter
Excludes 1: *fall from moving wheelchair (powered) (V00.811)*
fall from moving motorized mobility scooter (V00.831)
fall from nonmotorized scooter (V00.141)

The appropriate 7th character is to be added to each code from category W05:
  A   Initial encounter
  D   Subsequent encounter
  S   Sequela

W05.0xx- Fall from non-moving wheelchair
W05.1xx- Fall from non-moving nonmotorized scooter
W05.2xx- Fall from non-moving motorized mobility scooter

W06.xxx- Fall from bed
The appropriate 7th character is to be added to code W06:
  A   Initial encounter
  D   Subsequent encounter
  S   Sequela

W07.xxx- Fall from chair
The appropriate 7th character is to be added to code W07:
  A   Initial encounter
  D   Subsequent encounter
  S   Sequela

W08.xxx- Fall from other furniture
The appropriate 7th character is to be added to code W08:
  A   Initial encounter
  D   Subsequent encounter
  S   Sequela

W09- Fall on and from playground equipment
Excludes 1: *fall involving recreational machinery (W31)*
The appropriate 7th character is to be added to each code from category W09:
  A   Initial encounter
  D   Subsequent encounter
  S   Sequela

W09.0xx- Fall on or from playground slide
W09.1xx- Fall from playground swing
W09.2xx- Fall on or from jungle gym
W09.8xx- Fall on or from other playground equipment

W10- Fall on and from stairs and steps
Excludes 1: *Fall from stairs and steps due to ice and snow (W00.1)*
The appropriate 7th character is to be added to each code from category W10:
  A   Initial encounter
  D   Subsequent encounter
  S   Sequela

W10.0xx- Fall (on) (from) escalator
W10.1xx- Fall (on) (from) sidewalk curb
W10.2xx- Fall (on) (from) incline
  Fall (on) (from) ramp
W10.8xx- Fall (on) (from) other stairs and steps
W10.9xx- Fall (on) (from) unspecified stairs and steps

W11.xxx- Fall on and from ladder
The appropriate 7th character is to be added to code W11:
  A   Initial encounter
  D   Subsequent encounter
  S   Sequela

W12.xxx- Fall on and from scaffolding
The appropriate 7th character is to be added to code W12:
  A   Initial encounter
  D   Subsequent encounter
  S   Sequela

W
0
0
–
W
1
6

W13- <u>Fall</u> from, out of or through <u>building or structure</u>
The appropriate 7th character is to be added to each code from
   category W13:
  A <u>Initial</u> encounter
  D <u>Subsequent</u> encounter
  S <u>Sequela</u>
  W13.0xx- **Fall from, out of or through balcony**
    Fall from, out of or through railing
  W13.1xx- **Fall from, out of or through bridge**
  W13.2xx- **Fall from, out of or through roof**
  W13.3xx- **Fall through floor**
  W13.4xx- **Fall from, out of or through window**
    Excludes❷: fall with subsequent striking against sharp glass (W01.110)
  W13.8xx- **Fall from, out of or through other building or structure**
    Fall from, out of or through viaduct
    Fall from, out of or through wall
    Fall from, out of or through flag-pole
  W13.9xx- **Fall from, out of or through building, not otherwise specified**
    Excludes 1: collapse of a building or structure (W20.-)
     fall or jump from burning building or structure (X00.-)

W14.xxx- <u>Fall</u> from <u>tree</u>
The appropriate 7th character is to be added to code W14:
  A <u>Initial</u> encounter
  D <u>Subsequent</u> encounter
  S <u>Sequela</u>

W15.xxx- <u>Fall</u> from <u>cliff</u>
The appropriate 7th character is to be added to code W15:
  A <u>Initial</u> encounter
  D <u>Subsequent</u> encounter
  S <u>Sequela</u>

W16- <u>Fall</u>, jump or diving <u>into water</u>
  Excludes 1: accidental non-watercraft drowning and submersion not involving fall (W65-W74)
   effects of air pressure from diving (W94.-)
   fall into water from watercraft (V90-V94)
   hitting an object or against bottom when falling from watercraft (V94.0)
  Excludes❷: striking or hitting diving board (W21.4)
The appropriate 7th character is to be added to each code from
   category W16:
  A <u>Initial</u> encounter
  D <u>Subsequent</u> encounter
  S <u>Sequela</u>
  W16.0- <u>Fall</u> into <u>swimming pool</u>
    Fall into swimming pool NOS
    Excludes 1: fall into empty swimming pool (W17.3)
    W16.01- **Fall into swimming pool** <u>striking water surface</u>
     W16.011- **Fall into swimming pool striking water surface** <u>causing drowning and submersion</u>
      Excludes 1: drowning and submersion while in swimming pool without fall (W67)
     W16.012- **Fall into swimming pool striking water surface** <u>causing other injury</u>
    W16.02- **Fall into swimming pool** <u>striking bottom</u>
     W16.021- **Fall into swimming pool striking bottom** <u>causing drowning and submersion</u>
      Excludes 1: drowning and submersion while in swimming pool without fall (W67)
     W16.022- **Fall into swimming pool striking bottom** <u>causing other injury</u>
    W16.03- **Fall into swimming pool** <u>striking wall</u>
     W16.031- **Fall into swimming pool striking wall** <u>causing drowning and submersion</u>
      Excludes 1: drowning and submersion while in swimming pool without fall (W67)
     W16.032- **Fall into swimming pool striking wall causing other injury**
  W16.1- <u>Fall</u> into <u>natural body of water</u>
    Fall into lake
    Fall into open sea
    Fall into river
    Fall into stream
    W16.11- **Fall into natural body of water** <u>striking water surface</u>
     W16.111- **Fall into natural body of water striking water surface** <u>causing drowning and submersion</u>
      Excludes 1: drowning and submersion while in natural body of water without fall (W69)
     W16.112- **Fall into natural body of water striking water surface** <u>causing other injury</u>

W16.12- **Fall into natural body of** <u>water striking bottom</u>
  W16.121- **Fall into natural body of water striking bottom** <u>causing drowning and submersion</u>
   Excludes 1: drowning and submersion while in natural body of water without fall (W69)
  W16.122- **Fall into natural body of water striking bottom** <u>causing other injury</u>
W16.13- **Fall into natural body of** <u>water striking side</u>
  W16.131- **Fall into natural body of water striking side** <u>causing drowning and submersion</u>
   Excludes 1: drowning and submersion while in natural body of water without fall (W69)
  W16.132- **Fall into natural body of water striking side** <u>causing other injury</u>
W16.2- <u>Fall</u> in (into) <u>filled bathtub or bucket of water</u>
  W16.21- **Fall in (into) filled** <u>bathtub</u>
   Excludes 1: fall into empty bathtub (W18.2)
   W16.211- **Fall in (into) filled bathtub** <u>causing drowning and submersion</u>
    Excludes 1: drowning and submersion while in filled bathtub without fall (W65)
   W16.212- **Fall in (into) filled bathtub causing other injury**
  W16.22- **Fall in (into)** <u>bucket of water</u>
   W16.221- **Fall in (into) bucket of water** <u>causing drowning and submersion</u>
   W16.222- **Fall in (into) bucket of water** <u>causing other injury</u>
W16.3- <u>Fall</u> into <u>other water</u>
  Fall into fountain
  Fall into reservoir
  W16.31- **Fall into other water** <u>striking water surface</u>
   W16.311- **Fall into other water striking water surface** <u>causing drowning and submersion</u>
    Excludes 1: drowning and submersion while in other water without fall (W73)
   W16.312- **Fall into other water striking water surface** <u>causing other injury</u>
  W16.32- **Fall into other water** <u>striking bottom</u>
   W16.321- **Fall into other water striking bottom** <u>causing drowning and submersion</u>
    Excludes 1: drowning and submersion while in other water without fall (W73)
   W16.322- **Fall into other water striking bottom** <u>causing other injury</u>
  W16.33- **Fall into other water** <u>striking wall</u>
   W16.331- **Fall into other water striking wall** <u>causing drowning and submersion</u>
    Excludes 1: drowning and submersion while in other water without fall (W73)
   W16.332 **Fall into other water striking wall** <u>causing other injury</u>
W16.4- <u>Fall</u> into <u>unspecified water</u>
  W16.41x- **Fall into unspecified water** <u>causing drowning and submersion</u>
  W16.42x- **Fall into unspecified water** <u>causing other injury</u>
W16.5- <u>Jumping or diving</u> into <u>swimming pool</u>
  W16.51- **Jumping or diving into swimming pool** <u>striking water surface</u>
   W16.511- **Jumping or diving into swimming pool striking water surface causing drowning and submersion**
    Excludes 1: drowning and submersion while in swimming pool without jumping or diving (W67)
   W16.512- **Jumping or diving into swimming pool striking water surface** <u>causing other injury</u>
  W16.52- **Jumping or diving into swimming pool** <u>striking bottom</u>
   W16.521- **Jumping or diving into swimming pool striking bottom** <u>causing drowning and submersion</u>
    Excludes 1: drowning and submersion while in swimming pool without jumping or diving (W67)
   W16.522- **Jumping or diving into swimming pool striking bottom** <u>causing other injury</u>
  W16.53- **Jumping or diving into swimming pool** <u>striking wall</u>
   W16.531- **Jumping or diving into swimming pool striking wall** <u>causing drowning and submersion</u>
    Excludes 1: drowning and submersion while in swimming pool without jumping or diving (W67)
   W16.532- **Jumping or diving into swimming pool striking wall** <u>causing other injury</u>

W00-W16

© 2013 Channel Publishing, Ltd.

W16.6- <u>Jumping or diving</u> into <u>natural body of water</u>
  Jumping or diving into lake
  Jumping or diving into open sea
  Jumping or diving into river
  Jumping or diving into stream

W16.61-Jumping or diving into natural body of water <u>striking water surface</u>

  W16.611- Jumping or diving into natural body of water striking water surface <u>causing drowning and submersion</u>
    Excludes 1: drowning and submersion while in natural body of water without jumping or diving (W69)

  W16.612- Jumping or diving into natural body of water striking water surface <u>causing other injury</u>

W16.62-Jumping or diving into natural body of water <u>striking bottom</u>

  W16.621- Jumping or diving into natural body of water striking bottom <u>causing drowning and submersion</u>
    Excludes 1: drowning and submersion while in natural body of water without jumping ordiving (W69)

  W16.622- Jumping or diving into natural body of water striking bottom <u>causing other injury</u>

W16.7- Jumping or diving from <u>boat</u>
  Excludes 1: fall from boat into water — see watercraft accident (V90-V94)

W16.71-Jumping or diving from boat <u>striking water surface</u>

  W16.711- Jumping or diving from boat striking water surface <u>causing drowning and submersion</u>

  W16.712- Jumping or diving from boat striking water surface <u>causing other injury</u>

W16.72-Jumping or diving from boat <u>striking bottom</u>

  W16.721- Jumping or diving from boat striking bottom <u>causing drowning and submersion</u>

  W16.722- Jumping or diving from boat striking bottom <u>causing other injury</u>

W16.8- Jumping or diving into <u>other</u> water
  Jumping or diving into fountain
  Jumping or diving into reservoir

W16.81-Jumping or diving into other water <u>striking water surface</u>

  W16.811- Jumping or diving into other water striking water surface <u>causing drowning and submersion</u>
    Excludes 1: drowning and submersion while in other water without jumping or diving (W73)

  W16.812- Jumping or diving into other water striking water surface <u>causing other injury</u>

W16.82-Jumping or diving into other water <u>striking bottom</u>

  W16.821- Jumping or diving into other water striking bottom <u>causing drowning and submersion</u>
    Excludes 1: drowning and submersion while in other water without jumping or diving (W73)

  W16.822- Jumping or diving into other water striking bottom <u>causing other injury</u>

W16.83-Jumping or diving into other water <u>striking wall</u>

  W16.831- Jumping or diving into other water striking wall <u>causing drowning and submersion</u>
    Excludes 1: drowning and submersion while in other water without jumping or diving (W73)

  W16.832- Jumping or diving into other water striking wall <u>causing other injury</u>

W16.9- Jumping or diving into <u>unspecified water</u>

  W16.91x- Jumping or diving into unspecified water <u>causing drowning and submersion</u>

  W16.92x- Jumping or diving into unspecified water <u>causing other injury</u>

W17- <u>Other fall</u> <u>from one level to another</u>
  The appropriate 7th character is to be added to each code from category W17:
    A <u>Initial</u> encounter
    D <u>Subsequent</u> encounter
    S <u>Sequela</u>

W17.0xx- Fall into well

W17.1xx- Fall into storm drain or manhole

W17.2xx- Fall into hole
  Fall into pit

W17.3xx- Fall into empty swimming pool
  Excludes 1: fall into filled swimming pool (W16.0-)

W17.4xx- Fall from dock

W17.8- Other fall from one level to another

  W17.81x- Fall down embankment (hill)

  W17.82x- Fall from (out of) grocery cart
    Fall due to grocery cart tipping over

  W17.89x- Other fall from one level to another
    Fall from cherry picker
    Fall from lifting device
    Fall from mobile elevated work platform [MEWP]
    Fall from sky lift

W18- Other <u>slipping, tripping and stumbling and falls</u>
  The appropriate 7th character is to be added to each code from category W18:
    A <u>Initial</u> encounter
    D <u>Subsequent</u> encounter
    S <u>Sequela</u>

W18.0- Fall due to <u>bumping against object</u>
  Striking against object with subsequent fall
  Excludes 1: fall on same level due to slipping, tripping, or stumbling with subsequent striking against object (W01.1-)

  W18.00x- Striking against unspecified object with subsequent fall

  W18.01x- Striking against sports equipment with subsequent fall

  W18.02x- Striking against glass with subsequent fall

  W18.09x- Striking against other object with subsequent fall

W18.1- Fall from or off <u>toilet</u>

  W18.11x- Fall from or off toilet without subsequent striking against object
    Fall from (off) toilet NOS

  W18.12x- Fall from or off toilet with subsequent striking against object

W18.2xx- Fall in (into) <u>shower or empty bathtub</u>
  Excludes 1: fall in full bathtub causing drowning or submersion (W16.21-)

W18.3- Other and unspecified fall on same level

  W18.30x- Fall on same level, unspecified

  W18.31x- Fall on same level due to stepping on an object
    Fall on same level due to stepping on an animal
    Excludes 1: slipping, tripping and stumbling without fall due to stepping on animal (W18.41)

  W18.39x- Other fall on same level

W18.4- Slipping, tripping and stumbling <u>without falling</u>
  Excludes 1: collision with another person without fall (W51)

  W18.40x- Slipping, tripping and stumbling without falling, unspecified

  W18.41x- Slipping, tripping and stumbling without falling due to stepping on object
    Slipping, tripping and stumbling without falling due to stepping on animal
    Excludes 1: slipping, tripping and stumbling with fall due to stepping on animal (W18.31)

  W18.42x- Slipping, tripping and stumbling without falling due to stepping into hole or opening

  W18.43x- Slipping, tripping and stumbling without falling due to stepping from one level to another

  W18.49x- Other slipping, tripping and stumbling without falling

W19.xxx- <u>Unspecified fall</u>
  Accidental fall NOS
  The appropriate 7th character is to be added to code W19:
    A <u>Initial</u> encounter
    D <u>Subsequent</u> encounter
    S <u>Sequela</u>

**W
1
6
–
W
2
5**

Exposure to inanimate mechanical forces (W20-W49)

> *Excludes 1:   assault (X92-Y08)*
> *contact or collision with animals or persons (W50-W64)*
> *exposure to inanimate mechanical forces involving military or*
> *war operations (Y36-, Y37-)*
> *intentional self-harm (X71-X83)*

W20-   Struck by thrown, projected or falling object
Code first any associated:
   Cataclysm (X34-X39)
   Lightning strike (T75.00)
> *Excludes 1:   falling object in machinery accident (W24, W28-W31)*
> *falling object in transport accident (V01-V99)*
> *object set in motion by explosion (W35-W40)*
> *object set in motion by firearm (W32-W34)*
> *struck by thrown sports equipment (W21.-)*

The appropriate 7th character is to be added to each code from category W20:
   A   Initial encounter
   D   Subsequent encounter
   S   Sequela

W20.0xx-   Struck by falling object in cave-in
> *Excludes ❷: asphyxiation due to cave-in (T71.21)*

W20.1xx-   Struck by object due to collapse of building
> *Excludes 1:   struck by object due to collapse of burning building (X00.2, X02.2)*

W20.8xx-   Other cause of strike by thrown, projected or falling object
> *Excludes 1:   struck by thrown sports equipment (W21.-)*

W21-   Striking against or struck by sports equipment
> *Excludes 1:   assault with sports equipment (Y08.0-)*
> *striking against or struck by sports equipment with subsequent fall (W18.01)*

The appropriate 7th character is to be added to each code from category W21:
   A   Initial encounter
   D   Subsequent encounter
   S   Sequela

W21.0-   Struck by hit or thrown ball
   W21.00x-   Struck by hit or thrown ball, unspecified type
   W21.01x-   Struck by football
   W21.02x-   Struck by soccer ball
   W21.03x-   Struck by baseball
   W21.04x-   Struck by golf ball
   W21.05x-   Struck by basketball
   W21.06x-   Struck by volleyball
   W21.07x-   Struck by softball
   W21.09x-   Struck by other hit or thrown ball
W21.1-   Struck by bat, racquet or club
   W21.11x-   Struck by baseball bat
   W21.12x-   Struck by tennis racquet
   W21.13x-   Struck by golf club
   W21.19x-   Struck by other bat, racquet or club
W21.2-   Struck by hockey stick or puck
   W21.21-Struck by hockey stick
      W21.210-   Struck by ice hockey stick
      W21.211-   Struck by field hockey stick
   W21.22-Struck by hockey puck
      W21.220-   Struck by ice hockey puck
      W21.221-   Struck by field hockey puck
W21.3-   Struck by sports foot wear
   W21.31x-   Struck by shoe cleats
      Stepped on by shoe cleats
   W21.32x-   Struck by skate blades
      Skated over by skate blades
   W21.39x-   Struck by other sports foot wear
W21.4xx-   Striking against diving board
      Use additional code for subsequent falling into water, if applicable (W16.-)
W21.8-   Striking against or struck by other sports equipment
   W21.81x-   Striking against or struck by football helmet
   W21.89x-   Striking against or struck by other sports equipment
W21.9xx-   Striking against or struck by unspecified sports equipment

W22-   Striking against or struck by other objects
> *Excludes 1:   striking against or struck by object with subsequent fall (W18.09)*

The appropriate 7th character is to be added to each code from category W22:
   A   Initial encounter
   D   Subsequent encounter
   S   Sequela

W22.0-   Striking against stationary object
> *Excludes 1:   striking against stationary sports equipment (W21.8)*

   W22.01x-   Walked into wall
   W22.02x-   Walked into lamppost
   W22.03x-   Walked into furniture
   W22.04-Striking against wall of swimming pool
      W22.041-   Striking against wall of swimming pool causing drowning and submersion
      > *Excludes 1:   drowning and submersion while swimming without striking against wall (W67)*
      W22.042-   Striking against wall of swimming pool causing other injury
   W22.09x-   Striking against other stationary object
W22.1-   Striking against or struck by automobile airbag
   W22.10x-   Striking against or struck by unspecified automobile airbag
   W22.11x-   Striking against or struck by driver side automobile airbag
   W22.12x-   Striking against or struck by front passenger side automobile airbag
   W22.19x-   Striking against or struck by other automobile airbag
W22.8xx-   Striking against or struck by other objects
      Striking against or struck by object NOS
> *Excludes 1:   struck by thrown, projected or falling object (W20.-)*

W23-   Caught, crushed, jammed or pinched in or between objects
> *Excludes 1:   injury caused by cutting or piercing instruments (W25-W27)*
> *injury caused by firearms malfunction (W32.1, W33.1-, W34.1-)*
> *injury caused by lifting and transmission devices (W24.-)*
> *injury caused by machinery (W28-W31)*
> *injury caused by nonpowered hand tools (W27.-)*
> *injury caused by transport vehicle being used as a means of transportation (V01-V99)*
> *injury caused by struck by thrown, projected or falling object (W20.-)*

The appropriate 7th character is to be added to each code from category W23:
   A   Initial encounter
   D   Subsequent encounter
   S   Sequela

W23.0xx-   Caught, crushed, jammed, or pinched between moving objects
W23.1xx-   Caught, crushed, jammed, or pinched between stationary objects

W24-   Contact with lifting and transmission devices, not elsewhere classified
> *Excludes 1:   transport accidents (V01-V99)*

The appropriate 7th character is to be added to each code from category W24:
   A   Initial encounter
   D   Subsequent encounter
   S   Sequela

W24.0xx-   Contact with lifting devices, not elsewhere classified
      Contact with chain hoist
      Contact with drive belt
      Contact with pulley (block)
W24.1xx-   Contact with transmission devices, not elsewhere classified
      Contact with transmission belt or cable

W25.xxx-   Contact with sharp glass
      Code first any associated:
         Injury due to flying glass from explosion or firearm discharge (W32-W40)
         Transport accident (V00-V99)
> *Excludes 1:   fall on same level due to slipping, tripping and stumbling with subsequent striking against sharp glass (W01.10)*
> *striking against sharp glass with subsequent fall (W18.02)*

The appropriate 7th character is to be added to code W25:
   A   Initial encounter
   D   Subsequent encounter
   S   Sequela

W 1 6 - W 2 5

W26- Contact with <u>knife, sword or dagger</u>
   The appropriate 7th character is to be added to each code from
      category W26:
    A <u>Initial</u> encounter
    D <u>Subsequent</u> encounter
    S <u>Sequela</u>
  W26.0xx- **Contact with knife**
     Excludes 1: contact with electric knife (W29.1)
  W26.1xx- **Contact with sword or dagger**

W27- Contact with <u>nonpowered hand tool</u>
   The appropriate 7th character is to be added to each code from
      category W27:
    A <u>Initial</u> encounter
    D <u>Subsequent</u> encounter
    S <u>Sequela</u>
  W27.0xx- **Contact with <u>workbench tool</u>**
     Contact with auger
     Contact with axe
     Contact with chisel
     Contact with handsaw
     Contact with screwdriver
  W27.1xx- **Contact with <u>garden tool</u>**
     Contact with hoe
     Contact with nonpowered lawn mower
     Contact with pitchfork
     Contact with rake
  W27.2xx- **Contact with <u>scissors</u>**
  W27.3xx- **Contact with <u>needle (sewing)</u>**
     Excludes 1: contact with hypodermic needle (W46.-)
  W27.4xx- **Contact with <u>kitchen utensil</u>**
     Contact with fork
     Contact with ice-pick
     Contact with can-opener NOS
  W27.5xx- **Contact with <u>paper-cutter</u>**
  W27.8xx- **Contact with <u>other nonpowered hand tool</u>**
     Contact with nonpowered sewing machine
     Contact with shovel

W28.xxx-   **Contact with <u>powered lawn mower</u>**
     Powered lawn mower (commercial) (residential)
    Excludes 1: contact with nonpowered lawn mower (W27.1)
    Excludes:2 exposure to electric current (W86-)
   The appropriate 7th character is to be added to code W28:
    A <u>Initial</u> encounter
    D <u>Subsequent</u> encounter
    S <u>Sequela</u>

W29- Contact with <u>other powered hand tools and household machinery</u>
    Excludes 1: contact with commercial machinery (W31.82)
       contact with hot household appliance (X15)
       contact with nonpowered hand tool (W27.-)
       exposure to electric current (W86)
   The appropriate 7th character is to be added to each code from
      category W29:
    A <u>Initial</u> encounter
    D <u>Subsequent</u> encounter
    S <u>Sequela</u>
  W29.0xx- **Contact with powered <u>kitchen</u> appliance**
     Contact with blender
     Contact with can-opener
     Contact with garbage disposal
     Contact with mixer
  W29.1xx- **Contact with electric knife**
  W29.2xx- **Contact with other powered <u>household</u> machinery**
     Contact with electric fan
     Contact with powered dryer (clothes) (powered) (spin)
     Contact with washing-machine
     Contact with sewing machine
  W29.3xx- **Contact with powered <u>garden</u> and <u>outdoor</u> hand tools and machinery**
     Contact with chainsaw
     Contact with edger
     Contact with garden cultivator (tiller)
     Contact with hedge trimmer
     Contact with other powered garden tool
    Excludes 1: contact with powered lawn mower (W28)
  W29.4xx- **Contact with <u>nail gun</u>**
  W29.8xx- **Contact with <u>other</u> powered powered hand tools and household machinery**
     Contact with do-it-yourself tool NOS

W30- Contact with <u>agricultural</u> machinery
   Includes: Animal-powered farm machine
   Excludes 1: agricultural transport vehicle accident (V01-V99)
       explosion of grain store (W40.8)
       exposure to electric current (W86.-)
   The appropriate 7th character is to be added to each code from
      category W30:
    A <u>Initial</u> encounter
    D <u>Subsequent</u> encounter
    S <u>Sequela</u>
  W30.0xx- **Contact with combine harvester**
     Contact with reaper
     Contact with thresher
  W30.1xx- **Contact with power take-off devices (PTO)**
  W30.2xx- **Contact with hay derrick**
  W30.3xx- **Contact with grain storage elevator**
     Excludes 1: explosion of grain store (W40.8)
  W30.8- **Contact with other specified agricultural machinery**
    W30.81x- **Contact with agricultural transport vehicle in stationary use**
      Contact with agricultural transport vehicle under repair, not on public roadway
      Excludes 1: agricultural transport vehicle accident (V01-V99)
    W30.89x- **Contact with other specified agricultural machinery**
  W30.9xx- **Contact with unspecified agricultural machinery**
     Contact with farm machinery NOS

W31- Contact with <u>other and unspecified</u> machinery
    Excludes 1: contact with agricultural machinery (W30.-)
       contact with machinery in transport under own power or being towed by a vehicle (V01-V99)
       exposure to electric current (W86)
   The appropriate 7th character is to be added to each code from
      category W31:
    A <u>Initial</u> encounter
    D <u>Subsequent</u> encounter
    S <u>Sequela</u>
  W31.0xx- **Contact with mining and earth-drilling machinery**
     Contact with bore or drill (land) (seabed)
     Contact with shaft hoist
     Contact with shaft lift
     Contact with undercutter
  W31.1xx- **Contact with metalworking machines**
     Contact with abrasive wheel
     Contact with forging machine
     Contact with lathe
     Contact with mechanical shears
     Contact with metal drilling machine
     Contact with milling machine
     Contact with power press
     Contact with rolling-mill
     Contact with metal sawing machine
  W31.2xx- **Contact with powered woodworking and forming machines**
     Contact with band saw
     Contact with bench saw
     Contact with circular saw
     Contact with molding machine
     Contact with overhead plane
     Contact with powered saw
     Contact with radial saw
     Contact with sander
    Excludes 1: nonpowered woodworking tools (W27.0)
  W31.3xx- **Contact with prime movers**
     Contact with gas turbine
     Contact with internal combustion engine
     Contact with steam engine
     Contact with water driven turbine
  W31.8- **Contact with other specified machinery**
    W31.81x- **Contact with recreational machinery**
      Contact with roller coaster
    W31.82x- **Contact with other commercial machinery**
      Contact with commercial electric fan
      Contact with commercial kitchen appliances
      Contact with commercial powered dryer (clothes) (powered) (spin)
      Contact with commercial washing-machine
      Contact with commercial sewing machine
      Excludes 1: contact with household machinery (W29.-)
        contact with powered lawn mower (W28)
    W31.83x- **Contact with special construction vehicle in stationary use**
      Contact with special construction vehicle under repair, not on public roadway
      Excludes 1: special construction vehicle accident (V01-V99)
    W31.89x- **Contact with other specified machinery**

W
2
6
|
W
3
9

Excludes 1: = NOT CODED HERE! (Do not code both)   **872**   *Excludes❷:* = Not Included Here

W31.9xx- Contact with unspecified machinery
    Contact with machinery NOS

W32- Accidental handgun discharge and malfunction
    Includes: Accidental discharge and malfunction of gun for single hand use
                 Accidental discharge and malfunction of pistol
                 Accidental discharge and malfunction of revolver
         Handgun discharge and malfunction NOS
            Excludes 1:   accidental airgun discharge and malfunction (W34.010,
                               W34.110)
                       accidental BB gun discharge and malfunction
                               (W34.010, W34.110)
                       accidental pellet gun discharge and malfunction
                               (W34.010, W34.110)
                       accidental shotgun discharge and malfunction (W33.01,
                               W33.11)
                       assault by handgun discharge (X93)
                       handgun discharge involving legal intervention
                               (Y35.0-)
                       handgun discharge involving military or war
                               operations (Y36.4-)
                       intentional self-harm by handgun discharge (X72)
                       Very pistol discharge and malfunction (W34.09,
                               W34.19)

The appropriate 7th character is to be added to each code from
    category W32:
    A   **Initial** encounter
    D   **Subsequent** encounter
    S   **Sequela**

W32.0xx- Accidental handgun discharge
W32.1xx- Accidental handgun malfunction
    Injury due to explosion of handgun (parts)
    Injury due to malfunction of mechanism or component of
        handgun
    Injury due to recoil of handgun
    Powder burn from handgun

W33- Accidental rifle, shotgun and larger firearm discharge and malfunction
    Includes: Rifle, shotgun and larger firearm discharge and malfunction
                  NOS
    Excludes 1:   accidental airgun discharge and malfunction (W34.010,
                       W34.110)
                  accidental BB gun discharge and malfunction (W34.010,
                       W34.110)
                  accidental handgun discharge and malfunction (W32.-)
                  accidental pellet gun discharge and malfunction (W34.010,
                       W34.110)
                  assault by rifle, shotgun and larger firearm discharge (X94)
                  firearm discharge involving legal intervention (Y35.0-)
                  firearm discharge involving military or war operations
                       (Y36.4-)
                  intentional self-harm by rifle, shotgun and larger firearm
                       discharge (X73)

The appropriate 7th character is to be added to each code from
    category W33:
    A   **Initial** encounter
    D   **Subsequent** encounter
    S   **Sequela**

W33.0- Accidental rifle, shotgun and larger firearm discharge
    W33.00x- Accidental discharge of unspecified larger firearm
        Discharge of unspecified larger firearm NOS
    W33.01x- Accidental discharge of shotgun
        Discharge of shotgun NOS
    W33.02x- Accidental discharge of hunting rifle
        Discharge of hunting rifle NOS
    W33.03x- Accidental discharge of machine gun
        Discharge of machine gun NOS
    W33.09x- Accidental discharge of other larger firearm
        Discharge of other larger firearm NOS

W33.1- Accidental rifle, shotgun and larger firearm malfunction
    Injury due to explosion of rifle, shotgun and larger firearm (parts)
    Injury due to malfunction of mechanism or component of rifle,
        shotgun and larger firearm
    Injury due to piercing, cutting, crushing or pinching due to (by)
        slide trigger mechanism, scope or other gunpart
    Injury due to recoil of rifle, shotgun and larger firearm
    Powder burn from rifle, shotgun and larger firearm
    W33.10x- Accidental malfunction of unspecified larger firearm
        Malfunction of unspecified larger firearm NOS
    W33.11x- Accidental malfunction of shotgun
        Malfunction of shotgun NOS
    W33.12x- Accidental malfunction of hunting rifle
        Malfunction of hunting rifle NOS
    W33.13x- Accidental malfunction of machine gun
        Malfunction of machine gun NOS

W33.19x- Accidental malfunction of other larger firearm
    Malfunction of other larger firearm NOS

W34- Accidental discharge and malfunction from other and unspecified firearms and guns
    The appropriate 7th character is to be added to each code from
        category W34:
        A   **Initial** encounter
        D   **Subsequent** encounter
        S   **Sequela**

W34.0- Accidental discharge from other and unspecified firearms and guns
    W34.00x- Accidental discharge from unspecified firearms or gun
        Discharge from firearm NOS
        Gunshot wound NOS
        Shot NOS
    W34.01-Accidental discharge of gas, air or spring-operated guns
        W34.010- Accidental discharge of airgun
            Accidental discharge of BB gun
            Accidental discharge of pellet gun
        W34.011- Accidental discharge of paintball gun
            Accidental injury due to paintball discharge
        W34.018- Accidental discharge of other gas, air or spring-operated gun
    W34.09x- Accidental discharge from other specified firearms
        Accidental discharge from Very pistol [flare]

W34.1- Accidental malfunction from other and unspecified firearms and guns
    W34.10x- Accidental malfunction from unspecified firearms or gun
        Firearm malfunction NOS
    W34.11-Accidental malfunction of gas, air or spring-operated guns
        W34.110- Accidental malfunction of airgun
            Accidental malfunction of BB gun
            Accidental malfunction of pellet gun
        W34.111- Accidental malfunction of paintball gun
            Accidental injury due to paintball gun malfunction
        W34.118- Accidental malfunction of other gas, air or spring-operated gun
    W34.19x- Accidental malfunction from other specified firearms
        Accidental malfunction from Very pistol [flare]

W35.xxx- Explosion and rupture of boiler
    Excludes 1:   explosion and rupture of boiler on watercraft (V93.4)
    The appropriate 7th character is to be added to code W35:
        A   **Initial** encounter
        D   **Subsequent** encounter
        S   **Sequela**

W36- Explosion and rupture of gas cylinder
    The appropriate 7th character is to be added to each code from
        category W36:
        A   **Initial** encounter
        D   **Subsequent** encounter
        S   **Sequela**
    W36.1xx- Explosion and rupture of aerosol can
    W36.2xx- Explosion and rupture of air tank
    W36.3xx- Explosion and rupture of pressurized-gas tank
    W36.8xx- Explosion and rupture of other gas cylinder
    W36.9xx- Explosion and rupture of unspecified gas cylinder

W37- Explosion and rupture of pressurized tire, pipe or hose
    The appropriate 7th character is to be added to each code from
        category W37:
        A   **Initial** encounter
        D   **Subsequent** encounter
        S   **Sequela**
    W37.0xx- Explosion of bicycle tire
    W37.8xx- Explosion and rupture of other pressurized tire, pipe or hose

W38.xxx- Explosion and rupture of other specified pressurized devices
    The appropriate 7th character is to be added to code W38
        A   **Initial** encounter
        D   **Subsequent** encounter
        S   **Sequela**

W39.xxx- Discharge of firework
    The appropriate 7th character is to be added to code W39
        A   **Initial** encounter
        D   **Subsequent** encounter
        S   **Sequela**

W26 - W39

W40- Explosion of other materials
    Excludes 1: *assault by explosive material (X96)*
        explosion involving legal intervention (Y35.1-)
        explosion involving military or war operations (Y36.0-,
          Y36.2-)
        intentional self-harm by explosive material (X75)

    The appropriate 7th character is to be added to each code from
      category W40:
    A   Initial encounter
    D   Subsequent encounter
    S   Sequela

W40.0xx- Explosion of blasting material
    Explosion of blasting cap
    Explosion of detonator
    Explosion of dynamite
    Explosion of explosive (any) used in blasting operations

W40.1xx- Explosion of explosive gases
    Explosion of acetylene
    Explosion of butane
    Explosion of coal gas
    Explosion in mine NOS
    Explosion of explosive gas
    Explosion of fire damp
    Explosion of gasoline fumes
    Explosion of methane
    Explosion of propane

W40.8xx- Explosion of other specified explosive materials
    Explosion in dump NOS
    Explosion in factory NOS
    Explosion in grain store
    Explosion in munitions
    Excludes 1: *explosion involving legal intervention (Y35.1-)*
        explosion involving military or war operations
         (Y36.0-, Y36.2-)

W40.9xx- Explosion of unspecified explosive materials
    Explosion NOS

W42- Exposure to noise
    The appropriate 7th character is to be added to each code from
      category W42:
    A   Initial encounter
    D   Subsequent encounter
    S   Sequela

W42.0xx- Exposure to supersonic waves
W42.9xx- Exposure to other noise
    Exposure to sound waves NOS

W45- Foreign body or object entering through skin
    Excludes❷: *contact with hand tools (nonpowered) (powered) (W27-W29)*
        contact with knife, sword or dagger (W26.-)
        contact with sharp glass (W25.-)
        struck by objects (W20-W22)

    The appropriate 7th character is to be added to each code from
      category W45:
    A   Initial encounter
    D   Subsequent encounter
    S   Sequela

W45.0xx- Nail entering through skin
W45.1xx- Paper entering through skin
    Paper cut
W45.2xx- Lid of can entering through skin
W45.8xx- Other foreign body or object entering through skin
    Splinter in skin NOS

W46- Contact with hypodermic needle
    The appropriate 7th character is to be added to each code from
      category W46:
    A   Initial encounter
    D   Subsequent encounter
    S   Sequela

W46.0xx- Contact with hypodermic needle
    Hypodermic needle stick NOS
W46.1xx- Contact with contaminated hypodermic needle

W49- Exposure to other inanimate mechanical forces
    Includes: Exposure to abnormal gravitational [G] forces
        Exposure to inanimate mechanical forces NEC
    Excludes 1: *exposure to inanimate mechanical forces involving military or*
        war operations (Y36.-, Y37.-)

    The appropriate 7th character is to be added to each code from
      category W49:
    A   Initial encounter
    D   Subsequent encounter
    S   Sequela

W49.0- Item causing external constriction
W49.01x- Hair causing external constriction
W49.02x- String or thread causing external constriction
W49.03x- Rubber band causing external constriction
W49.04x- Ring or other jewelry causing external constriction
W49.09x- Other specified item causing external constriction
W49.9xx- Exposure to other inanimate mechanical forces

Exposure to animate mechanical forces (W50-W64)

    Excludes 1: *Toxic effect of contact with venomous animals and plants*
        (T63.-)

W50- Accidental hit, strike, kick, twist, bite or scratch by another person
    Includes: Hit, strike, kick, twist, bite, or scratch by another person NOS
    Excludes 1: *assault by bodily force (Y04)*
        struck by objects (W20-W22)

    The appropriate 7th character is to be added to each code from
      category W50:
    A   Initial encounter
    D   Subsequent encounter
    S   Sequela

W50.0xx- Accidental hit or strike by another person
    Hit or strike by another person NOS
W50.1xx- Accidental kick by another person
    Kick by another person NOS
W50.2xx- Accidental twist by another person
    Twist by another person NOS
W50.3xx- Accidental bite by another person
    Human bite
    Bite by another person NOS
W50.4xx- Accidental scratch by another person
    Scratch by another person NOS

W51.xxx- Accidental striking against or bumped into by another person
    Excludes 1: *assault by striking against or bumping into by another*
        person (Y04.2)
        fall due to collision with another person (W03)

    The appropriate 7th character is to be added to code W51:
    A   Initial encounter
    D   Subsequent encounter
    S   Sequela

W52.xxx- Crushed, pushed or stepped on by crowd or human stampede
    Crushed, pushed or stepped on by crowd or human stampede with
      or without fall

    The appropriate 7th character is to be added to code W52:
    A   Initial encounter
    D   Subsequent encounter
    S   Sequela

W53- Contact with rodent
    Includes: Contact with saliva, feces or urine of rodent
    The appropriate 7th character is to be added to each code from
      category W53:
    A   Initial encounter
    D   Subsequent encounter
    S   Sequela

W53.0- Contact with mouse
W53.01x- Bitten by mouse
W53.09x- Other contact with mouse
W53.1- Contact with rat
W53.11x- Bitten by rat
W53.19x- Other contact with rat
W53.2- Contact with squirrel
W53.21x- Bitten by squirrel
W53.29x- Other contact with squirrel
W53.8- Contact with other rodent
W53.81x- Bitten by other rodent
W53.89x- Other contact with other rodent

W
4
0
–
W
6
0

W54- Contact with dog
  Includes: Contact with saliva, feces or urine of dog
  **The appropriate 7th character is to be added to each code from
    category W54:**
    A Initial encounter
    D Subsequent encounter
    S Sequela
  W54.0xx- Bitten by dog
  W54.1xx- Struck by dog
        Knocked over by dog
  W54.8xx- Other contact with dog

W55- Contact with other mammals
  Includes: Contact with saliva, feces or urine of mammal
  Excludes 1: animal being ridden- see transport accidents
        bitten or struck by dog (W54)
        bitten or struck by rodent (W53.-)
        contact with marine mammals (W56.-)
  **The appropriate 7th character is to be added to each code from
    category W55:**
    A Initial encounter
    D Subsequent encounter
    S Sequela
  W55.0- Contact with cat
    W55.01x- Bitten by cat
    W55.03x- Scratched by cat
    W55.09x- Other contact with cat
  W55.1- Contact with horse
    W55.11x- Bitten by horse
    W55.12x- Struck by horse
    W55.19x- Other contact with horse
  W55.2- Contact with cow
        Contact with bull
    W55.21x- Bitten by cow
    W55.22x- Struck by cow
        Gored by bull
    W55.29x- Other contact with cow
  W55.3- Contact with other hoof stock
        Contact with goats
        Contact with sheep
    W55.31x- Bitten by other hoof stock
    W55.32x- Struck by other hoof stock
        Gored by goat
        Gored by ram
    W55.39x- Other contact with other hoof stock
  W55.4- Contact with pig
    W55.41x- Bitten by pig
    W55.42x- Struck by pig
    W55.49x- Other contact with pig
  W55.5- Contact with raccoon
    W55.51x- Bitten by raccoon
    W55.52x- Struck by raccoon
    W55.59x- Other contact with raccoon
  W55.8- Contact with other mammals
    W55.81x- Bitten by other mammals
    W55.82x- Struck by other mammals
    W55.89x- Other contact with other mammals

W56- Contact with nonvenomous marine animal
  Excludes 1: contact with venomous marine animal (T63.-)
  **The appropriate 7th character is to be added to each code from
    category W56:**
    A Initial encounter
    D Subsequent encounter
    S Sequela
  W56.0- Contact with dolphin
    W56.01x- Bitten by dolphin
    W56.02x- Struck by dolphin
    W56.09x- Other contact with dolphin
  W56.1- Contact with sea lion
    W56.11x- Bitten by sea lion
    W56.12x- Struck by sea lion
    W56.19x- Other contact with sea lion
  W56.2- Contact with orca
        Contact with killer whale
    W56.21x- Bitten by orca
    W56.22x- Struck by orca
    W56.29x- Other contact with orca

W56.3- Contact with other marine mammals
    W56.31x- Bitten by other marine mammals
    W56.32x- Struck by other marine mammals
    W56.39x- Other contact with other marine mammals
  W56.4- Contact with shark
    W56.41x- Bitten by shark
    W56.42x- Struck by shark
    W56.49x- Other contact with shark
  W56.5- Contact with other fish
    W56.51x- Bitten by other fish
    W56.52x- Struck by other fish
    W56.59x- Other contact with other fish
  W56.8- Contact with other nonvenomous marine animals
    W56.81x- Bitten by other nonvenomous marine animals
    W56.82x- Struck by other nonvenomous marine animals
    W56.89x- Other contact with other nonvenomous marine animals

W57.xxx- Bitten or stung by nonvenomous insect and other nonvenomous arthropods
  Excludes 1: contact with venomous insects and arthropods (T63.2-, T63.3-, T63.4-)
  The appropriate 7th character is to be added to code W57:
    A Initial encounter
    D Subsequent encounter
    S Sequela

W58- Contact with crocodile or alligator
  **The appropriate 7th character is to be added to each code from
    category W58:**
    A Initial encounter
    D Subsequent encounter
    S Sequela
  W58.0- Contact with alligator
    W58.01x- Bitten by alligator
    W58.02x- Struck by alligator
    W58.03x- Crushed by alligator
    W58.09x- Other contact with alligator
  W58.1- Contact with crocodile
    W58.11x- Bitten by crocodile
    W58.12x- Struck by crocodile
    W58.13x- Crushed by crocodile
    W58.19x- Other contact with crocodile

W59- Contact with other nonvenomous reptiles
  Excludes 1: contact with venomous reptile (T63.0-, T63.1-)
  **The appropriate 7th character is to be added to each code from
    category W59:**
    A Initial encounter
    D Subsequent encounter
    S Sequela
  W59.0- Contact with nonvenomous lizards
    W59.01x- Bitten by nonvenomous lizards
    W59.02x- Struck by nonvenomous lizards
    W59.09x- Other contact with nonvenomous lizards
        Exposure to nonvenomous lizards
  W59.1- Contact with nonvenomous snakes
    W59.11x- Bitten by nonvenomous snake
    W59.12x- Struck by nonvenomous snake
    W59.13x- Crushed by nonvenomous snake
    W59.19x- Other contact with nonvenomous snake
  W59.2- Contact with turtles
        Excludes 1: contact with tortoises (W59.8-)
    W59.21x- Bitten by turtle
    W59.22x- Struck by turtle
    W59.29x- Other contact with turtle
        Exposure to turtles
  W59.8- Contact with other nonvenomous reptiles
    W59.81x- Bitten by other nonvenomous reptiles
    W59.82x- Struck by other nonvenomous reptiles
    W59.83x- Crushed by other nonvenomous reptiles
    W59.89x- Other contact with other nonvenomous reptiles

W60.xxx- Contact with nonvenomous plant thorns and spines and sharp leaves
  Excludes 1: contact with venomous plants (T63.7-)
  The appropriate 7th character is to be added to code W60
    A Initial encounter
    D Subsequent encounter
    S Sequela

W
4
0
|
W
6
0

Excludes 1: = NOT CODED HERE! (Do not code both)   **875**   *Excludes* ❷: = Not Included Here

W61- **Contact with <u>birds (domestic) (wild)</u>**
     Includes: Contact with excreta of birds
     The appropriate 7th character is to be added to each code from
        category W61:
        A   <u>Initial</u> encounter
        D   <u>Subsequent</u> encounter
        S   <u>Sequela</u>
     W61.0- **Contact with <u>parrot</u>**
        W61.01x- **Bitten by parrot**
        W61.02x- **Struck by parrot**
        W61.09x- **Other contact with parrot**
           Exposure to parrots
     W61.1- **Contact with <u>macaw</u>**
        W61.11x- **Bitten by macaw**
        W61.12x- **Struck by macaw**
        W61.19x- **Other contact with macaw**
           Exposure to macaws
     W61.2- **Contact with <u>other psittacines</u>**
        W61.21x- **Bitten by other psittacines**
        W61.22x- **Struck by other psittacines**
        W61.29x- **Other contact with other psittacines**
           Exposure to other psittacines
     W61.3- **Contact with <u>chicken</u>**
        W61.32x- **Struck by chicken**
        W61.33x- **Pecked by chicken**
        W61.39x- **Other contact with chicken**
           Exposure to chickens
     W61.4- **Contact with <u>turkey</u>**
        W61.42x- **Struck by turkey**
        W61.43x- **Pecked by turkey**
        W61.49x- **Other contact with turkey**
     W61.5- **Contact with <u>goose</u>**
        W61.51x- **Bitten by goose**
        W61.52x- **Struck by goose**
        W61.59x- **Other contact with goose**
     W61.6- **Contact with <u>duck</u>**
        W61.61x- **Bitten by duck**
        W61.62x- **Struck by duck**
        W61.69x- **Other contact with duck**
     W61.9- **Contact with <u>other birds</u>**
        W61.91x- **Bitten by other birds**
        W61.92x- **Struck by other birds**
        W61.99x- **Other contact with other birds**
           Contact with bird NOS
W62- **Contact with <u>nonvenomous amphibians</u>**
     Excludes 1:   contact with venomous amphibians (T63.81-R63.83)
     The appropriate 7th character is to be added to each code from
        category W62:
        A   <u>Initial</u> encounter
        D   <u>Subsequent</u> encounter
        S   <u>Sequela</u>
     W62.0xx- **Contact with nonvenomous frogs**
     W62.1xx- **Contact with nonvenomous toads**
     W62.9xx- **Contact with other nonvenomous amphibians**
W64.xxx- **<u>Exposure to other animate mechanical forces</u>**
     Includes: Exposure to nonvenomous animal NOS
     Excludes 1:   contact with venomous animal (T63.-)
     The appropriate 7th character is to be added to code W64:
        A   <u>Initial</u> encounter
        D   <u>Subsequent</u> encounter
        S   <u>Sequela</u>

Accidental non-transport drowning and submersion (W65-W74)

Excludes 1:   accidental drowning and submersion due to fall into water
        (W16.-)
        accidental drowning and submersion due to water transport
        accident (V90.-, V92.-)
Excludes❷: accidental drowning and submersion due to cataclysm (X34-
        X39)

W65.xxx- **<u>Accidental drowning and submersion while in bath-tub</u>**
     Excludes 1:   accidental drowning and submersion due to fall in
        (into) bathtub (W16.211)
     The appropriate 7th character is to be added to code W65:
        A   <u>Initial</u> encounter
        D   <u>Subsequent</u> encounter
        S   <u>Sequela</u>
W67.xxx- **<u>Accidental drowning and submersion while in swimming-pool</u>**
     Excludes 1:   accidental drowning and submersion due to fall into
        swimming pool (W16.011, W16.021, W16.031)
        accidental drowning and submersion due to striking
        into wall of swimming pool (W22.041)
     The appropriate 7th character is to be added to code W67:
        A   <u>Initial</u> encounter
        D   <u>Subsequent</u> encounter
        S   <u>Sequela</u>
W69.xxx- **<u>Accidental drowning and submersion while in natural water</u>**
     Accidental drowning and submersion while in lake
     Accidental drowning and submersion while in open sea
     Accidental drowning and submersion while in river
     Accidental drowning and submersion while in stream
     Excludes 1:   accidental drowning and submersion due to fall into
        natural body of water (W16.111, W16.121,
        W16.131)
     The appropriate 7th character is to be added to code W69:
        A   <u>Initial</u> encounter
        D   <u>Subsequent</u> encounter
        S   <u>Sequela</u>
W73.xxx- **<u>Other specified cause of accidental non-transport drowning and</u>**
<u>submersion</u>
     Accidental drowning and submersion while in quenching tank
     Accidental drowning and submersion while in reservoir
     Excludes 1:   accidental drowning and submersion due to fall into
        other water (W16.311, W16.321, W16.331)
     The appropriate 7th character is to be added to code W73:
        A   <u>Initial</u> encounter
        D   <u>Subsequent</u> encounter
        S   <u>Sequela</u>
W74.xxx- **<u>Unspecified cause of accidental drowning and submersion</u>**
     Drowning NOS
     The appropriate 7th character is to be added to code W74:
        A   <u>Initial</u> encounter
        D   <u>Subsequent</u> encounter
        S   <u>Sequela</u>

W
6
1
-
X
0
0

Excludes 1: = NOT CODED HERE! (Do not code both)   **876**   *Excludes❷:* = Not Included Here

Exposure to electric current, radiation and extreme ambient air temperature and pressure (W85-W99)

Excludes 1:   exposure to:
lightning (T75.0-)
natural cold (X31)
natural heat (X30)
natural radiation NOS (X39)
radiological procedure and radiotherapy (Y84.2)
sunlight (X32)
failure in dosage of radiation or temperature during surgical and medical care (Y63.2-Y63.5)

W85.xxx-   Exposure to <u>electric transmission lines</u>
Broken power line
The appropriate 7th character is to be added to code W85:
A   <u>Initial</u> encounter
D   <u>Subsequent</u> encounter
S   <u>Sequela</u>

W86- Exposure to other specified electric current
The appropriate 7th character is to be added to each code from category W86:
A   <u>Initial</u> encounter
D   <u>Subsequent</u> encounter
S   <u>Sequela</u>

W86.0xx- Exposure to <u>domestic wiring and appliances</u>
W86.1xx- Exposure to <u>industrial wiring, appliances and electrical machinery</u>
Exposure to conductors
Exposure to control apparatus
Exposure to electrical equipment and machinery
Exposure to transformers

W86.8xx- Exposure to <u>other electric current</u>
Exposure to wiring and appliances in or on farm (not farmhouse)
Exposure to wiring and appliances outdoors
Exposure to wiring and appliances in or on public building
Exposure to wiring and appliances in or on residential institutions
Exposure to wiring and appliances in or on schools

W88- Exposure to <u>ionizing radiation</u>
Excludes 1: exposure to sunlight (X32)
The appropriate 7th character is to be added to each code from category W88:
A   <u>Initial</u> encounter
D   <u>Subsequent</u> encounter
S   <u>Sequela</u>

W88.0xx- Exposure to X-rays
W88.1xx- Exposure to radioactive isotopes
W88.8xx- Exposure to other ionizing radiation

W89- Exposure to <u>man-made visible and ultraviolet light</u>
Includes: Exposure to welding light (arc)
Excludes❷: exposure to sunlight (X32)
The appropriate 7th character is to be added to each code from category W89:
A   <u>Initial</u> encounter
D   <u>Subsequent</u> encounter
S   <u>Sequela</u>

W89.0xx- Exposure to <u>welding light (arc)</u>
W89.1xx- Exposure to <u>tanning bed</u>
W89.8xx- Exposure to <u>other</u> man-made visible and ultraviolet light
W89.9xx- Exposure to <u>unspecified</u> man-made visible and ultraviolet light

W90- Exposure to <u>other nonionizing radiation</u>
Excludes 1: exposure to sunlight (X32)
The appropriate 7th character is to be added to each code from category W90:
A   <u>Initial</u> encounter
D   <u>Subsequent</u> encounter
S   <u>Sequela</u>

W90.0xx- Exposure to radiofrequency
W90.1xx- Exposure to infrared radiation
W90.2xx- Exposure to laser radiation
W90.8xx- Exposure to other nonionizing radiation

W92.xxx-   Exposure to <u>excessive heat of man-made origin</u>
The appropriate 7th character is to be added to code W92:
A   <u>Initial</u> encounter
D   <u>Subsequent</u> encounter
S   <u>Sequela</u>

W93- Exposure to <u>excessive cold of man-made origin</u>
The appropriate 7th character is to be added to each code from category W93:
A   <u>Initial</u> encounter
D   <u>Subsequent</u> encounter
S   <u>Sequela</u>

W93.0- Contact with or inhalation of <u>dry ice</u>
W93.01x- Contact with dry ice
W93.02x- Inhalation of dry ice
W93.1- Contact with or inhalation of <u>liquid air</u>
W93.11x- <u>Contact</u> with liquid air
Contact with liquid hydrogen
Contact with liquid nitrogen
W93.12x- <u>Inhalation</u> of liquid air
Inhalation of liquid hydrogen
Inhalation of liquid nitrogen
W93.2xx- Prolonged exposure in <u>deep freeze unit or refrigerator</u>
W93.8xx- Exposure to other excessive cold of man-made origin

W94- Exposure to <u>high and low air pressure and changes in air pressure</u>
The appropriate 7th character is to be added to each code from category W94:
A   <u>Initial</u> encounter
D   <u>Subsequent</u> encounter
S   <u>Sequela</u>

W94.0xx- Exposure to prolonged high air pressure
W94.1- Exposure to prolonged low air pressure
W94.11x- Exposure to residence or prolonged visit at high altitude
W94.12x- Exposure to other prolonged low air pressure
W94.2- Exposure to rapid changes in air pressure during ascent
W94.21x- Exposure to reduction in atmospheric pressure while surfacing from deep-water diving
W94.22x- Exposure to reduction in atmospheric pressure while surfacing from underground
W94.23x- Exposure to sudden change in air pressure in aircraft during ascent
W94.29x- Exposure to other rapid changes in air pressure during ascent
W94.3- Exposure to rapid changes in air pressure during descent
W94.31x- Exposure to sudden change in air pressure in aircraft during descent
W94.32x- Exposure to high air pressure from rapid descent in water
W94.39x- Exposure to other rapid changes in air pressure during descent

W99.xxx-   Exposure to other man-made environmental factors
The appropriate 7th character is to be added to code W99:
A   <u>Initial</u> encounter
D   <u>Subsequent</u> encounter
S   <u>Sequela</u>

Exposure to smoke, fire and flames (X00-X08)

Excludes 1:   arson (X97)
Excludes❷: explosions (W35-W40)
lightning (T75.0-)
transport accident (V01-V99)

X00- Exposure to <u>uncontrolled fire</u> in <u>building or structure</u>
Includes: Conflagration in building or structure
Code first any associated cataclysm
Excludes❷: exposure to ignition or melting of nightwear (X05)
exposure to ignition or melting of other clothing and apparel (X06.-)
exposure to other specified smoke, fire and flames (X08.-)
The appropriate 7th character is to be added to each code from category X00:
A   <u>Initial</u> encounter
D   <u>Subsequent</u> encounter
S   <u>Sequela</u>

X00.0xx- Exposure to <u>flames</u> in uncontrolled fire in building or structure
X00.1xx- Exposure to <u>smoke</u> in uncontrolled fire in building or structure
X00.2xx- Injury due to <u>collapse</u> of burning building or structure in uncontrolled fire
Excludes 1: injury due to collapse of building not on fire (W20.1)
X00.3xx- <u>Fall</u> from burning building or structure in uncontrolled fire
X00.4xx- <u>Hit by object</u> from burning building or structure in uncontrolled fire
X00.5xx- <u>Jump</u> from burning building or structure in uncontrolled fire
X00.8xx- <u>Other</u> exposure to uncontrolled fire in building or structure

W
6
1
I
X
0
0

X01- Exposure to <u>uncontrolled fire</u>, <u>not in</u> building or structure
Includes: Exposure to forest fire
The appropriate 7th character is to be added to each code from category X01:
A <u>Initial</u> encounter
D <u>Subsequent</u> encounter
S <u>Sequela</u>

X01.0xx- Exposure to <u>flames</u> in uncontrolled fire, not in building or structure

X01.1xx- Exposure to <u>smoke</u> in uncontrolled fire, not in building or structure

X01.3xx- <u>Fall</u> due to uncontrolled fire, not in building or structure

X01.4xx- <u>Hit</u> by object due to uncontrolled fire, not in building or structure

X01.8xx- <u>Other</u> exposure to uncontrolled fire, not in building or structure

X02- Exposure to <u>controlled fire</u> in <u>building or structure</u>
Includes: Exposure to fire in fireplace
Exposure to fire in stove
The appropriate 7th character is to be added to each code from category X02:
A <u>Initial</u> encounter
D <u>Subsequent</u> encounter
S <u>Sequela</u>

X02.0xx- Exposure to <u>flames</u> in controlled fire in building or structure

X02.1xx- Exposure to <u>smoke</u> in controlled fire in building or structure

X02.2xx- Injury due to <u>collapse</u> of burning building or structure in controlled fire
Excludes 1: injury due to collapse of building not on fire (W20.1)

X02.3xx- <u>Fall</u> from burning building or structure in controlled fire

X02.4xx- <u>Hit by object</u> from burning building or structure in controlled fire

X02.5xx- <u>Jump</u> from burning building or structure in controlled fire

X02.8xx- <u>Other</u> exposure to controlled fire in building or structure

X03- Exposure to <u>controlled fire</u>, <u>not in</u> building or structure
Includes: Exposure to bon fire
Exposure to camp-fire
Exposure to trash fire
The appropriate 7th character is to be added to each code from category X03:
A <u>Initial</u> encounter
D <u>Subsequent</u> encounter
S <u>Sequela</u>

X03.0xx- Exposure to <u>flames</u> in controlled fire, not in building or structure

X03.1xx- Exposure to <u>smoke</u> in controlled fire, not in building or structure

X03.3xx- <u>Fall</u> due to controlled fire, not in building or structure

X03.4xx- <u>Hit by object</u> due to controlled fire, not in building or structure

X03.8xx- <u>Other</u> exposure to controlled fire, not in building or structure

X04.xxx- Exposure to ignition of highly flammable material
Includes: Exposure to ignition of gasoline
Exposure to ignition of kerosene
Exposure to ignition of petrol
Excludes❷: exposure to ignition or melting of nightwear (X05)
exposure to ignition or melting of other clothing and apparel (X06)
The appropriate 7th character is to be added to code X04:
A <u>Initial</u> encounter
D <u>Subsequent</u> encounter
S <u>Sequela</u>

X05.xxx- Exposure to <u>ignition or melting of nightwear</u>
Excludes❷: exposure to uncontrolled fire in building or structure (X00.-)
exposure to uncontrolled fire, not in building or structure (X01.-)
exposure to controlled fire in building or structure (X02.-)
exposure to controlled fire, not in building or structure (X03.-)
exposure to ignition of highly flammable materials (X04.-)
The appropriate 7th character is to be added to code X05:
A <u>Initial</u> encounter
D <u>Subsequent</u> encounter
S <u>Sequela</u>

X06- Exposure to <u>ignition or melting of other clothing and apparel</u>
Excludes❷: exposure to uncontrolled fire in building or structure (X00.-)
exposure to uncontrolled fire, not in building or structure (X01.-)
exposure to controlled fire in building or structure (X02.-)
exposure to controlled fire, not in building or structure (X03.-)
exposure to ignition of highly flammable materials (X04.-)
The appropriate 7th character is to be added to each code from category X06:
A <u>Initial</u> encounter
D <u>Subsequent</u> encounter
S <u>Sequela</u>

X06.0xx- Exposure to ignition of plastic jewelry

X06.1xx- Exposure to melting of plastic jewelry

X06.2xx- Exposure to ignition of other clothing and apparel

X06.3xx- Exposure to melting of other clothing and apparel

X08- Exposure to <u>other specified smoke, fire and flames</u>
The appropriate 7th character is to be added to each code from category X08:
A <u>Initial</u> encounter
D <u>Subsequent</u> encounter
S <u>Sequela</u>

X08.0- Exposure to <u>bed fire</u>
Exposure to mattress fire

X08.00x- Exposure to bed fire due to unspecified burning material

X08.01x- Exposure to bed fire due to burning cigarette

X08.09x- Exposure to bed fire due to other burning material

X08.1- Exposure to <u>sofa fire</u>

X08.10x- Exposure to sofa fire due to unspecified burning material

X08.11x- Exposure to sofa fire due to burning cigarette

X08.19x- Exposure to sofa fire due to other burning material

X08.2- Exposure to <u>other furniture fire</u>

X08.20x- Exposure to other furniture fire due to unspecified burning material

X08.21x- Exposure to other furniture fire due to burning cigarette

X08.29x- Exposure to other furniture fire due to other burning material

X08.8xx- Exposure to <u>other specified smoke, fire and flames</u>

Contact with heat and hot substances (X10-X19)

Excludes 1: exposure to excessive natural heat (X30)
exposure to fire and flames (X00-X09)

X10- Contact with <u>hot drinks, food, fats and cooking oils</u>
The appropriate 7th character is to be added to each code from category X10:
A <u>Initial</u> encounter
D <u>Subsequent</u> encounter
S <u>Sequela</u>

X10.0xx- Contact with hot drinks

X10.1xx- Contact with hot food

X10.2xx- Contact with fats and cooking oils

X11- Contact with <u>hot tap-water</u>
Includes: Contact with boiling tap-water
Contact with boiling water NOS
Excludes 1: contact with water heated on stove (X12)
The appropriate 7th character is to be added to each code from category X11:
A <u>Initial</u> encounter
D <u>Subsequent</u> encounter
S <u>Sequela</u>

X11.0xx- Contact with hot water in bath or tub
Excludes 1: contact with running hot water in bath or tub (X11.1)

X11.1xx- Contact with running hot water
Contact with hot water running out of hose
Contact with hot water running out of tap

X11.8xx- Contact with other hot tap-water
Contact with hot water in bucket
Contact with hot tap-water NOS

X12.xxx- Contact with <u>other hot fluids</u>
Contact with water heated on stove
Excludes 1: hot (liquid) metals (X18)
The appropriate 7th character is to be added to code X12:
A <u>Initial</u> encounter
D <u>Subsequent</u> encounter
S <u>Sequela</u>

Excludes 1: = NOT CODED HERE! (Do not code both)

Excludes❷: = Not Included Here

X01-X37

X13-   Contact with <u>steam and other hot vapors</u>
   The appropriate 7th character is to be added to each code from
      category X13:
   A   <u>Initial</u> encounter
   D   <u>Subsequent</u> encounter
   S   <u>Sequela</u>
   X13.0xx-   Inhalation of steam and other hot vapors
   X13.1xx-   Other contact with steam and other hot vapors

X14-   Contact with <u>hot air and other hot gases</u>
   The appropriate 7th character is to be added to each code from
      category X14:
   A   <u>Initial</u> encounter
   D   <u>Subsequent</u> encounter
   S   <u>Sequela</u>
   X14.0xx-   Inhalation of hot air and gases
   X14.1xx-   Other contact with hot air and other hot gases

X15-   Contact with <u>hot household appliances</u>
   Excludes 1:   contact with heating appliances (X16)
      contact with powered household appliances (W29.-)
      exposure to controlled fire in building or structure due to
         household appliance (X02.8)
      exposure to household appliances electrical current (W86.0)
   The appropriate 7th character is to be added to each code from
      category X15:
   A   <u>Initial</u> encounter
   D   <u>Subsequent</u> encounter
   S   <u>Sequela</u>
   X15.0xx-   Contact with hot stove (kitchen)
   X15.1xx-   Contact with hot toaster
   X15.2xx-   Contact with hotplate
   X15.3xx-   Contact with hot saucepan or skillet
   X15.8xx-   Contact with other hot household appliances
      Contact with cooker
      Contact with kettle
      Contact with light bulbs

X16.xxx-   Contact with <u>hot heating appliances, radiators and pipes</u>
   Excludes 1:   contact with powered appliances (W29.-)
      exposure to controlled fire in building or structure due
         to appliance (X02.8)
      exposure to industrial appliances electrical current
         (W86.1)
   The appropriate 7th character is to be added to code X16:
   A   <u>Initial</u> encounter
   D   <u>Subsequent</u> encounter
   S   <u>Sequela</u>

X17.xxx-   Contact with <u>hot engines, machinery and tools</u>
   Excludes 1:   contact with hot heating appliances, radiators and
         pipes (X16)
      contact with hot household appliances (X15)
   The appropriate 7th character is to be added to code X17:
   A   <u>Initial</u> encounter
   D   <u>Subsequent</u> encounter
   S   <u>Sequela</u>

X18.xxx-   Contact with <u>other hot metals</u>
      Contact with liquid metal
   The appropriate 7th character is to be added to code X18:
   A   <u>Initial</u> encounter
   D   <u>Subsequent</u> encounter
   S   <u>Sequela</u>

X19.xxx-   Contact with <u>other heat and hot substances</u>
   Excludes 1:   objects that are not normally hot, e.g., an object made
         hot by a house fire (X00-X09)
   The appropriate 7th character is to be added to code X19:
   A   <u>Initial</u> encounter
   D   <u>Subsequent</u> encounter
   S   <u>Sequela</u>

Exposure to forces of nature (X30-X39)

X30.xxx-   Exposure to <u>excessive natural heat</u>
      Exposure to excessive heat as the cause of sunstroke
      Exposure to heat NOS
   Excludes 1:   excessive heat of man-made origin (W92)
      exposure to man-made radiation (W89)
      exposure to sunlight (X32)
      exposure to tanning bed (W89)
   The appropriate 7th character is to be added to code X30:
   A   <u>Initial</u> encounter
   D   <u>Subsequent</u> encounter
   S   <u>Sequela</u>

X31.xxx-   Exposure to <u>excessive natural cold</u>
      Excessive cold as the cause of chilblains NOS
      Excessive cold as the cause of immersion foot or hand
      Exposure to cold NOS
      Exposure to weather conditions
   Excludes 1:   cold of man-made origin (W93.-)
      contact with or inhalation of dry ice (W93.-)
      contact with or inhalation of liquefied gas (W93.-)
   The appropriate 7th character is to be added to code X31:
   A   <u>Initial</u> encounter
   D   <u>Subsequent</u> encounter
   S   <u>Sequela</u>

X32.xxx-   Exposure to <u>sunlight</u>
   Excludes 1:   radiation-related disorders of the skin and
         subcutaneous tissue (L55-L59)
      man-made radiation (tanning bed) (W89)
   The appropriate 7th character is to be added to code X32:
   A   <u>Initial</u> encounter
   D   <u>Subsequent</u> encounter
   S   <u>Sequela</u>

X34.xxx-   Earthquake❷
   Excludes❷: tidal wave (tsunami) due to earthquake (X37.41)
   The appropriate 7th character is to be added to code X34:
   A   <u>Initial</u> encounter
   D   <u>Subsequent</u> encounter
   S   <u>Sequela</u>

X35.xxx-   Volcanic eruption
   Excludes❷: tidal wave (tsunami) due to volcanic eruption (X37.41)
   The appropriate 7th character is to be added to code X35:
   A   <u>Initial</u> encounter
   D   <u>Subsequent</u> encounter
   S   <u>Sequela</u>

X36-   Avalanche, landslide and other earth movements
   Includes: Victim of mudslide of cataclysmic nature
   Excludes 1:   earthquake (X34)
   Excludes❷: transport accident involving collision with avalanche or
         landslide not in motion (V01-V99)
   The appropriate 7th character is to be added to each code from
      category X36:
   A   <u>Initial</u> encounter
   D   <u>Subsequent</u> encounter
   S   <u>Sequela</u>
   X36.0xx-   Collapse of dam or man-made structure causing earth
      movement
   X36.1xx-   Avalanche, landslide, or mudslide

X37-   Cataclysmic storm
   The appropriate 7th character is to be added to each code from
      category X37:
   A   <u>Initial</u> encounter
   D   <u>Subsequent</u> encounter
   S   <u>Sequela</u>
   X37.0xx-   Hurricane
      Storm surge
      Typhoon
   X37.1xx-   Tornado
      Cyclone
      Twister
   X37.2xx-   Blizzard (snow)(ice)
   X37.3xx-   Dust storm
   X37.4-   Tidalwave
      X37.41x-   Tidal wave due to earthquake or volcanic eruption
         Tidal wave NOS
         Tsunami
      X37.42x-   Tidal wave due to storm
      X37.43x-   Tidal wave due to landslide
   X37.8xx-   Other cataclysmic storms
      Cloudburst
      Torrential rain
      Excludes❷: flood (X38)
   X37.9xx-   Unspecified cataclysmic storm
      Storm NOS
      Excludes 1:   collapse of dam or man-made structure causing earth
         movement (X39.0)

X 0 1 - X 3 7

Excludes 1: = NOT CODED HERE! (Do not code both)   *Excludes❷:* = Not Included Here

X38.xxx- **Flood**
Flood arising from remote storm
Flood of cataclysmic nature arising from melting snow
Flood resulting directly from storm
Excludes 1: collapse of dam or man-made structure causing earth movement (X39.0)
tidal wave NOS (X37.41)
tidal wave caused by storm (X37.2)
The appropriate 7th character is to be added to code X38:
A **Initial** encounter
D **Subsequent** encounter
S **Sequela**

X39- Exposure to <u>other forces of nature</u>
The appropriate 7th character is to be added to each code from category X39:
A **Initial** encounter
D **Subsequent** encounter
S **Sequela**
X39.0- Exposure to natural radiation
Excludes 1: contact with and (suspected) exposure to radon and other naturally occuring radiation (Z77.122)
exposure to man-made radiation (W88-W90)
exposure to sunlight (X32)
X39.01x- **Exposure to radon**
X39.08x- **Exposure to other natural radiation**
X39.8xx- Other exposure to forces of nature

Accidental exposure to other specified factors (X52-X58)

X52.xxx- **Prolonged stay in weightless environment**
Weightlessness in spacecraft (simulator)
The appropriate 7th character is to be added to code X52:
A **Initial** encounter
D **Subsequent** encounter
S **Sequela**

X58.xxx- **Exposure to other specified factors**
Accident NOS
Exposure NOS
The appropriate 7th character is to be added to code X58:
A **Initial** encounter
D **Subsequent** encounter
S **Sequela**

Intentional self-harm (X71-X83)

Purposely self-inflicted injury
Suicide (attempted)

X71- <u>Intentional self-harm</u> by <u>drowning and submersion</u>
The appropriate 7th character is to be added to each code from category X71:
A **Initial** encounter
D **Subsequent** encounter
S **Sequela**
X71.0xx- Intentional self-harm by drowning and submersion while in <u>bathtub</u>
X71.1xx- Intentional self-harm by drowning and submersion <u>while in swimming pool</u>
X71.2xx- Intentional self-harm by drowning and submersion after <u>jump into swimming pool</u>
X71.3xx- Intentional self-harm by drowning and submersion in <u>natural water</u>
X71.8xx- <u>Other</u> intentional self-harm by drowning and submersion
X71.9xx- Intentional self-harm by drowning and submersion, <u>unspecified</u>

X72xxx- <u>Intentional self-harm</u> by <u>handgun discharge</u>
Intentional self-harm by gun for single hand use
Intentional self-harm by pistol
Intentional self-harm by revolver
Excludes 1: Very pistol (X74.8)
The appropriate 7th character is to be added to code X72:
A **Initial** encounter
D **Subsequent** encounter
S **Sequela**

X73- <u>Intentional self-harm</u> by <u>rifle, shotgun and larger firearm discharge</u>
Excludes 1: airgun (X74.01)
The appropriate 7th character is to be added to each code from category X73:
A **Initial** encounter
D **Subsequent** encounter
S **Sequela**
X73.0xx- Intentional self-harm by shotgun discharge
X73.1xx- Intentional self-harm by hunting rifle discharge
X73.2xx- Intentional self-harm by machine gun discharge
X73.8xx- Intentional self-harm by other larger firearm discharge
X73.9xx- Intentional self-harm by unspecified larger firearm discharge

X74- <u>Intentional self-harm</u> by <u>other and unspecified firearm and gun discharge</u>
The appropriate 7th character is to be added to each code from category X74:
A **Initial** encounter
D **Subsequent** encounter
S **Sequela**
X74.0- Intentional self-harm by gas, air or spring-operated guns
X74.01x- **Intentional self-harm by airgun**
Intentional self-harm by BB gun discharge
Intentional self-harm by pellet gun discharge
X74.02x- **Intentional self-harm by paintball gun**
X74.09x- **Intentional self-harm by other gas, air or spring-operated gun**
X74.8xx- Intentional self-harm by other firearm discharge
Intentional self-harm by Very pistol [flare] discharge
X74.9xx- Intentional self-harm by unspecified firearm discharge

X75.xxx- <u>Intentional self-harm</u> by <u>explosive material</u>
The appropriate 7th character is to be added to code X75:
A **Initial** encounter
D **Subsequent** encounter
S **Sequela**

X76.xxx- <u>Intentional self-harm</u> by <u>smoke, fire and flames</u>
The appropriate 7th character is to be added to code X76:
A **Initial** encounter
D **Subsequent** encounter
S **Sequela**

Excludes 1: = NOT CODED HERE! (Do not code both)

Excludes ❷: = Not Included Here

X77- Intentional self-harm by steam, hot vapors and hot objects
The appropriate 7th character is to be added to each code from category X77:
A   Initial encounter
D   Subsequent encounter
S   Sequela

X77.0xx- Intentional self-harm by steam or hot vapors
X77.1xx- Intentional self-harm by hot tap water
X77.2xx- Intentional self-harm by other hot fluids
X77.3xx- Intentional self-harm by hot household appliances
X77.8xx- Intentional self-harm by other hot objects
X77.9xx- Intentional self-harm by unspecified hot objects

X78- Intentional self-harm by sharp object
The appropriate 7th character is to be added to each code from category X78:
A   Initial encounter
D   Subsequent encounter
S   Sequela

X78.0xx- Intentional self-harm by sharp glass
X78.1xx- Intentional self-harm by knife
X78.2xx- Intentional self-harm by sword or dagger
X78.8xx- Intentional self-harm by other sharp object
X78.9xx- Intentional self-harm by unspecified sharp object

X79.xxx- Intentional self-harm by blunt object
The appropriate 7th character is to be added to code X79:
A   Initial encounter
D   Subsequent encounter
S   Sequela

X80.xxx- Intentional self-harm by jumping from a high place
Intentional fall from one level to another
The appropriate 7th character is to be added to code X80:
A   Initial encounter
D   Subsequent encounter
S   Sequela

X81- Intentional self-harm by jumping or lying in front of moving object
The appropriate 7th character is to be added to each code from category X81:
A   Initial encounter
D   Subsequent encounter
S   Sequela

X81.0xx- Intentional self-harm by jumping or lying in front of motor vehicle
X81.1xx- Intentional self-harm by jumping or lying in front of (subway) train
X81.8xx- Intentional self-harm by jumping or lying in front of other moving object

X82- Intentional self-harm by crashing of motor vehicle
The appropriate 7th character is to be added to each code from category X82:
A   Initial encounter
D   Subsequent encounter
S   Sequela

X82.0xx- Intentional collision of motor vehicle with other motor vehicle
X82.1xx- Intentional collision of motor vehicle with train
X82.2xx- Intentional collision of motor vehicle with tree
X82.8xx- Other intentional self-harm by crashing of motor vehicle

X83- Intentional self-harm by other specified means
Excludes 1: intentional self-harm by poisoning or contact with toxic substance — see Table of Drugs and Chemicals
The appropriate 7th character is to be added to each code from category X83:
A   Initial encounter
D   Subsequent encounter
S   Sequela

X83.0xx- Intentional self-harm by crashing of aircraft
X83.1xx- Intentional self-harm by electrocution
X83.2xx- Intentional self-harm by exposure to extremes of cold
X83.8xx- Intentional self-harm by other specified means

Assault (X92-Y09)

Includes: Homicide
Injuries inflicted by another person with intent to injure or kill, by any means
*Excludes 1: injuries due to legal intervention (Y35.-)
injuries due to operations of war (Y36.-)
injuries due to terrorism (Y38.-)*

X92- Assault by drowning and submersion
The appropriate 7th character is to be added to each code from category X92:
A   Initial encounter
D   Subsequent encounter
S   Sequela

X92.0xx- Assault by drowning and submersion while in bathtub
X92.1xx- Assault by drowning and submersion while in swimming pool
X92.2xx- Assault by drowning and submersion after push into swimming pool
X92.3xx- Assault by drowning and submersion in natural water
X92.8xx- Other assault by drowning and submersion
X92.9xx- Assault by drowning and submersion, unspecified

X93.xxx- Assault by handgun discharge
Assault by discharge of gun for single hand use
Assault by discharge of pistol
Assault by discharge of revolver
Excludes 1: Very pistol (X95.8)
The appropriate 7th character is to be added to code X93:
A   Initial encounter
D   Subsequent encounter
S   Sequela

X94- Assault by rifle, shotgun and larger firearm discharge
Excludes 1: airgun (X95.01)
The appropriate 7th character is to be added to each code from category X94:
A   Initial encounter
D   Subsequent encounter
S   Sequela

X94.0xx- Assault by shotgun
X94.1xx- Assault by hunting rifle
X94.2xx- Assault by machine gun
X94.8xx- Assault by other larger firearm discharge
X94.9xx- Assault by unspecified larger firearm discharge

X95- Assault by other and unspecified firearm and gun discharge
The appropriate 7th character is to be added to each code from category X95:
A   Initial encounter
D   Subsequent encounter
S   Sequela

X95.0- Assault by gas, air or spring-operated guns
X95.01x- Assault by airgun discharge
Assault by BB gun discharge
Assault by pellet gun discharge
X95.02x- Assault by paintball gun discharge
X95.09x- Assault by other gas, air or spring-operated gun
X95.8xx- Assault by other firearm discharge
Assault by very pistol [flare] discharge
X95.9xx- Assault by unspecified firearm discharge

X96- Assault by explosive material
*Excludes 1: incendiary device (X97)
terrorism involving explosive material (Y38.2-)*
The appropriate 7th character is to be added to each code from category X96:
A   Initial encounter
D   Subsequent encounter
S   Sequela

X96.0xx- Assault by antipersonnel bomb
Excludes 1: antipersonnel bomb use in military or war (Y36.2-)
X96.1xx- Assault by gasoline bomb
X96.2xx- Assault by letter bomb
X96.3xx- Assault by fertilizer bomb
X96.4xx- Assault by pipe bomb
X96.8xx- Assault by other specified explosive
X96.9xx- Assault by unspecified explosive

X38 - X96

X97.xxx- **Assault** by <u>smoke, fire and flames</u>
Assault by arson
Assault by cigarettes
Assault by incendiary device
The appropriate 7th character is to be added to code X97:
  A   <u>Initial</u> encounter
  D   <u>Subsequent</u> encounter
  S   <u>Sequela</u>

X98- **Assault** by <u>steam, hot vapors and hot objects</u>
The appropriate 7th character is to be added to each code from category X98:
  A   <u>Initial</u> encounter
  D   <u>Subsequent</u> encounter
  S   <u>Sequela</u>
  X98.0xx- Assault by steam or hot vapors
  X98.1xx- Assault by hot tap water
  X98.2xx- Assault by hot fluids
  X98.3xx- Assault by hot household appliances
  X98.8xx- Assault by other hot objects
  X98.9xx- Assault by unspecified hot objects

X99- **Assault** by <u>sharp object</u>
Excludes 1: assault by strike by sports equipment (Y08.0-)
The appropriate 7th character is to be added to each code from category X99:
  A   <u>Initial</u> encounter
  D   <u>Subsequent</u> encounter
  S   <u>Sequela</u>
  X99.0xx- Assault by sharp glass
  X99.1xx- Assault by knife
  X99.2xx- Assault by sword or dagger
  X99.8xx- Assault by other sharp object
  X99.9xx- Assault by unspecified sharp object
         Assault by stabbing NOS

Y00.xxx- **Assault** by <u>blunt object</u>
Excludes 1: assault by strike by sports equipment (Y08.0-)
The appropriate 7th character is to be added to code Y00:
  A   <u>Initial</u> encounter
  D   <u>Subsequent</u> encounter
  S   <u>Sequela</u>

Y01.xxx- **Assault** by <u>pushing from high place</u>
The appropriate 7th character is to be added to code Y01:
  A   <u>Initial</u> encounter
  D   <u>Subsequent</u> encounter
  S   <u>Sequela</u>

Y02- **Assault** by <u>pushing or placing victim in front of moving object</u>
The appropriate 7th character is to be added to each code from category Y02:
  A   <u>Initial</u> encounter
  D   <u>Subsequent</u> encounter
  S   <u>Sequela</u>
  Y02.0xx- Assault by pushing or placing victim in front of motor vehicle
  Y02.1xx- Assault by pushing or placing victim in front of (subway) train
  Y02.8xx- Assault by pushing or placing victim in front of other moving object

Y03- **Assault** by <u>crashing of motor vehicle</u>
The appropriate 7th character is to be added to each code from category Y03:
  A   <u>Initial</u> encounter
  D   <u>Subsequent</u> encounter
  S   <u>Sequela</u>
  Y03.0xx- Assault by being hit or run over by motor vehicle
  Y03.8xx- Other assault by crashing of motor vehicle

Y04- **Assault** by <u>bodily force</u>
Excludes 1: assault by:
       submersion (X92.-)
       use of weapon (X93-X95, X99, Y00)
The appropriate 7th character is to be added to each code from category Y04:
  A   <u>Initial</u> encounter
  D   <u>Subsequent</u> encounter
  S   <u>Sequela</u>
  Y04.0xx- Assault by unarmed brawl or fight
  Y04.1xx- Assault by human bite
  Y04.2xx- Assault by strike against or bumped into by another person
  Y04.8xx- Assault by other bodily force
         Assault by bodily force NOS

Y07- **Perpetrator** of <u>assault, maltreatment and neglect</u>
Note: Codes from this category are for use only in cases of confirmed abuse (T74-)
Note: Selection of the correct perpetrator code is based on the relationship between the perpetrator and the victim
Includes: Perpetrator of abandonment
           Perpetrator of emotional neglect
           Perpetrator of mental cruelty
           Perpetrator of physical abuse
           Perpetrator of physical neglect
           Perpetrator of sexual abuse
           Perpetrator of torture

Y07.0- <u>Spouse or partner</u>, perpetrator of maltreatment and neglect
       Spouse or partner, perpetrator of maltreatment and neglect against spouse or partner
  Y07.01 Husband, perpetrator of maltreatment and neglect
  Y07.02 Wife, perpetrator of maltreatment and neglect
  Y07.03 Male partner, perpetrator of maltreatment and neglect
  Y07.04 Female partner, perpetrator of maltreatment and neglect

Y07.1- <u>Parent</u> (adoptive) (biological), perpetrator of maltreatment and neglect
  Y07.11 Biological father, perpetrator of maltreatment and neglect
  Y07.12 Biological mother, perpetrator of maltreatment and neglect
  Y07.13 Adoptive father, perpetrator of maltreatment and neglect
  Y07.14 Adoptive mother, perpetrator of maltreatment and neglect

Y07.4- <u>Other family member</u>, perpetrator of maltreatment and neglect
  Y07.41- <u>Sibling</u>, perpetrator of maltreatment and neglect
     Excludes 1: stepsibling, perpetrator of maltreatment and neglect (Y07.435, Y07.436)
     Y07.410 Brother, perpetrator of maltreatment and neglect
     Y07.411 Sister, perpetrator of maltreatment and neglect
  Y07.42- <u>Foster parent</u>, perpetrator of maltreatment and neglect
     Y07.420 Foster father, perpetrator of maltreatment and neglect
     Y07.421 Foster mother, perpetrator of maltreatment and neglect

  Y07.43- <u>Stepparent or stepsibling</u>, perpetrator of maltreatment and neglect
     Y07.430 Stepfather, perpetrator of maltreatment and neglect
     Y07.432 Male friend of parent (co-residing in household), perpetrator of maltreatment and neglect
     Y07.433 Stepmother, perpetrator of maltreatment and neglect
     Y07.434 Female friend of parent (co-residing in household), perpetrator of maltreatment and neglect
     Y07.435 Stepbrother, perpetrator of maltreatment and neglect
     Y07.436 Stepsister, perpetrator or maltreatment and neglect
  Y07.49- <u>Other family member</u>, perpetrator of maltreatment and neglect
     Y07.490 Male cousin, perpetrator of maltreatment and neglect
     Y07.491 Female cousin, perpetrator of maltreatment and neglect
     Y07.499 Other family member, perpetrator of maltreatment and neglect

Y07.5- <u>Non-family member</u>, perpetrator of maltreatment and neglect
  Y07.50 <u>Unspecified</u> non-family member, perpetrator of maltreatment and neglect
  Y07.51- <u>Daycare provider</u>, perpetrator of maltreatment and neglect
     Y07.510 At-home childcare provider, perpetrator of maltreatment and neglect
     Y07.511 Daycare center childcare provider, perpetrator of maltreatment and neglect
     Y07.512 At-home adultcare provider, perpetrator of maltreatment and neglect
     Y07.513 Adultcare center provider, perpetrator of maltreatment and neglect
     Y07.519 Unspecified daycare provider, perpetrator of maltreatment and neglect

X 9 7 - Y 3 1

Y07.52- <u>Healthcare provider</u>, perpetrator of maltreatment and neglect

    Y07.521 Mental health provider, perpetrator of maltreatment and neglect

    Y07.528 Other therapist or healthcare provider, perpetrator of maltreatment and neglect
        Nurse perpetrator of maltreatment and neglect
        Occupational therapist perpetrator of maltreatment and neglect
        Physical therapist perpetrator of maltreatment and neglect
        Speech therapist perpetrator of maltreatment and neglect

    Y07.529 Unspecified healthcare provider, perpetrator of maltreatment and neglect

Y07.53 <u>Teacher or instructor</u>, perpetrator of maltreatment and neglect
    Coach, perpetrator of maltreatment and neglect

Y07.59 <u>Other non-family</u> member, perpetrator of maltreatment and neglect

Y07.9 Unspecified perpetrator of maltreatment and neglect

Y08- <u>Assault</u> by <u>other specified means</u>
The appropriate 7th character is to be added to each code from category Y08:
  A <u>Initial</u> encounter
  D <u>Subsequent</u> encounter
  S <u>Sequela</u>

Y08.0- Assault by strike by sport equipment
  Y08.01x- Assault by strike by hockey stick
  Y08.02x- Assault by strike by baseball bat
  Y08.09x- Assault by strike by other specified type of sport equipment

Y08.8- Assault by other specified means
  Y08.81x- Assault by crashing of aircraft
  Y08.89x- Assault by other specified means

Y09 Assault by unspecified means
  Assassination (attempted) NOS
  Homicide (attempted) NOS
  Manslaughter (attempted) NOS
  Murder (attempted) NOS

Event of undetermined intent (Y21-Y33)

Note: Undetermined intent is only for use when there is specific documentation in the record that the intent of the injury cannot be determined. If no such documentation is present, code to accidental (unintentional).

Y21- Drowning and submersion, <u>undetermined intent</u>
The appropriate 7th character is to be added to each code from category Y21:
  A <u>Initial</u> encounter
  D <u>Subsequent</u> encounter
  S <u>Sequela</u>

Y21.0xx- Drowning and submersion while in bathtub, undetermined intent
Y21.1xx- Drowning and submersion after fall into bathtub, undetermined intent
Y21.2xx- Drowning and submersion while in swimming pool, undetermined intent
Y21.3xx- Drowning and submersion after fall into swimming pool, undetermined intent
Y21.4xx- Drowning and submersion in natural water, undetermined intent
Y21.8xx- Other drowning and submersion, undetermined intent
Y21.9xx- Unspecified drowning and submersion, undetermined intent

Y22.xxx- Handgun discharge, <u>undetermined intent</u>
  Discharge of gun for single hand use, undetermined intent
  Discharge of pistol, undetermined intent
  Discharge of revolver, undetermined intent
  Excludes❷: Very pistol (Y24.8)
The appropriate 7th character is to be added to code Y22:
  A <u>Initial</u> encounter
  D <u>Subsequent</u> encounter
  S <u>Sequela</u>

Y23- Rifle, shotgun and larger firearm discharge, <u>undetermined intent</u>
  Excludes❷: airgun (Y24.0)
The appropriate 7th character is to be added to each code from category Y23:
  A <u>Initial</u> encounter
  D <u>Subsequent</u> encounter
  S <u>Sequela</u>

Y23.0xx- Shotgun discharge, undetermined intent
Y23.1xx- Hunting rifle discharge, undetermined intent
Y23.2xx- Military firearm discharge, undetermined intent
Y23.3xx- Machine gun discharge, undetermined intent
Y23.8xx- Other larger firearm discharge, undetermined intent
Y23.9xx- Unspecified larger firearm discharge, undetermined intent

Y24- Other and unspecified firearm discharge, <u>undetermined intent</u>
The appropriate 7th character is to be added to each code from category Y24:
  A <u>Initial</u> encounter
  D <u>Subsequent</u> encounter
  S <u>Sequela</u>

Y24.0xx- Airgun discharge, undetermined intent
  BB gun discharge, undetermined intent
  Pellet gun discharge, undetermined intent
Y24.8xx- Other firearm discharge, undetermined intent
  Paintball gun discharge, undetermined intent
  Very pistol [flare] discharge, undetermined intent
Y24.9xx- Unspecified firearm discharge, undetermined intent

Y25.xxx- Contact with explosive material, <u>undetermined intent</u>
The appropriate 7th character is to be added to code Y25:
  A <u>Initial</u> encounter
  D <u>Subsequent</u> encounter
  S <u>Sequela</u>

Y26.xxx- Exposure to smoke, fire and flames, <u>undetermined intent</u>
The appropriate 7th character is to be added to code Y26:
  A <u>Initial</u> encounter
  D <u>Subsequent</u> encounter
  S <u>Sequela</u>

Y27- Contact with steam, hot vapors and hot objects, <u>undetermined intent</u>
The appropriate 7th character is to be added to each code from category Y27:
  A <u>Initial</u> encounter
  D <u>Subsequent</u> encounter
  S <u>Sequela</u>

Y27.0xx- Contact with steam and hot vapors, undetermined intent
Y27.1xx- Contact with hot tap water, undetermined intent
Y27.2xx- Contact with hot fluids, undetermined intent
Y27.3xx- Contact with hot household appliance, undetermined intent
Y27.8xx- Contact with other hot objects, undetermined intent
Y27.9xx- Contact with unspecified hot objects, undetermined intent

Y28- Contact with sharp object, <u>undetermined intent</u>
The appropriate 7th character is to be added to each code from category Y28:
  A <u>Initial</u> encounter
  D <u>Subsequent</u> encounter
  S <u>Sequela</u>

Y28.0xx- Contact with sharp glass, undetermined intent
Y28.1xx- Contact with knife, undetermined intent
Y28.2xx- Contact with sword or dagger, undetermined intent
Y28.8xx- Contact with other sharp object, undetermined intent
Y28.9xx- Contact with unspecified sharp object, undetermined intent

Y29.xxx- Contact with blunt object, <u>undetermined intent</u>
The appropriate 7th character is to be added to code Y29:
  A <u>Initial</u> encounter
  D <u>Subsequent</u> encounter
  S <u>Sequela</u>

Y30.xxx- Falling, jumping or pushed from a high place, <u>undetermined intent</u>
  Victim falling from one level to another, undetermined intent
The appropriate 7th character is to be added to code Y30:
  A <u>Initial</u> encounter
  D <u>Subsequent</u> encounter
  S <u>Sequela</u>

Y31.xxx- Falling, lying or running before or into moving object, <u>undetermined intent</u>
The appropriate 7th character is to be added to code Y31:
  A <u>Initial</u> encounter
  D <u>Subsequent</u> encounter
  S <u>Sequela</u>

X97 - Y31

Y32.xxx- **Crashing of motor vehicle, <u>undetermined intent</u>**
   The appropriate 7th character is to be added to code Y32:
   A   <u>Initial</u> encounter
   D   <u>Subsequent</u> encounter
   S   <u>Sequela</u>

Y33.xxx- **Other specified events, <u>undetermined intent</u>**
   The appropriate 7th character is to be added to code Y33:
   A   <u>Initial</u> encounter
   D   <u>Subsequent</u> encounter
   S   <u>Sequela</u>

Legal intervention, operations of war, military operations, and terrorism (Y35-Y38)

Y35-   <u>**Legal intervention**</u>
   Includes: Any injury sustained as a result of an encounter with any law enforcement official, serving in any capacity at the time of the encounter, whether on-duty or off-duty. Includes: injury to law enforcement official, suspect and bystander

   The appropriate 7th character is to be added to code Y35:
   A   <u>Initial</u> encounter
   D   <u>Subsequent</u> encounter
   S   <u>Sequela</u>

Y35.0-   Legal intervention involving <u>firearm discharge</u>
   Y35.00-   Legal intervention involving unspecified firearm discharge
      Legal intervention involving gunshot wound
      Legal intervention involving shot NOS
      Y35.001-   **Legal intervention involving <u>unspecified firearm</u> discharge, <u>law enforcement official injured</u>**
      Y35.002-   **Legal intervention involving unspecified firearm discharge, <u>bystander</u> injured**
      Y35.003-   **Legal intervention involving unspecified firearm discharge, <u>suspect</u> injured**
   Y35.01-   Legal intervention involving injury by <u>machine gun</u>
      Y35.011-   **Legal intervention involving injury by machine gun, <u>law enforcement official injured</u>**
      Y35.012-   **Legal intervention involving injury by machine gun, <u>bystander</u> injured**
      Y35.013-   **Legal intervention involving injury by machine gun, <u>suspect</u> injured**
   Y35.02-   Legal intervention involving injury by <u>handgun</u>
      Y35.021-   **Legal intervention involving injury by handgun, <u>law enforcement official injured</u>**
      Y35.022-   **Legal intervention involving injury by handgun, <u>bystander</u> injured**
      Y35.023-   **Legal intervention involving injury by handgun, <u>suspect</u> injured**
   Y35.03-   Legal intervention involving injury by <u>rifle pellet</u>
      Y35.031-   **Legal intervention involving injury by rifle pellet, <u>law enforcement official injured</u>**
      Y35.032-   **Legal intervention involving injury by rifle pellet, <u>bystander</u> injured**
      Y35.033-   **Legal intervention involving injury by rifle pellet, <u>suspect</u> injured**
   Y35.04-   Legal intervention involving injury by <u>rubber bullet</u>
      Y35.041-   **Legal intervention involving injury by rubber bullet, <u>law enforcement official injured</u>**
      Y35.042-   **Legal intervention involving injury by rubber bullet, <u>bystander</u> injured**
      Y35.043-   **Legal intervention involving injury by rubber bullet, <u>suspect</u> injured**
   Y35.09-   Legal intervention involving <u>other firearm discharge</u>
      Y35.091-   **Legal intervention involving other firearm discharge, <u>law enforcement official injured</u>**
      Y35.092-   **Legal intervention involving other firearm discharge, <u>bystander</u> injured**
      Y35.093-   **Legal intervention involving other firearm discharge, <u>suspect</u> injured**
Y35.1-   Legal intervention involving <u>explosives</u>
   Y35.10-   Legal intervention involving unspecified explosives
      Y35.101-   **Legal intervention involving unspecified explosives, <u>law enforcement official injured</u>**
      Y35.102-   **Legal intervention involving unspecified explosives, <u>bystander</u> injured**
      Y35.103-   **Legal intervention involving unspecified explosives, <u>suspect</u> injured**

Y35.11-   Legal intervention involving injury by <u>dynamite</u>
   Y35.111-   **Legal intervention involving injury by dynamite, <u>law enforcement official injured</u>**
   Y35.112-   **Legal intervention involving injury by dynamite, <u>bystander</u> injured**
   Y35.113-   **Legal intervention involving injury by dynamite, <u>suspect</u> injured**
Y35.12-   Legal intervention involving injury by <u>explosive shell</u>
   Y35.121-   **Legal intervention involving injury by explosive shell, <u>law enforcement official injured</u>**
   Y35.122-   **Legal intervention involving injury by explosive shell, <u>bystander</u> injured**
   Y35.123-   **Legal intervention involving injury by explosive shell, <u>suspect</u> injured**
Y35.19-   Legal intervention involving <u>other explosives</u>
   Legal intervention involving injury by grenade
   Legal intervention involving injury by mortar bomb
   Y35.191-   **Legal intervention involving other explosives, <u>law enforcement official injured</u>**
   Y35.192-   **Legal intervention involving other explosives, <u>bystander</u> injured**
   Y35.193-   **Legal intervention involving other explosives, <u>suspect</u> injured**
Y35.2-   Legal intervention involving <u>gas</u>
   Legal intervention involving asphyxiation by gas
   Legal intervention involving poisoning by gas
   Y35.20-   Legal intervention involving <u>unspecified</u> gas
      Y35.201-   **Legal intervention involving unspecified gas, <u>law enforcement official injured</u>**
      Y35.202-   **Legal intervention involving unspecified gas, <u>bystander</u> injured**
      Y35.203-   **Legal intervention involving unspecified gas, <u>suspect</u> injured**
   Y35.21-   Legal intervention involving injury by <u>tear gas</u>
      Y35.211-   **Legal intervention involving injury by tear gas, <u>law enforcement official injured</u>**
      Y35.212-   **Legal intervention involving injury by tear gas, <u>bystander</u> injured**
      Y35.213-   **Legal intervention involving injury by tear gas, <u>suspect</u> injured**
   Y35.29-   Legal intervention involving <u>other gas</u>
      Y35.291-   **Legal intervention involving other gas, <u>law enforcement official injured</u>**
      Y35.292-   **Legal intervention involving other gas, <u>bystander</u> injured**
      Y35.293-   **Legal intervention involving other gas, <u>suspect</u> injured**
Y35.3-   Legal intervention involving <u>blunt objects</u>
   Legal intervention involving being hit or struck by blunt object
   Y35.30-   Legal intervention involving <u>unspecified</u> blunt objects
      Y35.301-   **Legal intervention involving unspecified blunt objects, <u>law enforcement official injured</u>**
      Y35.302-   **Legal intervention involving unspecified blunt objects, <u>bystander</u> injured**
      Y35.303-   **Legal intervention involving unspecified blunt objects, <u>suspect</u> injured**
   Y35.31-   Legal intervention involving <u>baton</u>
      Y35.311-   **Legal intervention involving baton, <u>law enforcement official injured</u>**
      Y35.312-   **Legal intervention involving baton, <u>bystander</u> injured**
      Y35.313-   **Legal intervention involving baton, <u>suspect</u> injured**
   Y35.39-   Legal intervention involving <u>other blunt objects</u>
      Y35.391-   **Legal intervention involving other blunt objects, <u>law enforcement official injured</u>**
      Y35.392-   **Legal intervention involving other blunt objects, <u>bystander</u> injured**
      Y35.393-   **Legal intervention involving other blunt objects, <u>suspect</u> injured**
Y35.4-   Legal intervention involving <u>sharp objects</u>
   Legal intervention involving being cut by sharp objects
   Legal intervention involving being stabbed by sharp objects
   Y35.40-   Legal intervention involving <u>unspecified</u> sharp objects
      Y35.401-   **Legal intervention involving unspecified sharp objects, <u>law enforcement official injured</u>**
      Y35.402-   **Legal intervention involving unspecified sharp objects, <u>bystander</u> injured**
      Y35.403-   **Legal intervention involving unspecified sharp objects, <u>suspect</u> injured**

Y 3 2 - Y 3 6

© 2013 Channel Publishing, Ltd.

Y35.41- Legal intervention involving <u>bayonet</u>
    Y35.411- Legal intervention involving bayonet, <u>law enforcement official injured</u>
    Y35.412- Legal intervention involving bayonet, <u>bystander</u> injured
    Y35.413- Legal intervention involving bayonet, <u>suspect</u> injured
Y35.49- Legal intervention involving <u>other sharp objects</u>
    Y35.491- Legal intervention involving other sharp objects, <u>law enforcement official injured</u>
    Y35.492- Legal intervention involving other sharp objects, <u>bystander</u> injured
    Y35.493- Legal intervention involving other sharp objects, <u>suspect</u> injured
Y35.8- Legal intervention involving <u>other specified means</u>
  Y35.81- Legal intervention involving <u>manhandling</u>
    Y35.811- Legal intervention involving manhandling, <u>law enforcement official injured</u>
    Y35.812- Legal intervention involving manhandling, <u>bystander</u> injured
    Y35.813- Legal intervention involving manhandling, <u>suspect</u> injured
  Y35.89- Legal intervention involving <u>other specified means</u>
    Y35.891- Legal intervention involving other specified means, <u>law enforcement official injured</u>
    Y35.892- Legal intervention involving other specified means, <u>bystander</u> injured
    Y35.893- Legal intervention involving other specified means, <u>suspect</u> injured
Y35.9- Legal intervention, <u>means unspecified</u>
  Y35.91- Legal intervention, means unspecified, <u>law enforcement official injured</u>
  Y35.92- Legal intervention, means unspecified, <u>bystander</u> injured
  Y35.93- Legal intervention, means unspecified, <u>suspect</u> injured

Y36- Operations of war
  Includes: Injuries to military personnel and civilians caused by war, civil insurrection, and peacekeeping missions
  Excludes 1: injury to military personnel occurring during peacetime military operations (Y37.-)
  military vehicles involved in transport accidents with non-military vehicle during peacetime (V09.01, V09.21, V19.81, V29.81, V39.81, V49.81, V59.81, V69.81, V79.81)

The appropriate 7th character is to be added to each code from category Y36:
  A   <u>Initial</u> encounter
  D   <u>Subsequent</u> encounter
  S   <u>Sequela</u>

Y36.0- <u>War</u> operations involving <u>explosion of marine weapons</u>
  Y36.00- <u>War</u> operations involving explosion of <u>unspecified</u> marine weapon
    War operations involving underwater blast NOS
    Y36.000- <u>War</u> operations involving explosion of unspecified marine weapon, <u>military</u> personnel
    Y36.001- <u>War</u> operations involving explosion of unspecified marine weapon, <u>civilian</u>
  Y36.01- <u>War</u> operations involving explosion of <u>depth-charge</u>
    Y36.010- <u>War</u> operations involving explosion of depth-charge, <u>military</u> personnel
    Y36.011- <u>War</u> operations involving explosion of depth-charge, <u>civilian</u>
  Y36.02- <u>War</u> operations involving explosion of <u>marine mine</u>
    War operations involving explosion of marine mine, at sea or in harbor
    Y36.020- <u>War</u> operations involving explosion of marine mine, <u>military</u> personnel
    Y36.021- <u>War</u> operations involving explosion of marine mine, <u>civilian</u>
  Y36.03- <u>War</u> operations involving explosion of <u>sea-based artillery shell</u>
    Y36.030- <u>War</u> operations involving explosion of sea-based artillery shell, <u>military</u> personnel
    Y36.031- <u>War</u> operations involving explosion of sea-based artillery shell, <u>civilian</u>
  Y36.04- <u>War</u> operations involving explosion of <u>torpedo</u>
    Y36.040- <u>War</u> operations involving explosion of torpedo, <u>military</u> personnel
    Y36.041- <u>War</u> operations involving explosion of torpedo, <u>civilian</u>

Y36.05- <u>War</u> operations involving <u>accidental detonation of onboard marine weapons</u>
  Y36.050- <u>War</u> operations involving accidental detonation of onboard marine weapons, <u>military</u> personnel
  Y36.051- <u>War</u> operations involving accidental detonation of onboard marine weapons, <u>civilian</u>
Y36.09- <u>War</u> operations involving explosion of <u>other marine weapons</u>
  Y36.090- <u>War</u> operations involving explosion of other marine weapons, <u>military</u> personnel
  Y36.091- <u>War</u> operations involving explosion of other marine weapons, <u>civilian</u>
Y36.1- <u>War</u> operations involving <u>destruction of aircraft</u>
  Y36.10- <u>War</u> operations involving <u>unspecified</u> destruction of aircraft
    Y36.100- <u>War</u> operations involving unspecified destruction of aircraft, <u>military</u> personnel
    Y36.101- <u>War</u> operations involving unspecified destruction of aircraft, <u>civilian</u>
  Y36.11- <u>War</u> operations involving destruction of aircraft <u>due to enemy fire or explosives</u>
    War operations involving destruction of aircraft due to air to air missile
    War operations involving destruction of aircraft due to explosive placed on aircraft
    War operations involving destruction of aircraft due to rocket propelled grenade [RPG]
    War operations involving destruction of aircraft due to small arms fire
    War operations involving destruction of aircraft due to surface to air missile
    Y36.110- <u>War</u> operations involving destruction of aircraft due to enemy fire or explosives, <u>military</u> personnel
    Y36.111- <u>War</u> operations involving destruction of aircraft due to enemy fire or explosives, <u>civilian</u>
  Y36.12- <u>War</u> operations involving destruction of aircraft <u>due to collision with other aircraft</u>
    Y36.120- <u>War</u> operations involving destruction of aircraft due to collision with other aircraft, <u>military</u> personnel
    Y36.121- <u>War</u> operations involving destruction of aircraft due to collision with other aircraft, <u>civilian</u>
  Y36.13- <u>War</u> operations involving destruction of aircraft <u>due to onboard fire</u>
    Y36.130- <u>War</u> operations involving destruction of aircraft due to onboard fire, <u>military</u> personnel
    Y36.131- <u>War</u> operations involving destruction of aircraft due to onboard fire, <u>civilian</u>
  Y36.14- <u>War</u> operations involving destruction of aircraft due to <u>accidental detonation of onboard munitions and explosives</u>
    Y36.140- <u>War</u> operations involving destruction of aircraft due to accidental detonation of onboard munitions and explosives, <u>military</u> personnel
    Y36.141- <u>War</u> operations involving destruction of aircraft due to accidental detonation of onboard munitions and explosives, <u>civilian</u>
  Y36.19- <u>War</u> operations involving <u>other destruction of aircraft</u>
    Y36.190- <u>War</u> operations involving other destruction of aircraft, <u>military</u> personnel
    Y36.191- <u>War</u> operations involving other destruction of aircraft, <u>civilian</u>
Y36.2- <u>War</u> operations involving <u>other explosions and fragments</u>
  Excludes 1: war operations involving explosion of aircraft (Y36.1-)
  war operations involving explosion of marine weapons (Y36.0-)
  war operations involving explosion of nuclear weapons (Y36.5-)
  war operations involving explosion occurring after cessation of hostilities (Y36.8-)
  Y36.20- <u>War</u> operations involving <u>unspecified</u> explosion and fragments
    War operations involving air blast NOS
    War operations involving blast NOS
    War operations involving blast fragments NOS
    War operations involving blast wave NOS
    War operations involving blast wind NOS
    War operations involving explosion NOS
    War operations involving explosion of bomb NOS
    Y36.200- <u>War</u> operations involving unspecified explosion and fragments, <u>military</u> personnel
    Y36.201- <u>War</u> operations involving unspecified explosion and fragments, <u>civilian</u>

Y 3 2 - Y 3 6

Y36.21- War operations involving explosion of aerial bomb
   Y36.210- War operations involving explosion of aerial bomb, military personnel
   Y36.211- War operations involving explosion of aerial bomb, civilian
Y36.22- War operations involving explosion of guided missile
   Y36.220- War operations involving explosion of guided missile, military personnel
   Y36.221- War operations involving explosion of guided missile, civilian
Y36.23- War operations involving explosion of improvised explosive device [IED]
   War operations involving explosion of person-borne improvised explosive device [IED]
   War operations involving explosion of vehicle-borne improvised explosive device [IED]
   War operations involving explosion of roadside improvised explosive device [IED]
   Y36.230- War operations involving explosion of improvised explosive device [IED], military personnel
   Y36.231- War operations involving explosion of improvised explosive device [IED], civilian
Y36.24- War operations involving explosion due to accidental detonation and discharge of own munitions or munitions launch device
   Y36.240- War operations involving explosion due to accidental detonation and discharge of own munitions or munitions launch-device, military personnel
   Y36.241- War operations involving explosion due to accidental detonation and discharge of own munitions or munitions launch device, civilian
Y36.25- War operations involving fragments from munitions
   Y36.250- War operations involving fragments from munitions, military personnel
   Y36.251- War operations involving fragments from munitions, civilian
Y36.26 War operations involving fragments of improvised explosive device [IED]
   War operations involving fragments of person-borne improvised explosive device [IED]
   War operations involving fragments of vehicle-borne improvised explosive device [IED]
   War operations involving fragments of roadside improvised explosive device [IED]
   Y36.260- War operations involving fragments of improvised explosive device [IED], military personnel
   Y36.261- War operations involving fragments of improvised explosive device [IED], civilian
Y36.27- War operations involving fragments from weapons
   Y36.270- War operations involving fragments from weapons, military personnel
   Y36.271- War operations involving fragments from weapons, civilian
Y36.29- War operations involving other explosions and fragments
   War operations involving explosion of grenade
   War operations involving explosions of land mine
   War operations involving shrapnel NOS
   Y36.290- War operations involving other explosions and fragments, military personnel
   Y36.291- War operations involving other explosions and fragments, civilian
Y36.3- War operations involving fires, conflagrations and hot substances
   War operations involving smoke, fumes, and heat from fires, conflagrations and hot substances
   Excludes 1: war operations involving fires and conflagrations aboard military aircraft (Y36.1-)
      war operations involving fires and conflagrations aboard military watercraft (Y36.0-)
      war operations involving fires and conflagrations caused indirectly by conventional weapons (Y36.2-)
      war operations involving fires and thermal effects of nuclear weapons (Y36.53-)
Y36.30- War operations involving unspecified fire, conflagration and hot substance
   Y36.300- War operations involving unspecified fire, conflagration and hot substance, military personnel
   Y36.301- War operations involving unspecified fire, conflagration and hot substance, civilian

Y36.31- War operations involving gasoline bomb
   War operations involving incendiary bomb
   War operations involving petrol bomb
   Y36.310- War operations involving gasoline bomb, military personnel
   Y36.311- War operations involving gasoline bomb, civilian
Y36.32- War operations involving incendiary bullet
   Y36.320- War operations involving incendiary bullet, military personnel
   Y36.321- War operations involving incendiary bullet, civilian
Y36.33- War operations involving flamethrower
   Y36.330- War operations involving flamethrower, military personnel
   Y36.331- War operations involving flamethrower, civilian
Y36.39- War operations involving other fires, conflagrations and hot substances
   Y36.390- War operations involving other fires, conflagrations and hot substances, military personnel
   Y36.391- War operations involving other fires, conflagrations and hot substances, civilian
Y36.4- War operations involving firearm discharge and other forms of conventional warfare
Y36.41- War operations involving rubber bullets
   Y36.410- War operations involving rubber bullets, military personnel
   Y36.411- War operations involving rubber bullets, civilian
Y36.42- War operations involving firearms pellets
   Y36.420- War operations involving firearms pellets, military personnel
   Y36.421- War operations involving firearms pellets, civilian
Y36.43- War operations involving other firearms discharge
   War operations involving bullets NOS
   Excludes 1: war operations involving munitions fragments (Y36.25-)
      war operations involving incendiary bullets (Y36.32-)
   Y36.430- War operations involving other firearms discharge, military personnel
   Y36.431- War operations involving other firearms discharge, civilian
Y36.44- War operations involving unarmed hand to hand combat
   Excludes 1: war operations involving combat using blunt or piercing object (Y36.45-)
      war operations involving intentional restriction of air and airway (Y36.46-)
      war operations involving unintentional restriction of air and airway (Y36.47-)
   Y36.440- War operations involving unarmed hand to hand combat, military personnel
   Y36.441- War operations involving unarmed hand to hand combat, civilian
Y36.45- War operations involving combat using blunt or piercing object
   Y36.450- War operations involving combat using blunt or piercing object, military personnel
   Y36.451- War operations involving combat using blunt or piercing object, civilian
Y36.46- War operations involving intentional restriction of air and airway
   Y36.460- War operations involving intentional restriction of air and airway, military personnel
   Y36.461- War operations involving intentional restriction of air and airway, civilian
Y36.47- War operations involving unintentional restriction of air and airway
   Y36.470- War operations involving unintentional restriction of air and airway, military personnel
   Y36.471- War operations involving unintentional restriction of air and airway, civilian
Y36.49- War operations involving other forms of conventional warfare
   Y36.490- War operations involving other forms of conventional warfare, military personnel
   Y36.491- War operations involving other forms of conventional warfare, civilian

Y36 - Y37

Y36.5- <u>War</u> operations involving <u>nuclear weapons</u>
　　War operations involving dirty bomb NOS
　Y36.50- <u>War</u> operations involving <u>unspecified</u> effect of nuclear weapon
　　Y36.500- <u>War</u> operations involving unspecified effect of nuclear weapon, <u>military</u> personnel
　　Y36.501- <u>War</u> operations involving unspecified effect of nuclear weapon, <u>civilian</u>
　Y36.51- <u>War</u> operations involving <u>direct blast effect</u> of nuclear weapon
　　War operations involving blast pressure of nuclear weapon
　　Y36.510- <u>War</u> operations involving direct blast effect of nuclear weapon, <u>military</u> personnel
　　Y36.511- <u>War</u> operations involving direct blast effect of nuclear weapon, <u>civilian</u>
　Y36.52- <u>War</u> operations involving <u>indirect blast effect</u> of nuclear weapon
　　War operations involving being thrown by blast of nuclear weapon
　　War operations involving being struck or crushed by blast debris of nuclear weapon
　　Y36.520- <u>War</u> operations involving indirect blast effect of nuclear weapon, <u>military</u> personnel
　　Y36.521- <u>War</u> operations involving indirect blast effect of nuclear weapon, <u>civilian</u>
　Y36.53- <u>War</u> operations involving <u>thermal radiation effect</u> of nuclear weapon
　　War operations involving direct heat from nuclear weapon
　　War operation involving fireball effects from nuclear weapon
　　Y36.530- <u>War</u> operations involving thermal radiation effect of nuclear weapon, <u>military</u> personnel
　　Y36.531- <u>War</u> operations involving thermal radiation effect of nuclear weapon, <u>civilian</u>
　Y36.54- <u>War</u> operation involving <u>nuclear radiation effects</u> of nuclear weapon
　　War operation involving acute radiation exposure from nuclear weapon
　　War operation involving exposure to immediate ionizing radiation from nuclear weapon
　　War operation involving fallout exposure from nuclear weapon
　　War operation involving secondary effects of nuclear weapons
　　Y36.540- <u>War</u> operation involving nuclear radiation effects of nuclear weapon, <u>military</u> personnel
　　Y36.541- <u>War</u> operation involving nuclear radiation effects of nuclear weapon, <u>civilian</u>
　Y36.59- <u>War</u> operation involving <u>other</u> effects of nuclear weapons
　　Y36.590- <u>War</u> operation involving other effects of nuclear weapons, <u>military</u> personnel
　　Y36.591- <u>War</u> operation involving other effects of nuclear weapons, <u>civilian</u>
Y36.6- <u>War</u> operations involving <u>biological weapons</u>
　Y36.6x- <u>War</u> operations involving biological weapons
　　Y36.6x0- <u>War</u> operations involving biological weapons, <u>military</u> personnel
　　Y36.6x1- <u>War</u> operations involving biological weapons, <u>civilian</u>
Y36.7- <u>War</u> operations involving <u>chemical weapons and other forms of unconventional warfare</u>
　　Excludes 1:　war operations involving incendiary devices (Y36.3-, Y36.5-)
　Y36.7x- <u>War</u> operations involving <u>chemical weapons and other forms of unconventional warfare</u>
　　Y36.7x0- <u>War</u> operations involving chemical weapons and other forms of unconventional warfare, <u>military</u> personnel
　　Y36.7x1- <u>War</u> operations involving chemical weapons and other forms of unconventional warfare, <u>civilian</u>
Y36.8- <u>War</u> operations occurring <u>after cessation of hostilities</u>
　　War operations classifiable to categories Y36.0-Y36.8 but occurring after cessation of hostilities
　Y36.81- Explosion of <u>mine</u> placed during <u>war</u> operations but <u>exploding after</u> cessation of hostilities
　　Y36.810- Explosion of mine placed during <u>war</u> operations but exploding after cessation of hostilities, <u>military</u> personnel
　　Y36.811- Explosion of mine placed during <u>war</u> operations but exploding after cessation of hostilities, <u>civilian</u>

　Y36.82- Explosion of <u>bomb</u> placed during <u>war</u> operations but <u>exploding after</u> cessation of hostilities
　　Y36.820- Explosion of bomb placed during <u>war</u> operations but exploding after cessation of hostilities, <u>military</u> personnel
　　Y36.821- Explosion of bomb placed during <u>war</u> operations but exploding after cessation of hostilities, <u>civilian</u>
　Y36.88- <u>Other</u> <u>war</u> operations <u>occurring after</u> cessation of hostilities
　　Y36.880- Other <u>war</u> operations occurring after cessation of hostilities, <u>military</u> personnel
　　Y36.881- Other <u>war</u> operations occurring after cessation of hostilities, <u>civilian</u>
　Y36.89- <u>Unspecified</u> <u>war</u> operations <u>occurring after</u> cessation of hostilities
　　Y36.890- Unspecified <u>war</u> operations occurring after cessation of hostilities, <u>military</u> personnel
　　Y36.891- Unspecified <u>war</u> operations occurring after cessation of hostilities, <u>civilian</u>
Y36.9- Other and unspecified <u>war</u> operations
　Y36.90- <u>War</u> operations, <u>unspecified</u>
　Y36.91- <u>War</u> operations involving <u>unspecified weapon of mass destruction [WMD]</u>
　Y36.92- <u>War</u> operations involving <u>friendly fire</u>

Y37- 　Military operations
　Includes:　Injuries to military personnel and civilians <u>occurring during peacetime</u> on military property and <u>during routine military exercises and operations</u>
　Excludes 1:　military aircraft involved in aircraft accident with civilian aircraft (V97.81-)
　　　　military vehicles involved in transport accident with civilian vehicle (V09.01, V09.21, V19.81, V29.81, V39.81, V49.81, V59.81, V69.81, V79.81)
　　　　military watercraft involved in water transport accident with civilian watercraft (V94.81-)
　　　　war operations (Y36.-)

The appropriate 7th character is to be added to each code from category Y37:
　A　<u>Initial</u> encounter
　D　<u>Subsequent</u> encounter
　S　<u>Sequela</u>

Y37.0- 　Military operations involving <u>explosion of marine weapons</u>
　Y37.00- Military operations involving explosion of <u>unspecified</u> marine weapon
　　Military operations involving underwater blast NOS
　　Y37.000- Military operations involving explosion of unspecified marine weapon, <u>military</u> personnel
　　Y37.001- Military operations involving explosion of unspecified marine weapon, <u>civilian</u>
　Y37.01- Military operations involving explosion of <u>depth-charge</u>
　　Y37.010- Military operations involving explosion of depth-charge, <u>military</u> personnel
　　Y37.011- Military operations involving explosion of depth-charge, <u>civilian</u>
　Y37.02- Military operations involving explosion of <u>marine mine</u>
　　Military operations involving explosion of marine mine, at sea or in harbor
　　Y37.020- Military operations involving explosion of marine mine, <u>military</u> personnel
　　Y37.021- Military operations involving explosion of marine mine, <u>civilian</u>
　Y37.03- Military operations involving explosion of <u>sea-based artillery shell</u>
　　Y37.030- Military operations involving explosion of sea-based artillery shell, <u>military</u> personnel
　　Y37.031- Military operations involving explosion of sea-based artillery shell, <u>civilian</u>
　Y37.04- Military operations involving explosion of <u>torpedo</u>
　　Y37.040- Military operations involving explosion of torpedo, <u>military</u> personnel
　　Y37.041- Military operations involving explosion of torpedo, <u>civilian</u>
　Y37.05- Military operations involving <u>accidental detonation of onboard marine weapons</u>
　　Y37.050- Military operations involving accidental detonation of onboard marine weapons, <u>military</u> personnel
　　Y37.051- Military operations involving accidental detonation of onboard marine weapons, <u>civilian</u>

Y 3 6 I Y 3 7

Y37.09- Military operations involving explosion of <u>other marine weapons</u>
  Y37.090- Military operations involving explosion of other marine weapons, <u>military</u> personnel
  Y37.091- Military operations involving explosion of other marine weapons, <u>civilian</u>
Y37.1- Military operations involving <u>destruction of aircraft</u>
  Y37.10- Military operations involving <u>unspecified</u> destruction of aircraft
  Y37.100- Military operations involving unspecified destruction of aircraft, <u>military</u> personnel
  Y37.101- Military operations involving unspecified destruction of aircraft, <u>civilian</u>
  Y37.11- Military operations involving destruction of aircraft <u>due to enemy fire or explosives</u>
    Military operations involving destruction of aircraft due to air to air missile
    Military operations involving destruction of aircraft due to explosive placed on aircraft
    Military operations involving destruction of aircraft due to rocket propelled grenade [RPG]
    Military operations involving destruction of aircraft due to small arms fire
    Military operations involving destruction of aircraft due to surface to air missile
  Y37.110- Military operations involving destruction of aircraft due to enemy fire or explosives, <u>military</u> personnel
  Y37.111- Military operations involving destruction of aircraft due to enemy fire or explosives, <u>civilian</u>
  Y37.12- Military operations involving destruction of aircraft <u>due to collision with other aircraft</u>
    Y37.120- Military operations involving destruction of aircraft due to collision with other aircraft, <u>military</u> personnel
    Y37.121- Military operations involving destruction of aircraft due to collision with other aircraft, <u>civilian</u>
  Y37.13- Military operations involving destruction of aircraft <u>due to onboard fire</u>
    Y37.130- Military operations involving destruction of aircraft due to onboard fire, <u>military</u> personnel
    Y37.131- Military operations involving destruction of aircraft due to onboard fire, <u>civilian</u>
  Y37.14- Military operations involving destruction of aircraft <u>due to accidental detonation of onboard munitions and explosives</u>
    Y37.140- Military operations involving destruction of aircraft due to accidental detonation of onboard munitions and explosives, <u>military</u> personnel
    Y37.141- Military operations involving destruction of aircraft due to accidental detonation of onboard munitions and explosives, <u>civilian</u>
  Y37.19- Military operations involving <u>other destruction of aircraft</u>
    Y37.190- Military operations involving other destruction of aircraft, <u>military</u> personnel
    Y37.191- Military operations involving other destruction of aircraft, <u>civilian</u>
Y37.2- Military operations involving <u>other explosions and fragments</u>
  Excludes 1: *military operations involving explosion of aircraft (Y37.1-)*
    military operations involving explosion of marine weapons (Y37.0-)
    military operations involving explosion of nuclear weapons (Y37.5-)
  Y37.20- Military operations involving <u>unspecified</u> explosion and fragments
    Military operations involving air blast NOS
    Military operations involving blast NOS
    Military operations involving blast fragments NOS
    Military operations involving blast wave NOS
    Military operations involving blast wind NOS
    Military operations involving explosion NOS
    Military operations involving explosion of bomb NOS
    Y37.200- Military operations involving unspecified explosion and fragments, <u>military</u> personnel
    Y37.201- Military operations involving unspecified explosion and fragments, <u>civilian</u>
  Y37.21- Military operations involving explosion of <u>aerial bomb</u>
    Y37.210- Military operations involving explosion of aerial bomb, <u>military</u> personnel
    Y37.211- Military operations involving explosion of aerial bomb, <u>civilian</u>

Y37.22- Military operations involving explosion of <u>guided missile</u>
  Y37.220- Military operations involving explosion of guided missile, <u>military</u> personnel
  Y37.221- Military operations involving explosion of guided missile, <u>civilian</u>
Y37.23- Military operations involving explosion of <u>improvised explosive device [IED]</u>
    Military operations involving explosion of person-borne improvised explosive device [IED]
    Military operations involving explosion of vehicle-borne improvised explosive device [IED]
    Military operations involving explosion of roadside improvised explosive device [IED]
  Y37.230- Military operations involving explosion of improvised explosive device [IED], <u>military</u> personnel
  Y37.231- Military operations involving explosion of improvised explosive device [IED], <u>civilian</u>
Y37.24- Military operations involving explosion due to <u>accidental detonation and discharge of own munitions or munitions launch device</u>
  Y37.240- Military operations involving explosion due to accidental detonation and discharge of own munitions or munitions launch device, <u>military</u> personnel
  Y37.241- Military operations involving explosion due to accidental detonation and discharge of own munitions or munitions launch device, <u>civilian</u>
Y37.25- Military operations involving <u>fragments from munitions</u>
  Y37.250- Military operations involving fragments from munitions, <u>military</u> personnel
  Y37.251- Military operations involving fragments from munitions, <u>civilian</u>
Y37.26- Military operations involving <u>fragments of improvised explosive device [IED]</u>
    Military operations involving fragments of person-borne improvised explosive device [IED]
    Military operations involving fragments of vehicle-borne improvised explosive device [IED]
    Military operations involving fragments of roadside improvised explosive device [IED]
  Y37.260- Military operations involving fragments of improvised explosive device [IED], <u>military</u> personnel
  Y37.261- Military operations involving fragments of improvised explosive device [IED], <u>civilian</u>
Y37.27- Military operations involving <u>fragments from weapons</u>
  Y37.270- Military operations involving fragments from weapons, <u>military</u> personnel
  Y37.271- Military operations involving fragments from weapons, <u>civilian</u>
Y37.29- Military operations involving <u>other explosions and fragments</u>
    Military operations involving explosion of grenade
    Military operations involving explosions of land mine
    Military operations involving shrapnel NOS
  Y37.290- Military operations involving other explosions and fragments, <u>military</u> personnel
  Y37.291- Military operations involving other explosions and fragments, <u>civilian</u>
Y37.3- Military operations involving <u>fires, conflagrations and hot substances</u>
    Military operations involving smoke, fumes, and heat from fires, conflagrations and hot substances
  Excludes 1: *military operations involving fires and conflagrations aboard military aircraft (Y37.1-)*
    military operations involving fires and conflagrations aboard military watercraft (Y37.0-)
    military operations involving fires and conflagrations caused indirectly by conventional weapons (Y37.2-)
    military operations involving fires and thermal effects of nuclear weapons (Y36.53-)
  Y37.30- Military operations involving <u>unspecified</u> fire, conflagration and hot substance
    Y37.300- Military operations involving unspecified fire, conflagration and hot substance, <u>military</u> personnel
    Y37.301- Military operations involving unspecified fire, conflagration and hot substance, <u>civilian</u>
  Y37.31- Military operations involving <u>gasoline bomb</u>
    Military operations involving incendiary bomb
    Military operations involving petrol bomb
    Y37.310- Military operations involving gasoline bomb, <u>military</u> personnel
    Y37.311- Military operations involving gasoline bomb, <u>civilian</u>

Y37 - Y37

Y37.32- Military operations involving <u>incendiary bullet</u>
  Y37.320- Military operations involving incendiary bullet, <u>military</u> personnel
  Y37.321- Military operations involving incendiary bullet, <u>civilian</u>
Y37.33- Military operations involving <u>flamethrower</u>
  Y37.330- Military operations involving flamethrower, <u>military</u> personnel
  Y37.331- Military operations involving flamethrower, <u>civilian</u>
Y37.39- Military operations involving <u>other</u> fires, conflagrations and hot substances
  Y37.390- Military operations involving other fires, conflagrations and hot substances, <u>military</u> personnel
  Y37.391- Military operations involving other fires, conflagrations and hot substances, <u>civilian</u>
Y37.4- Military operations involving <u>firearm discharge and other forms of conventional warfare</u>
  Y37.41- Military operations involving <u>rubber bullets</u>
    Y37.410- Military operations involving rubber bullets, <u>military</u> personnel
    Y37.411- Military operations involving rubber bullets, <u>civilian</u>
  Y37.42- Military operations involving <u>firearms pellets</u>
    Y37.420- Military operations involving firearms pellets, <u>military</u> personnel
    Y37.421- Military operations involving firearms pellets, <u>civilian</u>
  Y37.43- Military operations involving <u>other</u> firearms discharge
      Military operations involving bullets NOS
      Excludes 1: military operations involving munitions fragments (Y37.25-)
      military operations involving incendiary bullets (Y37.32-)
    Y37.430- Military operations involving other firearms discharge, <u>military</u> personnel
    Y37.431- Military operations involving other firearms discharge, <u>civilian</u>
  Y37.44- Military operations <u>involving unarmed hand to hand combat</u>
      Excludes 1: military operations involving combat using blunt or piercing object (Y37.45-)
      military operations involving intentional restriction of air and airway (Y37.46-)
      military operations involving unintentional restriction of air and airway (Y37.47-)
    Y37.440- Military operations involving unarmed hand to hand combat, <u>military</u> personnel
    Y37.441- Military operations involving unarmed hand to hand combat, <u>civilian</u>
  Y37.45- Military operations involving <u>combat using blunt or piercing object</u>
    Y37.450- Military operations involving combat using blunt or piercing object, <u>military</u> personnel
    Y37.451- Military operations involving combat using blunt or piercing object, <u>civilian</u>
  Y37.46- Military operations involving <u>intentional restriction of air and airway</u>
    Y37.460- Military operations involving intentional restriction of air and airway, <u>military</u> personnel
    Y37.461- Military operations involving intentional restriction of air and airway, <u>civilian</u>
  Y37.47- Military operations involving <u>unintentional restriction of air and airway</u>
    Y37.470- Military operations involving unintentional restriction of air and airway, <u>military</u> personnel
    Y37.471- Military operations involving unintentional restriction of air and airway, <u>civilian</u>
  Y37.49- Military operations involving <u>other</u> forms of conventional warfare
    Y37.490- Military operations involving other forms of conventional warfare, <u>military</u> personnel
    Y37.491- Military operations involving other forms of conventional warfare, <u>civilian</u>

Y37.5- Military operations involving <u>nuclear weapons</u>
    Military operation involving dirty bomb NOS
  Y37.50- Military operations involving <u>unspecified</u> effect of nuclear weapon
    Y37.500- Military operations involving unspecified effect of nuclear weapon, <u>military</u> personnel
    Y37.501- Military operations involving unspecified effect of nuclear weapon, <u>civilian</u>
  Y37.51- Military operations involving <u>direct blast effect</u> of nuclear weapon
      Military operations involving blast pressure of nuclear weapon
    Y37.510- Military operations involving direct blast effect of nuclear weapon, <u>military</u> personnel
    Y37.511- Military operations involving direct blast effect of nuclear weapon, <u>civilian</u>
  Y37.52- Military operations involving <u>indirect blast effect</u> of nuclear weapon
      Military operations involving being thrown by blast of nuclear weapon
      Military operations involving being struck or crushed by blast debris of nuclear weapon
    Y37.520- Military operations involving indirect blast effect of nuclear weapon, <u>military</u> personnel
    Y37.521- Military operations involving indirect blast effect of nuclear weapon, <u>civilian</u>
  Y37.53- Military operations involving <u>thermal radiation effect</u> of nuclear weapon
      Military operations involving direct heat from nuclear weapon
      Military operation involving fireball effects from nuclear weapon
    Y37.530- Military operations involving thermal radiation effect of nuclear weapon, <u>military</u> personnel
    Y37.531- Military operations involving thermal radiation effect of nuclear weapon, <u>civilian</u>
  Y37.54- Military operation involving <u>nuclear radiation effects</u> of nuclear weapon
      Military operation involving acute radiation exposure from nuclear weapon
      Military operation involving exposure to immediate ionizing radiation from nuclear weapon
      Military operation involving fallout exposure from nuclear weapon
      Military operation involving secondary effects of nuclear weapons
    Y37.540- Military operation involving nuclear radiation effects of nuclear weapon, <u>military</u> personnel
    Y37.541- Military operation involving nuclear radiation effects of nuclear weapon, <u>civilian</u>
  Y37.59- Military operation involving <u>other</u> effects of nuclear weapons
    Y37.590- Military operation involving other effects of nuclear weapons, <u>military</u> personnel
    Y37.591- Military operation involving other effects of nuclear weapons, <u>civilian</u>
Y37.6- Military operations involving <u>biological weapons</u>
  Y37.6x- Military operations involving biological weapons
    Y37.6x0- Military operations involving biological weapons, <u>military</u> personnel
    Y37.6x1- Military operations involving biological weapons, <u>civilian</u>
Y37.7- Military operations involving <u>chemical weapons and other forms of unconventional warfare</u>
    Excludes 1: military operations involving incendiary devices (Y36.3-, Y36.5-)
  Y37.7x- Military operations involving <u>chemical weapons</u> and other forms of unconventional warfare
    Y37.7x0- Military operations involving chemical weapons and other forms of unconventional warfare, <u>military</u> personnel
    Y37.7x1- Military operations involving chemical weapons and other forms of unconventional warfare, <u>civilian</u>
Y37.9- Other and unspecified military operations
  Y37.90x- Military operations, <u>unspecified</u>
  Y37.91x- Military operations involving <u>unspecified weapon of mass destruction [WMD]</u>
  Y37.92x- Military operations involving <u>friendly fire</u>

Y37 - Y37

Y38- Terrorism
  Note: These codes are for use to identify injuries resulting from the
    unlawful use of force or violence against persons or property to
    intimidate or coerce a Government, the civilian population, or any
    segment thereof, in furtherance of political or social objective
  Use additional code for place of occurrence (Y92.-)
  **The appropriate 7th character is to be added to each code from
  category Y38:**
    A   Initial encounter
    D   Subsequent encounter
    S   Sequela

Y38.0- Terrorism involving explosion of marine weapons
    Terrorism involving depth-charge
    Terrorism involving marine mine
    Terrorism involving mine NOS, at sea or in harbor
    Terrorism involving sea-based artillery shell
    Terrorism involving torpedo
    Terrorism involving underwater blast
  Y38.0x- Terrorism involving explosion of marine weapons
    Y38.0x1- Terrorism involving explosion of marine weapons,
      public safety official injured
    Y38.0x2- Terrorism involving explosion of marine weapons,
      civilian injured
    Y38.0x3- Terrorism involving explosion of marine weapons,
      terrorist injured

Y38.1- Terrorism involving destruction of aircraft
    Terrorism involving aircraft burned
    Terrorism involving aircraft exploded
    Terrorism involving aircraft being shot down
    Terrorism involving aircraft used as a weapon
  Y38.1x- Terrorism involving destruction of aircraft
    Y38.1x1- Terrorism involving destruction of aircraft, public
      safety official injured
    Y38.1x2- Terrorism involving destruction of aircraft, civilian
      injured
    Y38.1x3- Terrorism involving destruction of aircraft, terrorist
      injured

Y38.2- Terrorism involving other explosions and fragments
    Terrorism involving antipersonnel (fragments) bomb
    Terrorism involving blast NOS
    Terrorism involving explosion NOS
    Terrorism involving explosion of breech block
    Terrorism involving explosion of cannon block
    Terrorism involving explosion (fragments) of artillery shell
    Terrorism involving explosion (fragments) of bomb
    Terrorism involving explosion (fragments) of grenade
    Terrorism involving explosion (fragments) of guided missile
    Terrorism involving explosion (fragments) of land mine
    Terrorism involving explosion of mortar bomb
    Terrorism involving explosion of munitions
    Terrorism involving explosion (fragments) of rocket
    Terrorism involving explosion (fragments) of shell
    Terrorism involving shrapnel
    Terrorism involving mine NOS, on land
    *Excludes 1: terrorism involving explosion of nuclear weapon
      (Y38.5)*
          terrorism involving suicide bomber (Y38.81)
  Y38.2x- Terrorism involving other explosions and fragments
    Y38.2x1- Terrorism involving other explosions and fragments,
      public safety official injured
    Y38.2x2- Terrorism involving other explosions and fragments,
      civilian injured
    Y38.2x3- Terrorism involving other explosions and fragments,
      terrorist injured

Y38.3- Terrorism involving fires, conflagration and hot substances
    Terrorism involving conflagration NOS
    Terrorism involving fire NOS
    Terrorism involving petrol bomb
    *Excludes 1: terrorism involving fire or heat of nuclear weapon
      (Y38.5)*
  Y38.3x- Terrorism involving fires, conflagration and hot substances
    Y38.3x1- Terrorism involving fires, conflagration and hot
      substances, public safety official injured
    Y38.3x2- Terrorism involving fires, conflagration and hot
      substances, civilian injured
    Y38.3x3- Terrorism involving fires, conflagration and hot
      substances, terrorist injured

Y38.4- Terrorism involving firearms
    Terrorism involving carbine bullet
    Terrorism involving machine gun bullet
    Terrorism involving pellets (shotgun)
    Terrorism involving pistol bullet
    Terrorism involving rifle bullet
    Terrorism involving rubber (rifle) bullet
  Y38.4x- Terrorism involving firearms
    Y38.4x1- Terrorism involving firearms, public safety official
      injured
    Y38.4x2- Terrorism involving firearms, civilian injured
    Y38.4x3- Terrorism involving firearms, terrorist injured

Y38.5- Terrorism involving nuclear weapons
    Terrorism involving blast effects of nuclear weapon
    Terrorism involving exposure to ionizing radiation from nuclear
      weapon
    Terrorism involving fireball effect of nuclear weapon
    Terrorism involving heat from nuclear weapon
  Y38.5x- Terrorism involving nuclear weapons
    Y38.5x1- Terrorism involving nuclear weapons, public safety
      official injured
    Y38.5x2- Terrorism involving nuclear weapons, civilian injured
    Y38.5x3- Terrorism involving nuclear weapons, terrorist injured

Y38.6- Terrorism involving biological weapons
    Terrorism involving anthrax
    Terrorism involving cholera
    Terrorism involving smallpox
  Y38.6x- Terrorism involving biological weapons
    Y38.6x1- Terrorism involving biological weapons, public safety
      official injured
    Y38.6x2- Terrorism involving biological weapons, civilian
      injured
    Y38.6x3- Terrorism involving biological weapons, terrorist
      injured

Y38.7- Terrorism involving chemical weapons
    Terrorism involving gases, fumes, chemicals
    Terrorism involving hydrogen cyanide
    Terrorism involving phosgene
    Terrorism involving sarin
  Y38.7x- Terrorism involving chemical weapons
    Y38.7x1- Terrorism involving chemical weapons, public safety
      official injured
    Y38.7x2- Terrorism involving chemical weapons, civilian
      injured
    Y38.7x3- Terrorism involving chemical weapons, terrorist
      injured

Y38.8- Terrorism involving other and unspecified means
  Y38.80x- Terrorism involving unspecified means
    Terrorism NOS
  Y38.81- Terrorism involving suicide bomber
    Y38.811- Terrorism involving suicide bomber, public safety
      official injured
    Y38.812- Terrorism involving suicide bomber, civilian injured
  Y38.89- Terrorism involving other means
    Terrorism involving drowning and submersion
    Terrorism involving lasers
    Terrorism involving piercing or stabbing instruments
    Y38.891- Terrorism involving other means, public safety official
      injured
    Y38.892- Terrorism involving other means, civilian injured
    Y38.893- Terrorism involving other means, terrorist injured

Y38.9- Terrorism, secondary effects
  Note: This code is for use to identify conditions occurring
    subsequent to a terrorist attack not those that are due to the
    initial terrorist attack.
  Y38.9x- Terrorism, secondary effects
    Y38.9x1- Terrorism, secondary effects, public safety official
      injured
    Y38.9x2- Terrorism, secondary effects, civilian injured

© 2013 Channel Publishing, Ltd.

Complications of medical and surgical care (Y62-Y84)

Includes: Complications of medical devices
            Surgical and medical procedures as the cause of abnormal
            reaction of the patient, or of later complication, without
            mention of misadventure at the time of the procedure

Misadventures to patients during surgical and medical care (Y62-Y69)

Excludes❷: *breakdown or malfunctioning of medical device (during*
               procedure) (after implantation) (ongoing use) (Y70-Y82)
               surgical and medical procedures as the cause of abnormal
               reaction of the patient, without mention of misadventure
               at the time of the procedure (Y83-Y84)

Y62-   Failure of sterile precautions during surgical and medical care
- **Y62.0**   Failure of sterile precautions during <u>surgical operation</u>
- **Y62.1**   Failure of sterile precautions during <u>infusion or transfusion</u>
- **Y62.2**   Failure of sterile precautions during <u>kidney dialysis and other perfusion</u>
- **Y62.3**   Failure of sterile precautions during <u>injection or immunization</u>
- **Y62.4**   Failure of sterile precautions during <u>endoscopic examination</u>
- **Y62.5**   Failure of sterile precautions during <u>heart catheterization</u>
- **Y62.6**   Failure of sterile precautions during <u>aspiration, puncture and other catheterization</u>
- **Y62.8**   Failure of sterile precautions during <u>other</u> surgical and medical care
- **Y62.9**   Failure of sterile precautions during <u>unspecified</u> surgical and medical care

Y63-   Failure in dosage during surgical and medical care
  Excludes❷: *accidental overdose of drug or wrong drug given in error (T36-T50)*
- **Y63.0**   <u>Excessive amount</u> of blood or other fluid given during transfusion or infusion
- **Y63.1**   <u>Incorrect dilution</u> of fluid used during infusion
- **Y63.2**   <u>Overdose of radiation</u> given during therapy
- **Y63.3**   <u>Inadvertent exposure</u> of patient to radiation during medical care
- **Y63.4**   Failure in dosage in <u>electroshock or insulin-shock therapy</u>
- **Y63.5**   <u>Inappropriate temperature</u> in local application and packing
- **Y63.6**   <u>Underdosing</u> and <u>nonadministration</u> of necessary drug, medicament or biological substance
- **Y63.8**   Failure in dosage during <u>other</u> surgical and medical care
- **Y63.9**   Failure in dosage during <u>unspecified</u> surgical and medical care

Y64-   Contaminated medical or biological substances
- **Y64.0**   Contaminated medical or biological substance, <u>transfused or infused</u>
- **Y64.1**   Contaminated medical or biological substance, <u>injected or used for immunization</u>
- **Y64.8**   Contaminated medical or biological substance <u>administered by other means</u>
- **Y64.9**   Contaminated medical or biological substance administered by <u>unspecified</u> means
       Administered contaminated medical or biological substance NOS

Y65-   Other misadventures during surgical and medical care
- **Y65.0**   <u>Mismatched</u> blood in transfusion
- **Y65.1**   <u>Wrong</u> fluid used in infusion
- **Y65.2**   <u>Failure in suture or ligature</u> during surgical operation
- **Y65.3**   <u>Endotracheal tube wrongly placed</u> during anesthetic procedure
- **Y65.4**   <u>Failure to introduce or to remove</u> other tube or instrument
- **Y65.5-**   Performance of <u>wrong procedure</u> (operation)
  - **Y65.51**   Performance of wrong procedure (operation) on correct patient
         Wrong device implanted into correct surgical site
         Excludes 1:   performance of correct procedure (operation) on wrong side or body part (Y65.53)
  - **Y65.52**   Performance of procedure (operation) on patient not scheduled for surgery
         Performance of procedure (operation) intended for another patient
         Performance of procedure (operation) on wrong patient
  - **Y65.53**   Performance of correct procedure (operation) on <u>wrong side or body part</u>
         Performance of correct procedure (operation) on wrong side
         Performance of correct procedure (operation) on wrong site
- **Y65.8**   <u>Other</u> specified misadventures during surgical and medical care

Y66   <u>Nonadministration</u> of <u>surgical and medical care</u>
       Premature cessation of surgical and medical care
       Excludes 1:   DNR status (Z66)
                     palliative care (Z51.5)

Y69   <u>Unspecified</u> misadventure during surgical and medical care

Medical devices associated with adverse incidents in diagnostic and therapeutic use (Y70-Y82)

Includes: Breakdown or malfunction of medical devices (during use) (after implantation) (ongoing use)
Excludes 1:   *misadventure to patients during surgical and medical care, classifiable to (Y62-Y69)*
               later complications following use of medical devices without breakdown or malfunctioning of device (Y83-Y84)

Y70-   Anesthesiology devices <u>associated with adverse incidents</u>
- **Y70.0**   Diagnostic and monitoring anesthesiology devices associated with adverse incidents
- **Y70.1**   Therapeutic (nonsurgical) and rehabilitative anesthesiology devices associated with adverse incidents
- **Y70.2**   Prosthetic and other implants, materials and accessory anesthesiology devices associated with adverse incidents
- **Y70.3**   Surgical instruments, materials and anesthesiology devices (including sutures) associated with adverse incidents
- **Y70.8**   Miscellaneous anesthesiology devices associated with adverse incidents, not elsewhere classified

Y71-   Cardiovascular devices <u>associated with adverse incidents</u>
- **Y71.0**   Diagnostic and monitoring cardiovascular devices associated with adverse incidents
- **Y71.1**   Therapeutic (nonsurgical) and rehabilitative cardiovascular devices associated with adverse incidents
- **Y71.2**   Prosthetic and other implants, materials and accessory cardiovascular devices associated with adverse incidents
- **Y71.3**   Surgical instruments, materials and cardiovascular devices (including sutures) associated with adverse incidents
- **Y71.8**   Miscellaneous cardiovascular devices associated with adverse incidents, not elsewhere classified

Y72-   Otorhinolaryngological devices <u>associated with adverse incidents</u>
- **Y72.0**   Diagnostic and monitoring otorhinolaryngological devices associated with adverse incidents
- **Y72.1**   Therapeutic (nonsurgical) and rehabilitative otorhinolaryngological devices associated with adverse incidents
- **Y72.2**   Prosthetic and other implants, materials and accessory otorhinolaryngological devices associated with adverse incidents
- **Y72.3**   Surgical instruments, materials and otorhinolaryngological devices (including sutures) associated with adverse incidents
- **Y72.8**   Miscellaneous otorhinolaryngological devices associated with adverse incidents, not elsewhere classified

Y73-   Gastroenterology and urology devices <u>associated with adverse incidents</u>
- **Y73.0**   Diagnostic and monitoring gastroenterology and urology devices associated with adverse incidents
- **Y73.1**   Therapeutic (nonsurgical) and rehabilitative gastroenterology and urology devices associated with adverse incidents
- **Y73.2**   Prosthetic and other implants, materials and accessory gastroenterology and urology devices associated with adverse incidents
- **Y73.3**   Surgical instruments, materials and gastroenterology and urology devices (including sutures) associated with adverse incidents
- **Y73.8**   Miscellaneous gastroenterology and urology devices associated with adverse incidents, not elsewhere classified

Y74-   General hospital and personal-use devices <u>associated with adverse incidents</u>
- **Y74.0**   <u>Diagnostic</u> and monitoring general hospital and personal-use devices associated with adverse incidents
- **Y74.1**   <u>Therapeutic</u> (nonsurgical) and rehabilitative general hospital and personal-use devices associated with adverse incidents
- **Y74.2**   <u>Prosthetic</u> and other implants, materials and accessory general hospital and personal-use devices associated with adverse incidents
- **Y74.3**   <u>Surgical</u> instruments, materials and general hospital and personal-use devices (including sutures) associated with adverse incidents
- **Y74.8**   <u>Miscellaneous</u> general hospital and personal-use devices associated with adverse incidents, not elsewhere classified

Y38 – Y74

Y75- Neurological devices associated with adverse incidents

Y75.0 Diagnostic and monitoring neurological devices associated with adverse incidents

Y75.1 Therapeutic (nonsurgical) and rehabilitative neurological devices associated with adverse incidents

Y75.2 Prosthetic and other implants, materials and neurological devices associated with adverse incidents

Y75.3 Surgical instruments, materials and neurological devices (including sutures) associated with adverse incidents

Y75.8 Miscellaneous neurological devices associated with adverse incidents, not elsewhere classified

Y76- Obstetric and gynecological devices associated with adverse incidents

Y76.0 Diagnostic and monitoring obstetric and gynecological devices associated with adverse incidents

Y76.1 Therapeutic (nonsurgical) and rehabilitative obstetric and gynecological devices associated with adverse incidents

Y76.2 Prosthetic and other implants, materials and accessory obstetric and gynecological devices associated with adverse incidents

Y76.3 Surgical instruments, materials and obstetric and gynecological devices (including sutures) associated with adverse incidents

Y76.8 Miscellaneous obstetric and gynecological devices associated with adverse incidents, not elsewhere classified

Y77- Ophthalmic devices associated with adverse incidents

Y77.0 Diagnostic and monitoring ophthalmic devices associated with adverse incidents

Y77.1 Therapeutic (nonsurgical) and rehabilitative ophthalmic devices associated with adverse incidents

Y77.2 Prosthetic and other implants, materials and accessory ophthalmic devices associated with adverse incidents

Y77.3 Surgical instruments, materials and ophthalmic devices (including sutures) associated with adverse incidents

Y77.8 Miscellaneous ophthalmic devices associated with adverse incidents, not elsewhere classified

Y78- Radiological devices associated with adverse incidents

Y78.0 Diagnostic and monitoring radiological devices associated with adverse incidents

Y78.1 Therapeutic (nonsurgical) and rehabilitative radiological devices associated with adverse incidents

Y78.2 Prosthetic and other implants, materials and accessory radiological devices associated with adverse incidents

Y78.3 Surgical instruments, materials and radiological devices (including sutures) associated with adverse incidents

Y78.8 Miscellaneous radiological devices associated with adverse incidents, not elsewhere classified

Y79- Orthopedic devices associated with adverse incidents

Y79.0 Diagnostic and monitoring orthopedic devices associated with adverse incidents

Y79.1 Therapeutic (nonsurgical) and rehabilitative orthopedic devices associated with adverse incidents

Y79.2 Prosthetic and other implants, materials and accessory orthopedic devices associated with adverse incidents

Y79.3 Surgical instruments, materials and orthopedic devices (including sutures) associated with adverse incidents

Y79.8 Miscellaneous orthopedic devices associated with adverse incidents, not elsewhere classified

Y80- Physical medicine devices associated with adverse incidents

Y80.0 Diagnostic and monitoring physical medicine devices associated with adverse incidents

Y80.1 Therapeutic (nonsurgical) and rehabilitative physical medicine devices associated with adverse incidents

Y80.2 Prosthetic and other implants, materials and accessory physical medicine devices associated with adverse incidents

Y80.3 Surgical instruments, materials and physical medicine devices (including sutures) associated with adverse incidents

Y80.8 Miscellaneous physical medicine devices associated with adverse incidents, not elsewhere classified

Y81- General- and plastic-surgery devices associated with adverse incidents

Y81.0 Diagnostic and monitoring general- and plastic-surgery devices associated with adverse incidents

Y81.1 Therapeutic (nonsurgical) and rehabilitative general- and plastic-surgery devices associated with adverse incidents

Y81.2 Prosthetic and other implants, materials and accessory general- and plastic-surgery devices associated with adverse incidents

Y81.3 Surgical instruments, materials and general- and plastic-surgery devices (including sutures) associated with adverse incidents

Y81.8 Miscellaneous general- and plastic-surgery devices associated with adverse incidents, not elsewhere classified

Y82- Other and unspecified medical devices associated with adverse incidents

Y82.8 Other medical devices associated with adverse incidents

Y82.9 Unspecified medical devices associated with adverse incidents

Surgical and other medical procedures as the cause of abnormal reaction of the patient, or of later complication, without mention of misadventure at the time of the procedure (Y83-Y84)

Excludes 1: misadventures to patients during surgical and medical care, classifiable to (Y62-Y69)

Y83- Surgical operation and other surgical procedures as the cause of abnormal reaction of the patient, or of later complication, without mention of misadventure at the time of the procedure

Y83.0 Surgical operation with transplant of whole organ as the cause of abnormal reaction of the patient, or of later complication, without mention of misadventure at the time of the procedure

Y83.1 Surgical operation with implant of artificial internal device as the cause of abnormal reaction of the patient, or of later complication, without mention of misadventure at the time of the procedure

Y83.2 Surgical operation with anastomosis, bypass or graft as the cause of abnormal reaction of the patient, or of later complication, without mention of misadventure at the time of the procedure

Y83.3 Surgical operation with formation of external stoma as the cause of abnormal reaction of the patient, or of later complication, without mention of misadventure at the time of the procedure

Y83.4 Other reconstructive surgery as the cause of abnormal reaction of the patient, or of later complication, without mention of misadventure at the time of the procedure

Y83.5 Amputation of limb(s) as the cause of abnormal reaction of the patient, or of later complication, without mention of misadventure at the time of the procedure

Y83.6 Removal of other organ (partial) (total) as the cause of abnormal reaction of the patient, or of later complication, without mention of misadventure at the time of the procedure

Y83.8 Other surgical procedures as the cause of abnormal reaction of the patient, or of later complication, without mention of misadventure at the time of the procedure

Y83.9 Surgical procedure, unspecified as the cause of abnormal reaction of the patient, or of later complication, without mention of misadventure at the time of the procedure

Y84- Other medical procedures as the cause of abnormal reaction of the patient, or of later complication, without mention of misadventure at the time of the procedure

Y84.0 Cardiac catheterization as the cause of abnormal reaction of the patient, or of later complication, without mention of misadventure at the time of the procedure

Y84.1 Kidney dialysis as the cause of abnormal reaction of the patient, or of later complication, without mention of misadventure at the time of the procedure

Y84.2 Radiological procedure and radiotherapy as the cause of abnormal reaction of the patient, or of later complication, without mention of misadventure at the time of the procedure

Y84.3 Shock therapy as the cause of abnormal reaction of the patient, or of later complication, without mention of misadventure at the time of the procedure

Y84.4 Aspiration of fluid as the cause of abnormal reaction of the patient, or of later complication, without mention of misadventure at the time of the procedure

Y84.5 Insertion of gastric or duodenal sound as the cause of abnormal reaction of the patient, or of later complication, without mention of misadventure at the time of the procedure

Y84.6 Urinary catheterization as the cause of abnormal reaction of the patient, or of later complication, without mention of misadventure at the time of the procedure

Y84.7 Blood-sampling as the cause of abnormal reaction of the patient, or of later complication, without mention of misadventure at the time of the procedure

Y84.8 Other medical procedures as the cause of abnormal reaction of the patient, or of later complication, without mention of misadventure at the time of the procedure

Y84.9 Medical procedure, unspecified as the cause of abnormal reaction of the patient, or of later complication, without mention of misadventure at the time of the procedure

Y75 I Y92

Supplementary factors related to causes of morbidity classified elsewhere (Y90-Y99)

Note: These categories may be used to provide supplementary information concerning causes of morbidity. They are not to be used for single-condition coding.

Y90- **Evidence of alcohol involvement determined by blood alcohol level**
Code first any associated alcohol related disorders (F10)

Y90.0   Blood alcohol level of less than 20 mg/100 ml

Y90.1   Blood alcohol level of 20-39 mg/100 ml

Y90.2   Blood alcohol level of 40-59 mg/100 ml

Y90.3   Blood alcohol level of 60-79 mg/100 ml

Y90.4   Blood alcohol level of 80-99 mg/100 ml

Y90.5   Blood alcohol level of 100-119 mg/100 ml

Y90.6   Blood alcohol level of 120-199 mg/100 ml

Y90.7   Blood alcohol level of 200-239 mg/100 ml

Y90.8   Blood alcohol level of 240 mg/100 ml or more

Y90.9   Presence of alcohol in blood, level not specified

Y92- **Place of occurrence** of the external cause
Note: The following category is for use, when relevant, to identify the place of occurrence of the external cause. Use in conjunction with an activity code.
Note: Place of occurrence should be recorded only at the initial encounter for treatment.

Y92.0- **Non-institutional (private) residence** as the place of occurrence of the external cause
Excludes 1: abandoned or derelict house (Y92.89)
home under construction but not yet occupied (Y92.6-)
institutional place of residence (Y92.1-)

Y92.00- **Unspecified** non-institutional (private) residence as the place of occurrence of the external cause

Y92.000   **Kitchen** of unspecified non-institutional (private) residence as the place of occurrence of the external cause

Y92.001   **Dining room** of unspecified non-institutional (private) residence as the place of occurrence of the external cause

Y92.002   **Bathroom** of unspecified non-institutional (private) residence single-family (private) house as the place of occurrence of the external cause

Y92.003   **Bedroom** of unspecified non-institutional (private) residence as the place of occurrence of the external cause

Y92.007   **Garden or yard** in unspecified non-institutional (private) residence as the place of occurrence of the external cause

Y92.008   **Other** place in unspecified non-institutional (private) residence as the place of occurrence of the external cause

Y92.009   **Unspecified** place in unspecified non-institutional (private) residence as the place of occurrence of the external cause
Home (NOS) as the place of occurrence of the external cause

Y92.01- **Single-family** non-institutional (private) house as the place of occurrence of the external cause
Farmhouse as the place of occurrence of the external cause
Excludes 1: barn (Y92.71)
chicken coop or hen house (Y92.72)
farm field (Y92.73)
orchard (Y92.74)
single family mobile home or trailer (Y92.02-)
slaughter house (Y92.86)

Y92.010   **Kitchen** of single-family (private) house as the place of occurrence of the external cause

Y92.011   **Dining room** of single-family (private) house as the place of occurrence of the external cause

Y92.012   **Bathroom** of single-family (private) house as the place of occurrence of the external cause

Y92.013   **Bedroom** of single-family (private) house as the place of occurrence of the external cause

Y92.014   **Private driveway** to single-family (private) house as the place of occurrence of the external cause

Y92.015   **Private garage** of single-family (private) house as the place of occurrence of the external cause

Y92.016   **Swimming-pool** in single-family (private) house or garden as the place of occurrence of the external cause

Y92.017   **Garden or yard** in single-family (private) house as the place of occurrence of the external cause

Y92.018   **Other** place in single-family (private) house as the place of occurrence of the external cause

Y92.019   **Unspecified** place in single-family (private) house as the place of occurrence of the external cause

Y92.02- **Mobile home** as the place of occurrence of the external cause

Y92.020   **Kitchen** in mobile home as the place of occurrence of the external cause

Y92.021   **Dining room** in mobile home as the place of occurrence of the external cause

Y92.022   **Bathroom** in mobile home as the place of occurrence of the external cause

Y92.023   **Bedroom** in mobile home as the place of occurrence of the external cause

Y92.024   **Driveway** of mobile home as the place of occurrence of the external cause

Y92.025   **Garage** of mobile home as the place of occurrence of the external cause

Y92.026   **Swimming-pool** of mobile home as the place of occurrence of the external cause

Y92.027   **Garden or yard** of mobile home as the place of occurrence of the external cause

Y92.028   **Other** place in mobile home as the place of occurrence of the external cause

Y92.029   **Unspecified** place in mobile home as the place of occurrence of the external cause

Y92.03- **Apartment** as the place of occurrence of the external cause
Condominium as the place of occurrence of the external cause
Co-op apartment as the place of occurrence of the external cause

Y92.030   **Kitchen** in apartment as the place of occurrence of the external cause

Y92.031   **Bathroom** in apartment as the place of occurrence of the external cause

Y92.032   **Bedroom** in apartment as the place of occurrence of the external cause

Y92.038   **Other** place in apartment as the place of occurrence of the external cause

Y92.039   **Unspecified** place in apartment as the place of occurrence of the external cause

Y92.04- **Boarding-house** as the place of occurrence of the external cause

Y92.040   **Kitchen** in boarding-house as the place of occurrence of the external cause

Y92.041   **Bathroom** in boarding-house as the place of occurrence of the external cause

Y92.042   **Bedroom** in boarding-house as the place of occurrence of the external cause

Y92.043   **Driveway** of boarding-house as the place of occurrence of the external cause

Y92.044   **Garage** of boarding-house as the place of occurrence of the external cause

Y92.045   **Swimming-pool** of boarding-house as the place of occurrence of the external cause

Y92.046   **Garden or yard** of boarding-house as the place of occurrence of the external cause

Y92.048   **Other** place in boarding-house as the place of occurrence of the external cause

Y92.049   **Unspecified** place in boarding-house as the place of occurrence of the external cause

Y92.09- **Other** non-institutional residence as the place of occurrence of the external cause

Y92.090   **Kitchen** in other non-institutional residence as the place of occurrence of the external cause

Y92.091   **Bathroom** in other non-institutional residence as the place of occurrence of the external cause

Y92.092   **Bedroom** in other non-institutional residence as the place of occurrence of the external cause

Y92.093   **Driveway** of other non-institutional residence as the place of occurrence of the external cause

Y92.094   **Garage** of other non-institutional residence as the place of occurrence of the external cause

Y92.095   **Swimming-pool** of other non-institutional residence as the place of occurrence of the external cause

Y92.096   **Garden or yard** of other non-institutional residence as the place of occurrence of the external cause

Y92.098   **Other** place in other non-institutional residence as the place of occurrence of the external cause

Y92.099   **Unspecified** place in other non-institutional residence as the place of occurrence of the external cause

Y7 5 - Y9 2

Y92.1- <u>Institutional (nonprivate) residence</u> as the place of occurrence of the external cause

Y92.10 <u>Unspecified</u> residential institution as the place of occurrence of the external cause

Y92.11- <u>Children's home and orphanage</u> as the place of occurrence of the external cause

Y92.110 <u>Kitchen</u> in children's home and orphanage as the place of occurrence of the external cause

Y92.111 <u>Bathroom</u> in children's home and orphanage as the place of occurrence of the external cause

Y92.112 <u>Bedroom</u> in children's home and orphanage as the place of occurrence of the external cause

Y92.113 <u>Driveway</u> of children's home and orphanage as the place of occurrence of the external cause

Y92.114 <u>Garage</u> of children's home and orphanage as the place of occurrence of the external cause

Y92.115 <u>Swimming-pool</u> of children's home and orphanage as the place of occurrence of the external cause

Y92.116 <u>Garden or yard</u> of children's home and orphanage as the place of occurrence of the external cause

Y92.118 <u>Other</u> place in children's home and orphanage as the place of occurrence of the external cause

Y92.119 <u>Unspecified</u> place in children's home and orphanage as the place of occurrence of the external cause

Y92.12- <u>Nursing home</u> as the place of occurrence of the external cause

Home for the sick as the place of occurrence of the external cause

Hospice as the place of occurrence of the external cause

Y92.120 <u>Kitchen</u> in nursing home as the place of occurrence of the external cause

Y92.121 <u>Bathroom</u> in nursing home as the place of occurrence of the external cause

Y92.122 <u>Bedroom</u> in nursing home as the place of occurrence of the external cause

Y92.123 <u>Driveway</u> of nursing home as the place of occurrence of the external cause

Y92.124 <u>Garage</u> of nursing home as the place of occurrence of the external cause

Y92.125 <u>Swimming-pool</u> of nursing home as the place of occurrence of the external cause

Y92.126 <u>Garden or yard</u> of nursing home as the place of occurrence of the external cause

Y92.128 <u>Other</u> place in nursing home as the place of occurrence of the external cause

Y92.129 <u>Unspecified</u> place in nursing home as the place of occurrence of the external cause

Y92.13- <u>Military base</u> as the place of occurrence of the external cause

Excludes 1: military training grounds (Y92.83)

Y92.130 <u>Kitchen</u> on military base as the place of occurrence of the external cause

Y92.131 <u>Mess hall</u> on military base as the place of occurrence of the external cause

Y92.133 <u>Barracks</u> on military base as the place of occurrence of the external cause

Y92.135 <u>Garage</u> on military base as the place of occurrence of the external cause

Y92.136 <u>Swimming-pool</u> on military base as the place of occurrence of the external cause

Y92.137 <u>Garden or yard</u> on military base as the place of occurrence of the external cause

Y92.138 <u>Other</u> place on military base as the place of occurrence of the external cause

Y92.139 <u>Unspecified</u> place military base as the place of occurrence of the external cause

Y92.14- <u>Prison</u> as the place of occurrence of the external cause

Y92.140 <u>Kitchen</u> in prison as the place of occurrence of the external cause

Y92.141 <u>Dining room</u> in prison as the place of occurrence of the external cause

Y92.142 <u>Bathroom</u> in prison as the place of occurrence of the external cause

Y92.143 <u>Cell</u> of prison as the place of occurrence of the external cause

Y92.146 <u>Swimming-pool</u> of prison as the place of occurrence of the external cause

Y92.147 <u>Courtyard</u> of prison as the place of occurrence of the external cause

Y92.148 <u>Other</u> place in prison as the place of occurrence of the external cause

Y92.149 <u>Unspecified</u> place in prison as the place of occurrence of the external cause

Y92.15- <u>Reform school</u> as the place of occurrence of the external cause

Y92.150 <u>Kitchen</u> in reform school as the place of occurrence of the external cause

Y92.151 <u>Dining room</u> in reform school as the place of occurrence of the external cause

Y92.152 <u>Bathroom</u> in reform school as the place of occurrence of the external cause

Y92.153 <u>Bedroom</u> in reform school as the place of occurrence of the external cause

Y92.154 <u>Driveway</u> of reform school as the place of occurrence of the external cause

Y92.155 <u>Garage</u> of reform school as the place of occurrence of the external cause

Y92.156 <u>Swimming-pool</u> of reform school as the place of occurrence of the external cause

Y92.157 <u>Garden or yard</u> of reform school as the place of occurrence of the external cause

Y92.158 <u>Other</u> place in reform school as the place of occurrence of the external cause

Y92.159 <u>Unspecified</u> place in reform school as the place of occurrence of the external cause

Y92.16- <u>School dormitory</u> as the place of occurrence of the external cause

Excludes 1: reform school as the place of occurrence of the external cause (Y92.15-)
school buildings and grounds as the place of occurrence of the external cause (Y92.2-)
school sports and athletic areas as the place of occurrence of the external cause (Y92.3-)

Y92.160 <u>Kitchen</u> in school dormitory as the place of occurrence of the external cause

Y92.161 <u>Dining room</u> in school dormitory as the place of occurrence of the external cause

Y92.162 <u>Bathroom</u> in school dormitory as the place of occurrence of the external cause

Y92.163 <u>Bedroom</u> in school dormitory as the place of occurrence of the external cause

Y92.168 <u>Other</u> place in school dormitory as the place of occurrence of the external cause

Y92.169 <u>Unspecified</u> place in school dormitory as the place of occurrence of the external cause

Y92.19- <u>Other specified residential institution</u> as the place of occurrence of the external cause

Y92.190 <u>Kitchen</u> in other specified residential institution as the place of occurrence of the external cause

Y92.191 <u>Dining room</u> in other specified residential institution as the place of occurrence of the external cause

Y92.192 <u>Bathroom</u> in other specified residential institution as the place of occurrence of the external cause

Y92.193 <u>Bedroom</u> in other specified residential institution as the place of occurrence of the external cause

Y92.194 <u>Driveway</u> of other specified residential institution as the place of occurrence of the external cause

Y92.195 <u>Garage</u> of other specified residential institution as the place of occurrence of the external cause

Y92.196 <u>Pool</u> of other specified residential institution as the place of occurrence of the external cause

Y92.197 <u>Garden or yard</u> of other specified residential institution as the place of occurrence of the external cause

Y92.198 <u>Other</u> place in other specified residential institution as the place of occurrence of the external cause

Y92.199 <u>Unspecified</u> place in other specified residential institution as the place of occurrence of the external cause

Y92 - Y92

© 2013 Channel Publishing, Ltd.

Y92.2- <u>School, other institution and public administrative area</u> as the place of occurrence of the external cause

Building and adjacent grounds used by the general public or by a particular group of the public

Excludes 1: *building under construction as the place of occurrence of the external cause (Y92.6)*

residential institution as the place of occurrence of the external cause (Y92.1)

school dormitory as the place of occurrence of the external cause (Y92.16-)

sports and athletics area of schools as the place of occurrence of the external cause (Y92.3-)

Y92.21- <u>School (private) (public) (state)</u> as the place of occurrence of the external cause

Y92.210 <u>Daycare center</u> as the place of occurrence of the external cause

Y92.211 <u>Elementary school</u> as the place of occurrence of the external cause

Kindergarten as the place of occurrence of the external cause

Y92.212 <u>Middle school</u> as the place of occurrence of the external cause

Y92.213 <u>High school</u> as the place of occurrence of the external cause

Y92.214 <u>College</u> as the place of occurrence of the external cause

University as the place of occurrence of the external cause

Y92.215 <u>Trade school</u> as the place of occurrence of the external cause

Y92.218 <u>Other</u> school as the place of occurrence of the external cause

Y92.219 <u>Unspecified</u> school as the place of occurrence of the external cause

Y92.22 <u>Religious institution</u> as the place of occurrence of the external cause

Church as the place of occurrence of the external cause

Mosque as the place of occurrence of the external cause

Synagogue as the place of occurrence of the external cause

Y92.23- <u>Hospital</u> as the place of occurrence of the external cause

Excludes 1: *ambulatory (outpatient) health services establishments (Y92.53-)*

home for the sick as the place of occurrence of the external cause (Y92.12-)

hospice as the place of occurrence of the external cause (Y92.12-)

nursing home as the place of occurrence of the external cause (Y92.12-)

Y92.230 <u>Patient room</u> in hospital as the place of occurrence of the external cause

Y92.231 <u>Patient bathroom</u> in hospital as the place of occurrence of the external cause

Y92.232 <u>Corridor</u> of hospital as the place of occurrence of the external cause

Y92.233 <u>Cafeteria</u> of hospital as the place of occurrence of the external cause

Y92.234 <u>Operating room</u> of hospital as the place of occurrence of the external cause

Y92.238 <u>Other</u> place in hospital as the place of occurrence of the external cause

Y92.239 <u>Unspecified</u> place in hospital as the place of occurrence of the external cause

Y92.24- <u>Public administrative building</u> as the place of occurrence of the external cause

Y92.240 <u>Courthouse</u> as the place of occurrence of the external cause

Y92.241 <u>Library</u> as the place of occurrence of the external cause

Y92.242 <u>Post office</u> as the place of occurrence of the external cause

Y92.243 <u>City hall</u> as the place of occurrence of the external cause

Y92.248 <u>Other</u> public administrative building as the place of occurrence of the external cause

Y92.25- <u>Cultural building</u> as the place of occurrence of the external cause

Y92.250 <u>Art Gallery</u> as the place of occurrence of the external cause

Y92.251 <u>Museum</u> as the place of occurrence of the external cause

Y92.252 <u>Music hall</u> as the place of occurrence of the external cause

Y92.253 <u>Opera house</u> as the place of occurrence of the external cause

Y92.254 <u>Theater (live)</u> as the place of occurrence of the external cause

Y92.258 <u>Other</u> cultural public building as the place of occurrence of the external cause

Y92.26 <u>Movie house or cinema</u> as the place of occurrence of the external cause

Y92.29 <u>Other</u> specified public building as the place of occurrence of the external cause

Assembly hall as the place of occurrence of the external cause

Clubhouse as the place of occurrence of the external cause

Y92.3- <u>Sports and athletics area</u> as the place of occurrence of the external cause

Y92.31- <u>Athletic court</u> as the place of occurrence of the external cause

Excludes 1: *tennis court in private home or garden (Y92.09)*

Y92.310 <u>Basketball</u> court as the place of occurrence of the external cause

Y92.311 <u>Squash</u> court as the place of occurrence of the external cause

Y92.312 <u>Tennis</u> court as the place of occurrence of the external cause

Y92.318 <u>Other</u> athletic court as the place of occurrence of the external cause

Y92.32- <u>Athletic field</u> as the place of occurrence of the external cause

Y92.320 <u>Baseball</u> field as the place of occurrence of the external cause

Y92.321 <u>Football</u> field as the place of occurrence of the external cause

Y92.322 <u>Soccer</u> field as the place of occurrence of the external cause

Y92.328 <u>Other</u> athletic field as the place of occurrence of the external cause

Cricket field as the place of occurrence of the external cause

Hockey field as the place of occurrence of the external cause

Y92.33- <u>Skating rink</u> as the place of occurrence of the external cause

Y92.330 <u>Ice skating</u> rink (indoor) (outdoor) as the place of occurrence of the external cause

Y92.331 <u>Roller skating</u> rink as the place of occurrence of the external cause

Y92.34 <u>Swimming pool (public)</u> as the place of occurrence of the external cause

Excludes 1: *swimming pool in private home or garden (Y92.016)*

Y92.39 <u>Other</u> specified sports and athletic area as the place of occurrence of the external cause

Golf-course as the place of occurrence of the external cause

Gymnasium as the place of occurrence of the external cause

Riding-school as the place of occurrence of the external cause

Stadium as the place of occurrence of the external cause

Y92.4- <u>Street, highway and other paved roadways</u> as the place of occurrence of the external cause

Excludes 1: *private driveway of residence (Y92.014, Y92.024, Y92.043, Y92.093, Y92.113, Y92.123, Y92.154, Y92.194)*

Y92.41- <u>Street and highway</u> as the place of occurrence of the external cause

Y92.410 <u>Unspecified</u> street and highway as the place of occurrence of the external cause

Road NOS as the place of occurrence of the external cause

Y92.411 <u>Interstate highway</u> as the place of occurrence of the external cause

Freeway as the place of occurrence of the external cause

Motorway as the place of occurrence of the external cause

Y92.412 <u>Parkway</u> as the place of occurrence of the external cause

Y92.413 <u>State road</u> as the place of occurrence of the external cause

Y92.414 <u>Local residential or business street</u> as the place of occurrence of the external cause

Y92.415 <u>Exit ramp or entrance ramp</u> of street or highway as the place of occurrence of the external cause

Y
9
2
–
Y
9
2

Excludes 1: = NOT CODED HERE! (Do not code both)

Excludes❷: = Not Included Here

Y92.48- Other paved roadways as the place of occurrence of the external cause

Y92.480 Sidewalk as the place of occurrence of the external cause

Y92.481 Parking lot as the place of occurrence of the external cause

Y92.482 Bike path as the place of occurrence of the external cause

Y92.488 Other paved roadways as the place of occurrence of the external cause

Y92.5- Trade and service area as the place of occurrence of the external cause

Excludes 1: garage in private home (Y92.015)
schools and other public administration buildings (Y92.2-)

Y92.51- Private commercial establishments as the place of occurrence of the external cause

Y92.510 Bank as the place of occurrence of the external cause

Y92.511 Restaurant or café as the place of occurrence of the external cause

Y92.512 Supermarket, store or market as the place of occurrence of the external cause

Y92.513 Shop (commercial) as the place of occurrence of the external cause

Y92.52- Service areas as the place of occurrence of the external cause

Y92.520 Airport as the place of occurrence of the external cause

Y92.521 Bus station as the place of occurrence of the external cause

Y92.522 Railway station as the place of occurrence of the external cause

Y92.523 Highway rest stop as the place of occurrence of the external cause

Y92.524 Gas station as the place of occurrence of the external cause

Petroleum station as the place of occurrence of the external cause

Service station as the place of occurrence of the external cause

Y92.53- Ambulatory health services establishments as the place of occurrence of the external cause

Y92.530 Ambulatory surgery center as the place of occurrence of the external cause

Outpatient surgery center, including that connected with a hospital as the place of occurrence of the external cause

Same day surgery center, including that connected with a hospital as the place of occurrence of the external cause

Y92.531 Health care provider office as the place of occurrence of the external cause

Physician office as the place of occurrence of the external cause

Y92.532 Urgent care center as the place of occurrence of the external cause

Y92.538 Other ambulatory health services establishments as the place of occurrence of the external cause

Y92.59 Other trade areas as the place of occurrence of the external cause

Office building as the place of occurrence of the external cause

Casino as the place of occurrence of the external cause

Garage (commercial) as the place of occurrence of the external cause

Hotel as the place of occurrence of the external cause

Radio or television station as the place of occurrence of the external cause

Shopping mall as the place of occurrence of the external cause

Warehouse as the place of occurrence of the external cause

Y92.6- Industrial and construction area as the place of occurrence of the external cause

Y92.61 Building [any] under construction as the place of occurrence of the external cause

Y92.62 Dock or shipyard as the place of occurrence of the external cause

Dockyard as the place of occurrence of the external cause

Dry dock as the place of occurrence of the external cause

Shipyard as the place of occurrence of the external cause

Y92.63 Factory as the place of occurrence of the external cause

Factory building as the place of occurrence of the external cause

Factory premises as the place of occurrence of the external cause

Industrial yard as the place of occurrence of the external cause

Y92.64 Mine or pit as the place of occurrence of the external cause

Mine as the place of occurrence of the external cause

Y92.65 Oil rig as the place of occurrence of the external cause

Pit (coal) (gravel) (sand) as the place of occurrence of the external cause

Y92.69 Other specified industrial and construction area as the place of occurrence of the external cause

Gasworks as the place of occurrence of the external cause

Power-station (coal) (nuclear) (oil) as the place of occurrence of the external cause

Tunnel under construction as the place of occurrence of the external cause

Workshop as the place of occurrence of the external cause

Y92.7- Farm as the place of occurrence of the external cause

Ranch as the place of occurrence of the external cause

Excludes 1: farmhouse and home premises of farm (Y92.01-)

Y92.71 Barn as the place of occurrence of the external cause

Y92.72 Chicken coop as the place of occurrence of the external cause

Hen house as the place of occurrence of the external cause

Y92.73 Farm field as the place of occurrence of the external cause

Y92.74 Orchard as the place of occurrence of the external cause

Y92.79 Other farm location as the place of occurrence of the external cause

Y92.8- Other places as the place of occurrence of the external cause

Y92.81- Transport vehicle as the place of occurrence of the external cause

Excludes 1: transport accidents (V00-V99)

Y92.810 Car as the place of occurrence of the external cause

Y92.811 Bus as the place of occurrence of the external cause

Y92.812 Truck as the place of occurrence of the external cause

Y92.813 Airplane as the place of occurrence of the external cause

Y92.814 Boat as the place of occurrence of the external cause

Y92.815 Train as the place of occurrence of the external cause

Y92.816 Subway car as the place of occurrence of the external cause

Y92.818 Other transport vehicle as the place of occurrence of the external cause

Y92.82- Wilderness area

Y92.820 Desert as the place of occurrence of the external cause

Y92.821 Forest as the place of occurrence of the external cause

Y92.828 Other wilderness area as the place of occurrence of the external cause

Swamp as the place of occurrence of the external cause

Mountain as the place of occurrence of the external cause

Marsh as the place of occurrence of the external cause

Prairie as the place of occurrence of the external cause

Y92.83- Recreation area as the place of occurrence of the external cause

Y92.830 Public park as the place of occurrence of the external cause

Y92.831 Amusement park as the place of occurrence of the external cause

Y92.832 Beach as the place of occurrence of the external cause

Seashore as the place of occurrence of the external cause

Y92.833 Campsite as the place of occurrence of the external cause

Y92.834 Zoological garden (Zoo) as the place of occurrence of the external cause

Y92.838 Other recreation area as the place of occurrence of the external cause

Y92.84 Military training ground as the place of occurrence of the external cause

Y92.85 Railroad track as the place of occurrence of the external cause

Y92.86 Slaughter house as the place of occurrence of the external cause

Y92.89 Other specified places as the place of occurrence of the external cause

Derelict house as the place of occurrence of the external cause

Y92.9 Unspecified place or not applicable

Y92 - Y93

Excludes 1: = NOT CODED HERE! (Do not code both)

Excludes ❷: = Not Included Here

Y93- Activity codes

Note: Category Y93 is provided for use to indicate the activity of the person seeking healthcare for an injury or health condition, such as a heart attack while shoveling snow, which resulted from, or was contributed to, by the activity. These codes are appropriate for use for both acute injuries, such as those from chapter 19, and conditions that are due to the long-term, cumulative effects of an activity, such as those from chapter 13. They are also appropriate for use with external cause codes for cause and intent if identifying the activity provides additional information on the event. These codes should be used in conjunction with codes for external cause status (Y99) and place of occurrence (Y92).

This section contains the following broad activity categories:

Y93.0 Activities involving walking and running
Y93.1 Activities involving water and water craft
Y93.2 Activities involving ice and snow
Y93.3 Activities involving climbing, rappelling, and jumping off
Y93.4 Activities involving dancing and other rhythmic movement
Y93.5 Activities involving other sports and athletics played individually
Y93.6 Activities involving other sports and athletics played as a team or group
Y93.7 Activities involving other specified sports and athletics
Y93.A Activities involving other cardiorespiratory exercise
Y93.B Activities involving other muscle strengthening exercises
Y93.C Activities involving computer technology and electronic devices
Y93.D Activities involving arts and handcrafts
Y93.E Activities involving personal hygiene and interior property and clothing maintenance
Y93.F Activities involving caregiving
Y93.G Activities involving food preparation, cooking and grilling
Y93.H Activities involving exterior property and land maintenance, building and construction
Y93.I Activities involving roller coasters and other types of external motion
Y93.J Activities involving playing musical instrument
Y93.K Activities involving animal care
Y93.8 Activities, other specified
Y93.9 Activity, unspecified

Y93.0- Activities involving walking and running
Excludes 1: activity, walking an animal (Y93.K1)
activity, walking or running on a treadmill (Y93.A1)

Y93.01 Activity, walking, marching and hiking
Activity, walking, marching and hiking on level or elevated terrain
Excludes 1: activity, mountain climbing (Y93.31)

Y93.02 Activity, running

Y93.1- Activities involving water and water craft
Excludes 1: activities involving ice (Y93.2-)

Y93.11 Activity, swimming
Y93.12 Activity, springboard and platform diving
Y93.13 Activity, water polo
Y93.14 Activity, water aerobics and water exercise
Y93.15 Activity, underwater diving and snorkeling
Activity, SCUBA diving
Y93.16 Activity, rowing, canoeing, kayaking, rafting and tubing
Activity, canoeing, kayaking, rafting and tubing in calm and turbulent water
Y93.17 Activity, water skiing and wake boarding
Y93.18 Activity, surfing, windsurfing and boogie boarding
Activity, water sliding
Y93.19 Activity, other involving water and watercraft
Activity involving water NOS
Activity, parasailing
Activity, water survival training and testing

Y93.2- Activities involving ice and snow
Excludes 1: activity, shoveling ice and snow (Y93.H1)

Y93.21 Activity, ice skating
Activity, figure skating (singles) (pairs)
Activity, ice dancing
Excludes 1: activity, ice hockey (Y93.22)
Y93.22 Activity, ice hockey
Y93.23 Activity, snow (alpine) (downhill) skiing, snow boarding, sledding, tobogganing and snowtubing
Excludes 1: activity, cross country skiing (Y93.24)
Y93.24 Activity, cross country skiing
Activity, nordic skiing
Y93.29 Activity, other involving ice and snow
Activity involving ice and snow NOS

Y93.3- Activities involving climbing, rappelling and jumping off
Excludes 1: activity, hiking on level or elevated terrain (Y93.01)
activity, jumping rope (Y93.56)
activity, trampoline jumping (Y93.44)
Y93.31 Activity, mountain climbing, rock climbing and wall climbing
Y93.32 Activity, rappelling
Y93.33 Activity, BASE jumping
Activity, Building, Antenna, Span, Earth jumping
Y93.34 Activity, bungee jumping
Y93.35 Activity, hang gliding
Y93.39 Activity, other involving climbing, rappelling and jumping off

Y93.4- Activities involving dancing and other rhythmic movement
Excludes 1: activity, martial arts (Y93.75)
Y93.41 Activity, dancing
Y93.42 Activity, yoga
Y93.43 Activity, gymnastics
Activity, rhythmic gymnastics
Excludes 1: activity, trampolining (Y93.44)
Y93.44 Activity, trampolining
Y93.45 Activity, cheerleading
Y93.49 Activity, other involving dancing and other rhythmic movements

Y93.5- Activities involving other sports and athletics played individually
Excludes 1: activity, dancing (Y93.41)
activity, gymnastic (Y93.43)
activity, trampolining (Y93.44)
activity, yoga (Y93.42)
Y93.51 Activity, roller skating (inline) and skateboarding
Y93.52 Activity, horseback riding
Y93.53 Activity, golf
Y93.54 Activity, bowling
Y93.55 Activity, bike riding
Y93.56 Activity, jumping rope
Y93.57 Activity, non-running track and field events
Excludes 1: activity, running (any form) (Y93.02)
Y93.59 Activity, other involving other sports and athletics played individually
Excludes 1: activities involving climbing, rappelling, and jumping (Y93.3-)
activities involving ice and snow (Y93.2-)
activities involving walking and running (Y93.0-)
activities involving water and watercraft (Y93.1-)

Y93.6- Activities involving other sports and athletics played as a team or group
Excludes 1: activity, ice hockey (Y93.22)
activity, water polo (Y93.13)
Y93.61 Activity, american tackle football
Activity, football NOS
Y93.62 Activity, american flag or touch football
Y93.63 Activity, rugby
Y93.64 Activity, baseball
Activity, softball
Y93.65 Activity, lacrosse and field hockey
Y93.66 Activity, soccer
Y93.67 Activity, basketball
Y93.68 Activity, volleyball (beach) (court)
Y93.6A Activity, physical games generally associated with school recess, summer camp and children
Activity, capture the flag
Activity, dodge ball
Activity, four square
Activity, kickball
Y93.69 Activity, other involving other sports and athletics played as a team or group
Activity, cricket

Y93.7- Activities involving other specified sports and athletics
Y93.71 Activity, boxing
Y93.72 Activity, wrestling
Y93.73 Activity, racquet and hand sports
Activity, handball
Activity, racquetball
Activity, squash
Activity, tennis
Y93.74 Activity, frisbee
Activity, ultimate frisbee
Y93.75 Activity, martial arts
Activity, combatives

Y92
-
Y93

Y93.79 Activity, other specified sports and athletics
Excludes 1:   sports and athletics activities specified in categories Y93.0-Y93.6

Y93.A- Activities involving <u>other cardiorespiratory exercise</u>
Activities involving physical training

Y93.A1 Activity, exercise machines primarily for cardiorespiratory conditioning
Activity, elliptical and stepper machines
Activity, stationary bike
Activity, treadmill

Y93.A2 Activity, calisthenics
Activity, jumping jacks
Activity, warm up and cool down

Y93.A3 Activity, aerobic and step exercise

Y93.A4 Activity, circuit training

Y93.A5 Activity, obstacle course
Activity, challenge course
Activity, confidence course

Y93.A6 Activity, grass drills
Activity, guerilla drills

Y93.A9 Activity, other involving cardiorespiratory exercise
Excludes 1:   activities involving cardiorespiratory exercise specified in categories Y93.0-Y93.7

Y93.B- Activities involving other <u>muscle strengthening</u> exercises

Y93.B1 Activity, exercise machines primarily for muscle strengthening

Y93.B2 Activity, push-ups, pull-ups, sit-ups

Y93.B3 Activity, free weights
Activity, barbells
Activity, dumbbells

Y93.B4 Activity, pilates

Y93.B9 Activity, other involving muscle strengthening exercises
Excludes 1:   activities involving muscle strengthening specified in categories Y93.0-Y93.A

Y93.C- Activities involving <u>computer technology and electronic devices</u>
Excludes 1:   activity, electronic musical keyboard or instruments (Y93.J-)

Y93.C1 Activity, computer keyboarding
Activity, electronic game playing using keyboard or other stationary device

Y93.C2 Activity, hand held interactive electronic device
Activity, cellular telephone and communication device
Activity, electronic game playing using interactive device
Excludes 1:   activity, electronic game playing using keyboard or other stationary device (Y93.C1)

Y93.C9 Activity, other involving computer technology and electronic devices

Y93.D- Activities involving <u>arts and handcrafts</u>
Excludes 1:   activities involving playing musical instrument (Y93.J-)

Y93.D1 Activity, knitting and crocheting

Y93.D2 Activity, sewing

Y93.D3 Activity, furniture building and finishing
Activity, furniture repair

Y93.D9 Activity, other involving arts and handcrafts

Y93.E- Activities involving <u>personal hygiene and interior property and clothing maintenance</u>
Excludes 1:   activities involving cooking and grilling (Y93.G-)
activities involving exterior property and land maintenance, building and construction (Y93.H-)
activities involving caregiving (Y93.F-)
activity, dishwashing (Y93.G1)
activity, food preparation (Y93.G1)
activity, gardening (Y93.H2)

Y93.E1 Activity, personal bathing and showering

Y93.E2 Activity, laundry

Y93.E3 Activity, vacuuming

Y93.E4 Activity, ironing

Y93.E5 Activity, floor mopping and cleaning

Y93.E6 Activity, residential relocation
Activity, packing up and unpacking involved in moving to a new residence

Y93.E8 Activity, other personal hygiene

Y93.E9 Activity, other interior property and clothing maintenance

Y93.F- Activities involving <u>caregiving</u>
Activity involving the provider of caregiving

Y93.F1 Activity, caregiving, bathing

Y93.F2 Activity, caregiving, lifting

Y93.F9 Activity, other caregiving

Y93.G- Activities involving <u>food preparation, cooking and grilling</u>

Y93.G1 Activity, food preparation and clean up
Activity, dishwashing

Y93.G2 Activity, grilling and smoking food

Y93.G3 Activity, cooking and baking
Activity, use of stove, oven and microwave oven

Y93.G9 Activity, other involving cooking and grilling

Y93.H- Activities involving <u>exterior property and land maintenance, building and construction</u>

Y93.H1 Activity, digging, shoveling and raking
Activity, dirt digging
Activity, raking leaves
Activity, snow shoveling

Y93.H2 Activity, gardening and landscaping
Activity, pruning, trimming shrubs, weeding

Y93.H3 Activity, building and construction

Y93.H9 Activity, other involving exterior property and land maintenance, building and construction

Y93.I- Activities involving <u>roller coasters and other types of external motion</u>

Y93.I1 Activity, roller coaster riding

Y93.I9 Activity, other involving external motion

Y93.J- Activities involving <u>playing musical instrument</u>
Activity involving playing electric musical instrument

Y93.J1 Activity, piano playing
Activity, musical keyboard (electronic) playing

Y93.J2 Activity, drum and other percussion instrument playing

Y93.J3 Activity, string instrument playing

Y93.J4 Activity, winds and brass instrument playing

Y93.K- Activities involving <u>animal care</u>
Excludes 1:   activity, horseback riding (Y93.52)

Y93.K1 Activity, walking an animal

Y93.K2 Activity, milking an animal

Y93.K3 Activity, grooming and shearing an animal

Y93.K9 Activity, other involving animal care

Y93.8- Activities, <u>other specified</u>

Y93.81 Activity, refereeing a sports activity

Y93.82 Activity, spectator at an event

Y93.83 Activity, rough housing and horseplay

Y93.84 Activity, sleeping

Y93.89 Activity, other specified

Y93.9 Activity, <u>unspecified</u>

Y95 Nosocomial condition

Y99- <u>External cause status</u>
Note: A single code from category Y99 should be used in conjunction with the external cause code(s) assigned to a record to indicate the status of the person at the time the event occurred.

Y99.0 Civilian activity done for income or pay
Civilian activity done for financial or other compensation
Excludes 1:   military activity (Y99.1)
volunteer activity (Y99.2)

Y99.1 Military activity
Excludes 1:   activity of off duty military personnel (Y99.8)

Y99.2 Volunteer activity
Excludes 1:   activity of child or other family member assisting in compensated work of other family member (Y99.8)

Y99.8 Other external cause status
Activity NEC
Activity of child or other family member assisting in compensated work of other family member
Hobby not done for income
Leisure activity
Off-duty activity of military personnel
Recreation or sport not for income or while a student
Student activity
Excludes 1:   civilian activity done for income or compensation (Y99.0)
military activity (Y99.1)

Y99.9 Unspecified external cause status

Excludes 1: = NOT CODED HERE! (Do not code both)

Excludes ❷: = Not Included Here

Chapter 21 – Factors influencing health status and contact with health services (Z00-Z99)

Note: Z codes represent reasons for encounters. A corresponding procedure code must accompany a Z code if a procedure is performed. Categories Z00-Z99 are provided for occasions when circumstances other than a disease, injury or external cause classifiable to categories A00-Y89 are recorded as "diagnoses" or "problems". This can arise in two main ways:

> (a) When a person who may or may not be sick encounters the health services for some specific purpose, such as to receive limited care or service for a current condition, to donate an organ or tissue, to receive prophylactic vaccination (immunization), or to discuss a problem which is in itself not a disease or injury.
>
> (b) When some circumstance or problem is present which influences the person's health status but is not in itself a current illness or injury.

This chapter contains the following blocks:

Z00-Z13	Persons encountering health services for examinations
Z14-Z15	Genetic carrier and genetic susceptibility to disease
Z16	Resistance to antimicrobial drugs
Z17	Estrogen receptor status
Z18	Retained foreign body fragments
Z20-Z28	Persons with potential health hazards related to communicable diseases
Z30-Z39	Persons encountering health services in circumstances related to reproduction
Z40-Z53	Encounters for other specific health care
Z55-Z65	Persons with potential health hazards related to socioeconomic and psychosocial circumstances
Z66	Do not resuscitate status
Z67	Blood type
Z68	Body mass index (BMI)
Z69-Z76	Persons encountering health services in other circumstances
Z77-Z99	Persons with potential health hazards related to family and personal history and certain conditions influencing health status

Persons encountering health services for examinations (Z00-Z13)

Note: Nonspecific abnormal findings disclosed at the time of these examinations are classified to categories R70-R94.
Excludes 1: examinations related to pregnancy and reproduction (Z30-Z36, Z39.-)

Z00- Encounter for general examination without complaint, suspected or reported diagnosis
Excludes 1: encounter for examination for administrative purposes (Z02.-)
Excludes❷: encounter for pre-procedural examinations (Z01.81-)
special screening examinations (Z11-Z13)

Z00.0- Encounter for general adult medical examination
Encounter for adult periodic examination (annual) (physical) and any associated laboratory and radiologic examinations
Excludes 1: encounter for examination of sign or symptom- code to sign or symptom
general health check-up of infant or child (Z00.12.-)

Z00.00 Encounter for general adult medical examination without abnormal findings
Encounter for adult health check-up NOS

Z00.01 Encounter for general adult medical examination with abnormal findings
Use additional code to identify abnormal findings

Z00.1- Encounter for newborn, infant and child health examinations
Z00.11- Newborn health examination
Health check for child under 29 days old
Use additional code to identify any abnormal findings
Excludes 1: health check for child over 28 days old (Z00.12-)

Z00.110 Health examination for newborn under 8 days old
Health check for newborn under 8 days old

Z00.111 Health examination for newborn 8 to 28 days old
Health check for newborn 8 to 28 days old
Newborn weight check

Z00.12- Encounter for routine child health examination
Encounter for development testing of infant or child
Health check (routine) for child over 28 days old
Excludes 1: health check for child under 29 days old (Z00.11-)
health supervision of foundling or other healthy infant or child (Z76.1-Z76.2)
newborn health examination (Z00.11-)

Z00.121 Encounter for routine child health examination with abnormal findings
Use additional code to identify abnormal findings

Z00.129 Encounter for routine child health examination without abnormal findings
Encounter for routine child health examination NOS

Z00.2 Encounter for examination for period of rapid growth in childhood

Z00.3 Encounter for examination for adolescent development state
Encounter for puberty development state

Z00.5 Encounter for examination of potential donor of organ and tissue

Z00.6 Encounter for examination for normal comparison and control in clinical research program
Examination of participant or control in clinical research program

Z00.7- Encounter for examination for period of delayed growth in childhood

Z00.70 Encounter for examination for period of delayed growth in childhood without abnormal findings

Z00.71 Encounter for examination for period of delayed growth in childhood with abnormal findings
Use additional code to identify abnormal findings

Z00.8 Encounter for other general examination
Encounter for health examination in population surveys

Z01- Encounter for other special examination without complaint, suspected or reported diagnosis
Includes: Routine examination of specific system
Note: Codes from category Z01 represent the reason for the encounter. A separate procedure code is required to identify any examinations or procedures performed.
Excludes 1: encounter for examination for administrative purposes (Z02.-)
encounter for examination for suspected conditions, proven not to exist (Z03.-)
encounter for laboratory and radiologic examinations as a component of general medical examinations (Z00.0-)
encounter for laboratory, radiologic and imaging examinations for sign(s) and symptom(s) — code to the sign(s) or symptom(s)
Excludes❷: screening examinations (Z11-Z13)

Z01.0- Encounter for examination of eyes and vision
Excludes 1: examination for driving license (Z02.4)

Z01.00 Encounter for examination of eyes and vision without abnormal findings
Encounter for examination of eyes and vision NOS

Z01.01 Encounter for examination of eyes and vision with abnormal findings
Use additional code to identify abnormal findings

Z01.1- Encounter for examination of ears and hearing
Z01.10 Encounter for examination of ears and hearing without abnormal findings
Encounter for examination of ears and hearing NOS

Z01.11- Encounter for examination of ears and hearing with abnormal findings
Z01.110 Encounter for hearing examination following failed hearing screening

Z01.118 Encounter for examination of ears and hearing with other abnormal findings
Use additional code to identify abnormal findings

Z01.12 Encounter for hearing conservation and treatment
Z01.2- Encounter for dental examination and cleaning
Z01.20 Encounter for dental examination and cleaning without abnormal findings
Encounter for dental examination and cleaning NOS

Z01.21 Encounter for dental examination and cleaning with abnormal findings
Use additional code to identify abnormal findings

Z01.3- Encounter for examination of blood pressure
Z01.30 Encounter for examination of blood pressure without abnormal findings
Encounter for examination of blood pressure NOS

Z01.31 Encounter for examination of blood pressure with abnormal findings
Use additional code to identify abnormal findings

Y93 - Z01

Z01.4-   Encounter for <u>gynecological examination</u>
Excludes❷: pregnancy examination or test (Z32.0-)
routine examination for contraceptive maintenance (Z30.4-)

Z01.41- Encounter for <u>routine</u> gynecological examination
Encounter for general gynecological examination with or without cervical smear
Encounter for gynecological examination (general) (routine) NOS
Encounter for pelvic examination (annual) (periodic)
Use additional code:
For screening for human papillomavirus, if applicable, (Z11.51)
For screening vaginal pap smear, if applicable (Z12.72)
To identify acquired absence of uterus, if applicable (Z90.71-)
Excludes 1: gynecologic examination status-post hysterectomy for malignant condition (Z08)
screening cervical pap smear not a part of a routine gynecological examination (Z12.4)

Z01.411   Encounter for gynecological examination (general) (routine) <u>with abnormal findings</u>

Z01.419   Encounter for gynecological examination (general) (routine) <u>without</u> abnormal findings
Use additional code to identify abnormal findings

Z01.42 Encounter for cervical smear to confirm findings of recent normal smear following initial abnormal smear

Z01.8-   Encounter for other specified special examinations

Z01.81- Encounter for <u>preprocedural examinations</u>
Encounter for preoperative examinations
Encounter for radiological and imaging examinations as part of preprocedural examination

Z01.810   Encounter for preprocedural <u>cardiovascular</u> examination

Z01.811   Encounter for preprocedural <u>respiratory</u> examination

Z01.812   Encounter for preprocedural <u>laboratory</u> examination
Blood and urine tests prior to treatment or procedure

Z01.818   Encounter for <u>other</u> preprocedural examination
Encounter for preprocedural examination NOS
Encounter for examinations prior to antineoplastic chemotherapy

Z01.82 Encounter for allergy testing
Excludes 1: encounter for antibody response examination (Z01.84)

Z01.83 Encounter for blood typing
Encounter for Rh typing

Z01.84 Encounter for antibody response examination
Encounter for immunity status testing
Excludes 1: encounter for allergy testing (Z01.82)

Z01.89 Encounter for other specified special examinations

Z02-   Encounter for <u>administrative examination</u>

Z02.0   Encounter for examination for admission to educational institution
Encounter for examination for admission to preschool (education)
Encounter for examination for re-admission to school following illness or medical treatment

Z02.1   Encounter for pre-employment examination

Z02.2   Encounter for examination for admission to residential institution
Excludes 1: examination for admission to prison (Z02.89)

Z02.3   Encounter for examination for recruitment to armed forces

Z02.4   Encounter for examination for driving license

Z02.5   Encounter for examination for participation in sport
Excludes 1: blood-alcohol and blood-drug test (Z02.83)

Z02.6   Encounter for examination for insurance purposes

Z02.7-   Encounter for issue of medical certificate
Excludes 1: encounter for general medical examination (Z00-Z01, Z02.0-Z02.6, Z02.8-Z02.9,)

Z02.71 Encounter for disability determination
Encounter for issue of medical certificate of incapacity
Encounter for issue of medical certificate of invalidity

Z02.79 Encounter for issue of other medical certificate

Z02.8-   Encounter for other administrative examinations

Z02.81 Encounter for paternity testing

Z02.82 Encounter for adoption services

Z02.83 Encounter for blood-alcohol and blood-drug test
Use additional code for findings of alcohol or drugs in blood (R78.-)

Z02.89 Encounter for other administrative examinations
Encounter for examination for admission to prison
Encounter for examination for admission to summer camp
Encounter for immigration examination
Encounter for naturalization examination
Encounter for premarital examination
Excludes 1: health supervision of foundling or other healthy infant or child (Z76.1-Z76.2)

Z02.9   Encounter for administrative examinations, unspecified

Z03-   Encounter for <u>medical observation for suspected diseases and conditions</u> <u>ruled out</u>
Note: This category is to be used when a person without a diagnosis is suspected of having an abnormal condition, without signs or symptoms, which requires study, but after examination and observation, is ruled out. This category is also for use for administrative and legal observation status.
Excludes 1: contact with and (suspected) exposures hazardous to health (Z77.-)
newborn observation for suspected condition, ruled out (P00-P04)
person with feared complaint in whom no diagnosis is made (Z71.1)
signs or symptoms under study — code to signs or symptoms

Z03.6   Encounter for observation for suspected toxic effect from ingested substance ruled out
Encounter for observation for suspected adverse effect from drug
Encounter for observation for suspected poisoning

Z03.7-   Encounter for <u>suspected maternal and fetal conditions</u> <u>ruled out</u>
Encounter for suspected maternal and fetal conditions not found
Excludes 1: known or suspected fetal anomalies affecting management of mother, not ruled out (O26.-, O35.-, O36.-, O40.-, O41.-)

Z03.71 Encounter for suspected problem <u>with amniotic cavity and membrane</u> <u>ruled out</u>
Encounter for suspected oligohydramnios ruled out
Encounter for suspected polyhydramnios ruled out

Z03.72 Encounter for suspected <u>placental problem</u> <u>ruled out</u>

Z03.73 Encounter for suspected <u>fetal anomaly</u> <u>ruled out</u>

Z03.74 Encounter for suspected <u>problem with fetal growth</u> <u>ruled out</u>

Z03.75 Encounter for suspected <u>cervical shortening</u> <u>ruled out</u>

Z03.79 Encounter for suspected <u>other</u> suspected maternal and fetal conditions <u>ruled out</u>

Z03.8-   Encounter for observation for other suspected diseases and conditions ruled out

Z03.81- Encounter for observation for suspected exposure to biological agents ruled out

Z03.810   Encounter for observation for suspected exposure to anthrax ruled out

Z03.818   Encounter for observation for suspected exposure to other biological agents ruled out

Z03.89 Encounter for observation for other suspected diseases and conditions ruled out

Z04-   Encounter for examination and observation for other reasons
Includes: Encounter for examination for medicolegal reasons
Note: This category is to be used when a person without a diagnosis is suspected of having an abnormal condition, without signs or symptoms, which requires study, but after examination and observation, is ruled out. This category is also for use for administrative and legal observation status.

Z04.1   Encounter for examination and observation following transport accident
Excludes 1: encounter for examination and observation following work accident (Z04.2)

Z04.2   Encounter for examination and observation following work accident

Z04.3   Encounter for examination and observation following other accident

Z04.4-   Encounter for examination and observation following <u>alleged rape</u>
Encounter for examination and observation of victim following alleged rape
Encounter for examination and observation of victim following alleged sexual abuse

Z04.41 Encounter for examination and observation following alleged <u>adult</u> rape
Suspected adult rape, ruled out
Suspected adult sexual abuse, ruled out

Z04.42 Encounter for examination and observation following alleged <u>child</u> rape
Suspected child rape, ruled out
Suspected child sexual abuse, ruled out

Z01 - Z13

Z04.6   Encounter for general psychiatric examination, requested by authority

Z04.7-   Encounter for examination and observation following <u>alleged physical abuse</u>

    Z04.71   Encounter for examination and observation following alleged <u>adult</u> physical abuse
        Suspected adult physical abuse, ruled out
        Excludes 1: confirmed case of adult physical abuse (T74.-)
                encounter for examination and observation following alleged adult sexual abuse (Z04.41)
                suspected case of adult physical abuse, not ruled out (T76.-)

    Z04.72   Encounter for examination and observation following alleged <u>child</u> physical abuse
        Suspected child physical abuse, ruled out
        Excludes 1: confirmed case of child physical abuse (T74.-)
                encounter for examination and observation following alleged child sexual abuse (Z04.42)
                suspected case of child physical abuse, not ruled out (T76.-)

Z04.8   Encounter for examination and observation for other specified reasons
    Encounter for examination and observation for request for expert evidence

Z04.9   Encounter for examination and observation for unspecified reason
    Encounter for observation NOS

Z08   Encounter for follow-up examination after completed treatment for malignant neoplasm
    Medical surveillance following completed treatment
    Use additional code to identify any acquired absence of organs (Z90.-)
    Use additional code to identify the personal history of malignant neoplasm (Z85.-)
    Excludes 1: aftercare following medical care (Z43-Z49, Z51)

Z09   Encounter for follow-up examination after completed treatment for conditions other than malignant neoplasm
    Medical surveillance following completed treatment
    Use additional code to identify any applicable history of disease code (Z86.-. Z87.-)
    Excludes 1: aftercare following medical care (Z43-Z49, Z51)
               surveillance of contraception (Z30.4-)
               surveillance of prosthetic and other medical devices (Z44-Z46)

Z11-   Encounter for screening for infectious and parasitic diseases
    Note: Screening is the testing for disease or disease precursors in asymptomatic individuals so that early detection and treatment can be provided for those who test positive for the disease.
    Excludes 1: encounter for diagnostic examination — code to sign or symptom

Z11.0   Encounter for screening for intestinal infectious diseases

Z11.1   Encounter for screening for respiratory tuberculosis

Z11.2   Encounter for screening for other bacterial diseases

Z11.3   Encounter for screening for infections with a predominantly sexual mode of transmission
    Excludes❷: encounter for screening for human immunodeficiency virus [HIV] (Z11.4)
               encounter for screening for human papillomavirus (Z11.51)

Z11.4   Encounter for screening for human immunodeficiency virus [HIV]

Z11.5-   Encounter for screening for other viral diseases
    Excludes❷: encounter for screening for viral intestinal disease (Z11.0)

    Z11.51   Encounter for screening for human papillomavirus (HPV)

    Z11.59   Encounter for screening for other viral diseases

Z11.6   Encounter for screening for other protozoal diseases and helminthiases
    Excludes❷: encounter for screening for protozoal intestinal disease (Z11.0)

Z11.8   Encounter for screening for other infectious and parasitic diseases
    Encounter for screening for chlamydia
    Encounter for screening for rickettsial
    Encounter for screening for spirochetal
    Encounter for screening for mycoses

Z11.9   Encounter for screening for infectious and parasitic diseases, unspecified

---

Z12-   Encounter for <u>screening for malignant neoplasms</u>
    Note: Screening is the testing for disease or disease precursors in asymptomatic individuals so that early detection and treatment can be provided for those who test positive for the disease.
    Use additional code to identify any family history of malignant neoplasm (Z80.-)
    Excludes 1: encounter for diagnostic examination — code to sign or symptom

Z12.0   Encounter for screening for malignant neoplasm of <u>stomach</u>

Z12.1-   Encounter for screening for malignant neoplasm of <u>intestinal tract</u>

    Z12.10   Encounter for screening for malignant neoplasm of intestinal tract, <u>unspecified</u>

    Z12.11   Encounter for screening for malignant neoplasm of <u>colon</u>
        Encounter for screening colonoscopy NOS

    Z12.12   Encounter for screening for malignant neoplasm of <u>rectum</u>

    Z12.13   Encounter for screening for malignant neoplasm of <u>small intestine</u>

Z12.2   Encounter for screening for malignant neoplasm of <u>respiratory organs</u>

Z12.3-   Encounter for screening for malignant neoplasm of <u>breast</u>

    Z12.31   Encounter for screening <u>mammogram</u> for malignant neoplasm of breast
        Excludes 1: inconclusive mammogram (R92.2)

    Z12.39   Encounter for <u>other screening</u> for malignant neoplasm of breast

Z12.4   Encounter for screening for malignant neoplasm of <u>cervix</u>
    Encounter for screening pap smear for malignant neoplasm of cervix
    Excludes 1: encounter for screening for human papillomavirus (Z11.51)
               when screening is part of general gynecological examination (Z01.4-)

Z12.5   Encounter for screening for malignant neoplasm of <u>prostate</u>

Z12.6   Encounter for screening for malignant neoplasm of <u>bladder</u>

Z12.7-   Encounter for screening for malignant neoplasm of other genitourinary organs

    Z12.71   Encounter for screening for malignant neoplasm of <u>testis</u>

    Z12.72   Encounter for screening for malignant neoplasm of <u>vagina</u>
        Vaginal pap smear status-post hysterectomy for non-malignant condition
        Use additional code to identify acquired absence of uterus (Z90.71-)
        Excludes 1: vaginal pap smear status-post hysterectomy for malignant conditions (Z08)

    Z12.73   Encounter for screening for malignant neoplasm of <u>ovary</u>

    Z12.79   Encounter for screening for malignant neoplasm of <u>other genitourinary organs</u>

Z12.8-   Encounter for screening for malignant neoplasm of other sites

    Z12.81   Encounter for screening for malignant neoplasm of <u>oral cavity</u>

    Z12.82   Encounter for screening for malignant neoplasm of <u>nervous system</u>

    Z12.83   Encounter for screening for malignant neoplasm of <u>skin</u>

    Z12.89   Encounter for screening for malignant neoplasm of <u>other</u> sites

Z12.9   Encounter for screening for malignant neoplasm, <u>site unspecified</u>

Z13-   Encounter for <u>screening for other diseases and disorders</u>
    Note: Screening is the testing for disease or disease precursors in asymptomatic individuals so that early detection and treatment can be provided for those who test positive for the disease.
    Excludes 1: encounter for diagnostic examination — code to sign or symptom

Z13.0   Encounter for screening for diseases of the blood and blood-forming organs and certain disorders involving the immune mechanism

Z13.1   Encounter for screening for diabetes mellitus

Z13.2-   Encounter for screening for nutritional, metabolic and other endocrine disorders

    Z13.21   Encounter for screening for nutritional disorder

    Z13.22-   Encounter for screening for metabolic disorder

        Z13.220   Encounter for screening for lipoid disorders
            Encounter for screening for cholesterol level
            Encounter for screening for hypercholesterolemia
            Encounter for screening for hyperlipidemia

        Z13.228   Encounter for screening for other metabolic disorders

Z 0 1 - Z 1 3

Z13.29   **Encounter for screening for other suspected endocrine disorder**
> *Excludes 1: encounter for screening for diabetes mellitus (Z13.1)*

Z13.4   **Encounter for screening for certain developmental disorders in childhood**
> Encounter for screening for developmental handicaps in early childhood
> *Excludes 1: routine development testing of infant or child (Z00.1-)*

Z13.5   **Encounter for screening for eye and ear disorders**
> *Excludes ❷: encounter for general hearing examination (Z01.1-)*
> *encounter for general vision examination (Z01.0-)*

Z13.6   **Encounter for screening for cardiovascular disorders**

Z13.7-   **Encounter for screening for genetic and chromosomal anomalies**
> *Excludes 1: genetic testing for procreative management (Z31.4-)*

Z13.71   **Encounter for nonprocreative screening for genetic disease carrier status**

Z13.79   **Encounter for other screening for genetic and chromosomal anomalies**

Z13.8-   **Encounter for screening for other specified diseases and disorders**
> *Excludes ❷: screening for malignant neoplasms (Z12.-)*

Z13.81-   **Encounter for screening for digestive system disorders**

Z13.810   **Encounter for screening for upper gastrointestinal disorder**

Z13.811   **Encounter for screening for lower gastrointestinal disorder**
> *Excludes 1: encounter for screening for intestinal infectious disease (Z11.0)*

Z13.818   **Encounter for screening for other digestive system disorders**

Z13.82-   **Encounter for screening for musculoskeletal disorder**

Z13.820   **Encounter for screening for osteoporosis**

Z13.828   **Encounter for screening for other musculoskeletal disorder**

Z13.83   **Encounter for screening for respiratory disorder NEC**
> *Excludes 1: encounter for screening for respiratory tuberculosis (Z11.1)*

Z13.84   **Encounter for screening for dental disorders**

Z13.85-   **Encounter for screening for nervous system disorders**

Z13.850   **Encounter for screening for traumatic brain injury**

Z13.858   **Encounter for screening for other nervous system disorders**

Z13.88   **Encounter for screening for disorder due to exposure to contaminants**
> *Excludes 1: those exposed to contaminants without suspected disorders (Z57.-, Z77.-)*

Z13.89   **Encounter for screening for other disorder**
> Encounter for screening for genitourinary disorders

Z13.9   **Encounter for screening, unspecified**

Genetic carrier and genetic susceptibility to disease (Z14-Z15)

Z14-   **Genetic carrier**

Z14.0-   **Hemophilia A carrier**

Z14.01   **Asymptomatic hemophilia A carrier**

Z14.02   **Symptomatic hemophilia A carrier**

Z14.1   **Cystic fibrosis carrier**

Z14.8   **Genetic carrier of other disease**

Z15-   **Genetic susceptibility to disease**
> Includes: confirmed abnormal gene
> Use additional code, if applicable, for any associated family history of the disease (Z80-Z84)
> *Excludes 1: chromosomal anomalies (Q90-Q99)*

Z15.0-   **Genetic susceptibility to malignant neoplasm**
> Code first, if applicable, any current malignant neoplasm (C00-C75, C81-C96)
> Use additional code, if applicable, for any personal history of malignant neoplasm (Z85-)

Z15.01   **Genetic susceptibility to malignant neoplasm of breast**

Z15.02   **Genetic susceptibility to malignant neoplasm of ovary**

Z15.03   **Genetic susceptibility to malignant neoplasm of prostate**

Z15.04   **Genetic susceptibility to malignant neoplasm of endometrium**

Z15.09   **Genetic susceptibility to other malignant neoplasm**

Z15.8-   **Genetic susceptibility to other disease**

Z15.81   **Genetic susceptibility to multiple endocrine neoplasia [MEN]**
> *Excludes 1: multiple endocrine neoplasia [MEN] syndromes (E31.2-)*

Z15.89   **Genetic susceptibility to other disease**

Resistance to antimicrobial drugs (Z16)

Z16-   **Resistance to antimicrobial drugs**
> Note: The codes in this category are provided for use as additional codes to identify the resistance and nonresponsiveness of a condition to antimicrobial drugs.
> Code first the infection
> *Excludes 1: methicillin resistant Staphylococcus aureus infection (A49.02)*
> *methicillin resistant Staphylococcus aureus infection in diseases classified elsewhere (B95.62)*
> *methicillin resistant Staphylococcus aureus pneumonia (J15.212)*
> *sepsis due to methicillin resistant Staphylococcus aureus (A41.02)*

Z16.1-   **Resistance to beta lactam antibiotics**

Z16.10   **Resistance to unspecified beta lactam antibiotics**

Z16.11   **Resistance to penicillins**
> Resistance to amoxicillin
> Resistance to ampicillin

Z16.12   **Extended spectrum beta lactamase (ESBL) resistance**

Z16.19   **Resistance to other specified beta lactam antibiotics**
> Resistance to cephalosporins

Z16.2-   **Resistance to other antibiotics**

Z16.20   **Resistance to unspecified antibiotic**
> Resistance to antibiotics NOS

Z16.21   **Resistance to vancomycin**

Z16.22   **Resistance to vancomycin related antibiotics**

Z16.23   **Resistance to quinolones and fluoroquinolones**

Z16.24   **Resistance to multiple antibiotics**

Z16.29   **Resistance to other single specified antibiotic**
> Resistance to aminoglycosides
> Resistance to macrolides
> Resistance to sulfonamides
> Resistance to tetracyclines

Z16.3-   **Resistance to other antimicrobial drugs**
> *Excludes 1: resistance to antibiotics (Z16.1-, Z16.2-)*

Z16.30   **Resistance to unspecified antimicrobial drugs**
> Drug resistance NOS

Z16.31   **Resistance to antiparasitic drug(s)**
> Resistance to quinine and related compounds

Z16.32   **Resistance to antifungal drug(s)**

Z16.33   **Resistance to antiviral drug(s)**

Z16.34-   **Resistance to antimycobacterial drug(s)**
> Resistance to tuberculostatics

Z16.341   **Resistance to single antimycobacterial drug**
> Resistance to antimycobacterial drug NOS

Z16.342   **Resistance to multiple antimycobacterial drugs**

Z16.35   **Resistance to multiple antimicrobial drugs**
> *Excludes 1: resistance to multiple antibiotics only (Z16.24)*

Z16.39   **Resistance to other specified antimicrobial drug**

Estrogen receptor status (Z17)

Z17-   **Estrogen receptor status**
> Code first malignant neoplasm of breast (C50-)

Z17.0   **Estrogen receptor positive status [ER+]**

Z17.1   **Estrogen receptor negative status [ER-]**

Retained foreign body fragments (Z18)

Z18-   **Retained foreign body fragments**
> Includes: Embedded fragment (status)
> Embedded splinter (status)
> Retained foreign body status
> *Excludes 1: artificial joint prosthesis status (Z96.6-)*
> *foreign body accidentally left during a procedure (T81.5-)*
> *foreign body entering through orifice (T15-T19)*
> *in situ cardiac device (Z95.-)*
> *organ or tissue replaced by means other than transplant (Z96.-, Z97.-)*
> *organ or tissue replaced by transplant (Z94.-)*
> *personal history of retained foreign body fully removed Z87.821*
> *superficial foreign body (non-embedded splinter) — code to superficial foreign body, by site*

Z18.0-   **Retained radioactive fragments**

Z18.01   **Retained depleted uranium fragments**

Z18.09   **Other retained radioactive fragments**
> Other retained depleted isotope fragments
> Retained nontherapeutic radioactive fragments

Excludes 1: = NOT CODED HERE! (Do not code both)   **902**   *Excludes ❷: = Not Included Here*

Z13-Z28

Z18.1- **Retained metal fragments**
Excludes 1: retained radioactive metal fragments (Z18.01-Z18.09)

Z18.10 **Retained metal fragments, unspecified**
Retained metal fragment NOS

Z18.11 **Retained magnetic metal fragments**

Z18.12 **Retained nonmagnetic metal fragments**

Z18.2 **Retained plastic fragments**
Acrylics fragments
Diethylhexylphthalates fragments
Isocyanate fragments

Z18.3- **Retained organic fragments**

Z18.31 **Retained animal quills or spines**

Z18.32 **Retained tooth**

Z18.33 **Retained wood fragments**

Z18.39 **Other retained organic fragments**

Z18.8- **Other specified retained foreign body**

Z18.81 **Retained glass fragments**

Z18.83 **Retained stone or crystalline fragments**
Retained concrete or cement fragments

Z18.89 **Other specified retained foreign body fragments**

Z18.9 **Retained foreign body fragments, unspecified material**

Persons with potential health hazards related to communicable diseases (Z20-Z28)

Z20- **Contact with and (suspected) exposure to communicable diseases**
Excludes 1: carrier of infectious disease (Z22.-)
diagnosed current infectious or parasitic disease — see Alphabetic Index
Excludes ❷: personal history of infectious and parasitic diseases (Z86.1-)

Z20.0- **Contact with and (suspected) exposure to intestinal infectious diseases**

Z20.01 **Contact with and (suspected) exposure to intestinal infectious diseases due to Escherichia coli (E. coli)**

Z20.09 **Contact with and (suspected) exposure to other intestinal infectious diseases**

Z20.1 **Contact with and (suspected) exposure to tuberculosis**

Z20.2 **Contact with and (suspected) exposure to infections with a predominantly sexual mode of transmission**

Z20.3 **Contact with and (suspected) exposure to rabies**

Z20.4 **Contact with and (suspected) exposure to rubella**

Z20.5 **Contact with and (suspected) exposure to viral hepatitis**

Z20.6 **Contact with and (suspected) exposure to human immunodeficiency virus [HIV]**
Excludes 1: asymptomatic human immunodeficiency virus [HIV] HIV infection status (Z21)

Z20.7 **Contact with and (suspected) exposure to pediculosis, acariasis and other infestations**

Z20.8- **Contact with and (suspected) exposure to other communicable diseases**

Z20.81- **Contact with and (suspected) exposure to other bacterial communicable diseases**

Z20.810 **Contact with and (suspected) exposure to anthrax**

Z20.811 **Contact with and (suspected) exposure to meningococcus**

Z20.818 **Contact with and (suspected) exposure to other bacterial communicable diseases**

Z20.82- **Contact with and (suspected) exposure to other viral communicable diseases**

Z20.820 **Contact with and (suspected) exposure to varicella**

Z20.828 **Contact with and (suspected) exposure to other viral communicable diseases**

Z20.89 **Contact with and (suspected) exposure to other communicable diseases**

Z20.9 **Contact with and (suspected) exposure to unspecified communicable disease**

Z21 **Asymptomatic human immunodeficiency virus [HIV] infection status**
HIV positive NOS
Code first human immunodeficiency virus [HIV] disease complicating pregnancy, childbirth and the puerperium, if applicable (O98.7-)
Excludes 1: acquired immunodeficiency syndrome (B20)
contact with human immunodeficiency virus [HIV] (Z20.6)
exposure to human immunodeficiency virus [HIV] (Z20.6)
human immunodeficiency virus [HIV] disease (B20)
inconclusive laboratory evidence of human immunodeficiency virus [HIV] (R75)

Z22- **Carrier of infectious disease**
Includes: Colonization status
Suspected carrier

Z22.0 **Carrier of typhoid**

Z22.1 **Carrier of other intestinal infectious diseases**

Z22.2 **Carrier of diphtheria**

Z22.3- **Carrier of other specified bacterial diseases**

Z22.31 **Carrier of bacterial disease due to meningococci**

Z22.32- **Carrier of bacterial disease due to staphylococci**

Z22.321 **Carrier or suspected carrier of methicillin susceptible Staphylococcus aureus**
MSSA colonization

Z22.322 **Carrier or suspected carrier of methicillin resistant Staphylococcus aureus**
MRSA colonization

Z22.33- **Carrier of bacterial disease due to streptococci**

Z22.330 **Carrier of Group B streptococcus**

Z22.338 **Carrier of other streptococcus**

Z22.39 **Carrier of other specified bacterial diseases**

Z22.4 **Carrier of infections with a predominantly sexual mode of transmission**

Z22.5- **Carrier of viral hepatitis**

Z22.50 **Carrier of unspecified viral hepatitis**

Z22.51 **Carrier of viral hepatitis B**
Hepatitis B surface antigen [HBsAg] carrier

Z22.52 **Carrier of viral hepatitis C**

Z22.59 **Carrier of other viral hepatitis**

Z22.6 **Carrier of human T-lymphotropic virus type-1 [HTLV-1] infection**

Z22.8 **Carrier of other infectious diseases**

Z22.9 **Carrier of infectious disease, unspecified**

Z23 **Encounter for immunization**
Code first any routine childhood examination
Note: Procedure codes are required to identify the types of immunizations given.

Z28- **Immunization not carried out and underimmunization status**
Includes: Vaccination not carried out

Z28.0- **Immunization not carried out because of contraindication**

Z28.01 **Immunization not carried out because of acute illness of patient**

Z28.02 **Immunization not carried out because of chronic illness or condition of patient**

Z28.03 **Immunization not carried out because of immune compromised state of patient**

Z28.04 **Immunization not carried out because of patient allergy to vaccine or component**

Z28.09 **Immunization not carried out because of other contraindication**

Z28.1 **Immunization not carried out because of patient decision for reasons of belief or group pressure**
Immunization not carried out because of religious belief

Z28.2- **Immunization not carried out because of patient decision for other and unspecified reason**

Z28.20 **Immunization not carried out because of patient decision for unspecified reason**

Z28.21 **Immunization not carried out because of patient refusal**

Z28.29 **Immunization not carried out because of patient decision for other reason**

Z28.3 **Underimmunization status**
Delinquent immunization status
Lapsed immunization schedule status

Z28.8- **Immunization not carried out for other reason**

Z28.81 **Immunization not carried out due to patient having had the disease**

Z28.82 **Immunization not carried out because of caregiver refusal**
Immunization not carried out because of guardian refusal
Immunization not carried out because of parent refusal
Excludes 1: immunization not carried out because of caregiver refusal because of religious belief (Z28.1)

Z28.89 **Immunization not carried out for other reason**

Z28.9 **Immunization not carried out for unspecified reason**

Z
1
3
-
Z
2
8

Excludes 1: = NOT CODED HERE! (Do not code both)   **903**   *Excludes ❷:* = Not Included Here

Persons encountering health services in circumstances related to reproduction (Z30-Z39)

Z30- Encounter for contraceptive management
    Z30.0- Encounter for general counseling and advice on contraception
        Z30.01- Encounter for initial prescription of contraceptives
            Excludes 1: encounter for surveillance of contraceptives (Z30.4-)
            Z30.011 Encounter for initial prescription of contraceptive pills
            Z30.012 Encounter for prescription of emergency contraception
                Encounter for postcoital contraception
            Z30.013 Encounter for initial prescription of injectable contraceptive
            Z30.014 Encounter for initial prescription of intrauterine contraceptive device
                Excludes 1: encounter for insertion of intrauterine contraceptive device (Z30.430, Z30.432)
            Z30.018 Encounter for initial prescription of other contraceptives
            Z30.019 Encounter for initial prescription of contraceptives, unspecified
        Z30.02 Counseling and instruction in natural family planning to avoid pregnancy
        Z30.09 Encounter for other general counseling and advice on contraception
            Encounter for family planning advice NOS
    Z30.2 Encounter for sterilization
    Z30.4- Encounter for surveillance of contraceptives
        Z30.40 Encounter for surveillance of contraceptives, unspecified
        Z30.41 Encounter for surveillance of contraceptive pills
            Encounter for repeat prescription for contraceptive pill
        Z30.42 Encounter for surveillance of injectable contraceptive
        Z30.43- Encounter for surveillance of intrauterine contraceptive device
            Z30.430 Encounter for insertion of intrauterine contraceptive device
            Z30.431 Encounter for routine checking of intrauterine contraceptive device
            Z30.432 Encounter for removal of intrauterine contraceptive device
            Z30.433 Encounter for removal and reinsertion of intrauterine contraceptive device
                Encounter for replacement of intrauterine contraceptive device
        Z30.49 Encounter for surveillance of other contraceptives
    Z30.8 Encounter for other contraceptive management
        Encounter for postvasectomy sperm count
        Encounter for routine examination for contraceptive maintenance
        Excludes 1: sperm count following sterilization reversal (Z31.42) sperm count for fertility testing (Z31.41)
    Z30.9 Encounter for contraceptive management, unspecified
Z31- Encounter for procreative management
    Excludes 1: complications associated with artificial fertilization (N98.-) female infertility (N97.-) male infertility (N46.-)
    Z31.0 Encounter for reversal of previous sterilization
    Z31.4- Encounter for procreative investigation and testing
        Excludes 1: postvasectomy sperm count (Z30.8)
        Z31.41 Encounter for fertility testing
            Encounter for fallopian tube patency testing
            Encounter for sperm count for fertility testing
        Z31.42 Aftercare following sterilization reversal
            Sperm count following sterilization reversal
        Z31.43- Encounter for genetic testing of female for procreative management
            Use additional code for recurrent pregnancy loss, if applicable (N96, O26.2-)
            Excludes 1: nonprocreative genetic testing (Z13.7-)
            Z31.430 Encounter of female for testing for genetic disease carrier status for procreative management
            Z31.438 Encounter for other genetic testing of female for procreative management

Z31.44- Encounter for genetic testing of male for procreative management
    Excludes 1: nonprocreative genetic testing (Z13.7-)
    Z31.440 Encounter of male for testing for genetic disease carrier status for procreative management
    Z31.441 Encounter for testing of male partner of patient with recurrent pregnancy loss
    Z31.448 Encounter for other genetic testing of male for procreative management
    Z31.49 Encounter for other procreative investigation and testing
Z31.5 Encounter for genetic counseling
Z31.6- Encounter for general counseling and advice on procreation
    Z31.61 Procreative counseling and advice using natural family planning
    Z31.62 Encounter for fertility preservation counseling
        Encounter for fertility preservation counseling prior to cancer therapy
        Encounter for fertility preservation counseling prior to surgical removal of gonads
    Z31.69 Encounter for other general counseling and advice on procreation
Z31.8- Encounter for other procreative management
    Z31.81 Encounter for male factor infertility in female patient
    Z31.82 Encounter for Rh incompatibility status
    Z31.83 Encounter for assisted reproductive fertility procedure cycle
        Patient undergoing in vitro fertilization cycle
        Use additional code to identify the type of infertility
        Excludes 1: pre-cycle diagnosis and testing — code to reason for encounter
    Z31.84 Encounter for fertility preservation procedure
        Encounter for fertility preservation procedure prior to cancer therapy
        Encounter for fertility preservation procedure prior to surgical removal of gonads
    Z31.89 Encounter for other procreative management
Z31.9 Encounter for procreative management, unspecified
Z32- Encounter for pregnancy test and childbirth and childcare instruction
    Z32.0- Encounter for pregnancy test
        Z32.00 Encounter for pregnancy test, result unknown
            Encounter for pregnancy test NOS
        Z32.01 Encounter for pregnancy test, result positive
        Z32.02 Encounter for pregnancy test, result negative
    Z32.2 Encounter for childbirth instruction
    Z32.3 Encounter for childcare instruction
        Encounter for prenatal or postpartum childcare instruction
Z33- Pregnant state
    Z33.1 Pregnant state, incidental
        Pregnant state NOS
        Excludes 1: complications of pregnancy (O00-O9A)
    Z33.2 Encounter for elective termination of pregnancy
        Excludes 1: early fetal death with retention of dead fetus (O02.1) late fetal death (O36.4) spontaneous abortion (O03)
Z34- Encounter for supervision of normal pregnancy
    Excludes 1: any complication of pregnancy (O00-O9A) encounter for pregnancy test (Z32.0-) encounter for supervision of high risk pregnancy (O09-)
    Z34.0- Encounter for supervision of normal first pregnancy
        Z34.00 Encounter for supervision of normal first pregnancy, unspecified trimester
        Z34.01 Encounter for supervision of normal first pregnancy, first trimester
        Z34.02 Encounter for supervision of normal first pregnancy, second trimester
        Z34.03 Encounter for supervision of normal first pregnancy, third trimester
    Z34.8- Encounter for supervision of other normal pregnancy
        Z34.80 Encounter for supervision of other normal pregnancy, unspecified trimester
        Z34.81 Encounter for supervision of other normal pregnancy, first trimester
        Z34.82 Encounter for supervision of other normal pregnancy, second trimester
        Z34.83 Encounter for supervision of other normal pregnancy, third trimester

Z30 - Z39

Excludes ❷: = Not Included Here

Z34.9-   Encounter for supervision of normal pregnancy, <u>unspecified</u>

    Z34.90   Encounter for supervision of normal pregnancy, unspecified, <u>unspecified trimester</u>

    Z34.91   Encounter for supervision of normal pregnancy, unspecified, <u>first trimester</u>

    Z34.92   Encounter for supervision of normal pregnancy, unspecified, <u>second trimester</u>

    Z34.93   Encounter for supervision of normal pregnancy, unspecified, <u>third trimester</u>

Z36   **Encounter for antenatal screening of mother**

    Excludes 1:   *abnormal findings on antenatal screening of mother (O28.-)*
        diagnostic examination- code to sign or symptom
        encounter for suspected maternal and fetal conditions ruled out (Z03.7-)
        suspected fetal condition affecting management of pregnancy — code to condition in Chapter 15

    Excludes ❷: *genetic counseling and testing (Z31.43-, Z31.5)*
        routine prenatal care (Z34)

Z3A-   <u>Weeks of gestation</u>

    Note: Codes from category Z3A are for use, only on the maternal record, to indicate the weeks of gestation of the pregnancy.
    Code first complications of pregnancy, childbirth and the puerperium (O00-O9A)

    Z3A.0-   Weeks of gestation of pregnancy, unspecified or less than 10 weeks

        Z3A.00   Weeks of gestation of pregnancy not specified

        Z3A.01   Less than 8 weeks of gestation of pregnancy

        Z3A.08   8 weeks of gestation of pregnancy

        Z3A.09   9 weeks of gestation of pregnancy

    Z3A.1-   Weeks of gestation of pregnancy, weeks 10-19

        Z3A.10   10 weeks of gestation of pregnancy

        Z3A.11   11 weeks of gestation of pregnancy

        Z3A.12   12 weeks of gestation of pregnancy

        Z3A.13   13 weeks of gestation of pregnancy

        Z3A.14   14 weeks of gestation of pregnancy

        Z3A.15   15 weeks of gestation of pregnancy

        Z3A.16   16 weeks of gestation of pregnancy

        Z3A.17   17 weeks of gestation of pregnancy

        Z3A.18   18 weeks of gestation of pregnancy

        Z3A.19   19 weeks of gestation of pregnancy

    Z3A.2-   Weeks of gestation of pregnancy, weeks 20-29

        Z3A.20   20 weeks of gestation of pregnancy

        Z3A.21   21 weeks of gestation of pregnancy

        Z3A.22   22 weeks of gestation of pregnancy

        Z3A.23   23 weeks of gestation of pregnancy

        Z3A.24   24 weeks of gestation of pregnancy

        Z3A.25   25 weeks of gestation of pregnancy

        Z3A.26   26 weeks of gestation of pregnancy

        Z3A.27   27 weeks of gestation of pregnancy

        Z3A.28   28 weeks of gestation of pregnancy

        Z3A.29   29 weeks of gestation of pregnancy

    Z3A.3-   Weeks of gestation of pregnancy, weeks 30-39

        Z3A.30   30 weeks of gestation of pregnancy

        Z3A.31   31 weeks of gestation of pregnancy

        Z3A.32   32 weeks of gestation of pregnancy

        Z3A.33   33 weeks of gestation of pregnancy

        Z3A.34   34 weeks of gestation of pregnancy

        Z3A.35   35 weeks of gestation of pregnancy

        Z3A.36   36 weeks of gestation of pregnancy

        Z3A.37   37 weeks of gestation of pregnancy

        Z3A.38   38 weeks of gestation of pregnancy

        Z3A.39   39 weeks of gestation of pregnancy

    Z3A.4-   Weeks of gestation of pregnancy, weeks 40 or greater

        Z3A.40   40 weeks of gestation of pregnancy

        Z3A.41   41 weeks of gestation of pregnancy

        Z3A.42   42 weeks of gestation of pregnancy

        Z3A.49   Greater than 42 weeks of gestation of pregnancy

Z37-   <u>Outcome of delivery</u>

    Note: This category is intended for use as an additional code to identify the outcome of delivery on the mother's record. It is not for use on the newborn record.

    Excludes 1:   *stillbirth (P95)*

Z37.0   **Single live birth**

Z37.1   **Single stillbirth**

Z37.2   **Twins, both liveborn**

Z37.3   **Twins, one liveborn and one stillborn**

Z37.4   **Twins, both stillborn**

Z37.5-   **Other multiple births, all liveborn**

    Z37.50   **Multiple births, unspecified, all liveborn**

    Z37.51   **Triplets, all liveborn**

    Z37.52   **Quadruplets, all liveborn**

    Z37.53   **Quintuplets, all liveborn**

    Z37.54   **Sextuplets, all liveborn**

    Z37.59   **Other multiple births, all liveborn**

Z37.6-   **Other multiple births, some liveborn**

    Z37.60   **Multiple births, unspecified, some liveborn**

    Z37.61   **Triplets, some liveborn**

    Z37.62   **Quadruplets, some liveborn**

    Z37.63   **Quintuplets, some liveborn**

    Z37.64   **Sextuplets, some liveborn**

    Z37.69   **Other multiple births, some liveborn**

Z37.7   **Other multiple births, all stillborn**

Z37.9   **Outcome of delivery, unspecified**
    Multiple birth NOS
    Single birth NOS

Z38-   <u>Liveborn infants according to place of birth and type of delivery</u>

    Note: This category is for use as the principal code on the initial record of a newborn baby. It is to be used for the initial birth record only. It is not to be used on the mother's record.

Z38.0-   <u>Single</u> liveborn infant, <u>born in hospital</u>
    Single liveborn infant, born in birthing center or other health care facility

    Z38.00   Single liveborn infant, delivered <u>vaginally</u>

    Z38.01   Single liveborn infant, delivered by <u>cesarean</u>

Z38.1   <u>Single</u> liveborn infant, born <u>outside hospital</u>

Z38.2   <u>Single</u> liveborn infant, <u>unspecified</u> as to place of birth
    Single liveborn infant NOS

Z38.3-   <u>Twin</u> liveborn infant, <u>born in hospital</u>

    Z38.30   <u>Twin</u> liveborn infant, delivered <u>vaginally</u>

    Z38.31   <u>Twin</u> liveborn infant, delivered by <u>cesarean</u>

Z38.4   <u>Twin</u> liveborn infant, born <u>outside hospital</u>

Z38.5   <u>Twin</u> liveborn infant, <u>unspecified</u> as to place of birth

Z38.6-   **Other multiple liveborn infant, born in hospital**

    Z38.61   <u>Triplet</u> liveborn infant, delivered <u>vaginally</u>

    Z38.62   <u>Triplet</u> liveborn infant, delivered by <u>cesarean</u>

    Z38.63   <u>Quadruplet</u> liveborn infant, delivered <u>vaginally</u>

    Z38.64   <u>Quadruplet</u> liveborn infant, delivered by <u>cesarean</u>

    Z38.65   <u>Quintuplet</u> liveborn infant, delivered <u>vaginally</u>

    Z38.66   <u>Quintuplet</u> liveborn infant, delivered by <u>cesarean</u>

    Z38.68   <u>Other multiple</u> liveborn infant, delivered <u>vaginally</u>

    Z38.69   <u>Other multiple</u> liveborn infant, delivered by <u>cesarean</u>

Z38.7   **Other multiple liveborn infant, born outside hospital**

Z38.8   **Other multiple liveborn infant, unspecified as to place of birth**

Z39-   **Encounter for maternal postpartum care and examination**

Z39.0   **Encounter for care and examination of mother immediately after delivery**
    Care and observation in uncomplicated cases when the delivery occurs outside a healthcare facility

    Excludes 1:   *care for postpartum complication — see Alphabetic index*

Z39.1   **Encounter for care and examination of lactating mother**
    Encounter for supervision of lactation

    Excludes 1:   *disorders of lactation (O92.-)*

Z39.2   **Encounter for routine postpartum follow-up**

Z30 - Z39

Encounters for other specific health care (Z40-Z53)

NOTE: Categories Z40-Z53 are intended for use to indicate a reason for care. They may be used for patients who have already been treated for a disease or injury, but who are receiving aftercare or prophylactic care, or care to consolidate the treatment, or to deal with a residual state.
Excludes❷: follow-up examination for medical surveillance after treatment (Z08-Z09)

Z40- Encounter for <u>prophylactic surgery</u>
Excludes 1: organ donations (Z52.-)
therapeutic organ removal — code to condition

Z40.0- Encounter for prophylactic surgery for risk factors related to malignant neoplasms
Admission for prophylactic organ removal
Use additional code to identify risk factor

Z40.00 Encounter for prophylactic removal of unspecified organ
Z40.01 Encounter for prophylactic removal of breast
Z40.02 Encounter for prophylactic removal of ovary
Z40.09 Encounter for prophylactic removal of other organ
Z40.8 Encounter for other prophylactic surgery
Z40.9 Encounter for prophylactic surgery, unspecified

Z41- Encounter for <u>procedures for purposes other than remedying health state</u>
Z41.1 Encounter for <u>cosmetic surgery</u>
Encounter for cosmetic breast implant
Encounter for cosmetic procedure
Excludes 1: encounter for plastic and reconstructive surgery following medical procedure or healed injury (Z42-)
encounter for post-mastectomy breast implantation (Z42.1)
Z41.2 Encounter for routine and ritual male circumcision
Z41.3 Encounter for ear piercing
Z41.8 Encounter for other procedures for purposes other than remedying health state
Z41.9 Encounter for procedure for purposes other than remedying health state, unspecified

Z42- Encounter for <u>plastic and reconstructive surgery following medical procedure or healed injury</u>
Excludes 1: encounter for cosmetic plastic surgery (Z41.1)
encounter for plastic surgery for treatment of current injury — code to relevent injury
Z42.1 Encounter for breast reconstruction following mastectomy
Excludes 1: deformity and disproportion of reconstructed breast (N65.1-)
Z42.8 Encounter for other plastic and reconstructive surgery following medical procedure or healed injury

Z43- Encounter for <u>attention to artificial openings</u>
Includes: Closure of artificial openings
Passage of sounds or bougies through artificial openings
Reforming artificial openings
Removal of catheter from artificial openings
Toilet or cleansing of artificial openings
Excludes 1: artificial opening status only, without need for care (Z93.-)
complications of external stoma (J95.0-, K94.-, N99.5-)
Excludes❷: fitting and adjustment of prosthetic and other devices (Z44-Z46)
Z43.0 Encounter for attention to tracheostomy
Z43.1 Encounter for attention to gastrostomy
Z43.2 Encounter for attention to ileostomy
Z43.3 Encounter for attention to colostomy
Z43.4 Encounter for attention to other artificial openings of digestive tract
Z43.5 Encounter for attention to cystostomy
Z43.6 Encounter for attention to other artificial openings of urinary tract
Encounter for attention to nephrostomy
Encounter for attention to ureterostomy
Encounter for attention to urethrostomy
Z43.7 Encounter for attention to artificial vagina
Z43.8 Encounter for attention to other artificial openings
Z43.9 Encounter for attention to unspecified artificial opening

Z44- Encounter for <u>fitting and adjustment of external prosthetic device</u>
Includes: Removal or replacement of external prosthetic device
Excludes 1: malfunction or other complications of device — see Alphabetical Index
presence of prosthetic device (Z97.-)
Z44.0- Encounter for fitting and adjustment of <u>artificial arm</u>
Z44.00- Encounter for fitting and adjustment of <u>unspecified</u> artificial arm
Z44.001 Encounter for fitting and adjustment of unspecified <u>right</u> artificial arm
Z44.002 Encounter for fitting and adjustment of unspecified <u>left</u> artificial arm
Z44.009 Encounter for fitting and adjustment of unspecified artificial arm, <u>unspecified</u> arm
Z44.01- Encounter for fitting and adjustment of <u>complete</u> artificial arm
Z44.011 Encounter for fitting and adjustment of complete <u>right</u> artificial arm
Z44.012 Encounter for fitting and adjustment of complete <u>left</u> artificial arm
Z44.019 Encounter for fitting and adjustment of complete artificial arm, <u>unspecified</u> arm
Z44.02- Encounter for fitting and adjustment of <u>partial</u> artificial arm
Z44.021 Encounter for fitting and adjustment of partial artificial <u>right</u> arm
Z44.022 Encounter for fitting and adjustment of partial artificial <u>left</u> arm
Z44.029 Encounter for fitting and adjustment of partial artificial arm, <u>unspecified</u> arm
Z44.1- Encounter for <u>fitting and adjustment of artificial leg</u>
Z44.10- Encounter for fitting and adjustment of unspecified artificial leg
Z44.101 Encounter for fitting and adjustment of unspecified <u>right</u> artificial leg
Z44.102 Encounter for fitting and adjustment of unspecified <u>left</u> artificial leg
Z44.109 Encounter for fitting and adjustment of unspecified artificial leg, <u>unspecified</u> leg
Z44.11- Encounter for fitting and adjustment of <u>complete</u> artificial leg
Z44.111 Encounter for fitting and adjustment of complete <u>right</u> artificial leg
Z44.112 Encounter for fitting and adjustment of complete <u>left</u> artificial leg
Z44.119 Encounter for fitting and adjustment of complete artificial leg, <u>unspecified</u> leg
Z44.12- Encounter for fitting and adjustment of <u>partial</u> artificial leg
Z44.121 Encounter for fitting and adjustment of partial artificial <u>right</u> leg
Z44.122 Encounter for fitting and adjustment of partial artificial <u>left</u> leg
Z44.129 Encounter for fitting and adjustment of partial artificial leg, unspecified leg
Z44.2- Encounter for <u>fitting and adjustment of artificial eye</u>
Excludes 1: mechanical complication of ocular prosthesis (T85.3)
Z44.20 Encounter for fitting and adjustment of artificial eye, <u>unspecified</u>
Z44.21 Encounter for fitting and adjustment of artificial <u>right</u> eye
Z44.22 Encounter for fitting and adjustment of artificial <u>left</u> eye
Z44.3- Encounter for <u>fitting and adjustment of external breast prosthesis</u>
Excludes 1: complications of breast implant (T85.4-)
encounter for adjustment or removal of breast implant (Z45.81-)
encounter for initial breast implant insertion for cosmetic breast augmentation (Z41.1)
encounter for breast reconstruction following mastectomy (Z42.1)
Z44.30 Encounter for fitting and adjustment of external breast prosthesis, <u>unspecified</u> breast
Z44.31 Encounter for fitting and adjustment of external <u>right</u> breast prosthesis
Z44.32 Encounter for fitting and adjustment of external <u>left</u> breast prosthesis
Z44.8 Encounter for fitting and adjustment of other external prosthetic devices
Z44.9 Encounter for fitting and adjustment of unspecified external prosthetic device

Z45-   Encounter for <u>adjustment and management of implanted device</u>
Includes: Removal or replacement of implanted device
*Excludes 1:   malfunction or other complications of device — see
        Alphabetical Index
        presence of prosthetic and other devices (Z95-Z97)*
*Excludes❷: encounter for fitting and adjustment of non-implanted device
        (Z46-)*

Z45.0-   Encounter for adjustment and management of <u>cardiac device</u>

Z45.01-   Encounter for adjustment and management of cardiac
    <u>pacemaker</u>
    *Excludes 1:   encounter for adjustment and management of
        automatic implantable cardiac defibrillator
        with synchronous cardiac pacemaker (Z45.02)*

Z45.010   Encounter for checking and testing of cardiac
    pacemaker <u>pulse generator [battery]</u>
        Encounter for replacing cardiac pacemaker pulse
        generator [battery]

Z45.018   Encounter for adjustment and management of <u>other
    part of cardiac pacemaker</u>

Z45.02   Encounter for adjustment and management of automatic
    implantable <u>cardiac defibrillator</u>
        Encounter for adjustment and management of automatic
        implantable cardiac defibrillator with synchronous cardiac
        pacemaker

Z45.09   Encounter for adjustment and management of other cardiac
    device

Z45.1   Encounter for adjustment and management of <u>infusion pump</u>
Z45.2   Encounter for adjustment and management of <u>vascular access
    device</u>
        Encounter for adjustment and management of vascular catheters
    *Excludes 1:   encounter for adjustment and management of renal
        dialysis catheter (Z49.01)*

Z45.3-   Encounter for <u>adjustment and management of implanted devices
    of the special senses</u>

Z45.31   Encounter for adjustment and management of implanted
    visual substitution device

Z45.32-   Encounter for adjustment and management of <u>implanted
    hearing device</u>
    *Excludes 1:   Encounter for fitting and adjustment of hearing
        aide (Z46.1)*

Z45.320   Encounter for adjustment and management of <u>bone
    conduction device</u>

Z45.321   Encounter for adjustment and management of
    <u>cochlear device</u>

Z45.328   Encounter for adjustment and management of <u>other</u>
    implanted hearing device

Z45.4-   Encounter for <u>adjustment and management of implanted
    nervous system device</u>

Z45.41   Encounter for adjustment and management of <u>cerebrospinal
    fluid drainage device</u>
        Encounter for adjustment and management of cerebral
        ventricular (communicating) shunt

Z45.42   Encounter for adjustment and management of
    <u>neuropacemaker</u> (brain) (peripheral nerve) (spinal cord)

Z45.49   Encounter for adjustment and management of <u>other</u>
    implanted nervous system device

Z45.8-   Encounter for adjustment and management of <u>other implanted
    devices</u>

Z45.81-   Encounter for <u>adjustment or removal of breast implant</u>
        Encounter for elective implant exchange (different material)
        (different size)
        Encounter removal of tissue expander without synchronous
        insertion of permanent implant
    *Excludes 1:   complications of breast implant (T85.4-)
        encounter for initial breast implant insertion for
        cosmetic breast augmentation (Z41.1)
        encounter for breast reconstruction following
        mastectomy (Z42.1)*

Z45.811   Encounter for adjustment or removal of <u>right</u> breast
    implant

Z45.812   Encounter for adjustment or removal of <u>left</u> breast
    implant

Z45.819   Encounter for adjustment or removal of <u>unspecified</u>
    breast implant

Z45.82   Encounter for adjustment or removal of myringotomy device
    (stent) (tube)

Z45.89   Encounter for adjustment and management of other
    implanted devices

Z45.9   Encounter for adjustment and management of unspecified
    implanted device

Z46-   Encounter for <u>fitting and adjustment of other devices</u>
Includes: Removal or replacement of other device
*Excludes 1:   malfunction or other complications of device — see
        Alphabetical Index*
*Excludes❷: encounter for fitting and management of implanted devices
        (Z45-)
        issue of repeat prescription only (Z76.0)
        presence of prosthetic and other devices (Z95-Z97)*

Z46.0   Encounter for fitting and adjustment of <u>spectacles and contact
    lenses</u>

Z46.1   Encounter for fitting and adjustment of <u>hearing aid</u>
    *Excludes 1:   encounter for adjustment and management of implanted
        hearing device (Z45.32-)*

Z46.2   Encounter for fitting and adjustment of <u>other devices related to
    nervous system and special senses</u>
    *Excludes❷: encounter for adjustment and management of implanted
        nervous system device (Z45.4-)
        encounter for adjustment and management of implanted
        visual substitution device (Z45.31)*

Z46.3   Encounter for fitting and adjustment of <u>dental prosthetic device</u>
        Encounter for fitting and adjustment of dentures

Z46.4   Encounter for fitting and adjustment of <u>orthodontic</u> device

Z46.5-   Encounter for fitting and adjustment of <u>other gastrointestinal
    appliance and device</u>
    *Excludes 1:   encounter for attention to artificial openings of
        digestive tract (Z43.1-Z43.4)*

Z46.51   Encounter for fitting and adjustment of <u>gastric lap band</u>

Z46.59   Encounter for fitting and adjustment of <u>other</u>
    gastrointestinal appliance and device

Z46.6   Encounter for fitting and adjustment of <u>urinary device</u>
    *Excludes❷: attention to artificial openings of urinary tract (Z43.5,
        Z43.6)*

Z46.8-   Encounter for fitting and adjustment of other specified devices

Z46.81   Encounter for fitting and adjustment of <u>insulin pump</u>
        Encounter for insulin pump titration
        Encounter for insulin pump instruction and training

Z46.82   Encounter for fitting and adjustment of <u>non-vascular
    catheter</u>

Z46.89   Encounter for fitting and adjustment of <u>other</u> specified
    devices
        Encounter for fitting and adjustment of wheelchair

Z46.9   Encounter for fitting and adjustment of unspecified device

Z47-   Orthopedic aftercare
*Excludes 1:   aftercare for healing fracture — code to fracture with 7th
        character D*

Z47.1   Aftercare following <u>joint replacement</u> surgery
    Use additional code to identify the joint (Z96.6-)

Z47.2   Encounter for <u>removal of internal fixation device</u>
    *Excludes 1:   encounter for adjustment of internal fixation device for
        fracture treatment — code to fracture with
        appropriate 7th character
        encounter for removal of external fixation device —
        code to fracture with 7th character D
        infection or inflammatory reaction to internal fixation
        device (T84.6-)
        mechanical complication of internal fixation device
        (T84.1-)*

Z47.3-   Aftercare following <u>explantation of joint prosthesis</u>
        Aftercare following explantation of joint prosthesis, staged
        procedure
        Encounter for joint prosthesis insertion following prior
        explantation of joint prosthesis

Z47.31   Aftercare following explantation of <u>shoulder</u> joint prosthesis
    *Excludes 1:   acquired absence of shoulder joint following prior
        explantation of shoulder joint prosthesis
        (Z89.23-)
        shoulder joint prosthesis explantation status
        (Z89.23-)*

Z47.32   Aftercare following explantation of <u>hip</u> joint prosthesis
    *Excludes 1:   acquired absence of hip joint following prior
        explantation of hip joint prosthesis (Z89.62-)
        hip joint prosthesis explantation status (Z89.62-)*

Z47.33   Aftercare following explantation of <u>knee</u> joint prosthesis
    *Excludes 1:   acquired absence of knee joint following prior
        explantation of knee joint prosthesis (Z89.52-)
        knee joint prosthesis explantation status (Z89.52-)*

Z40 – Z47

Excludes 1: = NOT CODED HERE! (Do not code both)   *Excludes❷:* = Not Included Here

Z47.8- Encounter for <u>other orthopedic aftercare</u>
    Z47.81 Encounter for orthopedic aftercare <u>following surgical amputation</u>
        Use additional code to identify the limb amputated (Z89.-)
    Z47.82 Encounter for orthopedic aftercare <u>following scoliosis surgery</u>
    Z47.89 Encounter for <u>other</u> orthopedic aftercare

Z48- Encounter for <u>other postprocedural aftercare</u>
    Excludes 1: encounter for follow-up examination after completed treatment (Z08-Z09)
    Excludes ❷: encounter for attention to artificial openings (Z43.-)
        encounter for fitting and adjustment of prosthetic and other devices (Z44-Z46)
    Z48.0- Encounter for attention to dressings, sutures and drains
        Excludes 1: encounter for planned postprocedural wound closure (Z48.1)
        Z48.00 Encounter for change or removal of nonsurgical wound dressing
            Encounter for change or removal of wound dressing NOS
        Z48.01 Encounter for change or removal of surgical wound dressing
        Z48.02 Encounter for removal of sutures
            Encounter for removal of staples
        Z48.03 Encounter for change or removal of drains
    Z48.1 Encounter for planned postprocedural wound closure
        Excludes 1: encounter for attention to dressings and sutures (Z48.0-)
    Z48.2- Encounter for <u>aftercare following organ transplant</u>
        Z48.21 Encounter for aftercare following <u>heart</u> transplant
        Z48.22 Encounter for aftercare following <u>kidney</u> transplant
        Z48.23 Encounter for aftercare following <u>liver</u> transplant
        Z48.24 Encounter for aftercare following <u>lung</u> transplant
        Z48.28- Encounter for aftercare following <u>multiple</u> organ transplant
            Z48.280 Encounter for aftercare following <u>heart-lung transplant</u>
            Z48.288 Encounter for aftercare following <u>multiple organ transplant</u>
        Z48.29- Encounter for aftercare following <u>other</u> organ transplant
            Z48.290 Encounter for aftercare following <u>bone marrow</u> transplant
            Z48.298 Encounter for aftercare following <u>other</u> organ transplant
    Z48.3 Aftercare following <u>surgery for neoplasm</u>
        Use additional code to identify the neoplasm
    Z48.8- Encounter for other specified postprocedural aftercare
        Z48.81- Encounter for surgical aftercare following surgery on specified body systems
            Note: These codes identify the body system requiring aftercare. They are for use in conjunction with other aftercare codes to fully explain the aftercare encounter. The condition treated should also be coded if still present.
            Excludes 1: aftercare for injury — code the injury with 7th character D
            aftercare following surgery for neoplasm (Z48.3)
            Excludes ❷: aftercare following organ transplant (Z48.2-)
            orthopedic aftercare (Z47.-)
        Z48.810 Encounter for surgical aftercare following surgery on the sense organs
        Z48.811 Encounter for surgical aftercare following surgery on the nervous system
            Excludes ❷: encounter for surgical aftercare following surgery on the sense organs (Z48.810)
        Z48.812 Encounter for surgical aftercare following surgery on the circulatory system
        Z48.813 Encounter for surgical aftercare following surgery on the respiratory system
        Z48.814 Encounter for surgical aftercare following surgery on the teeth or oral cavity
        Z48.815 Encounter for surgical aftercare following surgery on the digestive system
        Z48.816 Encounter for surgical aftercare following surgery on the genitourinary system
            Excludes 1: encounter for aftercare following sterilization reversal (Z31.42)
        Z48.817 Encounter for surgical aftercare following surgery on the skin and subcutaneous tissue
        Z48.89 Encounter for other specified surgical aftercare

Z49- Encounter for care involving renal dialysis
    Code also associated end stage renal disease (N18.6)
    Z49.0- Preparatory care for renal dialysis
        Encounter for dialysis instruction and training
        Z49.01 Encounter for fitting and adjustment of <u>extracorporeal dialysis catheter</u>
            Removal or replacement of renal dialysis catheter
            Toilet or cleansing of renal dialysis catheter
        Z49.02 Encounter for fitting and adjustment of <u>peritoneal dialysis catheter</u>
    Z49.3- Encounter for adequacy testing for <u>dialysis</u>
        Z49.31 Encounter for adequacy testing for <u>hemodialysis</u>
        Z49.32 Encounter for adequacy testing for <u>peritoneal dialysis</u>
            Encounter for peritoneal equilibration test

Z51- Encounter for other aftercare
    Code also condition requiring care
    Excludes 1: follow-up examination after treatment (Z08-Z09)
    Z51.0 Encounter for <u>antineoplastic radiation therapy</u>
    Z51.1- Encounter for antineoplastic chemotherapy and immunotherapy
        Excludes ❷: encounter for chemotherapy and immunotherapy for nonneoplastic condition — code to condition
        Z51.11 Encounter for <u>antineoplastic chemotherapy</u>
        Z51.12 Encounter for <u>antineoplastic immunotherapy</u>
    Z51.5 Encounter for <u>palliative care</u>
    Z51.8- Encounter for other specified aftercare
        Excludes 1: holiday relief care (Z75.5)
        Z51.81 Encounter for therapeutic drug level monitoring
            Code also any long-term (current) drug therapy (Z79.-)
            Excludes 1: encounter for blood-drug test for administrative or medicolegal reasons (Z02.83)
        Z51.89 Encounter for other specified aftercare

Z52- Donors of organs and tissues
    Includes: Autologous and other living donors
    Excludes 1: cadaveric donor — omit code
        examination of potential donor (Z00.5)
    Z52.0- <u>Blood donor</u>
        Z52.00- <u>Unspecified</u> blood donor
            Z52.000 Unspecified donor, whole blood
            Z52.001 Unspecified donor, stem cells
            Z52.008 Unspecified donor, other blood
        Z52.01- <u>Autologous</u> blood donor
            Z52.010 Autologous donor, whole blood
            Z52.011 Autologous donor, stem cells
            Z52.018 Autologous donor, other blood
        Z52.09- <u>Other blood</u> donor
            Volunteer donor
            Z52.090 Other blood donor, whole blood
            Z52.091 Other blood donor, stem cells
            Z52.098 Other blood donor, other blood
    Z52.1- <u>Skin</u> donor
        Z52.10 Skin donor, unspecified
        Z52.11 Skin donor, autologous
        Z52.19 Skin donor, other
    Z52.2- <u>Bone</u> donor
        Z52.20 Bone donor, unspecified
        Z52.21 Bone donor, autologous
        Z52.29 Bone donor, other
    Z52.3 Bone marrow donor
    Z52.4 Kidney donor
    Z52.5 Cornea donor
    Z52.6 Liver donor
    Z52.8- Donor of other specified organs or tissues
        Z52.81- Egg (Oocyte) donor
            Z52.810 Egg (Oocyte) donor <u>under age 35, anonymous recipient</u>
                Egg donor under age 35 NOS
            Z52.811 Egg (Oocyte) donor <u>under age 35, designated</u> recipient
            Z52.812 Egg (Oocyte) donor <u>age 35 and over, anonymous recipient</u>
                Egg donor age 35 and over NOS
            Z52.813 Egg (Oocyte) donor <u>age 35 and over, designated</u> recipient
            Z52.819 Egg (Oocyte) donor, <u>unspecified</u>
        Z52.89 Donor of other specified organs or tissues
    Z52.9 Donor of unspecified organ or tissue
        Donor NOS

Z53- Persons encountering health services for <u>specific procedures and treatment</u>, <u>not carried out</u>
  Z53.0- Procedure and treatment not carried out because of <u>contraindication</u>
    Z53.01 Procedure and treatment not carried out <u>due to patient smoking</u>
    Z53.09 Procedure and treatment not carried out <u>because of other contraindication</u>
  Z53.1 Procedure and treatment not carried out <u>because of patient's decision for reasons of belief and group pressure</u>
  Z53.2- Procedure and treatment not carried out <u>because of patient's decision for other and unspecified reasons</u>
    Z53.20 Procedure and treatment not carried out because of patient's decision for unspecified reasons
    Z53.21 Procedure and treatment not carried out due to patient leaving prior to being seen by healthcare provider
    Z53.29 Procedure and treatment not carried out because of patient's decision for other reasons
  Z53.8 Procedure and treatment <u>not carried out for other reasons</u>
  Z53.9 Procedure and treatment <u>not carried out</u>, <u>unspecified</u> reason

Persons with potential health hazards related to socioeconomic and psychosocial circumstances (Z55-Z65)

Z55- Problems related to education and literacy
  Excludes 1: disorders of psychological development (F80-F89)
  Z55.0 Illiteracy and low-level literacy
  Z55.1 Schooling unavailable and unattainable
  Z55.2 Failed school examinations
  Z55.3 Underachievement in school
  Z55.4 Educational maladjustment and discord with teachers and classmates
  Z55.8 Other problems related to education and literacy
    Problems related to inadequate teaching
  Z55.9 Problems related to education and literacy, unspecified
    Academic problems NOS

Z56- Problems related to employment and unemployment
  Excludes❷: occupational exposure to risk factors (Z57.-)
    problems related to housing and economic circumstances (Z59.-)
  Z56.0 Unemployment, unspecified
  Z56.1 Change of job
  Z56.2 Threat of job loss
  Z56.3 Stressful work schedule
  Z56.4 Discord with boss and workmates
  Z56.5 Uncongenial work environment
    Difficult conditions at work
  Z56.6 Other physical and mental strain related to work
  Z56.8- Other problems related to employment
    Z56.81 Sexual harassment on the job
    Z56.82 Military deployment status
      Individual (civilian or military) currently deployed in theater or in support of military war, peacekeeping and humanitarian operations
    Z56.89 Other problems related to employment
  Z56.9 Unspecified problems related to employment
    Occupational problems NOS

Z57- Occupational exposure to risk factors
  Z57.0 Occupational exposure to noise
  Z57.1 Occupational exposure to radiation
  Z57.2 Occupational exposure to dust
  Z57.3- Occupational exposure to other air contaminants
    Z57.31 Occupational exposure to environmental tobacco smoke
      Excludes❷: exposure to environmental tobacco smoke (Z77.22)
    Z57.39 Occupational exposure to other air contaminants
  Z57.4 Occupational exposure to toxic agents in agriculture
    Occupational exposure to solids, liquids, gases or vapors in agriculture
  Z57.5 Occupational exposure to toxic agents in other industries
    Occupational exposure to solids, liquids, gases or vapors in other industries
  Z57.6 Occupational exposure to extreme temperature
  Z57.7 Occupational exposure to vibration
  Z57.8 Occupational exposure to other risk factors
  Z57.9 Occupational exposure to unspecified risk factor

Z59- Problems related to housing and economic circumstances
  Excludes❷: problems related to upbringing (Z62.-)
  Z59.0 Homelessness
  Z59.1 Inadequate housing
    Lack of heating
    Restriction of space
    Technical defects in home preventing adequate care
    Unsatisfactory surroundings
    Excludes 1: problems related to the natural and physical environment (Z77.1-)
  Z59.2 Discord with neighbors, lodgers and landlord
  Z59.3 Problems related to living in residential institution
    Boarding-school resident
    Excludes 1: institutional upbringing (Z62.2)
  Z59.4 Lack of adequate food and safe drinking water
    Inadequate drinking water supply
    Excludes 1: effects of hunger (T73.0)
    inappropriate diet or eating habits (Z72.4)
    malnutrition (E40-E46)
  Z59.5 Extreme poverty
  Z59.6 Low income
  Z59.7 Insufficient social insurance and welfare support
  Z59.8 Other problems related to housing and economic circumstances
    Foreclosure on loan
    Isolated dwelling
    Problems with creditors
  Z59.9 Problem related to housing and economic circumstances, unspecified

Z60- Problems related to social environment
  Z60.0 Problems of adjustment to life-cycle transitions
    Empty nest syndrome
    Phase of life problem
    Problem with adjustment to retirement [pension]
  Z60.2 Problems related to living alone
  Z60.3 Acculturation difficulty
    Problem with migration
    Problem with social transplantation
  Z60.4 Social exclusion and rejection
    Exclusion and rejection on the basis of personal characteristics, such as unusual physical appearance, illness or behavior.
    Excludes 1: target of adverse discrimination such as for racial or religious reasons (Z60.5)
  Z60.5 Target of (perceived) adverse discrimination and persecution
    Excludes 1: social exclusion and rejection (Z60.4)
  Z60.8 Other problems related to social environment
  Z60.9 Problem related to social environment, unspecified

Z62- Problems related to upbringing
  Includes: Current and past negative life events in childhood
    Current and past problems of a child related to upbringing
  Excludes❷: maltreatment syndrome (T74.-)
    problems related to housing and economic circumstances (Z59.-)
  Z62.0 Inadequate parental supervision and control
  Z62.1 Parental overprotection
  Z62.2- Upbringing away from parents
    Excludes 1: problems with boarding school (Z59.3)
    Z62.21 Child in welfare custody
      Child in care of non-parental family member
      Child in foster care
      Excludes❷: problem for parent due to child in welfare custody (Z63.5)
    Z62.22 Institutional upbringing
      Child living in orphanage or group home
    Z62.29 Other upbringing away from parents
  Z62.3 Hostility towards and scapegoating of child
  Z62.6 Inappropriate (excessive) parental pressure
  Z62.8- Other specified problems related to upbringing
    Z62.81- <u>Personal history of abuse in childhood</u>
      Z62.810 Personal history of <u>physical and sexual</u> abuse in childhood
        Excludes 1: current child physical abuse (T74.12-, T76.12-)
        current child sexual abuse (T74.22-, T76.22-)
      Z62.811 Personal history of <u>psychological</u> abuse in childhood
        Excludes 1: current child psychological abuse (T74.32-, T76.32-)
      Z62.812 Personal history of <u>neglect</u> in childhood
        Excludes 1: current child neglect (T74.02, T76.02-)
      Z62.819 Personal history of <u>unspecified</u> abuse in childhood
        Excludes 1: current child abuse NOS (T74.92, T76.92-)

Z47 - Z62

Excludes 1: = NOT CODED HERE! (Do not code both)

Excludes❷: = Not Included Here

Z62.82- **Parent-child conflict**
    Z62.820   **Parent-biological child conflict**
        Parent-child problem NOS
    Z62.821   **Parent-adopted child conflict**
    Z62.822   **Parent-foster child conflict**
Z62.89- **Other specified problems related to upbringing**
    Z62.890   **Parent-child estrangement NEC**
    Z62.891   **Sibling rivalry**
    Z62.898   **Other specified problems related to upbringing**
Z62.9   **Problem related to upbringing, unspecified**

Z63- **Other problems related to primary support group, including family circumstances**
  Excludes❷: maltreatment syndrome (T74.-, T76)
    parent-child problems (Z62.-)
    problems related to negative life events in childhood (Z62.-)
    problems related to upbringing (Z62.-)
Z63.0   **Problems in relationship with spouse or partner**
  Excludes 1: counseling for spousal or partner abuse problems (Z69.1)
    counseling related to sexual attitude, behavior, and orientation (Z70.-)
Z63.1   **Problems in relationship with in-laws**
Z63.3- **Absence of family member**
  Excludes 1: absence of family member due to disappearance and death (Z63.4)
    absence of family member due to separation and divorce (Z63.5)
  Z63.31   **Absence of family member due to military deployment**
    Individual or family affected by other family member being on military deployment
    Excludes 1: family disruption due to return of family member from military deployment (Z63.71)
  Z63.32   **Other absence of family member**
Z63.4   **Disappearance and death of family member**
    Assumed death of family member
    Bereavement
Z63.5   **Disruption of family by separation and divorce**
    Marital estrangement
Z63.6   **Dependent relative needing care at home**
Z63.7- **Other stressful life events affecting family and household**
  Z63.71   **Stress on family due to return of family member from military deployment**
    Individual or family affected by family member having returned from military deployment (current or past conflict)
  Z63.72   **Alcoholism and drug addiction in family**
  Z63.79   **Other stressful life events affecting family and household**
    Anxiety (normal) about sick person in family
    Health problems within family
    Ill or disturbed family member
    Isolated family
Z63.8   **Other specified problems related to primary support group**
    Family discord NOS
    Family estrangement NOS
    High expressed emotional level within family
    Inadequate family support NOS
    Inadequate or distorted communication within family
Z63.9   **Problem related to primary support group, unspecified**
    Relationship disorder NOS

Z64- **Problems related to certain psychosocial circumstances**
Z64.0   **Problems related to unwanted pregnancy**
Z64.1   **Problems related to multiparity**
Z64.4   **Discord with counselors**
    Discord with probation officer
    Discord with social worker

Z65- **Problems related to other psychosocial circumstances**
Z65.0   **Conviction in civil and criminal proceedings without imprisonment**
Z65.1   **Imprisonment and other incarceration**
Z65.2   **Problems related to release from prison**
Z65.3   **Problems related to other legal circumstances**
    Arrest
    Child custody or support proceedings
    Litigation
    Prosecution
Z65.4   **Victim of crime and terrorism**
    Victim of torture
Z65.5   **Exposure to disaster, war and other hostilities**
  Excludes 1: target of perceived discrimination or persecution (Z60.5)

Z65.8   **Other specified problems related to psychosocial circumstances**
Z65.9   **Problem related to unspecified psychosocial circumstances**

Do not resuscitate status (Z66)

Z66   **Do not resuscitate**
    DNR status

Blood type (Z67)

Z67- **Blood type**
Z67.1- **Type A blood**
  Z67.10   **Type A blood, Rh positive**
  Z67.11   **Type A blood, Rh negative**
Z67.2- **Type B blood**
  Z67.20   **Type B blood, Rh positive**
  Z67.21   **Type B blood, Rh negative**
Z67.3- **Type AB blood**
  Z67.30   **Type AB blood, Rh positive**
  Z67.31   **Type AB blood, Rh negative**
Z67.4- **Type O blood**
  Z67.40   **Type O blood, Rh positive**
  Z67.41   **Type O blood, Rh negative**
Z67.9- **Unspecified blood type**
  Z67.90   **Unspecified blood type, Rh positive**
  Z67.91   **Unspecified blood type, Rh negative**

Body mass index [BMI] (Z68)

Z68- **Body mass index [BMI]**
    Kilograms per meters squared
    Note: BMI adult codes are for use for persons 21 years of age or older.
    Note: BMI pediatric codes are for use for persons 2-20 years of age. These percentiles are based on the growth charts published by the Centers for Disease Control and Prevention (CDC).
Z68.1   **Body mass index (BMI) 19 or less, adult**
Z68.2- **Body mass index (BMI) 20-29, adult**
  Z68.20   **Body mass index (BMI) 20.0-20.9, adult**
  Z68.21   **Body mass index (BMI) 21.0-21.9, adult**
  Z68.22   **Body mass index (BMI) 22.0-22.9, adult**
  Z68.23   **Body mass index (BMI) 23.0-23.9, adult**
  Z68.24   **Body mass index (BMI) 24.0-24.9, adult**
  Z68.25   **Body mass index (BMI) 25.0-25.9, adult**
  Z68.26   **Body mass index (BMI) 26.0-26.9, adult**
  Z68.27   **Body mass index (BMI) 27.0-27.9, adult**
  Z68.28   **Body mass index (BMI) 28.0-28.9, adult**
  Z68.29   **Body mass index (BMI) 29.0-29.9, adult**
Z68.3- **Body mass index (BMI) 30-39, adult**
  Z68.30   **Body mass index (BMI) 30.0-30.9, adult**
  Z68.31   **Body mass index (BMI) 31.0-31.9, adult**
  Z68.32   **Body mass index (BMI) 32.0-32.9, adult**
  Z68.33   **Body mass index (BMI) 33.0-33.9, adult**
  Z68.34   **Body mass index (BMI) 34.0-34.9, adult**
  Z68.35   **Body mass index (BMI) 35.0-35.9, adult**
  Z68.36   **Body mass index (BMI) 36.0-36.9, adult**
  Z68.37   **Body mass index (BMI) 37.0-37.9, adult**
  Z68.38   **Body mass index (BMI) 38.0-38.9, adult**
  Z68.39   **Body mass index (BMI) 39.0-39.9, adult**
Z68.4- **Body mass index (BMI) 40 or greater, adult**
  Z68.41   **Body mass index (BMI) 40.0-44.9, adult**
  Z68.42   **Body mass index (BMI) 45.0-49.9, adult**
  Z68.43   **Body mass index (BMI) 50-59.9 , adult**
  Z68.44   **Body mass index (BMI) 60.0-69.9, adult**
  Z68.45   **Body mass index (BMI) 70 or greater, adult**
Z68.5- **Body mass index (BMI) pediatric**
  Z68.51   **Body mass index (BMI) pediatric, less than 5th percentile for age**
  Z68.52   **Body mass index (BMI) pediatric, 5th percentile to less than 85th percentile for age**
  Z68.53   **Body mass index (BMI) pediatric, 85th percentile to less than 95th percentile for age**
  Z68.54   **Body mass index (BMI) pediatric, greater than or equal to 95th percentile for age**

Z 6 2 - Z 7 2

Persons encountering health services in other circumstances (Z69-Z76)

Z69-   **Encounter for mental health services for victim and perpetrator of abuse**
Includes: Counseling for victims and perpetrators of abuse

Z69.0-   **Encounter for mental health services for <u>child abuse problems</u>**

    Z69.01- **Encounter for mental health services for <u>parental child</u> abuse**

       Z69.010   **Encounter for mental health services for <u>victim</u> of parental child abuse**

       Z69.011   **Encounter for mental health services for <u>perpetrator</u> of parental child abuse**
          Excludes 1:   *encounter for mental health services for non-parental child abuse (Z69.02-)*

    Z69.02- **Encounter for mental health services for <u>non-parental child abuse</u>**

       Z69.020   **Encounter for mental health services for <u>victim</u> of non-parental child abuse**

       Z69.021   **Encounter for mental health services for <u>perpetrator</u> of non-parental child abuse**

Z69.1-   **Encounter for mental health services for <u>spousal or partner</u> abuse problems**

    Z69.11   **Encounter for mental health services for <u>victim</u> of spousal or partner abuse**

    Z69.12   **Encounter for mental health services for <u>perpetrator</u> of spousal or partner abuse**

Z69.8-   **Encounter for mental health services for victim or perpetrator of <u>other</u> abuse**

    Z69.81   **Encounter for mental health services for <u>victim</u> of other abuse**
         Encounter for rape victim counseling

    Z69.82   **Encounter for mental health services for <u>perpetrator</u> of other abuse**

Z70-   **Counseling related to sexual attitude, behavior and orientation**
Includes: Encounter for mental health services for sexual attitude, behavior and orientation
Excludes❷: contraceptive or procreative counseling (Z30-Z31)

Z70.0   **Counseling related to sexual attitude**

Z70.1   **Counseling related to patient's sexual behavior and orientation**
Patient concerned regarding impotence
Patient concerned regarding non-responsiveness
Patient concerned regarding promiscuity
Patient concerned regarding sexual orientation

Z70.2   **Counseling related to sexual behavior and orientation of third party**
Advice sought regarding sexual behavior and orientation of child
Advice sought regarding sexual behavior and orientation of partner
Advice sought regarding sexual behavior and orientation of spouse

Z70.3   **Counseling related to combined concerns regarding sexual attitude, behavior and orientation**

Z70.8   **Other sex counseling**
Encounter for sex education

Z70.9   **Sex counseling, unspecified**

Z71-   **Persons encountering health services for other counseling and medical advice, not elsewhere classified**
Excludes❷: contraceptive or procreation counseling (Z30-Z31)
sex counseling (Z70.-)

Z71.0   **Person encountering health services to consult on behalf of another person**
Person encountering health services to seek advice or treatment for non-attending third party
Excludes❷: anxiety (normal) about sick person in family (Z63.7)
expectant (adoptive) parent(s) pre-birth pediatrician visit (Z76.81)

Z71.1   **Person with feared health complaint in whom no diagnosis is made**
Person encountering health services with feared condition which was not demonstrated
Person encountering health services in which problem was normal state
"Worried well"
Excludes 1: medical observation for suspected diseases and conditions proven not to exist (Z03.-)

Z71.2   **Person consulting for explanation of examination or test findings**

Z71.3   **Dietary counseling and surveillance**
Use additional code for any associated underlying medical condition
Use additional code to identify body mass index (BMI), if known (Z68.-)

Z71.4-   **<u>Alcohol abuse counseling and surveillance</u>**
Use additional code for alcohol abuse or dependence (F10.-)

    Z71.41   **Alcohol abuse counseling and surveillance of <u>alcoholic</u>**

    Z71.42   **Counseling for <u>family member of alcoholic</u>**
         Counseling for significant other, partner, or friend of alcoholic

Z71.5-   **Drug abuse counseling and surveillance**
Use additional code for drug abuse or dependence (F11-F16, F18-F19)

    Z71.51   **Drug abuse counseling and surveillance of drug abuser**

    Z71.52   **Counseling for <u>family member of drug abuser</u>**
         Counseling for significant other, partner, or friend of drug abuser

Z71.6   **Tobacco abuse counseling**
Use additional code for nicotine dependence (F17.-)

Z71.7   **Human immunodeficiency virus [HIV] counseling**

Z71.8-   **Other specified counseling**
Excludes❷: counseling for contraception (Z30.0-)
counseling for genetics (Z31.5)
counseling for procreative management (Z31.6-)

    Z71.81   **Spiritual or religious counseling**

    Z71.89   **Other specified counseling**

Z71.9   **Counseling, unspecified**
Encounter for medical advice NOS

Z72-   **Problems related to lifestyle**
Excludes❷: problems related to life-management difficulty (Z73.-)
problems related to socioeconomic and psychosocial circumstances (Z55-Z65)

Z72.0   **Tobacco use**
Tobacco use NOS
Excludes 1: history of tobacco dependence (Z87.891)
nicotine dependence (F17.2-)
tobacco dependence (F17.2-)
tobacco use during pregnancy (O99.33-)

Z72.3   **Lack of physical exercise**

Z72.4   **Inappropriate diet and eating habits**
Excludes 1: behavioral eating disorders of infancy or childhood (F98.2.-F98.3)
eating disorders (F50.-)
lack of adequate food (Z59.4)
malnutrition and other nutritional deficiencies (E40-E64)

Z72.5-   **High risk sexual behavior**
Promiscuity
Excludes 1: paraphilias (F65)

    Z72.51   **High risk heterosexual behavior**

    Z72.52   **High risk homosexual behavior**

    Z72.53   **High risk bisexual behavior**

Z72.6   **Gambling and betting**
Excludes 1: compulsive or pathological gambling (F63.0)

Z72.8-   **Other problems related to lifestyle**

    Z72.81- **Antisocial behavior**
       Excludes 1: conduct disorders (F91.-)

       Z72.810   **Child and adolescent antisocial behavior**
          Antisocial behavior (child) (adolescent) without manifest psychiatric disorder
          Delinquency NOS
          Group delinquency
          Offenses in the context of gang membership
          Stealing in company with others
          Truancy from school

       Z72.811   **Adult antisocial behavior**
          Adult antisocial behavior without manifest psychiatric disorder

    Z72.82- **Problems related to sleep**

       Z72.820   **Sleep deprivation**
          Lack of adequate sleep
          Excludes 1: insomnia (G47.0-)

       Z72.821   **Inadequate sleep hygiene**
          Bad sleep habits
          Irregular sleep habits
          Unhealthy sleep wake schedule
          Excludes 1: insomnia (F51.0-, G47.0-)

    Z72.89   **Other problems related to lifestyle**
       Self-damaging behavior

Z72.9   **Problem related to lifestyle, unspecified**

Z62 - Z72

Z73- Problems related to life management difficulty
   Excludes❷: problems related to socioeconomic and psychosocial circumstances (Z55-Z65)
   Z73.0 Burn-out
   Z73.1 Type A behavior pattern
   Z73.2 Lack of relaxation and leisure
   Z73.3 Stress, not elsewhere classified
       Physical and mental strain NOS
       Excludes 1: stress related to employment or unemployment (Z56.-)
   Z73.4 Inadequate social skills, not elsewhere classified
   Z73.5 Social role conflict, not elsewhere classified
   Z73.6 Limitation of activities due to disability
       Excludes 1: care-provider dependency (Z74.-)
   Z73.8- Other problems related to life management difficulty
       Z73.81- Behavioral insomnia of childhood
           Z73.810 Behavioral insomnia of childhood, sleep-onset association type
           Z73.811 Behavioral insomnia of childhood, limit setting type
           Z73.812 Behavioral insomnia of childhood, combined type
           Z73.819 Behavioral insomnia of childhood, unspecified type
       Z73.82 Dual sensory impairment
       Z73.89 Other problems related to life management difficulty
   Z73.9 Problem related to life management difficulty, unspecified

Z74- Problems related to care provider dependency
   Excludes❷: dependence on enabling machines or devices NEC (Z99.-)
   Z74.0- Reduced mobility
       Z74.01 Bed confinement status
           Bedridden
       Z74.09 Other reduced mobility
           Chairridden
           Reduced mobility NOS
           Excludes❷: wheelchair dependence (Z99.3)
   Z74.1 Need for assistance with personal care
   Z74.2 Need for assistance at home and no other household member able to render care
   Z74.3 Need for continuous supervision
   Z74.8 Other problems related to care provider dependency
   Z74.9 Problem related to care provider dependency, unspecified

Z75- Problems related to medical facilities and other health care
   Z75.0 Medical services not available in home
       Excludes 1: no other household member able to render care (Z74.2)
   Z75.1 Person awaiting admission to adequate facility elsewhere
   Z75.2 Other waiting period for investigation and treatment
   Z75.3 Unavailability and inaccessibility of health-care facilities
       Excludes 1: bed unavailable (Z75.1)
   Z75.4 Unavailability and inaccessibility of other helping agencies
   Z75.5 Holiday relief care
   Z75.8 Other problems related to medical facilities and other health care
   Z75.9 Unspecified problem related to medical facilities and other health care

Z76- Persons encountering health services in other circumstances
   Z76.0 Encounter for issue of repeat prescription
       Encounter for issue of repeat prescription for appliance
       Encounter for issue of repeat prescription for medicaments
       Encounter for issue of repeat prescription for spectacles
       Excludes❷: issue of medical certificate (Z02.7)
           repeat prescription for contraceptive (Z30.4-)
   Z76.1 Encounter for health supervision and care of foundling
   Z76.2 Encounter for health supervision and care of other healthy infant and child
       Encounter for medical or nursing care or supervision of healthy infant under circumstances such as adverse socioeconomic conditions at home
       Encounter for medical or nursing care or supervision of healthy infant under circumstances such as awaiting foster or adoptive placement
       Encounter for medical or nursing care or supervision of healthy infant under circumstances such as maternal illness
       Encounter for medical or nursing care or supervision of healthy infant under circumstances such as number of children at home preventing or interfering with normal care
   Z76.3 Healthy person accompanying sick person
   Z76.4 Other boarder to healthcare facility
       Excludes 1: homelessness (Z59.0)
   Z76.5 Malingerer [conscious simulation]
       Person feigning illness (with obvious motivation)
       Excludes 1: factitious disorder (F68.1-)
           peregrinating patient (F68.1-)

Z76.8- Persons encountering health services in other specified circumstances
   Z76.81 Expectant parent(s) prebirth pediatrician visit
       Pre-adoption pediatrician visit for adoptive parent(s)
   Z76.82 Awaiting organ transplant status
       Patient waiting for organ availability
   Z76.89 Persons encountering health services in other specified circumstances
       Persons encountering health services NOS

Persons with potential health hazards related to family and personal history and certain conditions influencing health status (Z77-Z99)

   Code also any follow-up examination (Z08-Z09)

Z77- Other contact with and (suspected) exposures hazardous to health
   Includes: Contact with and (suspected) exposures to potential hazards to health
   Excludes❷: contact with and (suspected) exposure to communicable diseases (Z20.-)
       exposure to (parental) (environmental) tobacco smoke in the perinatal period (P96.81)
       newborn (suspected to be) affected by noxious substances transmitted via placenta or breast milk (P04.-)
       occupational exposure to risk factors (Z57.-)
       retained foreign body (Z18.-)
       retained foreign body fully removed (Z87.821)
       toxic effects of substances chiefly nonmedicinal as to source (T51-T65)
   Z77.0- Contact with and (suspected) exposure to hazardous, chiefly nonmedicinal, chemicals
       Z77.01- Contact with and (suspected) exposure to hazardous metals
           Z77.010 Contact with and (suspected) exposure to arsenic
           Z77.011 Contact with and (suspected) exposure to lead
           Z77.012 Contact with and (suspected) exposure to uranium
               Excludes 1: retained depleted uranium fragments (Z18.01)
           Z77.018 Contact with and (suspected) exposure to other hazardous metals
               Contact with and (suspected) exposure to chromium compounds
               Contact with and (suspected) exposure to nickel dust
       Z77.02- Contact with and (suspected) exposure to hazardous aromatic compounds
           Z77.020 Contact with and (suspected) exposure to aromatic amines
           Z77.021 Contact with and (suspected) exposure to benzene
           Z77.028 Contact with and (suspected) exposure to other hazardous aromatic compounds
               Aromatic dyes NOS
               Polycyclic aromatic hydrocarbons
       Z77.09- Contact with and (suspected) exposure to other hazardous, chiefly nonmedicinal, chemicals
           Z77.090 Contact with and (suspected) exposure to asbestos
           Z77.098 Contact with and (suspected) exposure to other hazardous, chiefly nonmedicinal, chemicals
               Dyes NOS
   Z77.1- Contact with and (suspected) exposure to environmental pollution and hazards in the physical environment
       Z77.11- Contact with and (suspected) exposure to environmental pollution
           Z77.110 Contact with and (suspected) exposure to air pollution
           Z77.111 Contact with and (suspected) exposure to water pollution
           Z77.112 Contact with and (suspected) exposure to soil pollution
           Z77.118 Contact with and (suspected) exposure to other environmental pollution

Z73 – Z80

© 2013 Channel Publishing, Ltd.

Z77.12- Contact with and (suspected) exposure to hazards in the physical environment

Z77.120 Contact with and (suspected) exposure to mold (toxic)

Z77.121 Contact with and (suspected) exposure to harmful algae and algae toxins
Contact with and (suspected) exposure to (harmful) algae bloom NOS
Contact with and (suspected) exposure to blue-green algae bloom
Contact with and (suspected) exposure to brown tide
Contact with and (suspected) exposure to cyanobacteria bloom
Contact with and (suspected) exposure to Florida red tide
Contact with and (suspected) exposure to pfiesteria piscicida
Contact with and (suspected) exposure to red tide

Z77.122 Contact with and (suspected) exposure to noise

Z77.123 Contact with and (suspected) exposure to radon and other naturally occuring radiation
Excludes❷: radiation exposure as the cause of a confirmed condition (W88-W90, X39.0-)
radiation sickness NOS (T66)

Z77.128 Contact with and (suspected) exposure to other hazards in the physical environment

Z77.2- Contact with and (suspected) exposure to other hazardous substances

Z77.21 Contact with and (suspected) exposure to potentially hazardous body fluids

Z77.22 Contact with and (suspected) exposure to environmental tobacco smoke (acute) (chronic)
Exposure to second hand tobacco smoke (acute) (chronic)
Passive smoking (acute) (chronic)
Excludes 1: nicotine dependence (F17.-)
tobacco use (Z72.0)
Excludes❷: occupational exposure to environmental tobacco smoke (Z57.31)

Z77.29 Contact with and (suspected) exposure to other hazardous substances

Z77.9 Other contact with and (suspected) exposures hazardous to health

Z78- Other specified health status
Excludes❷: asymptomatic human immunodeficiency virus [HIV] infection status (Z21)
postprocedural status (Z93-Z99)
sex reassignment status (Z87.890)

Z78.0 Asymptomatic menopausal state
Menopausal state NOS
Postmenopausal status NOS
Excludes❷: symptomatic menopausal state (N95.1)

Z78.1 Physical restraint status
Excludes 1: physical restraint due to a procedure — omit code

Z78.9 Other specified health status

Z79- Long term (current) drug therapy
Includes: Long term (current) drug use for prophylactic purposes
Code also any therapeutic drug level monitoring (Z51.81)
Excludes❷: drug abuse and dependence (F11-F19)
drug use complicating pregnancy, childbirth, and the puerperium (O99.32-)

Z79.0- Long term (current) use of anticoagulants and antithrombotics/antiplatelets
Excludes❷: long term (current) use of aspirin (Z79.82)

Z79.01 Long term (current) use of anticoagulants

Z79.02 Long term (current) use of antithrombotics/antiplatelets

Z79.1 Long term (current) use of non-steroidal anti-inflammatories (NSAID)
Excludes❷: long term (current) use of aspirin (Z79.82)

Z79.2 Long term (current) use of antibiotics

Z79.3 Long term (current) use of hormonal contraceptives
Long term (current) use of birth control pill or patch

Z79.4 Long term (current) use of insulin

Z79.5- Long term (current) use of steroids

Z79.51 Long term (current) use of inhaled steroids

Z79.52 Long term (current) use of systemic steroids

Z79.8- Other long term (current) drug therapy

Z79.81- Long term (current) use of agents affecting estrogen receptors and estrogen levels
Code first, if applicable:
Malignant neoplasm of breast (C50.-)
Malignant neoplasm of prostate (C61)
Use additional code, if applicable, to identify:
Estrogen receptor positive status (Z17.0)
Family history of breast cancer (Z80.3)
Genetic susceptibility to malignant neoplasm (cancer) (Z15.0-)
Personal history of breast cancer (Z85.3)
Personal history of prostate cancer (Z85.46)
Postmenopausal status (Z78.0)
Excludes 1: hormone replacement therapy (postmenopausal) (Z79.890)

Z79.810 Long term (current) use of selective estrogen receptor modulators (SERMs)
Long term (current) use of raloxifene (Evista)
Long term (current) use of tamoxifen (Nolvadex)
Long term (current) use of toremifene (Fareston)

Z79.811 Long term (current) use of aromatase inhibitors
Long term (current) use of anastrozole (Arimidex)
Long term (current) use of exemestane (Aromasin)
Long term (current) use of letrozole (Femara)

Z79.818 Long term (current) use of other agents affecting estrogen receptors and estrogen levels
Long term (current) use of estrogen receptor downregulators
Long term (current) use of fulvestrant (Faslodex)
Long term (current) use of gonadotropin-releasing hormone (GnRH) agonist
Long term (current) use of goserelin acetate (Zoladex)
Long term (current) use of leuprolide acetate (leuprorelin) (Lupron)
Long term (current) use of megestrol acetate (Megace)

Z79.82 Long term (current) use of aspirin

Z79.83 Long term (current) use of bisphosphonates

Z79.89- Other long term (current) drug therapy

Z79.890 Hormone replacement therapy (postmenopausal)

Z79.891 Long term (current) use of opiate analgesic
Long term (current) use of methadone for pain management
Excludes 1: methadone use NOS (F11.2-)
use of methadone for treatment of heroin addiction (F11.2-)

Z79.899 Other long term (current) drug therapy

Z80- Family history of primary malignant neoplasm

Z80.0 Family history of malignant neoplasm of digestive organs
Conditions classifiable to C15-C26

Z80.1 Family history of malignant neoplasm of trachea, bronchus and lung
Conditions classifiable to C33-C34

Z80.2 Family history of malignant neoplasm of other respiratory and intrathoracic organs
Conditions classifiable to C30-C32, C37-C39

Z80.3 Family history of malignant neoplasm of breast
Conditions classifiable to C50.-

Z80.4- Family history of malignant neoplasm of genital organs
Conditions classifiable to C51-C63

Z80.41 Family history of malignant neoplasm of ovary

Z80.42 Family history of malignant neoplasm of prostate

Z80.43 Family history of malignant neoplasm of testis

Z80.49 Family history of malignant neoplasm of other genital organs

Z80.5- Family history of malignant neoplasm of urinary tract
Conditions classifiable to C64-C68

Z80.51 Family history of malignant neoplasm of kidney

Z80.52 Family history of malignant neoplasm of bladder

Z80.59 Family history of malignant neoplasm of other urinary tract organ

Z80.6 Family history of leukemia
Conditions classifiable to C91-C95

Z80.7 Family history of other malignant neoplasms of lymphoid, hematopoietic and related tissues
Conditions classifiable to C81-C90, C96.-

Z80.8 Family history of malignant neoplasm of other organs or systems
Conditions classifiable to C00-C14, C40-C49, C69-C79

Z80.9 Family history of malignant neoplasm, unspecified
Conditions classifiable to C80.1

Z73 - Z80

Z81- Family history of mental and behavioral disorders
Z81.0   **Family history of intellectual disabilities**
Conditions classifiable to F70-F79
Z81.1   **Family history of alcohol abuse and dependence**
Conditions classifiable to F10.-
Z81.2   **Family history of tobacco abuse and dependence**
Conditions classifiable to F17.-
Z81.3   **Family history of other psychoactive substance abuse and dependence**
Conditions classifiable to F11-F16, F18-F19
Z81.4   **Family history of other substance abuse and dependence**
Conditions classifiable to F55
Z81.8   **Family history of other mental and behavioral disorders**
Conditions classifiable elsewhere in F01-F99

Z82- Family history of certain disabilities and chronic diseases (leading to disablement)
Z82.0   **Family history of epilepsy and other diseases of the nervous system**
Conditions classifiable to G00-G99
Z82.1   **Family history of blindness and visual loss**
Conditions classifiable to H54.-
Z82.2   **Family history of deafness and hearing loss**
Conditions classifiable to H90-H91
Z82.3   **Family history of stroke**
Conditions classifiable to I60-I64
Z82.4-   **Family history of ischemic heart disease and other diseases of the circulatory system**
Conditions classifiable to I00-I52, I65-I99
Z82.41   **Family history of sudden cardiac death**
Z82.49   **Family history of ischemic heart disease and other diseases of the circulatory system**
Z82.5   **Family history of asthma and other chronic lower respiratory diseases**
Conditions classifiable to J40-J47
Excludes❷: family history of other diseases of the respiratory system (Z83.6)
Z82.6-   **Family history of arthritis and other diseases of the musculoskeletal system and connective tissue**
Conditions classifiable to M00-M99
Z82.61   **Family history of arthritis**
Z82.62   **Family history of osteoporosis**
Z82.69   **Family history of other diseases of the musculoskeletal system and connective tissue**
Z82.7-   **Family history of congenital malformations, deformations and chromosomal abnormalities**
Conditions classifiable to Q00-Q99
Z82.71   **Family history of polycystic kidney**
Z82.79   **Family history of other congenital malformations, deformations and chromosomal abnormalities**
Z82.8   **Family history of other disabilities and chronic diseases leading to disablement, not elsewhere classified**

Z83- Family history of other specific disorders
Excludes❷: contact with and (suspected) exposure to communicable disease in the family (Z20.-)
Z83.0   **Family history of human immunodeficiency virus [HIV] disease**
Conditions classifiable to B20
Z83.1   **Family history of other infectious and parasitic diseases**
Conditions classifiable to A00-B19, B25-B94, B99
Z83.2   **Family history of diseases of the blood and blood-forming organs and certain disorders involving the immune mechanism**
Conditions classifiable to D50-D89
Z83.3   **Family history of diabetes mellitus**
Conditions classifiable to E08-E13
Z83.4-   **Family history of other endocrine, nutritional and metabolic diseases**
Conditions classifiable to E00-E07, E15-E88
Z83.41   **Family history of multiple endocrine neoplasia [MEN] syndrome**
Z83.49   **Family history of other endocrine, nutritional and metabolic diseases**

Z83.5- Family history of eye and ear disorders
Z83.51- **Family history of eye disorders**
Conditions classifiable to H00-H53, H55-H59
Excludes❷: family history of blindness and visual loss (Z82.1)
Z83.511   **Family history of glaucoma**
Z83.518   **Family history of other specified eye disorder**
Z83.52   **Family history of ear disorders**
Conditions classifiable to H60-H83, H92-H95
Excludes❷: family history of deafness and hearing loss (Z82.2)
Z83.6   **Family history of other diseases of the respiratory system**
Conditions classifiable to J00-J39, J60-J99
Excludes❷: family history of asthma and other chronic lower respiratory diseases (Z82.5)
Z83.7-   **Family history of diseases of the digestive system**
Conditions classifiable to K00-K93
Z83.71   **Family history of colonic polyps**
Excludes 1: family history of malignant neoplasm of digestive organs (Z80.0)
Z83.79   **Family history of other diseases of the digestive system**

Z84- Family history of other conditions
Z84.0   **Family history of diseases of the skin and subcutaneous tissue**
Conditions classifiable to L00-L99
Z84.1   **Family history of disorders of kidney and ureter**
Conditions classifiable to N00-N29
Z84.2   **Family history of other diseases of the genitourinary system**
Conditions classifiable to N30-N99
Z84.3   **Family history of consanguinity**
Z84.8-   **Family history of other specified conditions**
Z84.81   **Family history of carrier of genetic disease**
Z84.89   **Family history of other specified conditions**

Z85- Personal history of malignant neoplasm
Code first any follow-up examination after treatment of malignant neoplasm (Z08)
Use additional code to identify:
Alcohol use and dependence (F10.-)
Exposure to environmental tobacco smoke (Z77.22)
History of tobacco use (Z87.891)
Occupational exposure to environmental tobacco smoke (Z57.31)
Tobacco dependence (F17.-)
Tobacco use (Z72.0)
Excludes❷: personal history of benign neoplasm (Z86.01-)
personal history of carcinoma-in-situ (Z86.00-)
Z85.0- Personal history of malignant neoplasm of digestive organs
Z85.00   **Personal history of malignant neoplasm of unspecified digestive organ**
Z85.01   **Personal history of malignant neoplasm of esophagus**
Conditions classifiable to C15
Z85.02- **Personal history of malignant neoplasm of stomach**
Z85.020   **Personal history of malignant carcinoid tumor of stomach**
Conditions classifiable to C7A.092
Z85.028   **Personal history of other malignant neoplasm of stomach**
Conditions classifiable to C16
Z85.03- **Personal history of malignant neoplasm of large intestine**
Z85.030   **Personal history of malignant carcinoid tumor of large intestine**
Conditions classifiable to C7A.022-C7A.025, C7A.029
Z85.038   **Personal history of other malignant neoplasm of large intestine**
Conditions classifiable to C18
Z85.04- **Personal history of malignant neoplasm of rectum, rectosigmoid junction, and anus**
Z85.040   **Personal history of malignant carcinoid tumor of rectum**
Conditions classifiable to C7A.026
Z85.048   **Personal history of other malignant neoplasm of rectum, rectosigmoid junction, and anus**
Conditions classifiable to C19-C21
Z85.05   **Personal history of malignant neoplasm of liver**
Conditions classifiable to C22
Z85.06- **Personal history of malignant neoplasm of small intestine**
Z85.060   **Personal history of malignant carcinoid tumor of small intestine**
Conditions classifiable to C7A.01-
Z85.068   **Personal history of other malignant neoplasm of small intestine**
Conditions classifiable to C17
Z85.07   **Personal history of malignant neoplasm of pancreas**
Conditions classifiable to C25

Z
8
1
-
Z
8
6

Z85.09 Personal history of malignant neoplasm of other digestive organs

Z85.1- Personal history of <u>malignant neoplasm</u> of <u>trachea, bronchus and lung</u>

 Z85.11- Personal history of malignant neoplasm of bronchus and lung

  Z85.110 Personal history of malignant carcinoid tumor of bronchus and lung
   Conditions classifiable to C7A.090

  Z85.118 Personal history of other malignant neoplasm of bronchus and lung
   Conditions classifiable to C34

 Z85.12 Personal history of malignant neoplasm of trachea
  Conditions classifiable to C33

Z85.2- <u>Personal history</u> of <u>malignant neoplasm</u> of <u>other respiratory and intrathoracic organs</u>

 Z85.20 Personal history of malignant neoplasm of unspecified respiratory organ

 Z85.21 Personal history of malignant neoplasm of larynx
  Conditions classifiable to C32

 Z85.22 Personal history of malignant neoplasm of nasal cavities, middle ear, and accessory sinuses
  Conditions classifiable to C30-C31

 Z85.23- Personal history of malignant neoplasm of thymus

  Z85.230 Personal history of malignant carcinoid tumor of thymus
   Conditions classifiable to C7A.091

  Z85.238 Personal history of other malignant neoplasm of thymus
   Conditions classifiable to C37

 Z85.29 Personal history of malignant neoplasm of other respiratory and intrathoracic organs

Z85.3 <u>Personal history</u> of <u>malignant neoplasm</u> of <u>breast</u>
 Conditions classifiable to C50.-

Z85.4- <u>Personal history</u> of <u>malignant neoplasm</u> of <u>genital organs</u>
 Conditions classifiable to C51-C63

 Z85.40 Personal history of malignant neoplasm of unspecified female genital organ

 Z85.41 Personal history of malignant neoplasm of cervix uteri

 Z85.42 Personal history of malignant neoplasm of other parts of uterus

 Z85.43 Personal history of malignant neoplasm of ovary

 Z85.44 Personal history of malignant neoplasm of other female genital organs

 Z85.45 Personal history of malignant neoplasm of unspecified male genital organ

 Z85.46 Personal history of malignant neoplasm of prostate

 Z85.47 Personal history of malignant neoplasm of testis

 Z85.48 Personal history of malignant neoplasm of epididymis

 Z85.49 Personal history of malignant neoplasm of other male genital organs

Z85.5- <u>Personal history</u> of <u>malignant neoplasm</u> of <u>urinary tract</u>
 Conditions classifiable to C64-C68

 Z85.50 Personal history of malignant neoplasm of unspecified urinary tract organ

 Z85.51 Personal history of malignant neoplasm of bladder

 Z85.52- Personal history of malignant neoplasm of kidney
  Excludes 1: personal history of malignant neoplasm of renal pelvis (Z85.53)

  Z85.520 Personal history of malignant carcinoid tumor of kidney
   Conditions classifiable to C7A.093

  Z85.528 Personal history of other malignant neoplasm of kidney
   Conditions classifiable to C64

 Z85.53 Personal history of malignant neoplasm of renal pelvis

 Z85.54 Personal history of malignant neoplasm of ureter

 Z85.59 Personal history of malignant neoplasm of other urinary tract organ

Z85.6 <u>Personal history</u> of <u>leukemia</u>
 Conditions classifiable to C91-C95
 Excludes 1: leukemia in remission C91.0-C95.9 with 5th character 1

Z85.7- <u>Personal history</u> of other <u>malignant neoplasms</u> of <u>lymphoid, hematopoietic and related tissues</u>

 Z85.71 Personal history of Hodgkin lymphoma
  Conditions classifiable to C81

 Z85.72 Personal history of non-Hodgkin lymphomas
  Conditions classifiable to C82-C85

 Z85.79 Personal history of other malignant neoplasms of lymphoid, hematopoietic and related tissues
  Conditions classifiable to C88-C90, C96
  Excludes 1: multiple myeloma in remission (C90.01)
   plasma cell leukemia in remission (C90.11)
   plasmacytoma in remission (C90.21)

Z85.8- <u>Personal history</u> of <u>malignant neoplasms</u> of <u>other organs and systems</u>
 Conditions classifiable to C00-C14, C40-C49, C69-C79, C7A.098

 Z85.81- Personal history of malignant neoplasm of lip, oral cavity, and pharynx

  Z85.810 Personal history of malignant neoplasm of tongue

  Z85.818 Personal history of malignant neoplasm of other sites of lip, oral cavity, and pharynx

  Z85.819 Personal history of malignant neoplasm of unspecified site of lip, oral cavity, and pharynx

 Z85.82- <u>Personal history</u> of <u>malignant neoplasm</u> of <u>skin</u>

  Z85.820 Personal history of malignant melanoma of skin
   Conditions classifiable to C43

  Z85.821 Personal history of Merkel cell carcinoma
   Conditions classifiable to C4A

  Z85.828 Personal history of other malignant neoplasm of skin
   Conditions classifiable to C44

 Z85.83- <u>Personal history</u> of <u>malignant neoplasm</u> of <u>bone and soft tissue</u>

  Z85.830 Personal history of malignant neoplasm of bone

  Z85.831 Personal history of malignant neoplasm of soft tissue
   Excludes❷: personal history of malignant neoplasm of skin (Z85.82-)

 Z85.84- <u>Personal history</u> of <u>malignant neoplasm</u> of <u>eye and nervous tissue</u>

  Z85.840 Personal history of malignant neoplasm of eye

  Z85.841 Personal history of malignant neoplasm of brain

  Z85.848 Personal history of malignant neoplasm of other parts of nervous tissue

 Z85.85- <u>Personal history</u> of <u>malignant neoplasm</u> of <u>endocrine glands</u>

  Z85.850 Personal history of malignant neoplasm of thyroid

  Z85.858 Personal history of malignant neoplasm of other endocrine glands

 Z85.89 <u>Personal history</u> of <u>malignant neoplasm</u> of <u>other</u> organs and systems

Z85.9 <u>Personal history</u> of <u>malignant neoplasm, unspecified</u>
 Conditions classifiable to C7A.00, C80.1

Z86- <u>Personal history</u> of <u>certain other diseases</u>
Code first any follow-up examination after treatment (Z09)

 Z86.0- <u>Personal history</u> of <u>in situ and benign neoplasms</u> and <u>neoplasms of uncertain behavior</u>
  Excludes❷: personal history of malignant neoplasms (Z85.-)

  Z86.00- Personal history of <u>in situ neoplasm</u>

   Z86.000 Personal history of in situ neoplasm of breast

   Z86.001 Personal history of in situ neoplasm of cervix uteri

   Z86.008 Personal history of in situ neoplasm of other site

  Z86.01- Personal history of <u>benign neoplasm</u>

   Z86.010 Personal history of colonic polyps

   Z86.011 Personal history of benign neoplasm of the brain

   Z86.012 Personal history of benign carcinoid tumor

   Z86.018 Personal history of other benign neoplasm

  Z86.03 Personal history of neoplasm of uncertain behavior

 Z86.1- <u>Personal history</u> of <u>infectious and parasitic diseases</u>
  Conditions classifiable to A00-B89, B99
  Excludes 1: personal history of infectious diseases specific to a body system
   sequelae of infectious and parasitic diseases (B90-B94)

  Z86.11 Personal history of tuberculosis

  Z86.12 Personal history of poliomyelitis

  Z86.13 Personal history of malaria

  Z86.14 Personal history of methicillin resistant Staphylococcus aureus infection
   Personal history of MRSA infection

  Z86.19 Personal history of other infectious and parasitic diseases

 Z86.2 <u>Personal history</u> of <u>diseases of the blood and blood-forming organs and certain disorders involving the immune mechanism</u>
  Conditions classifiable to D50-D89

Excludes 1: = NOT CODED HERE! (Do not code both)

Excludes❷: = Not Included Here

Z86.3- <u>Personal history</u> of <u>endocrine, nutritional and metabolic diseases</u>
Conditions classifiable to E00-E88

Z86.31 **Personal history of diabetic foot ulcer**
Excludes❷: current diabetic foot ulcer (E08.621, E09.621, E10.621, E11.621, E13.621)

Z86.32 **Personal history of gestational diabetes**
Pesonal history of conditions classifiable to O24.4-
Excludes 1: gestational diabetes mellitus in current pregnancy (O24.4-)

Z86.39 **Personal history of other endocrine, nutritional and metabolic disease**

Z86.5- <u>Personal history</u> of <u>mental and behavioral disorders</u>
Conditions classifiable to F40-F59

Z86.51 **Personal history of combat and operational stress reaction**

Z86.59 **Personal history of other mental and behavioral disorders**

Z86.6- <u>Personal history</u> of <u>diseases of the nervous system and sense organs</u>
Conditions classifiable to G00-G99, H00-H95

Z86.61 **Personal history of infections of the central nervous system**
Personal history of encephalitis
Personal history of meningitis

Z86.69 **Personal history of other diseases of the nervous system and sense organs**

Z86.7- <u>Personal history</u> of <u>diseases of the circulatory system</u>
Conditions classifiable to I00-I99
Excludes❷: old myocardial infarction (I25.2)
personal history of anaphylactic shock (Z87.892)
postmyocardial infarction syndrome (I24.1)

Z86.71- **Personal history of venous thrombosis and embolism**

Z86.711 **Personal history of pulmonary embolism**

Z86.718 **Personal history of other venous thrombosis and embolism**

Z86.72 **Personal history of thrombophlebitis**

Z86.73 **Personal history of transient ischemic attack (TIA), and cerebral infarction without residual deficits**
Personal history of prolonged reversible ischemic neurological deficit (PRIND)
Personal history of stroke NOS without residual deficits
Excludes 1: personal history of traumatic brain injury (Z87.820)
sequelae of cerebrovascular disease (I69.-)

Z86.74 **Personal history of sudden cardiac arrest**
Personal history of sudden cardiac death successfully resuscitated

Z86.79 **Personal history of other diseases of the circulatory system**

Z87- <u>Personal history</u> of <u>other diseases and conditions</u>
Code first any follow-up examination after treatment (Z09)

Z87.0- **Personal history of diseases of the** <u>respiratory system</u>
Conditions classifiable to J00-J99

Z87.01 **Personal history of pneumonia (recurrent)**

Z87.09 **Personal history of other diseases of the respiratory system**

Z87.1- **Personal history of diseases of the** <u>digestive system</u>
Conditions classifiable to K00-K93

Z87.11 **Personal history of peptic ulcer disease**

Z87.19 **Personal history of other diseases of the digestive system**

Z87.2 **Personal history of diseases of the** <u>skin and subcutaneous tissue</u>
Conditions classifiable to L00-L99
Excludes❷: personal history of diabetic foot ulcer (Z86.31)

Z87.3- **Personal history of diseases of the** <u>musculoskeletal system and connective tissue</u>
Conditions classifiable to M00-M99
Excludes❷: personal history of (healed) traumatic fracture (Z87.81)

Z87.31- **Personal history of (healed) nontraumatic fracture**

Z87.310 **Personal history of (healed) osteoporosis fracture**
Personal history of (healed) fragility fracture
Personal history of (healed) collapsed vertebra due to osteoporosis

Z87.311 **Personal history of (healed) other pathological fracture**
Personal history of (healed) collapsed vertebra NOS
Excludes❷: personal history of osteoporosis fracture (Z87.310)

Z87.312 **Personal history of (healed) stress fracture**
Personal history of (healed) fatigue fracture

Z87.39 **Personal history of other diseases of the musculoskeletal system and connective tissue**

Z87.4- **Personal history of diseases of** <u>genitourinary system</u>
Conditions classifiable to N00-N99

Z87.41- **Personal history of** <u>dysplasia</u> of the <u>female genital tract</u>
Excludes 1: personal history of malignant neoplasm of female genital tract (Z85.40-Z85.44)

Z87.410 **Personal history of cervical dysplasia**

Z87.411 **Personal history of vaginal dysplasia**

Z87.412 **Personal history of vulvar dysplasia**

Z87.42 **Personal history of** <u>other</u> **diseases of the** <u>female genital tract</u>

Z87.43- **Personal history of diseases of** <u>male genital organs</u>

Z87.430 **Personal history of prostatic dysplasia**
Excludes 1: personal history of malignant neoplasm of prostate (Z85.46)

Z87.438 **Personal history of other diseases of male genital organs**

Z87.44- **Personal history of diseases of** <u>urinary system</u>
Excludes 1: personal history of malignant neoplasm of cervix uteri (Z85.41)

Z87.440 **Personal history of urinary (tract) infections**

Z87.441 **Personal history of nephrotic syndrome**

Z87.442 **Personal history of urinary calculi**
Personal history of kidney stones

Z87.448 **Personal history of other diseases of urinary system**

Z87.5- <u>Personal history</u> of <u>complications of pregnancy, childbirth and the puerperium</u>
Conditions classifiable to O00-O9A
Excludes❷: recurrent pregnancy loss (N96)

Z87.51 **Personal history of pre-term labor**
Excludes 1: current pregnancy with history of pre-term labor (O09.21-)

Z87.59 **Personal history of other complications of pregnancy, childbirth and the puerperium**
Personal history of trophoblastic disease

Z87.7- <u>Personal history</u> of **(corrected)** <u>congenital malformations</u>
Conditions classifiable to Q00-Q89 that have been repaired or corrected
Excludes 1: congenital malformations that have been partially corrected or repair but which still require medical treatment — code to condition
Excludes❷: other postprocedural states (Z98.-)
personal history of medical treatment (Z92.-)
presence of cardiac and vascular implants and grafts (Z95.-)
presence of other devices (Z97.-)
presence of other functional implants (Z96.-)
transplanted organ and tissue status (Z94.-)

Z87.71- **Personal history of (corrected)** <u>congenital malformations of genitourinary system</u>

Z87.710 **Personal history of (corrected) hypospadias**

Z87.718 **Personal history of other specified (corrected) congenital malformations ofgenitourinary system**

Z87.72- **Personal history of (corrected)** <u>congenital malformations of nervous system and senseorgans</u>

Z87.720 **Personal history of (corrected) congenital malformations of eye**

Z87.721 **Personal history of (corrected) congenital malformations of ear**

Z87.728 **Personal history of other specified (corrected) congenital malformations ofnervous system and sense organs**

Z87.73- **Personal history of (corrected)** <u>congenital malformations of digestive system</u>

Z87.730 **Personal history of (corrected) cleft lip and palate**

Z87.738 **Personal history of other specified (corrected) congenital malformations of digestive system**

Z87.74 **Personal history of (corrected)** <u>congenital malformations of heart and circulatory system</u>

Z87.75 **Personal history of (corrected)** <u>congenital malformations of respiratory system</u>

Z87.76 **Personal history of (corrected)** <u>congenital malformations of integument, limbs and musculoskeletal system</u>

Z87.79- **Personal history of** <u>other</u> **(corrected) congenital malformations**

Z87.790 **Personal history of (corrected) congenital malformations of face and neck**

Z87.798 **Personal history of other (corrected) congenital malformations**

Excludes 1: = NOT CODED HERE! (Do not code both)

Excludes❷ = Not Included Here

Z87.8- Personal history of <u>other</u> specified conditions
Excludes❷: *personal history of self harm (Z91.5)*

    Z87.81 Personal history of <u>(healed) traumatic fracture</u>
        Excludes❷: *personal history of (healed) nontraumatic fracture (Z87.31-)*

    Z87.82- Personal history of <u>other (healed) physical injury and trauma</u>
        Conditions classifiable to S00-T88, except traumatic fractures

        Z87.820 Personal history of traumatic brain injury
            Excludes 1: *personal history of transient ischemic attack (TIA), and cerebral infarction without residual deficits (Z86.73)*

        Z87.821 Personal history of retained foreign body fully removed

        Z87.828 Personal history of other (healed) physical injury and trauma

    Z87.89- Personal history of <u>other</u> specified conditions

        Z87.890 Personal history of sex reassignment

        Z87.891 Personal history of nicotine dependence
            Excludes 1: *current nicotine dependence (F17.2-)*

        Z87.892 Personal history of anaphylaxis
            Code also allergy status, such as:
                Allergy status to drugs, medicaments and biological substances (Z88-)
                Allergy status, other than to drugs and biological substances (Z91.0-)

        Z87.898 Personal history of other specified conditions

Z88- Allergy status to drugs, medicaments and biological substances
Excludes❷: *Allergy status, other than to drugs and biological substances (Z91.0-)*

    Z88.0 Allergy status to penicillin
    Z88.1 Allergy status to other antibiotic agents status
    Z88.2 Allergy status to sulfonamides status
    Z88.3 Allergy status to other anti-infective agents status
    Z88.4 Allergy status to anesthetic agent status
    Z88.5 Allergy status to narcotic agent status
    Z88.6 Allergy status to analgesic agent status
    Z88.7 Allergy status to serum and vaccine status
    Z88.8 Allergy status to other drugs, medicaments and biological substances status
    Z88.9 Allergy status to unspecified drugs, medicaments and biological substances status

Z89- <u>Acquired absence of limb</u>
    Includes: Amputation status
             Postprocedural loss of limb
             Post-traumatic loss of limb
    Excludes 1: *acquired deformities of limbs (M20-M21)*
             congenital absence of limbs (Q71-Q73)

    Z89.0- Acquired absence of thumb and other finger(s)

        Z89.01- Acquired absence of <u>thumb</u>
            Z89.011 Acquired absence of <u>right</u> thumb
            Z89.012 Acquired absence of <u>left</u> thumb
            Z89.019 Acquired absence of <u>unspecified</u> thumb

        Z89.02- Acquired absence of <u>other finger(s)</u>
            Excludes❷: *acquired absence of thumb (Z89.01-)*
            Z89.021 Acquired absence of <u>right</u> finger(s)
            Z89.022 Acquired absence of <u>left</u> finger(s)
            Z89.029 Acquired absence of <u>unspecified</u> finger(s)

    Z89.1- Acquired absence of hand and wrist

        Z89.11- Acquired absence of <u>hand</u>
            Z89.111 Acquired absence of <u>right</u> hand
            Z89.112 Acquired absence of <u>left</u> hand
            Z89.119 Acquired absence of <u>unspecified</u> hand

        Z89.12- Acquired absence of <u>wrist</u>
            Disarticulation at wrist
            Z89.121 Acquired absence of <u>right</u> wrist
            Z89.122 Acquired absence of <u>left</u> wrist
            Z89.129 Acquired absence of <u>unspecified</u> wrist

    Z89.2- Acquired absence of upper limb above wrist

        Z89.20- Acquired absence of <u>upper limb, unspecified level</u>
            Z89.201 Acquired absence of <u>right</u> upper limb, unspecified level
            Z89.202 Acquired absence of <u>left</u> upper limb, unspecified level
            Z89.209 Acquired absence of <u>unspecified</u> upper limb, unspecified level
                Acquired absence of arm NOS

Z89.21- Acquired absence of <u>upper limb below elbow</u>
    Z89.211 Acquired absence of <u>right</u> upper limb below elbow
    Z89.212 Acquired absence of <u>left</u> upper limb below elbow
    Z89.219 Acquired absence of <u>unspecified</u> upper limb below elbow

Z89.22- Acquired absence of <u>upper limb above elbow</u>
    Disarticulation at elbow
    Z89.221 Acquired absence of <u>right</u> upper limb above elbow
    Z89.222 Acquired absence of <u>left</u> upper limb above elbow
    Z89.229 Acquired absence of <u>unspecified</u> upper limb above elbow

Z89.23- Acquired absence of <u>shoulder</u>
    Acquired absence of shoulder joint following explantation of shoulder joint prosthesis, with or without presence of antibiotic-impregnated cement spacer
    Z89.231 Acquired absence of <u>right</u> shoulder
    Z89.232 Acquired absence of <u>left</u> shoulder
    Z89.239 Acquired absence of <u>unspecified</u> shoulder

Z89.4- Acquired absence of toe(s), foot, and ankle

    Z89.41- Acquired absence of <u>great toe</u>
        Z89.411 Acquired absence of <u>right</u> great toe
        Z89.412 Acquired absence of <u>left</u> great toe
        Z89.419 Acquired absence of <u>unspecified</u> great toe

    Z89.42- Acquired absence of <u>other toe(s)</u>
        Excludes❷: *acquired absence of great toe (Z89.41-)*
        Z89.421 Acquired absence of other <u>right</u> toe(s)
        Z89.422 Acquired absence of other <u>left</u> toe(s)
        Z89.429 Acquired absence of other toe(s), <u>unspecified</u> side

    Z89.43- Acquired absence of <u>foot</u>
        Z89.431 Acquired absence of <u>right</u> foot
        Z89.432 Acquired absence of <u>left</u> foot
        Z89.439 Acquired absence of <u>unspecified</u> foot

    Z89.44- Acquired absence of <u>ankle</u>
        Disarticulation of ankle
        Z89.441 Acquired absence of <u>right</u> ankle
        Z89.442 Acquired absence of <u>left</u> ankle
        Z89.449 Acquired absence of <u>unspecified</u> ankle

Z89.5- Acquired absence of <u>leg below knee</u>

    Z89.51- Acquired absence of leg below knee
        Z89.511 Acquired absence of <u>right</u> leg below knee
        Z89.512 Acquired absence of <u>left</u> leg below knee
        Z89.519 Acquired absence of <u>unspecified</u> leg below knee

    Z89.52- Acquired absence of <u>knee</u>
        Acquired absence of knee joint following explantation of knee joint prosthesis, with or without presence of antibiotic-impregnated cement spacer
        Z89.521 Acquired absence of <u>right</u> knee
        Z89.522 Acquired absence of <u>left</u> knee
        Z89.529 Acquired absence of <u>unspecified</u> knee

Z89.6- Acquired absence of leg above knee

    Z89.61- Acquired absence of <u>leg above knee</u>
        Acquired absence of leg NOS
        Disarticulation at knee
        Z89.611 Acquired absence of <u>right</u> leg above knee
        Z89.612 Acquired absence of <u>left</u> leg above knee
        Z89.619 Acquired absence of <u>unspecified</u> leg above knee

    Z89.62- Acquired absence of <u>hip</u>
        Acquired absence of hip joint following explantation of hip joint prosthesis, with or without presence of antibiotic-impregnated cement spacer
        Disarticulation at hip
        Z89.621 Acquired absence of <u>right</u> hip joint
        Z89.622 Acquired absence of <u>left</u> hip joint
        Z89.629 Acquired absence of <u>unspecified</u> hip joint

Z89.9 Acquired absence of limb, <u>unspecified</u>

Z
8
6
-
Z
8
9

Excludes 1: = NOT CODED HERE! (Do not code both)

Excludes❷: = Not Included Here

Z90- <u>Acquired absence</u> of organs, <u>not elsewhere classified</u>
Includes: Postprocedural or post-traumatic loss of body part NEC
Excludes 1: congenital absence — see Alphabetical Index
Excludes❷: postprocedural absence of endocrine glands (E89.-)

Z90.0- Acquired absence of part of head and neck

Z90.01 Acquired absence of eye

Z90.02 Acquired absence of larynx

Z90.09 Acquired absence of other part of head and neck
Acquired absence of nose
Excludes❷: teeth (K08.1)

Z90.1- Acquired absence of <u>breast and nipple</u>

Z90.10 Acquired absence of <u>unspecified</u> breast and nipple

Z90.11 Acquired absence of <u>right</u> breast and nipple

Z90.12 Acquired absence of <u>left</u> breast and nipple

Z90.13 Acquired absence of <u>bilateral</u> breasts and nipples

Z90.2 Acquired absence of lung [part of]

Z90.3 Acquired absence of stomach [part of]

Z90.4- Acquired absence of other specified parts of digestive tract

Z90.41 Acquired absence of pancreas
Use additional code to identify any associated:
Insulin use (Z79.4)
Diabetes mellitus, postpancreatectomy (E13.-)

Z90.410 Acquired total absence of pancreas
Acquired absence of pancreas NOS

Z90.411 Acquired partial absence of pancreas

Z90.49 Acquired absence of other specified parts of digestive tract

Z90.5 Acquired absence of kidney

Z90.6 Acquired absence of other parts of urinary tract
Acquired absence of bladder

Z90.7- Acquired absence of genital organ(s)
Excludes 1: personal history of sex reassignment (Z87.890)
Excludes❷: female genital mutilation status (N90.81-)

Z90.71- Acquired absence of cervix and uterus

Z90.710 Acquired absence of <u>both cervix and uterus</u>
Acquired absence of uterus NOS
Status post total hysterectomy

Z90.711 Acquired absence of <u>uterus with remaining cervical stump</u>
Status post partial hysterectomy with remaining cervical stump

Z90.712 Acquired absence of <u>cervix with remaining uterus</u>

Z90.72- Acquired absence of <u>ovaries</u>

Z90.721 Acquired absence of ovaries, <u>unilateral</u>

Z90.722 Acquired absence of ovaries, <u>bilateral</u>

Z90.79 Acquired absence of other genital organ(s)

Z90.8- Acquired absence of other organs

Z90.81 Acquired absence of spleen

Z90.89 Acquired absence of other organs

Z91- Personal risk factors, not elsewhere classified
Excludes❷: contact with and (suspected) exposures hazardous to health (Z77-)
exposure to pollution and other problems related to physical environment (Z77.1-)
personal history of physical injury and trauma (Z87.81, Z87.82-)
occupational exposure to risk factors (Z57-)

Z91.0- <u>Allergy status</u>, other than to drugs and biological substances
Excludes❷: allergy status to drugs, medicaments, and biological substances (Z88-)

Z91.01- <u>Food</u> allergy status
Excludes❷: food additives allergy status (Z91.02)

Z91.010 Allergy to peanuts

Z91.011 Allergy to milk products
Excludes 1: lactose intolerance (E73-)

Z91.012 Allergy to eggs

Z91.013 Allergy to seafood
Allergy to shellfish
Allergy to octopus or squid ink

Z91.018 Allergy to other foods
Allergy to nuts other than peanuts

Z91.02 <u>Food additives</u> allergy status

Z91.03- <u>Insect</u> allergy status

Z91.030 Bee allergy status

Z91.038 Other insect allergy status

Z91.04- <u>Nonmedicinal substance</u> allergy status

Z91.040 Latex allergy status
Latex sensitivity status

Z91.041 Radiographic dye allergy status
Allergy status to contrast media used for diagnostic X-ray procedure

Z91.048 Other nonmedicinal substance allergy status

Z91.09 <u>Other</u> allergy status, other than to drugs and biological substances

Z91.1- <u>Patient's noncompliance with medical treatment and regimen</u>

Z91.11 Patient's noncompliance with <u>dietary regimen</u>

Z91.12- Patient's <u>intentional underdosing</u> of medication regimen
Code first underdosing of medication (T36-T50) with fifth or sixth character 6
Excludes 1: adverse effect of prescribed drug taken as directed — code to adverse effect
poisoning (overdose) — code to poisoning

Z91.120 Patient's intentional underdosing of medication regimen <u>due to financial hardship</u>

Z91.128 Patient's intentional underdosing of medication regimen <u>for other reason</u>

Z91.13- Patient's <u>unintentional underdosing</u> of medication regimen
Code first underdosing of medication (T36-T50) with fifth or sixth character 6
Excludes 1: adverse effect of prescribed drug taken as directed — code to adverse effect
poisoning (overdose) — code to poisoning

Z91.130 Patient's unintentional underdosing of medication regimen <u>due to age-related debility</u>

Z91.138 Patient's unintentional underdosing of medication regimen <u>for other reason</u>

Z91.14 Patient's <u>other noncompliance</u> with medication regimen
Patient's underdosing of medication NOS

Z91.15 Patient's <u>noncompliance</u> with renal dialysis

Z91.19 Patient's <u>noncompliance</u> with other medical treatment and regimen

Z91.4- Personal history of psychological trauma, not elsewhere classified

Z91.41- Personal history of adult abuse
Excludes❷: personal history of abuse in childhood (Z62.81-)

Z91.410 Personal history of adult physical and sexual abuse
Excludes 1: current adult physical abuse (T74.11, T76.11)
current adult sexual abuse (T74.21, T76.11)

Z91.411 Personal history of adult psychological abuse

Z91.412 Personal history of adult neglect
Excludes 1: current adult neglect (T74.01, T76.01)

Z91.419 Personal history of unspecified adult abuse

Z91.49 Other personal history of psychological trauma, not elsewhere classified

Z91.5 Personal history of self-harm
Personal history of parasuicide
Personal history of self-poisoning
Personal history of suicide attempt

Z91.8- Other specified personal risk factors, not elsewhere classified

Z91.81 <u>History of falling</u>
At risk for falling

Z91.82 Personal history of military deployment
Individual (civilian or military) with past history of military war, peacekeeping and humanitarian deployment (current or past conflict)
Returned from military deployment

Z91.83 Wandering in diseases classified elsewhere
Code first underlying disorder, such as:
Alzheimer's disease (G30.-)
Autism or pervasive developmental disorder (F84.-)
Intellectual disabilities (F70-F79)
Unspecified dementia with behavioral disturbance (F03.9-)

Z91.89 Other specified personal risk factors, not elsewhere classified

Z92- <u>Personal history</u> of medical treatment
Excludes❷: postprocedural states (Z98-)

Z92.0 Personal history of <u>contraception</u>
Excludes 1: counseling or management of current contraceptive practices (Z30-)
long term (current) use of contraception (Z79.3)
presence of (intrauterine) contraceptive device (Z97.5)

Z92.2- Personal history of <u>drug therapy</u>
Excludes❷: long term (current) drug therapy (Z79-)

Z92.21 Personal history of antineoplastic chemotherapy

Z92.22 Personal history of monoclonal drug therapy

Z92.23 Personal history of estrogen therapy

Excludes 1: = NOT CODED HERE! (Do not code both)   **918**   *Excludes❷: = Not Included Here*

Z92.24- Personal history of steroid therapy
    Z92.240   Personal history of inhaled steroid therapy
    Z92.241   Personal history of systemic steroid therapy
      Personal history of steroid therapy NOS
Z92.25 Personal history of <u>immunosupression therapy</u>
    Excludes❷: personal history of steroid therapy (Z92.24)
Z92.29 Personal history of other drug therapy
Z92.3   Personal history of <u>irradiation</u>
    Personal history of exposure to therapeutic radiation
    Excludes 1: exposure to radiation in the physical environment
        (Z77.12)
        occupational exposure to radiation (Z57.1)
Z92.8- Personal history of <u>other</u> medical treatment
    Z92.81 Personal history of extracorporeal membrane oxygenation (ECMO)
    Z92.82 Status post administration of tPA (rtPA) in a different facility within the last 24 hours prior to admission to current facility
      Code first condition requiring tPA administration, such as:
        Acute cerebral infarction (I63-)
        Acute myocardial infarction (I21-, I22-)
    Z92.83 Personal history of failed moderate sedation
      Personal history of failed conscious sedation
      Excludes❷: failed moderate sedation during procedure
        (T88.52)
    Z92.89 Personal history of other medical treatment

Z93- <u>Artificial opening status</u>
    Excludes 1: artificial openings requiring attention or management (Z43.-)
        complications of external stoma (J95.0-, K94.-, N99.5-)
Z93.0   Tracheostomy status
Z93.1   Gastrostomy status
Z93.2   Ileostomy status
Z93.3   Colostomy status
Z93.4   Other artificial openings of gastrointestinal tract status
Z93.5- Cystostomy status
    Z93.50 Unspecified cystostomy status
    Z93.51 Cutaneous-vesicostomy status
    Z93.52 Appendico-vesicostomy status
    Z93.59 Other cystostomy status
Z93.6   Other artificial openings of urinary tract status
    Nephrostomy status
    Ureterostomy status
    Urethrostomy status
Z93.8   Other artificial opening status
Z93.9   Artificial opening status, unspecified

Z94- <u>Transplanted organ and tissue status</u>
    Includes: Organ or tissue replaced by heterogenous or homogenous transplant
    Excludes 1: complications of transplanted organ or tissue — see Alphabetical Index
    Excludes❷: presence of vascular grafts (Z95.-)
Z94.0   Kidney transplant status
Z94.1   Heart transplant status
    Excludes 1: artificial heart status (Z95.812)
        heart-valve replacement status (Z95.2-Z95.4)
Z94.2   Lung transplant status
Z94.3   Heart and lungs transplant status
Z94.4   Liver transplant status
Z94.5   Skin transplant status
    Autogenous skin transplant status
Z94.6   Bone transplant status
Z94.7   Corneal transplant status
Z94.8- Other transplanted organ and tissue status
    Z94.81 Bone marrow transplant status
    Z94.82 Intestine transplant status
    Z94.83 Pancreas transplant status
    Z94.84 Stem cells transplant status
    Z94.89 Other transplanted organ and tissue status
Z94.9   Transplanted organ and tissue status, unspecified

Z95- <u>Presence of cardiac and vascular implants and grafts</u>
    Excludes 1: complications of cardiac and vascular devices, implants and grafts (T82.-)
Z95.0   Presence of cardiac pacemaker
    Excludes 1: adjustment or management of cardiac pacemaker (Z45.0)
        presence of automatic (implantable) cardiac defibrillator with synchronous cardiac pacemaker (Z95.810)
Z95.1   Presence of aortocoronary bypass graft

Z95.2   Presence of prosthetic heart valve
    Presence of heart valve NOS
Z95.3   Presence of xenogenic heart valve
Z95.4   Presence of other heart-valve replacement
Z95.5   Presence of coronary angioplasty implant and graft
    Excludes 1: coronary angioplasty status without implant and graft (Z98.61)
Z95.8- Presence of other cardiac and vascular implants and grafts
    Z95.81- Presence of other cardiac implants and grafts
      Z95.810   Presence of automatic (implantable) cardiac defibrillator
        Presence of automatic (implantable) cardiac defibrillator with synchronous cardiac pacemaker
      Z95.811   Presence of heart assist device
      Z95.812   Presence of fully implantable artificial heart
      Z95.818   Presence of other cardiac implants and grafts
    Z95.82- Presence of other vascular implants and grafts
      Z95.820   Peripheral vascular angioplasty status with implants and grafts
        Excludes 1: peripheral vascular angioplasty without implant and graft (Z98.62)
      Z95.828   Presence of other vascular implants and grafts
        Presence of intravascular prosthesis NEC
Z95.9   Presence of cardiac and vascular implant and graft, unspecified

Z96- <u>Presence of other functional implants</u>
    Excludes❷: complications of internal prosthetic devices, implants and grafts (T82-T85)
        fitting and adjustment of prosthetic and other devices (Z44-Z46)
Z96.0   Presence of urogenital implants
Z96.1   Presence of intraocular lens
    Presence of pseudophakia
Z96.2- Presence of otological and audiological implants
    Z96.20 Presence of otological and audiological implant, unspecified
    Z96.21 Cochlear implant status
    Z96.22 Myringotomy tube(s) status
    Z96.29 Presence of other otological and audiological implants
      Presence of bone-conduction hearing device
      Presence of eustachian tube stent
      Stapes replacement
Z96.3   Presence of artificial larynx
Z96.4- Presence of endocrine implants
    Z96.41 Presence of insulin pump (external) (internal)
    Z96.49 Presence of other endocrine implants
Z96.5   Presence of tooth-root and mandibular implants
Z96.6- <u>Presence of orthopedic joint implants</u>
    Z96.60 Presence of unspecified orthopedic joint implant
    Z96.61- Presence of artificial <u>shoulder</u> joint
      Z96.611   Presence of <u>right</u> artificial shoulder joint
      Z96.612   Presence of <u>left</u> artificial shoulder joint
      Z96.619   Presence of <u>unspecified</u> artificial shoulder joint
    Z96.62- Presence of artificial <u>elbow</u> joint
      Z96.621   Presence of <u>right</u> artificial elbow joint
      Z96.622   Presence of <u>left</u> artificial elbow joint
      Z96.629   Presence of <u>unspecified</u> artificial elbow joint
    Z96.63- Presence of artificial <u>wrist</u> joint
      Z96.631   Presence of <u>right</u> artificial wrist joint
      Z96.632   Presence of <u>left</u> artificial wrist joint
      Z96.639   Presence of <u>unspecified</u> artificial wrist joint
    Z96.64- Presence of artificial <u>hip</u> joint
      Hip-joint replacement (partial) (total)
      Z96.641   Presence of <u>right</u> artificial hip joint
      Z96.642   Presence of <u>left</u> artificial hip joint
      Z96.643   Presence of artificial hip joint, <u>bilateral</u>
      Z96.649   Presence of <u>unspecified</u> artificial hip joint
    Z96.65- Presence of artificial <u>knee</u> joint
      Z96.651   Presence of <u>right</u> artificial knee joint
      Z96.652   Presence of <u>left</u> artificial knee joint
      Z96.653   Presence of artificial knee joint, <u>bilateral</u>
      Z96.659   Presence of <u>unspecified</u> artificial knee joint
    Z96.66- Presence of artificial <u>ankle</u> joint
      Z96.661   Presence of <u>right</u> artificial ankle joint
      Z96.662   Presence of <u>left</u> artificial ankle joint
      Z96.669   Presence of <u>unspecified</u> artificial ankle joint

Z90 - Z96

Z96.69-   Presence of <u>other</u> orthopedic joint implants

    Z96.691   Finger-joint replacement of <u>right</u> hand

    Z96.692   Finger-joint replacement of <u>left</u> hand

    Z96.693   Finger-joint replacement, <u>bilateral</u>

    Z96.698   Presence of other orthopedic joint implants

Z96.7   Presence of other bone and tendon implants
    Presence of skull plate

Z96.8-   Presence of other specified functional implants

    Z96.81   Presence of artificial skin

    Z96.89   Presence of other specified functional implants

Z96.9   Presence of functional implant, unspecified

Z97-   **Presence of other devices**
    Excludes 1: complications of internal prosthetic devices, implants and grafts (T82-T85)
        fitting and adjustment of prosthetic and other devices (Z44-Z46)
    Excludes❷: presence of cerebrospinal fluid drainage device (Z98.2)

Z97.0   Presence of artificial eye

Z97.1-   <u>Presence of artificial limb</u> (complete) (partial)

    Z97.10   Presence of artificial limb (complete) (partial), <u>unspecified</u>

    Z97.11   Presence of artificial <u>right</u> <u>arm</u> (complete) (partial)

    Z97.12   Presence of artificial <u>left</u> <u>arm</u> (complete) (partial)

    Z97.13   Presence of artificial <u>right</u> <u>leg</u> (complete) (partial)

    Z97.14   Presence of artificial <u>left</u> <u>leg</u> (complete) (partial)

    Z97.15   Presence of artificial <u>arms</u>, <u>bilateral</u> (complete) (partial)

    Z97.16   Presence of artificial <u>legs</u>, <u>bilateral</u> (complete) (partial)

Z97.2   Presence of dental prosthetic device (complete) (partial)
    Presence of dentures (complete) (partial)

Z97.3   Presence of spectacles and contact lenses

Z97.4   Presence of external hearing-aid

Z97.5   Presence of (intrauterine) contraceptive device
    Excludes 1: checking, reinsertion or removal of contraceptive device (Z30.43)

Z97.8   Presence of other specified devices

Z98-   <u>Other postprocedural states</u>
    Excludes❷: aftercare (Z43-Z49, Z51)
        follow-up medical care (Z08-Z09)
        postprocedural complication — see Alphabetical Index

Z98.0   Intestinal bypass and anastomosis status
    Excludes❷: bariatric surgery status (Z98.84)
        gastric bypass status (Z98.84)
        obesity surgery status (Z98.84)

Z98.1   Arthrodesis status

Z98.2   Presence of cerebrospinal fluid drainage device
    Presence of CSF shunt

Z98.3   Post therapeutic collapse of lung status
    Code first underlying disease

Z98.4-   Cataract extraction status
    Use additional code to identify intraocular lens implant status (Z96.1)
    Excludes 1: aphakia (H27.0)

    Z98.41   Cataract extraction status, <u>right</u> eye

    Z98.42   Cataract extraction status, <u>left</u> eye

    Z98.49   Cataract extraction status, <u>unspecified</u> eye

Z98.5-   Sterilization status
    Excludes 1: female infertility (N97.-)
        male infertility (N46.-)

    Z98.51   Tubal ligation status

    Z98.52   Vasectomy status

Z98.6-   <u>Angioplasty status</u>

    Z98.61   <u>Coronary</u> angioplasty status
        Excludes 1: coronary angioplasty status with implant and graft (Z95.5)

    Z98.62   <u>Peripheral vascular</u> angioplasty status
        Excludes 1: peripheral vascular angioplasty status with implant and graft (Z95.820)

Z98.8-   Other specified postprocedural states

    Z98.81-   Dental procedure status

        Z98.810   Dental sealant status

        Z98.811   Dental restoration status
           Dental crown status
           Dental fillings status

        Z98.818   Other dental procedure status

    Z98.82   Breast implant status
        Excludes 1: breast implant removal status (Z98.86)

    Z98.83   Filtering (vitreous) bleb after glaucoma surgery status
        Excludes 1: Inflammation (infection) of postprocedural bleb (H59.4-)

Z98.84   <u>Bariatric surgery status</u>
    Gastric banding status
    Gastric bypass status for obesity
    Obesity surgery status
    Excludes 1: bariatric surgery status complicating pregnancy, childbirth, or the puerperium (O99.84)
    Excludes❷: intestinal bypass and anastomosis status (Z98.0)

Z98.85   Transplanted organ removal status
    Transplanted organ previously removed due to complication, failure, rejection or infection
    Excludes 1: encounter for removal of transplanted organ — code to complication of transplanted organ (T86.-)

Z98.86   Personal history of breast implant removal

Z98.87-   Personal history of in utero procedure

    Z98.870   Personal history of in utero procedure during pregnancy
        Excludes❷: complications from in utero procedure for current pregnancy (O35.7)
           supervision of current pregnancy with history of in utero procedure during previous pregnancy (O09.82-)

    Z98.871   Personal history of in utero procedure while a fetus

Z98.89   Other specified postprocedural states
    Personal history of surgery, not elsewhere classified

Z99-   <u>Dependence on enabling machines and devices, not elsewhere classified</u>
    Excludes 1: cardiac pacemaker status (Z95.0)

Z99.0   Dependence on aspirator

Z99.1-   Dependence on respirator
    Dependence on ventilator

    Z99.11   Dependence on <u>respirator [ventilator] status</u>

    Z99.12   Encounter for <u>respirator [ventilator] dependence during power failure</u>
        Excludes 1: mechanical complication of respirator [ventilator] (J95.850)

Z99.2   Dependence on <u>renal dialysis</u>
    Hemodialysis status
    Peritoneal dialysis status
    Presence of arteriovenous shunt for dialysis
    Renal dialysis status NOS
    Excludes 1: encounter for fitting and adjustment of dialysis catheter (Z49.0-)
        noncompliance with renal dialysis (Z91.15)

Z99.3   Dependence on wheelchair
    Wheelchair confinement status
    Code first cause of dependence, such as:
    Muscular dystrophy (G71.0)
    Obesity (E66.-)

Z99.8-   Dependence on other enabling machines and devices

    Z99.81   Dependence on <u>supplemental oxygen</u>
        Dependence on long-term oxygen

    Z99.89   Dependence on other enabling machines and devices
        Dependence on machine or device NOS

Excludes 1: = NOT CODED HERE! (Do not code both)   *Excludes❷:* = Not Included Here

NOTES